The Cat

Clinical Medicine and Management

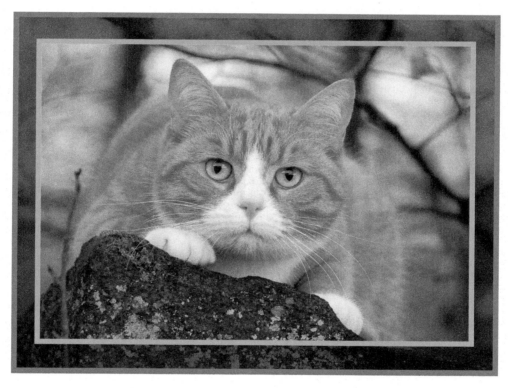

Susan E. Little, DVM, DABVP (Feline Practice)
Bytown Cat Hospital
Ottawa, Ontario, Canada

ELSEVIER

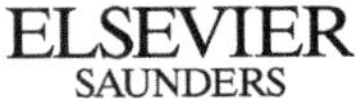

3251 Riverport Lane
St. Louis, Missouri 63043

THE CAT: CLINICAL MEDICINE AND MANAGEMENT ISBN: 978-1-4377-0660-4

Notices

International Standard Book Number: 978-1-4377-0660-4

Vice President and Publisher: Linda Duncan
Acquisitions Editor: Heidi Pohlman
Managing Editor: Shelly Stringer
Publishing Services Manager: Catherine Jackson
Senior Project Manager: David Stein
Designer: Margaret Reid
Cover and Section Opener Images: Mats Göran Hamnäs

Printed in the United States of America

Last digit is the print number: 9 8 7

Section Editors

Randolph M. Baral, BVSc, MACVSc (Feline Medicine)
Paddington Cat Hospital
Sydney, New South Wales, Australia
Feline Internal Medicine

Joe Bartges, BS, DVM, PhD, DACVIM, DACVN
Professor of Medicine and Nutrition
Acree Endowed Chair of Small Animal Research
Staff Internist and Nutritionist
Department of Small Animal Clinical Sciences
College of Veterinary Medicine
The University of Tennessee
Knoxville, Tennessee
Feline Nutrition

Jeffrey N. Bryan, DVM, MS, PhD, DACVIM (Oncology)
Associate Professor of Oncology
Department of Veterinary Medicine and Surgery
College of Veterinary Medicine
University of Missouri
Columbia, Missouri
Feline Internal Medicine (Chapter 28: *Oncology*)

Brenda Griffin, DVM, MS, DACVIM
Adjunct Associate Professor
Department of Small Animal Clinical Sciences
College of Veterinary Medicine
University of Florida
Gainesville, Florida
Population Medicine

Melissa Kennedy, DVM, PhD, DACVM
Associate Professor
Director of Clinical Virology
Department of Biomedical and Diagnostic Services
College of Veterinary Medicine
The University of Tennessee
Knoxville, Tennessee
Infectious Diseases and Zoonoses

Susan E. Little, DVM, DABVP (Feline Practice)
Bytown Cat Hospital
Ottawa, Ontario, Canada
Fundamentals of Feline Practice
Feline Internal Medicine
Special Considerations for the Senior Cat
Feline Reproduction and Pediatrics

Leslie A. Lyons, PhD
Professor
Department of Population Health and Reproduction
School of Veterinary Medicine
University of California, Davis
Davis, California
The Feline Genome and Clinical Genetics

Margie Scherk, DVM, DABVP (Feline)
Editor
Journal of Feline Medicine and Surgery;
CatsINK
Vancouver, British Columbia, Canada
Managing the Cat with Concurrent and Chronic Diseases

Kersti Seksel, BVSc (Hons), MRCVS MA (Hons), FACVSc, DACVB, CMAVA, DECVBM-CA
Registered Veterinary Specialist, Behavioural Medicine
Sydney Animal Behaviour Service
Seaforth, New South Wales, Australia
Adjunct Senior Lecturer
Charles Sturt University
Wagga Wagga, New South Wales, Australia
Feline Behavior

Contributors

Randolph M. Baral, BVSc, MACVSc (Feline Medicine)
Paddington Cat Hospital
Sydney, New South Wales, Australia
Approach to the Vomiting Cat
Approach to the Cat with Diarrhea
Diseases of the Intestines
Diseases of the Exocrine Pancreas
Approach to the Cat with Ascites and Diseases Affecting the Peritoneal Cavity
Endocrine Pancreatic Disorders
Thyroid Gland Disorders
Adrenal Gland Disorders
Disorders of Calcium Metabolism
Lower Respiratory Tract Diseases
The Thoracic Cavity
Bacterial Infections

Georgina Barone, DVM, DACVIM (Neurology)
Veterinary Medical Center of Long Island
West Islip, New York
Neurology

Joe Bartges, BS, DVM, PhD, DACVIM, DACVN
Professor of Medicine and Nutrition
Acree Endowed Chair of Small Animal Research
Department of Small Animal Clinical Sciences
College of Veterinary Medicine
The University of Tennessee
Knoxville, Tennessee
The Unique Nutritional Requirements of the Cat: A Strict Carnivore
Nutrition for the Normal Cat
Nutritional Disorders
Nutritional Management of Diseases
Current Controversies in Feline Nutrition

Marie-Claude Bélanger, DMV, MSc, DACVIM
Associate Professor
Department of Clinical Sciences
Faculty of Veterinary Medicine
University of Montreal
St-Hyacinthe, Quebec, Canada
Heart Failure and Chronic Kidney Disease

Scott A. Brown, VMD, PhD, DACVIM
Josiah Meigs Distinguished Professor
Department of Small Animal Medicine and Surgery
College of Veterinary Medicine
The University of Georgia
Athens, Georgia
Chronic Kidney Disease and Hypertension

Jane E. Brunt, DVM
Founder and Owner
Cat Hospital At Towson-CHAT
Baltimore, Maryland
Executive Director
Catalyst Council, Inc.
Annapolis, Maryland
The Cat-Friendly Practice

Jeffrey N. Bryan, DVM, MS, PhD, DACVIM (Oncology)
Associate Professor of Oncology
Department of Veterinary Medicine and Surgery
College of Veterinary Medicine
University of Missouri
Columbia, Missouri
Lymphoma

Jenna H. Burton, DVM
Assistant Professor
Animal Cancer Center
Department of Clinical Sciences
College of Veterinary Medicine and Biomedical Sciences
Colorado State University
Fort Collins, Colorado
Chemotherapy for the Feline Cancer Patient

Debbie Calnon, BSc, BVMS, MACVSc (Animal Behavior), CMAVA, Cert IV TAA
Behaviour Counselling Service
Mount Waverley, Victoria, Australia;
Good Pet Behaviour
Kingston, Victoria, Australia
Box Hill Institute TAFE
Box Hill, Victoria, Australia
Behavioral History Taking

Sarah Caney, BVSc PhD DSAM (Feline), MRCVS
Cat Professional Ltd.
Midlothian Innovation Centre
Pentlandfield, Roslin, Midlothian, United Kingdom
Hyperthyroidism and Chronic Kidney Disease

Kevin Choy, BVSc
Resident, Oncology
Department of Veterinary Clinical Sciences
College of Veterinary Medicine
Washington State University
Pullman, Washington
Lymphoma
Mammary Tumors

Melissa Clark, DVM
Resident, Clinical Pharmacology
Department of Veterinary Biosciences
College of Veterinary Medicine
University of Illinois at Urbana-Champaign
Urbana, Illinois
Monitoring Long-Term Therapy

Leah A. Cohn, DVM, PhD, DACVIM
Professor
Department of Veterinary Medicine and Surgery
College of Veterinary Medicine
University of Missouri
Columbia, Missouri
Immune Deficiency, Stress, and Infection
Immunosuppressive Drug Therapy

Steve Dale, CABC
Contributing Editor (pets)
USA Weekend;
Pet Columnist Tribune Media Services;
Host National Radio Shows
Black Dog Radio Productions
Chicago, Illinois
Kitten Socialization and Training Classes

Duncan C. Ferguson, VMD, PhD, DACVIM, DACVCP
Professor of Pharmacology and Head
Department of Comparative Biosciences
College of Veterinary Medicine
University of Illinois at Urbana-Champaign
Urbana, Illinois
Monitoring Long-Term Therapy

Brooke Fowler, DVM
Oncology Resident
Small Animal
Department of Veterinary Medicine and Science
College of Veterinary Medicine
University of Missouri
Columbia, Missouri
Basic Approach to the Feline Cancer Patient

Deborah S. Greco, DVM, PhD, DACVIM
Senior Medical Consultant
Nestle Purina Petcare
New York, New York
Diabetes Mellitus and Feline Lower Urinary Tract Disorders

Brenda Griffin, DVM, MS, DACVIM
Adjunct Associate Professor
Department of Small Animal Clinical Sciences
College of Veterinary Medicine
University of Florida
Gainesville, Florida
Care and Control of Community Cats
Population Wellness: Keeping Cats Physically and Behaviorally Healthy

Beth Hamper, DVM, DACVN
Department of Small Animal Clinical Sciences
College of Veterinary Medicine
The University of Tennessee
Knoxville, Tennessee
The Unique Nutritional Requirements of the Cat: A Strict Carnivore
Nutrition for the Normal Cat
Nutritional Disorders
Nutritional Management of Diseases
Current Controversies in Feline Nutrition

Greg L. G. Harasen, DVM
Animal Clinic of Regina
Regina, Saskatchewan, Canada
Musculoskeletal Diseases

Chamisa Herrera, DVM
Oncology Resident
Department of Small Animal Medicine and Surgery
College of Veterinary Medicine
University of Missouri
Columbia, Missouri
Paraneoplastic Syndromes

Margarethe Hoenig, DrMedVet, PhD
Professor
Department of Veterinary Clinical Medicine
College of Veterinary Medicine
University of Illinois
Urbana, Illinois
Hyperthyroidism and Diabetes Mellitus
Diabetes Mellitus and Obesity

Jan E. Ilkiw, BVSc, PhD, DECVAA
Associate Dean for Academic Programs
Professor
Department of Surgical and Radiological Sciences
School of Veterinary Medicine
University of California, Davis
Davis, California
Anesthesia and Perioperative Care

Katherine M. James, DVM, PhD, DACVIM
Veterinary Education Coordinator
Veterinary Information Network
Davis, California
Fluid Therapy

Edward Javinsky, DVM, DABVP (Canine/Feline)
Veterinary Medical Consultations
Ottawa, Ontario, Canada
Gastrointestinal Parasites
Hematology and Immune-Related Disorders

Anthony S. Johnson, BS, DVM, DACVECC
Assistant Clinical Professor
Emergency and Critical Care
Department of Veterinary Clinical Sciences
School of Veterinary Medicine
Purdue University
West Lafayette, Indiana
Fluid Therapy

Melissa Kennedy, DVM, PhD, DACVM
Associate Professor
Director of Clinical Virology
Department of Biomedical and Diagnostic Sciences
College of Veterinary Medicine
The University of Tennessee
Knoxville, Tennessee
Viral Diseases
Bacterial Infections

Claudia Kirk, DVM, PhD, DACVN, DACVIM
Professor of Medicine and Nutrition
Department Head
Department of Small Animal Clinical Sciences
College of Veterinary Medicine
The University of Tennessee
Knoxville, Tennessee
The Unique Nutritional Requirements of the Cat: A Strict Carnivore
Nutrition for the Normal Cat
Nutritional Disorders
Nutritional Management of Diseases
Current Controversies in Feline Nutrition

William C. Kisseberth, DVM, PhD, DACVIM (Oncology)
Associate Professor
Department of Veterinary Clinical Sciences
College of Veterinary Medicine
The Ohio State University
Columbus, Ohio
Injection-Site Sarcoma

Jennifer Dawn Kurushima, BS, PhD
Post-Doctoral Fellow
Population Health and Reproduction
School of Veterinary Medicine
University of California, Davis
Davis, California
A Short Natural History of the Cat and Its Relationship with Humans

Gary Landsberg, BSc, DVM, DACVB, DECVBM-CA
Veterinary Behaviorist
North Toronto Animal Clinic
Thornhill, Ontario, Canada;
Director Veterinary Affairs
CanCog Technologies, Inc.
Toronto, Ontario, Canada
Kitten Development
Behavioral Therapeutics

Michael R. Lappin, DVM, PhD, DACVIM
Professor
Small Animal Medicine
Department of Clinical Sciences
College of Veterinary Medicine and Biomedical Sciences
Colorado State University
Fort Collins, Colorado
The Upper Respiratory Tract
Molecular Assays Used for the Diagnosis of Feline Infectious Diseases

Sidonie Lavergne, DVM, PhD
Assistant Professor
Comparative Biosciences
College of Veterinary Medicine
University of Illinois at Urbana-Champaign
Urbana, Illinois
Managing Adverse Drug Reactions

Kristin M. Lewis, DVM
Internal Medicine Resident
Department of Veterinary Medicine and Surgery
College of Veterinary Medicine
University of Missouri
Columbia, Missouri
Immunosuppressive Drug Therapy

Jacqueline Mary Ley, BVSc (Hons), MACVSc (Veterinary Behavior), PhD
Research Assistant
Psychology
Monash University
Melbourne, Victoria, Australia;
Veterinary Behaviourist
Sydney Animal Behaviour Service
Sydney, New South Wales, Australia;
Veterinary Behaviourist
Veterinary Behavioural Medicine
Melbourne Veterinary Specialist Centre
Melbourne, Victoria, Australia
Kitten Development
Normal Behavior of Cats
Behavioral Therapeutics

Christine C. Lim, DVM, DACVO
Assistant Clinical Professor
Veterinary Clinical Sciences
College of Veterinary Medicine
University of Minnesota
St. Paul, Minnesota
Ophthalmology

Susan E. Little, DVM, DABVP (Feline Practice)
Bytown Cat Hospital
Ottawa, Ontario, Canada
Diseases of the Esophagus
Diseases of the Stomach
Endocrine Pancreatic Disorders
Musculoskeletal Diseases
Toxicology
The Lower Urinary Tract
Viral Diseases
Bacterial Infections
Managing the Senior Cat
Evaluation of the Senior Cat with Weight Loss
Male Reproduction
Female Reproduction
Pediatrics

Katharine F. Lunn, BVMS, MS, PhD, MRCVS, DACVIM
Assistant Professor
Department of Clinical Sciences
College of Veterinary Medicine and Biomedical Sciences
Colorado State University
Fort Collins, Colorado
Fluid Therapy

Leslie A. Lyons, PhD
Professor
Department of Population Health and Reproduction
School of Veterinary Medicine
University of California, Davis
Davis, California
A Short Natural History of the Cat and Its Relationship with Humans
The Feline Genome and Clinical Implications
Genetics of Feline Diseases and Traits

David J. Maggs, BVSc, DACVO
Professor
Department of Surgical and Radiological Sciences
School of Veterinary Medicine
University of California, Davis
Davis, California
Ophthalmology

Carolyn McKune, DVM, DACVA
Clinical Assistant Professor
Department of Large Animal Clinical Sciences
College of Veterinary Medicine
University of Florida
Gainesville, Florida
Analgesia

Karen A. Moriello, DVM, DACVD
Clinical Professor, Dermatology
Department of Medical Sciences
School of Veterinary Medicine
University of Wisconsin
Madison, Wisconsin
Feline Skin Diseases

Daniel O. Morris, DVM, DACVD
Associate Professor and Chief of Dermatology/Allergy
Department of Clinical Studies
School of Veterinary Medicine
University of Pennsylvania
Philadelphia, Pennsylvania
Human Allergies to Cats

Maryanne Murphy, DVM
Hill's Fellow in Clinical Nutrition and Doctoral Student
Department of Small Animal Clinical Sciences
College of Veterinary Medicine
The University of Tennessee
Knoxville, Tennessee
The Unique Nutritional Requirements of the Cat: A Strict Carnivore
Nutrition for the Normal Cat
Nutritional Disorders
Nutritional Management of Diseases
Current Controversies in Feline Nutrition

John C. New, Jr., DVM, MPH, DACVPM
Professor and Director of Public Health and Outreach
Department of Biomedical and Diagnostic Sciences
College of Veterinary Medicine
The University of Tennessee
Knoxville, Tennessee
Feline Zoonotic Diseases and Prevention of Transmission

Mark E. Peterson, DVM, DACVIM
Director
Department of Endocrinology and Nuclear Medicine
Animal Endocrine Clinic
New York, New York
Thyroid Gland Disorders
Adrenal Gland Disorders
Pituitary Disorders

Bruno H. Pypendop, DrMedVet, DrVetSci, DACVA
Professor
Department of Surgical and Radiological Sciences
School of Veterinary Medicine
University of California, Davis
Davis, California
Anesthesia and Perioperative Care

Jessica Quimby, DVM, DACVIM
Graduate Student
Department of Clinical Sciences
College of Veterinary Medicine and Biomedical Sciences
Colorado State University
Fort Collins, Colorado
The Upper Respiratory Tract

Donna Raditic, DVM, CVA
Adjunct Associate Clinician
Department of Animal Clinical Sciences
Integrative Medicine Service
College of Veterinary Medicine
The University of Tennessee
Knoxville, Tennessee
The Unique Nutritional Requirements of the Cat: A Strict Carnivore
Nutrition for the Normal Cat
Nutritional Disorders
Nutritional Management of Diseases
Current Controversies in Feline Nutrition

Alexander M. Reiter, Dipl. Tzt., Dr. med.vet., DAVDC, DEVDC
Associate Professor and Chief of Dentistry and Oral Surgery
Department of Clinical Sciences
School of Veterinary Medicine
University of Pennsylvania
Philadelphia, Pennsylvania
Dental and Oral Diseases

Jill A. Richardson, DVM
Pharmacovigilance Veterinarian
Merck Animal Health
Summit, New Jersey
Toxicology

Mark Rishniw, BVSc, MS, PhD, DACVIM
Visiting Scientist
Department of Clinical Sciences
College of Veterinary Medicine
Cornell University
Ithaca, New York;
Director of Clinical Research
Veterinary Information Network
Davis, California
Cardiovascular Diseases

Sheilah Robertson, BVMS (Hons), PhD, DACVA, DECVAA, MRCVS
Professor
Department of Large Animal Clinical Sciences
College of Veterinary Medicine
University of Florida
Gainesville, Florida
Analgesia
Palliative Medicine: Pain Assessment and Management

Ilona Rodan, DVM, DABVP (Feline)
Feline-Friendly Consulting
Medical Director
Cat Care Clinic
Madison, Wisconsin
Understanding the Cat and Feline-Friendly Handling
Preventive Health Care for Cats

Bernard E. Rollin, PhD
University Distinguished Professor
Department of Philosophy
College of Liberal Arts
Colorado State University
Fort Collins, Colorado
Palliative Medicine, Quality of Life, and Euthanasia Decisions

Margie Scherk, DVM, DABVP (Feline)
Editor
Journal of Feline Medicine and Surgery;
CatsINK
Vancouver, British Columbia, Canada
The Upper Urinary Tract
Palliative Medicine, Quality of Life, and Euthanasia Decisions

Kersti Seksel, BVSc (Hons), MRCVS MA (Hons), FACVSc, DACVB, CMAVA, DECVBM-CA
Registered Veterinary Specialist, Behavioural Medicine
Sydney Animal Behaviour Service
Seaforth, New South Wales, Australia
Adjunct Senior Lecturer
Charles Sturt University
Wagga Wagga, New South Wales, Australia
Normal Behavior of Cats
Kitten Socialization and Training Classes
Behavior Problems
Behavioral Therapeutics

Lisa M. Singer, VMD
Resident, Internal Medicine
Department of Internal Medicine, Small Animal
College of Veterinary Medicine
Michigan State University
East Lansing, Michigan
Immune Deficiency, Stress, and Infection

Marcy J. Souza, DVM, MPH, DABVP (Avian), DACVPM
Assistant Professor
Department of Biomedical and Diagnostic Sciences
College of Veterinary Medicine
The University of Tennessee
Knoxville, Tennessee
Feline Zoonotic Diseases and Prevention of Transmission

Andrew H. Sparkes, BVetMed, PhD, DECVIM, MRCVS
Veterinary Scientific Advisor
International Society for Feline Medicine
Tisbury, Wilts, United Kingdom
Preventive Health Care for Cats

Jennifer Stokes, DVM, DACVIM
Clinical Associate Professor
Department of Small Animal Clinical Sciences
College of Veterinary Medicine
The University of Tennessee
Knoxville, Tennessee
Fungal and Rickettsial Diseases

Vicki Thayer, DVM, DABVP (Feline)
Purrfect Practice PC
Lebanon, Oregon;
President
Winn Feline Foundation, Inc.
Hillsborough, New Jersey
Deciphering the Cat: The Medical History and Physical Examination

Lauren A. Trepanier, DVM, PhD, DACVIM, DACVCP
Professor
Department of Medical Sciences
School of Veterinary Medicine
University of Wisconsin
Madison, Wisconsin
Guidelines and Precautions for Drug Therapy in Cats

Julia Veir, DVM, PhD, DACVIM
Assistant Professor, Small Animal Medicine
Department of Clinical Sciences
College of Veterinary Medicine and Biomedical Sciences
Colorado State University
Fort Collins, Colorado
Molecular Assays Used for the Diagnosis of Feline Infectious Diseases

Katrina R. Viviano, DVM, PhD, DACVIM
Clinical Assistant Professor
Department of Medical Sciences
School of Veterinary Medicine
University of Wisconsin
Madison, Wisconsin
Therapeutics for Vomiting and Diarrhea

Angela L. Witzel, DVM, PhD, DACVN
Clinical Instructor
Department of Small Animal Clinical Sciences
College of Veterinary Medicine
The University of Tennessee
Knoxville, Tennessee
The Unique Nutritional Requirements of the Cat: A Strict Carnivore
Nutrition for the Normal Cat
Nutritional Disorders
Nutritional Management of Diseases
Current Controversies in Feline Nutrition

Jackie M. Wypij, DVM, MS, DACVIM (Oncology)
Assistant Professor
Department of Veterinary Clinical Medicine
College of Veterinary Medicine
University of Illinois at Urbana-Champaign
Urbana, Illinois
Palliative Care

Debra L. Zoran, DVM, MS, PhD, DACVIM-SAIM
Associate Professor
Chief of Medicine
Department of Small Animal Clinical Sciences
College of Veterinary Medicine and Biomedical Sciences
Texas A&M University
College Station, Texas
Diseases of the Liver
Management of Concurrent Pancreatitis and Inflammatory Bowel Disease

This book would not have been possible without the support and advice of many, including my colleagues at Bytown and Merivale Cat Hospitals (Ottawa, Ontario, Canada), most especially Dr. Douglas Boeckh who made it possible for me to become a feline specialist. My long-suffering family was integral in many ways (advice on the book cover from my son Benjamin, photographs from my daughter Tori-Rose, and expert writing from my husband Dr. Edward Javinsky) and they put up with the endless and exacerbating process of editing a textbook. And, finally, it would not have been possible without over two decades of feline patients—I hope I can continue to learn from them every day.

AN OUTLINE OF FELINE MEDICINE*

J. E. B. Graham†

This paper is an attempt to give a broad outline of feline medicine rather than to concentrate on any particular aspect of this field. No attempt will be made to cover the virus infections since they are familiar to most veterinarians.

Preliminary Examination

The following examination is the type done on any sick cat when the diagnosis is not obvious. It should require no more than ten minutes. An examination table with a slippery surface, such as stainless steel or arborite, facilitates handling. Since most cats are nervous after traveling, a few moments spent stroking their head and back to allay their suspicions is time well spent.

The anus and surrounding hair are checked for tapeworm segments and a well lubricated thermometer is inserted in the rectum. Cats resist a dry thermometer more than dogs do. While waiting for the thermometer to register, an accurate history is obtained from the owner. The next step is the examination of the skin paying particular attention to external parasites, dermatitis, excessive dryness of the skin or hair, quality of the coat and excessive hair shedding. The external lymph nodes are examined and any abnormality of the subcutaneous tissue or muscular system is noted.

The ears are then checked for mites, infection of the canal or excess wax production. The lips are examined for evidence of rodent ulcer, the gums and tongue are checked for evidence of ulceration, anemia, jaundice or cyanosis, the teeth are checked for tartar accumulation and loose roots, and the odor of the mouth is noted. After forward withdrawal of the tongue to see any infected spots, tumor formation, foreign body or tonsil infection, the back of the throat is checked.

The character of the respirations are observed and any abnormalities noted. All quadrants of the chest are examined with a stethoscope. Abnormal heart or lung sounds are determined. (A moment with a stethoscope will also give you some privacy to collect your thoughts.)

Palpation of the abdomen is easier in cats than in dogs. By palpation a pregnant uterus can be noted after the fourth week, and pyometra is readily discernable. Intestines are checked for foreign bodies, constipation, thick walls, gas pockets, tumors and enlarged lymph nodes.

Kidneys are palpated for size: they are small and hard in chronic interstitial nephritis, large and painful in acute nephritis, enlarged and knobby in kidney lymphosarcoma. The wall of the bladder is thick in cystitis. The spleen is often enlarged in anemia. If the border of the liver is palpable it is pathological.

*A paper presented at the Mid-Ontario Veterinary Association meeting held at Toronto on October 27, 1960.

†3206 Eglinton Avenue East, Toronto, Ontario.

FIGURE FM-1 In 1961, J.E.B. Graham presented an outline of all that was currently known about feline medicine in the Canadian Veterinary Journal in 10 pages. Today, 50 years later, we have advanced in knowledge to the point that we need one hundred times that many pages devoted to feline medicine. Undoubtedly, the cat has benefited from this expansion of knowledge but the clinician has the daunting task of learning and putting it into practice. *(From Graham JEB: An Outline of Feline Medicine,* Can Vet J *2:8, 1961.)*

Preface

As any veterinary clinician knows, it is a daunting task to work with cats! Over the years, I have found my experiences as a feline specialist humbling, but also have realized what a great learning opportunity feline medicine provides. Cats force us to be expert diagnosticians, relying more than ever on the "old school" skills of a good medical history and a thorough physical examination. Unfortunately, cats are still the "poor stepchild" in companion animal medicine, receiving less attention in research on common medical problems as well as improved diagnostic and treatment approaches than is given to their canine counterparts. It is therefore fitting that the Winn Feline Foundation has endorsed this book, as the organization has provided the research funding and support necessary to uncover an impressive amount of the information found in this text.

Fortunately, we know much more about feline medicine than we did 10 or 15 years ago. This book compiles the current state of knowledge from a group of talented and wise experts. These superb clinicians and diagnosticians share insights from their many combined years of feline practice, based on available evidence whenever possible, to bring together in one volume comprehensive information on state-of-the-art diagnostic tests, treatments, and techniques. I am grateful for their generosity in sharing and their desire to pass on their knowledge.

The focus of this book is first and foremost practical and concentrates on what most of us can and should accomplish in general practice. It is designed to give veterinarians information that can be used every day in an accessible format. It contains information on new topics (e.g., management of cats with chronic and concurrent diseases, feline life-stage medicine) and expanded information on emerging topics (e.g., genetics, feline-friendly practice, the importance of senior cat care, and the special needs of indoor cats). Throughout the book, algorithms, key points, and many photos are used to illustrate conditions and techniques. The book is also available electronically where the many illustrations will fully come alive.

Presenting the current state of knowledge about feline medicine in one volume presents challenges, but it has forced us to focus on the most important and clinically relevant aspects. Material is organized largely by body system to make finding information easy, and it has been kept concise and readable. In most cases, a logical "road map" for diagnosis and treatment has been provided, such as how to approach the vomiting cat or the cat with diarrhea. Common procedures, such as placing an esophagostomy tube, are described in detail with accompanying photos. Students, and those new to performing certain procedures, will find this approach invaluable. The reader will also find that some topics are covered more than once in different sections of the book. This allows different perspectives and even different points of view on important issues to be presented by experts in their areas of expertise.

The foundations of feline medicine are more important than ever, and thus a full section has been devoted to updated information and techniques for handling and physical examination, the art of taking the medical history, the idiosyncrasies of cats and drug therapy, the most effective drugs and techniques for analgesia, and detailed information on fluid therapy and anesthesia for many different medical situations. Special attention is paid to reducing the barriers that prevent so many of our feline companions from receiving regular veterinary care in a ground-breaking chapter on making your practice feline-friendly.

Veterinarians must continually strive to be open to learning from cats because cats do not give up their secrets easily. Clues are there for those who are willing to observe and listen. This textbook is a guide to that experience and it will enhance every veterinarian's feline practice skills, whether a new graduate or an "old hand." Our hope is that it will be your "go-to" reference for feline medicine, whether on your bookshelf or in electronic form.

Susan E. Little, DVM, DABVP (Feline)
Ottawa, Ontario, Canada

Acknowledgments

I owe a debt of gratitude to my support team at Elsevier—Shelly Stringer, David Stein, and Heidi Pohlman—for helping a novice editor survive. My thanks also go to Dr. Anthony Winkel, whose idea this was in the first place.

About the artist:
The cover and section opener images were provided by photographer Mats Göran Hamnäs. Mats was born in Stockholm, Sweden, in 1947. He works as a data programmer and lives and works in southern Sweden, Helsingborg, and Malmö. Mats interests include design, art, and architecture. His intent with his feline photographs is to portray cats in their natural environment.

Foreword

A new text in the field of feline medicine is always eagerly anticipated, especially in an era of rapidly increasing scientific knowledge and as more is learned about feline genetics and genetic diseases. An impressive group of authors have collaborated to present the latest information with the aim of improving feline health. This becomes more important as cats have longer lives and are increasingly selected to share the homes of people everywhere.

The Winn Feline Foundation is a not-for-profit organization founded by The Cat Fanciers' Association (CFA) in 1968, and it has been funding feline health studies for over 35 years. As a nonprofit foundation, Winn has funded over $3.3 million in direct research grants. Some of these projects have been basic science investigations; others have been aimed at immediate clinical impact. Examples of feline disease research supported by Winn Feline Foundation include studies that have investigated feline leukemia virus, feline immunodeficiency virus, feline infectious peritonitis, hypertrophic cardiomyopathy and other heart disorders, polycystic kidney disease and other kidney disorders, mammary and other cancers, hyperthyroidism, asthma, and inflammatory bowel disease. The Foundation also supports research into behavioral disorders. The emergence of feline genomic research in recent years is leading to an added focus in research at the molecular level. Grants are made to researchers at the leading research universities and institutions in the United States, and increasingly to researchers around the world.

Winn has been associated with some of the major breakthroughs in feline health. To name a few of these: identification of feline immunodeficiency virus, discovery of the link between taurine deficiency and dilated cardiomyopathy, development of methods to measure feline blood pressure, discovery of genes that cause several inherited diseases, and studies showing that early-age spays and neuters are safe.

Winn, in partnership with the American Veterinary Medical Association (AVMA), presents an annual Excellence in Feline Research Award and an annual scholarship award to an outstanding veterinary student with a special interest in feline medicine.

Winn welcomes this text as an important addition to the libraries of scientists, veterinarians, and veterinary students around the world.

Betty White
Winn Feline Foundation, Past President

Contents

V

INFECTIOUS DISEASES AND ZOONOSES

Editor: Melissa Kennedy

VI

MANAGING THE CAT WITH CONCURRENT AND CHRONIC DISEASES

Editor: Margie Scherk

VII

SPECIAL CONSIDERATIONS FOR THE SENIOR CAT

Editor: Susan E. Little

VIII

FELINE REPRODUCTION AND PEDIATRICS

Editor: Susan E. Little

IX

THE FELINE GENOME AND CLINICAL GENETICS

Editor: Leslie A. Lyons

X

POPULATION MEDICINE

Editor: Brenda Griffin

SECTION I

FUNDAMENTALS OF FELINE PRACTICE

Editor: Susan E. Little

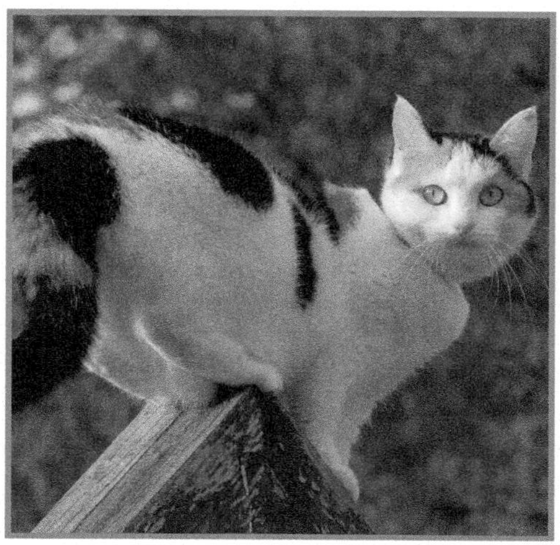

CHAPTER

1

Understanding the Cat and Feline-Friendly Handling

Ilona Rodan

OUTLINE

The cat has become the most popular pet in the United States, Canada, and Northern Europe, and its popularity continues to grow. Cats are fun, affectionate, beautiful, unique, and fascinating. Many people love their cats; 78% of us consider them family members.[38] As much as we help cats, they help us: by protecting human health, such as by decreasing their owners' blood pressure, reducing the probability of a second heart attack, and lessening the risk of depression or loneliness.

Nevertheless, and despite the great advances in feline medicine and surgery, many of us—veterinarians, veterinary teams, and cat owners—do not understand the nature of the cat and normal feline behavior. Among other issues, a lack of understanding of how cats react to fear and pain leads to difficulty during veterinary visits and a subsequent lack of routine veterinary care.[18] Compared with cat owners, dog owners take their pets to the veterinarian more often and are more likely to follow recommendations. In fact, in 2006 in the United States dog owners took their dogs to the veterinarian more than twice as often as cat owners brought their cats.[18] In addition, 72% of cats were seen by a veterinarian less often than once a year, compared with 42% of dogs.[18] Dog owners were also more likely than cat owners to procure vaccinations, physical examinations, and preventive dental care for their pets. In multipet households 33% of cats did not visit a veterinarian annually, compared with only 13% of dogs.[18] Feline diseases and pain thus go undetected, client relationships are not developed, and cats may suffer a reduced quality of life and decreased longevity. *This is an important issue involving feline welfare.*

We are all affected—our clients, the veterinary team, and the cats—by the challenges associated with feline veterinary visits. To understand the gravity of the problem and to find a solution, we must first understand several perspectives: that of the client, the veterinary team, and the cat.

THE CLIENT'S PERSPECTIVE

Many cat owners encounter practical difficulties in simply getting the cat to the veterinarian, such as putting the cat into a carrier.[40] Cat owners also worry that taking their cat to the veterinarian may damage the bond they have with their beloved feline. Some cat owners are embarrassed about their cat's behavior at the veterinary hospital, and others are upset about the way the veterinarian or veterinary team handles and interacts with their cat. They have often had a negative experience with their cat at a veterinary hospital, or when their cat returns home and is treated differently by the other cat (or cats). Some clients believe that the traumatic experience is more detrimental to the cat's health than a lack of veterinary care.

THE VETERINARY TEAM'S PERSPECTIVE

The challenges that the veterinary team faces with difficult feline patients include potential injury, zoonotic diseases (e.g., cat-scratch disease), decreased efficiency, increased use of resources (e.g., time and staff needed to handle a single cat), and an inability to properly educate clients because of their preoccupation with their cat's behavior or on how the clinicians handle their cat. Liability issues related to injury, zoonoses, and handling techniques are also cause for concern.[30]

In addition, performing a thorough physical examination or collecting laboratory samples from the cat may be difficult or impossible. Even when possible, feline stress associated with the veterinary visit may affect the results. Stress can result in the following examination abnormalities: tachycardia, bradycardia (if stress is prolonged), increased respiratory rate, dilated pupils, and hyperthermia. Some cats may evacuate anal sacs or bladder and bowel contents. The stool may be soft, blood tinged, and covered with mucus on account of colitis associated with the stressful experience.

Further, diagnostic test results can be markedly abnormal in a healthy but fearful patient. *Stress hyperglycemia is associated with patient struggling and can occur rapidly.*[32] Blood glucose levels can increase quickly and be as high as 613 mg/dL with or without glucosuria; this hyperglycemia can last for 90 to 120 minutes. Another blood chemistry abnormality is hypokalemia caused by epinephrine release.[6,10] Complete blood count (CBC) changes associated with epinephrine release include platelet hypersensitivity, lymphocytosis, and neutrophilia.[10] The author has seen lymphocytosis values of 8000 to 11,000 in fearful cats that have no underlying medical problems. In addition, "white-coat hypertension" can elevate the blood pressure well above 200 mm Hg (normal levels range from 104.5 to 159.3 mm Hg).[16]

THE CAT'S PERSPECTIVE

Imagine for a moment what a cat likely thinks and feels during the clinic visit and when traveling to and from the facility. The cat's perception differs significantly from that of the owner or the veterinarian. It is napping in a pool of sunlight when it sees its favorite person pulling out the cage that appears *only* when a veterinarian visit is imminent. The cat runs to hide, only to be pursued, then snatched from the safety of its hiding place. No matter how much the cat protests, it is shoved into the hated cage. The owner might be stressed, too, and might shout and grumble. Then comes the jostling, bumpy trip in the car, which might make the cat feel nauseated. If the cat urinates, defecates, or vomits, it must sit in the results, surrounded by the horrible stench. Even if the cat does not become sick, it may become so terrified in the car or at the clinic that it experiences increased gastrointestinal motility, leading to possible nausea, vomiting, or diarrhea. The cat might also salivate profusely because it is so nervous and uncomfortable.[22] Once the cat arrives at the clinic, strangers touch it and do things that make the cat feel uncomfortable. The cat is afraid and might scratch or bite in an attempt to protect itself. Worse yet, when the cat returns home, the other cats will probably give it a hard time because it smells different. Fortunately, the veterinarian can make the experience less stressful for the cat, the owner, and the veterinary team.

A BETTER WAY

Most clients cannot judge the veterinarian's knowledge of feline medicine, but they can judge the veterinarian's ability to work confidently, respectfully, and effectively with their cat. Having excellent surgical skills and medical knowledge is necessary but not sufficient; clients have higher needs and expectations. *Clients do not care how much the veterinarian knows until they know how much the veterinarian cares—for the client as well as the cat.*

By respecting and understanding the cat, veterinarians can build trusting relationships among cat owners, veterinary teams, and feline patients that will result in improved feline health and well-being through regular veterinary visits. Veterinary visits will be safer—and more relaxing—for all concerned. Examinations and diagnostic testing will yield more accurate results, and the veterinary team's job satisfaction will be enhanced while working with feline patients. Equally important, effective client education and communication can readily occur in this improved atmosphere. Finally, better practices attract new clients and feline patients, leading to more frequent veterinary visits—and the resultant better care—for cats.

Fortunately, veterinary visits can be made more pleasant for all involved. This chapter describes methods to better understand cats and how they perceive the world and react as they do. Further, this chapter addresses ways in which cat communication and learning can be used to help prevent aggression and fear. In addition, this chapter provides practical information regarding techniques to get the cat to the veterinary hospital, client education, and respectful handling of all feline patients during examinations and sample collections to prevent pain and distress.

UNDERSTANDING THE CAT

The History of the Cat

The earliest known ancestors of the Felidae family existed 45 million years ago. The modern cat, *Felis catus*, is descended from *Felis libyca*, also known as the *African wildcat* or *small African bush cat*. Recent discoveries indicate that cats began to live among humans when agriculture began in the Fertile Crescent (modern-day Western Asia and the Middle East) approximately 10,000 years ago.[8] The relationship between cats and humans likely began because it was mutually beneficial, with cats killing rodents attracted to stored grain. The earliest direct evidence of cat domestication occurred 9500 years ago, when a kitten was buried with its owner in Cyprus.[39] Archaeologists found a feline molar at a site in Israel dating to roughly 9000 years ago (7000 BCE) and also discovered an ivory cat statuette estimated to be 3700 years old (1700 BCE), also in Israel. Some 3600 years ago (1,600 BCE) in Egypt, cats were worshiped and mourned at their death. Mourners shaved off their eyebrows, and cats were mummified for burial in sanctified plots, often with mummified mice added for use in the afterlife. Egyptian paintings from that time depict cats poised under chairs, sometimes collared or tethered and often eating from bowls.[7] The cat population increased and spread to other countries, likely by people who prized cats' ability to control rodent populations.

The cat's good reputation in Europe began to plummet in the late Middle Ages, when Catholic leaders declared cats to be agents of the devil and associated them with witchcraft. From approximately 1400 to 1800, vast numbers of cats were exterminated, and individuals who kept them were accused of being witches and also killed. Louis Pasteur's discovery of microbes in the nineteenth century helped to reinstate cats to their former high regard; they were considered the cleanest of animals. By the late 1800s, the growing middle class became interested in cat shows and developing and establishing distinctive breeds, especially long-haired breeds. During the twentieth century, cats became even more cherished, often living long and comfortable lives.

Other domesticated species have undergone genetic selection. For example, there are specialized breeds of dogs for hunting, herding, and guarding. However, the mutually beneficial relationship between humans and cats made such genetic selection unnecessary. As a result, domestic cats have retained many aspects of their wild predecessors. Cats are true carnivores and have amazing athletic abilities and keen senses to allow them to hunt successfully. They can sense and avoid danger, and they possess a heightened fight-or-flight response.[11] Like their wild ancestors, they hide illness and pain as a protective mechanism, which adds to the mistaken impression that cats are independent and require little or no care.

Indeed, cats are social animals, but their social structure differs from that of humans and dogs. Given sufficient food resources, free-living cats will choose to live in social groups, called *colonies*.[20,27] The social organization of the colony is based on females cooperatively nursing and raising their young.[20] Within a colony, cats will choose preferred associates, or affiliates. These cats show affection toward one another by allogrooming: grooming one another, generally on the head and neck.[4,5] Because the head and neck are preferred areas for physical touch, cats may become upset and even aggressive when people try to pet them in other areas. Therefore, unless a person knows an individual cat's preferences, stroking or petting in other areas should be avoided in favor of rubbing or stroking the cat around the neck and head (e.g., under the chin).

Feral cat colonies are quite insular, and strangers are generally driven away. If a new cat continues to visit the colony, it may eventually be integrated into the group, but the process requires several weeks.[19] This is why gradually introducing a cat into a household with resident cats is so important.

Although social, cats are solitary hunters. They catch small prey and may need to hunt as often as 20 times a day. Because cats are solitary hunters, they must maintain their physical health and avoid fights with other cats whenever possible. Much of feline communication serves to prevent altercations over food and territory, and most cats try to avoid the risks associated with active fighting.

The Cat's Senses: How Cats Perceive the World

Because perception is everything, humans can better understand and interact with the cat by understanding how it perceives the world. Cats' perception is based on their senses, most of which are highly sensitive compared with ours.

The cat's sense of hearing is approximately four times more acute than a human's. Cats can hear a broad range of frequencies, including ultrasound, allowing them to perceive the ultrasonic calls or chattering of rodents.[11] Their movable pinnae help localize sounds. Because of their sensitive hearing, sources of stress at the clinic include ringing telephones, paging systems, and human voices, which sound uncomfortably loud even when we think we are talking in a normal tone.[29] The noise from centrifuges, x-ray machines, blood pressure monitors, and other medical equipment can startle feline patients. The sounds of other cats and other animals, such as barking, whining, growling, and yowling, can also generate stress.[29]

Cats can see well in dim light and are very sensitive to movement, abilities that help them hunt for prey. Consequently, rapid movements, especially if unanticipated, will likely heighten a cat's responses and can lead to a more reactive patient. In other words, veterinary staff members working with cats should remember that "slow is fast, and fast is slow."

Cats have an excellent sense of smell and have 5 to 10 times more olfactory epithelium than humans.[1] They also have vomeronasal organs (Jacobson's organ) located in the roof of the mouth behind the upper incisors. The flehmen response, wherein the cat grimaces and partially opens the mouth, occurs when the vomeronasal organs detect the odors of other cats.[36] Cats are also very sensitive to touch and use their whiskers to examine their environment. When aroused, they can be very sensitized and may respond aggressively even to gentle petting or stroking.

In summary, multiple stressors that come from auditory, visual, olfactory, and tactile stimuli typically occur at the veterinary hospital. The accumulated stress arising from these stimuli can be greater than the sum of the stress from the individual components.[29]

CAT COMMUNICATION

Cats communicate with us all the time, but are we listening? Before stressors at the clinic and home can be identified, it is necessary to understand that cats perceive the world through their senses and use vocal, visual, olfactory, and tactile means to communicate. Understanding this communication system is critical in preventing altercations with other felines. As solitary hunters, cats need to maintain their physical health and fitness. Clear communication helps them avoid injury and possible threats to their survival.[2,13] As a result, cats turn to fighting only as a last resort, after other attempts to communicate have failed. Being able to perceive and understand the cat's communication signals can prevent many aggressive acts at the veterinary hospital.

Visual Communication

Cats use a range of subtle body postures, facial expressions, and tail positions to communicate with other cats to defuse tension and avoid physical contact (Figures 1-1 and 1-2). Understanding body postures allows humans to recognize—and reward—calm behavior; if postures associated with fear are recognized in time, it is possible to keep that fear from escalating to a point at which injuries are likely (see Figures 1-1 and 1-2). Knowing how to recognize offensive and defensive behavior in cats is important because the purpose of most signaling and posturing is to avoid battle.

Familiarity with feline body postures helps humans identify whether the cat intends to flee, freeze, or fight. Although most cats do not want to fight, they may bluff, making themselves look much larger in an attempt to scare away others.[2] Figure 1-1 shows various body postures that cats use to communicate. The normal cat is in the top left corner. The cat becomes increasingly fearful in the subsequent illustrations (moving from top to bottom). The cat in the lower left-hand corner is extremely fearful but will become aggressive if no escape route is

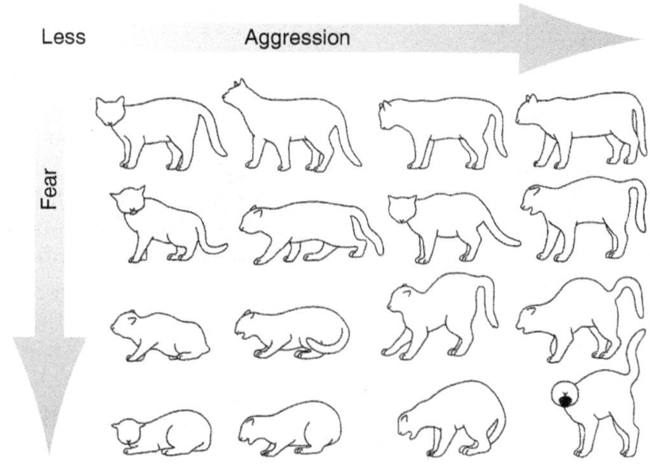

FIGURE 1-1 Recognizing body postures that communicate fear or aggression keeps fear from escalating to a situation that can lead to injuries to all involved. *(Adapted from Bowen J, Heath S: An overview of feline social behaviour and communication:* Behaviour problems in small animals: practical advice for the veterinary team, *ed 1, Philadelphia, 2005, Saunders. The original figure was adapted from Leyhausen P:* Cat behaviour, *New York, 1979, Garland STMP Press.)*

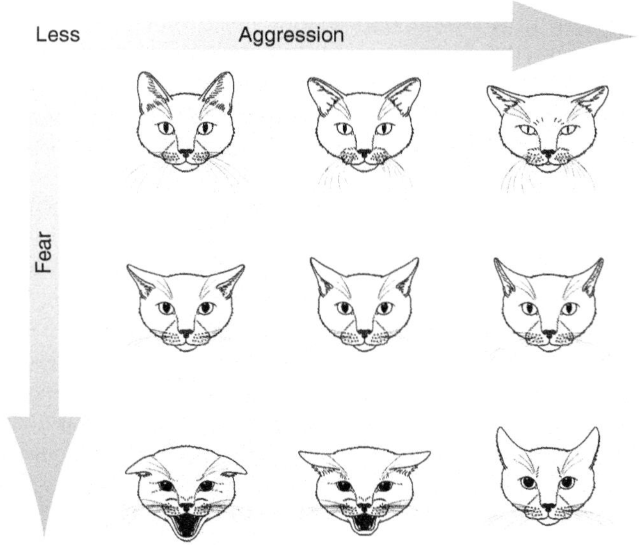

FIGURE 1-2 Facial signals change more quickly than body postures and provide more immediate indications of a cat's level of fear and aggression. *(Adapted from Bowen J, Heath S: An overview of feline social behaviour and communication:* Behaviour problems in small animals: practical advice for the veterinary team, *ed 1, 2005, Saunders Ltd. The original figure was adapted from P Leyhausen:* Cat behaviour, *1979, Garland STMP Press, New York.)*

available.[26] In the clinic a common example is a terrified cat that feels cornered and huddles in the back of a cage. As we move from left to right in the figure, the cat becomes increasingly aggressive. At first, the cat might be bluffing, but it may become aggressive if it cannot flee and continues to feel threatened. The cat in the lower right-hand corner is the most fearful and aggressive.

Whereas body postures effectively signal a cat's level of fear and aggression, even from a distance, facial signals (see Figure 1-2) change much more quickly and provide more immediate indications of a cat's level of fear and aggression. As with Figure 1-1, as we move from top to bottom in the figure, the cat becomes increasingly fearful, and as we move from left to right, the cat becomes increasingly aggressive.[26]

Ears are erect when the cat is alert and focusing on a stimulus *(top left corner)*. Ears are swiveled downward and sideways in a defensive cat *(bottom left)*; in the aggressive cat, the ears are swiveled, displaying the inner pinnae sideways *(bottom right)*.[26]

The pupils specifically are the most instructive feline signal. Slit pupils indicate the normal state *(top left corner)*, widely dilated pupils are associated with fear and the fight-or-flight response *(lower left corner)*, and oblong pupils signal aggression *(lower right)*.[26] Pupil size generally correlates to the intensity of the situation, as moving from top to bottom in Figure 1-2 illustrates. Cats understand these subtle differences and use them to help prevent fights. (It is important to recognize that ambient light can also affect pupil size.)

Two other eye communications are very important; knowing these can help to reduce the cat's stress levels. First, blinking is believed to signal that the cat is seeking reassurance in a tense environment. Fortunately, this behavior works for both intercat and human–cat communication.[2] Blinking slowly or making "winky-eyes" in the direction of the cat can help comfort the cat. Second, because prolonged eye contact, especially from an unknown cat or human, constitutes a threat to cats, people who are not well known to the cat should not stare. Veterinary team members should be taught to blink slowly in the cat's direction and refrain from staring to make the veterinary visit less stressful for the cat.

The cat's tail is remarkably expressive. When the tail is held up vertically or wrapped, it signals relaxed, friendly intentions. A tail held straight down or perpendicular to the ground indicates an offensive posture.[26] The cat lashes the tail vigorously from side to side when very agitated, annoyed, or aroused or during conflict. If this signal is unheeded, the cat's behavior can escalate to aggression.[2]

Olfactory Communication

Sebaceous glands that deposit the cat's scent are located around the lips and chin, interdigitally, and in the perianal area. Cats leave olfactory signals by rubbing the sebaceous glands of the face on objects, other cats, and humans; scratching (to deposit scent from the interdigital glands); and spraying. Spraying is usually a *normal* olfactory communication among cats (although intercat conflict in a household can induce spraying). Additionally, some cats communicate through urination and middening (fecal marking).

Olfactory signals play an important role in communication and social behavior. They enable hunting cats to communicate remotely, for example, by marking a territory as their own with a durable signal that lasts over a period of time.[2] Strategic use of olfactory signals means that hunting cats can protect their space without needing to meet or interact physically with other cats.

In veterinary hospitals the scent of unfamiliar cats, dogs, and humans can frighten and arouse feline patients. Because the cat's sense of smell is more acute than a human's, veterinarian staff members usually do not notice the olfactory signals left by another cat or even the scent of a cleaning solution that may be offensive to a cat. Often in an examination room that seems to be thoroughly cleaned, cats go directly to a specific area, sniff at that area, and then exhibit the flehmen response. When one cat is stressed, the feeling almost seems contagious, spreading quickly to other cats. This happens because distressed cats leave the scent of their distress, which affects the other cats.

Knowing the importance of olfactory communication among cats helps the staff in the veterinary hospital. Clients can be educated to put something that smells like home—the cat's basket, blanket, or a favorite person's clothing (that is not freshly laundered)—in the carrier when bringing the cat to the veterinary hospital. If the cat needs to stay at the hospital for any reason, the familiar item should also stay with the cat. In addition, when reintroducing cats after a veterinary visit or introducing new cats, the client can be taught to take simple precautions such as exchanging the bedding, or wiping the "at-home" cat with a towel and then wiping the returning cat with the same towel, to help reduce stress and conflict.

Vocal and Tactile Communication

Most feline vocalizations bring cats together. Cats also vocalize when communicating with humans, and they learn quickly how to make humans respond to their vocalizations for food and attention. Although cats purr when they are content, they may also purr when sick or fearful. The purr solicits contact and care. The trill and miaow are friendly greeting calls. Affiliate cats engage in allorubbing (rubbing against one another) and allogrooming, and they often lie close together.[4]

CAUSES OF MISBEHAVIOR AND AGGRESSION AT VETERINARY VISITS

Fear is the number-one cause of misbehavior and aggression in cats at the veterinary hospital. Punishment and poor socialization often lead to fear aggression.[15] Anxiety can also lead to misbehavior and aggression. It is *crucial* that all staff members understand the important role that fear plays in feline misbehavior and aggression. Further, giving negative labels to difficult patients (e.g., "evil" or "naughty)" can subtly influence the staff's behavior and attitude and further harm interactions with fearful patients.

Fear, defined as an emotional response that enables an animal to avoid situations and activities that could be potentially dangerous,[2] commonly occurs in cats in unfamiliar environments.[11] A common saying, "Cats don't like change without their consent," is only too apt. Having a sense of control, even if is not exerted, makes the cat more comfortable and reduces stress.[21] Giving the cat some control during the veterinary visit by letting it choose a comfortable position and place to be examined will significantly reduce stress associated with veterinary visits.

Box 1-1 provides a list of common causes of aggression at the veterinary hospital. The belief that dominance causes feline aggression at the veterinary hospital is a common misconception.[24]

Cats may experience anxiety, as well as fear, at the veterinary hospital. Anxiety is the emotional anticipation of an adverse event—which may or may not be real.[25] A cat that has had a previous painful experience at a veterinary hospital will likely be anxious during the next visit, anticipating pain. Using analgesia to prevent or treat pain and also prevent anxiety at future veterinary visits is critical.

Indeed, pain is the second most common reason for aggression in cats. Boxes 1-2 and 1-3 present some frequently underrecognized painful conditions and procedures. Cats tend to hide expressions of pain as a protective mechanism. *If there is any question regarding the presence of pain, administer an analgesic and then reassess the patient's response. Response to therapy is an appropriate and important tool in pain assessment.*[14] For a more detailed list and additional information about analgesia, see Chapter

BOX 1-1
Common Causes of Feline Aggression in the Veterinary Hospital

- Fear aggression: fear of unfamiliar places or people
- Pain-associated aggression
- Anxiety or memory of a previous negative (fearful or painful) experience at the veterinary hospital
- Getting attention for the behavior (e.g., "poor kitty")
- Play aggression
- Lack of socialization
- Forceful restraint
- Loud noises
- Unpleasant smells
- Fast or rushed movements toward cat
- Underlying medical problem (e.g., meningioma or other central nervous system problem)
- Petting intolerance or aggression
- Owner anxiety
- Physical punishment
- Redirected aggression

BOX 1-2
Frequently Overlooked Conditions that Cause Pain

- Anal sac impaction and evacuation
- Arthritis
- Cancer
- Chin acne, severe
- Chronic wounds
- Clipper burns
- Congestive heart failure
- Constipation
- Corneal ulcers and other corneal diseases
- Dental disease
- Otitis (from ear mites, yeast, and bacterial infections)
- Pleural effusion
- Pruritis
- Pulmonary edema
- Spondylosis
- Urine scalding
- Vomiting

BOX 1-3
Frequently Overlooked Procedures that Cause Pain

- Abdominocentesis
- Anal sac expression
- Bandaging
- Ear cleaning
- Handling—even gentle handling and hard surfaces can increase pain in animals with arthritis or other conditions that are painful
- Intravenous catheterization
- Manual extraction of stool
- Restraint and forceful handling procedures
- Thoracocentesis

6, as well as the Pain Management Guidelines developed by the American Animal Hospital Association and the American Association of Feline Practitioners.[14] Prompt provision of effective analgesia will both address the pain and eliminate or reduce pain-associated aggression. Buprenorphine is an excellent analgesic and is well absorbed when given transmucosally (0.02 mg/kg).[34] A prophylactic dose provides full effect within 30 minutes (although analgesia has been noted earlier), the same as that conferred by intravenous administration.[33] When buprenorphine is given before painful procedures and examinations, a prolonged, stressful, terrifying session can be transformed into a relatively quick, well-tolerated experience. Buprenorphine can also be administered subcutaneously, with full effect occurring at 60 minutes. Injectable delivery is preferred for cats that do not like to have their mouths handled.

Fear Responses

Because fear responses are among the more common causes of aggression, we will address them here. Any cat will try to defend itself if it feels threatened. Fearful animals engage in the fight-or-flight response. If cornered, most cats choose escape, or "flight," over "fight." However, if not allowed to leave, the cat will fight, which may involve biting and scratching. These are *normal* feline behaviors derived from predator-avoidance behaviors.

The fight or flight response includes the Four Fs:

- *Freeze*—the cat "freezes," crouching and becoming immobile. This immobility usually occurs at the beginning of the trigger stimulus or when the trigger stimulus is relatively low. This behavior is common in cats at the veterinary hospital, and it frequently expedites the examination.
- *Flight*—the cat actively avoids the trigger stimulus. For example, the cat may dart into a corner or under a chair to keep from being picked up.
- *Fight*—the cat exhibits defensive aggression to avoid or back away from a frightening stimulus. For example, when the veterinarian reaches for a cat that is cowering at the back of a cage, the cat may become aggressive to protect itself.
- *Fiddle or fidget*—the cat engages in a displacement activity, such as grooming, when faced with a fear-eliciting stimulus. Although the cat wishes to avoid the stimulus, it cannot do so.

LEARNING IN CATS

Kittens are excellent observational learners. This characteristic likely developed as an evolutionary adaptation, because kittens learn from the queen how to kill their prey.[4] Kittens learn quickly by observing an adult cat, generally the queen, performing a task before they attempt it. Thus, if an adult cat in the household is especially fearful at the veterinary clinic, scheduling separate appointments for the kitten is ideal.

A common misconception is that cats cannot learn tricks; in fact, they enjoy the interactions of training and can learn to "sit," "come," and follow other commands as long as they receive positive reinforcement (Figure 1-3). In fact, employing some useful and familiar commands or tricks in the veterinary hospital, along with treats, can help cats feel more comfortable and prevent reactivity.

Humans can influence what cats learn by affecting their experiences. For example, if a cat has a painful experience during its first visit to the veterinarian, it will almost certainly be fearful during subsequent visits. In contrast, if the cat learns to associate the carrier, car trip, and veterinary visit with treats and other positive experiences, it learns to enjoy everything associated with a trip to the vet.

People generally focus on preventing undesired behavior rather than rewarding desired behavior. Punishment inhibits learning and increases anxiety. If the cat does not understand what is wanted or why it is being punished, it may learn to associate pain or fear with the situation; eventually, this association can lead to overt aggression.[42] Verbal or physical punishment should *never* be used with cats.

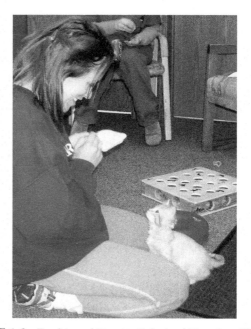

FIGURE 1-3 Teaching a kitten to sit during kitten class. Sit is easy: Slowly raise a treat from close to the nose slightly over the kitten's head. As the head goes up, the tail goes down. Softly say, "Sit" as the cat sits.

Consequently, it is important to teach team members and clients that positive reinforcement of desired behavior is the most effective way to teach a cat and unwanted behavior should be ignored or redirected to a desirable behavior. Desirable behavior is being calm, playing, purring, and accepting gentle handling. Positive reinforcement must be given within 3 seconds of the desired behavior so that the cat has no opportunity to engage in another, less desirable activity that might be inadvertently rewarded instead. At the veterinary hospital, the cat should always be rewarded with delicious treats and praise for calm behavior.

Because anxiety can inhibit learning, cats with a history of anxiety at the veterinary hospital may require anxiolytic medication. Alprazolam is a short-acting benzodiazepine that takes effect rapidly. This drug can both abort and prevent anxiety or distress associated with veterinary visits. Recommended doses for alprazolam are 0.125 to 0.25 mg/kg, PO, every 12 hours. It should be given 60 minutes before the scheduled appointment. Alprazolam works well in conjunction with food treats and other rewards. Further, alprazolam can be used concurrently with tricyclic antidepressants or selective serotonin reuptake inhibitors.

Although tranquilizers, such as acepromazine, have been used to prevent fear and aggression at the veterinary hospital, they do not relieve anxiety and can disinhibit aggression, resulting in a more aggressive cat.

Sensitive Period of Socialization

The socialization period is the age range during which particular events are especially likely to have long-term effects on the individual's development. In kittens the sensitive period is from 2 to 9 weeks (as a point of comparison, the sensitive period in dogs lasts until 16 weeks). Kittens that have positive handling experiences during this period are more resistant to stress, display less fear, and can learn some tasks faster than cats that are not handled.[26] Early enrichment and positive exposure to a wide variety of stimuli, especially the stimuli that the cat will commonly encounter during its lifetime (e.g., car travel, veterinary visits, children, dogs, vacuum cleaners), mean the kitten (and later the cat) will perceive these experiences as comfortable, even pleasant. The veterinary team should encourage clients to expose the kitten to people of different ages and gender, under calm conditions, and reinforce the pleasant experience appropriately (e.g., using treats, toys, massage, and praise).

Fortunately, the older cat can still learn, acclimate, and adapt to new experiences, although it is far easier to teach kittens during their sensitive period of socialization.

FELINE-FRIENDLY VETERINARY VISITS

The Situation Today

Historically, the education of veterinarians and technicians has focused on caring for sick, poisoned, and injured cats. Over the past several decades, the importance of preventive care has been recognized. More recently, education has emphasized communication and the business of veterinary medicine. Good business decisions include good communication with team members, clients, *and* patients. Unfortunately, listening to, understanding, and respecting the cat often receive little consideration. The current reality is that college instructional programs for veterinary students and technician trainees focus on the dog as the primary small animal companion, both in medical care (as the lecture ends, the professor might add, "...and yes, cats get arthritis, too") and patient handling and training. Because the primary patients that students encounter are dogs, they have little (or no) opportunity to learn appropriate handling techniques for feline patients or consider problems associated with excessive restraint. Schools typically teach technicians to overhandle cats, thus making visits unduly stressful for both feline patients and their owners.

Client Education

Client education starts with the phone call, before the client (whether a repeat or first-time client) even comes to the clinic. The veterinary staff member who answers the phone should ask all clients whether they expect difficulty in transporting the cat to the veterinary hospital. The staff member should provide information as needed regarding ways that the client can help make the visit as pleasant as possible. Because most people are visual learners and the busy clinic phone line precludes spending sufficient time to educate them effectively, it is a good idea to mail or e-mail handouts or videos explaining techniques to get the cat into the carrier and accustom the cat to car rides, as well as suggesting items that should accompany the cat to the veterinary hospital. Educational resources are listed in Box 1-4.

Getting the Cat to the Veterinary Hospital

The veterinary team can teach clients a simple way to make the carrier a feline haven: simply by keeping the carrier in a location that is easily accessible to the cat (Figure 1-4).[22] Placing familiar clothing from a favorite person in the carrier, along with treats or toys, will entice the cat to enter on its own. Rewarding the cat for entering the carrier with treats, food, and calm praise will positively reinforce the cat's favorable associations with

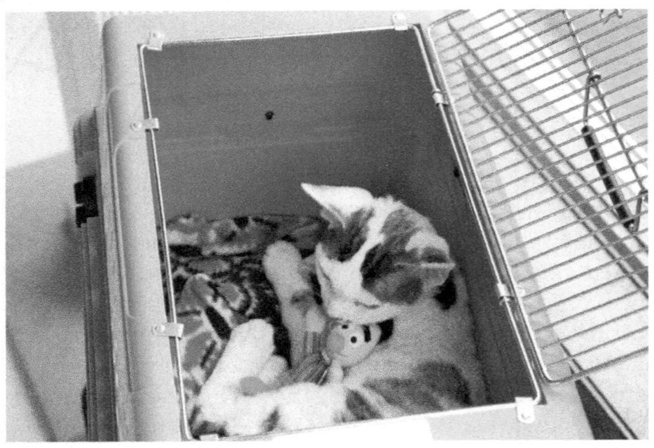

FIGURE 1-4 This kitten's carrier is always left out next to the cat tree. The kitten has learned to use the carrier as a safe haven, which greatly reduces or eliminates fear associated with travel and veterinary visits.

BOX 1-4
Educational Resources

For Veterinarians

1. American Association of Feline Practitioners Feline Behavior Guidelines: http://www.catvets.com
2. Feline Advisory Bureau: Creating a Cat Friendly Practice and Cat Friendly Practice 2, www.fabcats.org/catfriendlypractice/guides.html
3. Video: For veterinary professionals: Encourage cat visits, Ilona Rodan, http://www.catalystcouncil.org/enewsletter/february10/index.html
4. Healthy Cats for Life: http://www.healthycatsforlife.com/clinic.html

For Clients

1. Video: Tips for taking your cat to the veterinarian, Ilona Rodan, www.catalystcouncil.org/resources/video/?Id=89

the carrier. Once the cat regularly enters the carrier at home and uses it for resting, the owner can take the cat on car rides periodically, pairing the ride with positive experiences. Edible treats, favorite toys, and a comb or brush (if the cat enjoys being groomed) can be brought along to make the trip more pleasant and less strange. Fasting the cat for at least a few hours before car travel prevents motion sickness. The fasting also increases the cat's interest in treats both during the car ride and at the veterinary hospital, which creates a more positive experience. Spraying Feliway (Ceva Animal Health, St. Louis, Mo.), a synthetic feline pheromone that calms the cat, in the carrier 30 minutes before travel is very helpful.[28] Finally, draping a blanket or towel over the carrier helps prevent motion sickness.

Carriers designed to open from the top as well as from the front make it easier to move the cat into and out of the carrier in a nonstressful manner. The ideal carrier also allows for removal of the top half, so that an especially timid cat can remain in the bottom half of the carrier during as much of the veterinary examination as possible. Hard-sided carriers can be secured by the car's seatbelt to increase the cat's safety and prevent jostling during the car ride.

Receiving the Cat and Client

No matter how calm the reception area is, taking the cat directly to an examination room as soon as it arrives will reduce fear and anxiety caused by seeing, hearing, and smelling unfamiliar people and animals. Minimizing the waiting time is also important because most cats do not calm down as quickly as a dog might in the same circumstances.

First Veterinary Visits and Kitten Classes

First veterinary visits allow the veterinary team to set up the kitten or cat for success. If first veterinary visits are pleasant, future veterinary experiences are also likely to be positive.[23] Clients are more willing to bring back their cats for routine health care visits if they are not fraught with tension. Cat owners should be taught early about giving their cat positive exposure to normal feline maintenance procedures—such as claw trimming, combing, ear inspections and cleaning, and teeth brushing—so that these stimuli have little or no adverse impact during veterinary visits and home care. Clients should be encouraged to bring their kittens to the clinic between appointments for weight checks, increased socialization, and fun visits, especially during the first year of life.

Kitten classes are an excellent way to teach owners how to understand cats and their needs, to provide opportunities for family members to learn how to handle kittens for home maintenance procedures (e.g., claw trimming), and to allow kittens to socialize with other kittens.[37] See Chapter 11 for more information on kitten classes.

Getting the Cat Out of the Carrier

Once in the examination room, the cat should be allowed to initiate contact; cats are less apprehensive if they can control their environment. While greeting the client and reviewing the cat's history, the veterinarian should open the carrier door and allow the cat to sniff or explore the room. Tossing or quietly placing catnip or treats near the carrier can entice the cat to venture out on its own. While obtaining the history, the veterinarian can also assess the patient from a distance without making direct eye contact—which, as previously discussed, the cat may perceive as a threat—to evaluate respiratory pattern, gait, and overall behavior. Monitoring the patient's posturing and facial expressions and response to treats can reveal the cat's fear level. If the cat remains wary, the veterinarian may extend an index finger toward the cat that it may smell (and ideally rub against); most cats enjoy rubbing against protruding objects. The veterinarian should not touch the cat on its head or neck as it is exiting the carrier because this often causes the cat to retreat instinctively rather than move forward.

If the cat will not leave the carrier voluntarily, the top half of the carrier should be carefully removed, if possible, so that the cat can remain in the bottom half for as much of the examination as possible (Figures 1-5 and 1-6). If the cat is still fearful, the veterinarian may slowly slide a towel between the top and bottom of the carrier while the top is removed. The towel provides a safe hiding place for the cat and is in place for wrapping the towel around the cat (a feline "burrito wrap") if needed; the towel wrap helps calm and reassure the cat (Figure 1-7). When the cat must be removed from the bottom half of the carrier, lift the cat from underneath, supporting the caudal abdomen near the hind legs. *It is extremely important never to dump the cat out of the carrier.* Once the cat is out of the carrier, the carrier should be placed out of sight so that the cat will not attempt to return to it.

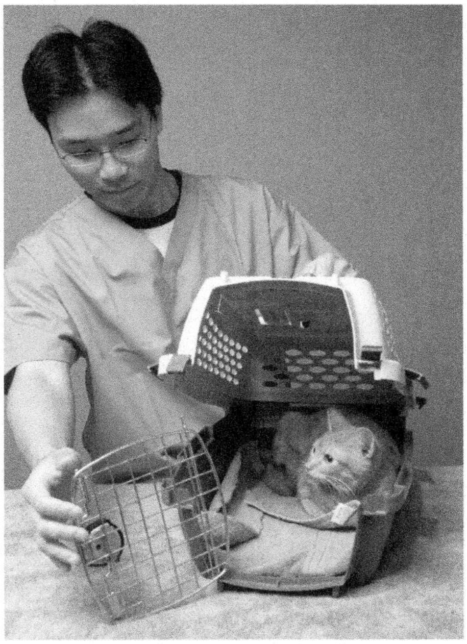

FIGURE 1-5 If the cat doesn't voluntarily leave the carrier, remove the top half. Ideally, have the front of the carrier facing the wall to prevent escape. *(Image courtesy Yin S:* Low stress handling, restraint and behavior modification of dogs & cats: techniques for developing patients who love their visits, *Davis, Calif, 2009, CattleDog.)*

Finally, once the examination is finished, the cat should be returned to its carrier as soon as possible.

Handling During Examination

1. The best place to examine the cat is wherever the cat wants to be; as previously explained, this gives the cat some control over its environment. Many cats do not like examination tables because they have been punished for climbing on tables at home. An examination room with perches or shelves, benches, and a small pet scale provides a

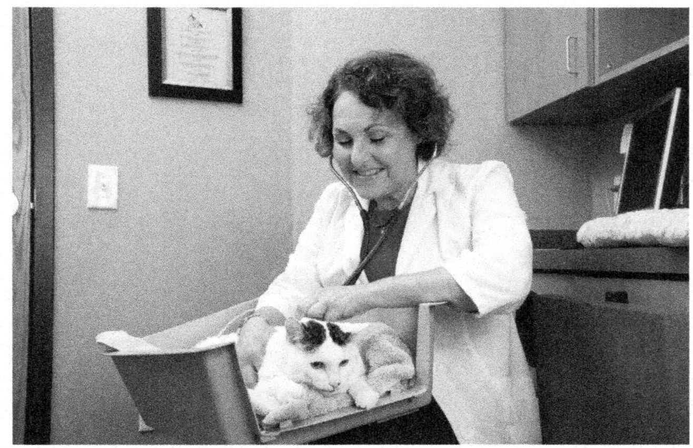

FIGURE 1-6 Examining the cat in the bottom half of the carrier often makes it feel more secure and is easier on everyone involved.

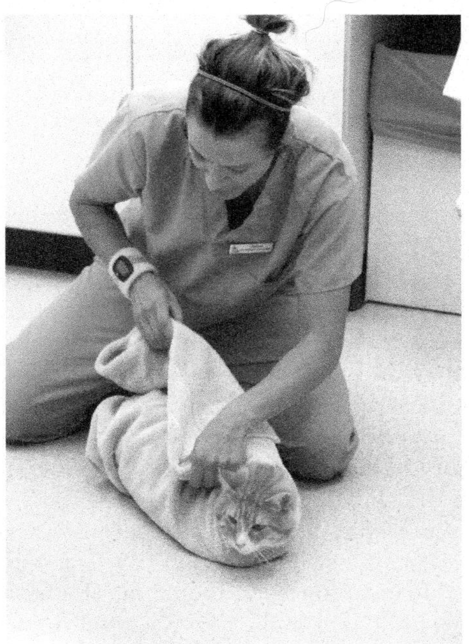

FIGURE 1-7 The "burrito" towel wrap often makes cats feel more secure and prevents scratching of those working with the patient. The best handler should educate other staff during staff meetings and assist with new employee training.

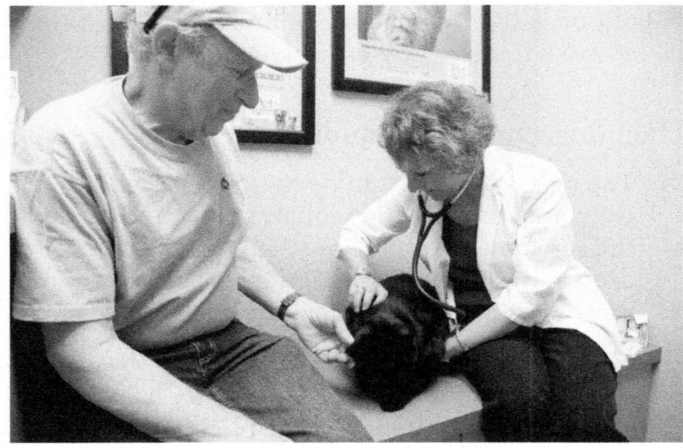

FIGURE 1-8 Cats often prefer to be with their people, either in their laps or sitting next to them. This cat is receiving positive reinforcement, the reward of attention, for good behavior at the veterinary hospital.

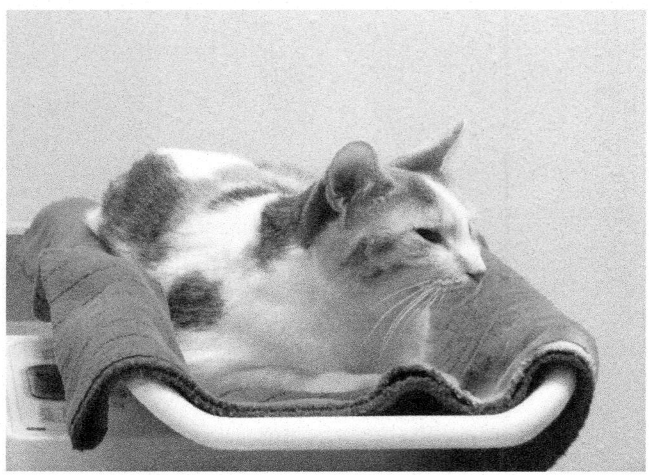

FIGURE 1-9 Many cats like to stay in a small pet scale after being weighed. The raised sides make them feel more secure.

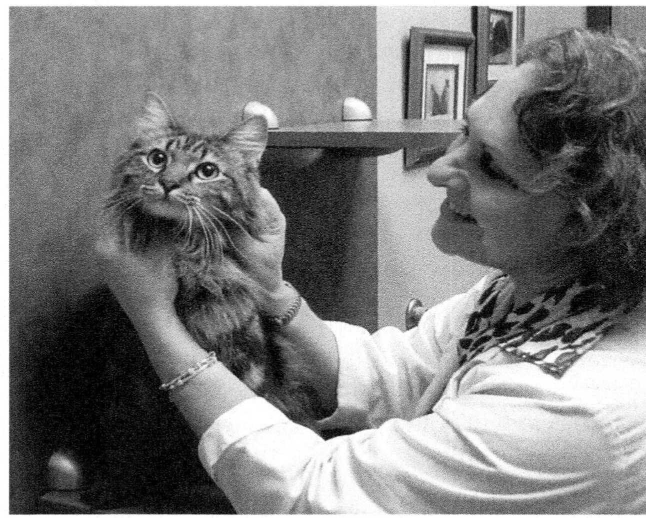

FIGURE 1-10 Some confident cats prefer to be higher up and enjoy the cat perches in this examination room.

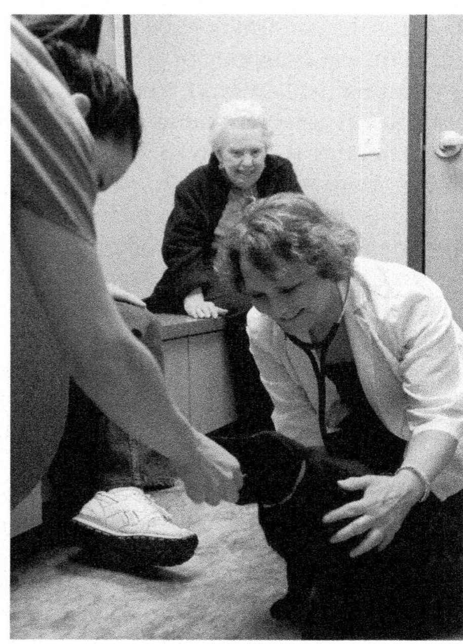

FIGURE 1-11 Some cats prefer to be examined on the floor. Just as children get stickers or treats when they go to the doctor, cats can receive treats or catnip.

good selection of options (Figures 1-8 through 1-10). Many cats prefer being examined when they are on a familiar blanket or item of clothing from the carrier, which already has the cat's scent. Often, it is easiest to have the cat stay next to the client or on the floor or a lap during the examination (Figure 1-11). Cats that like sitting on laps are often comfortable in the clinician's lap, but it should be in a position where it is facing away from the clinician and can see the family member. Further, it may help the cat feel more secure if it can lean against the clinician's body; otherwise, it might fear falling from the table. The following suggestions will make the examination far less stressful.

- If the table must be used for the examination and collection of laboratory samples, the cat should be placed on a fleece, towel, or other soft material that already has the scent of the cat, such as the padding or favorite person's clothing from the interior of the carrier.
- Slow motions should be used instead of fast ones.
- If possible, the cat should be allowed time to relax before the next part of the examination is performed.
- The cat should not be stretched out; it should be held in a relaxed manner, without pulling its feet (Figure 1-12).

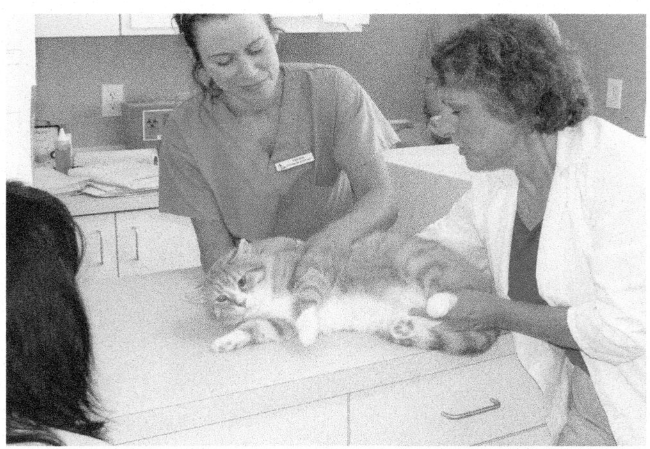

FIGURE 1-12 The cat should not be stretched out when being held on its side. See how the legs are held in a comfortable position, with the handler's fingers supporting the feet gently.

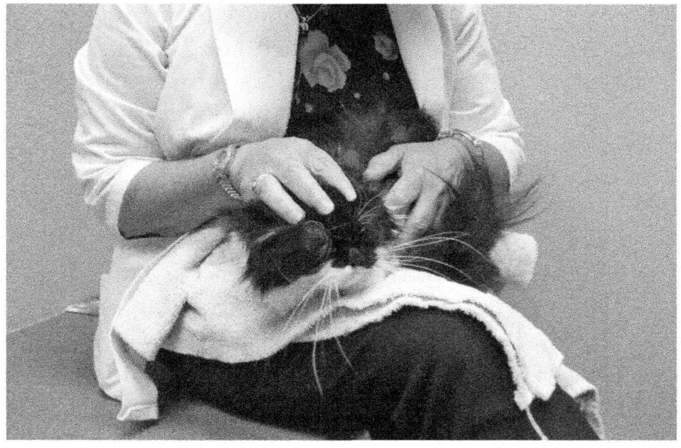

FIGURE 1-13 Slowly massaging the top of the head helps comfort the cat.

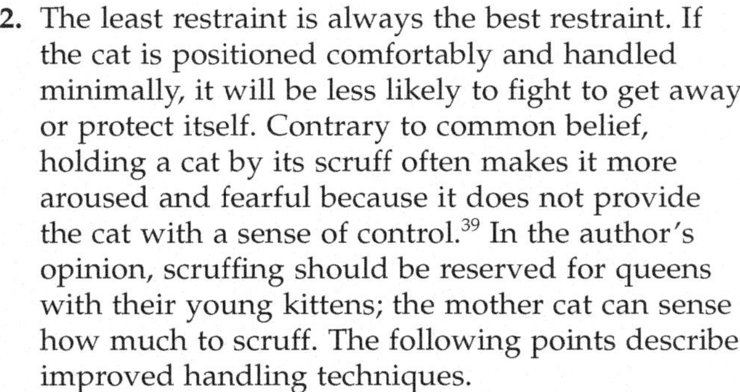

2. The least restraint is always the best restraint. If the cat is positioned comfortably and handled minimally, it will be less likely to fight to get away or protect itself. Contrary to common belief, holding a cat by its scruff often makes it more aroused and fearful because it does not provide the cat with a sense of control.[39] In the author's opinion, scruffing should be reserved for queens with their young kittens; the mother cat can sense how much to scruff. The following points describe improved handling techniques.
   - Rather than scruffing, many cats like to be massaged on their head, behind the ears, or under the chin. Such massage can both distract and calm the cat. Acupressure is another calming technique. The three middle fingers are used to slowly massage or stroke the top of the head, and the first and fifth digits (i.e., thumb and pinkie) are used to control the cat's head and thereby protect both examiner and cat (Figures 1-13 and 1-14).
   - The cat should not be stretched or extended; instead, it should be held in a relaxed manner, without pulling the feet.
   - The order of the examination should be modified to make it easier on the patient; it is not necessary to examine every cat starting at the head and working to the tail. In fact, performing the least stressful parts of the examination first and reserving areas that the cat does not like touched (for some, the teeth and mouth; for many arthritic cats, the feet; for cats with urinary tract problems, the abdomen) until the end of the examination will help the cat stay more relaxed.
3. Remember: "Slow is fast, and fast is slow." Fast or abrupt movements may alarm the cat and cause it to struggle, which may necessitate several holders. It is important to work slowly and confidently to make the cat comfortable.

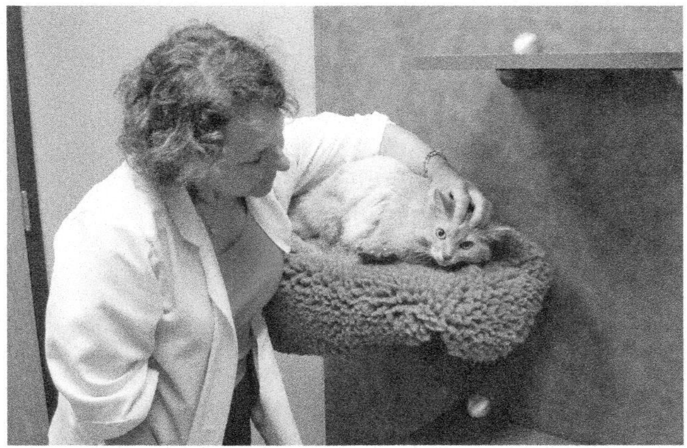

FIGURE 1-14 Notice how the thumb and fifth digit hold the cat's head in place while acupressure is used to calm the cat.

4. Desired behavior should be rewarded with treats, catnip toys, and soft praise. Rewards help reinforce desired behavior. Unwanted behavior should be ignored or redirected.
5. The clinician should try not to loom over the cat or grab for it; these actions can increase fear in the patient.
6. Anxious cats should be distracted by engaging them in alternative behaviors that are incompatible with fearful or anxious behavior, such as playing with an interactive toy, following a laser pointer, eating treats, or rubbing on catnip. Gently petting the cat behind the ears or rubbing it under the chin can also divert its attention from the procedures being performed.

7. Many towel-handling techniques can be used to successfully examine both fearful and fearfully aggressive cats and to collect laboratory samples.[43] In addition to the previously mentioned burrito-wrap method (see Figure 1-7), other common towel techniques include the following:
   - Covering the head with a towel to eliminate visual cues that might induce stress or anxiety
   - Moving a towel from one side of the cat to another to examine different parts of the cat (Figure 1-15)
   - Gently placing a towel around the ventral neck and one front leg to keep the cat snugly wrapped, with only one front leg exposed for placing an intravenous catheter or collecting blood from the cephalic vein (Figure 1-16)
8. Prolonged (more than 2 seconds) or repeated struggling is not advised.[43] If the cat struggles, the position should be changed, or toweling, sedation, or anesthesia can be used as needed. Analgesia is always recommended if the cat is in pain or might be in pain and if painful procedures are to be performed. Senior patients commonly have arthritis and may experience pain with physical manipulation, positioning for radiographs, or placement on hard surfaces. For a list of painful conditions and procedures, see the AAHA/AAFP Pain Management Guidelines[14] and Boxes 1-2 and 1-3.
9. Some cats behave more calmly when visual cues are eliminated. Most cats do not need a muzzle or similar device, but for those that do, several relatively gentle options are available, such as a soft cloth or plastic muzzle that both prevents biting and greatly reduces visual cues. When the veterinarian is working away from the head, an Elizabethan collar (E-collar) or air muzzle can also protect against biting. Some veterinarians, especially in Europe, find "clipnosis," or pinch-induced behavioral inhibition (e.g., placement of binder clips along the dorsum of the neck), helpful for restraint.[31]
10. Preparing all necessary equipment in advance helps reduce handling time and keeps the cat from being startled by people going in and out of the examination room.
11. Documenting in the medical record which handling methods work best for the individual patient (and those to avoid because they frighten the cat) improves future veterinary visits and decreases stress for all. When attempting to quiet or calm the cat, the clinician should refrain from making shushing sounds, which sound like hissing to the cat and may exacerbate the aroused state.
12. Clients and veterinary team members empathize with cats that are distressed. However, saying, "Poor kitty" or "It's OK" in a soothing voice may serve as an inadvertent reward for their fearfulness. The best way to help the cat be calm and less fearful is for the veterinary staff and client to remain calm.

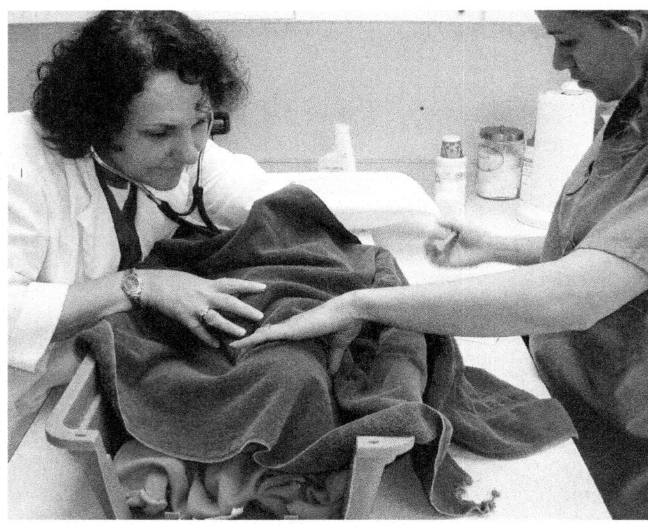

FIGURE 1-15 This cat is fearful and is much more comfortable with its head covered. Notice how the technician places her left hand to hold the head in place without scruffing or tight restraint.

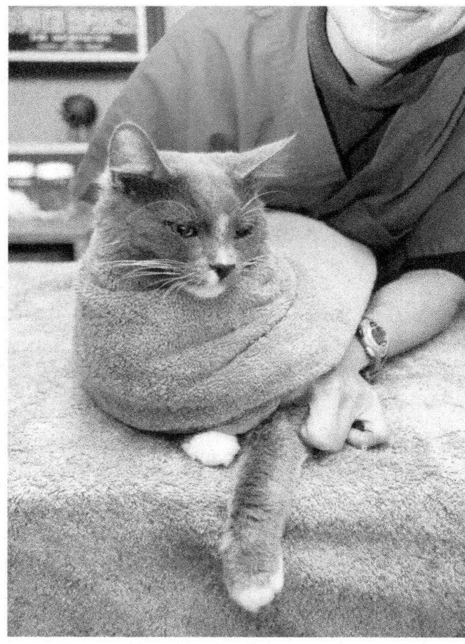

FIGURE 1-16 This towel technique provides comfort for the cat and a safe method of handling for venipuncture or catheter placement. *(Image courtesy Yin S:* Low stress handling, restraint and behavior modification of dogs & cats: techniques for developing patients who love their visits, *Davis, Calif, 2009, CattleDog.)*

Handling for Laboratory Sample Collection

Collecting laboratory samples from cats usually requires only minimal handling. The clinician should ensure that the patient is comfortable during sample collection by allowing the cat to remain in the most natural position possible, without stretching or holding legs tightly. A blanket or something soft for the cat to lie on, preferably an item that smells like home, should be provided. Older, arthritic, and underweight cats are especially uncomfortable on cold, hard surfaces and benefit from having soft padding underneath them. As previously discussed, cats can also be gently wrapped in a towel to help them feel more secure.

Many clients prefer to watch while laboratory samples are collected. Having owners present keeps them from worrying about what is happening to their cat, often calms the cat, and furthers client education and respect for the veterinary team.

Measuring Blood Pressure

Blood pressure measurements, when indicated, should be taken before other diagnostic tests, while the patient is kept as relaxed and calm as possible to minimize "white coat" hypertension. The environment should be quiet, away from other animals, and the owner should be present if possible.[3] Measuring blood pressure is usually best performed in the examination room rather than in the treatment area. The cat needs approximately 5 to 10 minutes to acclimate to a room; by the time the history is obtained and the physical examination is performed, the cat will have become accustomed to the examination room, reducing the likelihood of white-coat hypertension if blood pressure measurement is done there.[3,17]

The blood pressure readings can be taken from either front (antebrachium) or back (hock) legs or 1 inch from the base of the tail. The latter option is an excellent approach for arthritic cats and those cats that are more fearful when they see what is happening (Figure 1-17). If either the front or the back leg is used, the leg should not be extended excessively; instead, placing a hand gently behind the leg prevents the cat from withdrawing the leg during the procedure and keeps the cat comfortable. Blood pressure measurements should be taken wherever the cat is most comfortable, whether on a lap, in a carrier, or in some other comfortable place. The clinician should use headphones to prevent fear associated with monitor noise. In addition, using warmed gel precludes the startle response often seen with the application of cold gel. A free downloadable article, "Doppler Blood Pressure Measurement in Conscious Cats," (http://www.catprofessional.com/free_downloads.html) is an excellent educational resource for those new to taking blood pressure measurements.

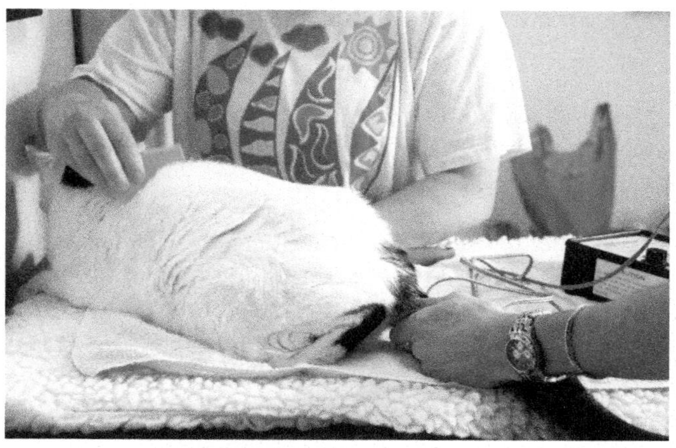

FIGURE 1-17 Blood pressure measurements from the tail work well with cats that do not like to have their feet handled. Notice that the client is distracting the cat with grooming, which is one of its favorite rewards.

Collecting Blood Samples

Most laboratories request a larger blood or serum sample than they actually need; it is helpful to contact the laboratory to find out how much blood is actually needed for the samples. If the laboratory will accept smaller samples, request microtainer or avian EDTA tubes so that a small blood volume is not overly diluted. Regardless of which vein is used to collect the blood sample, most patients require no more than one person to hold them during the collection; in fact, some veterinarians can collect samples from the jugular vein with no additional assistance (Figure 1-18). Many cats tolerate jugular collection very well; this collection site enables speedy collection of a large sample. Other cats prefer not seeing the sample collection and better tolerate collection from the medial saphenous or the cephalic veins; using a butterfly catheter will prevent collapse of these veins if a large blood sample is needed. For patients highly sensitive to needle pricks, lidocaine/prilocaine anesthetic cream (EMLA, AstraZeneca Pharmaceuticals) should be applied over the site at least 30 minutes before blood collection or intravenous catheterization. The site should then be covered with a bandage to prevent the cat from licking the cream. Minimal systemic absorption of lidocaine may occur in some cats, but it is substantially below toxic concentrations.[9] No other adverse effects have been reported, although struggling during catheter placement was not significantly reduced with use of EMLA cream in one study compared with placebo.[41]

Collecting Urine Samples

Urine should be collected by cystocentesis (except in rare cases). The cat should be held in as comfortable a position as possible, without extending the legs. Although most veterinarians and technicians prefer placing the cat

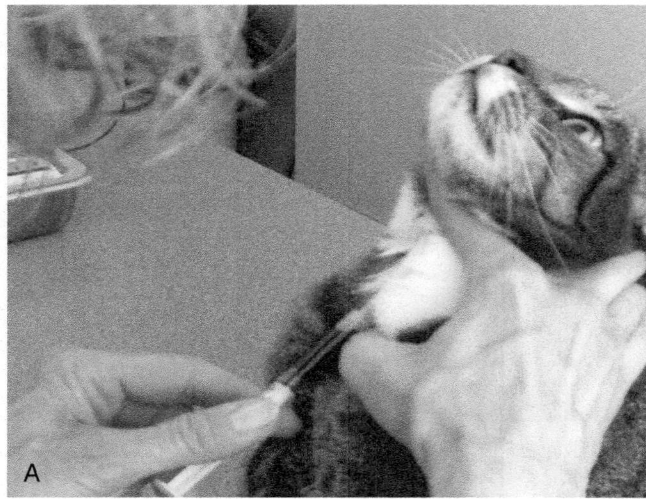

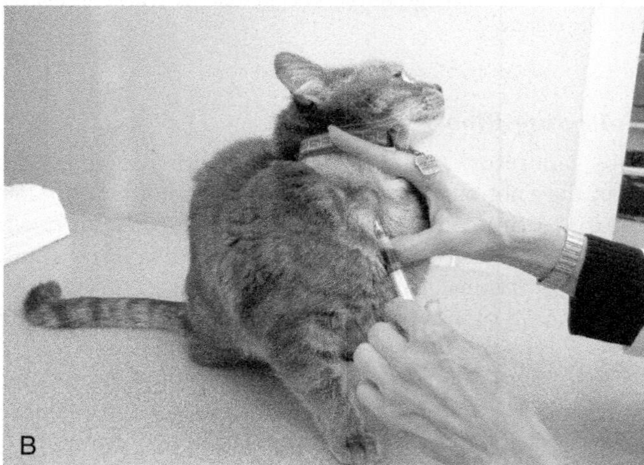

FIGURE 1-18 **A,** Blood sample being collected from the jugular vein single-handedly. **B,** Single-handed jugular collection (other view). *(Images courtesy Dr. Jane Brunt.)*

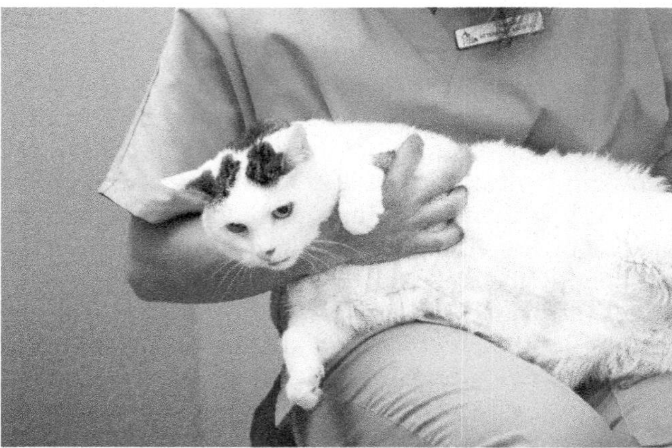

FIGURE 1-19 Cats often are more comfortable being held on someone's lap for cystocentesis.

on an examination or treatment table to perform cystocentesis, the procedure can also be performed with one person holding the cat in the lap (Figure 1-19). The free downloadable article "Cystocentesis in Cats" (http://www.catprofessional.com/free_downloads.html) is an excellent educational resource and illustrates how to perform cystocentesis with the cat in various positions.

Hospitalization

Whenever possible, it is best not to hospitalize cats; being away from home leads to disruption of the social network and lack of a sense of control, both of which can create fear and stress.[29] Hospitalized cats often withdraw and are inactive, leading to the misconception that the cat is not stressed. The high stress of the hospital inhibits normal behaviors such as eating, grooming, sleeping, and elimination.[11] This novel environment can be especially stressful for senior and geriatric cats and for cats that have not been well socialized.[11]

If hospitalization is essential, cats should be kept in a quiet area where they do not see other cats or dogs. Protecting the hospitalized cat from the sight and noise of barking dogs and hissing or screaming cats will greatly reduce stress. This goal can be achieved by providing both a separate hospitalized cat ward (see Chapter 2) and isolation areas for cats that hiss or scream and by covering the cat's cage with a towel or blanket to decrease the sight of hospital activities that may increase anxiety. Obviously, removing all scents of other animals or people is nearly impossible in a hospital or clinic environment. However, spraying Feliway in the cage at least 30 minutes before the patient is moved there will help calm the cat and increase food intake and grooming.[12]

Most veterinary clinic caging is too small for cats. Cages should be large enough so that the cat can stretch, groom, exercise, and have separate spaces for eating, sleeping, and eliminating (Figure 1-20).[11] Shelves and climbing opportunities can extend the available cage space (Figure 1-21). Indeed, by providing vantage points from which the cat can monitor its surroundings and detect the approach of people and other animals, such vertical space can make the patient feel more in control of its environment.[29]

In addition, providing materials the cat can use to make a hiding place can greatly reduce stress. Cats will hide when they are anxious or feel threatened[35]; hiding is an important coping strategy in response to change in environment.[13] Hiding places can be as simple as a paper bag, a cardboard box, or even a blanket or towel. Placing a blanket or padding on top of a sturdy cardboard box creates both a hiding place and perch.

Comfortable bedding should be provided in both the sleeping and hiding area. Cats prefer to rest on soft surfaces and experience longer periods of normal sleep

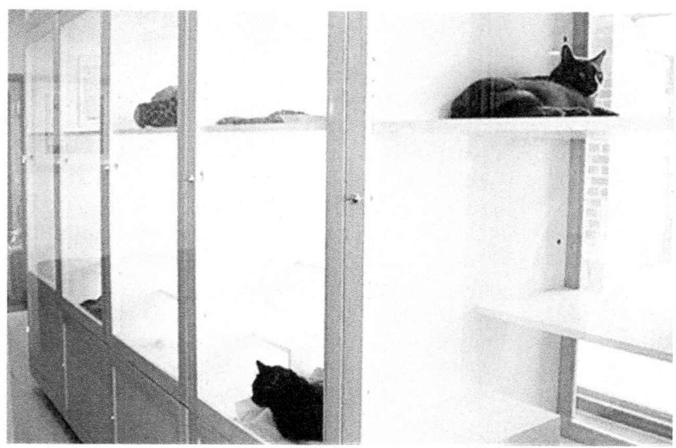

FIGURE 1-20 Cat condominiums with multiple shelves allow cats to choose where they wish to be.

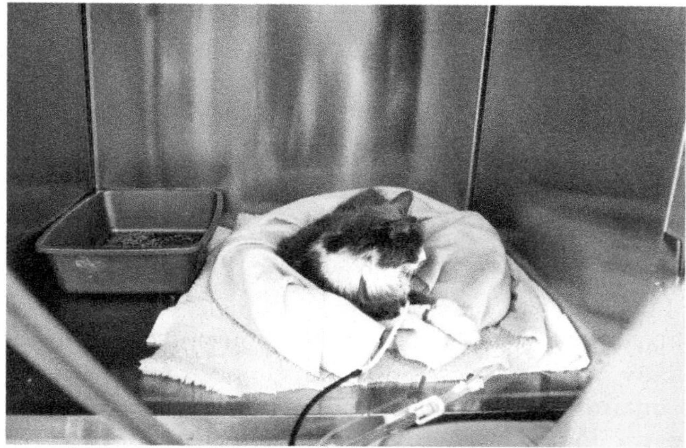

FIGURE 1-22 A towel twisted into a circle provides a convenient and comfortable bed that readily allows monitoring of intravenous catheters.

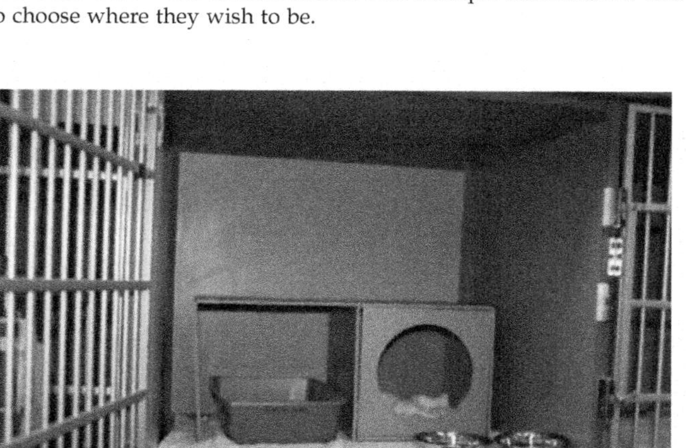

FIGURE 1-21 Cages that lack perches and hiding places can be modified by the addition of a sturdy box with space for hiding and being up high or a commercially made addition that allows hiding and perching. *(Image courtesy Drs. Peter and Kari Mundschenk.)*

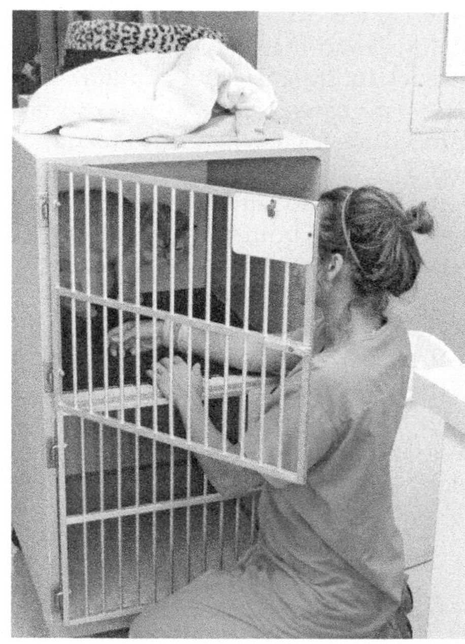

FIGURE 1-23 Standing or squatting to the side of the cage and gradually letting the cat approach or removing the cat while it remains in its basket or box is an excellent way to remove a cat from a cage.

when they lie on soft bedding.[11] A towel twisted into a circle (Figure 1-22) makes a good pet bed and allows visual monitoring of the status of intravenous catheters without disturbing the patient.[43]

Caged cats show signs of stress when the caretaking routine is unpredictable and when they have few or no human social interactions.[27] Consistent feeding and cleaning times are less stressful for feline patients,[29] as are consistent times for attention, grooming, and weight checks.

Because cats prefer contact with familiar people, the same staff member should, whenever possible, care for a cat being hospitalized or boarded. Also, the cat owner should be encouraged to visit the cat during hospitalization.[11]

Removing a fearful cat from a cage can be extremely challenging because the cat perceives that its opportunity to escape is restricted.[13] To reduce the fear response, the veterinarian or technician should stand to the side of the cage, not directly in front. From that position, the cat should be gently encouraged to approach or enter the carrier on its own (Figure 1-23). Reaching into the cage and trying to grab the cat will be counterproductive and is likely to exacerbate any fear responses.

Returning Home

In most situations a cat experiences no difficulty returning home from the veterinary hospital. Two situations should be addressed with clients, however: the aroused cat and other cats in the household that may not accept the returning cat.

An aroused cat may remain reactive for several hours or even days before it calms down.[13] If a cat is still aroused when sent home, it is important to explain the situation clearly to the client so that he or she knows what to expect. Until the cat becomes calm again at home, no one should handle the cat and—equally important—everyone should ignore the aroused behavior, so as not to not reinforce or cause it to escalate.

Regardless of how long the cat has been at the veterinary hospital, other cats in the household might not readily accept the returning cat because its scent will be unfamiliar.[36] In most situations, keeping the returning cat in the carrier until all cats are calm, which usually takes place within a few hours, is sufficient. Clients should be reminded to ignore any hissing or screaming and reward any positive interactions. If the re-introduction still causes problems, the client should first wipe the cat (or cats) that remained in the household with a towel and then wipe the returning cat with the same towel to transfer the familiar scent to the "stranger." In rare cases, cats will need to go through the same procedure used when introducing a new cat to a household.

One approach to prevent severe problems with the return home is taking both (or all) cats to the veterinarian at the same time, even when only one has a scheduled visit. As previously discussed, spraying Feliway in the carrier (or carriers) at least 30 minutes before travel to the veterinary hospital and including familiar clothing with your scent and the scent of the other cat (or cats) in the carrier (or carriers) will reduce stress and anxiety for the cats during the visit to the clinic.

CONCLUSION

Knowing how the cat perceives and communicates with its environment and other cats helps us to better comprehend the cat's signals at the veterinary hospital. Further, recognizing that fear and pain are the most common reasons for aggression at the veterinary hospital enables us to respect and understand the cat and provide analgesia as needed. It is now widely accepted that hissing and screaming cats are fearful cats trying to communicate with us to *prevent* escalation to outright aggression. Understanding the cat and working calmly with the cat will improve veterinary visits and feline health care. Working confidently with this knowledge means that veterinary team members are more relaxed and better able to help clients and cats relax during veterinary visits. This knowledgeable approach will improve the cat's (and the client's) visit and interactions at the veterinary hospital.

References

1. Beaver B: *Feline behavior: a guide for veterinarians*, ed 2, St Louis, 2003, Saunders.
2. Bowen J, Heath S: An overview of feline social behaviour and communication. In *Behaviour problems in small animals: practice advice for the veterinary team*, Philadelphia, 2005, Saunders, p 29.
3. Brown S, Atkins C, Bagley R et al: Guidelines for the identification, evaluation, and management of systemic hypertension in dogs and cats, *J Vet Intern Med* 21:542, 2007.
4. Crowell-Davis S: Social behaviour, communication and development of behaviour in the cat. In Horwitz D, Mills D, Heath S, editors: *BSAVA manual of canine and feline behavioural medicine*, ed 1, Gloucester, 2002, British Small Animal Veterinary Association, p 21.
5. Crowell-Davis S, Curtis T, Knowles R: Social organization in the cat: a modern understanding, *J Fel Med Surg* 6:19, 2004.
6. DiBartola S, de Morais H: Disorders of potassium. In diBartola SP, editor: *Fluid therapy in small animal practice*, ed 2, Philadelphia, 2000, Saunders, p 83.
7. Driscoll CA, Clutton-Brock J, Kitchener AC et al: The taming of the cat. Genetic and archaeological findings hint that wildcats became housecats earlier—and in a different place—than previously thought, *Sci Am* 300:68, 2009.
8. Driscoll CA, Menotti-Raymond M, Roca AL et al: The Near Eastern origin of cat domestication, *Science* 317:519, 2007.
9. Fransson B, Peck K, Smith J et al: Transdermal absorption of a liposome-encapsulated formulation of lidocaine following topical administration in cats, *Am J Vet Res* 63:1309, 2002.
10. Greco DS: The effect of stress on the evaluation of feline patients. In August J, editor: *Consultations in feline internal medicine*, ed 1, Philadelphia, 1991, Saunders, p 13.
11. Griffin B, Hume KR: Recognition and management of stress in housed cats. In August J, editor: *Consultations in feline internal medicine*, ed 5, St Louis, 2006, Saunders, p 717.
12. Griffith C, Steigerwald E, Buffington C: Effects of a synthetic facial pheromone on behavior of cats, *J Am Vet Med Assoc* 217:1154, 2000.
13. Heath S: Feline aggression. In Horwitz D, Mills D, Health S, editors: *BSAVA manual of canine and feline behavioural medicine*, ed 1, Gloucester, 2002, p 216.
14. Hellyer P, Rodan I, Brunt J et al.: AAHA/AAFP pain management guidelines for dogs and cats, *J Feline Med Surg* 9:466, 2007.
15. Landsberg G, Hunthausen W, Ackerman L: *Fear and phobias: Handbook of behaviour problems of the dog and cat*, ed 2, Philadelphia, 2003, Saunders.
16. Lin CH, Yan CJ, Lien YH et al: Systolic blood pressure of clinically normal and conscious cats determined by an indirect Doppler method in a clinical setting, *J Vet Med Sci* 68:827, 2006.
17. Love L, Harvey R: Arterial blood pressure measurement: physiology, tools, and techniques, *Compend Contin Educ Pract Vet* 28:450, 2006.
18. Lue TW, Pantenburg DP, Crawford PM: Impact of the owner-pet and client-veterinarian bond on the care that pets receive, *J Am Vet Med Assoc* 232:531, 2008.
19. Macdonald DW, Apps P, Carr G: Social dynamics, nursing coalitions and infanticide among farm cats, *Felis catus, Adv Ethology* 28, 1987.
20. Macdonald DW, Yamaguchi N, Kerby G: Group-living in the domestic cat: its sociobiology and epidemiology. In Turner DC,Bateson P, editors: *The domestic cat: the biology of its behaviour*, Cambridge, 2000, Cambridge University Press, p 95.
21. McMillan F: Development of a mental wellness program for animals, *J Am Vet Med Assoc* 220:965, 2002.
22. Milani M: Crate training as a feline stress reliever, *Feline Pract* 28:8, 2000.

23. Mills D: Training and learning protocols. In Horwitz D, Mills D, editors: *BSAVA manual of canine and feline behavioural medicine*, ed 2, Gloucester, 2009, British Small Animal Veterinary Association, p 49.
24. Moffat K: Addressing canine and feline aggression in the veterinary clinic, *Vet Clin North Am Small Anim Pract* 38:983, 2008.
25. Notari L: Stress in veterinary behavioural medicine. In Horwitz D, Mills D, editors: *BSAVA manual of canine and feline behavioural medicine*, ed 2, Gloucester, 2009, British Small Animal Veterinary Association, p 136.
26. Overall K: Normal feline behavior: *Clinical behavioral medicine for small animals*, St Louis, 1997, Mosby, p 45.
27. Overall K: Recognizing and managing problem behavior in breeding catteries. In Lawler D, editor: *Consultations in feline internal Medicine 3*, Philadelphia, 1997, Saunders.
28. Pageat P, Gaultier E: Current research in canine and feline pheromones, *Vet Clin North Am Small Anim Pract* 33:187, 2003.
29. Patronek G, Sperry E: Quality of life in long-term confinement. In August J, editor: *Consultations in feline internal medicine*, ed 4, Philadelphia, 2001, Saunders, p 621.
30. Patronek GJ, Lacroix CA: Developing an ethic for the handling, restraint, and discipline of companion animals in veterinary practice, *J Am Vet Med Assoc* 218:514, 2001.
31. Pozza ME, Stella JL, Chappuis-Gagnon AC et al: Pinch-induced behavioral inhibition ("clipnosis") in domestic cats, *J Feline Med Surg* 10:82, 2008.
32. Rand J, Kinnaird E, Baglioni A et al: Acute stress hyperglycemia in cats is associated with struggling and increased concentrations of lactate and norepinephrine, *J Vet Intern Med* 16:123, 2002.
33. Robertson S, Lascelles B, Taylor P et al: PK-PD modeling of buprenorphine in cats: intravenous and oral transmucosal administration, *J Vet Pharmacol Ther* 28:453, 2005.
34. Robertson S, Taylor P, Sear J: Systemic uptake of buprenorphine by cats after oral mucosal administration, *Vet Rec* 152:675, 2003.
35. Rochlitz I: Recommendations for the housing of cats in the home, in catteries and animal shelters, in laboratories and in veterinary surgeries, *J Feline Med Surg* 1:181, 1999.
36. Rochlitz I: Basic requirements for good behavioural health and welfare in cats. In Horwitz D, Mills D, editors: *BSAVA manual of canine and feline behavioural medicine*, ed 2, Gloucester, 2009, British Small Animal Veterinary Association, p 35.
37. Seksel K: Preventing behavior problems in puppies and kittens, *Vet Clin North Am Sm Anim Pract* 38:971, 2008.
38. Taylor P, Funk C, Craighill P: Gauging family intimacy: dogs edge cats (dads trail both): Pew Research Center Report, 2006.
39. Vigne J, Guilaine J, Debue K et al: Early taming of the cat in Cyprus, *Science* 304:259, 2004.
40. Vogt AH, Rodan I, Brown M et al: AAFP-AAHA: Feline life stage guidelines, *J Feline Med Surg* 12:43, 2010.
41. Wagner K, Gibbon K, Strom T et al: Adverse effects of EMLA (lidocaine/prilocaine) cream and efficacy for the placement of jugular catheters in hospitalized cats, *J Feline Med Surg* 8:141, 2006.
42. Yin S: Classical conditioning: learning by association, *Compend Contin Educ Pract Vet* 28:472, 2006.
43. Yin S: Low stress handling, restraint, and behavior modification of dogs and cats: techniques for developing patients who love their visits, Davis, Calif, 2009, CattleDog Publishing.

CHAPTER

2

The Cat-Friendly Practice

Jane E. Brunt

OUTLINE

The need for attention to cats' medical needs was first acknowledged by the American Association of Feline Practitioners (AAFP) in the early 1970s.[1] Since that time, increasing membership and programming in AAFP and other feline-oriented veterinary organizations, coupled with growth in the cat population, has allowed the areas of feline medicine and surgery to become increasingly mainstream and available through traditional companion animal veterinary hospitals and clinics, as well as feline-exclusive veterinary facilities. The addition of board certification for feline medicine specialists through the American Board of Veterinary Practitioners (ABVP) (http://www.abvp.com/categories_feline.htm. Accessed February 7, 2010) has further elevated the field of feline veterinary medicine. An increasing number of feline-specific scientific journals and consumer publications in print and online have provided more information to diverse audiences. Efforts to increase feline scientific and market research have been undertaken by foundations such as Winn Feline Foundation,[15] Morris Animal Foundation,[9] and the Cornell Feline Health Center.[4]

Despite the increased popularity of and knowledge about cats, recent statistics have shown that veterinary expenditures are declining even while the cat population continues to grow.[5] According to the American Veterinary Medical Association, the number of owned cats in the United States went from an estimated 59.1 million in 1996 to 81.7 million in 2006. Relative to veterinary care and services for dogs, cats receive far less medical care compared with dogs, and there was an 11% decline in feline veterinary visits between 2001 and 2006. In 2006 only 64% of owned cats visited the veterinarian, compared with 83% of dogs.[5] Reasons for this disparity range from the difficulty of transporting cats (e.g., putting them in a carrier) to a lack of awareness regarding cats' basic medical needs, a failure to recognize signs of illness, and the misperception that cats are able to take care of themselves.[8]

In response to the decline in veterinary care for cats, in February 2008 the AAFP hosted the CATalyst Summit, which featured representatives from more than 30 independent organizations across North America, including veterinary associations, shelter and welfare groups, foundations and cat fanciers, the media, and commercial industries. At this event more than 50 people united in their concern for the health and well-being of cats vowed to change the negative ways in which cats are often perceived and portrayed (http://catalystcouncil.org/newsroom/index.aspx?Id=9; accessed February 3, 2010).[3]

After the summit, leaders formed the CATalyst Council and set forth a vision of a future in which "all cats are valued and well cared for as pets."[3] Several collaborative and strategic initiatives were identified and implemented, including the development and publication of *Feline Life Stage Guidelines* by the AAFP and American Animal Hospital Association (AAHA) for veterinary health care teams.[14] These guidelines have also been made available online (http://www.catvets.com/uploads/PDF/Feline%20Life%20Stage%20Guidelines%20Final.pdf; accessed January 25, 2010) and are referenced in other areas of this textbook. A version of these guidelines for cat owners called *CATegorical Care: An Owner's Guide to America's #1 Companion* is also available (http://www.winnfelinehealth.org/Pages/CATegorical_Care.pdf).

FELINE VETERINARIANS

Any veterinarian who treats a single cat is a feline veterinarian and as such will benefit from a greater understanding of normal feline physiology and behavior, the ways in which cats respond to external stimuli, and the idiosyncrasies of domestic cats. Recent investigations regarding stimulation of the hypothalamic–pituitary–adrenal axis show that stressors placed on any individual cat can have negative consequences and play a role in development of disease.[2] This knowledge will help all veterinary health care team members to construct or modify physical and administrative features of their veterinary practices to enhance the comfort, care, and safety of cats, clients, and coworkers. By making the necessary modifications, incorporating proper handling techniques,[13] and implementing ongoing feline health education, virtually every veterinary facility can become a cat-friendly practice.

FOUNDATIONS OF A CAT-FRIENDLY PRACTICE

It is important to begin by engaging the entire health care team in the development of a cat-friendly practice. The framework for any new team and client communications, techniques, and physical or administrative changes can be provided in the following sequence:

- Education and commitment of staff; enlistment of a point person or team
- Adoption of AAFP–AAHA Feline Life Stage Guidelines[14] and development of practice protocols
- Scripting and role playing to communicate cats' needs to coworkers and clients
- Adherence to respectful feline handling techniques[13]

PHYSICAL FEATURES OF A CAT-FRIENDLY PRACTICE

Cats are more sensitive to sights, smells, and sounds, as well as touch, and arousal occurs through these senses, particularly in an unfamiliar setting. Heightened arousal subsequent to a change in routine and then travel frequently results in fear, and the *normal physiologic mechanisms* of fear can lead to aggression if the cat is unable to escape to a perceived safe area.[13] For example, if a cat is forced into an unfamiliar carrier and transported to the veterinary hospital, the stress generated by these activities has already initiated changes in heart rate, respiration, and other effects of epinephrine release by the time the cat arrives. In other words, the cat may be experiencing stress before it is even presented to the practice. With this understanding, the veterinary team can take the appropriate measures to mitigate this arousal or at least respond appropriately.[10]

Public Areas

Cat owners notice certain signs that cats are welcome at veterinary hospitals. Exterior features such as signage and cat statuary create an inviting appearance. Some facilities offer a separate entrance for cats. The reception area is usually the first place at which an owner interacts with a veterinary clinic or hospital, and a warm and calming environment contributes to a comfortable atmosphere for the client and cat (Figure 2-1). Cat-specific décor portraying cats in a positive manner is far more likely to encourage the cat owner to think, "This place likes and respects cats" than a design that focuses on dogs at the expense of cats. Posters or illustrations of staring cats are not recommended insofar as cats perceive this behavior as confrontational (Figure 2-2). Elevated counters or platforms near the reception desk allow space for cat carriers to be kept away from dogs. Segregated seating, which is less likely to result in visual and auditory arousal of the feline patient by dogs, other cats, or unfamiliar clients, is preferred (Figure 2-3)[12]; escorting the owner and cat into an examination room as soon as possible may help prevent further arousal. Some veterinary practices have adopted "cat-only" office hours to decrease the likelihood of interaction with canine patients. Providing cat-specific educational material in the reception area will also benefit both clients and cats.

Examination Rooms

Once the cat is inside the examination room, it should be allowed to come out of the carrier on its own and

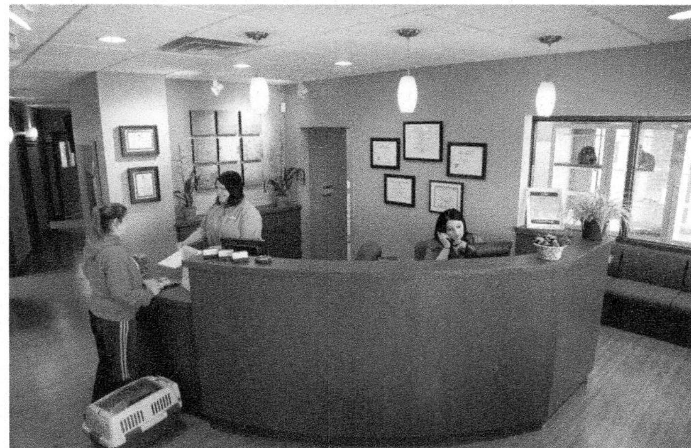

FIGURE 2-1 Calming environment of reception area. Cat Care Clinic, Madison, Wis. *(Image courtesy Dr. Ilona Rodan.)*

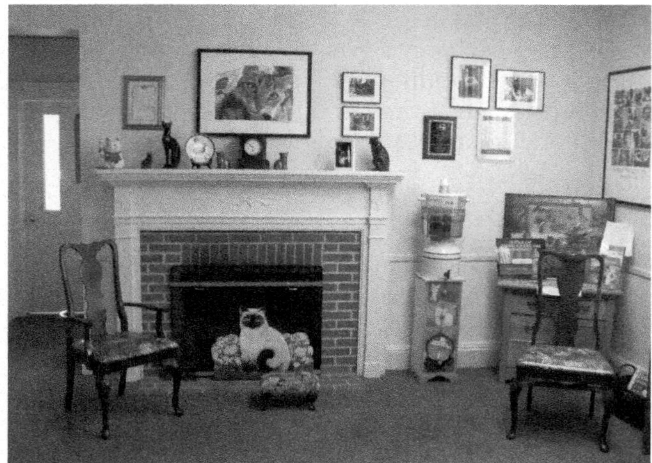

FIGURE 2-2 Reception area with cat décor. Nine Lives Cat Hospital, Sunrise, Fla. *(Image courtesy Dr. Samuel Frank.)*

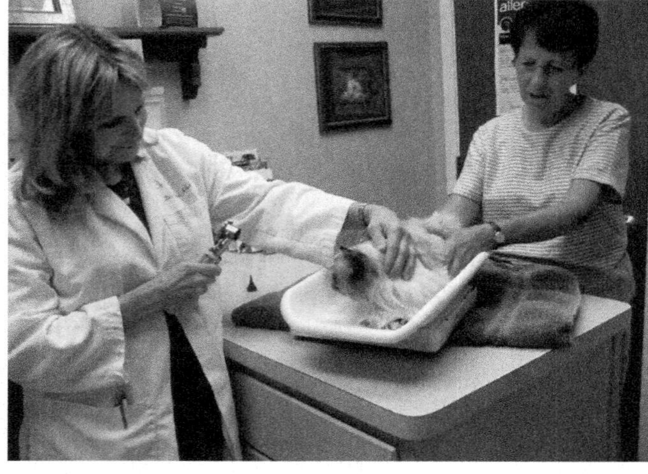

FIGURE 2-4 Performing examination on scale. Cat Hospital of Metairie, Metairie, La. *(Image courtesy Dr. Karen Miller-Bechnel.)*

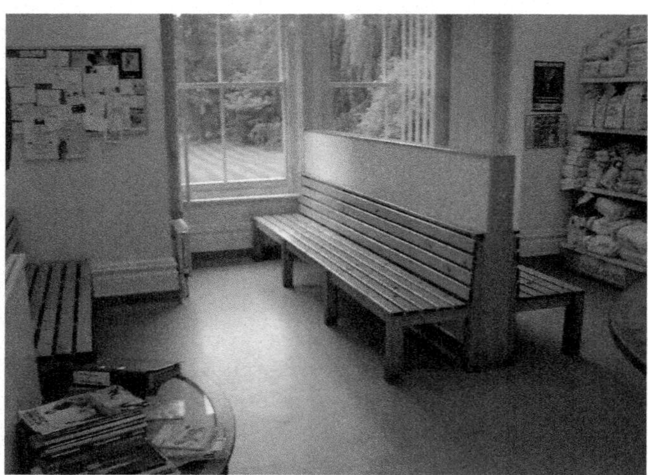

FIGURE 2-3 Segregated seating to minimize visual arousal.

explore its unfamiliar surroundings; this may help dispel the cat's anxiety. Controlling sounds, which includes voices in and around the examination room, often helps improve patient compliance. Examination tables covered with soft mats or towels increase the comfort of the patient on the table; bedding the cat has traveled with has its own scent and will help the environment seem more familiar. Many cats enjoy sitting on a tray-style pad or scale if available, and some veterinarians use these to perform the examination (Figure 2-4). Other cats prefer to sit on their owner's lap or stay on the floor while the veterinarian comes to their perceived safe area (see Figure 1-11). Being flexible and adjusting the examination to the individual cat's needs is critical and is addressed in Chapter 3.

The beneficial effects of synthetic facial pheromone have been documented, and this product should be considered for all areas of the hospital where cats will be present.[6,10]

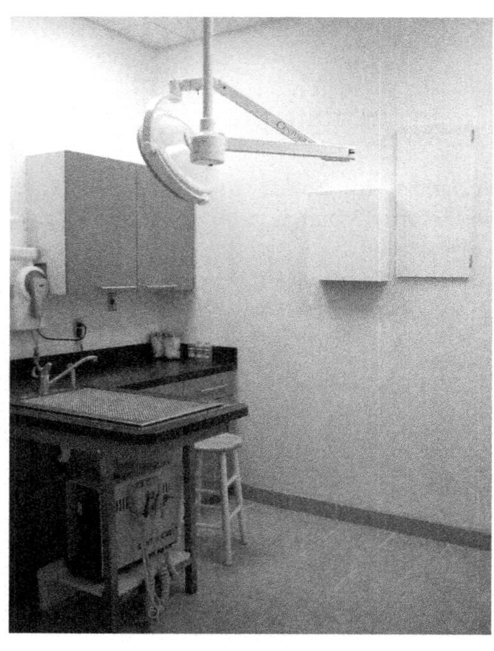

FIGURE 2-5 Treatment area adapted to cats' smaller size. Cat Hospital of Portland, Ore. *(Image courtesy Dr. Elizabeth Colleran.)*

Treatment Areas

Because cats are smaller than most dogs, the use of smaller tables and work areas may increase the ease of access to and handling of the feline patient. Treatment islands and peninsulas are preferred insofar as they provide space for the veterinarian, technician, and assistants to work comfortably with the patient on adjacent or opposite sides (Figure 2-5). As in the examination room, providing nonskid padding underneath the patient will help provide comfort and stability. Care should be taken not to overstimulate patients' senses.

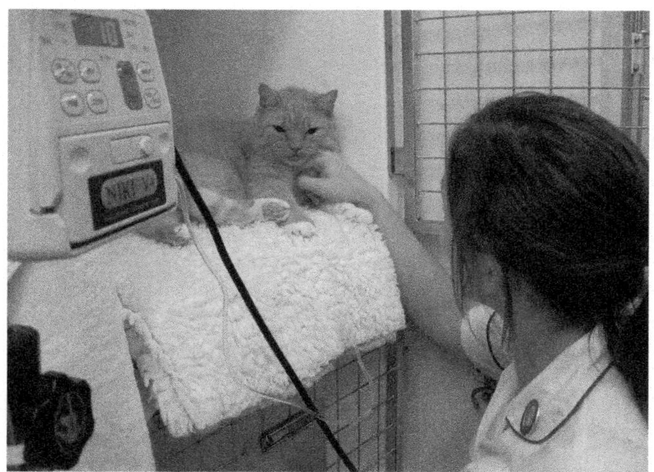

FIGURE 2-6 Feline patient with intravenous pump and comfortable bedding.

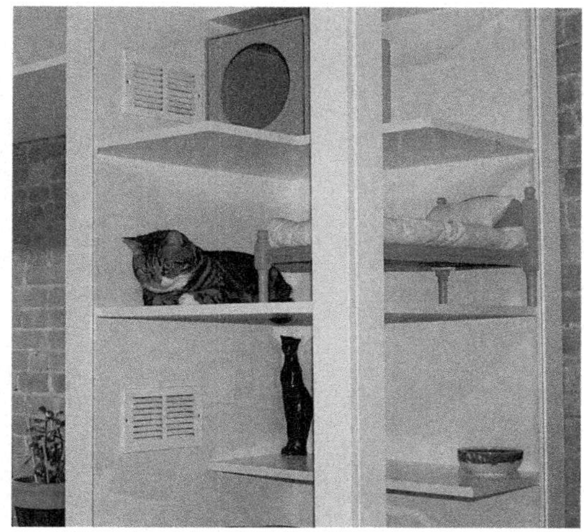

FIGURE 2-7 Many cats prefer access to a vertical space.

Calm and deliberate movement and treatment of unpleasant odors will minimize arousal; keeping the treatment area free of equipment that may make loud noises, such as dental tools, centrifuges, washers, and dryers, may help prevent fear caused by loud and unfamiliar sounds.

Equipment

The small size of feline patients is an important consideration when selecting supplies and equipment. Insulin syringes of various U-100 sizes (e.g., ½ and ⅓ mL) are helpful in administering accurate doses of injectable medications, and the small needle size decreases pain. Alternatively, 1-mL tuberculin syringes with a 23- to 25-gauge needle may be used. The use of small-volume blood collection supplies (e.g., microtubes) facilitates collection of the minimum sample size needed. Other supplies, such as endotracheal tubes in various sizes from 3.5 to 5 Fr, nasoesophageal feeding tubes (human infant feeding tubes), and esophageal feeding tubes, permit nutritional support of the ill or injured feline patient. Essential equipment includes safe warming blankets or other devices; intravenous and syringe pumps (Figure 2-6); blood pressure monitoring equipment; pulse oximetry and other anesthesia-monitoring devices; non-rebreathing anesthesia circuits; 0.5-L and 1-L rebreathing bags and resuscitation devices; general and dental radiography (digital equipment decreases the time the patient is under anesthesia and eliminates processing time and errors); refractometer and glucometer; human pediatric stethoscopes; and oxygen masks or cones, cage, or other means in which to deliver oxygen in a nonfrightening manner.[7] Soft muzzles to minimize visual stimulation and protect the safety of patient and handler may be used if appropriate training has been provided and the patient permits placement.

Housing

The housing of cats in veterinary hospitals follows the same principles of minimizing arousal of the senses. Having separate wards for cats and dogs is advised, and cages should be situated so that cats do not have visual contact with other patients (Figure 2-7). Areas such as an isolation room are important to separate cats suspected of having contagious diseases. Viral upper respiratory infections are most commonly disseminated by fomite transmission, and strict hygiene procedures associated with an isolation area should be implemented throughout the facility. Cats infected with feline leukemia virus and feline immunodeficiency virus that are otherwise healthy should be housed in regular cat wards, not in an isolation ward with other cats with contagious diseases.

Use of nonmetal cages decreases both sound and conduction of heat away from the body. Cats seek out vertical space and benefit from being able to move to other locations. Therefore condo-style cages can minimize stress by allowing the cat to hide or "escape" (Figure 2-8). Similarly, provision of hiding areas such as boxes, covered bedding, or the cat's own carrier with the door removed afford cats a sense of refuge while inside the cage (Figures 2-9 and 2-10).[7,12]

Because cats evolved as desert animals, providing an ambient temperature that is somewhat higher than the human comfort zone of approximately 21° C (70° F) and more in the range of 26° C (80° F) may be beneficial.[2a] At a minimum, bedding to provide insulation and allow burrowing will permit the cat to use its own body heat

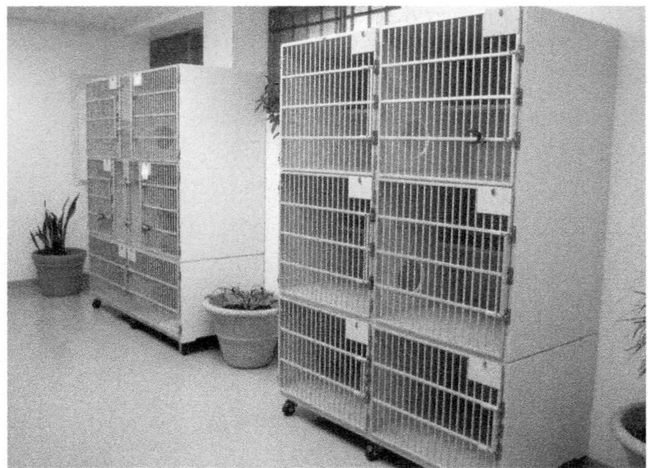

FIGURE 2-8 Cat condos allow for retreat. Cat Hospital of Portland, Ore. *(Image courtesy Dr. Elizabeth Colleran.)*

FIGURE 2-10 Patient housed with familiar carrier and bedding.

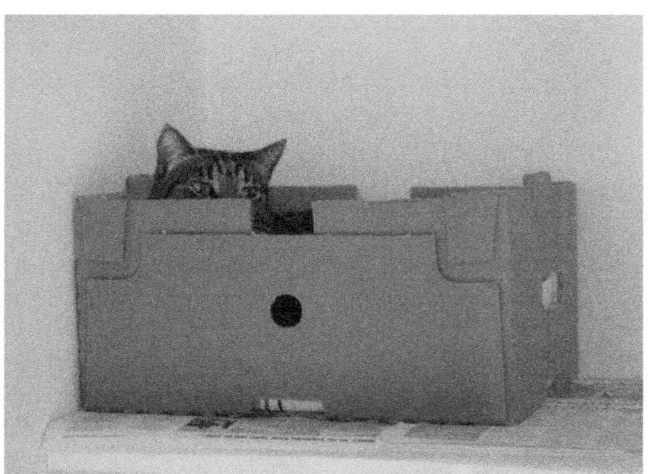

FIGURE 2-9 A cardboard box provides hiding space.

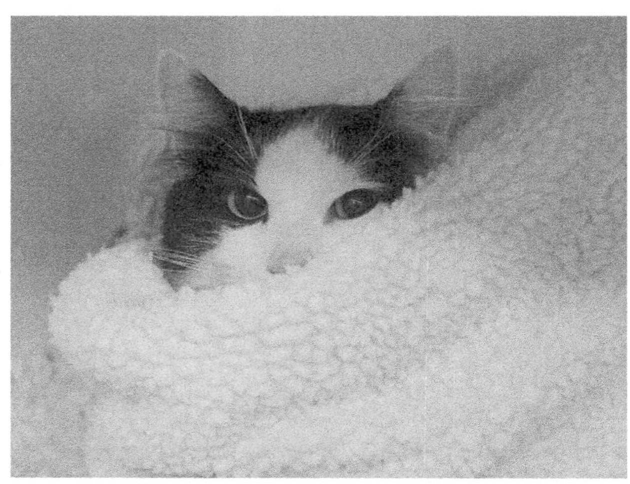

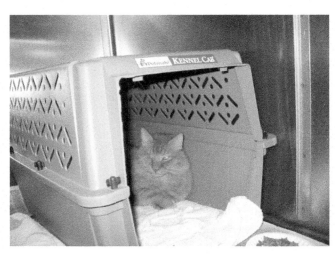

FIGURE 2-11 Tent-style plush bedding helps keep patients warm.

for increased warmth as well as serving as a hiding area (Figure 2-11).

CONCLUSION

By understanding and following the words of legendary feline veterinarian Dr. Barbara Stein ("Cats are not small dogs"), the veterinarian can ensure a cat-friendly veterinary practice regardless of the species being treated. The key to providing cat-friendly care lies in recognizing the unique nature of cats, educating team members and clients about cats' needs, and handling and treating feline patients according to those needs. When these fundamental points are observed, the development and implementation of procedures and adaptation of a facility become instinctive, like cats themselves.

References

1. American Association of Feline Practitioners. *About AAFP* (website): http://www.catvets.com/about/index.aspx?Id=239. Accessed January 23, 2010.
2. Buffington CA, Pacak K: Increased plasma norepinephrine concentration in cats with interstitial cystitis, *J Urol* 165:2051, 2001.

2a. Buffington CA: Personal communication. January 19, 2010.

3. CATalyst Council, Inc. Accessed January 23, 2010 at http://www.catalystcouncil.org.
4. Cornell Feline Health Center. College of Veterinary Medicine. Cornell University, Division W-3, Ithaca, NY 14853. Accessed January 23, 2010, at http://www.vet.cornell.edu/FHC/.
5. Flanigan J, Shepherd A, Majchrzak S et al: *US pet ownership & demographics sourcebook*, Schaumburg, Ill, 2007, American Veterinary Medical Association.
6. Griffith CA, Steigerwald ES, Buffington CA: Effects of a synthetic facial pheromone on behavior of cats, *J Am Vet Med Assoc* 217:1154, 2000.
7. Harvey A: *Cat friendly practice 2*. Accessed January 23, 2010, at http://fabcats.org/catfriendlypractice/cat%20friendly%2032pp.pdf.

8. Lue TW, Pantenburg DP, Crawford PM: Impact of the owner–pet and client–veterinarian bond on the care that pets receive, *J Am Vet Med Assoc* 232:531, 2008.
9. Morris Animal Foundation. 10200 East Girard Ave. B430, Denver, CO 80231. Accessed January 23, 2010, at http://www.morrisanimalfoundation.org/.
10. Overall K, Rodan I, Beaver B et al: Feline behavior guidelines from the American Association of Feline Practitioners, *J Am Vet Med Assoc* 227:70, 2005.
11. Pageat P, Gaultier E: Current research in canine and feline pheromones, *Vet Clin North Am Small Anim Pract* 33:187, 2003.
12. Riccomini F, Harvey A, Rudd S: Creating a feline friendly practice. Accessed January 23, 2010, at http://fabcats.org/catfriendlypractice/catfriendly44pp.pdf.
13. Rodan I, Folger B: *Respectful handling of cats to prevent fear and pain*. American Association of Feline Practitioners Position Statement. Accessed January 23, 2010, at http://catvets.com/uploads/PDF/Nov2009HandlingCats.pdf.
14. Vogt AH, Rodan I, Brown M et al: AAFP–AAHA: Feline life stage guidelines, *J Feline Med Surg* 12:43, 2010.
15. Winn Feline Foundation: Accessed January 23, 2010, at http://www.winnfelinehealth.org/.

CHAPTER

3

Deciphering the Cat: The Medical History and Physical Examination

Vicki Thayer

OUTLINE

Dr. Jim Richards, the late director of the Cornell Feline Health Center, said, "Cats are masters at hiding illness."[22] As veterinarians and cat lovers, clinicians must become masters at understanding and uncovering the illnesses so effectively hidden by cats. The purpose of this chapter is to assist veterinarians in developing techniques to decipher the obscure and sometimes confusing messages delivered by their feline patients. Preparing a complete medical history and performing a feline-centric physical examination are two essential tools for resolving patient issues and informing clients of the best means to keep their feline companions healthy.

Above all, by working together as a unit, the veterinary health care team can deliver a consistent message: that cats benefit from routine examinations, and wellness health care, along with early disease intervention, increases the length and quality of the feline companion's life.[31] Emphasizing this message should be the goal of the veterinarian during all interactions with the client and patient.

ESTABLISHING RELATIONSHIP-CENTERED CARE

All clients expect the veterinarian to care about cats and to care about their cat in particular. By using the cat's name and referring to its sex correctly and by eliciting and acknowledging the client's comments, the veterinarian builds on the bond between the client and cat and provides a strong foundation for meeting the client's expectations. Use of respectful and appropriate handling techniques further enhances the veterinarian's message while minimizing the stress and anxiety many cats exhibit during veterinary visits.

A model for demonstrating concern for the patient and enhancing the clinical interview through the use of distinctive, describable behaviors is well established in the field of human medicine. A similar concept in the veterinary field is called *relationship-centered care.*[28] Studies suggest that organizing these communication skills into a pattern of behaviors or habits is integral to the process and outcomes of medical care. The "Four Habits" model quickly establishes rapport and builds trust, facilitates the effective exchange of information, demonstrates caring and concern, and increases the likelihood of compliance and positive health outcomes for the patient (Box 3-1, Figure 3-1).[7]

THE MEDICAL HISTORY

Initial Information Phase

With today's electronic media, the veterinarian can obtain relevant information for building an initial history before the kitten or cat visits the hospital. For example, many owners use e-mail and social networks to communicate their observations and concerns. Sending a history questionnaire to the client, either electronically or by regular mail, is an effective way to

BOX 3-1

Four Habits: Enhancing the Clinical Encounter

Habit #1: Invest in the Beginning

- Create rapport quickly (use eye contact and appropriate terms of address, review record).
- Elicit client's concerns (use open-ended questions and continuers).
- Plan the visit (repeating concerns, checking understanding, stating what to expect).

Habit #2: Elicit the Client's Perspective

- What caused the problem from the client's perspective?
- What is the client's main worry?
- What are the client's expectations of the visit?
- What impact has the problem had for the patient and the client?

Habit #3: Demonstrate Empathy

- Be compassionate.
- Be open to the client's emotions.
- Be aware of nonverbal expressions of emotions.

Habit #4: Invest in the End

- Share results (deliver diagnostic information).
- Confirm understanding of shared information.
- Involve the client in decision making.
- Complete the visit (discuss treatment plan, check for adherence, provide support).

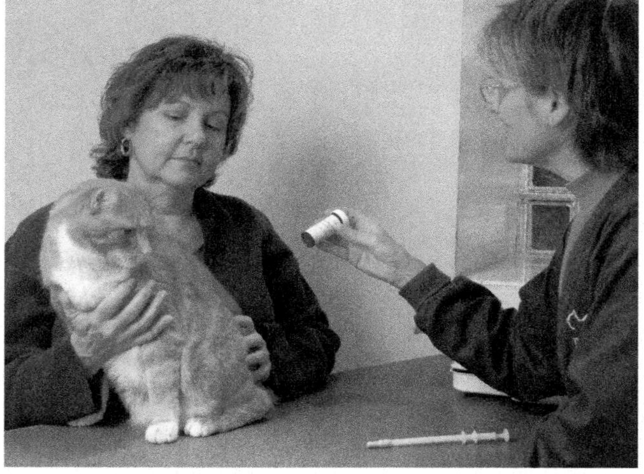

FIGURE 3-1 Relationship-centered care (e.g., taking time to discuss medication with the cat owner) aids in client compliance. *(Image courtesy Dr. Debra Givin.)*

gather information for a new or extended patient medical evaluation before the scheduled visit. Furthermore, this questionnaire can be used when an owner cannot be present for the history taking and physical examination (e.g., when patients are dropped off). Having correct contact information and a method or time for follow-up ensures accurate communication at the beginning of the client–veterinarian relationship. The veterinary team can also establish an initial history when the appointment is scheduled or during client and patient check-in. Specific questionnaires can also be developed for different medical issues, such as behavior or mobility problems and cognitive dysfunction.[19,23]

Histories must be consistent and comprehensive. Open-ended questions requiring a definitive response rather than a simple *yes* or *no* result in the best answers. The following are examples of open-ended questions: "What was the last day you noticed a normal appetite?"; "When did you last notice a normal volume and consistency of stool?"; "What other changes have you noticed?" The client's initial responses can lead to more specific questions or prompts to continue (e.g., "Please describe what you have seen"; "What else?"; "Go on") to help define a specific problem (Box 3-2).[3] By repeating key information provided by the client, veterinarians demonstrate that they are paying attention and care about the client's perspective. Additionally, a veterinarian who demonstrates the various behaviors and sounds cats make with certain conditions, such as when coughing or vomiting, can help owners better describe their cat's signs. By videotaping signs or behaviors and sharing the video with the veterinarian over the Internet, the client can communicate a complicated or an infrequently noted problem. This is also a useful way for the veterinarian to monitor the ongoing status of a case, especially when the cat becomes highly stressed during veterinary visits and is therefore difficult to examine. A good example is a series of videos posted online about "Cricket" (http://www.youtube.com/user/NLMACNEILL; accessed February 24, 2010). The patient had a slowly improving right tibial nerve and hock injury requiring a series of re-evaluations. Hospital visits were problematic, and video monitoring allowed effective and less stressful follow-up.

Adapting the communication style depending on the client's age group and individual preferences may be constructive. For example, some elderly clients require extra time and a sympathetic ear for their concerns. A more focused set of interview questions and additional attention to treatment compliance may be necessary to ensure understanding. On the other hand, some younger clients prefer to communicate using newer technologies and social media.

BOX 3-2

Sample Interview Questions

General	How has your cat been doing since the last visit? When did your cat last appear normal? Are there any hair coat changes? Has your cat changed its grooming habits? Are the signs intermittent or continuous?
Behavior	What behavior changes have you recently noticed? How frequently does the problem occur? When does it occur? Have there been any recent changes to the environment? Are there any changes to sleep patterns? Any changes in interactions with family or other pets? Are there any changes to the level of activity? Any fearful behavior noted? Is there decreased responsiveness? Is there increased vocalization?
Gait/Mobility	Is there any reluctance to move or to be handled? Any weakness noted? Is there any evidence of lameness? Any swelling? Any painful areas noted?
Appetite	When did your cat last eat a normal meal? Is the appetite normal, increased, or decreased? What type of food is fed and how much? Any recent food changes? Is there any pain or difficulty while eating? Any reluctance to eat or food avoidance?
Vomiting or regurgitation	Is there any vomiting or regurgitation? Describe the appearance of the vomitus. How often has it happened? How soon after eating?
Water Intake	Has water intake changed? Increased or decreased? For how long?
Urinary	Has the amount of urine changed? Increased or decreased? Has the frequency of urination increased or decreased? For how long? Is there any straining to urinate? What color is the urine? Is there evidence of pain while trying to urinate? Any vocalizing while urinating? Has there been any urinating in odd places or outside the litter box?
Defecation	Have bowel movements changed in appearance (color, consistency, size, or volume)? Is there any straining to defecate? Any crying out with defecation? Is there any defecation outside the litter box?
Continuers	Describe any changes you have noticed. Anything else? Please go on. Please describe. Hmm?

Routine History

Signalment collection is part of the initial informational stage and includes age, breed, sex, and reproductive status. There are different wellness and disease concerns for kittens (up to 6 months of age) and junior (7 months to 2 years), adult (3 to 6 years), mature (7 to 10 years), senior (11 to 14 years), and geriatric cats (15 years and older) (see Chapter 8).[31] Often, other factors, such as diet, behavior, and medication history, are more significant in light of the patient's age group. Including questions about where the cat was acquired (e.g., shelter, rescue group, found as a stray) or whether the cat previously lived in another geographic location helps define essential elements of the history.[27] Cats adopted from shelters are more likely to have been exposed to infectious disease agents (e.g., feline herpesvirus).[26] Veterinarians practicing in the Pacific Northwest are less likely to diagnose feline heartworm disease in a cat raised locally than in one that was recently relocated from the Gulf State region and is not on a heartworm preventive.[16]

An increasing number of kittens and cats adopted from shelters, as well as strays and owned cats, have been microchipped. Each new patient should be scanned, preferably with a universal microchip scanner, to confirm the presence of a microchip and document the radio-frequency identification (RFID) in the patient record. According to research, rescanning during annual examinations ensures that the microchip remains functional and has not migrated. Also, encouraging clients to keep their personal information current with their microchip registry helps reunite the client and cat in case of separation.[14] Established in 2009, the American Animal Hospital Association (http://www.petmicrochiplookup.org; accessed February 21, 2010) and Chloe Standard (http://www.checkthechip.com; accessed February 21, 2010) microchip websites are available for rapid association of a microchip number with a client's personal information. If no microchip is present, further discussion of the benefits of microchipping or another form of visual identification is warranted.

A new kitten or patient visit is a great opportunity to discuss behavior. An unaddressed behavior problem can lead to a diminished cat–human bond and increase the cat's risk of being relinquished to a shelter or euthanized. An initial set of behavior-based questions can help clients and veterinarians explore this issue. Some undesirable behaviors (e.g., urinating outside the litter box) may be the result of an undiagnosed medical condition. Further, a discussion of general litter-box habits is appropriate. Reviewing behavior during the kitten visits also helps the client understand the interactions required during the early (3 to 8 weeks) and late (9 to 16 weeks) socialization periods. Proper bonding early in the kitten's life leads to fewer behavioral problems later in life (Figure 3-2).[19]

A complete vaccination history documenting the types and dates of vaccinations, especially those given when the client first acquired the kitten or cat, is a critical step in building a complete patient medical history. It is important to note and highlight any past adverse reactions to vaccinations and follow up with a discussion of the potential disease risks and benefits associated with an immunization program. Age, health status, and whether the cat is kept indoors or has regular outdoor access are primary risk determinants. Even cats that are kept inside should not be considered strictly indoor creatures because outdoor pathogens and parasites can be brought inside and cats may periodically escape outside. Because of this possibility, rabies immunization remains a core vaccine recommendation for cats even in communities where it is not legally required.[24] Clients should be asked whether preventive drugs for heartworm, fleas, and other external and internal parasites are used; if they are, the veterinarian should note the product, dosage, and application interval in the medical record.[27,31]

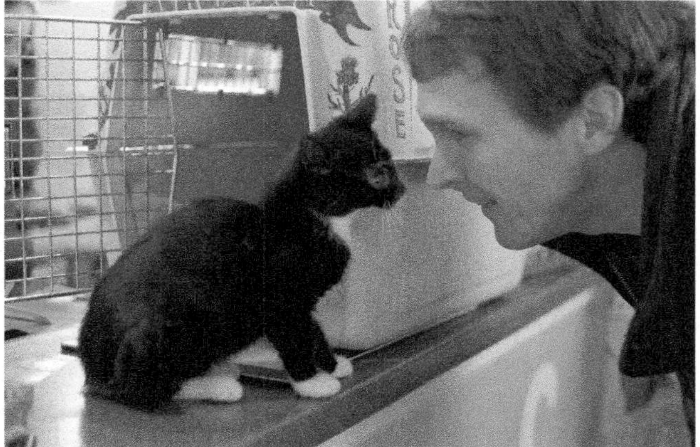

FIGURE 3-2 Early bonding enhances the veterinary visit and the owner's lifelong relationship with the pet. *(Image courtesy Dr. Debra Givin.)*

A cat's retroviral status (feline leukemia virus and feline immunodeficiency virus) is also an essential part of a complete history. Retrovirus testing is performed at different times in a cat's life, and the dates and results should be documented in the medical record. Depending on the responses and history obtained thus far, the key retrovirus risk factors (e.g., male sex, age, outdoor access) can be explored with the client to determine the need for initial testing or retesting.[12]

Nutrition, especially diet type and source (including treats), and daily caloric intake are other important components of a cat's medical history. Because a dietary change can either create or resolve an acute or chronic medical condition, updating the patient's nutritional history is an accepted and recommended practice. Further, because some clients do not know the brand, flavor, type, and amount of food consumed by their pet, persistent questioning and follow-up may be required. This issue becomes especially important when there is a significant change in the cat's weight and body condition score (BCS) (Figure 3-3). A change in weight may also affect the prescribed dosage of a medication. For example, because prednisolone does not appear to distribute to adipose tissue, the dosage for obese cats is based on ideal or lean body weight instead of current body weight.[4]

Questions regarding water sources, water intake, and the amount and type of urine and feces produced by the patient can follow. Using veterinary software to track the nutritional history and maintain contact information is beneficial in the event of a pet-food recall. The significance of the 2007 melamine contamination of pet food demonstrates the value of dietary information management.[5]

Prior and Existing Complaints

Additional history is required when the client seeks veterinary care for an existing complaint. Knowledge of current and past medications, as well as prior laboratory test results, may help clarify a medical problem or spur additional issue-oriented questions (e.g., "How did the cat respond to treatment?"; "Did anyone have difficulty giving the medication?"; "Were there any side effects, and if so, what were they?"). Three common general presenting signs are anorexia, lethargy, and a change in normal behavior (e.g., hiding). Clients regularly report one or more of these general signs when asked to describe their cat's problems. Specific questions should be asked about the dose and frequency of administration of prescribed medications because clients sometimes make changes without consulting the veterinarian. Moreover, clients may not report the use of nonprescription medications or supplements unless questioned directly.

Questions focusing on specific observations by the client before the onset of the problem and during the

Nestlé PURINA

BODY CONDITION SYSTEM

TOO THIN

1 Ribs visible on shorthaired cats; no palpable fat; severe abdominal tuck; lumbar vertebrae and wings of ilia easily palpated.

2 Ribs easily visible on shorthaired cats; lumbar vertebrae obvious with minimal muscle mass; pronounced abdominal tuck; no palpable fat.

3 Ribs easily palpable with minimal fat covering; lumbar vertebrae obvious; obvious waist behind ribs; minimal abdominal fat.

4 Ribs palpable with minimal fat covering; noticeable waist behind ribs; slight abdominal tuck; abdominal fat pad absent.

IDEAL

5 **Well-proportioned; observe waist behind ribs; ribs palpable with slight fat covering; abdominal fat pad minimal.**

TOO HEAVY

6 Ribs palpable with slight excess fat covering; waist and abdominal fat pad distinguishable but not obvious; abdominal tuck absent.

7 Ribs not easily palpated with moderate fat covering; waist poorly discernible; obvious rounding of abdomen; moderate abdominal fat pad.

8 Ribs not palpable with excess fat covering; waist absent; obvious rounding of abdomen with prominent abdominal fat pad; fat deposits present over lumbar area.

9 Ribs not palpable under heavy fat cover; heavy fat deposits over lumbar area, face and limbs; distention of abdomen with no waist; extensive abdominal fat deposits.

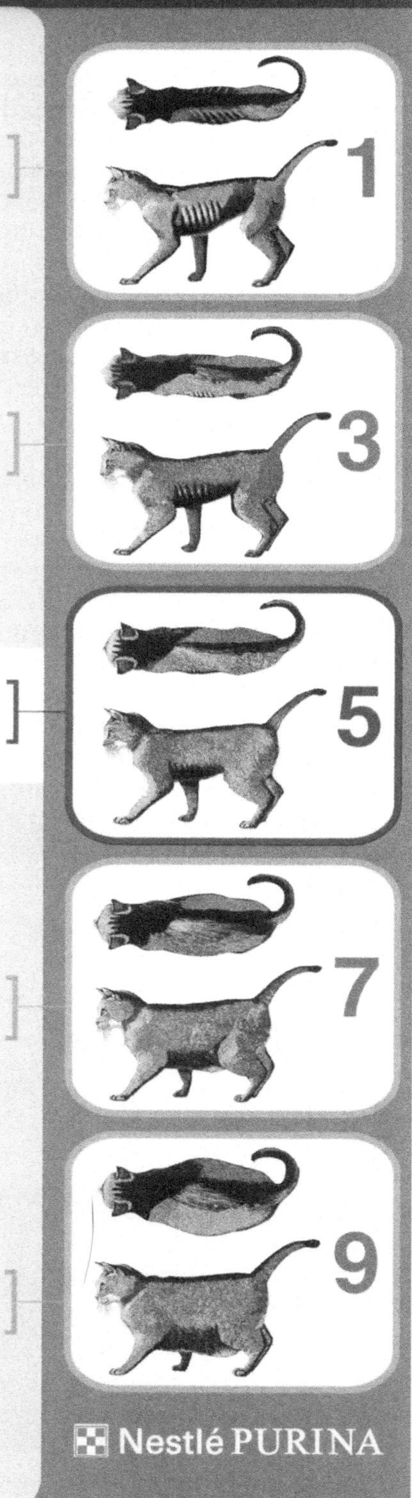

Call 1-800-222-VETS (8387), weekdays, 8:00 a.m. to 4:30 p.m. CT

FIGURE 3-3 An example of a 9-point body condition scoring chart for the cat. *(Image used by permission from Nestle Purina Petcare.)*

initial phase help the conversation move from generalizations to a specific description. Responses also help the veterinarian establish a timeline for additional intervening signs. The following are examples of questions that might prompt such responses: "Was the onset acute or gradual?"; "Were the signs steady or intermittent?"; "Has the problem occurred previously, and if so, what was the response?" Evaluating the client's answers helps the veterinarian determine the diagnosis, develop a list of possible causes, and decide on subsequent diagnostic planning. However, diagnosis can be fluid; new or different medical problems may emerge after the initial diagnosis. If so, the veterinarian may need to ask the client additional questions, further observe the patient, and re-evaluate the original diagnosis.[23,27]

An effective medical history summarizes the known health situation and the needs and potential problems of the patient (Box 3-3). The next step, a comprehensive physical examination, helps assemble the pieces of the puzzle.

THE PHYSICAL EXAMINATION

Initial Steps

History preparation is an opportune time for the patient to adjust to its surroundings. This gives the patient a chance to relax, thus enabling a more productive and less stress-inducing examination. Often, if given time and opportunity, cats voluntarily leave the carrier to explore (Figure 3-4). Although most patients will relax on the examination table, it is not unusual for others to find a comfortable perch elsewhere in the room. Performing the examination where the patient is most comfortable (e.g., on the floor, on a chair or bench) may be an effective tactic for the veterinarian. Further, providing familiar objects such as toys, towels, or a fleece bed can help make the cat more comfortable. Offering treats may calm the cat and entice it to leave the carrier. Spraying a towel or nearby surfaces with a synthetic feline pheromone (e.g., Feliway) or placing pheromone diffusers in the examination room may also help reduce stress.[25]

Conversely, some cats respond with more heightened senses if allowed to roam the room or hide under chairs or other furniture. Learning to recognize body postures associated with fear is fundamental for veterinarians and clients.[25] In these situations it is better to keep the cat in the carrier and minimize wait time and anxiety. The veterinarian should carefully observe the cat's behavior and demeanor while it is in the carrier or walking around the room. Detecting changes in gait, evidence of pain, types of respiratory patterns, or areas of asymmetry at this time can lead to additional questions for the client and specific issues to address in the

BOX 3-3

Medical History Components

Signalment	Age, breed, sex, and reproductive status
Locality	Disease prevalence in current and prior geographic locations
Acquisition	Private home, shelter, stray, pet store, or breeder
Environment	Primarily indoor, outdoor or both; other household pets; city, urban, or rural; possible toxin exposure; layout of home and yard
Vaccinations	History and any adverse reactions
Parasite Control	History and treatment, current and prior
Diet	Canned food, dry food, or both; brand and quantity; raw food; hunting prey; treats and supplements
Microchip	RFID number, registry information, periodic rescanning
Retroviral Testing	Dates, results, and risk evaluation
Prior Medical History	Illnesses, medications, adverse reactions, laboratory tests and results
Existing Complaints	Last known normal state
	Acute or gradual onset
	Progression (continuous or intermittent)
	Duration of problem
	Primary problem and prevailing secondary signs
	Present signs (attitude, appetite, activity, weight changes, water intake, behavioral changes, urination, defecation, and gait/mobility)

Modified with permission from Sherding RG: The medical history, physical examination, and physical restraint. In Sherding RG, editor: The cat: diseases and clinical management, *ed 2, Philadelphia, 1994, Saunders, p 7.*

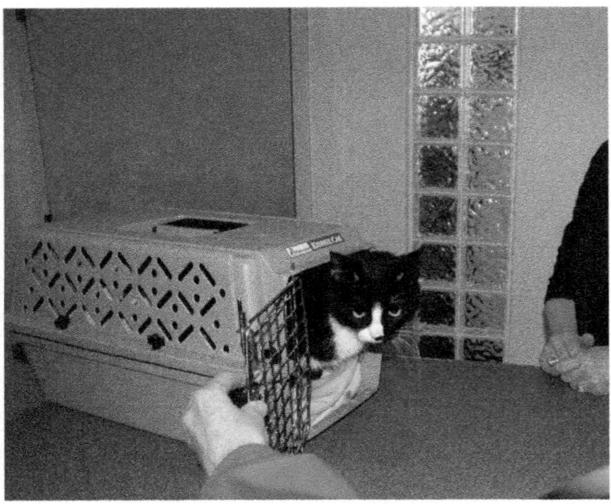

FIGURE 3-4 The cat should be allowed time to exit the carrier on its own before the examination when possible. *(Image courtesy Dr. Debra Givin.)*

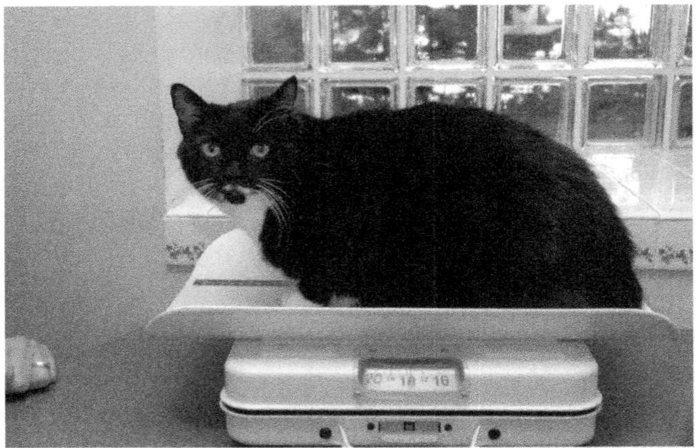

FIGURE 3-5 Cats should be weighed on a tabletop scale during every veterinary visit. *(Image courtesy Dr. Debra Givin.)*

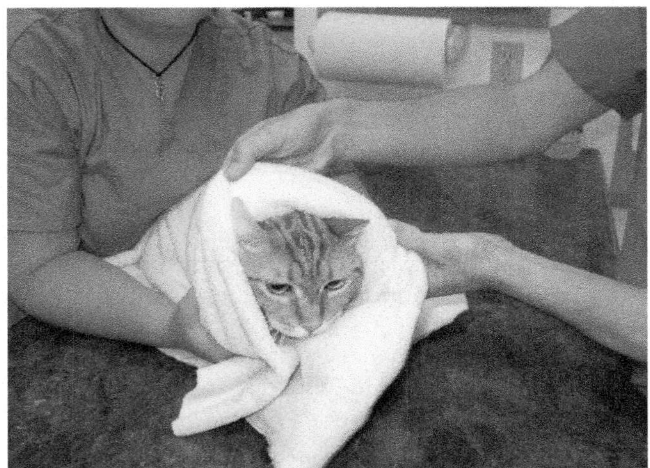

FIGURE 3-6 If needed, a towel can be used during the examination. *(Image courtesy Dr. Vicki Thayer.)*

physical examination. Some cats may be so ill during the initial observation that an assessment must be done quickly and the patient moved to a treatment area or enclosure. It is important to minimize stress and promptly stabilize ill patients before attempting a more detailed examination.[6]

An effective physical examination technique follows a routine, consistent pattern but allows for some flexibility. Cats perceive the world through their senses, and their response to a new setting and unfamiliar smells in the examination room is not predictable. If the cat prefers to remain in the carrier and exhibits signs of anxiety, the carrier top should be removed and a thick towel used to cover the cat. This is often a convenient time to weigh the cat, either after removing it from the carrier or while the cat is still in the carrier (with the carrier's weight subtracted from the total). A tabletop scale designed for small animals or human infants is the best equipment for weighing cats (Figure 3-5). The veterinarian can proceed by adjusting the towel as needed (Figure 3-6) while the cat remains in the carrier or after gently lifting and removing the cat from the carrier. Tipping the carrier and dumping the cat onto the examination table or floor is not recommended.[25]

As the examination continues, the veterinarian should move slowly and deliberately and speak quietly. The veterinarian should maintain physical contact with the cat by having examination tools close at hand. Losing physical contact may increase the cat's level of anxiety and lead to difficulty in completing the examination. The undeniable fact is that cats demand time and attention. A mindset of "less is more; more is less" and "slow is fast; fast is slow" pays dividends in both efficiency and effectiveness. The care, the time, and the examination should be tailored to the patient's needs.

Starting an examination at the tip of the nose and working toward the tip of the tail is a common and effective technique for some clinicians; others, especially during the initial examination, prefer to face the cat away to minimize eye contact, which some cats may find threatening. If the cat resists, the veterinarian can modify the routine to fit the patient and resume the examination in a less sensitive area, such as the head, over the hindquarters, or the abdomen and lumbar area. It is helpful to be flexible yet thorough and adapt to the cat's comfort level.

For most patients, obtaining an accurate rectal temperature reading is possible by slowly inserting a well-lubricated, quick-reading digital thermometer (Figure 3-7) while distracting the patient with treats or gentle massage of the head. If appropriate, the veterinarian can check for fecal impaction and anal tone at this time.

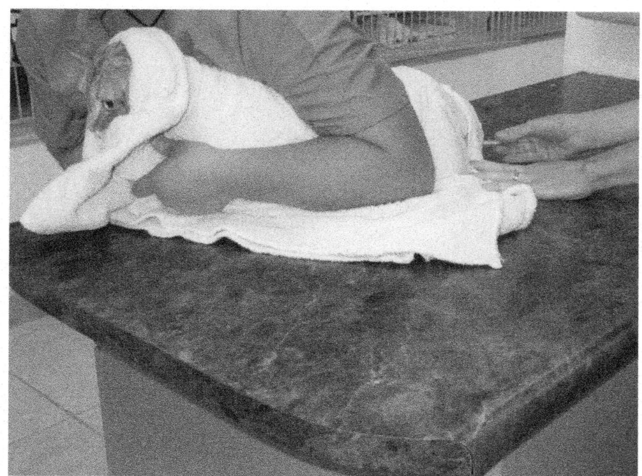

FIGURE 3-7 Using a digital thermometer to take a rectal temperature. *(Image courtesy Dr. Vicki Thayer.)*

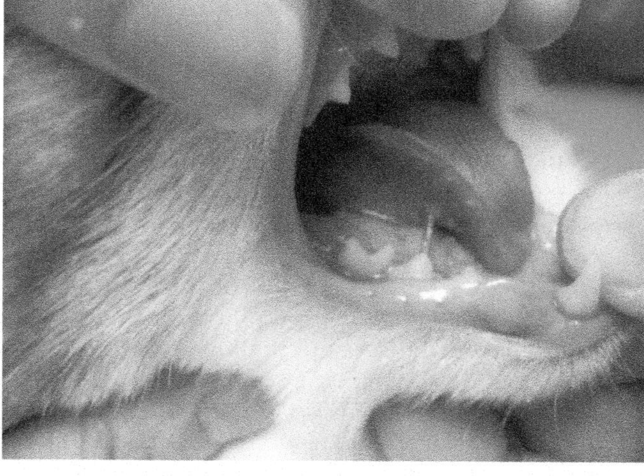

FIGURE 3-8 Gentle pressure in the intermandibular space elevates the tongue, allowing discovery of linear foreign bodies. *(Image courtesy Dr. Susan Little.)*

Forgoing temperature measurement during wellness examinations of less tolerant but healthy patients is acceptable. Using an ear thermometer for fractious cats is a reasonable alternative, although its accuracy, especially in ill cats, has been questioned.[11] It should be noted that a cat's body temperature can exceed 103° F (39.4° C) on warm days or as a result of travel stress.

According to current expert opinion, pain is considered the fourth vital sign after temperature, pulse, and respiration. Pain assessment is an essential part of every patient evaluation. Many conditions and procedures cause pain in cats, and veterinarians must remain aware of this potential and look for its signs. Because a change in behavior is the most common sign of pain, understanding a patient's normal behavior is important in identifying changes and making an appropriate choice to intervene. Several resources to aid in this process are available to the veterinary health care team.[9]

The Head

First, the nose is examined for any surface changes or lesions. Any lack of symmetry or the presence of discharge or an occasional foreign body, such as a blade of grass, can be more easily detected by shining a light on the nostrils. Ulcers on the nasal commissure may indicate an upper respiratory virus infection (e.g., feline calicivirus, feline herpesvirus).[15] Type and color of any nasal discharge should be documented, along with whether it is unilateral or bilateral; these signs can indicate inflammation, infection, or neoplasia. Unusual sound or air movement can denote obstruction or upper airway disease. Stertorous noise (e.g., snoring or snorting) may indicate changes involving the pharynx, whereas stridor (i.e., wheezing) is localized to the laryngeal area.[13]

As with the nose, the lips and chin are evaluated for lesions or skin changes. Next, the teeth are assessed, with any losses noted, along with oropharyngeal inflammation, periodontal disease, tooth resorption (formerly called *feline odontoclastic resorptive lesions* or *neck lesions*), and tooth fractures. The cat's mouth should be held open to examine the roof, both fauces, and the back of the throat (Figure 3-8). Common complaints include mouth odor, difficulty chewing, or pawing at the mouth. Jaundice is often most readily appreciated on the hard palate. The veterinarian should review the entire mouth for lesions consistent with inflammation. Applying gentle pressure with a thumb in the intermandibular space and elevating the tongue allow discovery of linear foreign material or other abnormalities in the sublingual area (see Figure 3-8).[27] A nonhealing inflammatory lesion requires evaluation for potential underlying neoplasia. Squamous cell carcinoma is the most common oral cancer in cats and is often seen as a mass under the tongue.[18] Further, color and appearance of the mucous membranes are indicators of anemia (pale), cyanosis (blue tint), and jaundice (yellow tint). A prolonged capillary refill time raises questions regarding the patient's tissue perfusion status.

Moving on to the eyes, the veterinarian should first appraise the status of or changes in the palpebral openings, pupils, eyelids, and nictitating membranes. The veterinarian should look for evidence of exophthalmus (may indicate retrobulbar lesions), retraction of the globe (may indicate weight loss or dehydration), excessive tearing, and blepharospasm. Next, the pupils are checked to confirm that they are equal in size and equally responsive to light. The patient's eyes should be examined for vascularization, cellular or fluid infiltrates, and ulceration in each cornea. The conjunctiva and sclera should be observed for signs of jaundice, anemia, and inflammation. The iris is assessed for change in color, thinning or thickening, and hyperemia, and hyperpigmented lesions should be monitored for changes in size or appearance during subsequent examinations. Uveal lesions may be the result of trauma, infectious disease (e.g., feline infectious peritonitis, feline immunodeficiency virus infection), or neoplasia. Senile nuclear sclerosis may occur as the cat ages. Cataracts may be congenital in some breeds, most commonly Persians and British Shorthairs, or subsequent to other problems, such as trauma or anterior uveitis.[1] Finally, the retina is evaluated by direct or indirect ophthalmoscopy for hemorrhage (may indicate hypertension), detachment (may indicate tumor, hypertension, or trauma), neoplasia (e.g., lymphoma), and degenerative (e.g., retinal atrophy) or inflammatory changes (e.g., toxoplasmosis).[27,32]

Proceeding to the ears, the surface of each pinna is examined for areas of alopecia or other skin lesions, including inflammation, ulceration, color changes, and crustiness. Each ear is checked for wounds or abscesses, especially if the cat engages in fighting, and aural hematomas. Evidence of jaundice or petechiae, if present, is typically observed in the medial lining of the pinnae. The ear canals are examined with an otoscope for changes and views of the tympanic membrane. The eardrum is normally flat and tense and the ear canal lining is generally smooth and devoid of wax or discharge. A cytologic examination of abnormal wax content or discharge can confirm preliminary diagnoses of ear mites *(Otodectes cyanotis)*, *Demodex* sp., bacterial infections, or yeast overgrowth (*Malassezia* sp.).[29] Abnormal growths or polyps may be the result of chronic inflammation or evidence of neoplasia. Pain on opening the mouth may be a sign of underlying external or middle ear disease when oral disease is not present.

The Neck and Forelimbs

Examination of the neck and forelimbs begins with palpation of the submandibular lymph nodes, salivary glands, and larynx. The paratracheal region, from the caudal larynx to the thoracic inlet, is checked for an enlarged thyroid gland. The normal thyroid gland may not be palpable. Although the classic technique to examine the thyroid gland is with the cat sitting and the neck and head extended upward for palpation, other effective techniques have been described (Figure 3-9).[20] The veterinarian should continue exploring the surface of the neck for lesions, changes since prior examinations, and evidence of pain. Ventroflexion of the neck may be evidence of a thiamine or potassium deficiency, polymyopathy, or polyneuropathy.

Gently flexing and extending the muscles, bones, and joints of the front legs help in detecting any swelling, discomfort, or lack of mobility. This can be accomplished through simultaneous palpation of both limbs and comparison of one limb with the other. The veterinarian should examine both front paws for the condition of the nails, nail beds, pads, and interdigital tissue while noting any unusual lesions or injury. Polydactyl and geriatric cats often have a nail that has grown into a digital pad. Nails that are split or torn completely from the nail bed can be evidence of trauma.

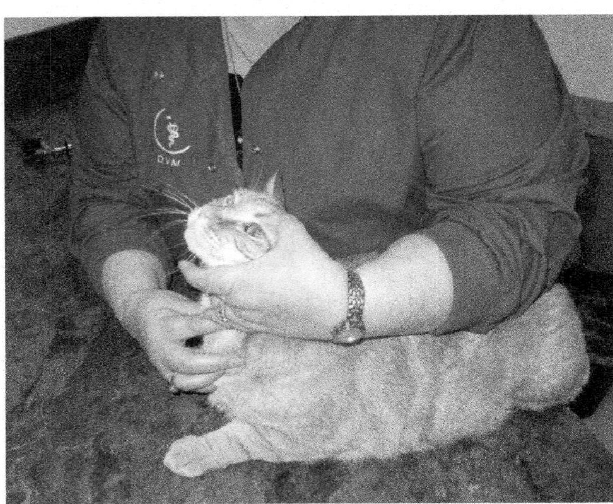

FIGURE 3-9 Thyroid gland palpation is an essential component of a senior cat examination. *(Image courtesy Dr. Vicki Thayer.)*

The Thorax and Trunk

Auscultation of the heart and lungs is a critical component of a complete thoracic examination. The veterinarian should position the cat so that it is facing forward and listen for rate, rhythm, and possible murmurs, using both the bell and diaphragm of the stethoscope (Figure 3-10). Auscultation is most effective in a quiet room. It may be necessary to ask the owner not to talk during thoracic auscultation. The presence of a cardiac murmur does not always signify underlying heart disease, nor does its absence preclude structural heart disease.[21] Murmurs may result from other physical states, such as anemia or the patient's hydration status.

Both sides of the thorax are auscultated to evaluate the heart from base to apex as well as along the sternum. The maximum intensity of cardiac sounds is usually from the third to fifth intercostal spaces on the left side. Loud cardiac murmurs will create palpable vibrations on the chest wall, referred to as a *precordial thrill*, and are experienced as a "buzzing" sensation typically at the point of maximum intensity. Gallop rhythms and other arrhythmias, such as bradycardia, are associated with forms of feline cardiomyopathy. In hyperdynamic states such as hyperthyroidism, sinus tachycardia is frequently

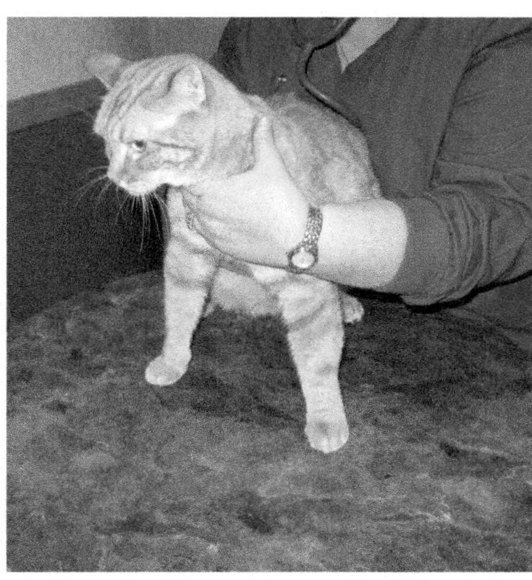

FIGURE 3-10 Cardiac auscultation should be performed in a quiet examination room. *(Image courtesy Dr. Vicki Thayer.)*

a prominent sign. Palpating the femoral pulse while auscultating the heart may help the veterinarian detect a pulse deficit or weakness. Diminished or no femoral pulse, along with cold, pale, and weak extremities, may indicate an aortic thromboembolism. Jugular vein distention or jugular pulses may be the result of right-sided heart failure; these are observed by wetting or shaving the hair over the jugular groove.[2,27]

Monitoring the respiratory rate and pattern, along with thoracic auscultation, can assist in detecting the presence of an underlying cardiac or respiratory disease. The normal respiratory rate is 20 to 40 breaths per minute. However, an increased respiratory rate can also be due to excitement, fever, pain, or fear. Dyspnea, or difficult or labored breathing, is primarily an observed state and usually causes anxiety for the cat. Pulmonary edema and pleural effusion may increase the respiratory rate with noticeable inspiratory and expiratory effort and no audible airway noise. Breath sounds are usually absent ventrally when pleural fluid is present. Careful percussion of the chest can identify areas of increased air or the presence of fluid or masses.

Prolonged expiration, an expiratory or abdominal push, or other increased respiratory efforts are indicators of lower airway disease caused by narrowing or obstruction of smaller airways. Lower airway disease (e.g., possible pulmonary edema or inflammatory airway disease) may produce harsh lung sounds such as inspiratory crackles and expiratory wheezes. Additional clinical signs of chronic respiratory disease may include a barrel-chested appearance and decreased chest compressibility. Patients with respiratory compromise may be unable to lie down comfortably and often sit hunched with the elbows abducted.[10]

As a final step in examining the thorax and trunk, the veterinarian should palpate the ribs, trunk, dorsum, ventrum, axillae, and mammary chains for lumps, abnormal lesions, and enlarged lymph nodes. Mammary neoplasia is not uncommon in female cats, and early detection is important for improving prognosis. Mammary masses should be considered neoplastic until proven otherwise.

Pectus excavatum or deformity of the xiphoid process of the sternum may be seen in younger cats. Focal lymph node enlargement signifies regional disease, usually subsequent to abscesses or skin disease, and diffuse lymphadenopathy may be the result of systemic disease, such as lymphoma.

The Abdomen

The veterinarian should visually evaluate the general size and appearance of the abdomen while palpating for fluid, fat, organ distention, or pain. Abdominal pain or discomfort during palpation may be due to an underlying pathology, although this type of reaction can also result from handling anxiety. Palpation is accomplished by moving front to back and from each side, using the tips of the fingers of one hand or both hands close together. Soft ballottement of the abdominal wall may indicate the presence of fluid or enable the veterinarian to detect other causes of abdominal distention. The liver is usually not palpable, but if hepatomegaly is present, the edge of the liver will be palpable past the costochondral arch. The veterinarian should note the shape of the palpable edge of the liver (e.g., sharp versus rounded edge or smooth versus irregular) because it may indicate abnormal changes. As with the liver, the stomach and pancreas are not usually palpable.

An enlarged spleen may denote hematopoietic or myeloproliferative disorders involving infiltration of the splenic tissue with abnormal type and numbers of lymphocytes and mast cells. In many cats it is possible to discern both kidneys, with the left kidney being more caudal than the right. Palpation helps in the detection of changes in size (larger or smaller) or shape (smooth versus irregular). A normal urinary bladder in the posterior abdomen has a thin wall and does not elicit pain on palpation. A larger, tense, and painful bladder may indicate a possible lower urinary tract obstruction.

The normal nonpregnant uterus is not palpable in cats. An enlarged uterus may be palpated as tubular structure(s) distinct from the intestinal tract and may be caused by pregnancy or uterine disease such as pyometra. A massively enlarged uterus may be due to late-stage pregnancy, pyometra, hydrometra, or mucometra and can occupy most of the abdominal space.

The small intestine is usually easily palpable, and the intestinal wall is typically symmetric throughout. A change in wall thickness, asymmetry, distention of intestinal segments, or pain on palpation often indicates an underlying pathology. Mesenteric lymph node enlargement may be associated with these signs and may result from inflammation or neoplasia. The various sections of colon are also palpable, and a colon full of feces is typically a sign of constipation or, more significantly, obstipation. Because obesity may mask significant changes to abdominal organs, successful palpation of obese cats requires extra attention by experienced veterinarians; in some cases, it may be impossible to perform a thorough abdominal palpation.

The Hindquarters and Tail

The hind legs and paws are evaluated and compared in the same manner as the front legs and paws. The veterinarian should gently flex and extend the coxofemoral, stifle, and hock joints to test for impaired mobility or pain, noting any swelling or other abnormalities. A tendency toward medial patellar luxation in one or both stifles may be detected in some younger cats. Acute lameness in cats, especially overweight cats, may be due to an anterior cruciate ligament rupture and requires testing for anterior drawer motion and noting any pain in the stifle joint. The skin, pads, and nails of the hind paws are examined for similar problems as the front, although ingrown nails are less frequent.

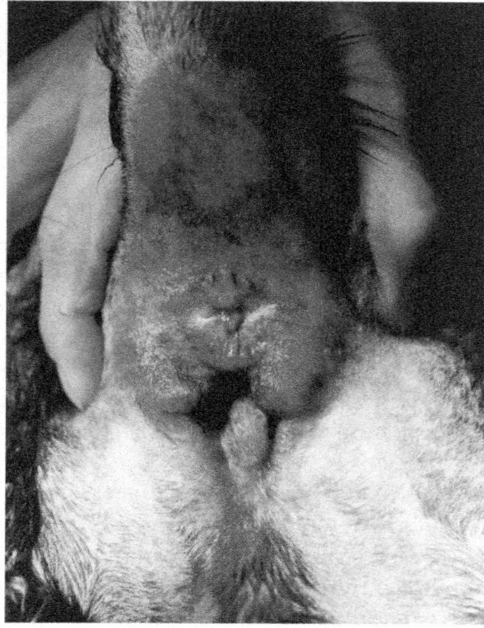

FIGURE 3-11 Perineal dermatitis is often seen in very obese patients. *(Image courtesy Dr. Susan Little.)*

Starting at the base of the tail and proceeding to the tip, the veterinarian palpates for possible wounds, pain, and swelling. Sacrococcygeal dislocations or fractures caused by trauma are most often discovered at the base. Next, the anal and perineal regions are assessed for appearance and cleanliness. Extra skin folds or the inability to clean the perineum often leads to hygienic issues and dermatitis in obese patients (Figure 3-11). Evidence of tapeworm infection, *Taenia taeniaeformis* or *Dipylidium caninum,* may be found in the hair surrounding the anus.

The anal glands are located at the 4 and 8 o'clock positions around the anus. Palpation of the anal glands may determine whether they need to be emptied, and anal gland abscesses are not uncommon in the cat. Cats can develop perineal hernias leading to fecal impaction. Rectal examination, when needed, may require patient sedation or general anesthesia in some cases. The vulva is normally free of discharge, even when a queen is in estrus.

The veterinarian should check unneutered male kittens and cats to confirm whether both testes are located in the scrotal sacs. If it is unknown whether a male cat has been neutered or is cryptorchid, the penis should be checked for spines. The presence of penile spines indicates a source of testosterone, typically a retained testicle.

Final General Assessment

Finally, the veterinarian examines, touches, and evaluates the skin and hair coat during the examination and discusses any issues with the client. Unusual odors may be the result of underlying problems, such as discharge from infected wounds and exposure to questionable agents (e.g., smoke, chemicals). Most cats prefer to be clean; a decreased desire to groom may reflect illness. Excessive saliva on the hair coat, especially the hair covering the lower extremities, may indicate significant oral disease.

Evidence of fleas or external parasites is found by combing sections of the hair coat at any time during the exam. The veterinarian should discuss noteworthy hair mats with the client and if needed, recommend removal (Figure 3-12). Matting of the hair coat can be uncomfortable for the cat and may reflect decreased grooming resulting from obesity, especially if the mats are evident on the caudal half of the body, in areas the cat can no longer reach. The veterinarian should monitor white cats and those with white or lightly pigmented areas on or around the pinnae, eyelids, and nasal philtrum for solar dermatitis or dysplastic changes.[17] Skin bumps or growths should be measured with a ruler or caliper, and these characteristics documented in the record. Alopecia, wounds, and other skin abnormalities should also

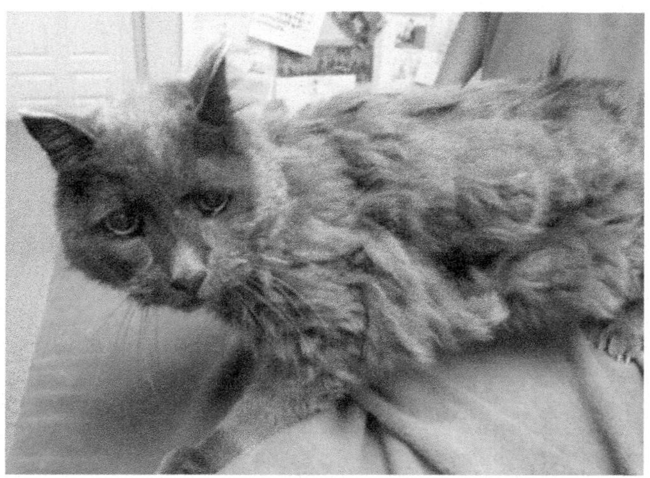

FIGURE 3-12 Matting of the hair can indicate decreased grooming habits, often resulting from underlying medical conditions. *(Image courtesy Dr. Susan Little.)*

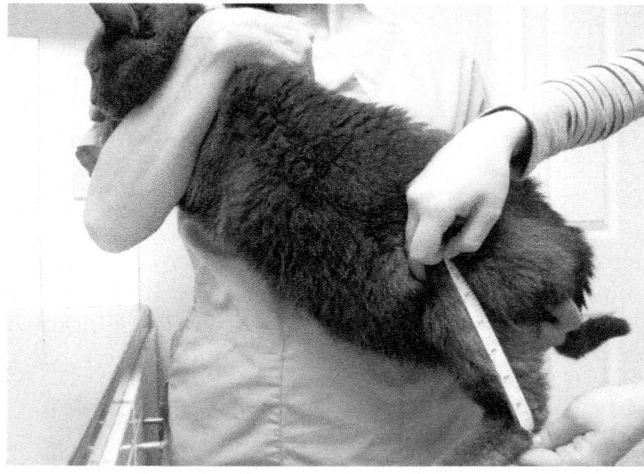

FIGURE 3-13 Leg index measurement (LIM) for the Feline Body Mass Index is the length (in cm) from the middle of the patella to the dorsal tip of the calcaneal process. *(Image courtesy Dr. Susan Little.)*

BOX 3-4

Formula for Calculation of the Feline Body Mass Index

$$\text{Percentage body fat} = \left(\frac{\left(\frac{\text{RCC}}{0.7062} \right) - \text{LIM}}{0.9156} \right) - \text{LIM}$$

Reprinted with permission from Waltham Focus, 10:32, 2000.
RCC, Rib cage circumference; *LIM,* leg index measurement.
All measurements in cm.

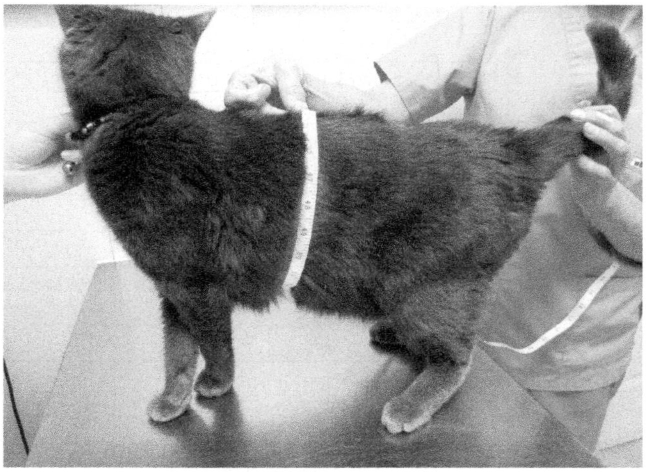

be noted. Alopecia over a joint may indicate pain, such as that associated with osteoarthritis. Alopecia on the ventral abdomen may indicate bladder pain. An area of fluctuant swelling with localized warmth often indicates an abscess, a common condition for cats.

During the final stages of the examination, the veterinarian scores general body condition by assigning a composite rating using either a 5-point or a 9-point scale (see Figure 3-3). Weight loss or weight gain is often best understood by the owner when it is expressed as a percentage of the cat's previous weight (e.g., the cat has gained 15% more than the previous weight recorded). Alternatively, the Feline Body Mass Index (FBMI) developed by the Waltham Center for Pet Nutrition provides an indicator of body fat content.[8] This valuable measurement tool helps clinicians and researchers better define the relationship between body fat content and disease risk in cats. The formula to determine FBMI is shown in Box 3-4. The equation uses rib cage circumference and the leg index measurement (the length of the lower hindlimb from the middle of the patella to the dorsal tip of the calcaneal process) (Figures 3-13 through 3-15).

FIGURE 3-14 Measurement of rib cage circumference (RCC) (in cm) for the Feline Body Mass Index. *(Image courtesy Dr. Susan Little.)*

If the cat has lost weight, muscle loss or wasting is evaluated. Specifically, a loss of muscle mass over the back (e.g., prominent vertebral spinous processes) or legs (e.g., prominent scapulae) and a pendulous abdomen or a large inguinal fat pad may indicate a serious underlying medical condition. Barring emaciation or the effects of aging, gauging skin turgor by tenting the skin over the back and monitoring its return to a resting position provides a rough assessment of hydration and assists in evaluating the patient's health status. Mild skin tenting may not occur until a cat is at least 5% dehydrated.

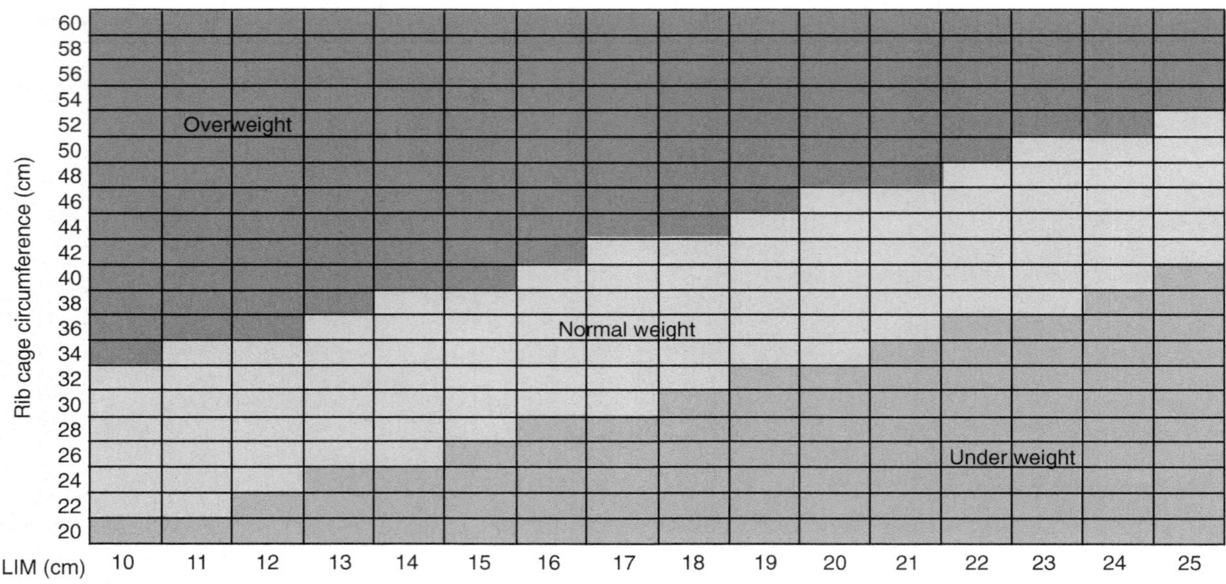

FIGURE 3-15 Use of the leg index measurement (LIM; in cm) and rib cage circumference (in cm) to determine Feline Body Mass Index. *(Image courtesy WALTHAM Center for Pet Nutrition.)*

Emotional Soap		
Medical variables		**Emotional variables**
How do you think this animal is doing?	**S|S**	How do you think this owner is doing?
–physical appearance		–physical appearance
–body language and demeanor	**Subjective**	–body language and demeanor
–interactions with the owner		–interactions with the pet
What is the reason for the visit?		What might the owner need from you?
What does your intuition tell you about this patient?	***What do you feel/ notice/suspect?***	What does your intuition tell you about this owner?
What does the owner tell you about this animal and the presenting problem?	**O|O**	What does the owner tell you about his/her feelings and relationship with this pet?
What is the important medical history?	**Objective**	What is the important emotional history?
What did you find on physical exam?	***What are the facts?***	What do you find on the Family-Pet Relationship Information Form?
What past experiences and knowledge can you draw on for this case?	**A|A**	What past experiences and knowledge can you draw on for this case?
What diagnosis can you rule in based on your collected information?	**Assessment**	What emotional needs and support-based services can you rule in as potentially applicable to this case?
	What can you conclude from an overall synthesis of the data?	
What options can you recommend and offer for treatment?	**P|P**	What options/resources (supportive people, finances, time) are available to this owner?
What is the time frame for treatment?	**Plan**	What is the time frame for support?
What is the cost of treatment?	***What treatment and support options are available to owners?***	What is the cost of the recommended support services?
What is the treatment follow-up?		What is the support follow-up?

FIGURE 3-16 Emotional Subjective Objective Assessment Plan.

Moderate skin tenting occurs when a cat is 6% to 8% dehydrated, and skin tenting that stays in place for a few seconds or longer indicates at least 10% dehydration. The appearance of sunken eyes or dry, tacky mucous membranes can further confirm dehydration.

A neurologic assessment is best performed when the history and physical examination indicate that it is necessary. A short version of a cranial nerve exam can be achieved while evaluating the head and neck area.

The final steps in a comprehensive and effective physical examination involve reviewing findings with the client and outlining treatment recommendations. A concise written "report card" for the patient is an accepted method of helping the client understand treatment recommendations. In fact, sharing examination findings, explaining treatment options, and providing a possible prognosis within a SOAP (*s*ubjective, *o*bjective *a*ssessment *p*lan) format increases owner compliance and satisfaction with the proposed regimen.[6] If a sick cat is being assessed, an Emotional SOAP technique (http://www.aah-abv.org, see Autumn 2002 newsletter; accessed February 24, 2010) can be used concurrently with the typical SOAP format to meet the client's emotional needs (Figure 3-16).[30] In many cases, listing differentials and so-called "rule outs" in the aforementioned format may also help explain the need for further diagnostic measures such as laboratory tests as part of a minimum database.

References

1. Barnett KC, Crispin SM: *Feline ophthalmology: an atlas and text*, London, 2002, Saunders, p 122.
2. Bonagura J: Cardiovascular diseases. In Sherding RG, editor: *The cat, diseases and clinical management*, ed 2, Philadelphia, 1994, Saunders, p 819.
3. Caney S: Weight loss in the elderly cat, *J Feline Med Surg* 11:730, 2009.
4. Center SA: Progress in characterization and management of the feline cholangitis/cholangiohepatitis syndrome, *Proc Am Assoc Feline Pract Fall Conf* 1-16, 2009.
5. Ciancolo RE, Bischoff K, Ebel JG et al: Clinicopathologic, histologic, and toxicologic findings in 70 cats inadvertently exposed to pet food contaminated with melamine and cyanuric acid, *J Am Vet Med Assoc* 233:729, 2008.
6. Ettinger SJ: The physical examination of the dog and cat. In Ettinger S, Feldman EC, editors: *Textbook of veterinary internal medicine*, ed 6, St Louis, 2005, Saunders, p 2.
7. Frankel M, Stein T: Getting the most out of the clinical encounter: the four habits model, *Perm J* 3:79, 1999.
8. Hawthorne A, Butterwick R: The feline body mass index: a simple measure of body fat content in cats, *Waltham Focus* 10:32, 2000.
9. Hellyer P, Rodan I, Brunt J et al: AAHA/AAFP pain management guidelines for dogs and cats, *J Am Anim Hosp Assoc* 43:235, 2007.
10. Henik R, Yeager A: Bronchopulmonary diseases. In Sherding RG, editor: *The cat: diseases and clinical management*, ed 2, Philadelphia, 1994, Saunders, p 979.
11. Kunkle G, Nicklin C, Sullivan-Tamboe D: Comparison of body temperature in cats using a veterinary infrared thermometer and a digital rectal thermometer, *J Am Anim Hosp Assn* 40:42, 2004.
12. Levy J, Crawford C, Hartmann K et al: AAFP feline retrovirus management guidelines, *J Feline Med Surg* 10:300, 2008.
13. Levy J, Ford R: Diseases of the upper respiratory tract. In Sherding RG, editor: *The cat: diseases and clinical management*, ed 2, Philadelphia, 1994, Saunders, p 947.
14. Lord L, Ingwersen W, Gray J et al: Characterization of animals with microchips entering animal shelters, *J Am Vet Med Assoc* 235:160, 2009.
15. Mansell J, Rees C: Cutaneous manifestations of viral disease. In August JR, editor: *Consultations in feline internal medicine*, ed 5, St Louis, 2006, Elsevier, p 11.
16. Nelson CT, Seward RL, McCall JW et al: 2007 guidelines for the diagnosis, treatment and prevention of heartworm *(Dirofilaria immitis)* infection in cats (website): www.heartwormsociety.org/veterinary-resources/feline-guidelines.html. Accessed February 21, 2010.
17. Ogilvie GK, Moore AS: Skin tumors. In Ogilvie GK, Moore AS, editors: *Feline oncology: a comprehensive guide to compassionate care*, Trenton, N.J., 2001, Veterinary Learning Systems, p 412.
18. Ogilvie G, Moore A: Tumors of the alimentary tract. In Ogilvie GK, Moore AS, editors: *Feline oncology: a comprehensive guide to compassionate care*, Trenton, NJ, 2001, Veterinary Learning Systems, p 271.
19. Overall K, Rodan I, Beaver B et al: Feline behavior guidelines of the American Association of Feline Practitioners, *J Am Vet Med Assoc* 227:70, 2005.
20. Paepe D, Smets P, van Hoek I et al: Within- and between-examiner agreement for two thyroid palpation techniques in healthy and hyperthyroid cats, *J Feline Med Surg* 10:558, 2008.
21. Paige CF, Abbott JA, Elvinger F et al: Prevalence of cardiomyopathy in apparently healthy cats, *J Am Vet Med Assoc* 234:1398, 2009.
22. Pittari J, Rodan I: Senior cats: untangling the problems of these special patients, *J Feline Med Surg* 11:737, 2009.
23. Pittari J, Rodan I, Beekman G et al: American Association of Feline Practitioners senior care guidelines, *J Feline Med Surg* 11:763, 2009.
24. Richards J, Elston TH, Ford RB et al: The 2006 American Association of Feline Practitioners Feline Vaccine Advisory Panel report, *J Am Vet Med Assoc* 229:1405, 2006.
25. Rodan I, Folger B: Respectful handling of cats to prevent fear and pain, American Association of Feline Practitioners Position Statement: http://catvets.com/uploads/PDF/Nov2009HandlingCats.pdf. Accessed February 21, 2010.
26. Scarlett J: Controlling feline respiratory disease in animal shelters. In August JR, editor: *Consultations in feline internal medicine*, ed 5, St Louis, 2006, Saunders, p 735.
27. Sherding RG: The medical history, physical examination, and physical restraint. In Sherding RG, editor: *The cat: diseases, and clinical management*, ed 2, Philadelphia, 1994, Saunders, p 7.
28. Suchman AL: A new theoretical foundation for relationship-centered care: complex responsive processes of relating, *J Gen Intern Med* (Suppl 1):S40, 2006.
29. Venker-van Haagen AJ: Diseases and surgery of the ear. In Sherding RG, editor: *The cat: diseases and clinical management*, ed 2, Philadelphia, 1994, Saunders, p 1999.
30. Villalobos A: Hospice "Pawspice." In August JR, editor: *Consultations in feline internal medicine*, ed 6, St Louis, 2010, Saunders, p 811.
31. Vogt AH, Rodan I, Brown M et al: AAFP-AAHA: feline life stage guidelines, *J Feline Med Surg* 12:43, 2010.
32. Wilkie D: Diseases and surgery of the eye. In Sherding RG, editor: *The cat: diseases and clinical management*, ed 2, Philadelphia, 1994, Saunders, p 2011.

CHAPTER

4

Guidelines and Precautions for Drug Therapy in Cats

Lauren A. Trepanier

OUTLINE

Drug therapy in feline patients has many potential roadblocks: differences in drug metabolism between cats and other species, which make dose extrapolations difficult; a paucity of good safety and dose optimization studies in cats; the relative lack of approved drugs with associated efficacy data in cats compared with dogs; the need for reformulation of many drugs designed for larger patients; and the difficulty in administering medications to many cats.

DIFFERENCES IN DRUG METABOLISM IN CATS

Cats have important differences in drug metabolism compared with humans and dogs, two species from which feline dosages are often extrapolated. It is well known that cats are deficient in glucuronidation of some xenobiotics; for example, UDP-glucuronosyltranferase (UGT) activity for acetaminophen is tenfold lower in cats compared with dogs and humans.[20] This is due to a nonfunctional feline pseudogene for UGT1A6,[21] the UGT isoform that metabolizes acetaminophen in humans. This same enzyme glucuronidates morphine and serotonin[48] and contributes to the metabolism of silybin (in milk thistle).[55] Glucuronidation is therefore deficient for many drugs in cats (Table 4-1). However, cats are able to normally glucuronidate endogenous compounds such as thyroxine[41] and bilirubin.[87]

Cats are also deficient in the enzyme thiopurine methyltransferase, which metabolizes thiopurine drugs such as azathioprine. The activity of this enzyme, which can be measured in red blood cells, is 80% to 85% lower in cats than in dogs.[29,79,100] This may explain why cats treated with azathioprine are especially sensitive to myelosuppression,[3] which is a dose-dependent side effect of this drug. Further individual variability in thiopurine methyltransferase among cats (almost tenfold) can be attributed to genetic polymorphisms in the feline gene, such that there is overlap between some "high-activity" cats and some "low-activity" dogs.[45,79] However, a relationship between polymorphisms in thiopurine methyltransferase and azathioprine response has not yet been established in either cats or dogs.

DOSAGE ADJUSTMENTS FOR RENAL INSUFFICIENCY

Renal insufficiency leads to decreased filtration of renally eliminated drugs and their active metabolites, as well as impaired tubular secretion of some drugs, including famotidine, ranitidine, trimethoprim, and digoxin.[86] These drugs are ionized at physiologic pH and in humans

TABLE 4-1 **Xenobiotic Glucuronidation Capacity in the Cat**

Compounds	UGT Enzyme Responsible in Humans	Glucuronidation in Cats	Clinical Consequences and Dosing in Cats
Acetaminophen	UGT1A6 (pseudogene in cats)[21]	Hepatic activities tenfold lower in cats compared with dogs and humans[20]	Acetaminophen toxicity at threefold to fourfold lower doses in cats (≥60 mg/kg) versus dogs (≥200 mg/kg)[81]
Morphine	UGT2B7 and others in humans	No glucuronide metabolites in dogs in vivo[50] Not evaluated in cats	Elimination half-life of morphine in cats (1-1.5 h)[91] is similar to that in dogs (1.2 h)[50]
Chloramphenicol	UGT2B7[15]	Not directly evaluated in cats	Slightly longer elimination half-life in cats (~4-8 h) compared with dogs (1.1-5 h)[71]
Aspirin	Several isoforms (UGT1A6 has high affinity)[49]	Not directly evaluated in cats	Longer elimination half-life in cats (22 h)[69] compared with dogs (5-6 h)[61] Dosed fourfold less frequently in cats versus dogs
Thyroxine	UGT1A1 and others[104]	Thyroxine is glucuronidated in cats[63]	Comparable daily thyroxine dosages in dogs and cats
Carprofen	Glucuronidated in humans[78]	Glucuronidated in dogs[78]	Oral elimination half-life in cats (20 h)[69] prolonged compared with dogs (8 h) (Rimadyl label)
	Isoform not identified	Not directly evaluated in cats	Increased susceptibility to carprofen toxicity in cats (gastrointestinal signs at 8 mg/kg in cats versus 20 mg/kg in dogs)[58]

require active transport in the renal tubules for elimination in the urine. Renal insufficiency is also associated with less obvious effects on drug disposition, such as decreased renal cytochrome P450 and conjugative metabolism of some drugs, impaired binding to albumin of acidic drugs (e.g., furosemide, sulfamethoxazole, and aspirin), and reduced tissue binding of digoxin.[97] All these effects can lead to drug accumulation in renal insufficiency.

Dosage reductions in renal insufficiency are indicated for any drug with a relatively narrow margin of safety that either is primarily eliminated by the kidneys or has an active metabolite that is eliminated by the kidneys (Table 4-2). There is little information in cats to guide dosage adjustments for renal insufficiency. In humans dose adjustments are typically made when glomerular filtration rate (GFR), as measured by creatinine clearance, drops to about 0.7 to 1.2 mL/kg/min, depending on the drug's therapeutic index.[66] Based on the demonstrated relationship between GFR and serum creatinine in cats,[60] this is equivalent to serum creatinine concentrations of approximately 2.5 to 3.5 mg/dL (221 to 309 μmol/L). In the absence of specific data in cats, it is therefore reasonable to consider dosage adjustments for renally cleared drugs when the serum creatinine reaches this range.

For many renally excreted drugs, a crude dose reduction can be made by multiplying the standard dose by a normal serum creatinine concentration (e.g., 1.0 mg/dL) divided by the patient's serum creatinine concentration. This results in less drug given at the same intervals and is based on the finding that serum creatinine is inversely related to GFR in early to moderate renal insufficiency in cats.[60] For example, in a cat with a serum creatinine concentration of 2 mg/dL (twice a typical normal value of 1 mg/dL), cephalothin would be given at 10 mg/kg every 8 hours rather than 20 mg/kg every 8 hours. An alternative approach is to multiply the dosing interval (e.g., every 12 hours) by the patient's serum creatinine concentration, divided by a normal creatinine level. This results in the same individual dose given at less frequent intervals. For example, for the same cat enrofloxacin would be given at a dosage of 5 mg/kg every 48 hours, rather than every 24 hours. Dosage adjustments using this method may be roughly accurate for serum creatinine concentrations up to 4 mg/dL (354 μmol/L), after which the relationship between creatinine concentration and GFR becomes nonlinear in cats.[60] In humans dosages for renally cleared drugs in renal failure are typically 25% to 75% of the standard daily dosage.[66]

Ampicillin and amoxicillin are renally excreted but have wide safety margins, so dose adjustments are probably not clinically necessary. Cephalothin can cause lipid peroxidation and nephrotoxicity in animal models[105] and can be nephrotoxic in combination with aminoglycosides in older human patients.[105] Therefore dosage reductions of this cephalosporin may be indicated in veterinary patients with renal insufficiency.

TABLE 4-2 **Drugs Requiring Precaution or Dosage Adjustment in Renal Insufficiency**

Drug	Adverse Outcome	Recommendations
Cephalothin	Possible dose-dependent nephrotoxin in humans[105]	Avoid or consider adjusting dosage
Aminoglycosides	Dose-dependent nephrotoxin in cats	Avoid in renal insufficiency If unavoidable, extend dosing interval Maintain hydration Monitor urine for granular casts Minimize duration of treatment
Fluoroquinolones	Dose-dependent retinotoxicity in cats	Use fluoroquinolones with wide safety margin for retinotoxicity (e.g., marbofloxacin or orbifloxacin) Extend dosing interval
Trimethoprim–sulfadiazine	Can precipitate as obstructive sulfadiazine crystals and uroliths in humans[14]	Use more soluble sulfamethoxazole Maintain hydration Avoid urinary acidifiers
Furosemide	Causes dehydration and hypokalemia	Avoid in renal insufficiency unless strong rationale (e.g., overt heart failure) Use careful clinical monitoring
H_2 blockers	Confusion or mania in elderly human patients	Extend dosing interval or reduce individual dose
Metoclopramide	Tremors resulting from dopamine antagonism	Empiric dosage reductions (decrease constant-rate infusion daily dose by ~50%)
Enalapril	May cause renal decompensation[98]	Consider using benazepril, which does not accumulate in moderate renal insufficiency in cats[46]
Nonsteroidal antiinflammatory drugs	Gastric ulceration, renal decompensation	Substitute other analgesics whenever possible

For more expensive beta lactam derivatives, such as meropenem, dose adjustments are recommended in humans when creatinine clearance dips below 0.7 mg/mL/kg; initial prolongation of the dosing interval is recommended.[105]

Aminoglycosides are dose-dependent nephrotoxins and should be avoided, whenever possible, in preexisting renal insufficiency. For patients with renal insufficiency that develop resistant gram-negative infections, other antimicrobials (e.g., fluoroquinolones, cefotetan, meropenem, ticarcillin) should be considered whenever possible. When aminoglycosides are necessary, rehydration and concurrent fluid therapy (intravenous or subcutaneous) are recommended because hypovolemia is a risk factor for aminoglycoside nephrotoxicity in humans.[65] In addition, amikacin should be considered (Figure 4-1) because it is less nephrotoxic than gentamicin in human patients[89] and may be less nephrotoxic in cats as well.[17]

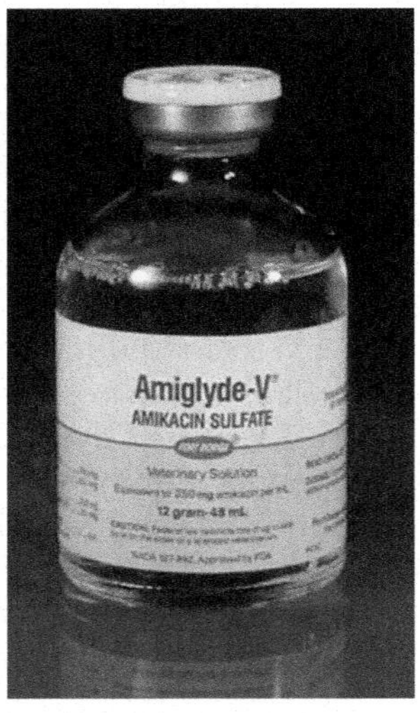

FIGURE 4-1 Aminoglycosides should be avoided whenever possible in cats with renal insufficiency. Administration of subcutaneous or intravenous fluids, avoidance of concurrent nonsteroidal antiinflammatory or furosemide therapy, and monitoring urine sediments daily for granular casts may decrease the risk of dose-dependent nephrotoxicity.

The dosage of aminoglycosides is routinely adjusted for human patients with renal insufficiency. Aminoglycosides are concentration-dependent antimicrobials (i.e., bacterial kill correlates with peak concentrations, not time above the minimum inhibitory concentration), and nephrotoxicity correlates with trough, not peak, drug concentrations.[74] Therefore aminoglycosides should be given at the same dose, but less frequently, in renal insufficiency.[92] For example, for a cat with a serum creatinine concentration of 2 mg/dL, amikacin or gentamicin would be dosed every 48 hours instead of every 24 hours, assuming that no alternative antimicrobials were available.

In humans aminoglycoside drug dosages are adjusted to keep trough plasma drug concentrations below 2 μg/mL.[36] Measurement of trough drug concentrations is ideal in patients with underlying renal insufficiency; however, rapid turnaround of serum drug concentrations is necessary for therapeutic drug monitoring to be useful in real-time clinical decision making. One practical monitoring alternative is to examine daily fresh urine sediments for granular casts, which can be seen days before azotemia develops.[82] Granular casts indicate renal proximal tubular damage and if observed suggest that the drug should be discontinued, unless the infection is life threatening. Toxicity in cats is lessened if aminoglycoside therapy can be limited to 5 days or less, whenever possible.[38] Aminoglycosides are contraindicated in combination with furosemide[1] or a nonsteroidal antiinflammatory drug (NSAID),[65] both of which can exacerbate nephrotoxicity.

Fluoroquinolones, like aminoglycosides, are renally cleared. Although they do not cause cartilage toxicity in growing kittens at the label dosage, they do cause dose-dependent retinal toxicity in cats.[101] Therefore dosage adjustments for fluoroquinolones may be important in cats with renal insufficiency, although this has not been directly evaluated. Dosage adjustments may be particularly important for enrofloxacin, which appears to be more retinotoxic in cats (retinal lesions at four times the label dosage) compared with other veterinary fluoroquinolones (orbifloxacin, retinal lesions at 18 times the label dose; marbofloxacin, no retinal lesions at 20 times the label dose).[101] Although the optimal method for dose adjustment is not established in cats, extending the dosing interval may be most appropriate,[23] insofar as fluoroquinolones are also concentration-dependent antimicrobials.

Potentiated sulfonamides should also be used with caution in azotemic patients, owing to decreased renal clearance and decreased protein binding. Dosage reductions for the human generic drug, trimethoprim–sulfamethoxazole, are recommended in human patients.[96] Dose reductions may be even more important for trimethoprim–sulfadiazine (found in Tribrissen) because sulfadiazine is reported to cause hematuria, urolithiasis, and even acute renal failure in humans.[14] This is due to the relative insolubility of sulfadiazine, which can precipitate as drug crystals in the renal tubules, especially at high concentrations or in acid urine.[66] Although comparable studies in feline patients are not available, this author recommends rehydration and discontinuation of urinary acidifiers before the use of trimethoprim–sulfadiazine in cats.

Furosemide is renally cleared and can cause significant dehydration and hypokalemia, which can lead to further renal decompensation. Furosemide should not be used in cats with underlying renal insufficiency unless there is a good rationale (e.g., fulminant congestive heart failure). Cats treated with furosemide should be monitored closely for dehydration, hypokalemia, and worsened azotemia, with routine evaluation of skin turgor, body weight, body condition score, packed cell volume and total protein values, serum potassium levels, and renal indices at each recheck.

Histamine 2 (H_2)–blocker antacids such as cimetidine, ranitidine, and famotidine are cleared by the kidneys, and dosage reductions are recommended for human patients with renal insufficiency.[62] H_2 blockers can also lead to central nervous system disturbances (mania, confusion), particularly in elderly patients, although it is not clear whether decreased GFR is a factor.[11] Therefore the dosage of H_2 blockers may merit reductions in cats with renal insufficiency, especially geriatric cats. Either reductions in the individual dose or extensions of the dosing interval are used in humans. Metoclopramide is also renally cleared. As a dopaminergic antagonist, metoclopramide can lead to tremors in some human patients.[85] Standard constant-rate infusion (CRI) dosages (1 to 2 mg/kg per day) can cause tremor and ataxia in azotemic patients (observed in dogs), and lower doses (e.g., 0.25 to 0.5 mg/kg/day as a CRI) appear anecdotally to be better tolerated.

Angiotensin-converting enzyme (ACE) inhibitors are recommended to reduce proteinuria in cats with renal insufficiency (International Renal Interest Society Guidelines; http://www.iris-kidney.com, accessed February 25, 2010). Benazepril does not depend solely on renal elimination and does not require dose adjustment in moderately azotemic cats.[46] Benazepril therefore may be preferable to enalapril in cats with substantial azotemia. Although ACE inhibitors typically do not cause systemic hypotension at therapeutic dosages in cats, they can adversely affect GFR at high dosages, particularly in a dehydrated patient or with concurrent furosemide administration. It is therefore important to monitor blood urea nitrogen, creatinine, and electrolytes in cats treated with ACE inhibitors: for example, initially after 1 week, after 1 month, and then every 3 months, depending on clinical status.

The use of NSAIDs can adversely affect GFR in patients with hypovolemia or underlying renal disease by blocking the elaboration of renal prostaglandins that otherwise autoregulate renal blood flow.[44] Although meloxicam was generally well tolerated for chronic use in cats with osteoarthritis in one study (at 0.01 to 0.03 mg/kg daily), relatively few cats with chronic renal disease (3 of 46 treated cats) were enrolled.[35] In addition, meloxicam has been implicated in episodes of acute renal failure in cats (Metacam label). Coxibs (cyclooxygenase-2 [COX-2]– selective NSAIDs) have the same potential for adverse renal events as do other NSAIDs.[70] This is because COX-2 is expressed in the kidney and is important for regulating renal blood flow.[39] For analgesia in renal insufficiency, buprenorphine provides an alternative to NSAIDs, with comparable analgesic efficacy in cats.[88] If an antiinflammatory effect is needed, NSAIDs should be dosed conservatively and cats should be monitored frequently for dehydration, inappetence, evidence of gastrointestinal ulceration, or increases in blood urea nitrogen and creatinine levels.

DRUG THERAPY CONSIDERATIONS IN HEPATIC INSUFFICIENCY

In humans with inflammatory liver disease without failure, hepatic drug metabolism appears to be fairly well conserved. With hepatic dysfunction or cirrhosis, however, drugs that are normally extensively metabolized by the liver are not efficiently cleared. This leads to decreased first-pass clearance and increased oral bioavailability of certain drugs, such as propranolol and benzodiazepines. For these drugs 50% dosage reductions are recommended for human patients with impaired liver function.[26] Other drugs that require dosage reductions (to 25% to 50% of regular dosages) in humans with cirrhosis are listed in Box 4-1. Although cirrhosis is uncommon in cats, significant hepatic dysfunction is common with fulminant hepatic lipidosis or portosystemic shunts. In these patients dosage reductions for the drugs listed in Box 4-1 may be indicated, although we do not have comparable studies in cats.

Some therapies can worsen hepatic encephalopathy and are not recommended for cats at risk. Stored whole blood generates ammonia, which increases with time of storage (Figure 4-2).[51] Although time-course studies of ammonia generation have not been performed for feline whole blood or packed red blood cell units, stored blood should be used with caution in cats with liver failure, such as those with lipidosis or acute hepatotoxicity. Screening blood units for high blood ammonia before transfusion, using an in-house analyzer, is one option, as is using an in-house blood donor to obtain fresh whole blood.

NSAIDs have the potential to exacerbate hepatic encephalopathy, either by causing gastrointestinal bleeding (which is a protein load in the gut) or renal decompensation (which increases blood urea nitrogen that subsequently recycles to ammonia).[28] Furosemide can cause hypokalemia, dehydration, azotemia, and alkalosis, all of which can worsen hepatic encephalopathy.[28] Finally, glucocorticoids, which lead to muscle catabolism,[28] can enhance deamination of proteins and release of ammonia (NH_3). Glucocorticoids also enhance peripheral lipolysis, which could exacerbate hepatic lipidosis, although this has never been directly evaluated in cats. The safest course is to stabilize clinical signs, control hepatic encephalopathy, and provide nutritional support before considering glucocorticoids in cats with any type of liver disease.

BOX 4-1

Drugs that Require Dosage Reductions in Humans with Severe Impairment in Hepatic Function[37]

Buspirone	Loratidine
Butorphanol	Metronidazole
Cisapride	Midazolam
Cyclophosphamide	Mirtazapine
Diazepam	Omeprazole
Doxorubicin	Prednisone
Fluconazole	Propranolol
Fluoxetine	Theophylline
Itraconazole	Vincristine
Lidocaine	

THERAPEUTIC CONSIDERATIONS IN NEONATES AND KITTENS

The neonatal period in dogs and cats has been defined as the first 4 weeks of life, with the pediatric period defined as up to 12 weeks of age.[34] Although drug therapy of neonates is common in human medicine, very few pharmacokinetic studies have been performed in newborns and infants. Given that neonatal pharmacology is even less well studied in cats, specific and valid recommendations are difficult to make. However, there

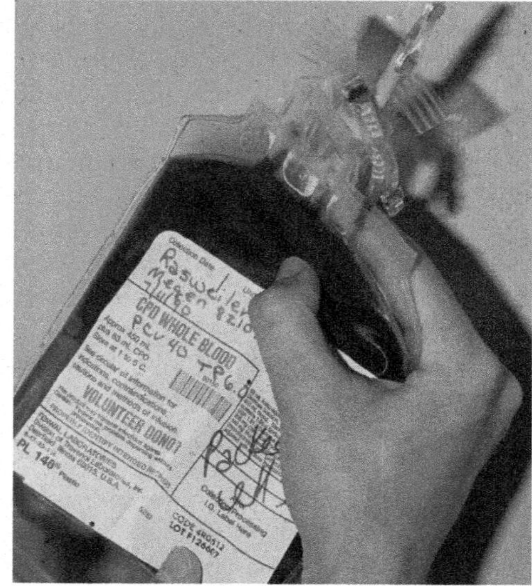

FIGURE 4-2 Whole blood and packed red blood cells can generate ammonia during storage. Transfusion of older units could exacerbate hepatic encephalopathy in cats with hepatic lipidosis or acute hepatotoxicities.

are certain physiologic differences between neonates and adults (based on studies in humans, dogs, rodents, and occasionally in cats) that can help guide rational drug therapy in these tiny and rapidly changing patients.

Oral absorption may be different in newborn kittens compared with adult cats. Immaturity of gastric parietal cells leads to a relatively high gastric pH in neonates; for example, gastric pH is greater than 3.0 through 5 weeks of age in puppies.[54] High gastric pH may decrease the bioavailability of drugs that require an acid environment for absorption, such as ketoconazole, itraconazole, and iron supplements.[54] Fluconazole may be better absorbed in these neonates because its absorption is not affected by gastric pH, at least in humans.[106] Oral absorption of some drugs may be affected by nursing because of the binding of drugs by milk components such as calcium. For example, the bioavailability of enrofloxacin, which is chelated by calcium, is low in nursing kittens, with overall bioavailability less than 35%.[84] The subcutaneous route provides more reliable absorption in nursing kittens, with bioavailability closer to 85% for enrofloxacin.[84]

Hepatic cytochrome P450 activities are low in newborns but approach and even exceed adult levels by 7 weeks of age, as shown in puppies[90]; this is likely an evolutionary response to a wider variety of dietary chemicals encountered at weaning. Immature cytochrome P450 content is associated with delayed hepatic clearance of some drugs in neonates. For example, lidocaine and theophylline have prolonged elimination half-lives in very young puppies (less than 1 to 2 weeks old).[2,40] However, by the time most feline patients are brought to the veterinarian for their first vaccination, hepatic function has greatly matured.

Newborn kittens have decreased GFR rates before 9 weeks of age, when GFR reaches rates found in adult cats.[43] Before this age, kittens may be at greater risk for fluid overload because of impaired solute and water excretion and for toxicity resulting from renally eliminated drugs such as aminoglycosides. Classic early warning signs of nephrotoxicity, such as granular casts, are not consistently observed in neonatal pups given gentamicin, despite the development of renal tubular lesions and impairment of GFR.[22] Aminoglycosides therefore should be avoided whenever possible in very young patients. In contrast, enrofloxacin, despite its renal excretion, is cleared efficiently in kittens as young as 2 weeks of age[84] and does not appear to require dosage reductions in this age group.

THERAPEUTIC CONSIDERATIONS IN SENIOR AND GERIATRIC CATS

Adverse drug reactions are reported to be two to three times higher in elderly human patients than in younger adults.[94] Some of this risk can be attributed to patient confusion and errors in self-dosing; however, pharmacokinetic and pharmacodynamic factors are also involved. Geriatric veterinary patients have been defined as those that have reached 75% of their expected life span (Figure 4-3).[12] In both geriatric cats and humans, changes in renal function, hepatic blood flow, body composition, and compensatory physiologic responses alter drug response.

Age-related renal insufficiency is the most important factor affecting drug dosing in geriatric human patients.[94] Even patients without overt azotemia are likely to have decreased GFR associated with aging. The prevalence of renal insufficiency in older cats has not been established but appears to be relatively high, at least according to anecdotal reports. This may lead to decreased elimination and increased toxicity of renally cleared drugs (see Table 4-2) in older cats. Enrofloxacin has been associated with retinal toxicity in elderly cats at the label dose of 5 mg/kg per day.[32] Because this ocular toxicity is dose-dependent,[101] cases seen in older cats are likely due to decreased renal clearance of the drug. Although orbifloxacin and marbofloxacin are also cleared by the kidneys, they are less retinotoxic at higher dosages in young healthy cats[101] and may be safer for geriatric cats. Older patients also tend to have decreased total body and interstitial water,[94] which may contribute to increased susceptibility to dehydration when elderly patients are given diuretics such as furosemide.

Aging is associated with decreased liver mass, with variable reductions in cytochrome P450 function in elderly human patients.[27] Decreased liver blood flow also occurs with aging and can lead to decreased clearance of certain drugs.[83] For example, propofol is a "blood flow–limited" drug, and its clearance is diminished in

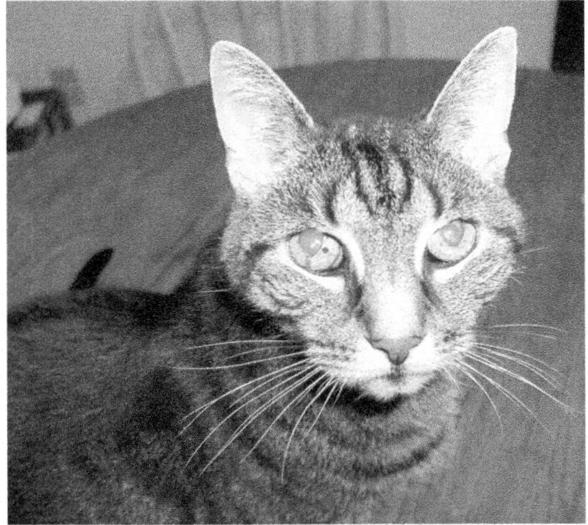

FIGURE 4-3 Geriatric cats have been defined as those that have reached 75% of their expected life span. This 17-year-old cat almost certainly has some degree of renal insufficiency, which may require dosing adjustments for some drugs.

older humans[95] and geriatric dogs, with higher plasma drug concentrations and apnea seen in some older dogs given standard dosages.[75] Other drugs that show impaired clearance in elderly human patients, owing to renal or liver impairment or other factors, are listed in Box 4-2. Although comparable feline studies are not available, these drugs probably should be dosed conservatively in older cats, and the owner should be taught to carefully monitor their pet for adverse effects.

Middle-aged to older cats may be overweight, which can affect drug distribution. For relatively polar drugs with poor fat distribution, such as digoxin, dosing should be based on lean body weight (ideal body weight).[16] For cats ideal body weight can be estimated from the patient's body conformation or from previous medical records when the patient had a normal body condition score. For the polar drug gentamicin, dose reductions of 15% to 20% are indicated in obese cats, based on differences in pharmacokinetics between obese and lean cats.[103] For lipid-soluble drugs, such as propofol and benzodiazepines, single or loading dosages are based on total body weight (lean body weight plus fat) in humans.[13]

DRUG COMPOUNDING FOR CATS

Custom veterinary pharmacies abound in the United States and provide reformulation options such as flavored liquid suspensions, capsules, chew tabs, and compressed minitablets. Pharmacists in the United States are legally allowed to compound veterinary or human drugs for individual veterinary patients if no appropriate approved veterinary formulation exists.[67] Pharmacists are not legally allowed to mass-produce compounded drugs, and as for all prescriptions, there must be a valid doctor–client–patient relationship.

Practitioners often assume that because a custom formulation is available, it must be safe and effective; this is not always true. Unfortunately, the stability and bioavailability of veterinary custom-compounded drugs are usually not tested. In addition, owners may perform their own reformulations at home to ease administration, such as crushing pills in food or water or combining medications in a capsule. Veterinarians usually have inadequate information to advise owners about these manipulations. However, some basic principles can help determine the advisability of a given reformulation.

Crushing medications is not always benign. Sustained-release tablets, such as theophylline (Theo-Dur), diltiazem (Cardizem CD), enteric-coated fluoxetine (Prozac Weekly), and tramadol (Ultram ER), should never be crushed. Crushing of extended-release formulations can lead to rapid, high peak plasma concentrations and potential side effects. In addition, tablets that are enteric coated should not be crushed because this may lead to a bitter taste and degradation in the stomach. Examples include budesonide (Entocort), erythromycin, omeprazole capsules, and potassium citrate tablets. Antineoplastic drugs, such as cyclophosphamide and chlorambucil, should never be crushed by clients or by clinic staff because this results in aerosols and dust that can lead to systemic exposure.[31] These drugs should be reformulated only by a licensed pharmacist, with an appropriate ventilated cabinet.

Mixing drugs with water can also cause problems. Drugs in a blister pack, which are often moisture sensitive, should not be mixed with water,[67] nor should lipophilic drugs, such as itraconazole and diazepam. The veterinarian should check the product insert to see whether a drug is highly lipophilic. Irritating drugs, such as doxycycline or clindamycin, should not be given as capsules to cats because capsules tend to lodge in the midcervical esophagus in cats.[33] This can lead to esophagitis and even esophageal stricture from doxycycline or clindamycin in cats (Figure 4-4).[4,6] Capsules can be chased with an ounce of food or a 6-mL bolus of water after each dose to ensure passage into the stomach.[33,99] However, this may be impractical in inappetent or fractious cats. In these cases oral suspensions of doxycycline or clindamycin may be safer.

Drugs that contain aluminum or other cationic minerals should not be crushed and combined with other drugs. For example, the aluminum in sucralfate or aluminum hydroxide forms complexes with many other drugs in the gastrointestinal tract and can markedly impair the absorption of fluoroquinolones, doxycycline, theophylline, digoxin, and amitriptyline.[56] In addition, aluminum can decrease peak plasma concentrations of azithromycin in humans.[30] Other cationic minerals, such as calcium, iron, zinc, and magnesium, found in multivitamins, may also chelate fluoroquinolones and impair their absorption.[52] Similarly, the

BOX 4-2

Drugs that Show Decreased Clearance (by 20% or More) in Elderly Human Patients[95]

Amikacin	Lidocaine
Amlodipine	Methylprednisolone
Atenolol	Metoclopramide
Ciprofloxacin	Midazolam
Diazepam	Omeprazole
Digoxin	Ondansetron
Diphenhydramine	Piroxicam
Famotidine	Propofol
Furosemide	Terbutaline
Gentamicin	Theophylline

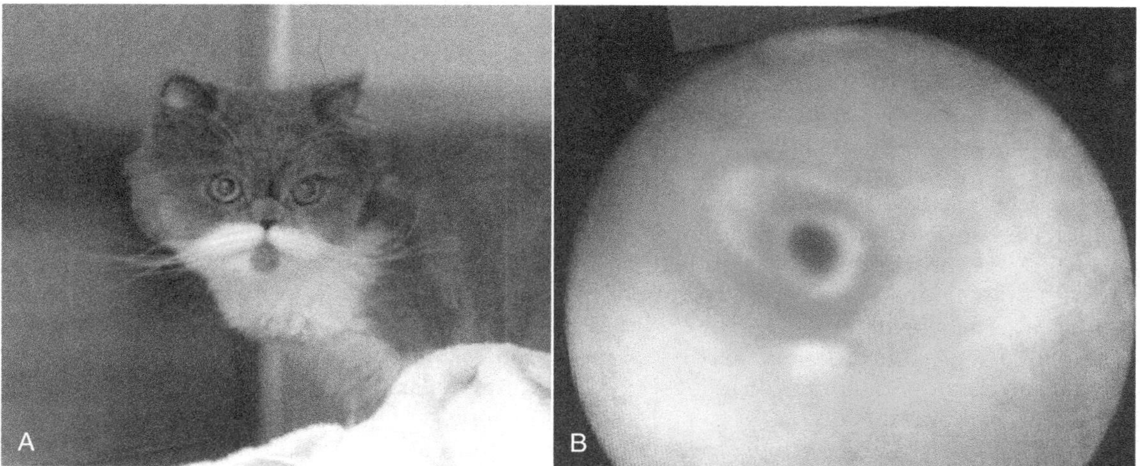

FIGURE 4-4 This male neutered Persian **(A)** developed an esophageal stricture **(B)** after administration of clindamycin capsules. *(From Trepanier L: Acute vomiting in cats, rational treatment selection,* J Feline Med Surg *12(3):225-230, 2010.)*

calcium in dairy products can decrease the absorption of doxycycline.[59]

Drugs that *can* be readily reformulated into capsules include cyclosporine emulsion, potassium chloride beads, omeprazole enteric-coated beads, and itraconazole beads; the number of beads in one original capsule can be counted and divided as needed for the desired dose. For cats with hypertension, amlodipine and benazepril can be reformulated in a single capsule without affecting bioavailability.[9] Fluoroquinolones are reportedly quite stable in most vehicles and flavorings, such as molasses, fish sauce, or corn syrup.[67] It is important, however, to make sure that the vehicle does not contain cationic minerals (e.g., iron, calcium) that will impair fluoroquinolone absorption. Other reformulated suspensions with demonstrated stability are summarized in Table 4-3.

TABLE 4-3 **Pediatric Suspensions with Demonstrated Stability[64]**

Drug	Formulation	Stability
Aminophylline	5 mg/mL in bacteriostatic water	1 week refrigerated
Chlorambucil	2 mg/mL in methylcellulose and syrup	1 week refrigerated; protect from light
Cyclophosphamide	2 mg/mL in aromatic elixir (from injectable)	2 weeks refrigerated
Hydralazine	2 mg/mL in bacteriostatic water	24 hours at room temperature
Metronidazole	20 mg/mL in purified water USP and syrup	10 days refrigerated
Phenobarbital	10 mg/mL in bacteriostatic water (from injection)	3 months refrigerated
Sucralfate	200 mg/mL in purified water USP	2 weeks refrigerated Shake well

ALTERNATIVE FORMULATIONS/ ROUTES FOR MEDICATING CATS

Transdermal drug formulations are a common compounding product in the United States. Transdermal administration, in which the goal is therapeutic drug concentrations in the systemic circulation, is distinct from topical administration, in which the goal is local therapeutic drug concentrations in surface organs (skin, eye, ear canal). Effective transdermal drug delivery is much harder to achieve.

Transdermal drugs are attractive because of their many potential advantages, which include better acceptance compared with pilling or injections, decreased gastrointestinal irritation, avoidance of first-pass intestinal and hepatic degradation, possible longer duration of action without peak side effects, and the ability to custom formulate the drug concentration to the patient's size. However, there are significant disadvantages and limitations to transdermal drug formulations as available through custom compounders. The transdermal route is inappropriate for drugs acting locally in the gastrointestinal tract and may be ineffective for prodrugs dependent on hepatic biotransformation for efficacy. There is a lack of immediate effect for most drugs needed in an emergency setting (nitroglycerin is an exception), and some cats resent the sensation of a transdermal gel. Compounding of transdermal drugs can add significantly to the prescription cost. Most important, many drugs are poorly absorbed transdermally and never reach therapeutic plasma concentrations.

Transdermal drugs that are effectively absorbed in humans tend to have relatively high lipid solubility (so that they can traverse the waxy stratum corneum) and a low melting point (i.e., they are readily converted from a solid to a liquid at body temperatures). Very polar compounds, such as aminoglycosides and many peptides, are poorly absorbed without additional interventions, such as an electric field, microneedles, or ultrasonic disruption of the stratum corneum.[73] Approved transdermal drugs for humans are typically small compounds (i.e., molecular weight less than 500 g/mol or 500 Da [daltons]).[7,8] Small drugs advertised for transdermal formulations in cats include methimazole (114 g/mol), nitroglycerin (227 g/mol), fentanyl (336 g/mol), and amitriptyline (277 g/mol). Larger drugs that are less likely to be absorbed but are still offered by veterinary compounding pharmacies include itraconazole (705 g/mol), ketoconazole (531 g/mol), and amikacin (585 g/mol). Amikacin has the additional disadvantage of being poorly lipid soluble.

Transdermal drugs that are approved for human patients tend to be those that are effective at very low dosages. For example, for fentanyl, lidocaine, nicotine, nitroglycerin, scopolamine, oxybutynin, and contraceptive hormones, total daily dosages range from 0.1 to 32 mg per day.[73] Transdermal dosing is constrained by the physical limitations of permeation enhancers, as well as by practical limitations in the amount of skin coverage that patients will accept. Transdermal formulations of veterinary drugs that require higher total daily dosages (i.e., more than 50 mg per patient per day) are unlikely to be adequately absorbed, especially through the relatively small surface area of a cat's pinna.

Veterinary transdermal drugs are typically formulated in a permeation enhancer such as pluronic lecithin organogel (PLO), which increases the fluidity of the stratum corneum and enhances the formation of drug micelles. PLO also leads to exfoliation of the stratum corneum and low-grade inflammation with chronic use, which likely contributes to drug penetration. PLO separates at cold temperatures and should be discarded if this occurs. Another available permeation enhancer is Lipoderm, a commercial product with proprietary ingredients. Lipoderm is comparable to PLO but is less greasy and does not separate at cold temperatures. A second proprietary permeation enhancer, VanPen, is used for more lipophilic drugs. There are essentially no data to compare the efficacy of PLO, Lipoderm, and VanPen in the delivery of veterinary drugs. Dimethyl sulfoxide (DMSO), although an excellent permeation enhancer, is not recommended because it can be quite irritating.

Several drugs have shown low bioavailability (less than 10% compared with oral) when given transdermally to cats as single doses: fluoxetine, diltiazem, dexamethasone, buspirone, and amitriptyline.[18,25,57,102] Glipizide in PLO has about 20% bioavailability (relative to oral administration) after a single dose in cats. Despite relatively low absorption, transdermal glipizide was associated with a delayed decrease in blood glucose in some cats,[5] and multiple-dose studies in diabetic cats are warranted. Multiple doses of transdermal methimazole in PLO were effective at lowering serum T_4 in hyperthyroid cats and had fewer gastrointestinal side effects than oral methimazole.[80] However, the risk of idiosyncratic drug toxicity (facial pruritus, hepatotoxicity, blood dyscrasias) appeared to be the same for both routes. Similar responses have been observed for transdermal carbimazole (a prodrug of methimazole) in Europe.[10] Modest efficacy has been reported for transdermal atenolol (6.25 mg once daily, in propylene glycol–glycerin–Tween) in reducing heart rate in cats[53] and for transdermal amlodipine (0.625 mg daily in Lipoderm) in reducing blood pressure in hypertensive cats (although the transdermal route was inferior to oral amlodipine).[42] The transdermal route is *not appropriate* for empiric dosing of antimicrobials because of the considerable risk of poor absorption, subtherapeutic plasma concentrations, and potential selection for resistant bacterial strains.

In contrast to transdermal administration, transmucosal drug delivery is typically associated with rapid absorption and relatively high bioavailability. This is because the mucous membranes are highly vascular and lack the stratum corneum. Drugs can be administered transmucosally by several routes (Table 4-4). Like transdermal administration, transmucosal administration bypasses first-pass intestinal and hepatic metabolism and may prevent gastrointestinal upset resulting from direct gastric irritation. However, this route cannot be used for irritating medications.

Buprenorphine is often given by the transmucosal (buccal) route in cats. It is well accepted at 0.01 mg/kg of injectable solution in the buccal pouch and is absorbed as well as that administered by the intravenous route, with equivalent analgesia.[76] It is hypothesized that the higher bioavailability in cats (compared to humans) is due to the relatively high pH in the feline mouth (pH 8 to 9), in which buprenorphine is mostly uncharged, which favors absorption across the mucosa.[77]

Fluticasone, a trifluorinated glucocorticoid with potent antiinflammatory activity, can also be administered by the transmucosal (pulmonary aerosol) route in cats, using a metered-dose inhaler with a spacer. The goal is high topical potency in the lungs with few systemic side effects. Inhaled fluticasone has been associated with decreased lower airway inflammation in cats with bronchitis,[47] and dosages up to 220 μg every 12 hours have not been associated with adrenal suppression in cats.[19] Although local irritation can lead to acute bronchospasm, inhaled fluticasone is anecdotally well tolerated by many cats with reactive airway disease.

TABLE 4-4 **Drugs that Are Effective When Given by the Transmucosal Route**

Drug	Route of Administration	Indication
Apomorphine	Conjunctival sac	Emesis (dogs only; emetic dosages in cats cause unacceptable central nervous system side effects)[93]
Buprenorphine	Buccal cavity[77]	Analgesia[76]
Desmopressin (DDAVP)	Nasal mucosa Conjunctival sac	Diabetes insipidus (rare in cats)
Diazepam	Intrarectal[68] Nasal mucosa	Cluster seizures (efficacy demonstrated in dogs)[72]
Epinephrine	Pulmonary Through endotracheal tube	Cardiopulmonary resuscitation
Fluticasone	Pulmonary Via metered-dose inhaler	Reactive airway disease/feline asthma[47]

Finally, human recombinant regular insulin was recently marketed for transmucosal (pulmonary aerosol) administration in human diabetic patients (Exubera, Pfizer). This formulation was shown to lower blood glucose in healthy cats at high dosages (25 U/kg), with hypoglycemia even seen in some cats.[24] Although this drug had a short duration of action and was recently discontinued because of poor market performance, it demonstrates proof of the principle that peptide drugs can be administered without injection to cats, which is an exciting development.

CONCLUSION

The differences between cats and humans require the feline practitioner to be quite savvy when it comes to feline therapeutics. Dosage extrapolations to cats should always be made with attention to whether the drug is cleared by glucuronidation in humans and dogs. Drugs with narrow safety margins should be dosed with attention to the primary route of clearance in adult cats (or in other species if data in cats are lacking), young kittens, geriatric cats, or cats with renal or hepatic insufficiency. Drug compounding, although very appealing, should be undertaken with a critical eye toward factors such as original formulation (enteric coated or extended release), water solubility of the drug, and drug–drug and drug–mineral interactions. Transdermal drug administration should be reserved for drugs with good evidence of absorption or efficacy (or both) in cats.

References

1. Adelman RD, Spangler WL, Beasom F et al: Furosemide enhancement of experimental gentamicin nephrotoxicity: comparison of functional and morphological changes with activities of urinary enzymes, *J Infect Dis* 140:342, 1979.
2. Alberola J, Perez Y, Puigdemont A et al: Effect of age on theophylline pharmacokinetics in dogs, *Am J Vet Res* 54:1112, 1993.
3. Beale KM, Altman D, Clemmons RR et al: Systemic toxicosis associated with azathioprine administration in domestic cats, *Am J Vet Res* 53:1236, 1992.
4. Beatty JA, Swift N, Foster DJ et al: Suspected clindamycin-associated oesophageal injury in cats: five cases, *J Feline Med Surg* 8:412, 2006.
5. Bennett N, Papich MG, Hoenig M et al: Evaluation of transdermal application of glipizide in a pluronic lecithin gel to healthy cats, *Am J Vet Res* 66:581, 2005.
6. Bissett SA, Davis J, Subler K et al: Risk factors and outcome of bougienage for treatment of benign esophageal strictures in dogs and cats: 28 cases (1995-2004), *J Am Vet Med Assoc* 235:844, 2009.
7. Bos JD, Meinardi MM: The 500 Dalton rule for the skin penetration of chemical compounds and drugs, *Exp Dermatol* 9:165, 2000.
8. Brown MB, Martin GP, Jones SA et al: Dermal and transdermal drug delivery systems: current and future prospects, *Drug Deliv* 13:175, 2006.
9. Budde J, Head Pharmacist UoW-M, Veterinary Medical Teaching Hospital: Personal Communication, 2009.
10. Buijtels JJ, Kurvers IA, Galac S et al: [Transdermal carbimazole for the treatment of feline hyperthyroidism], *Tijdschr Diergeneeskd* 131:478, 2006.
11. Cantu TG, Korek JS: Central nervous system reactions to histamine-2 receptor blockers, *Ann Intern Med* 114:1027, 1991.
12. Carpenter RE, Pettifer GR, Tranquilli WJ: Anesthesia for geriatric patients, *Vet Clin North Am Small Anim Pract* 35:571, 2005.
13. Casati A, Putzu M: Anesthesia in the obese patient: pharmacokinetic considerations, *J Clin Anesth* 17:134, 2005.
14. Catalano-Pons C, Bargy S, Schlecht D et al: Sulfadiazine-induced nephrolithiasis in children, *Pediatr Nephrol* 19:928, 2004.
15. Chen M, Leduc B, Kerr SG et al: Identification of human UGT2B7 as the major isoform involved in the O-glucuronidation of chloramphenicol, *Drug Metab Dispos* 38:368, 2010.
16. Cheymol G: Drug pharmacokinetics in the obese, *Fundam Clin Pharmacol* 2:239, 1988.
17. Christensen EF, Reiffenstein JC, Madissoo H: Comparative ototoxicity of amikacin and gentamicin in cats, *Antimicrob Agents Chemother* 12:178, 1977.
18. Ciribassi J, Luescher A, Pasloske KS et al: Comparative bioavailability of fluoxetine after transdermal and oral administration to healthy cats, *Am J Vet Res* 64:994, 2003.

19. Cohn LA, Declue AE, Cohen RL et al: Effects of fluticasone propionate dosage in an experimental model of feline asthma, *J Feline Med Surg* 12:91, 2010.
20. Court MH, Greenblatt DJ: Molecular basis for deficient acetaminophen glucuronidation in cats. An interspecies comparison of enzyme kinetics in liver microsomes, *Biochem Pharmacol* 53:1041, 1997.
21. Court MH, Greenblatt DJ: Molecular genetic basis for deficient acetaminophen glucuronidation by cats: UGT1A6 is a pseudogene, and evidence for reduced diversity of expressed hepatic UGT1A isoforms, *Pharmacogenetics* 10:355, 2000.
22. Cowan RH, Jukkola AF, Arant BS Jr: Pathophysiologic evidence of gentamicin nephrotoxicity in neonatal puppies, *Pediatr Res* 14:1204, 1980.
23. Czock D, Rasche FM: Dose adjustment of ciprofloxacin in renal failure: reduce the dose or prolong the administration interval? *Eur J Med Res* 10:145, 2005.
24. DeClue AE, Leverenz EF, Wiedmeyer CE et al: Glucose lowering effects of inhaled insulin in healthy cats, *J Feline Med Surg* 10:519, 2008.
25. DeFrancesco T: Transdermal cardiac therapy in cats: the NCSU experience. Annual Forum of the American College of Veterinary Internal Medicine, 2003.
26. Delco F, Tchambaz L, Schlienger R et al: Dose adjustment in patients with liver disease, *Drug Saf* 28:529, 2005.
27. El Desoky ES: Pharmacokinetic-pharmacodynamic crisis in the elderly, *Am J Ther* 14:488, 2007.
28. Faint V: The pathophysiology of hepatic encephalopathy, *Nurs Crit Care* 11:69, 2006.
29. Foster AP, Shaw SE, Duley JA et al: Demonstration of thiopurine methyltransferase activity in the erythrocytes of cats, *J Vet Intern Med* 14:552, 2000.
30. Foulds G, Hilligoss DM, Henry EB et al: The effects of an antacid or cimetidine on the serum concentrations of azithromycin, *J Clin Pharmacol* 31:164, 1991.
31. Gambrell J, Moore S: Assessing workplace compliance with handling of antineoplastic agents, *Clin J Oncol Nurs* 10:473, 2006.
32. Gelatt KN, van der Woerdt A, Ketring KL et al: Enrofloxacin-associated retinal degeneration in cats, *Vet Ophthalmol* 4:99, 2001.
33. Graham JP, Lipman AH, Newell SM et al: Esophageal transit of capsules in clinically normal cats, *Am J Vet Res* 61:655, 2000.
34. Grundy SA: Clinically relevant physiology of the neonate, *Vet Clin North Am Small Anim Pract* 36:443, 2006.
35. Gunew MN, Menrath VH, Marshall RD: Long-term safety, efficacy and palatability of oral meloxicam at 0.01-0.03 mg/kg for treatment of osteoarthritic pain in cats, *J Feline Med Surg* 10:235, 2008.
36. Hagen I, Oymar K: Pharmacological differences between once daily and twice daily gentamicin dosage in newborns with suspected sepsis, *Pharm World Sci* 31:18, 2009.
37. Hardman J, Limbard L: *Goodman and Gilman's the pharmacologic basis of therapeutics*, ed 10, New York, 2001, McGraw-Hill.
38. Hardy ML, Hsu RC, Short CR: The nephrotoxic potential of gentamicin in the cat: enzymuria and alterations in urine concentrating capability, *J Vet Pharmacol Ther* 8:382, 1985.
39. Harris RC: COX-2 and the kidney, *J Cardiovasc Pharmacol* 47(Suppl 1):S37, 2006.
40. Hastings CL, Brown TC, Eyres RL et al: The influence of age on lignocaine pharmacokinetics in young puppies, *Anaesth Intensive Care* 14:135, 1986.
41. Hays MT, Broome MR, Turrel JM: A multicompartmental model for iodide, thyroxine, and triiodothyronine metabolism in normal and spontaneously hyperthyroid cats, *Endocrinology* 122:2444, 1988.
42. Helms SR: Treatment of feline hypertension with transdermal amlodipine: a pilot study, *J Am Anim Hosp Assoc* 43:149, 2007.
43. Hoskins JD, Turnwald GH, Kearney MT et al: Quantitative urinalysis in kittens from four to thirty weeks after birth, *Am J Vet Res* 52:1295, 1991.
44. House AA, Silva Oliveira S, Ronco C: Anti-inflammatory drugs and the kidney, *Int J Artif Organs* 30:1042, 2007.
45. Kidd LB, Salavaggione OE, Szumlanski CL et al: Thiopurine methyltransferase activity in red blood cells of dogs, *J Vet Intern Med* 18:214, 2004.
46. King JN, Strehlau G, Wernsing J et al: Effect of renal insufficiency on the pharmacokinetics and pharmacodynamics of benazepril in cats, *J Vet Pharmacol Ther* 25:371, 2002.
47. Kirschvink N, Leemans J, Delvaux F et al: Inhaled fluticasone reduces bronchial responsiveness and airway inflammation in cats with mild chronic bronchitis, *J Feline Med Surg* 8:45, 2006.
48. Krishnaswamy S, Hao Q, Von Moltke LL et al: Evaluation of 5-hydroxytryptophol and other endogenous serotonin (5-hydroxytryptamine) analogs as substrates for UDP-glucuronosyltransferase 1A6, *Drug Metab Dispos* 32:862, 2004.
49. Kuehl GE, Bigler J, Potter JD et al: Glucuronidation of the aspirin metabolite salicylic acid by expressed UDP-glucuronosyltransferases and human liver microsomes, *Drug Metab Dispos* 34:199, 2006.
50. KuKanich B, Lascelles BD, Papich MG: Pharmacokinetics of morphine and plasma concentrations of morphine-6-glucuronide following morphine administration to dogs, *J Vet Pharmacol Ther* 28:371, 2005.
51. Latham JT, Jr, Bove JR, Weirich FL: Chemical and hematologic changes in stored CPDA-1 blood, *Transfusion* 22:158, 1982.
52. Lomaestro BM, Bailie GR: Absorption interactions with fluoroquinolones. 1995 update, *Drug Saf* 12:314, 1995.
53. Macgregor JM, Rush JE, Rozanski EA et al: Comparison of pharmacodynamic variables following oral versus transdermal administration of atenolol to healthy cats, *Am J Vet Res* 69:39, 2008.
54. Malloy MH, Morriss FH, Denson SE et al: Neonatal gastric motility in dogs: maturation and response to pentagastrin, *Am J Physiol* 236:E562, 1979.
55. Matal J, Jancova P, Siller M et al: Interspecies comparison of the glucuronidation processes in the man, monkey, pig, dog and rat, *Neuro Endocrinol Lett* 29:738, 2008.
56. McCarthy DM: Sucralfate, *N Engl J Med* 325:1017, 1991.
57. Mealey KL, Peck KE, Bennett BS et al: Systemic absorption of amitriptyline and buspirone after oral and transdermal administration to healthy cats, *J Vet Intern Med* 18:43, 2004.
58. Mensching D, Volmer P: Toxicology brief: managing acute carprofen toxicosis in dogs and cats, *Vet Med* 104(7):325, 2009.
59. Meyer FP, Specht H, Quednow B et al: Influence of milk on the bioavailability of doxycycline—new aspects, *Infection* 17:245, 1989.
60. Miyamoto K: Use of plasma clearance of iohexol for estimating glomerular filtration rate in cats, *Am J Vet Res* 62:572, 2001.
61. Morton DJ, Knottenbelt DC: Pharmacokinetics of aspirin and its application in canine veterinary medicine, *J S Afr Vet Assoc* 60:191, 1989.
62. Munar MY, Singh H: Drug dosing adjustments in patients with chronic kidney disease, *Am Fam Physician* 75:1487, 2007.
63. Myant NB: Excretion of the glucuronide of thyroxine in cat bile, *Biochem J* 99:341, 1966.
64. Nahata M, Hipple T: *Pediatric drug formulations*. ed 2, Cincinnati, 1992, Harvey Whitney Books.
65. Oliveira JF, Silva CA, Barbieri CD et al: Prevalence and risk factors for aminoglycoside nephrotoxicity in intensive care units, *Antimicrob Agents Chemother* 53:2887, 2009.

66. Olyaei AJ, Bennett WM: Drug dosing in the elderly patients with chronic kidney disease, *Clin Geriatr Med* 25:459, 2009.
67. Papich MG: Drug compounding for veterinary patients, *AAPS J* 7:E281, 2005.
68. Papich MG, Alcorn J: Absorption of diazepam after its rectal administration in dogs, *Am J Vet Res* 56:1629, 1995.
69. Parton K, Balmer TV, Boyle J et al: The pharmacokinetics and effects of intravenously administered carprofen and salicylate on gastrointestinal mucosa and selected biochemical measurements in healthy cats, *J Vet Pharmacol Ther* 23:73, 2000.
70. Pham K, Hirschberg R: Global safety of coxibs and NSAIDs, *Curr Top Med Chem* 5:456, 2005.
71. Plumb D: *Plumb's veterinary drug handbook*, ed 6, Ames, 2008, Blackwell.
72. Podell M: The use of diazepam per rectum at home for the acute management of cluster seizures in dogs, *J Vet Intern Med* 9:68, 1995.
73. Prausnitz MR, Mitragotri S, Langer R: Current status and future potential of transdermal drug delivery, *Nat Rev Drug Discov* 3:115, 2004.
74. Rea RS, Capitano B: Optimizing use of aminoglycosides in the critically ill, *Semin Respir Crit Care Med* 28:596, 2007.
75. Reid J, Nolan AM: Pharmacokinetics of propofol as an induction agent in geriatric dogs, *Res Vet Sci* 61:169, 1996.
76. Robertson SA, Lascelles BD, Taylor PM et al: PK-PD modeling of buprenorphine in cats: intravenous and oral transmucosal administration, *J Vet Pharmacol Ther* 28:453, 2005.
77. Robertson SA, Taylor PM, Sear JW: Systemic uptake of buprenorphine by cats after oral mucosal administration, *Vet Rec* 152:675, 2003.
78. Rubio F, Seawall S, Pocelinko R et al: Metabolism of carprofen, a nonsteroid anti-inflammatory agent, in rats, dogs, and humans, *J Pharm Sci* 69:1245, 1980.
79. Salavaggione OE, Yang C, Kidd LB et al: Cat red blood cell thiopurine S-methyltransferase: companion animal pharmacogenetics, *J Pharmacol Exp Ther* 308:617, 2004.
80. Sartor LL, Trepanier LA, Kroll MM et al: Efficacy and safety of transdermal methimazole in the treatment of cats with hyperthyroidism, *J Vet Intern Med* 18:651, 2004.
81. Savides MC, Oehme FW, Nash SL et al: The toxicity and biotransformation of single doses of acetaminophen in dogs and cats, *Toxicol Appl Pharmacol* 74:26, 1984.
82. Schentag JJ, Gengo FM, Plaut ME et al: Urinary casts as an indicator of renal tubular damage in patients receiving aminoglycosides, *Antimicrob Agents Chemother* 16:468, 1979.
83. Schmucker DL: Age-related changes in liver structure and function: implications for disease? *Exp Gerontol* 40:650, 2005.
84. Seguin MA, Papich MG, Sigle KJ et al: Pharmacokinetics of enrofloxacin in neonatal kittens, *Am J Vet Res* 65:350, 2004.
85. Sirota RA, Kimmel PL, Trichtinger MD et al: Metoclopramide-induced parkinsonism in hemodialysis patients. Report of two cases, *Arch Intern Med* 146:2070, 1986.
86. Somogyi A: Renal transport of drugs: specificity and molecular mechanisms, *Clin Exp Pharmacol Physiol* 23:986, 1996.
87. Spivak W, Carey MC: Reverse-phase h.p.l.c. separation, quantification and preparation of bilirubin and its conjugates from native bile. Quantitative analysis of the intact tetrapyrroles based on h.p.l.c. of their ethyl anthranilate azo derivatives, *Biochem J* 225:787, 1985.
88. Steagall PV, Taylor PM, Rodrigues LC et al: Analgesia for cats after ovariohysterectomy with either buprenorphine or carprofen alone or in combination, *Vet Rec* 164:359, 2009.
89. Sweileh WM: A prospective comparative study of gentamicin- and amikacin-induced nephrotoxicity in patients with normal baseline renal function, *Fundam Clin Pharmacol* 23:515, 2009.
90. Tanaka E, Narisawa C, Nakamura H et al: Changes in the enzymatic activities of beagle liver during maturation as assessed both in vitro and in vivo, *Xenobiotica* 28:795, 1998.
91. Taylor PM, Robertson SA, Dixon MJ et al: Morphine, pethidine and buprenorphine disposition in the cat, *J Vet Pharmacol Ther* 24:391, 2001.
92. Touw DJ, Westerman EM, Sprij AJ: Therapeutic drug monitoring of aminoglycosides in neonates, *Clin Pharmacokinet* 48:71, 2009.
93. Trulson ME, Crisp T: Behavioral and neurochemical effects of apomorphine in the cat, *Eur J Pharmacol* 80:295, 1982.
94. Turnheim K: Drug therapy in the elderly, *Exp Gerontol* 39:1731, 2004.
95. Turnheim K: Pharmacokinetic dosage guidelines for elderly subjects, *Expert Opin Drug Metab Toxicol* 1:33, 2005.
96. Van Scoy RE, Wilson WR: Antimicrobial agents in adult patients with renal insufficiency: initial dosage and general recommendations, *Mayo Clin Proc* 62:1142, 1987.
97. Verbeeck RK, Musuamba FT: Pharmacokinetics and dosage adjustment in patients with renal dysfunction, *Eur J Clin Pharmacol* 65:757, 2009.
98. Weinberg MS: Renal effects of angiotensin converting enzyme inhibitors in heart failure: a clinician's guide to minimizing azotemia and diuretic-induced electrolyte imbalances, *Clin Ther* 15:3, 1993.
99. Westfall DS, Twedt DC, Steyn PF et al: Evaluation of esophageal transit of tablets and capsules in 30 cats, *J Vet Intern Med* 15:467, 2001.
100. White SD, Rosychuk RA, Outerbridge CA et al: Thiopurine methyltransferase in red blood cells of dogs, cats, and horses, *J Vet Intern Med* 14:499, 2000.
101. Wiebe V, Hamilton P: Fluoroquinolone-induced retinal degeneration in cats, *J Am Vet Med Assoc* 221:1568, 2002.
102. Willis-Goulet HS, Schmidt BA, Nicklin CF et al: Comparison of serum dexamethasone concentrations in cats after oral or transdermal administration using pluronic lecithin organogel (PLO): a pilot study, *Vet Dermatol* 14:83, 2003.
103. Wright LC, Horton CR, Jr, Jernigan AD et al: Pharmacokinetics of gentamicin after intravenous and subcutaneous injection in obese cats, *J Vet Pharmacol Ther* 14:96, 1991.
104. Yoder Graber AL, Ramirez J, Innocenti F et al: UGT1A1*28 genotype affects the in-vitro glucuronidation of thyroxine in human livers, *Pharmacogenet Genomics* 17:619, 2007.
105. Zhanel GG: Cephalosporin-induced nephrotoxicity: does it exist? *DICP* 24:262, 1990.
106. Zimmermann T, Yeates RA, Riedel KD et al: The influence of gastric pH on the pharmacokinetics of fluconazole: the effect of omeprazole, *Int J Clin Pharmacol Ther* 32:491, 1994.

CHAPTER

5

Fluid Therapy

Katharine F. Lunn, Anthony S. Johnson, and Katherine M. James

OUTLINE

Fluid therapy should be approached with the same attention to detail as drug therapy, and the foundation for this approach is an understanding of body fluid balance and perfusion. Without understanding these concepts, the clinician risks taking a "cookbook" or one-size-fits-all approach to fluid therapy. Potential adverse effects of oversimplified approaches to fluid therapy include persistent dehydration, fluid overload, hypoperfusion, acid–base imbalance, and electrolyte disorders, all of which have profound effects on morbidity in patients.

BODY FLUID BALANCE

Body fluid balance depends on both salt and water balance and the relationship between them. When referring to salt balance, we primarily consider the sodium ion (Na^+) because it is the principal extracellular cation. *Water balance* refers to the amount of Na^+ present relative to water. The concepts of salt and water balance are challenging, but they are essential for understanding the types, amounts, and rates of fluids to administer. It is perhaps counterintuitive that disordered salt balance does not cause abnormalities of serum sodium concentration but rather results in abnormalities of extracellular fluid (ECF) volume. Disorders of sodium concentration result from abnormalities in water balance. Salt and water balance will be discussed in more depth in later sections.

STEADY STATE AND THE CONCEPT OF MAINTENANCE

With the exception of small, steady changes during growth, the amount of water coming into the body each day must equal the amount of water eliminated from the body over the same period. If not, the cat will have either a net water gain or a net water loss. Cats take in water by drinking, eating (food contains some water), and metabolizing nutrients to CO_2 and water. Physiologic water losses result from the following:

- Obligate urinary loss
- Fecal loss
- Salivary loss
- Evaporation from the respiratory tract and the skin surface (insensible losses)

Pathologic loss of water can result from the following:

- Vomiting or regurgitation
- Diarrhea

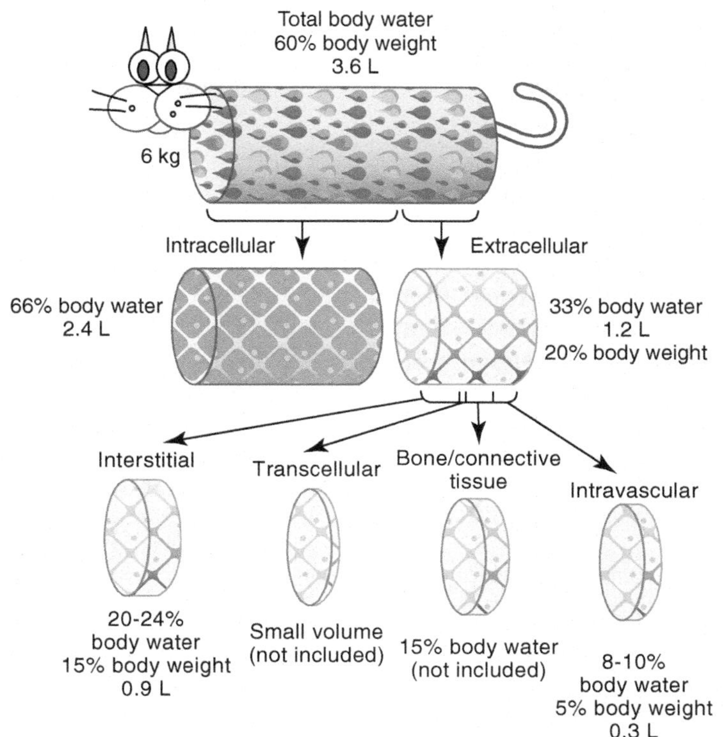

FIGURE 5-1 Body fluid compartments of the cat. The body's two main fluid compartments are the intracellular fluid (ICF) and the extracellular fluid (ECF). Approximately 66% of functional total body water is located within the ICF compartment, and 33% is in the ECF compartment.

- Bleeding
- Loss from wounds, burns, or drains
- Excessive urinary loss
- Excessive respiratory loss
- Excessive salivary loss

Electrolytes must also be consumed and eliminated in equal quantities on an approximately daily basis to maintain homeostasis. These continual losses that must be replaced promptly and nearly continually underlie the concept of "maintenance fluids." Maintenance needs, normally met by eating food and drinking water, are largely dependent on the cat's lean body mass. Sick animals that are no longer eating or drinking will continue to have daily obligatory fluid and electrolyte losses that can be addressed by fluid therapy to prevent negative fluid and electrolyte balance.

BODY FLUID COMPARTMENTS

Water is a major contributor to a cat's body weight. In healthy animals approximately 60% of body weight is water. This value can change slightly depending on age, lean body mass, degree of leanness or obesity, and gender. For example, neonatal and young kittens have a relatively higher percentage of water in their bodies than do adults.

Figure 5-1 depicts the cat's body fluid compartments. The body's two main fluid compartments are the intracellular fluid (ICF) and the ECF. Approximately 66% of functional total body water is located within the ICF compartment, and 33% is in the ECF compartment.

The ICF is, of course, not a single compartment but rather a conceptualization of the result of combining the very small volumes of a body's trillions of cells as one. This is useful for understanding physiology because of commonalities of ICF composition and behavior. The fluid inside cells is high in potassium (K^+) and magnesium (Mg^{++}) and low in Na^+ and chloride (Cl^-) ions. Additionally, fluid inside all cells will respond similarly to tonicity changes in the ECF.

The ECF space is composed of four main subcompartments: interstitial, intravascular, transcellular, and bone and dense connective tissue. The intravascular fluid is that which is contained within blood vessels; it contributes only 8% to 10% of total body water (5% of body weight) and has been estimated to be approximately 45 mL/kg in cats.[10]

The interstitial compartment refers to that portion of the ECF located outside of the vascular space. Like the ICF, this is not a single space but rather a conceptualization, or "virtual space," that would be created if all the interstitial fluid spaces were to be combined. It contributes approximately 22% to 24% to total body water (15% of total body weight).

The fluid of bone and dense connective tissue provides about 15% of the total body water. However, this fluid is mobilized very slowly, decreasing its importance when considering the effects of acute fluid interventions. Transcellular fluid is a normally small compartment that represents all those body fluids that are formed from the transport activities of cells. It is contained within epithelium-lined spaces. It includes cerebrospinal fluid (CSF), gastrointestinal fluids, urine in the bladder, aqueous humor, and joint fluid. The electrolyte compositions of the various transcellular fluids are dissimilar, but they are small in aggregate volume. However, fluid fluxes involving gastrointestinal fluid can be significant in disease.

The water in bone and dense connective tissue and the transcellular fluids, because of their slow mobilization, are subtracted from the total ECF volume to yield the functional ECF.

It is important to note that when excess fluid builds up in transcellular or interstitial compartments in which fluid volume are normally small, the process is termed *third spacing*. Excess fluid in the peritoneal space, pleural space, or gastrointestinal tract can add considerably to body weight, while diminishing the effective ECF volume.

BOX 5-1

Starling Forces

The Starling forces are defined by the equation $J_v = K_f([P_c - P_i] - \sigma[\pi_c - \pi_i])$ relating to the following six variables: capillary hydrostatic pressure (P_c), interstitial hydrostatic pressure (P_i), capillary oncotic pressure (π_c), interstitial oncotic pressure (π_i), filtration coefficient (K_f), reflection coefficient (σ).

In the equation, $([P_c - P_i] - \sigma[\pi_c - \pi_i])$ is the net driving force, K_f is the proportionality constant, and J_v is the net fluid movement between compartments.

By convention, outward force is defined as positive, and inward force is defined as negative. The solution to the equation is known as the net filtration or net fluid movement (J_v). If positive, fluid will tend to leave the capillary (filtration). If negative, fluid will tend to enter the capillary (absorption). This equation has a number of important physiologic implications, especially when pathologic processes grossly alter one or more of the variables.

Fluid Movement in the Extracellular Fluid Compartment

The water in the body's ECF compartments is in a constant state of flux. Fluid moves across the capillary membrane, which is composed of endothelial cells that contain gap junctions through which fluid and solutes can flow. Solutes dissolved in fluid move from an area of higher to lower concentration along concentration gradients by the process of passive diffusion. The factors that regulate this transport of fluid and the electrolytes and other molecules it contains are called *Starling forces* (Box 5-1). The key factors are the hydrostatic and colloid oncotic pressure gradients between the intravascular and extravascular spaces. The hydrostatic pressure is greater in the capillary than in the interstitium, and the gradient favors fluid movement (filtration) out of the capillary. The colloid oncotic pressure, determined by protein concentration, is also greater in the capillary, and this tends to draw fluid into the capillary. Simplistically, at the beginning of the capillary the high hydrostatic pressure results in fluid egress into interstitium. As the fluid leaves along the length of the capillary, the hydrostatic pressure falls and the colloid oncotic pressure increases, resulting in fluid reentry into the capillary lumen toward the end of the capillary. Fluid also leaves the interstitial compartment by way of the lymphatics.

Fluids in the ECF move continuously between the vascular space and the interstitial space across the capillary endothelium to achieve tissue perfusion. Edema results when the balance of the hydrostatic and colloid oncotic pressure gradients shifts such that fluid egress from the capillary is favored. All of the following promote edema formation: (1) decreased plasma oncotic pressure, (2) increased capillary hydrostatic pressure, (3) increased capillary permeability, and (4) lymphatic obstruction. The other key requirement for edema formation is Na^+ retention: an increase in the ECF Na^+ content.

Fluid Movement Between the Intracellular Fluid and Extracellular Fluid Compartments

The ICF and ECF are separated by cellular membranes. The protein components of these membranes give them substantial and rapid permeability to water while carefully controlling their permeability to solutes such as ions. Cell membranes are also flexible. Thus, when water flows into or out of cells, those cells expand or shrink, respectively. Hydrostatic pressure, therefore, does not play a significant role in fluid movement between ECF and ICF compartments, because osmosis results in water flow rather than the development of pressure. Osmotic water flow occurs wherever there is a gradient of impermeable solute (such as Na^+) across a water-permeable membrane (the body cell membranes).

In the body the ECF and ICF compartments are always in osmotic equilibrium, even though the composition of the fluids within them is very different. Water flows into or out of cells and changes their volume when an osmotic gradient exists between the ICF and ECF compartments.

PERFUSION

Perfusion refers to the process in which blood carries oxygen and nutrients to body tissues and organs and transports waste products of cellular metabolism away. Perfusion is optimized when an animal is in a state of normal fluid balance. Oxygen delivery is a critical part of perfusion and is dependent on the animal's cardiac output and the oxygen-carrying capacity of the blood. Cardiac output is a function of heart rate and stroke volume. Stroke volume depends on ventricular preload, ventricular afterload, and contractility. The amount of blood that enters the ventricle, causing the ventricular wall to stretch, thus affects the ventricular preload because the amount of wall stretch is directly proportional to the force of contraction. When there is adequate circulating volume, cardiac preload on the healthy ventricle results in a contraction of appropriate force. By contrast, in a cat with hypovolemia cardiac preload will be diminished, thus decreasing the force of ventricular contraction. Intravenous fluid therapy can affect cardiac preload by replenishing intravascular fluid volume in a hypovolemic animal.

SALT BALANCE: DISORDERS OF ECF VOLUME

Sodium Content

The Na^+ content of the body determines the volume of the ECF and total body fluid volume. It does this because the osmolality of body fluids is regulated within a very narrow range. If Na^+ ions (always with an accompanying anion) are added to the ECF space, more water molecules must be added to ECF space in the same proportion or the osmolality will increase beyond the relatively narrow range compatible with health and normal cellular function. Thus increasing the number of Na^+ ions in the ECF (the Na^+ content) increases the ECF volume. Similarly, if Na^+ ions are removed from the ECF space, water molecules must leave in proportion, resulting in a decreased ECF volume, or the fluid's osmolality would decrease beyond that which the body's regulatory mechanisms will allow in health. In that sense, the Na^+ content of the ECF fluid space determines its volume.

Regulation of Sodium Balance

Regulatory mechanisms exist to control both Na^+ content and Na^+ concentration ($[Na^+]$), and they are interrelated. Body Na^+ content is regulated by mechanisms that control the renal excretion of Na^+ and which operate in response to body fluid volume and not $[Na^+]$.[9] Control of $[Na^+]$ is determined by the osmoregulatory control mechanisms.

Evolutionarily, it appears that salt was a scarce commodity. Thus the kidney has evolved mechanisms to conserve salt. Na^+ excretion in the urine can vary over 500-fold depending on Na^+ intake and body need. The homeostatic mechanisms that control Na^+ content are poorly understood. Regulation is generally a comparatively slow process. For example, many hours will pass before excesses in Na^+ content (e.g., when isotonic saline is infused) are corrected by increased renal Na^+ excretion. In contrast, excesses or deficiencies of water relative to Na^+ (changes in $[Na^+]$) activate the osmoregulatory mechanisms and are dealt with very rapidly. Many physiologists believe that a set point for Na^+ regulation does not exist. Rather, Na^+ is retained in low volume states until the volume deficit is corrected.[12]

Sodium excess results in augmented ECF volume, which increases urinary Na^+ excretion. A useful analogy is a bucket with a hole in its side: When volume is at or below the hole, Na^+ excretion is minimal while the bucket fills to the level of the hole. Once there, the inflow equals the outflow. When the volume of the bucket is above the hole (ECF expansion), the pressure of fluid in the bucket drives the fluid to flow out of the hole more quickly. For example, when dietary Na^+ intake is increased, it takes several days to reach a new steady state of neutral Na^+ balance.

The following factors are known to affect renal Na^+ excretion:

1. Arterial hypertension
2. Tubuloglomerular feedback
3. Circadian rhythm

It is suspected that others also exist. The sensors (afferent signals) in the regulation of Na^+ excretion are thought to include intrathoracic volume receptors, atrial pressure receptors, arterial baroreceptors, intrarenal baroreceptors, the macula densa, hepatic volume receptors, CSF volume receptors, and possibly tissue receptors. The mediators of Na^+ conservation or excretion include the sympathetic nervous system, the renin–angiotensin–aldosterone system (RAAS), vasopressin, atrial natriuretic peptide (ANP), renal prostaglandins, the kallikrein–kinin system, nitric oxide, and renal pressure and flow phenomena (glomerular filtration rate [GFR], renal blood flow, and arterial pressure).

Salt excess states include congestive heart failure, nephrotic syndrome, hepatic cirrhosis, hyperaldosteronism, Na^+ channel defects, and pregnancy. In the pathogenesis of certain salt-retaining states, reference is made to the *effective plasma volume*. This is not a measurable quantity, and the concept lacks a precise definition.

It refers to the "fullness" of the vascular volume. It is the portion of the vascular volume that is being sensed by those mechanisms that regulate body fluid volume. An inadequate effective circulating volume is inferred when salt-retaining mechanisms are activated.

Salt-deficient states are secondary to a number of disease conditions that result in losses of Na^+ or inadequate intake. Extrarenal losses are localized to diseases of the gastrointestinal tract, skin, respiratory tract, and third space losses. Renal salt loss may occur with the following:

1. Diuresis (e.g., diuretic phase of acute tubular necrosis, postobstructive diuresis, or the use of diuretic medications)
2. Intrinsic renal disease (e.g., chronic renal failure, Fanconi syndrome, Bartter syndrome)
3. Defects in the RAAS system (e.g., hypoadrenocorticism, hyporeninemic hypoaldosteronism)
4. Disorders resulting in excesses of ANP

The use of high-sodium, isotonic fluid types in fluid therapy is thus primarily for the administration of Na^+. They augment the total ECF Na^+ content and thus expand the functional ECF volume, both vascular and interstitial.

WATER BALANCE: DISORDERS OF SODIUM CONCENTRATION

Permeant and Impermeant Solutes

The next important concept to be understood is that of water balance. Cells must be in osmotic equilibrium with the fluid that surrounds them, insofar as their membranes are permeable to water. Although extracellular and intracellular fluids have very different compositions, they must have the same total solute concentrations because of the free movement of water. Looking at this concept "in reverse," the water concentration of the ECF and the ICF must be the same. Inequalities of water concentrations in body fluid compartments can exist only transiently because water movement occurs rapidly to correct these inequalities. This basic concept underlies an understanding of fluid movement between intracellular and extracellular compartments during intravenous fluid therapy.

The concentration of solutes in fluid defines the solution's osmolality. Because cell membranes are water permeable and water movement will occur until solutions on either side of a membrane are iso-osmolar, the osmolality of plasma reflects the osmolality of the body fluid in total. It is important to distinguish between permeant and impermeant solutes. Permeant solutes (e.g., urea) move freely across cellular membranes and thus do not induce net water movement across cell membranes when they are introduced into a solution; they are termed *ineffective osmoles*. Impermeant solutes (e.g., Na^+) do not freely move across cell membranes and do induce water movement when introduced into a solution; thus they are effective osmoles.

Tonicity

The term *tonicity* refers to the effect a solution has on cellular volume. Hypertonicity results when impermeant solutes are added to the ECF; this promotes cellular dehydration. Hypotonicity results from a decrease in the concentration of impermeant solutions; this results in water movement into cells and cellular swelling. Hypertonic solutions are always hyperosmolar. The reverse is not always the case: Hyperosmolar solutions are not necessarily hypertonic because ineffective osmoles contribute to osmolality but not tonicity.

Plasma $[Na^+]$ is the key determinant of the osmolality of body fluids. Glucose and urea make minor contributions under normal circumstances. Plasma osmolality may be calculated using the following equation:

$$2[Na^+](mEq/l) + [glucose](mg/dL)/18 + [BUN](mg/dL)/2.8$$

The preceding equation is a simplification because it does not take into account the fact that plasma is only 93% water; that sodium salts are not completely dissociated in solution; or that calcium, magnesium, and potassium salts also contribute. However, these factors appear to cancel out because experimental evidence demonstrates that calculated osmolality and measured osmolality are in close agreement in normal patients.

Plasma $[Na^+]$ reflects the plasma tonicity very well in normal patients. Urea is an ineffective osmole because it equilibrates freely across cell membranes and does not induce fluid shifts. Glucose normally can move across cell membranes in normal patients in the presence of insulin; therefore it is usually an ineffective osmole, similar to urea. In diabetic patients lacking insulin, it becomes an effective osmole. Thus plasma $[Na^+]$ predicts plasma tonicity when the glucose concentration is known. In hyperglycemia water leaves the cells because of the hypertonicity of the ECF. This serves to dilute the Na^+, and hyponatremia is observed.

It is important to remember that serum $[Na^+]$ does not reflect body salt balance. Salt balance determines ECF volume. Serum $[Na^+]$, instead, reflects the state of water balance. The term *osmoregulation* refers to the control of body fluid tonicity. By stabilizing body fluid tonicity, osmoregulation thus controls cell volume. Osmoreceptors are, in fact, hypothalamic cells that sense their own cell volume. Changes in plasma osmolality sensed by these cells affect secretion of arginine vasopressin (antidiuretic hormone; ADH). ADH is the primary regulator of renal water excretion. Changes in plasma osmolality also strongly affect the thirst mechanism. This is why patients with central diabetes insipidus, who thus lack ADH, are able to maintain a relatively normal osmolality provided they have access to water and the ability to drink.

Regulation of Water Balance

In contrast to salt balance, which is controlled by many factors and has a relatively slow response to changes in effective plasma volume, plasma osmolality is very tightly regulated. When plasma osmolality is altered, changes in thirst and ADH secretion, and the resulting renal response, are brisk.

In addition to plasma osmolality, hypotension and hypovolemia also stimulate ADH release and thus this is a point where regulation of salt and water balance are interrelated. ADH release is not as sensitive to hemodynamic stimuli as it is to changes in osmolality; however, when the hemodynamic stimulus is sufficiently strong, the ADH response will be of higher magnitude. In the presence of a significant volume deficit, decreased water excretion by the kidney will in fact act to increase volume at the expense of a decrease in plasma osmolality.

The primary function of ADH is to increase the water permeability of the luminal membrane of the collecting duct of the nephron. ADH, through a second-messenger system, causes water channels called *aquaporins* to be inserted into the cell membrane. Water reabsorption in the collecting duct occurs through these channels, thus allowing the kidney to conserve water.

UNDERSTANDING FLUID LOSSES

Sensible and Insensible Fluid Losses

Sensible fluid losses are those that can be measured and include fluid lost in the form of urine, feces, vomitus, body cavity effusions, and wound exudates. It is important in seriously ill patients actually to quantify these losses and incorporate them into the fluid prescription. For example, urine output can be determined by collecting voided urine or by weighing the bedding or litter when dry and again after urination. Similarly, vomitus or diarrhea can be weighed to allow the clinician to estimate fluid loss, given that 1 g is approximately equivalent to 1 mL water. For wounds with large volumes of exudate, an animal's bandage material can be weighed before and after use to create a fluid loss estimate. For patients with drains or chest tubes in place, the amount of fluid produced from these devices can also be measured.

Insensible losses are those that cannot directly be measured. They include largely solute-free water in evaporative respiratory, sweat, and salivary losses. This classical definition of *insensible losses* is sometimes replaced with a clinical definition that includes fecal water loss. This is because the amount of normal daily fecal water loss is small and is rarely measured.[16]

As a gross approximation, sensible fluid losses account for half of a healthy animal's daily fluid requirement and insensible losses account for the other half. However, this partitioning is variable and is species and environment dependent. For example, dogs as a species may have a higher percentage of insensible losses compared with cats because of the greater use of panting for thermoregulation. However, cats may have considerable salivary losses if they have increased grooming or lick their fur to promote evaporative cooling in hot weather.[7]

Insensible fluid losses are generally considered to be solute-free water because respiratory losses are the major contributor in small animal species, including cats. Insensible losses are estimated to be 12 to 30 mL/kg/day, depending on the study and definition.[16]

In contrast to insensible losses, sensible fluid losses do contain solutes. Although a necessary oversimplification, this explains why maintenance fluid types are hypotonic. They replace the solute-free water of insensible losses and the solute-containing water of sensible losses. As a matter of practicality, given these estimates and variable definitions, it is reasonable to assume that half of daily maintenance fluids are to offset normal levels of obligate urine output required for daily solute excretion and are solute-containing fluid losses, and the other half, accounting for everything else, are solute-free water losses. This is important clinically when adjusting the fluid prescription for "ins and outs" because it provides a method to estimate how much of measured hourly urine production is abnormal losses in polyuric patients (who have excessive ongoing urinary fluid loss that must be met by the replacement portion of the fluid prescription) and how much is normal obligate urine (and thus met by maintenance portion of the fluid prescription).

Body Weight and Fluid Losses

Total body water remains essentially the same day to day in a healthy animal. However in disease, excessive loss of fluid can occur associated with hemorrhage, vomiting, diarrhea, burns, fever, effusions, wound exudates, polyuria, and panting. Because rapid changes in body weight, over the span of hours to a few days, are largely due to changes in total body water, changes in an animal's weight are an invaluable tool in the assessment of an animal's hydration status. Because of the relative small size of cats, weighing animals on scales that can accurately detect changes of a few ounces or several grams (human pediatric scales) are very important.

Relationship to Lean Body Mass

Because lean body mass is so important in determining an animal's daily fluid need, resting energy requirement (RER), or daily caloric requirement, is used to calculate an animal's metabolic water requirements: To metabolize 1 kilocalorie of energy, 1 mL of water is consumed. As such, calculation of an animal's RER can be extrapolated to determine the volume of fluid in mL required in a 24-hour period. Several equations may be used to calculate RER and hence water requirement.[5] The following is one of the most commonly used:

$$RER = 30(BW_{kg}) + 70$$

This formula is accurate for animals weighing more than 2 kg and less than 25 kg and thus is applicable to adult domestic cats. Kittens and cats weighing less than 2 kg require the use of a different formula:

$$RER = 70(BW_{kg})^{0.75}$$

Terminology of Body Fluid Balance

The terminology used to describe body fluid balance is at times unfortunately vague. *Dehydration* refers to a decrease in total body water: loss of fluid from the ICF and ECF compartments. However, the physical examination findings used to assess hydration, such as skin tenting and mucous membrane dryness, are specifically assessments of the ECF volume and subject to significant individual variation and inaccuracy. Thus when clinicians suggest that a patient "appears dehydrated," they are referring specifically to clinical signs of ECF volume depletion. This is to be distinguished from *hypovolemia,* which refers to inadequate circulating intravascular fluid volume. The distinction is important because hypovolemia is a much more time-sensitive condition requiring rapid, aggressive treatment.

Assessment of Fluid loss

Patients can be assumed to have a decrease in total body water in the presence of known excessive net losses, such as those produced by vomiting, diarrhea, anorexia, and marked polyuria, even without a demonstrable increase in skin tenting and mucous membrane dryness, which are detectable only when 4% to 5% of total body weight has been lost. Humans report headaches with dehydration, and presumably this may reflect some of the general lethargy seen in volume-depleted cats. At 7% total body weight loss, mild tachycardia could also be present. At 10% total body weight loss, the patient might also have a palpably decreased pulse pressure. Signs of very severe total body water loss are sunken eyes, dry corneas, and altered mentation. Overt hypovolemia will occur with severe fluid loss (>12% body weight), even when chronic. It is important to note at this time that lethargy can be present with both underhydration and overhydration. This is particularly important in cats with oliguria because they are readily susceptible to overhydration.

The aforementioned physical findings that are used to determine an animal's total body fluid status are not used to assess hypovolemia. Peripheral perfusion should instead be assessed by capillary refill time (CRT), mucous membrane color, arterial blood pressure, pulse quality and rate, and temperature of extremities.

The body responds to fluid loss by redistributing the functional ECF volume—that is, by pulling fluid into the intravascular space from the interstitial space to maintain circulating blood volume as the first priority. When the interstitial space can no longer replenish intravascular volume depletion, clinical signs of hypovolemia will result. In decompensated shock, severe hypovolemia results in a marked worsening of perfusion parameters. Hypotension, bradycardia, prolonged CRT, pale pink to gray or cyanotic mucous membranes, hypothermia, decreased central venous pressure, altered mentation, and decreased urine output will be present in decompensated shock. Table 5-1 gives examples of the types of fluid losses that would be expected with selected medical problems.

Assessment of Fluid Excess

Overhydration, like dehydration, is detrimental to patients and should be avoided in patients on fluid therapy. Human and canine patients with ECF volume excess can have pulmonary edema, ascites, and generalized peripheral edema. Unique to the cat, possibly because of a difference in the anatomy of pulmonary venous drainage, pleural effusion may develop more readily than pulmonary edema or ascites. Cats with preexisting cardiac disease are more susceptible to pleural effusion or pulmonary edema with volume overload, depending on their underlying disease. Cats with oliguria or markedly decreased GFRs are also particularly at risk for overhydration, and measurement of urinary output is essential in such patients. Early signs of overhydration may include the more subtle findings of loss of appetite and mental dullness. An astute clinician will notice tachypnea or crackles on auscultation, insofar as pleural effusion or pulmonary edema develops before the onset of overt dyspnea. Careful and repeated weighing is important for prevention of volume overload, particularly in cats, because of their small size.

TABLE 5-1 **Examples of the Types of Fluid Losses that Would Be Expected with Selected Medical Problems**

Condition	Dehydration	Hypovolemia
Blood loss		X
Vomiting	X	X (if severe)
Diarrhea	X	X (if severe)
Sepsis/vasodilation		X
Hypoadrenocorticism		X
Polyuria	X (depending on cause)	X (depending on cause)
Hypodipsia or water deprivation	X	

BODY RESPONSE TO HYPOVOLEMIA

Intravascular volume status is sensed by baroreceptors in the carotid body and aortic arch. In euvolemic cats, stimulation of the stretch receptors triggers the vagus nerve to maintain an appropriate heart rate. In hypovolemia the baroreceptors sense a decrease in wall tension, and the sympathetic nervous system is activated. Norepinephrine and epinephrine release results in vasoconstriction, improved cardiac contractility, and an increase in heart rate. These effects are designed to compensate for decreased intravascular fluid volume by improving cardiac output and maintaining systemic blood pressure and, ultimately, perfusion. Hypovolemic shock results when intravascular volume is sufficiently reduced that these compensatory mechanisms are overwhelmed and decreased tissue perfusion results. Perfusion parameters that can be assessed include capillary refill time, blood pressure, heart rate, and temperature of extremities.

Cats are unique in that the vasoconstrictor response to volume loss is blunted in the presence of hypothermia.[13,14] For this reason, cats are more prone than other species to fluid overload when they have been volume resuscitated while hypothermic. Once body temperature returns to normal, the vasoconstrictor response returns and intravascular pressure rises. For this reason, hypothermia in cats is a potentiator of shock, as well as a result of shock. Cautious fluid resuscitation must coincide with aggressive rewarming efforts to prevent volume overload. Specific therapy and therapeutic endpoints for resuscitation are discussed in subsequent sections.

GENERAL CONSIDERATIONS FOR FLUID THERAPY

Fluid therapy choices are often the product of educated guesswork. They certainly rely on the physiologic abilities of a normally functioning kidney for fine-tuning. Although there are many useful guidelines for selection of fluid types and rates, good fluid management demands careful monitoring of body weight, physical examination, and electrolyte concentrations. The veterinarian must be prepared to alter the fluid therapy prescription in response to changes in these parameters, and should understand that the initial fluid therapy plan merely provides a starting point. The clinician must also be more vigilant with fluid therapy monitoring in patients with cardiovascular or renal disease. It should be remembered that cats may have cardiac disease in the absence of a detectable murmur.

As fluid bag sizes are not scaled down to the size of feline patients, it is helpful to use fluid pumps, burettes, and other devices to prevent fluid overload and pulmonary edema or pleural effusion (Figure 5-2).

FLUID TYPES

The two main types of parenteral fluids, crystalloids and colloids, have fundamental differences that affect the way fluid distributes among body fluid compartments. Crystalloids are composed of smaller molecules that diffuse readily; therefore approximately 80% of the fluid infused will leave the intravascular space within 1 hour. Colloids, made of larger molecules, stay within the intravascular space longer, which is an important advantage when managing hypovolemia. The tonicity of fluids determines distribution rates to the intracellular and extracellular spaces. When the $[Na^+]$ of a fluid approximates that of plasma (145 mEq/L), it will equilibrate rapidly with the interstitial space. Remaining fluid that is not lost in urine or as other ongoing losses will distribute to the ICF in proportion to the normal size of those compartments: two thirds ICF and one third ECF.

Hypotonic fluids, with a $[Na^+]$ lower than that of plasma, will dilute the plasma and drive water into cells to equilibrate the water concentration inside and outside cells. The decreasing plasma osmolality (pOsm) will also result in a decreased ADH production and, thus, increased water excretion by the kidney. Most of the Na^+-free fluid thus either enters cells or is excreted. Hypertonic fluids with a $[Na^+]$ higher than plasma will draw water out of cells and into the ECF, thus increasing

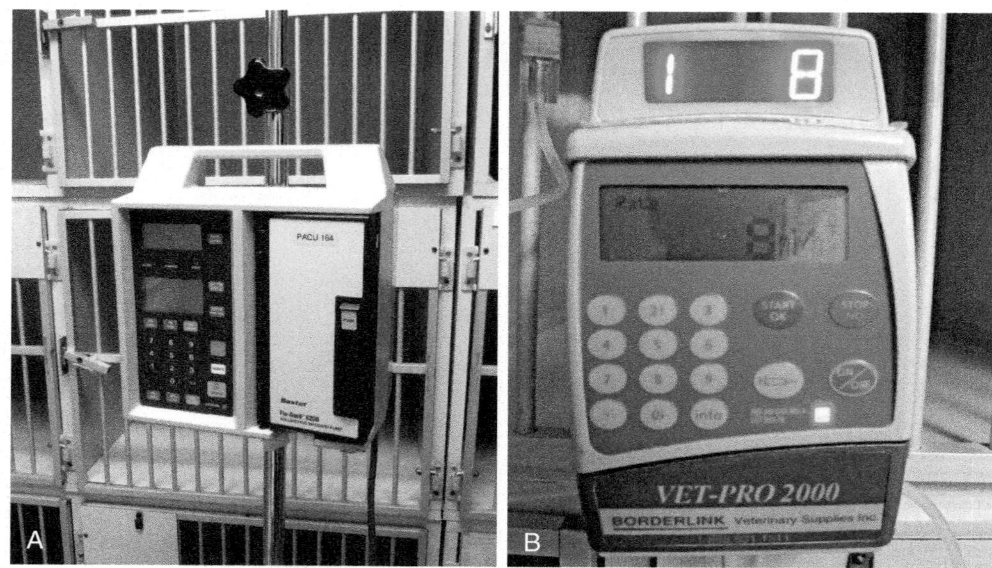

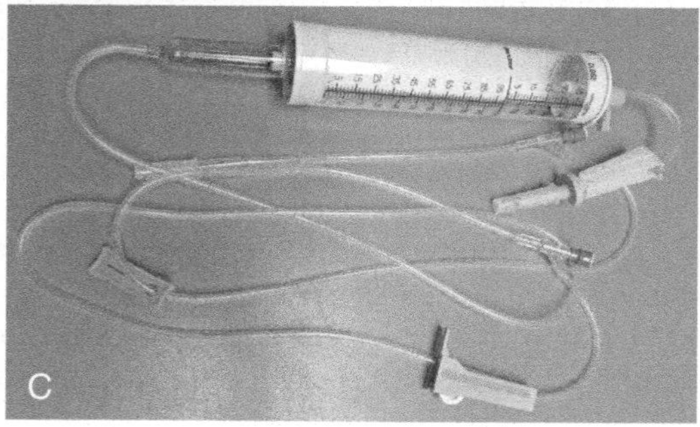

FIGURE 5-2 Because fluid bag sizes are not scaled down to the size of feline patients, it is helpful to use fluid pumps (**A** and **B**), burettes (**C**), and other devices to prevent fluid overdosing.

the intravascular and interstitial volumes but at the expense of taking water from the ICF compartment. Thus an understanding of which body compartments need to be replenished in any given patient is essential in fluid selection. This is true not only regarding fluid types selected but also in terms of route of administration. For example, fluids instilled into the subcutaneous space cannot be used readily to replenish the intravascular blood volume because they will be absorbed too slowly in a patient with hypovolemia.

Crystalloids

A crystalloid is a solution that is able to pass through a semipermeable membrane, including the vascular endothelium. The ability of crystalloids to pass through the capillary endothelium allows them to replenish fluid losses both in the intravascular and interstitial compartments, making them ideal for rehydration therapy. All crystalloid fluids are true solutions, meaning that they are homogeneous and transparent, diffuse rapidly, and do not settle. Substances that are dissolved in crystalloids are termed *solutes*; these are predominantly electrolytes and dextrose.

Solutes contained in crystalloid fluids move freely from the intravascular space to the interstitial space. Movement of impermeant solutes such as ions and glucose into the intracellular compartment is comparatively slower, occurring by facilitated diffusion or active transport. As parenteral fluid solutions, most crystalloids are formulated with a solute concentration close to that of plasma to avoid osmotic cell damage, particularly red blood cell damage from tonicity-induced osmotic water movement. Some parenteral intravenous solutions, such as 0.45% NaCl and 5% dextrose in water (D5W) are hypotonic and can cause hemolysis if given too rapidly.

The three categories of crystalloids are isotonic high-sodium, hypotonic low-sodium, and hypertonic saline; they differ primarily in their sodium concentrations.

Isotonic High-Sodium Crystalloids

GENERAL CHARACTERISTICS AND INDICATIONS FOR ISOTONIC HIGH-SODIUM CRYSTALLOIDS

Isotonic high-sodium fluids are commonly referred to as *replacement fluids* because they are often used for rapid replacement of ECF volume deficits caused by vomiting

TABLE 5-2 **Composition of Common Crystalloids***

	0/9% NaCl	Lactated Ringer's Solution	Ringer's Solution	Normosol-R	0.45% NaCl + 2.5% Dextrose	5% Dextrose	Plasma-Lyte 56 + 5% Dextrose
Na^+ (mEq/L)	154	130	147	140	77	0	40
Cl^- (mEq/L)	154	109	154	98	77	0	40
K^+ (mEq/L)	0	4	4	5	0	0	13
Ca^{++} (mEq/L)	0	3	4	0	0	0	0
Mg^{++} (mEq/L)	0	0	0	3	0	0	3
Osmolality (mOsm/L)	308	273	309	294	280	252	112
pH	5.6	6.6	5.4	6.6	4.3	4.3	5.5
Buffer (mEq/L)	0	28 (Lactate)	0	27 (Acetate), 23 (Gluconate)	0	0	16 (Acetate)
Dextrose (g/L)	0	0	0	0	25	50	50
Calories (Kcal/L)	0	9	0	15	85	170	175

*High-sodium "replacement" fluids are in red. Low-sodium "maintenance" fluids are in green.

and diarrhea. They have a [Na^+] near that of ECF, ranging from approximately 130 mEq/L (e.g., lactated Ringer's solution [LRS]) to a high of 154 mEq/L (e.g., 0.9% saline). Table 5-2 includes additional examples of replacement fluids, highlighted in red.

Isotonic high-sodium fluids are used both for hypovolemia and for less severe ECF volume depletion, such as dehydration. When given rapidly, they can be used to restore the intravascular fluid volume in cats with hypovolemia. They are also used, when administered more slowly, to replace ECF volume in states of isotonic dehydration that are not immediately life threatening, such as occurs in patients with gastrointestinal or urinary fluid losses when oral intake is insufficient to balance losses.

Isotonic high-sodium fluids are not suited for use as maintenance fluids. They lack sufficient solute-free water content to offset ongoing solute-free water loss, such as through respiratory evaporation. When used on a short-term basis, most patients with normal renal function will tolerate the excess Na^+ that these fluids contain when they are being used primarily to compensate normal daily ongoing hypotonic fluid loss. This is particularly true when patients are able to drink some water in addition to their intravenous fluid therapy. Some patients can become hypernatremic after therapy with high-sodium fluid. There are also some patients for whom the use of high-sodium fluids is contraindicated, including those with congestive heart failure, oliguric renal disease, and some edema states.

Isotonic high-sodium fluids are used to maintain patients with ongoing isotonic fluid losses, as, for example, in vomiting or diarrhea. However, in these patients the fluids are in fact being used for replacement of these losses, rather than for true maintenance. It is critical to understand this distinction. *Maintenance* is a term used to reflect what is needed to replace only normal sensible and insensible losses, and such losses are not isotonic. Isotonic fluids may work to maintain fluid balance in animals with additional pathologic losses because such patients need the additional sodium and chloride. However, such patients need to drink to provide solute-free water; otherwise, hypernatremia will develop. In addition to the relative solute-free water deficit of high-sodium isotonic fluids, all of these fluids are also too low in potassium to be used as true maintenance fluids, unless K^+ is added to the fluids. Patients with continuing ongoing losses for more than 1 to 2 days that stay on high-sodium fluids are likely to need nutritional support, which will also replace their hypotonic maintenance fluid needs.

Some patients with readily corrected deficits and no ongoing losses will need to be transitioned to a maintenance-type solution, such as Normosol-M-D5 or Plasmalyte-56-D5, after their rehydration and electrolyte needs have been corrected and before the start of enteral or parenteral nutrition. The need to change to a true maintenance fluid will be indicated by a progressive increase in serum [Na^+] in these patients. Changes should be made well in advance of the development of hypernatremia.

Sick cats that have been anorexic for 2 to 3 days or longer should receive nutritional support. Generally, the provision of enteral or parenteral nutrition sufficient to

TABLE 5-3 **Calculation Worksheet for Fluid Therapy***[†]

Components of the Fluid Plan		Type of Fluid	Volume of Fluid	
			mL/day	mL/h
Deficits	Isotonic			
	Hypertonic			
Maintenance	Normal ongoing losses			
	(Enteral contribution from feeding)		( )	( )
	Net normal loss to be provided by fluids			
Abnormal ongoing losses	GI			
	Urinary			
	Other sensible			
	Insensible			
Totals		1. 2. 3.	1. 2. 3.	1. 2. 3.

*The enteral contribution includes what the cat is eating or drinking on its own plus any provision of food or water through tube feeding. It is indicated in *parentheses* ( ) to signify that this volume is subtracted from the calculated maintenance fluid needs to yield the net that must be provided to the cat as part of intravenous fluid therapy plan.
[†]For a case example, see Table 5-8.

meet the patient's caloric needs will also provide maintenance fluid needs. Thus the use of additional isotonic, high-sodium fluids in this setting will be to replace excessive isotonic losses, such as those associated with gastrointestinal loss or polyuria. Intravenous fluid rates can be greatly reduced in patients receiving either enteral or parenteral nutrition to a rate sufficient to meet additional ongoing losses only. In other words, the fluid therapy recipe should account for all sources of fluid intake (Table 5-3; also see Table 5-8).

ACIDIFYING AND ALKALINIZING FLUIDS

Sick cats requiring fluid therapy may also have acid–base disorders, and fluid therapy can be used to mitigate these disturbances. Restoration of ECF volume will improve tissue perfusion and correct lactic acidosis. The replenishment of water and electrolytes in appropriate concentrations will also improve renal perfusion and normalize renal electrolyte handling, thus promoting an improved acid–base balance. The volume expansion and improved perfusion seen with appropriate fluid therapy will also promote the peripheral utilization of glucose and decrease production of lactate. The end result of this can be the normalization of acid–base balance without the need to resort to the use of sodium bicarbonate, which can have adverse effects, such as hypernatremia and central nervous system acidosis.

High-sodium crystalloids will have a primary effect on the patient's acid–base status, depending on their composition. As such, they can be classified as either acidifying or alkalinizing solutions. High-sodium fluids that contain more Cl^- than is present in the patient's ECF are acidifying. Although 0.9% saline has a high Na^+ content and thus is frequently used to restore intravascular fluid in hypovolemic patients, it also has a high Cl^- content and will be acidifying. This fluid is most appropriate for treatment of patients with hypochloremic metabolic alkalosis because it provides the necessary Cl^-. A common clinical scenario associated with hypochloremic metabolic acidosis is the vomiting of gastric contents. It is important to point out that although the measured pH of parenteral fluid solutions ranges from about 4 to 6.5, they are extremely weak acids. These low measured in vitro pH values will *not* reflect their effect on pH in the patient because of buffering.

Alkalinizing fluids, by contrast, do not have a higher Cl^- concentration than ECF fluid. Some of the chloride is replaced with another anion such as lactate, acetate, or gluconate. The anions are metabolized by the liver to bicarbonate. One example of a commonly used alkalinizing fluid is LRS.

SUPPLEMENTS

In some situations fluids must be supplemented with additional electrolytes; this decision is based on an assessment of the history, physical examination findings, and measured electrolyte values. Commonly added electrolytes are listed in Table 5-4. Electrolyte additives may be appropriate for replacing deficits, providing replacement for normal maintenance losses in anorexic patients, compensation for transcellular movement of ions, or replacement of ongoing gastrointestinal or urinary losses. Potassium and magnesium are found in some low-sodium hypotonic fluids formulated as maintenance fluids. If not, they can be added to fluids to maintain homeostasis in animals that are not depleted.

POTASSIUM All of the isotonic high-sodium fluids, apart from 0.9% NaCl, contain 4 or 5 mEq/L of potassium. Although this amount of potassium is within

TABLE 5-4. **Concentration of Common Fluid Additives**

Product	Concentration per mL
KCl	2 mEq each
KPO_4	4.4 mEq K^+, 3 mM PO_4
MgCl	1.97 mEq each
$MgSO_4$	4.06 mEq each
Ca gluconate 10%	0.465 mEq Ca^{++}
$CaCl_2$	1.36 mEq Ca^{++}
$NaPO_4$	4 mEq Na^+, 3 mM PO_4
Dextrose 50%	500 mg

From Abbott Animal Health Fluid Therapy Module 2, courtesy Dr. Steve Haskins.

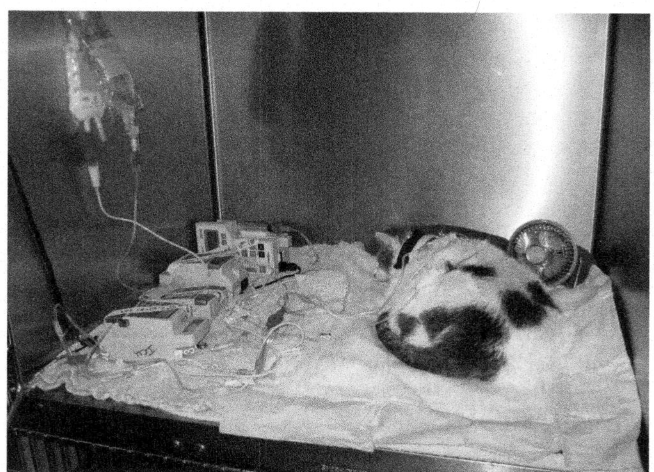

FIGURE 5-3 A constant-rate infusion is typically used to give K^+ separately when the patient seems resistant to "normal" amounts of K^+ supplementation, particularly in diabetic ketoacidosis.

TABLE 5-5 **Sliding Scale for the Amount of KCl Added to Intravenous Fluids Depending on the Serum [K^+]***

Measured Serum K^+ (mEq/L)	KCl Added (mEq/L)
>5.5	None
3.6-5.5	20
3.1-3.5	30
2.6-3	40
2-2.5	60
<2	80

*If the [K^+] of the fluid exceeds 5 mEq/L, the fluid must *not* be infused rapidly for intravascular volume restoration because of the risk of hyperkalemia.

the normal range of plasma [K^+], it is not in fact sufficient for maintenance of the patient. This is because therapy with intravenous isotonic high-sodium fluids typically causes a solute diuresis. The rate of flow of filtrate through the renal tubule is one of the factors regulating renal potassium excretion. As urine flow rate increases in response to intravenous fluid administration, K^+ loss in the urine will also increase. The loss of K^+ from the body will be further compounded by decreased intake in patients that are anorexic or hyporexic and by increased losses of K^+ in gastrointestinal secretions in patients with vomiting or diarrhea. Thus when isotonic high-sodium fluids are used for maintenance of patients that are drinking or for support of patients with ongoing isotonic fluid losses, it is necessary to supplement the fluids with additional K^+. A common level of supplementation for a cat that is normokalemic is the addition of 20 mEq/L of KCl to the isotonic high-sodium fluid. This amount is typically added to the K^+ already present in the fluids; it is not necessary to subtract the small amount that is already present in the fluid. If K^+ is not added to these fluids when they are used for more than a short time in normokalemic patients, hypokalemia will result.

For patients that are hypokalemic, a sliding scale is used to calculate how much potassium to add to the fluid. One such scale is shown in Table 5-5. When using the potassium-containing replacement fluids for fluid resuscitation, it must be remembered that if the K^+ concentration of the fluid exceeds 5 mEq/L, the fluid must not be infused rapidly for intravascular volume restoration because of the risk of hyperkalemia.

Cats with anorexia, gastrointestinal losses, or polyuria are particularly at risk for K^+ depletion. As an alternative to the sliding scale, a constant-rate infusion (CRI) is typically used to give K^+ separately when the patient seems resistant to "normal" amounts of K^+ supplementation, particularly in diabetic ketoacidosis (DKA) (Figure 5-3). This allows K^+ to be adjusted separately from the remainder of the fluid prescription. If CRI is used, it must be monitored very carefully. The usual dose range to replace normal ongoing losses of potassium is 0.05 to 0.1 mEq/kg per hour. The dosage for cats with severe whole body potassium depletion, severe symptomatic hypokalemia, or both can be as high as 0.5 mEq/kg per hour, known as KMax. Administration at rates higher than 0.5 mEq/kg per hour can cause serious or fatal cardiac arrhythmias. Administration of undiluted KCl (2 mEq/mL) through a programmable syringe pump is possible, but should only be done with extreme care, reserved for intensive care situations in patients with life-threatening hypokalemia (generally levels below 1.5 mEq/L).

PHOSPHATE Hypophosphatemia may develop rapidly during insulin therapy for DKA. For hypophosphatemia a portion or all of the phosphate (PO_4^-) can be administered as potassium phosphate (KPO_4) when the [PO_4^-] is less than 2 mEq/L or when serum [$PO4^-$] is observed to be decreasing rapidly and a drop below that level is expected. This also provides K^+ for concurrently hypokalemic patients. Hemolysis can occur when the $[PO_4^-]$ is less than approximately 1.5 mEq/L in cats. Sodium phosphate is used in the unusual case of phosphate-depleted patients that do not require potassium. The usual dose range to replace normal ongoing losses of phosphate is 0.01 to 0.03 mmol/kg per hour. Dose rates as high as 0.12 mmol/kg per hour may be necessary in some patients being treated for DKA.

MAGNESIUM Magnesium depletion is common in critically ill patients, particularly those with decreased dietary intake and polyuria, such as patients with diabetes mellitus. Supplementation is generally recommended when serum total magnesium concentration is less than 1.5 mg/dL. Because total serum magnesium concentration does not represent the physiologically active form of the element, measurement of ionized magnesium should be performed when possible; however, this assay is not readily available in most veterinary hospitals.

Replacement doses are 0.03 to 0.04 mEq/kg per hour for severe cases requiring rapid replacement and 0.013 to 0.02 mEq/kg/hour for more mild deficiency. $MgCl_2$ or $MgSO_4$ may be given but not mixed with calcium- or bicarbonate-containing fluids.[2] Patients with reduced GFR are at greater risk for hypermagnesemia during supplementation and require more frequent monitoring. Magnesium is a cofactor for potassium homeostasis, and magnesium supplementation should be considered in any patient with refractory hypokalemia.

CALCIUM Calcium gluconate 10% is used as a calcium source for animals with symptomatic hypocalcemia, such as that associated with eclampsia, hypoparathyroidism, acute pancreatitis, and renal failure. It may be administered on an emergency basis at a dosage of 0.5 to 1.5 mL/kg, diluted and given over several minutes, or it is added to fluid therapy and given more slowly and at a rate that is titrated to effect. Calcium chloride contains about three times the amount of calcium per mL compared with calcium gluconate and is administered at one third the volume of calcium gluconate. Calcium gluconate is preferred because it is less irritating if inadvertently given perivascularly. Renal failure patients often have hypocalcemia associated with hyperphosphatemia, and thus administration of calcium may lead to the formation of $CaPO_4$ in tissues. The latter occurs when the product of $[Ca^{++}]$ and $[PO_4^-]$ exceeds 70. Ideally, these patients should have their serum phosphate lowered as rapidly as possible to minimize this risk.

ELECTROLYTE INFUSIONS Because rapid infusion of any of these electrolytes can cause cardiac arrhythmias and other side effects, they should be added to fluids provided at a constant rate for maintenance to avoid inadvertent overdose. Delivery systems that guard against fluids being inadvertently left to run "wide open" are strongly recommended. Electrocardiographic monitoring is necessary when intravenous Ca^{++} or Mg^{++} are given rapidly.

When using these electrolyte additives, remember that divalent cation salts of phosphate are insoluble. They should not be added to fluids containing Ca^{++}, Mg^{++}, or PO_4^- to avoid precipitation of $CaPO_4$ or $MgPO_4$.

GLUCOSE Hypoglycemia may accompany critical illness and can be treated with dextrose supplementation. There is increasing evidence in humans that tight glycemic control improves outcomes in critically ill patients; whether this holds true in cats is unknown. Typically, 50% dextrose is added to intravenous fluids in concentrations from 2.5% to 5% to maintain blood glucose in the 80 to 120 mg/dL range. Final concentrations that are above 10% should be administered through central venous catheters to reduce the risk of thrombophlebitis. The concentration can be measured in percentage or g/dL. For example, to make 1 L of a 5% solution (5 g/dL or 50 g/L), 100 mL of fluid is removed from the bag and 100 mL (50 g) of 50% dextrose is added. For partial liters the amount of stock dextrose solution (usually 50% dextrose) to add can be calculated by the following means:

$$\frac{\text{Volume remaining in bag (mL)} \times \text{desired dextrose concentration (as a decimal)}}{\text{Concentration of stock solution (as a decimal)}}$$

For example, to make a 3% dextrose solution with 650 mL fluids using 50% dextrose:

$$\frac{650\ \text{mL} \times 0.03}{0.5} = 39\ \text{mL of 50\% dextrose}$$

The 39 mL of dextrose should be added after removing 39 mL of fluid from the bag.

Hypotonic Low-Sodium Crystalloids

MAINTENANCE

Low-sodium crystalloid fluids are indicated for the short-term support of water and electrolyte homeostasis by replacing normal ongoing losses in patients in which oral intake is not appropriate or possible. Thus hypotonic low-sodium fluids have historically been referred to as *maintenance fluids.* These crystalloids have a lower $[Na^+]$ than the ECF. Given that normal insensible fluid losses (respiratory and other evaporative loss) do not contain Na^+, these fluids are indicated when the patient needs a supply of solute-free water to replace daily requirements normally met through drinking and metabolism of food. The $[Na^+]$ concentration of low-sodium crystalloid fluids ranges from 0 mEq/L in the case of 5% dextrose in water to 77 mEq/L in the case of a half-strength, or 0.45%, saline solution. Solutions with less than 77 mEq/L of Na^+ contain 2.5 or 5% dextrose to raise the osmolality closer to that of ECF. Nonetheless, maintenance fluids are hypotonic and must be given slowly to allow for equilibration and to prevent hemolysis. It is important to note that dextrose, when present in these fluids, does not provide significant calories. The addition of dextrose is merely a way to raise the osmolality of the fluid (to make it isotonic with plasma) with a readily metabolized solute that will allow sodium-free water to be administered intravenously without causing hemolysis. It should be noted that the potassium content of the hypotonic low-sodium crystalloids is highly variable. As previously discussed, a potassium concentration of 20 mEq/L is the minimum that is usually considered necessary for true maintenance of a normokalemic patient.

Table 5-2 lists some examples of low-sodium crystalloid fluids in green. The rate of administration of IV fluids used for maintenance is based on the metabolic body size and will only change when patients begin to eat and drink. Low-sodium crystalloids are contraindicated in patients requiring rapid administration, such as for hypovolemia, as doing so will rapidly reduce the ECF [Na^+] and cause cell swelling due to rapid reduction in osmolality.

SUBCUTANEOUS ADMINISTRATION

Fluids administered to replace normal ongoing losses on a long-term basis are generally best provided orally, such as by means of an enteral feeding tube. This also allows for the essential provision of additional calories. These fluids can also be given subcutaneously in animals that are too ill to consistently maintain their hydration orally, such as cats with severe chronic kidney disease (CKD). Half-strength LRS with dextrose is an example of an appropriate fluid type for this type of subcutaneous administration. However the provision of fluids containing dextrose in the home setting may add risk, in that these fluids can support the growth of fungi and bacteria when single bags of fluid are generally reused for multiple days. LRS without dextrose is also an appropriate fluid type for this type of subcutaneous administration. Although classified as a high-sodium isotonic crystalloid, LRS is often used for subcutaneous fluid administration for cats that cannot maintain hydration orally. This fluid is slightly hypotonic to plasma and can provide some solute-free water. Anecdotally, LRS is better tolerated by patients during subcutaneous administration than is 0.9% sodium chloride or Normosol-R. However, LRS is still higher in [Na^+] than is optimal for maintenance use and may result in a higher Na^+ intake than is ideal. This may promote hypertension in predisposed patients and even hypernatremia when given chronically and at a high volume. An additional advantage of subcutaneous administration of LRS in cats with CKD is that this fluid is alkalinizing, which can be beneficial in managing the acidosis that often occurs in these patients.

OTHER USES

INFUSION VEHICLE Because the rate of administration of the maintenance component of a fluid therapy plan is often constant, these fluids may be used as a vehicle for the continuous administration of drugs provided they are physically compatible with the fluid. Several references exist that provide compatibility information for various medications and fluid compositions. If drugs are administered in this way, clinicians must remember that adjustments in the fluid rate to meet the patient's changing fluid needs will also affect the rate of delivery of medications.

HYPERTONIC DEHYDRATION Low-sodium crystalloid fluids are also used to treat hypertonic dehydration, which is loss of water in excess of solute. These patients are hypernatremic. This type of dehydration is comparatively rare in cats; heat stroke (one of the most common causes) is more frequently encountered in dogs. However, hypertonic dehydration may be seen in cats that are inadvertently locked in closets or basements without water or in animals with hypothalamic disease manifesting as hypodipsia. This type of dehydration may also be seen in cats with hyperglycemic hyperosmolar syndrome.

Combinations of High- and Low-Sodium Crystalloids

There is a common misconception that patients should only need to be given one intravenous fluid solution at any one time. There are many instances when both high- and low-sodium crystalloid fluids should be used concurrently. Patients that are not eating or drinking will need to have an ECF volume deficit replaced or will have ongoing excessive losses in addition to their maintenance needs. Combinations of fluids in these patients are often better able to meet their requirements than are prepackaged "maintenance" fluids.

Thus the cat will require a calculated amount of a high-sodium crystalloid to restore its ECF content back to normal baseline and replace any pathologic ongoing loss of high-sodium fluid, such as gastrointestinal losses or polyuria. The patient should also be given a low-sodium crystalloid to replace its normal daily losses of solute-free water. It is very important to remember that cats with inadequate caloric intake must also have those needs addressed very early in their hospitalization. Provision of nutrition through enteral or parenteral means will also meet maintenance fluid needs, as mentioned previously.

Hypertonic Saline Solutions

Hypertonic saline fluids contain sodium at concentrations substantially higher than the ECF; thus they facilitate rapid restoration of the ECF Na^+ content during treatment of hypovolemic shock. Increasing the [Na^+] in the ECF produces a rapid, although transient, osmotically driven movement of water from ICF to ECF, which can occur far more quickly than when infusing isotonic high Na^+ fluids alone. Because the ECF volume determines plasma volume, this fluid type is thus a rapid intravascular volume expander, at the expense of the ICF fluid volume. Hypertonic saline doses must be followed by infusions of isotonic high-sodium fluids to maintain their effect, insofar as they will rapidly equilibrate from the intravascular space into the ICF. Hypertonic saline will expand the intravascular volume by 2.5 to 3 mL for each mL infused.[15]

Clinical situations in which hypertonic saline may be useful in cats include resuscitation of animals with both hypovolemic shock and preexisting tissue edema, particularly cerebral edema resulting from traumatic brain injury. Hypertonic saline promotes rapid restoration of blood volume to improve blood flow to the brain while simultaneously decreasing cell volume, thus reducing brain edema. It also has positive inotropic effects on the myocardium. There are several contraindications to the use of hypertonic saline, including heart failure, uncontrolled hemorrhage, hypernatremia, and severe dehydration. Hypertonic saline is not appropriate as a treatment for chronic hyponatremia because of the risk for severe neurologic side effects that ensue when hyponatremia is corrected faster than 0.5mEq per hour.

Hypertonic saline solutions range in concentration from 3 to 23.4%. Solutions above 7.5% must be diluted before administration because they can cause phlebitis at the injection site. The dose in cats for the 7.5% solution is 2 to 4 mL/kg administered over 5 to 10 minutes.[3] Hypertonic saline may be given in combination with a colloid. One way to accomplish this is to add 1 part of 23.4% saline to 2 parts of a hetastarch; this yields a solution with a final concentration of just above 7.5%.

Colloids

General Characteristics of Colloids

Colloids are high-molecular-weight substances contained in a high-sodium solution, usually 0.9% saline. Unlike crystalloids, colloids will not readily diffuse through the vascular endothelium and will thus stay in the intravascular space longer than crystalloids. This effect is beneficial in achieving a sustained increase in intravascular volume when treating hypovolemia. In states of low oncotic pressure, such as is seen with sepsis, systemic inflammatory response syndrome (SIRS), and hypoalbuminemia, colloids can theoretically plug leaks in capillary endothelium and prevent extravasation of fluids and the resultant edema.

Colloids are often used to replace and maintain intravascular colloid osmotic pressure (COP) and decrease edema that can result from the use of crystalloid fluids. Colloids are rarely used alone, however; they are typically used in conjunction with crystalloid fluids. Because of their efficient volume expansion, colloids can produce volume overload and pulmonary edema at lower volumes than crystalloids.

The crystalloid-versus-colloid controversy for resuscitation of hypovolemic patients has been an ongoing discussion in human and veterinary medicine for many years. Results of studies have failed to show a clear benefit to colloids, despite numerous theoretical advantages. Some studies have concluded that colloids promote decreased mortality, whereas other studies have shown better results with crystalloid therapy. Until more veterinary studies have been undertaken, it is difficult to make specific recommendations. One clinical approach to hypovolemic feline patients would be to begin with crystalloid therapy, reserving colloid therapy for patients who fail to respond. As previously discussed, hypothermic feline patients should be aggressively rewarmed concurrently with fluid therapy. For the markedly hypotensive patient, crystalloids, colloids, and potentially blood products may have to be provided concurrently.[11]

Natural Colloids and Blood Products

Natural colloids include human albumin, blood products, and hemoglobin-based products. They are generally more expensive than the synthetic colloids, but there are certain situations in which they are preferred. The main use of fresh whole blood (FWB) and packed red blood cells (PRBCs) is in patients with symptomatic anemia. As a very general guideline, blood transfusion should be considered at a packed cell volume (PCV) below 20% (which corresponds to a hemoglobin concentration of 7 g/dL). However, the decision to transfuse should also be based on the patient's clinical signs and not on numeric values alone. More details on blood transfusion medicine are found in Chapter 25.

FWB contains all of the coagulation factors and platelets, so it can be used in patients with coagulation or platelet disorders. However, 6 to 8 hours after donation, platelet viability is markedly diminished. Fresh plasma, which is less than 6 to 8 hours old, has all of the coagulation factors but will not have platelets unless platelet-rich plasma is specifically prepared. Refrigerator storage of whole blood or plasma results in the gradual loss of the unstable or labile coagulation factors (factor VIII and von Willebrand's factor) within about 24 hours and factor V and factor XI after about 1 week. What remains are the stable coagulation factors: II, VII, IX, X, and XIII. Fresh frozen plasma (FFP) is created by freezing plasma within 4 to 6 hours of collection. Freezing destroys platelets but preserves all coagulation factors. FFP should not be used for thrombocytopenia or thrombocytopathia. Plasma can be frozen for up to 1 year with the unstable coagulation factors preserved. Plasma that has been frozen after 6 hours of collection or kept frozen for longer than 1 year does not provide coagulation factors, only albumin, and is known as frozen plasma (FP).

Plasma or concentrated human albumin can also be used primarily for albumin replacement, although the volumes of plasma needed may be prohibitive. Albumin, although it has many functions, is the principal protein responsible for COP. Fluids containing albumin include concentrated albumin and some blood products.

The discussion of human albumin must be prefaced with a statement that its use in cats is considered controversial by many. Concentrated human albumin solution typically contains 20% or 25% albumin (200 or 250 mg/mL). By contrast, whole blood and plasma contain about 2.5% albumin; thus they will not increase intravascular COP or albumin as effectively and will require higher volumes.

Plasma can be used for albumin replacement and oncotic pressure support at a dosage of 20 to 30 mL/kg, but the volumes needed can risk volume overload and incur considerable expense. Concentrated 25% albumin may be the more appropriate colloid for resuscitation in patients with symptomatic hypoalbuminemia, particularly in postoperative or septic critical care feline patients.

Cats must always be blood typed before any blood product administration (human serum albumin does not require blood typing for cats), and donors must always be typed. A cross-match should ideally be performed for all transfusions but may not always be feasible because of the typically limited number of donors against which to cross-match.

Simply replacing albumin because the measured value is low is not indicated in the absence of clinical signs and exposes the patient to unnecessary risk. If possible, nutritional support by way of enteral or parenteral nutrition is the preferred means for normalizing serum albumin through hepatic synthesis, but this may not always be feasible. It should also be noted that in patients with protein-losing disorders, such as protein-losing enteropathies or nephropathies, albumin that is administered therapeutically will quickly be lost by the same routes as the patient's own albumin.

Albumin dose for transfusion of concentrated albumin solutions can be calculated through the following formula:

1. Calculate the total body plasma volume in deciliters: 4.5% of body weight (kg) × 10.
2. Calculate the total plasma albumin in grams (patient and target value): This is the patient's measured serum albumin level × plasma volume, as well as the desired albumin level × plasma volume (typically a value of 2 g/dL is sufficient for a target level).
3. Calculate the plasma albumin deficit; this is the difference between the patient's albumin level and the target level.
4. Because only 40% of the total body albumin resides in the vascular space (60% is interstitial), divide the plasma albumin deficit by 0.4 to obtain the total body albumin deficit in grams.
5. Calculate the volume of albumin needed, given that 1 mL of 25% albumin contains 250 mg of albumin. This is equivalent to multiplying the albumin deficit in grams by a factor of 4 for 25% and a factor of 5 for 20%.

An example calculation is given in Box 5-2.

As a general rule, administration of 1 mL of whole blood per kg body weight will raise the PCV by 1%. Thus for a rise of 10%, one would administer 10 mL/kg whole blood. PRBCs can be dosed at 75% of the whole blood dose because of the higher PCV.

Risks of using concentrated human albumin and blood products in cats are allergic transfusion reactions and volume overload.[11] Signs of mild allergic transfusion reactions may include fever, vomiting, urticaria, and facial swelling. More serious transfusion reactions include acute respiratory difficulty, hypotension, and circulatory collapse. Urine, serum, or plasma can show signs of hemolysis. Fatal reactions to mismatched blood products can and do occur, particularly if a type B cat is administered type A blood. Delayed reactions up to

BOX 5-2

Calculation of Albumin Dose for Transfusion of Concentrated Albumin Solution: A Case Example

The patient is a 5-kg cat that is 2 days postsurgery for a septic abdomen caused by a penetrating injury. There is generalized edema and persistent vomiting. The serum albumin is 1.5 g/dL.

1. Plasma volume: 5 kg × 4.5% × 10 = 2.25 dL
2. Total plasma albumin: 1.5 g/dL × 2.25 dL = 3.375 g
3. Plasma albumin deficit using a target value of 2:
   a. Target: 2 g/dL × 2.25 dL = 4.5 g albumin
   b. Patient's albumin = 3.375 g
   c. Deficit is 4.5 − 3.375 = 1.125 g albumin
4. Total body albumin deficit is 1.125 g/0.4 = 2.8 g
5. Amount of 25% albumin solution to administer: 2.8 g/0.25 g/mL = 11.2 mL

several weeks later have also been reported with human albumin administration. Cats should have capillary refill time (CRT), mucous membrane color, temperature, pulse rate, and respiratory rate monitored initially every 15 minutes during the first hour of administration, then hourly until the transfusion is completed.

When side effects do occur, the transfusion should be immediately discontinued, and additional therapy considered, such as diphenhydramine (1 to 2 mg/kg intramuscularly) for mild reactions. Fast-acting corticosteroids, such as dexamethasone sodium phosphate (0.1 to 0.2 mg/kg intramuscularly or intravenously) may be used for severe transfusion reactions but are generally not needed for milder reactions. An assessment should be made to determine if there is a continued need for blood products but at a slower infusion rate. Re-evaluation of donor compatibility through further cross-matching should be considered. Because of the possibility that blood products may be contaminated with bacteria, submission of a sample for bacteriologic testing should be considered. Pretreatment with corticosteroids or antihistamines is not routinely indicated unless a patient has experienced a transfusion reaction in the past.

Once the unit of blood or plasma has been entered ("spiked" with the administration set), the transfusion should be completed within 4 hours to minimize the risk of bacterial contamination. Unused product should be refrigerated immediately and used within 24 hours, then discarded. (For instance, if a kitten were to receive a partial unit of blood, the volume to be administered would be drawn off under sterile conditions and transfused. The remainder of the unit could be refrigerated immediately, stored for 24 hours, and then administered.)

Oxyglobin (bovine hemoglobin glutamer-200, Hemopure) is another natural colloid. It is a hemoglobin-based oxygen-carrying solution used for the treatment of symptomatic anemia, and the dosages are the same as for whole blood. A benefit of Oxyglobin is that it has universal compatibility; therefore no blood typing or cross-matching is necessary.

There are considerable risks with the use of Oxyglobin in cats, and the veterinarian should carefully conduct a risk assessment for each patient before using it. When larger volumes are infused, it produces a dark plasma color, which interferes with enzyme-based chemistry analyzers (e.g., the Vet-Test Chemistry Analyzer, IDEXX Laboratories, Westbrook, Maine); thus these results may not be reliable. Side effects are most common in euvolemic patients, such as patients with immune-mediated hemolytic anemia. It is contraindicated in cats with known or suspected cardiac disease. Side effects include volume overload, pulmonary edema, vomiting, diarrhea, and hypertension. When side effects arise, the veterinarian should administer small quantities slowly and titrate to effect. Oxyglobin is not currently available commercially.

Synthetic Colloids

The most commonly used colloids are the synthetic hetastarch solutions. Hydroxyethyl starch is a synthetic polymer of glucose, a polysaccharide closely resembling glycogen. Available hydroxyethyl starch products include both hetastarch and pentastarch. 6% Hetastarch is formulated either in 0.9% sodium chloride or in LRS. The difference between the two is that hetastarch with LRS also contains calcium, magnesium, a small amount of dextrose, and a lower [Cl^-].

Hetastarch contains very large molecules that must be broken down before they leave the vasculature, which generates a long-lasting colloid osmotic pressure effect. Hetastarch may decrease inflammation in the intravascular space and decrease vascular membrane permeability by plugging leaks in vascular endothelium in cases such as septic shock and SIRS patients.[4]

Rapid infusions within 5 to 10 minutes in cats can result in vomiting and transient hypotension. This effect can be mitigated by using hetastarch in small volume increments to effect (on the order of 5 mL/kg) over 10 to 15 minutes. Total dose for use in shock and hypotension is 10 to 20 mL/kg.

Hetastarch can interfere with clotting; however, the presence of calcium in hetastarch with LRS may reduce this effect. Clinical evidence of bleeding has not been reported in patients receiving 6% hetastarch at doses up to 20 mL/kg/day. If the activated clotting time or partial thromboplastin time rises above 50% of the high end of the reference range, concurrent coagulation problems should be investigated. 10% Pentastarch contains a narrower range of hydroxyethyl starch molecule size. Without the largest molecule sizes present in hetastarch, pentastarch breaks down more quickly and is eliminated from the body more rapidly. It has less of an effect on blood coagulation than hetastarch does.

An important objective when using colloids is to infuse the smallest volume needed to achieve resuscitation endpoints, such as normalized heart rate, improved blood pressure, oxygen delivery, and lactate clearance. Cats are very susceptible to volume overload, which can result in serious and disastrous consequences, so careful monitoring is essential.

Because most patients receiving colloids are usually concurrently given isotonic crystalloids, the crystalloid volume for intravascular volume replacement and hydration can be decreased by 40% to 60% of the volume calculated for crystalloids alone.

When more than one type of colloid is indicated, the colloids are usually administered consecutively rather than simultaneously. For example, a patient with hemorrhagic shock caused by severe trauma may receive whole blood to correct hypotension and hypovolemia, then

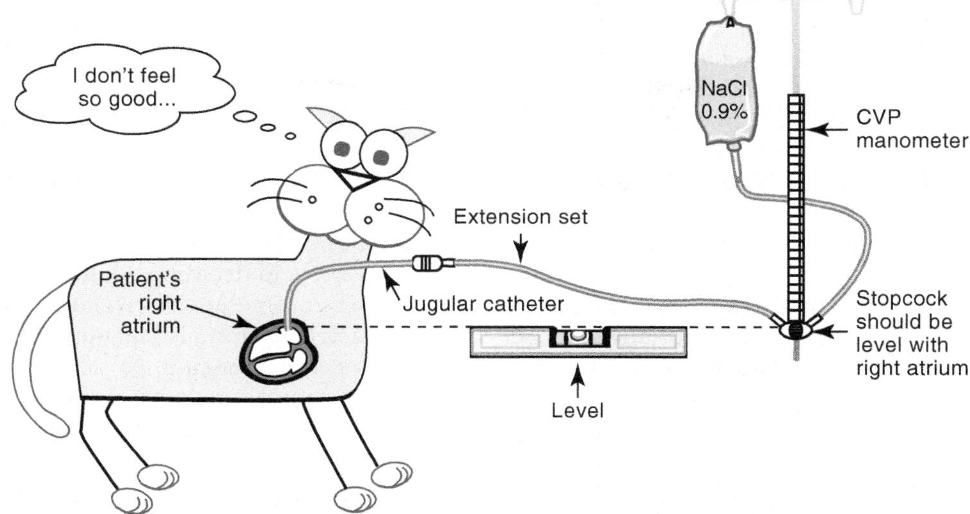

FIGURE 5-4 Monitoring of central venous pressure (CVP). A central catheter with the tip in the cranial or caudal vena cava can be used to guide fluid therapy and resuscitation. The normal CVP is 0 to 5 cm H_2O.

hetastarch for colloid maintenance during acute recovery. Bolus infusions of colloids are titrated in succession, and monitoring for endpoints of resuscitation is performed between boluses.

As previously discussed, cats should be monitored frequently for signs of volume overload, which include serous nasal discharge, jugular distention, chemosis, tachypnea, reduced lung sounds (suggestive of pleural effusion), moist lung sounds (suggestive of pulmonary edema), and subcutaneous edema. As shown in Figure 5-4, monitoring of central venous pressure (CVP) through a central catheter with its tip in the cranial or caudal vena cava (see section on vascular access later in this chapter) can also be used to guide fluid therapy and resuscitation. The normal range for CVP is 0 to 5 cm H_2O; marginal volume overload exists at 5 to 10 cm H_2O; serious volume overload occurs at amounts greater than 10 cm H_2O. Because of the considerable variability among operators, consistency in technique and positioning is vital. Trends in CVP are more clinically useful than any single measurement. CVP monitoring will be discussed in greater detail in the section on monitoring therapy for hypovolemia.

Colloids are relatively contraindicated in patients with active, uncontrolled hemorrhage because they may potentially interfere with platelet function and may exacerbate hemorrhage.

ROUTES OF ADMINISTRATION

Subcutaneous Fluid Therapy

Cats with mild illness or those requiring fluid therapy at home are candidates for subcutaneous fluid administration. Subcutaneous fluid therapy is not appropriate for cats with severe dehydration, hypovolemia, hypotension, or critical illness. Isotonic high-sodium crystalloid fluids (e.g., LRS) are most often used. The volume that can be delivered at any one site is limited by the distensibility of the subcutaneous tissue, which is generally favorable in the interscapular region of the upper torso. In most adult cats, fluid pockets of 50 to 150 mL can be accommodated without patient discomfort. Owners should be notified that fluid will settle ventrally with gravity and should disperse within a few hours. Just how much is too much is determined by the development of a painful, firm fluid pocket that leaks fluid from the hole created by the needle.

Although isotonic, high-sodium fluids are preferred, the following broader guidelines may apply to subcutaneous fluids. The osmolality of the fluid being administered should not exceed 450 mOsm/kg and the fluid should contain at least 40 mEq/L of sodium. The maximum concentration of K^+ should not exceed 40 mEq/L, although pain responses have been reported at even lower doses.[6] Fluids containing magnesium have also been observed to cause discomfort.

Intravenous Fluid Therapy

Venous Access

Vascular access is indicated for the following clinical scenarios:

- The patient needs fluid or colloid boluses to manage hypotension.
- The patient needs therapy for rehydration, nutrition, or electrolyte imbalances that cannot be met through enteral or subcutaneous means.

- The patient needs hemodynamic monitoring (CVP).
- The patient requires continuous infusions of analgesics or vasoactive substances.
- The patient requires other intravenous medications or transfusion of blood products.
- The patient needs frequent blood sampling (e.g., those with DKA).

If a particular patient does not fit into one of these scenarios, there may not be a need for intravenous access or intravenous fluids. Simply being hospitalized is not an indication for an intravenous catheter, unless the patient's status is uncertain and vascular access may be necessary. Consideration should be given to enteral provision of medications, nutrition, and fluids if the gastrointestinal tract is functional.

There are five main types of intravenous catheters: peripheral catheters, central venous catheters, peripherally inserted central catheters (PICC lines), intraosseous catheters, and winged infusion sets. Table 5-6 summarizes the features of these catheters.

Catheter gauge reflects the internal diameter of the catheter; the smaller the gauge number, the larger the diameter. If rapid fluid administration is required, it is advisable to choose the largest diameter catheter that fits within the vessel. Intravenous fluids can be administered most quickly through shorter, larger diameter catheters. For cats weighing less than 5 kg, 24- to 22-gauge catheters will be appropriate for routine fluid therapy, but smaller diameter catheters are prone to more technical problems. Most cats in the 5- to 7-kg weight range can accommodate a 22-gauge catheter for routine fluid therapy. Larger (18- to 20-gauge) catheters are useful for resuscitative therapy.

Venous catheters should not be placed in limbs that are traumatized or painful. Animals with severe coagulopathies, including hypercoagulability, should not have catheters placed in the jugular vein, if at all possible. A cat with an aortic thromboembolism should not have a catheter placed in either of the pelvic limbs.

The cephalic and accessory cephalic veins of the thoracic limbs or the lateral saphenous vein of the pelvic limbs are the most common peripheral veins catheterized in feline patients. Alternative vessels include the medial saphenous veins and the femoral veins. The peripheral vessels of hypotensive cats may not be easily observable, although the lateral and medial saphenous veins are often most visible on account of the thin overlying skin in these areas.

If the skin or subcutaneous tissues in the area of the catheter are compromised, that site should be avoided to decrease the risk of infection and thrombosis. If the leg and catheter wrap are likely to be soiled, the risk of a catheter-site infection is increased. Patients with diarrhea, urinary leakage, or vaginal discharge should have catheters placed in the thoracic limb. Vomiting patients should have the catheter adequately wrapped or have a hind limb catheter. The appropriate choice of vein should minimize the risk of the patient damaging or removing the catheter. Generally, a light wrap will be sufficient to prevent most cats from attempting to remove their catheters; however, some may require an Elizabethan collar to prevent premature removal.

Operator expertise and the temperament of the patient also play a role in deciding where the catheter should be placed. It can sometimes be a challenge to place intravenous catheters in animals that are extremely small, hypovolemic, or challenging to restrain. Newly trained veterinary professionals should place the catheter in a vessel that is readily visible and amenable to catheterization. Experienced veterinary professionals should make the initial catheter attempts when placing larger catheters in critically ill patients, especially if the vessels are difficult to visualize. Animals that are fractious should not have catheters placed in the thoracic limbs because it may be difficult to gain access to the catheter without risk of staff injury.

The overall treatment goal for the patient should be considered when deciding on catheter type and location. Any vein may be used for short-term administration of intravenous fluids. A centrally located catheter or PICC line may be required for the following:

- Long-term (>3 to 5 days) fluid or IV drug administration
- Parenteral nutrition
- Treatment with hypertonic or irritating fluids or drugs
- Concomitant delivery of incompatible drugs or fluids
- Frequent phlebotomy sampling
- CVP monitoring
- Transvenous pacing

How to Place an Intravenous Catheter

The jugular or saphenous veins are most commonly used to gain access to the central venous circulation. Preparation for placement of a catheter consists of several steps: gathering all necessary supplies, clipping the catheter insertion site with a well-lubricated 40 blade, applying a surgical prep to the catheter insertion site, and occluding the vein. When establishing intravenous access, caution should be used in very ill, dyspneic, or compromised patients, for whom the stress of physical restraint could cause an acute decompensation of their condition.

Sites for indwelling catheters should be aseptically scrubbed with sterile gauze squares freshly soaked with antimicrobial solution, alternating with either alcohol or sterile water. A total of three scrubs should be performed, and contact time of the scrub solution with the skin surface should be 3 to 5 minutes. Care should be taken

TABLE 5-6 **Features of Catheters that Are Used to Gain Vascular Access in Cats**

Type of Catheter	Indications	Advantages	Disadvantages	Comments
Peripheral	Short-term fluid and/or medication administration	Ease and speed of placement Low complication rate	Tip may fray, damaging vein Often becomes nonpatent May be resented or dislodged by patient	Available as over-the-needle or through-the-needle (former used more commonly)
Central venous	Hyperosmolar solutions (<600 mOsm/L) Parenteral nutrition Long-term fluid or medication administration Caustic drugs Frequent blood sampling CVP monitoring	Large gauge allows blood sampling Patency maintained longer	More difficult and time-consuming to place More expensive	Multiple lumen catheters can facilitate blood sampling and concurrent fluid and parenteral nutrition administration
Peripherally inserted central catheter (PICC)	Coagulopathy Hyperosmolar solutions (<600 mOsm/L) Parenteral nutrition Long-term fluid or medication administration Caustic drugs Frequent blood sampling CVP monitoring	Allows frequent blood sampling Patency maintained longer	More difficult and time-consuming to place More expensive	Inserted into a peripheral vein and terminating in a great vessel Positioning should be verified with radiographs
Intraosseous	Very small patients (e.g., kittens)	Avoid difficult catheter placement in small veins	Cannot use to take blood samples	18-gauge needle Sites include proximal humerus, intertrochanteric fossa of femur, and proximal tibia
Butterfly catheter	Very short-term administration of medications or small volumes of fluid	Ease and speed of placement	Tip may lacerate vein	Should not be bandaged in place or left unattended

CVP, Central venous pressure.

during shaving and scrubbing not to damage the skin surface; this can increase the chance of catheter-site infection.

Appropriate antiseptic agents include chlorhexidine gluconate 4%, chlorhexidine diacetate 2%, or povidone–iodine. The clinician should remove the residual scrub solution from the skin and surrounding hair with gauze sponges soaked in alcohol, sterile water, or sterile saline solution. Residual soap is removed from the skin to avoid irritation. The person placing the catheter should wash his or her hands and apply a germicidal lotion before catheter placement. Clean examination gloves are recommended during catheter placement of peripheral intravenous catheters, and sterile gloves are donned during PICC and central line placement.

For central lines or in patients with thick skin, it may be helpful to make a facilitating incision to ease catheter passage and decrease damage to the tip of the catheter associated with passage through tissue. To create a facilitating incision, the clinician should slide the skin overlying the venipuncture site to either side of the vein, make an incision about 0.5 mm long using a the bevel of a 20-gauge needle, and then let the skin return to its original position. The incision should now be ideally placed over the vein. The catheter is inserted through the newly created incision.

The final preparation step in catheter placement is to occlude the vein proximal to the anticipated insertion site. The assistant should make sure the vessel is in a position that will be conducive to catheterization. For cephalic catheterization, this is accomplished by rolling the vessel laterally (usually with the thumb that is occluding the vein). The assistant should also ensure that the patient's head is properly restrained so the cat cannot cause harm during the procedure. Trimming nails before catheterization may also help decrease scratch injuries. Some cats require at least two people to properly position and restrain them, whereas others are more compliant with less restraint. Chemical restraint may be needed for some cats. Caution should be used in very ill or compromised patients, for whom the stress of physical restraint could cause an acute decompensation of their condition.

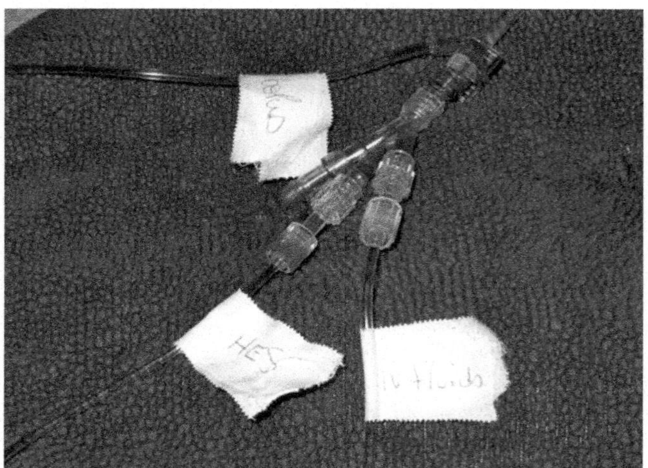

FIGURE 5-5 Multiple fluid lines can be attached to one intravenous catheter with the use of three-way connectors.

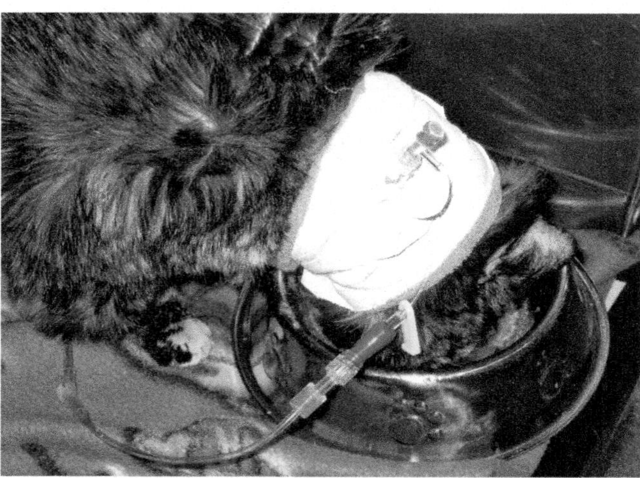

FIGURE 5-6 A properly wrapped jugular catheter will still allow the patient to eat and drink.

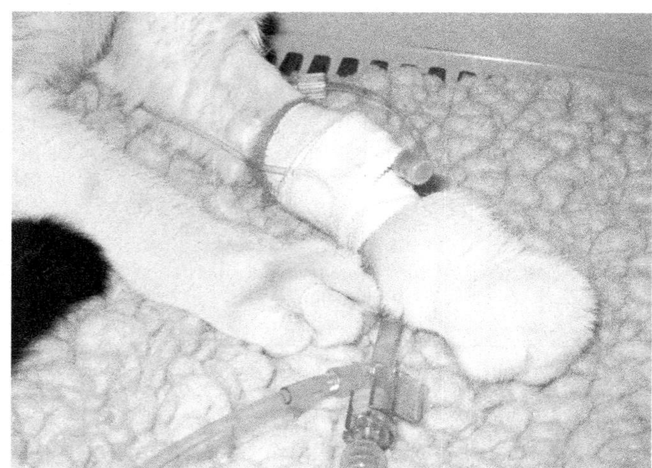

FIGURE 5-7 Swelling distal to a catheter is commonly caused by an excessively tight bandage or tape.

For peripheral catheter insertion, the limb is stabilized and the catheter inserted with the bevel up at an approximately 15-degree angle to the vessel. The catheter is then advanced into the vessel a few millimeters, making sure to stay parallel to the vessel so it does not penetrate the far vessel wall. When blood appears in the hub of the stylet or catheter, the needle and catheter are advanced together approximately 1 to 4 mm to ensure the end of the catheter is entirely inside the lumen of the vessel. The catheter is then advanced off of the stylet and into the vessel. The stylet is removed, and either an injection cap or T-connector is placed on the end of the catheter and flushed with saline. Multiple fluid lines can be attached to one intravenous catheter with the use of three-way connectors (Figure 5-5).

Signs that indicate the catheter is not in the vein include resistance to injection or a visual bleb of fluid forming in the subcutaneous space when a small volume of saline is injected.

Once the catheter has been inserted and the stylet removed, the catheter should be taped in place (for peripheral catheters) or sutured in place (for most central lines). Catheters that will be left in place for more than a few minutes should be covered with a light dressing that protects the catheter from traction, damage, or contamination (Figure 5-6). Addition of antibiotic ointment is not necessary. The catheter wrap should be thick enough to protect the catheter but not so occlusive that moisture will accumulate. The catheter wrap should allow daily visual inspection of the insertion site. For long-term peripheral catheters, typically a layer of cast padding is placed over the tape, followed by stretch gauze, and then adhesive or self-adhesive bandage material. The material should be wrapped snugly but should not occlude venous return or edema will result. Catheters intended for very short-term use (minutes to a few hours) can be wrapped with adhesive tape alone, if desired.

Once the catheter has been properly placed and secured, it is necessary to monitor and maintain it to ensure proper function and minimize the risk of infection. Indwelling venous catheters should be unwrapped and the insertion site examined and cleaned every 24 hours or more frequently if the catheter wrap is soiled. Swelling distal to a catheter is commonly caused by an excessively tight bandage or tape (Figure 5-7).

There is no evidence in veterinary patients that the common practice of routine catheter replacement every 72 hours is warranted. If a catheter is functional without any signs of thrombophlebitis, the catheter should be closely monitored and can be left in place. The purpose of catheter monitoring is to identify any of the following signs of thrombophlebitis:

- Thrombosis, or formation of a thrombus on the catheter or vessel wall
- Embolism, or breakage of a portion of the catheter into the circulation
- Subcutaneous fluid infiltration or leakage at the insertion site
- Infection or purulent discharge
- Pain on injection
- Otherwise unexplained fever

Should any of these complications be identified, removal of the catheter should be considered. Culture of the catheter tip is recommended in patients with evidence of catheter site infection or unexplained fever.

Catheters that are used for continuous fluid therapy do not need to be flushed routinely but should still be visually inspected. Catheters that are not in use should be either removed or flushed every 4 to 6 hours using 0.9% NaCl with or without the addition of 1 U/mL of heparin.

To decrease the risk of bacterial contamination, administration sets should be sterile and clean technique, including clean hands and disposable gloves, should be used to attach and detach the system when changing fluid bags. A T-connector should be used to help prevent the catheter from being pulled out from the insertion site and should be clamped whenever fluids are not flowing through the catheter. Needleless connection systems minimize contamination of the catheter and fluid lines by decreasing entry into the system, but these are considerably more expensive than conventional fluid sets.

The fluid administration tubing should be anchored to the catheter bandage with tape to prevent premature dislodgment. If the T-connector is securely taped to the leg, this may not be necessary, but it provides extra security in active patients. If a needleless connector is used, the fluid line should be disconnected before moving a patient, if possible.

Intravenous tubing and fluid bags should be changed every 24 to 72 hours. Injection ports and needleless connectors should be swabbed with 70% isopropyl alcohol before needle puncture or drug administration. All injection caps should be replaced after approximately 20 penetrations or if there is any observed fluid leakage.

FLUID THERAPY PLANS AND MONITORING

Management of Hypovolemia

Assessment of Hypovolemia

Several parameters can be used to estimate the adequacy of circulating blood volume, although it is a physiologic variable that is almost impossible to quantify in vivo. It is important to assess several parameters because no single one can accurately depict overall cardiovascular status. Any of the following clinical signs can be associated with hypovolemia:

- Decreased jugular venous distention
- Poor pulse quality
- Hypotension
- Low CVP
- Hypothermia
- Tachycardia
- Pale mucous membranes
- Prolonged CRT
- Cool extremities
- Oliguria or decreasing urine production
- Metabolic acidosis
- Hyperlactatemia
- Decreased central venous oxygen

Many of these parameters can also be influenced by abnormalities in other body systems and are neither sensitive nor specific for hypovolemia in cats. Tachycardia deserves special mention, insofar as cats can have profound hypovolemia without the tachycardia commonly seen in other species. Important considerations for cats in shock are listed in Box 5-3.

Therapy Options for Hypovolemia

Correction of hypovolemia and restoration of tissue perfusion are the primary and immediate goals of fluid therapy in any patient with decreasing intravascular volume resulting from blood loss, severe dehydration, or shock. This can be accomplished in different ways depending on the cause and degree of the hypovolemia and the patient's response to therapy. Correction of hypovolemia should be accomplished rapidly and, in cats, should be undertaken in concert with establishment of normothermia and aggressive rewarming, given the link between vasomotor tone and body temperature that is unique to this species.

BOX 5-3

Important Considerations for Cats in Shock

- Cats are not small dogs.
- Cats are less tolerant of volume overload than dogs.
- Cats in shock may not be tachycardic (as seen in dogs).
- Blood pressure is more difficult to measure accurately in cats.
- Hypothermic cats cannot regulate blood pressure and are therefore more prone to volume overload; external rewarming should occur before aggressive fluid therapy to avoid volume overload.

Hypovolemia may be treated initially with high-sodium isotonic replacement crystalloids, which are generally available in every practice and very economical. Most crystalloid fluids are redistributed to the interstitial space within 30 to 60 minutes of administration and thus can cause interstitial edema before an acceptable effective circulating blood volume is attained. When edema or hemodilution occur before hypovolemia has been corrected, it may be advisable to add an appropriate colloid or blood product depending on the cause of the hypovolemia.

When intravenous crystalloids redistribute to the interstitial space, the ensuing interstitial edema can result in decreased cellular perfusion. To mitigate this effect, the flow of fluid in the lymphatic system is increased in response to the higher hydrostatic pressure. High concentrations of albumin exist within the lymphatics, and this is rapidly returned to the systemic circulation. This is known as the *protein pump*. The resultant increase in plasma albumin concentration increases intravascular oncotic pressure, which reduces the interstitial fluid volume and increases the intravascular volume though changes in Starling's forces.

The feline blood volume is 50 to 60 mL/kg, which is often cited as both the daily fluid requirement (i.e., maintenance fluids) and the shock dose of fluids. Volumes and rates of fluid administered to treat hypovolemia and dehydration in cats must be considerably lower than those used in dogs because of the risk of fluid overload. To correct hypovolemia, a low dose of a replacement crystalloid is initially given, such as 25% of the shock dose, or roughly 10 to 15 mL/kg. A useful short-cut for calculating 25% of the shock dose of crystalloids for a cat is to add a "0" to the cat's body weight in kg. Thus 25% of the shock dose for a 5-kg cat would be 50 mL. Cardiovascular and physical examination parameters are then reassessed, and additional aliquots of fluid are administered until the cardiovascular status has improved or a full shock dose of fluids has been administered. Because of the risk for fluid overdose in cats, overly aggressive fluid therapy to rapidly achieve normal cardiovascular parameters cannot be recommended. The goal is to ensure resuscitation sufficient that the patient's status does not deteriorate as a result of hypovolemia, as well as prevent organ injury caused by poor perfusion. Any remaining deficit caused by dehydration can be corrected over the next 6 to 24 hours as part of rehydration fluid therapy.

An additional crystalloid that can be used to treat certain types of hypovolemia is hypertonic (usually 7%) saline. Hypertonic saline provides greater blood volume augmentation per volume administered than isotonic replacement crystalloids and has a positive effect on cardiac output. It has similarly transient effects to isotonic crystalloid fluids. It is most efficacious in patients with head injuries and those experiencing arrest because of its tendency to decrease cerebral edema. The efficacy of hypertonic saline is limited because repeated doses will cause significant hypernatremia, and electrolytes should be closely monitored during its use. Additionally, crystalloid fluids must be concurrently administered to offset the fluid shifts that take place from the interstitial space into the intravascular space. Hypertonic saline can be used in hypovolemia resuscitation at a dosage of 2 to 4 mL/kg, administered over 10 to 15 minutes. It is contraindicated with existing hypernatremia or severe dehydration.

Colloids can also be used to treat hypovolemia, with similar cautions regarding fluid overload in the feline patient as with crystalloid fluids. Colloids have the advantage of mobilizing interstitial fluid into the intravascular space and will actually increase the effective circulating volume by a greater amount than that infused. Additionally, colloids will remain in the intravascular space longer than crystalloids because they must be enzymatically degraded before elimination. For these reasons they are effective for the therapy of hypovolemia, low oncotic pressure, and shock. Total daily dose (typically used for oncotic support in hypoalbuminemic patients or those with vasculitis) as well as shock doses are in the range of 10 to 20 mL/kg. For shock, as for crystalloid therapy, 25% to 33% of the fluid dose (5 to 7 mL/kg) is administered rapidly over the first 5 to 10 minutes, and the patient's physical examination and hemodynamic parameters are reassessed.

Monitoring Response to Therapy in Patients with Hypovolemia

Monitoring is an essential component of fluid therapy and allows for ongoing adjustments in the fluid prescription to meet patient needs. Fluid therapy is a dynamic process requiring active and vigilant monitoring to ensure effectiveness, prevent complications, and meet treatment goals. Endpoints for resuscitation are given in Box 5-4.

BLOOD VOLUME STATUS PARAMETERS

Hypovolemia should be addressed in patients before therapy for dehydration. Volume status is classically divided into preload and forward flow parameters. The Frank–Starling law of the heart dictates that cardiac output is related to end-diastolic volume, a component of cardiac preload; for this reason adequate venous return is vital to ensuring appropriate perfusion. Preload parameters are indicators of the adequacy of venous return to the heart and include venous volume and cardiac chamber diameters. Venous volume cannot be directly measured in vivo and must be estimated by assessing the ease of venous distention, central venous pressure, and radiographic diameter of the caudal vena cava.

In a patient with normal blood volume, both jugular and peripheral veins should distend easily when

BOX 5-4

Resuscitation Endpoints

- Improved mentation
- Normal blood pressure (>90 mm Hg systolic)
- Normal heart rate
- Warm extremities
- Improved capillary refill time
- Urine output >1-2 mL/kg per hour
- SVO_2 >70% (mixed venous oxygen saturation): the SPO_2 of blood being returned to the heart—a measure of how much oxygen the tissues are extracting. Low SVO_2 indicates either excessive oxygen demand by the tissues or inadequate oxygen supply.

occluded. Lack of venous distention in vessels above the level of the heart may indicate hypovolemia. Obviously, this is a subjective assessment, but it can give some idea of relative volume status.

Venous volume can also be indirectly assessed by measuring CVP. CVP is the hydrostatic pressure of the blood entering the heart, as measured by a catheter with its tip in the right atrium or vena cava. CVP is proportional to the volume of blood in the anterior vena cava and venous tone. This pressure is decreased by hypovolemia or venodilation and is increased by fluid therapy or venoconstriction. Several other factors can contribute to the accuracy of CVP measurement, such as cardiac or respiratory pathology, making it a somewhat unreliable (but useful) physiologic variable.

CVP can be measured with a column manometer (the most common method) or a direct pressure transducer. The normal range is 0 to 10 cm H_2O. However, because of variations in venous tone and other technical factors, single CVP values are often difficult to interpret without the aid of other monitoring. Normal and abnormal values can overlap; for example, CVP can range from −5 to +5 cm of H_2O in hypovolemic animals and from 5 to 15 cm H_2O in animals with volume overload. Therefore measurements should be considered meaningful to the fluid therapy prescription only if they are below 0 or above 10 cm of water and, more important, if the overall trend in CVP is considered. Taking into account all available parameters, if a patient's CVP is consistently below 0 cm H_2O, consideration should be given to either a bolus of fluids or an increased rate of fluid administration. If a patient's CVP value is consistently above 10 cm H_2O, fluid administration should be slowed or discontinued, and diuretic administration should be considered.

CVP measurements are primarily indicated during volume restoration for shock and in patients for whom volume overload is a concern, such as patients in acute renal failure or those with concurrent cardiac disease.

Observation of correct technique for CVP measurement is very important, insofar as there is considerable interoperator variability. For the most accurate and clinically useful results, the patient's position should be recorded in the medical record and the same staff should perform the readings whenever possible.

To measure CVP (see Figure 5-4), the patient is positioned in right lateral recumbency and the level of the right atrium (near the manubrium—the cranial tip of the sternum) is identified. The clinician should ensure that the stopcock is level with the right atrium (this line is known as the *phlebostatic axis*) using a bubble level. This serves as the reference point and is the "zero" mark on the manometer.

With the stopcock closed towards the patient, the clinician opens the fluid bag line and fills the manometer to about 25 to 30 cm H_2O. The clinician then opens the stopcock toward the patient (turning it off toward the fluid bag) and allows the fluid in the manometer to run into the patient. At some point the fluid will begin to oscillate with the patient's heartbeat and will stop falling as it equilibrates with the pressure in the vena cava (usually about 25 to 30 seconds); this is the CVP measurement and should be noted in the patient's record.

Venous volume can also be very roughly estimated by evaluating the diameter of the caudal vena cava on a lateral thoracic radiograph. Normal diameter is roughly equivalent to one rib width. A small caudal vena cava diameter suggests hypovolemia, and further fluid administration may be indicated depending on the patient's status. A large caudal vena cava diameter may suggest hypervolemia or heart failure, and the fluid therapy prescription should be re-evaluated.

PARAMETERS RELATED TO LARGE ARTERIES

Physiologic parameters related to large arteries include pulse quality and arterial blood pressure. Pulse quality assessment through palpation is a reflection of stroke volume and the difference between systolic arterial pressure and diastolic arterial pressure, not a measure of blood pressure. For this reason, poor pulse quality does not always correlate with hypotension. Poor pulse quality can be associated with small stroke volumes, venoconstriction, or hypotension. Hypovolemia may be the most common cause of poor pulse quality, but it is also a feature of other conditions, such as poor cardiac contractility, tachycardia, restrictive heart disease, aortic stenosis, and positive pressure ventilation, none of which absolutely requires fluid therapy. If the cause of the poor pulse quality is determined to be hypovolemia by corroborating history, clinical signs, and other measurements, then fluid administration may be indicated.

Mean arterial blood pressure is the average pressure of the pulse pressure waveform. Systolic arterial blood pressure is the highest pressure of the waveform and is primarily determined by stroke volume and arterial wall compliance. Diastolic arterial blood pressure is the lowest pressure before the next stroke volume and is primarily determined by systemic vascular resistance and heart rate. Arterial blood pressure can be measured indirectly (with a Doppler transducer, occlusion cuff, and sphygmomanometer) or directly (with an arterial catheter by way of a pressure transducer). Normal systolic pressure measurements range between 100 and 160 mm Hg, mean pressure measurements between 80 and 120 mm Hg, and diastolic pressure measurements between 60 and 100 mm Hg.

The determinants of blood pressure (BP) are as follows:

$$BP = CO \times SVR, \text{ where CO is cardiac output in mL/min and SVR is systemic vascular resistance in dynes/sec/cm}^5.$$

Determinants of CO are stroke volume (SV) and heart rate (HR). Taken as a whole, the equation is as follows:

$$BP = (HR \times SV) \times SVR$$

From this relationship, it can be seen that in order to maintain constant BP (an analog for perfusion) in the face of falling cardiac output (as with hypovolemia), either the heart rate has to increase or the systemic vascular resistance (as mediated by catecholamine release) must rise.

Arterial blood pressure is not a very good measure of circulating blood volume because animals have a great ability to compensate for alterations in blood volume to preserve blood pressure. Eventually, however, severe hypovolemia will result in hypotension as heart rate may be maximized or the systemic vasculature may be maximally constricted.

Hypotension may be caused by hypovolemia, poor cardiac output, or excessive vasodilation, as illustrated by the previous formula. If the cause of the hypotension is hypovolemia, further fluid therapy is indicated. Hypotension resulting from vasodilation, as seen with hypothermia in cats, should be treated with cautious fluid therapy concomitantly with external rewarming. When inappropriate vasodilation is due to vasoplegia, as with sepsis or distributive shock, treatment should consist of fluid therapy coupled with vasoactive substances (pressors or catecholamines) such as phenylephrine or dopamine. It is important to remember that catecholamines should not be administered until the veterinarian is fairly certain that adequate circulating volume has been restored, because their use while the patient is hypovolemic will only worsen ischemia, not improve it. When hypovolemia is due to heart failure, further fluid therapy is not indicated and disease-specific therapy is required.

Another category of forward flow parameters is made up of variables that reflect precapillary arteriolar vasomotor tone. Increased vasomotor tone, or vasoconstriction, commonly occurs in conditions such as hypovolemia, heart failure, hypothermia, and administration of vasoconstrictors. Decreased vasomotor tone, or vasodilation, commonly occurs in conditions such as septic shock, hypothermia or hyperthermia, and administration of vasodilators and some anesthetics. Arteriolar tone can be assessed by monitoring mucous membrane color and CRT.

Normal mucous membrane color is pink. Vasoconstriction decreases capillary perfusion, causing the color of the mucous membrane to change from pink, to pale pink, and then to white as vasoconstriction progresses in severity. Vasodilation increases capillary perfusion, causing the color of the mucous membrane to change from pink to red as vasodilation progresses in severity. Ambient lighting, visual acuity, and patient pigmentation can make absolute assessment of mucous membrane color problematic, and it should be evaluated in concert with other variables and physiologic parameters. The most common sites to observe mucous membrane color are the unpigmented gingiva, tongue, and conjunctiva.

Deoxygenated hemoglobin causes a bluish discoloration of the capillary beds as cyanosis progresses in severity. Cyanosis is usually caused by hypoxemia, which should prompt an evaluation of pulmonary function, but it occasionally can be caused by sluggish capillary blood flow or diminished cardiac output, which necessitates further evaluation of cardiovascular function.

Anemia causes pale mucous membrane color and may warrant a hemoglobin infusion. Mucous membrane color is determined by the amount of oxygenated hemoglobin in the visible capillary beds. Arteriolar vasomotor tone determines the amount of blood in the observed capillary beds.

CRT is primarily determined by arteriolar vasomotor tone. CRT is assessed by using digital pressure on mucous membranes until they turn white and then noting how long it takes for normal color to return. Normal CRT is 1 to 2 seconds. The most common site to evaluate CRT is on unpigmented gingiva. Vasoconstriction, which prolongs CRT, may be caused by hypovolemia, heart failure, hypothermia, and administration of vasoconstrictors. If the patient's history and other cardiovascular parameters suggest hypovolemia, fluid therapy is indicated. Vasodilation shortens CRT. Vasodilation may be caused by septic shock, hyperthermia, and administration of vasodilators and some anesthetics. Vasodilation may cause hypotension, and blood pressure should be assessed in these patients.

Another forward flow category, tissue perfusion, includes extremity temperature, urine output, lactic acidosis, and central venous partial pressure of oxygen. Urine output can be used in cats with functioning kidneys as an indirect measure of renal perfusion and vital organ perfusion. Hypovolemia and dehydration reduce renal perfusion and GFR. In both situations there will be avid tubular reabsorption of Na^+ and glomerular filtrate, thus reducing the urine volume. A decrease in urine volume is thus expected with hypovolemia or dehydration if renal function and urine concentrating ability are normal.

Appendage temperature is a subjective assessment made by palpating the extremities. It can also be assessed by simultaneous measurement of core and toe web temperature. During vasoconstriction the extremities are not as well perfused as vital organs because of shunting of blood away from the periphery. Consequently, appendages cool toward ambient temperature. The normal core appendage temperature gradient is 2 to 4° C. Values in excess of this range suggest poor perfusion, most commonly caused by vasoconstriction or hypovolemia.

Metabolic acidosis has several causes, one of which is poor perfusion. This occurs when lactic acid is generated in poorly oxygenated tissues because of inadequate perfusion and anaerobic metabolism. Acidosis is best assessed by means of a venous blood gas and may be identified by an elevated blood lactate concentration not caused by lactated fluid administration, a decrease in measured bicarbonate or total CO_2 concentration, or a greater than normal base deficit. Normal blood lactate concentrations range between 0.5 and 2 mM/L. A point-of-care lactate monitor is available for veterinary patients (Accutrend, Roche Diagnostics), and lactate measurement should be considered for all hypotensive patients to help guide resuscitative measures. Rather than over-interpret any single value, normalization of elevated lactate after resuscitation can be used to indicate improved volume status and perfusion. Persistently elevated lactate values after initial fluid resuscitation should prompt a search for possible ischemic tissue (e.g., devitalized bowel) or a need for additional fluid therapy. Clinicians should not be overly surprised when finding elevated lactate in a compromised and hypotensive patient, but failure to normalize lactate should trigger a re-evaluation of the fluid prescription and possibly an evaluation for other causes of poor perfusion, such as cardiac disease or sepsis.

Central venous partial pressure of oxygen (CvO_2) is a measure of the relationship between oxygen delivery and oxygen consumption; alterations in either component will change CvO_2. When oxygen delivery is diminished for any reason, including poor perfusion, tissues will continue to extract oxygen to meet metabolic demand. Continued extraction in the face of diminished oxygen delivery results in a greater percentage of oxygen extraction from the blood, resulting in a reduction of CvO_2. Increased tissue demand for oxygen, as in a hypermetabolic state, will also decrease CvO_2 if oxygen delivery does not increase. CvO_2 can be assessed with point-of-care analyzers (such as the iSTAT, Abbott Laboratories; IRMA TruPoint, ITC Medical; or Stat Profile, Nova Biomedical) capable of performing blood gas analysis.

Jugular venous blood should be used to assess CvO_2 because peripheral venous values are highly variable and are considered unpredictable. Normal central venous CvO_2 values range between 40 and 50 mm Hg. Values between 30 and 40 are common in critically ill patients and have no known adverse consequences. Values between 20 and 30 mm Hg are progressively more worrisome, and values below 20 mm Hg are considered to indicate life-threatening tissue hypoxia.

If the cause of poor oxygen delivery is determined to be anemia, a hemoglobin infusion may be indicated. If the cause is determined to be hypoxemia, further evaluation of pulmonary function is indicated. If the cause is determined to be hypovolemia, further blood volume augmentation may be warranted. If the cause is determined to be heart failure or vasoconstriction, the underlying cause should be investigated and treated appropriately. Central venous PO_2 values above normal may represent hyperperfusion of the tissues but are more often taken to represent poor oxygen uptake by the tissues secondary to impaired oxygen metabolism, such as occurs in sepsis. No adjustments in fluid therapy are likely to be necessary.

The Hemodynamically Stable Patient

Development of a Fluid Therapy Plan

The patient's history, physical examination, laboratory results, and diagnosis are used to develop a fluid therapy plan by completing the following steps:

1. Determine the patient's fluid therapy needs, considering the component of these needs that will be met through the provision of the patient's nutritional requirements. This may occur if the patient is eating and drinking to meet some of its own needs or when parenteral or enteral nutritional support is provided.
2. Identify the ideal crystalloid(s) and/or colloid fluid to administer.
3. Determine the volume and rate of fluid administration for each fluid being administered.
4. Select the appropriate catheter type, size, and insertion site.
5. Develop a monitoring protocol, and make adjustments to the fluid therapy plan according to the patient's response to treatment.

HYDRATION STATUS VERSUS HYPOVOLEMIA

It is important to remember that hydration status is the total body water of the cat. It is reflected in the ECF volume (i.e., the crystalloid volume status of the ECF) and is determined by the ECF Na^+ content because of the equality of ICF and ECF osmolality. The vascular fluid compartment is an integral component of the ECF compartment, but the association between the volume of the ECF (and thus total body water) and hypovolemia can vary. Blood volume status and hydration status must be evaluated independently because changes in intravascular volume status can occur independently of hydration. Patients can be hypovolemic without being dehydrated. Patients on therapy can be made hypervolemic without correcting a total body water deficit. Patients with edema may be hypervolemic as a result of fluid overload or hypovolemic as a result of vasculitis or hypoproteinemia.

CREATING A FLUID PLAN

The fluid plan is generally divided into three categories, evaluated for each patient: deficits, maintenance, and ongoing losses. Within each category the clinician should determine the quantity and type of fluid to administer and also determine the fluid volume and rate for each type of fluid being administered. A worksheet such as that shown in Table 5-3 can be a useful tool for constructing a fluid plan. Although it is often preferable to use a single fluid because of cost considerations, it is not always appropriate to do this for complex cases or seriously ill cats.

CORRECTION OF EXTRACELLULAR FLUID VOLUME DEPLETION

The first element of the fluid plan should address preexisting dehydration. To determine the degree of total body water depletion (dehydration), the veterinarian should assess skin turgor, mucous membrane moistness, recent changes in body weight, urine output, and blood solute concentrations.

Most dehydrated patients have undergone isotonic fluid loss and thus have too low an ECF Na^+ content. The magnitude of the deficit is first assessed by changes in skin turgor and moistness of the mucous membranes. The skin along the back or shoulders is lifted into a fold and released. In ECF volume–replete patients, the skin will snap back rapidly to its resting position. If it is detectably slow, the animal is estimated to be about 5% dehydrated. If the skin stands in a fold, the animal has life-threatening ECF volume depletion of about 12% of body weight. Intermediate skin turgor between these two levels of detection is interpolated between 5% and 12% dehydration. These are just rough estimates because of individual variation. Poor skin turgor in emaciated cats may overestimate dehydration, whereas obesity may cause it to be underestimated. Mucous membrane moistness can be assessed to add further support for the initial estimation. Body weight change, especially in the short term, is an excellent way to estimate the percentage of dehydration, provided recent and highly accurate body weights have been recorded. When patients have a history consistent with the development of dehydration, such as vomiting, diarrhea, or polyuria coupled with poor intake, a 4% of body weight ECF volume depletion should be assumed even when skin turgor appears normal.

The volume deficit is calculated by multiplying the percentage of dehydration by the patient's body weight (in kg). For example, a 5-kg cat that is 5% dehydrated requires replacement of a fluid deficit of 250 mL, because 1 g equals 1 mL. This volume is then divided by the number of hours over which the deficit is to be restored to calculate the mL/hour fluid rate. Often, 24 hours is chosen for restoration of the deficit. However, the presence of azotemia believed to be prerenal or acute renal in origin requires a more rapid restoration of the deficit, such as within 4 to 6 hours. For a less critically ill patient or one with suspected or known heart disease, the clinician may elect to correct the deficit over as long as 36 hours or more. Again, it is important to recognize that these are merely guidelines, and the clinician should be prepared to periodically re-evaluate or change the rate of fluid administration in response to changes in the patient's clinical status.

When selecting the appropriate crystalloid, the clinician should always evaluate the history and clinical signs to understand how the deficit developed. This allows the clinician to make an educated guess as to the composition of the fluid that has been lost. When a serum chemistry panel with electrolytes becomes available, this can be used to confirm the best fluid composition for replacement. For example, fluids without calcium or potassium are indicated for patients with hypercalcemia or hyperkalemia. Fluids with a buffer will be indicated for patients with low serum bicarbonate. Table 5-7 illustrates the types of fluids recommended to replace specific types of losses.

The ideal way to determine the amount of KCl to add to the fluids would be to measure the serum $[K^+]$ and then use the sliding scale in Table 5-5. However, if the patient's current serum $[K^+]$ is not known, it is generally safe to use the empirical dosage of 20 mEq/L. When KCl is being added to parenteral fluids, it is important to mix the bag to distribute the KCl throughout the fluid.

CORRECTION OF INTRACELLULAR FLUID VOLUME DEPLETION

Although uncommon, some patients may have hypertonic dehydration. This develops when solute-free water is lost in excess of isotonic fluid loss. It is more commonly observed in dogs because they suffer from heat stroke more commonly than do cats because of the very high respiratory evaporative heat loss required for thermoregulation. However, cats can suffer heat stroke as well, losing water through respiratory and salivary losses. Cats trapped in basements and closets may experience hypertonic dehydration because they have been

TABLE 5-7 **Assessment of Typical Fluid and Electrolyte Losses for Various Clinical Syndromes**

Abnormality	Type of Losses	Type of Dehydration	Electrolyte Balance	Acid–Base Status	Fluid Therapy
Simple dehydration (water unavailable, stress, exercise fever)	Free water	Hypertonic Largely intracellular	Normal	Normal	Free water D5W
Heatstroke	Very hypotonic	Hypertonic	K^+ variable Na^+ variable	M Acidosis	0.45% NaCl, followed by balanced electrolyte solution
Anorexia (still drinking)	Hypertonic	Hypotonic	Na^+ lost K^+ lost	M Acidosis	Balanced electrolyte solution w/KCl supplement
Anorexia (unable to drink)	Hypotonic	Hypertonic Largely intracellular	Na^+ lost K^+ lost	M Acidosis	0.45% NaCl w/KCl
Vomiting (gastric contents)	Hypotonic or isotonic	Isotonic or mildly hypertonic	Na^+ lost K^+ lost H^+ lost Cl^- lost	M Alkalosis	0.9% NaCl w/KCl
Vomiting (duodenal contents)	Hypertonic or isotonic	Isotonic or mildly hypertonic	Na^+ lost Mg^{++} lost K^+ lost HCO_3^- lost	M Acidosis	Balanced electrolyte solution w/KCl
Diarrhea	Hypotonic or isotonic	Isotonic or hypertonic	HCO_3^- lost K^+ lost Mg^{++} lost Na^+ lost	M Acidosis	Balanced electrolyte solution w/KCl
Diabetes mellitus	Hypotonic	Hypertonic extracellular & intracellular	Na^+ lost PO_4^{--} lost K^+ lost Mg^{++} lost	M Acidosis HAG w/ DKA	Balanced electrolyte solutions w/KCl & Mg^{++} upon Rx, some need PO_4^{--}
Hypoadrenocorticism	Hypertonic	Hypotonic	Na^+ lost	M Acidosis	0.9% NaCl initially; if severe, balanced electrolyte solutions
Diabetes insipidus	Free water	Hypertonic largely intracellular	K^+ lost Mg^{++} lost	M Acidosis	0.45% NaCl
Hypercalcemia	Hypotonic	Isotonic or hypertonic	Na^+ lost	M Acidosis	0.9% NaCl w/KCl 0.45% NaCl if hypertonic
Chronic renal failure	Isotonic	Isotonic	Variable, depends on GFR H^+ retained	M Acidosis	Balanced electrolyte solutions usually w/KCl
Acute renal failure	Variable, depends on urine output	Variable, depends on urine output	K^+, H^+, PO_4^{--} retained Na^+, Mg^{++} variable	M Acidosis	Variable
Urethral obstruction	Isotonic or hypotonic	Isotonic or hypertonic	K^+, H^+, PO_4^{--} retained Na^+, Cl^- variable	M Acidosis	0.9% NaCl initially Followed by balanced electrolyte solution w/KCl
Congestive heart failure (untreated)	Isotonic gains	Isotonic Overhydration	Na^+ retention	R Alkalosis M Acidosis	D5W for KVO
Congestive heart failure (treated w/furosemide)	Dosage dependent	Variable	K^+ lost Na^+ variable	Variable, possible M alkalosis	Variable
Septic shock/SIRS	Isotonic	Isotonic	Na^+ lost	M Acidosis	0.9% or hypertonic NaCl, balanced electrolyte solutions, colloids
Hemorrhagic shock	Isotonic	Isotonic	Na^+ lost	M Acidosis	0.9% or hypertonic NaCl, balanced electrolyte solutions, colloids, blood

M, Metabolic; *R,* respiratory; *HAG,* high anion gap; *DKA,* diabetic ketoacidosis; *Rx,* prescription; *GFR,* glomerular filtration rate; *SIRS,* systemic inflammatory response syndrome.

Modified from Muir WW, DiBartola SP: Fluid therapy. In Kirk RW, editor: *Current veterinary therapy VIII,* Philadelphia, 1983, Saunders, p 31.

deprived of a source of oral water to replace losses. Hypertonic dehydration is detected by the presence of hypernatremia. The volume of a solute-free water deficit can be estimated from the plasma [Na^+] concentration as follows:

$$\text{Free water deficit (liters)} = 0.6 \times \text{body weight (kg)} \times [(\text{plasma } [Na^+]/148) - 1]^{8}$$

This type of volume deficit is given a separate line in the worksheet in Table 5-3 because the type of fluid required to replace the deficit is solute-free water. A water deficit can be replaced enterally or parenterally and is discussed in more detail in the section on fluid therapy for hypernatremia.

MAINTENANCE

Normal ongoing sensible and insensible losses must be balanced with maintenance fluid intake, provided either through fluid therapy or nutritional support. The cat's maintenance needs are calculated using the formula 30 × body weight (in kg) + 70. For example, for a 5-kg cat, this equals 220 mL. This is then divided by 24 hours to calculate a rate of 9 mL/hour. Maintenance fluid needs are replaced using a maintenance fluid type. Patients that are eating and drinking or are receiving enteral or parenteral nutrition support will have their maintenance fluid needs already fully or partially met.

ONGOING LOSSES

The fluid prescription must also offset any abnormal ongoing losses. The goal is to pick the best crystalloid that will most likely replace the electrolytes lost in the pathologic condition being treated; this is often the same fluid type being used for replacement. Typical losses associated with various clinical conditions are detailed in Table 5-7. Gastrointestinal and urinary losses can be measured. However, to prevent underestimating the losses, estimates are often used, based on client information (e.g., the volume and frequency of vomiting) for the first few hours of fluid therapy before such measurements are made.

Some patients also have abnormal insensible losses such as those due to increased respiratory loss or fever. These types of losses are insensible and replaced with solute-free water. Because they cannot be measured, they must be estimated. Allotting an additional one quarter to one third of maintenance rate, depending on severity, is a reasonable starting estimate.

ACID–BASE

Acid–base status is important in fluid selection because many crystalloid fluids contain buffers. The three most prevalent buffers found in commercial crystalloid solutions are lactate, acetate, and gluconate; they are bicarbonate (HCO_3^-) precursors.

The cat's acid–base status may be assessed from a serum total carbon dioxide concentration ([TCO_2]), or a venous blood gas. [TCO_2] provides an estimate of [HCO_3^-]. Metabolic acidosis occurs when the [TCO_2] is lower than normal, and metabolic alkalosis occurs when the [TCO_2] is higher than normal. It must be remembered that any metabolic acid–base derangement may be primary or compensatory. For example, a metabolic alkalosis may exist as a primary disorder owing to vomiting of gastric contents, or it may exist as a compensatory response to respiratory acidosis; thus [TCO_2] must always be assessed in light of the cat's history and clinical signs. For patients with severe or complex acid–base disorders, a blood gas is necessary for complete assessment.

Buffers are used for prevention and treatment of metabolic acidosis because they replace HCO_3^- deficit. However, buffered solutions are considered contraindicated in patients with metabolic alkalosis.

Cats rarely need to be treated for metabolic acidosis with HCO_3^- itself because the kidney is able to correct the acid–base imbalance after fluid replacement and treatment of the primary disease. However, when acidosis is severe ($pH < 7.1$), the mEq of sodium bicarbonate to administer is calculated by multiplying the body weight (in kg) by the base excess obtained from a blood gas sample and multiplying this by a value of 0.3, representing the ECF space to which the $NaHCO_3$ will redistribute. Only metabolic acidosis, and not respiratory acidosis, should be treated with $NaHCO_3$. Respiratory acidosis is treated by improving the cat's ventilation.

Typically, only one third to one half of the aforementioned calculated replacement dose of $NaHCO_3$ is given intravenously, over 15 to 30 minutes, once the intravascular volume has been restored. After administration and time for equilibration, another blood gas may be sampled to re-evaluate the patient's acid–base status. The goal is not to completely normalize the acidosis but to increase the pH to a value of 7.2.

Although this is not ideal, when blood gas measurement is not available, the [TCO_2] may be used to infer the severity of metabolic acidosis; [TCO_2] below 8 mEq/L after rehydration suggests a need for $NaHCO_3$ therapy.

DEXTROSE

Dextrose is added to fluids as a method to provide solute-free water isotonically (dextrose moving intracellularly in the presence of insulin) and *not* as an energy source. 5% Dextrose contains 170 kcal/L of solution and will not provide meaningful calorie support. Each mL will contain only 0.17 kcal. Using the formula of 30 × body weight (kg) + 70, the resting energy requirement for a 5-kg cat is 220 kcal. The amount of 5% dextrose needed to meet the basal requirements of a 5-kg cat would be 1294 mL, about 6 times the daily maintenance fluid requirement.

A CASE EXAMPLE

A case example, Table 5-8, illustrates how to develop a fluid plan for a 5-kg cat that is presented with a history of vomiting of 7 days' duration. The vomiting is thought to be due to a flare-up of previously diagnosed inflammatory bowel disease and is not thought to be gastric in origin. The cat is estimated to be 7% dehydrated. Thus the fluid deficit volume would be estimated to be 0.35 kg, which is equivalent to 350 mL. This is likely to be an isotonic loss in which Na^+, K^+, Mg^{++}, and HCO_3^- are lost. This is entered into the table as either 350 mL total or 14.5 mL/hour. Because the dehydration developed slowly over the past week, the plan is to restore it over 24 hours.

Until the measured electrolyte values are available from the laboratory, the clinician will assume a fluid concentration of 20 mEq/L K^+ and use a fluid that also contains Mg^{++} at approximately 3 mEq/L. Thus a reasonable choice would be Normosol with 15 mEq/L additional KCl added.

The next step is to determine the volume needed for normal ongoing losses for the cat and the most appropriate fluid to use for this purpose. This volume is meant to replace the normal ongoing sensible and insensible fluid losses, *not* including deficits or abnormal ongoing losses from persistent vomiting.

Using the formula (30 × body weight in kg) + 70 to estimate the total volume of fluids in mL per 24 hours required by the patient, the clinician determines that a 5-kg cat requires 220 mL/day, or 9 mL/hour. For maintenance a low Na^+ fluid such as Plasma-Lyte 56 + 5% dextrose is appropriate. It contains a buffer, Na^+ and Mg^{++}, and solute-free water for maintenance. The patient will be transitioned to partial parenteral nutrition to provide for its nutritional needs after approximately the first 24 hours of hospitalization, which will then provide its maintenance fluid needs.

Next, the clinician selects the type and rate type of fluid to administer to replace the abnormal ongoing loss. In talking with the client, the clinician estimates that the cat vomited about 40 mL in the previous 24 hours. The clinician will adjust the fluid plan if the measured volume differs from this estimate while the cat is observed over the next 12 hours. The cat does not have excess urinary or respiratory loss, diarrhea, fever, or known third spacing. Thus at present the only abnormal ongoing loss is vomiting. In anticipation of a similar amount of vomiting over the next 24 hours, an additional 40 mL (approximately 1.5 mL/hour) is added to the fluid plan. This will be provided as an isotonic fluid, such as the Normosol with supplemental potassium, as indicated previously for replacement therapy.

With duodenal vomiting, metabolic acidosis can be expected. However, because the cat will likely be able to correct this itself when fully rehydrated, the clinician will usually wait for the serum chemistry result before considering any specific therapy for an acid–base disorder.

Lastly, to calculate the drops per minute, the clinician takes the desired fluid rate (in mL/hour), multiplies it by the drops/mL designated for the particular fluid administration set, and then divides that number by 60 min/hour.

The completed worksheet represents the fluid prescription for the cat. Next, the prescription should be translated into an administration plan. The fluid types can be administered concurrently using a T-port.

Patient-Monitoring Recommendations

Repeated measurements of body weight are the best way to assess improving hydration status. Because changes in lean body and fat mass do not occur rapidly, short-term changes in body weight reflect changes in body fluid. Body weight measurements should be

TABLE 5-8 **Case Example Using the Calculation Worksheet for Fluid Therapy**

Components of the Fluid Plan		Type of Fluid	Volume of Fluid mL/day	Volume of Fluid mL/h
1. Deficits	Isotonic	Balanced crystalloid containing 20 mEq/L K^+ and Mg^{++}	350	14.5
	Hypertonic			
2. Maintenance	Normal ongoing losses	Low-Na^+ maintenance fluid	220	9
	(Enteral contribution from feeding)	Will be added on day 2	(0)	(0)
	Net normal loss to be provided by fluids		220	9
3. Abnormal ongoing losses	Gastrointestinal	Balanced crystalloid containing 20 mEq/L K^+ and Mg^{++}	Est 40	1.5
	Urinary		0	0
	Other sensible		0	0
	Insensible		0	0
Totals		1. Normosol + KCL	1. 390	1. 16
		2. Plasma-Lyte 56 + 5% Dextrose	2. 220	2. 9
		3. n/a	3. n/a	3. n/a

performed every 4 to 12 hours depending on the severity of the cat's condition and rate of fluid being given. It is important to use the same scale each time, and a human pediatric scale is likely to be the most accurate.

Skin turgor can be used serially to assess improvement in hydration status. The skin tenting tendency can also be used to determine the presence of subcutaneous edema. When the skin of a normally hydrated patient is released, it returns rapidly to its resting position. With severe subcutaneous edema, digital pressure to the skin surface will actually cause a transient pit or dimple in the skin surface when the finger is removed. Edematous patients are already overloaded with crystalloids, and further crystalloid therapy is not warranted.

Urine output can also be monitored to evaluate a patient's hydration status. Normal urine output varies between 0.5 and 2 mL/kg/hr. Oliguria (urine output <0.5 mL/kg per hour) associated with dehydration should respond rapidly to rehydration with crystalloid fluids.

Laboratory parameters, such as PCV, total protein, and serum electrolytes, must be monitored serially, often more than once daily depending on the severity of any detected derangements, to allow for necessary adjustments to the fluid therapy plan.

INTRAVENOUS FLUIDS DURING ANESTHESIA AND SURGERY

Fluid therapy is important during all anesthetic procedures. Cats given appropriate fluid therapy have better outcomes and show fewer adverse side effects. Recovery times and quality are improved after anesthesia. Human patients receiving fluids also report less nausea, dizziness, and thirst. Although some of these parameters are difficult to assess in cats, it is likely that similar benefits occur. Appropriate use of fluids helps maintain intravascular volume and acid–base balance and electrolyte normality, supports organ function, and provides cells with nutrients and oxygen. Maintenance of appropriate liver blood flow also facilitates metabolism of anesthetic drugs, which in turn will result in more rapid patient recovery. In addition to the cardiovascular benefits of fluid therapy during anesthesia, some patients need fluids to correct specific metabolic abnormalities in glucose and acid–base balance. Fluid therapy for surgery and anesthesia will be discussed in greater detail in Chapter 7.

SPECIFIC DISEASE CONDITIONS

Hypernatremia

Hypernatremic patients have a free water deficit, or water loss in excess of sodium. When hypernatremia is present, calculating the dehydration deficit alone, as is done for patients whose sodium is still within normal range, often underestimates the fluid volume needed because the loss is from the ICF compartment. Therefore the free water deficit, or water lost in excess of solute, must be calculated.

The volume of the deficit can be estimated as follows:

$$\text{Free water deficit (liters)} = 0.6 \times \text{body weight (kg)} \times [(\text{plasma }[Na^+]/148) - 1]$$ [8]

In cases of chronic hyperosmolality, the rate of replacement should be proportional to the duration of the hyperosmolality. Ideally, serum sodium should not be raised or lowered by more than 0.5 to 1 mEq/hour. For example, to decrease the serum [Na^+] from 168 mEq/L to 150 mEq/L, a difference of 18 mEq, divide 18 by 0.5 mEq/hour, which results in 36 hours. Using the example of a 5-kg cat, because the deficit is 405 mL, divide 405 by 36 hours to get a free water administration rate of 11 mL/hour. In patients that are eating on their own or have a feeding tube, this fluid can be given orally as water. When it must be given intravenously, it can be given as D5W.

For patients with hypernatremia, the ECF volume deficit, maintenance requirement, and any abnormal ongoing losses are also calculated as discussed earlier and included in the fluid therapy prescription. The rate at which the serum [Na^+] is decreasing should be monitored every 6 to 8 hours.

Optimal therapy for patients with acute salt toxicity (Na^+ overdose leading to hypervolemic hypernatremia) is unknown, and a more rapid correction may be advantageous. A correction rate of no faster than 1 mEq/hour is generally employed to prevent complications.[1] Furosemide may be given to increase renal Na^+ excretion. However, acute hypernatremia is unlikely to be encountered in felines because they are not inclined to ingest de-icers or water-softening compounds.

Azotemia and Renal Disease

Localization of Azotemia

Patients with azotemia should always be assessed to determine whether their azotemia is prerenal, renal, postrenal, or some combination thereof. Those patients without preexisting renal disease must have a severe ECF volume depletion to manifest an azotemia that is detectable as outside the normal reference range. By contrast, patients with preexisting functional renal disease (even when nonazotemic in the volume-replete state) may develop azotemia with only mild ECF volume depletion. Both situations warrant rapid restoration of the ECF volume, although total volume required may be different; thus the degree of ECF volume depletion, not the degree of azotemia, must be used to guide the amount of fluids necessary.

Urethral and ureteral obstructions are the most common causes of postrenal azotemia, although fluid therapy decisions are similar for ruptured urinary tract. The primary difference between urethral and ureteral obstruction is that the former is often acute and complete, whereas the latter is often partial or unilateral and some urine production remains. It should always be remembered that the cat's ability to void urine does not preclude azotemia being postrenal. Postrenal azotemia patients often have accompanying fluid deficits, varying from mild to severe enough to result in hypovolemia. Such deficits should be restored rapidly, even in patients with complete urethral obstruction. Leaving such patients in a state of volume depletion does not protect them from making further urine and does not prevent bladder rupture or kidney damage. Volume should be restored while the urethral obstruction is being corrected or the bladder emptied to remove the pressure preventing renal filtration. Cats that have existing or recently corrected postrenal azotemia need to have their urine output monitored because ongoing urinary loss can be high and unpredictable.

Primary renal azotemia should be suspected when prerenal and postrenal causes of azotemia have been eliminated. The cat with renal azotemia should then be assessed to determine whether the kidney disease is chronic or acute; this assessment is based largely on history. Patients with chronic renal failure typically have polyuria, although exceptions exist with advanced disease. Cats with acute renal failure may be polyuric or oliguric depending on the cause and severity of their disease. Assessment of the hourly rate of urine production is essential in cats with acute renal failure for determination of their fluid therapy plans. Sometimes it is difficult to determine if a patient has acute or chronic renal failure at initial presentation. When this is in doubt, the veterinarian should assume that it is acute and begin measuring urine output promptly. When managing a cat with azotemia, the veterinarian must always consider prerenal, postrenal, and acute renal azotemia, because each of these has the potential to be reversible.

Electrolyte Disorders

Cats with azotemia may have hypokalemia or hyperkalemia. Hypokalemia is most often seen with mild to moderate chronic renal failure. Hypokalemia can cause renal failure in cats, which is termed *hypokalemic nephropathy*.

Hyperkalemia is common with acute renal failure and postrenal azotemia. There may be a temptation to employ K^+-free solutions, such as 0.9% saline, initially. However, 0.9% saline may contribute to metabolic acidosis, which is also likely to be severe in these patients. Unfortunately, no studies exist comparing 0.9% saline with buffered balanced electrolyte solutions on the outcome of cats with life-threatening hyperkalemia caused by postrenal azotemia. It is postulated that the dilution provided by a balanced electrolyte solution, even one containing small amounts of K^+, will lower the cat's serum [K^+]. Once the obstruction is eliminated and renal filtration is restored, K^+ will be excreted. However, this may not occur rapidly enough in cats that have severe symptomatic hyperkalemia. Such patients will require insulin–dextrose therapy to shift K^+ intracellularly and possibly calcium gluconate if cardiac arrhythmias are present.

Critically ill cats with urethral obstruction and other forms of postrenal azotemia may have severe metabolic acidosis, and the blood pH may be below 7.1. This degree of acidosis can lead to ventricular arrhythmias and poor tissue perfusion. Treatment for metabolic acidosis in such cats requires prompt correction of the problem leading to the postrenal azotemia, fluid diuresis, and bicarbonate therapy, which has been discussed previously.

When the acidosis is not severe, resolution of obstruction and diuresis will allow the return of renal filtration and the kidney should correct the problem without supplemental HCO_3^-.

Hyperphosphatemia is common whenever the GFR is reduced and is seen with prerenal, renal, and postrenal azotemia. Severe hyperphosphatemia can lead to hypocalcemia, acidosis, and tissue deposition of calcium phosphate salts, potentially causing dysfunction of the kidney, heart, and other organs. In cats that are still eating, phosphate binders can be added to the food. In those that are not yet eating, only improvement in the GFR will rectify the situation. Intractable hyperphosphatemia is one factor that may necessitate dialysis in patients with severely compromised renal function. When hyperkalemia is present with hyperphosphatemia, the associated severe ionized hypocalcemia will accentuate the affect of hyperkalemia on membrane excitability and increase the risk for the development of arrhythmias. Nonetheless, treatment of ionized hypocalcemia with calcium gluconate is reserved for patients that have clinical signs of ionized hypocalcemia, because the additional calcium in the presence of hyperphosphatemia will potentiate tissue mineralization.

Diuresis After Resolution of Obstruction and in the Healing Phase of Acute Renal Failure

There are two clinical situations associated with azotemia in which urine output may be exceptionally high. Postobstructive diuresis is the most common and can be profound—greater than 120 mL/hour in some cats. All postobstructed cats must have their urine output and body weight measured frequently to allow adjustments in their fluid prescriptions so that the volume in always balances the volume out. Relying on shortcuts for fluid therapy calculations (e.g., twice maintenance, three times maintenance) can markedly underestimate the fluid needs in these patients. Cats that have been obstructed have also suffered a renal insult. During the healing phase, a second insult (e.g., the development of ECF volume depletion and hypoperfusion) will worsen the prognosis for full renal recovery. Hypokalemia may develop during the postobstructive diuresis; therefore serum [K^+] should also be monitored. Some cats may require K^+ supplementation as soon as a few hours after initial stabilization despite initially presenting with hyperkalemia.

As healing occurs, there is a danger that matching fluid intake with urine output will create a situation in which fluids being administered are driving the increased urine production. To prevent this, once the cat is stable and eating well, fluid rates are adjusted to just below output by approximately 5 mL per hour. If the body weight falls or the urine output does not drop accordingly, the decrease in fluid rate may have been premature. Weaning a cat with postobstructive diuresis off fluids requires careful monitoring and attention to detail.

The other situation in which azotemia may be accompanied by a considerable diuresis is in the healing phase of acute renal failure. Such patients may make large quantities of "bad-quality urine." This state may persist for as long as 1 week, and the considerations for weaning the patient off intravenous fluid therapy discussed for postobstructive diuresis apply. Some of these patients may be left with chronic renal failure as a result of the initial acute insult. Thus it is expected that they will remain polyuric as they are weaned off fluids. But as long as the patient is able to drink and is given the opportunity to do so, increased water intake should balance increased urine output. Fluid therapy should be weaned slowly and carefully so that the clinician can observe if in fact the patient is able to keep up with its increased urinary losses. If it cannot and fluids are weaned too quickly, then recovery from acute renal disease will be compromised.

Proteinuric Renal Disease

Although comparatively rare in cats, patients with primary proteinuric renal disease will generally have increased total body Na^+ content. They may not need fluid therapy, providing additional Na^+, despite the presence of azotemia. The veterinarian should always assess the volume status of the cat rather than assume that the azotemic patient requires fluid therapy.

Oliguric Renal Disease

Patients with oliguric or anuric renal failure have little or no urine production, respectively. They require careful monitoring for ECF volume overload. Signs of ECF volume overload were discussed earlier. Cats with oliguric renal failure require intensive nursing care and should have their urine output and body weight monitored very frequently, initially as often as every 1 to 2 hours. Normal urine output for a hydrated animal is 1 to 2 mL/kg/hour. Once interstitial and intravascular fluid deficits have been corrected, patients with oliguria must have their "ins and outs" monitored. That is, the clinician can measure the amount of fluid taken in, orally or by intravenous fluids, and compare it with the amount of fluid lost as urine, vomitus, or diarrhea, worsening third space fluid accumulation, and insensible losses (20 to 30 mL/kg per day). The clinician should adjust the fluid rate to match the fluid coming out in addition to the calculated insensible losses. Because all fluid need calculations are inherently educated guesses, a critical component of the monitoring plan will be to weigh the patient frequently using a highly accurate scale. This will help prevent overhydration and underhydration, both equal enemies of a cat in renal failure.

Chronic Renal Disease

Cats with mild to moderate stable chronic kidney disease are sometimes given prescriptions for subcutaneous fluids as diuresis, described as "flushing out the kidney." There is little justification for this practice. Most cats with mild and moderate stable disease eat and drink enough to offset their own losses, even in the presence of polyuria. Subcutaneous fluid therapy does not result in any sort of dialysis to lessen azotemia. The values for blood urea nitrogen and creatinine may fall slightly, but this is due to the increased Na^+ load increasing the GFR, essentially making the kidney work harder. Subcutaneous fluid therapy should be reserved for situations when the cat cannot keep up with losses, such as an episode of vomiting or diarrhea, and thus fluids are indicated to stave off ECF volume depletion. Cats with more severe chronic kidney disease may have trouble keeping up with losses through oral intake and may benefit from continuous subcutaneous fluid therapy. However, such cats may also not eat enough to meet their calories and may be better served with a feeding tube to allow provision of both fluids and calories.

Congestive Heart Failure

Congestive heart failure (CHF) is a volume overload state, in which the ECF Na^+ content is high, as is the intravascular fluid volume, with increased end-diastolic pressures leading to imbalance of Starling's forces across the capillary endothelium and resulting in edema. Depending upon the underlying pathology, the volume overload and edema can be largely localized to either the systemic or pulmonary circulations or may affect both. These patients have RAAS activation and high circulating levels of aldosterone, promoting renal Na^+ retention. Consequently, most patients with heart failure do not benefit from the further addition of Na^+ in the form of intravenous fluids. In fact, the clinical aim more often is to remove the excess Na^+ by use of diuretics that increase renal salt loss while simultaneously improving cardiac performance. Patients with pleural or abdominal effusion may need thoracocentesis or abdominocentesis to more rapidly and effectively remove excess Na^+ and fluid.

As a general rule, it is best not to administer significant amounts of intravenous fluids or Na^+. In most cases of acute left-sided CHF and in cats with significant pleural effusion, it is imperative to focus on treating the CHF and lowering end-diastolic pressures, often with diuretics; it is less important to correct measurable electrolyte or acid–base abnormalities. These can be addressed once the patient is stable.

Stable patients with compensated CHF may require fluid therapy to address acid–base or electrolyte disorders or ongoing excess losses. Some patients with CHF have poor tissue perfusion and metabolic acidosis and may have hypokalemia or hypomagnesemia. Further, they may need intravenous medications and possibly continuous intravenous isotonic dextrose infusions to keep their catheters patent. Additionally, they may need calories; parenteral nutrition may be required if they are unable or unwilling to eat.

If crystalloids are given, they should be low in Na^+, buffered, and potentially supplemented with K^+ or Mg^{++}. Often, improvement of cardiac performance will correct the metabolic acidosis, and thus supplemental sodium bicarbonate administration is rarely needed.

Although patients with CHF typically have volume overload and do not require rehydration therapy, they may have abnormal ongoing losses, such as vomiting or diarrhea, which must be replaced.

Cats with CHF that are receiving diuretics should be monitored: Parameters include urine output, improvement in respiratory character, and ability to rest and sleep. This minimizes the risk of overtreatment, dehydration, and marked decreases in GFR. Mild increases in blood urea nitrogen and creatinine are expected, but induction of renal failure through extreme prerenal lowering of GFR must be avoided. The veterinarian may be tempted to preemptively treat patients in cardiac failure with a conservative dose of intravenous fluids as a form of renal protection. However, this is not medically sound: Diuretics are given to promote renal Na^+ excretion; adding Na^+ in the form of intravenous fluids just counteracts the effect. Having a patient on a diuretic, such as furosemide, concurrently with intravenous fluids is typically counterproductive; it is not possible to simultaneously dehydrate and rehydrate a patient.

One situation in which Na^+-containing fluids may be needed is when the patient has been grossly dehydrated by overzealous diuretic use and needs to be brought back to euvolemia. However, even in these cases, it is often best to allow for slow rehydration by temporarily discontinuing or decreasing the dose of diuretic given while carefully monitoring respiratory rate and other clinical indications of developing pulmonary edema. In some cases oral rehydration (simply by allowing the patient to drink) will suffice.

Concurrent Cardiac and Renal Disease

Cats that have both heart disease and kidney disease pose a unique challenge. It is difficult to prescribe a therapy that will support one organ without harming the other, particularly when organ failure is present for either disease. Expanding the total body fluid will promote better renal perfusion and an improved GFR, but the addition of fluid also increases the risk of CHF. Reducing total body fluid, such as by giving diuretics, alleviates Na^+ and fluid retention in patients with heart failure, but this will lower the GFR and worsen renal failure. When both conditions are severe, the veterinarian aims to address and improve both conditions simultaneously: to improve cardiac function and perform the functions of the kidney through continual renal replacement therapy. However, when disease is relatively mild or advanced therapies such as continuous renal replacement therapy are unavailable, one condition is generally determined to be more severe from a clinical standpoint, on the basis of the physical examination and laboratory data. Identifying the more severe condition is often a straightforward, deliberative process. It is an essential first step for choosing the optimal treatment.

For example, if a cat with cardiomyopathy and chronic kidney disease presents with dyspnea and pulmonary edema, the most immediate problem is CHF; that patient will need a diuretic, regardless of the severity of its azotemia. In contrast, the patient with cardiomyopathy and kidney disease who presents with inappetence, lethargy, vomiting, and dehydration has a dominant problem of renal failure. This patient likely needs fluids or a reduction in the dose of diuretic given. Another consideration is removing ancillary medications such as angiotensin-converting enzyme (ACE) inhibitors. Often, cats will return to eating and drinking when pharmacotherapy is simplified; clinicians should resist the temptation to solve every problem with more medications.

For cats with cardiac disease, it should be pointed out that the urine specific gravity may be inadequately concentrated, even when azotemia is present, if the cat is taking diuretic medications or has hyperthyroidism or other causes of obligate polyuria. Thus azotemia together with isosthenuria (or minimally concentrated urine) is not synonymous with renal failure. Azotemia may, in these cases, be solely prerenal.

When a gallop sound appears for the first time during fluid therapy in a cat with heart disease, it may be a harbinger of fluid overload. Cats can have third heart sounds without being in CHF, so it is the newness of the gallop sound during fluid therapy that should alert the clinician to the impending clinical signs of fluid overload, including dyspnea. As a general rule, a cardiorenal patient that develops dyspnea during fluid therapy should be suspected of having progressed to CHF. Thoracic radiographs can be taken to confirm the condition and rule out other potential causes of dyspnea.

Replacement-type fluids such as LRS should not be given to cardiorenal patients once they are euvolemic because they result in administration of excess of Na^+ and a deficit of K^+. Such patients will either be eating or should be given a maintenance fluid type, although this should be supplanted by the provision of sufficient calories in patients that are not eating.

For cats with chronic renal disease that are being treated with subcutaneous fluids at home, extra vigilance is required when there is concurrent heart disease. Owners of these cats must be advised to watch for the development of dyspnea, often manifested as "belly breathing," because the abdominal effort of many dyspneic cats is apparent to clients.

Diabetic Ketoacidosis

Poorly regulated diabetic patients lose Na^+, Cl^-, and K^+ in their urine as a result of osmotic diuresis. The presence of ketosis will worsen these losses, and the cat may become unable to compensate through intake, particularly if appetite decreases with the onset of acidosis and dehydration. Electrolyte and fluid losses may be further compounded by vomiting, which can occur in patients with DKA. The components of therapy of DKA, in descending order of importance, are as follows:

1. Correction of volume and hydration deficits
2. Correction and monitoring of electrolyte and phosphorus abnormalities
3. Resolution of ketosis with insulin and dextrose therapy

Although insulin therapy is third on this list, this does not imply that it is not important. It simply serves as a reminder that it is the fluid and electrolyte derangements that are life threatening in these patients. Correction of acid–base abnormalities is also a component of therapy for DKA, but this is usually accomplished through fluid and insulin therapy.

Correction of Volume and Hydration Deficits

0.9% NaCl is generally the initial fluid of choice for the ketoacidotic diabetic patient with severe ECF volume depletion, insofar as this provides for the rapid re-expansion of the ECF volume. However, 0.9% NaCl is an acidifying solution and theoretically may contribute further to the acidosis in these patients. Once insulin therapy is initiated, a non-acidifying, buffered fluid such as Normosol-R is preferred. This fluid contains 140 mEq/L of sodium, gluconate, and acetate as buffers and small amounts of potassium and magnesium, both of which are generally depleted in patients with DKA. Fluids that employ lactate as their buffer may, at least in theory, not be the optimal choice for DKA. Metabolism of lactate to bicarbonate occurs in the liver, and cats with DKA may have significant hepatic lipidosis. Despite the acidifying potential of 0.9% NaCl and the concerns about lactate metabolism in cats with DKA, in the clinical situation any isotonic replacement fluid is suitable for initial therapy in these patients, as long as volume status, hydration, electrolytes, and acid–base parameters are closely monitored.

Correction and Monitoring of Electrolyte and Phosphorus Abnormalities

POTASSIUM

Although total body K^+ depletion exists, serum $[K^+]$ may initially be normal or even increased as a result of insulin deficiency and metabolic acidosis in the patient with DKA. Once insulin therapy is initiated, serum K^+ will move intracellularly and the serum $[K^+]$ will often drop precipitously. Thus cats with DKA are expected to need K^+ supplementation early in their treatment to stave off hypokalemia. Serum $[K^+]$ should be monitored frequently during management of DKA; ideally, at least every 4 hours. Table 5-5 can be used to determine the amount of potassium to be added to the fluids for these patients. However, clinicians should anticipate that hypokalemia in these patients can be severe and poorly responsive to "normal" levels of potassium supplementation. In some cases, administration of potassium by CRI, using the KMax value (0.5 mEq/kg per hour) is necessary. However, this should never be undertaken without the ability to frequently monitor serum $[K^+]$ values.

PHOSPHORUS

Serum phosphorus should be monitored every 8 to 12 hours during initial management of the patient with DKA. Serum phosphorus levels may initially be low or normal or may be increased if the patient's GFR is reduced. However, it is common for phosphorus levels to decrease with the initiation of fluid and insulin therapy. This is due to movement of phosphorus into the cells in the presence of insulin, dilution by intravenous fluid therapy, and improvement in GFR. If phosphorus levels fall below approximately 1.5 mg/dL, the patient is at risk for hemolytic anemia. Hypophosphatemia may also be clinically undetectable or may contribute to muscle weakness and ataxia. When phosphorus levels approach the low end of the reference range, supplementation is necessary, with ongoing monitoring to allow for dosage adjustments as necessary. Supplementation is provided by the addition of potassium or sodium phosphate to the intravenous fluids. Typical dose rates for phosphorus range from 0.01 to 0.03 mmol/kg per hour. Dose rates as high as 0.12 mmol/kg per hour may be necessary in some patients being treated for DKA. Potassium phosphate is more commonly used, and the amount of potassium provided in this way should be taken into account when calculating potassium supplementation rates in these patients. Some clinicians prefer to provide the patient's calculated potassium needs as a mixture of 50% KCl and 50% potassium phosphate, in anticipation of the development of hypophosphatemia. However, this is a shortcut that may not provide the correct amount of phosphorus in every patient.

MAGNESIUM

Hypomagnesemia is common in cats with DKA; however, its clinical significance has not been fully elucidated. Supplementation may be considered if serum total [Mg] approaches 1 mg/dL, and supplementation is also indicated when hypokalemia appears to be resistant to potassium supplementation. An initial dose of 0.5 to 1 mEq/kg every 24 hours is used in these situations. This dose may be given on the first day and then followed with half this dose on subsequent days. Magnesium may be provided as the chloride or sulfate. These salts are not compatible with solutions containing calcium or bicarbonate.

Resolution of Ketosis with Insulin and Dextrose Therapy

In the patient with DKA, the first goal is to restore ECF volume and improve renal perfusion and urine production. These alone will decrease blood glucose values. Insulin therapy in these patients is often not started until ECF volume deficits are being addressed. Insulin may be administered by CRI or intermittent subcutaneous or intramuscular techniques. The details of insulin therapy in DKA are beyond the scope of this chapter; however, the addition of dextrose to the intravenous fluids is an important part of fluid therapy in these patients. In general, the goal is to decrease serum glucose values by approximately 50 to 100 mg/dL per hour. The insulin dose is adjusted to achieve this goal. In addition, glucose is added to the intravenous fluids as the glucose levels fall. This prevents hypoglycemia and provides a substrate for the insulin, thus allowing the body to resume glucose metabolism and resolve the ketosis. Once ketoacidosis has resolved and the patient is eating, food intake will provide an energy source and the addition of dextrose to the fluids can be discontinued.

Acidosis

Aside from the electrolyte and glucose abnormalities in a patient with ketoacidosis, there is a considerable metabolic acidosis from the circulating ketoacids. In most cases, the acidosis of DKA is rapidly self-correcting. Rapid re-expansion of the ECF volume improves perfusion. Ketones, once their production is halted, will be lost in the urine or converted to bicarbonate. Thus specific therapy for acidosis generally is not required if fluid and insulin therapies are instituted appropriately. When a fluid containing a bicarbonate precursor, such as acetate, is being used, additional bicarbonate will not likely be necessary.

When the venous pH level is below 7.1, the administration of sodium bicarbonate may be considered to promote normal enzymatic functions. In these cases the previously outlined calculation may be used. Again, most clinicians will administer one third to one half of the amount needed over 20 minutes and then reassess the patient's acid–base status. It should be noted that the use of sodium bicarbonate in these patients is the subject of disagreement between clinicians. Potential adverse effects of sodium bicarbonate administration include exacerbation of hypokalemia, increased affinity of hemoglobin for oxygen, paradoxical central nervous system acidosis, delayed development of alkalosis, and sodium overload. Because of these risks, and particularly because of the lack of documented evidence of a clear benefit, many specialists do not advocate the use of sodium bicarbonate therapy in patients with DKA. One conservative approach would be to consider the use of sodium bicarbonate for patients with persistent metabolic acidosis despite fluid therapy for 12 to 24 hours if the pH is 7.1 or below and the [HCO_3^-] is 12 mEq/L or below.

Monitoring

Frequent monitoring is crucial for patients with ketoacidosis. Ideally, patients with diabetic ketoacidosis should have their blood glucose monitored every 2 hours and acid–base and electrolyte status evaluated every 4 to 6 hours. Serum phosphorus concentration and urine ketones should be measured twice daily. Serum ketone measurement may also be available in some hospitals. This level of close monitoring is particularly important in the early phases of rehydration and insulin supplementation. If the veterinary clinic is not able to provide this level of care, the feline patient with DKA should be referred to a specialty hospital whenever possible.

Hyperglycemic Hyperosmolar Syndrome

Hyperglycemic hyperosmolar syndrome (HHS) is an uncommon complication of diabetes mellitus in cats. It is less common than DKA and is often associated with a poorer prognosis. The pathogenesis of HHS is similar to

DKA, but low levels of insulin are present in patients with HHS; thus lipolysis and ketosis do not occur. Hyperglycemia is the predominant abnormality in these patients, with blood glucose levels in excess of 600 mg/dL. Hyperglycemia results in osmotic diuresis, and the patient incurs a significant water deficit. This worsens the hyperglycemia, and eventually the dehydration leads to a reduction in GFR. This is exacerbated by fluid losses caused by vomiting and decreased fluid intake in the sick patient. The decreased GFR then further exacerbates the hyperglycemia.

Patients with HHS are, by definition, hyperosmolar. Osmolality can be measured or calculated. Measurement is typically performed by the freezing point depression method, but this is not readily available to all clinicians. Osmolality is often calculated using the following equation:

$$2[Na^+](mEq/L)+[glucose](mg/dL)/18 \\ +[BUN](mg/dL)/2.8$$

Serum osmolality in patients with HHS is typically greater than 330 mOsm/kg, largely because of the contribution of the severe hyperglycemia. Normal osmolality in cats is around 300 mOsm/kg.

Cats with HHS may be hypernatremic, normonatremic, or hyponatremic. It is important to remember that these values reflect water balance, and not total body Na levels. The latter are likely to be low in patients with HHS. In the presence of hyperglycemia, water moves into the vasculature along an osmotic gradient, and this will reduce the serum [Na^+]. This is called dilutional hyponatremia. To determine if the degree of hyponatremia is appropriate for the patient's level of hyperglycemia, a corrected serum [Na^+] can be calculated:

$$[Na^+]_{Corrected}=[Na^+]_{Measured} \\ +1.6([measured\ glucose-normal\ glucose]/100$$

The equation essentially states that for every 100 mg/dL increase in glucose, there should be a 1.6 mg/dL decrease in [Na^+]. Thus if the patient has a normal corrected [Na^+], the measured serum [Na^+] should correct as hyperglycemia resolves. However, the patient with HHS may have significant ongoing free water loss, contributing to an increase in serum [Na^+]. Thus if a patient with HHS has a normal or elevated uncorrected serum [Na^+] in the face of hyperglycemia, the patient has a free water deficit.

Although patients with HHS are hyperosmolar, isotonic fluids are indicated in these cases; 0.9% NaCl is the fluid of choice. This will replenish total body Na, correct volume deficits, improve GFR, promote glycosuria, and reduce hyperglycemia. Potassium supplementation will also be required, depending on serum levels. As for patients with DKA, it should be expected that aggressive potassium supplementation will be needed once the patient has received adequate fluid therapy and insulin therapy has been initiated.

Fluid therapy in the patient with HHS should be approached conservatively. Rapid correction of long-standing hyperosmolality can lead to fluid shifts that can cause cerebral edema. It is recommended that the fluid deficits be replaced over 24 to 48 hours in these patients, beginning with 0.9% NaCl, as previously indicated. If hypotonic fluids are used initially, the hyperosmolality is likely to be corrected too quickly, and neurologic abnormalities could result. If hypernatremia persists and is not improving after 6 to 12 hours of 0.9% NaCl administration, the patient likely has a significant free water deficit and lower Na fluids such as 0.45% NaCl may be indicated. However, serum [Na^+] should be monitored carefully to ensure that the hypernatremia does not resolve too quickly. A decrease in serum [Na^+] of approximately 0.5 to 1 mEq per hour is a reasonable goal. Different combinations of 0.9% and 0.45% NaCl may be required to achieve this.

Insulin therapy should be withheld in patients with HHS for at least 4 to 6 hours to allow improvements in hypovolemia and dehydration. During this time the serum glucose will likely fall significantly as a result of dilution and an increase in GFR. Hypokalemia should also be addressed before insulin therapy is initiated. Insulin protocols that are used for cats with DKA can also be used for management of HHS, but the dose of insulin should be reduced by 50%. In the management of HHS the goal should be to decrease serum glucose levels by no more than 50 mg/dL per hour. Again, this is to avoid rapid changes in osmolality with resulting detrimental fluid shifts. As for DKA, dextrose should be added to the fluids as serum glucose levels approach 250 mg/dL.

Liver Disease

With severe liver disease it is difficult to predict the electrolyte and acid–base abnormalities in an individual patient. Some patients have elevated Na^+, Cl^-, and HCO_3^- concentrations; others have just the opposite. One consistent finding is that these patients are usually hypokalemic. If in doubt about the electrolyte and acid–base status of a patient with severe liver disease, the clinician should choose a fluid low in Na^+ and Cl^-. A fluid that does not contain lactate is recommended because the liver may not be able to convert the lactate to HCO_3^-. It is important not to confuse lactate with lactic acid. The lactate ion in LRS is a precursor of HCO_3^- and cannot be converted to lactic acid; 0.45% sodium chloride with 2.5% dextrose fits these requirements. Because cats with liver disease are generally hypokalemic, additional KCl usually must be added to the fluids. This is particularly important in liver disease because hypokalemia exacerbates the development of hepatic encephalopathy. Because patients with liver disease may also have an obligate polyuria, the clinician should be prepared to adjust the fluid prescription to account for additional urine output. This is a particular concern in patients that do not drink because of debility or hepatic encephalopathy associated with their primary disease.

References

1. Albi A, Baudin F, Matmar M et al: Severe hypernatremia after hypertonic saline irrigation of hydatid cysts, *Anesth Analg* 95:1806, 2002.
2. Bateman S: Disorders of magnesium: magnesium deficit and excess. In DiBartola SP, editor: *Fluid, electrolyte, and acid-base disorders in small animal practice*, ed 3, St Louis, 2006, Saunders, p 210.
3. Boag A: Shock and blood volume replacement. Proceedings of the 52nd British Small Animal Veterinary Association Congress 2009.
4. Dieterich HJ, Weissmuller T, Rosenberger P et al: Effect of hydroxyethyl starch on vascular leak syndrome and neutrophil accumulation during hypoxia, *Crit Care Med* 34:1775, 2006.
5. Freeman LM, Chan DL: Total parenteral nutrition. In Dibartola SP, editor: *Fluid, electrolyte, and acid-base disorders in small animal practice*, ed 3, St Louis, 2006, Saunders, p 589.
6. Hansen B: *Introduction to fluid types* (website): http://www.abbottanimalhealthce.com/fluid_therapy/index.htm. Accessed Sept. 13, 2010.
7. Haupt KA: *Domestic animal behavior*, ed 4, Ames, Iowa, 2005, Blackwell.
8. James KM, Lunn KF: Normal and abnormal water balance: hyponatremia and hypernatremia, *Compend Contin Edu Vet* 29:589, 2007.
9. Kirchner KA, Stein JH: Sodium metabolism. In Narins RG, editor: *Maxwell and Kleeman's clinical disorders of fluid and electrolyte metabolism*, New York, 1994, McGraw-Hill, p 45.
10. Kohn CW, DiBartola SP: Composition and distribution of body fluids in dogs and cats. In DiBartola SP, editor: *Fluid, electrolyte, and acid-base disorders in small animal practice*, ed 2, Philadelphia, 2000, Saunders, p 5.
11. Mathews KA: The therapeutic use of 25% human serum albumin in critically ill dogs and cats, *Vet Clin North Am Sm Anim Pract* 38:595, 2008.
12. Rose BD, Post TW: *Clinical physiology of acid-base and electrolyte disorders*, New York, 2001, McGraw-Hill.
13. Schwartz PJ, Pagani M, Lombardi F et al: A cardiocardiac sympathovagal reflex in the cat, *Circ Res* 32:215, 1973.
14. Schwartz PJ, Pagani M, Lombardi F et al: Reflex changes in cardiac vagal efferent nervous activity elicited by stimulation of afferent fibres in the cardiac sympathetic nerves, *Brain Res* 42:482, 1972.
15. Silverstein D: Past, present and future of fluid therapy. Proceedings of the 15th International Veterinary Emergency and Critical Care Symposium 2009.
16. Wellman ML, DiBartola SP, Kohn CW: Applied physiology of body fluids in dogs and cats. In DiBartola SP, editor: *Fluid, electrolyte, and acid-base disorders in small animal practice*, ed 3, St Louis, 2006, Saunders, p 16.

CHAPTER

6

Analgesia

Carolyn McKune and Sheilah Robertson

OUTLINE

Recognition and management of feline pain are increasingly prominent in veterinary medicine. Given the 63.3 million veterinary visits made annually by an estimated 82.4 million cats owned in the United States,[22,121] there is ample opportunity to include the assessment of pain as a routine component of a feline examination. Published surveys of analgesic use in cats over a 10-year span show a marked increase in the number of cats that now receive perioperative analgesics.[34,55,65,66] Continuing professional education and review articles contribute to this phenomenon.[55,65] Owners are also seeking and demanding appropriate pain management for their cats, both for surgical procedures and for chronic conditions such as degenerative joint disease.

However, there is room for improvement. Some cats continue to be denied analgesics for procedures such as castration, and very few cats receive analgesic agents in the postoperative period despite the fact that many procedures are likely to result in pain lasting several days.[55] The perception by veterinarians that owners will not pay for analgesia is often given as a reason for the undertreatment of pain in cats. This assumption was not supported in a survey of owners in Finland, where 77% of respondents agreed that the cost of treating pain was not a concern.[55,149] Between 78% and 98% of owners also agreed that treating their animal's pain was somewhat to very important to them.[149] The purpose of this chapter is to review the current state of knowledge on the recognition and treatment of acute pain in cats.

PAIN RECOGNITION AND ASSESSMENT

"Before we can treat something we first have to recognize it."
Sheilah Robertson

The American Animal Hospital Association (AAHA) and the American Association of Feline Practitioners (AAFP) have published guidelines for incorporating pain management into veterinary practice.[54] The first and pivotal step in the algorithm is assessing whether the animal is in pain. However, up to 42% of veterinarians consider their knowledge of pain assessment for both dogs and cats to be inadequate.[59,163]

The International Association for the Study of Pain (IASP) defines pain as "an unpleasant sensory or emotional experience associated with actual or potential tissue damage, or described in terms of such damage."[140] The emotional or affective aspects of pain are important but difficult to measure in nonverbal species. Assessment of pain in animals is based primarily on ethological quantification of behavior, but the wide range of feline "personalities" and variety of normal behaviors make this a challenge. Very subtle changes in behavior may indicate pain, and these can be easily overlooked by both owners and professional caregivers. Because the pain experience is unique to each individual, behaviors vary among cats, making standardization of assessment difficult. Behaviors related to fear and stress may be difficult to differentiate from those associated with pain. For example, one cat may be immobile and crouched in the back of a cage even when no painful procedure has been performed, whereas another cat displaying the same behavior may be in pain. For this reason understanding the individual patient's normal behavior is imperative. Owners can provide valuable insight into their cats "normal" behavior and should be consulted.

A structured assessment tool is necessary both as a baseline and to monitor response to therapy. The components of such a tool must be user friendly, accurate, reliable, and time-efficient. Objective data, such as heart rate and respiratory rate, are easy to collect; however, there is poor correlation between this type of information and observed behaviors in animals after surgery.[24] Blood pressure is a good objective indicator of pain in cats after ovariohysterectomy in a controlled environment, but in a clinical setting this tool is less reliable.[131,132] The use of multiple indicators to assess feline discomfort is beneficial for compiling an overall picture. Compared to dogs, there is currently no robustly tested or validated composite acute pain scale for cats[57,92]; however, such pain scales are currently being developed. Preliminary data suggest that cats in pain show consistent changes in psychomotor behavior (e.g., comfort, activity, mental status), "miscellaneous behaviors," and protective behaviors (e.g., response to surgical wound, abdominal or flank palpation) and that there is a correlation between pain and vocalization.[13] Specific postures are also associated with abdominal pain.[158]

Although visual analog scales and numeric rating scales are technically easier to use compared with a composite pain scale, they are unidimensional, and interobserver variation is large; in one study variability was 36%.[58] When a behavioral pain indicator is used, assigning a descriptor as well as a score assists in reproducibility and consistency of scoring.[92] For example, under the heading "posture," descriptors such as *relaxed, hunched,* and *rigid* could be added. The details of these descriptors and the weighting of scores are not fully worked out. Useful information in the hospital environment falls into several main categories, which are listed in Box 6-1.

A cat in pain shows little interest in interacting with caretakers, does not seek attention, has little interest in its surroundings, is more reclusive, has minimal interest in food, and may not groom itself normally (this may be exhibited either as lack of grooming or as excessive grooming, especially of the painful site). Cats in pain may urinate or defecate outside the litter box because it is too painful to move to or into it. The posture for a cat experiencing pain after abdominal surgery has been described as "half tucked up" or "crouching."[158]

Figure 6-1 shows an example of a pain-scoring system based on posture. Figure 6-2 shows clinical examples that correspond to various places along the scale.

BOX 6-1
Useful Information in the Hospital Environment for Assessing Pain

Behaviors and their deviation from normal
- Interaction with caretakers
- Interest in food
- Interest in grooming
- Interest in the environment
- Normal litter box usage

Posture
Location in the hospital cage
Response and severity of response to palpation

Facial expression has been used to assess pain in newborn infants[118] and may also be useful in cats. Cats in pain often hold their heads low with their eyes half or fully shut and in a slanted position (see Figure 6-2).

Response to palpation of a surgical or traumatic wound yields useful information. The response to palpation may be mild or may elicit a defensive behavior from the cat (e.g., hissing, growling, attempting to scratch or bite). If pain has been well managed, it is possible to apply firm pressure over a wound and the surrounding area without the patient resenting it. In some cases the cat is defensive before any contact is made because it anticipates pain when handled. Although this may be a normal reaction for some cats (reflecting fear rather than pain), it usually indicates pain that is poorly managed. In feral cats whose behavior makes interactions unlikely, the clinician is ethically obligated to treat with the assumption that an injury or surgery is painful and medicate appropriately. Even without palpation, the improvement in their observed behaviors can be obvious after intervention. No animal should be required to "earn" its analgesia.

The timing of assessments is also important. An assessment of the cat *before* a painful event such as surgery or another invasive procedure is often critical to assessing the cat appropriately after that event has occurred. The clinician is looking for changes in behavior, and the goal of treatment is to restore normal behaviors. Frequent observations after painful events are important because the choice of drug, dose, and dosing interval needed to keep each patient comfortable will vary. This decision must be balanced with the need of the animal to sleep and rest. Implementing a practical system of assessing the animal every 2 hours except when the animal is sleeping comfortably is a suitable compromise.

A review of the relevant literature on the treatment of feline pain yields varying methods of assessment. In

Observation	Score	Patient Criteria
Comfort	0	Asleep or calm
	1	Awake; interested in surroundings
	2	Mild agitation; obtunded and uninterested in surroundings
	3	Moderate agitation; restless and uncomfortable
	4	Extremely agitated; thrashing
Movement	0	Normal amount of movement
	1	Frequent position changes or reluctance to move
	2	Thrashing
Appearance	0	Normal
	1	Mild changes; eyelids partially closed; ears flattened or carried abnormally
	2	Moderate changes: eyes sunken or glazed; unthrifty appearance
	3	Severe changes: eyes pale; enlarged pupils; "grimacing" or other abnormal facial expressions; guarding; hunched-up position; legs in abnormal position; grunting before expiration; teeth grinding
Behavior (unprovoked)	0	Normal
	1	Minor changes
	2	Moderately abnormal: less mobile and less alert than normal; unaware of surroundings, very restless
	3	Markedly abnormal: very restless; vocalizing; self-mutilation; grunting; facing the back of cage
Interactive behavior	0	Normal
	1	Pulls away when surgical site is touched; looks at wound; mobile
	2	Vocalizing when wound is touched; somewhat restless; reluctant to move but will if coaxed
	3	Violent reaction to stimuli; vocalizing when wound is not touched; snapping; growling or hissing when approached; extremely restless; will not move when coaxed
Vocalization	0	Quiet
	1	Crying; responds to calm voice and stroking
	2	Intermittent crying or whimpering; no response to calm voice and stroking
	3	Continuous noise that is unusual for this animal
Heart rate	0	0% to 15% above presurgical value
	1	16% to 29% above presurgical value
	2	30% to 45% above presurgical value
	3	>45% above presurgical value
Respiration rate	0	0% to 15% above presurgical value
	1	16% to 29% above presurgical value
	2	30% to 45% above presurgical value
	3	>45% above presurgical value
Total score	(0 to 24)	

IT IS NOT THE INTENT OF THIS FORM TO REQUIRE THAT ANIMALS PROVE THEY ARE IN PAIN BEFORE THERAPY IS INITIATED. Instead, this form is intended to aid in the evaluation of dogs and cats that may be in pain following surgery or trauma. The exact score that will indicate that treatment for pain is appropriate will vary from individual to individual. Animals that are expected to be in moderate to severe pain, based on the surgical procedure performed, should be treated BEFORE assessment indicates severe pain. Many animals will receive analgesics before pain is detected based on this scoring system. Regardless of score, if there is evidence that the animal is in pain, a test dose of analgesic should be administered and changes in behavior noted.

FIGURE 6-1 Example of a pain scoring system based on posture and behavior. Following surgery or trauma the goal is to maintain a score of <1.0. See Figure 6-2 for examples of scoring. *(From Hellyer PW, Gaynor JS: How I treat: acute postsurgical pain in dogs and cats,* Comp Contin Educ *20:140-153, 1998.)*

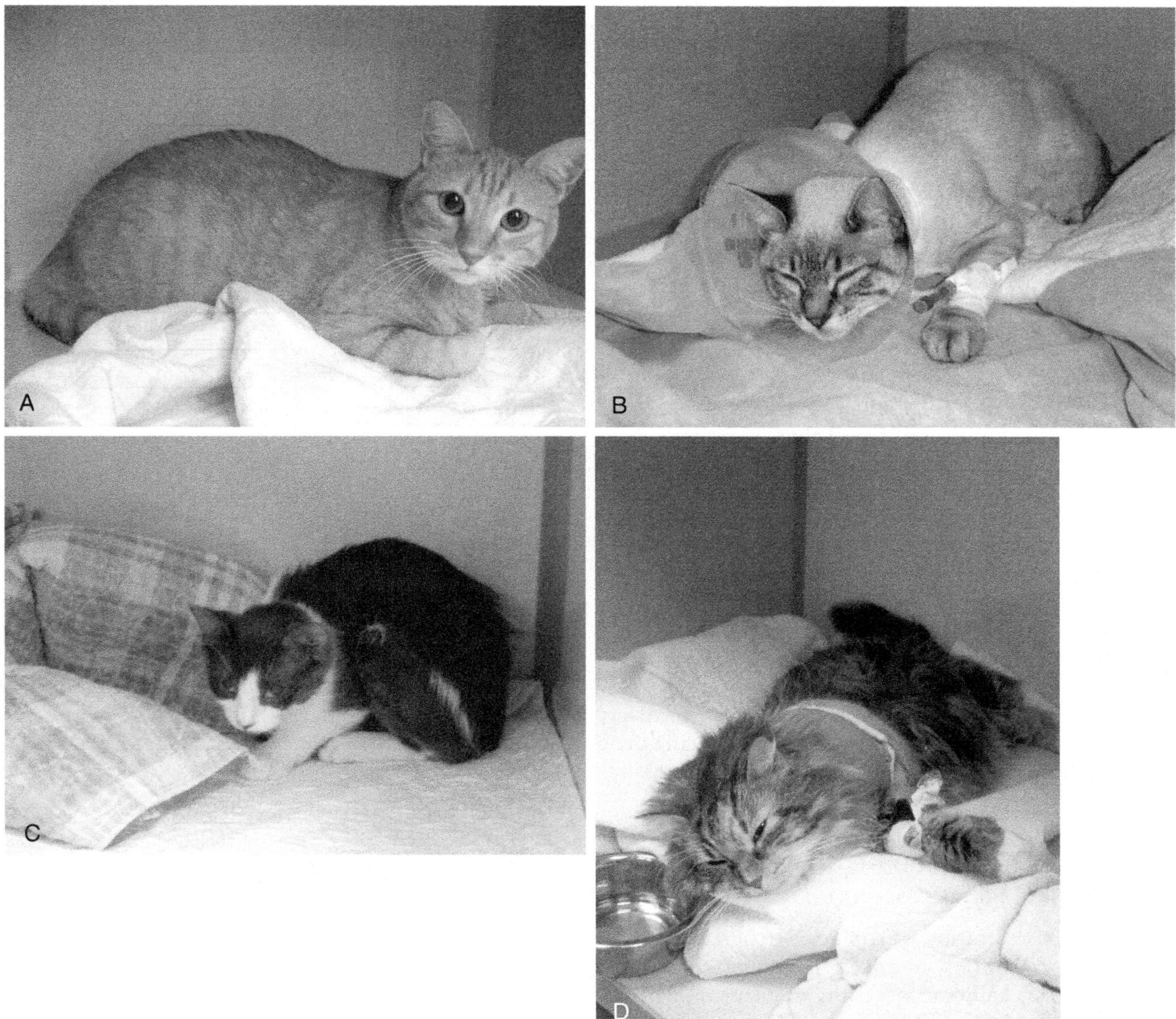

FIGURE 6-2 **A,** This cat falls in the range of 0.5 to 1.0. **B,** This cat displays the posture and facial expression often observed in cats with untreated acute pain. The cat's head is held low, with its eyes almost completely shut and in a slanted position, and it is hunched or "tucked up." This cat would receive a score of 2.5-3.0. **C,** This cat received a score of 2.5. **D,** This cat is painful and received a score of 3.5 before treatment.

addition to the clinically applicable techniques previously described, several nociceptive threshold testing devices have been successfully adapted for use in cats. These are often used in a laboratory setting to screen putative analgesics for onset, intensity, and duration of antinociceptive actions before clinical testing is performed. In addition, different routes of administration can be compared. Thermal, mechanical, electrical, and visceral stimulation models have all been used in cats.[10,31,32,35]

As with all nonverbal species, cats depend on their owners to seek care and treatment for their ailments, including pain. Differences are present not just among individual cats but also among caretakers. Owners range from novices with a first pet to experienced owners who may care for multiple cats at any one time. This variability in exposure and experience can influence the owner's understanding of a cat's need for analgesia. For example, when owners who currently owned a cat were compared with owners who had no cat ownership experience, members of the former group were more likely to agree with a statement suggesting a similar pain experience between animals and humans,[149] and this may lead to a higher value being placed on appropriate analgesia. In one survey of pet owners, 50% were concerned about postoperative pain,[153,154] so it seems logical that these same owners would be receptive to learning about recognizing and alleviating pain.

The goals of pain management are to minimize pain, not necessarily eliminate it. Only local anesthetics can completely abolish pain, and these are not applicable to all surgical procedures or types of trauma. The aims of the veterinarian are to make feline patients comfortable so that they can perform normal daily activities and to prevent any marked changes in their normal behavior or personality.

ROUTES AND METHODS OF DRUG ADMINISTRATION

Analgesic drugs are given by many different routes, including parenteral (intravenous, intramuscular, subcutaneous), transdermal, topical, oral, transmucosal, and epidural. Careful thought regarding choice of route, both for ease of administration and efficacy, is necessary. For example, the same dose of hydromorphone has very different antinociceptive and side effects depending on whether it is given intravenously, intramuscularly, or subcutaneously.[113]

Because some cats are difficult to medicate, compliance with a recommended treatment is often poor. Therefore the route of administration, number of drugs, and dosing schedules should be carefully evaluated for feasibility in each patient.

When individual drugs are administered by a variety of routes, they will be discussed under that specific drug section. Points pertinent to certain routes of administration deserve specific discussion.

Parenteral Administration (Intravenous, Intramuscular, Subcutaneous)

Parenteral administration of analgesic drugs is straightforward and commonly done in most veterinary settings. If there is a catheter in a cat who needs analgesics, it is logical to make use of the intravenous route. Additionally, familiarity with specific analgesics will help elucidate which parenteral route is appropriate.

Sustained-Release Formulations

Long-acting formulations of drugs are advantageous in some cats. A sustained-release formulation of buprenorphine that is injected subcutaneously has been evaluated in cats.[18]

Constant-Rate Infusions

Opioids, ketamine, and alpha$_2$-adrenergic agonists have all been administered to cats as constant-rate intravenous infusions (CRIs). The goal of a CRI is to achieve a steady-state concentration of the drug and avoid the peaks and troughs of intermittent treatment, thereby resulting in more consistent patient comfort. Selecting the loading and infusion rates to achieve a steady-state concentration requires species-specific pharmacokinetic data as well as plasma concentration–effect data that are not currently available for all analgesic drugs used in cats. However, pharmacokinetic and pharmacodynamic data are available for some opioids, such as fentanyl and remifentanil. Box 6-2 shows the steps for calculating a CRI.

Transdermal Administration

It is easy to understand why a "hands-off" approach for delivering drugs to cats is attractive to caregivers insofar as it precludes the need for intramuscular or intravenous injections and may provide constant and long-term pain relief. Several drugs are available in the form of a transdermal patch, including lidocaine, and the opioids fentanyl and buprenorphine, all of which have been used in cats with varying success.[71,82,96]

Transdermal gels containing a wide variety of drugs have been touted by compounding pharmacies as effective in cats, and the simplicity of this technique is very attractive. Unfortunately, there is little scientific evidence to support that this method of administration results in effective uptake (see Chapter 4). Fentanyl formulated in a pluronic lecithin gel and applied to the shaved skin of the neck or to the pinnae of cats' ears could not be detected in plasma,[112] and this method is not recommended by these authors.

Topical Administration

Cream and gel preparations of local anesthetics are available and have been used in cats; they are helpful for placement of intravenous catheters.[38,41,157]

Oral Administration

Administering a drug by way of the oral route results in absorption from the gastrointestinal tract. In cats the most common analgesic drugs given by this route are the nonsteroidal antiinflammatory drugs (NSAIDs). Tramadol and gabapentin have good oral bioavailability,[105,122] whereas first-pass metabolism of opioids limits their efficacy when given by this route. Palatability is a high priority with oral medications. The oral formulation of meloxicam, an NSAID, is highly palatable to cats,[23,52,79] whereas tramadol is not (in the authors' experience).

Oral Transmucosal Administration

Oral transmucosal, sometimes referred to as *buccal,* administration involves depositing the drug (usually liquid) onto the oral mucosa, where it is absorbed into the bloodstream, thereby avoiding first-pass metabolism. In cats the easiest approach is to deposit the drug in the cheek pouch or under the tongue. A variety of drugs can be administered this way in uncooperative

BOX 6-2

Constant-Rate Infusion Setup

Step 1: Preliminary Information

- Patient's weight in kilograms (kg)
- Analgesic drug and drug concentration
- Method of delivery (syringe pump or fluid bag)

Step 2: Determine Dosage and Time Period for Analgesic Drug

- Is the dose in milligrams (mg) or micrograms (μg)?
- Convert appropriately to desired concentration unit (mg or μg).
- Is there a range of dosages? If so, start out low with the possibility of increasing dose.
- Is the time administration rate per minute or per hour?
- Convert appropriately to desired time unit.

Step 3: Programming a Syringe Pump for Delivery

- Consult the manual about pump programming.
- Calculate the milliliters for delivery in 1 hour.
- Confirm that the pump is set to deliver above volume/h, or
- Recheck syringe pump in 15 minutes to ensure only 25% of the 1-hour volume has been administered, or
- Have appropriately trained staff double-check each other.

Step 4: Using Maintenance Fluids for Delivery

- Determine total volume of fluids per kilogram per hour for administration (mL/kg/h).
- Determine the rate of administration of the constant-rate infusion in milligrams per kilogram per hour (mg/kg/h).
- Determine the total volume for infusion in mL.
- Divide the number of mg/kg/h by the mL/kg/h, with the end result in mg/mL.
- Multiple this number (mg/mL) by the total volume for infusion, resulting in the mg needed to add to the fluids.
- Divide this mg by the drug concentration in mg/mL.
- Add this volume of drug to the predetermined volume of fluids.
- Administer the fluid containing the drug at the rate selected.

Example of using maintenance fluids for delivery in a 5-kg cat receiving 3 μg/kg/h of 50 μg/mL fentanyl*

- Cat will get 2 mL/kg/h of maintenance fluids.
- The drug will be administered at a rate of 0.003 mg/kg/h (= to 3 μg/kg/h).
- We will put 6 h of fluids in a buretrol (60 mL).
- (0.003 mg/kg/h)/(2 mL/kg/h) = 0.0015 mg/h.
- (0.0015 mg/h)/(0.05 mg/mL) = 0.03 mL.
- Add 0.03 mL of fentanyl to 60 mL of selected fluid.
- Administer at 2 mL/kg/h (10 mL/h).

*Bear in mind increasing fluids will increase analgesic drug delivery, so desired changes in fluid administration and drug administration will occur concurrently. The advantage of a syringe pump is the analgesic drug administration is independent of fluid rate and varying the drug delivery has minimal consequences on fluid administration.

patients, such as dexmedetomidine.[128] Buprenorphine, an opioid that is discussed in detail later, has almost 100% bioavailability after oral transmucosal administration.[109,111] Compared with other species that have a neutral oral pH, the more alkaline mouth of the cat may enhance absorption of this drug. Butorphanol has also been administered by the oral transmucosal route in cats, but it is not effective at maintaining the plasma concentrations that are achieved after intravenous dosing.[161]

Epidural

Administration of drugs into the epidural space can provide long-lasting analgesic benefit to the animal, with few systemic effects. The rate of complications for epidurals is low, although urinary retention was noted in 2 of 23 (8%) cats in one study.[148] However, with appropriate nursing care (e.g., observing for urination, expressing the bladder after the procedure, placing a urinary catheter), this complication can be minimized. The spinal cord ends at L7-S1 in the cat, so careful needle placement and observation for the presence of cerebrospinal fluid is necessary to avoid administration of drugs into the subarachnoid space. If the subarachnoid space is entered, the drug volume is halved.[73] Epidural catheters are available for use and have been used successfully in dogs[139] but are not widely used in cats. The epidural space is approached after the cat has been anesthetized. This space is easily palpable with the cat in sternal recumbency, with the hindlimbs pulled forward. The animal is appropriately clipped and prepped; a sterile approach is vital to avoid bacterial contamination of the epidural space. Infected skin is an absolute contraindication to an epidural. The wings of the ilium are palpated bilaterally with the thumb and third finger while wearing sterile gloves, while the index finger palpates the lumbosacral space. Once the space is palpated, it is approached with a 1.5-inch 22-gauge spinal needle at a 45- to 90-degree angle to the skin, targeting midline of the animal and the center of the epidural space. Often, practice is necessary for proficient placement of a spinal needle. Blood in the spinal needle necessitates aborting the procedure.

ANALGESIC DRUGS

The classic and most commonly used analgesic drugs include the opioids, NSAIDs, and local anesthetics. Historically, information on drug therapy in one species has been extrapolated to the cat without consideration of the ways in which the cat's unique metabolism may alter both the pharmacokinetic profile and pharmacodynamic effect of the drug. Drug metabolism is discussed in Chapter 4, and this information should be kept in mind before using a drug in a cat for any reason, including pain management.

Opioids

Opioids are the cornerstone for the treatment of acute pain in many species, including the cat. The reasons for its popularity include efficacy, high margin of safety,[9] and reversibility. Fortunately, there has been significant progress in dispelling the myth that opioid use in cats results in excitement, making their use inappropriate. So-called morphine mania was documented in the early literature, when doses as high as 20 mg/kg of morphine were used.[138] It is now recognized that when clinically relevant doses of opioids are given, cats frequently display some euphoric responses, such as purring, rubbing, and kneading with the forepaws, and are easy to handle.[109,112] Opioid administration is appropriate for trauma patients, cats undergoing surgery or invasive diagnostic procedures, and those with painful medical conditions (e.g., pancreatitis, cystitis).

Opioids are more effective when given before a painful procedure than after one because of their ability to decrease the development of central sensitization in response to surgical stimulation.[82] This preemptive effect has been demonstrated in many species, including the dog[77] and rat,[83] and there is no reason to believe that it does not also occur in the cat. Therefore opioids should be incorporated whenever possible into premedication protocols for elective surgery. This does not mean that postoperative administration is unnecessary; continued assessment for comfort is essential after surgery and administration of analgesic drugs. Opioids or other analgesic agents may be necessary for several days, depending on the severity of the surgical procedure.

Because of their abuse potential in humans, opioids for veterinary use are subject to strict regulations with regard to prescribing, storage, and dispensing. These rules and regulations differ among countries, and it is important that the clinician be aware of current relevant local statutes.

Side Effects of Opioids

Elevated body temperatures have been reported in cats given opioids between 1 and 5 hours after recovery from anesthesia.[97,102] Hydromorphone at clinically recommended doses (0.05 to 0.1 mg/kg subcutaneously, intramuscularly, or intravenously) was associated with an increase in rectal temperature above 40° C (104° F) in 75% of cats in one study,[97] and in one cat a rectal temperature of 42.5° C (108.5° F) was recorded. In another study most cats undergoing elective surgery that received hydromorphone, diazepam, and ketamine followed by isoflurane had postanesthetic temperatures that exceeded those recorded before anesthesia, with a peak rectal temperature of 41.6° C (107.0° F) reported in one cat.[102] In a clinical setting, one study[102] found that the lower a cat's temperature was during anesthesia and surgery, the more severe the "rebound" hyperthermia.

In a laboratory study, hydromorphone at 0.1 mg/kg (administered intravenously) was associated with a significant increase in body temperature, whereas doses of 0.025 and 0.05 mg/kg were not. However, the lower doses were found to have minimal antinociceptive effects compared with the 0.1 mg/kg dose.[159] Transdermal fentanyl patches resulted in higher rectal temperatures compared with butorphanol for cats undergoing onychectomy, although no temperature exceeded 40° C (104° F).[40] Alfentanil infusions during anesthesia were also associated with increased rectal temperatures in cats.[61]

Recent laboratory studies in cats with implanted thermistors that did not undergo surgery showed that intramuscular administration of the opioids hydromorphone (0.05 to 0.2 mg/kg), morphine (0.5 mg/kg), buprenorphine (0.02 mg/kg), and butorphanol (0.2 mg/kg) alone or in combination with ketamine or isoflurane caused a mild to moderate increase in body temperature (≤40.1° C, 104.2° F), which lasted several hours but was self-limiting.[103]

After the end of anesthesia, body temperature is usually measured until the cat becomes normothermic, but as noted previously, it is prudent to monitor beyond that point and for 5 hours or longer after the end of anesthesia. Using warm air or circulating water blankets can prevent intraoperative hypothermia, which may in turn limit severe "rebound" hyperthermia. If profound hyperthermia develops, treatment includes active cooling or administration of naloxone (0.01 mg/kg intramuscularly, subcutaneously) or both.[103]

Some opioids, including morphine and hydromorphone, may cause retching, vomiting, and nausea characterized by salivation,[110,113] especially when used alone and in pain-free cats (e.g., as a premedicant for an elective procedure). Vomiting and profuse salivation are common after subcutaneous administration of hydromorphone and appears distressing to the cats.[113] Vomiting and retching are best prevented in cats with increased intraocular pressure, penetrating corneal foreign bodies, and elevated intracranial pressure. In many cases of foreign body ingestion (e.g., needles or linear objects), vomiting and retching can cause penetration of the gastrointestinal tract.

In dogs the administration of acepromazine reduces opioid-related vomiting[151] and is potentially effective in cats. Clinically, vomiting occurs less commonly when opioids are combined with acepromazine than when they are used alone in cats. Maropitant, a neurokinin-1 antagonist, is highly effective against the emetic effects of xylazine in cats,[56] but there are no reports of its use in conjunction with opioids. If vomiting is contraindicated in a feline patient but an opioid is required to provide pain relief, appropriate choices would include buprenorphine or methadone (intramuscular or intravenous) or fentanyl as a CRI.

In the cat opioids induce marked mydriasis. Cats with dilated pupils often appear more agitated, perhaps as a result of reduced visual acuity, which causes them to bump into objects and become startled when approached. Dimming the lights and speaking softly to the cat as it is approached helps reduce these behaviors.

In humans decreased intestinal motility is a common, unpleasant, and problematic side effect of opioid administration.[120] In the authors' experience, it is uncommon to see constipation in cats being treated for acute pain or when opioids are only used for a few days.

Potential Drug Interactions

With the increasing use of psychoactive drugs (selective serotonin reuptake inhibitors, tricyclic antidepressants, monoamine oxidase inhibitors and serotonin agonists; see Chapter 14) in veterinary medicine as part of a treatment regimen for behavior problems, there is a growing concern for the possibility of adverse drug interactions.[9,90] Serotonin toxicity—which can range from mild signs such as salivation and diarrhea to severe signs such as myoclonus and hyperthermia resulting in death—can occur when two drugs that increase serotonin levels are co-administered. Meperidine (pethidine), fentanyl, remifentanil, pentazocine, and tramadol impair the reuptake of serotonin. Although not well documented in the veterinary literature, the addition of these analgesic agents to an established psychoactive drug protocol in humans has triggered serotonin toxicity.[85] Before an analgesic plan is drawn up for a cat, it is essential to establish a list of all current medications. This includes any supplements or herbs the owner is administering; St. John's wort *(Hypericum perforatum)*, for instance, alters serotonin reuptake.

Specific Opioid Drugs

Current nomenclature of opioid receptors is based on molecular cloning. The three types of receptors—OP_1, OP_2, and OP_3—were formerly known as delta (δ), kappa (κ), and mu (μ), respectively.[123] Opioid drugs are traditionally classified by their actions on these receptors into agonists, partial agonists, agonist-antagonists, and antagonists. Suggested doses of commonly used drugs are given in Table 6-1.

Butorphanol (Torbutrol, Torbugesic) is one of the few analgesic drugs to have market authorization for use specifically in the cat in some countries, including the United States and United Kingdom. It is an agonist at the OP_2 receptor, an antagonist at the OP_3 receptor, and exhibits a ceiling effect. This is clinically relevant, insofar as increasing doses do not produce further analgesia.[81] In one research model using a somatic thermal stimulus, the duration of action was approximately 90 minutes, regardless of dose,[81] whereas a similar study showed large intercat variability, with antinociception lasting up to 8 hours in some cats.[63] The response to butorphanol may vary depending on the source of pain. Visceral antinociception was demonstrated with 0.1 mg/kg of

TABLE 6-1 **Suggested Dose Ranges and Route of Administration for Analgesic Drugs Commonly Used to Treat Acute Pain***

Drug	Dose (Range)	Route of Administration
OPIOIDS		
Butorphanol	0.1-0.2 mg/kg	IV, IM
Buprenorphine	0.02-0.03 mg/kg	IV, IM, OTM
Fentanyl	2-10 μg/kg (bolus) 5-50 μg/kg/hour intraoperatively 2-10 μg/kg/hour postoperatively or in trauma patients	IV IV IV
Hydromorphone	0.05-0.1 mg/kg	IV, IM
Oxymorphone	0.05-0.1 mg/kg	IV, IM
Meperidine (pethidine)	5 mg/kg	IM—not to be given IV
Methadone	0.2-0.5 mg/kg	IV, IM
Morphine	0.2-0.5 mg/kg	IV (slow administration advised to prevent histamine release), IM
NSAIDs	*DOSES SUGGESTED FOR SINGLE USE*	
Carprofen	2-4 mg/kg	SC, IV
Ketoprofen	2 mg/kg	SC, IM
Meloxicam	0.1-0.3 mg/kg	SC

SC, Subcutaneous; *IM,* intramuscular; *OTM,* oral transmucosal; *NSAIDs,* nonsteroidal antiinflammatory drugs.
*For information on repeated dosing and dosing intervals, please see details in the text.

butorphanol, whereas somatic antinociception was unaffected in the same cats.[117]

A large multicenter study comparing the clinical usefulness of butorphanol with that of buprenorphine in more than 150 cats undergoing primarily, but not solely, ovariohysterectomy or castration found that buprenorphine resulted in lower pain scores for a greater duration than did butorphanol.[143] Current data suggest that butorphanol is a sensible choice for acute, visceral pain (e.g., cystitis), but in light of its relatively short duration of action and ceiling effect, it is a poor choice for somatic or visceral pain that is more than transient in nature, such as would occur with invasive surgery.[108]

Nalbuphine (Nubain), like butorphanol, is an opioid agonist–antagonist. Little has been published regarding the use of nalbuphine in cats. One study demonstrated visceral analgesia, with intravenous doses of 0.75, 1.5, and 3 mg/kg producing similar effects that lasted between 156 and 200 minutes.[117] None of these doses resulted in somatic analgesia.

Pentazocine (Talwin), another agonist–antagonist, only provided visceral analgesia when 3 mg/kg (intravenous) was administered.[117] No somatic antinociception was noted with this dose, and undesirable side effects such as ataxia and apprehension were described, which suggests that this drug has little utility in cats.

Buprenorphine (Buprenex) is a partial OP_3 agonist and has been widely studied in cats in both laboratory and clinical settings. It has market authorization for use in cats in some countries. Laboratory studies report varying times to onset of effect and duration of action, which appear partly related to dose and route of administration. For example, when antinociception is evaluated using a thermal threshold model, a dose of 0.01 mg/kg (intramuscular) required up to 2 hours for onset of action, and the duration of effect varied from 4 to 12 hours.[110] In the same model a dose of 0.02 mg/kg (intramuscular) resulted in a quicker onset of antinociception, which was significant at 35 minutes and lasted approximately 5 hours.[63] Intravenous administration of buprenorphine across a range of doses from 0.01 mg/kg to 0.04 mg/kg showed that onset of thermal antinociception time is short (15 minutes), with little difference in intensity or duration of effect. A different test of somatic analgesia (mechanical threshold) did show a dose-related effect; 0.01 mg/kg was ineffective, 0.02 mg/kg was effective but short acting, and 0.04 mg/kg had the longest duration of action.[135] These authors commented that another reason for the variability among studies was significant intercat variability, a reminder that pain and the efficacy of drugs used to relieve it are unique to each individual and that individual assessment is the key to success in each patient.

Similar to the reported effects of subcutaneous hydromorphone, this route also seems less effective when a single dose of buprenorphine is used.[43,134] In a laboratory setting, there was no difference in onset or duration of action (30 minutes and 6 hours, respectively) between oral transmucosal and intravenous administration of buprenorphine at 0.02 mg/kg. In a clinical trial intravenous and intramuscular administration of buprenorphine were more effective than the oral transmucosal route.[43] However, this could be a result of the low oral transmucosal dose used (0.01 mg/kg). Additional information gained from these studies is the time of peak effect, which consistently occurs between 60 and 90 minutes after administration. Pain is often most intense in the immediate postoperative period. Therefore the timing of preoperative (preemptive) buprenorphine administration should be planned to meet these needs.

In several clinical studies, the analgesia produced by buprenorphine (usually given intramuscularly) in cats undergoing a variety of invasive procedures was greater in magnitude and longer lasting than that produced by several other opioids, including butorphanol, levomethadone, morphine, oxymorphone, and pethidine.[33,91,129,133,143] However, it should be noted that equianalgesic doses of opioids were not necessarily used, and the methods of pain assessment were not standardized.

A sustained-release preparation of buprenorphine, available from ZooPharm (Fort Collins, Colo.), for subcutaneous administration has been evaluated in cats undergoing ovariohysterectomy. A single sustained-release dose of 120 μg/kg was as effective as 20 μg/kg buprenorphine by the oral transmucosal route given every 12 hours until 60 hours after the operation.[18] The sustained-release formulation is convenient to use, and in feral cats, which are often difficult to handle after procedures, this formulation is a viable option for providing postoperative analgesia of suitable duration.

Buprenorphine is available for use in humans as a matrix patch. In cats the plasma concentrations were quite variable after application of a 35 μg/h patch, and no analgesia was evident during a 4-day period in one study.[96] Until further studies are performed with different sizes of patches and perhaps using a loading dose of buprenorphine, this method of administration cannot be recommended.

The following conclusions can be drawn from the extensive published data on buprenorphine in cats: Doses for clinical use should be 0.02 mg/kg or greater; intravenous, intramuscular, and oral transmucosal routes of administration are effective, but the subcutaneous route is not; and individual variation is well documented.

OP_3 Opioid Agonists

Fentanyl is a potent opioid used in cats as an intravenous bolus, a CRI, and a transdermal patch (Duragesic).

Intravenous fentanyl (10 μg/kg IV) reaches peak effect in less than 5 minutes and provides significant antinociception for almost 2 hours with minimal to no adverse effects.[112] The pharmacokinetic profile of fentanyl makes it a suitable agent for use as a CRI. The plasma levels and therefore the degree of analgesia can be rapidly altered, and fentanyl is frequently used in this manner to provide analgesia in trauma cases both during and after surgery. A research model suggests that the effective plasma concentration in cats is 1 ng/mL.[112] The infusion rate required to maintain this plasma concentration has not been verified, and it is likely that requirements will vary depending on the individual and the severity of injury or extent of surgery. These authors have used infusion rates from 0.08 to 0.8 μg/kg per minute (5 to 50 μg/kg per hour) during surgery and from 0.03 to 0.16 μg/kg per minute (2 to 10 μg/kg per hour) postoperatively or in trauma patients.

After application of a transdermal patch, the plasma concentration of fentanyl is highly variable and undetectable in some cats. Many factors may account for this variability, including body weight (which dictates the dose/kg from a standard-size patch), subcutaneous fat, body temperature, and location and method of patch placement. Serum levels of fentanyl are higher in normothermic (38° C) than in hypothermic cats (35° C).[101] Cats weighing less than 4 kg have higher plasma concentrations when the full adhesive layer of a 25 μg/h patch is exposed, as opposed to half.[27] A steady state can be achieved within 6 to 12 hours and maintained for up to 72 hours after patch placement in some cats.[84] The cat's skin may act as a drug depot because, unlike in dogs, the serum concentrations can take as long as 20 hours to decline after the patch is removed.[84] Clinical reports suggest that the transdermal fentanyl patch has clinical utility in cats undergoing onychectomy and ovariohysterectomy,[37,40,47] but clinicians should be aware that just because the patch has been applied does not mean it is providing adequate analgesia in every case.

There is a case report of a dog that became extremely sedate after it punctured and presumably ingested or licked the contents of a transdermal fentanyl patch applied to its flank,[119] and it is highly plausible that this could also occur in a cat. The clinician should consider all consequences carefully before sending a cat home with a patch; this has caused some serious liability issues in human medicine, including diversion, abuse, and accidental ingestion by a child.[146,147]

Remifentanil (Ultiva) is rapidly metabolized and does not accumulate. It is used as an infusion in several species, including humans, because of the ability to change plasma concentrations very quickly. Currently, remifentanil is predominantly used to provide analgesia during anesthesia at rates of 1 to 2 μg/kg per minute (60 to 120 μg/kg per hour), which would cause dysphoric and sometimes frantic behavior in conscious cats.[14] However, if infusion rates are kept below 1 μg/kg per minute (<60 μg/kg per hour), these adverse effects can be avoided and antinociception can still be demonstrated,[14] making it suitable for postoperative use.

Hydromorphone is widely used in veterinary medicine because of its low cost.[5] Hydromorphone and oxymorphone (at 0.05 mg/kg) provide clinically equivalent analgesia in cats undergoing a variety of surgical procedures.[5] In a research model an intravenous dose of 0.05 mg/kg provided moderate antinociception for 80 minutes, whereas 0.1 mg/kg (administered intravenously) provided profound effects for 200 minutes in one study and for up to 7 hours in another.[159,160] Two independent studies noted that vomiting and nausea are a side effect of hydromorphone use.[5,113] The concerns related to hydromorphone-related hyperthermia were discussed previously.

Oxymorphone (Numorphan) is in wide clinical usage, but there is little published information regarding this drug in cats. In a small number of cats, oxymorphone at 0.05 mg/kg (administered intravenously) appeared as effective clinically as hydromorphone at the same dose.[5] In another study oxymorphone was not as effective an analgesic as buprenorphine for cats undergoing onychectomy with or without castration.[33] The published information suggests few adverse effects from oxymorphone, but evidence-based data supporting its use are largely lacking.

Meperidine (Demerol), also known as pethidine, can cause excitement when administered intravenously; therefore only subcutaneous or intramuscular administration is recommended. Both clinical and laboratory studies suggest that it is short acting,[83,88] and clinicians should expect it to be effective for only 1 to 2 hours. Because meperidine can result in sedation, it can be used for this purpose when a traditional sedative or tranquillizer is contraindicated, such as in a hemodynamically unstable patient.

Use of methadone is increasingly popular in veterinary medicine. No pharmacokinetic data are currently available for use in the cat. In addition to its opioid actions, methadone has other desirable properties, including action at the *N*-methyl *D*-aspartate (NDMA) receptor,[50] which is involved in the development of central sensitization. Methadone is available as an isomer (levomethadone) and a racemic mixture. The racemic mixture, at the relatively low dose of 0.2 mg/kg subcutaneously, increased thermal thresholds between 1 and 3 hours but had little effect on mechanical thresholds.[134] In a clinical setting, both racemic methadone (0.6 mg/kg intramuscularly) and levomethadone (0.3 mg/kg intramuscularly) given before ovariectomy provide effective postoperative analgesia, as assessed by palpation and behavior, with no adverse effects.[114] However, compared with buprenorphine or carprofen, levomethadone (0.3 mg/kg subcutaneously every 8 hours for 5 days) was not as effective for orthopedic surgery and was associated with excitement in some cats.[91] It is likely that better results may have been achieved with a shorter dosing interval; it is unlikely that the duration of action would be 8 hours at that dose.

Morphine has a long history of use in humans and animals and is often considered the gold standard for opioids. Because of the limited ability of cats to glucuronidate drugs, morphine may have less overall efficacy than in other species, insofar as glucuronidation is necessary for the production of morphine-6-glucuronide (M-6-G), a potent and active metabolite. This metabolite was not detected after intramuscular administration of morphine in cats and was detected in only three of six cats receiving intravenous morphine.[144] Because of the belief that morphine caused excitement in cats, lower doses (0.1 to 0.2 mg/kg) have historically been recommended and may have led to the impression that morphine is not an effective analgesic in cats. Owing to the lack of M-6-G production, it is possible that higher doses of the parent compound are necessary to produce analgesia in the cat equivalent to that in species able to produce this metabolite. Intramuscular doses of 0.5 mg/kg are used with success and minimal side effects[103] (in the authors' experience).

Intravenous morphine has been associated with histamine release in dogs in a dose-related manner, although no similar study has been performed in cats.[51] If morphine is used intravenously, slow administration is advised.

Combinations of Opioids

Co-administration of opioids has been proposed as a means of achieving the positive benefits of different drugs. Although mixing of opioids has been reported, the results are variable, ranging from a decrease in intensity of antinociception but prolongation of effect[80] to no measurable effect[63] to improved outcome.[10] Because of this unpredictability, simultaneous administration of different opioids is not recommended. On the basis of reports that ultralow doses of opioid antagonists enhanced the analgesic actions of opioids in rodents and humans,[72] a similar study was performed in cats. Combining low-dose naloxone with buprenorphine failed to show any benefits over buprenorphine alone,[126] which suggests that direct extrapolation of data among species is unwise without careful evaluation in the target species.

Epidural Administration of Opioids

When evaluated in a thermal threshold model, both buprenorphine (12.5 μg/kg) and morphine (0.1 mg/kg) provided analgesia by way of the epidural route, but morphine provided analgesia of greater intensity and longer duration (16 hours as opposed to 10 hours).[107] Meperidine, methadone, and fentanyl have all been evaluated after epidural injection.[35,64] These drugs are more lipophilic than morphine, resulting in systemic diffusion and actions that mimic those of the drug when given by the intravenous or intramuscular route. In contrast, hydrophilic drugs, such as morphine, do not readily diffuse, remaining in the epidural space and providing a long duration of action and minimal systemic effects.[74] Epidural morphine does not produce motor dysfunction and is an excellent choice of technique for perianal surgery and hindlimb surgery, including amputation.

Tramadol

Although not classified as a true opioid, tramadol (Ultram) is included here because much of its analgesia results from its opioid receptor site. Tramadol exerts its action at multiple sites, including opioid, serotonin, and adrenergic receptors.[60] It is available in injectable and oral formulations and is not currently a controlled drug. It has good oral bioavailability in cats, and its active metabolite O-desmethyl-tramadol was found after both systemic and oral administration. The half-life of tramadol is longer in cats than dogs, so dosing intervals can be extended.[105] In a research model, a subcutaneous dose of 1 mg/kg did not increase thermal threshold.[136] However, 4 mg/kg administered subcutaneously clinically improved postoperative comfort in cats undergoing ovariohysterectomy compared with the NSAID tolfenamic acid alone.[20] Similarly, the combination of the NSAID vedaprofen and tramadol at 2 mg/kg improved postoperative analgesia more than either drug given alone.[11,20] In a study done by the same group, no adverse effects with regard to platelet aggregation, vomiting, gastrointestinal function, or biochemical values were found.[12] Tramadol produced mild euphoria,[11] but this was not deemed an undesirable attribute of the drug.

NONSTEROIDAL ANTIINFLAMMATORY DRUGS

NSAIDs are widely used to combat acute pain because the basis of surgical and traumatic pain is inflammation. NSAIDs are convenient because they are not strictly regulated and most provide up to 24 hours of analgesia. However, unlike opioids and alpha$_2$-adrenergic agonists, NSAIDs are not reversible and have the potential to alter clotting function, renal perfusion, and gastrointestinal integrity.

Side Effects of Nonsteroidal Antiinflammatory Drugs

Cyclooxygenase (COX) enzymes are traditionally thought to exist in two major isoforms, COX-1 and

COX-2, but COX-3 and other subclasses are also reported. Initially, COX-1 was considered the constitutive "housekeeping" enzyme responsible for multiple essential physiologic functions, and COX-2 was considered an inducible enzyme that resulted from inflammation. Preferential blockade of the COX-2 enzyme was thought to increase the safety of NSAIDs. It is now understood that the COX enzymes are multifaceted, there is overlap in their functions, and it is unlikely that COX-2 can be inhibited without some impact on the COX-1 enzymes. COX-2 is also constitutive and required for normal function in many tissues—for example, in the kidney of dogs, rats, monkeys, and humans.[69,70,152]

NSAIDs have been used less in cats than other species because of their well-documented toxic side effects. A recent review outlines the challenges of using NSAIDs in cats but also concludes that with proper precautions these drugs can be part of successful acute pain management in this species.[75] Many NSAIDs are heavily dependent on glucuronidation for metabolism, and for this reason some NSAIDs have long half-lives in cats. Although aspirin is the classic example of one such drug, carprofen also has a relatively long half-life in the cat compared with the dog.[99,142] Conversely, NSAIDs that are oxidized (e.g., meloxicam) may have a shorter half-life.[75]

NSAIDs should not be used concurrently with corticosteroids or in cats with gastrointestinal compromise. Meloxicam does not the alter glomerular filtration rate in healthy, euvolemic conscious cats,[48] but in the face of hypotension, renal autoregulation is dependent on prostaglandins, and therefore decreased volume status, as may be seen after acute trauma, is considered a contraindication for NSAID use. Hypotension (a mean arterial blood pressure <60 mmHg or systolic blood pressure <90 mm Hg) is documented in between 10% and 33% of cats under anesthesia.[39,49] For this reason many experts recommend that NSAIDs not be administered before anesthesia and instead be reserved for use in the immediate postoperative period.

NSAIDs can alter hemostasis as a result of their effect on platelets and vascular endothelium. There is no evidence that the newer NSAIDs with market authorization for use in cats have a significant effect on surgical bleeding.[75]

When compared with one another, ketoprofen, carprofen, meloxicam, and tolfenamic acid were equally effective in cats undergoing routine soft tissue surgery,[130] and therefore the clinician may select one on the basis of personal preference, ease of administration (oral versus injection), and market authorization for each drug in different countries.

When a single dose of each drug was given in a clinical setting, carprofen provided better postoperative analgesia than meperidine, butorphanol, buprenorphine, and levomethadone[3,76,91]; this is likely due to the difference in duration of action of the two classes of drugs.

Specific Nonsteroidal Antiinflammatory Drugs

Although aspirin (acetylsalicylic acid) is readily available over the counter, its side effects (e.g., gastrointestinal ulceration, platelet inactivation, and decreased protective renal prostaglandins[15,100]) in combination with a half-life of up to 45 days[29] make aspirin an unsuitable perioperative analgesic.

Only the most widely used NSAIDs are discussed here; for complete information on these and other less commonly used agents, the reader is referred to the review by Lascelles and colleagues.[75] The individual NSAIDs discussed in this chapter have market authorization for use in cats in some but not all countries, and their labeled indication may also vary. Therefore it is strongly recommended that clinicians verify this data in each region before use.

Carprofen (Rimadyl) is a COX-1–sparing NSAID, although this selectivity appears to decrease as dosage increases in in vitro models.[46] Because the half-life in the cat is variable among individuals and ranges anywhere from 9 to 49 hours,[99] repeat dosing is not advised. In countries where it has market authorization for use in cats, it is for one-time use only. In cats that underwent ovariohysterectomy, doses ranging from 1 mg/kg to 4 mg/kg were more effective than meperidine (pethidine) from 2 to 20 hours after surgery.[77] An intravenous or subcutaneous dose of 1 to 2 mg/kg is most commonly recommended.[75]

Ketoprofen (Anafen) is not a selective COX inhibitor and has the potential to produce similar adverse effects as described for aspirin. However, obvious effects on hemostasis are not reported.[75] It is effective in alleviating the pain associated with soft tissue surgery and injury.[79,130] In cats with musculoskeletal pain, it was administered at 1 mg/kg orally for 5 days with beneficial effects.[79]

Meloxicam (Metacam) is a COX-1–sparing NSAID, and decreasing the dosage of the drug may decrease the incidence of COX-1-inhibition–mediated effects.[75] Meloxicam (0.3 mg/kg subcutaneously, given once only) is the only NSAID approved for postoperative control of pain related to soft tissue and orthopedic surgery in cats in the United States. On the basis of multiple behavioral assessments, cats receiving meloxicam appeared more comfortable after onychectomy compared with those receiving butorphanol.[17] Meloxicam was as effective as ketoprofen in alleviating pain in cats with musculoskeletal disease, but an advantage of meloxicam is its palatability.[79] Recent work indicates no measurable effect on glomerular filtration when meloxicam is administered once at 0.2 mg/kg followed by 0.1 mg/kg once daily PO for 4 additional days.[48] Although it is an off-label use, this dosing schedule is widely used to provide 5 days of postoperative analgesia in healthy cats that are normovolemic.

Robenacoxib (Onsior), a COX-1–sparing NSAID,[45] is the most recent NSAID and first coxib class NSAID approved for use in cats. It is available in both injectable and tablet formulations and is marketed for the alleviation of acute pain and inflammation associated with musculoskeletal disorders and soft tissue surgery. The injection is approved for preoperative use, and the tablets for up to 6 days in some countries. At a dose of 2 mg/kg, it was effective at reducing pain and swelling in an inflammatory paw model.[44] There are no published reports of its use in clinical patients at this time.

Tolfenamic acid has limited pharmacokinetic information available, and its status as a COX-1–sparing agent is controversial.[67] Although not licensed in the United States, tolfenamic acid is licensed and popular in many other countries.[75] At 4 mg/kg, it appears to be as effective as meloxicam (0.3 mg/kg subcutaneously) in the cat for control of postoperative pain.[6]

Local Anesthetic Agents

Local anesthetics are versatile agents that have multiple applications in the treatment of acute pain. Unlike the drugs discussed previously, local anesthetics can provide *complete* analgesia by blocking nociceptive transmission. Sadly, these techniques are underutilized, perhaps because cats are under general anesthesia for most surgical procedures and the potential benefits of adding a local anesthetic technique are overlooked. Although general anesthesia provides unconsciousness and immobility, transmission of noxious stimuli still occurs and reaches the spinal cord and brain of the anesthetized patient, where long-lasting effects such as central sensitization and secondary hyperalgesia can develop. Local anesthetics block nociception and transmission of painful stimuli, reducing these deleterious consequences.

Although a multitude of local anesthetics are available, lidocaine and bupivacaine are most frequently used in veterinary medicine. These local anesthetics differ from each other in their speed of onset, as well as potency and duration of action, but both undergo hepatic metabolism. Lidocaine is traditionally thought to have a rapid onset, whereas bupivacaine has a slower onset. Bupivacaine is more potent than lidocaine, and its duration of action is longer.[124] Often, these two local anesthetics are combined to reap the most desirable qualities of each (rapid onset and prolonged action); however, the efficacy of this approach has not been tested. When incorporating local anesthetics into the analgesic plan, the clinician must consider toxicity and calculate a safe dose based on mg/kg for each individual cat. For example, using 4 mg/kg of lidocaine for a 5-kg cat translates to no more than 1 mL of 2% lidocaine total for that animal. If the calculated dose provides insufficient volume for the intended block, the drug can be diluted. Toxic effects of local anesthetics include neurologic signs such as seizures and cardiovascular changes that can be mild or result in complete cardiovascular collapse. Doses reported to cause neurologic signs in cats are 11.7 ± 4.6 mg/kg for lidocaine and 3.8 ± 1 mg/kg for bupivacaine. Cardiotoxic doses of lidocaine and bupivacaine are 47.3 ± 8.6 mg/kg and 18.4 ± 4.9 mg/kg, respectively.[19]

Lidocaine administered by CRI is widely used in dogs to decrease the requirements for inhalant agents and provide intraoperative and postoperative analgesia, but this is not recommended in cats. Serious adverse effects, including cardiovascular depression and increased plasma lactate values, were reported in anesthetized cats with a wide variety of infusion rates,[104] which emphasizes the need to critically evaluate techniques that are successful in other species before applying them to the cat.

Topical application of local anesthetic creams to desensitize the skin can ease catheter placement and venipuncture, as well as aid in a variety of other minimally invasive procedures, such as skin biopsy. Two products are readily available: lidocaine in a liposome-encapsulated formulation (ELA-Max; Ferndale Laboratories, Ferndale, Michigan) and a eutectic mixture of lidocaine and prilocaine (EMLA cream; AstraZeneca LP, Willington, Delaware, and as a generic formulation). There is little systemic absorption after application of the liposome formulation, and no uptake of the components of the eutectic mixture.[38,41] The success rate of jugular catheterization increased by over 20% (from 38% to 60%) when the eutectic mixture was used as part of the catheterization process in one study.[157] The proposed skin site is clipped in advance and cleaned in a routine fashion. The cream is applied and covered with an occlusive dressing, which could be a small square cut from a plastic bag or surgery or examination glove, then covered by a light wrap for approximately 20 minutes. When it is time to place the catheter, the dressing is removed and a final cleansing of the skin performed.

Another method for delivery of local anesthesia is the lidocaine patch (Lidoderm 5%; Endo Pharmaceuticals, Chadds Ford, Pennsylvania). This patch produces high concentrations of lidocaine at the site of application with minimal systemic absorption and appeared effective for the 72-hour duration of assessment.[71] The patch can be cut to any desired size or shape without fear of altered drug delivery, making it a good option for wound management.

Other useful techniques that are worth learning include brachial plexus blocks, dental blocks, distal paw blocks, intercostal nerve blocks, and wound infusion ("soaker") catheters. These techniques are inexpensive, relatively easy to perform, and associated with minimal complications if done correctly.

Local Anesthetic Blocks

Cats are rarely tolerant of a local block performed while awake, and complications can arise if an animal moves at the wrong moment; therefore, heavy sedation or general anesthesia is recommended prior to performing local blocks. Some clinically useful blocks are described below.

Brachial Plexus Block

The aim of this procedure is to block the ventral branches of cervical nerves 6, 7, and 8 and thoracic nerve 1; this technique has been demonstrated to reduce intraoperative inhalant requirement, as well as early postoperative pain in the cat.[93] This is a useful technique for procedures that are located below the elbow joint. A block can be performed in three ways: with ultrasound guidance, with use of a nerve stimulator, or based on anatomic landmarks with no visualization. Ultrasound-guided nerve blocks are a relatively novel technique in animals. Instruction for this technique in dogs is available.[16] Use of peripheral nerve stimulation has been described in the rabbit as well as the dog but not yet in the cat.[8,162] This technique does increase the success rate when used in children[116] and has great potential in cats. Because the appropriate equipment for these two techniques is not yet widely available in general practice, the technique described here is based on anatomic landmarks (Figure 6-3).[73] The point of the shoulder (scapulohumeral joint), first rib, and cervical vertebrae are the anatomic landmarks that will assist with correctly performing this block. Once the hair coat has been clipped and the insertion site prepared using sterile technique, the patient's head and neck are placed in a neutral position (i.e., with minimal flexion or extension). The cervical transverse processes form a line that typically traverses the proximal brachial plexus at the first rib.[73] The first rib is followed dorsal as far as possible, and a 1.5-inch, 22-gauge sterile needle is inserted and advanced toward and caudal to this rib, below the scapula. A syringe containing lidocaine (4 mg/kg) or bupivacaine (2 mg/kg) is attached to the needle. It is critical to pull back on the plunger of the syringe after it is attached to the needle and before drug administration; complications of this block can include injection into the axillary vein or artery, as well as needle placement into the thoracic cavity. If blood or air is aspirated, the procedure is best aborted. If nothing is aspirated, approximately one quarter of the total volume is deposited at this location and the needle is withdrawn a short distance (0.5 cm). After aspirating again, more local anesthetic can be deposited. This continues until the needle is withdrawn from the skin.

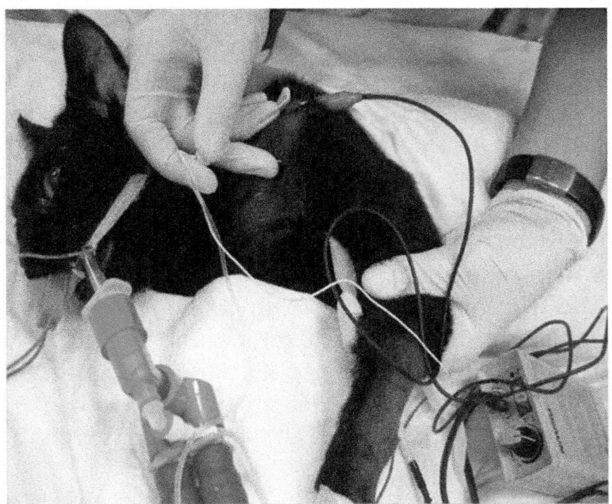

FIGURE 6-3 A cat receiving a brachial plexus block. *(Image courtesy Heidi Reicht and Martina Mosing.)*

Dental Blocks[73]

Dental blocks are often used to help manage pain associated with surgery of the jaw and face and dental procedures, targeting (as appropriate) the mental, inferior alveolar (mandibular), and infraorbital nerves. The mental nerve foramen can be palpated rostrally between the canine and the first premolar tooth, on the buccal side of the mandible. The inferior alveolar nerve is blocked intraorally, from either an external or internal approach, at the caudal aspect of the mandible. It is palpated on the lingual side of the mandible, ventrally and rostral to the angular process. Often, because of the small size of the cat mandible, it is necessary to approach this foramen from the external caudal aspect of the jaw. Skin over the site of needle entry must be appropriately clipped and prepped. The infraorbital canal in the cat is extremely shallow, so while this foramen is easily palpated, care should be taken to avoid inserting the needle more than a few millimeters into the canal. One can palpate the foramen ventral to the eye where the zygomatic arch meets the maxilla by lifting the lip and palpating along the buccal mucosa. It is important to aspirate before depositing local anesthetic at any of these foramens and not to exceed the total toxic dose of lidocaine or bupivacaine for the cat when performing multiple blocks. Occasionally, it is necessary to combine local anesthetic with saline to provide more volume.

Distal Paw Block[124]

Declawing of cats is an increasingly controversial procedure and not permitted in many countries. However, if it is performed, it is essential to provide adequate analgesia, often for several days after surgery. Preoperative and postoperative opioids are recommended in combination with an NSAID (e.g., meloxicam), as previously described. The addition of a regional block is widely used, although the postoperative benefits were not obvious in one study.[25] However, many clinicians comment on improved quality of recovery and postoperative comfort, lower intraoperative anesthetic requirements, and fewer changes in intraoperative heart rate and blood pressure after incorporating it into their perioperative plan. Often referred to as the four-point block, the superficial branches of the radial, the palmar and dorsal cutaneous ulnar, and the median nerves are selectively blocked. The radial nerves are located proximal to the carpal joint and on the dorsomedial aspect of the paw, where they are blocked. The ulnar nerve is blocked at two points: proximal and lateral to the accessory carpal bone. The medial carpal pad provides the landmark for blocking the median nerve, which is blocked proximal to this site (Figure 6-4).

Intercostal Nerve Block[73]

This block can alleviate the pain associated with a lateral thoracotomy incision or fractured rib. For an efficacious block, it is important to remember that the innervation supplied to an individual rib has contributions from the nerve roots of the ribs cranial and caudal to the affected nerve, and therefore it is prudent to block one to two intercostal spaces cranial and one to two intercostal spaces caudal to the affected rib. The nerve is blocked near the intervertebral foramen at the caudal border of the rib, with care taken to avoid the blood vessels coursing along the caudal boarder of the rib. When a thoracotomy is performed, the nerve(s) can be directly visualized. If the technique is performed percutaneously, as opposed to directly visualized, care must be taken not to enter the thoracic cavity.

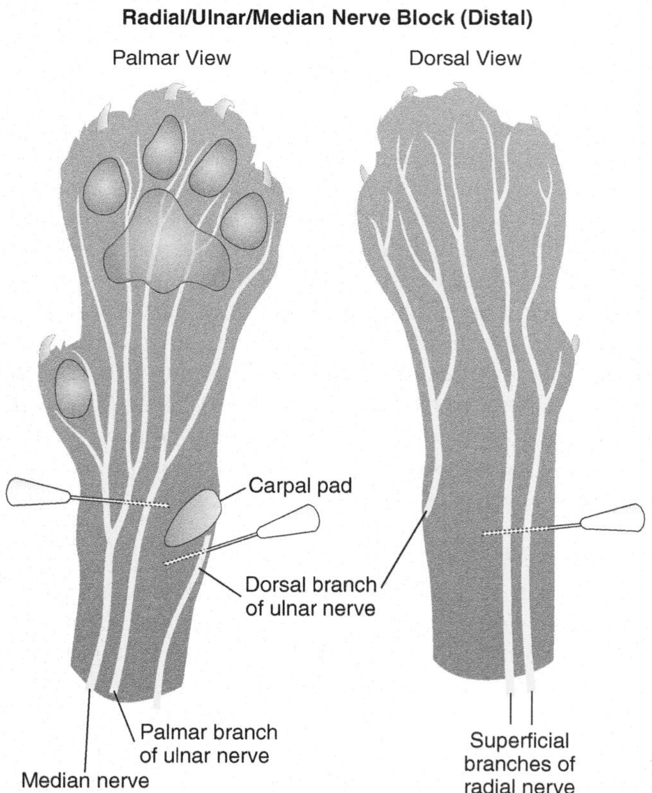

FIGURE 6-4 Targeted nerves for a distal paw block. *(Image courtesy John Spahr and Teton NewMedia.)*

Wound Infusion Catheters

Wound infusion ("soaker") catheters provide in situ continuous local analgesia of a wound. These catheters can be purchased as a "ready to use" product (ON-Q Pain Buster, I-Flow Co, Lake Forest, California) or can be made from a 5-french red rubber catheter, with alternating holes placed 5 mm apart starting 8 cm proximal to the end of the catheter. When wound infusion catheters were used as part of the pain management protocol after fibrosarcoma removal, cats were discharged from the hospital significantly earlier because they met the criteria for discharge (improved mobility and food consumption) sooner.[28] Fear of introducing infection has been cited as a reason for not using this technique, but a retrospective review of cats and dogs with wound soaker catheters did not support this concern.[1]

Alpha$_2$-Adrenergic Agonist Agents

Use of xylazine, detomidine, medetomidine, romifidine and dexmedetomidine are all reported in the cat. Dexmedetomidine (Dexdomitor) is currently the primary alpha$_2$-agonist used in cats and has market authorization in many countries. Alpha$_2$-agonists provide sedation, muscle relaxation, and analgesia. In a research model, the effects of dexmedetomidine (given as an intramuscular injection) on sedation appear to be dose related, but the analgesic effects may not be,[127] and the clinician should be aware that although sedation is obvious, analgesia may not be adequate. Dexmedetomidine also produces well-recognized cardiovascular effects, including bradycardia, decreased cardiac output, and hypertension.

Dexmedetomidine is primarily used as a premedicant before general anesthesia, for chemical restraint, and in combination with local anesthetics for minor procedures.

Oral transmucosal dexmedetomidine (40 μg/kg) provided sedation and measurable antinociceptive effects similar to the same dose given intramuscularly[128] and is a particularly useful technique when dealing with a cat that is in pain and difficult to handle.

The actions of dexmedetomidine are reversed with atipamezole (Antisedan), but it must be remembered that this reverses all effects, including analgesia. Therefore if an invasive procedure is performed, other analgesics (e.g., opioids, NSAIDs) should be given before reversal.

In an effort to utilize the analgesic properties but avoid heavy sedation and unwanted cardiovascular effects, low doses of dexmedetomidine can be given as a CRI. This strategy has been successful in dogs and was as effective as a CRI of morphine in the postoperative period.[150] Similar studies have not been reported in cats, but infusion rates of 0.5 to 2.0 μg/kg per hour are used in clinical settings with reports of success. The cat should be evaluated for pain, including wound palpation, to ensure that any sedative effects of the drug are not masking pain. A benefit of this technique is that the infusion rate can be increased before nursing interventions, such as a bandage change, and lowered over time to assess the patient's comfort level.

N-Methyl-D-Aspartate Receptor Antagonists

Drugs in this category include ketamine, amantadine, and memantine. The latter two drugs are more commonly used in patients with long-term pain conditions, and reliable information on these drugs in cats is lacking or at best anecdotal. Ketamine, however, has a potential role to play in acute pain management.

Ketamine, classified as a dissociative anesthetic, is widely used in cats for chemical restraint or in combination with dexmedetomidine, diazepam, or midazolam to induce general anesthesia (see Chapter 7). However, because of its interaction at the NMDA receptor, there is great interest in using ketamine to provide analgesia and prevent central sensitization and "wind up." In cats arousal (as measured by electroencephalography [EEG]) and autonomic responses during nociceptive stimulation were abolished by ketamine.[141] One clinical study found that cats undergoing ovariohysterectomy with ketamine as part of their anesthesia protocol had better analgesia postoperatively.[125] Experience with sub-anesthetic infusions of ketamine given as part of a multimodal analgesic protocol in dogs undergoing major surgery suggests that it has beneficial effects on postoperative pain.[156] The clinical impression is that doses of ketamine in the range of 5 to 10 μg/kg per minute (300 to 600 μg/kg per hour) during surgery and 2 to 5 μg/kg per minute after surgery (120 to 300 μg/kg per hour for up 24 hours) improve postoperative outcome in cats, but this has not been confirmed in a well-controlled study.

Like ketamine, amantadine is also a NMDA antagonist, but in contrast to ketamine, amantadine stabilizes the NMDA channels as opposed to blocking current flow through the channel.[7] Amantadine is a somewhat new addition to the veterinary analgesic arsenal, and as such there is little information about its use in cats. It was found to enhance the effect of NSAIDs in dogs with osteoarthritis,[78] but its role in acute pain management, especially in the feline, is unclear.

Epidural administration of ketamine has been reported in cats and, when combined with lidocaine, can provide prolonged analgesia.[30] However, a preservative-free formulation of ketamine is not commercially available, and drugs containing preservatives are not recommended for epidural use. Epidural morphine provides effective analgesia and is available in a preservative-free formulation, making this the preferred drug if this route of administration is chosen.

Other Analgesic Drugs

Gabapentin is an anticonvulsant that has utility in alleviating neuropathic pain in humans.[98] There is also interest in using it in the perioperative period to prevent persistent postsurgical pain, which is thought to result from nerve damage during surgery.[68]

In the cat oral bioavailability is high (92%).[122] Oral gabapentin produced no antinociceptive effects in a thermal threshold model,[106] but this is not surprising because its mechanism of action is on damaged nerves.[26] Gabapentin has been used as an "add-on" medication in dogs that underwent intervertebral disk surgery, and beneficial effects were seen on postoperative days 3 and 4.[2] Conversely, no benefit was detected when gabapentin was used as an adjunct analgesic in dogs that underwent forelimb amputation.[155] There are no published studies on the perioperative use of gabapentin in cats.

Maropitant, a neurokinin-1 (NK-1) antagonist commonly used in the cat for prevention of emesis,[56] has shown potential as an analgesic in other species, and investigation is under way in the cat for this purpose. In a research setting there was a marked variation in individual responses to this drug; in some cats thermal antinociception could be demonstrated, but not in others.[94]

MULTIMODAL ANALGESIA

Multimodal analgesia describes the combined use of drugs that work at different receptors and pathways with the assumption this will provide superior analgesia or allow lower doses of each drug to lessen adverse side effects. Although this sounds logical, further investigation is necessary to fully validate this in the cat and to determine which drugs, dosages, and combinations will be most beneficial. Synergism has been demonstrated between the NSAID vedaprofen and tramadol.[11] Buprenorphine may have a synergistic action with carprofen; cats given both drugs exhibited fewer signs of pain than when either drug was administered alone.[137]

"SEND HOME" MEDICATIONS

When intravenous fluid support and intensive nursing are not needed, cats can go home to recuperate from surgery; most fare better in familiar surroundings, away from the stressors of a veterinary clinic. Outpatient anesthetic and surgical techniques allow cats to return to normal function quickly; however, analgesics may be required for several days postoperatively. The liability issues associated with transdermal fentanyl patches have already been discussed. One popular take-home drug is buprenorphine (a less tightly controlled opioid), which most owners find easy to administer by the oral transmucosal route. Doses of 0.01 to 0.02 mg/kg twice or three times daily are administered depending on the severity of the surgery and the cat's behavior at home. Buprenorphine is usually no longer needed after 2 to 3 days. Oral meloxicam (0.025 to 0.05 mg/kg, once daily for 4 days) is also easy to use in a home setting because it is given once daily and is highly palatable; it is administered alone or with food.

INDIVIDUAL VARIATION IN RESPONSE TO ANALGESIC DRUGS

Pharmacogenetics (the study of genetic variation that results in different responses to drugs) is a major area of interest in the scientific community. Female humans and mice with the melanocortin-1 receptor gene (which is associated with red hair and fair skin in humans) have altered sensitivity to pentazocine compared with male subjects or female subjects with another hair color.[89] It is very likely that cats, with their many different genetic traits, also express individual variation in response to analgesic drugs. Gender differences in pain sensitivity are well documented in humans[36] but have not been well studied in animals other than rodents. Marked variations in response to butorphanol and buprenorphine have been reported in cats under well-controlled laboratory conditions.[63,81,117,135] Clinically, this is a concern because some cats may be "nonresponders" to a chosen opioid,[145] making their analgesic management more challenging. However, armed with this knowledge, good pain assessment skills, and a variety of analgesic drugs, clinicians have the ability to keep feline patients comfortable. Now that the feline genome has been mapped,[95] this opens up exciting possibilities for investigating pain and analgesia in cats.

SPECIAL POPULATIONS

There is limited information on the safety and efficacy of analgesic drugs in nursing queens, kittens, and senior cats.

Analgesics have often been withheld in young animals because of their organ immaturity and decreased ability to metabolize drugs. However, neonates do experience pain, and noxious stimuli can cause detrimental and permanent changes in the developing nervous system.[87] Carprofen can be used in kittens older than 6 weeks of age (see package insert in licensed countries), whereas meloxicam is not recommended until 16 weeks of age.[62] In kittens younger than 6 weeks, opioid agonists are the analgesic drugs of choice because they are reversible if an adverse event occurs. In neonates, cardiac output depends on heart rate; therefore opioid-related bradycardia is a concern. For this reason, and the observation that kittens may be more sensitive to the sedative and respiratory-depressant effects of opioids, it is suggested that lower doses be used initially with further treatment based on close observation. Co-administration of anticholinergics can reduce the incidence of opioid-mediated bradycardia.

Drugs administered to a dam may be excreted in milk. In species in which this has been studied, only a small percentage of the drug is detectable in milk. In cows carprofen was below detectable limits in milk after single or daily dosing[86]; no comparable study has been performed in lactating queens. There is concern that exposure of the fetus or neonates to NSAIDs may impair renal development or ductus arteriosus function[4]; therefore until more specific information becomes available, the use of NSAIDs should be restricted to a "one time only" basis in pregnant or lactating queens. It is unlikely that the concentration of opioid drugs present in milk after systemic administration to the queen will have any negative effect in nursing kittens. Epidural opioids that are hydrophilic (e.g., morphine) remain concentrated in the epidural space with minimal systemic distribution, making them a suitable choice for a queen undergoing a cesarean section. A local anesthetic line block is another simple and effective, albeit short-acting, analgesic technique for cesarean section. The review by Mathews[87] provides further information on these patient categories. With these infrequent but challenging cases, the clinician needs to tailor the analgesic plan to the specific patient.

Aging cats present a challenge in terms of treating pain because of co-existing disease(s) and Rollin reminds us that our duty is to preserve quality of life rather than just "quantity" of life in this population.[115] A full understanding of the patient's co-existing diseases and evaluation of liver and renal function are essential before a treatment regimen can be developed. Age-related neurodegeneration occurs in cats,[53] but it is not known how this relates to changes in neurotransmission, pain sensitivity, or analgesic requirements. Initially, it may be wise to use a reduced drug dose in elderly cats and base additional administration on careful evaluation.

OTHER ANALGESIC MODALITIES

Finally, not all pain management is pharmacologic. Other modalities, such as massage, physical therapy, and acupuncture, may provide benefit for the alleviation of acute pain in the cat. These modalities have not undergone robust scientific scrutiny in this species, but individual case reports are encouraging.[21,42] In addition, the contribution of warmth, comfortable dry bedding, quiet surroundings, and gentle and considerate caretakers to a cat's overall comfort should not be underestimated.

CONCLUSION

The unique characteristics of the cat make assessing and treating these patients for pain both rewarding and challenging. However, there is no doubt that incorporating newer approaches to pain assessment, understanding individual variation, and dispelling myths about some analgesic agents have all been significant in improving the care of cats after trauma and in the perioperative period. Veterinarians have a better understanding of how to use current knowledge and have identified specific areas that require further research. Although there is still progress to be made, veterinarians are confronting the issue of pain in the cat with evidence-based, logical, compassionate choices.

References

1. Abelson AL, McCobb EC, Shaw S et al: Use of wound soaker catheters for the administration of local anesthetic for postoperative analgesia: 56 cases, *Vet Anaesth Analg*, 36:597, 2009.
2. Aghighi SA, Tipold A, Kastner SBR: Effects of gabapentin as add on medication on pain after intervertebral disc surgery in dogs—preliminary results. In *10th World Congress of Veterinary Anaesthesia*, Glasgow, UK, 2009, p 133.
3. Balmer TV, Irvine D, Jones RS et al: Comparison of carprofen and pethidine as postoperative analgesics in the cat, *J Small Anim Pract* 39:158, 1998.
4. Baragatti BS, Sodini D, Uematsu S, Coceani F: Role of microsomal prostaglandin E synthase-1 (mPGES1)-derived PGE2 in patency of the ductus arteriosus in the mouse, *Pediatr Res* 64:523, 2008.
5. Bateman SW, Haldane S, Stephens JA: Comparison of the analgesic efficacy of hydromorphone and oxymorphone in dogs and cats: a randomized blinded study, *Vet Anaesth Analg* 35:341, 2008.
6. Benito-de-la-Vibora J, Lascelles BD, Garcia-Fernandez P et al: Efficacy of tolfenamic acid and meloxicam in the control of postoperative pain following ovariohysterectomy in the cat, *Vet Anaesth Analg* 35:501, 2008.
7. Blanpied TA, Clarke RJ, Johnson JW: Amantadine inhibits NMDA receptors by accelerating channel closure during channel block, *J Neurosci* 25:3312, 2005.
8. Boogaerts JG, Lafont ND, Luo H et al: Plasma concentrations of bupivacaine after brachial plexus administration of liposome-associated and plain solutions to rabbits, *Can J Anaesth* 40:1201, 1993.
9. Borron SW, Monier C, Risède P et al: Flunitrazepam variably alters morphine, buprenorphine, and methadone lethality in the rat, *Hum Exp Toxicol* 21:599, 2002.
10. Briggs SL, Sneed K, Sawyer DC: Antinociceptive effects of oxymorphone-butorphanol-acepromazine combination in cats, *Vet Surg* 27:466, 1998.
11. Brondani JT, Loureiro Luna SP, Beier SL et al: Analgesic efficacy of perioperative use of vedaprofen, tramadol or their combination in cats undergoing ovariohysterectomy, *J Feline Med Surg* 11:420, 2009.
12. Brondani JT, Luna SP, Marcello GC et al: Perioperative administration of vedaprofen, tramadol or their combination does not interfere with platelet aggregation, bleeding time and biochemical variables in cats, *J Feline Med Surg* 11:503, 2009.
13. Brondani JT, Luna SP, Padovani CR: Development and preliminary validation of a multidimensional composite pain scale for cats. In *10th World Congress of Veterinary Anaesthesia*, Glasgow, UK, 2009, p 151.
14. Brosnan RJ, Pypendop BH, Siao KT et al: Effects of remifentanil on measures of anesthetic immobility and analgesia in cats, *Am J Vet Res* 70:1065, 2009.
15. Bugat R, Thompson MR, Aures D et al: Gastric mucosal lesions produced by intravenous infusion of aspirin in cats, *Gastroenterology* 71:754, 1976.
16. Campoy L, Korich J, Bezuidenhout A: Peripheral nerve blocks in the dog. Accessed January 10, 2010, at http://www.partnersah.com/CAMPOY/CVM101_demo/index.html.
17. Carroll GL, Howe LB, Peterson KD: Analgesic efficacy of preoperative administration of meloxicam or butorphanol in onychectomized cats, *J Am Vet Med Assoc* 226:913, 2005.
18. Catbagan DL, Quimby JM, Mama KR et al: Comparison of the efficacy of subcutaneously administered sustained-release buprenorphine and oral transmucosal buprenorphine in cats post surgical ovariohysterectomy, *Am J Vet Res*, in press.
19. Chadwick HS: Toxicity and resuscitation in lidocaine- or bupivacaine-infused cats, *Anesthesiology* 63:385, 1985.
20. Chen HC, Radzi R, Rahman NA: Analgesic effect of tramadol combined with tolfenamic acid in cats after ovariohysterectomy. In *13th Annual IVECCS Conference*, New Orleans, 2007.
21. Choi KH, Hill SA: Acupuncture treatment for feline multifocal intervertebral disc disease, *J Feline Med Surg* 11:706, 2009.
22. Chu K, Anderson WM, Rieser MY: Population characteristics and neuter status of cats living in households in the United States, *J Am Vet Med Assoc* 234:1023, 2009.
23. Clarke SP, Bennett D: Feline osteoarthritis: a prospective study of 28 cases, *J Small Anim Pract* 47:439, 2006.
24. Conzemius MG, Hill CM, Sammarco JL et al: Correlation between subjective and objective measures used to determine severity of postoperative pain in dogs, *J Am Vet Med Assoc* 210:1619, 1997.
25. Curcio K, Bidwell LA, Bohart GV et al: Evaluation of signs of postoperative pain and complications after forelimb onychectomy in cats receiving buprenorphine alone or with bupivacaine administered as a four-point regional nerve block, *J Am Vet Med Assoc* 228:65, 2006.
26. Curros-Criado MM, Herrero JF: The antinociceptive effect of systemic gabapentin is related to the type of sensitization-induced hyperalgesia, *J Neuroinflammation* 4:15, 2007.
27. Davidson CD, Pettifer GR, Henry JDJ: Plasma fentanyl concentrations and analgesic effects during full or partial exposure to transdermal fentanyl patches in cats, *J Am Vet Med Assoc* 224:700, 2004.
28. Davis KM, Hardie EM, Martin FR et al: Correlation between perioperative factors and successful outcome in fibrosarcoma resection in cats, *Vet Rec* 161:199, 2007.
29. Davis LE, Westfall BA: Species differences in biotransformation and excretion of salicylate. *Am J Vet Res*, 33:1253, 1972.
30. DeRossi R, Benites AP, Ferreira JZ et al: Effects of lumbosacral epidural ketamine and lidocaine in xylazine-sedated cats, *J S Afr Vet Assoc* 80:79, 2009.
31. Dixon MJ, Robertson SA, Taylor PM: A thermal threshold testing device for evaluation of analgesics in cats, *Res Vet Sci* 72:205, 2002.

32. Dixon MJ, Taylor PM, Steagall PV et al: Development of a pressure nociceptive threshold testing device for evaluation of analgesics in cats, *Res Vet Sci* 82:85, 2007.
33. Dobbins S, Brown NO, Shofer FS: Comparison of the effects of buprenorphine, oxymorphone hydrochloride, and ketoprofen for postoperative analgesia after onychectomy or onychectomy and sterilization in cats, *J Am Anim Hosp Assoc* 38:507, 2002.
34. Dohoo SE, Dohoo IR: Postoperative use of analgesics in dogs and cats by Canadian veterinarians, *Can Vet J* 37:546, 1996.
35. Duke T, Cox AM, Remedios AM et al: The analgesic effects of administering fentanyl or medetomidine in the lumbosacral epidural space of cats, *Vet Surg* 23:143, 1994.
36. Fillingim RB: Sex, gender, and pain: women and men really are different, *Curr Rev Pain* 4:24, 2000.
37. Franks JN, Boothe HW, Taylor L et al: Evaluation of transdermal fentanyl patches for analgesia in cats undergoing onychectomy, *J Am Vet Med Assoc* 217:1013, 2000.
38. Fransson BA, Peck KE, Smith JK et al: Transdermal absorption of a liposome-encapsulated formulation of lidocaine following topical administration in cats, *Am J Vet Res* 63:1309, 2002.
39. Gaynor JS, Dunlop CI, Wagner AE et al: Complications and mortality associated with anesthesia in dogs and cats, *J Am Anim Hosp Assoc* 35:13, 1999.
40. Gellasch KL, Kruse-Elliott KT, Osmond CS et al: Comparison of transdermal administration of fentanyl versus intramuscular administration of butorphanol for analgesia after onychectomy in cats, *J Am Vet Med Assoc*, 220:1020, 2002.
41. Gibbon KJ, Cyborski JM, Guzinski MV et al: Evaluation of adverse effects of EMLA (lidocaine/prilocaine) cream for the placement of jugular catheters in healthy cats, *J Vet Pharmacol Ther* 26:439, 2003.
42. Ginman AA, Kline KL, Shelton GD: Severe polymyositis and neuritis in a cat, *J Am Vet Med Assoc* 235:172, 2009.
43. Giordano T, Steagall PVM, Ferreria TH et al: Postoperative analgesic effects of intravenous, intramusclar, subcutaneous or oral transmucosal buprenorphine administered to cats undergoing ovariohysterectomy. In *10th World Congress of Veterinary Anaesthesia*, Glasgow, UK, 2009, p 58.
44. Giraudel JM, King JN, Jeunesse EC et al: Use of a pharmacokinetic/pharmacodynamic approach in the cat to determine a dosage regimen for the COX-2 selective drug robenacoxib, *J Vet Pharmacol Ther* 32:18, 2009.
45. Giraudel JM, Toutain PL, King JN et al: Differential inhibition of cyclooxygenase isoenzymes in the cat by the NSAID robenacoxib, *J Vet Pharmacol Ther* 32:31, 2009.
46. Giraudel JM, Toutain PL, Lees P: Development of in vitro assays for the evaluation of cyclooxygenase inhibitors and predicting selectivity of nonsteroidal anti-inflammatory drugs in cats, *Am J Vet Res* 66:700, 2005.
47. Glerum LE, Egger CM, Allen SW et al: Analgesic effect of the transdermal fentanyl patch during and after feline ovariohysterectomy, *Vet Surg* 30:351, 2001.
48. Goodman LA, Brown SA, Torres BT et al: Effects of meloxicam on plasma iohexol clearance as a marker of glomerular filtration rate in conscious healthy cats, *Am J Vet Res* 70:826, 2009.
49. Gordon AM, Wagner AE: Anesthesia-related hypotension in a small-animal practice, *Vet Med* 101:22, 2006.
50. Gorman AL, Elliott KJ, Inturrisi CE: The d- and l-isomers of methadone bind to the non-competitive site on the N-methyl-D-aspartate (NMDA) receptor in rat forebrain and spinal cord, *Neurosci Lett* 223:5, 1997.
51. Guedes AG, Papich MG, Rude EP et al: Comparison of plasma histamine levels after intravenous administration of hydromorphone and morphine in dogs, *J Vet Pharmacol Ther* 30:516, 2007.
52. Gunew MN, Menrath VH, Marshall RD: Long-term safety, efficacy and palatability of oral meloxicam at 0.01-0.03 mg/kg for treatment of osteoarthritic pain in cats, *J Feline Med Surg* 10:235, 2008.
53. Gunn-Moore DA, McVee J, Bradshaw JM et al: Ageing changes in cat brains demonstrated by beta-amyloid and AT8-immunoreactive phosphorylated tau deposits, *J Feline Med Surg*, 8:234, 2006.
54. Hellyer P, Rodan I, Brunt J et al: AAHA/AAFP pain management guidelines for dogs and cats, *J Feline Med Surg* 9:466, 2007.
55. Hewson CJ, Dohoo IR, Lempke KA: Perioperative use of analgesics in dogs and cats by Canadian veterinarians in 2001, *Can Vet J* 47:352, 2006.
56. Hickman MA, Cox SR, Mahabir S et al: Safety, pharmacokinetics and use of the novel NK-1 receptor antagonist maropitant (Cerenia) for the prevention of emesis and motion sickness in cats, *J Vet Pharmacol Ther* 31:220, 2008.
57. Holton L, Reid J, Scott EM et al: Development of a behaviour-based scale to measure acute pain in dogs, *Vet Rec* 148:525, 2001.
58. Holton LL, Scott EM, Nolan AM et al: Relationship between physiological factors and clinical pain in dogs scored using a numerical rating scale, *J Small Anim Pract* 39:469, 1998.
59. Hugonnard M, Leblond A, Keroack S et al: Attitudes and concerns of French veterinarians towards pain and analgesia in dogs and cats, *Vet Anaesth Analg* 31:154, 2004.
60. Ide S, Minami M, Ishihara K et al: Mu opioid receptor-dependent and independent components in effects of tramadol, *Neuropharmacology* 51:651, 2006.
61. Ilkiw JE, Pascoe PJ, Fisher LD: Effect of alfentanil on the minimum alveolar concentration of isoflurane in cats, *Am J Vet Res* 58:1274, 1997.
62. Ingelheim B: Meloxicam Package Insert. Accessed January 10, 2010, at http://www.metacam.com/index.php/Package-Inserts.
63. Johnson JA, Robertson SA, Pypendop BH: Antinociceptive effects of butorphanol, buprenorphine, or both, administered intramuscularly in cats, *Am J Vet Res* 68:699, 2007.
64. Jones RS: Epidural analgesia in the dog and cat, *Vet J* 161:123, 2001.
65. Joubert KE: Anaesthesia and analgesia for dogs and cats in South Africa undergoing sterilisation and with osteoarthritis—an update from 2000, *J S Afr Vet Assoc* 77:224, 2006.
66. Joubert KE: The use of analgesic drugs by South African veterinarians, *J S Afr Vet Assoc* 72:57, 2001.
67. Kay-Mugford P, Benn SJ, LaMarre J et al: In vitro effects of nonsteroidal anti-inflammatory drugs on cyclooxygenase activity in dogs, *Am J Vet Res* 61:802, 2000.
68. Kehlet H, Jensen TS, Woolf CJ: Persistent postsurgical pain: risk factors and prevention, *Lancet* 367:1618, 2006.
69. Khan KN, Paulson SK, Verburg KM et al: Pharmacology of cyclooxygenase-2 inhibition in the kidney, *Kidney Int*, 61:1210, 2002.
70. Khan KN, Venturini CM, Bunch RT et al: Interspecies differences in renal localization of cyclooxygenase isoforms: implications in nonsteroidal antiinflammatory drug-related nephrotoxicity, *Toxicol Pathol* 26:612, 1998.
71. Ko JC, Maxwell LK, Abbo LA et al: Pharmacokinetics of lidocaine following the application of 5% lidocaine patches to cats, *J Vet Pharmacol Ther* 31:359, 2008.
72. La Vincente SF, White JM, Somogyi AA et al: Enhanced buprenorphine analgesia with the addition of ultra-low-dose naloxone in healthy subjects, *Clin Pharmacol Ther* 83:144, 2008.
73. Lamont LA: Feline perioperative pain management, *Vet Clin North Am Small Anim Pract* 32:747, 2002.

74. Lamont LA, Mathews KA: Opioids, non-steroidal anti-inflammatories, and analgesic adjuvants. In Tranquilli WJ, Thurmon JC, Grimm, KA, editors: *Lumb and Jones' veterinary anesthesia and analgesia*, ed 4, Ames, Iowa, 2007, Blackwell, p 246.
75. Lascelles BD, Court MH, Hardie EM et al: Nonsteroidal anti-inflammatory drugs in cats: a review, *Vet Anaesth Analg* 34:228, 2007.
76. Lascelles BD, Cripps P, Mirchandani S et al: Carprofen as an analgesic for postoperative pain in cats: dose titration and assessment of efficacy in comparison to pethidine hydrochloride, *J Small Anim Pract* 36:535, 1995.
77. Lascelles BD, Cripps PJ, Jones A et al: Post-operative central hypersensitivity and pain: the pre-emptive value of pethidine for ovariohysterectomy, *Pain* 73:461, 1997.
78. Lascelles BD, Gaynor JS, Smith ES et al: Amantadine in a multimodal analgesic regimen for alleviation of refractory osteoarthritis pain in dogs, *J Vet Intern Med* 22:53, 2008.
79. Lascelles BD, Henderson AJ, Hackett IJ: Evaluation of the clinical efficacy of meloxicam in cats with painful locomotor disorders, *J Small Anim Pract*, 42:587, 2001.
80. Lascelles BD, Robertson SA: Antinociceptive effects of hydromorphone, butorphanol, or the combination in cats, *J Vet Intern Med* 18:190, 2004.
81. Lascelles BD, Robertson SA: Use of thermal threshold response to evaluate the antinociceptive effects of butorphanol in cats, *Am J Vet Res* 65:1085, 2004.
82. Lascelles BD, Waterman A: Analgesia in cats, *In Pract* 19:203, 1997.
83. Lascelles BD, Waterman AE, Cripps PJ et al: Central sensitization as a result of surgical pain: investigation of the pre-emptive value of pethidine for ovariohysterectomy in the rat, *Pain* 62:201, 1995.
84. Lee DD, Papich MG, Hardie EM: Comparison of pharmacokinetics of fentanyl after intravenous and transdermal administration in cats, *Am J Vet Res* 61:672, 2000.
85. Looper KJ: Potential medical and surgical complications of serotonergic antidepressant medications, *Psychosomatics* 48:1, 2007.
86. Ludwig B, Jordan JC, Rehm WF et al: Carprofen in veterinary medicine. I. Plasma disposition, milk excretion and tolerance in milk-producing cows, *Schweiz Arch Tierheilkd* 131:99, 1989.
87. Mathews KA: Pain management for the pregnant, lactating, and neonatal to pediatric cat and dog, *Vet Clin North Am Small Anim Pract* 38:1291, 2008.
88. Millette VM, Steagall PV, Duke-Novakovski T et al: Effects of meperidine or saline on thermal, mechanical and electrical nociceptive thresholds in cats, *Vet Anaesth Analg* 35:543, 2008.
89. Mogil JS, Wilson SG, Chesler EJ, et al: The melanocortin-1 receptor gene mediates female-specific mechanisms of analgesia in mice and humans, *Proc Natl Acad Sci U S A*, 100:4867, 2003.
90. Mohammad-Zadeh LF, Moses L, Gwaltney-Brant SM: Serotonin: a review, *J Vet Pharmacol Ther* 31:187, 2008.
91. Möllenhoff A, Nolte I, Kramer S: Anti-nociceptive efficacy of carprofen, levomethadone and buprenorphine for pain relief in cats following major orthopaedic surgery, *J Vet Med A Physiol Pathol Clin Med* 52:186, 2005.
92. Morton CM, Reid J, Scott EM et al: Application of a scaling model to establish and validate an interval level pain scale for assessment of acute pain in dogs, *Am J Vet Res* 66:2154, 2005.
93. Mosing M, Reich H, Moens Y: Clinical evaluation of the anaesthetic sparing effect of brachial plexus block in cats, *Vet Anaesth Analg* 37:154, 2010.
94. Murison PJ, Waterman-Pearson AE, Murrell JC: Effect of maropitant on thermal and mechanical nociceptive thresholds in cats: preliminary results. In *10th World Congress of Veterinary Anaesthesia*, Glasgow, UK, 2009, p 130.
95. Murphy WJ: The feline genome, *Genome Dyn* 2:60, 2006.
96. Murrell JC, Robertson SA, Taylor PM et al: Use of a transdermal matrix patch of buprenorphine in cats: preliminary pharmacokinetic and pharmacodynamic data, *Vet Rec* 160:578, 2007.
97. Niedfeldt RL, Robertson SA: Postanesthetic hyperthermia in cats: a retrospective comparison between hydromorphone and buprenorphine, *Vet Anaesth Analg* 33:381, 2006.
98. O'Connor AB, Dworkin RH: Treatment of neuropathic pain: an overview of recent guidelines, *Am J Med* 122:S22, 2009.
99. Parton K, Balmer TV, Boyle J et al: The pharmacokinetics and effects of intravenously administered carprofen and salicylate on gastrointestinal mucosa and selected biochemical measurements in healthy cats, *J Vet Pharmacol Ther* 23:73, 2000.
100. Patrono C: Aspirin and human platelets: from clinical trials to acetylation of cyclooxygenase and back, *Trends Pharmacol Sci* 10:453, 1989.
101. Pettifer GR, Hosgood G: The effect of rectal temperature on perianesthetic serum concentrations of transdermally administered fentanyl in cats anesthetized with isoflurane, *Am J Vet Res* 64:1557, 2003.
102. Posner LP, Gleed RD, Erb HN et al: Post-anesthetic hyperthermia in cats, *Vet Anaesth Analg* 34:40, 2007.
103. Posner LP, Pavuk AA, Rokshar JL et al: Effects of opioids and anesthetic drugs on body temperature in cats, *Vet Anaesth Analg* 37:35, 2010.
104. Pypendop BH, Ilkiw JE: Assessment of the hemodynamic effects of lidocaine administered IV in isoflurane-anesthetized cats, *Am J Vet Res* 66:661, 2005.
105. Pypendop BH, Ilkiw JE: Pharmacokinetics of tramadol, and its metabolite O-desmethyl-tramadol, in cats, *J Vet Pharmacol Ther* 31:52, 2008.
106. Pypendop BH, Siao KT, Ilkiw JE: Effects of gabapentin on the thermal threshold in cats. In *10th World Congress of Veterinary Anaesthesia*, Glasgow, UK, 2009, p 129.
107. Pypendop BH, Siao KT, Pascoe PJ et al: Effects of epidurally administered morphine or buprenorphine on the thermal threshold in cats, *Am J Vet Res* 69:983, 2008.
108. Robertson SA: Managing pain in feline patients, *Vet Clin North Am Small Anim Pract* 38:1267, 2008.
109. Robertson SA, Lascelles BD, Taylor PM et al: PK-PD modeling of buprenorphine in cats: intravenous and oral transmucosal administration, *J Vet Pharmacol Ther* 28:453, 2005.
110. Robertson SA, Taylor PM, Lascelles BD et al: Changes in thermal threshold response in eight cats after administration of buprenorphine, butorphanol and morphine, *Vet Rec* 153:462, 2003.
111. Robertson SA, Taylor PM, Sear JW: Systemic uptake of buprenorphine by cats after oral mucosal administration, *Vet Rec* 152:675, 2003.
112. Robertson SA, Taylor PM, Sear JW et al: Relationship between plasma concentrations and analgesia after intravenous fentanyl and disposition after other routes of administration in cats, *J Vet Pharmacol Ther* 28:87, 2005.
113. Robertson SA, Wegner K, Lascelles BD: Antinociceptive and side-effects of hydromorphone after subcutaneous administration in cats, *J Feline Med Surg* 11:76, 2009.
114. Rohrer Bley C, Neiger-Aeschbacher G, Busato A et al: Comparison of perioperative racemic methadone, levo-methadone and dextromoramide in cats using indicators of post-operative pain, *Vet Anaesth Analg* 31:175, 2004.
115. Rollin BE: Ethical issues in geriatric feline medicine, *J Feline Med Surg* 9:326, 2007.

116. Rubin K, Sullivan D, Sadhasivam S: Are peripheral and neuraxial blocks with ultrasound guidance more effective and safe in children? *Paediatr Anaesth* 19:92, 2009.
117. Sawyer DC, Rech RH: Analgesia and behavioral effects of butorphanol, nalbuphine, and pentazocine in the cat, *J Am Anim Hosp Assoc* 23:438, 1987.
118. Schiavenato M, Byers JF, Scovanner P et al: Neonatal pain facial expression: evaluating the primal face of pain, *Pain* 138:460, 2008.
119. Schmiedt CW, Bjorling DE: Accidental prehension and suspected transmucosal or oral absorption of fentanyl from a transdermal patch in a dog, *Vet Anaesth Analg* 34:70, 2007.
120. Schwarzer A, Nauck F, Klaschik E: [Strong opioids and constipation]. *Schmerz* 19:214, 2005.
121. Shepherd AJ: Results of the 2007 AVMA survey of US pet-owning households regarding use of veterinary services and expenditures, *J Am Vet Med Assoc* 233:727, 2008.
122. Siao KT, Pypendop BH, Ilkiw JE: Pharmacokinetics of gabapentin in cats. In *10th World Congress of Veterinary Anaesthesia*, Glasgow, UK, 2009, p 129.
123. Singh VK, Bajpai K, Biswas S et al: Molecular biology of opioid receptors: recent advances, *Neuroimmunomodulation* 4:285, 1997.
124. Skarda RT, Tranquilli WJ: Local and regional anesthetic and analgesic techniques: cats. In Tranquilli WJ, Thurmon JC, Grimm KA, editor: *Lumb and Jones' veterinary anesthesia and analgesia*, ed 4, Ames, Iowa, 2007, Blackwell, p 597.
125. Slingsby LS, Lane EC, Mears ER et al: Postoperative pain after ovariohysterectomy in the cat: a comparison of two anaesthetic regimens, *Vet Rec* 143:589, 1998.
126. Slingsby LS, Taylor PM: Thermal and mechanical nociceptive thresholds in cats after adminstration of buprenorphine 10 mcg/kg, naloxone 0.67 mcg/kg or their 15:1 combination. In *10th World Congress of Veterinary Anesthesia*, Glasgow, UK, 2009, p 139.
127. Slingsby LS, Taylor PM: Thermal antinociception after dexmedetomidine administration in cats: a dose-finding study, *J Vet Pharmacol Ther* 31:135, 2008.
128. Slingsby LS, Taylor PM, Monroe T: Thermal antinociception after dexmedetomidine administration in cats: a comparison between intramuscular and oral transmucosal administration, *J Feline Med Surg* 11:829, 2009.
129. Slingsby LS, Waterman-Pearson AE: Comparison of pethidine, buprenorphine and ketoprofen for postoperative analgesia after ovariohysterectomy in the cat, *Vet Rec* 143:185, 1998.
130. Slingsby LS, Waterman-Pearson AE: Postoperative analgesia in the cat after ovariohysterectomy by use of carprofen, ketoprofen, meloxicam or tolfenamic acid, *J Small Anim Pract* 41:447, 2000.
131. Smith JD, Allen SW, Quandt JE: Changes in cortisol concentration in response to stress and postoperative pain in client-owned cats and correlation with objective clinical variables, *Am J Vet Res* 60:432, 1999.
132. Smith JD, Allen SW, Quandt JE et al: Indicators of postoperative pain in cats and correlation with clinical criteria, *Am J Vet Res* 57:1674, 1996.
133. Stanway G, Taylor P, Brodbelt D: A preliminary investigation comparing pre-operative morphine and buprenorphine for postoperative analgesia and sedation in cats, *Vet Anaesth Analg* 29:29, 2002.
134. Steagall PV, Carnicelli P, Taylor PM et al: Effects of subcutaneous methadone, morphine, buprenorphine or saline on thermal and pressure thresholds in cats, *J Vet Pharmacol Ther* 29:531, 2006.
135. Steagall PV, Mantovani FB, Taylor PM et al: Dose-related antinociceptive effects of intravenous buprenorphine in cats, *Vet J* 182:203, 2009.
136. Steagall PV, Taylor PM, Brondani JT et al: Antinociceptive effects of tramadol and acepromazine in cats, *J Feline Med Surg* 10:24, 2008.
137. Steagall PV, Taylor PM, Rodrigues LC et al: Analgesia for cats after ovariohysterectomy with either buprenorphine or carprofen alone or in combination, *Vet Rec* 164:359, 2009.
138. Sturtevant FM, Drill VA: Tranquilizing drugs and morphine-mania in cats, *Nature* 179:1253, 1957.
139. Swalander DB, Crowe DTJ, Hittenmiller DH et al: Complications associated with the use of indwelling epidural catheters in dogs: 81 cases (1996-1999), *J Am Vet Med Assoc* 216:368, 2000.
140. Taxonomy ITFo: Part III: Pain terms. A current list with definitions and notes on usagem ed 2. Accessed December 11, 2009, at http://www.iasp-pain.org/AM/Template.cfm?Section=Pain_Definitions&Template=/CM/HTMLDisplay.cfm&ContentID=1728#Pain.
141. Taylor JS, Vierck CJ: Effects of ketamine on electroencephalographic and autonomic arousal and segmental reflex responses in the cat, *Vet Anaesth Analg* 30:237, 2003.
142. Taylor PM, Delatour P, Landoni FM et al: Pharmacodynamics and enantioselective pharmacokinetics of carprofen in the cat, *Res Vet Sci* 60:144, 1996.
143. Taylor PM, Kirby JJ, Robinson C et al: A prospective multicentre clinical trial to compare buprenorphine and butorphanol for postoperative analgesia in cats, *J Feline Med Surg* 12(4):247, 2009.
144. Taylor PM, Robertson SA, Dixon MJ et al: Morphine, pethidine and buprenorphine disposition in the cat, *J Vet Pharmacol Ther* 24:391, 2001.
145. Taylor PM, Slingsby LS, Pypendop BH et al: Variable response to opioid analgesia, *Veterinary Anaesthesia and Analgesia* 34:6, 2007.
146. Teske J, Weller JP, Larsch K et al: Fatal outcome in a child after ingestion of a transdermal fentanyl patch, *Int J Legal Med* 121:147, 2007.
147. Tharp AM, Winecker RE, Winston DC: Fatal intravenous fentanyl abuse: four cases involving extraction of fentanyl from transdermal patches, *Am J Forensic Med Pathol* 25:178, 2004.
148. Troncy E, Junot S, Keroack S et al: Results of preemptive epidural administration of morphine with or without bupivacaine in dogs and cats undergoing surgery: 265 cases (1997-1999), *J Am Vet Med Assoc* 221:666, 2002.
149. Vaisanen MAM, Tuomikoski-Alin SK, Brodbelt DC et al: Opinions of Finnish small animal owners about surgery and pain management in small animals, *J Small Anim Pract* 49:626, 2008.
150. Valtolina C, Robben JH, Uilenreef J et al: Clinical evaluation of the efficacy and safety of a constant rate infusion of dexmedetomidine for postoperative pain management in dogs, *Vet Anaesth Analg* 36:369, 2009.
151. Valverde A, Cantwell S, Hernández J et al: Effects of acepromazine on the incidence of vomiting associated with opioid administration in dogs, *Vet Anaesth Analg* 31:40, 2004.
152. Vane JR, and Botting RM: New insights into the mode of action of anti-inflammatory drugs, *Inflamm Res* 44:10, 1995.
153. Wagner AE, Hellyer PW: Observations of private veterinary practices in Colorado, with an emphasis on anesthesia, *J Vet Med Educ* 29:176, 2002.
154. Wagner AE, Hellyer PW: Survey of anesthesia techniques and concerns in private veterinary practice, *J Am Vet Med Assoc* 217:1652, 2000.
155. Wagner AE, Hellyer PW, Mich PW et al: Perioperative gabapentin as an adjunct for post-operative analgesia in dogs undergoing amputation of a forelimb. In *American College of Veterinary Anesthesiologists*, Phoenix, 2008, p 2.
156. Wagner AE, Walton JA, Hellyer PW et al: Use of low doses of ketamine administered by constant rate infusion as an adjunct for postoperative analgesia in dogs, *J Am Vet Med Assoc* 221:72, 2002.

157. Wagner KA, Gibbon KJ, Strom TL et al: Adverse effects of EMLA (lidocaine/prilocaine) cream and efficacy for the placement of jugular catheters in hospitalized cats, *J Feline Med Surg* 8:141, 2006.
158. Waran N, Best L, Williams V et al: A preliminary study of behaviour-based indicators of pain in cats, *Anim Welf* 16:105, 2007.
159. Wegner K, Robertson SA: Dose-related thermal antinociceptive effects of intravenous hydromorphone in cats, *Vet Anaesth Analg* 34:132, 2007.
160. Wegner K, Robertson SA, Kollias-Baker C et al: Pharmacokinetic and pharmacodynamic evaluation of intravenous hydromorphone in cats, *J Vet Pharmacol Ther* 27:329, 2004.
161. Wells SM, Glerum LE, Papich MG: Pharmacokinetics of butorphanol in cats after intramuscular and buccal transmucosal administration, *Am J Vet Res* 69:1548, 2008.
162. Wenger S, Moens Y, Jäggin N et al: Evaluation of the analgesic effect of lidocaine and bupivacaine used to provide a brachial plexus block for forelimb surgery in 10 dogs, *Vet Rec* 156:639, 2005.
163. Williams VM, Lascelles BD, Robson MC: Current attitudes to, and use of, peri-operative analgesia in dogs and cats by veterinarians in New Zealand, *N Z Vet J* 53:193, 2005.

CHAPTER

7

Anesthesia and Perioperative Care

Bruno H. Pypendop and Jan E. Ilkiw

OUTLINE

ASSESSMENT OF RISK

In both medical and veterinary anesthesia, patients are often classified using the American Society of Anesthesiologists Physical Status Classification (ASA-PS), which attempts to give a subjective and relative risk based only on the patient's preoperative medical history (Table 7-1). In this classification ASA 1 is considered a healthy patient with no overt signs of disease, and 5 is considered a moribund patient who is considered likely to die in the next 24 hours with or without surgery. Addition of "E" to the classification indicates emergency surgery.[61]

Although anesthetic-related death in cats has decreased over the years, the most recent published mortality rate of 0.24%, or 1 in 453 anesthetics,[27] is still up to 10 times that found in human studies.[42] The "Confidential Enquiry into Perioperative Small Animal Fatalities"[26] was undertaken in 117 veterinary practices in the United Kingdom from 2002 to 2004. The study included 79,178 cats with overall risks of sedation and anesthetic-related deaths within 48 hours of procedure of 0.24%. In this study most cats were premedicated (70%), intubated (70%), and breathing spontaneously (92%). Procedures were short (25 to 30 minutes), and fluids were administered to only 26% of cats. Monitoring was rare, with pulse monitored in 38%, pulse oximetry in 16%, and both pulse and pulse oximetry in 25% of cats. Temperature was monitored intraoperatively in 1% to 2% of cats and postoperatively in 11% to 15% of cats. Specifically in cats, factors associated with increased odds of anesthetic-related death were poor health status (ASA-PS classification), increasing age, extremes of weight, increasing procedural urgency and complexity, endotracheal intubation, and fluid therapy. In this study the greater risk associated with anesthesia in cats compared with dogs was reported to be related to their size (relatively small with a large surface area to volume ratio), which predisposes them to hypothermia and drug overdosage, and a small airway and a sensitive larynx, which predisposes them to upper airway complications. Pulse monitoring and pulse oximetry were associated with reduced odds, related more to patient monitoring than to the specific equipment used. A total of 61% of cats died in the postoperative period, with 62% of those occurring in the first 3 hours after surgery. Factors considered important in reducing mortality risk are listed in Box 7-1.

SEDATION AND PREMEDICATION

Cats often require sedation to allow diagnostic or minor procedures to be performed. Although *sedation* is defined as the induction of a relaxed state, the goals may include decreased stress and anxiety, as well as depression of the central nervous system so that handling is easier, and analgesia. Drugs or drug combinations used for sedation in cats are often similar to those used for premedication before general anesthesia. Ideally, they should have minimal effect on cardiovascular and respiratory function. However, drugs producing moderate to profound sedation in cats produce significant cardiorespiratory effects, and in some cases general anesthesia may be a safer approach, even if only sedation is required for the procedure.

TABLE 7-1 **American Society of Anesthesiologists' Physical Status Classification**

Class*	Preoperative Health Status	Comments
PS 1	Normal healthy patient	No health problems; excludes the very young and very old
PS 2	Patients with mild systemic disease	Mild, well-controlled systemic disease
PS 3	Patients with severe systemic disease	Severe or poorly controlled systemic disease
PS 4	Patients with severe systemic disease that is a threat to life	At least one disease that is poorly controlled or end stage, possible risk of death
PS 5	Moribund patients not expected to live >24 hours with or without surgery	Imminent risk of death, multiorgan failure

*An *E* is added to the class to designate emergency surgery.
Adapted from http://www.asahq.org/clinical/physicalstatus.htm.

BOX 7-1

Factors Likely to Reduce Mortality

- Better preoperative evaluation of patients
- Better preparation of patients
- Better monitoring of patients both during anesthesia and in the early postoperative period

Premedication before general anesthesia is part of the overall anesthetic plan and should be planned in relation to it. Premedication may aim to produce one or several effects and may require the administration of a single drug or, more often, a combination of drugs. Goals of premedication include the following:

- Sedation to facilitate intravenous catheterization and induction of anesthesia
- Reduction of stress and anxiety
- Analgesia
- Reduction of anesthetic dose for induction and maintenance to reduce adverse effects due to anesthetic agents
- Prevention or treatment of adverse effects of other drugs given for premedication
- Anesthetic induction, or maintenance
- Improvement in quality of anesthetic induction and/or recovery
- Prevention or treatment of specific conditions

This latter effect will not be reviewed here; it would, for example, include the administration of antihistamine drugs in patients with mast cell tumors.

BOX 7-2

Advantages and Disadvantages of Acepromazine

Advantages

- It produces sedation.
- It may prevent the behavioral effects produced by opioids.
- It decreases anesthetic requirements.
- It has minimal impact on ventilation.

Disadvantages

- Sedation appears minimal and variable in cats.
- It produces vasodilation and hypotension.
- It interferes with thermoregulation, leading to hypothermia in most situations.

It is important to consider that premedication is not always necessary and that in some patients only some of the aforementioned effects may be desirable. For example, in the obtunded patient sedation is unnecessary, and agents producing sedation are often contraindicated because of the adverse effects they produce.

Agents used for premedication are usually administered parenterally. Subcutaneous administration is usually easy and causes minimal pain and stress; however, onset of effect is expected to be delayed, and the effect is more variable than after intramuscular or intravenous administration. Some agents may be administered orally (e.g., by the owners before going to the veterinary hospital). This may be advantageous in particularly anxious patients.

Agents commonly used for premedication belong to one of three classes: tranquilizers/sedatives, analgesics, and anticholinergics. The pharmacology of drugs commonly used for premedication is briefly reviewed in Table 7-2.

Tranquilizers and Sedatives

Acepromazine

Acepromazine is the prototype tranquilizer and is the only drug in that category commonly used in clinical practice (Box 7-2). Acepromazine is a phenothiazine compound. It antagonizes the actions of dopamine as a central neurotransmitter. It also blocks the effects of dopamine at peripheral D_1 and D_2 receptors. Its onset of action is long (15 minutes after intravenous administration, 30 to 45 minutes after intramuscular administration), and it has a long (3 to 6 hours) duration. Acepromazine is sometimes administered orally, but its bioavailability appears poor,[88] although data in cats are not available. High doses should therefore be used.

TABLE 7-2 **Drugs Commonly Used for Sedation and Premedication in the Cat**

Drug	Main Desired Effect	Suggested Dose Range and Route
Acepromazine	Sedation	0.02-0.05 mg/kg SC, IM, IV
Diazepam	Sedation	0.1-0.5 mg/kg IV
Midazolam	Sedation	0.1-0.3 mg/kg IM, IV
Xylazine	Sedation	0.5-2 mg/kg SC, IM, IV
Dexmedetomidine	Sedation	5-20 μg/kg SC, IM, IV
Morphine	Analgesia	0.1-0.2 mg/kg SC, IM
Hydromorphone	Analgesia	0.03-0.1 mg/kg SC, IM, IV
Oxymorphone	Analgesia	0.03-0.1 mg/kg SC, IM, IV
Methadone	Analgesia	0.2-0.5 mg/kg SC, IM, IV
Buprenorphine	Analgesia	10-30 μg/kg SC, IM, IV
Butorphanol	Analgesia	0.1-0.4 mg/kg SC, IM, IV
Ketamine	Sedation	5 mg/kg SC, IM; 2-5 mg/kg IV
Telazol	Sedation	3-5 mg/kg SC, IM; 2-3 mg/kg IV
Atropine	Prevention of bradycardia, decreased secretions	0.01-0.04 mg/kg SC, IM, IV
Glycopyrrolate	Prevention of bradycardia, decreased secretions	0.01 mg/kg SC, IM, IV

SC, Subcutaneous; *IM*, intramuscular; *IV*, intravenous.

Acepromazine produces sedation. Typically, patients are rousable by stimuli of sufficient intensity. The sedative effect is variable among individuals but may be improved by combining acepromazine and opioids (neuroleptanalgesia). Chlorpromazine, another phenothiazine, was shown to decrease morphine-induced excitement in cats,[48] and acepromazine is expected to have similar effects. Phenothiazines appear to suppress aggressive behaviors related to dominance rather than fear. Acepromazine is usually not thought to produce analgesia. However, in a recent study in cats, acepromazine produced mechanical antinociception and potentiated the effect of tramadol.[211] Acepromazine has been reported to decrease anesthetic requirements, both for injectable and inhaled anesthetics.[95,233] In a study in cats, however, acepromazine did not reduce the induction dose of propofol.[69] Phenothiazines may decrease the seizure threshold,[57,128] and acepromazine should be used with caution in patients with a history of seizures or during procedures or with drugs that may cause seizures.

Acepromazine produces minimal effects on the respiratory system. Respiratory rate may decrease, but blood gases remain normal, probably because of an increase in tidal volume. Acepromazine produces vasodilation and hypotension.[41] The effect is mainly due to alpha-adrenergic blockade; central sympatholysis, direct vasodilation, and/or stimulation of $beta_2$ adrenergic receptors may contribute. If a vasoconstrictor is used to treat hypotension in cats receiving acepromazine, an $alpha_1$ agonist devoid of $beta_2$ effect such as phenylephrine or norepinephrine should be used. Heart rate may decrease, but the effect is usually mild. Phenothiazines protect against epinephrine-induced arrhythmias.[153] They cause splenic sequestration of red blood cells and markedly reduce the hematocrit level.

Acepromazine interferes with temperature regulation. Hypothermia or hyperthermia may result, depending on ambient temperature, although hypothermia is more common. Acepromazine produces antiemetic effects because of its interaction with central dopaminergic receptors at the level of the chemoreceptor trigger zone. Acepromazine reduces gastroesophageal sphincter pressure, possibly increasing the incidence of esophageal reflux and regurgitation.[90] Acepromazine blocks histamine H_1 receptors and may affect the results of intradermal skin testing.[14] Acepromazine applied topically does not affect intraocular pressure in normal eyes but may reduce it when elevated.[94] Acepromazine reduces tear production in normal cats.[70]

According to the authors' clinical experience, cats treated with acepromazine appear sedated in the absence of stimulation, but the effects seem to disappear with handling. Acepromazine worsens the hypotensive effect of inhalant anesthetics in cats, and the authors do not commonly use this drug in feline patients.

Benzodiazepines

Three drugs in the benzodiazepine class are used in clinical practice as part of anesthetic management:

BOX 7-3

Advantages and Disadvantages of Benzodiazepines

Advantages

- They decrease anxiety.
- They produce muscle relaxation.
- They prevent convulsions.
- They may produce sedation.
- They reduce anesthetic requirements.
- They have minimal effects on the cardiovascular and respiratory systems.

Disadvantage

- They may produce dysphoria.

diazepam, midazolam, and zolazepam. Zolazepam is available only in combination with tiletamine (Telazol) and will not be discussed here (Box 7-3).

Benzodiazepines act by modulating $GABA_A$ (gamma-aminobutyric acid) receptors. GABA is the most prominent inhibitory neurotransmitter in the mammalian brain. Benzodiazepines have a short onset of effect, and their duration of action is drug dependent; the effects of diazepam last longer than those of midazolam, as a result of active metabolites with slow clearance.

Clinical effects relevant to anesthesia include sedation or dysphoria, decreased anxiety, inhibition of aggressive behavior, amnesia, muscle relaxation, anticonvulsant effects, and reduced anesthetic requirements. Benzodiazepines do not appear to produce analgesia after systemic administration. In cats 1 mg/kg of diazepam administered intramuscularly caused apparent sedation; however, when cats were restrained for handling, they vigorously objected.[93] A study examined the effects of midazolam, administered intravenously or intramuscularly, at various doses ranging from 0.05 to 5 mg/kg.[108] Restlessness was observed initially, followed by sedation, with most cats receiving the higher doses intravenously assuming a lateral recumbency. When cats were restrained, an approximately equal proportion responded more and less than normal, independent of dose and time. It therefore appears that benzodiazepines do not consistently produce sedation in cats, at least when administered alone. Combinations with opioids may improve the consistency of the sedative effect.

Benzodiazepines are commonly used with induction agents to improve muscle relaxation and/or reduce the anesthetic dose. Diazepam and midazolam have been reported to decrease the anesthetic dose of both inhaled and injectable anesthetics.* They are very effective at preventing and treating convulsions. In humans midazolam is useful in the treatment of status epilepticus refractory to phenobarbital, phenytoin, and diazepam.[227]

Benzodiazepines produce minimal cardiovascular and respiratory effects. Diazepam may decrease ventricular arrhythmias resulting from myocardial ischemia.[152] In hypovolemic patients high doses of midazolam may produce hypotension.[3] Hypotension, arrhythmias, and asystole have been reported after intravenous administration of diazepam; this is thought to be due to propylene glycol, which is used as a solvent in commercially available solutions.[79]

The main difference between diazepam and midazolam is related to their physicochemical characteristics and pharmacokinetics. Diazepam is highly hydrophobic, and studies in humans suggest that absorption may be poor after administration in some muscle groups. Midazolam is hydrophilic at low pH and lipophilic at higher pH; it may be better suited to intramuscular administration than diazepam. Its bioavailability after intramuscular administration is higher than 90% in humans and dogs. Onset of effect is short for both drugs. Diazepam undergoes oxidation to nordiazepam, an active metabolite, which is eliminated about 6 times more slowly than diazepam. The clearance of diazepam itself in cats is low. Diazepam is therefore expected to have long-lasting effects.[43] There are no published data on the pharmacokinetics of midazolam in cats. However, in dogs midazolam is rapidly eliminated, in contrast to diazepam.[44,126] In the species in which it has been examined, the metabolism of midazolam results in the production of hydroxymidazolams, which have pharmacologic activity but are usually rapidly eliminated. Clinically, the duration of effect of midazolam appears much shorter than that of diazepam.

Acute fulminant hepatic necrosis has been reported in cats following diazepam administration.[34] However, it followed repeated oral administration; similar toxicity has not been reported after occasional parenteral administration of the drug.

Clinically, benzodiazepines are sometimes used for premedication before general anesthesia, in combination with opioids, in an attempt to improve the sedation produced by the opioid.

Alpha$_2$-Adrenoceptor Agonists

Agonists of the alpha$_2$-adrenergic receptors (alpha$_2$ agonists) act mainly by modulating noradrenergic transmission in the central nervous system. They also have direct effects on various organs. Drugs in this class commonly used in cats include xylazine and dexmedetomidine (Box 7-4).

Alpha$_2$ agonists produce sedation; the effect is dose dependent.[214] At high doses sedation is profound, and patients are unresponsive to most stimuli, although

*References 84, 107, 111, 115, 133, 136, 169, 242, 243.

BOX 7-4

Advantages and Disadvantages of Alpha$_2$-Adrenoceptor Agonists

Advantages

- They produce dose-dependent sedation.
- At high doses, they produce profound sedation.
- They produce analgesia.
- They reduce anesthetic requirements in a dose-dependent manner.
- They have minimal effect on the respiratory system.

Disadvantages

- They produce bradycardia and decreased cardiac output.
- They produce vasoconstriction.
- They cause hyperglycemia.
- They cause diuresis.
- They cause hypothermia.

arousal and aggressive behavior is always possible. Alpha$_2$ agonists also produce analgesia.[228] The duration of the analgesic effect of both xylazine and dexmedetomidine appears short.[154,208] Alpha$_2$ agonists reduce anesthetic requirements in a dose-dependent manner. They induce hypothermia through an effect of the hypothalamic thermoregulatory center.

Respiratory effects produced by alpha$_2$ agonists are considered minimal in cats. Respiratory rate tends to decrease, but blood gases are usually unaffected.[78,117]

The typical cardiovascular response to the administration of alpha$_2$ agonists is biphasic. Initially, blood pressure and systemic vascular resistance increase, whereas heart rate and cardiac output decrease.[74,117,154] The increase in blood pressure may not be seen after intramuscular administration. These effects are followed by a decrease in arterial pressure; heart rate and cardiac output remain lower than normal. Systemic vascular resistance either returns progressively toward normal or remains elevated, depending on the drug and the dose considered. The bradycardia may be accompanied by other arrhythmias. The cardiovascular effects of alpha$_2$ agonists are usually considered to be dose dependent. The increase in systemic vascular resistance is due to stimulation of alpha$_2$ receptors on the vascular smooth muscle, resulting in vasoconstriction. The decrease in cardiac output is due to the decrease in heart rate. Myocardial contractility appears unaffected.

Because the decrease in cardiac output appears to be mainly related to the bradycardia, the combination with anticholinergics has been advocated. However, the concomitant use of anticholinergics with alpha$_2$ agonists is controversial. The effectiveness in increasing heart rate could depend on the timing of administration of the drugs. When given before the alpha$_2$ agonist, anticholinergics tend to increase heart rate, which decreases after the alpha$_2$ agonist is administered. When given simultaneously, there is an initial bradycardia followed by a return of heart rate toward baseline values. In both cases severe hypertension is produced, and cardiac performance further decreases.[6,50,206]

Alpha$_2$ agonists inhibit insulin release and cause an increase in glycemia. They also inhibit the release of antidiuretic hormone (ADH) and its effect on renal tubules, resulting in water diuresis. Alpha$_2$ agonists cause vomiting in cats and have been used for that purpose. The incidence of vomiting is higher after xylazine than after dexmedetomidine administration.

Xylazine is shorter acting, less potent, and less selective for the alpha$_2$ receptors than dexmedetomidine. Some of the effects following xylazine administration may be related to its action on alpha$_1$ receptors.

Clinically, xylazine and dexmedetomidine are used mainly for their sedative effect. They are sometimes used to improve analgesia. Combinations with opioids may reduce the dose required to produce sedation.[199] Because of their cardiovascular effects, they should be used with caution in geriatric patients or patients with significant organ dysfunction. The use of medetomidine in cats with hypertrophic cardiomyopathy and left ventricular outflow tract obstruction has been suggested to decrease the obstruction; dexmedetomidine is expected to produce similar effects.[118]

Dissociative Anesthetics

Ketamine and Telazol are sometimes used as premedication before general anesthesia. Their pharmacology is reviewed in the section on induction agents. Dissociative anesthetics produce dose-dependent effects ranging from mild or moderate sedation to anesthesia. They may be useful in the intractable cat, as long as an injection can be administered. Ketamine should not be used alone because of its effect on muscle tone and the risk for convulsions; it should be combined with acepromazine, a benzodiazepine, or an alpha$_2$ agonist (Box 7-5).

OPIOIDS

The pharmacology of opioids is reviewed in Chapter 6. Only their use in the context of premedication will be addressed here.

Opioids are used for their analgesic effect (Box 7-6). They are commonly given at the time of premedication to produce preemptive analgesia. Because they are considered to be the first line of treatment for acute (surgical) pain, they should be included in the anesthetic regimen for any procedure likely to cause pain. In addition to their analgesic effect, they reduce the effective dose of sedative and anesthetic drugs. They also produce some behavioral modification. Usually, at the doses

BOX 7-5
Advantages and Disadvantages of Dissociative Anesthetics

Advantages

- They produce dose-dependent sedation.
- At moderate doses they produce profound sedation.
- At high doses, they produce anesthesia.
- Their effects are consistent.

Disadvantages

- Ketamine can cause convulsions.
- Ketamine increases muscle tone.
- They should always be combined with an agent producing muscle relaxation.

BOX 7-6
Advantages and Disadvantages of Opioids

Advantages

- They produce analgesia.
- At moderate doses they produce euphoria.

Disadvantages

- They can produce dysphoria and excitement.
- Their efficacy may be variable.

recommended for clinical use, opioids produce euphoria in cats (i.e., cats do not appear sedated but are more playful and resist restraint less). At higher doses dysphoria may be produced, and cats become hyperactive, excitable, and more difficult to handle. Various drugs can be used. Typically, the full agonists (e.g., morphine, hydromorphone, oxymorphone, methadone) are considered to have a higher analgesic efficacy than the partial agonist buprenorphine. The agonists–antagonists such as butorphanol usually have low analgesic efficacy. However, buprenorphine, at the doses commonly used clinically, appears to produce good analgesia in cats.

ANTICHOLINERGICS

Anticholinergics antagonize the effects of acetylcholine at muscarinic receptors, which result in the blockade of transmission at parasympathetic postganglionic nerve terminals. They decrease overall parasympathetic tone (Box 7-7).

Two drugs in this class are used in clinical patients for premedication: atropine and glycopyrrolate. Glycopyrrolate is a quaternary ammonium and does not cross the blood–brain barrier or the placenta. It is therefore devoid of atropine's effect on the central nervous system, including on pupil size.

BOX 7-7
Advantages and Disadvantages of Anticholinergics

Advantages

- They prevent bradycardia due to high vagal tone.
- They decrease secretions.

Disadvantages

- They can cause arrhythmias.
- They decrease gastrointestinal motility.
- Excessive doses of atropine have effects on the central nervous system.

At high doses atropine causes central nervous system excitement followed by depression. Atropine causes mydriasis. It increases intraocular pressure in narrow-angle glaucoma and should therefore not be used in patients with this condition.

Anticholinergics inhibit nasal, pharyngeal, buccal, and bronchial secretions. They reduce mucous secretion and mucociliary clearance, sometimes resulting in the formation of mucus plugs. They cause relaxation of the bronchial smooth muscle and therefore bronchodilation.

Anticholinergics increase heart rate. There is sometimes a transient decrease in heart rate after administration of a low dose of atropine. Anticholinergics prevent the effects of vagal stimulation on heart rate. They are effective at treating some forms of second-degree atrioventricular block and sometimes increase ventricular rate in third-degree atrioventricular block.

Anticholinergics decrease salivary and gastric secretions. Gastric pH is increased. These drugs decrease motility of the stomach, duodenum, jejunum, ileum, and colon. They also decrease the tone of the gastroesophageal sphincter, increasing the risk for regurgitation and reflux.

The onset and duration of effect of glycopyrrolate are longer than those of atropine. Glycopyrrolate is considered to decrease the risk of producing tachycardia and may have higher efficacy in decreasing secretions.

The main desirable effects of anticholinergics are to prevent the bradycardia caused by other drugs that increase vagal tone or vagal reflexes and to decrease salivary and bronchial secretions. They are often used to prevent opioid-induced bradycardia and to block dissociative anesthetic-induced increase in secretions. Their use in premedication is controversial; some clinicians prefer to treat bradycardia and increased secretions if needed rather than preventing these effects. At clinical doses, their undesirable effects appear to be well tolerated in cats.

Induction Agents

The injectable anesthetic agents currently available to induce anesthesia in cats are ketamine, Telazol (a mixture of tiletamine and zolazepam), thiopental, propofol, and etomidate. Alphaxolone is available in some countries but not in the United States. Whereas ketamine and thiopental were the mainstay injectable anesthetic agents in veterinary practice for a number of years, it now appears that propofol is the most commonly used drug, with thiopental reported to have disappeared from the U.S. market by 2010. Telazol is usually restricted for use in feral cats, in which it is administered intramuscularly or subcutaneously, and the use of etomidate as an induction agent is generally restricted to sick or older cats. In countries where it is available, alphaxalone has increased in popularity.

Toxicity studies in cats allowed the therapeutic index of ketamine, thiopental, and alphaxalone to be derived.[36] In one study[36] the difference between the dose that caused recumbency and the fatal dose was 4 times for thiopental and 5 times for ketamine and alphaxalone.

Calculated intravenous induction doses, reported in Table 7-3, vary depending on the end point and whether the agent is administered after premedication or in conjunction with a benzodiazepine.

Thiopental

Thiopental is the oldest of the injectable anesthetic agents, having been introduced into veterinary practice in the early 1930s. It is a rapidly acting thiobarbiturate with an ultrashort duration of action. It is marketed as the sodium salt in powder form and is reconstituted with 0.9% sodium chloride or water for injection. The usual concentration for clinical use is 2.5%. The drug is a weak acid, and because the unionized form is poorly water soluble, concentrated solutions for administration are alkalinized so that the drug is restricted almost entirely to the water-soluble ionized form. The high pH of the solution is partly responsible for the irritancy of the drug if it is given perivascularly (Box 7-8).

CLINICAL USE

The dose reported in the literature varies from 5 to 20 mg/kg, depending on the desired end point. For induction of anesthesia, after premedication, the calculated dose is 12 mg/kg, whereas administration of adjuvant agents such as diazepam or midazolam, together with premedication, reduces the calculated dose to 10 mg/kg. The usual concentration is 2.5%; however, if the calculated volume is small (<6 mL), a more dilute solution will allow better titration. One quarter of the calculated dose is usually administered over 20 to 30 seconds and the patient observed for drug effects. If more of the drug is required, another quarter of the calculated dose is again administered over 20 to 30 seconds. In a cat with a normal circulation time, 30 seconds is the usual time between administrations of doses.

Generally, induction of anesthesia is rapid, smooth, and excitement-free. Central nervous system activation occurs initially, and this may translate into an excitement phase if insufficient thiopental is administered.

PHARMACODYNAMIC EFFECTS

Although thiopental has been used in veterinary anesthesia for many years, there are few reports concerning pharmacologic effects in cats. Early cardiopulmonary studies reported a decrease in respiratory rate and tidal volume, a fall in blood pressure, and a slowing of heart rate.[80] A dose of 20 mg/kg produced mild hypotension between 5 and 10 minutes after administration, with little change in heart rate. Approximately 30% of cats developed apnea lasting up to almost 1 minute, and arterial carbon dioxide tension was elevated and arterial oxygen tension decreased at 1.5 minutes.[143] A more in-depth study undertaken after acepromazine (0.2 mg/kg), meperidine (4 mg/kg), and atropine (0.05 mg/kg) premedication followed by induction with thiopental (10 mg/kg) reported minor respiratory depression but a significant fall in cardiac index with no change in heart rate.[51] Thiopental (6.8 mg/kg) had a negative effect on the cat myocardium, suggesting that the hypotension may be due to direct myocardial depression.[76]

TABLE 7-3 **Calculated Intravenous Doses for Induction Agents**

Induction Agents	Alone	After Premedication	After Premedication and with a Benzodiazepine
Thiopental	5-20 mg/kg	12 mg/kg	10 mg/kg
Ketamine	10 mg/kg*	5 mg/kg*	
Telazol	1-3 mg/kg		
Propofol	8 mg/kg	6 mg/kg	4 mg/kg
Etomidate	2 mg/kg*	2 mg/kg*	
Alfaxan	5 mg/kg	2-3 mg/kg	

*Must always be administered with a benzodiazepine.

BOX 7-8

Advantages and Disadvantages of Thiopental

Advantages

- It is a rapidly acting drug, with effects discernible within a circulation time. Thiopental lends itself to titration to effect and is especially useful when an airway needs to be secured quickly, such as in a cat with a full stomach or a history of vomiting.
- It has an ultrashort duration of action (5-10 minutes) depending on administered dose. Thiopental is an excellent induction agent before intubation and maintenance with inhalant agents. It is also suitable for nonpainful procedures of short duration (15-20 minutes), although propofol provides better recovery conditions.
- It decreases intracranial pressure (ICP) in patients with raised ICP and has protective cerebral effects if administered before a hypoxemic event. It is an effective anticonvulsant, although its anesthetic and anticonvulsant effects cannot be separated.
- It depresses laryngeal reflexes less than other induction agents, such as propofol and ketamine, and therefore facilitates examination of vocal cords and correct diagnosis of laryngeal paralysis.

Disadvantages

- It is not a suitable drug for maintenance of anesthesia because clearance is slow, leading to accumulation and prolonged recoveries.
- It is an irritant if given perivascularly, and treatment is important to prevent tissue necrosis and sloughing.
- It decreases packed cell volume and white blood cell and platelet counts and may decrease total protein concentration.
- It does not block autonomic responses to noxious stimuli and thus is not suitable for short painful procedures.
- Recovery can be rough, especially if the patient awakes from thiopental alone.
- It is a myocardial-depressant drug that induces tachycardia and an increased incidence of arrhythmias. In healthy animals these arrhythmias are rarely of clinical importance.
- Laryngeal reflexes are active, increasing the difficulty of intubation. Because of this, traumatic intubation may be more likely with thiopental than other agents.

Thiopental induces a dose-related depression of cerebral metabolic oxygen consumption rate and, presumably because of preserved cerebral autoregulation, reduces cerebral blood flow.[142] As a result of the reduced cerebral blood flow and accompanying fall in cerebral blood volume, cerebrospinal fluid pressure is reduced. With thiopental, as with etomidate, cerebral perfusion pressure is not compromised because intracranial pressure decreases more than mean arterial pressure. Thiopental is an effective anticonvulsant, although its hypnotic and anticonvulsant properties occur at similar doses.

No difference in the incidence of gastroesophageal reflux was reported in cats between thiopental and propofol, with an incidence of 16% and 12%, respectively.[66]

PHARMACOKINETIC EFFECTS

The pharmacokinetics of thiopental in cats has not been reported, although that of a very similar thiobarbiturate, thiamylal, has been described.[238] The rapid distribution half-life was 1.91 minutes, and a second, or slower, distribution half-life was 26.51 minutes. The elimination half-life was 14.34 hours. The apparent volume of distribution was 3.61 L/kg, whereas the apparent volume of the central compartment was 0.46 L/kg, and the total clearance was 0.135 L/kg/h. As in other species, initial wake-up is due to redistribution initially into vessel-rich tissues and muscle and later into fat.[28,29] Although the drug does not have a high clearance, metabolism does contribute to recovery.[192]

Ketamine

Ketamine is partly water soluble and is prepared in a slightly acidic (pH 3.5 to 5.5) solution. It is formulated for veterinary use as a 10% solution in sodium chloride with the preservative, benzethonium chloride (Box 7-9).

Ketamine is considered a dissociative anesthetic, a term used to describe a state in which there is functional and electrophysiologic dissociation between the thalamoneocortical and limbic systems.[240] This unique clinical state of hypnosis and analgesia is characterized by open eyes, dilated pupils, muscle hypertonus, and increased lacrimation and salivation. An anticholinergic drug, atropine or glycopyrrolate, is usually administered as a preanesthetic to decrease salivation.

Ketamine acts primarily through the *N*-methyl-D-aspartate (NMDA) receptor.[112,158]

CLINICAL USE

Induction of anesthesia with ketamine alone is unsatisfactory insofar as muscle tone is extreme and spontaneous movement virtually continuous.[246] Tranquilizers are often administered before ketamine, whereas the benzodiazepines, diazepam or midazolam, are usually administered in combination with ketamine to eliminate or minimize the deleterious side effects. When ketamine is used as an induction agent, the calculated dose in

BOX 7-9

Advantages and Disadvantages of Ketamine

Advantages

- Rapidly acting agent without excitement and with a duration of action that allows induction of anesthesia to proceed slowly
- Excellent analgesic agent even at subanesthetic doses with demonstrated preemptive analgesic properties
- Reported to induce less respiratory depression than thiopental or propofol, and respiratory responses to hypoxemia and hypercarbia are better maintained
- Potent bronchodilating drug that is a suitable induction agent in asthmatic patients or patients with reactive airways

Disadvantages

- It increases muscle tone and induces purposeless muscle movements, making it difficult to carry out certain procedures.
- Salivation and lacrimation are present and may be profuse.
- Intraocular pressure may increase, and eyes remain open and are susceptible to corneal abrasion.
- Cerebral blood flow and cerebral oxygen consumption increase, which may have serious adverse effects in patients with raised intracranial pressure.
- Ketamine depresses the myocardium, but central sympathetic stimulation leads to an increase in heart rate, blood pressure, and cardiac output. In diseases such as hypertrophic cardiomyopathy, these cardiovascular effects may prove fatal.

unpremedicated healthy cats is 10 mg/kg IV,[86] together with diazepam (0.5 mg/kg IV) or midazolam (0.3 to 0.5 mg/kg IV). Premedication reduces the dose of ketamine to 5 mg/kg, and the dose of diazepam or midazolam remains the same. Studies in cats using a calculated dose of 3 mg/kg of ketamine reported that the ED_{50} (effective dose in 50% of the population) of midazolam required for intubation and to prevent movement in response to a noxious stimulation was 0.286 mg/kg and 0.265 mg/kg, respectively. At that dose recovery to walking with ataxia took 41.50 ± 15.18 minutes and complete recovery 3.6 ± 1.3 hours.[107]

One quarter of the calculated dose of ketamine, followed by one half of the calculated dose of diazepam or midazolam, is usually administered over 10 to 20 seconds and the patient observed for drug effects after 1 minute. If more of the drug is required, another quarter of the calculated dose of ketamine and the remainder of the diazepam or midazolam is administered over another minute. Some veterinarians prefer to combine the drugs in the same syringe and then just administer in quarter-dose boluses.[86]

Recovery from ketamine anesthesia can be associated with hyperexcitability, especially in cats. General recommendations are to allow cats to recover in a quiet, dark room with minimal handling.

PHARMACODYNAMIC EFFECTS

Ketamine is reported to have sympathomimetic effects, which increase heart rate, cardiac output, and blood pressure, primarily by direct stimulation of central nervous system structures.[240] In the absence of autonomic control, ketamine has direct myocardial depressant properties.[223,245] The cardiopulmonary effects of intravenous administration of ketamine have been studied in cats.[143] At clinical doses (6.6 mg/kg intravenously), both heart rate and blood pressure increased, with peak effects generally occurring 2.5 minutes after administration. Transient respiratory depression was also reported.[143] In cats anesthetized with halothane, ketamine has been reported to decrease the arrhythmogenic threshold.[17] Respiration has been noted as apneustic, shallow, and irregular immediately after ketamine administration in cats.[37]

Ketamine has bronchodilating properties[167] and is often recommended as the induction agent of choice in cats with asthma.

Swallow, cough, and gag reflexes are relatively intact after ketamine, and in cats, but not humans, competent laryngeal protective reflexes are maintained, such that material that reaches the trachea is coughed up and swallowed.[188,221] In cats contrast radiography has been suggested as a diagnostic aid in ketamine-anesthetized cats suspected of laryngeal reflex abnormalities.[188]

Care is needed in interpretation of echocardiographic measurements in cats under light sedation doses (1.5 to 2.5 mg/kg intravenously) of ketamine, insofar as significant differences were reported in studies conducted using different drugs or in non-anesthetized cats.[64]

Although there are no specific published studies in cats, in other species ketamine increases cerebral blood flow and intracranial pressure, principally by cerebral vasodilation and elevated systemic arterial pressure.[200,218] Part of the vasodilation is due to increased arterial carbon dioxide tensions when ventilation is not controlled,[196] and the other most likely results from stimulation of cerebral metabolic rate. Thus the use of ketamine in patients with raised intracranial pressure is not recommended. Ketamine has been reported to cause seizures in cats,[15,186] although usually only after intramuscular administration of high doses.

Under ketamine anesthesia, segmental stretch and withdrawal reflexes are preserved even at levels that block electroencephalographic arousal and autonomic changes in response to nociceptive stimulation.[220]

Ketamine, compared with thiopental, propofol, and Saffan, had the least effect on gastroesophageal sphincter pressure and barrier pressure in cats.[89]

Administration of ketamine interferes with the results of glucose tolerance tests in cats and thus this test should be performed without chemical restraint.[102]

In cats a slight but significant increase in intraocular pressure occurs with ketamine,[82] so this agent should be avoided if the cat is at risk for corneal perforation. The increase is thought to be due to increases in extraocular muscle tone induced by ketamine.

Cats induced with ketamine (5 mg/kg intravenously) and diazepam (0.25 mg/kg intravenously) and maintained with halothane anesthesia were found to mount a normal response to an ACTH stimulation test, indicating adequate adrenocortical function.[147]

Various sedative protocols, including those containing ketamine, have been reported to produce significant effects on thyroid function and salivary gland uptake of technetium Tc 99m pertechnetate and, as such, may interfere with thyroid scintigraphic image interpretation.[194]

Sedation with ketamine results in a lower number of spermatozoa per ejaculate compared with medetomidine when semen was collected after electroejaculation.[249]

Ketamine has been reported to possess analgesic properties. Induction with ketamine or addition of ketamine to general anesthesia before surgical stimulation decreases postoperative pain and leads to better pain control.[156,191] It appears that the analgesic properties of ketamine reduce sensitization of pain pathways and extend into the postoperative period. Although ketamine appears to provide good somatic analgesia, its visceral analgesia is weak.[193]

PHARMACOKINETIC EFFECTS

Recovery from ketamine is due to both redistribution and metabolism. Several studies have reported the pharmacokinetic profile of ketamine in cats.[10,96] Ketamine has a rapid distribution with a brief distribution half-life of 5.2 minutes. The high lipid solubility is reflected in the large volume of distribution (3.21 L/kg). Clearance is also high (37.8 mL/kg/min), which accounts for the short elimination half-life (60.6 min).[96] Mean total body clearance is very similar to liver blood flow, which means that changes in liver blood flow affect clearance. This has been reported in the cat, where xylazine prolonged the duration of ketamine anesthesia by increasing the elimination half-life.[232] Ketamine is metabolized extensively in the liver to form norketamine (metabolite I), which has 20% to 30% of the activity of the parent drug. Cats, as a species, are unable to metabolize norketamine further, and elimination of norketamine is dependent on renal excretion. Thus duration of action may be prolonged in cats with severe renal dysfunction.

Telazol

Telazol is a combination of a dissociative anesthetic agent, tiletamine, and a benzodiazepine, zolazepam, and is currently marketed for intramuscular administration in dogs and cats. Once reconstituted for use, the solution contains 50 mg/mL of each compound or 100 mg/mL of the combination. The recommended dose is usually expressed in terms of the combined dose.

CLINICAL USE

Although Telazol is not registered for intravenous use in cats, it is a suitable induction agent. The reported dose is 1 to 3 mg/kg, and administration of an anticholinergic is recommended because salivation can be profuse.[129] A dose of 3 mg/kg is diluted to 1 mL with saline, and a 1 mg/kg bolus is administered intravenously every 1 minute until intubation is possible.

A dose of 9.9 mg/kg administered intravenously or intramuscularly resulted in a similar duration of anesthesia (20 minutes) and time to walking (174 to 180 minutes).[224]

PHARMACODYNAMIC EFFECTS

There is little published data on effects of Telazol, especially in cats, and it is presumed that the effects are similar to ketamine.[125,129] The cardiovascular and respiratory effects of intravenous administration of Telazol have been reported, although the doses (9.7, 15.8, and 23.7 mg/kg) were higher than those commonly used in practice.[98] An initial cardiovascular depressor response, with degree and duration depending on the dose, was then followed by a pressor response. In another study Telazol did not alter the arrhythmogenic threshold in cats.[16]

The degree of respiratory depression in cats appears to be dose dependent, with higher doses causing more depression. In one study respiratory rate decreased and was often characterized initially by an apneustic respiratory pattern.[248] Within 10 to 15 minutes, respiration had returned to a normal pattern.[224] Periods of apnea have been reported after intravenous administration of high doses (15.8 and 23.7 mg/kg), and arterial carbon dioxide tension was elevated.[98]

Telazol is considered a suitable intravenous agent for intradermal skin testing in cats.[149]

Telazol carries the same warning as other dissociative agents.[129] It is not recommended for cats with hypertrophic cardiac disease, hepatic or renal disease may prolong the actions, and dose-dependent respiratory

BOX 7-10

Advantages and Disadvantages of Propofol

Advantages

- Rapidly acting drug with minimal excitement, even after subanesthetic doses.
- Recovery is rapid, smooth, and complete, making it an ideal outpatient anesthetic.
- It can be used to induce anesthesia before intubation, or anesthesia can be maintained with propofol by either repeated bolus injections or constant-rate infusion.
- It decreases intracranial pressure in patients with raised intracranial pressure and has protective cerebral effects if administered before a hypoxemic event.
- It decreases intraocular pressure and is a good induction agent in cats with descemetoceles or corneal lacerations.
- It is the induction agent of choice in healthy queens requiring cesarean section if viability of the kittens is important.
- It induces bronchodilation and is a suitable agent in asthmatic patients.
- It is not irritant if administered perivascularly.

Disadvantages

- Apnea is the most common side effect in cats, and cyanosis is often observed during induction.
- Myoclonus sometimes occurs on induction and, if severe, may prevent surgery.
- It has myocardial-depressant and vasodilatory properties without altering heart rate and may cause hypotension, especially in hypovolemic and geriatric patients.
- Bacterial contamination of the solution can increase the incidence of surgical wound infection or cause sepsis.
- Autonomic responses to noxious stimuli are not blocked, and therefore it is not a suitable anesthetic agent for painful procedures.
- Cats have reduced capacity to conjugate propofol, and length of recovery increases with increasing duration of propofol anesthesia.
- Care should be taken if propofol is administered to cats over consecutive days because oxidative injury to feline red blood cells has been reported.

depression is reported when Telazol is administered intravenously with other anesthetic drugs. According to further information on the package insert, use in animals with severe cardiac or pulmonary dysfunction and those requiring cesarean section is not recommended.

PHARMACOKINETIC EFFECTS

The plasma half-life of tiletamine in cats was reported as 2 to 4 hours, with only 5% to 10% of the dose detected in urine, none in feces, and some in bile. Three metabolites were detected in the urine from cats.[125] The plasma half-life of zolazepam in cats was reported as 4.5 hours, with three metabolites detected in urine.[125]

The package insert recommends against the use of Telazol in animals with renal disease because tiletamine is excreted primarily by the kidneys.

Propofol

Propofol is a substituted isopropylphenol, which is only slightly soluble in water and is formulated as a 1% aqueous solution containing soybean oil, egg lecithin, and glycerol. It has a rapid onset, with a smooth, excitement-free induction (Box 7-10).

Patient infections related to the use of propofol have been reported. This is thought to be due to microbial contamination of propofol and has resulted in life-threatening sepsis and postoperative infections of clean wounds in both human and veterinary patients.[18,97] Propofol was found to be an excellent medium for rapid bacterial growth.[209] Current recommendations are to discard unused propofol 6 hours after a vial or ampule is opened.[73]

CLINICAL USE

Initial clinical studies in cats reported the induction dose as 6.8 mg/kg in unpremedicated cats and 7.2 mg/kg in premedicated cats.[24] In some studies, premedication reduced the dose by up to 60%,[148,201] while in other studies premedication did not affect the induction dose.[24,234] In a large clinical trial, the dose in unpremedicated cats was reported as 8.03 mg/kg and in premedicated cats as 5.97 mg/kg.[148] Apnea after induction has been reported in all animal studies and is minimized by slow administration. The time from administration of the last dose to walking was reported as 27 to 38 minutes, depending on premedication and top-up doses. Recovery was rapid and usually excitement free.

Side effects have been reported in all animal studies. In cats an incidence of 14% was reported, with retching, sneezing, and pawing at the eyes and mouth the most prominent effects.[24] The incidence was decreased by premedication with acepromazine.[24]

Because of the high incidence of apnea associated with propofol induction, oxygen should be delivered by face mask throughout the induction. If the patient will not tolerate the face mask before propofol administration, it can usually be placed after administration of the first quarter dose. One quarter of the calculated dose is usually administered over 1 minute and the patient observed for drug effects after 30 seconds. If more of the drug is required, a second quarter of the calculated dose is administered over another minute. When administering propofol to sick patients, the clinician should first administer a very small calculated dose (<0.5 mg/kg) and determine the onset time and effect.

PHARMACODYNAMIC EFFECTS

There are no in-depth studies reporting the cardiopulmonary effects in cats, although in an early clinical study no changes were reported in heart rate or respiratory rate.[234] In other species propofol is depressant, causing a fall in arterial blood pressure and cardiac output. It is not recommended for use in human patients with cardiac disease or hypovolemia. The arrhythmogenic threshold in cats induced and maintained with propofol increased compared with that of cats induced with either thiopental or propofol and maintained with halothane.[72]

Like thiopental and etomidate, propofol induces a dose-related depression of cerebral metabolic oxygen consumption rate and, presumably because of preserved cerebral autoregulation, reduces cerebral blood flow.[215] As a result of the reduced cerebral blood flow and accompanying fall in cerebral blood volume, cerebrospinal fluid pressure is reduced. With propofol cerebral perfusion pressure may decrease as a result of a fall in arterial blood pressure, and care is required to minimize the fall so that cerebral perfusion is not compromised.

Propofol, like ketamine, demonstrated bronchodilating properties in the isolated guinea pig trachea[167] and is considered a suitable induction agent for cats with asthma.

Propofol lowers gastroesophageal sphincter pressure and gastric pressure in cats, although this effect was less than reported with Saffan or thiopental.[89]

Propofol was reported to provide good conditions for semen collection by way of ejaculation in cats, in that ejaculation did not induce stress, onset of anesthesia was rapid, and recovery was smooth.[35]

Care should be taken if propofol is administered to cats over consecutive days because oxidative injury to cat red blood cells has been reported.[8] Administration of propofol daily for 6 days resulted in an increase in Heinz bodies on day 3. Five of the six cats developed generalized malaise, anorexia, and diarrhea, and two cats developed facial edema.[8] If anesthesia is restricted to a single induction dose, behavioral effects were not reported after daily administration for 4 weeks, although increases in methemoglobinemia and Heinz bodies were observed.[73]

PHARMACOKINETIC EFFECTS

Initial studies reported a lower utilization ratio (0.19 mg/kg/min) in cats compared with other species.[71] The utilization ratio was reported as the amount of drug administered divided by the duration of anesthesia. Differences in utilization ratio were likely related to differences in the rate of biotransformation and conjugation, insofar as the cat has a deficiency in its ability to conjugate phenols.[71] In laboratory animals the initial distribution volume was large and redistribution to other parts of the body was extremely rapid. The total apparent volume of distribution was large, as was metabolic clearance from the body, with elimination half-lives in the range 16 to 55 minutes.[2] In this study the slowest elimination was found in the cat.[2] In most species the drug is reported to be noncumulative, making it an excellent drug for maintenance of anesthesia. In cats, when recovery to walking was compared among an induction dose only, an induction and maintenance dose for 30 minutes, and an induction and maintenance dose for 150 minutes, a significant increase in recovery time was reported for the latter dose.[164] This provides further evidence that cats have reduced capacity to conjugate propofol, and thus recoveries will increase with increasing duration of propofol anesthesia.

Pulmonary extraction of propofol has been studied in cats and is substantial.[132] This uptake is decrease by concomitant administration of halothane or fentanyl.

Etomidate

Etomidate is an imidazole derivative that is soluble in water but not stable, so it is formulated as a 0.2% solution in propylene glycol (35% by volume) with a pH of 6.9 and an osmolality of 4640 mOsm/L. It is more expensive than other induction agents and therefore is not used extensively in veterinary practice. However, in certain circumstances it does offer advantages in cats (Box 7-11).

CLINICAL USE

The initial dose of etomidate is calculated on a body weight basis; however, the drug is titrated to effect. A calculated dose of 2 mg/kg is suitable and should be administered with an adjuvant agent such as diazepam (calculated dose, 0.5 mg/kg) or midazolam (calculated dose, 0.2 to 0.5 mg/kg) to facilitate induction.

One quarter of the calculated dose of etomidate is usually administered over 20 to 30 seconds, followed by one quarter to one half of the calculated dose of a benzodiazepine, and the patient is observed for drug effects after 30 seconds. If more drug is required, another quarter of the calculated dose of etomidate followed by a quarter to half of the calculated dose of benzodiazepine are administered over 20 to 30 seconds. To minimize side effects associated with injection of a solution with a high osmolality into a small peripheral vein, etomidate can be injected at the injection port of a fluid administration set through which a balanced electrolyte solution is being administered.

After 3 mg/kg intravenously, in which half was given rapidly and the remainder over 1 minute, induction of anesthesia was rapid and smooth. Recovery was also

BOX 7-11

Advantages and Disadvantages of Etomidate

Advantages

- It is a rapidly acting agent, with loss of consciousness occurring in 15 to 29 seconds. In situations in which a rapid sequence induction technique is required, etomidate is a suitable agent.
- It has an ultrashort duration of action, depending on administered dose, with a relatively rapid recovery. It is also suitable for nonpainful procedures of short duration.
- The relatively short elimination half-life and rapid clearance of etomidate make it a suitable drug for administration in a single dose, in multiple doses, or as a constant-rate infusion. Its adrenocortical suppression, however, limits its use to a single dose.
- It is the recommended induction agent when hemodynamic stability is important. It has been recommended in veterinary patients with preexisting cardiovascular disease or cardiac rhythm disturbances. It is a useful induction agent in cats with severe cardiac disease.
- It induces minimal respiratory depression and thus is a suitable agent when ventilatory stability is important.
- It decreases intracranial pressure in patients with raised intracranial pressure and is a good induction agent when there is concomitant cardiovascular disease or hypovolemia from trauma.
- Etomidate is an effective anticonvulsant; however, because it may activate a seizure focus, caution is advised in cats with epilepsy.
- It decreases intraocular pressure and is a good induction agent in cats with descemetoceles or corneal lacerations associated with other systemic trauma.

Disadvantages

- It is the most expensive of the injectable anesthetic agents.
- In the commercially available solution, the diluent is 35% propylene glycol, which can cause hemolysis, pain on injection, and thrombophlebitis.
- Induction and recovery may not be smooth and may include myoclonus and excitement.
- Adrenocortical suppression follows both induction and maintenance doses. Although its use as an induction agent is considered safe, it should not be administered as an infusion for maintenance of anesthesia.
- Some authors suggest that, in animals dependent on corticosteroids, a physiologic dose of dexamethasone or any other short-acting glucocorticoid should be administered if anesthesia is induced with etomidate.

rapid, although a brief period of myoclonia was observed in all cats early in recovery.[239]

PHARMACODYNAMIC EFFECTS

There are few reports concerning the pharmacologic effects of etomidate in cats. In all species etomidate has minimal effects on the cardiovascular and respiratory systems. In dogs heart rate, blood pressure, and cardiac output were unchanged after administration of 1.5 or 3 mg/kg of etomidate.[155] Similarly, 1 mg/kg of etomidate induced minimal changes in hypovolemic dogs.[165] It also appears that etomidate has minimal effects on the cardiovascular system in cats.[207]

Etomidate induces a dose-related depression of cerebral metabolic oxygen consumption rate and, presumably because of preserved cerebral autoregulation, reduces cerebral blood flow.[144] As a result of the reduced cerebral blood flow and accompanying fall in cerebral blood volume, cerebrospinal fluid pressure is reduced. With etomidate cerebral perfusion pressure is not compromised because intracranial pressure decreases more than mean arterial pressure.

Similar to other induction agents, etomidate decreases gastroesophageal sphincter pressure and barrier pressure and thus may predispose cats to regurgitation under anesthesia.[89]

Etomidate causes hemolysis, even after a single induction dose.[237] The mechanism is thought to be the rapid increase in osmolality caused by the propylene glycol, causing red blood cell rupture. Caution should be exercised in patients with renal insufficiency because of the increased pigment load brought about by hemolysis.[159]

Induction of anesthesia with etomidate (2 mg/kg intravenously) in cats caused suppression of adrenocortical function during 2 hours of halothane anesthesia and for 1 hour in recovery. An additional 2 hours were required for cortisol to return to baseline.[147] The impact of adrenocortical suppression after etomidate administration on long-term morbidity and mortality has not been determined. Some authors suggest that, in animals dependent on corticosteroids, a physiologic dose of dexamethasone or any other short-acting glucocorticoid should be administered if anesthesia is induced with etomidate.[129] Adrenocortical suppression, however, precludes the administration of etomidate as an infusion for maintenance of anesthesia.

BOX 7-12

Advantages and Disadvantages of Alfaxan

Advantages

- Rapid-acting drug with smooth induction
- Recovery is rapid, smooth, and complete, making it an ideal outpatient anesthetic
- Appears to be noncumulative in the cat at clinical dose rates

Disadvantages

- Currently not available in the United States
- Very little reported on its use in clinical patients

PHARMACOKINETIC EFFECTS

The pharmacokinetics of etomidate in cats has been reported.[239] The drug has a rapid distribution (half-life 0.05 hour); a large volume of distribution at steady state (4.88 L/kg); and rapid clearance (2.47 L/kg/h), which accounts for its short duration of action and rapid recovery.[239]

Steroid Anesthetics

The progesterone derivative, alphaxalone, is a neuroactive steroid anesthetic agent (Box 7-12). It was first introduced into veterinary anesthesia in 1971 as a component of the drug Saffan, an anesthetic agent in cats. Alphaxalone was insoluble in water and was mixed with alfadolone acetate to increase its solubility. Alfadolone also had anesthetic properties, with about half the potency of alphaxalone. Saffan is formulated such that the mixture contains 9 mg/mL of alphaxalone and 3 mg/mL of alfadolone, with the solubilizing agent as 20% polyethoxylated castor oil (Cremophor EL). The recommended dose is either expressed as mL of formulated solution/kg or mg of combined steroid/kg. Despite widespread use in other countries, Saffan or its medical counterpart, Althesin, were never available in the United States. Cremophor EL causes histamine release in animals by stimulating mast cell degranulation, and this was responsible for unacceptable adverse events.[40,49,62] In humans the incidence of anaphylactoid reactions was high, and Althesin was removed from the market.

Recently, an Australian company has reformulated alphaxalone in hydroxypropyl beta cyclodextrin (Alfaxan), and it is commercially available for use in dogs and cats in Australia, New Zealand, South Africa, and the United Kingdom.[150] Two recent publications have reported the pharmacokinetics and cardiorespiratory and anesthetic effects of this drug in cats.[150,241]

CLINICAL USE

The initial dose of Saffan is calculated on a body weight basis; however, the drug is titrated to effect. The intravenous induction dose is 0.75 mL/kg (9 mg/kg). Generally, one half of the calculated dose is administered over 20 to 30 seconds, and the patient is observed for drug effects. If more drug is required, a quarter of the calculated dose is administered over 20 to 30 seconds, and this is repeated until the desired anesthetic depth is accomplished. Intravenous injection produces unconsciousness in 10 to 25 seconds, and the depth and duration of surgical anesthesia is dose dependent. Return of righting reflex took 7, 17, 44, 75, and 136 minutes after doses of 1.2, 2.4, 4.8, 9.6, and 19.2 mg/kg, respectively.[37] After the recommended intravenous dose of 9 mg/kg, relaxation occurs in 9 seconds and surgical anesthesia in about 25 seconds. Anesthesia is usually maintained for about 10 minutes, and recovery is rapid.[116]

The calculated dose for the newly released, reformulated alphaxalone (Alfaxan) is 5 mg/kg, with premedicants decreasing the dose to 2 to 3 mg/kg.[114] After administration of 5 and 15 mg/kg doses, induction of anesthesia was characterized as quiet, uneventful, and relaxed. Time to lateral recumbency was inversely proportional to the dose of alphaxalone administered. The average time to lateral recumbency was approximately 15 to 30 seconds. Recovery scores for the 5 and 15 mg/kg doses of alphaxalone were excellent and not different from each other. Doses 10 times the induction dose were invariably fatal.[150]

PHARMACODYNAMIC EFFECTS

Initial cardiovascular and respiratory studies reported a decrease in blood pressure and a tachycardia.[37] The decrease in blood pressure was reported to be less than that found with comparable doses of ketamine. Greater cardiovascular depression was subsequently reported, with 9 mg/kg administered as a 12 mg/mL solution at 0.25 mL/sec inducing profound and sustained hypotension with clinical manifestations consistent of histamine release.[143] An in-depth study undertaken in cats, demonstrated significant depression in cardiac output at 45 and 60 minutes.[52] Although changes in respiratory pattern were observed, no changes in arterial blood gas tensions were found in the latter two studies.[52,143]

In primates Althesin induced a fall in cerebral blood flow and a decrease in cerebrospinal fluid pressure.[174]

In cats the risk of gastroesophageal reflux was reported to be higher with Saffan than with thiopental, if the lower esophageal sphincter pressure and gastric pressure are used as indicators of likely reflux.[89]

Administration of Saffan was reported to interfere with the results of glucose tolerance tests in cats, and this test should be performed without chemical restraint.[102]

Complications associated with Saffan anesthesia were recorded after 100 administrations of the anesthetic to cats.[49] Hyperemia or edema of the pinnae or forepaws was recorded in 69% of cats. Other common complications included coughing and partial laryngeal spasm at intubation, cyanosis, postoperative vomiting, and opisthotonos.

Despite the side effects reported for Saffan in cats, the survey undertaken to look at morbidity and mortality in veterinary practice in the late 1980s reported that Saffan seemed to be the safest agent for the induction of anesthesia in cats in veterinary general practice.[39]

More recently, cardiorespiratory and anesthetic effects of the new formulation have been reported in cats.[150] Alphaxalone produced dose-dependent anesthesia, cardiorespiratory depression, and unresponsiveness to noxious stimulation in unpremedicated cats. Hypoventilation and apnea were the most common side effects, and, other than occasional involuntary muscle movement, other common side effects reported after Saffan were not observed.[150]

PHARMACOKINETIC EFFECTS

Initial pharmacokinetic studies in cats reported a mean plasma half-life of 3.5 minutes[116] and demonstrated a lack of cumulative effect for Saffan.[36] Cats topped up with Saffan for 3 hours took 3 to 4 hours to return to normal behavior.[116]

More recently, the pharmacokinetic effects of the new formulation have been reported in cats.[241] In that report two doses were studied, 5 and 25 mg/kg, and the pharmacokinetics of alphaxalone in cats were reported to be nonlinear. Plasma clearance was 25.1 and 14.8 mL/kg/min, and elimination half-lives were 45.2 and 76.6 minutes, respectively. In a second experiment, alphaxalone was administered intravenously at 5 mg/kg followed by four doses each of 2 mg/kg, administered at onset of responsiveness to a noxious stimulus. A regression line through their peak plasma concentrations indicated that there was no clinically relevant pharmacokinetic accumulation. The duration of nonresponsiveness after each maintenance dose was similar at approximately 6 minutes, indicating a lack of accumulation of pharmacodynamic effect. Thus at clinical dose rates neither alphaxalone nor its anesthetic effects accumulated to a clinically relevant extent.

Induction with Inhalant Anesthetics

Some cats are not amenable to intravenous induction agents, and, rather than using drugs administered subcutaneously or intramuscularly, some veterinarians prefer to use inhalant anesthetics administered by way of a chamber. Advantages of inhalant inductions include reduced need to handle the patient, the ability to tailor the anesthetic dose and therefore depth to the individual patient, a relatively fast induction and recovery, and little reliance on renal and hepatic systems for removal of anesthetic and thus recovery.[226] Disadvantages of this technique include contamination of the environment with inhalant anesthetics, in some cases greater cost and greater cardiovascular and respiratory depression than some injectable agents. Because of the harmful effects of exposure of personnel to low concentrations of inhalant anesthetics, many recommend that mask or chamber inductions should be avoided whenever possible.[87,91]

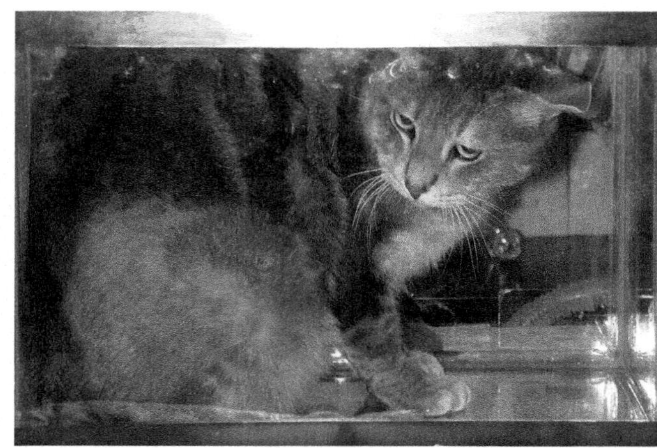

FIGURE 7-1 An airtight Plexiglas induction chamber that allows input of anesthetic gases; a non-rebreathing circuit, such as a Bain circuit, is attached to the chamber.

CLINICAL USE

The inhalant agents commonly used in veterinary practice for mask or chamber inductions are isoflurane and sevoflurane.

With chamber inductions the cat is placed in an airtight Plexiglas chamber that allows input of anesthetic gases (Figure 7-1). A non-rebreathing circuit, such as a Bain circuit, is attached to the chamber, and a high flow of oxygen is administered (5 L/min). Generally, the maximum vaporizer setting is used, and the patient is watched carefully until recumbency ensues. At that time the chamber is rocked gently, and when the cat no longer responds, it is removed from the chamber and induction continued using a face mask until intubation is possible. Once induction is continued by face mask, the oxygen flow is decreased to 2 L/min and the vaporizer setting to that required to maintain the desired anesthetic depth.

Mask techniques are not often used in cats given that they require good patient compliance and restraint. Generally, the cat is restrained by the scruff and a close-fitting mask attached to a non-rebreathing circuit is applied to the face. Usually, oxygen alone is administered at a flow of 2 L/min, and then the inhalant concentration is increased at 0.5% increments every 10 seconds until the vaporizer setting is 3% for isoflurane or 4% for sevoflurane. Induction is continued until the cat is at the desired anesthetic depth.

PHARMACOKINETIC AND PHARMACODYNAMIC EFFECTS

No specific studies have been undertaken to measure the pharmacodynamic effects of mask or chamber inductions in cats. Most published studies have determined induction and recovery times and the quality of induction and recovery utilizing different inhalant agents. No difference was reported in the qualitative induction and recovery characteristics when isoflurane and sevoflurane were compared for chamber induction in the cat.[110] Time to recumbency and intubation were shorter with sevoflurane compared with isoflurane.[110] Similar results were reported after mask induction in cats.[124] Desflurane administered by way of chamber induction was reported to result in an excellent quality of induction and recovery in cats, with airway irritant effects noticed only during recovery and manifested as a brief period of coughing after extubation.[12] A mask induction technique using sevoflurane with a 2:1 mixture of nitrous oxide has been described in cats.[226]

INTUBATION

The onset of unconsciousness produced by general anesthesia is associated with depression of other physiologic systems, such as airway, respiratory, and cardiovascular systems, which can cause immediate threats to the patient. Endotracheal intubation enables maintenance of a patent airway, administration of oxygen, delivery of inhalant anesthetics, protection of the airway from foreign material, application of positive pressure ventilation, and suction of the airway. Although these are all important advantages, endotracheal intubation in cats has been reported to increase anesthetic risk,[27] and therefore extra care is needed during endotracheal intubation in this species.

Respiratory complications represent a major cause of perioperative anesthetic-related deaths.[25] Problems with airway maintenance and inadequacy of ventilation were the principal factors resulting in death. Endotracheal intubation problems and respiratory obstruction represented a major cause of death in cats in at least three studies.[27,39,53] In one of these studies, more cats that were intubated died postoperatively than those that were not (63% versus 48%), suggesting that laryngeal trauma, spasm, or edema may have been a more common contributory cause than endotracheal tube obstruction.[27]

Sensitivity of the larynx and its response to external stimuli vary from species to species. The cat's larynx is reported to be very reactive, and spastic closure is relatively common.[187] For these reasons topical local anesthetics such as lidocaine should always be applied to desensitize the larynx, with at least 60 seconds left from application until intubation.

More recently, tracheal rupture has been recognized as an important clinical entity associated with endotracheal intubation in cats.[145] In all reported cases, incidence was high after procedures in which inadvertent overinflation of the endotracheal tube cuff was likely, such as dental procedures, oral surgery for mass removal, or bronchoalveolar lavage.[85,145] Clinical signs associated with tracheal rupture included subcutaneous emphysema, coughing, gagging, dyspnea, anorexia, and fever. In all cats that were radiographed, subcutaneous emphysema and pneumomediastinum without pneumothorax were present (Figure 7-2).[85,145] Medical treatment alone is successful for cats with moderate dyspnea, whereas surgical treatment should be considered for cats with severe dyspnea (open-mouth breathing despite treatment with oxygen) or worsening subcutaneous emphysema. Ruptures that extent into the carina are associated with a poor prognosis.[85] Prevention of tracheal rupture is considered possible provided that care is taken in endotracheal tube selection and cuff inflation. The largest endotracheal tube that will easily pass through the larynx should be selected (adult cat 3.5- to 4.5-mm internal diameter). Once the tube is placed in the trachea, it should be attached to a non-rebreathing circuit. Positive pressure should be applied to the reservoir bag to a circuit pressure of 10 to 15 cm H_2O for not more than 2 seconds while the clinician listens for escape of audible amounts of air past the endotracheal tube cuff. If escaping air is heard, the cuff should be inflated with 0.5-mL increment of air, and positive pressure again applied to the reservoir bag. This should be repeated until escaping air is no longer audible. In a cat cadaver study, the amount of air required to obtain an airtight seal ranged from 0 to 3 mL (mean ± SD, 1.6 ± 0.7 mL; median, 1.5 mL).[85] It is also recommended that each time a cat is turned under anesthesia, the endotracheal tube be disconnected from the breathing circuit to prevent further tracheal trauma.

MAINTENANCE

Inhalant Anesthetics

Inhalant anesthetic agents are widely used for maintenance of anesthesia in cats. Some advantages include the predictable and rapid adjustment of anesthetic depth along with rapid recovery that is not dependent on metabolism or excretion of drugs by the liver or kidneys. Oxygen is administered along with inhalant anesthetics, and ventilation can be easily controlled if needed. Both these components decrease morbidity and mortality.

Only three inhalant anesthetics are currently available for use in cats: isoflurane, sevoflurane, and desflurane. Of those, only isoflurane and sevoflurane are currently used in veterinary practice. Although nitrous oxide is

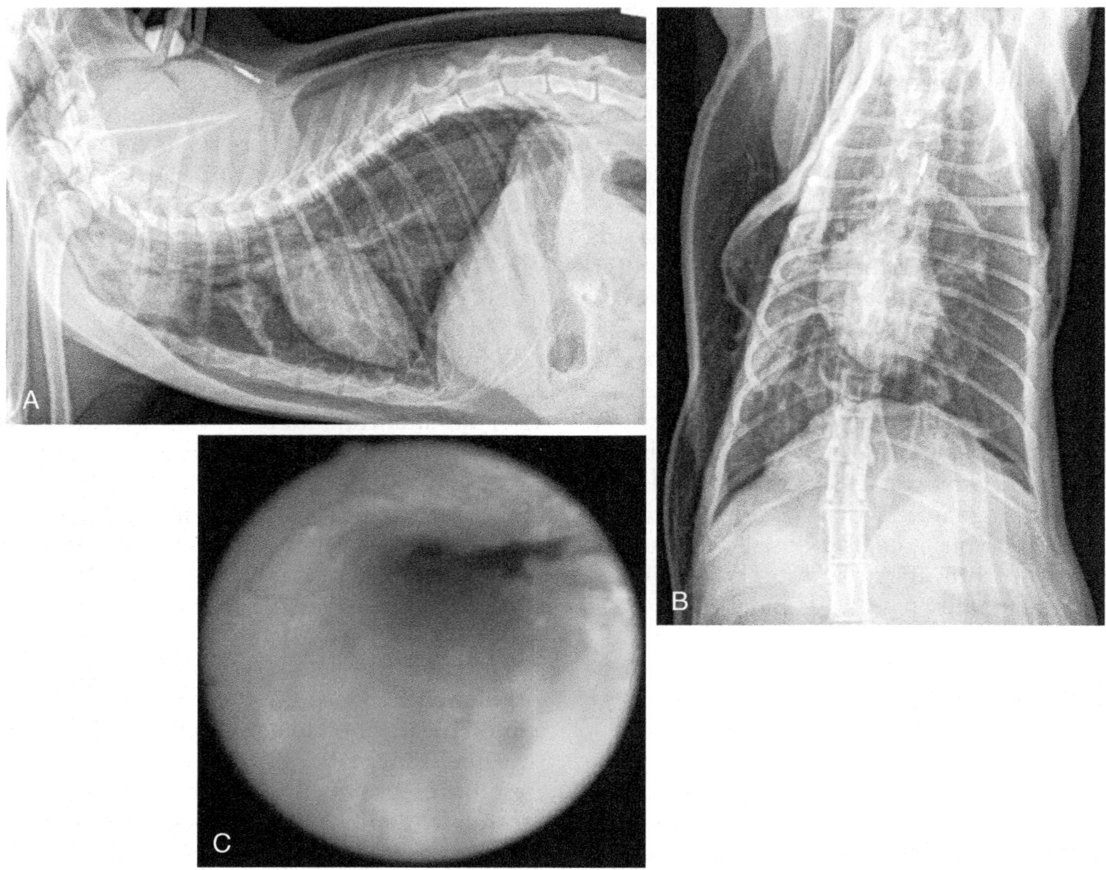

FIGURE 7-2 Lateral **(A)** and ventrodorsal **(B)** view of a cat with a tracheal tear showing subcutaneous emphysema and pneumomediastinum; **C,** bronchoscopic view of a tracheal tear.

still available, it does not induce unconsciousness alone in cats and therefore is used as part of a balanced anesthetic technique.

Isoflurane

Isoflurane is a fluorinated ether released for veterinary use in the late 1980s. It is stable in solution and does not require a preservative. It is easily vaporized (vapor pressure 250 mm Hg) and so is usually delivered through a precision, out-of-circuit vaporizer. It has low blood gas solubility (1.46), resulting in rapid induction and recovery, and undergoes minimal biotransformation (0.2%); thus the potential for toxic metabolites is reduced. It is a potent anesthetic, with a MAC (minimum anesthetic concentration required to prevent a response in 50% of the population) in the cat of 1.63%.[213] Cardiopulmonary studies at 1.3 MAC in cats reported minimal cardiopulmonary depression, especially if cats were allowed to breathe spontaneously.[101] At 2 MAC isoflurane caused hypotension and hypercapnia; however, cardiac index was maintained. When the hypercapnia was corrected by controlled ventilation, cardiac index decreased. In the cat respiratory rate tends to be maintained as dose is increased, whereas tidal volume decreases. The alveolar concentration that causes apnea is 2.4 MAC.[213] In another study mean arterial blood pressure fell from a conscious value of 95 ± 5 mm Hg to 60 ± 7 mm Hg at 1.5% inspired concentration and 40 ± 2 mm Hg at 2.5% inspired concentration.[175] Isoflurane does not sensitize the heart to catecholamines. It has a strong, pungent odor that many cats find aversive, which may lead to struggling or breath-holding during mask induction.

Sevoflurane

Sevoflurane is also a fluorinated ether released for veterinary use in the late 1990s. It is easily vaporized (vapor pressure 160 mm Hg) and so is usually delivered through a precision, out-of-circuit vaporizer. It has lower blood gas solubility (0.68) than isoflurane, resulting in rapid induction and recovery, and undergoes minimal biotransformation (2% to 5%); thus the potential for toxic metabolites is reduced. It is a potent anesthetic with a MAC in the cat of 2.58%. The cardiopulmonary effects of 1.25, 1.5, and 1.75 MAC of sevoflurane have been reported in cats.[178] Sevoflurane induced dose-dependent cardiovascular depression characterized by decreases in arterial blood pressure, cardiac index, and stroke index. Arterial blood pressure was better maintained than with isoflurane, thus limiting hypotension despite substantial myocardial depression. Sevoflurane also caused dose-dependent respiratory depression, although it appears less severe than reported in other species. Like isoflurane, sevoflurane does not sensitize the heart to catecholamines; however, it has a pleasant fruity odor, and thus mask inductions are better tolerated than with isoflurane. Compared with isoflurane, it is an expensive inhalant anesthetic.

TABLE 7-4 **Doses of Adjuvants Administered Intravenously as Part of a Balanced Anesthetic Technique**

Adjuvant Drug	Loading Dose	Infusion Dose
Fentanyl	2-5 μg/kg	0.4 μg/kg/min
Lidocaine	Not recommended	
Ketamine	0.5 mg/kg	10 μg/kg/min
Dexmedetomidine	0.5 μg/kg	0.5 μg/kg/h

Desflurane

Desflurane is also a fluorinated ether released only for human use. It is difficult to vaporize (vapor pressure 700 mm Hg) and requires a expensive precision, out-of-circuit vaporizer, which is heated to deliver accurate concentrations. This, together with its very rapid recovery, limits its use in veterinary anesthesia. It has the lowest blood gas solubility (0.42), resulting in very rapid induction and recovery, and because it undergoes minimal biotransformation (0.02%), the potential for toxic metabolites is much reduced. It is the least potent anesthetic, with an MAC in the cat of 9.79%. The cardiopulmonary effects of 1.3 and 1.7 MAC of desflurane have been reported in cats.[138] Desflurane at 1.7 MAC decreased mean arterial pressure and induced marked hypercapnia, although cardiac index was not affected. When the hypercapnia was corrected by controlled ventilation, cardiac index decreased. In the cat respiratory rate tends to be maintained as dose is increased, and tidal volume decreases. Like isoflurane and sevoflurane, desflurane does not sensitize the heart to catecholamines; however, it appears to be irritant to airways. Compared with isoflurane, it is an expensive inhalant anesthetic.

Balanced Anesthetic Techniques

Balanced anesthesia refers to the use of a combination of drugs, such that the advantages of small amounts of drugs are utilized without the need to contend with the disadvantages of large doses of any one drug. Often, specific drugs can be used for specific effects, such as analgesia. Although balanced anesthetic techniques are the usual maintenance technique in humans and sick dogs, their use in cats is rare, especially in veterinary practice. Doses that have been reported can be found in Table 7-4.

Balanced anesthetic techniques that have been investigated in cats include those discussed in the following sections.

Nitrous Oxide

Although nitrous oxide has been a component of more general anesthetic techniques than any other single inhalant[55] in human anesthesia, its use in veterinary anesthesia is controversial. Its widespread use resulted from many desirable properties, including low blood gas solubility, limited cardiovascular and respiratory depression, and minimal toxicity.[55] In veterinary anesthesia some report minimal advantages in supplementing more potent anesthetic agents,[212] whereas others agree that its analgesic properties enable excessive dosage of the more potent agents to be avoided and concurrent cardiopulmonary depression to be minimized.[83] More recently, the contribution of anesthetic-released nitrous oxide to global warming, the greenhouse effect, and ozone depletion has led some to call for its elimination from anesthetic practice.

In the cat 50% nitrous oxide has been reported to decrease halothane MAC by 19%, and 75% nitrous oxide decreased halothane MAC by 31%.[212] In a similar study undertaken with isoflurane, consistent MAC reduction properties of nitrous oxide in cats were not documented.[109] Instead, there were both responder and nonresponder groups to the anesthetic-sparing effect of nitrous oxide. A further study comparing the cardiovascular effects of equipotent doses of isoflurane alone versus isoflurane and 70% nitrous oxide in cats demonstrated improved arterial pressure owing to a vasoconstrictive effect.[182] In that study similar isoflurane concentrations were administered with and without nitrous oxide. Despite the lack of reported overall beneficial effects, our clinical impression is that addition of nitrous oxide to isoflurane will often stabilize mean arterial blood pressure within a normal range despite changes in surgical stimulation, especially in critically ill cats.

Because high concentrations of nitrous oxide are administered with oxygen and a potent inhalant, care must be taken to prevent the delivery of a hypoxemic mix. Because of an increase in the alveolar to arterial oxygen tension difference under anesthesia, an inspired oxygen concentration of at least 33% is recommended. With a non-rebreathing circuit, such as a Bain coaxial system, accurate measurement of the inspired oxygen concentration requires gas sampling within the endotracheal tube. Inexpensive monitoring devices can be used only to monitor the oxygen concentration at the fresh gas inflow. Generally, a total gas flow of 200 mL/kg/min is recommended for a Bain circuit, and this gas flow should be split such that oxygen is administered at a flow of 100 mL/kg/min and nitrous oxide at a flow of 100 mL/kg/min. When the nitrous oxide is discontinued, the oxygen flow must be increased to 200 mL/kg/min to avoid rebreathing of expired gases.

Precautions exist with the use of nitrous oxide. Because of the risk of hypoxemia, nitrous oxide should not be administered to patients with respiratory dysfunction unless the arterial oxygen tension can be measured. Potential problems associated with gas spaces can arise when an animal previously breathing air is given a gas mixture containing nitrous oxide. Given that nitrous oxide moves into the space more rapidly than nitrogen moves out, an increase in volume will occur in compliant spaces or an increase in pressure in noncompliant spaces. Thus nitrous oxide should not be administered to patients with pneumothorax or in situations when air embolus could occur (e.g., spinal surgery). At the end of anesthesia, the rapid outpouring of nitrous oxide from the blood into the lung results in a transient but marked decrease in alveolar oxygen tension with a resultant decrease in arterial oxygen tension. To prevent hypoxemia, 100% oxygen, rather than room air, should be administered to the patient during this period. Because nitrous oxide is not absorbed by activated charcoal canisters, active scavenging is necessary to prevent contamination of the environment.

Opioid Infusion

In human anesthesia administration of high doses of opioids, either as primary or sole anesthetics, has become popular because opioids produce or promote stable hemodynamics both in the presence and absence of noxious stimuli. In fact, opioids are said to be superior to most, if not all, other drugs in anesthesia in achieving this goal.[216] Similar beneficial effects have been documented in cats, in which administration during inhalant anesthesia has been shown to decrease the requirement for inhalant anesthesia and block autonomic responses to noxious stimuli, resulting in better hemodynamic stability.[104,163]

The most popular method to examine the anesthetic potential of opioids involves their ability to substitute for potent inhaled anesthetics. Variable results are reported, and it appears that the degree of inhalant MAC reduction induced by opioids is dependent on the dose administered, the specific receptor–opioid interaction, and the species to which the opioid is administered. Maximal inhalant MAC reduction is identified as the level where higher plasma opioid concentrations do not induce a statistically significant greater reduction in MAC. The beneficial effect of opioids on MAC reduction, or lack of, was studied initially in cats by screening a number of drugs at both high and low doses. The reason for this approach was that opioid administration, especially in high doses to cats, had been reported to induce mania, which could increase MAC through central transmitter release. Low and high doses of morphine, butorphanol, buprenorphine, and U50488H (kappa agonist) were found to induce significant MAC reductions of 12% and 28%, 18% and 19%, 11% and 14%, and 4% and 11%, respectively. However, only the MAC reductions induced by morphine (1 mg/kg) and butorphanol (0.08 and 0.8 mg/kg) were considered clinically important.[105] Further studies identified maximal MAC reduction for alfentanil in cats as 35%.[104] From these studies the veterinarian can conclude that when selecting a drug for a balanced opioid technique, a μ-agonist should be chosen. Beneficial cardiovascular effects were reported in cats when isoflurane alone was compared with an equipotent alfentanil–isoflurane MAC multiple.[163] In that study alfentanil was found to attenuate most of the hemodynamic and metabolic responses to a noxious stimulus. More recently, two studies have published the effect of remifentanil infusions on isoflurane MAC in cats.[30,58] In the first study, infusion doses of 0.25, 0.5, and 1.0 μg/kg/min induced significant MAC reduction (23%, 30%, 26%, respectively).[58] In the other, no significant decrease in MAC was reported.[30]

To accurately determine loading and constant-rate infusion doses for opioids in cats, pharmacokinetic data is necessary. The pharmacokinetic profiles of fentanyl,[121] alfentanil,[161] and the newer opioid remifentanil[177] have been reported in cats. Published pharmacokinetic data for fentanyl[121] predicts a loading dose of 2 μg/kg (calculated using the volume of the central compartment) with an infusion of 0.4 μg/kg/min. The authors currently administer a loading dose of 5 μg/kg followed by an infusion of 0.4 μg/kg/min. Anesthesia is induced with other agents and converted to a balanced anesthetic technique during maintenance of anesthesia. The infusion is discontinued about 30 minutes before the end of surgery. In cats, unlike in dogs, heart rate does not decrease and administration of an anticholinergic agent is not necessary. Although opioid infusion techniques induce less respiratory depression in cats than in dogs, ventilation is usually controlled. Cats maybe somewhat hypersensitive to touch and sound when awakening, but this is minimized by recovery in a quiet environment with minimal handling.

Epidural/Spinal Opioid

Opioids may be administered by injection into the epidural or subarachnoid (spinal) space to provide regional analgesia. Opioids such as morphine, oxymorphone and fentanyl selectively block pain conduction without interference to motor function. Although opioids are generally administered epidurally to provide postoperative analgesia,[184] their effects will be evident intraoperatively.

Epidural administration of morphine was found to reduce the inhalant anesthetic requirement in cats.[75] In that study epidural administration of 0.1 mg/kg morphine resulted in 31% isoflurane MAC reduction. More recently, a significant effect of epidural administration of morphine or buprenorphine on the MAC of isoflurane in cats could not be detected.[183]

Transdermal Opioid/Inhalant Anesthesia

Fentanyl administration using a transdermal patch provides postoperative analgesia. However, to be effective in the postoperative period, patches are placed before surgery. Thus plasma fentanyl levels within the analgesic range will also be present during surgery and add a balanced component to standard inhalant techniques.

Pharmacokinetic studies in cats have been reported with sustained plasma concentrations of fentanyl citrate throughout a 5-day period. However, variation of plasma drug concentrations with transdermal absorption for each cat was pronounced.[121]

The isoflurane MAC reduction after application of 25 and 50 μg/h patches to cats has been reported.[247] Both 25 and 50 μg/h patches reduced isoflurane MAC (17% and 18%, respectively), although the reduction was not different between the two doses.

Lidocaine

Lidocaine is an analgesic agent and in humans has been administered intravenously to provide postoperative analgesia.[137] When administered intraoperatively, the analgesia has been reported in humans to extend into the postoperative period, decreasing postoperative pain[47] and the amount of supplemental analgesia.[13] It also has been reported to reduce the requirement for both inhalant and injectable anesthetic agents.[100] Additionally, small dose of lidocaine administered intravenously are anticonvulsant and induce sedation.

In cats lidocaine was reported to decrease the isoflurane MAC in cats with target plasma concentrations of 1, 3, 5, 7, 9, and 11 μg/mL, linearly decreasing MAC by 3, 14, 24, 33, 40, and 52%, respectively.[181] Unfortunately, cardiovascular studies demonstrated that the decrease in inhalant requirements was associated with greater cardiovascular depression than an equipotent dose of isoflurane alone.[180] Oxygen delivery decreased, which could result in poor tissue perfusion. Therefore the administration of lidocaine as part of a balanced anesthetic technique in cats is not recommended.

Ketamine

Ketamine has been reported to decrease isoflurane MAC in cats by 45 ± 17%, 63 ± 18%, and 75 ± 17% at the infusion rates of 23, 46, and 115 μg/kg/min. These infusion rates corresponded to ketamine plasma concentrations of 1.75 ± 0.21, 2.69 ± 0.40, and 5.36 ± 1.19 μg/mL.[162] In-depth cardiovascular studies have not been reported in cats; however, in the MAC reduction study, both arterial blood pressure and heart rate increased significantly with ketamine infusion. Unfortunately, recovery was prolonged, and therefore further work is needed to better define infusion doses before this can be recommended in cats.

The effect of ketamine when combined with morphine and lidocaine (MLK) has been studied in dogs.[151] The MLK solution was prepared by mixing 10 mg (0.8 mL) of morphine sulfate, 150 mg (7.5 mL) of 2% lidocaine hydrochloride, and 30 mg (0.3 mL) of ketamine hydrochloride in the same syringe and injecting the final volume (8.6 mL) into a 500-mL bag of lactated Ringer's solution. The administration rate was set at 10 mL/kg/h, and isoflurane MAC reduction was compared with similar doses of morphine, ketamine, and lidocaine alone. Morphine, lidocaine, ketamine, and MLK significantly lowered isoflurane MAC by 48%, 29%, 25%, and 45%, respectively. The percentage reductions in isoflurane MAC for morphine and MLK were not significantly different but were significantly greater than for lidocaine and ketamine. This mixture has become a very common balanced anesthetic technique in veterinary practice, and its use has spread to cats, although some practitioners do not include lidocaine in the solution.

The effect of ketamine administration on intraoperative and postoperative analgesia has also been reported in dogs.[229] Ketamine was administered intravenously as a loading dose (0.5 mg/kg), 10 μg/kg/min as an infusion during surgery, and 2 μg/kg/min as an infusion postoperatively. Results suggested that perioperative administration of low doses of ketamine to dogs may augment analgesia and comfort in the postoperative surgical period. This technique has become common in veterinary practice, and its use has spread to cats.

Dexmedetomidine

Dexmedetomidine is an alpha$_2$-adrenergic agonist with sedative, analgesic, and anesthetic-sparing effects.[135] It also causes cardiovascular depression, characterized by bradycardia, decreased cardiac output, and increased systemic vascular resistance.[74,117,185] In dogs intravenous dexmedetomidine (0.5 μg/kg loading dose followed by 0.5 μg/kg/h) was reported to decrease isoflurane MAC by about 20% without producing significant cardiovascular depression.[160,166] Recently, the pharmacokinetics of dexmedetomidine in cats anesthetized with isoflurane has been studied (Escobar, Pypendop, and Ilkiw, unpublished data). Using pharmacokinetic data from that study, dexmedetomidine, at target plasma concentrations between 1.25 and 20 ng/mL, was found to decrease isoflurane MAC in a dose-dependent manner by approximately 25% to 80% (Escobar, Pypendop, and Ilkiw, unpublished data). In a follow-up study, researchers found that dexmedetomidine at target plasma concentrations of 2.5 ng/mL and higher produced significant cardiovascular depression (Pypendop, Barter, and Ilkiw, unpublished data). On the basis of these studies, it appears that intravenous dexmedetomidine administered to a target plasma concentration of 1.25 ng/mL (corresponding to a loading dose of 0.5 μg/kg followed by 0.5 μg/kg/h) produces about 25% reduction in isoflurane requirements without producing significant cardiovascular depression. However, hemodynamics were not improved compared with an equipotent (i.e., higher) concentration of isoflurane alone. The use of dexmedetomidine for balanced anesthesia in cats is therefore not supported by these data if the goal is to improve hemodynamics. It is nevertheless possible that dexmedetomidine would provide other benefits (e.g., analgesia, better hemodynamic stability).

Total Intravenous Anesthesia

Total intravenous anesthesia (TIVA) refers to induction and maintenance of anesthesia by intravenous agents only. The technique of TIVA anesthesia has gained popularity as a result of the introduction of injectable anesthetic agents that can be infused for long periods of time without resulting in excessively long recovery periods. Injectable anesthetic agents that result in unconsciousness and could be used for TIVA include thiopental, ketamine, propofol, and alphaxalone. Only propofol and alphaxalone offer acceptable recovery quality and times in cats. The drugs can be administered by intermittent bolus administration or as a constant-rate infusion, with constant-rate infusion offering many benefits, such as more stable anesthetic depth, lower total drug administration, and faster recoveries.

Propofol

Initial clinical studies in cats in which anesthesia was maintained by incremental doses of propofol reported a mean maintenance propofol requirement of 0.51 mg/kg/min (confidence limits 0.41 to 0.62 mg/kg/min). After a surgical duration of approximately 30 minutes, mean recovery time was 37.5 minutes (confidence limits 7 to 26 minutes).[24] This maintenance rate is much lower that the initial utilization ratio of 0.19 mg/kg/min[71] and may represent the difference between doses required for lateral recumbency versus surgery. Unfortunately, because of the cat's reduced capacity to conjugate propofol, recovery of anesthesia increases with duration of anesthesia.[164]

Although propofol provides hypnosis, immobility and muscle relaxation, it does not block autonomic responses to noxious stimuli in other species and must be administered at high infusion rates to induce a surgical plane of anesthesia.[140] Opioids have been administered with propofol in other species to provide better surgical conditions. Administration of fentanyl (0.1 μg/kg/min), sufentanil (0.01 μg/kg/min), or alfentanil (0.5 μg/kg/min) with propofol in cats was reported to result in satisfactory anesthesia with a reduction in infusion dose of propofol and no greater cardiovascular depression than that associated with infusion of propofol alone. Although the propofol infusion rates were not given in the text, the infusion rate to prevent movement in response to a noxious stimulus was approximately 0.25 mg/kg/min for propofol alone and between 0.1 and 0.15 mg/kg/min during opioid infusions.[140] Ketamine is another drug that can be administered in low doses to block autonomic responses to noxious stimulus. In cats the minimum infusion rate (MIR) required to stop movement in response to a tail clamp was 0.15 mg/kg/min for propofol alone and 0.11 mg/kg/min when either low-dose ketamine (loading dose, 2 mg/kg; constant-rate infusion, 23 μg/kg/min) or high-dose ketamine (loading dose, 4 mg/kg; constant-rate infusion, 46 μg/kg/min) were infused.[106] In this study a linear relationship, depending on the type of stimulus applied, was found between propofol doses and hemodynamic responses, such that as propofol dose increased, the magnitude of the hemodynamic response to stimulus decreased. Follow-up cardiovascular studies also supported that in the cat propofol alone provided stable hemodynamics irrespective of noxious stimuli and addition of ketamine was not beneficial.[103]

Ketamine

Two studies have reported infusion rates for ketamine anesthesia in cats. The first study measured electroencephalographic arousal and autonomic changes in response to tail clamping and reported that these were abolished when ketamine was administered intravenously at infusion rates between 10 and 22 mg/kg/h.[220] In the second study, the MIR in cats to prevent movement in response to tail clamp was reported as 0.41 mg/kg/min (range 0.32 to 0.52) for ketamine.[235]

Thiopental

The MIR in cats to prevent movement in response to tail clamp was reported as 0.37 mg/kg/min (range 0.29 to 0.42) for thiopental.[130]

Alphaxalone

The only reported study in cats compared recovery from incremental doses of Saffan and thiopental.[116] Cats topped up for 3 hours required 39 to 42 mg/kg of Saffan, which amounts to 0.22 to 0.23 mg/kg/min. Recovery from the last dose to normal behavior was 160 to 233 minutes. This contrasts to thiopental, wherein the total dose administered was 70 mg, amounting to 0.39 mg/kg/min and a recovery from last dose to normal of 45 to 47 hours.[116]

Anesthetic Options for Feral Cats

Feral cats are domesticated cats that have reverted to a wild state and for safety reasons should be regarded as wild animals. Attempts to reduce overpopulation by trapping and removal have been largely unsuccessful, insofar as the cats remaining in the colonies continue to breed, filling the void left by those that were removed. Feral cat neutering through trap–neuter–return (TNR; castration or spay) programs is a nonlethal method of feral cat population control. TNR programs are an increasingly popular alternative to removal, and veterinarians are frequently called on to participate in feral cat neutering either on an individual-cat basis or large-scale settings. The anesthetic protocol is an important component of these programs if they are to operative effectively.

An ideal anesthetic agent for feral cats would have a wide safety margin; provide rapid and predictable surgical anesthesia and postoperative analgesia; and be reversible, inexpensive, and simple to administer to trapped cats.[244] The most commonly reported anesthetic protocol consists of Telazol, ketamine, and xylazine (TKX). Each mL of TKX contains 100 mg of Telazol, 80 mg of ketamine, and 20 mg of xylazine. In a population of almost 7000 cats, the mean initial dose of TKX was 0.24 ± 0.04 mL/cat. The total mean dose of TKX was 0.27 ± 0.09 mL/cat. The drug was injected intramuscularly into either the lumbar or thigh muscles. After surgery yohimbine (0.5 mg) was administered intravenously to adult cats, and 0.3 mg was administered intravenously to kittens. Although total doses between males and females were not different, females received more injections than males. Cats were monitored by assessment of mucous membrane color and respiration and heart rate. Cats were not intubated, breathed room air, and were not supported by fluid administration. In this study the overall mortality was 0.35%, and the death rate attributable solely to potential anesthetic death was 0.23%.[244] In another study with almost 100 cats, a dose of 0.25 mL TKX was administered.[38] Lateral recumbency occurred in 4 ± 1 minutes, and anesthesia was adequate in 92% of cats to complete surgical procedure. Anesthesia was reversed with yohimbine (0.5 mg IV) at the completion of surgery. Time from anesthetic reversal to sternal recumbency was prolonged (72 ± 42 mins), although all cats recovered.

EQUIPMENT, MONITORING, AND FLUID THERAPY

Anesthesia equipment for use in cats is reviewed elsewhere.[123,157] Typically, Mapleson (non-rebreathing) systems are used in cats, and high fresh gas flows are therefore required. In North America the Bain coaxial system is most popular and offers good efficiency in carbon dioxide removal during both spontaneous and positive pressure ventilation (Figure 7-3). A minimum of 100 to 200 mL/kg/min of fresh gas flow is recommended with this system.[123] Higher fresh gas flow is more likely to actually prevent rebreathing of expired gas.

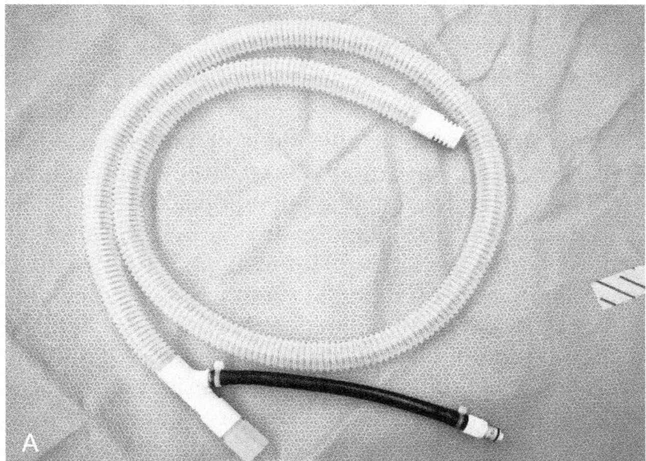

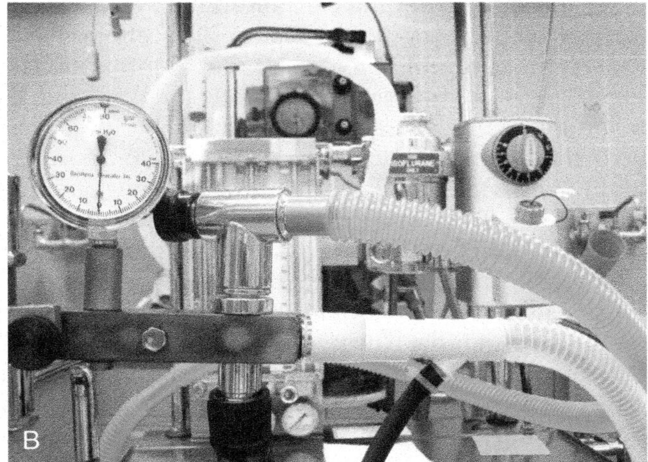

FIGURE 7-3 Bain circuit **(A)** and Bain circuit adaptor **(B)** with a low-pressure gauge; this setup helps detect increases in airway pressure if the exhaust system is obstructed for some reason and is also useful for mechanical ventilation.

The American College of Veterinary Anesthesiologists (ACVA) recently published Recommendations for Monitoring Anesthetized Patients (http://acva.org), and these should be used as a basis to determine the needs for personnel, equipment, and techniques.

Monitoring is directed at assessing vital functions and at detecting changes early so that treatment can be instituted as appropriate. The emphasis is on cardiovascular and respiratory functions. In addition, depth of anesthesia should be assessed so it is maintained at an appropriate level for the degree of stimulation, and body temperature should be measured and maintained as close as possible to normal.

The most critical role of the cardiovascular and respiratory systems is to deliver oxygen to tissues. Oxygen delivery depends on the amount of oxygen carried by arterial blood and cardiac output.[11,92] Because neither is routinely measured in anesthetized patients, indirect assessment based on observation of the patient and measurement of variables such as blood pressure and packed cell volume is necessary. Nevertheless, the anesthetist should always prioritize maintenance of oxygen delivery to tissues.

A trained, dedicated anesthetist should be available to monitor anesthesia continuously, particularly if the patient is not healthy. Depth of anesthesia requires direct observation of the patient and cannot be automated.[92] Because anesthetic drugs produce dose-dependent adverse effects, including cardiorespiratory depression, the lowest dose producing the desired effect should always be used. Monitoring of depth of anesthesia mainly relies on assessment of muscle tone and somatic or autonomic responses to stimulation.[92] The authors have found that the most useful signs for assessing depth of anesthesia are eye position, jaw tone, and palpebral reflex. The palpebral reflex is usually present only at light depth of anesthesia (some individual and drug variations). The eye rotates medioventrally in most individuals and with most anesthetic agents at surgical depth of anesthesia. The eye is central if anesthesia is light or too deep. Jaw tone gives a continuum in the assessment of CNS depression. At light depth of anesthesia, strong jaw tone can be felt; as anesthesia becomes deeper and deeper, jaw tone progressively decreases, to disappear at moderately deep surgical anesthesia. A notable exception is very young animals, which tend to lose jaw tone at light depth of anesthesia. If these signs cannot be used (e.g., surgery of the head), assessment is based on the autonomic response to noxious stimulation (i.e., increase in heart rate, blood pressure, and/or respiratory rate or ventilation), and movement or lack thereof. Clinicians should remember that inhalant anesthetics are not potent at blocking autonomic responses; therefore if anesthesia maintenance relies mainly on these drugs, some degree of response is expected. Lack of autonomic response to noxious stimulation in that situation would mean excessively deep anesthesia.

Pulse rate, respiratory rate, and body temperature should be measured at short intervals and recorded. Normal heart rate in cats ranges from 90 to 240 bpm[1]; because anesthesia causes myocardial depression, cardiac output becomes more rate-dependent than in conscious cats, and heart rate should be maintained within that range. Bradycardia is usually caused by excessive vagal tone or hypothermia.[92] Excessive vagal tone can be prevented or treated with anticholinergics (e.g., atropine 0.01 mg/kg intravenously or 0.02 mg/kg intramuscularly). External heat should be provided as necessary to prevent or treat hypothermia. Means of providing external heat should allow temperature to be controlled to prevent the risk of skin burns. Warm water–circulating blankets are commonly used, but these have limited efficacy because of the limited area available for heat exchange with the patient. Forced-air systems are more effective.[122] When these systems are used, caution should be exerted not to cause hyperthermia.

Blood pressure should be routinely measured. Noninvasive techniques are appropriate for most patients. If hemodynamic instability is expected or present, invasive monitoring of blood pressure is preferable. Noninvasive blood pressure measurement relies on the placement of an occluding cuff. Optimal width has been reported to be approximately 40% of the circumference of the appendage on which the cuff is placed.[77] Two techniques are commonly used: Doppler ultrasound and oscillometric. The Doppler ultrasound technique requires user intervention and can be used only to determine systolic blood pressure (Figure 7-4). It is usually considered to

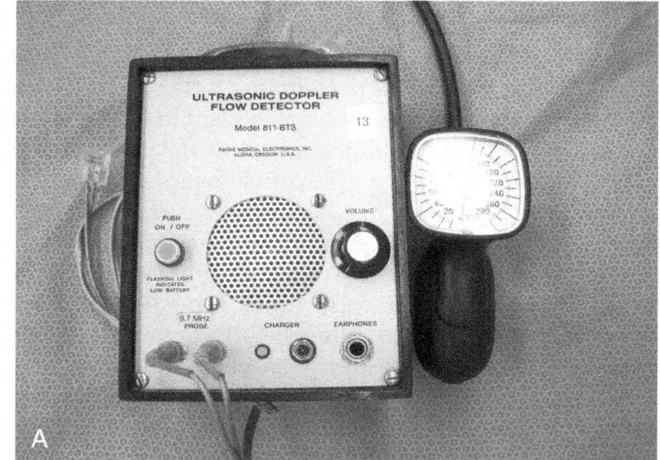

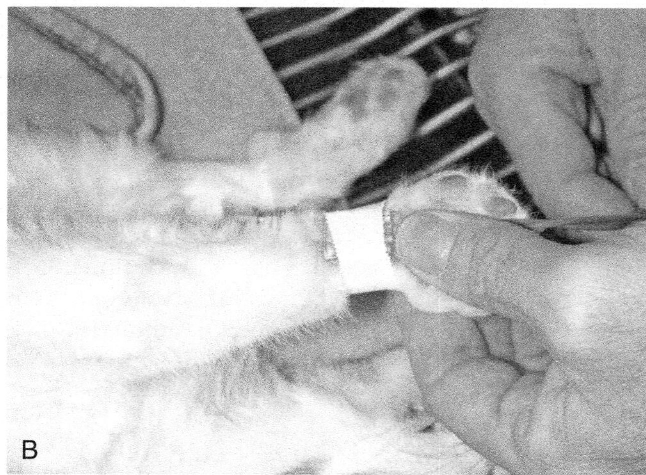

FIGURE 7-4 Doppler ultrasound units can be used only to determine systolic blood pressure but correlate well with invasive measurements. **A,** Parks Medical Ultrasonic Doppler Flow Detector. **B,** Parks Medical infant flat probe in place for blood pressure monitoring during anesthesia.

correlate well with invasive measurements but to underestimate invasive systolic blood pressure.[33,77] The Doppler ultrasound technique also provides an audible signal corresponding to blood flow, which can be used to count pulse rate and detect arrhythmias. The oscillometric technique allows automated measurement of systolic, diastolic, and mean arterial pressures. The accuracy appears to be highly dependent on the device.[19,23,33,168] Mean arterial pressure is expected to be the most accurate measurement with this technique. Most devices also measure pulse rate. Oscillometric measurements tend to be inaccurate in cases of movement, arrhythmias, or vasoconstriction. Systolic and mean arterial pressures should be maintained between 100 and 140, and 80 and 100 mm Hg, respectively.[92] Hypertension is uncommon and usually due to inadequate anesthesia or analgesia. Other causes include excessive treatment of hypotension, drugs causing vasoconstriction (e.g., alpha$_2$ agonists), and some diseases (e.g., hyperthyroidism, chronic renal failure). The treatment of hypertension is directed to the underlying cause. Hypotension is common, even in lightly anesthetized cats, particularly when there is no noxious stimulation. Treatment includes decreasing anesthetic depth if possible, administration of a fluid bolus (5 to 10 mL/kg, which can be repeated if some improvement is seen), and positive inotropes (dopamine or dobutamine, titrated to effect, starting at 5 μg/kg/min). Vasoconstrictors are preferred to positive inotropes in some disease states (e.g., hypertrophic cardiomyopathy, see relevant section later in this chapter).

Capnography and pulse oximetry may be useful additions to basic monitoring. Capnographs can either sample gas (side-stream) or measure carbon dioxide directly in the respiratory gases flowing to and from the patient, using an adapter connected between the patient and the circuit (mainstream, Figure 7-5). Measurement of end-tidal carbon dioxide partial pressure often yields lower than actual values in cats, particularly if the side-stream method is used, because of small tidal volume, and mixing of inspired and expired gas, in part related to the use of high fresh gas flows. End-tidal carbon dioxide partial pressure closely approximates alveolar carbon dioxide partial pressure,[63] which is usually 0 to 5 mm Hg lower than arterial carbon dioxide partial pressure. Capnography therefore allows noninvasive, continuous assessment of $PaCO_2$. End-tidal PCO_2 should ideally be maintained between 35 and 45 mm Hg. Higher values indicate hypoventilation. If inhalant anesthetics are used, hypoventilation is often related to excessive depth of anesthesia or the use of other drugs causing respiratory depression (or both). The main deleterious effect of high PCO_2 is its effect on pH (i.e., respiratory acidosis). Moderate to severe anesthesia-induced respiratory acidosis (pH < 7.2) is usually treated by mechanical ventilation. However, mechanical ventilation may cause or worsen cardiovascular depression and should be used with caution, particularly if the patient is deeply anesthetized or hypovolemic.[65,101]

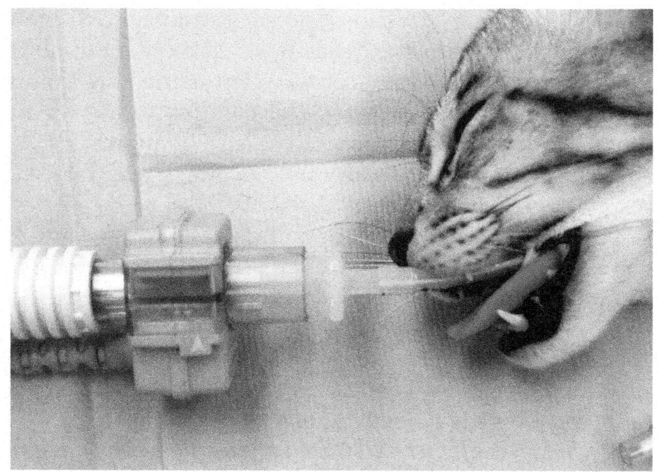

FIGURE 7-5 A mainstream capnograph sensor uses an adapter connected between the patient and the circuit to measure carbon dioxide.

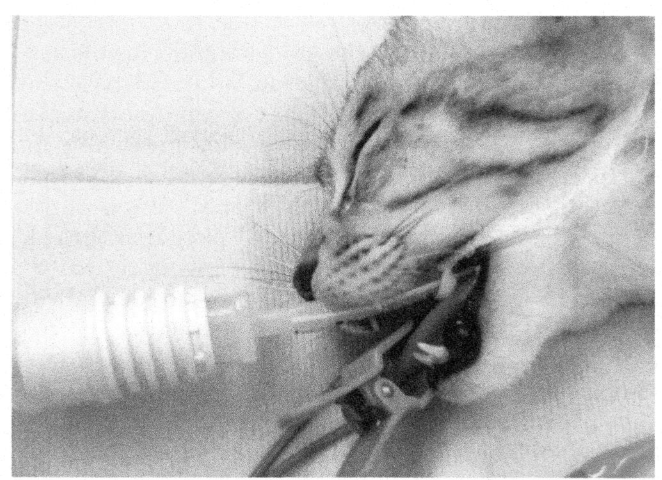

FIGURE 7-6 Pulse oximetry is a noninvasive, continuous assessment of oxygenation that performs variably in cats.

Pulse oximetry measures the fraction of hemoglobin saturated with oxygen in arterial blood. It is a noninvasive, continuous assessment of oxygenation (Figure 7-6). Pulse oximeters perform variably in cats.[134] It is not unusual to obtain erroneously low readings. The value of pulse oximetry is somewhat limited in patients receiving a high inspired oxygen fraction. This is due to the shape of the oxyhemoglobin dissociation curve. In normal cats breathing close to 100% oxygen, PaO_2 is expected to be 500 mm Hg or more. Hemoglobin oxygen saturation will be 99% to 100% when PaO_2 is higher than 120 mm Hg. Therefore, in patients receiving a high inspired oxygen fraction, pulse oximetry will detect only extremely severe deficiencies in oxygenation. This should be taken into account when using this monitor in these conditions. Conversely, a 95% saturation, which corresponds approximately to a PaO_2 of 80 mm Hg, in a patient breathing close to 100% oxygen, if accurate, indicates a serious problem.

Central venous pressure is the pressure measured in the thoracic vena cava. It results from the interaction of blood volume and capacity.[92] It is a measure of the relative ability of the heart to pump preload and may be helpful to guide fluid therapy, particularly when large fluid volumes are administered. Central venous pressure requires the placement of a catheter, the tip of which lies in the thoracic vena cava. The catheter is usually inserted through the jugular vein. The catheter can be connected to a water manometer or to an electronic transducer and monitor. Normal central venous pressure is 0 to 10 cm H_2O (0 to 7 mm Hg) and should be measured at the end of expiration.[92] Low values may indicate hypovolemia. High values may indicate excessive circulating volume.

Blood gas analysis is the gold standard for the assessment of oxygenation, ventilation, and acid–base status. Although it requires equipment not commonly available in veterinary practice, it may provide invaluable information in selected cases. Assessment of oxygenation requires the analysis of arterial blood. PaO_2 is normally approximately 5 times the inspired oxygen fraction in % (i.e., approximately 100 mm Hg if breathing room air; 500 mm Hg when breathing 100% oxygen). Lower values may be due to hypoventilation, ventilation–perfusion mismatching, anatomic right-to-left shunting, or impairment of the diffusion of oxygen through the alveolar–capillary membrane. Among these causes, hypoventilation and ventilation–perfusion mismatching are the most common in anesthetized patients. It should be noted that as long as PaO_2 is higher than 80 to 100 mm Hg, hemoglobin is almost fully saturated, and arterial oxygen content will be adequate if hemoglobin concentration is normal, even if PaO_2 is much lower than normal (e.g., if the patient is breathing 100% oxygen). Nevertheless, inadequate oxygen content may arise in these cases when inspired oxygen fraction is decreased (e.g., when recovering from anesthesia and breathing room air). Lower than expected PaO_2 should be treated by addressing the underlying cause or by increasing inspired oxygen fraction. Hypoventilation is managed by decreasing anesthetic depth or by using mechanical ventilation (as previously discussed). Ventilation–perfusion mismatching is treated by increasing inspired oxygen fraction (if possible), mechanical ventilation, and sometimes positive end-expiratory pressure. Alveolar recruitment maneuvers have also been described in humans and may restore better oxygenation.[119] Assessment of ventilation relies on the measurement of PCO_2. Although arterial PCO_2 is the gold standard, venous PCO_2 is an acceptable alternative, because it is only 3 to 6 mm Hg higher than $PaCO_2$ in most states. Normal $PaCO_2$ in cats has been reported to be approximately 33 mm Hg.[99] Anesthesia depresses ventilation, and normal $PaCO_2$ is commonly considered to range from 35 to 45 mm Hg in anesthetized patients.

For details on management of fluid therapy, the reader is referred to Chapter 5. Fluid therapy during anesthesia usually relies on the administration of isotonic crystalloids, colloids, or a combination of both. Fluids should be given intravenously or, if this is not possible, intraosseously. Preoperative dehydration or hypovolemia should be corrected before anesthetizing the patient (see Chapter 5). Intraoperative fluid therapy is directed at maintaining effective circulating volume and replacement solutions (i.e., solutions with electrolyte concentrations close to plasma concentrations), or solutions remaining in the vascular space are therefore used. If crystalloids are selected, lactated Ringer's solution or similar preparations or isotonic saline are most commonly used. The rate of administration is often set at 5 to 10 mL/kg/h.[197] The number is arbitrary and usually in excess of actual fluid losses because of metabolism, renal excretion, evaporation in the respiratory tract, and evaporation through open body cavities. However, using that rate rarely causes significant adverse effects in cats with normal cardiac function, and expanding vascular volume may partly compensate for anesthetic-induced vasodilation and surgical blood loss. In cats with abnormal cardiac function or structure, crystalloid administration rate is generally reduced to 3 to 5 mL/kg/h. Acute blood loss can be replaced by administering approximately a volume of crystalloid approximately 3 times that of blood lost. Blood loss of more than 20% of blood volume or hemorrhage in an anemic patient is best addressed by administration of whole blood or packed red blood cells. Colloids remain in the vascular volume longer than crystalloids and usually expand plasma volume in excess of the volume administered. Artificial colloids include dextrans and hetastarch. They increase colloid osmotic pressure and may increase blood pressure more reliably than crystalloids. However, they inhibit coagulation in a dose-dependent manner, may cause allergic reactions (dextrans), and may cause renal injury.[46] Natural colloids include whole blood, packed red cells, and plasma. Fresh whole blood contains erythrocytes, platelets, and all clotting factors and is the fluid of choice when these components are all needed. Packed red cells only contain erythrocytes. Fresh frozen plasma contains all clotting factors and is a source of albumin. Blood and blood products can cause transfusion reactions. Colloids are usually administered as a bolus (3 to 5 mL/kg) for the correction of hypotension or as an infusion (2 to 5 mL/kg/h) in place of or in combination with crystalloids.

ANESTHETIC CONSIDERATIONS FOR SPECIAL CONDITIONS

Neonatal Patients

There is little information regarding anesthetic considerations for neonatal and geriatric feline patients. Most information regarding the management of these patients is extrapolated from experience with adult animals and information obtained in dogs and humans. Cats are considered neonates from birth to weaning, which is approximately the first 4 weeks of life.[81] During that time many organ systems undergo important changes, which will influence anesthetic management (Box 7-13).

Physiologic Changes

The cardiovascular system is dramatically altered at birth, when the fetomaternal circulation is replaced by the neonatal circulation. Additional changes occur as the neonate ages. The neonatal circulation is characterized by low pressure, low volume, and low resistance.[4] This results in a high heart rate and low blood pressure. Heart rate progressively decreases, and blood pressure increases to reach values close to those observed in adults around 4 weeks of age.[4] Sympathetic innervation of the heart is incomplete at birth, while parasympathetic innervation is anatomically mature.[127] However, anticholinergic administration may have minimal effect on heart rate during the first few days of life, suggesting that the parasympathetic system is not functional yet. In very young animals hypoxemia results in bradycardia and hypotension, a response opposite to that seen in the adult animal. This response appears to be lost at 5 days of age.[60]

Neonates have high oxygen requirements, but their carotid body chemoreceptors are immature at birth. This may increase the risk for hypoxemia. In anesthetized kittens the ventilatory response to hypoxia appears biphasic, with an initial increase in respiratory rate and tidal volume, followed within 5 minutes by a decrease in respiratory rate below baseline, whereas tidal volume decreases but remains larger than baseline values.[21]

The hematocrit level is comparable to adult values at birth, decreases during the first 4 weeks, then increases to reach adult values around 10 weeks.[141] P450 enzyme activity is low at birth and increases over the first few months of life.[219] Maintenance of normal body temperature largely depends on ambient temperature; because of their high surface-to-volume ratio, neonates are particularly susceptible to hypothermia.[45]

BOX 7-13

Key Points of Neonatal Anesthesia

- Cardiac output is highly dependent on heart rate.
- Sympathetic responses may be immature.
- Blockade of parasympathetic responses is important.
- Blood pressure is lower than in adult patients.
- Preanesthetic fasting should be limited.
- Induction of anesthesia is preferably achieved by using propofol or an inhaled anesthetic.
- Fluids may need to be supplemented with dextrose.
- External heat should be provided from the start of anesthesia.

Anesthetic Management

Overall, neonatal and pediatric patients have limited physiologic reserves and are less able to compensate for homeostatic disturbances. Hydration status should be carefully assessed, and any fluid deficit should be corrected before anesthesia. Minimum preanesthetic blood work should include packed cell volume, total proteins, and blood glucose measurements. Additional laboratory work should be performed as indicated by the patient's condition. Preanesthetic fasting should be limited to between 2 and 4 hours in pediatric patients eating solid food. No fasting is indicated in neonatal patients still on a milk diet.

Anesthetic premedication should include an anticholinergic because cardiovascular function is highly dependent on heart rate and the parasympathetic nervous system appears to reach maturity before the sympathetic nervous system.[127] An opioid can be added for painful procedures. Tranquilizers and sedatives are best avoided because of their prolonged duration of action in these patients and because of the potential for adverse effects. If sedation with an opioid is inadequate, a combination with midazolam can be used, but it may have prolonged effects in neonates compared with adult patients.

Induction of anesthesia is preferably achieved with propofol, insofar as this agent does not rely solely on liver metabolism for its elimination. Nevertheless, duration of action is expected to be longer than in adults.[7] Alternatively, mask induction with an inhaled anesthetic can be used. Dissociative agents should be avoided because of evidence in rodents that they cause neurodegeneration in the developing brain.[139] Propofol and inhaled anesthetics produce dose-dependent cardiovascular and respiratory depression and should be carefully titrated to effect.

Maintenance of anesthesia is typically achieved using an inhaled anesthetic. Concurrent administration of analgesics should be performed if indicated. Fluid therapy with a balanced electrolyte solution is administered. Dextrose is added if hypoglycemia is present or if glycemia cannot be measured. Minimum monitoring should include heart rate, respiratory rate, depth of anesthesia, blood pressure, and body temperature. Hypothermia should be prevented or treated aggressively because neonates are highly susceptible to large decreases in body temperature.

Normal heart rate is approximately 200 beats per minute in neonatal cats, and bradycardia should be treated with diligence in neonates because cardiac output is highly rate dependent. Normal blood pressure is lower in neonates than adults and increases over the few first weeks of life; appropriate reference ranges should be used.[4] In canine neonates systolic blood pressure is 61 +/−5 mm Hg at birth, increasing to 139 +/−4 mm Hg at 4 weeks of age. Similar values have not been published for neonatal kittens.

Geriatric Patients

The definition of *geriatric* in the context of small animal patients has been debated; it is commonly accepted that an animal that has reached 66% to 75% of its life expectancy is geriatric.[32] Aging is a physiologic process characterized by decreasing organ reserve and functional capacity, increasing imbalance of homeostatic mechanisms, and increasing incidence of diseases.[236] However, there is a large variability in health status among geriatric patients. A high index of suspicion for diseases or conditions common in old age should be maintained, and appropriate tests should be performed to confirm or rule out these conditions (Box 7-14).

Physiologic Changes

Major organ systems in elderly animals have decreased functional reserve, which may alter the response to anesthetic drugs. Of particular interest to the anesthetist, the cardiovascular, respiratory, hepatic, renal, and central nervous systems are all affected. Drug dose requirements are usually decreased, and duration of effect is usually increased.[203] Careful consideration as to whether a drug is a necessary part of anesthetic management and cautious titration to effect should therefore be exerted.

Geriatric animals compensate less for cardiovascular changes produced by sedative and anesthetic drugs than younger patients, resulting in greater depression of normal hemodynamics.[203] Autonomic control is altered, with decreased response to beta-adrenoceptor stimulation and increased sympathetic nervous system activity.[190] Cardiac myocyte number decreases, leading to decreased contractility, decreased ventricular compliance, and increased ventricular filling pressures.[176] Clinically, these changes translate to a higher incidence and severity of hypotension in the anesthetized geriatric patient. The chronotropic response to hypotension is decreased. Geriatric animals are expected to be particularly sensitive to perioperative hypovolemia; however, because of the decreased ventricular compliance, they are also expected to be more sensitive to fluid overload than younger patients.

Drug-induced respiratory depression is increased in geriatric patients.[250] Aging causes structural changes in the lung. Loss of elastic recoil is due to collagen and elastin reorganization.[210] Compliance is increased. Small airway collapse may occur during expiration. Closing capacity increases in relation to functional residual capacity, leading to increased ventilation–perfusion mismatching. Ventilatory responses to hypoxia and hypercapnia are impaired.[250] Overall, these changes increase the risk for hypoxemia in the geriatric patient.

Liver mass and liver blood flow decrease with age.[195] This is accompanied by a decrease in the liver's intrinsic capacity to metabolize drugs. Clearance of drugs with both high and low extraction ratios is affected. Drug dose requirements, particularly for maintenance, are decreased.

Renal mass decreases with age, predominantly in the cortex.[56,131,205] This is related to a decrease in the number of glomeruli. Renal blood flow also decreases. Renal capacity to conserve sodium decreases with age, as is the ability to excrete concentrated urine. Overall, this makes the geriatric patient less tolerant of fluid deficits. In addition, the incidence of renal disease increases with age, and many geriatric cats have some degree of chronic renal disease.

Cerebral mass decreases with aging.[67,68] The risk for perioperative delirium and cognitive dysfunction is increased in geriatric humans. There may be altered balance between inhibitory and excitatory neurotransmission.[20] Brain dopamine concentration decreases with increasing age.[170] Serotonin and brain-derived neurotrophic factor levels also fall.[170] There may be calcium dysregulation, mitochondrial dysfunction, and production of reactive oxygen species. The density of NMDA receptors is decreased, and there are age-related changes in the interaction between glutamate and other neurotransmitters, such as GABA and dopamine.[198]

Anesthetic Management

Similar to neonatal patients, geriatric animals have limited functional organ reserve and have limited compensatory responses to homeostatic disturbances. A

BOX 7-14

Key Points of Geriatric Anesthesia

- Functional organ reserve is decreased.
- Geriatric patients tend to be more sensitive to the cardiovascular and respiratory depressant effects of anesthetic drugs.
- Careful titration of the lowest possible dose of anesthetic agent is important.
- Acepromazine and alpha$_2$ agonists should be avoided whenever possible.
- Balanced anesthetic techniques should be considered.

thorough physical examination, with an emphasis on hydration status and the cardiovascular and respiratory systems, should be performed. Complete blood count, biochemistry profile, urinalysis and total T_4 are usually recommended.

Anesthetic premedication usually includes an opioid and an anticholinergic, unless contraindicated. If additional sedation is desirable, a benzodiazepine can be added. Acepromazine appears to produce more severe hypotension in geriatric than in younger animals and is therefore preferably avoided. Similarly, $alpha_2$ agonists are better avoided due to their effects on the cardiovascular system and organ blood flow. Dissociative anesthetics may have prolonged effects in geriatric animals because of decreased renal elimination.

Preferred agents for induction of anesthesia include propofol and etomidate. Propofol produces significant cardiovascular and respiratory depression and should be carefully titrated to effect. The quality of induction with etomidate is not great, but this agent produces minimal cardiovascular depression. Etomidate should be combined with a benzodiazepine; a benzodiazepine can also be used with propofol to decrease the dose required for induction of anesthesia.

Maintenance of anesthesia usually relies on the administration of an inhaled anesthetic, such as isoflurane or sevoflurane. Balanced anesthetic techniques may be beneficial in geriatric patients that tolerate the cardiovascular depressant effects of inhalant anesthetics poorly.

Meticulous physiologic monitoring and support is particularly important in geriatric patients to ensure that their limited ability to compensate for changes is not overwhelmed. Minimum monitoring consists of assessments of depth of anesthesia, body temperature, noninvasive blood pressure, pulse rate, and respiratory rate. Additional monitoring tailored to the patient's condition should be used when indicated. External heat should be provided to prevent or limit hypothermia. Fluid therapy, aimed at maintaining extracellular fluid volume and electrolyte balance, should be administered.

Hyperthyroidism

Hyperthyroidism is the most common endocrine disorder in cats.[173] It is a multisystemic disorder resulting from excessive levels of the thyroid hormones T_4 and T_3. Hyperthyroid cats have increased metabolism, energy requirement, and heat production, resulting in increased appetite, weight loss, muscle wasting, weakness, heat intolerance and slightly elevated body temperature. Thyroid hormones also interact with the central nervous system; in particular, sympathetic nervous system tone is increased, which results in hyperexcitability or nervousness, behavioral changes, tremors, and tachycardia (Box 7-15).

BOX 7-15

Key Points of Anesthesia of the Hyperthyroid Patient

- Good sedation is necessary for handling the animal safely and avoiding sympathetic stimulation.
- If possible, antithyroid medication should be administered for 2 to 3 weeks minimum before anesthesia.
- If the procedure is emergent or urgent, beta-adrenergic blockers should be administered, ideally for 48 hours before anesthesia.
- Arrhythmogenic drugs and drugs causing sympathetic stimulation should be avoided.
- Premedication with an opioid combined with acepromazine or an $alpha_2$ agonist is indicated.
- Induction of anesthesia with propofol or etomidate is preferred.
- Balanced anesthetic techniques should be considered to blunt autonomic responses to noxious stimulation.
- Caution should be exerted in the treatment of hypotension with catecholamines.

Hyperthyroid cats most often require anesthesia for elective surgical management of hyperthyroidism, but occasionally they require anesthetic management as an emergency for problems unrelated to hyperthyroidism. The pathophysiology of hyperthyroidism is reviewed in Chapter 24; only the aspects directly relevant to anesthesia will be addressed here.

Clinical Signs and Laboratory Findings

Hyperthyroidism causes dysfunction of many organ systems. Of particular concern for anesthesia are the effects on cardiovascular, respiratory, gastrointestinal, and hepatic systems. Handling of hyperthyroid cats may be difficult because of the restlessness associated with the disease. Moreover, hyperthyroid cats may become aggressive when restrained. Good sedation is warranted to avoid excessive sympathetic stimulation. Respiratory distress, weakness, and development of cardiac dysrhythmias may occur when these cats are placed in stressful situations. Weight loss may affect the pharmacokinetics of some anesthetic agents (e.g., by changing the volume of distribution) and will worsen anesthesia-induced hypothermia. When present, muscle weakness may predispose to hypoventilation under anesthesia, which may predispose to dysrhythmias under anesthesia.

The cardiovascular system is affected by hyperthyroidism in important ways.[217] Heart rate is increased. The sympathoadrenal system appears hyperresponsive. Systemic vascular resistance is decreased, but systolic arterial pressure increases, resulting in systemic hypertension. Cardiac output is increased, as is plasma volume.

Systolic murmurs and gallop rhythms are frequent. Tachypnea is sometimes present but is not necessarily associated with congestive heart failure. Over time, most cats with hyperthyroidism will develop a cardiomyopathy with hypertrophy of the left ventricular free wall and ventricular septum. Dynamic left or right (or both) ventricular outflow tract obstruction is common. These cats are predisposed to cardiac arrhythmias.

Renal blood flow, glomerular filtration rate, and sodium excretion are increased in experimental and naturally occurring hyperthyroidism, possibly as a result of the activation of the renin–angiotensin–aldosterone system.[146,217] Sodium reabsorption also appears increased, so that blood sodium concentration is usually normal. Polyuria and polydipsia may be prominent signs, and experimental studies in thyrotoxic rats reveal impaired concentrating ability because of the downregulation of aquaporins.[222,230]

Dyspnea, panting, and hyperventilation have been reported in some cats with hyperthyroidism, often associated with stressful situations.[222] Respiratory muscle weakness has been reported in hyperthyroid humans.[202] Pulmonary hypertension may be present.[204] Respiratory depression induced by anesthetic drugs is common under general anesthesia, and control of ventilation in hyperthyroid cats is advisable. Dyspnea in cats with congestive heart failure may be caused by pulmonary edema or pleural effusion. If pleural effusion is extensive, thoracocentesis is advisable before induction of anesthesia.

Hematocrit levels may be increased, or hematologic changes may be minimal.[172,222] The most common serum biochemical abnormalities include elevated serum urea, alkaline phosphatase, lactate dehydrogenase, aspartate aminotransaminase, and alanine aminotransaminase.[172,222] Avoidance of hypoxemia and maintenance of liver blood flow are important anesthetic considerations.

Anesthetic Management

Thyrotoxic cats are often considered poor anesthetic candidates because they tend to be elderly, cachectic animals with organ system dysfunction. Preparation before anesthesia is important in the hyperthyroid cat to prevent serious complications, such as ventricular dysrhythmias and acute death. Cats not rendered euthyroid before anesthesia appear to be at high risk of perioperative mortality, and untreated cats should therefore be anesthetized only for emergency procedures.[171] Elective procedures should be postponed for 2 to 3 weeks and cats started on antithyroid medication. T_4 levels should be rechecked before anesthesia.

Because hyperthyroidism affects multiple organ systems and cardiovascular, respiratory, renal and liver functions may all be compromised, it is important that the laboratory data and other diagnostic tests accurately define the involvement of these body systems. A complete blood count and serum chemistry profile, an electrocardiogram and serum thyroid hormones are essential in all cases. Cats with cardiac abnormalities on auscultation or electrocardiography should have further cardiac workup, including thoracic radiography and echocardiography. Treatment should be instituted as appropriate.

If anesthesia is required without time to render the patient euthyroid and the cat does not have heart failure with poor contractility, the peripheral manifestations of hyperthyroidism can be dramatically improved within a few days of initiation of therapy with propranolol. The chronotropic and inotropic manifestations of excess hormone secretion are decreased, left ventricular efficiency is enhanced, and the risk of arrhythmias is reduced.

If the cat has been rendered euthyroid, the risk of anesthesia is likely similar to a normal patient, and many drugs can be tolerated if cardiac involvement is minimal. Good sedation is desirable to avoid sympathetic nervous system stimulation. In addition arrhythmogenic drugs should be avoided, and the electrocardiogram should be monitored.

In humans it has been reported that no drug has proved better than any other when outcome is examined.[189] It is therefore likely that preoperative stabilization is more critical than anesthetic drug selection.

An opioid is usually used for premedication. A low dose of acepromazine may be added for improved sedation. Medetomidine or dexmedetomidine may be useful to produce sedation and decrease sympathetic tone. Atropine is generally omitted because it may induce sinus tachycardia and enhance anesthetic-induced dysrhythmias. The authors generally administer glycopyrrolate because it has minimal effects on cardiac rate and rhythm.

Intravenous induction is preferred to mask or chamber induction. In cats without heart failure, a thiobarbiturate may be suitable because it provides a smooth induction without catecholamine release. Diazepam can be administered in combination with thiobarbiturates to decrease the dose of thiobarbiturate and slightly prolong the duration of action. Another possible benefit of thiopental is its antithyroid action.[231] However, thiopental is the most arrhythmogenic induction agent currently used in clinical patients. Propofol or etomidate are good alternatives. In particular, in cats with heart failure or dysrhythmias, etomidate combined with a benzodiazepine is expected to have minimal effects on cardiovascular and respiratory function. The dissociative agents ketamine and tiletamine are usually avoided because of the sympathetic stimulation they produce.

Anesthesia is typically maintained with inhalant anesthetics. The larynx should be sprayed with lidocaine to aid intubation and attenuate catecholamine release.

The goals during maintenance of anesthesia are to avoid administration of drugs that sensitize the heart to catecholamines and to provide a level of anesthesia or use a technique that prevents exaggerated responses to noxious stimulation. Isoflurane or sevoflurane are good choices. Because cats under inhalants alone respond to surgical stimulation with increases in heart rate and arterial blood pressure, nitrous oxide can be added to blunt these responses.

Hyperthyroid cats should be closely monitored during anesthesia, with particular emphasis on the cardiovascular system. Before induction, electrocardiogram limb leads and a Doppler crystal and occluding cuff are placed, without causing stress if possible. Hypoxemia should be prevented by oxygenation using a face mask during induction. Additional monitoring can be placed after induction of anesthesia, such as temperature probe, capnograph, and pulse oximeter. If heart failure is present, direct measurement of arterial blood pressure is useful to determine the need for more aggressive management and the response to treatment. In addition, an arterial catheter allows arterial blood to be sampled for blood gas analysis. This enables early recognition and treatment of hypoxemia and hypercarbia, two situations likely to increase the incidence of arrhythmias in hyperthyroid patients.

A balanced electrolyte replacement solution should be administered. The rate of fluid administration will depend on the cardiovascular status of the patient (conservative, 3 to 5 mL/kg/h, if heart failure is present) and the need of the patient (10 to 20 mL/kg bolus if significant blood loss occurs).

Catecholamines for the treatment of hypotension should be used with caution. Hyperthyroid patients may have exaggerated responsiveness to catecholamines, and reduced doses of direct-acting vasopressors such as phenylephrine may be a more logical selection than drugs such as ephedrine, which acts in part by provoking release of catecholamines. Arrhythmias are usually treated by administration of beta-adrenergic blocking agents, such as propranolol or esmolol.

Urethral Obstruction

Disease of the lower urinary tract is common in cats. Urethral obstruction is almost exclusively seen in male cats. Acute urethral obstruction can be life-threatening and can induce acute renal failure, whereas chronic partial obstruction can induce a reduction in renal function. The pathophysiology of urethral obstruction is reviewed elsewhere in this text, and only aspects directly relevant to anesthesia will be addressed here. Male cats presenting with acute urethral obstruction require some form of restraint, usually chemical, to enable urine flow to be restored (Box 7-16).

BOX 7-16

Key Points of Anesthesia of the Patient with Urethral Obstruction

- Dehydration should be corrected before anesthesia.
- Blood potassium concentration should be measured and hyperkalemia corrected.
- The electrocardiogram should be monitored for signs of hyperkalemia even if it is not present before anesthesia.
- Cardiac output and blood pressure should be maintained to prevent further renal injury.

Clinical Signs and Laboratory Findings

Acute urethral obstruction causes bladder distention with increased bladder wall tension and intravesical pressure. The increased intravesical pressure is transmitted to the renal tubules, where increased intratubular hydrostatic pressure reduces glomerular filtration rate, which persists for some time after relief of the obstruction. With chronic partial obstruction, renal blood flow decreases progressively, and after days to weeks glomerular filtration rate is variably reduced. Depending on the duration and degree of obstruction, renal function may be significantly reduced. Therefore an important anesthetic consideration in these patients is to preserve existing renal function and prevent further loss of function.

Hyperkalemia is the most important abnormality associated with complete obstruction because this electrolyte abnormality may cause life-threatening alterations in cardiac conduction. The first clinical signs of hyperkalemia are usually weakness, absence of reflexes and other neuromuscular dysfunction, eventually leading to muscular and respiratory paralysis. Potassium causes progressive depression in excitability and conduction velocity. The electrocardiographic abnormalities include peaking of the T wave, decreased amplitude and widening of the P wave, prolongation of the P-R interval, eventual disappearance of the P wave, widening of the QRS complex and irregular RR intervals, and sine wave type QRS complexes. Eventually, severe hyperkalemia culminates in ventricular fibrillation or asystole. Prompt recognition and treatment of hyperkalemia are critical. Exposure of hyperkalemic cats to anesthetic agents may further aggravate cardiovascular depression and result in cardiac arrest. An essential part of the preanesthetic preparation is to direct therapy toward normalizing the serum potassium concentration before administration of anesthetic agents.

Cats with urethral obstruction have varying degrees of dehydration. Correction of body fluid deficits before induction of anesthesia is necessary because anesthetic-induced peripheral vasodilation and myocardial depression accentuate preexisting fluid deficits and may cause profound hypotension.

Acidemia occurs in obstructive uropathy and causes various effects: decreased myocardial contractility, stroke volume, and cardiac output; excitable membrane alterations leading to dysrhythmias; central nervous system depression; dysfunction of metabolic pathways; alterations in transcellular potassium distribution; and changes in plasma protein binding and ionization of pharmacologic agents. Because of its far-reaching effects, acidemia should be corrected before inducing anesthesia.

Elevation of blood urea nitrogen concentration occurs in obstructive uropathy. Uremia causes central nervous system and myocardial depression. The effects of general anesthetic agents are potentiated, and drug dosages should be decreased.

Anesthetic Management

Fluid therapy and restoration of urine flow are the most important components of therapy for cats with urethral obstruction. It appears that relieving the obstruction as sole therapy results in poor outcome, and it is therefore essential also to correct for fluid deficits and electrolyte and acid base imbalances.[59]

Blood should be collected before anesthesia for hematocrit; total protein; blood urea nitrogen; creatinine; serum electrolytes; and, if possible, blood gas and acid–base status. A lead II electrocardiogram should be obtained and continuously monitored for signs of hyperkalemia. Any electrocardiographic sign of hyperkalemia warrants intervention. Calcium gluconate or chloride can be administered to restore normal cardiac excitability; however, the effect is short lived and does not address the primary problem. Insulin, dextrose, and sodium bicarbonate will cause extracellular potassium to move intracellularly. Potassium-free fluids will decrease blood potassium concentration by dilution.

Even in healthy patients, general anesthesia depresses renal function by decreasing renal blood flow, glomerular filtration rate, and electrolyte excretion, at least transiently.[31] After short uncomplicated anesthesia, renal blood flow and glomerular filtration rate return to normal within a few hours. However, in the obstructed patient in which renal blood flow and glomerular filtration are already decreased, the added depression induced by anesthesia may have profound effects, and every effort should be made to minimize these changes.

An opioid and anticholinergic are usually administered for premedication before general anesthesia. Cats with minimal abnormalities can usually be restrained by intravenous administration of low-dose ketamine and diazepam or midazolam to effect. The administration of the dissociative agents, ketamine and tiletamine, to cats with renal failure is controversial. Pharmacokinetic studies after ketamine administration to cats found that it is mainly eliminated unchanged by the kidney.[10] This drug should therefore be used with caution in cats with abnormal renal function. However, as for most injectable anesthetics, recovery occurs at least in part because of redistribution rather than elimination. Clinical experience indicates that ketamine, in low doses, is suitable for restraining cats with urethral obstruction, provided they do not have renal failure and that they receive fluids as part of their management. Increased toxicity of thiobarbiturates may be observed in cats with urethral obstruction because of an increase in the nonionized and nonbound portion of the drug from metabolic acidosis, as well as increased permeability of the blood–brain barrier. In addition, barbiturates are arrhythmogenic, and their use may make cardiac abnormalities more prominent. Mask or chamber induction with isoflurane is acceptable for these patients, provided excitement can be minimized.

In critically ill cats the authors prefer to induce anesthesia with a low dose of etomidate and midazolam.

Tracheal intubation is performed, and oxygen is administered. If necessary, isoflurane or sevoflurane is administered to prolong anesthesia. Mechanical ventilation is instituted if necessary. Both hypoxemia and hypercarbia should be avoided insofar as they are likely to increase the incidence of arrhythmias.

Monitoring should be directed toward recognition of arrhythmias and hypotension. As previously mentioned, electrocardiographic monitoring should be started before administration of anesthetic drugs. A Doppler crystal and occluding cuff can also be placed before induction and can be used to monitor systolic arterial blood pressure before and during maintenance of anesthesia. If systolic arterial blood pressure falls below 90 mm Hg, the anesthetic level should be decreased, a fluid bolus should be administered, and administration of an inotrope such as dopamine should be considered. Body temperature should be measured and hypothermia prevented. Measurement of urine production, using a closed technique, provides an index of renal function and should be above 1 mL/kg/h.

Idiopathic Hepatic Lipidosis

Clinical Signs and Laboratory Findings

Cats with hepatic lipidosis usually have significant weight loss. These changes in body weight and composition will make the cats more susceptible to hypothermia under anesthesia and in some cases change the pharmacokinetics of anesthetic agents (Box 7-17).

Many cats with hepatic lipidosis will present with dehydration. Vomiting, diarrhea, chronic anorexia, and reluctance to drink all contribute to the dehydration in these animals. Electrolyte abnormalities, including severe hypokalemia leading to muscle weakness, may

BOX 7-17

Key Points of Anesthesia of the Patient with Hepatic Lipidosis

- Dehydration should be corrected before anesthesia.
- Fluids should be administered to maintain adequate circulating blood volume.
- Acepromazine, $alpha_2$ agonists, and benzodiazepines should be avoided.
- Induction of anesthesia is preferably achieved using an inhaled anesthetic.
- Blood pressure should be monitored and hypotension treated aggressively.

be present.[9] Correction of body fluid deficits before induction of anesthesia is necessary to prevent profound hypotension from anesthetic-induced peripheral vasodilation and myocardial depression.

Many of these patients have a mild to moderate normocytic, normochromic, nonregenerative anemia.[9] Coagulation disorders may be present.

Cats with severe lipidosis may have hepatic encephalopathy with lethargy, behavioral changes, intermittent blindness, dementia, ptyalism, seizures, rage, and coma. Changes in response to anesthetic drugs can occur through changes in receptors such as GABA and opioid, as well as changes in neurotransmitters.

Cats with hepatic lipidosis have varying degrees of hepatic dysfunction. Increased activities of serum alkaline phosphatase, alanine aminotransferase, aspartate aminotransferase, and gamma-glutamyltransferase are common. Cats with moderate to severe disease usually are hyperbilirubinemic and appear icteric. These changes cause hepatocyte dysfunction, and drugs that rely heavily on the liver for metabolism or excretion should be avoided.

Anesthetic Management

Blood should be collected for a complete blood count and serum chemistry profile. The coagulation status must be evaluated before a procedure, especially if the patient is icteric. Prolonged clotting times should be corrected by preoperative administration of fresh frozen plasma. If dehydration is present, the patient should be rehydrated before induction of anesthesia by intravenous administration of a balanced electrolyte solution with appropriate potassium supplementation. Serum electrolyte concentrations should be monitored to guide fluid supplementation.

Maintenance of hepatic blood flow during anesthesia is an important goal in these patients. Anesthesia and surgery decrease hepatic blood flow, usually in proportion of the decrease in systemic pressure. Maintenance of an adequate circulating blood volume limits decreases in hepatic blood flow. Changes in arterial carbon dioxide tension also affect liver blood flow; hypocapnia has been reported to significantly decrease hepatic blood flow, whereas hypercapnia has the opposite effect.

Liver disease alters drug pharmacokinetics. The hepatic elimination of drugs can be affected by either changes in hepatic blood flow or changes in the ability of the liver cells to biotransform or excrete a given drug. Other mechanisms of altered pharmacokinetics in liver disease include changes in protein binding of drugs, as well as changes in volume of distribution.

Owing to alterations in pharmacokinetics and pharmacodynamics (in cases of hepatic encephalopathy), the response of the patient with hepatic disease to anesthetic drugs is virtually unpredictable. Therefore each drug must be carefully selected and, more important, carefully titrated to the desirable effect.

Premedication usually consists of a low dose of an opioid and an anticholinergic. Acepromazine and $alpha_2$ agonists should be avoided because of their effects on the cardiovascular system and on liver blood flow.[120,225] The use of benzodiazepines in hepatic encephalopathy is controversial.[5]

Induction of anesthesia is preferably achieved using an inhaled anesthetic such as isoflurane or sevoflurane. Alternatively, propofol or etomidate would be acceptable, although the latter is usually combined to a benzodiazepine to decrease the incidence of myoclonus. Anesthesia is usually maintained using an inhalant anesthetic.

Administration of a balanced electrolyte solution at 5 to 10 mL/kg/h during maintenance of anesthesia will help offset part of the drug-induced decrease in hepatic blood flow. Blood pressure should be monitored, and hypotension should be treated aggressively.

Hypertrophic Cardiomyopathy

Clinical Signs and Laboratory Findings

Many cats with mild to moderate disease have no clinical signs other than an auscultable gallop rhythm or systolic cardiac murmur. The murmur may be related to either mitral regurgitation or left ventricular outflow obstruction and may vary with changes in heart rate, ventilation, or body position. Audible crackles over the lung fields are suggestive of pulmonary edema. Laboratory tests are usually normal unless there is increased serum potassium or skeletal muscle enzymes caused by aortic obstruction secondary to aortic thromboembolism or unless renal infarction has occurred, resulting in azotemia (Box 7-18).

Anesthetic Management

Before sedating or anesthetizing a cat with hypertrophic cardiomyopathy, a current assessment of the severity of the disease should be obtained. Full hematologic and

BOX 7-18

Key Points of Anesthesia in the Patient with Hypertrophic Cardiomyopathy

- Acepromazine and anticholinergics should be avoided.
- Dissociative anesthetics, thiopental, and induction with inhaled anesthetics should be avoided.
- Electrocardiography and blood pressure should be monitored.
- Treatment of hypotension with vasoconstrictors may be preferable to the use of positive inotropes.

biochemical evaluation, thoracic radiographs, electrocardiogram, and cardiac ultrasound are recommended. Anemia can be exacerbated by anesthesia and should be corrected. Because of the sensitivity of some of these patients to fluid overload, correction of anemia is best carried out before anesthesia, using slow administration of packed red blood cells and monitoring the patient carefully. Cats on loop diuretics may have electrolyte imbalances that should be corrected before anesthesia. Arrhythmias and pulmonary edema should ideally be treated before anesthesia. Chronically administered medications such as beta-adrenergic blockers and calcium channel blockers should be given as usual on the day of anesthesia. However, it may be preferable to withdraw angiotensin-converting enzyme inhibitors because these drugs have been associated with severe, refractory hypotension in anesthetized humans. A study in cats suggests that enalapril significantly worsens isoflurane-induced hypotension.[113]

Cats with hypertrophic cardiomyopathy have poor ventricular compliance, and maintenance of cardiac output requires large ventricular volume and maintenance of (slow) sinus rhythm to improve diastolic filling. The atrial contribution to filling is important. If outflow tract obstruction is a component of the disease, increased myocardial contractility, decreased afterload, and decreased preload are predicted to decrease cardiac output by worsening the obstruction. However, factors that normally decrease cardiac output such as myocardial depression, increased systemic vascular resistance, and ventricular overdistention typically improve systolic function and cardiac output in these cases.

Cats with hypertrophic cardiomyopathy are commonly premedicated with a μ-opioid receptor agonist such as oxymorphone, hydromorphone, or methadone. Glycopyrrolate may be added if heart rate is excessively low. The use of the $alpha_2$-adrenergic agonist medetomidine has been shown to reduce left ventricular outflow tract obstruction in cats with left ventricular hypertrophy[118]; however, the effect has not been studied in anesthetized cats, and it is unclear whether the hemodynamic effects of $alpha_2$ agonists would prove beneficial during anesthesia in cats with hypertrophic cardiomyopathy. Induction of anesthesia is best performed using an injectable agent because induction with inhalation agents causes excitement and release of catecholamines. Etomidate and a benzodiazepine are preferred, particularly for the severe cases. For mild to moderate cases, propofol, either alone or in combination with a benzodiazepine, is an acceptable alternative, but it does cause systemic vasodilation and decreased afterload. Thiopental and dissociative agents (ketamine, tiletamine) should be avoided, the former because of the tachycardia and ventricular arrhythmias it may induce and the latter because of the sympathetic stimulation produced. Anesthesia is maintained with isoflurane or sevoflurane in oxygen. Sevoflurane may be slightly preferable, because data suggest that it reduces systemic vascular resistance to a lesser extent than isoflurane and that its vasodilatory effect may reach a ceiling at low to moderate concentrations.[178]

Balanced anesthetic techniques, most commonly based on utilizing an opioid infusion to reduce the amount of inhalant anesthetic and improve hemodynamics, have often been advocated in these patients. However, opioids decrease inhalant anesthetic requirements only moderately in cats[58,104,105] or may not even decrease them at all,[30] and at the doses required to achieve that effect, significant sympathetic stimulation has been reported,[163] which would be detrimental to cats with hypertrophic cardiomyopathy. Low doses of opioids could be used, but benefits remain to be demonstrated. Epidural morphine can be used to provide analgesia, but conflicting results on its effect on anesthetic requirements have been published.[75,183] Alternatives to opioids for balanced anesthesia that have been studied in cats include ketamine, nitrous oxide, and lidocaine. Ketamine and nitrous oxide produce sympathetic stimulation and may therefore not be good choices for cats with hypertrophic cardiomyopathy[22,54]; lidocaine produces significant cardiovascular depression in normal cats,[179] and caution should therefore be exerted in cats with cardiac disease. $Alpha_2$-adrenergic agonists at low doses may prove useful for balanced anesthesia in cats with hypertrophic cardiomyopathy; however, no study on their use for that purpose is available to date.

A lead II electrocardiogram, temperature, and blood pressure should be monitored during anesthesia. The electrocardiogram should ideally be assessed during induction of anesthesia as well. Blood pressure can be measured using noninvasive techniques; however, for long or invasive procedures, direct measurement is preferred. A catheter can be inserted in the dorsal pedal or femoral artery. Ventilation can be spontaneous, unless significant hypoventilation occurs, or in cases in which pulmonary edema interferes with oxygenation. In these cases intermittent positive pressure ventilation with or without positive end-expiratory pressure is usually indicated. Oxygenation should be assessed by blood gas analysis or by the use of a pulse oximeter. Fluid administration and replacement of blood loss must be judicious to optimize preload without causing pulmonary edema. Typically, crystalloids are administered at a slower rate than in the normal cat; however, hypovolemia should be adequately corrected, and large volumes of fluid should be administered if necessary. Treatment of hypotension not related to hypovolemia relies on decreasing the inhalant anesthetic concentration, and, if necessary, on the administration of vasoconstrictors. Phenylephrine may be preferable to norepinephrine in these patients because of the lack of effect on beta$_1$-adrenergic receptors. Tachyarrhythmias should be treated with a beta-adrenergic antagonist. Esmolol is commonly used in anesthetized patients because of its short duration of action.

References

1. Abbott JA: Heart rate and heart rate variability of healthy cats in home and hospital environments, *J Feline Med Surg* 7:195, 2005.
2. Adam HK, Glen JB, Hoyle PA: Pharmacokinetics in laboratory animals of ICI 35 868, a new i.v. anaesthetic agent, *Br J Anaesth* 52:743, 1980.
3. Adams P, Gelman S, Reves JG et al: Midazolam pharmacodynamics and pharmacokinetics during acute hypovolemia, *Anesthesiology* 63:140, 1985.
4. Adelman RD, Wright J: Systolic blood pressure and heart rate in the growing beagle puppy, *Dev Pharmacol Ther* 8:396, 1985.
5. Ahboucha S, Butterworth RF: Role of endogenous benzodiazepine ligands and their GABA-A–associated receptors in hepatic encephalopathy, *Metab Brain Dis* 20:425, 2005.
6. Alibhai HI, Clarke KW, Lee YH et al: Cardiopulmonary effects of combinations of medetomidine hydrochloride and atropine sulphate in dogs, *Vet Rec* 138:11, 1996.
7. Allegaert K, de Hoon J, Verbesselt R et al: Maturational pharmacokinetics of single intravenous bolus of propofol, *Paediatr Anaesth* 17:1028, 2007.
8. Andress JL, Day TK, Day D: The effects of consecutive day propofol anesthesia on feline red blood cells, *Vet Surg* 24:277, 1995.
9. Armstrong PJ, Blanchard G: Hepatic lipidosis in cats, *Vet Clin North Am Small Anim Pract* 39:599, 2009.
10. Baggot JD, Blake JW: Disposition kinetics of ketamine in the domestic cat, *Arch Int Pharmacodyn Ther* 220:115, 1976.
11. Barrett KE, Barman SM, Boitano S et al: Gas transport and pH in the lung. In Barrett KE, Barman SM, Boitano S et al, editors: *Ganong's review of medical physiology*, ed 23, New York, 2009, McGraw-Hill Medical, p 609.
12. Barter LS, Ilkiw JE, Pypendop BH et al: Evaluation of the induction and recovery characteristics of anesthesia with desflurane in cats, *Am J Vet Res* 65:748, 2004.
13. Bartlett EE, Hutserani O: Xylocaine for the relief of postoperative pain, *Anesth Analg* 40:296, 1961.
14. Beale KM, Kunkle GA, Chalker L et al: Effects of sedation on intradermal skin testing in flea-allergic dogs, *J Am Vet Med Assoc* 197:861, 1990.
15. Beck CC, Coppock RW, Ott BS: Evaluation of Vetalar (ketamine HCl): A unique feline anesthetic, *Vet Med Small Anim Clin* 66:993, 1971.
16. Bednarski RM, Muir WW: Ventricular arrhythmogenic dose of epinephrine in dogs and cats anesthetized with tiletamine/zolazepam and halothane, *Am J Vet Res* 51:1468, 1990.
17. Bednarski RM, Sams RA, Majors LJ et al: Reduction of the ventricular arrhythmogenic dose of epinephrine by ketamine administraton in halothane-anesthetized cats, *Am J Vet Res* 49:350, 1988.
18. Bennett SN, McNeil MM, Bland LA et al: Postoperative infections traced to contamination of an intravenous anesthetic, propofol, *N Engl J Med* 333:147, 1995.
19. Binns SH, Sisson DD, Buoscio DA et al: Doppler ultrasonographic, oscillometric sphygmomanometric, and photoplethysmographic techniques for noninvasive blood pressure measurement in anesthetized cats, *J Vet Intern Med* 9:405, 1995.
20. Bishop NA, Lu T, Yankner BA: Neural mechanisms of ageing and cognitive decline, *Nature* 464:529, 2010.
21. Blanco CE, Hanson MA, Johnson P et al: Breathing pattern of kittens during hypoxia, *J Appl Physiol* 56:12, 1984.
22. Bovill JG: Intravenous anesthesia for the patient with left ventricular dysfunction, *Semin Cardiothorac Vasc Anesth* 10:43, 2006.
23. Branson KR, Wagner-Mann CC, Mann FA: Evaluation of an oscillometric blood pressure monitor on anesthetized cats and the effect of cuff placement and fur on accuracy, *Vet Surg* 26:347, 1997.
24. Brearley JC, Kellagher RBE, Hall LW: Propofol anaesthesia in cats, *J Small Anim Pract* 28:315, 1988.
25. Brodbelt D: Perioperative mortality in small animal anaesthesia, *Vet J* 182:152, 2009.
26. Brodbelt DC, Blissitt KJ, Hammond RA et al: The risk of death: the confidential enquiry into perioperative small animal fatalities, *Vet Anaesth Analg* 35:365, 2008.
27. Brodbelt DC, Pfeiffer DU, Young LE et al: Risk factors for anaesthetic-related death in cats: results from the confidential enquiry into perioperative small animal fatalities (CEPSAF), *Br J Anaesth* 99:617, 2007.
28. Brodie BB: Physiological disposition and chemical fate of thiobarbiturates in the body, *Fed Proc* 11:632, 1952.
29. Brodie BB, Bernstein E, Mark LC: The role of body fat in limiting the duration of action of thiopental, *J Pharmacol Exp Ther* 105:421, 1952.
30. Brosnan RJ, Pypendop BH, Siao KT et al: Effects of remifentanil on measures of anesthetic immobility and analgesia in cats, *Am J Vet Res* 70:1065, 2009.
31. Burchardi H, Kaczmarczyk G: The effect of anaesthesia on renal function, *Eur J Anaesthesiol* 11:163, 1994.
32. Carpenter RE, Pettifer GR, Tranquilli WJ: Anesthesia for geriatric patients, *Vet Clin North Am Small Anim Pract* 35:571, 2005.
33. Caulkett NA, Cantwell SL, Houston DM: A comparison of indirect blood pressure monitoring techniques in the anesthetized cat, *Vet Surg* 27:370, 1998.
34. Center SA, Elston TH, Rowland PH et al: Fulminant hepatic failure associated with oral administration of diazepam in 11 cats, *J Am Vet Med Assoc* 209:618, 1996.
35. Chatdarong K, Ponglowhapan S, Manee-in S et al: The use of propofol for electroejaculation in domestic cats, *Theriogenology* 66:1615, 2006.
36. Child KJ, Currie JP, Dis B et al: The pharmacological properties in animals of CT1341—a new steroid anaesthetic agent, *Br J Anaesth* 43:2, 1971.
37. Child KJ, Davis B, Dodds MG et al: Anaesthetic, cardiovascular and respiratory effects of a new steroidal agent CT 1341: a comparison with other intravenous anaesthetic drugs in the unrestrained cat, *Br J Pharmacol* 46:189, 1972.
38. Cistola AM, Golder FJ, Centonze LA et al: Anesthetic and physiologic effects of tiletamine, zolazepam, ketamine, and xylazine combination (TKX) in feral cats undergoing surgical sterilization, *J Feline Med Surg* 6:297, 2004.

39. Clarke KW, Hall LW: A survey of anaesthesia in small animal practice: AVA/BSAVA report, *Journal of the Association of Veterinary Anaesthetists of Great Britain and Ireland* 17:4, 1990.
40. Clarke RS, Dundee J, Garrett FT et al: Adverse reactions to intravenous anaesthetics, *Br J Anaesth* 47:575, 1975.
41. Colby ED, Sanford TD: Blood pressure and heart and respiratory rates of cats under ketamine/xylazine, ketamine/acepromazine anesthesia, *Fel Pract* 11:19, 1981.
42. Cooper GM: Confidential enquiries into anaesthetic deaths, *Br J Anaesth* 99:606, 2007.
43. Cotler S, Gustafson JH, Colburn WA: Pharmacokinetics of diazepam and nordiazepam in the cat, *J Pharm Sci* 73:348, 1984.
44. Court MH, Greenblatt DJ: Pharmacokinetics and preliminary observations of behavioral changes following administration of midazolam to dogs, *J Vet Pharmacol Ther* 15:343, 1992.
45. Crighton GW, Pownall R: The homeothermic status of the neonatal dog, *Nature* 251:142, 1974.
46. Dart AB, Mutter TC, Ruth CA et al: Hydroxyethyl starch (HES) versus other fluid therapies: effects on kidney function, Cochrane Database Syst Rev:CD007594, 2010.
47. De Clive-Lowe SG, Desmond J, North J: Intravenous lignocaine anaesthesia, *Anaesthesia* 13:138, 1958.
48. Dhasmana KM, Dixit KS, Jaju BP et al: Role of central dopaminergic receptors in manic response of cats to morphine, *Psychopharmacologia* 24:380, 1972.
49. Dodman NH: Complications of saffan anaesthesia in cats, *Vet Rec* 107:481, 1980.
50. Dunkle N, Moise NS, Scarlett-Kranz J et al: Cardiac performance in cats after administration of xylazine or xylazine and glycopyrrolate: echocardiographic evaluations, *Am J Vet Res* 47:2212, 1986.
51. Dyson DH, Allen DG, Ingwersen W et al: Evaluation of acepromazine/meperidine/atropine premedication followed by thiopental anesthesia in the cat, *Can J Vet Res* 52:419, 1988.
52. Dyson DH, Allen DG, Ingwersen W et al: Effects of saffan on cardiopulmonary function in healthy cats, *Can J Vet Res* 51:236, 1987.
53. Dyson DH, Maxie MG, Schnurr D: Morbidity and mortality associated with anesthetic management in small animal veterinary practice in Ontario, *J Am Anim Hosp Assoc* 34:325, 1998.
54. Ebert TJ, Kampine JP: Nitrous oxide augments sympathetic outflow: direct evidence from human peroneal nerve recordings, *Anesth Analg* 69:444, 1989.
55. Eger EI: *Nitrous oxide/N2O*, ed 1, New York, 1985, Elsevier.
56. Epstein M: Aging and the kidney, *J Am Soc Nephrol* 7:1106, 1996.
57. Farver TB, Haskins SC, Patz JD: Cardiopulmonary effects of acepromazine and of the subsequent administration of ketamine in the dog, *Am J Vet Res* 47:631, 1986.
58. Ferreira TH, Aguiar AJ, Valverde A et al: Effect of remifentanil hydrochloride administered via constant rate infusion on the minimum alveolar concentration of isoflurane in cats, *Am J Vet Res* 70:581, 2009.
59. Finco DR, Cornelius LM: Characterization and treatment of water, electrolyte, and acid-base imbalances of induced urethral obstruction in the cat, *Am J Vet Res* 38:823, 1977.
60. Finley JP, Kelly C: Heart rate and respiratory patterns in mild hypoxia in unanaesthetized newborn mammals, *Can J Physiol Pharmacol* 64:122, 1986.
61. Fischer S, Bader AM, Sweitzer B: *Preoperative evaluation*, ed 7, Philadelphia, 2010, Churchill Livingstone.
62. Fisher MM: Severe histamine mediated reactions to intravenous drugs used in anaesthesia, *Anaesth Intensive Care* 3:180, 1975.
63. Fordyce WE, Kanter RK: Arterial-end tidal PCO2 equilibration in the cat during acute hypercapnia, *Respir Physiol* 73:257, 1988.
64. Fox PR, Bond BR, Peterson ME: Echocardiographic reference values in healthy cats sedated with ketamine hydrochloride, *Am J Vet Res* 46:1479, 1985.
65. Fujita Y, Yamamoto T, Sano I et al: A comparison of changes in cardiac preload variables during graded hypovolemia and hypervolemia in mechanically ventilated dogs, *Anesth Analg* 99:1780, 2004.
66. Galatos AD, Savas I, Prassinos NN et al: Gastro-oesophageal reflux during thiopentone or propofol anaesthesia in the cat, *J Vet Med A Physiol Pathol Clin Med* 48:287, 2001.
67. Ge Y, Grossman RI, Babb JS et al: Age-related total gray matter and white matter changes in normal adult brain. Part I: volumetric MR imaging analysis, *Am J Neuroradiol* 23:1327, 2002.
68. Ge Y, Grossman RI, Babb JS et al: Age-related total gray matter and white matter changes in normal adult brain. Part II: quantitative magnetization transfer ratio histogram analysis, *Am J Neuroradiol* 23:1334, 2002.
69. Geel JK: The effect of premedication on the induction dose of propofol in dogs and cats, *J S Afr Vet Assoc* 62:118, 1991.
70. Ghaffari MS, Malmasi A, Bokaie S: Effect of acepromazine or xylazine on tear production as measured by Schirmer tear test in normal cats, *Vet Ophthalmol* 13:1, 2010.
71. Glen JB: Animal studies of the anaesthetic activity of ICI 35 868, *Br J Anaesth* 52:731, 1980.
72. Glen JB, Hunter SC, Blackburn TP et al: Interaction studies and other investigations of the pharmacology of propofol ("Diprivan"), *Postgrad Med J* 61 (Suppl 3):7, 1985.
73. Glowaski MM, Wetmore LA: Propofol: application in veterinary sedation and anesthesia, *Clin Tech Small Anim Pract* 14:1, 1999.
74. Golden AL, Bright JM, Daniel GB et al: Cardiovascular effects of the alpha$_2$-adrenergic receptor agonist medetomidine in clinically normal cats anesthetized with isoflurane, *Am J Vet Res* 59:509, 1998.
75. Golder FJ, Pascoe PJ, Bailey CS et al: The effect of epidural morphine on the minimum alveolar concentration of isoflurane in cats, *J Vet Anaesth* 25:52, 1998.
76. Gordh T: The effect of Althesin on the heart in situ in the cat, *Postgrad Med J* 48:(Suppl 2):31, 1972.
77. Grandy JL, Dunlop CI, Hodgson DS et al: Evaluation of the Doppler ultrasonic method of measuring systolic arterial blood pressure in cats, *Am J Vet Res* 53:1166, 1992.
78. Granholm M, McKusick BC, Westerholm FC et al: Evaluation of the clinical efficacy and safety of dexmedetomidine or medetomidine in cats and their reversal with atipamezole, *Vet Anaesth Analg* 33:214, 2006.
79. Greenblatt DJ, Koch-Weser J: Adverse reactions to intravenous diazepam: a report from the Boston Collaborative Drug Surveillance Program, *Am J Med Sci* 266:261, 1973.
80. Gruber CM: The effects of anesthetic doses of sodium thiopentobarbital, sodium thio-ethamyl and pentothal sodium upon the respiratory system, the heart and blood pressure in experimental animals, *J Pharmacol Exp Ther* 60(2):143-173, 1937.
81. Grundy SA: Clinically relevant physiology of the neonate, *Vet Clin North Am Small Anim Pract* 36:443, 2006.
82. Hahnenberger RW: Influence of various anesthetic drugs on the intraocular pressure of cats, *Albrecht Von Graefes Arch Klin Exp Ophthalmol* 199:179, 1976.
83. Hall LW, Clarke KW: *Veterinary anaesthesia*, ed 9, London, 1991, Baillière Tindall.
84. Hall RI, Schwieger IM, Hug CC Jr: The anesthetic efficacy of midazolam in the enflurane-anesthetized dog, *Anesthesiology* 68:862, 1988.
85. Hardie EM, Spodnick GJ, Gilson SD et al: Tracheal rupture in cats: 16 cases (1983-1998), *J Am Vet Med Assoc* 214:508, 1999.

86. Hartsfield SM: Advantages and guidelines for using ketamine for induction of anesthesia, *Vet Clin North Am Small Anim Pract* 22:266, 1992.
87. Harvey RC: Precautions when using mask induction, *Vet Clin North Am Small Anim Pract* 22:310, 1992.
88. Hashem A, Kietzmann M, Scherkl R: The pharmacokinetics and bioavailability of acepromazine in the plasma of dogs, *Dtsch Tierarztl Wochenschr* 99:396, 1992.
89. Hashim MA, Waterman AE: Effects of thiopentone, propofol, alphaxalone-alphadolone, ketamine and xylazine-ketamine on lower oesophageal sphincter pressure and barrier pressure in cats, *Vet Rec* 129:137, 1991.
90. Hashim MA, Waterman AE: Effects of acepromazine, pethidine and atropine premedication on lower oesophageal sphincter pressure and barrier pressure in anaesthetised cats, *Vet Rec* 133:158, 1993.
91. Haskins SC: Inhalational anesthetics, *Vet Clin North Am Small Anim Pract* 22:297, 1992.
92. Haskins SC: Monitoring anesthetized patients. In Tranquilli WJ, Thurmon JC,Grimm KA, editors: *Lumb & Jones' veterinary anesthesia and analgesia*, ed 4, Ames, 2007, Blackwell Publishing, p 533.
93. Hatch RC, Kitzman JV, Zahner JM et al: Comparison of five preanesthetic medicaments in thiopental-anesthetized cats: antagonism by selected compounds, *Am J Vet Res* 45:2322, 1984.
94. Hayreh SS, Kardon RH, McAllister DL et al: Acepromazine. Effects on intraocular pressure, *Arch Ophthalmol* 109:119, 1991.
95. Heard DJ, Webb AI, Daniels RT: Effect of acepromazine on the anesthetic requirement of halothane in the dog, *Am J Vet Res* 47:2113, 1986.
96. Heavner JE, Bloedow DC: Ketamine pharmacokinetics in domestic cats, *Vet Anesthesia* 6:16, 1979.
97. Heldmann E, Brown DC, Shofer F: The association of propofol usage with postoperative wound infection rate in clean wounds: a retrospective study, *Vet Surg* 28:256, 1999.
98. Hellyer PW, Muir WW, III, Hubbell JAE et al: Cardiorespiratory effects of the intravenous administration of tiletamine-zolazepam to cats, *Vet Surg* 17:172, 1988.
99. Herbert DA, Mitchell RA: Blood gas tensions and acid-base balance in awake cats, *J Appl Physiol* 30:434, 1971.
100. Himes RS, Jr, DiFazio CA, Burney RG: Effects of lidocaine on the anesthetic requirements for nitrous oxide and halothane, *Anesthesiology* 47:437, 1977.
101. Hodgson DS, Dunlop CI, Chapman PL et al: Cardiopulmonary effects of anesthesia induced and maintained with isoflurane in cats, *Am J Vet Res* 59:182, 1998.
102. Hsu WH, Hembrough FB: Intravenous glucose tolerance test in cats: influenced by acetylpromazine, ketamine, morphine, thiopental, and xylazine, *Am J Vet Res* 43:2060, 1982.
103. Ilkiw JE, Pascoe PJ: Cardiovascular effects of propofol alone and in combination with ketamine for total intravenous anesthesia in cats, *Am J Vet Res* 64:913, 2003.
104. Ilkiw JE, Pascoe PJ, Fisher LD: Effect of alfentanil on the minimum alveolar concentration of isoflurane in cats, *Am J Vet Res* 58:1274, 1997.
105. Ilkiw JE, Pascoe PJ, Tripp LD: Effects of morphine, butorphanol, buprenorphine, and U50488H on the minimum alveolar concentration of isoflurane in cats, *Am J Vet Res* 63:1198, 2002.
106. Ilkiw JE, Pascoe PJ, Tripp LD: Effect of variable-dose propofol alone and in combination with two fixed doses of ketamine for total intravenous anesthesia in cats, *Am J Vet Res* 64:907, 2003.
107. Ilkiw JE, Suter C, McNeal D et al: The optimal intravenous dose of midazolam after intravenous ketamine in healthy awake cats, *J Vet Pharmacol Ther* 21:54, 1998.
108. Ilkiw JE, Suter CM, Farver TB et al: The behaviour of healthy awake cats following intravenous and intramuscular administration of midazolam, *J Vet Pharmacol Ther* 19:205, 1996.
109. Imai A, Ilkiw JE, Pypendop BH et al: Nitrous oxide does not consistently reduce isoflurane requirements in cats, *Vet Anaesth Analg* 29:98, 2002.
110. Imai A, Steffey E, Ilkiw J et al: Quantitative characteristics of anesthetic induction with and recovery from isoflurane and sevoflurane in cats, *Vet Anaesth Analg* 30:106, 2003.
111. Inagaki Y, Sumikawa K, Yoshiya I: Anesthetic interaction between midazolam and halothane in humans, *Anesth Analg* 76:613, 1993.
112. Irifune M, Shimizu T, Nomoto M et al: Ketamine-induced anesthesia involves the N-methyl-D-aspartate receptor-channel complex in mice, *Brain Res* 596:1, 1992.
113. Ishikawa Y, Uechi M, Ishikawa R et al: Effect of isoflurane anesthesia on hemodynamics following the administration of an angiotensin-converting enzyme inhibitor in cats, *J Vet Med Sci* 69:869, 2007.
114. Kastner SBR: *Intravenous anaesthetics*, ed 2, Gloucester, UK, 2007, British Small Animal Veterinary Association.
115. Kissin I, Vinik HR, Bradley EL, Jr: Midazolam potentiates thiopental sodium anesthetic induction in patients, *J Clin Anesth* 3:367, 1991.
116. Laboratories G: *A Glaxo guide to Saffan*, Greenford, Middlesex, 1974, Glaxo Laboratories, Ltd.
117. Lamont LA, Bulmer BJ, Grimm KA et al: Cardiopulmonary evaluation of the use of medetomidine hydrochloride in cats, *Am J Vet Res* 62:1745, 2001.
118. Lamont LA, Bulmer BJ, Sisson DD et al: Doppler echocardiographic effects of medetomidine on dynamic left ventricular outflow tract obstruction in cats, *J Am Vet Med Assoc* 221:1276, 2002.
119. Lapinsky SE, Mehta S: Bench-to-bedside review: Recruitment and recruiting maneuvers, *Crit Care* 9:60, 2005.
120. Lawrence CJ, Prinzen FW, de Lange S: The effect of dexmedetomidine on nutrient organ blood flow, *Anesth Analg* 83:1160, 1996.
121. Lee DD, Papich MG, Hardie EM: Comparison of pharmacokinetics of fentanyl after intravenous and transdermal administration in cats, *Am J Vet Res* 61:672, 2000.
122. Lenhardt R: Monitoring and thermal management, *Best Pract Res Clin Anaesthesiol* 17:569, 2003.
123. Lerche P, Muir WW, 3rd, Bednarski RM: Nonrebreathing anesthetic systems in small animal practice, *J Am Vet Med Assoc* 217:493, 2000.
124. Lerche P, Muir WW, Grubb TL: Mask induction of anaesthesia with isoflurane or sevoflurane in premedicated cats, *J Small Anim Pract* 43:12, 2002.
125. Lin HC, Thurmon JC, Benson GJ et al: Telazol: a review of its pharmacology and use in veterinary medicine, *J Vet Pharmacol Ther* 16:383, 1993.
126. Loscher W, Frey HH: Pharmacokinetics of diazepam in the dog, *Arch Int Pharmacodyn Ther* 254:180, 1981.
127. Mace SE, Levy MN: Neural control of heart rate: a comparison between puppies and adult animals, *Pediatr Res* 17:491, 1983.
128. Maly P, Olivecrona H, Almen T et al: Interaction between chlorpromazine and intrathecally injected non-ionic contrast media in non-anaesthetized rabbits, *Neuroradiology* 26:235, 1984.
129. Mama KR: New drugs in feline anesthesia, *Compendium on Continuing Education for the Practicing Veterinarian* 20:125, 1998.
130. Marroum PJ, Webb AI, Aeschbacher G et al: Pharmacokinetics and pharmacodynamics of acepromazine in horses, *Am J Vet Res* 55:1428, 1994.
131. Martin JE, Sheaff MT: Renal ageing, *J Pathol* 211:198, 2007.
132. Matot I, Neely CF, Katz RY et al: Pulmonary uptake of propofol in cats. Effect of fentanyl and halothane, *Anesthesiology* 78:1157, 1993.
133. Matthews NS, Dollar NS, Shawley RV: Halothane-sparing effect of benzodiazepines in ponies, *Cornell Vet* 80:259, 1990.

134. Matthews NS, Hartke S, Allen JC, Jr.: An evaluation of pulse oximeters in dogs, cats and horses, *Vet Anaesth Analg* 30:3, 2003.
135. Maze M, Tranquilli W: Alpha-2 adrenoceptor agonists: defining the role in clinical anesthesia, *Anesthesiology* 74:581, 1991.
136. McClune S, McKay AC, Wright PM et al: Synergistic interaction between midazolam and propofol, *Br J Anaesth* 69:240, 1992.
137. McLaughlin JA: The intravenous use of novocaine as a substitute for morphine in postoperative care, *Can Med Assoc* 52:383, 1945.
138. McMurphy RM, Hodgson DS: Cardiopulmonary effects of desflurane in cats, *Am J Vet Res* 57:367, 1996.
139. Mellon RD, Simone AF, Rappaport BA: Use of anesthetic agents in neonates and young children, *Anesth Analg* 104:509, 2007.
140. Mendes GM, Selmi AL: Use of a combination of propofol and fentanyl, alfentanil, or sufentanil for total intravenous anesthesia in cats, *J Am Vet Med Assoc* 223:1608, 2003.
141. Meyers-Wallen VN, Haskins ME, Patterson DF: Hematologic values in healthy neonatal, weanling, and juvenile kittens, *Am J Vet Res* 45:1322, 1984.
142. Michenfelder JD: The interdependency of cerebral functional and metabolic effects following massive doses of thiopental in the dog, *Anesthesiology* 41:231, 1974.
143. Middleton DJ, Ilkiw JE, Watson AD: Physiological effects of thiopentone, ketamine and CT 1341 in cats, *Res Vet Sci* 32:157, 1982.
144. Milde LN, Milde JH, Michenfelder JD: Cerebral functional, metabolic, and hemodynamic effects of etomidate in dogs, *Anesthesiology* 63:371, 1985.
145. Mitchell SL, McCarthy R, Rudloff E et al: Tracheal rupture associated with intubation in cats: 20 cases (1996-1998), *J Am Vet Med Assoc* 216:1592, 2000.
146. Montiel M, Jimenez E, Navaez JA et al: Aldosterone and plasma renin activity in hyperthyroid rats: effects of propranolol and propylthiouracil, *J Endocrinol Invest* 7:559, 1984.
147. Moon PF: Cortisol suppression in cats after induction of anesthesia with etomidate, compared with ketamine-diazepam combination, *Am J Vet Res* 58:868, 1997.
148. Morgan DW, Legge K: Clinical evaluation of propofol as an intravenous anaesthetic agent in cats and dogs, *Vet Rec* 124:31, 1989.
149. Mueller RS, Ihrke PJ, Kass PH et al: The effect of tiletamine-zolazepam anesthesia on the response to intradermally injected histamine in cats, *Vet Dermatol* 2:119, 1991.
150. Muir W, Lerche P, Wiese A et al: The cardiorespiratory and anesthetic effects of clinical and supraclinical doses of alfaxalone in cats, *Vet Anaesth Analg* 36:42, 2009.
151. Muir WW, 3rd, Wiese AJ, March PA: Effects of morphine, lidocaine, ketamine, and morphine-lidocaine-ketamine drug combination on minimum alveolar concentration in dogs anesthetized with isoflurane, *Am J Vet Res* 64:1155, 2003.
152. Muir WW, Werner LL, Hamlin RL: Antiarrhythmic effects of diazepam during coronary artery occlusion in dogs, *Am J Vet Res* 36:1203, 1975.
153. Muir WW, Werner LL, Hamlin RL: Effects of xylazine and acetylpromazine upon induced ventricular fibrillation in dogs anesthetized with thiamylal and halothane, *Am J Vet Res* 36:1299, 1975.
154. Murrell JC, Hellebrekers LJ: Medetomidine and dexmedetomidine: a review of cardiovascular effects and antinociceptive properties in the dog, *Vet Anaesth Analg* 32:117, 2005.
155. Nagel ML, Muir WW, Nguyen K: Comparison of the cardiopulmonary effects of etomidate and thiamylal in dogs, *Am J Vet Res* 40:193, 1979.
156. Ngan Kee WD, Khaw KS, Ma ML et al: Postoperative analgesic requirement after cesarean section: a comparison of anesthetic induction with ketamine or thiopental, *Anesth Analg* 85:1294, 1997.
157. Nicholson A: Monitoring techniques and equipment for small animal anaesthesia, *Aust Vet J* 74:114, 1996.
158. Oye I, Paulsen O, Maurset A: Effects of ketamine on sensory perception: evidence for a role of N-methyl-D-aspartate receptors, *J Pharmacol Exp Ther* 260:1209, 1992.
159. Pablo LS, Bailey JE: Etomidate and telazol, *Vet Clin North Am Small Anim Pract* 29:779, 1999.
160. Pascoe P: The cardiovascular effects of dexmedetomidine given by continuous infusion during isoflurane anesthesia in dogs, *Vet Anaest Analg* 32:9, 2005.
161. Pascoe PJ, Ilkiw JE, Black WD et al: The pharmacokinetics of alfentanil in healthy cats, *J Vet Anaest* 20:9, 1993.
162. Pascoe PJ, Ilkiw JE, Craig C et al: The effects of ketamine on the minimum alveolar concentration of isoflurane in cats, *Vet Anaesth Analg* 34:31, 2007.
163. Pascoe PJ, Ilkiw JE, Fisher LD: Cardiovascular effects of equipotent isoflurane and alfentanil/isoflurane minimum alveolar concentration multiple in cats, *Am J Vet Res* 58:1267, 1997.
164. Pascoe PJ, Ilkiw JE, Frischmeyer KJ: The effect of the duration of propofol administration on recovery from anesthesia in cats, *Vet Anaesth Analg* 33:2, 2006.
165. Pascoe PJ, Ilkiw JE, Haskins SC et al: Cardiopulmonary effects of etomidate in hypovolemic dogs, *Am J Vet Res* 53:2178, 1992.
166. Pascoe PJ, Raekallio M, Kuusela E et al: Changes in the minimum alveolar concentration of isoflurane and some cardiopulmonary measurements during three continuous infusion rates of dexmedetomidine in dogs, *Vet Anaesth Analg* 33:97, 2006.
167. Pedersen CM, Thirstrup S, Nielsen-Kudsk JE: Smooth muscle relaxant effects of propofol and ketamine in isolated guinea-pig trachea, *Eur J Pharmacol* 238:75, 1993.
168. Pedersen KM, Butler MA, Ersboll AK et al: Evaluation of an oscillometric blood pressure monitor for use in anesthetized cats, *J Am Vet Med Assoc* 221:646, 2002.
169. Perisho JA, Buechel DR, Miller RD: The effect of diazepam (Valium) on minimum alveolar anaesthetic requirement (MAC) in man, *Can Anaesth Soc J* 18:536, 1971.
170. Peters R: Ageing and the brain, *Postgrad Med J* 82:84, 2006.
171. Peterson ME, Birchard SJ, Mehlhaff CJ: Anesthetic and surgical management of endocrine disorders, *Vet Clin North Am Small Anim Pract* 14:911, 1984.
172. Peterson ME, Kintzer PP, Cavanagh PG et al: Feline hyperthyroidism: pretreatment clinical and laboratory evaluation of 131 cases, *J Am Vet Med Assoc* 183:103, 1983.
173. Peterson ME, Ward CR: Etiopathologic findings of hyperthyroidism in cats, *Vet Clin North Am Small Anim Pract* 37:633, 2007.
174. Pickerodt VW, McDowall DG, Coroneos NJ et al: Effect of althesin on cerebral perfusion, cerebral metabolism and intracranial pressure in the anaesthetized baboon, *Br J Anaesth* 44:751, 1972.
175. Poterack KA, Kampine JP, Schmeling WT: Effects of isoflurane, midazolam, and etomidate on cardiovascular responses to stimulation of central nervous system pressor sites in chronically instrumented cats, *Anesth Analg* 73:64, 1991.
176. Priebe HJ: The aged cardiovascular risk patient, *Br J Anaesth* 85:763, 2000.
177. Pypendop BH, Brosnan RJ, Siao KT et al: Pharmacokinetics of remifentanil in conscious cats and cats anesthetized with isoflurane, *Am J Vet Res* 69:531, 2008.
178. Pypendop BH, Ilkiw JE: Hemodynamic effects of sevoflurane in cats, *Am J Vet Res* 65:20, 2004.
179. Pypendop BH, Ilkiw JE: Assessment of the hemodynamic effects of lidocaine administered IV in isoflurane-anesthetized cats, *Am J Vet Res* 66:661, 2005.
180. Pypendop BH, Ilkiw JE: Assessment of the hemodynamic effects of lidocaine administered IV in isoflurane-anesthetized cats, *Am J Vet Res* 66:661, 2005.

181. Pypendop BH, Ilkiw JE: The effects of intravenous lidocaine administration on the minimum alveolar concentration of isoflurane in cats, *Anesth Analg* 100:97, 2005.
182. Pypendop BH, Ilkiw JE, Imai A et al: Hemodynamic effects of nitrous oxide in isoflurane-anesthetized cats, *Am J Vet Res* 64:273, 2003.
183. Pypendop BH, Pascoe PJ, Ilkiw JE: Effects of epidural administration of morphine and buprenorphine on the minimum alveolar concentration of isoflurane in cats, *Am J Vet Res* 67:1471, 2006.
184. Pypendop BH, Siao KT, Pascoe PJ et al: Effects of epidurally administered morphine or buprenorphine on the thermal threshold in cats, *Am J Vet Res* 69:983, 2008.
185. Pypendop BH, Verstegen JP: Hemodynamic effects of medetomidine in the dog: a dose titration study, *Vet Surg* 27:612, 1998.
186. Reid JS, Frank RJ: Prevention of undesirable side reactions of ketamine anesthetic in cats, *J Am Anim Hosp Assoc* 8:115, 1972.
187. Rex MA: The laryngeal reflex, *N Z Vet J* 15:222, 1967.
188. Robinson EP, Johnston GR: Radiographic assessment of laryngeal reflexes in ketamine-anesthetized cats, *Am J Vet Res* 47:1569, 1986.
189. Roizen MF, Fleisher LA: Anesthetic implications of concurrent diseases. In Miller RD, editor: *Miller's anesthesia*, Philadelphia, 2009, Churchill Livingstone.
190. Rooke GA: Cardiovascular aging and anesthetic implications, *J Cardiothorac Vasc Anesth* 17:512, 2003.
191. Roytblat L, Korotkoruchko A, Katz J et al: Postoperative pain: the effect of low-dose ketamine in addition to general anesthesia, *Anesth Analg* 77:1161, 1993.
192. Saidman LJ, Eger EI, 2nd: The effect of thiopental metabolism on duration of anesthesia, *Anesthesiology* 27:118, 1966.
193. Sawyer DC, Rech RH, Durham RA: Does ketamine provide adequate visceral analgesia when used alone or in combination with acepromazine, diazepam, or butorphanol in cats, *J Vet Anest* 18(S1):381, 1991.
194. Schaafsma IA, Pollak YW, Barthez PY: Effect of four sedative and anesthetic protocols on quantitative thyroid scintigraphy in euthyroid cats, *Am J Vet Res* 67:1362, 2006.
195. Schmucker DL: Age-related changes in liver structure and function: implications for disease? *Exp Gerontol* 40:650, 2005.
196. Schwedler M, Miletich DJ, Albrecht RF: Cerebral blood flow and metabolism following ketamine administration, *Can Anaesth Soc J* 29:222, 1982.
197. Seeler DC: Fluid, electrolyte, and blood component therapy. In Tranquilli WJ, Thurmon JC, Grimm KA, editors: *Lumb & Jones' veterinary anesthesia and analgesia*, ed 4, Ames, Iowa, 2007, Blackwell, p 185.
198. Segovia G, Porras A, Del Arco A et al: Glutamatergic neurotransmission in aging: a critical perspective, *Mech Ageing Dev* 122:1, 2001.
199. Selmi AL, Mendes GM, Lins BT et al: Evaluation of the sedative and cardiorespiratory effects of dexmedetomidine, dexmedetomidine-butorphanol, and dexmedetomidine-ketamine in cats, *J Am Vet Med Assoc* 222:37, 2003.
200. Shaprio HM, Wyte SR, Harris AB: Ketamine anaesthesia in patients with intracranial pathology, *Br J Anaesth* 44:1200, 1972.
201. Short CE, Bufalari A: Propofol anesthesia, *Vet Clin North Am Small Anim Pract* 29:747, 1999.
202. Siafakas NM, Alexopoulou C, Bouros D: Respiratory muscle function in endocrine diseases, *Monaldi Arch Chest Dis* 54:154, 1999.
203. Sieber FS, Pauldine R: Geriatric anesthesia. In Miller RD, editor: *Miller's anesthesia*, Philadelphia, 2009, Churchill Livingstone.
204. Silva DR, Gazzana MB, John AB et al: Pulmonary arterial hypertension and thyroid disease, *J Bras Pneumol* 35:179, 2009.
205. Silva FG: The aging kidney: a review—part I, *Int Urol Nephrol* 37:185, 2005.
206. Sinclair MD, O'Grady MR, Kerr CL et al: The echocardiographic effects of romifidine in dogs with and without prior or concurrent administration of glycopyrrolate, *Vet Anaesth Analg* 30:211, 2003.
207. Skovsted P, Sapthavichaikul S: The effects of etomidate on arterial pressure, pulse rate and preganglionic sympathetic activity in cats, *Can Anaesth Soc J* 24:565, 1977.
208. Slingsby LS, Taylor PM: Thermal antinociception after dexmedetomidine administration in cats: a dose-finding study, *J Vet Pharmacol Ther* 31:135, 2008.
209. Sosis MB, Braverman B: Growth of Staphylococcus aureus in four intravenous anesthetics, *Anesth Analg* 77:766, 1993.
210. Sprung J, Gajic O, Warner DO: Review article: age related alterations in respiratory function—anesthetic considerations, *Can J Anaesth* 53:1244, 2006.
211. Steagall PV, Taylor PM, Brondani JT et al: Antinociceptive effects of tramadol and acepromazine in cats, *J Feline Med Surg* 10:24, 2008.
212. Steffey EP, Gillespie JR, Berry JD et al: Anesthetic potency (MAC) of nitrous oxide in the dog, cat, and stump-tail monkey, *J Appl Physiol* 36:530, 1974.
213. Steffey EP, Howland D, Jr: Isoflurane potency in the dog and cat, *Am J Vet Res* 38:1833, 1977.
214. Stenberg D, Salven P, Miettinen MV: Sedative action of the alpha 2-agonist medetomidine in cats, *J Vet Pharmacol Ther* 10:319, 1987.
215. Stephan H, Sonntag H, Schenk HD et al: [Effect of Disoprivan (propofol) on the circulation and oxygen consumption of the brain and CO_2 reactivity of brain vessels in the human], *Anaesthesist* 36:60, 1987.
216. Stevens WC, Kingston HGG: *Inhalation anesthesia*, ed 1, Philadelphia, 1989, JB Lippincott.
217. Syme HM: Cardiovascular and renal manifestations of hyperthyroidism, *Vet Clin North Am Small Anim Pract* 37:723, 2007.
218. Takeshita H, Okuda Y, Sari A: The effects of ketamine on cerebral circulation and metabolism in man, *Anesthesiology* 36:69, 1972.
219. Tavoloni N: Postnatal changes in hepatic microsomal enzyme activities in the puppy, *Biol Neonate* 47:305, 1985.
220. Taylor JS, Vierck CJ: Effects of ketamine on electroencephalographic and autonomic arousal and segmental reflex responses in the cat, *Vet Anaesth Analg* 30:237, 2003.
221. Taylor PA, Towey RM: Depression of laryngeal reflexes during keatmine anaesthesia, *Br Med J* 2:688, 1971.
222. Thoday KL, Mooney CT: Historical, clinical and laboratory features of 126 hyperthyroid cats, *Vet Rec* 131:257, 1992.
223. Traber DL, Wilson RD, Priano LL: Differentiation of the cardiovascular effects of CI-581, *Anesth Analg* 47:769, 1968.
224. Tracy CH, Short CE, Clark BC: Comparing the effects of intravenous and intramuscular administration of Telazol, *Vet Med* 83:104, 1988.
225. Turner DM, Ilkiw JE, Rose RJ et al: Respiratory and cardiovascular effects of five drugs used as sedatives in the dog, *Aust Vet J* 50:260, 1974.
226. Tzannes S, Govendir M, Zaki S et al: The use of sevoflurane in a 2:1 mixture of nitrous oxide and oxygen for rapid mask induction of anaesthesia in the cat, *J Feline Med Surg* 2:83, 2000.
227. Ulvi H, Yoldas T, Mungen B et al: Continuous infusion of midazolam in the treatment of refractory generalized convulsive status epilepticus, *Neurol Sci* 23:177, 2002.
228. Vaha-Vahe T: Clinical evaluation of medetomidine, a novel sedative and analgesic drug for dogs and cats, *Acta Vet Scand* 30:267, 1989.
229. Wagner AE, Walton JA, Hellyer PW et al: Use of low doses of ketamine administered by constant rate infusion as an adjunct for postoperative analgesia in dogs, *J Am Vet Med Assoc* 221:72, 2002.

230. Wang W, Li C, Summer SN et al: Polyuria of thyrotoxicosis: downregulation of aquaporin water channels and increased solute excretion, *Kidney Int* 72:1088, 2007.
231. Wase AW, Foster WC: Thiopental and thyroid metabolism, *Proc Soc Exp Biol Med* 91:89, 1956.
232. Waterman AE: Influence of premedication with xylazine on the distribution and metabolism of intramuscularly administered ketamine in cats, *Res Vet Sci* 35:285, 1983.
233. Watney GC, Pablo LS: Median effective dosage of propofol for induction of anesthesia in dogs, *Am J Vet Res* 53:2320, 1992.
234. Weaver BM, Raptopoulos D: Induction of anaesthesia in dogs and cats with propofol, *Vet Rec* 126:617, 1990.
235. Webb AI: Minimum infusion rates (MIR) for ketamine and thiopentone in the cat, *J Vet Anaesth* 21:41, 1994.
236. Weinert BT, Timiras PS: Invited review: Theories of aging, *J Appl Physiol* 95:1706, 2003.
237. Wertz E: Does etomidate cause haemolysis? *Br J Anaesth* 70:490, 1993.
238. Wertz EM, Benson GJ, Thurmon JC et al: Pharmacokinetics of thiamylal in cats, *Am J Vet Res* 49:1079, 1988.
239. Wertz EM, Benson GJ, Thurmon JC et al: Pharmacokinetics of etomidate in cats, *Am J Vet Res* 51:281, 1990.
240. White PF, Way WL, Trevor AJ: Ketamine—its pharmacology and therapeutic uses, *Anesthesiology* 56:119, 1982.
241. Whittem T, Pasloske KS, Heit MC et al: The pharmacokinetics and pharmacodynamics of alfaxalone in cats after single and multiple intravenous administration of Alfaxan at clinical and supraclinical doses, *J Vet Pharmacol Ther* 31:571, 2008.
242. Wilder-Smith OH, Ravussin PA, Decosterd LA et al: Midazolam premedication and thiopental induction of anaesthesia: interactions at multiple end-points, *Br J Anaesth* 83:590, 1999.
243. Wilder-Smith OH, Ravussin PA, Decosterd LA et al: Midazolam premedication reduces propofol dose requirements for multiple anesthetic endpoints, *Can J Anaesth* 48:439, 2001.
244. Williams LS, Levy JK, Robertson SA et al: Use of the anesthetic combination of tiletamine, zolazepam, ketamine, and xylazine for neutering feral cats, *J Am Vet Med Assoc* 220:1491, 2002.
245. Wilson RD, Traber DL, McCoy NR: Cardiopulmonary effects of C1-581–the new dissociative anesthetic, *South Med J* 61:692, 1968.
246. Wright M: Pharmacologic effects of ketamine and its use in veterinary medicine, *J Am Vet Med Assoc* 180:1462, 1982.
247. Yackey M, Ilkiw JE, Pascoe PJ et al: Effect of transdermally administered fentanyl on the minimum alveolar concentration of isoflurane in cats, *Vet Anaesth Analg* 31:183, 2004.
248. Yoda Y, Mori N, Oka K et al: Intracytoplasmic localization of CD3 antigen in NKH1+ azurophilic granular T-lymphoblastic lymphoma cells, *Nippon Ketsueki Gakkai Zasshi* 52:740, 1989.
249. Zambelli D, Cunto M, Prati F et al: Effects of ketamine or medetomidine administration on quality of electroejaculated sperm and on sperm flow in the domestic cat, *Theriogenology* 68:796, 2007.
250. Zaugg M, Lucchinetti E: Respiratory function in the elderly, *Anesthesiol Clin North Am* 18:47, 2000.

CHAPTER

8

Preventive Health Care for Cats

Ilona Rodan and Andrew H. Sparkes

OUTLINE

Cats have become the most popular pet in the United States, Canada, and Northern Europe, and 78% of owners consider their cats to be family members (Figure 8-1).[93] Despite the popularity of and affection for the feline species, cats are still the underdog when it comes to veterinary care, especially preventive care. This chapter discusses the benefits of feline preventive health care, the barriers to feline veterinary care, the opportunities for improvement, and the components of a comprehensive feline preventive health care program for all feline life stages. The authors of this chapter were also members of the panel that developed the Feline Life Stage Guidelines by the American Association of Feline Practitioners (AAFP) and the American Animal Hospital Association (AAHA). Although more information is provided in this chapter, the outline for comprehensive care is taken from the guidelines.[99]

BENEFITS OF FELINE PREVENTIVE CARE

Cats, above all other species, need preventive care because they hide pain and illness, a protective mechanism derived from predator avoidance in the wild. Cat owners are more willing to seek veterinary care when they understand and appreciate its importance.[56] To achieve optimal feline health care, veterinarians must educate clients about the benefits of feline preventive care, which include the following:

- Improved quality of life and longevity
- Early disease detection, when diseases are easiest to treat or manage
- Pain prevention and early detection to prevent suffering
- Reduced expenses associated with urgent and sick care
- Development of a baseline of the individual cat's normal values for comparison when cats become ill (e.g., weight comparisons and minimum database), which helps in the early detection of disease and health concerns
- Increased owner–pet bond and decreased relinquishment and euthanasia of pet cats through prevention of undesirable behavior (often normal behavior in ways that owners consider undesirable) and behavioral problems
- Increased client–veterinarian bond and loyalty, which increase compliance with needed preventive care
- Increased quality of life for cat owners (e.g., the human–cat bond can decrease human blood pressure, reduce the chance of a second heart attack, decrease or prevent depression and loneliness, and increase confidence in children)
- Early detection of weight gain or loss

Wellness visits are also a good opportunity to educate owners about the needs of their cat. These visits should be structured to allow time to listen to the owner's concerns and address them.

Current Barriers to Feline Preventive Care: Understanding the Problems

Millions of cats in the United States alone do not receive the veterinary care they need. One of the biggest hurdles

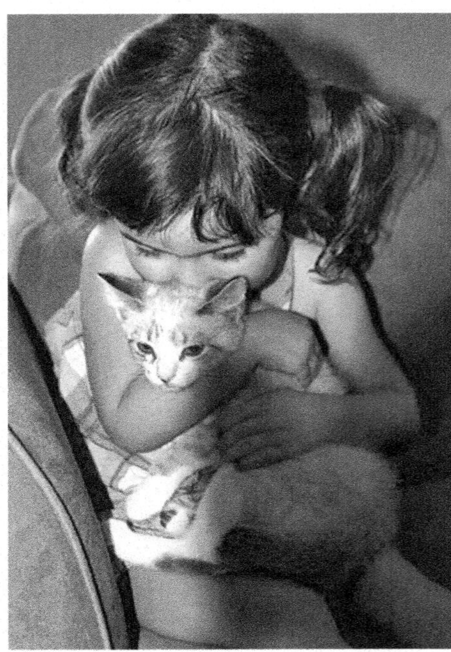

FIGURE 8-1 People consider their cats to be family members that provide companionship and affection. Cats are beneficial for the health of people of all ages and help prevent disease. *(Image courtesy Dr. Deb Given.)*

is that cat owners are often unaware of the medical needs of their cat and the importance of feline preventive care.[56] Troubling statistics indicate that dogs are taken to the veterinarian more than twice as often as cats; dogs generally visit the veterinarian 2.3 times per year, whereas cats see the veterinarian only 1.1 times per year.[56] From 33% to 36% cats do not see a veterinarian even once annually. In households with both cats and dogs, the cats received less veterinary care than the dogs, with adult cats especially lacking in preventive care.[56] Unfortunately, adult cats have many diseases that are overlooked, such as obesity, dental and lower urinary tract diseases, and behavioral problems. Adult cats are also more likely to be surrendered because of behavior problems. Lack of care has an impact on quality of life and longevity.

There is a common misconception that cats are independent and self-sufficient, which makes them easy to care for.[56] One reason for this misconception is that cats hide their pain and illness and may appear healthy or show only subtle signs that often go unnoticed by their owners until the condition is serious. The "Healthy Cats for Life" campaign from the AAFP and Boehringer Ingelheim lists the 10 subtle signs of sickness in cats (http://www.healthycatsforlife.com):

1. Inappropriate elimination behavior
2. Changes in interaction
3. Changes in activity
4. Changes in sleeping habits
5. Changes in food and water consumption
6. Unexplained weight loss or gain
7. Changes in grooming
8. Signs of stress
9. Changes in vocalization
10. Bad breath

Another important problem is the difficulty of getting cats to the veterinary hospital and the veterinary experience itself. This includes the practical difficulties of getting the cat into the carrier and feline fear or stress associated with the car ride and the veterinary visit. Cat owners may also be embarrassed by the way their cat behaves at the veterinary hospital, or they may not like how the veterinarian or veterinary staff handles their cat.[56]

One of the main obstacles to owner compliance is the lack of a clear recommendation by the veterinary team.[1] Cat owners often complain that they did not know the care was necessary, the veterinarian did not recommend the service, or that the need or benefit was not well explained.[56]

The Opportunities

Veterinarians and their staff have huge opportunities to improve feline preventive care and increase the number of feline patients and the frequency of feline veterinary visits in their hospitals. Many of these opportunities were identified in a large study on the impact of the owner–pet and client–veterinarian bond.[56] The AAFP and AAHA Feline Life Stage Guidelines provide evidence-based recommendations to help veterinary teams and clients understand each component of feline preventive care and the associated benefits.[99]

A veterinarian's communication skills, interaction with pets, and ability to educate owners about their pets' needs all drive clients' perceptions of the value of services and the quality of care. Study findings revealed that clear and thorough veterinarian communication with the client could ultimately *increase compliance by as much as 40%*.[56] For example, when the veterinarian recommends and clearly explains the service and benefits to the patient, preventive dental care increases by 64%.[56] Improved communication skills can enhance the way veterinarians and staff members communicate with clients. Lectures on communication are available at every major veterinary conference and through Internet seminars, as well as more general communication resources. Although the study addressed the veterinarian specifically, all members of our veterinary teams should have excellent communication skills.

The ways in which veterinarians interact with their feline patients and whether they encourage a feline-friendly hospital environment influence the the number

Adult (3-6 Years)	Mature (7-10 Years)	Senior (11-14 Years)	Geriatric (15+ Years)
This age group is often overlooked and would benefit from regular veterinary care.	Specific management of mature and older cats is described in the AAFP Senior Care Guidelines and AAHA Senior Care Guidelines for Dogs and Cats.	Specific management of mature and older cats is described in the AAFP Senior Care Guidelines and AAHA Senior Care Guidelines for Dogs and Cats.	Specific management of mature and older cats is described in the AAFP Senior Care Guidelines and AAHA Senior Care Guidelines for Dogs and Cats.
• Review environmental enrichment. • Teach techniques to increase the cat's activity (e.g., retrieve). • Encourage object and interactive play as a weight management strategy.	Increased importance of easy accessibility to litter box, bed, food.	• Environmental needs may change (e.g., with osteoarthritis): ensure easy accessibility to litter box, soft bed, food. • Educate clients about subtle behavior changes that are not "just old age."	• Ensure accessibility to litter box, bed, food. • Monitor cognitive function (vocalization/confusion), signs of pain/osteoarthritis. • Discuss quality-of-life issues.
Discuss baseline adult data to assess subsequent changes (e.g., weight, BCS, MDB)	• Monitor for subtle changes such as increased sleeping or decreased activity. • Increase focus on mobility, duration, and/or progression of any specific signs.	Increase focus on mobility, duration, and/or progression of any specific signs	Increasing importance for regular review of medications and supplements
	Review the size and edge height of litter box to ensure that the cat can enter easily as it ages.	Adjust litter box size, height, and cleaning regimens as necessary.	Adjust litter box size, height, and cleaning regimens as necessary.
Feed to moderate body condition. Monitor for weight changes, and modify food intake accordingly.	Feed to moderate body condition. Monitor for weight changes, and modify food intake accordingly.	Feed to moderate body condition. Monitor for weight changes, and modify food intake accordingly.	Feed to moderate body condition. Monitor food intake and BCS weight changes.
Moderate and discuss.	Moderate and discuss.	Monitor for oral tumors, inability to eat, and decreased quality of life from painful dental disease.	Monitor for oral tumors, inability to eat, and decreased quality of life from painful dental disease.
Conduct fecal exams 1 to 2 times per year, depending on health and lifestyle factors.	Conduct fecal exams 1 to 2 times per year, depending on health and lifestyle factors.	Conduct fecal exams 1 to 2 times per year, depending on health and lifestyle factors.	Conduct fecal exams 1 to 2 times per year, depending on health and lifestyle factors.
Continue core vaccines according to current guidelines. Evaluate risk assessment and use of noncore vaccines, if indicated, according to current guidelines.	Continue core vaccines according to current guidelines. Evaluate risk assessment and use of noncore vaccines, if indicated, according to current guidelines.	Continue core vaccines according to current guidelines. Evaluate risk assessment and use of noncore vaccines, if indicated, according to current guidelines.	Continue core vaccines according to current guidelines. Evaluate risk assessment and use of noncore vaccines, if indicated, according to current guidelines.

wellness examinations for cats at all life stages. Reasons include the following: Changes in health status may occur in a short period of time; ill cats often show no signs of disease; and earlier detection of poor health, body weight changes, dental disease, and other problems allows for earlier intervention. In addition, semiannual exams provide an opportunity for more frequent communication with the owner regarding behavioral and attitudinal changes and education about preventive health care. Both the AAFP Senior Care Guidelines[74] and the AAHA Senior Care Guidelines for dogs and cats[25] recommend semiannual examinations for apparently healthy cats 7 years of age and older. Cats with previously diagnosed health conditions may require more frequent examinations. Further research is needed to identify the optimal examination schedule to maximize the health and longevity of the cat.

General Preventive Care Recommendations

Meeting the Costs of Veterinary Care

The vast majority of cat owners do not leave a veterinarian because of the cost of care,[56] but clients do want value, which is all about the experience they have at the veterinary hospital. Financial realities must be considered. It is important to address the cost of care and give clients a schedule and treatment plan (including a cost estimate) for upcoming visits so that they can plan for these expenses. The AAHA strongly suggests that all pet-owning families consider their ability to meet unexpected expenses that may be incurred for veterinary care (Box 8-1). The expenses may be met through existing savings, credit card reserves, Care Credit or other medical payment cards, monthly budgeting for pet care expenses, or pet health insurance policies.

Pet health insurance has become a good method of mitigating health care expenses. The proportion of cats insured varies greatly among different countries, but it is almost invariably lower than the proportion of dogs insured. Pet insurance can provide excellent value for the cost and allow patients to receive highly expensive urgent care and crisis management that may not be feasible otherwise. Many policies now offer preventive health care coverage. Each insurance company works differently, and clients are encouraged to review policies carefully. Few clients are aware of pet insurance without a specific veterinary recommendation; the veterinary team should explain benefits and possible limitations of pet insurance. The National Commission on Veterinary Economic Issues (NCVEI) position paper, "A veterinarian's guide to pet health insurance," contains excellent information to help veterinarians and veterinary teams learn more about pet insurance.[100] In the United States there is also a website that helps consumers compare various pet health insurance companies (Pet Insurance Review, see Box 8-1).

Microchipping

Microchipping is recommended for cats of all lifestyles (indoor, indoor–outdoor, and fully outdoor) to ensure permanent identification that cannot be lost and increase the chance that lost cats will be returned to their owners. One study found that 41% of people looking for their lost cats considered them indoor-only pets,[55] which emphasizes the importance of microchipping all cats, regardless of lifestyle. According to the American Humane Association, only about 2% of lost cats ever find their way back from shelters, a major reason being the lack of tag or microchip identification (see Box 8-1). According to another study, owners of almost three quarters of microchipped cats were located because their cats had microchips.[54]

The wellness examination is the ideal time to discuss the importance of identification with owners. The benefits of both visible (e.g., collar and tag) and permanent identification should be explained; the AVMA provides an excellent resource for veterinarians in the United States to make decisions about the type of microchip and methods of microchip implantation (see Box 8-1). The veterinarian should note that the owner has complied with this identification and record the microchip number in the cat's medical history.

Microchip implantation is a minimally invasive procedure that can be done in the examination room without anesthesia or scheduled with an upcoming dental prophylaxis or routine surgical procedure. The standard site for subcutaneous injection of the microchip is on the dorsal midline, just cranial to the shoulder blade or scapula. In the United States microchip implantation should be performed by, or under the supervision of, a licensed veterinarian (see AVMA policy on electronic identification; see Box 8-1). In the United Kingdom microchip insertion is not considered a veterinary practice. Although risks are rare, any adverse reactions should be reported.

All major veterinary organizations endorse the use of electronic identification. The International Standards Organization (ISO) standards have been accepted by Canada, Europe, Asia, and Australia. Although the United States supports ISO standardization, at this time there is still no U.S. standard for microchip frequencies. Animals traveling to countries with adopted ISO regulations should be implanted with microchips that meet the standards, or the cat owner should carry a scanner that can read the non-ISO microchip.[55]

Every cat should be scanned during wellness examinations. Scanning new patients identifies whether they have been previously microchipped; scanning patients known to be microchipped ensures that the microchip is functioning properly and still in the proper location

BOX 8-1

Internet Resources

General Preventive Care Recommendations

- AAHA Statement on Meeting the Cost of Pet Care
  - http://www.aahanet.org/
- Pet Insurance Review
  - http://www.petinsurancereview.com
- AVMA policy on electronic identification
  - http://www.avma.org/issues/policy/electronic_identification.asp
- WSAVA microchip identification
  - http://www.wsava.org/MicrochipID.htm
- AAHA Pet Microchip Lookup Tool
  - http://www.petmicrochiplookup.org/
- Chloe Standard, Inc., Check the Chip
  - http://www.checkthechip.com/

Disaster Preparedness

- American Humane Association—Don't Leave Your Pet's Safety To Chance
  - http://www.americanhumane.org/about-us/who-we-are/american-humane-blog/blog-posts/dont-leave-your-pets-safety.html
- AVMA Saving the Whole Family booklet
  - http://www.avma.org/disaster/saving_family.asp
- Humane Society of the United States, Disaster Preparedness for Pets
  - http://www.hsus.org/hsus_field/hsus_disaster_center/resources/disaster_preparedness_for_pets.html
- ASPCA Disaster Preparedness
  - http://www.aspca.org/pet-care/disaster-preparedness/

Estate Planning

- AVMA Pet Estate Planning
  - http://www.avma.org/onlnews/javma/dec01/s120101e.asp
- Humane Society of the United States—Planning Your Estate?
  - http://www.hsus.org/press_and_publications/press_releases/planning_your_estate_the.html

Environmental Enrichment

- The Indoor Cat Initiative, The Ohio State University
  - http://www.vet.osu.edu/indoorcat.htm
- AAFP Feline Behavior Guidelines, 2004
  - http://www.catvets.com/professionals/guidelines/publications/?Id=177

Claw Care

- AAFP Position Statement on Declawing
  - http://www.catvets.com/professionals/guidelines/position/?Id=291
- AAHA Declawing (Onychectomy) Position Statement
  - http://www.aahanet.org
- AVMA Position Statement on the Declawing of Domestic Cats
  - http://www.avma.org/onlnews/javma/apr03/030415c.asp
- CVMA Position Statement on Declawing
  - http://canadianveterinarians.net/ShowText.aspx?ResourceID=28
- Cornell University, College of Veterinary Medicine: Trimming Your Cat's Claws
  - http://www.partnersah.vet.cornell.edu/pet/fhc/trimming_claws

Testing for Inherited Diseases

- University of California—Davis, Veterinary Genetics Laboratory
  - http://www.vgl.ucdavis.edu/services/cat/
- Washington State University, Veterinary Cardiac Genetics Lab
  - http://www.vetmed.wsu.edu/deptsVCGL/
- University of Pennsylvania, PennGen Laboratories
  - http://research.vet.upenn.edu/Default.aspx?alias=research.vet.upenn.edu/penngen

Dental Care

- American Veterinary Dental Society
  - http://www.avds-online.org/
- Cornell University, College of Veterinary Medicine—Brushing Your Cat's Teeth
  - http://partnersah.vet.cornell.edu/pet/fhc/brushing_teeth
- Veterinary Oral Health Council—Products awarded the VOHC Seal
  - http://www.vohc.org/accepted_products.htm

Parasite Control

- Companion Animal Parasite Council
  - http://www.capcvet.org/
- European Scientific Counsel Companion Animal Parasites
  - http://www.esccap.org/
- Centers for Disease Control and Prevention—Healthy Pets, Healthy People
  - http://www.cdc.gov/healthypets/index.htm
- American Heartworm Society
  - http://www.heartwormsociety.org/

(microchips occasionally migrate). The veterinarian should use a universal scanner that can read microchips of all commonly used frequencies. This routine scanning also reminds owners to keep their microchip database contact information current. More valuable information about microchip scanning is provided by the World Small Animal Veterinary Association (WSAVA; see Box 8-1).

Staff members should be trained to pass the scanner over the cat in different directions; it may be necessary to do this more than once. Scanning should be performed away from computers, metal tables, and fluorescent lighting, and metal collars should be removed first. Batteries should be checked or replaced regularly to ensure that the device is functioning properly.[55] The United States is the only country in which microchip implantation and registration are often separate processes.[54] This lack of a centralized database has led to concerns about the reduced ability to identify pets. To resolve the problem, the AAHA has created the AAHA Universal Pet Microchip Lookup Tool, and Chloe Standard, Inc. has also created a search engine, Check the Chip (see Box 8-1).

Disaster Preparedness and Estate Planning

Although most people are reluctant even to think about it, disaster can occur wherever one lives, whether a natural or other type of disaster. After the Hurricane Katrina disaster in 2005, a Zogby International poll found that 61% of pet owners would not evacuate if they could not bring their pets with them (http://www.zogby.com/news/readnews.cfm?ID=1029). In 2006 the United States Congress addressed this issue by passing the "Pets Evacuation and Transportation Standards (PETS) Act" (Public Law 109-308), which requires state and local emergency management agencies to make plans that take into account the needs of individuals with pets and service animals in the event of a major disaster or emergency. Box 8-1 lists websites that provide helpful information on disaster preparedness.

It is important that owners have a pet estate plan in case their pets outlive them. Clients can be provided with information to support them in making decisions about care in the event of their death or if they are no longer able to take care of their cats (see Box 8-1).

Behavior

Despite continued advances in feline health care, prevention of behavioral problems is the weakest area of most preventive health programs for cats. It is also the most serious problem when it comes to disruption of the human–animal bond and surrender, relinquishment, and euthanasia of pet cats. The following facts indicate the enormity of behavioral problems in cats:

- There is no greater threat to the human–animal bond than behavioral problems.[85]
- Behavioral problems continue to be the most common reason that pet cats are relinquished and euthanized.[87]
- *Normal* feline behaviors that cat owners consider unacceptable are among the most common reasons for abandonment.[2]
- Cats with inappropriate elimination habits have the highest risk of relinquishment, with about 4 million cats euthanized yearly in shelters in the United States.[92]
- Behavioral problems directly affect animal welfare[26] and cause decreased quality of life for cats and their owners.
- Unresolved behavioral problems cause veterinarians to lose approximately 15% of their client base annually.[70]
- Most pets surrendered to shelters were seen by a veterinarian at least once in the year preceding relinquishment.[83]
- Of owners of cats that marked urine vertically, 26% did not contact their veterinarian because they thought that the veterinarian could not help them with the problem; 93% reported that they consulted other sources (+/− the veterinarian).[8]

By preventing behavioral problems, veterinarians have the opportunity to protect and strengthen the human–pet–veterinary bond and increase the quality of life for both cats and cat lovers.[70] It is crucial that veterinarians educate their staff and clients, as well as themselves, about preventive-behavior health care. During wellness appointments there are two ways to help clients with cat behavior: identifying client concerns and behavior changes by taking and reviewing the history and educating clients to prevent behavioral problems.

The medical history is critical for early detection of behavioral problems and collection of information about the cat's lifestyle (i.e., indoor versus outdoor), other cats in the household and how they interact, and other potential stressors for the cat. An excellent question to ask is, "What changes in behavior or undesirable behavior have you noticed?" This allows the veterinarian to detect problems earlier, educate clients about the fact that behavioral changes are often due to underlying medical problems, and address client concerns about unwanted behavior.

The second opportunity to deal with behavioral issues during wellness appointments is by educating clients about normal cat behaviors and environmental enrichment. If owners are properly informed, cats can retain their normal behaviors in ways that are also acceptable to cat owners. Client education should begin at the first appointment and reviewed during each life stage. It has been shown that dog obedience training and the receipt of advice regarding companion animal behavior reduce the risk of relinquishment to an animal shelter and increase human–companion animal interactions.[87] If cat owners receive the same education, by participating in training or "Kitten Kindy" classes (see Chapter 11) that deal with normal feline behavior and prevention of behavioral problems, they are less likely to relinquish their cats and more likely to have a satisfying human–cat relationship. Veterinarians must also remind clients to call the veterinary hospital with any behavioral questions and concerns, which will, with any luck, keep them from acting on misinformation from other sources. If the veterinarian is unable to help, referring the client to an appropriate specialist is an important way to maintain the human–animal bond as well as the veterinarian–client relationship. A list of board-certified veterinary behavior specialists can be found through the American College of Veterinary Behaviorists (http://www.veterinarybehaviorists.org/); in areas where behavior specialists are not available, referral to those with a special interest and extensive training in feline behavior is a good alternative.

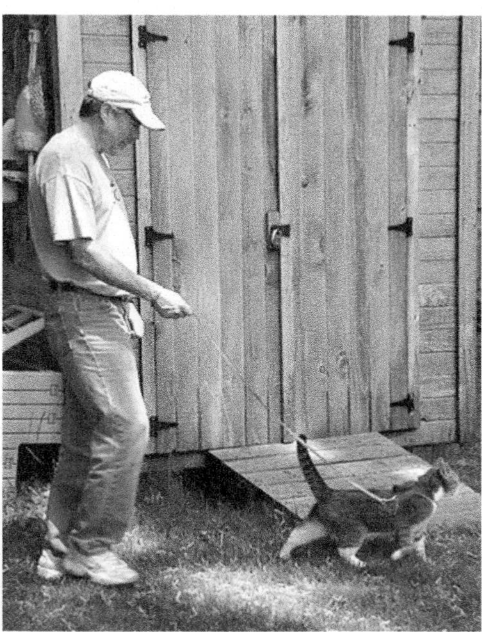

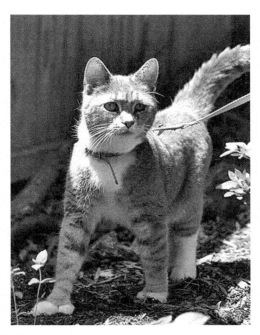

FIGURE 8-4 Indoor cats are often bored. Cats can be taught to walk on a leash, which may afford them a more enriched lifestyle than the cat that is indoors exclusively. *(Image courtesy Dr. Deb Given.)*

Indoor Versus Outdoor Lifestyle

Controversy exists over whether cats should be kept exclusively indoors or allowed to go outside sometimes. These debates usually reflect geographic and cultural differences.[12,17,67,95] An indoor–outdoor lifestyle may provide a more natural and stimulating environment for cats, but it also increases the cat's risk of contracting an infectious disease or experiencing trauma, and it has important environmental consequences, insofar as cats prey on wildlife. Supervised or controlled outdoor access (e.g., a safe outdoor cat enclosure, leash walking) has been recommended to reduce some of the risks associated with access to the outdoors (Figures 8-4 and 8-5). An indoor-only lifestyle may decrease the risks of infectious disease and trauma and increase longevity, but it also may increase the risks of compromised welfare and illness owing to stress associated with lack of environmental stimulation.

FIGURE 8-5 Note how interested this cat is in what it sees, hears, and smells outdoors. *(Image courtesy Dr. Deb Given.)*

Environmental Enrichment

Appropriate environmental enrichment is essential for maintaining the mental and physical well-being of cats housed indoors.[39,70] Environmental enrichment allows cats to carry out their normal behaviors, which are similar to those of their ancestors, in a manner that is acceptable to cat owners. Cats need resources in the home to allow them to perform their normal behavior: scratching posts in desirable locations and cat trees, perches, or shelves to allow for climbing and resting and to increase overall space in the home (Figure 8-6). Normal feeding behavior and multiple toileting (litter box) areas are also necessary. Many cats also like hiding spots, especially in multicat households, households with children, and when company visits. Queens teach kittens to play so that they learn to hunt for food and catch their prey; play is an important component of the cat's day. Cats are social animals and enjoy both interactive toys and hunting games. They also enjoy playing on

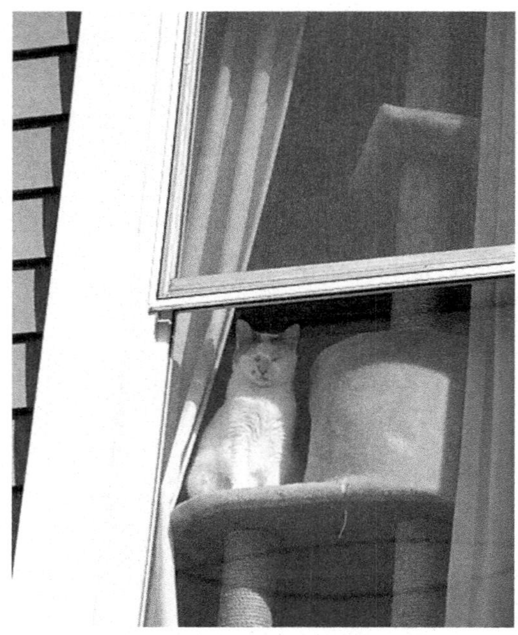

FIGURE 8-6 Cat trees placed next to windows increase space vertically and provide a view of the outdoors. *(Image courtesy Dr. Deb Given.)*

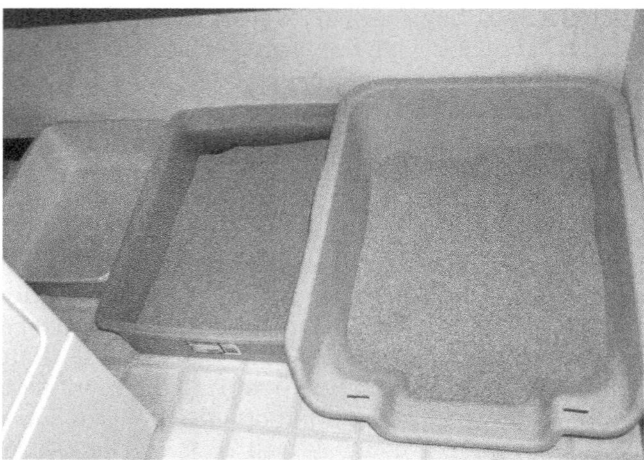

FIGURE 8-7 The commercial cat litter box *(left)* is often too small for fully grown cats. The sweater storage box *(middle)* and the dog litter box for animals up to 35 pounds *(right)* are better choices. *(Image courtesy Dr. Ilona Rodan.)*

their own; rotation of toys prevents boredom. There are excellent resources to educate veterinary teams and cat owners about cats' needs and environmental enrichment. The Indoor Cat Initiative (see Box 8-1) provides outstanding information, as does Chapter 46. Another client resource is the book *From the Cat's Point of View* (Bohnenkamp G, Perfect Paws Publishing, 1991; ISBN 0964460114).

Environmental enrichment prevents behavioral problems and is also needed for treatment of most behavioral problems, either as the only treatment or as an important component of the treatment plan. Multimodal environmental modification (MEMO) has also been shown to decrease clinical signs of interstitial cystitis and respiratory and gastrointestinal diseases.[12,14]

The more cats in the household, the more resources are needed to increase feline welfare and help prevent behavioral problems. Litter boxes are an excellent example showing why cats need multiple resources. The recommendation for the number of litter boxes is traditionally one litter box per cat plus one extra, so that a household with three cats should contain four litter boxes, placed in different locations. In a multiple-floor dwelling, a minimum of one box should be placed on each floor to which the cats have access. This allows cats to have easy access to a litter box regardless of where the cat is in the house and reduces the risk of another cat blocking access to the cat or bothering it while it is eliminating. Boxes should be located in easily accessible areas but not high-traffic areas. Most cats prefer unscented clumping litter,[65,70] and some cats may find scented litters aversive. Kittens may be offered a variety of litter box options from which to choose, with one choice being unscented clumping litter.[66] Litter boxes should be scooped at least once daily and changed completely once weekly for clay litter and once every 2 weeks for clumping litter. Cats also prefer litter boxes[66] large enough for them to turn around in; the ideal size is approximately 1.5 times the size of the cat, from the tip of the nose to the base of the tail.[70] Most commercial cat litter boxes are too small; plastic clothes storage boxes and dog litter boxes for dogs up to 35 pounds are excellent choices (Figure 8-7). Cats with arthritis and other health problems that make it difficult to jump over the edge of the box should be provided with a box that has a smaller lip or edge at the front of the box; dog litter boxes already have these. Otherwise, an opening can be cut in a sweater or other plastic box.

Cats learn best when desired behavior is reinforced and rewarded and when undesired behavior is redirected. Clients should be reminded that cats should never be punished verbally or physically.

Client communication should occur both verbally and with supporting client handouts or other educational materials. Excellent client educational handouts are available in the AAFP Feline Behavior Guidelines[70] (see Box 8-1) and include the following topics:

- Introducing a new cat into a household with resident cats
- Litter box care to prevent or treat elimination problems

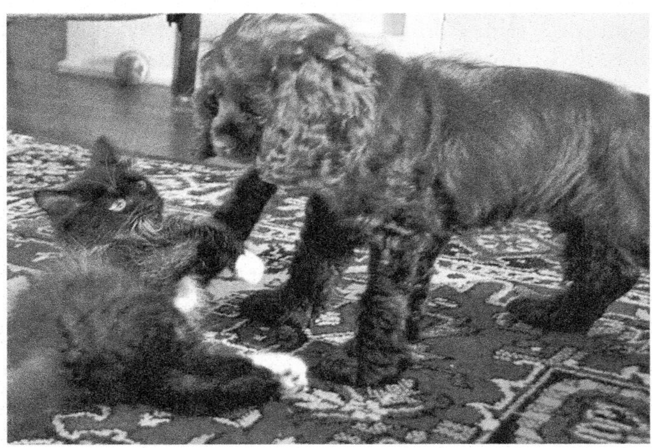

FIGURE 8-8 Cats and dogs can be great friends, playing and sleeping together. It is best to expose them to each other as kittens and puppies, with positive experiences. *(Image courtesy Dr. Deb Given.)*

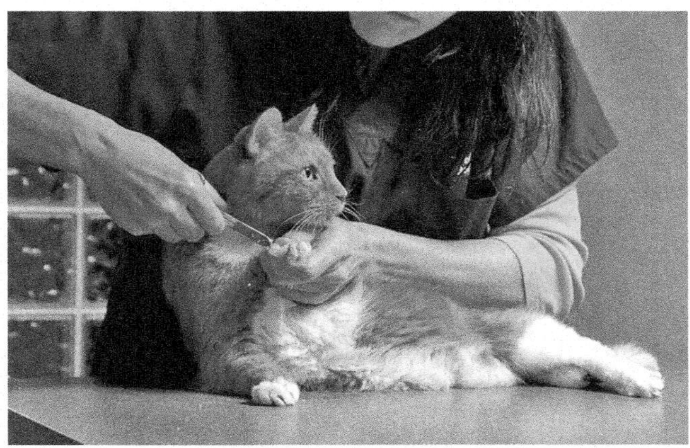

FIGURE 8-9 Teaching clients how to trim their cat's nails and to associate nail trimmings with rewards allows most clients to perform all grooming services at home. *(Image courtesy Dr. Deb Given.)*

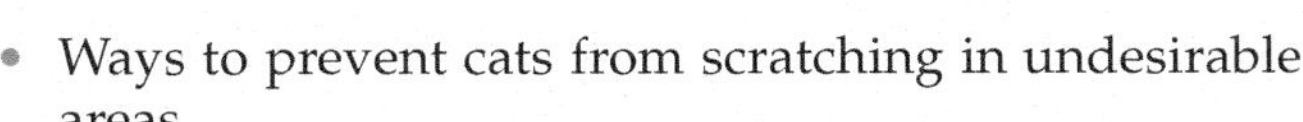

- Ways to prevent cats from scratching in undesirable areas
- Feeding tips to prevent obesity in your cat
- Ways to help your cat have pleasant veterinary visits
- Environmental enrichment to enhance the cat's quality of life

Behavior Needs by Life Stage

KITTEN (BIRTH TO 6 MONTHS)

Kittens have a strong drive to play. Intercat social play peaks at about 12 weeks of age,[16] after which object play becomes more prevalent. Toys offer an outlet for normal predatory sequences as part of play and help prevent play biting. The primary socialization period of cats to people is from 3 to 9 weeks of age. If kittens associate positive experiences with exposure to humans during this time, they will be more willing to approach people and be held by them later in life. Kittens should be handled gently and positively and exposed as early as possible to any stimuli or handling techniques the cat may encounter during their lifetime (e.g., children, dogs, nail trims, tooth brushing, car rides) (Figures 8-8 and 8-9). Positive carrier, car, and veterinary experiences that occur early in life can improve future veterinary visits (Figure 8-10). Positive behaviors should always be reinforced by using food or other appropriate rewards; kittens should never be punished because this may elicit defensive aggression.

JUNIOR (7 MONTHS TO 2 YEARS)

It is important during the junior life stage to continue training the young cat to allow manipulation of mouth, ears, and feet. Intercat relations may change when a cat reaches 1 to 2 years of age (the age at which free-living offspring leave the family unit), and intercat aggression may develop. Stress associated with the change in intercat relationships can lead to inappropriate urination or spraying. It is critical to provide needed resources in multiple areas. Synthetic feline pheromone (Feliway diffusers and spray) therapy is purported to assist in spatial organization, enhance intercat relations, and provide emotional stabilization.[66]

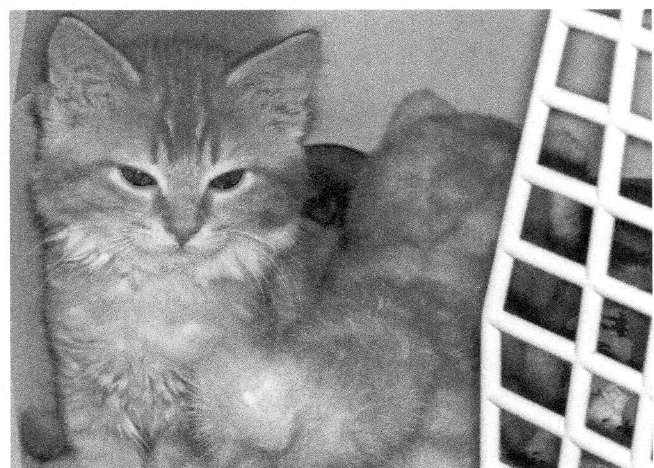

FIGURE 8-10 This kitten was trained during kitten class to get into the carrier.

ADULT (3 TO 6 YEARS) AND MATURE (7 TO 10 YEARS)

A decline in play activity in adult and mature cats increases susceptibility to weight gain. Three 10- to 15-minute play sessions daily can lead to a loss of approximately 1% of body weight in 1 month with no food intake restrictions.[18]

SENIOR (11 TO 14 YEARS)

Veterinarians should always evaluate senior cats with behavioral changes (e.g., vocalization, changes in litter box usage) for an underlying medical problem.[74] One study found that 28% of pet cats 11 to 14 years of age develop at least one behavioral problem, increasing to more than 50% cats over 15 years of age.[61] Clients should be educated about subtle behavior changes that are not just part of the normal aging process. Osteoarthritis is common in senior and geriatric cats; placement of ramps so that the cat can get to higher places, soft bedding, and a lower front lip on litter boxes decrease the risk of behavioral problems and improve the cat's quality of life.

GERIATRIC (15 YEARS AND OVER)

The client should be reminded to ensure the cat's accessibility to its litter box, bed, and food and to monitor the cat for signs of pain and osteoarthritis. Geriatric cats may also exhibit a decline of cognitive function, with confusion. Vocalization may be caused by several geriatric conditions (e.g., vision or hearing loss, hypertension, hyperthyroidism, and cognitive dysfunction). It is important to help clients assess quality-of-life issues. A mobility and cognitive dysfunction questionnaire is provided in the AAFP Senior Care Guidelines to help clients identify problems earlier.[74]

Grooming and Claw Care

Scratching is a normal feline behavior used for stretching, conditioning of claws, and marking of territory both visually and with scent. It is important to teach clients that scratching is a normal behavior that can be directed to areas that they consider appropriate. Scratching materials preferred by most cats are wood, sisal rope, and rough fabric. Because cats often stretch and scratch when they awaken, the posts should be placed near the cat's sleeping area. Many cats prefer vertical scratching posts; however, if a cat continues to scratch on carpets, horizontal scratching posts should be offered as well. Vertical posts should be sturdy and tall enough for the cat to be able to fully stretch. In multicat households there should be several scratching posts, both vertical and horizontal, located throughout the house.

Owners can train kittens and cats to use scratching posts by enticing them to the post with catnip, treats, or toys and rewarding behavior on the scratching post. If the cat scratches elsewhere, it should be picked up gently and taken to the scratching post and then rewarded. If the cat continues to go to the other area, the owner should use double-sided adhesive tape or a cover with a texture the cat that the cat finds unappealing. As previously stated, cats should be rewarded or positively reinforced for desirable behavior and never punished verbally or physically.

Feline onychectomy, or declawing, is illegal in Australia, New Zealand, Israel, and many European countries. Although declawing was once considered a routine procedure in the United States, it is now ethically controversial. The current position statements (see Box 8-1) of the AVMA, the Canadian Veterinary Medical Association, the AAFP, and the AAHA state that declawing should be considered only after efforts are made to prevent the cat from using the claws destructively (e.g., scratching posts, nail trimming) or for cats that live with immunocompromised people for whom clawing may present a zoonotic disease or injury risk. Zoonotic disease potential should be discussed and documented in the medical record. If declawing is performed, four-paw declawing is not recommended; keeping the hind claws allows the cat some means of protection, and property destruction and human injury occur less commonly with the rear claws. There are good alternatives to onychectomy, including training cats to use scratching posts and trimming their nails regularly. In most cases clients can be taught to trim nails, especially with kittens. Nails should be trimmed in a calm environment, and the cat should be positively reinforced. In addition to nail-trimming demonstrations, at-home education can be reinforced with client educational handouts or a video on nail trimming (see Box 8-1). The client educational handout "How To Prevent Cats from Scratching in Undesirable Areas" is provided at the end of the AAFP Feline Behavior Guidelines.[70] Another alternative is temporary synthetic nail caps that are usually applied every 4 to 6 weeks.

Although declawing is controversial, there is no scientific evidence that it leads to behavioral abnormalities. Declawed cats should be housed indoors or allowed outside only with strict supervision. If surgical onychectomy is performed, multimodal pain management, including local nerve blocks and perioperative analgesia for an appropriate length of time, is essential.

Although most cats do not need to be bathed, regular combing of the hair coat helps identify skin or coat problems more quickly, prevents matting, and decreases ingestion of excess fur. Certain types of coats may need more care. Brushing affects only the topcoat, but combing allows care of the undercoat as well. Overweight cats may have difficulty grooming themselves and require added attention, especially to the back half of the body.

Neutering

The benefits of ovariohysterectomy and castration are well known. They include prevention of feline overpopulation, infection, and neoplasia of reproductive organs and reduction in spraying and roaming tendencies. To further prevent the overpopulation problem, cats are often neutered at shelters before they are released to their new owners. Many studies show that pediatric neutering is safe and can be performed when the kitten is as young as 6 weeks of age.[44,88,91] A large study involving 1660 cats showed that early gonadectomy did not lead to significant medical or behavioral problems.[88] Steps should be taken to prevent hypoglycemia and hypothermia during anesthetic procedures in young kittens. For more on early-age spaying and neutering, see Chapter 41.

Minimum Database

The goal of the minimum database in apparently healthy cats is early disease detection and treatment. It is especially important in cats because they hide disease and may not show signs of illness until late in the disease process. The minimum database also serves to provide preanesthetic testing to identify problems that would otherwise not be detected, assisting in decisions about anesthesia. Early detection and treatment can lead to increased quality of life and longevity.

Performing an annual (or more frequent) minimum database allows veterinarians to establish a baseline for each individual patient and its normal values, which helps with early disease detection. A diagnostic test might fall within the normal range of the laboratory reference intervals but still be abnormal for the patient if there is an increasing trend. For example, a patient may have a normal serum creatinine concentration between 0.9 mg/dL and 1.1 mg/dL for several years, and then the creatinine may increase to 1.5 mg/dL the next year; although this value is still in the normal range, it is elevated for this individual patient, and further diagnostic testing and follow-up are indicated. Individual laboratory test comparisons can be made using summary sheets that provide results of all test results in chronologic order, allowing each specific test to be compared over years. Software is also available by which specific test results can be compared and graphed over time.

Laboratory profiles evaluate a number of tests at one time to better assess the overall health status of the patient. Although an individual test may provide some information, performing multiple tests at the same time often yields a more complete diagnostic assessment. Any one test result could be misleading without those from other tests and lead to misdiagnosis or partial diagnosis.[78] For example, serum alanine amino transferase (ALT) may be significantly elevated with hyperthyroidism, but if only ALT is analyzed, the veterinarian may focus on liver problems instead of the many other health conditions that may affect ALT.

There is high value to an individual cat when disease is found early, even when many tests yield normal results. However, routine laboratory testing of otherwise apparently normal animals increases the statistical likelihood of revealing test results that are outside of the normal range but not clinically significant. Interpretation of these values and decisions for further workup require clinical judgment in the context of the individual patient; additional workups are not always innocuous.[74]

The components of the minimum database for the different life stages can be found in Table 8-2. The incidence of many feline diseases increases with age.[74]

Although limited studies have been done to identify the age of onset of hyperthyroidism in cats, hyperthyroidism is considered to be the most common endocrine disorder in cats older than 8 years of age.[62] Total T_4 (TT_4) testing is recommended in all senior and geriatric cats, and veterinarians should strongly consider TT_4 testing in apparently healthy mature cats.[99] Many cats have concurrent chronic renal disease and hyperthyroidism, and each disease can affect the laboratory tests of the other; chronic kidney disease can decrease the TT_4 into the normal range, and hyperthyroidism can lead to a decreased serum creatinine value despite chronic renal disease.[37]

Hypertension, a common problem in senior cats, is most commonly associated with chronic renal disease or hyperthyroidism. Currently, Doppler ultrasound devices

TABLE 8-2 **Components of the Minimum Database for Different Life Stages**

	Kitten/Junior	Adult	Mature	Senior/Geriatric
Complete blood count + cytology	+/−	+/−	+	+
Chemistries + electrolytes	+/−	+/−	+	+
Urinalysis + sediment	+/−	+/−	+	+
Total T_4		+/−	+/−*	+
Blood pressure		+/−	+/−	+
FeLV/FIV testing	+	+/−	+/−	+/−
Fecal flotation	+	+	+	+

Adapted from Vogt AH, Rodan I, Brown M et al: AAFP-AAHA: feline life stage guidelines, *J Feline Med Surg* 12:43, 2010.

*The panel recommends that veterinarians strongly consider T_4 testing in apparently healthy mature cats. More incidence data are needed to make concrete recommendations.

are the most accurate blood pressure machine for small patients such as cats. To prevent "white-coat hypertension," the veterinarian should measure the cat's blood pressure in the examination room with the owner present. The cat should be allowed to acclimate to the room for at least 5 or 10 minutes; this can decrease anxiety-associated hypertension up to 20 mm Hg.[11] More information on sample collections is found in Chapter 1.

Retrovirus Testing

Feline leukemia virus (FeLV) and feline immunodeficiency virus (FIV) are among the most common infectious diseases of cats; in a study of more than 18,000 cats tested in the United States in 2004, 2.3% were seropositive for FeLV antigen and 2.5% were seropositive for FIV antibody.[50] A similar survey of more than 11,000 cats in Canada found that seroprevalence for FeLV antigen was 3.4% and seroprevalence for FIV antibody was 4.3%.[52] Although vaccines exist for both viruses, testing and segregation of infected cats are the cornerstone for prevention of spread to noninfected cats.

The FeLV and FIV status of all cats should be known. FeLV antigen and FIV antibody enzyme-linked immunosorbent assay (ELISA) tests are the screening tests of choice. Although these are excellent tests, no test is 100% accurate. However, negative test results for either FeLV or FIV are much more reliable than positive test results because of the low prevalence of infection in most cat populations. Positive test results should be confirmed. A cat with a confirmed-positive test result should be diagnosed as having a retroviral infection, not clinical disease; even in sickness, the cat infected with FeLV or FIV may not be sick as a result of the retrovirus infection. In fact, cats infected with FeLV or FIV may live for many years. A decision to euthanize should never be made solely on the basis of whether the cat is infected. Positive tests help identify infected cats so as to prevent exposure to others and influence patient management in preventive and illness care.

Two situations can cause false-positive FIV results: Cats vaccinated against FIV will be seropositive, and kittens younger than 6 months of age may test positive if the queen was infected or vaccinated and passed FIV antibodies to the kitten through the colostrum. Kittens that test positive for FIV antibodies should be retested every 60 days up to 6 months of age. If the kitten is seronegative at 6 months of age, it is unlikely to be infected.

All cats should be tested at appropriate intervals on the basis of risk assessment. This includes testing of all new cats entering a household or group housing (e.g., shelters). Cats with negative tests should be retested in 60 days or more; if retesting for FeLV and FIV separately, the veterinarian should retest for FeLV a minimum of 30 days after initial FeLV testing and a minimum of 60 days after initial FIV testing. This is especially helpful when clients cannot or will not keep the new cat separated from other cats in the household, because FeLV is more commonly transmitted among friendly cats. Testing should also occur before initial vaccination for FeLV or FIV, and annual retrovirus testing is recommended for cats that remain at risk of infection, regardless of vaccination status. Retrovirus testing is discussed in detail in the AAFP feline retrovirus management guidelines.[49]

Ringworm, especially that caused by *Microsporum canis,* is very common in cats housed in shelters; in one study up to 38% of cats housed in shelters were culture positive.[79] Fungal culture testing of all kittens and adult cats adopted from shelters can decrease the spread of this fungal agent to other pets and to people.

Genetic Testing

In the future genetic testing may become a more important part of wellness testing in veterinary medicine. Cats are subject to numerous genetic diseases, the most common being hypertrophic cardiomyopathy (various breeds as well as nonpedigreed cats) and polycystic kidney disease in Persians, Exotic Shorthairs, Himalayans, and any breeds with Persian ancestry.[9] Genetic testing can help breeders reduce the prevalence of genetic diseases (or eliminate them altogether) through informed breeding choices. Pet adopters also can identify cats with possible genetic problems before purchase, which is helpful for breeding and pet purposes. When clients want to purchase a cat of a breed with known genetic diseases, veterinarians can advise them to request results of genetic testing for both parents and, if available, the kitten. Many laboratories offering genetic testing accept samples collected with a cheek swab. Genetic test results should be recorded in the medical record in a location that is easy to find (e.g., master problem list).

For example, hypertrophic cardiomyopathy (HCM) genetic mutations have been identified in Maine Coon and Ragdoll cats. The prevalence of myosin-binding protein C mutation in Maine Coons worldwide is 34%.[29] In humans with this disease, there are many different causative genetic mutations, which also is likely to be the case in the cat, but to date most of these mutations have not been identified. It is important to recognize that absence of the identified mutations does not mean the cat will never develop HCM. The Veterinary Cardiac Genetics Laboratory of Washington State University and the University of California Veterinary Genetics Laboratory (see Box 8-1) offer HCM tests: one for the mutation found predominantly in Maine Coonss,[59] the other for Ragdolls.[60] Both the University of California and the University of Pennsylvania, Section of Medical Genetics, offer other feline genetic tests (see Box 8-1).

Blood typing is also recommended for breeds with a high prevalence of blood type B, such as Cornish and Devon Rex, Birmans, and British Shorthairs. If blood transfusion is needed for cats with blood type B, a donor with the same blood type is required to prevent a severe transfusion reaction (see Chapter 25). It makes sense to obtain the blood type of cats belonging to these breeds when they are kittens and to record the blood type prominently in the medical record.

More information about genetic testing is found in Chapter 44.

Dental Care

Dental disease is extremely common in cats and can affect feline health and welfare.[53] Client education about preventive dental care is crucial because the majority of cat owners do not understand the seriousness of this silent disease. As previously noted, cats rarely show signs of pain, and their difficulty chewing and other problems related to their dental disease may not be obvious. Left untreated, dental disease is often painful, can lead to inappetence, and can contribute to other local and systemic diseases. Fortunately, dental care allows for optimal health and quality of life.[41]

The compliance rate for preventive dental care in the United States is only 9% for cats,[56] which is less than that for any other needed preventive care.[1] As mentioned previously, cat owners generally have a higher level of education than dog owners and may become more compliant if they receive adequate information.[56] Incidence studies and other statistical information may help clients recognize that feline preventive dental care is necessary. In one study of 109 apparently healthy cats, 98.2% had periodontal disease.[34] The prevalence of tooth resorption lesions in cats in the same clinical environment showed lesions to be present in 70% of purebred cats and 38% of mixed-breed cats. These cats were fed only dry food and had annual dental scalings.[33]

Cats of all life stages need both home and veterinary dental care to allow for complete oral health—kittens for retained deciduous teeth and dentition problems and cats 2 years of age and older for periodontal disease and other problems.[41] The wellness examination is the ideal time to discuss dental health. An oral examination is included with each exam, and at least an annual examination is recommended for cats with healthy dentition. Semiannual examinations can help ensure optimal home care.[41] In addition, cats with gingivitis should be evaluated every 6 months, and more frequently if periodontitis is found.[41]

Evaluation of the oral cavity in the conscious feline patient allows the veterinarian to design a preliminary treatment plan[41]; anesthesia is required to perform a complete and thorough oral examination and formulate a precise treatment plan. Dental cleaning, periodontal probing with a dental explorer, and intraoral radiographs allow a complete assessment of the dental patient. Dental radiographs, and not skull films, are critical to evaluate the teeth and determine pathology when it is not otherwise apparent (Figure 8-11). Important pathology was found in one study in 41.7% of cats when no abnormal findings were noted in the awake patient.[98] When abnormal findings were noted in the conscious patient, dental radiographs revealed additional pathology in 53.9% of cats.[98]

Staff and client education is important to reinforce the concepts that most dental disease is hidden and that anesthesia with review of digital or intraoral radiographs is necessary for a complete oral examination. The veterinarian should discuss all safety measures taken to support the cat under anesthesia and pain management to prevent or control pain.

Terminology is also important; most people equate dental care with clean teeth and not oral health; this reduces compliance and client understanding of preventive dental care. Instead of saying, "Your cat needs a dental," veterinarians should explain to clients the benefits of oral health care and what is involved. For example, the veterinarian might say, "Dental prophylaxis is recommended for cats every year, starting at 1 year of age, to prevent periodontal disease."[41] Dental prophylaxis should be done in cats with an essentially healthy mouth or with mild gingivitis.[41] Patients with dental disease should undergo dental treatment or oral surgery. It is important to explain to clients that prophylaxis involves removing plaque and calculus both supragingivally (above the gum line) and subgingivally (below the gum line). Cleaning only above the gum line has no therapeutic effect; it is the plaque and calculus below the gum line that cause periodontal disease, the most common dental disease in cats. Dental prophylaxis includes several important steps, and the American Veterinary Dental Society has developed an excellent

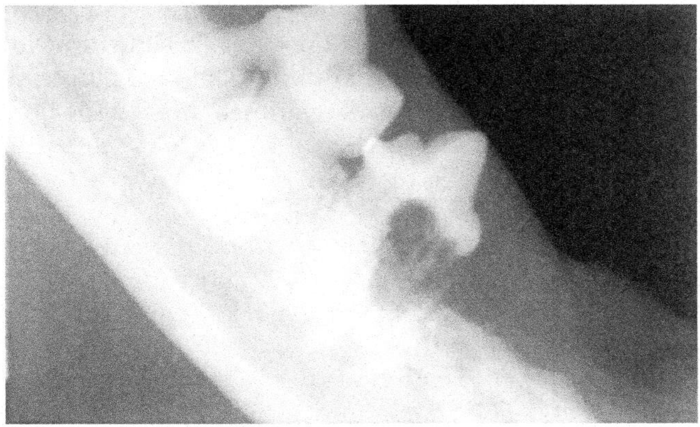

FIGURE 8-11 Dental radiographs identify tooth resorptive lesions that may not otherwise be evident and allow evaluation of other dental structures. *(Image courtesy Dr. Ilona Rodan.)*

educational piece that may be used to educate clients about the steps of dental prophylaxis and other needed dental care (see Box 8-1).

Home dental care should be addressed both at wellness appointments and after dental prophylaxis, with or without dental treatment. Home care can maintain or improve dental health.[77] Tooth brushing is the gold standard of home dental care. It is best to begin client education about tooth brushing when the patient is a kitten. However, even older cats can be trained to accept tooth brushing, and this should be recommended for them routinely. Client compliance for adult cats may increase if education follows dental prophylaxis or treatment because these clients are more aware of dental health problems. Tooth brushing should never be done in a forceful manner or when the client is at risk of being injured. It is best to train the cat with positive reinforcement, starting first by lifting the lips and immediately giving the cat a treat. Then the client can try to give the cat a little seafood or poultry toothpaste, which, with any luck, the cat will find palatable. The conditioning or training may take 1 week or more, but with continued positive reinforcement of the desired behavior, it is successful in most cats. Providing clients with verbal instruction and supplemental information on tooth brushing is helpful; the Cornell Feline Health Center has a helpful video (see Box 8-1).

Additional home care can include dental diets, treats, and chews that have been approved by the Veterinary Oral Health Council (VOHC), which certifies products as effective for plaque or calculus removal (or both); these products can be found on the VOHC website (see Box 8-1). This is especially helpful for clients who are unable or unwilling to brush teeth at home, but is likely not as effective as daily tooth brushing. (See Chapter 21 for more information on dental and oral diseases.)

Nutrition and Weight Management

Providing optimal nutrition is a crucial part of preventive health care for cats at all life stages. Feline nutrition and dietetics are covered in more detail in Chapters 15 to 19, but some of the basics relating to preventive health care are briefly reviewed here.

Diet Basics

Cats are obligate carnivores, with a predatory rather than scavenging natural lifestyle and a preference for consumption of frequent small meals. Their natural diet, which consists mainly of wild rodents, is relatively high in protein and fat, and in studies cats show a preference for synthetic diets that mimic this profile.[27,73] As obligate carnivores, cats have a high protein requirement, and a number of animal-derived nutrients (e.g., the amino acids taurine and arginine; vitamins A, D, and B_3 [niacin]; and the polyunsaturated fatty acids arachidonic acid and docosahexaenoic acid) are obligatory in their diets, although these may not be absolutely essential during all life stages.[6,64]

The precise energy and nutrient requirements of cats vary depending on various factors such as age (e.g., increased nutrient demand during growth and reduced digestibility in older cats), activity levels, neutering status, and pregnancy and lactation. Although home-prepared diets may be used to support all feline life stages, ensuring that all macronutritional and micronutritional needs are adequately provided in such foods can be problematic, and there may be risks associated with the use or feeding of raw foods (e.g., transmission of infectious diseases). Commercially available dry or wet foods that meet the specific nutritional requirements of cats at the appropriate life stage and have been tested in feeding trials are the best way to ensure that a diet is satisfactory.[99] Development of food preferences in cats is complex and incompletely understood. Studies of feeding behavior in cats have demonstrated a so-called monotony effect in which cats may develop an aversion to foods that have formed a large part of their diet. This may be a protective mechanism; eating a variety of foods may reduce the likelihood of an unbalanced or deficient diet. However, although the monotony effect has been demonstrated in both kittens and adults, it appears to be much stronger in free-ranging cats and can be abrogated, at least in part, in cats raised on nutritionally complete diets.[10] Kittens are also strongly influenced in their food preferences by their mothers,[10,101] and a primacy effect may be seen whereby adult cats develop a strong preference for their weaning or normal diet.[10,90]

Feeding Regimens

Many feeding regimens may be successful in maintaining feline nutritional health, including both free access to daily food rations and provision of food in meals. It is impossible to replicate the natural diet or feeding conditions of wild cats, but partially mimicking this by placing dry food in foraging devices (e.g., food balls or puzzles) or dispensing the food in multiple small meals in several widely dispersed places (which may include hiding the food) may help in slowing food intake and providing mental and physical stimulation.[99] Cats should be fed away from toileting areas (e.g., litter boxes), and quiet areas should be chosen, especially for nervous cats. For healthy cats there is no evidence to suggest that feeding a single diet or feeding a variety of diets (or flavors) is beneficial or detrimental, and the preferences of an individual cat may be determined in part by food exposure at the time of weaning.

Neither wet (canned) nor dry commercial foods mimic the texture, consistency, or energy density of the natural feline diet, but both have been demonstrated to be effective in maintaining optimal nutrition. For healthy cats there is no evidence to suggest that either dry or wet foods are preferable, and the choice depends largely on owner preference.[13,99] However, in certain conditions in which increased water intake is desirable, feeding wet rather than dry foods may help achieve this goal.

Factors to Consider When Changing Diets

A change of diet may be necessary for medical or other reasons at various times in the cat's life. Changing the diet can be problematic for a number of reasons, including those associated with food preference. In individual cats the monotony effect (i.e., the desire to explore alternative food sources) or the primacy effect (i.e., the desire to maintain the same food source) may dominate. Acceptance of a new food is generally easier in cats in which the monotony effect dominates, but because development of food preferences is complex, feeding patterns that would achieve this are difficult to recommend. Neither previous feeding of a single food nor previous feeding of a variety of foods is necessarily associated with increased ease in introducing a new food.

General considerations with the introduction of a new food are to provide an isocaloric intake comparable to that of the old food (unless specific adjustments are necessary) and to offer the new diet along with the old diet for a period of time, perhaps mixing the two and gradually increasing the proportion of the new diet. Mixing the diets may increase acceptance of the new diet, but this also may result in both food types being rejected. A gradual change to a different diet will help increase acceptance of a new diet and also minimize the risks of any gastrointestinal disturbance that might occur with a sudden change. Warming the new diet and increasing its palatability by adding fish juice may help.[99]

Weight Management

Obesity, generally defined as 20% or more above ideal body weight, is prevalent in cats in many Western countries. Estimates of the number of obese or overweight cats vary between 5% and 50%. Obesity is associated with a number of other diseases, such as diabetes mellitus, hepatic lipidosis, osteoarthritis, and lower urinary tract disease.[19,103] Obesity is most prevalent in middle-aged cats, and recognized risk factors include neutering, gender (it is more prevalent in males), lack of exercise (indoors only, no other animals in the house), and the owner's tendency to underestimate the cat's body condition.[4,19,81,82] Interestingly, a study from the Netherlands showed an association between the degree of obesity in dogs and the body mass index of the owners, but no such relationship was found for cats and their owners.[69] Nevertheless, the complex human–pet interactions associated with feeding are undoubtedly an important component in the high prevalence of obesity.[47]

Neutering appears to be a major contributory factor to the development of obesity, with both male and female cats being less active after neutering and undergoing hormonal changes that also contribute to obesity, such as reduced lipoprotein lipase, adiponectin activity, and insulin sensitivity and increased leptin, prolactin, and insulin-like growth factor-1 expression.[7,40,58]

Prevention of obesity after neutering is a crucial goal in preventive veterinary medicine, and careful discussions with clients should include the need to restrict caloric intake after neutering by carefully measuring daily food allocations and avoiding *ad libitum* feeding, the importance of encouraging activity, and the potential value of altering diet type (e.g., increased moisture, air, or fiber) to help control caloric intake. Regular monitoring of body weight and body condition score along with appropriate adjustments of caloric intake are vital. Neutered cats are likely to need approximately 30% fewer calories than typically indicated in feeding guidelines printed on cat food packaging.[103] Using food balls, hiding food, and encouraging foraging through other means can be valuable ways both to increase exercise and to prevent overeating at meal times (Figure 8-12).[99]

Parasite Control

Effective control and prevention of parasites is of considerable importance both to promote the health of kittens and cats and to prevent zoonotic infections. Control of ectoparasites is found in Chapter 22, and specific endoparasite infections are covered in Chapter 23. This section focuses on preventive health care as it relates to the major endoparasite infections.

Various studies have been published evaluating the prevalence of gastrointestinal parasites in cats by fecal or postmortem examination. Results of some of these

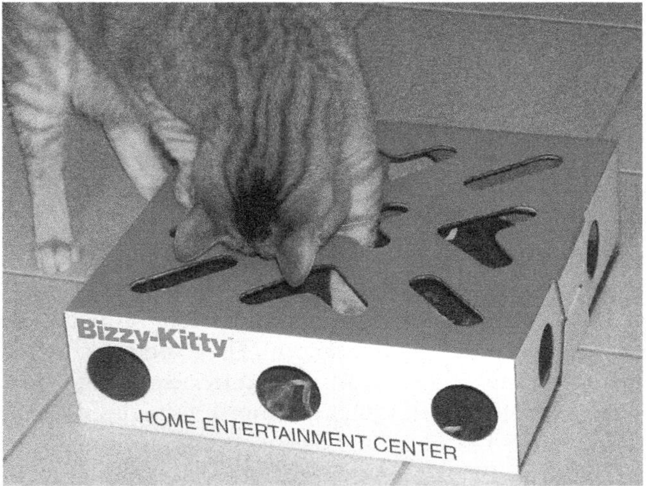

FIGURE 8-12 Hiding kibbles and toys in a puzzle box simulates hunting for food. *(Image courtesy Dr. Ilona Rodan.)*

TABLE 8-3 **Prevalence of Selected Gastrointestinal Parasites Found in Seven Different Studies**

	Gates & Nolan[32]	Gow et al[36]	Barutzki & Schaper[5]	Yamamoto et al[102]	Calvete et al[15]	Nichol et al[68]	Palmer et al[72]
Year	2009	2009	2003	2009	1998	1981	2007
Country	U.S.	U.K.	Germany	Japan	Spain	U.K.	Australia
Number of cats	1566	57	3167	1079	58	92	572
Toxocara cati	7.5%	15.7%	26.2%	21.8%	55.2%	53.3%	3.2%
Toxascaris leonina	0.1%	0	0			1.1%	0.3%
Ancylostoma spp.	0.5%	0	0.3%	13.2%	29.3%		0%
Isospora felis	3.7%	7%	15.3%	4.5%		4.3%	5.6%
Isospora rivolta	1.2%	0	7.9%	2.2%			2.7%
Taenia taeniaformis	0.3%	0	2.6%	0.2%	8.6%	12.0%	0
Dipylidium caninum	0.8%	0	0.1%	1.4%	20.7%	38.4%	0.2%

studies are shown in Table 8-3. The data from different countries and studies are clearly not comparable insofar as the prevalence of infection largely depends on the age, background, and lifestyle of the cats examined and is also affected by the detection technique used. In general, nematode (with the exception of hookworms) and protozoal infections are more common in young cats, whereas cestode and hookworm infections tend to be more common in adults. Infections are generally also more common in stray or feral cats and in cats from multicat environments. Also, there are geographic variations in the prevalence of parasites, with some having a restricted distribution.

Although a variety of diagnostic tests are valuable in assessing the presence of endoparasites, fecal flotation techniques are commonly employed in veterinary clinical practice to diagnose and demonstrate infection with common endoparasites such as helminths, nematodes, and coccidia. Commonly used solutions for fecal flotation techniques include zinc sulfate (331 g $ZnSO_4$ in 1 L water, for a specific gravity [SG] of 1.18 to 1.20), magnesium sulfate (450 g $MgSO_4$ in 1 L water, for a SG of 1.20), and saturated salt (350 g NaCL in 1 L water, for a SG of 1.18 to 1.20). However, studies in dogs (which can be assumed to be applicable to cats) indicate that using a modified Sheather's sugar solution that produces a higher SG of 1.27 (454 g granulated sugar dissolved in 355 mL hot water with 6 mL formaldehyde to prevent microbial growth) is considerably more efficient in diagnosing common infections. This method yields fewer false-negative results (studies used 2 g feces mixed with 10 mL flotation solution), especially when dealing with heavier worm eggs such as *Taenia* spp. Furthermore, the use of a centrifugation–flotation technique (280 g for 5 minutes) followed by a standing time of 10 minutes was also much more sensitive than using a simple standing flotation technique, even allowing up to 20 minutes standing time for the latter.[22] These studies emphasize the importance of using the correct techniques to optimize results from routine fecal examinations.

According to the CAPC (see Box 8-1) in the United States, client awareness of intestinal parasites is low, and knowledge of the zoonotic risks is even lower. Among the zoonotic parasites, *Toxocara cati* has recently been increasingly recognized as a potential cause of visceral and ocular larval migrans in humans.[28] Both the CAPC and the European Scientific Counsel Companion Animal Parasites (ESCCAP) (see Box 8-1) publish guidelines on the diagnosis and prevention of parasitic infections of dogs and cats. Together, the 2008 CAPC guidelines and the 2006 ESCCAP guidelines carry a number of recommendations, including the following:

- Parasite control should be guided by veterinarians and should be adapted to the individual needs of the animal (e.g., those dictated by regional and epidemiologic data, the lifestyle of the cat, such as access to intermediate and paratenic hosts, and the health status and history of the cat).
- Pet owners should be informed of the risks of parasitic infections to their pets and to humans, and responsible pet ownership should be promoted.
- Pet populations should be protected from the risks associated with increased travel of pets between geographic areas, and the impact this can have on the spread of parasites should be considered (ESCCAP, 2006).
- Regular year-round broad-spectrum parasite control (including heartworm, where indicated) should be undertaken for the life of the pet.

- Regular fecal examinations are recommended, two to four times in the first year of life and one to two times per year in adults (CAPC, 2008). Fecal testing can be used to monitor the effectiveness of preventive programs.
- Pets should be fed commercial diets or cooked foods to prevent raw meat–transmitted parasites.
- Good hygiene measures should be taken, including cleaning up feces regularly (at least daily) to reduce environmental contamination and zoonotic risks. Particular attention should be given to worm control in cats with free access to outdoors given the difficulty of controlling where they defecate (ESCCAP 2006), and children's sandboxes should always be covered when not in use.
- All staff within the veterinary clinic should be aware of protocols to control parasitic infections, and these protocols should be applied in a consistent way.
- Special care should be taken in giving accurate information to immunocompromised pet owners or caregivers and other groups that may be more susceptible to zoonotic disease, such as infants and young children, people with learning difficulties, and people with occupational risks.

Client-oriented information is available from both CAPC and ESCCAP to help educate owners, and the United States Centers for Disease Control website (see Box 8-1) also provides information on a variety of zoonoses. A detailed and comprehensive review of feline endoparasites is beyond the scope of this chapter, but a brief overview of the major worms of concern with routine prophylaxis is provided in the following sections.

Toxocara cati *and* Toxascaris leonina

Toxocara cati and *Toxascaris leonina* are prevalent ascarid (roundworm) nematode infections in cats, and most cats are thought to become infected at some point in their lives. Generally *T. cati* is more commonly encountered than *T. leonina*, and both are more common in kittens and young cats than adults. Adult worms measuring 8 to 15 cm in length are found in the small intestine, with ova being shed in the feces after a prepatent period of approximately 5 to 7 weeks for *T. cati* and around 9 to 12 weeks for *T. leonina*. The life cycle can be either direct (through ingestion of infective ova) or indirect (through ingestion of infected paratenic hosts such as rodents, birds, worms, or mollusks). In contrast to dogs, there is no transplacental migration with *Toxocara* spp. in cats, although infection with *T. cati* leads to liver–lung migration of larvae, and because larvae may also be present in the milk of queens, they can be transmitted to neonatal kittens. Diagnosis of infection is through fecal flotation techniques to demonstrate the presence of ova. However, routine fecal examination may not always detect the presence of an infection, and because these ascarids are prevalent and *T. cati* should be considered a zoonosis, routine prophylaxis (discussed later) is always recommended.

Dipylidium caninum

In general *Dipylidium caninum* is the most prevalent cestode infection of cats, although geographic and lifestyle variations exist. Mature worms are 20 to 50 cm in length and shed motile proglottids (containing egg sacs) in the feces. The proglottids, which resemble rice grains, may also be observed around the perineum, and egg packets can be seen microscopically in the feces. Flea larvae ingest eggs from the environment, and the life cycle is completed when cats ingest infected fleas during grooming. The prepatent period is approximately 3 weeks. Because fleas are the intermediate host, cats may be infected from a young age. Humans are occasionally infected also by ingesting infected fleas.

Taenia taeniaformis

Taenia taeniaformis is generally the most prevalent *Taenia* spp. infecting cats, although geographic variations occur. *Taenia* spp. are usually found in cats that are active hunters or are fed raw meat, which is the primary source of infection (intermediate hosts). Adult worms are approximately 60 cm in length and shed proglottids in the feces. Rodents and lagomorphs act as intermediate hosts for *T. taeniaformis*, and after ingestion there is a prepatent period of 4 to 11 weeks. Diagnosis is by observation of proglottids or identification of taeniid eggs in feces by flotation or sedimentation.

Ancylostoma *and* Uncinaria *spp.*

Cats are host to several hookworm species, the most widely distributed of which is *Ancylostoma tubaeforme*. Although *Uncinaria stenocephala* has a wide geographic distribution, cats are relatively resistant to infection with this worm. Adults in the small intestine are typically 1 to 3 cm long, eggs are passed in the feces, and larvae that develop are infective for either cats or paratenic hosts. Cats are infected by cutaneous penetration of larvae, ingestion of larvae, or ingestion of an infected paratenic host (e.g., rodents), and there is a prepatent period of 2 to 4 weeks. There is no evidence of transplacental or transmammary transmission of hookworms in cats, but humans can also be infected (cutaneous larva migrans). Infection can be demonstrated by detecting eggs in feces by flotation.

Dirofilaria immitis

Although more resistant to infection than dogs (the prevalence of infection in cats is generally approximately 10% of that seen in dogs), cats can host heartworm, with small numbers of adult worms developing in some (in the right ventricle and pulmonary artery). Infections in cats are usually more severe than in dogs, and *Dirofilaria immitis* is an important cause of morbidity and mortality in cats. There is a wide geographic distribution for *D. immitis*, with infection being more prevalent in tropical and subtropical climates where the mosquito intermediate hosts exist. Diagnosis of *D. immitis* infection in cats relies on a combination of antigen and antibody tests and also echocardiography, which may demonstrate adult worms in the right side of the heart, the caudal vena cava, or the pulmonary arteries.[51] Radiographs of the chest may show enlargement of the caudal lobar arteries and a bronchointerstitial lung pattern (heartworm-associated respiratory disease) that may mimic feline asthma. Treatment of cats infected with adult *D. immitis* is not recommended because this can induce fatal reactions, which underscores the importance of prophylaxis to prevent infection with this parasite in cats.

Routine Endoparasite Prophylaxis in Kittens

Because prenatal infection does not occur in kittens, both the CAPC and ESCCAP recommend starting prophylactic roundworm and hookworm therapy at 3 weeks of age, with treatment being repeated every 2 weeks until the kitten is 9 weeks of age. The CAPC then recommends that kittens receive monthly therapy along with the nursing queen. In heartworm-endemic areas, choosing a monthly preventive therapy for heartworm that also has efficacy against roundworms is a sensible approach to control.

Routine Endoparasite Prophylaxis for All Life Stages

The ESCCAP guidelines note that annual or twice-annual therapy for roundworms and hookworms does not have any significant impact on patent shedding of eggs, and continued monthly therapy is appropriate, especially in situations of increased risk, such as when the cat resides in a household with children or is allowed free access outdoors (where they may be defecating and contaminating the environment). Monthly therapy for hookworms and roundworms is also recommended by the CAPC as ideal for adults. In lower-risk situations, ESCCAP recommends a minimum therapy frequency of four times a year. Whether a narrow- or broad-spectrum anthelmintic is used depends on the risk of exposure to other parasites, and fecal testing two to four times a year not only helps monitor the effectiveness of the prophylaxis but also may allow identification of parasite infections not covered by the routine anthelmintics being used.

Infection with cestodes is more common in adults than kittens, and the risk is directly related to contact with, and access to, intermediate hosts. Prevention of predation, provision of commercial foods or fully cooked meat only, and avoidance or prevention of flea infestations will minimize the risk of cestode infection. However, when such risks cannot be completely controlled, routine prophylaxis is indicated and a broad-spectrum anthelmintic (rather than a narrow-spectrum type that controls only ascarids and hookworms) should be selected.

Both indoor and outdoor cats are at risk of infection with heartworm, and routine prophylaxis is important in areas where the parasite is endemic or when cats may move to such areas (e.g., cats that vacation with owners in such areas). In these cases monthly prophylaxis is recommended. Testing (serum antigen and antibody tests) of cats before commencement of therapy is recommended by both the CAPC and the ESCCAP to detect any cats already infected; using products that are adulticide in an infected cat may create a life-threatening reaction, and adulticide treatment is therefore not generally recommended for cats at this time. There is no evidence that it improves survival in infected cats, and the death of adult worms can be life threatening. However, the American Heartworm Society (see Box 8-1) recommends monthly doses of oral ivermectin or milbemycin oxime or topical moxidectin or selamectin as chemoprophylaxis against heartworm infection from 8 weeks of age in cats in endemic areas, and administration of these drugs is not precluded by a positive serum antigen or antibody test. Many heartworm preventives also provide control of other parasites, and the spectrum of activity of some anthelmintics used in cats is shown in Table 8-4.

TABLE 8-4 Spectrum of Activity of Selected Anthelmintics and Combinations of Anthelmintics

Drug	Ascarids	Hookworms	Cestodes	Heartworm
Piperazine	X	X		
Pyrantel	X	X		
Benzimidazoles	X	X	X*	
Praziquantel			X	
Milbemycin	X	X		X
Ivermectin		X		X
Pyrantel/ praziquantel	X	X	X	
Selamectin	X	X		X
Imidacloprid/ moxidectin	X	X		X
Milbemycin/ praziquantel	X	X	X	X

*Not *Dipylidium caninum*.

Vaccination

Prevention of disease is the ultimate goal of veterinarians, and the widespread use of vaccines undoubtedly has contributed greatly to achievement of that goal. However, the current prevalence of vaccination in cat populations is not sufficiently high to achieve a good level of herd immunity, and elimination of infectious agents,[42] with only an estimated 25% of cats in North America ever being vaccinated.[84] The practical implication of this statistic is that a more realistic goal is containment and control of infection in defined populations of cats (e.g., multicat environments), along with protection of the individual animal against disease and infection. However, the value of reaching a much wider population of cats with vaccination should not be underestimated, and the WSAVA Vaccine Guidelines Group (VGG) has stated that the aim should be to vaccinate *every* animal but each individual animal less frequently.[21]

Vaccination is not an entirely innocuous procedure, and side effects sometimes occur. The prevalence of adverse events associated with vaccination has recently been reported to be less than 1%, depending on the vaccine and method of data collection.[31,35,63] It is important to note that most of these reactions are mild and transient. In one study risk of an adverse reaction after vaccination was greatest for cats of approximately 1 year of age, and lethargy with or without fever was the most commonly reported reaction.[63] Female cats were at greater risk than male cats of the same neuter status. Although breed was not associated with increased risk in this study, in another report based on a passive surveillance system in the United Kingdom, some breeds were overrepresented.[31] Occasionally, though, severe and life-threatening events can occur, such as hypersensitivity reactions or injection-site sarcomas.[20,42] Such devastating effects, although rare, challenge the assumption that vaccine choice and vaccination intervals are not important considerations. Adverse events should be reported to both the product manufacturer and the appropriate regulatory authority. In the United States this is the Department of Agriculture, Center for Veterinary Biologics (http://www.aphis.usda.gov), in Canada this is the Canadian Food Inspection Agency (http://www.inspection.gc.ca), and in the United Kingdom this is the Veterinary Medicines Directorate (http://www.vmd.gov.uk).

Although in the past there was a tendency to recommend annual booster vaccinations for all or most vaccines, scientific data are increasingly becoming available to demonstrate the true duration of immunity (DOI) after the use of different vaccines, which provides a more rational basis for the recommendations regarding the frequency of booster inoculations. There has also been an interest in measurement of immune responses to predict resistance to infection and determine whether revaccination is required. For most feline infectious agents, the presence of serum antibodies indicates that the cat has the immunologic memory required to mount a rapid anamnestic response if exposed to the agent. Unfortunately, local immune responses, particularly important for certain respiratory and gastrointestinal tract pathogens, are not easily measured. Information about vaccine-induced serum antibody responses and resistance to infection has been collected primarily for feline panleukopenia virus (FPV), feline herpesvirus (FHV-1), and feline calicivirus (FCV). For FPV cats with serum antibodies from vaccination within the previous 7 years are protected against challenge.[80] However, the situation is not as clear for FHV-1 and FCV because vaccination against these pathogens does not reliably induce sterilizing immunity. The predictive value of serum antibody titers to determine the need for revaccination is unclear.[80] It is important to note that antibody tests offered by laboratories should not be assumed to be equivalent and virus neutralization assays are probably the best predictor of resistance to infection. Finally, failure to demonstrate serum antibodies against FPV, FCV, or FHV-1 does not necessarily indicate susceptibility to infection but should be taken as an indicator that revaccination is likely beneficial.

Three international panels have been established to provide guidelines on feline vaccination protocols (Table 8-5): the AAFP Vaccine Advisory Panel, which most recently reported in 2006[80]; the WSAVA VGG, which reported in 2007[21]; and the European Advisory Board on Cat Diseases (ABCD), which reported in 2009.* The major recommendations, made by all three of these bodies, are summarized as follows:

- Vaccines should not be given needlessly.
- An annual health examination is advisable irrespective of whether vaccines are given.
- Owners should be involved with discussions, and the risks and benefits of vaccination should be explained so that informed consent is given.
- Adverse reactions to vaccines should be properly reported to vaccine manufacturers and regulatory authorities.
- Vaccines should be classified as *core* (i.e., vaccination of *all* cats is justifiable) and *noncore* (i.e., vaccination can be justified only in certain circumstances).
- Booster vaccination schedules include extended intervals (beyond the traditional 12 months), especially for the core vaccines (for which more data are available), but choices should be made on an individual basis, and protocols cannot be formulated that are suitable for all cats in all circumstances.

Certain circumstances may influence a cat's ability to respond to vaccination. Cats and kittens should always receive a complete physical examination before

*References 3, 24, 30, 38, 43, 57, 76, 94, 97.

TABLE 8-5 **Summary of Feline Vaccination Recommendations from the AAFP, WSAVA, and ABCD Vaccine Guideline Groups**

Vaccine	Initial Series: Kittens (<16 Weeks)	Initial Series: Adults (>16 Weeks)	Boosters
CORE VACCINES			
FPV	First dose at 8 weeks (or as early as 6 weeks), booster every 3-4 weeks until 16 weeks old	Two doses, 3-4 weeks apart	Booster 1 year after last kitten vaccine, then no more often than every 3 years
FHV-1 + FCV	First dose at 8 weeks (or as early as 6 weeks), booster every 3-4 weeks until 16 weeks old	Two doses, 3-4 weeks apart	Booster 1 year after last kitten vaccine, then no more often than every 3 years
Rabies: Canarypox virus-vectored	Start as early as 8 weeks, revaccination 1 year later	Two doses, 1 year apart	Annually, or every 3 years, depending on local laws and product licensing
Rabies: Killed virus	Start as early as 12 weeks, revaccination 1 year later	Two doses, 1 year apart	Annually, or every 3 years, depending on local laws and product licensing
NONCORE VACCINES			
FeLV	Start as early as 8 weeks, booster 3-4 weeks later	Two doses, 3-4 weeks apart	Booster 1 year after last kitten vaccine, then annually for cats at ongoing risk (ABCD recommends booster vaccines every 2-3 years after 3-4 years of age)
FIV	Start as early as 8 weeks, booster every 2-3 weeks for 2 additional doses (3 doses required)	Three doses required, administered 2-3 weeks apart	Booster 1 year after last kitten vaccine, then annually for cats at ongoing risk
FIP	First dose at 16 weeks, booster 3-4 weeks later	Two doses, 3-4 weeks apart	Annual booster recommended by vaccine manufacturer
Chlamydophila felis	Start as early as 9 weeks, booster 3-4 weeks later	Two doses, 3-4 weeks apart	Annual booster for cats at ongoing risk
Bordetella bronchiseptica	Single dose as early as 8 weeks	Single dose	Annual booster for cats at ongoing risk

FPV, Feline panleukopenia virus; *FHV,* feline herpesvirus; *FCV,* feline calicivirus; *FeLV,* feline leukemia virus; *FIV,* feline immunodeficiency virus; *FIP,* feline infectious peritonitis.

vaccination to determine age, existence of illness, and factors that may affect the immune response. Maternally derived antibodies (MDAs) may affect the ability of kittens to respond to vaccination. In most kittens MDA is lost by 9 to 12 weeks of age, but this may occur either earlier (6 weeks of age or earlier) or later (as late as 16 weeks of age) depending on the individual and the pathogen. Little data exist to determine whether senior cats respond to vaccination as do younger cats. In the absence of data, healthy senior cats and those with stable chronic diseases should receive vaccinations as do younger cats.[80]

In cats with acute disease, high fevers, or debilitation, vaccination should be delayed until the cat has recovered.[80] Vaccination of cats with chronic but stable illnesses may be done at the discretion of the veterinarian. Another common situation facing veterinarians is vaccination of cats on chronic corticosteroid therapy. Corticosteroids may cause suppression of immune responses, but studies evaluating vaccine efficacy and safety in cats receiving corticosteroids are lacking. The concurrent use of corticosteroids at the time of vaccination should be avoided when practical.[80]

Core vaccines can be administered to healthy FIV- and FeLV-infected cats, and noncore vaccine should be used only if justified by risk of exposure. Cats with FeLV may not receive protection from vaccination comparable to that achieved in uninfected cats.[80] Healthy FIV-infected cats are able to mount an immune response to vaccination. It is not known if cats with FIV may develop vaccine-induced disease. The administration of killed virus vaccines is recommended when possible.

Generally, vaccines are administered at intervals of 3 to 4 weeks. The minimum interval between vaccinations is 2 weeks, and the maximum recommended interval is 4 weeks.[80] If a kitten is presented for a booster vaccination 6 weeks or longer after the previous dose, at least two doses of vaccine should be administered, 3 to 4 weeks apart.[80] Adult cats of unknown vaccination status may receive a single modified live virus core vaccination, with a booster 1 year later. If a killed virus core vaccine product is used, adult cats should receive two injections, 3 to 4 weeks apart, with a booster vaccination 1 year later. The exception is rabies vaccine, wherein one injection is given with a booster 1 year later. Any brand of vaccine is suitable as a booster; it is not necessary to use the same brand as for the previous immunization.

Kittens are typically enrolled in socialization classes between 7 and 14 weeks of age, too young to have received a complete set of vaccinations. Ideally class size should be limited to fewer than eight kittens, and kittens should receive at least one FPV, FHV-1, and FCV vaccine at least 10 days before the first class.[80]

Feline Panleukopenia Virus

Vaccination against FPV is usually highly effective, with most vaccinated cats being completely protected against disease and infection. Although vaccination is highly efficacious, FPV remains a prevalent virus and all three feline vaccine guideline groups (FVGGs) recommend FPV as a core vaccine. In kittens vaccination should start as early as 6 to 8 weeks of age, and inoculations should be repeated every 3 to 4 weeks until the cat is 16 to 20 weeks of age. Giving a final vaccine at 16 to 20 weeks of age helps ensure optimal vaccine efficacy in those cats in which high levels of MDAs may prevent an effective response at an earlier age. Modified live vaccines should not be used in kittens younger than 4 weeks of age or in pregnant queens because of the risk of cerebellar damage in the developing brain. In high-risk situations, modified live injectable vaccines may provide a more rapid onset of immunity, whereas intranasal vaccines may be less effective. In FeLV- and FIV-infected cats and in immunocompromised cats, using a killed rather than a modified live vaccine is recommended.

Studies have demonstrated a prolonged DOI after successful vaccination with FPV, and therefore all three FVGGs have recommended a booster at 1 year of age followed by boosters no more frequently than every 3 years.

Feline Herpesvirus and Feline Calicivirus

Both FHV-1 and FCV are ubiquitous viruses; infection is extremely common, and vaccination plays a major role in controlling disease. Vaccination is important in protecting cats from disease and reducing the severity of disease in infected cats, although it does not necessarily prevent infection with these viruses (partly because there are many different strains of FCV, and partly because of the inherent difficulty in inducing sterilizing immunity against these viruses). Vaccinated cats can also become carriers and pass infection to others. Because of the prevalent nature of these viruses and the severe disease they sometimes cause, all three FVGGs recommend these as core vaccines. Similar to FPV, recommendations are to start vaccination at 6 to 9 weeks of age and repeat every 3 to 4 weeks until 16 weeks of age. Early vaccination (from around 4 to 6 weeks of age) is particularly appropriate in high-risk situations or where MDA status is questionable. As with FPV, in FeLV- and FIV-infected cats and those that are immunocompromised, killed vaccines are recommended.

Both the AAFP and WSAVA guidelines suggest giving the first booster at 1 year of age, followed by booster inoculations every 3 years (although the AAFP suggests considering additional boosters if the cat is going to enter a known high-risk situation, such as a boarding cattery). In contrast, the ABCD guidelines generally recommend annual boosters for FHV-1 in all but low-risk situations and boosters every 3 years for FCV. However, the ABCD defines low-risk cats as those that are kept strictly indoors and have no contact with other cats; it might be arguable as to whether these cats should be defined as low risk insofar as their lifestyle affords little or no exposure to respiratory viruses and therefore little or no opportunity for natural boosting of immunity.

Although at least one commercial vaccine has been made available that has incorporated a virulent-strain FCV isolate, the AAFP has pointed out that because outbreaks of virulent systemic disease are caused by unique and variable mutations of existing FCV isolates, the incorporation of one such variant in a vaccine is unlikely to be of appreciable benefit in protecting against other virulent strains that may emerge.

Feline Leukemia Virus

Infection with FeLV has been one of the major infectious causes of death in domestic cat populations. For many years test-and-removal policies were the main way of controlling FeLV infection, and while this is still appropriate in breeding colonies, there is no doubt that the introduction of effective FeLV vaccines has played a very important role in controlling this disease among pet cats. A number of FeLV vaccines are available, and there are marked differences in the way a number of these vaccines have been developed, which may lead to appreciable differences in efficacy among them.[89,96] All three FVGGs regard FeLV vaccination as noncore insofar as not all cats are necessarily at risk for infection (the virus generally requires prolonged close contact between cats for efficient transmission). Vaccination of kittens is begun at 8 to 9 weeks of age, with a second vaccine given 3 to 4 weeks later. Testing for FeLV is recommended before vaccination, and because no FeLV vaccine can guarantee complete protection, vaccination should not be seen as a failproof way to protect FeLV-free cats living with FeLV-infected cats.

The AAFP has recommended that strong consideration be given to vaccinating all kittens against FeLV. This is a logical recommendation worthy of serious consideration because it is rarely, if ever, possible to predict with absolute certainty what environment and lifestyle a kitten will ultimately have (and therefore what the potential future risk of exposure may be) and because kittens are also the most susceptible age group to infection with the virus.

Where required, the AAFP and WSAVA groups recommend annual booster vaccinations for FeLV, whereas the ABCD group recommends annual boosters until 3 to 4 years of age and then boosters every 2 to 3 years. The latter recommendation has merit in that the DOI for FeLV vaccines may be longer than 12 months (although specific studies evaluating this are lacking), and traditionally it has been thought that there is an age-related natural resistance to infection, meaning that older cats are less likely to become infected than younger cats.

Rabies Virus

Vaccination against rabies virus is considered a core vaccine by all three FVGGs where rabies is endemic or where vaccination is required by statute, and this is a major zoonotic virus. Rabies vaccination is highly efficacious after a single inoculation and recombinant, vectored, and killed vaccines are available. The three FVGGs generally recommend vaccinating kittens at 12 to 16 weeks of age to avoid any risks of interference from MDA, although earlier vaccination (from 8 weeks) is possible with some vaccines. All three groups recommend a booster at 12 months followed by inoculations every 1 to 3 years depending on statutory regulations and vaccine licensing.

Feline Immunodeficiency Virus

The use of FIV vaccines remains controversial. One of the major difficulties with the currently available FIV vaccine is that it induces an antibody response that is indistinguishable from that induced by natural infection, and thus vaccinated cats will yield positive results on routinely used serologic diagnostic tests (and vaccine-induced antibodies are known to persist for at least 12 months). Some questions also have been raised regarding the efficacy of the vaccine, and although cross-protection with other strains or clades of FIV has been demonstrated in some studies,[45,46,48,75] the vaccine did not induce protection against a virulent United Kingdom–derived FIV isolate in one study,[23] and it has not been widely tested against European isolates of the virus. The AAFP has recommended the FIV vaccine be regarded as noncore, with use restricted to cats at high risk of infection, with antibody testing being carried out immediately before vaccination and vaccinated cats permanently identified as such (e.g., through microchipping). However, the WSAVA does not recommend the FIV vaccine, and the ABCD stipulates that the vaccine is not recommended in Europe for the reasons given.

Feline Infectious Peritonitis

Similar controversy surrounds the use of the currently available feline infectious peritonitis (FIP) vaccine. The AAFP states that this vaccine is not generally recommended, pointing out that although the vaccine (a temperature-sensitive modified live intranasal feline coronavirus [FCoV] vaccine) appears to be safe, significant questions have been raised regarding its efficacy, insofar as only cats seronegative (and potentially FCoV-naïve) are likely to respond to vaccination and show some protection. The vaccine is not licensed for use in kittens younger than 16 weeks of age, and kittens reared in environments where FCoV is endemic (i.e., the ones most likely to benefit from vaccination) are likely already to have been exposed to the virus at that age, making vaccination futile. The WSAVA similarly states that the FIP vaccine is not recommended, whereas the ABCD categorizes it as noncore and recommends that it be considered in kittens likely to be seronegative but that may subsequently enter a FCoV-endemic environment. The ABCD notes that vaccine-induced immunity is likely to be short-lived and recommends regular (annual) booster vaccinations when use is justified.

Chlamydophila felis *and* Bordetella bronchiseptica

Both *Chlamydophila felis* and *Bordetella bronchiseptica* may cause ocular and upper respiratory tract disease and are more prevalent in multicat environments. However, in contrast to FCV and FHV-1, both *C. felis* and *B. bronchiseptica* can be effectively treated with antibiotics, and these agents are not as prevalent as the viral causes of upper respiratory tract disease. Although vaccination may prevent or reduce the severity of clinical disease, and the onset of protection with the intranasal *B. bronchiseptica* vaccine may be very rapid, all three FVGGs recommend that these be regarded as noncore vaccines, with their use restricted to cats at risk of exposure in multicat environments (i.e., where these agents have been demonstrated to be endemic). Antibiotics should be avoided at the time of administering modified live bacterial vaccines, and the ABCD recommends that *B. bronchiseptica* vaccination be avoided in immunosuppressed cats.

Summary

Vaccination plays a vital role in the control of many diseases, but care needs to be exercised in developing vaccination programs tailored to the needs of the individual cat. Vaccination of all cats against certain common and important pathogens can be justified, but for other pathogens the choice of whether to vaccinate should be made carefully on the basis of local epidemiology, the lifestyle of the cat, and discussion of the risk and benefits of vaccination with the cat owner. The stated aim of the WSAVA—to vaccinate every animal

TABLE 8-6 **Additional Web Resources for Feline Health Care**

Category		Veterinarian	Client/Owner
GENERAL WELLNESS INFORMATION			
Feline Advisory Bureau (FAB)	http://www.fabcats.org	✓	✓
Morris Animal Foundation Healthy Happy Cat	http://www.research4cats.org		✓
Veterinary Partner	http://www.veterinarypartner.com		✓
CATalyst Council	http://www.catalystcouncil.org	✓	✓
AAHA Compliance Study (2003, 2009)	http://www.aahanet.org	✓	
Veterinary Information Network	http://www.vin.com	✓	
Felipedia	http://www.felipedia.org	✓	✓
The Cat Group	http://www.thecatgroup.org.uk	✓	✓
Cornell Feline Health Center	http://www.vet.cornell.edu/fhc	✓	✓
Winn Feline Foundation	http://www.winnfelinehealth.org	✓	✓
BEHAVIOR, ENVIRONMENT, AND THE VETERINARY ENCOUNTER			
OSU Indoor Cat Initiative	http://www.indoorcat.org	✓	✓
Humane Society of US—Indoor Cats	http://www.hsus.org	✓	✓
FAB Cat Friendly Practice	http://www.fabcats.org	✓	
Dumb Friends League: Playing With Your Cat	http://www.ddfl.org		✓
NUTRITION AND DIET			
American College of Veterinary Nutrition	http://www.acvn.org	✓	
MEDICAL/DENTAL CARE			
AAFP Vaccination Guidelines	http://www.catvets.com	✓	
AAFP Zoonoses Guidelines	http://www.catvets.com	✓	
AAFP Retrovirus Testing Guidelines	http://www.catvets.com	✓	
AAFP Feline Senior Care Guidelines	http://www.catvets.com	✓	✓
AAHA Senior Care Guidelines For Dogs & Cats	http://www.aahanet.org	✓	
AAHA Dental Care Guidelines for Dogs & Cats	http://www.aahanet.org	✓	
AAHA/AAFP Pain Management Guidelines	http://www.aahanet.org	✓	
International Veterinary Academy of Pain Management	http://www.ivapm.org	✓	
Veterinary Anesthesia and Analgesia Support Group	http://www.vasg.org	✓	
PARASITE PREVENTION			
Veterinary Parasitology Image Database	http://instruction.cvhs.okstate.edu	✓	
Companion Animal Parasite Council	http://www.petsandparasites.org		✓
VACCINATION			
European Advisory Board on Cat Diseases	http://www.abcd-vets.org	✓	

but each individual less frequently—is highly laudable. For many vaccines increasing data demonstrate a prolonged DOI, and clinicians should strive not to vaccinate more frequently than necessary. Perhaps of note is the fact that in the United States, since 1998, when the AAFP first introduced recommendations suggesting booster vaccination for core vaccines be given less frequently (i.e., every 3 years) and despite apparent widespread uptake of this recommendation, there have been no reports or suggestions of outbreaks of disease that would otherwise have been prevented by more frequent vaccination.

More information is still needed to reconcile some of the discrepancies among the recommendations of the three international FVGGs and to provide a greater evidence base for ongoing refinement and changes to these recommendations, but a growing international consensus is emerging regarding the way feline vaccines should be employed. It is also noteworthy that the AAFP has made recommendations about the site of administration of feline vaccines to help identify vaccines that may be associated with development of injection-site sarcomas and to enable more effective treatment of these on the rare occasions when they arise. The vaccine site recommendations are as follows:

- FPV, FHV-1, FCV (± *C. felis*): given subcutaneously on the lateral right forelimb below the elbow
- Rabies: given subcutaneously on the lateral right hindlimb below the stifle
- FeLV and/or FIV: given subcutaneously on the lateral left hindlimb below the stifle
- Site of other medications should be recorded

The value of this procedure has been emphasized by a recent publication showing that the use of such recommendations is indeed successful in altering the anatomic distribution of injection-site sarcomas and may therefore have a significant impact on disease management when this devastating side effect occurs.[86]

Client Communication and Resources

Clients face a potentially overwhelming amount of information at each visit to the veterinarian, so effective communication is essential if cats are to receive optimal health care. Studies in human medicine have demonstrated that after consultations with doctors, patients remember only a very limited amount of information accurately, which emphasizes the need for good communication and the use of ancillary aids such as client handouts, DVDs, and reliable websites.

In addition to the literature created by veterinarians for their own clients, a vast number of other resources are available to assist veterinarians and their clients. Websites may be oriented toward pet owners, veterinarians, or both; some useful resources for the feline clinician and cat owner are listed in Table 8-6.

References

1. AAHA: *Six steps to higher-quality patient care*, Lakewood, Colo, 2009, AAHA Press.
2. Adamelli S, Marinelli L, Normando S et al: Owner and cat features influence the quality of life of the cat, *Appl Anim Behav Sci* 94:89, 2005.
3. Addie D, Belák S, Boucraut-Baralon C et al: Feline infectious peritonitis. ABCD guidelines on prevention and management, *J Feline Med Surg* 11:594, 2009.
4. Allan FJ, Pfeiffer DU, Jones BR et al: A cross-sectional study of risk factors for obesity in cats in New Zealand, *Prev Vet Med* 46:183, 2000.
5. Barutzki D, Schaper R: Endoparasites in dogs and cats in Germany 1999-2002, *Parasitol Res* 90(Suppl 3):S148, 2003.
6. Bauer JE: Metabolic basis for the essential nature of fatty acids and the unique dietary fatty acid requirements of cats, *J Am Vet Med Assoc* 229:1729, 2006.
7. Belsito KR, Vester BM, Keel T et al: Impact of ovariohysterectomy and food intake on body composition, physical activity, and adipose gene expression in cats, *J Anim Sci* 87:594, 2009.
8. Bergman L, Hart B, Bain M et al: Evaluation of urine marking by cats as a model for understanding veterinary diagnostic and treatment approaches and client attitudes, *J Am Vet Med Assoc* 221:1282, 2002.
9. Biller D, DiBartola S, Eaton K et al: Inheritance of polycystic kidney disease in Persian cats, *J Hered* 87:1, 1996.
10. Bradshaw JW: The evolutionary basis for the feeding behavior of domestic dogs *(Canis familiaris)* and cats *(Felis catus)*, *J Nutr* 136:1927S, 2006.
11. Brown S, Atkins C, Bagley R et al: Guidelines for the identification, evaluation, and management of systemic hypertension in dogs and cats, *J Vet Intern Med* 21:542, 2007.
12. Buffington CA: External and internal influences on disease risk in cats, *J Am Vet Med Assoc* 220:994, 2002.
13. Buffington CA: Dry foods and risk of disease in cats, *Can Vet J* 49:561, 2008.
14. Buffington CA, Westropp JL, Chew DJ et al: Clinical evaluation of multimodal environmental modification (MEMO) in the management of cats with idiopathic cystitis, *J Feline Med Surg* 8:261, 2006.
15. Calvete C, Lucientes J, Castillo JA et al: Gastrointestinal helminth parasites in stray cats from the mid-Ebro Valley, Spain, *Vet Parasitol* 75:235, 1998.
16. Caro T: Predatory behaviour and social play in kittens, *Behaviour* 76:1, 1981.
17. Clancy E, Moore A, Bertone E: Evaluation of cat and owner characteristics and their relationships to outdoor access of owned cats, *J Am Vet Med Assoc* 222:1541, 2003.
18. Clarke DL, Wrigglesworth D, Holmes K et al: Using environmental and feeding enrichment to facilitate feline weight loss, *J Anim Physiol Anim Nutr (Berl)* 89:427, 2005.
19. Colliard L, Paragon B-M, Lemuet B et al: Prevalence and risk factors of obesity in an urban population of healthy cats, *J Feline Med Surg* 11:135, 2009.
20. Davis-Wurzler GM: Current vaccination strategies in puppies and kittens, *Vet Clin North Am Small Anim Pract* 36:607, 2006.
21. Day MJ, Horzinek MC, Schultz RD: Guidelines for the vaccination of dogs and cats. Compiled by the Vaccination Guidelines Group (VGG) of the World Small Animal Veterinary Association (WSAVA), *J Small Anim Pract* 48:528, 2007.
22. Dryden M, Payne P, Ridley R et al: Gastrointestinal parasites: the practice guide to accurate diagnosis and treatment, *Comp Contin Edu Pract Vet* 28:3, 2006.
23. Dunham SP, Bruce J, MacKay S et al: Limited efficacy of an inactivated feline immunodeficiency virus vaccine, *Vet Rec* 158:561, 2006.
24. Egberink H, Addie D, Belak S et al: *Bordetella bronchiseptica* infection in cats ABCD guidelines on prevention and management, *J Feline Med Surg* 11:610, 2009.
25. Epstein M, Kuehn NF, Landsberg G et al: AAHA senior care guidelines for dogs and cats, *J Am Anim Hosp Assoc* 41:81, 2005.

26. Fatjo J, Ruiz-de-la-Torre JL, Manteca X: The epidemiology of behavioural problems in dogs and cats: a survey of veterinary practitioners, *Animal Welfare* 15:179, 2006.
27. Fekete SG, Fodor K, Proháczik A et al: Comparison of feed preference and digestion of three different commercial diets for cats and ferrets, *J Anim Physiol Anim Nutr (Berl)* 89:199, 2005.
28. Fisher M: *Toxocara cati:* an underestimated zoonotic agent, *Trends Parasitol* 19:167, 2003.
29. Fries R, Heaney AM, Meurs KM: Prevalence of the myosin-binding protein C mutation in Maine Coon cats, *J Vet Intern Med* 22:893, 2008.
30. Frymus T, Addie D, Belak S et al: Feline rabies ABCD guidelines on prevention and management, *J Feline Med Surg* 11:585, 2009.
31. Gaskell R, Gettinby G, Graham S et al: Veterinary Products Committee working group report on feline and canine vaccination, *Vet Rec* 150:126, 2002.
32. Gates MC, Nolan TJ: Endoparasite prevalence and recurrence across different age groups of dogs and cats, *Vet Parasitol* 166:153, 2009.
33. Girard N, Servet E, Biourge V et al: Feline tooth resorption in a colony of 109 cats, *J Vet Dent* 25:166, 2008.
34. Girard N, Servet E, Biourge V et al: Periodontal health status in a colony of 109 cats, *J Vet Dent* 26:147, 2009.
35. Gobar G, Kass P: World Wide Web–based survey of vaccination practices, postvaccinal reactions, and vaccine site–associated sarcomas in cats, *J Am Vet Med Assoc* 220:1477, 2002.
36. Gow AG, Gow DJ, Hall EJ et al: Prevalence of potentially pathogenic enteric organisms in clinically healthy kittens in the UK, *J Feline Med Surg* 11:655, 2009.
37. Graves TK: Hyperthyroidism and the kidneys. In August J, editor: *Consultations in feline internal medicine*, ed 6, St Louis, 2010, Saunders Elsevier, p 269.
38. Gruffydd-Jones T, Addie D, Belak S et al: *Chlamydophila felis* infection ABCD guidelines on prevention and management, *J Feline Med Surg* 11:605, 2009.
39. Heidenberger E: Housing conditions and behavioural problems of indoor cats as assessed by their owners, *Appl Anim Behav Sci* 52:345, 1997.
40. Hoenig M, Ferguson DC: Effects of neutering on hormonal concentrations and energy requirements in male and female cats, *Am J Vet Res* 63:634, 2002.
41. Holmstrom SE, Bellows J, Colmery B et al: AAHA dental care guidelines for dogs and cats, *J Am Anim Hosp Assoc* 41:277, 2005.
42. Horzinek MC, Thiry E: Vaccines and vaccination: the principles and the polemics, *J Feline Med Surg* 11:530, 2009.
43. Hosie MJ, Addie D, Belák S et al: Feline immunodeficiency. ABCD guidelines on prevention and management, *J Feline Med Surg* 11:575, 2009.
44. Howe LM: Short-term results and complications of prepubertal gonadectomy in cats and dogs, *J Am Vet Med Assoc* 211:57, 1997.
45. Huang C, Conlee D, Gill M et al: Dual-subtype feline immunodeficiency virus vaccine provides 12 months of protective immunity against heterologous challenge, *J Feline Med Surg* 12:451, 2010.
46. Huang C, Conlee D, Loop J et al: Efficacy and safety of a feline immunodeficiency virus vaccine, *Anim Health Res Rev* 5:295, 2004.
47. Kienzle E, Bergler R: Human–animal relationship of owners of normal and overweight cats, *J Nutr* 136:1947S, 2006.
48. Kusuhara H, Hohdatsu T, Okumura M et al: Dual-subtype vaccine (Fel-O-Vax FIV) protects cats against contact challenge with heterologous subtype B FIV infected cats, *Vet Microbiol* 108:155, 2005.
49. Levy J, Crawford C, Hartmann K et al: 2008 American Association of Feline Practitioners' feline retrovirus management guidelines, *J Feline Med Surg* 10:300, 2008.
50. Levy J, Scott H, Lachtara J et al: Seroprevalence of feline leukemia virus and feline immunodeficiency virus infection among cats in North America and risk factors for seropositivity, *J Am Vet Med Assoc* 228:371, 2006.
51. Litster AL, Atwell RB: Feline heartworm disease: a clinical review, *J Feline Med Surg* 10:137, 2008.
52. Little S, Sears W, Lachtara J et al: Seroprevalence of feline leukemia virus and feline immunodeficiency virus infection among cats in Canada, *Can Vet J* 50:644, 2009.
53. Lommer MJ, Verstraete FJ: Radiographic patterns of periodontitis in cats: 147 cases (1998-1999), *J Am Vet Med Assoc* 218:230, 2001.
54. Lord LK, Ingwersen W, Gray JL et al: Characterization of animals with microchips entering animal shelters, *J Am Vet Med Assoc* 235:160, 2009.
55. Lord LK, Wittum TE, Ferketich AK et al: Search and identification methods that owners use to find a lost cat, *J Am Vet Med Assoc* 230:217, 2007.
56. Lue TW, Pantenburg DP, Crawford PM: Impact of the owner-pet and client-veterinarian bond on the care that pets receive, *J Am Vet Med Assoc* 232:531, 2008.
57. Lutz H, Addie D, Belak S et al: Feline leukaemia ABCD guidelines on prevention and management, *J Feline Med Surg* 11:565, 2009.
58. Martin LJ, Siliart B, Dumon HJ et al: Spontaneous hormonal variations in male cats following gonadectomy, *J Feline Med Surg* 8:309, 2006.
59. Meurs K, Sanchez X, David R et al: A cardiac myosin binding protein C mutation in the Maine Coon cat with familial hypertrophic cardiomyopathy, *Hum Mol Genet* 14:3587, 2005.
60. Meurs KM, Norgard MM, Ederer MM et al: A substitution mutation in the myosin binding protein C gene in ragdoll hypertrophic cardiomyopathy, *Genomics* 90:261, 2007.
61. Moffat K, Landsberg G: An investigation into the prevalence of clinical signs of cognitive dysfunction syndrome (CDS) in cats, *J Am Anim Hosp Assoc* 39:512, 2003.
62. Mooney CT: Hyperthyroidism. In Ettinger S, Feldman EC, editors: *Textbook of veterinary internal medicine diseases of the dog and cat*, ed 6, St Louis, 2005, Elsevier Saunders, p 1544.
63. Moore GE, DeSantis-Kerr AC, Guptill LF et al: Adverse events after vaccine administration in cats: 2,560 cases (2002-2005), *J Am Vet Med Assoc* 231:94, 2007.
64. Morris JG: Idiosyncratic nutrient requirements of cats appear to be diet-induced evolutionary adaptations, *Nutr Res Rev* 15:153, 2002.
65. Neilson J: Thinking outside the box: feline elimination, *J Feline Med Surg* 6:5, 2004.
66. Neilson JC: House soiling in cats. In Horwitz DF, Mills DS, editors: *BSAVA manual of canine and feline behavioural medicine*, ed 2, Cheltenham, UK, 2009, British Small Animal Veterinary Association, p 117.
67. Neville PF: An ethical viewpoint: the role of veterinarians and behaviourists in ensuring good husbandry for cats, *J Feline Med Surg* 6:43, 2004.
68. Nichol S, Ball S, Snow K: Prevalence of intestinal parasites in feral cats in some urban areas of England, *Vet Parasitol* 9:107, 1981.
69. Nijland ML, Stam F, Seidell JC: Overweight in dogs, but not in cats, is related to overweight in their owners, *Public Health Nutr* 13:102, 2010.
70. Overall K, Rodan I, Beaver B et al: Feline behavior guidelines from the American Association of Feline Practitioners, *J Am Vet Med Assoc* 227:70, 2005.
71. Overall KL: The veterinary importance of clinical behavior medicine. In *Clinical behavioral medicine for small animals*, St Louis, 1997, Mosby, p 1.

72. Palmer CS, Thompson RC, Traub RJ et al: National study of the gastrointestinal parasites of dogs and cats in Australia, *Vet Parasitol* 151:181, 2008.
73. Peachey SE, Harper EJ: Aging does not influence feeding behavior in cats, *J Nutr* 132:1735S, 2002.
74. Pittari J, Rodan I, Beekman G et al: American Association of Feline Practitioners. Senior Care Guidelines, *J Feline Med Surg* 11:763, 2009.
75. Pu R, Sato E, Coleman J et al: Dual-subtype FIV vaccine protection against virulent heterologous subtype virus. 7th International Feline Retrovirus Research Symposium 2004.
76. Radford AD, Addie D, Belak S et al: Feline calicivirus infection ABCD guidelines on prevention and management, *J Feline Med Surg* 11:556, 2009.
77. Ray JD, Jr., Eubanks DL: Dental homecare: teaching your clients to care for their pet's teeth, *J Vet Dent* 26:57, 2009.
78. Rebar A: Maximize diagnostic value: use laboratory profiling to establish baselines and follow trends in health and disease, *Dx Consult* 2:8, 2009.
79. Reberg SR, Blakemore JC, Thorpe RJ: *Dermatophytosis in shelter cats in northeastern Indiana: a survey of disease prevalence and the influence of shelter management practices*. AAVD/ACVD Proceedings 1999, p 39.
80. Richards JR, Elston TH, Ford RB et al: The 2006 American Association of Feline Practitioners Feline Vaccine Advisory Panel report, *J Am Vet Med Assoc* 229:1405, 2006.
81. Robertson ID: The influence of diet and other factors on owner-perceived obesity in privately owned cats from metropolitan Perth, Western Australia, *Prev Vet Med* 40:75, 1999.
82. Scarlett JM, Donoghue S, Saidla J et al: Overweight cats: prevalence and risk factors, *Int J Obes Relat Metab Disord* 18 (Suppl 1):S22, 1994.
83. Scarlett JM, Salman MD, New JG et al: The role of veterinary practitioners in reducing dog and cat relinquishments and euthanasias, *J Am Vet Med Assoc* 220:306, 2002.
84. Schultz RD, Thiel B, Mukhtar E et al: Age and long-term protective immunity in dogs and cats, *J Comp Pathol* 142 (Suppl 1):S102, 2010.
85. Seibert LM, Landsberg GM: Diagnosis and management of patients presenting with behavior problems, *Vet Clin North Am Small Anim Pract* 38:937, 2008.
86. Shaw SC, Kent MS, Gordon IK et al: Temporal changes in characteristics of injection-site sarcomas in cats: 392 cases (1990-2006), *J Am Vet Med Assoc* 234:376, 2009.
87. Shore ER, Burdsal C, Douglas DK: Pet owners' views of pet behavior problems and willingness to consult experts for assistance, *J Appl Anim Welf Sci* 11:63, 2008.
88. Spain C, Scarlett J, Houpt K: Long-term risks and benefits of early-age gonadectomy in cats, *J Am Vet Med Assoc* 224:372, 2004.
89. Sparkes AH: Feline leukaemia virus: a review of immunity and vaccination, *J Small Anim Pract* 38:187, 1997.
90. Stasiak M: The development of food preferences in cats: the new direction, *Nutr Neurosci* 5:221, 2002.
91. Stubbs WP, Bloomberg MS, Scruggs SL et al: Effects of prepubertal gonadectomy on physical and behavioral development in cats, *J Am Vet Med Assoc* 209:1864, 1996.
92. Sung W, Crowell-Davis SL: Elimination behavior patterns of domestic cats *(Felis catus)* with and without elimination behavior problems, *Am J Vet Res* 67:1500, 2006.
93. Taylor P, Funk C, Craighill P: Gauging family intimacy: dogs edge cats (dads trail both): Pew Research Center, 2006.
94. Thiry E, Addie D, Belak S et al: Feline herpesvirus infection ABCD guidelines on prevention and management, *J Feline Med Surg* 11:547, 2009.
95. Toribio J-ALM, Norris JM, White JD et al: Demographics and husbandry of pet cats living in Sydney, Australia: results of cross-sectional survey of pet ownership, *J Feline Med Surg* 11:449, 2009.
96. Torres AN, O'Halloran KP, Larson LJ et al: Feline leukemia virus immunity induced by whole inactivated virus vaccination, *Vet Immunol Immunopathol* 134:122, 2010.
97. Truyen U, Addie D, Belak S et al: Feline panleukopenia ABCD guidelines on prevention and management, *J Feline Med Surg* 11:538, 2009.
98. Verstraete FJ, Kass PH, Terpak CH: Diagnostic value of full-mouth radiography in cats, *Am J Vet Res* 59:692, 1998.
99. Vogt AH, Rodan I, Brown M et al: AAFP-AAHA: Feline life stage guidelines, *J Feline Med Surg* 12:43, 2010.
100. Volk J, Merle C: *A veterinarian's guide to pet health insurance*, Schaumberg, Ill, 2009, National Commission on Veterinary Economic Issues.
101. Wyrwicka W: Social effects on development of food preferences, *Acta Neurobiol Exp (Wars)* 53:485, 1993.
102. Yamamoto N, Kon M, Saito T et al: [Prevalence of intestinal canine and feline parasites in Saitama Prefecture, Japan], *Kansenshogaku Zasshi* 83:223, 2009.
103. Zoran DL: Feline obesity: clinical recognition and management, *Comp Contin Educ Vet* 31:284, 2009.

SECTION II

FELINE BEHAVIOR

Editor: Kersti Seksel

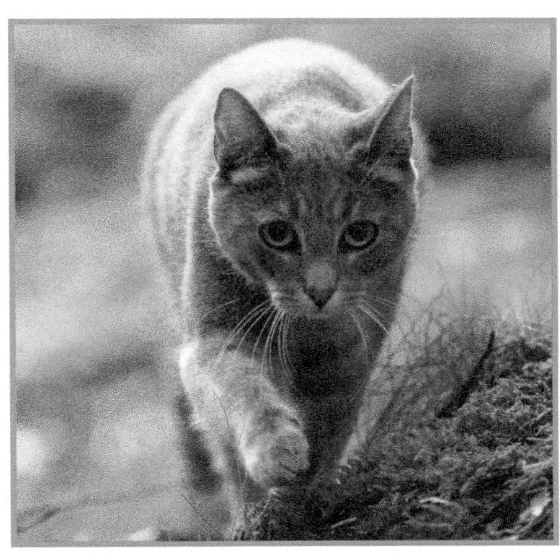

CHAPTER

9

Kitten Development

Gary Landsberg and Jacqueline Mary Ley

OUTLINE

The development of a kitten from a dependent neonate with a limited ability to perceive and respond to stimuli to an independent creature with a fully developed physiology that is able to care for itself, hunt, and interact with other cats is a rapid yet complex process that is affected by many factors. These include the genetics of the sire and dam, the environment of the uterus, and the kitten's environment after birth. There is a complex ballet of neurologic, physiologic, musculoskeletal, and psychologic development that must occur in the correct sequence if the kitten is to develop normally. One of the most important stages in a kitten's development is the socialization period, wherein kittens are most receptive to learning the things and individuals in their environment that they should avoid, ignore, or derive benefit from.

Problems can occur at any stage of development and can have far-reaching effects for the kitten, especially in the role of a companion cat. Cats whose behavior does not meet owner expectations are at risk of being surrendered to a shelter,[36] where they are likely to be euthanized. Understanding normal kitten development allows owners to provide the right environment for healthy kitten development. It is also important that veterinarians understand the behaviors that kittens normally display at various stages of development and educate owners accordingly.

INFLUENCE OF PARENTAL FACTORS ON BEHAVIORAL DEVELOPMENT

Genetics

Cats are unique among domesticated animals because the majority of their breeding is not controlled by humans.[11] Many kittens are the result of opportunistic matings wherein male social skills and female preferences dictate who sires the kittens. The breeding season for the modern domestic cat is based on multiple estrous cycles throughout the year, especially spring through summer, with a second peak in kitten numbers in late autumn. The modern domestic cat is capable of producing two or three litters annually, depending on the length of time that the kittens remain with the queen after weaning. Natural selection pressures are working, as opposed to human preferences for coat and eye color, size, and temperament. Although this works to keep the feline population relatively free of genetic diseases, it can have important effects on the suitability of kittens to be companion animals. Development of behavior is the result of the complex interrelationship between inherited factors (i.e., genetics) and noninherited environmental influences.[6]

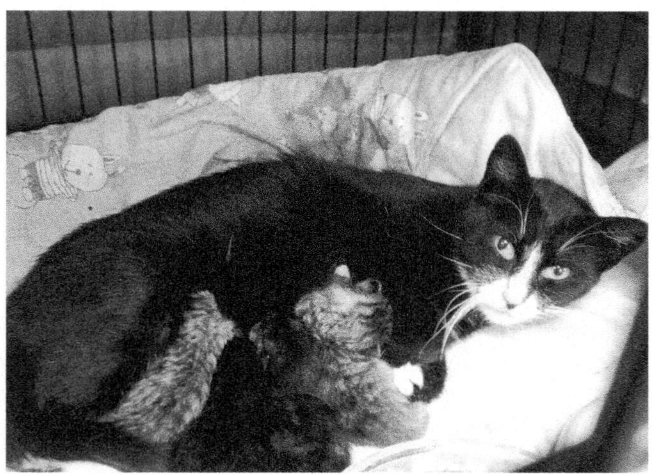

FIGURE 9-1 Newborn kittens are totally dependent on the queen.

In Utero Effects

The environment in the uterus during pregnancy can have far-reaching effects on the behavior and development of the individual kitten. Poor quality of nutrition for the queen during pregnancy has been shown to produce a wide variety of behavioral and physical abnormalities in kittens. Kittens from queens fed a low-protein diet during late gestation and through lactation have been found to be more emotional and move and vocalize more frequently than kittens from queens fed an adequately formulated diet.[20] These kittens also lost their balance more often and had poor social attachment and fewer social interactions with the queen. It is not clear if the restricted protein leads to the emotionality or if changes in the queen's behavior caused by the protein deficiency lead to the change in the kittens' behavior. In another study, when queens were restricted to half of their nutritional requirements, the kittens demonstrated growth deficits in some brain regions (e.g., cerebrum, cerebellum, and brain stem).[38] Delays were apparent in many areas of development, including suckling, eye opening, crawling, posture, walking, running, playing, and climbing.

Tactile sensitivity is present in the embryo by day 24 of prenatal life, and the vestibular righting reflex develops by approximately day 54 of gestation.[6] Kittens are generally born after a 63-day gestation.

Maternal Factors

Good maternal behavior is essential for healthy kitten development. In fact, because kittens are born blind, with limited ability to move and regulate body temperature, they are totally dependent on their mothers (Figure 9-1). Kittens may be communally reared by other female cats, especially in environments where food is abundant.[18] Kittens that were separated from their mother and hand raised from 2 weeks of age were more fearful and aggressive toward people and other cats, were more sensitive to novel stimuli, learned poorly, and developed poor social and parenting skills.[34,37] These effects may be attenuated, at least in part, if kittens are hand reared in a home with other cats.[15,34] When queens are fed a rationed diet, their kittens were more active, engaged in more object-directed play, and were more likely to hunt.[1,7] Stressors on the queen before and after the birth of her kittens can affect the behavior of her kittens. Kittens from queens fed a restricted-protein diet were found to vocalize more than kittens from queens fed a balanced diet.[7]

Paternal Factors

Though the tom is not involved in raising the kittens, he appears to have a strong effect on the kitten's social development. Studies of cat personality have identified three personality types: sociable, confident, and easy-going; timid and nervous; and active and aggressive.[29,32] Although maternal genetics and the influence of the mother and offspring on early development are important, paternal genetic factors appear to have the strongest influence on the development of personality. Kittens sired by toms considered to be "bold" have been found to be significantly friendlier to familiar people, less stressed by the approach of unfamiliar people, and more likely to spend time near a novel object.[32]

Of course, the socialization of kittens is a complex process that involves the interplay of genetics, environment, and learning. However, it is likely that some feral cats are genetically shy, which hinders their ability to live close to humans. Their kittens will be similarly affected, making their socialization to humans and their suitability as pets less certain.

BEHAVIORAL DEVELOPMENT

Development after Birth

Similar to the patterns identified in dogs during puppy development, kittens have several sensitive periods of intense development from birth to 6 months of age. They tend to have shorter sensitive periods than do puppies, and the 8-week-old kitten is quite different from the 8-week-old puppy with regard to its physical, mental, and social development. The earlier stages of development, the neonatal and transition period, tend to occur very quickly. Important milestones occur in each of the sensitive periods that correspond to the physical development of the kittens. For example, the myelination of nerves must occur before the kitten can show the fine motor control to send social signals by using changes in body posture or to practice hunting behaviors such as pouncing.

Sensitive Periods

Neonatal (0 to 7 Days)

The neonatal period is a time primarily of nursing and sleeping in which the kitten is fully dependent on its mother. During the first 2 weeks, nursing and eliminative behaviors are initiated by the queen, who provides food and warmth, cleans the kittens, and stimulates defecation and urination by licking the anogenital area of the kittens. The kitten is guided by tactile, thermal, and olfactory stimuli to find the queen and littermates. Kittens are unable to hear at birth, but hearing is present by the fifth day. Kittens maintain their body temperature by huddling together and with the queen. The actions of newborn kittens are initially very clumsy, but as the nervous system and muscles mature and behaviors are repeated, their actions become smoother and more efficient. For example, by 4 days after birth, most kittens are proficient at locating and attaching to their preferred teat.[9] Olfaction is present and highly developed at birth, insofar as kittens use their sense of smell to locate the queen's teats and find their preferred teats. This is important when kittens have upper respiratory tract infections because they will not actively suckle and may need artificial feeding. Even 2-day-old kittens will show pronounced avoidance of offensive odors.[8,27]

The neonatal kitten has a limited range of behaviors. It can orientate its body toward touch and warmth, move by squirming along with swimming movements of the forelimbs, suckle, and vocalize. Kittens begin vocalizing soon after birth. These sounds attract the queen and increase the likelihood that she will allow nursing. She will also locate a lost kitten by its vocalizations and carry it back to the nest.[9]

Kittens have several reflexes present at birth. If touched on the face, a kitten will turn toward the side that was touched (auriculonasocephalic reflex). A kitten will also turn to the side being touched when it is touched on the flank. The rooting reflex, wherein the kitten burrows into its mother, littermates, or any warm material, may be present for up to 16 days. This behavior is used to locate teats. Newborn kittens have a strong suckling reflex, which is initially stimulated by objects in the mouth or being touched on the face. The suckle reflex is strongest on waking. Kittens rapidly develop teat preferences and will preferentially feed from one or two teats.[24] The suckling reflex can be stimulated initially by touching a large area of the kitten's face or putting small objects in the mouth. However, as the kitten gains experience, the area that will produce this response is reduced to the lip area. At the same time, foreign bodies placed in the mouth will be rejected.[28] The suckling reflex usually disappears after approximately 20 days.[28]

Transitional (7 to 14 Days)

During the transitional period the kitten changes from expressing limited neonate behaviors to beginning to show adult behaviors in eating, elimination, locomotion, and social interactions. From about 2 weeks of age, kittens begin to raise their bodies off the ground and move with a slow, paddling gait. Between weeks 2 and 3, the eyes and ears open, allowing the kitten to process more information about the environment. The eyes open at around 7 to 10 days. Although hearing is present by the fifth day of age, the kitten does not begin to orient to sounds until approximately 2 weeks of age. Olfaction is fully mature by 3 weeks. Dental development commences between 2 and 3 weeks of age.

Communal nesting results in kittens leaving the nest earlier: 20 days compared with 30 days for kittens raised in single-litter nests.[19]

Socialization (14 Days to 7 Weeks)

During the socialization period, kittens begin to explore their environment and learn its hazards and pleasures. Visual orienting and following develop in the third week, but obstacle avoidance is not developed until 4 to 5 weeks of age. Full visual acuity may not be achieved until 3 to 4 months of age. Rudimentary walking begins at approximately 3 weeks and develops into brief episodes of running by 5 weeks; kittens use all gait patterns of adult locomotion by 6 to 7 weeks of age.[6] Between the third and sixth weeks, kittens develop air righting, which is the ability to land on their feet.[23]

By 4 weeks the kitten begins to move away from the nest and develops social relationships with people and other animals in its environment. Social play with siblings and the mother begins at approximately 4 weeks and includes wrestling, rolling, and biting. When there are no other kittens or cats present, these behaviors may be directed toward human hands and other moving body parts. Social play peaks at 7 to 9 weeks and continues at a relatively high level to approximately 16 weeks of age.

At 4 weeks weaning begins, and kittens begin to eat solid foods. By 7 to 8 weeks weaning is largely completed, although suckling may continue intermittently for several more weeks.[6,30] From about 4 weeks of age, the mother may begin to bring dead prey; over the next several weeks, the mother may bring home weakened and then live prey, which she releases at the nest, providing the kittens with an opportunity to hunt and kill.[13] Kittens generally share their mother's food choices and choice of prey.[13] Kittens that are weaned early (4 weeks) are more likely to be mouse killers, whereas late weaning (9 weeks) is associated with a delayed development of predation and reduced propensity to kill mice.[39] Time of weaning is associated with a change from social play to object play.[3] In fact, kittens weaned early showed higher rates of play.[7,31] Locomotor play also begins at around this age.

By 5 to 6 weeks of age, the kitten has full voluntary control of elimination, and digging and covering feces and urine on loose soil may begin.

Fearful reactions to threatening stimuli may begin to be displayed by 6 weeks of age.[27] Individual differences in behavior begin to be displayed during the second month of life, owing to both genetic influences and contrasting early environments.[2]

Juvenile (7 Weeks to Sexual Maturity at 6 to 12 Months)

The juvenile period is associated with kittens becoming ready to disperse from their queen's home range and become fully independent for their food needs. Play and exploration of inanimate objects and locomotory play begins to escalate at approximately 7 to 8 weeks of age and peaks at approximately 18 weeks of age. Social play, on the other hand, is most prevalent from about 4 weeks to 16 weeks of age. Social play begins to take on aspects of predation in the third month. Object play may be social or solitary and may consist of pawing, stalking, leaping, and biting of objects and securing them with the paws. This type of play simulates a variety of aspects of the predatory sequence.

Adult (Sexual and Social Maturity)

The adult period begins and the juvenile period ends with the development of sexual maturity. Female kittens may show their first signs of estrus between 3.5 and 12 months of age, although first estrus typically occurs at 5 to 9 months.[9] Earlier signs of estrus can be influenced by environmental factors such as being born in the early spring, exposure to mature tomcats, presence of other female cats in estrus, or periods of increasing light.[9,23] Although cats are able to reproduce at sexual maturity, sexual maturity is not equivalent to social maturity. *Social maturity* refers to the development of adult social behavior and interactions with other cats and is believed to occur between 36 and 48 months of age. Social maturity includes defense of territory. Male domestic kittens reach sexual maturity between 9 and 12 months of age. Wild or feral male cats may not reach sexual maturity until 18 months of age.

SPECIFIC BEHAVIOR PATTERNS

Play

Of all the behaviors in which kittens engage, play behaviors are probably the most fascinating to watch. Play is normal and possibly essential to the normal development of kittens. Play helps kittens develop physical fitness and practice behavior patterns essential for their survival as adults. Hunting, for example, is a complex behavior that has to be practiced to bring all the elements together successfully. Hunting inanimate objects such as leaves helps the kitten coordinate muscles and practice timing different elements of the hunting sequence. Play allows kittens to explore their environment and also make social contacts.[9]

Because the expression of play behaviors depends on the physical development of the kitten, play changes over time. Play can be divided into social play, which involves two or more cats, and individual or object-directed play, which appears to be independently organized and separately controlled.[3] A kitten's first play attempts are generally seen at approximately 2 weeks of age, when the kitten will attempt to bat at objects it finds.[9] At 3 weeks of age, social play takes the form of orientated pawing and occasional biting.[9] Development of leaping occurs from 2.5 weeks to 6 weeks. Between 5 and 6 weeks, stalking, chasing, and wrestling begin. Climbing and balancing on ledges begins at approximately 7 weeks (Figure 9-2).[9] Play behavior patterns contain elements of other behavior patterns, such as hunting, killing, and social behavior patterns.

Social play is seen most commonly between the ages of 4 and 16 weeks of age.[9,41] Eight different play behaviors, all occurring at different ages, have been identified (Table 9-1): belly up and stand up (3 weeks), side step and pounce (4.5 weeks), rearing (5 weeks), chase (5.5 weeks), horizontal leap (6 weeks), and face off (7 weeks). The general decline in social play between 12 and 16 weeks of age may coincide with the decrease in social interest before dispersal.[9] Sexual behaviors may be seen during play, beginning between 3 and 4 months of age, with some male kittens showing mounting, neck biting, and pelvic thrusting.[9]

Individual or object-directed play is also seen in kittens starting at 2 weeks of age and begins to increase with weaning, at approximately 7 weeks of age.[7,9,31] It

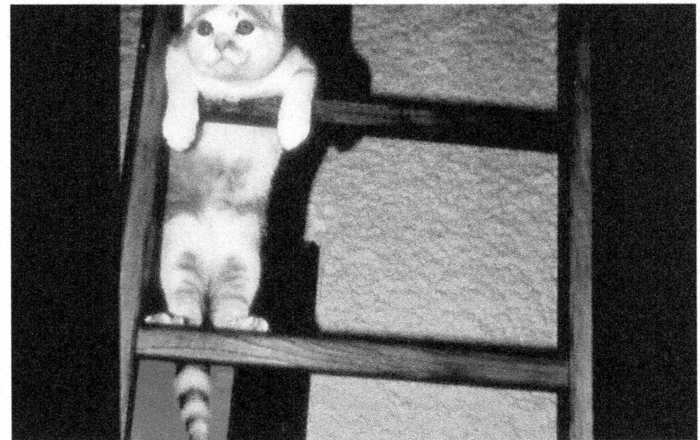

FIGURE 9-2 The ability to climb and balance on objects begins at approximately 7 weeks of age.

TABLE 9-1 **Play Behavior of Kittens**

	Age at Which Play Behavior Is First Seen and Percentage of Time Spent in Play							
Play behavior*	**2 Weeks**	**3 Weeks**	**4 Weeks**	**5 Weeks**	**6 Weeks**	**7-9 Weeks**	**12 Weeks**	**16 Weeks**
Belly up		21-23 days			13%		16%	
Stand up		23 days						
Side step			32 days		20%			
Pounce			33-35 days		42%		37%	
Rearing				35 days			25%	
Chase				38-41 days				
Horizontal leap					43 days			
Face off					48 days			
Object-directed play	14 days					Peaks at 50 days		

***Belly up:** Kitten is in dorsal recumbency with its forelimbs pawing and hind limbs treading. Its mouth may be open, with teeth exposed. **Stand up:** Kitten sits up on its hind limbs with forepaws pawing. **Side step:** Kitten stands by the side of its play partner with its back slightly arched and an upward curve in its tail. **Pounce:** This is similar to the ambush rush of the hunting sequence. The kitten crouches with its hind limbs under it and tail straight out. It shifts its weight between the hind limbs before rushing at the play partner. **Vertical stance/rearing:** This is similar to stand up, except the kitten pushes itself up so that it is standing on its hind limbs. **Chase:** This involves pursuit and flight between kittens. Sometimes one will run, but the play partner will not chase. **Horizontal leap:** From the side step posture, the kitten leaps off the ground. **Face off:** The kitten faces the play partner and directs pawing movements at the partner's face. The partner may also reciprocate the behavior. **Object-directed play:** This play is directed toward inanimate objects such as toys or leaves.
Adapted from Caro TM: The effects of experience on the predatory patterns of cats, *Behav Neural Biol* 29:1, 1980.

may be important for the development of hunting skills. Kittens are interested in moving objects and will leap, strike, and grab at small, erratically moving objects (Figure 9-3). At other times, kittens appear to play with imaginary objects and will leap at and bat at what seems to be an imaginary object. Another version of this exuberant play occurs when kittens dash wildly around the house, often in the evening, for no reason apparent to humans.

Single kittens play more with objects and with their mothers compared with kittens in litters.[35] Kittens need opportunities for social play, object play, and exploration that are acceptable to both the cat and the pet owner. Toys encourage normal development and prevent kittens from directing normal play behavior toward humans. The most attractive toys for cats and kittens have been shown to be small (mouse size) and appealing in texture and movement; play is increased by hunger.[21,22]

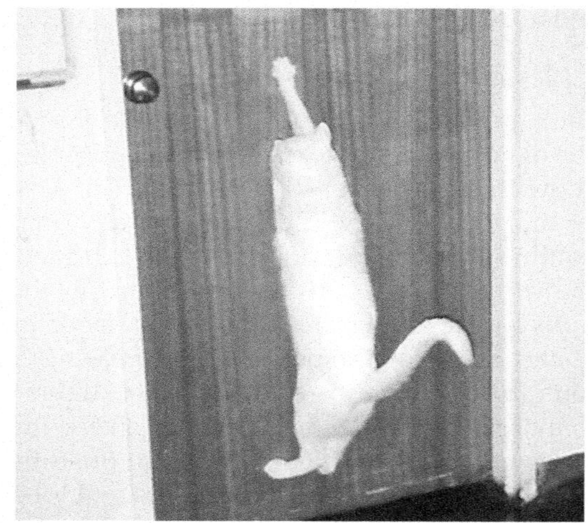

FIGURE 9-3 Laser toys simulate moving objects, and kittens will leap and grab in response to the erratic movement.

Social Behavior

Kittens begin to develop social responses when their eyes have opened and their muscles are sufficiently coordinated to send signals. This is first seen at the transitional period, at about 3 weeks of age. The most receptive time for socializing kittens to humans and other species is between 2 and 7 weeks of age, and the more handling by people, the less likely that fear of humans will develop.[6,25,26]

Adult-like responses to urine from strange cats begin to be seen at approximately 8 weeks of age in kittens, whereas fear responses to a black silhouette of a threatening cat are seen from 6 weeks of age.[27] Social behaviors associated with positive interactions between cats, such as mutual rubbing, have been recorded between 4-month-old kittens that are littermates.[29]

Feeding

Although the urge to suckle is an innate, natural behavior, newborn kittens are initially very clumsy when attempting to nurse; however, within 4 days they generally are proficient at locating the teat and attaching to

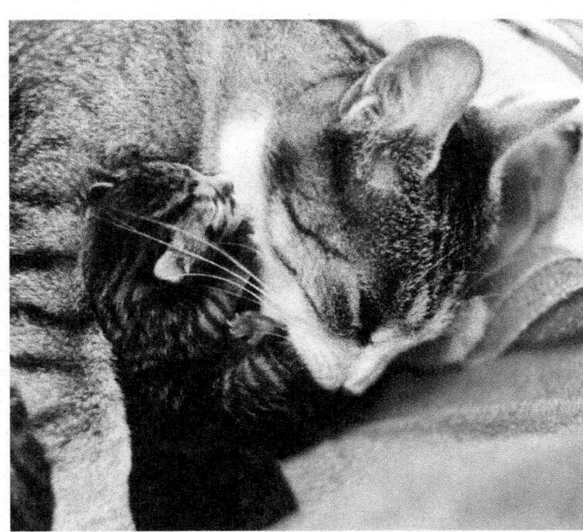

FIGURE 9-4 Newborn kittens cannot voluntarily eliminate urine and feces; the queen licks the anogenital area to stimulate elimination and ingests the waste products to keep the nest clean. *(Photo courtesy Susan Little.)*

suckle. The young kitten spends about 25% of its time nursing. By 5 weeks of age, this has decreased to 20% of the kitten's time.

Weaning usually begins at approximately 4 weeks of age and tends to be initiated by the queen. As the kittens become skilled and bold in initiating nursing bouts at approximately 4 weeks, the queen becomes increasingly evasive.[9] The kittens begin to show an interest in solid food—either prey items or food supplied for the queen by humans—and nonfood items such as dirt and kitty litter between 28 and 50 days.

The queen shows a distinct series of behaviors when she begins to introduce her kittens to prey, and encouragement by the mother could play a large part in the development of predation in cats.[13] Experience with specific types of prey as a young kitten affects the adult cat's preferences for prey species.[12] The queen's preferences for prey species also affect her kittens' preferences. The kittens start to follow the queen on hunts at 15 to 18 weeks of age and watch her locate, stalk, ambush, and kill prey. It is not clear if the queen's modeling acts to excite predatory responses already in the repertoire of the young animals[1] or if the kittens learn by direct observation of the queen's behavior. Feral kittens are generally hunting independently by 6 months of age.[13]

Toileting

Initially, the queen stimulates the kitten to void bowels and bladder by licking the anogenital area (Figure 9-4). She ingests the waste materials. The anogenital reflex disappears between 23 and 39 days. Voluntary control of the bowels and bladder begins to develop at 3 weeks. The queen may still clean up after the kittens until they are 6 weeks old because they remain close to the nest.[9] The nest must be clean and relatively free of odors to keep the kittens safe from predators.

At approximately 30 days the kittens start exploring loose, light toilet materials. They appear to be attracted to the queen's toileting area or litter tray by olfactory cues and will get into the tray or area and begin to dig around. Ingestion of the litter as a form of exploration is not uncommon at this age. Soon after this they begin to show adult elimination behaviors, such as using areas with loose, light material and covering feces and urine.

Many kittens are adopted into their new homes with the expectation that they are fully house trained. However, their litter box habits should not be considered reliable before 6 months of age because they are still forming location and substrate preferences for toileting.[9] Some kittens need to be shown the owner's preferred kitten toileting area and material. This is easily done by taking the kitten to the litter box or toilet area after eating, drinking, sleeping, and playing. Giving the kitten plenty of opportunities to use the litter box, keeping it clean and in a location that appeals to the kitten, and preventing accidents by watching the kitten or confining it with a litter box will generally result in a house-trained cat.

Grooming

During the first few weeks of life, feline newborns depend on the queen to meet their grooming needs. She conditions their coats, stimulates urination and defecation, and provides tactile stimulation. Self-grooming begins at approximately 2 weeks of age, but the kitten's efforts are clumsy and incomplete. The kitten's first efforts usually involve licking a front paw; within a few days the kitten is licking the rest of its body. Scratching with a hind limb occurs by 18 days of age. At approximately 4 weeks a kitten will begin to use its forepaws as a tool for grooming the head and neck after eating. By maturity a cat will devote 30% to 50% of its waking time budget to grooming.[9] The primary purpose of grooming is body hygiene, which includes removing loose hair and dander and minimizing external parasites. Most grooming is performed with the tongue (licking) or teeth and usually takes place after rest, sleep, or eating. In hot weather evaporative cooling is achieved by licking the skin and hair.

Grooming is also an affiliative behavior among cats. In addition to queen–kitten grooming, some female cats will groom both females and males in their social group; males generally groom only females.[4] Cats are likely to have closer proximity and are more likely to groom familiar cats (i.e., those within their social group). However, the most frequent allogrooming and closest proximity are likely to occur among related cats.[16] Mutual grooming may also be demonstrated by cats toward humans by licking and by humans toward cats by petting. However, it is not unusual for humans to extend petting sessions beyond what is acceptable to the cat or to pet areas of the body other than the head or neck, which sometimes results in aggression.

Cats may engage in increased grooming after a stressful event and may display displacement grooming in situations of conflict. Although grooming that leads to excessive hair loss may be associated with stress and compulsive disorders, most cases are likely to have a medical cause including external parasites such as fleas. On the other hand, grooming practices may decrease in situations of chronic or recurrent stress. This may be accompanied by concurrent signs, including alterations in appetite, a decreased interest in social interactions, and avoidance or hiding. Of course, because decreased grooming may be due to medical problems, including systemic illness such as gastrointestinal and dental disease, metabolic disorders, pain, and aging, these must be ruled out first.

LEARNING

Although operant learning principles apply to training cats, as they do in other domestic species, it can be particularly challenging to find an appropriate incentive or motivator for cats. In addition, species-typical behaviors influence what behaviors are more likely to be learned. Therefore it is important that cats, as both a predator and a prey species, be in an environment that is conducive to learning new tasks.

Kittens can learn immediately after birth on the basis of sensory development. They learn to locate the preferred teat by 10 days through trial and error and olfactory cues.[9] Conditioned responses to sounds are seen by 10 days. Active avoidance also begins at this age. Passive avoidance, in which the kitten learns to associate cues with noxious stimuli, develops between 25 and 50 days.[17]

Kittens are not capable of learning to respond to purely visual cues until at least 1 month of age. By 6 to 8 weeks, kittens begin to show adult-like responses to both visual and olfactory social threats.[6]

Cats learn well by observation of other cats; kittens learn best by observing their own mother, but they can also learn by observing siblings and other feline members of the colony.[14] Ideally, kittens learn instinctive imitations that are required for self-preservation, such as hunting behavior, from the queen. Adult cats also display social learning by observing other cats and perhaps even humans. It is more significant for cats to watch another cat acquire a skill than to watch a skill that has been previously learned.[6]

At 8 weeks kittens can begin to solve problems, but their attention span is not yet stable.[9] Experiences such as human interactions and exposure to new environments when the kitten is between 5 and 6.5 weeks can result in latent learning; later in life they are less fearful when exposed to new people and novel stimuli.[9] Another important process of learning is habituation, in which kittens learn about threats and things of no consequence to them. This is not the same as socialization.

SOCIALIZATION AND THE KITTEN

The process by which näive kittens learn to accept the close proximity of members of their own species and members of other species is termed *socialization.* The most receptive time for socializing kittens to humans and other species is between 2 and 7 weeks of age.[25,26] Fear of people may be decreased by nonthreatening, gentle handling and exposure to humans during this period, which may persist into adulthood.[5,10] Conversely, lack of human exposure during this time increases the chance that the cat will interact poorly with humans, although genetic variables also play an important role.

Socialization is repeated in each generation of kittens and is not the same as domestication. It is strongly tied to the neurologic and physical development of the kitten. However, the socialization process is not just confined to kittenhood but continues throughout the life of the cat. A cat's socialization as a kitten can play a role in how they socialize to new individuals as adults. Problems can arise in the behavior of the adult cat if their socialization was inadequate, but poor socialization as a kitten is not insurmountable. Attachments can be formed at other times outside the sensitive period, although the process is much slower and involves extensive exposure.

Hand-raised kittens may still develop social attachments to other kittens, but this occurs much more slowly (Figure 9-5). However, a recent study found that kittens reared by hand were no more likely to display human and conspecific-directed aggression and fear, provided that there was a second cat in the home and wand-type toys were used to stimulate play and chase.[15]

Early handling of kittens by humans not only is beneficial for improving social relationships between kittens and humans but also leads to accelerated physical and central nervous system development and a general reduction of fearfulness. Kittens that were held and lightly stroked daily for the first few weeks of life opened their eyes earlier and began to explore earlier.[33] Kittens handled daily from birth to 45 days approached strange toys and people more frequently and were slower to learn avoidance.[42]

Social contact with the mother is also important for normal social development of kittens. Insufficient maternal care can result in cats that are fearful of humans and other cats. However, with sufficient human handling and care, the presence of another cat during the kitten's social development, and the use of wand-type play toys, problems may be minimized or prevented.[15]

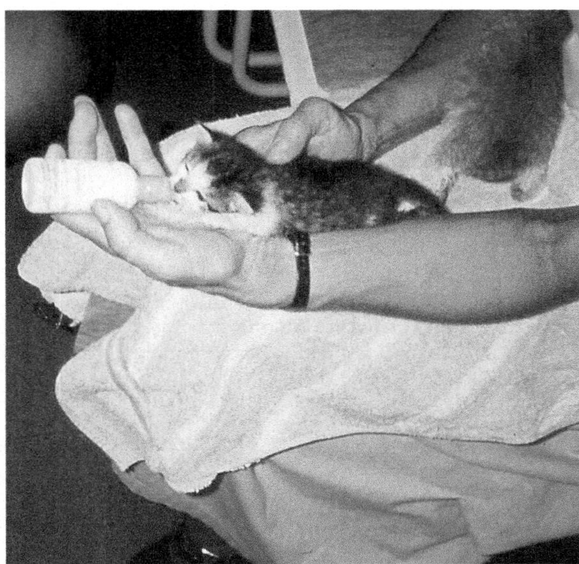

FIGURE 9-5 Hand-raised kittens may suffer from poor socialization, which can be overcome by sufficient handling and care, the presence of another cat during social development, and the use of wand-type play toys.

Cats, like other social species, are born with the capacity for species-specific social skills but need experience with their own species during the sensitive period of development to refine their social and communication skills with other cats. A kitten separated from its mother and littermates and kept as a sole cat in a household may be unable to form functional social attachments with other cats later in life, having missed opportunities for future socialization during this early developmental period.

What is not known in detail is how much handling is required to socialize a kitten to humans and human environments or what kinds of experiences are necessary for kittens to develop normally. For example, should all experiences be positive, or does the kitten need to have some moderately unpleasant experiences to develop fully? Research is hinting at the answers to some of these questions, but detailed investigation is necessary to determine the best socialization process for domestic kittens. In fact, studies in which kittens were handled from 1 minute to 5 hours daily suggest that in general, the more handling, the friendlier the kitten, although there may be an upper limit of approximately 1 hour above which no further benefit is seen.[40]

References

1. Adamec RE, Stark-Adamec C, Livingston KE: The development of predatory aggression and defense in the domestic cat *(Felis catus)*. I. Effects of early experience on adult patterns of aggression and defense, *Behav Neural Biol* 30:389, 1980.
2. Baerands van Room J, Baerands G: *The morphogenesis of the behaviour of the domestic cat*, Amsterdam, 1978, Elsevier Science.
3. Barrett P, Bateson P: The development of play in cats, *Behaviour* 66:106, 1978.
4. Barry KJ, Crowell-Davis SL: Gender differences in the social behavior of the neutered indoor-only domestic cat, *Appl Anim Behav Sci* 64:193, 1999.
5. Bateson P: How do sensitive periods arise and what are they for? *Anim Behav* 27:470, 1979.
6. Bateson P: Behavioural development in the cat. In Turner D,Bateson P, editors: *The domestic cat: the biology of its behaviour*, ed 2, Cambridge, 2000, Cambridge University Press, p 9.
7. Bateson P, Mendl M, Feaver J: Play in the domestic cat is enhanced by rationing of the mother during lactation, *Anim Behav* 40:514, 1990.
8. Beaver B: Reflex development in the kitten, *Appl Anim Ethol* 4:93, 1978.
9. Beaver B: *Feline behavior: a guide for veterinarians*, ed 2, St Louis, 2003, Saunders Elsevier.
10. Bradshaw J, Horsfield G, Allen J et al: Feral cats: their role in the population dynamics of *Felis catus*, *Appl Anim Behav Sci* 65:273, 1999.
11. Budiansky S: *The character of cats: the origins, intelligence, behavior, and stratagems of Felis silvestris catus*, New York, 2002, Viking.
12. Caro TM: The effects of experience on the predatory patterns of cats, *Behav Neural Biol* 29:1, 1980.
13. Caro TM: Effects of the mother, object play, and adult experience on predation in cats, *Behav Neural Biol* 29:29, 1980.
14. Chesler P: Maternal influence in learning by observation in kittens, *Science* 166:901, 1969.
15. Chon E: The effects of queen *(Felis sylvestris)*-rearing versus hand-rearing on feline aggression and other problematic behaviors. In Mills D, Levine E, editors: *Current issues and research in veterinary behavioral medicine*, West Lafayette, Ind., 2005, Purdue University Press, p 201.
16. Curtis T, Knowles R, Crowell-Davis S: Influence of familiarity and relatedness on proximity and allogrooming in domestic cats *(Felis catus)*, *Am J Vet Res* 64:1151, 2003.
17. Davis J, Jensen R: The development of passive and active avoidance learning in cats, *Dev Psychogiol* 9:175, 1976.
18. Deag J, Manning A, Lawrence C: Factors influencing the mother-kitten relationship. In Turner D, Bateson P, editors: *The domestic cat: the biology of its behaviour*, ed 2, Cambridge, 2000, Cambridge University Press, p 24.
19. Feldman H: Maternal care and differences in the use of nests in the domestic cat, *Anim Behav* 45:13, 1993.
20. Gallo PV, Werboff J, Knox K: Protein restriction during gestation and lactation: development of attachment behavior in cats, *Behav Neural Biol* 29:216, 1980.
21. Hall SL, Bradshaw JWS: The influence of hunger on object play by adult domestic cats, *Appl Anim Behav Sci* 58:143, 1998.
22. Hall SL, Bradshaw JWS, Robinson IH: Object play in adult domestic cats: the roles of habituation and disinhibition, *Appl Anim Behav Sci* 79:263, 2002.
23. Houpt K: *Domestic animal behavior*, ed 4, Ames, Iowa, 2005, Blackwell Publishing.
24. Hudson R, Raihani G, Gonzalez D et al: Nipple preference and contests in suckling kittens of the domestic cat are unrelated to presumed nipple quality, *Dev Psychobiol* 51:322, 2009.
25. Karsh E: *The effects of early and late handling on the attachment of cats to people. The pet connection: its influence on our health and quality of life: proceedings of conferences on the human-animal relationships and human-animal bond*, University of Minnesota, 1983, p 207.
26. Karsh E: The effects of early handling on the development of social bonds between cats and people. In Katcher A, Beck A, editors: *New perspectives on our lives with companion animals*, Philadelphia, 1983, University of Pennsylvania Press, p 22.
27. Kolb B, Nonneman AJ: The development of social responsiveness in kittens, *Anim Behav* 23:368, 1975.

28. Kovach JK, Kling A: Mechanisms of neonate sucking behaviour in the kitten, *Anim Behav* 15:91, 1967.
29. Lowe SE, Bradshaw JW: Ontogeny of individuality in the domestic cat in the home environment, *Anim Behav* 61:231, 2001.
30. Martin P: An experimental study of weaning in the domestic cat, *Behavior* 99:221, 1986.
31. Martin P, Bateson P: The influence of experimentally manipulating a component of weaning on the development of play in domestic cats, *Anim Behav* 33:511, 1985.
32. McCune S: The impact of paternity and early socialisation on the development of cats' behaviour to people and novel objects, *Appl Anim Behav Sci* 45:109, 1995.
33. Meier G: Infantile handling and development in Siamese kittens, *J Comp Physiol Psychol* 54:284, 1961.
34. Mellen J: Effects of early rearing experience on subsequent adult sexual behavior using domestic cats *(Felis catus)* as a model for exotic small felids, *Zoo Biol* 11:17, 1992.
35. Mendl M: The effects of litter-size variation on the development of play behaviour in the domestic cat: litters of one and two, *Anim Behav* 36:20, 1988.
36. Patronek G, Glickman L, Beck A et al: Risk factors for relinquishment of cats to an animal shelter, *J Am Vet Med Assoc* 209:582, 1996.
37. Seitz PFD: Infantile experience and adult behavior in animal subjects: II. Age of separation from the mother and adult behavior in the cat, *Psychosom Med* 21:353, 1959.
38. Smith B, Jensen G: Brain development in the feline, *Nutr Rep Int* 16:487, 1977.
39. Tan PL, Counsilman JJ: The influence of weaning on prey-catching behaviour in kittens, *Z Tierpsychol* 70:148, 1985.
40. Turner D: The human–cat relationship. In Turner D, Bateson P, editors: *The domestic cat: the biology of its behaviour*, ed 2, Cambridge, 2000, Cambridge University Press, p 194.
41. West M: Social play in the domestic cat, *Am Zool* 14:427, 1974.
42. Wilson M, Warren JM, Abbott L: Infantile stimulation, activity, and learning by cats, *Child Dev* 36:843, 1965.

CHAPTER

10

Normal Behavior of Cats

Jacqueline Mary Ley and Kersti Seksel

OUTLINE

The behavior displayed at any time by an individual cat is the result of the interplay of genetic predisposition, what the cat has learned from previous experiences, and the current environment in which the cat finds itself. Although some behavioral patterns are common to all members of a species, others are unique to each individual. It is essential to understand the normal or common behavioral patterns of cats to assess the behaviors that owners are concerned about. Sometimes owners are concerned about behaviors that are normal for cats to express, such as spraying or predatory behavior. At other times, knowledge of the normal range of expression of a behavior pattern (e.g., grooming behavior) will help the veterinarian determine whether the behavior is normal and adaptive or abnormal and maladaptive.

THE BIOLOGY OF CATS

To understand the behavior of cats, the veterinarian must first look at the physical characteristics of the cat, such as its size and sensory capabilities, because these are intertwined with behavior. Only by appreciating the behavioral biology of the domestic cat is it possible to understand their behavioral needs.

The domestic cat is a small, crepuscular, solitary hunter of the felid family. Whether the domestic cat is a unique species or a subtype of the wild cat *(Felis silvestris)* of northern Africa remains controversial.[16] The cat evolved in arid areas and hunts small animals such as rodents, frogs, birds, and reptiles. They are small, tending to weigh between 2 kg (4.4 lb) and 8 kg (17.6 lb) and have large, forward-facing eyes; large, mobile ears; and sensitive vibrissae on the face that aid in detecting prey in dim light. They have large, ventrally flattened canine teeth and sharp retractable claws on all toes to catch, hold, and kill prey. The cat is an ambush hunter. It locates prey using its sensitive hearing, vision, and sense of smell. It then stalks the prey silently until it is close enough for a sudden rush and grab. Cats do not possess the stamina to chase prey for long periods. However, they are able to climb and jump up to five times their own height.[16] Being small, they are potential prey for larger animals, so their agility is an advantage not only for hunting but also for escaping when being hunted.

SENSE ORGANS

Vision

One of the reasons that cats are so appealing to people is their large, prominent eyes. Large eyes are necessary for seeing (and hunting) in dim light. Cats' eyes have many characteristics to maximize the visual field and the collection of light entering the eye and stimulating the retinal cells.[3] The cornea is large and bulges outward, which allows about five times more light to enter the eye than does the human cornea.[16] The retina has approximately 25 light-sensitive rod cells for every color-sensitive cone cell. When rod cells in a cluster are stimulated by light, they all stimulate one nerve fiber. This results in cats being able to see in very dim light, albeit a fuzzy image.[16] The tapetum lucidum under the retina reflects light back to maximize the chance of rods being stimulated. This layer is what makes cat eyes glow yellowish green when light is shone into them. Cats have little need for color vision because they hunt mainly at night, and most prey species do not have a wide range of coat colors. It appears that cats can see yellow and blue wavelengths of light and can be taught to distinguish among red and other colors. However, this is difficult for them to learn, which suggests that cats are just not interested in colors.[16]

The lens of the eye has a limited capacity for accommodation. This means that a cat's vision is best at approximately 2 to 6 meters (6.5 to 19.7 feet) from the viewed object.[16] This is why cats have trouble taking treats from an owner's hand. To maximize visual acuity, they have multifocal lenses that focus light at particular wavelengths. The slit pupil prevents the loss of visual fields that can focus at set wavelengths and maximizes the cat's vision.[27]

Binocular vision aids the cat in judging distances for catching prey, climbing, and jumping. The binocular overlap is about 98 degrees, which allows cats to judge distances very accurately.[3,16] Their accuracy is even more amazing in light of how short sighted they are. Cats are very attuned to even small movements in their visual field.

The eyes of cats are not functional at birth. The eyelids open between days 14 and 21. Vision develops with experience. If kittens are deprived of vision through blindfolding before their eyes open[30] or are housed in environments that are altered to show no horizontal lines, the kittens do not develop normal vision, even though the eyes are structurally and functionally normal.[21,29]

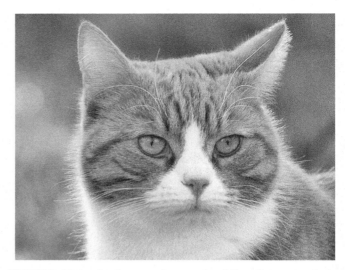

FIGURE 10-1 Cats' ears are large and mobile and can move independently, as well as swivel almost 180 degrees. *(Photo courtesy Mats Hamnas.)*

Hearing

The large, mobile pinnae of cats act to collect and funnel sounds into the ear canal. Each ear can move independently of the other, and the ears can swivel almost 180 degrees, effectively giving them surround sound (Figure 10-1).

When tracking a sound, such as that of a prey animal, cats use a combination of the interaural time differences for sounds to reach both pinnae, level differences between the pinnae, and directional amplification effects of the pinnae to localize the sound and orientate their head.[4] They are able to do this as both the prey animal and the cat are moving.

Olfaction

Cats have a well-developed sense of smell at birth. These nerves are myelinated at birth, in contrast to most other neurons in the nervous system. This allows signals to pass rapidly to the brain. The kittens use their sense of smell and touch to find the queen's nipples. If they are unable to smell, because of an upper respiratory tract infection, for instance, kittens cannot find the queen's nipples and feed.[24]

Cats use their sense of smell for locating prey and evaluating communication signals left by other cats. Odors play an important role in the social organization of cats and in reproduction. The feline nasal mucosa is between 20 and 40 square centimeters, small when compared with dogs, although it still eclipses the human nasal epithelium. To further aid in scent detection, the cat has two structures: the subethmoid shelf[16] and the vomeronasal organ (VMO).[22]

The subethmoid shelf traps air and scent particles taken into the nasal cavity allowing more time for them to stimulate receptors in the olfactory mucosa.[11,28] The VMO sits between the oral cavity and the nasal cavity. It has connections with the nasal cavity and the oral cavity. The receptors of the VMO are different from those of the nasal epithelium. The gape or flehmen response may be performed after the cat has sniffed or even licked at a scent source. By wrinkling the upper lip and opening the mouth, the cat opens the ducts of the VMO and pumps saliva and the scent into the VMO.[22] Cats cannot fully evert their upper lip as horses and cattle can because of the frenulum between the upper lip and upper jaw. The gape reaction is seen when tomcats encounter urine from another cat. However, queens and neutered cats also exhibit this behavior when investigating odors.

Touch

Anyone who has petted a cat knows how important physical contact is to cats. Touch is used as a means to build social bonds within feline social groups. The response of cats to touch and temperature varies across their bodies. Cats do not react to temperature on their bodies until the temperatures reach 51° to 54° C (124 to 129° F). However, the skin around the nasal area is exquisitely sensitive to temperature changes, reacting to temperature increases of 0.2° C and decreases of 0.5° C. This ability is an advantage for locating prey. Cats have individual differences in their preferences regarding petting and handling. Some like very strong pressure, whereas others prefer a light touch.

Cats have specialized tactile vibrissae on their faces and forelegs. The vibrissae are long, thick hairs that are obvious against the coat of the cat. They sit in a large follicle with a sebaceous gland attached. Striated muscle attached to the follicle allows the vibrissae to be voluntarily moved. The follicle has several nerve receptors associated with it. These are sensitive to pressures on the vibrissae as light as 2 mg or 5 Angstrom,[15] and they are sensitive to movement of the vibrissae from the normal position.

The facial vibrissae, better known as the whiskers, are synonymous with cats. These are arranged in rows on the upper lips. The upper rows move independently of the lower rows. Cats fold the whiskers back when relaxed and spread them when walking or showing interest in something. Because cats cannot see things that are close, their whiskers are important for the location of prey, food, water, and other objects close to the face. Whiskers also aid in spatial awareness. Cats have a superciliary tuft above each eye and two tufts between the ear and point of mandible known as genal tuft 1 and 2. Genal tuft 1 is dorsal to genal tuft 2. These vibrissae also help in spatial awareness. There are also vibrissae on the back of both carpi just dorsal to the accessory pad. It is thought that these tufts aid the cat in using its forelimbs for activities such as hunting.

Taste

The sense of taste is important to cats. They have two types of taste buds on their tongues: mushroom-shaped papillae at the front and sides of the tongue and cup-shaped papillae at the back of the tongue. Cats can taste salty, bitter, and acid. They have little reaction to sucrose and tend to drink sweet water only if the sugar is masked by salt. In fact, cats lack the ability to taste sweetness, unlike other mammals. The taste receptor for sweetness is made up of two proteins generated by two genes, *Tas1r2* and *Tas1r3*. In cats the *Tas1r2* gene does not code for the normal mammalian protein, thereby impairing the function of taste receptors for sweetness.[26]

COMMUNICATION

Cats send signals using body language—that is, by changing their posture, the position of their limbs and ears, and the size of their pupils and by puffing up their fur to appear larger. Cats are very expressive, and it can help when learning cat communication signals to look at each area of the body separately.

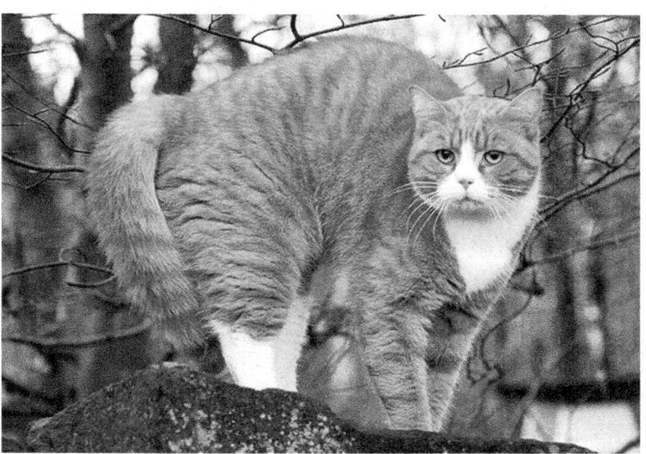

FIGURE 10-2 When a cat feels threatened, it will arch its back and puff up the hair coat in an attempt to appear larger. *(Photo courtesy Mats Hamnas.)*

Body Language

Body

Cats send messages to other cats and animals and humans by using their bodies. The size of the body, the shape of the body, the position of ears, size of pupils, size and position of the tail, and visibility of weapons such as teeth all convey important messages to others. In general terms a confident cat stands tall and evenly on all four feet, with its tail up or level with its back and its ears facing forward. An attacking cat usually makes itself appear larger by standing at its full height and bristling its hair coat. The tail will also be raised, with its fur puffed out. When a cat really wants to convey a message to an opponent that it is ready to fight if the other does not back down, the cat will arch its back (Figure 10-2). The more fearful a cat is feeling, the lower its body gets to the ground. An uncertain cat may take the middle road, often lowering its rump while keeping its forelegs available for striking.

Ears

An interested cat will have its ears rotated forward. A frightened cat will have its ears flat and facing backward. Cats that are attempting to bluff another cat or that are uncertain will hold their ears halfway between forward facing and flat and backwards.

Eyes

Interested cats will look at the person or object of their interest. Cats will stare at other cats or people as an aggressive signal. This should not be confused with making friendly eye contact. Aggressive stares are intense. Friendly eye contact can be soft and often the cat may blink in an exaggerated manner. Less confident cats and cats that wish to avoid a physical altercation will avoid looking at another cat or a person who is staring at them. In avoiding the eye contact, the cat may simply look away or, if it is feeling very uncomfortable, may engage in intensive grooming—hence the important feline rule of thumb: "When in doubt, wash." Often, other cats will avoid looking at a cat that is engaged in a bout of composure grooming. In scientific language the grooming strategy is a displacement behavior that occurs when a cat feels threatened but is unsure if it should run away or stay put.

Tail

Cat tails are extremely expressive and rarely still. Vertical tails are seen at greetings, during play, and in the female during sexual approaches. It is thought that cats raise their tails in acknowledgment of the higher social status of another cat.[5] For example, kittens show the behavior toward their queens. Horizontal tails are seen during amicable approaches. A lowered tail is seen in aggressive incidents, and a tail held between the legs is seen when a cat wants to avoid any altercation. The concave tail position, in which the tail is held vertically from the base and then curves over so that the tip points at the ground, is often used in aggressive incidents but may also be seen during play.

Vocalizations

The noises cats make have been studied for many years because their sense of hearing is more sensitive than that of humans and because cats were used as the animal model for the development of the cochlear implant, or bionic ear.[8] The sounds cats make can be divided into three main categories: sounds made with the mouth shut, sounds made with the mouth initially open but then closing, and sounds made with the mouth held open. Some sounds are specific to particular circumstances, such as the sounds a queen makes for her kittens.

Closed Mouth

There are two sounds included in the closed-mouth category. They are the purr and the trill/chirrup/greeting meow. Purring has fascinated people for a long time. It is a monotone sound made by cats in a wide range of situations. However, the common feature of all situations appears to be cat-to-cat or cat-to-human contact. Interestingly, cats also purr when in extreme pain. There is little information to explain why this occurs, but some think it may be the cat's attempt to calm itself. The trill/chirrup/greeting meow is, as its name suggests, uttered on contact with a known and liked cat or person.

Open–Closing Mouth

There are four sounds included in the open–closing mouth group: the meow, the long meow, the female call, and the mowl (a male call, also known as *caterwaul*). Only the meow and long meow will be considered here, insofar as they are social communications that are often directed at humans.

The meow is a general communication sound for cats, with the long meow being a high-intensity version of the ordinary meow. Many cats have expressive meows that can be identified as having different meanings by humans. The variety in the meows of cats appears to be due to individual differences among cats and, for meows directed at people, the result of interactions with humans. The role of the long meow in cat-to-cat communication is unclear at present, but many cat owners know what their cat means when it directs a long meow at them (e.g., "Open the door, please!"; "Hurry up with the food already!").

Open Mouth

Open-mouth sounds are the sounds of aggression—that is, the growl, the yowl, the snarl, the hiss, and the spit. Growling, yowling, and snarling are used when the cat signals that it is threatening or actively attacking, whereas hissing and spitting tend to be used in defensive aggression when the cat is threatened or attacked.

Odor Signals

Cats recognize members of their social group or a cat with which they have fought by appearance and smell. Each cat has its own particular smell, the result of secretions from glands in the skin of the corners of the mouth, sides of the forehead, and along the tail. Feline greeting behavior involves sniffing these areas and around the anus. Cats will rub or bump their faces against objects, people, familiar dogs, and other cats to spread their scent. It has been suggested that this behavior forms a group scent, which identifies members of a particular social group. Members who go missing from the group may initially be rejected until they smell "right" again. This is why it can be useful in multicat households to rub a newcomer or a recently absent feline family member with a towel that has been rubbed over the other cat members of the family. The fact the cat smells "right" can speed its acceptance into the group.

Urine

Long-term odor signals are posted prominently using urine sprayed on vertical surfaces. The urine can be very pungent and serves to inform other cats as to the gender and sexual status of the cat claiming the territory. Before spraying, the cat may sniff the area and may show a flehmen response. It will then back up to the vertical surface and eject a small, strong jet of urine onto the surface. The tail is held upright and typically quivers as the urine is voided.

Cat urine owes its characteristic odor to volatile chemicals, some of which have the precursor felinine, a unique sulfur-containing amino acid. Felinine is unique to certain *Felidae* species, such as the bobcat and domestic cat. Felinine concentrations are highest in intact male cats, lower in castrated male cats, and lowest in female cats.[18] It takes about 5 days after castration for felinine levels to decrease in urine.[18] The biological function of felinine is unknown, but it is believed to be a pheromone precursor.

Spraying behavior differs between the sexes, with intact male cats spraying more than castrated male cats and intact queens. Spayed queens are the group least likely to spray. Spraying increases when queens are in season (estrus). Some cats also spray if they feel worried or anxious. However, cats do not spray because they are angry, spiteful, or mean.

LEARNING

Cats are born with behavior patterns for feeding, hunting, grooming, marking, and reproduction already hard-wired in the brain. Another way of describing these behaviors is being instinctive. Instinctive behavior in cats is refined through learning and experience. Kittens instinctively orient themselves toward high-pitched sounds, and experience helps them learn how to localize the sound; identify it; and then potentially stalk, pounce, and catch the small rodent.

Experience is gained largely through trial-and-error learning. This type of learning describes the way cats learn about their environment by interacting with objects of interest. When cats are repeatedly exploring and manipulating objects, one of the following occurs: they receive a payoff (positive reinforcement); something aversive occurs (positive punishment); or nothing happens, in which case they learn there is no value in interacting with the object.

Cats use trial-and-error learning when learning how to apply instinctive behavior patterns. Thus naïve cats know how to catch new prey species, but their technique improves with experience.[6,7] However, kittens are capable of some observational learning. Cats also appear able to learn by watching other cats acquire a new skill.[20] Kittens can learn by watching the queen demonstrate hunting and killing behaviors.[6]

HUNTING AND FEEDING

The cat is an obligate carnivore that evolved to hunt small animal species—mostly mice and rats but also lizards, frogs, birds, and insects. Cats will also scavenge food from human rubbish.

Cats show distinct behavioral patterns when offered palatable and unpalatable foods.[32] When the cat is investigating food, it sniffs at palatable foods and generally licks its lips and sniffs around the food before consuming it. When presented with an unpalatable food, the cat behaves differently, possibly sniffing at the food and then licking its nose. It may then groom its chest and body. After eating, the cat usually grooms its face and body.

GROOMING

The grooming behavior of cats is familiar to most people. Grooming plays a very important role in the self-care and maintenance of cats but can also be performed when the cat is anxious; when performed on another cat, an activity called *allogrooming,* it helps create or reinforce a social bond.

Cats spend approximately 8% of their time awake engaged in grooming behavior.[13] Most of this time is spent licking multiple areas of the body. A very small percentage of grooming time is spent scratching at a single area with the hind leg.[13] Grooming removes dead hair and skin parasites. When cats are prevented from grooming, they have higher numbers of fleas than cats that are not prevented from grooming.[12] Cats with fleas groom themselves at a much higher rate than cats that do not have fleas. Cats ingest about two thirds of the hair that they lose annually.[19]

As previously mentioned, grooming can be used as a displacement behavior when cats are anxious or after acute stress.[31] It is not surprising that a common presentation of anxiety in cats is overgrooming, which can lead to hair loss and skin damage.[25] Grooming may also be used as a cutoff signal to avoid an aggressive encounter with another cat. Allogrooming is seen among bonded members of a social group.[9]

SOCIAL ORGANIZATION AND DENSITY

The normal social organization of cats is variable, which may be one reason that cats have been so successful as a species. Rather than being easily described by one social system, they are highly variable as to how they can live and organize themselves socially.[23] Cats can be found living as solitary animals, intolerant of other cats, and as members of large, crowded colonies, as well as every variation between those extremes.

Although cats are solitary hunters, insofar as their prey are small animals best caught by a single hunter, it is generally accepted that cats are a social species that form complex social groups.[9] Cats can live in a variety of social group structures. These include being solitary

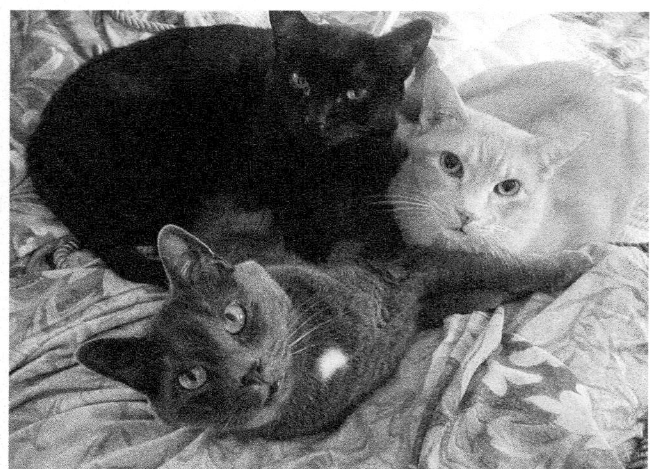

FIGURE 10-3 Long-term associates will often be found together and will share sleeping and resting places. *(Photo courtesy Susan Little.)*

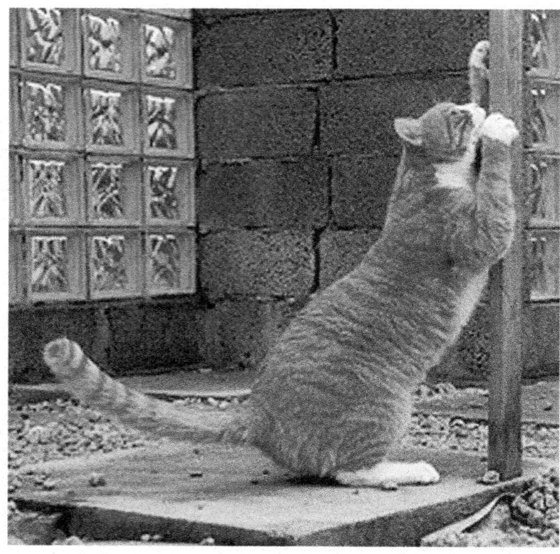

FIGURE 10-4 Territorial boundaries are maintained by visual and olfactory signals left by scratching on vertical surfaces. *(Photo courtesy Mats Hamnas.)*

unless mating or raising young to forming stable social groups. The composition of the groups varies in part with the distribution and abundance of food and the sex of the cats. Where food is abundant, cats will gather together and form structured groups.

A population of cats within an area can be considered a colony.[9] Within a colony the cats will form affiliative and antagonistic relationships. Affiliated cats greet one another, rub heads and bodies, and sometimes twine their tails; as previously discussed, they may groom one another.[9] It is thought that this behavior helps create a group odor that identifies all members. Long-term associates will generally be found together and may share sleeping spaces and food (Figure 10-3).[1] There are differences between the sexes with regard to social contact, with one study of 60 two-cat households finding that male cats spent more time in close proximity than did female cats[2] and another study finding a lack of affiliative behavior among feral male cats.[10] Antagonistic encounters are rare in a stable colony. Cats that do not get along tend to avoid each other and use time-sharing arrangement to access shared areas.

Queens generally form groups with their kittens. Queens may raise their kittens with other queens. These kittens have been found to leave the nest sooner than kittens raised by the dam alone: 20 days for group-reared kittens compared with 30 days for single-reared kittens.[14]

Intact male cats may join groups briefly. For intact male cats, spending time with queens is important to increase the chance of being able to mate when the queens are next in heat. However, spending too much time with one group of queens reduces the time available to spend with other queens. There is a trade-off depending on how closely the groups of cats live. Neutered male cats often form close bonds with other cats.

Cats are territorial. Territory boundaries are maintained with visual and olfactory signals in the form of scratching on vertical surfaces and depositing urine, feces, or both (Figure 10-4). Surrounding the territory is the home range, which may be shared in part with other cats. The size of the home range is directly related to the density of food sources. Where food is abundant, home ranges may be as small as 0.2 acre for female cats and 2.1 acres for male cats. In areas with less abundant food, ranges have been measured at 667 acres for females and 1038 acres for males.[3]

TIME BUDGETS: WHAT DO CATS DO ALL DAY?

Although cats are thought of as nocturnal, they are better classified as crepuscular animals, insofar as they are most active at dawn and dusk. They tend to spend most of their time resting.[10] Laboratory cats have been found to sleep approximately 10 hours a day, with short intervals of activity adding up to approximately 1 and ½ hours.

During hot weather cats spend more time lying stretched out, whereas in colder weather they spend more time curled up. One study of urban cats found a positive relationship between nighttime activity of cats and nighttime weather, with cats being less active on colder nights.[17] Rain decreased cat activity, and cat activity increased in spring, before waning in autumn.[17]

Grooming and self-care behaviors such as hunting, foraging, and feeding take 50% of cats' time.[13] The time spent in social interactions has not been measured.

References

1. Alger JM, Alger SF: *Cat culture: the social world of a cat shelter*, Philadelphia, 2005, Temple University Press.
2. Barry KJ, Crowell-Davis SL: Gender differences in the social behavior of the neutered indoor-only domestic cat, *Appl Anim Behav Sci* 64:193, 1999.
3. Beaver B: *Feline behavior: a guide for veterinarians*, ed 2, St Louis, 2003, Saunders Elsevier.
4. Beitel RE: Acoustic pursuit of invisible moving targets by cats, *J Acoust Soc Am* 105:3449, 1999.
5. Cafazzo S, Natoli E: The social function of tail up in the domestic cat *(Felis silvestris catus)*, *Behav Processes* 80:60, 2009.
6. Caro TM: The effects of experience on the predatory patterns of cats, *Behav Neural Biol* 29:1, 1980.
7. Caro TM: Effects of the mother, object play, and adult experience on predation in cats, *Behav Neural Biol* 29:29, 1980.
8. Clark G: Research directions for future generations of cochlear implants, *Cochlear Implants Int* 5 Suppl 1:2, 2004.
9. Crowell-Davis S, Curtis T, Knowles R: Social organization in the cat: a modern understanding, *J Feline Med Surg* 6:19, 2004.
10. Dards JL: The behavior of dockyard cats: interactions of adult males, *Appl Anim Ethol* 10:133, 1983.
11. Done SH, Goody PC, Stickland NC et al: *Color atlas of veterinary anatomy: the dog and cat*, Barcelona, 2003, Elsevier Science.
12. Eckstein RA, Hart BL: Grooming and control of fleas in cats, *Appl Anim Behav Sci* 68:141, 2000.
13. Eckstein RA, Hart BL: The organization and control of grooming in cats, *Appl Anim Behav Sci* 68:131, 2000.
14. Feldman H: Maternal care and differences in the use of nests in the domestic cat, *Anim Behav* 45:13, 1993.
15. Fitzgerald O: Discharges from the sensory organs of the cat's vibrissae and the modification in their activity by ions, *J Physiol* 98:163, 1940.
16. Fogle B: *The cat's mind*, London, 1991, Pelham Books.
17. Haspel C, Calhoon RE: Activity patterns of free-ranging cats in Brooklyn, New York, *J Mammal* 74:1, 1993.
18. Hendriks WH, Rutherfurd-Markwick KJ, Weidgraaf K et al: Testosterone increases urinary free felinine, N-acetylfelinine and methylbutanolglutathione excretion in cats *(Felis catus)*, *J Anim Physiol Anim Nutr (Berl)* 92:53, 2008.
19. Hendriks WH, Tarttelin MF, Moughan PJ: Seasonal hair loss in adult domestic cats *(Felis catus)*, *J Anim Physiol Anim Nutr (Berl)* 79:92, 1998.
20. Herbert MJ, Harsh CM: Observational learning by cats, *J Comp Psychol* 37:81, 1944.
21. Hirsch HV, Spinelli DN: Visual experience modifies distribution of horizontally and vertically oriented receptive fields in cats, *Science* 168:869, 1970.
22. Houpt KA: *Domestic animal behavior for veterinarians and animal scientists*, Ames, Iowa, 1998, Iowa State University Press.
23. Izawa M, Doi T: Flexibility of the social system of the feral cat, *Felis catus*, *Physiol Ecol Japan* 29:237, 1993.
24. Kovach JK, Kling A: Mechanisms of neonate sucking behaviour in the kitten, *Anim Behav* 15:91, 1967.
25. Landsberg G, Hunthausen W, Ackerman L: *Handbook of behavior problems of the dog and cat*, ed 2, St Louis, 2003, Elsevier Saunders.
26. Li X, Li W, Wang H et al: Cats lack a sweet taste receptor, *J Nutr* 136:1932S, 2006.
27. Malmstrom T, Kroger RH: Pupil shapes and lens optics in the eyes of terrestrial vertebrates, *J Exp Biol* 209:18, 2006.
28. Negus VE: Observations on the comparative anatomy and physiology of olfaction, *Acta Otolaryngol* 44:13, 1954.
29. Olson CR, Pettigrew JD: Single units in visual cortex of kittens reared in stroboscopic illumination, *Brain Res* 70:189, 1974.
30. Pettigrew JD: The effect of visual experience on the development of stimulus specificity by kitten cortical neurones, *J Physiol* 237:49, 1974.
31. Van den Bos R: Post-conflict stress-response in confined group-living cats *(Felis silvestris catus)*, *Appl Anim Behav Sci* 59:323, 1998.
32. Van den Bos R, Meijer MK, Spruijt BM: Taste reactivity patterns in domestic cats *(Felis silvestris catus)*, *Appl Anim Behav Sci* 69:149, 2000.

CHAPTER

11

Kitten Socialization and Training Classes

Kersti Seksel and Steve Dale

OUTLINE

It is now well accepted that puppies benefit from attending socialization and training classes. So if puppies can attend school, why not kittens? There are many positive outcomes when kittens and people attend kitten socialization classes, which were first developed in Australia as Kitten Kindy.[13]

The idea of training cats, let alone holding kitten socialization and training classes, is a foreign concept to most people.[13] However, kitten classes can be just as successful and deliver many of the same benefits to owners, kittens, and the veterinary practice as puppy classes (Box 11-1). Kitten classes are designed to be an early socialization, training, and education program to help owners and kittens start off on the right track. Kitten classes aim to help prevent behavioral problems, as well as educate owners on all aspects of raising a kitten and then living with a cat in the family. The aim is also to establish a close bond among the cat, the owner, and the veterinary practice. It is yet another valuable service that veterinarians should offer their patients and clients.

Although the issue has not been formally studied, kitten classes are likely to save lives, insofar as some of the recognized potential risk factors for relinquishment could be addressed in well-run kitten classes. These risk factors include harboring unrealistic or inappropriate expectations about the cat's role in the household, allowing the cat outdoors, owning a sexually intact cat, and never having read a book about cat behavior; cats that eliminate inappropriately on a daily or weekly basis are also at risk.[11] The most frequent explanations for surrender are behavioral problems—problems that might have been prevented.[9,10]

Most veterinary behaviorists now believe that kitten socialization classes (when properly taught) are beneficial,[9,10,12] and kitten socialization classes are suggested in the American Association of Feline Practitioners Feline Behavior Guidelines.[10]

On average, cats visit the veterinarian less than half as often as dogs,[7] yet cats outnumber dogs by approximately 20%.[1] Given that most socialization classes require a sign-off form from the veterinarian, enrollment in such a class ensures at least one veterinary visit and so establishes a relationship with a veterinarian.[10]

There are many reasons that cats may visit the veterinarian less often than dogs, and these range from the cat's fear of the carrier and the corresponding car ride to difficulties with handling the cat for even minor procedures. Kitten class instructors can address some of these issues in the class, as well as provide instructions regarding the best ways to desensitize kittens to carriers and car rides even before the first kitten class.

Dog trainers who teach puppy classes often remark that educating the owner is the most important aspect of the classes. Kitten classes are no different, offering an opportunity to educate clients about their kitten's behavior and set up realistic expectations of living with a cat in the household.

Getting to know a cat better might help when a cat is not feeling well. This is even more imperative with cats than dogs because cats often mask signs of illness. The more connected families are to their cats, the more likely they are to detect these subtle signs.

BOX 11-1

The Value of Kitten Socialization Classes

- All kittens are examined before attending, which requires establishing a relationship with a veterinarian.
- Kittens are desensitized to the carrier.
- Kittens are habituated to travel.
- Kittens are habituated to unfamiliar people.
- Owners learn about proper care, which enhances cat health: nail clipping, brushing the coat, and brushing teeth.
- Owners who have a stronger bond with their cats may be more likely to note subtle signs of illness and visit the veterinarian proactively for wellness exams.
- Many behavioral problems can be prevented.
- The class provides a veterinary resource for behavior-related problems.
- The instructor can provide information on feline heartworm prevention and what to do to control fleas and ticks (where applicable).
- The class helps to dispel common myths about cats (e.g., cats are antisocial).
- Owners learn that they *can* exercise their cats and provide an interesting enriched life indoors. They also discover that cats can learn and be trained.
- The class boosts the confidence of kittens and owners alike, and the sessions are fun for kittens, owners, and instructors.

GETTING STARTED

Planning Classes

For maximum benefit the classes should be held at a veterinary clinic so that the kittens and their owners can meet veterinarians and staff and become familiar with the practice. These classes should be planned carefully. The aim and outcome for running the classes should be considered in advance.

The classes should be fun and also provide a relaxed and safe environment for both pets and owners to learn. The objectives of kitten classes will differ with each veterinary practice, but the aim should be to accomplish the following:

- Inform owners about normal feline behavior.
- Allow kittens to socialize in a safe and controlled environment.
- Teach kittens to accept gentle handling from humans.
- Habituate kittens to a variety of stimuli so that they grow into manageable, easily handled adult cats.
- Identify problem behaviors, and provide possible solutions to common issues such as litter training, biting, and scratching.
- Provide advice on how to modify unacceptable behavior, and refer to a veterinary behaviorist if necessary.
- Help owners to have realistic expectations for their pet.
- Help owners build a strong bond with the veterinary practice.
- Educate owners on all aspects of kitten development, pet care, and living with a cat in the family—fostering socially responsible pet ownership.

Recruitment and Promotion

Ideally, kittens are recruited at the time of their first vaccination or health examination. This visit should include provision of written material on kitten care and kitten classes. Because classes for kittens are a novelty, the local media are often interested in covering the story and thereby help advertise the classes. There are also some veterinarians who work in tandem with local shelters that support the concept of kitten classes. Working together with a shelter has benefits because it provides a partner to help promote the classes and also helps rehome kittens. However, the success of the program depends on the support of all personnel at the veterinary practice. Everyone needs to understand what the classes involve to recruit the kittens effectively.

Kittens

All kittens attending classes should be between 8 and 14 weeks of age and must have started their vaccination and worming program. Kittens should be no more than 14 weeks old when they complete the course to prevent potential fighting. The recommended minimum number of kittens for a class is three and the optimal maximum number is six, so that all kittens and their owners get suitable attention.

Attendees

The whole family, including children, should be encouraged to attend. If young children are attending, one adult must accompany each child so that they are adequately supervised. Owners of cats older than 14 weeks are encouraged to attend *without* their cat so that they too can benefit from the information provided.

Staff

So that the classes are functional and owners and kittens derive value from attending, at least two people should run each class. This allows for better observation of the kittens and more effective control of the class. At least one instructor should be well versed in normal feline behavior so that up-to-date advice regarding medical and behavioral matters can be given.

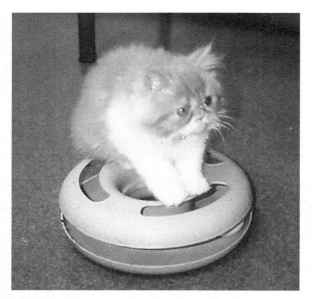

FIGURE 11-1 Track-type toys have a ball inside a box or circular plastic cylinder and are popular with kittens.

Equipment

The following items can be used and demonstrated in kitten kindergarten class:

- Cat-safe collars, harnesses, and leashes
- Clickers (if the instructor wants to demonstrate their use)
- Several different types of scratching posts (vertical and horizontal)
- Empty cardboard boxes
- A range of toys:
  - Tunnels (e.g., air conditioning tubing, ready-made cat tunnels)
  - Track-type toys in which a ball is held inside a box or plastic track, allowing the kitten to bat at it; can be as simple as an empty tissue box with a ball inside (Figure 11-1)
  - Balls
  - Kitten-safe toys on elastic or fishing poles
  - Homemade toys that children can make or paint
- Assortment of cat carriers: top opening, front opening, and so forth, so that the advantages and disadvantages of each can be explained
- Selection of litter boxes (e.g., covered, uncovered, liners) so that the advantages and disadvantages of each can be explained. (Standard litter boxes or inexpensive disposable cardboard litter boxes should always be available for kittens to use during class. These should be disposed of and replaced or disinfected after each class.)
- An indoor garden with samples of cat grass, catnip, and other kitten-safe greens so that the instructors can explain which plants are suitable and the potential hazards of certain toxic house plants

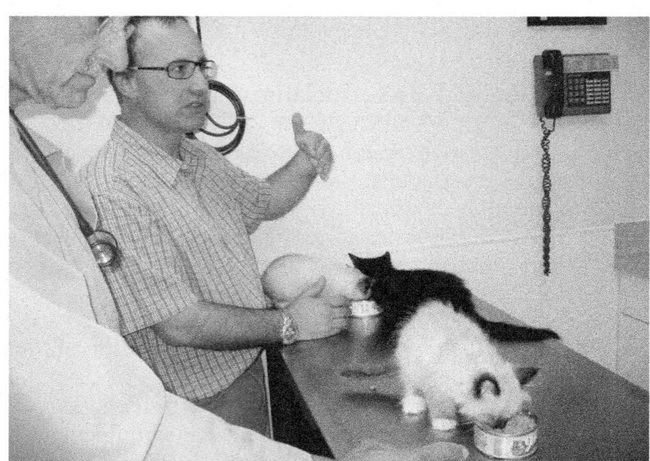

FIGURE 11-2 A kitten class held at a veterinary clinic allows kittens to become accustomed to veterinary visits; relaxed behavior should be rewarded with praise and treats.

Although all participants enjoy watching kittens interact with one another, the class should not resemble a playground setting. Too much kitten play may be overstimulating and ultimately not enjoyable for the kittens. Additionally, because people are easily distracted by the antics of playing kittens, they may not listen to the instructors.

Location

As previously mentioned, the veterinary clinic is the ideal location for the classes because the aim is to familiarize the kitten and the owner with the practice and its staff (Figure 11-2). Although other locations allow kittens to socialize and owners to be educated about cats, these places do not allow optimal familiarization with the veterinary practice or its staff.

The space should be of appropriate size: Too large a space offers kittens too much freedom; too small a space may not allow for adequate spacing between chairs for people to sit comfortably, and if the kittens themselves are too crowded, that may also lead to problems. A safe, secure environment with closed doors is imperative so that kittens cannot escape. A diffuser with a synthetic analog of a feline facial pheromone (e.g., Feliway; Ceva) should be plugged in to help reduce potential anxiety and enhance comfort.

TEACHING KITTENS

Kittens are not small puppies. Although the basic principles of training are the same as those for puppies or any other animal (i.e., rewarding appropriate and acceptable behaviors), the classes cannot be conducted in the same way as puppy socialization and training classes. Cat communication and body language are very different, and the socialization period ends much earlier than that of dogs. As the kittens are interacting, the instructors can point out and discuss the differences in signaling and body language between cats and dogs.

When teaching any exercise, instructors must be very patient, remain consistent, and keep each training session short. Just 5 minutes of teaching at any one time is sufficiently long because a kitten's concentration span is short. Training should occur when the kitten is most responsive (e.g., just before a meal).

Rewards

Small tasty treats such as dehydrated liver, barbecue chicken, cheese, minced meat, or Vegemite work well. Food rewards should be varied because some kittens are very timid and may not be used to eating from the hand. The food rewards should also be very small so that the kitten does not become satiated early in class and lose interest in the treat.

Some kittens respond more to toys and games, so these also work well as rewards.

Verbal and visual cues can be taught in each class. For example, cats can be taught to come, walk on a lead, sit, and even perform tricks such as "Give me five." However, the main aim is to help owners understand their cats, prevent problem behaviors from developing, and recognize behavioral problems (behavioral illness or pathology) so that appropriate intervention and management programs can be recommended and kittens referred to a veterinary behaviorist if necessary.

It is always important to offer encouragement to owners about their kitten's progress, even if this progress is not apparent in class. Instructors should explain that there are many distractions in class that make learning more difficult and that all exercises should be repeated in different places at varying times so the kitten can learn them.

Punishment

Punishment should not be used when teaching a new behavior in any species. Punishment does not teach the kitten what behavior is expected and can lead to fear and a breakdown in the bond between the cat and the owner.

CLASS STRUCTURE

Because there is so much room for variation, each practice should decide what structure works best for each class. Ideally, kitten classes are run for 1 hour each week, and the course is conducted over 2 to 3 weeks. One option is to have owners attend the first class without their kittens so that they can listen without being distracted by the kittens.

Ideally, each 1-hour class is scheduled for 2 consecutive weeks (for example, 2 consecutive Tuesday nights). However, other options include two 1-hour classes on 2 consecutive days (e.g., a Tuesday evening and again on the next day, Wednesday, same time, same place). Another option, which might work for some practices, is a one-time 90-minute class, although this does not allow for any follow-up, except over the phone.

Topics to Cover

Litter Training

Inappropriate elimination is, according to some data, the most frequently given reason for relinquishment.[11] One newspaper column[2] on pet behavior reported that over a period of 15 years, feline inappropriate elimination was by far the most common topic for questions (followed by canine aggression).

Many owners need to be taught about litter box care: how often to change litter boxes, how to clean them, how many are needed, and where to place them. The following is a summary that can be covered in class:

- One litter box per kitten (cat) plus one extra is a good rule of thumb.
- Litter boxes should be at least 1½ times the length of the cat, so bigger ones may be needed as the kitten grows.
- Litter boxes should be placed in readily accessible locations. For example, a litter box in a downstairs bathroom is not convenient for a kitten that spends most of the day upstairs.
- Litter boxes should be cleaned at least once daily.
- Offer a selection of different litters (e.g., clumping litter, sand, sawdust, recycled paper) to find the one that the kitten prefers.
- Schedule feeding times (this makes elimination times more predictable).
- Place litter boxes in a low-traffic zone, one that provides privacy. If the kitten is frightened while in the litter box, it may be discouraged from using the box. For example, if the kitten is cornered by a dog or an older cat or the washing machine jumps into full spin cycle just as the kitten is using the litter box, the kitten is unlikely to want to go back there to toilet.

Handling

Cats that are handled frequently at a younger age benefit physically and emotionally, showing less fear and greater confidence and friendliness as adults.[5] It has been shown that socialized cats that were handled between 2 and 12 weeks of age were at 1 year of age quicker to approach, touch, and rub familiar and unfamiliar test persons; this is likely to increase the bond between owner and cat.[7a] Owners should be taught how to handle kittens. Instructors should demonstrate how to hold kittens, clip nails, and medicate, using rewards for good behavior. They should also show owners how to groom and brush the kitten and discuss bathing when necessary.

If the class is being conducted at a veterinary clinic, instructors should take one kitten at a time to be handled on an examination table, rewarding relaxed behavior with quiet praise and tasty treats. The instructor should wear a laboratory coat or usual staff uniform for this exercise to make it seem as much like a real veterinary visit as possible. External parasite control, heartworm prevention, nutrition, and dental care can be discussed in these sessions.

Scratching

Scratching furniture is a common complaint of many cat owners. The importance of scratching as a means of communication should be explained, as well as advising on suitable placement of scratching posts, appropriate material for cats to scratch, and a discussion of what to do if kittens have begun to scratch inappropriately.

More information about enriched environments for indoor cats is found in Chapter 46.

SAMPLE CURRICULUM

The following is a sample kitten class curriculum. The order and topics discussed may vary in each practice according to regional differences in the incidence of disease and individual preferences.[4,10,12,13] Questions from owners are always encouraged. Information sheets should be handed out that repeat the advice given in each of the lessons. Additional resources are listed in Box 11-2.

BOX 11-2
Additional Resources

1. Seksel K: Kitten Kindy video, Melbourne, 1998, Malcolm Hunt Productions; available by contacting sabs@sabs.com.au.
2. Seksel K: *Training your cat,* Victoria, Australia, 2001, Hyland House Publishing.
3. Kitty-K: A kitten's mind is a terrible thing to waste: http://www.stevedalepetworld.com/kitty-k. Last accessed March, 28, 2011.
4. Pryor K: *Getting started: clicker training for cats,* Waltham, Mass, 2003, Sunshine Books.
5. Yin S: *Low stress handling, restraint and behavior modification of dogs and cats,* Davis, Calif, 2009, Cattle Dog Publishing.
6. Rodan I, Sundahl E, Carney H, et al: AAFP and ISFM feline-friendly handling guidelines, *J Feline Med Surg* 13:364, 2011.

Week One

1. Registration: Check vaccination certificates, and perform a brief examination for any signs of illness such as weepy eyes or runny noses.
2. Welcome:
   - Ask all the owners to be seated. All kittens should still be in their carriers, because people tend to pay more attention while the kittens are confined.
   - Introduce the instructors, and ask the owners to introduce themselves and their kittens.
   - Set out house rules, and outline the course objectives and content. Introductory remarks should explain why kitten classes are important. Congratulate clients for caring enough about their kittens to attend.
   - Stress that class attendees should follow up with their veterinarian as a future resource for any future behavior issue, and proactively visit the veterinarian for exams twice a year, even if cats appear healthy.
3. Interaction:
   - Various kitten toys and scratchers are strewn randomly throughout the play zone (Figure 11-3).
   - Release kittens one by one from their carrier to interact, but if the group is large, not all should be out of the carriers at the same time (Figure 11-4).
   - Some kittens may feel more comfortable sitting on their owner's laps. It is important not to force kittens to interact; no hissing should occur.
   - Kittens should be left to investigate their surroundings for 15 minutes while various topics are discussed. It is important to observe the kittens' behavior carefully and intervene to prevent kittens from being frightened or bullied.

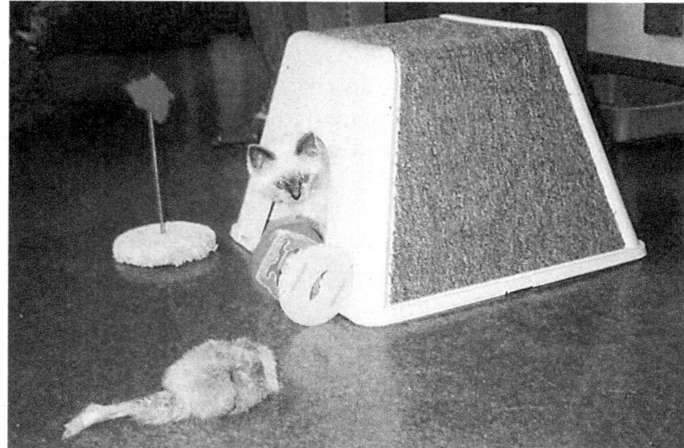

FIGURE 11-3 Various types of toys should be provided in a play zone for kitten classes.

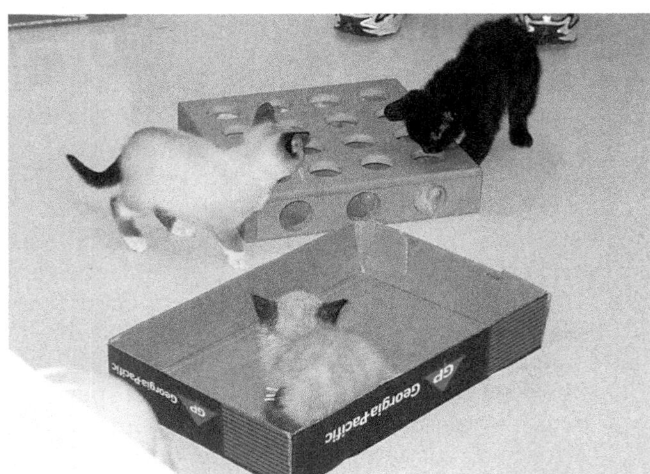

FIGURE 11-4 During kitten classes kittens can be released from their carriers to interact with one another, but careful supervision is required.

- Discuss each of the toys, and show owners how to interact and play with their kittens appropriately.
- Explain various aspects of feline communication. Owners love to learn why their cat is behaving the way it is.
- Allow time for owners to ask questions. Children attending the class should be taught to play appropriately with kittens.

4. Training:
    - There are limitations as to what people can do with their cats (although there are now agility competitions for cats), but training a cat is widely assumed to lead to a stronger bond with the family.[9,10] A cohesive bond is also important if a behavioral problem, such as elimination in unacceptable places, or an illness occurs. More cats than dogs are surrendered to shelters by owners.[8] It is possible that by becoming more tightly connected with the owner through training and "teamwork," the cat is more likely to be treated rather than surrendered.
    - Many owners seem genuinely surprised that cats can be trained in the first place. People smile when an instructor demonstrates how a cat can be clicker trained to sit within a minute. The instructor offers an explanation of operant conditioning.
    - Training offers cats both mental and physical exercise. Attendees can be taught to clicker train their cats to do something, such as to sit on cue.
    - Teaching the cat to come: Teaching kittens to come on cue is generally not difficult. The kitten should always be rewarded for coming in response to its name and the word "come." It helps if the kitten is hungry, interested in the treats, and willing to eat from a hand. Demonstrate by offering the kitten a treat, and slowly back up a few paces. Call the kitten's name, and say "Come" as it is walking toward you. Reward the kitten immediately. Repeat this exercise a few times. Then, one at a time, the class participants should practice with their own kittens. Encourage owners to do this exercise at home before every meal, when there are fewer distractions.
    - Handling exercises: Spend a few minutes showing owners how to hold and gently handle their kitten. Discuss how to gently massage the kitten to relax it (Figure 11-5). The instructor might also demonstrate how to clip nails and how to medicate using rewards for relaxed behavior. Demonstrate how to groom, brush, and, if necessary, bathe the kitten. This discussion might include topics such as flea control, nutrition, and dental care. Encourage owners to check their kitten's mouth and teeth daily. The importance of dental hygiene and toothbrushing (using pet toothbrushes, finger brushes, and pet toothpastes) could also be discussed.

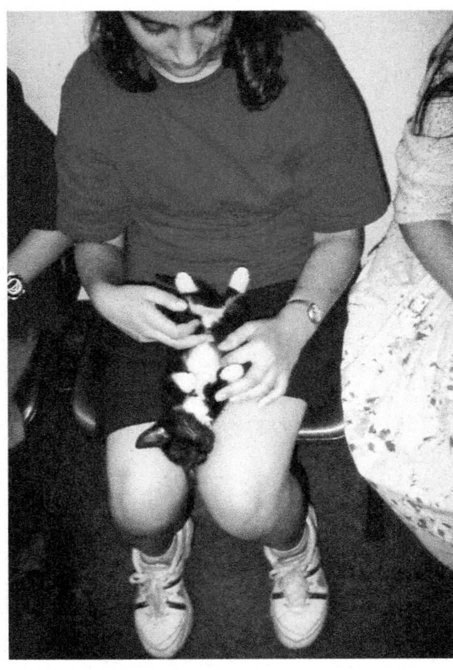

FIGURE 11-5 Owners should be taught how to hold and gently handle the kitten, as well as massage and relaxation techniques.

5. Discussion topics:
    - Indoor cats and environmental enrichment: Some people still believe that keeping cats inside is cruel. It is important to explain that because indoor cats do not get lost, do not get run over, and do not get into cat fights, they are generally

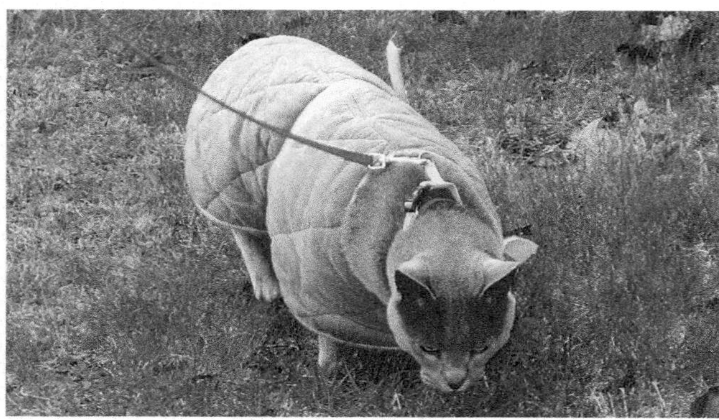

FIGURE 11-6 Cats can be trained from a young age to accept a harness and leash as a way to provide exercise and stimulation out of doors in a safe manner.

healthier. Indoor cats rely on their owners to provide them with a physically and mentally stimulating environment. A demonstration of how to leash and harness train kittens can be followed by ideas on how to allow cats outside safely (e.g., using cat strollers and cat fencing) (Figure 11-6).

- Modifying unwanted normal behaviors: Unwanted behaviors may include scratching furniture or jumping onto counters. It is always better to teach the kitten desirable behaviors rather than punish undesirable ones. Scratching is another way that cats communicate. They leave a visual and scent marker when they scratch. Appropriate and correctly placed scratching posts will help prevent damage to furniture.
- Owners are often concerned about their cat's predatory instincts, but not all cats hunt. Some cats do like to stalk and pounce, so owners can be taught appropriate ways to manage the behavior, such as interactive games that allow the kitten to exercise. A cord or string tied around the owner's waist, with a toy on the other end trailing along the floor, allows owners to divert the cat from an owner's ankles or feet.

6. Conclusion: Hand out information sheets that reinforce the advice given in the lessons. Encourage owners to ask questions.

Week Two

1. Welcome: Greet owners, and answer any questions that may have arisen since the previous week. Kittens are given another brief physical examination. Outline the lesson plan for this class.
2. Interaction: Kittens are allowed out of the carriers so that they can explore the room and interact with one another if they are amenable. Kittens often appear more confident on their second visit.
3. Review: "Come" and handling exercises are reviewed. Ask owners to demonstrate one at a time with their own kittens. Remember that this is a strange environment for young kittens because there are many distractions and smells. Therefore some kittens may find it difficult to concentrate, and fear may override the desire to eat a treat, let alone come when called. Encourage the owner to practice at home.
4. Discussion: Other topics that can be covered this week include the following:
   - Routine health care: The importance of spay/neuter, vaccination, and deworming can be discussed. The importance of identification (i.e., microchips and collars with tags) should also be discussed during this time. Local legislation regarding licensing/registration, curfews, and so forth should also be discussed.[6] Grooming, bathing, and flea and tick control should be discussed, if they were not covered the first week.
   - Feline behavior: Feline social systems, communication, and the importance of a predictable routine should be reviewed. Advise owners to have regular times to feed, groom, and play with their kitten. Daily play sessions are important for young kittens to use up energy and promote a strong bond with the owner.
5. Training:
   - "Sit": Call the kitten to come, and offer it a treat. Hold the treat directly above the kitten's nose and then slowly direct your hand back over the kitten's head toward its rear end. As the head goes up and backward, the rear is lowered to the ground. The kitten is rewarded as soon as its bottom hits the ground. Repeat this a few times. Once the kitten is sitting consistently, start saying the word "sit" as the action and the word are paired together (Figure 11-7).
   - "Give me five": This is a fun exercise that is similar to teaching a dog to shake hands. Kittens naturally lift their paws in response to food being offered, so this behavior can be slowly shaped into "Give me five" or "Give me ten" in response to the verbal cue.
   - Walking on a lead: The kitten should be habituated to wearing a collar or harness. Once the kitten has become used to the collar or the harness, allow the kitten to drag the leash around so that the kitten gets used to the weight of the collar or the harness and the clip on the leash. Encourage the kitten to walk and follow by using treats or wiggling a toy in front of the kitten as you walk along.
6. Common behavior concerns: Any behavior that owners find unacceptable should be addressed now,

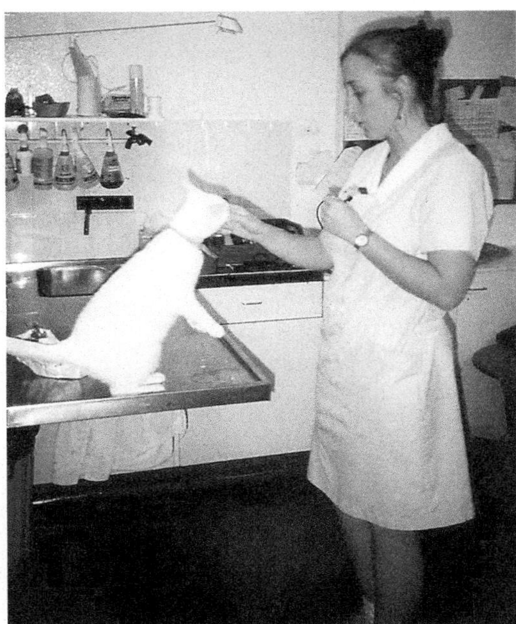

FIGURE 11-7 Kittens and cats can be taught to sit by holding a treat directly above the kitten's nose, encouraging the head to go up and the rear end to go down.

as cats do not "grow out of it." Methods of modifying or managing unacceptable behaviors should be discussed and the owners should be made aware of normal behaviors so that they have realistic expectations of their cat.

7. Graduation: Kitten classes come to an end with a small ceremony. Every owner receives a certificate of attendance, some samples of products, and a list of resources. Final questions and comments are answered. Owners should be advised that they can always come back to the clinic or consult the instructor if problems occur in the future. If a problem is too complicated and requires expert help, they should be referred to a qualified applied animal behaviorist or veterinary behaviorist.

References

1. American Veterinary Medical Association: *U.S. pet demographic sourcebook*, Schaumberg, Ill, 2007, American Veterinary Medical Association.
2. Dale S: *My pet world*, Tribune Media Services.
3. Horwitz DF: House soiling cats. In Horwitz DF, Mills DS, Heath S, editors: *BSAVA manual of canine and feline behavioural medicine*, ed 1, Gloucester, UK, 2002, British Small Animal Veterinary Association, p 97.
4. Hunthausen W, Seksel K: Preventive behavioural medicine. In Horwitz DF, Mills DS, Heath S editors: *BSAVA manual of canine and feline behavioural medicine*, ed 1, Gloucester, UK, 2002, British Small Animal Veterinary Association.
5. Karsh E: The effects of early handling on the development of social bonds between cats and people. In Katcher A, Beck A, editors: *New perspectives on our lives with companion animals*, Philadelphia, 1983, University of Pennsylvania Press, p 22.
6. Lord LK, Wittum TE, Ferketich AK, et al: Search and identification methods that owners use to find a lost cat, *J Am Vet Med Assoc* 230:217, 2007.
7. Lue TW, Pantenburg DP, Crawford PM: Impact of the owner–pet and client–veterinarian bond on the care that pets receive, *J Am Vet Med Assoc* 232:531, 2008.

7a. McCune S: The impact of paternity and early socialisation on the development of cats' behaviour to people and novel objects, *Appl Anim Behav Sci* 45:109, 1995.

8. National Council on Pet Population Study and Policy: The shelter statistics survey, 1994-1997: http://www.petpopulation.org/statsurvey.html. Accessed December 12, 2010.
9. Overall K: *Clinical behavioral medicine for small animals*, St Louis, 1997, Mosby.
10. Overall K, Rodan I, Beaver B et al: Feline behavior guidelines from the American Association of Feline Practitioners, *J Am Vet Med Assoc* 227:70, 2005.
11. Patronek G, Glickman L, Beck A et al: Risk factors for relinquishment of cats to an animal shelter, *J Am Vet Med Assoc* 209:582, 1996.
12. Seksel K: *Training your cat*, Victoria, Australia, 2001, Hyland House Publishing.
13. Seksel K: Preventative behavioural medicine for cats. In Horwitz DF, Mills DS, editors: *BSAVA manual of canine and feline behavioural medicine*, ed 2, Gloucester, UK, 2009, British Small Animal Veterinary Association.

CHAPTER

12

Behavioral History Taking

Debbie Calnon

OUTLINE

The first step in making a behavioral diagnosis, or list of differential diagnoses, is collection of a thorough and accurate history. Taking a thorough behavioral history is arguably the most important part of dealing with animal behavioral issues.[5]

Although the primary focus in veterinary medicine is generally the patient itself, behavioral problems invariably require a much broader base. This history should include more detailed information about not only the patient, people, and other animals in the household but also characteristics of the cat's physical environment. Less tangible aspects of that environment, including the client's emotional responses to the cat's behavior, are essential to a good understanding of the problem behavior. It is not simply a matter of making a behavioral diagnosis—what that diagnosis *means* for the client can be just as important as the diagnosis itself.

IT'S NOT JUST ABOUT THE CAT

Good communication skills with clients are particularly important in behavioral medicine, and history taking is no exception. It is not just the content of questions that matters, but also the way in which these questions are asked and the answers more fully explored. Behavioral disorders can cause clients significant distress and may lead to disharmony among household members.[4]

Many clients greatly appreciate the opportunity to talk about their cat's behavioral problem with someone whom they recognize as objective and understanding. This is particularly important given that many owners feel guilty about their pet's behavioral problem.[3] The time taken to collect an oral history can help build a strong relationship between the veterinarian and the client and allow for clarification of any complex issues.

EMPATHY

Empathy underpins all counseling. Empathy is a skill that "creates a climate for acceptance, support, disclosure and a working alliance. It is crucial for the building of a trusting relationship."[13] Empathy includes being sensitive to the feelings of the client without making judgments. It requires respect and interest in the client and constructive honesty to enhance the cat–human bond. The veterinarian must remain sufficiently objective to make rational and well-informed decisions.

COUNSELING SKILLS

Many of the basic counseling skills employed in various forms of psychological counseling are appropriate for history taking in a veterinary context. The need to develop rapport and understanding with the client is critical in both instances. These skills include the following[13]:

1. *Reflective listening:* This skill involves paying full attention to what the client has said and

summarizing the main message. It can be useful to allow the client to express anything the client feels is critical to the veterinarian's understanding of the situation at the beginning of the consultation. For instance, if the client is concerned that the veterinarian does not fully understand the sentimental value of an item that was ruined after the cat urinated on it, then this may reduce the client's desire to collaborate in formulating a useful treatment plan for the cat. Later in the consultation it will be necessary to add more shape and structure to the conversation. The veterinarian should take time at the outset to reflect on the following:

- What has been happening: Much of this may be contained in a behavioral questionnaire (discussed later).
- The thoughts, feelings, and reactions of the client: This may vary among household members.
- Apparent themes: These can often give the veterinarian a sense of why the clients contacted the veterinarian and their current understanding of the situation. The same presentation can uncover different themes for different clients. For instance, for one family a urine-spraying cat may be causing great distress because the cat is failing to fulfill their expectations of fastidious cleanliness; for another family the main issue may be that they recognize the spraying as a sign of anxiety for their cat, and this becomes a recurring theme throughout the consultation.
- The significance of the situation for the client: For instance, the point at which a toileting issue becomes a concern for a client varies significantly among clients. Some may consider finding feces outside the litter box once a week tolerable, whereas others may consider finding feces outside the box once a month a reason for euthanasia if the problem is not resolved.

2. *Sensitive questioning:* This allows clarification of the situation and permits a greater level of understanding by the veterinarian.
3. *Accurate summarizing:* A behavioral history requires collection of a great deal of information. Summarizing the major events, themes, and reactions as they relate to the client's current situation can be very useful. It helps ensure that the veterinarian and client are on the same wavelength before moving on.
4. *Focusing and structuring:* This part of the consultation allows time to focus on the key concerns, clarify expectations, and set realistic goals.
5. *Collaboratively formulating a management and treatment plan:* Behavioral medicine is always interesting and challenging because no two situations are the same for any particular behavior problem. The veterinarian will be in the best position to recommend an effective treatment plan if the preceding steps have been taken in collecting a history that encompasses client concerns and expectations, as well as patient behaviors.

ORGANIZING A CONSULTATION

The type, duration, and intensity of behavioral problems vary enormously. This chapter focuses on issues that require a behavioral consultation to be addressed appropriately. A good starting point for behavioral issues is a thorough physical examination and, generally speaking, a blood profile and urine test to help rule out medical issues that could be contributing to the behavioral problem and that may also have an impact on the treatment plan.[7] One case study showed the importance of a full medical workup of a cat presenting with feline idiopathic cystitis that could be successfully controlled with behavioral therapy alone.[12] It is not uncommon for there to be a crossover between medical and behavioral issues, with both needing to be addressed. The results of such investigations will form part of the collected history and are addressed elsewhere (see Chapter 3).

A behavioral questionnaire can be used to allow clients time to consider and answer a number of questions about the cat before they arrive for the consultation. Many clients will not have undertaken a behavioral consultation with their cat before. A cover letter provided with the questionnaire explaining the likely duration of the consultation, topics that will be covered, and an estimate of cost is useful to demystify the process and can be given at the same time as the questionnaire.

A questionnaire not only provides structure for the veterinarian so that critical areas are covered but also helps clients see their cats' issues more clearly. Encouraging input from all household members affords the best chance of obtaining an accurate history and identifying potential areas for disagreement that may need to be addressed. A number of textbooks have behavioral history templates that can be modified according to the style and preferences of the attending veterinarian (Box 12-1).[6,8,10]

The location of the consultation can also influence the type of information that is asked of the client. For instance, a plan of the house and any enclosures may be useful if the consultation takes place in the veterinary clinic. Points of interest, such as areas of elimination, position of litter boxes, favored resting areas, and feeding areas, can be marked on the plan. If a home visit is undertaken, then the veterinarian can see these things firsthand.

There are advantages and disadvantages to clinic versus home visit consultations, and both can be successful. Behavioral consultations will generally last

BOX 12-1

Sample Behavioral Questionnaire

Owner's Details:

Cat's Details:

- Main reason for consultation:
- Any other behavioral problems:
- Medical history (if not readily available within practice):
- Name the people living in your household (including ages of children):
- Do you have any physical ailment(s) that influences your ability to interact with your cat?
- Have you owned a pet before you owned this cat?
- Where and at what age was your current cat acquired?
- Did your cat have any previous owners? If so, do you know why it was given up?
- Do you know any details about its parents or siblings?
  - If so, do they have any behavioral problems?
- Why did you choose this breed?
- Why did you choose this individual?
- Where does your cat sleep?
- What, when, and where is your cat fed?
- List your cat's favorite food treats and toys, in order of preference:
- How much time does your cat spend indoors/outdoors?
- How does your cat react with:
  - Other cats
  - Strangers
  - Children
  - Friends
  - Groomer
  - Veterinarian
- Are there other pets in the household? If so, how do they get along with one another?
- What is your cat's typical daily routine?
- What is your typical daily routine?
- How long ago did the problem begin? Can you describe the first episode?
- Describe the last three episodes in which the problem behavior occurred:
- How often does the problem behavior occur?
- Has the problem changed over time in frequency or intensity? If so, how quickly has the change occurred?
- Can you identify any factors that may have triggered or coincided with the onset of the problem behavior?
- Can you predict when a problem is likely to occur?
- What has been tried to correct the problem? How successful have these measures been?
- What are your goals for treatment?
- Provide the following information if your cat is urinating or defecating inappropriately:
  - Number of litter boxes provided
  - Type of litter box (shape, depth, size, any covering, any lining)
  - Type of litter material used in the box
  - Location of the litter boxes
  - Cat's typical use of the box (e.g., feces is covered/left uncovered, cat scratches before elimination, cat stands while eliminating, cat squats while eliminating)
- Please note any other information that may be relevant to this problem.

significantly longer than a standard consultation, so it is important that clients be seated comfortably and that the veterinarian allow sufficient time to obtain an adequate history without rushing through the questions. The cat's stress level should be reduced as much as possible. Ideally, waiting time is short and exposure to other animals at the clinic is minimal.

Asking clients to provide video footage of their cat can also be useful. Even in a long consultation, the cat will be observed only in one particular context, which will be influenced by the presence of the veterinarian, whether this takes place at the clinic or during a home visit. It is very important that the client not provoke the cat to perform behaviors that may be deleterious to the cat's welfare. For instance, if two cats in the household are engaging in aggressive behavior with each other, the client should not videotape them fighting. This may seem obvious, but many clients need to be educated about the fact that certain behaviors are better described than demonstrated.

BASIC PATIENT INFORMATION

As previously discussed, many veterinarians use a questionnaire to help make the consultation time more productive. The written information provided by the client should always be reviewed during the face-to-face part of the consultation. The terminology that clients use to describe their cat's behavior may be ambiguous. A client may consider their cat to be spraying but then reveal, on further questioning, that the cat is simply voiding urine outside of the litter box rather than actually spraying urine. One study found that almost a third of veterinarians did not seem to distinguish correctly between urine marking (spraying) and inappropriate urination.[2] Because the treatment approaches for these two conditions are likely to be quite different, the importance of asking the right questions is critical. Another example of a need for further clarification is when clients report that their cat has bitten them. A bite can vary from making contact with the skin but leaving no mark or bruise to multiple deep puncture wounds; the implications of each are clearly quite different.

The client's details should be collected, as for any veterinary consultation. The identifying details for the cat can also be useful from a behavioral perspective. Even the cat's name may give some indication of its relationship with the owner. The cat's age at presentation may coincide with sexual or social maturity or suggest the possible role of senility in the disorder. Gender and reproductive status influence the expression of many behaviors such as urine spraying.[11] Breed predispositions occur for many behavioral disorders; Siamese cats, for example, are overrepresented for ingestive behavior problems.[1] Finally, the cat's weight is relevant when dispensing medications and is particularly important with regard to eating disorders such as pica.

The age and gender of the other animals and people living with the cat should be determined. Asking about any physical ailments that may have an impact on the client's ability to interact with the cat is useful because this may not be immediately evident during the consultation. The occupation of employed household members can help the veterinarian provide examples or descriptions to which the clients can readily relate. Asking whether the client has owned cats in the past can also assist in understanding the potential challenges of the current situation. For instance, although new cat owners might have difficulty interpreting feline body language, experienced owners might have difficulty understanding why they are having problems with their current cat when previous cats did not have similar issues. Occasionally, individuals from outside the home should also be considered. For instance, the routines of neighborhood cats can have a significant impact on the resident cat.

The primary presenting behavioral complaint, as perceived by the client, should be provided in the questionnaire. Because clients are sometimes concerned about more than one behavioral problem, allowing space for other issues to be listed is recommended. The veterinarian may become aware of other problems that were not perceived as such by the client or may decide that secondary issues should take precedence to the one cited as primary by the client.[3] It can take some time to work through such issues and reach an agreement about prioritizing interventions.

The cat's age at acquisition and the place from which it was acquired should be ascertained. If the cat had previous owners, the veterinarian should ask if the client knows why it was surrendered. The reasons for the choice of a particular breed or an individual cat may assist in defining the relationship between cat and client. If available, any information about the behavior of close relatives can also provide clues about etiology. It is known that early experiences can have a significant impact on the adult cat's behavior. Although such information can be very useful, it is often impossible to obtain. Stray cats and those adopted from shelters often have an unknown early history.

A client may suspect that one cat in the household is scratching or soiling inappropriately but not be certain which cat (or cats) is the offender. A third party (e.g., a neighbor) may report that the client's cat is eliminating in their garden, but the client may not have witnessed this behavior firsthand.

Invariably, some facts will be missing or questionable in any behavioral history. Ongoing observation and data collection can help compensate for any deficiency at the time of the consultation. For example, a videocamera could be set up to identify a urine sprayer in the household.

SELF-MAINTENANCE BEHAVIORS

The cat's diet, water intake, grooming and sleeping habits, and elimination behaviors all need to be reviewed. The level of detail that is collected about any of these is likely to vary depending on the presenting complaint. For instance, for a cat with toileting problems, the following questions could be included:

- How many litter boxes are provided?
- What type of litter box is used (e.g., shape, depth, size, any covering, any lining)?
- What kind of litter material is used in the box?
- When are the boxes cleaned, and what is used for cleaning?
- Where are the litter boxes located?
- How is the tray used? Is the feces usually covered or uncovered? Does the cat scratch before elimination? Does the cat stand or squat?

SOCIAL ENVIRONMENT

The amount of time the cat spends indoors or outdoors can play a significant role in the etiology of some behavioral disorders and also have an impact on the type of intervention that is selected. Detailed information can also be obtained regarding the way the cat responds to other cats (both within and outside the home), adult strangers and friends, children, groomer (if applicable), the veterinarian, other animals (if applicable), and the client.

Learning the cat's and the client's daily routines assists in defining the relationship they have together, the time that might be available to work on the problem, and some of the management strategies that could be practical.

THE PROBLEM BEHAVIORS

In the "Problem Behaviors" section of the history, clients are likely to have given an initial brief description of the problematic behavior. Having them fill out a questionnaire with the additional details often helps them understand that the behavior does not stand alone but is influenced by many factors in the environment. After understanding this, clients usually are more willing to implement strategies that address some of the broader issues, rather than expect to learn a simple method to suppress the problematic behavior. For example, an owner may initially think that a good way to address the problem of a cat vocalizing at night may be to squirt it with a water pistol. Once the bigger picture becomes clear, the client is more likely to consider some of the underlying causes of the vocalization and address these instead of simply trying to stop the behavior. Invariably, this approach protects the cat's welfare and improves the cat–client relationship over the long term.

The following questions can be asked to elucidate the problem behavior:

- How long ago did the problem begin?
- Can you describe what happened the first time the behavior occurred?
- Can you describe the last three episodes in which the problem behavior occurred?
- How often does the problem behavior occur?
- Has the problem changed with time in frequency or intensity? If so, how quickly has the change occurred?
- Can you identify any factors that may have triggered or coincided with the onset of the problem behavior?
- Can you predict when a problem is likely to occur?
- What has been tried to correct the problem? How successful have these measures been?
- Is there anything else that may be important and that has not been covered elsewhere?

Again, further details could be provided regarding specific behavior details. For instance, a feline aggression screening tool has been formulated by Overall[10] to more accurately assess a cat presenting with aggression issues. It is also useful to ask clients to describe particular features, such as the cat's body language before, during, and after an event such as a fight.[9] Requesting specific details can be a useful way to counter the subjective interpretation that clients often give when first questioned about such incidents (e.g., describing the cat as angry, jealous, or spiteful or otherwise anthropomorphizing its behavior).

FORMULATING A TREATMENT PLAN

See Chapters 13 and 14 for details regarding treatment options for various behavioral disorders. One last question on the history form is particularly important. Both the client and the veterinarian must be absolutely clear about the goals for implementation of the treatment plan. A thorough history, collected in a way that is supportive of the client, is the best starting point to making a behavioral diagnosis. The veterinarian can then identify and confirm the client's strengths, offer fresh avenues to approach the problem, and build on this foundation to formulate a collaborative treatment plan that the client will be willing and able to implement.

References

1. Bamberger M, Houpt KA: Signalment factors, comorbidity, and trends in behavior diagnoses in cats: 736 cases (1991-2001), *J Am Vet Med Assoc* 229:1602, 2006.
2. Bergman L, Hart B, Bain M et al: Evaluation of urine marking by cats as a model for understanding veterinary diagnostic and treatment approaches and client attitudes, *J Am Vet Med Assoc* 221:1282, 2002.
3. Crowell-Davis S, Murray T: *Veterinary psychopharmacology*, Ames, Iowa, 2005, Blackwell.
4. Dehasse J: The role of the family in behavioral therapy. In Horwitz D, Mills D, Heath S, editors: *BSAVA manual of canine and feline behavioural medicine*, Gloucester, UK, 2002, British Small Animal Veterinary Association.
5. Horwitz D: Behavior fundamentals. In *Atlantic Coast Veterinary Conference*, Atlantic City, NJ, 2001.
6. Horwitz DF, Mills DS, Heath S: *BSAVA manual of canine and feline behavioural medicine*, ed 1, Gloucester, UK, 2002, British Small Animal Veterinary Association.
7. Juarbe-Diaz SV. Behavioral triage: treat or refer. *North American Veterinary Conference*, Orlando, FL, 1999.
8. Landsberg G, Hunthausen W, Ackerman L: *Handbook of behavior problems of the dog and cat*, ed 2, St Louis, 2003, Elsevier Saunders.
9. Luescher UA: Feline aggression to people, *Western Veterinary Conference*, Las Vegas, 2004.
10. Overall K: *Clinical behavioral medicine for small animals*, St Louis, 1997, Mosby.
11. Pryor P, Hart B, Bain M et al: Causes of urine marking in cats and effects of environmental management on frequency of marking, *J Am Vet Med Assoc* 219:1709, 2001.
12. Seawright A, Casey R, Kiddie J et al: A case of recurrent feline idiopathic cystitis: The control of clinical signs with behavior therapy, *J Vet Behav* 3:32, 2008.
13. *Lifeline—it's a fine line training manual*, session 2, p 2, Melbourne, Australia, 2009, Wesley Mission.

CHAPTER

13

Behavior Problems

Kersti Seksel

OUTLINE

Behavioral concerns of cat owners can be categorized into two main areas: problem behaviors and behavioral problems. It is important that veterinarians distinguish between the two so that they can recommend appropriate management and treatment programs.

Problem behaviors are classified as behaviors that are part of the cat's normal behavioral repertoire but are unacceptable to the owner or community. Although it is considered problematic by owners, the behavior itself is normal. The behavior may be exhibited because of the owner's failure to understand feline behavioral needs, lack of knowledge of feline social structure, or insufficient training of the cat. For example, a cat that jumps onto a kitchen counter may be doing this as part of the cat's normal preference to be up high, and there may be a lack of other, more appropriate locations in the house (e.g., shelves). It is also possible that the cat has never been taught that sitting elsewhere, such as on a scratching post or play center, is the behavior preferred by the owner.

Behavioral problems, on the other hand, fall into two categories: (1) behaviors that may be normal for the cat to exhibit but are excessive in duration or intensity and exhibited in response to stimuli that should not elicit this response and (2) behaviors that are abnormal and thus indicate that the cat is unwell and should be considered as mental health issues. Behavioral problems are generally maladaptive for the cat as well as problematic for the owner or community. Examples include compulsive disorders, self-mutilation, and phobias.

Although these two categories are not mutually exclusive, classifying any unacceptable behavior in this way helps determine not only what advice should be given but also where to refer the client, if necessary.

The most common problems that cat owners report include some of the risk factors for surrender. These problems include aggression, house soiling, scratching, and fear- and anxiety-related behaviors.[14] Some of these are normal behaviors and as such cannot be eliminated entirely. In fact, it is possibly detrimental to the cat's welfare to try to stop these normal behaviors. However, steps can be taken to manage the behaviors.

Some of these unacceptable, destructive, and nuisance behaviors are exacerbated by a lack of physical as well as mental activity. Cats are highly intelligent, active, social animals that need activity, company, and stimulation. Educating owners about the basic needs of cats should help address many behavioral concerns.

Veterinarians working in companion animal practice are increasingly recognizing that fear and anxiety are the underlying factors for many of the behavioral problems presented. The actual prevalence of anxiety-related conditions is unknown, but they are probably the most common class of behavioral disorders in pets. Anxiety disorders make up well over 90% of veterinary patients presented for referral.[4] Many cases that present in general practice with recurrent medical issues such as vomiting, diarrhea, or skin problems may be caused or influenced by underlying anxiety issues.

The way an animal behaves depends on three key factors: its genetic predisposition, previous experiences, and its environment. None of these factors acts in isolation. All need to be taken into consideration when dealing with animals that have behavioral issues.

All behavioral problems require a systematic approach so that the best outcome is achieved for the patient. Use of a questionnaire, which is sent to the owner and filled in before the consultation, is one useful approach. The veterinarian is then prepared to ask specific questions about the behaviors during the consultation and begin to evaluate the environment, social interactions, and behavior of the cat. This permits the veterinarian to determine the possible cause (or causes) and prognosis (likelihood of success) and devise a treatment and management program.

The more detailed the information that is provided, the more specific the recommendations that can be made. The process of evaluating this behavioral history in the context of other clinical information about the cat may take a significant amount of time, often 2 to 3 hours. Most cats that have behavioral problems cannot be cured much as diabetes is managed not cured. However, with environmental management, behavior modification, and sometimes medication, the cat's quality of life can be greatly improved and the bond with its owners restored.

ANXIETY, FEAR, AND PHOBIA

Overview

Although the terms *anxiety* and *fear* are often used interchangeably, they are not the same. Fear is related to the specific behaviors of escape and avoidance, whereas anxiety is the result of threats that are perceived to be uncontrollable or unavoidable. Both fear and anxiety may be adaptive in some circumstances, whereas phobias are maladaptive. The prefrontal cortex, amygdala and limbic system, and hypothalamus (hypothalamic–pituitary–adrenal axis) is thought to be involved in the regulation of fear. Serotonin, noradrenaline, dopamine, and gamma-aminobutyric acid (GABA) are neurotransmitters involved in the development of fear and anxiety. Serotonin has been identified as a mediator of fear and anxiety.

Fear

Fear is a physiologic, behavioral, and emotional reaction to potentially injurious stimuli. The fear response is a complex physiologic response that involves several areas of the brain. Cognitive, musculoskeletal, and neuroendocrine responses occur when an animal perceives a frightening situation.[3] Experiencing fear is a survival mechanism and an adaptive response that usually occurs in response to a specific stimulus. Fear is often connected to pain or a traumatic event. For example, if a cat falls down a flight of stairs, it may develop a fear of stairs.

Fear-evoking situations lead to activation of the locus ceruleus, the key noradrenergic area of the brain. This stimulates neurotransmission in the noradrenergic pathways projecting to the cerebral cortex, limbic system, and spinal cord and prepares the cat physiologically to deal with the threat.

Various emotional stages of fear correspond with the physiologic effects of the sympathetic nervous system: the flight, fight, or freeze responses. The muscles used for physical movement are tightened and primed with oxygen and glucose in preparation for a physical fight-or-flight response. For example, a cat may try to run away from a fear-evoking stimulus (e.g., a veterinarian). However, if cornered, it may freeze or become defensively aggressive. There is also a fourth emotional response: the fiddle response (displacement behavior). In this case the cat faced with the fear-evoking stimulus may yawn or lick its lips.

The physiologic reaction results in increased heart rate, increased respiratory rate (panting), sweating, trembling, pacing, and possibly urination and defecation.

Cats exhibit changes in body posture and activity when afraid and may engage in an avoidance response such as fleeing or hiding. A fearful animal may assume body postures that are protective, such as lowering the body and head, placing the ears closer to the head, widening the eyes, and tucking the tail under the body. If the animal perceives a threat, the response can also include elements of defensive aggression. Whether an animal fights or flees when fearful or defensive depends on its genetic predisposition, its previous experiences, and its current environment. Normal fear is adaptive and transient.

Phobia

A *phobia* is defined as an irrational, intense, persistent fear of certain situations, activities, things, or people. The fear (or panic) response is out of proportion to the stimulus and is maladaptive. Animals with phobias do not habituate to the stimulus, even after many harmless contacts, and the response does not decrease with time.

Common phobias in animals involve noises and places. Phobic responses are physiologic, behavioral, and emotional responses similar to fear, but they are extremely exaggerated.

Anxiety

Fear should be distinguished from anxiety, which typically occurs without any external threat. *Anxiety* is defined as the anticipation of future danger or misfortune. The threat may be real or imagined, and the response of the cat may be normal or abnormal depending on the context. Anxiety may also be an adaptive response to a specific threat in some circumstances. However, whereas fear is usually of acute onset and transient in duration, anxiety is a more chronic state of nonspecific apprehension. Dysregulation of fear pathways plays a key role in anxiety. The changes in the activity of neurotransmitters in anxiety disorders results in changes across many neurochemical systems, including the seratonergic, noradrenergic, dopaminergic, and GABAergic systems. Because these systems are closely integrated, changes in one system elicit effects in another. Corticotrophin-releasing factor (CRF) has been identified as a stress neurotransmitter that effects changes in the serotonergic system through changes to receptor function that contribute to the onset of anxiety.[9]

Chronic anxiety leads to sympathetic arousal and is usually accompanied by signs of hypervigilance, such as scanning; autonomic hyperactivity, such as gastrointestinal upsets; and increased motor activity, such as pacing.

Anxiety can occur after sensitization to a specific stimulus and can then become generalized to other situations. It may also be nonspecific in origin. It is problematic to the cat when it is out of context and occurs at a constant and elevated level or interferes with normal functioning. Although panic attacks are not experienced by every animal that suffers from anxiety, they are relatively common. Panic attacks usually come without warning, and although the fear is generally irrational, the perceived danger is very real.

Anxiety-Related Disorders

Anxiety-related disorders in cats may include excessive self-grooming, changes in appetite, and inappropriate elimination (e.g., urine spraying). Stress or anxiety in cats may manifest in many ways. The following are the most commonly seen behavioral signs:

- Changes in appetite (e.g., a decrease in appetite, pica)
- Changes in grooming habits (i.e., an increase or decrease)
- Changes in elimination (e.g., urine spraying, nonspraying marking)
- Changes in social interactions (e.g., vocalization)
- Changes in physical activity (i.e., an increase or decrease)

Many factors are reported to result in anxiety in cats. These include environmental changes such as moving house, a new baby or spouse, separation from the owner, an excessive number of cats in the household or area, presence of new cats in the area, loss of territory, punishment by the owner, lack of stimulation, and even the presence of attacking birds (e.g., magpies). However, it may not be possible to determine all factors. Medical conditions such as hyperthyroidism have also been associated with feline anxiety, as have some medications.

Feline anxiety disorders include some types of aggression, separation anxiety, noise phobias, pica, and obsessive–compulsive disorders (OCDs). Diagnosis is based on a complete behavioral history and thorough physical examination. It may involve complete blood work, dermatologic and neurologic workup, and radiography or other imaging modalities to rule out contributing or concurrent medical factors.

Treatment usually involves behavior-modification techniques, environmental management, and the use of psychotropic medications. Medications that influence serotonin metabolism, such as the selective serotonin reuptake inhibitors (SSRIs) and the tricyclic antidepressants (TCAs) have been used in the treatment of anxiety-related disorders (see Chapter 14). Anxiolytic medication (e.g., benzodiazepines) has also proved useful in some cases in combination with TCAs and SSRIs, especially if the cat has phobias or experiences panic attacks. The owner should set realistic goals and recognize that in most cases the behavioral problem can be successfully managed but not necessarily eliminated. This will require a lifetime commitment from the owner. Punishment is not recommended because it serves to further increase the anxiety as well as impede learning of appropriate behavior.

Obsessive–Compulsive Disorders

In cats OCDs include stereotypes and self-directed behaviors. These are defined as being constant and repetitive in form, appearing to serve no obvious purpose, and interfering with the animal's normal functioning. OCDs are often derived from otherwise normal behaviors such as grooming, eating, or walking, but they are abnormal in that they are excessive in duration, frequency, or intensity in the context in which they are performed. Thus some causes of overgrooming, pica, and vocalization may be considered part of the OCD complex.

The anatomic focus of OCD is believed to be the limbic system. Computed tomography indicates that the basal ganglia near the caudate nucleus are involved. Dopaminergic, serotonergic, and opioid pathways are thought to be involved in compulsive and self-injurious behaviors. Aberrant serotonin metabolism and possibly endorphin metabolism are also thought to contribute. Increased dopamine in the basal ganglia and relative increase in serotonin metabolite 5-hydroxyindoleacetic acid (5-HIAA) in the cerebrospinal fluid (CSF) have also been detected.[12,15b]

Diagnosis is based on a complete behavioral history and thorough physical examination. It may involve complete blood work, dermatologic and neurologic workup, and radiography or other imaging modalities to rule out contributing or concurrent medical factors (e.g., seizures).

Treatment usually involves behavior-modification techniques; environmental management; and in most cases, the use of psychotropic medications. Medications that influence serotonin metabolism, such as the SSRIs and the TCAs, have been used in the treatment of OCD (see Chapter 14).[12a,15a]

The cat should not be punished because its behavior is not deliberate and it may serve to further increase the anxiety and thus the behavior.

Overgrooming

Grooming is a normal behavior of cats and serves many purposes, including cleaning, removing parasites, regulating body temperature, and alleviating stress. It is often seen after punishment or after aggressive encounters between cats. Normal adult cats spend about 30% to 50% of their waking hours grooming. Currently, feline hyperesthesia, overgrooming, self-mutilation, and psychogenic alopecia are considered to be part of the anxiety response.

CLINICAL SIGNS

Hair loss and discoloration occur only on the parts of the body that can be reached by the teeth and tongue. This hair loss is usually most noticeable around the sides and rump, back legs, and groin. The head and back of the neck may still have a normal hair coat. Usually, the alopecia is nonsymmetrical, and the skin may look normal.

Hair can be removed by plucking, barbering, or just licking and excoriation. The plucked hair has evidence of shearing. In some cats the grooming becomes excessive, and self-mutilation and ulceration occur in the affected areas. Secondary bacterial infections may then occur that also need treatment. Occasionally, the overgrooming is so severe that ulcers develop in the mouth (tongue and pharynx), making eating very difficult or even impossible.

DIFFERENTIAL DIAGNOSES

Many conditions, such as flea allergy, dietary allergy, and sensitivity to dust mites, have been known to trigger the initial grooming episodes. These must be eliminated as causes or contributing factors. In the case of fleas, treatment must be instigated even when no evidence of fleas is seen.[18]

Conditions causing pain, such as feline lower urinary tract disease (which may lead to abdominal grooming), as well as any source of trauma or infection, must be eliminated as contributing factors.

MANAGEMENT

Treatment of any concurrent or underlying medical problem, such as fleas, or resolution of food allergy by changing the diet is essential. If anxiety is suspected as a factor, the cause of the anxiety should be minimized or removed, if possible. Pain should always be a consideration in feline patients and should be addressed in any management program.

The cat should be provided with a regular, predictable routine. This includes feeding and playing at a set time each day. In many cases medication is also necessary. Medications that influence serotonin metabolism, such as the SSRIs and the TCAs, have been used in the treatment of anxiety-related disorders. Other anxiolytic medications have also proved useful in some cases. At this stage the comparative effectiveness of each medication remains to be evaluated and may depend on the underlying factors or eliciting causes.

Complete blood work, including a biochemistry panel, should be done before administering medication to determine a baseline, especially for liver and kidney parameters. Many cats may require medication for a prolonged period (at least 6 to 12 months, to allow hair regrowth and for the condition to be assessed), and then slow withdrawal of medication should be attempted. If cats require longer-term or lifetime medication, monitoring of a biochemistry panel should be carried out every 6 to 12 months or more often if indicated by clinical signs.

Punishment is not effective in changing these behaviors. It serves only to increase the anxiety, as well as impede learning of non-anxious behavior, and should be avoided.

Pica

Pica involves the ingestion of non-nutritive substances. However, eating substances other than food is not always abnormal. Consumption of plant material may be caused by lack of access to grass or vegetation or normal investigatory behavior. Young cats in particular may chew, but not necessarily ingest, nonfood substances as part of their normal exploratory behavior.

CLINICAL SIGNS

Cats have been reported to ingest many substances, including soil, rubber, paper, wood, string, house plants, wool, and fabric. Individual cats tend to ingest one type of substance only. Some of these behaviors may be more annoying than damaging until they start interfering with the cat's normal functioning.

Fabric-eating cats appear to start by eating woolen fabrics (Figure 13-1). They may then proceed to other fabrics, such as cotton, silk, and synthetics, but this is not

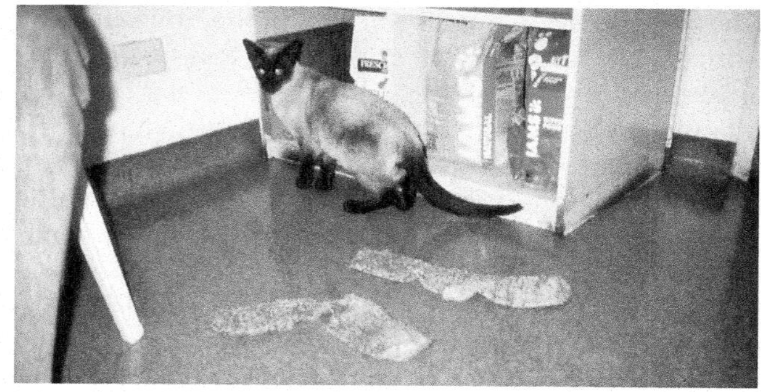

FIGURE 13-1 Fabric eating is a form of pica often seen in Siamese cats. If large quantities are ingested, intestinal obstruction may occur.

always the case. While the cat is chewing, it appears to be totally engrossed. The cat pulls and tugs on the wool and then grinds it with its molars. Quite large quantities can be ingested, and this is a problem if blankets, socks, and sweaters are eaten because these items may cause an intestinal obstruction.

This behavior is reportedly more common in oriental breeds such as Siamese and Burmese, although it has been reported in all breeds, as well as nonpedigreed cats. No gender predisposition for wool eating has been reported, and the behavior can occur between the ages of 2 to 8 months to 1 to 2 years. It is believed to be more common in cats that are kept exclusively indoors. Some cats appear to grow out of it, and the problem resolves during early adulthood without treatment.[2a]

The following are among the many postulated causes:

- Early weaning (at 2 to 4 weeks; feral cats may suckle until 6 months of age)
- Insufficient handling of kittens before homing
- Insufficient fiber in the diet
- Separation anxiety
- Lack of opportunity to develop exploratory and hunting behaviors
- A malfunction in the neural control of appetitive behavior

DIFFERENTIAL DIAGNOSES

Several medical conditions can also lead to pica. These include hyperthyroidism, lead intoxication, dietary deficiencies, intestinal parasites, and anemia. It may also be normal investigative behavior, which is more common in young cats.

MANAGEMENT

It is important that medical conditions be addressed. If the behavior is causing problems, the cat must be kept away from potentially harmful ingestible materials. Taste deterrents such as Grannick's Bitter Apple or chili pepper have been reported as helpful in deterring some cats. These substances may be more potent if they are paired with a distinctive scent such as eucalyptus oil or cologne to provide an additional (olfactory) cue that the substance is to be avoided. The cat learns to associate the smell of the oil with an unpleasant taste, and eventually the scent alone is sufficient to make the cat avoid the material. This technique appears to deter some cats if the behavior is of recent origin and the substances ingested are limited.

Establishing a predictable routine appears to help many cats by minimizing stress. This may mean having set times to feed the cat and play or otherwise interact with the cat. Providing an enriched environment by supplying the cat with toys and other forms of mental and physical stimulation has also been reported to be helpful. Planting an indoor garden with grass, catnip, or cat mint can provide a safe source of vegetation (fiber), as well as a means of enriching the cat's environment. The following suggestions may also help:

- Allowing the cat access to dried food all day
- Increasing the fiber content of the diet by adding bran or vegetables
- Providing gristly meat and raw bones to chew on to increase time spent chewing and eating

Direct punishment is not helpful; it may increase anxiety and exacerbate the problem.

Treatment with psychotropic medication such as SSRIs and TCAs may be necessary if a diagnosis of OCD is made. Premedication blood work (complete blood count and serum biochemistry panel) is recommended to provide baseline values, especially if the cat stays on long-term or lifetime medication. These tests should be repeated every 6 to 12 months depending on the age and health status of the cat. A minimum treatment period of 6 months is recommended because some medications may take 6 to 8 weeks to reach therapeutic levels. Gradual weaning off medication may be attempted when the behavior has been successfully managed for at least 3 months.

Separation Anxiety

Separation anxiety is a term that is used to describe cats that are overly attached or dependent on people, especially family members. They become extremely anxious and show distress behaviors of vocalization, destruction, house soiling, inappetence, inactivity, and even vomiting or diarrhea when separated from their owners.

CLINICAL SIGNS

Cats with separation anxiety tend to follow their owners from room to room and begin to display signs of anxiety as soon as their owners prepare to leave. This can occur as early as when the alarm clock rings in the morning. Some affected cats also exhibit excessive attention-seeking behaviors and may seek physical contact with their owners. During these separations the cat may vocalize, eliminate, and refuse to eat or become very quiet and withdrawn. Not all cats exhibit all of the signs; however, in general, the more signs that are exhibited, the more difficult it is to manage the case. Although the behavior usually occurs every time the owner leaves, it sometimes happens only on selected departures, such as when the owner leaves for work or when the owner leaves again after coming home from work.

DIFFERENTIAL DIAGNOSES

Because the separation anxiety complex involves many different signs, a complete physical examination is necessary to rule out other causes for the signs exhibited. For example, this should include other causes of elimination outside the litter box or any condition causing pain that may lead to vocalization.

MANAGEMENT

The aim of management is to teach the cat to cope without human company. This process may be very slow, and the owner must be patient as well as consistent. The earlier steps are taken to reduce the cat's anxiety, the easier it should be to manage.

The first step involves teaching the cat to be relaxed while the owner is present. When the cat learns to be relaxed in one place (e.g., in its bed or special mat) rather than constantly following the owner around, it will be possible to teach the cat to accept even the shortest of separations. It can also be useful to help the cat associate a particular scent or odor with the bed or mat and being calm. Whenever the cat is lying quietly anywhere, it should always be rewarded with quiet praise.

The owner should establish a predictable routine, feeding and playing with the cat at a set time each day, and enrich the cat's environment by providing toys (and rotating them regularly), hiding places, and play opportunities. However, care should be taken not to provide too many choices, which may exacerbate the anxiety.

Medication is often needed, especially in severe cases. Medication is often best started early in treatment rather than after the anxiety has increased to a level that makes it difficult to manage. According to studies, dogs improve about three to four times faster when antidepressant medication (e.g., clomipramine) is used in combination with behavior modification than when behavior modification is used alone.[6a] The same is likely to be true for cats.

Medications that influence serotonin metabolism, such as the SSRIs and the TCAs, have been used in the treatment of anxiety-related disorders. Anxiolytic medication (e.g., benzodiazepines) has also proved useful in some cases in combination with TCAs and SSRIs, especially if the cat exhibits panic attacks. They should be given before the potentially stressful event. However, long-term use is not recommended.

The synthetic facial pheromone analog Feliway has been reported to be useful in decreasing anxiety in some cats. Physical or verbal punishment is discouraged because it increases anxiety and impedes learning of more appropriate behavior.

Complete blood work should be done before medication is administered to determine a baseline, especially for liver and kidney parameters. The cat may require medication for prolonged periods (up to 12 months) or even for life. Owners should be informed of the possibility of lifelong medication at the outset of a management program.

Excessive Vocalization

Vocalization is a normal behavior of cats. Cats make many sounds, including purring, trilling, and meowing, and each may indicate a different purpose or function, such as a need for social contact, attention, or food. Excessive vocalization may be a normal innate behavior in some breeds, such as the Siamese. It has also been reported in cats that are on restricted calorie diets, which may indicate hunger.

CLINICAL SIGNS

The problem vocalization is of changed duration, frequency, or intensity. It may be a nocturnal behavior, or perhaps it is just more noticeable to owners at night. It is relatively common in older cats with decreased perceptual and locomotor abilities. Anxiety is also said to increase in older animals in general. It may also be due to reduced cognitive function (e.g., senility).

DIFFERENTIAL DIAGNOSES

Vocalization may be a normal behavioral response to physical stressors such as cold and hunger. Hyperthyroidism, cognitive dysfunction (e.g., aging, senility), feline hyperesthesia syndrome, and any condition leading to pain should be considered as contributing factors. Cats in estrus also vocalize. The presence of classical behavioral signs of restlessness, frequent urination, spraying, rolling, and lordosis during the breeding season help differentiate this as a diagnosis.

MANAGEMENT

Concurrent or underlying medical problems should be treated. Normal feline behavior should be explained to owners to help them understand that some vocalizations cannot be eliminated but may be managed. Ignoring the cat when it is vocalizing may decrease some attention-seeking behavior. Concurrent or underlying medical problems should be treated. If possible, triggers for anxiety should be removed or minimized. A regular, predictable routine should be established, with the owner feeding and playing with the cat at a set time each day. The cat's environment should be enriched by providing toys (and rotating them regularly), hiding places, and play opportunities.

In cases of severe anxiety, treatment may also include medication. Medications that influence serotonin metabolism, such as the SSRIs and the TCAs, have been used in the treatment of anxiety-related disorders. Treatment for cognitive decline may also be necessary with natural supplements such as Senilife (CEVA Animal Health), the nutraceutical Aktivait (a combination of phosphatidylserine and antioxidants), or S-adenosylmethionine (SAMe). Selegiline (Anipryl, Pfizer Animal Health [also known as L-deprenyl]) at 0.5 to 1 mg/kg per day orally has been reported to be effective but is not licensed for use in cats. Other anxiolytic medication has proved useful in some cases. It should be noted that the benzodiazepines can lead to increased vocalization in some cats. Feliway has been reported to be useful in decreasing anxiety in some cats. Physical or verbal punishment should not be used because it increases anxiety and impedes learning of appropriate behavior.

Complete blood work should be done before medication is administered to determine a baseline, especially for liver and kidney parameters. The cat may require medication for prolonged periods (up 12 months).

Elimination in Unacceptable Locations[15c]

Elimination problems are the most common behavioral condition reported in cats, accounting for between 40% and 75% of reported behavioral problems. Both males and females, neutered and intact, present with elimination problems, and elimination problems have been reported in all breeds and across all age groups. Elimination problems must be differentiated from spraying or marking behavior.

CLINICAL SIGNS

Clinical signs include urination, defecation, or both outside the litter box. The elimination is of changed amount, frequency, or location and may be associated with an underlying medical condition. It may also be a normal response. Urination or defecation outside the litter box is generally unacceptable to owners. It usually involves the cat passing normal amounts of urine or feces and is associated with the elimination of waste. The cat usually squats to produce a normal quantity of urine. The cat uses a horizontal surface and often scratches afterwards. Defecation outside the litter box is only rarely a marking behavior. Predisposing factors include the following:

1. Litter box aversion (substrate and/or location)
   - This may be due to a new type of litter or a dirty box.
   - Cats that experience pain while urinating or defecating (e.g., because of constipation, arthritic pain) may develop an aversion to using the litter box.
   - Aversion can also be induced by "catching" the cat in the litter box before performing potentially unpleasant procedures such as medicating or grooming.
2. Litter box preference (substrate and/or location)
   - This may be influenced by fear and/or anxiety.
   - Separation anxiety can lead to elimination problems, and this is usually seen when the owner is absent. The cat may choose to eliminate on the objects associated with the owner (e.g., clothes, bedding, briefcases, shoes). It is usually seen after separation longer than 12 hours or immediately after the owner returns.
   - Fearful cats may eliminate in the place where they are frightened because they often are too frightened to go to the litter box.
   - The presence of another cat can also lead to elimination problems, as they may increase anxiety or block access to litter boxes.

DIFFERENTIAL DIAGNOSES

Medical conditions such as arthritis, diarrhea, constipation, lower urinary tract disease, and any cause of polyuria have been implicated as factors contributing to elimination problems.

MANAGEMENT

Careful questioning of the owner is important to differentiate urine marking from urination in inappropriate locations. After obtaining a complete behavioral history, the veterinarian should perform a thorough physical examination, complete blood cell count and biochemistry panel, urinalysis, and possibly radiography or other imaging procedures to exclude medical causes.

After any concurrent or contributing medical problems are addressed, the treatment involves two aspects:

1. Increasing the attractiveness of the area the owner wants the cat to use
2. Decreasing the attractiveness of the area that the cat wants to use

Punishment is discouraged because it increases the cat's anxiety and impedes learning of appropriate behavior.

LITTER BOX PROBLEMS The following recommendations have proved useful to help make the litter box more attractive to the cat:

- Change the type of litter by changing brand, or to sawdust, shredded newspaper (or recycled paper litter), clumping litter, or sand.
- Increase the frequency with which the litter box is cleaned and changed.
- Change the cleaning agent used to clean the litter box, and avoid disinfectants or bleaches when cleaning the litter box.
- Increase the number of litter boxes (a good rule of thumb is one litter box per cat and one extra).
- Place litter boxes in easily accessible, separate locations separated from food and water bowls.
- Provide a litter box that is large enough for the cat (at least 1½ times the length of the cat).
- Make sure the cat can enter the litter box. For example, if the sides are too high, small cats or older cats may have trouble climbing inside.

LOCATION PROBLEMS To make the location of the litter box more acceptable to the cat, the following suggestions may be helpful:

- Place a litter box over the area that is being used by the cat. Then very gradually change the location of

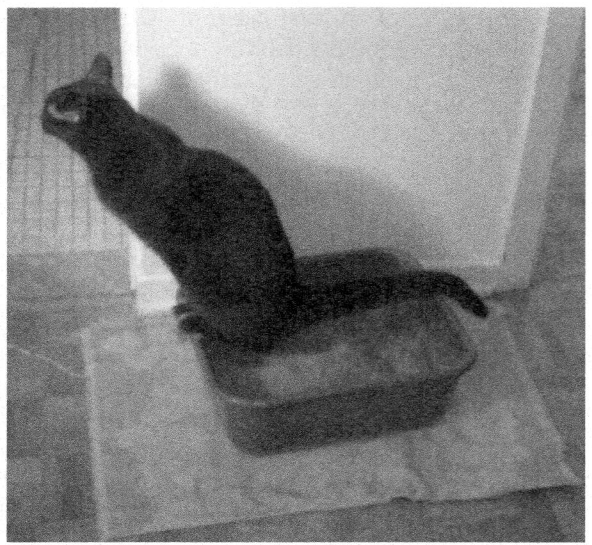

FIGURE 13-2 A cat with substrate aversion perches on the sides of the litter box to keep from touching the litter. *(Courtesy Dr. Susan Little.)*

the litter box until it is in an area that is more acceptable to the owner. This may mean gradual increments of movement as small as 5 cm (2 inches) daily.

- Cover the litter box to make it more private for the cat. For example, put a cardboard box, with appropriate openings, over the litter box.
- Change the type of litter box (e.g., one with higher or lower sides).
- Place the box away from noisy or high-traffic areas.

Cats may be discouraged from using specific locations to eliminate by the following suggestions:

- Feed or play with the cat in these areas.
- Place dry cat food in these areas (because it takes longer to consume than canned food).
- Leave the cat's toys or bedding in the area.
- Make the area less accessible and less pleasant to the cat by covering the area with thick plastic, aluminum foil, or double-sided sticky tape.

SUBSTRATE PROBLEMS Make the substrate the owner wants the cat to use more readily acceptable to the cat by implementing the following suggestions:

- Changing the litter type to one the cat prefers
- Cleaning the litter box as soon as it is used
- Using an empty litter box for cats that prefer smooth surfaces such as bathtubs and sinks (Figure 13-2)

ANXIETY-RELATED PROBLEMS Removing or minimizing the cause of the anxiety, if possible, is important. Providing a predictable routine, such as feeding and playing at a set time each day, can be helpful. In some cases the cat must be confined to a small area to be retrained. However, because this can increase anxiety in some cats, it must be carefully managed. Access to larger areas should happen very gradually, when the cat starts to use the litter box consistently.

CLEANING The soiled areas should be cleaned with non–ammonia-based products such as enzymatic washing powders. Additionally, neutralizers such as A.O.E. Animal Odor Eliminator (Thornell Corporation; Smithville, Missouri) or Urine Off (Bio-Pro Research; Hickory, North Carolina) used after cleaning the area with water can be effective in removing the odor.

Urine Spraying

Urine spraying is a marking behavior and is often associated with anxiety. It may be territorial, sexual, or agonistic. In multicat households it may be associated with overt or covert aggression. Intact cats spray more than neutered cats, and male cats spray more than female cats. It is estimated that 10% of castrated males and 5% of spayed females spray.[6] Spraying appears to be more common in multicat households, with a reported 100% chance of at least one cat spraying in a household with more than 10 cats. Male cats that live with a female cat are reported to be more likely to spray than those living with another male cat.

CLINICAL SIGNS

Cats that spray usually stand (but may squat), usually produce only a small quantity of urine, and frequently use vertical surfaces (but may use horizontal surfaces), and rarely scratch afterwards.

DIFFERENTIAL DIAGNOSES

Predisposing factors include medical conditions ranging from those associated with the urogenital system (e.g., renal calculi, renal failure, lower urinary tract disease), viral diseases (e.g., feline immunodeficiency virus, feline leukemia virus), to impacted anal glands. It is reported that up to 30% of cats that present for spraying may have a concurrent medical condition.[5]

Territorial, agonistic encounters or any highly arousing circumstances such as environmental stimuli (e.g., the sight, sound, or smell of another cat, within the household as well as outside) have been reported to be associated with spraying. Anxiety-related problems, including separation anxiety, and changes in routine (e.g., moving house, the introduction of a new spouse, new baby, or new cat in the area) have also been implicated.[15a]

MANAGEMENT

After a complete behavioral history and a thorough physical examination, diagnostic testing such as a complete blood cell count and biochemistry panel, urinalysis, and radiography (or other imaging or diagnostic techniques) may be required to exclude medical causes.

Careful questioning of the owner is important to differentiate urine marking from urination in unacceptable locations. Medical problems must be dealt with before, or at least concurrently with, any behavioral therapy that is instigated. Neutering the intact cat has been shown to be successful in many cases of spraying.

Educating owners about normal feline behavior is important so that they understand the behavior may not be completely eliminated but can usually be managed successfully. If possible, any anxiety-provoking stimuli should be removed or minimized. Provision of a regular predictable routine, such as feeding the cat or playing with the cat at a set time each day, has proved helpful in many cases. Punishment is not recommended because it increases the anxiety and impedes the learning of appropriate behavior.

ENVIRONMENTAL MANAGEMENT Environmental manipulation may be difficult to achieve in practice, although in theory it should work well. It is rarely possible or practical to remove the cat next door, the new baby, or the new spouse or entirely prevent other anxiety-provoking circumstances, such as moving house. Other recommendations that have been suggested include the following:

- Decreasing the number of cats in the household
- Decreasing access to windows and doors to decrease sight, sound, and smell stimuli
- Changing the amount of time spent indoors or outdoors
- Preventing access to arousing stimuli
- Making the sprayed areas less attractive to the cat by making them feeding or play areas instead
- Using Feliway (Ceva Animal Health) diffuser or spray

PHARMACOLOGIC TREATMENTS Pharmacologic treatments are generally aimed at reducing the anxiety level of the cat by altering the neurochemical environment in conjunction with behavior modification and environmental management. Potential side effects should be explained to the owner before instigating any therapy because most of the medications are not registered for use in cats. Complete blood work should be carried out before beginning drug therapy. All medication should be gradually withdrawn under veterinary supervision. The most commonly used medications are TCAs such as clomipramine and SSRIs such as fluoxetine. However, benzodiazepines, azapirones, and antihistamines have proved useful in some cases.

CLEANING The soiled areas should be cleaned with non–ammonia-based products such as enzymatic washing powders. Additionally, neutralizers such as A.O.E. Animal Odor Eliminator (Thornell Corporation; Smithville, Missouri) or Urine Off (Bio-Pro Research; Hickory, North Carolina) used after cleaning can be effective in removing the odor.

AGGRESSION

Overview

Aggression is not a diagnosis but a description of what is happening at a particular time. *Aggression* can be defined as a threat, challenge, or attack that is directed toward one or more individuals. It can be intraspecific (between cats) or interspecific (between a cat and another animal).[15] Aggression may be normal or abnormal depending on the context in which it occurs.[12]

Aggression is a nonspecific sign—that is, it may be exhibited in many different situations. It may be passive (covert) or active (overt), and it is important to recognize that several different "categories" of aggression may occur concurrently. The more "categories" of aggression that co-occur, generally the more guarded the prognosis, unless there is a common underlying trigger (e.g., pain).

The signs of aggression may be visual (e.g., changes in body posture, changes in ear and eye position, piloerection), auditory (e.g., growling, hissing, spitting), olfactory (e.g., spraying, scratching), or tactile (e.g., scratching) and may involve use of teeth and claws (Figure 13-3).

Although many diagnostic categories of aggression are recognized, there is some variation in the classification of aggression into various categories among authors,

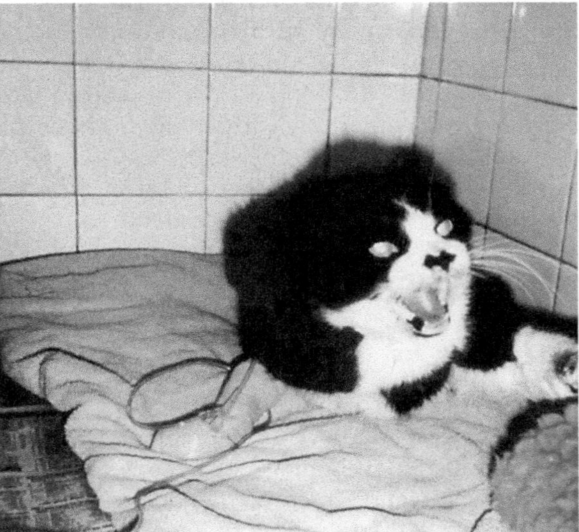

FIGURE 13-3 Signs of aggression include changes in body position, ear and eye position, piloerection, and growling.

countries, and continents. Aggression may be classified by its target or by its presumed function. The actual prevalence of each category of aggression in the cat population is unknown.

Medical conditions such as toxoplasmosis, ischemic vascular problems, hepatoencephalopathy, encephalitis, meningioma, lead poisoning, arthritis, sensory (hearing, sight) deficits, hyperthyroidism, epilepsy, lower urinary tract disease, feline immunodeficiency virus infection, rabies, and any condition leading to pain or discomfort have all been associated with aggression, as has the use of medications such as anesthetic agents and corticosteroids. A thorough physical examination and appropriate medical workup is therefore always necessary.

Fear Aggression

Clinical Signs

Cats can be fearful of people, places, other cats, and various stimuli such as noises and odors. The signs of aggression may be a combination of offense and defense. The fearful cat will initially attempt to avoid the stimulus and exhibit many warning signals. Fearful cats typically hiss, spit, growl, piloerect, or flatten their ears against the head and show a low or crouched body position. Pupillary dilation is common. They may try to flee, but if they have learned that this has not been successful in the past, they may attack. Aggression is usually the last resort but is generally very violent, and the behavior may become learned.

Differential Diagnoses

Genetically, two types of cat personalities have been recognized—timid, fearful cats and confident, friendly cats—and it appears that the temperament of the tom may have the greatest influence on the personality of kittens. This may account for some fearful behavior seen in cats. Inadequate or lack of socialization and handling before 12 weeks of age may also contribute to the cat's responses to people. Inadequate or lack of socialization with other cats early in life may contribute to the cat's responses to other cats. Cats learn to be fearful in certain situations, especially if they have had a bad experience with no opportunity to escape (e.g., rough handling, loud noises, unpleasant odors at veterinary hospitals).

Management Options

Depending on the severity of the problem, the cat may need no treatment or may need behavior modification, such as desensitization and counterconditioning, in combination with psychopharmacologic intervention in severe or long-standing cases. Behavior modification includes desensitization and counterconditioning, which involves slowly introducing the cat to the fearful situation in a gradual, controlled sequence.

The first step is to teach the cat to be calm and relaxed. This can be done by offering the cat a tasty treat such as Vegemite (Kraft Foods, Australia), chicken, baby food, or dehydrated liver. If the cat eats, it is usually a good indication that it is not too anxious. Then, while the cat is eating, the fearful stimulus (e.g., a person) is gradually introduced at a distance. The initial distance should be great enough not to elicit a fearful response from the cat. If the cat continues to take food, the person may approach the cat very slowly. The time frame for the gradual approach may vary from days to months depending on the severity of the problem. The cat should not be forced to interact in any way because that will exacerbate its fear.

Anxiolytic medication may also be needed. TCAs, SSRIs, or benzodiazepines may be necessary. The cat may require medication for a prolonged period (up to 12 months). Attempts to wean the cat off medication should be slow, and some cats may need lifelong treatment. A serum biochemistry panel should be obtained before prescribing medication. Feliway (spray and diffuser) may also be beneficial. Feliway can be used at home, as well as in the veterinary hospital. It can be sprayed onto wrists and hands before handling to help decrease arousal levels. The diffuser is useful in the environment. Punishment or forced restraint will aggravate the situation and should not be used to manage fearful cats.[1a] It may increase the cat's anxiety and impede learning.

Intercat Aggression

Clinical Signs

Intercat aggression is a very common problem. In intact male cats, it usually starts at approximately 2 to 4 years of age, when they reach social maturity. In some cases it may be normal male–male aggression associated with mating. This increases during the breeding season and with overcrowding. In male–male aggression, the cat flattens its ears, howls, hisses, piloerects, and uses both the teeth and claws in fights (Figure 13-4). Male–male aggression involves hormonal changes associated with sexual maturity and neurochemical changes associated with social maturity.

In neutered cats it tends to appear later in life and may be associated with social role. The signs depend on the mode and may be active (threatening) or passive (blocking access). Outright fighting appears to be rare.

Management Options

Prepubertal and postpubertal castration reduces or stops the frequency of fights in about 90% of cases occurring between intact males.[6] Management may involve changing the social environment. Cats in the same household should be reintroduced slowly, as described later in this chapter with regard to redirected aggression. It is important not to try to introduce them too quickly or too soon.

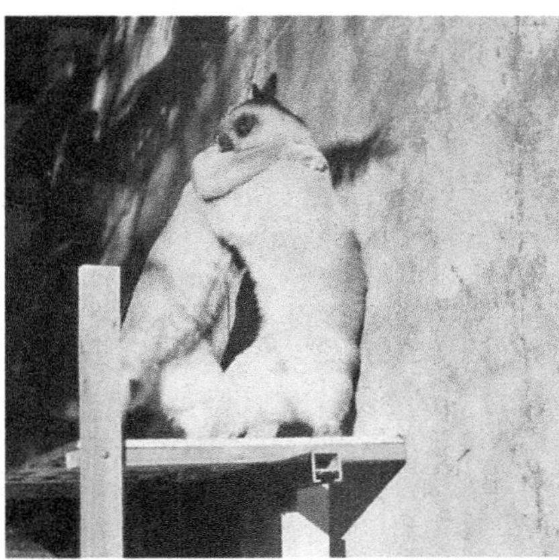

FIGURE 13-4 Intercat aggression is common between intact male cats and may lead to fighting with use of teeth and claws.

Anxiolytic medication may also be necessary for one or both cats to alter the neurochemical environment. Blood biochemistry analysis should be obtained before prescribing medication to determine a baseline, especially for liver and kidney parameters, and these levels should be checked every 6 to 12 months depending on the age and general health status of the cat. Patients may require medication for a prolonged period (up to 12 months) and then should be slowly weaned off. Feliway, has been anecdotally reported to be beneficial in managing intercat aggression in multicat households.

Maternal Aggression

Clinical Signs

The queen will threaten, hiss, and give other long-distance signals when she, the kittens, or the nesting area are approached. She will attack if cornered. Maternal aggression usually involves threatening behavior more than actual attack and usually is directed toward unfamiliar individuals. Attack tends to be a last resort when the queen is cornered.

Some queens may cannibalize their own kittens, and this is considered to be abnormal. This may happen if the queen is stressed or malnourished, and the incidence has been reported to increase with very large litters, second pregnancies, or sickly kittens. However, it can be normal if the queen eats stillborn or aborted fetuses. Cannibalization may also occur during overzealous eating of the placenta after birth.

Maternal aggression occurs in the periparturient period and may involve protecting the nest area as well as the kittens. This aggression may be the normal result of hormonal influences on the hypothalamus and is associated with the presence and the proximity of the kittens. The queen may be aggressive in the presence of male cats, and this may be related to the fact that free-ranging males have been reported to kill kittens. The response may also be anxiety related.

Management

People should avoid approaching the queen during this period to minimize her stress. She should be separated from other cats, especially males, at this time. Queens that kill their kittens should not be used for breeding. The aggression should resolve when the kittens are removed from the queen but may recur with the next litter.

Play Aggression

Clinical Signs

A cat may stalk, chase, pounce, and lie in wait for people to pass by while playing, but it rarely vocalizes. Play aggression may involve biting as well as scratching. Targets are usually moving objects or people and may be another cat, especially an older one, in the household. Young cats, especially those that are orphaned, hand raised, or weaned early, are more likely to show this type of aggression, and in many cases it may be normal behavior.[2b,12]

It is sometimes difficult to recognize play aggression because some cats play more roughly than others and do not retract their claws when they swat. In cats social play is seen between 4 and 12 weeks of age, and by 14 weeks of age may progress to social fighting.

Management Options

The aim of treatment is to redirect the play behavior onto more suitable objects, rather than trying to stop the behavior completely. One way to redirect the behavior is to provide the cat with appropriate toys (e.g., toys on poles) so that the cat can pounce without hurting anyone. However, the toys must be changed at regular intervals, even daily, for the cat to maintain interest. Additionally, the cat may need to be taught how to play with toys and then encouraged to do so.

Rough play, especially involving hands or other body parts, is discouraged. Whenever the cat plays in this manner, play should be interrupted or suspended and the cat's attention directed to appropriate toys instead.

Any punishment, such as smacking or squirting the cat with a water pistol, may actually encourage the behavior and increase the cat's arousal. Punishment is discouraged because it may lead to other problems, such as fear aggression. Providing the cat with a regular routine that involves interactive play involving toys 2 to 3 times daily for 5 to 10 minutes is important to provide a natural outlet for the behavior. In some cases a second kitten, preferably one that is not very young, may also help teach more appropriate play behavior, but this is not recommended unless the clients really want another cat, because the introduction of another cat may lead to additional problems.

Redirected Aggression

Clinical Signs

Redirected aggression occurs when the original target of the aggression is not accessible and the cat directs its aggression toward an unrelated target. This target may be a person or another cat that enters the area soon after the provocative event. The eliciting factors of the aggression are different in the initial and subsequent episodes. The first episode is triggered by a stimulus that the cat is in some way thwarted in its attempt to respond. This episode is commonly missed. The highly aroused cat now may direct its attention to the next (usually moving) thing that it encounters. For example, a cat may see another cat through the window and be unable to reach it. Another cat in the household then enters the room, and the cat redirects the aggression to the second cat. In the second and subsequent episodes, the initial stimulus no longer has to be present to elicit the aggression, just the target of the first attack. Commonly, the behavior of the target also changes, and this then results in a prolonged conflict, with the second cat now acting warily, running away, and showing avoidance behavior (victim behavior) whenever the first cat enters the room or approaches.

Cats have been used as models for "kindling" (a change in brain function in which seizures may be induced by repeated chemical or electrical stimuli). Once stimulated, the cells of the nervous system then have a very low threshold for stimulation, and cats may stay reactive for up to 48 hours (or even longer).

Management Options

The cat should be left alone until it is calmer. It is never advisable to approach any highly aroused cat, especially to try to calm or reassure it. If another cat is involved, the cats should be separated immediately (provided it is safe to do so) regardless of which cat is the victim or the instigator of the aggression. Treatment then involves slowly reintroducing the cats to each other. They should be placed in separate rooms so that they can hear and smell each other, but no visual contact should occur. The cats should be rotated around all the rooms until they have left their scent in all the rooms. This may take up to 2 weeks. While the cats are separated, a regular routine should be established with each cat so that certain events, such as feeding and playing, occur at a set time each day. Ideally, the cats are fed 5 or 6 small meals daily.

The cats are then slowly re-introduced but only after they are calm and displaying no signs of anxiety to the sounds and odors of the other cat. The aim is for them to have a positive association with each other. This essentially means that "good" things such as play or feeding happen only in the presence of the other cat. Initially they are in the same room only during meal times. They are placed in cages at opposite ends of the room and are fed at this time. This should create a positive association with food and the presence of the other cat, although it has been suggested that food may not always be a suitable reward insofar as cats do not share food. If no hissing or spitting occurs and the cats eat the food, the cages are gradually brought closer and closer to each other over a period of days and meals. This may take several weeks or even months. Then one cat at a time is allowed out of its cage to explore, and if no aggression occurs, both are allowed to interact under supervision. The re-introduction must be very gradual.

In some cases anxiolytic medication may also be needed to treat one or both cats to help decrease the reactivity. Blood biochemistry analysis should be obtained before prescribing medication to determine a baseline, especially for liver and kidney parameters. TCAs such as amitriptyline and clomipramine or SSRIs such as fluoxetine may be useful for the aggressor. Benzodiazepines such as diazepam or an azapirone such as buspirone may be necessary for the victim. The owners should be informed that the cats may require medication for a prolonged period, up to 12 months or even lifelong if the anxiety induced by the presence of the other cat persists. Gradual reduction and weaning off medication can be attempted only if the cats have learned to tolerate each other's presence for at least 6 months.

When sprayed into the cages during the desensitization process, Feliway can also be beneficial to decrease anxiety. Additionally, the Feliway diffuser can be plugged into the rooms in which the cats spend most of their time, which may also help decrease anxiety. Feliway should be used for at least 2 to 3 months.

Aggression Directed Toward Owners

Clinical Signs

The signs of aggression directed toward owners may be active (overt) or passive (covert). The cat may bite when the owner attempts to approach, lift, move, or handle the cat (overt aggression). It may also involve behaviors, such as soliciting attention by biting. The cat may bite when approached or handled or solicit attention and then bite if it is or is not given. Biting may also occur when the attention ceases. The cat may also block access to areas, possibly by sitting in doorways and staring (covert aggression). This type of aggression may be anxiety based when the cat is not given clear and consistent signals by owners.

Management Options

The veterinarian's role is to help the owner identify all situations that may be provocative and provide advice re strategies so that these situations can be avoided (e.g., approaching, stroking, handling the cat). Then it is important to instigate a behavior modification program where the cat is taught to perform a behavior (such as come or sit) to gain attention. The cat should come or sit at the owner's request before any interaction with the owner. If the cat solicits attention, the owner should completely ignore the cat or walk away. No reward or attention is given until the cat defers and responds to a verbal cue (e.g., "sit" or "come"; see Chapter 11).

Desensitization and counterconditioning to handling, moving, and other provoking actions can be done and the cat rewarded for appropriate acceptable behavior. If the cat shows any sign of aggression, the owner should move away and stop all interactions. The cat should not be physically punished because that will exacerbate the problem. Psychotropic medication may also be needed to manage the cat. Feliway can also be helpful in decreasing reactivity in some cats.

Territorial Aggression

Clinical Signs

Territorial aggression can be intraspecific as well as interspecific, and this includes aggression toward people. The cat may patrol its territory and mark it by rubbing or spraying to maintain social distance as well as define hierarchy. The aggression may be directed toward another cat, or a person, that approaches or enters its territory. The behavior may be more marked in intact toms during the breeding season. Unfamiliar cats are less well tolerated than familiar or neighboring cats. The aggression decreases with increased distance away from the cat's core (home) territory.

Management Options

Management options involve attempting to avoid all potentially provocative situations so as not to reinforce the behavior. If the aggression is directed toward another cat within the home, the cats should be separated and slowly re-introduced, as described in a previous section. A Feliway diffuser plugged into the room in which the cats spend most of their time may also be helpful. Psychotropic medication to decrease any associated anxiety may also be necessary.

If the aggression is directed toward people, the cat should be denied access to all areas that may be guarded. If the cat shows any signs of aggression, the owner should move away slowly and stop all interactions. Physical punishment is never recommended because it may exacerbate the problem.

Petting Aggression

Clinical Signs

Some cats have a very low tolerance to being patted or stroked. Although the cat may seek out attention and jump on the owner's lap, it may still not tolerate being stroked. The cat may suddenly bite or scratch after tactile stimulation of variable duration. The cat may swipe or bite if the petting stops or if the stroking is carried out for a prolonged period. The cat may stiffen, lash its tail, or give a warning bite while being patted. Some cats appear to enjoy sitting on a lap as long as no stroking or other tactile stimulation occurs. Owners are most commonly bitten or scratched on the hands and arms. The behavior is reported to be more common in intact males and is thought to relate to social grooming behavior.

Management Options

Some of these cats can be taught to gradually tolerate longer periods of stroking, but this takes time and patience. Some cats never learn to tolerate patting, and this must be explained to owners. It is also important to teach owners how to stroke or pat cats in an appropriate way, where to stroke the cat, and how to keep from overstimulating the cat. Medical conditions that cause pain or skin irritation should be investigated and treated.

Once owners understand that some cats never tolerate handling, no treatment may be necessary. What owners find distressing is that some of these cats actually solicit attention and then attack when it is given.

Before starting a desensitization program, the veterinarian must determine how long the cat can tolerate attention. If the cat usually tolerates a short period of stimulation (e.g., 3 minutes but not 4 minutes), the cat should be slowly stroked for only 2 minutes. The period of time used should always be below the cat's current stimulation threshold. The cat should be rewarded with food treats or play. The time can be gradually increased over a period of days to weeks until the cat tolerates increasingly longer periods. The owner should be instructed always to stop the stroking before the cat shows signs of arousal. The training session should be held at a predictable time each day. Punishment is not effective because it tends to lead to more aggression, insofar as the cat is already aroused and overstimulated.

Anxiolytic medication has been used to treat some cats. Feliway has been useful in some cases when sprayed on the owner's hands before handling the cat.

Pain Aggression

Clinical Signs

When the aggression is due to pain, the cat may respond to being handled or approached in an aggressive manner. The cat may show signs of offensive (e.g., direct eye contact; forward body position; back-and-forth tail flagging, especially of the tail tip) or defensive (e.g. "Halloween" cat posture—arched back, piloerection, flattened ears, dilated pupils) aggression or avoidance with handling, or the signs may be exhibited before any manipulation or when the cat is approached.

Management Options

The aim of treatment is to relieve the source of the pain (e.g., by using analgesics). Then the anxiety associated with the pain should be treated. This may require the use of anxiolytics, TCAs, or other agents. All potentially painful situations should be avoided. Inadvertent reinforcement by patting, telling the cat "It's okay" in an effort to calm it, and similar responses should be avoided, unless it helps decrease the cat's arousal level. Unfortunately, in many of these cases some learned aggression may result. In other words, the cat has associated previous handling with pain, so desensitization and counterconditioning may be necessary so that the cat learns to relax when handled.

Prevention is more practical than resolution. Ideally, aggression should be prevented from developing by providing appropriate analgesia with all potentially painful manipulations, especially surgery. Punishment is never recommended because it may exacerbate the aggression.

Predatory Aggression

Clinical Signs

Although the behaviors are the same as those exhibited in predatory behavior, which is normal, the context in which predatory aggression is exhibited make this behavior abnormal. Signs of predatory behavior include stalking in silence, a lowered body posture, and a sudden lunge or pounce when the target moves suddenly, but the aggression is directed toward nonprey. The cat stalks and lies in wait for the "victim," then pounces when the target moves. No preceding threat is apparent. In other words, the cat shows all the contextual behaviors of predatory behavior, but it is out of context. There are no warning signs, and it may be directed toward people as well as other animals. Predatory aggression must be differentiated from predatory behavior, which is normal and instinctive. The focus of predatory aggression (e.g., nonprey item, body part) and outcome (the "victim" is not eaten) are different.

Management Options

The aim is to avoid all potentially problematic situations. The following options may help minimize predatory behavior directed toward prey:

- Confine the cat indoors to prevent predation.
- Confine the cat outdoors in runs and tunnels, such as modular cat parks or cat enclosures.
- Supervise when outside with the use of a harness or collar and lead.
- Provide appropriate toys for mental stimulation (see the section on enrichment in Chapter 14).
- If the cat is outside unsupervised, place several bells at intervals on the cat's collar to provide warning to prey.
- Use distracters such as loud noises when the cat is about to pounce. Then reward the cat for relaxed behavior. Please note this is *not* used to punish the cat, and the cat may learn only that it should not hunt while in the owner's presence.

In cases of predatory aggression directed toward nonprey (e.g., humans or other cats), the following suggestions may be helpful:

- Provide appropriate toys for mental stimulation.
- Place several bells on the cat's collar at varying intervals so that the victim is warned of the cat's presence.
- Use distracters such as loud noises when the cat is about to pounce. Then reward the cat for relaxed behavior.

Predatory aggression can be dangerous, especially when the targets are children and elderly people, on whom a cat can inflict severe damage. Euthanasia or careful rehoming may be necessary in some cases.

Idiopathic Aggression

Clinical Signs

Idiopathic aggression is unpredictable and appears to be unprovoked. Sudden mood changes and aggressive episodes, with neither provocation nor predictability, have been reported. It has been described as "toggle-switch" aggression, insofar as it may start suddenly, as if a switch has been turned on. This is a diagnosis of exclusion, and it is very rare. It is not well understood, but it reflects truly abnormal behavior. It may reflect seizure activity.

Management Options

Idiopathic aggression is difficult to treat using standard behavior-modification techniques because it is unpredictable. Additionally, it is impossible to avoid potentially provocative situations because there is no true provocation. Treatment with anticonvulsants such as phenobarbital should be considered if seizures are likely. No physical punishment should be used.

ONYCHECTOMY AND BEHAVIOR

Onychectomy (declawing) is a controversial surgery that is allowed in some countries and banned in others. Many owners and veterinarians are concerned that the procedure causes permanent physical and behavioral changes. Common reasons for considering onychectomy are to prevent damage from scratching and to prevent injury to humans (particularly seniors and people with diabetes, cancer, and compromised immune systems) or other pets. For some owners onychectomy may be an alternative to relinquishment to a shelter, a change to an outdoor lifestyle, or euthanasia.[7,10] Studies have shown that owners of declawed cats have a positive attitude about the procedure and perceive an increase in the quality of the bond to their pet.[7,8,13,19] Numerous studies have failed to show an increase in behavioral problems in declawed cats.[1,2,11,13] In countries where onychectomy is not performed, the ability to resolve behavioral problems associated with the cat's use of its claws appears to be no less successful than in countries where onychectomy is performed. Onychectomy should not be routinely recommended as a solution to scratching and clawing behaviors. It should be recommended only when all other means of addressing the problem have been attempted. Furthermore, onychectomy does not address the underlying reasons for the problem behavior.

Onychectomy is a painful procedure, and adequate analgesia must be provided both in the immediate postoperative period and for as long afterward as the patient requires. Complications associated with onychectomy include pain, lameness, hemorrhage, wound dehiscence, claw regrowth, paralysis, wound infection, and ischemia of the paw and distal limb caused by improper bandaging.[8,13,17] However, these are almost entirely avoidable with proper attention to instrumentation and technique.

Alternatives to onychectomy include behavior modification and the provision of suitable scratching materials, frequent claw trimming, and nail caps. Deep digital flexor tenectomy is an alternative surgical procedure that is similar to onychectomy in terms of recovery time but is not as well accepted by owners.[19] The claws may overgrow if they are not regularly trimmed. In addition, long-term complications have been reported, such as stiff and painful forelimbs.[16]

Both the American Veterinary Medical Association (AVMA) and the Canadian Veterinary Medical Association recommend that onychectomy be performed only after other options have been exhausted or when the risk of an injury presents a human health risk. For more information, the reader is referred to the AVMA's 2009 background article on the welfare implications of declawing of domestic cats (http://www.avma.org/issues/animal_welfare/declawing_bgnd.asp).

References

1. Bennett M, Houpt KA, Erb HN: Effects of declawing on feline behavior, *Comp Anim Pract* 2:7, 1988.

1a. American Association of Feline Practitioners: Feline friendly handing guidelines, *J Feline Med Surg* Volume 13, May 2011.

2. Borchelt PL, Voith VL: Aggressive behavior in cats, *Comp Contin Educ Pract Vet* 9:49, 1987.

2a. Bradshaw JWS, Neville PF, Sawyer D: Factors affecting pica in the domestic cat, *Applied Animal Behaviour Science* 52:373-379, 1997.

2b. Caro TM: Predatory behaviour and social play in kittens, *Behaviour* 76:1-24, 1981.

3. Casey R: Fear and stress. In Horwitz D, Mills D, Heath S, editors: *BSAVA manual of canine and feline behavioural medicine*, Gloucester, UK, 2002, British Small Animal Veterinary Association, p 144.

4. Denenberg S, Landsberg GM, Horwitz D et al: A comparison of cases referred to behaviorists in three different countries. In Mills D, Levine E, editors: *Current issues and research in veterinary behavioral medicine: papers presented at the fifth veterinary behavior meeting*, West Lafayette, Ind, 2005, Purdue University Press, p 56.

5. Frank DF, Erb HN, Houpt KA: Urine spraying in cats: presence of concurrent disease and effects of a pheromone treatment, *Appl Anim Behav Sci* 61:263, 1999.

6. Hart BL, Cooper L: Factors relating to urine spraying and fighting in prepubertally gonadectomized cats, *J Am Vet Med Assoc* 184: 1255, 1984.

6a. King JN, Simpson KL, Overall D, et al: Treatment of separation anxiety in dogs with clomipramine: results from a prospective, randomized, double-blind, placebo-controlled, parallel-group, multicenter clinical trial, *Appl Anim Behav Sci* 67:255-275, 2000.

7. Landsberg GM: Cat owners' attitudes toward declawing, *Anthrozoos* 4:192, 1991.

8. Landsberg GM: Feline scratching and destruction and the effects of declawing, *Vet Clin North Am Small Anim Pract* 21:265, 1991.

9. Leonard BE: The HPA and immune axes in stress: the involvement of the serotonergic system, *Eur Psychiatry* 20(Suppl 3):S302, 2005.

10. McKeown D, Luescher A, Machum M: The problem of destructive scratching by cats, *Can Vet J* 29:1017, 1988.

11. Morgan M, Houpt KA: Feline behavior problems: the influence of declawing, *Anthrozoos* 3:50, 1989.

12. Overall K: *Clinical behavioral medicine for small animals*, St Louis, 1997, Mosby.

12a. Overall KL, Dunham AE: Clinical features and outcome in dogs and cats with obsessive-compulsive disorder: 126 cases (1989-2000), *J Am Vet Med Assoc* 221:1445-1452, 2001.

13. Patronek G: Assessment of claims of short- and long-term complications associated with onychectomy in cats, *J Am Vet Med Assoc* 219:932, 2001.

14. Patronek G, Glickman L, Beck A et al: Risk factors for relinquishment of cats to an animal shelter, *J Am Vet Med Assoc* 209:582, 1996.

15. Seksel K: Aggression, cat. In Cote E, editor: *Clinical veterinary advisor*, ed 2, St Louis, 2011, Elsevier, p 46.

15a. Seksel K, Lindeman MJ: Use of clomipramine in the treatment of anxiety-related and obsessive-compulsive disorders in cats, *Austral Vet J* 76:317-321, 1998.

15b. Stein DJ: Neurobiology of the obsessive—compulsive spectrum disorders, *Biological Psychiatry* 47(4):296-304, 2000.

15c. Sung W, Crowell-Davis SL: Elimination behavior patterns of domestic cats (*Felis catus*) with and without elimination behavior problems, *Am J Vet Res* 67:1500-1504, 2006.

16. Swiderski J: Onychectomy and its alternatives in the feline patient, *Clin Tech Small Anim Pract* 17:158, 2002.

17. Tobias K: Feline onychectomy at a teaching institution: a retrospective study of 163 cases, *Vet Surg* 23:274, 1994.

18. Waisglass S, Landsberg G, Yager J et al: Underlying medical conditions in cats with presumptive psychogenic alopecia, *J Am Vet Med Assoc* 228:1705, 2006.

19. Yeon S, Flanders J, Scarlett J et al: Attitudes of owners regarding tendonectomy and onychectomy in cats, *J Am Vet Med Assoc* 218:43, 2001.

CHAPTER

14

Behavioral Therapeutics

Kersti Seksel, Gary Landsberg, and Jacqueline Mary Ley

OUTLINE

After diagnosing a behavioral problem, the veterinarian must plan a treatment and management program that is both practical and rational from the owner's perspective. If the program is too complex or time consuming, owners will have difficulty incorporating it into their daily lives and routines. If the program does not make sense to the owner, the owner is likely to disregard the advice. In either case, if the issue is not satisfactorily resolved, the cat may be relinquished or euthanized. It is essential that veterinarians spend time helping owners understand the problem and the reason it has occurred (the underlying causes) and then develop reasonable expectations.

The initial approach is to modify the environment and manage the owner's expectations so that further problems can be prevented. This may be a short-term remedy, but it may also be the best or only practical long-term solution for some owners and some problems. The owner can then be educated about how cats learn and how their behavior can be effectively modified; this knowledge will help the owner implement the program so that there is some resolution of their concerns.

There is no one-size-fits-all approach in resolving behavioral problems. Therefore every treatment and management program must be tailored to the individual pet and the household where it resides. If there is a safety issue, prevention of further injury is the first concern. Therefore an assessment of the owner, cat, problem, and household is essential not only for determining the prognosis but also for developing an effective treatment and management program.

In general, treatment and management programs for most behavioral problems consist of three key areas, the three M's: behavior modification, environmental management, and psychotropic medication. Medication is not always necessary, but long-standing, recurrent, or severe cases are unlikely to improve without medication. It should also be noted that delaying the use of medication has serious welfare implications for the cat, so if medication is indicated, then the sooner the medication is started the better.

BEHAVIOR MODIFICATION

Since first coined by Thorndike in 1911,[43] the term *behavior modification* has been used in many ways. Currently, it mainly refers to techniques for increasing adaptive behavior through reinforcement and decreasing maladaptive behavior through extinction or punishment (with much more emphasis on the former). This is because when aversive punishments are used (or misused), they can lead to more emotional distress and behavioral problems involving fear and anxiety. Most aversive techniques are inappropriate in context, duration, intensity, or time of application. Recent studies have confirmed that punishment-based training and confrontational techniques are more likely to lead to increased aggression and avoidance behaviors.

The aim of any behavior-modification program should always be to reward appropriate behaviors rather than to punish unwanted behaviors. Therefore rather than focusing on how to stop what is undesirable, the owner should first focus on providing a desirable alternative (e.g., where to sleep, where to climb, where to scratch).

Behavior modification in cats generally involves reward-based training, desensitization, counterconditioning, and response substitution. Therefore an understanding of learning theory and the effects of operant and classical conditioning is essential before recommending treatment.

Classical conditioning is the pairing of an unconditioned stimulus with a neutral stimulus that results in a conditioned stimulus and a conditioned response. It does not use rewards, but the cat learns to pair an involuntary behavior with another neutral stimulus.

Classical conditioning can occur in both positive and negative ways. Examples of a positive conditioned emotional response are the pairing of a clicker with favored treats (for clicker training) or any sounds associated with feeding (e.g., filling the food bowl, opening the food cupboard, opening the refrigerator, shaking the package of treats).

Problems arise when a fearfully conditioned emotional response is established toward a previously neutral stimulus (visual, olfactory, auditory, animate, or inanimate) by repeatedly pairing it with a fear-producing stimulus. Once this occurs, the stimulus itself will elicit the fear response. Some examples might be the sound of a doorbell or a car pulling into the driveway that becomes paired with the visit of unfamiliar people (for cats that are fearful of visitors). Another example might be the sight of a grooming brush or nail clipper for a cat that is frightened by those procedures.

Operant conditioning involves the way actions result in consequences. The results either increase or decrease the likelihood of future responses. There are four types of behavior–consequence relationships. Reinforcement increases the likelihood that a behavior will be repeated, and punishment decreases the likelihood that the behavior will be exhibited. There can be both positive and negative reinforcement and punishment techniques. *Negative* refers to the removal of a stimulus, and *positive* refers to the application of a stimulus.

Counterconditioning occurs when a stimulus that evokes an unpleasant response is consistently and repeatedly paired with something that is highly positive until a positive association is made. To be successful, counterconditioning should be coupled with desensitization, wherein the intensity of the stimulus is minimized to a level that does not incite the fear response, such as by reducing volume, increasing distance, changing the environment, or modifying the stimulus to something less threatening.

Desensitization and counterconditioning are extremely time consuming. The exercises must be constantly repeated so that the response is altered to one that is positive. Clients often want both a quick fix and less work. However, moving too quickly provokes anxiety and sabotages any behavior-modification program.

Response substitution involves replacing an undesirable response with a desirable one. The process would be to use high-value rewards to teach desirable behaviors that have been selected as an acceptable and practical alternative to the undesirable behavior. However, if the behavior is part of the cat's natural repertoire (e.g., scratching), it can be particularly difficult to train the cat to perform alternative behaviors.

Training should always begin in the environment where success can be most readily achieved. The target behavior is for the cat to be quiet and calm. Therefore the owner must learn to read the look in the cat's eyes, its body posture, its facial expressions, and its breathing to be able to gradually shape the desired behavior. Training could then move to environments with increasing distractions and places where the problem is most likely to arise.

To replace the undesirable behavior with a desirable behavior, response substitution should be coupled with desensitization, by setting up exposure to low levels of the stimulus and practicing the target behaviors and relaxation exercises while reinforcing with the highest-valued rewards. If the cat is fearful or anxious, the focus should also be on classical counterconditioning so that each exposure to the stimulus is associated with only highly positive outcomes and no negative outcomes.

ENVIRONMENTAL MANAGEMENT

Environmental management is usually necessary to prevent exposure to the stimulus, prevent access to locations where problems might arise, or provide outlets for expression of the behavior. For example, cats may need to be confined to avoid exposure or access to other cats, so cat enclosures made of metal or mesh can be attached to a door or window to allow the cat access to outdoors and some or all of the yard (Figure 14-1). Another option might be to fence off the garden to keep the cat enclosed.

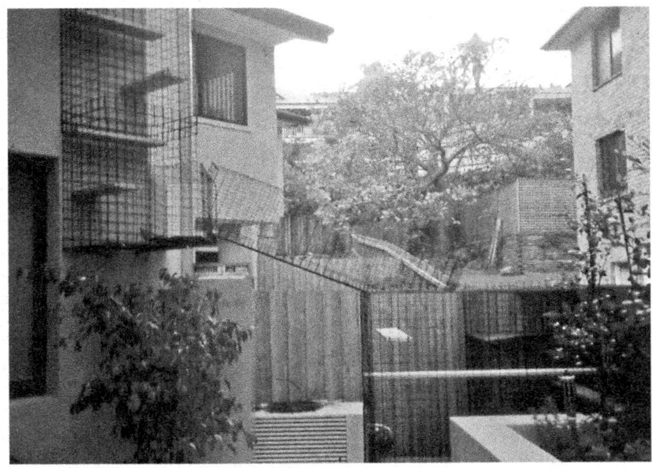

FIGURE 14-1 A cat enclosure attached to a door or window allows for safe access to a stimulating environment outdoors.

Management may also include physical and mental stimulation in the form of enrichment, which may reduce stress as well as help the cat cope with potential stressors in day-to-day living. There are many types of environmental enrichments that allow the cat to express normal behaviors in an acceptable way.

Any environmental enrichment program should be designed to provide sufficient outlets and opportunities for species-specific normal behavioral patterns, while offering the individual cat sufficient control and choices to be able to cope with challenges in a normal way. Therefore motivation, novelty, and complexity are important considerations when developing enrichment strategies.

The goal is an environment that the cat can use in a positive way, while reducing or eliminating abnormal behaviors. The enrichment program suggested must be individually tailored to the cat, its personality, and its behavioral problem so that the behavior is not inadvertently exacerbated. It should also be noted that too much enrichment (i.e., too many choices) can lead to increased stress in already anxious cats.

Studies have investigated disease rates among animals in enriched environments versus those in standard housing. Enriched environments were found to decrease the incidence of gastric ulcers in rats[35] and urinary tract disorders in cats[4] and to improve the immune functioning of animals.[39] Conversely, stress may alter immune function and has been shown to be a contributing or aggravating factor in gastrointestinal diseases, dermatologic conditions, respiratory and cardiac conditions, behavioral disorders, and a shortened life span.[12,31,44]

Enrichment might also delay the onset or lessen the effects of feline cognitive dysfunction. Studies in dogs and humans have shown that continued learning; physical exercise; and a change to a diet rich in antioxidants, essential fatty acids, and mitochondrial cofactors can have a positive effect on well-being,[26,29] and the same may be true for cats.[16]

Appropriate enrichment may prevent some behaviors that are of concern to owners[33,46] and lower stress, which may in turn lessen the chances of stress-related diseases such as interstitial cystitis.[3-5]

Enrichment can alleviate boredom and may play a role in preventing obesity and associated medical problems such as diabetes mellitus, hepatic lipidosis, and osteoarthritis.[33] Stress has a negative role in the development of skin conditions such as infections and pruritus, feline lower urinary tract disease (FLUTD), and conditions such as irritable bowel syndrome.[31,44] Addressing the environment of affected cats may help in reducing the number and severity of outbreaks of chronic diseases such as FLUTD.[21]

Any enrichment that is added to a cat's environment must take into account the species-specific behavior of cats and the preferences of the individual cat. An elderly cat that has lived most of its life without feline company will have different needs than a young cat living in a multicat household. As discussed in previous chapters, cats are small, solitary, ambush hunters that have a crepuscular activity pattern. They have complex and highly variable social systems, depending on the spread and amount of resources such as food and shelter.[9,11] Cats are territorial, with male territories overlapping several female territories.[10] Enrichment devices and activities must address the biological needs of cats as well as the individual preferences to have a positive effect on feline welfare.

Hunting and Foraging Behavior

Wild and feral cats spend a significant amount of their waking hours foraging and hunting for food. It is therefore unsurprising that pet cats investigate new objects in their environments and engage in play with small, prey-size objects.[17] Cats should not be allowed to play with human hands or feet because of the potential for injury resulting from their claws and teeth. However, toys that encourage the behaviors of the hunting sequence, such as stalking, rushing, pouncing, and biting, are popular with cats and their caregivers and provide opportunities for cats to engage in these normal behaviors. There are many types of toys that foster this type of play, including fishing rod–style toys and laser pointers. However, because the cat can never catch the light, some cats find laser toys frustrating. It can also be an issue for cats with the potential of developing an obsessive-compulsive disorder. Providing treats periodically during the game or afterwards may reduce frustration.

Cats hunt in short bursts, so play sessions should mimic this natural behavior. The owner should provide toys of a size and texture that motivate the cat. Cats may quickly become habituated to and lose interest in a particular toy; studies have shown that play intensity may be heightened in the short term if play is repeated with three or four different toys that have slightly different characteristics. Owners should try to maintain the cat's role as the predator with the toy as prey by using sudden changes of speed and direction when manipulating the toy. Toys on strings should be used for supervised play only as when alone the cat may ingest the string, leading to severe intestinal damage and possible death. After play sessions the cat's interest in further play may remain heightened for 15 minutes or more, so it might be advisable to give the cat some food or treats to keep it occupied and perhaps simulate the feeding that might logically follow predatory activity in the wild.

Cats that hunt for food will chase, capture, and eat several small meals a day. Therefore some cats may benefit from more play sessions and multiple smaller, prey-size meals. This might be accomplished by using timed feeding dishes or making meal feeding more complex by placing canned food in ice cube trays, small

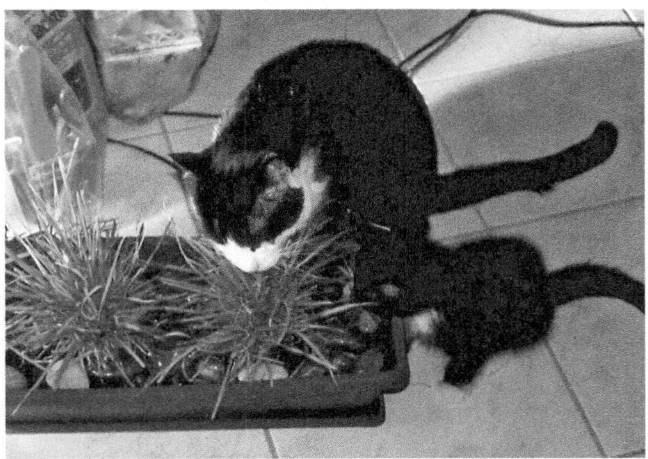

FIGURE 14-2 Feral cats frequently eat grass. Indoor cat gardens allow cats to carry out this normal behavior.

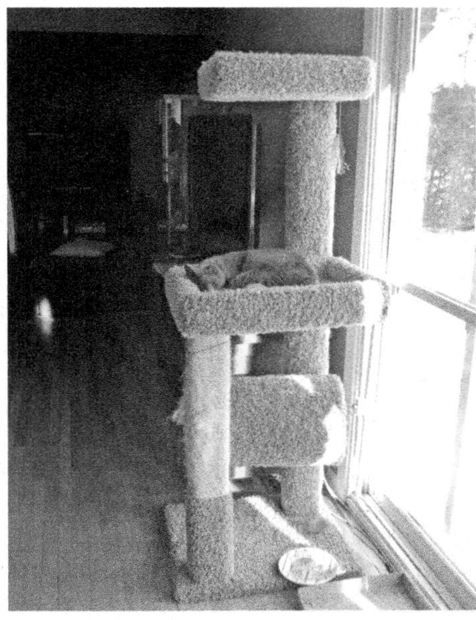

FIGURE 14-3 Appropriate hiding and perching places can reduce stress. If perches are placed near windows, cats can watch birds, butterflies, and other outdoor activities, which can be enriching for them. *(Courtesy Dr. Susan Little.)*

containers, or toys that require manipulation with paws or teeth to extract the food. A number of commercial toys are now available that require varying degrees of batting and rolling, dexterity, and mental activity to release the food.

Wild and feral cats frequently eat grass.[1] Cat grass offers a safe grazing choice for cats kept indoors (Figure 14-2). If the owner periodically moves the cat grass throughout the home, the cat will have to seek out the forage and therefore replicate natural behavior.

Resting Places

Cats spend an average of 2.8 hours resting and 7.8 hours sleeping during the day.[1] Comfortable, protected areas should be provided for cats to sleep and rest. Many cats like high positions and will gravitate to beds in high places, such as in cupboards or on shelves. In multicat homes cats are less likely to compete over prime space when there are several choices, such as window ledges, cat climbing frames, and furniture to which cats are allowed access. Every room that cats visit frequently should offer them appropriate hiding and perching places, which can reduce stress (Figure 14-3).[23] Cats are both predator and prey and may feel more secure in a place where they can watch activities without being watched themselves.

Scratching

Scratching is a normal behavior for cats. A cat's motivation to scratch includes maintenance grooming of the claws and deposition of an olfactory mark to convey temporal cues regarding the cat's proximity or passage.[25] Cats often scratch when they are excited (e.g., when their owners come home or during play) and after sleeping.[25] Old and new objects will be scratched, although older, frequently used scratching posts seem to continue to maintain interest for many cats.[25]

Owners should provide suitable outlets for scratching that are easily accessible and attractive and make unacceptable targets, such as furniture, less attractive. When a cat's scratching appears to be excessive in frequency, location, or duration, the possibility that the marking is related to stress or anxiety (as with urine marking) should be considered. In this case increased environmental enrichment, identification and removal of potential stressors, and possibly pheromone therapy may be necessary.

It is advisable to have at least one scratching post in the room most frequented by family members and in other well-traveled places in the home. More posts are needed in multicat homes. Ideally, vertical scratching posts should be tall enough for the cat to stand on its back legs and reach up to scratch. Posts should also be sturdy and stable. Cats have individual preferences regarding the materials and orientation (vertical or horizontal) of the posts. Therefore owners can be both proactive and reactive in providing scratching posts that appeal to the cat's tastes in type, texture, and location.

Cats can be encouraged to scratch by using an interactive toy (e.g., a fishing pole–type toy with feathers) and waving it over the post or attaching a dangling toy to the post. Once a cat's scent is deposited on the post, the cat is more likely to return. Cats can also be clicker trained to scratch at the posts.

Viewing Places

Watching birds, butterflies, and other things can be enriching for cats. However, the presence of other free-roaming cats in the vicinity can be stressful for some indoor cats and result in frustration and redirected aggression toward other family members, both human and feline.[26]

Novelty

For cats that have all of their basic needs met, exploratory behavior becomes a greater priority.[46] Because most pet cats do not have to spend several hours a day hunting, novelty plays an important role in enriching a well-fed and rested cat's time. The owner can increase this novelty by using different feeding techniques, such as placing food in treat balls, scattering dry food over a wide area for the cat to hunt, and putting food in different locations; offering new toys; and rotating toys every few days. Another option is providing new objects with which the cat can interact, such as a box or tunnel. Objects and toys can be moved around the space the cat occupies to create the appearance of a new environment. Cats can become used to hunt-and-chase toys within a few minutes, necessitating the introduction of a few different items within and between play sessions.[17]

Social Interaction

Cats are social creatures[3] and are often found in the vicinity of people with whom they are bonded. Cats enjoy not only human companionship but also that of members of their own and other species. However, there can be extensive individual variation depending on genetics, early experiences, and previous encounters. Just because a cat has a healthy social relationship with one or more cats does not mean that the cat will tolerate an unfamiliar cat being added to the household.

Brushing and hand grooming can be a form of enrichment for cats that enjoy physical contact and attention. Positive reinforcement training can also be enriching to cats[45] and can be used to train a number of simple behaviors, such as "sit," "roll over," and "come here." One useful and effective form of training for cats is clicker training. Training enhances the human–animal bond in dogs[2] and is likely to do the same in cats.

Environmental enrichment takes effort but should be considered as an important part of caring for companion cats, regardless of whether they have behavioral problems.

PSYCHOTROPIC MEDICATION

Medication for behavioral problems should not be viewed as a quick fix or a silver bullet. The decision to use medication depends on the diagnosis, and this should include a thorough physical workup, blood work, and a behavioral assessment. Medications are not generally indicated for problem behaviors (often normal behaviors that are problematic for the owners), only for behavioral problems, so it is important that veterinarians understand the rationale for prescribing psychotropic medication.[40]

Many of the medications in common usage are not registered for this purpose in animals. As more and more medications are registered for use in animals, it is increasingly important that veterinarians be familiar with these medications and the research that supports their use. This allows veterinarians to make an informed decision about which medication to use, as well as why and when to use it.

Much information regarding psychotropic medication is derived from human-medicine literature. When used in animals, the medication may have different effects, different side effects, and different therapeutic and toxic levels, and these factors may also vary with the species. It is the veterinarian's responsibility to be familiar with these factors before prescribing medication.

Medications do not change the relationship with the stimulus, and concurrent behavior modification will also be necessary to desensitize, countercondition, and train the cat in desirable responses. Clients must understand that behavior modification and environmental management are necessary if medication is used. Clients should be informed that the cat may require medication for the rest of its life, similar to chronic therapy for diseases such as diabetes. Once the behavior is managed to the owner's satisfaction, a lifelong commitment from the owner and continued support from the veterinarian may be necessary.

In veterinary medicine there is limited opportunity to perform evidence-based studies on the use of medication in cats, and much of the information has therefore been extrapolated from human-medicine literature.[24] This information should be interpreted with care because drug metabolism and receptor effects vary among species. This variation can lead to inaccurate assumptions with respect to dose, duration of effect, contraindications, and side effects. Therefore medications that are licensed for use in cats (e.g., clomipramine) should be considered first because data regarding safety, efficacy, side effects, contraindications, toxicity, and pharmacokinetics are available. In addition, the manufacturer can provide additional expertise, which is especially important should an adverse event occur.

When medication is used for longer than 8 weeks, it is prudent to consider a gradual weaning to determine the lowest effective dose and minimize potential withdrawal effects.

Why Use Psychotropic Medication?

The rationale for using psychotropic medications is based on their purported neurochemical actions in the brain. Many medications have now been used to modify behavior in humans and companion animals. Medications may influence neurotransmitters in three main ways:

1. They may act presynaptically and affect the presynaptic action potential, synthesis, storage, metabolism, release, or reuptake.
2. They may act on the enzymes that deactivate the neurotransmitter.
3. They may act postsynaptically and affect binding to receptors by acting as agonists or antagonists or actually modify receptors.

Obtaining the results of blood tests before prescribing medication is always recommended, especially in very old or young animals and those with a previous history of medical problems. A minimum database should include a complete blood count (CBC), biochemistry panel, and urinalysis. Because most of the medications are metabolized through the liver and then excreted through the renal system, liver and kidney function monitoring is important both before and during treatment.

It may be necessary to repeat these tests, often at 4 to 6 weeks after starting medication, depending on the cat, the medication, and the effects seen. All cats on long-term medication should be reassessed and have blood work re-evaluated every 6 to 12 months, depending on the cat's age and medical history.

It is also important to question owners about any other medications that they may be administering to their cat. This includes the use of natural remedies or homeopathic medications; many owners do not realize that these may also have significant effects on their pet and interact with the medications prescribed by the veterinarian.

When to Use Psychotropic Medication

Psychotropic medications have proved to be useful in several categories of behavioral problems. These include anxiety-related problems (including fears and phobias), obsessive–compulsive behaviors, some types of aggression, and geriatric behavioral problems.

The treatment of nonspecific signs (e.g., excessive vocalization, aggression, inappropriate elimination) by using medication is not acceptable, and this approach will ultimately lead to treatment failures.

What if the Medication Does Not Work?

Owners may sometimes believe that the medication has been ineffective. Reasons include the following:

- No diagnosis was made.
- An incorrect diagnosis was made.
- The incorrect medication was selected.
- An inadequate length of time was allowed for the treatment program to take effect.
- Medication has been used as stand-alone therapy when it should have been combined with a behavior-modification program.
- The owner was unable to medicate the pet.
- The owner has unrealistic expectations regarding the influence of the medication.

In some cases the effects of medication can be seen only when the medication has been stopped. It is important to advise owners that medication should never be suddenly stopped except under veterinary advice. The patient should always be weaned off the medication slowly and monitored by a veterinarian.

What Owners Need to Know About Psychotropic Medication

- Medication may take 6 to 8 weeks to reach therapeutic blood levels. Owners must understand that the effects will not be immediate.
- It may be necessary to change the medication or the dose as the management and treatment progresses.
- The minimum time required for a cat to receive medication is usually 6 months.
- Medication may be needed for the duration of the cat's life. This should be discussed with the owner before the medication is prescribed.
- Medication should never be suddenly stopped. The cat should always be weaned off it gradually to avoid a rebound affect. Owners should be warned of the danger of sudden cessation whenever medication is prescribed.
- Changing the dose, discontinuing the medication, or changing the type of medication should occur only with veterinary advice and under veterinary supervision.

Dosing and Compliance

Because many owners cannot administer pills, they are often reformulated into compounded liquids, flavored tablets, and transdermal medications. For compounded medications it is necessary to determine the stability and storage of these products. To date, no data support the efficacy of transdermal medication for behavior-modifying drugs in cats. One study found that the bioavailability of transdermal doses of fluoxetine was 10%

compared with oral dosing.[7] In another study systemic absorption of both amitriptyline and buspirone was poor compared with that conferred by the oral route.[28]

Common Psychotropic Medications

Medications that have anxiolytic action include the benzodiazepines, tricyclic antidepressants (TCAs), antihistamines, barbiturates, selective serotonin reuptake inhibitors (SSRIs), and beta blockers, and these have proved useful in some cases. Commonly used medications and dosing are summarized in Table 14-1 and Box 14-1.

Antidepressants cause little or no sedation and are unlikely to inhibit learning or memory. There is extensive evidence on the efficacy of clomipramine and fluoxetine for treating anxiety disorders, obsessive–compulsive disorders, and urine marking in dogs and cats; however, despite their use in the treatment of aggression, there is minimal evidence supporting efficacy.

TABLE 14-1 **Drug Doses for Behavior-Modification Therapy in Cats**

Drug	Dose
Alprazolam	0.125 to 0.25 mg/cat every 8, 12, or 24 hours
Diazepam	0.2 to 0.5 mg/kg every 8 to 12 hours
Oxazepam	0.2 to 0.5 mg/kg every 12 to 24 hours
Clonazepam	0.02 to 0.2 mg/kg every 12 to 24 hours
Lorazepam	0.025 to 0.05 mg/kg every 12 to 24 hours
Amitriptyline	0.5 to 1 mg/kg every 24 hours
Clomipramine	0.3 to 0.5 mg/kg every 24 hours
Fluoxetine	0.5 to 1 mg/kg every 24 hours
Paroxetine	0.5 to 1 mg/kg every 24 hours
Buspirone	0.5 to 1 mg/kg every 12 hours

BOX 14-1

Characteristics of Commonly Used Behavior-Modifying Medications in Cats

Tricyclic Antidepressants

- Clinical uses: urine spraying, feline lower urinary tract disease, overgrooming, anxiety, intercat aggression, impulsivity, obsessive–compulsive disorders[22,27,41]
- Side effects: short-term lethargy or sedation, mild and intermittent vomiting (usually transient), increases or decreases in appetite, dry mouth, constipation, urine retention (especially at higher doses),[37] tachycardia, cardiac arrhythmia, decreased tear production; high doses have been associated with increased liver enzymes, hepatotoxicity
- Contraindications and precautions: cardiac dysrhythmias, urinary retention, narrow-angle glaucoma, seizures, or within 2 weeks of a monoamine oxidase inhibitor drug; these medications may interfere with thyroid function and should be used with caution in affected patients
- Examples: amitriptyline, clomipramine, doxepin

Selective Serotonin Reuptake Inhibitors

- Clinical uses: urine spraying, some types of aggression, obsessive–compulsive disorders
- Side effects: liver changes, gastrointestinal disturbances, rashes; nausea, weight loss, tremors, and agitation have been reported in humans
- Contraindications and precautions: should not be used concurrently with monoamine oxidase inhibitors (may cause serotonin syndrome), and at least 2 weeks should be allowed as a washout period between selective serotonin reuptake inhibitor and monoamine oxidase inhibitor therapy (a 5-week washout period should be allowed for fluoxetine)
- Examples: fluoxetine, paroxetine

Benzodiazepines

- Clinical uses: urine spraying, overgrooming, fear-related aggression
- Side effects: increased appetite, transient ataxia, paradoxical hyperactivity, increased friendliness, increased vocalization, fatal idiopathic hepatic necrosis, interference with memory and learning, disinhibition of suppressed behaviors such as aggression
- Contraindications and precautions: not recommended for patients with liver or kidney failure or in obese cats, and use with caution in aggressive cats
- Examples: diazepam, alprazolam, oxazepam, clonazepam

Azapirones

- Clinical uses: mild fear; long-standing anxiety-related problems, including urine marking or spraying and inappropriate urination[19] and overgrooming
- Side effects: bradycardia and tachycardia, nervousness, gastrointestinal disturbances, stereotypic behaviors; restlessness has been reported in humans
- Contraindications and precautions: may lead to increased aggression as the disinhibitory effects of fear are decreased
- Example: buspirone

Although antidepressants reach peak plasma levels within hours, this does not reflect their therapeutic effect because reuptake inhibition may induce downregulation of postsynaptic receptors. Therefore 4 to 8 weeks of therapy is generally recommended to fully assess therapeutic effects.

TCAs and SSRIs should not be used concurrently with other antidepressants or monoamine oxidase (MAO) inhibitors such as selegiline and amitraz and should be used cautiously in pets with seizures. Because SSRIs inhibit cytochrome P450 enzymes, they can lead to increased toxicity if combined with other drugs that are metabolized by these enzymes.

Tricyclic Antidepressants

The primary mechanism of action of TCAs such as clomipramine and amitriptyline is to block the reuptake of serotonin and, to a lesser extent, noradrenaline. The degree of serotonin and noradrenaline reuptake blockade, as well as anticholinergic, antihistaminic, and alpha-adrenergic effects, varies among TCAs. Clomipramine is the most selective inhibitor of serotonin reuptake of the TCAs. It also inhibits noradrenaline reuptake and has mild anticholinergic and antihistaminic effects, which might account for some its side effects, such as lethargy, dry mouth, and gastrointestinal upset.

Clomipramine may help facilitate training in cats that are fearful of unfamiliar people or animals and may be useful for a variety of fear- and anxiety-based behavioral problems, alone or in combination with other anxiolytic agents.

Selective Serotonin Reuptake Inhibitors

As the name implies, SSRIs are selective for serotonin and lack the anticholinergic and cardiovascular side effects of the TCAs.

SSRIs are selective in their blockade of the reuptake of the neurotransmitter 5-hydroxytryptamine (5-HT) into the presynaptic neurons. Because they are selective for serotonin reuptake, they may have fewer side effects than TCAs, including fewer cardiac effects and less hypotension.[42] They may also be preferable where urine retention, increased intraocular pressure, sedation, or anticholinergic effects might be a concern. Paroxetine is mildly anticholinergic.

In a study of generalized anxiety disorders, fluoxetine and paroxetine were effective when combined with behavioral therapy. The primary side effect is decreased appetite, which may resolve with decreased dose.

For intercat aggression sertraline, paroxetine, or an anxiolytic might be used to increase confidence in the victim cat, and the aggressor may be treated with fluoxetine. Fluoxetine may also be effective in the treatment of feline urine marking.[18,38]

Benzodiazepines

Benzodiazepines potentiate the effects of gamma-aminobutyric acid (GABA), an inhibitory neurotransmitter. They cause a decrease in anxiety and hyperphagia and induce muscle relaxation. They reach peak effect shortly after each dose and can be used alone or in combination with other drugs on an as-needed basis. Diazepam may be effective for feline urine marking.[8] Because clonazepam, oxazepam, and lorazepam have no active intermediate metabolites, they may be safer when hepatic function is compromised. Benzodiazepines must be dosed frequently, and there may be a rebound effect if withdrawal is not gradual. They can cause paradoxical excitability and can have an amnesic effect. They are useful for counterconditioning because they decrease anxiety and increase appetite; however, diazepam has been reported to cause rare cases of fatal hepatotoxicity in cats.[6] Benzodiazepines can also be used for drug desensitization.

Azapirones

Buspirone, an azapirone, is a serotonin (5HT1A) receptor agonist and a dopamine (D_2) agonist. It is nonsedating, does not stimulate appetite, and does not appear to inhibit memory. It takes a week or more to reach effect and is therefore not useful for situational anxieties. Higher doses may have more immediate effect. Adding buspirone to an SSRI or a TCA might help ensure an adequate serotonin pool.

Synthetic Pheromone Analogs

Pheromones are released during facial rubbing on objects when cats feel comfortable in their environment. A synthetic feline facial pheromone (Feliway, Ceva Animal Health) has been developed as an aid in the treatment for anxiety-related disorders. Several studies have documented a significant decrease in urine-spraying behavior when the pheromone is sprayed in a cat's environment.[13,20,30,32] Other documented uses include reduction of stress during handling, hospitalization, or transport and treatment of intercat aggression in multicat households.[14,15,34,36] There are no reported side effects associated with use of Feliway, although caution should be exercised when using the product around cats with asthma or in the presence of birds.

References

1. Beaver B: *Feline behavior: a guide for veterinarians*, ed 2, St Louis, 2003, Saunders Elsevier.
2. Bennett PC, Rohlf VI: Owner–companion dog interactions: relationships between demographic variables, potentially problematic behaviours, training engagement and shared activities, *Appl Anim Behav Sci* 102:65, 2007.
3. Buffington CA: External and internal influences on disease risk in cats, *J Am Vet Med Assoc* 220:994, 2002.
4. Buffington CA, Westropp JL, Chew DJ et al: Clinical evaluation of multimodal environmental modification (MEMO) in the

management of cats with idiopathic cystitis, *J Feline Med Surg* 8:261, 2006.
5. Cameron ME, Casey RA, Bradshaw JW et al: A study of environmental and behavioural factors that may be associated with feline idiopathic cystitis, *J Small Anim Pract* 45:144, 2004.
6. Center SA, Elston TH, Rowland PH et al: Fulminant hepatic failure associated with oral administration of diazepam in 11 cats, *J Am Vet Med Assoc* 209:618, 1996.
7. Ciribassi J, Luescher A, Pasloske K et al: Comparative bioavailability of fluoxetine after transdermal and oral administration to healthy cats, *Am J Vet Res* 64:994, 2003.
8. Cooper L, Hart BL: Comparison of diazepam with progestin for effectiveness in suppression of urine-spraying behavior in cats, *J Am Vet Med Assoc* 200:797, 1992.
9. Crowell-Davis S, Curtis T, Knowles R: Social organization in the cat: a modern understanding, *J Feline Med Surg* 6:19, 2004.
10. Crowell-Davis SL, Barry K, Wolfe R: Social behavior and aggressive problems of cats, *Vet Clin North Am Small Anim Pract* 27:549, 1997.
11. Curtis T, Knowles R, Crowell-Davis S: Influence of familiarity and relatedness on proximity and allogrooming in domestic cats *(Felis catus)*, *Am J Vet Res* 64:1151, 2003.
12. Dreschel NA: Anxiety, fear, disease, and lifespan in domestic dogs, *J Vet Behav* 4:249, 2009.
13. Frank DF, Erb HN, Houpt KA: Urine spraying in cats: presence of concurrent disease and effects of a pheromone treatment, *Appl Anim Behav Sci* 61:263, 1999.
14. Gaultier E, Pageat P, Tessier Y: Effect of a feline appeasing pheromone analogue on manifestations of stress in cats during transport. In *Proceedings 32nd Congress of the International Society for Applied Ethology*, Clermont-Ferrand, 1998, p. 198.
15. Griffith CA, Steigerwald ES, Buffington CA: Effects of a synthetic facial pheromone on behavior of cats, *J Am Vet Med Assoc* 217:1154, 2000.
16. Gunn-Moore D, Moffat K, Christie LA et al: Cognitive dysfunction and the neurobiology of ageing in cats, *J Small Anim Pract* 48:546, 2007.
17. Hall SL, Bradshaw JWS, Robinson IH: Object play in adult domestic cats: the roles of habituation and disinhibition, *Appl Anim Behav Sci* 79:263, 2002.
18. Hart B, Cliff K, Tynes V et al: Control of urine marking by use of long-term treatment with fluoxetine or clomipramine in cats, *J Am Vet Med Assoc* 226:378, 2005.
19. Hart B, Eckstein R, Powell K et al: Effectiveness of buspirone on urine spraying and inappropriate elimination in cats, *J Am Vet Med Assoc* 203:254, 1993.
20. Hunthausen W: Evaluating a feline facial pheromone analogue to control urine spraying, *Vet Med* 95:151, 2000.
21. Ibanez M, Dominguez C, Martin M: Cats showing comfort or well-being in cages with an enriched and controlled environment. In *Proceedings of the 3rd International Congress on Veterinary Behavioural Medicine*, 2001, p. 50.
22. King J, Steffan J, Heath S et al: Determination of the dosage of clomipramine for the treatment of urine spraying in cats, *J Am Vet Med Assoc* 225:881, 2004.
23. Kly K, Casey R: The effects of hiding enrichment on stress levels, behaviour and time to homing of domestic cats in a rescue shelter in the UK. In *Proceedings of the Companion Animal Behaviour Therapy Study Group study day*, Birmingham, England, 2004.
24. Kochevar DT, Fajt V: Evidence-based decision making in small animal therapeutics, *Vet Clin North Am Small Anim Pract* 36:943, 2006.
25. Landsberg G: Feline behavior and welfare, *J Am Vet Med Assoc* 208:502, 1996.
26. Landsberg G, Hunthausen W, Ackerman L: *Handbook of behavior problems of the dog and cat*, ed 2, St Louis, 2003, Elsevier Saunders.
27. Landsberg GM, Wilson AL: Effects of clomipramine on cats presented for urine marking, *J Am Anim Hosp Assoc* 41:3, 2005.
28. Mealey KL, Peck KE, Bennett BS et al: Systemic absorption of amitriptyline and buspirone after oral and transdermal administration to healthy cats, *J Vet Intern Med* 18:43, 2004.
29. Milgram NW, Head E, Zicker SC et al: Long-term treatment with antioxidants and a program of behavioral enrichment reduces age-dependent impairment in discrimination and reversal learning in beagle dogs, *Exp Gerontol* 39:753, 2004.
30. Mills DS, Mills CB: Evaluation of a novel method for delivering a synthetic analogue of feline facial pheromone to control urine spraying by cats, *Vet Rec* 149:197, 2001.
31. Nagata M, Shibata K, Irimajiri M et al: Importance of psychogenic dermatoses in dogs with pruritic behavior, *Vet Derm* 13:211, 2002.
32. Ogata N, Takeuchi Y: Clinical trial of a feline pheromone analogue for feline urine marking, *J Vet Med Sci* 63:157, 2001.
33. Overall K, Rodan I, Beaver B et al: Feline behavior guidelines from the American Association of Feline Practitioners, *J Am Vet Med Assoc* 227:70, 2005.
34. Pageat P, Tessier Y: Usefulness of the F3 synthetic pheromone Feliway in preventing behaviour problems in cats during holidays. In *Proceedings 1st International Veterinary Behavior Meeting*, Birmingham, 1997, p 231.
35. Pare WP, Kluczynski J: Developmental factors modify stress ulcer incidence in a stress-susceptible rat strain, *J Physiol Paris* 91:105, 1997.
36. Patel G, Health S, Coyne K et al: Pilot study to investigate whether a feline pheromone analogue reduces anxiety-related behavior during clinical examination of cats in a rescue shelter, *J Vet Behav* 5:33, 2010.
37. Pfeiffer E, Guy N, Cribb A: Clomipramine-induced urinary retention in a cat, *Can Vet J* 40:265, 1999.
38. Pryor P, Hart B, Cliff D et al: Effects of a selective serotonin reuptake inhibitor on urine spraying behavior in cats, *J Am Vet Med Assoc* 219:1557, 2001.
39. Schapiro SJ, Nehete PN, Perlman JE et al: A comparison of cell-mediated immune responses in rhesus macaques housed singly, in pairs, or in groups, *Appl Anim Behav Sci* 68:67, 2000.
40. Seksel K: Behaviour modifying drugs. In Maddison J, Page S, Church D, editors: *Small animal clinical pharmacology*, St Louis, 2008, Saunders.
41. Seksel K, Lindeman M: Use of clomipramine in the treatment of anxiety-related and obsessive-compulsive disorders in cats, *Aust Vet J* 76:317, 1998.
42. Steinberg MI, Smallwood JK, Holland DR et al: Hemodynamic and electrocardiographic effects of fluoxetine and its major metabolite, norfluoxetine, in anesthetized dogs, *Toxicol Appl Pharmacol* 82:70, 1986.
43. Thorndike E: *Animal intelligence*, Cambridge, Mass, 1911, Harvard University Press.
44. Westropp JL, Kass PH, Buffington CA: Evaluation of the effects of stress in cats with idiopathic cystitis, *Am J Vet Res* 67:731, 2006.
45. Yin S: *Low stress handling, restraint and behavior modification of dogs and cats*, Davis, Calif, 2009, Nerd Books.
46. Young R: *Environmental enrichment for captive animals*, Oxford, 2003, Blackwell Science.

SECTION III

FELINE NUTRITION

Editor: Joe Bartges

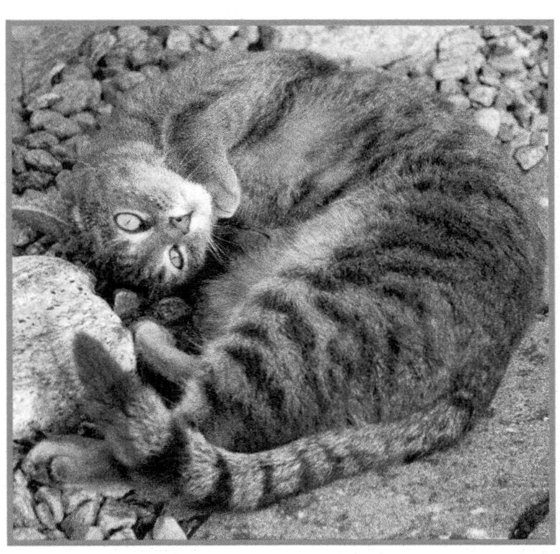

CHAPTER

15

The Unique Nutritional Requirements of the Cat: A Strict Carnivore

Beth Hamper, Joe Bartges, Claudia Kirk, Angela L. Witzel, Maryanne Murphy, and Donna Raditic

OUTLINE

The domestic cat is believed to have evolved from the African wild cat *Felis sylvestris libyca* between 4000 and 10,000 years ago.[4,20] Cats belong to the order Carnivora, meaning "flesh eating," and the family Felidae. The felids diverged from the other carnivorous groups early in the evolutionary tree.[16] Other members of the order Carnivora include canids/canines, bears, pandas, weasels, raccoons, and hyenas. There is a wide diversity of feeding patterns within the order Carnivora. Canids and bears are considered omnivores, whereas pandas are strict herbivores. All felids are meat eaters, or strict carnivores. This specialized and exclusive meat diet has led to unique metabolic and nutritional adaptations not seen in canids/canines or other members of the order Carnivora. A great deal of knowledge has been gained regarding the cat's unique metabolic and nutritional requirements over the past 60 years, thanks to the work of Dr. James Morris and Dr. Quinton Rodgers, along with many other nutritionists and researchers around the world. The goal of this chapter is to review these findings and provide a review of the unique requirements of the cat.[16,18] Some highlights of this research in feline nutrition and metabolism include:

- A limited ability to downregulate enzymes of nitrogen catabolism and urea cycle enzymes
- A strict requirement for the amino acid arginine, which, if lacking in the diet for longer than 24 hours, can lead to life-threatening consequences
- An inability to synthesize taurine from cysteine
- Limited capabilities in handling carbohydrates in the diet
- An inability to synthesize vitamin A from beta carotenes
- An inability to synthesize niacin from the amino acid tryptophan

Arginine, taurine, niacin, and vitamin A are abundant in an all-flesh diet, along with high levels of protein and amino acids and very limited carbohydrates.

ANATOMY AND PHYSIOLOGY

Cats have fewer teeth than dogs. They have the same number of incisors, canine, and carnassial teeth but fewer premolar and molar teeth with fissured surfaces. Their dentition is more specialized for shearing flesh rather than grinding it. Cats lack salivary amylase, the enzyme that is involved in early starch digestion.[19] Because cats evolved to eat small, frequent meals throughout the day, their stomach capacity is smaller than that of dogs. The cat's maximum stomach capacity is between 45 and 60 mL/kg of body weight, compared with 90 mL/kg in the dog.

Relative intestinal length is determined by the ratio of intestinal length to body length. Intestinal length is one of the factors that influence the amount of time for digestion and absorption to occur. Cats have a shorter intestinal length than dogs and other omnivores and herbivores. In the cat, this ratio is 4:1 compared with 6:1 in dogs.[19] In herbivorous species this ratio is much higher due to the lower digestibility of their foodstuffs: 12:1 in the horse, 20:1 in the ox, and 27:1 in the sheep.[19]

Cobalamin, or vitamin B_{12}, requires binding to intrinsic factor for its absorption and uptake in the ileum. Most mammals manufacture and secrete intrinsic factor from both the stomach and pancreas. In the cat, intrinsic factor is produced only in the pancreas.[7]

Very little is known about companion animals' microbiome. The effect of small intestinal microbes on nutrient requirements in dogs and cats has yet to be established. The human microbiome contains approximately 10^{14} microorganisms, ten times the number of human cells.[28] The metabolic functions of the microbiota within the gastrointestinal tract include production of metabolites such as short-chain fatty acids used as an energy source for colonocytes, degradation of potentially toxic compounds, enhanced metabolism of amino acids and nondigestible carbohydrates, and synthesis of vitamins and lipids.[29] A study in clinically healthy cats demonstrated that cats have large numbers of bacteria in their proximal small intestine compared to dogs. Cats show unique numbers of microbes within the intestinal tract. The total bacterial counts from duodenal cultures in cats ranged from 10^5 to 10^8 colony-forming units (CFU)/mL, compared with a maximum of 10^4 CFU/mL in dogs.[10] Higher bacterial levels in the gut may be another adaption to a carnivorous diet. Relying on culturing methods alone has greatly limited identification of microbial species. Newer molecular techniques show promise in evaluating these ecosystems in both the cat and dog and their effect on diet, and vice versa.[27]

FEEDING BEHAVIOR

In the wild cats hunt small prey such as mice, rats, rabbits, birds, frogs, reptiles, and insects. Mice are the most common prey for the cat, with a caloric density of approximately 30 kcal per mouse. The small size and low kcal of their prey dictate that cats need to eat many small meals throughout the day to meet their energy and nutritional requirements. Cats prefer to ingest freshly killed prey rather than carrion. Domestic cats will have 7 to 20 small meals a day if given free access to food. Predatory behavior is a strong drive in the cat and will even take precedence over feeding. Cats will stop eating a meal to kill prey and then go back to eating the original meal rather than the freshly killed rat.[1]

Food preferences are influenced by the diet of the queen during pregnancy and lactation. Particularly important to later food preferences and choices are the flavors kittens experience between 1 and 6 months of age.[32] Owners should be encouraged to feed kittens a variety of flavors and textures at this stage with the hope that it will lead to more flexibility in the adult.

Smell, taste, and texture all play important roles in the cat's dietary preferences. The most abundant taste receptors (neurons of the facial nerve) are those for amino acids, particularly those amino acids that are described as sweet.[3] These include proline, cysteine, ornithine, lysine, histidine, and alanine. Cats reject bitter-tasting amino acids such as arginine, isoleucine, phenylalanine, and tryptophan. The second most abundant taste receptors are for acidic foods. These receptors are stimulated by phosphoric acid, carboxylic acids, and nucleotide dipeptides and tripeptides.[3] Cats will avoid monophosphate nucleotides, which accumulate in tissues after death. This may be why cats dislike carrion. Cats have no taste receptors for sucrose/sugar.[3,14] Temperature is also important, with cats preferring food at body or room temperature. Cats will generally reject foods at temperatures colder than 15° C or greater than 50° C.[32] Food preferences are strongly correlated with the amount of protein in the diet, particularly animal protein. Liver, blood, and red meat are highly palatable to cats. Besides protein, fat has been shown to have positive palatability in cat. Fats applied to the outside of dry kibble are positive flavor enhancers, but it is believed that the positive influence of fat is more related to textural changes rather than flavor. Despite this, cats do show a strong aversion to medium-chain fatty acids.[16] Cats will generally select moist foods similar in water content to animal tissue, compared to dry, extruded diets. Cats that have been fed exclusively dry foods for an extended period of time can develop a strong preference for only dry foods.

Stressful situations can result in learned aversions to new or novel foods; therefore starting a new therapeutic diet in hospitalized cats is inadvisable. Cats are intermediate in their ability to avoid foods that can result in deficiencies over a long period of time; for example, cats will consistently eat taurine-free diets despite development of cardiac, reproductive, and retinal diseases. Similar to other species, cats will learn to avoid foods that are toxic.

The cat is believed to have evolved as a desert animal because of its ability to highly concentrate its urine (specific gravity up to 1.080 to 1.085). Cats will drink less water than dogs under the same conditions. Cats on canned or moist diets may not drink any additional water, although it should always be available. Besides the water content of the food, the protein and mineral content of the diet may affect water intake. High-protein diets increase the solute load, with increased water production and urination. The weak thirst drive in the cat has been implicated in some aspects of lower urinary tract health, particularly in cats fed dry foods, because of the propensity of minerals to crystallize in concentrated solutions.

SPECIFIC NUTRIENTS

Protein and Amino Acids

Protein

Dietary protein is required for two reasons. The first is for amino acids (AAs) the cat cannot synthesize, called the essential amino acids. The second is for nitrogen and carbon skeletons for the synthesis of nonessential AAs and other necessary compounds containing nitrogen (i.e., purines, pyrimidines, heme, hormones, and neurotransmitters). Both essential and nonessential AAs become part of the AA pool for protein synthesis in the tissues. The essential AAs for both dogs and cats are arginine (Arg), histidine (His), isoleucine (Ile), leucine (Leu), lysine (Lys), methionine (Met), phenylalanine (Phe), threonine (Thr), tryptophan (Trp), and valine (Val).[19] Cats have an additional requirement for taurine, which they cannot synthesize from cysteine compared to dogs.

The protein requirement for the kitten is approximately 1.5 times the protein requirement for the puppy. Adult cats require 2 to 3 times as much protein as adult dogs.[19] The increased protein requirement in the cat is not for increased levels of essential AAs but rather for a dietary source of nitrogen. Excess nitrogen from proteins and other sources is removed by way of the urea cycle in the liver. Most omnivorous species, when given a low-protein diet, will conserve AAs by decreasing enzyme levels involved in AA catabolism. Omnivorous species can also conserve AAs and nitrogen when given low-protein diets by altering the activity of the urea cycle enzymes. In cats given low-protein diets, enzymes for both AA catabolism and the urea cycle are not downregulated.[23] Therefore cats cannot conserve nitrogen when given low-protein diets and will begin to catabolize protein sources within the body (i.e., muscle) to supply tissue needs. Endogenous urinary nitrogen losses in animals fed protein-free diets have been found to be 360 mg N/kg in cats, compared with 210 mg N/kg in dogs, 128 mg N/kg in rats, and 62 mg N/kg in humans, indicating lack of enzyme adaptation in the cat.[19] Protein is also being continually utilized for gluconeogenesis in the cat. Because of the very limited number of carbohydrates they ingest in their wild diet, cats are very efficient at synthesizing glucose from proteins by gluconeogenesis. In other species, gluconeogenesis occurs several hours after a meal, whereas in cats it occurs immediately after a meal and is permanently "switched on" to maintain blood glucose levels. The benefit of these adaptations is the immediate ability to catabolize high levels of protein without developing hyperammonemia and the rapid ability to make glucose from protein for energy through gluconeogensis.[18]

Arginine

Arginine is a key intermediate in the urea cycle involved in the excretion of nitrogen via urea. A single meal without the AA arginine can result in life-threatening events in the cat. Arginine-deficient cats develop emesis, hypersalivation, hyperactivity, and hyperesthesia eventually leading to death as a result of ammonia intoxication. This is due to the cat's inability to synthesize arginine from other dietary precursors. Arginine can be produced from ornithine and citrulline in the intestine in humans and rats and to some degree in dogs. The cat has lost this ability because of the lack of two enzymes in the pathway, pyrroline-5-carboxylate synthase and ornithine aminotransferase. Overnight food deprivation results in a low concentration of plasma arginine and urea cycle intermediates. When the cat eats a meal with protein that includes arginine, the arginine replenishes the level in the liver for urea cycle function with subsequent disposal of nitrogen and ammonia. If arginine is missing from the meal, the cat cannot replenish its urea cycle intermediates and severe hyperammonemia develops.[17] Animal tissue is high in arginine content, making its de novo synthesis redundant in carnivores on all meat diets. Also, depletion of urea cycle intermediates after a meal results in conserving nitrogen needed for synthesis of disposable AAs.

Methionine and Cysteine

The dietary requirement for the sulfur AAs, methionine, and cysteine is higher in cats than in other mammals.[19] Methionine can be converted to cysteine; therefore the sulfur AA requirement can be met with either methionine alone or methionine and cysteine. Methionine is a methyl group donor important for DNA and RNA synthesis and is a component of many proteins. Cysteine is a component of many proteins and is an important component of hair/fur. Cysteine is also the precursor for glutathione, a major antioxidant in mammalian systems, and a precursor for the synthesis of felinine. Felinine is a branched-chain AA found in the urine of domestic cats. The biological function of felinine is not fully known, although it is believed to function as a pheromone and is important in territorial marking. It can be found in the urine of cats as young as 2 months of age, with levels being quite high in intact male cats (0.4 to 8 grams/L of urine).[8] Felinine concentrations in females are only 20% to 25% of that in intact males. The high requirement for sulfur AAs in cats has been attributed to their dense hair and the need to synthesize felinine.[16]

Taurine

Taurine is a beta-sulfonic AA that is not used in protein synthesis but is found as a free AA in tissues. The highest concentrations of taurine are found in the heart, muscle, brain, and retina. Taurine serves numerous important functions, including osmoregulation, calcium channel modulation, as an antioxidant, and bile acid conjugation.[9] Many mammals are able to use either glycine or taurine for bile acid conjugation. Cats and dogs are only able to utilize taurine to conjugate bile acids. Dogs are able to synthesize sufficient taurine from cysteine. Cats are also able to synthesize taurine from cysteine, but the activity of two enzymes in the pathway is so low that taurine synthesis is negligible and therefore taurine must be provided in the diet.[18] Taurine deficiency can be due to:

- Inadequate dietary supply
- Loss of taurine in the enterohepatic circulation associated with increases in bacterial flora that degrade taurine or processing effects

Taurine deficiency in the cat is well documented as being associated with dilated cardiomyopathy (see Chapter 20), feline central retinal degeneration (see Chapter 29, Figures 29-61 and 29-62), and reproductive failure. Insofar as taurine is abundant in animal tissue, the need to synthesize taurine would be redundant in the cat's normal metabolic pathways.

Fat and Fatty Acids

Fats and fatty acids have four major physiologic roles[26]:

1. As a concentrated source of energy for storage and utilization
2. As structural components of cell membranes
3. As lubricants
4. As important signaling molecules (i.e., eicosanoids, cholesterol-derived hormones)

Cats are able to tolerate high levels of fat in their diet.

Dietary fats are fatty acids linked to either a glycerol backbone as triglycerides or fatty acids linked to cholesterol or retinol as cholesterol or retinyl esters. Free fatty acids are long-chain hydrocarbons with (unsaturated) or without (saturated) double bonds. Fatty acids can be classified in either of two ways on the basis of the position of these double bonds in comparison to the carboxyl end or the methyl end of the hydrocarbon chain. The delta system utilizes counting from the carboxyl end. The 18 carbon linoleic acid with two double bonds is notated as 18:2 Δ9,12 in the delta system. If counted from the methyl end as in the omega system, linoleic acid is 18:2 n-6.

Cats are able to synthesize nonessential saturated and monounsaturated fatty acids from glucose or AAs. However, cats, like other mammals, are unable to introduce double bonds between carbon 12-13 and carbon 15-16 via Δ12 and carbon Δ15 desaturase enzymes. This is the basis for the essential nature of the fatty acids linoleic (18:2n-6), and linolenic (18:3n-3).[2] Most mammals can subsequently convert linoleic (n-6) and linolenic (n-3) to their respective longer-chain derivatives, arachidonic and eicosapentaenoic acid/docosahexaenoic acid (EPA/DHA), through a Δ6 desaturase. Arachidonic acid is a precursor for eicosanoid synthesis and is an abundant component of cell membranes. Cats are unique in that they have low Δ6 desaturase activity. Initially, it was believed that cats lacked any Δ6 desaturase activity and thus had an absolute requirement for arachidonic acid as well as linoleic acid. Further studies have shown that cats may have an alternative pathway for arachidonic acid synthesis,[2] and studies have shown that they are able to synthesize sufficient quantities for maintenance but have an absolute requirement for arachidonic acid during reproduction and early growth.[2] Similarly, for the n-3 or omega 3 fatty acids EPA/DHA, cats have limited synthesis from the precursor alpha-linolenic acid. High levels of DHA are required for neural and retinal tissue development in kittens, so DHA becomes conditionally essential for cats at this life stage. Flaxseed oil is an 18 carbon n-3 fatty acid typically added to foods to increased EPA/DHA levels. This 18 carbon n-3 fatty acid is not significantly converted to EPA/DHA in dogs or cats and should not be considered as a source.[19]

Carbohydrates

Cats that eat only animal flesh have a diet low in carbohydrates. As with protein, cats have evolved several unique adaptations to metabolism of carbohydrates compared with omnivores or herbivores. These include:

- An absence of glucokinase activity in the liver
- Lower levels of amylase and the disaccharidases sucrase and lactase in the pancreas and intestine
- Little adaptation in amylase activity with increased carbohydrate diets
- High levels of gluconeogenesis from proteins and fats

Cats have no dietary requirement for carbohydrates but do have a dietary requirement for energy. As long as their diet contains fats and gluconeogenic proteins, they are able to synthesize glucose and energy sufficient for maintenance. A study in dogs demonstrated that lactating dogs given a carbohydrate-free diet became hypoglycemic, with a low survival rate among the puppies.[24] It is probable that although cats have no absolute carbohydrate requirement, queens with some carbohydrate in the diet are better able to support lactation and nursing kittens.

Mammals have up to four isoenzymes in the liver that catalyze the conversion of glucose to glucose-6-phosphate, the first step in glucose utilization. The hexokinase responsible for operating under high glucose loads is hexokinase D, or glucokinase. The cat does not have glucokinase activity, in line with a diet containing low levels of carbohydrates.[30] In contrast, dogs do possess glucokinase activity and are able to handle larger carbohydrate loads. In contrast, enzymes involved in gluconeogenesis such as pyruvate carboxylase, fructose 1,6-bisphosphate, and glucose-6-phosphatase are much higher in feline than canine liver.[30] It was previously believed that cats do not express fructokinase activity as high-sucrose diets resulted in fructosuria and fructosemia. A recent study found that cats do have fructokinase enzyme activity in their liver producing frucose-1-phosphate.[25] Fructose-1-phosphate is then catalyzed into dihydroxyacetone and glyceraldehyde by way of the enzyme aldolase. It is believed that fructose intolerance in humans is due to a defect in this enzyme. The level of aldose activity has not been analyzed in the cat but low levels would support their low tolerance for elevated levels of fructose with resulting fructosuria.

Amylase activity, the enzyme responsible for hydrolysis of starch to glucose, is low in cats compared with dogs. The cat lacks salivary amylase,[19] with pancreatic amylase levels only 5% of those found in dogs, and intestinal values only 10% of those found in dogs.[11] The activity of the sugar transporters in the intestine is also not adaptable to higher levels of carbohydrate in the diet, compared with the dog. Compared with other species, cats have much lower levels of maltase, isomaltase, and sucrase activity in the small intestinal mucosa.[12] Lactase activity is high in newborn kittens but rapidly declines at weaning, as has been found in other mammals. Compared with puppies, however, kittens exhibit a more rapid decrease in lactase.[12] Despite limited enzymatic breakdown of sugars, once absorbed, the digestibility of all the sugars, with the exception of lactose is high, between 98% and 100%.[12] Apparent protein digestibility was found to be reduced in the diets containing lactose or sucrose by 4% to 5% compared with the carbohydrate-free diet.[13] This was believed to be due to the accelerated rate of passage of the food resulting from the osmotic effects of the soluble sugars and increased bacterial carbohydrate fermentation with increased bacterial nitrogen fixation.

There has been much speculation recently regarding high-carbohydrate diets and the increasing incidence of obesity and diabetes mellitus in cats. Dry foods can contain up to 40% carbohydrate on a dry matter basis. Although this seems feasible given the cat's unique metabolic pathways, long-term studies are needed to fully evaluate long term carbohydrate feeding effects in the cat.

Vitamins

The cat has several unique vitamin requirements, both quantitatively and qualitatively different from those of other mammals, including the following:

- An absolute requirement for preformed vitamin A
- An increased tolerance for high levels of vitamin A in the diet
- An absolute requirement for niacin
- A higher level of requirement for thiamine (four times higher that of the dog), pyridoxine (four times that of the dog), and folate (four times higher than that of the dog)

Vitamin A

Cats are able to absorb carotenoids but cannot convert these to the active form of vitamin A because of the lack the enzyme 15,15′-dioxygenase.[18] Carotenoids are vitamin A precursors synthesized in plant lipids. Preformed vitamin A occurs naturally only in animal tissues where high levels occur within the viscera. It would therefore be redundant to convert carotenoids when the preformed vitamin is already present in the diet. Vitamin A, being lipid soluble, can become toxic if given in large doses. Vitamin A toxicity occurs in cats given mainly all liver diets or given high dosages of vitamin A supplements. Chronic hypervitaminosis A in cats is characterized by the formation of exostoses on the cervical vertebrae causing ankylosis, deformity, and crippling.[21] Cats are believed to be more tolerant of high vitamin A levels than are rodents or humans. In a study comparing effects of high levels of vitamin A given during gestation in cats and rats, the incidence of malformations in the rat offspring was 80% compared with 2.9% in the kittens.[6] Unlike rodents and humans, cats transport vitamin A primarily as retinyl esters rather than retinol and are able to excrete large amounts of retinyl esters in the urine.[22] Cats are also able to store higher concentrations of vitamin A in their livers compared with humans, rats, and dogs. A smaller amount is also stored in the kidneys. As animal viscera can be high in vitamin A content, increased storage and the ability to excrete large amounts in the urine would be protective mechanisms for minimizing vitamin A toxicity.

Vitamin D

Vitamin D is conditionally essential for most mammals dependent on their exposure to sunlight. Both cats and dogs are unable to convert the precursor of vitamin D in the skin, 7-dehydrocholesterol to pre-vitamin D via ultraviolet radiation. This is not due to their thick hair coat, but rather to high levels of an enzyme in an alternative pathway that converts 7-dehydrocholesterol to cholesterol rather than pre-vitamin D.[19] Insofar as a carnivorous diet has adequate amounts of vitamin D, pathways for synthesis would be unnecessary.

Niacin (B_3)

Niacin can be endogenously synthesized from the AA tryptophan, but the efficiency of this conversion varies among mammals. Rats are able to do this conversion very well, whereas cats are able to synthesize only negligible amounts of niacin. This is due to the high activity of an enzyme at a branching point in the pathway. The enzyme picolinic carboxylase dominates this branching point in the cat and directs it to the production of acetyl CoA and CO_2 rather than niacin synthesis.[18] Because muscle tissue is well supplied with niacin, de novo synthesis is unnecessary, and the production of acetyl CoA for ATP production is more energetically advantageous.

Pyridoxine (B_6)

One of the major biological functions of pyridoxine is to serve as a coenzyme in transamination reactions or amino group removal from amino acids.[26] Cats have high transaminase activity because of their constant state of gluconeogenesis. Therefore they have a high pyridoxine requirement, approximately four times higher than that of the dog.

Thiamine (B_1)

Thiamine is one of the water-soluble B vitamins that is required for the formation of the coenzyme thiamin pyrophosphate (TPP). TPP serves as a coenzyme in decarboxylation reactions in both carbohydrate and AA catabolism. Cats require four times as much thiamine in their diet compared with dogs. This may be due to their higher level of AA catabolism and gluconeogenesis. TPP is a coenzyme in branched-chain keto acid dehydrogenase complex involved in the catabolism of leucine, isoleucine, and valine. These reactions result in the production of acetyl CoA, which can enter the tricarboxylic acid cycle for ATP production.

Thiamine deficiency can be seen in cats fed raw or undercooked fish diets. Certain raw fish contain enzyme thiaminases.[15] Thiaminase enzymes have also been found in certain species of the bacteria *Clostridium* spp. and *Bacillus* spp. Thiaminase bacterial production has been found in the contents of ruminant animals with resulting neurological deficits.[5] It has been documented that cats have higher numbers of bacteria within their intestinal tract compared with dogs. Whether there are thiaminase bacteria within these populations resulting in a higher requirement for thiamine is unknown at this time. Clinical signs of thiamine deficiency include anorexia, weight loss, and depression, progressing to neurological signs of dilated pupils, ataxia, weakness, seizures and eventually death.

Folate

Folate, similar to the other B vitamins, is an important coenzyme in several metabolic pathways. Folate is used in metabolic reactions involving one-carbon transfers. It is important in AA metabolism, DNA synthesis, and protein synthesis.[26] Specifically, folate is involved in histidine catabolism, thymidylate synthesis, interconversion of the AAs serine and glycine, and methionine catabolism. Cats have a fourfold higher requirement for folate compared with dogs. This is probably due to higher amino acid catabolic activity. In histidine metabolism, folate is required for the conversion of the intermediate, formiminoglutamate to glutamate. Folate deficiency has been shown to result in increased urinary formiminoglutamic acid (FIGLU) secretion in cats.[31]

CONCLUSION

The unique nutritional requirements of cats reflect their adaptation to an all-meat diet. Their high protein requirement reflects their high level of gluconeogenic activity and amino acid catabolism and their inability to downregulate the nitrogen catabolic enzyme pathways. Their unique requirement for arginine, taurine, vitamin A, vitamin D, and niacin are due to adaptations in their enzyme systems secondary to deletion or downregulation of enzymes for synthesis of nutrients found abundantly in their diet.[18]

References

1. Adamec RE: The interaction of hunger and preying in the domestic cat *(Felis catus)*: an adaptive hierarchy? *Behav Biol* 18:263, 1976.
2. Bauer JE: Metabolic basis for the essential nature of fatty acids and the unique dietary fatty acid requirements of cats, *J Am Vet Med Assoc* 229:1729, 2006.
3. Bradshaw JW, Goodwin D, Legrand-Defretin V et al: Food selection by the domestic cat, an obligate carnivore, *Comp Biochem Physiol A Physiol* 114:205, 1996.
4. Driscoll CA, et al: The Near Eastern origin of cat domestication, *Science* 317:519, 2007.
5. Edwin EE, Jackman R: Ruminant thiamine requirement in perspective, *Vet Res Commun* 5:237, 1982.
6. Freytag TL: *Vitamin A metabolism and toxicity in the domestic cat*, Davis, Calif, 2001, University of California.
7. Fyfe JC: Feline intrinsic factor is pancreatic in origin and mediates ileal cobalamin absorption (abstract), *J Vet Intern Med* 7:133, 1993.
8. Hendriks WH, Rutherfurd-Markwick KJ, Weidgraaf K et al: Urinary felinine excretion in intact male cats is increased by dietary cystine, *Br J Nutr* 100:801, 2008.
9. Huxtable RJ: Physiological actions of taurine, *Physiol Rev* 72:101, 1992.
10. Johnston K, Lamport A, Batt RM: An unexpected bacterial flora in the proximal small intestine of normal cats, *Vet Rec* 132:362, 1993.
11. Kienzle E: Carbohydrate metabolism of the cat 1. Activity of amylase in the gastrointestinal tract of the cat, *J Anim Physiol Anim Nutr (Berl)* 69:92, 1993.
12. Kienzle E: Carbohydrate metabolism of the cat. 3. Digestion of sugars, *J Anim Physiol Anim Nutr (Berl)* 69:203, 1993.
13. Kienzle E: Effect of carbohydrates on digestion in the cat, *J Nutr* 124:2568S, 1994.
14. Li X, Li W, Wang H et al: Cats lack a sweet taste receptor, *J Nutr* 136:1932S, 2006.
15. Lonsdale D: A review of the biochemistry, metabolism and clinical benefits of thiamin(e) and its derivatives, *Evid Based Complement Alternat Med* 3:49, 2006.

16. MacDonald ML, Rogers QR, Morris JG: Nutrition of the domestic cat, a mammalian carnivore, *Annu Rev Nutr* 4:521, 1984.
17. Morris JG: Nutritional and metabolic responses to arginine deficiency in carnivores, *J Nutr* 115:524, 1985.
18. Morris JG: Idiosyncratic nutrient requirements of cats appear to be diet-induced evolutionary adaptations, *Nutr Res Rev* 15:153, 2002.
19. National Research Council: *Nutrient requirements of dogs and cats*, Washington, DC, 2006, National Academies Press.
20. O'Brien SJ, Yuhki N: Comparative genome organization of the major histocompatibility complex: lessons from the Felidae, *Immunol Rev* 167:133, 1999.
21. Polizopoulou Z, Kazakos G, Patsikas M et al: Hypervitaminosis A in the cat: a case report and review of the literature, *J Fel Med Surg* 7:363, 2005.
22. Raila J, Mathews U, Schweigert FJ: Plasma transport and tissue distribution of beta-carotene, vitamin A and retinol-binding protein in domestic cats, *Comp Biochem Physiol A Mol Integr Physiol* 130:849, 2001.
23. Rogers QR, Morris JG, Freedland RA: Lack of hepatic enzymatic adaptation to low and high levels of dietary protein in the adult cat, *Enzyme* 22:348, 1977.
24. Romsos DR, Palmer HJ, Muiruri KL et al: Influence of a low carbohydrate diet on performance of pregnant and lactating dogs, *J Nutr* 111:678, 1981.
25. Springer N, Lindbloom-Hawley S, Schermerhorn T: Tissue expression of ketohexokinase in cats, *Res Vet Sci* 87:115, 2009.
26. Stipanuk M: *Biochemical, physiological and molecular aspects of human nutrition*, ed 2, St Louis, 2006, Saunders.
27. Swanson KS: Using molecular techniques to study canine and feline gut microbial ecology, *Comp Contin Edu Pract Vet* 29:34, 2007.
28. Turnbaugh PJ, Ley RE, Hamady M et al: The human microbiome project, *Nature* 449:804, 2007.
29. Verberkmoes NC, Russell AL, Shah M et al: Shotgun metaproteomics of the human distal gut microbiota, *ISME J* 3:179, 2009.
30. Washizu T, Tanaka A, Sako T et al: Comparison of the activities of enzymes related to glycolysis and gluconeogenesis in the liver of dogs and cats, *Res Vet Sci* 67:205, 1999.
31. Yu S, Morris JG: Folate requirement of growing kittens to prevent elevated formiminoglutamic acid excretion following histidine loading, *J Nutr* 128:2606S, 1998.
32. Zaghini G, Biagi G: Nutritional peculiarities and diet palatability in the cat, *Vet Res Commun* 29(Suppl 2):39, 2005.

CHAPTER

16

Nutrition for the Normal Cat

Angela L. Witzel, Joe Bartges, Claudia Kirk, Beth Hamper, Maryanne Murphy, and Donna Raditic

OUTLINE

NORMAL FEEDING BEHAVIOR

The domestic cat, *Felis catus,* evolved from the north African wildcat *Felis silvestris lybica* and began cohabitating with Egyptians as early as 2300 BCE.[29] Although cats have lived closely with humans for many years, when domestication is defined as cultivation and breeding to create a reproductively isolated group, only pedigree cats qualify.[4] Common domestic cats usually choose their own mates and can still reproduce with wild *F. sylvestris* when they share common territory.[4,9] With relatively little breeding interference from humans, most pet cats retain adept hunting skills and feeding patterns similar to those of their wild ancestors. Cats are solitary hunters and eat 7 to 20 small prey meals spread evenly over 24 hours.[17,23] Examples of prey include rodents, lagomorphs, birds, and reptiles.[14]Although domestic cats retain many innate hunting behaviors, they adapt well to controlled feeding situations and can be fed either *ad libitum* or by meals. Free-choice feeding more closely resembles natural feeding patterns but may be a risk factor for obesity. In addition, *ad libitum* feeding makes it more difficult for owners to assess their cat's appetite, and periods of anorexia may go unnoticed until significant weight loss has occurred. Cats are hunters; therefore placing food in different locations and using devices to hide food so that it must be sought (e.g., puzzle balls) not only stimulates predatory drive but also encourages exercise.

Food preferences in cats are both instinctive and acquired. Taste receptors in cats are specialized for eating meat. For example, taste buds of the facial nerve are very reactive to amino acids but do not respond to many monosaccharides and disaccharides.[5] Acquired taste preferences in kittens have been demonstrated through prenatal and postnatal exposure of certain flavors in amniotic fluid and milk of queens.[2] Kittens also learn appropriate food choices by imitating their mothers. One study demonstrated that when weanling kittens (5 to 8 weeks of age) accompanied their mothers as they ate bananas and mashed potatoes, the kittens would later eat the inappropriate foods on their own.[32] Preferences for food texture also appear to be a learned behavior. In a study comparing house cats and outdoor farm cats, the house cats avoided raw meat whereas the outdoor cats shunned dry kibble.[6] Although cats can develop preferences for certain food types on the basis of their experience, they also can grow tired of the same food (known as the "monotony effect") and often prefer a novel diet as long as it has a familiar texture.[4,6]

CARNIVOROUS ADAPTATIONS

Mark Twain once said, "If man could be crossed with the cat it would improve the man, but it would deteriorate the cat."[30] Cats are unique creatures with novel evolutionary adaptations. The carnivorous nature of the cat has led to anatomic and metabolic modifications. Cats are designed to hunt small prey. Their ears are more attuned to the high-pitched sounds of rodents; they have a large optic cortex to focus on small, quick movements; their retractable claws allow them to stalk prey with soft pads and then attack; they have fewer molars and premolars than do omnivorous dogs; and their jaws have little side-to-side motion for grinding.[1] Because feline prey species comprise mostly protein and fat, cats lack salivary amylase for carbohydrate digestion. Because cats evolved eating a highly digestible diet with little fiber and complex carbohydrates, they have shorter intestinal length and absorptive capacity than do dogs and humans.[1]

The most notable metabolic difference between cats and more omnivorous species such as human beings and dogs is that cats have a much higher requirement for protein. Adult cats require about 4 grams of protein per kilogram of body weight compared with 2.6 grams in dogs and 0.8 grams in humans.[16,24] Because cats have evolved eating a diet plentiful in protein and low in carbohydrates, gluconeogenesis from amino acids is used to maintain blood glucose levels. Dietary protein is also a potent stimulator of insulin release in the cat. Although most animals suppress gluconeogenesis during meals, cats actually increase hepatic glucose production during the absorptive phase to offset increased levels of insulin. Because cats are so dependent on protein for gluconeogenesis, they continue metabolizing amino acids for energy even when protein malnourished. As a result, cats lack the ability to downregulate the production of aminotransferases and urea cycle enzymes in response to low protein intake and can become protein malnourished quickly when anorexic.[26,33] Deficiencies in essential amino acids can lead to severe disease and death. The most dramatic response to an amino acid deficiency is caused by a lack of arginine. Arginine is required by the urea cycle to convert toxic ammonia to urea. Ammonia is a by-product of protein metabolism, and if cats are fed even one meal without arginine, hyperammonemia can occur. Symptoms include vocalization, vomiting, ataxia, apnea, cyanosis, and death within a few hours.[23] Taurine is technically a sulfonic acid rather than an amino acid and can be synthesized from cysteine in most species. Cats have minimal activity of enzymes necessary to synthesize taurine and must obtain it from the diet. Taurine is used exclusively to conjugate bile salts into bile acids in cats, and this causes an obligatory loss of taurine even when dietary intake is deficient.[18] The most notable symptoms of taurine deficiency in cats are dilated cardiomyopathy and retinal degeneration.[1,25]

The carnivorous nature of the wild feline has also led to modifications in fatty acid and vitamin requirements. Arachidonic acid is a fatty acid abundant in animal tissues. Because it is plentiful in the natural feline diet, cats do not have the canine or human ability to synthesize arachidonic acid from linoleic acid. Arachidonic acid is especially important for growth, pregnancy, and lactation.[1,23] Cats and dogs are unable to synthesize vitamin D from sunlight because they lack adequate 7-dehydrocholesterol in the skin. Vitamin D is abundant in animal fat and tissues such as the liver, so deficiencies rarely occur.[15] Vitamin A is found only in animal tissues, whereas its precursor, beta-carotene, is synthesized by plants. Cats have limited ability to convert beta-carotene to vitamin A and must ingest the retinol or retinyl ester form of the vitamin (e.g., retinyl acetate or retinyl palmitate).[24]

ENERGY NEEDS

The cat's caloric requirement, or daily energy requirement (DER), is a combination of several factors. In the average housecat, most energy is devoted to maintaining basal metabolic functions, known as resting energy requirement (RER). Energy is also expended for exercise, digestion, and temperature regulation. To estimate how many kilocalories a cat should be fed daily, RER is estimated using a cat's ideal body weight. Unlike muscle tissue, fat tissue utilizes little caloric energy. Therefore an overweight cat that carries 3 lb (1.4 kg) of extra fat does not need additional calories to support the excess fat mass. RER can be estimated using an exponential or linear equation:

$$\text{RER (kcal/day)} = (\text{Body weight}_{\text{kg}})^{0.75} \times 70$$

or

$$\text{RER (kcal/day)} = (\text{Body weight}_{\text{kg}} \times 30) + 70$$

For example, a 10-lb or 4.5-kg cat would have an RER of 217 kcal/day with the exponential equation and 205 kcal/day with the linear equation. Once the RER has been estimated, it is necessary to consider the age, activity, and neuter status of the cat to determine its DER. Life stage factors by which RER can be multiplied to estimate DER can be found in Table 16-1. For example, for an intact male cat, its RER is calculated at ideal weight using one of the preceding equations above and then multiplying that number by 1.4 or 1.6.

LIFE STAGE NUTRITION

Adult Maintenance

The first step when developing a nutritional plan for adult cats is to assess the patient's health status. A complete history, physical examination, and necessary

TABLE 16-1 **Estimated Energy Requirements for Cats at Different Life Stages***

Life Stage	Factor to Multiply by Resting Energy Requirement
Intact	1.4-1.6
Neutered	1.2-1.4
Obese prone	1
Weight loss	0.8
Senior	1.1-1.4
Geriatric	1.1-1.6
Gestation	1.6-2
Lactation	2-6
Growth	
<50% of adult weight	3
50%-70% of adult weight	2.5
70% to adult weight	2
Active	1.8-2.5

*The resting energy requirement (RER) is calculated and the result multiplied by the appropriate factor to estimate daily energy requirements (DER).

TABLE 16-2 **Body Condition Scoring Systems (5- And 9-Point) with Correlated Body Fat Content***

5-Pt Scale	9-Pt Scale	% Body Fat	Body Condition Scoring
1	1	≤5	Emaciated—ribs and bony prominences are visible from a distance. No palpable body fat. Loss of muscle mass.
2	2	6-9	Very thin—ribs and bony prominences visible. Minimal loss of muscle mass but no palpable fat.
	3	10-14	Thin—ribs easily palpable, tops of lumbar are visible. Obvious waist and may have an abdominal tuck.
3	4	15-19	Lean—ribs easily palpable, waist visible from above. Abdominal fat may be present or absent. If present, it is made up of loose skin and no fat within.
	5	20-24	Ideal—ribs palpable without excess fat covering. Cats have a waist and a minimal abdominal fat pad.
4	6	25-29	Slightly overweight—ribs have slight excess fat covering. Waist is discernible from above but not obvious. Abdominal fat pad is apparent but not obvious in cats.
	7	30-34	Overweight—difficult to palpate ribs. Moderate abdominal fat pad and rounding of the abdomen.
5	8	35-39	Obese—ribs not palpable, and abdomen may be rounded. Prominent abdominal fat pad and lumbar fat deposits. Fat deposit may be obvious in shoulder or abdominal area.
	9	40-45+	Morbidly obese—heavy fat deposits over lumbar area, face, and limbs. Large abdominal fat pad and rounded abdomen. Body appears broadened from above.

*Also see Figure 3-3.

laboratory testing should be performed to rule out diseases responsive to specific nutritional modifications (see Chapter 18). A key component of the physical examination should be assessment of body condition. Body condition scoring is a semiquantitative method for estimating body fat mass using a combination of visual assessment and palpation (Table 16-2; also see Figure 3-3). The veterinarian can use either a 5- or 9-point scale in which 1 is cachexic and 5 or 9 is obese (see Chapter 3). Once a body condition is assigned, body fat mass can be estimated. Ideally, cats should be between 20% and 25% fat mass. If the body condition score is 5/5 or 9/9, then the fat mass is estimated to be 40% to 45%. For example, a 15-lb (6.8 kg) cat that is 45% body fat is 55% lean mass: 15 lb × 0.55 = 8.25 lb (3.7 kg) of lean tissue. At an ideal body condition (20% fat mass), 8.25 lb (3.7 kg) of lean tissue is 80% of the cat's total body weight: 8.25 lb × 100/80 = 10.3 lb (4.7 kg) would be the cat's ideal weight. Once the ideal weight is estimated, it is possible to calculate RER from the preceding equations and use a DER factor (see Table 16-1) to approximate daily caloric requirements.

Once the DER is estimated, an appropriate food must be chosen. The most common forms of available commercial food are moist foods, canned foods, and dry kibble. However, frozen, refrigerated, freeze-dried, and semimoist foods are also available forms. Many owners also choose to cook for their cats or feed them raw diets (see Chapter 19). The best form of food to feed cats is debatable. Dry foods tend to be calorically dense, very palatable, and higher in carbohydrates (see Chapter 19 for a discussion of low-carbohydrate diets) and may contribute to feline obesity, especially when fed free choice. Canned foods are more expensive and less convenient to feed. However, they help increase water intake and seem more satiating to many cats.

Assessing the quality of diets on the basis of packaging claims is difficult. The Association of American Feed Control Officials (AAFCO) has established standards and regulations regarding animal feed. One method for assessing the quality of a cat food brand is to look for an AAFCO statement on the package. Foods can either undergo a standard AAFCO feeding trial or be chemically tested to meet AAFCO nutrient requirements. Feeding trials are considered the gold standard because they test nutrient content, digestibility, and bioavailability. In addition to looking for AAFCO statements before recommending a food brand, the cat owner should also rely on company reputation and look for those with good quality control and safety measures.

Pregnancy and Lactation

The physical demands of pregnancy and lactation can be immense for queens. Therefore optimal nutrition is important for reproducing females before conception. They should not be underweight or overweight and should receive a diet with high-quality protein and plentiful essential fatty acids. Malnourished cats can have difficulty conceiving, produce fetuses more likely to have abnormalities or abort, and give birth to underweight kittens.[11] On the opposite end of the spectrum, obese queens are more likely to experience stillbirths and cesarean sections.[3]

Pregnant queens gain weight in a steady, linear fashion from conception to parturition. This is different from most other species, such as dogs, which gain the majority of pregnancy weight in the last trimester. The weight gained by queens initially goes toward building maternal fat reserves, rather than fetal or reproductive tissue growth.[21] The average weight gain of queens during pregnancy is 40% of prepregnancy weight.[11,21] Cats typically lose only 40% of their excess pregnancy weight during parturition. The remainder is used to sustain lactation.[11]

Queens should produce milk at the time of parturition. For the first 24 to 72 hours, colostrum will be produced. After birth, kittens have a short window (12 to 18 hours) for colostral antibody absorption through the gastrointestinal tract.[8] Lactation peaks 3 to 4 weeks after birth. The best way to assess milk production in queens is through kitten growth and weight gain. Newborn kittens should gain 10 to 15 grams daily. If they are gaining less than 7 g per day, milk supplementation is needed.[11,20]

Information regarding the specific nutritional needs of pregnant and lactating cats is scarce.[11,31] Most nutritional recommendations are based on the requirements of growing kittens. Pregnant queens typically need 25% to 50% more calories than maintenance needs. This can be achieved by feeding 1.6 times RER at breeding and gradually increasing to 2 times RER at parturition (see Table 16-1). Lactating cats require the most energy of any life stage and need 2 to 6 times RER. High-quality, energy-dense growth formulas or formulas designated for pregnancy and lactation should be fed free choice to pregnant and lactating queens.[11] Vegetarian diets are especially hazardous for pregnant and lactating cats because animal-based essential amino acids and fatty acids are needed for fetal and kitten development. In addition, milk production requires increased fluid intake. All cats, lactating cats in particular, should have access to clean, fresh water at all times.[11]

Growth

Kittens usually begin weaning at 3 to 4 weeks of age and complete the process by 6 to 9 weeks. Moist or dry kitten food moistened with water should be offered at the onset of weaning. Kittens will continue to receive most of their calories from milk for the first 2 weeks of weaning and by 5 to 6 weeks of age should be eating about 30% of their calories from solid food.[10] For information on feeding orphan kittens, see Chapter 41.

After weaning, kittens should be placed on a kitten food or a variety of foods that have passed AAFCO feeding trials for feline growth. Estimations for DER can be made using Table 16-1. Kittens can be fed free choice until they are approximately 5 months of age. After this time, owners should monitor their cat's food intake to prevent obesity from developing. Gonadectomy also influences the caloric requirements of juvenile cats. Neutered male cats require 28% fewer calories than do intact male cats, and spayed females require 33% fewer calories than do intact females.[27] Teaching owners to perform body condition scoring is one method to help prevent obesity in the young adult (see Table 16-2). Cats typically reach their adult weight by about 10 months of age and can be switched from kitten to adult food at this time.

Senior and Geriatric Cats

The population of senior and geriatric cats in the United States has nearly doubled in recent years.[28] Many authors consider cats to be senior when they reach 7 years of age. However, metabolic and digestive changes are not usually detected until later in life. For this discussion, cats are considered senior by 11 years and geriatric by 15 years of age.[7]

The nutritional requirements of older cats are unique compared with those of humans and dogs. Whereas the DERs of most animals decrease later in life, elderly cats require more energy to maintain their body weight. There are a couple of explanations for this difference. The activity patterns of cats remain similar throughout their lives.[13] They spend most of their time sleeping and grooming. Therefore a 5-year-old cat may not move much more than a 15-year-old cat. Elderly cats also require more dietary energy because their fat and protein digestion is impaired. Approximately 30% of cats older than 12 years of age have decreased fat absorption, and 20% have decreased protein digestibility.[19] This attenuated digestion can also lead to deficiencies in other vitamins and minerals.[19] To compensate for impaired nutrient absorption, elderly cats tend to eat more food relative to their body weight than younger cats.[12]

Choosing an appropriate diet for senior and geriatric cats should be based on individual needs. Health screenings should be routinely conducted to look for kidney, gastrointestinal, endocrine, and oncologic disease (see Chapter 18). Healthy, geriatric cats with weight loss benefit from highly digestible, calorically dense diets that are higher in fat and protein. Feline growth diets can be used for this purpose. Protein should not be restricted in elderly cats that do not have underlying renal disease. Obesity is a major nutritional concern in cats and tends to peak in middle-aged cats (5 to 10 years old).[22] After approximately 11 years of age, obesity rates decline dramatically. Many senior feline diets are marketed for cats older than 7 years of age and may be designed to minimize weight gain. Therefore senior diets may not be appropriate for all geriatric patients, and the veterinarian should assess body condition and overall health status before making a dietary recommendation.

References

1. Armstrong P, Gross K, Becvarova I et al: In Hand M, Thatcher C, Remillard R et al, editors: *Small animal clinical nutrition*, ed 5, Topeka, Kan, 2010, Mark Morris Institute, p 361.
2. Becques A, Larose C, Gouat P et al: Effects of pre- and postnatal olfactogustatory experience on early preferences at birth and dietary selection at weaning in kittens, *Chem Senses* 35:41, 2010.
3. Bilkei G: Effect of the nutrition status on parturition in the cat, *Berl Munch Tierarztl Wochenschr* 103:49, 1990.
4. Bradshaw JWS: The evolutionary basis for the feeding behavior of domestic dogs *(Canis familiaris)* and cats *(Felis catus)*, *J Nutr* 136:1927S, 2006.
5. Bradshaw JWS, Goodwin D, Legrand-Defrétin V et al: Food selection by the domestic cat, an obligate carnivore, *Comp Biochem Physiol A Physiol* 114:205, 1996.
6. Bradshaw JWS, Healey LM, Thorne CJ et al: Differences in food preferences between individuals and populations of domestic cats *Felis silvestris catus*, *Appl Anim Behav Sci* 68:257, 2000.
7. Caney S: Weight loss in the elderly cat. Appetite is fine and everything looks normal, *J Feline Med Surg* 11:738, 2009.
8. Casal M, Jezyk P, Giger U: Transfer of colostral antibodies from queens to their kittens, *Am J Vet Res* 57:1653, 1996.
9. Daniels MJ, Johnson PJ, Balharry D et al: Ecology and genetics of wild-living cats in the north-east of Scotland and the implications for the conservation of the wildcat, *J Appl Ecol* 38:146, 2001.
10. Gross K, Becvarova I, Debraekeleer J: Feeding nursing and orphaned kittens from birth to weaning. In Hand M, Thatcher C, Remillard R et al, editors: *Small animal clinical nutrition*, ed 5, Topeka, Kan, 2010, Mark Morris Institute, p 415.
11. Gross K, Becvarova I, Debraekeleer J: Feeding reproducing cats. In Hand M, Thatcher C, Remillard R et al, editors: *Small animal clinical nutrition*, ed 5, Topeka, Kan, 2010, Mark Morris Institute, p 401.
12. Harper EJ: Changing perspectives on aging and energy requirements: aging and digestive function in humans, dogs and cats, *J Nutr* 128:2632S, 1998.
13. Harper EJ: Changing perspectives on aging and energy requirements: aging and energy intakes in humans, dogs and cats, *J Nutr* 128:2623S, 1998.
14. Horwitz D, Soulard Y, Junien-Castagna A: The feeding behavior of the cat. In Pibot P, Biourge V, Elliott DA, editors: *Encyclopedia of feline clinical nutrition*, Aimargues, France, 2008, Direction Communication Royal Canin Group, p 439.
15. How KL, Hazewinkel HAW, Mol JA: Dietary vitamin D dependence of cat and dog due to inadequate cutaneous synthesis of vitamin D, *Gen Comp Endocrinol* 96:12, 1994.
16. Institute of Medicine of the National Academies: *Dietary reference intakes for energy, carbohydrate, fiber, fat, fatty acids, cholesterol, protein, and amino acids*, Washington, DC, 2005, The National Academies Press.
17. Kane E, Rogers QR, Morris JG: Feeding behavior of the cat fed laboratory and commercial diets, *Nutr Res* 1:499, 1981.
18. Knopf K, Sturman JA, Armstrong M et al: Taurine: an essential nutrient for the cat, *J Nutr* 108:773, 1978.
19. Laflamme DP: Nutrition for aging cats and dogs and the importance of body condition, *Vet Clin North Am Sm Anim Pract* 35:713, 2005.
20. Lawlor DA, Bebiak D: Nutrition and management of reproduction in the cat, *Vet Clin North Am Sm Anim Pract* 16:495, 1986.
21. Loveridge G, Rivers J: Bodyweight changes and energy intakes of cats during pregnancy and lactation. In Burger I, Rivers J, editors: *Nutrition of the dog and cat*, Cambridge, UK, 1989, Cambridge University Press, p 113.
22. Lund E, Armstrong P, Kirk C et al: Prevalence and risk factors for obesity in adult cats from private US veterinary practices, *Intern J Appl Res Vet Med* 3:88, 2005.
23. MacDonald ML, Rogers QR, Morris JG: Nutrition of the domestic cat, a mammalian carnivore, *Annu Rev Nutr* 4:521, 1984.
24. National Research Council: *Nutrient requirements of dogs and cats*, Washington, DC, 2006, National Academies Press.
25. Novotny MJ HP, Flannigan G: Echocardiographic evidence for myocardial failure induced by taurine deficiency in domestic cats, *Can J Vet Res* 58:6, 1994.
26. Rogers Q, Morris J, Freedland R: Lack of hepatic enzymatic adaptation to low and high levels of dietary protein in the adult cat, *Enzyme* 22:348, 1977.
27. Root MV, Johnston SD, Olson PN: Effect of prepuberal and postpuberal gonadectomy on heat production measured by indirect calorimetry in male and female domestic cats, *Am J Vet Res* 57:371, 1996.
28. Stratton-Phelps M: AAFP and AFM panel report of feline senior health care, *Compend Contin Educ Pract Vet* 21:531, 1999.
29. Turner DC, Bateson P: *The domestic cat*, ed 2, New York, 2000, Cambridge University Press.
30. Twain M: *Notebook*, 1894.
31. Wichert B, Schade L, Gebert S et al: Energy and protein needs of cats for maintenance, gestation, and lactation, *J Feline Med Surg* 11:808, 2009.
32. Wyrwicka W: Imitation of mother's inappropriate food preference in weanling kittens, *Pavlov J Biol Sci* 13:55, 1978.
33. Zoran DL: The carnivore connection to nutrition in cats, *J Am Vet Med Assoc* 221:1559, 2002.

CHAPTER

17

Nutritional Disorders

Joe Bartges, Donna Raditic, Claudia Kirk, Angela L. Witzel, Beth Hamper, and Maryanne Murphy

OUTLINE

Providing nutrition to companion animals is relatively easy and safe; however, an adverse reaction to a diet or nutrient or exposure to a food hazard occasionally occurs. A complete and balanced diet is a diet that contains the appropriate ingredients in the appropriate amounts so that animals remain clinically healthy. It provides complete nutrition, and the nutrients are balanced with one another, especially the energy density of the diet. Nutritional disorders may result from imbalances in diet formulation or from specific food components.

FOOD COMPONENTS

Hazardous food components encompass dietary components that are present in the food. These may be components that should be present but are present in an unbalanced manner, or these may be components that should not be present. *Nutrient imbalances* may occur when there is a problem in the formulation or manufacture of a diet or if the owner supplements a complete and balanced diet with an incomplete and unbalanced food or supplements. Generic foods are more likely to be unbalanced and result in clinical disease.[26]

Excesses

Food components may be present in greater than recommended amounts. For example, consumption of energy in excess of expenditure is one potential mechanism for development of obesity (see Chapter 18). Other food components present in excess may pose serious health concerns and are discussed in the subsequent sections and in Table 17-1.

Hypervitaminosis A

Cats require preformed vitamin A in the diet because beta-carotene, the plant precursor of vitamin A, cannot be converted to vitamin A by cats (see Chapter 15).[6] Hypervitaminosis A is uncommonly seen but results in ankylosing spondylosis, particularly of the cervical vertebrae in cats; it can also induce growth retardation, abnormal dentition, and neurologic deficits as a result of nerve entrapment from hyperostoses.[10,16,44,51,52] It occurs when excessive vitamin A is present in the diet in the form of raw liver or cod liver oil or as a vitamin supplement.* Hyperostoses resulting from hypervitaminosis A include primarily cervical stiffness and forelimb lameness. Affected cats resist movement, particularly neck flexion. Clinical signs are attributed to new periosteal bone formation at sites of ligament and tendon attachment, which restrict joint movements and may impinge on nerves exiting vertebral foramina. With continued exposure to high levels of vitamin A, bony changes may extend to sternebrae, ribs, scapulae, other long bones, and pelvis. Ankylosis of cervical vertebrae and elbow joints may occur. Affected cats typically have an unkempt appearance because of an inability to groom. On presentation adult cats typically have a prolonged history of malaise, poor appetite, and a diet consisting mainly of liver or other concentrated source (or sources) of vitamin A. Physical examination often reveals muscle wasting, cutaneous hyperesthesia, inability to move neck, and a tendency to sit on the hindlimbs in a "kangaroo" position. Cervical radiography is diagnostic for ankylosing

*References 3, 10, 16, 44, 51, 52.

TABLE 17-1 **Nutrient Excesses**

Nutrient Class/Elements	Associated Diseases/Conditions
Energy	Obesity Increased risk for other diseases
Protein	May result in imbalanced or deficient diet
Carbohydrate	Lactose intolerance Diarrhea, bloating
Minerals	
Magnesium	Struvite-related urolithiasis and urethral plugs
Phosphorus	Secondary nutritional hyperparathyroidism
Sodium	Hypertension Congestive heart failure
Vitamins	
Vitamin A	Cervical osteocartilaginous hyperplasia
Vitamin D	Soft tissue calcification
Trace elements	
Iron	Vomiting, diarrhea, neurological signs
Copper	Chronic active hepatitis
Zinc	Hemolytic anemia
Iodine	Hyperthyroidism

spondylosis. Plasma vitamin A can be measured. Normal plasma vitamin A concentrations are 960 ± 770 ng/mL[2]; plasma concentrations of vitamin A in cats with hypervitaminosis A have been reported to be higher than 4500 ng/mL.[9,16,44,51] Treatment for hypervitaminosis A includes discontinuing the high vitamin A diet or supplement, changing the diet to one containing recommended vitamin A levels, and administering an analgesic and possibly antiinflammatory medication. If caught early, changing the diet may result in resolution of early ankylosis; however, when ankylosis has been present for some time, it will not resolve. Affected cats may have difficulty eating and drinking because of their inability to flex their neck. It may be necessary for the owner to provide food and water at a height that does not require neck flexion, or a feeding tube may be required.

Hypervitaminosis D

The dietary vitamin D requirement of adult cats is fairly low, although cats require a dietary source because sunlight is not required for activation of vitamin D.[46] Hypervitaminosis D is uncommon but may occur if complete diets are supplemented with vitamin D or when manufacturing errors occur. In 2006 a major pet food manufacturer recalled canine and feline canned diets because of excessive levels of vitamin D_3 contained in the vitamin–mineral premix. Affected cats developed gastrointestinal signs, hypercalcemia, and renal disease. More commonly, hypervitaminosis D results from ingestion of vitamin D containing rodenticides and causes an acute disease manifested as hypercalcemia, polyuria–polydipsia, muscle fasciculations, vomiting, diarrhea, anorexia, seizures, and possibly renal failure (see Chapter 31). Chronic hypervitaminosis D results in musculoskeletal deformities, although cats appear to be relatively resistant.[53]

Excessive Intake of Polyunsaturated Fatty Acids

Steatitis, a painful inflammatory condition of adipose tissue, may result from excessive intake of polyunsaturated fatty acids or ingestion of rancid fat. Hard, painful masses can be palpated in adipose tissue of affected cats.* Although this condition is uncommon, it may occur if the antioxidant activity of the food is not adequate, if the food is fed beyond the effective time of included antioxidants, or with homemade diets that are stored for long periods without added antioxidants. Fish oil is particularly susceptible to oxidation and requires higher levels of antioxidants compared with vegetable or animal fat sources. Treatment involves analgesic therapy, antioxidant supplementation, and possibly surgical excision of necrotic fat.

Deficiencies

Diets may be deficient in required nutrients, including macronutrients and micronutrients. Important deficiencies are described in the subsequent sections and in Table 17-2.

Thiamin

Thiamin is a B vitamin that is involved with neurologic function. Classic thiamin deficiency occurs with ingestion of large amounts of raw fish that contain thiaminase, an enzyme that destroys thiamin. Cooking the fish destroys thiaminase and eliminates the problem. Thiamin deficiency has been reported with sulfur dioxide preservation of dietary meat and in cats fed commercial cat food.[11,30,31,55,57] A small cluster of thiamin-deficiency cases associated with commercial cat foods occurred in the eastern part of the United States in 2009, and another limited precautionary recall of canned cat foods owing to inadequate thiamin content occurred in 2010. Clinical signs of thiamin deficiency include decreased food intake, hypersalivation, ventral flexion of the neck (see Figure 26-19), and seizures. Myocardial degeneration has also been associated with thiamin deficiency.[1] Fundic examination may reveal retinal venous dilation and hemorrhages. Treatment includes discontinuing the offending diet, changing to a complete and balanced cat food, and supplementing with thiamin (5 mg orally or 1 mg parenterally). Thiamin supplementation results in resolution of clinical signs, usually within 24 hours.

*References 6, 17, 27, 34, 37, 38, 62, 67.

TABLE 17-2 **Nutrient Deficiencies**

Nutrient Class/ Elements	Associated Diseases/Conditions
Energy	Malnutrition Poor growth and body condition
Protein	Poor hair coat Hypoproteinemia Edema/ascites Vacuolar hepatopathy
Taurine	Dilated cardiomyopathy Retinal degeneration Poor reproductive performance
Fat: linoleic, arachidonic	Poor hair coat Fat-soluble vitamin deficiencies
Minerals	
Calcium, phosphorus	Nutritional secondary hyperparathyroidism
Magnesium	Calcium oxalate urolithiasis (?) Cardiac dysfunction
Sodium	Poor appetite
Potassium	Polymyopathy
Vitamins	
Vitamin A	Dermatologic and ophthalmologic disease
Vitamin D	Rickets
Thiamine	Seizures
Niacin	Pellagra/black tongue
Biotin	Poor hair coat
Vitamin E	Pansteatitis
Trace elements	
Iron	Anemia
Copper	Anemia Depigmentation of skin
Zinc	Parakeratosis, poor hair coat
Iodine	Goiter, alopecia
Selenium	Muscular weakness

Vitamin E

Ingestion of large quantities of raw fish may also result in vitamin E deficiency. Fish contains polyunsaturated fatty acids that are easily oxidized. Vitamin E is an antioxidant that prevents oxidation of fatty acids in cell membranes. Signs of vitamin E deficiency include pansteatitis (discussed previously), decreased appetite, hyperesthesia, fever, and myositis.[13,15,64] Treatment consists of changing the diet with vitamin E supplementation (vitamin E acetate 100 mg/kg daily by mouth). Glucocorticoids may help decrease inflammation.

Taurine

Taurine is a beta-sulfonic amino acid that is an essential nutrient for cats, and deficiency has been associated with heart disease. Cats cannot make taurine from other amino acids and lose taurine in bile. Taurine is found primarily in animal-based products, and commercial cat foods have added taurine. Taurine deficiency occurs in cats when loss exceeds intake. This usually occurs when homemade vegetarian diets are fed or when cats are fed primarily dog food. In cats taurine deficiency is associated with retinal degeneration and blindness (see Figures 29-61 and 29-62), dilated cardiomyopathy (see Figure 18-1), reproductive problems, and abnormal skeletal development in kittens.* In pregnant queens taurine deficiency is associated with abortions, stillbirths, and birthing of kittens that do not survive. If neonatal kittens are born live to queens that are taurine deficient, they often have skeletal abnormalities, such as curved spines and small stature.

With dilated cardiomyopathy the diagnosis of taurine deficiency is made by radiography and echocardiography (see Chapter 20). In cats with retinal degeneration, a thorough ophthalmic examination should be performed (see Chapter 29). If reproductive problems are present, evaluation for other causes of decreased conception rates or stillbirths is undertaken (see Chapter 40). In kittens with skeletal abnormalities, radiography should be performed. In cats plasma taurine concentration can decrease below the normal range after less than 24 hours of fasting; therefore whole blood is preferred for evaluation of taurine levels.[22,36,54] Although taurine deficiency is now a rare cause of dilated cardiomyopathy in cats, taurine is inexpensive and safe and is often empirically administered (250 to 500 mg orally every 12 hours) for 8 weeks to patients with presumed deficiency. Commercial dry cat foods are required to contain 0.1% taurine on a dry matter basis, and canned foods are required to contain 0.2% on a dry matter basis. Canned diets are required to contain more taurine than dry diets because canned diets promote bacterial growth in the intestines that degrade taurine.

Inappropriate Food Components

Occasionally, foods and ingredients that are not toxic to other species may induce toxicity in cats. Examples include onion and garlic ingestion, which can cause Heinz body hemolytic anemia.[5,47] The primary toxic principle in members of the *Allium* genus is n-propyl disulfide, which causes oxidative damage to erythrocytes. Toxicoses have been reported with fresh, cooked, dried, or powdered material. Feeding commercial baby food containing onion powder has also been reported to cause toxicity in cats. Clinical signs include vomiting, weakness, and pallor. Affected cats may also have hemoglobinuria. Therapy involves inducing emesis and administering activated charcoal if ingestion is recent, along with supportive care. Patients with severe anemia may require whole blood transfusions, and fluid diuresis is recommended for cats with hemoglobinuria.

*References 19-21, 24, 42, 43, 48-50, 58-61.

FOOD CONTAMINANTS

Occasionally, food may become contaminated. This may occur if the manufacturer uses contaminated foodstuffs, or the food may become contaminated after production. Bacterial contamination with *Salmonella, Campylobacter,* and *Escherichia coli* have been reported in cats, and clinical signs usually include vomiting, diarrhea, and inappetence.[12,23,56]

In 2007, melamine and cyanuric acid contamination of cat food resulted in renal failure, death, and the largest cat and dog food recall in U.S. history, involving about 150 brands of food.[8,29,40,45] Melamine and cyanuric acid were likely added to increase the nitrogen content of imported wheat flour or wheat gluten. Although it is illegal to add melamine to human or animal food in the United States, it is a common additive in other countries, such as China. Clinical signs varied in severity and included inappetence with or without vomiting, polydipsia, polyuria, dehydration, vomiting, lethargy, and anorexia. Abdominal palpation often revealed renomegaly. Affected cats became azotemic, with decreased urine specific gravity within 2 weeks of ingesting the contaminated food. Although some cats appeared to recover renal function, others developed chronic renal disease. Cats with severe azotemia, hyperphosphatemia, and hyperkalemia were unlikely to survive. Microscopic examination of the urine of some cats revealed goldish brown crystals, and at necropsy kidneys were found to contain such crystals. Renal tubular necrosis was also present. Kidney and urine samples contained melamine and cyanuric acid.

In 1996 an outbreak of food-associated peripheral neuropathy in cats occurred in the Netherlands and Switzerland.[41,63] The outbreak was related to feeding two brands of dry food contaminated by the coccidiostatic drug salinomycin. Affected cats had acute onset of lower motor neuron signs of variable severity. The clinical signs varied from paraparesis to tetraplegia, were symmetric and bilateral, and progressed from the pelvis to thoracic limbs. Dyspnea occurred in some severely tetraplegic cats. The majority of reported cases recovered with withdrawal of the diet and supportive care, although the most severely affected cats died or were euthanized.

FOOD HYPERSENSITIVITY

An *adverse reaction* to food is defined as a clinically abnormal response attributed to an ingested food or food substance. It may be immunologic or nonimmunologic.

A food hypersensitivity or allergic reaction is an immunologically mediated reaction to an ingested food or food ingredient. This is different from food intolerance, which is a nonimmunologically mediated adverse reaction. Food hypersensitivity reactions appear to cause primarily dermatologic and gastrointestinal clinical signs.

Throughout their lives cats are exposed to a variety of potential dietary allergens; however, after a variable period of time, some animals may develop an immune response against a particular food that activates one or more immunopathogenic pathways. After development of this response, subsequent ingestion of this foodstuff results in clinical signs. These dietary antigens do not normally cause problems because the intestinal mucosa forms a barrier that limits absorption of macromolecules, but this mechanism is imperfect. There is evidence that antigens are absorbed through both normal and abnormal gut. Indeed, antibodies to food allergens, usually IgG, are often demonstrable in normal individuals, but they do not result in clinical disease. On initial presentation of the antigen to the gut mucosa, there is generally an immune response involving IgA. This reduces the amount of antigenic material that is absorbed. Immune complexes of antigen and IgA antibody are transported across hepatocytes, into bile, and are recirculated to the intestine. This local IgA response may be followed by a transitory systemic immune response, but immunologic tolerance follows. Thus there is an apparent paradox of a vigorous local immune response followed by a systemic tolerance. Absorption of macromolecules can be altered in either direction by local immunity. Decreased uptake has been demonstrated experimentally after oral or parenteral immunization in rats, and increased absorption occurs in IgA-deficient human beings. Absorption is also enhanced by vasodilation in the gut mucosa, such as that resulting from a local allergic reaction. In this case the patient becomes caught in an immunologic vicious circle because local hypersensitivity reactions favor access of allergens, which in turn heightens the antibody response.[14,33,65]

Factors that lead to the development of hypersensitivity to ingested antigens are the subject of speculation. Those most frequently implicated are heat- and acid-stable glycoproteins with molecular weights of 18,000 to 30,000 daltons. Hypersensitivity reactions involved in food allergies have been shown to involve types I, III, and IV reactions. However, studies indicate that IgE is implicated in most instances, and the reactions involved include both the classic, immediate type I reaction and the late-phase IgE-mediated reactions.[4,39] The factors that determine the extent of absorption of allergens by the intestine are not fully understood, although local vasodilation is clearly facilitatory. Once local vasodilation is stimulated by local reactions, the cycle feeds on itself. What initiates the original immunologic reaction is not clear. Certainly, if clinical or subclinical gastrointestinal disease occurs that alters mucosal integrity, absorption of antigenic proteins may occur, which may initiate the

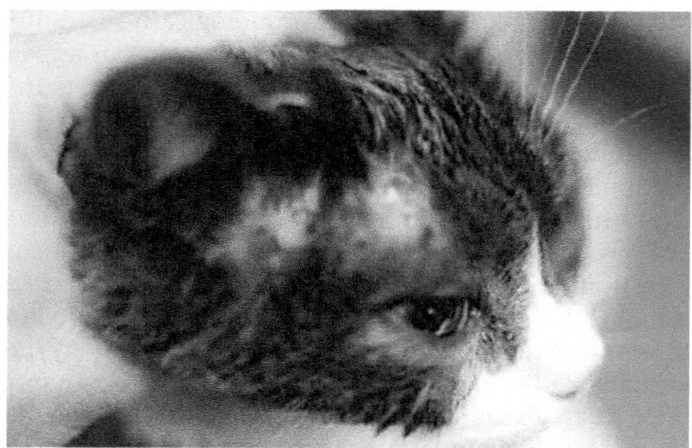

FIGURE 17-1 Facial pruritus and excoriation in a cat with presumed food allergy.

processes. Inflammatory mediators involved in food allergy may include interleukins, platelet-activating factor, histamine and other products of mast cells and basophils, and cytokines.

No age, gender, or breed predisposition has been identified for food hypersensitivities in cats. Clinical signs of food hypersensitivity reaction in cats include dermatologic and gastrointestinal signs.* Dermatologic signs include nonseasonal pruritus; alopecia and erythema, particularly around the face and ears (Figure 17-1); and secondary bacterial pyoderma. Other dermatologic signs include eosinophilic granuloma complex and miliary dermatitis. Gastrointestinal signs usually include vomiting, but diarrhea and inappetence may be present. Whether food hypersensitivity reaction is involved with feline asthma, cholangitis–cholangiohepatitis complex, and idiopathic cystitis is subject to speculation.

Most basic food ingredients have the potential to induce an allergic response, although proteins cause the majority of reactions. Dietary components reported to cause food sensitivity in cats include cow's milk, beef, mutton, pork, chicken, rabbit, horse meat, fish, eggs, oatmeal, wheat, corn, soy, rice flour, potatoes, kidney beans, canned foods, cod liver oil, dry food, pet treats, and food additives.

Diagnosis of food hypersensitivity involves first ruling out other potential causes of the clinical signs (Box 17-1). This may be complicated by concurrent diseases with similar clinical signs (e.g., the cat with flea allergy dermatitis and food hypersensitivity). Intradermal skin testing and serologic testing are unreliable for the diagnosis of food allergies in cats. The most useful and reliable aid in diagnosis of dietary sensitivity is the procedure of feeding a restricted or elimination diet followed by dietary challenge with a test meal; however, this is difficult in cats, especially in multicat households.

*References 25, 32, 35, 65, 66, 68, 69.

BOX 17-1

Diagnosis of Food Hypersensitivity

1. Rule out other potential causes for the clinical signs; start with a minimum database (CBC, chemistry panel, urinalysis [and total T_4 for senior cats]) as well as basic system-specific tests such as fecal parasite analysis and skin scrapings; further testing is performed as required.
2. Obtain a full dietary history, including all treats and table food; include food used to administer medications, such as Greenies Pill Pockets, and any flavored medications or supplements.
3. Choose an elimination diet (home prepared or commercial); ideally, the diet should contain a single protein and carbohydrate source to which the cat has not been exposed in the past; introduce the diet gradually (see Box 18-5), and counsel the owner to be patient because some cats will require several weeks to respond.
4. Once the clinical signs have resolved, attempt to identify the offending antigen by introducing foodstuffs one at a time to the elimination diet; if the owner is unwilling to attempt identification, the cat can be fed a commercially prepared limited-protein-source diet that does not provoke clinical signs.

CBC, Complete blood count; T_4, thyroxine.

Elimination diets must be individualized on the basis of previous dietary exposure and may be commercial or home-prepared diets. By definition, elimination diets contain protein and carbohydrate sources to which the cat has not been exposed. A detailed study of the cat's diet (including all treats, table food, and flavored medications and supplements) will allow identification of foods that have not been fed before and that could be used to formulate a nutritionally balanced elimination diet that will be hypoallergenic.[18,28,32] As the variety of protein sources in commercial diets has expanded over the years, it has become more difficult to find a novel protein. If it is not possible to formulate a suitable elimination diet, then a restricted diet may be used that contains only one or two potential allergens, preferably ones that the animal has not eaten in the preceding month. A canned diet may be preferable to a dry diet. Many homemade diets that are used as elimination diets are not complete and balanced (e.g., cottage cheese and rice, or chicken and rice) and therefore are not suitable for long-term use (i.e., more than 4 weeks). Supplementation of a homemade diet with vitamins and minerals is encouraged, but use of supplements that contain potentially offending foodstuffs (e. g., beef or pork) is not recommended. In one study use of a homemade diet resulted in better resolution of clinical signs than did commercially available diets.[28] The owner should also be instructed not to give treats and table food to the cat and restrict the cat's access to food intended for other pets in the home. Good client education and communication are critical to the success of a diet trial, especially in multicat homes. Scheduling follow-up telephone calls and a follow-up visit in the first 1 to 2 weeks may help identify problems that can be corrected early. Gastrointestinal signs may subside in 3 to 5 days, but if the signs are chronic, this may take 4 to 6 weeks or longer. Resolution of dermatologic signs may take 8 weeks or longer. Once clinical improvement is noted, the veterinarian should try to identify the offending antigen by introducing foodstuffs one at a time to the elimination diet. Most cats will relapse within a few days or within 2 weeks when the triggering allergen is reintroduced. However, not all owners are willing to perform this step because it is time-consuming and tedious, and the owner may be reluctant to risk recurrence of the cat's clinical signs.

Because proteins with molecular weights over 18,000 daltons are incriminated as being antigenic, modification of proteins to compounds having lower molecular weight may be of benefit. Protein modification is a process that alters the physical characteristics of protein molecules, presumably reducing the antigenicity and rendering them less able to elicit an immune response. By reducing the average weight of the protein molecule, this process can result in a protein that may be truly hypoallergenic. To be effective, it must reduce the molecular weight of the protein below 18,000 daltons.[7,18] Recently, several commercially available diets containing protein hydrolysates have been introduced. These diets appear to be effective as elimination diets, and they have the advantage of being complete and balanced.

If the client has been cooperative, the presumptive food antigen has been identified. If this has occurred, or if it is not possible to identify the antigen, then long-term management procedures should be instituted. If the elimination diet is a commercially prepared, complete, and balanced diet, it can be used long term. If the elimination diet is a home-prepared diet, it should be changed to a commercially prepared diet of selected protein or a protein hydrolysate diet. This not only provides a nutritionally balanced and complete diet but also is more convenient for owners. There are many single-protein source diets available including diets that contain duck, venison, lamb, rabbit, and kangaroo. If the cat continues to do well, the owner should be strongly advised not to feed the cat table scraps or treats and not to switch the diet even if clinical signs have not recurred. A few cats with dietary hypersensitivity may eventually develop sensitivities to ingredients in the new diet, and the procedure to identify the offending ingredient must be repeated. Dietary hypersensitivity is poorly responsive to corticosteroid therapy, and because of the risks of long-term corticosteroid treatment, emphasis should be placed on dietary management rather than drug therapy.

FOOD INTOLERANCE

Food intolerance is a nonimmunologic abnormal physiologic response to a food item and may involve toxic, pharmacologic, or metabolic reactions or dietary idiosyncrasies, in which the animal is unable to digest or otherwise process a dietary component. Examples of food intolerance include lactose intolerance, gluten intolerance, reactions to vasoactive amines in diet, reactions to histamine-containing foods or foods that stimulate histamine release, reactions to foods that contain opiates or additives, and toxic reaction to food substances. For diagnosis and management of food intolerances, the veterinarian should follow the same steps as for food hypersensitivities.

References

1. Anderson WI, Morrow LA: Thiamine deficiency encephalopathy with concurrent myocardial degeneration and polyradiculoneuropathy in a cat, *Cornell Vet* 77:251, 1987.
2. Baker H, Schor SM, Murphy BD et al: Blood vitamin and choline concentrations in healthy domestic cats, dogs, and horses, *Am J Vet Res* 47:1468, 1986.
3. Bennett D: Nutrition and bone disease in the dog and cat, *Vet Rec* 98:313, 1976.
4. Bircher AJ, Van Melle G, Haller E et al: IgE to food allergens are highly prevalent in patients allergic to pollens, with and without symptoms of food allergy, *Clin Exp Allergy* 24:367, 1994.
5. Botha CJ, Penrith ML: Potential plant poisonings in dogs and cats in southern africa, *J S Afr Vet Assoc* 80:63, 2009.
6. Burger I, Edney A, Horrocks D: Basics of feline nutrition, *In Practice* 9, 1987.
7. Cave NJ: Hydrolyzed protein diets for dogs and cats, *Vet Clin North Am Small Anim Pract* 36:1251, 2006.
8. Cianciolo RE, Bischoff K, Ebel JG et al: Clinicopathologic, histologic, and toxicologic findings in 70 cats inadvertently exposed to pet food contaminated with melamine and cyanuric acid, *J Am Vet Med Assoc* 233:729, 2008.
9. Clark L: Hypervitaminosis A: A review, *Aust Vet J* 47:568, 1971.
10. Clark L, Seawright AA: Skeletal abnormalities in the hindlimbs of young cats as a result of hypervitaminosis A, *Nature* 217:1174, 1968.
11. Davidson MG: Thiamin deficiency in a colony of cats, *Vet Rec* 130:94, 1992.
12. Deming MS, Tauxe RV, Blake PA et al: Campylobacter enteritis at a university: transmission from eating chicken and from cats, *Am J Epidemiol* 126:526, 1987.
13. Dennis JM, Alexander RW: Nutritional myopathy in a cat, *Vet Rec* 111:195, 1982.
14. Farhadi A, Banan A, Fields J et al: Intestinal barrier: An interface between health and disease, *J Gastroenterol Hepatol* 18:479, 2003.
15. Gershoff SN: Nutritional problems of household cats, *J Am Vet Med Assoc* 166:455, 1975.
16. Goldman AL: Hypervitaminosis A in a cat, *J Am Vet Med Assoc* 200:1970, 1992.
17. Griffiths RC, Thornton GW, Willson JE: Eight additional cases of pansteatitis ("yellow fat") in cats fed canned red tuna, *J Am Vet Med Assoc* 137:126, 1960.

18. Guilford WG, Matz ME: The nutritional management of gastrointestinal tract disorders in companion animals, *N Z Vet J* 51:284, 2003.
19. Hayes KC: Nutritional problems in cats: Taurine deficiency and vitamin a excess, *Can Vet J* 23:2, 1982.
20. Hayes KC, Carey RE, Schmidt SY: Retinal degeneration associated with taurine deficiency in the cat, *Science* 188:949, 1975.
21. Hayes KC, Trautwein EA: Taurine deficiency syndrome in cats, *Vet Clin North Am Small Anim Pract* 19:403, 1989.
22. Heinze CR, Larsen JA, Kass PH et al: Plasma amino acid and whole blood taurine concentrations in cats eating commercially prepared diets, *Am J Vet Res* 70:1374, 2009.
23. Hill SL, Cheney JM, Taton Allen GF et al: Prevalence of enteric zoonotic organisms in cats, *J Am Vet Med Assoc* 216:687, 2000.
24. Hilton J: The biosynthesis, function and deficiency signs of taurine in cats, *Can Vet J* 29:598, 1988.
25. Hirt R, Iben C: Possible food allergy in a colony of cats, *J Nutr* 128:2792s, 1998.
26. Huber TL, Laflamme DP, Medleau L et al: Comparison of procedures for assessing adequacy of dog foods, *J Am Vet Med Assoc* 199:731, 1991.
27. Kolata RJ: Feline steatitis (a case report), *Vet Med Small Anim Clin* 66:1028, 1971.
28. Leistra M, Willemse T: Double-blind evaluation of two commercial hypoallergenic diets in cats with adverse food reactions, *J Feline Med Surg* 4:185, 2002.
29. Lewin-Smith MR, Kalasinsky VF, Mullick FG et al: Melamine-containing crystals in the urinary tracts of domestic animals: sentinel event? *Arch Pathol Lab Med* 133:341, 2009.
30. Loew FM, Martin CL, Dunlop RH et al: Naturally-occurring and experimental thiamin deficiency in cats receiving commercial cat food, *Can Vet J* 11:109, 1970.
31. Malik R, Sibraa D: Thiamine deficiency due to sulphur dioxide preservative in "pet meat"—a case of deja vu, *Aust Vet J* 83:408, 2005.
32. Medleau L, Latimer KS, Duncan JR: Food hypersensitivity in a cat, *J Am Vet Med Assoc* 189:692, 1986.
33. Merchant SR, Taboada J: Food allergy and immunologic diseases of the gastrointestinal tract, *Semin Vet Med Surg (Small Anim)* 6:316, 1991.
34. Merchant SR, Taboada J: Systemic diseases with cutaneous manifestations, *Vet Clin North Am Small Anim Pract* 25:945, 1995.
35. Messinger LM: Therapy for feline dermatoses, *Vet Clin North Am Small Anim Pract* 25:981, 1995.
36. Muhlum A, Meyer H: Influence of taurine intake on plasma taurine values and renal taurine excretion of cats, *J Nutr* 121:S175, 1991.
37. Munson TO, Holzworth J, Small E et al: Steatitis (yellow fat) in cats fed canned red tuna, *J Am Vet Med Assoc* 133:563, 1958.
38. Niza MM, Vilela CL, Ferreira LM: Feline pansteatitis revisited: hazards of unbalanced home-made diets, *J Feline Med Surg* 5:271, 2003.
39. Orhan F, Karakas T, Cakir M et al: Prevalence of immunoglobulin e-mediated food allergy in 6-9-year-old urban schoolchildren in the eastern black sea region of turkey, *Clin Exp Allergy* 39:1027, 2009.
40. Osborne CA, Lulich JP, Ulrich LK et al: Melamine and cyanuric acid-induced crystalluria, uroliths, and nephrotoxicity in dogs and cats, *Vet Clin North Am Small Anim Pract* 39:1, 2009.
41. Pakozdy A, Challande-Kathman I, Doherr M et al: Retrospective study of salinomycin toxicosis in 66 cats, *Vet Med Int* 147:142, 2010.
42. Pion PD, Kittleson MD, Rogers QR et al: Myocardial failure in cats associated with low plasma taurine: a reversible cardiomyopathy, *Science* 237:764, 1987.
43. Pion PD, Kittleson MD, Rogers QE et al: Taurine deficiency myocardial failure in the domestic cat, *Prog Clin Biol Res* 351:423, 1990.
44. Polizopoulou ZS, Kazakos G, Patsikas MN et al: Hypervitaminosis A in the cat: a case report and review of the literature, *J Feline Med Surg* 7:363, 2005.
45. Puschner B, Poppenga RH, Lowenstine LJ et al: Assessment of melamine and cyanuric acid toxicity in cats, *J Vet Diagn Invest* 19:616, 2007.
46. Rivers JP, Frankel TL, Juttla S et al: Vitamin D in the nutrition of the cat, *Proc Nutr Soc* 38:36a, 1979.
47. Robertson JE, Christopher MM, Rogers QR: Heinz body formation in cats fed baby food containing onion powder, *J Am Vet Med Assoc* 212:1260, 1998.
48. Schmidt SY: Biochemical and functional abnormalities in retinas of taurine-deficient cats, *Fed Proc* 39:2706, 1980.
49. Schmidt SY, Berson EL, Hayes KC: Retinal degeneration in the taurine-deficient cat, *Trans Sect Ophthalmol Am Acad Ophthalmol Otolaryngol* 81:Op687, 1976.
50. Schuller-Levis G, Mehta PD, Rudelli R et al: Immunologic consequences of taurine deficiency in cats, *J Leukoc Biol* 47:321, 1990.
51. Seawright AA, English PB: Hypervitaminosis A and deforming cervical spondylosis of the cat, *J Comp Pathol* 77:29, 1967.
52. Seawright AA, Hrdlicka J: Severe retardation of growth with retention and displacement of incisors in young cats fed a diet of raw sheep liver high in vitamin A, *Aust Vet J* 50:306, 1974.
53. Sih TR, Morris JG, Hickman MA: Chronic ingestion of high concentrations of cholecalciferol in cats, *Am J Vet Res* 62:1500, 2001.
54. Sisson DD, Knight DH, Helinski C et al: Plasma taurine concentrations and m-mode echocardiographic measures in healthy cats and in cats with dilated cardiomyopathy, *J Vet Intern Med* 5:232, 1991.
55. Steel RJ: Thiamine deficiency in a cat associated with the preservation of "pet meat" with sulphur dioxide, *Aust Vet J* 75:719, 1997.
56. Stiver SL, Frazier KS, Mauel MJ et al: Septicemic salmonellosis in two cats fed a raw-meat diet, *J Am Anim Hosp Assoc* 39:538, 2003.
57. Studdert VP, Labuc RH: Thiamin deficiency in cats and dogs associated with feeding meat preserved with sulphur dioxide, *Aust Vet J* 68:54, 1991.
58. Sturman JA: Dietary taurine and feline reproduction and development, *J Nutr* 121:S166, 1991.
59. Sturman JA, Gargano AD, Messing JM et al: Feline maternal taurine deficiency: effect on mother and offspring, *J Nutr* 116:655, 1986.
60. Sturman JA, Messing JM: Dietary taurine content and feline reproduction and outcome, *J Nutr* 121:1195, 1991.
61. Sturman JA, Messing JM: High dietary taurine effects on feline tissue taurine concentrations and reproductive performance, *J Nutr* 122:82, 1992.
62. Summers BA, Sykes G, Martin ML: Pansteatitis mimicking infectious peritonitis in a cat, *J Am Vet Med Assoc* 180:546, 1982.
63. van der Linde-Sipman JS, van den Ingh TS, van Nes JJ et al: Salinomycin-induced polyneuropathy in cats: morphologic and epidemiologic data, *Vet Pathol* 36:152, 1999.
64. van Vleet JF, Ferrans VJ: Etiologic factors and pathologic alterations in selenium–vitamin E deficiency and excess in animals and humans, *Biol Trace Elem Res* 33:1, 1992.
65. Verlinden A, Hesta M, Millet S et al: Food allergy in dogs and cats: A review, *Crit Rev Food Sci Nutr* 46:259, 2006.
66. Wasmer ML, Willard MD, Helman RG et al: Food intolerance mimicking alimentary lymphosarcoma, *J Am Anim Hosp Assoc* 31:463, 1995.
67. Watson AD: More on feline pansteatitis, *Can Vet J* 21:321, 1980.
68. Zoran D: Is it IBD? Managing inflammatory disease in the feline gastrointestinal tract, *Vet Med* 95:128, 2000.
69. Zoran DL: Nutritional management of feline gastrointestinal diseases, *Top Companion Anim Med* 23:200, 2008.

CHAPTER

18

Nutritional Management of Diseases

Joe Bartges, Donna Raditic, Claudia Kirk, Angela L. Witzel, Beth Hamper, and Maryanne Murphy

OUTLINE

The American College of Veterinary Nutrition recommends a three-step approach to patient assessment that includes assessment of patient factors, dietary factors, and feeding factors. After the assessment phase, a nutritional treatment plan is developed and instituted, and serial monitoring and adjustment ensue (an iterative process).[259] This chapter focuses on the nutritional management of feline disorders. Additional information on each disorder can be found in other chapters in this book.

CARDIOVASCULAR DISEASES

Cardiovascular disease commonly occurs in cats with myocardial disease, occurring more commonly than valvular disease. The prevalence of dilated cardiomyopathy has decreased after the discovery of its association with taurine deficiency[213]; hypertrophic and restrictive cardiomyopathies occur most frequently. Systemic arterial hypertension may also result in left ventricular hypertrophy and myocardial failure. Cats with myocardial disease may be asymptomatic or may present with evidence of venous congestion, usually pleural effusion. For more information on cardiac disease, see Chapter 20.

Animal Factors

Cats with myocardial disease may be optimally conditioned or may be underconditioned or overconditioned depending on the severity and chronicity of the disease. Obesity results in blood volume expansion with elevated cardiac output, increased plasma and extracellular fluid volume, increased neurohumoral activation, reduced urinary sodium and water excretion, tachycardia, abnormal systolic and diastolic ventricular function, exercise intolerance, and systemic arterial hypertension.[86] This may result in progression of the disease. Likewise, cachexia may occur with myocardial failure. Cachexia associated with heart disease or failure results in negative nitrogen and energy balance.[89] The pathogenesis of cardiac cachexia is multifactorial, involving increased sympathetic tone, increased tumor necrosis factor and interleukin-1 levels, decreased physical activity with an increased resting energy requirement (RER), decreased tissue perfusion, venous congestion, and adverse effects of medications. Decreased nutrient intake and possibly increased nutrient losses (e.g., potassium loss with diuretic therapy) and loss of body weight and, more important, lean body mass occurs, resulting in an inability to respond to medical therapy and an increase in morbidity and mortality rates.

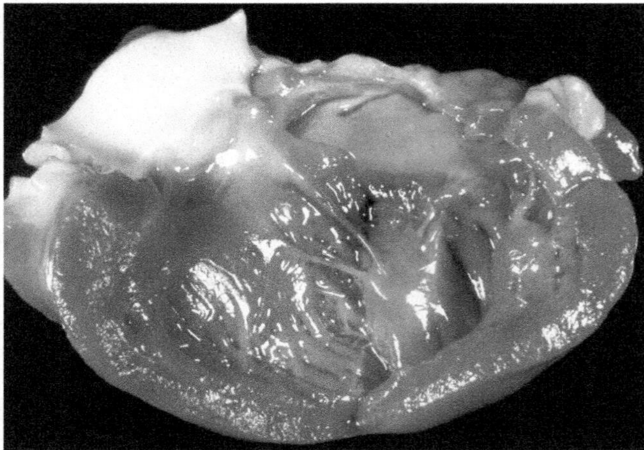

FIGURE 18-1 Dilated cardiomyopathy in a 4-year-old spayed female domestic shorthair cat with taurine deficiency.

Cats have a dietary requirement for taurine because they have limited ability to synthesize it from cysteine and methionine and because it is used exclusively for bile acid conjugation. Taurine deficiency results in dilated cardiomyopathy in predisposed cats (Figure 18-1). The mechanism of heart failure in taurine-deficient cats is poorly understood. Taurine may function in osmoregulation, calcium modulation, and inactivation of free radicals.[213] Other factors are likely involved because many cats fed taurine-deficient foods for prolonged periods fail to develop myocardial dysfunction. Additionally, there is an association between taurine and potassium balance.[67] Inadequate potassium intake may induce significant taurine depletion, resulting in myocardial dysfunction. Male cats may be more prone to developing taurine deficiency–associated myocardial failure than are female cats, or male cats may be more prone to developing clinical signs at higher plasma taurine concentrations.[83]

L-Carnitine is a conditionally essential nutrient involved with transport of long-chain fatty acids from the cytosol into the mitochondria, where they undergo beta oxidation for energy production. L-Carnitine deficiency has been associated with dilated cardiomyopathy in some dogs[132]; however, it has not been associated with this condition in cats.

Sodium intake is often restricted with heart disease; however, this may not be necessary until later in the course of the disease. Sodium restriction should occur concurrently with chloride restriction because chloride salt of sodium has more effect on blood pressure and plasma volume than non-chloride sodium salts.[26] Salt sensitivity has not been documented to occur in cats. Hypokalemia and hypomagnesemia are associated with arrhythmias, decreased myocardial contractility, and muscle weakness. Additionally, inadequate potassium intake may be associated with taurine deficiency.

BOX 18-1

Dietary Recommendations for Cats with Cardiac Disease

1. Restrict calories if obese; however, increase caloric intake if cachectic.
2. Protein content must be adequate or greater than normal (30% to 45% protein on a dry matter basis).
3. Omega-3 fatty acids may be beneficial in an omega-6:omega-3 ratio of 5:1.
4. Sodium restriction (0.07% to 0.3% on a dry matter basis) with chloride restriction (to 1.5 times the sodium content) is indicated with congestive heart failure.
5. Adequate potassium (>0.5% on a dry matter basis), phosphorus (0.3% to 0.7% on a dry matter basis), magnesium (>0.04% on a dry matter basis). With diuretic therapy, additional potassium supplementation may be required to prevent hypokalemia.
6. Taurine should be present in the diet at >0.3% on a dry matter basis but can be supplemented at 250 to 500 mg by mouth every 12 to 24 hours.

Dietary Factors

Dietary recommendations for cats with cardiac disease are designed to optimize body condition and are summarized in Box 18-1. Commercial diets formulated for cats with cardiovascular disease are available.

Feeding Factors

Some cats require feeding of frequent small meals because of decreased appetite. Pharmacologic appetite stimulation (Table 18-1) or assisted feeding through the use of feeding tubes may be required. Additional nutrients that may be beneficial include coenzyme Q10, which is required for energy reactions and is an antioxidant, and other antioxidants, which may decrease oxidative stress with dilated cardiomyopathy.

DENTAL AND ORAL DISEASES

Primary oral diseases are subdivided into conditions affecting the tooth, periodontium, and other oral tissues. In many cases dental disease is secondary to a systemic condition such as chronic renal disease in cats, although primary disorders such as lymphoplasmacytic gingivitis–stomatitis, tooth resorption, and neoplasia occur in cats. For more information, see Chapter 21.

Animal Factors

Oral disease occurs more commonly in older cats and usually is associated with systemic disease; therefore

TABLE 18-1 **Appetite Stimulants for Use in Cats**

Agent	Dose	Route	Frequency
Mirtazapine	⅛-¼ of 15 mg tab	PO	q72h
Maropitant	2-4 mg/kg	PO	q24h × 5 days
Diazepam	1-2 mg/cat 0.05-0.1 mg/kg 0.5-2.0 mg	PO IV IV	As needed As needed As needed
Oxazepam	0.3-0.4 mg/kg 2-2.5 mg	PO PO	q12-24h q12-24h
Flurazepam	0.2-0.4 mg/kg	PO	q4-7d
Chlordiazepoxide	2 mg	PO	q12-24h
Cyproheptadine	2 mg	PO	q8-12h
Prednisone	0.25-0.5 mg/kg	PO	q48h
Boldenone undecylenate	5 mg	IM/SC	q 7 days
Nandrolone decanoate	10 mg	IM	q 7 days
Stanozolol	1-2 mg 25-50 mg	PO IM	q12h q 7 days
B vitamins	1 mL/L fluids	IV	—
Cobalamin	0.5 mg/kg	SC	q24h
Elemental zinc	1 mg/kg	PO	q24h
Potassium	0.5-1 mEq KCl/kg 3 mEq K gluconate	PO PO	q12h q6-8h
Interferon alfa 2b	3-30 IU	PO	q12h

PO, By mouth; *IV*, intravenously; *IM*, intramuscularly; *SC*, subcutaneously.

oral disease may be related to systemic effects of those disorders and to nutritional imbalances caused by those disorders or eating difficulties. Historical information should include diet, eating behavior, and access to toys and other foreign bodies. The veterinarian should perform a complete oral examination, which may require sedation or anesthesia, in addition to a physical examination to evaluate for systemic disease.

Dietary Factors

Several dietary factors have been implicated with oral disease. Food texture and composition can directly affect oral cavity health through the following:

- Maintenance of tissue integrity
- Alteration of bacterial plaque metabolism
- Stimulation of salivary flow
- Cleaning of tooth and oral surfaces by physical contact
- Chelation of calculogenic constituents[162]

Claims of dry food being better for prevention of dental plaque than moist foods are unsubstantiated.[30] Likewise, there are no data to support the notion that natural diets and foods are better for oral health than commercial foods. Dietary texture can be modified by increasing fiber content with a size and texture that promotes chewing and mechanical cleansing of teeth.[30,161,272] Dental treats do not offer an advantage over dry foods; however, some contain hexametaphosphate, a calcium chelator, which may decrease calculus formation, although data are contradictory.[114,256] Hexametaphosphate has not been evaluated in cats. Many oral diseases are inflammatory, and modification of the inflammatory process may be beneficial. Antioxidants, vitamins E and C, and selenium may be beneficial, but data are lacking in cats. Nutritional deficiencies of such elements as calcium and vitamins A, B, C, D, and E are associated with oral cavity disease, but these are uncommon (see Chapter 17).

Nutrition has been implicated as a cause of feline tooth resorption. Acid coating of foods has been suggested to cause tooth resorption, although this has not been proved.[5,226,278] Dry food may cause microfractures that predispose teeth to infection and inflammation; however, this has not been proved. Dietary vitamin D has been implicated in tooth resorption. Evidence to support this assertion includes correlation between cats with tooth resorption and increased blood levels of 25-hydroxyvitamin D and histologic comparisons of the effects of excessive intake of vitamin D to the effects of bone resorption.[226,227] Although a direct effect of vitamin D has not been established, there is evidence of an active vitamin D signaling in the pathophysiology of tooth resorption.[27,28]

Feeding Factors

Feeding a "dental" diet that carries the Veterinary Oral Health Council (http://www.vohc.org/) seal for plaque control may be beneficial for cats that are prone to periodontal disease. Additional recommendations include the following:

1. Vitamin E: >500 IU/kg
2. Vitamin C: 100 to 200 mg/kg
3. Selenium: 0.5 to 1.3 mg/kg
4. Phosphorus: 0.5% to 0.8% on a dry matter basis
5. Sodium: 0.2% to 0.5% on a dry matter basis
6. Magnesium: 0.04% to 0.1% on a dry matter basis

SKIN DISORDERS

The most common feline skin disorders are abscesses, parasitic dermatoses, allergy (flea bite hypersensitivity and atopic dermatitis), miliary dermatitis, eosinophilic granuloma complex, fungal dermatitis, adverse reactions to food, psychogenic dermatoses, seborrheic conditions, neoplasia, and immune-mediated dermatoses.[116,243]

Animal Factors

Clinical signs associated with nutritional abnormalities include a sparse, dry, dull, and brittle hair coat that epilates easily; slow hair growth; abnormal scale accumulation; alopecia; erythema; crusting; decubital ulcers; and slow wound healing. Other clinical signs may be present with nutrient-deficient dermatoses (see Chapter 17). For more information on skin diseases, see Chapter 22.

Dietary Factors

Inadequate energy intake is associated with keratinization abnormalities, depigmentation, changes in epidermal and sebaceous glands, and increased susceptibility to trauma. Protein deficiency is associated with similar clinical signs. Essential omega-6 fatty acids include linoleic acid (>0.5% on a dry matter basis) and arachidonic acid (>0.02% on a dry matter basis).[169] Omega-3 fatty acids can supply part of the omega-6 fatty acid component. Clinical signs of essential fatty acid deficiency include scaling, matting of hair, loss of skin elasticity, dry and dull hair coat, erythema, epidermal peeling, otitis externa, and slow hair growth. Certain mineral deficiencies may affect the skin (see Chapter 17). Copper deficiency is associated with loss of normal hair coloration, decreased density or lack of hair, and rough or dull hair coat. Many dermatologic conditions may occur with zinc deficiency and respond to zinc supplementation. Dietary phytate binds zinc, resulting in clinical signs of deficiency. Clinical signs of zinc deficiency include erythema, alopecia, and hyperkeratosis. Certain vitamin deficiencies may affect the skin. Vitamin A deficiency is associated with skin lesions and focal sloughing of skin. Vitamin E deficiency occurs in cats in association with steatitis. Clinical signs include erythema and keratinization defects. Vitamin E–responsive dermatoses include discoid lupus erythematosus, systemic lupus erythematosus, pemphigus erythematosus, sterile panniculitis, acanthosis nigricans, dermatomyositis, and ear margin vasculitis. Dermatologic conditions also arise from food allergies (see Chapter 17).

Feeding Factors

In cats with dermatologic disease, the veterinarian should evaluate the quality and quantity of the diet fed, including treats, snacks, and table food. A complete and balanced diet may be made incomplete or unbalanced when fed with other food stuffs. Homemade diets must be evaluated carefully.[228] If a nutritional deficiency is suspected, the veterinarian should discuss with the owner the possibility of changing the diet to one of a higher quality. With suspected adverse food reaction, a diet change should be considered (see Chapter 17). If a specific nutrient deficiency is identified, the diet might be changed or supplemented accordingly. Zinc is supplemented for zinc-responsive dermatoses (zinc sulfate: 10 to 15 mg/kg per day by mouth; zinc methionine: 2 mg/kg per day by mouth). Vitamin A is supplemented for vitamin A–responsive dermatoses (tretinoin topically every 12 to 24 hours; isotretinoin: 1 to 3 mg/kg per day by mouth; etretinate: 0.75 to 1 mg/kg per day by mouth).

Fatty acid supplementation is often recommended for managing inflammatory skin disease. Cats have a limited capacity to convert 18-carbon long-chain fatty acids to 20-carbon long-chain fatty acids owing to low activity of delta-6-desaturase.[201] It is 20-carbon long-chain fatty acids that are incorporated into cellular membranes and subsequently metabolized to prostaglandins, leukotrienes, and thromboxanes. To alter levels of these cytokines in cats, it is necessary to supplement 20-carbon long-chain fatty acids. Insertion of omega-3 fatty acid (eicosapentaenoic acid [EPA]) into cell membranes results in production of cytokines of the odd-number series (e.g., prostaglandin E_3, leukotriene B_5) in place of the even-number series of cytokines produced from omega-6 long chain fatty acid, arachidonic acid (e.g., prostaglandin E_2, leukotriene B_4). These odd-numbered cytokines promote less inflammation and are more vasodilatory than the even-numbered cytokines. Cats being supplemented with omega-3 fatty acids must receive 20- and 22-carbon fatty acids owing to their limited ability to convert 18-carbon to 20-carbon fatty acids. The 20-carbon omega-3 fatty acid is EPA, and the 22-carbon omega-3 fatty acid is docosahexaenoic acid (DHA). Oils derived from marine life are high in EPA and DHA. Oils derived from plant life, such as flax seed and borage, contain primarily 18-carbon fatty acids, therefore limiting their conversion to the required 20-carbon fatty acid and their effectiveness in managing inflammation. There are no data on the effectiveness of omega-3 fatty acids in managing inflammatory skin diseases in cats.[41]

GASTROINTESTINAL DISEASES

Many disorders of the gastrointestinal system may respond to dietary management, whether or not the disorder is due to diet. For more information on gastrointestinal diseases, see Chapter 23. For information on adverse reactions to food, see Chapter 17.

Types of Foods Used in Managing Gastrointestinal Disease

Gastrointestinal Diets

Gastrointestinal diets are highly digestible with consistent ingredient and nutrient profiles. Highly digestible implies protein digestibility above 87% and fat and carbohydrate digestibility above 90%. These diets contain refined meat and carbohydrate sources with carbohydrates in the largest amount, fortified with fat-soluble vitamins, and contain less than 5% fiber (dry matter basis). The fiber is usually a soluble fiber or mixed fiber source providing substrate for intestinal microbial fermentation.

Fiber-Enhanced Diets

Fiber-enhanced diets contain 15% to 25% fiber (dry matter basis), often insoluble fiber. Soluble fiber increases the viscosity of intestinal contents, delays gastric emptying, slows intestinal transit time, undergoes microbial fermentation, and binds toxins and bile acids. Insoluble fiber is slowly fermentable, has little to no effect on gastric emptying, normalizes intestinal transit time, and increases fecal bulk.

Restricted- and Moderate-Fat Foods

Dietary fat is more digestible and more energy dense than carbohydrate. Average fat digestibility is 74% to 91% in cats. Moderate-fat diets containing 15% to 22% (dry matter basis) are tolerable. Low-fat diets (<10% dry matter basis) necessitate increased food intake to meet caloric needs.

Elimination Foods

Many diets are available with novel protein sources, including protein hydrolysates, duck, venison, rabbit, kangaroo, lamb, and fish.

Gluten- and Gliadin-Free Foods

Several potential antigens are found in flour when cereal grains are processed. Gliadin, a polypeptide, is responsible for gluten-sensitive enteropathies and is found in wheat, barley, rye, buckwheat, and oat flours. It is not present in whole grains and flours produced from rice and corn.

Monomeric Foods

Monomeric foods are water-soluble liquid foods containing nutrients in simple forms. They are hypoallergenic because they require minimal digestion for absorption; however, they are expensive and not very palatable.

Animal Factors

Cats with pharyngeal or esophageal disease have difficulty swallowing food; these diseases are, however, uncommon in cats. Cats with gastric or small intestinal disease often vomit, and they may have diarrhea characterized by large-volume watery feces or inappetence. Poor body condition and weight loss may occur because of the inability to eat, vomiting, or loss of nutrients with diarrhea. Inflammatory bowel disease is the most common cause of small intestinal disease; however, other conditions, such as neoplasia and foreign body obstruction, may occur. Large intestinal disease is usually associated with small-volume firm feces with mucous and/or blood or with constipation or obstipation.

Dietary Factors

Cats with pharyngeal and esophageal disease should be given a high-protein food (>40% on a dry matter basis) because protein increases lower esophageal tone. Feeding a high-fat (>25% on a dry matter basis) diet increases the caloric density of the diet; however, it delays gastric emptying. Therefore if gastric motility and emptying is a concern, a high-fat diet may not be indicated.

Several options exist for nutritional management of cats with inflammatory gastroenteritis.[106,280] In addition to pharmacologic therapy, cats may respond to elimination diets, whether it is a diet containing a novel protein source, a protein hydrolysate diet, or a homemade simple-ingredient diet. Inflammatory reactions are thought to occur through interaction of a protein with an antibody directed against it. *Novel protein* refers to a single dietary protein source that the cat has not been fed before; therefore an inflammatory response would not be evoked.[106] A protein hydrolysate diet involves feeding a diet where the protein has been hydrolyzed to a size that is not recognized by antigen processing cells and antibodies, typically below 12,000 daltons.[43] A homemade diet often comprises single unprocessed ingredients. In processing of foods, glycated protein end-products may be produced through the Mallard reaction and these glycated end-products may induce an inflammatory response. Feeding unprocessed foods decreases exposure to these glycation end products and subsequent inflammatory response.[156]

Cats with large intestinal disease may respond to an elimination diet or to a higher fiber (>5% on a dry matter basis) diet.[63,202,247,280] Dietary fiber increases fecal bulk, which stimulates colonic contraction; however, it increases fecal volume, which could exacerbate constipation.[247] Dietary recommendations for cats with inflammatory bowel disease are summarized in Box 18-2.[61]

Feeding Factors

A change of diet or formulation of diet, including a homemade diet, may be necessary to manage cats with intestinal disease. Feeding smaller meals or restricting the amount consumed at a meal may be beneficial.

HEPATIC DISEASE

The liver is a metabolically active organ involved with digestion and nutrient metabolism, synthesis (e.g. albumin), storage (e.g., glycogen), removal of environmental and endogenous noxious substances, and

BOX 18-2

Dietary Recommendations for Cats with Inflammatory Bowel Disease

1. Fat: 15% to 25% when feeding a highly digestible diet or 9% to 18% on a dry matter basis when feeding a fiber-enhanced diet.
2. Protein: >35% on a dry matter basis. When using a limited protein (elimination) diet, restrict protein to one or two sources and use a protein source that the cat has not consumed previously (novel protein).
3. Fiber: <5% on a dry matter basis for highly digestible diet or 7% to 15% for foods with increased fiber.
4. Digestibility: >87% for protein and >90% for fat and digestible carbohydrate for highly digestible diet, or >80% for protein and fat and >90% for carbohydrate for high fiber diet.

BOX 18-3

Dietary Recommendations for Cats with Hepatobiliary Disease

1. An energy-dense diet containing >4.2 kcal/g
2. Protein: 30% to 45% on a dry matter basis unless hepatoencephalopathy is present: 25% to 30% on a dry matter basis
3. Arginine: 1.5% to 2% on a dry matter basis
4. Taurine: >0.3% on a dry matter basis
5. Potassium: 0.8% to 1.0% on a dry matter basis
6. L-carnitine: >0.02% on a dry matter basis
7. Vitamin E: >500 IU/kg
8. Vitamin C: 100 to 200 mg/kg

metabolism of drugs and toxins. The liver influences nutritional status through bile acid synthesis and excretion into the gastrointestinal tract and its central role in intermediary metabolism of proteins, carbohydrates, fat, and vitamins. The most common causes of feline liver disease include inflammatory conditions (cholangitis–cholangiohepatitis complex), lipidosis, neoplasia (particularly lymphoma), and portovascular anomalies.[194] For more information on liver diseases, see Chapter 23. Nutritional management of hepatobiliary disease is usually directed at clinical manifestations of the disease rather than the specific cause. Goals of nutritional management of cats with liver disease include the following:

- Maintaining normal metabolic processes and homeostasis
- Avoiding and managing hepatoencephalopathy
- Providing substrates to support hepatocellular repair and regeneration
- Decreasing further oxidative damage to damaged hepatic tissue
- Correcting electrolyte disturbances[45]

Animal Factors

Animals with liver disease may demonstrate a variety of clinical signs, from none to hepatoencephalopathy (characterized by ptyalism, vomiting, depression, and possibly seizures). Weight loss and poor body condition may or may not be present depending on the severity and chronicity of the underlying disease. Cats may or may not have hyperbilirubinemia.

Dietary Factors

Maintenance of body condition and weight is important; therefore adequate caloric intake is paramount. Hepatic lipidosis is a result of negative energy balance with mobilization of peripheral adipose tissue and accumulation of intrahepatic lipid.[46] In managing cats with hepatic lipidosis, reversing the negative energy balance is most important in reversing the disease process. Protein restriction is not necessary unless hepatoencephalopathy and hyperammonemia are present. Hypokalemia may occur with liver disease and has been reported in approximately one third of cats with hepatic lipidosis[46]; therefore diet should be potassium replete. Many hepatic diseases are associated with oxidative stress that may induce further hepatocellular damage. Feeding diets with additional antioxidants or supplementing with antioxidants may be beneficial. Hepatic dysfunction entails a dysregulation of lipid metabolism; this is particularly prominent with hepatic lipidosis. L-Carnitine is involved with lipid metabolism, and although L-carnitine deficiency does not occur with hepatic lipidosis,[126] L-carnitine supplementation at 250 to 500 mg daily may be beneficial in cats with hepatic lipidosis.[44]

Dietary recommendations for cats with hepatobiliary disease are summarized in Box 18-3.[194]

Feeding Factors

Feeding small meals or facilitating food intake using pharmacologic stimulation or feeding tubes may be required. Caution must be exercised with administration of medications that require hepatic metabolism, such as appetite stimulants, because side effects may occur.

ENDOCRINOLOGIC DISEASES: OBESITY

Obesity is the most important nutritional disease of cats. With prevalence rate estimates of up to 40%,[8,166,242] obesity must be considered a significant hazard to cats. Increased emphasis on pet health and preventive health programs makes obesity prevention an important aspect of health maintenance programs in dogs and cats. Treatment for obesity varies from frustrating to rewarding, and evaluating and prescribing for successful, long-term weight loss and maintenance usually require management of multiple, interrelated patient and client factors. Diagnosis of disease secondary to obesity and the major task of client education and motivation are the province of the veterinarian.

Obesity is a condition of positive energy balance and excess adipose tissue accumulation that adversely affects the quality and quantity of life. *Obesity* literally means increased body fatness, but measurement of fat fractions of body composition is difficult in practice. Therefore *obesity* can be defined as body weight in excess of 15% to 20% of ideal, owing to the accumulation of body fat.[281] Negative health manifestations often begin at this level of weight excess and are a virtual certainty at a 30% excess over ideal weight. Associated health risks include musculoskeletal and cardiovascular disease, diabetes mellitus, hyperlipidemia, hepatic lipidosis, higher incidence of cancer, possible anesthetic and surgical complications, decreased heat tolerance and stamina, and reproductive problems. Obesity is a proinflammatory condition, and adipose tissue is an active endocrine organ that produces cytokines called adipokines.[168,221] This may explain in part the association of obesity with inflammatory conditions such as osteoarthritis.

The pathogenesis of obesity is multifactorial and is more than just "too much energy in and not enough energy out."[145] There are genetic, gender, and environmental influences. Apartment dwelling, inactivity, middle age, being male, neutered status, mixed parentage, and certain dietary factors are associated with being overweight.[166,242] The pet owner's contribution to the problem may be significant and must be understood and addressed. In one survey of more than 18,000 dog and cat owners in Australia and the United States, almost a third of owners reported their pets as overweight or obese, but fewer than 1% felt that obesity was a health problem.[87] In another study of 120 German owners of indoor cats, questionnaire responses of owners of cats with normal body weight were compared with responses from owners of overweight cats.[133] Owners of overweight cats were more likely to watch their cats eat and relented more frequently when their cats begged for food. Owners of overweight cats were less likely to spend time playing with their cats and appeared to have a different relationship with them, being more likely to anthropomorphize them and consider them a substitute for human companionship.

Diagnosis of obesity is the first step in managing the disease. Determining whether a cat is overweight is not difficult; however, accurately determining the degree of overweight and the cat's ideal weight is challenging. Many owners underestimate their cat's body condition, and veterinarians may overlook obesity. Documenting body weight in the medical record is important; in fact, veterinarians may be part of the problem. In one study medical records dramatically underreported overweight and obesity in cats when body condition scoring (BCS) results were compared to reported diagnoses.[166] For example, the prevalence of obesity defined by BCS in the population studied was 6.4% compared with 2.2% when defined by a recorded diagnostic code in the medical record. In addition to recording the body weight, it may be helpful to calculate the percentage change in weight since the last visit and compare it to a similar weight gain in a person. For example, an 8.8-lb (4-kg) cat that has gained 1 lb (0.5 kg) has increased its body weight by approximately 12%; this is equivalent to a 14-lb weight gain for a 120-lb person.

Muscle condition scoring and BCS provide additional information regarding the appropriateness of the cat's body weight to its overall condition.* Several BCS systems are available; the most widely used are the 5-point and 9-point scales (see Table 16-2).† In both scales the middle value (3/5 or 5/9) is considered optimal condition, and these cats have 15% to 25% body fat. Lower values on the scale are degrees of undercondition (cats having 2/5 or 3/9 have 5% to 15% body fat, and cats having 1/5 or 1/9 have <5% body fat), whereas higher values on the scale are degrees of overcondition (cats having 4/5 or 7/9 have 25% to 35% body fat, and cats having 5/5 or 9/9 have higher than 35% body fat).[265] As additional data are generated, it is likely that revisions of the scales will occur.[265] Muscle condition scoring assesses muscle mass and tone.[196] Evaluation of muscle mass includes visual examination and palpation over the temporal bones, scapulae, lumbar vertebrae, and pelvic bones. Decreased muscle mass may increase morbidity and mortality rates associated with disease.[52]

Animal Factors

The most important step is to recognize that a cat is overweight or obese. The veterinarian should compare the BCS with body weight, especially with historical data from annual examinations. Often a cat's ideal body weight can be determined by finding its weight at about 1 year of age in the medical record. Cats that are obese may show clinical signs of related conditions such as diabetes mellitus, hepatic lipidosis, and osteoarthritis. The veterinarian should take a good dietary history, including the type(s) of food fed, amount(s), and frequency.[195] It is important to gather information about snacks, treats, and table foods that may be fed, as well as access to food in the outdoors if the cat is allowed

*References 10, 40, 56, 144, 145, 167, 239, 241, 242, 274.

†References 10, 40, 143-145, 239, 241.

BOX 18-4

Questions to Ask When Taking a Diet History

1. What types and amounts of food are fed?
   - Include all treats and table food, other pets' food that may be eaten, prey, and food fed by neighbors for outdoor cats.
   - Include food or treats (e.g., Greenies Pill Pockets) used to administer medication.
2. How is the food measured?
   - Who feeds the cat its regular meals? Who gives the cat treats?
   - When and where is the cat fed?
   - Are there other pets in the home? If so, does each pet have a separate feeding station, or can they access each other's food?

access (Box 18-4). It may be helpful to have the owner keep a food diary for 1 or 2 weeks before the weight loss program is initiated. Collecting the information may help make owners aware of the role they play in the cat's obesity, as well as provide useful information.

Dietary Factors

To achieve weight loss to ideal body weight, a change in diet is necessary. Feeding less of the same food is usually unsuccessful because the cat is used to eating the diet, it does not induce a shift in metabolism, and it may lead to deficiencies. There are two dietary strategies for inducing weight loss in cats:

1. Increased-fiber/high-carbohydrate diets:
   - Carbohydrates: <40% on a dry matter basis. Avoid simple sugars and starch.
   - Fiber: 7% to 18% on a dry matter basis
   - Fat: <15% to 17% on a dry matter basis
   - Protein: 30% to 55% on a dry matter basis
   - Food form: Avoid semi-moist foods. Canned foods may facilitate weight loss better than dry foods.
2. Increased-protein/low-carbohydrate diets[267]:
   - Carbohydrates: <20% on a dry matter basis. Avoid simple sugars and starch.
   - Fiber: Usually <5% on a dry matter basis
   - Fat: 12% to 25% on a dry matter basis
   - Protein: 30% to 55% on a dry matter basis
   - Food form: Avoid semi-moist foods. Canned foods may facilitate weight loss better than dry foods.

Which dietary strategy will work in an individual cat is unknown. If one dietary strategy does not work, the veterinarian should switch to the other.

Recently, the first drug licensed for weight loss in veterinary medicine was approved for dogs. Dirlotapide (Slentrol, Pfizer Animal Health) is a selective microsomal triglyceride transfer protein inhibitor. The drug reduces fat absorption and increases satiety signals. However, dirlotapide is contraindicated in cats because it increases the risk of hepatic lipidosis. In multi-pet households in which a dog may be receiving the drug, client education is important to avoid administration of the drug to overweight or obese resident cats.

Feeding Factors

Weight-reduction programs are a multistep approach involving owner commitment, a feeding plan, and repeated communications and monitoring.[145,281] Owners must recognize that their cat is obese and understand associated health risks. Before instituting a weight loss program, the veterinarian should perform a thorough physical examination and obtain a minimum database (complete blood count, chemistry panel, urinalysis) to detect concurrent diseases. Then a feeding plan should be instituted. The veterinarian should first set the amount of calories to be fed on the basis of known or estimated energy requirements (see Chapter 15). Calculate the RER:

$$\text{RER (kcal/day)} = (\text{Body weight}_{\text{kg}})^{0.75} \times 70$$

or

$$\text{RER (kcal/day)} = (\text{Body weight}_{\text{kg}} \times 30) + 70$$

This number is multiplied by a factor of 0.8 to induce a weight loss of 1% to 2% body weight per week. The veterinarian should compare this estimated energy requirement with current caloric intake because some animals require further restriction to induce weight loss.[268] The calculations for an 8-kg cat with an ideal body weight of 5 kg would be as follows:

$$(8\ \text{kg} \times 30) + 70 = 310 \times 0.8 = 248\ \text{kcal/day}$$

Achieving a safe weight loss of 3 kg will take 5 to 9 months.

The veterinarian should choose a commercial diet, as previously described, and recommend that it be fed to meet the energy requirements estimated to induce weight loss. The veterinarian should eliminate or account for additional food and treats in the caloric intake, which should be less than 5% of total daily caloric intake. Some animals tolerate an abrupt change in diet with little problem, although some appear to have fewer gastrointestinal issues if food is gradually changed over a 7- to 10-day period. A new diet may be readily accepted by some cats, but patience will be required with others (Box 18-5).

BOX 18-5
How to Change a Cat's Diet

A transition to a new diet should be performed slowly, especially in cats that have become accustomed to one type or flavor of food. It is easiest to transition cats to a new food that is similar in texture and shape to the old food. Avoid changing a cat's diet when it is stressed by pain, illness, or separation from the owner (e.g., while hospitalized or boarding). Wait until the cat's condition is improved, it is eating normally, and it is at home before switching to a new diet. Patience is a virtue when changing diets; it may take 1 or 2 months for a successful transition in some cases. Educating owners about realistic expectations can help improve compliance. Monitor the cat's body weight during diet transitions, and intervene by returning to the old diet for a few weeks if weight loss greater than 10% occurs.

1. Meal feeding may make the transition to a new diet easier than *ad libitum* feeding because the cat is more likely to be hungry at mealtime. The transition to meal feeding can be made by leaving food out for 1 hour two to three times per day. It is often easiest to start this during the time of day when the owner is normally away from home and cannot be tempted to feed the cat off schedule.
2. Offer the new food along with the old food, rather than abruptly discontinuing the old food. Ideally, both foods should be in the same type of familiar bowl. It may be necessary to offer the new food for several days to a week or even longer before the cat will try it. Once the cat starts consuming the new food, decrease the amount of the old food offered by a small amount each day, with the aim of transitioning totally to the new diet over a 1- to 2-week period.
3. Another method of introducing a new diet involves mixing the old and new foods together. For the first few days, the cat is offered a mix of 75% current food and 25% new food. Then the ratio is changed to 50:50 for the next few days. By the end of the first week, it may be possible to offer 25% current diet and 75% new diet. The amount of the new food is increased thereafter until the cat is consuming 100% of the intended diet.
4. Cats must be exposed to both the smell and the taste of a new food to overcome neophobia. If the new diet is a canned food, it may be helpful to smear a small amount on a front paw to encourage the cat to lick and taste the food.
5. Enhancing the smell and flavor of the new food can be accomplished by warming it slightly or adding small quantities (approximately 1 tablespoon) of tuna or clam juice or low-salt chicken broth.

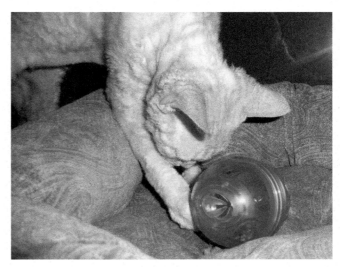

FIGURE 18-2 Food puzzle to encourage energy expenditure by a cat to acquire food. *(Courtesy Steve Dale.)*

The goal of weight reduction is to reduce the cat's excess adipose tissue; however, loss of lean muscle mass occurs as well.[98] Feeding a high-protein diet is associated with less lean muscle loss.[267] Additionally, increased dietary fiber is associated with decreased protein digestibility[75]; therefore high-fiber diets are formulated to account for this. It is important that owners ensure that the obese cat continues to eat because of the risk of hepatic lipidosis. L-Carnitine (250 to 500 mg/day, by mouth) has been shown to be beneficial in preventing hepatic lipidosis with weight loss in obese cats.[24,48] Diets should contain more than 500 ppm.

Although meal feeding is associated with more consistent weight loss, this may not be possible depending on the cat. Providing a measured amount of food during a 24-hour period achieves the same goal. Using food puzzles or hiding food in various locations both provides a more stimulating environment and encourages energy expenditure (Figures 18-2 and 18-3). When feeding dry diets, some owners find using pre-weighed portions of food more acceptable than measuring the amount of food daily in a cup.[23] In multicat households the owner should strive to keep the obese cat from eating food provided for nonobese cats. This can be accomplished by separating the cats and limiting the time for meal consumption. Another strategy is to provide food for the nonobese cats in an area that the obese cat cannot enter (e.g., a box with a hole that only the nonobese cats can fit through). Many owners have become accustomed to using food and treats to enhance the bond with their cat and mistakenly believe that eating is a social event for cats, as it is for humans. In addition, owners often mistake any vocalization as a cry for food. Teaching owners to interact with their cats through play or training sessions may be an important part of the program.

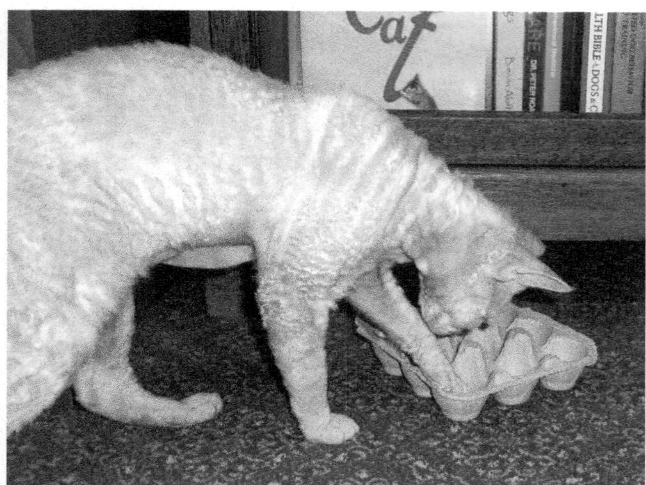

FIGURE 18-3 Placing small amounts of food in different compartments of an egg carton encourages cats to expend energy to acquire food. *(Courtesy Steve Dale.)*

Environmental enrichment for indoor cats can be an integral part of a weight loss program.

Communication and monitoring are important. The cat should be weighed every other week and the body weight charted. Owners should be aware that it may be necessary to adjust the amount of food, especially given that cats often lose weight steadily at the outset of the diet and then plateau. Many obese cats will require up to 12 months for safe weight loss. Many owners find that the cat's learned hunger behaviors (e.g., vocalizing, attention seeking) increase in frequency and intensity once a weight loss plan is in place, and some are unable to cope with this. It is important for the owner to have realistic expectations and to understand and anticipate some of the problems that may arise.

The veterinarian should use positive reinforcement with the client and reward successes. Charting the cat's weight loss on a graph will make progress more apparent. A photograph of the cat can be taken before and after weight loss is achieved and then displayed in the waiting room. Some clients are motivated by certificates of achievement. Once the target body weight has been achieved, the food intake should be adjusted to maintain that weight. It is important that the owner does not revert to old habits, such as letting the cat eat *ad libitum,* feeding it treats, and not ensuring that it get exercise. Owners must understand that long-term portion control will be necessary.

Prevention of obesity is easier than treating obesity in cats. The veterinarian should teach owners how to keep their cat's body condition from lean to optimally conditioned during growth.[9,19,111,120,182] It will be necessary to adjust food intake after neutering because gonadectomy reduces energy requirements, although food intake increases within weeks of surgery. At every veterinary visit, a cat's body weight and BCS should be recorded in the medical record.[111,129,233]

ENDOCRINOLOGIC DISEASES: DIABETES MELLITUS

Diabetes mellitus is the most common endocrine disease in cats. It may be insulin-dependent diabetes mellitus (IDDM), in which absolute insulin deficiency occurs, or non–insulin-dependent diabetes mellitus (NIDDM), in which insulin antagonism occurs; between 50% and 70% of cats with newly diagnosed diabetes mellitus have NIDDM. The goals of managing a cat with diabetes mellitus include achieving and maintaining optimal body condition and maintaining euglycemia. Obese cats with NIDDM may become nondiabetic with weight loss and dietary management.[20,85,135,231] For more information on diabetes mellitus, see Chapter 24.

Animal Factors

Insulin is a major anabolic hormone involved with energy, protein, carbohydrate, and lipid metabolism. With insulin deficiency or insulin antagonism, anabolic metabolic pathways are disrupted, resulting in polyuria/polydipsia, polyphagia, weight loss, muscle mass loss, decreased body condition, and clinical signs of ketoacidosis with progression of IDDM (e.g., vomiting, anorexia, seizures). Cats with NIDDM are typically obese and do not generally develop ketoacidosis. Risk factors identified for NIDDM in cats include indoor confinement and decreased physical activity, likely resulting in obesity and insulin resistance; type of food consumed is not necessarily a risk.[223,248]

Dietary Factors

Dietary management of cats with diabetes mellitus depends in part on whether IDDM or NIDDM is present. For cats with IDDM, timing of meals with insulin administration is advantageous; however, some cats with diabetes mellitus eat small meals even when fed *ad libitum.*[180] Diets that are higher in fiber may increase insulin sensitivity and blunt postprandial hyperglycemia.[135,203] In cats that are underconditioned as a result of unregulated IDDM, feeding a calorically dense diet to increase body weight and condition may be necessary while regulating the IDDM with insulin.

Because cats with NIDDM are typically obese, weight loss is an important component of management. Many cats can go into diabetic remission with a combination of weight loss and insulin treatment[178] or weight loss alone. Traditional diabetic cat diets have been fortified with fiber to reduce postprandial glucose absorption and control weight.[135,203] Many cats respond to being fed

BOX 18-6

Dietary Recommendations for Cats with Diabetes Mellitus

Increased-Fiber/High-Carbohydrate Diets:

1. Carbohydrates: <40% on a dry matter basis. Avoid simple sugars and starch.
2. Fiber: 7% to 18% on a dry matter basis
3. Fat: <15% to 17% on a dry matter basis
4. Protein: 30% to 55% on a dry matter basis
5. Food form: Avoid semi-moist foods

Increased-Protein/Low-Carbohydrate Diets:

1. Carbohydrates: <20% on a dry matter basis. Avoid simple sugars and starch.
2. Fiber: Usually <5% on a dry matter basis
3. Fat: 12% to 25% on a dry matter basis
4. Protein: 30% to 55% on a dry matter basis
5. Food form: Avoid semi-moist foods

low-carbohydrate, high-protein diets. In studies so far, low-carbohydrate, high-protein diets are associated with improved remission rates compared with higher-fiber diets (68% versus 41%) and maintain more lean body mass during weight loss.* However, in cats that do not go into remission and require long-term therapy, there appears to be little difference between the diets. In addition, some cats respond better to high-fiber diets, and weight control may be easier with a less calorically dense food. Canned food is preferred in diabetic cats to maintain hydration, lower carbohydrate content, and improve satiety. Dietary recommendations for cats with diabetes mellitus are summarized in Box 18-6.[279]

The following supplements have been suggested for the management of cats with diabetes mellitus, although they are for the most part unproven:

- Carnitine (250 to 500 mg per day, orally) is important for the breakdown of long-chain fatty acids. By facilitating energy utilization of fats, carnitine protects against muscle catabolism during weight loss. Carnitine has also been shown to suppress ketogenesis and acidosis in starving dogs and protect liver function in fasting cats.[24,48,124]
- Chromium is thought to increase insulin receptor numbers and activity. There are no studies in cats with diabetes, only in healthy cats.[6]
- Vanadium is thought to have insulin-like activity. One study showed vanadium lowered fructosamine, insulin requirements, and clinical signs in diabetic cats; however, vomiting and anorexia were significant side effects.[179]
- The role of taurine in diabetes is still controversial. Taurine is thought to exert antioxidant and antiinflammatory properties that decrease the incidence of diabetic complications such as neuropathy, retinopathy, and cardiovascular disease. Little research has evaluated taurine for use in diabetic cats.
- Supplementation with omega fatty acids in human studies has shown improved lipid metabolism and increased glycolysis in cells; however, they have not been evaluated in cats with diabetes mellitus.

*References 20, 85, 135, 185, 200, 260.

Feeding Factors

The goal is to achieve and maintain optimal body condition and body weight. For cats with IDDM, dietary intake should be matched with insulin administration. For cats with NIDDM, body weight should be decreased from obese body condition to optimal body condition.

ENDOCRINOLOGIC DISEASES: HYPERTHYROIDISM

Animal Factors

Hyperthyroidism is a clinical condition associated with excessive production and secretion of thyroxine (T_4). Most cats are older, with an average age at diagnosis of 13 years. Clinical signs associated with hyperthyroidism are usually polyphagia with weight loss, loss of muscle mass, polyuria/polydipsia, and hyperactivity; hyperthyroidism is also associated with cardiomyopathy. Because hyperthyroidism occurs in older cats, it may be associated with other diseases, most commonly chronic kidney insufficiency, which may become unmasked when the hyperthyroidism is treated. For more information on hyperthyroidism, see Chapter 24.

Dietary Factors

Most cats with hyperthyroidism are underweight and underconditioned; therefore feeding a calorically dense diet may be helpful in restoring body condition and weight. Increasing the fat content of the diet increases the caloric content. Underweight cats should receive a diet containing higher levels of protein; however, caution is necessary because of the association of renal disease with hyperthyroidism. Concentrations of blood urea nitrogen and creatinine should be monitored. If renal azotemia develops with treatment of hyperthyroidism, then dietary protein should be restricted (see the section on renal disease). Nutritional recommendations for feeding underweight cats with hyperthyroidism are summarized in Box 18-7.[279]

BOX 18-7

Dietary Recommendations for Feeding Underweight Cats with Hyperthyroidism

1. Calories: Feed to adult maintenance requirements at estimated or known optimal weight; typically, 1.2 × resting energy requirement
2. Fat: 15% to 25% on a dry matter basis
3. Protein: 30% to 55% on a dry matter basis unless renal disease is present or unmasked with treatment of hyperthyroidism
4. Fiber: <5% on a dry matter basis

Nutritional factors have been implicated in the pathogenesis of hyperthyroidism, although the etiopathogenesis is not known. Epidemiologic studies have identified consumption of commercial canned foods, especially fish or liver and giblets, as a risk for development of hyperthyroidism, which suggests that a goitrogenic compound may be present in the diet.[130,181,207,270] However, no specific goitrogenic factor has been identified. Iodine is one potential dietary goitrogen; however, most commercially prepared cat foods contain adequate amounts of iodine. It is important to note that such studies show association but not necessarily a cause-and-effect relationship. Additional non-nutritional risk factors have been identified, including use of cat litter; being an indoor cat; sleeping on the floor; presence of dental disease; presence of a smoker in the house; use of flea products; and exposure to herbicides, pesticides, or plant pesticides.[130,181,207,270]

Feeding Factors

Cats with untreated hyperthyroidism are often ravenous, although some may show hyporexia (so-called "apathetic hyperthyroidism"), and they often vomit. With treatment appetite often decreases; therefore clients must ensure adequate dietary intake during treatment. Additionally, medical therapy with methimazole or unmasking of renal disease with therapy may occur, resulting in hyporexia or anorexia.

MUSCULOSKELETAL DISEASES: OSTEOARTHRITIS

Osteoarthritis (OA) has multiple etiologies and is characterized by pathologic changes of synovial or diarthrodial joints that are accompanied by pain and disability. Although the prevalence of OA in cats is unknown, radiographic evidence was found in 63 of 292 cats (22%) in one study.[101] Clinical signs of OA in cats include decreased activity, reluctance to jump or climb stairs, decreased grooming, lameness, inappropriate elimination, decreased appetite, and lethargy.[18] For more information on osteoarthritis, see Chapter 26.

Animal Factors

OA occurs more commonly in cats older than 10 years of age. In one study of cats older than 12 years that were examined for reasons other than lameness, 90% of radiographs taken demonstrated OA.[109] Overweight cats are approximately 3 times more likely to present for lameness not associated with cat bite abscess.[241] Obesity may cause excessive forces on joints and articular cartilage, resulting in inactivity and further weight gain; however, obesity is a proinflammatory condition.[38,69,105,282] Therefore obesity may result not only in abnormal mechanical forces on joints but also in production of adipokines, and upregulation of inflammatory pathways associated with obesity may promote joint inflammation and progression of OA.[222]

Dietary Factors

There is a paucity of information concerning nutritional management of OA in cats. Weight loss is an important component of nutritionally managing OA in cats (see the section on obesity). In one study consumption of a diet containing high levels of n3 fatty acids (eicosapentaenoic and docosahexaenoic acid) and supplemented with green-lipped mussel extract and glucosamine/chondroitin sulfate improved activity in cats with OA.[149] There are no studies evaluating supplementation with n3 fatty acids, glucosamine/chondroitin sulfate, antioxidants, or nutraceuticals in cats with OA. As mentioned, n3 fatty acids may alter inflammation through production of odd-numbered cytokines.[15,38,246] Antioxidants scavenge free radicals that are increased with OA and may be beneficial.[17,38] Chondromodulating agents such as chondroitin sulfate and glucosamine may slow progression or alter processes involved with OA, including stimulating cartilage matrix synthesis, inhibiting catabolic enzymes, and increasing fluidity of synovial fluid.[17,38]

Feeding Factors

Obesity should be managed if present. This may require changing from *ad libitum* feeding to meal feeding or changing the diet.

ONCOLOGY

Cancer is among the most common causes of nonaccidental death in cats. Nutritional management of cats with cancer has several goals. Nutritional support can reduce or prevent toxicosis associated with cancer therapy (medical, surgical, radiation, or combination) and ameliorate presumed alterations in metabolism associated with cancer; possibly, specific nutrients can be used to treat cancer directly or indirectly.[240] There are four stages of metabolic alterations that may occur with cancer:

1. Phase 1 is a preclinical phase with no obvious clinical signs; metabolic changes include hyperlactatemia, hyperinsulinemia, and altered amino acid profiles.
2. Phase 2 is associated with early clinical signs, such as anorexia, lethargy, and weight loss; metabolic changes are similar to those of phase 1.
3. Phase 3 is associated with advanced clinical signs, such as cachexia, anorexia, lethargy, and increased morbidity associated with cancer treatment; metabolic changes are more profound than in phases 1 and 2.
4. Phase 4 is recovery and remission; metabolic changes usually persist.[240]

Cancer may cause alterations in metabolism.[206,276] Abnormalities in carbohydrate metabolism include glucose intolerance, insulin resistance, delayed glucose clearance, abnormal insulin secretion, increased glucose turnover, increased gluconeogenesis, hyperlactatemia, and increased Cori cycle activity (the pathway where lactic acid is recycled). Abnormalities of fat metabolism include excessive depletion of body fat relative to protein loss, decreased total body lipid content, increased lipolysis, decreased lipogenesis, hyperlipidemia, increased free fatty acid and glycerol turnover rates, failure of glucose to suppress free fatty acid oxidation, and decreased serum lipoprotein lipase activity. Abnormalities in protein metabolism include increased whole-body protein turnover, increased liver protein fractional synthetic rates, reduced muscle fractional synthetic rates, decreased incorporation of amino acids into muscle, increased hepatic protein synthesis, muscle breakdown, and decreased plasma branched-chain amino acids. Depending on the location and distribution of the cancer, malnutrition may result from interference with eating and digestion (Figure 18-4).

Treatment of cancer also induces problems. Surgery increases nutritional requirements, especially for energy and protein, and may impair food intake or result in malassimilation. Chemotherapy may induce anorexia, vomiting, mucositis, infections, and organ injury. Radiation therapy may cause mucositis or dermatitis. Complications may increase if multimodality therapy is used. For more information on feline oncology, see Chapter 28.

Animal Factors

Depending on the type of cancer, whether it is disseminated, and what treatments are undertaken, a cat with cancer may be optimally conditioned or extremely underconditioned; however, obesity may be associated with certain cancers.[282] In one study of feline cancer patients, fat mass was reduced in 60% and muscle mass was reduced in 91%; cats with suboptimal body condition had a median survival time that was approximately 5 times less than cats that were at least optimally conditioned.[10]

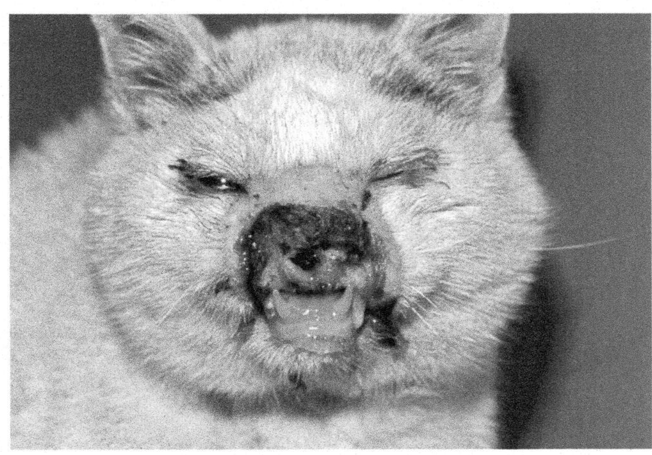

FIGURE 18-4 A 15-year-old castrated male domestic shorthair cat with inability to eat because of facial squamous cell carcinoma.

> **BOX 18-8**
> **Dietary Recommendations for Cats with Cancer**
>
> 1. Carbohydrates: <25% on a dry matter basis
> 2. Fat: 25% to 40% on a dry matter basis
> 3. n3 fatty acids: >5% on a dry matter basis with an n6:n3 fatty acid ratio of approximately 1:1
> 4. Protein: 40% to 50% on a dry matter basis
> 5. Arginine: >2% on a dry matter basis

Dietary Factors

There are no studies on nutritional requirements of cats with cancer. Information on nutritional factors for cats with cancer is derived from information generated primarily from dogs with lymphoma.[205] Cats with cancer may not utilize carbohydrates efficiently but may utilize fat preferentially; therefore a low-carbohydrate, high-fat diet may be beneficial. Protein requirements may be higher to help maintain lean muscle mass. Other nutrients that may be of benefit include n3 fatty acids, antioxidants, and arginine. Nutritional recommendations for cats with cancer are summarized in Box 18-8.[240]

Preventing obesity decreases the risk of cancer in general and of certain types of cancer (e.g., mammary cancer).[117,282]

Feeding Factors

Because many animals have decreased appetite or anorexia, a good dietary history is important. Getting an animal to eat may involve changing food type, texture, or feeding patterns, or it may involve stimulating appetite. Nutritional support is individualized. If possible, the cat should be fed enterally; however, parenteral nutrition may be required. Goals of nutrition include maintaining body condition and lean muscle mass and minimizing nutritional support of the actual cancer.[10]

OPHTHALMOLOGIC DISEASES: HERPESVIRUS INFECTION

Nutritional association with ophthalmologic diseases in cats is minimal, other than those associated with nutrient deficiencies (see Chapter 17); however, lysine and probiotics are associated with management of cats with herpesvirus infection.[68,148,175] For more information on herpesvirus infections, see Chapter 29.

Animal Factors

Cats with active herpesvirus infection usually present for upper respiratory signs and punctate keratitis.[97,172,261] Many cats infected with herpesvirus have latent infections with occasional flare-ups, particularly of ocular disease.[230] During active infections, cats may be anorexic.

Dietary Factors

Lysine, an amino acid, has been shown to be beneficial in managing cats with herpesvirus, although data are contradictory.[68,173-175,224,252] An oral dose of 400 to 500 mg of L-lysine every 12 to 24 hours has been recommended.[174,252] Two studies have been published evaluating L-lysine addition to diets at 5% on a dry matter basis; neither showed benefit.[68,175] There is one small study evaluating a probiotic (*Enterococcus faecium* SF68) in cats with herpesvirus infection; data were inconclusive, although some cats had lessened morbidity.[148]

Feeding Factors

Dietary change is not usually necessary, although cats that are anorexic with active herpesvirus infection may require a calorically dense and palatable diet. Supplemental lysine may be beneficial in some cats.

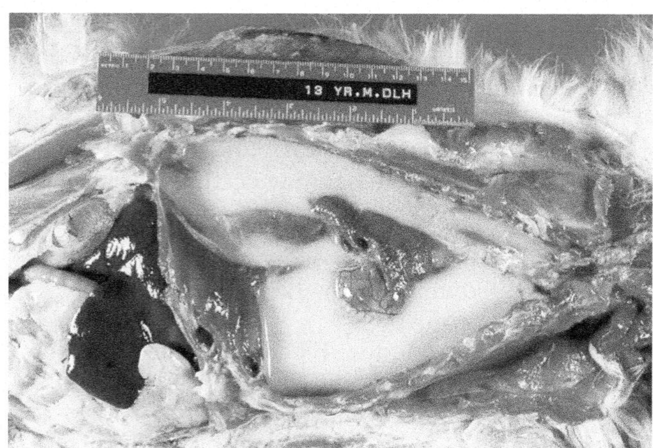

FIGURE 18-5 Chylous pleural effusion in a 13-year-old castrated male domestic longhair cat with idiopathic chylothorax.

PULMONARY AND THORACIC MEDICINE: CHYLOTHORAX

Chylothorax refers to the accumulation of high-fat fluid in the thoracic cavity (Figure 18-5). It may occur as an idiopathic disease or in association with cardiac or intrathoracic disease.* Management of the underlying condition, if identified, may be all that is required to manage chylothorax in a cat. In some cats, however, no identifiable cause is found, and the condition is termed *idiopathic chylothorax*.[21,22,80] Nutritional management of cats with idiopathic chylothorax is directed at decreasing lymphatic flow from the intestinal tract and decreasing accumulation of chyle in the thoracic cavity. For more information on chylothorax, see Chapter 30.

Animal Factors

Cats with idiopathic chylothorax are typically middle-aged.[21,81] Depending on length of duration of chylothorax, the cat may or may not be in optimal body condition.

Dietary Factors

Dietary fat restriction may decrease lymphatic drainage and amount of chyle accumulation in the thoracic cavity. Diets should contain less than 12% to 15% fat on a dry matter basis. Rutin is a citrus flavonoid glycoside found in buckwheat that has been shown to benefit some cats with idiopathic chylothorax and is dosed orally at every 8 hours until resolution of chylothorax; in some cases, indefinitely.[102,139,264] Suggested mechanisms of action for rutin include reduced leakage of lymph from lymphatic vessels, increased protein removal by

*References 21, 78, 81, 82, 113, 118, 157, 189, 191, 271.

lymphatics, increased phagocytosis by stimulation of macrophages, increased recruitment of macrophages in tissues, and increased proteolysis and removal of protein from tissues.[264]

Feeding Factors

Cats with idiopathic chylothorax require a dietary change to a low-fat diet, unless the cat is severely underconditioned. Feeding smaller amounts may decrease chylous effusion. Rutin is beneficial in some cats.

TOXICOLOGY

Foods, whether for human or animal consumption, are supposed to provide nutrients for maintenance of health; however, sometimes the food may be the source of the problem. There are basically two types of toxicities that can occur with pet foods, as with human foods: infectious agents and toxins. Additional adverse food reactions may occur as a result of immunologic and nonimmunologic reactions, such as consumption of an incomplete or unbalanced food or immunologic reaction to a food-borne allergen. Aflatoxin involved in a recent pet food recall was primarily hepatotoxic and often fatal; however, not all dogs exposed to aflatoxin develop disease.[251] Potentially pathogenic and zoonotic bacteria have been identified in dog food, including *Escherichia coli* O157:H7 (enterotoxigenic E. coli),[88] *Salmonella*,[253] *Yersinia enterocolitica, Campylobacter, Clostridium*, and *Listeria*.[280] Additionally, parasites may be transmitted in food, especially uncooked food, such as *Echinococcus, Taenia, Toxocara, Toxoplasma, Trichinella*, and *Neospora*. The Centers for Disease Control and Prevention (CDC) (http://www.cdc.gov) provides information on infectious disease–related food problems (http://www.cdc.gov/ncidod/diseases/food/index.htm). Toxins may be inadvertently or intentionally added to a pet food, or a pet may consume them independent of its diet. Examples of ingested toxins include onions,[232] lilies,[32,107,146,238,254] and melamine–cyanuric acid.[55,155,220,275]

Recognizing food-associated illness can be difficult because cases often present sporadically with no apparent connection. Recognizing clusters of cases geographically (e.g., regionally) or during the same time period (e.g., animals in the same household) is important. The veterinarian should take a good diet history from the owners. Introduction of a new food or a new bag of food, poor palatability, or acceptance of the food by the pet(s), and pets eating the same food whether in the same household or different households may provide clues to problems with diet. The veterinarian should keep in mind that animals may present with similar clinical signs and histories but consume different diets and snacks or treats. The veterinarian should discuss cases with colleagues because they may be having similar experiences. Guidelines for reporting food-related illnesses and adverse effects are summarized in Box 18-9.

> **BOX 18-9**
>
> **Reporting Food-Related Illnesses and Adverse Effects**
>
> 1. Contact the manufacturer. A representative should be willing to listen and take information as well as answer questions regarding other complaints, if any.
> 2. In the United States, contact the Food and Drug Administration (FDA): http://www.fda.gov/AnimalVeterinary/default.htm. Pet food safety issues can be reported to the Safety Reporting Portal: https://www.safetyreporting.hhs.gov
> 3. Contact the American Veterinary Medical Association (AVMA) to report adverse events with drugs, vaccines, and pet food: http://www.avma.org/animal_health/reporting_adverse_events.asp
> 4. To report an adverse event associated with pet food (or other animal feed), contact your state FDA consumer complaint coordinator(s). Contact information can be found at http://www.fda.gov/Safety/ReportaProblem/ConsumerComplaintCoordinators/default.htm. When reporting, include as much information as possible, including the specific product name, lot numbers, veterinarian's report and diagnosis, and any other pertinent information.

It is important to gather as much information as possible and to save as much as food as possible. The veterinarian should document the product name, type of food, manufacturer/distributer information, and date code or best-by code. A copy of the packaging should be retained if possible. If the owner has a copy of the purchase receipt, this may be helpful. The veterinarian should retain samples of the food, keeping at least four cans or pouches of canned or semi-moist food and 1 kg of dry food. The veterinarian should not send all of the samples for analysis but should instead keep or have the owner keep some. The owner should be asked to document consumption of the food by pet(s) with as much detail as he or she can recall. Thorough records, including signalment, clinical signs, and test results, should be kept. If a pet dies, the veterinarian should perform a necropsy or have a necropsy performed, making sure to tell the diagnostic laboratory performing the necropsy that toxicity is suspected. Tissue and fluid samples should be taken, if possible. All communication with the manufacturer and with the Food and Drug Administration (FDA) and the American Veterinary Medical Association (AVMA) should be documented. If other pets may have been exposed, they should also be tested.

Pet food toxicities occur commonly, although less so than in human beings. The CDC estimates that 76 million Americans get sick, more than 300,000 are hospitalized, and 5000 die from food-borne illnesses annually. After eating contaminated food, people can develop anything from a short, mild illness, often mistakenly referred to as "food poisoning," to a life-threatening illness. The veterinarian should be suspicious of a food-related disease, especially if trends in households, food consumed, or clusters of cases geographically are evident. Food and information should be saved as described. Owners should be instructed to discontinue feeding the suspected food immediately. As a short-term solution, owners can give their pets home-prepared meals, if they wish. To minimize risk of food poisoning in pets, owners should do the following:

- Prevent pets from eating garbage or carrion.
- Cover and refrigerate unused portions of wet food.
- Refrain from feeding pets foods that have a suspicious appearance or odor.
- Use stainless steel bowls and utensils, and clean them well.
- Store dry foods in a cool, dry location free of pests.

The Veterinary Information Network (http://www.vin.com) has a list of frequently asked questions and information about homemade pet foods. It was developed during the pet food crisis triggered by the melamine–cyanuric acid recall (Box 18-10).

CRITICAL CARE

Critical illnesses may be caused by factors such as trauma and acute or chronic disease and often result in inappetence. Nutritional support is indicated in animals that have not eaten for 3 to 5 days, have poor body condition, or have increased needs for nutrition.[49,50,212] A few days of food deprivation is not detrimental to healthy cats; however, it may be detrimental to a sick cat. Short periods of not eating are not a problem because the body is able to utilize endogenous energy substrates such as glycogen. During prolonged food deprivation, the body shifts to a hypometabolic state to conserve structural and functional proteins as much as possible; thus glucose and fatty acids become the major energy sources. During periods of food deprivation associated with stress and illness, however, the body cannot utilize fatty acids or glucose efficiently. Therefore amino acids are mobilized and used for gluconeogenesis, for DNA and RNA synthesis, and for acute phase protein production. Malnutrition occurs rapidly.[123,190,193,217] It is important to remember

BOX 18-10
Generic Adult Dog and Cat Homemade Food Recipe*

This recipe should be fed for not more than 2 months. Clinicians are advised to set up a consultation with the client at the end of this period to revisit feeding requirements and consider either re-instituting commercial food products or consulting with a clinical nutritionist.

This diet is adequate for healthy dogs and cats over 6 months of age:

- 1 pound fresh boneless skinless chicken breast
- 2⅔ cups cooked white rice
- 1 tablespoon safflower oil
- ¼ teaspoon Morton Lite Salt (Morton International, Inc.)
- ¼ teaspoon iodinated salt
- 3 grams of calcium carbonate without vitamin D: Use Tums Regular Strength (GlaxoSmithKline), 6 tablets (each contains 500 mg calcium carbonate, which provides 200 mg of elemental calcium). Other calcium preparations contain different amounts of calcium. For example, Tums 500 contains 1200 mg of calcium carbonate, providing 500 mg of elemental calcium.
- 1 Centrum (Wyeth Consumer Healthcare) adult multivitamin–mineral supplement (do not use Silver, Ultra Women's, Ultra Men's, or any other version)
- ¼ teaspoons taurine powder (or 500-mg tablet) (Taurine is optional for dogs but essential for cats.)

Sauté chopped chicken breast in oil until thoroughly cooked. Add rice and salt. Grind Tums (calcium carbonate), multivitamin–mineral tablet, and taurine supplement together. Add to cooled mixture. Store in refrigerator. Larger batches may be prepared in advance and stored in the freezer.

Nutritional Profile

- 40% protein (dry matter basis [DMB])
- 12% fat DMB
- 6% calcium DMB
- 4.3% phosphorus
- 1.4:1 calcium:phosphorus
- Calories: 1046 kcal per batch or 1.12 kcal/g
- Batch size: 932 g

To feed, calculate caloric needs, and divide into two or more daily feedings. One recipe batch should provide adequate intake for a 40- to 45-pound dog for 1 day. Adjust intake to maintain ideal body weight.

*Courtesy Veterinary Information Network, http://www.vin.com.

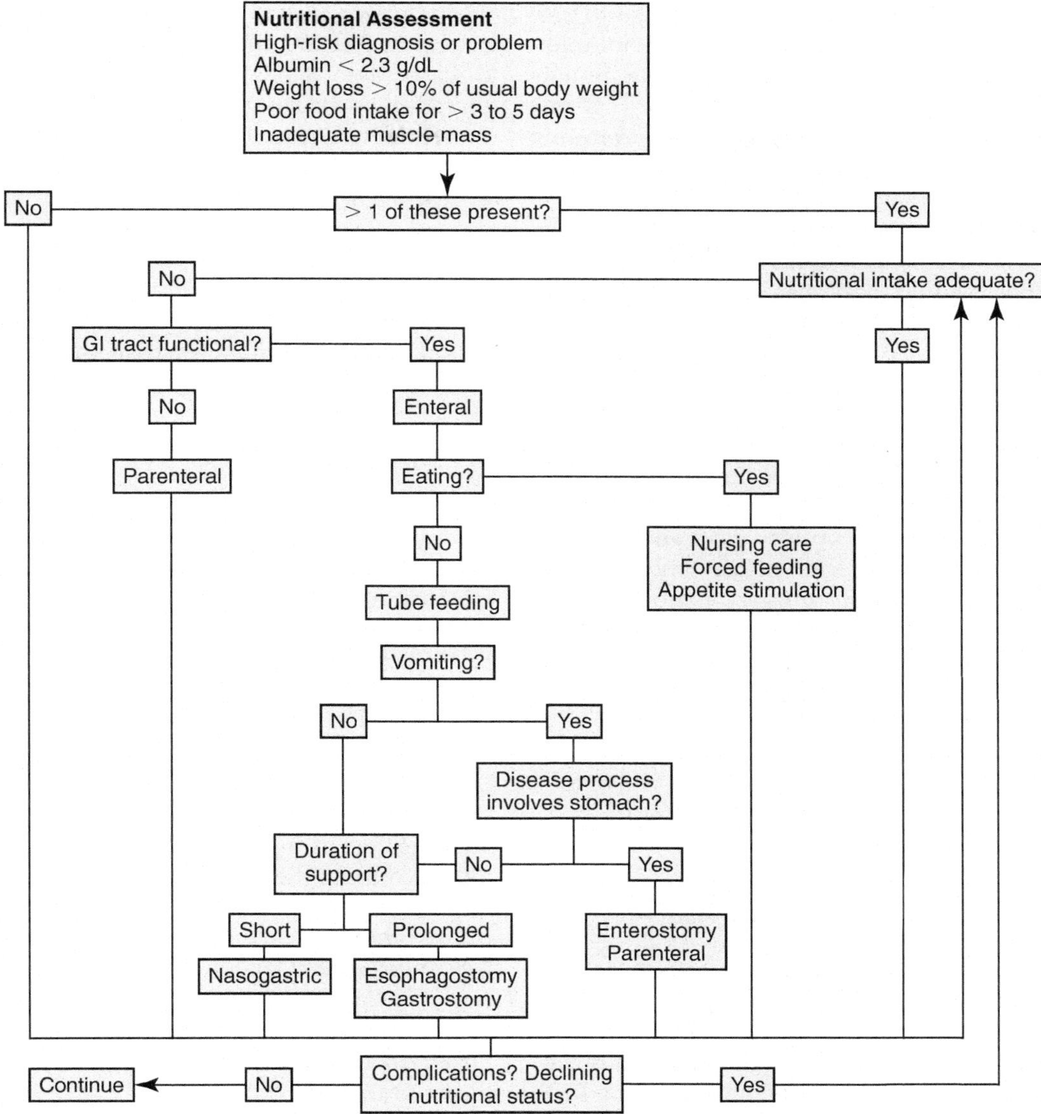

FIGURE 18-6 Algorithm for nutritional support.

that administration of parenteral fluids containing 5% dextrose does not provide nutritional support as 1 mL of 5% dextrose provides 0.17 kcal. For a 5-kg cat, it would require 1294 mL of 5% dextrose per day to meet RERs.

Goals of nutritional support for critical care patients are as follows:

1. To minimize metabolic derangements
   - Maintain hydration
   - Attenuate acid-base disorders
   - Attenuate electrolyte disturbances
   - Provide disease-specific nutrients
2. To provide nutrients to facilitate recovery
   - Suppress hypermetabolic response
   - Restore or reverse protein catabolism and negative nitrogen balance
   - Maintain gastrointestinal tract integrity and function
   - Optimize immune function
3. To maintain lean body mass and body weight
4. To avoid complications associated with refeeding

There are two main "Golden Rules" of nutrition: (1) If the gut works, use it; and (2) keep it simple (Figure 18-6). Nutrition should be provided enterally, when possible, because it is the easiest, safest, and most physiologic route. As much of the gastrointestinal tract should be used as possible. Not only does the enteral route provide nutrients for the whole animal; it also provides nutrition to enterocytes. Maintenance of enterocyte health is important to prevent bacterial translocation from the gastrointestinal tract into the systemic circulation or lymphatics and to facilitate recovery by the animal.[62] There are some potential disadvantages to providing nutritional enterally: Some patients cannot tolerate enteral feeding, some patients cannot assimilate nutrients when provided enterally, and there is a risk of aspiration pneumonia if regurgitation or vomiting occurs. Parenteral nutrition is limited to comatose or paralyzed patients or those with severe gastrointestinal dysfunction such as intractable vomiting, malassimilation syndromes, severe pancreatitis, and peritonitis. Parenteral nutrition should be considered in animals in which provision of nutrients is not feasible using the enteral route.

Animal Factors

The first step in providing nutritional support is to determine whether nutritional support is indicated (see Figure 18-6). This decision is based on historical and physical examination findings. A thorough history and complete physical examination with appropriate diagnostic testing is required before initiating nutritional support. It is important to ensure that the cat is able to eat. Severe periodontal disease and oral cancer are examples of reasons that cats may be unable to eat.

The RER is estimated by the following:

$$\text{RER (kcal/day)} = (\text{body weight}_{kg})^{0.75} \times 70$$

or

$$\text{RER (kcal/day)} = (\text{body weight}_{kg} \times 30) + 70$$

In critical care, hospital, or illness-associated conditions, RER is multiplied by 1. In other words, the goal is to provide RER to most patients. Exceptions to this include cases of severe trauma, head injury, and burns, in which energy requirements are greater than RER, often being more than twice the RER.[57,76,186,225] Protein requirements vary depending on whether enteral nutritional support or parenteral nutritional support is provided. For enteral nutritional support, adult cats should be fed 6 g of protein/body weight$_{kg}$ per day. Cats requiring protein restriction (e.g., renal failure or hepatoencephalopathy) are fed less (3 to 5 g of protein/body weight$_{kg}$ per day), whereas cats requiring protein supplementation (e.g., those with protein-losing nephropathy or peritonitis) are fed more (>6 g of protein/body weight$_{kg}$ per day).[158,159,212,229,262] For parenteral nutritional support, protein requirements are based on caloric intake. Adult cats should be provided 6 g of protein/100 kcal per day, whereas cats requiring protein restriction are provided 3 to 5 g of protein/100 kcal per day and cats requiring protein supplementation are provided more than 6 g of protein/100 kcal per day. Taurine is an essential amino acid for cats and is not provided in parenteral solutions. Water is provided by nutritional support because most anorexic cats do not drink. Maintenance fluid requirements for adult cats are approximately 60 mL/kg per day but may be more with diseases associated with fluid loss (e.g., renal failure, diarrhea, peritonitis).[183] Finally, the veterinarian should determine whether there are other nutrients of interest such as taurine and n3 fatty acids that should be added or restricted from nutritional support.

Dietary Factors

Choice of diet depends on several factors, including provision or exclusion of disease-specific nutrients and route of nutritional support.

Feeding Factors

Nutritional support may be accomplished using the enteral or parenteral routes. The route chosen depends on the individual patient and its ability to use the gastrointestinal tract (see Figure 18-6).

Enteral Route

Enteral nutrition may be accomplished by several means.

NURSING CARE AND COAXING

Sometimes good nursing care is all that is necessary to stimulate an animal to eat. This may include hand feeding the cat, using a highly palatable energy-dense food, warming the food to body temperature (especially important for cats), adding water to food, providing praise when the cat eats, and feeding the cat in a stress-free environment that is away from competition. Many cats will not eat while hospitalized but will eat voluntarily at home. Although anorectic cats often require hospitalization for diagnostic and therapeutic purposes, they should be hospitalized for the least amount of time possible. When food is offered, the cat should be stroked and given vocal reassurance to encourage voluntary food consumption. Although changing the diet or mixing diets may stimulate appetite, some cats may not accept a change in diet texture. If a cat has a nasal discharge, the nares should be cleaned. Sometimes these efforts are successful, particularly if it is an acute disease that is transient; however, if anorexia persists, other means should be considered.

APPETITE STIMULANTS

Some drugs may stimulate appetite (see Table 18-1). They do not work all the time, but when they do work, more aggressive means of nutritional support may not be necessary. Several pharmacologic agents have been used with variable success in veterinary medicine. Mirtazapine is, in part, a serotonin antagonist that has antiemetic and appetite-stimulatory properties. Diazepam[171] may cause sedation and should be used cautiously in cats with liver disease because it may induce hepatic

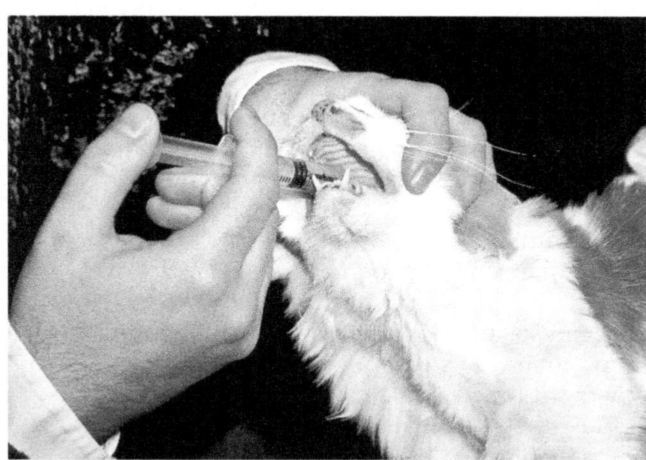

FIGURE 18-7 Administration of a bolus of a homogeneous canned food using a syringe.

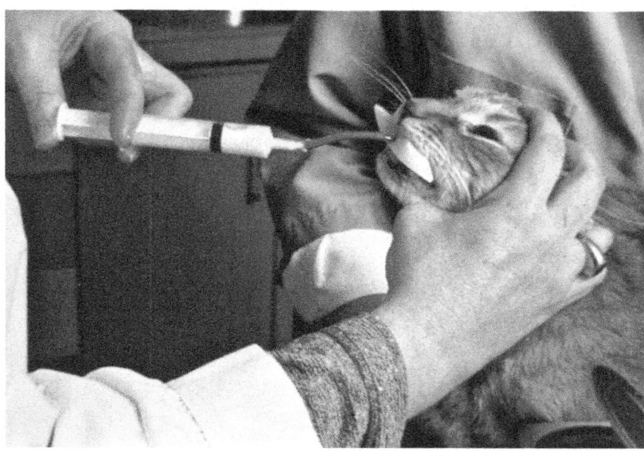

FIGURE 18-8 Nutritional support using an orogastric feeding tube in a 4-year-old castrated male cat.

failure.[47] Glucocorticoids are associated with side effects such as catabolism and insulin antagonism, which limits their usefulness as appetite stimulants.[197] Anabolic steroids are not as effective as benzodiazepines and may be associated with hepatotoxicity when used for prolonged periods.[110] Also, there may be a lag phase between beginning their administration and onset of appetite stimulation. Megestrol acetate[58] may induce diabetes mellitus, adrenal suppression, and mammary neoplasia in cats.[54,119,170,197,219] None of these drugs works consistently, and none has been evaluated under controlled conditions.

FORCED FEEDING

Boluses of food in the oropharynx will stimulate swallowing. This may be accomplished by forming the canned food into a meatball shape or using a syringe. Canned food gruels or convalescent canned veterinary products may be administered through a syringe (Figure 18-7). Forced feeding is easy to perform; however, it may add additional stress to a sick animal. Furthermore, it is difficult to do for more than a few days, and most cats do not tolerate it well.

TUBE FEEDING

Enteral feeding may be done by placing a tube within the gastrointestinal tract.[7,49,212] Such tubes include orogastric, nasoesophageal, pharyngostomy, esophagostomy, gastrostomy, and enterostomy tubes.

OROGASTRIC FEEDING TUBE

Passing a feeding tube through the mouth into the distal esophagus or stomach is technically easy to do (Figure 18-8); however, it is usually stressful to adult cats. It is often used to provide nutrition to orphaned kittens.

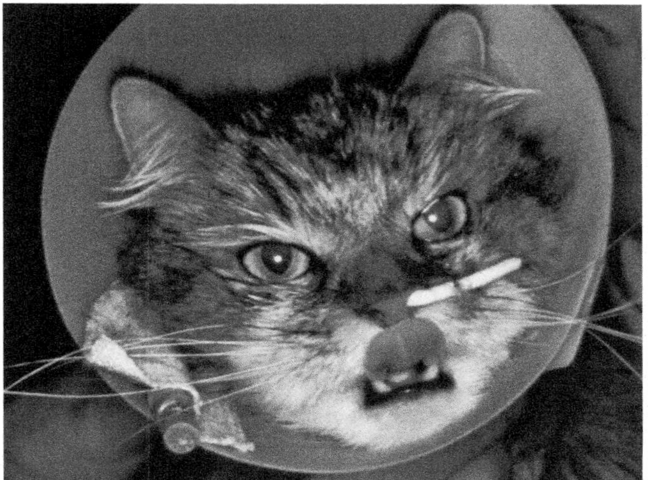

FIGURE 18-9 Nasoesophageal feeding tube.

NASOESOPHAGEAL FEEDING TUBE

Nasoesophageal feeding tubes are technically easy to place and can be used safely in many animals (Figure 18-9).[1] They should not be used if the patient is comatose or lacks a gag reflex because of risk of aspiration. Nasoesophageal feeding tubes probably should not be used in animals with esophageal motility disorders. These tubes may be placed without general anesthesia. Complications of nasoesophageal feeding tubes include rhinitis, dacryocystitis, esophageal reflux, vomiting, aspiration, pneumonia, inadvertent tube removal, and obstruction of the tube.

PLACEMENT[29]

- Place 0.5 to 1 mL 0.5% proparacaine hydrochloride into one of the nasal cavities of the cat. Tilt the head up to encourage the local anesthetic to coat the nasal

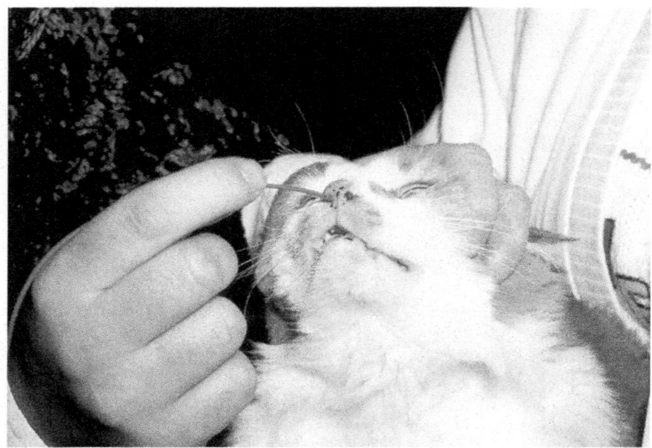

FIGURE 18-10 Insertion of a red rubber feeding tube into the ventral nasal cavity of a cat for nutritional support using a nasoesophageal feeding tube.

mucosa. Repeat the application to ensure adequate local anesthesia.

- If the cat is too stressed to place the tube, induce light sedation or a light plane of anesthesia.
- In general, for cats weighing less than 3 kg, choose a 5 Fr tube. For cats above 4 kg, an 8 Fr tube can often be inserted. Polyvinyl chloride feeding tubes or red rubber catheters are best because of their flexibility. Polyurethane tubes may be preferable for long-term feedings because of their resistance to degradation.[245] Use a tube that is radiopaque to facilitate radiographic confirmation of placement.
- Measure the length of the tube on the side of the animal from the nasal planum to the last rib. If the tube is to terminate in the stomach, mark the tube at the proximal end with tape as a butterfly. If the tube is to terminate in the thoracic esophagus, pull the tube back 1 to 5 cm and place the butterfly tape at the proximal end. Nasogastric intubation is not usually associated with complications because of the small diameter of the tube.
- Lubricate the tube with 5% lidocaine jelly before insertion. Maintain the cat's head in a normal position to avoid tracheal intubation. A guidewire may be used for small and flexible tubes.
- Insert the tube caudoventrally and medially into the nasal cavity (Figure 18-10). Flex the cat's head to facilitate passage into the oropharynx and esophagus. The tube should pass into the oropharynx and stimulate a swallowing reflex. When the cat swallows, pass the tube into the esophagus to the predetermined distance.
- Inject 3 to 5 mL of sterile saline into the tube to confirm placement in the esophagus. If a cough is elicited, remove the tube and attempt placement again. For additional confirmation, inject 6 to 12 mL of air in the tube and auscult for borborygmus at the xiphoid. If there is still uncertainty or if the cat is under general anesthesia, a lateral thoracic radiograph gives definitive confirmation.
- Secure the correctly positioned tube to the lateral aspect of the nose with the preplaced butterfly tape and again at the zygomatic arch. This can be done with sutures. Most cats will tolerate the tube without an Elizabethan collar.
- Place a column of water in the tube and cap it when not in use, and occlude the end with an infusion cap, three-way stopcock, or hypodermic needle cap (without the needle). This prevents intake of air, reflux of esophageal contents, and occlusion of the tube by diet.

ESOPHAGOSTOMY FEEDING TUBE

Esophagostomy tubes are easy to place, and a large-bore (>12 Fr) feeding tube may be placed in most animals.* Advantages of an esophagostomy feeding tube are that there is no interference with voluntary consumption of food, and gruels may be used because of diameter of the tube. Esophagostomy tubes must be placed under heavy sedation or general anesthesia. The distal tip of the tube should terminate in the distal esophagus and not the stomach to prevent gastroesophageal reflux and esophagitis.[59] They should not be used in cats with esophageal motility disorders. Additional complications include inflammation and infection at the tube exit site and vomiting.[154] Vomiting may occur as a result of the underlying disorder, overly rapid administration of food, or failure to warm food to almost body temperature.

PLACEMENT[266]

- Anesthetize and intubate the cat, and position it in right lateral recumbency; shave and prep the cervical area from the base of the ear to the point of the shoulder (Figure 18-11, *A*).
- Insert a speculum to hold the mouth open.
- Pass the curved end of a curved Carmalt forceps through the oral cavity and into the mid to proximal esophagus.
- Palpate the curved end of the forceps, and make a 1-cm skin incision over the end (see Figures 18-11, *B* and *C*).
- Continue the incision through the subcutaneous tissue and esophageal wall, and exteriorize the curved tips of the forceps.
- Grab the distal end of the feeding tube with the curved forceps, and pull the tube through the incision into the oral cavity and out of the mouth (see Figures 18-11, *D* and *E*).

*References 60, 64, 108, 125, 128, 154, 269.

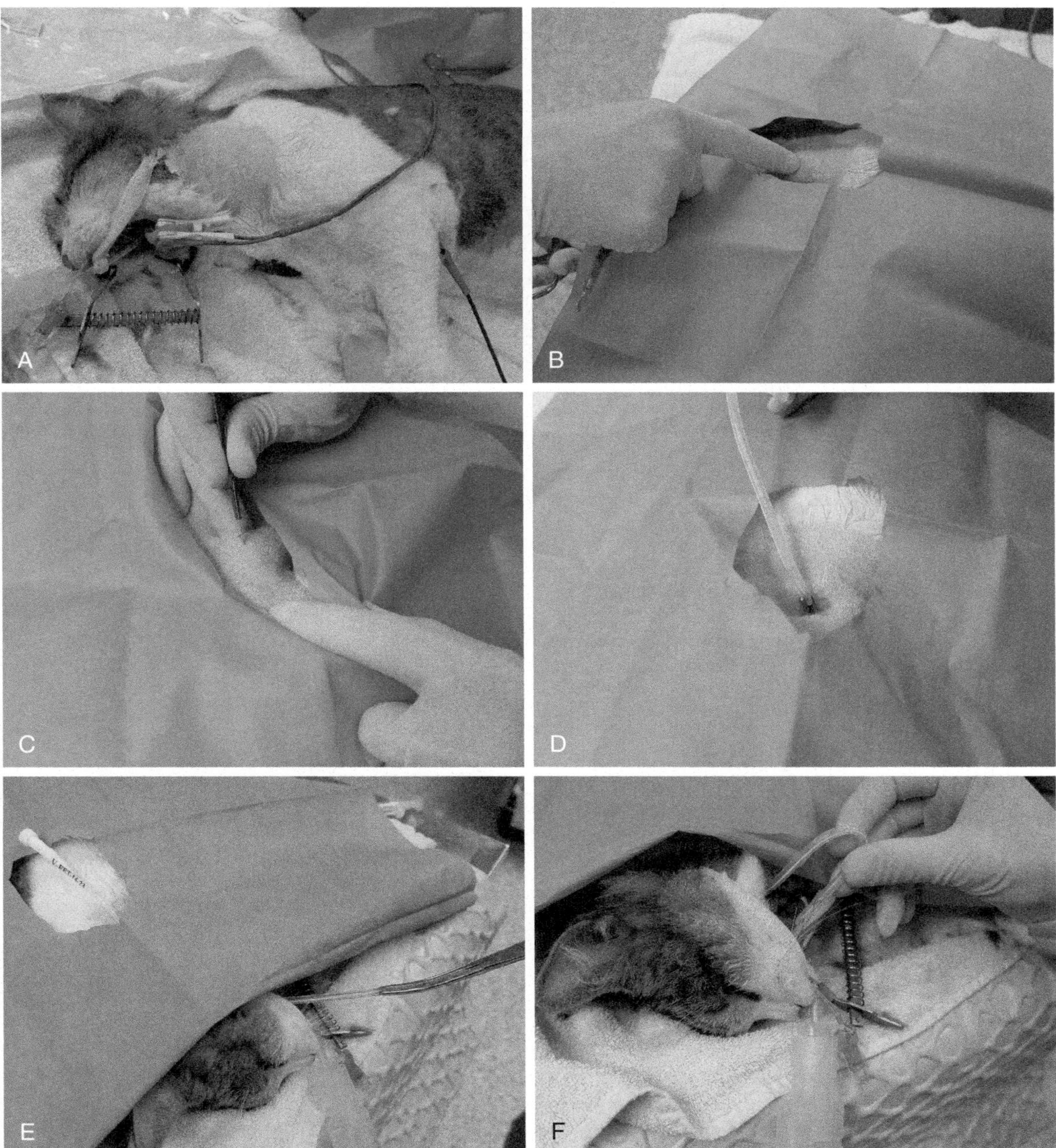

FIGURE 18-11 **A,** Placement of an esophagostomy feeding tube. Anesthetize and intubate the cat, and position in right lateral recumbency; shave and prep the cervical area from the base of the ear to the point of the shoulder; insert a speculum to hold the mouth open. **B** and **C,** After passing the end of a curved Carmalt forceps through the oral cavity and into the mid-esophagus, palpate the end of the forceps through the skin and make a 1-cm incision. **D** and **E,** Grab the distal end of the feeding tube with the forceps, and pull the tube through the incision into the oral cavity and out of the mouth. **F,** Redirect the distal end of the feeding tube into and down the esophagus by hand or using the forceps to the premeasured mark.

Continued

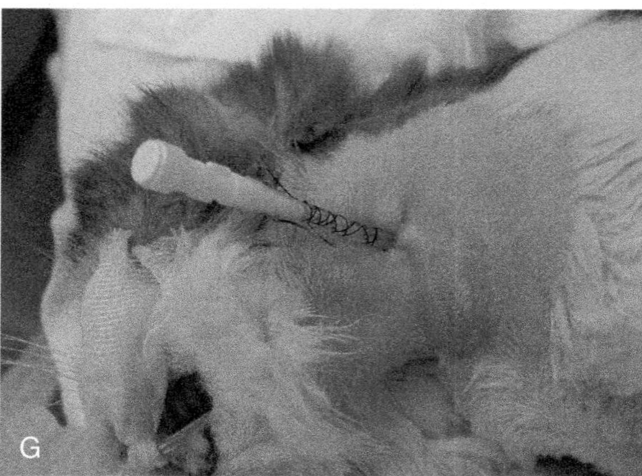

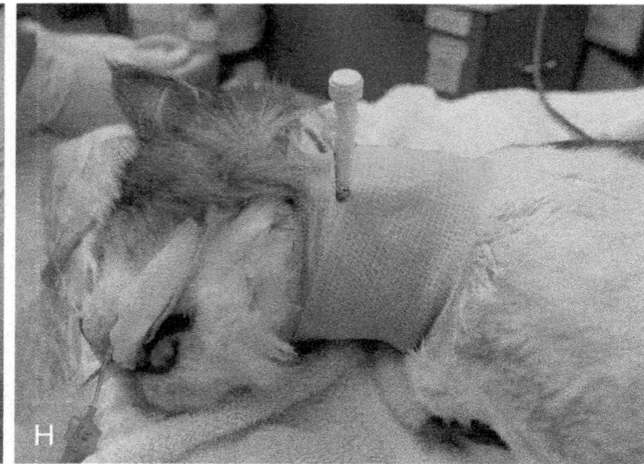

FIGURE 18-11, cont'd **G** and **H,** Secure the tube to the patient's neck at the exit point with a finger trap suture and bandage lightly. *(From Chan DL: The inappetent hospitalised cat: clinical approach to maximising nutritional support,* J Feline Med Surg *11:925, 2009.)*

- Redirect the distal end of the feeding tube into and down the esophagus to the premeasured mark. The distal end is grasped as it exits the oral cavity and is inserted down the esophagus by hand or using the forceps (see Figure 18-11, *F*).
- Secure the tube to the patient's neck at its exit point with a finger trap friction suture (see Figures 18-11 *G* and *H*). The tube may be incorporated into a light neck bandage,
- A column of water is placed in the tube after food administration and the end closed with a three-way stopcock, infusion plug, or hypodermic needle cap (without the needle),
- When the tube is ready to be removed, no sedation is required. The sutures are removed, and the tube is gently pulled out. The stoma site is left to close by second intention.

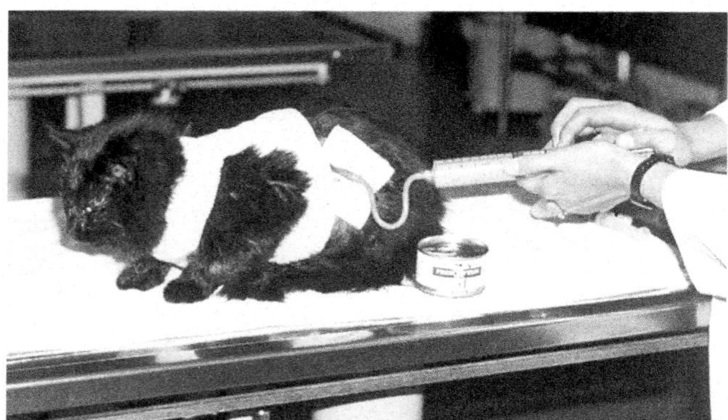

FIGURE 18-12 Providing nutritional support to a 6-year-old spayed female domestic shorthair cat with idiopathic hepatic lipidosis using a percutaneous endoscopically placed gastrostomy feeding tube.

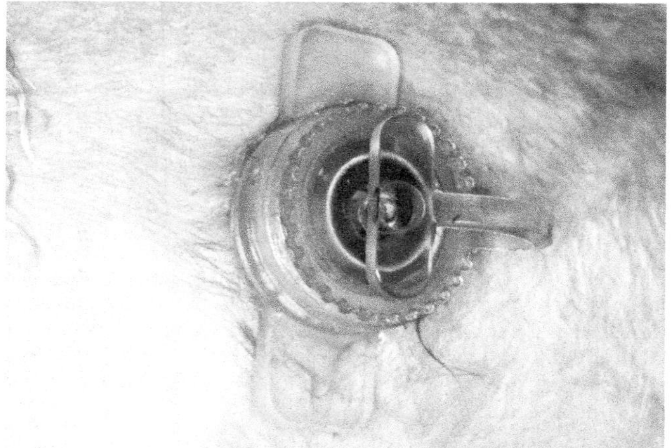

FIGURE 18-13 Low-profile gastrostomy feeding tube.

GASTROSTOMY FEEDING TUBE

Gastrostomy feeding tubes may be placed surgically through a small laparotomy incision or at the time of abdominal surgery, or non-surgically using an endoscope (percutaneous endoscopic gastrostomy tube) or nonendoscopically.* Advantages of a gastrostomy tube are that they can be used in animals with esophageal or higher disease, a large bore feeding tube (16 to 24 French) can be used so pet food gruels may be administered, they can be used for extended periods of time (months to years), and there is no mechanical inhibition of voluntary food consumption (Figure 18-12). Cats tend to tolerate gastrostomy feeding tubes well. In addition, a low profile gastrostomy feeding tube device may be used for extended periods of time (Figure 18-13). Complications with use of gastrostomy feeding tubes include vomiting with risk of aspiration pneumonia (often associated with administering cold food or with administering food too quickly), dislodgement of the tube which may result in peritonitis or cellulitis, peristomal infections, and difficulties in maintaining bandages on cats.

*References 7, 33, 90, 100, 127, 164, 192, 250, 263.

ENTEROSTOMY FEEDING TUBE

Enterostomy feeding tubes are usually 5 Fr tubes that are placed directly into the duodenum or jejunum either surgically or percutaneously using endoscopy.[7,84,115,127,176] Placement of an enterostomy feeding tube can be done at the time of surgery; therefore careful planning is necessary to avoid a second surgery. Advantages of an enterostomy feeding tube are that they bypass the stomach and therefore can be used in animals undergoing gastric surgery or in cats with pancreatitis. Usually, liquid enteral diets are administered through a 5 Fr feeding tube using constant-rate infusion.

Selection of a diet administered through a feeding tube depends on the diameter of the feeding tube and location of its termination within the gastrointestinal tract. Liquid diets or homogenous gruels of canned foods can be administered through 5 Fr and larger feeding tubes. Gruels of canned foods can be administered through 10 Fr and larger feeding tubes. When using gruels, the veterinarian should ensure that no large pieces of food or dietary constituents are present that may clog the tube.

Begin tube feeding by administering warm water through the tube. If this is well tolerated, then divide the first day's administration of diet into 6 meals, and administer every 4 hours. If this is tolerated, increase the volume of food administered and decrease the frequency of feeding. Many cats can tolerate 2 to 3 bolus feedings daily by feeding tube. Constant-rate infusions are used for enterostomy tubes and are begun at one half the calculated administration rate for the first 6 to 12 hours and then increased to full rate if well tolerated. Ensure that the feeding tube is properly situated before feeding by infusing approximately 6 to 12 mL of warm water through the tube and observing for clinical signs of discomfort. After administration of the meal, flush the tube with 6 to 12 mL of warm water and cap the tube, leaving a column of water inside the tube; this will help prevent occlusion of the tube with food.

Parenteral Nutrition

Parenteral nutrition may be used for short-term nutritional support, if enteral nutrition cannot be used or to supplement enteral food intake.* Parenteral nutrition is often considered to be "total" if all components are used and "partial" if selected components are used. In reality, parenteral nutrition in veterinary medicine is not complete and is therefore not "total." It is better to consider parenteral nutrition as either centrally administered, in which the solution is hypertonic, or peripherally administered, in which the solution is isotonic to plasma. Components of parenteral nutrition include 3.5% to 10% amino acids with or without electrolytes (protein source); 5% to 50% dextrose (carbohydrate source); 20% lipid emulsion (fat source); and vitamins, minerals, and electrolytes (Figure 18-14). Frequently, vitamins, other than B-complex vitamins (1 mL per liter of parenteral fluids), and minerals are excluded from parenteral nutrition formulations in cats.[198] Isotonic fluids used in parenteral nutrition are 3.5% amino acids and 5% dextrose. Lipid emulsions do not exert tonicity, although they can decrease the tonicity of the final solution. As a general rule, solutions that are above 600 mOsm/kg (approximately two times plasma osmolality) should be administered only through a centrally placed venous catheter.

Parenteral nutritional solutions must be prepared aseptically and are administered for no longer than 3 days owing to potential contamination and breakdown of the lipid emulsion. Prepared parenteral nutritional solutions may be refrigerated for up to 7 days. Venous catheters used for administration of parenteral nutritional solutions should be used only for nutritional support; they should not be used for blood sample collection or administration of medications.

CENTRALLY ADMINISTERED PARENTERAL NUTRITION

Centrally administered parenteral nutrition solutions are formulated and compounded to provide amino acids, dextrose, lipids, electrolytes, and B-complex vitamins; they may contain trace minerals and other vitamins (total admixture). They are hypertonic and must be administered through a centrally located venous catheter. Energy requirements are calculated as previously explained, and dextrose and lipid are used to meet these energy requirements; some recommend including calories provided by amino acids. The caloric content of 50% dextrose is 1.7 kcal/mL and that of 20% lipid is 2 kcal/mL. In most cases the ratio of dextrose to lipid ranges from 40:60 to 60:40, although other ratios may be used depending on the patient.[158,159,229] Protein requirements

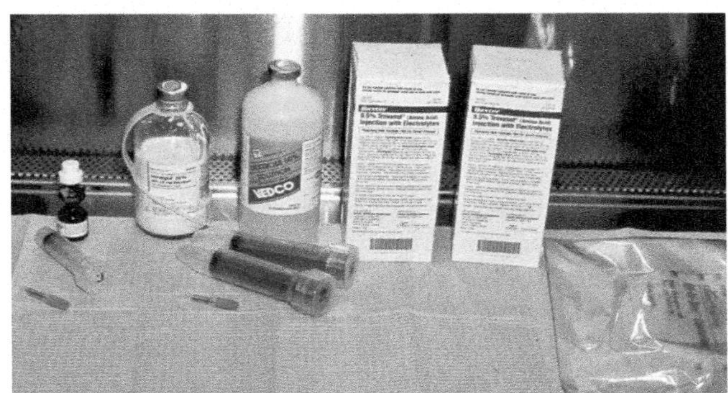

FIGURE 18-14 Components of parenteral nutrition, including multivitamin for infusion, lipid emulsion, dextrose, and amino acid solution.

*References 49, 51, 53, 158-160, 212, 262.

are calculated as previously described, and volume of amino acid infused is determined by the solution used; 8.5% amino acid solution provides 0.085 g/mL, and 10% amino acid solution provides 0.1 g/mL. Electrolytes are provided as a component of the amino acid solution, added as a supplement, or added as a balanced crystalloid to the parenteral nutrition solution. Vitamins are added as 1 mL of B-complex vitamins/L solution, although multivitamin and trace mineral solutions are available for addition to parenteral nutrition solutions.[198] Begin the infusion at ½ of estimated rate for the first 8 to 12 hours. At that time, check concentrations of blood glucose and urea nitrogen and inspect the plasma for lipemia; if concentrations are within normal reference range and lipemia is not apparent, increase the rate to full administration and re-evaluate a biochemical panel after an additional 8 to 12 hours. Do not abruptly cease administration of centrally administered parenteral nutrition; decrease the rate by ½ for 8 to 12 hours, and then discontinue. Complications of centrally administered parenteral nutrition are related to the catheter or solution (e.g., sepsis, thrombophlebitis, inadvertent catheter removal) or to metabolic complications (e.g., hyperglycemia or hypoglycemia, azotemia, metabolic acidosis, electrolyte imbalances).[51,160,184,199]

PERIPHERALLY ADMINISTERED PARENTERAL NUTRITION

Peripherally administered parenteral nutrition refers either to administration of one or two components, such as lipids alone, or administration of total admixture at less than what is required for the maintenance of the patient.[53,212,229] Peripherally administered parenteral nutrition solutions may be administered alone or used in combination with enteral nutrition. Commonly, 20% lipid is administered as a calorie source, or 5% dextrose with 3.5% amino acid solution is administered as a caloric and protein source. Peripherally administered parenteral nutrition solutions must be less than 2 times plasma osmolality (<600 mOsm/kg), or thrombophlebitis may occur.[229]

Refeeding syndrome may occur in cats that have experienced prolonged anorexia, such as cats with hepatic lipidosis. Prolonged anorexia induces a hypometabolic state, as described previously. Refeeding stimulates the release of insulin, causing dramatic shifts in electrolytes from the extracellular to the intracellular space. This affects primarily phosphorus, potassium and magnesium. Hypophosphatemia may also induce hemolytic anemia in cats. To prevent refeeding syndrome, identify patients at risk, especially those that have experienced anorexia for more than 5 to 7 days. Initial feeding rates should not exceed the patient's basic RER. Serum phosphorus, potassium, and magnesium should be monitored at least daily for the first few days of refeeding, and supplemental therapy should be provided as needed. Patients should also be monitored carefully for fluid overload.

URINARY TRACT DISORDERS: CHRONIC RENAL DISEASE

Animal Factors

Cats with chronic renal disease may show clinical signs consistent with a chronic disease such as weight loss, loss of muscle mass, poor hair coat, and pale mucous membranes; however, they may appear clinically normal.[70,104,150,215] Chronic renal disease may occur in association with other conditions, such as hyperthyroidism.[4,25,138,147] A staging system and recommended treatment plan were developed by the International Renal Insufficiency Society (http://iris-kidney.com/). Staging of chronic kidney disease (CKD) is undertaken after the diagnosis of CKD to facilitate appropriate treatment and monitoring of the patient. Staging is based initially on fasting plasma creatinine, assessed on at least two occasions in the stable patient. The patient is then substaged on the basis of proteinuria and systemic blood pressure. This staging system has been shown to correlate with survival.[31] Additional variables associated with decreased survival in cats with chronic renal failure include degree of azotemia, proteinuria, leukocytosis, anemia, systemic arterial hypertension, and ureteral calculi.* Nephrolithiasis is not associated with progression of renal failure.[236] For more information on CKD, see Chapter 32.

Dietary Factors

Dietary modification has been shown to improve survival and quality of life of cats with CKD.† Because cats with CKD have polyuria and polydipsia, feeding them a canned diet may be beneficial. Fresh water should be available at all times. Some cats with CKD do not drink adequately and require supplemental subcutaneously administered crystalloid solutions (75 to 150 mL per day). If subcutaneous fluid administration is not possible, placement of a feeding tube (esophagostomy or gastrostomy) provides a means to administer supplemental fluids, nutrition, and medications. Some cats with CKD have decreased appetite; therefore they should be fed a calorically dense diet (i.e., a high-fat diet). Restrict dietary protein to 3.8 to 4.4 g/kg per day or 28% to 32% on a dry matter basis. Hypokalemia may occur in cats with CKD (Figure 18-15); therefore a diet replete in potassium (0.8% to 1.2% on a dry matter basis) should

*References 72, 134, 140, 142, 257, 258.

†References 2, 3, 11, 73, 74, 112, 214, 216, 218, 235.

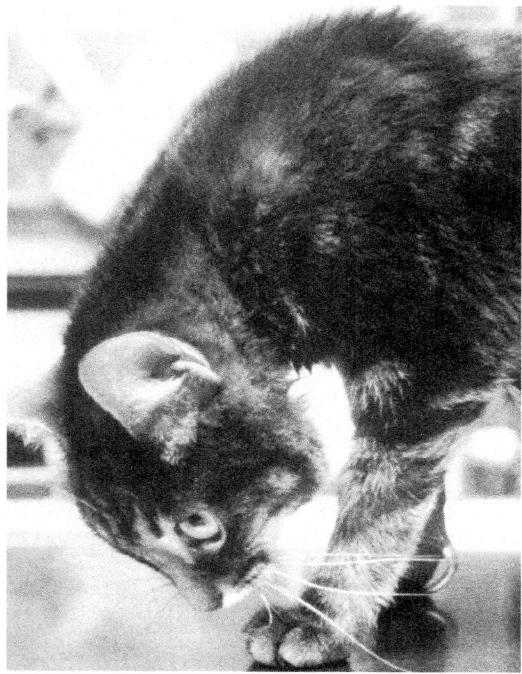

FIGURE 18-15 Hypokalemic polymyopathy in a 16-year-old castrated male domestic shorthair cat with chronic kidney disease.

be fed, or supplementation provided using potassium gluconate or potassium citrate. Renal disease diets are typically sodium restricted, which may be beneficial with associated fluid retention and systemic arterial hypertension; however, there is evidence that it may contribute to hyperkalemia.[39] Metabolic acidosis occurs with CKD, although it may not occur until late in the course of the disease. Feed an alkalinizing diet to offset metabolic acidosis or supplement with an alkalinizing agent (e.g., potassium citrate). Phosphorus restriction has been shown to modify progression of CKD.[234] Modification of dietary fatty acids, including increased n3 fatty acid intake, has been shown to be beneficial in dogs,[16,35-37] but the efficacy has not been proved in cats. CKD is a pro-oxidative condition, and antioxidants may be beneficial.[34,131,277]

The recommended dietary formulation for feeding cats with chronic renal failure is summarized in Box 18-11.[77]

Feeding Factors

Decreased appetite may result from uremic gastroenteritis. Management includes feeding a highly palatable, calorically dense diet, administering histamine$_2$ receptor antagonists or antacids, feeding small meals frequently, and using feeding tubes.[71]

BOX 18-11

Dietary Recommendations for Cats with Chronic Renal Disease

1. Protein: 28% to 35% on a dry matter basis
2. Phosphorus: 0.3% to 0.6% on a dry matter basis
3. Sodium: <0.4% on a dry matter basis, if hypertensive
4. Chloride: 1.5 times sodium level on a dry matter basis
5. Potassium: 0.7% to 1.2% on a dry matter basis
6. n3 fatty acids: 0.4% to 2.5% on a dry matter basis. Ratio of n6:n3 fatty acids in the diet should be 1.1-7:1
7. Vitamin E: >500 IU/kg of diet
8. Vitamin C: 100 to 200 mg/kg of diet

URINARY TRACT DISORDERS: UROLITHIASIS

Animal Factors

Uroliths may be composed of several different types of minerals; struvite and calcium oxalate occur most commonly in adult cats.[42,121,210] In kittens, infection-induced struvite and urate uroliths occur most commonly. In young adults struvite uroliths are typically not associated with a bacterial urinary tract infection. In older cats infection-induced struvite and calcium oxalate occur more commonly.[12] Uroliths occurring in the upper urinary tract are typically composed of calcium oxalate.[141,151,237]

Urolith formation is associated with varying underlying causes. Sterile struvite uroliths are associated with the feeding of meals versus *ad libitum* feeding, dry foods, increased carbohydrate, certain protein sources, and alkaluria.* Conditions necessary for the formation of struvite crystals and uroliths include sufficient concentration of the composite minerals (i.e., magnesium, ammonium, and phosphate) and retention of the components in the urinary tract for sufficient time to allow crystallization. Thus production of small volumes of concentrated urine would seem to be a contributing factor. In addition, a pH favorable for struvite precipitation must exist (7 and above). However, many cats with struvite urolithiasis have a neutral or acidic urine pH at presentation.

Calcium oxalate uroliths are associated with hypercalcemia (idiopathic hypercalcemia is the most common cause in cats) or hypercalciuria. The factors predisposing cats without hypercalcemia to hypercalciuria are not well understood and may involve consumption of high

*References 14, 65, 91-96, 211, 249.

BOX 18-12

Dietary Recommendations for Dissolution of Sterile Struvite Uroliths in Cats

1. Water: Canned foods induce polyuria and excretion of minerals
2. Magnesium: 0.04% to 0.09% on a dry matter basis
3. Phosphorus: 0.45% to 1.1% on a dry matter basis
4. Protein: 30% to 50% on a dry matter basis
5. Sodium: 0.3% to 0.6% on a dry matter basis
6. Urinary pH: 5.5 to 6.5

BOX 18-13

Dietary Recommendations for Prevention of Sterile Struvite Uroliths in Cats

1. Water: Canned diet may increase urine volume and dilute potential calculogenic compounds
2. Magnesium: 004% to 0.14% on a dry matter basis
3. Phosphorus: 0.5% to 0.9% on a dry matter basis
4. Protein: 30% to 50% on a dry matter basis
5. Urinary pH: 6 to 6.8

levels of sodium (discussed later) and the vitamin D and ascorbic acid levels in the diet. Some cats with calcium oxalate uroliths are mildly acidemic, which may result in mobilization of calcium that is excreted in the urine. Most cats with calcium oxalate uroliths have normal serum calcium, but some have moderate hypercalcemia, which may promote urinary calcium excretion. Urate uroliths are associated with liver disease or an underlying defect in uric acid metabolism.[13,188] Cystine uroliths are associated with an inborn error of cystine reabsorption in the renal proximal tubule.[66] For more information on urolithiasis, see Chapter 32.

Dietary Factors

Struvite uroliths can be dissolved medically with a calculolytic diet. For dissolution of struvite uroliths, feed a low-magnesium, low-phosphorus, low-protein, acidifying (pH 5.5 to 6.5), and diuretic diet, and administer antibiotics if the uroliths are associated with infection.[13,208,209] The average time for dissolution of sterile struvite uroliths is 2 to 4 weeks.[13,209]

The recommended dietary formulation for inducing dissolution of sterile struvite uroliths in cats is summarized in Box 18-12.[79]

At the time of this writing, no therapeutic diets are available for dissolution of calcium oxalate uroliths in cats. Other methods of urolith removal from the lower urinary tract must be employed, such as cystoscopic basket retrieval, voiding urohydropropulsion, and cystotomy.

Prevention of uroliths may involve dietary changes insofar as many types of feline uroliths are recurrent.

For infection-induced struvite uroliths, no dietary change is required. Infection-induced struvite uroliths result from a microbial infection with an organism that produces urease. Therefore if an infection does not recur, infection-induced struvite uroliths will not recur.[13,244] Sterile struvite uroliths are recurrent if diet is not modified. The recommended dietary formulation for prevention of sterile struvite uroliths in cats is summarized in Box 18-13.[79]

BOX 18-14

Dietary Recommendations for Prevention of Calcium Oxalate Uroliths in Cats

1. Water: Canned diets increase urine volume and dilute potential calculogenic compounds
2. Magnesium: 0.07% to 0.14% on a dry matter basis
3. Phosphorus: 0.5% to 1% on a dry matter basis
4. Calcium: 0.6% to 1% on a dry matter basis
5. Protein: 30% to 40% on a dry matter basis
6. Urinary pH: >7
7. Crude fiber: >7% on a dry matter basis if idiopathic hypercalcemia is present

Dietary management to prevent recurrence of calcium oxalate uroliths depends on whether the cat is normocalcemic or hypercalcemic. In cats that are normocalcemic, feed an oxalate-preventive diet that is low in calcium and replete in magnesium and that induces a neutral to alkaline urine pH (>7).[13,14,99,165] Cats with idiopathic hypercalcemia should be fed a higher-fiber diet supplemented with potassium citrate.[187] The recommended dietary formulation for prevention of calcium oxalate uroliths in cats is summarized in Box 18-14.[79]

A current controversy in the management of calcium oxalate uroliths is dietary content of sodium. Consumption of high levels of sodium may augment renal calcium excretion in human beings. Epidemiologic evidence suggests that low dietary sodium levels in cat and dog foods increase the risk for calcium oxalate urolithiasis, and diets containing high dietary sodium levels decrease the risk.[152,153] Recent studies in healthy cats did not find increased urine calcium excretion in response to high dietary salt intake (minimum 1.2% sodium dry matter basis).[137] In humans with hypocitraturia, sodium supplementation increased urine volume and decreased urinary saturation for calcium oxalate[255]; however, in a study of humans with hypercalciuria, sodium restriction decreased urinary calcium excretion and risk of stone formation.[204] In one study cats with naturally occurring

BOX 18-15

Dietary Recommendations for Prevention of Urate Uroliths in Cats

1. Protein: 28% to 35% on a dry matter basis
2. Phosphorus: 0.3% to 0.6% on a dry matter basis
3. Sodium: <0.4% on a dry matter basis, if hypertensive
4. Chloride: 1.5 times sodium level on a dry matter basis
5. Potassium: 0.7% to 1.2% on a dry matter basis
6. Urinary pH: >7

calcium oxalate uroliths excreted less urine calcium when fed a food lower in sodium.[165] In healthy cats or those with marginal renal function and hypercalciuria, increased dietary sodium exacerbated calcium excretion with[136] and without[39,122,163,273] increasing azotemia or blood pressure. Furthermore, in another study restriction of dietary sodium was associated with kaliuresis, an increased risk of hypokalemia, and a decrease in glomerular filtration rate in cats with induced chronic renal failure.[39] Until further data are available, orally administered sodium chloride or loop diuretics, which promote renal sodium excretion, for diuresis should be used cautiously and with careful monitoring because they may increase the risk of calcium oxalate urolith formation or worsening azotemia in some patients. Recommended levels of sodium in foods for cats predisposed to calcium oxalate formation is unknown; diets containing as low as 0.4 g/1000 kcal sodium and as high as 3.5 g/1000 kcal sodium are available commercially.

For urate uroliths not associated with underlying liver disease, cats should be fed a low-protein, alkalinizing, and diuretic diet. Allopurinol has not been evaluated in cats. The recommended dietary formulation for prevention of urate uroliths in cats is summarized in Box 18-15.

For management of cystine uroliths, cats should be fed a low-protein, alkalinizing, and diuretic diet similar to that used to manage cats with urate uroliths.

Feeding Factors

Free-choice feeding is associated with persistent aciduria because ingesting multiple small meals per day reduces the magnitude of the postprandial alkaline tide. As the size of the meal increases, so does the postprandial urine pH. Therefore *ad libitum* feeding may be most appropriate for management of struvite urolithiasis. Feeding a canned diet may decrease the risk of recurrence of sterile struvite, calcium oxalate, urate, and cystine uroliths by decreasing concentrations of calculogenic compounds in the urine. For cats that will not eat a canned diet, other methods may be employed to increase water intake (Box 18-16). Monitor response to dietary therapy using urine specific gravity, urine pH, and absence of crystalluria.

BOX 18-16

How to Increase Water Consumption

1. Fresh water should be provided every day.
   - Some cats will drink more water if offered filtered water rather than tap water.
   - Water can be flavored with ice cubes made from tuna or clam juice.
2. Provide water in more than one location.
   - Ensure that water bowls are placed away from food dishes, if possible, and definitely away from litter boxes.
3. Try a different type of water bowl.
   - Wide or shallow bowls may be preferred by some cats; try using a dog water bowl.
   - Keep the water filled to near the top; some cats dislike putting their face into a bowl.
   - Clean food and water bowls at least every other day.
   - Use stainless steel or ceramic bowls; plastic is more difficult to clean and retains odors.
4. Try providing a source of running water, such as a dripping tap or a pet water fountain.
   - Pet water fountains require meticulous cleaning.
5. Increase the frequency of meals.
   - Feed a larger number of small meals, ensuring that the total quantity fed is not increased.
6. Add water to canned food, but do not make it too thin; some cats will even accept water added to dry diets.

URINARY TRACT DISORDERS: IDIOPATHIC CYSTITIS

Animal Factors

Idiopathic cystitis is a sterile inflammatory process that usually occurs in young adult cats and is the most common diagnosis for young cats with lower urinary tract disease signs. Clinical signs include pollakiuria, dysuria, hematuria, and periuria. Clinical signs tend to be self-limiting, resolving in 3 to 7 days. However, recurrence is common. Males may obstruct from matrix-crystalline urethral plugs that are often composed of struvite. The pathophysiology of idiopathic cystitis is not well understood but appears to involve derangements of the interactions between the central nervous system and the endocrine system, with the bladder as target organ. For more information on idiopathic cystitis, see Chapter 32.

Dietary Factors

Dry diets may result in concentrated urine and increased concentration of crystallogenic compounds. Although cats consuming dry diets may drink more water than cats consuming canned diets, they do not increase water intake in sufficient amounts to compensate for the lower moisture content of dry diets. This is an important concept for owners to understand. Canned diets increase water intake and urine volume and decrease urine specific gravity, which may be beneficial.[13,103,177] Increased water intake may also dilute noxious components in urine that could irritate the bladder mucosa. The treatment goal should be to decrease the cat's urine specific gravity to 1.030 or less. Acidifying diets per se are of no value in treating idiopathic cystitis unless significant struvite crystalluria is present.

Feeding Factors

Cats fed *ad libitum* may have increased frequency of urination and greater total urine volume than meal-fed cats. Feeding a canned diet also increases volume and frequency of urination and may be beneficial in cats with idiopathic cystitis. Changing diets is a stressor and must be approached carefully for cats with idiopathic cystitis (see Box 18-5). For cats that will not eat a canned diet, other methods may be employed to increase water intake (see Box 18-16).

References

1. Abood SK, Buffington CA: Enteral feeding of dogs and cats: 51 cases (1989-1991), *J Am Vet Med Assoc* 201:619, 1992.
2. Adams LG, Polzin DJ, Osborne CA et al: Effects of dietary protein and calorie restriction in clinically normal cats and in cats with surgically induced chronic renal failure, *Am J Vet Res* 54:1653, 1993.
3. Adams LG, Polzin DJ, Osborne CA et al: Influence of dietary protein/calorie intake on renal morphology and function in cats with 5/6 nephrectomy, *Lab Invest* 70:347, 1994.
4. Adams WH, Daniel GB, Legendre AM et al: Changes in renal function in cats following treatment of hyperthyroidism using 131I, *Vet Radiol Ultrasound* 38:231, 1997.
5. Anderson JG, Harvey CE, Flax B: Clinical and radiographic evaluation of external odontoclastic resorptive lesions in cats (abstract), *J Vet Intern Med* 7:134, 1993.
6. Appleton DJ, Rand JS, Sunvold GD et al: Dietary chromium tripicolinate supplementation reduces glucose concentrations and improves glucose tolerance in normal-weight cats, *J Feline Med Surg* 4:13, 2002.
7. Armstrong PJ, Hand MS, Frederick GS: Enteral nutrition by tube, *Vet Clin North Am Small Anim Pract* 20:237, 1990.
8. Armstrong PJ, Lund EM: Changes in body composition and energy balance with aging, *Vet Clinical Nutr* 3:83, 1996.
9. Backus RC, Cave NJ, Keisler DH: Gonadectomy and high dietary fat but not high dietary carbohydrate induce gains in body weight and fat of domestic cats, *Br J Nutr* 98:641, 2007.
10. Baez JL, Michel KE, Sorenmo K et al: A prospective investigation of the prevalence and prognostic significance of weight loss and changes in body condition in feline cancer patients, *J Feline Med Surg* 9:411, 2007.
11. Barber PJ, Rawlings JM, Markwell PJ et al: Effect of dietary phosphate restriction on renal secondary hyperparathyroidism in the cat, *J Small Anim Pract* 40:62, 1999.
12. Bartges JW: Lower urinary tract disease in older cats: What's common, what's not? In *Health and nutrition of geriatric cats and dogs*, Proceedings, North American Veterinary Conference, Orlando, Fla, 1996.
13. Bartges JW, Kirk CA: Nutrition and lower urinary tract disease in cats, *Vet Clin North Am Small Anim Pract* 36:1361, 2006.
14. Bartges JW, Kirk CA, Moyers T: Influence of alkalinization and acidification on urine saturation with calcium oxalate and struvite and bone mineral density in healthy cats, *Urol Res* 32:172, 2004.
15. Bauer JE: Responses of dogs to dietary omega-3 fatty acids, *J Am Vet Med Assoc* 231:1657, 2007.
16. Bauer JE, Markwell PJ, Rawlings JM et al: Effects of dietary fat and polyunsaturated fatty acids in dogs with naturally developing chronic renal failure, *J Am Vet Med Assoc* 215:1588, 1999.
17. Beale BS: Use of nutraceuticals and chondroprotectants in osteoarthritic dogs and cats, *Vet Clin North Am Small Anim Pract* 34:271, 2004.
18. Beale BS: Orthopedic problems in geriatric dogs and cats, *Vet Clin North Am Small Anim Pract* 35:655, 2005.
19. Belsito KR, Vester BM, Keel T et al: Impact of ovariohysterectomy and food intake on body composition, physical activity, and adipose gene expression in cats, *J Anim Sci* 87:594, 2009.
20. Bennett N, Greco DS, Peterson ME et al: Comparison of a low carbohydrate-low fiber diet and a moderate carbohydrate-high fiber diet in the management of feline diabetes mellitus, *J Feline Med Surg* 8:73, 2006.
21. Birchard SJ, McLoughlin MA, Smeak DD: Chylothorax in the dog and cat: a review, *Lymphology* 28:64, 1995.
22. Birchard SJ, Smeak DD, McLoughlin MA: Treatment of idiopathic chylothorax in dogs and cats, *J Am Vet Med Assoc* 212:652, 1998.
23. Bissot T, Servet E, Vidal S et al: Novel dietary strategies can improve the outcome of weight loss programmes in obese client-owned cats, *J Feline Med Surg* 12:104, 2010.
24. Blanchard G, Paragon BM, Milliat F et al: Dietary L-carnitine supplementation in obese cats alters carnitine metabolism and decreases ketosis during fasting and induced hepatic lipidosis, *J Nutr* 132:204, 2002.
25. Boag AK, Neiger R, Slater L et al: Changes in the glomerular filtration rate of 27 cats with hyperthyroidism after treatment with radioactive iodine, *Vet Rec* 161:711, 2007.
26. Boegehold MA, Kotchen TA: Relative contributions of dietary Na^+ and Cl- to salt-sensitive hypertension, *Hypertension* 14:579, 1989.
27. Booij-Vrieling HE, Ferbus D, Tryfonidou MA et al: Increased vitamin D-driven signalling and expression of the vitamin D receptor, MSX2, and RANKL in tooth resorption in cats, *Eur J Oral Sci* 118:39, 2010.
28. Booij-Vrieling HE, Tryfonidou MA, Riemers FM et al: Inflammatory cytokines and the nuclear vitamin D receptor are implicated in the pathophysiology of dental resorptive lesions in cats, *Vet Immunol Immunopathol* 132:160, 2009.
29. Bosworth C, Bartges JW, Snow P: Nasoesophageal and nasogastric feeding tubes, *Vet Med* 99:590, 2004.
30. Boyce EN, Logan EI: Oral health assessment in dogs: study design and results, *J Vet Dent* 11:64, 1994.
31. Boyd LM, Langston C, Thompson K et al: Survival in cats with naturally occurring chronic kidney disease (2000-2002), *J Vet Intern Med* 22:1111, 2008.

32. Brady MA, Janovitz EB: Nephrotoxicosis in a cat following ingestion of Asiatic hybrid lily *(Lilium* sp), *J Vet Diagn Invest* 12:566, 2000.
33. Bright RM: Percutaneous endoscopic gastrostomy, *Vet Clin North Am Small Anim Pract* 23:531, 1993.
34. Brown SA: Oxidative stress and chronic kidney disease, *Vet Clin North Am Small Anim Pract* 38:157, 2008.
35. Brown SA, Brown CA, Crowell WA et al: Does modifying dietary lipids influence the progression of renal failure? *Vet Clin North Am Small Anim Pract* 26:1277, 1996.
36. Brown SA, Brown CA, Crowell WA et al: Effects of dietary polyunsaturated fatty acid supplementation in early renal insufficiency in dogs, *J Lab Clin Med* 135:275, 2000.
37. Brown SA, Finco DR, Brown CA: Is there a role for dietary polyunsaturated fatty acid supplementation in canine renal disease? *J Nutr* 128:2765S, 1998.
38. Budsberg SC, Bartges JW: Nutrition and osteoarthritis in dogs: does it help? *Vet Clin North Am Small Anim Pract* 36:1307, 2006.
39. Buranakarl C, Mathur S, Brown SA: Effects of dietary sodium chloride intake on renal function and blood pressure in cats with normal and reduced renal function, *Am J Vet Res* 65:620, 2004.
40. Burkholder WJ: Use of body condition scores in clinical assessment of the provision of optimal nutrition, *J Am Vet Med Assoc* 217:650, 2000.
41. Campbell KL: Fatty acid supplementation and skin disease, *Vet Clin North Am Small Anim Pract* 20:1475, 1990.
42. Cannon AB, Westropp JL, Ruby AL et al: Evaluation of trends in urolith composition in cats: 5,230 cases (1985-2004), *J Am Vet Med Assoc* 231:570, 2007.
43. Cave NJ: Hydrolyzed protein diets for dogs and cats, *Vet Clin North Am Small Anim Pract* 36:1251, 2006.
44. Center SA: Hepatic lipidosis, glucocorticoid hepatopathy, vacuolar hepatopathy, storage disorders, amyloidosis and iron toxicity. In Guilford WG, Center SA, Strombeck DR et al, editors: *Strombeck's small animal gastroenterology*, ed 3, Philadelphia, 1996, Saunders, p 766.
45. Center SA: Nutritional support for dogs and cats with hepatobiliary disease, *J Nutr* 128:2733S, 1998.
46. Center SA, Crawford MA, Guida L et al: A retrospective study of 77 cats with severe hepatic lipidosis: 1975-1990, *J Vet Intern Med* 7:349, 1993.
47. Center SA, Elston TH, Rowland PH et al: Fulminant hepatic failure associated with oral administration of diazepam in 11 cats, *J Am Vet Med Assoc* 209:618, 1996.
48. Center SA, Harte J, Watrous D et al: The clinical and metabolic effects of rapid weight loss in obese pet cats and the influence of supplemental oral L-carnitine, *J Vet Intern Med* 14:598, 2000.
49. Chan DL: The inappetent hospitalised cat: clinical approach to maximising nutritional support, *J Feline Med Surg* 11:925, 2009.
50. Chan DL, Freeman LM: Nutrition in critical illness, *Vet Clin North Am Small Anim Pract* 36:1225, 2006.
51. Chan DL, Freeman LM, Labato MA et al: Retrospective evaluation of partial parenteral nutrition in dogs and cats, *J Vet Intern Med* 16:440, 2002.
52. Chandler ML: Nutritional support for the hospitalised small animal patient, *Practice* 30:442, 2008.
53. Chandler ML, Guilford WG, Payne-James J: Use of peripheral parenteral nutritional support in dogs and cats, *J Am Vet Med Assoc* 216:669, 2000.
54. Chastain CB, Graham CL, Nichols CE: Adrenocortical suppression in cats given megestrol acetate, *Am J Vet Res* 42:2029, 1981.
55. Cianciolo RE, Bischoff K, Ebel JG et al: Clinicopathologic, histologic, and toxicologic findings in 70 cats inadvertently exposed to pet food contaminated with melamine and cyanuric acid, *J Am Vet Med Assoc* 233:729, 2008.
56. Colliard L, Paragon BM, Lemuet B et al: Prevalence and risk factors of obesity in an urban population of healthy cats, *J Feline Med Surg* 11:135, 2009.
57. Cook AM, Peppard A, Magnuson B: Nutrition considerations in traumatic brain injury, *Nutr Clin Pract* 23:608, 2008.
58. Cooper JH: Megestrol acetate and appetite gain, *Vet Rec* 102:45, 1978.
59. Crowe DT, Downs MO: Pharyngostomy complications in dogs and cats and recommended technical modifications: Experimental and clinical investigations, *J Am Anim Hosp Assoc* 22:493, 1986.
60. Crowe DT, Jr, Devey JJ: Esophagostomy tubes for feeding and decompression: clinical experience in 29 small animal patients, *J Am Anim Hosp Assoc* 33:393, 1997.
61. Davenport DJ, Jergens AE, Remillard RL: Inflammatory bowel disease. In Hand MS, Thatcher CD, Remillard RL et al, editors: *Small animal clinical nutrition*, ed 5, Topeka, Kan, 2010, Mark Morris Institute, p 1065.
62. De-Souza DA, Greene LJ: Intestinal permeability and systemic infections in critically ill patients: effect of glutamine, *Crit Care Med* 33:1125, 2005.
63. Dennis JS, Kruger JM, Mullaney TP: Lymphocytic/plasmacytic colitis in cats: 14 cases (1985-1990), *J Am Vet Med Assoc* 202:313, 1993.
64. Devitt CM, Seim HB III: Clinical evaluation of tube esophagostomy in small animals, *J Am Anim Hosp Assoc* 33:55, 1997.
65. Devois C, Biourge V, Morice G et al: Struvite and oxalate activity product ratios and crystalluria in cats fed acidifying diets. In *Urolithiasis 2000*, Capetown, South Africa, 2000.
66. DiBartola SP, Chew DJ, Horton ML: Cystinuria in a cat, *J Am Vet Med Assoc* 198:102, 1991.
67. Dow SW, Fettman MJ, Smith KR et al: Taurine depletion and cardiovascular disease in adult cats fed a potassium-depleted acidified diet, *Am J Vet Res* 53:402, 1992.
68. Drazenovich TL, Fascetti AJ, Westermeyer HD et al: Effects of dietary lysine supplementation on upper respiratory and ocular disease and detection of infectious organisms in cats within an animal shelter, *Am J Vet Res* 70:1391, 2009.
69. Eckersley RM: Losing the battle of the bulge: causes and consequences of increasing obesity, *Med J Aust* 174:590, 2001.
70. Elliott DA: Nutritional management of chronic renal disease in dogs and cats, *Vet Clin North Am Small Anim Pract* 36:1377, 2006.
71. Elliott DA, Riel DL, Rogers QR: Complications and outcomes associated with use of gastrostomy tubes for nutritional management of dogs with renal failure: 56 cases (1994-1999), *J Am Vet Med Assoc* 217:1337, 2000.
72. Elliott J, Barber PJ: Feline chronic renal failure: clinical findings in 80 cases diagnosed between 1992 and 1995, *J Small Anim Pract* 39:78, 1998.
73. Elliott J, Barber PJ, Rawlings JM et al: Effect of phosphate and protein restriction on progression of chronic renal failure in cats, *J Vet Intern Med* 12:221(abstract), 1998.
74. Elliott J, Rawlings JM, Markwell PJ et al: Survival of cats with naturally occurring chronic renal failure: effect of dietary management, *J Small Anim Pract* 41:235, 2000.
75. Fekete S, Hullar I, Andrasofszky E et al: Reduction of the energy density of cat foods by increasing their fibre content with a view to nutrients' digestibility, *J Anim Physiol Anim Nutr (Berl)* 85:200, 2001.
76. Flynn MB: Nutritional support for the burn-injured patient, *Crit Care Nurs Clin North Am* 16:139, 2004.
77. Forrester SD, Adams LG, Allen TA: Chronic kidney disease. In Hand MS, Thatcher CD, Remillard RL et al, editors: *Small animal clinical nutrition*, ed 5, Topeka, Kan, 2010, Mark Morris Institute, p 865.

78. Forrester SD, Fossum TW, Rogers KS: Diagnosis and treatment of chylothorax associated with lymphoblastic lymphosarcoma in four cats, *J Am Vet Med Assoc* 198:291, 1991.
79. Forrester SD, Kruger JM, Allen TA: Feline lower urinary tract diseases. In Hand MS, Thatcher CD, Remillard RL et al, editors: *Small animal clinical nutrition*, ed 5, Topeka, Kan, 2010, Mark Morris Institute, p 925.
80. Fossum TW: Chylothorax in cats: is there a role for surgery? *J Feline Med Surg* 3:73, 2001.
81. Fossum TW, Forrester SD, Swenson CL et al: Chylothorax in cats: 37 cases (1969-1989), *J Am Vet Med Assoc* 198:672, 1991.
82. Fossum TW, Miller MW, Rogers KS et al: Chylothorax associated with right-sided heart failure in five cats, *J Am Vet Med Assoc* 204:84, 1994.
83. Fox PR, Trautwein EA, Hayes KC et al: Comparison of taurine, alpha-tocopherol, retinol, selenium, and total triglycerides and cholesterol concentrations in cats with cardiac disease and in healthy cats, *Am J Vet Res* 54:563, 1993.
84. Francis H, Bartges JW, Tobias K et al: Enterostomy feeding tubes, *Vet Med* 99:627, 2004.
85. Frank G, Anderson W, Pazak H et al: Use of a high-protein diet in the management of feline diabetes mellitus, *Vet Ther* 2:238, 2001.
86. Freeman LM: Interventional nutrition for cardiac disease, *Clin Tech Small Anim Pract* 13:232, 1998.
87. Freeman LM, Abood SK, Fascetti AJ et al: Disease prevalence among dogs and cats in the United States and Australia and proportions of dogs and cats that receive therapeutic diets or dietary supplements, *J Am Vet Med Assoc* 229:531, 2006.
88. Freeman LM, Michel KE: Evaluation of raw food diets for dogs, *J Am Vet Med Assoc* 218:705, 2001.
89. Freeman LM, Rush JE: Nutrition and cardiomyopathy: lessons from spontaneous animal models, *Curr Heart Fail Rep* 4:84, 2007.
90. Fulton RB, Jr, Dennis JS: Blind percutaneous placement of a gastrostomy tube for nutritional support in dogs and cats, *J Am Vet Med Assoc* 201:697, 1992.
91. Funaba M, Matsumoto C, Matsuki K et al: Comparison of corn gluten meal and meat meal as a protein source in dry foods formulated for cats, *Am J Vet Res* 63:1247, 2002.
92. Funaba M, Oka Y, Kobayashi S et al: Evaluation of meat meal, chicken meal, and corn gluten meal as dietary sources of protein in dry cat food, *Can J Vet Res* 69:299, 2005.
93. Funaba M, Tanak T, Kaneko M et al: Fish meal vs. corn gluten meal as a protein source for dry cat food, *J Vet Med Sci* 63:1355, 2001.
94. Funaba M, Uchiyama A, Takahashi K et al: Evaluation of effects of dietary carbohydrate on formation of struvite crystals in urine and macromineral balance in clinically normal cats, *Am J Vet Res* 65:138, 2004.
95. Funaba M, Yamate T, Hashida Y et al: Effects of a high-protein diet versus dietary supplementation with ammonium chloride on struvite crystal formation in urine of clinically normal cats, *Am J Vet Res* 64:1059, 2003.
96. Funaba M, Yamate T, Narukawa Y et al: Effect of supplementation of dry cat food with D,L-methionine and ammonium chloride on struvite activity product and sediment in urine, *J Vet Med Sci* 63:337, 2001.
97. Gaskell R, Dawson S, Radford A et al: Feline herpesvirus, *Vet Res* 38:337, 2007.
98. German AJ, Holden S, Bissot T et al: Changes in body composition during weight loss in obese client-owned cats: loss of lean tissue mass correlates with overall percentage of weight lost, *J Feline Med Surg* 10:452, 2008.
99. Gisselman K, Langston C, Palma D et al: Calcium oxalate urolithiasis, *Compend Contin Educ Vet* 31:496, 2009.
100. Glaus TM, Cornelius LM, Bartges JW et al: Complications with non-endoscopic percutaneous gastrostomy in 31 cats and 10 dogs: a retrospective study, *J Small Anim Pract* 39:218, 1998.
101. Godfrey DR: Osteoarthritis in cats: a retrospective radiological study, *J Small Anim Pract* 46:425, 2005.
102. Gould L: The medical management of idiopathic chylothorax in a domestic long-haired cat, *Can Vet J* 45:51, 2004.
103. Grant DC: Effect of water source on intake and urine concentration in healthy cats, *J Feline Med Surg* 12:431, 2009.
104. Grauer GF: Early detection of renal damage and disease in dogs and cats, *Vet Clin North Am Small Anim Pract* 35:581, 2005.
105. Greenberg AS, Obin MS: Obesity and the role of adipose tissue in inflammation and metabolism, *Am J Clin Nutr* 83:461S, 2006.
106. Guilford WG, Matz ME: The nutritional management of gastrointestinal tract disorders in companion animals, *N Z Vet J* 51:284, 2003.
107. Hadley RM, Richardson JA, Gwaltney-Brant SM: A retrospective study of daylily toxicosis in cats, *Vet Hum Toxicol* 45:38, 2003.
108. Han E: Esophageal and gastric feeding tubes in ICU patients, *Clin Tech Small Anim Pract* 19:22, 2004.
109. Hardie EM, Roe SC, Martin FR: Radiographic evidence of degenerative joint disease in geriatric cats: 100 cases (1994-1997), *J Am Vet Med Assoc* 220:628, 2002.
110. Harkin KR, Cowan LA, Andrews GA et al: Hepatotoxicity of stanozolol in cats, *J Am Vet Med Assoc* 217:681, 2000.
111. Harper EJ, Stack DM, Watson TD et al: Effects of feeding regimens on bodyweight, composition and condition score in cats following ovariohysterectomy, *J Small Anim Pract* 42:433, 2001.
112. Harte JG, Markwell PJ, Moraillon RM et al: Dietary management of naturally occurring chronic renal failure in cats, *J Nutr* 124:2660S, 1994.
113. Hayes G: Chylothorax and fibrosing pleuritis secondary to thyrotoxic cardiomyopathy, *J Small Anim Pract* 46:203, 2005.
114. Hennet P, Servet E, Soulard Y et al: Effect of pellet food size and polyphosphates in preventing calculus accumulation in dogs, *J Vet Dent* 24:236, 2007.
115. Heuter K: Placement of jejunal feeding tubes for post-gastric feeding, *Clin Tech Small Anim Pract* 19:32, 2004.
116. Hill PB, Lo A, Eden CA et al: Survey of the prevalence, diagnosis and treatment of dermatological conditions in small animals in general practice, *Vet Rec* 158:533, 2006.
117. Hill RC: Conference on "Multidisciplinary approaches to nutritional problems". Symposium on "Nutrition and health." Nutritional therapies to improve health: lessons from companion animals, *Proc Nutr Soc* 68:98, 2009.
118. Hinrichs U, Puhl S, Rutteman GR et al: Lymphangiosarcomas in cats: a retrospective study of 12 cases, *Vet Pathol* 36:164, 1999.
119. Hinton M, Gaskell CJ: Non-neoplastic memmary hypertrophy in the cat associated either with pregnancy or with oral progestagen therapy, *Vet Rec* 100:277, 1977.
120. Hoenig M, Ferguson DC: Effects of neutering on hormonal concentrations and energy requirements in male and female cats, *Am J Vet Res* 63:634, 2002.
121. Houston DM, Moore AE: Canine and feline urolithiasis: examination of over 50 000 urolith submissions to the Canadian veterinary urolith centre from 1998 to 2008, *Can Vet J* 50:1263, 2009.
122. Hughes KL, Slater MR, Geller S et al: Diet and lifestyle variables as risk factors for chronic renal failure in pet cats, *Prev Vet Med* 55:1, 2002.
123. Iapichino G, Radrizzani D, Destrebecq A et al: Metabolic support of the critically ill: 2008 update, *Minerva Anestesiol* 74:709, 2008.
124. Ibrahim WH, Bailey N, Sunvold GD et al: Effects of carnitine and taurine on fatty acid metabolism and lipid accumulation in the liver of cats during weight gain and weight loss, *Am J Vet Res* 64:1265, 2003.
125. Ireland LM, Hohenhaus AE, Broussard JD et al: A comparison of owner management and complications in 67 cats with

esophagostomy and percutaneous endoscopic gastrostomy feeding tubes, *J Am Anim Hosp Assoc* 39:241, 2003.

126. Jacobs G, Cornelius L, Keene B et al: Comparison of plasma, liver, and skeletal muscle carnitine concentrations in cats with idiopathic hepatic lipidosis and in healthy cats, *Am J Vet Res* 51:1349, 1990.
127. Jergens AE, Morrison JA, Miles KG et al: Percutaneous endoscopic gastrojejunostomy tube placement in healthy dogs and cats, *J Vet Intern Med* 21:18, 2007.
128. Kahn SA: Placement of canine and feline esophagostomy feeding tubes, *Lab Anim (NY)* 36:25, 2007.
129. Kanchuk ML, Backus RC, Calvert CC et al: Neutering induces changes in food intake, body weight, plasma insulin and leptin concentrations in normal and lipoprotein lipase-deficient male cats, *J Nutr* 132:1730S, 2002.
130. Kass PH, Peterson ME, Levy J et al: Evaluation of environmental, nutritional, and host factors in cats with hyperthyroidism, *J Vet Intern Med* 13:323, 1999.
131. Keegan RF, Webb CB: Oxidative stress and neutrophil function in cats with chronic renal failure, *J Vet Intern Med*, 2010.
132. Keene BW, Panciera DL, Atkins CE et al: Myocardial L-carnitine deficiency in a family of dogs with dilated cardiomyopathy, *J Am Vet Med Assoc* 198:647, 1991.
133. Kienzle E, Bergler R: Human-animal relationship of owners of normal and overweight cats, *J Nutr* 136:1947S, 2006.
134. King JN, Tasker S, Gunn-Moore DA et al: Prognostic factors in cats with chronic kidney disease, *J Vet Intern Med* 21:906, 2007.
135. Kirk CA: Feline diabetes mellitus: low carbohydrates versus high fiber? *Vet Clin North Am Small Anim Pract* 36:1297, 2006.
136. Kirk CA, Jewell DE, Lowry SR: Effects of sodium chloride on selected parameters in cats, *Vet Ther* 7:333, 2006.
137. Kirk CA, Ling GV, Osborne CA et al: Clinical guidelines for managing calcium oxalate uroliths in cats: medical therapy, hydration, and dietary therapy. In *Managing urolithiasis in cats: recent updates and practice guidelines*, Topeka, Kan, 2003, Hill's Pet Nutrition Inc, p 10.
138. Kobayashi DL, Peterson ME, Graves TK et al: Hypertension in cats with chronic renal failure or hyperthyroidism, *J Vet Int Med* 4:58, 1990.
139. Kopko SH: The use of rutin in a cat with idiopathic chylothorax, *Can Vet J* 46:729, 2005.
140. Kuwahara Y, Ohba Y, Kitoh K et al: Association of laboratory data and death within one month in cats with chronic renal failure, *J Small Anim Pract* 47:446, 2006.
141. Kyles AE, Hardie EM, Wooden BG et al: Clinical, clinicopathologic, radiographic, and ultrasonographic abnormalities in cats with ureteral calculi: 163 cases (1984-2002), *J Am Vet Med Assoc* 226:932, 2005.
142. Kyles AE, Hardie EM, Wooden BG et al: Management and outcome of cats with ureteral calculi: 153 cases (1984-2002), *J Am Vet Med Assoc* 226:937, 2005.
143. Laflamme D: Development and validation of a body condition score system for cats: a clinical tool, *Feline Pract* 25:13, 1997.
144. Laflamme DP: Nutrition for aging cats and dogs and the importance of body condition, *Vet Clin North Am Small Anim Pract* 35:713, 2005.
145. Laflamme DP: Understanding and managing obesity in dogs and cats, *Vet Clin North Am Small Anim Pract* 36:1283, 2006.
146. Langston CE: Acute renal failure caused by lily ingestion in six cats, *J Am Vet Med Assoc* 220:49, 2002.
147. Langston CE, Reine NJ: Hyperthyroidism and the kidney, *Clin Tech Small Anim Pract* 21:17, 2006.
148. Lappin MR, Veir JK, Satyaraj E et al: Pilot study to evaluate the effect of oral supplementation of *Enterococcus faecium* SF68 on cats with latent feline herpesvirus 1, *J Feline Med Surg* 11:650, 2009.
149. Lascelles BD, Depuy V, Thomson A et al: Evaluation of a therapeutic diet for feline degenerative joint disease, *J Vet Intern Med* 24(3):487, 2010.
150. Lees GE: Early diagnosis of renal disease and renal failure, *Vet Clin North Am Small Anim Pract* 34:867, 2004.
151. Lekcharoensuk C, Osborne CA, Lulich JP et al: Increased frequency of calcium oxalate uroliths in the upper urinary tract of cats: 1981 to 1999. In *Managing urolithiasis in cats: recent updates and practice guidelines*, Davis, Calif, 2003.
152. Lekcharoensuk C, Osborne CA, Lulich JP: Epidemiologic study of risk factors for lower urinary tract diseases in cats, *J Am Vet Med Assoc* 218:1429, 2001.
153. Lekcharoensuk C, Osborne CA, Lulich JP et al: Association between dietary factors and calcium oxalate and magnesium ammonium phosphate urolithiasis in cats, *J Am Vet Med Assoc* 219:1228, 2001.
154. Levine PB, Smallwood LJ, Buback JL: Esophagostomy tubes as a method of nutritional management in cats: a retrospective study, *J Am Anim Hosp Assoc* 33:405, 1997.
155. Lewin-Smith MR, Kalasinsky VF, Mullick FG et al: Melamine-containing crystals in the urinary tracts of domestic animals: sentinel event? *Arch Pathol Lab Med* 133:341, 2009.
156. Lin L: RAGE on the Toll Road? *Cell Mol Immunol* 3:351, 2006.
157. Lindsay FE: Chylothorax in the domestic cat—a review, *J Small Anim Pract* 15:241, 1974.
158. Lippert AC: Enteral and parenteral nutritional support in dogs and cats with gastrointestinal disease, *Semin Vet Med Surg (Small Anim)* 4:232, 1989.
159. Lippert AC, Faulkner JE, Evans AT et al: Total parenteral nutrition in clinically normal cats, *J Am Vet Med Assoc* 194:669, 1989.
160. Lippert AC, Fulton RB, Jr, Parr AM: A retrospective study of the use of total parenteral nutrition in dogs and cats, *J Vet Intern Med* 7:52, 1993.
161. Logan EI: Dietary influences on periodontal health in dogs and cats, *Vet Clin North Am Small Anim Pract* 36:1385, 2006.
162. Logan EI, Wiggs RB, Scherl DS et al: Periodontal disease. In Hand MS, Thatcher CD, Remillard RL et al, editors: *Small animal clinical nutrition*, ed 5, Topeka, Kan, 2010, Mark Morris Institute, p 979.
163. Luckschander N, Iben C, Hosgood G et al: Dietary NaCl does not affect blood pressure in healthy cats, *J Vet Intern Med* 18:463, 2004.
164. Luhn A, Bartges JW, Snow P: Gastrostomy feeding tubes: percutaneous endoscopic placement, *Vet Med* 99:612, 2004.
165. Lulich JP, Osborne CA, Lekcharoensuk C et al: Effects of diet on urine composition of cats with calcium oxalate urolithiasis, *J Am Anim Hosp Assoc* 40:185, 2004.
166. Lund EM, Armstrong PJ, Kirk CA et al: Prevalence and risk factors for obesity in adult cats from private veterinary practices, *Int J Appl Res Vet Med* 3:88, 2005.
167. Lund EM, Armstrong PJ, Kirk CA et al: Health status and population characteristics of dogs and cats examined at private veterinary practices in the United States, *J Am Vet Med Assoc* 214:1336, 1999.
168. Lusby AL, Kirk CA, Bartges JW: The role of key adipokines in obesity and insulin resistance in cats, *J Am Vet Med Assoc* 235:518, 2009.
169. MacDonald ML, Rogers QR, Morris JG: Role of linoleate as an essential fatty acid for the cat independent of arachidonate synthesis, *J Nutr* 113:1422, 1983.
170. MacDougall LD: Mammary fibroadenomatous hyperplasia in a young cat attributed to treatment with megestrol acetate, *Can Vet J* 44:227, 2003.
171. Macy DW, Gasper PW: Diazepam-induced eating in anorexic cats, *J Am Anim Hosp Assoc* 21:17, 1985.

172. Maggs DJ: Update on pathogenesis, diagnosis, and treatment of feline herpesvirus type 1, *Clin Tech Small Anim Pract* 20:94, 2005.
173. Maggs DJ, Collins BK, Thorne JG et al: Effects of L-lysine and L-arginine on in vitro replication of feline herpesvirus type-1, *Am J Vet Res* 61:1474, 2000.
174. Maggs DJ, Nasisse MP, Kass PH: Efficacy of oral supplementation with L-lysine in cats latently infected with feline herpesvirus, *Am J Vet Res* 64:37, 2003.
175. Maggs DJ, Sykes JE, Clarke HE et al: Effects of dietary lysine supplementation in cats with enzootic upper respiratory disease, *J Feline Med Surg* 9:97, 2007.
176. Marks SL: The principles and practical application of enteral nutrition, *Vet Clin North Am Small Anim Pract* 28:677, 1998.
177. Markwell PJ, Buffington CA, Chew DJ et al: Clinical evaluation of commercially available urinary acidification diets in the management of idiopathic cystitis in cats, *J Am Vet Med Assoc* 214:361, 1999.
178. Marshall RD, Rand JS, Morton JM: Treatment of newly diagnosed diabetic cats with glargine insulin improves glycaemic control and results in higher probability of remission than protamine zinc and lente insulins, *J Feline Med Surg* 11:683, 2009.
179. Martin G, Rand J: Current understanding of feline diabetes: part 2, treatment, *J Feline Med Surg* 2:3, 2000.
180. Martin GJ, Rand JS: Food intake and blood glucose in normal and diabetic cats fed ad libitum, *J Feline Med Surg* 1:241, 1999.
181. Martin KM, Rossing MA, Ryland LM et al: Evaluation of dietary and environmental risk factors for hyperthyroidism in cats, *J Am Vet Med Assoc* 217:853, 2000.
182. Martin L, Siliart B, Dumon H et al: Leptin, body fat content and energy expenditure in intact and gonadectomized adult cats: a preliminary study, *J Anim Physiol Anim Nutr (Berl)* 85:195, 2001.
183. Mathews KA: The various types of parenteral fluids and their indications, *Vet Clin North Am Small Anim Pract* 28:483, 1998.
184. Mazzaferro EM: Complications of fluid therapy, *Vet Clin North Am Small Anim Pract* 38:607, 2008.
185. Mazzaferro EM, Greco DS, Turner AS et al: Treatment of feline diabetes mellitus using an alpha-glucosidase inhibitor and a low-carbohydrate diet, *J Feline Med Surg* 5:183, 2003.
186. McCarthy MS, Fabling J, Martindale R et al: Nutrition support of the traumatically injured warfighter, *Crit Care Nurs Clin North Am* 20:59, 2008.
187. McClain HM, Barsanti JA, Bartges JW: Hypercalcemia and calcium oxalate urolithiasis in cats: a report of five cases, *J Am Anim Hosp Assoc* 35:297, 1999.
188. McCue J, Langston C, Palma D et al: Urate urolithiasis, *Compend Contin Educ Vet* 31:468, 2009.
189. Meadows RL, MacWilliams PS, Dzata G et al: Chylothorax associated with cryptococcal mediastinal granuloma in a cat, *Vet Clin Pathol* 22:109, 1993.
190. Mehta NM, Duggan CP: Nutritional deficiencies during critical illness, *Pediatr Clin North Am* 56:1143, 2009.
191. Meincke JE, Hobbie WV, Jr, Barto LR: Traumatic chylothorax with associated diaphragmatic hernias in the cat, *J Am Vet Med Assoc* 155:15, 1969.
192. Mesich ML, Bartges JW, Tobias K et al: Gastrostomy feeding tubes: surgical placement, *Vet Med* 99:604, 2004.
193. Mesotten D, Van den Berghe G: Clinical benefits of tight glycaemic control: focus on the intensive care unit, *Best Pract Res Clin Anaesthesiol* 23:421, 2009.
194. Meyer HP, Twedt DC, Roudebush P et al: Hepatobiliary disease. In Hand MS, Thatcher CD, Remillard RL et al, editors: *Small animal clinical nutrition*, ed 5, Topeka, Kan, 2010, Mark Morris Institute, p 1155.
195. Michel KE: Focus on nutrition, *Compend Contin Educ Vet* 31:22, 2009.
196. Michel KE, Anderson W, Cupp C et al: Validation of a subjective muscle mass scoring system for cats, *J Anim Physiol Anim Nutr (Berl)* 93:806, 2009.
197. Middleton DJ, Watson AD: Glucose intolerance in cats given short-term therapies of prednisolone and megestrol acetate, *Am J Vet Res* 46:2623, 1985.
198. Miller CC, Bartges JW: Parenteral feeding products. In Kirk RW,Bonagura JD, editors: *Current veterinary therapy XIII*, Philadelphia, 1999, Saunders, p 80.
199. Miller CC, Bartges JW: Refeeding syndrome. In Kirk RW, Bonagura JD, editors: *Current veterinary therapy XIII*, Philadelphia, 1999, Saunders, p 89.
200. Mori A, Sako T, Lee P et al: Comparison of three commercially available prescription diet regimens on short-term post-prandial serum glucose and insulin concentrations in healthy cats, *Vet Res Commun* 33:669, 2009.
201. Morris JG: Idiosyncratic nutrient requirements of cats appear to be diet-induced evolutionary adaptations, *Nutr Res Rev* 15:153, 2002.
202. Nelson RW, Dimperio ME, Long GG: Lymphocytic-plasmacytic colitis in the cat, *J Am Vet Med Assoc* 184:1133, 1984.
203. Nelson RW, Scott-Moncrieff JC, Feldman EC et al: Effect of dietary insoluble fiber on control of glycemia in cats with naturally acquired diabetes mellitus, *J Am Vet Med Assoc* 216: 1082, 2000.
204. Nouvenne A, Meschi T, Prati B et al: Effects of a low-salt diet on idiopathic hypercalciuria in calcium-oxalate stone formers: a 3-mo randomized controlled trial, *Am J Clin Nutr* 91:565, 2010.
205. Ogilvie GK, Fettman MJ, Mallinckrodt CH et al: Effect of fish oil, arginine, and doxorubicin chemotherapy on remission and survival time for dogs with lymphoma: a double-blind, randomized placebo-controlled study, *Cancer* 88:1916, 2000.
206. Ogilvie GK, Vail DM: Nutrition and cancer. Recent developments, *Vet Clin North Am Small Anim Pract* 20:969, 1990.
207. Olczak J, Jones BR, Pfeiffer DU et al: Multivariate analysis of risk factors for feline hyperthyroidism in New Zealand, *N Z Vet J* 53:53, 2005.
208. Osborne CA, Lulich JP, Bartges JW et al: Medical dissolution and prevention of canine and feline uroliths: diagnostic and therapeutic caveats, *Vet Rec* 127:369, 1990.
209. Osborne CA, Lulich JP, Kruger JM et al: Medical dissolution of feline struvite urocystoliths, *J Am Vet Med Assoc* 196:1053, 1990.
210. Osborne CA, Lulich JP, Kruger JM et al: Analysis of 451,891 canine uroliths, feline uroliths, and feline urethral plugs from 1981 to 2007: perspectives from the Minnesota Urolith Center, *Vet Clin North Am Small Anim Pract* 39:183, 2009.
211. Palma D, Langston C, Gisselman K et al: Feline struvite urolithiasis, *Compend Contin Educ Vet* 31:542, 2009.
212. Perea SC: Critical care nutrition for feline patients, *Top Companion Anim Med* 23:207, 2008.
213. Pion PD, Kittleson MD, Rogers QR et al: Myocardial failure in cats associated with low plasma taurine: A reversible cardiomyopathy, *Science* 237:764, 1987.
214. Plantinga EA, Beynen AC: A case-control study on the intake of polyunsaturated fatty acids and chronic renal failure in cats, *J Appl Res Vet Med* 1:127, 2003.
215. Plotnick A: Feline chronic renal failure: long-term medical management, *Compend Contin Educ Vet* 29:342, 2007.
216. Polzin DJ, Osborne CA, Ross S et al: Dietary management of feline chronic renal failure: where are we now? In what direction are we headed? *J Feline Med Surg* 2:75, 2000.
217. Powell-Tuck J: Nutritional interventions in critical illness, *Proc Nutr Soc* 66:16, 2007.
218. Pratt A: Effect of commercial diets on cats with chronic renal insufficiency, *Vet Rec* 157:455, 2005.
219. Pukay BP: A hyperglycemia-glucosuria syndrome in cats following megestrol acetate therapy, *Can Vet J* 20:117, 1979.

220. Puschner B, Poppenga RH, Lowenstine LJ et al: Assessment of melamine and cyanuric acid toxicity in cats, *J Vet Diagn Invest* 19:616, 2007.
221. Radin MJ, Sharkey LC, Holycross BJ: Adipokines: a review of biological and analytical principles and an update in dogs, cats, and horses, *Vet Clin Pathol* 38:136, 2009.
222. Rajala MW, Scherer PE: Minireview: The adipocyte—at the crossroads of energy homeostasis, inflammation, and atherosclerosis, *Endocrinology* 144:3765, 2003.
223. Rand JS, Fleeman LM, Farrow HA et al: Canine and feline diabetes mellitus: nature or nurture? *J Nutr* 134:2072S, 2004.
224. Rees TM, Lubinski JL: Oral supplementation with L-lysine did not prevent upper respiratory infection in a shelter population of cats, *J Feline Med Surg* 10:510, 2008.
225. Reid CL: Nutritional requirements of surgical and critically-ill patients: do we really know what they need? *Proc Nutr Soc* 63:467, 2004.
226. Reiter AM, Lewis JR, Okuda A: Update on the etiology of tooth resorption in domestic cats, *Vet Clin North Am Small Anim Pract* 35:913, 2005.
227. Reiter AM, Lyon KF, Nachreiner RF et al: Evaluation of calciotropic hormones in cats with odontoclastic resorptive lesions, *Am J Vet Res* 66:1446, 2005.
228. Remillard RL: Homemade diets: attributes, pitfalls, and a call for action, *Top Companion Anim Med* 23:137, 2008.
229. Remillard RL, Saker KE: Parenteral-assisted feeding. In Hand MS, Thatcher CD, Remillard RL et al, editors: *Small animal clinical nutrition*, ed 5, Topeka, Kan, 2010, Mark Morris Institute, p 477.
230. Richter M, Schudel L, Tobler K et al: Clinical, virological, and immunological parameters associated with superinfection of latently with FeHV-1 infected cats, *Vet Microbiol* 138:205, 2009.
231. Rios L, Ward C: Feline diabetes mellitus: diagnosis, treatment, and monitoring, *Compend Contin Educ Vet* 30:626, 2008.
232. Robertson JE, Christopher MM, Rogers QR: Heinz body formation in cats fed baby food containing onion powder, *J Am Vet Med Assoc* 212:1260, 1998.
233. Root MV, Johnston SD, Olson PN: Effect of prepuberal and postpuberal gonadectomy on heat production measured by indirect calorimetry in male and female domestic cats, *Am J Vet Res* 57:371, 1996.
234. Ross LA, Finco DR, Crowell WA: Effect of dietary phosphorus restriction on the kidneys of cats with reduced renal mass, *Am J Vet Res* 43:1023, 1982.
235. Ross SJ, Osborne CA, Kirk CA et al: Clinical evaluation of dietary modification for treatment of spontaneous chronic kidney disease in cats, *J Am Vet Med Assoc* 229:949, 2006.
236. Ross SJ, Osborne CA, Lekcharoensuk C et al: A case-control study of the effects of nephrolithiasis in cats with chronic kidney disease, *J Am Vet Med Assoc* 230:1854, 2007.
237. Ross SJ, Osborne CA, Lulich JP et al: Canine and feline nephrolithiasis. Epidemiology, detection, and management, *Vet Clin North Am Small Anim Pract* 29:231, 1999.
238. Rumbeiha WK, Francis JA, Fitzgerald SD et al: A comprehensive study of Easter lily poisoning in cats, *J Vet Diagn Invest* 16:527, 2004.
239. Russell K, Sabin R, Holt S et al: Influence of feeding regimen on body condition in the cat, *J Small Anim Pract* 41:12, 2000.
240. Saker KE, Selting KA: Cancer. In Hand MS, Thatcher CD, Remillard RL et al, editors: *Small animal clinical nutrition*, ed 5, Topeka, Kan, 2010, Mark Morris Institute, p 588.
241. Scarlett JM, Donoghue S: Associations between body condition and disease in cats, *J Am Vet Med Assoc* 212:1725, 1998.
242. Scarlett JM, Donoghue S, Saidla J et al: Overweight cats: prevalence and risk factors, *Int J Obes Relat Metab Disord* 18(Suppl 1):S22, 1994.
243. Scott DW, Paradis M: A survey of canine and feline skin disorders seen in a university practice: Small Animal Clinic, University of Montreal, Saint-Hyacinthe, Quebec (1987-1988), *Can Vet J* 31:830, 1990.
244. Seaman R, Bartges JW: Canine struvite urolithiasis, *Compen Contin Educ Pract Vet* 23:407, 2001.
245. Seim HB, Bartges JW: Enteral and parenteral nutrition. In Tams TR, editor: *Handbook of small animal gastroenterology*, ed 2, Philadelphia, 2003, Saunders, p 416.
246. Simopoulos AP: Omega-3 fatty acids in inflammation and autoimmune diseases, *J Am Coll Nutr* 21:495, 2002.
247. Simpson JW: Diet and large intestinal disease in dogs and cats, *J Nutr* 128:2717s, 1998.
248. Slingerland LI, Fazilova VV, Plantinga EA et al: Indoor confinement and physical inactivity rather than the proportion of dry food are risk factors in the development of feline type 2 diabetes mellitus, *Vet J* 179:247, 2009.
249. Smith BH, Stevenson AE, Markwell PJ: Urinary relative supersaturations of calcium oxalate and struvite in cats are influenced by diet, *J Nutr* 128:2763S, 1998.
250. Smith SA, Ludlow CL, Hoskinson JJ et al: Effect of percutaneous endoscopic gastrostomy on gastric emptying in clinically normal cats, *Am J Vet Res* 59:1414, 1998.
251. Stenske KA, Smith JR, Newman SJ et al: Aflatoxicosis in dogs and dealing with suspected contaminated commercial foods, *J Am Vet Med Assoc* 228:1686, 2006.
252. Stiles J, Townsend WM, Rogers QR et al: Effect of oral administration of L-lysine on conjunctivitis caused by feline herpesvirus in cats, *Am J Vet Res* 63:99, 2002.
253. Stiver SL, Frazier KS, Mauel MJ et al: Septicemic salmonellosis in two cats fed a raw-meat diet, *J Am Anim Hosp Assoc* 39:538, 2003.
254. Stokes JE, Forrester SD: New and unusual causes of acute renal failure in dogs and cats, *Vet Clin North Am Small Anim Pract* 34:909, 2004.
255. Stoller ML, Chi T, Eisner BH et al: Changes in urinary stone risk factors in hypocitraturic calcium oxalate stone formers treated with dietary sodium supplementation, *J Urol* 181:1140, 2009.
256. Stookey GK, Warrick JM, Miller LL: Effect of sodium hexametaphosphate on dental calculus formation in dogs, *Am J Vet Res* 56:913, 1995.
257. Syme HM, Barber PJ, Markwell PJ et al: Prevalence of systolic hypertension in cats with chronic renal failure at initial evaluation, *J Am Vet Med Assoc* 220:1799, 2002.
258. Syme HM, Markwell PJ, Pfeiffer D et al: Survival of cats with naturally occurring chronic renal failure is related to severity of proteinuria, *J Vet Intern Med* 20:528, 2006.
259. Thatcher CD, Hand MS, Remillard RL: Small animal clinical nutrition: an iterative process. In Hand MS, Thatcher CD, Remillard RL et al, editors: *Small animal clinical nutrition*, ed 5, Topeka, Kan, 2010, Mark Morris Institute.
260. Thiess S, Becskei C, Tomsa K et al: Effects of high carbohydrate and high fat diet on plasma metabolite levels and on i.v. glucose tolerance test in intact and neutered male cats, *J Feline Med Surg* 6:207, 2004.
261. Thiry E, Addie D, Belak S et al: Feline herpesvirus infection. ABCD guidelines on prevention and management, *J Feline Med Surg* 11:547, 2009.
262. Thomovsky E, Reniker A, Backus R et al: Parenteral nutrition: uses, indications, and compounding, *Compend Contin Educ Vet* 29:76, 2007.
263. Thompson K, Bartges JW, Snow P: Gastrostomy feeding tubes: percutaneous, nonsurgical, nonendoscopic placement, *Vet Med* 99:619, 2004.
264. Thompson MS, Cohn LA, Jordan RC: Use of rutin for medical management of idiopathic chylothorax in four cats, *J Am Vet Med Assoc* 215:345, 1999.

265. Toll PW, Yamka RM, Schoenherr WD et al: Obesity. In Hand MS, Thatcher CD, Remillard RL et al, editors: *Small animal clinical nutrition*, ed 5, Topeka, Kan, 2010, Mark Morris Institute, p 501.
266. Vannatta M, Bartges JW, Snow P: Esophagostomy feeding tubes, *Vet Med* 99:596, 2004.
267. Vasconcellos RS, Borges NC, Goncalves KN et al: Protein intake during weight loss influences the energy required for weight loss and maintenance in cats, *J Nutr* 139:855, 2009.
268. Villaverde C, Ramsey JJ, Green AS et al: Energy restriction results in a mass-adjusted decrease in energy expenditure in cats that is maintained after weight regain, *J Nutr* 138:856, 2008.
269. von Werthern CJ, Wess G: A new technique for insertion of esophagostomy tubes in cats, *J Am Anim Hosp Assoc* 37:140, 2001.
270. Wakeling J, Everard A, Brodbelt D et al: Risk factors for feline hyperthyroidism in the UK, *J Small Anim Pract* 50:406, 2009.
271. Walberg J: Idiopathic chylothorax in a cat, *J Am Vet Med Assoc* 182:525, 1983.
272. Watson AD: Diet and periodontal disease in dogs and cats, *Aust Vet J* 71:313, 1994.
273. Xu H, Laflamme DP, Long GL: Effects of dietary sodium chloride on health parameters in mature cats, *J Feline Med Surg* 11:435, 2009.
274. Yang VK, Freeman LM, Rush JE: Comparisons of morphometric measurements and serum insulin-like growth factor concentration in healthy cats and cats with hypertrophic cardiomyopathy, *Am J Vet Res* 69:1061, 2008.
275. Yhee JY, Brown CA, Yu CH et al: Retrospective study of melamine/cyanuric acid-induced renal failure in dogs in Korea between 2003 and 2004, *Vet Pathol* 46:348, 2009.
276. Young CD, Anderson SM: Sugar and fat—that's where it's at: metabolic changes in tumors, *Breast Cancer Res* 10:202, 2008.
277. Yu S, Paetau-Robinson I: Dietary supplements of vitamins E and C and beta-carotene reduce oxidative stress in cats with renal insufficiency, *Vet Res Commun* 30:403, 2006.
278. Zetner K, Steurer I: The influence of dry food on the development of feline neck lesions, *J Vet Dent* 9:4, 1992.
279. Zicker SC, Nelson RW, Kirk CA et al: Endocrine disorders. In Hand MS, Thatcher CD, Remillard RL et al, editors: *Small animal clinical nutrition*, ed 5, Topeka, Kan, 2010, Mark Morris Institute, p 559.
280. Zoran D: Is it IBD? Managing inflammatory disease in the feline gastrointestinal tract, *Vet Med* 95:128, 2000.
281. Zoran DL: Feline obesity: recognition and management, *Compend Contin Educ Vet* 31:284, 2009.
282. Zoran DL: Obesity in dogs and cats: a metabolic and endocrine disorder, *Vet Clin North Am Small Anim Pract* 40:221, 2010.

CHAPTER

19

Current Controversies in Feline Nutrition

Maryanne Murphy, Joe Bartges, Claudia Kirk, Angela L. Witzel, Beth Hamper, and Donna Raditic

OUTLINE

When thinking about feeding the domestic cats in your client's household, the veterinarian may need to make recommendations that are more involved than merely prescribing a certain amount of commercially available food for the specific life stage of each cat. Many clients are now taking matters into their own hands, sifting through information they find on the Internet, in books, on television, or by word of mouth, and making their own dietary decisions. How should the responsible veterinarian respond when owners say they plan to feed their cat a raw food diet or a homemade one based on a recipe they found online?

This chapter explores current controversial issues in feline nutrition. By the end of this section, the reader will be familiar with the most recent research and should be able to make confident, informed recommendations (at least until the next new diet fad appears).

RAW FOOD DIETS

Proponents of raw food diets have a very basic philosophy: Cats are obligate carnivores designed to eat raw meat similar to what their ancestors consumed. Traditional extruded and canned commercially available diets have been heat processed, which can degrade vitamins, minerals, and enzymes inherently contained in the preprocessed form. The ancestors of domestic cats were not affected by nutrient degradation because they hunted live prey and ingested meat from fresh carcasses. In addition to maintaining the natural nutrient balance, proponents also claim that these diets offer benefits such as improved immune function, general health, energy, coat and skin condition, and behavior. It has also been said that general body odors (breath, body, and feces) will be minimized and the incidence of various medical conditions reduced.[17]

Published in 1993, *Give Your Dog a Bone,* by Dr. Ian Billinghurst,[5] was one of the first widely publicized and referenced manuals on feeding raw diets. Dr. Billinghurst followed this with another book, *The BARF Diet: Raw Feeding for Dogs and Cats Using Evolutionary Principles,*[6] which catapulted raw food diets to an area of prominence in 2001. With this book Dr. Billinghurst provided an "introductory primer" to allow cat and dog owners to return their pets to "their evolutionary diet." He coined the acronym *BARF,* meaning either "biologically appropriate raw food" diet or "bone and raw food" diet. The basis of Dr. Billinghurst's diet plan is that a feline diet should mimic the carcass of a small mammal or bird and should contain 75% raw meaty bones, 15% crushed offal (internal organs), and 5% crushed vegetables and supplements to mimic feces and soil. Although individual meals can be balanced, Billinghurst contends that achieving nutrient balance over many meals is preferable.[6]

He may have been instrumental in starting the raw food evolution, but Dr. Billinghurst is not alone. A quick Internet search garners a wide variety of raw food producers and promoters. There are also many owner testimonials and other anecdotal reports claiming that raw diets improved animals' health problems, behavior, and appearance (to name a few). At the time of manuscript preparation there were no peer-reviewed research publications with data in accordance with or in opposition to these reports. However, there are published data regarding concerns voiced by raw diet opponents, including the possibility of bacterial and nonbacterial contamination with zoonotic potential, nutritional inadequacies, and clinical diseases.

Contamination Concerns

Salmonella

Salmonella has gained the most attention regarding bacterial contamination concerns of raw food diets. In humans the national rate of reported *Salmonella* isolates in 2006 was 13.6 per 100,000 in the United States.[9] A large proportion of *Salmonella typhimurium* isolates, the most commonly isolated subtype, have also been found to be resistant to multiple antimicrobials. In 2004 39% of nationally reported *S. typhimurium* isolates in the United States were resistant to one or more drugs, and 23% had a five-drug resistance pattern.[10]

Symptoms of salmonellosis are similar across species and include fever, vomiting, abdominal pain, and diarrhea. Severe cases, especially in previously immunocompromised individuals or in individuals with systemic disease, can be fatal. It is common, however, for *Salmonella* to be present in the feces of asymptomatic animals. According to published estimates, 1% to 36% of healthy dogs and 1% to 18% of healthy cats are asymptomatic fecal shedders. Fecal shedding of *Salmonella* can wax and wane after the first week of infection, and clinical signs are seen in conjunction with stress and immunosuppression.[35]

Whereas most human *Salmonella* infections originate from food animals, food sources include eggs, meat, poultry, and produce. Human infections are also seen involving direct contact with animals and their environments.[8] It is the combined risk of using raw meat and poultry while in close contact with pets and their environments that has raw food opponents concerned for human safety.

There are multiple published reports of pet dogs and cats testing positive for *Salmonella* isolates that were indistinguishable from isolates obtained from humans. In these cases both symptomatic and asymptomatic animals were linked to humans in multiple capacities. Some were staff in veterinary clinics, individual pet owners, children of owners, or neighbors of infected pets. A connection was also found between children attending a day care center with a child living with two asymptomatic positive cats.[11,36,53] Only one of these reports mentioned diets consumed by *Salmonella*-positive pets. In this case a symptomatic infant was positive for a *Salmonella* Virchow isolate that was indistinguishable from isolates found in two of three asymptomatic dogs living in the same home. All three dogs were fed a commercial diet supplemented with boiled chicken 2 to 3 times per week.[36] *Salmonella* isolates in all of the previous reports were also resistant to multiple antimicrobials, with flouroquinolones and third-generation cephalosporins included in some cases. This is significant because these classes of antimicrobials are commonly used to treat human salmonellosis.[53]

Risk of zoonosis is an important consideration with salmonellosis, especially because in all the aforementioned reports, multiple pets in a household were infected with variation in the presence of symptomatic and asymptomatic pets.[11,36,53] After an investigation in one veterinary clinic, 5 of 43 hospitalized cats tested positive for *Salmonella,* including the asymptomatic blood donor cat. The floor of the boarding area and floor and door handles to the isolation ward in this clinic also tested positive.[53] In another veterinary clinic, three previously healthy pets developed transient diarrhea after prophylactic dental procedures performed by a veterinary technician later determined to be *Salmonella* positive. One of the three pets had a positive stool sample with an isolate indistinguishable from that of the veterinary technician.[11]

These reports underscore the importance of training veterinary staff to recognize, address, and learn to avoid situations that can place themselves and others at risk of *Salmonella* infection. On the basis of a list of factors contributing to four of the aforementioned outbreaks, pertinent reminders for all veterinary staff can be made (Box 19-1).[53]

One recommendation on the list involves environmental contamination concerns. A small study by Weese and Rousseau[50] evaluated survival of *Salmonella* spp. in pet food bowls using a *Salmonella* Copenhagen isolate previously obtained from a commercial raw food product. They inoculated multiple bowls and left them at room temperature for 7 days. The average concentration of *Salmonella* spp. was 5.4×10^5 colony-forming units per gram, and *Salmonella* was isolated from all bowls on days 1, 2, 4 and 7. They then took six stainless steel and six plastic food bowls and inoculated them with the

BOX 19-1

Reminders of *Salmonella* Risk in Veterinary Facilities

1. There is a risk of occupational zoonotic transmission of *Salmonella* spp.
2. There is a risk of zoonotic transmission of *Salmonella* spp. to clients and pet owners.
3. There is a risk of nosocomial transmission of *Salmonella* spp. among animals in veterinary facilities and animal shelters.
4. Environmental contamination can serve as an ongoing source of infection, especially when eating and drinking from contaminated work surfaces.

TABLE 19-1 Bacteria Types Recovered from 25 Commercial Raw Food Diets Purchased in Ontario, Canada

Bacterium type	Total result
Escherichia coli	16/25
Salmonella spp.	5/25
Campylobacter spp.	0/25
Spore-forming bacteria	4/25 (direct culture), 25/25 (enriched medium)
Clostridium perfringens	5/25
Clostridium difficile	1/25
Staphylococcus aureus	1/25

From Weese JS, Rousseau J, Arroyo L: Bacteriological evaluation of commercial canine and feline raw diets, *Can Vet J* 46:513, 2005.

same *Salmonella* strain. After assigning the bowls to various disinfectant treatment groups, the researchers evaluated them for *Salmonella* persistence. No significant difference was noted among disinfection methods for the plastic bowls. Scrubbing the stainless steel bowl with soap and then soaking it in bleach was significantly more effective than no cleaning, warm water rinse, and warm water rinse with scrubbing. None of the cleaning techniques used was able to eradicate all traces of bacteria, including use of a dishwasher. Some of this may have been due to the amount of organic debris used to inoculate the dishes, but the risk of food bowl contamination is an important concept to discuss with owners participating in raw feeding.

Other Pathogens

In addition to *Salmonella,* other bacterial species common in raw meat include *Campylobacter* spp., *Escherichia coli, Yersinia enterocolitica, Listeria monocytogenes, Clostridium perfringens, Staphylococcus aureus,* and *Bacillus cereus.*[24] In a study of raw food diets purchased in Ontario, Canada, coliforms were present in all 25 raw diets sampled, with a mean value of 8.9×10^5 colony-forming units per gram.[51] Table 19-1 illustrates the total number and types of bacteria isolated from these raw food diets, which contain enteropathogens of both animals and humans.

Another study evaluated bacterial and protozoal contamination of commercially available raw, dry, and canned dog food diets. Of 233 samples 153 (53%) were positive for non–type-specific *E. coli,* including dry and canned food varieties. *Salmonella enterica* was found in 17 of 233 (5.9%) samples from raw products, and 3 of 144 (2.1%) samples contained *Cryptosporidium* spp. in raw and canned products. Unfortunately, the design of this study did not allow for direct comparison of the degree of bacterial contamination in raw versus dry and canned diets.[42]

A third study compared two commercial raw diets and three homemade raw diets. *E. coli* O157:H7 was found in one of the homemade diets, whereas all three of the homemade diets were negative for *Salmonella* spp.[17] These data are especially troubling because *E. coli* O157:H7 is an important human pathogen causing hemorrhagic colitis in all ages and hemolytic–uremic syndrome in children and the elderly, with mortality rates between 3% and 5%. There is also no current recommended antimicrobial therapy in humans for this specific bacterial agent.[12]

Nutritional Inadequacies

As previously discussed, according to the recommendations for Dr. Billinghurst's BARF diet, nutritional balance should be achieved over the course of many meals rather than each meal being individually balanced.[6] Logistically, it is difficult to determine the complete nutritive value of a home-prepared diet over many days owing to the large amount of variability. There are, however, canine data regarding three raw diet meals (two for adults, one for a puppy) prepared at home by three owners and two commercially available raw preparations. The two adult homemade diets and both commercial diets were compared to nutrient standards for canine adult maintenance developed by the Association of American Feed Control Officials (AAFCO). One commercial diet and both adult home-cooked diets were low in calcium and phosphorus, with an unbalanced calcium:phosphorus ratio. The same home-prepared diets and the second commercial diet had high vitamin D levels. There were also inappropriate variations in zinc, iron, magnesium, and vitamin E noted in these diets. Using AAFCO standards for canine growth, all the puppy homemade diets and both commercial diets had nutrient imbalances, especially in relation to calcium, phosphorus, and vitamin D.[17]

While there are no similar data published for feline diets, these results suggest that home-prepared diets (whether raw or cooked) are unbalanced until evaluated by a veterinary nutritionist. Further discussion of unbalanced diets is included in the homemade diet section later in this chapter.

Clinical Disease Concerns

Animal

When nutritional inadequacies are present in a diet, clinical disease may be a consequence depending on the affected nutrients, the duration of feeding the deficient diet, and the life stage of the animal. One of the most commonly reported nutritionally related clinical diseases is osteodystrophy attributed to derangements of calcium, phosphorus, or vitamin D. Even though the incidence of such musculoskeletal diseases is reportedly low in cats,[49] it is not unheard of, and all owners of affected animals should be asked about the specific diet being fed so that the likelihood of this etiology can be assessed. There are multiple case reports involving both suspected and definitively diagnosed cases of nutritional secondary hyperparathyroidism[19,45,46,52] and vitamin D–dependent rickets[18,38,43] manifested as bone abnormalities in domestic and wild cats. Although not all of these cases were specifically linked to raw diets, most of them involve animals fed unbalanced diets. Therefore, as previously explained, it is important to remember that any raw food diet (even those commercially obtained) should be considered unbalanced until evaluated by a veterinary nutritionist.

Arguably the most severe consequence to feeding a raw-prepared diet involves the risk of septicemic salmonellosis. A case report involving diagnosed septicemic salmonellosis in two cats originating in the same household recounted the diagnostics and results obtained. Both were fed a homemade raw beef diet. The first, a 14-year-old Exotic Shorthair, was presented deceased with a 1 week history of weight loss, soft stools, and anorexia. Histopathologic evidence of necrotizing hepatitis, chronic enteritis, and interstitial pneumonia was noted on necropsy, with *S. typhimurium* isolated from the lung, liver, spleen, and kidney. Nine months later, a 10-week-old Exotic Shorthair kitten from the same household was presented moribund with a history of possible respiratory obstruction. After euthanasia, gross evidence of reduced fat and muscle stores, serous nasal discharge, corneal opacity, and consolidated lungs was noted along with histopathologic signs of suppurative pneumonia and enteritis with villi erosion and blunting. *Bordetella bronchiseptica* was isolated from the lungs, and *Salmonella newport* was identified in the lung and small intestine. Samples of the raw beef fed to the kitten yielded *S. newport* and *Salmonella bardo* and *E. coli* among many other bacterial isolates.[40]

Human

The public health concerns associated with raw diets deal with possible human exposure to *Salmonella* spp. and *E. coli*, among other pathogens. Some raw food proponents believe that the risk of human bacteriosis such as salmonellosis is inconsequential because there are so few documented cases of direct transfer from raw-fed pets to their owners. For the average healthy adult who is aware of foodborne pathogen risk and prevention, the chance of salmonellosis may be low. It is important to remember, however, that unless the gastrointestinal signs are severe, this same average healthy adult is unlikely to submit fecal culture samples from themselves and their pets, and many veterinarians reserve use of fecal cultures to those animals with refractory diarrhea. In many of the case reports referenced in the preceding sections, regulatory health officials actively obtained diagnostic fecal cultures only after the diagnostic laboratory noticed an outbreak pattern between a small subset of human or animal samples.[11,36,53]

The Bottom Line

The veterinarian's educational efforts should be focused especially on those raw-fed pet households containing immunocompromised people (children, elderly, those with chronic diseases) because these are higher risk individuals more likely to become infected. Disinfection of contaminated kitchen work surfaces and food bowls should be of paramount importance. Clients should consider using dishwasher-safe dishes and implementing a bleach soak into the disinfection regimen. Proper handwashing should be performed after every animal interaction, especially just before food preparation and consumption. If cats in the household are known to jump on kitchen counters, all of those surfaces should be considered contaminated at all times and food (human or animal) should be prepared only on other work surfaces such as cutting boards.

At this point sufficient evidence does not exist to determine whether raw diets affect immune function, general health, energy, coat and skin condition, behavior, metabolic diseases, or fecal odor. Although anecdotal reports may seem convincing, clinically based peer-reviewed studies are necessary before any definitive conclusions can be drawn. Until that occurs, veterinarians are advised to instruct owners to cook all meat included in home-prepared diets.

CATS AND CARBOHYDRATES

Cats are obligate carnivores that have naturally evolved to maintain blood glucose in the face of a low carbohydrate intake. The classic example of a low-carbohydrate feline diet is the rat carcass, which is 55% protein, 38.1% fat, 9.1% carbohydrate, and 1.2% fiber on a dry matter basis.[54] Because cats are carnivores, the adaptation to a high-protein diet such as the rat carcass is necessary because adult cats require 2 to 3 times more protein than adult omnivores, and kittens require 1.5 times more protein than do young of noncarnivorous species.[31] Cats also have constant hepatic glucose production from amino acids (gluconeogenesis) and a delay in dietary carbohydrate use (low glucokinase activity).[25] The combination of the natural adaptation to a high-protein diet and delay in dietary carbohydrate use has shaped the recent argument that carbohydrates should make up a small fraction of the average domesticated cat's diet. The one caveat to keep in mind regarding this argument is that most carbohydrates in pet foods are composed of complex carbohydrates, not simple sugars, as is common in processed human foods.[22] This is an important distinction because diets high in sucrose and simple sugars are

TABLE 19-2 **Percent Dry Matter (%DM) Macronutrient Composition of Various Diets in Referenced Studies**

	Hoenig et al[21]		*Mazzaferro et al*[28]	*Thiess et al*[44]		*Michel et al*[30]		*Bennett et al*[4]*		*Backus et al*[3]				*Frank et al*[17]		*Verbrugghe et al*[47]		
	HC	**HP**	**LC**	**HC**	**HF**	**HC**	**LC**	**MC, HFb**	**LC, LFb**	**LC**	**LMC**	**MHC**	**HC**	**HFb**	**HP**	**LP**	**LF**	**LC**
Protein	31	48	49	37	50	39	63	46	42	47	41	36	33	42	57	19	32	30
Fat	18	17	36	15	30	10	20	19	24	40	24	12	4	17	24	12	8	13
Carbohydrate	43	26	7	40	13	44	16	30	14	4	27	45	56	24	8	19	16	4
Crude fiber	1	1	—	2	1	7	1	12	0.4	—	—	—	—	11	4	0.2	0.2	0.3

HC, High carbohydrate; *LMC,* low to moderate carbohydrate; *MC,* moderate carbohydrate; *MHC,* moderate to high carbohydrate; *LC,* low carbohydrate; *HP,* high protein; *HFb,* high fiber; *LFb,* low fiber; *HF,* high fat; *LF,* low fat.
Dashes (—) indicate information not provided in referenced study.
*Caloric density of diets was not provided in study so dry matter calculations were made with the assumption of a 4000 kcal ME/kg DM diet.

not efficiently metabolized in the cat, but complex carbohydrates used in processed pet foods can be fully metabolized.

Fate of Carbohydrates in the Cat

With a diet high in carbohydrates, blood glucose rises, causing an increase in insulin requirements. Lipoprotein lipase activity increases as more glucose enters adipose cells for conversion into fatty acids, with subsequent storage as fat. With a low-carbohydrate diet, blood glucose and insulin levels are lower and enzyme pathways are altered to conserve glucose, limit gluconeogenesis from amino acids (to conserve body proteins), and mobilize fats. There is higher fat and protein consumption, and higher protein levels are needed to support increased hepatic gluconeogenesis. The hepatic glucose production is responsible for a slow and steady rate of glucose being released into the bloodstream, maintaining a consistent glucose level.[21]

The aforementioned concept is the basis of the human Atkins diet, with the idea that low dietary carbohydrate will cause a shift in metabolic drive from glucose oxidation to fat metabolism as the primary energy source. This leads to a lower serum glucose and limited drive for insulin secretion from pancreas. Purported benefits of this low-carbohydrate, high-protein diet in people are appetite control, increased calorie loss by way of futile cycling and ketone loss, improved insulin sensitivity, shift from glucose oxidation and lipogenesis to lipolysis, and weight loss.[2]

Whether discussing the low-carbohydrate concept in cats or humans, it is important to keep in mind that fat, protein, or both must increase to account for the loss of energy that would have been provided by carbohydrates.[21] Several published reports (Table 19-2) have evaluated the implications of replacing a low-carbohydrate diet with one higher in fat. One of these studies found that during growth, fat deposition was 2.5 times greater when a high-fat diet was fed to mice, and fat deposition was lower in the high-carbohydrate group.[7] Another found that total fat deposition is much less when a high-carbohydrate diet is fed compared with a high-fat diet.[3] A third study evaluated healthy cats fed three dry diets: low-carbohydrate, high-protein diet versus high carbohydrate, high-fat diet versus high-carbohydrate, high-fiber diet. The low-carbohydrate, high-protein diet resulted in a lower postprandial serum glucose concentration over a short period of time (10 hours) compared with preprandial levels, but it also resulted in twice as much postprandial insulin as the high-carbohydrate, high-fiber diet over the same period. This effect may have been due to the low-carbohydrate, high-protein diet's higher fat content, which can lead to insulin resistance, or its higher arginine level, which also increases insulin in cats.[30]

The problem with a direct cross-correlation of the aforementioned studies is that the diets varied in more than just the protein, fat, and carbohydrate content in that they were formulated by different manufacturers with different base ingredients. Thiess and colleagues[44] studied isonitrogenous diets in healthy male cats to diminish unwanted variation between diets. A high-carbohydrate diet was compared with a high-fat diet (see Table 19-2), resulting in a slightly elongated glucose clearance and decreased acute insulin response to glucose administration. These results suggest diminished pancreatic insulin secretion, beta cell responsiveness to glucose, or both with a high-fat diet.[44] Backus and colleagues[3] also limited for unwanted variability between experimental diets. The researchers studied 24 cats before and after gonadectomy with *ad libitum* feeding of one of four diets differing in carbohydrate content (see Table 19-2). Any difference in carbohydrate content among the diets was replaced with fat, whereas the same protein level remained across all diets. Metabolizable energy (ME) intake and body weight increased in all groups after gonadectomy, especially in females. The highest-fat diet (64% ME)/lowest-carbohydrate diet combination was associated with weight gain and increased insulin concentration, potentially indicating a risk factor for insulin resistance and subsequent diabetes mellitus (DM).

It is possible that less insulin resistance will be seen when feeding a high-protein diet because of increased heat production. Hoenig and colleagues[21] noted increased heat production in lean cats consuming isocaloric amounts of a high-protein diet compared with those consuming a high-carbohydrate diet (see Table 19-2). A long-term study is necessary to investigate whether cats with the same caloric intake develop less obesity and show less insulin resistance when fed a high-protein diet compared with high-carbohydrate diet.

Canned Versus Dry Carbohydrates

Canned food typically contains fewer carbohydrates, but specific differences between outcomes of feeding canned carbohydrates versus dry carbohydrates have not been studied. Despite this lack of data, many veterinarians now recommend that cat owners feed canned diets exclusively in an effort to limit carbohydrate intake. Most domesticated cats are neutered, which, as previously discussed, is associated with decreased metabolic rate and increased food intake. In owner-based surveys, owners are more likely to provide cats with dry food *ad libitum* rather than feed a specific amount of food in discrete meals, as they would with canned food.[23] Some veterinarians have expressed the concern that dry food may be a risk factor for development of obesity and DM. A survey based study of 96 diabetic cats versus 192 matched controls showed indoor confinement and physical inactivity are risk factors for DM, not the proportion of dry food consumed.[39]

Clinical Disease Concerns

Obesity

Obesity is one of the most prevalent conditions affecting domestic cats worldwide, which has led to widespread interest in nutritional intervention to limit its occurrence. Epidemiologic data have suggested that high-fat, rather than high-carbohydrate, foods play a role in obesity.[37] Further data show that total energy intake affects weight change in cats, with high-fat diets promoting excessive calorie intake, not high-carbohydrate content.[22] Crossover research was conducted involving 12 lean and 16 obese neutered cats fed either a high-carbohydrate (38.1 g/100 g) or a high-protein (45.2 g/100 g) diet each for 4 months to maintain weight (see Table 19-2). After this 8-month period, obese cats remained on their current experimental diet and intake was decreased to obtain approximately 1.5% body weight loss weekly to return to original lean weight. When obese cats on the high-protein diet lost weight, it comprised more total fat than cats on high-carbohydrate diet, but both groups lost same total amount of weight. It was noted that obesity, not protein or carbohydrate level of the diet, led to severe insulin resistance and a marked decrease of glucose effectiveness. The authors calculated each kilogram increase in weight led to approximately 30% loss in insulin sensitivity and glucose effectiveness, which is instrumental in DM development.[20] In another study using 24 group-housed adult cats, high-carbohydrate versus low-carbohydrate diets from different manufacturers were fed (see Table 19-2). Body condition and energy intake, not type of diet, influenced weight, but the cats were group housed and individual energy intake was not assessed.[28]

As mentioned previously, it is difficult to make direct correlations between studies because of the variation in ingredients used and final macronutrient composition of the diets. The data do, however, shape an argument that the amount of calories fed is inherently more important in weight gain with potential predisposition to DM than the specific nutrient composition of the food.

Diabetes Mellitus

The goals of nutritional management of DM are to blunt postprandial hyperglycemia, control body weight, support altered nutrient needs, improve peripheral insulin sensitivity, avoid diabetic complications, coordinate peak nutrient uptake, and achieve diabetic remission when possible.[21] To achieve these goals, using the metabolic adaptations mentioned in the preceding section, it has been hypothesized that a low-carbohydrate diet (<10% to 20% dry matter) is best.[54] Multiple authors have reported improved glycemic control in healthy and diabetic cats fed low-carbohydrate (<15% dry matter) diets (see Table 19-2).[4,16,26] Weight control and subsequent improved insulin sensitivity are also critical to the success of low-carbohydrate food.[21]

Feeding a low-carbohydrate canned food to 18 diabetic cats with or without acarbose (an α-amylase inhibitor) resulted in declines of blood glucose and serum fructosamine levels along with exogenous insulin requirements. More than 60% of cats fed the low-carbohydrate food reverted to a nondiabetic state.[26] Low-carbohydrate versus high-fiber, high-carbohydrate diets were studied in 63 cats with naturally occuring DM. Within 4 months of diet change, approximately 68% of cats consuming low-carbohydrate diets and 41% of cats in the high-fiber group discontinued insulin, but none of the cats that had been diabetic for longer than 36 months reverted to a non–insulin-dependent state. The authors concluded that diabetic cats fed low-carbohydrate foods are three times more likely to discontinue insulin and revert to a nondiabetic state.[4] To the author's knowledge, there are currently no published studies showing a benefit to feeding less than 12% (dry matter) of dietary calories as carbohydrate, which is the level in the aforementioned study. It is also interesting to note the similarity of 9.1% dry matter to the carbohydrate content of the average rat carcass.

Both of the aforementioned studies used variations in carbohydrate and fat in their diet formulations. Because fat is known to increase insulin resistance and decrease glucose tolerance, Thiess and colleagues suggested that it is logical to replace carbohydrates with protein. Anecdotal evidence that a high-protein diet leads to improved glucose homeostasis and lowering of insulin requirements was not found, insofar as the diet had no effect on insulin sensitivity.[44] The research team did find that the high-protein group exhibited significantly higher heat production, which may have eventually led to decreased food intake. Further study into this subject is warranted before making such conclusions.

Diabetic ketoacidosis (DKA) can be a complication of uncontrolled DM. The production of β-hydroxybutyrate is favored in cats with increased fat metabolism. However, urine ketone sticks react only with acetoacetate and acetone, so a positive reaction is not seen until ketones increase significantly, as with uncontrolled DM. Low-carbohydrate food improves weight loss and increases blood ketone levels because these diets also invariably have a higher fat level. It is important to keep in mind that diet-mediated ketosis is minimal compared with poor diabetic regulation, meaning that a positive urine ketone stick should not be considered a result of a low-carbohydrate diet.[21]

Contraindications for Low-Carbohydrate Diets

Any condition requiring protein or fat restriction should be carefully considered before recommending low-carbohydrate diets. This includes renal disease, severe hepatic disease, hepatoencephalitis, and possibly pancreatitis. Diet recommendations for cats with pancreatitis are somewhat controversial, with some experts advising moderate protein, low-fat, high-carbohydrate diets and others calling for high-protein, high-fat, low-carbohydrate diets.[21]

Recent Research

Using three isoenergetic homemade diets (low-protein versus low-fat versus low-carbohydrate), effects on glucose and insulin response were evaluated. Every 3 weeks, nine lean cats were exposed to one of three diets in a Latin square design until all cats had consumed each diet. There was no difference in glucose levels among diets. Although all diets did exhibit a bimodal insulin peak, the second peak insulin was delayed with the low-carbohydrate diet (45% DM protein, 48% DM fat). If followed long-term, this diet may have led to an insulin-resistant state that could have produced beta cell exhaustion. The authors also suggest the effect of carbohydrate on insulin sensitivity might be a U-shaped response in which extremely low- and extremely high-carbohydrate levels cause diminished insulin sensitivity. It is possible that a long-term evaluation of both diet conditions would exhibit eventual beta cell exhaustion.[47]

Another recent thought-provoking study examined kittens fed diets differing only in carbohydrate and protein content while in utero and after weaning during growth. Although the difference was not significant, kittens fed the high-protein diet tended to have a higher total average physical activity level. This trend may be related to the high thermal effect of protein consumption in lean cats noted by Hoenig and coworkers. The kittens fed the high-protein diet also tended to have more lean body mass compared with the kittens receiving the high-carbohydrate diets, but there was no difference in body fat mass between groups at 8 months of age. The trends lend themselves to a conclusion that food intake had greater influence on body composition than dietary macronutrient composition.[48] It will be interesting to compare results from these cats as adults in the future. Will the high-carbohydrate group become more obese than the high-protein group, or will long-term follow-up dispel all of our current thoughts on cats and carbohydrates?

The Bottom Line

As of this writing, there is still not enough concrete evidence to mandate the ideal carbohydrate content of a domestic cat's diet. Although cats are obligate carnivores requiring meat-containing diets to provide all the essential dietary nutrients, they are also able to effectively metabolize complex carbohydrates. Certain metabolic conditions will necessitate limited protein or fat with an unavoidable increase in dietary carbohydrate. The burden is still on the veterinarian's shoulders to consider each individual patient and determine the ideal nutritional strategy depending on that patient's life stage and disease status.

At this point it should be possible to reach a consensus that total energy consumption and weight management are paramount for both prevention of DM and induction of diabetic remission along with overall health. Perhaps in the future, when more long-term studies are published, there will be a standard recommendation for macronutrient composition of the average healthy cat's diet. For now it seems wise for the veterinarian to focus on helping the cat achieve a lean body weight rather than concentrating on the carbohydrate content or on whether the food is coming from a can or bag.

HOMEMADE DIETS

Cat owners may want to prepare meals for their pets in their own home for several reasons that fall in the following general categories:

1. Wariness regarding additives, preservatives, and contaminants
2. An inability to understand pet food label ingredients and subsequent distrust
3. A lack of suitable commercial products that meet the medical needs of the pet[33]

Many such owners also refer to their pets as their children, and they see an obligation to provide the best care possible, just as they would for a human child.

In a telephone-based survey in the United States and Australia, it was found that 13.1% of cats were fed non-commercial food such as table scraps, leftovers, and homemade diets as part of the main diet, and at least one quarter of the total diet for 6.2% of cats. The same survey also found 98.8% of cats were fed at least half their daily intake in the form of a commercial diet and were more likely to be fed *ad libitum* compared with dogs.[23] A separate report using the same telephone survey data noted that owners who fed their pets 50% to 75% home-prepared foods reflected greater mistrust of commercial pet foods, food processing, and the pet food industry and had more positive opinions about raw and home-prepared diets.[29]

Safety

In general, the most common safety concern voiced by owners unwilling to use a commercially available pet food product is the risk of contamination necessitating a diet recall, as occurred with the melamine contamination scare of 2007. From March 2009 through March 2010, the Food and Drug Administration (FDA) Center for Veterinary Medicine listed 10 reports of national pet food recalls. The reasons for these recalls ranged from possible *Salmonella* contamination of a nationally available raw food product to thiamine deficiency.[15] In the month of March 2010, there were more than 45 recalls of human food products with *Salmonella* contamination listed as a common inciting cause.[14] These statistics emphasize the point that all nationally produced food, whether for human or animal consumption, is closely scrutinized for contamination and safety of ingredients and that humans are much more likely to encounter a recall with a food item intended for their own consumption rather than one for their pet's consumption.

Other safety concerns owners have voiced regarding commercial diets include the use of artificial additives, especially preservatives, colorings, and flavorings, leading to long-term intake of these items.[27] Many fear that food additives play a role in carcinogenesis and development of dietary hypersensitivity or autoimmune disorders.[13] When evaluating the safety of a substance and whether it should be approved, the FDA considers the following factors:

- The composition and properties of the substance
- The amount that would typically be consumed
- The immediate and long-term health effects
- Various safety factors

All substances are approved in conjunction with an appropriate level of use that is much lower than what would be expected to produce an adverse effect.[32] Adverse events with a suspected association to specific food additives are reported to the FDA for investigation, allowing for ongoing safety reviews even after initial ingredient approval.

Despite this regulation process, foods free of artificial additives or with ingredients that are perceived to be more wholesome and safe can be appealing to the homemade diet enthusiast.[27] Even those looking for a more natural commercial diet must be educated about the regulations involving labeling of specific commercial diets. According to the AAFCO definition, a natural product is one in which all ingredients are derived solely from plant, animal, or mined sources that were not subjected to a chemically synthetic process and not containing any additives or processing aids that are chemically synthetic. Organic products must be produced and handled in compliance with requirements of the U.S. Department of Agriculture National Organic Program.[1] All commercial pet foods with labeling using the words *natural* or *organic* must meet the preceding definition.

From a public health standpoint, the most important documented safety concern related to use of homemade diets is the increasing popularity of raw food diets. There are also a growing number of commercially available raw food products. These feeding plans were discussed in preceding sections.

Complete and Balanced

All commercially available diets in the United States that are designed for long-term feeding must contain an AAFCO nutritional adequacy label on the packaging. This label will state that the diet either has been formulated to meet the needs of the specific life stage of the animal or has gone through an AAFCO feeding trial.[1] Homemade diet formulations are not governed by AAFCO regulation, and there is currently no standardized system in place regulating the nutritional adequacy of published home-prepared diet recipes. This lack of standardized regulation leads to concerns regarding the nutritional adequacy of homemade diets. Even if the diet is developed by a veterinary nutritionist, that diet is only as good as the database the nutritionist uses for individual ingredient evaluation, how well the client follows the instructions, and if the client deviates from the diet by substituting other ingredients over time.[33]

In a report analyzing 49 maintenance and 36 growth diets from six publications (compared with

AAFCO recommendations), 55% of the diets contained inadequate amounts of protein and 62% were inadequate in vitamins. Taurine or choline supplementation would have resolved the deficiency for 77% of the cases. Many of the ingredients in the databases used for ingredient nutrient levels are not analyzed for taurine and choline, meaning that diets determined as inadequate or deficient may have actually been adequate. Of these diets 86% were inadequate in various minerals and 8% were inadequate in essential amino acids.[34] In a separate study 44 commercial versus 35 home-prepared canine diets were compared. The diets were not different in energy content, but vitamin and mineral differences were noted. Home-prepared diet calcium to phosphorus ratios, vitamin A and E levels, along with potassium, copper, and zinc quantities were below AAFCO recommendations, whereas all commercial diet nutrients were above AAFCO minimums, except the calcium to phosphorus ratio, which was within the recommended range.[41]

Excessive protein is common in home-cooked diets, with many recipes recommending a ratio of greater than 1 part meat to 1 part grain. Excessively high protein levels can lead to a calcium imbalance with high phosphorus levels. Addition of bone, bone meal, or calcium does not resolve the calcium to phosphorus ratio issue of a diet that is also disproportionately high in phosphorus. Owners must also be educated that the vast majority of over-the-counter pet supplements do not contain vitamins and minerals in sufficient concentrations to balance and complete a homemade diet.[33] For all these reasons, homemade diets must be evaluated by a veterinary nutritionist to determine the risk or merit of feeding each individual diet.

The Bottom Line

For owners who have a strong desire to cook food for their pets at home, education is the major obligation of their veterinarian. There is currently no supportive information in the literature for safety concerns associated with FDA-approved food additives in the levels allowed in diets. Although occasional issues such as the widespread recall initiated by melamine contamination in 2007 do occur, they are rare in pet foods, especially compared with recalls of human food items.

There is minimal inherent risk of an owner feeding a homemade diet that is formulated by a veterinary nutritionist as long as the owner is diligent in following all specific ingredient and supplementation instructions. Many veterinary nutritionists are available for phone consultation and are able to analyze individual diets for nutritional adequacy. This will help to take this complicated burden off the shoulders of general practitioners while giving the owners access to accurate nutrition information.

References

1. AAFCO: Official Publication of Association of American Feed Control Officials, 2010
2. Atkins R: *Dr. Atkins' new diet revolution, revised edition*, New York, 2002, M Evans and Company.
3. Backus RC, Cave NJ, Keisler DH: Gonadectomy and high dietary fat but not high dietary carbohydrate induce gains in body weight and fat of domestic cats, *Br J Nutr* 98:641, 2007.
4. Bennett N, Greco DS, Peterson ME et al: Comparison of a low-carbohydrate low-fiber diet and a moderate carbohydrate-high fiber diet in the management of feline diabetes mellitus, *J Feline Med Surg* 8:73, 2006.
5. Billinghurst I: *Give your dog a bone: the practical commonsense way to feed dogs for a long healthy life*, Alexandria, Australia, 1993, Ian Billinghurst.
6. Billinghurst I: *The BARF diet: raw feeding for dogs and cats using evolutionary principles*, Alexandria, Australia, 2001, Ian Billinghurst.
7. Brunengraber DZ, McCabe BJ, Kasumov T et al: Influence of diet on the modeling of adipose tissue triglycerides during growth, *Am J Physiol Endocrinol Metab* 285:E917, 2003.
8. Centers for Disease Control and Prevention, Foodborne Diseases Active Surveillance Network (FoodNet): *FoodNet surveillance final report for 2005*, Atlanta, 2008, U.S. Department of Health and Human Services.
9. Centers for Disease Control and Prevention: *Salmonella surveillance: annual summary*, Atlanta, 2006, U.S. Department of Health and Human Services, Centers for Disease Control.
10. Centers for Disease Control: *National Antimicrobial Monitoring System for Enteric Bacteria (NARMS): Human isolates final report, 2006*, Atlanta, 2009, US Department of Health and Human Services, Centers for Disease Control and Prevention.
11. Center for Food Safety and Applied Nutrition: Food Ingredients and Colors, 2010.
12. Cherry B, Burns A, Johnson GS et al: *Salmonella typhimurium* outbreak associated with veterinary clinic, *Emerg Infect Dis* 10:2249, 2004.
13. DuPont HL: Clinical practice. Bacterial diarrhea, *N Engl J Med* 361:1560, 2009.
14. Dzanis DA: Safety of ethoxyquin in dog foods, *J Nutr* 121:S163, 1991.
15. Food and Drug Administration: 2010 recalls, market withdrawals and safety alerts, 2010.
16. Food and Drug Administration: *Pet food recalls and withdrawals*, March 2010.
17. Frank G, Anderson W, Pazak H et al: Use of a high-protein diet in the management of feline diabetes mellitus, *Vet Ther* 2:238, 2001.
18. Freeman LM, Michel KE: Evaluation of raw food diets for dogs, *J Am Vet Med Assoc* 218:705, 2001.
19. Geisen V, Weber K, Hartmann K: Vitamin D–dependent hereditary rickets type I in a cat, *J Vet Intern Med* 23:196, 2009.
20. Herz V, Kirberger RM: Nutritional secondary hyperparathyroidism in a white lion cub *(Panthera leo)*, with concomitant radiographic double cortical line, *J S Afr Vet Assoc* 75:49, 2004.
21. Hoenig M, Thomaseth K, Waldron M et al: Insulin sensitivity, fat distribution, and adipocytokine response to different diets in lean and obese cats before and after weight loss, *Am J Physiol Regul Integr Comp Physiol* 292:R227, 2007.
22. Kirk CA: Feline diabetes mellitus: low carbohydrates versus high fiber? *Vet Clin North Am Small Anim Pract* 36:1297, 2006.
23. Laflamme DP: Letter to the editor: cats and carbohydrates, *Top Companion Anim Med* 23:159, 2008.
24. Laflamme DP, Abood SK, Fascetti AJ et al: Pet feeding practices of dog and cat owners in the United States and Australia, *J Am Vet Med Assoc* 232:687, 2008.

25. Lauten S, Kirk CA: Computer analysis of nutrient sufficiency of published home-cooked diets for dogs and cats [abstract], *J Vet Intern Med* 19:476, 2005.
26. LeJeune JT, Hancock DD: Public health concerns associated with feeding raw meat diets to dogs, *J Am Vet Med Assoc* 219:1222, 2001.
27. MacDonald ML, Rogers QR, Morris JG: Nutrition of the domestic cat, a mammalian carnivore, *Annu Rev Nutr* 4:521, 1984.
28. Mazzaferro EM, Greco DS, Turner AS et al: Treatment of feline diabetes mellitus using an alpha-glucosidase inhibitor and a low-carbohydrate diet, *J Feline Med Surg* 5:183, 2003.
29. Michel KE: Unconventional diets for dogs and cats, *Vet Clin North Am Small Anim Pract* 36:1269, 2006.
30. Michel KE, Bader A, Shofer FS et al: Impact of time-limited feeding and dietary carbohydrate content on weight loss in group-housed cats, *J Feline Med Surg* 7:349, 2005.
31. Michel KE, Willoughby KN, Abood SK et al: Attitudes of pet owners toward pet foods and feeding management of cats and dogs, *J Am Vet Med Assoc* 233:1699, 2008.
32. Mori A, Sako T, Lee P et al: Comparison of three commercially available prescription diet regimens on short-term post-prandial serum glucose and insulin concentrations in healthy cats, *Vet Res Commun* 33:669, 2009.
33. Morris JG: Idiosyncratic nutrient requirements of cats appear to be diet-induced evolutionary adaptations, *Nutr Res Rev* 15:153, 2002.
34. Remillard RL: Homemade diets: attributes, pitfalls, and a call for action, *Top Companion Anim Med* 23:137, 2008.
35. Sanchez S, Hofacre CL, Lee MD et al: Animal sources of salmonellosis in humans, *J Am Vet Med Assoc* 221:492, 2002.
36. Sato Y, Mori T, Koyama T et al: Salmonella virchow infection in an infant transmitted by household dogs, *J Vet Med Sci* 62:767, 2000.
37. Scarlett JM, Donoghue S: Associations between body condition and disease in cats, *J Am Vet Med Assoc* 212:1725, 1998.
38. Schreiner CA, Nagode LA: Vitamin D–dependent rickets type 2 in a four-month-old cat, *J Am Vet Med Assoc* 222:337, 2003.
39. Slingerland LI, Fazilova VV, Plantinga EA et al: Indoor confinement and physical inactivity rather than the proportion of dry food are risk factors in the development of feline type 2 diabetes mellitus, *Vet J* 179:247, 2009.
40. Stiver SL, Frazier KS, Mauel MJ et al: Septicemic salmonellosis in two cats fed a raw-meat diet, *J Am Anim Hosp Assoc* 39:538, 2003.
41. Streiff EL, Zwischenberger B, Butterwick RF et al: A comparison of the nutritional adequacy of home-prepared and commercial diets for dogs, *J Nutr* 132:1698S, 2002.
42. Strohmeyer RA, Morley PS, Hyatt DR et al: Evaluation of bacterial and protozoal contamination of commercially available raw meat diets for dogs, *J Am Vet Med Assoc* 228:537, 2006.
43. Tanner E, Langley-Hobbs SJ: Vitamin D-dependent rickets type 2 with characteristic radiographic changes in a 4-month-old kitten, *J Feline Med Surg* 7:307, 2005.
44. Thiess S, Becskei C, Tomsa K et al: Effects of high carbohydrate and high fat diet on plasma metabolite levels and on i.v. glucose tolerance test in intact and neutered male cats, *J Feline Med Surg* 6:207, 2004.
45. Tomsa K, Glaus T, Hauser B et al: Nutritional secondary hyperparathyroidism in six cats, *J Small Anim Pract* 40:533, 1999.
46. van Rensburg IB, Lowry MH: Nutritional secondary hyperparathyroidism in a lion cub, *J S Afr Vet Assoc* 59:83, 1988.
47. Verbrugghe A, Hesta M, Van Weyenberg S et al: The glucose and insulin response to isoenergetic reduction of dietary energy sources in a true carnivore: the domestic cat *(Felis catus)*, *Br J Nutr* 104:214, 2010.
48. Vester BM, Liu KJ, Keel TL et al: In utero and postnatal exposure to a high-protein or high-carbohydrate diet leads to differences in adipose tissue mRNA expression and blood metabolites in kittens, *Br J Nutr* 102:1136, 2009.
49. von Pfeil DJ, Decamp CE, Abood SK: The epiphyseal plate: nutritional and hormonal influences; hereditary and other disorders, *Compend Contin Educ Vet* 31:E1, 2009.
50. Weese JS, Rousseau J: Survival of *Salmonella Copenhagen* in food bowls following contamination with experimentally inoculated raw meat: effects of time, cleaning, and disinfection, *Can Vet J* 47:887, 2006.
51. Weese JS, Rousseau J, Arroyo L: Bacteriological evaluation of commercial canine and feline raw diets, *Can Vet J* 46:513, 2005.
52. Won DS, Park C, In YJ et al: A case of nutritional secondary hyperparathyroidism in a Siberian tiger cub, *J Vet Med Sci* 66:551, 2004.
53. Wright JG, Tengelsen LA, Smith KE et al: Multidrug-resistant *Salmonella typhimurium* in four animal facilities, *Emerg Infect Dis* 11:1235, 2005.
54. Zoran DL: The carnivore connection to nutrition in cats, *J Am Vet Med Assoc* 221:1559, 2002.

SECTION IV

FELINE INTERNAL MEDICINE

Editors: Randolph M. Baral, Susan E. Little, and Jeffrey N. Bryan (Chapter 28: Oncology)

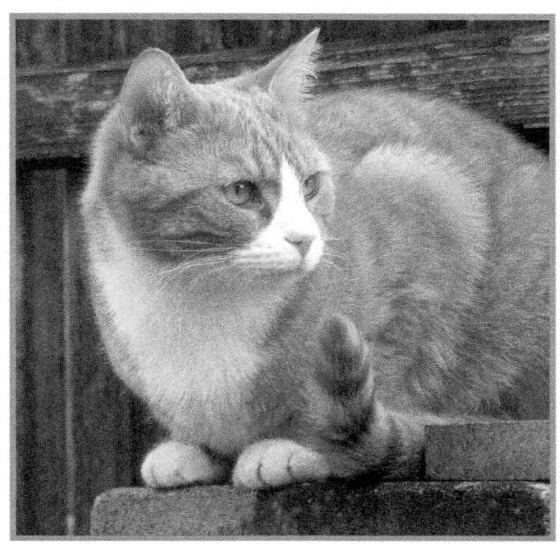

CHAPTER

20

Cardiovascular Diseases

Mark Rishniw

OUTLINE

PREVALENCE AND RISK FACTORS

Prevalence

The prevalence of cardiac disease in the general feline population is not currently determined. Stalis and coworkers[83] found that myopathic heart disease was identified in approximately 9% of 1472 feline necropsies from 1986 to 1992 at the University of Pennsylvania. More recently, two small studies (approximately 200 cats in total) have examined the prevalence of cardiac disease in apparently healthy cats.[18,61] Côté and colleagues[18] examined the prevalence of heart murmurs in apparently healthy cats and detected murmurs in 22 of 103 cats examined. Of these 22 cats, seven had echocardiographic evaluations, and six were considered to have evidence of myocardial hypertrophy (one was normal). Paige and coworkers[61] examined 103 apparently healthy cats: 16 of 103 had murmurs, and five of these had evidence of myocardial hypertrophy. Additionally, 11 of 103 cats had evidence of myocardial hypertrophy but no murmurs.

On the basis of these small epidemiologic studies, approximately 20% of apparently healthy cats examined at random will have cardiac murmurs, and a similar percentage might have myocardial hypertrophy. Of these, half will have murmurs, and half will have occult disease. Similarly, 50% or more of the cats with murmurs will not have identifiable cardiac disease; dynamic physiological murmurs likely account for some of these. It is important to note that both studies examined small numbers of cats. Furthermore, no longitudinal evaluation was performed to determine if the myocardial hypertrophy was transient (e.g., secondary to dehydration, thyroid disease or as yet unidentified causes of transient hypertrophy) or persistent. Only the latter would be consistent with hypertrophic cardiomyopathy. Thus the prevalence of cardiac disease in the general feline population remains unknown. However, a large longitudinal study of cats presenting to shelters in London is currently under way and may better define the prevalence of feline myocardial diseases.

Relative prevalence of cardiac disease has been examined by Harpster[31] at a single referral institution. Of 500 cats presenting to the cardiology department at Angell Memorial Animal Hospital from 1987 to 1989, 22% had hypertrophic cardiomyopathy, 15% had unclassified cardiomyopathy, 14% had mitral valve disease, 12% had dilated cardiomyopathy, 10% had thyrotoxic heart disease, and approximately 7% had congenital diseases. Systemic hypertension was identified in 1%. It should be obvious that these percentages do not represent true prevalence (or incidence) but rather describe the distribution of heart diseases in patients presenting for evaluation of heart disease. Additionally, substantial changes in feline nutrition (namely taurine supplementation) and early detection and management of hyperthyroidism have greatly reduced the percentage of cats presenting with either dilated cardiomyopathy or thyrotoxic heart disease.

Similarly, the prevalence of congenital cardiac diseases in cats is much less comprehensively reported than that of dogs. Frequency of congenital heart disease has not been examined in the last 30 years. Buchanan[11] estimated that atrioventricular valve malformations were the most common congenital defect in cats, followed by ventricular septal defect (VSD), endocardial fibroelastosis and patent ductus arteriosus (PDA).

Côté and Jaeger[17] examined the incidence of structural heart disease in 106 cats presenting with ventricular arrhythmias. Almost all cats with ventricular tachyarrhythmias had echocardiographic evidence of structural heart disease (102 of 106). Prior studies by Fox and associates[26] and Fox and Harpster[25] suggested substantially lower incidence rates of ventricular tachyarrhythmias in cats with hypertrophic cardiomyopathy (HCM) (10% to 40%). However, both studies reported all arrhythmias in cats with HCM at much higher rates (25% to 70%).

Risk Factors

Certain risk factors are associated with some feline heart disease. HCM has specific breed predispositions, and at least one identified genetic cause in each of two breeds (Maine Coons and Ragdolls).[53,55] Sphynx, Norwegian Forest Cats, American Shorthairs, Scottish Folds, Persians, Siamese, Abyssinians, Himalayans, and Birmans are all breeds considered to be predisposed to cardiomyopathies.[23] Whether there are any gender differences in expression of genetic traits or in prevalence of congenital disorders is not well defined.

Taurine deficiency was identified as a major cause of dilated cardiomyopathy in cats in the mid 1980s.[64] Subsequent supplementation of commercial diets with taurine has led to the almost complete disappearance of taurine-deficient myocardial failure in cats. However, homemade diets can still occasionally lead to taurine deficiency, resulting in dilated cardiomyopathy.

Hyperthyroidism is a risk factor for cardiac disease in cats. However, the prevalence of thyrotoxic heart disease has likely decreased since hyperthyroidism was first recognized, as clinicians have become more adept at identifying cats with hyperthyroidism earlier in the disease course, often before the development of severe cardiac remodeling and high-output heart failure. Other risk factors, such as acromegaly, appear to be extremely uncommon, and descriptions of these are limited to small case series or case reports.

HISTORY AND PHYSICAL EXAMINATION

Although history taking can offer insights to the clinician about the patient, the uncanny ability of cats to mask their disease status until the condition is critical prevents many owners from providing diagnostically useful information. Owners might report findings such as panting, hiding, or reluctance to participate in usual activities in the days preceding presentation for severe disease. With mild subclinical disease, no changes will be apparent to the owners. Dietary history is useful only if taurine deficiency is suspected; however, a homemade diet might be a clue to the clinician to examine the patient for taurine deficiency.

Systemic thromboembolism is often accompanied by a history of acute paralysis or paresis and apparent excruciating pain. Owners often report that their cat screamed or yowled loudly at the onset of the event, without any apparent evidence of trauma. Cats presenting later in the course of the disease often have a history of being missing for a period of time and being found paralyzed or paretic.

Murmurs

The physical examination of cats with heart disease is often only modestly revealing. Many cats with cardiac disease have no indicative clinical signs or physical examination findings. In one small study, only 5 of 16 of cats with cardiomyopathy had murmurs at initial examination; 11 had occult disease.[61] This number increased to 11 of 16 cats when dynamic murmurs (not necessarily ausculted at the time of examination but provoked during echocardiographic evaluation) were examined. Conversely, many cats with a murmur have no identifiable heart disease. Paige and coworkers[61] also identified murmurs in 16 of 103 healthy cats but found cardiac disease in only 5 of these; 11 had no evidence of structural disease.

Dynamic murmurs are common findings in cats with and without heart disease. Paige and coworkers[61] identified dynamic murmurs in 28 of 103 apparently healthy cats. Dynamic murmurs change in intensity or appear only after provocation (e.g., fear, aggression). They are generally parasternal murmurs (either right or left) and can be extremely transient, lasting only a few beats in some cats. Rishniw and Thomas[71] identified a dynamic right ventricular outflow tract obstruction in 50 cats between 1994 and 1996 that was only occasionally associated with structural heart disease. The most common diseases associated with this physiologic murmur were chronic kidney disease and nasal squamous cell carcinoma (SCC), but these cats were examined in California, where nasal SCC is highly prevalent. Cats younger than 4 years of age with dynamic right ventricular outflow tract obstruction most often had HCM.

Systolic anterior motion of the mitral valve and the associated dynamic left ventricular obstruction account for most of the remainder of identifiable dynamic murmurs in cats. This phenomenon is observed predominantly in cats with HCM but can occasionally be observed in cats without any identifiable structural heart disease. Midventricular obstructions have also been identified in cats with HCM or other feline cardiac diseases[49] and might account for some dynamic murmurs in cats. In one study only 36% of provocable murmurs had an identifiable etiology; thus many dynamic murmurs might not have an easily identifiable cause.[61]

Heart Sounds and Arrhythmias

The most commonly observed abnormal heart sound in feline heart disease (excluding murmurs) is the gallop sound. This can be intermittent or sustained and results from an increased intensity of the third or fourth heart sound (or a summation of the two). A true gallop sound is indicative of severe heart disease in cats, associated with marked diastolic dysfunction. However, because of the almost identical systolic and diastolic time intervals in cats, feline gallop sounds are auscultably indistinguishable from systolic clicks. Systolic clicks are uncommon, and, as in dogs, they are thought to be associated with mild mitral valve disease in older cats. They can be distinguished from gallop sounds only by high-fidelity phonocardiograms that have electrocardiographic timing, which demonstrate that the extra heart sound occurs in midsystole. Finally, ventricular extrasystoles (ventricular bigeminy) can sometimes produce a gallop sound if the ventricular extrasystolic beat occurs close to the sinus beat. In these cases the mitral valve opens and then closes during the extrasystole, but the aortic valve fails to open (causing only one heart sound from the extrasystole and two heart sounds from the preceding sinus beat). This can be identified by electrocardiography (ECG). Thus the presence of an additional heart sound in a cat warrants further diagnostic investigation.

Arrhythmias occur frequently in cats with heart disease. In one retrospective study, 96% of cats with ventricular tachyarrhythmias had echocardiographic evidence of structural heart disease. Thus auscultation of extrasystoles warrants further investigation. It is, however, more difficult to define sustained tachyarrhythmias in cats presenting to clinicians for physical evaluation. Feline heart rates can easily reach 240 to 260 beats per minute (bpm) in stressful situations and can do so in a matter of seconds. Cats stressed by a hospital visit or because of other systemic disease can have sustained heart rates above 220 bpm.[1] The astute clinician should note heart rates from prior visits in regular patients to determine whether the rate is appropriate for that patient. Unexpectedly high heart rates, especially those that deviate from rates obtained at prior visits, might warrant further investigation.

Bradyarrhythmias are less commonly ausculted but occur especially in older cats. The author considers any heart rate persistently lower than 130 bpm in a cat during a clinical examination to be unexpectedly low, warranting further diagnostic testing. However, healthy young (mostly) male cats occasionally appear to have low resting heart rates.

Sinus arrhythmias are uncommon in cats in the hospital environment and have been associated mostly with extracardiac disease.[69] However, some healthy young cats can have a mild sinus arrhythmia as an incidental finding. Additionally, most cats exhibit brief periods of sinus arrhythmia during sleep.[86]

Clinical Signs of Congestive Heart Failure

Cats are extremely adept at hiding signs of heart disease until they reach a critical stage. Often, clinical signs such as mild tachypnea and reduced activity are not apparent to the owner, and cats present to the clinician with profound dyspnea. Thoracic auscultation might reveal signs of congestive heart failure (CHF). A murmur or gallop sound coupled with dyspnea increases the index of suspicion for CHF. Muffled or absent breath sounds or dorsally displaced breath sounds (absent ventrally) are suggestive of pleural effusion. On the other hand, coughing and gagging, wheezing, or auscultable crackles are rarely associated with CHF but are almost always indicative of primary respiratory disease. Extremities may be somewhat cool because of vasoconstriction that occurs with CHF, but this is an unreliable sign of CHF.

Physical Examination Procedures of Limited Value in Diagnosis of Feline Heart Disease

Peripheral Pulse Quality

With the exception of systemic thromboembolic disease, assessment of peripheral pulses in cats with heart disease offers little in the general cardiovascular assessment of the patient. Pulses are rarely altered with most feline cardiac disease, and clinicians' ability to discern minor changes in pulse quality is limited. Thus the author advises evaluating feline pulses only if paresis or paralysis of limbs is suspected.

Mucous Membrane Color and Capillary Refill Time

Most cats have mucosal color that is somewhat "anemic" or "cyanotic looking." Severe heart disease and even CHF often fail to alter mucosal color or capillary refill time, and interpretation of the findings is questionable enough that performing these procedures in cats with suspected heart disease is not recommended.

Murmur Localization and Characterization

Although localization of murmurs in dogs can help with identification of the underlying heart disease, this approach is much more difficult in cats. First, many clinicians use stethoscopes with large diaphragms, and the area of the diaphragm is similar to the area of the cardiac silhouette. This effectively limits the ability to localize to an area smaller than the entire heart. Second, many cats with (and without) heart disease have parasternal murmurs, which are often dynamic. These can occur for various reasons and do not help in further defining the nature of the heart disease.

In some instances murmur localization and description can assist with diagnosis. VSDs and tricuspid valve defects are generally ausculted on the right side, whereas PDA murmurs are suprabasilar continuous murmurs.

Thus clinicians should, in practice, limit their auscultation to detection of a murmur and possible description of location but not expect to derive a diagnosis solely on the basis of this physical examination procedure.

DIAGNOSIS OF FELINE HEART DISEASE

As previously explained, the history and physical examination, although important, generally fail to provide a definitive diagnosis of heart disease or the type of heart disease. In most cases, when heart disease is suspected, additional diagnostics are required to confirm the suspicion before any therapy can be instituted.

Electrocardiography

ECG is largely limited to diagnosis of arrhythmias and conduction disturbances in cats. It is best reserved for those patients that have auscultable arrhythmias. Arrhythmias are relatively uncommon in cats, with the exception of sinus tachycardia. However, their frequency increases substantially with the presence of heart disease.

In eupneic cats the ECG is recorded in right lateral recumbency. However, sternal recumbency alters few electrocardiographic parameters of clinical interest.[29,32] Therefore assessment in sternal recumbency in fractious, dyspneic, or fragile patients is acceptable.

Continuous 24-hour ambulatory ECG (Holter) monitoring has historically been less successful in cats than dogs, largely because of the size of the recording systems. New digital Holter systems are small enough to be attached to the cat with adhesive bandaging. Holter monitoring can provide diagnostic information in cats with syncope.[22] Additionally, small event recorders can be surgically implanted into syncopal patients to increase the probability of arrhythmia detection.[20,38] Holter monitors should not be used on cats with severe structural heart disease or CHF because the stress of monitoring can result in the death of the patient.

Electrocardiography as a Screening Test for Subclinical Heart Disease

ECG is ineffective as a screening tool for occult cardiac disease in cats. The basis for using ECG as a screening tool relies on its ability to detect either chamber enlargement or shifts in the mean electrical axis (MEA). However, ECG is extremely insensitive and relatively imprecise in detecting chamber enlargement (or myocardial concentric hypertrophy), and although it can identify deviations in the MEA, these occur relatively infrequently in the general population and can occur in cats with and without underlying structural disease. Only one study has examined the ability of ECG to identify left atrial enlargement in cats.[76] This study showed poor sensitivity (12% to 60%) and good specificity (72% to 100%), suggesting that very few cats with p-wave abnormalities have normal left atria. No equivalent studies exist that specifically examine the sensitivity and specificity of ECG in detecting ventricular enlargement in cats; however, studies in humans and other species suggest sensitivities of approximately 50% and specificities of 80% (similar to those found by Schober and coworkers[76] for left atrial enlargement). Two studies have examined ECG abnormalities in cats with heart disease. Ferasin and coworkers[21] identified 106 cats with varying degrees of HCM; of these 41 (39%) had no identifiable ECG abnormalities. Riesen and coworkers[68] examined 395 cats with various symptomatic heart diseases, including 169 cats with HCM; of these 35 (21%) had no identifiable ECG abnormalities. Riesen and coworkers identified morphologic changes (i.e., chamber enlargement patterns) in only 15 of 169 (10%) cats with HCM, whereas Ferasin and coworkers found morphologic changes in 30 of 61 (50%) cats with HCM. If these data are combined, morphologic changes indicative of chamber enlargement occur in fewer than 20% of cats with HCM. However, this may be an overestimation, because individual animals in these studies might have had more than one morphologic change; we have assumed that each observation is independent, which gives the "best-case scenario." Thus the sensitivity of ECG in detecting morphologic changes consistent with chamber enlargement or HCM, on the basis of these two studies, is 20%. If one assumes that 15% of the general feline population has heart disease, the positive predictive value of morphologic changes on the ECG is approximately 15%, and the negative predictive value is approximately 85%. Thus a clinician is six times as likely to find a false-positive result as a true-positive result when screening cats by ECG, resulting in substantial expense to clients in pursuit of nonexistent disease. With lower prevalence the probability of a false-positive finding only increases. A negative result would strongly suggest that the cat is "unaffected" because most cats examined are going to be normal. However, most cats with HCM that are examined will also have normal ECG results; these will not be identified.

Presence of pathologic arrhythmias (ventricular premature contraction [VPC], atrial premature contraction [APC], atrial fibrillation) occurred in 17 of 169 (10%) of HCM cats in one study,[68] and 8 of 106 (8%) in another study[21]—again, whether these were independent observations or whether multiple arrhythmias were present in the same cat was not apparent. However, this again results in a sensitivity of 10%, preventing the clinician from effectively ruling out the presence of HCM in the absence of arrhythmias.

Radiography

Radiography has been used for diagnosis of feline heart disease since the early 1970s. More recently, it has been supplanted by echocardiography for diagnosis of heart disease, but it is still a valuable diagnostic test for identification of CHF or discrimination of causes of dyspnea in cats.

Identification of cardiomegaly from radiographs in cats is difficult. Enlargement patterns most amenable to radiographic evaluation are *left atrial* or *biatrial enlargement* and *left ventricular volume overload.* Mild enlargement (as defined echocardiographically) is generally not detectable radiographically; chambers must be at least moderately enlarged before they are radiographically detectable. Right-sided heart changes are both uncommon and difficult to identify in cats (and dogs). Similarly, left ventricular concentric hypertrophy, as occurs with HCM, is not radiographically identifiable; cats can have profoundly thickened left ventricular walls that are radiographically undetectable.

Both lateral and dorsoventral (DV) or ventrodorsal (VD) views are required for the diagnosis of feline heart disease because atrial enlargement is best appreciated in the DV/VD view. There is little difference between VD or DV views. Cats that are dyspneic or tachypneic are best imaged in sternal recumbency to reduce the stress of restraint, which can result in severe clinical deterioration. End-inspiratory films are preferred, although this is not essential in most cases. In the author's experience of evaluating feline thoracic radiographs obtained by general practitioners, most cats provide films of sufficient quality for interpretation. Obese cats can be problematic because of their reluctance to take deep breaths; in such patients, interpretation of the pulmonary parenchyma can be problematic.

Most traditional rules of cardiac mensuration (measurement) are of little value in cats. Comparisons of the cardiac silhouette to the thoracic cavity or degree of cardiosternal contact have no value in assessing feline thoracic radiographs for cardiac disease. Sternal contact is prominent in many cats and increases with age in cats with normal hearts.[57,59] Similarly, aortic "redundancy" or "undulation," wherein the ascending aorta forms a prominent silhouette on thoracic films, along with a more sternally positioned heart, is commonly observed in older cats and is an incidental finding.[57] One study suggested that this finding is associated with systemic hypertension.[60]

Vertebral heart scale (VHS) has been developed for assessment of cardiac size in cats[46] and can help with identification of atrial enlargement or generalized cardiomegaly. A VHS greater than 8.1 is consistent with cardiomegaly in the cat (Figures 20-1 and 20-2). However, clinicians should recognize that the most common adult-onset feline disease (HCM) often does not cause radiographically detectable ventricular enlargement, so a normal VHS does not rule out the presence of significant heart disease in cats.

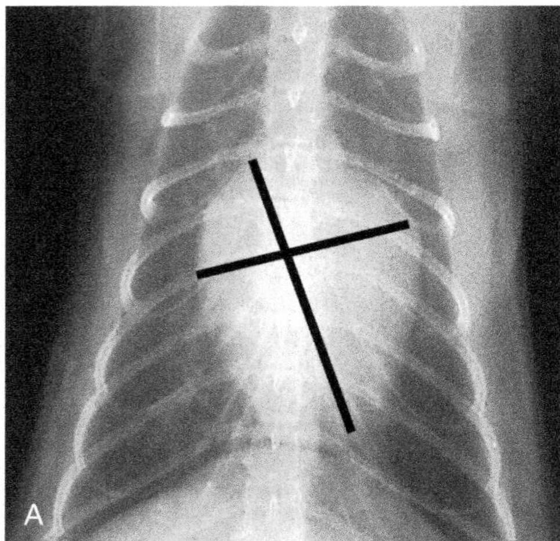

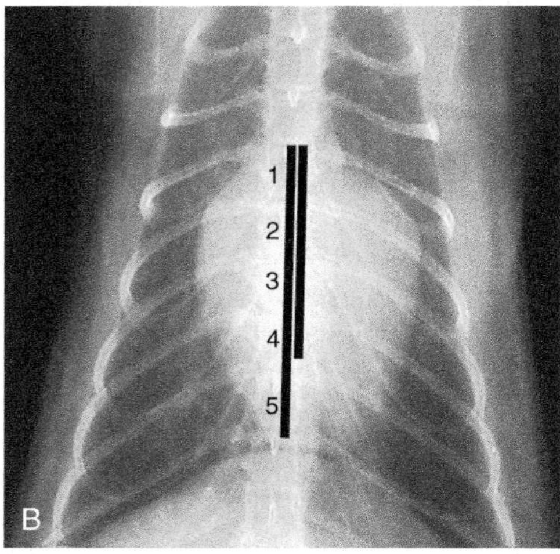

FIGURE 20-1 Measurement of vertebral heart scale on the dorsoventral radiographic view. **A,** A line is drawn along the long axis of the heart from right atrium to left ventricular apex. A second line is drawn perpendicular to the long axis, spanning the atria. **B,** These lines are then transferred to the cranial edge of the fourth thoracic vertebra, and the number of vertebrae spanned by the two lines is summed. In this example the vertebral heart scale is approximately 9 vertebrae.

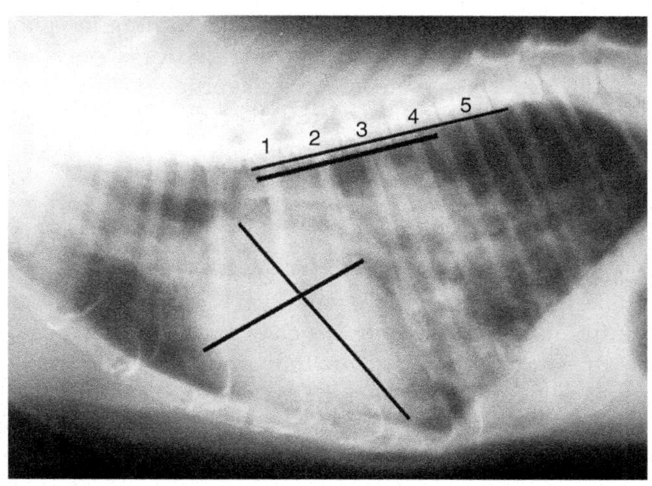

FIGURE 20-2 Measurement of vertebral heart scale on the lateral radiographic view. The same method is used as for the dorsoventral view. In this example the vertebral heart scale measures 9 vertebrae. Note the marked interstitial–alveolar pattern in the caudal and accessory lung lobes, consistent with congestive heart failure (pulmonary edema).

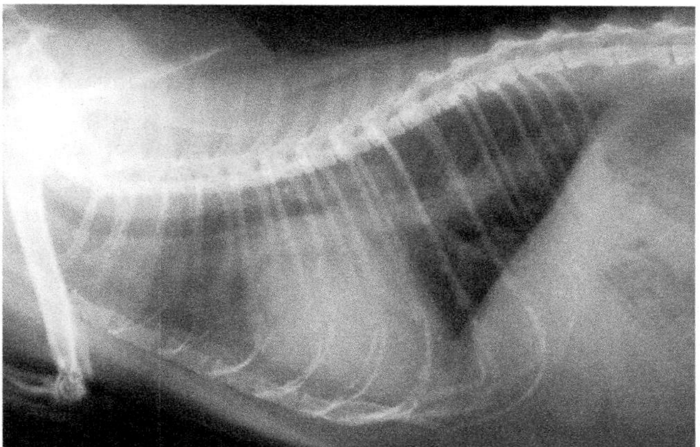

FIGURE 20-3 Lateral radiograph showing congestive heart failure secondary to hypertrophic cardiomyopathy in a cat. Note the prominent caudal lobar vessels with perivascular interstitial pattern. The left atrium is markedly enlarged.

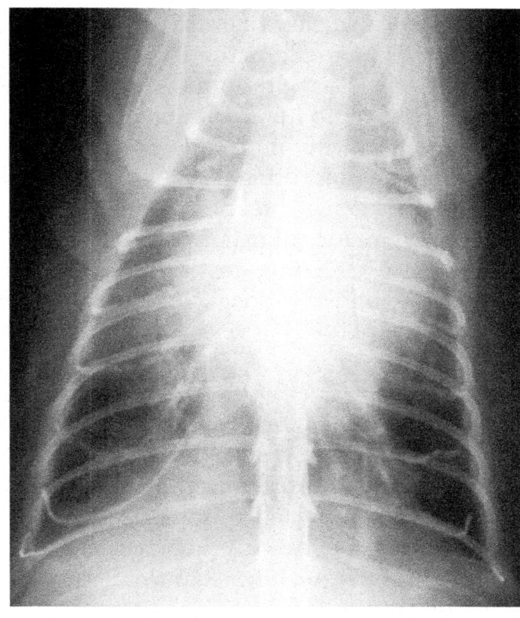

FIGURE 20-4 Dorsoventral radiograph showing congestive heart failure secondary to hypertrophic cardiomyopathy in a cat. Note the marked cardiomegaly and heavy interstitial pattern throughout the lung fields.

Assessment of pulmonary vasculature is substantially less reliable in cats than in dogs. Venous or arterial enlargement is subject to considerable misinterpretation and rarely accurately reflects the pulmonary hemodynamic state. In some cats with CHF, the pulmonary vasculature on the lateral projection appears to be pronounced, but this is subjective and unreliable.

Diagnosis of CHF in cats is aided by thoracic radiographs. Clinicians should not make a diagnosis of CHF in the absence of supportive clinical signs (i.e., radiographs should not be the primary means by which the diagnosis is made). Ideally, marked cardiomegaly is apparent radiographically to support the hypothesis of severe heart disease underlying the pulmonary changes. However, in many cats severe pulmonary changes (pulmonary edema or pleural effusion) obscure the cardiac silhouette, making interpretation of cardiac size impossible. In contrast to dogs, pulmonary edema in cats has little radiographic consistency.[50] One study of 23 cats with CHF showed at least six distinct pulmonary parenchymal patterns indicative of pulmonary edema (Figures 20-3 and 20-4).[7] Thus pulmonary edema cannot be excluded on the basis of a radiographic pattern that is different from that seen in most dogs. This can complicate the diagnosis of CHF in cats when the cardiac silhouette is not clearly visible.

Echocardiography

Echocardiography remains the most useful tool in identifying feline heart disease. Feline echocardiography requires substantial skill in both acquisition and interpretation of data. Additionally, many of the more common conditions require spectral and color Doppler analysis. Thus feline echocardiography remains largely a specialist diagnostic test. It is important to recognize these requirements when considering echocardiography for a patient because an incomplete or substandard echocardiographic evaluation can impoverish the client without providing a diagnosis.

Because of the cat's high heart rate and small heart size, imaging is usually performed with a high-frequency transducer (7 to 10 MHz). Advances in processing capabilities of ultrasound machines over the last 20 years have allowed most measurements of chamber and wall dimensions to be made from two-dimensional images rather than M-mode images. This also allows the echocardiographer to measure dimensions in regions not measurable by M-mode echocardiography (e.g., anterior and posterior aspects of the left ventricular wall). Linear and area chamber dimensions can be obtained.

A detailed explanation of echocardiographic technique is beyond the scope of this chapter, and readers should consult cardiology or echocardiography textbooks for additional details.

Biomarkers

Most recently, biochemical indicators of heart disease have been developed and marketed. These include cardiac troponin I; atrial natriuretic peptide (ANP) and its prohormone, NT-proANP; and B-type natriuretic peptide (BNP) and its prohormone, NT-proBNP. These are proteins either secreted or released by cardiomyocytes in response to stretch or injury and can be measured in serum or plasma. In humans these biomarkers have allowed early, rapid identification of acute myocardial injury and stratification of patients for appropriate acute interventions or additional diagnostic testing.

Use of biomarkers in feline medicine has been restricted largely to identification of subclinical heart disease (i.e., as a screening test) and differentiation of causes of acute dyspnea (cardiogenic versus pneumogenic/other).

NT-proBNP as a Screening Test

Several studies have examined the use of NT-proBNP as a screening test for cardiac disease in cats, namely HCM. While the test showed a difference in NT-proBNP concentrations between "affected" and "unaffected" cats in these studies and good or very good sensitivities and specificities for distinguishing "affected" and "unaffected" cats, most of the studies did not stratify the cats according to severity of subclinical disease. Only two small studies have looked at the ability of NT-proBNP to identify cats with HCM with varying degrees of subclinical disease.[35,78] The authors of the first study showed that only cats with severe myocardial hypertrophy (but not moderate or equivocal changes) could be somewhat confidently identified as being "affected." However, when the authors repeated the study with a new version of the assay, even this ability to detect severely affected cats was compromised. Thus, on the basis of these data, a high NT-proBNP might be expected to help rule in a cat with severe subclinical disease (not many false-positive results) but would not be able to rule out cats with HCM (many false-negative results). Additionally, personal observations by the author suggest that false-positive findings in cats are more common than reported in these studies. Finally, the assay has undergone substantial modifications since these studies were performed and has not yet been re-evaluated. Therefore substantially larger cross-sectional studies are needed, with patients stratified into degrees of subclinical severity and the modified version of the assay used.

NT-proBNP as a Diagnostic Test for Congestive Heart Failure

An alternative use for this assay has been directed at discriminating causes of dyspnea or respiratory distress. Several studies have shown that populations of unaffected cats or cats with dyspnea resulting from acute respiratory disease have lower NT-proBNP concentrations than cats with dyspnea from CHF. However, some overlap exists. One study, by Connolly and coworkers[16] showed that approximately 80% of cats would be correctly diagnosed on the basis of NT-proBNP concentrations. However, this also suggests that one in five cats would be incorrectly diagnosed and potentially inappropriately treated, with possible life-threatening consequences.

Diagnosis of the cause of tachydyspnea in cats can be difficult when the cardiac silhouette is obscured by pleural effusion, fat, or other pulmonary parenchymal changes. When the "probability of CHF" equals the "probability of not CHF," an NT-proBNP measurement might increase the odds of correct diagnosis. However, because such clinical situations are acute and demand rapid intervention, until the assay becomes available as an in-house rapid assay, it will have little value in diagnosis or treatment of acute tachydyspnea in cats, insofar as a therapeutic decision will likely have been made well before test results become available.

Whether the assay can improve the probability of correct diagnosis beyond what is achieved with current diagnostic tests (physical examination, history, echocardiography, radiography) is not known. Further studies are needed to demonstrate the true clinical efficacy of biomarkers in feline medicine.

Abuses of Biomarker Assays

Any screening test should only be applied to an "at-risk" population, rather than being performed indiscriminately. Furthermore, a screening test should be either specific or sensitive (depending on whether the veterinarian wishes either to rule in a disease or to rule out a disease), or both (which is rare). It should be affordable. An early diagnosis should allow intervention that either alters disease outcome or reduces risk of adverse events. It could be argued that every adult cat is at risk for having subclinical heart disease. However, there are currently no therapies known to alter disease progression in cats with heart disease (with the exception of the almost extinct taurine-deficient myocardial failure). Thus identifying HCM early in the course of the disease does not allow the clinician to alter the outcome for that patient. Because of this, random testing is not recommended, insofar as the probability of false-positive results (with consequent costly further investigations) far exceeds the probability of true-positive results. One could argue for the use of NT-proBNP as a preanesthetic test, although, as stated earlier, additional studies are required to better evaluate the validity of the assay.

FELINE HYPERTENSION AND HEART DISEASE

Definitions

Systemic hypertension is well documented in cats and can result in significant morbidity and potentially mortality. Clinically, systolic hypertension is identified most commonly, whereas diastolic hypertension has not been reported routinely. Systolic hypertension has been defined as a systolic blood pressure (BP) greater than 160 mm Hg. A grading scheme has been devised, with increasing levels of hypertension presumably associated with worse outcomes (Table 20-1).[10]

Causes

Feline systemic hypertension is generally thought to be associated with underlying systemic diseases, such as renal disease and hyperthyroidism. Essential hypertension and geriatric hypertension (the most common causes of hypertension in humans) have not been recognized as distinct entities in domestic animals. These forms of hypertension are secondary to various, mostly genetic factors (compounded by environmental factors, such as obesity) in the former case and loss of vascular elastance in the latter case. Thus any feline patient diagnosed with systemic hypertension should have an underlying etiology identified. Renal disease is the most common cause of systemic hypertension in cats, resulting in hyperreninemic hypertension. However, measurement of plasma renin activity is not routinely available to document a renal etiology. Because renal disease in cats most commonly manifests initially as a loss of urine-concentrating ability, the majority of older cats with hypertension would be expected to have suboptimal urine-concentrating ability.

TABLE 20-1 **Classification of Systolic Blood Pressure by Risk of Target Organ Damage in the Cat**

Risk Category	Systolic Blood Pressure (mm Hg)	Risk of Target Organ Damage
I	<150	Minimal
II	150-159	Mild
III	160-179	Moderate
IV	>180	Severe

Modified from Brown S, Atkins C, Bagley R et al: Guidelines for the identification, evaluation, and management of systemic hypertension in dogs and cats, *J Vet Intern Med* 21:542, 2007.

Clinical Signs

Systemic hypertension has been described as a "silent killer" in humans because clinical signs of disease are often inapparent while end-organ damage is occurring. Similarly, in feline patients, few clinical signs are apparent, and they may be subtle and nonspecific, such as anorexia and lethargy. Renal disease can be extremely mild and not clinically apparent. The most common clinical presentation with severe systemic hypertension is acute retinopathy (retinal separation or hemorrhage) (see Figure 29-59).[52] Ocular signs may also include dilated pupils and hyphema. Experimentally, acute severe hypertension has resulted in hemorrhagic encephalopathy ("stroke"), but this is not commonly identified in cats with spontaneous disease. Neurologic signs may include head tilt, ataxia, disorientation, and seizures. Cardiac murmurs have been associated with hypertension; however, there is no physiologic reason for systemic hypertension to produce turbulence that would result in a murmur. Thus it is likely that this association is coincidental rather than causal. Several authors have reported cardiac changes in cats with hypertension, including concentric left ventricular hypertrophy and redundancy of the ascending aorta.[12,14,34,60] These changes are generally mild but can be confused with a diagnosis of HCM.

Diagnosis

The diagnosis of systemic hypertension in cats is problematic for several reasons. First, the equipment currently available for noninvasive blood pressure (NIBP) measurement is neither accurate nor precise. Despite multiple studies claiming to validate NIBP systems, most have not compared to a true gold standard (direct, invasive telemetric instantaneous BP monitoring). Additionally, many of these studies have examined systems in anesthetized cats rather than conscious animals. Recently, a study comparing oscillometric systems with direct measurements in anesthetized cats found that no system was sufficiently accurate or precise to be useful.[2] Recommendations for measuring NIBP in cats have been made by multiple investigators who suggest that four measurements should be made, with the first measurement discarded and the remaining three measurements averaged. However, this method does not guarantee either accuracy or precision of the measurement.

Several NIBP systems are currently marketed and used for measuring systolic blood pressure (SBP) in cats:

traditional oscillometric systems; Doppler systems; and, most recently, high-definition oscillometric (HDO) systems. Anecdotal perceptions among clinicians suggested that Doppler-based methodology was more accurate than oscillometric methodology, but unpublished studies comparing both systems in the same animals against invasive measurements have failed to support this perception; both methodologies are equally inaccurate.[18b] No studies exist detailing performance of HDO systems in cats. However, studies in dogs suggest that these systems would perform no better than standard oscillometric and Doppler systems.[87]

Complicating the accurate measurement of SBP is the lability of feline BP. The author has observed conscious cats, gently restrained and accustomed to handling, with SBP measurements that vary by as much as 100 mm Hg in the space of a few seconds with little change in heart rate or perceived stress level. Many clinicians attempt to measure SBP at the patient's home to reduce the impact of stress, but no studies have demonstrated that this strategy results in more accurate measurement. One study examining the effect of conditioning on SBP in dogs showed that repeated measurements over several weeks resulted in a significant gradual reduction in measured BP as the "white-coat" effect subsided in these patients.[73] A similar pattern might be anticipated in cats. A study in cats demonstrated a significant white-coat effect in cats that would result in substantially higher SBP measurements than those obtained at rest.[6]

Sustained SBP above 200 mm Hg generally results in end-organ damage. This can often be appreciated in retinal vascular pathology because retinal blood vessels are exquisitely susceptible to hypertensive injury. Vascular engorgement and tortuosity or retinal hemorrhage should be searched for if repeated SBP measurements exceed 200 mm Hg. If the retinas appear normal, the diagnosis of systemic hypertension should be questioned. However, repeated measurements above 220 mm Hg are likely indicative of true hypertension. Similarly, evidence of severe hypertension in patients with acute retinopathy increases the probability of an accurate diagnosis.

Clinicians should adopt several steps in the diagnosis of feline systemic hypertension:

1. Examine the appropriate target population. Hypertension is mostly a geriatric disorder in cats. Cats younger than 8 or 9 years of age rarely have systemic hypertension. Therefore BP should not be measured in healthy young to middle-aged cats because the prior probability of these patients actually having hypertension is very low, unless they have renal disease. Indeed, the value of routine BP screening in cats is questionable; it might be more prudent to perform routine urinalysis and an ophthalmic examination and restrict BP measurement to those patients with either inappropriate urine concentrating ability or retinopathy.
2. Obtain multiple measurements over several weeks if an apparently healthy patient is presumptively diagnosed with hypertension on a routine examination. Because hypertension is a chronic progressive disorder, rapid diagnosis is generally not required (unless there is apparent end-organ damage). This can be laborious for both clinician and client, but it reduces the risk of a false-positive diagnosis.
3. Obtain measurements in a quiet environment, using the same technique each time. BP measurement should be performed before the physical examination or any diagnostic procedures, such as blood or urine collection, are performed. Some Doppler machines allow the use of headphones to minimize noise (Figure 20-5). The width of the BP cuff should be 30% to 40% of the circumference of the leg, and it should be positioned at the level of the heart (Figure 20-6). Use the same trained personnel for each measurement to prevent interoperator variability. Record the cuff size and location of the measurement in the medical record along with the BP readings.
4. Accept the lowest reading obtained over several sessions as the most likely.
5. Examine the patient for underlying renal disease (including a urinalysis) and other endocrine

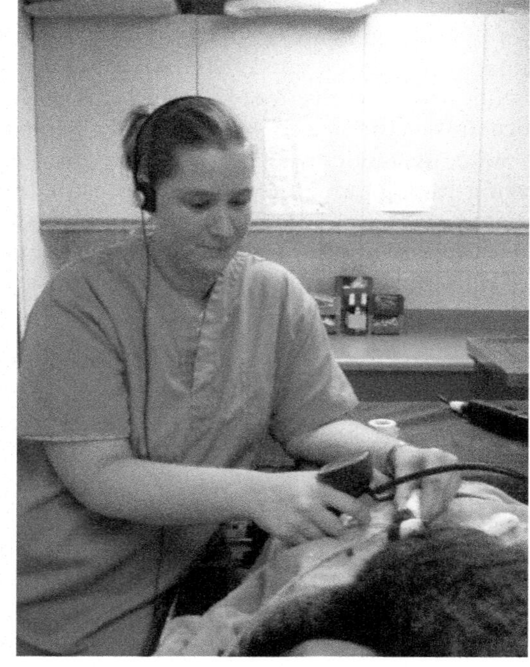

FIGURE 20-5 Use of headphones with Doppler blood pressure units minimizes noise that might be stressful to the patient.

disorders that might result in systemic hypertension. If no underlying cause can be identified, reconsider the diagnosis of hypertension.
6. Perform a retinal examination to identify hypertensive retinopathies, especially if the SBP is consistently above 200 mm Hg.
7. Remain skeptical of the diagnosis in every patient in which the diagnosis was unexpected or unexplained.

One study recently evaluated the use of NT-proBNP in hypertensive cats with chronic kidney disease (CKD).[44] These authors found elevated NT-proBNP concentrations in hypertensive cats with CKD and occasionally in normotensive cats with severe CKD. Thus NT-proBNP might help identify hypertension in cats with CKD in the absence of cardiac disease. Additional larger studies would be necessary to confirm this initial observation.

Treatment

Treatment of systemic hypertension generally involves administration of arteriodilators (Table 20-2). The most common drug used for management of feline hypertension is amlodipine. This is usually administered at 0.625 mg per cat, every 12 to 24 hours, by mouth. The medication can be administered transdermally, but reductions in SBP are less predictable and of lesser magnitude than with oral administration.[33] Reductions in SBP of 20 to 50 mm Hg can be anticipated with oral amlodipine therapy.

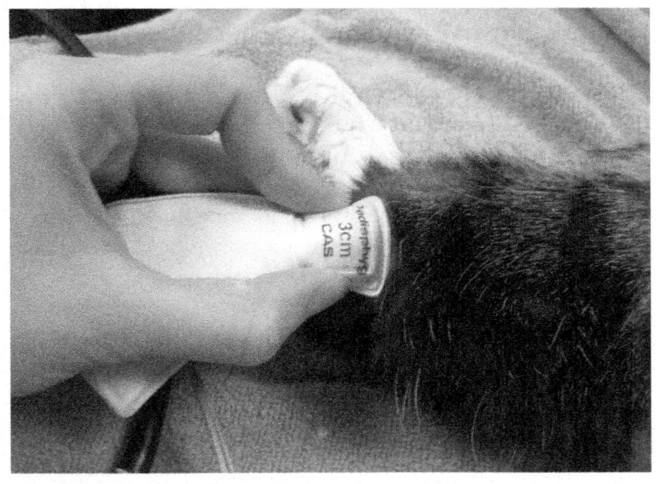

FIGURE 20-6 The width of the blood pressure cuff should be 30% to 40% of the circumference of the leg.

Other drugs that have been examined in management of hypertension include angiotensin-converting enzyme (ACE) inhibitors, beta blockers, and hydralazine. None of these medications has proved to be effective in routine control of SBP or has been associated with undesirable side effects. In cases of hypertension that are refractory to high-dose amlodipine therapy, clinicians can consider adding ACE inhibitors or beta blockers to the therapeutic protocol, although the outcomes are not predictable.

Despite the popularity of both diagnosis and treatment of feline hypertension over the last 10 to 15 years, no studies have documented decreased morbidity or increased survival rates in treated spontaneously hypertensive cats. One study examining the effect of good and poor control of hypertension in cats with renal disease failed to show any increase in survival of cats with good control compared with cats with poor control of SBP, suggesting that management of hypertension in this population of cats might not result in improved clinical outcomes.[39] These authors examined survival factors and found that the only variable that predicted survival was proteinuria. The author is unaware of any studies examining rates of nonfatal complications (e.g., retinopathies, progressive renal disease, encephalopathies) in cats with well-controlled versus poorly controlled hypertension. Thus whether morbidity is affected by antihypertensive therapies is unknown. Clinicians should consider that therapy in many patients presumptively diagnosed with hypertension might be of no clinical value. Additionally, therapy of cats with borderline hypertension should be questioned both because of the inherent inaccuracy of diagnosis and the lack of any documented benefit to such therapy.

TABLE 20-2 **Drugs Used in the Treatment of Feline Hypertension**

Drug	Dose	Mechanism	Comments
Amlodipine	0.625 to 1.25 mg/cat, every 12 to 24 hours, orally	Calcium channel blocker	Preferred first-line therapy; may be combined with ACE inhibitor or beta blocker in refractory cases
Benazepril	0.25 to 0.5 mg/kg, every 12 to 24 hours, orally	ACE inhibitor	Adjunctive therapy, especially for cats with proteinuric renal disease
Hydralazine	1 to 3 mg/kg, every 12 hours, orally	Direct arterial dilator	Primarily used for acute control of hypertension in the hospital setting
Atenolol	6.25 to 12.5 mg/cat, every 24 hours, orally	Beta-adrenoceptor blocker	Primarily used in hyperthyroid cats or as adjunctive therapy for refractory cases

ACE, Angiotensin-converting enzyme.

CARDIOMYOPATHIES

Cardiomyopathies account for most acquired feline cardiac disease. Several types of cardiomyopathy have been described in cats: hypertrophic, dilated, restrictive, unclassified, arrhythmogenic right ventricular cardiomyopathy, excess moderator band, and endomyocardial fibroelastosis. Instances of isolated atrial cardiomyopathy have also been described. Of these, HCM is the most commonly diagnosed.

Hypertrophic Cardiomyopathy

HCM is a concentric hypertrophy of the ventricular myocardium, either diffuse or localized, that is not attributable to any identifiable cause such as hypertension, hyperthyroidism, neoplasia, or increased afterload (e.g., aortic stenosis). Causes of feline HCM are mostly unknown, although, as in humans, genetic mutations likely account for some percentage of cases. Most mutations in humans with HCM have been detected in sarcomeric proteins (proteins associated with the contractile apparatus). A genetic mutation in myosin-binding protein C has been proposed as a cause of HCM in Maine Coons[53] and Ragdolls,[55] although two subsequent studies have disputed the initial observation.[13,88]

Prevalence of HCM in cats is also poorly estimated. Relatively small studies of apparently healthy cats have identified left ventricular hypertrophy in 7% to 15% of cats.[18,61] These estimates seem alarming, especially given the fact that most cats with HCM in these studies were random-source, unrelated, domestic shorthair or longhair cats, rather than breeds predisposed to HCM, and that similar studies in people put the estimate at 0.2% of the general population. Such an "epidemic" of HCM is difficult to explain through genetic causes and requires invoking of either infectious or other environmental etiologies. Indeed, authors have proposed nongenetic causes for feline HCM. Alternatively, because the diagnosis is based on echocardiographic evaluation and measurement, and given that many, if not most, of these cats remain subclinical for their entire life, it is possible that current diagnostic criteria are insufficiently stringent for accurate diagnosis of this condition, resulting in a high percentage of false-positive diagnoses. Furthermore, no studies have examined a large cohort of apparently healthy cats longitudinally to determine whether initial observations of hypertrophy persist over time. Such studies are currently being conducted, but results cannot be expected for several years.

The median survival rate of cats from the time of diagnosis of HCM approaches 5 years. Some studies have suggested an 80% survival rate at 5 years of cats diagnosed with subclinical HCM.[3,72] Thus the outcome appears to be highly variable. This further supports the hypothesis that not all idiopathic left ventricular hypertrophy, diagnosed echocardiographically, is HCM. Alternatively, this finding could be attributed to a wide range of expression of the disease in affected individuals; in humans with HCM, identical mutations can cause a wide range of phenotypes, ranging from apparently unaffected to severely affected.

Clinical Signs

Cats with HCM can present with a variety of clinical signs and physical examination findings. Murmurs are present in approximately 50% of cats with HCM. Conversely, cats with murmurs do not necessarily have HCM or even cardiac disease. Therefore presence or absence of a murmur is not useful in identifying cats with HCM. Murmurs in cats with HCM are often associated with systolic anterior mitral valve motion, which produces both a dynamic left ventricular outflow obstruction and mitral regurgitation (Figure 20-7). Some cats with HCM can develop dynamic right ventricular outflow tract obstruction.

Arrhythmias are commonly observed in cats with subclinical HCM. A recent study has suggested that most apparently healthy cats with ventricular arrhythmias have evidence of structural heart disease; however, this study requires additional validation with larger sample populations.[17]

Most commonly, cats with clinical HCM present with left-sided CHF. Cats often display subtle signs of CHF until they reach a critical tipping point, at which time they decompensate rapidly. Subtle clinical signs can include mild tachypnea, altered grooming behavior or activity, and decreased appetite. Coughing is a rare clinical finding in cats with CHF; the vast majority of cats with cough have noncardiac disorders, such as asthma. CHF in cats with HCM manifests as pulmonary edema,

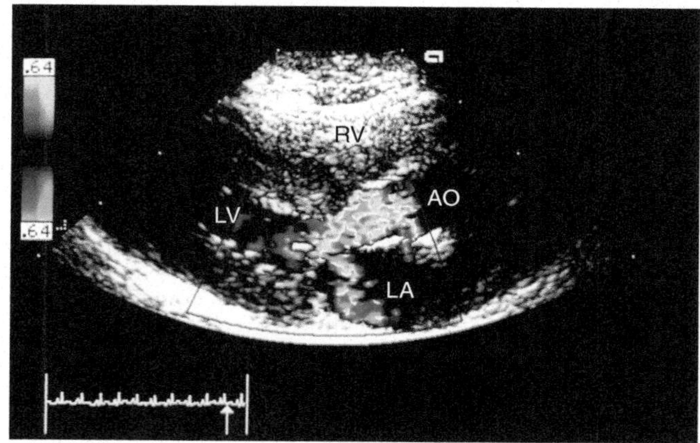

FIGURE 20-7 Right-parasternal long-axis color Doppler echocardiographic image demonstrating the divergent jets characteristic of systolic anterior motion of the mitral valve. Turbulence is seen extending into the aorta, and a second discrete jet is seen extending towards the posterior wall of the left atrium.

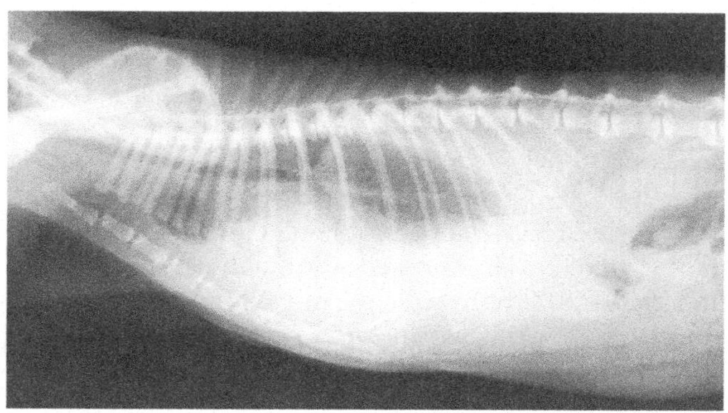

FIGURE 20-8 Pleural effusion often accompanies pulmonary edema in cats with congestive heart failure and may make it difficult to visualize the heart as well as the lung fields.

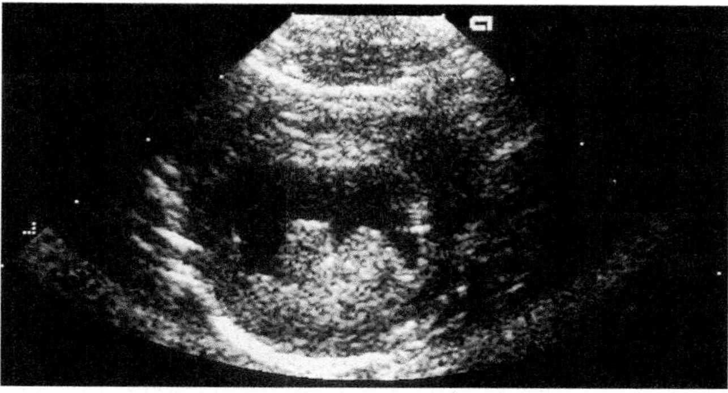

FIGURE 20-9 Right-parasternal long-axis echocardiographic image demonstrating marked papillary hypertrophy and fusion of a cat with hypertrophic cardiomyopathy. Note that the septum and lateral walls do not appear markedly thickened in this patient.

pleural effusion, or both. Rarely, pericardial effusion can be detected, but this is generally mild and of no clinical hemodynamic consequence. Distribution and radiographic pattern of pulmonary edema in cats with CHF is highly variable.[7] Therefore clinicians should not rely on identification of "typical" radiographic findings when making the diagnosis of CHF. Pleural effusion often accompanies pulmonary edema (Figure 20-8), but substantial effusion will obscure the radiographic pattern of pulmonary edema. Pleural effusion can be a modified transudate or chylous.

Cats with severe CHF exhibit marked tachydyspnea or respiratory distress. Body temperature can be normal or low; hypothermia with CHF is a poor prognostic indicator. Similarly, cats can be tachycardic, have atrial or ventricular arrhythmias, or be normocardic. Cats with an absence of tachycardia at diagnosis of CHF also carry a worse prognosis than those with tachycardia.

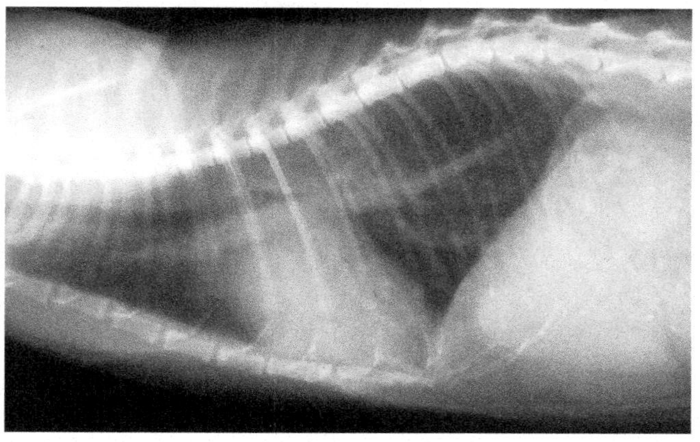

FIGURE 20-10 Lateral radiograph of a cat with severe hypertrophic cardiomyopathy. Note the cardiomegaly, enlarged pulmonary veins, and the moderate generalized interstitial pulmonary pattern, consistent with congestive heart failure.

Diagnosis

Diagnosis of HCM requires echocardiography. Left ventricular wall thicknesses (either globally or regionally), measured at the standard submitral location, that exceed 6 mm constitute a tentative diagnosis of HCM (Figure 20-9). Cats with wall thicknesses exceeding 7 mm are considered to have moderate left ventricular hypertrophy. Hypertrophy can be focal or diffuse. More controversy exists regarding basilar septal bulges or thickening. This is a common finding in older cats and can cause dynamic left ventricular outflow tract obstruction. However, whether this constitutes HCM or simply is a consequence of aging changes is unclear.

A diagnosis of HCM cannot be made on the basis of ECG and radiography. Many cats with subclinical disease have a normal electrocardiographic reading and a normal cardiac silhouette on thoracic radiographs. Conversely, changes on radiographs consistent with left atrial enlargement (especially on the DV view) are not pathognomonic for HCM but merely indicate cardiomegaly and left-sided heart disease (Figures 20-10 and 20-11). ECG is both insensitive and nonspecific for diagnosis of cardiomegaly and should be reserved for diagnosis of arrhythmias.

Biomarkers do not currently appear to be of use in diagnosis of subclinical HCM. Their use in diagnosis of CHF is also unresolved at this time; studies demonstrating true clinical utility of the assay do not exist. However, when ECG is unavailable and radiographs cannot demonstrate cardiomegaly (e.g., owing to obscuring of the cardiac silhouette by pleural effusion or pulmonary edema), NT-proBNP might provide useful information in a subset of cats with CHF, allowing clinicians to increase the probability of a correct diagnosis and institute timely and appropriate therapy.

Genetic testing is available for specific cardiac mutations associated with HCM. These tests are reserved for specific breeds in which the mutations have been identified rather than as a general screening tool. Two

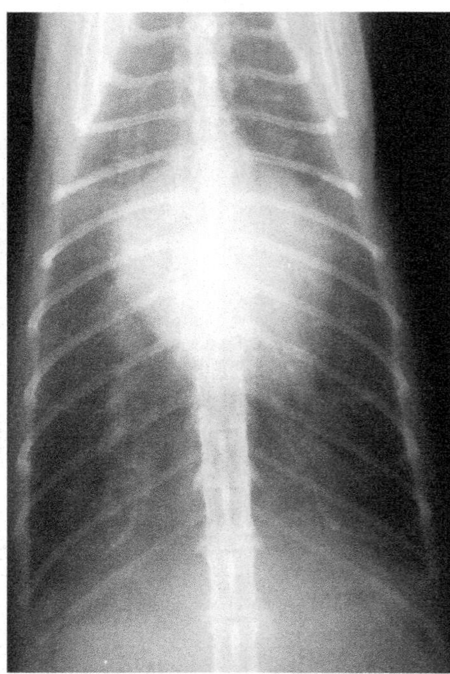

FIGURE 20-11 Dorsoventral radiograph of a cat with severe hypertrophic cardiomyopathy. Note the marked left atrial enlargement and moderate generalized interstitial pulmonary pattern, consistent with congestive heart failure. Note also that left atrial enlargement is significantly more apparent than on the corresponding lateral radiograph seen in Figure 20-10.

mutations have been identified in myosin-binding protein C that have been associated with HCM in Maine Coons and Ragdolls.[53,55] The investigators who identified these mutations have suggested that cats homozygous for the mutation die in utero (i.e., the mutation is embryonically lethal when both alleles express the mutation). However, recent studies from investigators in Europe have contested these claims, having identified cats homozygous for the mutation both with and without echocardiographic evidence of HCM.[13,88] These investigators have further contested the hypothesis that the proposed mutation in Maine Coons is associated with HCM in that breed. However, the European investigators used different methodology to identify and determine genotype in their cats and examined predominantly younger cats, in which the disease might not yet be apparent. Thus whether the mutation is causal and differences in phenotype merely reflect expressivity of the trait or whether the mutation is a noncausal polymorphism is still subject to debate. Additional evidence for causality has been proposed in a recent study by the investigators who originally identified the mutation, in which the authors demonstrated altered methylation of CpG sites within the MyBPC gene.[54]

Additionally Maine Coons without the MyBPC mutation have been identified with HCM, both in the colony where the mutation was initially identified and in the general Maine Coon population.[13,88] Therefore a normal genotype in this breed does not exclude the diagnosis of HCM.

Treatment

Treatment of HCM is controversial. Currently, no therapeutic studies exist demonstrating clinically important outcomes in cats with subclinical HCM. No drugs have demonstrated a delay in progression or reversal of hypertrophy in cats with subclinical HCM. One study examining ACE inhibitor therapy in subclinical disease failed to show regression of hypertrophy over 1 year; however, the study did not examine whether long-term therapy with ACE inhibitors prevented or delayed the onset of CHF or arterial thromboembolism (ATE).[51] One unpublished study showed that beta blockers reduced the dynamic outflow obstruction in cats with subclinical disease better than calcium channel blockers.[74] However, whether reducing the obstruction alters clinical outcomes, such as progression to CHF, was not examined. Arguments that reducing obstruction alters "demeanor" or "behavior" are difficult to accept because these cats are, by definition, without clinical signs ("subclinical"). Furthermore, beta blockers have psychotropic effects, so attributing any change in behavior to reduction in left ventricular outflow tract obstruction without a controlled study is improper.

Treatment of CHF in cats is similarly devoid of published evidence. Diuretics are the mainstay of therapy, both in acute and chronic settings. One unpublished study that compared addition of beta blockers, calcium channel blockers, ACE inhibitors, or placebo with furosemide on survival of cats with chronic CHF failed to demonstrate a benefit of any therapy.[24] In that study ACE inhibitors tended to improve outcomes, and beta blockers worsened outcomes, compared with placebo. A prior study of calcium channel blockers (diltiazem) and beta blockers in cats with CHF and HCM suggested a survival benefit of diltiazem; however, no placebo group was included in that study to determine whether the difference was due to a benefit of diltiazem or harm from beta blockade.[9] Recent anecdotal evidence from several investigators has suggested that pimobendan does not appear to dramatically worsen clinical outcomes in cats with HCM and CHF, despite initial concerns of administering a positive inotrope to a cat with HCM. However, no controlled studies have demonstrated a clear benefit of pimobendan therapy in HCM. Thus clinicians should carefully consider their treatment strategies for cats with CHF, remembering that polypharmacy in cats is often substantially more difficult than in dogs and that adding drugs may not improve clinical outcomes and may worsen quality of life for both client and patient.

Acute treatment of CHF in cats is best accomplished by adhering to several simple rules:

- Undue stress can kill a cat with respiratory distress. Therefore physical restraint for diagnostic procedures should be minimal, brief, and gentle. Consider obtaining DV and standing lateral films if necessary (and do not worry excessively about positioning). Do not perform diagnostic tests that require sedation or extensive manual restraint.
- Before any imaging studies, especially if echocardiography is not available, perform a bilateral diagnostic (and potentially therapeutic) pleurocentesis. This can be done with the patient in either sternal recumbency or sitting on the examination table (Figure 20-12). A 23G butterfly needle, coupled to a 10 mL syringe and three-way stopcock, is sufficient for most cases (Figure 20-13). This procedure allows quick and easy identification of severe pleural effusion (especially if prior thoracic auscultation is suggestive) and evacuation of fluid. Even removal of 50% of the volume of pleural effusion can dramatically alleviate dyspnea in feline patients with CHF, allowing further diagnostic tests to be performed in a hemodynamically more stable patient.

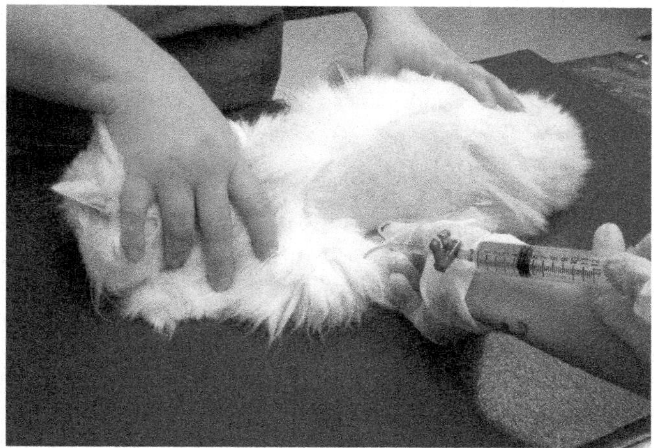

FIGURE 20-12 Pleurocentesis should be performed on patients with respiratory distress before imaging studies. The patient can be positioned in sternal recumbency; undue stress should be avoided.

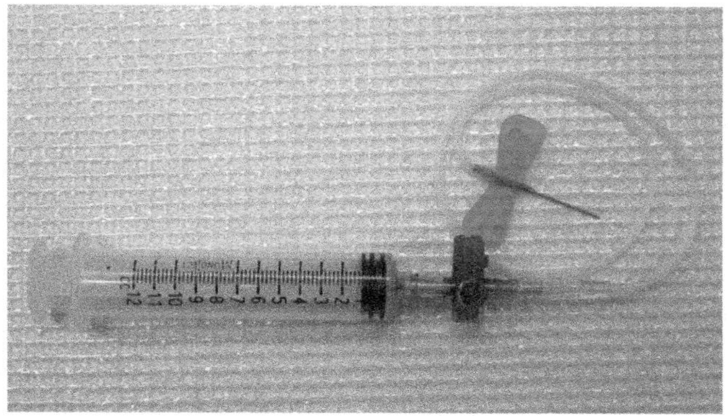

FIGURE 20-13 Pleurocentesis can be performed with a 23G butterfly needle coupled to a 10-mL syringe and three-way stopcock.

- Do not provide oxygen by face mask; this is generally too stressful for a cat. Consider placing the patient in an oxygen cage to improve oxygenation, and then stage diagnostic procedures such that the patient can be allowed time to recover in the oxygen cage.
- If intravenous catheterization is not easily achievable with minimal patient restraint, administer furosemide intramuscularly. Doses for severe respiratory distress should approach 4 mg/kg every 2 to 4 hours until substantial improvement in respiratory effort and rate are noted. Doses should then be tapered to prevent excessive dehydration and electrolyte depletion.
- If unsure of the diagnosis of CHF, perform a brief echocardiogram with the patient on your lap to determine if there is marked left atrial enlargement. Most cats with HCM and CHF have enlarged left atria. A complete echocardiogram is not required during the acute management period, but a brief gentle evaluation of left atrium size is often beneficial in establishing the diagnosis and directing appropriate therapy.
- Resist the temptation to perform repeated physical examinations of the patient; observe the patient's respiratory character through the cage, and handle the patient only when absolutely necessary.
- *Do not* administer fluids to *any* cat with CHF while initially attempting to reduce pulmonary edema acutely. It is impossible to dehydrate the pulmonary parenchyma and pleural space while hydrating the rest of the body. Instead, provide water *ad libitum* to allow the patient to drink at will.
- *Do not* evaluate electrolytes repeatedly; this will stress the patient. Such tests can be performed once the patient is stable.
- Do not become concerned by temporary anorexia. Cats with CHF are often anorexic but will generally begin eating within 3 or 4 days of stabilization. Although potassium depletion is possible during this period, it is rarely of major clinical concern.
- Do not worry about development of mild or moderate azotemia. Acute dehydration is expected to result in azotemia; you are not inducing renal failure or damaging kidneys by dehydrating your patient. Treatment of cats with preexisting chronic kidney disease that develop CHF is difficult, insofar as specific therapies for each condition are diametrically opposed. Such cases are best managed by specialists, or clients should be advised of the difficulty associated with this situation so that informed decisions can be made about both acute and chronic management. For more information on

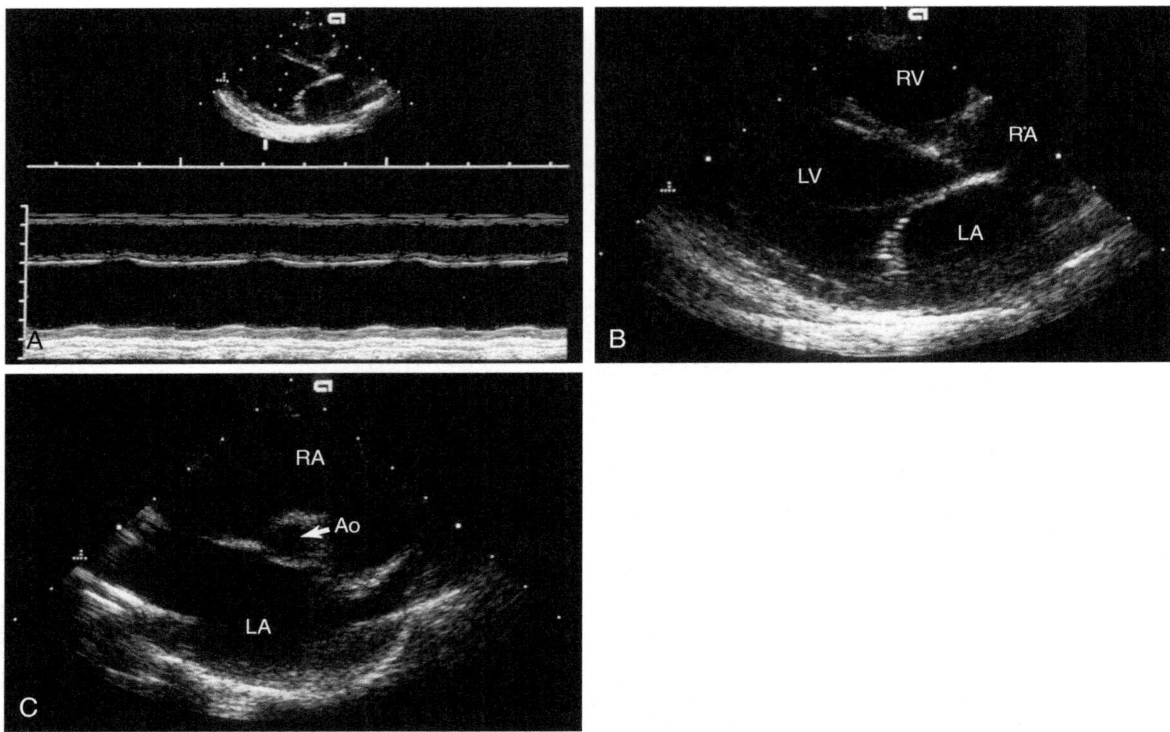

FIGURE 20-14 Echocardiographic images of a cat with dilated cardiomyopathy. **A,** M-mode of the left ventricle showing marked eccentric hypertrophy and myocardial failure. **B,** Right-parasternal long-axis image demonstrating left ventricular and left atrial enlargement (and some right-sided enlargement). **C,** Right-parasternal short-axis image demonstrating a large left atrium.

the management of cats with CHF and chronic renal disease, see Chapter 35.

Clinicians who adhere to these guidelines are likely to resolve an acute CHF crisis in most of their feline patients.

Dilated Cardiomyopathy

Dilated cardiomyopathy (DCM) is an uncommon disease in cats. It is identified echocardiographically as a hypocontractile (usually large) left ventricle (with occasional right ventricular involvement) (Figure 20-14). Subsequent to the identification of taurine-associated DCM in the late 1980s, the prevalence of DCM decreased dramatically. Currently, most DCM in cats is not related to taurine deficiency. However, after the 2008 incident of melamine contamination of pet foods, many clients opted to avoid commercial pet foods and resorted to homemade diets. It is possible that if these diets continue to be fed for prolonged periods, incidence of taurine-associated DCM could increase in cats on homemade diets. Thus clinicians should consider testing any cat diagnosed with DCM for taurine deficiency insofar as such a diagnosis could result in complete cure of the patient. Taurine testing requires specific blood collection if analysis is to be performed on plasma. Heparinized plasma tubes should be prechilled on ice. Blood should be placed into the chilled tubes and then centrifuged immediately to separate plasma and cells. Plasma can then be drawn off and placed into a regular serum tube (not a separator tube) and shipped cold to laboratories performing taurine analysis.

Cats with DCM present similarly to those with HCM. Many remain subclinical for substantial periods of time. Diagnosis requires echocardiography. Treatment of subclinical disease is controversial; no drugs have been studied for their ability to delay onset of clinical signs or reverse disease. Treatment of CHF is the same as for HCM: diuretics, ACE inhibitors, or both. Digoxin can improve contractility in a minority of patients but is associated with substantial risk of toxicity because of its long half-life in cats. Pimobendan has not been critically evaluated in cats with DCM. Anecdotal reports suggest that responses in contractility and clinical picture are underwhelming; however, it can be considered as adjunct therapy if desired.

Other Cardiomyopathies

Several less easily characterized cardiomyopathies exist in cats. Restrictive and unclassified cardiomyopathies (Figure 20-15) are largely indistinguishable antemortem; both result in primary diastolic dysfunction owing to either altered relaxation or altered compliance of the

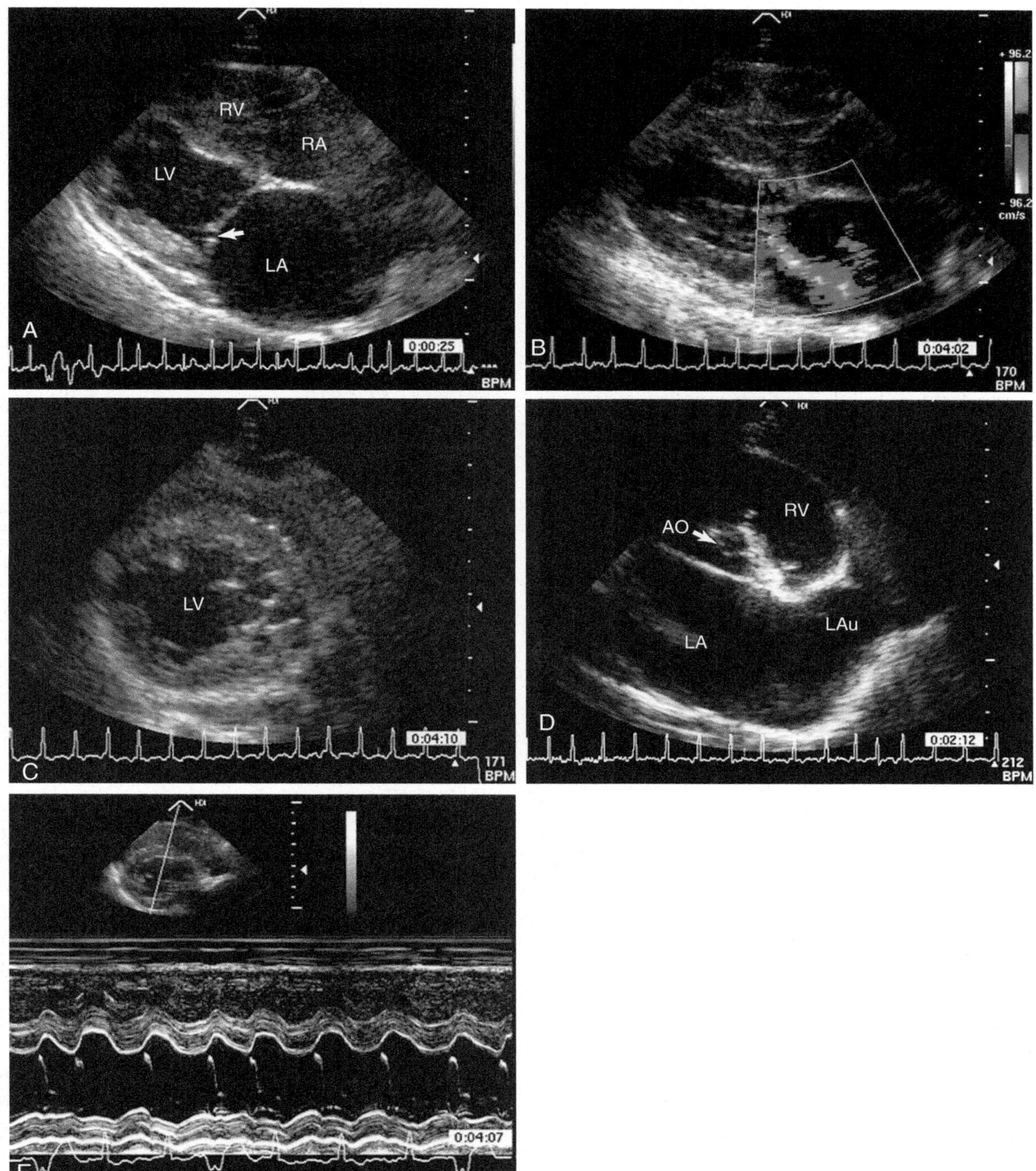

FIGURE 20-15 Echocardiographic images of a cat with unclassified cardiomyopathy. **A,** Right parasternal long-axis view of the heart. Note the four-chamber enlargement. The *arrow* is pointing to a gap in the coaptation point of the mitral valve, consistent with annular distention. **B,** Color Doppler showing mitral regurgitation. **C,** Right parasternal short-axis view of the left ventricle, showing a normal wall thickness, with marked heterogeneity of the endocardial surface. **D,** Right parasternal short-axis view showing marked left atrial enlargement. **E,** M-mode of the left ventricle at the level of the mitral valve showing moderate chamber enlargement and mild hypokinesis, especially evident in the posterior wall.

ventricles. These two conditions often affect both ventricles, resulting in biatrial enlargement. Diagnosis is by echocardiography. Cats with these cardiomyopathies present with CHF, and personal and anecdotal impressions are that the chance of survival among patients with these cardiomyopathies is worse than that of patients with HCM.

Arrhythmogenic right ventricular cardiomyopathy (ARVC) is a relatively recently described disorder characterized by fibrofatty infiltration of the right ventricular wall.[27] This results in severe contractile dysfunction of the right ventricle, dilation of the tricuspid annulus, and severe tricuspid regurgitation. The name of this disease is somewhat of a misnomer, insofar as arrhythmias are *not* a feature of the disease; the name was based on a histopathologic similarity to ARVC in humans. Cats with ARVC tend to be older and present with severe right-sided CHF (ascites and pleural effusion). Treatment is generally directed at reducing the effusions by abdominocentesis and thoracocentesis. Survival rates of cats with ARVC have not been extensively examined; however, personal impressions suggest that these patients are relatively resistant to therapy and have a poor quality of life, usually resulting in euthanasia.

Excess moderator band cardiomyopathy is a rare disease of unknown etiology or pathophysiology. It is usually characterized by a rete or network of fibrous bands that traverse the left ventricular chamber and, presumably, alter compliance of the ventricle. Endocardial thickening can be observed in some cases. Additionally, substantial presence of false tendons in cats without apparent heart disease makes the diagnosis of this condition difficult. Treatment is directed against CHF, as described previously.

Atrial standstill has been described in a cat. This is a rare disorder, characterized by atrial enlargement and loss of atrial electrical and mechanical activity with subsequent right-sided CHF. Heart rate is dependent on junctional or ventricular pacemakers. It is different from depressed atrial activity secondary to hyperkalemia in that the latter does not inhibit sinus node activation but merely depresses atrial myocardial depolarization, resulting in a sinoventricular rhythm. Hyperkalemic atrial depression is reversible, whereas atrial standstill is ultimately a fatal condition.

Arterial Thromboembolism

Cardiogenic arterial thromboembolism (ATE) is an uncommon complication of cardiomyopathies in cats.[4,45,77,82] ATE manifests as sudden occlusive vasculopathy of the systemic arteries. Although the exact pathophysiology of the syndrome is not completely understood, most cardiologists believe that the condition arises when thrombi from the left atrium enter the systemic circulation and lodge in distal locations, with subsequent occlusion of the affected vessels. The distal aorta is the most commonly recognized site of arterial occlusion, and occlusion can be partial or complete. Secondary thrombosis can develop, extending cranially up the aorta to occlude visceral arteries (intestinal, renal). Occasionally, direct splanchnic infarction can occur. Less commonly, thromboemboli will occlude forelimb arteries (right more commonly than left), resulting in unilateral forelimb paresis or paralysis. Cerebrovascular arterial occlusion is thought to occur on occasion but is difficult to document or substantiate.

Cardiogenic ATE occurs almost exclusively in cats with large left atria. However, atrial enlargement alone is insufficient for development of ATE; this is apparent in the fact that most cats with HCM that develop CHF (and therefore have markedly enlarged left atria) do not develop ATE and that cats with other cardiac diseases, such as VSD and mitral valve disease, can also develop markedly enlarged atria without increased risk of ATE. Thus ATE requires atrial dysfunction, which produces blood stasis or decreased blood flow within the left auricle.[75] Additionally, alterations in either platelet function or coagulation (or both) might play a role in development of ATE.[5,84] To date, studies have failed to identify specific risk factors for development of ATE. However, anecdotally, spontaneous echocardiographic contrast (SEC) within the LA is considered by most cardiologists to be a risk factor, insofar as this finding suggests intraatrial blood stasis and aggregation of red blood cells. SEC has been associated with decreased left auricular blood flow and clinicopathologic evidence of hypercoagulability, further supporting the hypothesis that it is a risk factor for ATE.[75,84] However, not all cats with SEC develop ATE, and cats without SEC can also develop ATE. Presence of an intraatrial thrombus is considered to be a strong risk factor for cardiogenic ATE (Figures 20-16 and 20-17).

Clinical Signs

Clinical signs of ATE depend on the vascular bed occluded and the degree of occlusion. Most commonly, clients observe acute paresis or paralysis, which is accompanied by acute and severe pain in the absence of obvious trauma. The acute pain response is a hallmark of ATE. Pain can persist for several hours and subsides

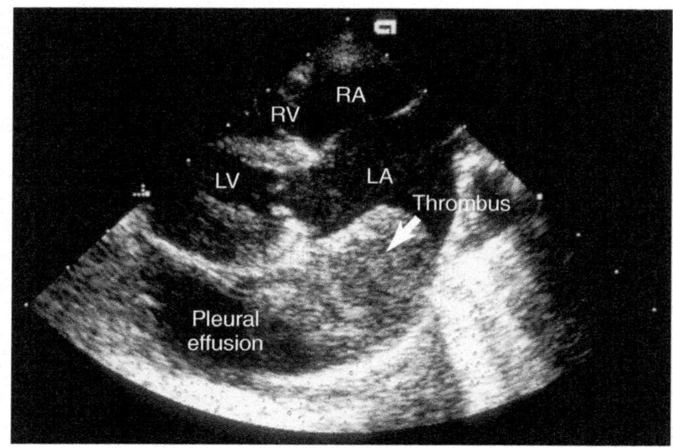

FIGURE 20-16 Right-parasternal long-axis echocardiographic image demonstrating a large left atrial thrombus. A pleural effusion can be observed distal to the heart on the image.

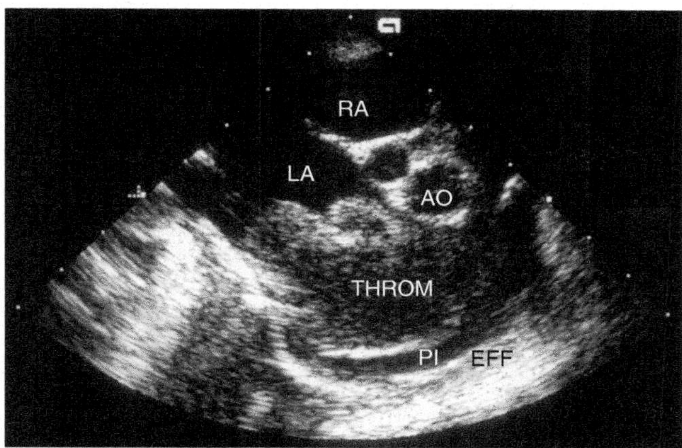

FIGURE 20-17 Right-parasternal short-axis echocardiographic image demonstrating a huge left atrial thrombus.

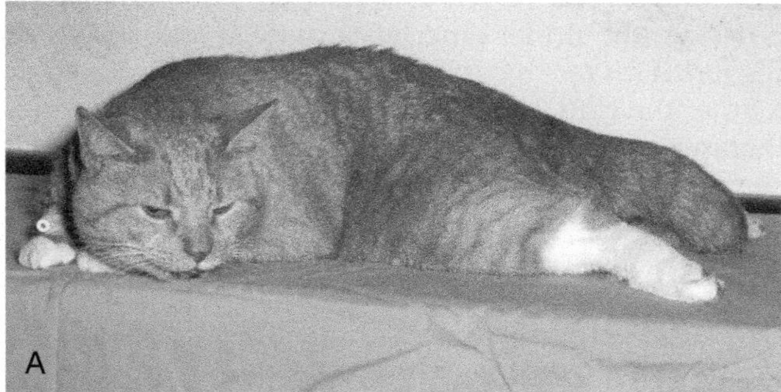

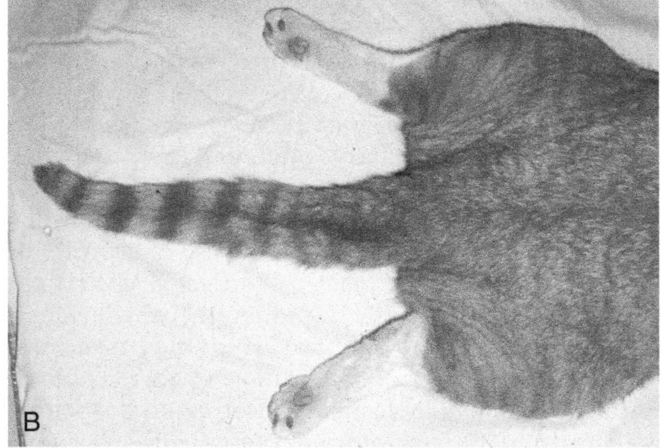

FIGURE 20-18 **A,** A cat with hindlimb paresis secondary to aortic thromboembolism. **B,** Note the cyanotic pads.

as neuronal ischemia develops. Typically, the pain subsides after 24 to 48 hours of complete ischemia. Reperfusion or incomplete occlusion can produce ongoing or recurrent pain. Ultimately, anesthesia of the affected limb (or limbs) ensues. Physical examination can reveal a loss of pulse in the affected limb. Depending on the severity and duration of occlusion, affected limbs can feel hypothermic, with loss of motor and sensory function (Figure 20-18). Nail beds and foot pads can appear cyanotic. Clipping a toenail on the affected limb to the quick will result in no bleeding or oozing of dark deoxygenated blood. Over several hours swelling and rigidity of affected limb musculature (e.g., gastrocnemius, biceps) can be palpated if the occlusion is severe and persistent. Clinical chemistry analysis will usually reveal elevated creatine kinase and aspartate aminotransferase owing to the ischemic myonecrosis.

CHF is not a necessary feature of ATE; however, in some cats CHF can develop secondary to the stress of the occlusive episode and subsequent hospitalization and therapy. Thus clinicians should carefully monitor respiratory rate and effort in cats presenting and hospitalized for ATE for the possible development of CHF during hospitalization. However, an elevated respiratory rate or mild tachydyspnea could be associated with pain rather than CHF.

If the thromboembolism progresses, renal and gastrointestinal ischemia can ensue. Patients in which this occurs or those with primary splanchnic infarction harbor a grave prognosis and warrant consideration of euthanasia.

The clinical course of ATE is variable. Rarely, complete resolution can be observed in 24 to 48 hours. More commonly, paresis or paralysis persists, with slow return of function or sensation. Occasionally, the larger thromboembolus fragments and dislodges to occlude more distal arteries, resulting in a change in the clinical picture. The more rapidly and completely that function and sensation are regained, the better the short-term prognosis. A partial return of function (sensory or motor) in 48 to 72 hours is encouraging and can be expected in many cases. Persistent complete paralysis beyond this period carries a more guarded prognosis; however, the author has seen cats with complete paralysis that lasted for more than 10 days eventually regain partial motor and sensory function. Provided that the owners are willing to nurse a cat with complete paralysis, including potential bladder expression, clinicians should consider delaying euthanasia in such cases. In general, if complete gangrenous ischemia is not apparent and the toes or foot pads are not completely devoid of blood (black–blue) after 72 hours, the author recommends persisting with therapy if the owners are willing. Additionally, once the acute phase of the syndrome has passed (usually in less than 48 hours), home care can be instituted to minimize stress and costs, with owners being taught to observe for signs of progressive or nonresolving ischemia of the affected limbs.

Treatment

Treatment of ATE is entirely anecdotal and without substantial clinical trials to demonstrate benefit or harm. Most studies of acute therapy consist of small case series. Treatment of acute ATE can be divided into several aims: thrombolysis, promotion of collateral circulation, prevention of additional thrombosis, control of pain, and treatment of any underlying heart disease.

Thrombolytic therapy has been attempted with various chemical and mechanical approaches, including streptokinase[58]; urokinase[43]; tissue plasminogen activator[63]; and, most recently, intravascular thrombectomy.[67] All these approaches resulted in either substantial periinterventional mortality (e.g., reperfusion injury) or failure to resolve the thrombus. Thus this author finds it difficult to recommend aggressive thrombolytic therapy in acute ATE.

Fluid therapy is theoretically of benefit (to promote collateral circulation). However, because most of these cats have severe heart disease underlying the ATE, fluid therapy should be used judiciously for fear of producing CHF. Other approaches for improving collateral circulation, such as the use of vasodilators (e.g., acepromazine), have not proved effective. No reports exist regarding the use of more potent arteriodilators such as amlodipine, nitroprusside, and hydralazine, so their use cannot be recommended at this time. Clopidogrel therapy before experimental ATE has been shown to maintain collateral circulation by an as yet unknown mechanism[34a]; however, whether prophylactic treatment with clopidogrel will reduce episodes of ATE is currently unknown and under investigation.

Prevention of additional thrombosis during the acute phase of the disease has been promoted by various authors. Most commonly, unfractionated heparin can be administered (300 IU/cat, every 12 hours, subcutaneously).[19] However, no clinical studies have demonstrated any benefit to such heparin therapy. Oral antithrombotic therapies have not been shown to be useful in the acute setting of feline ATE.[82] Experimentally, pretreatment with antithrombotics can reduce ATE; however, this does not reflect the clinical scenario of ATE, in which thrombosis exists at the time of presentation.[62]

Pain management is paramount in acute ATE. Cats should have routine pain control with fentanyl patches (applied over the more cranial body to ensure absorption) or other acute analgesic therapy such as buprenorphine. Pain control can be reduced after 48 to 72 hours, provided that the patient is comfortable.

Treatment of the underlying heart disease is performed as necessary. Unless there is overt CHF, treatment of the heart disease should be delayed until the patient recovers from the acute ATE episode.

Published case series of ATE suggested that up to 65% of patients can be discharged from the hospital alive (what percentage recovered, and to what degree, was not detailed).[45,82] Presence of CHF does not appreciably alter these statistics. Hypothermia, loss of anal sphincter, and loss of tail tone are considered poor prognostic indicators (because they demonstrate more profound thromboembolism). Additional studies of prognostic indicators (e.g., return of function) are needed to allow the clinician to better advise clients before they incur substantial costs.

Once circulation begins to return, clinicians should monitor the color of the foot pads or temperature of the limbs. Furthermore, reperfusion can be painful and associated with hyperkalemia. Therefore serum potassium should be evaluated if clinical signs suggest hyperkalemia is likely.

Chronic therapy of ATE during the recuperative period can include physical therapy. Gentle limb massage and manipulation might help improve circulation or return of function (although there are no studies demonstrating any benefit); in any case, they have little potential for harm, provided the patient tolerates it. Clinicians should advise clients to watch for gangrenous necrosis, the presence of which necessitates either limb amputation or euthanasia. Permanent loss of function in a single limb can be addressed with amputation; however, the underlying heart disease and strong predisposition to recurrent thromboembolism should temper the clinician's eagerness to perform such radical therapy. Clients can be taught to monitor foot pads for changes of color or temperature that might indicate a return of circulation.

Recurrence and Prevention

Limited case series have examined the recurrence of ATE in cats that survive the initial episode.[45,82] Some of these suggest that most cats will suffer a second event within 6 months of the first, even if they fully recover from the first. There are some patients that have had multiple episodes from which they recovered; however, this is uncommon, at least in part because most owners are unwilling to endure multiple bouts of ATE. Most patients are euthanized if they suffer a second bout of ATE.

Therapy to prevent or delay the occurrence of subsequent episodes of ATE includes the use of aspirin, low-molecular-weight (fractionated) heparin (LMWH)[79] and clopidogrel. Of these only clopidogrel is being evaluated critically in a randomized trial. This study is currently ongoing at the time of publication of this chapter, so results are not available. One concern with this study is that the comparative group was prescribed aspirin rather than placebo. However, given the lack of evidence of the efficacy of aspirin (low-dose or high-dose), one might argue that aspirin is, in effect, a placebo. Similarly, no clinical studies of the efficacy of LMWH are available. This, coupled with the expense of LMWH therapy and the need for daily injections, makes it difficult to recommend such therapy in cats without additional evidence of efficacy. Some clinicians have considered combining aspirin with clopidogrel to reduce ATE recurrence or occurrence, but no evidence supports this approach.

Prevention of initial episodes of ATE involves the use of the same drugs as for prevention of recurrence: aspirin, clopidogrel, and LMWH, either alone or in combination.

As with recurrent ATE prevention, no clinical trials have demonstrated the value of any of these approaches. Furthermore, clear identification of patients at high risk of ATE that would benefit from preventive therapy has not been studied. Studies evaluating putative risk factors are warranted to help define the subpopulation of cats with cardiac disease that might benefit from early intervention (assuming that early intervention is effective in reducing the risk).

Myocardial Infarction

Myocardial infarction has been documented on necropsy in cats with HCM.[23] However, more recently, cardiologists have recognized what appears to be myocardial infarction in cats without evidence of HCM. Often, these patients have no clinical signs associated with the lesion, which is identified by echocardiography. Affected cats are often older and commonly have other diseases, such as chronic kidney disease. Echocardiographic features include regional thinning of the left ventricular wall or interventricular septum associated with regional dyskinesia or hypokinesia of the affected wall segment. Compensatory eccentric hypertrophy can occasionally occur if the affected region is large. The etiology is usually unknown, and currently no pathologic evidence exists in the veterinary literature to support this antemortem observation. Moreover, no treatment exists to specifically address such presumptive myocardial injury.

ARRHYTHMIAS

Ventricular tachyarrhythmias—ventricular premature contraction (VPC), ventricular tachycardia (VT)—appear to be the most common form of arrhythmias associated with feline heart disease (Figures 20-19 and 20-20). These occur with HCM, unclassified cardiomyopathy, dilated cardiomyopathy, and arrhythmogenic right ventricular cardiomyopathy. Ventricular arrhythmias appear to be common in healthy adult cats. One study of 23 cats showed that 80% had VPCs detectable by 24-hour ambulatory electrocardiography, but 50% of these had less than four VPCs in 24 hours (with a range of 0 to 146 VPCs/24 hours).[30] These findings corroborated a previous study of 20 cats wherein VPCs were observed in most healthy cats and increased in frequency with age.[86]

Nonsinus supraventricular tachyarrhythmias are less commonly observed in cats than in dogs. Supraventricular premature complexes, supraventricular tachycardia (Figure 20-21), and atrial fibrillation often require profound atrial enlargement to allow impulse propagation, and in most feline heart disease, unless the disease is severe, the atrial size is insufficient to sustain these arrhythmias. The aforementioned study of 23 healthy cats showed that only one cat had a single atrial premature contraction (APC) over a 24-hour period. The study of 20 apparently healthy cats mentioned previously found a higher rate of APC occurrence, with more APCs

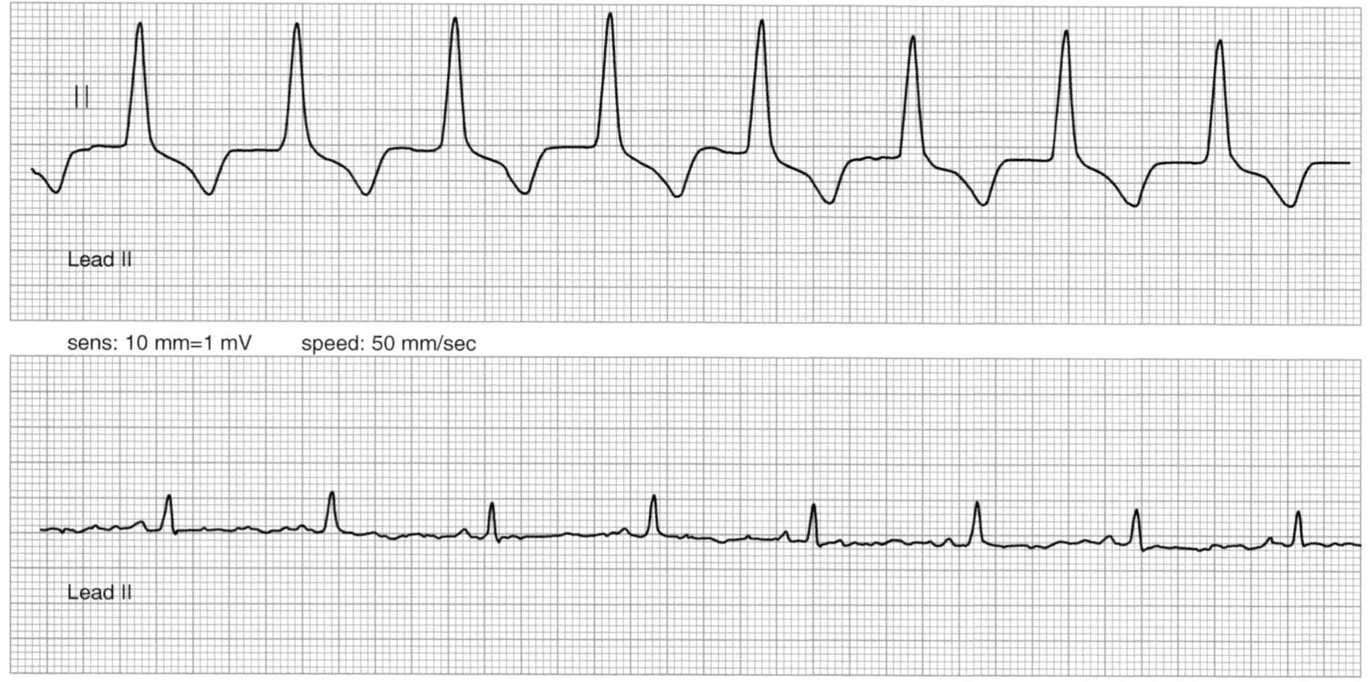

FIGURE 20-19 Electrocardiographic tracing of slow ventricular tachycardia (accelerated idioventricular rhythm) *(top strip)*. The rhythm converted spontaneously to sinus rhythm *(bottom strip)*.

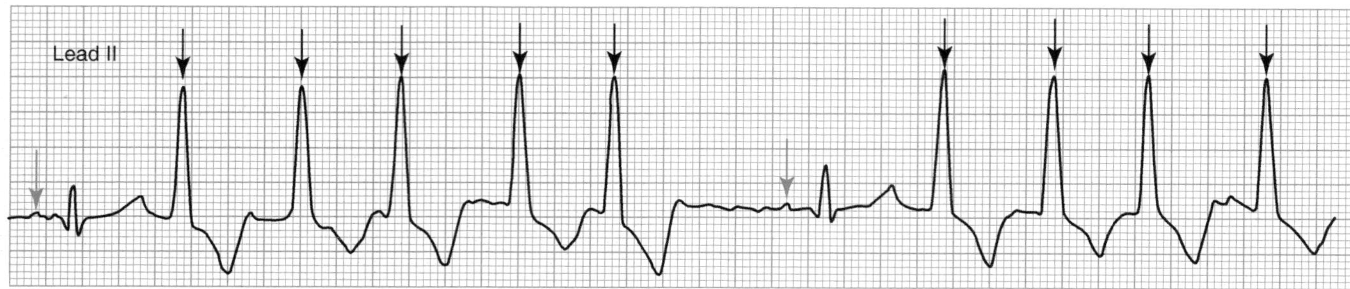

FIGURE 20-20 Electrocardiographic tracing of nonsustained ventricular tachycardia. *Black arrows* denote normally conducted p-waves; *blue arrows* denote ventricular ectopic complexes.

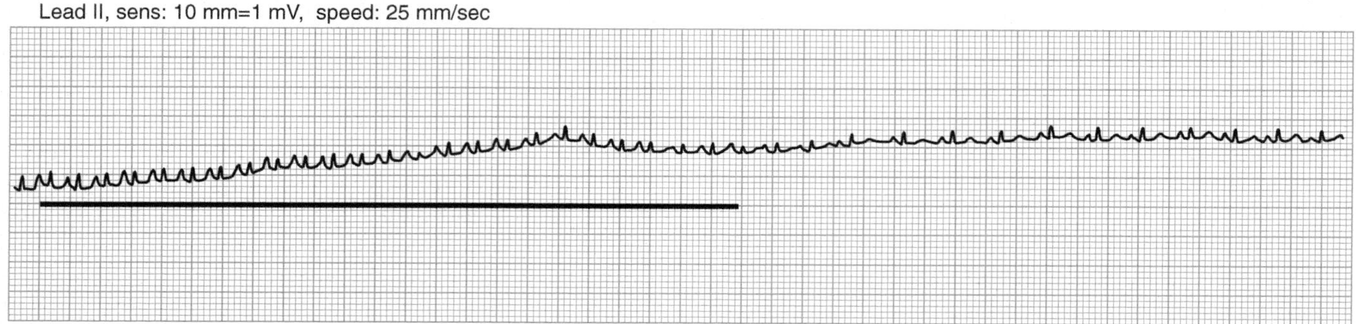

FIGURE 20-21 Electrocardiographic tracing of a supraventricular tachycardia *(underlined)*, which converts spontaneously into a sinus rhythm.

being detected in older cats. Whether these differences can be explained by differences in methodology (at-home monitoring versus in-hospital monitoring) is not clear.

Atrial fibrillation (AF) is almost always associated with severe heart disease in cats,[18] but rare instances of lone or primary atrial fibrillation have been documented.[15] In a study of 50 cats with AF, Côté and coworkers[18a] identified structural disease in all cases, but 14 of 39 cats (36%) for which left atrial data were available had questionable or mild atrial enlargement, suggesting that factors other than just left atrial size determine the probability of AF in cats. Atrial fibrillation in cats is almost always characterized by a high ventricular response rate, resulting in a tachycardia. Diagnosis is identical to that in other species: a supraventricular tachycardia with no apparent p-waves and an unpatterned irregularity. Diagnosis is complicated in cats because the ventricular rate is often so fast that beat-to-beat irregularity is quite small, and the arrhythmia appears to be regular at first glance. Furthermore, cats often have ventricular conduction disturbances (e.g., left axis deviation), which can make the QRS complexes appear ventricular rather than supraventricular.

Bradyarrhythmias are uncommon in cats. One study of bradyarrhythmias in cats found that cats with complete atrioventricular block could develop escape rates as high as 130 bpm.[41] Thus any cat with a heart rate less than 130 bpm during a physical examination warrants an ECG investigation.

Atrial standstill has also been documented in cats. Commonly, severe hyperkalemia results in an electrocardiographic reading that resembles atrial standstill; indeed, this term is used by many to describe the sinoventricular rhythm that develops with severe hyperkalemia. In these cases the atrial myocardium fails to depolarize sufficiently to produce a p-wave, but impulses continue to arise in the sinus node and are propagated to the atrioventricular node and then into the ventricles. The ventricular depolarization is often abnormal, resulting in a wide and bizarre QRS complex. Correction of the hyperkalemia resolves the atrial dysfunction. True, persistent atrial standstill has also been identified in cats and results in a junctional or ventricular escape rhythm.[28] It is thought that these cases represent either an atrial cardiomyopathy or right ventricular cardiomyopathy, with progression from the right ventricle to the right atrium.

Conduction Disturbances

Cats frequently have deviations in the overall direction of ventricular depolarization. These usually deviate to the left, with a mean electrical axis of 0 degree to −90 degree—the so-called *left anterior fascicular block (LAFB) type pattern*. Whether such deviations truly represent a block of conduction through the left anterior fascicle or some other conduction abnormality is not known. This conduction abnormality has traditionally been equated with left-sided heart disease, usually HCM or thyrotoxic heart disease; however, the author has observed this pattern of depolarization in echocardiographically normal cats. Ferasin and coworkers[21] reported LAFB-type patterns in 17 of 61 (28%) cats with HCM (these were part of a total of 19 of 106 cats with various forms of cardiomyopathy that demonstrated this conduction abnormality). However, Riesen and coworkers[68] found a lower prevalence of LAFB-type patterns in a study of cats with symptomatic HCM (9 of 169; 5%).

Right axis deviations are less commonly seen in cats; the author has not recognized incidental right bundle branch block (RBBB) in cats that are echocardiographically normal, as occurs in dogs. Ferasin and coworkers[21] identified RBBB in only 3% of 106 cats with cardiomyopathies.

Atrioventricular Blocks

Atrioventricular blocks are commonly observed in cats and increase in prevalence with increasing age, with 95% of affected cats in one study older than 10 years of age.[41] Second- and third-degree atrioventricular blocks have been described in cats with and without structural heart disease or secondary heart disease (i.e., as a result of systemic disease such as thyrotoxicosis).[40] These are usually evident by routine electrocardiographic analysis but can occasionally be intermittent and require ambulatory ECG recording to be detected (Figure 20-22). Although pacemaker implantation is advised for cats with clinically significant atrioventricular block, one retrospective study of cats with third-degree atrioventricular block calculated a median survival of 400 days in the absence of pacemaker implantation.[41] In the study 14 of 21 cats died by the time of publication: six died or were euthanized for unknown reasons, five were euthanized for noncardiac causes, one was euthanized because of aortic thromboembolism, and two were euthanized because of quality-of-life issues. No cats were known to have died suddenly. Additionally, 6 of 21 cats in that study had no clinical signs at presentation. The author's personal experience supports this finding; many, if not most, cats with third-degree atrioventricular block are diagnosed on routine examination, rather than because of specific clinical signs, and appear to require no specific interventions in most cases. The likely cause for this is that the escape rates in cats are often higher than those in dogs (80 to 140 bpm versus 20 to 60 bpm), and old cats are largely sedentary, so a modest bradycardia has little impact on hemodynamics.

Isorhythmic Dissociation

Isorhythmic dissociation is a form of conduction disturbance that is prevalent in cats. It is frequently observed during anesthesia but is occasionally identified in conscious cats and is not necessarily associated with structural cardiac disease. Isorhythmic dissociation is identified by observing a p-wave that "wanders" into and out of the adjacent QRS complex over several seconds, indicating that the two complexes are unassociated; the ventricular depolarizations are independent of the atrial depolarizations but occur at essentially the same rate (Figure 20-23). If the atrial depolarization occurs early enough after the preceding ventricular depolarization, "sinus capture" can occur with a sinus rhythm resuming for an unspecified length of time (and identified because of a shortened R-R interval). Atropine will generally correct the arrhythmia by accelerating the sinus rate above the junctional escape rate; however, the arrhythmia is considered benign and does not warrant therapy.

Treatment of Arrhythmias

Surprisingly little information exists regarding the treatment of feline arrhythmias (Table 20-3). Acute therapy of ventricular arrhythmias requires administration of intravenous agents, most commonly lidocaine. However,

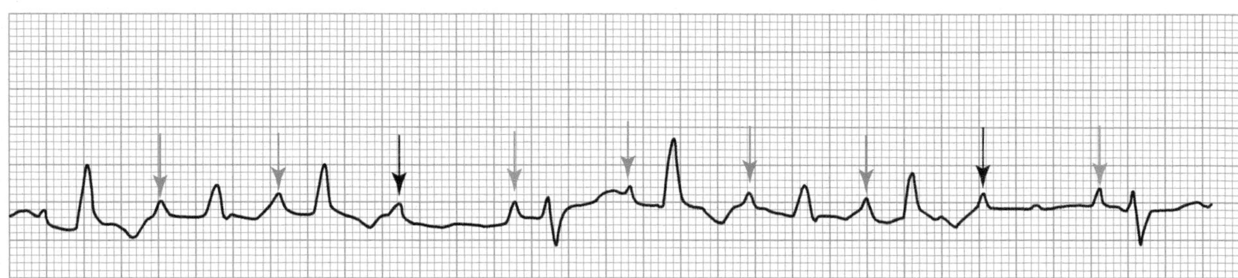

FIGURE 20-22 Electrocardiographic tracing of second-degree atrioventricular block. *Black arrows* indicate unconducted p-waves (buried in the preceding T-wave); *green arrows* denote normally conducted p-waves; *blue arrows* denote p-waves conducted with aberrancy (note the longer PR interval—first-degree atrioventricular block—and wide QRS complex).

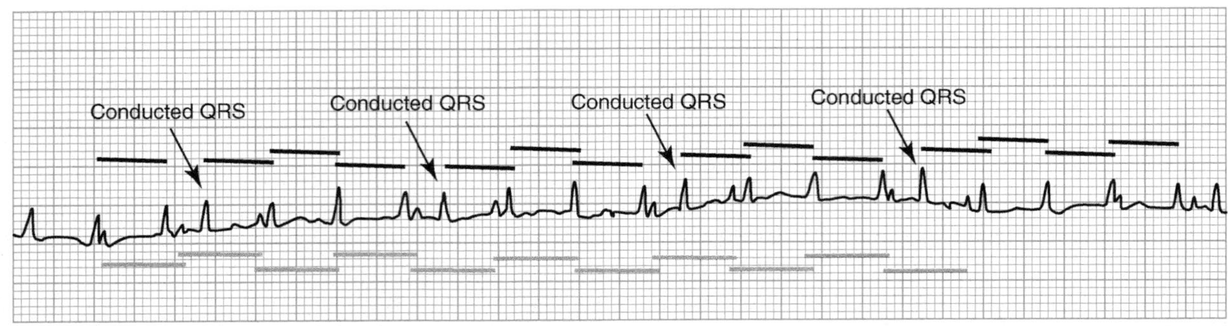

FIGURE 20-23 Electrocardiographic tracing of isorhythmic dissociation. The P-P interval is denoted by the *gray bars* below the electrocardiographic tracing. R-R intervals of nonconducted QRS complexes are denoted by the *black bars* above the electrocardiographic tracing. Sinus complexes are highlighted as "conducted QRS," with the preceding p-wave being conducted in a normal manner.

TABLE 20-3 **Drugs Used in the Treatment of Arrhythmias in the Cat**

Drug	Dose	Indications
Atenolol	6.25 to 12.5 mg/cat, PO, once daily	Ventricular tachyarrhythmias
Digoxin	0.005 to 0.008 mg/kg/day, orally, divided twice daily	Atrial tachyarrhythmias
Diltiazem	7.5 mg/cat, orally, every 8 hours	Atrial tachyarrhythmias
Esmolol	Loading dose 200 to 500 µg/kg, slow IV; followed by CRI 25 to 200 µg/kg/minute	Acute management of ventricular arrhythmias
Lidocaine	0.25 to 0.5 mg/kg, slow IV; repeat up to 2 more times if needed	Acute management of ventricular arrhythmias
Propranolol	0.02 mg/kg, slow IV; repeat up to 4 times if needed	Acute management of ventricular arrhythmias
Sotalol	2 mg/kg, orally, every 12 hours	Ventricular tachyarrhythmias

lidocaine has a relatively small therapeutic window in cats and can easily induce neurologic events such as seizures. Acute beta blockade with intravenous propranolol or esmolol can also be attempted, but there is no published literature supporting these strategies.

Atrial tachycardias are often amenable to treatment with diltiazem or digoxin, although the latter drug also has a small therapeutic window in cats and should be administered cautiously.

Beta blockade provides the most common strategy for ventricular tachyarrhythmias. Atenolol has been used extensively in cats and requires twice-daily administration. More recently, sotalol has gained popularity in the management of feline ventricular tachyarrhythmias. However, no studies have demonstrated the natural history of ventricular tachyarrhythmias in cats, so it is impossible to determine if treating these arrhythmias prevents or reduces the risk of sudden cardiac death in these patients.

Feline bradyarrhythmias can, on occasion, require therapy. Pacemaker implantation most commonly resolves clinically apparent atrioventricular block (high-grade second degree or third degree), and can be attempted in cases of persistent atrial standstill.

Isorhythmic dissociation does not require specific therapy because the ventricular rate is sufficient to meet the demands of the patient.

CONGENITAL HEART DISEASES

Very little is known about the prevalence of congenital heart diseases in cats. No studies have examined breed predispositions. In the author's experience, the most common congenital defect presented for diagnostic evaluation is the VSD. Most congenital defects seen in dogs have also been reported in cats, with a few exceptions. For example, the author knows of no cases of cor triatriatum dexter in cats but has seen several cats with a similar defect affecting the left atrium (cor triatriatum sinister, or supravalvular mitral stenosis), which has not been reported in dogs. Treatment of common congenital defects is similar to that in dogs.

Ventricular Septal Defect

VSDs in cats are similar to those in other species (Figure 20-24). Most are perimembranous (situated just under the aortic valve), and their hemodynamic consequences are determined by the size of the defect. In the author's experience, many VSDs are incidental findings in cats and cause little hemodynamic perturbation, other than a loud murmur. Most VSDs have a loud right-sided systolic murmur. Larger VSDs generally result in a left-to-right shunt, with pulmonary overcirculation and left-sided heart enlargement. If sufficiently large, left

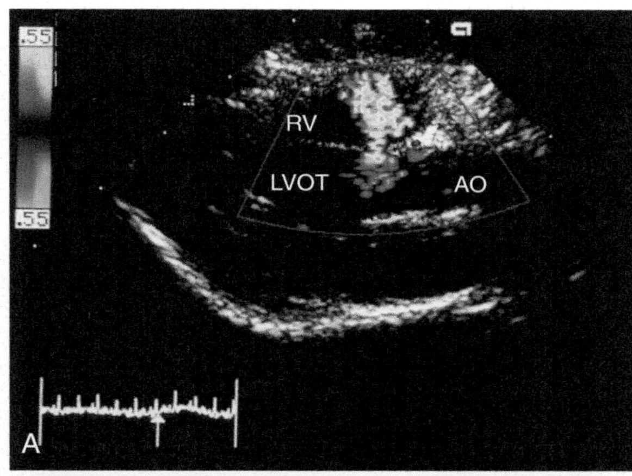

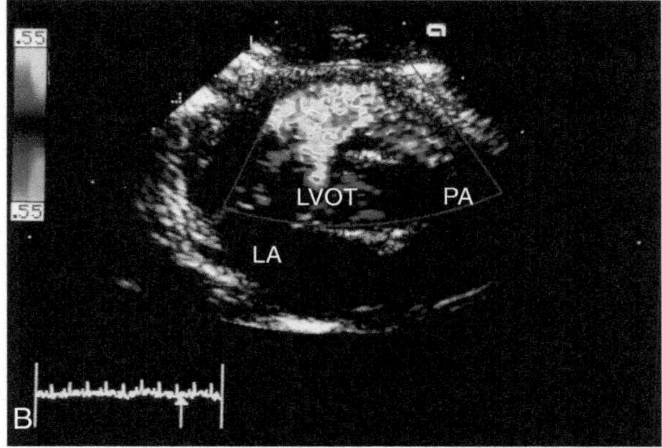

FIGURE 20-24 Echocardiographic images of a cat with a ventricular septal defect. **A,** Right-parasternal long-axis color Doppler image demonstrating left-to-right shunting of blood across the ventricular septal defect. **B,** Right-parasternal short-axis color Doppler image demonstrating left-to-right shunting of blood across the ventricular septal defect. Note that the turbulent jet is directed out into the right ventricular outflow tract in systole.

ventricular and atrial diastolic pressures can increase to the point of CHF (pulmonary edema and pleural effusion). Right-sided changes are uncommon, unless the VSD is extremely large or more ventrally located (in the muscular septum, rather than membranous septum). Because the defect is present at birth and does not generally increase in size as the patient grows, a clinically inconsequential VSD at 3 months of age will not become clinically compromising as the patient matures.

Treatment of VSDs also depends on the size of the shunt. In most instances treatment is reserved for cases with evidence of CHF. Standard diuretic and ACE inhibitor therapy is usually prescribed. Additionally, afterload reduction with arteriodilators, such as hydralazine or amlodipine, can decrease the shunt fraction and reduce left ventricular preload. Surgical correction is generally not possible in cats because of the inability to perform open-heart procedures in this species and the lack of suitable endovascular devices that could close the defect by way of a venous approach.

Atrioventricular valvular malformations (so-called "endocardial cushion defects") are also found in cats, although in the author's experience, these are less common than VSDs. Signs vary considerably with these defects and depend on the extent of involvement of the valves and the septa. In most cases these defects result in left-sided CHF.

Atrial Septal Defect

Atrial septal defects (ASDs) are relatively uncommonly diagnosed in cats. Septum primum defects appear to be more common than septum secundum defects. Occasionally, ASDs can be seen with supravalvular mitral stenosis. Complete absence of an atrial septum is also described.[42a] Finally, ASDs can be seen as part of the endocardial cushion defect complex.

Most ASDs do not cause clinical problems. However, with large ASDs, right-sided volume overload occurs (shunting from the left atrium to the right atrium and right ventricle in diastole), resulting in increased end-diastolic right ventricle pressures and right-sided CHF (ascites, pleural effusion). Pulmonary blood flow increases, resulting in pulmonary arterial hypertension.

Closure of clinically relevant ASDs is not currently feasible in most cats. Treatment includes diuretic therapy and abdominocentesis as required.

Supravalvular Mitral Stenosis (Cor Triatriatum Sinister)

Supravalvular mitral stenosis (also identified in some cats as cor triatriatum sinister) is an uncommon defect in which the left atrium has a perforated intraatrial membrane just dorsal to the mitral valve annulus, effectively producing a hemodynamic perturbation similar to mitral valvular stenosis. Flow to the left ventricle is severely restricted. In some cases atrial septal defects can result in left-to-right shunting at the atrial level. An interesting consequence of this defect is the development of severe pulmonary hypertension, rather than left-sided CHF, despite markedly elevated left atrial and pulmonary venous pressures in some cats. Other cats can develop pulmonary edema or pleural effusion.

Surgical correction has been described in one case, where the membrane was torn to allow normal transatrial flow.[85] The author was involved in an unsuccessful attempt at surgical correction in another case. Medical treatment of the CHF is generally unrewarding because diuretic therapy sufficient to reduce pulmonary venous pressures generally results in underloading of the left ventricle and output failure.

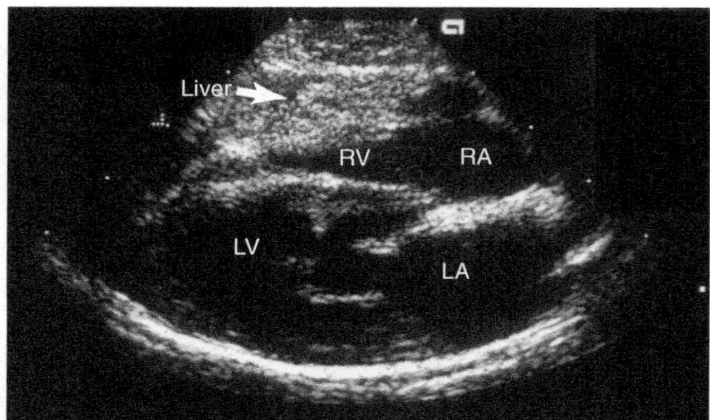

FIGURE 20-25 Echocardiographic right-parasternal long-axis image demonstrating the intrapericardial presence of liver tissue secondary to a peritoneopericardial diaphragmatic hernia.

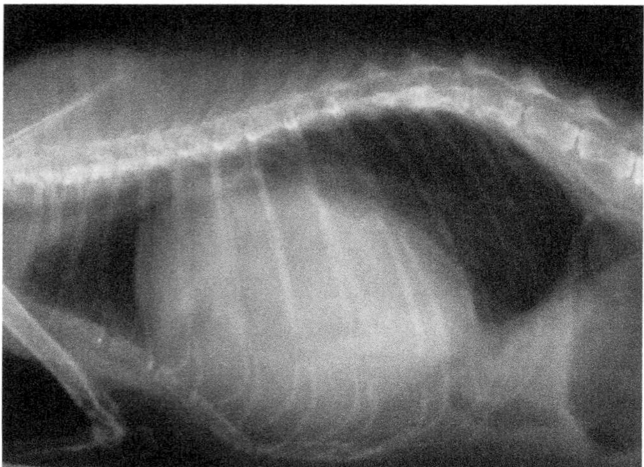

FIGURE 20-26 Lateral radiograph of a cat with a peritoneopericardial diaphragmatic hernia. Note the marked cardiomegaly with heterogeneous opacity of the cardiac silhouette, suggesting presence of fat and soft tissue within the pericardium. Also note the absence of the liver on the abdominal side of the diaphragm.

Peritoneopericardial Diaphragmatic Hernias

Peritoneopericardial diaphragmatic hernias (PPDHs) are congenital defects that are found most commonly as an incidental finding on routine radiography of older patients. Most PPDHs cause no clinical signs. The precordial impulse, or point of maximal intensity of the heart sounds on auscultation, can be displaced (e.g., absent on the left or positioned extremely dorsally in the chest) as a consequence of abdominal viscera displacing the heart within the pericardium. Falciform fat is often found prolapsing through the hernia; however, other organs can also prolapse into the pericardium (Figure 20-25). This can occasionally cause visceral entrapment or strangulation of organs. Some cats develop dyspnea or tachypnea, which is thought to be secondary to PPDH. Radiographic findings usually include a massive cardiac silhouette within which multiple soft tissue structures can be seen (Figures 20-26 and 20-27). Abdominal viscera (e.g., falciform fat, liver silhouette) might be missing from their usual locations. More specific radiographic signs have been described.[8]

Treatment of PPDH generally relies on development of clinical signs that can be attributed to the defect. Elective closure of the defect in cats that have no clinical signs (but where the defect was detected incidentally) is questionable, insofar as the risk associated with this procedure is not minimal. One study showed that postoperative hyperthermia was commonly seen in these cases and perioperative mortality was 14%—not an insignificant complication.[66] In this author's opinion, surgical correction therefore should be performed if clinical signs warrant intervention or if the patient is undergoing other elective abdominal surgery (e.g., spay) but should not be performed on cats (especially older cats) in which the finding is incidental. One study suggested that only a small percentage of these cases subsequently develop clinical signs requiring intervention,[66] so the risks

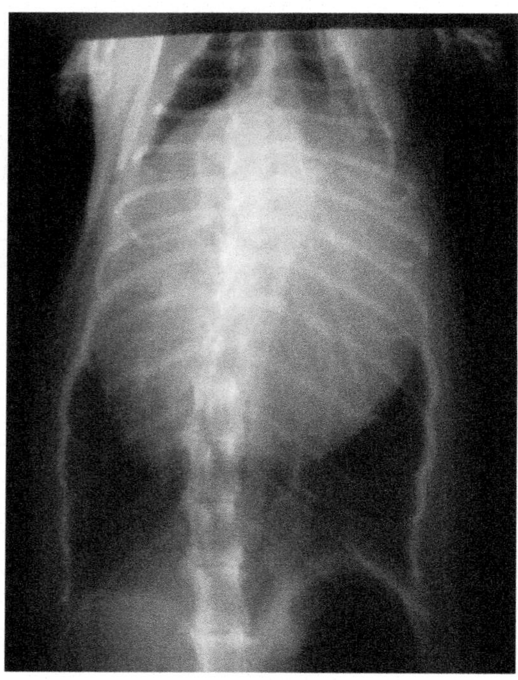

FIGURE 20-27 Dorsoventral radiograph of a cat with a peritoneopericardial diaphragmatic hernia. Note the marked cardiomegaly with heterogeneous opacity of the cardiac silhouette, suggesting presence of fat and soft tissue within the pericardium. Also note the absence of the liver on the abdominal side of the diaphragm.

associated with surgery outweigh the risks of the untreated abnormality in most patients.

Patent Ductus Arteriosus

PDA is less commonly diagnosed in cats than in dogs. However, the hemodynamic consequences of this defect are identical to those in dogs—namely, volume overload of the pulmonary circulation and left side of the heart. Physical examination findings include a left-sided continuous murmur cranial to the cardiac base, strong pulses and potentially CHF. Treatment of PDA in cats requires surgical thoracotomy and ligation as transvascular occlusion devices are too large to be used in cats. Successful ligation of the PDA will result in resolution of clinical signs and should allow the patient to lead a normal life.

Right-to-left shunting PDA is rarely identified in cats; again, affected cats suffer hemodynamic consequences similar to those of dogs with this defect. Hypoxemia and polycythemia result from blood bypassing the pulmonary circulation. Physical examination findings include a normal auscultation (no murmur) and exercise-induced hindlimb weakness and shortness of breath. Cyanotic mucous membranes can be observed caudally (genital mucosa), but oral mucosa appears normal (differential cyanosis). Treatment can include phlebotomy, although this can be difficult to accomplish in some cats. No other treatment is effective in controlling clinical signs.

MISCELLANEOUS HEART DISEASES

Glucocorticoid-Associated Congestive Heart Failure

In recent years investigators have postulated the possible causal association between the administration of glucocorticoids and subsequent development of CHF in cats. Initial reports found that cats with HCM presented for CHF shortly after either undergoing an anesthetic procedure or being administered glucocorticoids for various unassociated disorders (e.g., asthma, dermatopathies).[81] A subsequent case series reported on 13 cats over a 10-year period that presented to a referral institution with CHF after administration of various glucocorticoids.[80] Several of these cats succumbed to the CHF, whereas others were reported to have a reversible left ventricular hypertrophy. These authors subsequently suggested that glucocorticoid administration resulted in a hyperosmolar increase in plasma volume (up to 44% in some cats), which could account for the occurrence of CHF. However, they failed to document any changes in cardiac chamber dimensions that would have been anticipated with such increases in plasma volume. Other authors subsequently administered glucocorticoids to healthy cats and performed serial echocardiograms but also failed to document any change in cardiac dimensions that acute volume overload might be expected to produce.[70]

The mechanism by which glucocorticoids could produce CHF remains unresolved. One group of investigators documented an increase in plasma volume secondary to mild hyperglycemia.[65] However, this hypothesis is unconvincing. First, glucose is a weak osmole, with an osmotic effect approximately 5% that of sodium or potassium. The plasma glucose concentration that was documented in these cats was less than the renal threshold (180 mg/dL). Thus the osmotic effect would be minimal and would not be able to increase plasma volume by 44%. Second, the hypothesis does not explain the observation of reversible left ventricular hypertrophy. Furthermore, although one study claimed an association between CHF and diabetes mellitus in cats,[47] this paper has substantial flaws that preclude this author from reaching similar conclusions. Given that CHF is not a common feature of diabetic cats or cats with DKA and up to 20% of diabetic cats would be expected to have subclinical HCM, it is difficult to accept a hypothesis that invokes hyperglycemia as the cause. A mineralocorticoid effect can be excluded because most cats reported with CHF secondary to glucocorticoid administration were injected with methylprednisolone acetate (Depo-Medrol, Pfizer), which has virtually no mineralocorticoid effect.

In all the reports, there is a confounding factor that has not been considered: the hospital visit that accompanies each glucocorticoid prescription. It is possible that the stress of the hospital visit in a cat with subclinical but critical HCM could precipitate an onset of CHF shortly after the visit. The author has observed exactly this situation multiple times. Thus the possibility exists that, in some cats with severe subclinical heart disease, glucocorticoids, through some as yet undefined mechanism, can induce the onset of CHF. However, the evidence is unconvincing and could be an effect of selection bias. Additionally, the incidence appears to be rare (13 cats over 10 years at a single referral institution were identified), so clinicians should continue to use glucocorticoids when indicated in cats. Minimizing the use of glucocorticoids has a clinical rationale (e.g., decreasing the risk of diabetes mellitus) other than avoidance of CHF, so clinicians should prescribe these drugs judiciously in cats regardless of their cardiac status. It might be prudent to avoid glucocorticoids, if possible, in cats with preexisting severe heart disease (e.g., cats with prior episodes of CHF).

Hyperthyroidism and Heart Disease

Hyperthyroidism is the most commonly diagnosed endocrine disease in cats. The increased metabolic demands produced by hyperthyroidism result in cardiac hypertrophy. Additionally, direct stimulation of cardiomyocytes by thyroid hormone results in expression of myocardial genes encoding structural and contractile proteins, again resulting in hypertrophy. Consequently, the heart of a patient with hyperthyroidism has increased wall thickness, left ventricular chamber volume, and contractility. These changes, when coupled with the tachycardia that is induced by hyperthyroidism, increase cardiac output two to three times above baseline. Thus the heart of a cat with hyperthyroidism is working at a near-maximal capacity, even at rest. "High output failure" can result from prolonged hyperthyroidism because left ventricular diastolic pressures rise because of an increase in preload and blood volume and produce pulmonary edema or pleural effusion.

Reports exist of hyperthyroidism causing HCM in cats.[48,56] However, there is no rational basis for cats with hyperthyroidism to develop HCM. Instead, these cases likely represent independent comorbidities. Often, the increased preload induced by the hyperthyroid state results in CHF secondary to the previously subclinical HCM. Thus true concentric hypertrophy in a hyperthyroid cat should be considered evidence of HCM independent of the thyroid disease, and regression of the myocardial hypertrophy would not be anticipated in these cases once the thyroid disease is controlled. However, any CHF might resolve after the euthyroid state is achieved because of the reduction in preload and cardiac output.

A single report exists of myocardial failure in cats with hyperthyroidism.[36] This presentation is rarely encountered today because the disorder is recognized much more quickly than it was 30 years ago. It is likely that the myocardial failure observed in those cases was a late-stage finding; however, some of the cats in that report might also have had taurine-deficient cardiomyopathy as an independent comorbidity (because the association of taurine and myocardial failure had not yet been made).

Heart rate control in hyperthyroidism is often advocated and is warranted if the rate is exceedingly high or if CHF exists.[42] In these cases beta blockade is recommended, often resulting in improved clinical signs and hemodynamic stabilization. This is important if the patient is to be admitted to a facility for I-131 therapy, which requires several days of hospitalization because the stress can increase the likelihood of CHF developing. Clinicians should note that propranolol has a *longer* duration of action in hyperthyroid cats than in healthy cats and should adjust doses accordingly.[37] Whether similar changes in pharmacokinetics exist for atenolol is not known.

Endocarditis

Endocarditis is a rare condition in cats. Infection of cardiac valves has been reported in several case reports or case series, with the left-sided cardiac valves (aortic, mitral) involved more often than right-sided valves. Infectious agents that have most commonly been associated with feline endocarditis include *Bartonella* species *(B. henselae)* and gram-positive organisms *(Streptococcus)*.[14a,52a,61a] Clinical signs include malaise, fever, and a new murmur with or without CHF (which depends on the degree of valvular damage). Diagnosis requires culture or amplification of the organism along with echocardiographic evidence of valvular proliferative vegetative or erosive lesions, especially of the aortic or mitral valve. Treatment generally requires aggressive intravenous antibiotic therapy. Prognosis is guarded, although one case report suggested that early and aggressive intervention in endocarditis caused by *B. henselae* infections can have a complete resolution.[61a] However, most other reports were associated with either acute mortality or persistent clinical signs (e.g., CHF) and requirement for ongoing antibiotic therapy.

References

1. Abbott JA: Heart rate and heart rate variability of healthy cats in home and hospital environments, *J Feline Med Surg* 7:195, 2005.
2. Acierno MJ, Seaton D, Mitchell MA et al: Agreement between directly measured blood pressure and pressures obtained with three veterinary-specific oscillometric units in cats, *J Am Vet Med Assoc* 237:402, 2010.
3. Atkins CE, Gallo AM, Kurzman ID et al: Risk factors, clinical signs, and survival in cats with a clinical diagnosis of idiopathic hypertrophic cardiomyopathy: 74 cases (1985-1989), *J Am Vet Med Assoc* 201:613, 1992.
4. Baty C, Malarkey D, Atkins C et al: Natural history of hypertrophic cardiomyopathy and aortic thromboembolism in a family of domestic shorthair cats, *J Vet Intern Med* 15:595, 2001.
5. Bedard C, Lanevschi-Pietersma A, Dunn M: Evaluation of coagulation markers in the plasma of healthy cats and cats with asymptomatic hypertrophic cardiomyopathy, *Vet Clin Pathol* 36:167, 2007.
6. Belew A, Barlett T, Brown S: Evaluation of the white-coat effect in cats, *J Vet Intern Med* 13:134, 1999.
7. Benigni L, Morgan N, Lamb CR: Radiographic appearance of cardiogenic pulmonary oedema in 23 cats, *J Small Anim Pract* 50:9, 2009.
8. Berry CR, Koblik PD, Ticer JW: Dorsal peritoneopericardial mesothelial remnant as an aid to diagnosis of feline congenital peritoneopericardial diaphragmatic hernia, *Vet Radiol Ultrasound* 31:239, 1990.
9. Bright JM, Golden AL, Gompf RE et al: Evaluation of the calcium channel-blocking agents diltiazem and verapamil for treatment of feline hypertrophic cardiomyopathy, *J Vet Intern Med* 5:272, 1991.
10. Brown S, Atkins C, Bagley R et al: Guidelines for the identification, evaluation, and management of systemic hypertension in dogs and cats, *J Vet Intern Med* 21:542, 2007.
11. Buchanan JW: Prevalence of cardiovascular disorders. In Fox PR, Sisson DD, Moise NS editors: *Textbook of canine and feline cardiology*, ed 2, Philadelphia, 1999, Saunders, p 457.
12. Carlos Sampedrano C, Chetboul V, Gouni V et al: Systolic and diastolic myocardial dysfunction in cats with hypertrophic cardiomyopathy or systemic hypertension, *J Vet Intern Med* 20:1106, 2006.
13. Carlos Sampedrano C, Chetboul V, Mary J et al: Prospective echocardiographic and tissue Doppler imaging screening of a population of Maine Coon cats tested for the A31P mutation in the myosin-binding protein C gene: a specific analysis of the heterozygous status, *J Vet Intern Med* 23:91, 2009.
14. Chetboul V, Lefebvre H, Pinhas C et al: Spontaneous feline hypertension: clinical and echocardiographic abnormalities, and survival rate, *J Vet Intern Med* 17:89, 2003.

14a. Chomel BB, Wey AC, Kasten RW et al: Fatal case of endocarditis associated with *Bartonella henselae* type I infection in a domestic cat, *J Clin Microbiol* 41:5337, 2003.
15. Connolly DJ: A case of sustained atrial fibrillation in a cat with a normal sized left atrium at the time of diagnosis, *J Vet Cardiol* 7:137, 2005.
16. Connolly DJ, Magalhaes RJS, Fuentes VL et al: Assessment of the diagnostic accuracy of circulating natriuretic peptide concentrations to distinguish between cats with cardiac and non-cardiac causes of respiratory distress, *J Vet Cardiol* 11:S41, 2009.
17. Côté E, Jaeger R: Ventricular tachyarrhythmias in 106 cats: associated structural cardiac disorders, *J Vet Intern Med* 22:1444, 2008.
18. Côté E, Manning A, Emerson D et al: Assessment of the prevalence of heart murmurs in overtly healthy cats, *J Am Vet Med Assoc* 225:384, 2004.
18a. Côté E, Harpster N, Laste N et al: Atrial fibrillation in cats: 50 cases (1979-2002), *J Am Vet Med Assoc* 225:256, 2004.
18b. Cowgill L: Personal communication, *Feb* 2009.
19. Falconer L, Atwell R: Feline aortic thromboembolism, *Aust Vet Pract* 33:20, 2003.
20. Ferasin L: Recurrent syncope associated with paroxysmal supraventricular tachycardia in a Devon Rex cat diagnosed by implantable loop recorder, *J Feline Med Surg* 11:149, 2009.
21. Ferasin L, Sturgess C, Cannon M et al: Feline idiopathic cardiomyopathy: a retrospective study of 106 cats (1994-2001), *J Feline Med Surg* 5:151, 2003.
22. Ferasin L, van de Stad M, Rudorf H et al: Syncope associated with paroxysmal atrioventricular block and ventricular standstill in a cat, *J Small Anim Pract* 43:124, 2002.
23. Fox PR: Feline cardiomyopathies. In Fox PR, Sisson DD, Moise NS, editors: *Textbook of canine and feline cardiology*, ed 2, Philadelphia, 1999, Saunders, p 623.
24. Fox PR: Prospective, double-blinded, multicenter evaluation of chronic therapies for feline diastolic heart failure: interim analysis (abstract), *J Vet Intern Med* 17:398, 2003.
25. Fox PR, Harpster NK: Diagnosis and management of feline arrhythmias. In Fox PR, Sisson DD, Moise NS, editors: *Textbook of canine and feline cardiology*, ed 2, Philadelphia, 1999, Saunders, p 387.
26. Fox PR, Liu SK, Maron BJ: Echocardiographic assessment of spontaneously occurring feline hypertrophic cardiomyopathy. An animal model of human disease, *Circulation* 92:2645, 1995.
27. Fox PR, Maron BJ, Basso C et al: Spontaneously occurring arrhythmogenic right ventricular cardiomyopathy in the domestic cat: A new animal model similar to the human disease, *Circulation* 102:1863, 2000.
28. Gavaghan BJ, Kittleson MD, McAloose D: Persistent atrial standstill in a cat, *Aust Vet J* 77:574, 1999.
29. Gompf RE, Tilley LP: Comparison of lateral and sternal recumbent positions for electrocardiography of the cat, *Am J Vet Res* 40:1483, 1979.
30. Hanås S, Tidholm A, Egenvall A et al: Twenty-four hour Holter monitoring of unsedated healthy cats in the home environment, *J Vet Cardiol* 11:17, 2009.
31. Harpster NK: Feline arrhythmias: diagnosis and management. In Kirk RW, Bonagura JD editors: *Current veterinary therapy XI small animal practice*, Philadelphia, 1992, Saunders, p 732.
32. Harvey AM, Faena M, Darke PG et al: Effect of body position on feline electrocardiographic recordings, *J Vet Intern Med* 19:533, 2005.
33. Helms SR: Treatment of feline hypertension with transdermal amlodipine: a pilot study, *J Am Anim Hosp Assoc* 43:149, 2007.
34. Henik R, Stepien R, Bortnowski H: Spectrum of m-mode echocardiographic abnormalities in 75 cats with systemic hypertension, *J Am Anim Hosp Assoc* 40:359, 2004.
34a. Hogan DF: Unpublished data, June 2009.
35. Hsu A, Kittleson MD, Paling A: Investigation into the use of plasma NT-proBNP concentration to screen for feline hypertrophic cardiomyopathy, *J Vet Cardiol* 11:S63, 2009.
36. Jacobs G, Hutson C, Dougherty J et al: Congestive heart failure associated with hyperthyroidism in cats, *J Am Vet Med Assoc* 188:52, 1986.
37. Jacobs G, Whittem T, Sams R et al: Pharmacokinetics of propranolol in healthy cats during euthyroid and hyperthyroid states, *Am J Vet Res* 58:398, 1997.
38. James R, Summerfield N, Loureiro J et al: Implantable loop recorders: a viable diagnostic tool in veterinary medicine, *J Small Anim Pract* 49:564, 2008.
39. Jepson RE, Elliott J, Brodbelt D et al: Effect of control of systolic blood pressure on survival in cats with systemic hypertension, *J Vet Intern Med* 21:402, 2007.
40. Johnson L, Sisson DD: Atrioventricular block in cats, *Comp Contin Edu Pract Vet* 15:1356, 1993.
41. Kellum HB, Stepien RL: Third-degree atrioventricular block in 21 cats (1997-2004), *J Vet Intern Med* 20:97, 2006.
42. Kienle RD, Bruyette D, Pion PD: Effects of thyroid hormone and thyroid dysfunction on the cardiovascular system, *Vet Clin North Am Small Anim Pract* 24:495, 1994.
42a. Kittleson MD: Septal defects. In Kittleson MD, Kienle RD editors: *Small animal cardiovascular medicine*, St. Louis, 1998, Mosby, p 231.
43. Koyama H, Matsumoto H, Fukushima RU et al: Local intra-arterial administration of urokinase in the treatment of a feline distal aortic thromboembolism, *J Vet Med Sci* 72:1209, 2010.
44. Lalor SM, Connolly DJ, Elliott J et al: Plasma concentrations of natriuretic peptides in normal cats and normotensive and hypertensive cats with chronic kidney disease, *J Vet Cardiol* 11:S71, 2009.
45. Laste NJ, Harpster NK: A retrospective study of 100 cases of feline distal aortic thromboembolism: 1977-1993, *J Am Anim Hosp Assoc* 31:492, 1995.
46. Litster A, Buchanan J: Vertebral scale system to measure heart size in radiographs of cats, *J Am Vet Med Assoc* 216:210, 2000.
47. Little CJ, Gettinby G: Heart failure is common in diabetic cats: findings from a retrospective case-controlled study in first-opinion practice, *J Small Anim Pract* 49:17, 2008.
48. Liu SK, Peterson ME, Fox PR: Hypertropic cardiomyopathy and hyperthyroidism in the cat, *J Am Vet Med Assoc* 185:52, 1984.
49. Liu SK, Tilley LP: Animal models of primary myocardial diseases, *Yale J Biol Med* 53:191, 1980.
50. Lord PF, Zontine WJ: Radiologic examination of the feline cardiovascular system, *Vet Clin North Am* 7:291, 1977.
51. MacDonald KA, Kittleson MD, Larson RF et al: The effect of ramipril on left ventricular mass, myocardial fibrosis, diastolic function, and plasma neurohormones in Maine Coon cats with familial hypertrophic cardiomyopathy without heart failure, *J Vet Intern Med* 20:1093, 2006.
52. Maggio F, DeFrancesco TC, Atkins CE et al: Ocular lesions associated with systemic hypertension in cats: 69 cases (1985-1998), *J Am Vet Med Assoc* 217:695, 2000.
52a. Malik R, Barrs V, Church D et al: Vegetative endocarditis in six cats, *J Feline Med Surg* 1:171, 1999.
53. Meurs K, Sanchez X, David R et al: A cardiac myosin binding protein C mutation in the Maine Coon cat with familial hypertrophic cardiomyopathy, *Hum Mol Genet* 14:3587, 2005.
54. Meurs KM, Kuan M: Differential methylation of CpG sites in two isoforms of myosin binding protein C, an important hypertrophic cardiomyopathy gene, *Environ Mol Mutagen* 52:161, 2011.
55. Meurs KM, Norgard MM, Ederer MM et al: A substitution mutation in the myosin binding protein C gene in ragdoll hypertrophic cardiomyopathy, *Genomics* 90:261, 2007.
56. Miyamoto T, Kato M, Kuwamura M et al: A first feline case of cardiomyopathy associated with hyperthyroidism due to thyroid adenoma in Japan, *Feline Pract* 26:6, 1998.

57. Moon M, Keene BW, Lessard P et al: Age related changes in the feline cardiac silhouette, *Vet Radiol Ultrasound* 34:315, 1993.
58. Moore KE, Morris N, Dhupa N et al: Retrospective study of streptokinase administration in 46 cats with arterial thromboembolism, *J Vet Emerg Crit Care* 10:245, 2000.
59. Myer CW, Bonagura JD: Survey radiography of the heart, *Vet Clin North Am Small Anim Pract* 12:213, 1982.
60. Nelson O, Reidesel E, Ware W et al: Echocardiographic and radiographic changes associated with systemic hypertension in cats, *J Vet Intern Med* 16:418, 2002.
61. Paige CF, Abbott JA, Elvinger F et al: Prevalence of cardiomyopathy in apparently healthy cats, *J Am Vet Med Assoc* 234:1398, 2009.
61a. Perez C, Hummel JB, Keene BW et al: Successful treatment of *Bartonella henselae* endocarditis in a cat, *J Feline Med Surg* 12:483, 2010.
62. Piegras DG, Sundt TM Jr, Didisheim P: Effect of anticoagulants and inhibitors of platelet aggregation on thrombotic occlusion of endarterectomized cat carotid arteries, *Stroke* 7:248, 1976.
63. Pion PD: Feline aortic thromboemboli: t-PA thrombolysis followed by aspirin therapy and rethrombosis, *Vet Clin North Am Small Anim Pract* 18:262, 1988.
64. Pion PD, Kittleson MD, Rogers QR et al: Myocardial failure in cats associated with low plasma taurine: a reversible cardiomyopathy, *Science* 237:764, 1987.
65. Ployngam T, Tobias AH, Smith SA et al: Hemodynamic effects of methylprednisolone acetate administration in cats, *Am J Vet Res* 67:583, 2006.
66. Reimer S, Kyles A, Filipowicz D et al: Long-term outcome of cats treated conservatively or surgically for peritoneopericardial diaphragmatic hernia: 66 cases (1987-2002), *J Am Vet Med Assoc* 224:728, 2004.
67. Reimer SB, Kittleson MD, Kyles AE: Use of rheolytic thrombectomy in the treatment of feline distal aortic thromboembolism, *J Vet Intern Med* 20:290, 2006.
68. Riesen SC, Kovacevic A, Lombard CW et al: Prevalence of heart disease in symptomatic cats: an overview from 1998 to 2005, *Schweiz Arch Tierheilkd* 149:65, 2007.
69. Rishniw M, Bruskiewicz K: ECG of the month. Respiratory sinus arrhythmia and wandering pacemaker in a cat, *J Am Vet Med Assoc* 208:1811, 1996.
70. Rishniw M, Center SA, Randolph JF et al: Methylprednisolone acetate fails to alter echocardiographic variables in healthy cats. Proceedings European College of Veterinary Internal Medicine—Companion Animals Congress, 2008.
71. Rishniw M, Thomas WP: Dynamic right ventricular outflow obstruction: a new cause of systolic murmurs in cats, *J Vet Intern Med* 16:547, 2002.
72. Rush J, Freeman L, Fenollosa N et al: Population and survival characteristics of cats with hypertrophic cardiomyopathy: 260 cases (1990-1999), *J Am Vet Med Assoc* 220:202, 2002.
73. Schellenberg S, Glaus TM, Reusch CE: Effect of long-term adaptation on indirect measurements of systolic blood pressure in conscious untrained beagles, *Vet Rec* 161:418, 2007.
74. Schober KE, Bonagura JD, Fuentes VL: Atenolol versus diltiazem for LV diastolic function in cats with occult HCM. *Proceedings American College of Veterinary Internal Medicine Forum*, 2007.
75. Schober KE, Maerz I: Assessment of left atrial appendage flow velocity and its relation to spontaneous echocardiographic contrast in 89 cats with myocardial disease, *J Vet Intern Med* 20:120, 2006.
76. Schober KE, Maerz I, Ludewig E et al: Diagnostic accuracy of electrocardiography and thoracic radiography in the assessment of left atrial size in cats: comparison with transthoracic 2-dimensional echocardiography, *J Vet Intern Med* 21:709, 2007.
77. Schoeman J: Feline distal aortic thromboembolism: a review of 44 cases (1990-1998), *J Feline Med Surg* 1:221, 1999.
78. Singh MK, Cocchiaro MF, Kittleson MD: NT-proBNP measurement fails to reliably identify subclinical hypertrophic cardiomyopathy in Maine Coon cats, *J Feline Med Surg* 12:942, 2010.
79. Smith C, Rozanski E, Freeman L et al: Use of low molecular weight heparin in cats: 57 cases (1999-2003), *J Am Vet Med Assoc* 225:1237, 2004.
80. Smith S, Tobias A, Fine D et al: Corticosteroid-associated congestive heart failure in 12 cats, *Intern J Appl Res Vet Med* 2:159, 2004.
81. Smith S, Tobias A, Fine D et al: Corticosteroid-associated congestive heart failure in 29 cats (abstract), *J Vet Intern Med* 16:371, 2002.
82. Smith S, Tobias A, Jacob K et al: Arterial thromboembolism in cats: acute crisis in 127 cases (1992-2001) and long-term management with low-dose aspirin in 24 cases, *J Vet Intern Med* 17:73, 2003.
83. Stalis IH, Bossbaly MJ, Van Winkle TJ: Feline endomyocarditis and left ventricular endocardial fibrosis, *Vet Pathol* 32:122, 1995.
84. Stokol T, Brooks M, Rush JE et al: Hypercoagulability in cats with cardiomyopathy, *J Vet Intern Med* 22:546, 2008.
85. Wander K, Monnet E, Orton E: Surgical correction of cor triatriatum sinister in a kitten, *J Am Anim Hosp Assoc* 34:383, 1998.
86. Ware W: Twenty-four-hour ambulatory electrocardiography in normal cats, *J Vet Intern Med* 13:175, 1999.
87. Wernick M, Doherr M, Howard J et al: Evaluation of high-definition and conventional oscillometric blood pressure measurement in anaesthetised dogs using ACVIM guidelines, *J Small Anim Pract* 51:318, 2010.
88. Wess G, Schinner C, Weber K et al: Association of A31P and A74T polymorphisms in the myosin binding protein C3 gene and hypertrophic cardiomyopathy in Maine Coon and other breed cats, *J Vet Intern Med* 24:527, 2010.

CHAPTER

21

Dental and Oral Diseases

Alexander M. Reiter

OUTLINE

Resorption of multiple teeth is very common in cats. However, its etiology remains a mystery up to this day. Similarly, stomatitis has been described for many decades, but progress in identifying its cause and providing effective treatment continues to be challenging. Oral and maxillofacial trauma also manifests somewhat uniquely in the cat in that the mandibular symphysis, the temporomandibular joints, and the hard palate are typically affected, but rarely the midportion of the mandibular body. Squamous cell carcinoma is the most common tumor of the oral cavity in the cat, and curative surgical treatment is usually reserved for those tumors affecting the lower jaw. A comprehensive review of dental and oral diseases in the cat has recently been published.[8]

ORAL ANATOMY

Eruption of Deciduous and Permanent Teeth

Cats have two sets of teeth, the deciduous and permanent dentitions. Deciduous incisors erupt at 2 to 3 weeks, canines at 3 to 4 weeks, and premolars at 3 to 6 weeks of age. There should be 26 deciduous teeth. Permanent incisors erupt at 3 to 4 months, canines at 4 to 5 months, premolars at 4 to 6 months, and molars at 4 to 5 months of age. There should be 30 permanent teeth. At 7 months of age, the young cat should have 30 fully erupted permanent teeth in place (Table 21-1).

There are four specific types of teeth, each serving a distinct purpose. The incisors are designed to cut, prehend, and groom. The canines are used to penetrate and grasp prey or food and also function as defensive weapons in protection. The cheek teeth (premolars and molars) assist in the ability to hold and carry, in addition to the breaking and tearing of food into smaller pieces in preparation for digestion. The so-called carnassials refer to the maxillary fourth premolar and mandibular first molar teeth, which serve a shearing function in carnivores.[66]

Tooth Formula in the Domestic Cat

The total number of teeth in the cat is greatly decreased compared with that of the dog, and the shapes of the crowns of feline teeth reflect the function of a true carnivore.[90] Accepted dental formulas for the deciduous and permanent dentition in the domestic cat are shown in Tables 21-2 and 21-3. Using the modified Triadan

TABLE 21-1 Eruption of the Deciduous and Permanent Dentitions in the Domestic Cat

	Deciduous Teeth	Permanent Teeth
Incisors	2-3 weeks	3-4 months
Canines	3-4 weeks	4-5 months
Premolars	3-6 weeks	4-6 months
Molars	No deciduous molars	4-5 months

TABLE 21-2 Formula for the Deciduous Dentition in the Domestic Cat

Deciduous	Incisors	Canines	Premolars	Total
Maxilla	3	1	3	× 2 = 26
Mandible	3	1	2	

TABLE 21-3 Formula for the Permanent Dentition in the Domestic Cat

Permanent	Incisors	Canines	Premolars	Molars	Total
Maxilla	3	1	3	1	× 2 = 30
Mandible	3	1	2	1	

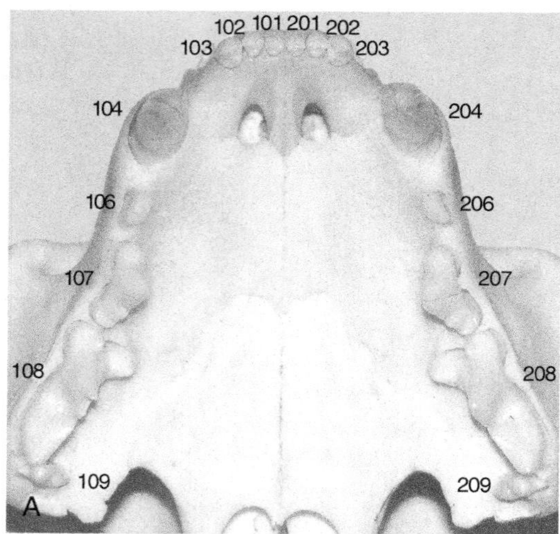

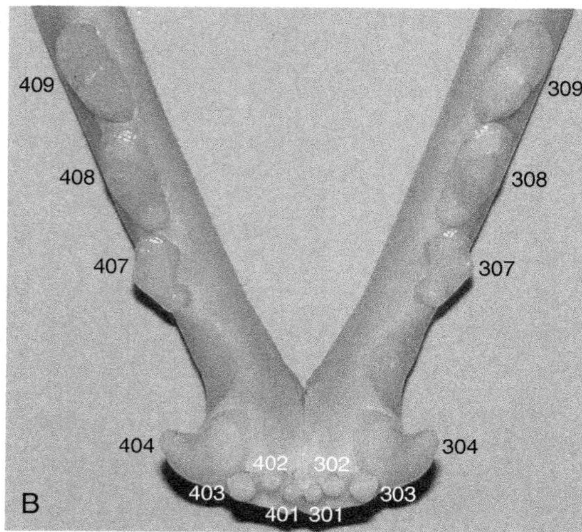

FIGURE 21-1 Modified Triadan tooth-numbering system for the maxillary **(A)** and mandibular **(B)** permanent teeth of the domestic cat. Note that there are no permanent maxillary first premolars or mandibular first and second premolars. *(Copyright 2010 Dr. Alexander M. Reiter; used with permission.)*

tooth-numbering system, each jaw quadrant is numbered as follows: right maxillary quadrant 100 (500 when referring to deciduous teeth), left maxillary quadrant 200 (600 when referring to deciduous teeth), left mandibular quadrant 300 (700 when referring to deciduous teeth), and right mandibular quadrant 400 (800 when referring to deciduous teeth).[66]

Beginning with 01 for the first incisor (the one closest to the midline), teeth are consecutively numbered from mesial (the surface of the tooth that faces the midline of the dental arch) to distal (the surface of the tooth that faces away from the midline of the dental arch). Several premolars and molars have been evolutionarily lost in the permanent dentition of the cat. The canine (04) and the first molar (09) are present as reference teeth to allow counting forward or backward when numbering teeth. The permanent maxillary first (05) premolar and the permanent mandibular first (05) and second (06) premolars are absent in the cat. Because the maxillary fourth premolar (08) and mandibular first molar (09) are the largest cheek teeth of the upper and lower jaws, counting forward identifies the premolars between the maxillary canine and fourth premolar as the maxillary second and third premolars (teeth 06 and 07). Similarly, the premolars between the mandibular canine and first molar are identified as the mandibular third and fourth premolars (teeth 07 and 08).[66]

Taking the quadrant and tooth number into consideration, three numbers are used to identify a specific tooth. For example, the permanent right maxillary canine is tooth 104. The permanent right maxillary fourth premolar is tooth 108. The permanent left maxillary second premolar is tooth 206. The permanent left mandibular third and fourth premolars are teeth 307 and 308. The permanent right mandibular first molar is tooth 409 (Figure 21-1). The deciduous right maxillary canine is tooth 504. The deciduous right mandibular fourth premolar is tooth 808 (Figure 21-2).

Teeth

The tooth consists of a crown and one or more roots. Enamel (with >95% mineralization, the hardest tissue of the body) covers the crown, and cementum covers the

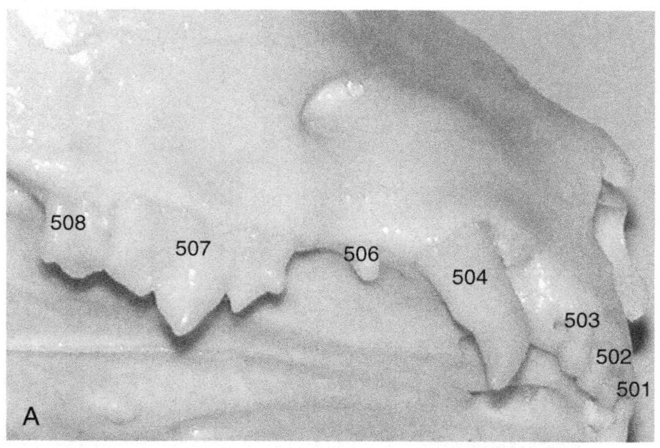

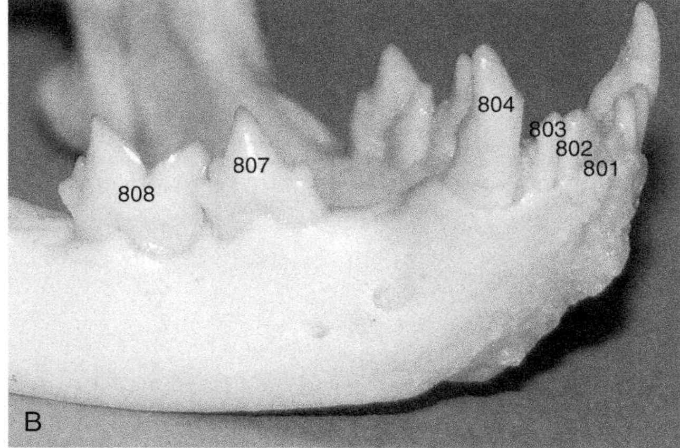

FIGURE 21-2 Modified Triadan tooth-numbering system for the maxillary **(A)** and mandibular **(B)** deciduous teeth of the domestic kitten. Note that the number of deciduous teeth differs from that of permanent teeth because there are no deciduous maxillary and mandibular first molars. *(Copyright 2010 Dr. Alexander M. Reiter; used with permission.)*

root(s). The borderline between the anatomic crown and root(s) is the cementoenamel junction.[21] The incisors and canine teeth have one root. The maxillary second premolars and first molars have two roots that are often fused to each other, giving the appearance of only one root.[114] The mandibular third and fourth premolars and first molars and the maxillary third premolars have two roots. The maxillary fourth premolar has three roots. The furcation is where two or more roots meet at the crown.[66]

Dentin makes up the bulk of the adult tooth. It is approximately 70% mineralized and porous, and consists of thousands of dentinal tubules per square millimeter radiating outward from the pulp to the enamel in the crown and cementum in the root.[90] Odontoblasts line the periphery of the pulp cavity and produce dentin, which—in a vital tooth—is laid down throughout life. Dentinal tubules contain cytoplasmic processes of odontoblasts, fluid, and nerves extending from the pulp. Tooth pain may result from fluid movement and nerve stimulation in the area of exposed tubules. Odontoblasts adjacent to exposed dentinal tubules may respond by producing tertiary dentin to halt the progression of an external insult.[66]

The pulp cavity consists of the pulp chamber in the crown and the root canal(s) in the root(s) of the tooth. It contains the pulp, which is made up of undifferentiated mesenchymal cells, fibroblasts, odontoblasts, blood and lymph vessels, and nerves.[90] Odontoblasts line the inside of the pulp cavity at the periphery of the pulp, initially producing nonmineralized predentin, which later becomes mineralized dentin. Unlike human teeth that have only one apical foramen, the pulp of cat teeth connects with periapical tissues through several foramina in the root apex (forming the apical delta). Secondary, accessory, lateral, and furcation canals also may connect pulp tissue with the periodontal ligament.[80] Therefore entrance into the pulp cavity can be through exposed dentinal tubules, direct pulp exposure, and apical and non-apical ramifications.

The tooth "grows" toward the inside. The dentin becomes continually thicker in a vital tooth. Dentin apposition along the inside of the pulp cavity continues throughout life, unless irreversible pulpitis or pulp necrosis occurs. Therefore teeth of young adult cats have a fairly wide pulp cavity (Figure 21-3). In older cats the pulp cavity of teeth with vital pulps is usually very narrow (Figure 21-4). The narrower the pulp cavity, the thicker are the dentinal walls, and thus the stronger and more aged is the tooth.

Periodontium

The periodontium is a functional unit and consists of the gingiva, periodontal ligament, cementum, and alveolar bone.[90] The gingiva surrounds the tooth like a collar and is firmly attached to the alveolar bone and cervical portion of the tooth. The most coronal edge of the gingiva is the gingival margin. A normal space between the tooth and most coronal gingiva is called the gingival sulcus, which should not be deeper than 0.5 mm in cats. The periodontal ligament acts as shock absorber and attaches the tooth to the alveolar bone by means of Sharpey's fibers. Some fibers connect adjacent teeth by traveling through or coronal to the alveolar septum. Radiographically, the periodontal ligament space appears as a dark line surrounding the root.

The cementum covers the root(s) and is produced by cementoblasts. It is similar in mineral composition and histologic appearance to bone. Cementum width increases with age.[66] An excessive production of cementum (hypercementosis) is often seen in cat teeth, most commonly at the apical portion of the root. Alveolar bone surrounds the alveolar socket. An increased radiodensity of alveolar bone is visible adjacent to the periodontal ligament space, referred to as the *lamina dura,* which is an extension of cortical bone into the

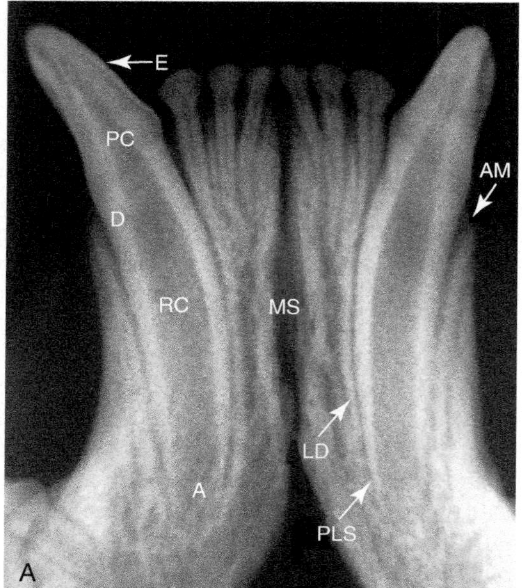

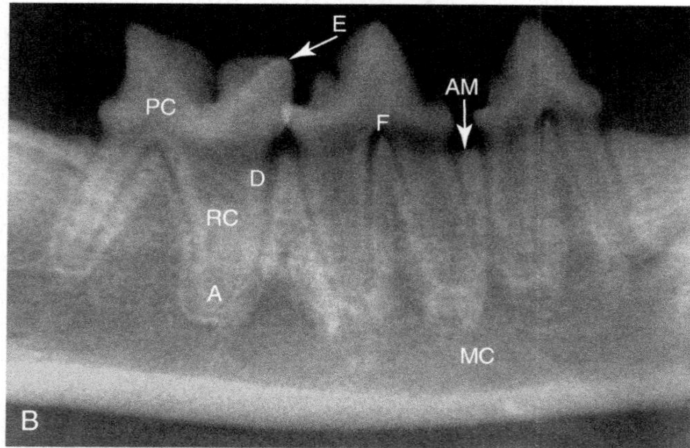

FIGURE 21-3 Radiographs of the mandibular incisors and canines **(A)** and the right mandibular cheek teeth **(B)** in a cat younger than 1 year of age. Note the thin dentinal walls, wide pulp cavities, and open root apices. *E*, Enamel; *PC*, pulp chamber; *D*, dentin; *RC*, root canal; *A*, apex; *MS*, mandibular symphysis; *AM*, alveolar margin; *LD*, lamina dura; *PLS*, periodontal ligament space; *F*, furcation; *MC*, mandibular canal. *(Copyright 2010 Dr. Alexander M. Reiter; used with permission.)*

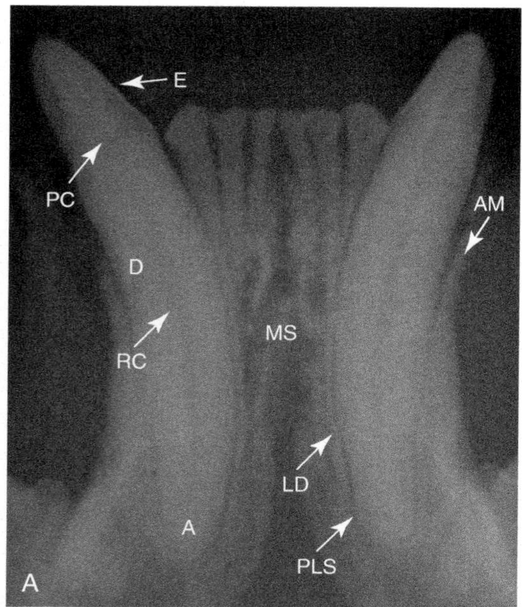

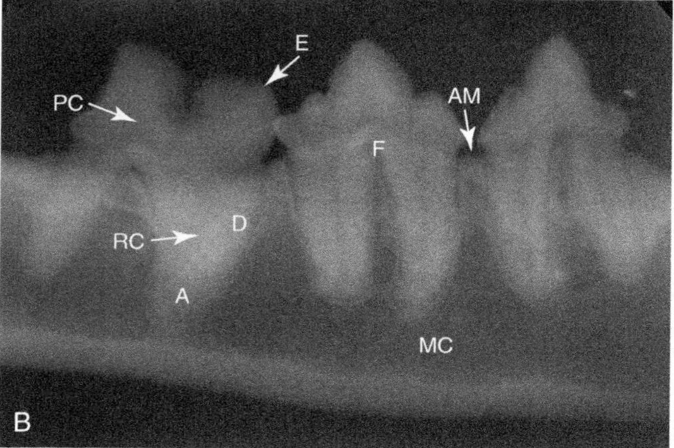

FIGURE 21-4 Radiographs of the mandibular incisors and canines **(A)** and the right mandibular cheek teeth **(B)** in a cat older than 3 years of age. Note the thicker dentinal walls, narrower pulp cavities, and closed root apices, compared with Figure 21-3. *E*, Enamel; *PC*, pulp chamber; *D*, dentin; *RC*, root canal; *A*, apex; *MS*, mandibular symphysis; *AM*, alveolar margin; *LD*, lamina dura; *PLS*, periodontal ligament space; *F*, furcation; *MC*, mandibular canal. *(Copyright 2010 Dr. Alexander M. Reiter; used with permission.)*

alveolus. The most coronal edge of the alveolar bone is the alveolar margin.[66] Alveolar bone is constantly remodeling in response to use and the forces placed on it.

Oral Mucosa

Oral mucosa other than gingiva includes the very flexible and elastic alveolar mucosa, which covers the alveolar bone and is separated from the gingiva by the mucogingival junction; the labial and buccal mucosae, which line the inside of the lip and cheek; the loose sublingual mucosa, the mucosa covering the dorsal and ventral tongue surfaces; the mucosa of the hard palate, which is firmly attached to underlying maxillae and palatine bones; and the mucosa of the soft palate.[66] The oral mucosa is separated from the skin by the mucocutaneous junction (Figure 21-5).

Bones and Joints

Most cats are mesaticephalic; in other words, their heads are of medium proportions. Brachycephalic cats, such as the Persian, have short, wide heads. Dolichocephalic cats, such as the Siamese, have long, narrow heads. The

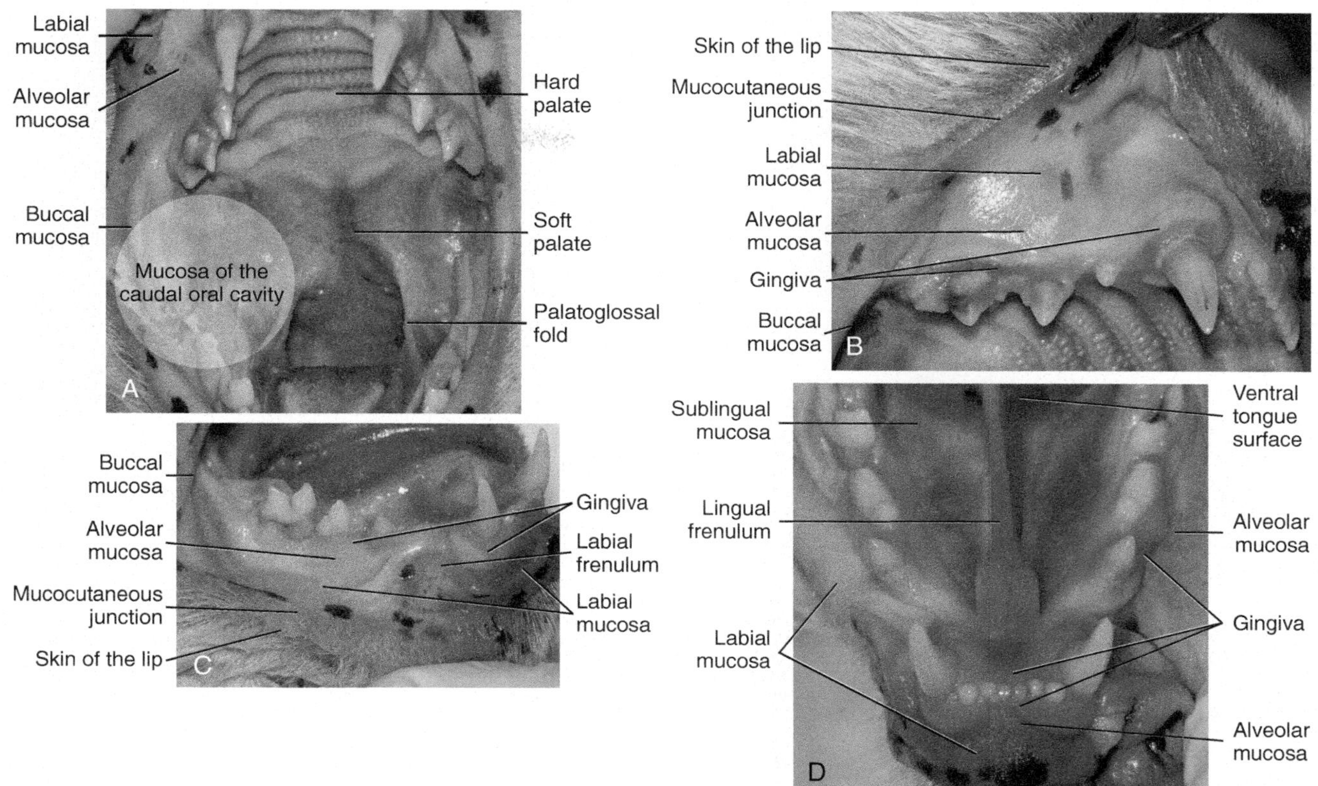

FIGURE 21-5 Oral mucosa of the roof of the mouth and caudal oral cavity **(A)**, the upper jaw **(B)**, the lower jaw **(C)**, and the sublingual region **(D)**. *(Copyright 2010 Dr. Alexander M. Reiter; used with permission.)*

upper jaw and the face consist of the paired incisive bones; maxillae; palatine, nasal, zygomatic, and temporal bones; and the unpaired vomer bone. The incisive bones carry the maxillary incisor teeth, and the maxillae carry the maxillary canines, premolars, and molars. The infraorbital canal (containing the infraorbital artery, vein, and nerve) penetrates the maxillary bone in the area of the fourth premolar and molar teeth.[66]

The lower jaw consists of the paired mandibular bones. The ventral third of each mandible includes the mandibular canal, which contains the inferior alveolar artery, vein, and nerve. Right and left mandibles are separated rostrally by a fibrocartilaginous synchondrosis (mandibular symphysis) and carry all mandibular teeth. The temporomandibular joint is formed by the condylar process of the mandible and the mandibular fossa and retroarticular process of the temporal bone (Figure 21-6). A thin fibrocartilagenous disk lies between the hyaline cartilage–covered articular surfaces. A thick band of fibrous tissue on the lateral aspect of the joint capsule forms the lateral ligament, which tightens when the jaw opens.[66]

Muscles, Cheeks, and Lips

The masticatory musculature includes the masseter, temporal, and pterygoid (medial and lateral) muscles, which close the mouth, and the digastricus muscle, which opens the mouth.[90] The lips and cheeks of cats are "tighter" and their oral vestibules less spacious than in dogs, making their labial and buccal mucosae less available for closure of large intraoral wounds. The commissure is where the upper and lower lips meet. There are three important structures within the soft tissues of the cheek that run nearly parallel over the masseter musle in a rostrocaudal direction: the dorsal and ventral buccal branches of the facial nerve and the parotid duct traversing between the two nerves and opening into the mouth at the parotid papilla in the buccal mucosa near the maxillary fourth premolar.[66]

Palate

The primary palate is made up of the rostral upper lip and the most rostral hard palate. The majority of the

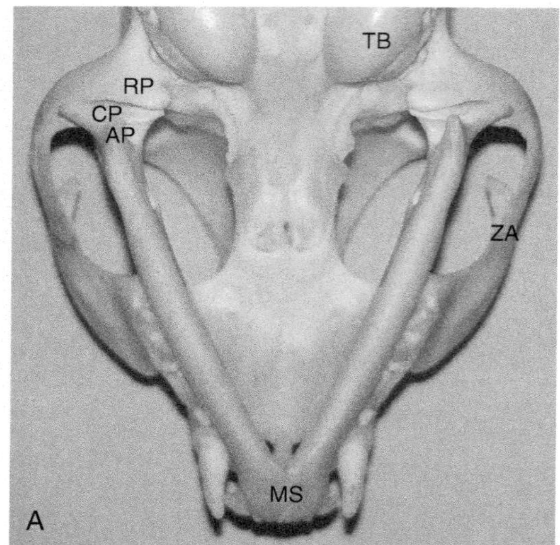

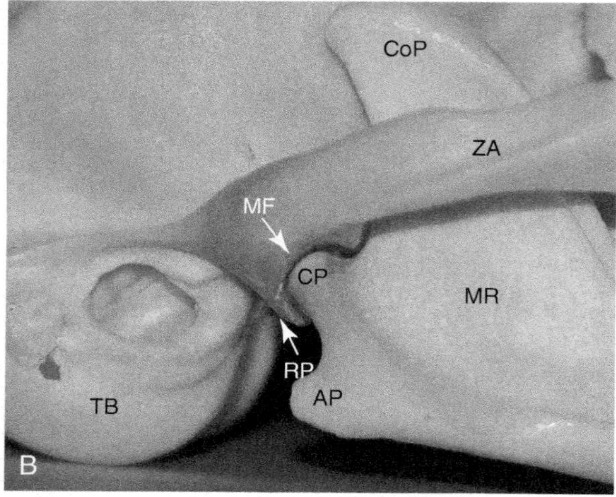

FIGURE 21-6 Ventral **(A)** and lateral **(B)** views of the feline skull, showing the temporomandibular joints and the mandibular symphysis. *CP,* Condylar process; *RP,* retroarticular process; *AP,* angular process; *TB,* tympanic bulla; *ZA,* zygomatic arch; *MS,* mandibular symphysis; *CoP,* coronoid process; *MR,* mandibular ramus. *(Copyright 2010 Dr. Alexander M. Reiter; used with permission.)*

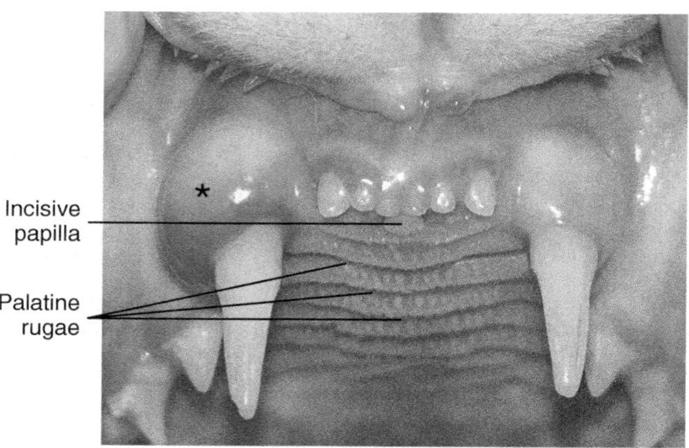

FIGURE 21-7 Note the incisive papilla just caudal to the maxillary first incisor teeth and the palatine rugae of the hard palate. The right maxillary canine tooth appears extruded and shows periodontal inflammation and severe alveolar bone expansion *(asterisk). (Copyright 2010 Dr. Alexander M. Reiter; used with permission.)*

hard palate and the soft palate constitute the secondary palate. The hard palate mucosa is non-elastic and has several transverse ridges (palatine rugae) and depressions. On the midline rostral to the first palatine ruga and just caudal to the maxillary first incisor teeth is the incisive papilla, which should not be confused with an abnormal proliferative lesion (Figure 21-7).[90] The main blood supply to the hard palate mucosa is provided by the paired major palatine arteries, which pass through the palatine canals and emerge at the major palatine foramina palatal to the level of the maxillary fourth premolar teeth about halfway toward the midline, from where they run rostrally in the palatine sulci to the palatine fissures.[66]

When the tongue is withdrawn from the mouth, palatoglossal folds can be seen that run from the body of the tongue to the rostrolateral aspect of the muscular and elastic soft palate, which receives its main blood supply from the paired minor palatine arteries. The soft palate is elevated and closes off the nasopharynx during swallowing, and it is depressed and closes off the oropharynx during nose breathing.

Tongue

The tongue has a complex muscular structure and is used to lap fluids, form food boluses, and groom the cat's fur. The body of the tongue constitutes the rostral two thirds, and the root of the tongue constitutes the caudal one third. The lateral margins of the tongue separate the dorsal and ventral surfaces.

The lingual mucosa is thick and heavily cornified dorsally but thin and less cornified ventrally. The cat's dorsal tongue surface is very rough, with firm papillae that point caudally (Figure 21-8). The lingual frenulum, which is part of the sublingual mucosa whose submucosa contains the paired sublingual veins and mandibular and sublingual gland ducts, connects the body of the tongue to the floor of the mouth. The sublingual caruncles are situated at the frenulum's rostroventral aspect and contain the orifices of mandibular and sublingual gland ducts. The lingual artery is the major blood supply to the tongue.[66]

Salivary Glands

There are four pairs of major salivary glands in cats: the parotid gland surrounding the horizontal ear canal; the mandibular gland situated in the Viborg's triangle, near the maxillary and linguofacial veins; the sublingual gland, with its monostomatic part intimately attached to the mandibular gland and its polystomatic part located

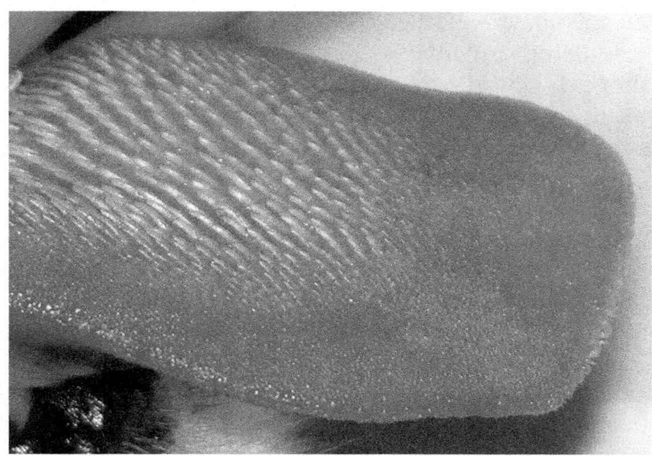

FIGURE 21-8 Caudally pointing firm papillae on the cat's rough dorsal tongue surface. *(Copyright 2010 Dr. Alexander M. Reiter; used with permission.)*

more rostrally between the mandible and the tongue; and the zygomatic gland, located on the floor of the orbit, whose ducts open on the buccal mucosa near the maxillary first molar tooth.[90] Scattered glandular tissue is present submucosally in the lips (ventral and dorsal buccal glands). A small lingual molar gland is situated caudolingually to each mandibular first molar tooth and should not be confused with an abnormal proliferative lesion.[88]

Lymph Nodes and Tonsils

There are three lymph centers in the head (parotid, mandibular, and retropharyngeal).[66] The parotid lymph node is located at the rostral base of the ear. Several mandibular lymph nodes lie ventral to the angle of the jaw above and below the linguofacial vein. The medial retropharyngeal lymph node is an elongated, transversely compressed node and lies along the craniodorsal wall of the pharynx. The paired small palatine tonsil is attached to the lateral pharyngeal wall.

Neurovascular Structures

The maxillary and mandibular branches of the trigeminal nerve are sensory, but the mandibular branch also supplies motor function to the masticatory musculature and other muscles. The lingual nerve is a branch of the mandibular nerve and provides sensory function to the rostral two thirds of the tongue. The facial nerve provides motor function to many cutaneous facial muscles and the caudal belly of the digastricus muscle and is responsible for taste in the rostral two thirds of the tongue.

The maxillary artery provides blood supply to the upper jaw by way of the infraorbital, palatine (major and minor), and sphenopalatine arteries. The inferior alveolar artery (running in the mandibular canal) is a branch of the maxillary artery and provides blood supply to the lower jaw. It exits at the caudal, middle, and rostral mental foramina to supply the lower lips. Veins often exist concurrently with arteries and empty by way of the maxillary and linguofacial veins into the external jugular vein.[66]

Common Terminology

Rostral refers to the direction toward the tip of the nose, *caudal* to the direction toward the tail, *ventral* to the direction toward the lower jaw, and *dorsal* to the direction toward the top of the head or muzzle. *Mesial* is the surface of a tooth facing the midline of the dental arch, and *distal* is the surface of a tooth facing away from the midline of the dental arch. *Labial* is the surface of a tooth facing the lip, and *buccal* is the surface of a tooth facing the cheek. *Lingual* refers to the surface of mandibular teeth facing the tongue, and *palatal* refers to the surface of maxillary teeth facing the hard palate (Figure 21-9). *Occlusal* refers to the surface of a tooth facing an opposing dental arch, *coronal* refers to a location or direction toward the crown of a tooth, and *apical* refers to a location or direction toward the apex of a tooth's root. *Subgingival* refers to an area that is apical to the gingival margin, and *supragingival* refers to an area that is coronal to the gingival margin.[66]

ORAL EXAMINATION

Patient History and Clinical Signs

Age, breed, and sequence of development of clinical signs often are useful indicators. A full patient history is essential and should include questions about appetite; eating and drinking patterns; prehending, chewing, and swallowing; preference for soft or hard food; behavioral idiosyncrasies; access to treats and toys; vomiting, diarrhea, and weight loss; coughing and sneezing; polydipsia and polyuria; scratching, head shaking; presence of rapid lower jaw motions; previous and current medications (and responsiveness to medications); the animal's environment; and the type and frequency of home oral hygiene.[46]

The presence of halitosis, preferential chewing on one side of the mouth, inability or reluctance to open or close the mouth, dropping food from the mouth, drooling of saliva, inappetence, weight loss, sneezing, nasal discharge, pawing at the face, enophthalmos or exophthalmos, oral and maxillofacial swellings, pain on palpation of oral and maxillofacial tissues, atrophy of masticatory muscles, malocclusion, and other abnormal clinical signs should be assessed. It is often helpful for the examiner

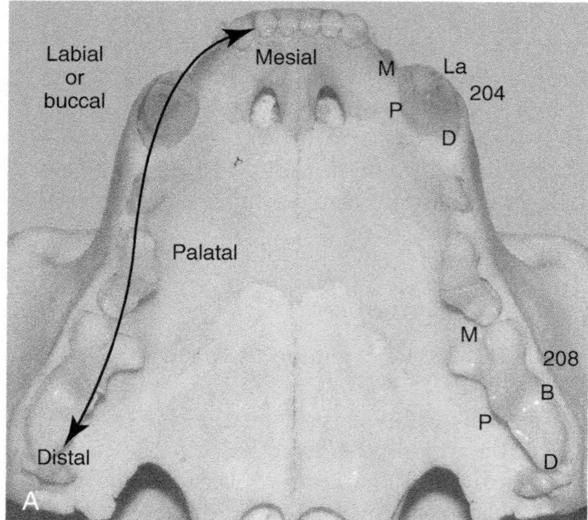

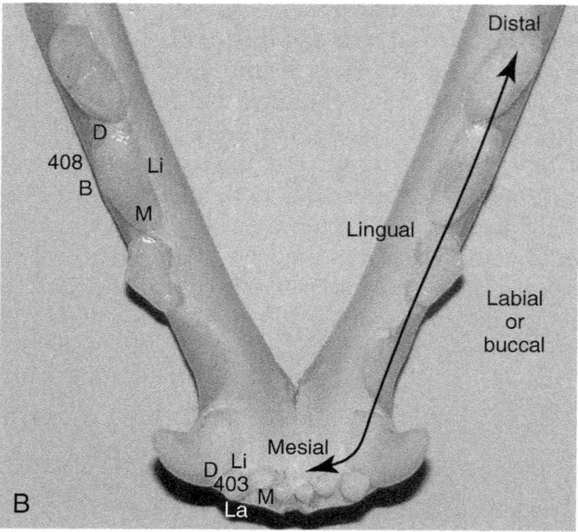

FIGURE 21-9 Directions and surfaces of maxillary **(A)** and mandibular **(B)** teeth. *M,* Mesial; *La,* labial; *B,* buccal; *D,* distal; *P,* palatal; *Li,* lingual. *(Copyright 2010 Dr. Alexander M. Reiter; used with permission.)*

to watch the animal eat and drink if the owner reports any abnormal behavior during eating and drinking.[46]

Halitosis may be caused by oral disease (e.g., periodontal disease, stomatitis, neoplasia), nonoral diseases (e.g., uremia, respiratory or gastrointestinal disease), and the diet. Inappetence may result from pain associated with inflammation and ulceration in the oral cavity. This may progress to unwillingness or inability to drink, which in turn leads to dehydration. Pawing at the mouth and rubbing the mouth on furnishings are indications of oral or facial pain. Drooling usually results from the reluctance or inability to swallow rather than from increased salivary production. It also may be caused by the reluctance or inability to close the mouth. Saliva may be blood stained if ulceration is present in the mouth. Dysphagia (i.e., difficulty in or pain on swallowing) may result from inflamed, ulcerated, or traumatized tissues that cause local pain or from obstruction to the mechanics of swallowing by a mass lesion, neurologic disease, or palate defects. Rapid lower jaw motions ("jaw chattering") often indicate oral pain in cats with tooth resorption. Nasal discharge may be related to rhinitis, endodontic disease, neoplasia, or a palate defect.[46]

The cat may be unable or unwilling to eat or chew on the side of the mouth that has a problem. Teeth on the affected side may then show increased plaque and calculus accumulation compared with those on the healthy side. Differential diagnoses for a cat that is unable or unwilling to open the mouth include oral ulceration, temporomandibular joint ankylosis, maxillofacial fractures, tetanus, ocular disease, space-occupying retrobulbar lesion, ear disease, and neoplasia. Differential diagnoses for a cat that is unable or unwilling to close the mouth include temporomandibular joint luxation or fracture of bones forming the joint, open-mouth jaw locking, maxillary and (bilateral) mandibular fractures, and neoplasia.[46]

Extraoral Examination

The eyes, ears, nose, face, lips, jaws, masticatory muscles, lymph nodes, and salivary glands should be examined. Attention should be paid to the nostrils (one nostril is closed with a thumb while airflow from the other nostril is evaluated); any discharge from oral, nasal, and ocular orifices and sinus tracts; facial lacerations; asymmetry and facial swellings; presence of exophthalmos or enophthalmos; the ability to retropulse the eye globes (assessed by gently pushing them into their orbits); and swelling or atrophy of masticatory muscles.

The jaws, intermandibular tissues, zygomatic arches, and neck should be palpated for pain, asymmetry, discontinuity, crepitus, and emphysema. The range of mouth opening is assessed, which also provides information about abnormalities of the temporomandibular joints and muscles of mastication.[46]

Intraoral Examination

The skin and mucocutaneous areas should be examined before opening the cat's mouth. The labial and buccal mucosa is examined by lifting the cat's upper and lower lips. The oral mucosa should be moist, intact, and nonpainful on touch and may be pigmented. The color, size, location, thickness, surface characteristics, and symmetry of any oral lesions should be noted.[46] The incisors, canines, and most cheek teeth can be evaluated without opening the mouth. Opening the mouth is greatly facilitated when the cat's head is rotated dorsally. One hand holds the entire head (in the area of the zygomatic arches) and then rotates it dorsally. The other hand

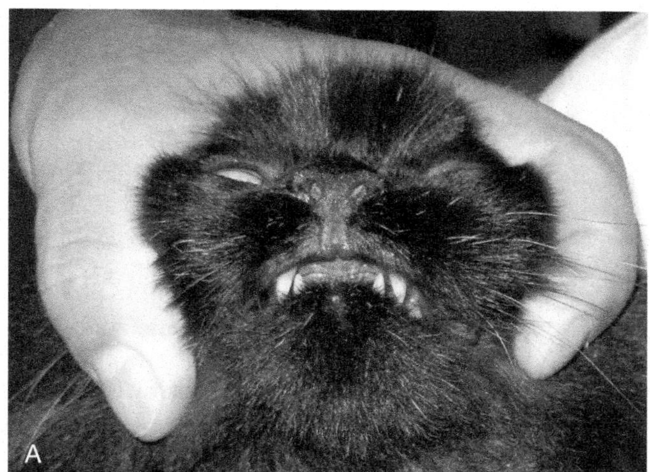

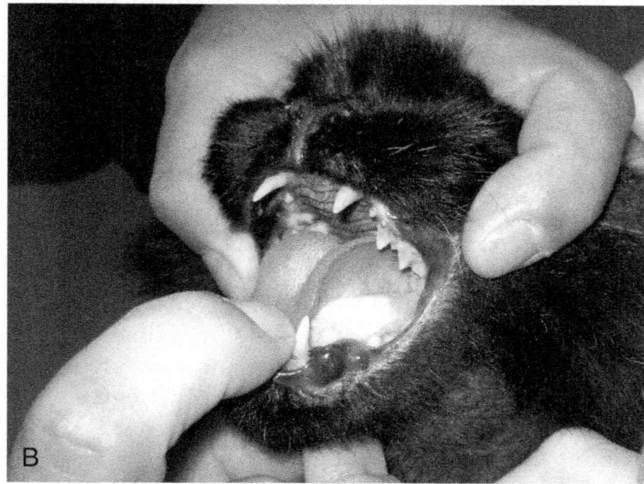

FIGURE 21-10 Note that the cat already starts opening the mouth after slight dorsal rotation of its head with one hand **(A).** The index finger of the other hand opens the mouth by pushing the lower jaw ventrally. Gently forcing the thumb of the same hand into the intermandibular area will raise the tongue, allowing inspection of its ventral surface and the sublingual tissues **(B).** *(Copyright 2010 Dr. Alexander M. Reiter; used with permission.)*

opens the mouth by pushing the lower jaw ventrally (Figure 21-10). The ventral surface of the tongue and sublingual tissues can be inspected by gently forcing the thumb of the second hand into the intermandibular area. This raises the tongue. The hard palate can also be inspected.[46] Obvious lesions such as fractured teeth, moderate to severe periodontal disease, stomatitis, and oral masses can often be identified in the conscious patient. However, sedation or general anesthesia is usually required for a thorough intraoral examination.

The two most important instruments for evaluation of dental and periodontal tissues are the dental explorer and periodontal probe (Figure 21-11). The structural integrity of teeth is assessed with a dental explorer whose pointed tip can detect irregularities of the crown surface. It is also used to determine the presence of pulp

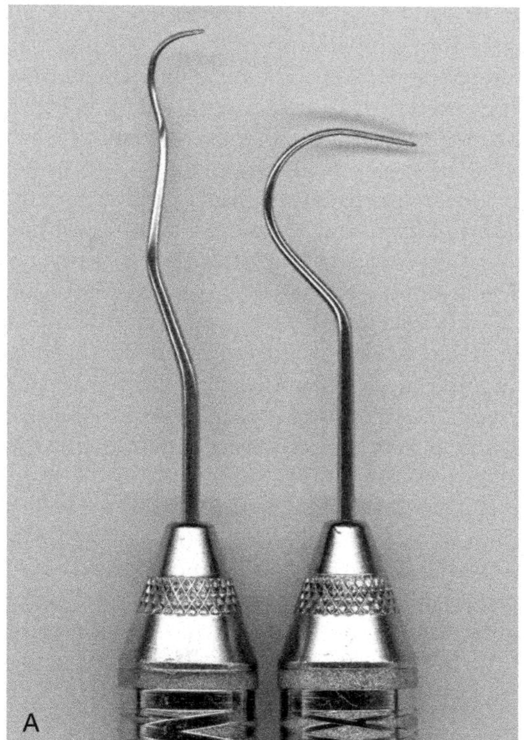

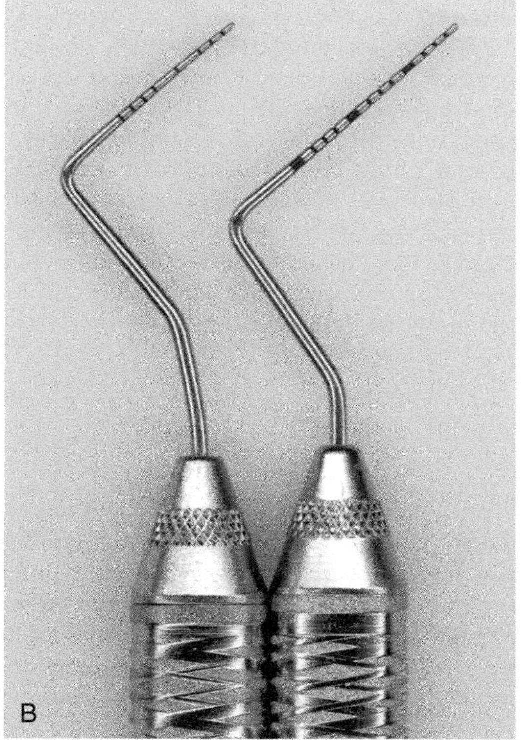

FIGURE 21-11 Dental explorers **(A)** are used for tactile exploration of the tooth's surfaces; the 11/12 ODU explorer on the left is preferred over the sphepherd's hook on the right for exploration of feline teeth. Periodontal probes **(B)** are used for measuring of gingival sulcus and periodontal pocket depths; the Williams probe on the left (with markings at 1, 2, 3, then 5, then 7, 8, 9, and 10 mm) is preferred over the CP-15 UNC on the right (with millimeter markings and a wide, black marking at 5, 10, and 15 mm) for probing of feline teeth. *(Copyright 2010 Dr. Alexander M. Reiter; used with permission.)*

exposure in a fractured tooth. The alveolar mucosa over the roots of the teeth should be inspected and palpated for the presence of swellings and sinus tracts (the latter are often located near the mucogingival junction), which may indicate endodontic disease or neoplasia.[46] The periodontal probe is invaluable for an accurate periodontal examination. The probe is gently inserted into the gingival sulcus, and measurements are obtained at several locations around the entire circumference of each tooth. The gingival sulcus of cat teeth should not be deeper than 0.5 mm. Greater measurements indicate the presence of a periodontal pocket or, in the case of gingival enlargement, a pseudopocket. Other periodontal parameters include plaque and calculus (tartar) accumulation, gingival index, gingival recession or enlargement, total attachment loss, tooth mobility, and missing teeth. Any other abnormalities should be recorded in the dental chart, such as persistent (retained) deciduous teeth, supernumerary teeth, dental or skeletal malocclusion, circumscribed ulcers, widespread oral inflammation, palate defects, oral masses, lacerations, and other signs of trauma.[46]

Laboratory Examination

Examination for systemic disease is important to assess anesthetic risk or determine the possibility of dental and oral lesions being secondary to a systemic condition.[46] Preanesthetic blood tests should include a complete blood cell count and biochemical profile. Blood typing and cross-matching may occasionally be indicated. Urinalysis and cardiac examination are performed as necessary. Cats with acute or chronic oral inflammation (beyond gingivitis) should be tested for feline leukemia virus (FeLV), for feline immunodeficiency virus (FIV), and occasionally for feline bartonellosis.

DIAGNOSTIC IMAGING

Dental Radiography

Dental radiographs should always be obtained before tooth extraction to assess alveolar bone health and variations in root anatomy and to determine the presence of dentoalveolar ankylosis or replacement resorption of roots that could complicate the extraction procedure. They are also essential during all steps of endodontic procedures, including assessment of treatment outcome at follow-up visits. In addition to dental-related conditions, most jaw pathology can be satisfactorily assessed with dental (nonscreen) film and intraoral and extraoral imaging techniques.[28]

Needed equipment includes a dental radiography machine, dental (nonscreen) films, a chairside film processor, developer and fixer solutions, and a view box. Digital imaging uses sensor pads or phosphor plates (instead of films) that transfer the image to a computer. The digital system requires less radiation to produce an image, which may also be modified with software programs. Exposure time often is the only adjustment to be made and depends on the size of the patient and tissue thickness to be imaged.[82,84] Dental film is available in several sizes and speeds, with sizes 0, 2, and 4 and D film (ultra speed) most commonly used (Figure 21-12). The largest dental film (size 4) is very useful to evaluate diseases of the nasal cavity, orbit, zygomatic arch, mandibular ramus, temporomandibular joint, and tympanic bulla in cats. The films are inside a moisture-resistant packet and surrounded by black paper. A layer of lead foil is located at the back of the packet next to the tab opening, protecting the film from secondary radiation. A dimple is located in one corner of the film packet and also on the film and is used to distinguish images obtained from the left and right sides of the mouth on the processed radiographs. The convex (raised) surface of the dimple must face the radiographic beam during exposure. Dental rapid developer and fixer solutions are placed in small containers within a chairside film processor (from left to right: developer, water, fixer, and water).[47]

All personnel should leave the room while radiographs are exposed. If this is not possible, anyone remaining in the room should stand at least 6 feet from the radiographic cone and at a 90- to 135-degree angle to the tube head. Gauze or paper may be used to hold the films in proper position inside the mouth of an

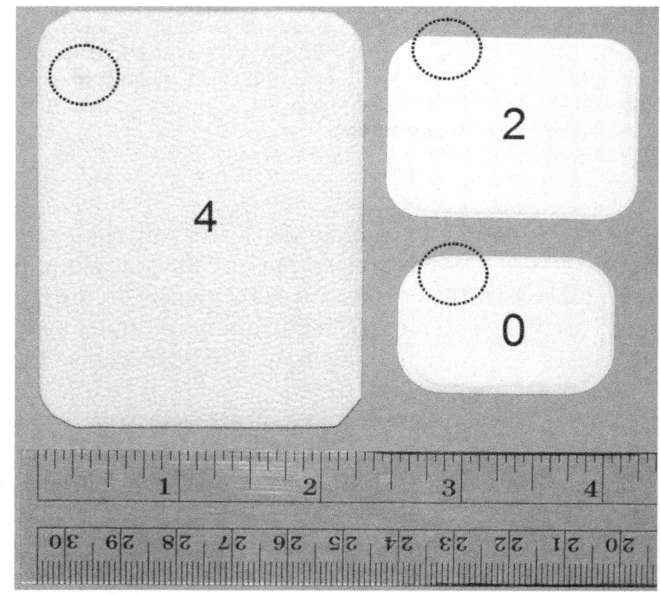

FIGURE 21-12 Sizes 0, 2, and 4 dental film; note the convex (raised) surface of the dimple *(circled)* that must face the radiographic beam during exposure. *(Copyright 2010 Dr. Alexander M. Reiter; used with permission.)*

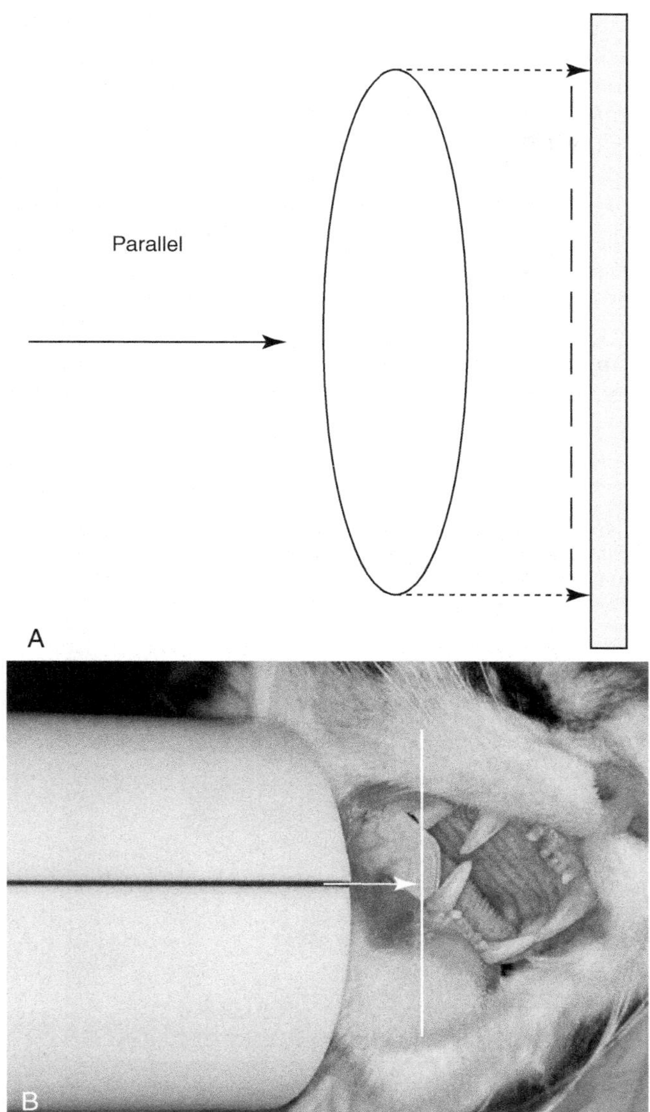

FIGURE 21-13 Parallel technique with the film placed parallel to the tooth and the radiographic beam directed perpendicular (90 degrees) to the film and tooth **(A),** shown for imaging the mandibular cheek teeth in a cat **(B).** (**A** *copyright 2010 Dr. Alexander M. Reiter; used with permission;* **B** *from Harvey CE, Flax BM: Feline oral-dental radiographic examination and interpretation,* Vet Clin North Am Small Anim Pract *22:1279, 1992.)*

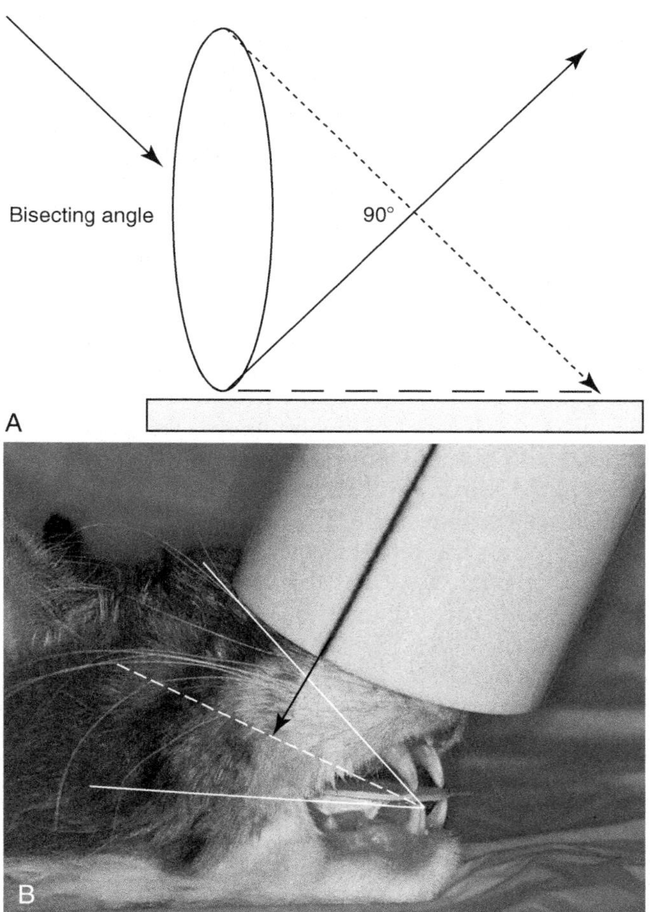

FIGURE 21-14 Bisecting angle technique with the radiographic beam directed perpendicular (90 degrees) to an imaginary line that bisects the angle formed between the long axis of the teeth and the plane of the film **(A),** shown for imaging the maxillary canine and incisor teeth in a cat **(B).** (**A** *copyright 2010 Dr. Alexander M. Reiter; used with permission;* **B** *from Harvey CE, Flax BM: Feline oral-dental radiographic examination and interpretation,* Vet Clin North Am Small Anim Pract *22:1279, 1992.)*

intubated cat. The parallel technique is used for imaging the mandibular molars and the caudal mandibular premolars, with the film placed parallel to the teeth and the radiographic beam directed perpendicular (90 degrees) to the film and teeth (Figure 21-13).[84] The bisecting angle technique minimizes distortion when obtaining radiographs of all maxillary teeth and the mandibular canines, incisors, and rostral premolars (Figure 21-14).[42] The film is placed as close to the teeth as possible. The angle that is formed between the long axis of the teeth and the plane of the film is bisected by an imaginary line. The tube head is positioned perpendicular to this imaginary line. An extraoral technique has also been suggested for imaging the maxillary cheek teeth to avoid overlapping of the teeth with the zygomatic arch of the cat.[28,47,83]

The lid of the chairside film processor must be closed when processing dental radiographs. One hand holds the film, the other hand a film clip. Both hands are slid through the front windows of the processor. The exposed film is removed from the packet and placed in the film clip. The film is first placed into developer for about 30 seconds, then briefly rinsed in water, and placed in fixer for at least 60 seconds before viewing. After another brief water rinse, the film may be viewed using a dental view box. After initial viewing the film should be placed for another 15 minutes in the fixer solution. This is followed by thorough rinsing under running water for 20 minutes before air drying the film. Films dried over night are stored in a labeled envelope and kept as part of the patient's medical record.[28,86]

Dental radiographs should be viewed in labial mounting (all of the radiographs in this chapter were obtained with dental film and are arranged in labial mounting), which requires that the processed film be placed on the view box with the raised dot facing the viewer.[28] It is determined whether the image is of the upper or lower jaw and of the left or right side. The only three-rooted teeth are the maxillary fourth premolars. The palatine fissure is also located in the upper jaw. The ventral mandibular cortex or mandibular canal is often visible on films of the lower jaw. Films of teeth of the left jaws are placed on the right side of the view box, and those of the right jaws on the left side of the view box. Each film should be rotated so that the crowns of the maxillary teeth face downward and those of the mandibular teeth face upward.

The enamel, dentin, cementum (visible radiographically only when thickened), alveolar margin, periodontal ligament space, lamina dura, and pulp cavity are evaluated. The mandibular canal is visible as a radiolucent tubular structure in the mandible. Mental foramina and palatine fissures may sometimes be mistaken for periapical pathology.[28,47]

Computed Tomography

Computed tomography is a useful imaging modality for the diagnosis and treatment planning of oral and maxillofacial trauma, neoplasia, and many other conditions.[3,108] It is of great value for exploration of a large volume of soft and hard tissue in a significantly shorter examination time and at a much lower cost than magnetic resonance imaging. This is particularly important when a rapid diagnosis is needed for patients with head trauma or uncertain head pathology and for those that are less than optimal anesthesia candidates. Computed tomography is of great value for detection of hard tissues, which is imperative when defining tumor margins and planning radical surgical excision. It also allows three-dimensional reconstruction, which facilitates understanding of the overall appearance of lesions, and can help guidance of a needle aspiration to establish a cytologic diagnosis.

The patient is placed on the couch in sternal recumbency with the head extended and secured in position and the forelimbs flexed caudally. Fluid lines and other extraneous structures are kept out of the gantry field to prevent artifacts. After a precontrast scan, an intravenous iodinated contrast medium is administered and a postcontrast scan is performed. Precontrast and postcontrast image series of the entire head and cranial neck should be obtained in an axial scanning mode, with slice thickness of 1 mm and interval of 2 to 3 mm for bone and slice thickness of 3 mm and interval of 3 mm for soft tissue. If lesions are located in surgically inaccessible locations, a fine needle aspirate can be obtained with an appropriate needle, which is inserted into the skin and advanced under subsequent computed tomography guidance (scan, advance, scan) to the lesion.

Soft tissue structures are evaluated on soft tissue algorithm images, and the teeth, bones, and joints of the head are evaluated on bone algorithm images (Figure 21-15). Window levels and widths are adjusted manually as needed. Maxillofacial soft tissue structures of interest

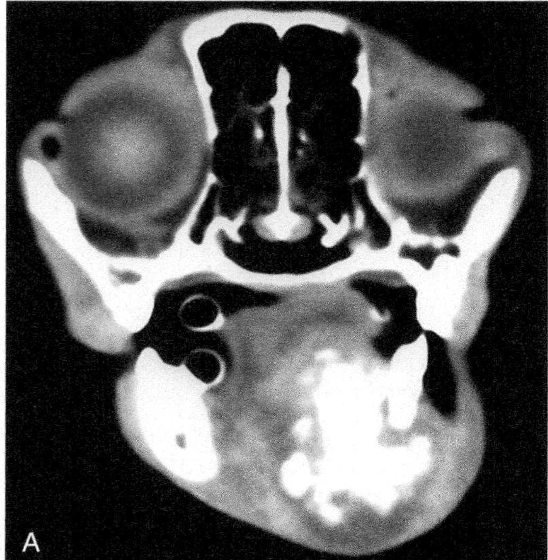

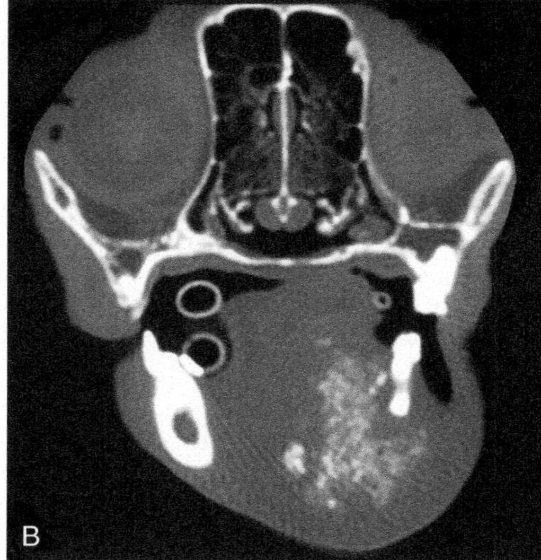

FIGURE 21-15 Computed tomography performed in a cat with left mandibular squamous cell carcinoma. Soft tissue structures are evaluated on a soft tissue algorithm image **(A),** and the teeth, bones, and joints of the head are evaluated on a bone algorithm image **(B).** *(Copyright 2010 Dr. Alexander M. Reiter; used with permission.)*

include the masticatory muscles, salivary glands, soft tissue coverings of the nasal and oral cavity, soft palate, pharynx and larynx, and head and neck lymph nodes. These soft tissues can be evaluated for their size, precontrast tissue attenuation and shape of abnormal densities, and degree and distribution of contrast enhancement. Enlarged soft tissues are consistent with edema, inflammation, or neoplasia. Abnormally small soft tissue structures are indicative of atrophy, necrosis, or fibrosis. Precontrast tissue hypoattenuation indicates increased fluid content consistent with edema. Irregular contrast enhancement is indicative of areas of increased vascularity consistent with inflammation or neoplasia, and nonenhancing cores are suggestive of necrosis or abscess. Bones and joints of the head are evaluated for any evidence of periosteal reaction or periarticular new bone formation, fractures, osteolysis, deformity, masses, and joint pathology.[37] The teeth are evaluated for structural defects, abnormal root canal widths, and changes to the periodontal attachment apparatus.

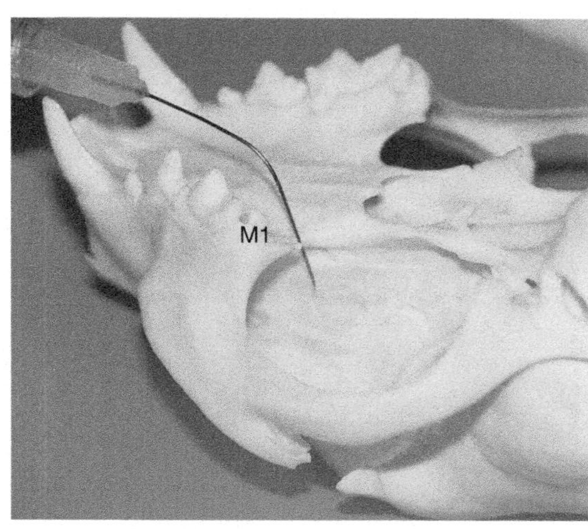

FIGURE 21-16 Maxillary nerve block demonstrated on a cat skull. Note the location of the needle in relation to the maxillary first molar tooth (M1). *(Copyright 2010 Dr. Alexander M. Reiter; used with permission.)*

LOCAL AND REGIONAL ANESTHESIA

Local and regional anesthesia allows reduction in the concentration of an inhalant anesthetic, which minimizes complications from hypotension, bradycardia, and hypoventilation. Patients consequently recover more quickly and with fewer complications. Furthermore, local and regional anesthesia continues to provide analgesia in the postoperative period, thus increasing patient comfort and decreasing the need for systemic administration of analgesics.[6,43,59,103]

Local anesthesia (e.g., infiltration anesthesia, use of topical anesthetic gels, and splash block) is less commonly performed in dentistry and oral surgery. *Regional anesthesia* (nerve blocks) refers to injection of a local anesthetic solution around a major nerve, utilizing 27-gauge, 1½-inch needles on 1-mL syringes (22-gauge needles when going through skin).[53,59,103] Commonly used local anesthetics in dentistry and oral surgery include bupivacaine 0.5% (effective for 6 to 10 hours) and lidocaine 2% without epinephrine (effective for less than 2 hours). The onset time for analgesia is longer with longer-acting local anesthetics (a few minutes for lidocaine, up to 30 minutes for bupivacaine). The total maximum dosage in cats is 2 mg/kg for bupivacaine and 1 mg/kg for lidocaine.[53,59] There are 5 mg of bupivacaine in 1 mL of a 0.5% solution (bupivacaine 0.5%).

The maxillary nerve block is given just caudal to the first molar tooth where the maxillary nerve enters the infraorbital canal through the maxillary foramen (Figure 21-16). Care must be taken not to inject anesthetic into the eye globe. The areas blocked include the incisive bone, maxilla and palatine bone, all maxillary teeth on that side, and adjacent soft tissues. Because the infraorbital canal is very short in the cat and the maxillary nerve can easily be reached by a needle advanced through the infraorbital canal, an infraorbital approach is usually chosen to perform a maxillary nerve block. The infraorbital nerve block is given at the infraorbital foramen or inside the infraorbital canal (Figure 21-17). The areas blocked include the incisive bone and maxilla, maxillary incisors, canine, and premolars/molars (depending how far the needle is advanced into the infraorbital canal) and adjacent soft tissues. The major palatine nerve block is given through the thick palatal

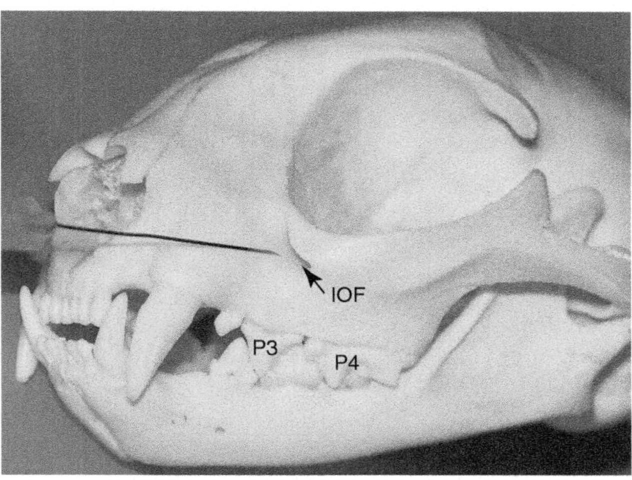

FIGURE 21-17 Infraorbital nerve block demonstrated on a cat skull. Note the location of the infraorbital foramen (IOF) in relation to the maxillary third (P3) and fourth (P4) premolars. The needle may also be advanced into the infraorbital canal to block hard and soft tissues caudal to the infraorbital foramen. *(Copyright 2010 Dr. Alexander M. Reiter; used with permission.)*

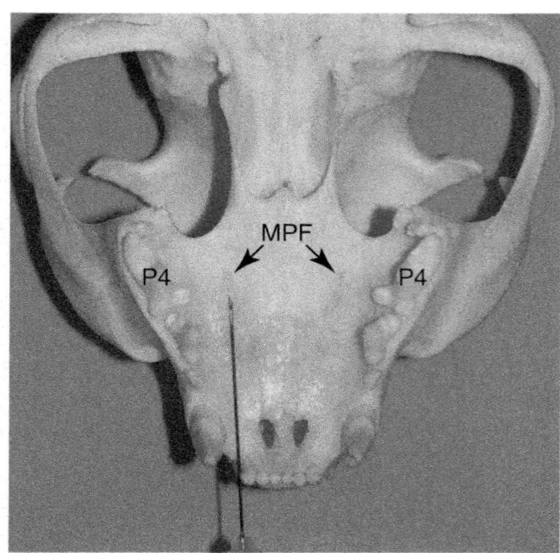

FIGURE 21-18 Major palatine nerve block demonstrated on a cat skull. Note the location of the major palatine foramina *(arrow)* in relation to the maxillary fourth premolar teeth (P4). *(Copyright 2010 Dr. Alexander M. Reiter; used with permission.)*

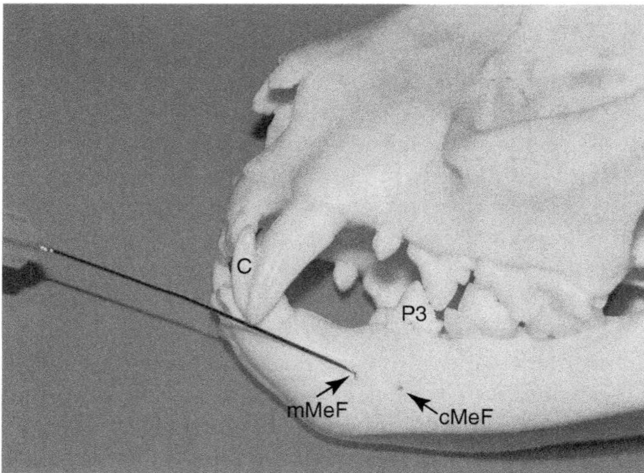

FIGURE 21-20 Middle mental nerve block demonstrated on a cat skull. Note the location of the middle mental foramen (mMeF) in relation to the mandibular canine (C) and third premolar (P3) teeth and the caudal mental foramen (cMeF). *(Copyright 2010 Dr. Alexander M. Reiter; used with permission.)*

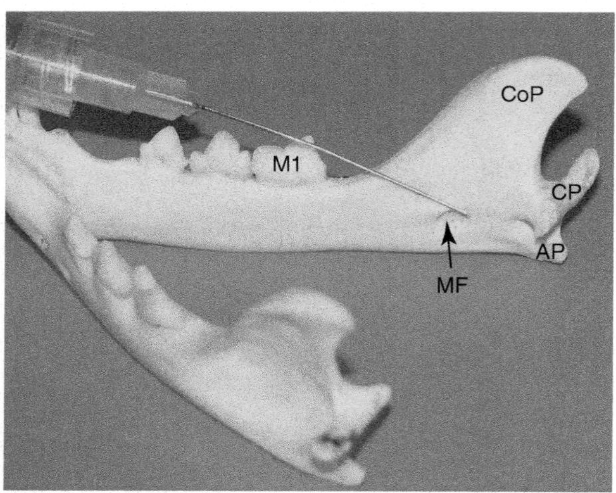

FIGURE 21-19 Inferior alveolar nerve block demonstrated on a cat skull. Note the location of the mandibular foramen (MF) in relation to the mandibular first molar tooth (M1) and the processes of the mandibular ramus. *CoP,* Coronoid process; *CP,* condylar process; *AP,* angular process. *(Copyright 2010 Dr. Alexander M. Reiter; used with permission.)*

mucosa just rostral to the major palatine foramen (Figure 21-18). The areas blocked include the palatine shelf of the maxilla and adjacent soft tissues. The inferior alveolar nerve block can be given intraorally (at a relatively flat angle through the alveolar mucosa at the lingual surface of the mandible) (Figure 21-19) or extraorally through the skin slightly rostral to the angular process at the medial side of the mandible. The areas blocked include the mandibular body, all mandibular teeth, and adjacent soft tissues. The middle mental nerve block is given through the lateral labial frenulum at the middle mental foramen halfway between the canine and third premolar (Figure 21-20). The areas blocked include the rostral mandibular body, teeth rostral to the injection site, and adjacent soft tissues.[6,53,59,103]

PERIODONTAL DISEASE

Periodontal disease affects a majority of adult cats and involves inflammation and infection of the periodontium (gingiva, periodontal ligament, alveolar bone, and cementum) caused by plaque bacteria and the host's response to the bacterial insult. Its systemic effects have been well documented in humans (heart disease and stroke, diabetes, respiratory disease, and increased risk of premature delivery and low-birth-weight infants) and are being increasingly investigated in companion animals.[98]

Gingivitis and Periodontitis

Gingivitis is reversible, affecting gingiva only (Figure 21-21). The gingiva may detach from the tooth, creating a periodontal pocket, and a shift occurs in the gingival flora from a gram-positive aerobic to a gram-negative anaerobic spectrum. Treatment of gingivitis requires plaque control, and daily toothbrushing can resolve gingivitis. In adolescent cats a particular form of gingivitis has been recognized. This so-called juvenile hyperplastic gingivitis occurs after eruption of the permanent dentition at about 6 to 8 months of age, with the inflamed gingiva being enlarged to a degree that it can cover the crowns of the teeth (Figure 21-22). It is not known whether juvenile hyperplastic gingivitis is a precursor form of more severe oral inflammation or whether it can

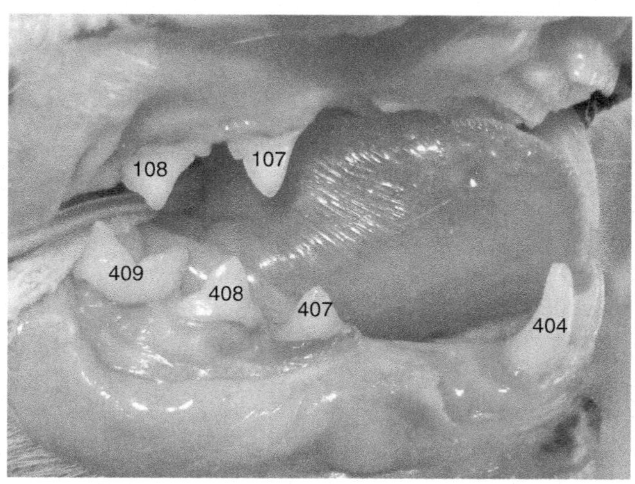

FIGURE 21-21 Gingivitis (worst at tooth 407) in a cat. The right maxillary canine and second premolar teeth are missing. *(Copyright 2010 Dr. Alexander M. Reiter; used with permission.)*

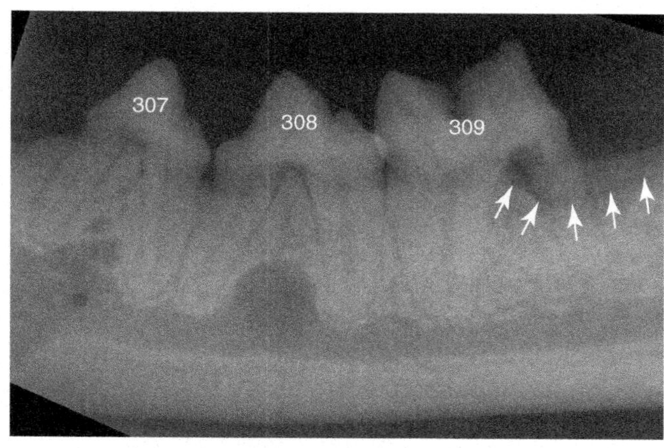

FIGURE 21-23 Dental radiograph showing the left mandibular cheek teeth in an adult cat. Note loss of alveolar bone particularly around the distal root *(arrows)* of tooth 309. *(Copyright 2010 Dr. Alexander M. Reiter; used with permission.)*

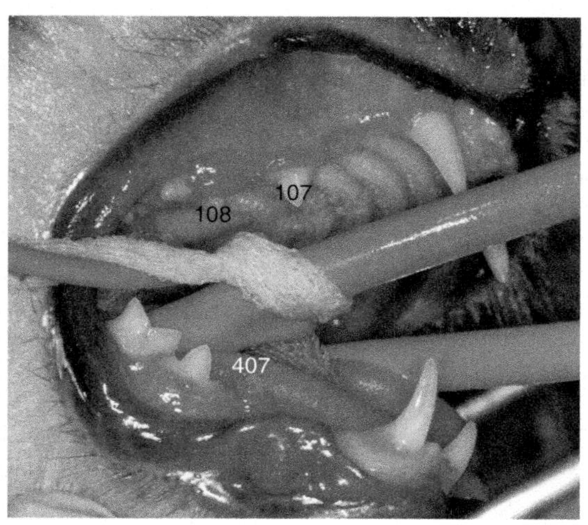

FIGURE 21-22 Juvenile hyperplastic gingivitis in an adolescent cat. Note inflamed and enlarged gingiva partially covering the crowns of teeth 107, 108, and 407. *(Copyright 2010 Dr. Alexander M. Reiter; used with permission.)*

progress to stomatitis in the adult cat. Gingival enlargement is also caused after administration of anticonvulsants, cyclosporine, and calcium channel blockers. Treatment of gingival hyperplasia involves cessation of its cause and removal of excess gingiva. Because most cat teeth have less than 2 mm of attached gingiva, gingival surgery should be carefully executed and is often reserved for canine teeth and teeth with significant gingival enlargement.[8]

Periodontitis is the more severe form of periodontal disease, affecting all periodontal tissues and resulting in attachment loss, gingival recession, furcation exposure, periodontal pocket formation, and alveolar bone loss (Figure 21-23).[69] Bacterial infection of the pulp is possible in areas devoid of cementum and through apical and non-apical ramifications. Alveolar bone loss is usually irreversible, causing the tooth to become mobile and ultimately to exfoliate.[45] Similar to juvenile hyperplastic gingivitis, a so-called juvenile-onset periodontitis has been described in cats younger than 1 year of age.[8] The teeth of such adolescent cats often are severely mobile on digital palpation and show most other clinical and radiographic signs associated with periodontitis.

Periodontal Therapy

Closed treatment may be sufficient when periodontal pocket depths do not exceed 2 mm in cats. Professional dental cleaning is performed with power scalers, followed by the use of hand scalers to remove residual calculus in pits, fissures, and developmental grooves of the crowns supragingivally and hand curettes to clean and plane exposed root surfaces subgingivally (Figure 21-24).[64] Prevention of hypothermia is particularly important when water is used to cool power instruments or rinse debris from the mouth.[44] Hand curettes can also be used for gingival curettage that removes the inflamed and infected soft tissue lining of the periodontal pocket. Once scaling is completed, the tooth surfaces are polished with fine polishing paste and a rubber cup on a prophy angle that is attached to a low-speed handpiece. Debris and polishing paste are rinsed from the tooth surface with water from an air–water syringe.[45]

Open treatment is usually indicated when pocket depths exceed 2 mm and is performed after reflection of a mucoperiosteal flap with or without vertical releasing incisions made into gingiva and alveolar mucosa. Osseous surgery and placement of implants are possible with this flap design.[7] The flap is sutured closed with

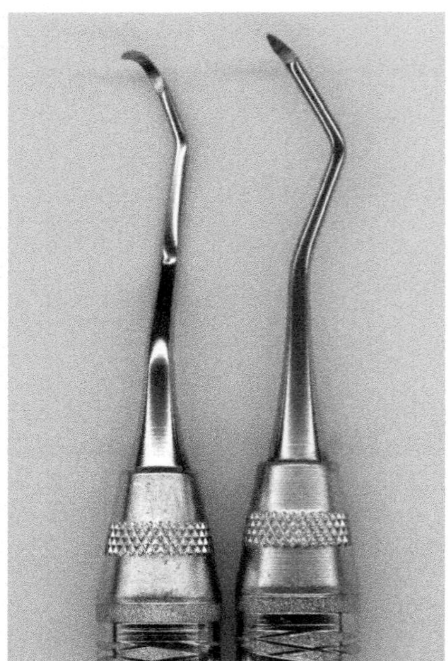

FIGURE 21-24 Note the different working ends between a scaler *(right)* and a curette *(left)*. The scaler has a pointed tip for removal of residual calculus in pits, fissures, and developmental grooves in supragingival areas of the tooth, while the curette has a rounded tip to avoid soft tissue injury in subgingival areas of the tooth. *(Copyright 2010 Dr. Alexander M. Reiter; used with permission.)*

synthetic absorbable monofilament material such as poliglecaprone 25 (e.g., Monocryl, Ethicon). Lateral sliding flaps and free gingival graft techniques are available for treatment of gingival clefts. Medical therapy includes the use of topical rinsing solutions (e.g., 0.2% chlorhexidine) or systemic antimicrobials (e.g., amoxicillin–clavulanic acid, clindamycin). Because of potential side effects and the possibility of bacterial resistance, systemic antimicrobials should be used only in selected cases to serve as an adjunct to local treatment.[25] Low-dose doxycycline gel (e.g., Doxirobe Gel, Pfizer Animal Health) may be inserted into cleaned periodontal pockets greater than 4 mm after root planing and gingival curettage.

Home Oral Hygiene

Plaque control is a critical component of periodontal disease prevention and in the maintenance of treatment success.[17,18,25,104] The owner is given instructions on daily tooth brushing with a soft-bristled toothbrush and pet dentifrice.[92] In addition, oral hygiene is enhanced by the use of treats, diets, and products that meet established criteria for effectiveness in mechanically or chemically controlling plaque or calculus deposition.[36,40,56,115] For a list of approved products, please visit the website of the Veterinary Oral Health Council (http://vohc.org).

TOOTH RESORPTION

Tooth resorption (previously called *feline odontoclastic resorptive lesion [FORL])* affects 25% to 75% of cats, depending on the population of cats investigated and diagnostic tools applied. The condition usually involves multiple permanent teeth and can start anywhere on the tooth's root surface.[101] Chronic dietary intake of excess vitamin D has been suggested as one potential cause of tooth resorption in cats.[99,100]

Replacement Resorption and Inflammatory Resorption

Feline teeth may appear clinically healthy, but they often show histologic and radiographic changes of periodontal and dental tissues, such as periodontal ligament degeneration, hypercementosis, and hyperosteoidosis. Narrowing of the periodontal space may result in ankylotic fusion (dentoalveolar anylosis) between the tooth and alveolar bone. These findings demonstrate events that occur before obvious tooth resorption and suggest that the very early lesion is probably noninflammatory.[41] Ankylosed roots are at risk of being incorporated into the normal bone remodeling process, resulting in gradual resorption of the root and replacement by bone (replacement resorption) (Figure 21-25).[100,101]

Resorption of enamel may occur when root resorption has progressed coronally into the crown. The enamel may then become undermined or penetrated by the resorption process. When such lesions emerge at the gingival margin, they become exposed to oral bacteria, which results in formation of inflamed granulation tissue (Figure 21-26). These defects are painful and bleed easily when probed with a dental instrument. One common feature of inflammatory root resorption is that the alveolar bone adjacent to the tooth defect is also resorbed.[100,101]

Several other peculiarities are noted in the permanent teeth of cats that could be associated with tooth resorption, including unusual thickening of alveolar bone (alveolar bone expansion), with or without periodontal pocket formation, and abnormal extrusion of canine teeth (supereruption).[65,100,101]

Etiologic Considerations

Cats with tooth resorption were shown to have significantly lower urine specific gravity and significantly higher serum concentrations of 25-hydroxyvitamin D (25OHD) compared with cats without tooth resorption.[99] These findings, together with the fact that multiple teeth are affected, indicate that tooth resorption in cats may have a systemic rather than a local cause. Cats are not able to produce vitamin D in skin,[54] and their minimum dietary vitamin D requirement may be low when

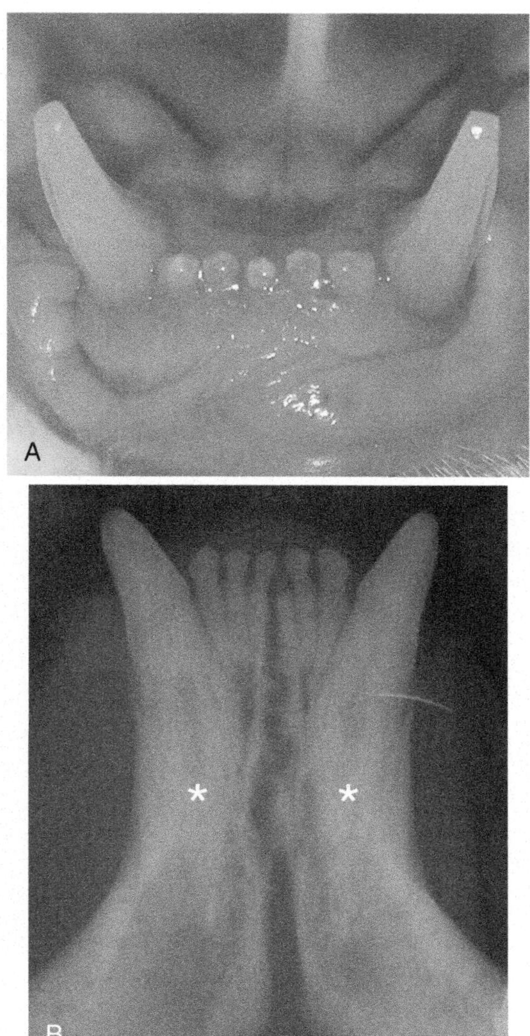

FIGURE 21-25 Replacement resorption in a cat. Clinical photograph **(A)** shows mandibular canine teeth that have mild gingivitis. Radiograph **(B)** reveals severe replacement resorption *(asterisks)* of the roots of both canines. *(Copyright 2010 Dr. Alexander M. Reiter; used with permission.)*

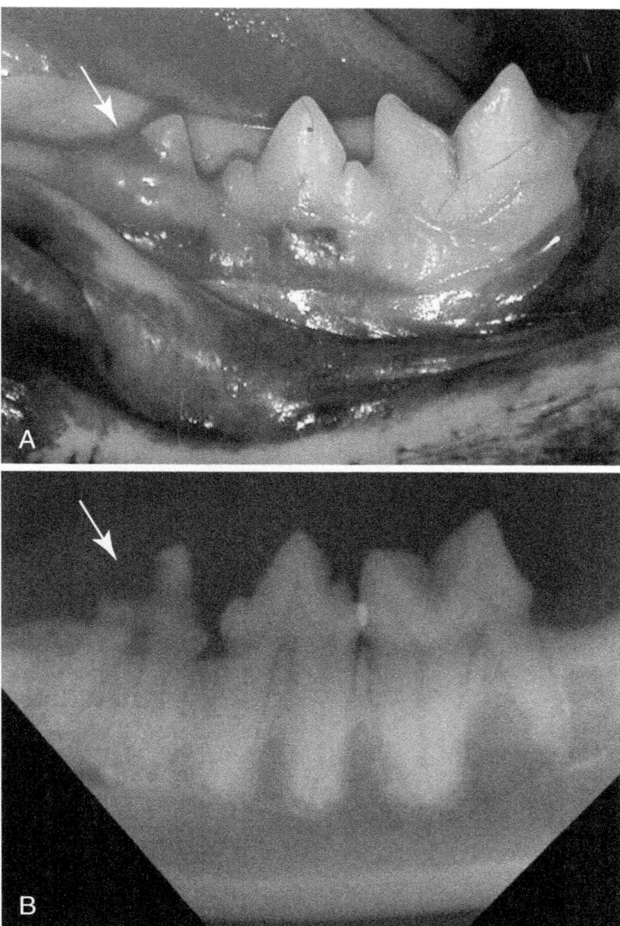

FIGURE 21-26 Inflammatory resorption in a cat. Clinical photograph **(A)** and radiograph **(B)** of the left mandibular cheek teeth in a cat, showing an inflammatory resorption *(arrows)* coronal to the gingival attachment of the left mandibular third premolar tooth. *(Copyright 2010 Dr. Alexander M. Reiter; used with permission.)*

compared with that of other species.[78] Commercial cat foods often contain vitamin D in excess of the maximal allowance.[77] Because a direct linear relationship exists between 25OHD serum concentrations and dietary intake of vitamin D,[79] cats with higher 25OHD serum concentrations must have ingested larger amounts of vitamin D or vitamin D metabolites. Significantly decreased urine specific gravity in cats with tooth resorption[99] also indicates that this condition might not just be a local oral disease but is probably associated with pathology in other areas of the body, such as abnormal mineralization of kidneys resulting from excessive dietary intake of vitamin D.[99,100] Recent studies also demonstrated that the nuclear vitamin D receptor is implicated in the pathophysiology of tooth resorption in cats.[13,14]

Numerous studies demonstrate the effects of excess vitamin D and vitamin D metabolites on the periodontium in experimental animals.[100] These changes in periodontal tissues resemble histologic features of teeth from cats with tooth resorption and include periodontal ligament degeneration, hypercementosis, hyperosteoidosis, narrowing of the periodontal ligament space, dentoalveolar ankylosis, and resorption of dental hard tissues. Loss of biological width (the distance between the bottom of the gingival sulcus and the alveolar margin) and coronal displacement of transseptal fibers have also been reported in these experimental animals, which may provide explanations for two other phenomena commonly seen in the mouth of cats (i.e., thickening of alveolar bone and extrusion of canine teeth).[65,100]

Clinical Signs

Tooth resorption is rarely seen in cats younger than 2 years of age, and clinically obvious disease may not be noted before the cat is 4 to 6 years of age. An increase in prevalence is seen with increasing age. There is no obvious predisposition with regard to gender, breed, or neuter status. The most commonly affected teeth include the mandibular third premolars; however, any tooth can be affected. Multiple teeth—in some cases the entire dention—are likely to be affected throughout a cat's life.[99,101]

Many affected cats will not show clinical signs. Some cats present with oral discomfort, lethargy, anorexia, dehydration, and weight loss. Halitosis, plaque and calculus accumulation, gingivitis, and gingival enlargement in areas of crown defects may be noted. Nasal discharge and sneezing are occasionally observed when there is severe resorption of maxillary teeth. Repetitive lower jaw motions may be seen during eating, drinking, and grooming or on palpation of oral and dental tissues.[101] Alveolar bone expansion (Figure 21-27) and extrusion of canine teeth (Figure 21-28) can frequently be observed in cats with tooth resorption.[100]

When tooth resorption progresses from the root into the crown and becomes exposed to the oral environment, an inflammatory component will join the initially noninflammatory process, filling the defect with inflamed granulation tissue. Resorption coronal to the gingival attachment is palpable by means of a dental explorer and, if large enough, visible as a red spot on the crown surface.[101] Affected crowns often break off, leaving resorbing root remnants in the alveolar bone. Retained root remnants can irritate the surrounding tissues, resulting in abscessation and local osteomyelitis with or without sinus tracts in gingiva, alveolar mucosa, or skin. A bulge may be seen in areas where gingiva has completely covered remnants of resorbing dental tissue.[101]

Exposed dentin surface—although covered by inflamed granulation tissue—is sensitive to mechanical and thermal stimuli. Therefore tooth resorption emerging at the gingival margin is considered to be painful. In the absence of pulpitis and periapical inflammation, however, tooth resorption apical to the gingival attachment is thought to be asymptomatic.

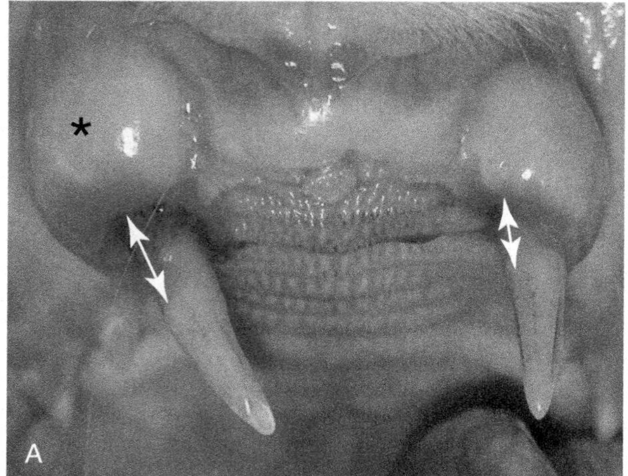

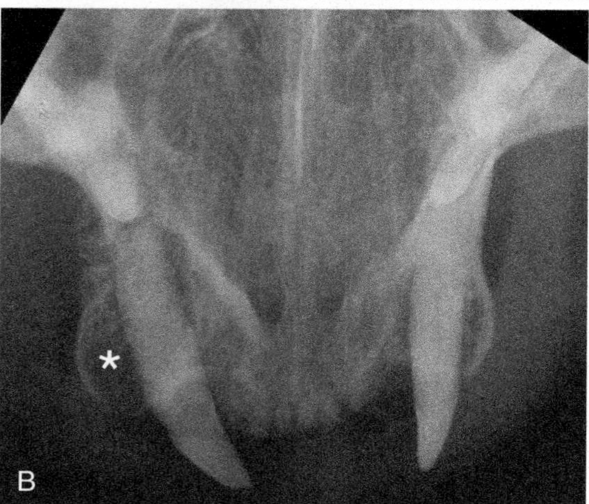

FIGURE 21-27 Clinical photograph **(A)** and radiograph **(B)** of the rostral upper jaw in a cat, showing alveolar bone expansion—more severe on the right *(asterisk)*—and extrusion of both maxillary canine teeth *(double-ended arrows* indicate exposure of root surface). The crown of the right maxillary canine is displaced palatally, and there are retained root remnants in areas of missing maxillary incisors. *(Copyright 2010 Dr. Alexander M. Reiter; used with permission.)*

Radiographic Signs

On the basis of the radiographic appearance of the root(s) of affected teeth, two presentations are distinguished. In type 1 lesions, unaffected root areas are surrounded by a radiographically visible periodontal space.[27] Notched radiolucencies with sharp or scalloped margins are usually found in cervical root or crown areas of the tooth, where they are exposed to inflammatory stimuli of the oral environment. Pathognomonic of inflammatory resorption is that the alveolar bone adjacent to the tooth defect is also resorbed.[100] However, pulpal involvement associated with these lesions does not appear to be associated with development of radiographically detectable periapical lucencies.[68] Tooth resorption that emerges at the gingival margin often appears small clinically but may exhibit advanced replacement resorption of the root(s) with disappearance of the lamina dura, often giving the tooth a diffusely moth-eaten or striated appearance. Ankylosed roots and those with replacement resorption have been categorized radiographically as type 2 lesions.[27] It is important to understand that both types of resorption can be present on a single tooth. The Nomenclature Committee of the American Veterinary Dental College (http://

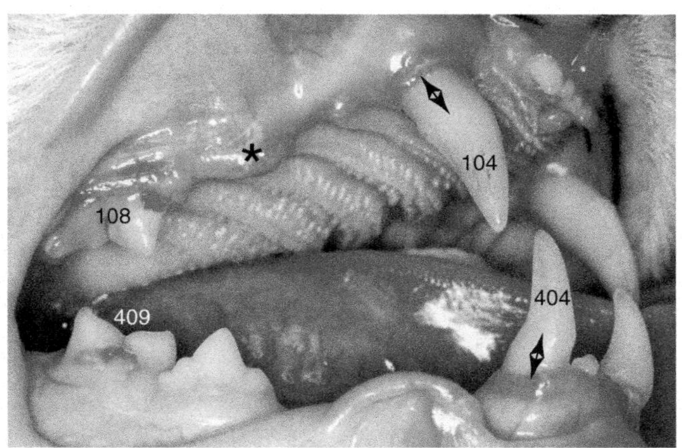

FIGURE 21-28 Mouth of a cat, showing vascular granulation tissue filling areas of resorption at the mesiobuccal aspect of tooth 108 and buccal aspect of tooth 409. The maxillary and mandibular third premolars are missing. There is a bulge with inflamed gingiva *(asterisk)* in the area of the missing third premolar, indicating the presence of retained root fragments. The right maxillary and mandibular canines (teeth 104 and 404) appear to be extruded *(double-ended arrows* indicating exposure of root surface). *(From Reiter AM, Mendoza KA: Feline odontoclastic resorptive lesions. An unsolved enigma in veterinary dentistry,* Vet Clin North Am Small Anim Pract *32:791, 2002.)*

avdc.org) proposed a staging system from 1 to 5 (with 4a, b, and c) for the classification of tooth resorption (Box 21-1).

Histologic Features

Histologic studies provide compelling evidence that the very early tooth resorption in cats is noninflammatory.[41] Clinically and radiographically normal teeth of cats with obvious resorption of other teeth showed a loss of the physiologic periodontal ligament architecture, a narrowing of the periodontal ligament space (caused by hypercementosis along the root surface, hyperosteoidosis along the alveolar bone surface, or mineralization within the periodontal ligament), fusion of the tooth root with alveolar bone (dentoalveolar ankylosis), and areas of resorption of cementum and dentin.[41]

Teeth with dentoalveolar ankylosis are at risk of being incorporated into the normal bone remodeling process and are ultimately resorbed and replaced by new bone (replacement resorption). When this process occurs close to the gingival attachment, the defect may emerge at the gingival margin, and the histologic picture may change to that of an inflammatory resorption; pathognomonic of which is that the adjacent alveolar bone often is resorbed as well.[100] Attempts at repair may be noted by production of bone or cementum-like material; however, tooth resorption in cats usually progresses until the roots are completely resorbed or the crown breaks off, leaving root remnants behind.[101]

BOX 21-1

Classification of Tooth Resorption Proposed by the American Veterinary Dental College

Stage 1

Mild dental hard tissue loss (cementum or cementum and enamel)

Stage 2

Moderate dental hard tissue loss (cementum or cementum and enamel with loss of dentin that does not extend to the pulp cavity)

Stage 3

Deep dental hard tissue loss (cementum or cementum and enamel with loss of dentin that extends to the pulp cavity); most of the tooth retains its integrity

Stage 4

Extensive dental hard tissue loss (cementum or cementum and enamel with loss of dentin that extends to the pulp cavity); most of the tooth has lost its integrity

- 4a: Crown and root are equally affected
- 4b: Crown is more severely affected than the root
- 4c: Root is more severely affected than the crown

Stage 5

Remnants of dental hard tissue are visible only as irregular radiopacities, and gingival covering is complete

Treatment

Topical fluoride treatment has never been evaluated for prevention of tooth resorption in cats, and it is highly doubtful whether fluoride application on the crowns of teeth has any effect on resorption of roots apical to the gingival attachment.[101] Systemic alendronate therapy has been suggested on the basis of results of a very small sample of cats[75]; however, studies in mice provide evidence that dentoalveolar ankylosis and extensive tooth resorption actually result from bisphosphonate administration.[116,117] Restorative therapy also does not address pathology located apical to the gingival attachment and has repeatedly been shown to fail over both the short and long term.[101] If increased vitamin D activity ever proves to be the causative factor of tooth resorption in cats, feeding a diet less rich in vitamin D would be recommended.

Extraction and crown amputation with intentional root retention are the current treatment options. Feline teeth are best extracted using an open technique. A mucoperiosteal flap is raised, alveolectomy is performed, multirooted teeth are sectioned, and teeth or crown-root segments are elevated and extracted.[12,106] Retained root remnants are removed in a similar fashion. Root remnants under intact and healthy gingiva and without endodontic or periapical pathology on dental radiographs may be left where they are. Ankylosed teeth and those with replacement resorption of their roots often make complete extraction impossible. Crown amputation with intentional retention of resorbing root tissue (discussed later in this chapter) is a viable treatment option for such teeth.[26]

DENTOALVEOLAR TRAUMA

Rapid tooth wear can result in chronic irritation of the pulp or even pulp exposure. However, abrasion and attrition are fairly uncommon in cats. Tooth fracture can be either uncomplicated (without pulp exposure) or complicated (with pulp exposure).[98] Fracture of canine teeth is common in cats after motor-vehicle trauma, falls from heights, kicks, and hits. If dentin is exposed in an uncomplicated fracture, a pathway can still exist for stimuli to pass through the dentinal tubules to the pulp, resulting in formation of tertiary dentin or endodontic disease. Pulp exposure in complicated fractures will always result in endodontic disease (pulpitis and pulp necrosis). Extension of endodontic disease into the periapical tissues will cause apical periodontitis or granuloma or abscess formation, often manifesting in facial swelling and formation of sinus tracts. Localized or widespread infection of the bone and bone marrow (osteomyelitis) can arise from an endodontic infection.[98] Tooth resorption starting on external root surfaces and progressing into root or crown dentin is often the cause of fracture of feline teeth. Tooth displacement injuries (luxation and avulsion) can be seen in cats whose canine teeth are affected by alveolar bone expansion and supereruption.

Clinical Signs and Diagnosis

Reluctance to eat hard food may be noted in the patient with dentoalveolar trauma. The teeth on the affected side may then show increased plaque and calculus accumulation and gingival inflammation. Regional lymphadenopathy and fever may be present with an acute apical abscess. Endodontic disease may result in crown discoloration (pink, red, purple, gray, or brown), which can be interpreted as indicative of pulp necrosis.[98] The integrity of the dental crowns is evaluated with a dental explorer, the fine and pointed tip of which may catch in an open pulp chamber. Recent pulp exposures reveal red tissue at or bleeding from the fracture site (Figure 21-29), whereas old pulp exposures show black debris and

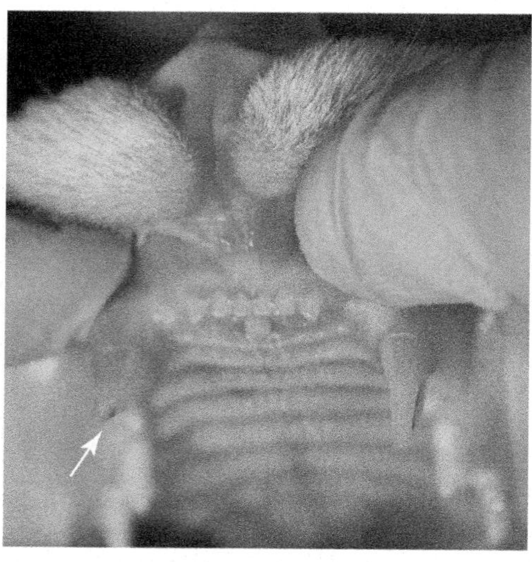

FIGURE 21-29 Upper jaw of a cat, showing complicated fracture of the right maxillary canine tooth *(arrow)*. Note the bleeding from exposed pulp tissue after evaluation of the fracture site with a dental explorer. *(Copyright 2010 Dr. Alexander M. Reiter; used with permission.)*

necrotic pulp tissue. Endodontically diseased maxillary canine or cheek teeth may result in maxillofacial swelling and formation of extraoral or intraoral sinus tracts that often have a history of responsiveness to antibiotics and recurrence when antibiotic therapy is discontinued. Sinus tracts can be traced with a gutta-percha cone (root canal filling material), and a radiograph is obtained to locate their source.[98]

Treatment

Vital pulp therapy is primarily performed on teeth with acute complicated crown fractures (of less than 2 days' duration in animals older than 18 months of age and of less than 2 weeks' duration in animals younger than 18 months of age) to preserve pulp vitality and increase the strength of the tooth by allowing continued dentin formation.[85] Intentional crown reduction with vital pulp therapy may be performed in cats with unilateral mandibulectomies when medial drift of the remaining mandible results in the mandibular canine tooth puncturing the palate on closure of the mouth. Instruments and materials in contact with vital pulp must be sterile to prevent iatrogenic bacterial infection. Intentional crown reduction is followed by partial pulpectomy, direct pulp capping, and restoration. Dental radiographs are obtained in 6 months to confirm pulp vitality and then once annually.

If the pulp is exposed for longer periods of time or has become necrotic, standard root canal therapy is performed and includes accessing the pulp cavity; débriding, shaping, disinfecting, and obturating the root canal; and restoring access and fracture sites (Figure 21-30).[52,81]

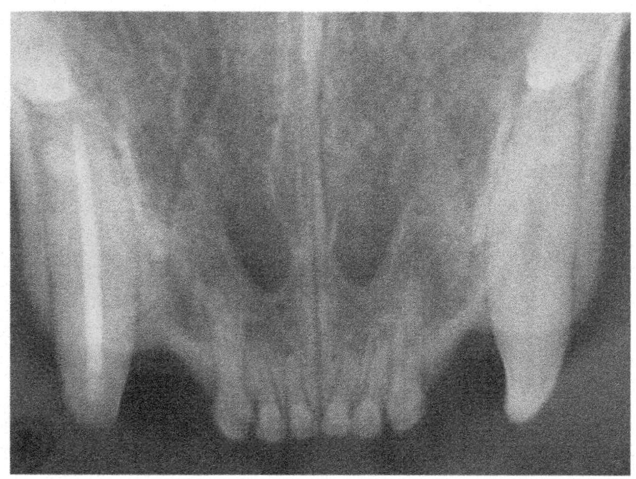

FIGURE 21-30 Radiograph obtained following standard root canal therapy of the right maxillary canine tooth shown in Figure 21-29. *(Copyright 2010 Dr. Alexander M. Reiter; used with permission.)*

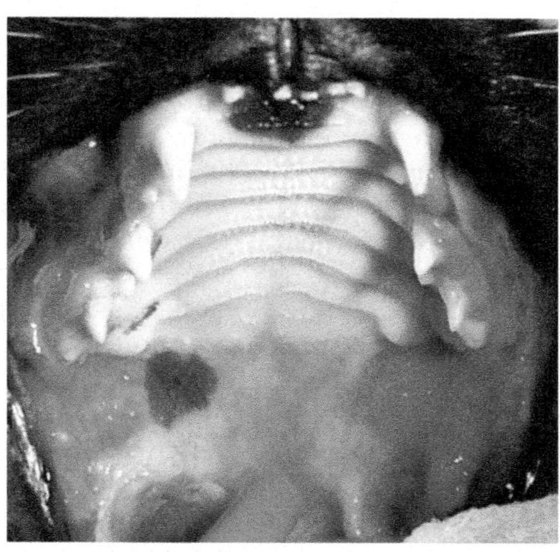

FIGURE 21-31 Cat with inflammation of the gingiva, alveolar mucosa, labial and buccal mucosa, and mucosa of the caudal oral cavity lateral to the palatoglossal folds. Note that the hard palate mucosa is usually not inflamed in cats with stomatitis. *(From Harvey CE: Stomatitis. In Cote E, editor:* Clinical veterinary advisor, *ed 1, St Louis, 2007, Mosby, p 1039.)*

Perioperative dental radiography is essential, and an armamentarium of instruments and materials are required to perform the various steps of root canal therapy. Surgical root canal therapy is performed when standard root canal therapy has failed and includes access through oral mucosa (maxillary canine) or skin (mandibular canine), alveolectomy, apicoectomy, and retrograde filling. With either technique, the treated tooth should be reexamined radiographically in 6 months and then once annually.[4,39] Luxated and avulsed teeth have lost their blood supply and should be extracted in cats rather then repositioned or replanted.

STOMATITIS

Stomatitis is recognized mainly in adult cats and characterized by persistent inflammation of the oral mucosa. One investigation found that 88% of cats with stomatitis were shedding both feline calicivirus (FCV) and feline herpesvirus-1 (FHV-1) in saliva, which suggests that these two viruses may play a role in feline stomatitis.[70] Evidence for a cause-and-effect relationship between *Bartonella* and feline stomatitis has not been provided.[24,91]

Clinical Signs and Diagnosis

Cats with stomatitis often have a long history of inappetence, weight loss, pawing at the face, and oral pain. Clinical signs usually include focal or diffuse oral inflammation involving the gingiva, alveolar mucosa, labial and buccal mucosa, sublingual mucosa, and the area of or lateral to the palatoglossal folds (Figure 21-31).[71] In severe cases the inflamed tissues become proliferative and ulcerated and bleed spontaneously. Various degrees of dental and periodontal disease may be present (tooth resorption, gingival recession, periodontal pockets, mobile or missing teeth). Mandibular lymphadenopathy; oral, nasal, and ocular discharge; and focal ulceration of the lips may also be present.

A complete blood count, biochemical profile, and urinalysis are performed to identify concurrent or contributory diseases. An increase in total protein usually is due to elevated gamma globulin concentrations. Leukocytosis caused by mild to moderate neutrophilia may be present. Serologic evaluation for FeLV antigen and FIV antibody should be performed. Testing for *Bartonella* infection is controversial. A biopsy specimen should be obtained to rule out neoplasia or other causes of oral inflammation. Histopathology typically shows ulceration with subepithelial lymphocytic–plasmacytic infiltration, which may reflect a chronic response to the presence of an overwhelming bacterial load rather than being an indicator of the primary cause of the condition.[71]

Treatment

Stomatitis presents a therapeutic challenge, and management is often frustrating for both the veterinarian and owner. Many cases are refractory to treatment. A multimodal treatment approach is imperative in patients with stomatitis, often requiring a combination of medical and surgical therapies for resolution of clinical signs and occasional placement of an esophageal feeding tube for nutritional management. Plaque control is achieved with professional dental cleaning, topical and systemic antimicrobial therapy, and tooth extraction. Systemic antibiotic therapy (e.g., amoxicillin–clavulanic acid and clindamycin) often provides only short-term clinical benefit or can be ineffective in the initial management of inflammation. Topical 0.12% chlorhexidine products may be used for adjunctive therapy in the initial management.[71]

Glucocorticosteroids are often required to decrease inflammation, reduce pain, and stimulate appetite. Administration of oral prednisolone (starting at 1 to 2 mg/kg orally every 12 hours initially for 1 week, followed by tapering it to the lowest effective dose over a period of 4 to 8 weeks) can be challenging in the patient experiencing pain. Therefore some cats may initially benefit from subcutaneous injections of methylprednisolone (4 mg/kg) that, after a few weeks, is followed by oral administration of prednisolone.[71] The presence of lymphocytes in affected tissues suggests that antilymphocyte drugs such as cyclosporines may be useful (starting at 2.5 mg/kg of Neoral [Novartis] solution orally every 12 hours; given for 6 weeks before judging effectiveness; monitoring of trough drug levels [should be 250 to 500 ng/mL], kidney values, and other blood parameters).[112] Clinical improvement was reported in cats with stomatitis that were given bovine lactoferrin (bacteriocidal immunomodulator that may inhibit adhesion of periodontopathogens; 250 mg orally once daily).[1] Low-dose doxycycline (antiinflammatory, anticollagenolytic, and antimetalloproteinolytic effects; 1 mg/kg orally once daily) and feline interferon omega (Virbagen Omega, Virbac; 5 MU are diluted and divided as necessary to submucosally inject all inflamed areas; the remaining 5 MU are injected into a 100-mL bag of sodium chloride and frozen in ten 10-mL aliquots; client gives 1 mL orally every 24 hours for 100 days; the 10 mL fraction in use is refrigerated and the other aliquots are kept frozen until needed) have also been suggested as medical treatment options for cats with stomatitis.[109,120]

Tooth extraction appears to be the best long-term therapeutic strategy because it removes the surfaces that are available for plaque retention.[50] Teeth with periodontitis or resorption and retained roots must be extracted. Plaque seems to play a role in perpetuating stomatitis even if teeth are located relatively distant from the actual site of inflammation (e.g., in cases of stomatitis of the caudal oral cavity). Therefore reasonably healthy teeth may be extracted in cats with severe stomatitis that do not respond to medication. Extraction of all teeth caudal to the canine teeth is often sufficient. If inflammation also occurs adjacent to the canines and incisors, a full-mouth extraction procedure may be necessary. Débridement of friable and inflamed soft tissue and bone before wound closure with an absorbable monofilament suture material (e.g., poliglecaprone 25) will aid in resolution of inflammation. The response to tooth extraction ranges from complete resolution of inflammation (60%), minimal residual inflammation, and no oral pain (20%); to initial improvement requiring continued medical therapy to control clinical signs (13%); to no improvement (7%). Cats tolerate extractions, even full-mouth extractions, very well and can eat moist and even dry food without teeth.[50]

Laser surgery may be used as an adjunct in patients with refractory stomatitis not responding to extractions and medical therapy.[67] The CO_2 laser is used in excision and ablation modes. Fibrosis formation is enhanced when lased areas are left to heal by second intention. Follow-up oral examination typically shows granulation tissue and striations of fibrous tissue spanning the previously treated areas. Laser treatments are repeated in intervals of several weeks to months, increasing the amount of fibrous tissue and decreasing interspersed areas of continued inflammation. The patient should be seen for reexaminations every few weeks to monitor improvement, obtain body weight measurements, and slowly taper oral glucocorticosteroids. Sublingual and oropharyngeal tissues around the endotracheal tube can often become swollen from intubation and handling. Dexamethasone (0.25 mg/kg intravenously) may be administered to minimize swelling that could affect breathing after extubation.[67]

TOOTH EXTRACTION

Tooth extraction is most frequently performed in cats with periodontal disease, tooth resorption, stomatitis, and traumatized teeth. Other indications include roots retained in the jaws; persistent deciduous teeth; teeth causing malocclusion; unerupted teeth; teeth near jaw fracture lines, in areas of osteomyelitis, and osteonecrosis or surrounded by oral neoplasia; and client preference.[94] The client must have given permission for extraction of any tooth before the procedure is undertaken. To prevent complications such as local or systemic infection,[97] the entire tooth must be removed, without leaving any root structure in the alveolus.

Instruments and Mechanics

Dental luxators have sharp, flat-tipped blades that can penetrate into the periodontal space. Dental elevators have less sharp, more curved blades that fit the shape of the tooth. Luxating elevators often combine the benefits of the two basic designs. They are grasped with the butt of the handle seated in the palm, and the index finger is extended along the blade to act as a stop in case the instrument slips. Smaller luxating elevators, root tip picks, root tip forceps, bone curettes, periosteal elevators, and extraction forceps are available for use in cats (Figure 21-32).[94]

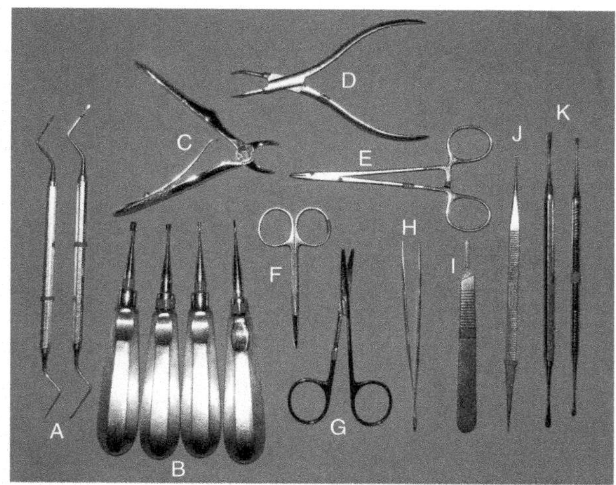

FIGURE 21-32 Set of smaller-sized instruments for extraction of feline teeth, including root fragment elevators *(A)*, winged luxating elevators *(B)*, extraction forceps *(C)*, root fragment forceps *(D)*, needle holder *(E)*, suture scissors *(F)*, curved Metzenbaum scissors *(G)*, Adson thumb forceps *(H)*, scalpel handle *(I)*, spoon curette *(J)*, and periosteal elevators *(K)*. *(Copyright 2010 Dr. Alexander M. Reiter; used with permission.)*

Teeth are secured to the alveolar bone of the incisive bone, maxilla, and mandible by the gingiva and periodontal ligament. The roots of the incisors and canine teeth in cats are slightly curved and flattened oval in cross-section, thus providing antirotational retention. The maximum circumference of canine teeth is not at the cementoenamel junction or the alveolar margin but rather at some distance apical to them, thus locking the roots into the jaw. The roots of the premolars and molars diverge, which also aids in retention. The maxillary fourth premolars in cats have three roots. The cheek teeth of many cats often have bulbous root apices as a result of hypercementosis.[94]

Closed Extraction

A no. 15 scalpel blade is inserted into the gingival sulcus, and the gingival attachment is incised around the tooth. The blade of a luxating elevator is then worked vertically into the space between the tooth and alveolar bone, and the handle is rotated along its long axis to create gentle and steady pressure on the tooth. This wedging force will widen the periodontal ligament space until the instrument can be inserted further apically. Rotational pressure with the instrument is then applied and maintained for at least 10 seconds to cause the periodontal ligament fibers to tear. The luxating elevator should be moved around the entire tooth, while also progressing toward the root apex. Extraction forceps should be used only when the tooth is already mobile and applied as far apically as possible to reduce the chances of tooth fracture. The tooth should be examined visually and by means of digital palpation, verifying that the entire root was extracted. The alveolus is then débrided and lavaged, sharp bony edges are smoothed, and the extraction site is sutured closed with a synthetic absorbable monofilament (e.g., 5-0 poliglecaprone 25) in a simple interrupted pattern. A blood clot should remain in the alveolus to allow for proper healing.[22,94]

Multirooted teeth must be sectioned before extraction to prevent root fracture. This provides multiple single-rooted crown-root segments, the extraction of which is no more difficult than that of multiple single-rooted teeth. Sectioning is performed with a fissure bur in a water-cooled high-speed handpiece, starting from the furcation through the tooth crown. Two-rooted teeth are separated into one mesial and one distal single-rooted crown-root segment. Three-rooted teeth are separated into three one-rooted crown-root segments. The luxating instrument can also be placed perpendicular to the tooth between the crown-root segments to lever them out of their alveoli.[22,94]

Open Extraction

When firmly seated deciduous canine teeth, large and periodontally intact permanent teeth, or multiple permanent teeth in one jaw quadrant need to be extracted, a mucoperiosteal flap is raised with one or two releasing incisions that extend from the gingival margin beyond the mucogingival junction into alveolar mucosa. Round or pear-shaped carbide burs attached to a water-cooled high-speed handpiece are used to remove alveolar bone at the vestibular tooth surfaces by as much as one third to two thirds of the length of the root(s). Sectioning of multirooted teeth, extraction of crown-root segments, and débridement of the alveoli are performed as for the closed extraction technique.[22,94]

The flap margins are trimmed with fine gingival scissors or curved Metzenbaum scissors. A scalpel blade is used on the connective tissue side to incise the periosteum in a distomesial direction across the base of the flap. The flap will advance as the inelastic periosteal layer is cut. The back of a scalpel blade can also be used to "strum" and weaken the periosteal layer without cutting into or through the flap, followed by blunt dissection with a scissors. Alternatively, a small incision can be made in the periosteum with a scalpel blade. Then the tips of a closed Metzenbaum scissors are inserted through the opening and opened to undermine the periosteal layer mesially and distally, carefully avoiding injury to adjacent neurovascular structures. The flap is sutured to the palatal or lingual gingiva with synthetic absorbable monofilament in a simple interrupted pattern (Figure 21-33).[12,108]

Root remnants with sinus tracts, roots fractured during the extraction procedure, and roots remaining after mandibulectomies and maxillectomies should be removed to prevent infection and inflammation of the

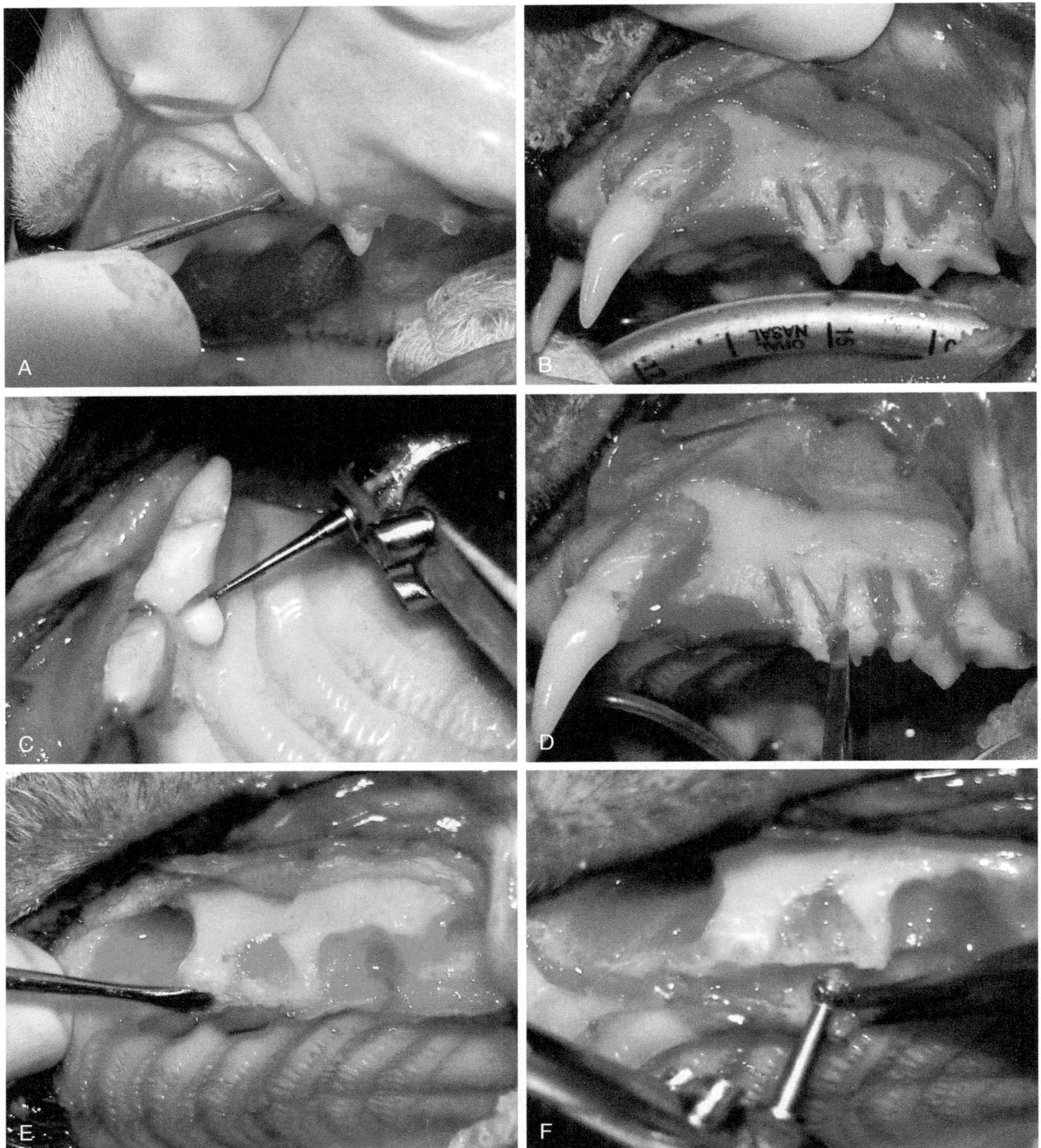

FIGURE 21-33 Clinical photographs showing extraction of multiple maxillary teeth in a cat. A periosteal elevator is used to elevate a mucoperiosteal flap **(A)**. This is followed by alveolectomy with a round carbide bur **(B)** and sectioning of teeth with the same bur or a fissure carbide bur **(C** and **D)**. Following elevation and removal of all teeth and crown-root segments, the palatal gingiva is elevated as an envelope flap **(E)** to allow for alveoloplasty of exposed alveolar margins with a diamond grit-coated round bur **(F)**.

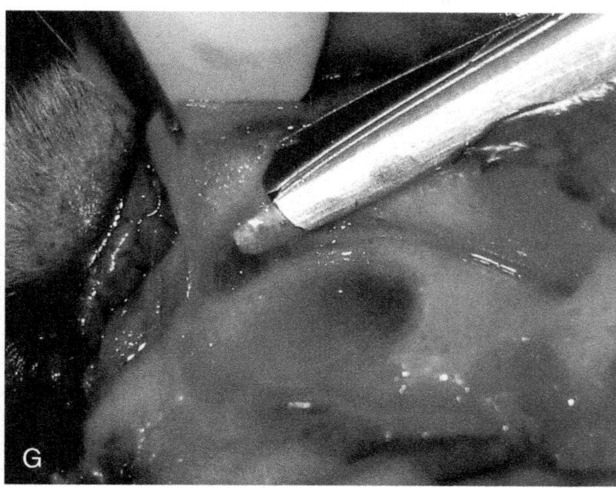

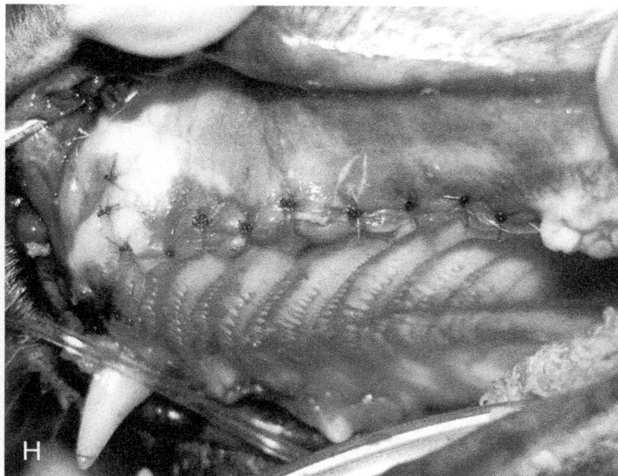

FIGURE 21-33, cont'd A small incision is made in the periosteum with a scalpel blade, and closed Metzenbaum scissors are inserted through the opening to bluntly undermine the periosteal layer mesially, labially, buccally, and distally **(G)**. The extraction sites are rinsed before wound closure with a tension-free flap **(H)**. *(From Blazejewski S, Lewis JR, Reiter AM: Mucoperiosteal flap for extraction of multiple teeth in the maxillary quadrant of the cat,* J Vet Dent *23:200, 2006; used with permission.)*

bone. Special root tip elevators, picks, and extraction forceps are available. Creation of a mucoperiosteal flap and partial alveolectomy will facilitate removal of a root fragment. If a root fragment cannot be retrieved, the surgical site should be evaluated periodically by means of clinical and radiographic follow-up examination. Retrieval of root fragments from the nasal cavity or infraorbital or mandibular canal after their accidental repulsion into these spaces may be made through soft tissue and bone away from the extraction site.[94]

Crown amputation with intentional retention of resorbing root tissue can be performed on teeth that show radiographic dentoalveolar ankylosis and root replacement resorption. It is contraindicated for mobile teeth with periodontitis, endodontic disease, and periapical pathology and not recommended when closed or open extraction can be accomplished.[94] The gingival attachment is incised, a mucoperiosteal flap with or without releasing incisions is made, and the crown is amputated with a round or fissure bur attached to a water-cooled high-speed handpiece at the level of the cervical root portion of the tooth. The resorbing root is further reduced with a round diamond grit–coated bur to about 1 to 2 mm below the level of the alveolar margin to allow for alveolar bone to grow over it. The gingiva is then sutured closed over the wound (Figure 21-34). Postoperative radiographs must be obtained for future monitoring (Figure 21-35).[26]

EOSINOPHILIC GRANULOMA COMPLEX

Eosinophilic granuloma complex entails a group of lesions that can affect the oral cavity, lips, and skin. There is no breed predisposition. Lesions have been recognized in several cats of multicat households, and experimental transmission was demonstrated from one area of a cat to another. Therefore an infectious or allergic etiology has been suggested, with lesions resulting from a hypersensitivity reaction caused by fleas or mosquitos, food, and contact or environmental allergies.[46] Eosinophilic granulomas manifest in the mouth, often at the mucosa of the hard and soft palate, dorsal tongue surface, and sublingual region. The surface of oral lesions may be speckled with small dense white areas (Figure 21-36). The eosinophilic ulcer ("rodent ulcer") is usually seen in the rostral portion of the upper lip, well-demarcated with raised edges that surround a pink-yellow ulcerated surface (Figure 21-37). Both lesions are more commonly found in young female cats and characterized by eosinophilic infiltrates on histopathology. One major differential diagnosis is squamous cell carcinoma, and biopsy should be performed before treatment.[46]

Treatment of eosinphilic lesions consists of glucocorticosteroid therapy (1 to 2 mg/kg prednisolone orally every 12 hours initially for 1 week, followed by tapering it to the lowest effective dose over a period of 4 to 8 weeks). Injectable drugs (4 mg/kg methylprednisolone subcutaneously) may also be attempted 2 to 3 times, several weeks apart. Intralesional injection of triamcinolone is sometimes helpful.[46] Oral cyclosporine may be an effective alternative to steroids.[112] Secondary infection may be treated with amoxicillin–clavulanic acid at 14 mg/kg orally every 12 hours for 2 to 3 weeks. Surgical excision and laser therapy have also been suggested for single oral lesions. In the case of flea infestation, a flea control program should be started. A strict elimination diet should be attempted when an adverse food reaction is suspected as an underlying cause.

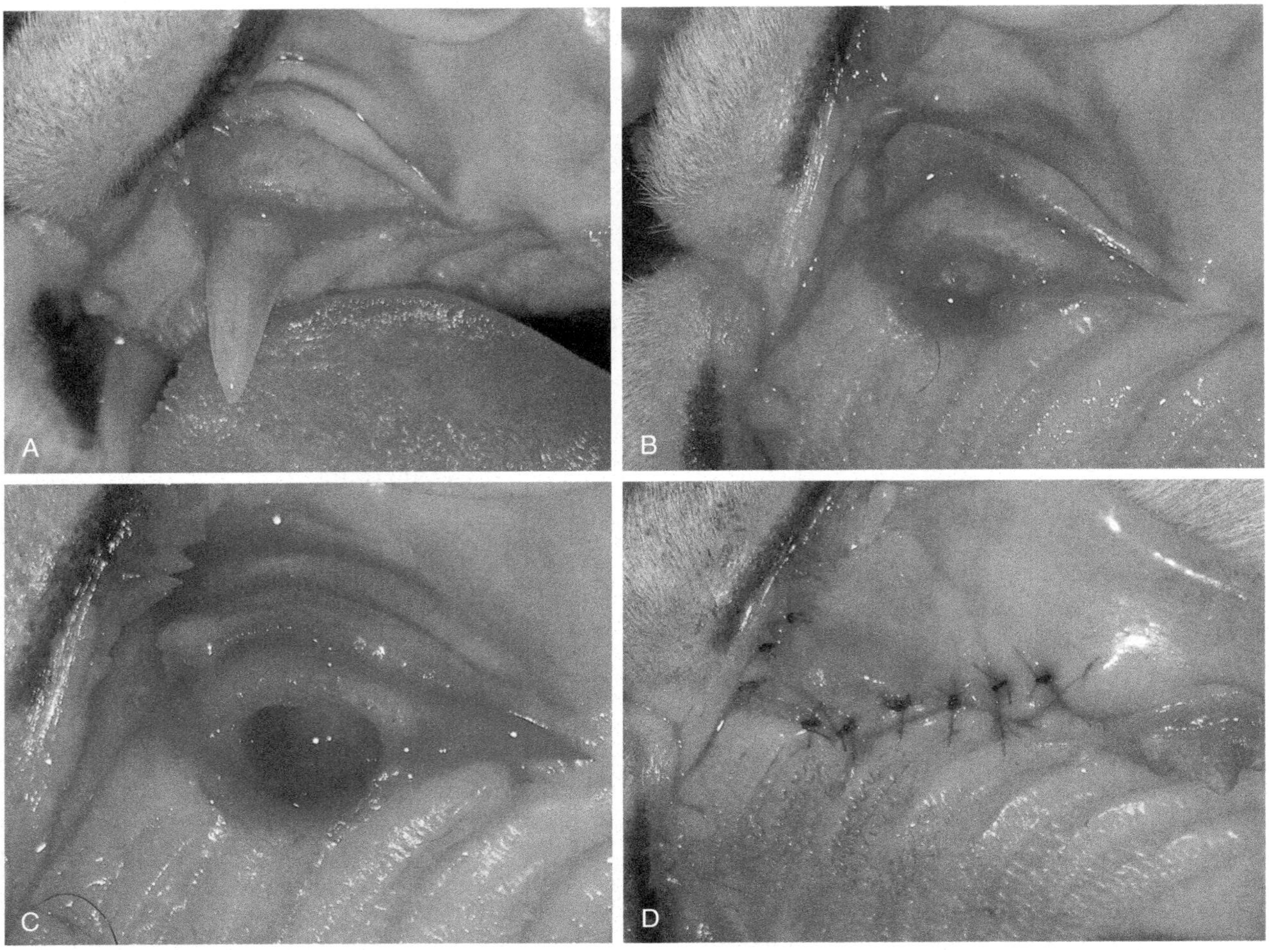

FIGURE 21-34 Clinical photographs showing crown amputation of the left maxillary canine tooth with intentional retention of resorbing root tissue. A mucoperiosteal flap is raised **(A)**. The crown is amputated with a dental bur at the level of the cervical root portion of the tooth **(B)**. The resorbing root is further reduced with a dental bur to about 1 or 2 mm below the level of the alveolar margin **(C)**. The gingiva is sutured closed over the wound **(D)**. *(Copyright 2010 Dr. Alexander M. Reiter; used with permission.)*

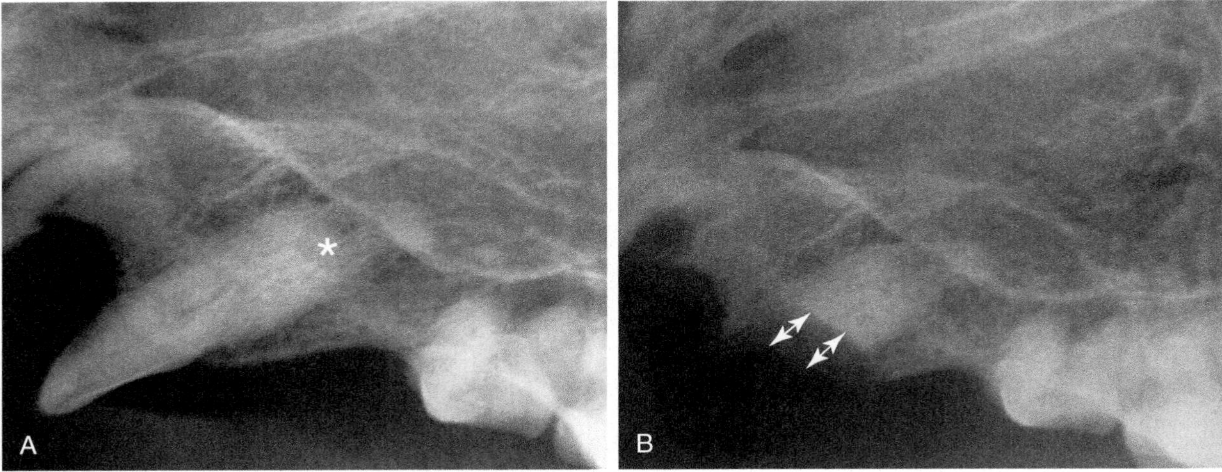

FIGURE 21-35 Preoperative radiograph **(A)** of the left maxillary canine tooth from Figure 21-34, showing root replacement resorption *(asterisk)*. Postoperative radiograph **(B)** following crown amputation and intentional retention of root tissue, showing reduction of the resorbing root about 1 or 2 mm below the level of the alveolar margin *(double-ended arrows)*. *(Copyright 2010 Dr. Alexander M. Reiter; used with permission.)*

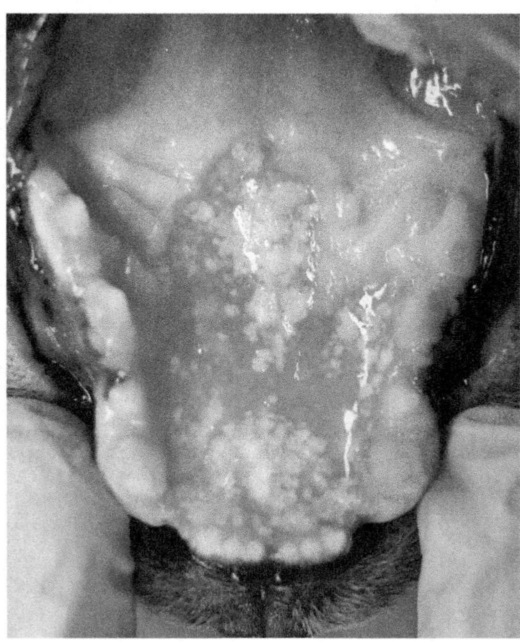

FIGURE 21-36 Eosinophilic granuloma of the hard palate mucosa in a cat. Note the mucosal surface speckled with small dense white areas. *(Copyright 2010 Dr. Alexander M. Reiter; used with permission.)*

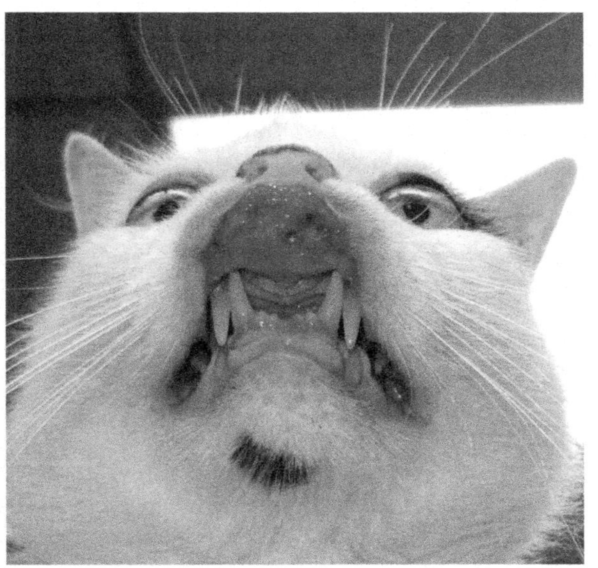

FIGURE 21-37 Eosinophilic ulcer in the rostral portion of the upper lip in a cat. Note the well-demarcated lesion with raised edges that surround a pink-yellow ulcerated surface. *(Copyright 2010 Dr. Alexander M. Reiter; used with permission.)*

FELINE OROFACIAL PAIN SYNDROME

Feline orofacial pain syndrome (FOPS) is considered to be an episodic neuropathic pain disorder caused by a dysfunction of central or ganglion processing of sensory trigeminal information. Affected cats usually exhibit exaggerated licking, unusual chewing movements, and pawing at the mouth. More severe cases have acute oral pain (with pain-free intervals) confined to one side of the mouth and face (or worse on one side). Mutilation of the tongue, lips, and labial and buccal mucosa may also be seen. The disease has predominantly been seen in Burmese cats in the United Kingdom, suggesting an inherited disorder, and can affect cats at any age. Many cats showed first signs of FOPS at the time of eruption of the permanent dentition, often redeveloping the syndrome as they mature. The discomfort is reported to be triggered by movements of the mouth, including those associated with eating, drinking, and grooming. Cats may be anorexic and unwilling to eat. The disease is often recurrent and unremitting, and some cats are euthanized as a consequence of the condition.[105]

Sensitization of trigeminal nerve endings from tooth eruption and oral disease and environmental stress appear to be important precipitating factors in the etiology of the disease, suggesting that the disease may be a pain disorder analogous to trigeminal neuralgia and glossodynia (burning mouth syndrome) in humans. Diagnosis is by elimination of other causes of oral pain or trigeminal nerve dysfunction. Oral disease must be treated appropriately, and social incompatibility in a multicat household should be identified. Antiepileptic drugs with analgesic effects (e.g., phenobarbital, diazepam, carbamazepine, gabapentin) appear to be better pain relievers in FOPS than traditional analgesics (e.g., opioids, antiinflammatory drugs). Periodic monitoring of liver function and drug serum concentrations is recommended for cats treated with antiepileptic drugs.[105]

PALATE DEFECTS

Congenital lip and palate defects are rarely encountered in cats. Palate defects acquired after birth usually are located in the hard palate and result from chronic infection (e.g., severe periodontal disease), trauma (e.g., high-rise syndrome, electrical cord and gunshot injury, dog bites, foreign body penetration, and pressure wounds secondary to a maloccluding tooth), neoplasia, and surgical or radiation therapy. Such oronasal defects do not heal because of the continuous passage of air and food, leading to chronic rhinitis and nasal discharge.[96]

The choice of repair technique depends on the location and size of the defect and the amount of tissue available for flap procedures. There may be considerable bleeding during hard palate surgery, but digital pressure with gauze sponges is often sufficient to control hemorrhage. The best chance of success is with the first attempt at repair. Teeth at the surgical site and those that could traumatize flaps should be extracted. Electrocautery for hemostasis must be avoided. The flaps should be larger than the defect they will cover. The blood supply to the flaps must be maintained, and flaps should be handled as carefully as possible. Rather than using tissue forceps, the veterinarian should make stay sutures at the flap edges for tissue manipulation. Connective tissue surfaces or cut edges should be sutured together, and a two-layer closure should be employed if practical. Longer-lasting synthetic absorbable monofilament suture material (e.g., 4-0 polydioxanone [PDS]) and simple interrupted or mattress sutures are recommended. Suture lines should not be located over a void if possible, and closure must be accomplished without tension.[96,102]

Congenital Palate Defects

Cleft lip appears as a defect of the lip (harelip) and most rostral hard palate. Cleft lips rarely result in clinical signs beyond mild rhinitis, and repair may be performed for cosmetic reasons. The most rostral palate and the floor of the nasal vestibule are reconstructed. This is accomplished by creating overlapping double flaps and advancement, rotation, or transposition flaps of both oral and nasal tissue or flaps that are harvested from oral soft tissue only. Reconstructive cutaneous surgery completes the repair.[96]

Cleft palate is almost always in the midline and usually associated with a midline soft palate abnormality. Soft palate defects without hard palate defects may occur in the midline or are unilateral. Clinical signs and history of patients with cleft palate include failure to create negative pressure for nursing, nasal discharge, coughing, gagging, sneezing, nasal reflux, tonsillitis, rhinitis, aspiration pneumonia, poor weight gain, and general unthriftiness. Management requires nursing care by the owner, which includes tube feeding to avoid aspiration pneumonia.[96,102]

Surgical correction is performed in 3- to 4-month-old cats, preferably using the overlapping flap technique because there is less tension on the suture line (which is not located directly over the defect) and the area of opposing connective tissues is larger, which results in a stronger scar. It provides more reliable results compared with the medially positioned flap technique. Incisions are made in the mucoperiosteum to the bone (full-thickness flaps) at the medial margin of the defect on one side (envelope flap) and along the dental arch about 1 to 2 mm palatal to the teeth to the rostral and caudal margins of the defect on the other side (overlapping flap). The tissues are undermined with a periosteal elevator, ensuring that the major palatine arteries are not transected. The overlapped flap is folded on itself, turned, and sutured under the envelope flap so that the connective tissue surfaces are in contact. The sutures are placed in a horizontal mattress pattern. Granulation and epithelialization of exposed tissues are completed in 3 to 4 weeks.[96,102]

Midline soft palate defects are corrected by making incisions along the medial margins of the defect to the level of the caudal end of the tonsils. The palatal tissue is separated with a Metzenbaum scissors to form a dorsal (nasopharyngeal) and ventral (oropharyngeal) flap on each side. The two dorsal and the two ventral flaps are sutured separately in a simple interrupted pattern to the midpoint or caudal end of the tonsils.[96,102]

Acquired Palate Defects

An oronasal fistula may result from loss of incisive and maxillary bone associated with severe periodontal disease or tooth extraction, typically in the area of a maxillary canine tooth. An acute oronasal fistula following tooth extraction is diagnosed by direct visualization of the nasal cavity and bleeding from the ipsilateral nostril. Clinical signs of a chronic oronasal fistula include sneezing and ipsilateral nasal discharge, and a defect that communicates with the nasal cavity in the area of a missing tooth may be noted on oral examination. Elevating and positioning a labial-based mucoperiosteal flap over the defect repairs the oronasal fistula.[96,102]

Traumatic cleft palate is an acute midline soft or hard tissue defect of the hard palate (Figure 21-38) typically associated with high-rise syndrome[95] and less often with road-traffic trauma in cats. Although these clefts may sometimes heal spontaneously in 2 to 4 weeks with conservative management, the benefit of surgical management with medially positioned flaps outweighs the risk of developing a persistent oronasal communication. An acute traumatic cleft palate is managed by débriding the torn palatal tissue edges, undermining the palatal mucoperiosteum on either side of the defect (carefully avoiding transection of the major palatine arteries), approximating the displaced bony structures with digital pressure, and apposing and suturing of the two palatal flaps in a simple interrupted or mattress pattern. Tension on the suture line can be minimized by creating relieving incisions along the dental arches about 1 to 2 mm palatal to the teeth, allowing the flaps to be moved medially into apposition with each other (Figure 21-39). The exposed bone next to the teeth is left to granulate and epithelialize. If the palatal defect is extensive, inter-quadrant fixation is performed by securing a twisted wire between the maxillary canines (or other maxillary teeth if the crowns of the canines are missing) and covering the wire with bis-acryl composite.[96,102]

The modified split palatal U-flap is useful for large caudal defects.[96,102] The epithelial margins of the defect are débrided with a scalpel blade. One flap of slightly longer and another of slightly shorter length are created. The shorter flap is rotated through 90 degrees and transposed to cover the defect. Its medial aspect is sutured to

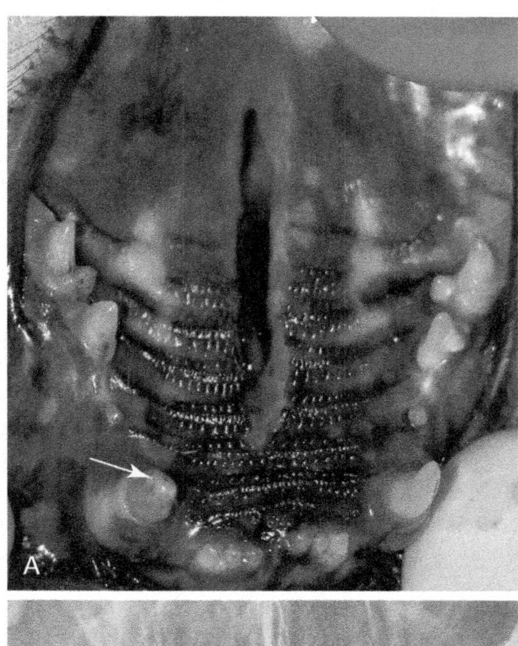

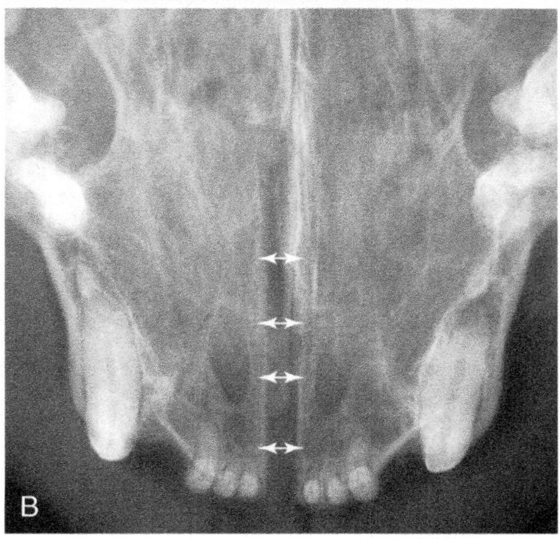

FIGURE 21-38 Clinical photograph **(A)** and radiograph **(B)** showing a traumatic cleft palate in a cat as a result of falling from a height. Note the wide separation of left and right incisive and maxillary bones *(double-ended arrows)* and the fractured left maxillary canine tooth *(arrow)*. *(Copyright 2010 Dr. Alexander M. Reiter; used with permission.)*

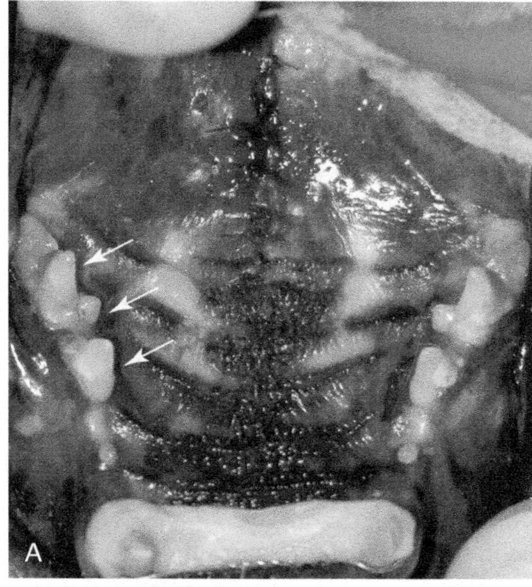

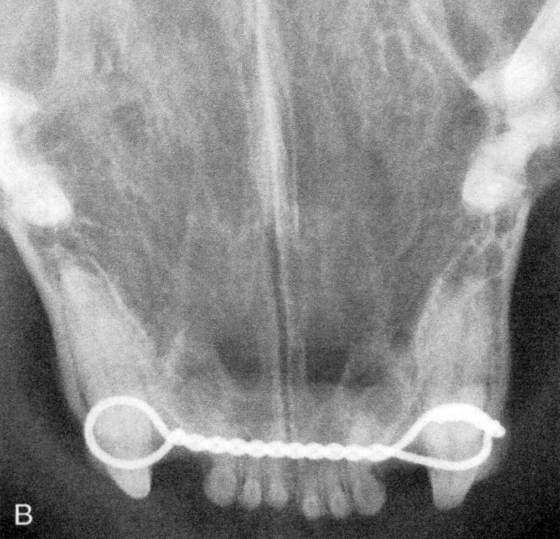

FIGURE 21-39 Clinical photograph **(A)** and radiograph **(B)** showing repair of the traumatic cleft palate in Figure 21-38, accomplished by means of approximation and suturing of medially positioned flaps after creation of bilateral releasing incisions *(arrows)* into palatal mucoperiosteum along the dental arches. Note interquadrant fixation (twisted wire covered with composite resin) between the maxillary canine teeth. *(Copyright 2010 Dr. Alexander M. Reiter; used with permission.)*

the caudal aspect of the palatal defect. The longer flap is rotated through 90 degrees and transposed rostral to shorter flap. Its medial aspect is sutured to the lateral edge of the shorther flap. The denuded rostral aspect of the palate from which the flaps were harvested is left to granulate and epithelialize.[72,96,102]

Other techniques for repair of large palate defects include combinations of overlapping flaps and buccal- or labial-based pedicle or axial pattern flaps, which are created and sutured across the defect 4 to 6 weeks after extraction of several teeth. These flaps are supplied by major palatine or infraorbital blood vessels. The use of auricular cartilage grafts underneath flaps has also been described.[20] An alternative for repair of defects in the rostral or midportion of the hard palate is the use of a tongue flap. The edges of the dorsal aspect of the tongue are excised and apposed to the débrided edges of the palatal defect. The tongue is separated from the palate several weeks later, leaving enough tongue tissue with the palate to close the defect without tension. Another alternative is to create a permanent or removable silicone or acrylic obturator.[110]

OROFACIAL SOFT TISSUE INJURY

Penetration of the oral cavity may result from animal bites or, less commonly, foreign bodies; linear foreign bodies (such as dental floss) can get caught around the tongue and saw through to the lingual frenulum. Penetrating wounds can be deep and contaminated and are often located in the sublingual area, palate, tonsils, floor of the orbit, or pharyngeal walls. Management of these injuries requires surgical exploration; cleansing; and, if appropriate, suturing. Trauma to the mandibular or sublingual salivary gland ducts with subsequent sublingual mucocele (ranula) formation is rare in the cat. Lacerations of the cheek or lip are débrided and sutured for apposition of the mucosa and skin.

Lip avulsion is a degloving injury frequently associated with road-traffic trauma or when someone steps on the lip of a usually young cat. The lower lip is more frequently involved than the upper lip.[73] The wound is débrided, and the lip is repositioned. Simple interrupted sutures are made in areas with sufficient remaining gingiva and alveolar mucosa. Large horizontal mattress sutures can be passed around the tooth crowns. Securing the connective tissue side of the degloved lower lip to intermandibular tissues and the mandibular symphysis will decrease dead space and will reduce the likelihood of seroma formation (Figure 21-40).

Electric-cord injury occurs most often in young cats that chew on power cords.[60] Life-threatening airway compromise can result from pulmonary edema, which is caused by smoke inhalation or electrical exposure. Initially, the patient is managed conservatively (lavage with lactated Ringer's solution), and the injured tissues are left to necrose so that the maximum amount of tissue is retained. It can take several days before the extent of

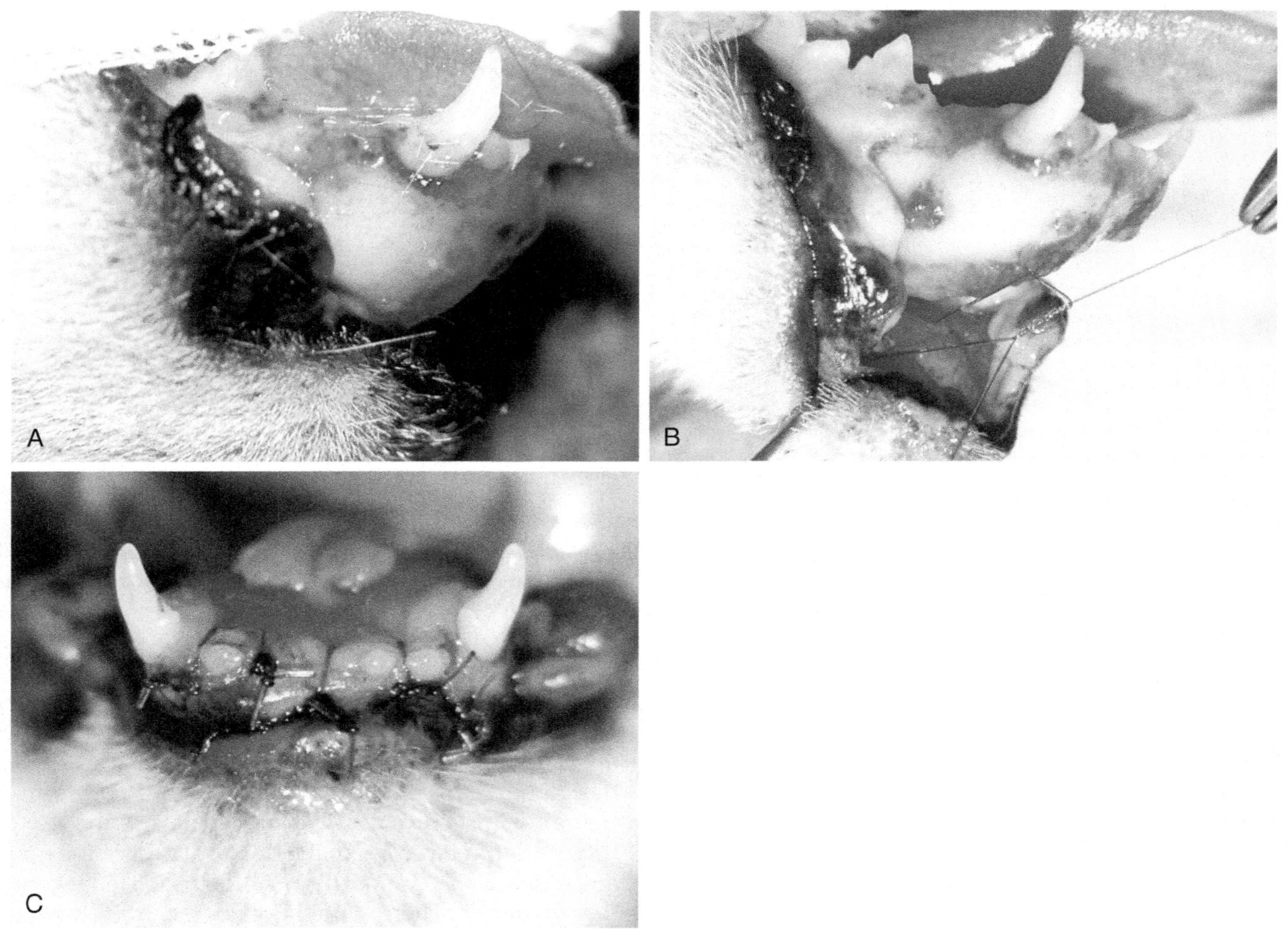

FIGURE 21-40 Kitten with lower lip avulsion. Note the exposed surface of the mandibles **(A)**. Securing the connective tissue side of the degloved lower lip to intermandibular tissues and the mandibular symphysis will decrease dead space and reduce the likelihood of seroma formation **(B)**. Large horizontal mattress sutures can be passed around the tooth crowns **(C)**. *(Copyright 2010 Dr. Alexander M. Reiter; used with permission.)*

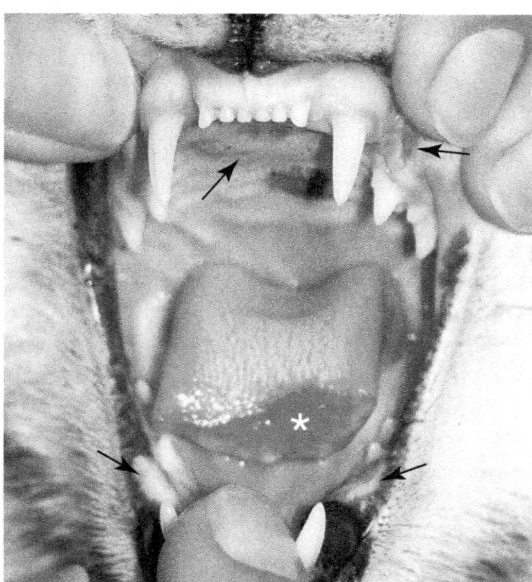

FIGURE 21-41 Kitten presenting for the 1-week reexamination after electric-cord injury. Note that a rostral portion of the lingual body has been lost *(asterisk)*. There are multiple incompletely healed electric burns on the hard palate, alveolar mucosa of the left maxilla, and mucocutaneous junction areas of the lower lips *(arrows)*. *(Copyright 2010 Dr. Alexander M. Reiter; used with permission.)*

local injury is clearly defined. Necrosis of the lips, cheeks, tongue, and hard palate is common (Figure 21-41); more extensive electric burns cause necrosis of dental pulp tissue and maxillary, palatal, or mandibular bones. Once the necrotic tissue is evident, surgical débridement is initiated, which should be conservative to the level of bleeding tissue, allowing time for definitive demarcation of devitalized tissue. Formation of osteonecrosis or oronasal fistula requires further surgery.[60] Possible causes for chemical burns are corrosive chemicals (the cat's skin should also be evaluated) or gastric reflux. The lesions are acute-onset ulcers covered by necrotic debris; initial therapy is lavage with lactated Ringer's solution, followed by conservative management.

Multiple factors influence tissue destruction in cats with gunshot trauma, including projectile mass, velocity, flight instability, and secondary projectiles formed by the primary projectile. Projectiles damage tissue by means of laceration and crushing, shock waves, and cavitation. Bones are shattered, and soft tissue damage can occur well beyond the visible injury as a result of progressive vascular compromise. Control of bleeding and maintenance of airway are initial considerations, followed by careful débridement, removal of projectiles and projectile fragments, and wound closure. Larger wounds may be only temporarily sutured closed to allow tissue swelling to decrease and sloughing of necrotic tissue to take place. Treating the patient conservatively for a few days allows determination of viable tissues available for definitive repair at a later time.

JAW FRACTURES

After stabilization of life-threatening injuries, jaw fractures are evaluated by inspection and palpation of mandibular and maxillary bones and the temporomandibular joints. The head is examined for asymmetry and discontinuity, exophthalmos or enophthalmos, lip avulsions, and facial wounds, and the oral cavity is inspected for mucosal lacerations, fractured and displaced teeth, malocclusion, hematomas, and hemorrhage.

Most mandibular and maxillary fractures can be satisfactorily assessed with size 2 and 4 dental radiographic film. The largest dental radiographic film can also be used in the cat to evaluate injuries to the zygomatic arch, mandibular ramus, and temporomandibular joint and tympanic bulla. Computed tomography is indicated for caudal mandibular fractures, maxillary fractures, and temporomandibular joint injury that cannot be assessed adequately with radiography. Imaging studies of intracranial structures should be considered in any patient with moderate to severe head trauma on presentation, failure to improve, or deterioration of clinical signs.

Mandibular Fractures

Mandibular fractures in cats are typically located in the area of the mandibular symphysis (symphyseal separation or parasymphyseal fracture) or the mandibular ramus (fracture of the condylar process or coronoid process). The midportion of the mandibular body is less often fractured in cats. However, iatrogenic mandibular fracture occurs after extraction of teeth, particularly in the area of the mandibular canines. Unilateral mandibular fractures often result in the lower jaw being deviated toward the side of injury, causing malocclusion. Bilateral mandibular fractures may result in a dropped lower jaw appearance. An oblique mandibular body fracture, with the fracture line running in a rostroventral direction, is relatively stable, insofar as the masticatory muscle forces may hold the fracture segments in apposition (favorable fracture). A mandibular body fracture with the fracture line running in a caudoventral direction is unstable because the muscular forces will lead to displacement of the fracture segments (unfavorable fracture).[63]

Mandibular ramus fractures are relatively stable because the surrounding muscle mass often prevents gross displacement of the fracture segments. Some say that condylar process fractures should be treated with condylectomy. Others suggest letting them heal as pain-free and functional nonunion, but immature and young adult cats with such injuries are at risk to develop temporomandibular joint ankylosis.

Maxillary Fractures

Fractures of the upper jaw are less frequent in cats. Epistaxis, facial swelling, subcutaneous emphysema, pain, and asymmetry are the usual clinical findings. Some cats with head trauma present with an acute traumatic cleft palate, zygomatic arch fracture, or a unilateral separation of the temporal bone from the parietal bone (the latter may often go unnoticed). Combined fractures of the zygomatic arch and the mandibular ramus can result in excess callus formation and ankylotic fusion in young animals, resulting in inability to open the mouth.

Minimally displaced upper jaw fractures may not require surgical repair other than suturing of torn soft tissues. Severely comminuted, depressed, and grossly unstable fractures require surgical intervention. Airway obstruction caused by displaced bones, swelling, or blood can be life-threatening. Cats with respiratory compromise should be placed in an oxygen cage, and the nostrils should be cleaned of blood and discharge and kept unobstructed.

Jaw Fracture Repair

Surgical treatment is aimed at repairing hard and soft tissue injuries, establishing normal masticatory function and providing acceptable cosmesis. Initially, the mouth is flushed with dilute chlorhexidine (0.12%), and the fracture sites are carefully débrided to remove blood clots, food particles, foreign material, small bone fragments, and necrotic tissue. Severely mobile teeth, teeth with advanced periodontitis or periapical disease, and those that interfere with reduction of the jaw fracture should be extracted. If teeth with fracture lines extending along the periodontal ligament space toward the root apex are retained, they should be carefully monitored for evidence of periodontal or endodontic pathology, and appropriate treatment must be instituted as soon as either is recognized. Soft tissue lacerations are sutured or closed after orthopedic repair. Most mandibular and some maxillary fractures are open to the oral cavity, and antibiotic therapy may be considered in selected cases to prevent infection.

Tape or nylon muzzles[55,118] can be used as temporary first-aid treatment while awaiting definitive repair for most mandibular fractures and represent a means of additional support in active patients in which the healing mandible may be subjected to excessive forces. Muzzles may be the sole means of stabilization for mandibular fractures in young cats, minimally displaced mandibular ramus fractures, and pathologic mandibular fractures when the owner declines surgical repair. However, they are contraindicated for maxillary fractures (airway compromise) and maybe also for temporomandibular joint injury (joint immobility may promote temporomandibular joint ankylosis). The tape muzzle is applied snugly enough to maintain the dental interlock but loosely enough (leaving a gap of about 0.5 to 1 cm between the incisal edges of the maxillary and mandibular incisors) to permit the tongue to protrude and lap water and semiliquid food (Figure 21-42).[55,118] Occlusal alignment and stabilization of midbody and caudal mandibular fractures may also be achieved with bis-acryl composite bridges between the maxillary and mandibular canines (or other teeth) (Figure 21-43).[9] Similar to the muzzling technique, a small gap between the maxillary and mandibular incisors should provide space for the tongue to protrude. If the distance between maxillary and mandibular incisors is too wide, the cat may experience difficulty in swallowing food. Other complications of maxillomandibular fixation techniques include dermatitis (only for muzzling), dyspnea, and aspiration pneumonia.[9,63]

Mandibular symphyseal separation or parasymphyseal fractures are repaired with circumferential wiring.[63] A stab incision is made in the chin at the ventral midline. An 18-gauge needle is inserted between bone and soft tissues to exit into the mouth distal to the canine teeth. A 20- to 22-gauge orthopedic wire is passed through the needle. The needle is removed and reinserted on the other side, and the oral wire end is passed through the needle opening. The needle is again removed, the symphysis is held in proper alignment, and the wire ends are twisted below the chin until the lower jaw is stable. The twisted wire is trimmed, and the 0.5- to 1-cm portion of twisted wire is bent caudally so that the skin covers

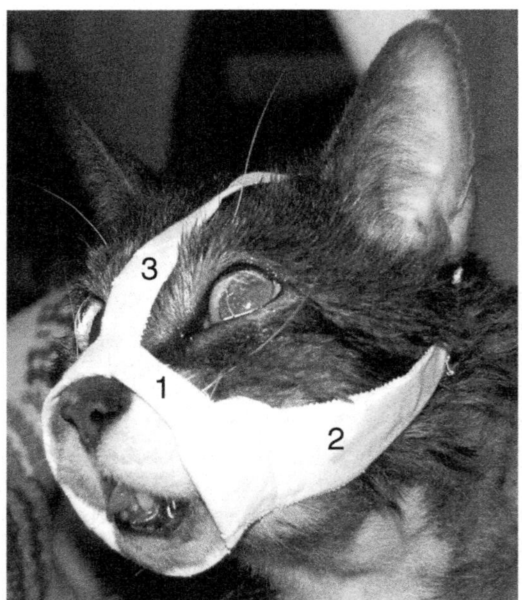

FIGURE 21-42 Cat with mandibular fracture and adhesive tape muzzle in place. Note the three parts of the muzzle: *(1)* loop encircling the upper and lower jaws, *(2)* loop ventral to the ears and around the neck, and *(3)* an additional middle layer running over the forehead. *(Copyright 2010 Dr. Alexander M. Reiter; used with permission.)*

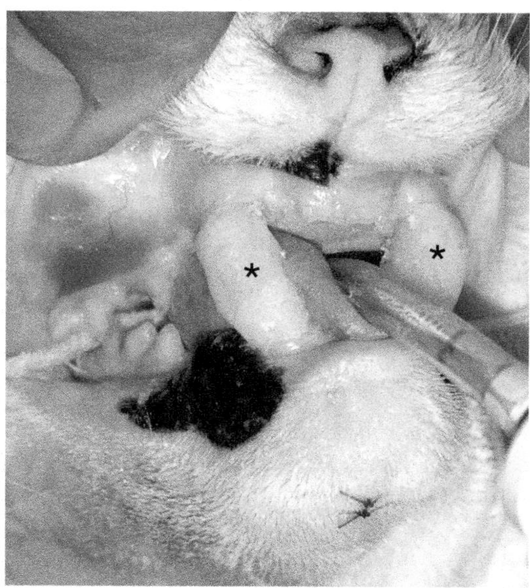

FIGURE 21-43 Cat with mandibular fracture and bis-acryl composite bridges *(asterisks)* between the maxillary and mandibular canines. Note the space between the incisal edges of the maxillary and mandibular incisors to permit the tongue to protrude and lap water and soft food. *(Copyright 2010 Dr. Alexander M. Reiter; used with permission.)*

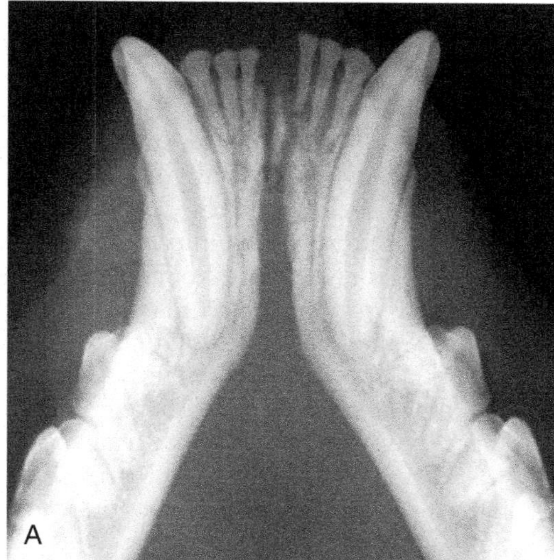

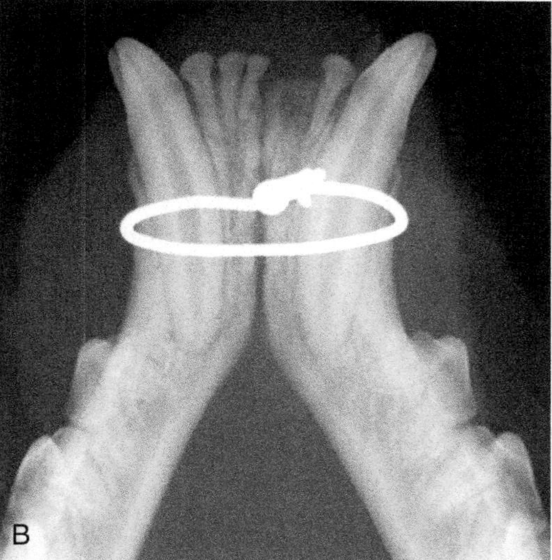

FIGURE 21-44 Dental radiographs of a cat with separation of the mandibular symphysis before treatment **(A)** and after circumferential wiring **(B)**. Note that two mobile incisor teeth had been extracted. *(Copyright 2010 Dr. Alexander M. Reiter; used with permission.)*

it. The wire is removed in about 4 weeks by cutting it intraorally and pulling it out from below the chin (Figure 21-44). Leaving the wire in place for extended periods or overtightening the wire bears the risk of necrosis and resorption of bone around the canine tooth roots. A twisted intraoral wire can be applied between the crowns of the mandibular canine teeth to give additional stabilization.[61] A figure-of-eight wire pattern around the mandibular canine teeth is not recommended because twisting of the wire ends can result in linguoverted canine teeth and long-term malocclusion.

Effective alignment of fracture segments is achieved with interdental wiring techniques, making use of the tooth crowns as anchoring points and providing additional retention surface for splint materials.[53,63] Interdental wiring should never be a stand-alone treatment, but rather should always be followed by intraoral splinting with resin. The teeth should be cleaned with hand or ultrasonic scalers and their surface slightly roughened with course pumice before maxillofacial repair. The Stout multiple-loop wiring technique includes at least two teeth in each fracture segment into the wiring procedure. The size of the orthopedic wire used in cats may range from 24 to 28 gauge. Wire slippage from the teeth can be prevented by using a 20- or 22-gauge needle and placing the wire subgingivally between the teeth. Alternatively, drops of composite can be placed at the gingival third of the mesial and distal crown surfaces of the teeth to create overhangs that allow the wire to remain in position. Loops are situated on the buccal side of the interdental spaces of the maxillary teeth and lingual (or buccal—depending on evaluation of occlusion) sides of the interdental spaces of the mandibular teeth. The wire can be twisted in areas of missing teeth, and looping is continued with the next teeth in line. Once sufficient teeth have been looped, the "static" wire end is threaded through all loops so that both wire ends can be twisted in a pull-and-twist fashion. Finally, all loops are twisted (slight ventral pull for mandibular teeth and dorsal pull for maxillary teeth) and bent interdentally. The modified Risdon wiring technique uses a wire whose middle portion is initially anchored to one tooth. The two wire ends are twisted along the dental arch and anchored again to another tooth. The twisted wire is sutured to gingiva at several locations between the two anchor teeth, which effectively aligns displaced fracture segments before placement of an intraoral resin splint.

Bis-acryl composite is used to fabricate intraoral resin splints. The cleaned teeth are acid etched (to improve attachment of the resin) and air dried. The resin is applied with an applicator gun (syringe with mixing tip) primarily to the lingual surface of mandibular teeth and the labial and buccal surface of maxillary teeth, preferably coronal to the mucogingival junction.[62] Once the material has set, the splint is trimmed and shaped with acrylic burs on low-speed handpieces, allowing for closure of the mouth, and finally polished (Figure 21-45).[53] Because food particles may become trapped between the splint and oral tissues, home oral hygiene is instituted (repeated flushing with dilute chlorhexidine and regular tooth and splint brushing). The splint is removed by interdental sectioning with a bur and detaching the material in segments, using an extraction forceps or luxating elevator. After splint removal, the teeth are cleaned and polished. Gingival inflammation from splint and wire trauma usually subsides within a few days.

Other less commonly employed techniques include osseous wiring, external fixation, and bone plating.[11] Regardless of whether a noninvasive or invasive technique is used to repair a jaw fracture, the occlusion should be assessed and radiographs of the surgical sites obtained before extubation. The cat is discharged on adequate pain control, an Elizabethan collar, and proper feeding instructions. Repair devices are removed after radiographic confirmation of fracture healing, usually 3 (immature and adolescent cats) to 7 weeks postoperatively. Minor occlusal discrepancies after device removal can be corrected by odontoplasty. If malocclusion is severe and prevents closure of the mouth, extraction of one or more teeth will be necessary to restore acceptable masticatory function. Affected jaws and teeth should be reevaluated in 6 and 12 months to determine appropriate healing and ensure periodontal and endodontic health of teeth near jaw fracture lines. Severe jaw fractures in kittens can disturb normal skeletal growth and development of the teeth, resulting in facial deformities and dental abnormalities in the growing cat.

TEMPOROMANDIBULAR JOINT DISORDERS

There are three temporomandibular joint disorders relevant to the cat: temporomandibular joint luxation, open-mouth jaw locking, and temporomandibular joint ankylosis. Luxation of the temporomandibular joint is often confused with open-mouth jaw locking. Both

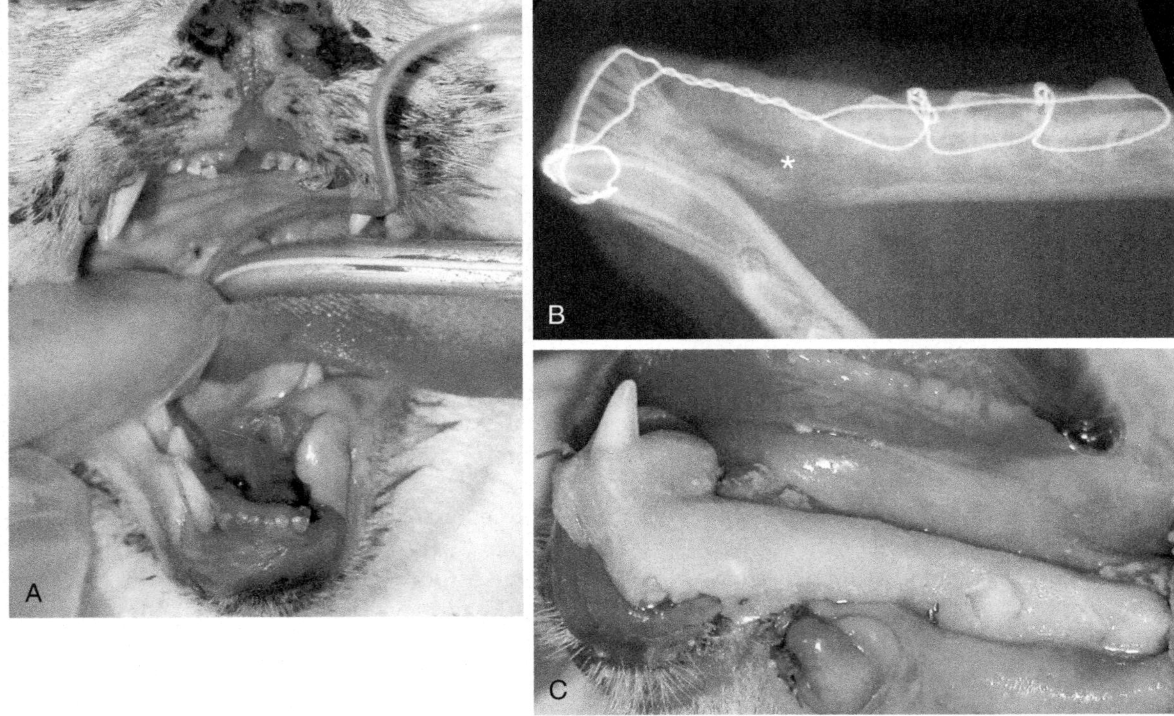

FIGURE 21-45 Clinical photographs and radiograph of cat with severe head trauma. There are maxillary and mandibular fractures **(A).** Jaw fracture repair in the area of the injured and extracted left mandibular canine tooth involved interdental wiring using the Stout multiple-loop technique and twisting *(asterisk)* of the wire ends in edentulous areas **(B)** and intraoral splinting using bis-acryl composite resin **(C).** *(Copyright 2010 Dr. Alexander M. Reiter; used with permission.)*

conditions usually present with inability to close the mouth, but their etiologies, pathophysiologies and treatments are completely different. A definitive diagnosis can be made on the basis of clinical examination and radiography (dorsoventral view). Knowing which condition is present is paramount when formulating a treatment plan. Although temporomandibular joint luxation often may be resolved with a wooden dowel (e.g., a pencil) placed between the maxillary and mandibular carnassial teeth and then closing the jaws, the same treatment will cause further trauma and pain to the cat with open-mouth jaw locking. It should be noted that any trauma to the temporomandibular joint in young cats can lead to joint ankylosis.

Temporomandibular Joint Luxation

Luxation typically occurs as a result of trauma. With rostrodorsal luxation the mandibular condyle moves rostrally and dorsally.[58] As a result, the lower jaw shifts laterorostrally to the contralateral side. Malocclusion will be a presenting clinical sign, resulting in the inability of the animal to close its mouth fully owing to abnormal contact between the maxillary and mandibular teeth. Very well-developed retroarticular processes resist caudal displacement of the mandibular condyle. Consequently, fracture of this structure may be obligatory for caudal luxation to occur (which is rare).

A dorsoventral radiographic view best demonstrates rostrodorsal temporomandibular joint luxation, usually showing an increased width of the joint space and a rostral displacement of the mandibular condyle (Figure 21-46). Lateral oblique views are also useful in establishing a diagnosis. Reduction of rostrodorsal temporomandibular joint luxation in the cat is obtained by placing a pencil between the maxillary fourth premolar and mandibular first molar teeth on the affected side only (pencil acts as a fulcrum) and closing the lower jaw against the pencil while simultaneously easing the jaw caudally. The reduction is often unstable, and a tape muzzle for 2 to 4 weeks may be indicated to prevent the cat from opening the mouth wide, thus reducing the likelihood of recurring displacement. Chronic luxation is treated by condylectomy.[29]

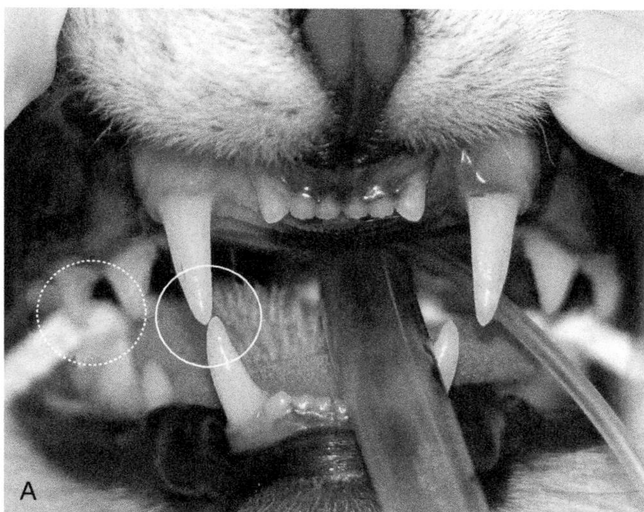

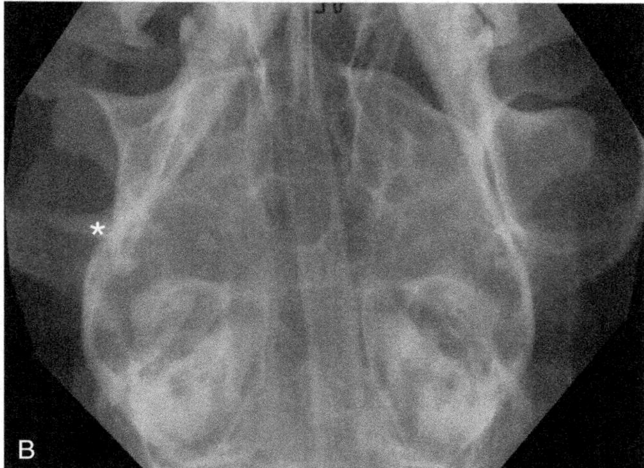

FIGURE 21-46 Cat with rostrodorsal luxation of the left temporomandibular joint. Note inability to fully close the mouth because of contact between maxillary and mandibular canines *(full circle)* and cheek teeth *(interrupted circle)* after shifting of the lower jaw towards the unaffected side **(A)**. Dorsoventral radiographic view shows the condylar process *(asterisk)* of the left mandible being displaced rostrally **(B)**. *(Copyright 2010 Dr. Alexander M. Reiter; used with permission.)*

Open-Mouth Jaw Locking

Dysplasia of the bony or soft tissues of the temporomandibular joint is congenital or acquired during life and has primarily been reported in Persian cats.[93] It may result in increased laxity of the temporomandibular joint capsule and open-mouth jaw locking. Yawning often precipitates an event. The coronoid process of the mandible can flare laterally, locking onto or ventrolateral to the zygomatic arch. In contrast to rostrodorsal temporomandibular joint luxation, there is no contact between maxillary and mandibular teeth, and the cat presents with its mouth wide open (Figure 21-47). The addition of computed tomography is of academic interest and may not be necessary for establishing a diagnosis (Figure 21-48).[93,108]

An ipsilateral protuberance on the ventrolateral aspect of the zygomatic arch may be palpable. Locking occurs on the opposite side of the dysplastic joint. However, both joints can be affected (warranting bilateral surgery), and manual locking of the apparently unaffected side should be attempted under chemical restraint before surgical treatment. Open-mouth jaw locking can also occur without temporomandibular joint dysplasia as a result of traumatic events that caused

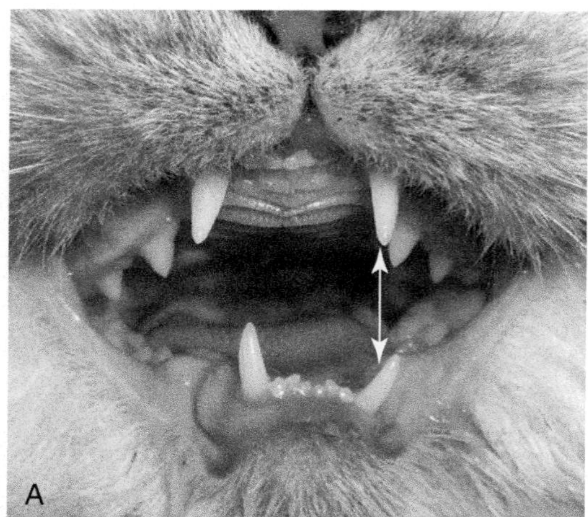

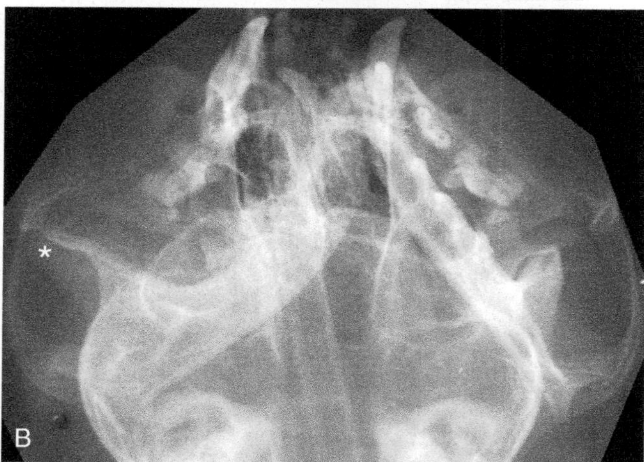

FIGURE 21-47 Cat with open-mouth jaw locking on the left side. Note shifting of the lower jaw toward the affected side (with the left mandibular dental arch farther ventral compared with that on the right) and inability to close the mouth, which is held wide open *(double-ended arrow)* without any contact between maxillary and mandibular teeth **(A)**. Dorsoventral radiographic view shows the coronoid process *(asterisk)* of the left mandible being locked ventrolateral to the zygomatic arch **(B)**. *(Copyright 2010 Dr. Alexander M. Reiter; used with permission.)*

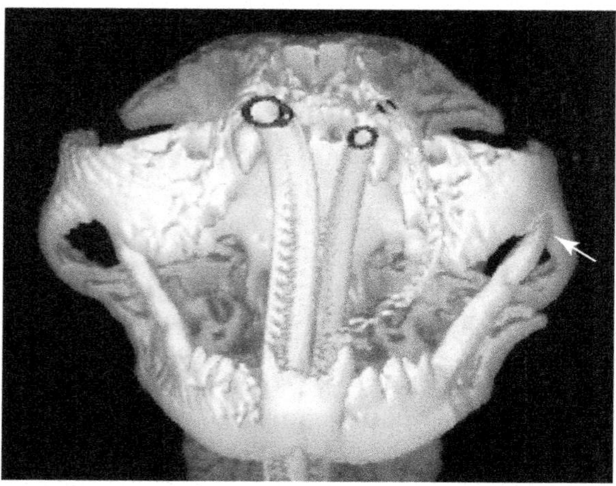

FIGURE 21-48 Computed tomography (three-dimensional reconstruction) performed in a cat with open-mouth jaw locking, demonstrating the coronoid process of the left mandible being locked ventrolateral to the zygomatic arch *(arrow)*. *(From Reiter AM: Symphysiotomy, symphysiectomy and intermandibular arthrodesis in a cat with open-mouth jaw locking: case report and literature review,* J Vet Dent *21:147, 2004; used with permission.)*

flattening of or excessive callus formation at the zygomatic arch, malunion fracture of the mandibular body, and increased mandibular symphyseal laxity.[93]

Acute treatment of open-mouth jaw locking consists of opening the mouth further (sedation may be needed) to release the coronoid process from the ventrolateral aspect of the zygomatic arch and then closing the mouth. Tape muzzling is a temporary solution. Definitive surgical treatment involves partial coronoidectomy, partial zygomectomy, or preferably a combination of both.[93] A curvilinear incision is made parallel to the zygomatic arch, muscle attachments are dissected from the bone with a periosteal elevator, and the coronoid process locked ventrolateral to it is identified. A segment of the zygomatic arch is removed with a rongeur. The same instrument is then used to remove a portion of the coronoid process, followed by closure of the surgical site. It is helpful to grab the coronoid process, once identified, with a small towel clamp so that it can be readily found after partial zygomectomy.[93]

Temporomandibular Joint Ankylosis

Progressive inability to open the mouth usually occurs as a complication after trauma to the temporomandibular joint. True or intracapsular ankylosis is fusion of hard tissues within the temporomandibular joint capsule. Radiographic features are loss of temporomandibular joint space, irregular mandibular condyle contour, and extensive new bone formation. Treatment consists of condylectomy and excision of all associated callus (which often extends extracapsularly).[2,74,89] Transposing adjacent muscle tissue or packing fat transplants into the space between the cut bony surfaces may be helpful in avoiding or reducing reankylosis. Postoperative care includes physical therapy (repeated mouth opening several times a day) and use of glucocorticosteroids (that slow down healing capacity of connective tissue such as bone). Oral prednisolone is given at 1 to 2 mg/kg daily divided in two doses for 1 week and then tapered to 0.25 to 0.5 mg/kg once a day over a 4-week period. Injection of repository triamcinolone into each surgery site can be used if oral prednisolone is not satisfactory.

Excessive callus formation during healing of fractures of the zygomatic arch and mandibular ramus can also lead to progressive inability to open the mouth without temporomandibular joint involvement. Such false or extracapsular ankylosis may also be a sequela of extensive new bone formation associated with otitis media. Surgical treatment depends on the nature and location of the ankylotic lesion and often requires resection of zygomatic arch, coronoid process, condylar process, and excessive new bone.

ORAL AND MAXILLOFACIAL TUMORS

Oral and maxillofacial tumors may be benign (noninvasive or invasive with no metastasis) or malignant (invasive and with metastasis) and may be of dental (odontogenic; epithelial, mesenchymal, or mixed) or nondental origin.[102] Geriatric cats are generally predisposed to oral and maxillofacial tumors, but there are certain tumors that typically occur in adolescent and young adult cats (e.g., inductive fibroameloblastoma typically in the rostral maxilla of cats younger than 2 years old). Odontogenic tumors can occur at any age, but tumors in young cats are more likely to be of odontogenic origin.

Clinical complaints may be absent with benign tumors, but dysphagia, drooling, bloody oral discharge, halitosis, and weight loss are often reported with malignant tumors. There may be an obvious proliferative mass or swelling of the mandible or maxilla. Daily home oral hygiene by the owner and professional oral examination at every patient visit by the veterinarian is imperative in early tumor detection.

Benign Lesions

Benign oral and maxillofacial tumors are less common in cats, but osteoma, lipoma, peripheral odontogenic fibroma, giant cell epulis, ameloblastoma, inductive fibroameloblastoma (feline inductive odontogenic tumor), amyloid-producing odontogenic tumor, and plasmacytoma are occasionally seen.[32,34,35] *Epulis* (plural, *epulides)* is a nonspecific, clinical term referring to a local, exophytic growth on the gingiva that could present non-neoplastic or neoplastic disease (benign or malignant). Therefore its use is discouraged without the addition of descriptive adjectives. The nature and origin of so-called multiple feline epulides are controversial. Some consider these gingival proliferations to be benign neoplasms[16,19]; others suggest that they arise from the periosteum and represent inflammatory lesions (reacting to plaque, calculus, and other irritation).[33]

Malignant Lesions

The predominant malignant oral and maxillofacial tumor in cats is squamous cell carcinoma (SCC),[111] which—if occurring on the lower jaw—often presents as mandibular swelling (with bone invasion and "sunburst" formation) (Figure 21-49), but often without significant intraoral soft tissue proliferation. If occurring on the upper jaw (there often is a history of a nonhealing tooth extraction site), SCC usually is nonprotuberant, with severe bone invasion into the maxilla, orbit, and zygomatic arch. SCC tends to be more proliferative and ulcerated when located on the lips, cheeks, tongue, and sublingual region. Lingual and sublingual SCC often extends into the caudal body or the root of the tongue, making it firm and non-elastic on palpation. Metastasis to regional lymph nodes is common, and distant metastasis may occur late in the disease process. The average age of onset is 10 years, and occurrence of SCC in cats has been associated with exposure to flea collars, high intake of canned food, regular ingestion of canned tuna, and environmental tobacco smoke.[10,107] History and clinical signs include mobile teeth, nonhealing extraction sites, swelling of the mandible or maxilla, oral ulceration and bleeding, halitosis, and dysphagia if

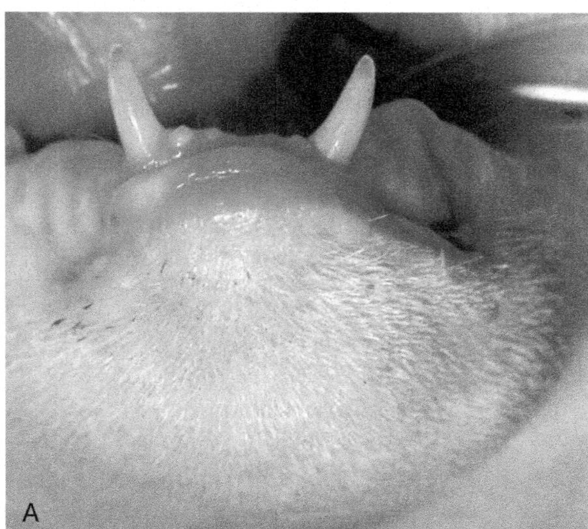

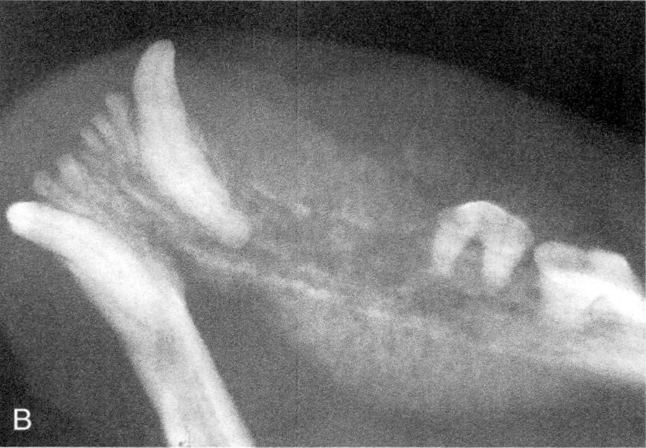

FIGURE 21-49 Cat with mandibular squamous cell carcinoma. Swelling of the lower jaw without significant intraoral soft tissue proliferation is commonly seen with this type of tumor **(A)**. Radiograph of the left mandible showing bone destruction and sunburst effect, and the third premolar tooth is missing **(B)**. *(Copyright 2010 Dr. Alexander M. Reiter; used with permission.)*

the mass is large enough to affect masticatory function. Fibrosarcoma, osteosarcoma, hemangiosarcoma, and lymphosarcoma are less common oral and maxillofacial tumors, and malignant melanoma is very rare in the mouths of cats.[102]

Differential Diagnoses

Many differential diagnoses can mimic oral and maxillofacial tumors. Normal anatomy should be distinguished from pathology (e.g., incisive papilla caudal to maxillary incisors, lingual molar gland caudolingual to the mandibular first molar teeth). If the suspicious lesion is located directly on the midline or bilateral, an anatomy textbook should be consulted and normal structures ruled out before performing a biopsy.

Other non-neoplastic differential diagnoses include scar tissue (usually on oral mucosa along bite planes or the tongue), eosinophilic lesions (granuloma and ulcer), healing wounds (granulation tissue), inflammatory lesions (e.g., ulcers), foreign bodies, apical abscess, cellulitis, osteomyelitis, gingival hyperplasia (abnormal increase in the number of normal cells in a normal arrangement that results clinically in gingival enlargement), dentigerous cyst (arising in an area of a tooth that has not erupted), odontomas (conglomerate of disorganized normal tissue cells), edema, and sialoceles (extravasation of saliva into submucosal or subcutaneous tissues as a result of trauma to salivary ducts or gland capsule).[38]

Staging, Oral Examination, and Biopsy

Thoracic radiographs should be obtained of any patient in which oral and maxillofacial cancer is suspected. Abdominal ultrasound may be added in selected cases. Regional lymph node enlargement indicates either tumor metastasis or reactivity related to oral inflammation. Enlarged lymph nodes should be evaluated by fine-needle aspiration or excisional biopsy. A negative lymph node biopsy does not preclude the possibility of regional metastasis, which may occur along perineural or vascular routes, or metastasis to other, less accessible lymph nodes.[51]

Oral examination focuses on the location, size, extent, and surface characteristics of the lesion, which may be smooth, irregular, pigmented, inflamed, ulcerated, bleeding, or necrotic. Teeth may be displaced or missing. Some cats have difficulty opening (when rostral movement of the coronoid process of the mandible is inhibited or the temporomandibular joint is involved) or fully closing the mouth (when opposing teeth bite into the intraoral tumor), and appetite and activity level may be affected. Decreased ability to retropulse the eye globes is often noted in the case of maxillary, retroorbital, and caudal pharyngeal masses. Radiography of the jaws and head (using standard film or sizes 2 and 4 dental film) will further define the extent of oral and maxillofacial tumors. Computed tomography is particularly helpful in cats with maxillary and caudal mandibular tumors and for the assessment of regional lymph nodes.

Suspect lesions should be sampled for examination.[102] A biopsy is preferably obtained from an area that can be included in the definitive resection. If cytologic or histologic results do not match the clinical findings, a second, deeper, and larger specimen is obtained. Cytologic techniques are often performed with a 22-gauge needle by means of a needle biopsy ("woodpecker method") or needle aspiration. Impression smears and scrapings may be of value only if obtained from the cut surface of a tumor. Instruments for histologic sampling include rongeurs, disposable open-ended skin biopsy punches, and cold scalpel blades for incisional or excisional biopsy. Multiple samples should be obtained. Hemostasis is achieved by digital pressure, and biopsy sites of more deeply invading tumors are sutured. For adequate fixation the specimen is placed in 10% buffered formalin at a ratio of one part tissue to 10 parts fixative.[102]

Laboratory workup before definitive surgery should include complete blood cell count and biochemical profile. Urinalysis, blood typing and cross-matching, coagulation profiles, and buccal mucosa bleeding time are performed in selected cases. The client must be informed about intraoperative and postoperative complications, follow-up care, long-term function, quality of life, and prognosis.

Treatment

Marginal resection with small amounts of unaffected surrounding tissue is restricted to small and benign oral and maxillofacial tumors. Radical surgery (mandibulectomy, maxillectomy, glossectomy, and wide lip and cheek resection) of invasive and malignant tumors should include at least 1 cm of apparently healthy tissue (including skin) surrounding the neoplastic lesion.[113] The use of electrocautery along wound edges that will be sutured is to be avoided. Wound closure depends on tissues available for creation of flaps (mucosa, skin, local, and distant). Combined therapy (surgery plus radiotherapy or chemotherapy or both) may be indicated, particularly for tumors with regional or distant metastasis.[76] When surgical excision is not an option, efforts should be made to decrease the rate of growth (radiotherapy, chemotherapy) and provide relief from discomfort (extraction of teeth impinging on the tumor, administration of pain medications).* Expression of cyclooxygenase (COX) in feline oral SCC has been

*References 15, 30, 31, 49, 57, 76, 119.

determined,[23,48] and the use of COX inhibitors such as piroxicam and meloxicam for cancer palliation may thus provide a survival advantage. Concurrent use of corticosteroids should be avoided, and gastric protectants such as misoprostol should be considered.

The relatively small size of the head of the cat, the proximity of the upper jaw to the nasal cavity and orbit, and the rather short and tight upper lips (limiting the amount of soft tissue available for wound closure) make radical maxillectomy far more challenging in the cat than in the dog. Therefore maxillectomy in the cat is often reserved to small and rostrally located tumors of the upper jaw. Mid and caudal maxillary malignancies could appear small on clinical examination, but they have a tendency to invade the nasal cavity, orbit, and zygomatic arch. In addition to that, surgical efficiency is critical when performing maxillectomies because bleeding may not be controlled effectively until the affected piece of jaw is removed. Bone should initially be scored with power instruments (rotating burs; sagittal and oscillating saws) or an osteotome and mallet, followed by the use of leverage with an appropriate instrument to break the remaining bony attachments. This approach prevents injury to nasal mucosa and allows for safe ligation of vessels within the infraorbital (or mandibular, in the case of partial mandibulectomy) canals. Diffuse bleeding from nasal mucosa may respond to wound irrigation with 0.05 to 0.1 mL/kg of a mixture of 0.25 mL phenylephrine 1% and 50 mL lidocaine 2%. When there is insufficient lip and cheek mucoperiosteum available for wound closure, distant flaps will be necessary to close the maxillectomy site.

Unilateral and bilateral rostral mandibulectomy just distal to the canine teeth provides good function and cosmesis in cats.[87] Bilateral resection caudal to this level or unilateral mandibular body resection results in loss of the mandibular symphysis, "floating" of the remaining mandibular sections, and progressively greater problems with tongue retention, eating, and grooming. In the case of unilateral total mandibulectomy,[113] the mandibular symphysis is separated with a scalpel blade. Incisions are made well away from the tumor in the oral mucosa and skin, and the mandible is undermined by blunt dissection. The lateral attachments of the tongue are separated, and mandibular and sublingual salivary ducts are ligated when transected. This frees the mandible for further dissection of the masseter and pterygoid muscles from their attachments. The inferior alveolar artery and vein entering and exiting the mandibular canal through the mandibular foramen at the medial aspect of the mandible are ligated and transected. The temporomandibular joint capsule is incised, temporal muscle attachments on the coronoid process are dissected free, and the mandible is lifted out. The incision is closed with synthetic absorbable monofilament sutures, apposing connective tissue and oral mucosal edges (Figure 21-50). After more

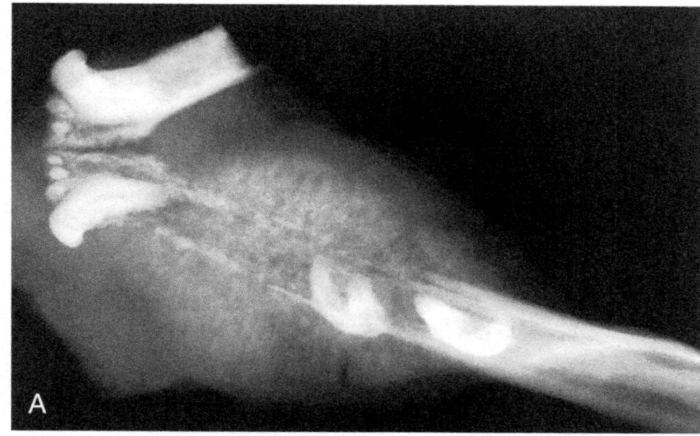

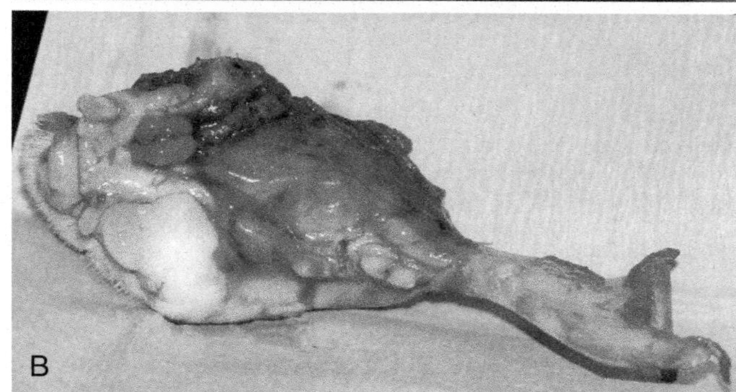

FIGURE 21-50 Radiograph **(A)** and clinical photograph of resected specimen **(B)** of cat in Figure 21-49 undergoing left total and right partial mandibulectomy. *(Copyright 2010 Dr. Alexander M. Reiter; used with permission.)*

involved unilateral mandibulectomy procedures, two complications should be addressed, preferably at the time of resective surgery. The opposite mandible will swing over toward the midline, which may result in the remaining mandibular canine tooth to impinge on the palate when the mouth is closed; to avoid this, the tooth is extracted or its crown surgically reduced, followed by vital pulp therapy. The tongue also may lose its ventrolateral support and hang out of the mouth, resulting in drooling and chronic dermatitis. This can be prevented by ipsilateral, rostral advancement of the lip commissure to form a fold that contains the tongue (commissuroplasty).

Wound dehiscence 2 to 3 days after surgery usually results from tension on suture lines or compromised vascularity of flaps. Freshly dehisced flaps are resutured after further undermining to eliminate tension. Closure of chronic oronasal defects should be performed after complete healing of surrounding soft tissues has occurred. Postoperative pain is controlled with a combination of centrally acting opioids and nonsteroidal antiinflammatory medications. Injectable or oral opioids are supplemented until fentanyl from a transdermal patch achieves an adequate level in the blood.[5] Antibiotic treatment is not required after oral and maxillofacial

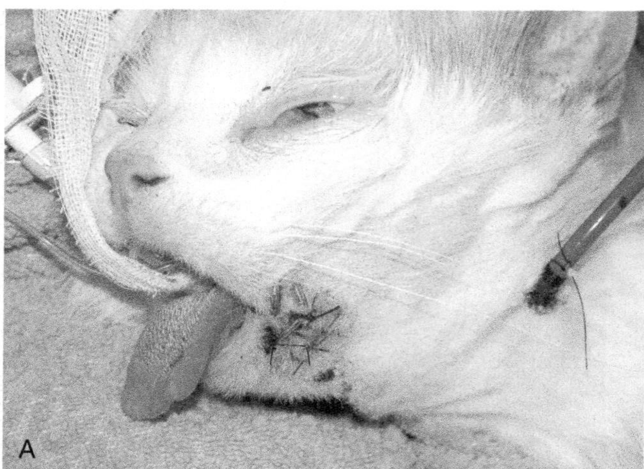

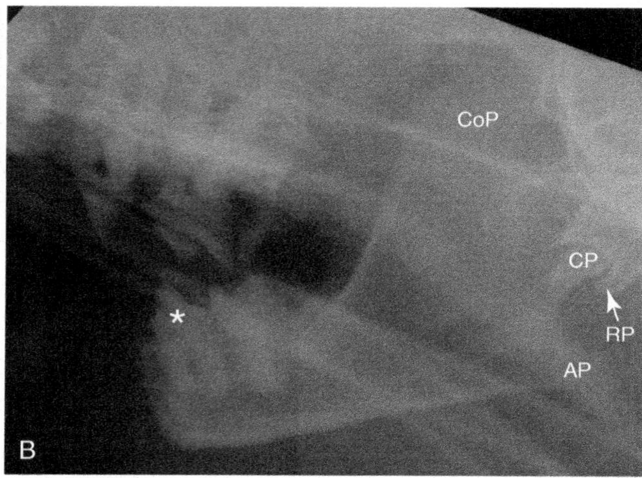

FIGURE 21-51 Clinical photograph of cat in Figure 21-49 2 weeks after left total and right partial mandibulectomy, left commissuroplasty (tension-relieving sutures still in place), and esophageal feeding tube placement **(A)**. Radiograph **(B)** revealing extent of mandibular resection just rostral to the right mandibular fourth premolar tooth *(asterisk)*. *CoP,* Coronoid process; *CP,* condylar process; *RP,* retroarticular process; *AP,* angular process. *(Copyright 2010 Dr. Alexander M. Reiter; used with permission.)*

surgeries in the otherwise healthy cat. Broad-spectrum antibiotics are given perioperatively in debilitated and immunosuppressed patients and those suffering from organ disease, endocrine disorders, cardiovascular disease, severely contaminated wounds, and systemic infections.

Water is offered once the animal has recovered from anesthesia. Soft food is offered 12 to 24 hours after surgery and maintained for about 2 weeks.[102] The cat may require several days to adapt to the changed circumstances in its mouth before being willing to eat normally. An esophageal feeding tube will provide proper nutrition during the immediate postoperative period. Chlorhexidine digluconate solution or gel (0.12%) is administered into the mouth for 2 to 3 weeks. An Elizabethan collar may be used to prevent disruption of the surgical sites. Reexaminations (including palpation of head and neck lymph nodes) are scheduled at 2 weeks (removal of skin sutures) and 2, 6, and 12 months postoperatively and then once annually (Figure 21-51). After the histopathologic results arrive, collaboration with an oncologist is helpful to discuss the need for further treatment (surgery, radiation therapy, and chemotherapy). Thoracic radiographs are repeated as necessary to monitor for distant metastasis.

References

1. Addie DD, Radford A, Yam PS et al: Cessation of feline calicivirus shedding coincident with resolution of chronic gingivostomatitis in a cat, *J Small Anim Pract* 44:172, 2003.
2. Anderson MA, Orsini PG, Harvey CE: Temporomandibular ankylosis: treatment by unilateral condylectomy in two dogs and two cats, *J Vet Dent* 13:23, 1996.
3. Bar-Am Y, Pollard RE, Kass PH et al: The diagnostic yield of conventional radiographs and computed tomography in dogs and cats with maxillofacial trauma, *Vet Surg* 37:294, 2008.
4. Beckman BW: Engine driven rotary instrumentation for endodontic therapy in a cat, *J Vet Dent* 21:88, 2004.
5. Beckman BW: Pathophysiology and management of surgical and chronic oral pain in dogs and cats, *J Vet Dent* 23:50, 2006.
6. Beckman B, Legendre L: Regional nerve blocks for oral surgery in companion animals, *Comp Cont Ed Pract Vet* 24:439, 2002.
7. Beebe DE, Gengler WR: Osseous surgery to augment treatment of chronic periodontitis of canine teeth in a cat, *J Vet Dent* 24:30, 2007.
8. Bellows J: *Feline dentistry—oral assessment, treatment, and preventative care*, ed 1, Ames, Iowa, 2010, Wiley-Blackwell.
9. Bennett JW, Kapatkin AS, Marretta SM: Dental composite for the fixation of mandibular fractures and luxations in 11 cats and 6 dogs, *Vet Surg* 23:190, 1994.
10. Bertone ER, Snyder LA, Moore AS: Environmental and lifestyle risk factors for oral squamous cell carcinoma in domestic cats, *J Vet Intern Med* 17:557, 2003.
11. Bilgili H, Kurum B: Treatment of fractures of the mandible and maxilla by mini titanium plate fixation systems in dogs and cats, *Aust Vet J* 81:671, 2003.
12. Blazejewski S, Lewis JR, Reiter AM: Mucoperiosteal flap for extraction of multiple teeth in the maxillary quadrant of the cat, *J Vet Dent* 23:200, 2006.
13. Booij-Vrieling HE, Ferbus D, Tryfonidou MA et al: Increased vitamin D-driven signalling and expression of the vitamin D receptor, MSX2, and RANKL in tooth resorption in cats, *Eur J Oral Sci* 118:39, 2010.
14. Booij-Vrieling HE, Tryfonidou MA, Riemers FM et al: Inflammatory cytokines and the nuclear vitamin D receptor are implicated in the pathophysiology of dental resorptive lesions in cats, *Vet Immunol Immunopathol* 132:160, 2009.
15. Bregazzi VS, LaRue SM, Powers BE et al: Response of feline oral squamous cell carcinoma to palliative radiation therapy, *Vet Radiol Ultrasound* 42:77, 2001.
16. de Bruijn ND, Kirpensteijn J, Neyens IJ et al: A clinicopathological study of 52 feline epulides, *Vet Pathol* 44:161, 2007.
17. Clarke DE: Clinical and microbiological effects of oral zinc ascorbate gel in cats, *J Vet Dent* 18:177, 2001.

18. Clarke DE: Drinking water additive decreases plaque and calculus accumulation in cats, *J Vet Dent* 23:79, 2006.
19. Colgin LM, Schulman FY, Dubielzig RR: Multiple epulides in 13 cats, *Vet Pathol* 38:227, 2001.
20. Cox CL, Hunt GB, Cadier MM: Repair of oronasal fistulae using auricular cartilage grafts in five cats, *Vet Surg* 36:164, 2007.
21. Crossley DA: Tooth enamel thickness in the mature dentition of domestic dogs and cats—preliminary study, *J Vet Dent* 12:111, 1995.
22. DeBowes LJ: Simple and surgical exodontia, *Vet Clin North Am Small Anim Pract* 35:963, 2005.
23. DiBernardi L, Dore M, Davis JA et al: Study of feline oral squamous cell carcinoma: potential target for cyclooxigenase inhibitor treatment, *Prostaglandins Leukot Essent Fatty Acids* 76:245, 2007.
24. Dowers KL, Hawley JR, Brewer MM et al: Association of *Bartonella* species, feline calicivirus, and feline herpesvirus 1 infection with gingivostomatitis in cats, *J Feline Med Surg* 12:314, 2010.
25. DuPont GA: Prevention of periodontal disease, *Vet Clin North Am Small Anim Pract* 28:1129, 1998.
26. DuPont GA: Crown amputation with intentional root retention for dental resorptive lesions in cats, *J Vet Dent* 19:107, 2002.
27. DuPont GA, DeBowes LJ: Comparison of periodontitis and root replacement in cat teeth with resorptive lesions, *J Vet Dent* 19:71, 2002.
28. DuPont GA, DeBowes LJ: *Atlas of dental radiography in dogs and cats*, ed 1, St Louis, 2009, Saunders.
29. Eisner ER: Bilateral mandibular condylectomy in a cat, *J Vet Dent* 12:23, 1995.
30. Fidel JL, Sellon RK, Houston RK et al: A nine-day accelerated radiation protocol for feline squamous cell carcinoma, *Vet Radiol Ultrasound* 48:482, 2007.
31. Fox LE, Rosenthal RC, King RR et al: Use of cis-bis-neodecanoato-trans-R,R-1,2-diaminocyclohexane platinum (II), a liposomal cisplatin analogue, in cats with oral squamous cell carcinoma, *Am J Vet Res* 61:791, 2000.
32. Gardner DG: Ameloblastoma in cats: a critical evaluation of the literature and the addition of one example, *J Oral Pathol Med* 27:39, 1998.
33. Gardner DG: Odontogenic tumors in animals with emphasis on dogs and cats, *Proc Eur Cong Vet Dent* 11:16, 2002.
34. Gardner DG, Dubielzig RR: Feline inductive odontogenic tumor (inductive fibroameloblastoma)—a tumor unique to cats, *J Oral Pathol Med* 24:185, 1995.
35. Gardner DG, Dubielzig RR, McGee EV: The so called calcifying epithelial odontogenic tumour in dogs and cats (amyloid-producing odontogenic tumour), *J Comp Pathol* 111:221, 1994.
36. Gawor JP, Reiter AM, Jodkowska K et al: Influence of diet on oral health in cats and dogs, *J Nutr* 136:2021S, 2006.
37. Gendler A, Lewis JR, Reetz JA et al: Computed tomographic features of oral squamous cell carcinoma in cats: 18 cases (2002-2008), *J Am Vet Med Assoc* 236:319, 2010.
38. Gioso MA, Gomes Carvalho VG: Maxillary dentigerous cyst in a cat, *J Vet Dent* 20:28, 2003.
39. Girard N, Southerden P, Hennet P: Root canal treatment in dogs and cats, *J Vet Dent* 23:148, 2006.
40. Gorrel C, Inskeep G, Inskeep T: Benefits of a "dental hygiene chew" on the periodontal health of cats, *J Vet Dent* 15:135, 1998.
41. Gorrel C, Larsson A: Feline odontoclastic resorptive lesions: unveiling the early lesion, *J Small Anim Pract* 43:482, 2002.
42. Gracis M: Radiographic study of the maxillary canine tooth of four mesaticephalic cats, *J Vet Dent* 16:115, 1999.
43. Gross ME, Pope ER, Jarboe JM et al: Regional anesthesia of the infraorbital and inferior alveolar nerves during noninvasive tooth pulp stimulation in halothane-anesthetized cats, *Am J Vet Res* 61:1245, 2000.
44. Hale FA, Anthony JMG: Prevention of hypothermia in cats during routine oral hygiene procedures, *Can Vet J* 38:297, 1997.
45. Harvey CE: Management of periodontal disease: understanding the options, *Vet Clin North Am Small Anim Pract* 35:819, 2005.
46. Harvey CE, Emily PP: *Small animal dentistry*, ed 1, St Louis, 1993, Mosby.
47. Harvey CE, Flax BM: Feline oral-dental radiographic examination and interpretation, *Vet Clin North Am Small Anim Pract* 22:1279, 1992.
48. Hayes A, Scase T, Miller J et al: COX-1 and COX-2 expression in feline oral squamous cell carcinoma, *J Comp Pathol* 135:93, 2006.
49. Hayes AM, Adams VJ, Scase TJ et al: Survival of 54 cats with oral squamous cell carcinoma in United Kingdom general practice, *J Small Anim Pract* 48:394, 2007.
50. Hennet P: Chronic gingivo-stomatitis in cats: long-term follow-up of 30 cases treated by dental extractions, *J Vet Dent* 14:15, 1997.
51. Herring ES, Smith MM, Robertson JL: Lymph node staging of oral and maxillofacial neoplasms in 31 dogs and cats, *J Vet Dent* 19:122, 2002.
52. Holmstrom SE: Feline endodontics, *Vet Clin North Am Small Anim Pract* 22:1433, 1992.
53. Holmstrom SE, Frost PF, Eisner ER: *Veterinary dental techniques for the small animal practitioner*, ed 3, Philadelphia, 2004, Saunders.
54. How KL, Hazewinkel AW, Mol JA: Dietary vitamin D dependence of cat and dog due to inadequate cutaneous synthesis of vitamin D, *Gen Comp Endocrinol* 96:12, 1994.
55. Howard PE: Tape muzzle for mandibular fractures, *Vet Med Small Anim Clin* 76:517, 1981.
56. Ingham KE, Gorrel C, Bierer TL: Effect of a dental chew on dental substrates and gingivitis in cats, *J Vet Dent* 19:201, 2002.
57. Jones PD, de Lorimier LP, Kitchell BE et al: Gemcitabine as a radiosensitizer for nonresectable feline oral squamous cell carcinoma, *J Am Anim Hosp Assoc* 39:463, 2003.
58. Klima LJ: Temporomandibular joint luxation in the cat, *J Vet Dent* 24:198, 2007.
59. Lantz GC: Regional anesthesia for dentistry and oral surgery, *J Vet Dent* 20:181, 2003.
60. Legendre LFJ: Management and long term effects of electrocution in a cat's mouth, *J Vet Dent* 10(3):6, 1993.
61. Legendre L: Use of maxillary and mandibular splints for restoration of normal occlusion following jaw trauma in a cat: a case report, *J Vet Dent* 15:179, 1998.
62. Legendre L: Intraoral acrylic splints for maxillofacial fracture repair, *J Vet Dent* 20:70, 2003.
63. Legendre L: Maxillofacial fracture repairs, *Vet Clin North Am Small Anim Pract* 35:985, 2005.
64. Lewis JR, Miller BR: Dentistry and oral surgery, In Bassert JM, McCurnin DM, editors: *McCurnin's clinical textbook for veterinary technicians*, ed 7, St Louis, 2010, Saunders, p 1093.
65. Lewis JR, Okuda A, Pachtinger G et al: Significant association between tooth extrusion and tooth resorption in domestic cats, *J Vet Dent* 25:86, 2008.
66. Lewis JR, Reiter AM: Anatomy and physiology, In Niemiec BA, editor: *Small animal dental, oral and maxillofacial disease*, ed 1, London, 2010, Manson Publishing Ltd., p 9.
67. Lewis JR, Tsugawa AJ, Reiter AM: Use of CO_2 laser as an adjunctive treatment for caudal stomatitis in a cat, *J Vet Dent* 24:240, 2007.
68. Lommer MJ, Verstraete FJ: Prevalence of odontoclastic resorption lesions and periapical radiographic lucencies in cats: 265 cases (1995-1998), *J Am Vet Med Assoc* 217:1866, 2000.
69. Lommer MJ, Verstraete FJ: Radiographic patterns of periodontitis in cats: 147 cases (1998-1999), *J Am Vet Med Assoc* 218:230, 2001.
70. Lommer MJ, Verstraete FJ: Concurrent oral shedding of feline calicivirus and feline herpesvirus 1 in cats with chronic gingivostomatitis, *Oral Microbiol Immunol* 18:131, 2003.
71. Lyon KF: Gingivostomatitis, *Vet Clin North Am Small Anim Pract* 35:891, 2005.

72. Marretta SM, Grove TK, Grillo JF: Split palatal U-flap: a new technique for repair of caudal hard palate defects, *J Vet Dent* 8(1):5, 1991.
73. Masztis PS: Repair of labial avulsion in a cat, *J Vet Dent* 10(1):14, 1993.
74. Meomartino L, Fatone G, Brunetti A et al: Temporomandibular ankylosis in the cat: a review of seven cases, *J Small Anim Pract* 40:7, 1999.
75. Mohn KL, Jacks TM, Schleim KD et al: Alendronate binds to tooth root surfaces and inhibits progression of feline tooth resorption: a pilot proof-of-concept study, *J Vet Dent* 26:74, 2009.
76. Moore A: Treatment choices for oral cancer in cats. What is possible? What is reasonable? *J Feline Med Surg* 11:23, 2009.
77. Morris JG: Vitamin D synthesis by kittens, *Vet Clin Nutr* 3(3):88, 1996.
78. Morris JG: Ineffective vitamin D synthesis in cats is reversed by an inhibitor of 7-dehydrocholesterol-delta7-reductase, *J Nutr* 129:903, 1999.
79. Morris JG, Earle KE, Anderson PA: Plasma 25-hydroxyvitamin D in growing kittens is related to dietary intake of cholecalciferol, *J Nutr* 129:909, 1999.
80. Negro VB, Hernandez SZ, Maresca BM et al: Furcation canals of the maxillary fourth premolar and the mandibular first molar teeth in cats, *J Vet Dent* 21:10, 2004.
81. Niemiec BA: Fundamentals of endodontics, *Vet Clin North Am Small Anim Pract* 35:837, 2005.
82. Niemiec BA: Digital dental radiography, *J Vet Dent* 24:192, 2007.
83. Niemiec BA, Furman R: Feline dental radiography, *J Vet Dent* 21:252, 2004.
84. Niemiec BA, Gilbert T, Sabatino D: Equipment and basic geometry of dental radiography, *J Vet Dent* 21:48, 2004.
85. Niemiec BA, Mulligan TW: Vital pulp therapy, *J Vet Dent* 18:154, 2001.
86. Niemiec BA, Sabatino D, Gilbert T: Developing dental radiographs, *J Vet Dent* 21:116, 2004.
87. Northrup NC, Selting KA, Rassnick KM et al: Outcomes of cats with oral tumors treated with mandibulectomy: 42 cases, *J Am Anim Hosp Assoc* 42:350, 2006.
88. Okuda A, Inouc E, Asari M: The membranous bulge lingual to the mandibular molar tooth of a cat contains a small salivary gland, *J Vet Dent* 13:61, 1996.
89. Okumura M, Kadosawa T, Fujinaga T: Surgical correction of temporomandibular joint ankylosis in two cats, *Aust Vet J* 77:24, 1999.
90. Orsini P, Hennet P: Anatomy of the mouth and teeth of the cat, *Vet Clin North Am Small Anim Pract* 22:1265, 1992.
91. Quimby JM, Elston T, Hawley J et al: Evaluation of the association of *Bartonella* species, feline herpesvirus 1, feline calicivirus, feline leukemia virus and feline immunodeficiency virus with chronic feline gingivostomatitis, *J Feline Med Surg* 10:66, 2008.
92. Ray JD, Eubanks DL: Dental homecare: teaching your clients to care for their pet's teeth, *J Vet Dent* 26:57, 2009.
93. Reiter AM: Symphysiotomy, symphysiectomy and intermandibular arthrodesis in a cat with open-mouth jaw locking—case report and literature review, *J Vet Dent* 21:147, 2004.
94. Reiter AM: Dental surgical procedures. In Tutt C, Deeprose J, Crossley D, editors: *BSAVA manual of canine and feline dentistry*, ed 3, Gloucester, 2007, British Small Animal Veterinary Association, p 178.
95. Reiter AM: High-rise syndrome. In Cote E, editor: *Clinical veterinary advisor*, ed 1, St Louis, 2007, Mosby, p 518.
96. Reiter AM: Palate defect. In Bojrab MJ, Monnet E, editors: *Mechanisms of disease in small animal surgery*, ed 3, Jackson, 2010, Teton NewMedia, p 118.
97. Reiter AM, Brady CA, Harvey CE: Local and systemic complications in a cat after poorly performed dental extractions, *J Vet Dent* 21:215, 2004.
98. Reiter AM, Harvey CE: Periodontal and endodontic disease. In Bojrab MJ, Monnet E, editors: *Mechanisms of disease in small animal surgery*, ed 3, Jackson, 2010, Teton NewMedia, p 125.
99. Reiter AM, Lyon KF, Nachreiner RF et al: Evaluation of calciotropic hormones in cats with odontoclastic resorptive lesions, *Am J Vet Res* 66:1446, 2005.
100. Reiter AM, Lewis JR, Okuda A: Update on the etiology of tooth resorption in domestic cats, *Vet Clin North Am Small Anim Pract* 35:913, 2005.
101. Reiter AM, Mendoza KA: Feline odontoclastic resorptive lesions. An unsolved enigma in veterinary dentistry, *Vet Clin North Am Small Anim Pract* 32:791, 2002.
102. Reiter AM, Smith MM: The oral cavity and oropharynx. In Brockman DJ, Holt DE, editors: *BSAVA manual of canine and feline head, neck and thoracic surgery*, ed 1, Gloucester, 2005, British Small Animal Veterinary Association, p 25.
103. Rochette J: Regional anesthesia and analgesia for oral and dental procedures, *Vet Clin North Am Small Anim Pract* 35:1041, 2005.
104. Roudebush P, Logan E, Hale FA: Evidence-based veterinary dentistry: a systematic review of homecare for prevention of periodontal disease in dogs and cats, *J Vet Dent* 22:6, 2005.
105. Rusbridge C, Heath S, Gunn-Moore DA et al: Feline orofacial pain syndrome (FOPS): a retrospective study of 113 cases, *J Feline Med Surg* 12:498, 2010.
106. Smith MM: Extraction of teeth in the mandibular quadrant of the cat, *J Vet Dent* 25:70, 2008.
107. Snyder LA, Bertone ER, Jakowski RM et al: p53 expression and environmental tobacco smoke exposure in feline oral squamous cell carcinoma, *Vet Pathol* 41:209, 2004.
108. Soukup JW, Snyder CJ, Gengler WR: Computed tomography and partial coronoidectomy for open-mouth jaw locking in two cats, *J Vet Dent* 26:226, 2009.
109. Southerden P, Gorrel C: Treatment of a case of refractory feline chronic gingivostomatitis with feline recombinant interferon omega, *J Small Anim Pract* 48:104, 2007.
110. Souza de HJ, Amorim FV, Corgozinho KB et al: Management of the traumatic oronasal fistula in the cat with a conical silastic prosthetic device, *J Feline Med Surg* 7:129, 2005.
111. Stebbins KE, Morse CC, Goldschmidt MH: Feline oral neoplasia: a ten-year survey, *Vet Pathol* 26:121, 1989.
112. Vercelli A, Raviri G, Cornegliani L: The use of oral cyclosporin to treat feline dermatoses: a retrospective analysis of 23 cases, *Vet Dermatol* 17:201, 2006.
113. Verstraete FJ: Mandibulectomy and maxillectomy, *Vet Clin North Am Small Anim Pract* 35:1009, 2005.
114. Verstraete FJM, Terpak CH: Anatomical variations in the dentition of the domestic cat, *J Vet Dent* 14:137, 1997.
115. Vrieling HE, Theyse LRF, Winkelhoff van AJ et al: Effectiveness of feeding large kibbles with mechanical cleaning properties in cats with gingivitis, *Tijdschr Diergeneeskd* 130:136, 2005.
116. Wesselink PR, Beertsen W: Ankylosis of the mouse molar after systemic administration of 1-hydroxyethylidene-1,1-bisphosphonate (HEBP), *J Clin Periodontol* 21:465, 1994.
117. Wesselink PR, Beertsen W: Repair processes in the periodontium following dentoalveolar ankylosis: the effect of masticatory function, *J Clin Periodontol* 21:472, 1994.
118. Withrow SJ: Taping of the mandible in treatment of mandibular fractures. *J Am Anim Hosp Assoc* 17:27, 1981.
119. Wypij JM, Fan TM, Fredrickson RL et al: In vivo and in vitro efficacy of zoledronate for treating oral squamous cell carcinoma in cats, *J Vet Intern Med* 22:158, 2008.
120. Zetner K, Stoian C, Benetka V et al: Influence of omega-interferon on the chronic gingivostomatitis of the cat, *Prakt Tierarzt* 85:798, 2004.

CHAPTER

22

Dermatology

OUTLINE

FELINE SKIN DISEASES

Karen A. Moriello

This chapter focuses on the common skin diseases encountered in clinical practice. Information is arranged in a problem-oriented format. The most commonly encountered feline dermatologic problems are pruritus, scaling and crusting, alopecia, ulcers and erosions, paw and nail disorders, otitis, anal sac diseases, and fragile skin. The chapter concludes with a brief discussion of human allergies to cats. The more uncommon skin diseases of cats are discussed in several excellent encyclopedic sources.[40,43,55,66]

DIAGNOSTIC APPROACH

For appropriate management of a cat with skin disease, the ultimate goal is to make a definitive diagnosis and outline a therapeutic plan. There are three major points the veterinarian should discuss with owners. The first is that skin diseases of cats involve either an easy diagnosis or a complicated diagnosis. Secondly, feline skin diseases are either "treated and cured" or "treated and managed." Finally, the ease or difficulty of diagnosis in no way predicts whether the disease is curable or just manageable. From a practical point of view, the first thing the clinician should establish through the history and physical examination is whether the cat is pruritic. Pruritus is the most common problem of cats.

The clinic visit is less stressful for all involved parties if the cat is made as comfortable as possible. Some veterinarians prefer to examine cats on clean white towels that have been sprayed with feline pheromones. If the situation allows, the history is obtained first and the carrier is placed on the towel, allowing the cat to relax. The use of prepared diagnostic kits (Figure 22-1) allows specimens to be collected easily once the examination starts. Good lighting and magnification are important because examination of the skin requires close inspection. Handheld magnifying lenses work just as well as magnification examination loops. The amount of light needed for a thorough examination of the skin is similar to that needed for surgery. If high-power spotlights are not available, handheld battery-operated flashlights are an excellent option.

Taking the History

The value of a thorough history with any disease is obvious. The following information should be obtained through either a preprinted history form or an interview:

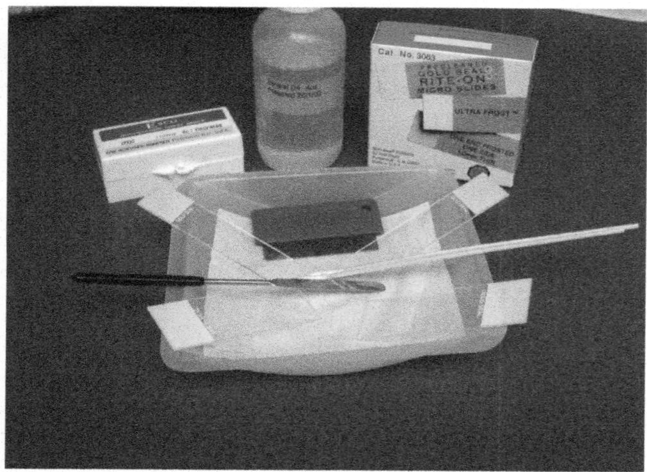

FIGURE 22-1 Diagnostic dermatology kit. This preorganized diagnostic kit makes the clinical examination and collection of specimens much more efficient. *(Photo courtesy University of Wisconsin School of Veterinary Medicine.)*

1. Client complaint: This may or may not help determine the dermatologic problem.
2. Signalment information:
   - Age: Many skin diseases are common in certain age groups. Ear mites, contagious parasites, and dermatophytosis are more common in kittens than adult cats. Allergic diseases tend to be first noted in cats 6 months to 2 years of age. Older cats are more likely to have immune-mediated skin diseases, tumors, or diseases associated with systemic diseases.
   - Sex: Intact male cats, especially if they are free roaming, are more prone to abscesses and other infections.
   - Breed: This is less important than in dogs, but there are some breed-related diseases such as *Malassezia* dermatitis of Rex cats.
   - Lifestyle and presence or absence of other cats in the house: Cats with access to the outdoors are more likely to contract contagious skin diseases, and knowledge of whether the skin problem is present in other cats in the household can help determine whether the skin disease is contagious.
   - Origin: Recently acquired pets from breeders, shelters, pet stores, or rescue organizations are at increased risk for contagious and infectious skin diseases.

With regard to the skin disease itself, the veterinarian should establish the following key elements:

1. Date of onset: This helps establish the age of onset and duration of the skin disease.
2. Acute or chronic development: Acute onset may suggest drug reactions or irritant reactions in contrast to a chronic problem that is more compatible with allergic diseases or tumors.
3. Seasonality: Seasonal skin diseases include fleas, flea allergy, atopic dermatitis, and parasitic diseases. Food allergies are not seasonal.
4. What did it look like originally?
5. Is the disease pruritic? This is important and often difficult to establish because many behaviors associated with pruritus in cats may not be recognized as such by owners. When in doubt, the veterinarian should assume that the cat is pruritic.

In cats with known or suspect pruritus, there are five key points to establish:

1. Did the pruritus develop before, at the same time as, or after the lesions developed?
2. How severe is the pruritus, and how frequently does it occur? It is often more helpful to use adjectives rather than a 1-to-10 scale at the initial visit. Terms such as *frantic, severe, constant, intermittent,* and *occasional* are more meaningful than a number.
3. How does the pruritus manifest itself (e.g., biting, chewing on nails, hair pulling, rubbing)?
4. Which parts of the body are affected?
5. Does the pruritus respond to treatment with corticosteroids?

Physical Examination

It is easy to focus on just the skin, so a general health examination should be performed before the dermatologic examination. Quite commonly, information from the general physical examination can be helpful in the diagnostic process. When performing a dermatologic examination on a cat, the clinician should focus on the following:

- Whiskers: Are they blunted or broken? This can be sign of pruritus and is common in atopic cats.
- Chin and lips: Is there hair loss? Are comedones or furuncles present? These are signs of facial rubbing.
- Ears and preauricular area: Is there excessive exudate in the ears? What is the consistency? Preauricular hyperpigmentation may be due to inflammation or comedones. Is there evidence of prior auricular hematoma? Are lesions present on the inner pinnae? Is there hair loss or crusting on the pinnae? Dermatophytosis and pemphigus affect the ear pinnae. Are the ear margins normal? Irregular ear margins may be due to trauma, frostbite, or neoplasia. If white hair is present on the head, is the skin normal? If abnormal, this may be due to solar damage, and squamous cell carcinomas or early actinic changes may be evident.
- Nose and face: Hair loss? Crusting? Ulceration?

- Oral cavity: Look for ulcers or erosions.
- Paws and nail beds: Pruritic cats often bite their nails, which will appear as broken and split. Is there black waxy debris near the nail bed or in the interdigital area? This is often a sign of yeast overgrowth associated with allergies or systemic illnesses.[77] Pemphigus will cause nail bed exudation and crusting. Are the foot pads normal? Crusting and thickening of the foot pads are abnormal and can be caused by immune-mediated diseases, dermatophytosis, and hepatocutaneous syndrome. Are corns present on the foot pads? This may suggest a disorder of keratinization or a developmental abnormality, or it may explain lameness. Do the foot pads appear puffy? This is common in plasma cell pododermatitis.
- Coat quality: Cats are meticulous groomers, and a matted, unkempt hair coat is abnormal. Is there excessive scaling? Are hairs pierced by scales? This is common in cats with bacterial pyoderma. If scaling is present, is it thick and adherent? This is seriously abnormal and most commonly associated with neoplastic or immune-mediated diseases. It can also be seen in severe dermatophytosis. Do the hairs easily epilate? Is there hair loss? If so, are the hairs blunted, suggesting barbering? What is the overall pattern of hair loss?
- Ventrum: Closely inspect the nipples. Are pustules or crusts present? Pustules around the nipples are rare and most commonly seen in cases of pemphigus. Examine the tail and base of the tail. Excessively oily hair on the tail suggests inflammation of sebaceous glands, poor grooming, or both. Hair loss at the tail base is commonly a sign of pruritus caused by fleas, tapeworms, or both. Closely inspect the skin for primary and secondary lesions. Many lesions are not easily found except by palpation of the skin.

BOX 22-1

Equipment List for a Dermatology Mini-Laboratory

Frosted glass microscope slides
Glass cover slips
Scalpel blade
Skin-scraping spatula (metal weighing spatula used in chemistry labs)
Mineral oil in a dropper bottle
Cotton-tipped swabs
5- and 10-mL syringes
22- to 23-gauge needles
Wood's lamp (optional)
Inexpensive new toothbrushes (unopened)
Lactophenol cotton blue stain
Dermatophyte test media
Sterile culture swabs with transport media
Sterile 25- to 27-gauge needles
Matches or lighter
Small forceps
20% potassium hydroxide in a dropper bottle
Alcohol or alcohol swabs
Flea comb
Clear acetate adhesive tape
Microscope with 4×, 10×, and oil immersion objectives
Diff-Quik stains

Skin Biopsy Equipment

Lidocaine hydrochloride
Needles and syringes
#10 or #11 scalpel blades
Suture material or skin staples
Adson–Brown forceps
Sterile surgical instruments
Wooden tongue depressors
4-, 6-, and 8-mm skin biopsy punches (optional)
Bottles containing 10% neutral buffered formalin
Camera

Core Diagnostic Tests

As the examination proceeds, the veterinarian should collect samples at the time a lesion is seen rather than later. This is more efficient and less stressful to the cat. For this reason it is a good idea to keep the dermatology kit (see Figure 22-1) close at hand. Core diagnostic tests include skin scrapings, flea combings, mineral oil ear swab, ear swab cytology, skin cytology (glass slide or tape), hair trichograms, and toothbrush fungal cultures. Box 22-1 contains a list of equipment for in-house dermatologic diagnostic testing.

Skin Scrapings

The primary parasites identified by skin scrapings are feline *Demodex* mites, *Cheyletiella* mites, and *Notoedres* mites. *Otodectes* mites can sometimes be found on skin scrapings. Positive skin scrapings rule in a parasite, but negative skin scrapings do not necessarily rule out these parasites. Skin scrapings in cats should only be performed with a skin-scraping spatula (Figure 22-2). Skin-scraping spatulas are safer and less expensive and provide better sample material than dulled scalpel blades. Optimal samples are obtained by putting several drops of mineral oil on the skin and using the length of the spatula (not the tip) to dislodge material from the surface and follicular material by gently scraping with short sweeping movements. Using the length of the spatula allows the veterinarian to gently scrape large or small areas of the skin. The mites of interest are more superficial in the cat's skin than in the dog's, so unless there is thickening of the skin, it is rarely necessary to scrape until capillary bleeding is apparent. It is more

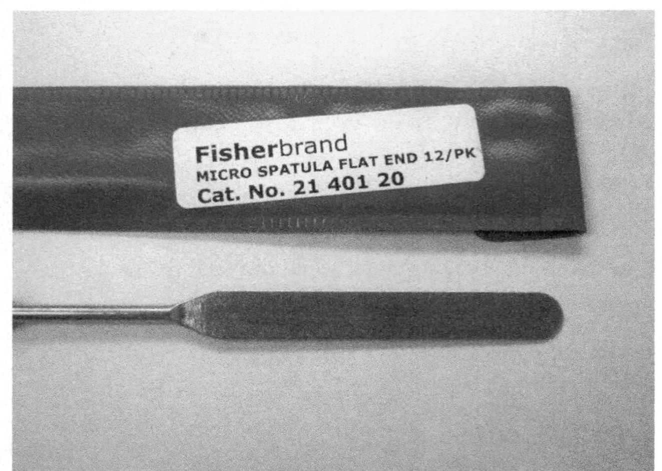

FIGURE 22-2 Skin-scraping spatula used for collecting cytologic specimens. This tool makes collection of specimens much easier and safer than doing so with a scalpel blade. *(Photo courtesy University of Wisconsin School of Veterinary Medicine.)*

fruitful to scrape more frequently and over larger areas when dealing with cats with skin disease.

After obtaining the sample, the material is transferred to a clean glass microscope slide and cover slipped. The latter is important because the pressure from the cover slip "pushes" mites to the margins of the slide. Examine the slides using 10× magnification and starting at the margins of the cover slip. It is often helpful to move the condenser down to increase contrast and scan first for movement. *Demodex* spp. mites can vary in shape, and the short, fat *Demodex gatoi* mite is easily overlooked, particularly at 4× magnification. The following are artifacts: red-brown globules (blood cells), brown-black granules (melanin granules), colored threads, broken hair shafts, and plant pollen or mold spores (usually darkly pigmented). *Microsporum canis* macroconidia are never seen on skin scrapings.

Flea Combing

Flea combing is indicated in any cat with hair loss, scaling, or pruritus. The fine-tooth combs can be used to find fleas, flea excreta, ticks, lice, and *Cheyletiella* spp. mites. The hair coat is combed using a fine metal- or plastic-tooth comb. The material can be examined with a handheld magnifying lens or under a microscope. Soil particles can be confused with flea excreta, and water can be used to distinguish between the two substances; the flea excreta dissolve, leaving a reddish brown smear. Shampoo residue (usually uncommon in cats) may mimic excessive scaling. It appears as fine, powdery debris on the distal tips of the hairs.

Acetate Tape Preparations

Acetate tape preparations can be used to capture fleas and flea excreta and ticks and to collect scales to look for *Cheyletiella* spp. mites. *Cheyletiella* spp. mites are more often found on skin scrapings or flea combings; the usefulness of this technique is greatly overemphasized. The sticky side of a clear piece of acetate tape is pressed against the object of interest and then placed on a glass microscope slide over a drop of mineral oil. Another drop of mineral oil is placed on top of the tape, and then a cover slip is added. This enhances visualization of mites. The slide is examined under increasing magnification. Common artifacts include crinkling of the tape, frosted tape, clothing treads, pigmented fungal spores, and plant matter.

Ear Swab Cytology

It is important to collect specimens for ear swab cytology *before* collecting specimens for mineral oil examination. Ear swab cytology examines debris, wax, and exudate from the ear canal. It is indicated in all cases of otitis or head and neck pruritus. A dry cotton-tipped swab is used to collect material and rolled onto a clean glass microscope slide. The slide is heat fixed and stained using a rapid Giemsa stain. Slides should be examined at low power (4× or 10× magnification) to find areas of cellularity for closer scrutiny. Bacteria and yeast are best seen under oil immersion. If rods are evident, an ear culture is indicated.

Mineral Oil Ear Swab Cytology

Mineral oil ear swab cytology is most commonly used when *Otodectes* spp. mites are suspected; however, it is an underused diagnostic test in cats. *D. gatoi* and *Demodex cati* can cause pruritic otitis in young and adult cats. Ear swabs are indicated whenever ear mites are suspected, debris is in the ear, or the cat has head and neck or ear pruritus. A dry cotton-tipped swab is used to collect ear debris. To look for mites, the veterinarian should roll the tip of the swab in a drop of mineral oil on a glass microscope slide and then place a cover slip over the oil drop.

Skin Cytology and Nail Bed Cytology

Skin cytology and nail bed cytology is an underused diagnostic test in feline dermatology. It is most commonly used to identify bacterial and yeast overgrowth. It can also be used to help identify acantholytic cells that are seen in pemphigus foliaceus (PF). There are three common methods for taking samples from the skin: glass slide impressions, clear acetate tape, and spatula collection:

- Glass slide impression smears: Using a clean glass slide, the veterinarian gently pinches up the skin lesions, making a small fold of target skin, and presses a glass slide firmly over the area. Pressure should be applied directly above the sample site using a thumb or index finger. If this is not done, the slide may break.

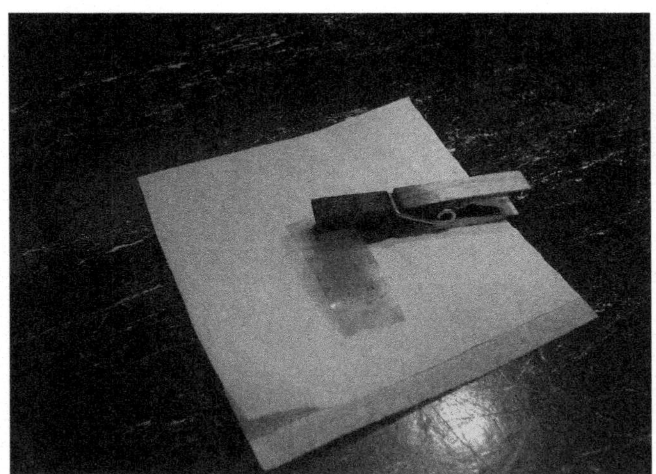

FIGURE 22-3 Acetate tape cytology specimen. Clear acetate tape facilitates the collection of cytologic specimens from the skin of cats. *(Photo courtesy University of Wisconsin School of Veterinary Medicine.)*

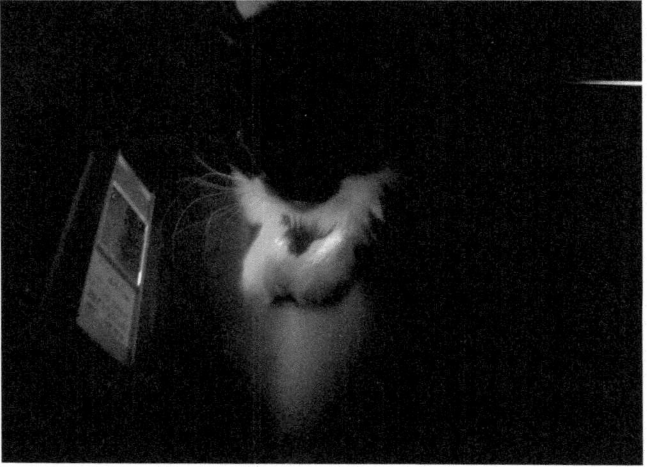

FIGURE 22-4 Wood's lamp positive hairs. Note the apple-green fluorescence of the hairs. *(Photo courtesy University of Wisconsin School of Veterinary Medicine.)*

- Clear adhesive tape: Using clear adhesive tape, the veterinarian presses the sticky side on the target area and gently pulls up. This is especially useful for small areas of the skin or if the cat is fractious, in which case the owner can be instructed as to where to place the tape. It is critical to skip the fixative step when staining tape cytology specimens because this will damage the tape. Using forceps or clothespins, the tape is dipped is stained and allowed to dry (Figure 22-3). To view the specimen, the veterinarian places a drop of immersion oil on a glass slide and then places the tape over this drop.
- Spatula collection: Using a clean skin-scraping spatula, the veterinarian gently scrapes the skin and smears the material onto a glass slide. This is useful when the target area is small (e.g., focal area of comedones) or when the area is greasy. Nail bed debris or material from between crevices in the skin can be scooped out using a skin-scraping spatula or the wooden end of a cotton swab. This material can then be smeared onto a glass microscope slide.
- Samples collected onto glass slides should be gently heat fixed. This enhances the ability to find yeast. It is important *not* to heat fix slides if structural architecture is important (e.g., examination of exudate).

Two common normal findings are easily mistaken for bacteria: melanin granules (darkly pigmented and slightly refractile) and surface lipids (very small and slightly basophilic, granular in appearance). Cocci, diplococci, rods, and yeast stain deeply basophilic and are not refractile.

Wood's Lamp Examination

A Wood's lamp is an ultraviolet light with a wavelength of 273.7 nm filtered through a cobalt or nickel filter. The light interacts with a metabolite on the surface of infected hairs, resulting in an apple-green fluorescence (Figure 22-4). *M. canis* is the only species of importance in veterinary medicine that fluoresces with a Wood's lamp. After allowing the lamp to warm up for several minutes, the veterinarian should turn off the room lights and hold the light over suspected lesions for several minutes. The hair examination should continue for at least 3 or 4 minutes to ensure that the examiner's eyes have adapted to the light. Positive hairs can be plucked for fungal culture or hair trichogram. Not all strains of *M. canis* fluoresce. Any topical medication can cause a false-positive or false-negative test. The most common false-positive result occurs with the blue-white fluorescence of dust and scales.

Hair Trichograms

Hair trichograms are used to examine hair shafts and hair bulbs for evidence of fungal infections, stage of growth (anagen or telogen), and *Demodex* mites. Target hairs should be plucked in the direction of growth, placed on a drop of mineral oil, cover slipped, and examined. Mites will be found around the hair bulb. When examining hairs for fungal spores, the veterinarian does not need to use a clearing agent such as potassium hydroxide. Infected hairs will have a cuff of spores around the shaft and appear wider and more filamentous than normal hairs (Figure 22-5). Fungal spores are more refractile. If suspicious glowing hairs cannot be found on a microscope slide, the Wood's lamp can be used to locate them on the glass slide. The veterinarian should turn out the lights again and hold the lamp over the glass slide to locate them.

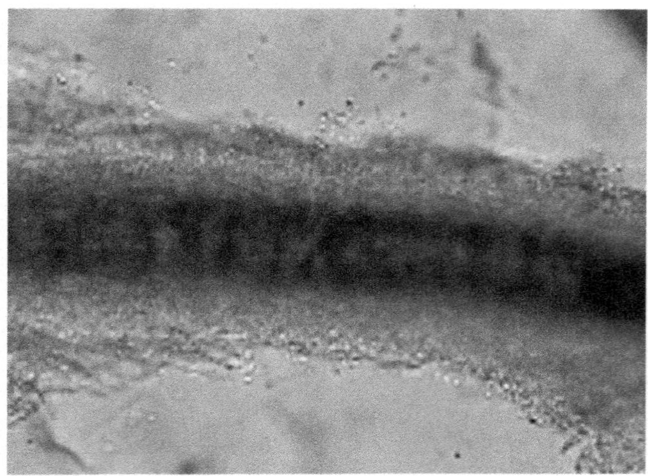

FIGURE 22-5 Hair trichogram of *M. canis*–infected hair. Note the large cuff of spores seen around the base of the hair. This is a mineral oil mount of an infected hair. *(Photo courtesy University of Wisconsin School of Veterinary Medicine.)*

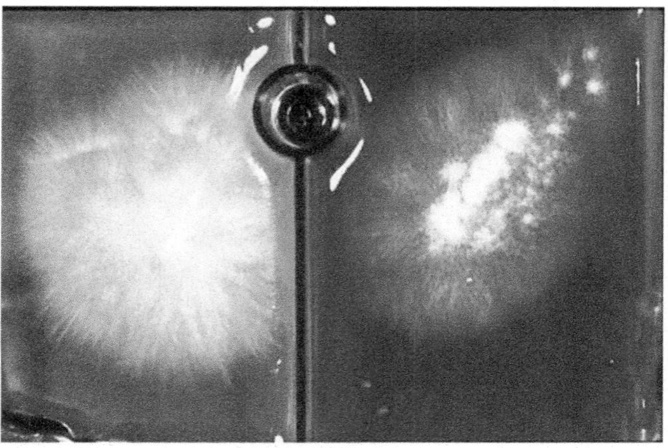

FIGURE 22-6 Positive culture of *M. canis*. This is a dual culture plate with DTM on one side (note red color change around the growing colony) and Sabouraud dextrose agar on the other side. The difference in gross characteristics is because the phenol color indicator in the DTM changes gross colony morphology. *(Photo courtesy University of Wisconsin School of Veterinary Medicine.)*

Dermatophyte Cultures

A fungal culture is the best way to diagnose a dermatophyte infection. It is indicated whenever a Wood's lamp examination yields a positive result or the veterinarian suspects a dermatophyte infection.

Samples are most commonly collected by way of a toothbrush combing of suspect lesions or plucking of suspected hairs. A newly wrapped toothbrush is combed over the coat for several minutes to obtain a specimen. This is a particularly useful technique for obtaining samples from cats. Alternatively, broken hairs from the margin of a lesion can be gently plucked in the direction of growth. Plucked hair samples are firmly pressed to the surface of the fungal culture plate.

Toothbrush samples are inoculated by gently stabbing the surface of the plate 10 to 20 times with the bristles, taking care not to lift the media off the plate. Commercial media plates should be placed in a self-closing zip-lock bag and labeled. The plastic bag will help minimize cross-contamination of samples, help keep the plate moist, and prevent media mite infestations. Plates are incubated at 21° C to 23.8° C (70° F to 75° F).[99] The most commonly used fungal culture media are Dermatophyte Test Media (DTM), which contain a color indicator and plain Sabouraud dextrose agar. It is important to remember that the red color change in the DTM media is only suggestive of, not diagnostic of, a pathogen. Definitive diagnosis requires microscopic examination. If DTM is used, suspect colonies are those that are pale with a red color change surrounding them as they are growing (Figure 22-6). Most pathogens will grow by day 14 of culture. All suspect cultures should be identified microscopically using lactophenol cotton blue stain or new methylene blue stain. A piece of clear acetate tape is pressed to the surface of the growth and placed over a drop of stain. A second drop of stain is placed on top of the tape, and a cover slip is added. Additional information can be found at http://www.doctorfungus.org regarding the identification of common pathogens, particularly *M. canis*.

Skin Biopsy

Skin biopsy specimens can be obtained using a scalpel blade or a skin biopsy punch (Figure 22-7). Primary lesions (e.g., pustules, vesicles) should be sampled. If these are not found, several representative samples should be obtained. When multiple skin biopsy specimens are being obtained, lesions should be circled with a black marker so that the veterinarian can identify the sites to biopsy after the local anesthetic has been injected. The skin is not washed or scrubbed because surface pathology is very important in the diagnostic evaluation. A local anesthetic is injected subcutaneously directly beneath the sample. Skin biopsy punches are placed directly over the lesion and twisted in one direction, using gentle pressure; twisting clockwise and counterclockwise produces shear, which ruins the specimen. Because cat skin is very thin, the veterinarian must be careful to cut through to the dermis without penetrating the underlying musculature. Using fine-tipped forceps, the veterinarian harvests the sample by grabbing the subcutaneous fat pedicle; the sample is harvested in the same manner as a flower is plucked (see Figure 22-7, *B*). If junctional samples are desired, an elliptical biopsy is collected. Blood is gently blotted from the sample, and the subcutaneous side is placed on a piece of tongue depressor and fixed in 10% neutral buffered formalin. If there is a particular lesion or lesions that the clinician wants cut into the block, he or she can place a small black dot on the site and tell the pathologist to section over

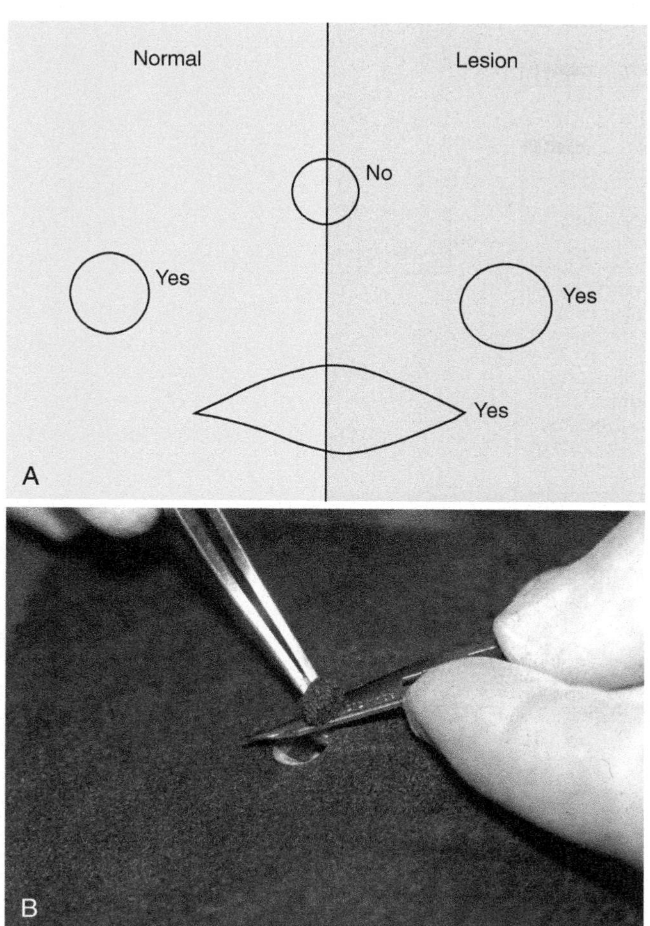

FIGURE 22-7 **A,** Collection of skin biopsy specimen. This diagram shows the correct placement of a skin biopsy punch for harvesting a sample of tissue. Given the small size of the punch, marginal lesions are not recommended because there is no way to ensure that the pathologist will know how to section the sample. Take a sample from an abnormal area and normal area. If it is important to see margins, use an elliptical incision. **B,** It is important to grasp the biopsy specimen by the subcutaneous pedicle and cut it free from the skin without crushing the specimen. *(**A** and **B** courtesy University of Wisconsin School of Veterinary Medicine.)*

this site since discriminating features such as erythema can be lost by tissue in fixative. The veterinarian should always include digital pictures and a complete history. The samples should be sent to a laboratory where there are veterinary pathologists with a declared interest in dermatopathology.

PRURITUS

The most common skin problem in cats is pruritus, and the diagnosis either is obvious or requires a systematic work up (Figure 22-8). The three most common causes of pruritus in cats are parasites, infections, and allergic skin diseases. Behaviors and clinical findings associated with pruritus include, but are not limited to, obvious scratching and biting at the body, facial rubbing, broken and bent whiskers, hair loss on the chin, comedone formation on the lips and chin, head shaking, overgrooming in symmetric or asymmetric patterns of hair loss, broken or stubbly hair, salivary staining of the paws, self-mutilation, focal areas of exudation compatible with eosinophilic plaques, twitching, and irritability when petted.

Parasitic Causes of Pruritus

The general workup of a cat with pruritus starts with eliminating parasites as the cause even if the cat is receiving flea control and even if other cats in the household are not affected. Parasite infestations can be very difficult to diagnose in cats because of their meticulous grooming habits. Fecal flotation examinations may be helpful in diagnosing mite infestations in cats insofar as the mites are ingested when grooming.

Otodectes

The most common mite infestation of cats is the ear mite, *Otodectes*. Ear mites live on or in the ears. Eggs are cemented to the hairs and skin on the margin of the ears. Mites feed on the epithelium, and the ear canal fills with black-brown crumbly material. Kittens are recognized as a high-risk group, but any cat can be affected; adult animals should be examined with the same care as kittens. The classic clinical signs are a coffee-ground discharge and pruritus. Hypersensitivity reactions in cats can develop secondary to mite infestations. Pruritus will be severe, yet mites are often not found. Untreated or inappropriately treated ear mite infestations can lead to secondary infections, purulent otitis externa (OE) or otitis media (OM), and aural hematomas and may be involved in the development of chronic OM in adult cats. Severe mite infestations can occur over the entire body, leading to a pruritic, papular skin disease that can mimic many other parasitic and nonparasitic diseases (Figure 22-9).

Diagnosis of ear mite infestations is made by finding mites either by direct examination with an otoscope or, more commonly, on mineral oil ear swab cytology. One mite or egg is diagnostic for an infestation. Positive pinna–pedal reflexes are common in cats with gross or subclinical infestations; when the ear is manipulated or swabbed, the cat scratches with the ipsilateral hind limb. Mites can often be found on skin scrapings of ear margins in animals in which mites are suspected but cannot be found on ear swab cytology.

There are many well-accepted and effective treatment protocols for ear mite infestations. The key treatment points are as follows:

- Debris is gently removed from the ear canal because no topical ear treatments or topical spot-on

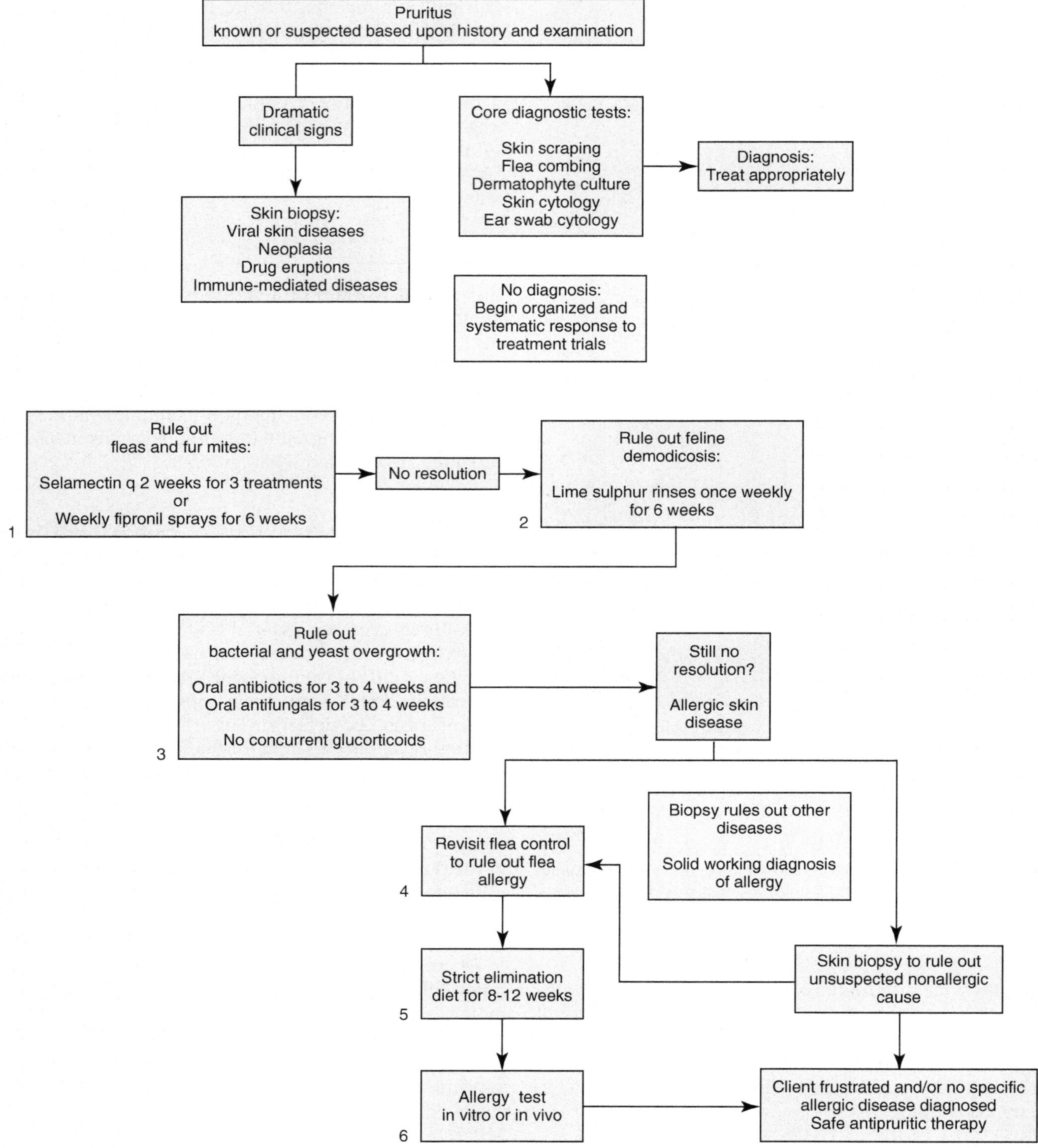

FIGURE 22-8 Pruritus flow chart. Pruritus is known or suspected based on history and examination. *(Image courtesy University of Wisconsin School of Veterinary Medicine.)*

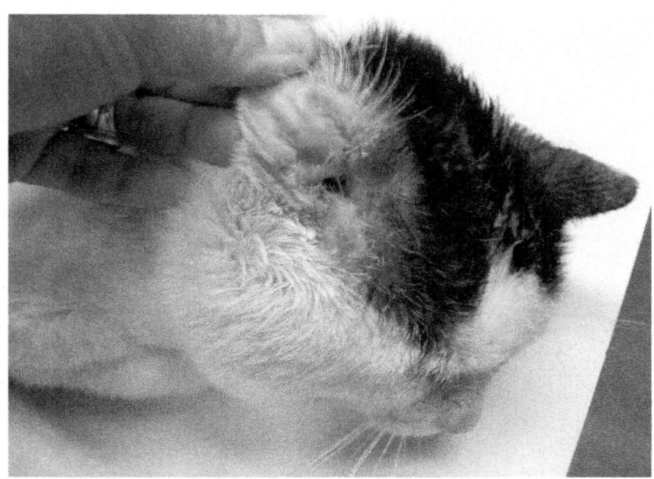

FIGURE 22-9 Adult cat with intense otic pruritus due to hypersensitivity reaction to *Otodectes*. *(Photo courtesy University of Wisconsin School of Veterinary Medicine.)*

treatments (e.g., selamectin) can penetrate this material, which can contain a large number of mites and eggs. The mineral oil is useful to soften material.

- Humane relief of ear pruritus is provided by the topical application of an otic steroid.
- A whole-body treatment is used to prevent re-infestation from migrating mites. The concurrent use of an otic miticide and a whole-body flea control product is recommended.
- Treatment of all affected animals (and those with which they are in contact) should be continued for at least 4 weeks.

The application of otic ear mite preparations at night has been recommended on the basis of a report from a human infested with ear mites. This person reported that the mites were more active at night than during the day. In this fascinating report, a veterinarian self-inoculated his ears three times with ear mites.[50]

Fur Mites and Lice

The most common fur mites of cats include *Dermanyssus gallinae, Lynxacarus radovskyi,* chiggers *(Eutrombicula* spp., *Walchia americana),* and *Cheyletiella* spp. (see below).[40,43,55,66] *D. gallinae,* or the poultry mite, is most common in wild birds and pet birds. Pet birds can be affected if they are in contact with wild birds. Contact need not be direct; mites can be mechanically transmitted to pet birds through contact with contaminated material or close exposure to nests. Clinical signs vary from none to pruritic papular eruptions. Contact with poultry or exposure to wild birds is an important part of the history. Pet cats are most commonly exposed when homes have wild birds nesting near screened porches. The diagnosis can be difficult, but one helpful finding in the history is if the owner reports finding dead baby birds near these nests.

L. radovskyi infestations have been reported in Hawaii, Texas, and Florida.[22] Clinical signs varied from mild to severe pruritus and papular eruption. Mite infestations were generalized and produced large amounts of scale. In the few cases seen by the authors, the mites were not difficult to find.

Chiggers are an underdiagnosed cause of pruritus in cats. Chiggers live in organic material, and it is the larvae that are parasitic and feed on animals. Bites can occur anywhere but are most common in areas in contact with grass or soil. The most common clinical sign is a papular eruption. In the cases seen by the authors, both owners and cats were affected. The infestations are seasonal and tend to occur in the late summer and fall.

Cheyletiella mites are the most well-known and common fur mite infestation of cats. These mites can also affect dogs, rabbits, and other small mammals. The mites are highly contagious and of zoonotic importance. There are several species but all have the same general appearance. Infested animals can be asymptomatic and not identified until people or other cats become affected. The classic clinical presentation is dorsal scaling with mild to moderate pruritus that can be severe.

Notoedres cati, also known as "feline scabies," is an intensely pruritic skin disease of cats. It is uncommon and is most often found in catteries and multiple-cat households. Affected cats present with intensely pruritic crusting and scaling on the face, ears, head, neck, paws, and perineum. If left untreated, the skin becomes lichenified, hyperpigmented, alopecic, and excoriated. These mites are easily found on skin scraping, and the mite is similar in appearance to *Sarcoptes* spp.

Lice are species specific and are contracted by direct contact with another infected host. Cats are afflicted with only one species of lice, *Felicola subrostratus.* Infested animals may be asymptomatic or more commonly present with restlessness, pruritus, scaling, hair loss, and irritability. Lice cement their eggs to the hairs, and these eggs are often referred to as *nits.*

Definitive diagnosis of lice and fur mite infestations can be difficult because there is no single best diagnostic test to find these parasites. Skin scrapings, flea combings, hair trichograms, acetate tape preparations, and fecal examinations are recommended. In many cases, however, definitive diagnosis or ruling out of mite infestations can be done only by identifying a response to treatment trial. Lice infestations are most often made by finding the lice or nits (or both) while making a visual inspection of the cat's hair coat.

Treatment options for lice, fur mites, *Cheyletiella,* and *Notoedres* infestations are similar. The key to successful treatment is use of a product that is applied to the entire hair coat. If possible, the cat should be bathed to remove debris, excess scales, egg cases, and nits from the hair

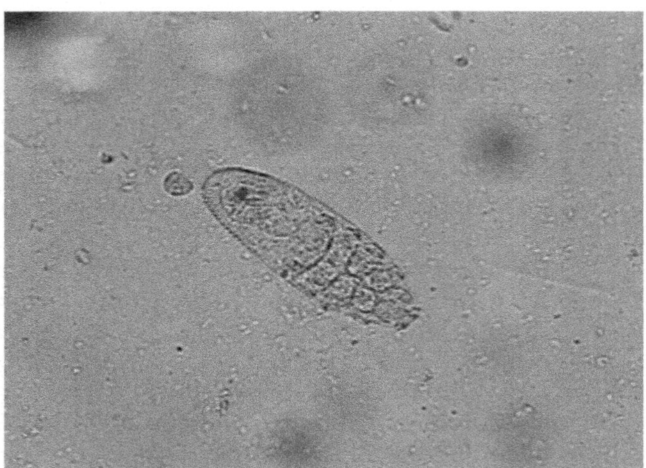

FIGURE 22-10 *Demodex gatoi* mite. This mite lives in the superficial layers of the skin and can be difficult to find. This mite was found on a fecal examination of an intensely pruritic cat (400× magnification). *(Photo courtesy University of Wisconsin School of Veterinary Medicine.)*

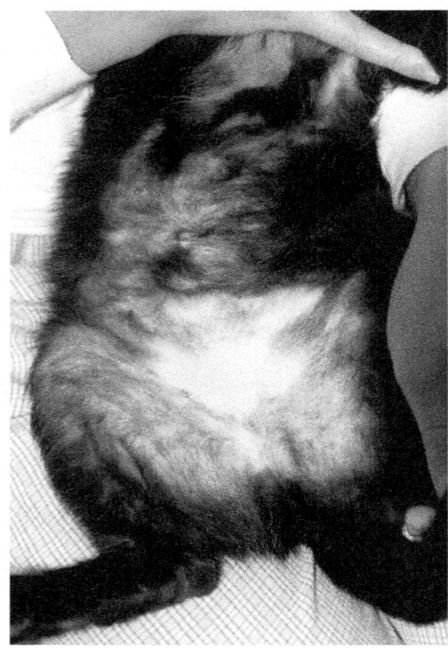

FIGURE 22-11 *D. gatoi*–infested cat. This cat was presented for the problem of over grooming and feline symmetric alopecia. *D. gatoi* mites were found, and the pruritus resolved with treatment. *(Photo courtesy University of Wisconsin School of Veterinary Medicine.)*

coat. Nits can be loosened from the hair coat with a 1:4 dilution of white household vinegar in water. The solution is applied to the coat for 2 to 3 minutes, and then the hair coat is rinsed. If the cat has long hair and the infestation is severe or if soaking the hair coat is difficult, it may be necessary to clip the coat. These parasites generally have a life cycle of 3 weeks, so a treatment plan of 4 weeks is recommended. Whole-body treatments include lime sulfur rinses, fipronil spray, and pyrethrin sprays.[23] Water-based pyrethrin sprays labeled as safe to use in kittens are recommended to minimize the risks of toxicity from pyrethrins. Permethrins are very toxic in cats and should never be used. Whole-body treatments should be done at least once weekly. Concurrent systemic treatment options include ivermectin (0.2 mg/kg to 0.4 mg/kg orally, once daily for 4 weeks) and milbemycin (0.5 to 2 mg/kg orally, once daily for 4 weeks). Selamectin used every 2 weeks for three treatments is also effective; however, it is important to mechanically remove debris, scales, and nits from the hair coat if selamectin is used.

Demodicosis

Demodicosis is increasingly being recognized as a cause of skin disease and pruritus in cats. The disease is caused by *D. cati*, a long slender mite, or *D. gatoi* (Figure 22-10), a short, rounded mite. Skin disease may be limited to the ears, causing pruritic otitis. Localized or generalized skin lesions may also be seen. As with dermatophytosis, the clinical presentation is highly variable. Localized lesions are usually characterized by patchy hair loss, scaling, and erythema around the eyes or on the head or neck. Erythema, scales, crusts, easily epilated hairs, symmetric alopecia, or just intense pruritus mimicking feline "hyperesthesia-like" quivering may be all that is found. *D. cati* is most commonly found in cats with pruritic ears or in cats with skin lesions and concurrent disease such as diabetes mellitus, feline hyperadrenocorticism, feline immunodeficiency virus (FIV), feline leukemia virus (FeLV), toxoplasmosis, systemic lupus or other immune-mediated diseases, and neoplasia.[70]

D. cati is not considered to be a contagious mite. *D. gatoi* is increasingly being recognized as a pruritic skin disease of cats and is a known contagion; it can be difficult to find on skin scrapings.[87] The mite lives in the superficial layers of the stratum corneum, and routine grooming of cats often removes the mite. It is increasingly being found in cats with symmetric alopecia, which suggests that this mite is an overlooked and underdiagnosed cause of this reaction pattern in cats (Figure 22-11).[32] Diagnosis is made by demonstration of the mite on skin scrapings, fecal flotation, ear swab cytology, or hair trichogram. In cats with symmetric alopecia, diagnosis is often made by response to treatment.[32] *D. cati* often resolves without treatment if the underlying disease can be identified or managed. It has been successfully treated with lime sulfur rinses every 4 to 7 days for to 8 weeks.[23] Feline demodicosis responds well to a number of treatment options, including twice-weekly lime sulfur rinses (e.g., Lime Sulfur Dip, Vet Solutions, Fort Worth, Texas) alone or paired with daily oral ivermectin (200 μg/kg) for 4 to 8 weeks or oral daily milbemycin (0.5 mg/kg) for 4 to 8 weeks. If lime sulfur is not an option, the author (KM) has used topical fipronil spray once weekly. Cats with a suspected or known *D. gatoi* infestation must be isolated during treatment. All cats in contact with the afflicted cat should be treated.

Tick and Flea Infestations and Flea Bite Hypersensitivity

Flea infestations are common ectoparasites of cats. Flea infestations are most common in the warm weather months but can be found year round, even in climates with well-defined seasons and cold winters. Foxes, raccoons, opossums, and other small mammals are the reservoirs of infestations in these climates. Flea infestations can lead to severe flea bite anemia. Young, old, and severely debilitated cats are most at risk. Table 22-1 provides a summary of commonly used flea control products.[89]

Cats that are not allergic to fleas may show no signs of disease even if their hair coat is heavily infested with fleas. This represents a state of tolerance and is not common in pet cats. Most cats with a flea infestation are pruritic. Hair loss, scaling, papular eruptions with or without crusting, and areas of self-trauma (i.e., eosinophilic plaques) are common. The severity of pruritus in a flea-allergic cat is disproportionate to the number of fleas found. No fleas may be found because flea-allergic cats will bite, nibble, hunt, and ingest fleas. Hair loss over the lumbosacral area, hind legs, and neck is common (Figure 22-12). Miliary dermatitis (small red crusts of serum and blood) are common, especially on the face and abdomen. Ulcerated lips and symmetric alopecia are common. "Rodent ulcer" lesions are frequently the result of flea bites around the lips.

The diagnosis of fleas or flea allergy dermatitis can be made on the basis of clinical signs and suspicion. Evidence of a flea infestation can be found using a flea comb. Fleas, flea eggs, and flea excreta are common findings. The finding of tapeworms in a fecal specimen is also suggestive of fleas because tapeworms may result from flea ingestion. Both cats and dogs with flea infestations and flea allergy dermatitis often have secondary bacterial infections. Treatment of flea infestations is strongly encouraged, not only because of the discomfort fleas cause for the animal and the distress they cause the owners but also because fleas transmit zoonotic diseases such as bartonellosis (cat scratch fever).

The diagnosis of a flea infestation may be easy or difficult depending on whether fleas or flea excreta are found. If fleas are not found, many owners are often hesitant (if not adamantly opposed) to a trial of flea control treatment, especially if the cat is a strictly indoor cat. What many owners do not realize is that fleas can invade their home and infest their cats even if the cats do not go outdoors. Further complicating the situation is that cats will groom and ingest fleas, making it difficult to find them. A trial of a flea control product (e.g., fipronil) every 2 weeks for 3 to 4 treatments is an excellent approach as a treatment trial to eliminate fleas, ear mites, and fur mites.

Treatment of obvious infestations can start with oral nitenpyram (1 mg/kg orally, every 24 to 48 hours for 1 to 2 weeks until no more fleas are seen). At the same time, monthly spot-on treatments can be started. Anecdotal reports about regional efficacy are common, and the clinician should use products known to be effective in his or her practice area. Owners should be advised to use only products labeled as safe for use in kittens and cats and warned that focal areas of hair loss at the site of spot-on products can occur.

Treatment of kittens requires aggressive removal of fleas as they can cause life-threatening anemia. Bathing with a pet shampoo or a dilute baby shampoo (1:4) product may be needed to enhance removal of fleas. After a complete drying and combing of the hair coat, a thorough application of water-based pyrethrin spray labeled for kittens is recommended, followed by aggressive flea combing. If the infestation is severe or the kitten is too young to be safely sprayed, the author (KM) uses a "tent" to remove fleas. The veterinarian places the kitten on a clean towel, soaks a paper towel with a knockdown spray, and places the towel in a tentlike fashion over the kitten, taking care to keep the spray out of the kitten's eyes and ensuring that the kitten does not inhale the spray. Fleas will fall off the neonate, facilitating removal. A spot-on product can be used, and the author has safely used selamectin in kittens as young as 6 weeks of age in flea-endemic areas.

Tick infestations can and do occur in cats and are important to control because they can transmit infectious diseases. Owners often do not notice infestations or believe they can occur because ticks are mechanically removed by self-grooming in many cases. Tick bites can lead to small nodular reactions in the skin at the site of attachment. The lesions tend to occur several weeks after the tick bite. Another common complication of tick infestations is invasion of the ear canal. An affected cat may present with otitis or possibly severe vestibular disease.

Infectious Causes of Pruritus

Infectious causes of pruritic skin in cats include bacterial overgrowth (pyoderma), yeast overgrowth, and dermatophytosis. (See the section on scaling, crusting, and greasy skin for a detailed discussion.)

Pyoderma

Until recently, bacterial pyoderma in cats was considered rare. The clinical signs of bacterial infections or overgrowth are more subtle than in dogs and are easily overlooked. The most commonly isolated pathogens are *Staphylococcus* spp. Clinical signs of feline bacterial pyoderma include papules, pustules (rare), miliary dermatitis–like lesions, epidermal collarettes, and scaling

TABLE 22-1 **Summary of Commonly Used Flea Control Products in Cats**

Drug	Class	Mode of Action	Application	Target Parasites	Age of Use
Imidacloprid (Advantage) Primarily an adulticide Larvicidal activity	Neonicotinoid	Acts as agonist at polysynaptic nicotinic acetylcholine receptors; results in paralysis and death of adult fleas	Spot-on treatment that spreads over the skin by translocation and is not absorbed systemically; must be applied to skin, not hair coat	Fleas	Labeled for use in cats 8 weeks of age or older
Imidacloprid with moxidectin (Advantage multi, Advocate)	Neonicotinoid and avermectin	Is an avermectin and causes paralysis	Spot-on	Fleas, heartworm prevention, ear mites, hookworms, and roundworms	Labeled for use in cats 9 weeks of age or older
Fipronil (Frontline) Also available with methoprene (Frontline Plus) Adulticide	Phenylpyrazole	Binds at GABA-gated chloride channel, causing excessive neuronal stimulation, paralysis, and death of adult fleas	Spray or spot-on Spreads over skin by translocation by way of the surface lipids on the skin and is stored in sebaceous glands, where it is constantly resecreted onto the hair and skin Not absorbed systemically Must be applied to skin	Fleas and ticks	Labeled for use in cats 8 weeks of age or older and is safe in breeding, pregnant, and lactating cats
Selamectin (Revolution, Stronghold) Adulticide but has ovicidal and larvicidal activity	Semisynthetic avermectin	Binds to receptors on glutamate-gated (and possibly GABA) chloride channels, leading to flaccid paralysis and death	Topical spot-on Absorbed through skin into the blood and then is redistributed to sebaceous glands	Fleas, heartworm prevention, control of ear mite infestations, control of hookworms and roundworms	Labeled for use in cats 6 weeks of age or older and is safe for breeding, pregnant, and lactating cats
Nitenpyram (Capstar) Adulticide	Systemically active neonicotinoid	See imidacloprid	Orally administered	Adult fleas	Labeled as safe for cats 4 weeks of age or older weighing at least 2 pounds Safe in breeding, pregnant, or lactating cats Can be used with imidacloprid, fipronil, pyrethrins, lufenuron
Dinotefuran (Vectra)	Neonicotinoid	See imidacloprid	Spot-on formulation combined with insect growth regulator pyriproxifen Spreads over body and adheres to skin and hair, absorbed on contact with fleas	Fleas	Labeled for use in cats 8 weeks of age or older
Pyrethrins and pyrethroids	Pyrethrin and synthetic pyrethroids	Affect voltage-dependent sodium channels of neurons and cause paralysis	Sprays and sponge-ons	Adult fleas, ticks, lice, *Cheyletiella*, ear mites, fur mites	Important to read label of each product Pyrethroids, especially >2%, can be extremely toxic to cats

GABA, Gamma-aminobutyric acid.
Table reprinted with permission from Schwassman M, Logas D: How to treat common parasites safely. In August J, editor: *Consultations in feline internal medicine*, ed 6, St Louis, 2010, Saunders Elsevier, p 390.

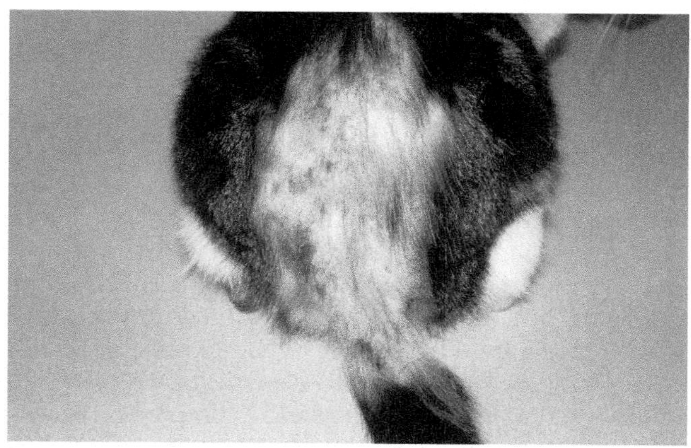

FIGURE 22-12 Cat with classic flea allergy pattern. Note the hair loss over the lumbosacral area. Palpation of skin in this area reveals widespread crusted papules. *(Photo courtesy University of Wisconsin School of Veterinary Medicine.)*

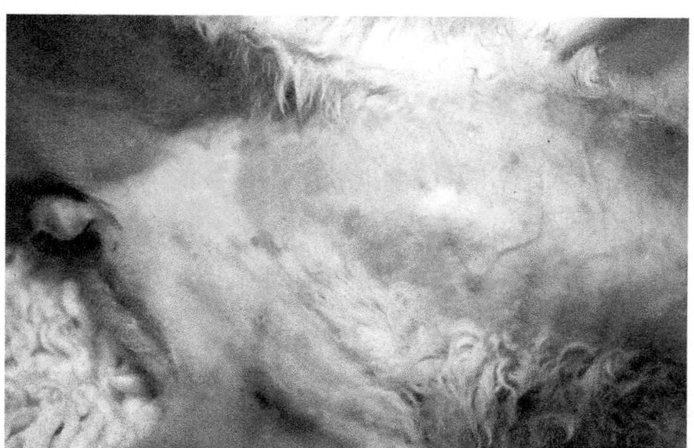

FIGURE 22-13 Pyoderma. Intact pustules, papules and small epidermal collarettes are present in this Rex cat. *(Photo courtesy University of Wisconsin School of Veterinary Medicine.)*

(Figure 22-13). Epidermal collarettes are very subtle and small, often only 1 to 2 mm in size.[41,104] The most common clinical presentation encountered is excessive scaling (Figure 22-14), especially over the lumbosacral areas. Close inspection of the hairs reveals scales pierced by hairs. Another common antibiotic-responsive skin lesion in cats is areas of self-trauma that have the clinical appearance of eosinophilic plaques[105] (Figure 22-15). Before recognition of the antimicrobial responsiveness of these lesions, corticosteroid therapy was used.

The diagnosis of feline bacterial pyoderma is similar to that in the dog: It is primarily a clinical diagnosis with confirmation most often based on response to antibiotic therapy. Glass slide skin impression smears are excellent for exudative or ulcerative skin lesions; however, acetate tape cytology preparations are much easier to use on other areas of the body. Exudative skin lesions will show neutrophils, eosinophils, bacteria, or *Malassezia* spp. However, samples from sites with predominant scaling may show only shed keratinocytes.

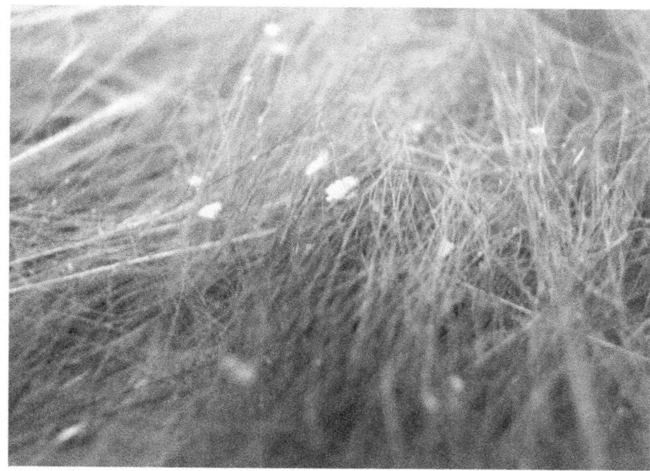

FIGURE 22-14 Pyoderma. Note the excessive scaling typical of this condition. *(Photo courtesy University of Wisconsin School of Veterinary Medicine.)*

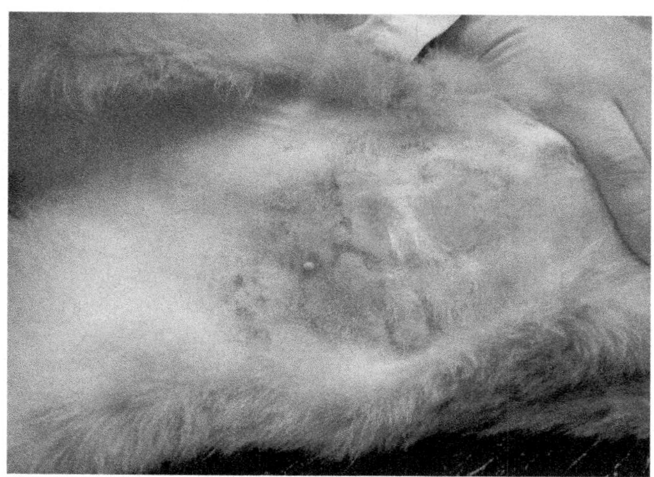

FIGURE 22-15 Eosinophilic plaque. This lesion was triggered by flea allergy and resolved not with glucocorticoid therapy but with combined bacterial and yeast therapy. *(Photo courtesy University of Wisconsin School of Veterinary Medicine.)*

Appropriate drugs for treatment are listed in Table 22-2. It is important to treat for at least 21 days and possibly longer. It is also important to remember that bacterial infections of the skin are often complicated by concurrent *Malassezia* overgrowth, and concurrent treatment of both is often needed. Feline pyoderma occurs because of an underlying trigger, and although it is important to treat these infections, there should always be a search for the underlying cause. The trigger may be a one-time event that has passed (e.g., flea infestation) or, more commonly, an underlying chronic skin disease or systemic disease.

Malassezia *Overgrowth*

As with bacterial pyoderma, overgrowth of *Malassezia* organisms is an underrecognized and underdiagnosed

TABLE 22-2 **Select Antimicrobial Drugs for Treatment of Skin Disease in Cats**

ANTIBIOTICS		
Drug	**Dose Range**	**Route**
Amoxicillin–clavulanic acid	12.5-25 mg/kg q12h	PO, IM, SC
Cephalexin	15-30 mg/kg q12h	PO
Cefadroxil	20 mg/kg q12h	PO
*Cefpodoxime	5-10 mg/kg q24h	PO
Clindamycin	5.5 mg/kg q12h	PO
Doxycycline	5-10 mg/kg q12h	PO
Enrofloxacin	5 mg/kg q24h	PO, SC
Marbofloxacin	2-5 mg/kg q24h	PO
Lincomycin	20 mg/kg q12h	PO
Trimethoprim–sulfadiazine	15-30 mg/kg q12h	PO
ANTIFUNGALS		
Drug	**Dose**	**Route**
†Itraconazole	5-10 mg/kg q24h	PO
†Terbinafine	40 mg/kg q24h	PO
Fluconazole	10 mg/kg q24h	PO

PO, Orally; *IM*, intramuscularly; *SC*, subcutaneously.
*This is a third-generation cephalosporin, and use should be reserved for infections that cannot be treated with another drug. To minimize the development of methicillin-resistant infections, the drug should be used at the higher dosage range.
†These drugs can be used daily or as a pulse therapy on a 1 week on/1 week off basis until the target infection is resolved.

cause of pruritic skin disease in cats. It is caused by overgrowth of *Malassezia* spp. yeast, which is part of the normal flora of the ear canals, mucosal surfaces (oral and anal), and anal sacs. There is a wide diversity in the species of *Malassezia* that vary in size and shape.

The most commonly encountered clinical presentations include pruritic recurrent OE, recurrent chin acne, paronychia, and scaly and waxy seborrhea.[1-2] Ears may contain a waxy black material or just excessive ceruminous debris. Waxy debris around the nail beds of cats is uncommon and is typical of *Malassezia* dermatitis. The one unifying clinical sign is pruritus that varies from mild to severe. *Malassezia* dermatitis is a common complication of allergic skin diseases, poor grooming, immunosuppression resulting from FIV or FELV, diabetes mellitus, and neoplasia.[77]

It is important to remember that the pathophysiology of *Malassezia* dermatitis includes a hypersensitivity reaction. Therefore the number of organisms seen may be disproportionate to the severity of the clinical signs. The author's (KM) rule of thumb is that if the cat is symptomatic and clinical signs are compatible, any number of organisms seen is significant, and the cat should be treated for yeast overgrowth. The sampling technique depends on the anatomic site affected: ear swabs for ears, spatula scrapings for nail beds and areas of follicular plugging and chin acne, and acetate tape preparation for skin sites. Samples should be examined carefully under oil immersion. It is important to remember that there are many species of yeast, and some species of yeast and recently divided organisms can resemble cocci. The major differentiating factor is the size of the organism. Cocci are approximately 0.2 to 2 μm in diameter, and yeast are much larger. When looking at a slide or describing the difference to clients, the veterinarian may find that a "moon versus earth" comparison works well. This is easiest to determine if there is a mixed population of organisms in the field for the purpose of comparison.

Bathing is an important part of treatment in dogs and can be used in cats if the cat is cooperative. In most cases this is not a treatment option; however, grooming, whether by a professional or the owner, is very helpful in cats with yeast dermatitis. Removal of shed hairs, mats, and accumulated oils, combined with systemic therapy, is very helpful. If yeast overgrowth is localized to a focal area such as nail beds, chin, or ears, application of a topical combined antibacterial and antifungal shampoo or solution may be possible. In general, the use of products containing phytosphingosine (e.g., Douxo Calm Micro-emulsion Spray and Shampoo, Sogeval Laboratories, Coppell, Texas) is strongly recommended. This molecule is part of skin lipids responsible for maintaining normal skin cohesion, controlling local flora, and regulating moisture balance. These products may be used as shampoo substitutes. Most cats, however, require systemic treatment with an oral antifungal drug (see Table 22-2) such as itraconazole or terbinafine. Ketoconazole is not recommended because cats do not tolerate this drug well. Fluconazole has been used successfully by the author (KM) at 10 mg/kg orally, once daily for 30 days. Pharmacokinetic studies with itraconazole and terbinafine have shown that pulse therapy protocols can be used with these drugs. The most common protocol is 1 week on and 1 week off for two to three cycles.[35,101] Yeast otitis is very pruritic, and an otic glucocorticoid is recommended. The author's (KM) otic glucocorticoid of choice is a compounded solution of propylene glycol and dexamethasone injectable (2 mg/mL) in equal concentrations applied once daily to the ears.

Cat breeds with abnormal hair coats (e.g., Rex, Sphynx) have increased oil production on the skin and are at increased risk for yeast overgrowth. This may involve the whole body, the nail folds, or both. Otherwise, it is important to remember that yeast overgrowth is always the result of an underlying skin disease or medical condition. Lack or response to therapy may be the result of an undiagnosed concurrent bacterial infection or persistent underlying skin disease.

Dermatophytosis

This is the most common infectious and contagious skin disease of cats, and pruritus can vary. This skin disease is discussed in the section on scaling, crusting, and greasy skin.

Allergic Causes of Pruritus

The most common allergic skin diseases of cats include flea allergy dermatitis, food allergy, feline atopic dermatitis, and feline insect bite hypersensitivity. The pathogenesis of these allergic diseases involves combinations of type 1 and type 4 hypersensitivity reactions to allergens. The diagnosis is based on history; compatible clinical signs; ruling out of other, more common causes of allergic disease; and response to treatment trials. In the case of feline atopic dermatitis, it is important to remember that allergy testing (in vitro or intradermal) reflects exposure and is not a definitive diagnostic test. In other words, it does not answer the question "Is this cat atopic or not?"

Flea Allergy Dermatitis

Flea allergy dermatitis is a very common feline skin disease caused by a hypersensitivity reaction to flea bites. Depending on the geographic region, the clinical signs can be seasonal or occur year round. Seasonal clinical signs are most common in regions where there are defined cold weather seasons; flea allergy tends to occur in the warm weather months, but not always. A viable population of fleas, sufficiently large to perpetuate flea bite dermatitis, can exist in homes over the winter months. Furthermore, small mammals living in or around homes can be a source of flea exposure year round.

The clinical signs of flea allergy dermatitis are highly variable and can cause any of the well-recognized skin reaction patterns of cats (Box 22-2). The classic pattern is hair loss and miliary dermatitis over the lumbosacral region and hind legs; however, this may not be what is observed in clinical practice (see Figure 22-12). Clients are increasingly aware of the importance of flea control in cats, and the use of spot-on products has made this practice much easier. Flea allergy dermatitis is a common cause of symmetric alopecia, recurrent papular pruritic lesions, recurrent bacterial and yeast overgrowth, eosinophilic diseases, and odd behaviors. Flea allergy is a major differential diagnosis in cats presented for frequent twitching of the skin; sudden, frantic attacks of the skin; and sudden episodes of hyperactive behavior wherein the cat appears to be chased or trying to escape. The author (KM) has noticed one consistent presentation of flea allergy in obese or geriatric cats that cannot groom themselves, particularly their abdomen or lumbosacral area. In response to pruritic areas of the skin that the cat cannot reach, the cat may overgroom or mutilate areas that it can reach (e.g., the tip of the tail, the paws). These behaviors can often be triggered in the examination room by scratching the lumbosacral area of the cat. Care must be taken because sometimes the pruritus is so intense that the cat will bite. Another presentation of possible flea allergy is unilateral, and often intermittent, small eosinophilic lip ulcers. The "rodent ulcer" reaction pattern of cats can be triggered by almost any trauma or inflammatory reaction, including a flea bite.

Diagnosis of flea allergy dermatitis can be an easy or a difficult diagnosis. The presence of a compatible history, clinical signs, and fleas or flea excreta is compelling. Unfortunately, the latter are not commonly found on cats that are able to groom effectively. Intradermal testing with flea antigen and observation of a positive reaction are suggestive but not diagnostic. The best diagnostic tool is response to flea control. This can be met with resistance by clients because it involves treatment of all pets in the home and because "having fleas" still carries a stigma. In these cases it is often helpful to discuss the expense of a diagnostic workup for skin disease and to emphasize that even if the underlying cause is not fleas, year-round flea control is part of the management of cats with chronic skin diseases. Chronic skin diseases are expensive and time consuming to manage and tend to relapse, and it is important to know that the relapse is not caused by something as simple as fleas.

One change in the response to treatment trials for flea allergy dermatitis in cats is that clinicians should be prepared to treat concurrently for secondary bacterial and yeast overgrowth; if left untreated, it may give the false impression that the flea control trial is unsuccessful. It is very common for the author (KM) to encounter cats referred for second opinions after having "failed" excellent flea control and food trials, only to find that the cat has an undiagnosed bacterial and yeast infection.

BOX 22-2

Feline Skin Reaction Patterns

- Head and neck pruritus
- Recurrent otitis
- Symmetric alopecia
- Self-induced alopecia with self-trauma
- Overgrooming without self-trauma
- Twitchy–itchy cat
- Eosinophilic patterns (often chronic and recurrent)
  - Indolent ulcer
  - Eosinophilic plaque
  - Eosinophilic granuloma
  - Miliary dermatitis

Insect Bite Hypersensitivity

Insect bite hypersensitivity is a skin disease caused by hypersensitivity reactions to bites from small biting

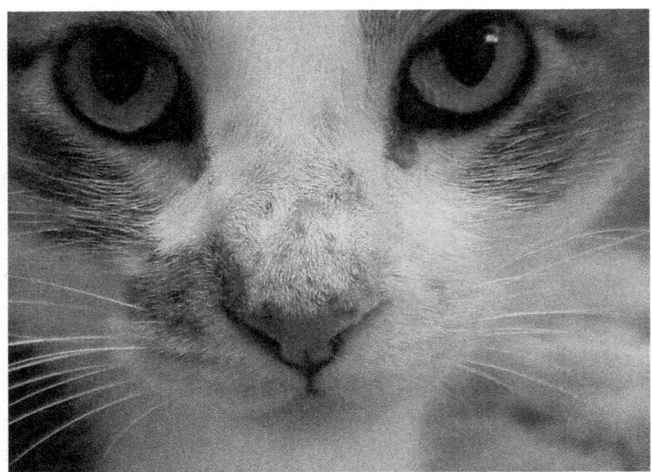

FIGURE 22-16 Insect bite hypersensitivity. Note the multifocal areas of hair loss on the nose and muzzle. This is a common presentation of this syndrome. *(Photo courtesy University of Wisconsin School of Veterinary Medicine.)*

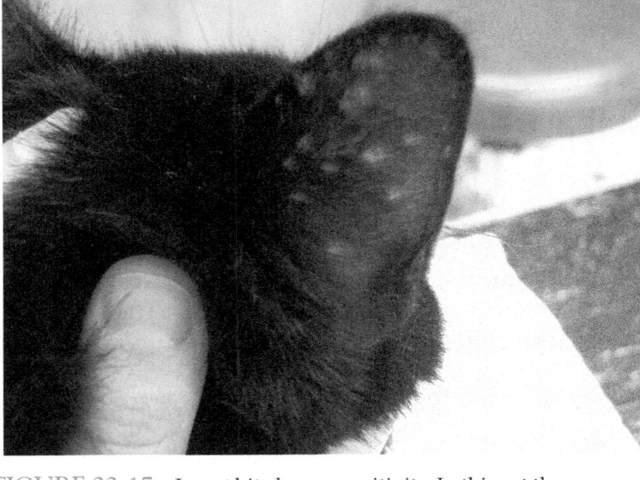

FIGURE 22-17 Insect bite hypersensitivity. In this cat the ears were attacked, and insect bites resulted in the rapid development of small eosinophilic granulomas. *(Photo courtesy University of Wisconsin School of Veterinary Medicine.)*

insects such as mosquitoes, *Culicoides* midges, and gnats.[8] Insect bite hypersensitivity may occur in cats that freely roam outdoors or cats that have access to the outdoors on porches that are screened or have screens that allow entry of the insects. Clinical signs can occur year round depending on geography and the life cycle of the biting insect.

Insect bites occur on the thinly haired areas of the cat, including the nose, inner and outer pinnae, periocular area, and foot pads near the junction of the haired and hairless areas.[53] The insect bites result in papules that vary in severity from mild to severe. Clinical signs become more dramatic as the severity of the pruritus increases and can include widespread ulceration, hair loss, hyperpigmentation, or hypopigmentation (Figures 22-16 and 22-17). Foot pads may become hyperkeratotic, swollen, painful, or ulcerated. The author (KM) has observed regional to generalized lymphadenopathy and peripheral eosinophilia.

Diagnosis is primarily based on history and clinical signs. Exposure to the outdoors, particularly in the morning or evening, should raise suspicion. Lesions will resolve within 1 week without treatment if the cat is confined indoors.

Treatment is not necessary unless the pruritus is severe. Possible treatment options include antiinflammatory doses of prednisolone (0.5 mg/kg orally, once daily until lesions heal) or alternate-day doses of prednisolone if the cat cannot be housed indoors. Some evidence suggests that prednisolone is better absorbed in cats than prednisone.[39] Alternately, repositol methylprednisolone acetate can be used every 6 to 8 weeks throughout the affected season (20 mg/cat subcutaneously or intramuscularly). Chronic prednisolone use is not appropriate for long-term therapy. Localized lesions can be treated with topical glucocorticoids. Another useful drug is cyclosporine (5 mg/kg orally, once daily for 30 days and then every other day). It comes as two formulations: modified and unmodified. The modified formulation has improved absorption and is the only formulation recommended for use in cats (e.g., Atopica, Novartis).

The disease can be prevented by keeping the cat indoors. If this is not possible, the cat should be kept indoors during the dawn and dusk periods. In homes where screened porches are areas of family congregation during the evening, this may be impossible or unreasonable. Improving the screening of porches is an option. The use of citronella candles is very helpful. The application of water-based pyrethrin products can also be used. Pyrethroid products must be used with care in cats, and products marketed for humans as repellants are commonly toxic to cats.

The lesions of insect bite hypersensitivity can mimic feline atopy; food allergy; dermatophytosis; and, most important, feline plasma cell pododermatitis and PF. Cats that do not respond quickly to simple confinement or are refractory to low doses of prednisolone should be more aggressively investigated for other diseases.

Food Allergy

Food allergies in cats are caused by a hypersensitivity reaction to a food or food additive.[100] Food allergies can develop at any age. At this time there are no studies documenting whether food allergies in cats are more common than atopy, as is anecdotally reported.

The clinical signs of a food allergy are highly variable, and there is no classic presentation. Food allergies can present with or without gastrointestinal signs; however, in one study the presence of concurrent signs was the most common presentation.[44] Food allergies can be the cause of any of the commonly recognized skin reaction patterns of cats. What is unique about food allergies is that they are associated with nonseasonal pruritus, and response to glucocorticoid therapy is variable.

Common questions about feline food allergies include the following: When is a diet trial indicated? Can it be diagnosed by allergy testing? What type of diet is best? In the author's (KM) practice, a diet trial is pursued only after more common differential diagnoses have been ruled out. These include the following:

- Response to treatment trial for demodicosis
- Response to flea control
- Negative fungal culture for dermatophytosis
- Lack of response to therapy for a combined bacterial and yeast infection

Using lime sulfur as a response to therapy for feline demodicosis will also rule out other parasite infestations, except for fleas. If the cat is still pruritic at this point, the most likely causes in an otherwise healthy cat are food allergy and feline atopic dermatitis.

Food allergies in cats cannot be diagnosed by blood allergy tests or intradermal skin tests. One of the most difficult aspects of referral of the itchy cat is dealing with a client who is holding the results of a blood allergy test that has positive reactions to every test ingredient. These tests reflect exposure to the allergen, and positive reactions do not correlate with diagnosis. The only way to diagnose a food allergy is by implementing a strict diet trial followed by a provocative test.[46] A dietary hypersensitivity is diagnosed when the target clinical sign (i.e., pruritus) resolves while the trial diet is being fed and recurs when the cat is fed its original diet. Diet trials must be conducted over extended periods of time (8 to 12 weeks) to be certain, and during this time there could be a change of season or another factor. Therefore positive proof by way of a challenge is required.

There is no consensus among veterinary dermatologists regarding the best diet, nor studies to support one in particular. There are three major types of diets used for food trials: home-cooked diets, novel protein diets, and hydrolyzed diets. Whatever diet is used, it should be complete and balanced because this may be the cat's diet for the remainder of its life. Client compliance increases with ease of feeding, which would suggest that commercial diets are superior; however, this is not necessarily the case. If a home-cooked diet is selected, the owner can devote 1 day a month to making the diet and freezing portions for the remainder of the month. The major drawback of home-cooked diets is that if a food allergy is confirmed, the owner either needs to continue to prepare the diet or search for a suitable alternative diet.

Success of a diet trial is directly related to addressing a number of key issues. The test must be indicated and performed at the appropriate time in the workup. The differential diagnoses must be narrowed to allergy (food or atopy). The client needs to be able and willing to do the diet trial, and questions regarding whether they can adhere to the feeding plan must be asked and positively answered. Food trials can be impossible in multiple-pet households if there is any chance that the cat will eat other food. Cats are less likely to be fed table scraps than dogs, but this is not always the case. For example, cats can and do climb on tables and chairs and can reach unwashed dinner plates and pans, and some cats steal food. The cat also must be kept indoors during the entire period of the food trial.

The change from the original diet to the new diet can take several weeks in cats that are persnickety eaters. Palatability is an issue for many cats, and owners and veterinarians may have to use one diet type rather than another depending on what the cat will eat. Another major hurdle is the cat's comfort during the trial. If the cat is severely pruritic, some type of antipruritic agent must be used during the trial. The author (KM) commonly uses cyclosporine modified (5 mg/kg, up to 25 mg/cat, PO, once daily) for the first 4 to 6 weeks of the trial. Once the cat is comfortable and eating the trial diet, the drug is gradually withdrawn between weeks 6 and 8. If the cat becomes pruritic after the cyclosporine is withdrawn, this particular diet is a failure. If not, the diet is continued for several weeks, and then provocative challenge is performed.

It is important that clients understand that they may need to repeat a food trial with another type of diet if the original diet trial is a failure and all other causes of pruritus have been ruled out or if the cat is diagnosed with atopic dermatitis and there is inadequate response to immunotherapy.

It is not uncommon for clients to stop food trials if the cat responds to cyclosporine. Clients want relief of pruritus for the cat, and if cyclosporine provides this relief, the client may not want to proceed with any further diagnostics. The author (KM) does not use glucocorticoid therapy during the first few weeks of the food trial for several reasons. First, if allergy testing is needed after the food trial, cyclosporine will not interfere with test results. Second, glucocorticoid therapy for long-term management of pruritus is fraught with well-known problems. Cyclosporine has been used successfully with few adverse effects and can be used for long periods. Third, if the client completes the food trial and a food allergy is diagnosed, the client has the option of feeding the cat the diet used in the trial, pursuing identification of the individual offending food allergen and then avoiding it, or using cyclosporine therapy for long-term management.

Atopic Dermatitis

The name of the skin disease caused by a type 1 hypersensitivity to environmental allergens in cats is a topic of much debate because the disease has not been as well characterized in cats as it has in dogs. In this discussion the term *feline atopic dermatitis* will be used; however, the reader may see other terms, such as *feline atopic-like dermatitis, feline hypersensitivity dermatitis,* and *feline allergic dermatitis.*

There is no known sex or breed predilection for feline atopic dermatitis. In the author's (KM) experience, owners usually report the development of clinical signs in their cats between the ages of 6 months and 3 years of age, although the cat may not be brought to the veterinarian for evaluation until it is much older. The author (KM) has documented a family of cats with atopy, and others have anecdotally reported a genetic component, but there is not as much evidence for a breed or genetic predisposition in cats as there is in dogs.[59] It is rare to have information on the family of any particular cat. The hallmark of the disease is pruritus that is responsive to glucocorticoid therapy. If there are complicating factors such as a secondary bacterial and yeast overgrowth, response may not be complete. Clinical signs may be seasonal or year round and are variable.

A working diagnosis of feline atopic dermatitis is made by ruling out other common causes of pruritus (i.e., parasites, infections, flea allergy, and food allergy) and having a compatible history and clinical signs. Owners may have difficulty confirming the presence of pruritus because they may not recognize it or notice behaviors associated with pruritus (e.g., licking). A history of vomiting hairballs or constipation may suggest overgrooming. Atopic dermatitis is a differential diagnosis for many feline reaction patterns. In addition to feline symmetric alopecia, some of the most common clinical signs include, but are not limited to, recurrent eosinophilic lesions (plaques, linear granuloma, miliary dermatitis, lip ulcers), "overall itchy cat complaint," patchy alopecia, biting of the hair coat (Figure 22-18), hair loss on the medial and lateral aspects of the limbs (Figure 22-19), pedal pruritus (Figure 22-20), yeast overgrowth at the nail beds, recurrent yeast otitis, increased ceruminous discharge from the ears, symmetric alopecia, broken whiskers, hair loss on the chin and lips, and development of comedones. The hair coat may be dull, rough, or even damp. Nondermatologic signs may include rhinitis, sneezing, conjunctivitis, chronic coughing, and lymphadenopathy.

The question always arises, "Where does allergy testing fit into the diagnosis of feline atopic skin disease?" It is important to remember that allergy tests reflect exposure and are not diagnostic for atopic dermatitis. Allergy testing is appropriate for cats in which immunotherapy is indicated as a treatment modality. It is also indicated in cats that fail food trials or for owners who will not do a food trial until the results of an allergy test are negative. Allergen identification can be done by way of intradermal skin testing or in vitro testing. As is the

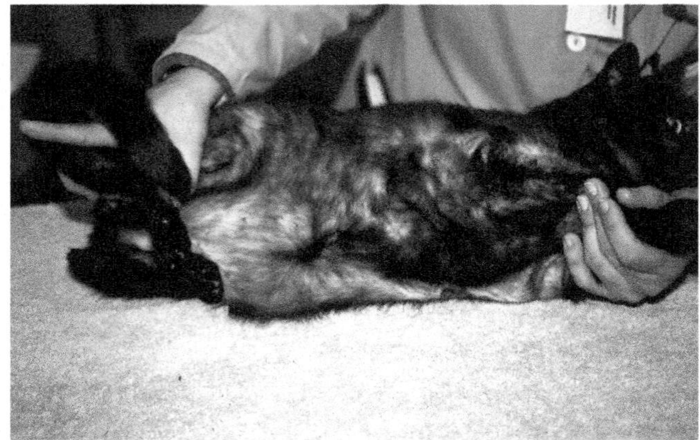

FIGURE 22-18 Atopic cat. This cat had generalized pruritus, and the owner complained about the cat "madly biting itself." *(Photo courtesy University of Wisconsin School of Veterinary Medicine.)*

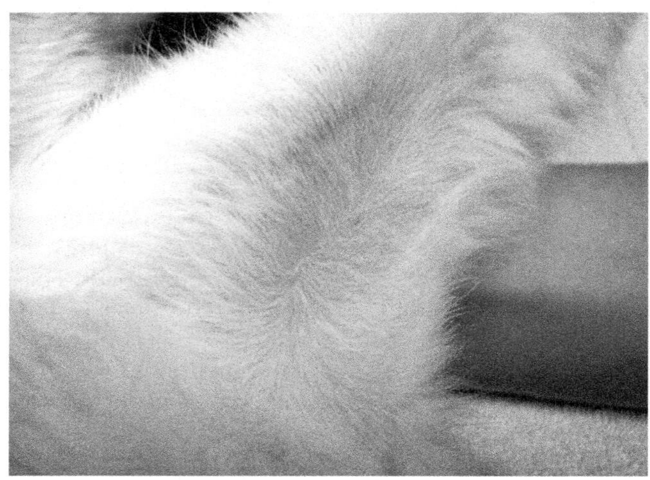

FIGURE 22-19 Atopic cat: Note the hair loss on the medial foreleg. Cytology by tape preparation revealed a combined bacterial and yeast infection, intensifying the pruritus. *(Photo courtesy University of Wisconsin School of Veterinary Medicine.)*

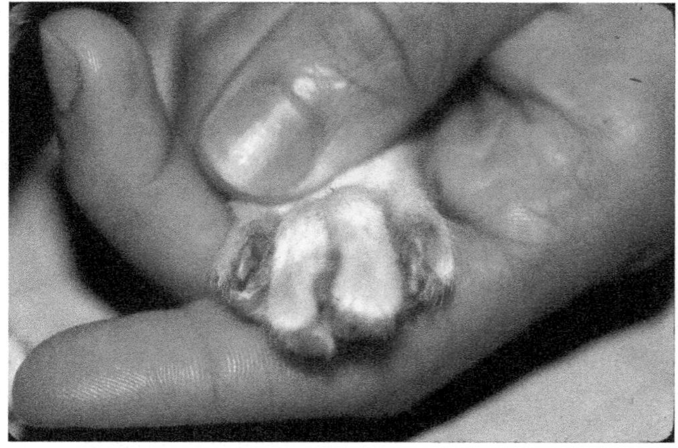

FIGURE 22-20 Atopic cat with pedal pruritus. This cat chewed its nails and had waxy debris at the nail base. Cytology revealed large numbers of yeast organisms. *(Photo courtesy University of Wisconsin School of Veterinary Medicine.)*

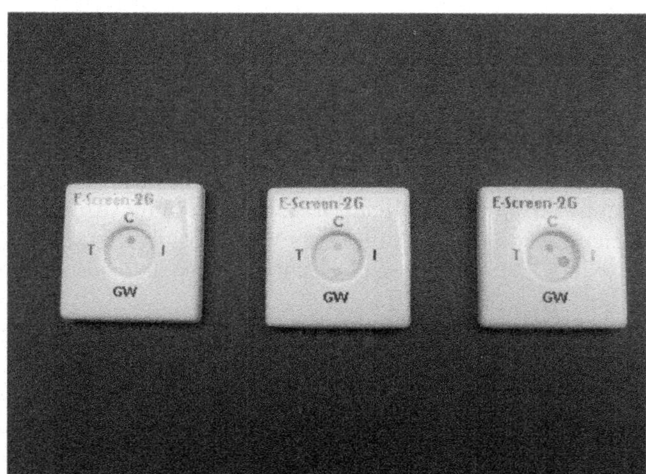

FIGURE 22-21 Heska 2nd Generation E-Screen Test. This test can be used as a screening test to determine if a cat with clinical atopy is likely to have positive reactions on a full panel. If negative, an intradermal skin test should be considered. *(Photo courtesy University of Wisconsin School of Veterinary Medicine.)*

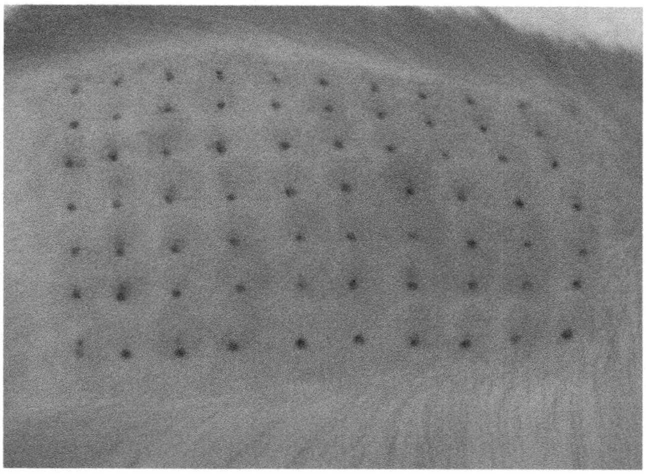

FIGURE 22-22 Positive intradermal test in a cat. Note the large number of wheal and flare reactions. Unlike what is commonly reported in cats, this cat had a strong easily identified skin test reactions. *(Photo courtesy University of Wisconsin School of Veterinary Medicine.)*

case in dogs, there is much debate as to which test is best. Because intradermal skin testing requires drug withdrawals and a referral to a veterinary dermatologist, is more costly, and entails a more involved procedure, the author (KM) recommends in vitro allergy testing first. In the author's (KM) practice, cats are screened with Heska 2nd Generation E-Screen (Heska Corp. Fort Collins, Colorado) (Figure 22-21), which is a miniscreen serum allergy test. In addition to positive and negative controls, there are three wells (for trees, weeds, and indoor allergens). If there is a positive reaction on this screening test, serum is submitted for a full screening. In a recent study in cats, there was strong agreement between a positive E-screen and in vitro allergy test (88%).[30] If the test is negative, an intradermal skin test is performed.

Preparation for intradermal skin testing in cats requires steroid and antihistamine drug withdrawals; however, cyclosporine need not be withdrawn before skin testing.[37] Antihistamines must be stopped 7 days before testing. The time required for steroid withdrawal is varied, but generally it is no less than 4 weeks for a cat receiving an oral glucocorticoid and no less than 8 weeks after a single injection of a repositol glucocorticoid, and possibly longer. Intradermal skin test reactions in cats are typically, but not always, less dramatic than those seen in dogs (Figure 22-22). This makes interpretation more difficult.

Feline atopic dermatitis can be managed but not cured. Management of the disease depends on whether the clinical signs are seasonal or year round; the severity of the pruritus during the cat's allergy season; the distribution of affected sites; concurrent medical conditions; and, of course, what the owner is able or willing to do for the cat.

Avoidance of the offending allergen is rarely possible or feasible. However, if the cat regularly goes outdoors, keeping it indoors will decrease direct exposure to various seasonal allergens. Pollens can be decreased in the home by regular cleaning of household heating ducts and use of high-quality disposable furnace filters. For cats with allergies to house dust mites, old cat beds should be replaced by new beds that are washed at least once weekly. Carpets, mattresses, clothes, and furniture can be treated with benzyl benzoate (e.g., Acarosan Dust Mite Spray and Dust Mite Control Power, Bissell) once a month for 3 months and then every 3 months thereafter to kill and control house dust mite populations. Benzyl benzoate is not difficult to find and is the common ingredient in most over-the-counter products marketed to remove or kill house dust mites. It is important to use a high-quality vacuum cleaner to remove mites. Mites do not thrive well in dry environments, and decreasing relative humidity (<40%) will decrease house dust mite, flea, and mold allergens in the home. Owners may need to purchase several dehumidifier units and should get the most energy-efficient models possible.

All pets in the household should be treated with year-round flea control so that fleas do not aggravate the affected cat's pruritus. Many clients will object, arguing that they never see fleas on the cat or that the cat does not go outdoors. As mentioned previously, the grooming behavior of cats makes finding fleas difficult, and indoor cats can encounter fleas. Management of atopic dermatitis can be complex, and something as simple as flea control can make evaluation and treatment of relapses much easier and quicker to resolve. One of the most compelling counterarguments for these clients is an explanation of the pruritic threshold. Cats may be comfortable with their allergies if less aggressive treatment modalities are used as long as other factors such as flea infestations and secondary infections are controlled.

It is now recognized that part of the pathogenesis of allergic skin disease involves abnormal barrier functioning. From a treatment perspective, this means that greater attention to the health of the hair coat and skin is necessary. Replacement and maintenance of the barrier function in cats can be enhanced by the use of spot-on products that contain ceramides and fatty acids normally found on skin (e.g., Allerderm Spot-On, Virbac Animal Health). In addition, this can also be accomplished with the use of sprays and shampoos with similar ingredients. Spray formulations are undoubtedly more tolerable for most cats than weekly baths.

Recurrent bacterial and yeast overgrowth is common in atopic animals. As mentioned previously, the signs of feline bacterial pyoderma and yeast overgrowth are less dramatic than in dogs. These overgrowths are underrecognized, underdiagnosed, and undertreated. Signs of a bacterial pyoderma may first start with excessive scaling and shedding. In some cats yeast overgrowth occurs most commonly in the ears and nail beds. Cats that develop recurrent *Malassezia* overgrowth in the nail beds may tolerate and benefit from bathing of the paws.

Management of the cat's pruritus is the primary problem with atopic dermatitis. Some cats have focal areas of pruritus that can be managed with topical treatments only. Periocular pruritus can be managed with topical ophthalmic steroids if it is severe. Once the severe pruritus has been resolved or if the ocular pruritus is less severe, other options include ophthalmic cyclosporine or with some of the newer over-the-counter topical ophthalmic drops marketed for people with pruritic eyes caused by allergies. For long-term management of pruritic otitis or ceruminous otitis, the author (KM) uses a compounded steroid ear drop containing a 1 : 1 mixture of propylene glycol and dexamethasone injectable (2 mg/mL). This is very inexpensive and well tolerated by cats.

Options for systemic management of pruritus include essential fatty acids, antihistamines, glucocorticoid therapy, cyclosporine, and immunotherapy. In the author's (KM) experience, essential fatty acids and antihistamines are beneficial in only a small number of patients. These tend to be cats with very mild, seasonal pruritus. The author uses essential fatty acid liquid formulations that can be applied to foods. Antihistamines that can be used in cats are listed in Table 22-3[95,96]; there is no consensus as to which one is most effective. It is important to tell owners that it can take 7 to 10 days before the full benefit of an antihistamine is determined. Lack of response to one drug does not necessarily predict whether other drugs will be effective. Side effects of antihistamines can vary from none to sleepiness, decreased appetite, and hyperexcitability. Glucocorticoid therapy is usually quite effective in managing pruritus in cats, and this may be a cost-effective choice if the cat has seasonal allergies and is otherwise healthy. Treatment options are listed in Table 22-3. In addition to the well-recognized adverse effects of glucocorticoid therapy, there is increasing evidence that methylprednisolone acetate may predispose some cats to congestive heart failure.[80,91] Cyclosporine is another medical option for the management of feline atopic dermatitis. Up to 30 days may elapse before the maximum benefit of the drug is attained, but it can be used in cats with seasonal (>1 month) or year-round allergies as the primary treatment for the pruritus or in conjunction with other treatments. If therapeutic response is good, the dose can be tapered to every other day. Glucocorticoid therapy can be used concurrently to provide a more immediate response.

Immunotherapy is indicated in cats that do not respond to medical management. Currently, there are two protocols for administration of immunotherapy in

TABLE 22-3 **Commonly Used Antipruritic Drugs for Atopic Cats**

Drug	Common Dose	Common Adverse Effects
ANTIHISTAMINES		
Cetirizine HCl (e.g., Zyrtec, Reactine)	5 mg/cat, PO, q24h	None reported
Chlorpheniramine maleate (e.g., Chlor-Tripolon)	2-4 mg/kg, PO, q12h	Drowsiness, salivation from bitter tablets
Clemastine fumarate (e.g., Tavist)	0.68 mg/cat, PO, q12h	Diarrhea, lethargy
Diphenhydramine HCl (e.g., Benadryl)	0.5 mg/kg, PO, q12h	Hyperexcitability
Hydroxyzine HCl (e.g., Atarax)	5-10 mg/cat, PO, q12h	Depression, behavioral changes
CORTICOSTEROIDS		
Prednisolone	0.5-1.0 mg/kg, PO, q24h	Polyuria, polydipsia, polyphagia
Methylprednisolone acetate	5 mg/kg or 20 mg/cat, SC/IM	
Cyclosporine modified* (e.g., Atopica)	5 mg/kg, PO, q24h; can be tapered to q48h	Vomiting, diarrhea

PO, Orally; *SC,* subcutaneously; *IM,* intramuscularly.
*Only the modified formulations of this drug should be used.

cats (traditional and rush therapy), and these are discussed in detail in other sources.[95,96] Briefly, the difference is the administration of allergens in increasing amounts until a maintenance dose is reached over approximately 1 month (traditional) versus several days (rush). Afterwards, a maintenance dose of allergen is administered at regular intervals (e.g., every 7 to 10 days). In the author's (KM) experience, a favorable response is seen in two out of three cats. For some cats it may be the sole therapy, whereas for others intermittent use of some type of adjunct antipruritic therapy may be necessary. On the basis of information from studies of dogs, maximum benefit may not be seen for up to 12 months. However in the author's (KM) experience, some evidence of efficacy usually occurs in 3 to 6 months. Cyclosporine or glucocorticoid therapy can be used to manage the cat's pruritus during this time and provide significant antipruritic relief.[74,106] If the cat responds to cyclosporine therapy, the cost of immunotherapy versus cyclosporine therapy should be considered, insofar as cyclosporine therapy is inexpensive in small patients and may be less expensive for long-term management.[85] Cats receiving long-term cyclosporine therapy should be screened for *Toxoplasma* spp. because this drug may predispose cats to fatal systemic toxoplasmosis.[48] Owners should also take precautions to prevent new infections. The key precautions are to keep the cat indoors to limit exposure through predation of rodents and other potential intermediate hosts and consumption of water from the environment. Other important precautions are to clean the litter box daily, avoid feeding the cat raw meat or unpasteurized milk, control indoor rodent populations safely, and practice good hygiene when handling food for human consumption.

SCALING, CRUSTING, AND GREASY SKIN

Scaling ("dandruff") and crusts are common client complaints. Widespread crusting and exfoliation are uncommon and are usually associated with a medical problem or more serious dermatologic disease. Greasy hair coat can be focal or generalized. As with other dermatologic problems, the history can often provide key information that will narrow the possible differential diagnoses. Young cats and cats that roam freely are more likely to contract dermatophytosis and parasitic infestations. Older cats are more likely to have immune-mediated diseases and skin tumors. Evidence of transmission to other animals or people is compatible with a contagion. Prior treatments may help rule in or out drug eruptions. Response to glucocorticoid therapy may suggest allergic skin diseases. The cat's breed may also provide useful information. The association of longhaired cats with dermatophytosis is the classic example.

Excessive Scaling

In general, the most common causes of scaling and crusting in cats are ectoparasites, bacterial and yeast infections of the skin, and dermatophytosis. Flea combing, skin scraping, and response to flea control are key core diagnostic tests and treatment trials (see previous discussion). As previously mentioned, excessive scaling with scales pierced by hairs is common in cats with bacterial infections of the skin. Response to antibiotic therapy is important to establish. Careful examination of skin impression smears and skin cytology are needed to determine if a concurrent yeast infection is present (see previous discussion). Finally, a dermatophyte culture is indicated at the first presentation to rule in or out the presence of a dermatophyte infection.

It is not uncommon to encounter cats that start to shed hairs or scales excessively when stressed during an examination. Undoubtedly, this is biological in nature but is not a pathologic problem that requires treatment. Some clients report that their cat's hair coat scales excessively when the relative humidity is low (e.g., in winter). This is most likely related to heat-seeking behavior and can be corrected by increasing humidity in the home and using humectants on the hair coat. Cats that cannot groom (e.g., because of obesity) may develop excessive scaling; this can sometimes be corrected by having the owner brush the hair coat on a regular basis. The largest collection of sebaceous glands is located on the cat's dorsum, and routine grooming helps disperse these oils.

Dermatophytosis

Dermatophytosis is the most common infectious and contagious skin disease of cats. The most commonly isolated pathogen is *M. canis;* however, cats can be infected with *Trichophyton* spp. and *Microsporum gypseum*. Because *M. canis* is the primary pathogen of cats, this discussion will focus on *M. canis* dermatophytosis, unless otherwise specified. Although cats are often referred to as the "reservoirs of infection" for *M. canis,* it is important to note that *M. canis* is not part of the normal fungal flora of cats.[61,62] The clinical significance is that isolation of *M. canis* from the hair coat of cats is associated with one of the following situations: mechanical carriage of the spores, subclinical infection, or overt clinical disease. A decision about some type of action is required when a positive fungal culture result is obtained.

The prevalence of the disease is not known because it is not reportable. In general practice, it accounts for approximately 2% of skin diseases presented to a primary care veterinarian.[56] In a multiple-animal facility, prevalence depends on a number of factors, including, but not limited to, use of the facility (cattery, home, closed shelter, open shelter, rescue organization), number of cats present, geographic region (dermatophytosis is more common in warm, humid climates or seasons), age of the animals (dermatophytosis is more common in kittens than adults), health of the population (sick cats do not groom, which predisposes them to disease), and overall animal care practices and philosophies.

Dermatophytosis is transmitted through contact with contaminated environments or other infected animals. For an infection to successfully establish itself, the arthrospores (infective material formed from segmentation and fragmentation of fungal hyphae) have to evade both mechanical, physiologic, and immunologic protective mechanisms. The cat's most important protective mechanism is a healthy hair coat coupled with routine grooming. Infective spores are readily removed from the hair coat of cats. Fungal spores are small and can be carried on air currents. In addition, the author (KM) has isolated "culture-positive fleas," and recently the common housefly was found to mechanically transmit spores.[14] The dose of infective spores necessary to establish an infection is unknown; however, under experimental conditions at least 100 are required.[25] Once the spores penetrate the hair coat and reach the skin surface, some type of trauma is needed to establish infection because spores cannot penetrate intact skin. Increased hydration and maceration of the skin favor penetration and germination of spores. In general, the normally dry skin and hair combined with fungistatic properties of serum and sebum are natural physiologic host defenses. Normal grooming behavior of cats distributes sebum from areas of high concentration and production (chin and dorsum) to other areas. It is easy to understand how flea infestations, pruritus from other causes, or even lack of grooming can predispose a cat to a dermatophyte infection. The incubation period is approximately 1 to 3 weeks from time of exposure to development of lesions. Recovery from infection depends on a strong cellular immune response; stress and immunosuppression compromise recovery.

Dermatophytosis is a pleomorphic disease and cannot be diagnosed on the basis of clinical signs alone. The disease affects the hair follicle, and the most common clinical findings include hair loss, hair breakage, scaling, and crusting (Figure 22-23). Consequences of pruritus vary from none to self-mutilation. In cats, lesions may be focal, multifocal, or generalized in appearance. Because spores are easily spread over the entire body, the lesion distribution may be markedly more limited than the amount of infective material on the hair coat and skin. Hyperpigmentation is uncommon in feline skin diseases but is seen commonly in cats with dermatophytosis. Scaling may be focal or generalized and vary from fine scales to marked exfoliation. In severe cases the cat may look as if it has PF.

The typical presenting complaint is hair loss, but because the disease is zoonotic, owners may complain of lesions that they or other family members have contracted. Cats with generalized dermatophytosis often ingest large amounts of hair while grooming and may have a history of vomiting, constipation, hairball problems, or any combination of these. Erythema and scaling of the inner or outer pinnae (or both) are also common presenting symptoms in adult cats. Patches of scale with minor alopecia or hair breakage is one of the most common presentations in longhaired cats. Feline skin reaction patterns for which dermatophytosis should be considered as a differential diagnosis include miliary dermatitis, symmetric alopecia, eosinophilic plaques, and indolent ulcers, especially unilateral ulcers in young cats. Dermatophyte lesions in kittens tend to consist of areas of hair loss and scaling; erythema is variable and is often difficult to detect in dark-haired cats. Lesions are often first seen as areas of hair loss on the muzzle, face, ears, and forelegs. Depending on the overall health of the kitten, lesions may be focal, multifocal, or generalized. Kittens with limited dermatophyte lesions that develop upper respiratory infections, gastrointestinal diseases, or both are at increased risk for the development of generalized lesions. *M. canis* can cause comedone-like lesions (i.e., chin acne) in young cats.

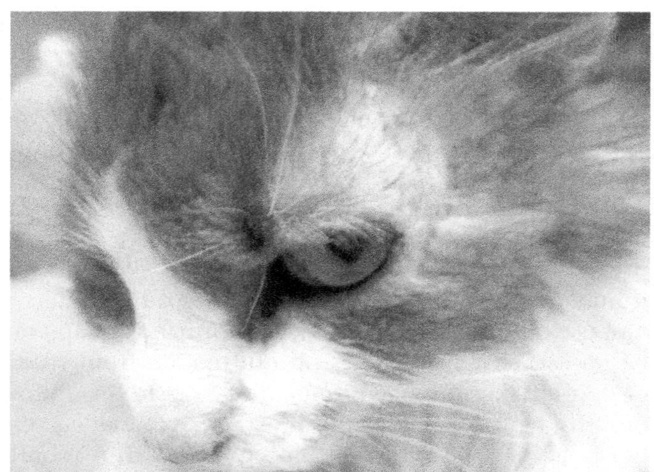

FIGURE 22-23 Cat with dermatophytosis. This is a follicular disease, and the hallmark is hair loss. In this case lesions were present on the face and preauricular area. *(Photo courtesy University of Wisconsin School of Veterinary Medicine.)*

Uncommon presentations of feline dermatophytosis include an appearance clinically identical to that of PF, with scaling and crusting over the bridge of the nose and the face, crusting exudative paronychia, or both. Unilateral or bilateral pinnal pruritus is another underrecognized presentation of *M. canis*. In the cats examined by one of the authors (KM), infected hairs were limited to the ear margin or long hairs within the "bell" of the ear (or both). *M. canis* is uncommonly a cause of recurrent OE.[26] Granulomatous dermatitis, in the form of well-circumscribed, ulcerated dermal nodules, is infrequently recognized in cats. The lesions occur on cats afflicted with more generalized typical *M. canis* infections. These lesions have been called *mycetomas, pseudomycetomas,* and *Majocchi's granulomas.*

Diagnostic testing was described earlier in the chapter. All cats with skin lesions should be screened with a Wood's lamp, and a fungal culture should be obtained. Again, a positive Wood's lamp examination is suggestive, but not diagnostic, of an infection. The value of this test is that it allows the veterinarian to select hairs for direct examination or culture; toothbrush fungal cultures are the preferred culture technique. If spores are seen on direct examination, this is confirmation of infection, and treatment can start pending culture. Culture is always recommended to confirm the infection and species even if spores are seen on direct examination. It is also necessary to obtain a pretreatment culture so that the number of colony-forming units (CFUs) per plate can be monitored. This is an increasingly important method for monitoring response to therapy, particularly when there are multiple cats or screening programs in place.

It is important to remember that this is a self-curing disease in otherwise healthy cats. The reason cats are treated is to speed resolution of the disease, limit spread to other animals and people, and minimize contamination of the environment. Without treatment cats and kittens will be cured in 60 to 100 days, whereas with treatment this time can be significantly shortened. Optimal treatment involves topical, systemic, and environmental modalities, each of which has a different role. Topical treatment reduces contamination on the hair coat, helps minimize re-infection of the host, and decreases spread of spores into the environment. Systemic treatment benefits the cat by reducing the number of weeks to complete cure by affecting the growth of the dermatophyte at the hair follicle stage. Environmental cleaning reduces the chances of re-infection and spread to other susceptible hosts.

Clipping of the hair coat will mechanically remove fragile hairs that tend to fracture and spill spores onto the hair coat and into the environment. It also allows for more thorough application of a topical rinse and decreases the amount and duration of treatment. If the clipping is to be performed in a veterinary clinic, it is important to minimize spread of infective material. The only time that hair coat clipping would be done in a veterinary clinic would be if the entire cat needs to be clipped. The procedure should be done in an area where the cat is confined, such as a transport cage or an open animal carrier. After the cat is sedated (cats should not be clipped without sedation because of the risk of injury), it is placed on a large sheet of disposable surgical drape and clipped. The technician should wear protective clothing that can be removed and washed. Once the cat is clipped, it is immediately treated with a topical antifungal solution. All material in contact with the cat is then disposed of in a biohazard bag. The physical area used to confine the cat is mechanically cleaned. Instead of vacuuming, the veterinarian or staff member should use 3M Easy Trap Duster Sheets (3M, St. Paul, Minn.), which are similar to Swiffer Sweeper dry cloths but are sticky, thereby trapping hair and spores. Then the area should be washed with a detergent several times, finishing with a dilute bleach solution (1:10 to 1:100) and allowing 10 minutes of contact time. Clipping of the hair coat does put the cat at risk for thermal burns from the electric clippers. It may require sedation, which may not be possible or practical in some situations. It also may not be possible in multiple-cat situations. Finally, microtrauma can temporarily worsen the lesions. Clipping of localized lesions can be easily accomplished using disposable children's scissors. For more generalized lesions, clipping of the hair coat with a No. 10 clipper blade is usually adequate. One of the authors (KM) has successfully treated shelter cats for mild to severe generalized dermatophytosis without clipping of the hair coat by using a combination of twice-weekly topical therapy and itraconazole.[64,71,72] However, it is important to note that there was thorough application of the topical solution, concurrent use of a systemic drug, and confinement of the cats.

Consistently effective topical antifungal rinses include lime sulfur, enilconazole, and miconazole. Lime sulfur (1:16 dilution) administered twice weekly is effective as an adjunct or sole therapy. There are many formulations of lime sulfur available, and no difference in the sporicidal efficacy against *M. canis* was found among them when the products were tested in vitro.[31] Adverse effects include staining of the hair coat and drying of the foot pads and skin. Oral ulceration has not been observed in cats treated with lime sulfur by one of the authors (KM), even when cats were allowed to lick the diluted solution. Oral ulcerations anecdotally attributed to lime sulfur were more likely caused by viruses associated with upper respiratory infections.

Enilconazole is not licensed for use in cats and is not available in the United States. The safety and efficacy of enilconazole have been evaluated in cats. In general, it is well tolerated, but some adverse reactions were noted, including hypersalivation, anorexia, weight loss, emesis, idiopathic muscle weakness, and slightly elevated serum alanine aminotransferase concentrations. Anecdotal reports of severe adverse reactions and death are uncommon but do exist, and cats should be prevented from grooming the wet solution from the hair coat. Miconazole is an effective antifungal agent, and synergism between miconazole and chlorhexidine has been demonstrated.[78] This combination is available in shampoo and rinse formulations.

Systemic antifungal drugs must be cost effective and well tolerated in cats. The two antifungal drugs of choice for systemic therapy in cats are itraconazole and terbinafine because both have been shown to have residual activity in the stratum corneum of cats. Both drugs are very effective and well tolerated by cats and can be used in pulse therapy, which is highly tolerable to both cats and owners. Itraconazole (5 to 10 mg/kg orally) can be administered daily or on a 1 week on/1 week off basis until the mycologic cure.[101] Terbinafine (40 mg/kg orally) can be administered similarly.[35] Adverse effects of either drug include vomiting, diarrhea, inappetence, elevations in serum liver enzymes, and facial pruritus (terbinafine). Fluconazole has been used by one of the authors (KM) at 10 mg/kg orally, but whether this drug can be used in pulse therapy is unknown. Lufenuron has been shown to be ineffective both as a treatment and preventive in feline dermatophytosis.[27,60,63] Given the widespread availability of alternative drugs that are safer and better tolerated by cats, griseofulvin is not recommended for systemic antifungal therapy.

Concurrent topical and systemic antifungal therapy should continue until mycologic cure, as defined by a minimum of two consecutive negative fungal cultures. Ideally, cultures should be performed at weekly intervals. Owners can be taught to perform toothbrush fungal cultures at home. It is important to stress application of the topical antifungal solution to the face, periocular area (Figure 22-24), and interior of the ears because these sites are often undertreated and persistent infections or apparent failure to cure is commonly traced to this problem.

A common dilemma is what to do about other pets in the home. All animals should be examined for lesions and fungal cultured. Pending cultures, all animals should be treated topically with lime sulfur rinses twice weekly. If lesions and fungal cultures indicate that another animal is infected, that pet should receive concurrent systemic antifungal therapy. Otherwise, the veterinarian should continue to treat all animals topically until the infected cat is cured. The approach to management of dermatophytosis is not unlike that needed for contagious mites or fleas; all in-contact animals are to be treated.

Ideally, cats should be examined every 2 to 4 weeks. Most cats with a healthy immune system will require 30 to 60 days to reach mycologic cure; longer treatment may be necessary in ill cats or those with severe infections. Fungal cultures should be observed daily, and instead of simply reporting the results as positive or negative, the veterinarian should record the number of CFUs. A successful treatment should show a decrease in the number of CFUs from one week to the next. Persistence of high numbers of CFUs indicates environmental contamination, persistence of lesions, or development of new lesions. As previously mentioned, seemingly resistant infections are almost always due to issues related to treatment. If there is any concern about an owner's ability to thoroughly apply a topical antifungal rinse, daily antifungal therapy may be the best choice.

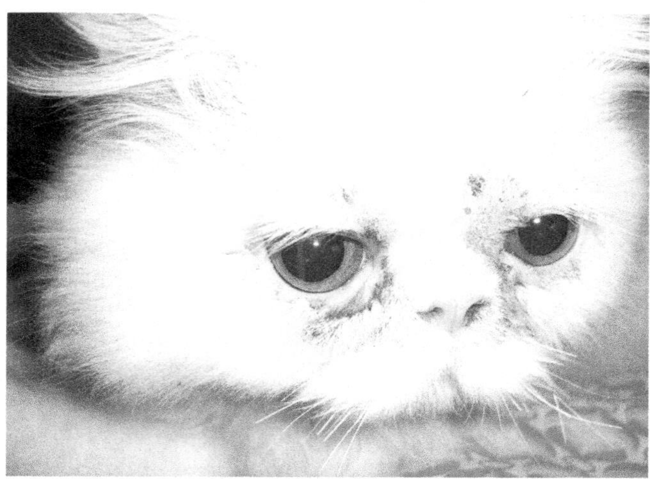

FIGURE 22-24 Persistent dermatophytosis in a Persian cat. This cat was referred for "resistant infection," but careful examination revealed glowing hairs in the periocular area. The client had not treated the face of the cat with the topical antifungal rinse. *(Photo courtesy University of Wisconsin School of Veterinary Medicine.)*

The following strategies will minimize contamination of the home:

- As soon as an infected animal is identified, isolate the cat to an easily cleaned room.
- Remove clutter from the room, and keep closet doors closed.
- Remove contaminated toys, and wash bedding.
- Remove infected hairs by clipping, combing, or using a lint roller.
- Use a topical antifungal rinse twice weekly. Lime sulfur is particularly safe and effective.
- Routinely clean the home and use a triple-cleaning technique in the room where the cat is being confined. Specifically:
  - Mechanically remove gross debris by vacuuming.
  - Wash the area with a detergent that is safe to use around cats.
  - Repeat washing of an area is very effective in the mechanical removal of infected hairs and spores.
  - On nonporous areas use a 1:100 dilution of household bleach in water.
- After the cat has been cured, the home should be thoroughly cleaned using the triple-cleaning technique. Surfaces that can be damaged by household bleach should be repeatedly cleaned with a cleanser indicated as safe for that surface.
- If confirmation of decontamination is needed, the following sampling technique can be used. Wait 1 hour after an area or room has been cleaned, and then when surfaces are dry, wipe the area with a small section of sterile gauze sponge until soiled.

Seal the sample in a plastic bag, label it, and submit it for culture. This technique will readily detect spores and help identify areas that need additional cleaning.

Special Considerations for Infected Multiple-Animal Facilities[56]

Space does not allow a detailed discussion of the management of dermatophytosis in animal shelters, and the reader is referred to recommended sources[58,64] for more details; however, the major points are discussed in the subsequent paragraphs.

Endemic dermatophytosis has a profound effect on the health, community reputation, and economic status of animal breeding colonies and animal shelters. Breeding programs must be interrupted because newborn animals are rapidly and easily infected, leading to debilitation and sometimes death. Adoption of shelter pets must be temporarily halted to prevent spread of the infection to new owners. Eradication of dermatophytosis from such a facility is completely possible but requires a commitment to a screening and treatment program and may not be practical or affordable in many facilities. It is important to do the job correctly the first time and institute preventive measures against future outbreaks. Using a standardized system of evaluation, culture, and treatment, eradication has been reported in as little as 2 months.[16]

It is important to recognize that animals with visible, obvious lesions represent only *the tip of the iceberg* in an endemic colony, particularly in a *M. canis*–infected facility. Many animals also have subclinical infections, and many more will be innocently carrying dermatophyte spores on their hair coats. Therefore the eradication process must begin by toothbrush culturing every animal in the facility, regardless of the animal's clinical appearance. While the initial culture results are pending, the staff members should quarantine any animals with obvious or suspected infection. This precaution requires isolation in a separate *contaminated* room or building, with floor surfaces that can be disinfected easily. A Wood's lamp is very helpful here, if the outbreak is caused by a fluorescing strain. A separate *clean* room or building must also be prepared, into which cured animals will be gradually moved. If new animals must be introduced into the colony during the eradication effort, a third intake room is recommended. Pending the results of the fungal cultures, all animals should be treated with topical lime sulfur 1:16 dilution twice weekly. This is very safe and easily and rapidly applied to animals using a garden sprayer. It is important to use warm water because this makes the application less objectionable, and the sprayer should be held as close to the skin as possible so that the skin and hair are thoroughly coated. Environmental decontamination procedures should begin immediately in all three rooms and continued indefinitely because the introduction of dermatophytosis into a shelter or multiple animal facility is always a risk.

Once the initial culture results are known, the animals can be divided into two groups on the basis of culture results, assuming that the two groups of animals can be kept separate and cross-contamination is not likely. The first group consists of cats that are culture negative and are kept in the clean room. The second group consists of cats that are culture positive with or without lesions. All culture-positive cats should be treated with either itraconazole (10 mg/kg orally, once daily) for 21 days or terbinafine (40 mg/kg orally, once daily) for 21 days. In addition, twice-weekly application of lime sulfur should be continued until two negative consecutive fungal cultures are obtained. A 1 week on/1 week off dosing schedule for itraconazole is quite acceptable; however, if large numbers of cats are involved or multiple people are involved in the medication of the cats, the week on/week off protocol becomes confusing and treatment lapses can occur.

Animals in the clean room should be recultured once after being transferred to that room, as a precautionary measure. Animals in the contaminated room are cultured every week until each animal has a negative result on at least two successive times. Animals that initially had positive culture results but carried only a few spores (as opposed to being actively infected) will develop negative results rapidly, and when they achieve two cultures with negative results, they can be transferred to the clean room. This is easily recognized by a marked and rapid reduction in the number of CFUs on each fungal culture plate. It will soon become obvious which animals are truly infected because they will have multiple successive positive culture results even during treatment. Treatment is continued in the contaminated room until all animals are cured and moved to the clean room. At this point, the contaminated room should be thoroughly cleaned and decontaminated before further use.

During the treatment period, it is important to watch for animals that have persistently positive fungal culture results with too many CFUs to count on the culture plate and little apparent resolution despite treatment. These animals, which will typically be only one or a few, may be chronically infected because of their failure to develop an appropriate cell-mediated immune response, and they represent a potent threat to the continued health of the entire colony. Testing these cats for FeLV and FIV is appropriate insofar as it may explain the lack of response, but test results will not change the treatment protocol unless the owners want to remove the infected cats from the population. If the hair coat has not been clipped, this is recommended. It is also recommended that daily antifungal treatment be started. In addition, these chronically infected animals should be either euthanized or removed to a separate facility for treatment.

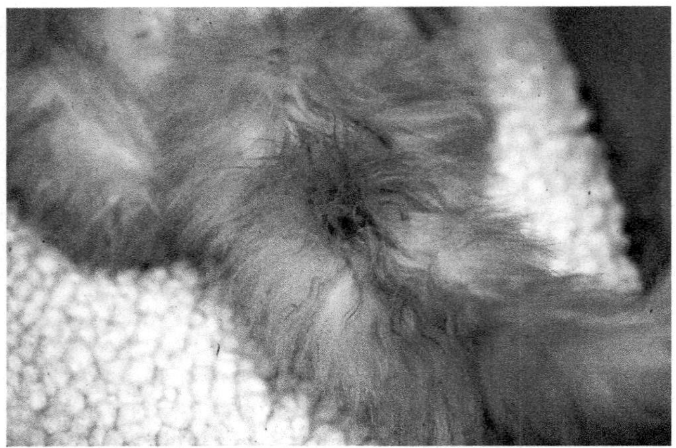

FIGURE 22-25 Disorder of keratinization. Increased greasy hair on the dorsal tail is a common form of disorder of keratinization in cats. *(Photo courtesy University of Wisconsin School of Veterinary Medicine.)*

If new animals are entering by way of the intake room, as each animal enters, it should be immediately toothbrush cultured and then given an antifungal bath and dip. Most animals will have negative culture results and can be transferred to the clean room as the culture results become known. Any animal that has a positive culture result is transferred to the contaminated room and treated as previously noted. After the eradication effort is concluded, this intake procedure should be maintained indefinitely.

Greasy Seborrhea Syndromes

In general, it is uncommon for cats to have greasy hair coats because of their fastidious grooming habits; however, there are several well-recognized clinical presentations that clinicians should recognize. Cats do not simply stop grooming. Cats that develop greasy, unkempt hair coats do so because of illness or pain, and a careful physical examination and medical evaluation is needed. Greasy hair coats are common findings in cats with hyperthyroidism or diabetes mellitus, but they can occur in any cat that does not feel well. Another common presentation in healthy cats is a focal area of greasy hair on the proximal third of the tail (Figure 22-25). Sebaceous glands are present in large numbers on the dorsum of the cat and in particular in this area. This condition is called "stud tail" by lay people, which implies that it occurs more commonly in intact male cats; however, it can occur in intact or neutered male or female cats. This area can become secondarily infected. Depending on the severity of the greasy tail, management can vary from grooming the cat's tail to bathing and grooming. Persian and Himalayan cats can develop an idiopathic facial dermatitis characterized by moderate to severe accumulations of adherent debris. This idiopathic facial fold dermatitis has been reported to be nonpruritic, but pruritus is variable depending on whether secondary infections develop (Figure 22-26).[9,11] These cats should be thoroughly evaluated because some may have underlying treatable diseases. They also need to be differentiated from cats with facial lesions caused by herpes virus.[45] Management of these cats is difficult, but tacrolimus ointment has recently been reported to be useful, and there are anecdotal reports of cyclosporine therapy being helpful.[18] However, it is important that clients understand that cleansing of the face may be a lifelong part of therapy. Greasy skin is a common finding in Rex and Sphynx cats.[1,2,10] *Malassezia* overgrowth can be a chronic problem in some cats. Primary seborrhea can also be seen in some longhaired breeds as a primary disorder of keratinization. Bathing with Douxo Seborrhea Shampoo (Sogeval, Coppell, Texas), and use of the companion spray product (Douxo Seborrhea Micro-emulsion Spray, Sogeval, Coppell, Texas) is very successful in managing these cats. The spray can also be used as a shampoo substitute.

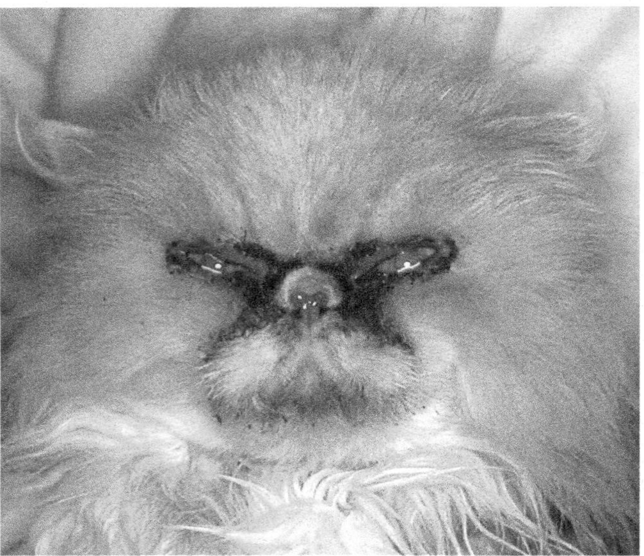

FIGURE 22-26 Greasy-faced Persian cat: Persian cat with symmetric periocular and facial sebum-rich exudates. *(From Rest J: Controversial and emerging diseases. In August J, editor:* Consultations in feline internal medicine, *ed 5, St Louis, 2006, Saunders Elsevier, p 270.)*

Sebaceous Adenitis

Sebaceous adenitis is an immune-mediated disease in which the sebaceous glands are destroyed. It is more common in dogs than in cats, but this may be due to differences in presentation. The few cases described in the literature presented with either noninflammatory alopecia on the body, patchy areas of hair loss, or a periocular brown-black exudation around the eyelids and vulva.[75] The disease is diagnosed using skin biopsy and can be managed with cyclosporine.

Pemphigus Foliaceus

PF is an immune-mediated skin disease characterized by the loss of intercellular adhesion of cells in the epidermis. Autoantibodies attack the adhesion molecules causing the epidermal cells to detach (acanthocytes). Neutrophils invade the spaces in response to inflammatory mediators. The disease can occur spontaneously, or it can be the result of drug reactions.

The disease is most common in middle-aged cats; however, the author (KM) has seen one case in a 6-month-old Siamese kitten. Clinically, the disease is characterized by waves of intact pustules that rupture and crust, resulting in crusting and scaling of affected areas.[17,83] In cats lesions are most commonly seen on the face, nose, and inner pinnae (Figure 22-27). Lesions can also involve the paws, resulting in exudative paronychia and foot pad crusting (Figure 22-28). Lesions can become widespread and are more easily palpated than seen; small crusts covering areas of exudation are felt throughout the hair coat. Intact pustules are difficult to find and are most common on the inner pinnae and around the mammae. As mentioned before, lesions tend to develop in waves, and cats may become depressed and febrile just before the start of a wave of lesion development.

Definitive diagnosis is made through histologic examination of skin biopsy specimens. A careful search for intact pustules must be made. In the absence of finding these lesions, numerous skin biopsies of crusted areas of the skin should be sampled. Micropustules are often found within characteristic lesions. Cytologic examination of exudate from an intact pustule can often provide a working diagnosis if large rafts of acanthocytes are seen (Figure 22-29).

This is a disease that can be managed but not cured. Most cats do very well with therapy. Treatment options include glucocorticoid therapy; chlorambucil; adjunct topical steroids; and, most recently, cyclosporine. Corticosteroids are usually the first drug of choice insofar as remission can be rapidly induced. Oral prednisolone (2 to 4 mg/kg, once daily or divided) is administered until the lesions are in remission. The dose is then administered every other day and gradually reduced until the lowest possible dose is found that will maintain the cat in remission. It is important to note that in rare cases even short courses of prednisolone can cause diabetes mellitus in cats. Also, although rare, corticosteroid use has been associated with congestive heart failure in cats.[81,91] Some cases of feline PF do not respond to prednisolone, and dexamethasone may be very effective in these cases. In cases where corticosteroids cannot be

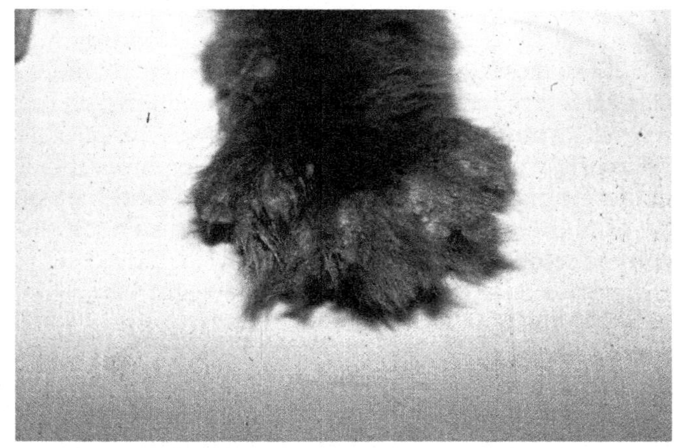

FIGURE 22-28 Paw of cat with pemphigus foliaceus. Note the crusting on the paws. This is an excellent site to obtain cytology. Exudate can often be removed from beneath the crust to reveal acanthocytes. *(Photo courtesy University of Wisconsin School of Veterinary Medicine.)*

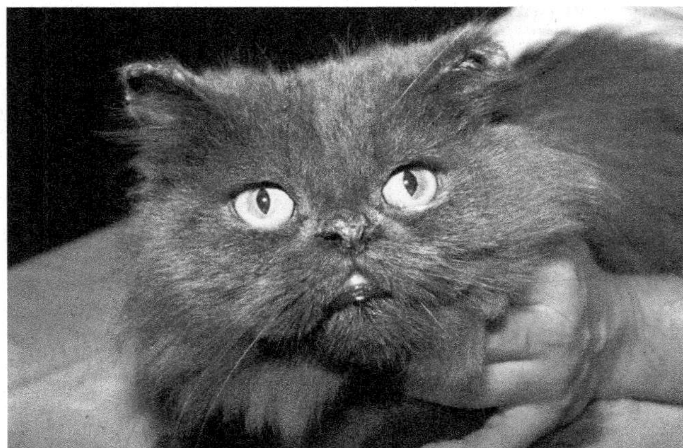

FIGURE 22-27 Cat with pemphigus foliaceus. Note the lesions on the nose and ear tips. This disease presentation can mimic dermatophytosis. *(Photo courtesy University of Wisconsin School of Veterinary Medicine.)*

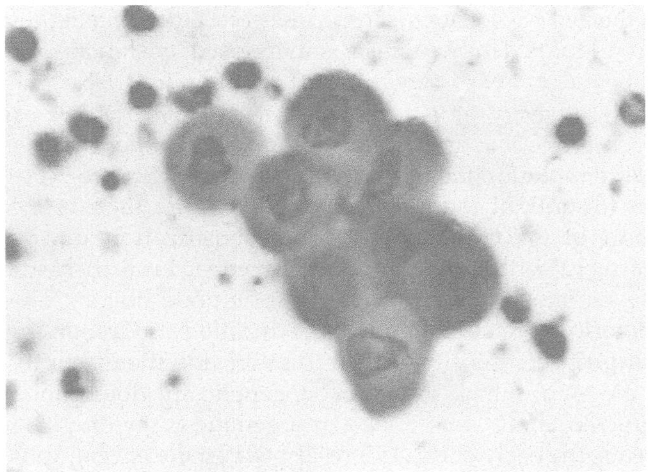

FIGURE 22-29 Cytology from paw in Figure 22-28. The large, deeply staining cells are rounded keratinocytes or acanthocytes and are strongly suggestive of pemphigus foliaceus. *(Photo courtesy University of Wisconsin School of Veterinary Medicine.)*

used long term or do not provide adequate control, chlorambucil (0.1 mg/kg orally, once daily, or 0.2 mg/kg orally, every other day) can be given concurrently with a glucocorticoid. There is a lag time of 2 to 4 weeks before maximum benefit may be seen. Complete blood counts should be monitored every week for the first month and then every 2 to 4 weeks thereafter because this drug can cause bone marrow suppression. Azathioprine is contraindicated in cats because of serious bone marrow toxicity.[5] Another option is the use of cyclosporine (5 mg/kg orally, once daily). Given that this drug has a lag period of 30 days before maximum benefit is seen, concurrent use of prednisolone therapy to induce remission is necessary.

Paraneoplastic Exfoliative Dermatitis

The clinical signs of paraneoplastic exfoliative dermatitis may precede the development of the tumor in the thymus gland. Lesions start as a nonpruritic, erythematous dermatitis that rapidly becomes markedly exfoliative on the head, neck, pinnae, and body. Overgrowth of yeast is very common and present in alarmingly large numbers, and these organisms are readily found on skin biopsy. This skin presentation may be the only sign of the thymoma. Nondermatologic signs may include coughing, dyspnea, anorexia, lethargy, and weight loss. Thymectomy typically results in resolution of all clinical signs (including paraneoplastic signs) and results in prolonged survival.[13,34,36,86,97]

Epitheliotropic Lymphoma

Epitheliotropic lymphoma is an uncommon cutaneous T-cell lymphoma characterized by pruritic exfoliative erythroderma with hair loss and scaling (Figure 22-30). Lesions can start with excessive scaling or just diffuse erytherma.[90,94] Lesions can progress to areas of plaques and nodules. This neoplasia is diagnosed by skin biopsy.

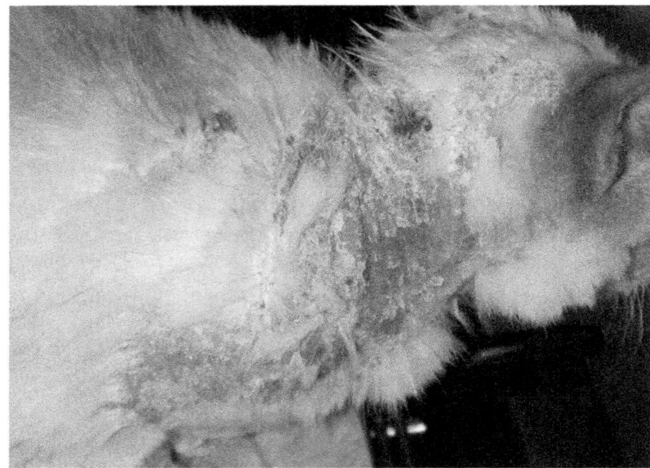

FIGURE 22-30 Exfoliation. This cat has severe exfoliation and *Malassezia* overgrowth. The cat had a thymoma. *(Photo courtesy University of Wisconsin School of Veterinary Medicine.)*

Solar or Actinic Dermatitis

Solar or actinic changes occur as a result of chronic exposure to sunlight and ultraviolet light; further, there is one report of a cat developing photosensitization during treatment with clofazimine for mycobacterial disease.[6] This emphasizes the importance of a good history. The deleterious effects depend on the duration and frequency of exposure, intensity of the radiation, and the reactivity of the skin, which is based on genetically determined skin color, hair coat density, and genetic susceptibility.[12] In cats, the early clinical signs appear on the ear margins of sparsely haired pinnae as erythema and fine scaling. As the lesions progress, erythema increases with crusting and scaling, pain, and ear twitching. Further progression of untreated lesions leads to ulceration and hemorrhage. In addition to the lesions on the ear, solar or actinic lesions can occur on the eyelid and dorsal aspects of the nose. Major differential diagnoses include immune-mediated diseases; however, a history of chronic sun exposure and slow progression are compelling. Definitive diagnosis is made with biopsy. A key finding on biopsy is the presence of apoptotic epidermal keratinocytes.[102] Clinical management ranges from limiting sun exposure to surgical excision of the affected area. Given the difficulty in limiting cats' sun exposure, ultraviolet-blocking sun shades are more practical to use. Sunscreen can be used, but it is likely to be removed during grooming. If a sunscreen is applied, it should be one that is safe to use on infants, with the highest possible sun protection factor (SPF) available. Lip balm products are safe and easy to apply. For maximum benefit, the sunscreen needs to be applied 30 minutes before sun exposure. If actinic lesions are left untreated, transformation into malignant squamous cell carcinoma (SCC) is likely. Cats with SCC tend to be white or light colored, and lesions are most common on the nose, eyelids, and ears.

CHIN ACNE AND CHIN FURUNCULOSIS

Chin acne has recently been extensively reviewed.[47] Acne is considered a follicular disorder and varies in presentation from scattered comedones to severe chin furunculosis. This is a clinical diagnosis (Figures 22-31 and 22-32). It is important to remember that facial pruritus is a common clinical sign in cats with many diseases, and repeated rubbing of the face will result in hair loss and plugging of sebaceous glands or comedones. Useful diagnostic tests include cytology of the skin to

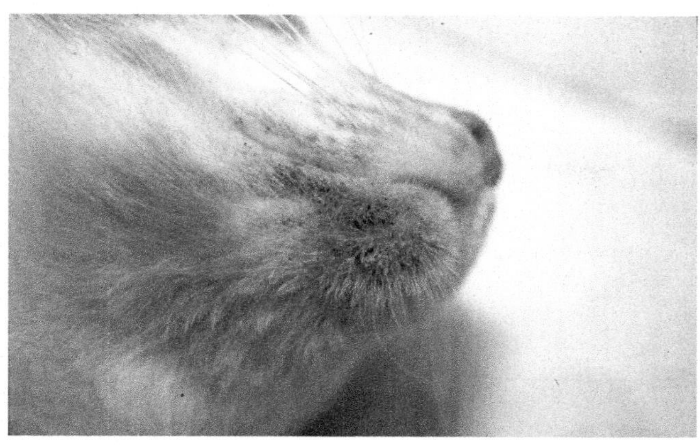

FIGURE 22-31 Chin acne. This is a classical presentation with comedones and black debris. *(Photo courtesy University of Wisconsin School of Veterinary Medicine.)*

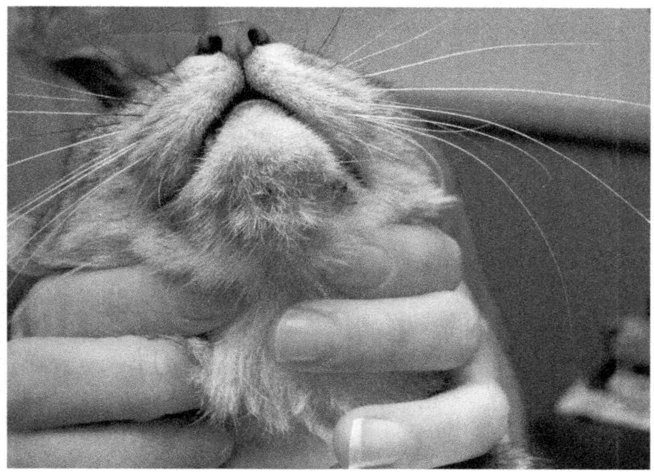

FIGURE 22-32 Chin pyoderma. This is a more purulent form of chin acne and is characterized by pustules and furuncles. *(Photo courtesy University of Wisconsin School of Veterinary Medicine.)*

look for bacterial and yeast overgrowth; often, the underlying trigger of the disease is gone, and the clinical signs will resolve with treatment. Skin scrapings and hair plucking should be performed to look for demodicosis. Rapid onset of chin acne in a household of cats can be caused by a bacterial infection, dermatophytosis, or *D. gatoi*. Oddly, the latter can develop in a stable population of pet cats in the home. Skin biopsy is not often necessary for diagnosis or as a part of the diagnostic evaluation but may be helpful in refractory cases. Facial washing with a mild antibacterial and antifungal shampoo can be helpful; in many cases, washing with plain warm water combined with systemic antimicrobial therapy is effective. Topical mupirocin ointment is very effective, but cats will lick this solution off the face, causing rupture of the hair follicles in the dermis and worsening the disease. Some cats have been reported to respond to cyclosporine. Manual expression of the lesions is never helpful.

ALOPECIA

After pruritus, alopecia is the most common reason that cats are brought to the veterinarian for dermatologic examination. The most common cause of alopecia in cats is self-induced by licking. The diagnostic evaluation for most cases of alopecia should include a careful history, thorough examination, and a methodical diagnostic plan (Figure 22-33).

Feline Symmetric Alopecia

Feline symmetric alopecia (FSA) is a clinical reaction pattern in which the cat presents with symmetric alopecia over the thorax, flanks, ventral abdomen, or pelvic regions. In most cases the underlying etiology is a pruritic disease that may be complicated by a secondary bacterial and yeast overgrowth. FSA can also develop after exposure to irritants or topical drugs; in one report two cats developed FSA within 2 weeks of exposure to diesel oil.[28] Early in the diagnostic evaluation, it is important to determine if the overgrooming is associated with pain or a medical illness so that the cat does not suffer needlessly.[103] Radiographs of the affected area may reveal fractures, particularly over the lumbosacral area (Figure 22-34). Excessive overgrooming of the ventral abdomen may indicate abdominal pain, particularly pain associated with the bladder. Increasingly, the author (KM) is seeing older cats with no history of prior skin disease being brought in for overgrooming of anatomic areas where radiographs reveal arthritic changes, particularly intervertebral arthritis. Resolution of the overgrooming and regrowth of the hair after alleviation of chronic pain provide compelling evidence that pain was the trigger.

True behavioral causes of overgrooming are rare[103] and, in this author's (KM) experience, commonly associated with other behavioral problems (e.g., inappropriate urination or defecation). Treatment with behavior-modifying drugs should be a last resort because these drugs are not without risk. Treatment should alleviate the overgrooming, allowing the hair to regrow and return once the behavior-modifying drug is withdrawn. A very common scenario with obsessive–compulsive grooming in cats that have FSA is a history of a flea infestation that was successfully treated and followed by persistent grooming. The cats are referred for consultation when the behavior-modifying drugs are no longer effective; invariably, these cats respond to a treatment trial of combined antimicrobial therapy.

Telogen Effluvium

Telogen effluvium is a nonpruritic and noninflammatory hair loss pattern characterized by easily epilated hairs.

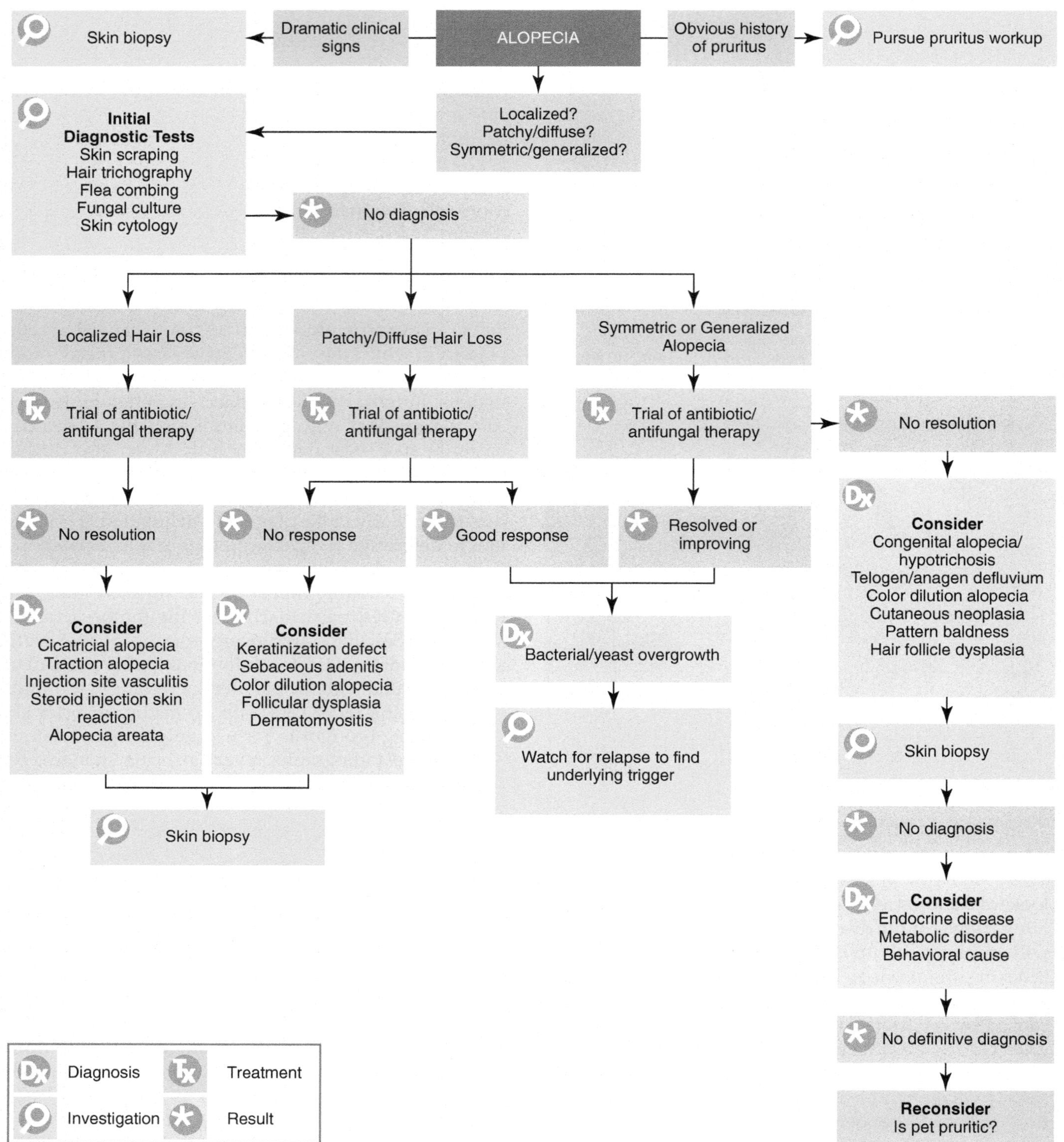

FIGURE 22-33 Diagnostic flow chart for alopecia in cats. *(From Moriello K: Alopecia in cats,* Clinicians Brief *7:19, 2009.)*

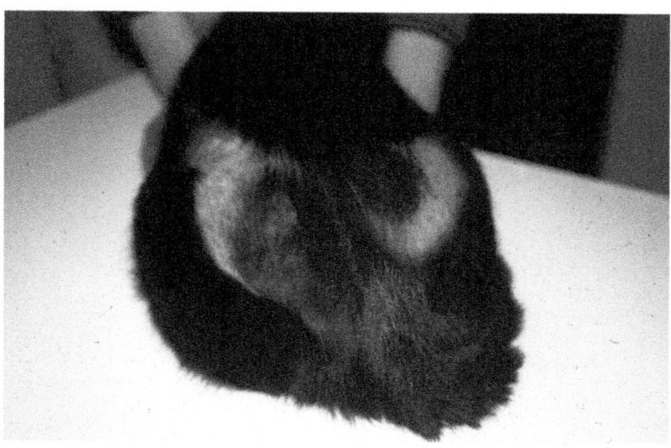

FIGURE 22-34 Symmetric alopecia. This is an unusual form of symmetric alopecia; however, this site and pattern are common in cats that have suffered pelvic fracture. *(Photo courtesy University of Wisconsin School of Veterinary Medicine.)*

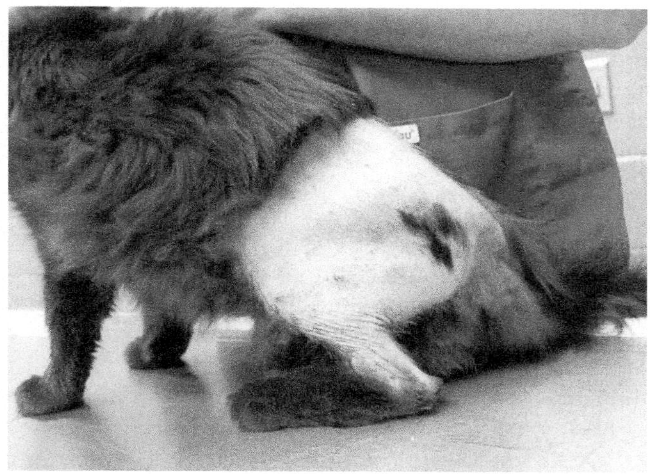

FIGURE 22-35 Telogen effluvium. This cat was from a shelter, and large amounts of hair were easily epilated. The hair coat regrew. *(Photo courtesy University of Wisconsin School of Veterinary Medicine.)*

Close inspection of the hair bulbs reveals that they are in telogen. Clinically, the hairs are easily removed with gentle traction, and often it appears as if the hair coat could almost be peeled off (Figure 22-35). This condition is common in cats or kittens from animal shelters that have a history of severe respiratory infection, especially accompanied by fever (Figure 22-36). The cause is unknown but may be related to a viral infection or overall debilitation. The nonpruritic hair loss resolves without treatment. In practice, the most common presentation of this would be a kitten with a sudden loss of hair that grows back quickly. Dermatophytosis is a major differential diagnosis, insofar as severe infection can result in massive hair loss caused by breakage of the hair shafts; however, usually the hair shafts are stubbly and the skin is inflamed in cats with dermatophytosis.

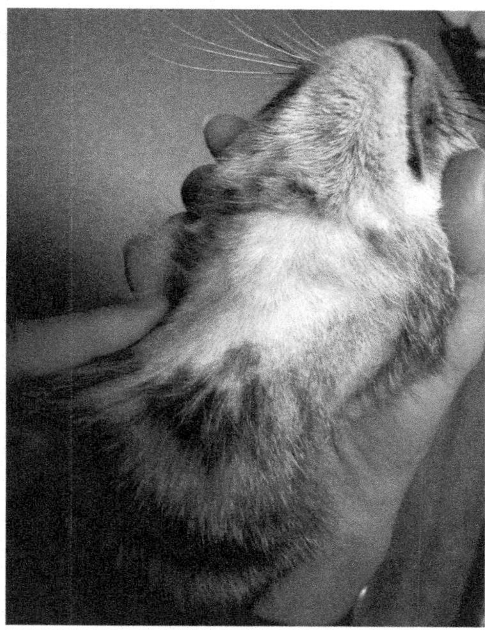

FIGURE 22-36 Focal telogen effluvium. Approximately 2 weeks after recovery from a severe upper respiratory infection, this cat developed focal areas of easily epilated hairs. *(Photo courtesy University of Wisconsin School of Veterinary Medicine.)*

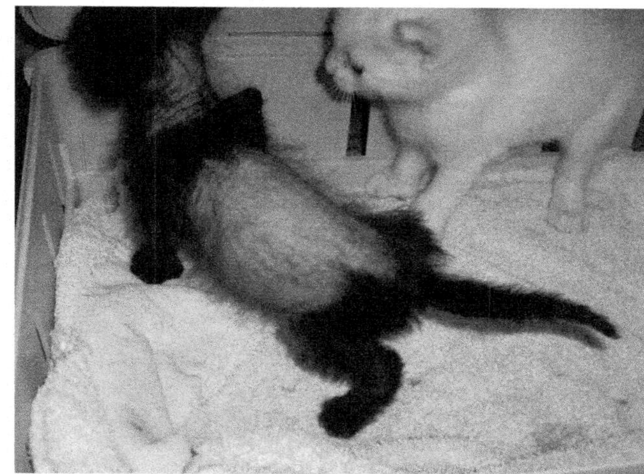

FIGURE 22-37 Congenital hair loss in a kitten. One kitten in a litter was born without hair follicles on the trunk. *(Photo courtesy University of Wisconsin School of Veterinary Medicine.)*

Congenital Hypotrichosis

Congenital hypotrichosis is a rare disease in which one or more kittens in a litter are affected. Kittens are either born alopecic or lose their hair coats over the first month of life (Figure 22-37). Skin biopsy reveals absence of, or markedly atrophic, hair follicles. The problem is cosmetic, but care must be taken that the skin is not damaged owing to the lack of protection from the hair coat. Whether these cats are more susceptible to actinic changes in the skin or solar-associated skin neoplasia remains unknown.

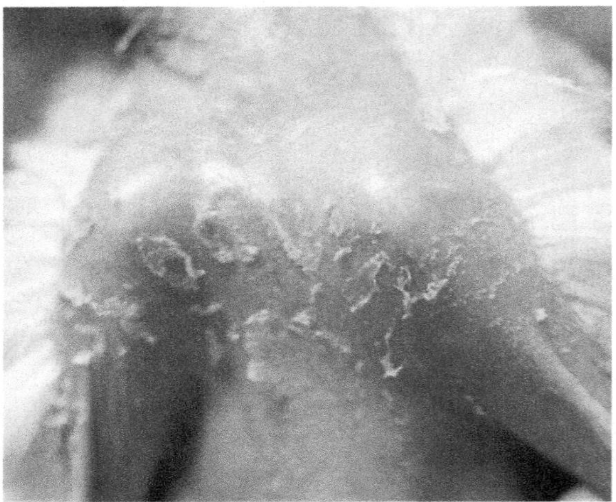

FIGURE 22-38 Paraneoplastic neoplasia. Note the alopecia, fine scales, and shiny skin. *(Photo courtesy Dr. Susan Little.)*

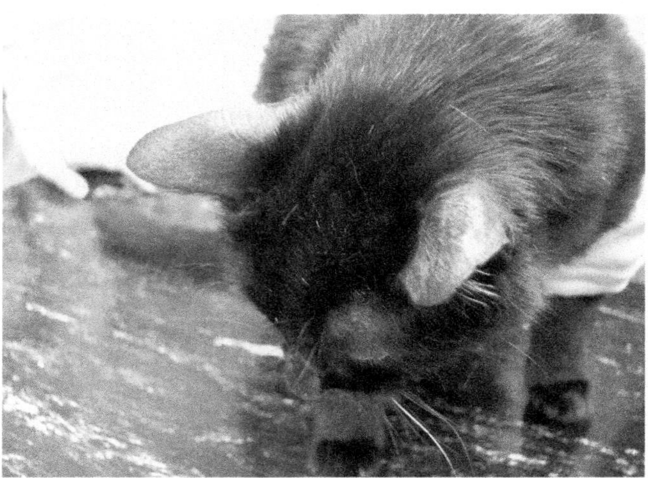

FIGURE 22-39 Pinnal alopecia. Bilaterally symmetric hair loss is present on the ears of a middle-aged cat. *(Photo courtesy University of Wisconsin School of Veterinary Medicine.)*

Paraneoplastic Alopecia

Paraneoplastic alopecia is a rare skin disease in cats in which there is widespread alopecia. A unique feature of the skin is that it is shiny in appearance and remaining hairs easily epilate (Figure 22-38). It can be associated with overgrowth of bacteria and *Malassezia* organisms.[79,93] It is seen most commonly in cats with systemic neoplasms and is reversible if the original neoplasm is removed. This is a clinical sign of systemic disease.[97]

Inflammatory Focal Alopecia

The most common causes of inflammatory focal alopecia in cats are dermatophytosis, pyoderma with or without a secondary yeast infection, demodicosis, and self-trauma secondary to a parasite infestation. Close inspection of the skin reveals that these lesions are rarely solitary. Core diagnostics include fungal culture, skin cytology, trichogram, and skin scraping.

Preauricular and Pinnal Alopecia

Preauricular hair loss is normal in cats but is most dramatic in dark-colored cats. Pinnal alopecia is uncommon and is characterized by episodic episodes of hair loss on the ear pinna (Figure 22-39). Siamese cats may be predisposed. This is a cosmetic problem, and no treatment is necessary.

Noninflammatory Focal Alopecia Associated with Treatments

Focal areas of noninflammatory hair loss are typically well demarcated. A common presentation is a lesion in the interscapular area. These are increasingly common with the widespread use of spot-on flea control products. Focal areas of hair loss can occur at the site of an injection of glucocorticoids. The author (KM) has not observed focal areas of noninflammatory alopecia at the site of vaccinations.

Alopecia Areata

Alopecia areata is an immune-mediated skin disease that presents as single or multiple areas of noninflammatory alopecia. The areas are well demarcated and can occur anywhere on the body. Diagnosis is made by ruling out other causes of focal noninflammatory hair loss and by skin biopsy. Early lesions are rarely observed in the cat, but skin biopsy may reveal peribulbar and intrabulbar accumulations of inflammatory cells affecting anagen hairs. Older lesions reveal atrophic hairs or hairs in telogen or catagen. Chronic lesions may reveal an absence of hairs. There is no successful treatment; it is important to rule out infectious or contagious causes of hair loss.

ULCERS AND EROSIONS

The most common causes of ulcers and erosions in cats are diseases that are pruritic or associated with scaling and crusting. These lesions can be very dramatic in appearance, and the immediate goal of the history and physical examination is to determine if the lesions are due to an infectious, contagious, immune-mediated, or otherwise life-threatening cause. In general, it is rare for cats with skin diseases to exhibit signs of systemic illness such as fever, anorexia, or weight loss. These signs warrant an aggressive medical workup in addition to dermatologic tests.

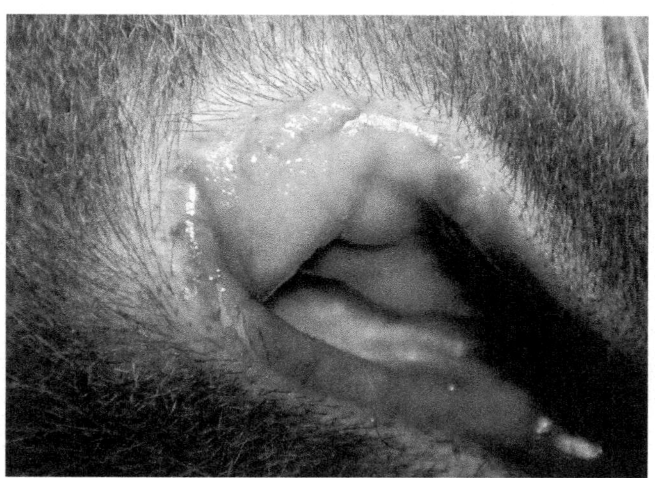

FIGURE 22-40 Mucocutaneous ulceration. Mucocutaneous ulceration is uncommon in cats and is suggestive of severe infectious disease, gingival disease, or immune-mediated diseases. *(Photo courtesy University of Wisconsin School of Veterinary Medicine.)*

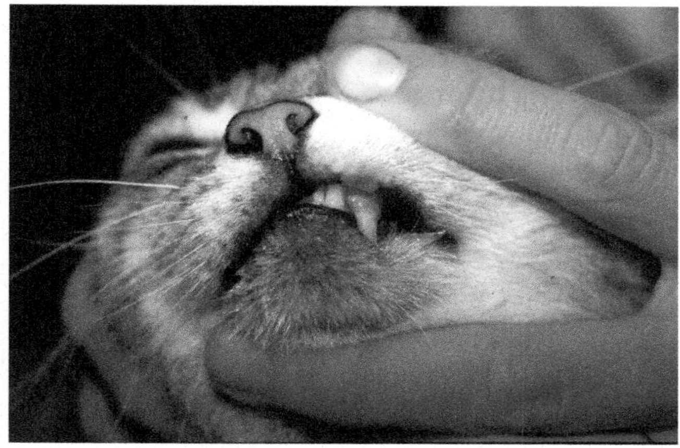

FIGURE 22-41 Focal indolent ulcer. This lesion is at the site of several *M. canis*–infected hairs. *(Photo courtesy University of Wisconsin School of Veterinary Medicine.)*

In most cases the most useful diagnostic tests in cats with ulcers or erosions are cytology of the lesion and exudate, fungal cultures, and skin biopsy. Dermatophytosis can mimic any skin disease, and one of the major differential diagnoses for ulcerative and erosive skin diseases is an immune-mediated disease or a disease that calls for glucocorticoid therapy. Diseases worsened by the use of corticosteroid therapy should be solidly eliminated from the differential diagnoses. For example, the lesions in the cat shown in Figure 22-40 reveal an erosive process suggestive of an immune-mediated disease, but this was a bacterial infection of the lip folds. Multiple skin cytology samples obtained with a glass microscope slide should be obtained. It is important not to heat fix these to prevent damage to cell integrity. Several slides should remain unfixed and unstained for submission to a reference laboratory if needed. Slides should be examined for the presence or absence of neutrophils, eosinophils, bacteria (intracellular and extracellular), neoplastic cells, and other infectious agents. In the absence of systemic signs of illness, septic neutrophilic or eosinophilic inflammation of the skin may be compatible with an antibiotic-responsive skin disease. Definitive diagnosis of many of the erosive and ulcerative skin lesions can be made only by histologic examination of skin biopsy specimens. It is important to include a list of differential diagnoses with the submission and to remember that knowing what a lesion is not may be as helpful as having a definitive diagnosis. In other words, lesions not compatible with neoplasia, immune-mediated diseases, infections agents, and drug eruptions are important as rule outs.

A few conditions warrant special mention. Oral ulceration in cats is most commonly associated with viral diseases, and the immediate diagnosis is not usually difficult. Although rare, pemphigus vulgaris and systemic lupus can occur in cats. The most likely presentation of either of these two diseases will be a middle-aged cat. In both diseases affected cats will show signs of systemic illness, and other mucocutaneous areas will be involved (e.g., eyelids, nasal area, genital and anal areas). Another rare disease is idiopathic ulcerative dermatitis. Affected cats have focal areas of intense pruritus, often in the scapular area. The diagnosis is one of exclusion after other causes of focal ulceration have been ruled out. The etiology is unknown, and the lesions are very difficult to manage. Some are so refractory to treatment that surgical excision is the only option. If neuropathic pain is involved, gabapentin may be a possible therapeutic option.

EOSINOPHILIC LESIONS

Eosinophilic lesions are skin lesions characterized by eosinophils on cytologic examination of skin or histologic examination of skin biopsy findings. Peripheral eosinophilia is variable. In severe cases cats may have lymphadenopathy, and fine-needle aspiration may reveal reactive lymph nodes with a large number of eosinophils. Lesions tend to be pruritic and are most commonly associated with allergic skin disease.

Indolent Ulcer

The term *indolent ulcer*[108] describes a unilateral or bilateral erosive lesion on the upper lip of cats of any age (Figure 22-41). Recently, there is emerging evidence that some cats may have a genetic predisposition to develop lesions when exposed to allergic triggers, particularly fleas.[8,82] Another interesting finding is that these lesions can also occur as a result of foreign bodies (e.g., cactus

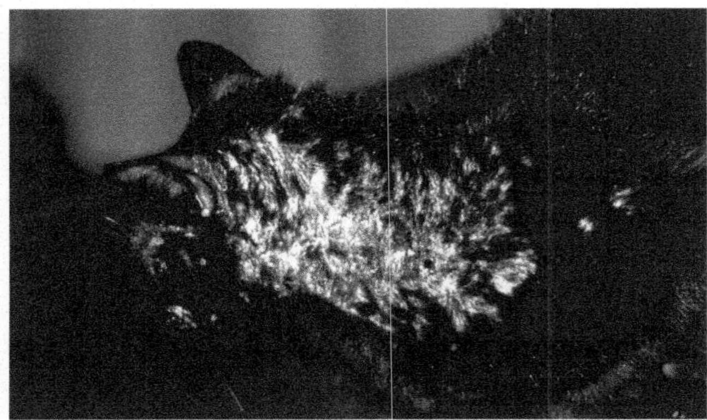

FIGURE 22-42 Miliary dermatitis. This papular crusted lesion is a common reaction pattern for many diseases of cats. Typical cutaneous cytology shows neutrophils and eosinophils. *(Photo courtesy University of Wisconsin School of Veterinary Medicine.)*

spines) or at the site of a focal insult, such as on the lip margins at the sites where dermatophyte-infected hairs, sticktight fleas, or ticks have previously been found.[21] Indolent ulcers as a result of focal trauma are transient and often one-time occurrences and may explain why in some cats, particularly young kittens, lesions may develop and resolve without treatment and not recur. Lesions that persist or are recurrent are caused by a persistent trigger such as atopy or food allergies. Initial therapy with antibiotics is recommended. It may be necessary to treat lesions not responding completely to antibiotics with glucocorticoids until lesions resolve.

Miliary Dermatitis and Eosinophilic Plaques

Miliary dermatitis refers to an erythematous crusted reaction pattern of the skin.[108] Eosinophilic plaques are intensely pruritic, erosive, exudative raised lesions of varying size.[108] Close inspection of many eosinophilic plaques often reveals that cats have concurrent miliary dermatitis–like lesions or that the plaques are a coalescence of these papulocrusted lesions (Figure 22-42). The most important new clinical finding is that these lesions are increasingly being recognized as the feline equivalent of canine pyotraumatic lesions (i.e., "hot spots"), and secondary overcolonization by bacteria or *Malassezia* spp. are common cytologic findings. Lesions are the direct result of self-trauma and are commonly seen on the face, abdomen, inguinal region, medial and caudal thigh areas, and neck (Figures 22-43 and 22-44). These lesions are most commonly triggered by an itch–scratch event, and recurrent lesions are often the hallmark of an underlying allergic disease, although this is not always the case. These lesions can also develop as a result of infections resulting from dermatophytosis, bacteria, and *Malassezia* spp.

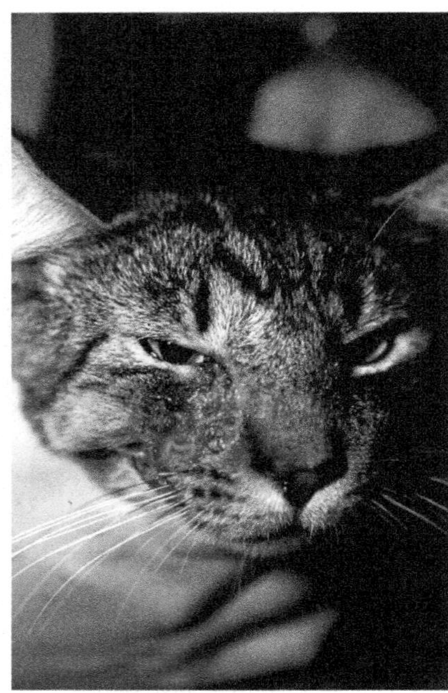

FIGURE 22-43 Facial ulceration. This is an area of self-trauma. The lesion is an eosinophilic plaque triggered by any disease that is pruritic. *(Photo courtesy University of Wisconsin School of Veterinary Medicine.)*

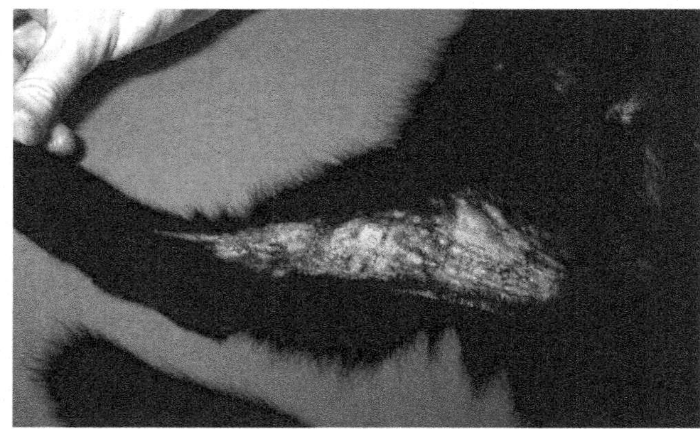

FIGURE 22-44 Eosinophilic plaque. This is a raised, intensely pruritic lesion that is common in feline allergic diseases. *(Photo courtesy University of Wisconsin School of Veterinary Medicine.)*

Eosinophilic Granuloma

Eosinophilic granulomas[108] are the only true granuloma variant of feline eosinophilic diseases. There are two recognized clinical variations. The first is an ulcerated, proliferative lesion often present in the oral cavity (Figure 22-45). Depending on the location of the mass, dysphagia, drooling, abnormal mastication, and coughing may be present. The other form is characterized by a hard, noninflammatory swelling. Alopecia is variable, and the cat seems unperturbed by the lesion. Clinical presentations include linear pencil-thick lesions on the

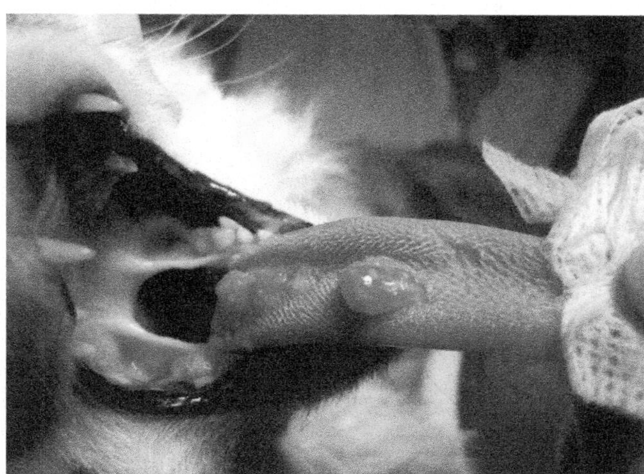

FIGURE 22-45 Oral eosinophilic granuloma. Oral proliferative lesions in the mouth may resemble oral neoplasia; biopsy is indicated. *(Photo courtesy Dr. Susan Little.)*

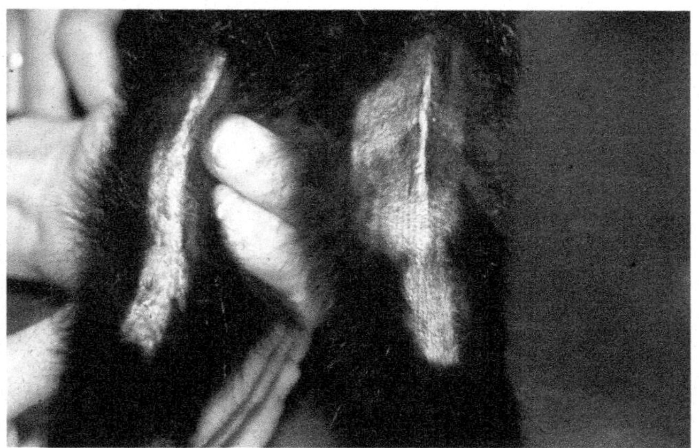

FIGURE 22-46 Linear granuloma. Linear granulomas on the hind legs of cats are a classic presentation of the true granuloma complex. *(Photo courtesy University of Wisconsin School of Veterinary Medicine.)*

caudal thigh of young cats; linear lesions on limbs (Figure 22-46); "fat lips" or asymptomatic chin swelling (Figure 22-47); 1- to 5-mm firm, papular lesions on the ears of cats; and interdigital masses. The origin of these lesions has long been thought to be the result of collagen degeneration and degenerate eosinophils. Recently, a study was conducted in which the ultrastructure of these lesions was investigated, and the researchers found that collagen fibrils were not damaged but were separated from one another by edema and surrounded by eosinophils undergoing degranulation. In this study the authors demonstrated that the eosinophil recruitment and degranulation are the primary event triggers in this disease and the collagen fibers do not play an active role in the development of these lesions.[4,33] This is a major challenge to the long-held belief that these lesions are caused by collagen degeneration; the lesions are the

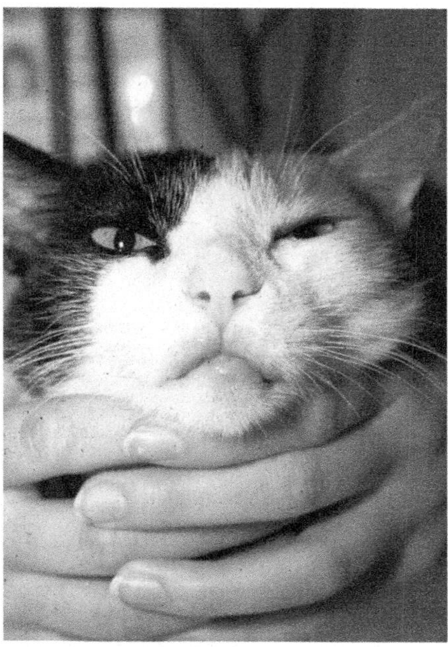

FIGURE 22-47 Chin granuloma. Fat lip syndrome is characterized by a hard swelling on the chin. The lesions are rarely bothersome to the cat. *(Photo courtesy University of Wisconsin School of Veterinary Medicine.)*

result of massive eosinophil infiltration and degranulation. Diagnosis of the underlying trigger is most important in these cases. These lesions are rarely problematic to the cat but are very corticosteroid responsive; lesions will recur if the underlying trigger is not identified.

Mosquito and Insect Bite Hypersensitivity

Mosquito and insect bite hypersensitivity[108] is characterized by a papular erosive eruption on the face, ear tips, nose, and foot pads of cats. Lesions tend to start in the thinly haired areas and may be more common in dark-coated cats. The lesions are intensely pruritic, and depigmentation, crusting, and exudates may occur. The lesions were first noted in cats exposed to mosquitoes but can result from the bites of other small flying insects, such as black flies and *Culicoides* species. Typically, affected cats have access to the outdoors, especially during the early morning or evening hours when these insects are feeding. It is important to remember that many of these biting insects are small enough to get through the holes used to screen most outdoor porches and windows. Although symmetric ulcerative facial lesions are the most commonly described clinical signs in individual case reports, a study of 26 cats from Japan found that the most commonly observed lesions were miliary dermatitis–like lesions on the ear pinnae.[67] Crusty patches on the ear margins are common client complaints, and this report suggests that the prevalence of insect bite hypersensitivity may be underrecognized.

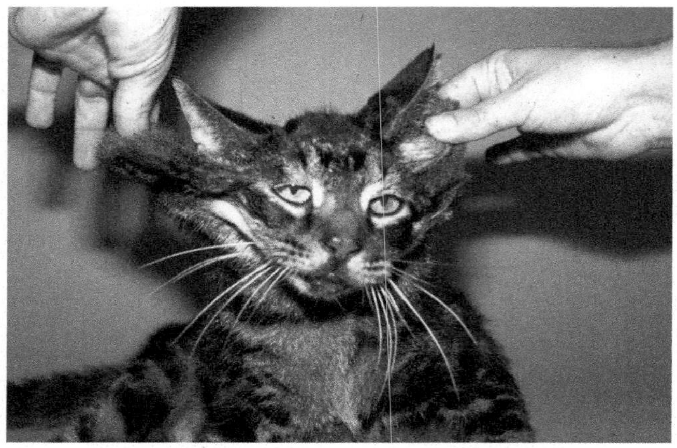

FIGURE 22-48 Ehlers–Danlos syndrome. This is a congenital collagen defect characterized by stretchy skin. *(Photo courtesy University of Wisconsin School of Veterinary Medicine.)*

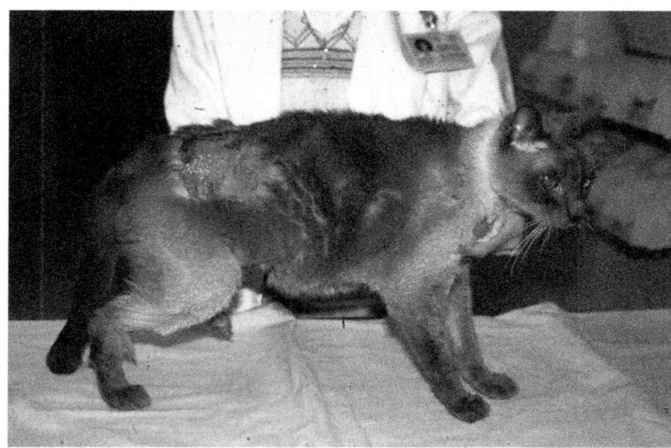

FIGURE 22-49 Skin fragility syndrome. This cat has naturally occurring feline hyperadrenocorticism, and the skin was easily torn. *(Photo courtesy University of Wisconsin School of Veterinary Medicine.)*

Familial Eosinophilic Lesions

Familial eosinophilic lesions[108] have been described in specific pathogen-free laboratory cats by at least two investigators.[19,82] These cats developed lesions between 4 and 18 months of age, and the lesions were observed to recur until the cats were at least 4 years of age. In one study 21 of 24 cats descended from these cats also developed lesions. The lesions tended to be most common during the spring and summer, suggesting a possible seasonal allergen, insect, hormonal, or reproductive trigger. A hereditary predisposition to eosinophilic lesions is not unexpected, particularly with regard to lesions that have allergic etiologies. Canine atopy has long been recognized to be heritable, and feline atopy was recently described in three littermates.[59]

FRAGILE SKIN

Easily torn skin is uncommon in cats. The most common causes are Ehlers–Danlos syndrome (EDS), spontaneously occurring feline hyperadrenocorticism, excessive use of exogenous glucocorticoids, and drug reactions. EDS is most common in domestic shorthair and Himalayan cats (Figure 22-48). These cats are young and healthy, with hyperextensible skin usually noticed within the first year of life and gradually worsening as the cat gets older. The skin tears easily, with minimal pain associated with the injuries, and will heal. Diagnosis is clinical, with the skin being unnaturally stretchy. There is no treatment. Affected cats commonly die as a result of disease-related problems (e.g., ruptured aortic vessels) or are euthanized by their owners.

Spontaneously occurring hyperadrenocorticism occurs in older cats. Affected cats exhibit signs of systemic illness, including, but not limited to, depression, lethargy, obesity or weight loss, anorexia, muscle weakness or wasting, hepatomegaly, and easily torn skin (Figure 22-49). (See Chapter 24, the section on Adrenal Diseases.) In addition to the unkempt coat of cats with systemic illnesses, another early dermatologic clue may be easy bruising.

Fragile skin as a result of excessive glucocorticoid use is not usually a difficult diagnosis.[49] Invariably, there is a history of exogenous glucocorticoid use, and careful history taking almost always reveals that the glucocorticoids were being used to treat pruritus. The author (KM) has seen acute onset of skin fragility in a cat receiving sulfa antibiotics for gastrointestinal problems. In addition, the author (KM) has seen several cats with toxic epidermal necrolysis present with the complaint of "torn skin." In these latter cats, the skin was tender and exudative. Skin biopsy may or may not identify an underlying cause for easily torn skin depending on the cause. Whether the condition is reversible depends on the underlying cause and treatment response. In the author's (KM) experience, gentle handling of the cat and use of surgical stockinettes over the skin to provide protection from further tearing have been helpful. Until the underlying problem is resolved, the major problems that are encountered are infection and the need to protect the underlying granulation tissue.

HARD SKIN

Focal areas of hard skin are most likely going to present as nodules and can be caused by bacterial or fungal infections, neoplasia, foreign bodies (e.g., bird shot), or sterile nodular panniculitis with pansteatitis. The most common cause of noninflammatory nodules in the skin is collagen degeneration; the most common trigger is insect bite hypersensitivity. Biopsy is indicated for diagnosis.

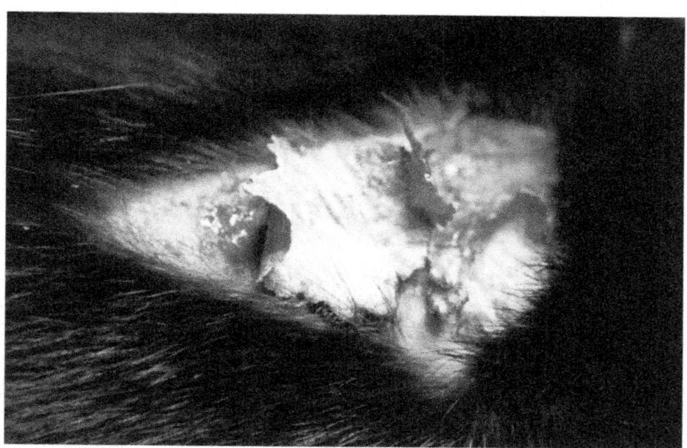

FIGURE 22-50 Skin eschar that developed over an area of trauma. *(Photo courtesy Dr. Susan Little.)*

Linear or more diffuse areas are most likely to be caused by a true eosinophilic granuloma. Biopsy is diagnostic. A less common cause of hard skin is an eschar from a burn or traumatic injury. Careful examination of the lesion usually reveals a hardened plaque of dead tissue overlying a bed of granulation tissue. Eschars protect the underlying granulation tissue and will dislodge as the tissue beneath heals. Burns are underrecognized in cats because the hair coat hides the injury. Eschars can also develop as a result of trauma (Figure 22-50). Furthermore, the most common type of burn in cat is a radiant burn from close but not direct contact with a heat source such as a wood-burning stove. Many days to weeks may elapse before the injury is discovered. Although uncommon in cats, focal areas of calcification (calcinosis circumscripta) can occur at the site of injections or injury.[76]

PIGMENTARY CHANGES

Postinflammatory Hyperpigmentation

Postinflammatory hyperpigmentation is uncommon in cats. In the author's (KM) experience, it is most common in cats with dermatophytosis. Focal areas of hyperpigmentation in inflamed skin should be closely examined because they are almost always due to follicular plugging. Skin scrapings, skin cytology, and fungal culture are indicated in feline patients with postinflammatory hyperpigmentation of an unknown cause. Skin cytology may reveal bacterial or yeast overgrowth. It can be difficult to sample areas near or around ears; acetate tape preparations or dry spatula collection techniques are helpful.

Lentigo

The most commonly encountered focal area of noninflammatory hyperpigmentation is lentigo simplex of orange cats. Flat, nonindurated macules ranging in size from 1 mm to 10 mm develop on the nose, lips, gingiva, ears, eyelids, or hard palate. These lesions may become more widespread as the cat ages. This is a cosmetic change, and no treatment is needed. The major differential diagnosis is melanoma; if there is a change in the size or nature of a lesion, a biopsy is indicated.

Depigmentation

Depigmentation is uncommon in cats, although idiopathic leukoderma of the pads of Siamese cats has been reported. In addition, Siamese cats may develop periocular leukotrichia (goggle syndrome) after pregnancy, dietary deficiency, or systemic illness.

Acromelanism

Acromelanism is seen in Siamese, Himalayan, Balinese, and Burmese kittens that are born white and develop pigmented points as they mature owing to the influence of external temperatures. High temperatures produce light hairs, and low temperatures produce dark hairs. This is caused by a temperature-dependent enzyme involved in melanin synthesis. The temperature-dependent pigmentary change is most commonly encountered in practice when the hair coat is clipped and the hairs that regrow appear as a different color (usually darker). The normal coat color returns with the next hair cycle.

DISEASES OF PAW PADS, PARONYCHIA, AND ANAL SACS

Paw Pads

In cats, diseases of the paw pads are uncommon, but when they do occur, scaling and crusting, swelling, digital calluses and horns, and ulceration are the most common problems. The underlying causes are variable and include trauma, allergic diseases, infections, immune-mediated diseases, tumors, and viral diseases. The most common causes are discussed in this section.

If scaling and crusting is present, the most common causes are dermatophytosis and PF. The author (KM) has noted that the paw pads of cats treated with lime sulfur may become dry and scaly. Although uncommon, scaling and crusting can be an early manifestation of hepatocutaneous syndrome in cats. Less commonly, pox virus infections can cause scaling.

Ulcerations of one or more paws may be due to self-trauma, injuries, irritant reactions, plasma cell pododermatitis, infections, eosinophilic granulomas, tumors (Figure 22-51), and drug reactions. Diagnosis depends on history, thorough dermatologic and medical examination, and biopsy.

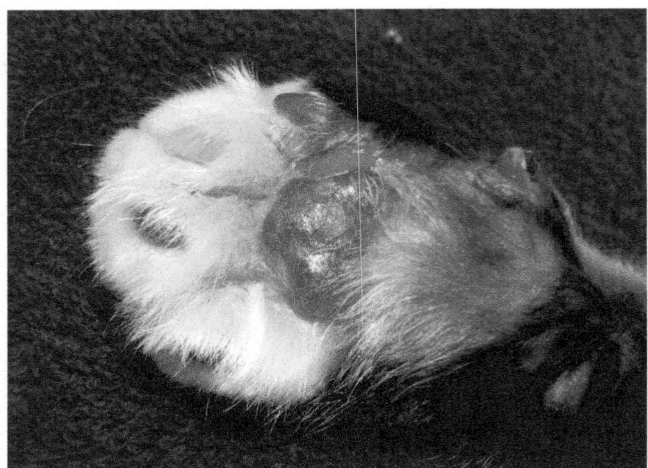

FIGURE 22-51 Cutaneous lymphoma. This is a case of cutaneous lymphoma presenting as foot pad swelling and crusting. *(Photo courtesy Dr. Susan Little.)*

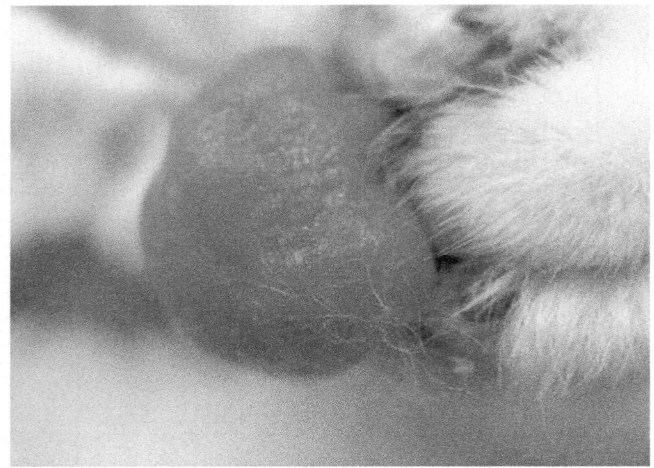

FIGURE 22-52 Plasma cell pododermatitis. This is a benign infiltrative skin disease that affects the paw pads. Note the swelling and "pillowlike" appearance. *(Photo courtesy University of Wisconsin School of Veterinary Medicine.)*

The most common cause of swelling of the foot pads is plasma cell pododermatitis (Figure 22-52). The swelling may or may not be painful. The color of the foot pads may appear red to purple, and clients may describe them as "pillowlike." In the author's (KM) experience, these lesions wax and wane and may ulcerate and crust. Definitive diagnosis is made by biopsy. Foot pads are painful to biopsy, and samples should be obtained from non–weight-bearing pads if at all possible. Alternatively, the veterinarian can use a 4-mm punch biopsy to obtain the specimen. If the pads are not tender or ulcerative, it is reasonable to make a clinical diagnosis, insofar as no treatment is needed. Tender or ulcerated pads require treatment. Prednisolone (4 mg/kg orally, once daily) induces the most rapid remission of lesions. Once lesions have resolved, the dose can be tapered while an alternative drug for long-term use (doxycycline or cyclosporine) is used. Doxycycline (5 to 10 mg/kg orally, every 12 hours) or cyclosporine (5 mg/kg orally, every 24 hours) can be used to keep lesions in remission or induce remission in less severe cases. It can take 1 to 2 months to see maximum benefit.

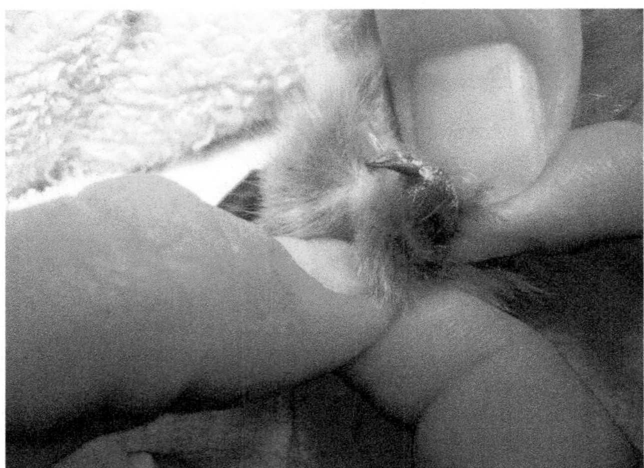

FIGURE 22-53 Digital pad callus. *(Image courtesy Dr. Susan Little.)*

Digital pad calluses are common and may be bothersome to the cat (Figure 22-53). These can occur anywhere on the paws. Management varies from none to surgical excision of the lesion.

Paronychia

The two most common presentations of paronychia in cats are crusting and exudation and pedal pruritus with waxy exudate. The most common causes of crusting and exudation of the nail bed are bacterial infections, *Notoedres* infestation, dermatophytosis, and PF. Pruritic nail beds are almost always due to yeast overgrowth (Figure 22-54).[20,68]

Bacterial infections are characterized by swollen nail beds, which are painful for the cat. Exudation is common and malodorous. Multiple digits are typically involved, and causative agents include *Staphylococcus* spp., *Streptococcus* spp., *Pseudomonas* spp., and *Proteus* spp. In rare cases this can be a presentation of cryptococcosis. The diagnosis is based on clinical signs. Skin cytology and culture are used to guide therapy.

Notoedres infestation is characterized by severe crusting with mild to severe pruritus. Similar clinical signs are usually present on the face and ears. Skin scrapings reveal mites. All in-contact cats should be treated with an appropriate miticide. Bathing and mechanical removal of crusts facilitates treatment. Ivermectin (0.2 to 0.4 mg/kg orally or subcutaneously) every 2 weeks for three treatments is effective; see previous discussion for other treatment options.

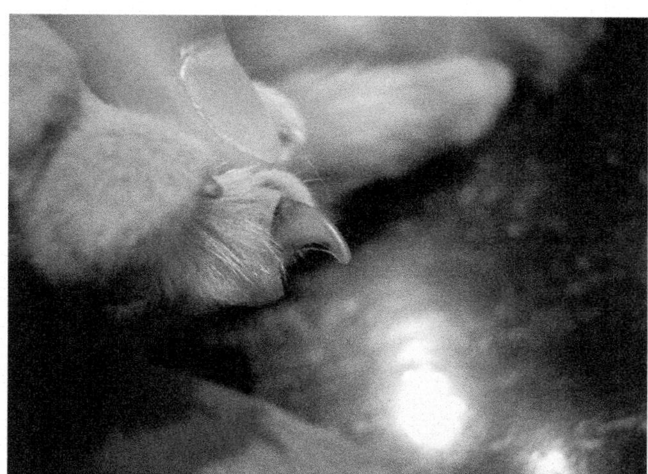

FIGURE 22-54 Nail bed. Accumulations of nail bed debris around the base of the nails is typical in cats with yeast pododermatitis. Yeast pododermatitis can result from a wide range of causes. *(Photo courtesy University of Wisconsin School of Veterinary Medicine.)*

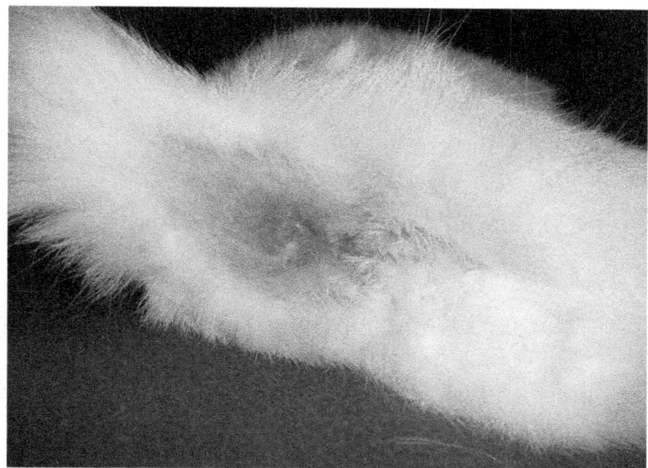

FIGURE 22-55 Perianal pruritus. This was an atopic cat with chronic anal sacculitis. The area became colonized with microbial overgrowth, magnifying the pruritus. The cat's anal sacs were chemically cauterized, but this did not resolve the pruritus. The cat was diagnosed with atopy, and the perineal pruritus resolved with therapy for allergies. *(Photo courtesy University of Wisconsin School of Veterinary Medicine.)*

PF in cats can begin with crusting of the nail beds and foot pads. Almost always, all the digits are involved. Careful examination of the cat may reveal other lesions compatible with PF, such as crusting on the face, ears, and body. Cytologic examination of exudate reveals neutrophils and rafts of acanthocytes. Intracellular or extracellular bacteria may also be present. Cats with a bacterial infection that does not respond to appropriate therapy and cats with negative cultures are highly suspect for PF. Definitive diagnosis is made by histologic examination of a skin biopsy.

Severe dermatophytosis involving all of the digits can be indistinguishable from PF or bacterial infections. Discriminating criteria may be found in the history (e.g., age of the animal, other affected animals in the household). Wood's lamp examination may reveal glowing hairs for direct examination or fungal culture. Close inspection of the whole cat almost always reveals other lesions suggestive of or diagnostic for dermatophytosis.

The nail beds and proximal portions of the nails should be examined in cats that have severe pedal pruritus. Accumulations of waxy debris are not a normal finding on the nails of cats and are typical of *Malassezia* overgrowth (see Figure 22-54). This is a common problem in cat breeds with abnormal hair coats (e.g., Devon and Cornish Rex, Sphynx), cats with systemic illnesses (e.g., diabetes mellitus), and cats with allergic skin diseases. Large numbers of yeast organisms are readily apparent on cytologic examination of debris. Treatment with systemic antifungal agents will resolve the pruritus or significantly minimize it. If the condition is caused by an underlying disease, this must be treated or else the problem will recur. Management of breed-related *Malassezia* overgrowth is more difficult and requires a combination of systemic therapy and a lifelong regimen of bathing the paws and nail beds.

Tumors and other Swellings of Individual Toes

Swelling of individual digits can be caused by neoplasia, foreign bodies, or infection. Biopsy is the most rapid way to diagnose the problem.

Anal Sac Diseases

Anal sac diseases are uncommon in cats compared with dogs. The most common cause of anal sac problems in cats is perineal pruritus caused by allergies. The skin surrounding the perineal area becomes inflamed, the small superficial ducts become swollen, and excretions cannot be evacuated when the cat defecates. Cats with recurrent anal sac impactions or cats whose owners complain about excessive anal licking should be carefully examined for allergic skin diseases, including flea allergy, food allergy, and atopic dermatitis (Figure 22-55). The perineal skin is easily overcolonized by bacteria and yeast, which magnify the pruritus. Combined systemic antimicrobial therapy may be necessary to resolve this inflammation. Cats with uncomplicated perineal pruritus caused by allergies can be managed with topical glucocorticoid therapy, short courses of oral steroids if the problem is seasonal, or cyclosporine.

Anal sac impaction is typically bilateral. The affected anal sac is distended and may elicit pain on palpation, and the contents, which are thick and dark in color, are not easily expressed. Discomfort may cause the cat to

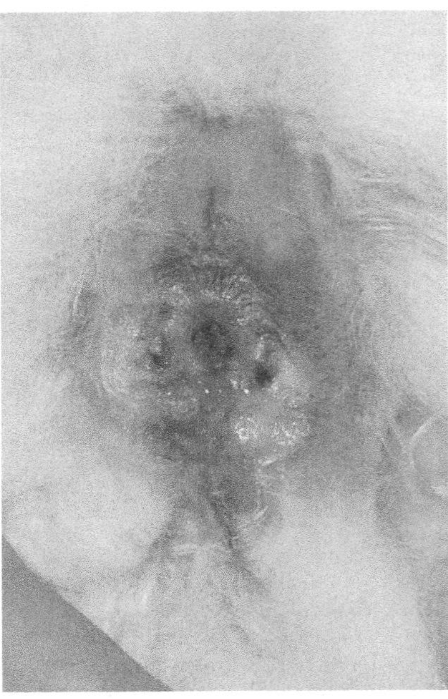

FIGURE 22-56 Anal sac abscess. This cat had chronic anal sac abscesses and exudates as a result of allergies. *(Photo courtesy University of Wisconsin School of Veterinary Medicine.)*

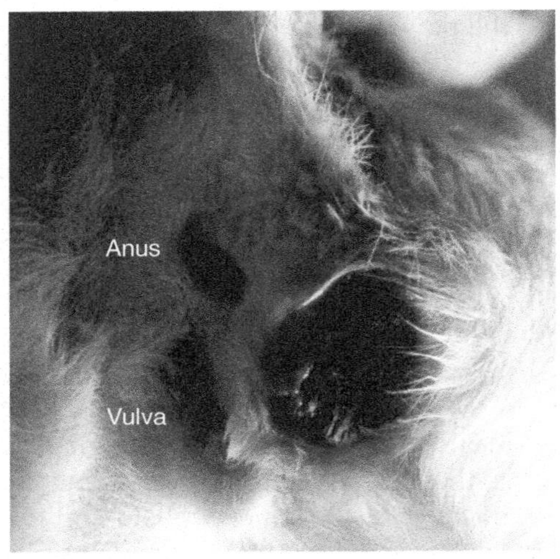

FIGURE 22-57 Anal sac abscess. *(Photo courtesy Dr. Susan Little.)*

scoot the hind end on the floor. Tenesmus and licking at the perineum may also occur. The cause for anal sac impaction is not well understood. The contents normally empty during defecation. Retention of anal sac contents may lead to inflammation and infection. Anal sac abscesses and rupture can and do occur in cats. Typically, the problem is unilateral. Owners may complain of blood, vocalizing, and other indications of pain. Clinical signs are typical of an abscess (Figure 22-56), with swelling, pain, exudation, and possible rupture (Figures 22-57 and 22-58). Management varies from conservative (e.g., antibiotics, stool softeners, cleansings) to surgical

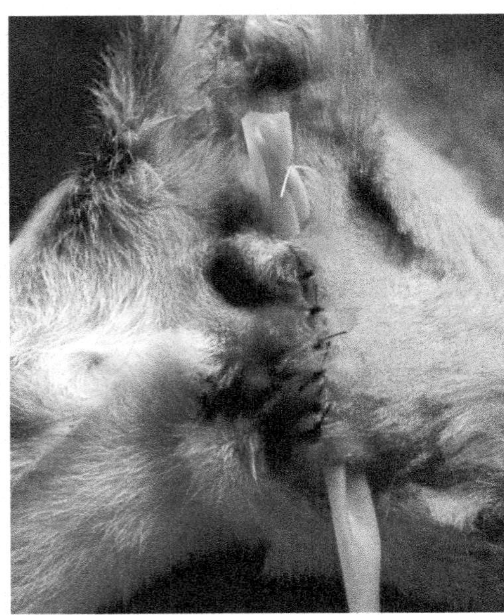

FIGURE 22-58 Anal sac abscess, after surgical débridement. This was a severe abscess that required placement of a surgical drain. *(Photo courtesy Dr. Susan Little.)*

débridement and irrigation with povidone–iodine solution. Laxatives that contain polyethylene glycol (e.g., Miralax, Schering-Plough HealthCare Products, Inc.) are effective stool softeners. These are tasteless powders that can be sprinkled on a small amount of food; approximately one-quarter of a teaspoon is administered daily for constipation and stool softening. Recurrent cases of anal sac abscess that are refractory to conservative management may be treated with anal sacculectomy, once inflammation and infection have resolved.

OTITIS

There are three clinical presentations of otitis[57] in cats depending on anatomic location: OE, OM, and otitis interna (OI).[38,65] The underlying etiology and pathogenesis of feline otitis involves the interplay of predisposing factors, primary diseases, and secondary or perpetuating factors.

Predisposing factors to consider in cats include, but are not limited to, living in a humid climate and increased maceration of the ear tissue caused by frequent grooming.[38] Stenosis of the ear canal and deformed ear pinna secondary to aural hematomas may predispose cats to overgrowth of microbial organisms if the ear canal is occluded or if pain and secondary self-trauma are present. Cats can develop otitis secondary to overly aggressive or frequent ear cleanings. Predisposing factors unique to cats include OM secondary to acute or chronic upper respiratory infections or chronic sinusitis.[29,88] Another factor is OE caused by a fixed drug reaction or allergic contact reaction as a result of transdermal drug administration. Finally, in some cats with chronic otitis the only abnormal finding is retrovirus infection.

Primary causes are diseases that directly cause ear disease.[38] These include but are not limited to parasitic diseases, allergies, autoimmune diseases, neoplasia, keratinization disorders, facial dermatitis of Persian cats, congenital diseases (hairless cat breeds), foreign bodies, polyps, trauma (including thermal injuries and frostbite), and neoplasia.

Perpetuating factors prevent the ear disease from healing.[38] The most common perpetuating factors are bacteria and yeast. The most common causes of recurrent otitis in cats are undiagnosed OM, resistant infections, and obstructions of the ear canal.

OE in cats includes, but is not limited to, any combination of the following clinical signs: erythema; hair loss; scaling; crusting; pruritus; pain; deformed ear pinna; thickening of the external pinna; odor; and exudate of variable color, amount, and consistency. The owner may report head shaking, ear twitching, fits of ear scratching after manipulation of the ear, changes in eating habits, changes in behavior (e.g., hiding or aggression) or changes in vocalization. Clinical signs may be unilateral or bilateral, persistent or intermittent, and acute or chronic. The initial presenting complaint may be unrelated to the ears; some cats are brought to the veterinarian because of facial lesions. OM is a common complication in cats with severe OE.

OM is inflammation of the middle ear cavity, including the tympanic membrane and bulla. Many, but not all, cats with OM have concurrent OE. OM should always be suspected when cats exhibit severe purulent OE and chronic recurrent OE. Cats with OM without signs of OE may be brought to the veterinarian for head shaking, pawing at the ear, pain when the head is touched, changes in eating habits or appetite, pain when the mouth is opened, depression, and loss of hearing. Clinical signs may be unilateral or bilateral. Otoscopic examination of the ear canal typically reveals exudate and inflammatory changes in the canal when OE is also present. Manual manipulation of the ear is usually painful, and a "squishing" sound is common, indicating fluid in the canal. If the tympanic membrane can be visualized, bulging, discoloration, or rupture may be evident. OM can be present without signs of OE, but the tympanic membrane almost always appears abnormal. Cats with OM and a ruptured tympanic membrane often have copious malodorous liquid discharge on otoscopic examination. This may also be seen on the floor of the horizontal canal. Mucus may be seen with OM. It is important to note that mucus is not normally present anywhere along the external ear canal, but it does ooze from tympanic bulla through any tear in the tympanic membrane. If mucus is present on otoscopic examination of the external canal, there is a tear in the tympanic membrane. OM is underrecognized in cats. Chronic sinusitis can lead to bulla effusion and OM in cats.[29]

OI involves inflammation of the bony labyrinth, where the organs of hearing (cochlea) and vestibular apparatus (semicircular canals and vestibule) are located.[7] Loss of hearing, head tilt, circling, falling, generalized incoordination, difficulty rising and ambulating, nystagmus, facial nerve paralysis, and Horner's syndrome are common signs in cats with OI. In cases of concurrent OM, head tilt is toward the affected side, and the cat may circle and fall toward the affected side. Nystagmus may be spontaneous, horizontal, or rotary, with the fast phase away from the affected side and head tilt. OI caused by an infection can be the result of an ascending infection through the eustachian tube or secondary to OM with or without complicating OE. When vestibular signs are associated with concurrent signs of OE or OM, it is reasonable to assume that the cat's OI is the result of this infection. Cats that exhibit signs of OI in the absence of signs of OE or OM present more of a challenge. These cats require an aggressive workup to determine if the vestibular signs are peripheral or central.

In addition to a careful and thorough history and physical examination, there are a number of useful diagnostic tests to help diagnose the cause of the otitis. Mineral oil microscopy can be used for *Otodectes* spp. and demodicosis; it is an often overlooked diagnostic test in adult cats with pruritic ears. Dermatophyte cultures are recommended, especially when cats are young, free roaming, or recently acquired. Dermatophytosis is highly variable, and PF and dermatophytosis in longhaired cats can look very similar.[84] Furthermore, early infections in cats often start on the face and ears; the hairs within the pinnae may be the first site of infection. Cytologic examination of ear exudate is mandatory regardless of the number of times that the cat is brought in for ear disease. It is not appropriate to assume that what was seen in the past is what is present at the current examination. Otic cytology helps guide further diagnostics and is a useful tool for monitoring therapy. Heat fixing slides before staining improves visualization of yeast.

Bacterial overgrowth is generally uncommon in cats; when bacteria (rods or cocci) are seen, culture is indicated. The presence of leukocytes signals suppurative otitis (SO) and a need for aggressive medical therapy. Culture is indicated in SO. Yeast is a common finding in normal cats, and the determining factor as to their significance is whether the cat is symptomatic at the time of sampling.[68,69] A recent study on the prevalence of *Malassezia* spp. in cats found that yeast was present in 23% of normal cats and 64% of cats with OE.[69]

Bacterial cultures should be performed by a reference laboratory. In addition, the laboratory should be able and willing to speciate pathogens and investigate sensitivities of multiple strains of a pathogen when indicated or requested. This becomes important in cases of chronic bacterial otitis. The presence of multistrain pathogens with variable sensitivities is common, especially when *Pseudomonas* spp. are isolated. Skin biopsy of the ear is an underused diagnostic test. It is strongly recommended when an immune-mediated skin disease, tumor, or proliferative disease is present. Depending on the location of the skin lesions, skin biopsy can be performed using a 4-mm skin biopsy punch, Tru-Cut biopsy needle, or otoscopic endoscope. Diagnostic imaging of the bullae can be helpful in diagnosing underlying OM, space-occupying lesions (i.e., tumors, polyps), or other obstruction in the ear canal. In cases of chronic OM, it may identify underlying sinonasal disease.

Otodectes Infestations

Ear mite infestations are one of the most common causes of otitis in cats and one of the most successfully "treatable and curable" ear diseases of cats (see previous discussion). In one survey it was found to be the cause of otitis in 25% of cats presented for otitis.[92] Complications are uncommon when proper treatment has been administered. Complications with the treatment of ear mite infestations include the following:

- Suppurative OE and OM
- Severe head and neck pruritus
- Otodectic whole body mange
- Classic infestation treatment failures
- Subclinical infestations
- Aural hematomas
- Deformed ear pinnae and chronic recurrent yeast infections (Figure 22-59)

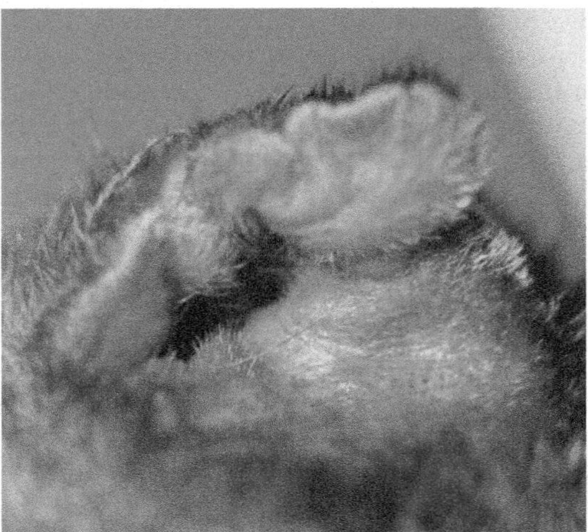

FIGURE 22-59 Deformed pinna. Lack of appropriate treatment or chronic recurrent aural hematomas can lead to deformed pinnae. This will predispose the cat to chronic ear infections. *(Photo courtesy Dr. Susan Little.)*

- Concretions in the external ear canal, middle ear, or both

The most common complication of ear mite infestations is an aural hematoma. Optimal management that will minimize recurrence and deformation of the ears includes surgical drainage of the blood and through-and-through suturing of the pinna to close the dead space. Obviously, the underlying cause must be addressed. Unlike the situation in dogs, atopic dermatitis does not appear to be a common trigger in cats.

Otic Demodicosis

D. cati (long and slender) and *D. gatoi* (short and fat) both can be found on mineral oil microscopy from the ears of cats with pruritic OE. The two most common presentations encountered are young cats with pruritic ears and older cats with pruritic ears. It has also been reported to be the cause of ceruminous otitis in cats.[42,98] In the latter case a concurrent systemic illness was either already diagnosed or diagnosed shortly thereafter. In young cats it is not uncommon to find concurrent *Otodectes* infestations and *Demodex* mites. There are no products licensed for the treatment of feline otic demodicosis. Successful treatments include milbemycin (0.5 mg/kg orally, once daily or on a week on/week off basis for 30 days), otic ivermectin, otic milbemycin, and otic preparations labeled for the treatment of ear mites in cats. Amitraz is not recommended for use in cats because it can be toxic. In young animals attention to general pediatric care will usually prevent recurrences. In older animals otic demodicosis can be difficult to resolve if the underlying disease process (e.g., neoplasia, hyperthyroidism, and diabetes mellitus) is not properly managed. Concurrent topical otic steroids may be helpful in relieving the pruritus.

Obstructive Otitis

The most common causes of obstructive otitis in cats are ear polyps (Figure 22-60), ear tumors, stenosis secondary to inflammation, ear deformity caused by untreated aural hematomas, and ear debris concretions. The most common clinical signs associated with space-occupying obstructive lesions are chronic recurrent OE or OM, head shaking, and malodorous suppurative discharge. These lesions tend to be unilateral but can be bilateral with ear polyps. Mast cell tumors in young cats, particularly Siamese cats, can present as obstructive lesions. In the case of space-occupying lesions, resolution of the problem requires imaging of the ear to locate the obstruction and surgical removal of the obstruction. Because these cases tend to be chronic, cats usually have a concurrent OM and need postoperative systemic and topical antimicrobial treatment based on culture and

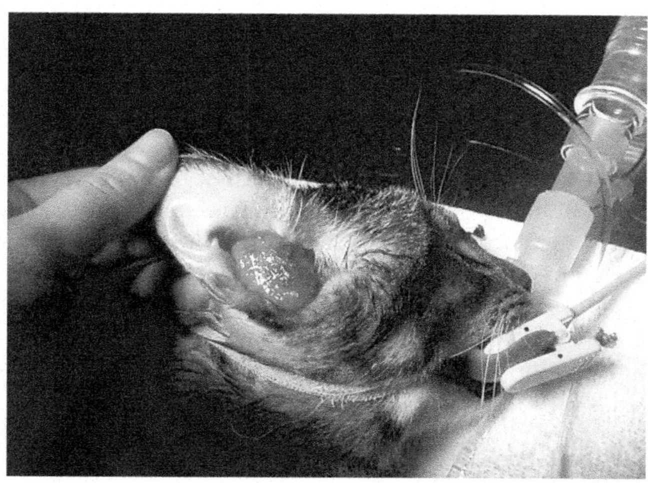

FIGURE 22-60 Ear polyp. This is an obvious polyp; however, polyps are not always so obvious, and sometimes surgical exploration or imaging (or both) are required to visualize them. *(Photo courtesy Dr. Carol Tice.)*

susceptibility testing. Irrigation of the ear canal and bulla may also be needed. It is important to remember to perform otic cytology because this may help guide initial antibiotic selection and may be able to identify concurrent yeast otitis that may not be otherwise diagnosed. Concurrent treatment of both bacterial and yeast OM is common.

Stenosis of the external ear canal of cats is most commonly, but not exclusively, seen as a result of aural hematomas that have healed without surgical intervention. If the obstruction is causing clinical discomfort and resulting in SO, intervention is needed. If the cat is not otherwise bothered by the problem, it is best left untreated.

Allergic Otitis

Allergic otitis in cats is a common complication of atopy and food allergy. The ideal treatment is appropriate management of the underlying allergy (food or atopy). Seasonal atopy is common, and otic pruritus may be the only clinical sign. Owners may complain about an increase in ceruminous discharge. Otic cytology will often reveal a concurrent yeast otitis; treatment of the yeast otitis may diminish but does not fully eliminate the pruritus, and otic glucocorticoids will be needed.

Yeast Otitis

Recurrent chronic yeast otitis in cats is most commonly seen in cats with allergic ear disease caused by atopy or food allergy, mild obstructive ear disease, and congenital hair coat abnormalities (e.g., Devon Rex and Sphynx). The most common treatment of choice is itraconazole (2 to 5 mg/kg orally, once daily) for 30 days or once daily on a 1 week off/1 week on protocol for 30 days. Fluconazole is increasingly being used as a treatment option because it is much less expensive than itraconazole. Ketoconazole is commonly used in dogs, but cats do not tolerate this drug; because of the increased potential for hepatotoxicity, its use is discouraged in cats. In mild cases or acute cases that are likely to be seen in primary care, combination antifungal and antiinflammatory topical products may be very suitable and appropriate.

Chronic recurrent yeast otitis may be due to *Malassezia* OM. Definitive diagnosis may be made by way of diagnostic imaging or myringotomy with culture and cytology of exudate from the bulla. In the authors' (KM) experience, these cases require aggressive ear irrigation and systemic therapy for resolution. A careful reassessment of the case history should be made to determine whether there is an underlying disease (e.g., allergies).

Otitis Media

OM can be a sequela to an upper respiratory infection, it can occur as a complication of ear mite infestation or obstructive lesion such as a polyp, or it can be a primary disease when organisms from the retropharynx ascend through the eustachian tube into the tympanic bulla.

The clinical signs of OM are described in the preceding sections, but it cannot be emphasized enough that OM should be suspected whenever there is recurrent unilateral or bilateral OE, especially if the cytology reveals septic inflammation.

Core diagnostics include ear cytology and bacterial culture. Bacterial culture is particularly important if rods are seen; recurrent *Pseudomonas* spp. infections in the ear are difficult to treat. Opinions vary as to when diagnostic imaging is needed or cost effective. Conventional radiographs are widely available, and a major strength of this type of imaging is that it provides a global view of skull, nasal cavity, and bulla. The major problem, of course, is that there is superimposition of overlying structures. Computed tomography (CT) provides cross-sectional views, allowing for localization of lesions. If soft tissue opacity in seen in the tympanic bulla, it is either tissue or fluid, and differentiation on radiographs is not possible; CT imaging can make this differentiation because fluid will not contrast enhance. In general, diagnostic imaging is indicated when an obstruction is suspected (unilateral or bilateral); when otitis exists concurrent with signs of nasopharyngeal polyps, when there is a head tilt, or when septic otitis fails to respond to therapy.

Medical Management for Otitis Media

Not all cases of OM require the aggressive medical treatment described in this section. Middle ear irrigation is not without risk and cost. It is very reasonable to treat OM with systemic and topical antibiotics and antifungal drugs for 4 to 6 weeks. A gentle lavage of the ear may be necessary. In all cases antiinflammatory drugs and pain medication should be provided. The most common causes of otitis media in cats in one author's (KM) experience are *Malassezia* and *Pseudomonas*.

The following treatment plan is appropriate for OM:

1. Administer general anesthesia and analgesics in preparation for sample collection and flushing of the bulla. Perform an otoscopic examination of the ear canal to determine whether the tympanic membrane is ruptured.
2. If the tympanic membrane is intact, a myringotomy should be performed to collect cytology and culture specimens. This can be done with a video otoscope or with an operating head otoscope. Using an operating head otoscope, a sterile urethral catheter or 22-gauge, 6-inch spinal needle attached to a 3-mL syringe containing 1 mL of sterile saline is inserted through the tympanic membrane; the fluid is flushed into the bulla, loosening debris and exudates that can be aspirated for sampling (Figure 22-61). This fluid can be used for both cytology and culture. Another technique that is equally useful is to use a minitip culturette to perform both the stab incision and collect the sample. The minitip culture swab is passed through a sterile ear cone attached to the operating head otoscope. It is used to puncture the tympanic membrane and then pushed into the bulla. The tip is rotated to collect specimens. This is repeated to collect specimens for cytologic examination. The needle, catheter, or swab is inserted through the tympanic membrane at the 5 to 7 o'clock position. The caudal–ventral part of the tympanic membrane is the largest and safest area to pass tubes and instruments insofar as it avoids the important vasculature, nerves, and the hearing apparatus (which are located cranial–dorsal).
3. If the tympanic membrane cannot be visualized, it will be necessary to thoroughly clean and dry the ear canal using suction before collection of samples from the bulla. The cat's face and eyes should be protected from ear cleaners and flushing fluid by gently wrapping the cat's head in a towel. If the tympanic membrane is ruptured, samples can be collected from the bulla through the rent in the tympanic membrane for both cytology and culture. Care must be taken not to contaminate the tips of the instruments with debris from the external ear canal. This can be accomplished by using a double catheter technique in which a large lumen catheter is used to shroud a small catheter inside it. Once the large catheter is safely in the bulla, the tip of the smaller catheter is pushed into the bulla to collect a sample. If liquid cannot be aspirated, 1 mL of sterile saline is flushed into the bulla. The same "shrouding" technique can be done using a sterile ear cone attached to operating otoscope. A sterile urinary catheter is then passed through the cone and used to collect a specimen by aspirating fluid. Again, if no fluid is obtained, 1 mL of sterile saline can be flushed into the bulla and aspirated.
4. Once samples have been collected, the bulla is flushed with copious amounts of warm sterile lavage fluid. Dilute povidone–iodine solution is commonly used. Suction is used to remove the fluid. This process is continued until the fluid is clear. This process frequently dislodges large chunks of debris. A small amount of hemorrhage is also possible.
5. After flushing, instill an enrofloxacin otic drop and dimethyl sulfoxide–fluocinolone otic solution into the bulla to decrease inflammation and deliver a high concentration of antibiotics to the target area.
6. After the procedure patients are treated with oral prednisolone (1 to 2 mg/kg orally, daily for 2 weeks and then gradually tapered over the next 2 weeks). Steroids decrease inflammation, secretions, and exudation in the bulla. If oral medication is difficult, alternatives include the use of injectable methylprednisolone acetate or intravenous dexamethasone (0.2 mg/kg) at the time of treatment and then once weekly.
7. Many cases of OM in cats are due to *Malassezia* spp. or a combined bacterial infection. Pending culture and sensitivity results, the author (KM) often prescribes marbofloxacin (3 to 5 mg/kg orally, once daily) and itraconazole or fluconazole (3 to 5 mg/kg orally, once daily).

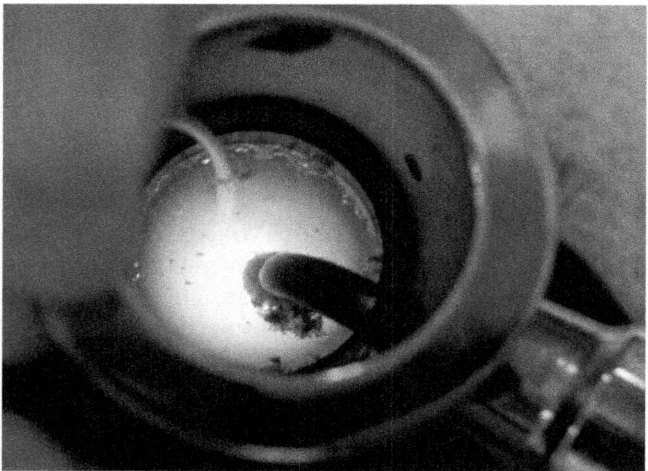

FIGURE 22-61 Exudate from middle ear irrigation. Sterile saline was flushed into the tympanic membrane and loosened debris that can be used for culture or an aspirate. This technique can be used when video otoscopy is not available or possible. *(Photo courtesy University of Wisconsin School of Veterinary Medicine.)*

8. Severe OM necessitating middle ear irrigation and flushing of the bulla is best treated with concurrent topical antibiotics. Most commonly, one of the following is used: fluoroquinolones (e.g., ciprofloxacin, enrofloxacin, orbifloxacin), ticarcillin, or ceftazidime. It may be necessary to request that a compounding pharmacy make these otic solutions.
9. Most cats will require pain medication after ear flushing for at least 5 to 7 days. Tramadol (1 to 4 mg/kg orally, every 8 hours) is effective.
10. Long-term antibiotic therapy will be determined by the results of the cytology and culture results. It is not uncommon for the cytology to reveal large numbers of yeast organisms that are not evident on culture. Total treatment time varies, but owners should be expected to administer medication for at least 4 to 8 weeks.
11. Complications that can occur after flushing include head tilt, nystagmus, potential OI, and pain. Owners should be warned that small amounts of blood-tinged fluid may be seen after the procedure. This procedure is best done early in the day and the patient released as late as possible in the day. Overnight hospitalization is ideal because it allows the cat to recover fully and the clinician to monitor the cat for adverse effects. Neurologic side effects are often transient and gone within 24 hours of flushing.
12. Cats with OM should be reexamined every 2 to 4 weeks during the treatment period.

Vestibular Disease and Otitis Media and Otitis Interna[57]

Space does not allow a detailed discussion of vestibular disease in cats; however, there are several important points to remember. Cats with vestibular disease need a careful physical and neurologic examination to determine if the vestibular signs are peripheral or central in cause. If clinical signs of OE or OM are present, it is likely that the vestibular signs are associated with the OM. OM can occur without obvious signs of otitis, making this determination difficult. Neurologic examination and imaging are usually indicated in these situations. Diagnostic imaging is needed in cats with vestibular signs to ensure that there is no obstructive lesion (e.g., polyp) causing the signs and, it is to be hoped, to confirm the presence of OM.

Animals with central vestibular disease (CVD) have a brainstem dysfunction. In peripheral vestibular disease (PVD), animals have a rotary or horizontal nystagmus that does not change with the animal's head position. Although the nystagmus may not be a constant finding in chronic cases, sudden head movements usually can trigger the nystagmus, and its direction is constant. The head tilt is always toward the side with the otitis, but the fast phase of the nystagmus is away from the ear with the disease. Proprioception is normal in animals with PVD. In addition, PVD caused by OM or OI may be accompanied by ipsilateral facial nerve paresis and Horner's syndrome. Animals with CVD can have any type of nystagmus, but vertical nystagmus is more common with CVD than with PVD. It has been reported that animals with CVD have a nystagmus that changes in character or direction with a change in head position. Most often the nystagmus does not change, but central disease is present if it does. Abnormalities of cranial nerves other than VII and VIII are suggestive of CVD, as is the presence of proprioceptive deficits. The most reliable signs to look for in CVD are proprioceptive deficits and changes in mentation. Proprioceptive deficits can be difficult to assess in cats, even more so if they are ataxic.

The three major differential diagnoses for cats with PVD are OI, OM, nasopharyngeal polyps, and idiopathic feline vestibular disease. The latter is most common in the summer and fall and can affect cats of any age, but it seems to be more common in cats that go outside. There is a sudden onset of ataxia, nystagmus, and head tilt consistent with a peripheral vestibular lesion. Facial paralysis, Horner's syndrome, and proprioceptive deficits are not features of this disease. It is important to rule out OM and OI. Neurologic signs typically improve spontaneously in approximately 2 weeks; this will not occur in cats with bacterial otitis. Some cats may have a mild persistent head tilt and ataxia. The cause is unknown, but it may be due to a virus or aberrant migration of *Cuterebra* larvae.

Otitis causes vestibular disease by one of two mechanisms. Bacteria that infect the middle ear can produce toxins that inflame the labyrinth (OM), or bacteria may invade the labyrinth itself (OI). Bacterial OM or OI should be treated for at least 4 to 6 weeks with systemic antibiotics based on culture and sensitivity findings. Topical antibiotics are insufficient. Given that OM and OI can be difficult to diagnose by otoscopic examination and imaging, a treatment trial is recommended even if OM or OI cannot be identified conclusively. Owing to damage to the neuronal structures, some residual head tilt, facial paralysis, or Horner's syndrome may be apparent.

Ototoxicity Concerns

Aminoglycoside antibiotics (i.e., gentamicin, amikacin) have been shown to cause ototoxicity in particularly sensitive animals. The drug can reach very high concentrations in the ear, leading to toxic side effects. In general, the development of ototoxicity depends on the duration of treatment, cumulative dose, average daily dose, peak and trough serum concentrations, concurrent diuretic use, underlying disease status, and previous use of aminoglycoside antibiotics. The ototoxic effects are generally preceded by nephrotoxicity insofar as the drug is

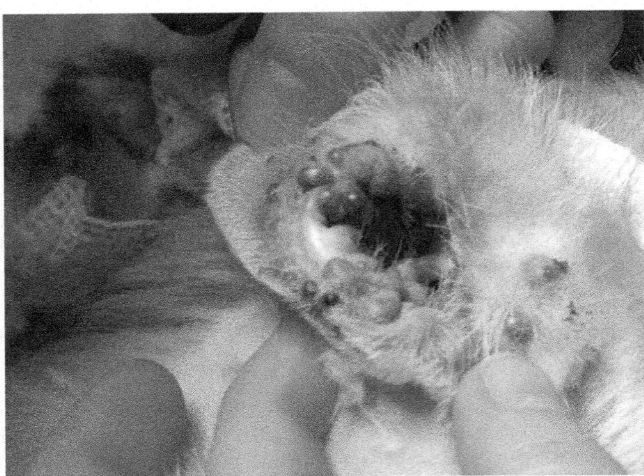

FIGURE 22-62 Apocrine hidrocystoma. This is a common presentation of this benign disease in the ears. *(Photo courtesy University of Wisconsin School of Veterinary Medicine.)*

also readily accumulated in kidney tissue. In dogs hearing loss is the most common presentation. Cats, however, generally show vestibular symptoms when ototoxicity occurs. Symptoms may eventually resolve once the medication is withdrawn, although in some cases, the adverse effects are irreversible. Other drugs that have the potential to cause ototoxicity include chlorhexidine, polymyxin B, ethacrynic acid, furosemide, salicylates, and cisplatin. The use of chlorhexidine as an ear cleaner is not recommended for this reason.

Apocrine Hidrocystoma

This is an uncommon, non-neoplastic condition in which cats have multiple or numerous nodules or vesicles in the external ear canal, inner pinnae, or eyelid (Figure 22-62). The vesicles are small, measuring less than 2 mm on average. These lesions are deeply colored (dark blue, brown, or black) and may be mistaken for pigmented neoplasms. Biopsy of the lesions will confirm the diagnosis. The condition has been seen in cats of all ages. Surgical removal or laser ablation may be beneficial in symptomatic animals. Other treatments include lancing the cysts with a needle or blade and using silver nitrate sticks as a chemical cautery. Within several weeks the cysts will dry and involute. After several weeks the remaining cysts can be treated. Chemical ablation with trichloroacetic acid has been used successfully to treat these cysts when they occur around the eyelids.[15,73] Cysts are surgically débrided and then treated topically with 20% trichloroacetic acid.[107]

Proliferative Necrotizing Otitis Externa

Young kittens between 2 and 6 months of age are primarily affected by proliferative necrotizing OE, a visually distinctive condition. One case report, however, diagnosed the disorder in three young adult domestic shorthair cats between 3 and 5 years of age.[54] It is a rare condition with unknown etiology. The disorder is characterized by well-demarcated, erythematous plaques with annular or serpiginous (wavy) borders. Thick keratinous debris is also present. Biopsy of the lesions will confirm the diagnosis. Lesions appear on the inner aspect of the pinnae, external ear canal, and sometimes the preauricular region on the face. Lesions develop rapidly and often progress to erosion and ulceration. The animal may be pruritic. Often, secondary bacterial and yeast infections may be present. Lesions generally regress spontaneously by the time the animal is 12 to 24 months of age. However, the disease may be more persistent in older cats. One study reported beneficial results when the animal was treated with once-daily tacrolimus ointment.[54]

BOX 22-3

Differential Diagnosis of Nonhealing Wounds in Cats

- Parasites
  - Cuterebra
  - Leishmaniasis
  - Disseminated infections with Protista
  - Leishmaniasis
- Fungal
  - *Microsporum canis* subcutaneous granuloma
  - Sporotrichosis
  - Opportunistic fungal infections (e.g., mycetoma, phaehyphomycosis)
  - Cutaneous involvement of systemic mycoses: cryptococcosis, coccidioidomycosis, blastomycosis, histoplasmosis
- Foreign bodies
- Neoplastic disease
- Bacterial infections
  - Bacterial furunculosis
  - *Actinomyces/Nocardia* infections
  - Cutaneous bacterial granuloma
  - Cutaneous mycobacterial infections
  - Feline leprosy

NONHEALING WOUNDS

The term *nonhealing wound* simply describes any lesion that does not resolve with what initially seems to be appropriate care. The causes of nonhealing wounds in cats are legion, and some of the more important differential diagnoses are listed in Box 22-3. Successful resolution of these lesions depends on using a cost-effective diagnostic approach. In general, the following are core diagnostic tests for nonhealing wounds: skin scrapings, skin cytology, fine-needle aspirate of mass or tissue, culture of the tissue by excisional wedge, and skin biopsy. Depending on the geographic region of the veterinarian's practice, some diseases may be more or less likely, and additional tests based on a high index of suspicion may be warranted. Because some of the agents are potential zoonoses, all cats with nonhealing wounds should be handled with gloves at all times.

Special stains are often needed to identify infectious agents. It is critical to include a list of differential diagnoses so that these tests can be ordered promptly. Submission of several unfixed cytology specimens is helpful, as is submission of tissue imprints from the biopsy site. In order to maximize the usefulness of the latter, the excised tissue should be blotted on a paper towel until the blood is removed. Then the veterinarian makes several impressions of the tissue on a glass microscope slide and submits that with the biopsy specimen. The most diagnostic biopsy specimens are deep wedge sections; many pathogens are few in number in the skin and are found deep in the tissue.

Feline Leprosy Syndromes

Feline leprosy refers to a mycobacterial disease in which multiple granulomas form in the skin or subcutaneous tissue.[24] These organisms are difficult to culture and very slow growing, requiring special growth conditions. Three patterns of disease have been recognized.[51] *Mycobacterium lepraemurium* occurs in young cats with nodular to ulcerative lesions on the legs. Lesions rapidly progress. There may be sparse to moderate numbers of acid-fast bacteria (AFB) seen on cytology or histopathology. Confirmation of the diagnosis is based on polymerase chain reaction (PCR) testing. A second clinical presentation of feline leprosy is seen in old cats. Cats may have localized or disseminated disease, and disease progression is slow and protracted. In contrast to the case in young cats, large numbers of AFB are found on cytology or histopathology. Again, definitive diagnosis is made with PCR testing. Finally, a third presentation seen in western Canada and the United States called *feline multisystemic granulomatous mycobacteriosis* has been described.[3] This is caused by the slow-growing *Mycobacterium visibilis*, which causes diffuse cutaneous disease and widespread dissemination to internal organisms. Treatment is challenging, and surgical excision, rifabutin, sulfa drugs, and clofazimine have been used.[51]

Rapidly Growing Mycobacterial Infections

Atypical or rapidly growing mycobacterial infections[52] are caused by the *Mycobacterium fortuitum* group, which grow within 7 days on appropriate culture medium. In cats the most common clinical presentation is a nonhealing wound in the inguinal area, often at the site of a cat bite abscess. The infection invades the surrounding skin and subcutaneous tissue. Affected areas are alopecic and have fistulous tracts and a watery discharge. Diagnosis can be made by cytologic examination of exudates and culture of exudates, but histologic confirmation may be needed. Treatment involving a combination of surgical excision and antimicrobial therapy with drugs such as clarithromycin may be required, although some species are susceptible to more routine antibiotics such as doxycycline or fluoroquinolones.

References

1. Ahman S, Perrins N, Bond R: Carriage of *Malassezia* spp. yeasts in healthy and seborrhoeic Devon Rex cats, *Med Mycol* 45:449, 2007.
2. Ahman S, Perrins N, Bond R: Treatment of *Malassezia pachydermatis*–associated seborrhoeic dermatitis in Devon Rex cats with itraconazole: a pilot study, *Vet Dermatol* 18:171, 2007.
3. Appleyard GD, Clark EG: Histologic and genotypic characterization of a novel *Mycobacterium* species found in three cats, *J Clin Microbiol* 40:2425, 2002.
4. Bardagi M, Fondati A, Fondevila D et al: Ultrastructural study of cutaneous lesions in feline eosinophilic granuloma complex, *Vet Dermatol* 14:297, 2003.
5. Beale KM, Altman D, Clemmons RR et al: Systemic toxicosis associated with azathioprine administration in domestic cats, *Am J Vet Res* 53:1236, 1992.
6. Bennett S: Photosensitisation induced by clofazimine in a cat, *Aust Vet J* 85:375, 2007.
7. Bensignor E: An approach to otitis externa and otitis media. In Foster AP, Foil CS, editors: *BSAVA manual of small animal dermatology*, ed 2, Gloucester, 2003, British Small Animal Veterinary Association, p 102.
8. Bloom PB: Canine and feline eosinophilic skin diseases, *Vet Clin North Am Small Anim Pract* 36:141, 2006.
9. Bond R, Curtis CF, Ferguson EA et al: An idiopathic facial dermatitis of Persian cats, *Vet Dermatol* 11:35, 2000.
10. Bond R, Stevens K, Perrins N et al: Carriage of *Malassezia* spp. yeasts in Cornish Rex, Devon Rex and Domestic short-haired cats: a cross-sectional survey, *Vet Dermatol* 19:299, 2008.
11. Bond RC, Mason C: An idiopathic facial dermatitis of thirteen Persian cats. In Thoday KL, Foil C, Bond R, editors: *Advances in veterinary dermatology*, ed 4, Oxford, 2002, Blackwell Publishing, p 307.
12. Burrows M: An approach to nodules and draining tracts. In Foster AP, Foil CS, editors: *BSAVA manual of small animal dermatology*, ed 2, Gloucester, 2003, British Small Animal Veterinary Association, p 213.
13. Byrne KP: Metabolic epidermal necrosis–hepatocutaneous syndrome, *Vet Clin North Am Small Anim Pract* 29:1337, 1999.
14. Cafarchia C, Lia RP, Romito D et al: Competence of the housefly, *Musca domestica*, as a vector of *Microsporum canis* under experimental conditions, *Med Vet Entomol* 23:21, 2009.
15. Cantaloube B, Raymond-Letron I, Regnier A: Multiple eyelid apocrine hidrocystomas in two Persian cats, *Vet Ophthalmol* 7:121, 2004.
16. Carlotti DN, Guinot P, Meissonnier E et al: Eradication of feline dermatophytosis in a shelter: a field study, *Vet Dermatol* 21(3):259-266, 2010.
17. Chapelin F, Cadiergues MC, Delverdier M et al: Feline pemphigus foliaceus: a clinical case and literature review, *Rev Med Vet* 155:87, 2004.
18. Chung TH, Ryu MH, Kim DY et al: Topical tacrolimus (FK506) for the treatment of feline idiopathic facial dermatitis, *Aust Vet J* 87:417, 2009.

19. Colombini S, Hodgin EC, Foil CS et al: Induction of feline flea allergy dermatitis and the incidence and histopathological characteristics of concurrent indolent lip ulcers, *Vet Dermatol* 12:155, 2001.
20. Colombo S, Nardoni S, Cornegliani L et al: Prevalence of *Malassezia* spp. yeasts in feline nail folds: a cytological and mycological study, *Vet Dermatol* 18:278, 2007.
21. Cornegliani L: Collagenolytic granuloma in three domestic shorthaired cats following foreign body penetration, *Vet Dermatol* 11:30, 2000.
22. Craig TM, Teel PD, Dubuisson LM et al: *Lynxacarus radovskyi* infestation in a cat, *J Am Vet Med Assoc* 202:613, 1993.
23. Curtis CF: Current trends in the treatment of *Sarcoptes, Cheyletiella* and *Otodectes* mite infestations in dogs and cats, *Vet Dermatol* 15:108, 2004.
24. Davies JL, Sibley JA, Myers S et al: Histological and genotypical characterization of feline cutaneous mycobacteriosis: a retrospective study of formalin-fixed paraffin-embedded tissues, *Vet Dermatol* 17:155, 2006.
25. DeBoer DJ, Moriello KA: Development of an experimental model of *Microsporum canis* infection in cats, *Vet Microbiol* 42:289, 1994.
26. DeBoer DJ, Moriello KA: Inability of two topical treatments to influence the course of experimentally induced dermatophytosis in cats, *J Am Vet Med Assoc* 207:52, 1995.
27. DeBoer DJ, Moriello KA, Blum JL et al: Effects of lufenuron treatment in cats on the establishment and course of *Microsporum canis* infection following exposure to infected cats, *J Am Vet Med Assoc* 222:1216, 2003.
28. Declercq J, De Bosschere H: Diesel oil-induced alopecia in two cats, *Vet Dermatol* 20:135, 2009.
29. Detweiler DA, Johnson LR, Kass PH et al: Computed tomographic evidence of bulla effusion in cats with sinonasal disease: 2001-2004, *J Vet Intern Med* 20:1080, 2006.
30. Diesel ADD: Allergen specific IgE in atopic and healthy cats—comparison of rapid screening immunoassay and complete panel analysis, *Vet Dermatol* 20:216, 2009.
31. Diesel A, Verbrugge M, Moriello KA: Efficacy of eight commercial formulations of lime sulphur on in vitro growth inhibition of M. canis, *Vet Dermatol* 19:107, 2008.
32. Ferrer-Canals G, Beale KM, Fadok V: Demodex gatoi infestation in cats presenting with noninflammatory alopecia, *Vet Dermatol* 20:224, 2009.
33. Fondati A, Fondevila D, Ferrer L: Histopathological study of feline eosinophilic dermatoses, *Vet Dermatol* 12:333, 2001.
34. Forster-Van Hijfte MA, Curtis CF, White RN: Resolution of exfoliative dermatitis and Malassezia pachydermatis overgrowth in a cat after surgical thymoma resection, *J Small Anim Pract* 38:451, 1997.
35. Foust AL, Marsella R, Akucewich LH et al: Evaluation of persistence of terbinafine in the hair of normal cats after 14 days of daily therapy, *Vet Dermatol* 18:246, 2007.
36. Godfrey DR: Dermatosis and associated systemic signs in a cat with thymoma and recently treated with an imidacloprid preparation, *J Small Anim Pract* 40:333, 1999.
37. Goldman C, Rosser Jr E, Petersen A et al: Investigation on the effects of ciclosporin (Atopica®) on intradermal skin test reactivity in dogs, *Vet Dermatol* 20:215, 2009.
38. Gotthelf LN: Diagnosis and treatment of otitis media in dogs and cats, *Vet Clin North Am Small Anim Pract* 34:469, 2004.
39. Graham CA, Rosser EJ: Bioavailabity and activity of prednisone and prednisolone in the feline patient, *Vet Dermatol* 15:7, 2004.
40. Gross TL, Ihrke PJ, Walder EJ et al: *Skin diseases of the dog and cat: clinical and histopathologic diagnosis*, ed 2, Ames, Iowa, 2005, Blackwell Science.
41. Guaguere E: Topical treatment of canine and feline pyoderma, *Vet Dermatol* 7:145, 1996.
42. Guaguere E MA, Degorce-Rubiales F: Feline demodicosis: retrospective study of 12 cases, *Vet Dermatol* 15:34, 2004.
43. Guaguere E, Pascal P: *A practical guide to feline dermatology*, Paris, 1999, Merial.
44. Guilford WG, Jones BR, Markwell PJ et al: Food sensitivity in cats with chronic idiopathic gastrointestinal problems, *J Vet Intern Med* 15:7, 2001.
45. Hargis AM, Ginn PE: Feline herpesvirus 1–associated facial and nasal dermatitis and stomatitis in domestic cats, *Vet Clin North Am Small Anim Pract* 29:1281, 1999.
46. Jackson HA: Diagnostic techniques in dermatology: the investigation and diagnosis of adverse food reactions in dogs and cats, *Clin Tech Small Anim Pract* 16:233, 2001.
47. Jazic E: Acne. In August J, editor: *Consultations in feline internal medicine*, vol 6, St Louis, 2010, Saunders Elsevier, p 375.
48. Last RD, Suzuki Y, Manning T et al: A case of fatal systemic toxoplasmosis in a cat being treated with cyclosporin A for feline atopy, *Vet Dermatol* 15:194, 2004.
49. Lien YH, Huang HP, Chang PH: Iatrogenic hyperadrenocorticism in 12 cats, *J Am Anim Hosp Assoc* 42:414, 2006.
50. Lopez RA: Of mites and man, *J Am Vet Med Assoc* 203:606, 1993.
51. Malik R, Hughes MS, Martin P, Wigney D: Feline leprosy syndrome. In Greene CE, editor: *Infectious diseases of the dog and cat*, ed 3, St Louis, 2005, Saunders Elsevier, p 477.
52. Malik R, Martin P, Wigney D, Foster S: Infections caused by rapidly growing mycobacteria. In Greene CE, editor: *Infectious diseases of the dog and cat*, ed 3, St Louis, 2005, Saunders Elsevier, p 482.
53. Mason KV, Evans AG: Mosquito bite–caused eosinophilic dermatitis in cats, *J Am Vet Med Assoc* 198:2086, 1991.
54. Mauldin EA, Ness TA, Goldschmidt MH: Proliferative and necrotizing otitis externa in four cats, *Vet Dermatol* 18:370, 2007.
55. Medleau L, Hnilica KA: *Small animal dermatology: a color atlas and therapeutic guide*, ed 2, St Louis, 2006, Saunders Elsevier.
56. Moriello K, DeBoer DJ: Dermatophytosis. In Greene CE, editor: *Infectious diseases of the dog and cat*, ed 4, 2012, Saunders Elsevier (in press).
57. Moriello K, Diesel A: Medical management of otitis. In August J, editor: *Consultations in feline internal medicine*, vol 6, St Louis, 2010, Saunders Elsevier, p 347.
58. Moriello K, Newbury S: Dermatophytosis. In Hurley KF, Miller L, editors: *Management of infectious diseases in animal shelters*, Ames, 2009, Wiley Blackwell, p 243.
59. Moriello KA: Feline atopy in three littermates, *Vet Dermatol* 12:177, 2001.
60. Moriello KA: Treatment of dermatophytosis in dogs and cats: review of published studies, *Vet Dermatol* 15:99, 2004.
61. Moriello KA, DeBoer DJ: Fungal flora of the coat of pet cats, *Am J Vet Res* 52:602, 1991.
62. Moriello KA, DeBoer DJ: Fungal flora of the haircoat of cats with and without dermatophytosis, *J Med Vet Mycol* 29:285, 1991.
63. Moriello KA, DeBoer DJ, Schenker R et al: Efficacy of pretreatment with lufenuron for the prevention of *Microsporum canis* infection in a feline direct topical challenge model, *Vet Dermatol* 15:357, 2004.
64. Moriello KA, Newbury S: Recommendations for the management and treatment of dermatophytosis in animal shelters, *Vet Clin North Am Small Anim Pract* 36:89, 2006.
65. Morris DO: Medical therapy of otitis externa and otitis media, *Vet Clin North Am Small Anim Pract* 34:541, 2004.
66. Muller GH, Kirk RW, Scott DW et al: *Muller & Kirk's small animal dermatology*, ed 6, Philadelphia, 2001, Saunders.
67. Nagata M, Ishida T: Cutaneous reactivity to mosquito bites and its antigens in cats, *Vet Dermatol* 8:19, 1997.
68. Nardoni S, Corazza M, Mancianti F: Diagnostic and clinical features of animal malasseziosis, *Parassitologia* 50:81, 2008.
69. Nardoni S, Mancianti F, Rum A et al: Isolation of *Malassezia* species from healthy cats and cats with otitis, *J Feline Med Surg* 7:141, 2005.

70. Neel JA, Tarigo J, Tater KC et al: Deep and superficial skin scrapings from a feline immunodeficiency virus–positive cat, *Vet Clin Pathol* 36:101, 2007.
71. Newbury S, Moriello K, Verbrugge M et al: Use of lime sulphur and itraconazole to treat shelter cats naturally infected with Microsporum canis in an annex facility: an open field trial, *Vet Dermatol* 18:324, 2007.
72. Newbury S, Moriello KA: Skin diseases of animals in shelters: triage strategy and treatment recommendations for common diseases, *Vet Clin North Am Small Anim Pract* 36:59, 2006.
73. Newkirk KM, Rohrbach BW: A retrospective study of eyelid tumors from 43 cats, *Vet Pathol* 46:916, 2009.
74. Noli C, Scarampella F: Prospective open pilot study on the use of ciclosporin for feline allergic skin disease, *J Small Anim Pract* 47:434, 2006.
75. Noli C, Toma S: Three cases of immune-mediated adnexal skin disease treated with cyclosporin, *Vet Dermatol* 17:85, 2006.
76. O'Brien CR, Wilkie JS: Calcinosis circumscripta following an injection of proligestone in a Burmese cat, *Aust Vet J* 79:187, 2001.
77. Ordeix L, Galeotti F, Scarampella F et al: *Malassezia* spp. overgrowth in allergic cats, *Vet Dermatol* 18:316, 2007.
78. Perrins N, Bond R: Synergistic inhibition of the growth in vitro of *Microsporum canis* by miconazole and chlorhexidine, *Vet Dermatol* 14:99, 2003.
79. Perrins N, Gaudiano F, Bond R: Carriage of *Malassezia* spp. yeasts in cats with diabetes mellitus, hyperthyroidism and neoplasia, *Med Mycol* 45:541, 2007.
80. Ployngam T, Tobias AH, Smith SA et al: Hemodynamic effects of methylprednisolone acetate administration in cats, *Am J Vet Res* 67:583, 2006.
81. Ployngam T, Tobias AH, Smith SA et al: Hemodynamic effects of methylprednisolone acetate administration in cats, *Am J Vet Res* 67:583, 2006.
82. Power HT, Ihrke PJ: Selected feline eosinophilic skin diseases, *Vet Clin North Am Small Anim Pract* 25:833, 1995.
83. Preziosi DE, Goldschmidt MH, Greek JS et al: Feline pemphigus foliaceus: a retrospective analysis of 57 cases, *Vet Dermatol* 14:313, 2003.
84. Preziosi DE, Goldschmidt MH, Greek JS et al: Feline pemphigus foliaceus: a retrospective analysis of 57 cases, *Vet Dermatol* 14:313, 2003.
85. Robson DC, Burton GG: Cyclosporin: applications in small animal dermatology, *Vet Dermatol* 14:1, 2003.
86. Rottenberg S, von Tscharner C, Roosje PJ: Thymoma-associated exfoliative dermatitis in cats, *Vet Pathol* 41:429, 2004.
87. Saari SA, Juuti KH, Palojarvi JH et al: *Demodex gatoi*–associated contagious pruritic dermatosis in cats—a report from six households in Finland, *Acta Vet Scand* 51:40, 2009.
88. Schlicksup MD, Van Winkle TJ, Holt DE: Prevalence of clinical abnormalities in cats found to have nonneoplastic middle ear disease at necropsy: 59 cases (1991-2007), *J Am Vet Med Assoc* 235:841, 2009.
89. Schwassman M, Logas D: How to treat common parasites safely. In August J, editor: *Consultations in feline internal medicine*, ed 6, St Louis, 2010, Saunders Elsevier, p 390.
90. Skorinsky I, Papadogiannakis E, Horowitz I et al: Epitheliotropic cutaneous lymphoma (mycosis fungoides) in a coati, *J Small Anim Pract* 49:204, 2008.
91. Smith S, Tobias A, Fine D et al: Corticosteroid-associated congestive heart failure in 12 cats, *Intern J Appl Res Vet Med* 2:159, 2004.
92. Sotiraki ST, Koutinas AF, Leontides LS et al: Factors affecting the frequency of ear canal and face infestation by *Otodectes cynotis* in the cat, *Vet Parasitol* 96:309, 2001.
93. Tasker S, Griffon DJ, Nuttall TJ et al: Resolution of paraneoplastic alopecia following surgical removal of a pancreatic carcinoma in a cat, *J Small Anim Pract* 40:16, 1999.
94. Tobey JC, Houston DM, Breur GJ et al: Cutaneous T-cell lymphoma in a cat, *J Am Vet Med Assoc* 204:606, 1994.
95. Trimmer AM, Griffin CE, Rosenkrantz WS: Feline immunotherapy, *Clin Tech Small Anim Pract* 21:157, 2006.
96. Trimmer AM, Newton HM: Rush and conventional immunotherapy. In August J, editor: *Consultations in feline internal medicine*, ed 6, St Louis, 2010, Saunders Elsevier, p 357.
97. Turek MM: Cutaneous paraneoplastic syndromes in dogs and cats: a review of the literature, *Vet Dermatol* 14:279, 2003.
98. Van Poucke S: Ceruminous otitis externa due to *Demodex cati* in a cat, *Vet Rec* 149:651, 2001.
99. Verbrugge M, Kettings R, Moriello K: Effects of light and temperature variations on time to growth of dermatophytes using commercial fungal culture media, *Vet Dermatol* 19:110, 2008.
100. Verlinden A, Hesta M, Millet S et al: Food allergy in dogs and cats: a review, *Crit Rev Food Sci Nutr* 46:259, 2006.
101. Vlaminck KMJA, Engelen MACM: Overview of the pharmokinetic and pharmodynamic studies on the development of itraconazole for feline *Microsporum canis* dermatophytosis. In Hillier A, Foster AP, Kwochka K, editors: *Advances in veterinary dermatology*, ed 5, Oxford, 2005, Blackwell Publishing, p 130.
102. Vogel JW, Scott DW, Erb HN: Frequency of apoptotic keratinocytes in the feline epidermis: a retrospective light-microscopic study of skin-biopsy specimens from 327 cats with normal skin or inflammatory dermatoses, *J Feline Med Surg* 11:963, 2009.
103. Waisglass SE, Landsberg GM, Yager JA et al: Underlying medical conditions in cats with presumptive psychogenic alopecia, *J Am Vet Med Assoc* 228:1705, 2006.
104. Wildermuth BE, Griffin CE, Rosenkrantz WS: Feline pyoderma therapy, *Clin Tech Small Anim Pract* 21:150, 2006.
105. Wildermuth BE, Griffin CE, Rosenkrant, WS: Response of feline eosinophilic cutaneous plaques and eosinophilic lip ulcers to amoxicillin-clavulanate therapy, *Vet Dermatol* 20:223, 2009.
106. Wisselink MA, Willemse T: The efficacy of cyclosporine A in cats with presumed atopic dermatitis: a double blind, randomised prednisolone-controlled study, *Vet J* 180:55, 2009.
107. Yang SH, Liu CH, Hsu CD et al: Use of chemical ablation with trichloroacetic acid to treat eyelid apocrine hidrocystomas in a cat, *J Am Vet Med Assoc* 230:1170, 2007.
108. Young KM, Moriello, KA: Eosinophils and eosinophilic diseases. In August J, editor: *Consultations in feline internal medicine*, ed 5, St Louis, 2006, Elsevier Saunders, p 238.

HUMAN ALLERGIES TO CATS

Daniel O. Morris

GENERAL INFORMATION

The prevalence of human allergy to pet dander has risen rapidly over the past several decades as a consequence of lifestyle changes that have enhanced the exposure of people to pet-source allergens. During this time the popularity of cats as companion animals has increased substantially in industrialized nations, and changes in indoor climate control systems, furnishings, and hygiene practices have magnified the retention of allergens in public and private buildings. The net effect has been a rise in ambient exposure to cat dander in both the domestic and public environs.[49,52,68] Human allergy to pet dander is a problem of global public health importance, insofar as the morbidity associated with allergic diseases disproportionately affects socioeconomically disadvantaged populations, particularly children.[16,70] It is also an occupational hazard for some workers, such as animal health care professionals. Although the public often seeks advice from veterinary professionals regarding healthy pet ownership practices, including strategies for reducing pet dander exposure in the home, many misconceptions persist in the public domain regarding pet dander allergy. Perhaps the most prevalent is the belief that certain dog and cat breeds are "hypoallergenic" as a result of their hair coat type.

The human diseases most commonly associated with sensitization to environmental allergens include allergic asthma, atopic dermatitis, urticaria, and allergic rhinitis–conjunctivitis ("hay fever"). Collectively referred to as *atopic reactions,* these diseases result from immediate or type 1 hypersensitivity responses and are characterized by production of elevated levels of allergen-specific immunoglobulin E (IgE) that can be detected by either serologic or skin-prick testing.[79] Although atopic reactions likely evolved as protective mechanisms against parasites, they are purely pathogenic when directed against otherwise harmless allergens such as ubiquitous pollens and dander. A genetic predisposition is obvious from familial studies, although the atopic state is a complex trait that is likely influenced by multiple genes.[42,54] Still, the rapid increase in the incidence of allergic diseases in human populations cannot be explained by genetic models alone; shifts in exposure or immunoreactivity must also be in play. Assuming exposure to be equal, failure to develop clinical allergy must result from either a lack of immune response to allergens (anergy) or a response that induces immunologic tolerance.[61] Tolerance is the ability of an active immune response to prevent or redirect sensitization to an allergen and is thought to occur most commonly through natural or induced production of IgG4-blocking antibodies.[61] Induction of blocking antibodies by immunization with allergen vaccines (also known as allergen-specific immunotherapy or "allergy shots") may be an important medical treatment strategy for individuals with pet dander allergies.[25] Similarly, natural exposure to high levels of environmental allergen (e.g., cat dander) may promote specific tolerance in some individuals (discussed later).

The term *dander* refers to particles that are sloughed from animal skin. Although composed primarily of skin flakes, its physical properties cannot be standardized and defined accurately; hence the term is used in a generic sense. Dander serves as a vehicle for animal allergens, which are typically low-molecular-weight proteins or glycoproteins that arise from ubiquitous plant or animal sources. Allergens are designated by a systematic nomenclature maintained by a subcommittee of the World Health Organization/International Union of Immunological Societies. The designation is derived from the first three letters of the source organism's genus name, the first letter of the species name, and an Arabic numeral that indicates the chronology of the allergen's discovery.[14] For example, the first allergen purified from domestic cat *(Felis domesticus)* dander is Fel d 1. Allergens such as Fel d 1 can be carried on a diverse array of particles,[24] many of which are of an aerodynamic size (less than 3 μm in diameter) such that attached allergens remain airborne for long periods after disturbance (i.e., continuously in occupied homes).[11]

Most organisms produce more than one type of allergen that can be recognized by an allergic person's immune system, and when more than 50% of the allergic population is reactive to a particular allergen, it is referred to as a *major allergen; minor allergens* are recognized by less than 50% of the allergic population.[66] Fel d 1 is a globulin secreted by the feline salivary,[6,29] sebaceous,[6,15,29] and perianal glands,[22] with the skin and hair serving as reservoirs.[15,22] Its physiologic function remains unknown. It is recognized by specific IgE produced by 85% to 95% of cat-sensitized people,[49] and its production may be influenced by testosterone, as the sebaceous gland output of male cats is reduced after castration.[81] In fact, a study of Fel d 1 levels in reservoir house dust showed reproductive status to be the only cat-dependent variable associated with allergen levels in homes. However, this was the opposite of what would be expected: The homes of sterilized cats harbored significantly *more* allergen than those housing sexually intact animals (effect size greater for males than females).[56] Coat length, age, body mass, and time spent indoors showed no effect in a multivariable regression model.[58] Allergen production did, however, vary with anatomic site, with the face producing dramatically higher levels than the chest.[12] This makes sense considering the greater glandular distribution and secretory activity of the facial skin.

Other minor (yet defined) cat allergens include Fel d 2, a serum albumin protein with extensive cross-antigenicity to other mammalian serum albumins, and Fel d 3, a cysteine protease inhibitor produced in the skin (exact structure of origin unknown).[37] These allergens are recognized by specific IgE of about 20% and 10% of cat-sensitized people, respectively.[49] Finally, a lipocalin salivary protein designated Fel d 4, which was bound by specific IgE in 64% of sera from cat-allergic subjects, was characterized recently.[69] Although the majority of these sera samples harbored relatively low titres of anti–Fel d 4 IgE, 47% of them exceeded the corresponding titers of anti–Fel d 1 IgE. The clinical relevance of Fel d 4 allergen therefore merits additional investigation, insofar as it could be the most relevant allergen for some allergic individuals.

The bulk of epidemiologic research on the topic of pet dander allergy has focused on Fel d 1, which is present ubiquitously in the human environment, and because cats are the dominant source of animal-origin allergy of people. Whereas levels of Fel d 1 are much higher in households with current cat residence,[27,33] it can be detected in homes without resident cats.[7,33,34,55] In homes where there has never been a resident cat, there is a direct correlation of indoor allergen level with the prevalence of cat ownership in the community at large.[33] The average level of allergen contamination in reservoir dust of U.S. homes, regardless of cat ownership,[7] should be sufficient to both sensitize and elicit symptoms in genetically predisposed individuals based on current estimates of dose–response relationships.[60,72]

Fel d 1 is also detectible in many public places at levels capable of sensitizing susceptible individuals. This is especially relevant and problematic for children in schools and day care centers[1,4,38,65,78] but also occurs in the workplace,[51] automobiles,[55] airplanes,[51] cinemas,[51] and even human hospitals.[18] Secondary exposure (e.g., to a room where a cat has been previously) can be high enough not only to sensitize individuals but also to provoke acute allergic inflammation.[80] The evidence for sensitization and exacerbation of cat dander allergy in school children is compelling. Epidemiologic studies have demonstrated that sensitization of children without regular cat contact may increase in a dose–response fashion according to the degree of contact experienced by their classmates.[4,65] Elicitation of symptoms is also possible: non–cat-owning asthmatic children in classrooms with high cat ownership experienced a doubling of asthmatic symptoms and medication use in the 2 weeks after their return to school from holiday break. Those in classrooms with low cat ownership showed no such increases.[4] Because of the risk to asthmatic children, reduced-allergen school environments have been studied.[25,40,78] Measures such as banning pet ownership[40,78] or providing school-issued clothing for students during the school day[40] were successful in reducing ambient Fel d 1 concentrations, although the effects on allergic symptoms were not assessed.

In schools and day care centers, mattresses have been shown to be a source of higher in-school allergen levels than settled dust.[8,38] Mattresses are a known reservoir for dust mite and pet allergens, and the quantity of Fel d 1 increases with the advancing age of the mattress.[26] Even newly purchased mattresses can contain detectible and relevant cat and dog allergen levels, although those wrapped in plastic when purchased are of less concern.[21,23] A study in which customers in Swedish stores were allowed to try out floor model mattresses showed highly statistically significant increases in the deposition of dog, cat, and horse allergens. For cat and horse allergens, the concentrations detected strongly correlated with the duration of in-store display.[23] In non–cat-owning homes, a combination of the presence of stuffed animals on the bed, lack of mattress and pillow encasements, and infrequent sheet washing were associated with significantly increased Fel d 1 levels in children's bedrooms.[58] The net experience suggests that use of allergen-impermeable encasements for mattresses and pillows may be useful components of allergen avoidance strategies, although the efficiency of Fel d 1 exclusion by such materials varies widely,[57] and controlled trials have not been reported. Also of interest is the finding that pillows stuffed with synthetic fibers trap significantly more pet allergens than feather pillows, an effect likely to be due to the tighter weave used in pillow covers to prevent extrusion of feathers.[19]

Sources of secondary exposure extend beyond the indoor environment. The clothing of classmates, playmates, and coworkers is commonly implicated.[20,55] In fact, clothing is often the point source for indoor contamination, insofar as levels of Fel d 1 in the homes of people who do not own cats have correlated with the level of exposure experienced by their children in school, with the vehicle being clothing.[3] Even human hair has been shown to serve as a vehicle for Fel d 1 dispersal.[41,50] In societies where keeping of indoor pets is rare, the prevalence of sensitization to cat allergens is still similar to the rates observed in Western countries, which suggests that feral outdoor cats provide a sufficient degree of dander exposure to induce human allergy.[13,32]

MITIGATION STRATEGIES

Avoidance Through Environmental Interventions

Indoor lifestyle changes that may have contributed to the rise of human allergic diseases over the past several decades include the increasing prevalence of wall-to-wall fixed carpeting that cannot be removed for laundering[24,46,60] and improved efficiency of indoor climate control systems. The latter reduces air exchange with the outdoor environment (reducing dilution of indoor allergens), whereas upholstery and carpeting trap indoor allergens and complicate cleaning regimens.[49] Because of the ubiquity of pet allergen dispersal, household and classroom intervention presents a difficult challenge. Randomized trials have shown that environmental reduction of pet dander allergens can be achieved, in some instances with modest clinical benefits.[2,43,67] However, the measures necessary—such as extensive home-cleaning regimens, removal of carpeting and upholstered furniture, and encasement of mattresses and pillows with impermeable membranes—can be quite costly and burdensome to sustain. In addition, socioeconomic status is highly associated with environmental factors (e.g., housing characteristics, number of residents, pet ownership, and general home hygiene) that strongly influence allergic sensitization,[10,16,70] and it is apparent that the populations bearing the greatest burden of disease are often those with least access to health care and other resources.

Vacuuming can actually exacerbate dispersal of pet allergens from carpet reservoirs, and allergen leakage from the machine and the vacuum bag is of major concern.[60] However, in the past decade improvements such as two- and three-layer microfiltration vacuum bags and high-efficiency particulate arresting (HEPA) filters in both vacuum machines and room air cleaners (which claim to capture 99.9% of particles 0.3 μm diameter or larger) have increased allergen uptake and reduced leakage.[30,31,62,77] The use of such units has been correlated with decreased allergen in reservoir dust and improvements in asthmatic patients,[62] although an evaluation of cat allergen levels after HEPA-filtrated vacuuming showed an actual increase in inhaled Fel d 1 when measured by nasal air sampling.[30,31]The authors attribute this to disturbance of allergen adhered to walls and other surfaces by all vacuum models caused by beater bar action, the back-and-forth motion of the cleaning head, and air exhaust flow from the machine. With regard to HEPA-filtered air cleaners, results have also been mixed, with some suggesting excellent utility in reducing airborne pet allergen levels,[28,30,31,74] but not in reservoir dust, and not to a degree where they are likely to be effective alone.[71,74-76] The effect of furniture dusting has also been evaluated in simulation studies; as might be expected, dry dusting of wood surfaces releases allergen, whereas application of a spray polish to the dusting cloth or wood surface significantly reduces aerosolization of Fel d 1.[39,40,44]

In addition to housekeeping regimens, laundering of clothing plays an important role in allergen reduction. Washing cotton fabrics in water is a simple and highly effective method for Fel d 1 removal,[47] and use of detergents is a superior method for removing Fel d 1 compared with use of soap or water alone.[73] It has also been demonstrated that removal of dog allergen from cotton sheets by mechanical washing machines can be highly effective at all temperatures. However, removal is significantly better at high temperature (60° C or 140° F) and when two rinse cycles are used.[17] Dry cleaning of woolens significantly reduces Fel d 1 concentrations but does not abolish it entirely, and allergen-free items can actually become contaminated during the dry cleaning process.[48]

Pet-Directed Interventions

It might seem that the most effective pet-directed intervention would be to remove the pet from the household. This recommendation has been part of several interventional studies, and not surprisingly, compliance has been low. Some physicians and public health professionals will also suggest banishing pets to the outdoors, a recommendation that, especially for cats, is unacceptable to most veterinarians and pet owners. In addition, time spent indoors does not correlate with Fel d 1 levels in reservoir house dust.[58] Also, it is known that some degree of cross-reactivity occurs between canine and feline dander allergens, and there is a high prevalence of human co-sensitization to dogs and cats.[45,53,63,64] Finally, although removal of a pet is likely to reduce the overall allergen burden in a home, levels still may not fall below the sensitization or elicitation thresholds.

In light of these facts, studies have been performed to assess the utility of pet bathing in reducing allergen burden. For both dogs and cats, bathing removes significant amounts of allergen from the pet, but it must be performed at least twice weekly to maintain a relevant reduction.[9,36] For dogs this regimen achieves only a modest reduction of Can f 1 in room air.[36] Commercial products Allerpet/C (for cats) and Allerpet/D (for dogs) (Allerpet, New York), available as shampoos and as moistened wipes for cats, claim to substantially reduce the quantity of pet-related allergens in the home. However, an evaluation study showed that Allerpet/C solution removed significantly less allergen than submersion in water and no more allergen than application of damp towels.[59]

Perhaps the most prevalent, but essentially irrelevant, question presented to veterinary health care professionals in relation to human allergies of pet origin is, which breed or hair coat type will be "hypoallergenic"? The widely held assumption that breeds that shed less produce less allergen has been disproved for dogs, and coat length of cats was not correlated with reservoir dust levels in homes.[56]

Recently, Allerca Lifestyle Pets (San Diego, California) has produced and marketed so-called hypoallergenic cats. These have been developed not through genetic engineering but rather by natural breeding of individuals deficient in Fel d 1 as a result of putative gene mutations. Although no refereed scientific reports have surfaced to date, the company offers many testimonials from satisfied clients and claims that blinded clinical trials conducted by a reputable allergist have proven efficacy (http://www.allerca.com; accessed December 31, 2009). Clearly, this is not a public health solution (especially at a price ranging from $6950 to $27,000 for a cat), but from a personal health perspective, it could be a welcome solution for individuals who are symptomatic only with direct pet exposure. However, as discussed previously, Fel d 1 is not the only dander allergen recognized by all cat-allergic people, so it is conceivable that these purpose-bred pets will not provide complete benefit for affected people.

The human–animal bond is an undeniable facet of human health, both psychiatric and physical,[35] and it is clear that pets are in our hearts and homes to stay. Despite significant advances in understanding of the epidemiology and immunology of pet dander allergies over the past two decades, little progress has occurred in mitigating this problem on a population-wide basis. Fortunately, medical therapies for use on an individual basis have improved significantly over this same time frame,[5] although access to health care remains a major roadblock in many human populations. Considering the sheer magnitude of morbidity that allergic diseases create—especially pediatric asthma—the primary focus for public health professionals, now and in the foreseeable future, should be the elimination of disparities in health care access. As a significant amount of misinformation persists among the general public and human health care providers, the primary role of veterinarians will, for the foreseeable future, continue to be education regarding healthy pet ownership practices.

References

1. Abramson SL, Turner-Henson A, Anderson L et al: Allergens in school settings: results of environmental assessments in 3 city school systems, *J School Health* 76:246, 2006.
2. Adgate JL, Ramachandran G, Cho SJ et al: Allergen levels in inner city homes: baseline concentrations and evaluation of intervention effectiveness, *J Exp Sci Env Epidemiol* 18:430, 2008.
3. Almqvist C, Larsson PH, Egmar AC et al: School as a risk environment for children allergic to cats and a site for transfer of cat allergen to homes, *J Allergy Clin Immunol* 103:1012, 1999.
4. Almqvist C, Wickman M, Perfetti L et al: Worsening of asthma in children allergic to cats, after indirect exposure to cat at school, *Am J Resp Crit Care Med* 163:694, 2001.
5. Alvarez-Cuesta E, Berges-Gimeno P, Mancebo EG et al: Sublingual immunotherapy with a standardized cat dander extract: evaluation of efficacy in a double blind placebo controlled study, *Allergy* 62:810, 2007.
6. Anderson MC, Baer H, Ohman JL: A comparative study of the allergens of cat urine, serum, saliva, and pelt, *J Allergy Clin Immunol* 76:563, 1985.
7. Arbes SJ, Cohn RD, Yin M et al: Dog allergen (Can f 1) and cat allergy (Fel d 1) in US homes: results from the National Survey of Lead and Allergens in Homes, *J Allergy Clinical Immunol* 114:111, 2004.
8. Arbes SM, Sever M, Mehta J et al: Exposure to indoor allergens in day-care facilities: results from 2 North Carolina counties, *J Allergy Clin Immunol* 116:133, 2005.
9. Avner DB, Perzanowski MS, Platts-Mills TAE et al: Evaluation of different techniques for washing cats: quantitation of allergen removal from the cat and the effect on airborne Fel d 1, *J Allergy Clin Immunol* 100:307, 1997.
10. Bjornsdottir JS, Jakobinudottir S, Runarsdottir V et al: The effect of reducing levels of cat allergen (Fel d 1) on clinical symptoms in patients with cat allergy, *Ann Allergy Asthma Immunol* 91:189, 2003.
11. Bousquet J, Demoly P: Allergens in 1998: from molecular biology to improved patient care, *Allergy* 53:549, 1998.
12. Carayol N, Birnbaum J, Magnan A et al: Fel d 1 production in the cat skin varies according to anatomical sites, *Allergy* 55:570, 2000.
13. Chan-Yeung M, McClean PA, Sandell PR et al: Sensitization to cat without direct exposure to cats, *Clin Exp Allergy* 29:762, 1999.
14. Chapman MD, Pomes A, Breiteneder H et al: Nomenclature and structural biology of allergens, *J Allergy Clin Immunol* 119:414, 2007.
15. Charpin C, Mata P, Charpin D et al: Fel d 1 allergen distribution in cat fur and skin, *J Allergy Clin Immunol* 88:77, 1991.
16. Chen CM, Mielck A, Fahlbusch B et al: Social factors, allergen, endotoxin, and dust mass in mattress, *Indoor Air* 17:384, 2007.
17. Choi SY, Lee IY, Sohn JH et al: Optimal conditions for the removal of house dust mite, dog dander, and pollen allergens using mechanical laundry, *Ann Allergy Asthma Immunol* 100:583, 2008.
18. Custovic A, Fletcher A, Pickering CA et al: Domestic allergens in public places. III: House dust mite, cat, dog and cockroach allergens in British hospitals, *Clin Exp Allergy* 28:53, 1998.
19. Custovic A, Hallam C, Woodcock H et al: Synthetic pillows contain higher levels of cat and dog allergen than feather pillows, *Ped Allergy Immunol* 11:71, 2000.
20. D'Amato G, Liccardi G, Russo M et al: Clothing is a carrier of cat allergens, *J Allergy Clin Immunology* 99:577, 1997.
21. de Boer R: Allergens, Der p 1, Der f 1, Fel d 1, and Can f 1 in newly bought mattresses for infants, *Clin Exp Allergy* 32:1602, 2002.
22. Dornelas De Andrade A, Birnbaum J, Magalon C et al: Fel d 1 levels in cat anal glands, *Clin Exp Allergy* 26:178, 1996.
23. Egmar AC, Almqvist C, Emenius G et al: Deposition of cat (Fel d 1), dog (Can f 1), and horse allergen over time in public environments—a model of dispersion, *Allergy* 53:957, 1998.
24. Erwin EA, Woodfolk JA, Custis N et al: Animal dander, *Immunol Allergy Clin North Amer* 23:469, 2003.
25. Ewbank PA, Murray J, Sanders K et al: A double-blind, placebo controlled immunotherapy dose-response study with standardized cat extract, *J Allergy Clin Immunol* 111:155, 2003.
26. Fahlbusch B, Gehring U, Richter K et al: Predictors of cat allergen (Fel d 1) in house dust of German homes with/without cats, *J Invest Allergol Clin Immunol* 12:12, 2002.
27. Giovanangelo M, Nordling E, Gehring U et al: Variation of biocontaminant levels within and between houses—the AIRALLERG study, *J Exp Sci Environ Epidemiol* 17:134, 2007.
28. Green R, Simpson A, Custovic A et al: The effect of air filtration on airborne dog allergen, *Allergy* 54:484, 1999.
29. Griffith IJ, Craig S, Pollock J et al: Expression and genomic structure of the genes encoding Fd1, the major allergen from the domestic cat, *Gene* 113:263, 1992.
30. Gore RB, Bishop S, Durrell B et al: Air filtration units in homes with cats: can they reduce personal exposure to cat allergen? *Clin Exp Allergy* 33:765, 2003.
31. Gore RB, Durrell B, Bishop S et al: High-efficiency particulate arrest-filter vacuum cleaners increase personal cat allergen exposure in homes with cats, *J Allergy Clin Immunol* 111:784, 2003.
32. Gulbahar O, Sin A, Mete N et al: Sensitization to cat allergens in non-cat owner patients with respiratory allergy, *Ann Allergy Asthma Immunol* 90:635, 2003.
33. Heinrich J, Bedada GB, Zock JP et al: Cat allergen level: its determinants and relationship to specific IgE to cat across European centers, *J Allergy Clin Immunol* 18:674, 2006.
34. Heissenhuber A, Heinrich J, Fahlbusch B et al: Health impacts of second-hand exposure to cat allergen Fel d 1 in infants, *Allergy* 58:154, 2003.
35. Hines L, Fredrickson M: Perspectives on animal-assisted activities and therapy. In Wilson CC, Turner DC, editors: *Companion animals in human health*, Thousand Oaks, Calif, 1998, Sage Publications, p 23.
36. Hodson T, Custovic A, Simpson A et al: Washing the dog reduces dog allergen levels but the dog needs to be washed twice a week, *J Allergy Clin Immunol* 103:581, 1999.
37. Ichikawa K, Vailes LD, Pomes A et al: Molecular cloning, expression and modelling of cat allergen, cystatin (Fel d 3), a cysteine protease inhibitor, *Clin Exp Allergy* 31:1279, 2001.
38. Instanes C, Hetland G, Berntsen S et al: Allergens and endotoxin in settled dust from day-care centers and schools in Oslo, Norway, *Indoor Air* 15:356, 2005.
39. Jerrim KL, Whitmore LF, Hughes JF et al: Airborne dust and allergen generation during dusting with and without spray polish, *J Allergy Clin Immunol* 109:63, 2002.

40. Karlsson AS, Andersson B, Renstrom A et al: Airborne cat allergen reduction in classrooms that use special school clothing or ban pet ownership, *J Allergy Clin Immunol* 113:1172, 2004.
41. Karlsson AS, Renstrom A: Human hair is a potential source of cat allergen contamination of ambient air, *Allergy* 60:961, 2005.
42. Kere J, Laitinen T: Positionally cloned susceptibility genes in allergy and asthma, *Current Opin Immunol* 16:689, 2004.
43. Kitch BT, Chew G, Burge HA et al: Socioeconomic predictors of high allergen levels in homes in the greater Boston area, *Env Health Perspect* 108:301, 2000.
44. Ko G, Burge HA: Effects of furniture polish on release of cat allergen-laden dust from wood surfaces, *Indoor Air* 14:434, 2004.
45. Konieczny A, Morgenstern JP, Bizinkauskas CB et al: The major dog allergens, *Can f* 1 and *Can f* 2, are salivary lipocalin proteins: cloning and immunological characterization of the recombinant forms, *Immunol* 92:577, 1997.
46. Lewis RD, Breysse PN: Carpet properties that affect the retention of cat allergen, *Ann Allergy Asthma Immunol* 84:31, 2000.
47. Liccardi G, Russo M, Barber D et al: Washing the clothes of cat owners is a simple method to prevent can allergen dispersal, *J Allergy Clin Immunol* 102:143, 1998.
48. Liccardi G, Russo M, Barber D et al: Efficacy of dry-cleaning in removing Fel d 1 allergen from wool fabric exposed to cats, *Ann Allergy Asthma Immunol* 88:301, 2002.
49. Liccardi G, D'Amato G, Russo M et al: Focus on cat allergen (Fel d 1): Immunological and aerodynamic characteristics, modality of airway sensitization and avoidance strategies, *Int Archives Allergy Immunol* 132:1, 2003.
50. Liccardi G, Barber D, Russo M et al: Human hair: an unexpected source of cat allergen, *Int Archives Allergy Immunol* 137:141, 2005.
51. Martin IR, Wickens K, Patchett K et al: Cat allergen in public places in New Zealand, *New Zealand Med J* 111:356, 1998.
52. Matricardi PM: Prevalence of atopy and asthma in eastern versus western Europe: why the difference? *Ann Allergy Asthma Immunol* 87(suppl):24, 2001.
53. Mattson L, Lundgren T, Everberg H et al: Prostatic kallikrein: a new major dog allergen, *J Allergy Clin Immunol* 123:362, 2009.
54. Morar N, Willis-Owen SAG, Moffatt MR et al: The genetics of atopic dermatitis, *J Allergy Clin Immunol* 118:24, 2006.
55. Neal JS, Arlian LG, Morgan MS: Relationship among house-dust mites, Der 1, Fel d 1, and Can f 1 on clothing and automobile seats with respect to densities in houses, *Ann Allergy Asthma Immunol* 88:410, 2002.
56. Nicholas C, Wegienka G, Havstad S et al: Influence of cat characteristics on Fel d 1 levels in homes, *Ann Allergy Asthma Immunol* 101:47, 2008.
57. Peroni DG, Ress M, Pigozzi R et al: Efficacy in allergen control and air permeability of different materials used for bed encasement, *Allergy* 59:969, 2004.
58. Perry TT, Wood RA, Matsui EC et al: Room-specific characteristics of suburban homes as predictors of indoor allergen concentrations, *Ann Allergy Asthma Immunol* 97:628, 2006.
59. Perzanowski MS, Wheatley LM, Avner DB et al: The effectiveness of Allerpet/C in reducing the cat allergen Fel d 1, *J Allergy Clin Immunol* 100:428, 1997.
60. Platts-Mills TAE, Vaughan JW, Carter MC et al: The role of intervention in established allergy: avoidance of indoor allergens in the treatment of chronic allergic disease, *J Allergy Clin Immunol* 106:787, 2000.
61. Platts-Mills TA, Woodfolk JA, Erwin EA et al: Mechanisms of tolerance to inhalant allergens: the relevance of modified Th2 response to allergens from domestic animals, *Springer Semin Immunopathol* 25:271, 2004.
62. Popplewell EJ, Innes VA, Lloyd-Hughes S et al: The effect of high-efficiency and standard vacuum cleaners on mite, cat and dog allergen levels and clinical progress, *Ped Allergy Immunol* 11:142, 2000.
63. Ramadour M, Guetat M, Guetat J et al: Dog factor differences in Can f 1 allergen production, *Allergy* 60:1060, 2005.
64. Reininger R, Varga EM, Zach M et al: Detection of an allergen in dog dander that cross-reacts with the major cat allergen, Fel d 1, *Clin Exp Allergy* 37:116, 2007.
65. Ritz BR, Hoelscher B, Frye C et al: Allergic sensitization owing to "second-hand" cat exposure in schools, *Allergy* 57:357, 2002.
66. Schaub B, Lauener R, von Mutius E: The many faces of the hygiene hypothesis, *J Allergy Clin Immunol* 117:969, 2006.
67. Simpson A, Simpson B, Custovic A et al: Stringent environmental control in pregnancy and early life: the long-term effects on mite, cat and dog allergen, *Clin Exp Allergy* 33:1183, 2003.
68. Sly RM: Changing prevalence of allergic rhinitis and asthma, *Ann Allergy Asthma Immunol* 82:233, 1999.
69. Smith W, Butler AJL, Hazell LA et al: Fel d 4, a cat lipocalin allergen, *Clin Exp Allergy* 34:1732, 2004.
70. Stevenson LA, Gergen PJ, Hoover DR et al: Sociodemographic correlates of indoor allergen sensitivity among United States children, *J Allergy Clin Immunol* 108:747, 2001.
71. Sulser C, Schulz G, Wagner P et al: Can the use of HEPA cleaners in homes of asthmatic children and adolescents sensitized to cat and dog allergens decrease bronchial hyperresponsiveness and allergen contents in solid dust? *Int Archives Allergy Immunol* 148:23, 2009.
72. Torrent M, Sunyer J, Garcia R et al: Early-life exposure and atopy, asthma, and wheeze up to 6 years of age, *Am J Resp Crit Care Med* 176:446, 2007.
73. Tovey ER, Taylor DJ, Mitakakis TZ et al: Effectiveness of laundry washing agents and conditions in the removal of cat and dust mite allergen from bedding dust, *J Allergy Clin Immunol* 108:369, 2001.
74. van der Heide S, Kauffman JF, Dubois AE et al: Allergen reduction measures in houses of allergic asthma patients: Effects of air-cleaners and allergen-impermeable mattress covers, *Eur Resp J* 10:1217, 1997.
75. van der Heide S, Kauffman JF, Dubois AE et al: Allergen reduction measures in houses of allergic asthma patients: Effects of air-cleaners and allergen-impermeable mattress covers, *Eur Resp J* 10:1217, 1997.
76. van der Heide S, van Aalderen WM, Kauffman HF et al: Clinical effects of air cleaners in homes of asthmatic children sensitized to pet allergens, *J Allergy Clin Immunol* 104:447, 1999.
77. Vaughan JW, Woodfolk JA, Platts-Mills TA: Assessment of vacuum cleaners and vacuum cleaner bags recommended for allergic subjects, *J Allergy Clin Immunol* 104:1079, 1999.
78. Wickman M, Egmar A, Emenius G et al: Fel d 1 and Can f 1 in settled dust and airborne Fel d 1 in allergen avoidance day-care centres for atopic children in relation to number of pet-owners, ventilation, and general cleaning, *Clin Exp Allergy* 29:626, 1999.
79. Woodfolk JA: T-cell responses to allergens, *J Allergy Clin Immunol* 119:280, 2007.
80. Zeidler MR, Goldin JG, Kleerup EC et al: Small airways response to naturalistic cat allergen exposure in subjects with asthma, *J Allergy Clinical Immunol* 118:1075, 2006.
81. Zielonka TM, Charpin D, Berbis P et al: Effects of castration and testosterone on Fel d 1 production by sebaceous glands of male cats: I. Immunological assessment, *Clin Exp Allergy* 24:1169, 1994.

CHAPTER

23

Digestive System, Liver, and Abdominal Cavity

OUTLINE

APPROACH TO THE VOMITING CAT

Randolph M. Baral

Vomiting can be defined as the ejection of part or all of the contents of the stomach and/or upper intestine through the mouth, usually in a series of involuntary spasmodic movements. The disturbances in gastrointestinal (GI) motility are coordinated with respiratory and abdominal muscle contractions and mediated by the central nervous system (CNS).

Vomiting begins with retching, a series of brief negative intrathoracic pressure pulses that coincide with positive abdominal contractions. These pressure changes occur as a result of repeated herniations of the abdominal esophagus and cardiac portion of the stomach into the esophagus. During retching, food freely moves back and forth in the esophagus, which is now dilated because of the ingesta. Ultimately, the diaphragm rapidly moves cranially, resulting in positive intrathoracic pressure that leads to expulsion of these contents.[12] Vomiting is such an active process that it seems to involve the whole cat, and so it is little wonder that it concerns owners so much.

Since vomiting is mediated by the CNS with input and influence from just about anywhere in the body, it is important to summarize this physiology so it can be appreciated when managing clinical cases. Vomiting results from stimulation of the "vomiting center," which is located in the brainstem; there are four main pathways that stimulate the vomiting center,[12] and these are summarized below and in Figure 23-1.

1. Peripheral sensory receptors
   a. Intraabdominal
      i. From stomach, intestines, pancreas, liver, peritoneum, kidneys, bladder
      ii. Via visceral afferent fibers in sympathetic and vagal nerves
   b. Heart and large vessels
      i. Via vagus nerve
   c. Pharynx
      i. Via glossopharyngeal nerve
2. Bloodborne substances can stimulate the chemoreceptor trigger zone (CTZ). The CTZ lacks a blood-brain barrier so that substances diffuse to it freely.
   a. Uremia
   b. Electrolyte imbalances
   c. Bacterial toxins
   d. Drugs (e.g., antibiotics, nonsteroidal antiinflammatories, chemotherapeutics)
3. Vestibular input
   a. Inflammatory processes
   b. Motion sickness
      i. Via acoustic nerve
4. Higher CNS centers
   a. Psychogenic
      i. Fear, stress, excitement by catecholamine release
   b. Inflammatory CNS lesions

These complex pathways highlight the need to consider the *whole* cat and not just the cat's gastrointestinal

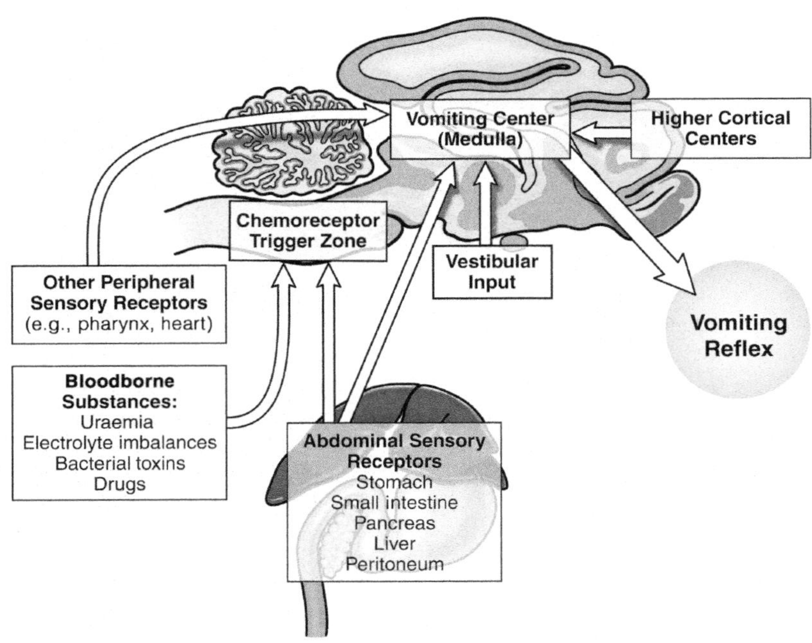

FIGURE 23-1 Summary of the main pathways that stimulate the vomiting center.

tract when assessing a cat presenting for vomiting. The approach to managing a cat with vomiting must follow logical steps. When the underlying cause is gastrointestinal disease, a precise diagnosis can only be reached after obtaining biopsy samples. A summary of diagnostic steps and possible underlying causes is shown in Figure 23-2.

The diagnostic steps are

1. Signalment and clinical history
2. Physical examination

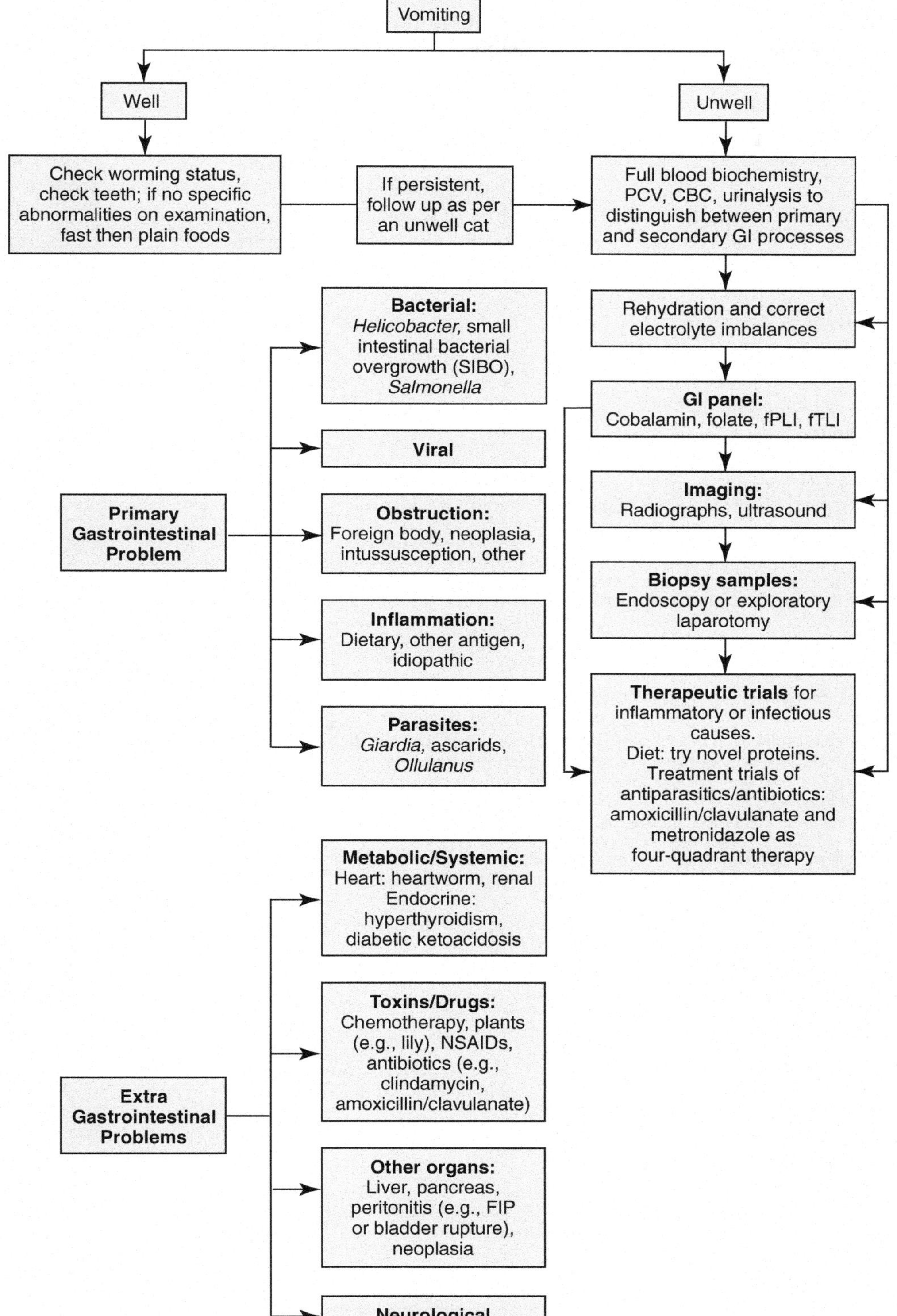

FIGURE 23-2 Summary of diagnostic steps and possible underlying causes of vomiting.

3. Blood and urine testing
4. Imaging (radiography, ultrasonography)
5. Biopsy samples
6. Treat and manage underlying problem

The decision to proceed to steps 4 and 5 is based on the assumption that the prior steps have narrowed down the underlying cause as gastrointestinal, pancreatic, or hepatic in origin.

STEP 1: SIGNALMENT AND CLINICAL HISTORY

The important aspects of the clinical history are given in Table 23-1. Signalment is important, because younger cats are more likely to have ingested foreign bodies (though not all older cats have grown out of this habit). Some extragastrointestinal problems, such as hyperthyroidism and renal disease are more likely to occur in older cats.

Most texts and references instruct clinicians to distinguish between vomiting and regurgitation, with the latter noted as being quite passive.[3,11,12] In practice, it can be hard to make this distinction, because it is the author's experience that cats with esophageal disease can have quite forceful, spasmodic movements when ejecting ingesta by regurgitation—although it is also possible for regurgitation to be a passive process. Given that the physiology of vomiting, as described above, results in ingesta being forced to and then evacuated from the esophagus, it is hardly surprising that it can resemble regurgitation. Fortunately, regurgitation and esophageal disease do vary from vomiting in other ways! Vomiting

TABLE 23-1 **Clinical History for Vomiting Cats**

Question	Interpretation
Signalment	Younger cats more likely to ingest foreign bodies, hunt prey; older cats more likely to have systemic or chronic diseases
Diet	Regular diet, any dietary change; potential of food intolerance, food hypersensitivity, food sensitivity
Environment	Presence of various plants and foreign bodies, seen with prey, access to toxins; health status of other cats in the household
Duration and frequency	Regular vomiter? Acute versus chronic, and severity
Relationship to eating	Immediately after eating, some gluttonous cats will engorge themselves with a meal and vomit immediately thereafter If greater than 8 hours after eating, implies gastric outlet obstruction or a gastric motility disorder No relationship to eating implies a systemic or metabolic disease
Describe vomiting process	Vomiting (licking lips, salivation, multiple swallowing) versus regurgitation (can be passive but not always); nature of ingesta also helps distinguish
Appearance of vomitus	Blood–gastric mucosal damage, state of digestion, neoplasia, or ulcer Bile: reflux from small intestine, rules out complete pyloric obstruction Parasitism: adults in vomitus (*Ollulanus tricuspis, Physaloptera* spp.) Food: state of digestion Hair: hairballs, motility disorder Fecal odor: GI obstruction or bacterial overgrowth
Deworming history	Rules in/out GI parasites
Previous illnesses	Organ system affected, recurrence
Current medications	Drug reaction or toxicity
Behavioral changes	Ptyalism or repeated licking lips/swallowing implies nausea Anorexia implies increased severity Hyperactivity suggests hyperthyroidism Star-gazing, unresponsiveness suggests hepatic encephalopathy Polydipsia/polyuria suggests inability to concentrate urine
Co-existing systemic signs	Diarrhea and weight loss are consistent with GI disease (but can also suggest hyperthyroidism) Polydipsia, polyuria, or coughing suggest polysystemic disorders

Adapted from Hall JE: Clinical approach to chronic vomiting. In August JR, editor: *Consultations in feline internal medicine,* ed 3, Philadelphia, 1997, Saunders, p 63.

is usually preceded by the cat licking its lips, salivating, or making attempts to swallow. Regurgitated ingesta is often in a tubelike structure and if undigested can be covered with frothy saliva. Partially digested food suggests vomitus, and the presence of bile or digested blood confirms this.

It is important to determine if the cat vomits regularly. Many owners have seen their cats vomit on a regular basis with no evidence of the cat being unwell, and this is noted frequently in the veterinary literature.[3,12] Hairballs can cause gastric irritation, and it may be that eating quickly also stimulates the peripheral sensory receptors that contribute to vomiting. If a cat *does* vomit regularly, it is important to assess if the cat is presenting for a change in the vomiting pattern (e.g., frequency or timing in relation to eating) and if the cat is unwell in any way, such as anorexia or weight loss.

The pattern of vomiting is important in all cases, because cats presenting with acute gastritis usually have a sudden onset of frequent vomiting compared with those with chronic disease processes that may vomit every few days. The timing in relation to eating can be helpful, because the stomach should empty by 6 to 8 hours after a meal; so, vomiting longer than 8 hours after a meal can suggest motility or retention disorders. The description of the vomitus can be helpful. If bile is present, the pylorus is not obstructed; the presence of blood (digested or fresh) indicates ulceration. Hair in the vomitus can indicate hairball gastritis, and the possibility of trichobezoar obstruction should be considered.

Access to foreign bodies or toxins is an important aspect of the clinical history. Has the cat been seen playing with an insect, mouse, or other prey? Are there any medications unaccounted for (e.g., a dropped aspirin tablet)? Are lilies present in the house?

STEP 2: PHYSICAL EXAMINATION

Vomiting is the major sign of gastric disease, but given the number of potential organ systems that can be involved, a thorough physical examination should be undertaken. Because linear foreign bodies are a common cause of vomiting, *all cats presenting for anorexia or vomiting should have the underside of the tongue evaluated for the presence of string caught there.* Applying gentle pressure with a thumb in the intermandibular space to elevate the tongue is an effective way to visualize lesions or foreign bodies in the sublingual area (see Figure 3-8).

A thorough examination may reveal specific signs, such as a palpable thyroid nodule and tachycardia in the case of hyperthyroidism or palpably small kidneys with chronic kidney disease. The author has found that some cats with dental disease can gorge their food, resulting in vomiting; so, paying attention to the state of the teeth and gums is important. Of course, some cats have multiple problems, and correction of dental disease may not resolve vomiting if there is another process. In the examination, it is also important to note consequences of both the underlying process and the vomiting itself; these include the demeanor of the cat, hydration status, and abdominal pain.

The physical examination findings, together with the clinical history, help determine the next appropriate steps. Well cats that are not continually vomiting and are appropriately hydrated, with no other specific signs, may be treated as outpatients by fasting them for 24 hours, then returning to food with a bland diet, such as plain cooked chicken or commercial, low-residue prescription diets designed for this purpose. Follow-up is important to ensure signs do not progress. Cats with nonspecific signs may require supportive care with subcutaneous or intravenous fluids and perhaps analgesia (with opioids). If clinical signs do not resolve, the pursuit of a specific diagnosis should be attempted. The practitioner must ask the following important questions:

- Are ancillary tests appropriate?
- Is supportive care necessary?
- Are any medications required?

STEP 3: BLOOD AND URINE TESTING

Routine Tests

Routine serum/plasma biochemistries, hematology, urinalysis, and total thyroxine (T_4) (for older cats) testing is not only important to distinguish primary from secondary gastrointestinal disease but to look for consequences of vomiting that may need to be addressed, such as hydration status and electrolyte abnormalities. Careful interpretations should be made. Severe azotemia, even with hyperphosphatemia, can occur as a result of primary gastrointestinal disease, and the distinction from renal disease usually requires an assessment of urine specific gravity.

Blood Tests for Gastrointestinal Disease

Cobalamin, folate, feline trypsin-like immunoreactivity (fTLI), and feline pancreatic lipase immunoreactivity (fPLI) tests are useful markers of intestinal and pancreatic disease,[7,8,9,10] but it is important to note that they mostly do not give a precise diagnosis. More detail about the utility of these tests is noted below in the section Approach to the Cat with Diarrhea.

STEP 4: IMAGING: ULTRASONOGRAPHY AND RADIOLOGY

Radiography is most useful for identifying foreign bodies or signs of intestinal obstruction from other causes. The major findings are noted below in the section Intestinal Obstruction. Contrast radiography can aid the diagnosis for both discrete and linear foreign bodies but should be used with caution, because intestinal perforation may be present. Nonionic iodinated agents that are typically used for myelography (such as iopamidol or iohexol) should be used, since barium irritates the peritoneum and oral iodine compounds are hypertonic. Hypertonic compounds may draw fluid into the stomach and intestines after oral administration, with the potential of creating further fluid and electrolyte imbalances in an already compromised patient.[6]

Ultrasonography is a useful diagnostic adjunct and helps to detect and characterize localized thickening of the stomach or intestinal wall, lymphadenopathy, radiolucent foreign bodies, and changes in the size and echogenicity of the pancreas, liver, kidneys, or spleen. Abdominal effusions can be assessed and sampled. Ultrasound-guided fine-needle aspiration can be used to sample masses, bile, or peritoneal fluid. It should be recognized that in most cases of gastrointestinal disease, imaging will not give a definitive diagnosis and biopsy will be required, usually using either endoscopy or laparotomy. Ultrasonography can be a considered as a means to "survey the field," assessing

- The nature of the underlying disease, such as
  - Thickened intestines with or without discrete layers
  - Lymph node involvement
  - Other organ involvement
- The location of disease, for example,
  - Diffuse or focal
  - Proximal duodenum (reachable by endoscope) versus distal ileum

These factors may be used to assess the appropriateness of endoscopy versus laparotomy to obtain diagnostic samples.

STEP 5: INTESTINAL (AND OTHER ORGAN) BIOPSIES

Histologic evaluation of affected tissue is usually needed for diagnosis of most chronic gastrointestinal diseases. Intestinal biopsy samples can be obtained by the use of endoscopy, laparotomy, or laparoscopy, each of which has advantages and disadvantages. Laparotomy allows gross examination of and access to the entire intestinal tract as well as other abdominal organs. Laparotomy is the most invasive alternative, but with careful anesthesia and analgesia, many cats recover uneventfully. One survey assessed that 83% of cats undergoing exploratory laparotomy survived the hospitalization, and although complications occurred in 26% of cats, these were more likely to be associated with the underlying disease process and not surgery or anesthesia.[4]

Laparoscopy is not readily available in all veterinary clinics. This alternative is less invasive and allows exploration of the abdomen but not as thoroughly as with laparotomy. Organs are usually exteriorized for biopsy. There is the possibility of anesthetic complications associated with insufflating the abdomen.

Endoscopy is the least invasive procedure and is the only alternative that allows examination of the intestinal lumen. This option limits the parts of the gastrointestinal tract that can be biopsied; it does not allow examination or sampling of any other part of the gastrointestinal tract and does not enable full-thickness biopsy samples. One study found that, of cats investigated for gastrointestinal disease, 9 of 33 cats (27%) had no pathology recognized proximal to the jejunum (i.e., the effective length of diagnostic endoscopes would have precluded diagnosis), and other organs were affected in 9 of 10 cats with inflammatory bowel diseases and 7 of 8 cats with intestinal small cell lymphoma.[1] Careful case selection for endoscopy from survey ultrasonography can reduce the number of missed diagnoses from endoscopy, but the possibility still remains.

The quality of endoscopically obtained biopsy samples varies greatly with the skill of the endoscopist. It has been stated that "it is exceedingly easy to take inadequate tissue samples with a flexible endoscope."[5] In an assessment of endoscopically obtained biopsy samples, two laboratories were compared, one that received samples from any practitioner and the other that received samples ONLY from practitioners trained to take, mount, and submit endoscopy samples. All slides were reviewed by three pathologists who found that, of samples from the first laboratory, 15% of the slides were considered inadequate for diagnosis, 71% were considered questionable, and only 14% were adequate. By comparison, in the second laboratory (with samples from experienced practitioners) 0% of slides were inadequate, 21% were questionable, and 79% were considered adequate for diagnosis.[13] In the case of distinguishing between lymphocytic intestinal infiltrates (commonly known as inflammatory bowel disease) and lymphocytic neoplasia (small cell lymphoma), endoscopically obtained samples can give an incorrect diagnosis.[2] Many of these problems can be minimized with experienced operators and careful case selection from prior ultrasonography.

References

1. Baral RM: Laparotomy for gastro-intestinal biopsies, Science Week Conference Proceedings (Small Animal Medicine chapter), Gold

Coast, Queensland, Australia, 2006, Australian College of Veterinary Scientists, p 70.
2. Evans SE, Bonczynski JJ, Broussard JD et al: Comparison of endoscopic and full-thickness biopsy specimens for diagnosis of inflammatory bowel disease and alimentary tract lymphoma in cats, *J Am Vet Med Assoc* 229:1447, 2006.
3. Hall J: Clinical Approach to chronic vomiting. In August J, editor: *Consultations in feline internal medicine*, ed 3, Philadelphia, 1997, Saunders, p 61.
4. Lester S, Welsh E, Pratschke K: Complications of exploratory coeliotomy in 70 cats, *J Small Anim Pract* 45:351, 2004.
5. Mansell J, Willard MD: Biopsy of the gastrointestinal tract, *Vet Clin North Am Small Anim Pract* 33:1099, 2003.
6. Shaiken L: Radiographic appearance of linear foreign bodies in cats, *Vet Med* 94:417, 1999.
7. Simpson KW, Fyfe J, Cornetta A et al: Subnormal concentrations of serum cobalamin (vitamin B12) in cats with gastrointestinal disease, *J Vet Intern Med* 15:26, 2001.
8. Steiner JM, Williams DA: Serum feline trypsin-like immunoreactivity in cats with exocrine pancreatic insufficiency, *J Vet Intern Med* 14:627, 2000.
9. Steiner JM, Wilson BG, Williams DA: Development and analytical validation of a radioimmunoassay for the measurement of feline pancreatic lipase immunoreactivity in serum, *Can J Vet Res* 68:309, 2004.
10. Suchodolski JS, Steiner JM: Laboratory assessment of gastrointestinal function, *Clin Tech Small Anim Pract* 18:203, 2003.
11. Tams TR: A diagnostic approach to vomiting in dogs and cats, *Vet Med* 87:785, 1992.
12. Twedt DC: Diseases of the stomach. In Sherding RG, editor: *The cat: clinical diseases and management*, ed 2, New York, 1994, Churchill Livingstone, p 1181.
13. Willard MD, Lovering SL, Cohen ND et al: Quality of tissue specimens obtained endoscopically from the duodenum of dogs and cats, *J Am Vet Med Assoc* 219:474, 2001.

THERAPEUTICS FOR VOMITING AND DIARRHEA

Katrina R. Viviano

Therapeutic strategies used in the treatment of feline gastrointestinal diseases include nonspecific supportive therapies and targeted therapies based on the primary underlying disease process identified. The most effective therapies for treating feline vomiting and diarrhea are those directed at treating the primary underlying disease process. However, symptomatic supportive care is often necessary prior to arriving at a definitive diagnosis at the onset of targeted therapy or during periods of clinical relapse.

NONSPECIFIC SUPPORTIVE THERAPIES FOR VOMITING

Antiemetics and Prokinetics

Antiemetics and prokinetics are used to control or prevent vomiting through specific receptor interactions mediated either centrally or peripherally, making some more effective in cats than others. The five most commonly used antiemetics all control vomiting by different mechanisms and include mirtazapine, metoclopramide, dolasetron/ondansetron, maropitant, and the phenothiazines (Tables 23-2 and 23-3). Metoclopramide functions both as an antiemetic and prokinetic in cats, while cisapride functions solely as a prokinetic.

Mirtazapine

Mirtazapine, a piperazinoazepine, antagonizes the presynaptic alpha$_2$-adrenergic receptor, increasing noradrenergic and serotonergic neurotransmission; the primary mechanism targeted for its use is as an antidepressant in humans. Mirtazapine is also a potent antagonist of the postsynaptic serotonergic receptors (5-HT$_2$ and 5-HT$_3$) and histamine H$_1$ receptors. Because of its antiserotonergic and antihistaminic effects, mirtazapine is used as an entiemetic and appetite stimulant in cats.

Anorexia is a common clinical problem in ill cats, and in some anorexic or partially anorexic cats the use of an appetite stimulant as adjunctive therapy to nutritional support (i.e. feeding tubes) may be of clinical benefit. Prior to the development of mirtazapine, cyproheptadine was used as an appetite stimulant in cats, with variable clinical results.

Recently, the pharmacokinetics and pharmacodynamics of mirtazapine have been reported in cats. In a group of healthy cats, mirtazapine was found to be an effective appetite stimulant, with a shorter half-life than that reported in humans. The recommended oral dose is 1.88 mg/cat every 48 hours.[55a] In humans, age and kidney and liver dysfunction affect mirtazapine metabolism (hepatic CYP 450 enzymes) and clearance (excreted in urine and feces), suggesting that dose adjustment may be necessary.[69a] Side effects reported in cats treated with mirtazapine include behavior changes (vocalization and interaction), tremors, muscle twitching, and hyperactivity.[9a,55a]

Metoclopramide

Metoclopramide is both an antiemetic and prokinetic drug that acts peripherally on the gastrointestinal tract and centrally within the central nervous system (CNS). At low doses metoclopramide inhibits dopaminergic (D$_2$) transmission, and at higher doses it inhibits serotonergic 5-HT$_3$ receptors in the chemoreceptor trigger zone (CRTZ).[15,23] Metoclopramide also acts peripherally as a prokinetic at the level of the gastrointestinal smooth muscle of the stomach and duodenum, triggering gastric emptying and duodenal contractions. Multiple mechanisms mediate metoclopramide's prokinetic activity, including augmentation of acetylcholine release and increased smooth muscle sensitivity to cholinergic neurotransmission, which may in part be because of antagonism of dopamine, but more recently, serotonergic 5HT$_4$ receptor activation has been suggested.[23,56] Metoclopramide has been reported to increase the lower

TABLE 23-2 **Mechanism of Action and Adverse Effects of the Common Antiemetic and Prokinetic Drugs Used to Treat Vomiting in Cats**

Drug	Mechanism of Action	Adverse Effects
Metoclopramide (antiemetic and prokinetic)	D_2 antagonism 5-HT_3 antagonism 5-HT_4 agonist	Extrapyramidal signs
Dolasetron (antiemetic) Ondansetron (antiemetic)	5-HT_3 antagonism	Prolongation QT interval Arrhythmias
Maropitant (antiemetic)	NK-1 antagonist	
Phenothiazines (antiemetic) Prochlorperazine Chlorpromazine	D_2 antagonism H_1, H_2 antagonism Cholinergic antagonism $alpha_1$, $alpha_2$ antagonism	Extrapyramidal signs Sedation Decreases seizure threshold Hypotension
Cisapride (prokinetic)	5-HT_4 agonist	Prolongation QT interval Arrhythmias
Mirtazapine (appetite stimulant and antiemetic)	5-HT_2 , 5-HT_3 antagonism H_1 antagonism	Behavior changes Tremors, muscle twitching Hyperactivity

TABLE 23-3 **Dosage Recommendations, Contraindications, Potential Drug Interactions, and Clinical Indications for Dosage Adjustments for the Common Antiemetic and Prokinetic Drugs Used to Treat Vomiting in Cats**

Drug	Dosage (Cats)	C: Contraindications DI: Drug Interactions DA: Dosage Adjustments
Metoclopramide	0.2-0.4 mg/kg SC, PO q8h 1-2 mg/kg/day CRI	C: GI obstruction DI: Phenothiazines: extrapyramidal signs DA: Azotemia
Dolasetron Ondansetron	0.5-1.0 mg/kg IV, SC, PO q12-24h 0.22-0.5 mg/kg IV, PO q8-12h	DI: Cisapride: prolonged QT interval and arrhythmias
Maropitant	1 mg/kg IV, SC, PO q24h (up to 5 days)	
Phenothiazines prochlorperazine chlorpromazine	0.2-0.4 mg/kg SC q8h	C: Dehydration; hypotension; seizure hx DI: Metoclopramide: extrapyramidal signs
Cisapride	1.5 mg/kg PO q12h	C: GI obstruction DI: Dolasetron: prolonged QT interval and arrhythmias; azole antifungals: inhibition CYP3A isoenzyme
Mirtazapine	1.88 mg/cat PO q48h	DI: Concurrent administration with other MAO inhibitors (i.e., selegiline, amitraz, tramadol, amitriptyline, clomipramine) and/or SSRIs (i.e., fluoxetine) contraindicated DA: Kidney or liver dysfunction

CRI, Constant rate infusion; *hx*, history.

esophageal sphincter tone in humans,[20] although in cats metoclopramide's affect on the lower esophageal sphincter is reported to be weak.[32]

Adverse central nervous system, extrapyramidal signs occur secondary to dopamine (D_2) antagonism, including excitement and behavior changes. Extrapyramidal signs are most often seen at the higher doses needed to block 5-HT_3 receptors. Because of metoclopramide's prokinetic properties, an intestinal obstruction should be ruled out prior to its use.

Dopamine is a less important neurotransmitter in the chemoreceptor trigger zone of cats than $alpha_2$-adrenergic and 5-HT_3-serotonergic receptors, suggesting that D_2-dopaminergic antagonist may be a less effective antiemetic in cats. Clinically metoclopramide commonly controls vomiting in cats, although this clinical response may be secondary to 5-HT_3 antagonism and/or its prokinetic effects.[32,44]

Extrapolated from the short elimination half-life of metoclopramide in dogs (90 minutes), frequent intermittent dosing or delivery by a constant rate infusion (CRI) is necessary. Empirical dosing in cats is 0.2 to 0.4 mg/kg subcutaneously or orally every 8 hours or 1 to 2 mg/kg/day as a CRI. Approximately 25% of metoclopramide is excreted in the urine, thus dose reduction is recommended in cats with underlying renal azotemia.[42]

Dolasetron and Ondansetron

Dolasetron and ondansetron are selective serotonin antagonists that inhibit central and peripheral 5-HT_3 receptors. Their main antiemetic effect is through antagonism of the peripheral 5-HT_3 receptors in the gastrointestinal tract. In cats 5-HT_3 antagonism of the CRZT is also likely important in the antiemetic effect of dolasetron and ondansetron. Dolasetron and ondansetron were originally used for vomiting secondary to chemotherapy because of their superior clinical efficacy.

The clinical use of dolasetron and ondansetron in cats has not been associated with reported side effects, and experimental studies report minimal toxicity in animals at doses 30 times the antiemetic dose.[15] Side effects reported in humans include headaches, elevated liver enzymes, rare hypersensitivity reactions, prolongation of the QT interval, and arrhythmias.[14,24]

Dolasetron is commonly used for parenteral administration and ondansetron for oral administration, dictated primarily based on the tablet sizes available and cost. Recommended dosing of dolasetron is 0.5 to 1 mg/kg intravenously every 24 hours and ondansetron 0.5 mg/kg orally every 12 hours.

Maropitant

Maropitant is a neurokinin-1 (NK-1) receptor antagonist, blocking the binding of substance P to the NK-1 receptors located in the emetic center, CRTZ, and the enteric plexus.[55] In cats maropitant has been reported to be efficacious in treating xylazine-induced vomiting and motion sickness.[31] Recommended dosing in cats is 1 mg/kg intravenously, subcutaneously or orally every 24 hours for up to 5 days.[31] Maropitant is reported to be well tolerated in cats.

Phenothiazines

Prochlorperazine and chlorpromazine are considered broad-spectrum antiemetics by antagonism of D_2-dopaminergic, histaminergic (H_1 and H_2), and cholinergic (muscarinic) receptors within the CRTZ and, at high doses, the alpha-adrenergic receptors (alpha$_1$ and alpha$_2$) within the vomiting center. In cats alpha$_2$-receptors play a key role in emesis (recall xylazine is the emetic of choice in cats), suggesting cats may be more sensitive to the antiemetic effects of the phenothiazines.

Prochlorperazine and chlorpromazine produce an antiemetic effect at relatively low doses, thus avoiding profound sedation; although, because of antagonism of the alpha-receptors, vasodilation and hypotension can be clinically significant side effects. Phenothiazines have the potential to lower the seizure threshold; their use is not recommended in patients with a known seizure history. Other CNS-associated side effects linked to D_2 antagonism occur at higher doses and produce extrapyramidal signs, including rigidity, tremors, weakness, and restlessness. Antagonism of the histaminergic receptors carries the risk of sedation.

Because of the need for frequent dosing (0.2 to 0.4 mg/kg subcutaneously every 8 hours) and the risk of hypotension and sedation, the clinical use of phenothiazine antiemetics is limited to hospitalized patients with refractory vomiting and should be avoided in patients who are dehydrated or hypotensive.

Cisapride

Cisapride is a serotonergic 5-HT_4 agonist that increases propulsive gastrointestinal motility from the lower esophageal sphincter to the colon. Cisapride binds serotonergic 5-HT_4 receptors in the myenteric plexus, increasing the release of acetylcholine in gastrointestinal smooth muscle. In dogs cisapride has greater prokinetic activity in the stomach relative to metoclopramide.[29] Cisapride has no direct antiemetic effect, although it is indicated in a vomiting cat with colonic dysmotility secondary to megacolon. Colonic distention can trigger the vomiting reflex in cats. Cisapride induces colonic smooth muscle contractions in cats with megacolon that is dependent on the influx of extracellular calcium and is only partially cholinergic dependent.[30] Other potential indications include refractory generalized ileus or gastroesophageal reflux. Dosage recommendations based on the pharmacokinetics in healthy cats is 1.5 mg/kg orally every 12 hours.[41] Prior to the use of cisapride, an intestinal obstruction should be ruled out because of its strong prokinetic effects.

Side effects reported in humans are cramping and diarrhea. Potentially life-threatening side effects include QT prolongation and ventricular arrhythmias, the primary concern in humans that led to cisapride's removal from the market in the United States.[47] In cats QT prolongation associated with cisapride administration requires 20 times the therapeutic dose.[37] Because of the risk of prolongation of the QT interval and ventricular arrhythmias, the concurrent use of cisapride and dolasetron is not recommended.[14] Other potential drug interactions associated with cisapride include concurrent therapy with azole antifungals (ketoconazole and itraconazole), because of their inhibition of hepatic CYP3A isoenzyme system and the inhibition of cisapride metabolism.[47]

Dietary Modification

Diet trials are commonly used in cats with idiopathic gastrointestinal signs or in cats with suspected or known food hypersensitivities. Dietary strategies used to control vomiting in cats focus on either a highly digestible diet or an elimination (novel protein/carbohydrate or hydrolyzed protein) diet.[72] The empirical use of elimination diets in cats is reported to be relatively successful, with approximately 50% of cats with idiopathic gastrointestinal signs responsive to a novel protein/carbohydrate diets within 2 to 3 days.[28] Interestingly, traditional diet trials are recommended for a minimum of 8 to 12 weeks, but in this group of diet-responsive cats with chronic gastrointestinal disease, clinical improvement was reported within days.[28] Thus if a cat is going to be diet responsive, clinical improvement to a diet trial should be noted relatively early.

Highly Digestible Diets

Highly digestible diets enable more effective absorption and assimilation of nutrients in the face of a compromised digestive tract. These diets contain highly digestible proteins and carbohydrates, moderate to low fat, soluble fiber but low concentrations of insoluble fiber, and are supplemented with omega-3 fatty acids.

Novel Protein/Carbohydrate or Elimination Diets

These diets are recommended when food allergy or intolerance is suspected. These diets contain a single highly digestible novel carbohydrate source and novel protein source. Alternatively, diets formulated with hydrolyzed proteins can be used as an alternative to novel protein/carbohydrate diets.

TARGETED THERAPIES WITH SPECIFIC INDICATIONS FOR VOMITING

Gastrointestinal Ulcers

See Tables 23-4 and 23-5 for information on gastrointestinal ulcers.

TABLE 23-4 **Mechanism of Action and the Adverse Effects of the Common Drugs Used to Treat Gastric Ulcers in Cats**

Drug	Mechanism of Action	Adverse Effects
Famotidine (increases gastric pH)	H_2 antagonism	
Ranitidine (increases gastric pH) (prokinetic)	H_2 antagonism Anticholinesterase	Hypotension (IV)
Omeprazole (increased gastric pH)	H^+/K^+ ATPase inhibitor	
Sucralfate (gastric ulcer healing)	Prevents H^+ back diffusion, inactivates pepsin, absorbs bile acids, and increases gastric mucosal prostaglandin synthesis	

TABLE 23-5 **Dosage Recommendations, Contraindications, Potential Drug Interactions, and Clinical Indications for Dosage Adjustments for the Common Drugs Used to Treat Gastric Ulcers in Cats**

Drug	Dosage (Cats)	C: Contraindications DI: Drug Interactions DA: Dosage Adjustments
Famotidine	0.5 mg/kg IV, SC, PO q12-24h	DA: azotemia
Ranitidine	2.5 mg/kg IV q12h 3.5 mg/kg PO q12h	DA: azotemia
Omeprazole	0.5-1 mg/kg PO q24h	DI: inhibition CYP2C: diazepam Do not crush enteric coated tablets
Sucralfate	250 mg PO q12h	DI: decreases oral absorption of fluoroquinolones, tetracyclines, and digoxin

Famotidine

Famotidine has no direct antiemetic effect but is a competitive inhibitor of the histamine (H_2) receptors associated with the gastric parietal cells. The H_2-receptor is the dominant receptor involved in gastric acid secretion. H_2-receptor antagonism is reported to result in a 70% to 90% reduction in acid production.[13] Famotidine is more effective at suppressing gastric acid secretion relative to ranitidine. Famotidine is well tolerated, although, with chronic therapy, there is the potential for hypoacidity and gastric bacterial overgrowth. In humans dose reduction is recommended in association with renal dysfunction.[21] Famotidine is not an inhibitor of the hepatic microsomal cytochrome P-450 enzyme system, therefore significant drug interactions are not anticipated.

Hyperacidity alone is not considered a common cause for vomiting in cats, but famotidine is effective in treating vomiting in cats associated with gastric ulcers or gastritis. Recommended dosage in cats is 0.5 mg/kg every 12 to 24 hours.

Ranitidine

Ranitidine is also a competitive inhibitor of the H_2 receptor associated with gastric parietal cells. In addition, ranitidine increases lower esophageal sphincter tone and functions as a prokinetic agent (increasing gastric emptying and stimulating intestinal motility, including colonic motility), because of its anticholinesterase activity.[40,54] Significant drug interactions associated with hepatic microsomal cytochrome P-450 enzyme system inhibition are not a clinical concern with ranitidine.[46] An adverse effect to be aware of in cats treated with ranitidine is transient hypotension associated with ranitidine administered as an IV bolus.[19] In humans dose reduction is recommended in patients with renal azotemia.[39]

Ranitidine is effective in decreasing gastric acid in cats.[22] Ranitidine would be a logical choice in a cat with gastrointestinal ulceration and/or atony. The reported dosage recommendation for ranitidine in cats is 3.5 mg/kg orally every 12 hours or 2.5 mg/kg intravenous every 12 hours.[19]

Omeprazole

Omeprazole is a proton pump inhibitor that targets the H^+/K^+ ATPase pump on the luminal surface of partial cells. Omeprazole is effective at suppressing parietal cell acid secretion, and its effects persist for ≈24 hours after drug withdrawal because of drug accumulation in the parietal cell (by ion trapping). Indications for omeprazole therapy are for the treatment and prevention of nonsteroidal antiinflammatory drug (NSAID)–induced ulcers.[9] Omeprazole is enteric coated to prevent its degradation by gastric acid; therefore oral formulations should not be crushed. Based on human studies, omeprazole is a hepatic microsomal cytochrome P-450 enzyme inhibitor with known drug interactions with diazepam.[2] The extent of clinically significant drug interactions in cats has yet to be studied.

Omeprazole is reported to be effective in reducing gastric acid secretion in cats.[22] The recommended empirical dosage in cats is 0.5 to 1 mg/kg orally once daily. Long-term use in humans[33] and dogs[11] is associated with gastric polyps and parietal cell hyperplasia, respectively, but the effect of long-term use in cats is currently unknown.

Sucralfate

Sucralfate is a disaccharide complexed with aluminum that dissociates to sucrose octasulfate and aluminum hydroxide upon exposure to gastric acid. The sucrose octasulfate spontaneously polymerizes, producing a viscous material capable of binding ulcerative lesions in the gastric mucosa. Once bound to the exposed mucosa, it prevents back diffusion of H^+, inactivates pepsin, absorbs bile acids, and increases mucosal prostaglandin synthesis, collectively supporting ulcer healing.

Sucralfate is not systemically absorbed but does prevent the absorption of drugs capable of chelating with aluminum, including fluoroquinolones, tetracyclines, and digoxin. If sucralfate is indicated in a cat being treated concurrently with fluoroquinolones, tetracyclines, or digoxin, the recommendation is to administer the other drug 2 hours prior to the administration of sucralfate to optimize drug absorption.

Clinical indications for the use of sucralfate in cats are for the treatment of gastric ulcers and esophagitis.[36] Dosage recommendation in cats is 250 mg orally every 12 hours. Sucralfate can be crushed, suspended in water, and administered as slurry.

NONSPECIFIC SUPPORTIVE THERAPIES FOR DIARRHEA

Dietary Modification

Diet trials are used in some cats with diarrhea if the underlying cause is from known or suspected food hypersensitivities. Dietary management includes either a highly digestible diet, an elimination (novel protein/carbohydrate or hydrolyzed protein) diet (see above for both), or a diet high in fiber.[72]

High-Fiber Diets

High-fiber diets contain a mixture of both soluble and insoluble fiber that can be beneficial in patients with signs of large bowel diarrhea. Insoluble fiber, such as cellulose, functions to increase the bulk of the stool, bind fluid, and regulate intestinal motility. Soluble fiber, including fruit and vegetable pectins and beet pulp, functions as a source of butyric acid that can be used by the colonic mucosa and decreases proinflammatory cytokines.[69,72]

Vitamin Supplementation

Cobalamin

Cobalamin (vitamin B_{12}) is an essential vitamin needed by a number of different enzymes, including key enzymes involved in methionine metabolism and the conversion of methylfolate to tetrahydrofolate needed for DNA synthesis. Cobalamin and folate are intimately linked, and hypocobalaminemia can lead to a functional deficiency of folate.[57] Ingested cobalamin requires intrinsic factor binding for enterocyte absorption at the level of the ileum.

Hypocobalaminemia is commonly associated with distal small intestine diseases in cats, including inflammatory bowel disease. In addition, low cobalamin has a negative impact on enterocyte function; therefore in many cats with intestinal disease and hypocobalaminemia, cobalamin supplementation is necessary for resolution of clinical signs.[60,64] Quantification of serum cobalamin levels is recommended in cats with clinical signs of small bowel diarrhea, ones suspected to have an infiltrative disease of the small intestine (inflammatory bowel disease or gastrointestinal lymphoma), or ones with pancreatic dysfunction. When hypocobalaminemia is identified, supplementation is recommended

(250 μg/cat every 7 days) while the underlying cause of cat's malabsorption is being investigated and at initiation of targeted therapy.

Probiotics and Prebiotics

Probiotics

Probiotics are ingested live microorganisms intended to benefit the host, specifically to support the microflora environment of the gastrointestinal tract as well as to provide an overall benefit to the body's immune function by immunomodulation.[8,18,51] Probiotics chemically modify ingesta and intestinal mucus, as well as affect immune cells, enterocytes, and goblet cells within the intestinal mucosa through direct receptor interactions and indirectly through the action of cytokines.

The microorganisms commonly used are nonpathogenic bacteria and yeast that have a vital role in gastrointestinal health, including *Lactobacillus* spp., *Enterococcus faecium*, *Bifidobacterium* spp., and *Saccharomyces* spp. For example, lactobacilli synthesize B vitamins, digestive enzymes, and folate coenzymes.[63] Clinical indications for the use of probiotics are diverse, including primary gastrointestinal disease, chronic renal disease, and pancreatitis.[71]

The rational use of probiotics in the treatment of gastrointestinal diseases include their ability to modulate gastrointestinal flora, minimize colonization by pathogenic bacteria, and decrease the likelihood of bacterial translocation.[17] In healthy cats, *Lactobacillus acidophilus* is reported to reduce fecal *Clostridium* counts.[45] When *Lactobacillus acidophilus* was used adjunctively with antimicrobial therapy, fecal shedding of *Campylobacter* was reduced in cats with *Campylobacter*-induced diarrhea relative to cats treated with antimicrobials alone.[3] Specifically, in cats with gastrointestinal disease, available research supports the probiotic *Enterococcus faecium* as clinically beneficial in resolving diarrhea in kittens.[16] Relative to the control group, the kittens treated with probiotics had increased fecal *Bifidobacteria* and blood IgA concentrations and decreased fecal counts of *Clostridium perfringens*.

Prebiotics

Prebiotics are dietary supplements used to select for the more beneficial enteric flora, support gastrointestinal function, and prevent the overgrowth of pathogenic bacteria, including *Salmonella*, *Escherichia coli*, *Clostridium*, or *Campylobacter*. For a food additive to be considered a prebiotic, it must be nondigestible by the gastrointestinal tract (resistant to gastric acidity, gastrointestinal hydrolysis and absorption), yet fermentable by gastrointestinal microflora to short-chain fatty acids to stimulate the growth of "good" intestinal bacterial.[72]

Prebiotics include nondigestible oligosaccharides—commonly, oligofructose, fructo-oligosaccharides, mannanoligosaccharides, inulin, chicory, and lactosucrose.[72] Reports on the use of prebiotics in cats are limited to their use in healthy cats; healthy cats fed fructo-oligosaccharides were reported to have a trend toward an increase in fecal concentrations of *Lactobacilli* and a decrease in concentration of *C. perfringens* and *E. coli* relative to the controls.[65] To date no reports are available on the use of prebiotics in cats with gastrointestinal disease.

Probiotics and prebiotics potentially have a supportive role in the treatment of gastrointestinal disease in cats. The important clinical consideration in the use of probiotics as an adjunctive therapy is to ensure the use of live nonpathogenic microorganisms that have been documented to colonize the intestinal tract of cats. Gastrointestinal flora co-evolve with their host. Gastrointestinal microorganism colonization varies among species and within each individual animal. The distribution of fecal microflora for a given individual is considered unique but stable over time.[68]

TARGETED THERAPIES WITH SPECIFIC INDICATIONS FOR DIARRHEA

Antimicrobials and Antiparasitics

Antimicrobial and antiparasitic therapies for the treatment of feline diarrhea are indicated based on the specific diagnosis of infectious diarrhea, bacterial enteritis, or as adjunctive therapy for inflammatory bowel disease. Infectious pathogens more commonly associated with feline diarrhea include bacterial enteropathies (*Clostridium, Campylobacter*), protozoal enteropathies (*Tritrichomonas foetus*, *Giardia* spp.), and helminthic enteropathies associated with ascarids, hookworms, whipworms, and tapeworms. Only the more common anthelminthic, antimicrobial, and antiprotozoal therapies are discussed below (Tables 23-6 and 23-7). More information about antimicrobials and antiparasitics is found under specific infections in the discussions of Infectious Enteritis and Gastrointestinal Parasites.

Fenbendazole

Fenbendazole is an anthelmintic used to treat common helminth infections, including ascarids, hookworms, whipworms, and a single species of tapeworm, *Taenia pisiformis*. *Giardia* spp. are also considered susceptible to fenbendazole. Fenbendazole binds beta-tubulin subunits of microtubules, interfering with their polymerization. Side effects include vomiting and diarrhea, although both are considered rare. Fenbendazole is not approved for use in cats in North America but is commonly used clinically, and an empirical dosage of 50 mg/kg

TABLE 23-6 **Mechanism of Action and Adverse Effects of the Common Antimicrobials and Antiparasitics Used to Treat Specific Causes of Diarrhea in Cats**

Drug	Mechanism of Action	Adverse Effects
Fenbendazole (anthelmintic)	Binds microtubule beta-tubulin subunits preventing polymerization	Vomiting Diarrhea
Pyrantel pamoate (anthelmintic)	Targets nicotinic acetylcholine receptors of parasites: depolarization and spastic paralysis	
Metronidazole (antimicrobial)	Anaerobic environment: converted to unstable intermediates that disrupt bacterial DNA synthesis	Inappetence, anorexia Nausea, vomiting Hypersalivation Cerebellovestibular ataxia
Ronidazole (antimicrobial)	Anaerobic environment: converted to unstable intermediates that disrupt bacterial DNA synthesis	Hepatotoxicity Neurotoxicity

TABLE 23-7 **Dosage Recommendations and Spectrum of Activity of the Common Antimicrobial and Antiparasitic Drugs Used to Treat Specific Causes of Diarrhea in Cats**

Drug	Dosage (Cats)	Spectrum
Fenbendazole	50 mg/kg PO every 24h × 5 days	Ascarids, hookworms, whipworms, *Taenia pisiformis*
Pyrantel pamoate	5 mg/kg PO once, repeat in 3 weeks	Ascarids, hookworms, *Physaloptera*
Metronidazole Metronidazole benzoate	10-15 mg/kg/day 20 mg/kg/day	Anaerobes, *Giardia* spp.
Ronidazole	30 mg/kg PO q24h	*T. foetus*

orally every 24 hours for 5 consecutive days is recommended.

Pyrantel Pamoate

Pyrantel pamoate is a nicotinic anthelmintic used primarily for the treatment of ascarids, but its spectrum of activity also includes hookworms and the stomach worm, *Physaloptera* spp. Pyrantel is toxic to susceptible parasites through its selective action on their nicotinic acetylcholine receptors, resulting in depolarization and spastic paralysis. Pyrantel is not approved for use in cats but is considered safe in cats and is commonly used clinically. The dosage recommendation in cats is 5 mg/kg orally once, repeat in 3 weeks, and finally repeated in 3 months.

Metronidazole

Metronidazole is a nitroimidazole antibiotic with an anaerobic antibacterial spectrum with antiprotozoal activity against *Giardia* spp. In an anaerobic environment, metronidazole is converted to unstable intermediates (nitroso free radicals) that disrupt bacterial DNA synthesis. Immunomodulatory properties capable of inhibiting cell-mediated immunity have been described for metronidazole, although its immunomodulatory properties are reported at dosages well beyond what is recommended for clinical use,[62] raising questions about the clinical use of metronidazole as an adjunctive therapy for treating inflammatory bowel disease.[34,43]

Resistance to metronidazole is considered rare.[43] The most common adverse reaction is gastrointestinal upset, including inappetence, anorexia, nausea, and vomiting. Profuse salivation can occur in cats after oral administration of metronidazole base (formulation used in standard tablets), which has lead to the use of metronidazole benzoate (a compounded formulation not approved by the Food and Drug Administration) in some cats because of its better oral palatability.[61] At high doses (>200 mg/kg/day) benzoic acid is reported to be neurotoxic in cats, but with appropriate clinical dosing of metronidazole benzoate benzoic acid toxicity is unlikely.[6] Dose-related metronidazole toxicity in cats results in cerebellovestibular ataxia secondary to gamma-aminobutyric acid (GABA) inhibition at dosages greater than or equal to 58 mg/kg/day[12,52]; clinical signs include nystagmus, head tilt, ataxia, seizures, and obtundation.

In cats with inflammatory bowel disease, the dosage recommendation for the metronidazole base is 10 to 15 mg/kg/day. Metronidazole benzoate contains approximately 60% metronidazole base by weight, translating to an empirical dosage of 20 mg/kg/day of metronidazole benzoate (equivalent to 12.4 mg/kg/day of metronidazole base).[61] Little is known about the safety of chronic metronidazole use in cats, but oral metronidazole has been reported to disrupt DNA within feline peripheral mononuclear cells following 7 days of therapy.[61] This metronidazole-induced genotoxicity is reversible and is no longer detected 6 days after antibiotic therapy is discontinued.

Ronidazole

Ronidazole is a nitroimidazole antibiotic (similar to metronidazole) and available as a powder-on-feed antibiotic. Ronidazole is not approved for use in cats but has been used off-label to effectively treat tritrichomoniasis in naturally and experimentally infected cats (30 mg/kg orally every 12 hours for 14 days).[25] *T. foetus* reduces nitroimidazoles to their nitroso free radicals. Ronidazole has been reported to have better in vitro and 10-fold higher in vivo activity against *T. foetus* relative to metronidazole.[25,35,49] Ronidazole resistance is beginning to be reported in *T. foetus* isolates from cats with diarrhea.[26]

Side effects include hepatoxicity and neurotoxicity. Neurotoxicity is associated with high doses and has been reported in cats.[59] The use of ronidazole is recommended only for confirmed cases of *T. foetus*, and dosing should not exceed 30 mg/kg once daily in cats, especially in cats at risk for neurotoxicity. Ronidazole is not registered for human or veterinary use in the United States; therefore its use in cats requires owner informed consent and client education of the potential human hazards.

Immunosuppressive Therapies

Immunosuppressive therapies are considered the standard of care for cats with gastrointestinal biopsies consistent with inflammatory bowel disease (lymphoplasmacytic or eosinophilic inflammation). The common immunosuppressive therapies used in cats with inflammatory bowel disease include glucocorticoids, cyclosporine, and chlorambucil (Tables 23-8 and 23-9). More information on the treatment of inflammatory bowel disease is found elsewhere in this chapter.

Glucocorticoids

Glucocorticoids are considered first-line therapy in the treatment of cats with inflammatory bowel disease. Glucocorticoids bind their intracellular glucocorticoid receptors, modifying the expression of genes with glucocorticoid response elements. Immunomodulation is achieved through inhibition of cytokine release and response, including decreasing leukocyte phagocytosis, chemotaxis, and antigen expression. The more common side effects in cats include gastrointestinal ulceration, opportunistic infections (e.g., urinary tract infections), pancreatitis, and diabetes mellitus. Cats are less susceptible to iatrogenic hyperadrenocorticism than dogs.

Initial therapy is usually with oral prednisone or prednisolone. Prednisone is a prodrug that is metabolized to its active form prednisolone. Cats are reported to be less efficient in the conversion of prednisone to

TABLE 23-8 **Mechanism of Action and Adverse Effects of the Common Immunosuppressive Drugs Used to Treat Inflammatory Bowel Disease in Cats**

Drug	Mechanism of Action	Adverse Effects
Glucocorticoids	Immunomodulation: decreasing leukocyte phagocytosis, chemotaxis, and antigen expression	Gastrointestinal ulceration Secondary infections Pancreatitis Diabetes mellitus Hyperadrenocorticism
Cyclosporine	Attenuates T-lymphocyte activation and proliferation by inhibition of interleukin-2	Vomiting Secondary infections Hepatotoxicity
Chlorambucil	Alkylates and cross links DNA Lymphocyte cytotoxicity	Bone marrow suppression Neurotoxicity

TABLE 23-9 **Dosage Recommendations and Drug Interactions for the Common Immunosuppressive Drugs Used to Treat Inflammatory Bowel Disease in Cats**

Drug	Types	Dosage (Cats)	Drug Interactions
Glucocorticoids	Prednisone/prednisolone		NSAIDs: gastrointestinal ulceration
	Antiinflammatory	0.5-1 mg/kg/day	
	Immunosuppressive	2-4 mg/kg/day	
	Dexamethasone	Prednisone dose divided by 7	
	Budesonide	0.5-1 mg/cat/day	
Cyclosporine	Cyclosporine modified (microemulsion)	4 mg/kg PO q12-24h	Ketoconazole: CYP3A inhibition
Chlorambucil	—	<4-kg cat: 2 mg/cat q72h >4-kg cat: 2 mg/cat q48h	—

NSAIDs, Nonsteroidal antiinflammatory drugs.

prednisolone[27]; therefore prednisolone may be preferred in cats, especially in cats refractory to prednisone therapy.

Alternative forms of glucocorticoids can be considered in specific patient populations. In patients with severe malabsorption, injectable dexamethasone may provide improved bioavailability and clinical response. Also dexamethasone maybe preferred in patients with a history of heart failure, fluid retention, or hypertension because of its lack of mineralocorticoid activity relative to prednisone/prednisolone. Dexamethasone's potency is 4 to 10 times that of prednisolone; therefore a dose reduction is necessary when prescribing dexamethasone (the dexamethasone dose is one seventh that of prednisolone).[4,10] Budesonide is an oral, locally active, high-potency glucocorticoid that is formulated to be released in the distal gastrointestinal tract (based on the pH differential between the proximal and distal small intestine), where it is absorbed and is locally immunomodulating at the level of the enterocyte. The amount of systemically absorbed budesonide is minimized, because 80% to 90% of the budesonide absorbed from the gastrointestinal tract undergoes first-pass metabolism in the liver. Some systemic absorption does occur, as evidenced by a blunted adrenocorticotropic hormone (ACTH) stimulation test in dogs treated with budesonide at 3 mg/m^2 for 30 days.[66,70] The use of budesonide in cats remains anecdotal, with a suggestive empirical dose of 0.5 to 1 mg/cat/day.

Initial glucocorticoid therapy for cats with inflammatory bowel disease consists of antiinflammatory (0.5 to 1 mg/kg/day) to immunosuppressive (2 to 4 mg/kg/day) dosages, with dosages based on the potency of prednisone/prednisolone. The goal of therapy is to achieve clinical remission and slowly taper the dose of glucocorticoids to the lowest dose that will control the cat's clinical signs.[67] Some cats may be completely weaned off therapy, while others require long-term low-dose therapy. The tapering of therapy should be slow, with a 25% to 50% dose reduction every 3 to 4 weeks.

Cyclosporine

Cyclosporine is considered a second-tier immunosuppressive drug used to treat inflammatory bowel disease in cats. Use of cyclosporine in the treatment of diarrhea associated with inflammatory bowel disease in cats is extrapolated from its use in dogs to treat glucocorticoid refractory inflammatory bowel diarrhea.[1] Cyclosporine suppresses T-lymphocyte–mediated inflammation in the gastrointestinal tract secondary to suppression of inflammatory cytokines. Specifically, cyclosporine attenuates T-lymphocyte activation and proliferation through the inhibition of interleukin-2 (IL-2) production. Side effects of cyclosporine in cats include dose-dependent inappetence and vomiting, which may occur at the onset of therapy and are generally responsive to dose reduction. Other less common side effects reported in cats are opportunistic infections, including toxoplasmosis[5] and hepatoxicity.

The microemulsion formulation of cyclosporine has higher oral bioavailability and less variable pharmacokinetics.[58] A suggested initial dosage of cyclosporine is 4 mg/kg every 12 or 24 hours. Serum cyclosporine levels can be used to monitor for excessive trough plasma concentration (>400 ng/mL) as determined using a high-performance liquid chromotography (HPLC) analytical method.[53]

Chlorambucil

Chlorambucil is a slow-acting nitrogen mustard that alkylates and effectively cross links DNA, leading to altered protein production. The immunosuppressive effects of chlorambucil are the result of its cytotoxic effect on lymphocytes, similar to other nitrogen mustards. Bone marrow suppression is considered mild to moderate and is rapidly reversible. Neurotoxicity and myoclonus has been reported in a cat accidently overdosed with chlorambucil.[7]

Chlorambucil is used as a second-tier drug in cats to treat immune-mediated disorders, in part because of ease of administration and its low risk of myelosuppression. For the treatment of inflammatory bowel disease, the recommended dosing in cats is 2 mg/cat every 48 hours in cats greater than 4 kg and 2 mg/cat every 72 hours in cats less than 4 kg.[50] Chlorambucil is commonly used in combination with glucocorticoids in the treatment of immune-mediated diseases, including inflammatory bowel disease,[48,50] and as a chemotherapeutic agent in the treatment of gastrointestinal small cell lymphoma in cats.[38]

References

1. Allenspach K, Rufenacht S, Sauter S, et al: Pharmacokinetics and clinical efficacy of cyclosporine treatment of dogs with steroid-refractory inflammatory bowel disease, *J Vet Intern Med* 20:239, 2006.
2. Andersson T: Omeprazole drug interaction studies, *Clin Pharmacokinet* 21:195, 1991.
3. Baillon ML, Butterwick RF: The efficacy of a probiotic strain, *Lactobacillus acidophilus* DSM, in the recovery of cats from clinical *Campylobacter* infection [abstract], *J Vet Intern Med* 17:416, 2003.
4. Ballard PL, Carter JP, Graham BS, et al: A radioreceptor assay for evaluation of the plasma glucocorticoid activity of natural and synthetic steroids in man, *J Clin Endocrinol Metab* 41:290, 1975.
5. Barrs VR, Martin P, Beatty JA: Antemortem diagnosis and treatment of toxoplasmosis in two cats on cyclosporin therapy, *Aust Vet J* 84:30, 2006.
6. Bedford PG, Clarke EG: Experimental benzoic acid poisoning in the cat, *Vet Rec* 90:53, 1972.
7. Benitah N, de Lorimier LP, Gaspar M, et al: Chlorambucil-induced myoclonus in a cat with lymphoma, *J Am Anim Hosp Assoc* 39:283, 2003.
8. Benyacoub J, Czarnecki-Maulden GL, Cavadini C, et al: Supplementation of food with *Enterococcus faecium* (SF68) stimulates immune functions in young dogs, *J Nutr* 133:1158, 2003.

9. Bersenas AM, Mathews KA, Allen DG, et al: Effects of ranitidine, famotidine, pantoprazole, and omeprazole on intragastric pH in dogs, *Am J Vet Res* 66:425, 2005.
9a. Cahil C: Mirtazapine as an antiemetic, *Vet Forum* 23:34, 2006.
10. Cantrill HL, Waltman SR, Palmberg PF, et al: In vitro determination of relative corticosteroid potency, *J Clin Endocrinol Metab* 40:1073, 1975.
11. Carlsson E: A review of the effects of long-term acid inhibition in animals, *Scand J Gastroenterol Suppl* 166:19, 1989.
12. Caylor KB, Cassimatis MK: Metronidazole neurotoxicosis in two cats, *J Am Anim Hosp Assoc* 37:258, 2001.
13. Coruzzi G, Bertaccini G, Noci MT, et al: Inhibitory effect of famotidine on cat gastric secretion, *Agents Actions* 19:188, 1986.
14. Cubeddu LX: Iatrogenic QT abnormalities and fatal arrhythmias: mechanisms and clinical significance, *Curr Cardiol Rev* 5:166, 2009.
15. Cunningham RS: 5-HT3-receptor antagonists: a review of pharmacology and clinical efficacy, *Oncol Nurs Forum* 24:33, 1997.
16. Czarnecki-Maulden G, Cavadini C, Lawler D, et al: Incidence of naturally occurring diarrhea in kittens fed *Enterococcus faecium* SF68. *Supplement to Compend Contin Edu Vet* 29:37, 2007.
17. Damaskos D, Kolios G: Probiotics and prebiotics in inflammatory bowel disease: microflora "on the scope", *Br J Clin Pharmacol* 65:453, 2008.
18. Dotan I, Rachmilewitz D: Probiotics in inflammatory bowel disease: possible mechanisms of action, *Curr Opin Gastroenterol* 21:426, 2005.
19. Duran S, Jernigan A, Ravis W, et al: Pharmacokinetics of oral and intravenous ranitidine in cats [abstract], *Proceedings of 9th Annual ACVIM Forum* 1991, p 902.
20. Durazo FA, Valenzuela JE: Effect of single and repeated doses of metoclopramide on the mechanisms of gastroesophageal reflux, *Am J Gastroenterol* 88:1657, 1993.
21. Echizen H, Ishizaki T: Clinical pharmacokinetics of famotidine, *Clin Pharmacokinet* 21:178, 1991.
22. Fandriks L, Jonson C: Effects of acute administration of omeprazole or ranitidine on basal and vagally stimulated gastric acid secretion and alkalinization of the duodenum in anaesthetized cats, *Acta Physiol Scand* 138:181, 1990.
23. Freeman AJ, Cunningham KT, Tyers MB: Selectivity of 5-HT3 receptor antagonists and anti-emetic mechanisms of action, *Anticancer Drugs* 3:79, 1992.
24. Goodin S, Cunningham R: 5-HT(3)-receptor antagonists for the treatment of nausea and vomiting: a reappraisal of their side-effect profile, *Oncologist* 7:424, 2002.
25. Gookin, JL, Copple, CN, Papich, MG, et al: Efficacy of ronidazole for treatment of feline Tritrichomonas foetus infection, *J Vet Intern Med* 20:536, 2006.
26. Gookin JL, Stauffer SH, Dybas D, et al: Documentation of in vivo and in vitro aerobic resistance of feline *Tritrichomonas foetus* isolates to ronidazole, *J Vet Intern Med* 24:1003, 2010.
27. Graham-Mize CA, Rosser EJ Jr: Comparison of microbial isolates and susceptibility patterns from the external ear canal of dogs with otitis externa, *J Am Anim Hosp Assoc* 40:102, 2004.
28. Guilford WG, Jones BR, Markwell PJ, et al: Food sensitivity in cats with chronic idiopathic gastrointestinal problems, *J Vet Intern Med* 15:7, 2001.
29. Gullikson GW, Loeffler RF, Virina MA: Relationship of serotonin-3 receptor antagonist activity to gastric emptying and motor-stimulating actions of prokinetic drugs in dogs, *J Pharmacol Exp Ther* 258:103, 1991.
30. Hasler AH, Washabau RJ: Cisapride stimulates contraction of idiopathic megacolonic smooth muscle in cats, *J Vet Intern Med* 11:313, 1997.
31. Hickman MA, Cox SR, Mahabir S, et al: Safety, pharmacokinetics and use of the novel NK-1 receptor antagonist maropitant (Cerenia) for the prevention of emesis and motion sickness in cats, *J Vet Pharmacol Ther* 31:220, 2008.
32. Hillemeier C, McCallum R, Oertel R, et al: Effect of bethanechol and metoclopramide on upper gastrointestinal motility in the kitten, *J Pediatr Gastroenterol Nutr* 5:134, 1986.
33. Jalving M, Koornstra JJ, Wesseling J, et al: Increased risk of fundic gland polyps during long-term proton pump inhibitor therapy, *Aliment Pharmacol Ther* 24:1341, 2006.
34. Jergens A: Feline idiopathic inflammatory bowel disease, *Compend Contin Educ Prac Vet* 14:509, 1992.
35. Kather EJ, Marks SL, Kass PH: Determination of the in vitro susceptibility of feline *Tritrichomonas foetus* to 5 antimicrobial agents, *J Vet Intern Med* 21:966, 2007.
36. Katz PO, Ginsberg GG, Hoyle PE, et al: Relationship between intragastric acid control and healing status in the treatment of moderate to severe erosive oesophagitis, *Aliment Pharmacol Ther* 25:617, 2007.
37. Kii Y, Nakatsuji K, Nose I, et al: Effects of 5-HT(4) receptor agonists, cisapride and mosapride citrate on electrocardiogram in anaesthetized rats and guinea-pigs and conscious cats, *Pharmacol Toxicol* 89:96, 2001.
38. Kiselow MA, Rassnick KM, McDonough SP, et al: Outcome of cats with low-grade lymphocytic lymphoma: 41 cases (1995-2005), *J Am Vet Med Assoc* 232:405, 2008.
39. Koch KM, Liu M, Davi, IM, et al: Pharmacokinetics and pharmacodynamics of ranitidine in renal impairment, *Eur J Clin Pharmacol* 52:229, 1997.
40. Kounenis G, Koutsoviti-Papadopoulou M, Elezoglou A, et al: Comparative study of the H2-receptor antagonists cimetidine, ranitidine, famotidine and nizatidine on the rabbit stomach fundus and sigmoid colon, *J Pharmacobiodyn* 15:561, 1992.
41. LeGrange SN, Boothe DM, Herndon S, et al: Pharmacokinetics and suggested oral dosing regimen of cisapride: a study in healthy cats, *J Am Anim Hosp Assoc* 33:517, 1997.
42. Lehmann CR, Heironimus JD, Collins CB, et al: Metoclopramide kinetics in patients with impaired renal function and clearance by hemodialysis, *Clin Pharmacol Ther* 37:284, 1985.
43. Lofmark S, Edlund C, Nord CE: Metronidazole is still the drug of choice for treatment of anaerobic infections, *Clin Infect Dis* 50(Suppl 1):S16, 2010.
44. Mangel AW, Stavorski JR, Pendleton RG: Effects of bethanechol, metoclopramide, and domperidone on antral contractions in cats and dogs, *Digestion* 28:205, 1983.
45. Marshall-Jones ZV, Baillon ML, Croft JM, et al: Effects of *Lactobacillus acidophilus* DSM13241 as a probiotic in healthy adult cats, *Am J Vet Res* 67:1005, 2006.
46. Martinez C, Albet C, Agundez JA, et al: Comparative in vitro and in vivo inhibition of cytochrome P450 CYP1A2, CYP2D6, and CYP3A by H2-receptor antagonists, *Clin Pharmacol Ther* 65:369, 1999.
47. Michalets EL, Williams CR: Drug interactions with cisapride: clinical implications, *Clin Pharmacokinet* 39:49, 2000.
48. Miller E: The use of cytotoxic agents in the treatment of immune-mediated diseases of dogs and cats, *Semin Vet Med Surg (Small Anim)* 12:157, 1997.
49. Miwa GT, Wang R, Alvaro R, et al: The metabolic activation of ronidazole [(1-methyl-5-nitroimidazole-2-yl)-methyl carbamate] to reactive metabolites by mammalian, cecal bacterial and *T. foetus* enzymes, *Biochem Pharmacol* 35:33, 1986.
50. Moore L: Beyond corticosteroids for therapy of inflammatory bowel disease in dogs and cats [abstract], Proceedings 22nd Am Coll Vet Intern Med Forum 2004, p 611.
51. Nomoto K: Prevention of infections by probiotics, *J Biosci Bioeng* 100:583, 2005.
52. Olson EJ, Morales SC, McVey AS, et al: Putative metronidazole neurotoxicosis in a cat, *Vet Pathol* 42:665, 2005.
53. Papich MG: Immunnosuppressive drug therapy, Proceedings of 14th Annual Members Meeting of the American Academy of Veterinary Dermatology and American College of Veterinary Dermatology 1998, p 41.

54. Petroianu GA, Arafat K, Schmitt A, et al: Weak inhibitors protect cholinesterases from strong inhibitors (paraoxon): in vitro effect of ranitidine, *J Appl Toxicol* 25:60, 2005.
55. Prommer E: Aprepitant (EMEND): the role of substance P in nausea and vomiting, *J Pain Palliat Care Pharmacother* 19:31, 2005.
55a. Quimby JM, Gustafson DL, Samber BJ et al: Studies on the pharmacokinetics and pharmacodynamics of mirtazapine in healthy young cats, *J Vet Pharmacol Ther* (in press).
56. Rao AS, Camilleri M: Review article: metoclopramide and tardive dyskinesia, *Aliment Pharmacol Ther* 31:11, 2010.
57. Reed N, Gunn-Moore D, Simpson K: Cobalamin, folate and inorganic phosphate abnormalities in ill cats, *J Feline Med Surg* 9:278, 2007.
58. Robson D: Review of the pharmacokinetics, interactions and adverse reactions of cyclosporine in people, dogs and cats, *Vet Rec* 152:739, 2003.
59. Rosado TW, Specht A, Marks, SL: Neurotoxicosis in 4 cats receiving ronidazole, *J Vet Intern Med* 21:328, 2007.
60. Ruaux CG, Steiner JM, Williams DA: Early biochemical and clinical responses to cobalamin supplementation in cats with signs of gastrointestinal disease and severe hypocobalaminemia, *J Vet Intern Med* 19:155, 2005.
61. Sekis I, Ramstead K, Rishniw M, et al: Single-dose pharmacokinetics and genotoxicity of metronidazole in cats, *J Feline Med Surg* 11:60, 2009.
62. Sen P, Chakravarty AK, Kohli J: Effects of some imidazoles on cellular immune responses—an experimental study, *Indian J Exp Biol* 29:867, 1991.
63. Shahani KM, Ayebo AD: Role of dietary lactobacilli in gastrointestinal microecology, *Am J Clin Nutr* 33:2448, 1980.
64. Simpson KW, Fyfe J, Cornetta A, et al: Subnormal concentrations of serum cobalamin (vitamin B12) in cats with gastrointestinal disease, *J Vet Intern Med* 15:26, 2001.
65. Sparkes AH, Papasouliotis K, Sunvold G, et al: Effect of dietary supplementation with fructo-oligosaccharides on fecal flora of healthy cats, *Am J Vet Res* 59:436, 1998.
66. Stroup ST, Behrend EN, Kemppainen RJ, et al: Effects of oral administration of controlled-ileal-release budesonide and assessment of pituitary-adrenocortical axis suppression in clinically normal dogs, *Am J Vet Res* 67:1173, 2006.
67. Tams TR: Feline inflammatory bowel disease, *Vet Clin North Am Small Anim Pract* 23:569, 1993.
68. Tannock GW: New perceptions of the gut microbiota: implications for future research, *Gastroenterol Clin North Am* 34:361, vii, 2005.
69. Tedelind S, Westberg F, Kjerrulf M, et al: Anti-inflammatory properties of the short-chain fatty acids acetate and propionate: a study with relevance to inflammatory bowel disease, *World J Gastroenterol* 13:2826, 2007.
69a. Timmer CJ, Sitsen JM, Delbressine LP: Clinical pharmacokinetics of mirtazapine, *Clin Pharmacokinet* 38:461, 2000.
70. Tumulty JW, Broussard JD, Steiner JM, et al: Clinical effects of short-term oral budesonide on the hypothalamic-pituitary-adrenal axis in dogs with inflammatory bowel disease, *J Am Anim Hosp Assoc* 40:120, 2004.
71. Wynn SG: Probiotics in veterinary practice, *J Am Vet Med Assoc* 234:606, 2009.
72. Zoran DL: Nutritional management of feline gastrointestinal diseases, *Top Companion Anim Med* 23:200, 2008.

DISEASES OF THE ESOPHAGUS

Susan E. Little

Esophageal disease is uncommon in the cat when compared with dogs, but it is also likely that problems such as esophagitis and esophageal strictures are often overlooked. Awareness about feline esophageal diseases is low, the clinical signs are often not specific, and imaging beyond survey radiographs may be required for diagnosis.

The esophagus is composed of four layers (from inner to outer): mucosa, submucosa, muscularis, and adventitia (there is no serosal layer). In the dog, the muscle layer is entirely composed of skeletal muscle, but in cats, the distal third of the esophagus is composed of smooth muscle. The upper esophageal sphincter prevents reflux of esophageal contents into the pharynx and minimizes aerophagia. The lower esophageal sphincter prevents gastroesophageal reflux and relaxes during swallowing to allow food and fluid to enter the stomach.

CLINICAL PRESENTATION

Clinical signs of esophageal disease include drooling, dysphagia, pain on swallowing (odynophagia), and, most classically, regurgitation. Weight loss may occur secondary to inadequate food intake when disease is severe or chronic. Other clinical signs, such as anorexia, cough, dyspnea, and fever, may occur if complications such as aspiration pneumonia or esophageal perforation occur.

Regurgitation is passive expulsion of food or fluid from the esophagus. The food is undigested and often accompanied by mucus and saliva. Mucosal erosions may produce frank blood in the regurgitated material. Regurgitation must be differentiated from vomiting (Table 23-10). Vomiting is typically preceded by

TABLE 23-10 **How to Differentiate Vomiting from Regurgitation**

Sign	Regurgitation	Vomiting
Prodromal nausea (salivation, licking lips, anxiety)	No	Usually
Retching (dry heaves)	No	Usually
Material produced:		
Food	Sometimes	Sometimes
Bile	No	Sometimes
Blood	Sometimes undigested	Sometimes (undigested or digested)
Volume produced	Variable	Variable
Timing relative to eating	Variable	Variable
Distention of cervical esophagus	Sometimes	No

Adapted from Willard MD: Clinical manifestations of gastrointestinal disorders. In Nelson RW, Couto CG, editors: *Small animal internal medicine*, St Louis, 2009, Mosby Elsevier, Table 28-1, p 354.

salivation, retching, and abdominal contractions. The vomitus consists of partially digested food from the stomach and/or intestines and may be mixed with bile-stained fluid. Some cats will have both vomiting and regurgitation. Expectoration may also be confused with vomiting or regurgitation. Expectoration is associated with coughing, but cats that cough excessively may also stimulate vomition so that a careful history is needed to characterize the clinical signs correctly. Coughing may also occur in cats that have aspirated as a result of regurgitation.

Drooling, dysphagia, and odynophagia are most commonly seen with conditions of the oropharynx and/or proximal esophagus. Odynophagia is most commonly associated with esophagitis and foreign bodies. Dysphagia and regurgitation together most commonly indicate oral or pharyngeal dysfunction; if regurgitation is not accompanied by dysphagia, esophageal dysfunction is likely.[55] Regurgitation in cats with esophageal disease is caused by obstruction or muscular dysfunction. Causes of obstruction include vascular ring anomaly, foreign object, stricture, and neoplasia. Causes of muscular dysfunction include congenital disease, esophagitis, myopathies, neuropathies, and dysautonomia.

Regurgitation may occur immediately after eating if the lesion is in the proximal esophagus. However, a dilated esophagus provides a reservoir for food and fluid so that regurgitation may not be associated in time with eating.

Young cats with signs of esophageal disease should be suspected of congenital defects, such as vascular ring anomaly, or a foreign body. Adult cats with esophageal disease may have a recent history of general anesthesia, administration of certain oral medications, or ingestion of irritant chemicals. Acute onset of clinical signs may suggest a foreign body, while chronic, slowly worsening signs may indicate a stricture or tumor.

DIAGNOSTIC APPROACH

All cats suspected of esophageal disease should have a minimum database as part of the diagnostic plan (complete blood cell count, serum chemistries, urinalysis, and other tests as indicated by age or concurrent diseases, such as serum total T_4 and blood pressure measurement). An important part of diagnosis is observation of the cat while eating food, to localize the location of the dysfunction. If the cat is unwilling to eat while in the veterinary clinic, the owner can make a video of the cat eating at home for the clinician to view.

The general diagnostic approach to regurgitation in cats is found in Figure 23-3. Plain and contrast radiography and endoscopy are important diagnostic tools for esophageal disease. Fluoroscopy is valuable for the diagnosis of motility disorders, but availability is limited to universities and referral centers because of the cost of equipment. Ultrasonography is limited to evaluation of

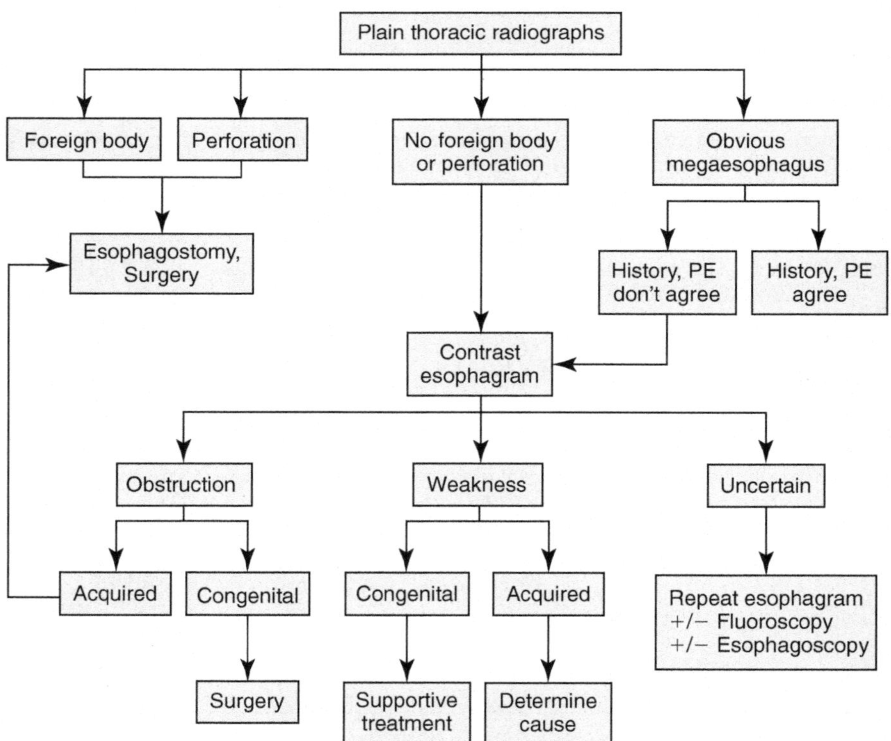

FIGURE 23-3 Diagnostic approach to regurgitation. *(Adapted from Willard MD: Clinical manifestations of gastrointestinal disorders. In Nelson RW, Couto CG, editors:* Small animal internal medicine, *St Louis, 2009, Mosby Elsevier, Figure 28-1, p 354.)*

the cervical esophagus and a small segment of abdominal esophagus between the cardia of the stomach and the diaphragm.

The entire esophagus should be evaluated with cervical and thoracic radiographs. Thoracic radiographs may also show evidence of complications such as aspiration pneumonia or esophageal perforation. The normal esophagus is not visualized on plain radiographs, but may be seen if food or fluid are retained or a foreign body or mass is present. Radiographic contrast agents useful for esophagrams in cats include liquid or paste barium. A water-soluble iodinated contrast agent (e.g., iohexol, Gastrografin) is preferred if there is any risk the esophagus is perforated, because these agents are less irritating and more rapidly reabsorbed. Esophagrams are most useful for diagnosis of luminal obstructions, extraluminal compression, mucosal irregularities, and possibly alterations in motility.

Dilute liquid barium can be administered with a syringe or it may be mixed with canned food, especially if a motility disorder or stricture is suspected. Multiple lateral radiographs are taken rapidly, starting within 10 seconds of swallowing the contrast agent. Contrast is rapidly cleared from the normal esophagus by peristalsis. If the contrast in the esophagus terminates abruptly, an obstruction is likely. If the contrast is retained throughout the esophagus, muscular dysfunction is suspected. Some conditions, such as esophagitis, are difficult to diagnose radiographically, because contrast agents may or may not adhere to ulcerated mucosa.

Flexible endoscopy is a noninvasive diagnostic tool for esophageal disorders and is often used if plain and contrast radiographs have failed to establish a diagnosis. It is most sensitive for diagnosis of masses, ulcers, perforations, and obstructions. In addition, it is often possible to retrieve foreign bodies using endoscopy as well as to assist with dilatation of strictures or placement of gastrostomy feeding tubes if required. Biopsy of the esophageal mucosa is more difficult than biopsy of gastric or intestinal mucosa and is not commonly performed with the exception of mass lesions.

SPECIFIC DISEASES

Esophagitis and Esophageal Strictures

Esophagitis may result from various causes of inflammation, such as contact irritation from foreign bodies (including trichobezoars lodged in the esophagus), chemical irritants or caustic medications, gastroesophageal reflux, persistent vomiting, hiatal hernia, or general anesthesia. Inflammation disrupts the esophageal mucosa and exposes the submucosa. An important part of the treatment plan is identification and treatment of the underlying cause.

Clinical signs include dysphagia, regurgitation, salivation, and repeated swallowing, although signs may be absent in cats with mild esophagitis. Cats with odynophagia may repeatedly extend the head and neck while swallowing. If the esophagitis or underlying disease is severe, weight loss and dehydration may occur secondary to anorexia.

If the submucosa and muscularis are damaged, strictures may form as a result of the production of fibrous connective tissue and compromise the esophageal lumen.[54] Neoplasia is an important cause of esophageal stricture in humans, but not in cats. Most cases have single strictures, but multiple strictures are possible. In two studies, the mean stricture diameter was reported as 5 mm.[26,32] Most strictures are less than 1 cm in length. Clinical signs associated with strictures appear 5 to 14 days after the esophageal injury and may be present for weeks before definitive treatment is pursued. Regurgitation typically occurs immediately after eating, although if the stricture is long standing, a pouch may form cranial to the lesion where food accumulates.

Survey radiographs may be normal in cats with esophagitis and strictures, but are useful to rule out other causes for the clinical signs, such as a foreign body, or to detect related problems, such as aspiration pneumonia. In some patients, dilation of the esophagus with fluid or air may be seen.[45] A contrast esophagram may disclose irregularities of the mucosa in cats with severe esophagitis. Segmental dilation may occur with severe inflammation. Strictures may be diagnosed with an esophagram (Figure 23-4); however, in some cases, it may be difficult to differentiate a stricture from intramural thickening (e.g., because of neoplasia).

Endoscopy is useful for diagnosis of esophagitis; findings include mucosal erythema, hemorrhage, and erosions or ulcerations. If gastroesophageal reflux is present, the lesions will be most severe in the distal esophagus, and the lower esophageal sphincter may be dilated. Endoscopy is often used for definitive diagnosis of esophageal stricture as well as to visualize the lesion during treatment by bougienage or balloon catheter dilation. Strictures appear as a ring of white fibrous tissue that narrows the esophageal lumen. If endoscopy is performed after a barium esophagram, 24 hours should be allowed to elapse between the procedures or the barium will obscure visualization with the endoscope.[19]

General anesthesia is an important cause of esophagitis (sometimes leading to stricture formation) in cats, probably because gastroesophageal reflux appears to occur commonly in anesthetized cats.* For example, in a series of seven cats with benign esophageal stricture, recent anesthesia for ovariohysterectomy was the suspected cause in five cases.[1] Clinical signs appeared up to 21 days after anesthesia.

*References 1, 8, 11, 15, 38, 43.

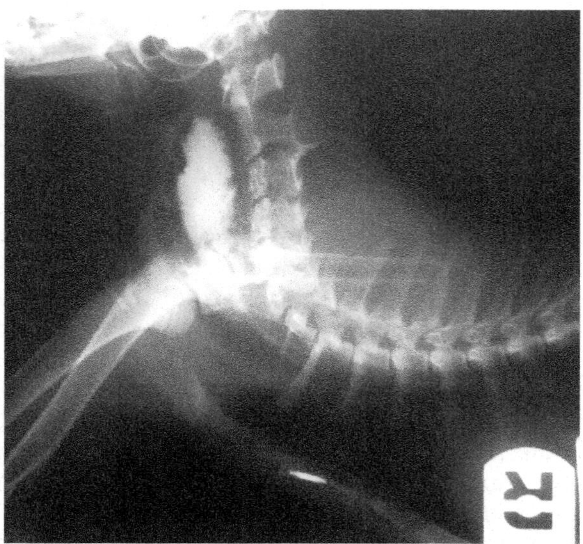

FIGURE 23-4 Lateral barium contrast esophagram of a 4-month-old domestic shorthair (DSH) cat with an esophageal stricture associated with administration of doxycycline tablets. *(Courtesy Dr. Emma Thom.)*

Many preanesthetic drugs and induction agents reduce lower esophageal sphincter pressure.[27,28] Other predisposing factors may be intraabdominal surgery and a head-down position on the surgery table. Reflux fluid with a pH less than 4 is likely to cause esophageal mucosal damage, as is prolonged contact time. Esophageal defense mechanisms include clearance of the reflux fluid by peristalsis and neutralization of the acidic pH by the bicarbonate present in saliva.

In a study of 40 kittens less than 15 weeks of age, risk of gastroesophageal reflux during anesthesia was evaluated with use of a laryngeal airway mask versus endotracheal intubation.[47] Gastroesophageal reflux was observed in 50% of kittens with use of the laryngeal airway mask but more importantly in 22% of kittens with endotracheal intubation. The reflux episodes occurred shortly after anesthesia induction. In a study of 50 cats anesthetized with thiopentone or propofol, gastroesophageal reflux occurred in 14%.[16] Reflux also occurred shortly after anesthesia was induced and lasted for a mean of 23 minutes. It is unknown why esophageal strictures form only in a small number of cats that experience gastroesophageal reflux during anesthesia.

Gastroesophageal reflux disease (GERD) is a commonly reported cause of esophagitis in humans, but it is rarely reported in cats when not associated with general anesthesia.[24,33] The true incidence is unknown, and diagnosis may be hampered by scant knowledge about the clinical presentation and diagnosis. Clinical signs and diagnostic procedures are as for other causes of esophagitis. In one case series of three cats, diagnosis of GERD was based on clinical signs, contrast radiography, and endoscopic findings.[24] Biopsy and histopathology of abnormal esophageal tissue was performed in two cases. The authors noted that the esophageal mucosa may appear grossly normal, but submucosal inflammation may be found on histopathologic examination of biopsies.

A consequence of chronic severe GERD in humans is the development of metaplastic columnar epithelium (Barrett esophagus) that replaces the normal squamous epithelium. One case series reported on Barrett-like esophagus in three cats.[23] Two cases were associated with hiatal hernia and one with cardial incompetence.

Drug-induced esophageal damage and stricture formation is well known in humans and cats (see Figure 4-4). In humans over 70 drugs have been implicated, and most are antibacterials or NSAIDs.[30] Implicated drugs in the cat include tetracycline, doxycycline, and clindamycin in tablet or capsule form administered without a food or water bolus.[4,17,32,36,37] Clinical signs (dysphagia, regurgitation, salivation, anorexia) appear 3 to 16 days after drug treatment is started. Strictures commonly form in the midcervical esophagus or over the heart base in the thoracic esophagus. Doxycycline hyclate is most commonly associated with esophageal strictures in cats, and the principle reason for its irritating properties is an acidic pH. The monohydrate salt of doxycycline is less irritating and is marketed as tablets and a palatable paste licensed for use in dogs and cats in some countries.[48] In humans esophageal ulceration after doxycycline therapy is more common than stricture formation. Although the development of strictures in cats would appear to be uncommon, it seems possible the incidence of esophagitis is underestimated, because the clinical signs (e.g., odynophagia, chest pain) may go unrecognized.

Esophageal transit studies of normal cats have shown that the passage time of dry-swallowed tablets and capsules is often prolonged (longer than 30 seconds).[20,53] Complete entrapment (retention for more than 4 minutes) in the midcervical region occurs commonly. However, a small bolus of food or water is sufficient to ensure immediate passage of the medication into the stomach.[20,53] The risk of esophageal retention can also be lessened by coating a tablet or capsule with butter or a gel dietary supplement (Nutri-Cal; Vétoquinol, Fort Worth, Tex.).[21] One study determined that tablets or capsules administered using a one-step pill gun with flavored liquid (FlavoRx Pill Glide; FLAVORx, Columbia, Md.) or a pill delivery treat (Greenies Pill Pockets; Nutro Products, Franklin, Tenn.) ensured an average transit time of 60 seconds or less.[6]

Delayed esophageal transit of medications allows tablets and capsules to disintegrate within the esophagus, exposing the mucosa to irritating chemicals. Cats may be at risk of delayed esophageal transit, because they do not typically drink water with medication, and they do not have an upright posture. In addition, medications are often given to sick or dehydrated patients that may be at greater risk of esophageal retention of medication. All oral medication given to cats in tablet or capsule form should be followed with food or a liquid.

Mild esophagitis will resolve on its own, especially if an underlying cause can be removed or treated. Frequent meals of canned food should be provided. Cats with moderate to severe esophagitis will require medical therapy, and those with difficulty eating or weight loss may also require gastrostomy tube feeding. Esophagostomy or pharyngostomy feeding tubes should be avoided in these patients. Treatment is provided to control inflammation and promote healing while reducing gastric acid secretion and increasing lower esophageal sphincter tone. The length of medical treatment will vary from about one week to several weeks, depending on the underlying cause and severity of disease. Medications indicated for esophagitis include prokinetics, H_2-receptor antagonists, proton pump inhibitors, and sucralfate (Table 23-11).

Prokinetic drugs enhance gastric emptying and increase lower esophageal sphincter tone. Metoclopramide also has antiemetic effects, which may be beneficial in patients with chronic vomiting. It can be administered by the subcutaneous (SC) route, an advantage in a vomiting or regurgitating patient. Cisapride may be more effective at enhancing both gastric emptying and lower esophageal sphincter tone, but it must be obtained from a compounding pharmacy in most countries and can only be given orally.

TABLE 23-11 **Drugs Used in the Treatment of Esophagitis and Esophageal Strictures**

Drug	Dose	Mechanism
Cisapride	1.5 mg/kg, q12h, PO	Prokinetic; increases lower gastroesophageal sphincter pressure, promotes gastric emptying
Famotidine	0.5-1.0 mg/kg, q12-24h, PO or IV	H_2-receptor antagonist; reduces gastric acid secretion
Metoclopramide	0.2-0.4 mg/kg, q6h, SC or PO	Prokinetic; increases lower gastroesophageal sphincter pressure, promotes gastric emptying
Omeprazole	0.5-1.0 mg/kg, q24h, PO	Proton pump inhibitor; reduces gastric acid secretion
Ranitidine	2.5 mg/kg, q12h, IV or 3.5 mg/kg, q12h, PO	H_2-receptor antagonist; reduces gastric acid secretion
Sucralfate	0.25 g/cat, q6-8h, PO	Adheres to and protects damaged mucosa

Drug doses from Trepanier L: Acute vomiting in cats: rational treatment selection, *J Feline Med Surg* 12:225, 2010.

H_2-receptor antagonists are competitive inhibitors that block parietal H_2 receptors and decrease the amount of gastric acid produced. Proton pump inhibitors are noncompetitive inhibitors that act on the H^+/K^+ ATPase enzyme system at the secretory surface of gastric parietal cells. They are considered superior for decreasing gastric acid secretion and are therefore the first choice, despite their greater cost.[45] A drawback of proton pump inhibitors is that they must be administered orally. Sucralfate may be beneficial for reflux esophagitis, because it binds to mucosal erosions in an acid environment and provides a protective barrier. It is given as oral slurry, ideally separate from meals or other medications.

Antibiotics are not commonly recommended unless aspiration pneumonia is present or the eroded mucosa is at risk of bacterial infection in a patient with severe disease or a compromised immune system. Corticosteroids are often recommended for cats with esophagitis to reduce esophageal inflammation and impair the formation of fibrous connective tissue. However, the benefit of corticosteroids in cats with esophagitis has not been investigated and administration must be weighed against potential adverse effects, especially in patients with aspiration pneumonia.

Treatment of esophageal stricture typically requires dilation with either bougienage or a balloon catheter; both are used with endoscopic visualization under general anesthesia. Appropriate analgesia should be provided, because dilating the stricture is painful. It does not appear that placement of a gastrostomy feeding tube is specifically required to recover from dilation procedures, although a tube may be placed in some anorexic cats to ensure nutritional intake and administer oral medications.

A bougie is a long, narrow, oblong, mechanical dilator available in various sizes (typically 9- to 12-mm sizes are used in cats) that is gently passed through the stricture, usually over a guide wire. Established criteria for selection of bougie diameter and dilation end points are not available. In one study, the initial bougie chosen was approximately the same size as the estimated diameter of the stricture, or no more than 2 mm larger.[8] Once the first bougie is passed, subsequent bougies of increasing diameter are employed. Two to four bougies of increasing size may be passed in a single session, with the goal of dilating the stricture without causing esophageal tear or perforation. Determining when dilation should be stopped is a matter of clinical judgment. The procedure may be repeated as needed to maintain improvement; the total number of procedures required is variable. In one retrospective case series of eight cats treated with bougienage, the median number of procedures was 4.5, and a good outcome was achieved in 75% of the cases.[8] In some cases, the endoscope tip itself has been used for bougienage when bougies or balloon catheters were not available.

Balloon catheter dilation has become a popular method in recent years.[26,32,38] Although some clinicians feel this is a safer procedure than bougienage, there is no data in the literature to support this assumption. The catheter can be placed through the endoscope biopsy channel, alongside the endoscope, or with the aid of a preplaced guide wire. As for bougienage, established criteria for selection of balloon diameter and dilation end points are not available, and the clinician's best judgment must be used. Various balloon sizes are available; in one study, the size was selected so that the inflated diameter was 4 mm larger than the stricture diameter.[32] The balloon is passed into the stricture with endoscopic guidance. It is then inflated to a predetermined pressure for 1 to 2 minutes to stretch the stricture, usually with saline, but contrast agents may also be used if fluoroscopy is used. As for bougienage, some cases may require more than one dilation procedure (typically two to four). Cuffed endotracheal tubes are not appropriate substitutes for balloon catheters.

Regardless of the method used, after the dilation procedure, the endoscope should be used to look for other strictures and should be passed into the stomach to look for potential causes, such as causes of chronic vomiting. After treatment, medical management to decrease ongoing gastroesophageal reflux, resolve inflammation, and prevent further stricture formation should be instituted (as described previously). Most cats are able to eat the day following the dilation procedure. Corticosteroid treatment after dilation is controversial, and no controlled studies in animals are available. Antibiotics are not routinely recommended.

The prognosis for cats undergoing esophageal dilation is generally good based on the ability to eat canned food with minimal episodes of regurgitation. However, published studies show 10% to 30% of cats died or were euthanized despite multiple episodes of dilation, and up to 30% could only be fed liquid diets.[1,8,32,38] Even among cats with good outcomes, a return to a dry kibble diet may not be possible.

The dilation technique employed may be dictated by the clinician's experience, the equipment available, and the cost. Potential complications of both methods include esophageal tear or perforation, hemorrhage, infection, and aspiration. Esophageal tears or perforations may lead to pneumothorax or pneumomediastinum. Repeated stricture formation is also possible, leaving only less desirable treatment options, such as long-term percutaneous gastrostomy tube feeding or surgery.

Esophageal surgery is generally avoided whenever possible, because it is difficult and invasive (requiring a thoracotomy), with risk of serious complications, such as failure of anastomosis, necrosis, and stricture formation. Closure of incisions in the esophagus is difficult, because there is no serosa, and the muscles are oriented longitudinally. Indications for esophageal surgery include repair of perforations, treatment of strictures that fail to respond to dilation, and tumor resection.

Stent placement has recently been described in cats with esophageal strictures with variable results. A 1-year-old cat presented with a 4-week history of dysphagia and regurgitation caused by a single cervical esophageal stricture after treatment with oral clindamycin.[18] Guided balloon dilation was performed 6 times over a period of 3 weeks, but stricture formation always recurred. A self-expanding metal stent was placed using endoscopy and fluoroscopy after another dilation procedure. The cat did well eating a canned diet from an elevated position for 10 months, but by 12 months, the cat was no longer able to eat even liquid food and was euthanized. On necropsy, the stent had migrated and was obstructed by swallowed hair.

In another case, a biodegradable self-expanding stent was used to successfully treat an 11-year-old cat that presented with a stricture in the cervical esophagus after anesthesia for dentistry.[3] Balloon dilation was performed twice, but regurgitation recurred 5 days after the last procedure. The stricture was dilated a third time with a balloon catheter, and a tubular self-expanding polydioxanone stent was placed with fluoroscopic guidance. The life span of the stent was estimated to be 10 to 12 weeks, sufficient time to allow healing of the esophagus.

Foreign Bodies

Foreign bodies are less commonly found in the esophagus of the cat than in other gastrointestinal locations. Reported foreign bodies include string, needles, fish hooks, and bones. Trichobezoars may cause obstruction when they become lodged in the esophagus during vomiting (Figure 23-5). Recurrent esophageal trichobezoars have been infrequently reported in the literature.[12,51] It is not known if an esophageal motility disorder is the underlying cause for recurrent obstructions. In one case, an esophageal diverticulum developed in association with recurrent trichobezoars.[12] Treatment for recurrent trichobezoars includes prokinetic drug therapy (e.g., cisapride), moderate to high-fiber diets, and shaving of long-haired cats.

Common areas for foreign bodies to lodge include the thoracic inlet, the heart base, and the esophageal hiatus in the diaphragm.[5] Obstruction of the esophageal lumen may be complete or partial. Clinical signs include acute onset of gagging, salivation, repeated swallowing, dysphagia, and regurgitation. However, chronic esophageal foreign bodies have been reported in cats with dysphagia, intermittent regurgitation, and weight loss over a period of weeks or months.[2]

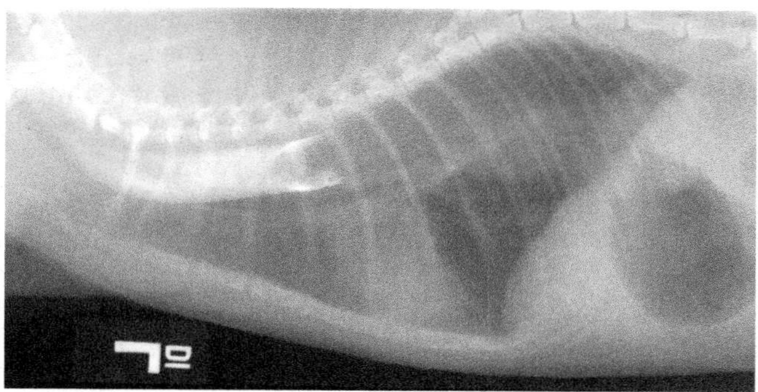

FIGURE 23-5 Lateral esophagram of a cat with a trichobezoar esophageal foreign body. Trichobezoars may cause obstruction when they become lodged in the esophagus during vomiting. *(Courtesy Dr. John Graham.)*

Cough, mucopurulent nasal discharge, and fever may be found if aspiration has occurred. Trauma to the esophagus may cause esophagitis and even esophageal stricture. Perforation of the esophagus by the foreign body may lead to pneumothorax, pneumomediastinum, or pyothorax with signs of depression, anorexia, fever, and dyspnea. If the perforation occurs in the cervical esophagus, swelling, cellulitis, and drainage of serous or purulent material may be noted.

Many foreign bodies are readily diagnosed with survey radiographs, especially if they are radiopaque. Other radiographic findings include an esophagus dilated with fluid or air. Radiolucent objects may be detected with an esophagram. Care must be taken when performing esophagrams on cats that may have an obstruction, because aspiration is a concern. If abnormalities that could be consistent with an esophageal perforation (e.g., periesophageal gas or fluid, pleural effusion) are detected on survey radiographs, an aqueous iodine contrast solution should be used.

Removal of esophageal foreign bodies should be performed as soon as possible to minimize esophageal trauma and pressure necrosis. Endoscopy can be used to confirm the diagnosis and often to remove the object. Both rigid and flexible endoscopes may be used along with accessories such as various forceps and Foley catheters. Care should be taken to remove the object as atraumatically as possible, especially if the object is sharp or pointed. If the object is in the caudal esophagus and it cannot be grasped and removed, an attempt should be made to gently push it into the stomach, where it can be retrieved using laparotomy and gastrotomy. If esophageal perforation has occurred, esophagotomy is recommended and is described elsewhere.[5,14]

Removal of fish hooks may require a combination of surgery and endoscopy.[5,39] A surgical approach to the esophagus is made, but the esophagus is not incised; rather, the portion of the hook protruding through the esophagus is cut and removed, and the endoscope is used to retrieve the remainder.

Following uncomplicated foreign body removal, the esophagus should be carefully inspected for lesions and bleeding before the endoscope is withdrawn. Food and water should be withheld for 24 to 48 hours. Supportive care includes fluid therapy and analgesia; a gastrostomy feeding tube may be required in selected cases for nutritional support. Broad-spectrum antibiotics are administered to control bacterial infection and therapy for esophagitis should be instituted as described previously. Careful follow-up should include evaluation for stricture formation.

If an esophageal perforation has occurred, conservative management may be sufficient if the defect is small. A broad-spectrum antibiotic should be administered along with other supportive care, such as fluid therapy and analgesia. Feeding through a gastrostomy tube for several days is recommended as well as close monitoring for complications such as pleuritis. Large perforations require thoracotomy for surgical repair.

Megaesophagus

Megaesophagus is a diffuse hypomotility disorder that may be classified as congenital versus acquired or idiopathic versus secondary to other diseases. It is uncommon in cats compared with dogs. At least two dog breeds have been identified with heritable congenital megaesophagus. A heritable form of megaesophagus has been suggested for cats, particularly for Siamese cats, although no detailed studies have been performed.[13,29] It is often frustrating to determine the underlying cause of acquired megaesophagus. Megaesophagus may be a manifestation of neuromuscular diseases, such as dysautonomia or myasthenia gravis (see Chapter 27). Megaesophagus may also develop secondary to esophagitis from chronic vomiting or GERD.[24,43]

Other uncommon causes of megaesophagus are found in the literature. One case report describes a young cat with megaesophagus secondary to a large nasopharyngeal polyp that extended into the cervical esophagus.[10] Megaesophagus resolved once the polyp was removed. In another report, a young cat with diaphragmatic hernia was diagnosed with megaesophagus and gastric dilation.[31] Megaesophagus resolved with medical treatment and surgical correction of the diaphragmatic defect.

Clinical signs are typically those of esophageal dysfunction; regurgitation is the most consistently found sign. Regurgitation may not be closely related in time to eating if the esophagus is markedly distended and holds food. Cats with long-standing disease may suffer from weight loss or secondary rhinitis. The appetite is typically normal or increased. Additional signs may occur if systemic neuromuscular disease is present. Aspiration pneumonia may cause fever, dyspnea, and cough. Two case reports describe cats with idiopathic

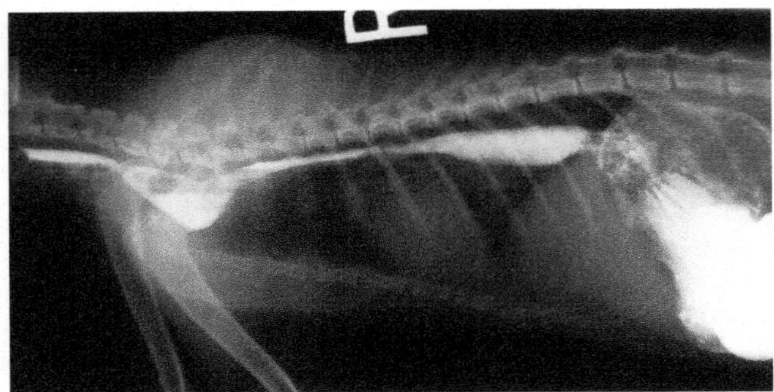

FIGURE 23-6 Lateral esophagram of a 5-month-old kitten with megaesophagus. *(Courtesy Dr. Emilia Monachino.)*

megaesophagus and chronic vomiting associated with intermittent gastroesophageal intussusception.[35,50] Survey and contrast radiographs may identify a dilated esophagus (Figure 23-6), but contrast fluoroscopy is the diagnostic tool of choice when available, because it allows for assessment of peristalsis. Care must be taken with contrast studies because of the risk of aspiration.

Treatment of megaesophagus is largely symptomatic and supportive unless an underlying disorder can be identified and treated. Frequent small meals are offered with the cat feeding in an upright position. The upright position should be maintained for at least 10 minutes after eating to allow for gravity-assisted passage of food into the stomach. This is best accomplished by having the owner hold the cat over their shoulder so that the esophagus is in a vertical position.[44] Different types of diets should be offered to determine which is best for the individual patient; calorically dense diets may be beneficial for patients with weight loss. Prokinetic drugs, such as cisapride, stimulate smooth muscle, but since most of the esophagus is skeletal muscle, the efficacy of such drugs is questionable for treatment of megaesophagus. Prokinetic drugs also increase lower esophageal sphincter tone and may increase esophageal transit time, neither of which is desirable in patients with megaesophagus.

Vascular Ring Anomaly

Vascular ring anomalies are congenital malformations of the great vessels that entrap the thoracic esophagus and cause obstruction. The most commonly reported anomaly is persistent right aortic arch. The esophagus is entrapped by the aorta on the right, the ligamentum arteriosum and the pulmonary trunk on the left, and the heart base ventrally. Other vascular anomalies are rarely described in cats, such as a double aortic arch described in a Siamese cat.[56]

Onset of clinical signs occurs around the time of weaning to solid food so that most affected cats are presented at less than 6 months of age. The most common clinical sign is regurgitation, and most patients are underweight. A distended cervical esophagus may be palpated, and secondary aspiration pneumonia may occur.

A history of regurgitation since weaning is very suggestive of a vascular ring anomaly, but other causes of regurgitation must be ruled out. Survey radiographs show a dilated esophagus cranial to the heart, while the caudal esophagus is usually normal. The bulge of the aortic arch normally seen on a ventrodorsal radiographic view is absent. An esophagram is used to confirm the location of the obstruction and the severity of disease.

Definitive treatment is surgical repair of the vascular defect (i.e., ligation and transection of the ligamentosum arteriosum). Some patients will require nutritional support through gastrostomy tube feeding and treatment for aspiration pneumonia before surgery. Early diagnosis and surgical intervention brings the best prognosis for return of normal esophageal function. Some affected cats are left with residual esophageal hypomotility, which is managed as for idiopathic megaesophagus.

Neoplasia

Esophageal neoplasia is rare in the cat as in the dog. Although parasitic granulomas caused by *Spirocerca lupi* are associated with esophageal neoplasia in dogs, this parasite does not infect cats. Both primary and metastatic esophageal tumors can occur in the cat. Squamous cell carcinoma is the most common primary esophageal tumor in cats and is often found in the caudal two thirds of the esophagus.[7,22,25,46] Affected cats are middle aged or older. Clinical signs are typically those associated with esophageal obstruction, such as regurgitation, dysphagia, odynophagia, and salivation. Patients with advanced disease may suffer anorexia, depression, and weight loss. On physical examination, an esophageal mass may or may not be palpable.

Survey and contrast radiographs reveal esophageal dilation, a soft tissue mass, or periesophageal lesions that displace the esophagus. Computed tomography is useful to identify periesophageal or intraluminal masses. Definitive diagnosis is made with endoscopy and biopsy. Mucosal biopsies are difficult to obtain, because the esophageal mucosa is tough; exfoliative cytology may also be helpful. Treatment is rarely undertaken, because disease is often advanced at the time of diagnosis, and many patients have complications such as aspiration pneumonia. Palliation may be attempted with chemotherapy or radiation, although data on efficacy is unavailable. In general, squamous cell carcinomas in other anatomic locations respond poorly to treatment. Surgical resection may be attempted if anastomosis can be accomplished without excessive tension.

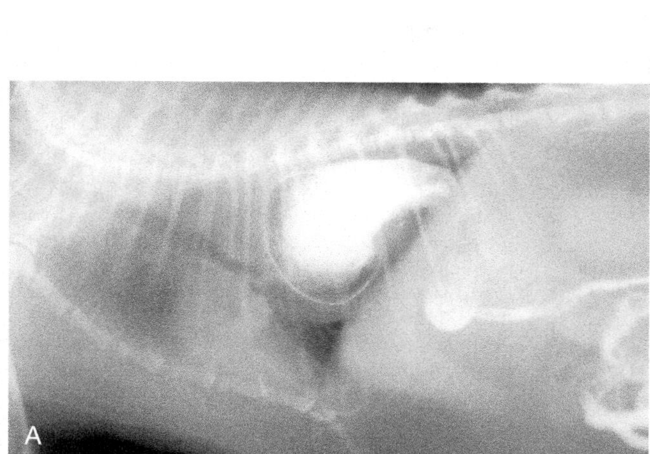

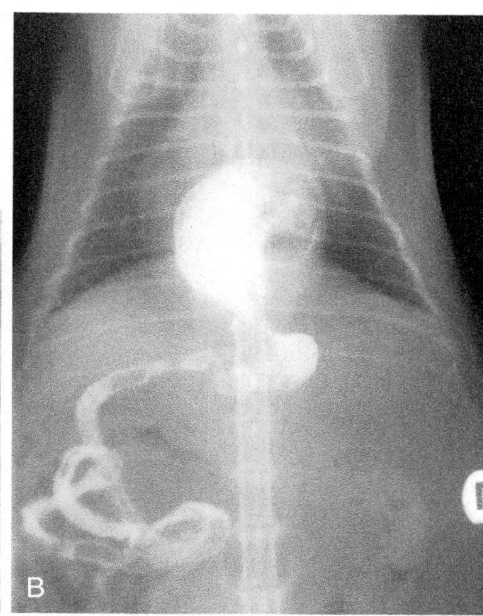

FIGURE 23-7 Lateral (**A**) and ventrodorsal (**B**) esophagrams of a cat with a hiatal hernia showing protrusion of the distal esophagus and stomach through the esophageal hiatus of the diaphragm into the thoracic cavity. *(Courtesy Dr. John Graham.)*

Hiatal Hernia

Disorders of the hiatus are rare in cats. Hiatal hernia is protrusion of the distal esophagus and stomach through the esophageal hiatus of the diaphragm into the thoracic cavity; the protrusion may be intermittent ("sliding") or persistent. Other organs are occasionally involved, such as the omentum.[40] This is distinct from a gastroesophageal intussusception where the stomach is prolapsed into the lumen of the distal esophagus.[35,49] Both congenital and traumatic hiatal hernias have been described in cats.[9,23,41,42,52] Congenital hernias appear to be more common than acquired hernias, and affected cats typically present with clinical signs before 1 year of age. It is suspected that increased inspiratory effort associated with upper airway obstruction, such as a nasopharyngeal polyp, may also lead to development of hiatal hernia.[23]

Hiatal herniation reduces lower esophageal sphincter pressure. Clinical signs associated with hiatal hernia, such as intermittent vomiting and regurgitation, may be because of reflux esophagitis, hypomotility, or obstruction. Large hernias and secondary aspiration pneumonia may be associated with respiratory distress. Survey radiographs may reveal a gas-filled soft tissue density in the caudal dorsal mediastinum. An esophagram will show the gastroesophageal junction and gastric rugae cranial to the diaphragm (Figure 23-7). Both fluoroscopy and endoscopy may be useful for diagnosis but are not typically necessary.

The prognosis for cats with hiatal hernia is considered to be good. A trial of medical management (as for reflux esophagitis) for 1 month has been recommended before surgery.[34] Surgery is the treatment of choice for large defects, especially in young cats with congenital disease or cats that have failed medical management. Various reconstructive surgical techniques have been described.[14]

References

1. Adamama-Moraitou KK, Rallis TS, Prassinos NN et al: Benign esophageal stricture in the dog and cat: a retrospective study of 20 cases, *Can J Vet Res* 66:55, 2002.
2. Augusto M, Kraijer M, Pratschke KM: Chronic oesophageal foreign body in a cat, *J Feline Med Surg* 7:237, 2005.
3. Battersby I, Doyle R: Use of a biodegradable self-expanding stent in the management of a benign oesophageal stricture in a cat, *J Small Anim Pract* 51:49, 2009.
4. Beatty JA, Swift N, Foster DJ et al: Suspected clindamycin-associated oesophageal injury in cats: five cases, *J Feline Med Surg* 8:412, 2006.
5. Bebchuk TN: Feline gastrointestinal foreign bodies, *Vet Clin North Am Small Anim Pract* 32:861, 2002.
6. Bennett AD, MacPhail CM, Gibbons DS et al: A comparative study evaluating the esophageal transit time of eight healthy cats when pilled with the FlavoRx pill glide versus pill delivery treats, *J Feline Med Surg* 12:286, 2010.
7. Berube D, Scott-Moncrieff JC, Rohleder J et al: Primary esophageal squamous cell carcinoma in a cat, *J Am Anim Hosp Assoc* 45:291, 2009.
8. Bissett SA, Davis J, Subler K et al: Risk factors and outcome of bougienage for treatment of benign esophageal strictures in dogs and cats: 28 cases (1995-2004), *J Am Vet Med Assoc* 235:844, 2009.
9. Brinkley CH: Hiatus hernia in a cat, *Vet Rec* 127:46, 1990.
10. Byron JK, Shadwick SR, Bennett AR: Megaesophagus in a 6-month-old cat secondary to a nasopharyngeal polyp, *J Feline Med Surg* 12:322, 2010.
11. Cottrell BD: Post anaesthetic oesophageal stricture in the cat, *Vet Rec* 118:645, 1986.

12. Durocher L, Johnson SE, Green E: Esophageal diverticulum associated with a trichobezoar in a cat, *J Am Anim Hosp Assoc* 45:142, 2009.
13. Forbes DC, Leishman DE: Megaesophagus in a cat, *Can Vet J* 26:354, 1985.
14. Fossum T, Hedlund C: Surgery of the digestive system. In Fossum TW, editor: *Small animal surgery*, ed 3, St Louis, 2007, Mosby Elsevier, p 339.
15. Galatos AD, Rallis T, Raptopoulos D: Post anaesthetic oesophageal stricture formation in three cats, *J Small Anim Pract* 35:638, 1994.
16. Galatos AD, Savas I, Prassinos NN et al: Gastro-oesophageal reflux during thiopentone or propofol anaesthesia in the cat, *J Vet Med A Physiol Pathol Clin Med* 48:287, 2001.
17. German AJ, Cannon MJ, Dye C et al: Oesophageal strictures in cats associated with doxycycline therapy, *J Feline Med Surg* 7:33, 2005.
18. Glanemann B, Hildebrandt N, Schneider MA et al: Recurrent single oesophageal stricture treated with a self-expanding stent in a cat, *J Feline Med Surg* 10:505, 2008.
19. Glazer A, Walters P: Esophagitis and esophageal strictures, *Comp Contin Edu Pract Vet* 30:281, 2008.
20. Graham J, Lipman A, Newell S et al: Esophageal transit of capsules in clinically normal cats, *Am J Vet Res* 61:655, 2000.
21. Griffin B, Beard DM, Klopfenstein KA: Use of butter to facilitate the passage of tablets through the esophagus in cats [abstract], *J Vet Intern Med* 17:445, 2003.
22. Gualtieri M, Monzeglio MG, Di Giancamillo M: Oesophageal squamous cell carcinoma in two cats, *J Small Anim Pract* 40:79, 1999.
23. Gualtieri M, Olivero D: Reflux esophagitis in three cats associated with metaplastic columnar esophageal epithelium, *J Am Anim Hosp Assoc* 42:65, 2006.
24. Han E, Broussard J, Baer K: Feline esophagitis secondary to gastroesophageal reflux disease: clinical signs and radiographic, endoscopic, and histopathologic findings, *J Am Anim Hosp Assoc* 39:161, 2003.
25. Happe RP, van der Gaag I, Wolvekamp WT et al: Esophageal squamous cell carcinoma in two cats, *Tijdschr Diergeneeskd* 103: 1080, 1978.
26. Harai BH, Johnson SE, Sherding RG: Endoscopically guided balloon dilatation of benign esophageal strictures in 6 cats and 7 dogs, *J Vet Intern Med* 9:332, 1995.
27. Hashim MA, Waterman AE: Effects of thiopentone, propofol, alphaxalone-alphadolone, ketamine and xylazine-ketamine on lower oesophageal sphincter pressure and barrier pressure in cats, *Vet Rec* 129:137, 1991.
28. Hashim MA, Waterman AE: Effects of acepromazine, pethidine and atropine premedication on lower oesophageal sphincter pressure and barrier pressure in anaesthetised cats, *Vet Rec* 133:158, 1993.
29. Hoenig M, Mahaffey MB, Parnell PG et al: Megaesophagus in two cats, *J Am Vet Med Assoc* 196:763, 1990.
30. Jaspersen D: Drug-induced oesophageal disorders: pathogenesis, incidence, prevention and management, *Drug Saf* 22:237, 2000.
31. Joseph R, Kuzi S, Lavy E et al: Transient megaoesophagus and oesophagitis following diaphragmatic rupture repair in a cat, *J Feline Med Surg* 10:284, 2008.
32. Leib MS, Dinnel H, Ward DL et al: Endoscopic balloon dilation of benign esophageal strictures in dogs and cats, *J Vet Intern Med* 15:547, 2001.
33. Lobetti R, Leisewitz A: Gastroesophageal reflux in two cats, *Feline Pract* 24:5, 1996.
34. Lorinson D, Bright RM: Long-term outcome of medical and surgical treatment of hiatal hernias in dogs and cats: 27 cases (1978-1996), *J Am Vet Med Assoc* 213:381, 1998.
35. Martinez NI, Cook W, Troy GC et al: Intermittent gastroesophageal intussusception in a cat with idiopathic megaesophagus, *J Am Anim Hosp Assoc* 37:234, 2001.
36. McGrotty Y, Knottenbelt C: Oesophageal stricture in a cat due to oral administration of tetracycline, *J Small Anim Pract* 43:221, 2002.
37. Melendez L, Twedt D, Wright M: Suspected doxycycline-induced esophagitis with esophageal stricture formation in three cats, *Feline Pract* 28:10, 2000.
38. Melendez LD, Twedt DC, Weyrauch EA et al: Conservative therapy using balloon dilation for intramural, inflammatory esophageal strictures in dogs and cats: a retrospective study of 23 cases (1987-1997), *Eur J Comp Gastroenterol* 3:31, 1998.
39. Michels G, Jones B, Huss B et al: Endoscopic and surgical retrieval of fishhooks from the stomach and esophagus in dogs and cats: 75 cases (1977-1993), *J Am Vet Med Assoc* 207:1194, 1995.
40. Mitsuoka K, Tanaka R, Nagashima Y et al: Omental herniation through the esophageal hiatus in a cat, *J Vet Med Sci* 64:1157, 2002.
41. Owen MC, Morris PJ, Bateman RS: Concurrent gastro-oesophageal intussusception, trichobezoar and hiatal hernia in a cat, *N Z Vet J* 53:371, 2005.
42. Papazoglou L, Patsikas M, Rallis T et al: Hiatal hernia with esophageal stricture in a cat, *Feline Pract* 28:10, 2000.
43. Pearson H, Darke PG, Gibbs C et al: Reflux oesophagitis and stricture formation after anaesthesia: a review of seven cases in dogs and cats, *J Small Anim Pract* 19:507, 1978.
44. Ridgway MD, Graves TK: Megaesophagus, *Clin Brief* 8:43, 2010.
45. Sellon RK, Willard MD: Esophagitis and esophageal strictures, *Vet Clin North Am Sm Anim Pract* 33:945, 2003.
46. Shinozuka J, Nakayama H, Suzuki M et al: Esophageal adenosquamous carcinoma in a cat, *J Vet Med Sci* 63:91, 2001.
47. Sideri AI, Galatos AD, Kazakos GM et al: Gastro-oesophageal reflux during anaesthesia in the kitten: comparison between use of a laryngeal mask airway or an endotracheal tube, *Vet Anaesth Analg* 36:547, 2009.
48. Trumble C: Oesophageal stricture in cats associated with use of the hyclate (hydrochloride) salt of doxycycline [letter], *J Feline Med Surg* 7:241, 2005.
49. Van Camp S, Love N, Kumaresan S: Gastroesophageal intussusception in a cat, *Vet Radiol Ultrasound* 39:190, 1998.
50. Van Geffen C, Saunders JH, Vandevelde B et al: Idiopathic megaoesophagus and intermittent gastro-oesophageal intussusception in a cat, *J Small Anim Pract* 47:471, 2006.
51. Van Stee EW, Ward CL, Duffy ML: Recurrent esophageal hairballs in a cat (a case report), *Vet Med* 75:1873, 1980.
52. Waldron DR, Moon M, Leib MS et al: Oesophageal hiatal hernia in two cats, *J Small Anim Pract* 31:259, 1990.
53. Westfall D, Twedt D, Steyn P et al: Evaluation of esophageal transit of tablets and capsules in 30 cats, *J Vet Intern Med* 15:467, 2001.
54. Weyrauch E, Willard M: Esophagitis and benign esophageal strictures, *Comp Contin Edu Pract Vet* 20:203, 1998.
55. Willard M: Clinical manifestations of gastrointestinal disorders. In Nelson RW, Couto CG, editors: *Small animal internal medicine*, ed 4, St Louis, 2009, Mosby Elsevier, p 351.
56. Yarim M, Gultiken ME, Ozturk S et al: Double aortic arch in a Siamese cat, *Vet Pathol* 36:340, 1999.

DISEASES OF THE STOMACH

Susan E. Little

The stomach is a frequent site for gastrointestinal problems in cats, and the most common gastric problems are described in this chapter. Some conditions such as gastric dilatation-volvulus are often reported in dogs but rarely reported in cats. In one report of three feline cases, all were associated with diaphragmatic hernia.[15] Gastric parasites, the diagnostic approach to the vomiting cat,

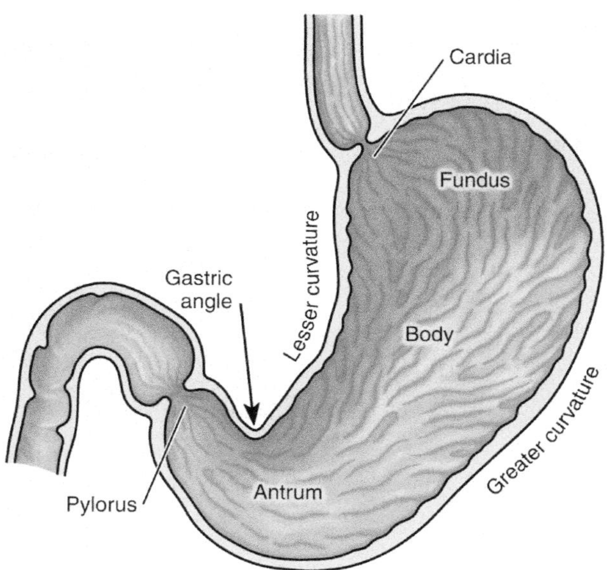

FIGURE 23-8 The five regions of the feline stomach. *(From Twedt DC: Diseases of the stomach. In Sherding RG, editor:* The cat: diseases and clinical management, *ed 2, Philadelphia, 1994, Saunders, Figure 38-1, p 1182.)*

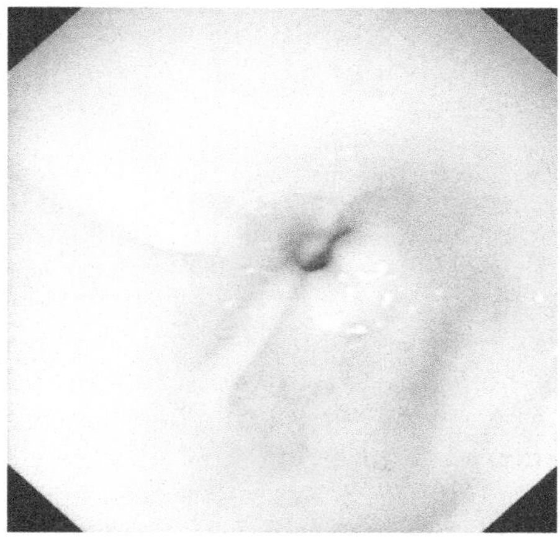

FIGURE 23-9 Endoscopic view of the normal feline pylorus. The pylorus is readily visible during endoscopic examination, and may be open or closed. *(Courtesy Prof. Danièlle Gunn-Moore.)*

and therapeutics for vomiting are covered elsewhere in this chapter.

The anatomy of the feline stomach is similar to that of other mammals having a simple glandular stomach. Most of the stomach is situated on the left side of the abdominal cavity. It has five regions, starting from the lower esophageal sphincter: cardia, fundus, body, antrum, and pylorus (Figure 23-8). The pylorus of the cat is unique compared with other species in that it is narrow and has high resistance in order to maintain a tight seal (Figure 23-9). The normal stomach has a characteristic appearance when viewed using endoscopy (Figure 23-10) or ultrasonography (Figure 23-11).

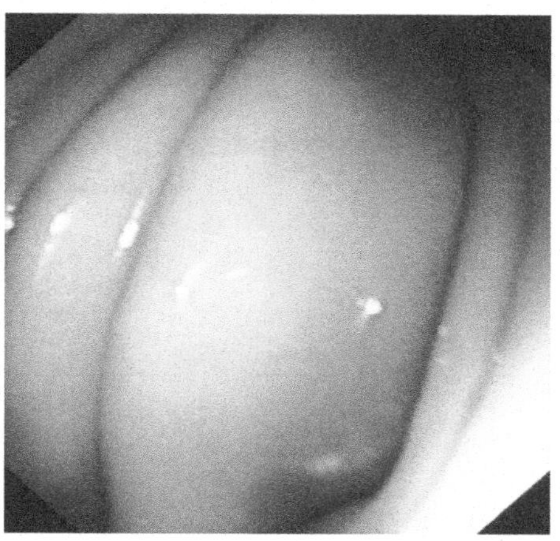

FIGURE 23-10 Endoscopic appearance of normal gastric folds in the cat. Prominent rugal folds are visible in the greater curvature of the stomach. *(Courtesy Prof. Danièlle Gunn-Moore.)*

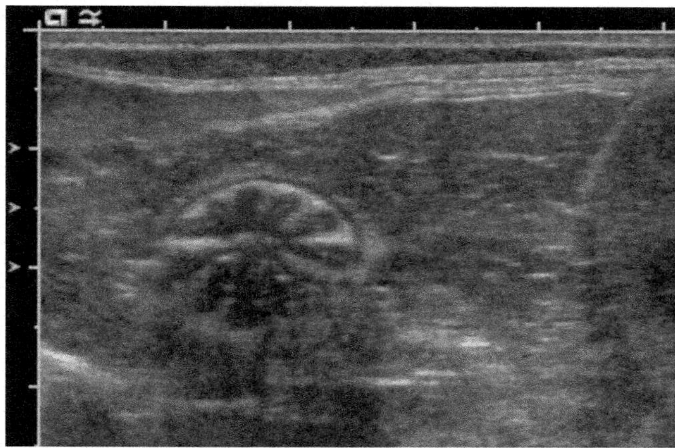

FIGURE 23-11 Ultrasonographic appearance of the normal feline stomach showing the characteristic rosette or wagon wheel appearance. *(Courtesy Dr. John Graham.)*

The gastric emptying time of normal cats is shorter than that of other mammals. In one study, the gastric emptying half-time for solid food in normal cats was 1.4 to 3.6 hours.[53] This implies prolonged fasting (longer than 8 hours) in preparation for anesthesia and surgery is unnecessary.

CLINICAL PRESENTATION

The main clinical sign of gastric disease is vomiting, but it is important to note that vomiting is also associated with many nongastric problems, including concurrent intestinal disease, such as enteritis or colitis. Vomiting patients therefore require a thorough physical examination and diagnostic plan to determine the cause. Vomiting must be distinguished from regurgitation, which is primarily associated with esophageal disease (see Table 23-10). Vomitus often contains food, hair, refluxed bile, or blood. Fresh blood may appear as large or small clots. Older blood clots have a brown "coffee ground" appearance. Gastric bleeding may also cause melena. Other clinical signs may be associated with gastric disease, such as anorexia, weight loss, pain, lethargy, bloating, and nausea.

SPECIFIC DISEASES

Gastritis

Gastritis may be acute or chronic in nature, and this distinction may be useful in assessing the potential cause. For example, cats with acute gastritis may be suspected of foreign body or plant ingestion, drug or toxin exposure (see Chapter 31), or dietary indiscretion. Cats with chronic gastritis may be suspected of parasitism, *Helicobacter* spp. infection, or dietary intolerance or hypersensitivity (see Chapter 17). Chronic lymphocytic plasmacytic gastritis of unknown etiology is also a common cause of chronic vomiting. Whenever possible, a specific underlying cause should be sought and treated.

Acute Uncomplicated Gastritis

Patients with sudden onset of vomiting may have an obvious cause in the history (e.g., dietary indiscretion), but in many cases, the cause is not apparent. Abdominal radiographs should be taken if foreign body ingestion is possible, especially in a young cat. If the patient is systemically well, further diagnostic testing may be postponed pending response to therapy. Treatment for uncomplicated acute gastritis is symptomatic and supportive. Clinical signs are expected to resolve in 24 to 48 hours; if signs persist, re-evaluation and further investigation is warranted. Subcutaneous fluid therapy using an isotonic balanced electrolyte solution may be used to correct mild fluid deficits (<5%). Oral intake of fluids and food should be discontinued for up to 24 hours. A highly digestible diet, either commercial or homemade, is introduced with a gradual transition back to the normal diet over the next several days.

Antiemetic therapy may be indicated for acute uncomplicated gastritis if the vomiting is frequent or the cat has signs of nausea (see Table 23-3). Protectants, such as kaolin and pectin, are difficult to administer to cats and are without proven efficacy. Bismuth subsalicylate is controversial; it is considered contraindicated by some experts, because of the cat's sensitivity to salicylates,[39] yet is commonly used in clinical practice.

Foreign Body Ingestion

Cats ingest foreign bodies less commonly than dogs. In one study of 208 cases of gastrointestinal foreign body ingestion, only 12% were in cats.[22] Foreign body ingestion is most likely to be seen in young cats and may involve a wide variety of objects, including linear objects (e.g., dental floss, thread with or without a needle, tinsel, string). The owner may or may not be aware of the ingestion. Ingestion of multiple foreign bodies may be seen in cats with pica (Figure 23-12). In one case report, a young domestic shorthair cat required gastrotomy for removal of 32 copper pennies.[43] Some patients require multiple surgeries, because of repeated foreign body ingestion.[22] In such cases, a behavioral diagnosis should be sought and treatment instituted (see Chapter 13).

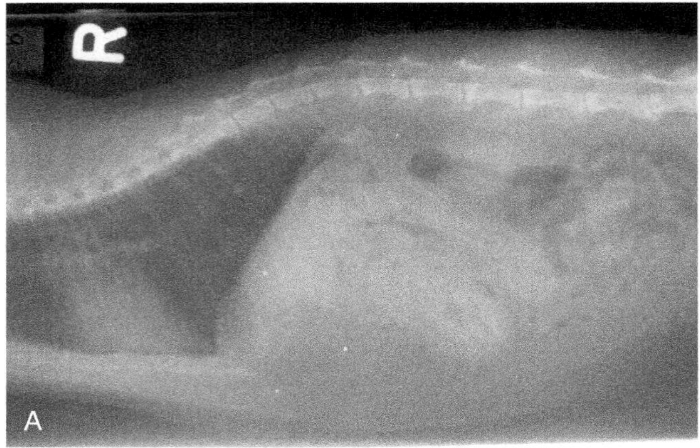

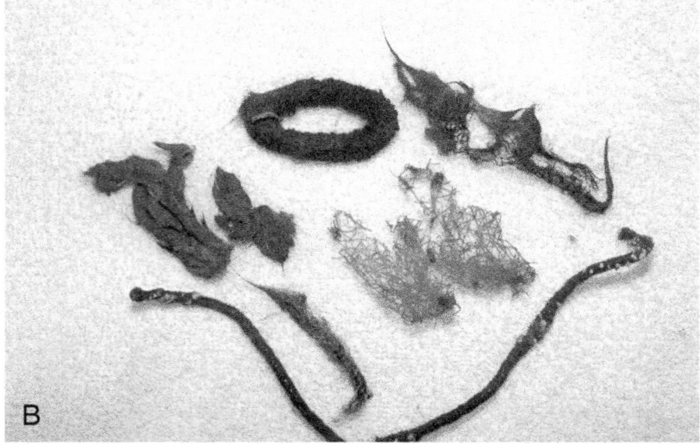

FIGURE 23-12 **A**, Abdominal radiograph of a 4-year-old female Siamese cat presented for vomiting pieces of hair elastics. **B**, Variety of objects removed by gastrotomy from the same cat; this was the second surgery for this patient for ingesting multiple foreign objects.

Trichobezoars (large masses of hair) also represent a type of foreign object. Both long- and shorthaired cats may be affected. Hair is normally ingested during grooming and is eliminated in vomitus and feces. Cats lack the strong peristaltic contractions ("housekeeper" contractions) that clear the stomach of undigested contents normally found in other species. This may explain why cats seem to be susceptible to gastric trichobezoars. Gastric motility dysfunction is suspected to cause repeated gastric trichobezoars in some cats. Intestinal[3,22] and esophageal[14,59] obstruction with trichobezoars has also been documented. Traditional treatments for cats with recurrent trichobezoars include regular grooming, shaving the hair coat of long-haired cats, flea control,

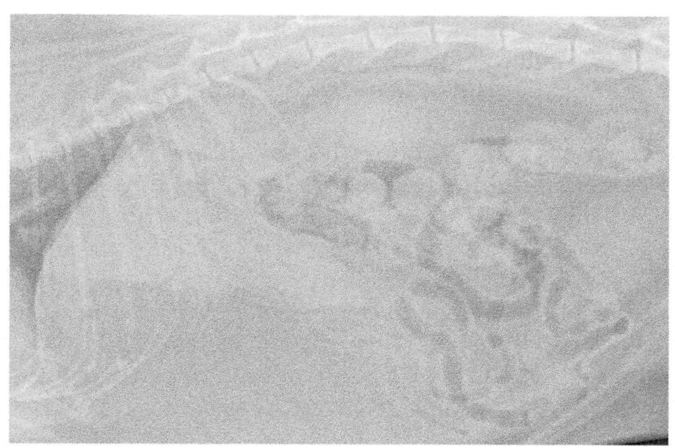

FIGURE 23-13 Abdominal radiograph of a cat with a large gastric trichobezoar. *(Courtesy Dr. John Graham.)*

treatment of underlying dermatologic disorders, and administration of semisolid petroleum laxatives. More recently, commercial diets have been formulated for control of trichobezoars. Cats with recurrent trichobezoars causing illness and suspected motility disorders may benefit from treatment with prokinetic drugs such as cisapride.

Clinical signs of gastric foreign bodies are variable but typically involve intermittent or persistent vomiting because of gastric outflow obstruction, distention, and mucosal irritation. Gastric obstruction may be partial or total. Patients with complete obstruction will present with more dramatic signs, including anorexia and depression. The base of the tongue should always be examined, because linear foreign bodies are sometimes anchored either in this location, or they may be lodged in the pylorus, causing intestinal plication. Gastric foreign bodies may also be asymptomatic and found incidentally.[5] Physical examination may be unremarkable or may reveal dehydration or abdominal pain. If the stomach is markedly distended, the foreign body may be palpable in some patients.

Survey radiographs are always indicated when foreign body ingestion is suspected. Radiopaque foreign bodies may be readily diagnosed, although some, along with radiolucent objects, will require a contrast study for diagnosis (Figure 23-13). Barium is commonly used as a contrast agent, although if gastric perforation is suspected, an aqueous iodinated agent is preferred. Ultrasonography is also useful for detection of gastrointestinal foreign bodies.[56]

Removal of some foreign bodies can be attempted endoscopically, particularly if the object does not have sharp edges and is not too large. Successful removal of fish hooks, particularly single-barb hooks, using endoscopy has been described.[35] Otherwise, foreign objects are best removed using gastrotomy through a ventral midline laparotomy. A radiograph should always be taken just before surgery to ensure the object has not moved further down the gastrointestinal tract.

Postoperative management after gastrotomy includes maintenance of hydration and electrolyte balance. Hypokalemia is common with anorexia and vomiting and should be treated by supplementation of IV fluids with 20 to 40 mEq/L potassium chloride (not to exceed 0.5 mEq/kg/hour). Refractory vomiting should be treated with an antiemetic. A highly digestible diet can be introduced the day after surgery. In general, the prognosis for recovery is good. In one study, 88% of cats with gastrointestinal foreign bodies survived to discharge.[22] Those cats that did not survive had linear foreign bodies of long-standing duration with subsequent peritonitis.

Helicobacter *Gastritis*

Helicobacter are spiral or curved gram-negative bacteria that inhabit the glands, parietal cells, and mucus of the gastric antrum and fundus. *Helicobacter* contain large amounts of urease, which alters the pH in the vicinity of the bacteria and allows for colonization of the acidic environment of the stomach. In the early 1980s, the discovery of the association of *Helicobacter pylori* with gastric disease (gastritis, peptic ulcers, and neoplasia) in humans revolutionized treatment of those diseases. Since then, *Helicobacter* spp. have been associated with gastric disease in various veterinary species, including cats and dogs. Several *Helicobacter* spp. (e.g., *H. heilmannii, H. bizzozeronii, H. felis*) have been identified in cats, some of which have the potential to infect humans, although transmission is thought to be rare.[19,48] The prevalence of *Helicobacter* infection in cats varies geographically and may be very high (>40%) in some locations.[1,27,37,47,58]

The importance of *Helicobacter* as a cause of gastric disease is cats is unclear; the bacteria may be found in the stomach of both clinically normal cats and cats with gastritis. The prevalence of *Helicobacter* infection is not higher in cats with gastritis compared with normal cats.[61] Determination of the role of *Helicobacter* is also hampered by the paucity of controlled clinical trials that evaluate eradication of gastritis and clinical signs in infected cats.

An immune response to infection characterized by gastric lymphoid hyperplasia is common, although the local immune response in cats is generally less severe than the response in humans infected with *H. pylori*. To date gastrointestinal ulcers have not been associated with *Helicobacter* infection in cats. Recent studies have suggested a possible association between *Helicobacter* infection and gastric lymphoma in cats, although more research is needed to confirm the association and understand the pathogenesis.[7,32] *Helicobacter* spp. may be commensal in most cats, and perhaps loss of tolerance explains the development of gastritis in some individuals.[49] Another possibility is that the inflammatory response is normally well managed and disease may result when there is an abnormality of the immunoregulatory system.[21]

The most commonly used methods for diagnosis of *Helicobacter* infection in cats are based on gastric specimens obtained during endoscopy (or laparotomy): exfoliative cytology, histopathologic examination of biopsy specimens, and rapid urease testing of biopsy specimens.[28] However, it is important to note that even when *Helicobacter* organisms are identified, the infection may not be the cause of the patient's clinical signs, and other causes of vomiting should always be evaluated.

Exfoliative cytology is the least expensive and most easily performed diagnostic test. In one study, it was also the most sensitive diagnostic method when compared with urease testing and histologic examination.[20] Brush cytology samples gathered during endoscopy are air-dried on microscope slides and stained with Wright's stain. The slide is examined at 100× magnification under oil immersion. Spiral bacteria are readily seen if present. At least 10 oil-immersion fields on two slides should be examined before determining a specimen is negative for *Helicobacter*-like organisms.[28]

Since *Helicobacter* produce abundant urease, a rapid urease test (e.g., CLOtest, Ballard Medical Products, Draper, Utah) may be used for diagnosis.[38] The kit consists of an agar gel impregnated with urea and a pH indicator. A gastric biopsy sample is applied to the gel, and if urease is present, ammonia will form and change the pH (and thus the color) of the gel. The gel may change color rapidly (within 30 minutes), but 24 hours must elapse before the test can be considered negative.[28] The more rapidly the color changes, the higher the bacterial load. Both false-positive and false-negative results are possible with rapid urease testing for various reasons, giving the test a sensitivity of 70% to 90%.[28,37]

Histopathologic examination of gastric biopsy samples using hemotoxylin and eosin (H&E) or silver stains is highly sensitive and specific in human studies for detection of *Helicobacter*-like organisms. The organisms are not equally distributed; so, examination of biopsy specimens from multiple sites will increase sensitivity. The bacteria may be seen in mucus on the surface epithelium as well as in the gastric pits, glandular lumen, and parietal cells. Organisms may also be seen submucosally within gastric lymphoid follicles.[46] Histopathologic examination of biopsy samples also allows for assessment of other abnormalities. Mild to severe lymphocytic-plasmacytic or lymphocytic gastritis may be present.

In humans combination therapy with antibiotics and antisecretory drugs is recommended to reduce the risk of gastric ulcers and cancer from *H. pylori* infection. Treatment is highly successful at eradicating both clinical signs and histologic changes in the gastric mucosa. Since *Helicobacter* infection is common in cats, yet no clear pathogenic role has been established, it is difficult to know when treatment should be attempted. One expert recommends treating only patients with clinical signs of gastritis that have biopsy-confirmed *Helicobacter* infection with a treatment regimen of amoxicillin (20 mg/kg, every 12 hours, PO), clarithromycin (7.5 mg/kg, every 12 hours, PO) and metronidazole (10 mg/kg, every 12 hours, PO) for 14 days.[49] A common dilemma would be determining the treatment of choice for patients with lymphoplasmacytic inflammation of the stomach and small intestine and confirmed *Helicobacter* infection. Are such patients best treated for inflammatory bowel disease, *Helicobacter* infection, or both? Currently, guidelines for determining the best treatment approach are lacking.

Also, few studies on the efficacy of combination therapy have been conducted in cats. Long-term eradication of infection may be difficult, and histopathologic resolution of gastritis may not be possible, which raises the question of whether *Helicobacter* is the true underlying cause.[38,41] In one study, two cats with clinical gastritis and *Helicobacter* infection were treated with oral metronidazole, amoxicillin, and bismuth subsalicylate for 3 weeks and were also fed a commercial elimination diet.[25] Posttreatment gastric biopsies were obtained a mean of 7 weeks after the cessation of treatment. Resolution of clinical signs occurred rapidly, and clearance of *Helicobacter* spp. was achieved at that time point, but gastric inflammation persisted in post-treatment biopsies. In another study, 13 cats with asymptomatic *Helicobacter* infection were treated with oral omeprazole, amoxicillin, metronidazole, and clarithromycin for 14 days.[26] Treatment failed to eradicate infection in 4 of the cats based on molecular analysis of post-treatment gastric biopsies. It is unclear if treatment failure is because of recrudescence or reinfection.

The reader is referred to excellent reviews of *Helicobacter* in cats for more information.[27,38,48]

Chronic Gastritis

Chronic gastritis is common in cats with chronic intermittent vomiting. *Ollulanus tricuspis* is a worm that infects the stomach of cats, causing chronic gastritis, and it is difficult to diagnose (see below, Gastrointestinal Parasites). The worm is occasionally found on histologic examination of gastric biopsy samples.[9] It is reasonable to treat empirically (fenbendazole 10 mg/kg, once daily, PO × 2 days) for this parasite when the cause of gastritis is not apparent.[49]

The frequency of vomiting in cats with chronic gastritis is highly variable, ranging from once or twice per week (and not necessarily every week) to more than once daily. Most patients are otherwise well, although other clinical signs (inappetence, anorexia, depression, or weight loss) are possible depending on disease severity. Results of routine laboratory testing are typically normal but may show neutrophilic leukocytosis,

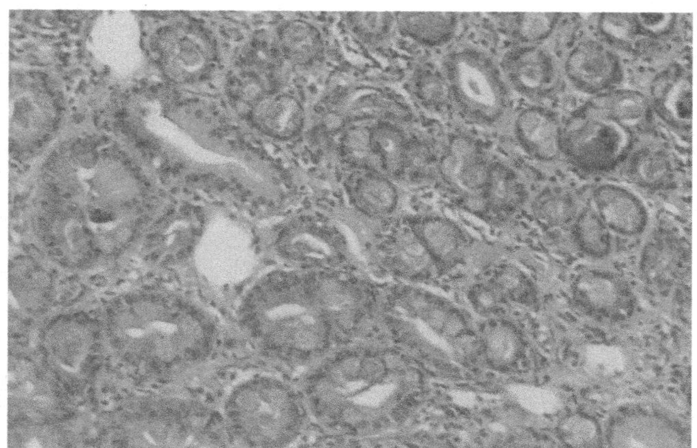

FIGURE 23-14 Histopathologic image (40×) of a stomach biopsy from a 10-year-old cat with a history of chronic vomiting. Small lymphocytes are increased in number in the lamina propria; cellular debris is evident within some gastric glands. *(Courtesy Dr. Sally Lester.)*

eosinophilia, or hypoproteinemia. Survey and contrast radiographs are often normal.

The most common finding on histopathologic examination of biopsy samples is lymphocytic plasmacytic (LP) gastritis (Figure 23-14). Some patients will also have concurrent evidence of LP inflammation in the small intestine, pancreas, and/or liver. Such patients will be treated for their concurrent problem; treatment of inflammatory bowel disease, pancreatitis, and cholangiohepatitis is covered elsewhere in this chapter.

Some cats with chronic LP gastritis respond to treatment for dietary intolerance or hypersensitivity with a limited antigen diet (see Chapter 17). Patients with moderate to severe LP gastritis may be best treated with a limited antigen diet and immunosuppressive therapy (prednisolone 1 to 2 mg/kg/day, PO tapering to every other day at the lowest dose that controls clinical signs). Patients that fail this initial treatment approach may require additional immunosuppressive therapy, such as chlorambucil (see Table 23-9).

Occasionally, cats with chronic gastritis are diagnosed with eosinophilic inflammation on histopathologic examination of biopsy specimens. Treatment is similar to that for LP gastritis, although such patients should be evaluated for evidence of hypereosinophilic syndrome and eosinophilic enteritis. Eosinophilic fibrosing gastritis was suspected to be caused by toxoplasmosis in one case report.[33]

Gastric Ulceration

Gastric or gastroduodenal ulcerations are uncommon in the cat compared with the dog and may be caused by a variety of disorders, both gastric and nongastric.[29] Classical clinical signs include vomiting, hematemesis, and melena. However, in one review of eight cats, hematemesis and melena were present in less than one third of cases.[29] Depending on the underlying cause and severity of disease, abdominal pain, anorexia, lethargy, pale mucous membranes, and drooling may also be seen. Cats with neoplastic disease may have prolonged clinical signs and are more likely to present with anorexia and weight loss.[29] Cats with perforated ulcers may or may not present with signs of shock. Diagnosis may be problematic because the clinical signs and physical examination findings are often not specific, even in cats with perforated ulcerations.[8]

The causes of gastric ulceration in cats are not well characterized. In dogs the most common cause is the administration of ulcerogenic drugs, particularly NSAIDs, either alone or in combination with corticosteroids. Several cases of NSAID-induced gastroduodenal ulceration or perforation have been reported in cats.[8,34,45] Additional cases may be reported in the future, because long-term administration of these drugs is gaining in popularity for treatment of chronic diseases such as osteoarthritis. NSAIDs cause direct mucosal damage and interfere with prostaglandin synthesis. Although inhibition of the COX-1 enzyme is thought to be the cause of adverse effects, such as gastric ulceration, even COX-2–selective drugs have been associated with adverse effects, and safety in sick cats is not well evaluated. Recently, guidelines for the long-term use of NSAIDs in cats were published by the International Society of Feline Medicine and the American Association of Feline Practitioners.[51] The recommendations include administering NSAIDs either with or shortly after food, withholding therapy if inappetence or anorexia develops, determining dose based on lean body weight, and titrating to the lowest effective dose.

Neoplastic causes of gastric ulceration include systemic mastocytosis, mast cell tumor, lymphosarcoma, adenocarcinoma, and gastrinoma (Zollinger-Ellison syndrome). Cats with chronic renal disease may suffer mucosal damage from uremic toxins and increased gastric acid production secondary to hypergastrinemia (because of decreased renal metabolism of gastrin).[18] Hepatic disease is a cause of gastric ulceration in dogs but is uncommonly reported in cats.[23] Recent anesthesia and surgery have been implicated as a cause of gastric ulceration and perforation, perhaps through hypovolemia, hypoperfusion, or stress.[8,29] Other non-neoplastic causes reported for gastric or gastroduodenal ulceration in cats include parasites (e.g., *Ollulanus tricuspis*, *Toxocara cati*, *Aonchotheca putorii*, *Gnathostoma* spp.), bacterial infections, toxins, inflammatory bowel disease, and foreign bodies. One case report describes a cat with severe gastric ulceration caused by intoxication with *Dieffenbachia* leaves.[36] In some case reports, the cause for the gastric ulcerations could not be determined.

A minimum database should be collected for cats suspected of gastric ulceration, to identify underlying diseases. Anemia, usually regenerative, may be present.

Other findings will be dependent on the presence of underlying diseases; for example, azotemia and isosthenuria may indicate renal disease. Electrolyte and acid–base abnormalities may be because of chronic vomiting and anorexia.

Survey and contrast radiographs and ultrasonography are primarily useful to rule out other causes for the clinical signs, such as foreign bodies. Cats with perforated ulcers may have evidence of pneumoperitoneum (sometimes severe) on plain radiographs or ultrasonographs, and this is an indication for surgical exploration.[6,8,24,31,34] Evidence of peritonitis on imaging studies should be followed with peritoneal fluid analysis. A definitive diagnosis may be made using endoscopy, which allows direct visualization of lesions and collection of biopsy samples. However, some cats with gastric ulceration present in poor condition, which may preclude the use of endoscopy because of anesthetic risk and risk of ulcer perforation.[29] The location of ulcers is typically pyloroantral or fundic in cats with non-neoplastic disease.[8,29] Areas of erosion may appear pale or hemorrhagic; the mucosa is often friable and bleeds easily. Fresh or clotted blood may be seen in the stomach lumen. In some cases, mucosal ulceration must be distinguished from ulcerated tumors. NSAID-induced ulcers are typically found in the antrum and do not have marked mucosal thickening; ulcerated tumors frequently have thickened edges and surrounding mucosa.[49] Biopsy samples should be taken at the periphery of the ulcer to avoid perforation.

Treatment should be directed at any underlying disorder. Treatment for NSAID toxicity is described in Chapter 31. General supportive measures include fluid therapy and electrolyte replacement; blood transfusion may also be required (see Chapter 25). Gastric acid production can be decreased with the use of H_2-receptor blockers or proton pump inhibitors, and sucralfate is used as a mucosal protectant (see Table 23-5). Sucralfate may inhibit absorption of other oral medications and should be given 2 hours apart from other drugs. If vomiting is severe or persistent, antiemetic therapy is warranted (see Table 23-3). Analgesia should be provided for painful patients; a good choice is the opioid buprenorphine (see Table 6-1). Broad-spectrum antibiotic therapy is indicated for patients with significant mucosal barrier dysfunction, perforation, leukopenia and/or neutrophilia, fever, and melena.

Surgical intervention is warranted for patients with life-threatening hemorrhage, failure to respond to medical management, or evidence of perforation.[29] The entire abdominal cavity and gastrointestinal tract should be thoroughly explored to locate extragastrointestinal lesions, non-perforated ulcers, and multiple ulcers. In one case series, nonperforated ulcers were detected at laparotomy by association with adhesions or a gastric mass.[29] Surgical management includes débridement and suturing of the ulcer site as well as collection of biopsy samples for histopathologic examination. The prognosis for recovery was excellent in two studies, particularly for cats with non-neoplastic causes of gastric or gastroduodenal ulceration.[8,29] In one study of seven cats with perforated gastric or duodenal ulcers, the survival rate was low (14%).[23]

Gastric Motility Disorders and Delayed Gastric Emptying

Disorders of gastric motility are better characterized in dogs than in cats. The most common clinical sign is vomiting of undigested food 8 hours or more after a meal. If outflow obstruction is present, vomiting may be projectile. There may also be a history of recurrent trichobezoars. Various disorders are associated with impaired gastric motility, such as chronic gastritis, drug therapy (e.g., anticholinergic and narcotic drugs), dysautonomia, gastric neoplasia, metabolic disorders (e.g., hypokalemia), and temporary postsurgical gastroparesis. In some cases of chronic motility dysfunction, no cause can be identified. Outflow obstruction may be caused by neoplasia, foreign bodies, and extragastric masses. Pyloric stenosis is infrequently documented in young cats, often Siamese cats.[4,40,55]

Since the range of underlying disorders is diverse, the diagnostic approach should allow for detection of both gastric and nongastric disorders. A minimum database (CBC, serum chemistries, urinalysis, feline leukemia virus [FeLV] and feline immunodeficiency virus [FIV] serology) is used to establish overall health status. Radiographs are used to confirm presence of food in the stomach for longer than 8 hours. Ultrasonography may detect gastric lesions, such as masses. Endoscopy is used to identify outflow obstruction as well as other lesions, such as ulcers, and evidence of gastritis.

Assessment of gastric emptying using nuclear scintigraphy is the most accurate method but is limited to referral centers. Gastric emptying times for liquids, canned food, and dry diets have been established using nuclear scintigraphy.[11,16,17] However, emptying times are variable, depending on the amount and type of diet fed as well as the amount of water ingested. Even the shape of kibble affects emptying time.[2] Radiographic contrast series are widely used, but gastric emptying times are variable for barium in either liquid form or mixed with canned food. Contrast radiography using liquid barium (8 to 10 mL/kg) is performed in a fasted patient. Radiographs are taken immediately after administration of the barium and again at 15 and 30 minutes, in some cases, also at 1 and 3 hours. Liquid barium is expected to enter the duodenum no more than 30 minutes after administration, and the stomach should be completely empty of barium within 3 hours. The clinician should be aware that some cats with gastric motility disorders will have a normal gastric emptying time with liquid barium. Barium can also be mixed with canned food and fed as a meal; retention of barium-containing food in the stomach for more than 8 to 12 hours is abnormal.

Gastric emptying time may also be established with the use of barium impregnated polyspheres (BIPS; Med I.D. Systems, Grand Rapids, Mich.) and radiography. Gastric emptying times for BIPS have been established in healthy fasted and fed cats as well as in sedated cats,[10,52] but the values do not correlate well with scintigraphic studies.[17] A mixture of small (1.5 mm) and large (5 mm) spheres are administered with food, and two to four radiographs are taken over the next 24 hours. The small spheres are intended to mimic liquid transit time and the large spheres solid transit time. However, studies assessing the clinical relevance of this method are lacking. One review concluded that BIPS are probably sufficiently sensitive to detect grossly delayed gastric emptying.[60]

Treatment of gastric emptying disorders is directed at identifiable causes. Treatment for gastric ulcers, chronic gastritis, and foreign bodies is described elsewhere in this chapter. Pyloric stenosis is managed surgically. If no outflow obstruction exists, treatment with prokinetic agents, such as metoclopramide or cisapride, may be beneficial (see Table 23-3).

Gastric Neoplasia

Gastric tumors account for less than 1% of malignancies in dogs and cats.[30] Benign gastric tumors are even less common than gastric malignancies. Gastric smooth muscle hamartoma has been reported in one 11-year-old cat.[50] Although adenocarcinoma is the most common gastric cancer of the dog, lymphoma is the most common gastric cancer in the cat. Feline gastrointestinal lymphoma occurs as two major types: small cell (lymphocytic) and the more aggressive large cell (lymphoblastic) form. Small cell lymphomas are more frequently enteric.[57] In one study of 12 cats with gastric lymphoma, diffuse large B-lymphocyte tumors of immunoblastic nuclear type predominated.[42] Gastric lymphoma is not associated with FeLV, and the role of *Helicobacter* in the development of gastric lymphoma in cats requires investigation.[7] Adenocarcinoma,[12,13,54] plasmacytoma,[62] and gastric carcinoid[44] have also been described. The Siamese cat may be predisposed to adenocarcinoma.[12,54] As would be expected, most cats with gastric neoplasia are older cats.

As for most gastric diseases, vomiting is the most common clinical sign of neoplasia. The vomitus may contain blood and melena may be present. Other clinical signs include anorexia, weight loss, bloating, and depression. Perforation of the tumor may occur, leading to pneumoperitoneum or septic peritonitis. Clinical signs present gradually and are often present for weeks to months. Physical examination findings are nonspecific, although occasionally a gastric mass or gastric thickening may be palpated if the stomach is markedly enlarged.

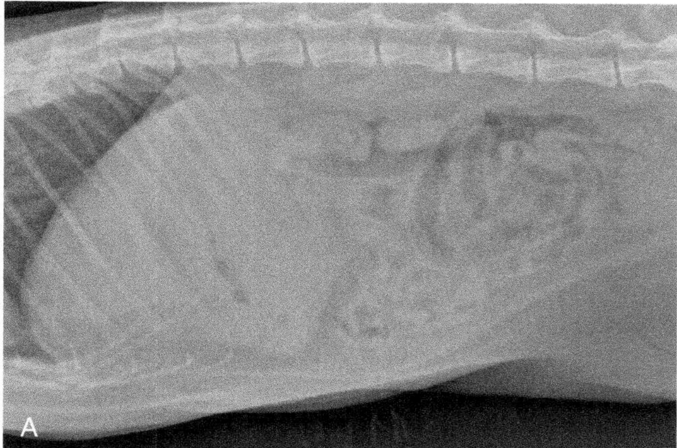

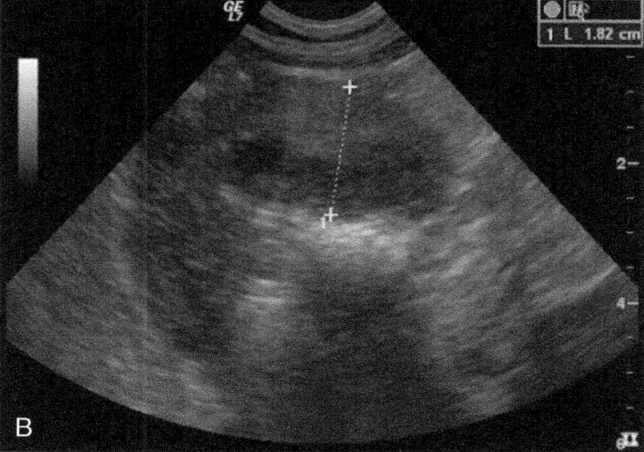

FIGURE 23-15 Radiographic (**A**) and ultrasonographic (**B**) images of a cat with a gastric mass that was determined to be lymphoma on biopsy. *(Courtesy Dr. John Graham.)*

Results of routine diagnostic testing are generally nonspecific; anemia may be associated with ulceration. Survey or contrast radiography may reveal a mass (Figure 23-15, *A*); other findings include delayed gastric emptying, impaired motility, and mucosal ulceration. Ultrasonography is also useful for diagnosis and can be used to guide needle aspirates of masses (Figure 23-15, *B*). Endoscopy allows for visualization of lesions as well as the ability to obtain partial thickness biopsy samples. Problems with interpretation of endoscopic biopsy samples include detection of necrosis, inflammation, and ulceration rather than the primary lesion. In dogs some neoplastic lesions are submucosal, making it very difficult to obtain diagnostic samples by endoscopy. Therefore several biopsies should be taken and masses should be biopsied multiple times in the same place to sample deeper tissues. The center of ulcerated lesions should not be biopsied. Surgical biopsies are more reliable for diagnosis.

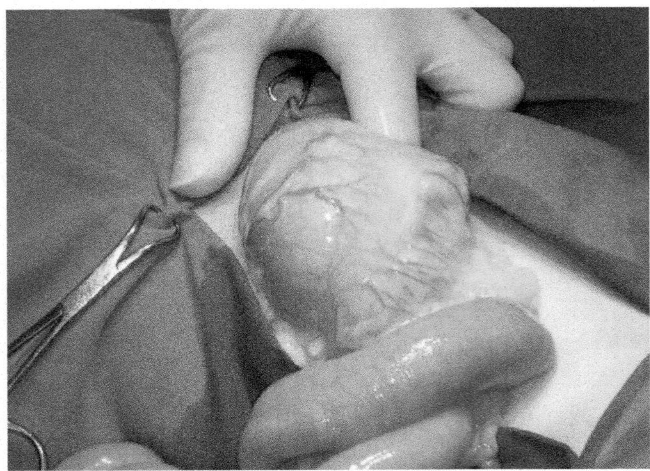

FIGURE 23-16 Surgical appearance of a gastric mass caused by small cell lymphoma. *(Courtesy Dr. Randolph Baral.)*

Surgical resection is the most common treatment for gastric neoplasia other than lymphoma (Figure 23-16). The prognosis for most patients is poor, typically because of debilitation, concurrent diseases, and recurrent or metastatic disease.[30] The success of chemotherapy for lymphoma depends on cell type, with small cell tumors carrying a better prognosis than large cell tumors.

References

1. Araujo IC, Mota SB, de Aquino MHC et al: *Helicobacter* species detection and histopathological changes in stray cats from Niterói, Brazil, *J Feline Med Surg* 12:509, 2010.
2. Armbrust LJ, Hoskinson JJ, Lora-Michiels M et al: Gastric emptying in cats using foods varying in fiber content and kibble shapes, *Vet Radiol Ultrasound* 44:339, 2003.
3. Barrs VR, Beatty JA, Tisdall PL et al: Intestinal obstruction by trichobezoars in five cats, *J Feline Med Surg* 1:199, 1999.
4. Baumberger A: [Pyloric dysfunction as a cause of chronic vomiting in the cat], *Schweiz Arch Tierheilkd* 119:415, 1977.
5. Bebchuk TN: Feline gastrointestinal foreign bodies, *Vet Clin North Am Small Anim Pract* 32:861, 2002.
6. Boysen SR, Tidwell AS, Penninck DG: Ultrasonographic findings in dogs and cats with gastrointestinal perforation, *Vet Radiol Ultrasound* 44:556, 2003.
7. Bridgeford EC, Marini RP, Feng Y et al: Gastric *Helicobacter* species as a cause of feline gastric lymphoma: a viable hypothesis, *Vet Immunol Immunopathol* 123:106, 2008.
8. Cariou MPL, Halfacree ZJ, Lee KCL et al: Successful surgical management of spontaneous gastric perforations in three cats, *J Feline Med Surg* 12:36, 2010.
9. Cecchi R, Wills SJ, Dean R et al: Demonstration of *Ollulanus tricuspis* in the stomach of domestic cats by biopsy, *J Comp Pathol* 134:374, 2006.
10. Chandler M, Guilford G, Lawoko C: Radiopaque markers to evaluate gastric emptying and small intestinal transit time in healthy cats, *J Vet Intern Med* 11:361, 1997.
11. Costello M, Papasouliotis K, Barr FJ et al: Determination of solid- and liquid-phase gastric emptying half times in cats by use of nuclear scintigraphy, *Am J Vet Res* 60:1222, 1999.
12. Cribb AE: Feline gastrointestinal adenocarcinoma: a review and retrospective study, *Can Vet J* 29:709, 1988.
13. Dennis MM, Bennett N, Ehrhart EJ: Gastric adenocarcinoma and chronic gastritis in two related Persian cats, *Vet Pathol* 43:358, 2006.
14. Durocher L, Johnson SE, Green E: Esophageal diverticulum associated with a trichobezoar in a cat, *J Am Anim Hosp Assoc* 45:142, 2009.
15. Formaggini L, Schmidt K, De Lorenzi D: Gastric dilatation-volvulus associated with diaphragmatic hernia in three cats: clinical presentation, surgical treatment and presumptive aetiology, *J Feline Med Surg* 10:198, 2008.
16. Goggin JM, Hoskinson JJ, Butine MD et al: Scintigraphic assessment of gastric emptying of canned and dry diets in healthy cats, *Am J Vet Res* 59:388, 1998.
17. Goggin JM, Hoskinson JJ, Kirk CA et al: Comparison of gastric emptying times in healthy cats simultaneously evaluated with radiopaque markers and nuclear scintigraphy, *Vet Radiol Ultrasound* 40:89, 1999.
18. Goldstein R, Marks S, Kass P et al: Gastrin concentrations in plasma of cats with chronic renal failure, *J Am Vet Med Assoc* 213:826, 1998.
19. Haesebrouck F, Pasmans F, Flahou B et al: Gastric helicobacters in domestic animals and nonhuman primates and their significance for human health, *Clin Microbiol Rev* 22:202, 2009.
20. Happonen I, Saari S, Castren L et al: Comparison of diagnostic methods for detecting gastric *Helicobacter*-like organisms in dogs and cats, *J Comp Pathol* 115:117, 1996.
21. Harbour S, Sutton P: Immunogenicity and pathogenicity of *Helicobacter* infections of veterinary animals, *Vet Immunol Immunopathol* 122:191, 2008.
22. Hayes G: Gastrointestinal foreign bodies in dogs and cats: a retrospective study of 208 cases, *J Small Anim Pract* 50:576, 2009.
23. Hinton L, McLoughlin M, Johnson S et al: Spontaneous gastroduodenal perforation in 16 dogs and seven cats (1982-1999), *J Am Anim Hosp Assoc* 38:176, 2002.
24. Itoh T, Nibe K, Naganobu K: Tension pneumoperitoneum because of gastric perforation in a cat, *J Vet Med Sci* 67:617, 2005.
25. Jergens AE, Pressel M, Crandell J et al: Fluorescence in situ hybridization confirms clearance of visible *Helicobacter* spp. associated with gastritis in dogs and cats, *J Vet Intern Med* 23:16, 2009.
26. Khoshnegah J, Jamshidi S, Mohammadi M, Sasani F: The efficacy and safety of long-term *Helicobacter* species quadruple therapy in asymptomatic cats with naturally acquired infection, *J Feline Med Surg* 13:88, 2011.
27. Lecoindre P, Chevallier M, Peyrol S et al: Gastric heliocbacters in cats, *J Feline Med Surg* 2:19, 2000.
28. Leib M, Duncan R: Diagnosing gastric *Helicobacter* infections in dogs and cats, *Comp Contin Edu Pract Vet* 27:221, 2005.
29. Liptak J, Hunt G, Barrs V et al: Gastroduodenal ulceration in cats: eight cases and a review of the literature, *J Feline Med Surg* 4:27, 2002.
30. Liptak JM, Withrow SJ: Cancer of the gastrointestinal tract. In Withrow SJ, Vail DM, editors: *Withrow & MacEwen's small animal clinical oncology*, ed 4, St Louis, 2007, Saunders Elsevier, p 455.
31. Lykken JD, Brisson BA, Etue SM: Pneumoperitoneum secondary to a perforated gastric ulcer in a cat, *J Am Vet Med Assoc* 222:1713, 2003.
32. Marini RP, Fox JG, White H et al: *Helicobacter* spp. influences the development of primary gastric lymphoma in cats: a viable hypothesis, *Gut* 49:A52, 2001.
33. McConnell JF, Sparkes AH, Blunden AS et al: Eosinophilic fibrosing gastritis and toxoplasmosis in a cat, *J Feline Med Surg* 9:82, 2007.
34. Mellanby RJ, Baines EA, Herrtage ME: Spontaneous pneumoperitoneum in two cats, *J Small Anim Pract* 43:543, 2002.
35. Michels G, Jones B, Huss B et al: Endoscopic and surgical retrieval of fishhooks from the stomach and esophagus in dogs and cats: 75 cases (1977-1993), *J Am Vet Med Assoc* 207:1194, 1995.

36. Muller N, Glaus T, Gardelle O: [Extensive stomach ulcers because of *Dieffenbachia* intoxication in a cat], *Tierarztl Prax Ausg K Klientiere Heimtiere* 26:404, 1998.
37. Neiger R, Dieterich C, Burnens A et al: Detection and prevalence of *Helicobacter* infection in pet cats, *J Clin Microbiol* 36:634, 1998.
38. Neiger R, Simpson K: *Helicobacter* infection in dogs and cats: facts and fiction, *J Vet Intern Med* 14:125, 2000.
39. Papich MG, Davis CA, Davis LE: Absorption of salicylate from an antidiarrheal preparation in dogs and cats, *J Am Anim Hosp Assoc* 23:221, 1987.
40. Pearson H, Gaskell CJ, Gibbs C et al: Pyloric and oesophageal dysfunction in the cat, *J Small Anim Pract* 15:487, 1974.
41. Perkins SE, Yan LL, Shen Z et al: Use of PCR and culture to detect *Helicobacter pylori* in naturally infected cats following triple antimicrobial therapy, *Antimicrob Agents Chemother* 40:1486, 1996.
42. Pohlman LM, Higginbotham ML, Welles EG et al: Immunophenotypic and histologic classification of 50 cases of feline gastrointestinal lymphoma, *Vet Pathol* 46:259, 2009.
43. Poortinga E: Copper penny ingestion in a cat, *Can Vet J* 36:634, 1995.
44. Rossmeisl JH Jr, Forrester SD, Robertson JL et al: Chronic vomiting associated with a gastric carcinoid in a cat, *J Am Anim Hosp Assoc* 38:61, 2002.
45. Runk A, Kyles A, Downs M: Duodenal perforation in a cat following the administration of nonsteroidal anti-inflammatory medication, *J Am Anim Hosp Assoc* 35:52, 1998.
46. Serna JH, Genta RM, Lichtenberger LM et al: Invasive *Helicobacter*-like organisms in feline gastric mucosa, *Helicobacter* 2:40, 1997.
47. Shojaee Tabrizi A, Jamshidi S, Oghalaei A et al: Identification of *Helicobacter* spp. in oral secretions vs. gastric mucosa of stray cats, *Vet Microbiol* 140:142, 2010.
48. Simpson K, Neiger R, DeNovo R et al: The relationship of *Helicobacter* spp. infection to gastric disease in dogs and cats, *J Vet Intern Med* 14:228, 2000.
49. Simpson KW: Diseases of the stomach. In Ettinger SJ, Feldman EC, editors: *Textbook of veterinary internal medicine*, ed 6, St Louis, 2005, Saunders Elsevier, p 1310.
50. Smith TJ, Baltzer WI, Ruaux CG et al: Gastric smooth muscle hamartoma in a cat, *J Feline Med Surg* 12:334, 2010.
51. Sparkes AH, Heiene R, Lascelles BDX et al: ISFM and AAFP consensus guidelines: Long-term use of NSAIDs in cats, *J Feline Med Surg* 12:521, 2010.
52. Sparkes AH, Papasouliotis K, Barr FJ et al: Reference ranges for gastrointestinal transit of barium-impregnated polyethylene spheres in healthy cats, *J Small Anim Pract* 38:340, 1997.
53. Steyn PF, Twedt D, Toombs W: The scintigraphic evaluation of solid phase gastric emptying in normal cats, *Vet Radiol Ultrasound* 36:327, 1995.
54. Turk MA, Gallina AM, Russell TS: Nonhematopoietic gastrointestinal neoplasia in cats: a retrospective study of 44 cases, *Vet Pathol* 18:614, 1981.
55. Twaddle AA: Congenital pyloric stenosis in two kittens corrected by pyloroplasty, *N Z Vet J* 19:26, 1971.
56. Tyrrell D, Beck C: Survey of the use of radiography vs. ultrasonography in the investigation of gastrointestinal foreign bodies in small animals, *Vet Radiol Ultrasound* 47:404, 2006.
57. Valli VE, Jacobs RM, Norris A et al: The histologic classification of 602 cases of feline lymphoproliferative disease using the National Cancer Institute working formulation, *J Vet Diagn Invest* 12:295, 2000.
58. Van den Bulck K, Decostere A, Baele M et al: Identification of non-*Helicobacter pylori* spiral organisms in gastric samples from humans, dogs, and cats, *J Clin Microbiol* 43:2256, 2005.
59. Van Stee EW, Ward CL, Duffy ML: Recurrent esophageal hairballs in a cat (a case report), *Vet Med* 75:1873, 1980.
60. Wyse CA, McLellan J, Dickie AM et al: A review of methods for assessment of the rate of gastric emptying in the dog and cat: 1898-2002, *J Vet Intern Med* 17:609, 2003.
61. Yamasaki K, Suematsu H, Takahashi T: Comparison of gastric lesions in dogs and cats with and without gastric spiral organisms, *J Am Vet Med Assoc* 212:529, 1998.
62. Zikes CD, Spielman B, Shapiro W et al: Gastric extramedullary plasmacytoma in a cat, *J Vet Intern Med* 12:381, 1998.

APPROACH TO THE CAT WITH DIARRHEA

Randolph M. Baral

OVERVIEW

Diarrhea can be defined as increased volume and/or increased frequency of defecation of stools with increased water content. Approaches to diarrhea, as for any clinical sign, need to take into account the individual animal. For example, neoplasia is much less likely to occur in a kitten than in a geriatric cat. In many cases, the precise diagnosis of gastrointestinal disease cannot be reached without biopsy samples. The decision to obtain biopsy samples should follow a logical pathway that is appropriate to the cat's condition. These are summarized in Figure 23-17. For example, many cases of acute diarrhea in a well cat can resolve with limited or no intervention, and so do not require a precise diagnosis.

The diagnostic steps are

1. Signalment and clinical history
2. Physical examination
3. Fecal assessment
4. Blood and urine testing
5. Imaging (radiography, ultrasonography)
6. Biopsy samples

These steps do not include treatment/diet trials or other empiric therapies that are appropriate in many cases. Steps 3 and 4 are often undertaken at the same time, and there is no definite order for these steps. They are divided here for reasons of clarity. In a younger cat, where infectious causes are more likely, thorough fecal testing is more important; in an older cat, extragastrointestinal diseases, such as hyperthyroidism, are more likely; so, blood and urine testing is more important, but fecal assessment should not be neglected.

The decision to proceed to Step 4 (and each subsequent step) should take into account several considerations. The main considerations in assessing and managing a cat with diarrhea are

- Is there an acute onset or a chronic time course?
- Are there any dietary changes or indiscretion?

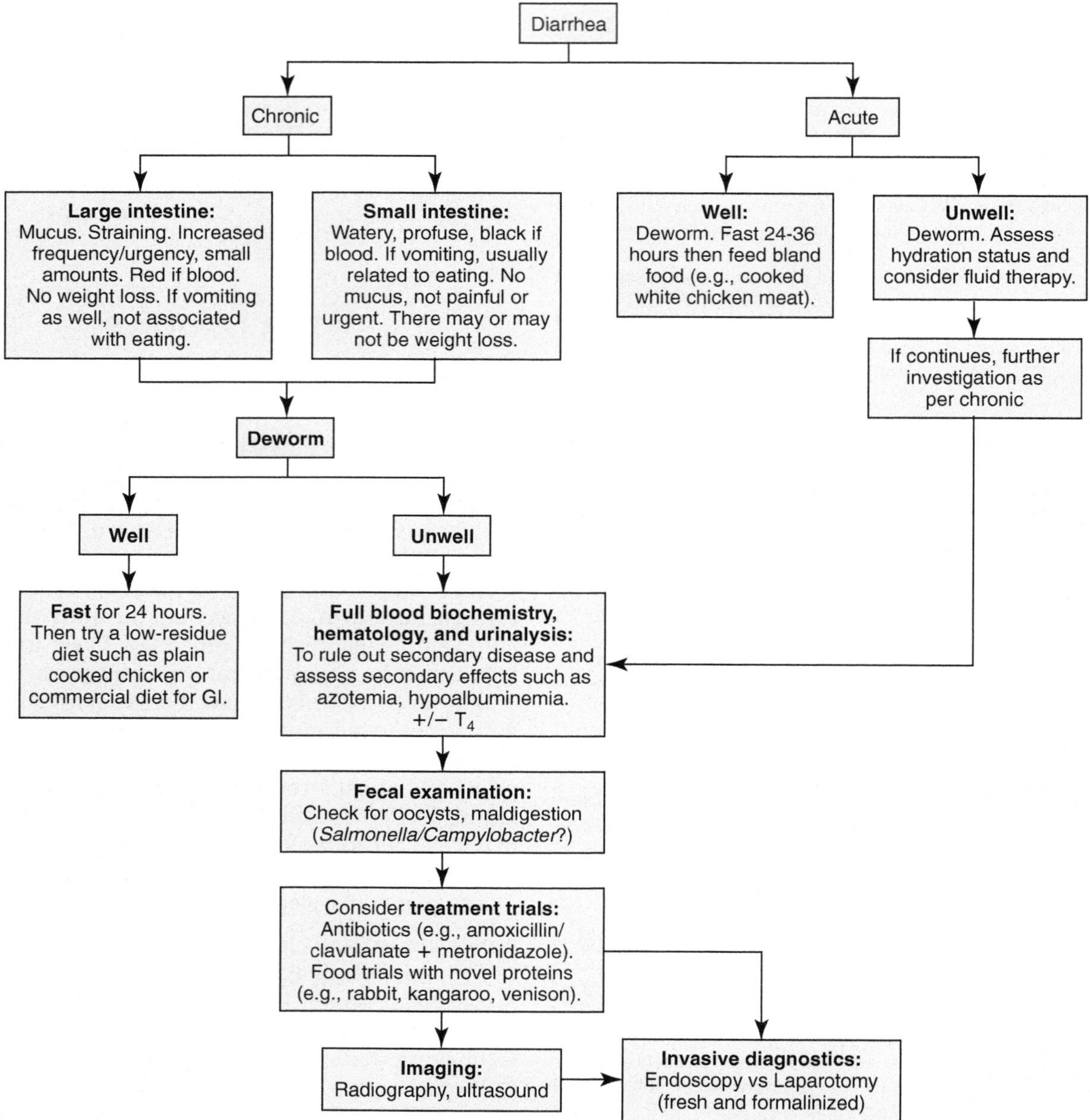

FIGURE 23-17 Diagnostic approach to the cat with diarrhea.

- Is the cat well or unwell?
- Is there primary or secondary gastrointestinal disease?
- Is there small or large bowel diarrhea?

STEP 1: SIGNALMENT AND CLINICAL HISTORY

The components of the clinical history for cats with diarrhea are detailed in Table 23-12. After establishing the cat's age, breed, vaccination, and deworming history, it is important to establish the duration and nature of the diarrhea. Chronic diarrhea is usually defined as greater than 3 weeks in duration and mostly warrants at least some degree of a diagnostic workup, whereas acute diarrhea is often self-limiting in a well cat.

A description of the feces helps determine whether the diarrhea is small or large bowel in origin (Table 23-13); this will affect how any investigations might proceed. Important questions to ask concern frequency of defecation (and how this compares with the normal state), tenesmus (straining usually indicates large bowel diarrhea, since an irritated colon leads to urgency), volume of feces (smaller volumes are typical of large bowel diarrhea; larger volumes are more typical of small

TABLE 23-12 **Clinical History for Cats with Diarrhea**

Signalment	Age? Young cats are prone to dietary, infectious, and parasitic causes of diarrhea; older cats are more likely to have inflammatory, metabolic, and neoplastic causes of diarrhea.
Vaccination status	Appropriate panleukopenia, FeLV vaccination?
Diet	Detailed dietary history as well as recent dietary changes. Adverse reactions to food are common causes of diarrhea. Diarrhea that ceases when an animal is not fed suggests osmotic diarrhea.
Environment	Presence of various plants, chemicals, and foreign objects? Health status of cats in the household? Outdoor cats are more likely to develop parasitic, toxic, and infectious disorders.
Travel history	Infectious potential or enzootic area (fungal or parasitic diarrhea)?
Current medications	Drug reaction or toxicity? Drug therapies that can cause diarrhea should be noted (e.g., antibiotics, anti-inflammatory agents, cardiac glycosides).
Past medical and surgical problems	Organ system affected? Recurrence? Response to previous treatment?
Onset and duration of diarrhea	Acute versus chronic? Acute diarrheas are abrupt in onset and of short duration, and generally they are self-limiting. Chronic diarrheas persist usually longer than 3 weeks and fail to respond to symptomatic therapy.
Appearance of diarrhea	Quantity and quality of the stool (color, consistency, character, presence of blood or mucus)? Loose to watery feces that contain fat droplets, undigested food, melena, and variable colors suggests small intestinal disease. The volume is always increased with small intestinal disease. Loose to semisolid feces containing excess mucus and fresh blood (hematochezia) indicates large intestinal disease. The volume may be normal to slightly decreased with large intestinal disease.
Description of defecation process	Tenesmus (straining) and dyschezia (painful defecation)? These are hallmarks of large intestinal disease (e.g., inflammatory or obstructive lesions of the colon, rectum, or anus).
Frequency of defecation	Frequency is normal to slightly increased with small bowel disease, but greatly increased with large bowel disease.
Associated physical signs	Vomiting, anorexia, weight loss, and dyschezia may help localize the disorder to a specific part of the gastrointestinal tract. Clinical signs relating to problems in other organs or body systems should be noted and may suggest a more generalized disease. Vomiting may occur as a consequence of small intestinal inflammation in some cats with diarrhea. Weight loss may result from decreased caloric intake (anorexia), decreased nutrient assimilation (maldigestion/malabsorption), or excessive caloric loss (protein-losing enteropathy or nephropathy). Weight loss is observed uncommonly with large bowel disease.

FeLV, Feline leukemia virus.
From Hall JE: Clinical approach to chronic diarrhea In August JR, editor: *Consultations in feline internal medicine,* ed 4, Philadelphia, 2001, Saunders, p 130.

TABLE 23-13 **Distinctions Between Small and Large Bowel Diarrhea**

Observation	Small Bowel Diarrhea	Large Bowel Diarrhea
Frequency of defecation	Normal to slightly increased	Very increased
Fecal output	Large volumes	Small volumes frequently
Urgency or tenesmus	Absent	Present
Dyschezia	Absent	Present with rectal disease
Mucus in feces	Absent	Present
Exudate in feces	Absent	Present sometimes
Hematochezia (red blood)	Absent	Present sometimes
Melena (digested blood)	Present sometimes	Absent
Steatorrhea	Present sometimes	Absent
Flatulence and borborygmus	Present sometimes	Absent
Weight loss	Present sometimes	Rare
Vomiting	Present sometimes	Rare

From Sherding RG: Diseases of the intestines. In Sherding RG, editor: *The cat: diseases and clinical management,* ed 2, New York, 1994, Churchill Livingstone, p 1215.

bowel), how formed the stool is (from soft stool to cow-pat consistency to liquid tea; usually more watery stool relates to small intestinal disease), color (darker indicates digested blood), and presence of any mucus or blood (presence relates to large bowel).

Most household toxins, such as plants, cause signs additional to diarrhea such vomiting or neurological signs,[11] but it is important to ascertain if the cat has had access to anything unusual. Likewise, it is important to find out if the cat has had any possible exposure to dietary indiscretions; this can include if the cat has been seen with or is known to hunt prey including insects. Cockroaches carry pathogenic bacteria[12,18] and other prey such as birds and rats can carry *Salmonella*; salmonellosis in cats has been dubbed songbird fever.[6]

Simple causes of self-limiting diarrhea include dietary change (either a new flavor or a new style of food, such as dry food for the first time); so, the owner must also be quizzed if anything new has been offered, either new cat food or treats (such as greasy fish or chicken).

Although the physical examination will usually determine how unwell a cat is, the owner's impressions are also important, because cats can hide signs from strangers, particularly in a practice setting. Lethargy and inappetence are important signs, as ill cats typically do not eat well.

STEP 2: PHYSICAL EXAMINATION

The cat's general demeanor can be an indicator of how unwell a cat is and therefore dictate the extent of diagnostic testing required. This can be noted by assessing how interested the cat is in its surroundings or any behavior changes from previous visits, such as if a normally difficult-to-handle cat is placid. Body weight should be assessed and, if possible, compared with that of previous visits (even those noted on a clinical record from another veterinarian). The body condition score (BCS) should also be assessed and can be very important when there is no prior weight information.

Dehydration is usually a sign that a cat needs more involved management. Abdominal palpation should be performed to assess pain (where?), any masses (foreign bodies, lymph nodes, or even focally thickened intestines, such as with neoplasia), or turgid intestines. Fever often indicates infection but can also reflect neoplasia or other inflammatory changes. A thorough examination of all body systems should always be performed, no matter what a cat presents for. In the case of diarrhea, extragastrointestinal signs can be of vital importance, such as a palpable thyroid and tachycardia suggesting hyperthyroidism. After the clinical history has been taken and the physical examination performed, the veterinarian must make the important decisions of whether any interventions are required and whether the patient should be managed as an inpatient or outpatient. The veterinarian should be asking

- Are ancillary tests appropriate?
- Is supportive care necessary?
- Are any medications required?

In many cases, the answers to these questions are obvious. For example, a cat may seem well but has had access to lilies (the author has seen diarrhea as a primary presenting sign for this!) or has a palpable abdominal mass. Substantial weight loss is an indicator that further investigations are warranted sooner rather than later. If the decision is made for empiric management and outpatient care, it is vital to follow up either by scheduling a recheck visit or calling the client, because simple acute problems can turn into complicated chronic problems.

The Well Cat with Acute Onset Diarrhea

If the diarrhea has been present for less than a week and the cat has no weight loss, dehydration, fever, or palpable abdominal abnormalities, it is appropriate to manage the cat as an outpatient. Even in the absence of fecal testing, it is appropriate to deworm the cat (see the section Gastrointestinal Parasites). The cat should be fasted for 24 hours (12 hours, if less than 4 months old) and then fed a bland diet (such as plain, cooked, skinless chicken, or low-residue prescription diets designed for cats with gastrointestinal problems). It is appropriate to maintain the cat on the low-residue diet for at least 7 to 10 days and then slowly reintroduce the regular diet.

STEP 3: FECAL ASSESSMENT +/– CULTURE

Fecal assessment is mostly used to assess infectious agents, such as parasite-associated diarrhea, but the importance of assessing feces, even when parasitic or bacterial infections are not suspected, should not be underestimated. Gross examination of feces can determine if melena or fresh blood or mucus are present to help distinguish large from small bowel disease when the owner's observations may be misleading. Occult fecal blood can be an indicator of gastrointestinal inflammation in cases of subtle disease, and undigested starches and fats can indicate maldigestion or malabsorption.[8]

For assessment of feces for parasites, the fecal sample should ideally be fresh (<1 hour old). Refrigeration (for no longer than one week) can preserve ova, oocysts, and cysts but not protozoal trophozoites. Feces should be assessed by

1. Direct wet preparation
   a. To assess for trophozoites

BOX 23-1

Methods of Fecal Analysis

Direct Wet Preparation

Used to evaluate the smear for the presence of trophozoites, such as *Giardia* spp. and *Tritrichomonas foetus*.

1. Place peppercorn size amount of feces on a warm slide and mix with a drop of 0.9% saline (smear must not be too thick, because trophozoites will be easily missed).
2. Apply coverslip.
3. Evaluate systematically for motile organisms using the 10× magnification.
4. Confirmation at 40× magnification.

Stained Fecal Smear

Adding iodine to a wet mount through the edge of the coverslip can aid in the visualization of internal structures of some protozoa. The direct wet preparation must be examined without any stain for motility first, because staining the preparation kills the organism. Methylene blue is useful for identifying trophozoites, particularly those of *Entamoeba histolytica*. This method has little to no diagnostic value for the diagnosis of bacterial-associated diarrhea.

Fecal Flotation

Used to find cysts, oocysts, and ova in feces. Standing (gravitational) flotation methods are easier and quicker but have much poorer sensitivity than centrifugation methods.[2] Solutions used in centrifugation flotation methods include zinc sulfate and Sheather sugar.

Procedure for Single Centrifugal Flotation[3]

1. Weigh out 2 to 5 g of feces.
2. Mix feces with approximately 10 mL of flotation solution.
3. Pour mixture through a tea strainer into a beaker or fecal cup.
4. Pour strained solution into a 15-mL centrifuge tube.
5. Fill tube with flotation solution so that a slight positive meniscus forms, being sure not to overfill the tube.
6. Place a coverslip on the tube, and put the tube in the centrifuge.
7. Make sure the centrifuge is balanced.
8. Centrifuge at 1200 rpm (280× g) for 5 minutes.
9. Remove the tube and let stand 10 minutes.
10. Remove the coverslip, and place it on a glass slide. Systematically examine the entire area under the coverslip at 100× magnification (i.e., 10× objective). You may wish to use the 40× objective lens to confirm your diagnosis and make measurements; however, *with practice, most parasites can be identified using the 10× objective (100× magnification).*

Citations are from the references in the section Approach to the Cat with Diarrhea.

Adapted from Marks SL: The scoop on poop—maximizing the diagnostic yield of the fecal examination. *WSAVA Conference Proceedings* 2007; Dryden MW, Payne PA, Smith V: Accurate diagnosis of *Giardia* spp. and proper fecal examination procedures, *Vet Ther* 7:4, 2006.

2. Stained fecal smear
   a. Can aid in the visualization of internal structures of some protozoa
3. Fecal flotation (preferably with centrifugation)
   a. To find cysts, oocysts, and ova

These techniques are described in Box 23-1. Specific fecal analyses can be performed to assess for

1. Tritrichomonas foetus
   a. InPouch TF (Biomed Diagnostics, White City, Ore.)[5]
   b. Polymerase chain reaction (PCR) assessment[4]
2. *Giardia:* SNAP *Giardia* Test Kit (IDEXX Laboratories, Westbrook, Me.)[10]
3. *Cryptosporidium* enzyme-linked immunosorbent assay (ELISA) (but care should be taken, since different ELISAs have varying sensitivity and specificity)[9]

Fecal culture should be undertaken with the understanding that bacteria *will* be cultured; so, interpretation is based on the relevance of the positive culture result. Factors affecting interpretation include whether the growth is a heavy and pure growth of a known pathogen, such as *Salmonella, Campylobacter, Yersinia,* or *Clostridium difficile*. Further information about the relevance of culture and PCR results is contained below in the section Infectious Enteritis.

STEP 4: BLOOD AND URINE TESTING

Routine Tests

Investigations begin by assessing if the diarrhea is the result of primary gastrointestinal disease or secondary to another process, by performing routine serum/plasma biochemistries, hematology, urinalysis, and total T_4 (for older cats). In most cases of secondary gastrointestinal disease, diarrhea is *not* usually the primary presenting complaint, but since the approach to investigations and management diverge so much, this is an important step to take. Biochemistry and urine tests may also show the consequences of diarrhea, such as dehydration and electrolyte abnormalities.

TABLE 23-14 **Sample Handling Factors for Tests Used to Assess Gastrointestinal Function**

Parameter	Cobalamin	Folate	fTLI	fPLI
Stable at room temperature?	Yes	No	Yes	Yes
Hemolysis interferes?	No	Yes	No	No
Lipemia interferes?	No	No	Yes	Yes
Fasting required?	No	No	Yes (12-18 h)	Yes (12-18 h)
Species-specific?	No	No	Yes	Yes

fPLI, Feline pancreatic lipase immunoreactivity; *fTLI,* feline trypsin-like immunoreactivity.

Hematology can be normal in some cats, with changes expected, and so should not be used to rule out any condition. It can be useful, for example, if there is a left shift neutrophilia, indicating acute infection, or eosinophilia, reflecting parasitism. Monocytosis can suggest chronic disease that was not suggested by the clinical history.

The Unwell Cat with Acute Onset Diarrhea

In the case of acute onset diarrhea, the cat may be unwell as a consequence of the diarrhea (e.g., from dehydration) and not because of the cause of the diarrhea. If rehydration is required (with intravenous or subcutaneous fluids, depending on severity of illness), then it is important that biochemistry tests are performed before fluid administration so that any diagnostic clues are not lost by alteration of the profile from the fluid therapy. Fever and neutrophilia may indicate the need for antibiotic therapy. If infection is suspected, fecal sampling (see Step 4) should occur before starting antibiotics. If a cat is unwell from dehydration, then further testing may not be warranted. The clinician should be alert that linear foreign bodies can result in diarrhea (see the section Intestinal Obstruction).

The Well Cat with Chronic Diarrhea but No Weight Loss

Diarrhea of chronic duration (greater than 3 weeks) does require a more thorough investigation at the outset. However, if clinically well, the cat can be managed as an outpatient in the first instance, at least while waiting for results of diagnostic testing. A diet trial with a novel protein is appropriate for a well cat with stable weight. As with any patient managed as an outpatient, follow-up is vital and, in this scenario, includes scheduling revisits.

Blood Tests for Gastrointestinal Disease

Cobalamin, folate, feline trypsin-like immunoreactivity (fTLI), and feline pancreatic lipase immunoreactivity (fPLI) are useful markers of intestinal and pancreatic disease,[14-17] but it is important to note that they typically do not give a precise diagnosis.

Cobalamin and folate are water-soluble vitamins and are readily found in commercial cat foods so that dietary insufficiency is rare, and decreased levels are almost always because of GI disease. These vitamins are taken up by specific receptors in different areas of the small intestine. Chronic inflammatory gastrointestinal disease may damage the receptors and lead to decreased serum concentrations of one or both vitamins, provided the disease process is severe and long standing enough to deplete body stores. Serum cobalamin and folate concentrations may also be decreased in cats with exocrine pancreatic insufficiency (EPI).

Trypsin-like immunoreactivity is a pancreas-specific marker, and assessment of serum TLI is used for diagnosis of EPI and pancreatitis in the cat, although the sensitivity of the assay for pancreatitis is low. PLI is a marker for pancreatic inflammation and is more sensitive than TLI for the diagnosis of pancreatitis. Since inflammation of the small intestine may be seen concurrently with pancreatitis, serum TLI and PLI are useful adjunctive tests in the diagnosis of diarrhea.

TLI, PLI, and cobalamin are stable in serum at room temperature for several days, but folate is unstable so that samples for cobalamin/folate analysis should be frozen (Table 23-14). Samples submitted for folate concentration should not be hemolyzed, because red blood cells contain high levels of folate. In addition, folate is light-sensitive, and samples should be wrapped to exclude light. Severe lipemia may interfere with common assays for TLI and PLI.

The main utility of these tests are

1. To indicate that further investigation of gastrointestinal disease is warranted.
   When a cat presents for weight loss with no overt signs of GI disease, decreased cobalamin or folate can indicate that further investigations with imaging and, ultimately, biopsy sampling are warranted. Many clients are more willing to proceed with

alkaline phosphatase (ALP).[27,40,43,84] As with IBDs, these liver enzyme changes may or may not represent overt hepatic disease.[67] Albumin may be reduced[43] but is normal in most cases[27,43,84]; azotemia may be present and may be of prerenal origin or represent concurrent renal disease. In one study, 25 of 32 cats were hypocobalaminemic; 1 of 27 cats had low folate, but 10 of 27 had elevated folate; and 12 of 16 cats had increased fTLI.[73]

Hematologically, a mature neutrophilia with or without monocytosis is sometimes present, representing the inflammatory response; lymphopenia may be present as a stress response. Anemia may be present and may occur as a result of chronic slow GI blood loss, and in some cases, ulceration, or it may be because of chronic disease; hemoconcentration is also possible, reflecting dehydration.[27,40,43,84]

Palpable or ultrasonographically visible thickened intestines (30% to 41% of cases)[27,40,43,84] or mesenteric lymph nodes (20% to 50% of cases)[27,40,43,84] are no more or less likely to be present in comparison with IBDs. There are no defined ultrasound guidelines for cats with intestinal small cell lymphoma, because most prior papers do not distinguish between small cell and lymphoblastic neoplasia.[54,113] A more recent paper found 9 of 15 cats undergoing ultrasound examination had diffuse small intestinal wall thickening, with a mean of 4.3 mm (range, 3.4 to 5.0 mm; median, 4.5 mm), and focal mural thickening of 20 mm was noted in one cat.[84] In many cases, against expectations, intestinal wall layering was preserved. These findings also mean that 5 of 15 cats had ultrasonographically normal intestinal wall thickness (≤2.8 mm for the duodenum and ≤3.2 mm for the ileum).[50] If affected, jejunal lymph nodes may appear as hypoechoic and enlarged; in the same study, 12 of 15 cats had lymph node changes with a mean diameter of 15.9 mm (range, 6.5 to 30 mm; median, 10 mm)[84] compared with the normal diameter of less than or equal to 5.0 mm.[132] None of these findings can definitively distinguish small cell lymphoma from IBDs; although one recent paper has suggested that ultrasonographic thickening of the muscularis layer is more likely in cats with intestinal small cell lymphoma (Figure 23-20) than those with IBD, this change was also seen in 12% of cats with a normal small intestine. However, thickening of the muscularis layer together with lymphadenopathy was recognized in 26% of those cats with small cell lymphoma compared with 4% of those with IBD and 2% of cats with no small intestinal pathology.[177]

Biopsy samples and histopathology are required for definitive diagnosis. An example of jejunal and mesenteric lymph node appearance at laparotomy is shown in Figure 23-21. As noted for IBDs, it is important to work with the pathologist by providing good quality samples and a thorough clinical history, as well as having an open dialogue if the findings are not within expectations.

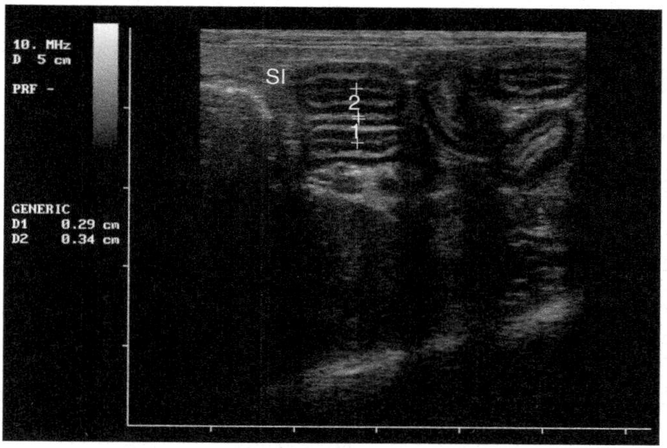

FIGURE 23-20 Ultrasonographic findings of small cell lymphoma; duodenal wall measurements at the two locations numbered D1 and D2 are 2.9 mm and 3.4 mm, respectively. Note that the prominence of the muscularis propria layer in the second measurement compared with the ultrasonographic appearance of inflammatory bowel disease (IBD) in Figure 23-19, in concordance with findings of Zwingenberger et al.[177]

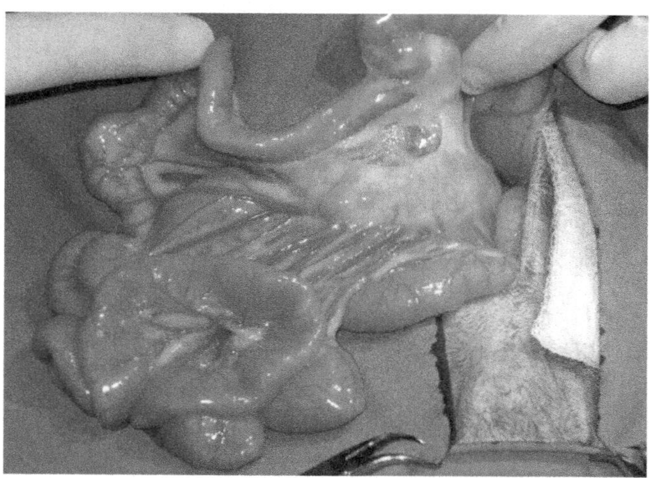

FIGURE 23-21 The appearance of intestinal small cell lymphoma at laparotomy. Note the erythematous and generally thickened intestines and prominent mesenteric lymph nodes.

It is difficult to distinguish between lymphocytic inflammation and small cell lymphocytic neoplasia in any location; some histopathologic features that might help in differentiating the ends of the spectrum may include

1. Demonstration of small lymphocyte domination (sometimes referred to as monotonous or monomorphous population) in small cell lymphoma, compared with morphologically mixed cell populations in IBD[27,40]
2. Infiltration into deeper layers (submucosa and muscle wall) in lymphocytic neoplasia[27,40,43]

3. No mucosal congestion, edema, or fibrosis in lymphocytic neoplasia,[43] compared with IBD
4. Epitheliotropism, or homing of neoplastic T lymphocytes to the mucosal epithelium in lymphocytic neoplasia[27]

These features can be seen in Figure 23-22. Each of these criteria may be useful but are unlikely to be definitive. Further studies that may not be routinely available but which may be helpful are

1. Immunophenotyping; most reports have found purely T lymphocytes in most cases of intestinal small cell lymphoma[27,73,84,116] (Figure 23-23).
2. Clonality; the detection of a clonal population of cells, as recently described for intestinal lymphocytic lymphosarcoma,[101] would be closest to providing the basis for definitive diagnosis.

Drug Therapy

Effective treatment of feline intestinal small cell lymphoma was brought to light by Fondacaro et al[43] and has therefore become known as the Fondacaro protocol. This consists of a combination of prednisolone and chlorambucil given orally by the client at home (Table 23-15). The rationale is that a slow alkylating agent, such as chlorambucil, is more appropriate to use for the slowly dividing, well-differentiated lymphocytes that cause disease. This can be contrasted to the aggressive chemotherapeutic agents required for the rapidly proliferating cells in lymphoblastic neoplasia that is typically associated with lymphosarcoma.

Reported response rates to this protocol are excellent, with 59% to 76% of cats achieving complete clinical remission, reported median survival times ranging from 20 to 30 months for those cats responding to therapy, and reports of individual cats surviving as long as 76 months.[43,73,84] The original reported protocol comprised prednisolone (10 mg/cat, PO or 2 mg/kg, PO) given daily with chlorambucil pulsed by administration of 15 mg/m^2 for 4 days every 3 weeks. A more recent study[73] dosed prednisolone similarly, but chlorambucil was given as continuous therapy of 2 mg/cat, PO every second or third day.

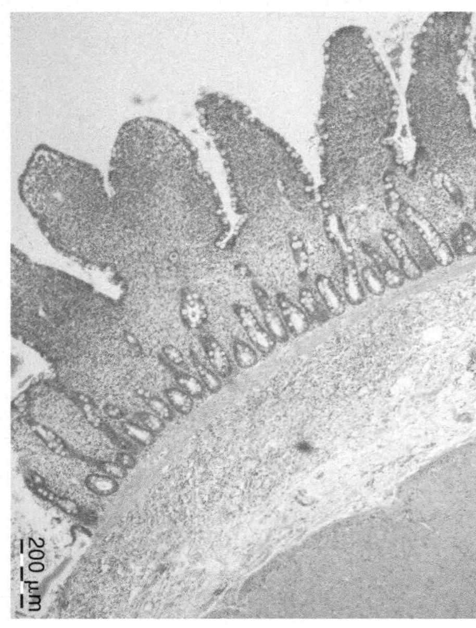

FIGURE 23-22 Photomicrograph of small intestinal mucosa in a cat with intestinal small cell lymphoma. There is marked cellular infiltrate of the lamina propria, extending through the lamina muscularis into the submucosa. Villous morphology is distorted by the infiltrate.

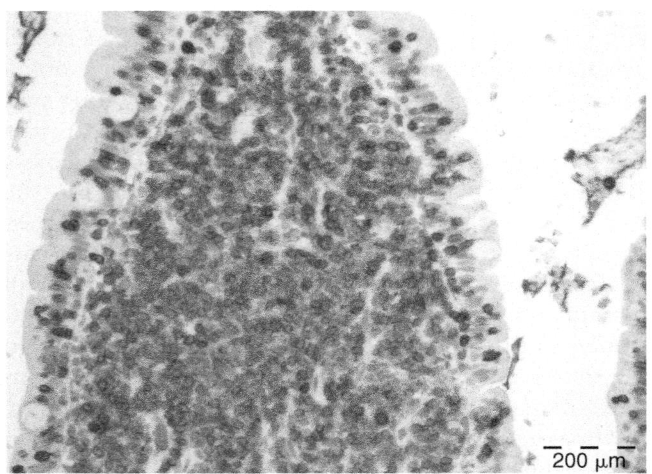

FIGURE 23-23 Photomicrograph of small intestinal mucosa in a cat with intestinal small cell lymphoma. Immunohistochemical labeling with a pan–T-lymphocyte marker reveals positive labeling of the infiltrating cells, consistent with a T-lymphocyte origin. CD3-positive cells can be seen in the mucosal epithelium but no Pautrier abscesses are evident.

TABLE 23-15 **Comparison of Small Cell Lymphoma Protocols, All Drugs Dosed Orally**

Protocol	Chlorambucil	Prednisolone	Median Survival (Months)
Pulsed	15 mg/m^2/24h for 4 days every 3 weeks[43]	10 mg/cat/24h[43] *or* 3 mg/kg/24h[84]	17 (range 0.33-50)[43] 15 (range 0.5-77)[84]
Continuous	2 mg/cat/48h[73] *or* 1 mg/cat/24h	10 mg/cat/24h[73] *or* 5 mg/cat/12-24h[73]	25 (range 1.5-67)[73]

Reference citations are from the section Diseases of the Intestines.

Similar protocols are used in humans with both low-grade (i.e., lymphocytic) lymphosarcoma and chronic lymphocytic leukemia.[117,151] Some studies with humans have indicated that continuous therapy with chlorambucil results in prolonged survival,[64] although meta-analyses have not been able to determine optimum dosing and scheduling of administration of chlorambucil or other alkylating agents in these conditions in humans.[20,72]

Although we do not have enough data to critically compare pulsed therapy to continuous dosing, the study assessing continuous dosing appeared to have a lower number of cats completely responding, although those cats that did respond had a longer median survival[73] than those in the studies assessing pulsed chlorambucil dosing.[43,84] The differences may also relate to the definitions used for complete response. The chlorambucil dose of 2 mg/cat, PO every second day (or third day) is often chosen because of the ready availability of 2 mg coated tablets, the breaking of which can expose the owner to these cytotoxic medications. Chlorambucil can be compounded into smaller doses, thus allowing daily dosing of 1 mg capsules. The author has used this dose to apparent good effect, but there has been no critical assessment.

It is unknown whether involvement of lymph nodes or other organs, such as the liver, affects prognosis. The only study of substantial size to include extra-GI locations found anatomic location was not prognostic for response or survival time.[73] In another study, of the five cats with liver involvement, two cats did not survive more than 5 months, yet the other three lived longer than 2½ years, with two surviving longer than 4½ years.[84] A study of hepatic small cell lymphoma suggests the density of neoplastic lymphocytes may influence survival, and density may relate to the stage of the disease when diagnosis occurs.[7]

Adverse effects of chlorambucil are rare, but gastrointestinal signs, myelosuppression, and myoclonus have all been reported. Gastrointestinal signs, such as vomiting, diarrhea, or inappetence, can be difficult to distinguish from continuation of the gastrointestinal disease diagnosed. These signs are usually self limiting. Myelosuppression is also possible with thrombocytopenia reported.[57,84] Monoclonus has been reported on one occasion.[17] It is ideal to check hematologic parameters every 2 months for cats receiving chlorambucil. Continuous therapy using lower doses of chlorambucil may be less likely to lead to these adverse effects.

High doses of corticosteroids can induce diabetes mellitus, and thus blood glucose should be checked regularly. If diabetes occurs, the author has found that budesonide (1 mg budesonide is generally considered to be equivalent of 5 mg prednisolone) can be substituted for prednisolone, since it has reputed lower systemic effects (though no assessments of this drug's effectiveness in cats have been made). An alternative is for the cat to be weaned off corticosteroids, with chlorambucil continued as monotherapy (as is often the case with humans). Iatrogenic diabetes mellitus usually needs to be managed with insulin therapy, at least initially (see Chapter 24).

Intestinal High-Grade (Lymphoblastic) Lymphoma

High-grade lymphoma or lymphosarcoma is the traditional style of aggressive, rapidly dividing lymphoid neoplasia that carries a much poorer prognosis than small cell lymphoma.

Prevalence

Most early studies do not distinguish grade of neoplasia; so, the prevalence of low-grade and high-grade alimentary lymphoma are difficult to assess. Several recent studies found a similar prevalence of each,[84,116] but the seminal paper describing small cell lymphoma found only 17 cases of lymphoblastic lymphoma compared with 50 cases of small cell lymphoma.[43] This ratio of approximately one high-grade GI lymphoma case for every three low-grade cases more closely approximates the rate found in the author's practice.

Patient Signalment and Risk Factors

The reported median ages of affected cats range from 10 to 12 years, but cats as young as 1 year old have been diagnosed. Most papers note that males are overrepresented, and Siamese cats may also be overrepresented although most affected cats are domestic shorthairs.[43,49,90,116,176] Precise signalment is difficult to determine from the literature, because many papers assess all anatomic locations of lymphoma without necessarily breaking down epidemiologic data for each anatomic site. Also, there are few comparisons to a reference population.

Pathophysiology

The association of lymphoma with FeLV infection is well established and documented[139] and is covered in Chapter 28; FIV has also been shown to be lymphomagenic.[12,139] Since the control of FeLV through vaccination began in the 1980s, nonretroviral-associated lymphoid neoplasia has become more common, and the rates of intestinal lymphoma have, in fact, increased since FeLV infection rates have decreased.[86] The underlying causes for this increase are not known. The association with inflammation from IBDs was noted for small cell lymphomas, and perhaps there is a spectrum from lymphocytic IBD to small cell lymphoma to high-grade lymphoma. That some cats are more likely to have inflammatory changes become neoplastic is suggested by a paper noting higher lymphoma rates in cats with vaccine-associated sarcomas (a neoplastic condition where the role of chronic inflammation is well noted).[89]

Whether the underlying cause is retroviral or chronic inflammation or anything else, the pathogenesis of high-grade intestinal lymphoma, as with small cell lymphoma and other neoplasia, depends on chromosomal changes that affect regulation of cell growth and death, resulting in malignant transformation and clonal expansion of immature lymphocytes.[152]

Metastasis can occur in one third to two thirds of cases,[90,92] with involvement of mesenteric lymph nodes most commonly noted, but spread to liver, spleen, kidneys, and thorax is also possible.[90]

A recent survey of gastrointestinal lymphoma found that most cases (37 of 50) involved the small intestine (including 3 that also involved the stomach and 4 that also involved the large intestine), and 4 of 50 cases involved the large intestine only.[116]

Clinical Signs

Cats with high-grade alimentary lymphoma often present similarly to those with other gastrointestinal diseases. Typical clinical signs are weight loss, anorexia, lethargy, vomiting, diarrhea, or a combination of these signs. Repeated studies have found cats with no vomiting or diarrhea; in one study, 13 of 28 cats had only anorexia or weight loss on presentation.[90]

Cats with large bowel pathology usually present, as with other causes of colitis, with increased urgency, and small, frequent amounts of diarrhea, often with blood or mucus. Cats with large bowel neoplasia of any form can present for constipation caused by intestinal obstruction.

Palpation of an abdominal mass has been recognized in 59% to 85% of cases,[43,90] but the corollary of this is that 15% to 41% of cases did not have a palpable mass. It is also important to note that up to 50% of cats with intestinal small cell lymphoma, and a number with IBDs, have palpable mesenteric lymph nodes; so, a palpable abdominal mass is not a specific indication of high-grade neoplasia. Many cats have palpably thickened bowel loops.[124]

Diagnosis

Hematology and plasma or serum biochemistry findings are also nonspecific. Increased liver enzymes may or may not indicate liver involvement. Anemia may be recognized and can be non-regenerative, reflecting chronic disease or slow blood loss, or regenerative if there is more substantial blood loss associated with mucosal ulceration. Hypoalbuminemia can be because of blood loss or intestinal protein loss. Hypercalcemia of malignancy is a possibility but not commonly reported. Despite nonspecific signs, laboratory testing is important to rule out extra-GI diseases and help manage consequences of enteric disease, as with small cell lymphoma and IBDs.

Ultrasonography commonly shows a focal intestinal thickening (of 5 to 25 mm) with partial or complete loss of distinction of intestinal layering as shown in Figure 23-24. The area of lymphomatous infiltration is hypoechoic, because it contains a uniform cell population without much reactionary fibrous tissue. Mesenteric lymphadenomegaly is common (Figure 23-25), as are changes in other organs, such as kidney, liver, or pancreas. Ascites may also be seen.[54,113] Although ultrasonographic distinctions predominate, there is considerable overlap between ultrasonographic findings with small cell lymphoma and high-grade lymphoma. The clinician must not lose sight of the fact that microscopic distinctions are required to diagnose either condition.

Cytologic diagnosis of high-grade lymphoma from fine-needle aspirates (FNA) is much more likely than with small cell lymphoma. This is because there is usually a focal lesion, and the neoplastic cells are a monomorphic population of large, immature cells (i.e., that are not normally seen in tissue). Sometimes, mixed lymphoid

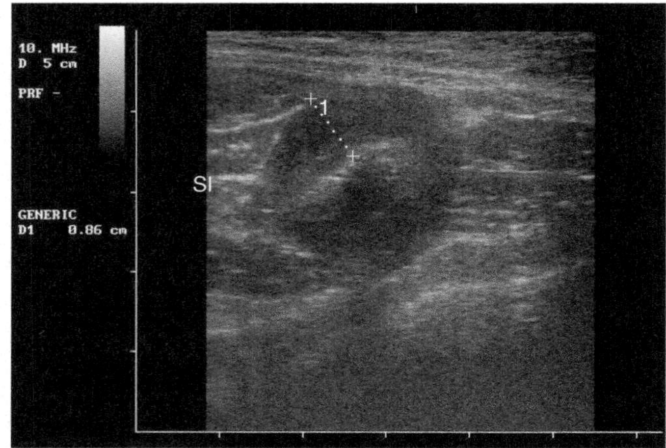

FIGURE 23-24 Ultrasonographic image of intestinal lymphoblastic lymphoma; the intestinal wall measurement is 8.6 mm. Note the total loss of layering.

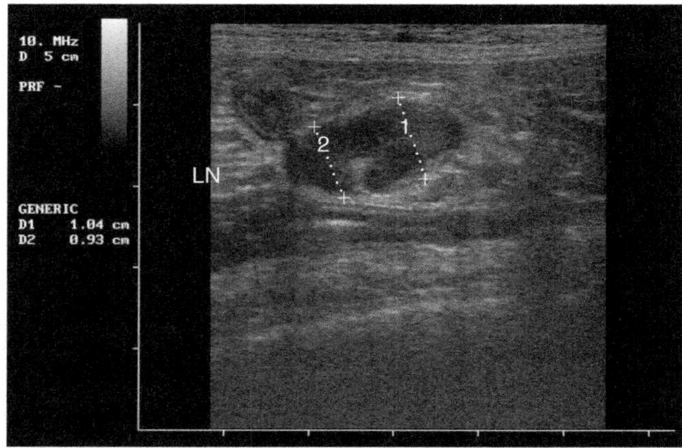

FIGURE 23-25 Ultrasonographic image of lymph node of a cat with intestinal lymphoblastic lymphoma, measurements are 10.4 mm and 9.3 mm (normal lymph nodes are <5 mm).

populations (of immature lymphoblasts and mature lymphocytes) are seen if a germinal lymphoid follicle is aspirated, and precise diagnosis may be difficult if there are a large number of lymphoblasts.[160] FNA samples are best obtained with ultrasound guidance. The cytologic sample quality is greatly improved by not aspirating when the needle is visualized in the mass but merely "pecked" into the mass so that the needle is merely acting to finely "core" the mass. On removing the syringe and needle, the hub of the needle is removed before drawing air into the syringe, the hub is replaced, and the sample within the needle is expressed onto a slide.

Usually, the decision to diagnose by cytology from FNA is based on the ultrasonographic appearance of a mass. Since there is substantial crossover of ultrasonographic appearance of intestinal masses, laparotomy for excision is often performed with the affected bowel submitted for histology. Except when intestinal obstruction has resulted, there is no therapeutic benefit of excising a gastrointestinal lymphoma (which requires excision and anastomosis), but there is minimal room for doubt when a histologic diagnosis is achieved.

Chemotherapy

The response to therapy for high-grade intestinal lymphoma is significantly worse than that for small cell lymphoma.[43,124] Further, response to therapy for high-grade intestinal lymphoma appears to be worse than for lymphoma in other anatomic locations.[142] Precise remission rates and survival times are difficult to quantify, because many studies assess lymphoma from multiple locations and do not necessarily differentiate response of gastrointestinal lymphoma or report the grade of lymphoma. With remission rates reported from 18% to 80%[43,92,176] and a median survival time of up to 41 weeks (range, 4 to 120 weeks),[176] it can be said with some certainty that *some* cats respond to therapy for reasonable durations. Multiple authors have noted that the best prognostic indicator is response to an initial treatment cycle,[92,100,176] which should prompt clinicians to encourage owners to start therapy and decide whether to continue based on the cat's response.

There are several published chemotherapeutic protocols,[43,92,100,142,176] but all follow the same principles of using medications to target specific phases of the cell division cycle (such as L-asparaginase and vincristine) with other medications that interrupt multiple phases of the cell cycle (cyclophosphamide and doxorubicin). Targeting the cancer cell in different ways enables more cells to be killed, reduces the toxicity of the individual drug used, and reduces the likelihood of resistance to a specific drug. Several authors have noted increased success with the addition of L-asparaginase and doxorubicin to protocols.[92,162,176]

Chemotherapy for lymphoma is covered in more detail in Chapter 28, Oncology.

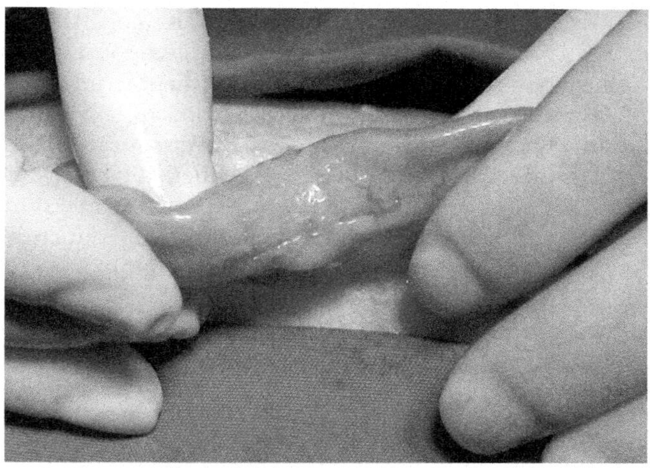

FIGURE 23-26 Appearance of the infiltrative form of intestinal adenocarcinoma at surgery; the thickened, annular, stenotic lesion can be seen.

Adenocarcinoma

Although noted as the next most common intestinal neoplasia, after the various forms of lymphoma, adenocarcinoma is seen relatively infrequently in practice. Most cats are more than 10 years old,[32,76,126] males may be overrepresented, and several studies have recognized a distinct overrepresentation of Siamese cats.[32,76]

Three distinct forms have been described[140]:

1. Infiltrative: characterized by a thickened, annular, stenotic lesion (Figure 23-26) that ultimately results in intestinal obstruction
2. Ulcerative: characterized by a deep, indurated mucosal ulcer with raised edges
3. Proliferative: characterized by a lobulated, expanding intestinal mass

Cats typically present with nonspecific signs of gastrointestinal disease but can present with obstructive signs. Cats with large bowel neoplasia can present for tenesmus or hematochezia and even constipation, if the lesion is obstructive (or partially obstructive). On physical examination, an abdominal mass is palpable in approximately 50% of cases, but other findings are usually nonspecific. Anemia can be found if mucosal ulceration has occurred, but there are no distinctive laboratory findings.

Lesions can occur anywhere along the intestinal tract. One study of 100 cases found 40% of feline intestinal adenocarcinoma lesions were present at the ileum or ileocolic junction.[32] Twenty-five to 50 percent of cases have metastasis at the time of the diagnosis, and this is a poor prognostic indicator.[32,76,145]

Radiology may show a mass lesion or intestinal obstruction, and ultrasonography can localize lesions to an intestinal origin. The ultrasonographic appearance of the proliferative, circumferential, outwardly expansile form is better described than the annular, constricting-band form with minimal outward enlargement. In these cases, sonographically, a solitary segmental intestinal mural mass is present and characterized by circumferential bowel wall thickening with transmural loss of normal sonographic wall layers. The thickening can vary in echogenicity but may be hypoechoic and may be symmetric or asymmetric. There is no definitive distinction, however, from lymphosarcoma, mast cell tumor, smooth muscle origin tumors, or even segmental benign inflammatory bowel disease.[126]

Surgical resection is the treatment of choice. There seem to be two distinct groups in terms of survival time postresection:

1. Short-duration survival (euthanasia or death within 2 weeks of surgery)
2. Long-duration survival (mean survival time of 15 months,[76] with a number of cats surviving greater than 2 years)[76,109]

Because clean margins improve prognosis, for large bowel adenocarcinoma, subtotal colectomy may be required for complete excision.[145] Because of the potential for success after resection, it is recommended to excise unidentified masses at the time of surgery.[145]

Other Intestinal Neoplasia

Other forms of intestinal neoplasia are recognized infrequently, and include intestinal mast cell tumors, adenomatous polyps, eosinophilic sclerosing fibroplasia, gastrointestinal stromal tumors (leiomyosarcoma), and hemangiosarcoma.

Intestinal Mast Cell Tumors

Mast cell tumors (MCT) are often cited as the third most common form of feline gastrointestinal tumor,[85] but the intestines are a far less common site than cutaneous, splenic, or hepatic mast cell neoplasia.[85,124] Masses are usually segmental nodular thickenings that occur in older cats.[140] The masses are indistinguishable ultrasonographically from other tumors, such as lymphoblastic lymphosarcoma.[126] A recent series of 50 cases described a variant of feline intestinal mast cell tumor, dubbed sclerosing mast cell tumor, for which neoplastic cells form a trabecular pattern with dense stromal collagen. Additionally, eosinophilic infiltrates were moderate to marked in most cases. These cases can be confused histologically with eosinophilic enteritis, gastrointestinal stromal tumor, or fibrosarcoma.[56] Surgical resection is recommended, but lesions are commonly infiltrative or metastasize widely, and there are few reports of successful treatment. Lomustine (dosed 50 to 60 mg/m^2, PO every 4 to 6 weeks) has recently been assessed as adjunctive chemotherapy for mast cell neoplasia in various locations,[123] and results look promising, but only two cats assessed had gastrointestinal mast cell neoplasia. Lomustine was used unsuccessfully in one cat with sclerosing MCT; another cat with sclerosing MCT received eight treatments of vinblastine and had a survival time of greater than 4 years.[56]

Adenomatous Polyps

Adenomatous polyps have been reported in the duodenum[87] and ileum[106] and can result in intussusception.[133] Cats of Asian ancestry, predominantly Siamese, are greatly overrepresented, and most reported cases have been males.[87] Cats usually present for vomiting or hematemesis that, surprisingly, can be very acute in onset; complete intestinal obstruction may result.[87,106,133] Resection is curative, with survival times of more than 4 years reported.[87]

Gastrointestinal Eosinophilic Sclerosing Fibroplasia

Eosinophilic sclerosing fibroplasia has recently been described in a series of 25 cases and is not strictly neoplasia.[29] The ulcerating mass lesions that can occur anywhere from the stomach to the colon are often grossly and histologically mistaken for neoplasia. There appears to be no breed predisposition or age predisposition (with ages ranging from 14 weeks to 16 years), but 18 of 25 cases (72%) were castrated males cats compared with 7 of 25 (28%) female spayed cats. Eighty-four percent of cats presented for vomiting, 68% presented for weight loss, and 7 of 12 (58%) cats had peripheral eosinophilia. All cases had a palpable abdominal mass. The pyloric sphincter was the most common site, and lesions in this location were mostly considered unresectable. Fourteen of 25 cats (56%) had bacterial colonies within microabscesses and necrotic foci within the lesion. The bacteria recognized were predominantly gram-negative rods, but antibiotics did not seem to be clinically effective. The bacteria are suspected to initiate the lesions, having been embedded after foreign body penetration. There are no specific treatment recommendations, but excision, where possible, would be prudent; corticosteroids appear to be helpful adjunctive therapy. Survival times are difficult to estimate since many cats were euthanized because neoplasia was suspected and follow-up times were short (up to 6 months) for the remaining cats.[29]

Gastrointestinal Stromal Tumors (Leiomyosarcoma)

There are very few reports of intestinal leiomyosarcomas in cats,[8,159] which have been reclassified as gastrointestinal stromal tumors.[99] These tumors may be more likely to arise from the ileocecocolic junction. Resection, if possible, is usually recommended, with survival times of 3 to 4 months reported before recurrence. The author owns a cat with this tumor where resection was not

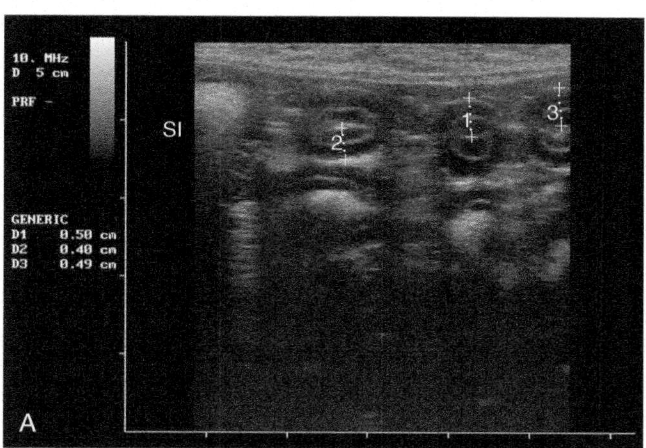

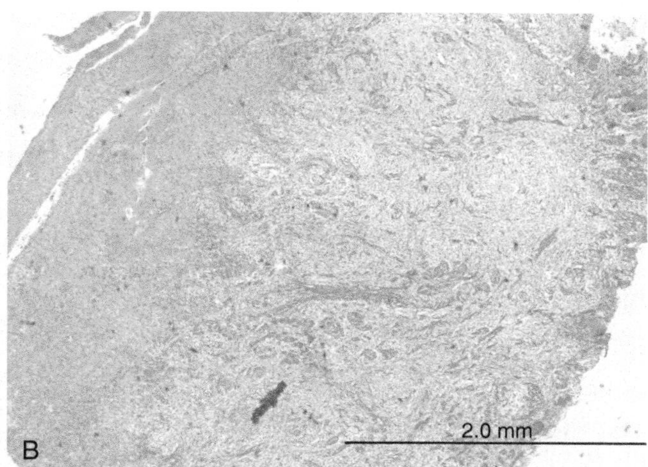

FIGURE 23-27 Ultrasonographic image (**A**) and photomicrograph (**B**) of a cat with gastrointestinal stromal tumor (leiomyosarcoma). The ultrasonographic image (**A**) demonstrates that notable thickening of both mucosal and muscularis layers. The histology (**B**) shows spindle cell proliferation extending between the smooth muscle bundles of the tunic muscularis.

possible, and the cat appears healthy 24 months past diagnosis (Figure 23-27).

Hemangiosarcoma

Cats with intestinal hemangiosarcoma often present with anemia, and the disease appears to be highly metastatic.[33] The intestines appear grossly thickened by dark red tissue.[138] The small and large intestines seem to be affected with similar frequency. Removal of macroscopic disease is recommended, but often the full extent of the severity is only recognized at surgery.[33] The prognosis is poor.

TABLE 23-16 **Common Intestinal Pathogens Differentiated by Most Likely Location**

Small Intestine	Both	Large Intestine
Coronavirus	*Campylobacter* spp.	Parvovirus (panleukopenia)
Toxocara cati	*Escherichia coli*	*Trichuris vulpis*
Toxascaris leonina	*Salmonella*	*Tritrichomonas foetus*
Ancylostoma tubaeforme		*Campylobacter* spp.
Giardia spp.		*Clostridium* spp.
Cryptosporidium parvum		*Yersinia enterocolitica*

INFECTIOUS ENTERITIS

Approach to Diagnosis

Suspicions of infectious causes of diarrhea should be aroused in younger cats, cats from shelters, or cats with immune suppression. When considering infectious causes of diarrhea, clinicians should assess whether the diarrhea is large bowel or small bowel in origin and correlate this with specific pathogens that are likely to cause clinical signs as shown in Table 23-16. To increase the diagnostic yield of fecal examination for parasitic causes of diarrhea, wet smears and appropriate fecal flotations should be performed on fresh fecal samples (<1 hour old). It is appropriate to administer broad-spectrum anthelminthics, even if fecal tests are negative.

Bacterial and viral causes of diarrhea should be considered when the cat is systemically unwell with fever. Fecal culture should be performed in these circumstances, but the limitations of this testing need to be recognized in that many intestinal bacteria can be found in healthy animals.[70] Further antibiotic administration can result in increase of other bacteria.[69]

Fungal causes of diarrhea are usually recognized from histology of biopsy samples.

It remains to be seen whether the recent ready availability of PCR panels looking at a number of infectious causes of diarrhea will be beneficial for recognizing pathogens that had previously been misdiagnosed or a hindrance for readily recognizing commensal organisms not necessarily causative of the clinical signs being investigated.

The most common viral, bacterial, and mycotic causes of diarrhea in cats are described below. Parasitic gastrointestinal diseases are covered later in this chapter.

Viral Enteritis

Viral causes of diarrhea are not usually specifically diagnosed, since, with the exception of the canine fecal ELISA for parvovirus, routine definitive tests are not available.

Panleukopenia/Parvovirus

Clinical signs of panleukopenia (feline parvovirus infection) are more likely to occur in kittens, with the highest morbidity and mortality occurring between 3 and 5 months of age. Subclinical cases in older (susceptible) cats probably go unrecognized. The organism is very stable in most environments, and infections mostly occur from environmental contact.

Peracute cases can result in death within 12 hours, with little or no warning signs. Acute cases often have fever, depression, and anorexia, with signs beginning approximately 3 to 4 days before presentation. Vomiting is usually bile tinged and unrelated to eating. Diarrhea does not always occur, and when it does, it is usually later in the course of the illness. Leukopenia is not pathognomonic, because this can also occur with acute bacterial infection (e.g., salmonellosis can present identically).[53]

Commercially available ELISA tests for canine parvovirus antigen in feces can detect feline parvovirus; however, shedding may have ceased by the time clinical signs occur, and vaccination can result in positive test results for up to 2 weeks.[111]

Aggressive fluid therapy, usually at twice maintenance rates, is usually required. Broad-spectrum antibiotic coverage is used to prevent or treat secondary bacterial infection from viral injury of intestinal mucosa. Parenteral antibiotics are preferred to prevent the possibility of further gastrointestinal irritation. The author recommends calculating IV doses and introducing appropriate amounts of antibiotics to the fluids bag to create a constant rate infusion (CRI); cefazolin can be used in this way at 100 mg/kg/24 hours, and beta-lactam CRIs are commonly used in human medicine.[127] Aminoglycosides or fluoroquinolones can be used concurrently at routine doses if fever persists after 24 hours or the cat is moribund on presentation, but care must be used with these agents. Aminoglycosides are potentially nephrotoxic, and fluoroquinolones have been reported to result in cartilage damage in growing animals, although this has not been demonstrated clinically in cats.[134] Fluoroquinolone retinal toxicity has been seen in all animals. Cats that survive the first week usually recover, and prior infection imparts lifelong immunity.[28] Vaccinations are highly effective for disease prevention.

Coronavirus

Feline enteric coronavirus (FECV) mostly causes mild, self-limiting diarrhea and must be distinguished from feline infectious peritonitis coronavirus (FIPCV), which is essentially always fatal and for which diarrhea is not a typical sign (but is possible). The most widely accepted current theory of FIP pathogenesis involves initial infection with FECV and then mutation to FIPCV in small numbers of susceptible individuals.[112,165]

Routine serologic testing for FECV in cats with diarrhea would neither prove correlation with the clinical signs nor affect how the disease is managed and so is not recommended. Cats with FECV diarrhea should be managed with symptomatic therapy of fasting, then reintroducing a bland diet and supportive care with fluid therapy if necessary.

Other Viral Enteridities

Other viruses, such as astrovirus, reovirus, rotavirus, and torovirus-like agent, have been recognized to cause diarrhea in cats, but their roles as pathogens are unclear. They are not routinely recognized in practice, since electron microscopy of fecal samples is necessary for diagnosis and is not routinely performed. Management is supportive care with appropriate fasting, then reintroduction of bland diets and fluid and electrolyte replacement if necessary.[51]

Bacterial Enteritis

Successful identification of a known bacterial pathogen from a fecal sample does not necessarily mean that the agent found is the cause of disease in the cat. Although a number of bacterial pathogens have been demonstrated to cause diseases when specific pathogen-free (SPF) cats are experimentally infected,[42] these same organisms can be found in healthy cats.[93] The differences between healthy and diarrheic cats that have bacteria found in their feces may relate to virulence factors of the organism, or host factors (local or systemic immunity) of the cat. There is no definitive answer for this quandary. The author's opinion is that

- If a diarrheic cat is systemically unwell and has a fever, then feces should be cultured.
- If an organism is isolated that is known to cause signs consistent with those the cat is showing, the cat should be treated appropriately.

Campylobacter

Campylobacter diarrhea is usually caused by *C. jejuni*. Clinical signs of infection are poorly documented, but most cats are asymptomatic. Younger cats are more likely to have clinical signs and hemorrhagic, mucoid diarrhea has been reported. Diagnosis can be from culture of feces or swabs, and the organism is quite hardy; so, it usually survives transport to the laboratory.[28] In individual cases, the organism has not been cultured after antibiotic treatment,[45,46] but it is not definitively proven that antibiotic therapy affects the natural course of the disease. Antibiotics that can be used are amoxicillin-clavulanate (15 mg/kg, every 12 hours, PO) or fluoroquinolones, such as enrofloxacin (5 mg/kg, once daily, PO) for durations of 14 to 21 days.[44] Macrolides, such as erythromycin (10 to 15 mg/kg, every 8 hours, PO), are regarded as the drug of choice for humans but can cause gastrointestinal side effects.[93]

Clostridium

Clostridium difficile has been recognized in up to 5% of diarrheic cats.[93] Clinical signs are typically acute onset watery diarrhea and anorexia. Diagnosis has been made with detection of toxin A or toxin B in fecal samples using ELISA. Although these tests have not yet been validated for cats, they may prove to be a useful aid to diagnosis[94] and are available for testing of equine feces at some commercial laboratories. Nontoxigenic strains exist; so, positive culture alone does not ensure diagnosis. Metronidazole (10 mg/kg, every 12 hours, PO) for approximately 7 days is the treatment of choice.[93]

Clostridium perfringens typically results in large bowel diarrhea with tenesmus, mucus, and hematochezia, but small bowel signs can also be seen.[42] PCR testing for enterotoxin A is commercially available and may prove to be a useful adjunct in diagnosis. Antibiotics that can be used include metronidazole (10 mg/kg, every 12 hours, PO), tylosin (10 to 20 mg/kg, twice daily, PO), or amoxicillin-clavulanate (22 mg/kg, every 12 hours, PO) for 7 days.[94]

Escherichia coli

Escherichia coli is a ubiquitous organism within the feline intestinal tract, and it would be unusual not to successfully culture *E. coli* from the feces of both healthy and unwell cats. When *E. coli* is associated with clinical signs of gastrointestinal disease, it is mostly as an opportunistic pathogen, with overgrowth resulting from changed environmental conditions, such as inflammation from other pathology or another pathogen. There are also specific strains of *E. coli* that are true pathogens because of virulence factors not present in commensal *E. coli*; these include enteropathogenic *E. coli* and enterotoxigenic *E. coli*, which both induce a watery diarrhea, and enterohemorrhagic *E. coli*, which produces a diarrheal syndrome with copious bloody discharge and no fever.[77] PCR testing is commercially available to identify pathogenic strains of *E. coli*[16,148]; although not offered at routine veterinary laboratories, this testing is available to veterinarians, and laboratories offering these services can readily be found online. Diagnosis should also document histologic lesions corresponding to the strain of *E. coli* identified.[77] There is emerging resistance to *E. coli* worldwide in all species of animals, including humans. This includes the typical therapies for gram-negative bacteria of beta-lactam–enhanced penicillins and fluoroquinolones.[167] A major risk factor is prior antibiotic usage, because commensal organisms are exposed to antibiotics. PCR testing does not enable antibiotic sensitivity testing, and fecal culture may not be able to distinguish pathogenic from nonpathogenic strains; so, sensitivities may not be an accurate reflection of the pathogenic organism. PCR testing for genes that impart resistance to *E. coli* have recently been described but are not yet commercially available.[34] In some circumstances, supportive care with fluid and electrolyte replacement may be all that is required while the cat's immune system combats the infection. Empiric therapy could include beta-lactam–enhanced penicillins (such as amoxicillin-clavulanate at 20 mg/kg, every 12 hours, PO), fluoroquinolones (such as enrofloxacin at 5 mg/kg, once daily, PO), or cefovecin (8 mg/kg, every 2 weeks, SC), but the clinician must be aware of possible drug resistance.

Salmonella

Salmonella typhimurium infection is possible from ingestion of infected prey, infected food sources, or from a contaminated environment, including the veterinary hospital. The resulting clinical signs depend on the number of infecting organisms, the immune status of the cat, and the presence of concurrent diseases. Infection rates in cats (and humans) have been correlated with seasonal bird migrations,[153] and the illness has been dubbed songbird fever,[52] but there is no distinction between this and other *Salmonella* infections. Clinical signs usually begin 3 to 5 days after exposure, starting with fever (often >40° C [104° F]), malaise and anorexia, and progressing to diarrhea, vomiting, and abdominal pain. Hematology can show leukopenia with a left shift and nonregenerative anemia, and biochemistry results are usually nonspecific. Diagnosis is based on isolation of the organism by culture or identification with PCR, but care should be taken to correlate pathogen identification with clinical signs since, as with most GI pathogens, the organism can be isolated from healthy animals.[147] As with *E. coli*, antibiotic resistance is widespread,[120] with one United Kingdom survey finding the multiple drug-resistant strain DT104 to be the most frequent bacteriophage type identified.[115] Treatment should be reserved only for those cats showing systemic signs, because routine antibiotic use in treating salmonellosis induces drug-resistant strains and prolongs the convalescent excretion period.[52] Antibiotic choice should be based solely on sensitivity findings, since resistances are so widespread and unpredictable.[98] This means that if the organism has been identified by PCR, then culture of feces must also be undertaken. The duration of treatment must be long enough to eliminate fecal excretion of the organism, prevent the chance of relapse, and reduce the chance of resistance developing; up to 28 days has been advocated.[4,164] These cautions are particularly important because of the zoonotic potential of salmonellosis.

Other Bacterial Enteridities

Other bacterial causes of diarrhea have been reported in cats, such as *Yersinia enterocolitica*,[48] *Yersinia pseudotuberculosis*,[63] *Clostridium piliforme* (Tyzzer's disease),[71] and *Anaerobiospirillum* sp.[36] Specific diagnosis of these (and other bacterial infections) may be found in the course of investigation. Management follows the principles of supportive care and appropriate antibiosis based on sensitivity testing.

Small Intestinal Bacterial Overgrowth

Small intestinal bacterial overgrowth (SIBO) has not been specifically described in cats. The criteria defined for dogs is a fasting bacterial count in duodenal juice of greater than 10^5 organisms/mL[11] and is often recognized with other chronic gastrointestinal diseases.[130] Healthy cats appear to have at least this number of upper intestinal bacterial with a range of 10^5 to 10^8/mL recognized.[68] Bacterial overgrowth could potentially occur with ileus or intestinal inflammation of any underlying cause. Foul-smelling small bowel diarrhea with no specific pathogen recognized may be an indicator of this condition, as could an increase in bacterial metabolites, such as folate. If suspected, it is appropriate to manage with broad-spectrum antibiotics, such as metronidazole (10 to 15 mg/kg, every 12 hours, PO) or amoxicillin (10 mg/kg, every 12 hours, PO) for an extended duration such as 21 to 28 days. Alterations in intestinal flora have been recognized after such treatment[69]; however, any advice for this "condition" is entirely empirical. All efforts should be directed at identifying a precise underlying cause.

Mycotic Enteritis

Mycotic and other infectious agents are only rarely recognized as intestinal pathogens in cats. Diagnosis is made by histologic and microbial analysis of samples obtained at biopsy. Possible agents include *Histoplasma capsulatum*,[24] *Aspergillus* spp., *Candida albicans*,[140] and *Pythium insidiosum*.[119]

INTESTINAL OBSTRUCTION

Intestinal obstructions arise most commonly as a result of neoplasia in older cats and foreign body ingestion predominantly in younger cats.[10,41,60] Less common causes include intussusception[83] and granulomatous inflammation (e.g., from FIP)[59]; tapeworm infection, with greater than 30 worms acting as a linear foreign body, has also been reported.[173] Other listed causes are volvulus, intestinal torsion, incarceration of bowel in a hernia, adhesions or stricture, intramural abscess or hematoma, and congenital malformations.[140]

Intestinal Foreign Bodies

Patient Signalment and Risk Factors

Linear foreign bodies have traditionally been considered more common than discrete foreign bodies in cats,[10,14,41] but a study from a primary care facility indicated only 33% of foreign body cases were because of linear foreign bodies.[60] The larger case load of linear foreign bodies at referral institutions noted in earlier studies may indicate the abilities of primary care practitioners to recognize and effectively deal with discrete foreign body obstructions.

Most studies have found that cats with intestinal foreign bodies are generally younger (mean, 1.0 to 2.7 years), with a notable exception being obstruction from trichobezoars where three of five cats in one study were 10 years or older; the greatest risk factor appears to be length of hair coat.[9] No specific breed predispositions have been described but Siamese and Siamese-related cats have been noted to have oral fixations[13] and so may be expected to be overrepresented with intestinal foreign bodies.

Clinical Signs

Clinical signs will vary depending on the type of foreign body (linear or discrete), the position of obstruction, and the time since obstruction. Most cats present for anorexia or vomiting. Partial obstruction can result in diarrhea (which can be bloody). Foreign body obstruction is typically considered an acute condition, with duration of obstruction because of a linear foreign body, measured from the onset of clinical signs to diagnosis, reported to range from 1 to 10 days.[10,41,60] However, one paper demonstrated chronic, intermittent, gastrointestinal disease from a linear foreign body of a 1-month duration[175] demonstrating that partial obstruction can result in a chronic course.

Physical examination may or may not reveal abdominal pain, palpable abdominal mass (or plication), dehydration, or fever. *All cats presenting for anorexia or vomiting should have the underside of the tongue evaluated for the presence of a linear foreign body.* Applying gentle pressure with a thumb in the intermandibular space to elevate the tongue is an effective way to visualize lesions or foreign bodies in the sublingual area (see Figure 3-8).

Pathophysiology

Life-threatening consequences can result from the interactions of local and systemic factors that arise from intestinal obstruction. Locally, damage to the mucosa from traction and pressure of the foreign object can cause hemorrhage, ischemia, and necrosis. Systemically, hypovolemia, toxemia, and acid–base and electrolyte imbalances can ensue.

Complete intestinal obstruction by discrete masses results in gas and fluid distention of the lumen proximal to the obstruction. Most gas accumulation is a result of swallowed air, which is predominantly nitrogen that cannot be absorbed by the intestinal mucosa. Gas also arises from bacterial fermentation. Fluid accumulates as a result of increased secretions (saliva, bile, and secretions of gastric, pancreatic, and small intestinal origin) and retention of fluid already ingested, and it can be augmented by local hemorrhage.[39] Since most intestinal obstructions in cats do not reach the midjejunum,[60] reabsorption of fluids that normally occurs at the jejunum and ileum is impaired.[39]

Linear foreign bodies, such as string, dental floss, or elastic toys, require proximal anchoring, usually under the tongue or in the pylorus (for example, by part of a toy attached to elastic). Peristalsis moves the free end of the "string" through the intestinal tract, resulting in pleats of intestines around the foreign body. As the foreign body is forced against the intestinal mucosa, the mucosa becomes edematous, and even partial penetration affects mucosal integrity, allowing systemic entry of bacteria.

Intraluminal bacterial populations increase for both discrete and linear foreign bodies as a result of stasis. Mucosal permeability can be affected by prolonged luminal distention, allowing entry of bacteria and toxins systemically or into the peritoneal cavity. Direct entry of bacteria to the peritoneal cavity, causing septic peritonitis, can result from perforation of the intestinal wall from linear foreign bodies or sharp discrete foreign bodies, such as toothpicks or plastic toys.

Diagnosis

Definitive diagnosis requires identification of the foreign body retrieved at surgery or in some cases, by endoscopy. This may be aided greatly prior to surgery by diagnostic imaging. However, imaging findings, particularly in the case of partial obstructions, may be subtle enough that obstruction of no identifiable cause is recognized or no overt signs are apparent. Laboratory findings are not helpful in the precise diagnosis but are important to assess fluid and electrolyte balances that must be corrected.

Cats rarely help practitioners by ingesting radiopaque objects, but on the rare occasions that they do, these can be observed easily on plain radiographs. Nonopaque foreign bodies depend on dilatation of the intestine from gas and fluid accumulation proximal to the obstruction for radiographic recognition (Figure 23-28). One study has suggested that if the jejunal diameter is greater than 2.5 times the length of the cranial end plate of the second lumbar vertebra, then intestinal obstruction is the most likely abnormality. Care must be taken that the jejunal and not duodenal diameter is measured and that the radiographs must be positioned strictly lateral, because an oblique view can alter the measurement of the lumbar vertebra.[1] However, dilatation of an obstructed intestine

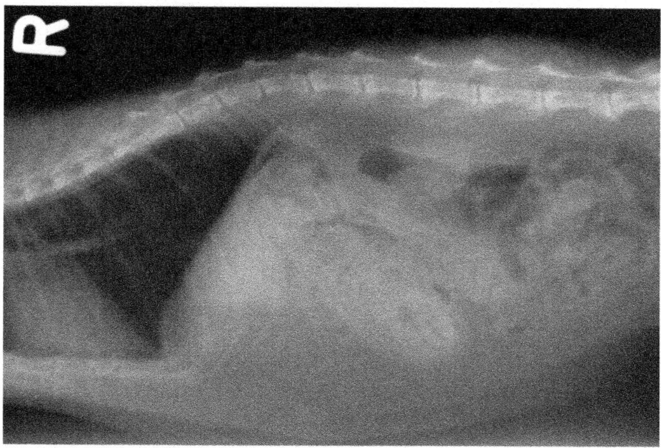

FIGURE 23-28 Radiography of discrete foreign body. Note that the dilatation of the intestine from gas and fluid accumulation proximal to the foreign body appears caudal to the obstruction. The foreign body was a piece of leather, and the obstruction was in the duodenum. The gross appearance is shown in Figure 23-33.

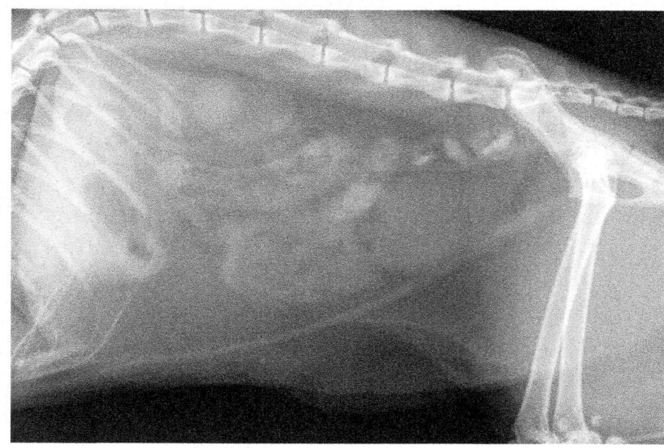

FIGURE 23-29 Radiographic appearance of a linear foreign body (lateral view). Note that most of the small intestine is localized in midventral region of the abdominal cavity instead of being dispersed uniformly throughout the peritoneal cavity.

may not occur if the obstruction is partial or intermittent, or if vomiting results in less fluid present. Since most foreign body obstructions in cats are proximal, identifiable dilatation may not be recognized for this reason.[78] Linear foreign bodies present further challenges for radiographic recognition; the following typical radiographic signs[129,137] may or may not be present:

- Accordion-like pleating or gathering (plication) of the jejunum
- Most of the small intestine localized in midventral region of the abdominal cavity instead of being dispersed uniformly throughout the peritoneal cavity on the lateral view (Figure 23-29)
- Gathering of small intestine to the right side of the midline in the ventrodorsal view (Figure 23-30)

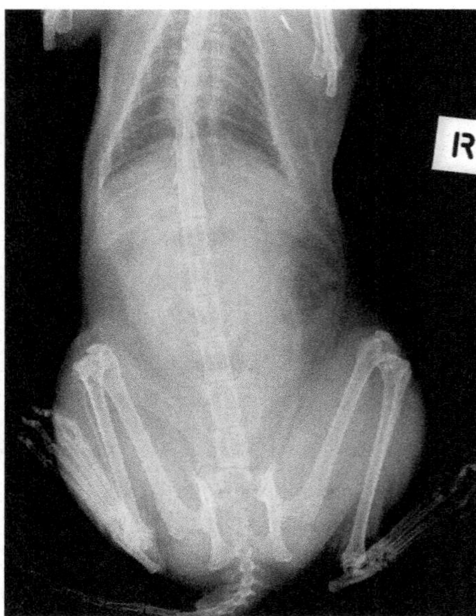

FIGURE 23-30 Radiographic appearance of a linear foreign body (ventrodorsal view). Note the gathering of most of the small intestine to the right side of the midline.

- Altered gas pattern with luminal gas collecting in small bubbles instead of normal curved tubular columns. This can be subtle when there is only minimal involvement of the intestine but overt when involving the entire small intestine. Comma-shaped gas patterns are more likely to occur with linear foreign bodies.[1]

Contrast radiography can aid diagnosis for both discrete and linear foreign bodies but should be used with caution because intestinal perforation may be present. Nonionic iodinated agents that are typically used for myelography (such as iopamidol or iohexol) should be used, since barium is irritating to the peritoneum and oral iodine compounds are hypertonic. Hypertonic compounds may draw fluid into the stomach and intestines after oral administration, with the potential of creating further fluid and electrolyte imbalances in an already compromised patient.[137]

Ultrasonography is a very useful diagnostic tool, particularly for discrete foreign bodies, where, in most cases, there is overt distention of the small intestines with intraluminal fluid apparent (Figure 23-31). This modality has not been extensively assessed as an adjunct to diagnosis of foreign body intestinal obstruction in cats specifically, although there are several papers assessing dogs and small numbers of cats that agree with its utility.[114,156,161] Linear foreign bodies are more difficult to assess ultrasonographically, but plicated bowel can be recognized, sometimes with the foreign body seen as a hyperechoic line centrally.[156]

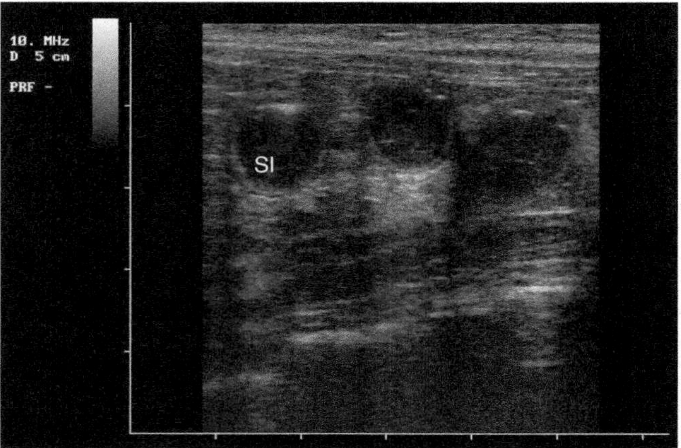

FIGURE 23-31 Ultrasonographic image of a grossly distended intestinal lumen because of intestinal obstruction with a discrete foreign body.

Conservative Management

Successful treatment of foreign body obstruction requires evacuation or removal of the foreign body as well as correction of any bacteremia or endotoxemia, acid–base or fluid imbalances. Discrete foreign body obstruction requires surgery or endoscopy to remove the object. In some specific circumstances, linear foreign body obstruction *may* be managed conservatively by cutting the anchor point below the tongue and allowing the cat to pass the foreign body by peristalsis. However, the decision to manage a cat conservatively must be done with the cat hospitalized, with fluid therapy and antibiotic coverage and a clear recognition on behalf of the practitioner and the owner that surgery may subsequently be required.

Cutting a sublingual linear foreign body may be achieved in a conscious cat by applying pressure with the thumb of one hand in the intermandibular space to elevate the tongue and gently grasping it using gauze with the other hand while a second person cuts the line with a suture cutter. There is a chance of a small nick on the sublingual surface. If the cat will not tolerate the procedure, sedation is appropriate. When cutting the line, the nature of the linear foreign body should be assessed (i.e., is it more or less likely to cut mucosa). In one study,[10] 19 cats with linear foreign bodies were managed conservatively with 10 cats subsequently requiring surgery. The authors of that paper created guidelines that will be adapted here.

Conservative management should be attempted if the cat

- Is presented acutely (within 2 days) after known ingestion of a linear foreign body
- Has a sublingually fixed linear foreign body that can be cut
- Has no overt signs of peritonitis

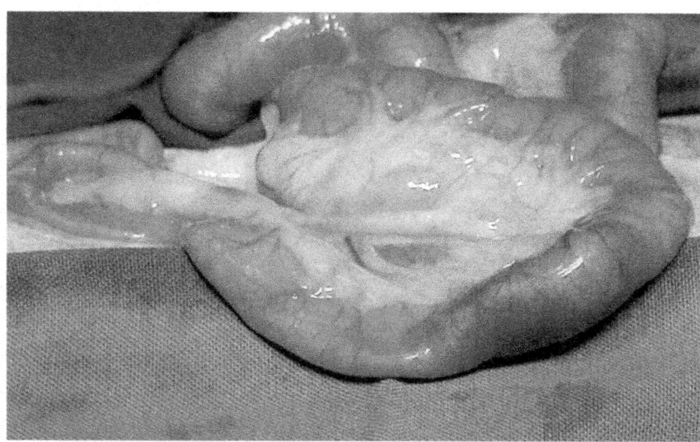

FIGURE 23-32 Appearance of a discrete foreign body at laparotomy. Note intestines are distended distal to obstruction (top and right of picture) but not proximally (to the left and bottom of picture).

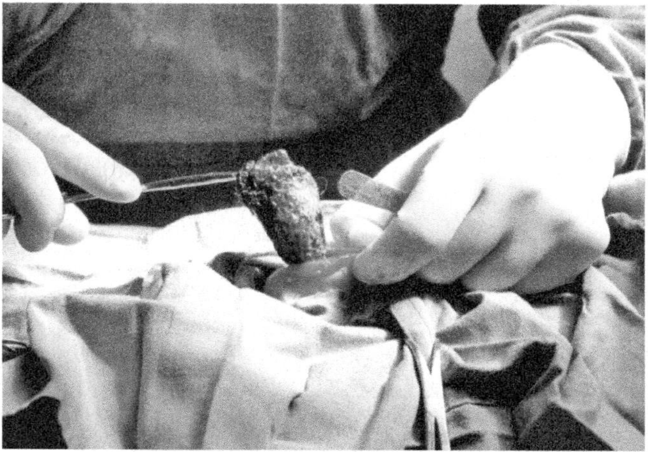

FIGURE 23-33 Removal of a discrete foreign body (a piece of leather) at laparotomy. Enterotomy to remove discrete foreign bodies should always be distal to the obstruction, because the intestine is likely to be compromised proximal to as well as overlying the obstruction. This is the same cat as in the radiology image in Figure 23-28.

Surgical intervention is mandatory if

- Clinical signs (e.g., vomiting or anorexia) persist or deterioration occurs with conservative management
- The cat has overt signs of peritonitis
- The linear foreign body is fixed at the pylorus

Some authors disagree with attempting conservative management, since a perforated intestine from a linear foreign body reportedly carries a 50% mortality rate,[41,88] and early surgical intervention is never an incorrect decision. This should be balanced with the observation that cats can carry a linear intestinal foreign body, such as an elastic cord for a 1-month duration without intestinal perforation.[175] However, fishing line, for example, would not be so forgiving!

Surgical Management

Surgery to remove an intestinal foreign body (Figures 23-32 and 23-33) should be considered an exploratory laparotomy. That is, the aim of the surgery is not only to remove the foreign body but to assess the entire intestinal tract and abdomen for other foreign bodies or pathology.

Enterotomy to remove discrete foreign bodies should always be distal to the obstruction, because the intestine is likely to be compromised proximal to as well as overlying the obstruction, thus delaying healing and creating the potential for surgical dehiscence. Linear foreign bodies require multiple enterotomy incisions, since pulling the object out through a single incision could create iatrogenic intestinal perforation. The anchor point (either sublingual or pylorus by gastrotomy) *must* be released in the first instance. Enterotomy incisions are closed with 5/0 synthetic, monofilament, absorbable suture material, such as polydioxyanone (PDS) or equivalent, in either a simple interrupted or simple continuous pattern.[14,88]

A technique has been described for removal of linear foreign bodies by making a single enterotomy incision proximally and passing a red rubber catheter over the linear foreign body aborally, milking the foreign body within the catheter through the colon for retrieval from the cat's anus by an assistant.[2] This technique is not always effective, because it can be hampered if the foreign body is knotted or does not run smoothly through the red rubber catheter.[102]

If the affected bowel segment demonstrates evidence of necrosis or perforation on the mesenteric border of the intestine, resection and anastomosis should be performed. Necrosis is indicated by dark discoloration, thin intestinal wall, poor arterial pulsation, poor capillary bleeding, or lack of peristalsis. End-to-end anastomosis can be accomplished using a simple interrupted appositional pattern or a modified simple continuous appositional pattern with the same type of suture material used for enterotomy closure.[14,88]

Mass Obstruction

Intraabdominal masses causing intestinal obstruction are often presumed to be neoplastic but can also be of infectious origin. Resection, where possible, is always recommended, because resection of neoplasia (if no metastasis) can offer a good prognosis,[76,87,109,145] and infectious causes may be managed with adjunctive therapy after definitive diagnosis.

Neoplasia

Intestinal obstruction in older cats is more likely to be secondary to neoplasia. Any neoplasia can cause obstruction, but adenocarcinoma[32,76] and adenomatous polyps[88,106] are reported to cause obstruction more often than other types of neoplasia. Please refer to the sections on intestinal neoplasia earlier in this chapter for more details.

Granulomatous Inflammation

Granulomatous inflammation causing a single focal intestinal lesion can lead to obstruction in the same way that neoplastic change can. Feline infectious peritonitis (FIP) can present as focal lesions,[59] often in the colon or ileocecocolic junction. In the case of FIP, the focal lesion is usually an indicator of multisystemic disease; so, resection does not help prognosis.

The fungus-like organism, *Pythium insidiosum* has also been reported to cause granulomatous lesions, resulting in intestinal obstruction[119] from large extraluminal masses that are approximately fist sized. Resection with adjunctive itraconazole (10 mg/kg) for 2 months after surgery was a successful treatment.

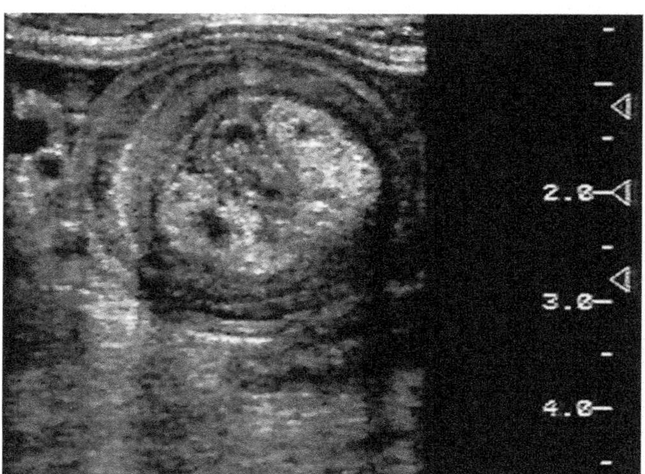

FIGURE 23-34 Ultrasonographic image of ileocolic intussusceptions. Note concentric circles alternating increased and decreased echogenicity within grossly distended intestines. *(Courtesy Dr. Karon Hoffmann, University of Sydney.)*

Intussusception

Intussusception refers to invagination or prolapse of one portion of the intestine into the part of the tract that either precedes or follows it. There is a bimodal age distribution with intussusceptions in older cats, most likely associated with neoplasia (or IBD in some cases)[25]; underlying causes for younger cats are ill defined and may be idiopathic in many cases,[15,25] but associations with parasitism and, in one case, a linear foreign body, have been made. Siamese and Burmese cats seem to be overrepresented. The most common locations are the ileocolic region and the jejunum.[15,25,83,110]

Affected cats present with nonspecific signs of gastrointestinal disease, such as anorexia and lethargy. Vomiting is not necessarily a presenting sign; diarrhea may occur. Abdominal palpation reveals a mass in most cases. Plain and contrast radiography only show evidence of obstruction and usually do not help define that the bowel has intussuscepted.[15,25,83,110]

Ultrasonography is very useful for diagnosis, because a distinctive pattern of alternating hypoechoic and hyperechoic concentric rings (Figure 23-34) is present in transverse sections.[25,110] Sometimes, the target lesion seen can be hard to distinguish from the pathology of other intraabdominal masses, such as lymph nodes, and in these cases, the size of the lesions can help, because the width will always be greater than 11 mm with an intussusception (because the sum of at least four intestinal wall widths cannot be less) and is often greater than16 mm.[110]

Surgical correction is always required, and manual reduction is typically not possible because there is usually significant venous infarction, edema, and congestion (Figure 23-35) as well as adhesions from fibrin and effusions from the affected bowel.[15,25] If the intussusception *does not* reduce manually, resection of the

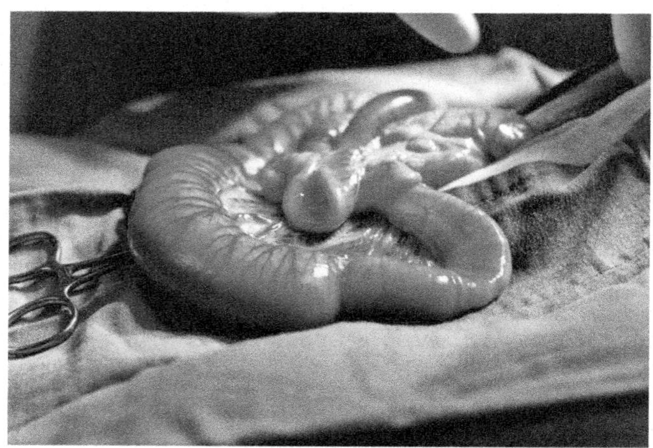

FIGURE 23-35 Gross appearance of ileal intussusception at laparotomy.

affected bowel is required, with anastomosis of the healthy tissue. There appears to be no benefit to enteroplication, which can result in significant ileus. There is no benefit to performing resection-anastomosis if the intussusception *does* reduce manually.[15,25]

The prognosis depends on the underlying disease process and the chronicity of the intussusception, and therefore how debilitated the cat is at presentation, However, prognosis is mostly good, with survival reported in up to 80% of cases, though recurrence can occur in some cats with idiopathic disease, often at different locations of the intestinal tract.[15]

CONSTIPATION AND MEGACOLON

Constipation is defined as infrequent or difficult defecation associated with retention of feces within the colon and rectum. Prolonged constipation results in harder and drier feces that become impacted, and this is known as *obstipation.*[140] Chronic, recurrent constipation and obstipation can result in *megacolon,* which refers to persistent increased bowel diameter that is not responsive to therapy. Megacolon is not a specific disease entity; it may be considered the most advanced stage in the spectrum of chronic constipation.[18]

In most cases, constipation can be managed quite simply if the underlying cause is determined and dealt with. A comprehensive list of causes of constipation is noted in Table 23-17, but the underlying causes can usually be attributed to

1. Reticence to defecate, because of
   a. Colorectal or anal pain
   b. Difficulty squatting
2. Inability to defecate, because of
   a. Fecal factors (including dehydration and fecal bulk)
   b. Colon factors (poor peristalsis)
3. Physical obstruction (less common), such as
   a. Mass (discrete foreign bodies do not obstruct distally in cats)
   b. Trauma resulting in pelvic canal narrowing

Of course, multiple factors can interact. For example, an older cat may have renal disease and so will be dehydrated to some degree and have arthritic hips and so be reticent to squat.

Clinical Signs

The presenting signs of constipation are usually evident to owners and include straining in the litter box and producing hard dry feces, if at all. Sometimes, however, owners can misinterpret signs. Cats can strain because of lower urinary tract problems, and, if no urine is produced, some owners assume the problem is because of constipation. Some constipated cats can intermittently have diarrhea because of direct colonic irritation from hard dry feces and so may present for diarrhea and not constipation. Cats can also present for less specific signs, such as anorexia, lethargy, weight loss, and even vomiting.[140,170] Vomiting can occur because of colonic receptors stimulating vagal afferent endings, which, in turn, can stimulate the chemoreceptor trigger zone.[61] Sometimes owners are concerned that their cat is defecating less, but the cat has just changed its diet to a much lower–residue diet and so is producing less feces. A full dietary history is an important aspect of the initial assessment.

Physical examination should confirm presence of feces in the colon and assess the degree of impaction. The presence of feces can usually be confirmed by abdominal palpation. In constipated cats, the colon is often palpated as a long firm tube extending cranially; sometimes, feces can be palpated to and around the colic flexure. Alternatively, the feces may be palpated as large, discrete fecal concretions (that can sometimes be hard to distinguish from intraabdominal masses such as lymph nodes). If there is any doubt of the presence or degree of fecal impaction, survey abdominal radiographs should be taken. A lateral view taken in a conscious cat should be adequate to confirm the diagnosis.

The physical examination should also assess for contributing causes, including musculoskeletal conditions. Any recent trauma should be taken into account. The hips and lumbosacral region should be assessed for pain. The degree of flexion and extension of the hips should be gently assessed. The lumbosacral spine can be assessed by running two fingers on either side of the spinous processes. The cat will flinch in painful areas. Any arthritic change is magnified in an underweight cat, since there may be less muscle mass and the joints may bear a heavier load. Any suspicions of underlying musculoskeletal abnormalities can be confirmed with radiographs.

Neurologic assessment should also be performed. Subtle changes just affecting colonic innervation will not be apparent on physical examination alone. However, an assessment of proprioception, placing reflexes, and gait should at least be performed to assess for lumbosacral spinal cord disease. Anorectal abnormalities or lesions should be evaluated. Impacted or infected anal sacs can lead to reticence to defecate; and therefore anal sacs should be assessed and expressed. Because this is painful for most cats, the cat should be held by an experienced assistant. The author prefers expressing one anal sac at a time with well-lubricated gloves and the index finger within the rectum and the thumb positioned externally. A rectal exam can be performed with a well-lubricated (gloved!) middle finger, feeling over the pelvic rim for masses as well as assessing if the colon closes over (squeezes) the finger. If the colon feels open around the finger, this can be an indicator of impaired colonic innervation but does not imply that this is a permanent change. If there are impacted feces continuing to the anus, rectal examination is not possible until this has been cleared. If a cat finds anal gland expression or rectal examination too painful to tolerate (based on the clinician's judgment), these procedures should be done under sedation.

Hydration and electrolyte status are also important factors in the constipated cat. Chronic renal disease is defined by azotemia (in conjunction with inadequately concentrated urine), which means the cat must be dehydrated to some degree. Plasma or serum biochemistry and urinalysis can be used to diagnose renal disease, assess degree of renal disease, or recognize prerenal dehydration. Electrolyte changes including hypokalemia and hypocalcemia may also contribute to reduced colonic smooth muscle function.[140] In young to middle-aged cats of apparent good health and hydration, blood

TABLE 23-17 **Classifications and Causes of Constipation**

Category	Cause
Dietary factors	Ingestion of foreign material (e.g., impaction of hair, bones, rodent, or bird carcasses, cloth, litter, plant material) Inadequate daily water intake
Environmental/psychological factors	Dirty litter box Prolonged inactivity Confinement (hospitalization, boarding) Change in habitat or daily routine Territorial competition with other cats
Difficulty posturing for defecation	Paraplegia Orthopedic diseases (spine, pelvis, or caudal limbs)
Painful anorectal disorders	Anal sac impaction, infection, or abscess Anorectal stricture, tumor, or foreign body Myiasis Perianal bite wound cellulitis or abscess Pseudocoprostasis
Anorectal obstruction	Extramural Malunion of pelvic and sacroiliac fractures Pelvic collapse attributable to nutritional bone disease Perianal tumor Pseudocoprostasis Intramural or intraluminal Anorectal stricture, tumor or foreign body Perineal hernia (rectal diverticulum) Rectal prolapse Fecalith
Neuromuscular dysfunction	Lumbosacral spinal cord disease (trauma, disc disease, deformity, degeneration, infection, neoplasia) Bilateral pelvic nerve injury Dysautonomia (Key-Gaskell syndrome) Hypothyroidism Idiopathic megacolon
Fluid and electrolyte abnormalities	Dehydration Hypokalemia Hypercalcemia (hyperparathyroidism) Combination of imbalances (e.g., chronic renal disease)
Drug-related effects	Aluminum hydroxide–containing antacids Anticholinergics Antihistamines Adrenergic blockers Barium sulfate Calcium channel blockers Diuretics Iron Kaolin-pectin Narcotic analgesics (opiates and opioids) Phenothiazines and benzodiazepines Sucralfate

From Sherding R: Diseases of the intestines. In Sherding R, editor: *The cat: diseases and clinical management,* ed 2, New York, 1994, Churchill Livingstone, p 1211.

and urine assessments are usually not required at an initial presentation for constipation.

Management

In all cases, the same principles of management apply:

1. Ensure removal of obstructing feces
2. Ensure colonic motility and smooth passage of feces
3. Reduce fecal bulk
4. Ensure adequate hydration
5. Manage underlying problems

Management of the First Episode in a Well Cat with Minimal Obstructing Feces

The first step is to ensure obstructing feces are removed. In simple cases, the cat will evacuate feces after use of a glycerin or sorbitol pediatric rectal suppository. Another option is administration of a microenema, such as Microlax (McNeil Consumer Healthcare, Fort Washington, Pa.), which contains 5 mL of sodium lauryl sulfoacetate. These products act to lubricate the colon wall and therefore facilitate the passage of feces. The author prefers to use one or two of these within the consult room to observe the cat defecating (the cat must be provided with a litter tray!). The outside tube should be lubricated with the suppository contents before carefully inserting and then expressing the rest of the contents. There are also stimulant laxatives (containing bisacodyl) and emollient laxatives (containing sodium docusate) that have reportedly been used.[140]

If a rectal suppository vial cannot easily be inserted because hardened fecal content obstructs its entry, a more substantive enema will be required (sometimes requiring sedation or anesthesia), and this is covered in the next section on management. Some cats present for difficulty defecating and pass hard, dry stools but do not have fecal impaction at the time of examination.

After the obstructing feces have been removed, steps must be taken to ensure colonic motility and smooth passing of feces. Medical management of constipation traditionally involves laxatives and prokinetic agents. These may not be required in straightforward cases. As long as there is no obstructive lesion, cisapride at 2.5 mg/cat, every 12 hours, PO[82] is very safe and can be instituted with a view to reducing the dose to once daily after 10 to 14 days and discontinuing if signs remain abated. Doses of up to 7.5 mg/cat, every 8 hours, PO have been reported. Cisapride is only available from compounding agencies in most countries. An osmotic or lubricant laxative (Table 23-18) may be used concurrently at reduced doses as necessary.

Reducing the fecal bulk produced is an important part of long-term management. Traditional dietary recommendations are to increase the amount of fiber.[18,26,140,170] Increased dietary fiber results in production of short-chain fatty acids, which have been demonstrated to stimulate feline colonic smooth muscle contractions.[128] However, dietary fiber is also classified as a bulk laxative and so, by definition, will increase fecal bulk. In humans dietary fiber has been considered a mainstay of therapy for constipation, but a recent review concluded that many patients with more severe constipation have worsening symptoms when increasing dietary fiber intake.[103] Because megacolon is believed to be the end result of chronic dilatation,[140,170] it is the author's firm belief that initial dietary efforts should be directed to reducing fecal bulk and thus introducing a low-residue diet. Reduced dry matter intake reduces stool volume,[31] and the author has found that recurrence rates of constipation reduce greatly when cats are transitioned to entirely wet food diets. Wet food diets also help ensure adequate water

TABLE 23-18 **Medical Management of Constipation**

Classification	Examples	Comment
Lubricant laxatives	Petrolatum Mineral oil	Over-the-counter pet products, very safe AVOID, risk of inhalation lipid pneumonia
Hyperosmotic laxatives	Lactulose Polyethylene glycol (e.g., MiraLAX, Schering-Plough Healthcare Products, Kennilworth, NJ)	Starting dose 2 mL/cat q12h Starting dose ¼ tsp q12h No controlled data
Emollient laxatives	Docusate (e.g., Colace, Purdue Products, Stamford, Conn.)	50 mg/cat PO q12h
Bulk laxatives	High fiber diets Psyllium (Metamucil, Procter & Gamble, Cincinnati, Ohio)	Increase colonic motility but also increase bulk of feces
Stimulant laxatives	Bisacodyl (Dulcolax, Boehringer Ingelheim, Ridgefield, Conn.)	5 mg/cat PO q24h
Prokinetic agents	Cisapride	2.5-5.0 mg/cat q12-24h Must be compounded

intake and therefore help maintain hydration. However, increased dietary fiber is beneficial for some cats, and trial and error may be required to determine whether a high-fiber or low-residue diet will be of benefit to each individual cat. In one report, 15 cats with recurrent constipation refractory to traditional medical and dietary management were successfully treated with a psyllium-enriched dry extruded diet.[48a] After 1 month on the diet, 14 cats had no clinical signs of constipation. The remaining cat was clinically normal after 2 months on the diet. Improvement was noted in 10 of 15 cats after only 7 days of dietary therapy.

Measures should be taken to ensure adequate hydration. Maintaining adequate hydration is particularly relevant for cats with chronic kidney disease that have impaired ability to conserve water. Changing to wet food diets helps increase water intake. Some cats with chronic kidney disease may need additional fluid support, such as subcutaneous fluids administered by the owner at home on a regular basis.

Underlying problems may be minor and simple to manage, such as an anal gland abscess, or more involved, such as reduced pelvic outflow, as a result of prior trauma. Arthritis is a common underlying factor in many older cats and may be managed with prudent use of nonsteroidal agents (see Chapter 26).

Management of Cats with Repeat Episodes and Obstipation

In cases of obstipation, the cat is more likely to be debilitated to some degree; so, laboratory investigations to assess plasma or serum biochemistry parameters as well as hematology and urinalysis are ideal. Any hydration deficit or electrolyte abnormalities should be corrected before the anesthesia that is often required to remove the obstructing feces. Rectal suppositories and microenemas are usually ineffective in obstipated cats. Enemas are often required to remove impacted feces in such circumstances. The enema solution must be warmed and introduced slowly to avoid vomiting. The typical volume required is 5 to 10 mL/kg (so, up to approximately 50 mL/cat). The enema solution can be an isotonic electrolyte solution or tap water, and mild soap can be added (but any soap used must *not* contain hexachlorophene, which is neurotoxic if absorbed); mineral oil can be used (5 to 10 mL/cat) as a lubricant or docusate as an emollient (5 to 10 mL/cat), but the two agents must not be used together since docusate promotes mucosal absorption. Sodium phosphate–containing enemas must not be used, because they can induce severe hypernatremia, hyperphosphatemia, and hypocalcemia in cats.

Often, the enema solution alone is insufficient to reduce the fecal mass, and manual manipulation of the feces by abdominal palpation is required. Sometimes the feces must be broken down by a gloved finger per-rectum while the colon is massaged manually through the abdominal wall with the other hand, but great care must be taken with this maneuver, because the devitalized colon can be perforated more easily.[140,170] Enemas as described are painful for the cat, and opioid analgesia is recommended at the time of anesthesia. Opioids can reduce peristalsis in humans,[96] but having evacuated the bowel, the pain relief is more important than this transient effect.

An alternative to enemas is administration of an oral polyethylene glycol (PEG 3350) solution (e.g., CoLyte, GoLytely). A nasoesophageal tube is placed and the solution is given as a slow trickle (6 to 10 mL/kg/hour) over 4 to 18 hours. Defecation usually results in 6 to 12 hours. In a retrospective study of 9 cats, median time to defecation was 8 hours and the median total dose of PEG 3350 was 80 mL/kg.[26a] No adverse effects were noted.

A cat that has been obstipated needs supportive therapy when discharged. There are no controlled comparisons of the various therapies noted in Table 23-21; the author prefers cisapride 2.5 mg, every 12 hours to every 8 hours, PO[82] (first thing in the morning, when the owner returns from work, when the owner goes to bed), and lactulose syrup 2 mL/cat, every 12 hours, PO. A cat that has been so severely obstipated that an enema under anesthesia is required can be expected to continue these medications lifelong.

To reduce fecal bulk and decrease the opportunity for recurrence, low-residue canned foods (or sachets) are preferred for cats that have become obstipated. Some cats may benefit from high-fiber diets. As with simple initial episodes, canned food helps maintain adequate hydration, and at home subcutaneous fluids may be used additionally in cats with chronic kidney disease. With repeat episodes or severe obstipation, investigations for an underlying cause should be thorough and include evaluation for colonic mass obstructions. A review of published cases indicated that 96% of cases of megacolon are accounted for by idiopathic megacolon (62%), pelvic canal stenosis (23%), nerve injury (6%), or Manx sacral spinal cord deformity (5%).[170] Although most cases are idiopathic, an attempt should be made to identify and treat any specific underlying causes.

Megacolon

Megacolon is not specifically defined in cats. It has been described as "generalized colonic dysfunction manifesting as severe colonic dilation and fecal impaction," or a "severely and irreversibly dilated and hypomotile" colon[140] and "a subjective evaluation of the diameter of the colon, usually based on radiographic assessment."[18] There are specific radiographic guidelines for humans with megacolon, in that a colonic diameter of more than 6.5 cm at the level of the pelvic brim is considered diagnostic.[118]

Radiographically, in the lateral view, the normal colon should be approximately the same diameter as the length of the body of the second lumbar vertebra.[81] In cats, however, "there are no published guidelines for determining megacolon, so, diagnosis of abnormal colonic dilatation is subjective."[75] However, one author has suggested that "as a rule of thumb, the diameter of the colon should be less than the length of the body of the seventh lumbar vertebra (L7)."[105] This author continues, "Enlargement of the diameter of the colon beyond 1½ times the length of the body of L7 is indicative of chronic large bowel dysfunction and an explanation must be sought."[105] A recent paper found that 15 of 20 cats with no gastrointestinal disease had a colon diameter greater than the length of L7; however, no assessment of constipated cats was made.[1] In practice, many cats with megacolon have a colonic diameter far exceeding this guideline (Figure 23-36). One study of 11 cats with megacolon found the mean diameter of the colon was 2.7 times greater than the length of the seventh lumbar vertebra (median, 2.4; range, 1.8 to 3.3),[107] but in general, objective descriptions of this condition are lacking in the veterinary literature.

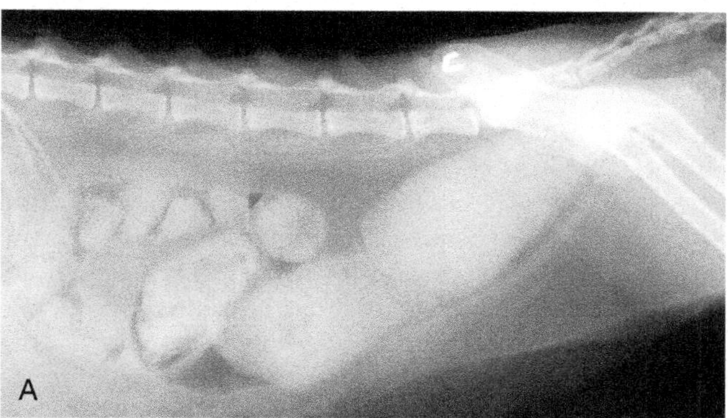

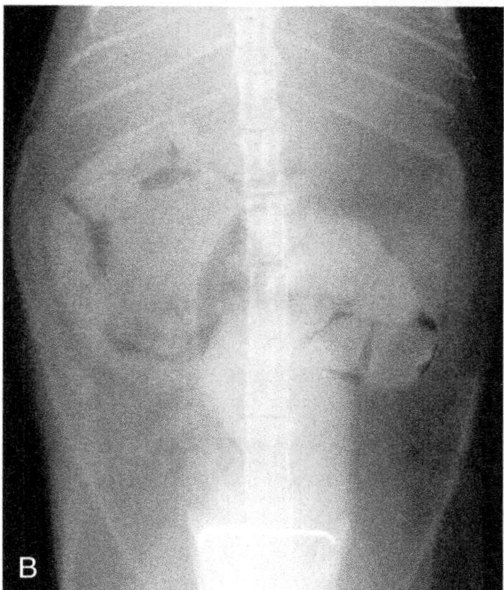

FIGURE 23-36 Radiographic appearance of an obstipated cat with megacolon, lateral (**A**) and ventrodorsal (**B**) views.

The definition of megacolon in cats should include functional as well as radiographic guidelines. In the absence of broadly recognized radiographic recommendations, the author proposes that the O'Brien rule-of-thumb guidelines[105] (as noted above) be introduced until a more comprehensive study can establish other radiographic diagnostic criteria (or confirm these). The author therefore proposes to define megacolon as dilatation of the colon, to more than 1.5 times the length of the seventh lumbar vertebra, which is refractory to medical and dietary management. Practitioners can expect the radiographic assessment of colonic dilatation to exceed this guideline in cats with megacolon and, conversely, there are likely to be cats having colonic distention greater than this amount that will respond to medical and dietary management and can therefore not be defined as having megacolon.

Management of Megacolon

By the definition used above, megacolon is refractory to medical and dietary therapy; so, to be defined as having megacolon, a cat may have had several episodes of obstipation managed by enema as well as dietary trials (with both low-residue and high-fiber diets) and medical therapy with cisapride and an osmotic or emollient laxative; yet the cat will still obstruct with feces. In these circumstances, the only possible therapy is subtotal colectomy.

Subtotal colectomy refers to surgical excision of 95% to 98% of the colon, whether it is grossly diseased or not with preservation of the ileocolic junction (ICJ). This approach has resulted in a more favorable clinical response than when the ICJ is also excised.[22,170] When preserving the ICJ, it has been noted that, in some rare cases, it can be difficult to join the proximal segment of colon to the distal piece of descending colon because of the tethering effect of the ileocecocolic blood vessels. In these cases, sacrificing these vessels and removing the ICJ (i.e., total colectomy) is recommended to facilitate approximation of the ileum to the distal colonic segment.[21] A recently described technique using a biofragmentable anastomosis ring, compared with sutured anastomoses, showed no discernible effect on prognosis.[131] Prognosis following subtotal colectomy is generally good. A review of multiple papers, totaling over 100 cats that had undergone subtotal colectomy, found the most commonly reported perioperative complication was diarrhea or loose stools immediately after surgery. In the majority of individuals, stool consistency improves without further treatment so that within 1 to 6 weeks of the surgery soft, formed stools are developed. Diarrhea can persist in a small number of cases. In the longer term, in some cats, constipation can eventually return, but this can usually be managed by dietary and medical therapies.[172]

ANORECTAL DISEASES

Pathology of the rectum or anus is relatively rare in cats and therefore poorly described in the veterinary literature. Consequently, published information is often not referenced, suggesting it expresses the authors' opinions. Readers are directed to surgical texts for details and approaches about surgical corrections.

Anal Sac Diseases

The anal sacs are paired cutaneous evaginations situated between the internal and external sphincter muscles. These sacs store secretions from alveolar and sebaceous glands that reside within the sacs. Each anal gland has an associated duct that opens to the skin surface just lateral to the anus.[136,155] Normal anal gland secretions have only very recently been described[47] and vary markedly; the color can be white, brown, orange, yellow, tan or gray, and consistency can range from watery to thick and creamy, with two thirds of cats having solid portions within the secretion. On microscopic examination, epithelial cells are commonly seen, with most cats having some neutrophils present. Bacteria are commonly recognized as are, on some occasions, yeasts. Bacteria seen in this study were mainly gram-positive cocci (63%) or gram-negative cocci (30%). Gram-negative or gram-positive rods were also seen but were rarely the dominant bacterial population.[47] With such a wide range of normal secretions, it is difficult to diagnose any pathology from the nature of the secretion alone. However, blood is infrequently recognized, and neutrophils are typically present in only small numbers in normal secretions.

Anal sac diseases described in cats include impaction, inflammation (sacculitis), infection, abscessation, and neoplasia (essentially the same as in dogs).[140,155]

Anal Sac Impaction/Inflammation/ Infection/Abscessation

It has been contended in dogs that sacculitis and abscessation are an extension of impaction. It is not known in dogs or cats what the predisposing causes are, but suggested underlying reasons are loose stools (that are less effective at expressing the sac during defecation), local swelling or edema occluding the duct, and obesity.[155] The author's observations have also indicated that constipation can result in anal sac impaction because of less frequent expulsion of the sac contents; the resultant pain of the anal sac impaction can lead to further constipation, thus establishing a cycle. The retention of secretions may predispose to sacculitis, but impacted anal sacs do not always result in inflammation. Abscessation is a likely sequel to sacculitis.[155]

Cats usually present for licking, scratching, or biting at the perineal area and can present for scooting (or dragging their anus) as dogs do. Other presenting signs can be inability to sit or settle, a lump seen by the owner, or a generally unwell state.

Expression is the only management required for impacted (and not infected) anal sacs. The author prefers expressing one anal sac at a time with well-lubricated gloves and the index finger within the rectum and the thumb externally. This is painful for most cats; so, the cat should be held by an experienced assistant, and it is sometimes not possible without some degree of sedation. With frequent episodes, underlying causes should be investigated. Sometimes, trial-and-error diet change to manipulate the nature of the feces to either more (high-fiber diets) or less (low-residue diets) bulk help reduce the frequency of episodes. Obesity should be managed by reduced caloric intake, but dietary management for this should also take into account the nature of the feces.

Overt infection may be recognized by pus secretion from the anal sacs, which will have a high numbers of neutrophils. This can be managed by broad-spectrum antibiotics, such as amoxicillin/clavulanate or cephalosporins. A single treatment with a nonsteroidal antiinflammatory drug, such as meloxicam, can be given in animals with appropriate hydration and without other illness.

Anal sac abscesses often present already open and draining. Many heal well by secondary intention with antibiotic treatment until they are closed over; so rechecks are required before the completion of an antibiotic course. Large abscesses may require surgical drainage with the insertion of a Penrose drain and management as for a cat fight abscess. It must be remembered that wounds in this area are easily re-infected by fecal contamination. Recurrent impaction, sacculitis, or infection may require anal sacculectomy (as in dogs). This procedure should be delayed until infection is cleared. The procedure is similar to that performed in dogs.

Neoplasia

Reports of anal sac/gland neoplasia were confined to sporadic case reports,[97,108] until a large case series was recently published.[141] In this study, 64 cases of anal gland carcinoma were recognized at a private diagnostic laboratory during a 12-year period, with submissions from 62 practices. This indicates that, for most practices, this condition will be seen, at most, once every 12 years. Affected cats ranged in age from 6 to 17 years (median and mean, 12 years); female (mostly spayed) cats were overrepresented (61% of cases), and Siamese cats may have been over-represented (7.8% of cases). The number of Siamese cats with anal sac neoplasia was 3 times greater than the number of Siamese cats in the laboratory reference population. Affected cats presented for dyschezia, recurrent constipation, change in the nature or volume of feces, and/or perineal swelling or ulceration, sometimes with purulent or hemorrhagic discharge. Most tumors were originally interpreted as and initially managed as anal sac abscess. Presumptive metastasis in liver, lung, or abdominal lymph nodes was recognized by physical examination or radiography in six cats; one cat was hypercalcemic. Excision appeared to be curative (with a 3- to 4-year follow-up period) in 3 of 29 cats undergoing surgery for resection or debulking (others had only incisional biopsy performed). For the remaining 36 cats with known postsurgical outcome, median survival was only 3 months, with a 19% 1-year survival rate (with none of these cats surviving to 2 years).[141]

Anal Diseases

Atresia Ani

Atresia ani is a developmental defect of the anal opening or terminal rectum (see Figure 41-4). Kittens usually present within days or weeks of birth with abdominal distention, discomfort, tenesmus, restlessness, vomiting, and/or loss of appetite. There are several anatomic variations[22]:

- *Type I*: A membrane over the anal opening remains, with the rectum ending as a blind pouch just cranial to the closed anus.
- *Type II:* The anus is closed as in type I, but the rectal pouch is located somewhat cranial to the membrane overlying the anus.
- *Type III*: The rectum ends as a blind pouch cranially within the pelvic canal (rectal atresia), whereas the terminal rectum and anus are normal.
- *Type IV*: Occurs in females and atresia ani exists with a persistent communication between the rectum and the vagina (rectovaginal fistula). This fistula can occur with a normal anal opening as well.

Most reported cases have been type IV,[23,146,150,158,166] and this has also been recognized with concurrent sacrococcygeal agenesis.[3] Surgical correction has been described for type II[157] and type IV[19,91] atresia ani in cats. The reader should consult these references for surgical advice; possible complications include megacolon after prolonged obstruction, postsurgical anal stricture, and fecal incontinence because of sphincter dysfunction.

Fecaliths

Foreign bodies in cats rarely obstruct the gastrointestinal tract distal to the jejunum[60]; however, large fecal balls resulting from constipation can, additional to constipation or obstipation, cause distention of the anus. This distention can result in inflammation of the anal sphincter with loss of tone (Figure 23-37, *A*), which, in the author's experience, is temporary with correction of the underlying cause of constipation. It can take some weeks for the dilated anus to return to normal (Figure 23-37, *B*). A low-residue wet diet is recommended to reduce fecal bulk during the healing period.

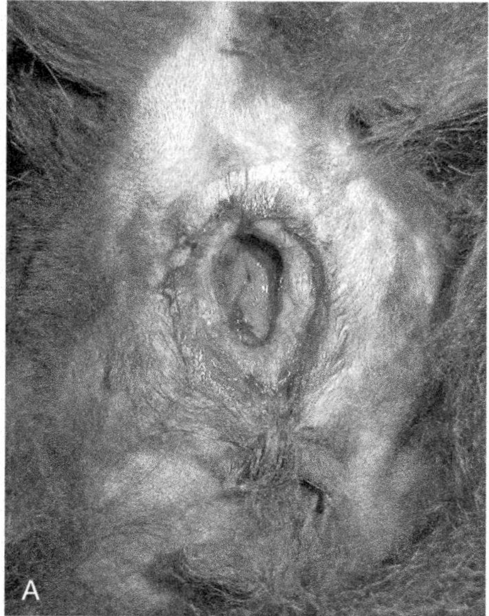

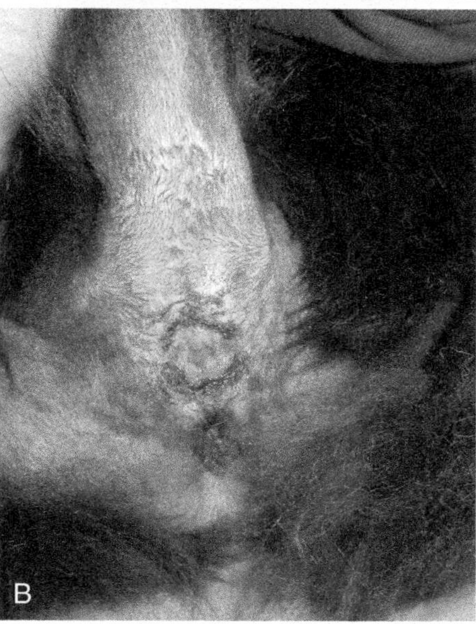

FIGURE 23-37 **A**, Dilated anus with loss of anal tone after removal of a fecalith. **B**, This is the same cat as in **A** 2 weeks later. Note the reduction in anal dilation. The cat's anal tone returned to entire normalcy in the following week. The only management used was feeding of a low-residue diet.

Rectal Prolapse

Rectal prolapse occurs as a result of a disease process that causes chronic straining, such as

1. Intestinal conditions that result in diarrhea and tenesmus
2. Conditions that result in constipation or other intestinal obstruction
3. Lower urinary tract diseases
4. Dystocia

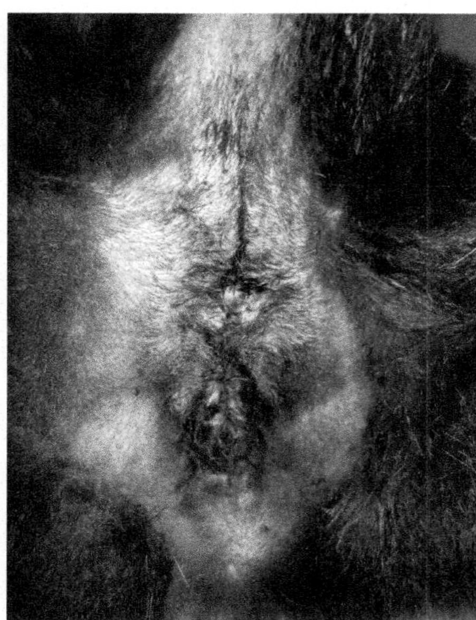

FIGURE 23-38 Perineal/skin fold dermatitis associated with obesity. Antibiotics were needed to manage the pyoderma while the cat was on a diet during a 12-week period. The condition resolved with weight loss, and no further management was required.

Prolapses are usually classified in three ways.[62]

1. First degree: prolapse of only mucous membrane
2. Second degree: prolapse of full rectal wall thickness
3. Third degree: prolapse is sufficient to bring mesorectum outside the anus

The prolapsed rectum is obvious but must be differentiated from ileocolic intussusceptions, which have been described with neoplasia.[37] This distinction can be made by inserting a thermometer through the anus alongside the prolapsed mass. Insertion will not be possible for an intussusception but will be for an anorectal prolapse.

The prolapsed tissue must be assessed for viability, and management must include determining and managing the underlying cause as well as management of the prolapse. In simple cases where the mucosa is viable, the prolapse can be reduced with lubrication and gentle pressure. A temporary purse-string suture may be required to prevent recurrence.

Perineal Dermatitis

Perineal dermatitis is often confused with gastrointestinal or urogenital disease, because there are often copious sebaceous secretions that can mimic fecal or urinary secretions. Perineal dermatitis can result from flea or other allergies but also fecal or urine scalding associated with diarrhea or urinary incontinence, respectively. Skin fold dermatitis can also occur in obese cats (Figure 23-38). Episioplasty has been described to correct this,[121] but the author has found that stringent dieting can result in improvement while managing the skin fold dermatitis with antibiotics, such as cephalosporins, and regular cleansing.

References

1. Adams WM, Sisterman LA, Klauer JM et al: Association of intestinal disorders in cats with findings of abdominal radiography, *J Am Vet Med Assoc* 236:880, 2010.
2. Anderson S, Lippincott C, Gill P: Single enterotomy removal of gastrointestinal linear foreign bodies, *J An Anim Hosp Assoc* 28:487, 1992.
3. Araújo FPD, Araújo BM, Kemper B et al: Sacrococcygeal agenesis association and anal atresia in mixed breed cats, *Ciencia Rural* 39:1893, 2009.
4. Asperilla MO, Smego RA, Scott LK: Quinolone antibiotics in the treatment of *Salmonella* infections, *Rev Infect Dis* 12:873, 1990.
5. Baez J, Hendrick M, Walker L et al: Radiographic, ultrasonographic, and endoscopic findings in cats with inflammatory bowel disease of the stomach and small intestine: 33 cases (1990-1997), *J Am Vet Med Assoc* 215:349, 1999.
6. Baral RM: Laparotomy for gastro-intestinal biopsies, Science Week Conference Proceedings (Small Animal Medicine chapter), Gold Coast, Queensland, Australia, 2006, Australian College of Veterinary Scientists, p 70.
7. Baral RM, Krockenberger MB, Foster DJ et al: Hepatic small cell lymphosarcoma in four cats, *J Feline Med Surg*, in press.
8. Barrand KR, Scudamore CL: Intestinal leiomyosarcoma in a cat, *J Small Anim Pract* 40:216, 1999.
9. Barrs VR, Beatty JA, Tisdall PL et al: Intestinal obstruction by trichobezoars in five cats, *J Feline Med Surg* 1:199, 1999.
10. Basher AW, Fowler JD: Conservative versus surgical management of gastrointestinal linear foreign bodies in the cat, *Vet Surg* 16:135, 1987.
11. Batt RM, Needham JR, Carter MW: Bacterial overgrowth associated with a naturally occurring enteropathy in the German Shepherd dog, *Res Vet Sci* 35:42, 1983.
12. Beatty J, Terry A, MacDonald J et al: Feline immunodeficiency virus integration in B-cell lymphoma identifies a candidate tumor suppressor gene on human chromosome 15q15, *Cancer Res* 62:7175, 2002.
13. Beaver BV: Disorders of behavior. In Sherding RG, editor: *The cat: diseases and clinical management*, ed 2, New York, 1994, Churchill Livingstone, p 191.
14. Bebchuk TN: Feline gastrointestinal foreign bodies, *Vet Clin North Am Small Anim Pract* 32:861, 2002.
15. Bellenger CR, Beck JA: Intussusception in 12 cats, *J Small Anim Pract* 35:295, 1994.
16. Bellin T, Pulz M, Matussek A et al: Rapid detection of enterohemorrhagic *Escherichia coli* by real-time PCR with fluorescent hybridization probes, *J Clin Microbiol* 39:370, 2001.
17. Benitah N, de Lorimier L-P, Gaspar M et al: Chlorambucil-induced myoclonus in a cat with lymphoma, *J Am Anim Hosp Assoc* 39:283, 2003.
18. Bertoy RW: Megacolon in the cat, *Vet Clin North Am Small Anim Pract* 32:901, 2002.
19. Bornet JP: Recto-vaginal fistula and anal imperforation in a cat: surgical treatment, *Bull Acad Vet Fr* 63:53, 1990.
20. Brandt L, Kimby E, Nygren P et al: A systematic overview of chemotherapy effects in indolent non-Hodgkin's lymphoma, *Acta Oncol* 40:213, 2001.
21. Bright RM: GI surgery. In *Proc Am Assoc Feline Pract Fall Meeting*, Atlanta, Ga, 1997.
22. Bright RM, Bauer MS: Surgery of the digestive system. In Sherding RG, editor: *The cat: diseases and clinical management*, ed 2, New York, NY, 1994, Churchill Livingstone, p 1353.
23. Broek AHM, Else RW, Hunter MS: Atresia ani and urethrorectal fistula in a kitten, *J Small Anim Pract* 29:91, 1988.

24. Brömel C, Sykes JE: Histoplasmosis in dogs and cats, *Clin Tech Small Anim Pract* 20:227, 2005.
25. Burkitt JM, Drobatz KJ, Saunders HM et al: Signalment, history, and outcome of cats with gastrointestinal tract intussusception: 20 cases (1986-2000), *J Am Vet Med Assoc* 234:771, 2009.
26. Byers C, Leasure C, Sanders NA: Feline idiopathic megacolon, *Comp Contin Edu Pract Vet* 28:658, 2006.
26a. Carr AP, Gaunt MC: Constipation resolution with administration of polyethylene glycol solution in cats (abstract), *J Vet Intern Med* 24:753, 2010.
27. Carreras JK, Goldschmidt M, Lamb M et al: Feline epitheliotropic intestinal malignant lymphoma: 10 Cases (1997-2000), *J Vet Intern Med* 17:326, 2003.
28. Cook AK: Feline infectious diarrhea, *Top Companion Anim Med* 23:169, 2008.
29. Craig LE, Hardam EE, Hertzke DM et al: Feline gastrointestinal eosinophilic sclerosing fibroplasia, *Vet Pathol* 46:63, 2009.
30. Crandell J, Jergens A, Morrison J et al: Development of a clinical scoring index for disease activity in feline inflammatory bowel disease, *J Vet Intern Med* 20:788, 2006
31. Crane SW, Griffin RW, Messent PR: Introduction to commercial pet Ffoods. In Hand MS, Thatcher CD, Remillard RL et al, editors: *Small animal clinical nutrition*, ed 4, Topeka, Kans, 2000, Mark Morris Institute, p 111.
32. Cribb A: Feline gastrointestinal adenocarcinoma: A review and retrospective study, *Can Vet J* 29:709, 1988.
33. Culp WTN, Drobatz KJ, Glassman MM et al: Feline visceral hemangiosarcoma, *J Vet Intern Med* 22:148, 2008.
34. Dallenne C, Da Costa A, Decre D et al: Development of a set of multiplex PCR assays for the detection of genes encoding important beta-lactamases in Enterobacteriaceae, *J Antimicrob Chemother* 65:490, 2010.
35. Day MJ, Bilzer T, Mansell J et al: Histopathological standards for the diagnosis of gastrointestinal inflammation in endoscopic biopsy samples from the dog and cat: a report from the World Small Animal Veterinary Association Gastrointestinal Standardization Group, *J Comp Pathol* 138(Suppl 1):S1, 2008.
36. De Cock HEV, Marks SL, Stacy BA et al: Ileocolitis associated with *Anaerobiospirillum* in cats, *J Clin Microbiol* 42:2752, 2004.
37. Demetriou J, Welsh E: Rectal prolapse of an ileocaecal neoplasm associated with intussusception in a cat, *J Feline Med Surg* 1:253, 1999.
38. Dennis JS, Kruger JM, Mullaney TP: Lymphocytic/plasmacytic colitis in cats: 14 cases (1985-1990), *J Am Vet Med Assoc* 202:313, 1993.
39. Ellison G: Intestinal obstruction. In Bojrab M, editor: *Disease mechanisms in small animal surgery*, ed 2, Philadelphia, 1993, Lea & Febiger, p 252.
40. Evans SE, Bonczynski JJ, Broussard JD et al: Comparison of endoscopic and full-thickness biopsy specimens for diagnosis of inflammatory bowel disease and alimentary tract lymphoma in cats, *J Am Vet Med Assoc* 229:1447, 2006.
41. Felts J, Fox P, Burk R: Thread and sewing needles as gastrointestinal foreign bodies in the cat: a review of 64 cases, *J Am Vet Med Assoc* 184:56, 1984.
42. Foley J, Hirsh DC, Pedersen NC: An outbreak of *Clostridium perfringens* enteritis in a cattery of Bengal cats and experimental transmission to specific pathogen free cats, *Feline Pract* 24:31, 1996.
43. Fondacaro JV Richter KP, Carpenter JL: Feline gastrointestinal lymphoma: 67 cases (1988-1996), *Eur J Comp Gastroenterol* 4:5, 1999.
44. Fox JG: *Campylobacter* infections. In Greene CE, editor: *Infectious diseases of the dog and cat*, ed 3, St Louis, 2006, Saunders Elsevier, p 339.
45. Fox JG, Ackerman JA, Newcomer CE: The prevalence of *Campylobacter jejuni* in random-source cats used in biomedical research [correspondence], *J Infect Dis* 151:743, 1985.
46. Fox JG, Claps M, Beaucage CM: Chronic diarrhea associated with *Campylobacter jejuni* infection in a cat, *J Am Vet Med Assoc* 189:455, 1986.
47. Frankel JL, Scott DW, Erb HN: Gross and cytological characteristics of normal feline anal-sac secretions, *J Feline Med Surg* 10:319, 2008.
48. Fredriksson-Ahomaa M, Korte T, Korkeala H: Transmission of *Yersinia enterocolitica* 4/O:3 to pets via contaminated pork, *Lett Appl Microbiol* 32:375, 2001.
48a. Freiche V, Deswarte G, Soulard Y et al: A psyllium-enriched dry extruded diet improves recurrent feline constipation (abstract), *J Vet Intern Med* 24:1547, 2010.
49. Gabor LJ, Malik R, Canfield PJ: Clinical and anatomical features of lymphosarcoma in 118 cats, *Aust Vet J* 76:725, 1998.
50. Goggin JM, Biller DS, Debey BM et al: Ultrasonographic measurement of gastrointestinal wall thickness and the ultrasonographic appearance of the ileocolic region in healthy cats, *J Am Anim Hosp Assoc* 36:224, 2000.
51. Greene CE: Feline enteric viral infections. In Greene CE, editor: *Infectious diseases of the dog and cat*, ed 3, St Louis, 2006, Saunders Elsevier, p 103.
52. Greene CE: Salmonellosis. In Greene CE, editor: *Infectious diseases of the dog and cat*, ed 3 St Louis, 2006, Saunders Elsevier, p 355.
53. Greene CE, Addie DD: Feline parvovirus infections. In Greene CE, editor: *Infectious diseases of the dog and cat*, ed 3, St Louis, 2006, Elsevier, p 78.
54. Grooters AM, Biller DS, Ward H et al: Ultrasonographic appearance of feline alimentary lymphoma, *Vet Radiol Ultrasound* 35:468, 1994.
55. Guilford WG, Jones BR, Markwell PJ et al: Food sensitivity in cats with chronic idiopathic gastrointestinal problems, *J Vet Intern Med* 15:7, 2001.
56. Halsey CH, Powers BE, Kamstock DA: Feline intestinal sclerosing mast cell tumour: 50 cases (1997-2008), *Vet Comp Oncol* 8:72, 2010.
57. Handagma PJ, Feldman BF: Drug-induced thrombocytopenia, *Vet Res Commun* 10:1, 1986.
58. Hart J, Shaker E, Patnaik A et al: Lymphocytic-plasmacytic enterocolitis in cats: 60 cases (1988-1990), *J Am Anim Hosp Assoc* 30:505, 1994.
59. Harvey CJ, Lopez JW, Hendrick MJ: An uncommon intestinal manifestation of feline infectious peritonitis: 26 cases (1986-1993), *J Am Vet Med Assoc* 209:1117, 1996.
60. Hayes G: Gastrointestinal foreign bodies in dogs and cats: a retrospective study of 208 cases, *J Small Anim Pract* 50:576, 2009.
61. Hicks GA, Coldwell JR, Schindler M et al: Excitation of rat colonic afferent fibres by 5-HT3 receptors, *J Physiol* 544:861, 2002.
62. Holt P: Anal and perianal surgery in dogs and cats, *In Pract* 7:82, 1985.
63. Iannibelli F, Caruso A, Castelluccio A et al: *Yersinia pseudotuberculosis* in a persian cat, *Vet Record* 129:103, 1991.
64. Jaksic B, Brugiatelli M: High dose continuous chlorambucil vs intermittent chlorambucil plus prednisone for treatment of B-CLL–IGCI CLL-01 trial, *Nouv Rev Fr Hematol* 30:437, 1988.
65. Janeczko S, Atwater D, Bogel E et al: The relationship of mucosal bacteria to duodenal histopathology, cytokine mRNA, and clinical disease activity in cats with inflammatory bowel disease, *Vet Microbiol* 128:178, 2008.
66. Jergens A, Moore F, Haynes J et al: Idiopathic inflammatory bowel disease in dogs and cats: 84 cases (1987-1990), *J Am Vet Med Assoc* 201:1603, 1992.

67. Jergens AE, Moore FM, Haynes JS et al: Idiopathic inflammatory bowel disease in dogs and cats: 84 cases (1987-1990), *J Am Vet Med Assoc* 201:1603, 1992.
68. Johnson K, Lamport A, Batt RM: An unexpected bacterial flora in the proximal small intestine of normal cats, *Vet Record* 132:362, 1993.
69. Johnston KL, Lamport AI, Ballèvre OP et al: Effects of oral administration of metronidazole on small intestinal bacteria and nutrients of cats, *Am J Vet Res* 61:1106, 2000.
70. Johnston KL, Swift NC, Forster-van Hijfte MF et al: Comparison of the bacterial flora of the duodenum in healthy cats and cats with signs of gastrointestinal tract disease, *J Am Vet Med Assoc* 218:48, 2001.
71. Jones BR, Greene CE: Tyzzer's disease. In Greene CE, editor: *Infectious diseases of the dog and cat*, ed 3 St Louis, 2006, Saunders Elsevier, p 362.
72. Kimby E, Brandt L, Nygren P et al: A systematic overview of chemotherapy effects in B-cell chronic lymphocytic leukaemia, *Acta Oncol* 40:224, 2001.
73. Kiselow MA, Rassnick KM, McDonough SP et al: Outcome of cats with low-grade lymphocytic lymphoma: 41 cases (1995-2005), *J Am Vet Med Assoc* 232:405, 2008.
74. Kleinschmidt S, Harder J, Nolte I et al: Chronic inflammatory and non-inflammatory diseases of the gastrointestinal tract in cats: diagnostic advantages of full-thickness intestinal and extraintestinal biopsies, *J Feline Med Surg* 12:97 2010.
75. Konde LJ, Pugh CR: Radiology and sonography of the digestive system. In Tams TR, editor: *Handbook of small animal gastroenterology*, Philadelphia, 1996, Saunders, p 75.
76. Kosovsky J, Matthiesen D, Patnaik A: Small intestinal adenocarcinoma in cats: 32 cases (1978-1985), *J Am Vet Med Assoc* 192:233, 1988.
77. Kruth SA: Gram-negative bacterial infections. In Greene CE, editor: *Infectious diseases of the dog and cat*, ed 3, St Louis, 2006, Elsevier, p 320.
78. Lamb CR, Hansson K: Radiological identification of nonopaque intestinal foreign bodies, *Vet Radiol Ultrasound* 35:87, 1994.
79. Lecoindre P: Chronic inflammatory bowel diseases, etiopathogeny, diagnosis, *Bull Acad Vét France* 159:333, 2006.
80. Lecoindre P, Chevallier M: Contribution to the study of feline inflammatory bowel disease: 51 cases (1991-1994). *Rev Méd Vét* 11:893, 1997
81. Lee R, Leowijuk C: Normal parameters in abdominal radiology of the dog and cat, *J Small Anim Pract* 23:251, 1982.
82. LeGrange S, Boothe D, Herndon S et al: Pharmacokinetics and suggested oral dosing regimen of cisapride: a study in healthy cats, *J Am Anim Hosp Assoc* 33:517, 1997.
83. Levitt L, Bauer MS: Intussusception in dogs and cats: a review of thirty-six cases, *Can Vet J* 33:660, 1992.
84. Lingard AE, Briscoe K, Beatty JA et al: Low-grade alimentary lymphoma: clinicopathological findings and response to treatment in 17 cases, *J Feline Med Surg* 11:692, 2009.
85. Litster AL, Sorenmo KU: Characterisation of the signalment, clinical and survival characteristics of 41 cats with mast cell neoplasia, *J Feline Med Surg* 8:177, 2006.
86. Louwerens M, London CA, Pedersen NC et al: Feline lymphoma in the post-feline leukemia virus era, *J Vet Intern Med* 19:329, 2005.
87. MacDonald J, Mullen H, Moroff S: Adenomatous polyps of the duodenum in cats: 18 cases (1985-1990), *J Am Vet Med Assoc* 202:647, 1993.
88. MacPhail C: Gastrointestinal obstruction, *Clin Tech Small Anim Pract* 17:178, 2002.
89. Madewell BR, Gieger TL, Pesavento PA et al: Vaccine site-associated sarcoma and malignant lymphoma in cats: a report of six cases (1997-2002), *J Am Anim Hosp Assoc* 40:47, 2004.
90. Mahony OM, Moore AS, Cotter SM et al: Alimentary lymphoma in cats: 28 cases (1988-1993), *J Am Vet Med Assoc* 207:1593, 1995.
91. Makkena S, Suryawanshi RV, Rambabu K: Management of atresia ani and recto-vaginal fistula in a Persian cat, *Indian Vet J* 85:985, 2008.
92. Malik R, Gabor LJ, Foster SF et al: Therapy for Australian cats with lymphosarcoma, *Aust Vet J* 79:808, 2001.
93. Marks SL: *Critical appraisal of infectious diarrhea in cats*. Proceedings 80th Western Veterinary Conference, Las Vegas, Nev, 2008.
94. Marks SL, Kather EJ: *Clostridium perfringens*- and *Clostridium difficile*-associated diarrhea. In Greene CE, editor: *Infectious diseases of the dog and cat*, ed 3, St Louis, 2006, Saunders Elsevier, p 363.
95. McManus P: Lymphoma in veterinary medicine: no longer a one-word diagnosis, *Vet Clin Pathol* 37:360, 2008.
96. Mehendale SR, Yuan CS: Opioid-induced gastrointestinal dysfunction, *Dig Dis* 24:105, 2006.
97. Mellanby RJ, Foale R, Friend E et al: Anal sac adenocarcinoma in a Siamese cat, *J Feline Med Surg* 4:205, 2002.
98. Michael GB, Butaye P, Cloeckaert A et al: Genes and mutations conferring antimicrobial resistance in *Salmonella*: an update, *Microbes Infect* 8:1898, 2006.
99. Miettinen M, Lasota J: Gastrointestinal stromal tumors—definition, clinical, histological, immunohistochemical, and molecular genetic features and differential diagnosis, *Virchows Archiv* 438:1, 2001.
100. Mooney SC, Hayes AA, MacEwen EG et al: Treatment and prognostic factors in lymphoma in cats: 103 cases (1977-1981), *J Am Vet Med Assoc* 194:696, 1989.
101. Moore PF, Woo JC, Vernau W et al: Characterization of feline T cell receptor gamma (TCRG) variable region genes for the molecular diagnosis of feline intestinal T cell lymphoma, *Vet Immunol Immunopathol* 106:167, 2005.
102. Muir P, Rosin E: Failure of the single enterotomy technique to remove a linear intestinal foreign body from a cat, *Vet Rec* 136:75, 1995.
103. Müller-Lissner SA, Kamm MA, Scarpignato C et al: Myths and misconceptions about chronic constipation, *Am J Gastroenterol* 100:232, 2005.
104. Nguyen Van N, Taglinger K, Helps CR et al: Measurement of cytokine mRNA expression in intestinal biopsies of cats with inflammatory enteropathy using quantitative real-time RT-PCR, *Vet Immunol Immunopathol* 113:404, 2006.
105. O'Brien T: Large intestine. In O'Brien TR, editor: *Radiographic diagnosis of abdominal disorders in the dog and cat*, Philadelphia, 1978, Saunders, p 352.
106. Orr CM, Gruffydd-Jones TJ, Kelly DF: Ileal polyps in Siamese cats, *J Small Anim Pract* 21:669, 1980.
107. Özak A, Beşaltı Ö, Gökçe P et al: Megacolon in cats: 11 cases (1995-2001), *Veteriner Cerrahi Dergisi* 7:28, 2001.
108. Parry NMA: Anal sac gland carcinoma in a cat, *Vet Pathol* 43:1008, 2006.
109. Patnaik A, Johnson G, Greene R et al: Surgical resection of intestinal adenocarcinoma in a cat, with survival of 28 months, *J Am Vet Med Assoc* 178:479, 1981.
110. Patsikas MN, Papazoglou LG, Papaioannou NG et al: Ultrasonographic findings of intestinal intussusception in seven cats, *J Feline Med Surg* 5:335, 2003.
111. Patterson EV, Reese MJ, Tucker SJ et al: Effect of vaccination on parvovirus antigen testing in kittens, *J Am Vet Med Assoc* 230:359, 2007.
112. Pedersen NC, Allen CE, Lyons LA: Pathogenesis of feline enteric coronavirus infection, *J Feline Med Surg* 10:529, 2008.
113. Penninck DG, Moore AS, Tidwell AS et al: Ultrasonography of alimentary lymphosarcoma in the cat, *Vet Radiol Ultrasound* 35:299, 1994.

114. Penninck DG, Nyland TG, Kerr LY et al: Ultrasonographic evaluation of gastrointestinal diseases in small animals, *Vet Radiol Ultrasound* 31:134, 1990.
115. Philbey AW, Brown FM, Mather HA et al: Salmonellosis in cats in the United Kingdom: 1955 to 2007, *Vet Rec* 164:120, 2009.
116. Pohlman LM, Higginbotham ML, Welles EG et al: Immunophenotypic and histologic classification of 50 cases of feline gastrointestinal lymphoma, *Vet Pathol* 46:259, 2009.
117. Portlock CS, Fischer DS, Cadman E et al: High-dose pulse chlorambucil in advanced, low-grade non-Hodgkin's lymphoma, *Cancer Treat Rep* 71:1029, 1987.
118. Preston D, Lennard-Jones J, Thomas B: Towards a radiologic definition of idiopathic megacolon, *Abdom Imaging* 10:167, 1985.
119. Rakich PM, Grooters AM, Tang KN: Gastrointestinal pythiosis in two cats, *J Vet Diagn Invest* 17:262, 2005.
120. Randall LP, Cooles SW, Osborn MK et al: Antibiotic resistance genes, integrons and multiple antibiotic resistance in thirty-five serotypes of *Salmonella enterica* isolated from humans and animals in the UK, *J Antimicrob Chemother* 53:208, 2004.
121. Ranen E, Zur G: Perivulvar dermatitis in a cat treated by episioplasty, *J Small Anim Pract* 46:582, 2005.
122. Rappaport H: Tumors of the hematopoietic system. Atlas of tumor pathology, *Ann Intern Med* 67:686, 1967.
123. Rassnick KM, Williams LE, Kristal O et al: Lomustine for treatment of mast cell tumors in cats: 38 cases (1999-2005), *J Am Vet Med Assoc* 232:1200, 2008.
124. Richter K: Feline gastrointestinal lymphoma. In Bonagura J, Twedt D, editors: *Kirk's current veterinary therapy XIV*, St Louis, Saunders Elsevier, 2009.
125. Richter KP: Feline gastrointestinal lymphoma, *Vet Clin North Am Small Anim Pract* 33:1083, 2003.
126. Rivers BJ, Walter PA, Feeney DA et al: Ultrasonographic features of intestinal adenocarcinoma in five cats, *Vet Radiol Ultrasound* 38:300, 1997.
127. Roberts JA, Webb S, Paterson D et al: A systematic review on clinical benefits of continuous administration of beta-lactam antibiotics, *Crit Care Med* 37:2071, 2009.
128. Rondeau M, Meltzer K, Michel K et al: Short-chain fatty acids stimulate feline colonic smooth muscle contraction, *J Feline Med Surg* 5:167, 2003.
129. Root CR, Lord PF: Linear radiolucent gastrointestinal foreign bodies in cats and dogs: their radiographic appearance, *Vet Radiol Ultrasound* 12:45, 1971.
130. Rutgers HC, Batt RM, Kelly DF: Lymphocytic-plasmacytic enteritis associated with bacterial overgrowth in a dog, *J Am Vet Med Assoc* 192:1739, 1988.
131. Ryan S, Seim H 3rd, Macphail C et al: Comparison of biofragmentable anastomosis ring and sutured anastomoses for subtotal colectomy in cats with idiopathic megacolon, *Vet Surg* 35:740, 2006.
132. Schreurs E, Vermote K, Barberet V et al: Ultrasonographic anatomy of abdominal lymph nodes in the normal cat, *Vet Radiol Ultrasound* 49:68, 2008.
133. Schwandt CS: Low-grade or benign intestinal tumours contribute to intussusception: a report on one feline and two canine cases, *J Small Anim Pract* 49:651, 2008.
134. Seguin MA, Papich MG, Sigle KJ et al: Pharmacokinetics of enrofloxacin in neonatal kittens, *Am J Vet Res* 65:350, 2004.
135. Selting KA: Intestinal tumors. In Withrow SJ, Vail DM, editors: *Withrow and MacEwen's small animal clinical oncology*, ed 4, St Louis, 2007, Saunders Elsevier, p 491.
136. Shabadash SA, Zelikina TI: Unknown hepatoid glands of certain cats and deer, *Biol Bull Russ Acad Sci* 30:383, 2003.
137. Shaiken L: Radiographic appearance of linear foreign bodies in cats, *Vet Med* 94:417, 1999.
138. Sharpe A, Cannon MJ, Lucke VM et al: Intestinal haemangiosarcoma in the cat: clinical and pathological features of four cases, *J Small Anim Pract* 41:411, 2000.
139. Shelton GH, Grant CK, Cotter SM et al: Feline immunodeficiency virus and feline leukemia virus infections and their relationships to lymphoid malignancies in cats: a retrospective study (1968-1988), *J Acquir Immune Defic Syndr* 3:623, 1990.
140. Sherding R: Diseases of the intestines. In Sherding R, editor: *The cat: diseases and clinical management*, ed 2, New York, 1994, Churchill Livingstone, p 1211.
141. Shoieb AM, Hanshaw DM: Anal sac gland carcinoma in 64 cats in the United Kingdom (1995-2007), *Vet Pathol* 46:677, 2009.
142. Simon D, Eberle N, Laacke-Singer L et al: Combination chemotherapy in feline lymphoma: treatment outcome, tolerability, and duration in 23 cats, *J Vet Intern Med* 22:394, 2008.
143. Simpson KW, Dogan B, Rishniw M et al: Adherent and invasive *Escherichia coli* is associated with granulomatous colitis in Boxer dogs, *Infect Immun* 74:4778, 2006.
144. Simpson KW, Fyfe J, Cornetta A et al: subnormal concentrations of serum cobalamin (vitamin B12) in cats with gastrointestinal disease, *J Vet Intern Med* 15:26, 2001.
145. Slawienski M, Mauldin G, Mauldin G et al: Malignant colonic neoplasia in cats: 46 cases (1990-1996), *J Am Vet Med Assoc* 211:878, 1997.
146. Souza HJM, Corgozinho KB, Rosário JMP et al: Rectovaginal fistula and atresia ani in a kitten: case report, *Clin Vet (Milano)* 5:26, 2000.
147. Spain CV, Scarlett JM, Wade SE et al: Prevalence of enteric zoonotic agents in cats less than 1 year old in Central New York State, *J Vet Intern Med* 15:33, 2001.
148. Stacy-Phipps S, Mecca JJ, Weiss JB: Multiplex PCR assay and simple preparation method for stool specimens detect enterotoxigenic *Escherichia coli* DNA during course of infection, *J Clin Microbiol* 33:1054, 1995.
149. Suchodolski JS, Steiner JM: Laboratory assessment of gastrointestinal function, *Clin Tech Small Anim Pract* 18:203, 2003.
150. Suess RP Jr, Martin RA, Moon ML et al: Rectovaginal fistula with atresia ani in three kittens, *Cornell Vet* 82:141, 1992.
151. Summerfield GP, Taylor PR, Mounter PJ et al: High-dose chlorambucil for the treatment of chronic lymphocytic leukaemia and low-grade non-Hodgkin's lymphoma, *Br J Haematol* 116:781, 2002.
152. Sweetenham J: Lymphoblastic lymphoma in adults, *Curr Hematol Malig Rep* 1:241, 2006.
153. Tauni MA, Österlund A: Outbreak of *Salmonella typhimurium* in cats and humans associated with infection in wild birds, *J Small Anim Pract* 41:339, 2000.
154. Thieblemont C, Nasser V, Felman P et al: Small lymphocytic lymphoma, marginal zone B-cell lymphoma, and mantle cell lymphoma exhibit distinct gene-expression profiles allowing molecular diagnosis, *Blood* 103:2727, 2004.
155. Thompson MS: Diseases of the anal sacs. In Bonagura J, editor: *Current veterinary therapy XIII small animal practice*, Philadelphia, 2000, Saunders, p 591.
156. Tidwell AS, Penninck DG: Ultrasonography of gastrointestinal foreign bodies, *Vet Radiol Ultrasound* 33:160, 1992.
157. Tsioli V, Papazoglou LG, Anagnostou T et al: Use of a temporary incontinent end-on colostomy in a cat for the management of rectocutaneous fistulas associated with atresia ani, *J Feline Med Surg* 11:1011, 2009.
158. Tudury EA, Lorenzoni OD: Colostomy in persian female cat with atresia ani and rectovaginal fistula, *Rev Centr Cienc Rurai* 19:155, 1989.
159. Turk M, Gallina A, Russell T: Nonhematopoietic gastrointestinal neoplasia in cats: a retrospective study of 44 cases, *Vet Pathol* 18:614, 1981.

160. Twomey L, Alleman, AR: Cytodiagnosis of feline lymphoma, *Comp Contin Educ Pract Vet* 27:17, 2005.
161. Tyrrell D, Beck C: Survey of the use of radiography vs. ultrasonography in the investigation of gastrointestinal foreign bodies in small animals, *Vet Radiol Ultrasound* 47:404, 2006.
162. Vail DM, Moore AS, Ogilvie GK et al: Feline lymphoma (145 cases): proliferation indices, cluster of differentiation 3 immunoreactivity, and their association with prognosis in 90 cats, *J Vet Intern Med* 12:349, 1998.
163. Valli V, Jacobs R, Norris A et al: The histologic classification of 602 cases of feline lymphoproliferative disease using the National Cancer Institute working formulation, *J Vet Diagn Invest* 12:295, 2000.
164. van Duijkeren E, Houwers DJ: A critical assessment of antimicrobial treatment in uncomplicated *Salmonella enteritis*, *Vet Microbiol* 73:61, 2000.
165. Vennema H, Poland A, Foley J et al: Feline infectious peritonitis viruses arise by mutation from endemic feline enteric coronaviruses, *Virology* 243:150, 1998.
166. Waknitz D, Greer DH: Urethrorectal fistula in a cat, *Vet Med Small Anim Clin* 78:1551, 1983.
167. Warren AL, Townsend KM, King T et al: Multi-drug resistant *Escherichia coli* with extended-spectrum β-lactamase activity and fluoroquinolone resistance isolated from clinical infections in dogs, *Aust Vet J* 79:621, 2001.
168. Washabau RJ: 2005 Report from: WSAVA Gastrointestinal Standardization Group. Available at http://www.wsava.org/GIStandards1.htm. Accessed January 17, 2010.
169. Washabau RJ, Day MJ, Willard MD et al: Endoscopic, biopsy, and histopathologic guidelines for the evaluation of gastrointestinal inflammation in companion animals, *J Vet Intern Med* 24:10, 2010.
170. Washabau RJ, Hasler AH: Constipation, obstipation, and megacolon. In August JR, editor: *Consultations in feline internal medicine*, ed 3, Philadelphia, 1997, Saunders, p 104.
171. Weiss DJ, Gagne JM, Armstrong PJ: Relationship between inflammatory hepatic disease and inflammatory bowel disease, pancreatitis, and nephritis in cats, *J Am Vet Med Assoc* 209:1114, 1996.
172. White R: Surgical management of constipation, *J Feline Med Surg* 4:129, 2002.
173. Wilcox RS, Bowman DD, Barr SC et al: Intestinal obstruction caused by *Taenia taeniaeformis* infection in a cat, *J Am Anim Hosp Assoc* 45:93, 2009.
174. Willard MD: Feline inflammatory bowel disease: a review, *J Feline Med Surg* 1:155, 1999.
175. Willis SE, Farrow CS: Partial gastrointestinal obstruction for one month because of a linear foreign body in a cat, *Can Vet J* 32:689, 1991.
176. Zwahlen CH, Lucroy MD, Kraegel SA et al: Results of chemotherapy for cats with alimentary malignant lymphoma: 21 cases (1993-1997), *J Am Vet Med Assoc* 213:1144, 1998.
177. Zwingenberger AL, Marks SL, Baker TW et al: Ultrasonographic evaluation of the muscularis propria in cats with diffuse small intestinal lymphoma or inflammatory bowel disease, *J Vet Intern Med* 24:289, 2010.

GASTROINTESTINAL PARASITES

Edward Javinsky

A common theme when discussing the prevalence of most gastrointestinal parasites in cats is that they occur more commonly in younger cats and in cats housed in crowded conditions, such as catteries and shelters. It is likely an increased chance for transmission exists in these populations.[48] The reported prevalence for each parasite varies greatly with the population studied, the geographic location of the population, and the sensitivity of the diagnostic test used to study that population.[48]

The presence or absence of diarrhea is not a reliable predictor of whether a particular cat is infected with or shedding a parasite.[42] In fact, most cats with diarrhea do not harbor enteric protozoa.[48] On the other hand, most cats with diarrhea because of enteric pathogens will shed those organisms, often intermittently.

It is important to remember that infection with most gastrointestinal parasites may not cause clinical signs. Therefore detection of a pathogenic parasite in a cat with diarrhea does not necessarily prove causation.[48] A search should always be undertaken to identify other causes of diarrhea prior to convicting a cat of having diarrhea because of a particular parasite. In addition, co-infections or the presence of other noninfectious causes of diarrhea can result in more severe diarrhea that is often refractory to treatment for the parasite. Treatment will be more rewarding if all potential causes of diarrhea are identified in the patient.

Enteric parasites with zoonotic potential occur commonly enough that cats, particularly those with diarrhea and who are owned by immunocompromised persons, should be evaluated for those pathogens.[26,27] The following is a discussion of the most common enteric parasites found in cats. For more on parasite prevention and control, see Chapter 8, and for more on zoonotic enteric parasites, see Chapter 34.

NEMATODES

Ollulanus tricuspis

Ollulanus tricuspis is an almost microscopic nematode worm infecting the stomach of domestic and wild cats.[5] The worm measures less than 1 mm long.[3]

Life Cycle

The larvae of *O. tricuspis* develop and hatch within the uterus of the female worm. They develop to maturity in the stomach of the cat where it is capable of re-infecting the host.[3] The worm is transmitted to other cats that ingest the vomitus of an infected cat.[41]

Clinical Signs and Pathophysiology

Clinical signs shown by infected cats include vomiting, anorexia, and weight loss.[2,5] Histologic findings in infected cats include lymphocytic-plasmacytic gastritis, lymphoid hyperplasia, and mucosal fibrosis. Gross lesions may be absent, or the cat may develop nodular gastritis.[41] One report suggested the parasite may have been a contributing factor in the carcinogenesis of a gastric adenocarcinoma in an infected cat.[10]

Diagnosis and Treatment

The diagnosis of infection with *O. tricuspis* is difficult, because ova are not shed in the feces; rather, the vomitus must be examined for worms or larvae. The worms may also appear in gastric mucosal biopsy samples.[41] A report of 131 cats undergoing endoscopic examinations found the parasite in gastric biopsy samples from 4 cats.[5]

Fenbendazole may be effective in treating infections with *O. tricuspis*.[41] Preparations with febantel may also be expected to successfully treat these infections.

Prevention and Zoonotic Potential

Transmission can be prevented by appropriately treating infected cats. Other cats should not be allowed to ingest infected vomit. This parasite is of no zoonotic concern.

Physaloptera

Another parasite rarely inhabiting the stomach in cats is in the genus *Physaloptera*. Larger than *Ollulanus tricuspis*, this blood-sucking worm infects cats that have ingested intermediate hosts, such as cockroaches, crickets, or flour beetles.[11] Preying on transport hosts, such as mice that have eaten an intermediate host, is another way cats become infected with this parasite. Clinical signs of infection with *Physaloptera* spp. include vomiting, anorexia, and melena. A diagnosis of *Physaloptera* infection can be made after identifying the ova in the patient's feces or adult worms in the vomitus. Occasionally, the worms may be seen during gastroscopy. The adult worms must be differentiated from ascarids.[11] Infection can be treated with ivermectin, pyrantel pamoate, or fenbendazole.[3] Because there is no migratory phase of the life cycle, the treatment does not need to be repeated.[11]

Strongyloides

Three species of *Strongyloides* infect cats. *Strongyloides felis* infects cats in India and tropical Australia,[1,43] *S. tumefaciens* is a rare parasite of cats in the southeastern United States,[3] and *S. planiceps* is found in cats in Malaya and Japan.[1] *Strongyloides stercoralis*, found in dogs and humans, produces experimental infections in cats, but natural infection with this species has not been observed.[1] Feline infection with *Strongyloides* spp. is considered by most to be rare. However, one report from Australia identified *S. felis* in 169 of 504 necropsied cats.[43]

Life Cycle

Infection with *Strongyloides* spp. occurs after ingestion of infective larvae. Infection can also take place after the larvae penetrate the skin of the cat.[11] Ingested larvae penetrate the intestinal wall and migrate through the diaphragm into the lungs. After cutaneous penetration, the larvae enter the venous circulation and enter the lungs. After further development in the lungs, the parasite migrates up the trachea and is swallowed. Adult *S. felis* and *S. planiceps* burrow into the wall of the small intestine, while adult *S. tumefaciens* lives in the colonic mucosa. Ova may be shed in the feces or hatch in the intestinal tract. Autoinfection occurs if larvae become infective and penetrate the intestinal wall before being shed. Ova and larvae that are shed develop into free-living adult worms.[11] The prepatent period is between 7 and 10 days.[1,11]

Clinical Signs and Diagnosis

Signs of a *Strongyloides* spp. infection are usually absent.[1,40] Lung migration may cause cough or respiratory distress. The presence of the parasite in the intestinal tract may result in diarrhea and weight loss.[11] *Strongyloides tumefaciens* is associated with the formation of small, worm-filled nodules in the colon.[40]

Identification of *Strongyloides* spp. larvae using the Baermann fecal concentration technique is required to diagnose most infections. Unless the infection is heavy, examination of a fresh fecal smear is insensitive for identification of these larvae.[1] The nodules formed by *S. tumefaciens* infection can be visualized during colonoscopy. Histopathology of the biopsied nodules should reveal many adult worms.[40]

Treatment and Prevention

Infection with *Strongyloides* spp. can be treated with fenbendazole,[11] pyrantel pamoate,[40] thiabendazole,[1,11] or ivermectin.[3] To evaluate efficacy, repeat a fecal examination 2 to 3 days after the treatment ends. Because of the presence of free-living adult worms in the environment and the ability of larvae to cause infection by penetrating intact skin, prevention is difficult. Keeping cats indoors in warm, humid climates may be an owner's only means of preventing infection with *Strongyloides* spp. parasites.

Whipworms

Infections with *Trichuris vulpis* rarely occur in cats and are considered to be clinically unimportant.[3,14]

Roundworms

The two species of roundworms commonly infecting cats are *Toxocara cati* (Figure 23-39) and *Toxascaris leonina* (Figure 23-40). The latter also has the ability to infect dogs.[14]

Life Cycle

Cats are infected with *T. cati* in several ways. Most commonly, infection is by ingestion of contaminated food, water, or infected paratenic hosts such as rodents. Transuterine transmission has not been reported.[14]

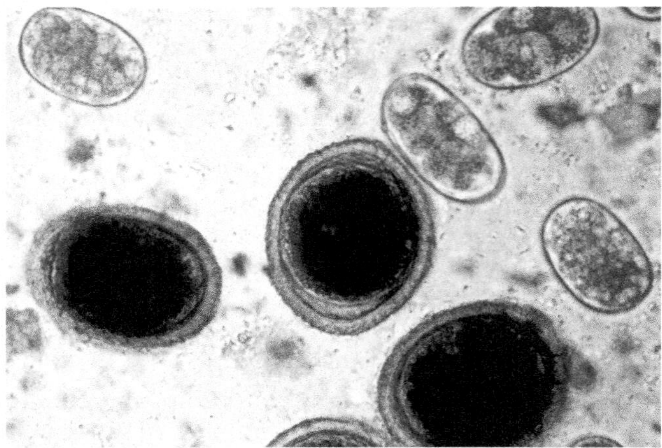

FIGURE 23-39 Fecal flotation showing the large, brown, thick-walled ova of *Toxocara cati*. The other ova are of *Ancylostoma caninum* (magnification 400×). *(From Marks SL, Willard MD: Diarrhea in kittens. In August JR, editor:* Consultations in feline internal medicine, *ed 5, St Louis, 2006, Saunders Elsevier, p 138.)*

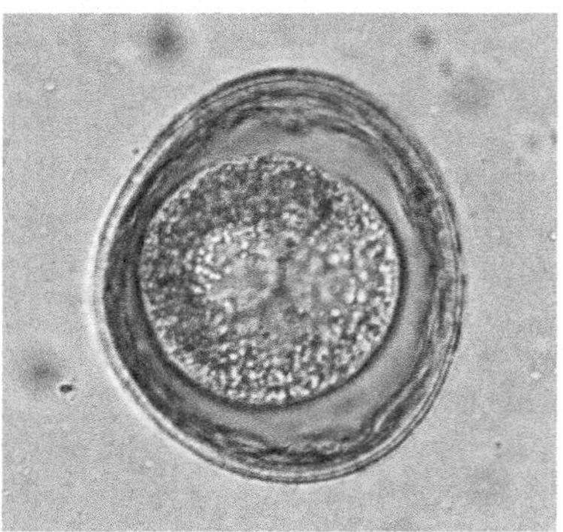

FIGURE 23-40 Ovum from *Toxascaris leonina* (magnification 400×). *(From Bowman DD: Helminths. In Bowman DD, editor:* Georgis' parasitology for veterinarians, *ed 9, St Louis, 2009, Saunders Elsevier, p 313.)*

Transmammary infection occurs, but only if the queen is acutely infected late in pregnancy. Chronically infected queens do not pass *T. cati* ova in their milk.[14]

After ingestion, *T. cati* larvae migrate through the small intestinal wall, into the liver, and then to the lungs where they are coughed up and swallowed. These larvae then infect the small intestine. Some of the migrating larvae become encysted in the cat's muscle tissue. Larvae from ova ingested through the milk tend not to undergo migration and mature directly in the small intestine.[14] The prepatent period is approximately 8 weeks.

Infection with *T. leonina* occurs after ingestion of infective ova or an infected paratenic host. Unlike *T. cati*, very few *T. leonina* larvae migrate through the cat's tissues. Most develop in the wall of the small intestine. The prepatent period is 7 to 10 weeks. *Toxascaris leonina* ova can become infective within 8 days of being passed in the feces when the ambient temperature is 27° C but normally require 3 to 4 weeks.[14]

Clinical Signs

Clinical illness because of roundworm infection is uncommon. Illness, when it does happen, most often occurs in kittens[26] Signs may be mild and can include vomiting,[14] diarrhea, weight loss, poor growth, and a "pot belly."[26] A heavy infection with *T. cati* can result in catarrhal enteritis. Severe infections can lead to intestinal obstruction and, possibly, perforation.[26] Much less dramatic changes arise after infection with *T. leonina*, although enteritis may occur.[14]

Diagnosis and Treatment

Roundworms are frequently diagnosed with a fecal floatation. The centrifugal floatation technique is more sensitive than the simple fecal floatation technique many hospitals use.[14] Occasionally, adult worms will be passed with the feces.

The goals of treating roundworms include disease prevention in an individual cat or kitten, prevention of environmental contamination by cats defecating outside, and the prevention of zoonotic infections. Many effective and safe anthelmintics are available (Table 23-19). Benzimidazoles, such as fenbendazole, act on the parasite's microtubular structure, leading to disintegration of the worm's intestines, muscular layer, and hypodermis.[14] Pyrantel in the pamoate formulation is poorly absorbed and causes paralytic parasite death. Macrocyclic lactones, such as milbemycin, also lead to paralytic parasite death. These compounds act on the parasite's gamma-aminobutyric acid (GABA)– and glutamate-controlled ion channels. These channels are lacking in tapeworms, accounting for the lack of efficacy against these parasites.[14] Lastly, emodepside (a cyclic octadepsipeptide) has been combined with praziquantel in the product Profender (Bayer Animal Health). This topical parasiticide has been shown to be both safe and effective.[14]

These drugs appear to be so safe that overdosing is almost impossible.[14] Kittens can be dewormed starting at two weeks of age and again at 4, 6, 8, 12, and 16 weeks.[26] Older kittens and adults can be dewormed every month to 4 months.[14] Because of the safety of these drugs, the possibility of false-negative tests and, more importantly, the zoonotic potential of these infections, perhaps all kittens should be dewormed, not just those testing positive.

Prevention

Roundworm ova are very hardy and can remain infective for years.[14] They survive sewage treatment and composting, and there is no practical means of decreasing the ova population once the environment is contaminated. Thus it is best to attempt to prevent contamination in the first place. When practical, keeping cats indoors allows appropriate control of potentially

TABLE 23-19 Anthelmintic Drugs

Drug	Trade Name	Dosage	Route and Duration	Susceptible Parasites
Emodepside	*Profender (Bayer Animal Health)	3 mg/kg	Topical, once	Roundworms Hookworms Tapeworms
Epsiprantel	Cestex (Pfizer)	2.75 mg/kg	PO, once	Tapeworms *Alaria marcianae*
Febantel	†Drontal Plus (Bayer Animal Health)	15 mg/kg	PO	Roundworms Hookworms Tapeworms
Fenbendazole	Panacur (Intervet)	50 mg/kg q24h	PO, 3-5 days	Roundworms Hookworms *Taenia* spp. *Strongyloides* spp.
Flubendazole	Flubenol (Janssen)	22 mg/kg q24h	PO, 2-3 days	Roundworms Hookworms Tapeworms
Ivermectin	Various	200 μg/kg	PO, once	Roundworms Hookworms *Strongyloides* spp.
Milbemycin	Interceptor, Milbemax* (Novartis)	2 mg/kg	PO, once	Roundworms Hookworms Tapeworms (with praziquantel)
Piperazine	Pipa-Tabs (Vet-A-Mix)	110 mg/kg	PO, repeat in 3 weeks	Roundworms
Praziquantel	Droncit (Bayer)	20 to 25 mg/kg	PO, SC, once	Flukes
Praziquantel	Droncit (Bayer)	5 mg/kg	PO, SC, once daily for 3 to 5 days	Tapeworms
Pyrantel pamoate	Nemex (Pfizer), Strongid (Pfizer)	5-20 mg/kg	PO, repeat in 3 weeks	Roundworms Hookworms *Strongyloides* spp.
Pyrantel plus praziquantel	Drontal (Bayer)	1 tablet/4 kg	PO, once	Roundworms Hookworms Tapeworms
Selamectin	Revolution, Stronghold (Pfizer)	6 mg/kg	Topical, once	Roundworms Hookworms

*Combined with praziquantel.
†Combined with praziquantel and pyrantel.

contaminated fecal material. If the pet cat is allowed outdoors, attempts at preventing hunting may reduce the possibility of infection. Keep children's play areas, such as sand boxes, inaccessible to cats when children are not at play. Feeding only well-cooked food can prevent infection by contaminated food. Finally, empirical, preventative deworming for cats that go outdoors should be performed 3 to 4 times yearly. Any less frequently does not lead to an appreciable decrease in the prevalence of the parasite.[7]

Zoonotic Potential

Roundworms easily infect humans who ingest the ova, particularly children. Visceral larval migrans occurs after infection with *Toxocara canis* in humans. Infection can lead to the formation of nodules in the brain, liver, lungs, and kidneys. Ocular larval migrans results in granulomatous retinitis that is often misdiagnosed as retinoblastoma in older children.[3] This can lead to unnecessary enucleation. *Toxocara cati* appears, however, to be less important than *T. canis* as an infection in humans.[3]

Hookworms

The species of hookworms that infect cats are *Ancylostoma tubaeforme* and *Ancylostoma braziliense* (see Figure 23-39). They are reported to be an uncommon infection in cats.[26,34] *Ancylostoma braziliense* can also infect dogs.

Life Cycle

Hookworm infections occur after ingesting food or water contaminated with hookworm larvae or eating infected paratenic hosts. The larvae can survive for months in the tissues of paratenic hosts.[14] Infection also occurs after larval migration through the skin. In either case, the worm matures in the small intestine.[14] Unlike dogs, transmammary infection has not been reported in cats.[3,14]

The prepatent period is between 19 and 28 days, depending on the route of infection. The time to patency after transcutaneous infection is longer than for direct colonization. Infective L3 larva develop 2 to 7 days after the ova are passed.[3]

Clinical Signs

Developing larvae attach to the mucosa of the small intestine where they ingest copious amounts of blood. Because the worms can remove a significant volume of blood from kittens, weakness from iron-deficiency anemia[34] or blood-loss anemia may be noted.[14] Melena and diarrhea may also be recognized. Signs are uncommon in adult cats.

Diagnosis and Treatment

Identification and treatment of hookworm infections are similar to that for roundworm infections (see Table 23-19).

Prevention

Hookworm larvae are not as hardy as roundworm eggs. Soil contamination may be a temporary problem in areas that experience a hard frost.[3] Hookworm larvae will not develop in temperatures less then 15° C or greater than 37° C. Frequent, appropriate disposal of feces, cleaning surfaces with a 1% bleach solution, and deterring hunting may prevent infections.

Zoonotic Potential

Migration through the skin of persons coming into contact with the larvae of *A. braziliense* is the most common cause of cutaneous larval migrans, particularly in the southeastern United States.[3] This is an erythematous, pruritic skin eruption often found on the soles of the feet of infected children.

CESTODES

The tapeworms most commonly found in cats are *Dipylidium caninum* and *Taenia taeniaeformis*. *Diphyllobothrium latum*, *Spirometra* spp., and *Echinococcus multilocularis* occasionally infect cats. The latter is important, because it can lead to alveolar echinococcosis in humans.[8] *Spirometra* tapeworms are found in North America (*S. mansonoides*) and far-East Asia (*S. mansoni* and *erinacei*), while *D. latum* prefers temperate climates.[11]

Life Cycle

The life cycle of tapeworms is indirect. This means a cat must ingest the tissues of an infected intermediate host. For *D. caninum*, this is the flea *Ctenocephalides felis*.[3] The intermediate hosts for *T. taeniaeformis* are small mammals such as rodents. Both *D. latum* and *Spirometra* spp. require two intermediate hosts for complete development. The first host for both is an aquatic copepod. The second intermediate host for *D. latum* is freshwater fish, while *Spirometra* tapeworms use tadpoles, snakes, mammals,[11] and birds as second intermediate hosts.[3] Cats become infected with these tapeworms only after ingesting the second intermediate host. After ingestion, the parasite attaches to the wall of the small intestine and begins to produce segments. These tapeworms rarely migrate through host tissues, but when they do, the infection can be life threatening. Patent infections become apparent in 17 days for *D. caninum*[8], 34 to 80 days for *T. taeniaeformis*,[3] 5 to 6 weeks for *D. latum*, and 10 days for *Spirometra* spp.[3] Segment shedding may last for years unless the infection is treated. *Taenia taeniaeformis* eggs are immediately infective and survive for variable periods of time depending on the environment. The eggs prefer low temperatures and high humidity and may live up to a year in these conditions.[8] Both *D. latum* and *Spirometra* spp. pass ova in the feces, not segments.[11]

Clinical Signs

Tapeworm infections are well tolerated by the cat. Usually there are no signs of infection other than finding segments on the feces or attached to perianal hair. Because both *D. latum* and *Spirometra* tapeworms absorb vitamin B_{12} across the cuticle, megaloblastic anemia is possible, but unlikely.[11]

Diagnosis and Treatment

Tapeworm infections are diagnosed by identifying the typical appearance of the segments[8] or the egg packets within the segments.[26] The segments of *T. taeniaeformis* are flat, while those of *D. caninum* have been described as appearing like a grain of rice. The segments should be handled carefully, because they are friable and rupture may result in exposure of the handler.[8] The operculated ova of *D. latum* and *Spirometra* spp. must be differentiated from trematode ova.

Even though tapeworm infections are well tolerated, cats should be treated for reasons of owner discomfort and public health concerns (see Table 23-19). These infections are easily treated, because drug treatment is highly effective. Re-infection must be controlled using preventative measures, especially flea control to prevent re-infection with *D. caninum*. Praziquantel and epsiprantel are safe and effective. Fenbendazole is effective against *T. taeniaeformis*, but not *D. caninum*.

Prevention

Without controlling exposure to intermediate hosts, tapeworm infections are difficult to eliminate. Flea control is imperative in eradicating infections with *D. caninum*. Controlling predation helps prevent ingestion of *T. taeniaeformis*–infected rodents.

Zoonotic Potential

Infection with *D. caninum* occurs in young children who are most likely to eat fleas. Infection results in only minimal signs of illness.[8] The larval stage of *T. taeniaeformis* is of little zoonotic importance.[3] Although cats are uncommonly infected with *Echinococcus multilocularis*, potentially life-threatening alveolar damage occurs in North American humans infected with this tapeworm.[8] Plerocercoids of *Spirometra* spp. can penetrate the mucous membranes or open skin wounds of humans and migrate around the subcutaneous connective tissue, forming nodules, a condition called sparganosis.[3] Megaloblastic anemia, as a result of vitamin B_{12} deficiency, may occur in humans infected with *D. latum* or *Spirometra* spp. tapeworms.[11]

TREMATODES

Alaria

Alaria marcianae flukes reside in the intestinal tract of cats and the mammary glands of lactating queens. Miracidia hatch underwater from ova shed in the feces and penetrate the skin of a snail. After further development, cercariae penetrate the skin of leopard frog tadpoles and are able to survive the metamorphosis to the adult frog.[3] If the tadpole is eaten by a snake, bird, or mammal, the parasite enters the host's tissues but does not undergo further development. After a male or nonlactating female cat ingests the infected intermediate host, the parasite penetrates the wall of the small intestine, passes through the diaphragm, and enters the lungs for further development. Finally, the parasite is coughed up and swallowed to complete maturation and reproduce in the small intestine.

If, however, an infected host is ingested by a lactating queen, the parasite migrates through the tissues to the mammary glands, rather than the lungs.[3] Once shed in the milk, the parasites develop into mature adults in the kittens. Some of the mesocercariae remain in the mammary glands to infect future litters. Clinical signs associated with worms in the small intestine are uncommon.[11] Migration through the lungs often goes unnoticed, but the cat may cough or experience hemoptysis.[3] Diagnosis involves demonstration of fluke ova in the feces. Although therapy may be unnecessary,[11] praziquantel or epsiprantel are effective in eliminating the intestinal population of the fluke.

Platynosomum

Platynosomum spp. are flukes living in the gall bladder, bile ducts,[46] and pancreatic ducts.[3] These flukes are most prevalent in the southeast United States and Caribbean islands[3] and require two intermediate hosts. The first host is a snail, while the second intermediate host is a lizard, toad, gecko, or skink.[46] Cats become infected with this fluke after ingesting an infected second intermediate host. The prepatent period for the fluke is 8 weeks.[46] Most infections are subclinical. If clinical signs do occur, they may include weight loss, vomiting, diarrhea, icterus, hepatomegaly, or abdominal distention. Diagnosis involves identification of ova shed in the feces using a fecal sedimentation method[46] or by finding adult flukes in the gall bladder or bile ducts during abdominal surgery. Treatment involves administering praziquantel (20 mg/kg, q24h, PO for 3 to 5 days) and/or surgical removal of the flukes.[3]

PROTOZOA

Coccidia

Two species of coccidians are the most common to infect cats, *Isospora felis* and *Isospora rivolta* (Figure 23-41). The genus *Isospora* may be renamed *Cystoisospora*. These are

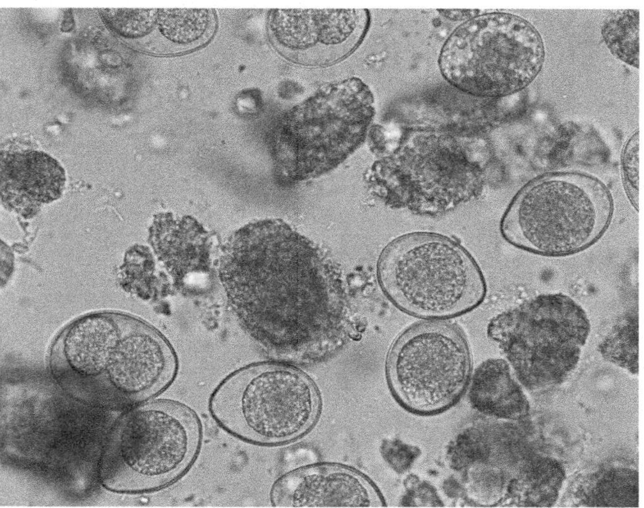

FIGURE 23-41 Zinc sulfate fecal flotation showing *Isospora* spp. oocysts from a kitten with diarrhea (magnification 1000×). *(From Marks SL, Willard MD: Diarrhea in kittens. In August JR, editor:* Consultations in feline internal medicine, *ed 5, St Louis, 2006, Saunders Elsevier, p 138.)*

species-specific obligate intracellular parasites.[4,13] They are able to survive in the environment for months.[13]

Life Cycle

A detailed description of the coccidial life cycle can be found elsewhere.[4,13] Simply put, direct transmission is by ingesting oocyst-contaminated food or water or by grooming contaminated body parts. Indirect transmission occurs after ingesting a mechanical vector or the infected tissues of paratenic hosts.[39] After ingestion by a cat, the oocyst excysts in the small intestine and enters the enterocyte where further development occurs.[26]

The parasite may also migrate through the intestinal wall to form cysts in mesenteric lymph nodes. These cysts may serve as a source for reinfection.[4,13] The prepatent period is 4 to 11 days[26] and the shed oocyst becomes infective after several days of exposure to warmth and moisture.[13]

Clinical Signs

Infection with *Isospora* spp. is usually subclinical.[26] Signs, if they occur, range from mild, transient watery diarrhea to severe mucohemorrhagic diarrhea with vomiting and resultant dehydration and weight loss.[4,13] Signs are most commonly recognized in severely infected neonatal kittens,[26] particularly those with concurrent illness, and arise because of small intestinal congestion, mucosal erosion, or villus atrophy.[39] Signs may also be noted in immunosuppressed adult cats.[26]

Diagnosis and Treatment

Isospora species are readily found in fecal floatation or wet-mount examinations. Shedding can be intermittent, but most cats with diarrhea caused by coccidial infection shed large numbers of oocsyts.[39]

Fortunately, in most cats, the diarrhea from *Isospora* spp. infection is self-limiting.[26] In fact, if a kitten is persistently shedding oocysts despite appropriate treatment[13] or the parasite is identified in an adult cat with chronic diarrhea, attempts should be made to identify co-infections or other diseases that may cause diarrhea.[39]

Anticoccidial drugs are either coccidiostatic or coccidiocidal (Table 23-20). Coccidiostatic drugs are the most commonly used drugs for individual pet cats. Trimethoprim-augmented sulfadiazine (Tribrissen; Intervet/Schering-Plough Animal Health, Summit, NJ) or another sulfa-containing antibiotic, sulfadimethoxine (Albon; Pfizer Animal Health, Madison, NJ), can be used. Supportive care for severely affected kittens, such as parenteral rehydration, should be used as needed.

Coccidiocidal drugs are often reserved for use in densely populated situations such as catteries or shelters.[26] However, many veterinarians are now using them

TABLE 23-20 **Antiprotozoal Drugs**

Drug	Trade Name	Dosage	Route, Duration	Susceptible Parasites
Azithromycin	Zithromax (Pfizer)	10 mg/kg q24h	PO, 10 days minimum; 28 days for *T. gondii*	*Cryptosporidium* spp., *Toxoplasma gondii*
Clindamycin	Antirobe (Pfizer)	25 mg/kg q12h	PO, 14 to 21 days	*Toxoplasma gondii* shedding
Clindamycin	Antirobe (Pfizer)	10 mg/kg q12h	PO, 28 days	*Toxoplasma gondii*
Febantel	†Drontal Plus (Bayer)	56.5 mg/kg q24h	PO, 5 days	*Giardia* spp.
Fenbendazole	Pancur (Intervet)	50 mg/kg q24h	PO, 5 days	*Giardia* spp.
Metronidazole	Flagyl (Pharmacia)	25 mg/kg q12h	PO, 7 days	*Giardia* spp.
Nitazoxanide	Alinia (Romark Laboratories)	25 mg/kg q12h	PO, 5-28 days	*Giardia, Cryptosporidium*
Paromomycin	Humatin (Parke-Davis)	125-165 mg/kg q12h	PO, 5 days	*Giardia, Cryptosporidium*
Ponazuril	*Marquis (Bayer)	20-50 mg/kg q24h	PO, 1-2 days	*Isospora* spp., *Toxoplasma gondii* shedding
Ronidazole	None	30 mg/kg q24h	PO, 14 days	*Tritrichomonas foetus*
Sulfadimethoxine	Albon (Pfizer Animal Health)	50 mg/kg once, then 25 mg/kg q24h	PO, 14-21 days	*Isospora* spp.
Trimethoprim-Sulfa	Tribrissen (Schering-Plough)	30 mg/kg q12h	PO, 14 days	*Isospora* spp.
Trimethoprim-Sulfa	Tribrissen (Schering-Plough)	15 mg/kg q12h	PO, 28 days	*Toxoplasma gondii*

*Dilute 1 gram of the paste in 3 mL of water to yield 37.5 mg of ponazuril per mL of solution.[39]
†Combined with praziquantel and pyrantel.

as a first-line defense against *Isospora* spp. infection.[13] Ponazuril (Marquis Oral Paste; Bayer Animal Health, Shawnee Mission, Kan.), formulated for horses, is effective and can be safely administered to cats. For more on the use of ponazuril in cats, see Chapter 46. A related drug, diclazuril, is also available and may be administered once at 25 mg/kg PO.[13] While not available in North America, toltrazuril (Baycox, Bayer Animal Health) may be administered once at 30 mg/kg PO or 15 mg/kg PO once daily for 3 days.[32a] A second course of therapy 10 days later may be required to completely eliminate the oocysts.

Prevention

Sanitation is very important, because the oocyst requires several days to become infective. Frequent removal of feces, preferably daily, is recommended to prevent re-infection and transmission to other cats.[39] Controlling a cat's ability to hunt reduces the chance of ingesting an *Isospora*-infected rodent. Control of mechanical vectors, such as cockroaches and flies, is also useful.[13] Since a cat can become infected after grooming an infected cat's perineum, consideration should be given to treating all cats in contact with the patient.[39]

In addition, catteries and shelters should ensure all food is well cooked, litter boxes are cleaned daily, and surfaces are well cleaned with steam[13] or 10% ammonia.[39] Where recurrent *Isospora* spp. infections are a problem, prophylactic treatment of all 2- to 3-week-old kittens with ponazuril should be considered.[13] Despite all well-intentioned efforts at hygiene and treatment, *Isospora* spp. infection can still be transmitted to other cats.[13]

Zoonotic Potential

Because these are species-specific parasites, transmission of *I. felis* and *I. rivolta* from cats to humans does not occur.

Giardia

The flagellated protozoal parasite, *Giardia duodenalis*, has seven microscopically indistinguishable genotypes or assemblages.[26] Assemblages A and B infect humans, while assemblage F is harbored by cats. Cats will occasionally harbor assemblages A and B.[39]

Life Cycle

Infection with *G. duodenalis* occurs after ingesting cyst-contaminated feces, by grooming an infected cat or from contaminated fomites.[37] Re-infection may occur by self-grooming. Only a small number of cysts need be ingested to establish an infection. In humans as few as 10 cysts are required to cause infection.[37]

After ingestion of infective cysts, trophozoites begin to excyst in the stomach.[37] This process is completed in the proximal duodenum.[26] The trophozoites adhere to enterocytes along the length of the small intestine using the ventral suction disk. Intermittent shedding of immediately infective cysts begins 5 to 16 days after infection.[28] Proteins released during encystment of the trophozoites are detected by the fecal antigen tests.[37] Cysts may adhere to the perianal region, facilitating re-infection by self-grooming.[28] Occasionally, trophozoites are found in examinations of fresh, watery feces. These do not survive for long and are not infective.[4]

Pathogenesis

The mechanisms of disease induced by *G. duodenalis* are still unclear. After the trophozoite attaches to the brush border of the enterocyte, the tight junction between cells is disrupted, increasing intestinal permeability.[37] The brush border becomes attenuated, further exacerbating malabsorption of water, electrolytes, and other nutrients.[39] The alteration in intercellular adhesion results in T-lymphocyte activation and mucosal cell injury.[37] Infection also promotes mucosal cell apoptosis (preprogrammed cell death).[28] In addition, small intestinal bacterial overgrowth may accompany *G. duodenalis* infections, resulting in more severe clinical signs.[39]

Clinical Signs

Fortunately, most cats infected with *G. duodenalis* show no clinical signs.[28,39] The most common sign is acute, transient, small bowel diarrhea[28] without systemic illness, such as fever or vomiting.[39] Less commonly, a cat might have profuse, watery malodorous diarrhea[37] with mucus.[39] Also possible, but uncommon, is weight loss[26,28] or abdominal pain.[37] The severity of clinical signs exhibited in an individual cat depends on the age and general health of the cat.[37] Cats co-infected with *Cryptosporidium felis* or *Tritrichomonas foetus* may have more severe diarrhea that is more difficult to control,[39] as will the presence of bacterial overgrowth.

Diagnosis

The diagnosis of *G. duodenalis* requires demonstration of trophozoites or cysts in a fecal examination, or detection of encystment proteins or giardial DNA in a fecal sample. A reliable diagnosis may be difficult to obtain for several reasons. Cysts are small, easily missed, and must be differentiated from plant debris or yeast.[37] Trophozoites are short lived outside the body and can only be found in very fresh, watery feces or, better yet, in diarrheic feces collected directly from the cat's rectum.[37] Shedding of cysts is usually intermittent, and the intensity of shedding varies greatly.[28,37] Because of these difficulties, the absence of the organism in a fecal sample does not eliminate it as the cause of diarrhea. It is often necessary to test multiple fecal samples, using at least two different techniques in order to find the organism.[37,39]

The easiest test to perform is a fecal smear or wet mount examination to identify trophozoites or cysts

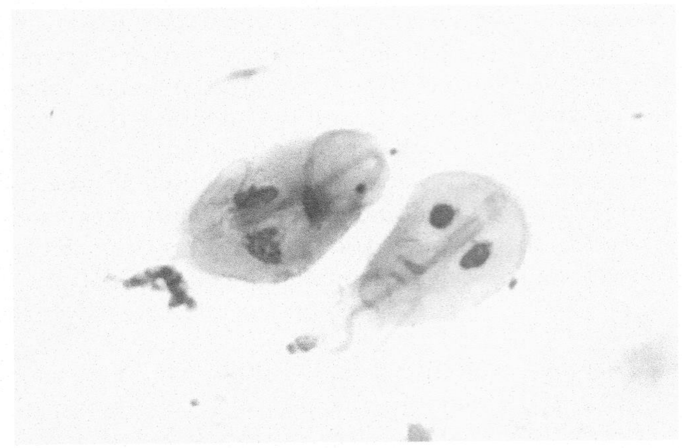

FIGURE 23-42 Giemsa-stained fecal smear showing two trophozoites of *Giardia duodenalis*. The trophozoite on the right, viewed from the top, displays the characteristic pear-shaped face appearance with the bilateral symmetry, two nuclei, posterior median bodies, and fibrils running the length of the parasite. *(From Marks SL, Willard MD: Diarrhea in kittens. In August JR, editor:* Consultations in feline internal medicine, *ed 5, St Louis, 2006, Saunders Elsevier, p 136.)*

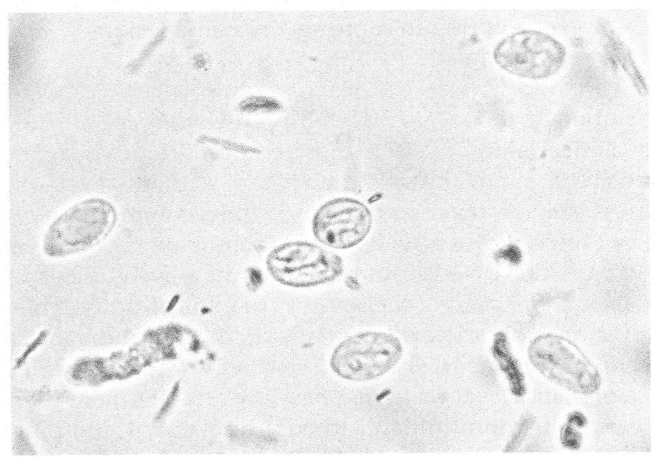

FIGURE 23-43 Zinc sulfate fecal flotation showing *Giardia duodenalis* cysts (magnification 400×). *(From Marks SL, Willard MD: Diarrhea in kittens. In August JR, editor:* Consultations in feline internal medicine, *ed 5, St Louis, 2006, Saunders Elsevier, Figure 15-6, p 137.)*

(Figures 23-42 and 23-43). The sample examined should be very fresh, warm, diarrheic feces.[39] One drop of feces is placed on a slide along with a drop of 0.9% saline or Lugol iodine.[28] Trophozoites are identified by their characteristic structure (Table 23-21). The motile trophozoites have a motion described as appearing like the back and forth rolling motion of a falling leaf. Since Lugol iodine stain kills the trophozoite, there will be no motion to detect.[28] This test is not very sensitive; however, with trained examiners, the test has a high specificity.

Increased sensitivity can be gained by performing a centrifugal flotation using zinc sulfate. The sample should be warm, fresh feces or feces refrigerated for no

TABLE 23-21 Physical Characteristics of *Tritrichomonas foetus* versus *Giardia duodenalis*

Characteristic	*Tritrichomonas foetus*	*Giardia duodenalis*
Size	15 μm × 5 μm	15 μm × 8 μm
Motility	Erratic, forward motion	Falling leaf, rolling motion
Structures	Undulating membrane	Ventral disk, median bodies
Flagellae	3 anterior, 1 posterior	8
Nuclei	1	2

more than 2 days.[28] The processed sample is examined for the same structures as the wet mount. The sensitivity of examining one sample is 70%[28] and increases as more samples are examined. The sensitivity of looking at three samples is 95%[26,28]; therefore the test is not considered negative until three specimens have been found free of the organism.[39]

A fecal antigen test that identifies the encystment protein is available. The SNAP *Giardia* antigen test (IDEXX Laboratories) uses fresh or frozen feces, or feces refrigerated for less than 7 days.[34] Since the antigen is continuously shed, this test avoids the problem of intermittent shedding of the whole organism.[28] The sensitivity of the test is 85%, with a specificity of 100%.[35] By combining the antigen test with a zinc sulfate fecal centrifugal flotation, the sensitivity improves to 97.8%.[11] It is unknown how long the antigen remains in the feces after treatment. Thus a zinc sulfate centrifugal flotation examination should be used to evaluate therapeutic efficacy.[28,39] The use of this test in cats without diarrhea is controversial, because these cats are unlikely to shed cysts. The zoonotic significance of a positive antigen test in a cat not shedding cysts is unknown and may cause confusion.[39]

Polymerase chain reaction detection of *Giardia* DNA is available, but the test has not been standardized across all diagnostic laboratories. One needs to ensure the laboratory performing the test has validated it for assemblage F. The test may also be used to identify cats harboring the zoonotic assemblages A and B. The sensitivity of this test is unknown.[39]

Treatment

Two commonly available drugs are used most frequently to treat infections with *G. duodenalis* (see Table 23-20). Fenbendazole may be effective and can be used in pregnant queens[28] and in cats co-infected with roundworms, hookworms, and *Taenia* spp. tapeworms.[39] However, in one small study, only four of eight cats infected with both *G. duodenalis* and *Cryptosporidium felis* stopped shedding *Giardia* permanently after receiving fenbendazole.[29] Febantel, in the combination product Drontal Plus

(Bayer Animal Health), is converted to fenbendazole. When six experimentally infected cats received 56.5 mg/kg of febantel q24h PO for 5 days, four of them stopped shedding *G. duodenalis* cysts.[39]

Metronidazole has been the traditional drug used to treat *G. duodenalis* in pets.[28] The drug is also useful for treating concurrent small intestinal bacterial overgrowth and clostridial infections.[39] The administration of metronidazole may eliminate shedding in 67% of cats.[26] Neurologic side effects may occur at the dose recommended for treatment of *Giardia* (see above, Therapeutics for Vomiting and Diarrhea). The use of a *Giardia* vaccine was ineffective in clearing infection by itself.[44]

The combination of fenbendazole and metronidazole has been suggested as the initial treatment of choice for *G. duodenalis* infections.[39] Although controlled studies are lacking, they may work synergistically by acting on two different targets within the parasite.[28] Febantel would be expected to have the same synergism with metronidazole.

Drug therapy may not be necessary in cats without diarrhea that are infected with *G. duodenalis*,[37] because it is uncommon for a cat to carry the assemblages required to infect humans. The veterinarian may be obligated to treat a healthy cat if the owner wants to treat, the owner is immunocompromised, or the goal is eradication of an infection from a multicat home or prevention of parasite transmission to *Giardia*-naïve cats is attempted.[28]

What may appear to be treatment failure is more likely to be re-infection. In addition to drug therapy, steps should be taken to prevent re-infection. All cats with diarrhea positive for *G. duodenalis* should be treated along with their housemates.[37] Sanitation is imperative in the fight against re-infection and transmission of *G. duodenalis*. Dispose of old litter pans and scoops and use disposable litter boxes during treatment. When the infection is eliminated, not just controlled, new litter boxes and scoops may be purchased. Bathe all cats during treatment to remove cysts from the hair coat. Since *Giardia* spp. cysts are susceptible to desiccation,[28] blow-dry all cats using a warm air blower, paying particular attention to the perineal area. Disinfect bowls, housing, and other utensils with bleach.[28]

In addition to antiprotozoal drugs and sanitation, supportive care may become necessary. Probiotics and a highly digestible, bland diet may be offered to cats with small bowel diarrhea, while a high-fiber diet may be useful for those few cats with large bowel diarrhea.[39] Where required, hydration and electrolyte imbalances must be corrected and antiemetics used to control vomiting.

Therapy can be evaluated by retesting feces with a zinc sulfate centrifugal flotation examination 1 to 3 days after the end of treatment and again 3 weeks later. A positive test immediately posttreatment is most likely because of therapeutic failure. If the cat is negative immediately after treatment ends, but is positive 3 weeks later, re-infection is likely.[28] Since the fecal antigen test may remain positive long after the infection is eradicated, this test is inappropriate for evaluating therapy.[28,39]

Re-treatment of fecal flotation-positive, recovered cats may be handled in a manner similar to the positive healthy cat mentioned above.[28] Cats with diarrhea that continue to shed cysts may be re-treated for *G. duodenalis* infection along with dietary modification and empirical treatment for other common intestinal parasites. However, serious consideration should be given to investigation into other potential causes of diarrhea.[28]

Prevention

The *Giardia* vaccine has been found to be ineffective in preventing infection[37] and production has been discontinued.[39] This means prevention of *Giardia* infection involves avoiding exposure, stress and re-infections. Providing a clean environment, feeding only processed foods, and controlling potential transport hosts will help reduce the chances of exposure. Isolation of cats with diarrhea may be important, too.[39] Municipal sanitation control is difficult as the cyst survives for weeks in cool, moist environments.[28] Cysts are also able to survive water treatment and can pass through attempts at water filtration.[37]

Zoonotic Potential

Giardiasis is associated with debilitating diarrhea in some humans, particularly those who are immunocompromised.[35] However, cats do not commonly carry the assemblages needed to infect humans. Transmission of *G. duodenalis* from cats to humans is rare and unproven.[28] Still, it seems prudent to consider the owner's health when contemplating management of giardial infections in cats. To avoid human health risks, cats with diarrhea that test positive for *G. duodenalis* should be treated with the goal of controlling the diarrhea.[39] Since no treatment for *G. duodenalis* is completely effective or 100% safe, treatment of positive cats without diarrhea should only begin after a discussion of the benefits and risks of the treatment with the owner.[39]

Tritrichomonas foetus

Tritrichomonas foetus is best known for causing bovine reproductive infections. It is an obligate anaerobic parasite[26] that also colonizes the lower intestinal tract of cats. There are enough differences between the two isolates that the feline isolate does not cause disease in heifers and vice versa.[39] The parasite depends on the host's normal intestinal flora and secretions for obtaining nutrition.[7] A report from the United States of purebred cats tested at an international cat show found *T. foetus* in 36 of the 117 cats tested, a prevalence of 31%.[23] This parasite seems to have a higher prevalence in purebred cats than nonpurebred cats. A study of pet cats visiting veterinary hospitals across the United States reported 12 of 32 purebred cats were positive for *T. foetus*, while only 5 of 141 nonpurebred cats were positive. In this same study, 12 of the 17 positive tests were from purebred cats.[45] A study from the United Kingdom of diarrheic fecal samples sent to a veterinary diagnostic laboratory reported similar results. Purebred cats represented 14 of the 16 cats testing positive for *T. foetus*. The U.K. study also found the Siamese and Bengal breeds each represented 6 of 14 positive cats; only two other breeds tested positive.[25]

Transmission

Like most other protozoal parasites, *T. foetus* is transmitted by ingestion of the parasite, in this case, the trophozoite. Unlike most of the other parasites, *T. foetus* does not form cysts and only survives up to 3 days outside the body in moist feces.[47] A cat becomes infected through the use of a shared litter box with an infected cat. After walking into the box, the parasite is transferred from the infected feces of one cat to the paws of the other. Infection then occurs through ingestion of the trophozoites during grooming.[47] After infection, *T. foetus* colonizes the distal ileum and colon,[15] followed by shedding of infective trophozoites 2 to 7 days later.[19]

Clinical Signs

There are several mechanisms by which *T. foetus* causes diarrhea. These include alteration of the cat's normal bacterial flora population, increases in local inflammatory cytokine concentrations, production of enzymes, and direct mucosal injury. The resulting injury leads to plasmacytic-lymphocytic[49] and neutrophilic colitis.[37] Although most infections involve only the mucosa of the colon, one study reported two of seven cats with diarrhea and *T. foetus* infections as having trophozoites in deeper layers of the colonic wall.[49] Co-infection with *Cryptosporidium felis*[17] or *Giardia duodenalis*[39] can be associated with increased numbers of *T. foetus* trophozoites and increased severity of diarrhea.

Signs of infection are most frequent in kittens and young cats, although infections without clinical signs can occur.[39] Adult cats, however, may also show signs of *T. foetus* infection. The most common sign is a foul-smelling large bowel diarrhea with increased frequency of defecation,[39] mucus, blood,[15] and flatulence.[37] The consistency of the diarrhea may wax and wane, but the presence of diarrhea does not.[47] Cats with diarrhea are otherwise in good health and maintain their body condition.[15,39] Severe diarrhea can result in anal swelling and fecal incontinence.[39] Diarrhea may respond to the use of antibiotics because of changes in the cat's intestinal microbial flora. However, it always returns at the cessation of therapy.[39,47] Many cats experience a spontaneous resolution of the diarrhea within 2 years of diagnosis.[15,38]

Since *T. foetus* causes reproductive infections in heifers and bulls, there is speculation the parasite also infects the reproductive tract in cats. *Tritrichomonas foetus* was found in the uterus of a queen with pyometra.[9] However, in a study of 60 breeding male and female cats from 33 catteries, no cytologic or molecular evidence of *T. foetus* was found in the reproductive tract. The authors reported colonic infection with *T. foetus* in 15 of the 60 cats representing 22 of the 33 catteries.[24]

Diagnosis

Detection of the trophozoites in a sample of feces is the most expedient means of diagnosing an infection with *T. foetus* (Figure 23-44). An index of suspicion is required, because the clinical presentation of *T. foetus* infection is often mistaken for infection with *Giardia duodenalis*. If a cat is not responding to treatment for that parasite, consider *T. foetus* as a cause of the diarrhea.

The sample required for the diagnosis of *T. foetus* is a fresh, nonrefrigerated sample of watery feces. Refrigeration kills the trophozoites, and they are not found in normal feces.[34] The sample may be freshly passed diarrhea, feces collected using a wire loop passed into the colon, or collected by a colonic flush using a red rubber catheter and 10 mL of saline.[47]

A wet mount or smear examination of the feces should be performed on all cats with diarrhea. Examination of multiple samples may be required to find the *T. foetus* trophozoites with this technique because it is insensitive.[39] The trophozoites must be differentiated from *Giardia duodenalis* based on structural differences and motility patterns (see Table 23-21).

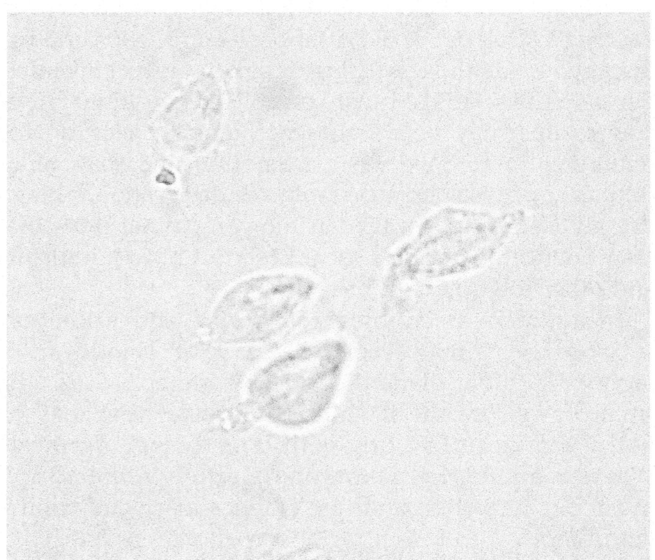

FIGURE 23-44 *Tritrichomonas foetus* trophozoites from culture. Notice the undulating membrane on the trophozoite on the right. *(From Scorza AV, Lappin MR: Gastrointestinal protozoal infections. In August JR, editor:* Consultations in feline internal medicine, *ed 6, St Louis, 2010, Saunders Elsevier, p 207.)*

The trophozoites of *T. foetus* can be cultured using the InPouch TF system (Biomed Diagnostics). This test is more sensitive than the fecal wet mount examination and detects 1000 trophozoites per sample.[15] The number of parasites shed by a cat with diarrhea is high enough to be routinely detected with this method.[18] The test should be performed in-house, because the parasite is unlikely to survive the trip to the laboratory.[47] The test pouch is inoculated with 50 µg of freshly collected feces, about the size of a peppercorn.[18] Any more than this increases the chances of bacterial overgrowth.[15] The pouch is incubated at 25° C and examined under the microscope for motile trophozoites every other day for 12 days. The pouch should be tapped gently to dislodge the parasites, which tend to collect along the seams.[15] The test is considered negative if parasites are not found after 12 days. One benefit of this system is that it does not support growth of *Giardia duodenalis* or *Pentatrichomonas hominis*.[18]

If a fecal wet mount examination and culture are both negative and infection with *T. foetus* is still under consideration, a PCR test can be performed. This test detects DNA from live or dead trophozoites, but is more expensive than other diagnostic methods.[47] This test is more sensitive than the other two methods and can detect 10 parasites per sample.[16] The sample size is 200 mg of feces not contaminated by litter preserved in 3 to 5 mL of rubbing alcohol shipped at room temperature.[15] Trophozoites of *T. foetus* are sometimes found in colonic biopsy samples adhered to the surface or in the lumen of crypts.[15]

Treatment

The most effective drug for the treatment of *T. foetus* in cats is ronidazole.[17] The drug has a bitter taste and should be compounded into capsules. Veterinary staff and owners should use gloves when handling ronidazole.[15] If a confirmed relapse occurs, another course of treatment may eliminate the parasite.[39] Diarrhea may take several weeks to resolve after elimination of the parasite, because significant colitis is often present.[47] Effectiveness of treatment can be evaluated by performing fecal PCR tests 2 and 20 weeks after the end of treatment.[15] Apparent treatment failures may occur because of re-infection, co-infection with *Giardia duodenalis* or *Cryptosporidium felis*, or the presence of another concurrent diarrhea-causing disorder. A more worrisome cause for treatment failure is a recent report of parasite resistance to ronidazole in two cats.[22] Fortunately, diarrhea ultimately resolved in both cats despite the continued presence of the parasite. If the cat retests negative and the diarrhea is not improving after 2 weeks, consider the possibility that another disease may exist.

Nonspecific treatment for diarrhea is unhelpful[37] and may prolong the duration of diarrhea.[15] Diarrhea may respond to antibiotics as they alter the intestinal flora population; however, once treatment is stopped, the diarrhea will return.[47]

An important and potentially serious adverse effect of ronidazole administration in cats is a reversible neurotoxicity. Onset of signs often begins within 1 week of the onset of therapy and may last between 1 and 4 weeks after cessation of therapy.[38] These signs can include depression, ataxia, seizures,[47] behavioral changes, weakness, hyperesthesia, and trembling.[38] Neurotoxicosis usually requires only supportive care along with discontinuation of the drug. The neurologically affected cat should be retested for the parasite, because it may have been eliminated.[38] Because of the potential for neurotoxicity, the use of ronidazole should be restricted to cats with confirmed infections with *T. foetus*.[47]

Prevention and Zoonotic Potential

Crowded conditions should be avoided, because transmission of *T. foetus* trophozoites is more efficient in these settings.[39] Cats testing positive should be isolated from other cats during treatment.[37] Providing a clean environment will help prevent transmission of trophozoites.

Although there is a report of an infection in one immunocompromised person, transmission of *T. foetus* trophozoites from cats to healthy humans has not been reported.[39] Still, prudence dictates handling feces infected with *T. foetus* trophozoites carefully.

Cryptosporidium felis

Recent genetic evaluations have shown that most feline infections with *Cryptosporidium* spp. are with *C. felis*; not, as previously thought, with *C. parvum*.[36] *Cryptosporidium parvum* seems to be limited to farm animals.[4] *Cryptosporidium felis* is an obligate intracellular parasite infecting the small intestine.[4]

Life Cycle

Infective oocysts are ingested from contaminated feces during self-grooming of contaminated body parts and from contaminated food and water.[32,39] After infection, the parasite attaches to the brush border of the enterocyte. The prepatent period is 3 to 6 days,[39] and the oocysts are infective as soon as they are shed, making this a very contagious disease.[20] Like most intestinal parasites, shedding is often intermittent.

Clinical Signs

The pathogenic effects of *C. felis* infections are not well understood. Direct cytotoxicity and inflammation causes villus atrophy and decreased surface area for absorption of water, electrolytes, and other nutrients.[20,32] Apoptosis (preprogrammed cell death) of the mucosal cells may be accelerated, adding to the malabsorption.[20]

Most infections with *C. felis* are subclinical.[39] Signs, if present, range from a mild, self-limiting small bowel diarrhea[33] to chronic intermittent small bowel diarrhea.[32] Severe diarrhea with weight loss and anorexia may also occur.[32,33] Clinically apparent infections are most common in kittens, adult cats with concurrent gastrointestinal diseases, and cats co-infected with *Giardia duodenalis* or *Tritrichomonas foetus*.[39] Cats with co-infections may experience more severe clinical signs.[32]

Diagnosis

A fecal flotation, which should be performed on all cats with diarrhea, may reveal *C. felis* if there are large numbers of oocysts (Figure 23-45). The fecal floatation test, however, is often negative[39] because of intermittent shedding. The parasite is small and floats in a higher plane than helminth ova; the high-power lens and appropriate adjustment of the microscope stage is required to find the parasite.[32] The small size of the oocyst makes identification difficult, particularly if the examiner is not specifically looking for them.[34]

A modified Ziehl-Neelsen stain of a thin fecal smear may help in the identification of the oocysts.[39] This technique works well in humans with large numbers of oocysts.[33] Once signs resolve or the oocyst numbers decline, a single examination of a stained smear becomes insensitive. When only one sample is available, testing for *C. felis* antigen is a good choice.[34] The ProSpecT Microplate Assay (Alexon Biomedical, Sunnyvale, Calif.) is more sensitive and specific for the diagnosis of *C. felis* than is the examination of a stained smear.[6] Immunofluorescent antibody testing is available from some laboratories.

Fecal *C. felis* DNA can be detected using PCR testing. This test is available at many veterinary diagnostic laboratories; however, at present, there is no test

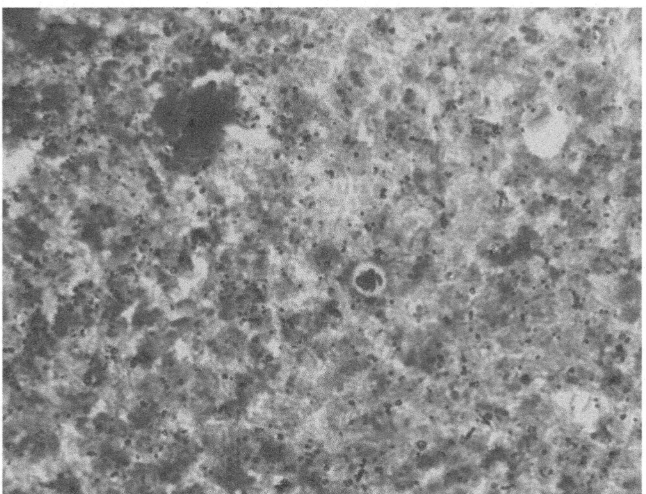

FIGURE 23-45 Fecal smear from a cat with diarrhea showing a single oocyst of *Cryptosporidium felis* colored with a modified Ziehl-Neelsen stain (magnification 1000×). *(From Marks SL, Willard MD: Diarrhea in kittens. In August JR, editor:* Consultations in feline internal medicine, *ed 5, St Louis, 2006, Saunders Elsevier, p 135.)*

standardization among laboratories.[39] The clinical and zoonotic significance of a positive PCR test combined with an oocyst negative test is unknown.[39] Therefore a positive PCR test in a cat without diarrhea presents a confusing situation for the attending veterinarian with regard to recommendations for the owner.

Treatment

Unfortunately, there are no completely effective and safe treatment protocols available for *C. felis*.[32,39] A concerted attempt to find other causes of diarrhea should take place prior to convicting a cat of having diarrhea solely from *C. felis* infection. Most reports on therapy for *C. felis* are uncontrolled and anecdotal. A number of drugs have been discussed. Azithromycin for at least 10 days appears safe but produces variable results.[39] Paromomycin, an oral aminoglycoside, may be effective. However, one study reported acute renal failure in 4 of 32 cats receiving the drug. Deafness also occurred in three of those four cats.[21] Nitazoxanide is a drug approved for treating humans with diarrhea caused by *Cryptosporidium* spp. infections. The administration of nitazoxanide to cats at 25 mg/kg q12h PO for at least 5 days[39] up to 28 days[32] may be effective. However, nitazoxanide is a gastrointestinal irritant and commonly results in vomiting and foul-smelling diarrhea.

Co-infections with *Giardia duodenalis* and/or *Tritrichomonas foetus* are more difficult to control. If diarrhea from *C. felis* infection improves but does not resolve at the end of therapy, the duration of treatment may be prolonged.[39] Additional diagnostic testing should also be performed to ensure the only cause of the diarrhea is infection with *C. felis*.

Prevention

Environmental control of *C. felis* is difficult, because it is extremely hardy. It is resistant to chlorination and most disinfectants.[32] Oocysts remain viable at temperatures above freezing up to 65° C.[4] The parasite is difficult to filter and survives treatment at municipal water treatment facilities.[20] Steam-cleaned housing and utensils may be beneficial in controlling parasite numbers, and they are susceptible to 5% ammonia solutions; however, the required contact time is 18 hours.[39]

Zoonotic Potential

Cryptosporidium spp. are relatively species specific, and there are no reports of waterborne outbreaks of human cryptosporidiosis associated with *C. felis*.[32] Cryptosporidiosis can cause life-threatening diarrhea in HIV-positive persons.[20] Fortunately, humans are rarely infected with *C. felis*.[39] In fact, the zoonotic species most commonly found in humans (often veterinary students), is *C. parvum* found in young heifers.[4] Regardless of a person's health, feces from a cat with diarrhea should be handled carefully. If a cat infected with *Cryptosporidium* spp. is owned by an immunocompromised person, a PCR test may be useful in determining the species of the parasite and its zoonotic risk.

Toxoplasma gondii

Like other coccidians, *Toxoplasma gondii* is an obligate intracellular parasite.[12] Domestic cats and other felids are the only animals that shed oocysts. Any warm-blooded animal, including humans, can be infected with this parasite.

Life Cycle

Toxoplasma gondii can be transmitted by ingestion of infective oocysts in fecally contaminated food or water after ingestion of tissue cysts through carnivorism, or by transplacental or trans-mammary transmission of the parasite. The parasite enters into one of two cycles, depending on the host species. The enteroepithelial cycle only occurs in cats and results in shedding of oocysts after sexual reproduction of the parasite. After a cat ingests an infective oocyst or a tissue cyst, the parasite enters the mucosal cells of the small intestine, where it may undergo development and sexual reproduction, after which oocysts are shed.[12] The prepatent period after ingesting an infective oocyst is 19 to 48 days, while shedding after ingesting tissue cysts starts in 3 to 10 days.[4] Fecal shedding, which occurs only after initial infection, lasts for 2 to 3 weeks[4,31] and the oocysts become infective 1 to 5 days after they are shed.[12]

The extraintestinal cycle occurs in any animal, including cats. After ingestion, the parasite penetrates the cells of the small intestine and rapidly replicates in the enterocytes and associated lymph nodes into tachyzoites. After hematogenous and lymphatic spread, tachyzoites infect cells in all tissues of the body.[4] Tissues most commonly infected include the brain, liver, pancreas, and lungs.[30] If a pregnant queen becomes infected, tachyzoites cause placentitis, after which they infect the fetus.[13] In 3 weeks, the host's immune response slows parasite replication, and the resultant bradyzoites form tissue cysts[30] in the brain, striated muscle, and liver, and they remain viable for the life of the animal.[4] Immunosuppressive drugs or disease may dull the suppression of parasite division by the host immune system and allow the slowly dividing bradyzoites in tissue cysts to begin rapid division, thereby reactivating the infection with tachyzoites.[30]

Pathogenesis

None of the forms of *T. gondii* produces a toxin. Rapid replication of tachyzoites within a cell leads to rupture of the cell and necrosis of the tissue in which they are located.[12] The most commonly injured tissues are the brain, lungs, liver, and pancreas. Prenatal infection leads to more severe illness, because the immature immune system is unable to slow down replication by tachyzoites, allowing continued damage to tissues. Prenatal infection is more likely to result in ocular infections, and neonatal death is usually caused by pulmonary or hepatic infection.[30] Type II and IV hypersensitivities may be involved in the pathogenesis of chronic disease from bradyzoites in tissue cysts.[30]

Clinical Signs

Kittens infected perinatally can be stillborn or die shortly after birth. They may also suffer from hepatomegaly and ascites, central nervous system signs resulting from encephalitis, respiratory distress, or uveitis.[12,13]

Clinical signs of infection in healthy adult cats are uncommon (Box 23-2).[31] Diarrhea from enteroepithelial development of the parasite is rare.[39] Cats that develop clinical disease often have an episodic course with vague signs[30] that depend on the body system affected. Onset of illness may be acute or chronic, and the most commonly affected organs include the brain, lungs, liver, heart, pancreas, and the eyes.[13] Signs are the result of spread of tachyzoites after initial infection or after reactivation of tissue cysts. Cats suffering from uveitis may develop lens luxation and glaucoma.

Diagnosis

The best way to identify a cat shedding *T. gondii* oocysts is to demonstrate them with a centrifugal fecal flotation technique using Sheather sugar solution. The oocysts are about a quarter of the size of *Isospora felis* oocysts (Figure 23-46).[12] Oocysts of *T. gondii* are morphologically indistinguishable from *Hammondia* or *Besnoitia* spp. oocysts.[13] Detection of fecal *T. gondii* DNA using a PCR test can be used to definitively differentiate *T. gondii* oocysts from similar coccidians.[31] It is probably best, however, to assume suspicious oocysts are those of *T. gondii* until proven otherwise.

Proving infection with *T. gondii* is responsible for a cat's systemic illness is also difficult. Finding tachyzoites in cytology samples is uncommon. They are most likely to be identified from body cavity effusions.[13] The most common method of identifying an infected cat is by detecting *T. gondii*–associated immunoglobulins using immunofluorescent antibody or ELISA techniques. Since cats are infected for life, a seropositive cat has been infected at some point in its life. However, use of serology alone is insufficient to diagnose an active *T. gondii* infection.

Serum immunoglobulin M (IgM) is produced within 1 to 2 weeks after infection, but increased IgM titers may persist for months to years. Serum immunoglobulin G (IgG) begins to rise later; in some cats, IgG may not be detectable for 4 to 6 weeks.[12] By the time IgG is detectable, shedding will have ceased. Maternally acquired IgG persists in kittens for 8 to 12 weeks.[13] A rising IgG titer is associated with an active infection, but the degree of increase is not associated with the severity of the

BOX 23-2

Clinical Findings in Feline Toxoplasmosis

Fever
Anorexia, lethargy
Weight loss
Muscle pain, hyperesthesia
Respiratory tract disease
- Conjunctivitis
- Rhinitis
- Coughing
- Respiratory distress, tachypnea
- Diffuse harsh lung sounds

Vomiting, diarrhea
Abdominal discomfort
Icterus
Abdominal effusion
Arthritis, joint pain, shifting lameness
Cardiac arrhythmias, sudden death
Splenomegaly
Lymphadenomegaly
Pyogranulomatous dermatitis
Neurologic signs
- Ataxia
- Circling
- Behavioral changes
- Twitching
- Tremors

Ocular signs
- Retinochoroiditis, retinal hemorrhages
- Optic neuritis
- Optic nerve atrophy
- Anisocoria
- Blindness
- Anterior uveitis, aqueous flare, hyphema, velvety iris
- Glaucoma
- Lens luxation
- Retinal detachment

Neonatal disease (after transplacental transmission)
- Stillbirth
- Fading kittens
- Organ dysfunction
  - Liver: hepatomegaly, icterus, ascites
  - Lung: respiratory distress
  - Central nervous system: excessive sleep, crying

Adapted from Dubey JP, Lappin MR: Toxoplasmosis and neosporosis. In Greene CE, editor: *Infectious diseases of the dog and cat*, ed 3, St Louis, 2006, Saunders Elsevier, p 759.

clinical signs. If a cat becomes seronegative, it is more likely the titer has fallen below the sensitivity of the test rather than the parasite has been eliminated from the body.[31] Because of the vague nature of the clinical signs, many cats are presented later in the course of the disease. By this time, they may have switched from IgM to IgG production or passed the time of maximal IgG production. Thus a negative IgM titer or a lack of rising IgG titer does not rule out *T. gondii* infection.[30] Also, reactivation of tissue cysts is rarely associated with rising IgG titers.[31]

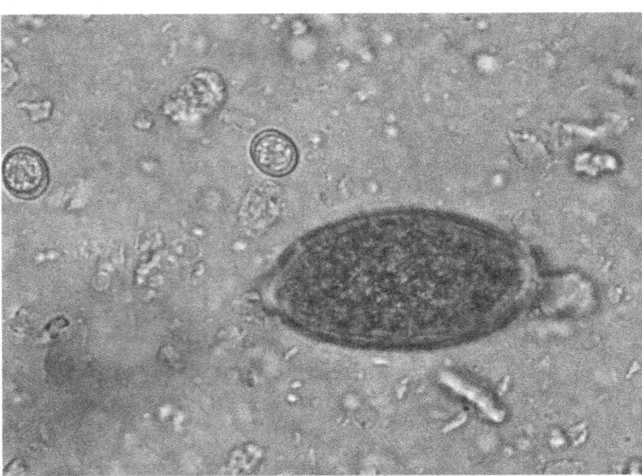

FIGURE 23-46 An unstained fecal sample from a naturally infected cat showing oocysts of *Toxoplasma gondii* compared with a *Capillaria* spp. ovum (magnification 400×). *(From Dubey JP, Lappin MR: Toxoplasmosis and neopsporosis. In Greene CE, editor:* Infectious diseases of the dog and cat, *ed 3, St Louis, 2006, Saunders Elsevier, p 756.)*

Ultimately, the diagnosis of an active systemic *T. gondii* infection requires demonstration of an IgM titer greater than 1 : 64 or a fourfold increase in IgG titers over a 2- to 3-week period *along with* signs consistent with toxoplasmosis, the exclusion of other disorders that may cause the clinical signs, and response to appropriate anti–*T. gondii* treatment.[31] Although serum IgM titers may be increased in otherwise healthy cats, increased IgM titers in cerebrospinal fluid or aqueous humor only occurs in cats with active CNS or ocular infections.[30]

Treatment

The goals of treating a cat infected with *T. gondii* are to reduce shedding of oocysts and to control the clinical signs in sick cats. Shedding can be reduced by using ponazuril,[13] toltrazuril, or high doses of clindamycin.

The drug options for treating a sick cat include clindamycin, trimethoprim-augmented sulfadiazine, or azithromycin for at least 4 weeks (see Table 23-20). Recurrences are more common if the cat is treated for less than 4 weeks.[13,30] The antifolate drug pyrimethamine may be more effective than trimethoprim, but megaloblastic anemia develops in many cats. Supplementation with folinic acid (5 mg/cat, once daily, PO) or brewer's yeast (100 mg/kg, once daily, PO) may prevent or reverse the anemia.[12] No drug clears all of the tissue cysts; so, cats remain infected for life. If uveitis is also present, use appropriate topical, oral, or parenteral corticosteroids. For a cat with proven *T. gondii*–associated uveitis alone, a topical ocular glucocorticosteroid is the only required treatment; no antibiotics are necessary unless the uveitis is persistent or recurrent.[31]

BOX 23-3

Guidelines for Cat Owners to Avoid Acquiring Toxoplasmosis

- Wash hands after handling cats, especially if you are pregnant or immunocompromised.
- Remove fecal material from the home environment daily, since shed oocysts require a minimum of 24 hours to become infective.
- Do not have immunocompromised persons clean the litter box. If they must clean the litter box, they should wear gloves and wash hands thoroughly when finished.
- Use litter box liners, and periodically wash the litter box with scalding water and detergent.
- Wear gloves when gardening, and wash hands thoroughly when finished.
- Cover children's sandboxes when not in use to avoid fecal contamination by outdoor cats.
- Only feed cats cooked or commercially processed food.
- Control potential transport hosts, such as flies and cockroaches, that may bring the organism into the home.
- Filter or boil water from sources in the environment.
- Cook meat for human consumption to 80° C for 15 minutes minimum (because of uneven heating, microwave cooking does not kill all *T. gondii*[12]).
- Freeze meat at −12° C for 24 hours.[12]
- Wear gloves when handling meat, and wash hands thoroughly with soap and water when finished.

Citation 12: Dubey JP, Lappin MR: Toxoplasmosis and neopsporosis. In Greene CE, editor: *Infectious diseases of the dog and cat*, ed 3, St Louis, 2006, Saunders Elsevier, p 754.
Adapted from Box 274-1 in Lappin MR: Toxoplasmosis. In Bonagura JD, Twedt DC, editors: *Kirk's current veterinary therapy XIV*, St Louis, 2009, Saunders Elsevier, p 1257.

Clinical signs such as malaise, fever, and muscle pain should begin to resolve in 2 to 3 days.[30] If there is no response within 7 days, switch to or add another drug.[31] If there is still no response, search for another condition that may cause the observed clinical signs. However, ocular and CNS signs resolve more slowly and thoracic radiographic changes may take weeks to resolve.[30] Some CNS changes may never completely resolve. Cats co-infected with feline immunodeficiency virus (FIV) do not respond to anti–*T. gondii* treatment as well as FIV-negative cats respond.[12]

Prevention

Feeding cats commercially processed cat food and avoiding undercooked or raw meat can prevent exposure to *T. gondii*. Controlling hunting reduces access to paratenic hosts with infective tissue cysts. Access to mechanical carriers of *T. gondii,* such as earthworms or cockroaches, should be minimized.

Zoonotic Potential

Human infection with *T. gondii* is common, more so in warm, humid climates where the prevalence of *T. gondii* seropositive persons approaches 100%. The number of persons seropositive for *T. gondii* is estimated to be around 500,000,000 worldwide.[12] Infective oocysts are hardy and may remain viable in the environment for up to 18 months.[12] Human infection most often occurs after eating raw or undercooked meat infected with tissue cysts or by transplacental infection.[31] Seropositive cats are finished shedding and are unlikely to resume shedding even if the infection becomes reactivated.[31] Cats found to be shedding oocysts should be quarantined at a veterinary hospital until shedding ends. Oocysts of *T. gondii* have not been found on the hair coat[13]; so, transmission of toxoplasmosis does not occur after touching a cat.[31]

Pregnant women infected with *T. gondii* for the first time, or chronically infected women who are also HIV positive, can transmit the parasite to their unborn child. Transplacental infection can result in stillbirths, CNS, or ocular disease.[30] More severe fetal disease may occur if the infection happens in the first half of the woman's pregnancy.[12] *Toxoplasma gondii* infection of immunocompetent humans usually results in a self-limiting fever and malaise.[30] Steps useful in preventing transmission of *T. gondii* to humans can be found in Box 23-3.

References

1. Bowman D, Hendrix C, Lindsay D et al: *Strongyloides* species. In *Feline clinical parasitology*, ed 1, Ames, Iowa, 2002, Iowa State University Press, p 235.
2. Bowman DD: Diagnostic parasitology. In Bowman DD, editor: *Georgis' parasitology for veterinarians*, ed 9, St Louis, 2009, Saunders Elsevier, p 295.
3. Bowman DD: Helminths. In Bowman DD, editor: *Georgis' parasitology for veterinarians*, ed 9, St Louis, 2009, Saunders Elsevier, p 115.
4. Bowman DD: Protozoans. In Bowman DD, editor: *Georgis' parasitology for veterinarians*, ed 9, St Louis, 2009, Saunders Elsevier, p 84.
5. Cecchi R, Wills SJ, Dean R et al: Demonstration of *Ollulanus tricuspis* in the stomach of domestic cats by biopsy, *J Comp Pathol* 134:374, 2006.
6. Cirak VY, Bauer C: Comparison of conventional coproscopical methods and commercial coproantigen ELISA kits for the

detection of *Giardia* and *Cryptosporidium* infections in dogs and cats, *Berl Munch Tierarztl Wochenschr* 117:410, 2004.
7. Coati N, Hellmann K, Mencke N et al: Recent investigation on the prevalence of gastrointestinal nematodes in cats from France and Germany, *Parasitol Res* 90(Suppl 3):S146, 2003.
8. Conboy G: Cestodes of dogs and cats in North America, *Vet Clin North Am Small Anim Pract* 39:1075, 2009.
9. Dahlgren SS, Gjerde B, Pettersen HY: First record of natural *Tritrichomonas foetus* infection of the feline uterus, *J Small Anim Pract* 48:654, 2007.
10. Dennis MM, Bennett N, Ehrhart EJ: Gastric adenocarcinoma and chronic gastritis in two related Persian cats, *Vet Pathol* 43:358, 2006.
11. Dimski DS: Helminth and noncoccidial protozoan parasites of the gastrointestinal tract. In Sherding RG, editor: *The cat: diseases and clinical management*, ed 2, Philadelphia, 1994, Saunders, p 585.
12. Dubey JP, Lappin MR: Toxoplasmosis and neosporosis. In Greene CE, editor: *Infectious diseases of the dog and cat*, ed 3, St Louis, 2006, Saunders Elsevier, p 754.
13. Dubey JP, Lindsay DS, Lappin MR: Toxoplasmosis and other intestinal coccidial infections in cats and dogs, *Vet Clin North Am Small Anim Pract* 39:1009, 2009.
14. Epe C: Intestinal nematodes: biology and control, *Vet Clin North Am Small Anim Pract* 39:1091, 2009.
15. Gookin JL: Tritrichomonas. In Bonagura JD, Twedt DC, editors: *Kirk's current veterinary therapy XIV*, St Louis, 2009, Saunders Elsevier, p 509.
16. Gookin JL, Birkenheuer AJ, Breitschwerdt EB et al: Single-tube nested PCR for detection of *Tritrichomonas foetus* in feline feces, *J Clin Microbiol* 40:4126, 2002.
17. Gookin JL, Copple CN, Papich MG et al: Efficacy of ronidazole for treatment of feline *Tritrichomonas foetus* infection, *J Vet Intern Med* 20:536, 2006.
18. Gookin JL, Foster DM, Poore MF et al: Use of a commercially available culture system for diagnosis of *Tritrichomonas foetus* infection in cats, *J Am Vet Med Assoc* 222:1376, 2003.
19. Gookin JL, Levy MG, Law JM et al: Experimental infection of cats with *Tritrichomonas foetus*, *Am J Vet Res* 62:1690, 2001.
20. Gookin JL, Nordone SK, Argenzio RA: Host responses to *Cryptosporidium* infection, *J Vet Intern Med* 16:12, 2002.
21. Gookin JL, Riviere JE, Gilger BC et al: Acute renal failure in four cats treated with paromomycin, *J Am Vet Med Assoc* 215:1821, 1999.
22. Gookin JL, Stauffer SH, Dybas D et al: Documentation of in vivo and in vitro aerobic resistance of feline *Tritrichomonas foetus* isolates to ronidazole, *J Vet Intern Med* 24:1003, 2010.
23. Gookin JL, Stebbins ME, Hunt E et al: Prevalence of and risk factors for feline *Tritrichomonas foetus* and *Giardia* infection, *J Clin Microbiol* 42:2707, 2004.
24. Gray SG, Hunter SA, Stone MR et al: Assessment of reproductive tract disease in cats at risk for *Tritrichomonas foetus* infection, *Am J Vet Res* 71:76, 2010.
25. Gunn-Moore DA, McCann TM, Reed N et al: Prevalence of *Tritrichomonas foetus* infection in cats with diarrhoea in the UK, *J Feline Med Surg* 9:214, 2007.
26. Hall EJ, German AJ: Diseases of the small intestine. In Ettinger SJ, Feldman EC, editors: *Textbook of veterinary internal medicine*, ed 7, St Louis, 2010, Saunders Elsevier, p 1526.
27. Hill SL, Cheney JM, Taton-Allen GF et al: Prevalence of enteric zoonotic organisms in cats, *J Am Vet Med Assoc* 216:687, 2000.
28. Janeczko S, Griffin B: *Giardia* infection in cats, *Compend Contin Educ Vet* 32:E1, 2010.
29. Keith CL, Radecki SV, Lappin MR: Evaluation of fenbendazole for treatment of *Giardia* infection in cats concurrently infected with *Cryptosporidium parvum*, *Am J Vet Res* 64:1027, 2003.
30. Lappin MR: Toxoplasmosis. In Bonagura JD, Twedt DC, editors: *Kirk's current veterinary therapy XIV*, St Louis, 2009, Saunders Elsevier, p 1254.
31. Lappin MR: Update on the diagnosis and management of *Toxoplasma gondii* infection in cats, *Top Companion Anim Med* 25:136, 2010.
32. Lindsay DS, Zajac AM: *Cryptosporidium* infections in cats and dogs, *Compend Contin Educ Vet* 26, 2004.
32a. Lloyd S, Smith J: Activity of toltrazuril and diclazuril against *Isospora* species in kittens and puppies, *Vet Rec* 148:509, 2001.
33. Marks SL, Hanson TE, Melli AC: Comparison of direct immunofluorescence, modified acid-fast staining, and enzyme immunoassay techniques for detection of *Cryptosporidium* spp in naturally exposed kittens, *J Am Vet Med Assoc* 225:1549, 2004.
34. Marks SL, Willard MD: Diarrhea in kittens. In August JR, editor: *Consultations in feline internal medicine*, ed 5, St Louis, 2006, Saunders Elsevier, p 133.
35. Mekaru SR, Marks SL, Felley AJ et al: Comparison of direct immunofluorescence, immunoassays, and fecal flotation for detection of *Cryptosporidium* spp. and *Giardia* spp. in naturally exposed cats in 4 Northern California animal shelters, *J Vet Intern Med* 21:959, 2007.
36. Palmer CS, Traub RJ, Robertson ID et al: Determining the zoonotic significance of *Giardia* and *Cryptosporidium* in Australian dogs and cats, *Vet Parasitol* 154:142, 2008.
37. Payne PA, Artzer M: The biology and control of *Giardia* spp and *Tritrichomonas foetus*, *Vet Clin North Am Small Anim Pract* 39:993, 2009.
38. Rosado TW, Specht A, Marks SL: Neurotoxicosis in 4 cats receiving ronidazole, *J Vet Intern Med* 21:328, 2007.
39. Scorza AV, Lappin MR: Gastrointestinal protozoal infections. In August JR, editor: *Consultations in feline internal medicine*, ed 6, St Louis, 2010, Saunders Elsevier, p 201.
40. Sherding RG, Johnson S: Diseases of the intestines. In Birchard S, Sherding RG, editors: *Saunders manual of small animal practice*, ed 3, St Louis, 2006, Saunders Elsevier, p 702.
41. Simpson KW: Diseases of the stomach. In Ettinger SJ, Feldman EC, editors: *Textbook of veterinary medicine*, ed 7, St Louis, 2010, Saunders Elsevier, p 1504.
42. Spain CV, Scarlett JM, Wade SE et al: Prevalence of enteric zoonotic agents in cats less than 1 year old in central New York State, *J Vet Intern Med* 15:33, 2001.
43. Speare R, Tinsley DJ: Survey of cats for *Strongyloides felis*, *Aust Vet J* 64:191, 1987.
44. Stein JE, Radecki SV, Lappin MR: Efficacy of *Giardia* vaccination in the treatment of giardiasis in cats, *J Am Vet Med Assoc* 222:1548, 2003.
45. Stockdale HD, Givens MD, Dykstra CC et al: *Tritrichomonas foetus* infections in surveyed pet cats, *Vet Parasitol* 160:13, 2009.
46. Tams TR: Hepatobiliary parasites. In Sherding RG, editor: *The cat: diseases and clinical management*, ed 2, Philadelphia, 1994, Saunders, p 607.
47. Tolbert MK, Gookin J: *Tritrichomonas foetus*: a new agent of feline diarrhea, *Compend Contin Educ Vet* 31:374, 2009.
48. Tzannes S, Batchelor DJ, Graham PA et al: Prevalence of *Cryptosporidium*, *Giardia* and *Isospora* species infections in pet cats with clinical signs of gastrointestinal disease, *J Feline Med Surg* 10:1, 2008.
49. Yaeger MJ, Gookin JL: Histologic features associated with *Tritrichomonas foetus*-induced colitis in domestic cats, *Vet Pathol* 42:797, 2005.

DISEASES OF THE EXOCRINE PANCREAS

Randolph M. Baral

PANCREATITIS

Pancreatitis refers to inflammation of the pancreas only, with no implication of the underlying cause or pathology. For example, acute necrotizing pancreatitis (ANP) with pancreatic auto-digestion, requiring predominantly supportive care by maintaining fluid and electrolyte balances and pain relief, must not be confused with chronic pancreatitis (CP) caused by lymphocytic infiltration, and commonly associated with lymphocytic inflammatory bowel disease (IBD), and often requires corticosteroids to manage. These two conditions (and others) can only be definitively distinguished histologically. In many cases, the clinical signs of cats with acute pancreatitis will resolve with supportive care before a precise diagnosis is reached and will thus remain undiagnosed.

There are no formal classifications for feline pancreatitis, but most authors[78,89,90] use the terms

- Acute pancreatitis
  - Acute necrotizing pancreatitis, characterized by severe peri-pancreatic fat necrosis
  - Acute suppurative pancreatitis, characterized by neutrophilic infiltration
- Chronic pancreatitis, characterized by lymphocytic infiltration

Prevalence

The exact prevalence of feline pancreatitis is unknown. Necropsy studies from the 1970s to 1990s reported prevalence of feline pancreatitis ranging from 0.45% to 2.4%.[21,67] A more recent study[17] found 67% of 115 cats had evidence of pancreatitis. However, this included pancreatic pathology in 45% of apparently healthy cats, which suggests that mild pathology is unlikely to cause clinical signs. These studies all show lymphocytic pancreatitis to be significantly more prevalent than acute pancreatitis. This may underestimate the true prevalence of acute pancreatitis, since it is understood that no permanent histopathologic changes are present after resolution of acute pancreatitis.[89] It is also possible that studies assessing pathology in necropsy cases do not reflect clinical practice.

Patient Signalment and Risk Factors

There are no specific age, breed, or sex predispositions. Although one study reported Siamese cats to be at increased risk of acute pancreatitis,[33] subsequent studies have recognized the majority of cases are domestic shorthair cats, suggesting no specific breed predispositions.[22,29,60,71] Most studies have indicated older cats (8 to 10 years of age) are more likely to be affected,[22,29,60,71] but these studies most likely underrepresent cats with less severe clinical disease for which definitive diagnosis may not be reached and which may be younger. No association has been made with a high-fat diet or obesity.

Etiology and Disease Associations

In most cases of both acute and chronic pancreatitis, no specific cause is found, and the disease is primarily considered to be idiopathic.[22,90] There are, however, some specific underlying causes that are sporadically recognized. These include infections with herpesvirus,[75] calicivirus,[37,49] feline infectious peritonitis (FIP),[44] liver fluke[58] and pancreatic fluke,[26,77] and toxoplasmosis.[20] However, a recent paper found no association between serum feline pancreatic lipase immunoreactivity (fPLI) concentrations and *Toxoplasma gondii* serology.[8] Pancreatitis has also been recognized subsequent to trauma[81] and organophosphate poisoning.[33]

The association of pancreatitis with inflammatory bowel disease and cholangitis is frequently mentioned (triaditis) but poorly described in the literature.[80] One study found 30% of IBD cases to have histologic evidence of pancreatic involvement,[6] and another found fPLI concentrations were elevated in 70% of cases with histologically confirmed IBD.[3] It is the author's experience that many cases of pancreatitis recognized with IBD have no specific clinical signs attributable to pancreatitis and should therefore be diagnosed and treated as intestinal disease.

Diabetes mellitus is a recognized co-morbidity of pancreatitis in cats. A recent study found fPLI concentrations were significantly higher in 29 diabetic cats compared with 23 non-diabetics. No association could be made between fPLI concentrations and the degree of diabetic control.[23]

One study found 5 of 13 cats (38%) histologically diagnosed with hepatic lipidosis were also histologically diagnosed with acute pancreatitis. It is not known if pancreatitis is a cause, consequence, or coincident disease of hepatic lipidosis. For example, anorexia associated with acute pancreatitis could predispose to fatty infiltration of the liver. However, the high rate of concurrent disease has important implications for ensuring cats with pancreatitis receive adequate caloric intake.[1]

Ongoing or recurrent pancreatitis may lead to pancreatic cysts[10] or exocrine pancreatic insufficiency,[74] which are both covered later in this chapter.

Pathophysiology

Although pancreatitis has been experimentally induced in cats,[18,41,56] the pathophysiology of spontaneous pancreatitis remains unknown. Acute pancreatitis is initiated by an increase in secretion of pancreatic enzymes that leads to inappropriate cellular activation of trypsin and subsequently other digestive zymogens. These activated digestive enzymes lead to local effects including inflammation, hemorrhage, acinar cell necrosis, and peripancreatic fat necrosis.[43,78,86] Chronic pancreatitis may result from any of several underlying processes: ongoing, low-grade acute pancreatitis episodes may instigate chronicity; chronic pancreatitis, with a predominance of lymphocytic inflammation has been induced experimentally within 5 weeks by narrowing the main pancreatic duct to approximately 25% of its normal diameter[18]; and the association with IBD[80] may suggest an immune-mediated cause.

Clinical Signs

The clinical signs of pancreatitis in cats are nonspecific. A review of eight prior series totaling 159 cases of acute pancreatitis in cats found anorexia (87% of cases) and lethargy (81%) to be the most common historical findings.[78] Vomiting was recognized in 46% of cases, diarrhea in 12%, and weight loss in 47%. Physical examination findings were similarly nonspecific with dehydration (54%) being the major finding; fever was recognized in only 25% of cases and abdominal pain in 19%. It is important to note that vomiting and abdominal pain, key features of pancreatitis in dogs, are not consistently recognized in cats. Similar, nonspecific findings indistinguishable from IBD are recognized in cats with chronic pancreatitis.[3,6]

Diagnosis

Because the presenting signs and physical examination findings are nonspecific, the diagnosis of pancreatitis can be challenging, requiring not only clinical suspicion but a combination of diagnostic modalities. For the most part, hematology and plasma biochemistry findings are unremarkable, although a combination of findings may increase clinical suspicion. For example, moderate elevations in liver enzymes, bilirubin, and glucose are present in approximately 50% of cases and hypocalcemia in approximately two of three of cases; hypocalcemia infers a poorer prognosis. Hypoalbuminemia is seen in approximately one of three of cases and has important implications for fluid therapy.[78] Amylase and lipase elevations are not reflective of pancreatitis in cats.[47] Feline trypsin-like immunoreactivity (fTLI) is the diagnostic test of choice of exocrine pancreatic insufficiency, but elevations in pancreatitis are not seen consistently enough to warrant use of this test for this purpose.[29,47,71]

The biggest recent advance in feline pancreatic diagnostics has been the characterization of feline pancreatic lipase,[69] leading to the development of a radioimmunoassay for the measurement of feline pancreatic lipase immunoreactivity (fPLI).[70] It must be remembered, however, that an increase in fPLI only tells the clinician that pancreatic pathology is present, but not the cause of pathology, which may be, for example, neutrophilic or lymphocytic pancreatitis or neoplasia, and it may or may not involve the intestines or liver. fPLI should therefore be used as a screening test, with elevated results not suggesting a diagnostic end point. Further, the high interassay variability of this test[70] would suggest that mild cases may be missed as shown in one study[24] and that the test may not be appropriate for serial monitoring. fPLI is currently available as "Spec fPL" from commercial laboratories and has a sensitivity of 79% and a specificity of 82% when 5.4 μg/L is used as the diagnostic cut off[25] compared with 3.5 μg/L, which is the listed reference range high point.

In an acutely unwell cat (less than 2 days) with only mild to moderate signs of disease, further diagnostics may not be warranted, and many cats will improve with supportive therapy of balancing fluid and electrolytes, pain relief, and antinausea/vomiting therapy.

Cats with chronic duration of signs and acutely unwell cats that do not improve with supportive therapy warrant further diagnostics. The underlying disease process cannot be assumed from an elevated fPLI; in one study of 63 cases, acute necrotizing pancreatitis could not be distinguished from chronic nonsuppurative pancreatitis by signalment, duration of signs, or clinical findings.[22]

The major utility of diagnostic imaging is to rule out other differential diagnoses, such as an intestinal foreign body, and perhaps confirm that the pancreas is affected. Radiography is non-specific for diagnosis of pancreatitis, but findings may include decreased abdominal detail (sometimes associated with ascites), soft tissue density in the right cranial quadrant of the abdomen, hepatomegaly, or gas-filled intestines[22,60,64] (see Figure 23-47).

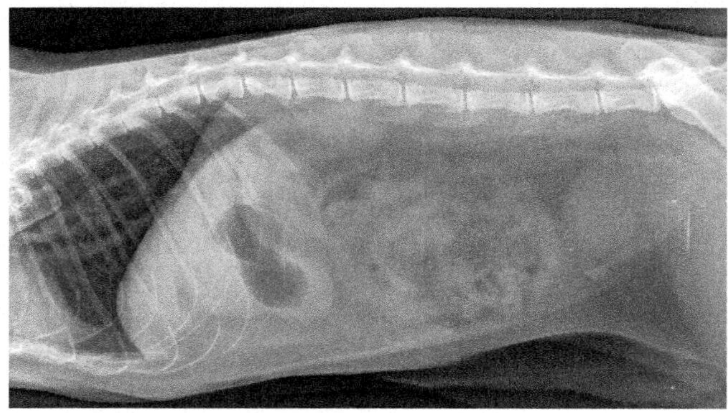

FIGURE 23-47 Abdominal radiograph (lateral view) of a cat with acute pancreatitis. The findings are essentially unremarkable; there is increased gas in the stomach and minor loss of serosal detail cranially. *(Courtesy Small Animal Specialist Hospital, North Ryde, Sydney, Australia.)*

Additionally, thoracic radiographs may show pleural effusion. One study found 5 of 20 cats with pancreatic necrosis had such a change[60]; the mechanisms resulting in pleural effusion are not precisely defined. Ultrasonography has high specificity (>85%) but low sensitivity (<35%) for recognizing pancreatitis in cats,[22,29,60,71] with findings dependent on operator skills, quality of equipment, and severity of lesions. Typical findings are hypoechogenicity of the pancreas, which may be enlarged or irregular; hyperechogenicity of the peripancreatic fat; the possible presence of abdominal effusion; and abnormal findings with other organs, such as liver or intestine, may add to the clinical picture[22,60,64,71] (Figure 23-48). One study indicated that contrast-enhanced Doppler ultrasonography can provide further diagnostic insights.[54] A recent study suggested that endosonography may be useful in cases where transabdominal ultrasonography is difficult, for example, because of obesity, hyperechoic mesentery, or excessive intestinal gas.[61]

For more than 20 years, computed tomography (CT) has been a commonly used modality to confirm pancreatitis in humans,[55] but this reliability has not been demonstrated in cats, where sensitivity may be as low as 20%.[24,29]

Definitive diagnosis of pancreatitis, including differentiation of the inflammatory process, can only be made by cytologic assessment of pancreatic tissue. In most cases, ultrasound-guided fine-needle aspiration (FNA) of the pancreas is technically difficult because of the small dimension of the feline pancreas; there appears to be no assessment of feline pancreatic FNA findings in the literature. Gross inspection of the pancreas and samples for histologic assessment can be obtained during laparotomy[22,64] (see Figures 23-49 and 23-50) or laparoscopy.[16,79] Because pancreatitis often occurs concurrently with pathology of other organs,[22] thorough evaluation of the abdomen by ultrasonography or gross inspection is recommended, as are multiple biopsies of, for example, intestines, liver, and mesenteric lymph nodes, where appropriate. Clinicians may be reluctant to biopsy the pancreas because of perceived risks of deleterious effects. Studies of pancreatic biopsy in healthy cats dispel the concern that the pancreas is unforgiving to mild manipulation and biopsy[16,42a] and the author's clinical experience is consistent with these findings.

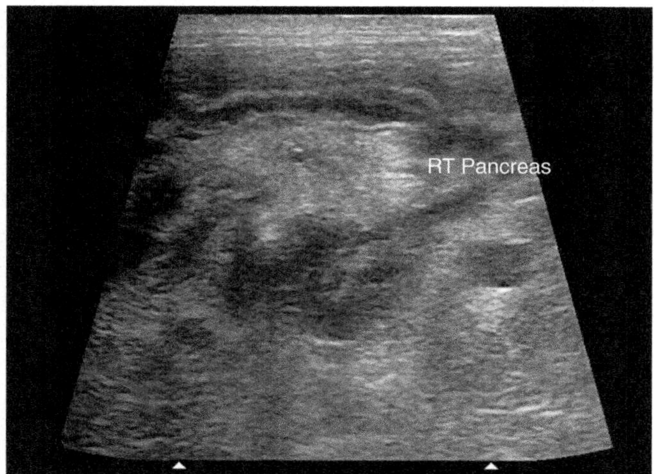

FIGURE 23-48 Ultrasonography of the right limb of the pancreas of a cat with acute pancreatitis. The pancreas is outlined by the duodenum (above) and the presence of abdominal effusion (to the sides and below); the hyperechoic areas (for example, to the right of the image, near the text) are most likely peripancreatic fat. *(Courtesy Small Animal Specialist Hospital, North Ryde, Sydney, Australia.)*

Therapy

Supportive care comprising correction of fluid/electrolyte imbalances, pain management, and nutritional support are the mainstay of therapy for cats with

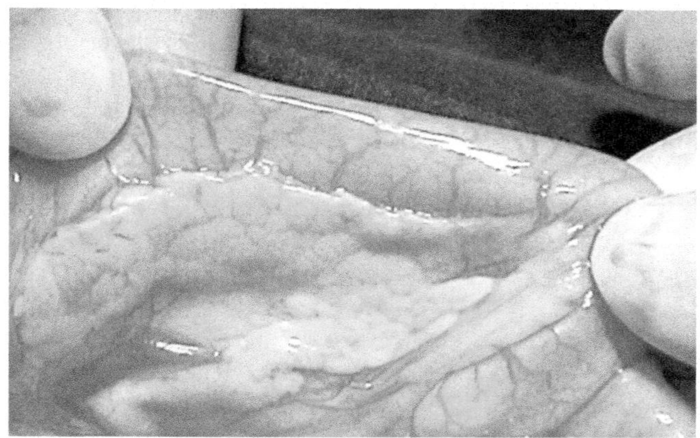

FIGURE 23-49 Gross appearance of pancreas at laparotomy; this was histologically diagnosed as chronic pancreatitis (i.e., lymphocytic infiltration was recognized).

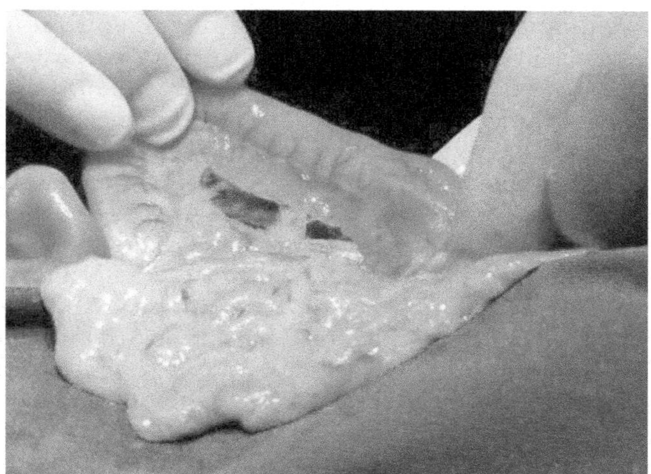

FIGURE 23-50 Gross appearance of pancreas at laparotomy; this pancreas was found to be histologically normal. It does look smaller than is typically seen; pancreatic atrophy can look similar to this, grossly.

pancreatitis.[78,86,89] Specific underlying causes, when diagnosed, should be managed, as should concurrent diseases. Follow-up evaluation is determined on a case-by-case basis; reduction or resolution of clinical signs is the main criterion for success of therapy. Serial fPLI values may be monitored when initial results are extremely high but are of limited value for mild increases because of assay variability.

Fluid Therapy

Dehydration, acid–base and electrolyte abnormalities should be corrected during the first 12 to 24 hours. Hypocalcemia, if present, should be treated with a calcium gluconate infusion of 50 to 150 mg/kg during 12 to 24 hours, with continued assessment of plasma calcium concentrations.

Plasma transfusions can be considered in cats with hypoalbuminemia.[78,86,90]

Pain Management

Although abdominal pain is not commonly described in cats with pancreatitis, it is likely to be present in most cases and may contribute to anorexia. Historical concern about exacerbation of pancreatitis with opioids is no longer accepted, and this class of drugs is considered appropriate. Meperidine (1 to 2 mg/kg SC or IM) every 1 to 2 hours, butorphanol (0.2 to 0.4 mg/kg SC) every 6 hours, or sustained-release buprenorphine (120 µg/kg SC) every 72 hours are alternatives.[67,78,86] The author uses one dose of methadone (0.1 to 0.2 mg/kg SC, IM, or IV) initially and places a fentanyl patch for longer-term pain management.

Nutritional Support

The traditional recommendation for management of pancreatitis across all species has been nil per os for several days. This recommendation is appropriate for cats with severe vomiting, but there is no evidence to support this approach in cats that are not vomiting and that are eating normally. Further, nutritional support is vital for those cats with concurrent hepatic lipidosis. If the cat is not eating voluntarily, nutritional support by tube feeding is often warranted.[67,78,86] A recent paper found nasogastric tube feeding of cats with pancreatitis was tolerated well and resulted in few clinically significant complications.[42] Other reported nutritional strategies for cats with pancreatitis incorporate partial parenteral nutrition (PPN; 8.5% amino acids, 20% lipids), or total parenteral nutrition (TPN; 6% amino acids, 20% lipids, 50% dextrose), or both instead of enteral feeding.[14,39,53] Cats do not seem to benefit from feeding of specially formulated low-fat diets; commercially available, veterinary liquefied diets appear to be well tolerated despite their high-fat contents.[86]

Drug Therapy

Other therapy may be appropriate in individual cases.

ANTIEMETICS

All cats with pancreatitis that are vomiting should be treated with antiemetics. Examples of drugs that can be used are 5-HT_3 antagonists, such as dolasetron (0.5 to 1.0 mg/kg IV or PO, once to twice daily); ondansetron (0.1 to 0.2 mg/kg IV every 6 to 12 hours); and maropitant, an NK_1-inhibitor (0.5 to 1.0 mg/kg SC once daily). These drugs are covered in detail earlier in this chapter under Therapeutics for Vomiting and Diarrhea. Dopaminergic antagonists, such as metoclopramide, are less effective antiemetic agents in cats than the other choices mentioned.[78,89]

ANTIBIOTICS

In most cases, pancreatitis begins as a sterile process, and antibiotic therapy is controversial. Pancreatic necrosis and inflammation may predispose to bacterial colonization of the pancreas as demonstrated in experimental models.[82,84] This has not been demonstrated in spontaneous disease, and no comparison of outcomes has been made of cats with pancreatitis treated with or without antibiotics. Cefotaxime (20 to 80 mg/kg IV, IM) has been used to prevent bacterial colonization in experimental models.[83] Other broad-spectrum cephalosporins or ampicillin may act similarly. Antibiotic considerations are possibly more important for acute pancreatitis than for treatment of chronic disease.

CORTICOSTEROIDS

Cats with demonstrated lymphocytic pancreatitis, with or without concurrent IBD or lymphocytic cholangitis, should be treated with corticosteroids (e.g., prednisolone, 1 to 2 mg/kg once to twice daily) with tapering to the lowest effective dose. There is no justification for use of corticosteroids in cats with acute necrotizing or acute suppurative pancreatitis, or cats for which the cause of pancreatitis has not been diagnosed histologically. Use of corticosteroids in cats with pancreatic disease creates a risk of iatrogenic diabetes mellitus.

Surgical Intervention

Surgical intervention is warranted to relieve any bile duct obstruction that may result or for the débridement of pancreatic abscesses or necrotic tissue; in many cases, cats will survive multiple years after such corrective surgery.[65]

PANCREATIC CYSTS, PSEUDOCYSTS, AND BLADDERS

Pancreatic cysts, pseudocysts, and bladders have been described sporadically in cats.* Pancreatic cysts are lined by a single layer of cuboidal epithelium and do not

*References 4, 9, 10, 15, 28, 34, 76, 88.

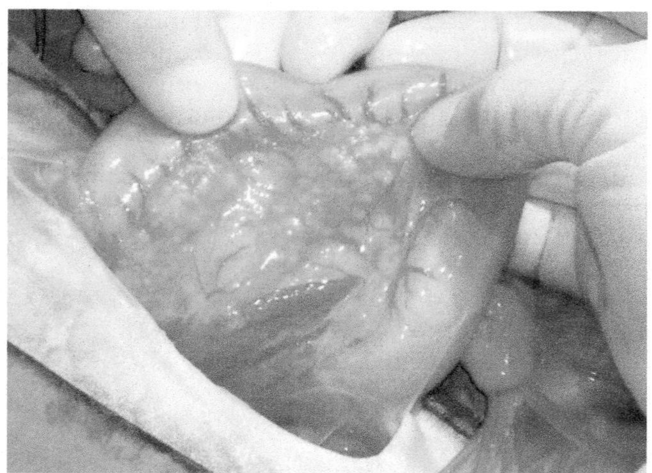

FIGURE 23-51 Gross appearance of pancreatic nodular hyperplasia at laparotomy; this was an incidental finding.

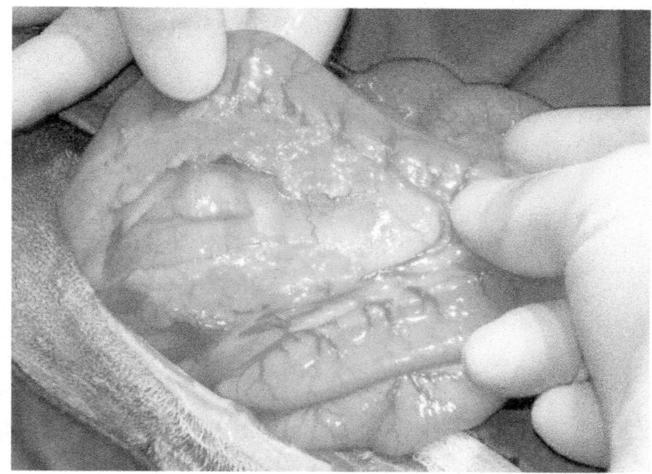

FIGURE 23-52 Gross appearance of pancreatic nodular hyperplasia at laparotomy; this was an incidental finding. Note the changes are more subtle than those in Figure 23-51.

communicate with the pancreatic duct; pseudocysts are enclosed by a wall of fibrous tissue, lacking the epithelial lining characteristic of true cysts and can form secondary to pancreatic inflammation; cystic dilations of the pancreatic duct are referred to as pancreatic bladder. True pancreatic cysts have been described in three cats[9,10,15]; a congenital pancreatic cyst with associated inflammation was described as an incidental finding in an adult cat[15]; multiple pancreatic cysts were described in a cat with concurrent polycystic disease in the kidney and liver[9]; and a another cat had multiple recurrent pancreatic cysts with concurrent mild pancreatic inflammation and atrophy associated a with rapid clinical course resulting in diabetes mellitus.[10]

Cysts, pseudocysts, and bladders may be identified ultrasonographically or by CT. They may be benign, but the associated pancreatic inflammation and other sequelae, such as diabetes mellitus, may need to be managed. Pancreatic bladders may result in biliary obstruction, and surgical correction may be required.

PANCREATIC NODULAR HYPERPLASIA

Pancreatic nodular hyperplasia is recognized quite frequently as an incidental finding in older cats or at necropsy.[45,67] Disseminated small nodules can be found throughout the exocrine portion of the pancreas (Figures 23-51 and 23-52). These lesions can be differentiated from pancreatic adenomas by the absence of a capsule in cases of nodular hyperplasia.[45,67] Nodular hyperplasia does not lead to functional changes and so does not cause any clinical signs unless the bile duct is obstructed.[38] Choledochenterostomy or cholenterostomy are feasible options in this circumstance[13] with survival much longer than reported when these procedures are performed in cats with neoplastic disease.

PANCREATIC NEOPLASIA

Neoplasia of the exocrine pancreas is rare in cats. Its frequency was assessed in the 1970s when one study estimated 12.6 cases per 100,000 patients per year at risk,[52] and another found pancreatic tumors in 5 of 800 feline necropsies.[45] A more recent study recognized, from 15,764 feline admissions over a 20-year study period, only two cats with pancreatic adenomas (0.013% of admissions) and eight with pancreatic adenocarcinomas (0.05% of admissions).[62]

Adenomas appear as small, solitary or multifocal nodules and are not typically associated with adjacent pancreatic inflammation. They do not cause clinical signs, unless large, when any clinical signs result from the physical size and are usually an incidental finding.[45,86]

Few generalities can be made about the presentation for pancreatic adenocarcinoma. The age range is large (4 to 20 years), there is no sex predisposition, and no clear breed predispositions are present.[62,86] Only cytology or histopathology can distinguish pancreatitis from pancreatic carcinoma in cats antemortem, yet it is important to differentiate the two conditions, because, in contrast to adenomas, pancreatic adenocarcinoma is associated with a grave prognosis.

The presence of lesions consistent with metastases on radiography or ultrasonography may suggest malignancy, but one study could not distinguish neoplasia from pancreatic nodular hyperplasia ultrasonographically based on the appearance of the pancreas alone[32] (Figures 23-53 and 23-54).

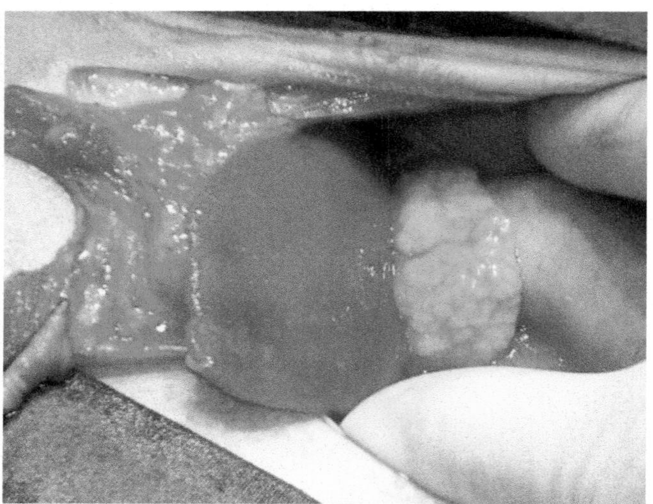

FIGURE 23-53 Gross appearance of pancreatic adenocarcinoma at laparotomy. Note that the appearance of the pancreas is very similar to that of pancreatic nodular hyperplasia in Figure 23-51. Additionally, ascites can be seen between the surgeon's thumb and the pancreas, and the mesentery is very inflamed.

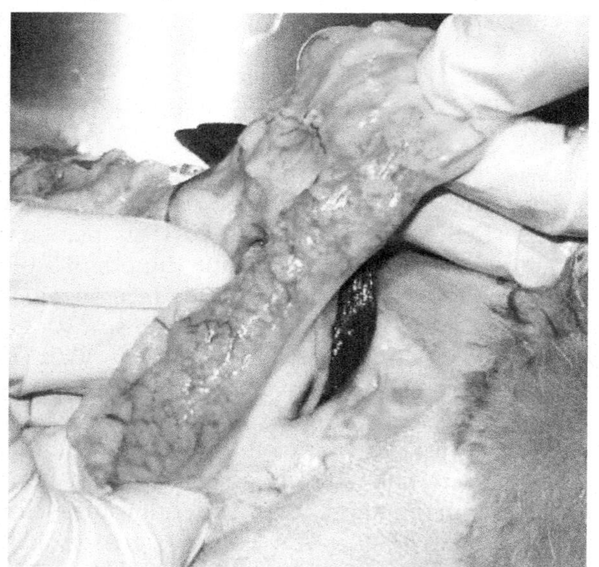

FIGURE 23-54 Gross appearance of pancreatic adenocarcinoma at necropsy. Note that the appearance of the pancreas is very similar to that of pancreatic nodular hyperplasia in Figure 23-51.

Pancreatic adenocarcinomas in cats can result in a paraneoplastic dermatologic condition consisting of nonpruritic, symmetric alopecia affecting the face, ventral body, and medial aspect of the limbs of cats. The skin is usually glistening but not fragile, and there can be crusty lesions on the footpads.* The pathogenesis of this dermatologic disease is unknown. In one case, surgical excision of the pancreatic carcinoma resulted in resolution of dermatologic disease, indicating that the process is reversible (although signs recurred as the tumor re-emerged).[73]

*References 5, 11, 30, 48, 50, 62, 73.

Diabetes mellitus is a recognized complication of pancreatic adenocarcinoma. The mechanism is unknown and may simply be secondary to compression or invasion of islet cells by the tumor. In some cats, diabetes is recognized ahead of pancreatic neoplasia.[31,40,62]

Obstructive jaundice has also been described with pancreatic adenocarcinoma.[13]

Most cases of pancreatic adenocarcinoma in cats have metastasized by the time of diagnosis, and most reported cases die or are euthanized within 7 days of diagnosis.[62] Surgical excision is a potential option if neoplasia is confined to one limb of the pancreas, but recurrence is possible even if there is no evidence of metastasis and excision seems complete at the time of surgery.[73]

EXOCRINE PANCREATIC INSUFFICIENCY

Exocrine pancreatic insufficiency (EPI) is a condition caused by insufficient synthesis and secretion of pancreatic digestive enzymes from the exocrine portion of the pancreas.[66] In humans it has been reported that 90% of pancreatic acinar cells must be lost before clinical signs of EPI are seen.[19]

Prevalence and Patient Signalment

EPI is considered rare in cats but is perhaps being recognized more frequently because of increased awareness. There are less than fifty cases described in the veterinary literature* with one of these papers describing only 16 cases from five institutions, with prevalence described as 0.01% to 0.1% of cats seen over a 15-year period.[74] In contrast to this, the Gastrointestinal Laboratory at Texas A&M University recognized 1342 samples with serum fTLI concentrations at or less than 8.0 μg/L, which is diagnostic for EPI, out of 84,523 submissions,[66] which equates to 1.6% *of cats with known or suspected gastrointestinal disease.*

All studies indicate a wide age range of cats can be affected, from kittens less than 6 months of age to cats more than 15 years old, with a median age of approximately 7 years. There is no apparent breed predisposition.[66,68,74] One paper recognized 10 of 16 (62.5%) cats to be male,[74] and another recognized 15 of 20 (75%) male cats,[68] suggesting a possible sex predisposition.

Etiology and Disease Associations

Chronic pancreatitis is believed to be the most common cause of EPI in cats,[66,85] although most reported cases have not had histologic confirmation of this. Pancreatic

*References 2, 12, 26, 35, 36, 46, 51, 57, 63, 68, 72, 74, 87.

acinar atrophy (PAA) is recognized as the most common cause of EPI in dogs, and has been definitively described in two feline cases[74] and mentioned as a cause for three other cases.[85] Other potential causes of EPI include disruption of pancreatic enzyme flow at the duodenal papilla following duodenal resection[72] and pancreatic fluke infection *(Eurytrema procyonis)*,[2,26] and amyloid deposition and neoplasia are other possible causes of pancreatic cell damage that have not definitively been described in cats.[66] Congenital pancreatic hypoplasia or aplasia has not definitively been reported in cats, but reports of EPI in cats as young as 3 months of age[63,74] suggest this possibility.

Since chronic pancreatitis is a common cause of EPI and chronic pancreatitis has a strong association with IBD, many cats may have concurrent lymphocytic pancreatitis and enteritis.[66,74,85] Therefore cats failing to respond to therapy for EPI may require further diagnostics and management of an underlying condition. Further, destruction of functional exocrine pancreatic tissue can also affect pancreatic endocrine tissue, resulting in concurrent diabetes mellitus.[35]

Clinical Signs

Several studies have indicated that all cats with EPI will have weight loss when diagnosed, unless a kitten, in which case ill-thrift is recognized.[68,74] Diarrhea is not necessarily present, being described in 50% to 75% of cats; the nature of feces can vary from voluminous, malodorous stools that can be discolored (yellow or pale), sometimes with steatorrhea, to normal feces in other cats. Increased frequency of defecation and the presence of mucus in the feces of some cats can lead to the diarrhea being characterized as large bowel. Only about 20% to 30% of cats are polyphagic, some described as having a ravenous appetite; conversely, some cats present with anorexia. Vomiting has also been described. Since cats with EPI often have concurrent disorders, such as IBD, the clinical signs recognized may reflect the concurrent disease and not necessarily EPI alone. Physical examination findings are similarly nonspecific, with thin/emaciated body condition being the most common finding. Hematologic findings are non-specific, but a mild nonregenerative, normocytic, normochromic anemia may be recognized as well as lymphopenia or neutrophilia. Plasma biochemistry results may show a mild to moderate increase in alanine aminotransferase (ALT) and a mild increase in alkaline phosphatase in some cats. Mild to moderate hyperglycemia may be seen, as may mild hypoglycemia or normoglycemia.[66,68,74] Hypocobalaminemia is recognized in nearly all cats with EPI.[66,68,74,85,87] This may be because of insufficient production of intrinsic factor, a cobalamin-binding protein only produced by the pancreas in cats and necessary for ileal absorption of cobalamin[27]; it may also be because of failure of pancreatic enzymes to liberate cobalamin from binding by R protein in the duodenum or small intestinal bacterial overgrowth (SIBO), not yet specifically described in cats.[74] Folate concentrations may be reduced (because of concurrent intestinal malabsorption),[68] normal,[68,74] or increased,[74] which may relate to reduced pancreatic bicarbonate secretion, secondary to severe hypocobalaminemia,[59] or associated with SIBO.[7]

None of these presenting complaints, physical examination findings, or routine testing results are specific to EPI. Therefore EPI requires a degree of clinical suspicion and/or thorough diagnostics to ensure the diagnosis is not missed.

Diagnosis

A low level of serum fTLI is diagnostic for EPI.[66,68,74] Samples can be sent to the Gastrointestinal Laboratory at Texas A&M University from anywhere worldwide (with instructions about sample handling requirements on their website: http://vetmed.tamu.edu/gilab/). The reference range for serum fTLI is 12 to 82 μg/L, with concentrations at or less than 8.0 μg/L diagnostic for EPI.

Since the clinical signs and routine laboratory findings are nonspecific for EPI, it is ideal to test serum for fTLI in any cat with weight loss or ill-thrift. The Texas A & M gastrointestinal panel also includes testing for levels of cobalamin, folate, and fPLI, ensuring concurrent hypocobalaminemia will not be missed and potentially providing indications of other gastrointestinal disease.

Conversely, although a low level of serum fTLI confirms a diagnosis of EPI, it is not necessarily a diagnostic end point, since EPI is so often recognized concurrently with other gastrointestinal disease. Failure to respond to therapy should prompt the clinician to consider and investigate further for concurrent processes.

Management

Most cats with EPI can be successfully managed with dietary supplementation of pancreatic enzymes. Commercial products (e.g., Viokase [Axcan Pharma, Birmingham, Ala.], Pancrezyme [Virbac, Fort Worth, Tex.], and Creon [Abbott Laboratories, Abbott Park, Ill.]) are available, and powder is considered more effective than tablets or capsules (some capsules can be opened and the contents sprinkled onto food, like powder). The required dose can vary quite substantially from cat to cat. It is appropriate to start with one teaspoon of powder with food twice daily, and adjustments can be made depending on the response; most cats accept the powder readily if it is mixed thoroughly through canned food, but other flavors (e.g., fish oil or brine from canned tuna) can be used to disguise the taste if necessary. Raw pancreas (e.g., from beef or pork) may also be used, with 30 to 60 g twice daily an appropriate starting dose.[66]

Since most cats with EPI are hypocobalaminemic, supplementation by subcutaneous injection is required (oral supplementation is not effective since cobalamin deficiency leads to cobalamin malabsorption). An appropriate dose for most cats is 250 μg, and it is usually given weekly for 6 weeks, then every second week for a further six doses; it is appropriate to continue dosing every month beyond that. Owners can be taught to inject their cats at home (as owners of diabetic animals are taught to do with insulin).[66] Because some cats may have SIBO, antibiotics such as metronidazole (15 to 25 mg/kg PO every 12 hours for 14 days) may be warranted. An elevation of folate may arouse suspicion of SIBO, but it is appropriate to try antibiotics in a cat failing to respond to enzyme and cobalamin supplementation.

Concurrent diseases, such as lymphocytic, chronic pancreatitis, or IBD may need to be managed with corticosteroids, or diabetes mellitus with insulin. No studies have assessed specific dietary requirements in cats with EPI.

Most cats respond to appropriate treatment, with a return to normal weight and normal feces. With ongoing therapy, cats can lead normal lives for a full life span.

References

1. Akol KG, Washabau RJ, Saunders HM et al: Acute pancreatitis in cats with hepatic lipidosis, *J Vet Intern Med* 7:205, 1993.
2. Anderson W, Georgi M, Car B: Pancreatic atrophy and fibrosis associated with *Eurytrema procyonis* in a domestic cat, *Vet Rec* 120:235, 1987.
3. Bailey S, Benigni L, Eastwood J et al: Comparisons between cats with normal and increased fPLI concentrations in cats diagnosed with inflammatory bowel disease, *J Small Anim Pract* 51:484, 2010.
4. Bailiff NL, Norris CR, Seguin B et al: Pancreatolithiasis and pancreatic pseudobladder associated with pancreatitis in a cat, *J Am Anim Hosp Assoc* 40:69, 2004.
5. Banner BF, Alroy J, Kipnis RM: Acinar cell carcinoma of the pancreas in a cat, *Vet Pathol* 16:543, 1979.
6. Baral RM: Laparotomy for gastro-intestinal biopsies, Science Week Conference Proceedings (Small Animal Medicine chapter), Gold Coast, Queensland, Australia, 2006, Australian College of Veterinary Scientists, p 70.
7. Batt RM, Rutgers HC, Sancak AA: Enteric bacteria: friend or foe? *J Small Anim Pract* 37:261, 1996.
8. Bayliss DB, Steiner JM, Sucholdolski JS et al: Serum feline pancreatic lipase immunoreactivity concentration and seroprevalences of antibodies against *Toxoplasma gondii* and *Bartonella* species in client-owned cats, *J Feline Med Surg* 11:663, 2009.
9. Bosje JT, van den Ingh TS, van der Linde-Sipman JS: Polycystic kidney and liver disease in cats, *Vet Q* 20:136, 1998.
10. Branter EM, Viviano KR: Multiple recurrent pancreatic cysts with associated pancreatic inflammation and atrophy in a cat, *J Feline Med Surg* 12:822, 2010.
11. Brooks DG, Campbell KL, Dennis JS et al: Pancreatic paraneoplastic alopecia in three cats, *J Am Anim Hosp Assoc* 30:557, 1994.
12. Browning T: Exocrine pancreatic insufficiency in a cat, *Aust Vet J* 76:104, 1998.
13. Buote NJ, Mitchell SL, Penninck D et al: Cholecystoenterostomy for treatment of extrahepatic biliary tract obstruction in cats: 22 cases (1994-2003), *J Am Vet Med Assoc* 228:1376, 2006.
14. Chan DL, Freeman LM, Labato MA et al: Retrospective evaluation of partial parenteral nutrition in dogs and cats, *J Vet Intern Med* 16:440, 2002.
15. Coleman MG, Robson MC, Harvey C: Pancreatic cyst in a cat, *N Z Vet J* 53:157, 2005.
16. Cosford KL, Shmon CL, Myers SL et al: Prospective evaluation of laparoscopic pancreatic biopsies in 11 healthy cats, *J Vet Intern Med* 24:104, 2010.
17. De Cock HEV, Forman MA, Farver TB et al: Prevalence and histopathologic characteristics of pancreatitis in cats, *Vet Pathol* 44:39, 2007.
18. De Giorgio R, Sternini C, Widdison AL et al: Differential effects of experimentally induced chronic pancreatitis on neuropeptide immunoreactivities in the feline pancreas, *Pancreas* 8:700, 1993.
19. DiMagno EP, Go VLW, Summerskill WHJ: Relations between pancreatic enzyme outputs and malabsorption in severe pancreatic insufficiency, *N Engl J Med* 288:813, 1973.
20. Dubey JP, Carpenter JL: Histologically confirmed clinical toxoplasmosis in cats: 100 cases (1952-1990), *J Am Vet Med Assoc* 203:1556, 1993.
21. Duffell SJ: Some aspects of pancreatic disease in the cat, *J Small Anim Pract* 16:365, 1975.
22. Ferreri JA, Hardam E, Kimmel SE et al: Clinical differentiation of acute necrotizing from chronic nonsuppurative pancreatitis in cats: 63 cases (1996-2001), *J Am Vet Med Assoc* 223:469, 2003.
23. Forcada Y, German AJ, Noble PJ et al: Determination of serum fPLI concentrations in cats with diabetes mellitus, *J Feline Med Surg* 10:480, 2008.
24. Forman MA, Marks SL, De Cock HE et al: Evaluation of serum feline pancreatic lipase immunoreactivity and helical computed tomography versus conventional testing for the diagnosis of feline pancreatitis, *J Vet Intern Med* 18:807, 2004.
25. Forman MA, Shiroma J, Armstrong PJ et al: Evaluation of feline pancreas-specific lipase (Spec fPLTM) for the diagnosis of feline pancreatitis [abstract], *J Vet Intern Med* 23:733, 2009.
26. Fox JN, Mosley JG, Vogler GA et al: Pancreatic function in domestic cats with pancreatic fluke infection, *J Am Vet Med Assoc* 178:58, 1981.
27. Fyfe JC: Feline intrinsic factor (IF) is pancreatic in origin and mediates ileal cobalamin (CBL) absorption [abstract], *J Vet Intern Med* 7:133, 1993.
28. Garvey MS, Zawie DA: Feline pancreatic disease, *Vet Clin North Am Small Anim Pract* 14:1231, 1984.
29. Gerhardt A, Steiner JM, Williams DA et al: Comparison of the sensitivity of different diagnostic tests for pancreatitis in cats, *J Vet Intern Med* 15:329, 2001.
30. Godfrey DR: A case of feline paraneoplastic alopecia with secondary *Malassezia*-associated dermatitis, *J Small Anim Pract* 39:394, 1998.
31. Goossens MMC, Nelson RW, Feldman EC et al: Response to insulin treatment and survival in 104 cats with diabetes mellitus (1985-1995), *J Vet Intern Med* 12:1, 1998.
32. Hecht S, Penninck DG, Keating JH: Imaging findings in pancreatic neoplasia and nodular hyperplasia in 19 cats, *Vet Radiol Ultrasound* 48:45, 2007.
33. Hill RC, Van Winkle TJ: Acute necrotizing pancreatitis and acute suppurative pancreatitis in the cat, *J Vet Intern Med* 7:25, 1993.
34. Hines B, Salisbury S, Jakovljevic S et al: Pancreatic pseudocyst associated with chronic-active necrotizing pancreatitis in a cat, *J Am Anim Hosp Assoc* 32:147, 1996.
35. Holzworth J, Coffin DL: Pancreatic insufficiency and diabetes mellitus in a cat, *Cornell Vet* 43:502, 1953.

36. Hoskins JD, Turk JR, Turk MA: Feline pancreatic insufficiency, *Vet Med Small Anim Clin* 77:1745, 1982.
37. Hurley KF, Pesavento PA, Pedersen NC et al: An outbreak of virulent systemic feline calicivirus disease, *J Am Vet Med Assoc* 224:241, 2004.
38. Kelly DF, Baggott DG, Gaskell CJ: Jaundice in the cat associated with inflammation of the biliary tract and pancreas, *J Small Anim Pract* 16:163, 1975.
39. Kerry H: Placement of jejunal feeding tubes for post-gastric feeding, *Clin Tech Small Anim Pract* 19:32, 2004.
40. Kipperman BS, Nelson RW, Griffey SM et al: Diabetes mellitus and exocrine pancreatic neoplasia in two cats with hyperadrenocorticism, *J Am Anim Hosp Assoc* 28:415, 1992.
41. Kitchell BE, Strombeck DR, Cullen J et al: Clinical and pathologic changes in experimentally induced acute pancreatitis in cats, *Am J Vet Res* 47:1170, 1986.
42. Klaus JA, Rudloff E, Kirby R: Nasogastric tube feeding in cats with suspected acute pancreatitis: 55 cases (2001-2006), *J Vet Emer Crit Car* 19:337, 2009.
42a. Lutz TA, Rand JS, Watt P, et al: Pancreatic biopsy in normal cats, *Aust Vet J* 17:223, 1994.
43. Mansfield CS, Jones BR: Review of feline pancreatitis part one: the normal feline pancreas, the pathophysiology, classification, prevalence and aetiologies of pancreatitis, *J Feline Med Surg* 3:117, 2001.
44. Montali RJ, Strandberg JD: Extraperitoneal lesions in feline infectious peritonitis, *Vet Pathol* 9:109, 1972.
45. Owens JM, Drazner FH, Gilbertson SR: Pancreatic disease in the cat, *J Am Anim Hosp Assoc* 11:83, 1975.
46. Packer RA, Cohn LA, Wohlstadter DR et al: D-Lactic acidosis secondary to exocrine pancreatic insufficiency in a cat, *J Vet Intern Med* 19:106, 2005.
47. Parent C, Washabau RJ, Williams DA et al: Serum trypsin-like immunoreactivity, amylase, lipase in the diagnosis of feline acute pancreatitis [abstract], *J Vet Intern Med* 9:194, 1995.
48. Pascal-Tenorio A, Olivry T, Gross TL et al: Paraneoplastic alopecia associated with internal malignancies in the cat, *Vet Derm* 8:47, 1997.
49. Pedersen NC, Elliott JB, Glasgow A et al: An isolated epizootic of hemorrhagic-like fever in cats caused by a novel and highly virulent strain of feline calicivirus, *Vet Microbiol* 73:281, 2000.
50. Perrins N, Gaudiano F, Bond R: Carriage of *Malassezia* spp. yeasts in cats with diabetes mellitus, hyperthyroidism and neoplasia, *Med Mycol* 45:541, 2007.
51. Perry LA, Williams DA, Pidgeon GL et al: Exocrine pancreatic insufficiency with associated coagulopathy in a cat, *J Am Anim Hosp Assoc* 27:109, 1991.
52. Priester WA: Data from eleven United States and Canadian colleges of veterinary medicine on pancreatic carcinoma in domestic animals, *Cancer Res* 34:1372, 1974.
53. Pyle SC, Marks SL, Kass PH: Evaluation of complications and prognostic factors associated with administration of total parenteral nutrition in cats: 75 cases (1994-2001), *J Am Vet Med Assoc* 225:242, 2004.
54. Rademacher N, Ohlerth S, Scharf G et al: Contrast-enhanced power and color doppler ultrasonography of the pancreas in healthy and diseased cats, *J Vet Intern Med* 22:1310, 2008.
55. Ranson J, Shamamian P: Diagnostic standards for acute pancreatitis, *World J Surg* 21:136, 1997.
56. Reber PU, Lewis MP, Patel AG et al: Ethanol-mediated neutrophil extravasation in feline pancreas, *Dig Dis Sci* 43:2610, 1998.
57. Root MV, Johnson KH, Allen WT et al: Diabetes mellitus associated with pancreatic endocrine insufficiency in a kitten, *J Small Anim Pract* 36:416, 1995.
58. Rothenbacher H, Lindquist WD: Liver cirrhosis and pancreatitis in a cat infected with *Amphimerus Pseudofelineus*, *J Am Vet Med Assoc* 143:1099, 1963.
59. Ruaux CG, Steiner JM, Williams DA: Early biochemical and clinical responses to cobalamin supplementation in cats with signs of gastrointestinal disease and severe hypocobalaminemia, *J Vet Intern Med* 19:155, 2005.
60. Saunders HM, VanWinkle TJ, Drobatz K et al: Ultrasonographic findings in cats with clinical, gross pathologic, and histologic evidence of acute pancreatic necrosis: 20 cases (1994-2001), *J Am Vet Med Assoc* 221:1724, 2002.
61. Schweighauser A, Gaschen F, Steiner J et al: Evaluation of endosonography as a new diagnostic tool for feline pancreatitis, *J Feline Med Surg* 11:492, 2009.
62. Seaman RL: Exocrine pancreatic neoplasia in the cat: a case series, *J Am Anim Hosp Assoc* 40:238, 2004.
63. Sheridan V: Pancreatic deficiency in the cat [letter], *Vet Rec* 96:229, 1975.
64. Simpson KW, Shiroma JT, Biller DS et al: Ante mortem diagnosis of pancreatitis in four cats, *J Small Anim Pract* 35:93, 1994.
65. Son TT, Thompson L, Serrano S et al: Retrospective study: surgical intervention in the management of severe acute pancreatitis in cats: 8 cases (2003-2007), *J Vet Emer Crit Car* 20:426, 2010.
66. Steiner JM: Exocrine pancreatic insufficiency. In August JR, editor: *Consultations in feline internal medicine*, ed 6, St Louis, 2010, Saunders Elsevier, p 225.
67. Steiner JM, Williams DA: Feline exocrine pancreatic disorders, *Vet Clin North Am Small Anim Pract* 29:551, 1999.
68. Steiner JM, Williams DA: Serum feline trypsin-like immunoreactivity in cats with exocrine pancreatic insufficiency, *J Vet Intern Med* 14:627, 2000.
69. Steiner JM, Wilson BG, Williams DA: Purification and partial characterization of feline classical pancreatic lipase, *Comp Biochem Physiol B Biochem Mol Biol* 134:151, 2003.
70. Steiner JM, Wilson BG, Williams DA: Development and analytical validation of a radioimmunoassay for the measurement of feline pancreatic lipase immunoreactivity in serum, *Can J Vet Res* 68:309, 2004.
71. Swift NC, Marks SL, MacLachlan NJ et al: Evaluation of serum feline trypsin-like immunoreactivity for the diagnosis of pancreatitis in cats, *J Am Vet Med Assoc* 217:37, 2000.
72. Tangner CH, Turrel JM, Hobson HP: Complications associated with proximal duodenal resection and cholecystoduodenostomy in two cats, *Vet Surg* 11:60, 1982.
73. Tasker S, Griffon DJ, Nuttall TJ et al: Resolution of paraneoplastic alopecia following surgical removal of a pancreatic carcinoma in a cat, *J Small Anim Pract* 40:16, 1999.
74. Thompson KA, Parnell NK, Hohenhaus AE et al: Feline exocrine pancreatic insufficiency: 16 cases (1992-2007), *J Feline Med Surg* 11:935, 2009.
75. Van Pelt CS, Crandell RA: Pancreatitis associated with a feline herpesvirus infection, *Compan Anim Pract* 1:7, 1987.
76. VanEnkevort BA, O'Brien RT, Young KM: Pancreatic pseudocysts in 4 dogs and 2 cats: ultrasonographic and clinicopathologic findings, *J Vet Intern Med* 13:309, 1999.
77. Vyhnal KK, Barr SC, Hornbuckle WE et al: *Eurytrema procyonis* and pancreatitis in a cat, *J Feline Med Surg* 10:384, 2008.
78. Washabau RJ: Acute necrotizing pancreatitis. In August JR, editor: *Consultations in feline internal medicine*, ed 5, St Louis, 2006, Saunders Elsevier, p 109.
79. Webb CB, Trott C: Laparoscopic diagnosis of pancreatic disease in dogs and cats, *J Vet Intern Med* 22:1263, 2008.
80. Weiss DJ, Gagne JM, Armstrong PJ: Relationship between inflammatory hepatic disease and inflammatory bowel disease, pancreatitis, and nephritis in cats, *J Am Vet Med Assoc* 209:1114, 1996.
81. Westermarck E, Saario E: Traumatic pancreatic injury in a cat: a case history, *Acta Vet Scand* 30:359, 1989.
82. Widdison AL, Alvarez C, Chang Y-B et al: Sources of pancreatic pathogens in acute pancreatitis in cats, *Pancreas* 9:536, 1994.

83. Widdison AL, Karanjia ND, Reber HA: Antimicrobial treatment of pancreatic infection in cats, *Br J Surg* 81:886, 1994.
84. Widdison AL, Karanjia ND, Reber HA: Routes of spread of pathogens into the pancreas in a feline model of acute pancreatitis, *Gut* 35:1306, 1994.
85. Williams DA: Feline exocrine pancreatic insufficiency. In Bonagura JD, editor: *Kirk's current veterinary therapy XII*, St Louis, 1995, Saunders, p 732.
86. Williams DA: Feline exocrine pancreatic disease. In Bonagura JD, Twedt DC, editors: *Kirk's current veterinary therapy XIV*, St Louis, 2009, Saunders Elsevier, p 538.
87. Williams DA, Reed SD, Perry L: Fecal proteolytic activity in clinically normal cats and in a cat with exocrine pancreatic insufficiency, *J Am Vet Med Assoc* 197:210, 1990.
88. Wolff A: An unusual unidentified abdominal mass in a cat, *Vet Med Small Anim Clin* 74:162, 1979.
89. Xenoulis PG, Steiner JM: Current concepts in feline pancreatitis, *Top Companion Anim Med* 23:185, 2008.
90. Zoran DL: Pancreatitis in cats: diagnosis and management of a challenging disease, *J Am Anim Hosp Assoc* 42:1, 2006.

DISEASES OF THE LIVER

Debra L. Zoran

The feline liver is a large, complex organ involved in a variety of essential metabolic, functional, and detoxification processes that can be affected, individually or collectively, by disease or dysfunction. Cats have a unique set of liver diseases that occur more commonly in this species compared with the typical diseases that occur in dogs, and these include hepatic lipidosis, feline cholangitis syndrome, and infectious hepatopathies (e.g., FIP, flukes, histoplasmosis, toxoplasmosis).[2,15,34,58,61] Nevertheless, these conditions often present with characteristic clinical, laboratory, and histopathologic changes that are necessary for proper diagnosis and management. The goal of this section is to review the interpretation of clinical and laboratory changes that occur in these feline liver diseases, provide an approach for separating the more common diseases by their clinical footprint, and then discuss therapy of each liver disease based on our current level of understanding of hepatoprotectants, antioxidants, and drugs used for specific therapeutic purposes.

CLINICAL SIGNS

The clinical signs of liver disease in cats are often vague and nonspecific; however, recognition of certain clinical and laboratory abnormalities and their association with liver disease can greatly aid the diagnostic process. The most common early clinical signs observed in cats with liver disease are anorexia, lethargy, and weight loss, which are signs present in many (if not most!) feline diseases.[2,15] Because these early indicators of disease do not point specifically toward liver disease, a delay in diagnosis will occur unless the clinician carefully considers all possibilities and performs other tests to further evaluate the situation. For example, feline hepatic lipidosis is the most common form of liver disease in cats in the United States, United Kingdom, Japan, and Western Europe, occurring with a prevalence of nearly 16% in one study.[2] However, the most common, and often only, clinical sign associated with onset of this condition is anorexia; the signs of serious hepatic disease (especially jaundice and vomiting) do not occur until later (days or weeks) in the course of the disease.[2,21] Recognition that anorexia in a cat, even for a few days, is a risk factor for development of hepatic lipidosis is essential, and this risk is increased in obese cats.[11,21] Further, the clinical signs of liver failure develop much more slowly; many cats with hepatic lipidosis present alert and responsive until much later in the course of the disease, thus delaying onset of appropriate therapy. A similar clinical situation exists for the second most common form of liver disease in cats, feline cholangitis syndrome.[15,28,58] This complex of diseases in the cat can be associated with signs ranging from anorexia and lethargy to vomiting and jaundice, and these signs can vary in severity and prevalence. The key point is that except for development of jaundice, there is no constellation of clinical signs that are classic clinical indicators of liver disease in cats.[15,28] As with many feline diseases, the subtle clinical signs of anorexia, lethargy, or inactivity are often the only signs of illness and should be further investigated.

ROUTINE LABORATORY TESTS

There are few changes that occur in the complete blood count that are specific indicators of primary liver disease in cats. The most common finding is the presence of poikilocytes, which are red blood cells with an irregular shape, speculated to be caused by changes in membrane lipids as a result of liver dysfunction.[14] Other abnormalities may occur, such as anemia of chronic disease or neutrophilia, but these findings are nonspecific and occur with variable frequency. Perhaps the most important reason for obtaining a hemogram is in icteric cats, because this test is essential to help rule out hemolysis as the cause of the hyperbilirubinemia.

The serum chemistry profile can be very helpful, but there are several critical points in interpretation of these values that are important to review. The hepatic transaminases (alanine aminotransferase [ALT] and aspartate aminotransferase [AST]) are leakage enzymes but do not discriminate among hepatobiliary disorders, nor do they provide an indicator of severity or disease origin. Thus although increases in ALT may be noted in cats with liver disease, they are also present in a variety of other systemic infectious, inflammatory, neoplastic, and endocrine diseases, including hyperthyroidism, feline heartworm disease, FIP, and neoplasia.* Alternatively, the cholestatic membrane–associated enzymes alkaline phosphatase (ALP) and gamma glutamyltransferase (GGT) are especially useful for recognizing disorders involving biliary or pancreatic ductal components. Unlike the dog, these enzymes will only increase modestly in cats, even in severe disease, and there is no glucocorticosteroid or drug induction of the enzymes to influence interpretation.[14,37] Thus increases in ALP in the adult cat represent a release of enzyme from the hepatobiliary tree and should be considered clinically important. Both ALP and GGT are produced in other tissues than the liver, with the highest GGT activity present in the kidney and pancreas; however, sources other than the liver do not contribute to the activity of these enzymes in health. Recent studies of the effects on these enzymes in cats with pancreatitis, cholangitis, extrahepatic bile duct obstruction (EHBDO), and hepatic lipidosis reveal some important characteristics in interpreting increases in these enzymes.[14] First, both ALP and GGT are increased in cats with pancreatitis, cholangitis, or EHBDO, because inflammation in the biliary tree also affects the pancreatic ducts (and vice versa, Figure 23-55), and if the fold increases in these enzymes are similar, the diagnosis is likely one of the three.[15] Conversely, in cats with hepatic lipidosis (without concurrent inflammatory disease of the biliary or pancreatic duct system), large increases in ALP are observed, but GGT will remain normal or only slightly increased. Thus if the increase in ALP is 5 to 10 times, while GGT is not increased or is only increased 1 to 2 times, then the likely diagnosis is hepatic lipidosis.[14-16]

Other than enzymes on the biochemistry panel, which are of limited value for assessing liver function, there are several key tests that can be used to help assess liver function cats with elevated liver enzymes. These five tests found on most routine biochemistry panels are helpful functional indicators: cholesterol, bilirubin, glucose, albumin, and urea nitrogen (BUN). However, none are immune to outside influences on their interpretation, including bilirubin and cholesterol, which are the most liver specific. In cats with severe liver disease or failure, bilirubin levels tend to be quite elevated, while BUN, albumin, cholesterol, and glucose concentrations tend to be significantly decreased, reflecting inability to metabolize urea (lack of arginine), inability to produce albumin or cholesterol, and abnormal metabolization of glucose. However, these changes represent severe loss of liver function and thus are not sensitive indicators of liver function because the changes occur quite late in the course of the disease. Nevertheless, in cats with elevated liver enzymes and clinical signs of liver disease, these values should be carefully assessed. Because GI disease

*References 4, 14, 31, 34, 45, 58.

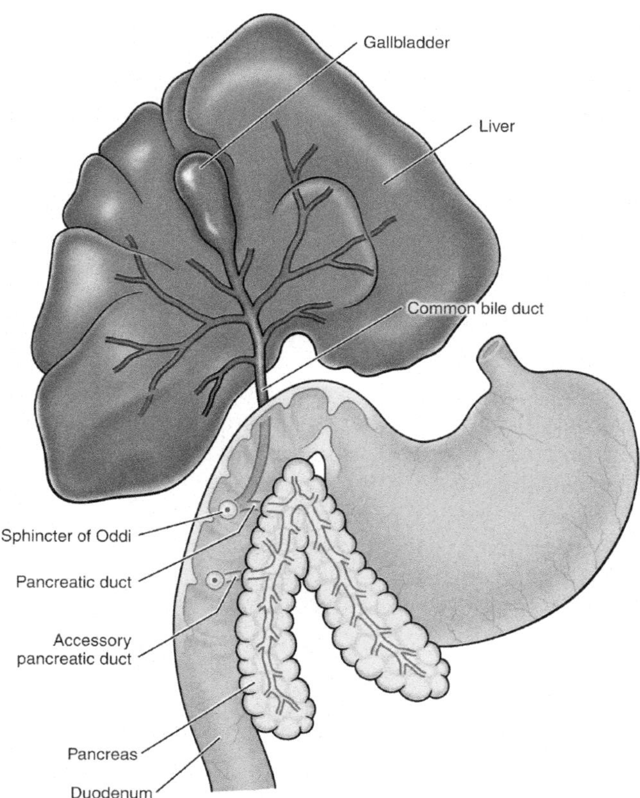

FIGURE 23-55 Diagram of feline anatomy of the biliary tree, pancreatic ducts, and connection to the duodenum. *(Available at http://media.gradvet.com/show10MinuteTopUp.php?type=&Entity=10MinuteTopUps&ID=31.)*

and protein-losing nephropathies can also cause loss of albumin and affect cholesterol, it is essential to evaluate the cat for these problems when interpreting these results. Finally, bilirubin metabolism is a critical function of the liver, but interpretation of hyperbilirubinemia requires a careful consideration of bilirubin disposition. Hyperbilirubinemia develps because of one of three possible causes: (1) excessive hemolysis of red blood cells (RBC) (also known as prehepatic icterus)—high bilirubin in the blood stream occurs because of an overload of the mononuclear/phagocyte system with heme pigments from RBC destruction, (2) hepatic parenchymal disease or insufficiency (also known as hepatic icterus)—resulting in lack of normal bilirubin metabolism in hepatocytes and regurgitation of the pigments into the blood stream when they are not taken up into cells and excreted in bile, and (3) disease of gall bladder, biliary tract, or pancreatic duct (also known as posthepatic icterus)—resulting in obstruction of the bile ducts or loss of bile into the abdomen (duct or gall bladder rupture and bile peritonitis).[41] The bottom line is that in any cat with hyperbilirubinemia, an assessment of the packed cell volume and RBC morphology should be completed to determine whether icterus is caused by hemolysis. Once hemolysis is ruled out, then assessment of primary parenchymal disease versus disease of the biliary tree is completed by evaluating the clinical presentation, laboratory values, and imaging of the biliary tree and abdomen for possible evidence of biliary or pancreatic disease.

A urinalysis is also an important part of the minimum database, and it is no different in a sick cat with suspected liver disease. In cats the presence of hyperbilirubinuria is abnormal at any urine concentration, because they do not conjugate bilirubin in their renal tubules.[14] However, like bilirubinemia, presence of bilirubin in the urine can occur because of any of the three possible causes of hyperbilirubinemia: prehepatic, hepatic, and posthepatic; thus further evaluation is necessary once bilirubin is detected. Ammonium biurate crystalluria suggests the presence of hyperammonemia, which in the cat is either because of a congenital portosystemic shunt (less common in cats than in dogs) or because of severe, end-stage liver disease resulting in portal hypertension, which is typically caused by cirrhosis or advanced polycystic liver disease.[6,41]

LIVER FUNCTION TESTS

The most common feline liver diseases are hepatic lipidosis and feline cholangitis syndrome, which are two diseases that often result in development of clinical or biochemical icterus. Thus because hyperbilirubinemia is a more sensitive indicator of liver function than bile acids or other liver function tests, the need for further testing is moot. However, there will be circumstances when further assessment of liver function is indicated, and for this, serum bile acids, blood ammonia levels, and urine bile acids may be needed. There are several situations where liver function testing may be indicated, but the most common indications for additional testing would be a cat with persistently elevated liver enzymes of unknown origin, a cat that develops urethral obstruction because of urate stones (suggestive of portosystemic shunting) or a cat with possible polycystic liver disease.[5] One of the oldest tests of liver function, because of its association with development of hepatoencephalopathy, is measurement of blood ammonia levels.[38] However, although this test is the only practical way to diagnose hepatoencephalopathy in dogs, the test has a number of limitations, including differences in ammonia levels between arterial and venous (lower) samples and significant sample handling issues (ammonia is labile and results are affected by improper sample handling or lack of immediate measurement) that make its use difficult in practice.[43] In cats hyperammonemia is even less common than in dogs likely because of their high-functioning urea cycle pathways[14]; the assays have not been validated for feline blood in most laboratories, and as such, the test is not recommended as the sole indicator of hepatic failure. In nonicteric cats with severe liver disease or in young cats suspected of having a portosystemic shunt, serum bile acids are the more reliable indicator of hepatic insufficiency.[18]

The measurement of serum bile acid concentrations, preprandially and postprandially, is the most reliable, readily available, and sensitive test of hepatic function in nonicteric cats.[5,14] That being said, although increases in bile acids are accurate indicators of hepatic insufficiency, the levels cannot be used to assess severity of disease or the type of dysfunction. Further, bile acid assays are most effective when paired samples (preprandial- and postprandial) are compared, because single, fasting, or random bile acid samples can result in a false-negative (normal) result. However, cats will often not eat in the hospital or when they are sick, and this prevents collection of a postprandial sample. However, this does not invalidate the results, because if the result of the single bile acid sample is abnormal, it does reliably indicate liver dysfunction.

An alternative to using serum for testing bile acids in cats is urine bile acid analysis. Healthy cats excrete a small percentage of conjugated bile acids in the urine[14]; however, in cats with liver disorders that cause increased serum bile acids (and especially cholestatic liver diseases) a significant increase in urine bile acid excretion occurs. When urine bile acids (UBA) were collected 4 to 8 hours after a meal and measured (normalizing the value with urine creatinine: UBA/UCr) and compared with serum bile acids in a study of 54 cats with hepatic disease, 17 cats with nonhepatic disease, and 8 normal cats, the results were highly correlated.[47] The utility of the urine bile acid test is that it does not require a paired sample (postprandial test), and it is not as affected as the serum test is by hemolysis or lipemia of the blood sample. Normal cats will have an UBA/UCr of less than 4.4 μmol/mg, while values greater than 4.4 are considered evidence of significant hepatic dysfunction.[47]

It is well known that the liver plays a central role in coagulation homeostasis and is the single site of synthesis of many coagulation proteins, anticoagulant proteins, and fibrinolytic factors. Vitamin K is one of the most common factors found to be inactive or deficient in cats with liver dysfunction, and it is essential for normal functioning of factors II, VII, IX, and X; protein C and S; and thrombin. Insufficient or inactive vitamin K can occur for a variety of reasons, including dietary restriction (e.g., anorexia or diet deficiency), disruption of the enteric microflora that synthesize vitamin K (e.g., chronic antibiotic therapy), diseases causing fat malabsorption (e.g., IBD, exocrine pancreatic insufficiency), ingestion of vitamin K antagonists, or liver dysfunction.[20] For example, in cats with hepatic lipidosis, approximately 25% will have an increased prothrombin time (PT), 35% will have an increased partial thromboplastin time (PTT), but 60% of cats will have increased PIVKA (proteins induced by vitamin K antagonists or absence).[20] Nevertheless, although PIVKA is a very sensitive test for abnormalities of vitamin K function, most cats with liver disease that have a normal PT/PTT, but abnormal PIVKA do not represent clinical evidence of bleeding. In any case, abnormalities in the clotting cascade related to vitamin K deficiency in cats with liver disease are common, whether or not they show evidence of active bleeding. And because the balance of the coagulation system in a cat with liver disease can be disrupted by a procedure that initiates small amounts of bleeding (e.g., a biopsy), all cats with liver disease should be given vitamin K as a precautionary measure before and after invasive procedures, even if the clotting times (PT and PTT) are normal. This may be especially important in cats with hepatic lipidosis, because their vitamin K clotting status is likely to be even more affected by the concurrent anorexia and disruption of enteric microflora.[14] The dose of vitamin K_1 (phytonadione, aquaMEPHYTON [Merck, West Point, Pa.]) used prophylactically is 2.5 mg SC, IM, or PO q12h for 3 to 5 days, then weekly until recovered.

CHOLESTASIS AND ICTERUS

See Box 23-4 for a summary of the causes of icterus. Cholestasis is the reduction of bile flow, which can occur at any point along the biliary tree; bile production occurs in hepatocytes, and flow is connected to the distal concentrating components (gallbladder and common bile duct) by the bile ductules. Thus cholestasis can occur inside the liver's biliary tree (intrahepatic cholestasis) or outside the liver in the gallbladder and common bile duct (extrahepatic cholestasis). Intrahepatic cholestasis most often occurs in diseases involving hepatocellular damage, leakage, or swelling, such as infections (e.g., bacterial cholangiohepatitis, toxoplasmosis, FIP, or other diseases causing inflammation), infiltrative diseases (e.g., lymphoma), metabolic diseases (e.g., hepatic lipidosis), or diseases causing disruption of architecture (e.g., cirrhosis or severe polycystic disease).[41] Intrahepatic cholestasis occurs in zone 1 of the liver lobules (periportal zone); at the level of hepatocytes, canaliculi or bile ductules; and is damaging to cells because of the emulsifying properties of lipid on membrane lipids. However, because the liver has a large reserve capacity, clinical icterus (e.g., jaundice) only occurs in the most severe cases when the liver is affected diffusely. Thus severe or persistent intrahepatic cholestasis can serve to perpetuate the inflammation and cell damage if it is not corrected.

Extrahepatic cholestasis or extrahepatic bile duct obstruction (EHBDO) is less common than intrahepatic cholestasis and is most commonly associated with obstruction of the common bile duct. Since gallstones are uncommon in cats, the most common causes are neoplasia (primarily of the pancreas, but cholangiocarcinomas can occur) or chronic pancreatitis, which can occur concurrently with cholangitis in cats, resulting in both intrahepatic and extrahepatic cholestasis in some cats.[23,41] The bile ducts are affected in cats with chronic pancreatitis, because the feline biliary system and pancreatic duct system merge at the level of the pancreas to form a single duct that empties into the duodenum. Thus in cats with either pancreatitis or biliary disease, recent evidence has shown that the inflammation affects both organs.[54,59] Further, in chronic pancreatitis, either persistent inflammation or development of fibrosis can result in dilation or obstruction of the common bile duct.[33] In cats with chronic EHBDO, the common bile duct will become widely dilated and tortuous, a finding easily seen on abdominal ultrasonography but a problem not easily managed (Figures 23-56 and 23-57). Interestingly, the gallbladder is often not enlarged, and may in fact be small in cats with this condition, because the remaining fluid in the gallbladder is white bile (highly concentrated mucinous bile from which the pigment has been resorbed).[41] In addition, variable filling of the gall bladder is a normal phenomenon; thus gallbladder size is not an indicator of EHBDO.

BOX 23-4

Summary of the Causes of Icterus

Icterus is the result of cholestasis, and the underlying cause can be either hemolysis or hepatobiliary disease, for which further clinical examination will be needed to determine if RBC destruction or liver disease is occurring. In most hepatobiliary diseases of cats, cholestasis is occurring, but there may be no clinically apparent icterus because the degree of hyperbilirubinemia must be at least 2 to 3 times greater than the normal values to exceed the capacity of the liver to process the excess bilirubin. In cats with hyperbilirubinemia not caused by hemolysis, whether it is clinical or subclinical, there is no need for further evaluation of liver function (e.g., bile acid assays), because bilirubin is a more sensitive indicator of liver function than bile acids. The degree of hyperbilirubinemia does not suggest differentiation of intrahepatic versus extrahepatic cholestasis; however, the presence of acholic feces (white feces) is diagnostic for extrahepatic bile duct obstruction (EHBDO), because lack of stercobilinogen (the brown/black pigment in feces) is only found in cats with complete obstruction of the bile duct. Finally, the presence of intrahepatic cholestasis and clinical icterus in a cat indicates a diffuse hepatobiliary disease, such as cholangitis or hepatic lipidosis, as focal liver disease, even if severe, will not cause clinical hyperbilirubinemia because of the tremendous reserve capacity of the liver for bilirubin uptake.

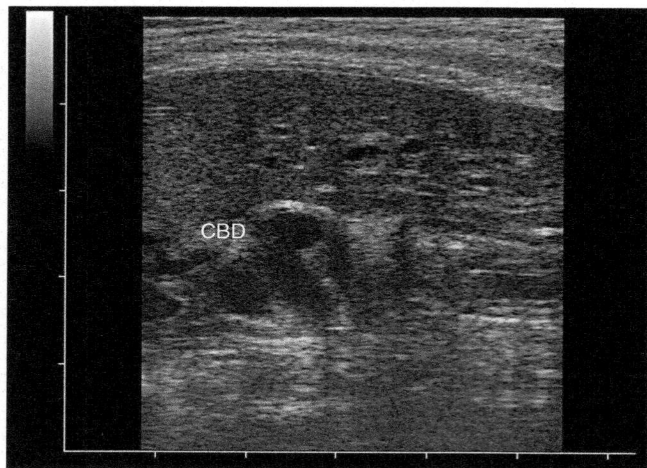

FIGURE 23-56 Ultrasonographic appearance of distended tortuous common bile duct (labeled CBD) in a cat with infectious cholangitis. *(Courtesy Dr. Randolph Baral.)*

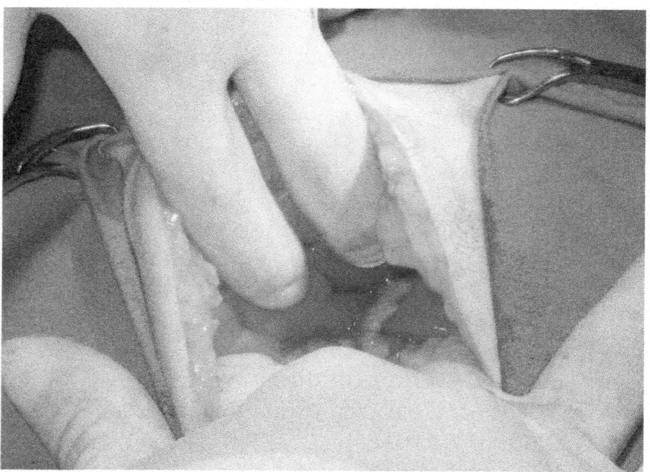

FIGURE 23-57 Appearance of distended bile duct at laparotomy of cat with infectious cholangitis (same cat as in Figure 23-56). *(Courtesy Dr. Randolph Baral.)*

PORTAL HYPERTENSION AND HEPATIC ENCEPHALOPATHY, ASCITES, AND ACQUIRED PORTOSYSTEMIC SHUNTING

Portal hypertension is an abnormally high venous pressure in the portal system and is typically caused by increased resistance to portal blood flow. There are potentially three regional causes of portal hypertension: prehepatic (disease in the portal vein itself), hepatic (intrahepatic diseases causing compression or decreased flow), and posthepatic (diseases of the caudal vena cava, right heart or pulmonary vasculature). The most common cause of portal hypertension in the cat is cirrhosis or portal venous thrombosis, because portal vein hypoplasia (formerly known as microvascular dysplasia) is known to occur only in the dog, and the other causes of portal hypertension (Budd-Chiari syndrome, heartworm caval syndrome, pulmonary hypertension) are rare and more likely to occur in the dog.[41,44] In any case, the clinically recognizable effects of portal hypertension are development of ascites (unusual in the cat), acquired portosystemic shunting (reported in cats), and development of hepatic encephalopathy (less common in cats than in dogs, because of their profound ability to handle protein wastes).[5,36,41] Most cats and dogs that develop hepatic encephalopathy (HE) secondarily to portal hypertension do so because of reduced liver function (because of portosystemic vascular shunting [PSS] or cirrhosis and the acquired shunting that develops). Cats can develop another form of chronic HE because of hepatic lipidosis, but this is believed to be because of the combination of liver failure and prolonged fasting, resulting in arginine deficiency and impaired ammonia detoxification.[2]

Portosystemic vascular anomalies, also called portosystemic shunts or portovenous shunts (PSS), although less common than in dogs, also occur in cats. These vascular anomalies can be either congenital or acquired, single or multiple in number, and occur as extrahepatic vascular shunts or within the liver itself (intrahepatic shunts).[5] The shunting of blood around the liver is the cause of hepatic atrophy and reduced hepatic function that results in an accumulation of toxins, particularly ammonia that leads to the development of hepatoencephalopathy. The two most common veins that serve as the connection point for the shunting portal venous blood are the caudal vena cava and the azygous.[5] In cats a single, extrahepatic, portocaval shunt is the most commonly reported form, and occurs in 75% of cats with PSS.[5] As in dogs, specific breeds of cats may have PSS more commonly, and these include domestic shorthair cats, Burmese, Siamese, Persian, and Himalayan breeds.[5] In contrast to dogs, males may be more predisposed to PSS than females, but the clinical signs relate to the three body systems most affected: the central nervous system, GI tract, and urinary tract. The most common presenting complaints in cats are weight loss or poor/stunted growth, and dull, bizarre or lethargic behavior, especially after eating. Signs of GI disease common in dogs, such as vomiting, diarrhea, or inappetence, are less common in cats, but in one report, 75% of cats with PSS drooled.[5] Finally, cats with PSS often present with signs of lower urinary tract disease (e.g., hematuria, stranguria, or even obstruction) because of the development of urate uroliths (which are radiolucent, thus difficult to detect).[5]

Because the most common signs of HE are apathy, listlessness, and decreased mental alertness, they are often not recognized specifically as indicative of brain dysfunction but as part of the constellation of signs of the liver disease. However, with progression of the disease, other signs will develop, including ataxia, salivation, stupor, or coma. The best and only practical diagnostic test for HE is plasma measurement of ammonia levels.[43] However, as previously noted, the test has many technical issues that make its clinical utility in the practice setting difficult at best, and there are few laboratories that have validated ammonia measurement in the cat.

MISCELLANEOUS DISEASES: HEPATOBILIARY NEOPLASIA AND AMYLOIDOSIS

Cancer of the liver can occur as a primary disease (Table 23-22) or as a result of metastasis of neoplastic disease occurring elsewhere and, most typically, the abdominal cavity. The most common neoplastic infiltration of the liver that is not a primary liver tumor is lymphoma (Figures 23-58 and 23-59), followed by visceral mastocytosis.[4] As with many other types of cancer, hepatobiliary neoplasia is most common in middle-aged to older cats, and it is relatively rare, with a reported incidence of 1.5% to 2.3%.[4] Benign tumors, such as biliary cystadenoma (Figure 23-60), carry a good prognosis if they are amenable to surgical resection. The incidence of metastatic neoplasia (including lymphoma and mast cell tumors) has not been reported. The clinical presentation is typically nonspecific (the most common signs are vomiting, lethargy, and anorexia), and there are no laboratory changes that are suggestive of hepatic neoplasia. Thus the diagnosis must be made by identification of

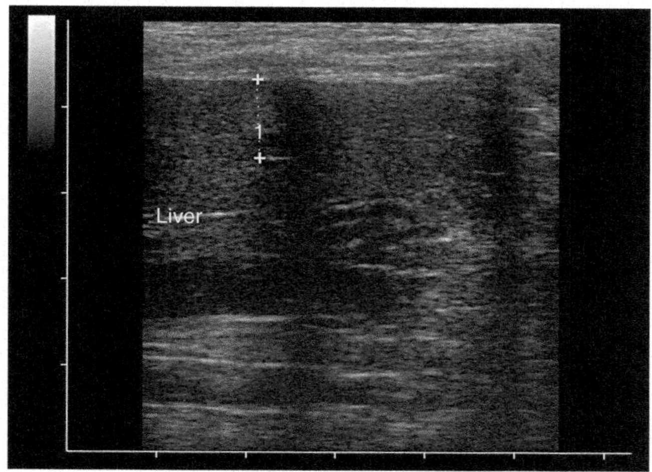

FIGURE 23-58 Ultrasonographic image of nodular lesion associated with hepatic small cell lymphoma. The nodule appears as a target lesion, being hypoechoic peripherally, yet hyperechoic centrally. Hypoechogenicity typically occurs with inflammatory cell infiltration, and dense hyperechogenicity as seen here is often associated with fibrosis. *(Courtesy Dr. Randolph Baral.)*

TABLE 23-22 **Hepatobiliary Neoplasia**

Tumor Type	Incidence/Species	Comments
Hepatocyte Tumors:		
Hepatocellular adenoma Hepatocellular carcinoma	Cats > dogs Most common primary tumor in dogs	Diagnosis by biopsy (FNA cannot differentiate normal from adenoma) Surgical removal is curative
Tumors of Bile Duct Epithelium:		
Adenoma (biliary cystadenoma [see Figure 23-60]) Bile duct carcinoma (cholangiocarcinoma)	Adenoma most common bile duct tumor in cats and frequent cause of cholestasis (rare in dogs) Carcinoma more common in dogs	Carcinomas (both species) are highly metastatic (lymph nodes and lung) and 80% have metastasized at the time of diagnosis in cats
Neuroendocrine Tumors:		
Carcinoma or carcinoid	Unusual in cats but carcinoid tumors reported occasionally	Can be intrahepatic or extrahepatic; if solitary can be excised, but no therapy if diffuse (more common in dogs)
Stromal Cell Tumors:		
Sarcomas (hemangiosarcoma, leiomyosarcoma, osteosarcoma, fibrosarcoma)	All are rare, but reported occasionally in cats (<13% of all hepatic tumors in dogs)	All behave aggressively and likely represent metastatic disease
Other Common Tumors:		
Lymphosarcoma Histiocytic sarcoma Mastocytosis	Most common round cell tumor in liver of cats (can be multicentric, alimentary, or hepatosplenic), followed by mast cell tumor (typically metastasis from spleen) Histiocytic tumors are more common in dogs	Both low-grade lymphocytic (small cell) and high-grade (large cell, blastic) lymphoma occur; the prognosis varies with the tumor type Prognosis with splenectomy and lomustine therapy is very good

FNA, Fine-needle aspiration.
Data from Balkman C: Hepatobiliary neoplasia in dogs and cats, *Vet Clin North Am Small Anim Pract* 39:617, 2009.

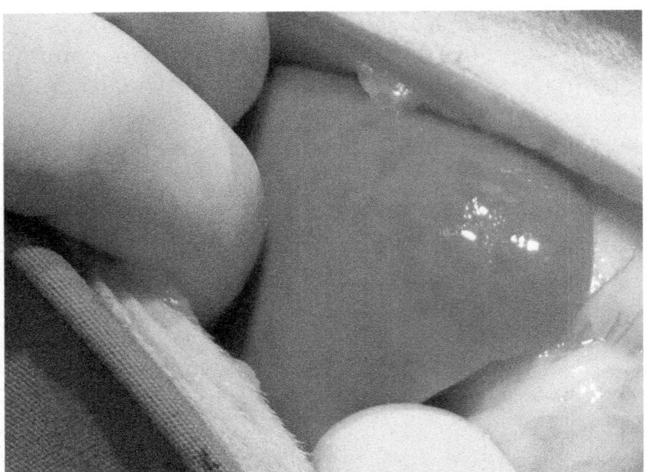

FIGURE 23-59 Gross appearance of liver from a cat diagnosed with hepatic small cell lymphoma. Note the mottled patchiness. *(Courtesy Dr. Randolph Baral.)*

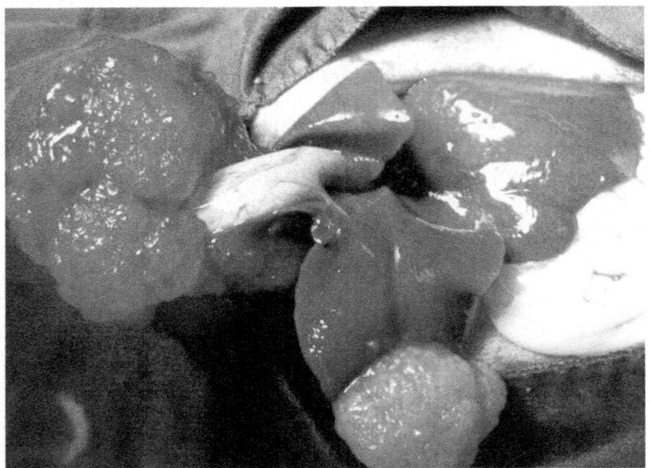

FIGURE 23-60 Gross appearance of a biliary cystadenoma (bile duct adenoma). These tumors account for more than 50% of all feline hepatobiliary tumors and may reach a large size by the time of diagnosis. *(Courtesy Dr. Susan Little.)*

structural abnormalities by hepatobiliary imaging and subsequent examination of the tissue either by FNA or biopsy techniques.

Historically, amyloidosis has been recognized as primarily a renal disease, especially in Abyssinian cats. More recently, cases of hepatic amyloidosis without renal involvement have been diagnosed in Siamese and related breeds, as well as in nonpedigreed cats.[4a,10a,30a] The majority of cases have been described in Australia, the United Kingdom, and Europe. Amyloid A is deposited in the liver, probably in response to chronic inflammation in another organ. In the Siamese breed, a genetic component may contribute.[48a] The amyloid A protein occurring in the Siamese breed differs from that known in the Abyssinian breed.[48a]

The most common clinical signs are related to spontaneous rupture of the enlarged and friable liver. Affected cats may present with lethargy, anorexia, pale mucous membranes, and a heart murmur secondary to anemia. Clinical signs of liver disease are usually absent. Hepatomegaly and hypotension may also be found. Results of routine laboratory testing (mild to marked increases in ALT and globulins while ALP and GGT are typically normal) and ultrasonographic examination (hepatomegaly, generalized increase in hepatic parenchymal echogenicity)[4a] of the liver may be supportive, but definitive diagnosis relies on histopathologic examination of a liver biopsy. FNA of the liver is not helpful because amyloid is rarely detected with this method. Hemostasis should be evaluated carefully before any biopsy procedure is planned. The most important differential diagnoses are FIP, hepatic lipidosis, and hepatic lymphoma. Scintigraphic imaging using I-123 serum amyloid P component has potential as a noninvasive test.[39a] There is no specific treatment for amyloidosis in cats, so therapy is primarily supportive care (antioxidants, vitamin K, blood transfusion). Attention should be paid to identification and control of any underlying chronic inflammatory disease. Unfortunately, the long-term prognosis is poor as most affected cats die of intra-abdominal bleeding.

HEPATOBILIARY IMAGING

Survey abdominal radiography is the simplest and most readily available imaging modality to assess structures in the abdominal cavity. Radiographs are most useful to assess liver size, will reveal large hepatic masses, and provide evidence of radiopaque masses or other abnormalities in the abdomen. However, the preferred imaging modality used to assess hepatic structures in cats with suspected liver disease is abdominal ultrasonography (AUS). The reasons why ultrasonography is a more useful tool for assessment of the liver in cats are numerous, but because feline liver diseases are primarily diffuse, infiltrative, or metabolic diseases that also affect the biliary tree, ultrasonography is the only imaging tool that will give reliable diagnostic information. This widely available diagnostic tool can be helpful in determining liver size and parenchymal echogenicity, in identifying mass lesions, evaluating the biliary tree and gallbladder, quantifying flow (Doppler techniques), and identifying vascular anomalies.[29] As with all diagnostic modalities, the skill and experience of the operator is vital to accurate procurement and interpretation of the images. Further, it is important to remember that although ultrasonographic images are extremely useful in the clinical evaluation of a cat with possible liver disease, the images themselves do not represent a histologic diagnosis.

For the most common liver diseases of cats (hepatic lipidosis, feline cholangitis syndrome, and neoplasia/lymphoma), AUS examination provides a useful means of obtaining clinical clues and tissue to support or refute the differentials. For example, in cats with hepatic lipidosis, the liver is quite enlarged and typically diffusely hyperechoic, while in cholangitis or other inflammatory diseases, the liver is more often diffusely hypochoic.[29] However, these sonographic findings are very nonspecific and can easily lead to errors in diagnosis if the tissue is not subsequently sampled for confirmation.[24,35] Thus one of the most important utilities of the AUS is the ability to obtain liver tissue (either by aspiration or guided-needle biopsy) and for aspiration of the gallbladder to obtain bile for culture.[24,49] These techniques alone have made the AUS an extremely important diagnostic tool in the evaluation of liver disease in cats.

LIVER HISTOPATHOLOGY (ASPIRATES AND BIOPSIES)

The diagnosis of most liver diseases requires a histopathologic sample of liver tissue, and this is particularly true in the most common feline liver diseases, which tend to be diffuse diseases affecting the entire liver. Cats with one of these diffuse diseases can be sampled randomly using any one of these commonly employed techniques: ultrasound-guided fine-needle aspirates (FNA), ultrasound-guided needle biopsy, laparoscopic biopsies, or biopsies obtained surgically. Some types of neoplasia (particularly round cell tumors) and vacuolar hepatopathies (hepatic lipidosis) can often be diagnosed by cytology using FNA techniques. However, differentiation of liver cell tumors (adenomas and carcinomas) and inflammatory diseases of the liver cannot be diagnosed without a larger sample of tissue and histopathologic examination.[30,50] Further, even in cats with classic hepatic lipidosis changes, concurrent diseases such as cholangitis or lymphoma can be missed if only FNA techniques are employed.[60] Thus it is essential to consider that in many liver diseases the lesions, although typically diffuse, may also have focal components; for example, inflammation may be throughout the liver, but fibrosis will be present only in focal areas. Thus the results of FNA or Tru-Cut needle biopsies should always be considered in the light of the clinical, laboratory, and ultrasonographic evidence.

Prior to scheduling a cat for a biopsy, the risk-to-benefit ratio of performing a liver biopsy should always be considered. This is primarily because heavy sedation or anesthesia will be essential in most cats undergoing a liver FNA, and for all cats undergoing a liver biopsy (needle or otherwise). In addition to anesthesia risks, the use of automatic spring-loaded biopsy guns to obtain ultrasound-guided biopsies of liver tissue is contraindicated in cats, because they may cause a lethal shock reaction.[40] A similar reaction may be seen with penetration of the larger bile ducts or gallbladder with a large-bore biopsy needle, because these tissues have a significant autonomic innervation in the cat that may result in bradycardia and shock following the procedure.[40,48,54] It is particularly important to recognize this as a risk in cats with EHDBO or dilated bile ducts, and this risk factor reiterates the need for ultrasound examination of the liver prior to making biopsy decisions. Nonetheless, owners should be informed of these potential risks, in addition to the risk of bleeding from biopsy sites in any cat undergoing liver sampling.[7,48]

Biopsy Techniques

Liver biopsies, whether they are obtained by needle, laparoscopy, or surgical means, should be taken from a location that represents the primary liver pathology, handled appropriately to ensure accurate interpretation of the sample, and the histopathologic description should be interpreted according to the guidelines set by the WSAVA Standards for Clinical and Histologic Diagnosis of Canine and Feline Liver Disease.[42,61] Guidelines for obtaining and handling surgical biopsies of the liver are reviewed elsewhere[27] and will not be further discussed. Because needle aspirates/biopsies, Tru-Cut–type biopsies, and laparoscopic biopsies are commonly used to obtain liver tissue in cats, the benefits and limitations of each of these techniques will be discussed. As a general rule, the more tissue that can be obtained, the better the pathologist's interpretation of the tissue abnormalities will be. For example, most pathologists believe that at least six portal areas are necessary to make a diagnosis of inflammation liver disease in cats.[42] This will require either a 16- or 18-gauge needle size or larger piece of tissue than is obtained with smaller needles or an aspirate. The amount of tissues required to view at least six portal areas is approximately 15 mg, and 5 mg will be required for culture of the tissue.[42] If other analyses of the tissues are considered (e.g., metal analysis), approximately 20 to 40 mg of liver is needed.[42] A typical laparoscopic cup biopsy forceps will provide 45 mg of liver tissue, a 14-g Tru-Cut–type biopsy needle provides 15 to 20 mg, and an 18-g needle biopsy provides only 3 to 5 mg of liver tissue.[42] Thus, depending on the clinical circumstances and considered differentials, the best approach for obtaining the needed tissue must be considered prior to planning the procedure.

Fine-needle aspiration to obtain liver tissue for cytologic examination is commonly performed in cats with liver disease for good reason. The procedure is inexpensive, easy to do, is relatively low risk, and often requires only sedation to complete.[57] Further, samples obtained by this method can be diagnostic for hepatic lipidosis, hepatic lymphoma or other round cell tumors, and in areas where appropriate, definitive diagnosis of certain infectious diseases (e.g., histoplasmosis).[57] However, even with these relatively straightforward diseases, FNA of liver tissue has significant limitations, the most important of which is the failure to accurately identify the primary disease. For example, although it is easy to make a diagnosis of hepatic lipidosis using this technique, a paper recently showed four cats that were incorrectly diagnosed with hepatic lipidosis instead of lymphoma because the FNA samples were obtained from areas that did not have lymphoma infiltration.[60] In another study, reviewing the agreement between FNA cytologic samples of liver and the histopathologic diagnosis, only 51% of the cases had overall agreement.[50] Thus although cytology of FNA samples of liver tissue in cats with diffuse hepatic disease remains a useful first step, it is important for the clinician to carefully interpret the results and discuss the potential limitations of this technique with owners.

There are several needle biopsy techniques available for sampling liver tissue, but not all are suitable or safe for use in cats. The Menghini technique is one such approach that is not suitable for use in cats, because it is a blind procedure using a large-bore needle that cannot be used with ultrasound guidance.[42] The second option among the needle biopsy techniques that is not recommended for cats is the biopsy gun device. Tru-Cut biopsy guns are operated by a triggering device that can result in the induction of a lethal vagotonic shock reaction in the cat immediately following the procedure.[40] For most ultrasound-guided liver biopsy procedures, either the manual or, preferably, the semiautomatic Tru-Cut device is recommended for use in obtaining needle biopsies from cats. As a general rule, the Tru-Cut device will advance into the liver to a depth of 2 cm; so, it is essential to carefully note the amount of liver tissue available during the ultrasound assessment before advancing the needle for tissue collection. Properly obtained Tru-Cut needle biopsies are a valuable technique for obtaining a representative sample of liver tissue[61]; however, because of the risk for bleeding or liver fracture with any movement, it is essential that cats be anesthetized for this procedure.

Laparoscopy is an intermediate step between needle biopsy and surgical laparotomy for obtaining liver tissue for histopathology in cats.[48,54] This technique is becoming more widely used as more specialists are trained for this procedure that allows visualization of tissues to be biopsied without opening the entire abdomen. Although this technique does require general anesthesia, the limited degree of invasiveness, the large biopsy sample size, and rapid patient recovery make laparoscopy a valuable tool for obtaining liver tissue,[48] and it can be used to obtain biopsies from the spleen, pancreas, kidneys, lymph nodes, or to aspirate the gallbladder. For a detailed discussion of laparoscopic techniques and equipment, the interested reader is referred to several recent reviews on the subject.[48,54] To maximize the histopathologic accuracy, biopsies taken at laparoscopy or surgically should be taken from both normal-appearing and abnormal areas in the liver. Further, if there is a need to obtain samples from the deeper tissues, the laparoscope can be used to direct a Tru-Cut needle biopsy to the best location for sampling. One of the major advantages of the laparoscopic technique is that it allows the operator to observe the biopsy sites for excessive bleeding, which is unusual, but if observed can be staunched by using pressure on the site, gelatin coagulation material placement, or electrocautery. With experienced operators, the complication rate for laparoscopy is very low (less than 2%), and most complications were because of anesthesia, bleeding, or air embolism.[48] Finally, although not necessary to have direct visualization to obtain an aspirate of gallbladder bile, laparoscopy allows easy sampling of bile for culture, which is important in all cats with suspected inflammatory liver disease or hepatobiliary disease.

THERAPY OF LIVER DISEASE

Once a diagnosis of liver disease is made in the cat, specific therapy for the cause (if available) should be instituted; however, for many feline liver diseases, no specific therapy is available, and thus hepatoprotective therapy is used concurrently to aid in the recovery of the liver from the insult. In this section, therapy of two of the most common diseases of the feline liver will be considered, with a special emphasis on nutritional aspects of treatment, nutraceutical therapy, and the unique needs of cats.

Idiopathic Hepatic Lipidosis

The most common liver disease of cats is idiopathic hepatic lipidosis (Figures 23-61 and 23-62), a disease that results in liver failure because of a combination of factors including hepatic lipid accumulation, insulin resistance, fasting, and protein (especially arginine) deficiency.[2,8,9,11] Thus, unlike many diseases of the liver, the primary focus of therapy and the essential component for recovery is nutritional support. As in any patient with serious liver disease, initial therapy is always aimed at correction of any fluid or electrolyte abnormalities that may exist, because these may be profound if the cat has been vomiting. In addition, normalization of electrolytes is particularly important in cats that have been anorexic for an especially long time (1 to 2 weeks), because refeeding syndrome may be triggered with the initiation of feeding, resulting in sudden drops in potassium, phosphate, and magnesium.[1] Although this phenomenon is less common and usually less profound in cats fed enterally versus

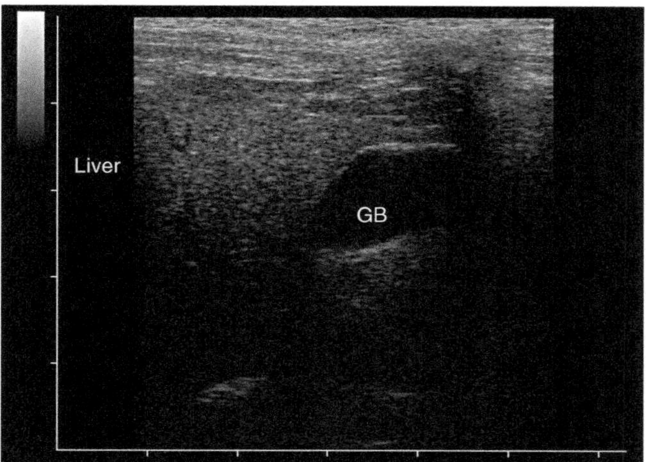

FIGURE 23-61 Ultrasonographic appearance of liver with hepatic lipidosis. The echogenicity of the parenchyma is uniformly increased, which is more apparent when compared with other ultrasonographic images presented in this chapter. Additionally, the gall bladder is distended. Hepatic lipidosis in this cat was secondary to anorexia associated with primary intestinal disease. *(Courtesy Dr. Randolph Baral.)*

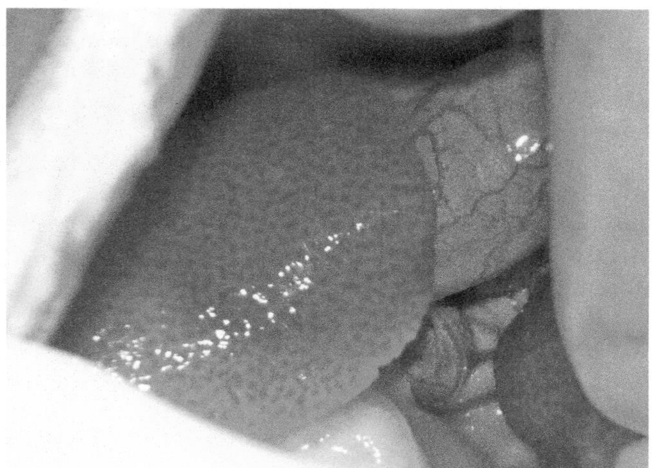

FIGURE 23-62 Gross appearance of liver from a cat with hepatic lipidosis. Note the pale tan and exaggerated reticular pattern. In most cases, the edges appear more rounded than is evident here. Hepatic lipidosis in this cat was secondary to anorexia associated with primary intestinal disease (same cat as in Figure 23-61). *(Courtesy Dr. Randolph Baral.)*

those started on intravenous nutrition, it can be a significant source of morbidity if electrolyte replacement and monitoring are not carefully attended.

Once the cat is hemodynamically stable, the next step in treatment planning in cats with hepatic lipidosis is re-introduction of nutrition, which must include placement of a feeding tube (Box 23-5). However, because many of these cats are extremely ill and are not good candidates for anesthesia, placement of a nasoesophageal (NE) tube to allow initiation of enteral feeding is often the most appropriate step for the first few days.

BOX 23-5

Considerations for Feeding Tubes in Patients with Liver Disease

When administering food through a feeding tube, there are several important points:

1. The food should be room temperature (not too hot or cold).
2. The tube should be flushed with water following feeding, to remove any particles of food or medication that may cause the tube to clog.
3. If the cat is volume sensitive, it is important to carefully calculate how much water is used for flushing the tube, because a significant volume of fluid can be infused, creating a potential fluid overload. If the cat is fluid sensitive, the total amount of fluids (amount in the food, amount added to food if blenderized, and amount of flush) must be determined, and the amount of fluid used in flushes or food preparation may have to be reduced.

Force feeding is to be strongly discouraged in these sick cats for several reasons:

- It is highly stressful and will further increase the stress response and insulin resistance phenomena that are perpetuating the hepatic lipidosis.
- It can be dangerous to the cat (aspiration) or operator (scratches/biting).
- It is rarely able to meet the necessary nutritional goals set for the patient.
- It may induce food aversion, a phenomenon unique to cats, but creating a profound aversion to the chosen food that can be lifelong.[12]

Although NE tubes are excellent choices for short-term feeding of cats unwilling to eat, there are several disadvantages to their long-term use, including the nasal irritation that occurs, the relative ease with which cats can (and will) remove them, and the need to use liquid enteral diets.[62] Thus once the cat is deemed stable enough for general anesthesia, a long-term feeding tube solution is needed, and this typically is either an esophageal (E) tube (Figure 23-63) or percutaneous endoscopic gastrostomy (PEG) tube.[22,62] Both feeding options are generally well tolerated methods for providing long-term feeding, but E tubes have the advantage of being placed without the need for any specialized equipment, and if complications occur, they are generally easily addressed, because the most common complications are infection at the tube site or premature removal of the tube by the cat. Placement of a PEG tube, although relatively easy to learn to place, requires having the appropriate endoscopic equipment, and if complications occur as a result of infection or tube removal, more significant morbidity can result. Because there is no advantage to placement of PEG tubes

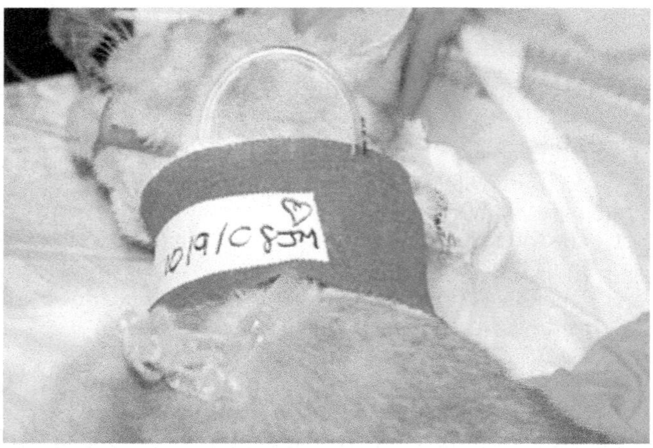

FIGURE 23-63 Esophageal feeding tubes are ideal for enteral nutrition in the cat, because they are easily placed and are associated with few serious complications.

TABLE 23-23 **Medications and Supplements Used in the Treatment of Hepatic Lipidosis**

Medication	Dose
Antiemetics:	
Maropitant	1 mg/kg, IV/SC/PO, q24h
Ondansetron	0.22-0.50 mg/kg, IV/PO, q8-12h
Dolasetron	0.5-1.0 mg/kg, IV/SC/PO, q12-24h
Vitamin K_1	2.5 mg/cat/day for 1 week, then weekly until recovered, PO, SC
Vitamin B_{12}	250 μg/cat weekly for 6 weeks, then monthly until blood values are normal, SC
L-carnitine	250 mg/cat/day, PO
SAMe	20 mg/kg, PO, q24h

SAMe, S-adenosylmethionine.

in cats versus E tubes, placement of E tubes is advocated as the best approach for most practice situations. Interested readers are referred to several recent reviews on tube placement for specific details on each method and to Chapter 18.[22,62]

Diet selection is the next step in treatment planning for cats with hepatic lipidosis. In contrast to the belief that animals in liver failure need lower quantities of protein to reduce the workload on the liver, cats with hepatic lipidosis actually need protein to recover. In fact, the work of Biourge and coworkers showed that protein was the essential nutrient in reducing hepatic lipid accumulation, was essential to eliminate the negative nitrogen balance, and also appeared to minimize muscle catabolism.[9] Further, diets high in protein can improve insulin sensitivity and assist weight loss in recovery from obesity.[8,11] Conversely, although carbohydrates are a readily available energy source, they are often associated with gastrointestinal distress (diarrhea, abdominal cramping) and hyperglycemia (secondary to the insulin resistance in place as a result of obesity and hepatic lipidosis).[2] Thus diets selected for cats with hepatic lipidosis should ideally be high in protein (>40% metabolizable energy [ME]) and have lower amounts of carbohydrates (<20% ME), with the remaining calories coming from fat. The diets that best fit this profile are the diets formulated for diabetic cats; however, kitten food, many adult cat foods, and some of the enteral recovery diets have this high protein/low carbohydrate profile. Many of the intestinal diets are not higher protein and are higher in carbohydrates, and so would not be the ideal choice. The key to using any of the foods that are not designed for use in a feeding tube is to blenderize them (and if necessary, strain the food) so that the food will easily go through the 14- or 16-g feeding tube without clogging it. Enteral diets designed for use in feeding tubes are the easiest to use, and are an acceptable choice in most situations. Finally, because many cat stomachs are volume sensitive with initiation of feeding, it is very important to start conservatively with small-volume feeding on a more frequent schedule. With prolonged fasting, the stomach volume of a cat with hepatic lipidosis may be reduced dramatically, preventing normal expansion and limiting intake to as little as 10% of normal. Thus to avoid vomiting when feeding, the starting volume may have to be as small as 10 to 15 mL every 2 to 3 hours. A good rule of thumb is to start with estimation of resting energy requirement (RER) (40 to 50 kcal/kg is a good estimate of RER), and then attempt to meet 25% of RER the first day. If no problems are encountered, increase the amount to 50% of RER the second day, and so on, but during this period, keep the frequency as high as possible (feed four to six meals per day) so that the volume remains relatively small at each meal. Once full RER has been achieved with multiple meals per day, the frequency of feeding can be gradually reduced to three to four meals per day. Most cats will eventually tolerate three meals per day well, and some can tolerate two meals per day, but this is quite variable and should not be attempted during the first weeks of feeding. In general, most cats with hepatic lipidosis will require tube feeding for a minimum of 3 to 6 weeks before they will show interest in food and begin eating again on their own. The tube should be retained until the cat has been eating on his or her own for at least 1 week or longer and can be maintained for a longer duration if it is being used to administer medications, because cats can eat normally with the E tube in place.

The other therapeutic considerations for cats diagnosed with hepatic lipidosis are directed toward dealing with the complications of the disease and reducing the oxidative stress on the liver with hepatoprotective therapy (Table 23-23). In cats that are vomiting, antiemetic therapy is beneficial, because it is imperative that the cat continues to receive some food, and vomiting will complicate this. Metoclopramide is often used in cats because of its ready availability and low cost, but it is a very weak antiemetic in cats and thus may not be the best choice. In most cats, the novel NK-1 receptor antagonist maropitant has been a safe and effective choice.[32] The most commonly used antiemetics in the author's feline practice are maropitant (1 mg/kg IV, SC or through the E tube q24h), ondansetron (0.22 mg/kg IV q8-12h), or dolasetron (0.5 mg/kg IV, SC q24h). In addition to control of vomiting, all cats with hepatic lipidosis should be given vitamin K_1 (2.5 mg/cat PO, SC) daily for a week, then weekly until the cat has recovered, and vitamin B_{12} (cobalamin) (250 μg/cat SC) weekly for 6 weeks, then monthly until blood values are normal.[46] Other vitamins may become deficient, such as some of the B vitamins and vitamin E; however, feeding is likely to rapidly replenish these deficiencies if they exist. This is also likely true of amino acid deficiencies, but supplementation of L-carnitine (250 mg/day PO) may be beneficial by improving fatty acid oxidation.[10] Finally, hepatoprotectant and antioxidant therapy with S-adenosylmethionine (SAMe) (20 mg/kg PO q24h) has been advocated to increase glutathione and may be beneficial in cats with hepatic lipidosis.[13,19,56] It is important to note that if SAMe is given through the tube (and thus the tablets must be crushed), the dose must be increased by approximately 50% to allow for the loss of absorption from loss of the enteric coating.

Because drug metabolism is often impaired in cats with hepatic lipidosis, appetite stimulants, such as mirtazapine, cyproheptadine, and clonazepam, should not be used in cats because dosing and side effects can be unpredictable. Benzodiazepine agonist drugs (e.g., diazepam) should be completely avoided in cats with possible lipidosis-induced hepatoencephalopathy, because they will exacerbate the signs and may cause fulminant liver failure.[2,14] Fortunately, most cats with idiopathic hepatic lipidosis that receive immediate and aggressive therapy and feeding for their disease will recover completely. Cats that develop hepatic lipidosis secondary to other serious diseases (e.g., lymphoma) have a much lower chance of complete recovery and often die of their disease or its complications.

Feline Cholangitis Syndrome

The most common inflammatory liver disease in the cat is a complex syndrome with multiple subgroups of disease previously termed cholangitis/cholangiohepatitis complex (CCH) but currently recognized under the terminology feline cholangitis syndrome.[61] This disease is quite variable in both its presentation and severity, and it may occur as a primary process or secondary to/concurrent with other diseases (e.g., pancreatitis, IBD). Because the primary starting point of the inflammatory disease in cats is the bile ducts (cholangitis), with inflammation extending to the hepatic parenchyma (cholangiohepatitis) only with time and severity, the term cholangitis syndrome has become the preferred terminology. The disease syndrome has been further classified by the WSAVA Liver Diseases Group into one of three primary types: neutrophilic or suppurative, chronic lymphoplasmacytic (Figures 23-64 and 23-65), and lymphocytic (non-suppurative).[61] Each of the forms appears to behave quite differently clinically as well as in their progression and outcome. In general, cats with the suppurative form of CCH typically have an acute onset of illness, which often includes fever, anorexia, and vomiting, and they may become icteric quite quickly (Figure 23-66).[28,52] The nonsuppurative form of CCH (lymphocytic form) tends to be a more chronic condition, with affected cats showing nonspecific signs of illness that may include partial anorexia and lethargy, but the signs may wax and wane or are non-progressive.[28,52] Because of the feline pancreatic and bile duct anatomy, it is common for cats with CCH to have pancreatitis and vice versa, and in some cases, cats will also have concurrent IBD; the constellation of the three conditions occurring together is called triaditis.[59] This combination is increasingly recognized in cats, and recent reports suggest from 50% to 85% of cats with one syndrome have all three diseases.[25,51,54,59] At this time, the etiology of each of these syndromes and the pathogenesis is not well understood; however, the enteric microflora are presumed to play an important role in the suppurative form, and immune mechanisms are presumed to be the cause of the chronic inflammation found in the chronic nonsuppurative

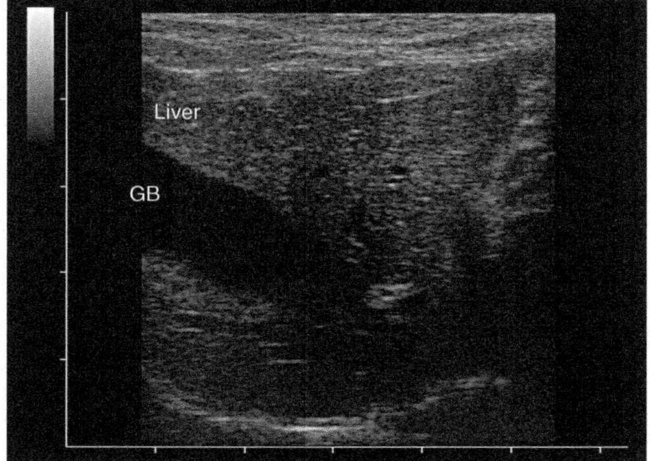

FIGURE 23-64 Ultrasonographic appearance of liver with lymphocytic/plasmacytic inflammation. Note the varying echogenicity throughout the hepatic parenchyma; areas of hypoechogenicity likely reflect inflammatory cell infiltration. The gall bladder is distended; its shape is distorted by pressure from the transducer. *(Courtesy Dr. Randolph Baral.)*

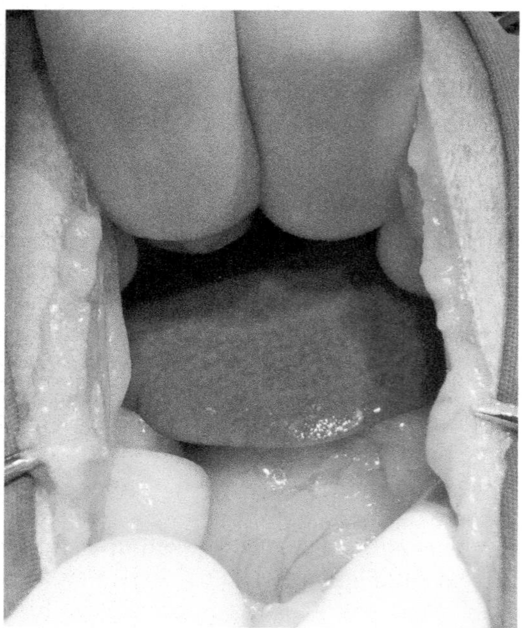

FIGURE 23-65 Gross appearance of liver from a cat diagnosed with lymphocytic/plasmacytic inflammation. Note the liver appears thickened with rounded edges and has a reticular pattern. *(Courtesy Dr. Randolph Baral.)*

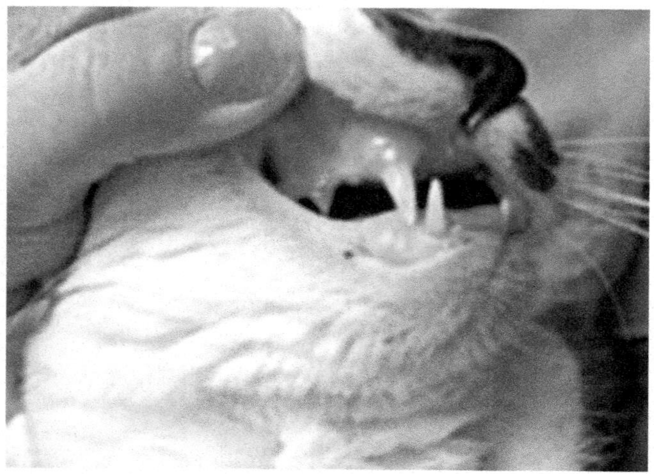

FIGURE 23-66 Icterus is the result of cholestasis and will only be apparent clinically when bilirubin levels are 2 to 3 times normal values.

forms. However, whether or not these syndromes are related, a continuum of disease or completely different diseases remains undetermined.

Once a definitive diagnosis is obtained by histopathology of the liver tissue and culture of bile, treatment can be tailored to needs of the cat. Cats with the more aggressive suppurative form of cholangitis often require intravenous fluid therapy, antibiotic therapy (based on results of culture whenever possible), and supportive therapy (antiemetics, vitamin K_1, hepatoprotectants such as SAMe [20 mg/kg PO q24h] and ursodeoxycholic acid [10 mg/kg PO q24h]), and if pancreatitis is concurrent, pain control with opioid pain relievers (e.g., buprenorphine 0.05 to 0.1 mg/kg PO, SQ q8-12h).[52] If culture is not possible, combination therapy with enrofloxacin (4 mg/kg PO q24h) and metronidazole (5 mg/kg PO q12h) is reasonable. In cats with chronic lymphoplasmacytic forms of cholangitis, management must be tailored to the individual situation and often requires therapy with either immunosuppressive doses of prednisolone (2 to 4 mg/kg PO q24h) or chlorambucil (4 mg/m^2 PO q2d), along with the hepatoprotectants and cholerectics, and concurrent treatment of other diseases (pancreatitis or IBD) that may be occurring.[52] The lymphocytic or lymphoplasmacytic forms of cholangitis may wax and wane in intensity over time, and may require long-term continuous or intermittent therapy to control the disease. There is no specific diet that is recommended for cats with inflammatory liver disease, but protein restriction should not be initiated unless the cat has clear evidence of severe hepatoencephalopathy. The diet should be selected based on other conditions (such as IBD), for which the diet may be more critical in the management. Monitoring of serum chemistry values (especially glucose), clotting times, cobalamin levels, and PLI/TLI concentrations are recommended every few months, as well as careful monitoring of the CBC for all cats on chlorambucil. In all cats with chronic inflammatory liver disease, prior to initiation of immunosuppressive therapy, a careful assessment of the cat for other possible causes of inflammation should be completed (Box 23-6).

BOX 23-6

Infectious Diseases Associated with Hepatopathy or Inflammation in the Feline Liver

Bacterial agents: hepatic abscess, ascending infection/bacterial translocation, leptospirosis, *Clostridium* spp., *Helicobacter* spp., bartonellosis
Viral agents: feline infectious peritonitis, feline herpesvirus, virulent calicivirus
Protozoal agents: toxoplasmosis, visceral leishmaniasis
Parasitic agents: flukes (*Platynosomum*), visceral migrans (*Toxocara*), heartworm (*Dirofilaria*)
Fungal agents: histoplasmosis, paecilomycosis

From Kearns S: Infectious hepatopathies in dogs and cats, *Top Comp Anim Med* 24:189, 2009.

Hepatoencephalopathy/Portosystemic Shunting

As in dogs, if a cat with PSS can have surgical closure of the shunting vessel (ligation, placement of an ameroid constrictor, intravenous coiling), the long-term

TABLE 23-24 **Medical Management of Hepatoencephalopathy in Cats**

Specific Problem to Address	Therapeutic Options
Decreasing bacterial production of ammonia	Emergent: enemas with warm water or lactulose Chronic: (1) oral lactulose (0.5-1 mL/kg q8h: based on stool softness), (2) antibiotics: metronidazole (5-10 mg/kg, PO, q12h) or ampicillin (20 mg/kg, PO q8h or IV q6h)
Coagulopathy (postoperative or if symptomatic)	Emergent: plasma therapy (fresh frozen) 10 mL/kg over 4 h (can be repeated) Vitamin K_1 1-2 mg/kg SC or PO daily for 3 days, then as needed
Gastrointestinal ulcers and gastritis	Famotidine (0.5-1 mg/kg PO q12-24h) Omeprazole (0.5-1 mg/kg PO q24h) Sucralfate (0.25 g/5 kg PO q8h in slurry)
Seizures	Benzodiazepines are controversial Phenobarbital 4 mg/kg loading dose: Can be given q6h during 24 hr if needed Levetiracetam (20 mg/kg PO q8h, increase to effect)
Nutritional support	Place E tube if needed Protein at least 35% (DM basis), only restrict further if ammonia/signs not improved B vitamin supplementation (1 mL/L fluids or can give 0.25 mL SC daily)
Hepatoprotectants	See Table 23-25 SAMe/silymarin alone or in combination N-acetylcysteine (if want to give IV) Vitamin E

SAMe, S-adenosylmethionine.
From Berent AC, Tobias KM: Portosystemic vascular anomalies, *Vet Clin North Am Small Anim Pract* 39:513, 2009.

prognosis for function and quality of life is generally very good.[5] However, even if surgical correction is anticipated, and especially if surgical correction is impossible or not completely successful, medical management of HE is indicated. See Table 23-24 for the basic therapeutic approach to medical management of cats with HE resulting from PSS.

Nutraceutical Therapy

Because hepatocytes, by their position in the body between the GI tract and rest of the body, as well as their critical role in metabolism and detoxification, are uniquely susceptible to oxidative injury and reactive intermediates of metabolism, they must be able to protect themselves. The natural defenses of the liver include superoxide dismutase and glutathione, free-radical scavengers such as vitamin E and ascorbate, and other prosurvival signaling pathways that are controlled by hormones and growth factors.[56] However, in injury or overwhelming infection or inflammation, the natural defenses of the liver can be overwhelmed, and then it is essential for medicines and nutraceutical therapy to be included in the treatment plan to help reduce inflammation and fibrosis, protect against oxidant injury, and enhance bile flow. The cytoprotective agents most commonly used in liver diseases to assist in these processes (Table 23-25) are:

- S-Adenosylmethionine (SAMe)—a precursor in the synthesis of glutathione and an important methyl donor to DNA and proteins, is an important antioxidant and stabilizes membrane functions
- N-acetylcysteine—a precursor to glutathione and antioxidant, also improves tissues oxygen delivery
- Ursodeoxycholic acid (tertiary bile acid)—used to replace hepatotoxic, hydrophobic bile acids and increase bile flow
- Silymarin (milk thistle)—a free radical scavenger and anti-inflammatory/antifibrotic agent
- Vitamin E—an antioxidant and antiinflammatory vitamin*

Although few clinical trials of these nutraceuticals have been performed in feline liver disease, a few studies have recently appeared showing that SAMe, ursodeoxycholic acid, silymarin, and N-acetylcysteine all are hepatoprotective, have few adverse side effects, and may be beneficial in many types of liver disease in cats.[3,26,39,53,55]

SUMMARY

Feline liver disease is a common problem that requires careful consideration of the presenting complaint, clinicopathologic findings, imaging results, and, if available, histopathologic interpretation to be able to provide an accurate diagnostic and therapeutic plan. A variety of insults can be responsible for liver dysfunction or failure, but hepatic lipidosis and feline cholangitis syndrome remain the most common reasons for cats to present

*References 13, 19, 21, 26, 53, 55, 56.

TABLE 23-25 **Dosages and Indications of Commonly Used Hepatoprotective Agents in Feline Liver Disease**

Agent	Indications	Dosage	Veterinary Products
S-Adenosylmethionine (SAMe)	Inflammatory hepatopathies, hepatic lipidosis, cholestatic hepatopathies, acetaminophen toxicity	20 mg/kg/day PO Breaking/crushing enteric coated tablets reduces bioavailability	Denosyl-SD4 or Denomarin (Nutramax Labs, Edgewood, Md.) Zentonil (Vetoquinol, Buena, New Jersey)
N-Acetylcysteine (NAC)	Acute liver failure, acetaminophen toxicity	140 mg IV once, then 70 mg/kg IV q6h or 100 mg/kg/24h in CRI	No veterinary products, but powder is widely available and is used in a 10% solution with saline
Silymarin (Milk thistle has four isomers: isosilybin, silydianin, silychristin, and silybin; this is the active component of silymarin)	Toxic hepatopathies, metabolic hepatopathies (hepatic lipidosis), and inflammatory hepatopathies	20-50 mg/kg/day PO divided q8h	Marin or Denomarin (Nutramax Labs)
Ursodeoxycholic acid (UDCA)	Cholestatic and inflammatory hepatopathies, and metabolic hepatopathies	10-15 mg/kg/day PO	No veterinary products
Vitamin E	Cholestatic and inflammatory hepatopathies	10-15 IU/kg/day PO	No veterinary products

CRI, Constant rate infusion; *IU,* international units.
From Webster CRL, Cooper J: Therapeutic use of cytoprotective agents in canine and feline hepatobiliary disease, *Vet Clin North Am Small Anim Pract* 39:631, 2009.

with icterus or liver failure. Therapy must be tailored to the individual, but nutritional support is critical in the management of hepatic lipidosis, and appropriate supportive therapy with hepatoprotectants may be crucial to treatment success.

References

1. Armitage-Chan E, O' Toole T, Chan DL: Management of prolonged food deprivation, hypothermia, and refeeding syndrome in a cat, *J Vet Emerg Crit Care* 16:S34, 2006.
2. Armstrong PJ, Blanchard G: Hepatic lipidosis in cats, *Vet Clin North Am Small Anim Pract* 39:599, 2009.
3. Avizeh R, Najafzadeh H, Razijalali M et al: Evaluation of prophylactic and therapeutic effects of silymarin and N-acetylcysteine in acetaminophen-induced hepatotoxicity in cats, *J Vet Pharmacol Therap* 33:95, 2009.
4. Balkman C: Hepatobiliary neoplasia in dogs and cats, *Vet Clin North Am Small Anim Pract* 39:617, 2009.

4a. Beatty JA, Barrs VR, Martin PA et al: Spontaneous hepatic rupture in six cats with systemic amyloidosis, *J Small Anim Pract* 43:355, 2002.

5. Berent AC, Tobias KM: Portosystemic vascular anomalies, *Vet Clin North Am Small Anim Pract* 39:513, 2009.
6. Bertolini G: Acquired portal collateral circulation in dogs and cats, *Vet Radiol* 51:25, 2010.
7. Bigge LA, Brown DJ, Pennick DG: Correlation between coagulation profile findings and bleeding complications after ultrasound guided biopsy: 434 cases (1993-1996), *J Am Anim Hosp Assoc* 37:228, 2001.
8. Biourge V, Nelson RW, Feldman EC, et al: Effect of weight gain and subsequent weight loss on glucose tolerance and insulin response in healthy cats, *J Vet Int Med* 11:86, 1997.
9. Biourge V, Massat B, Groff JM, et al: Effects of protein, lipid or carbohydrate supplementation on hepatic lipid accumulation during rapid weight loss in obese cats, *Am J Vet Res* 55:1406, 1994.
10. Blanchard G, Paragon BM, Mullat F, et al: Dietary L-carnitine supplementation in obese cats alters carnitine metabolism and decreases ketosis during fasting and induced hepatic lipidosis, *J Nutr* 132:204, 2002.

10a. Blunden A, Smith A: Generalized amyloidosis and acute liver haemorrhage in four cats, *J Small Anim Pract* 33:566, 1992.

11. Brown B, Mauldin GF, Armstrong PF, et al: Metabolic and hormonal alterations in cats with hepatic lipidosis, *J Vet Int Med* 14:20, 2000.
12. Brunetto MA, Gomes MOS, Andre MR, et al: Effects of nutritional support on hospital outcomes in dogs and cats, *J Vet Emerg Crit Care* 20:224, 2010.
13. Center SA: Metabolic, antioxidant, nutraceutical, probiotic, and herbal therapy relating to the management of hepatobiliary disorders, *Vet Clin North Am Small Anim Pract* 34:67, 2004.
14. Center SA: Current considerations for evaluating liver function in the cat. In August JR, editor: *Consultations in feline internal medicine*, ed 5, Philadelphia, 2006, Elsevier, p 89.
15. Center SA: Diseases of the gallbladder and biliary tree, *Vet Clin North Am Small Anim Pract* 39:543, 2009.
16. Center SA, Baldwin BH, Dillingham S et al: Diagnostic value of serum gamma glutamyl transferase and alkaline phosphatase in hepatobiliary disease in the cat: 1975-1990, *J Am Vet Med Assoc* 188:507, 1986.
17. Center SA, Crawford MA, Guida L et al: Retrospective study of 77 cats with severe hepatic lipidosis: 1975-1990, *J Vet Int Med* 7:349, 1993.
18. Center SA, Erb HN, Joseph SA: Measurement of serum bile acids concentrations for diagnosis of hepatobiliary disease in cats, *J Am Vet Med Assoc* 207:1048, 1995.

19. Center SA, Randolph JF, Warner KL et al: The effects of s-adenosylmethionine on clinical pathology and redox potential in the red blood cell, liver and bile of normal cats, *J Vet Int Med* 19:303, 2005.
20. Center SA, Warner D, Corbett J et al: Proteins invoked by vitamin K absence in clotting times in clinically ill cats, *J Vet Int Med* 14:292, 2000.
21. Center SA, Warner KL, Erb HN: Liver glutathione concentrations in dogs and cats with naturally occurring liver disease, *Am J Vet Res* 63:1187, 2003.
22. Chan DL: Critical care nutrition. In August JR, editor: *Consultations in feline internal medicine*, ed 6, Philadelphia, 2010, Elsevier, p 116.
23. Fahie MA, Martin RA: Extrahepatic biliary tract obstruction, a retrospective study of 45 cases (1983-1993), *J Am Anim Hosp Assoc* 31:478, 1995.
24. Feeney DA, Anderson KL, Ziegler LE, et al: Statistical relevance of ultrasound criteria in the assessment of different liver diseases in dogs and cats, *Am J Vet Res* 69:212, 2008.
25. Ferrari J, Hardam E, Van Winkle TJ, et al: Clinical differentiation of acute and chronic feline pancreatitis, *J Am Vet Med Assoc* 223:469, 2003.
26. Flora K, Hahn M, Rosen H, et al: Milk thistle (*Silybum marianum*) for the therapy of liver disease, *Am J Gastroenterol* 93:139, 1998.
27. Fossum TW, Hedlund CS: Surgery of the liver. In Fossum TW, editor: *Small animal surgery*, St Louis, 1997, Mosby, p 367.
28. Gagne JM, Armstrong PF, Weiss DJ: Clinical features of inflammatory liver disease in cats: 41 cases (1983-1993), *J Am Vet Med Assoc* 214:513, 1999.
29. Gaschen L: Update on hepatobiliary imaging, *Vet Clin North Am Small Anim Pract* 39:439, 2009.
30. Giordano A, Paltrinieri S, Bertazzolo W: Sensitivity of tru-cut and fine needle aspirate biopsies of liver and kidney for the diagnosis of feline infectious peritonitis, *Vet Clin Path* 34:368, 2004.
30a. Godfrey D, Day M: Generalised amyloidosis in two Siamese cats: spontaneous liver haemorrhage and chronic renal failure, *J Small Anim Pract* 39:442, 1998.
31. Haney DR, Christiansen JS, Toll J: Severe cholestatic liver disease secondary to liver fluke (*Platynosomum concinnum*) infection in three cats, *J Am Anim Hosp Assoc* 42:234, 2006.
32. Hickman MA, Cox SR, Mahabir S et al: Safety, pharmacokinetics and use of the novel NK-1 antagonist maropitant (Cerenia) for the prevention of emesis and motion sickness in cats, *J Vet Pharmacol Ther* 31:220, 2008.
33. Karanjia ND, Singh SM, Widdison AL et al: Pancreatic ductal and interstitial pressures in cats with chronic pancreatitis, *Gastroenterol* 37: 268, 1992.
34. Kearns S: Infectious hepatopathies in dogs and cats, *Top Comp Anim Med* 24:189, 2009.
35. Lewis KM, O'Brien RT: Abdominal ultrasonographic findings associated with feline infectious peritonitis: a retrospective review of 16 cases, *J Am Anim Hosp Assoc* 46:152, 2010.
36. Lipscomb VL, Jones HJ, Brockman DJ: Complications and long-term outcomes of the ligation of congenital portosystemic shunts in 49 cats, *Vet Rec* 160:465, 2007.
37. Lowe AD, Campbell KL, Barger A, et al: Clinical, clinicopathological, and histological changes observed in 14 cats treated with glucocorticoids, *Vet Rec* 162:777, 2009.
38. Maddison JE: Hepatic encephalopathy. Current concepts of the pathogenesis, *J Vet Int Med* 6:341, 1992.
39. Nicolson BT, Center SA, Randolph JF: Effects of oral ursodeoxycholic acids in healthy cats on clinicopathological parameters, serum bile acids and light microscopic and ultrastructural features of the liver, *Res Vet Sci* 61:258, 1996.
39a. Piirsalu K, McLean R, Zuber R et al: Role of I-123 serum amyloid protein in the detection of familial amyloidosis in Oriental cats, *J Small Anim Pract* 35:581, 1994.
40. Proot SJM, Rothuizen J: High complication rate of an automatic tru-cut biopsy gun device for liver biopsy in cats, *J Vet Int Med* 20:1327, 2006.
41. Rothuizen J: Important clinical syndromes associated with liver disease, *Vet Clin North Am Small Anim Pract* 39:419, 2009.
42. Rothuizen J, Twedt D: Liver biopsy techniques, *Vet Clin North Am Small Anim Pract* 39:469, 2009.
43. Rothuizen J, van den Ingh TS: Arterial and venous ammonia concentrations in the diagnosis of canine hepatoencephalopathy, *Res Vet Sci* 33:17, 1982.
44. Rogers CL, O'Toole TE, Keating JH, et al: Portal vein thrombosis in cats: 6 cases (2001-2006), *J Vet Int Med* 22:282, 2008.
45. Sergeeff JS, Armstrong PJ, Bunch SE: Hepatic abscesses in cats: 14 cases (1985-2002), *J Vet Int Med* 18:295, 2004.
46. Simpson KW, Fyfe I, Cornetta A, et al: Subnormal concentrations of serum cobalamin (vitamin B12) in cats with gastrointestinal disease, *J Vet Int Med* 15:26, 2001.
47. Trainor D, Center SA, Randolph JF, et al: Urine sulfated and non-sulfated bile acids as a diagnostic test for liver disease in cats, *J Vet Int Med* 17:145, 2003.
48. Twedt DC: Laparoscopy of the liver and pancreas. In Tams TR, editor: *Small animal endoscopy*, ed 2, St Louis, 1999, Mosby, p 44.
48a. van der Linde-Sipman J, Niewold T, Tooten P et al: Generalized AA-amyloidosis in Siamese and Oriental cats, *Vet Immunol Immunopathol* 56:1, 1997.
49. Wagner KA, Hartman FA, Trepanier LA: Bacterial culture results from liver, gallbladder, or bile in 248 dogs and cats evaluated for hepatobiliary disease: 1998-2003, *J Vet Int Med* 21:417, 2007.
50. Wang KY, Panciera DL, Al Rukivati RK, et al: Accuracy of ultrasound guided fine needle aspirate of the liver and cytologic finding in dogs and cats: 97 cases (1990-2000), *J Am Vet Med Assoc* 224:75, 2004.
51. Washabau RJ: Acute necrotizing pancreatitis. In August JR, editor: *Consultations in feline internal medicine*, ed 5, St Louis, 2006, Elsevier, p 109.
52. Webb C: Feline cholangitis syndrome. In Cote EC, editor: *Veterinary clinical advisor*, ed 2, Philadelphia, 2010, Elsevier, p 196.
53. Webb CB, McCord KW, Twedt DC: Oxidative stress and neutrophil function following oral supplementation of a silibinin-phophatidylcholine complex in cats, *J Vet Int Med* 22: 808A, 2008.
54. Webb CB, Trott C: Laparoscopic diagnosis of pancreatic disease in dogs and cats, *J Vet Intern Med* 22:1263, 2008.
55. Webb CB, Twedt DC, Fettman MJ, et al: S-adenosylmethionine in a feline acetominophen model of oxidative injury, *J Feline Med Surg* 38:246, 2003.
56. Webster CRL, Cooper J: Therapeutic use of cytoprotective agents in canine and feline hepatobiliary disease, *Vet Clin North Am Small Anim Pract* 39:631, 2009.
57. Weiss DJ, Moritz A: Liver cytology, *Vet Clin North Am Small Anim Pract* 32:1267, 2002.
58. Weiss DJ, Armstrong PJ, Gagne MJ: Inflammatory liver disease, *Sem Vet Med Surg* 12:22, 1997.
59. Weiss DJ, Gagne JM, Armstrong PJ, et al: Relationship between feline inflammatory liver disease and inflammatory bowel disease, pancreatitis, and nephritis, *J Am Vet Med Assoc* 209:1114, 1996.
60. Willard MD: Fine needle aspiration cytology suggests hepatic lipidosis in 4 cats with infiltrative hepatic disease, *J Feline Med Surg* 1:215, 1999.
61. WSAVA Liver Standardization Group, editors: *WSAVA Standards for clinical and histological diagnosis of canine and feline liver diseases*, Edinburgh, 2006, Churchill Livingston.
62. Zoran DL: Nutrition for anorectic, critically ill or injured cats. In August JR, editor: *Consultations in feline internal medicine*, ed 5, Philadelphia, 2006, Elsevier, p 145.

APPROACH TO THE CAT WITH ASCITES AND DISEASES AFFECTING THE PERITONEAL CAVITY

Randolph M. Baral

The peritoneum is the serous membrane lining the abdominal cavity, as well as covering the organs of the abdomen. It comprises a single layer of squamous mesothelial cells resting on a deeper layer of loose connective tissue. The layer of peritoneum that lines the inner surface of the abdomen is called parietal peritoneum; the abdominal organs are lined by visceral peritoneum. The total surface area of the peritoneum is one to one-and-a-half times that of the total cutaneous area of the body.[5,30]

The peritoneal cavity contains a small amount of fluid (less than 1 mL/kg body weight) that reduces friction between the abdominal organs as they slide over each other. The fluid is a pure transudate and contains solutes in the same concentration as serum (Box 23-7). This fluid is absorbed from the abdominal cavity predominantly through lymphatic vessels lying beneath the mesothelial basement membrane on the surface of the diaphragm. Lymphatic drainage occurs predominantly to the sternal lymph nodes.[5,30] Ascites is the abnormal effusion and accumulation of fluid in the abdominal cavity.

PATHOPHYSIOLOGY OF ASCITES

Fluid exchange across the capillary bed is determined by Starling forces, that is, the balance between hydrostatic pressure, which causes transudation of fluid out of blood vessels, and the colloid osmotic pressure, which acts to retain fluid within blood vessels. The amount of peritoneal fluid is therefore determined by the balance of these, as well as vascular permeability, with excess fluid drained by the lymphatic system. Accumulation of fluid within a body cavity results when the rate of filtration of fluid into a space is greater than the rate of fluid resorption from that space. Effusion accumulation is therefore correlated to increased capillary hydrostatic pressure, widening of the oncotic pressure gradient, increased endothelial permeability, increased interstitial hydrostatic pressure, or loss of effective lymphatic drainage or a combination of these factors.[10,23,32]

Peritonitis of any cause results in vascular dilation, increased capillary permeability, and the migration of inflammatory cells into the peritoneum in response to immunomodulatory mediators. The inflamed peritoneum becomes a freely diffusible membrane, allowing a massive outpouring of fluid and plasma proteins from the circulation.[5,30]

BOX 23-7

Characteristics of Normal Peritoneal Fluid

- Clear, slightly yellow
- Specific gravity <1.016
- Protein: 20 g/L (mainly albumin)
- Total white cell count: 2000 to 2500/mL
  - 50% macrophages
  - Some eosinophils, mast cells
  - Few neutrophils
- No fibrinogen (does not clot on standing)
- Fibronectin (a bacterial opsonizing protein)

From Bray J: Diagnosis and management of peritonitis in small animals, *In Practice* 18:403, 1996.

CLINICAL EVALUATION OF ASCITES

Ascites is not commonly seen in practice; one study recognized ascites in only three cats out of 1000 admissions to an American veterinary teaching hospital,[34] but the prevalence may be greater in primary care practice. In that study, dilated cardiomyopathy (DCM) was the most common disease associated with peritoneal effusion; however, DCM was diagnosed in most of these cats before 1987, when taurine deficiency was found to be a primary cause of this form of cardiomyopathy in cats. Neoplasia was the most common cause after 1987.[34] Feline infectious peritonitis (FIP) was by far the most common cause of feline ascites diagnosed over a 10-year period at the Feline Centre at the University of Bristol, comprising 50% of all cats with recognized ascites.[32]

Presentation and Clinical Signs

Cats with ascites usually present with nonspecific clinical signs, such as anorexia or lethargy. The owners may present the cat because they recognize abdominal enlargement (Figure 23-67), but in many cases, owners perceive this as weight gain. Clinicians should be aware that sudden weight gain in a chronically underweight cat may be because of fluid accumulation (which can be intrathoracic fluid if ascites is not present), particularly if muscle mass seems reduced. Ascitic cats presenting subsequent to trauma may have intraabdominal hemorrhage or urinary tract rupture. Fever in a young ascitic cat will often suggest FIP, and cats with FIP may or may not be jaundiced. Presence of jugular distention or even a jugular pulse can suggest right-sided heart failure.

A palpable fluid thrill can help to distinguish ascites from other causes of abdominal enlargement, such as organomegaly, abdominal masses, bladder distention, abdominal wall weakness, obesity or, occasionally, accumulations of gas within the abdominal cavity[27] (Table 23-26). Recognizing a fluid thrill involves gently tapping one side of the abdominal wall with the fingers of one hand while feeling for a sensation of fluid movement

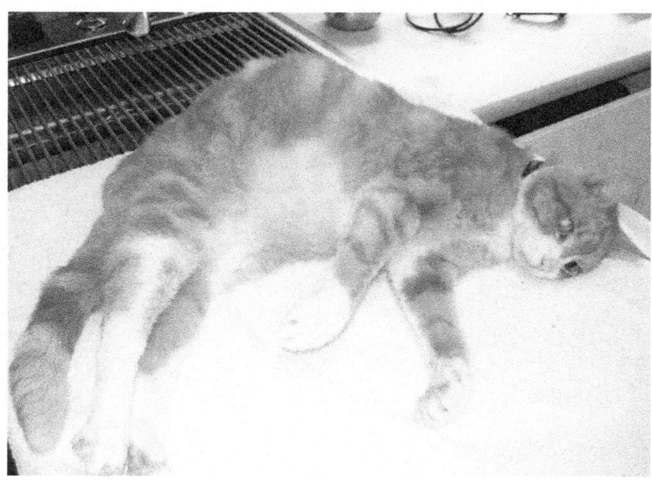

FIGURE 23-67 Abdominal distention because of ascites in an elderly cat. This cat had reduced muscle mass, despite weight gain because of the abdominal fluid.

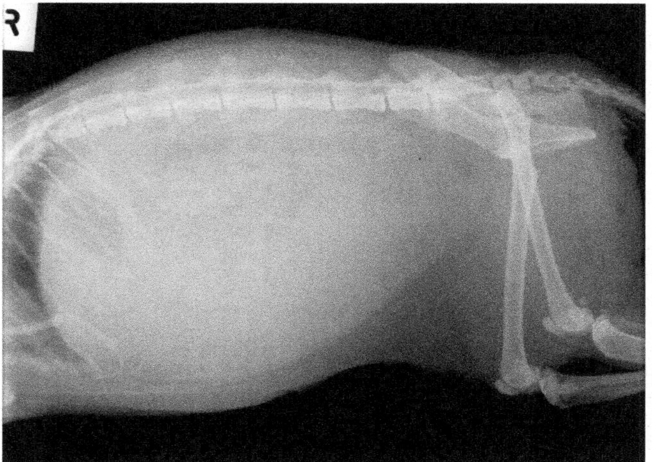

FIGURE 23-68 Radiographic appearance (right lateral view) of the same cat as in Figure 23-67. Note that, additional to the abdominal distention, the loss of serosal detail creates difficulty to discern abdominal organs.

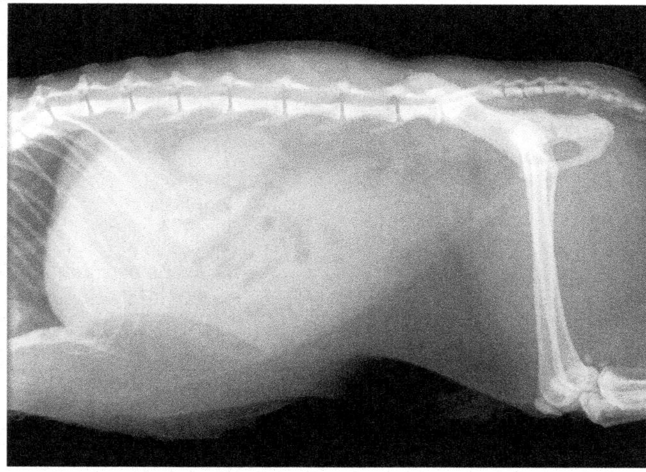

FIGURE 23-69 Radiographic appearance (right lateral view) of the same cat as in Figure 23-67 after drainage of a substantial amount of fluid. The abdominal distention is reduced but the remaining fluid still somewhat obscures the midabdominal organs.

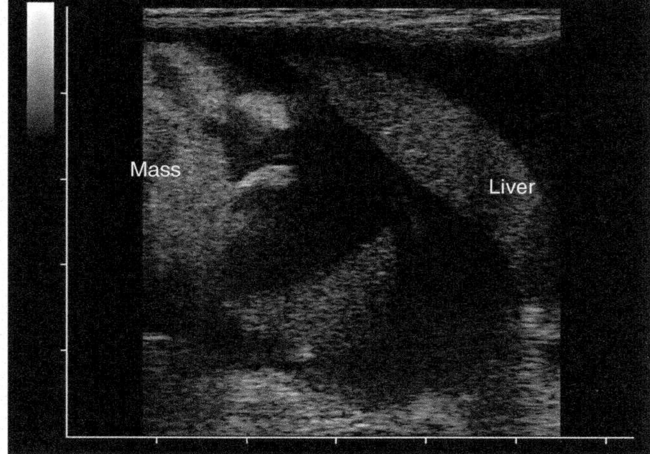

FIGURE 23-70 Ultrasonographic appearance of ascites. Note that organs are highlighted by the dark background of the hypoechoic fluid. This is particularly emphasized with the low cellularity of this particular effusion.

with the fingers of the other hand positioned on the opposite side of the abdomen.

Diagnostic Approaches

Hematology, Biochemistry, and Urinalysis

Routine laboratory findings are usually nonspecific but may provide clues to the underlying cause of ascites. For example, neutrophilia may point towards septic peritonitis but can also occur with FIP; most cats with hemoperitoneum are anemic at presentation[8]; uroperitoneum often results in azotemia and electrolyte abnormalities; hypoglycemia may reflect sepsis with septic peritonitis, and a recent study recognized 83% of cases of septic peritonitis had ionized hypocalcemia[17]; elevated liver enzymes may be associated with inflammatory, infectious or neoplastic hepatopathies including FIP; elevation of serum globulins occurs in many cats with FIP but can also be associated with neoplasia or septic peritonitis; and a finding of hypoalbuminemia (which can cause a pure transudate) should prompt for an assessment of urine protein:creatinine ratio to assess if there is renal protein loss.

Imaging

Imaging may be required to confirm the presence of fluid as well as to aid in diagnosis of the underlying cause. Radiographic findings can vary greatly depending on the amount of abdominal fluid present and the underlying etiology. Loss of normal detail or presence of a "ground glass" appearance to the abdominal cavity is suggestive of the presence of fluid (Figures 23-68 and 23-69). Very young, thin or dehydrated cats may also have a loss of detail that can mimic the presence of fluid. Ultrasonography of the abdomen (Figures 23-70 and

TABLE 23-26 **Causes of Abdominal Distention**

Weak abdominal wall	Hyperadrenocorticism
Organomegaly	Hepatomegaly/renomegaly/splenomegaly Mesenteric lymphadenopathy Gastric distention/bladder distention/advanced obstipation Pregnancy/pyometra Neoplasia Obesity
Gas accumulation (pneumoperitoneum)	Traumatic penetration of abdominal wall Rupture of the stomach or bowel Gas-forming bacterial infection Extension from pneumomediastinum or pneumothorax
Fluid Accumulation (Ascites)	
Transudates	
Pure transudate*	Hypoproteinemia: glomerular disease, intestinal malabsorption or protein loss, severe chronic liver disease (Neoplasia) (Obstruction of lymphatic drainage/lymphangiectasia)
Modified transudate	Congestive heart failure Hepatic disease: cirrhosis, neoplasia Neoplasia: obstruction of blood vessels and/or lymphatics Portal hypertension/obstruction of posterior vena cava
Exudates	
Nonseptic exudates	Feline infectious peritonitis Hepatitis (particularly lymphocytic cholangitis) Bile or urine peritonitis Pancreatic peritonitis Diaphragmatic or pericardial hernia Steatitis Neoplasia
Septic exudates	Extension of infection from elsewhere Intestinal perforation/bowel rupture Ruptured pyometra Penetrating wound Migrating foreign body Hematogenous spread
Caused by a Ruptured Vessel	
Hemorrhagic effusion	Organ or major blood vessel rupture; associated with trauma or secondary to ruptured neoplasm Perforation of stomach or intestine Bleeding disorders Splenic or gastric torsion Thrombosis
Chyle	Ruptured lymphatic drainage Obstruction of lymphatic drainage/lymphangiectasia Neoplasia Congestive heart failure Steatitis
Caused by a Ruptured Viscus	
Urine	Ruptured urinary tract. Since urine is irritant it usually results in a secondary nonseptic exudate.
Bile	Ruptured biliary tract. Since bile is irritant it usually results in a secondary nonseptic exudate.

*When present for any length of time, a pure transudate will become modified. This is particularly true of transudates that develop slowly, such as those associated with congestive heart failure or portal hypertension. Modified transudates are therefore more common than pure transudates.
Adapted from Tasker S, Gunn-Moore D: Differential diagnosis of ascites in cats, *In Practice* 22:472, 2000.

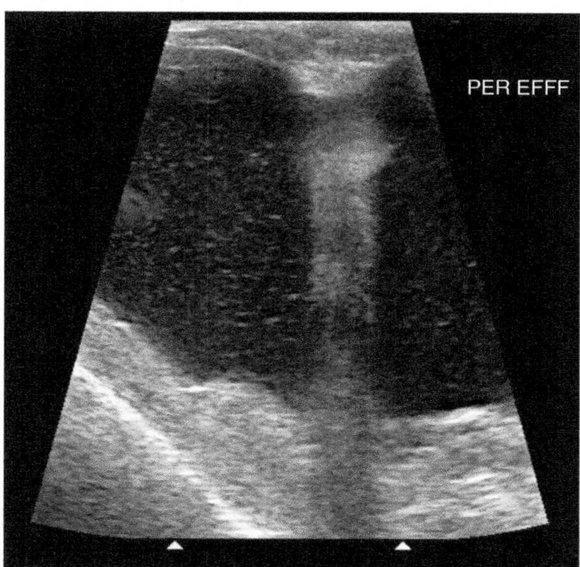

FIGURE 23-71 Ultrasonographic appearance of ascites, note the echogenic debris through the fluid that reflects the cellular nature of this chylous effusion. *(Courtesy Small Animal Specialist Hospital, North Ryde, Sydney, Australia.)*

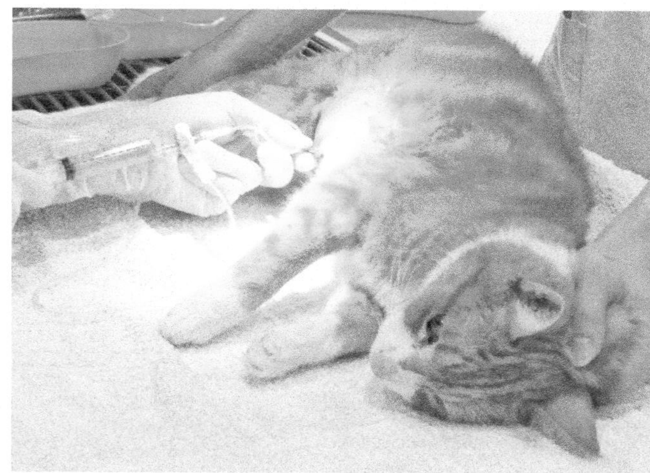

FIGURE 23-72 Drainage of large-volume abdominal effusion using a butterfly catheter, three-way stopcock, and 10-mL syringe.

23-71) can allow the detection of even very small volumes of fluid. It also enables evaluation of the size and structure of intraabdominal organs, such as the liver and spleen, which can help determine the underlying cause of ascites.

Abdominocentesis

Abdominocentesis confirms the presence of abdominal fluid (in cases of low-volume effusion) and assessment of the fluid is required to diagnose the underlying cause of ascites. Most cats tolerate abdominocentesis without sedation and the cat can be held in a standing position or in lateral recumbency (whichever is more comfortable for the cat and familiar to the clinician). The abdomen is clipped and aseptically prepared. A 20- to 22-gauge butterfly needle may be used with a 5- to 10-mL syringe. In cases with low-volume effusion, ultrasonography can help to guide fine needle aspiration from small pockets of abdominal fluid. Diagnostic peritoneal lavage can be used if ultrasound-guided aspiration is unsuccessful. For this procedure, 10 to 20 mL/kg of warmed, sterile fluid is infused into the abdomen over 2 to 5 minutes after aseptic preparation of the site. The cat is gently rolled from side to side or allowed to stand; gentle massage of the abdomen also helps distribute the fluid. The fluid is allowed to dwell for a minimum of 2 to 5 minutes before aseptic preparation is repeated before paracentesis. No attempt is made to remove all the fluid. It must be remembered that, since the recovered fluid has been diluted by this procedure, cell counts and biochemical analyses will be affected.[33]

If a large volume effusion causes discomfort because of abdominal distention, a three-way stopcock may be used so large volumes can be drained from one puncture (Figure 23-72). However, removal of large volumes of ascitic fluid can be detrimental, because it may prevent the subsequent reabsorption of valuable protein and/or red blood cells; the resulting reduction in intraabdominal pressure may encourage further accumulation of fluid; and rapid removal of large volumes can lead to fluid shifts causing cardiovascular collapse.[32] Fluid can be collected into ethylenediaminetetraacetic acid (EDTA) tubes (for total nucleated cell count, packed cell volume, total protein, and cytology), serum tubes (for biochemistry, such as albumin, bilirubin, creatinine, potassium, triglyceride, glucose, lactate, and lipase), sterile tubes for culture, and/or other tubes for effusion-specific tests such as PCR. Samples should be prioritized according to the volume of fluid available and to the suspected underlying disease process.[10]

FLUID ANALYSIS AND CLASSIFICATION

Initial assessment of fluid retrieved is made on the basis of color and protein concentration, and much information can be gleaned from this simple assessment, even before cell numbers and types are assessed. Although this brief, initial assessment is useful to refine the differential diagnoses, a thorough assessment based on underlying etiology and pathophysiology is required for definitive diagnosis and therefore appropriate management (Table 23-27). Ascitic fluid, classified according to its pathophysiologic cause, can be divided into transudates, modified transudates, exudates (septic or nonseptic), or effusions (chylous or hemorrhagic).[10,23]

TABLE 23-27 **Characteristics of Peritoneal Effusion Fluid**

	Pure Transudate	Modified Transudate	Exudate	Chyle	Hemorrhage
Appearance of fluid	Usually clear and colorless or occasionally amber-colored	Yellow or blood tinged, can be turbid	Turbid fluid	Milky or pinkish opaque	Red (blood)
Total protein (g/L)	<25	>25	>25, usually >30	25-60	35-75
Specific gravity	<1.015	1.015-1.025	>1.025	Not applicable	Not applicable
Nucleated cells ($\times 10^9$/L)	<1	1-7	>5	0.25-20	1-20, depending on peripheral count
Predominant cell types	Macrophages Mesothelial cells	Macrophages Mesothelial cells Lymphocytes Erythrocytes Neutrophils (nondegenerate) +/−Neoplastic cells	Neutrophils (non-degenerate, or degenerate, if bacterial) Macrophages Erythrocytes +/− Neoplastic cells	Small lymphocytes Neutrophils Macrophages	Erythrocytes Neutrophils Macrophages Mesothelial cells Neoplastic cells

Adapted from Tasker S, Gunn-Moore D: Differential diagnosis of ascites in cats, *In Practice* 22:472, 2000.

Transudates

Transudates are a consequence of altered fluid dynamics. Protein-poor transudates (commonly referred to as pure transudates) form predominantly as a result of severe hypoalbuminemia, which causes a lowered colloid osmotic pressure. Since there is no change in endothelial or mesothelial permeability, as fluid accumulates, there is no concurrent cell leakage; so, there is a decrease in the cell count through a dilutional effect. Consequently, transudative effusions are typically clear and colorless.[10,23,32] Other pathologic causes of protein-poor transudates include cirrhosis, lymphatic obstruction, and noncirrhotic portal hypertension (presinusoidal and sinusoidal). Since hypoalbuminemia is the most common cause of transudates, serum albumin concentrations must be measured to guide further diagnostics. If the serum albumin concentration is normal (or only minimally decreased), then radiographs, abdominal ultrasonography, and/or echocardiography are indicated to assess cardiac function and for urinary bladder rupture.[10] One review of feline ascitic cases found 24% of effusions were protein-poor transudates, of which 82% were the result of hepatic failure or primary renal disease.[34]

Modified Transudates

Modified transudates can result from increased hydrostatic pressure within the postsinusoidal vessels of the liver secondary to right-sided congestive heart failure (e.g., tricuspid insufficiency) or potentially from mass lesions (such as neoplastic masses) obstructing blood flow from the hepatic vein or caudal vena cava into the right side of the heart. The increase in hydrostatic pressure within the vessels of the liver causes a protein-rich fluid to leach out of the liver into the abdominal cavity. Since cell membrane permeability does not change, cells do not accumulate in the effusion.[10] Modified transudates can also result from increased vascular permeability in the early stages of an inflammatory process, in which case cellularity will be increased. Modified transudates were described as the most common type of ascitic effusion identified in cats in one study, with most being resulting from neoplasia and congestive cardiac failure; however, this study partially included cases prior to 1987, when right-sided heart failure associated with dilated cardiomyopathy (DCM) was prevalent.[34] The recognition of the role of taurine deficiency in this condition and the subsequent addition of this amino acid to feline diets now means that right-sided heart failure is only rarely encountered as a cause of ascites in cats.

Exudates

Exudates are a consequence of altered mesothelial and/or endothelial permeability. This permeability results from a cytokine-mediated inflammatory response of any underlying cause (e.g., infectious, neoplastic, immune mediated). Exudates have high protein and moderate to high cell concentrations and are classified as nonseptic or septic.

Exudates are often primarily composed of neutrophils. Nondegenerate neutrophils (and the absence of organisms) points to a nonseptic exudate (mostly FIP but also neoplasia). FIP is the most common cause of exudative effusion in cats and was the most common cause of feline ascites diagnosed over a 10-year period at the Feline Centre at the University of Bristol.[32] The presence of neoplastic cells rules in neoplasia, but the absence of such cells does not rule out this diagnosis since many cases of neoplastic ascites are not associated with exfoliated neoplastic cells. Other causes of nonseptic exudates include pancreatitis, lymphocytic cholangitis, and viscus rupture, such as the gall bladder or urinary bladder.

Degenerate neutrophils typify septic exudates (i.e., septic peritonitis), and their presence should instigate investigation for causes of infection (mostly leakage of gastrointestinal contents).[34]

Chylous Effusions

Chylous effusions appear as milky or pink opaque fluid, and small mature lymphocytes initially predominate in cell counts. After drainage, more macrophages and nondegenerate neutrophils may be found. Chyle is typically classified as an exudate, but its physical characteristics can be consistent with a modified transudate (protein content between 25 and 40 g/L); biochemical analysis of triglyceride and cholesterol levels in the fluid are required to confirm the diagnosis. Pseudochylous effusions resemble true chyle both in appearance and cytology but do not contain fat. Similar conditions result in both chylous and pseudochylous effusions. Chylous abdominal effusions are rarely reported in the cat and only accounted for 7% of cases of ascites in one study.[34] The described causes of chylous ascites in cats are predominantly neoplastic. In a series of nine cats, chylous ascites was associated with nonresectable abdominal neoplasia in four cases (i.e., hemangiosarcoma and paraganglioma), with intestinal and mesenteric lymphoma in two cases and lymphangiosarcoma of the abdominal wall in another.[13] One described case in a 10-year-old cat was thought to be because of FIP.[28] Figure 23-71 shows an ultrasonographic image of a cat with chylous abdominal effusion associated with pancreatitis. Other potential causes include right-sided congestive cardiac failure, steatitis (inflammation of fat), biliary cirrhosis, and lymphangiectasia.

Hemorrhagic Effusions

Hemoperitoneum in companion animals is categorized as traumatic or spontaneous. Traumatic hemoperitoneum is further divided into blunt causes of trauma (i.e., motor vehicle accidents and high-rise falls) and penetrating trauma (i.e., gunshot wounds and bite wounds).[8,21]

Inadvertent splenic aspiration, venipuncture, or acute severe hemorrhage should be suspected if the cytology is consistent with peripheral blood including platelets but without erythrophagocytosis or if the blood clots readily.

When there is no history of trauma, coagulopathy or spontaneous rupture of a vascular neoplasm should be considered. In one study of 16 feline cases of spontaneous hemoperitoneum, 12 cases (75%) were associated with hepatic pathology such as neoplasia, necrosis, and amyloidosis.[21] In another study of 65 cases of spontaneous hemoperitoneum, 46% (30 of 65) of cats had abdominal neoplasia, and 54% (35 of 65) had non-neoplastic conditions. Cats with neoplasia were significantly older and had significantly lower packed cell volumes (PCVs) than cats with non-neoplastic disease. Hemangiosarcoma was the most often diagnosed neoplasm (18 of 30, 60%), and the spleen was the most common location for neoplasia (11 of 30, 37%). Coagulopathies (8 of 35, 23%) and hepatic necrosis (8 of 35, 23%) were the most common causes of non-neoplastic hemoperitoneum.[8] Other non-neoplastic causes of hemoperitoneum include ruptured bladder, hepatic rupture secondary to hepatic amyloidosis, gastric/duodenal ulcer, hepatic hematoma, hepatitis, perinephric pseudocyst, feline infectious peritonitis–induced liver rupture, and feline infectious peritonitis–induced nephritis.[8,21]

The prognosis of cats with spontaneous hemoperitoneum is poor. In two studies, only approximately 12% of cases survived to be discharged from hospital.[8,21] Median survival time for cats that were discharged in one of those studies was 54 days (range, 5 to 1825 days).[8]

SPECIFIC CAUSES OF ASCITES

Feline Infectious Peritonitis

Feline infectious peritonitis (FIP) comprised 50% of cats with recognized ascites over a 10-year period at the Feline Centre at the University of Bristol,[32] and, as a rule of thumb, when ascites is recognized in a younger cat, FIP should be considered the major rule-out. The abdominal effusion found with FIP is typically straw to golden yellow (although the color can be very variable, for example, chyle may be present), may contain fibrin clots, and has a high protein concentration. The total protein content is greater than 35 g/L and often greater than 45 g/L, with globulins comprising 50% or more.[31] One study described an effusion with total protein greater than 80 g/L as 90% specific, 55% sensitive, and having a 0.78 positive predictive value to diagnose FIP.[31] The Rivalta test evaluates the fluid's globulin content, and was found to be very sensitive but only 80% specific; this test is performed by adding one drop of acetic acid (98%) to 5 mL of distilled water. This fluid is mixed thoroughly, and then one drop of effusion is gently placed on the surface of the mixture. If the drop stays at the top of the fluid or slowly floats to the bottom, the test is considered to be positive. This test can give inaccurate results if inappropriate technique is used or if there is a significant temperature difference between the fluid sample and the acetic acid solution. A positive Rivalta test can result from lymphosarcoma, septic, or FIP effusions; these can be distinguished by cytology and culture.

Immunofluorescence staining of coronavirus antigen in macrophages had a positive predictive value of 1.00 but a negative predictive value of 0.57.[15] The potential clinical presentations, diagnosis, and management of FIP are covered in detail in Chapter 33.

Neoplasia

One study found neoplasia to be the most common cause of ascites in cats,[34] and neoplasia should be considered the major rule-out in older cats with ascites. The effusion from cats with ascites resulting from neoplasia may be a modified transudate, resulting from compression of hepatic veins or the caudal vena cava, or metastases to the peritoneum; hemorrhage from neoplasia can cause hemoperitoneum; chylous effusions may result from reduced lymphatic drainage or rupture of lymphatic vessels; and raised vascular permeability caused by neoplastic infiltration can result in an exudative effusion. Carcinomas, mesotheliomas, and discrete (round) cell neoplasms (e.g., lymphoma, mast cell tumors, malignant histiocytosis) exfoliate cells into effusions more readily than sarcomas, and of these, lymphosarcoma is the most common malignancy of cats. Cytology of ascitic fluid reveals neoplastic cells in less than a quarter of cases; so the absence of such cells does not rule out a diagnosis of neoplasia. In these circumstances, the diagnosis may be achieved by ultrasound-guided fine-needle aspiration of affected organs, or even biopsy samples obtained at laparotomy. The specific approaches will depend on the specific neoplasia diagnosed.

Septic Peritonitis

Exudates caused by septic inflammation usually result from bacterial contamination of the peritoneal cavity secondary to gastrointestinal tract leakage or penetrating wounds associated with trauma. Gastrointestinal tract leakage may occur as a result of ulceration associated with neoplasia or inflammatory disease or as a result of penetration of a sharp object ingested (such as a toothpick), it can also occur subsequent to prior abdominal surgery.[7,9,17,24] Primary septic peritonitis in which no apparent cause can be identified has also been described in cats.[26]

Septic exudates are usually yellow to tan in color, with yellow particulate matter and are foul-smelling. Microscopically, the fluid is characterized by the presence of degenerate neutrophils and bacteria. Bacteria are often seen intracellularly within neutrophils. The condition is associated with high morbidity and mortality rates, with survival rates reported between 32% and 80%.[7,9,17,24,26] The history and clinical signs are often vague and nonspecific but can include abdominal pain, vomiting, lethargy/depression, and anorexia. Abdominal pain is an inconsistent finding, being recognized in only 62% of cats in one study[7] and 43% in another.[24] Some cats may have an inappropriately low heart rate.[7,26] Hematologic and serum biochemistry findings are also inconsistent; neutrophilia with a left shift may be present, as may neutropenia or a normal neutrophil count. Similarly, cats may be hypoglycemic, hyperglycemic, or normoglycemic, and they may be hypoalbuminemic.[7,24,26] One study recognized ionized hypocalcemia in 89% of cats with septic peritonitis at the time of diagnosis,[17] and another suggested hyperlactatemia, when present, may be associated with a poorer prognosis.[24] Radiographic findings are usually typical of ascites of any cause, but presence of pneumoperitoneum in a cat that has not undergone recent surgery may suggest the presence of gas-forming bacteria or rupture of an abdominal viscus and warrants immediate surgical intervention. Ultrasonography does not directly aid the diagnosis of septic peritonitis.[7] Exploratory laparotomy to determine and correct an underlying problem, such as full-thickness gastrointestinal perforation (often requiring partial resection) is required, as is copious abdominal lavage with sterile, warmed fluids (Figure 23-73). There are no statistically significant survival differences between postsurgical primary closure, open peritoneal drainage, or closed suction drainage postsurgical lavage; however, a trend toward a higher survival rate has been seen in cats treated with primary closure.[24,26] Treatment also involves antibiotics, initially parenterally, based on culture and sensitivity findings. Consistent with intestinal contents, most bacteria recognized are gram-negative aerobes, such as *E. coli* or *Enterobacter* spp., but mixed infections are usually found.[7,24] Anaerobes seem more common in cats with primary septic peritonitis,[26] which perhaps suggests these cases may result from healed over-bite wounds into the abdomen. Amoxicillin/clavulanate would be an appropriate empirical choice of

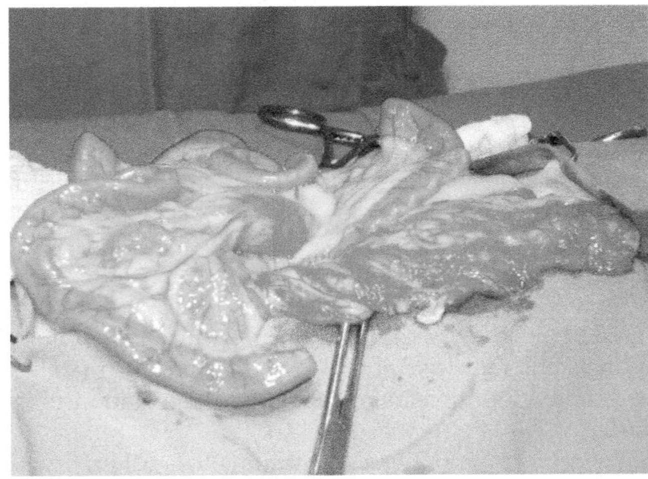

FIGURE 23-73 Fulminant peritonitis associated with gastrointestinal perforation. In this case, the effusion volume was low but the high degree of serosal inflammation is evident.

antibiotics while awaiting sensitivity results. There are no definitive guidelines for duration of antibiotic treatment; the author uses extended treatment courses of 4 to 6 weeks. Supportive care with intravenous fluids to maintain fluid and electrolyte balances is also required perioperatively.

Bile Peritonitis

Bile peritonitis is infrequently reported in cats but has been recognized in association with gunshot[20] or motor vehicle[2] trauma, with biliary obstruction from gall stones[2,22] and subsequent to percutaneous ultrasound-guided cholecystocentesis in a cat with infectious cholangitis.[4] Concurrent bacterial infection was recognized in each case; this increases severity of inflammation and worsens the prognosis, although full recovery was achieved in most reported cases.[2,4,20] Bile peritonitis has the potential to result in small-volume effusions; so, if abdominocentesis does not yield a sample of effusion but bile peritonitis is high on the differential list, then diagnostic peritoneal lavage is appropriate. Since repair of or removal of the gall bladder and abdominal lavage are required, exploratory laparotomy is an appropriate means to diagnose this condition. Management should be considered as for septic peritonitis of other causes.

Uroabdomen

Trauma, including blunt abdominal trauma, urethral catheterization, and bladder expression, is the most common cause of uroperitoneum in cats.[1] It is also recognized as a complication of ureteral surgery.[18] The bladder is the most frequent site of urine leakage after blunt abdominal trauma, whereas the urethra is most commonly injured following catheterization. Cats with ruptured bladders may still have a palpable bladder and the ability to urinate. Common historical complaints are anuria (53.8%) and vomiting (50%). Azotemia is a common finding, and hyperkalemia is seen in around 50% of cases. Drainage of urine from the peritoneal cavity seems to improve patient stabilization. Morbidity and mortality depended largely on the severity of associated injuries.[1] Regardless of the site of injury or the cause of uroabdomen, the first goal of treatment is patient stabilization. Isotonic replacement fluids are used for initial resuscitation. Treatment of hypovolemic shock, if present, is the first order of fluid therapy. After fluid resuscitation, drainage of urine from the abdomen should be established. Continuous passive drainage of the urine is necessary for stabilization and allows effective diuresis to occur. Indwelling catheterization of the urinary bladder is recommended to keep the bladder decompressed and reduce urine flow into the abdominal cavity in patients with bladder and proximal urethral injury. If the urethra is traumatized and a catheter cannot be placed, prepubic tube cystostomy may be necessary to achieve temporary urinary diversion. The decision to treat the uroabdomen patient surgically or conservatively should be based on the location and severity of the underlying injury, the condition of the patient at presentation, and the patient's response to initial stabilization.[1,12]

Right-Sided Congestive Heart Failure

Congestive heart failure has become an uncommon cause of ascites in cats since the late 1980s/early 1990s, from which time dilated cardiomyopathy has been largely eradicated.[32,34] Ascites does still result from right-sided congestive heart failure in conditions such as tricuspid insufficiency,[6] arrhythmogenic right ventricular cardiomyopathy,[16] myocardial fibrofatty infiltration,[14] or restrictive cardiomyopathy.[29,34] Concurrent pleural effusion or pulmonary edema is often, but not necessarily, present with cardiac induced ascites. A heart murmur is not necessarily noted. Noting a jugular pulse or thrill is helpful diagnostically, if present. The ascitic fluid is typically a modified transudate, but a chylous effusion is also possible. Cardiac diseases are covered in Chapter 20.

Hepatopathies

In some cases, hepatic lipidosis has been reported to cause ascites, particularly in association with pancreatitis. These cats are often hypoalbuminemic, with the possibility of intravenous fluid therapy contributing to the ascites by raising hydrostatic pressure.[11] Other liver diseases which can result in ascites include lymphocytic cholangitis,[19,25] neutrophilic cholangitis, cirrhosis,[13] necrosis, neoplasia, and suppurative cholangiohepatitis.[34] Portosystemic shunts in cats rarely result in ascites, compared with dogs.[3] Hypoalbuminemia and hepatic failure result in transudates; portal hypertension and cirrhosis cause higher protein ascites because of raised capillary hydrostatic pressure causing leakage of high protein lymph. Hepatopathies are covered in detail elsewhere in this chapter.

References

1. Aumann M, Worth L, Drobatz K: Uroperitoneum in cats: 26 cases (1986-1995), *J Am Anim Hosp Assoc* 34:315, 1998.
2. Bacon NJ, White RAS: Extrahepatic biliary tract surgery in the cat: a case series and review, *J Small Anim Pract* 44:231, 2003.
3. Blaxter AC, Holt PE, Pearson GR et al: Congenital portosystemic shunts in the cat: a report of nine cases, *J Small Anim Pract* 29:631, 1988.
4. Brain PH, Barrs VR, Martin P et al: Feline cholecystitis and acute neutrophilic cholangitis: clinical findings, bacterial isolates and response to treatment in six cases, *J Feline Med Surg* 8:91, 2006.
5. Bray J: Diagnosis and management of peritonitis in small animals, *In Practice* 18:403, 1996.

6. Closa J, Font A: Traumatic tricuspid insufficiency in a kitten, *J Am Anim Hosp Assoc* 35:21, 1999.
7. Costello MF, Drobatz KJ, Aronson LR et al: Underlying cause, pathophysiologic abnormalities, and response to treatment in cats with septic peritonitis: 51 cases (1990-2001), *J Am Vet Med Assoc* 225:897, 2004.
8. Culp WTN, Weisse C, Kellogg ME et al: Spontaneous hemoperitoneum in cats: 65 cases (1994-2006), *J Am Vet Med Assoc* 236:978, 2010.
9. Culp WTN, Zeldis TE, Reese MS et al: Primary bacterial peritonitis in dogs and cats: 24 cases (1990-2006), *J Am Vet Med Assoc* 234:906, 2009.
10. Dempsey SM, Ewing PJ: A review of the pathophysiology, classification, and analysis of canine and feline cavitary effusions, *J Am Anim Hosp Assoc* 47:1, 2011.
11. Dimski DS: Feline hepatic lipidosis, *Clin Tech Small Anim Pract* 12:28, 1997.
12. Gannon KM, Moses L: Uroabdomen in dogs and cats, *Compend Contin Educ Vet* 24:604, 2002.
13. Gores BR, Berg J, Carpenter JL et al: Chylous ascites in cats: nine cases (1978-1993), *J Am Vet Med Assoc* 205:1161, 1994.
14. Harjuhahto TAI, Leinonen MR, Simola OTM et al: Congestive heart failure and atrial fibrillation in a cat with myocardial fibrofatty infiltration, *J Feline Med Surg* 13:109, 2011.
15. Hartmann K, Binder C, Hirschberger J et al: Comparison of different tests to diagnose feline infectious peritonitis, *J Vet Int Med* 17:781, 2003.
16. Harvey AM, Battersby IA, Faena M et al: Arrhythmogenic right ventricular cardiomyopathy in two cats, *J Small Anim Pract* 46:151, 2005.
17. Kellett-Gregory LM, Mittleman Boller E, Brown DC et al: Retrospective study: ionized calcium concentrations in cats with septic peritonitis: 55 cases (1990-2008), *J Vet Emerg Crit Care* 20:398, 2010.
18. Kyles AE, Hardie EM, Wooden BG et al: Management and outcome of cats with ureteral calculi: 153 cases (1984-2002), *J Am Vet Med Assoc* 226:937, 2005.
19. Lucke VM, Davies JD: Progressive lymphocytic cholangitis in the cat, *J Small Anim Pract* 25:249, 1984.
20. Ludwig LL, McLoughlin MA, Graves TK et al: Surgical treatment of bile peritonitis in 24 dogs and 2 cats: a retrospective study (1987-1994), *Vet Surg* 26:90, 1997.
21. Mandell DC, Drobatz K: Feline hemoperitoneum 16 cases (1986-1993), *J Vet Emerg Crit Care* 5:93, 1995.
22. Moores AL, Gregory SP: Duplex gall bladder associated with choledocholithiasis, cholecystitis, gall bladder rupture and septic peritonitis in a cat, *J Small Anim Pract* 48:404, 2007.
23. O'Brien PJ, Lumsden JH: The cytologic examination of body cavity fluids, *Semin Vet Med Surg (Small Anim)* 3:140, 1988.
24. Parsons KJ, Owen LJ, Lee K et al: A retrospective study of surgically treated cases of septic peritonitis in the cat (2000-2007), *J Small Anim Pract* 50:518, 2009.
25. Prasse KW, Mahaffey EA, DeNovo R et al: Chronic lymphocytic cholangitis in three cats, *Vet Path* 19:99, 1982.
26. Ruthrauff CM, Smith J, Glerum L: Primary bacterial septic peritonitis in cats: 13 cases, *J Am Anim Hosp Assoc* 45:268, 2009.
27. Saunders WB, Tobias KM: Pneumoperitoneum in dogs and cats: 39 cases (1983-2002), *J Am Vet Med Assoc* 223:462, 2003.
28. Savary KC, Sellon RK, Law JM: Chylous abdominal effusion in a cat with feline infectious peritonitis, *J Am Anim Hosp Assoc* 37:35, 2001.
29. Saxon B, Hendrick M, Waddle JR: Restrictive cardiomyopathy in a cat with hypereosinophilic syndrome, *Can Vet J* 32:367, 1991.
30. Seim HB: Management of peritonitis. In Bonagura JD, Kirk RW, editors: *Kirk's current veterinary therapy XII: small animal practice*, Philadelphia, 1995, Saunders, p 764.
31. Sparkes A, Gruffydd-Jones T, Harbour D: Feline infectious peritonitis: a review of clinicopathological changes in 65 cases, and a critical assessment of their diagnostic value, *Vet Rec* 129:209, 1991.
32. Tasker S, Gunn-Moore D: Differential diagnosis of ascites in cats, *In Practice* 22:472, 2000.
33. Walters JM: Abdominal paracentesis and diagnostic peritoneal lavage, *Clin Tech Small Anim Pract* 18:32, 2003.
34. Wright KN, Gompf RE, DeNovo RC Jr: Peritoneal effusion in cats: 65 cases (1981-1997), *J Am Vet Med Assoc* 214:375, 1999.

CHAPTER

24

Endocrinology

OUTLINE

ENDOCRINE PANCREATIC DISORDERS

Randolph M. Baral and Susan E. Little

OVERVIEW

The endocrine pancreas comprises multitudes of islands of cells within the exocrine pancreas known as the *islets of Langerhans*. The islets represent only 2% of the pancreas and comprise several types of cell. Each cell type secretes a different hormone. The major cell types and the hormones they produce are found in Table 24-1. The close interrelationship among these different cell types allows for direct control of secretion of some hormones by other hormones. For example, insulin inhibits glucagon secretion and somatostatin inhibits the secretion of both insulin and glucagon. Activity of beta cells and production of insulin are of main importance for diabetes mellitus (DM).[24]

DIABETES MELLITUS

Epidemiology

The prevalence of feline DM is in the order of 1 in 100 to 1 in 200 cases, with higher numbers of cases seen in referral practice than in first opinion practice.[5,62,93,95] The number of diabetes cases in cats appears to be increasing (Figure 24-1), and this may relate to higher obesity rates and more cats being fed high-carbohydrate diets.[93] Male cats appear to be at greater risk, representing approximately 60% to 70% of all diabetics.[5,62,89,93,95] Increasing age also correlates with increasing risk of DM, with approximately 20% to 30% of diabetics diagnosed at 7 to 10 years of age and 55% to 65% of diabetics diagnosed when older than 10 years of age.[5,89,93,95] Numerous studies have indicated that Burmese are at higher risk of diabetes than other cats in Australia and New Zealand,[5,62,95,114,121] and a United Kingdom survey has indicated likewise.[77] This does not appear to be the case in North America, where the Burmese breed appears to be genetically distinct. One North American study indicated an overrepresentation of Siamese cats,[89] but a subsequent study did not confirm this.[93]

Clinical Signs and Diagnosis

According to one authority, "Currently, there are no internationally accepted criteria for the diagnosis of diabetes in cats."[94] Despite this statement, DM is usually recognized as persistent hyperglycemia above the renal threshold for normal cats, which is blood glucose (BG) greater than 16 mmol/L (288 mg/dL), with consistent clinical signs (polyuria, polydipsia, and weight loss). Elevations of BG above the renal threshold result in glycosuria. Caution must be taken to rule out stress hyperglycemia (reportedly as high as 60.4 mmol/L [1087mg/dL]).[59] In many cases serum fructosamine concentration will be normal with stress hyperglycemia. Ruling out stress hyperglycemia can also be achieved by treating underlying conditions and then rechecking blood and urine glucose on a subsequent day. This is particularly important if the BG is less than 20 mmol/L (360 mg/dL), intercurrent disease is present that could cause stress hyperglycemia, or typical clinical signs of DM are absent. A second test is not usually required if BG is greater than 20 mmol/L (360 mg/dL).

Evidence of gluconeogenesis (ketosis or ketonuria) supports a diagnosis of DM.[94] All diabetic cats in a recent study had at least some elevation of the plasma ketone, beta-hydroxybutyrate. Using a plasma value of 0.22 mmol/L beta-hydroxybutyrate as the cutoff value for diagnosis of DM gave a false positive rate of 9%, whereas 0.58 mmol/L reduced the false positive rate to 1.2%. No cat with moderate or severe stress-related hyperglycemia had beta-hydroxybutyrate concentrations above 0.22 mmol/L.[132]

Fructosamine is the term used to describe glycated plasma proteins, and serum concentration of fructosamine is related to BG concentration. Serum fructosamine concentration may be used to aid the diagnosis of DM, but care must be taken because in cats a single serum fructosamine concentration measurement most likely reflects the mean BG concentration for approximately the past week (compared with longer durations in other species). Further, serum fructosamine may not exceed the reference range in cats with moderate hyperglycemia of less than 17 mmol/L (306 mg/dL),[64] making serial BG testing a more reliable indicator of diabetes. Most cats with newly diagnosed DM will have serum fructosamine levels higher than 400 μmol/L.[16]

Other serum or plasma biochemistry changes in DM are variable but commonly include elevations in the hepatic enzymes, alanine aminotransferase (ALT), and alkaline phosphatase (ALP). These values return to normal on successful treatment of diabetes.

Hematology is typically normal but a stress leukogram of mild neutrophilia and lymphopenia may be recognized. Concurrent infection resulting in a more pronounced neutrophilia, perhaps with a left shift, can

TABLE 24-1 **The Major Cell Types of the Endocrine Pancreas and the Hormones They Produce**

Cell Type	Hormone
Alpha cells (20%-25% of each islet)	Glucagon
Beta cells (60%-80% of each islet)	Insulin
Delta cells (10% of each islet)	Somatostatin
Gamma cells have two subtypes: PP (or F) cells	Pancreatic polypeptide
D cells	Vasoactive intestinal peptide
EE (or enterochromaffin) cells	Serotonin, motilin, substance P

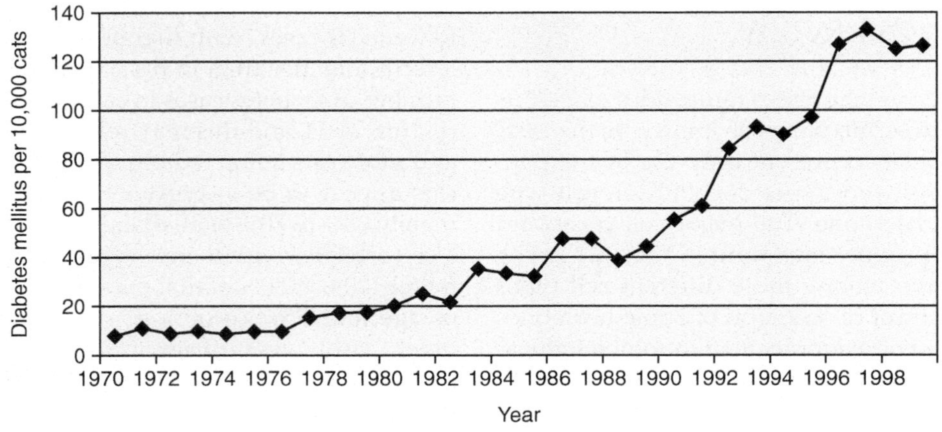

FIGURE 24-1 Hospital prevalence of feline diabetes mellitus. Veterinary Medical Data Base, 1970-1999. *(From Prahl A, Guptill L, Glickman NW et al: Time trends and risk factors for diabetes mellitus in cats presented to veterinary teaching hospitals,* J Feline Med Surg *9:351, 2007.)*

be present, and successful management of diabetes requires treatment of underlying infection.

Glycosuria should be considered as part of the diagnostic criteria because this arises as a result of BG above the renal threshold. Urine may be dilute and associated with polydipsia but not necessarily so as some affected cats have concentrated urine. One study showed that 13% of cats with DM had urinary tract infection (UTI),[4] and as with other infections, UTI must be treated to aid diabetic control.

Pathophysiology

Successful management of DM requires an understanding of its pathophysiology. Hyperglycemia resulting in DM comprises three processes:

1. Lack of insulin production
2. Lack of insulin receptivity (insulin resistance)
3. Hepatic gluconeogenesis

In the healthy individual, for most organs, insulin must bind to insulin receptors at the periphery of cells to allow entry of glucose from the bloodstream into the cell. When insulin binds to the receptor, intracellular mechanisms are activated that result in glucose transporters (contained within intracellular vesicles) moving to the cell membrane. At least 12 glucose transporter proteins (GLUTs) have been described. GLUT4 is responsible for insulin-mediated glucose uptake. GLUT4 vesicles dock on the cell membrane, and then GLUT4 fuses to the cell membrane to allow intracellular diffusion of glucose. This is a complex process mediated by at least three genes in all mammals. Glucose in the bloodstream is mostly from metabolized food.[63] These processes have been simplified, as depicted in Figure 24-2. There are two major organs with important differences in glucose metabolism:

1. The *liver* has enhanced uptake of glucose that is mediated as described previously but also *stores* glucose in the form of glycogen. In most species hepatic glycogen is split back into glucose (gluconeogenesis) in times of fasting, such as between meals. In cats gluconeogenesis is reported to be active even in the fed state.[38] Cats have low levels of glucokinase, an enzyme that facilitates conversion of glucose to glucose 6-phosphate, but high levels of glucose 6-phosphate. Glucose 6-phosphate plays a vital role in glycogen production and glycolysis (energy production).[43] The full implications of these feline-specific differences are not yet understood but may prove vital in our evolving understanding of the pathogenesis of feline diabetes.
2. *Brain* cells are permeable to glucose and can use glucose without the intermediation of insulin. The brain normally uses only glucose for energy and can use other substrates (e.g., fat) for energy only with difficulty (as opposed to other organs). For these reasons it is essential that BG concentration does not fall too low because hypoglycemic shock can result.[38]

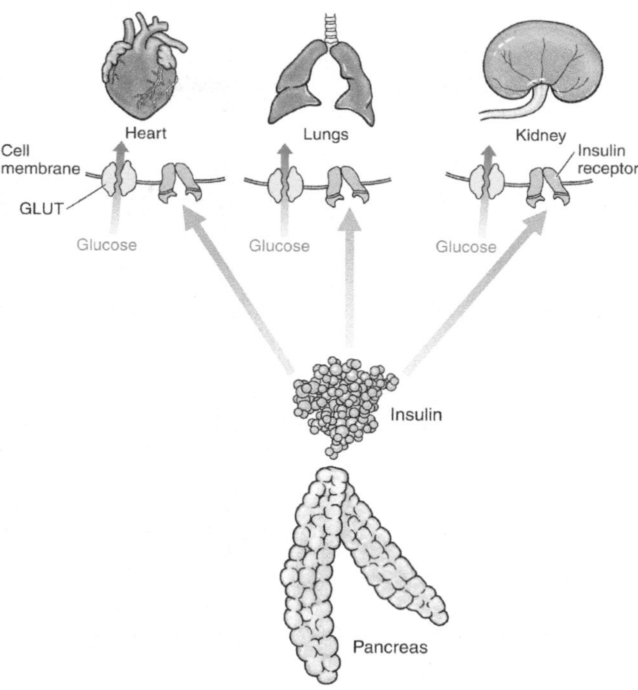

FIGURE 24-2 Normal physiology of glucose metabolism; beta islet cells of pancreas produce and secrete insulin, insulin binds to insulin receptors at cells of organs around body (e.g., heart, lungs, kidney), which increases the number of plasma membrane glucose transporters (GLUTs). GLUTs enable glucose uptake by cells.

With insulin deficiency or lack of insulin receptivity, cells become deprived of glucose; glucose remains in the bloodstream; and, once the renal threshold is reached, glucose spills into the urine. Because cells are deprived of glucose, negative feedback from the cells drives appetite, resulting in polyphagia, but insofar as there is reduced cellular metabolism, concurrent weight loss also results. Weight loss is also contributed to by muscle and protein catabolism to provide substrates for gluconeogenesis. Glycosuria results in osmotic loss of water from the kidneys, so polyuria occurs. To maintain hydration the animal has a compensatory polydipsia. Because there is less cellular recognition of glucose, another negative feedback mechanism stimulates gluconeogenesis in the liver. Ketones are a by-product of gluconeogenesis, and there is a resultant increase in ketone concentrations in the blood and urine. However, ketones can create nausea and, paradoxically, make the animal inappetent.

Type 1 DM is due to lack of insulin (Figure 24-3). It is rarely described in cats. It is most often associated with

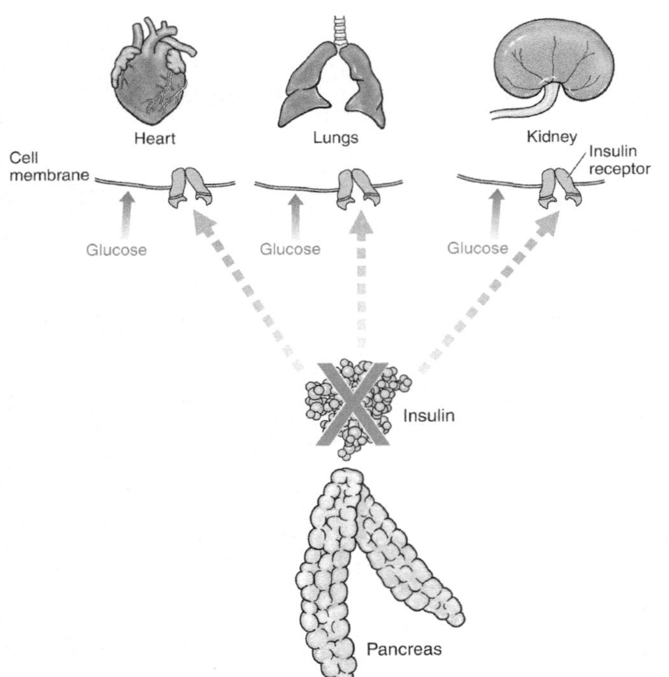

FIGURE 24-3 Type 1 diabetes mellitus, rarely described in cats; lack of production of insulin results in reduced number of plasma membrane glucose transporters (GLUTs). Fewer GLUTs means that glucose is less able to enter cells.

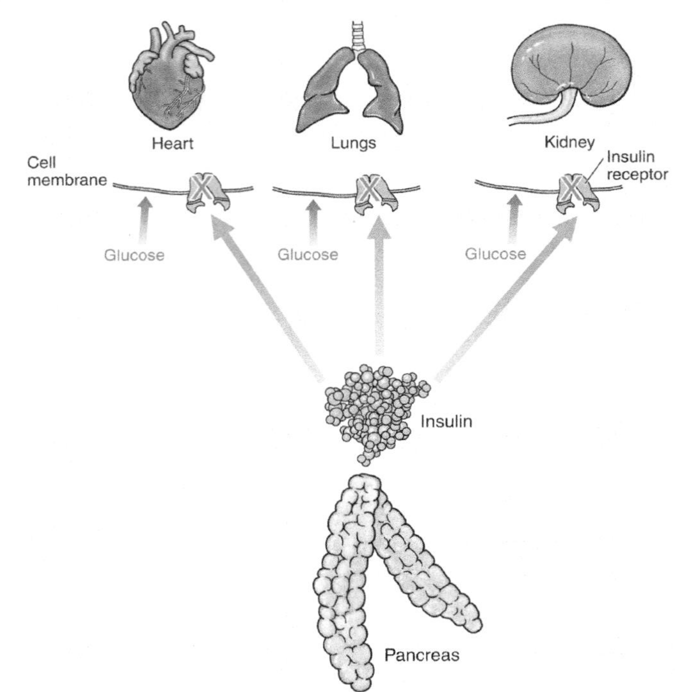

FIGURE 24-4 Type 2 diabetes mellitus is instigated by insulin resistance. The insulin receptor processes do not function appropriately, so fewer plasma membrane glucose transporters (GLUTs) are formed. Fewer GLUTs means that glucose is less able to enter cells. The body initially responds by producing more insulin. Chronic hyperfunction of the beta islet cells contributes to their eventual failure and the inability to secrete sufficient insulin.

immune-mediated destruction of beta islet cells but has also been described with exocrine pancreatic insufficiency.[107,118,131] Type 2 DM is far more common in cats.[94] The initiating factor is insulin resistance (Figure 24-4). This may be associated with decreased number of insulin receptors,[110] reduced receptor activity,[115] direct effect on GLUT4,[9] or a combination of factors. Initially, the body responds by producing more insulin. This chronic hyperfunction of the beta islet cells contributes to their eventual failure and the inability to secrete sufficient insulin.

Insufficient insulin production may affect potassium metabolism, insofar as insulin allows potassium to enter cells. In DM the lack of insulin or the lack of receptors means that less potassium is able to get into the cells. Hence there is an increase of potassium in the blood, which is cleared by the kidneys, especially with polyuria. Therefore serum/plasma potassium is even less reflective of the total body potassium than usual. In addition, insufficient insulin production may affect lipoprotein lipase (LPL) activity. LPL works in conjunction with insulin in fatty acid metabolism. The reduced LPL activity may be significant enough to result in lipemia. The lipemia may be due to triglycerides (TGs) or cholesterol, but TGs are more governed by chylomicrons (CMs) and very low-density lipoprotein (VLDL), which have more dependence on LPL activity.[127]

Underlying Causes

Pancreatic Factors

Even without any overt exocrine pancreatic dysfunction, diabetic cats produce amylin (an amyloid precursor) that is deposited in islet cells, leading to decreased insulin production. In humans genetic assessments have indicated that many of the genes associated with type 2 diabetes are associated with insulin secretion from beta islet cells.[102] Additionally, exocrine pancreatic disease occurs as a comorbidity with diabetes, and elevated serum feline pancreatic lipase immunoreactivity (fPLI) has been recognized in diabetic cats.[31] Pancreatic diseases such as pancreatitis, pancreatic adenocarcinoma,[94] and genetic associations may play a role.[61]

Peripheral Factors

DM arises as a consequence of complex interactions of both pancreatic and multiple peripheral factors in any individual. The most common peripheral causes cited are age, gender, and breed predispositions as well as obesity, dietary carbohydrates, corticosteroid administration, and concurrent conditions such as infection.

Epidemiologic studies in cats consistently show DM to be a disease of older cats, with the incidence increasing markedly in cats over the age of 8 years.[5,89,93,95] Age associations with insulin resistance are controversial in people with discordant results, most likely because of general health, physical training, and changes in liver size.[10,28] Multiple studies have indicated increased insulin resistance in male cats (in particular after neutering) that is consistent with the overrepresentation of males among diabetic cats.[3,44,46]

There are now several studies indicating that Burmese are more at risk of DM than other cats in Australia, New Zealand, and the United Kingdom.* Breed predispositions are likely to be analogous to the situation for humans, wherein DM is more prevalent in various indigenous groups such as Australian Aborigines, African Americans, and Pima Indians.[17,55,67] Genetic studies in humans have identified 20 common genetic variants associated with type 2 diabetes. Most of these genes are associated with regulation of insulin secretion from beta islet cells in response to insulin resistance, but there are also genes related to glucose transport and insulin sensitivity. Many associated genes have unknown roles. In most instances multiple genes are affected in individuals.[102] The increasing availability of genome-wide assessments will make searches for specific genes easier in cats, but the complex interactions of multiple genes in humans may make interpretation more difficult in cats, wherein the number of cases assessed will be far less than in studies of people.

Obesity has been directly related to insulin resistance in cats as well as humans[3,9] and specifically reduces GLUT4 expression.[9] Other consequences of obesity in people, such as decreased insulin signaling and glucose disposal rates,[63] are also likely to be relevant in cats. For obesity (and insulin resistance generally) to be associated with type 2 diabetes, the beta islet cells must be unable to compensate fully for the decreased insulin sensitivity.[63] Weight loss is therefore an important component of diabetes management.

In comparison to most mammals, cats have very low hepatic activity of the enzyme glucokinase, which plays the important role of acting as a "glucose sensor." Cats are able to compensate by having elevated levels of glucose 6-phosphate. This altered glucose-sensing pathway in the feline liver may represent an evolutionary adaptation to a low-carbohydrate diet.[43] These changes create challenges for all cats to handle the high glucose loads provided by high-carbohydrate diets and, if coupled with insulin resistance (from any cause), can result in diabetes. Recent studies have demonstrated improved remission rates when cats are fed low-carbohydrate/high-protein diets compared with high-fiber diets.[7,32,76]

Specific infections in people (e.g., hepatitis C) have been correlated with insulin resistance,[47] although the reasons for the associations are not elucidated. Additionally, tumor necrosis factor-alpha (TNF-alpha), a cytokine involved in systemic inflammation and the regulation of immune cells, has been demonstrated to play a role in the pathophysiology of insulin resistance.[8] Managing underlying infections is an important component of reducing insulin resistance. Azotemia associated with renal disease[18] and hyperthyroidism,[50] both common diseases in older cats, have also been demonstrated to contribute to insulin resistance. Management of concurrent conditions can therefore aid diabetic control.

Glucocorticoids impair insulin-dependent glucose uptake by peripheral cells and enhance hepatic gluconeogenesis as well as inhibiting insulin secretion from beta islet cells.[2] A recent study found that high doses of corticosteroids increased serum glucose in all 14 study cats assessed, but clinical signs were seen in only one cat.[68]

Catecholamines and a number of other hormones released during stress states contribute to the development of hyperglycemia by directly stimulating glucose production and interfering with tissue disposal of glucose. In a normal individual hyperglycemia stimulates the secretion of insulin and inhibits the secretion of glucagon, effects that will diminish the degree of hyperglycemia resulting from direct actions of stress hormones on glucose production and disposal. Cats with impaired islet responses to glucose will be particularly prone to the development of marked hyperglycemia during stress states because they may be unable to respond to the influence of hyperglycemia.[39]

Hyperglycemia itself suppresses the insulin response in three distinct ways that relate to chronicity of hyperglycemia:

1. Glucose desensitization: a normal physiologic response that is a rapid and reversible refractoriness of beta cells after short exposure to hyperglycemia
2. Beta cell exhaustion: a reversible depletion of the readily releasable pool of intracellular insulin caused by more prolonged hyperglycemia
3. Glucotoxicity: the slow and progressively irreversible direct toxicity of the beta cells induced by chronic hyperglycemia through functional change and cell death

A continuum exists between beta cell exhaustion and glucotoxicity in that the changes are reversible until a particular point in time.[92]

Treatment Principles

It was not so long ago that the principle aims of therapy for diabetic cats were simply to control hyperglycemia safely (reduce the chance of ketosis) and resolve clinical signs of disease (e.g., polyuria, polydipsia, weight loss). Now the aim is to induce diabetic remission for as long as possible. Clinicians have better

*References 5, 62, 77, 95, 114, 121.

tools than ever (e.g., improved insulin and dietary therapy, home monitoring techniques) to achieve this more stringent goal. However, it must not be forgotten that successful treatment of DM includes an assessment of impact on quality of life for both cat and owner. Owners that perceive the treatment will have a negative impact on quality of life may be more likely to choose euthanasia over treatment.

Recently, a series of 29 specific DM-associated questions centered on both owner and animal were designed as a quality-of-life tool for diabetic cats. The tool was tested with 221 owners of diabetic cats predominantly in the United States and the United Kingdom, about half of whom performed home BG measurements. Nine of the top 10 items judged by owners to have negative impact were related to their own quality of life rather than that of the cat. These were issues such as difficulty boarding the cat, difficulty leaving the cat with family or friends, worry about the disease, worry about hypoglycemia, and changes to work and social life.[86]

In a review of the pathophysiologic factors of type 2 DM detailed in the previous section, those factors that are unable to be influenced can be struck off, leaving those that should be addressed:

- Pancreatic factors
  - Reduced insulin
- Peripheral factors:
  - ~~Age predispositions~~
  - ~~Sex predispositions~~
  - ~~Breed predispositions~~
  - Obesity
  - High-carbohydrate diet
  - Underlying infection
  - Corticosteroid usage
  - Concurrent conditions (e.g., azotemia, hyperthyroidism)

Therefore management of the diabetic cat should be a multipronged approach incorporating insulin, dietary therapy (to reduce carbohydrate load and induce weight loss if the cat is overweight), weaning off corticosteroids when possible, and management of any infection or concurrent condition. If peripheral insulin resistance factors can be overcome, the cat may be weaned from insulin *as long as the beta islet cells have not suffered irreversible damage from chronic glucotoxicity.* With early intervention and good glycemic control, diabetic remission was achieved in 84% to 100% of cats in two recent studies.[73,104] Loss of control of peripheral factors such as a return to a high-carbohydrate diet, recurrence of obesity, or azotemia may result in a return to an insulin-dependent state.

Two recent studies have looked at factors associated with an increased chance of achieving remission. In one questionnaire-based study of owners of diabetic cats treated with glargine insulin participating in an Internet forum, strict glycemic control, administration of corticosteroids before diagnosis, and absence of polyneuropathy were more likely in cats that achieved remission. Factors that were not useful predictors of remission included age, sex, body weight, and presence of chronic renal disease or hyperthyroidism. Cats that achieved remission had a lower mean maximum insulin dose (0.43 U/kg, every 12 hours) than cats that did not achieve remission (0.66 U/kg, every 12 hours).[104]

In another study of 90 cats with newly diagnosed diabetes, 50% of cats achieved remission after a median time of 48 days. The maintenance insulin was glargine for 47% of cats and protamine zinc insulin (PZI) for 53% of cats. The median duration of remission was 151 days for cats still alive at the end of the study. Insulin was resumed in 29% of cats that had achieved remission, but six of the cats achieving remission did not require insulin again for more than 1000 days. In this study age and cholesterol levels were predictive of remission in multivariate analysis. Increased serum cholesterol decreased the chance of remission by about 65%. For each year of age, the chance of remission increased by approximately 25%. Duration of remission was longer with higher body weight and shorter with higher serum glucose. Cats treated with glargine insulin had an increased chance of remission based on univariate analysis.[135]

Specifics of Treatment in the "Well" Cat with Diabetes Mellitus

Insulin therapy and dietary management are the mainstays for management of the basically "well" cat with DM that is not anorexic. The importance of weaning off corticosteroids when possible and management of any underlying infections or concurrent diseases should not be underestimated, but they are not specific to diabetic management.

Insulin Therapy

Insulin therapy provides the most effective and reliable means of achieving glycemic control in diabetic cats. The sooner glycemic control is reached, the higher the likelihood that diabetic remission can be achieved. A variety of insulin types can be used in cats for maintenance insulin therapy. It is difficult to predict in advance which cats will do better with which insulin, so the clinician must be knowledgeable about the insulin choices for treatment of feline diabetes. Although there are guidelines for choosing the starting dose of insulin for cats, the appropriate maintenance dose for each patient will be the dose that controls clinical signs and hyperglycemia. Most cats require twice-daily administration, regardless of the type of insulin selected. Because of the

TABLE 24-2 **Characteristics of Insulins Commonly Used to Treat Feline Diabetes Mellitus**

Insulin	Licensed in Cats	Manufacturer	Formulation	Action	Dose*
ProZinc	Yes	Boehringer Ingelheim Vetmedica	U40 recombinant PZI	Nadir 5-7 hours Duration 8-9 hours	Start 0.25-0.5U/kg, every 12 hours; Median maintenance dose 0.6 U/kg, every 12 hours
Vetsulin, Caninsulin	Yes	Intervet/Schering Plough	U40 Porcine zinc	Nadir 4 hours Duration 8-12 hours	Start 0.25-0.5 U/kg, every 12 hours; Median maintenance dose 0.5 U/kg, every 12 hours
Lantus	No	Sanofi Aventis	U100 Insulin glargine (recombinant human analog)	Nadir and duration not determined in diabetic cats	Start 0.25-0.50 U/kg, every 12 hours Median maintenance dose 2.5 U/cat, every 12 hours
Levemir	No	Novo Nordisk	U100 Insulin detemir (recombinant human analog)	Nadir and duration not determined in diabetic cats	Start 0.25-0.50 U/kg, every 12 hours Median maintenance dose 1.75 U/cat, every 12 hours

*Based on lean body weight.

unpredictability of the individual response to different insulins, it is important to be conservative when selecting insulin doses, either initially or when switching a cat from one type of insulin to another.

It is critical for veterinary staff and owners to be aware of the concentration of the insulin being used for a given patient and to use the correct syringes for the insulin to prevent dosing error. Most human insulins are 100 units/mL (U100), and micro-fine or ultra-fine U100 syringes should be used. Because cats often require very small doses of insulin, many owners find it helpful to use 3/10 cc (0.3 mL) syringes for U100 insulins. However, Caninsulin/Vetsulin and ProZinc are U40 insulin, and U40 syringes must be used. U40 insulins are often more suitable than U100 insulins for administration of the small doses that diabetic cats require.

The types of insulins most commonly used in cats can be summarized as follows (Table 24-2):

Long-acting insulins:
- Glargine (Lantus, Sanofi Aventis)
- Detemir (Levemir, Novo Nordisk)
- Protamine Zinc Insulin (ProZinc, Boehringer Ingelheim Vetmedica)

Intermediate-duration insulins:
- Porcine Lente (Vetsulin or Caninsulin, Intervet Schering Plough)
- Neutral Protamine Hagedorn (NPH; e.g., Humulin-N, Eli Lilly or Novolin-N, Novo Nordisk)

Rapidly acting, soluble insulin will be discussed below with therapy of diabetic ketoacidosis.

PZI-Vet (IDEXX Pharmaceuticals, Inc.), a 90% beef/10% pork U40 insulin, was commonly used in cats but is no longer commercially available because of the lack of a U.S. Food and Drug Administration–approved source of bovine pancreas. Compounded PZI cannot be recommended because the potency varies from batch to batch, making long-term regulation difficult. A replacement product based on recombinant human PZI insulin was developed and approved for cats as ProZinc (Boehringer Ingelheim Vetmedica) in 2009. One study that compared recombinant PZI (PZI-R, now sold as ProZinc) to PZI-Vet was conducted in six private feline specialty clinics. A total of 50 cats with DM and stable glycemic control on PZI-Vet (for at least 90 days) were switched to PZI-R for 30 days at the same dose rate and interval. In the 47 cats completing the study, there were no significant differences in body weight or serum fructosamine concentrations at days 15 or 30 compared with day 0. The researchers concluded that PZI-R provides glycemic control that is comparable to that of PZI-Vet when used at the same dose and dosing interval.[87]

A prospective, uncontrolled 45-day clinical trial evaluating the efficacy of PZI-R (ProZinc) for controlling glycemia in cats with newly diagnosed, untreated diabetes (n = 120) and cats with previously treated, poorly controlled diabetes (n = 13) was also published recently. Treatment was started at 1 to 3 U/cat every 12 hours (0.22 to 0.66 U/kg every 12 hours), and the dose was adjusted at re-evaluations on the basis of the history and results of physical examination, body weight, and BG curves. Feeding the same diet to all cats was not attempted, although most cats were fed a high-protein/low-carbohydrate diet. The mean time of BG nadir was between 5 and 7 hours, and subsequent BG concentrations were rising in most cats by 9 hours after administration. By day 45 the owner's subjective assessment of polyuria and polydipsia had improved in 79% of cats; 89% of cats had good body weight; and 9-hour mean BG concentration, serum fructosamine concentration, or both had improved in 84% of the cats compared with day 0. Biochemical hypoglycemia (BG less than 4.4 mmol/L [80 mg/dL]) occurred at least once in 64% of cats, and clinical signs of hypoglycemia were confirmed in two cats.[83]

Vetsulin/Caninsulin, a porcine lente insulin, is a mixed insulin zinc suspension containing 30% amorphous zinc insulin (which is rapidly absorbed and has a short duration of activity) and 70% crystalline zinc insulin (which is absorbed more slowly and has a longer duration of activity). The onset and duration of action are shorter than that of PZI in cats, with a BG nadir at about 4 hours after injection, and a duration of about 8 to 12 hours.[72,74]

A 12-month prospective study of Vetsulin/Caninsulin was conducted with 25 cats, most of which were newly diagnosed (n = 15), whereas the remainder were poorly controlled on other therapies. Cats with BG over 19 mmol/L (over 342 mg/dL) were started at 0.5 U/kg every 12 hours and cats with BG less than 19 mmol/L (less than 342 mg/dL) were started at 0.25 U/kg every 12 hours. No specific diet was fed. After an initial 6-day examination period, the cats were re-examined at 4, 8, 12, 26, and 52 weeks. Increases in insulin dose were made as needed, with a target BG nadir of 5 to 9 mmol/L (90 to 162 mg/dL). The median insulin dose was 0.5 U/kg every 12 hours (range 0.1 to 1.9 U/kg every 12 hours), and only two cats required doses higher than 1 U/kg every 12 hours. During the study period seven cats went into remission within 15 weeks, and none relapsed during the 12 months. Of the 18 cats that did not go into remission, 13 reached the water intake target established for ideal diabetic control (less than 20 mL/kg per day for canned diets, less than 70 mL/kg per day for dry diets). The control of clinical signs in the cats that did not achieve remission was deemed either excellent or good. It took approximately 3 months for significant resolution of clinical signs.[75]

Another recent prospective, multicenter, nonblinded, open study followed 46 cats with diabetes (either newly diagnosed [n = 39], or previously treated but poorly controlled [n = 7]) during treatment with Vetsulin/Caninsulin. The cats were monitored for about 16 weeks (stabilization phase), with additional monitoring of some cats (n = 23) for a variable period. The starting dose for each cat was based on the initial BG concentration: 0.25 U/kg if the BG was less than 20 mmol/L (360 mg/dL), and 0.5 U/kg if greater than 20 mmol/L (360 mg/dL). The maximum starting dose did not exceed 2 U/dose, and dose rates greater than 0.5 U/kg twice daily were not recommended during the first 3 weeks of treatment. No specific diet was used for all cats. At the end of the stabilization phase, 15% of cats achieved clinical remission. None of these cats had been treated previously for diabetes. Approximately 60% of the remaining cats were clinically stable after 3 to 4 months of treatment, a finding in line with studies published previously using a variety of insulins. Clinical signs of hypoglycemia were observed in nine cats during the stabilization period and were significantly associated with a dose of 3 U/cat or over 0.5 U/kg administered every 12 hours.[79]

PZI and lente insulins, when administered twice daily, resulted in marked hyperglycemia (>18 mmol/L, 324 mg/dL) for several hours before each insulin injection in one study using nine healthy cats.[72] The continued (though intermittent) hyperglycemia of such therapy most likely contributes to continued glucotoxic effects of permanently damaging beta islet cells and would explain why higher remission rates have been seen with glargine[73,104] and detemir.[106]

Glargine is a genetically engineered human insulin analog that has hormonal action identical to native insulin. When glargine is injected, it precipitates because of a pH change and forms microcrystals, which cause sustained release of the product. In humans glargine achieves long-lasting glycemic control and minimizes fluctuations in BG concentrations.

The recommended starting dose of glargine is 0.25 U/kg every 12 hours for cats with BG less than 20 mmol/L (less than 360 mg/dL), and 0.50 U/kg every 12 hours when the BG is over 20 mmol/L (over 360 mg/dL). One study in nine healthy cats showed that the nadir with glargine occurs approximately 12 to 16 hours after injection,[72] whereas another study in five healthy cats using a euglycemic clamp showed the peak effect occurred between 2 and 9.75 hours.[33] Although it may appear that there is a discrepancy in reported time to peak action for glargine, it is likely a result of the very different study designs and different parameters each study used to define time to peak insulin action (nadir versus maximal glucose infusion rate). Put simply, the first study reported the time that nadir glucose occurred (based on actual BG concentration), whereas the second study reported the time of peak glucose infusion rate (to maintain normoglycemia). Further, these studies were performed with small numbers of healthy cats, and whether a similar response would be seen in diabetic cats is unknown. Individual cats with a glargine nadir after 12 hours may achieve adequate glycemic control with once-daily dosing, but twice-daily dosing is associated with better glycemic control and higher remission rates.[73,124] Hence twice-daily dosing is recommended for most cats.

Detemir is an insulin analog that binds to albumin and is released slowly for a long duration of action. On the basis of studies by the manufacturer in humans, variations in BG with detemir may be even less pronounced than with glargine. The duration of action and peak effect of detemir and glargine were evaluated in a study of five healthy cats. Definitive conclusions are hard to reach with small numbers of healthy cats, but the authors assessed that although glargine has a more rapid peak effect than detemir, it was more variable from cat to cat than detemir (glargine: 120 to 585 minutes; detemir: 370 to 575 minutes). The duration of action was longer for detemir in three cats but longer for glargine in two cats.[33]

It is important not to mix or dilute detemir or glargine insulin because the duration of action depends on the pH of the product. Glargine (Lantus) is available in 10-mL vials and a 3-mL SoloSTAR pen that measures in 1-unit increments. However, the pen is expensive, cannot be refrigerated, and expires in 1 month. The cartridges for the pen can be dispensed to be used as individual 3-mL vials. If refrigerated, open vials of glargine or detemir can be used for approximately 6 months.[96] Detemir is available in 10-mL vials and a 3-mL FlexPen that measures in 1-unit increments. Once in use, the FlexPen is stored at room temperature and expires in 42 days. These insulins should be clear and colorless; if cloudiness, discoloration, or clumping is noted, the product should be discarded. It is not necessary to shake or rotate the vial before use. Glargine and detemir are not licensed for use in veterinary patients.

Two studies with the same protocols, except varying insulin type, found similar remission rates for glargine (84%)[104] and detemir (81%)[106] in diabetic cats starting therapy within 6 months of diagnosis. Remission rates were much lower if insulin therapy was started more than 6 months after diagnosis. The insulins were administered twice daily, and a low-carbohydrate diet was fed. Median time to remission was 1.7 months for cats receiving detemir and 1.9 months for cats receiving glargine. Most of the cats achieving remission were able to stay off insulin, and the median duration of remission was 10.8 months for glargine and 1 year for detemir. Although biochemical hypoglycemia was common, clinical hypoglycemia was rare, with only a single event with mild signs in one cat on each insulin. The median detemir dose was 1.75 U/cat every 12 hours, and the median glargine dose was 2.5 U/cat every 12 hours.

A direct comparison of insulin therapies in 24 newly diagnosed diabetic cats found remission rates were higher in those cats receiving glargine (100%) than PZI (38%) and lente insulin (25%) during the 16-week study period.[73] The initial dose of insulin was 0.5 U/kg ideal body weight if the BG on admission was greater than or equal to 360 mg/dL (20 mmol/L), and 0.25 U/kg if BG was less than 20 mmol/L (360 mg/dL). BG was measured every 2 hours for 12 hours for each cat for the first 3 days of treatment to ensure that cats did not become hypoglycemic. No increase in insulin dose was made during the first 3 days, even if persistent hyperglycemia was present. During the study two cats treated with lente insulin and one cat treated with PZI had severe clinical hypoglycemia requiring intravenous glucose therapy. None of the glargine-treated cats exhibited signs of hypoglycemia, although many had biochemical hypoglycemia (BG less than 3 mmol/L [less than 54 mg/dL]) without clinical signs. By 16 weeks all eight cats in the glargine group had achieved remission, whereas two of eight cats in the porcine lente group and three of eight cats in the PZI group had achieved remission. The probability of remission in newly diagnosed patients fed a low-carbohydrate/high-protein diet was significantly greater for cats treated with glargine than cats treated with PZI or lente in this study.

One 12-week study of 13 diabetic cats found no significant difference in remission rates in cats receiving lente insulin (three of seven, 43%) compared to glargine (one of six, 17%). However, approximately half the cats enrolled in this study were not newly diagnosed with diabetes, cats received glargine only once daily but lente insulin twice daily, and monitoring was only every 4 weeks (after the initial 4 weeks).[124]

The findings of these studies indicate that the greatest chance of achieving diabetic remission is prompt initiation of therapy with glargine or detemir insulin twice daily combined with dietary therapy and intensive monitoring to enable dose adjustments. However, remission has been achieved with all of the insulin types previously listed, and clinicians should become familiar with the usage of more than one type of insulin for feline patients. In countries where a legal obligation exists to use a product with a veterinary license first, PZI would be the first choice, if available, and porcine lente would be the second choice. Many factors must be considered when choosing insulin, such as product availability and affordability, convenience and ease of dosing, legal and licensing issues, and product support. In general, clinicians can expect good product support when using veterinary-licensed products in cats but no product support when using products licensed for use in human medicine.

INSULIN DOSING AND MONITORING PROTOCOLS

Managing diabetic cats with insulin with the objective of diabetic remission is a balancing act requiring sufficient insulin for glycemic control without causing hypoglycemia. The recommended starting dose for most insulins is 0.25 U/kg to 0.5 U/kg, with higher doses preferred for those cats with higher BG (more than 20 mmol/L [360mg/dL]) recognized at diagnosis.[71,104,106] Frequent re-evaluations are required during the initial stabilization period, as outlined later and in Box 24-1. Typically, most cats first go through a phase where insulin dose is increasing, then stabilize when insulin dose is consistent, and then for cats achieving remission, a phase of decreasing insulin dose.

BOX 24-1

Suggested Treatment and Management Protocol for Cats with Nonketotic Diabetes Mellitus

At diagnosis

- Evaluate for concurrent diseases with minimum database (complete blood count, serum biochemistry profile, urinalysis, urine culture, total T_4, feline pancreatic lipase immunoreactivity).
- Hospitalize for 1 day to begin insulin therapy; measure blood glucose every 3-4 hours, monitor for hypoglycemia.
- Consultation with owner to demonstrate insulin handling and injection techniques, discharge with written instructions on diet, monitoring for hypoglycemia, monitoring appetite and water intake, and so on. Introduce the concept of home blood glucose monitoring.

Three days later (this step not necessary for Lente insulin).

- Hospitalize for 1 day; measure blood glucose every 3-4 hours, and monitor for hypoglycemia.
- Consult with owner to confirm insulin handling and injection techniques.

One week later

- Re-evaluate body weight and condition, and perform full physical examination.
- Hospitalize to perform blood glucose curve, and adjust insulin dose as needed; preferably use the same portable blood glucose meter that the owners would eventually use at home, and validate by comparison to in-hospital chemistry analyzer.
- Consult with owner on home management of diet, and identify and correct any problems with insulin administration.

Repeat weekly in hospital blood glucose curves.

- Until owner feels confident to perform at home (can show owner each week)
- *Or* until appropriate nadir is achieved
- Confirm appropriate nadir 1 month later.

One month later

- Re-evaluate body weight and condition, and perform full physical examination.
- Hospitalize to perform blood glucose curve, and adjust insulin dose as needed.
- Consult with owner on any problems encountered with home care or monitoring.
- Discuss home blood glucose monitoring; demonstrate techniques, and provide supplies and written instructions.

Home monitoring

- Owner performs 12-hour blood glucose curve weekly until stabilized and telephones hospital to provide results.

Three months later and every 3 months subsequently

- Re-evaluate body weight and condition, and perform full physical examination.
- Evaluate home monitoring, including blood glucose measurements.
- Hospitalize for blood glucose curve.
- Compare hospital blood glucose curve and home blood glucose curve.
- Make insulin dose adjustments as required.
- Make adjustments to dietary therapy as required.
- Owner performs home blood glucose curve once monthly.
- Periodically repeat minimum database.

In human medicine, specialized educators provide most of the information on disease management, insulin injection and handling, BG monitoring, and so forth. In the veterinary setting this function is performed by the veterinarian or often by the veterinary nurse/technician. Owners must be properly trained to give insulin injections and educated on the important aspects of the disease in cats. For example, if some of the insulin dose is spilled during injection, the owner should be warned not to give additional insulin to avoid overdose. Whenever there is uncertainty about whether a dose has been administered, it is safest to wait until the next scheduled dose, because the consequences of missing one dose are negligible. Close contact with owners during the initial weeks of insulin therapy can help identify and correct any problems or misconceptions.

The owner and all members of the household should be aware of the clinical signs of hypoglycemia, which include lethargy, trembling, ataxia, altered mentation, seizures, and coma. If signs suspected to be caused by hypoglycemia are noted at home, the owner should be instructed to give high glucose syrup orally. Suitable products are marketed for use by human diabetics. If the cat is unable to swallow, the syrup can be rubbed on the oral mucosa. When an episode of hypoglycemia occurs or is suspected, the owner should also seek veterinary care and discontinue insulin dosing in the meantime.

It is the authors' experience that hypoglycemia is rare initially, and if it is recognized biochemically within the first few days of therapy, there is a very low probability of clinical signs. Starting most diabetic cats at 0.5 U/kg increases the chance of establishing timely glycemic control. However, starting a cat on this dose of insulin requires close monitoring from day 1. When glargine was first introduced to management of feline diabetes, initial protocols called for BG testing every 4 hours for each of the first 3 days and then weekly.[71] It is usually more practical to perform BG curves on day 1 and day 3. Long-acting insulins are marketed in human medicine as being peakless; this is not the case (at the very least in cats),[72] and *"spot" checks of BG are not adequate or appropriate to maintain glycemic control of diabetic cats*. Serial BG measurements (BG curves) are the most effective monitoring technique to establish what is happening with the cat's glucose homeostasis. Fructosamine assays are a crude measure reflecting the mean BG concentration for approximately the past week (compared with longer time periods in other species)[64] and are not an effective measure for tight management of glycemic control. High serum fructosamine concentrations indicate poor glycemic control but give no information about the nadir BG concentration and cannot be used to determine whether the insulin dose must be increased or decreased. In addition, some disease states, such as hyperthyroidism, affect fructosamine concentrations. Cats with overt, uncontrolled hyperthyroidism may have fructosamine concentrations below the normal range, probably as a result of metabolic changes.[101]

There is no uniformly recognized BG monitoring protocol for diabetic cats. High remission rates have been achieved with weekly in-hospital monitoring of BG curves (stretching to every 2 weeks after 4 weeks)[73] as well as with home monitoring up to daily and insulin dose changes instituted as often as every 3 days.[104,106] The following schedule is suggested for BG monitoring either at home or in the hospital (serial measurements are taken on each day):

Long-acting insulins (see also Box 24-1):

- Day 1 (to monitor for early hypoglycemia)
- Day 3
- Day 10 (1 week later)
- Weekly until appropriate nadir (can be twice a week if monitored at home)
- Then confirm 1 week later
- 1 month later
- If monitored at home, once monthly
- In-hospital evaluation every 3 months for all cats (including those monitored at home)

BG can be evaluated every 3 to 4 hours. After an owner obtains a BG curve at home, especially during the stabilization period, the results should be reported to the clinician or veterinary nurse/technician. An appropriate BG curve for a stable diabetic cat being treating with long-acting insulin (e.g., glargine or detemir) is shown in Figure 24-5. A cat with a curve similar to the one illustrated needs no dose adjustment. However, cats can have such a curve yet need a dosage reduction (or increase) at a subsequent evaluation. In the early stages of treatment with long-acting insulins, the BG curve may resemble a curve obtained with lente insulin (Figure 24-6) with more distinct peaks but will usually flatten within 2 to 3 weeks. The slow absorption of glargine and detemir can result in atypical shaped curves with elevations of BG in the middle of the day (but this usually only occurs when there is minimal change in BG). Any dose adjustment decisions should be based on the lowest BG level of the day and should always take into account

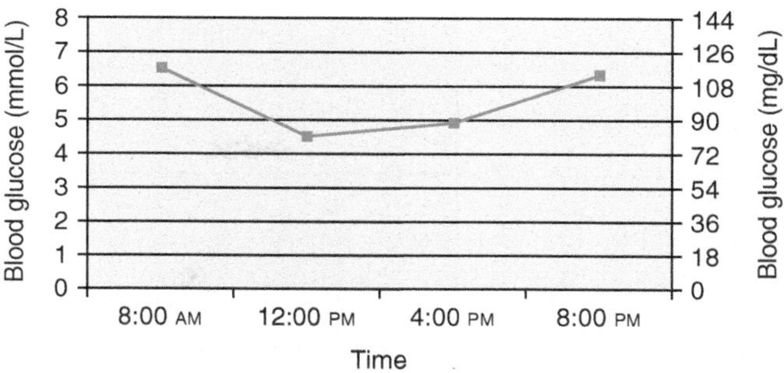

FIGURE 24-5 Ideal blood glucose curve for stable diabetic cat using long-acting insulin (e.g., glargine, detemir). Note that there typically is a nadir, but the variation from preinsulin blood glucose to nadir is not great.

the patient's clinical assessment (e.g., body weight, body condition score, appetite, water intake, and urine output).

Intermediate-acting insulins (e.g., lente) (see Box 24-1):

- Day 1 (to monitor for early hypoglycemia)
- Day 7
- Weekly until appropriate nadir (can be twice a week if monitored at home)
- Then confirm 1 week later
- 1 month later
- Every 3 months

An appropriate curve for a stable diabetic cat being treating with an intermediate-acting insulin (e.g., Vetsulin/Caninsulin or Humulin-N) is shown in Figure 24-6. Note the extended periods of time that BG remains above 15 mmol/L (above 260 mg/dL).

Common sense should be used when making any insulin dose adjustments. Suggested guidelines for dosage adjustments are shown in Table 24-3. Some guidelines for long-acting insulin dose adjustments also include recommendations based on the pre-insulin BG. The reason for monitoring is to assess the effect that particular dose of insulin has had, so changing the dose on the morning of testing defeats that purpose. The exception to this rule is when BG concentration is low before administration of insulin, in which case that dose should be skipped and the dose administered 12 hours later should be lower. As for long-acting insulins, dose adjustments should always take into account the patient's clinical assessment (e.g., body weight, body condition score, appetite, water intake, and urine output).

Once a cat achieves remission, ongoing BG monitoring should continue for the first month. Over the long term, urine glucose, body condition, appetite, and water intake can be monitored to detect loss of euglycemia. If hyperglycemia is detected, insulin therapy should be restarted promptly to avoid further damage to pancreatic beta cells. A low-carbohydrate, calorie-controlled diet often helps prevent obesity, minimize the demand on beta cells, and lower the risk of relapse.

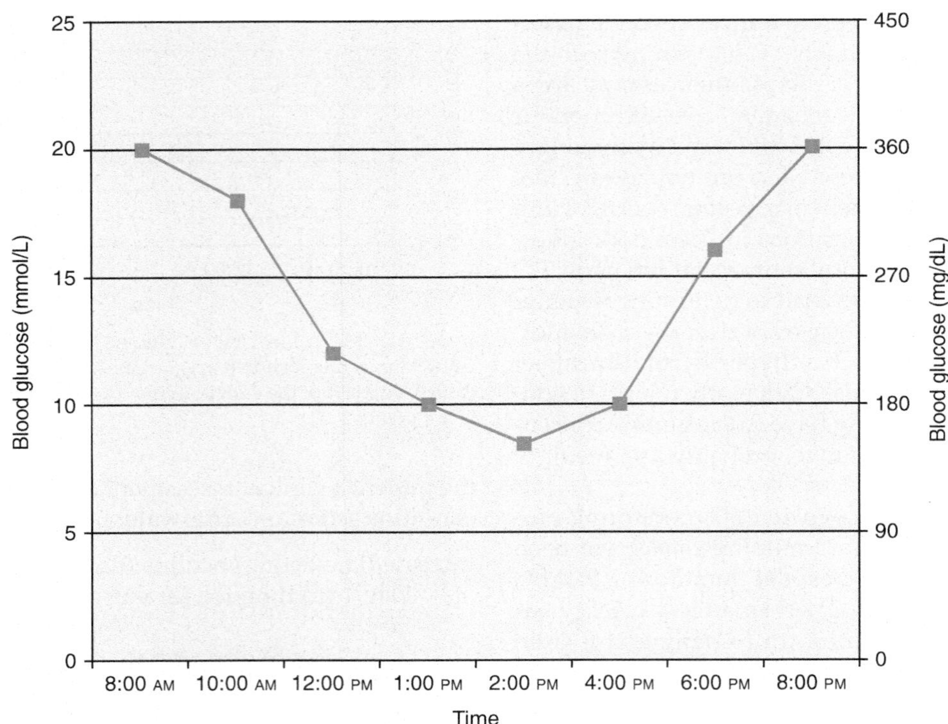

FIGURE 24-6 Ideal blood glucose curve for stable diabetic cat using intermediate-acting insulin (e.g., lente). Note the extended periods of time that blood glucose remains above the renal threshold.

TABLE 24-3 **Suggested Guidelines for Insulin Dose Adjustment Based on Blood Glucose Curve Results**

Insulin Type	Glucose Concentration	Insulin Dose Recommendation
Vetsulin	Nadir <3 mmol/L (54 mg/dL)	Reduce by 50%
Caninsulin	Nadir 3-4.5 mmol/L (54-81 mg/dL)	Reduce by 1 U
	Nadir 4.5-7 mmol/L (81-126 mg/dL)	Reduce by 0.5 U
	Nadir 7-10 mmol/L (126-180 mg/dL)	No change
	Nadir 10-12 mmol/L (180-216 mg/dL)	Increase by 0.5 U
	Nadir >13 mmol/L (234 mg/dL)	Increase by 1 U
	Pre-insulin <12mmol/L (216 mg/dL)	Withhold and check for remission
Lantus	Nadir 4.5-9 mmol/L (81-162 mg/dL)	No change
Levemir	Nadir <4.5 mmol/L (81 mg/dL)	Reduce by 0.5 U
ProZinc	Clinical hypoglycemia	Reduce by 50%
	Pre-insulin <4.5mmol/L (81 mg/dL)	Withhold and check for remission

Adapted from Rand J, Marshall R: Feline diabetes mellitus: which insulin do I choose & how do I adjust the dose? *Proc ACVIM Forum*, 2006; Nelson RW, Henley K, Cole C: Field safety and efficacy of protamine zinc recombinant human insulin for treatment of diabetes mellitus in cats, *J Vet Intern Med* 23:787, 2009; Marshall RD, Rand JS, Morton JM: Treatment of newly diagnosed diabetic cats with glargine insulin improves glycaemic control and results in higher probability of remission than protamine zinc and lente insulins, *J Feline Med Surg* 11:683, 2009.

CHANGING INSULINS

No washout period is needed to change insulin type. The new insulin can be substituted at the next scheduled dose. Recommendations for changing from one product to another for well-regulated cats include the following examples:

- From compounded PZI to ProZinc: Reduce the dose slightly, and perform a BG curve after 1 week and re-evaluate every 1 to 2 weeks until stable.
- From PZI-Vet to ProZinc: No dose adjustment is required; perform a BG curve 1 week later.
- From Vetsulin to ProZinc, Lantus, or Levemir or from PZI to Lantus or Levemir: It is not possible to extrapolate a dose, so the patient must be regulated on the new insulin as for a newly diagnosed patient; it is appropriate to start with 0.5 U/kg every 12 hours for most insulins.

In all cases, if a patient is currently not well regulated, the new insulin should be started at the recommended starting dose for the product and regulated as for a newly diagnosed patient.

GLUCOMETER CHOICE

Handheld glucometers to assess BG at the point of care have become standard in the management of DM in animals as well as humans. Only a limited number of glucometers have been critically assessed in the veterinary literature, with varying results.[15,22,65,125,136] Accuracy is assessed by precision (variation of the individual glucometer for a particular sample) and bias (variation from a reference laboratory measurement). Accuracy is most often poor when very low or very high BG concentrations are measured.

Most glucometers are calibrated for human use. The distribution of glucose between plasma and red blood cells is different in feline blood compared with human blood. Glucometers for human use generally read lower (approximately 1 to 2 mmol/L [18 to 36 mg/dL]) than measurements from an automated chemistry analyzer. To further confuse matters, whole BG (measured with a glucometer) is approximately 10% lower than glycolysis-inhibited plasma glucose ("gray-top" tube samples); also compared with whole BG measurements, serum glucose reduces by approximately 5% to 7% per hour as a result of continued metabolism of glucose by the red blood cells.[97] Even glycolysis inhibitors contained in gray-top blood tubes (e.g., sodium fluoride/potassium oxalate) result in reduced plasma glucose readings when compared with promptly spun serum samples.[122] Additionally, capillary BG measurements can be between 10% and 24% higher than venous whole BG in a nonfasted state.[58] Despite these multiple variations, studies in cats have shown minimal variation between samples obtained from the pinna versus peripheral vein,[117,126] and a further study assessed glucometers by directly comparing capillary pinna samples to venipuncture collected samples.[136]

The highest degree of accuracy among the glucometers tested to date has been shown with the AlphaTRAK glucometer (Abbott Laboratories), one of the few machines calibrated for use in veterinary patients. Although the AlphaTRAK is not as easy to use as human-medicine glucometers, it requires a very small sample volume (0.3 μL) and the test time is only 15 seconds. However, care must be taken with this glucometer insofar as it may be calibrated for canine or feline blood and accuracy is greatly diminished if it is set incorrectly.[136] The Ascencia Elite (Bayer Healthcare) glucometer has also been demonstrated to be accurate[125,136] but reads lower than the AlphaTRAK and reference laboratory samples,[136] which potentially means that lower nadirs will be recognized.[104,106] Other veterinary glucometers include GlucoPet and GlucoVet (Animal Diabetes Management, Janesville, Wisconsin), although they have not been critically assessed as of this writing. Glucometers should be selected carefully for use in practice and owners' use at home, with the clinician and owner having an awareness of the bias of the glucometer compared with laboratory measurements of glucose. Ideally, the clinician would calibrate each glucometer used at home against the hospital's own blood chemistry analyzer or calibrated glucometer.

HOME MONITORING

Home monitoring is often used to refer to monitoring of BG values, but all owners also need to assess how well their cat is eating (either increased or decreased appetite) and drinking and whether its general behavior is normal. Ideally, all diabetic cats would receive daily monitoring at a minimum. The ability to record body weight at home is a very valuable monitoring tool. Owners should be encouraged to buy inexpensive scales suitable for measuring small patients (e.g., scales used to weigh human infants) and to keep a weekly log of body weight.

Most owners of diabetic cats are initially very concerned about their cat's diagnosis, and many are concerned about their ability to use syringes to inject insulin (although most soon find it is easier than giving oral medications to their cats), let alone take BG measurements. Home monitoring of BG is the goal, but clinicians should introduce these concepts to their clients and demonstrate how to obtain blood samples in a stepwise manner during visits in the stabilization period.

Perceived benefits of home BG curves include obtaining samples in a less stressful environment where the cat's food intake should be normal and the ability to perform more frequent BG monitoring. Many owners have the dedication and the ability to perform BG curves at home, but many do not realize this at first and can be intimidated by this prospect. As already noted, success is most likely when additional tasks for the owner of a newly diagnosed diabetic cat are sequentially introduced. Showing owners how to take a BG sample at the same time they are shown how to give an insulin injection for the first time is likely to reduce compliance. Some owners are happy to proceed with sampling their cat's BG after being shown only once; others need reassurance and multiple demonstrations. Common reasons for their initial reluctance to attempt home BG monitoring include fear of hurting the cat, fear of taking a blood sample, and concern over cost and time commitment. Watching an owner perform the procedure allows the clinician to identify and correct problems. Providing reliable and easy to understand educational resources as well as ready access to telephone support is also important.[119] Long-term compliance with home BG monitoring is reportedly good, with 65% of owners performing it regularly in one study. Most owners in that study performed home BG curves every 2 to 4 weeks. Home monitoring provides owners with more confidence in their ability to manage their cat's disease.[54]

Alternatively, some owners become overconfident in their interpretive abilities and will not seek continued veterinary care until dramatic signs arise. It is important for owners to understand that information about protocols used to treat human diabetics cannot be applied to cats. In veterinary medicine, unlike human medicine, the goal in treating diabetes is not normoglycemia, because even some well-controlled diabetics can be at least slightly hyperglycemic at some time during the day.

In one study 12% of owners made changes to their cat's insulin dose without consulting the clinician. Owners should be cautioned against the temptation to make frequent changes to insulin dose and should make changes only after consultation with a veterinarian.[54] Another study found that approximately one fourth of cats had *higher* BG concentrations for 2 to 3 days after a glargine insulin dose increase.[104] The reasons for this are not known but may be associated with a lag time before feedback mechanisms adjust glucose homeostasis. The authors' experience is that the instinct of most owners is to further increase the insulin in this circumstance, sometimes on three consecutive days, which leads to an increased risk of hypoglycemia.

It must be emphasized that management of the diabetic cat is a team effort that includes the owner, the clinician, and often support staff such as veterinary technicians and nurses. Regular re-evaluations should be established to monitor weight and body condition score, look for underlying issues (e.g., dental infection), and confirm BG findings and discuss the owner's findings at home (see Box 24-1). One study has shown that the number of re-evaluations did not differ significantly between cats managed with and without home monitoring.[54] Once glycemic control has been achieved, diabetic cats should be re-evaluated approximately every 3 months.

BG concentrations measured at home have been compared with those measured in hospital in one study; surprisingly, hospital measurements were lower than those obtained at home.[13] This may have been due to inappetence in hospital or stress from the less experienced owner taking the sample at home. In about 40% of cats, the hypothetical treatment decisions based on the two methods of generating BG curves did not agree. Alternatively, it has been demonstrated that BG readings can be significantly higher in hospital (Figure 24-7).[100]

Another study compared paired BG curves generated at home on 2 consecutive days in seven diabetic cats. In the second part of the study, two BG curves generated at home and one BG curve generated in hospital were compared. The results demonstrated considerable day-to-day variation in BG curves, even those obtained at home. The day-to-day variability between the home and hospital BG curves was not larger than between the paired home BG curves. There was less variability in the home BG curves obtained from cats with good glycemic control than from cats with moderate to poor glycemic control. These findings would indicate that a single BG curve may not always be reliable for making treatment decisions, whether performed in the hospital or at home.[1]

In humans variations in BG concentrations occur within a 24-hour period as well as day to day and can be associated with activity level, meal size and type, stress, and some medications. Even when those factors are controlled, other factors, such as varying rates of insulin absorption from different injection sites and variation in length of insulin activity, cause day-to-day variability in BG concentrations. Many of these factors probably play a role in the variability of BG curves in cats as well. In particular, the role of absorption from different injection sites has not been investigated in cats. As more about day-to-day variability in BG measurements in cats becomes known, it is important not to rely solely on BG values but also to take into account the physical examination and other laboratory findings (e.g., weight loss or gain, urine specific gravity) and the owner's observations (e.g., appetite, water intake, activity level) when considering insulin dose adjustments.

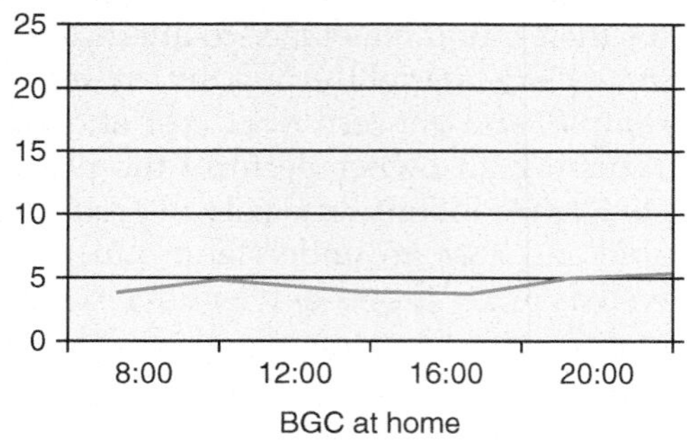

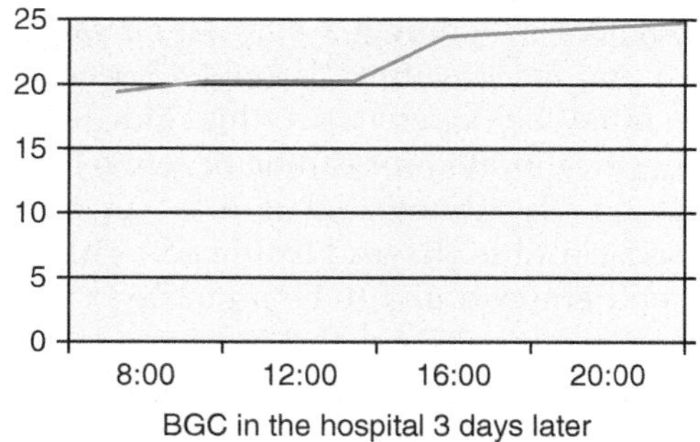

FIGURE 24-7 Blood glucose curve (BGC) at home and in the hospital 3 days later in a cat with diabetes mellitus (spayed female domestic shorthair, 4.7 kg). The cat was diabetic for 1 year and received 0.5 U/cat Caninsulin/Vetsulin every 12 hours at the time when the two curves were generated. According to the owner, the cat was doing well and had no signs of diabetes mellitus. The high blood glucose levels measured in the hospital were assumed to be stress-induced. Insulin dosage was not changed and the cat continued to do well. Blood glucose is noted in mmol/L; to convert to mg/dL, multiply by 18. *(From Reusch C, Kley S, Casella M: Home monitoring of the diabetic cat,* J Feline Med Surg *8:119, 2006.)*

Sites that may be used for home BG sampling are the ear[54,100,126] and the foot pads.[134] The pinnae (either the haired or nonhaired surface) are most commonly used to obtain samples (Figure 24-8). The ear should be warmed by rubbing or holding a heated cotton ball against the ear (the cotton ball can be heated by placing in a standard microwave for 10 seconds). The ear should not be cleaned or disinfected with alcohol. In longhaired cats, it may be helpful to shave a small portion of the pinna to improve visibility or to apply a thin film of petroleum jelly (petrolatum) to prevent the blood from dissipating into the fur. The opposite side of the ear can be stabilized with a cylindrical object, such as a roll of bandage tape. Then a lancet device or a 25-g hypodermic needle (without a syringe attached) can be used just near (but not directly over) the marginal ear vein to produce a blood drop. The test strip of the glucometer is then touched to the drop to absorb blood. While the machine is processing the sample, a piece of gauze or cotton ball can be used to apply pressure to the site to stop bleeding.

The main carpal (or tarsal) foot pads are usually easiest to use for sampling because they are the largest. Again, the pad should be warmed before a lancing device or hypodermic needle is used to prick the pad. Regardless of the site used for sampling, it can be helpful to place the cat in a favorite and comfortable spot for blood collection. The puncture site is usually not painful or visible.

Lancet devices are readily available from most pharmacists, and it is appropriate for the clinicians to have several brands in stock to try on individual cats because cats react differently. Two methods of capillary sampling from the ear have been described.[126] One method, using a conventional lancing device, was evaluated only in dogs but has also been used in cats. Alternatively, a lancing device that uses negative pressure (Ascensia Microlet Vaculance, Bayer Diagnostics) to help ensure a blood drop of adequate size can be used.[99]

As may be expected, certain difficulties are commonly encountered when owners initially begin home BG monitoring, such as the need for assistance to restrain the cat, numerous attempts to produce a blood drop of sufficient size, and resistance from the cat. These difficulties tend to decrease over time as the owner gains experience with the technique.[119]

Continuous glucose monitoring systems have been designed to help human diabetics improve glycemic control and have recently been introduced in veterinary medicine. These devices measure interstitial glucose concentrations through a subcutaneously placed sensor. The sensor and transmitter are secured to the patient's back or side by bandaging. The data are relayed to a monitor that must be placed within several feet of the patient to record readings. Glucose readings are taken every 5 minutes, allowing for a large number of readings

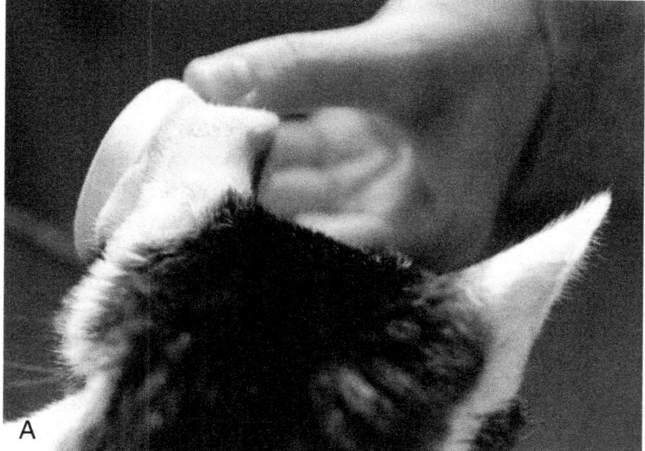

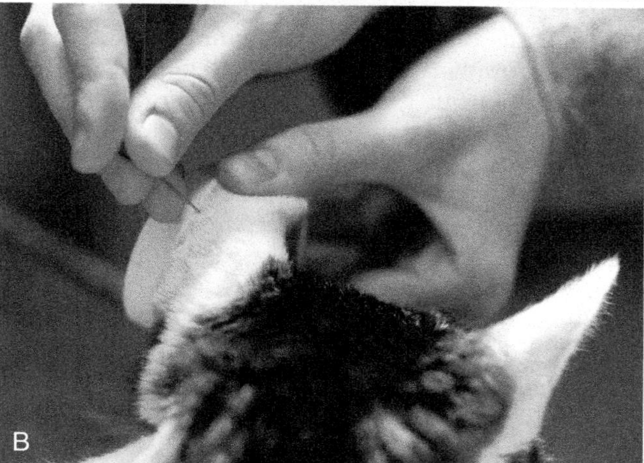

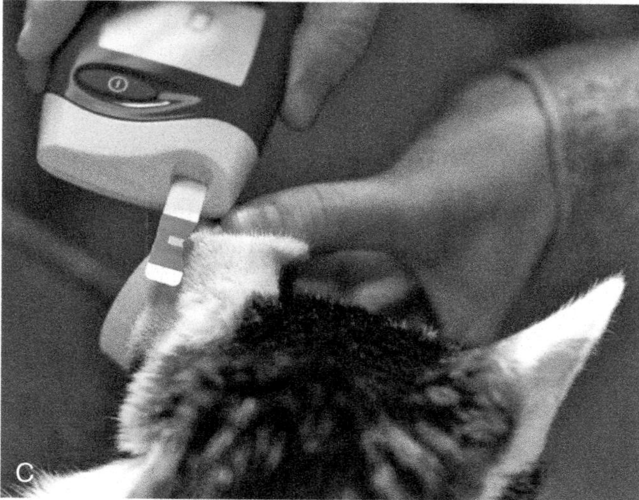

FIGURE 24-8 **A,** The pinnae are commonly used to obtain blood glucose samples. The opposite side of the ear can be stabilized with a cylindrical object, such as a roll of bandage tape. **B,** Then, a lancet device or a 25-g hypodermic needle (without a syringe attached) can be used just near (but not directly over) the marginal ear vein to produce a blood drop. **C,** The test strip of the glucometer is then touched to the drop and to absorb blood.

in a 24-hour period. Validation and use of these devices in cats have been described for both in-hospital and at-home use. Currently, drawbacks include the need for calibration every 12 hours and the need to remove the sensor after 72 hours, as well as the cost.*

Home monitoring urine for glucose and ketones may be an appropriate additional form of monitoring for some patients, particularly management of fractious cats. The main purpose of once- or twice-weekly urine monitoring is detection of uncontrolled hyperglycemia through persistently high urine glucose readings or, conversely, the detection of hypoglycemia through persistently negative urine glucose readings for cats receiving PZI or lente insulin. Persistently negative urine glucose readings may also indicate that diabetic remission is imminent. Negative urine glucose readings are commonly seen in well-controlled cats on glargine or detemir insulin. Owners should be cautioned never to change insulin dose solely on the basis of urine glucose readings.

Glucotest granules (Purina Veterinary Diagnostics) are a litter additive designed to detect glucosuria through a color change. In one study of the Glucotest granules, the glucose concentration was measured accurately in 29 of 48 feline urine samples. Of the inaccurate measurements, most were overestimates in the 2.8 to 16.6 mmol/L (50 to 300 mg/dL) range. Measurements taken at 8 hours were more accurate than immediate measurements. However, the researchers used frozen urine with added glucose rather than urine from diabetic cats, which may affect results.[30]

Urine dipsticks are commonly used to measure glucose as well as other urine chemistries and may be used by owners at home. The accuracy of these sticks for feline urine is not well investigated. The ability of one brand (Bayer Multistix) to detect glucosuria in feline urine was determined by comparison to a chemistry analyzer. Sensitivity (73%), specificity (97%), and positive (73%) and negative (97%) predictive values were calculated. Overall, the accuracy of the test strip for classifying the urine glucose concentration in the correct interval was 91% (compared with 59% in dogs). Inaccuracies tended to be underestimates. The study was performed on urine samples submitted to a laboratory, however, whereas most owners are testing urine voided into a litter box, which may affect results.[6] Well-regulated diabetic cats receiving PZI or lente insulin should have urine glucose readings between trace and 1+, although well-regulated cats on glargine or detemir insulin may have negative or trace readings. Persistent values outside this range should prompt the owner to seek veterinary advice.

Monitoring the fractious diabetic cat is a problem well known to most veterinarians. Fortunately, home BG monitoring can often be performed for these patients, even if they require sedation to obtain BG samples in the hospital. Some difficult-to-handle cats can be restrained enough for safe access to the pinna or the saphenous vein or for placement of a heparinized catheter for repeat blood sampling. Results should be interpreted in light of stress, but it is the author's (RMB) experience that results consistent with clinical signs (and at-home results) can be achieved in most cases in these circumstances. Other tools owners can use for monitoring of these difficult patients include measuring water consumption, monitoring body weight and condition, and measuring urine glucose. Close attention should be paid to appetite, behavior, and so on. Periodic re-evaluation in the hospital, even if sedation is required, should include a full physical examination, serum fructosamine, and minimum database testing (complete blood count, serum chemistries, urinalysis, urine culture, total T_4) as required.

*References 19, 82, 98, 103, 128-130.

Oral Hypoglycemic Agents

Oral treatments for diabetes such as sulfonylurea agents (e.g., glipizide, glyburide) act by stimulating the pancreatic beta cells to produce insulin as well as potentiating insulin action.[60] These agents have been assessed in veterinary practice, with glycemic control reported in as many as 35% of diabetic cats.[26,85] Unfortunately, there are no parameters that predict which cats will respond to sulfonylureas. The intrinsic problem with these agents is that the stimulation of any remaining functional beta islet cells to produce insulin can lead to beta cell exhaustion, which in turn leads to persistent hyperglycemia and possibly irreversible damage to beta cells. In addition, glipizide treatment may cause progressive amyloid deposition. Adverse effects include nausea, vomiting, anorexia, icterus, and elevated liver enzymes.[45]

Oral hypoglycemics have no advantage over insulin therapy in terms of cost, time commitment, or frequency of re-evaluation. However, some owners that are initially unwilling to give insulin injections may be prevented from euthanizing their cat in a forced life-or-death decision when they are given the option of oral treatment. Some of these owners can eventually be persuaded to try insulin therapy. Within these parameters glipizide may be administered orally to nonketotic and otherwise healthy diabetic cats at a starting dose of 2.5 mg/cat, every 12 hours with a meal. If no adverse effects have occurred after 2 weeks of therapy, the oral dose may be increased to 5 mg/cat, every 12 hours.

Diet

Dietary management is an intrinsic part of therapy for diabetic cats (see Box 18-6). Three studies have specifically demonstrated better glycemic control and higher remission rates when canned low-carbohydrate diets were fed.[7,32,76] Other studies assessing insulin type and dosage have found high rates of remission when such diets are used.[70,104,106] The optimal dietary level of carbohydrate for diabetic cats has not been defined, but all of these studies used diets with less than 12% carbohydrate as dry matter. By limiting dietary carbohydrate, BG is maintained primarily from hepatic gluconeogenesis, which releases glucose into the circulation at a slow and steady rate.[53]

An earlier study showed that fiber-supplemented diets can improved glycemic control.[84] One study assessing both low-carbohydrate diets and fiber-supplemented diets found diabetic remission in cats eating each diet but notably higher remission rates for those eating low-carbohydrate diets.[7] Remission in those cats eating the higher-fiber diets shows that carbohydrate load is only one aspect of glycemic control, as previously noted, with peripheral factors that contribute to diabetes.

More information about maintenance dietary requirements and weight loss strategies can be found in Chapter 18.

When It's Just Not Working! Insulin Resistance

As described in the previous sections, development of type 2 diabetes requires some degree of insulin resistance. The same term is used when the patient is resistant to exogenous insulin. There is no set dose that indicates insulin resistance; sometimes the required dose increases relatively quickly but then drops as glycemic control is gained. Suspicion of insulin resistance is raised when the insulin dose reaches 8 U/cat at each injection (just over 1.5 U/kg for a 5-kg/11-lb cat). This recommendation varies depending on the cat's weight; for example, a lean 7-kg cat receiving 8 U is receiving approximately 1 U/kg. The cat's body condition should also be taken into account, and U/kg should be based on the cat's normal weight. The BG nadir must also be taken into account, insofar as 1.5 U/kg may be an acceptable dose if the BG nadir is appropriate but may not be if there is minimal impact on BG levels. At approximately 1.5 U/kg at each injection in a poorly regulated cat, the clinician should start considering insulin resistance in earnest.

The following approach can be used for a cat when insulin resistance is suspected (Table 24-4). First, review the history, physical examination findings, and results from previous blood and urine testing. Were there uninvestigated clinical signs or biochemical abnormalities? Examples may include tachycardia and increased ALT (suggesting hyperthyroidism), hypercalcemia (suggesting malignancy, but having other causes as well), neutrophilia (suggesting underlying infection or inflammation), and hematuria (suggesting a urinary tract infection). Review of history and physical examination findings is important because mild changes may be initially overlooked in the face of a persistent, significant hyperglycemia and glucosuria.

TABLE 24-4 **Recognized Causes of Insulin Ineffectiveness or Insulin Resistance**

Caused by Insulin Therapy	Caused by Concurrent Disorder
Inactive insulin	Diabetogenic drugs
Dilute insulin	Infection (oral and urinary especially)
Improper administration technique	Acromegaly
Inadequate dose	Hyperadrenocorticism
Somogyi phenomenon	Pancreatic pathology
Inadequate administration frequency	Hyperthyroidism
Impaired insulin absorption	Renal insufficiency
Anti-insulin antibody excess	Liver insufficiency
	Cardiac insufficiency
	Hyperlipidemia
	Pheochromocytoma

Adapted from Nelson RW: Insulin resistance in diabetic dogs and cats. In Bonagura JD, editor: *Kirk's current veterinary therapy XII*, Philadelphia, 1995, Saunders, p 390.

Ensure that the owner is administering insulin properly. Have the owner demonstrate insulin handling and injection technique using sterile saline, and correct any problems. Doses of U100 insulin less than 2 U can be difficult to measure reliably, and the minimum accurate dose for U40 insulin is 1 U. Owners with poor vision or arthritis may have difficulty measuring very small insulin doses. In households with more than one owner, ensure that all caregivers are administering insulin properly and consider the use of a chart that is filled out when a dose is given so that no insulin doses are missed. Ensure the insulin is kept in the refrigerator (if there is any doubt, start a new bottle) and that expired product is not in use.

Ensure that no nonprescribed medications are being given (consider medications from concurrent or previous veterinarians as well as nutritional or botanical supplements the owner may be administering). Re-examine the cat thoroughly. Look for obvious signs of infection, such as in the mouth, but also check nail beds, ears, and anal glands. Palpate the abdomen thoroughly, particularly for cranial abdominal masses (e.g., pancreatic adenocarcinoma), and note the size of organs (enlargement may suggest acromegaly). A urine sample (obtained by cystocentesis) should be submitted for culture and sensitivity testing, particularly if there is turbidity or hematuria. A serum biochemistry panel and total T_4 may be repeated depending on previous results and physical examination findings.

In the absence of any findings, start the cat on a course of broad-spectrum antibiotics (e.g., amoxicillin–clavulanic acid), start a new bottle of insulin, and continue weekly BG curves. If glycemic control is still not achieved, consider changing the type of insulin. Perform thorough abdominal ultrasonography (looking for pancreatic pathology, liver changes other than fatty changes expected of diabetes, adrenal gland changes, or even generalized organomegaly that may be suggestive of acromegaly). Other tests that may be considered include a low-dose dexamethasone suppression test for hyperadrenocorticism and insulin-like growth factor 1 (IGF-1) assay or computed tomography (CT) for acromegaly. More information regarding hyperadrenocorticism and acromegaly are found elsewhere in this chapter.

Complications and Concurrent Conditions

Somogyi Effect

The *Somogyi effect* refers to rebound hyperglycemia that occurs as a counterregulatory response to hypoglycemia through the effects of adrenaline, cortisol, growth hormone (GH), and glucagon. It was first described by Dr. Michael Somogyi in 1938[111]; this condition remains controversial in human medicine[12,37] and is poorly described in cats.

A recent study has documented previously well-controlled diabetic cats with BG less than 2.2 mmol/L (40 mg/dL) followed by a fast, steep rise in BG concentration above 22 mmol/L (400 mg/dL) and/or concentrations that were at least 8 mmol/L (150 mg/dL) above the usually measured higher concentrations.[105] A similar scenario was recognized in cats that had not yet been well regulated but in which the preceding "hypoglycemia" was approximately 3.8 mmol/L (70 mg/dL). In both scenarios two subsequent insulin doses showed almost no effect, and the glucose concentration remained elevated for more than 24 hours. Four cats were recognized with one or other of these scenarios out of 55 cats assessed.

There are no specific guidelines for such a rare phenomenon, but if it is suspected, a prudent approach would be to withdraw insulin for 24 hours and then reintroduce it at a much lower dose, such as 50% of the previous dose.

Diabetic Neuropathy

Chronic hyperglycemia associated with uncontrolled diabetic mellitus results in neurologic structural abnormalities. Histologically, Schwann cell injury is most prevalent and includes myelin defects, such as splitting and ballooning and demyelination; axonal degeneration occurs in more severely affected cats.[81] These changes are associated with microvascular pathology.[25] The most common clinical signs are a plantigrade posture when standing or walking, but a range of clinical signs is possible.[81] The condition does not seem to be overtly painful, but most cats are irritable when their feet are touched or manipulated. The mainstay of treatment of diabetic neuropathy is achievement of glycemic control. Most animals have significant clinical improvement once consistent euglycemia is achieved; however, persistent deficits are common.[20] Acetyl-l-carnitine has been shown to improve neurologic function in experimental animals and human patients,[69] but no clinical assessment has been made in cats.

Pancreatitis and Exocrine Pancreatic Insufficiency in Diabetic Cats

Given that the location of the insulin producing beta islet cells is within the exocrine pancreas, it is hardly surprising to expect exocrine pancreatic disease as a comorbidity. Direct associations of the endocrine and exocrine pancreas in cats have been recognized.[29,31,34,109] Elevated serum fPLI in diabetic cats compared with nondiabetic cats was recently documented, but no association was made with degree of glycemic control.[31] Another study found no association between glycemic control and pancreatic pathology.[34] Despite these findings, individual cats may have episodes of loss of glycemic control associated with pancreatitis, and the clinician should have a high index of suspicion if glycemic control is lost intermittently. There is no specific management to reduce this possibility in susceptible cats, and each episode must be managed on its own merits. The only overt clue of an episode of pancreatitis may be loss of glycemic control because clinical signs of pancreatitis in cats are nonspecific.[123]

Exocrine pancreatic insufficiency (EPI) has been recognized concurrently with diabetes on few occasions.[46a,90,112,116] This is hardly surprising because EPI is very uncommon in cats. A series of 16 cats with EPI found four nondiabetic cats with hyperglycemia (as well as a diabetic cat).[116] BG should be assessed on a regular basis (e.g., every 3 months) in cats with recognized EPI. Pancreatic diseases are discussed further in Chapter 23.

Diabetic Crises

Diabetic crises result from relative or complete lack of insulin, an increase in counterregulatory hormones leading to gluconeogenesis and insulin resistance, a reduction in glucose utilization by peripheral tissues, hyperglycemia, and glycosuria with obligatory diuresis. The two most common diabetic crises are diabetic ketoacidosis (DKA) and hyperosmolar hyperglycemic syndrome (HHS), which is nonketotic.[56] Both conditions are initiated by a relative insulin lack, as with uncomplicated DM, but occur as a culmination of the cascade of events initiated by the body's response. Insulin retards lipolysis so that without insulin, adipocytes undergo lipolysis to release free fatty acids (FFAs) into the circulation. Circulating FFAs are taken up by the liver for TG production as well as for the manufacture of ketone bodies, which can become an additional energy source for most cells in the body. In uncomplicated diabetes TG production predominates and ketone production occurs slowly enough that the ketones can be used by tissues for energy and will not cause hyperketonemia. In DKA relative increases of glucagon, epinephrine, cortisol, and GH occur compared with the decrease of appropriate insulin activity. An elevated glucagon : insulin ratio is characteristic of DKA. This change is usually caused by a stressful event; however, the inciting event may not be identifiable in every patient.[51] In the far less common nonketotic HHS, it is believed that hepatic glucagon resistance and the presence of small amounts of insulin may inhibit lipolysis, thereby preventing ketosis.[56]

Diabetic Ketoacidosis

Cats with DKA usually present for anorexia and lethargy. Cats are typically dehydrated on examination, and other signs are inconsistent. DM may not have been previously recognized. The key laboratory finding is ketosis, but cats are also acidotic and, of course, hyperglycemic.[51] Ketones can be recognized in urine with urine dipsticks, and there are also plasma ketone dipsticks available. Plasma ketone dipsticks are unlikely to give a false-negative result, but the false-positive rate may be as high as 33%; conversely, urine ketone dipsticks are unlikely to give a false-negative result, but false-positive results may occur in 18% of cases. The tests can be used concurrently if there is any doubt about the result.[133] Some human glucometers (e.g., Optimum Xceed, Precision Xtra; Abbott Laboratories Ltd.) also have ketone test strips available. The latter monitor has been assessed in dogs, and although it tended to overestimate serum/whole blood beta-hydroxybutyrate levels, it still had good correlation with a reference laboratory analyzer and is recommended for use[41]; the use of such monitors in cats has not been critically evaluated.

In a recent study, 7 of 12 cats with DKA subsequently went into diabetic remission,[108] indicating that once DKA has been controlled, the overall prognosis for successful diabetic management is not necessarily worse.

Hyperglycemic Hyperosmolar Syndrome

The standard criteria for diagnosis of HHS (also known as *nonketotic hyperosmolar diabetes*) in veterinary medicine are documentation of a serum glucose concentration greater than 33 mmol/L (600 mg/dL), absence of urine ketones, and serum osmolality exceeding 330 mOsm/kg (or effective serum osmolality exceeding 320 mOsm/kg).[56] More information on calculating serum osmolality is found in Chapter 5.

Affected cats present similarly to those with DKA, with the exception that neurologic signs such as stupor and coma are more likely to be present. Azotemia is usually more severe. The only substantive study of HHS in cats (17 cases) found that cats with HHS were more likely to be older than DKA cats (mean age 12.6 years); more likely to be previously diagnosed as diabetic and receiving insulin for several months (but not necessarily so); and more likely to have serious concurrent disease such as chronic renal disease, infection, congestive heart failure, neoplasia, and gastrointestinal tract disease. Prognosis was poor with 11 of 17 cats not surviving the emergency admission, and of these six survivors, only two lived longer than 1 year.[56]

Management of Diabetic Ketoacidosis and Hyperglycemic, Hyperosmolar Syndrome

Management of DKA and HHS (Box 24-2) follow similar principles of correction of fluid and electrolyte imbalances and administration of soluble insulin such as Humulin-R (Eli Lilly), Novolin-R (Novo Nordisk), and Actrapid (Novo Nordisk). These insulins may also be referred to as "regular insulin" or "Toronto insulin," and although rapidly acting, they have a short duration of action. Parenteral fluid therapy, as well as correction of

BOX 24-2

Suggested Treatment and Management Protocol for Cats with Diabetic Ketoacidosis

1. Replace fluid and electrolyte deficits:
   - Fluid therapy: 0.9% saline for first hour, and *then* change to 0.45% saline (because most patients are hyperosmolar and there is potential for cerebral edema) or start with 0.45% saline
   - Administer fluids at 150 mL/kg every 24 hours, which is approximately 28 mL per hour for 4.5-kg (10-lb) cat.
   - Potassium: Add 30-40 mmol/L. (Note: This is approximately four times the maintenance amount for this rate of fluids.)
2. Insulin constant-rate infusion (use a separate bag of fluids, intravenous set, fluid pump):
   - Add 25 units of soluble/regular insulin to 500 mL fluids.
   - Run 50 mL of the insulin-containing fluid through the drip set.
   - Attach insulin infusion bag to Y-piece of fluid-replacement bag.
   - Administer insulin infusion at 1 mL/kg per hour.
3. Monitor:
   - Glucose and potassium every 4 hours until blood glucose is 10-12 mmol/L (180-216 mg/dL).
4. Maintenance, after blood glucose is 10-12 mmol/L (180-216 mg/dL):
   - Change the main fluid bag to 0.45% NaCl *and* 2.5% dextrose with 30 mmol/L KCl.
   - Reduce insulin infusion to 0.5 mL/kg per hour.
5. Discontinue infusion when the cat is eating, and manage as a stable diabetic.

Data from Church DB: Diabetes mellitus. In Kirk RW, editor: *Current veterinary therapy VIII*, Philadelphia, 1983, Saunders, p 838.

electrolyte abnormalities, for cats with DKA and HHS is covered in Chapter 5.

PARENTERAL FLUID THERAPY

DKA and HHS patients, by virtue of their poorly controlled diabetes, have relatively high fluid maintenance requirements. Consequently, providing intravenous fluids at approximately 150 mL/kg every 24 hours generally will provide some replacement and adequate maintenance; this works out to approximately 28 mL per hour for a 4.5-kg (10-lb) cat. The optimum fluid composition has not been determined for cats with DKA or HHS, and 0.9% saline has been advocated for initial use,[35,52,56] with a change to 0.45% NaCl after the first hour. In most cases it is not only more convenient to start with 0.45% NaCl but may be more appropriate insofar as many DKA patients are also hyperosmolar (and HHS cats are by definition). The addition of 30 to 40 mmol/L of potassium chloride (KCl) reduces the hypotonicity of the solution. Note that this is approximately four times the maintenance amount of potassium for this rate of fluid administration; this is important because the lack of relative insulin means that potassium is being restricted from entering cells, as well as glucose. Plasma measurements are always of extracellular potassium, and in a diabetic cat this provides an even further underestimation of total body potassium than is normally the case. Whereas one aim is to rehydrate the patient, the other must be to provide some measure of diabetic control, or at least inhibit ongoing peripheral lipolysis and hence start to reduce the potential for ketoacidosis.

INTRAVENOUS INSULIN THERAPY

For treatment of clinically significant ketoacidosis, insulin may be administered by constant-rate infusion (CRI) or by intramuscular injection. In both situations the insulin should be in a soluble and hence relatively rapidly acting form. Although an intravenous insulin infusion may sound daunting, it is certainly the simplest and least labor-intensive means of treating diabetic patients who are inappetent.

One method for administering insulin by CRI is to add 25 units of soluble insulin to 500 mL fluids, producing an insulin concentration of 50 μU/mL. Insulin adheres to glass and plastic surfaces, so approximately 50 mL of the insulin-containing fluid should be run through the drip set before it is attached to the patient. This ensures that the animal receives a constant insulin concentration in the administered fluid.[91] Because the standard insulin infusion rate to inhibit gluconeogenesis, but not unduly enhance extrahepatic glucose utilization, is 40 to 60 μU/kg per hour,[14] the CRI can be administered at 1 mL/kg per hour of this solution. Obviously, a flow rate of approximately 1 mL/kg per hour is inadequate for maintenance fluid requirements. Consequently, the insulin CRI must be administered through a second infusion line (Figure 24-9), usually attached to the Y-piece of the maintenance fluid line.

The insulin is infused at a rate of 1 mL/kg per hour until plasma glucose concentrations fall to 10 to 12 mmol/L (180 to 216 mg/dL). At this time the flow rate should be halved (0.5 mL/kg per hour), and a concurrent dextrose infusion introduced through the maintenance fluid line. One simple and effective means of achieving a balance between the insulin and glucose infused is to change the maintenance fluids from 0.45% sodium chloride (NaCl) and 30 mmol/L KCl to 0.45% NaCl *and* 2.5% dextrose with 30 mmol/L KCl and administering this combination at 150 mL/kg every 24 hours. This will produce a glucose infusion rate of approximately 150 mg/kg per hour, which should balance the insulin being infused at 0.5 mL/kg per hour.

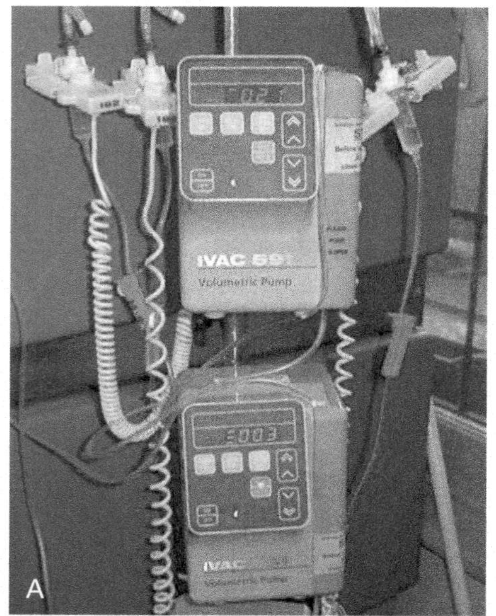

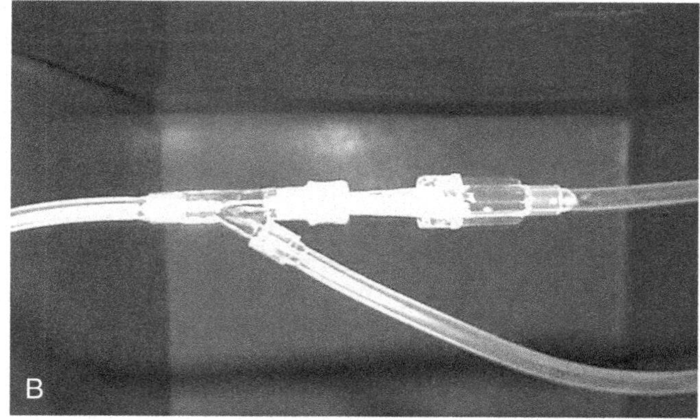

FIGURE 24-9 **A,** Two fluid pumps used to treat a cat with diabetic ketoacidosis. The cat weighs 3 kg, and the pump set at 21 mL per hour is delivering 0.45% NaCl with 40 mmol/L of potassium added. The pump set at 3 mL per hour has 25 units of soluble insulin added to a 500-mL bag of fluids. **B,** This second pump runs to a Y-piece so that only one intravenous catheter is needed.

During this time the patient's BG and serum potassium (and other electrolytes) are checked regularly. Over a period of 48 to 72 hours, the BG should remain relatively steady, ketonemia should disappear in DKA cats, and generally these patients should return to normal water and nutrient intake. Prognosis is more guarded in HHS cats, and management of concurrent conditions can affect how smoothly this protocol can be followed. For example, congestive heart failure is a contraindication to administering high fluid rates. Once initial abnormalities resolve, it is likely that, at least in the short term, the patient will be stabilized on a regular feeding regimen and an insulin dose regime appropriate for a stable diabetic cat, as outlined earlier in the chapter.

Other adjustments (e.g., of magnesium and bicarbonate) should be made only on the basis of measurement of these parameters. Acidosis usually resolves without addition of bicarbonate. Magnesium can be infused at 1 mEq/kg every 24 hours if hypomagnesemia is recognized.[42] Magnesium toxicity has been reported when administered unnecessarily.[48]

INTRAMUSCULAR INSULIN

Intramuscular (IM) protocols have been described and can be used as alternatives to the CRI insulin protocol outline in the preceding section; however, they are far more labor intensive. Two protocols have been described: hourly IM insulin[27] and intermittent IM insulin.[11]

For the *hourly IM insulin* protocol, soluble insulin should be administered at an initial IM dose of 0.2 U/kg, then 0.1 U/kg hourly thereafter. BG should be monitored hourly. When BG concentration falls below 16.5 mmol/L (approximately 300 mg/dL), 5% dextrose solution should be added to the intravenous fluids and insulin dosing frequency should be reduced to 4- to 6-hour intervals, administered intramuscularly.[27]

For the *intermittent IM insulin* protocol, 0.25 U/kg soluble insulin should be administered intramuscularly as a test dose, with subsequent doses based on the patient's response to initial treatment. In obese cats the initial dose should be based on estimated lean body weight to avoid overdosage and hypoglycemia. BG should be rechecked at 4- to 6-hour intervals; the goal is to reduce BG by 3 to 4 mmol/L per hour (54 to 72 mg/dL per hour). If this goal is surpassed, the next insulin dose should be reduced by 25% to 50%. If this goal is not met, the next dose should be increased by 25% to 50%. If the BG level reaches 10 to 12 mmol/L (180 to 216 mg/dL), 2.5% to 5% dextrose should be added to the intravenous fluids.[11]

As with the CRI insulin protocol, once BG returns to normal and the ketonemia resolves, the cat should be started on a dietary and insulin therapy appropriate for a stable diabetic.

GASTRINOMA

Functional pancreatic islet tumors that secrete gastrin have been infrequently described in cats.* Gastrin secretion results in the release of hydrochloric acid by the gastric parietal cells, and increased gastrin production typically results in gastroduodenal ulceration and potentially perforation. Reported cases were 8 to 12 years of age, with no sex or breed predispositions recognized in such a small sample. All cases presented with vomiting, weight loss, and poor body condition. Clinical and ancillary test results were not consistent, but possible findings include anemia (mild or severe and regenerative or nonregenerative, depending on the degree and rate of blood loss), a palpable abdominal mass, and an ultrasonographically visible pancreatic mass. One or several pancreatic masses were recognized at surgery or necropsy in all cases. Resected masses immunostain positive for gastrin. Fasting serum gastrin levels were elevated (as expected) in all cases evaluated. Surgical resection of pancreatic masses may be curative, but lifetime ancillary treatment with H_2-receptor antagonists such as cimetidine or ranitidine or, perhaps better, proton pump inhibitors such as omeprazole is warranted. Two cats were alive when their cases were described at 12 months[23] and 17 months, respectively,[21] after surgery. Another case survived 18 months until omeprazole was discontinued.[66]

INSULINOMA

Insulinoma is an islet cell carcinoma that secretes insulin, and very few cases have been described in cats.† Elevated insulin results in hypoglycemia, and resultant clinical signs include seizures, weakness, and localized muscle twitching. Documented cases have been 12 to 17 years of age, and three of the six described cases have been Siamese cats. Diagnosis is suspected by recognition of hypoglycemia with concurrent hyperinsulinemia and confirmed by finding pancreatic islet carcinoma on histologic examination of biopsy samples. The tumor should stain positive for insulin by immunocytochemistry. Only one published case has had prolonged survival beyond surgical resection, being 32 months after surgery when reported.[36] Recurrence of clinical signs occurred at 5 days, 6 days, 1 month, 7 months, and 18 months postoperatively in other cases.[40,57,78,88] In one of these cats, metastases to the pancreatic lymph nodes and liver were found at postmortem examination.[40] Frequent feeding and oral prednisolone allowed successful management

*References 21, 23, 66, 80, 88, 113, 120.

†References 36, 40, 49, 57, 78, 88.

for an additional 8 and 24 months in two cats[40,88] but was unsuccessful in another.[78] Cellular and molecular characterization in a recent case determined that the tumor secreted several peptide hormones in addition to insulin—namely, chromogranin A and somatostatin—but not glucagon or pancreatic polypeptide. It was also recognized that the tumor expressed several genes characteristic of pancreatic beta cells, including insulin (*INS*), glucose transporter 2 (*GLUT2*), and glucokinase (*GCK*). The tumor also expressed hexokinase 1 (*HK1*), a glycolytic enzyme not normally expressed in beta cells. GCK expression was higher in the insulinoma than in normal pancreas from the same cat. The GCK: HK1 ratio was twentyfold higher in insulinoma tissue than in normal pancreas. These findings suggest insulinoma cells may have an increased sensitivity to glucose that could contribute to the abnormal insulin secretory response observed at low serum glucose concentrations.[49]

References

1. Alt N, Kley S, Haessig M et al: Day-to-day variability of blood glucose concentration curves generated at home in cats with diabetes mellitus, *J Am Vet Med Assoc* 230:1011, 2007.
2. Andrews RC, Walker BR: Glucocorticoids and insulin resistance: old hormones, new targets, *Clin Sci (Lond)* 96:513, 1999.
3. Appleton D, Rand J, Sunvold G: Insulin sensitivity decreases with obesity, and lean cats with low insulin sensitivity are at greatest risk of glucose intolerance with weight gain, *J Feline Med Surg* 3:211, 2001.
4. Bailiff NL, Nelson RW, Feldman EC et al: Frequency and risk factors for urinary tract infection in cats with diabetes mellitus, *J Vet Intern Med* 20:850, 2006.
5. Baral RM, Rand JS, Catt MJ et al: Prevalence of feline diabetes mellitus in a feline private practice, *J Vet Intern Med* 17:433, 2003.
6. Behrend EN, Tapia J, Welles EG et al: Evaluation of a conventional urine glucose test strip method for detection of glucosuria in dogs and cats (abstract), *J Vet Intern Med* 22:790, 2008.
7. Bennett N, Greco D, Peterson M et al: Comparison of a low carbohydrate-low fiber diet and a moderate carbohydrate-high fiber diet in the management of feline diabetes mellitus, *J Feline Med Surg* 8:73, 2006.
8. Borst SE: The role of TNF-alpha in insulin resistance, *Endocrine* 23:177, 2004.
9. Brennan CL, Hoenig M, Ferguson DC: GLUT4 but not GLUT1 expression decreases early in the development of feline obesity, *Domest Anim Endocrinol* 26:291, 2004.
10. Broughton DL, Taylor R: Deterioration of Glucose Tolerance with Age: The Role of Insulin Resistance, *Age Ageing* 20:221, 1991.
11. Broussard JD, Wallace MS: Insulin treatment of diabetes mellitus in the dog and cat. In Bonagura JD, editor: *Kirk's current veterinary therapy XII: small animal practice*, Philadelphia, 1995, Saunders, p 393.
12. Campbell I: The somogyi phenomenon. A short review, *Acta Diabetol* 13:68, 1976.
13. Casella M, Hassig M, Reusch C: Home-monitoring of blood glucose in cats with diabetes mellitus: evaluation over a 4-month period, *J Feline Med Surg* 7:163, 2005.
14. Church DB: Diabetes mellitus. In Kirk RW, editor: *Current veterinary therapy VIII*, Philadelphia, 1983, Saunders, p 838.
15. Cohn LA, McCaw DL, Tate DJ et al: Assessment of five portable blood glucose meters, a point-of-care analyzer, and color test strips for measuring blood glucose concentration in dogs, *J Am Vet Med Assoc* 216:198, 2000.
16. Crenshaw KL, Peterson ME, Heeb LA et al: Serum fructosamine concentration as an index of glycemia in cats with diabetes mellitus and stress hyperglycemia, *J Vet Intern Med* 10:360, 1996.
17. Daniel M, Rowley KG, McDermott R et al: Diabetes and impaired glucose tolerance in Aboriginal Australians: prevalence and risk, *Diabetes Res Clin Pract* 57:23, 2002.
18. Davis TA, Klahr S, Karl IE: Glucose metabolism in muscle of sedentary and exercised rats with azotemia, *Am J Physiol Renal Physiol* 252:F138, 1987.
19. DeClue AE, Cohn LA, Kerl ME et al: Use of continuous blood glucose monitoring for animals with diabetes mellitus, *J Am Anim Hosp Assoc* 40:171, 2004.
20. Dickinson PJ, LeCouteur RA: Feline neuromuscular disorders, *Vet Clin North Am Small Anim Pract* 34:1307, 2004.
21. Diroff JS, Sanders NA, McDonough SP et al: Gastrin-secreting neoplasia in a cat, *J Vet Intern Med* 20:1245, 2006.
22. Dobromylskyj MJ, Sparkes AH: Assessing portable blood glucose meters for clinical use in cats in the United Kingdom, *Vet Rec* 167:438, 2010.
23. Eng J, Du B-H, Johnson GF et al: Cat gastrinoma and the sequence of cat gastrins, *Regul Pept* 37:9, 1992.
24. Engelking LR: Physiology of the endocrine pancreas, *Semin Vet Med Surg (Small Anim)* 12:224, 1997.
25. Estrella JS, Nelson RN, Sturges BK et al: Endoneurial microvascular pathology in feline diabetic neuropathy, *Microvasc Res* 75:403, 2008.
26. Feldman E, Nelson R, Feldman M: Intensive 50-week evaluation of glipizide administration in 50 cats with previously untreated diabetes mellitus, *J Am Vet Med Assoc* 210:772, 1997.
27. Feldman EC, Nelson RW: Diabetic ketoacidosis. In Feldman EC, Nelson RW, editors: *Canine and feline endocrinology and reproduction*, ed 2, Philadelphia, 1996, Saunders, p 392.
28. Ferrannini E, Vichi S, Beck-Nielsen H et al: Insulin action and age. European Group for the Study of Insulin Resistance (EGIR), *Diabetes* 45:947, 1996.
29. Ferreri J, Hardam E, Kimmel S et al: Clinical differentiation of acute necrotizing from chronic nonsuppurative pancreatitis in cats: 63 cases (1996-2001), *J Am Vet Med Assoc* 223:469, 2003.
30. Fletcher JM, Behrend EN, Lee HP et al: Accuracy of Purina Glucotest for monitoring of glucosuria in cats (abstract), *J Vet Intern Med* 20, 2006.
31. Forcada Y, German AJ, Noble PJ et al: Determination of serum fPLI concentrations in cats with diabetes mellitus, *J Feline Med Surg* 10:480, 2008.
32. Frank G, Anderson W, Pazak H et al: Use of a high-protein diet in the management of feline diabetes mellitus, *Vet Ther* 2:238, 2001.
33. Gilor C, Keel T, Attermeier KJ et al: Hyperglycemic-euglycemic clamps using insulin detemir and insulin glargine in health cats [abstract], *J Vet Intern Med* 22:729, 2008.
34. Goossens MMC, Nelson RW, Feldman EC et al: Response to insulin treatment and survival in 104 cats with diabetes mellitus (1985-1995), *J Vet Intern Med* 12:1, 1998.
35. Greco DS: Complicated diabetes mellitus. In Bonagura JD, Twedt DC, editors: *Kirk's current veterinary therapy XIV*, St Louis, 2009, Saunders Elsevier, p 214.
36. Greene SN, Bright RM: Insulinoma in a cat, *J Small Anim Pract* 49:38, 2008.
37. Guillod L, Comte-Perret S, Monbaron D et al: Nocturnal hypoglycaemias in type 1 diabetic patients: what can we learn with continuous glucose monitoring? *Diabetes Metab* 33:360, 2007.
38. Guyton AC, Hall JE: Insulin, glucagon and diabetes mellitus. In Guyton AC, Hall JE, editors: *Textbook of medical physiology*, ed 11, Philadelphia, 2006, Elsevier-Saunders, p 961.

39. Halter JB, Beard JC, Porte D, Jr: Islet function and stress hyperglycemia: plasma glucose and epinephrine interaction, *Am J Physiol Endocrinol Metab* 247:E47, 1984.
40. Hawks D, Peterson ME, Hawkins KL et al: Insulin-secreting pancreatic (islet cell) carcinoma in a cat, *J Vet Intern Med* 6:193, 1992.
41. Henderson DW, Schlesinger DP: Use of a point-of-care beta-hydroxybutyrate sensor for detection of ketonemia in dogs, *Can Vet J* 51:1000, 2010.
42. Hess RS: Diabetic emergencies. In August JR, editor: *Consultations in feline internal medicine 6*, St Louis, 2010, Saunders Elsevier, p 297.
43. Hiskett E, Suwitheechon O-u, Lindbloom-Hawley S et al: Lack of glucokinase regulatory protein expression may contribute to low glucokinase activity in feline liver, *Vet Res Comm* 33:227, 2009.
44. Hoenig M, Ferguson DC: Effects of neutering on hormonal concentrations and energy requirements in male and female cats, *Am J Vet Res* 63:634, 2002.
45. Hoenig M, Hall G, Ferguson D et al: A feline model of experimentally induced islet amyloidosis, *Am J Pathol* 157:2143, 2000.
46. Hoenig M, Wilkins C, Holson JC et al: Effects of obesity on lipid profiles in neutered male and female cats, *Am J Vet Res* 64:299, 2003.
46a. Holzworth J, Coffin DL: Pancreatic insufficiency and diabetes mellitus in a cat, *Cornell Vet* 43:502, 1953.
47. Hui JM, Sud A, Farrell GC et al: Insulin resistance is associated with chronic hepatitis C and virus infection fibrosis progression, *Gastroenterology* 125:1695, 2003.
48. Jackson CB, Drobatz KJ: Iatrogenic magnesium overdose: 2 case reports, *J Vet Emerg Crit Care* 14:115, 2004.
49. Jackson TC, Debey B, Lindbloom-Hawley S et al: Cellular and molecular characterization of a feline insulinoma, *J Vet Intern Med* 23:383, 2009.
50. Jenkins RC, Valcavi R, Zini M et al: Association of elevated insulin-like growth factor binding protein-1 with insulin resistance in hyperthyroidism, *Clin Endocrinol* 52:187, 2000.
51. Kerl M: Diabetic ketoacidosis: pathophysiology and clinical laboratory presentation, *Comp Contin Edu Pract Vet* 23:220, 2001.
52. Kerl M: Diabetic ketoacidosis: treatment recommendations, *Comp Contin Edu Pract Vet* 23:330, 2001.
53. Kirk C: Feline diabetes mellitus: low carbohydrates versus high fiber? *Vet Clin North Am Small Anim Pract* 36:1297, 2006.
54. Kley S, Casella M, Reusch C: Evaluation of long-term monitoring of blood glucose concentrations in cats with diabetes mellitus: 26 cases (1999-2002), *J Am Vet Med Assoc* 225:261, 2004.
55. Knowler WC, Bennett PH, Hamman RF et al: Diabetes incidence and prevalence in Pima Indians: a 19-fold greater incidence than in Rochester, Minnesota, *Am J Epidemiol* 108:497, 1978.
56. Koenig A, Drobatz KJ, Beale AB et al: Hyperglycemic, hyperosmolar syndrome in feline diabetics: 17 cases (1995-2001), *J Vet Emerg Crit Care* 14:30, 2004.
57. Kraje A: Hypoglycemia and irreversible neurologic complications in a cat with insulinoma, *J Am Vet Med Assoc* 223:812, 2003.
58. Kuwa K, Nakayama T, Hoshino T et al: Relationships of glucose concentrations in capillary whole blood, venous whole blood and venous plasma, *Clin Chim Acta* 307:187, 2001.
59. Laluha P, Gerber B, Laluhová D et al: Stress hyperglycaemia in sick cats: a retrospective study over 4 years, *Schweiz Arch Tierheilkd* 146:375, 2004.
60. Lebovitz HE, Feinglos MN: Mechanism of action of the second-generation sulfonylurea glipizide, *Am J Med* 75:46, 1983.
61. Lederer R, Rand JS, Hughes IP et al: Pancreatic histopathology of diabetic Burmese and non-Burmese cats (abstract), In *ACVIM Proceedings*, Charlotte, NC, 443, 2004.
62. Lederer R, Rand JS, Jonsson NN et al: Frequency of feline diabetes mellitus and breed predisposition in domestic cats in Australia, *Vet J* 179:254, 2009.
63. Lin Y, Sun Z: Current views on type 2 diabetes, *J Endocrinol* 204:1, 2010.
64. Link KR, Rand JS: Changes in blood glucose concentration are associated with relatively rapid changes in circulating fructosamine concentrations in cats, *J Feline Med Surg* 10:583, 2008.
65. Link KR, Rand JS, Hendrikz JK: Evaluation of a simplified intravenous glucose tolerance test and a reflectance glucose meter for use in cats *Vet Rec* 140:253, 1997
66. Liptak J, Hunt G, Barrs V et al: Gastroduodenal ulceration in cats: eight cases and a review of the literature, *J Feline Med Surg* 4:27, 2002.
67. Lipton RB, Uao Y, Cao G et al: Determinants of incident non-Insulin-dependent diabetes mellitus among blacks and whites in a national sample: the NHANES I epidemiologic follow-up study, *Am J Epidemiol* 138:826, 1993.
68. Lowe AD, Campbell KL, Barger A et al: Clinical, clinicopathological and histological changes observed in 14 cats treated with glucocorticoids, *Vet Rec* 162:777, 2008.
69. Lowitt S, Malone JI, Salem AF et al: Acetyl—carnitine corrects the altered peripheral nerve function of experimental diabetes, *Metabolism* 44:677, 1995.
70. Marshall R, Rand J: Treatment with insulin glargine results in higher remission rates than lente or protamine zinc insulins in newly diagnosed diabetic cats (abstract), *J Vet Intern Med* 19:425, 2005.
71. Marshall RD, Rand JS: Insulin glargine and a high protein–low carbohydrate diet are associated with high remission rates in newly diagnosed diabetic cats [abstract], *J Vet Intern Med* 18:401, 2004.
72. Marshall RD, Rand JS, Morton JM: Glargine and protamine zinc insulin have a longer duration of action and result in lower mean daily glucose concentrations than lente insulin in healthy cats, *J Vet Pharmacol Ther* 31:205, 2008.
73. Marshall RD, Rand JS, Morton JM: Treatment of newly diagnosed diabetic cats with glargine insulin improves glycaemic control and results in higher probability of remission than protamine zinc and lente insulins, *J Feline Med Surg* 11:683, 2009.
74. Martin GJ, Rand JS: Pharmacology of a 40 IU/ml porcine lente insulin preparation in diabetic cats: findings during the first week and after 5 or 9 weeks of therapy, *J Feline Med Surg* 3:23, 2001.
75. Martin GJ, Rand JS: Control of diabetes mellitus in cats with porcine insulin zinc suspension, *Vet Rec* 161:88, 2007.
76. Mazzaferro E, Greco D, Turner A et al: Treatment of feline diabetes mellitus using an alpha-glucosidase inhibitor and a low-carbohydrate diet, *J Feline Med Surg* 5:183, 2003.
77. McCann TM, Simpson KE, Shaw DJ et al: Feline diabetes mellitus in the UK: the prevalence within an insured cat population and a questionnaire-based putative risk factor analysis, *J Feline Med Surg* 9:289, 2007.
78. McMillan FD, Barr B, Feldman EC: Functional pancreatic islet cell tumor in a cat, *J Am Anim Hosp Assoc* 21:741, 1985.
79. Michiels L, Reusch CE, Boari A et al: Treatment of 46 cats with porcine lente insulin—a prospective, multicentre study, *J Feline Med Surg* 10:439, 2008.
80. Middleton DJ, Watson AD, Vasak E et al: Duodenal ulceration associated with gastrin-secreting pancreatic tumor in a cat, *J Am Vet Med Assoc* 183:461, 1983.
81. Mizisin AP, Shelton GD, Burgers ML et al: Neurological complications associated with spontaneously occurring feline diabetes mellitus, *J Neuropathol Exp Neurol* 61:872, 2002.
82. Moretti S, Tschuor F, Osto M et al: Evaluation of a novel real-time continuous glucose-monitoring system for use in cats, *J Vet Intern Med* 24:120, 2010.
83. Nelson R, Henley K, Cole C et al: Field safety and efficacy of protamine zinc recombinant human insulin for treatment of diabetes mellitus in cats, *J Vet Intern Med* 23:787, 2009.

84. Nelson R, Scott-Moncrieff J, Feldman E et al: Effect of dietary insoluble fiber on control of glycemia in cats with naturally acquired diabetes mellitus, *J Am Vet Med Assoc* 216:1082, 2000.
85. Nelson RW, Feldman EC, Ford SL et al: Effect of an orally administered sulfonylurea, glipizide, for treatment of diabetes mellitus in cats, *J Am Vet Med Assoc* 203:821, 1993.
86. Niessen S, Powney S, Guitian J et al: Evaluation of a quality-of-life tool for cats with diabetes mellitus, *J Vet Intern Med* 24:1098, 2010.
87. Norsworthy G, Lynn R, Cole C: Preliminary study of protamine zinc recombinant insulin for the treatment of diabetes mellitus in cats, *Vet Ther* 10:24, 2009.
88. O'Brien TD, Norton F, Turner TM et al: Pancreatic endocrine tumor in a cat: clinical, pathological, and immunohistochemical evaluation, *J Am Anim Hosp Assoc* 26:453, 1990.
89. Panciera D, Thomas C, Eicker S et al: Epizootiologic patterns of diabetes mellitus in cats: 333 cases (1980-1986), *J Am Vet Med Assoc* 197:1504, 1990.
90. Perry LA, Williams DA, Pidgeon G et al: Exocrine pancreatic insufficiency with associated coagulopathy in a cat, *J Am Anim Hosp Assoc* 27:109, 1991.
91. Peterson L, Caldwell J, Hoffman J: Insulin adsorbance to polyvinylchloride surfaces with implications for constant-infusion therapy, *Diabetes* 25:72, 1976.
92. Poitout V, Robertson RP: Minireview: Secondary β-cell failure in type 2 diabetes—a convergence of glucotoxicity and lipotoxicity, *Endocrinology* 143:339, 2002.
93. Prahl A, Guptill L, Glickman NW et al: Time trends and risk factors for diabetes mellitus in cats presented to veterinary teaching hospitals, *J Feline Med Surg* 9:351, 2007.
94. Rand J: Current understanding of feline diabetes. Part 1: Pathogenesis, *J Feline Med Surg* 1:143, 1999.
95. Rand J, Bobbermien L, Henkrikz J et al: Over representation of Burmese cats with diabetes mellitus, *Aust Vet J* 75:402, 1997.
96. Rand JS, Marshall RD: Diabetes mellitus in cats, *Vet Clin North Am Small Anim Pract* 35:211, 2005.
97. Ravel R: Tests for diabetes and hypoglycemia. In Ravel R, editor: *Clinical laboratory medicine*, ed 6, St Louis, 1995, Mosby, p 454.
98. Reineke EL, Fletcher DJ, King LG et al: Accuracy of a continuous glucose monitoring system in dogs and cats with diabetic ketoacidosis, *J Vet Emerg Crit Care (San Antonio)* 20:303, 2010.
99. Reusch C, Wess G, Casella M: Home monitoring of blood glucose concentrations in the management of diabetes mellitus, *Comp Contin Edu Pract Vet* 23:544, 2001.
100. Reusch CE, Kley S, Casella M: Home monitoring of the diabetic cat, *J Feline Med Surg* 8:119, 2006.
101. Reusch CE, Tomsa K: Serum fructosamine concentration in cats with overt hyperthyroidism, *J Am Vet Med Assoc* 215:1297, 1999.
102. Ridderstrale M, Groop L: Genetic dissection of type 2 diabetes, *Mol Cell Endocrinol* 297:10, 2009.
103. Ristic JM, Herrtage ME, Walti-Lauger SM et al: Evaluation of a continuous glucose monitoring system in cats with diabetes mellitus, *J Feline Med Surg* 7:153, 2005.
104. Roomp K, Rand J: Intensive blood glucose control is safe and effective in diabetic cats using home monitoring and treatment with glargine, *J Feline Med Surg* 11:668, 2009.
105. Roomp K, Rand JS: The Somogyi effect is rare in diabetic cats managed using glargine and a protocol aimed at tight glycemic control (abstract), *J Vet Intern Med* 22:790, 2008.
106. Roomp K, Rand JS: Evaluation of detemir in diabetic cats managed with a protocol for intensive blood glucose control (abstract), *J Vet Intern Med* 23:697, 2009.
107. Root M, Johnson K, Allen W et al: Diabetes mellitus associated with pancreatic endocrine insufficiency in a kitten, *J Small Anim Pract* 36:416, 1995.
108. Sieber-Ruckstuhl NS, Kley S, Tschuor F et al: Remission of diabetes mellitus in cats with diabetic ketoacidosis, *J Vet Intern Med* 22:1326, 2008.
109. Simpson KW, Shiroma JT, Biller DS et al: Ante mortem diagnosis of pancreatitis in four cats, *J Small Anim Pract* 35:93, 1994.
110. Soh I, Mamoru T, Masashige S: Decreased skeletal muscle insulin receptors in high-fat-diet–related hypertensive rats, *Nutr Res* 22:1049, 2002.
111. Somogyi M, Kirstein M: Insulin as a cause of extreme hyperglycemia and instability, *Bull St Louis Med Society* 32:498, 1938.
112. Steiner J, Williams D: Serum feline trypsin-like immunoreactivity in cats with exocrine pancreatic insufficiency, *J Vet Intern Med* 14:627, 2000.
113. Straus E, Raufman JP: The Brooklyn gastrinomas, *Mt Sinai J Med* 59:125, 1992.
114. Swinney G: Diabetes mellitus in the cat: A retrospective study 1984-1994 at Sydney University Veterinary Teaching Hospital. In *Australian Veterinary Association Conference Proceedings*, Melbourne, 84, 1995.
115. Taniguchi CM, Emanuelli B, Kahn CR: Critical nodes in signalling pathways: insights into insulin action, *Nat Rev Mol Cell Biol* 7:85, 2006.
116. Thompson KA, Parnell NK, Hohenhaus AE et al: Feline exocrine pancreatic insufficiency: 16 cases (1992-2007), *J Feline Med Surg* 11:935, 2009.
117. Thompson M, Taylor S, Adams V et al: Comparison of glucose concentrations in blood samples obtained with a marginal ear vein nick technique versus from a peripheral vein in healthy cats and cats with diabetes mellitus, *J Am Vet Med Assoc* 221:389, 2002.
118. Thoresen S, Bjerkas E, Aleksandersen M et al: Diabetes mellitus and bilateral cataracts in a kitten, *J Feline Med Surg* 4:115, 2002.
119. Van de Maele I, Rogier N, Daminet S: Retrospective study of owners' perception on home monitoring of blood glucose in diabetic dogs and cats, *Can Vet J* 46:718, 2005.
120. van der Gaag I, van den Ingh TS, Lamers CB et al: Zollinger-Ellison syndrome in a cat, *Vet Q* 10:151, 1988.
121. Wade C, Gething M, Rand J: Evidence of a genetic basis for diabetes mellitus in Burmese cats (abstract), *J Vet Intern Med* 13:269, 1999.
122. Waring WS, Evans LE, Kirkpatrick CT: Glycolysis inhibitors negatively bias blood glucose measurements: potential impact on the reported prevalence of diabetes mellitus, *J Clin Pathol* 60:820, 2007.
123. Washabau RJ: Acute necrotizing pancreatitis. In August JR, editor: *Consultations in feline internal medicine 5*, St Louis, 2006, Elsevier Saunders, p 109.
124. Weaver KE, Rozanski EA, Mahony OM et al: Use of glargine and lente insulins in cats with diabetes mellitus, *J Vet Intern Med* 20:234, 2006.
125. Wess G, Reusch C: Assessment of five portable blood glucose meters for use in cats, *Am J Vet Res* 61:1587, 2000.
126. Wess G, Reusch C: Capillary blood sampling from the ear of dogs and cats and use of portable meters to measure glucose concentration, *J Small Anim Pract* 41:60, 2000.
127. Whitney MS: Evaluation of hyperlipidemias in dogs and cats, *Semin Vet Med Surg (Small Anim)* 7:292, 1992.
128. Wiedmeyer CE, DeClue AE: Continuous glucose monitoring in dogs and cats, *J Vet Intern Med* 22:2, 2008.
129. Wiedmeyer CE, Johnson PJ, Cohn LA et al: Evaluation of a continuous glucose monitoring system for use in dogs, cats, and horses, *J Am Vet Med Assoc* 223:987, 2003.

130. Wiedmeyer CE, Johnson PJ, Cohn LA et al: Evaluation of a continuous glucose monitoring system for use in veterinary medicine, *Diabetes Technol Ther* 7:885, 2005.
131. Woods J, Panciera D, Snyder P et al: Diabetes mellitus in a kitten, *J Am Anim Hosp Assoc* 30:177, 1994.
132. Zeugswetter F, Handl S, Iben C et al: Efficacy of plasma β-hydroxybutyrate concentration as a marker for diabetes mellitus in acutely sick cats, *J Feline Med Surg* 12:300, 2010.
133. Zeugswetter F, Pagitz M: Ketone measurements using dipstick methodology in cats with diabetes mellitus, *J Small Anim Pract* 50:4, 2009.
134. Zeugswetter FK, Rebuzzi L, Karlovits S: Alternative sampling site for blood glucose testing in cats: giving the ears a rest, *J Feline Med Surg* 12:710, 2010.
135. Zini E, Hafner M, Osto M et al: Predictors of Clinical Remission in Cats with Diabetes Mellitus, *J Vet Intern Med* 24:1314, 2010.
136. Zini E, Moretti S, Tschuor F et al: Evaluation of a new portable glucose meter designed for the use in cats, *Schweiz Arch Tierheilkd* 151:448, 2009.

THYROID GLAND DISORDERS

Randolph M. Baral and Mark E. Peterson

HYPERTHYROIDISM

Hyperthyroidism refers to an increase in the functional thyroid hormones, thyroxine (T_4) and tri-iodothyronine (T_3), most commonly due to benign thyroid adenoma or adenomatous hyperplasia present in one or both lobes of the thyroid gland. Resultant clinical signs are variable but typically include weight loss, often with increased appetite, hyperactivity and cardiovascular signs; at least one lobe of the thyroid gland is palpable in most cases.

Epidemiology

Hyperthyroidism is commonly cited as the most common endocrinopathy of cats[28,63,89,130] and most clinicians' anecdotal experience would bear this out. However, different studies have used different measures of disease rates, and there are also likely to be geographical variations in disease occurrence rates. In one study, reported in 2005, an annualized incidence rate of 11.92% was recognized in cats older than 9 years of age at a primary accession practice in London compared with 1.53% in Spanish practices.[143] The hospital prevalence among cats older than 8 years of age in an urban population of cats in Germany was noted as 11.4% in 2006.[112] In Japan, in 2002, a prevalence of 8.9% was noted in cats older than 9 years,[70] and in Hong Kong, in 2009, a prevalence of 3.93% was recorded in cats older than 10 years.[24]

Despite these high disease rates, hyperthyroidism is a new disease that was first described in 1979.[93] Before this time enlargement of the thyroid gland had been found at necropsy in cats and nodules were observed histopathologically, but these abnormalities were relatively rare and were not associated with the clinical signs relating to hyperthyroidism.[61,62] Since this first description, several studies have documented marked increases worldwide with time—for example, from 0.3% in 1979 to 4.5% in 1985 in North America[113]; from 0.1% in 1978 to 1982 to 2% in 1993 to 1997, also in North America[27]; and from 0.2% in 1987 to 1994 to 2.6% in 1998 in Germany.[59]

The sudden appearance and subsequent increase in rates of this condition have led to investigations of potential underlying causes. These studies have indicated that numerous environmental and nutritional factors play a role in the pathology of this disorder.

A number of studies have pointed to consumption of canned food as a risk factor,* which is ironic because dry food consumption is considered a risk factor for DM, the next most common endocrinopathy in cats. "Pop-top" cans may pose more of a risk than cans for which a can opener is required[27,142] or packets.[142] This is potentially because of the release of chemicals such as bisphenol-A and bisphenol-F from the lacquer linings of the cans during the heating process. Higher amounts of these two chemicals have been found in high-fat foods from pop-top cans than in high-fat foods from other types of cans. The two studies that found pop-top cans to increase risk also found fish consumption (canned or home cooked) to provide increased risk of hyperthyroidism.[27,142] This is compared with other studies that did not find an association with fish consumption.[27,53,79,113] Soy protein in the diet has been demonstrated to increase thyroxine concentrations in cats,[148] and soy isoflavones were identified in nearly 60% of cat foods tested (dry, moist, and semimoist).[20] One study found that cats that consumed commercial foods without iodine supplementation were more than four times as likely to develop hyperthyroidism as cats that ate iodine-supplemented foods.[26a]

Environmental factors that have been associated with increased risk of developing hyperthyroidism include use of insecticidal products such as antiflea products[53,79,113] for the cat or fly sprays[79,113] within the household; exposure to herbicides, fertilizers (e.g., from water from puddles in households where these are used)[79,113]; and flame retardants that were introduced into routine use for building materials, electronics, furnishings, foams, and textiles at approximately the time hyperthyroidism was first recognized.[26]

Pathogenesis

The increases in T_4 and T_3 that cause clinical hyperthyroidism result from normal thyrocytes becoming

*References 27, 53, 65, 79, 113, 142.

hyperfunctional because of adenomatous hyperplasia or adenoma.[84] Thyroid carcinoma is relatively rare, occurring in up to only approximately 4% of cases,[47,74] and it has been suggested that such malignant thyroid tumors could have a different pathogenesis[102] than the typical benign lesions.

The feline thyroid gland normally contains a subpopulation of the follicular cells that have a high, intrinsic growth potential. In the thyroid gland eventually destined to develop adenomatous hyperplasia, this subpopulation of thyrocytes may replicate in an autonomous fashion. Once these rapidly dividing cells are present in sufficient numbers, they may continue to grow in the absence of extrathyroidal stimulation, such as thyroid-stimulating hormone (TSH). Therefore these thyroid adenomatous hyperplastic cells show autonomy of growth, as well as the ability to function and secrete thyroid hormone in an autonomous fashion.[84] Large case series have consistently demonstrated that bilateral thyroid involvement is present in more than 70% of hyperthyroid cats. This may be important in pathogenesis insofar as no physical connection exists between the two thyroid lobes in cats.[6,98]

In normal thyroid cells, after the TSH binds to its receptor, G proteins are activated that control the initiation of adenylate cyclase activation and cyclic adenosine monophosphate (cAMP) levels. G proteins couple to the TSH receptor and can be stimulatory (Gs), resulting in an increase in cAMP, or inhibitory (Gi), resulting in a decrease in cAMP. The relative amounts of Gs and Gi proteins determine the ultimate levels of cAMP in the cell. If the balance is altered in favor of Gs, by overexpression of Gs or underexpression of Gi, it results in overproduction of cAMP and overactivation of the thyroid cell. One study looked at eight hyperthyroid cats and four age-matched euthyroid cats and examined them for Gs and Gi protein expression. Gs expression was identical in both hyperthyroid and euthyroid cats, but Gi expression was significantly decreased in the hyperthyroid cats, suggesting that G protein expression regulating cellular cAMP levels may play a role in the pathogenesis of feline hyperthyroidism.[41]

TABLE 24-5 **Clinical Findings in Cats with Hyperthyroidism**[13]

Finding	Percentage of Cats
HISTORICAL OWNER COMPLAINTS	
Weight loss	88
Polyphagia	49
Vomiting	44
Polyuria/polydipsia	36
Increased activity	31
Decreased appetite	16
Diarrhea	15
Decreased activity	12
Weakness	12
Dyspnea	10
Panting	9
Large fecal volume	8
Anorexia	7
PHYSICAL EXAMINATION FINDINGS	
Large thyroid gland	83
Thin	65
Heart murmur	54
Tachycardia	42
Gallop rhythm	15
Hyperkinesis	15
Aggressiveness	10
Unkempt hair coat	9
Increased nail growth	6
Alopecia	3
Congestive heart failure	2
Ventral neck flexion	1

Clinical Signs

Hyperthyroidism most commonly occurs in middle-aged to older cats. Most large series of cases have found a mean or median age of 12 or 13 years, with only 5% of cases diagnosed in cats younger than 10 years of age. There is no definitive breed or sex susceptibility, but some papers have shown a skew to increased numbers of females.[69,100]

The typical historical findings and clinical signs of hyperthyroidism, together with indicative frequencies, are shown in Table 24-5. These frequencies are noted from a 1995 paper that assessed changes in clinical and laboratory findings in cats with hyperthyroidism from 1983 to 1993, finding lower frequency and severity of signs in the latter year[13]; similarly, the severity of cardiac changes reduced over a similar duration, though the percentage of cats with a murmur remained similar.[34] This reduction in frequency and severity of signs most likely arose from veterinarians' awareness of this new condition, and there may well have been further changes in clinical awareness, and therefore clinical signs that are seen, since 1993. Though reduced in frequency and severity, the general signs recognized remain the same.

Thyroid hormones regulate metabolic processes, so increased circulating levels of these hormones result in the increased appetite, weight loss, and muscle wastage that are typical of hyperthyroidism in cats. Thyroid hormones also appear to interact with the central nervous system, increasing sympathetic drive and resulting in the hyperexcitability, nervousness, tachycardia, and perhaps tremor that are also characteristic for hyperthyroidism.[101]

Weight Loss

Hyperthyroidism should be considered in all middle-aged to older cats that have lost weight. The differential diagnoses for weight loss are extensive, including primary gastrointestinal disease, neoplasia of any origin, and renal disease. Hyperthyroidism, however, is so common that it should always be considered, whether or not supporting signs such as tachycardia are present. Further, weight loss is the most commonly recognized sign of hyperthyroidism.[13] Weight loss is often associated with increased appetite, but some cats have the same, or even reduced, appetite.

Heart Murmur and Other Cardiac Signs

Cardiac signs of some description are present in approximately 50% of cats with hyperthyroidism.[34,69] Therefore, as for weight loss, hyperthyroidism should be considered in any older cat with cardiac signs. The most commonly auscultated change is a murmur or tachycardia; also, the intensity of each heartbeat is often more pronounced and feels almost like a pounding on the clinician's eardrums. Typical echocardiographic abnormalities include hypertrophy of the left ventricular free wall (approximately 70% of cats), left atrial and ventricular dilation (70% and 45% of cats, respectively), and hypertrophy of the interventricular septum (40% of cases). Myocardial hypercontractility, manifested by increased fractional shortening and velocity of circumferential fiber shortening, is often found.[9] These changes can (uncommonly) result in congestive heart failure and even aortic thromboembolism.

Mild to moderate hypertension, reversible upon induction of euthyroidism, was originally considered important in hyperthyroid cats.[58,118] However, it is now clear that hyperthyroid cats are typically only mildly hypertensive, if at all, and when present may simply reflect the reduced tolerance of hyperthyroid cats to stressful situations such as veterinary examinations ("white-coat phenomenon").[117] In accordance with this, hypertension-associated blindness and obvious ocular abnormalities are uncommon in hyperthyroid cats even in the presence of documented hypertension.[132] Although hyperthyroidism is associated with increased cardiac output, there is a decrease in systemic vascular resistance mitigating against the development of significant hypertension.[119] If moderate to severe hypertension and its effects are demonstrated in a hyperthyroid cat, other potential causes such as chronic renal disease should be considered. Interestingly, some cats appear to develop hypertension after successful treatment of hyperthyroidism, and this may result, at least in part, from the increase in systemic vascular resistance as thyroid hormone concentrations decrease or from the associated decline in renal function.[119,120]

Cardiac and blood pressure changes, like most other signs of hyperthyroidism, are mostly reversible on treatment of the underlying endocrinopathy.[101] In some cases, however, cardiac changes may persist or worsen after treatment, suggesting a preexisting cardiac defect or thyroid hormone–induced irreversible structural damage.[9]

Palpable Thyroid Gland(s)

At least 80% of hyperthyroid cats have at least one palpable thyroid lobe.[13] The normal thyroid lobes are not palpable because they are flat (2 to 3 mm thick) and lie ventrolateral to the trachea and dorsal to the medial borders of the sternothyroideus and sternohyoideus muscles.[28] There are several techniques to palpate thyroids:

- *Classic technique:* The cat is restrained in sitting position and the front legs held still. The neck of the cat is extended, and the clinicians' thumb and index finger are placed on each side of the trachea and swept downward from the larynx to the sternal manubrium (Figure 24-10). Palpation of a mobile subcutaneous nodule or a "blip" that slips under the fingertips determines the presence of a goiter.[101]

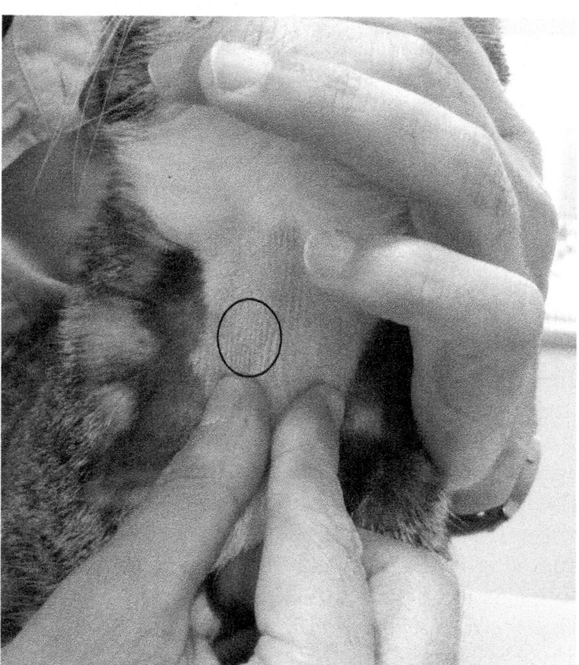

FIGURE 24-10 Classic thyroid palpation technique: The neck of the cat is extended, and the clinician's thumb and index finger are placed on each side of the trachea and swept downward from the larynx to the sternal manubrium. The thyroid is *circled*.

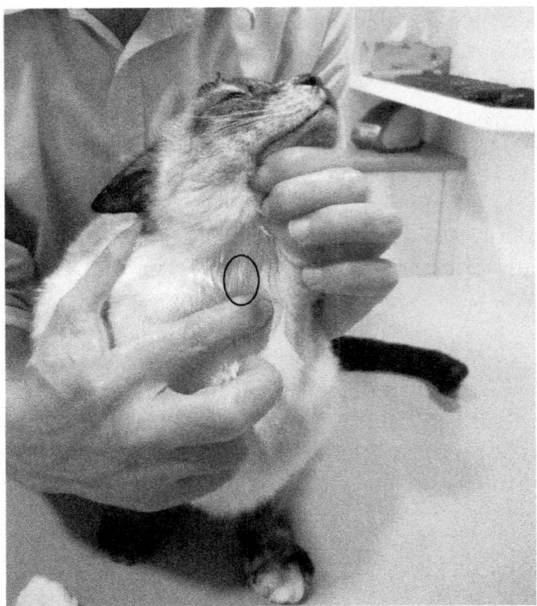

FIGURE 24-11 Norsworthy thyroid palpation technique: The cat's head is turned (45 degrees) from the side being assessed. The clinician's index finger is placed in the groove formed by the trachea and sternothyroid muscle just below the larynx and then moved downward in the groove to the thoracic inlet. The position of the thyroid lobe is circled. The technique is more successful when just the index finger runs down the jugular groove.

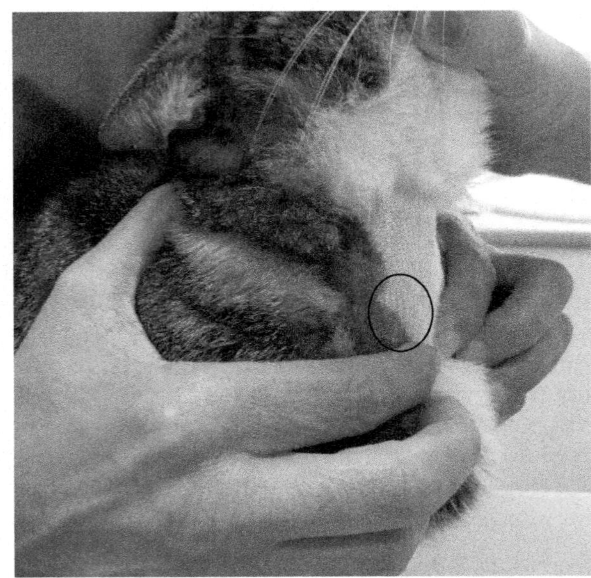

FIGURE 24-12 Two-handed thyroid palpation technique: A helper (possibly cat's owner) elevates the cat's chin to extend the neck. The clinician runs both index fingers, on either side of the trachea, from the larynx down to thoracic inlet. The thyroid is *circled*.

- *Norsworthy technique:* The clinician is positioned directly behind the cat, which is placed in standing position or sternal recumbency. The head of the cat is elevated and turned (45 degrees) alternatively to the right or left, away from the side being assessed (i.e., to palpate the right thyroid lobe, turn the cat's head to the left). The clinician's index finger is placed in the groove formed by the trachea and sternothyroid muscle just below the larynx and then moved downward in the groove to the thoracic inlet (Figure 24-11). If the thyroid lobe is enlarged, a characteristic "blip" is felt as the index finger passes the goiter.[77]
- *Two-handed technique:* The clinician is placed behind the sitting cat. A helper (which can be the cat's owner) elevates the cat's chin to extend the neck. The clinician runs both index fingers, on either side of the trachea, from the larynx down to thoracic inlet (Figure 24-12). As with the other techniques, a "blip" is felt as the index finger passes the goiter. This technique allows bilateral assessment with fingers of similar sensitivity.

The Norsworthy and classic techniques were compared, and both techniques were found to have a very good within- and good between-examiner agreement. The classic technique proved to be slightly more sensitive and specific in this study, but the authors were more familiar with it.[81] In one author's (RMB) practice, multiple techniques are used, and it seems that some thyroids that are more subtle to palpate are more noticeable with different techniques in different cats. All practitioners should be encouraged to practice all three techniques routinely.

Hyperactivity, Behavioral Changes, and General Appearance

The hyperactivity shown by hyperthyroid cats can be misconstrued by their owners as a sign of healthiness. In many cases the veterinarian may need to explain that older cats are usually quite sedentary and the increased activity is a manifestation of underlying processes causing agitation. Anxiety and restlessness can be obvious to owners if the cat yowls; the major differential diagnoses for night yowling are hyperthyroidism and hypertension (or both) as well as cognitive dysfunction. In clinical practice the restlessness shown may be manifested as an impaired tolerance for restraint for blood sampling (for example).

The hair coat of hyperthyroid cats is often dull and may be matted. Many hyperthyroid cats groom obsessively, resulting in alopecia and even miliary dermatitis; this may be associated with an underlying allergy (e.g., flea allergy dermatitis), but the response is magnified by apparent obsessive–compulsive behavior.

The increased activity in generally thin cats with dull coats has led to the description of hyperthyroid cats as "acting like they are alive, looking like they are dead."

Gastrointestinal Signs

Aside from weight loss, usually seen with increased or stable appetite, many hyperthyroid cats show other gastrointestinal signs, such as vomiting and diarrhea. Vomiting may be associated with rapid overeating; diarrhea is most likely due to intestinal hypermotility, although malabsorption is also a factor.

Urinary Signs

Polyuria and polydipsia are frequent signs of hyperthyroidism.[13] Thyroid hormones have a diuretic action that was recognized in the 1930s and 1940s,[104] and so hyperthyroidism (with renal disease and DM) is one of the three major rule-outs for a cat presenting with polyuria and polydipsia. Of course, conditions can occur concurrently, and diagnosing renal disease with hyperthyroidism may be difficult, insofar as hyperthyroidism can mask underlying renal disease.[8,38,133] Lower urinary tract signs may also be seen in hyperthyroid cats; a recent study demonstrated urinary tract infection in 12% of hyperthyroid cats assessed,[66] and one of the authors (RMB) has recognized noninfectious hematuria and dysuria in hyperthyroid cats that resolve on management of the hyperthyroidism.

Apathetic Hyperthyroidism

A percentage of hyperthyroid cats show atypical signs in which hyperexcitability or restlessness is replaced by depression or weakness. Although weight loss is present in these cats, it is accompanied by anorexia instead of increased appetite. Most studies have recognized these atypical signs in 5% to 10% of hyperthyroid cats,[13,123] but one (smaller) study found 20% of hyperthyroid cats to be lethargic and 28% to be inappetent.[14] Along these lines, although cardiac changes in hyperthyroid cats usually result in tachycardia, right bundle branch block and incomplete atrioventricular block, resulting in bradycardia, have been observed.[34] These disparate signs emphasize the need for clinicians to have a high index of suspicion for this common disease.

Diagnosis

The diagnosis of hyperthyroidism is usually straightforward, insofar as 90% of hyperthyroid cats have an elevated serum total T_4.[100] However, screening plasma (or serum) biochemistry and hematology are important to assess concurrent conditions that may affect the management if hyperthyroidism is diagnosed, as well as provide baseline values for parameters that can be affected by treatment (e.g., urea and creatinine or leukocytes). Thorough screening tests also aid in diagnosis if a cat with typical clinical signs of hyperthyroidism is not, in fact, hyperthyroid.

Hematologic Findings

Hematologic findings are usually nonspecific and mostly not clinically important. However, it is important to note baseline hematologic values because hematologic adverse reactions are possible when treating hyperthyroid cats with methimazole or carbimazole.[73,99] Some studies have found erythrocytosis and macrocytosis in approximately 50% of cats,[13,98] thought to be associated with direct bone marrow effects of thyroid hormones. Stress leukograms are sometimes recognized; eosinophilia and lymphocytosis have also been described.[13,98,123]

Biochemistry Findings

The liver enzymes, ALT, ALP, lactate dehydrogenase (LDH), and aspartate aminotransferase (AST) are increased in most hyperthyroid cats.[13,98,123] These liver enzyme changes and total T_4 concentrations are significantly correlated.[33,73] Despite sometimes very high increases, histologic examination of the liver usually reveals only mild, nonspecific changes. Liver enzymes return to normal on successful treatment of hyperthyroidism.[73]

Concurrent renal disease is common in hyperthyroid cats; however, the diagnosis of renal disease in hyperthyroid cats is not necessarily straightforward because of the interactions between the two diseases.* Blood urea nitrogen (BUN or urea) can be elevated in hyperthyroid cats as a result of excessive protein catabolism[37] but can also be decreased as a result of the increase in glomerular filtration rate (GFR) that occurs in hyperthyroidism.[1,5] Creatinine is usually reduced in hyperthyroid cats because of both increased GFR and reduced muscle mass.[133] One study found that most cats that have concurrent (masked) renal disease have urine specific gravities (USGs) that are below 1.040.[136] However, another study found that some cats with renal disease unmasked after treatment of hyperthyroidism had pretreatment USGs that were above 1.040, which suggests that USG cannot always predict concurrent renal disease.[108] Predicting which hyperthyroid cats will develop overt azotemia after treatment of hyperthyroidism can be difficult to impossible. The determination of GFR is clearly the best predictor of posttreatment chronic renal disease (CRD), with a low to low-normal GFR indicating that a hyperthyroid cat is at increased risk for posttreatment azotemia. However, techniques for assessment of GFR are not widely used in practice, and even GFR determinations are not a 100% perfect predictor of CRD. Routine pretreatment parameters such as serum urea or creatinine concentrations and

*References 1, 5, 38, 133, 135, 137.

USG are certainly useful, but they cannot consistently predict impending azotemia.[108] Similarly, treatment trials with methimazole or carbimazole can be very useful in unmasking concurrent renal disease, but these evaluations are not perfect predictors of CRD either. The interactions between CRD and hyperthyroidism are covered in more depth in Chapter 35.

Should methimazole trials be performed in all hyperthyroid cats? Again, determining which untreated hyperthyroid cats have clinically significant underlying CRD is sometimes difficult. Use of methimazole or carbimazole can provide a "preview" of how the cat will be after curing hyperthyroidism. Thus many veterinarians attempt trial therapy with methimazole or carbimazole to help test what renal function might remain after treating the hyperthyroidism. If no marked deterioration occurs, then a more permanent therapeutic option for hyperthyroidism may be recommended.

Except for advanced (IRIS Stage 3-4) CRD, the necessity of this approach in cats without pretreatment azotemia is questionable, given that treatment for the hyperthyroidism is required whatever the outcome. In support of this reasoning, the survival of nonazotemic cats that do develop CRD is not shorter than those that do not develop azotemia after treatment of hyperthyroidism. In one study the medium survival time of cats that developed azotemia (595 days) was similar to that of cats that remained nonazotemic (584 days) after treatment.[145]

Hyperphosphatemia, independent of azotemia, has been recognized in hyperthyroid cats.[2,4,13,98,123] This, with the recognized increase in the bone isoenzyme of ALP (which contributes to liver enzyme increases) suggests altered bone metabolism. Circulating osteocalcin concentration, a measure of osteoblastic activity and bone remodeling, is increased in hyperthyroid people, and this was recognized in nearly half of hyperthyroid cats in one study.[2] Coincident with this change, decreased blood ionized calcium and increased parathyroid hormone can be seen. The reasons for these changes are not entirely clear; they may be associated with increased tubular resorption of phosphate together with increased phosphate loads from exaggerated bone resorption and muscle catabolism.[4]

Blood glucose concentrations may be increased in some hyperthyroid cats, in many cases reflecting a stress response; however, hyperthyroidism is also associated with glucose intolerance characterized by delayed clearance of administered glucose from the plasma despite increased secretion of insulin.[46]

Thyroid Function Testing

Serum total T_4 is preferable as a screening test for hyperthyroidism because although total T_3 concentrations are highly correlated to total T_4,[13,98,100] 25% to 30% of hyperthyroid cats have serum total T_3 within the reference range.[13,100]

Most total T_4 assays available have been independently assessed and found to be comparable in ability to diagnose hyperthyroidism. Practitioners should have some awareness of the techniques available and being used by their commercial laboratories (or in house).

- Radioimmunoassay (RIA) validated for feline serum,[107,124] such as Coat-A-Count Total T_4 (Diagnostic Products Corp), is considered to be the preferred technique.[54,64,88]
- Chemiluminescent enzyme immunoassays such as Immulite Total T_4 (Diagnostic Products Corp) have also been validated for feline serum.[54,114] Many commercial laboratories prefer this technique because it is more automated.
- An enzymatic chemistry method (DRI thyroxine assay, Microgenics Corporation) is also now being used by some laboratories. This technique has the advantage for the laboratory of being fully automated, which benefits the practitioner and patient because results are available sooner. However, this technique does not appear to have been independently validated for cats.
- In-house enzyme-linked immunosorbent assay (ELISA) test kits are also available. One study found discrepancies with this in-house testing method compared with RIA,[64] but two more recent studies have found clinical agreement between the same in-house testing and validated techniques.[54,85]

Difficulties in Diagnosing Hyperthyroidism

Difficulties arise with the diagnosis of hyperthyroidism when a cat is hyperthyroid but total T_4 is not elevated or a cat has a palpably enlarged thyroid lobe (or both lobes) but does not have functional hyperthyroidism.

Hyperthyroid Cat with Normal T_4

Some cats with overt clinical signs of hyperthyroidism can have normal total T_4 believed to be due to either of the following:

1. Fluctuation of T_4 and T_3 concentrations in and out of the normal range. T_4 and other thyroid hormones have been shown to fluctuate considerably over time in hyperthyroid cats. These fluctuations seem to be relevant only in cats with mild hyperthyroidism in which a fluctuation downward can lower T_4 to within the reference range.[96]
2. Suppression of serum T_4 and T_3 concentrations into the normal range because of concurrent nonthyroidal illness.[67,95,100] Diseases that suppress T_4 include chronic renal disease, DM, neoplasia, gastrointestinal disorders, and primary hepatic

disease.[100] One of the authors (RMB) has also recognized infection as suppressing T_4, such as that acquired through a cat fight injury or dental disease. In the case of renal disease, hyperthyroidism can mask renal disease concurrent with the renal disease suppressing T_4[100,144]; thus cats with mild kidney disease and mild hyperthyroidism may have neither azotemia nor elevated total T_4. Occasionally, hyperthyroid cats that are extremely ill may have clinical signs of hyperthyroidism but serum total T_4 concentrations suppressed to the low end of the normal reference range.[100,126] In such cases the concurrent illness dictates the prognosis, and the existence of hyperthyroidism is of lesser clinical significance.[88]

Because there is no definitive approach to diagnose hyperthyroidism when total T_4 is normal, the practitioner has several options:

1. *Repeat total T_4:* When overt, manageable underlying disease, such as a cat fight abscess, is present, this should be managed in the first instance. If signs of hyperthyroidism are recognized when a cat presents for such a problem, the practitioner may elect not to test for hyperthyroidism until after successful treatment. When no overt underlying disease is present, the practitioner should wait at least 1 to 2 weeks because thyroid hormone fluctuations are greater over days than hours.[96]
2. *Scintigraphy:* Thyroid scintigraphy is a nuclear medicine procedure that produces a visual display of functional thyroid tissue based on the selective uptake of various radionuclides by thyroid tissue. Thyroid scintigraphy is able to identify thyroid disease and define the degree of disease relatively unaffected by the presence of concurrent nonthyroidal illness. Technetium (^{99m}Tc) as pertechnetate ($^{99m}TcO_4$) is a radioactive iodine isotope that has increased uptake in hyperthyroid cats. The cat is injected intravenously or subcutaneously with pertechnetate, and then images are taken with a gamma camera 20 minutes later. The uptake by the thyroid gland is compared with the uptake by the salivary glands (Figure 24-13). It is generally accepted that the thyroid-to-salivary uptake ratio in healthy cats is less than 1. Scintigraphy is also useful in identifying ectopic thyroid tissue (Figure 24-14), which may be present anywhere from the base of the tongue caudally to within the thoracic cavity.[11,43,82] Although scintigraphy is highly sensitive in diagnosis of hyperthyroid cats, one study questioned its specificity, with 3 of 14 cats proving to be false positives (by histologic assessment of the thyroids).[127]

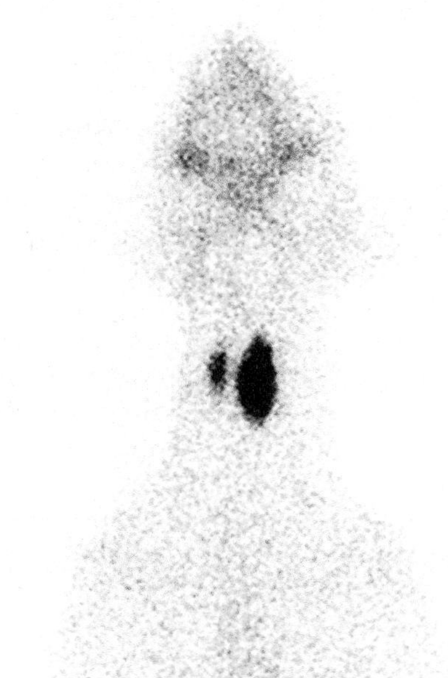

FIGURE 24-13 Scintigraphy indicating bilateral asymmetric pertechnetate uptake by thyroid glands. *(Courtesy Dr. Max Zuber, Gladesville Veterinary Hospital, Sydney, Australia.)*

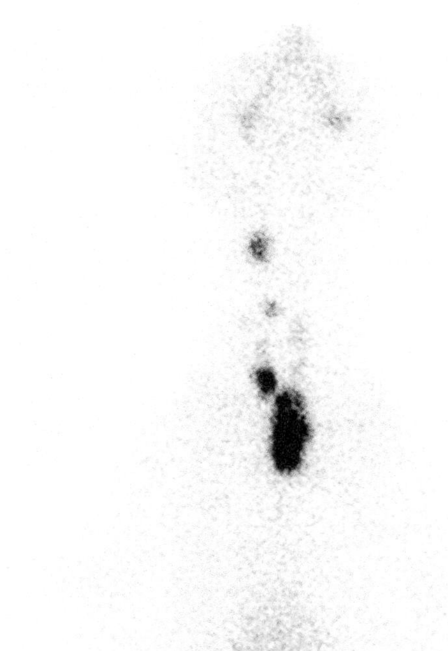

FIGURE 24-14 Scintigraphy indicating pertechnetate uptake ectopically at the thoracic inlet. *(Courtesy Dr Max Zuber, Gladesville Veterinary Hospital, Sydney, Australia.)*

Methimazole administration may also affect scintigraphy findings, resulting in a significant increase in the percentage uptake of pertechnetate,[75] although this is not a consistent finding.[30]

Scintigraphy requires specialized equipment and handling of radioisotopes so is not readily available.

In addition, sedation may be required, especially in fractious cats.

3. *Free T_4 values (tested by equilibrium dialysis):* The free T_4 value is more sensitive than total T_4 in hyperthyroid cats, with one large study demonstrating 98.5% having elevated free T_4 compared with 91.3% having elevated total T_4.[100] Free T_4 cannot, however, be used as a routine screening test because nonthyroidal disease can cause an elevation of free T_4 in up to 12% of nonhyperthyroid cats.[72,100] Free T_4 testing provides very useful information when used in conjunction with simultaneous total T_4 testing. A middle to high reference range total T_4 concentration and an elevated free T_4 concentration are consistent with hyperthyroidism.[100] By contrast, a low total T_4 value and elevated free T_4 value are usually associated with nonthyroidal illness.[72,100] Care must be taken that the laboratory measures free T_4 by equilibrium dialysis, insofar as other techniques are considered less accurate.[88]
4. *TSH:* As hyperthyroidism develops, TSH is suppressed.[57,144,146] Theoretically, as in humans, it could be expected that TSH levels should be low in the early stages of hyperthyroidism before T_4 is elevated or that TSH will remain low if T_4 is suppressed by nonthyroidal illness. Although there is currently no feline TSH test, because canine TSH has 96% homology with feline TSH, canine tests have been used.[36,110,144,146] This is controversial because the canine TSH assays are considered first-generation assays (there are more sophisticated human TSH assays) and normal concentrations cannot reliably be distinguished from undetectable values.[29] This claim is supported by one study in which not only all hyperthyroid but also 5 of 40 of the nonhyperthyroid cats had undetectable levels of TSH.[144] Feline TSH has recently been expressed and purified *in vitro*,[106] and if this work leads to the availability of a feline-specific TSH, this assay may prove useful in diagnosing hyperthyroidism in cats with equivocal T_4 levels.
5. *Dynamic testing:* In the majority of hyperthyroid cats with normal total T_4 concentrations, identification of concurrent disease, repeat total T_4 analysis, or simultaneous measurement of free T_4 allows confirmation of the diagnosis. Further diagnostic tests are rarely required. Although dynamic thyroid function tests have been recommended in the past as helpful in confirming a diagnosis of hyperthyroidism, the current consensus is that these tests should be considered only in cats with clinical signs suggestive of hyperthyroidism when repeated total T_4 concentration remains within reference range or free T_4 analysis is unavailable or diagnostically unhelpful. The authors rarely, if ever, use these tests. The protocols for these tests are shown in Table 24-6.
   - *T_3 suppression:* In a nonhyperthyroid cat, administration of T_3 should suppress TSH secretion and therefore T_4 secretion. In hyperthyroid cats, thyroidal function is autonomous so T_3 administration has little effect on serum T_4 concentration. T_3 (liothyronine, Cytomel, Jones Medical Industries, Pointe Claire, Quebec) must be given orally every 8 hours for seven doses (i.e., over 3 days). Failure to adhere to this protocol means T_3 will not rise and therefore T_4 will not be suppressed.[97]
   - *Thyroid releasing hormone (TRH) stimulation:* In clinically normal cats the administration of TRH causes an increase in TSH secretion and serum T_4

TABLE 24-6 **Commonly Used Protocols for Dynamic Thyroid Function Tests in Cats**[88]

	T_3 Suppression	TRH Stimulation	TSH Stimulation	
Drug	Liothyronine (Cytomel)	TRH	Bovine TSH	Human TSH
Dose	25 μg every 8 hours for 7 doses	0.1 mg/kg	0.5 IU/kg	0.025-0.20 mg/cat
Route	Oral	Intravenous	Intravenous	Intravenous
Sampling times	0 and 2-4 hours after last dose	0 and 4 hours	0 and 6 hours	1 and 6-8 hours
Assay	Total T_4 Total T_3	Total T_4	Total T_4	Total T_4
INTERPRETATION				
Euthyroidism	>50% suppression	>60% increase	>100% increase	>100% increase
Hyperthyroidism	<35% suppression	<50% increase	Minimal/no increase	Not determined

TRH, Thyrotropin-releasing hormone; *TSH*, thyroid-stimulating hormone.

concentrations, whereas in cats with hyperthyroidism the TSH and serum T_4 response to TRH is blunted or totally absent. T_4 is collected and sampled before and 4 hours after intravenous administration of 0.1 mg/kg TRH. Cats with mild hyperthyroidism show little, if any, rise in serum T_4 values after administration of TRH, whereas a consistent rise in serum T_4 concentrations (approximately a twofold rise) occurs after TRH administration in both clinically normal cats and cats with nonthyroidal disease. Side effects such as salivation, vomiting, tachypnea, and defecation almost invariably occur immediately after administration of the TRH.[94]

- *TSH stimulation:* Exogenous TSH should be a potent stimulator of thyroid hormone secretion; however, serum total T_4 concentrations show little or no increase after exogenous bovine TSH administration in hyperthyroid cats. Recombinant human TSH has been evaluated in healthy cats, and although it appears to be a safe and effective replacement for bovine TSH, it has not yet been evaluated in hyperthyroid cats. TSH stimulation testing is not recommended to diagnose hyperthyroidism.[88]

Enlarged Thyroid Gland But Not Hyperthyroid

Nonfunctional enlargement of thyroid glands (goiter) has been recognized since the 1960s[61,62] but has taken on new significance since functional hyperthyroidism arose as an entity in the late 1970s.[93] Nonfunctional goiter was recognized again in the late 1990s[17] but rose to prominence in 2002.[76,77] Many authors agree that clinical hyperthyroidism has a prodromal period (also called *subclinical hyperthyroidism* or *prehyperthyroidism*).* One paper claimed to have defined subclinical hyperthyroidism by depressed TSH concentrations,[146] but this has been contested because of the lack of sensitivity of the canine TSH assay.[29] It is not clear whether all goiters indicate that the cat will develop hyperthyroidism. Thyroidectomy of nonfunctional goiters has been proposed[28,76] as a preventive measure. This strategy appears benign,[28,76] but there is no definitive evidence to support this approach.

Treatment

Medical management with methimazole or carbimazole, surgical thyroidectomy, and radioactive iodine (I^{131}) are all appropriate modalities to manage hyperthyroid cats. Each has advantages and disadvantages that can be used to integrate them when formulating a treatment plan for each individual hyperthyroid cat. Medical management is considered reversible, and thyroidectomy and I^{131} are considered permanent treatments. Recent studies have indicated that a newly introduced iodine-restricted diet (Hill's Prescription Diet y/d Feline–Thyroid Health) may provide a further option for medical management.[67b,150]

Treatment Considerations

CONCURRENT CONDITIONS

RENAL Because CRD is very common in older cats, it is hardly surprising that it is commonly found concurrent with hyperthyroidism. As noted in the discussion of diagnosis, the increased GFR and reduced muscle mass that hyperthyroidism induces can mask underlying renal disease.* Because it is not possible to predict which hyperthyroid cats have renal disease, it is ideal to perform a treatment trial of hyperthyroid cats with a reversible therapy (e.g., methimazole, carbimazole) and then reassess renal parameters when rechecking total T_4.[37] Because the biggest reductions in GFR occur within the first month and then remain stable for the following 5 months,[135] a 30-day methimazole–carbimazole trial is appropriate. The practitioner should use discretion to assess whether the cat's hyperthyroidism seems controlled before testing; if, for example, the cat has not gained weight and tachycardia is still apparent, the methimazole–carbimazole dose can be increased and the cat can be tested for T_4 and renal parameters a month later.

If, when T_4 has normalized, renal parameters are normal, planning for a permanent therapy such as thyroidectomy or radioactive iodine can proceed. Mild to moderate kidney disease should not preclude permanent treatment of hyperthyroidism.

Immediate permanent therapy without a methimazole–carbimazole trial is appropriate for relatively young cats with completely normal BUN and creatinine, and USG above 1.035. Moreover, some owners may prefer immediate permanent therapy because of their reluctance to medicate their cat.

Figure 24-15 shows how T_4 is inversely related to urea and creatinine in one particular cat as carbimazole dose was changed over a 40-month period. This case also shows very nicely how the azotemia worsens over time. Although this is likely due to the expected progression of CRD in cats with time, it is important to realize that the hyperthyroid state in itself may be damaging to renal function. Recent research provides evidence that hyperthyroidism may contribute to the development or progression of CRD in cats. First of all, a number of recent reports indicate that many untreated hyperthyroid cats develop proteinuria, which resolves within 4 weeks of

*References 28-29, 76, 77, 140, 141.

*References 1, 5, 37, 38, 133, 135, 137.

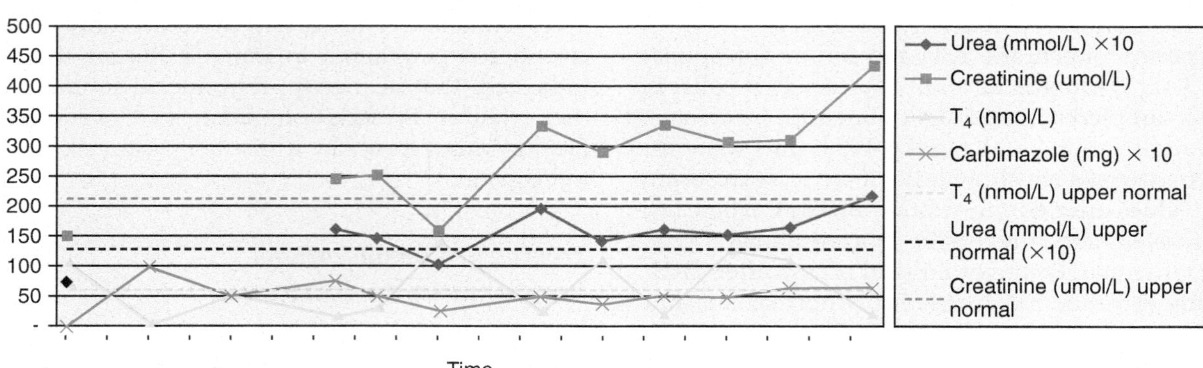

FIGURE 24-15 Variations in T_4 and renal parameters as carbimazole dose was changed multiple times over a 40-month period. The units are shown in the figure key, but more important is the inverse relationship between serum total T_4 (*yellow*) and renal parameters (creatinine is *pink*, and urea is *dark blue*). As carbimazole dose (*pale blue*) is reduced, T_4 (*yellow*) elevates and creatinine (*pink*) and urea (*dark blue*) decrease. As carbimazole increases, T_4 is suppressed but creatinine and urea increase. The clinical pathology results must be balanced with the cat's clinical responses. A mild elevation of T_4 may be tolerable if there are no cardiac signs and weight loss is not substantial. Conversely, mild azotemia often does not result in clinical signs.

successful treatment.[136,149] This proteinuria could be a reflection of glomerular hypertension and hyperfiltration, changes in tubular protein handling, or a change in the structure of the glomerular barrier. Secondly, cats with untreated hyperthyroidism have high levels of retinol-binding protein (RBP), a urinary marker for tubular dysfunction or damage.[134,138] This high urinary RBP excretion may reflect tubular damage or dysfunction resulting from the thyroid-induced hypertrophy and hyperplasia of the tubular cells. After treatment these high urinary RBP levels fall in cats without azotemia but may remain slightly high in cats with preexisting CRD. This too suggests that hyperthyroidism can cause reversible renal dysfunction; however, the renal tubular changes may become irreversible with time as CRD progresses. Thirdly, many cats with untreated hyperthyroidism have high values for urinary N-acetyl-b-D-glucosaminidase (NAG), a lysosomal glycosidase found primarily in epithelial cells of the proximal convoluted tubule.[60] Like RBP, NAG is a specific marker of active proximal tubular damage. After treatment these high urinary NAG levels decrease, again suggesting that these renal changes can be reversed, at least in cats without preexisting CRD.

Overall, these studies suggest that leaving a hyperthyroid cat untreated (or poorly regulated with methimazole) may be detrimental to long-term kidney function. Treating and curing hyperthyroidism may help both to reverse renal damage and to preserve remaining kidney function.

Concurrent hyperthyroidism and CRD are covered in more detail in Chapter 35.

CARDIAC The cardiac changes for most cats with hyperthyroidism are mild. Murmurs and tachycardia are not often associated with clinical signs of heart disease. However, some hyperthyroid cats initially present for severe cardiac-related disease. On the occasions when cats show more severe cardiac changes, such as congestive heart failure and aortic thromboembolism, these should be stabilized before a cat undergoes thyroidectomy or is isolated after I^{131} therapy.

HYPERTENSION Mild to moderate hypertension appears to develop in approximately 10% to 20% of untreated hyperthyroid cats and is generally reversible on induction of euthyroidism.[119] If hypertension is severe or persists after treatment of hyperthyroidism; however, these cats should be managed with amlodipine. In many cases amlodipine can be discontinued when the cat becomes euthyroid. Conversely, some cats are normotensive when hyperthyroidism is diagnosed but may become hypertensive after becoming euthyroid.[120] In the authors' experience, these cats invariably have some degree of renal disease.

HEPATIC As previously noted, cats often have benign elevations in liver enzymes when diagnosed with hyperthyroidism. Therefore it is not possible to know at the time of diagnosis if increased liver enzymes are due to hepatic pathology unrelated to hyperthyroidism or merely a manifestation of hyperthyroidism. If it is the latter, a treatment trial with methimazole–carbimazole should result in a reduction of liver enzymes, and a permanent treatment should be considered. If, with normalization of T_4, liver enzymes remain elevated, permanent treatment is not ideal and investigations should proceed to diagnose an underlying hepatopathy. However, a reversible hepatopathy can result *from* methimazole[99] or carbimazole (not reported except anecdotally, by one of the authors' [RMB]) therapy. In this circumstance the practitioner should discontinue medical therapy and, after the cat's recovery, consider whether, on balance, a permanent therapy is appropriate.

OTHER Because hyperthyroid patients are elderly, multiple other concurrent conditions are possible. UTI has been recognized in 12% of hyperthyroid cats[66] and should be treated before a cat goes into isolation after I^{131} therapy.

If, for example, an abdominal mass is recognized at the time of diagnosis, it is not appropriate for a cat to undergo thyroidectomy or I^{131} therapy until this has been investigated. Medical therapy is appropriate in this circumstance.

CLIENT CIRCUMSTANCES

Cost of therapy is a major consideration for many clients. Medical therapy costs far less initially. However, the cost of ongoing monitoring can equal that of thyroidectomy or I^{131} therapy over a several years. Many (most) cats treated with methimazole or carbimazole are remarkably stable and do not show side effects. All cats should have an initial assessment after 1 month of starting therapy to recheck total T_4, renal parameters, and hematology (and liver enzymes if they were elevated), as well as to assess for weight gain and improvement of any other clinical signs initially shown. Beyond this time cats should be checked every 3 months. It is ideal to recheck total T_4 at each visit, but if the client is concerned about the cost, a thorough physical examination should establish whether the clinical signs of hyperthyroidism are controlled and the testing may be performed less frequently.

Pregnancy and children in the household should be considered and discussed with the client before I^{131} therapy because cats will continue to emit radiation for some weeks after returning home. If isolation from pregnant women or children is not possible when the cat returns home, I^{131} therapy should not be considered as a treatment option.

Medical Therapy

Methimazole blocks thyroid hormone synthesis by inhibiting thyroid peroxidase, an enzyme involved in the oxidation of iodide to iodine, incorporation of iodine into thyroglobulin, and coupling of tyrosine residues to form T_4 and T_3. Methimazole does not block the release of preformed thyroid hormone, so there is a delay of 2 to 4 weeks before serum T_4 concentrations return to normal after initializing therapy.[99] Methimazole does not decrease goiter size, and because hyperplasia or adenomatous growth continues, goiters may become larger over time despite therapy. In most cats 2.5 mg twice daily is an appropriate dose to manage clinical signs. In one study of 40 hyperthyroid cats, 5 mg once daily was less effective than 2.5 mg twice daily, with only 54% of cats euthyroid after 2 weeks of once-daily treatment, compared with 87% of cats treated with divided daily dosing.[129] Doses can be titrated upward if the cat does not respond to the initial dose.

Carbimazole is a derivative of methimazole that is converted to methimazole *in vivo*.[90] It is available in Australia and Europe. Because a 5-mg carbimazole dose is equivalent to a 3-mg methimazole dose, 5 mg twice daily is an appropriate dose to manage hyperthyroidism in most cats.[73] For initial control 5 mg three times daily has been advocated,[73] but 5 mg twice daily is adequate in most cats, and if the dose needs to be titrated upward, 7.5 mg twice daily achieves the same result as 5 mg three times daily.

Adverse effects can be seen with both methimazole and carbimazole, although these may be less common and less severe with carbimazole.[63] Transient, self-limiting anorexia, vomiting, and lethargy are the most common side effects, occurring in approximately 10% of cats treated with methimazole.[99] Halving the dose and titrating to the lowest effective dose may be helpful to reduce these side effects.[130] More serious side effects include blood dyscrasias such as neutropenia and thrombocytopenia in 3% to 9% of treated cats; hepatopathy in approximately 2% of cats[99,111]; and excoriations of the face and neck in 2% to 3% of cats.[99] All these adverse effects are reversible on discontinuation of the medication.[130]

Methimazole or carbimazole is adequate to manage 99% of hyperthyroid cats.[99] Some cats, however, will not tolerate the dose of methimazole or carbimazole necessary to control their hyperthyroidism. In these cases a permanent therapy is recommended. For cats that are not good candidates for permanent therapy (e.g., moderate to severe azotemia, advanced age with other debilitating problems), lower doses of methimazole or carbimazole can be used, and adjunctive medical therapy can be used to manage other problems—for example, a beta blocker such as atenolol to control tachycardia or amlodipine for hypertension. These cats need to be monitored for changes in renal function or continued weight loss.[130]

Transdermal preparations of methimazole[48,49,111] and, more recently, carbimazole[15] have proved to be effective alternatives to the oral versions of these medications. Transdermal preparations must be prepared by a compounding pharmacy and, to ensure drug stability, should be dispensed in quantities lasting for no more than 1 month. They may be used when the owner has difficulty medicating the cat and may result in reduced gastrointestinal side effects.[111]

Recent studies have indicated that diets with restricted iodine levels (Hill's Prescription Diet y/d Feline–Thyroid Health) can result in normalization of T_4 levels in hyperthyroid cats.[67b,150] In one study, cats were fed diets with sequentially reduced iodine contents; an iodine restricted food with 0.28 ppm iodine resulted in euthyroidism in 8 of 9 cats and a diet with an iodine content of 0.17 ppm resulted in euthyroidism in all cats tested.[67b] The one cat that required the lower iodine level for euthyroidism had a notably higher total T_4 than the other cats tested, suggesting this therapy may be more appropriate for cats with only moderate elevations of T_4. Another study by the same investigators found that a dietary iodine level of 0.32 ppm also resulted in euthyroidism in cats with moderate elevations of T_4 (up to 84 nmol/L [6.5 μg/dL]).[150] Continued control of total T_4 levels was not possible when iodine content was increased to 0.39 ppm.[67a,67b] These interesting findings may change management of hyperthyroidism in the future. Ironically, a recent publication showed varying levels of available iodine in commercially available foods and suggested that hyperthyroidism in cats may be reduced by providing diets that are adequately supplemented with iodine.[26b] In humans, it is recognized that both high-iodine[115a] and low-iodine[60a] diets can contribute to hyperthyroidism; similar associations in cats are unproven but, if so, restricted dietary iodine therapy would not be expected to be helpful in all hyperthyroid cats. Further, cats with very high total T_4 levels may not be manageable with dietary therapy alone. Additionally, low-iodine diets may increase the percentage uptake of I^{131}; some authors believe that low-iodine diets in humans can increase radioiodine uptake in thyroid tissue as much as twofold.[52a] The reduced total I^{131} dose required would shorten the necessary hospitalization time after such therapy.

Once euthyroidism has been achieved, it is ideal for the cat to undergo permanent therapy. Thyroidectomy can be performed immediately. Antithyroid drugs appear to interfere with the thyroid's ability to uptake and concentrate radioactive iodine.[10] This is controversial: One study did not find such an association,[18] and another indicated that uptake can be enhanced,[75] which may create a risk of subsequent hypothyroidism. One recommendation is to discontinue methimazole or carbimazole for at least 1 week before treatment with radioiodine.[89] This solution is inappropriate for cats with serious consequences of their hyperthyroidism (e.g., congestive heart failure). These circumstances must be addressed on a case-by-case basis. Cats in these circumstances can continue with medical therapy, undergo thyroidectomy, or proceed with radioiodine therapy (perhaps with less predictable results but without apparent problems in many cases).

Those cats whose owners choose to continue with medical therapy should have ongoing monitoring; every 3 months is an appropriate interval. It is important to assess the cat for clinical signs of hyperthyroidism, but also, ideally, serum total T_4 should be checked. If renal parameters are normal, these need to be checked only every 6 months.

Thyroidectomy

Thyroidectomy is a straightforward procedure that most surgeons can learn relatively quickly. It is ideal to achieve euthyroidism before surgery, as already outlined, so the cardiac effects of hyperthyroidism are reduced (and preferably eliminated) to reduce anesthetic risk. The major postsurgical complication is hypocalcemia, which results from damage to the parathyroid glands. To reduce the chances of hypocalcemia, it has been recommended *not* to perform bilateral thyroidectomy but instead to stage surgery and perform surgery on the second side some weeks later.[31,32] This is not necessary for cats in which one thyroid gland is more prominent. Although disease is bilateral in 70% of cases, one of the authors (RMB) has found that most of these have a dominant side, and it often takes years for hyperthyroidism to recur from the remaining gland, if it does at all. However, the client must be warned that the condition could recur sooner or even immediately.

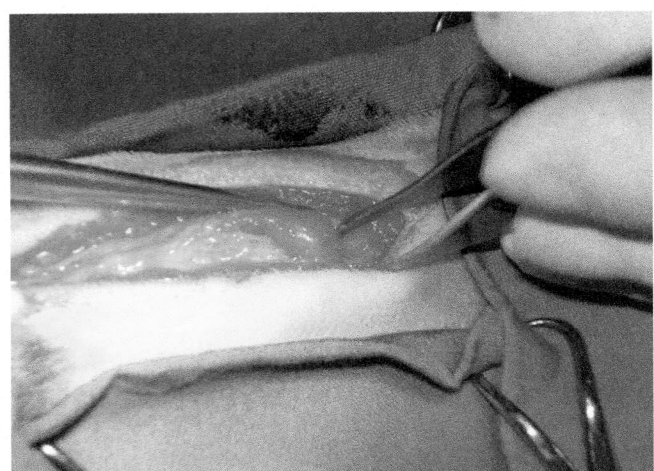

FIGURE 24-16 Thyroidectomy: Blunt dissection is required to free the affected thyroid lobe from surrounding fascia.

To further reduce the chances of hypocalcemia, the parathyroid glands should be preserved. This is best achieved by the modified extracapsular technique with parathyroid autotransplantation: After a ventral midline cervical approach, the affected thyroid lobe is dissected free from surrounding fascia, working from caudal to cranial (Figure 24-16). The external parathyroid gland is identified at the cranial aspect of the thyroid gland (Figure 24-17). The thyroid gland capsule is incised adjacent to the parathyroid gland. The parathyroid gland is then carefully separated from the thyroid using sterile cotton-tipped applicators. Once the parathyroid gland is completely separated from the thyroid, the thyroid gland is completely removed, using blunt and sharp dissection and taking care to ligate vasculature. The parathyroid gland is divided with two thirds inserted into a small pocket made in the cervical musculature. Revascularization can occur, and resumption of parathyroid function may result, decreasing the severity and time of postoperative hypocalcemia. Hypocalcemia is a

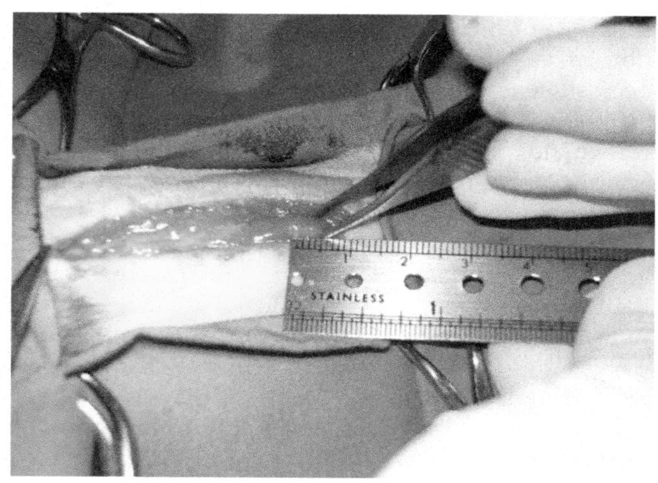

FIGURE 24-17 Identification of the parathyroid while performing thyroidectomy. The parathyroid gland is to the right of the thyroid, just in front of the ruler and measuring approximately 4 to 5 mm. Not all external parathyroids are as easily recognizable as this.

rare consequence of unilateral thyroidectomy. The remaining third of the parathyroid gland is sent for histology with the thyroid gland for confirmation that it is, in fact, parathyroid tissue.[80] Closure of the incision is by simple continuous suture pattern in the sternohyoideus muscle using absorbable suture, a simple continuous pattern in the subcutaneous tissues with absorbable suture, and interrupted sutures in the skin with nonabsorbable sutures.

Serum total T_4 should be checked 1 month after surgery, again 6 months later, and then annually to check for disease recurrence. The owner should be warned of the possibility of recurrence and return sooner if clinical signs of hyperthyroidism return.

Radioactive Iodine (I^{131})

Radioactive iodine (I^{131}) therapy is considered the gold-standard treatment of hyperthyroidism in cats. Treatment involves either oral dosing or subcutaneous injection and is without associated morbidity or mortality. A single treatment restores euthyroidism in most cats with hyperthyroidism. Although therapy is simple and relatively stress-free for cats, it does require special licensing and hospitalization facilities and extensive compliance with local and state radiation safety laws. The administered radioactive iodine concentrates in and destroys hyperactive thyroid tissue within the cat's body, whether in the normal cervical area or in ectopic sites. The major drawback is that after administration of radioiodine, the cat must be kept hospitalized for a period (7 to 10 days in most treatment centers), and visiting is not allowed. Most cats are very settled during their stay after (I^{131}) therapy (Figures 24-18 and 24-19). Some cats do become depressed with the long isolation, and, more importantly, the isolation period is not appropriate

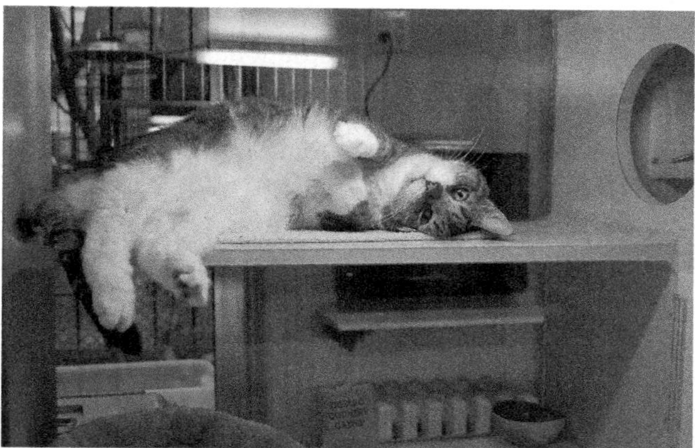

FIGURE 24-18 After administration of radioiodine, the cat must be kept hospitalized for 7 to 10 days and visiting is not allowed.

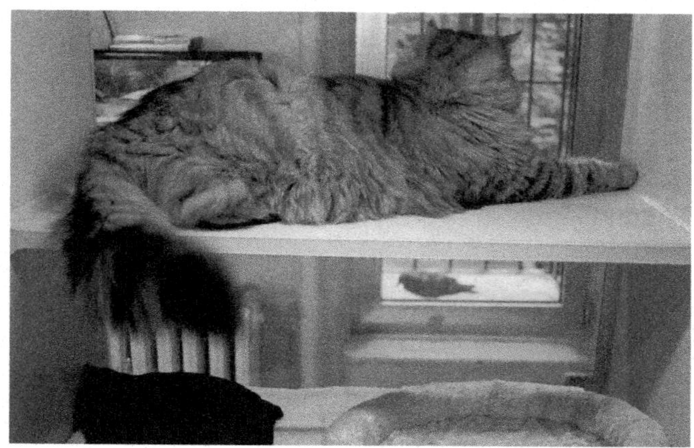

FIGURE 24-19 Environmental enrichment helps most cats feel content and settled during their stay.

for cats with any concurrent condition. Less than 5% do not respond adequately to a single treatment; most of these cases respond well to a repeat treatment with resolution of their hyperthyroidism.

Thyrocytes do not differentiate between stable and radioactive iodine; therefore radioiodine, like stable iodine, is concentrated by the thyroid gland after administration.[12,44,92] In cats with hyperthyroidism, radioiodine is concentrated primarily in the hyperplastic or neoplastic thyroid cells, where it irradiates and destroys the hyperfunctioning tissue.[91,92] Normal thyroid tissue, however, tends to be protected from the effects of radioiodine because the uninvolved thyroid tissue is suppressed and receives only a small dose of radiation (unless very large doses are administered).

When administered to a cat with hyperthyroidism, a large percentage of radioiodine accumulates in the thyroid gland (i.e., most cats extract between 20% and 60% of the administered radioiodine dose from the circulation).[12,44] The remainder of the administered I^{131} is excreted primarily in the urine and, to a lesser degree, the feces.[12,44] I^{131} has a half-life of 8 days and emits both beta particles and gamma radiation. The beta particles, which cause 80% of the tissue damage, travel a maximum of 2 mm in tissue and have an average path length of 400 μm. Therefore, beta particles are locally destructive but spare adjacent hypoplastic thyroid tissue, parathyroid glands, and other cervical structures.[89]

There is no definitive method to determine the most appropriate dose of I^{131}. Fixed doses are not recommended because they can provide too low a dose and not adequately treat the disease or they can provide too high a dose, resulting not only in hypothyroidism but also in a greater radiation hazard than is necessary for veterinary staff attending the cat in hospital. A more precise dose can be estimated by scoring systems that take into account the severity of clinical signs, the degree of elevation of T_4, and the size of the palpable gland.[71,92] Yet more precision can be gained with scintigraphy because it can also recognize ectopic thyroid tissue.

While hospitalized, cats should be housed in cages that shield radiation emission and allow safe collection of urine and feces. The ward should be restricted to staff properly trained in radiation safety. Proper attention cannot be given to cats that become unwell, and samples (e.g., blood, urine) cannot safely be submitted to laboratories. The cat's level of radiation emission must be assessed (usually by Geiger counter) before the cat can be discharged from hospital. Even when home, the cat continues to emit minimal residual radiation for several weeks; therefore close contact with owners should be limited to periods not exceeding 30 minutes and soiled cat litter should be discarded in sanitary sewer systems for about 2 weeks. Contact with pregnant women or children is entirely prohibited in this time.

The most notable side effect of radioactive iodine is hypothyroidism induced by too large a dose. In many cases there may be a laboratory decrease in serum T_4 without clinical signs.

Serum total T_4 should be rechecked 1 month after therapy, although it can take several more months for clinical signs of hyperthyroidism to resolve entirely. Relapse after I^{131} is possible but rare, and if it does occur may be 3 or more years after treatment; because of this possibility, rechecking serum total T_4 annually is ideal.[92]

Diagnosis and Treatment of Thyroid Adenocarcinoma

In most cases, cats with thyroid adenocarcinoma present similarly to those with hyperthyroidism as a result of adenomatous hyperplasia or thyroid adenoma.[40,45,131]

Histopathologic evaluation is generally considered the gold standard for the diagnosis of thyroid carcinoma, and definitive identification of thyroid carcinoma on histopathology often requires identification of vascular or capsular invasion and frequently necessitates that excisional biopsy be performed.[11] Scintigraphy can be used adjunctively, especially in recognizing regional and distance metastasis,[11] but scintigraphy alone cannot reliably distinguish whether the thyroid tissue is malignant.[45]

Thyroid carcinoma may be suspected if the palpable goiter is particularly big, serum total T_4 is particularly high (the authors have seen values greater than eight times the upper limit of normal), or hyperthyroidism persists despite high doses of methimazole or carbimazole. In some cases none of these criteria will apply, and each of these criteria may also apply to benign hyperthyroidism. Failure of a routine treatment approach (e.g., routine doses of methimazole, carbimazole, or I^{131}) should alert the clinician to the possibility of malignancy. In these circumstances thyroidectomy is recommended so that a histologic diagnosis can be achieved. Some thyroid carcinomas are highly vascular, and excision may be difficult without a high risk of hemorrhage; in these cases a biopsy sample should be taken for diagnostic purposes only.

Thyroid carcinomas sometimes concentrate and retain iodine less efficiently than thyroid adenomas (adenomatous hyperplasia), and the size of carcinomas is usually much larger; therefore extremely high doses of radioiodine are almost always needed for destruction of all malignant tissue.[40] The combination of surgical debulking followed by administration of high-dose radioactive iodine is the treatment of choice for thyroid carcinoma in humans[42,50,51] and also has been reported to be successful in cats with thyroid carcinoma.[40,45,92] If surgical debulking is not possible, higher doses of I^{131} will be needed, necessitating a longer hospital stay and a greater risk of subsequent hypothyroidism.

HYPOTHYROIDISM

In cats, as in other species, hypothyroidism is the clinical syndrome that results from the chronic deficient secretion of the two thyroid hormones: thyroxine (T_4) and triiodothyronine (T_3). This syndrome rarely develops spontaneously. Most commonly, feline hypothyroidism is iatrogenic, secondary to overtreatment of hyperthyroidism.

Causes of Hypothyroidism

Adult-Onset (Spontaneous) Hypothyroidism

Surveys of the histologic evaluation of the feline thyroid gland have revealed several pathologic abnormalities consistent with hypothyroidism (thyroid atrophy, lymphocytic thyroiditis, and goiter).[16,19,62] However, there are only two well-documented reports of adult cats with spontaneous primary hypothyroidism. In the first cat thyroid biopsy identified a marked lymphocytic infiltrate, consistent with lymphocytic thyroiditis.[105] The second cat had idiopathic atrophy of the thyroid gland.[7]

There are no reports of cats with naturally occurring secondary or tertiary hypothyroidism. One report describes a cat with secondary hypothyroidism (i.e., pituitary thyrotropin [TSH] deficiency) secondary to head trauma.[68]

Congenital Hypothyroidism

Congenital primary hypothyroidism is a rare disease, and only a few cases have been described.* A recessive mode of inheritance for the disorder has been reported in a family of Abyssinian cats and a family of Japanese cats.[52,122] All cases of congenital disease in cats have been primary, (i.e., defect at the level of the thyroid gland). There are no reports of pituitary (secondary) or hypothalamic (tertiary) forms of congenital hypothyroidism in cats.

Although still rare, congenital hypothyroidism develops more commonly than spontaneous hypothyroidism in adult cats. However, its prevalence is likely underestimated. Because most affected kittens die soon after birth, the condition is commonly misdiagnosed.

Congenital primary hypothyroidism can be divided into two main categories: thyroid dyshormonogenesis and thyroid dysgenesis. Thyroid dyshormonogenesis is a defect in any step of iodine uptake or thyroid hormone synthesis. As in all forms of primary hypothyroidism, the low circulating T_4 concentrations lead to increased pituitary TSH secretion. Because the thyroid follicles remain intact in cats with thyroid dyshormonogenesis, the high circulating TSH concentrations induce hyperplasia of the thyroid gland. Therefore the veterinarian can sometimes palpate an enlarged thyroid gland (bilateral goiter) in cats with this type of congenital hypothyroidism.[3,52,103,115]

Thyroid dysgenesis is a developmental defect of the thyroid gland, sometimes resulting from TSH receptor abnormalities. Opposite to dysmorphogenesis, thyroid dysgenesis leads to hypoplasia or aplasia of the thyroid gland; this is a nongoitrous form of congenital hypothyroidism.[101,122,128]

Iatrogenic Hypothyroidism

Iatrogenic hypothyroidism is a well-recognized side effect of treating hyperthyroidism, and it is the most common form of hypothyroidism diagnosed in cats.[87,101] Any of the treatment options for hyperthyroid cats, including antithyroid drugs, surgical thyroidectomy, and I^{131}, can potentially produce hypothyroidism.

Although cats treated with methimazole or carbimazole frequently develop a subnormal serum T_4 concentration, they generally do not develop clinical signs associated with hypothyroidism.[73,99] In such cats the corresponding serum T_3 concentration tends to remain within the reference range. This may explain why these cats generally remain clinically euthyroid. However, cats can develop clinical hypothyroidism with a prolonged overdose of an antithyroid drug.

Most cats will develop hypothyroidism a few days after surgical thyroidectomy. Supplementing with levothyroxine (L-T_4) for a few weeks to months postoperatively can sometimes be beneficial. Even after bilateral thyroidectomy, iatrogenic hypothyroidism is generally temporary, usually resolving within 6 months.[147] Thyroid hormone replacement can then be stopped.

Up to 30% of hyperthyroid cats treated with I^{131} are reported to develop iatrogenic hypothyroidism.[78] However, this prevalence appears greatly overestimated because most cats were diagnosed by a low serum T_4 concentration alone; they did not usually show the clinical features of hypothyroidism.[109] In other reports individualized radioiodine dosing methods reduced the prevalence of permanent iatrogenic hypothyroidism to less than 5%.[92]

Clinical Features of Hypothyroidism

Although many of the signs that develop in hypothyroid cats are similar to those seen in dogs with the disorder, there are a few major differences.[22,39] First, hypothyroid cats rarely develop total alopecia, a common sign in dogs. Second, cats may develop a poor appetite, a sign also not reported in hypothyroid dogs. Profound lethargy and mental dullness develops in some cats. Other cats, especially kittens with congenital hypothyroidism, may present with severe constipation as a primary complaint.

Adult-Onset (Spontaneous) and Iatrogenic Hypothyroidism

The major clinical signs of hypothyroidism in adult cats include progressive lethargy, dullness, decreased appetite, and dermatologic changes.[22,39,87,101] Weight gain, hypothermia, and bradycardia are less common (Table 24-7).

Common dermatologic signs include nonpruritic seborrhea sicca; a dull, dry hair coat; and matting of hair on the back caused by lack of grooming. Hair is easily epilated and regrows poorly after clipping. Some cats will develop alopecia of the pinnae. One cat with spontaneous hypothyroidism developed myxedema. Although obesity may develop, it is not a consistent sign. The cats that do become obese usually have iatrogenic hypothyroidism.[22,87,101]

*References 3, 21, 52, 101, 103, 115, 121, 122, 125, 128.

TABLE 24-7 **Clinical Features of Iatrogenic, Congenital, and Adult-Onset (Spontaneous) Hypothyroidism in Cats**

	Iatrogenic	Congenital	Adult Onset
Lethargy	+	+++	++
Dermatologic signs	+	+	++
Weight gain or obesity	++	+	+
Poor appetite	+	+	++
Constipation	+	+++	+
Goiter	– or +	– or +++	–
Disproportionate dwarfism	–	+	–
Delayed closure of growth plates	–	+	–

(+) Present; (–) absent.

Congenital Hypothyroidism

Thyroid hormones affect the function of all organs and are essential for normal growth, skeletal maturation, and brain development. Therefore congenital hypothyroidism is characterized by disproportionate dwarfism and neurologic abnormalities (see Table 24-7).* Hypothyroid kittens develop many signs similar to those observed in adult cats.

The clinical signs of congenital hypothyroidism vary in severity depending on the nature of the defect. Severely affected, untreated kittens rarely survive beyond 16 weeks of age.[122] At birth the kittens usually appear normal but exhibit retarded growth by 4 to 6 weeks of age. These kittens typically develop signs of disproportionate dwarfism, which is characterized by an enlarged, broad head and short neck and limbs, over the next few months.

Most hypothyroid kittens have severe lethargy and mental dullness, in part because their brain does not develop properly. Left untreated, human babies with congenital hypothyroidism can develop mental retardation. Similarly, some of these hypothyroid kittens are definitively mentally deficient.

On physical examination the veterinarian may detect hypothermia, bradycardia, or palpable goiter (with thyroid dyshormonogenesis).† Many kittens suffer from severe, recurrent episodes of constipation. Hair is usually present all over the body, but it consists mainly of undercoat with primary guard hairs scattered throughout. Unlike adult cats with iatrogenic hypothyroidism, hypothyroid kittens are generally not obese. They may exhibit weight loss, particularly if constipated. Eruption of the permanent teeth may be delayed.

Survival of untreated hypothyroid kittens varies. Many affected kittens die undiagnosed as part of the "fading kitten" syndrome. However, other kittens with milder degrees of goitrous hypothyroidism have clinical signs that partially resolve as they grow to adulthood.[52] It is thought that their enlarging goiter compensates for the deficient thyroid function in order to achieve a euthyroid state.

*References 3, 21, 52, 101, 103, 115, 121, 122, 125, 128.

†References 3, 21, 52, 101, 103, 115, 121, 122, 125, 128.

Diagnosing Hypothyroidism

Diagnosing feline hypothyroidism can be challenging, regardless of its etiology. A presumptive diagnosis is based on a combination of the history, clinical signs, physical examination findings, and routine laboratory tests. The veterinarian can confirm the diagnosis by use of thyroid function testing or by thyroid imaging techniques.

Diagnosing iatrogenic hypothyroidism in cats starts with determining if the cat has a history of treatment for hyperthyroidism, especially with radioiodine or surgical thyroidectomy. However, a number of factors can make the diagnosis of hypothyroidism difficult to confirm. First, the concomitant presence of another disease (e.g., CRD) in these middle-aged to geriatric cats is common. These concurrent diseases can result in euthyroid sick syndrome, which is characterized by falsely low serum thyroid hormone concentrations. Second, the veterinarian should expect weight gain and a decreasing activity level after successfully treating a cat with hyperthyroidism. Therefore the clinical signs of iatrogenic hypothyroidism and the expected return to a euthyroid status can overlap. Finally, many cats develop a marked transient decrease in total T_4, within the first month of therapy with I^{131}. This transient hypothyroid state is followed by a return to euthyroidism over the next 3 to 6 months as the remaining normal thyroid tissue recovers and starts to function once again.[92]

For most cats veterinarians are advised to wait 3 months before making a definitive diagnosis of iatrogenic hypothyroidism after I^{131} treatment, especially if the cat is not presenting with the clinical features of hypothyroidism. However, the veterinarian should diagnose or exclude hypothyroidism as soon as possible in cats with renal disease because hypothyroidism, treatment for hyperthyroidism, and chronic renal disease all lower the GFR.[25,83] The combined effect of these three factors can lead to severe azotemia or even total renal failure. Treating the hypothyroidism can raise the GFR to an acceptable level.[35]

Routine Hematology, Chemistry Panel, and Urinalysis

The most important reason to perform a routine panel in all cats with suspected hypothyroidism is to exclude nonthyroidal illness. In adult cats with hypothyroidism (both spontaneous and iatrogenic), mild normochromic, normocytic anemia and hypercholesterolemia are the most common routine laboratory findings. Unfortunately, these changes are inconsistent, especially in kittens with congenital hypothyroidism.

Serum Thyroxine Concentration

By definition, cats with hypothyroidism have deficient thyroid hormone secretion. Therefore finding a low serum T_4 concentration is key in diagnosing feline hypothyroidism. A normal T_4 concentration virtually excludes hypothyroidism.

Although important, a subnormal T_4 concentration alone is not definitive. The serum T_4 concentration can also be low in cats with nonthyroidal illness, such as DM, hepatic disease, renal disease, and systemic neoplasia.[86,95] In general, the severity of the illness correlates inversely with the serum T_4 concentration (i.e., sicker cats have lower serum T_4 concentrations). Because multiple diseases and other factors can falsely lower the serum T_4 concentration in cats, the veterinarian must first rule out nonthyroidal disease before considering a diagnosis of hypothyroidism.

Cats with suspected hypothyroidism and a low T_4 concentration still require additional testing before the veterinarian can make a definitive diagnosis. Further tests such as serum free T_4 (FT_4) concentration, canine TSH (cTSH) concentration, recombinant human TSH (rhTSH) stimulation test, or thyroid scintigraphy are indicated to confirm the disease.

Serum Free Thyroxine (FT_4) Concentration

Free T_4 (FT_4) is the nonprotein-bound fraction of circulating T_4 that can enter cells, producing the biologic effect of thyroid hormone and regulating the pituitary feedback mechanism. FT_4 accounts for less than 1% of circulating T_4. Because only the FT_4 is biologically active, measuring free T_4 is a more sensitive test for diagnosing hypothyroidism. In addition, nonthyroidal illness influences FT_4 less than it influences the total T_4.[86] Therefore FT_4 is better at distinguishing a euthyroid cat with nonthyroidal disease from a hypothyroid cat. However, only FT_4 assays that use equilibrium dialysis appear reliable, and most commercial laboratories measure FT_4 by inferior analog methods.

Although measuring FT_4 concentration by equilibrium dialysis is a more accurate stand-alone test than total T_4 concentration, FT_4 is far from perfect for confirming feline hypothyroidism for three reasons. First, moderate to severe nonthyroidal illness can falsely lower the FT_4 concentration, although to a lesser degree than seen with total T_4.[86] Second, up to 15% of cats with nonthyroidal disease develop a falsely high FT_4 concentration, further confusing the interpretation.[72,86] Finally, the test is approximately twice as expensive in most commercial laboratories as the total T_4.

Serum Thyroid-Stimulating Hormone Concentrations

In dogs with hypothyroidism, a high serum TSH concentration confirms that the disease is primary (located within the thyroid gland). A specific assay for feline TSH is not yet available. However, the commercially available cTSH assay cross-reacts with feline TSH sufficiently to enable its use as a diagnostic test for hypothyroid cats. In one of the reported adult cats with spontaneous hypothyroidism, the serum TSH concentration was high when measured with the cTSH assay.[7] Similarly, most cats with iatrogenic hypothyroidism will also develop high serum TSH concentration as measured by the cTSH assay.[22,39]

Normal cats and cats with nonthyroidal illness generally maintain normal values for serum TSH. Therefore the finding of a low total T_4 or FT_4 in combination with a high TSH concentration greatly improves the diagnostic sensitivity for hypothyroidism.

Thyroid-Stimulating Hormone Stimulation Test

The TSH stimulation test provides important information for diagnosing hypothyroidism because it directly tests the thyroid's secretory reserve. In normal cats administering exogenous TSH produces a consistent rise in total serum T_4 concentration. In contrast, hypothyroid cats show little, if any, rise in the low basal total serum T_4 concentrations after TSH stimulation.[22,39,87] As in dogs with hypothyroidism, the TSH stimulation test appears to be an effective, noninvasive means of confirming the diagnosis in hypothyroid cats.

In the past bovine TSH was the preferred preparation for TSH stimulation testing in cats. However, bovine TSH is no longer available. Recently, a recombinant human TSH (rhTSH) preparation was validated for TSH stimulation testing in cats.[116,139] The testing protocol involves collecting samples for total serum T_4 concentration before and 6 hours after the intravenous administration of 25 to 200 μg of rhTSH (Thyrogen, Genzyme Corporation). Administrating rhTSH to clinically normal cats generally increases the basal total T_4 concentration by at least twofold. Further studies are needed to validate the use of this test for diagnosing feline hypothyroidism, but one would expect that these cats would experience little to no rise in total serum T_4.

The major disadvantage of this test is that rhTSH is extremely expensive. The vial of rhTSH powder is reconstituted with sterile water (900 μg/vial), and the diluted

TSH can be aliquoted into vials and stored frozen for later use in other dogs and cats. Freezing at –20 degrees C maintains the biological activity of rhTSH for up to 12 weeks.[23] Unfortunately, it is unlikely that most hospitals would perform the test often enough to use the entire supply of rhTSH before it expires.

Radiology

Radiography can be a particularly useful aid in diagnosing congenital feline hypothyroidism because retarded skeletal development, particularly epiphyseal dysgenesis of the vertebrae and long bones, is pathognomonic for the disease.[39]

Thyroid Scintigraphy

Thyroid scintigraphy (thyroid scanning by nuclear imaging) provides valuable information regarding both thyroid anatomy and physiology, and it can play an integral role in the diagnosis and staging of thyroid disease in cats.[56,101] Thyroid scintigraphy is considered the gold standard for diagnosing mild hyperthyroidism in cats. Although most veterinarians diagnose hypothyroidism with serum thyroid tests, thyroid scanning is a valuable test as well.

To perform thyroid imaging, a small dose of radionuclide (most commonly, technetium-99m; ^{99m}Tc) is administered subcutaneously. The cats are laid on their abdomen (ventral view) or side (lateral view) 20 minutes later, while a gamma camera acquires the thyroid image.

In normal cats the thyroid gland appears as two well-defined, focal (ovoid) areas of radionuclide accumulation in the cranial to middle cervical region. The two thyroid lobes are symmetrical in size and shape and are located side by side. Activity in the normal thyroid closely approximates activity in the salivary glands, with an expected brightness ratio of 1:1.

Thyroid scintigraphy is considered the best imaging technique for dogs with suspected hypothyroidism because it can distinguish between hypothyroid dogs and dogs with a falsely low serum thyroid hormone concentration. In hypothyroid dogs thyroid imaging typically reveals decreased or even absent radionuclide uptake (thyroid gland is not visible on the scan). In contrast, dogs with a falsely low serum thyroid hormone concentration secondary to illness or drug therapy will have a normal thyroid image.

Thyroid scintigraphy is also a powerful tool for diagnosing adult hypothyroid cats (both spontaneous and iatrogenic). As in hypothyroid dogs, thyroid imaging shows minimal to zero uptake of the radionuclide.[7]

Although few studies have been done, thyroid scanning also appears to be helpful for kittens with congenital hypothyroidism because it can distinguish between thyroid dysgenesis and thyroid dyshormonogenesis. A kitten with thyroid dysgenesis will appear similar to a hypothyroid adult cat or dog—the thyroid should be dim or not visible. Conversely, a kitten with thyroid dyshormonogenesis will have normal to increased uptake of the radionuclide.[103] Furthermore, thyroid scanning with radioiodine (I^{131}) can help reveal the mechanism of the dyshormonogenesis. For example, a perchlorate discharge test can reveal a defect in iodine organification.[52,115]

Treating Hypothyroidism

The recommended treatment for feline hypothyroidism is L-T_4, at an initial dose of 10 to 20 μg/kg daily or 100 μg/cat daily. This dose is adjusted as needed on the basis of a cat's clinical response and postpill total serum T_4 concentration. With proper treatment clinical signs of hypothyroidism can be expected to resolve completely in adult cats. In contrast, kittens have a more variable response to treatment. Their prognosis depends on the severity and duration of time that the condition went untreated.

References

1. Adams WH, Daniel GB, Legendre AM et al: Changes in renal function in cats following treatment of hyperthyroidism using 131I, *Vet Radiol Ultrasound* 38:231, 1997.
2. Archer FJ, Taylor SM: Alkaline phosphatase bone isoenzyme and osteocalcin in the serum of hyperthyroid cats, *Can Vet J* 37:735, 1996.
3. Arnold U, Opitz M, Grosser I et al: Goitrous hypothyroidism and dwarfism in a kitten, *J Am Anim Hosp Assoc* 20:753, 1984.
4. Barber PJ, Elliott J: Study of calcium homeostasis in feline hyperthyroidism, *J Small Anim Pract* 37:575, 1996.
5. Becker TJ, Graves TK, Kruger JM et al: Effects of methimazole on renal function in cats with hyperthyroidism, *J Am Anim Hosp Assoc* 36:215, 2000.
6. Birchard SJ, Peterson ME, Jacobson A: Surgical treatment of feline hyperthyroidism: results of 85 cases, *J Am Anim Hosp Assoc* 20:705, 1984.
7. Blois SL, Abrams-Ogg AC, Mitchell C et al: Use of thyroid scintigraphy and pituitary immunohistochemistry in the diagnosis of spontaneous hypothyroidism in a mature cat, *J Feline Med Surg* 12:156, 2010.
8. Boag AK, Neiger R, Slater L et al: Changes in the glomerular filtration rate of 27 cats with hyperthyroidism after treatment with radioactive iodine, *Vet Rec* 161:711, 2007.
9. Bond BR, Fox PR, Peterson ME et al: Echocardiographic findings in 103 cats with hyperthyroidism, *J Am Vet Med Assoc* 192:1546, 1988.
10. Bonnema SJ, Bennedbaek FN, Veje A et al: Continuous methimazole therapy and its effect on the cure rate of hyperthyroidism using radioactive iodine: an evaluation by a randomized trial, *J Clin Endocrinol Metab* 91:2946, 2006.
11. Broome MR: Thyroid scintigraphy in hyperthyroidism, *Clin Tech Small Anim Pract* 21:10, 2006.
12. Broome MR, Hays MT, Turrel JM: Peripheral metabolism of thyroid hormones and iodide in healthy and hyperthyroid cats, *Am J Vet Res* 48:1286, 1987.
13. Broussard JD, Peterson ME, Fox PR: Changes in clinical and laboratory findings in cats with hyperthyroidism from 1983 to 1993, *J Am Vet Med Assoc* 206:302, 1995.

14. Bucknell DG: Feline hyperthyroidism: spectrum of clinical presentions and response to carbimazole therapy, *Aust Vet J* 78:462, 2000.
15. Buijtels JJ, Kurvers IA, Galac S et al: [Transdermal carbimazole for the treatment of feline hyperthyroidism], *Tijdschr Diergeneeskd* 131:478, 2006.
16. Carpenter JL, Andrews LK, Holzworth J: Tumors and tumor-like lesions. In Holzworth J, editor: *Diseases of the cat: medicine and surgery*, Philadelphia, 1987, Saunders, p 406.
17. Chaitman J, Hess R, Senz R et al: Thyroid adenomatous hyperplasia in euthyroid cats [abstract], *J Vet Intern Med* 13:242, 1999.
18. Chun R, Garrett LD, Sargeant J et al: Predictors of response to radioiodine therapy in hyperthyroid cats, *Vet Radiol Ultrasound* 43:587, 2002.
19. Clark ST, Meier H: A Clinico-pathological study of thyroid disease in the dog and cat, *Zentralbl Veterinarmed* 5:17, 1958.
20. Court M, Freeman L: Identification and concentration of soy isoflavones in commercial cat foods, *Am J Vet Res* 63:181, 2002.
21. Crowe A: Congenital hypothyroidism in a cat, *Can Vet J* 45:168, 2004.
22. Daminet S: Feline hypothyroidism. In Mooney CT, Peterson ME, editors: *BSAVA manual of canine and feline endocrinology*, ed 4, Shurdington, Cheltenham, 2011, British Small Animal Veterinary Association (in press).
23. Daminet S, Fifle L, Paradis M et al: Use of recombinant human thyroid-stimulating hormone for thyrotropin stimulation test in healthy, hypothyroid and euthyroid sick dogs, *Can Vet J* 48:1273, 2007.
24. De Wet CS, Mooney CT, Thompson PN et al: Prevalence of and risk factors for feline hyperthyroidism in Hong Kong, *J Feline Med Surg* 11:315, 2009.
25. DiBartola SP, Broome MR, Stein BS et al: Effect of treatment of hyperthyroidism on renal function in cats, *J Am Vet Med Assoc* 208:875, 1996.
26. Dye JA, Venier M, Zhu L et al: Elevated PBDE levels in pet cats: sentinels for humans? *Environ Sci Technol*, 2007.
26a. Edinboro CH, Scott-Moncrieff JC, Glickman LT: Review of iodine recommendations for commercial cat foods and potential impacts of proposed changes, *Thyroid* 14:722, 2004.
26b. Edinboro CH, Scott-Moncrieff JC, Glickman LT: Feline hyperthyroidism: potential relationship with iodine supplement requirements of commercial cat foods, *J Feline Med Surg* 12:672, 2010.
27. Edinboro C, Scott-Moncrieff J, Janovitz E et al: Epidemiologic study of relationships between consumption of commercial canned food and risk of hyperthyroidism in cats, *J Amer Vet Med Assoc* 224:879, 2004.
28. Ferguson DC, Freeman R: Goiter in apparently euthyroid cats. In August JR, editor: *Consultations in feline internal medicine*, ed 5, St Louis, 2006, Elsevier Saunders, p 207.
29. Ferguson DC, Hoenig M, Kaptein EM et al: Comments regarding "subclinical hyperthyroidism in cats: a spontaneous model of subclinical toxic nodular goiter in humans?" *Thyroid* 18:1339, 2008.
30. Fischetti AJ, Drost WT, DiBartola SP et al: Effects of methimazole on thyroid gland uptake of 99mTc-Pertechnate in 19 hyperthyroid cats, *Vet Radiol Ultrasound* 46:267, 2005.
31. Flanders J: Surgical options for the treatment of hyperthyroidism in the cat, *J Fel Med Surg* 1:127, 1999.
32. Flanders JA, Harvey HJ, Erb HN: Feline thyroidectomy: a comparison of postoperative hypocalcemia associated with three different surgical techniques, *Vet Surg* 16:362, 1987.
33. Foster DJ, Thoday KL: Tissue sources of serum alkaline phosphatase in 34 hyperthyroid cats: a qualitative and quantitative study, *Res Vet Sci* 68:89, 2000.
34. Fox P, Peterson M, Broussard J: Electrocardiographic and radiographic changes in cats with hyperthyroidism: comparison of populations evaluated during 1992-1993 vs. 1979-1982, *J Am Anim Hosp Assoc* 35:27, 1998.
35. Gommeren K, van Hoek I, Lefebvre HP et al: Effect of thyroxine supplementation on glomerular filtration rate in hypothyroid dogs, *J Vet Intern Med* 23:844, 2009.
36. Graham PA, Refsal KR, Nachreiner RF et al: The measurement of feline thyrotropin (TSH) using a commercial canine immunoradiometric assay [abstract], *J Vet Intern Med* 14:342, 2000.
37. Graves TK: Hyperthyroidism and the kidneys. In August JR, editor: *Consultations in feline internal medicine*, ed 6, St Louis, 2009, Saunders Elsevier, p 268.
38. Graves TK, Olivier NB, Nachreiner RF et al: Changes in renal function associated with treatment of hyperthyroidism in cats, *Am J Vet Res* 55:1745, 1994.
39. Greco DS: Diagnosis of congenital and adult-onset hypothyroidism in cats, *Clin Tech Small Anim Pract* 21:40, 2006.
40. Guptill L, Scott-Moncrieff CR, Janovitz EB et al: Response to high-dose radioactive iodine administration in cats with thyroid carcinoma that had previously undergone surgery, *J Am Vet Med Assoc* 207:1055, 1995.
41. Hammer K, Holt D, Ward C: Altered expression of G proteins in thyroid gland adenomas obtained from hyperthyroid cats, *Am J Vet Res* 61:874, 2000.
42. Handkiewicz-Junak D, Wloch J, Roskosz J et al: Total thyroidectomy and adjuvant radioiodine treatment independently decrease locoregional recurrence risk in childhood and adolescent differentiated thyroid cancer, *J Nucl Med* 48:879, 2007.
43. Harvey AM, Hibbert A, Barrett EL et al: Scintigraphic findings in 120 hyperthyroid cats, *J Feline Med Surg* 11:96, 2009.
44. Hays MT, Broome MR, Turrel JM: A multicompartmental model for iodide, thyroxine, and triiodothyronine metabolism in normal and spontaneously hyperthyroid cats, *Endocrinology* 122:2444, 1988.
45. Hibbert A, Gruffydd-Jones T, Barrett EL et al: Feline thyroid carcinoma: diagnosis and response to high-dose radioactive iodine treatment, *J Feline Med Surg* 11:116, 2009.
46. Hoenig M, Ferguson DC: Impairment of glucose tolerance in hyperthyroid cats, *J Endocrinol* 121:249, 1989.
47. Hoenig M, Goldschmidt MH, Ferguson DC et al: Toxic nodular goitre in the cat, *J Small Anim Pract* 23:1, 1982.
48. Hoffman G, Marks S, Taboada J et al: Transdermal methimazole treatment in cats with hyperthyroidism, *J Fel Med Surg* 5:77, 2003.
49. Hoffman S, Yoder A, Trepanier L: Bioavailability of transdermal methimazole in a pluronic lecithin organogel (PLO) in healthy cats, *J Vet Pharmacol Ther* 25:189, 2002.
50. Holzer S, Reiners C, Mann K et al: Patterns of care for patients with primary differentiated carcinoma of the thyroid gland treated in Germany during 1996. U.S. and German Thyroid Cancer Group, *Cancer* 89:192, 2000.
51. Hundahl SA, Cady B, Cunningham MP et al: Initial results from a prospective cohort study of 5583 cases of thyroid carcinoma treated in the united states during 1996. U.S. and German Thyroid Cancer Study Group. An American College of Surgeons Commission on Cancer Patient Care Evaluation study, *Cancer* 89:202, 2000.
52. Jones BR, Gruffydd-Jones TJ, Sparkes AH et al: Preliminary studies on congenital hypothyroidism in a family of Abyssinian cats, *Vet Rec* 131:145, 1992.
52a. Kalinyak JE, McDougall IR: Whole-body scanning with radionuclides of iodine, and the controversy of'thyroid stunning, *Nucl Med Commun* 25:883, 2004.
53. Kass PH, Peterson ME, Levy J et al: Evaluation of environmental, nutritional, and host factors in cats with hyperthyroidism, *J Vet Intern Med* 13:323, 1999.

54. Kemppainen RJ, Birchfield JR: Measurement of total thyroxine concentration in serum from dogs and cats by use of various methods, *Am J Vet Res* 67:259, 2006.
55. Reference deleted in pages.
56. Kintzer PP, Peterson ME: Nuclear medicine of the thyroid gland. Scintigraphy and radioiodine therapy, *Vet Clin North Am Small Anim Pract* 24:587, 1994.
57. Kirby R, Scase T, Wakeling J et al: Adenomatous hyperplasia of the thyroid gland is related to TSH concentration in cats, *J Vet Intern Med* 20:1522, 2006.
58. Kobayashi DL, Peterson ME, Graves TK et al: Hypertension in cats with chronic renal failure or hyperthyroidism, *J Vet Intern Med* 4:58, 1990.
59. Kraft W, Buchler F: Hyperthyroidism: incidence in the cat., *Tierarztl Prax KH* 27:386, 1999.
60. Lapointe C, Bélanger MC, Dunn M et al: N-Acetyl-β-d-glucosaminidase index as an early biomarker for chronic kidney disease in cats with hyperthyroidism, *J Vet Intern Med* 22:1103, 2008.
60a. Laurberg P, Pedersen KM, Vestergaard H et al: High incidence of multinodular toxic goitre in the elderly population in a low iodine intake area vs. high incidence of Graves' disease in the young in a high iodine intake area: comparative surveys of thyrotoxicosis epidemiology in East-Jutland Denmark and Iceland, *J Intern Med* 229:415, 1991.
61. Leav I, Schiller AL, Rijnberk A et al: Adenomas and carcinomas of the canine and feline thyroid, *Am J Pathol* 83:61, 1976.
62. Lucke VM: A histological study of thyroid abnormalities in the domestic cat, *J Small Anim Prac* 5:351, 1964.
63. Lurye JC: Update on treatment of hyperthyroidism. In August JR, editor: *Consultations in feline internal medicine*, ed 5, St Louis, 2006, Elsevier Saunders, p 199.
64. Lurye JC, Behrend EN, Kemppainen RJ: Evaluation of an in-house enzyme-linked immunosorbent assay for quantitative measurement of serum total thyroxine concentration in dogs and cats, *J Am Vet Med Assoc* 221:243, 2002.
65. Martin KM, Rossing MA, Ryland LM et al: Evaluation of dietary and environmental risk factors for hyperthyroidism in cats, *J Am Vet Med Assoc* 217:853, 2000.
66. Mayer-Roenne B, Goldstein RE, Erb HN: Urinary tract infections in cats with hyperthyroidism, diabetes mellitus and chronic kidney disease, *J Feline Med Surg* 9:124, 2007.
67. McLoughlin MA, DiBartola SP, Birchard SJ et al: Influence of systemic nonthyroidal illness on serum concentration of thyroxine in hyperthyroid cats, *J Am Anim Hosp Assoc* 29:227, 1993.
67a. Melendez LM, Yamka RM, Burris PA: Titration of dietary iodine for maintaining serum thyroxine concentrations in hyperthyroid cats [abstract], *J Vet Intern Med* 25:683, 2011.
67b. Melendez LM, Yamka RM, Forrester SD et al: Titration of dietary iodine for reducing serum thyroxine concentrations in newly diagnosed hyperthyroid cats [abstract], *J Vet Intern Med* 25:683, 2011.
68. Mellanby RJ, Jeffery ND, Gopal MS et al: Secondary hypothyroidism following head trauma in a cat, *J Feline Med Surg* 7:135, 2005.
69. Milner R, Channell C, Levy J et al: Survival times for cats with hyperthyroidism treated with iodine 131, methimazole, or both: 167 cases (1996-2003), *J Am Vet Med Assoc* 228:559, 2006.
70. Miyamoto T, Miyata I, Kurobane K et al: Prevalence of feline hyperthyroidism in Osaka and the Chugoku Region, *J Jpn Vet Med Assoc* 55:289, 2002.
71. Mooney CT: Radioactive iodine therapy for feline hyperthyroidism: efficacy and administration routes, *J Small Anim Pract* 35:289, 1994.
72. Mooney CT, Little CJL, Macrae AW: Effect of illness not associated with the thyroid gland on serum total and free thyroxine concentrations in cats, *J Am Vet Med Assoc* 208:2004, 1996.
73. Mooney CT, Thoday KL, Doxey DL: Carbimazole therapy of feline hyperthyroidism, *J Small Anim Pract* 33:228, 1992.
74. Naan EC, Kirpensteijn J, Kooistra HS et al: Results of thyroidectomy in 101 cats with hyperthyroidism, *Vet Surg* 35:287, 2006.
75. Nieckarz JA, Daniel GB: The effect of methimazole on thyroid uptake of pertechnetate and radioiodine in normal cats, *Vet Radiol Ultrasound* 42:448, 2001.
76. Norsworthy G, Adams V, McElhaney M et al: Palpable thyroid and parathyroid nodules in asymptomatic cats, *J Fel Med Surg* 4:145, 2002.
77. Norsworthy G, Adams V, McElhaney M et al: Relationship between semi-quantitative thyroid gland palpation and total thyroxine concentration in cats with an without hyperadrenocorticism, *J Fel Med Surg* 4:139, 2002.
78. Nykamp SG, Dykes NL, Zarfoss MK et al: Association of the risk of development of hypothyroidism after iodine 131 treatment with the pretreatment pattern of sodium pertechnetate Tc 99m uptake in the thyroid gland in cats with hyperthyroidism: 165 cases (1990-2002), *J Am Vet Med Assoc* 226:1671, 2005.
79. Olczak J, Jones BR, Pfeiffer DU et al: Multivariate analysis of risk factors for feline hyperthyroidism in New Zealand, *N Z Vet J* 53:53, 2005.
80. Padgett SL, Tobias KM, Leathers CW et al: Efficacy of parathyroid gland autotransplantation in maintaining serum calcium concentrations after bilateral thyroparathyroidectomy in cats, *J Am Vet Med Assoc* 34:219, 1998.
81. Paepe D, Smets P, van Hoek I et al: Within- and between-examiner agreement for two thyroid palpation techniques in healthy and hyperthyroid cats, *J Feline Med Surg* 10:558, 2008.
82. Page RB, Scrivani PV, Dykes NL et al: Accuracy of increased thyroid activity during pertechnetate scintigraphy by subcutaneous injection for diagnosing hyperthyroidism in cats, *Vet Radiol Ultrasound* 47:206, 2006.
83. Panciera DL, Lefebvre HP: Effect of experimental hypothyroidism on glomerular filtration rate and plasma creatinine concentration in dogs, *J Vet Intern Med* 23:1045, 2009.
84. Peter HJ, Gerber H, Studer H et al: Autonomy of growth and of iodine metabolism in hyperthyroid feline goiters transplanted onto nude mice, *J Clin Invest* 80:491, 1987.
85. Peterson M, DeMarco D, Sheldon K: Total thyroxine testing: comparison of an in-house test-kit with radioimmuno and chemiluminescent assays, *J Vet Intern Med* 17:396, 2003.
86. Peterson M, Melian C, Nichols R: Measurement of serum concentrations of free thyroxine, total thyroxine, and total triiodothyronine in cats with hyperthyroidism and cats with nonthyroidal disease, *J Am Anim Hosp Assoc* 218:529, 2001.
87. Peterson ME: Feline hypothyroidism In Kirk RW, Bonagura JD, editors: *Current veterinary therapy X*, Philadelphia, 1989, Saunders, p 1000.
88. Peterson ME: Diagnostic tests for hyperthyroidism in cats, *Clin Tech Small Anim Pract* 21:2, 2006.
89. Peterson ME: Radioiodine treatment of hyperthyroidism, *Clin Tech Small Anim Pract* 21:34, 2006.
90. Peterson ME, Aucoin DP: Comparison of the disposition of carbimazole and methimazole in clinically normal cats, *Res Vet Sci* 54:351, 1993.
91. Peterson ME, Becker DV: Radionuclide thyroid imaging in 135 cats with hyperthyroidism, *Vet Radiol Ultrasound* 25:23, 1984.
92. Peterson ME, Becker DV: Radioiodine treatment of 524 cats with hyperthyroidism, *J Am Vet Med Assoc* 207:1422, 1995.
93. Peterson ME, Becker DV, Hurley JR. Spontaneous hyperthyroidism in the cat [abstract], In *Proceedings of the American College of Veterinary Internal Medicine* Seattle, 1979, p 108.

94. Peterson ME, Broussard JD, Gamble DA: Use of the thyrotropin releasing hormone stimulation test to diagnose mild hyperthyroidism in cats, *J Vet Intern Med* 8:279, 1994.
95. Peterson ME, Gamble DA: Effect of nonthyroidal illness on serum thyroxine concentrations in cats: 494 cases (1988), *J Am Vet Med Assoc* 197:1203, 1990.
96. Peterson ME, Graves TK, Cavanagh I: Serum thyroid hormone concentrations fluctuate in cats with hyperthyroidism, *J Vet Intern Med* 1:142, 1987.
97. Peterson ME, Graves TK, Gamble DA: Triiodothyronine (T_3) suppression test, *J Vet Intern Med* 4:233, 1990.
98. Peterson ME, Kintzer PP, Cavanagh PG et al: Feline hyperthyroidism: pretreatment clinical and laboratory evaluation of 131 cases, *J Am Vet Med Assoc* 183:103, 1983.
99. Peterson ME, Kintzer PP, Hurvitz AI: Methimazole treatment of 262 cats with hyperthyroidism, *J Vet Intern Med* 2:150, 1988.
100. Peterson ME, Melian C, Nichols R: Measurement of serum concentrations of free thyroxine, total thyroxine, and total triiodothyronine in cats with hyperthyroidism and cats with nonthyroidal disease, *J Am Vet Med Assoc* 218:529, 2001.
101. Peterson ME, Randolph JF, Mooney CT: Endocrine diseases. In Sherding RG, editor: *The cat: diseases and clinical management*, ed 2, New York, 1994, Churchill Livingstone, p 1403.
102. Peterson ME, Ward CR: Etiopathologic findings of hyperthyroidism in cats, *Vet Clin North Am Small Anim Pract* 37:633, 2007.
103. Quante S, Fracassi F, Gorgas D et al: Congenital hypothyroidism in a kitten resulting in decreased IGF-I concentration and abnormal liver function tests, *J Feline Med Surg* 12:487, 2010.
104. Radcliffe CE: Observations on the relationship of the thyroid to the polyuria of experimental diabetes insipidus, *Endocrinology* 32:415, 1943.
105. Rand JS, Levine J, Best SJ et al: Spontaneous adult-onset hypothyroidism in a cat, *J Vet Intern Med* 7:272, 1993.
106. Rayalam S, Eizenstat LD, Davis RR et al: Expression and purification of feline thyrotropin (fTSH): immunological detection and bioactivity of heterodimeric and yoked glycoproteins, *Domest Anim Endocrinol* 30:185, 2006.
107. Reimers TJ, Cowan RG, Davidson HP et al: Validation of radioimmunoassay for triiodothyronine, thyroxine, and hydrocortisone (cortisol) in canine, feline, and equine sera, *Am J Vet Res* 42:2016, 1981.
108. Riensche MR, Graves TK, Schaeffer DJ: An investigation of predictors of renal insufficiency following treatment of hyperthyroidism in cats, *J Feline Med Surg* 10:160, 2008.
109. Romatowski J: Questions incidence of posttreatment hypothyroidism in cats, *J Am Vet Med Assoc* 227:32, 2005.
110. Rutland BE, Nachreiner RF, Kruger JM: Optimal testing for thyroid hormone concentration after treatment with methimazole in healthy and hyperthyroid cats, *J Vet Intern Med* 23:1025, 2009.
111. Sartor L, Trepanier L, Knoll M et al: Efficacy and safety of transdermal methimazole in the treatment of cats with hyperthyroidism, *J Vet Intern Med* 18:651, 2004.
112. Sassnau R: Epidemiological investigation on the prevalence of feline hyperthyroidism in an urban population in Germany, *Tierarztl Prax K H* 34:450, 2006.
113. Scarlett JM, Moise NS, Rayl J: Feline hyperthyroidism: a descriptive and case control study, *Prev Vet Med* 7:295, 1988.
114. Singh A, Jiang Y, White T et al: Validation of nonradioactive chemiluminescent immunoassay methods for the analysis of thyroxine and cortisol in blood samples obtained from dogs, cats, and horses, *J Vet Diagn Invest* 9:261, 1997.
115. Sjollema BE, den Hartog MT, de Vijlder JJ et al: Congenital hypothyroidism in two cats due to defective organification: data suggesting loosely anchored thyroperoxidase, *Acta Endocrinol (Copenh)* 125:435, 1991.
115a. Stanbury JB, Ermans AE, P Bourdoux P et al: Iodine-induced hyperthyroidism: occurrence and epidemiology, *Thyroid* 8:83, 1998.
116. Stegeman JR, Graham PA, Hauptman JG: Use of recombinant human thyroid-stimulating hormone for thyrotropin-stimulation testing of euthyroid cats, *Am J Vet Res* 64:149, 2003.
117. Stepien RL, Rapoport GS et al: Effect of measurement method on blood pressure findings in cats before and after therapy for hyperthyroidism [abstract], *J Vet Intern Med* 17:754, 2003.
118. Stiles J, Polzin DJ, Bistner SI: The prevalence of retinopathy in cats with systemic hypertension and chronic renal failure or hyperthyroidism, *J Am Anim Hosp Assoc* 30:564, 1994.
119. Syme HM: Cardiovascular and renal manifestations of hyperthyroidism, *Vet Clin North Am Small Anim Pract* 37:723, 2007.
120. Syme HM, Elliott J: The prevalence of hypertension in hyperthyroid cats at diagnosis and following treatment [ECVIM abstract], *J Vet Intern Med* 17:754, 2003.
121. Szabo SD, Wells KL: What is your diagnosis? Congenital hypothyroidism, *J Am Vet Med Assoc* 230:29, 2007.
122. Tanase H, Kudo K, Horikoshi H et al: Inherited primary hypothyroidism with thyrotrophin resistance in Japanese cats, *J Endocrinol* 129:245, 1991.
123. Thoday KL, Mooney CT: Historical, clinical and laboratory features of 126 hyperthyroid cats, *Vet Rec* 131:257, 1992.
124. Thoday KL, Seth J, Elton RA: Radioimmunoassay of serum total thyroxine and triiodothyronine in healthy cats: assay methodology and effects of age, sex, breed, heredity and environment, *J Small Anim Pract* 25:457, 1984.
125. Tobias S, Labato MA: Identifying and managing feline congenital hypothyroidism., *Vet Med* 96:719, 2001.
126. Tomsa K, Glaus T, Kacl G et al: Thyrotropin-releasing hormone stimulation test to assess thyroid function in severely sick cats, *J Vet Intern Med* 15:89, 2001.
127. Tomsa K, Hardeggar R, Glaus T et al: 99mTc-pertechnetate scintigraphy in hyperthyroid cats with normal serum thyroxine concentrations [abstract], *J Vet Intern Med* 15:299, 2001.
128. Traas AM, Abbott BL, French A et al: Congenital thyroid hypoplasia and seizures in 2 littermate kittens, *J Vet Intern Med* 22:1427, 2008.
129. Trepanier L, Hoffman S, Kroll M et al: Efficacy and safety of once versus twice daily administration of methimazole in cats with hyperthyroidism, *J Am Vet Med Assoc* 222:954, 2003.
130. Trepanier LA: Medical management of hyperthyroidism, *Clin Tech Small Anim Pract* 21:22, 2006.
131. Turrel JM, Feldman EC, Nelson RW et al: Thyroid carcinoma causing hyperthyroidism in cats: 14 cases (1981-1986), *J Am Vet Med Assoc* 193:359, 1988.
132. van der Woerdt A, Peterson ME: Prevalence of ocular abnormalities in cats with hyperthyroidism, *J Vet Intern Med* 14:202, 2000.
133. van Hoek I, Daminet S: Interactions between thyroid and kidney function in pathological conditions of these organ systems: a review, *Gen Comp Endocrinol* 160:205, 2009.
134. van Hoek I, Daminet S, Notebaert S et al: Immunoassay of urinary retinol binding protein as a putative renal marker in cats, *J Immunol Methods* 329:208, 2008.
135. van Hoek I, Lefebvre HP, Kooistra HS et al: Plasma clearance of exogenous creatinine, exo-iohexol, and endo-iohexol in hyperthyroid cats before and after treatment with radioiodine, *J Vet Intern Med* 22:879, 2008.
136. van Hoek I, Lefebvre HP, Peremans K et al: Short- and long-term follow-up of glomerular and tubular renal markers of kidney function in hyperthyroid cats after treatment with radioiodine, *Domest Anim Endocrinol* 36:45, 2009.
137. van Hoek I, Lefebvre HP, Peremans K et al: Short- and long-term follow-up of glomerular and tubular renal markers of kidney

function in hyperthyroid cats after treatment with radioiodine, *Domest Anim Endocrinol* 36:45, 2009.

138. Van Hoek I, Meyer E, Duchateau L et al: Retinol-binding protein in serum and urine of hyperthyroid cats before and after treatment with radioiodine, *J Vet Intern Med* 23:1031, 2009.
139. van Hoek IM, Peremans K, Vandermeulen E et al: Effect of recombinant human thyroid stimulating hormone on serum thyroxin and thyroid scintigraphy in euthyroid cats, *J Feline Med Surg* 11:309, 2009.
140. Wakeling J, Elliott J, Petrie A et al: Urinary iodide concentration in hyperthyroid cats, *Am J Vet Res* 70:741, 2009.
141. Wakeling J, Elliott J, Syme H: Does subclinical hyperthyroidism exist in cats? *J Vet Intern Med* 20:726, 2006.
142. Wakeling J, Everard A, Brodbelt D et al: Risk factors for feline hyperthyroidism in the UK, *J Small Anim Pract* 50:406, 2009.
143. Wakeling J, Melian C, Font A et al: Evidence for differing incidences of feline hyperthyroidism in London UK and Spain [abstract], In *Congress Proceedings, 15th ECVIM-CA*, Glasgow, Scotland, 220, 2005.
144. Wakeling J, Moore K, Elliott J et al: Diagnosis of hyperthyroidism in cats with mild chronic kidney disease, *J Small Anim Pract* 49:287, 2008.
145. Wakeling J, Rob C, Elliott J et al: Survival of hyperthyroid cats is not affected by post-treatment azotaemia [abstract], *J Vet Intern Med* 20:1523, 2006.
146. Wakeling J, Smith K, Scase T et al: Subclinical hyperthyroidism in cats: a spontaneous model of subclinical toxic nodular goiter in humans? *Thyroid* 17:1201, 2007.
147. Welches CD, Scavelli TD, Matthieson DT et al: Occurrence of problems after three techniques of bilateral thyroidectomy in cats, *Vet Surg* 18:392, 1989.
148. White H, Freeman L, Mahony O et al: Effect of dietary soy on serum thyroid hormone concentrations in healthy adult cats, *Am J Vet Res* 65:586, 2004.
149. Williams T, Elliott J, Syme H: Association of iatrogenic hypothyroidism with azotemia and reduced survival time in cats treated for hyperthyroidism, *J Vet Intern Med* 24:1086, 2010.
150. Yu S, Wedekind KJ, Burris PA et al: Controlled level of dietary iodine normalizes serum total thyroxine in cats with naturally occurring hyperthyroidism [abstract], *J Vet Intern Med* 25:683, 2011.

ADRENAL GLAND DISORDERS

Mark E. Peterson and Randolph M. Baral

HYPERADRENOCORTICISM

Hyperadrenocorticism (Cushing's syndrome) is the constellation of clinical signs resulting from chronic glucocorticoid excess.[14,17,41] Hyperadrenocorticism can be naturally occurring as a result of primary hyperfunction of either the pituitary or adrenal gland or iatrogenic subsequent to administration of synthetic glucocorticoids. Of naturally occurring disease, pituitary-dependent hyperadrenocorticism is due to excessive secretion of adrenocorticotropic hormone (ACTH), from an adenoma arising in the pituitary gland (pars distalis or pars intermedia), which induces bilateral adrenocortical hyperplasia.[14,29-30,41] A unilateral adenoma or carcinoma of the adrenal cortex secretes excessive cortisol autonomously, resulting in suppression of pituitary ACTH secretion and atrophy of the contralateral adrenal cortex.

Although naturally occurring hyperadrenocorticism is rare in cats, both pituitary-dependent hyperadrenocorticism and cortisol-secreting adrenal tumors have been well characterized.[14,17,30,41] Approximately 75% to 80% of cats with hyperadrenocorticism have the pituitary-dependent form of the disorder; the remaining 20% to 25% have unilateral adrenal tumors. Of the cats with functional adrenocortical tumors, approximately two thirds have unilateral adenoma; the others have adrenal carcinoma.

Cats tend to be more resistant to the effects of exogenous glucocorticoid excess than dogs, but iatrogenic hyperadrenocorticism is a well-recognized disorder in cats.[25,26]

Progesterone-secreting adrenal tumors have also been recognized in cats, albeit rarely.[7,12,32,42,47] Clinical signs are similar to those in cats with cortisol-secreting tumors, but measurement of cortisol precursors is necessary for diagnosis.

Clinical Features

Hyperadrenocorticism is a disease of middle-aged to older cats, with a median age of 10 to 11 years. Most case series of cats with hyperadrenocorticism have shown no sex predilection,[15,17,18,54] but a slight female sex predilection has been suggested.[14] There is no reported breed predilection.

The most common clinical signs (Table 24-8) associated with hyperadrenocorticism include the following (Figures 24-20 and 24-21):

- Polyuria
- Polydipsia
- Polyphagia
- Pendulous abdomen
- Cutaneous changes

Other signs typical for the disease in dogs, such as bilateral symmetric hair loss, weight gain, and muscle atrophy, can be seen in cats with advanced or long-term untreated hyperadrenocorticism.[14,17,18,54]

Differences in Clinical Presentation Between Cats and Dogs

Despite the apparent similarity between cats and dogs with hyperadrenocorticism, there are major differences in clinical presentation.

POLYURIA AND POLYDIPSIA

In contrast to dogs with hyperadrenocorticism, the onset of polyuria and polydipsia both in cats treated with large doses of glucocorticoids and in cats that develop naturally occurring hyperadrenocorticism is often delayed;

TABLE 24-8 Clinical Signs and Abnormal Laboratory Findings in Cats with Hyperadrenocorticism

Clinical and Laboratory Findings	Approximate % of Cats
CLINICAL SIGNS	
Polyuria and polydipsia	85-90
Pot-bellied appearance	70-85
Increased appetite	65-75
Unkempt, seborrheic hair coat	60-70
Muscle wasting	60-65
Bilateral symmetric hair thinning or alopecia	40-60
Lethargy	40-60
Insulin resistance (high daily insulin dose)	45-55
Weight loss	50-60
Fragile, tearing skin	30-50
Infection or sepsis	30-40
Obesity or weight gain	20-40
Hepatomegaly	25-35
Calcinosis cutis	0
COMPLETE BLOOD COUNT	
Lymphopenia	60-65
Eosinopenia	55-60
Mature leukocytosis	45-55
Monocytosis	20-25
SERUM BIOCHEMICAL ANALYSIS	
Hyperglycemia	80-90
Hypercholesterolemia	30-45
High alanine aminotransferase activity	35-40
High alkaline phosphatase activity	10-20
URINALYSIS	
Glycosuria	85-90
Urine specific gravity <1.015	5-10
Ketonuria	5-10

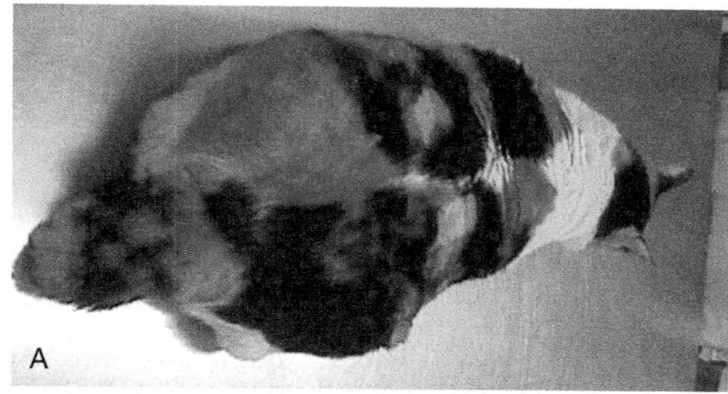

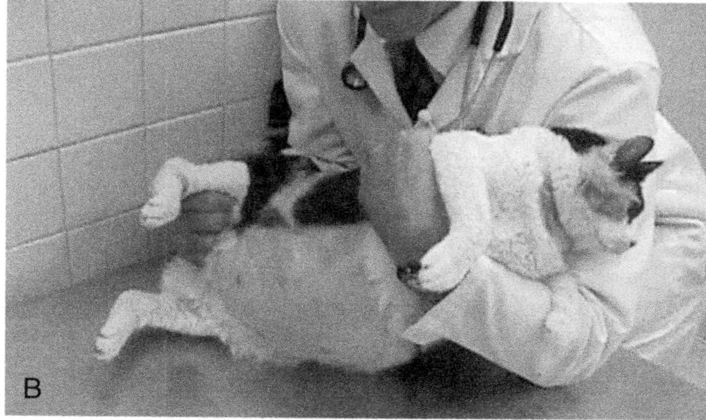

FIGURE 24-20 Cat with hyperadrenocorticism caused by a unilateral adrenal adenoma. Note the unkempt hair coat, pot belly, and alopecia on the ventral abdomen and tail.

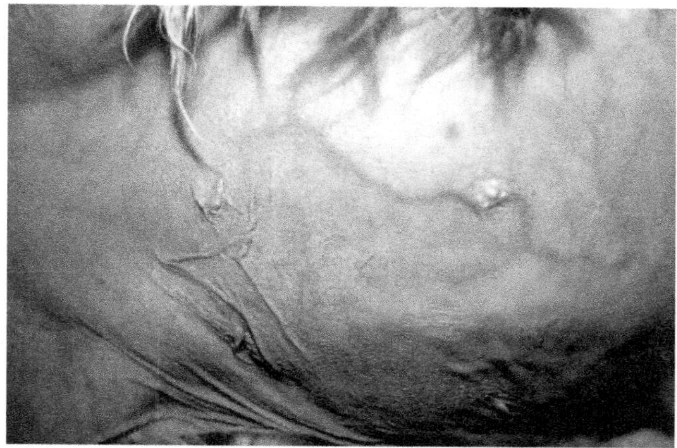

FIGURE 24-21 Ventral abdomen of a cat with advanced pituitary-dependent hyperadrenocorticism. Notice the alopecia, prominent abdominal veins, thin skin, and loss of cutaneous elasticity.

polyuria usually coincides with the development of moderate to severe hyperglycemia and glucosuria with subsequent osmotic diuresis.[14,21,28,41] Therefore these signs are not present in most cats during the less advanced stages of hyperadrenocorticism when glucose tolerance is still normal (i.e., before development of DM).

Although they are rare in cats with hyperadrenocorticism, it is important to realize that polyuria and polydipsia can also develop either without concurrent diabetes or before the progression of overt DM.[17,54] The mechanism for the development of polyuria and polydipsia in these nondiabetic cats is unclear, but it appears be related to concurrent renal disease in most.

SKIN FRAGILITY

Up to half of all cats with hyperadrenocorticism develop fragility of the skin, somewhat resembling that seen in cats with cutaneous asthenia (Ehlers–Danlos syndrome).

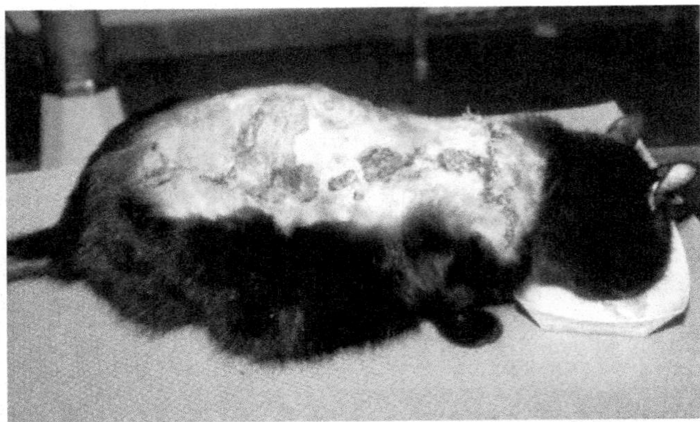

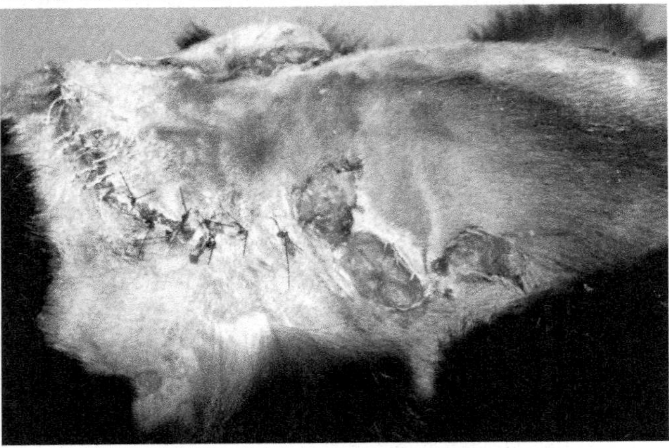

FIGURE 24-22 Cat with pituitary-dependent hyperadrenocorticism and diabetes mellitus. Note the multiple open wounds on the dorsal back. A large wound above the shoulder has been sutured by the referring veterinarian. This cat did not have alopecia, but the dorsal truncal area was shaved to facilitate treatment. The nonhealing wound is secondary to severe thinning of the skin.

This sign only rarely, if at all, develops in hyperadrenocorticoid dogs.[10,14,28,41,54] In affected cats the skin tends to tear with routine handling or when the cat plays with other cats, leaving large denuded areas (Figure 24-22). Many of the other cutaneous features of hyperadrenocorticism in cats are similar to those reported in dogs (e.g., unkempt hair coat, bilateral symmetric hair loss, atrophic thin skin, and bruising of the skin), but skin fragility appears to be a unique though serious manifestation of the disease in cats (see Table 24-8).

WEIGHT LOSS

Many cats with hyperadrenocorticism have a history of weight loss rather than weight gain or obesity as is seen in dogs with this disease (see Table 24-8). In most cases this weight loss occurs secondary to poorly controlled DM, which occurs in up to 90% of cats with hyperadrenocorticism. This concurrent diabetes may be slightly *insulin resistant* in some cats, but most are not receiving extremely high doses of insulin. Insulin resistance, even when present, is never as severe as in cats with acromegaly, in which extremely high insulin doses are sometimes required to control the GH-induced diabetes (see the section on Pituitary Disorders in this chapter).

Diagnosis

Routine Laboratory Tests

Routine laboratory results are variable and not necessarily specific for the disease.[14,17,21,41,54] The classic hematologic changes of mature leucocytosis, eosinopenia, lymphopenia, and monocytosis (see Table 24-8) may be reported, but these findings are inconsistent. By far the most striking serum biochemical abnormality reported is severe hyperglycemia and glycosuria (see Table 24-8). Hypercholesterolemia is seen in about half of affected cats and may be caused, at least in part, by a poorly controlled diabetic state. High serum ALT levels are also seen in a third of affected cats, probably related to the hepatic lipidosis associated with diabetes. In dogs with hyperadrenocorticism, steroid induction of a specific hepatic isoenzyme of ALP causes increases in the serum activity of this enzyme in 85% to 90% of cases; whereas only 10% to 20% of cats with hyperadrenocorticism have high ALP activity (see Table 24-8). The mild increase in serum ALP activity found in some cats probably results from the poorly regulated diabetic state rather than from a direct effect of glucocorticoid excess, insofar as it may normalize with insulin treatment alone, despite progression of the hyperadrenocorticism.

Cats with hyperadrenocorticism usually maintain urine specific gravity above 1.020 in spite of clinical polyuria and polydipsia. The dilute urine concentrations commonly seen in dogs with hyperadrenocorticism are rarely seen in cats. Again, this difference in urine concentration probably reflects the fact that polyuria in most cats is the result of hyperglycemia and glycosuria rather than being a direct inhibitory effect on secretion or action of antidiuretic hormone (ADH), as in dogs.

Pituitary-Adrenal Function Tests

Endocrinologic evaluation of cats suspected of hyperadrenocorticism is a two-step process:

1. Screening tests to confirm the diagnosis
2. Differentiating tests to distinguish pituitary-dependent disease from adrenal tumors

Test results can be difficult to interpret because clinical signs are often less dramatic in cats than in dogs, and results of individual tests are often inconsistent with poor sensitivity or specificity. In many cases it is necessary to use a combination of tests to determine if hyperadrenocorticism is present, as well as to determine the cause of the disorder.

SCREENING TESTS FOR HYPERADRENOCORTICISM

There are three endocrine tests that can be used for diagnosis of cats suspected of hyperadrenocorticism:

1. ACTH response test
2. Urine cortisol:creatinine ratio
3. Low-dose dexamethasone screening test

None of these tests is perfect, and each has its advantages and disadvantages. It is therefore recommended that the diagnosis of hyperadrenocorticism be reserved for cats with clinical signs of the disease, as well as endocrine test results consistent with that diagnosis.

ACTH RESPONSE TEST The ACTH stimulation test is commonly used as a screening test for hyperadrenocorticism in dogs and has also been recommended as a diagnostic test for cats suspected of having hyperadrenocorticism. This is the only test that can be used to distinguish iatrogenic from naturally occurring hyperadrenocorticism; it requires relatively little time (1 hour) and only two venipunctures.

Regardless of the basal cortisol value obtained, diagnosis of naturally occurring hyperadrenocorticism depends on demonstration of a post-ACTH cortisol concentration that is higher than the reference range for post-ACTH cortisol values. In contrast, cats with iatrogenic hyperadrenocorticism would be expected to have a subnormal response to exogenous ACTH administration.

In cats the main problem with the ACTH response test as a screening test for hyperadrenocorticism is poor sensitivity. Only 35% to 50% of cats with naturally occurring hyperadrenocorticism show an exaggerated serum cortisol response, whereas up to two thirds of cats with the disease have "normal" test results. Therefore the ACTH response test is not nearly as useful for detecting naturally occurring hyperadrenocorticism in cats as it is in dogs, where the test sensitivity is approximately 85%. However, if iatrogenic hyperadrenocorticism is suspected, the ACTH response test remains the screening test of choice to document secondary adrenocortical suppression.[14,17,21]

A variety of chronic illnesses (not associated with hyperadrenocorticism) also appear to influence ACTH-stimulated cortisol secretion in cats.[41,56] Stress associated with chronic illness most likely results in some degree of bilateral adrenocortical hyperplasia in sick cats, which could account for an exaggerated cortisol response to ACTH. Therefore the diagnosis of hyperadrenocorticism should not be based solely on the results of basal or ACTH-stimulated serum cortisol concentrations but also the cat's history, clinical signs, and routine laboratory findings.

Sex hormone–secreting adrenal tumors have also been rarely recognized in cats.[7,9,12,32,47] Clinical signs are similar to those in cats with cortisol-secreting tumors but, as in the dog, measurement of cortisol precursors is necessary for diagnosis. In these cats measurement of serum or plasma sex hormones (e.g., progesterone, 17-hydroxyprogesterone, androstenedione, testosterone, estradiol) before and after ACTH stimulation is an aid to diagnosis. However, ACTH stimulation testing is of limited value in diagnosis of these cats because most are found to have high basal serum concentrations of the sex steroid (or steroids), making stimulation tests unnecessary.

One commonly employed protocol for this test (Table 24-9) is to collect blood for determination of serum (or plasma) cortisol concentration before and 60 minutes after administration of 125 μg synthetic ACTH (tetracosactrin or cosyntropin) intravenously.[41] In cats intravenous administration of ACTH induces greater and more prolonged adrenocortical stimulation than the intramuscular route and is therefore preferred.[41] Lower doses of synthetic ACTH (1.25 and 12.5 μg per cat) produce comparable cortisol stimulation.[39] However, more prolonged stimulation is attained after administration of higher doses, and doses as high as 250 μg have been recommended for obese cats, particularly if sampling is delayed for any reason.[48]

Overall, the ACTH stimulation test is *not* recommended as the initial screening test for hyperadrenocorticism in cats because of two important reasons: (1) The test lacks sensitivity, and most cats with hyperadrenocorticism will have normal results; and (2) the other two screening tests (urine cortisol: creatinine ratio and low-dose dexamethasone suppression test) are clearly superior tests because of their increased test sensitivity.

URINE CORTISOL:CREATININE RATIO The urine cortisol: creatinine ratio is a valuable, highly sensitive screening test that can be used to help diagnose hyperadrenocorticism in cats.[17,18] As a diagnostic test, the test sensitivity for the urine cortisol:creatinine ratio ranges from 80% to 90%. However, as with the ACTH response test, the finding of a high (false-positive) urine cortisol:creatinine ratio is common in cats with moderate to severe nonadrenal illness.[11,20] This is especially true in cats with illnesses that are not usually associated with hyperadrenocorticism.

It is best to have the owner collect the urine specimen from the cat at home and bring the sample to the veterinary clinic for submission to the laboratory (see Table 24-9) to avoid the stress of travel or hospitalization (which could falsely increase the urine cortisol:creatinine ratio). The use of nonabsorbable cat litter or replacement of the cat litter with nonabsorbent aquarium gravel[18] will help owners collect a urine sample from their cats.

Overall, the urine cortisol:creatinine ratio is a sensitive diagnostic test for distinguishing cats with hyperadrenocorticism from those that do not have the disease. However, because the specificity of this test appears to be low, the veterinarian must carefully evaluate the cat's history and results of physical examination when

TABLE 24-9 **Diagnostic Tests Used in Cats with Suspected Hyperadrenocorticism**

Test	Test Protocol
SCREENING TESTS	
ACTH response test	Collect baseline blood sample for serum cortisol measurement Administer synthetic ACTH (tetracosactrin at 0.125 mg intravenously) Collect post-ACTH sample for cortisol determination 1 hour later
Urine cortisol : creatinine ratio	Owner collects urine specimen from cat at home and brings to veterinary clinic for submission to laboratory
Low-dose dexamethasone suppression test	Collect baseline blood sample for serum cortisol measurement Administer dexamethasone (0.1 mg/kg intravenously) Collect postdexamethasone sample for cortisol determination 4 and 8 hours later
Combined dexamethasone suppression/ACTH response test	Collect baseline blood sample for serum cortisol determination Administer dexamethasone at the dosage of 0.1 mg/kg intravenously Collect blood for postdexamethasone cortisol concentration 4 hours later Immediately after collecting the 4-hour sample, administer synthetic ACTH (tetracosactrin at 0.125 mg intravenously) Collect post-ACTH sample for cortisol determination at 5 hours (1 hour after ACTH administration)
DISCRIMINATION TESTS	
High-dose dexamethasone suppression test (serum cortisol measurements)	Collect baseline blood sample for serum cortisol measurement Administer dexamethasone (1.0 mg/kg intravenously) Collect post-dexamethasone sample for cortisol determination 4 and 8 hours later
High-dose dexamethasone suppression test (urine cortisol : creatinine measurements)	Owner collect urine from cat at home on two consecutive mornings for determination of baseline cortisol : creatinine ratios Owner then administers three oral doses of dexamethasone to the cat at the dosage of 0.1 mg/kg every 8 hours (e.g., 0800, 1600, and 2400 hours) Owner collects urine sample at home for postdexamethasone sample the next morning (e.g., 0800 hours)
Plasma endogenous ACTH concentration	Collect plasma in chilled tube with protease inhibitor added if available Immediately separate and freeze plasma until assayed
Abdominal ultrasonography	Equipment and skilled operator required to perform procedure

ACTH, Adrenocorticotropic hormone.

interpreting the test result. If the results of the urine cortisol : creatinine ratio are suggestive of hyperadrenocorticism and hyperadrenocorticism is strongly suspected clinically, the diagnosis is best confirmed with another follow-up screening test, such as the low-dose dexamethasone suppression test (discussed in the following section).

LOW-DOSE DEXAMETHASONE SUPPRESSION TEST For cats the low-dose (screening) dexamethasone suppression test is performed using a tenfold higher dose of dexamethasone than is required in dogs.[14,17,21,24,40] Blood samples for serum (or plasma) cortisol determination are collected before and 4 and 8 hours after administration of dexamethasone at an intravenous dose of 0.1 mg/kg (see Table 24-9).

This low-dose (screening) dexamethasone dosage will consistently suppress serum cortisol concentrations to below approximately 40 nmol/L at 4 and 8 hours in healthy cats and in those with nonadrenal illness. Inadequate serum cortisol suppression at both 4 and 8 hours is diagnostic for hyperadrenocorticism and is found in all cats with cortisol-secreting adrenal tumors. The vast majority of cats with pituitary-dependent hyperadrenocorticism will also fail to suppress serum cortisol concentration at 4 hours or 8 hours.[14,21,41] Again, this lack of normal serum cortisol suppression is diagnostic for hyperadrenocorticism.

Overall, the low-dose (0.1 mg/kg) dexamethasone suppression test is an excellent screening test, with close to 100% sensitivity and acceptable specificity. Because this test is clearly better than the ACTH stimulation test and has better test specificity than does baseline urine cortisol : creatinine ratios, this is the test of choice for evaluating a cat with suspected hyperadrenocorticism.

COMBINED ACTH RESPONSE/DEXAMETHASONE SUPPRESSION TEST It is possible to combine the ACTH response test and the low-dose (screening) dexamethasone suppression test (0.1 mg/kg) and perform them in a single day, insofar as only three blood samples must be collected over a 5-hour period (see Table 24-9).

To perform the combined test, a baseline blood sample for serum cortisol determination is collected and dexamethasone administered at an intravenous dose of 0.1 mg/kg, with collection of a further blood sample for cortisol measurement 4 hours later. Immediately after the 4-hour blood sample has been taken, synthetic ACTH (tetracosactrin or cosyntropin) is administered at an intravenous dose of 125 μg, and a post-ACTH sample for cortisol determination is collected at 5 hours (1 hour after ACTH administration).

Almost all cats with hyperadrenocorticism fail to show serum cortisol suppression after dexamethasone administration, and up to one half have an exaggerated response to ACTH administration. By contrast, healthy cats and almost all diabetic cats without hyperadrenocorticism exhibit marked serum cortisol suppression after dexamethasone and have a normal cortisol response after ACTH stimulation.[14,21,41]

Overall, because of the low sensitivity of the ACTH stimulation portion of this test, the combined ACTH response–dexamethasone suppression test is *not* recommended as a screening test for hyperadrenocorticism. Use of the 8-hour dexamethasone suppression test, as previously outlined, is a better diagnostic test for cats with suspected hyperadrenocorticism.

TESTS TO DETERMINE CAUSE OF HYPERADRENOCORTICISM

Once a diagnosis of hyperadrenocorticism has been confirmed, pituitary-dependent must be distinguished from adrenal-dependent (due to adrenocortical tumors) hyperadrenocorticism. This distinction can have important implications in providing the most effective method of management for the disease. An accurate test is therefore required to determine the cause of the cat's hyperadrenocorticism.

Endocrine tests in this category include the high-dose dexamethasone suppression test and endogenous plasma ACTH measurements. Imaging techniques such as abdominal radiography, ultrasonography, CT, and magnetic resonance imaging (MRI) can also be extremely helpful in determining the cause. In addition, it is only possible to detect metastatic lesions from an adrenal carcinoma by use of these imaging techniques, in the absence of adrenal biopsy and histopathology.

HIGH-DOSE DEXAMETHASONE SUPPRESSION TEST (SERUM CORTISOL MEASUREMENTS) To perform a high-dose dexamethasone suppression test in cats, blood is collected for serum (or plasma) cortisol determination before and 4 and 8 hours after the administration of dexamethasone at 1.0 mg/kg intravenously (see Table 24-9). Note that as with the low-dose dexamethasone suppression test, this dose is 10 times higher than is required in dogs.

After administration of high-dose dexamethasone, adequate cortisol suppression is generally defined as a serum cortisol concentration of less than 30 nmol/L or a cortisol concentration of less than 50% of the baseline value at 4 or 8 hours. In cats with functional adrenocortical neoplasia, high-dose dexamethasone never adequately suppresses cortisol concentration, whereas it suppresses serum cortisol concentration in approximately 50% of cats with pituitary-dependent hyperadrenocorticism.[14,17,41] This is unlike the situation in dogs with pituitary-dependent hyperadrenocorticism, in which 85% will show adequate cortisol suppression after administration of this high dose of dexamethasone.

Overall, this in-hospital, high-dose dexamethasone suppression test is relatively easy to perform. Suppression of serum cortisol concentrations, when demonstrated, is consistent with pituitary-dependent hyperadrenocorticism. Unfortunately, this test cannot reliably determine the cause of the disorder because one half of cats with pituitary-dependent hyperadrenocorticism fail to demonstrate cortisol suppression with this test. In these cases either plasma ACTH should be measured or abdominal ultrasonography should be performed to determine the cause of the hyperadrenocorticism.

HIGH-DOSE DEXAMETHASONE SUPPRESSION TEST (MEASUREMENT OF URINE CORTISOL: CREATININE RATIOS) The protocol for performing this high-dose dexamethasone suppression test, with monitoring of the percentage of suppression of urine cortisol:creatinine ratios, is as follows. Owners collect urine from the cat on two consecutive mornings (e.g., at 0700 to 0800 hours) for determination of baseline cortisol:creatinine ratios. The owners then administer three oral doses of dexamethasone to the cat at the dosage of 0.1 mg/kg every 8 hours. In other words, immediately after collection of the second basal urine sample, the first dexamethasone dose is administered; the second and third doses are administered in the afternoon and evening of the same day, respectively. The third urine sample is collected 8 hours after administration of the final dexamethasone dose, which would be the next morning. Thus for this test urine is collected on three consecutive mornings, and the three dexamethasone doses are all administered on the second day (see Table 24-9).

The finding that the urinary cortisol:creatinine ratio after dexamethasone administration is suppressed by more than 50% of the average basal cortisol: creatinine ratio is diagnostic for pituitary-dependent hyperadrenocorticism. If suppression is less than 50%, no discrimination is possible, as is the case for the standard high-dose dexamethasone suppression test described above.

Approximately 75% of cats with pituitary-dependent hyperadrenocorticism will demonstrate suppression with this at-home, urine high dose dexamethasone suppression test.[18,30] This makes this test more reliable than the standard high-dose dexamethasone suppression test for distinguishing the cause of hyperadrenocorticism in cats.

Overall, the at-home high-dose dexamethasone suppression test is generally easier to perform and is better at determining the cause of the disorder than the standard in-hospital test. Therefore for those owners who can administer the dexamethasone, this protocol can be recommended both as a screening test (the baseline urine cortisol:creatinine ratios) and discrimination test (postdexamethasone urine cortisol:creatinine ratio).

ENDOGENOUS ACTH DETERMINATIONS In cats with clinical signs and screening test results diagnostic for hyperadrenocorticism, the basal endogenous ACTH concentration is a valuable test for differentiating the origin of disease.[14,41] The endogenous ACTH concentration is high to high-normal in cats with pituitary-dependent hyperadrenocorticism, whereas the concentration in cats with functional adrenocortical tumors is low to undetectable.

It is important to remember that blood samples for determination of endogenous ACTH concentration must be handled carefully because ACTH can degrade rapidly in plasma after collection. Special handling requirements (see Table 24-9) include the addition of a protease inhibitor (e.g., aprotinin) when blood is collected, rapid separation of plasma, and proper storage temperatures until the assay is performed. Mishandling of samples may result in a falsely low value that could erroneously suggest an adrenal tumor.

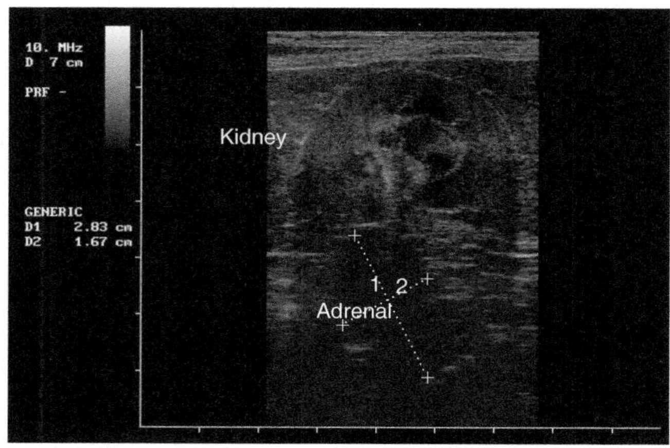

FIGURE 24-23 Ultrasonographic appearance of an enlarged adrenal gland showing proximity to kidney. Note that the adrenal gland appears hypoechoic. The kidney is at an oblique angle and is thus foreshortened.

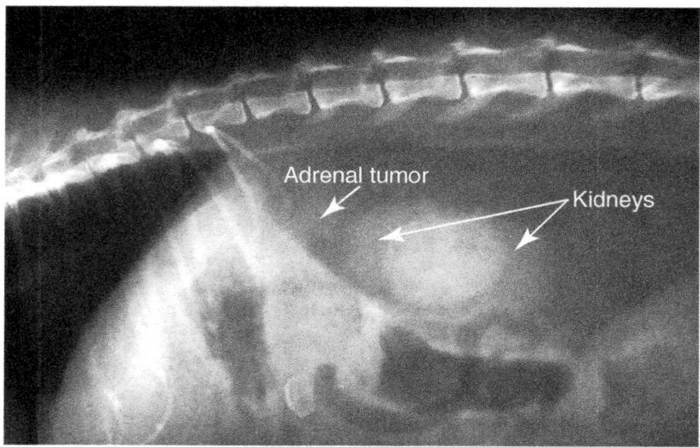

FIGURE 24-24 Lateral abdominal radiograph of a cat with hyperadrenocorticism. Notice the soft tissue mass cranial to the kidneys. Surgical exploration confirmed a right adrenal mass with atrophy of the contralateral left adrenal gland. Histopathology of the adrenal tumor confirmed adrenal adenoma.

DIAGNOSTIC IMAGING

Of the diagnostic imaging modalities, ultrasonographic evaluation of adrenal size and morphology is most commonly used and extremely useful in determining the cause of the hyperadrenocorticism in cats (Figure 24-23). Adrenal glands are relatively easy to identify in cats. In contrast to the dog, in which the left and right adrenal glands differ in shape, in cats both the adrenal glands are oblong and oval to bean shaped.[57] In cats with hyperadrenocorticism, if both adrenal glands are large or of equal size, the diagnosis is pituitary-dependent hyperadrenocorticism. If, on the other hand, one adrenal gland is large or misshapen and the contralateral adrenal is small or cannot be visualized on ultrasonographic evaluation, a cortisol-secreting adrenal tumor is diagnosed.[14,17,24,41]

Although a large adrenocortical tumor can sometimes be visualized on abdominal radiographs, radiography is of no value in confirming bilateral adrenocortical hyperplasia in cats with pituitary-dependent hyperadrenocorticism (Figure 24-24). Bilateral calcification of the adrenal gland can occasionally be detected in clinically normal cats, but this should not be interpreted as evidence of an adrenal tumor as it is in dogs.[41]

CT and MRI have also proven useful in the detection of pituitary tumors (>3 mm diameter) as well as unilateral adrenal tumors, but both require specialized equipment, are expensive to perform and are not widely available.

Treatment

In cats hyperadrenocorticism is difficult to treat successfully (Table 24-10). From collected experience over the last two decades, adrenalectomy has proved to be the most successful mode of treatment in cats, whereas medical management and use of pituitary radiotherapy

TABLE 24-10 **Treatment Options for Cats with Hyperadrenocorticism**

Treatment	Indication	Comments
MEDICAL THERAPY		
Mitotane (o,p′-DDD)	PDH or adrenal tumor	Initial dose 25-50 mg/kg daily Drug fails to adequately suppress adrenocortical function in most cats Adverse effects common Not strongly recommended
Ketoconazole	PDH or adrenal tumor	Ineffective in suppressing adrenocortical function in most cats Adverse effects common Not recommended
Metyrapone	PDH or adrenal tumor	Initial dose 250-500 mg daily Potential adverse effects include vomiting and anorexia Beneficial effects on suppressing adrenocortical function may be transient Most useful as preoperative preparation for adrenalectomy Unavailability of drug is a frequent problem
Trilostane	PDH or adrenal tumor	Initial dose 15-30 mg daily; increase to 60-90 mg daily if needed Adverse effects uncommon Effective in suppressing adrenocortical function Useful as preoperative preparation for adrenalectomy and possibly for long-term use Drug licensed for use only in dogs in the United Kingdom (not licensed for use in the United States)
RADIATION THERAPY		
Pituitary cobalt radiation treatment	PDH	Offers a potential cure for pituitary-dependent hyperadrenocorticism May be the only treatment for cats with a large or invasive pituitary tumor Treatment response typically delayed, so use of concurrent medical therapy or bilateral adrenalectomy recommended Limited availability and expense disadvantages
SURGERY		
Unilateral adrenalectomy	Adrenal tumor	Presurgical medical stabilization (e.g., metyrapone, trilostane) helpful Postoperative complications may include pancreatitis and wound dehiscence Clinical signs resolve by 2-4 months postoperatively Glucocorticoid supplementation required for approximately 2 months postoperatively, until function of the atrophied remaining adrenal gland recovers With complete removal of adrenal tumor, cure of disease accomplished
Bilateral adrenalectomy	PDH	Presurgical medical stabilization (e.g., metyrapone, trilostane) helpful Postoperative complications common Clinical signs resolve by 2-4 months postoperatively Lifelong replacement of both mineralocorticoid and glucocorticoid hormones required Pituitary defect (e.g., pituitary adenoma) remains; may later develop pituitary macroadenoma
Hypophysectomy	PDH	Offers potential cure for hyperadrenocorticism Presurgical medical stabilization (e.g., metyrapone, trilostane) helpful Requires highly skilled surgeon and advanced imaging facilities Postoperative complications (diabetes insipidus) common Recurrence of disease possible

PDH, Pituitary dependent hyperadrenocorticism.

have yielded mixed results.* Potential options for medical treatment include the use of the adrenocorticolytic agent mitotane (o,p′-DDD) or drugs that block one or more of the enzymes involved in cortisol synthesis (e.g., ketoconazole, metyrapone, trilostane). The more widespread use of the drug trilostane has resulted in reasonable medical control for at least a few weeks to months for most cats with hyperadrenocorticism.

Surgical treatment for cats with pituitary-dependent hyperadrenocorticism includes bilateral adrenalectomy or hypophysectomy, whereas unilateral adrenalectomy is indicated in cats with an adrenocortical tumor. Finally, external radiation therapy can also be used for pituitary-dependent hyperadrenocorticism, especially when the cat has a large pituitary adenoma.

*References 10, 14, 15, 33, 34, 41, 49, 54.

Medical Therapy

MITOTANE

Mitotane (o,p'-DDD) is an adrenocortical cytolytic agent that has been used extensively for the treatment of hyperadrenocorticism in dogs. Long-term results from a number of different protocols for mitotane treatment of cats with hyperadrenocorticism have been generally discouraging, although limited short-term success is sometimes obtained.[14,17,41,49] The standard daily dosages of mitotane (25 to 50 mg/kg per day, orally) used for dogs with pituitary-dependent hyperadrenocorticism neither effectively suppresses adrenocortical function nor alleviates clinical signs of the disease, even after prolonged daily treatment periods in most cats.[14,41] Adverse effects such as anorexia, vomiting, and lethargy are relatively common, even in cats in which the drug has not lowered serum cortisol concentrations (see Table 24-10). Because of the drug's poor effectiveness and high rate of adverse effects, mitotane is not recommended in cats with hyperadrenocorticism.

KETOCONAZOLE

Ketoconazole, a drug used principally for treatment of mycotic disease, inhibits the first step in cortisol biosynthesis (cholesterol side-chain cleavage to pregnenolone) and, to a lesser extent, the conversion of 11-deoxycortisol to cortisol. Although ketoconazole has been used successfully in both humans and dogs with hyperadrenocorticism, the drug does not reliably suppress adrenocortical function in normal cats or cats with hyperadrenocorticism and may cause serious side effects such as thrombocytopenia.[14,17,41] Therefore ketoconazole cannot be recommended for treatment of cats with hyperadrenocorticism (see Table 24-10).

METYRAPONE

Metyrapone inhibits the action of 11-beta-hydroxylase (the enzyme that converts 11-desoxy-cortisol [11-DOC] to cortisol). It has been used with mixed results in cats with hyperadrenocorticism. Total dosages ranging from 250 to 500 mg per day have been used.[10,14,33,41] Most cats appear to tolerate the drug reasonably well, but it can induce vomiting and anorexia, necessitating the discontinuation of the drug in some cats (see Table 24-10). If effective, metyrapone reduces both basal and ACTH-stimulated cortisol concentrations and ameliorates the clinical signs of disease. Overall, the effectiveness of metyrapone in cats with hyperadrenocorticism is variable and may be transient, so the drug is best used over the short term to prepare for surgical adrenalectomy. However, metyrapone is difficult to obtain, precluding its widespread use for cats with hyperadrenocorticism.

TRILOSTANE

Trilostane reversibly inhibits the 3-beta-hydroxysteroid dehydrogenase enzyme system in the adrenal cortex, which decreases the synthesis of both glucocorticoids and mineralocorticoids. Trilostane is an effective medical treatment for dogs with hyperadrenocorticism, and experience collected over the last few years indicates that it is also a valuable treatment for cats with the disorder (see Table 24-10).

Thus far, trilostane treatment has been reported in seven cats with hyperadrenocorticism (six with pituitary-dependent disease and one with an adrenal tumor), using a daily dose of 4.2 to 13.6 mg/kg.[6,34,51] Clinical signs of hyperadrenocorticism resolved to varying degrees after trilostane administration in all these cats.

Based on both the reported studies and personal experience, the recommended starting dose in cats with hyperadrenocorticism is 20 to 30 mg/cat per day, administered once daily or divided at the time of feeding. The daily trilostane dose frequently needs to be adjusted in cats treated with the drug, depending on resolution of clinical signs, serum chemistry results, and repeat ACTH stimulation testing.

Cats on trilostane treatment should be evaluated at 2 weeks, 1 month, 2 to 3 months, and every 1 to 3 months thereafter. At each recheck (scheduled at approximately 3 to 4 hours after the morning trilostane dose was given), the owner should be questioned and the cat examined. Blood is then collected for a hemogram and serum chemistry panel, and an ACTH stimulation test is performed. Although the ideal target range for the post-ACTH cortisol concentration for cats receiving trilostane has yet to be determined, a post-ACTH cortisol concentration of 50 to 150 nmol/L should be the goal. In cats with persistent clinical signs and serum cortisol values higher than this ideal range, the dose of trilostane is increased to 30 to 60 mg/cat per day, administered once daily or divided at the time of feeding. Additional dosage adjustments are made as needed depending on subsequent recheck examinations and ACTH stimulation testing. In some cats daily doses as high as 90 to 120 mg have been needed to control clinical signs and lower ACTH-stimulated cortisol concentrations into the ideal range.

If a cat on trilostane presents with clinical signs consistent with hypocortisolism, trilostane should be stopped and an ACTH stimulation test performed to confirm whether clinical signs are due to low cortisol concentrations. If hypoadrenocorticism is confirmed but serum electrolytes are normal, the veterinarian should stop trilostane and administer glucocorticoids as needed. If hypoadrenocorticism is associated with hyperkalemia or hyponatremia, the veterinarian should discontinue trilostane for 1 month and treat with both glucocorticoids and mineralocorticoids.

Overall, although further investigation is necessary, trilostane appears to be a valuable option for treatment of cats with hyperadrenocorticism and provides a useful medical alternative to metyrapone. Trilostane should be extremely useful in the preoperative preparation of cats with hyperadrenocorticism, before unilateral or bilateral adrenalectomy, but the drug may also be useful as sole agent in the long-term management of some cats.

Radiation Therapy

PITUITARY RADIOTHERAPY

Pituitary-dependent hyperadrenocorticism has been treated with radiation therapy in a number of cats with partial success.[14,17,27,41,50] Large or invasive pituitary tumors may become smaller, resulting in prolonged survival, and radiotherapy also offers a potential cure for cats with pituitary-dependent hyperadrenocorticism. However, because there is often a delay in reduction in both tumor size and ACTH secretion after therapy, cats can die as a result of complications attributable to hyperadrenocorticism before radiotherapy can adequately control the disease. Veterinarians are therefore recommended to use medical therapy (e.g., trilostane) to help control hyperadrenocorticism before performing radiotherapy in cats with pituitary-dependent hyperadrenocorticism.

Other disadvantages of radiotherapy for treatment of cats with hyperadrenocorticism include its limited availability and high expense, as well as the frequent anesthesia and extended hospitalization periods required to perform the treatment (see Table 24-10). Additionally, some cats require multiple radiation treatments.[50]

Surgery

UNILATERAL AND BILATERAL ADRENALECTOMY

The most successful method of treating cats with hyperadrenocorticism appears to be adrenalectomy (Figure 24-25).*

- Unilateral adrenalectomy should be performed in cats with a unilateral, cortisol-secreting adrenocortical tumor.
- Bilateral adrenalectomy must be performed in cats with pituitary-dependent bilateral adrenocortical hyperplasia.

The chronic hypersecretion of glucocorticoids with hyperadrenocorticism increases the risk of infection and delayed wound healing postoperatively. Postoperative complications also include pancreatitis, thromboembolic phenomena, wound dehiscence, and hypoadrenocorticism. Postoperative outcome is improved with presurgical medical stabilization (e.g., trilostane) of cats with severe clinical signs. The clinician must not lose sight of the fact that those cats with pituitary-dependent hyperadrenocorticism undergoing successful bilateral adrenalectomy will still have the pituitary defect (e.g., pituitary adenoma) remaining; these cats may later develop neurologic signs associated with a compressive pituitary tumor.

*References 14, 15, 17, 21, 33, 41, 54.

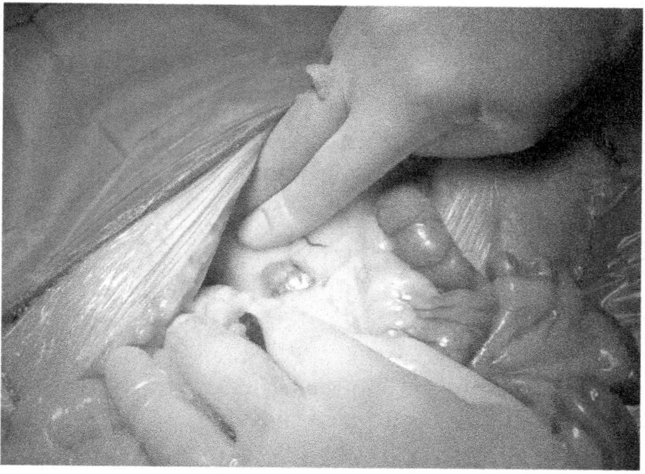

FIGURE 24-25 Appearance of adrenal cortical adenoma at surgery. Note the large amount of fat present in the surgical field that was present despite the cat being muscle wasted.

Unilateral adrenalectomy cases generally require glucocorticoid supplementation for approximately 2 months postoperatively (see Table 24-10), until there is recovery of the glucocorticoid secretory function of the atrophied contralateral adrenal gland. Lifelong replacement of both mineralocorticoid and glucocorticoid hormones is required for cats undergoing bilateral adrenalectomy.

When surgical treatment is successful, resolution of clinical signs (polyuria, polydipsia, polyphagia, lethargy) and physical abnormalities (pot belly, muscle wasting, alopecia, thin skin, hepatomegaly, infection) occurs 2 to 4 months after adrenalectomy.[15,17,54] In addition, many cats have decreased requirements for exogenous insulin therapy.

HYPOPHYSECTOMY

Microsurgical transsphenoidal hypophysectomy has been reported to be an effective method of treatment for cats with pituitary-dependent hyperadrenocorticism.[30] However, because this procedure requires an experienced, highly skilled veterinary surgeon and advanced CT imaging facilities, it remains a highly specialized form of treatment.

Hypophysectomy appears to be highly effective, at least in cats with a small pituitary tumor, but is associated with significant morbidity, and the procedure is not likely to be effective in cats with a large pituitary adenoma. Another disadvantage of this treatment is that hypopituitarism develops during the immediate postoperative period, resulting in hypocortisolism, hypothyroidism, and transient diabetes insipidus (DI); therefore substitution therapy with glucocorticoids, thyroxine, and desmopressin are required for at least 2 to 4 weeks or lifelong after hypophysectomy.

Prognosis

Hyperadrenocorticism is a serious disease with a guarded to grave prognosis. Without treatment most cats will succumb to complications of the disease within a few weeks to months of diagnosis.[14,17,41] One common reason for death of untreated cats is the deleterious effects of glucocorticoid excess on skin fragility, which leads to tearing of skin, open wounds, and delayed wound healing. The immunosuppressive effects of glucocorticoid excess also predispose cats to infection. Finally, chronic hypercortisolism can affect the cardiovascular system, resulting in hypertension, pulmonary thromboembolism, or congestive heart failure.

CATECHOLAMINE-SECRETING ADRENAL TUMORS

Pheochromocytoma is a catecholamine-producing tumor derived from the chromaffin cells of the adrenal medulla that is extremely rare in cats.[2,41] Clinical signs and physical examination findings develop as a result of the space-occupying nature of the tumor and its metastases or as a result of excessive secretion of catecholamines and their impact on blood pressure and cardiac function. A diagnosis of pheochromocytoma before surgery is usually one of exclusion. Unlike a cortisol-secreting adrenal tumor, the contralateral adrenal gland should be normal in size and shape with a catecholamine-producing adrenal tumor. Catecholamine secretion by the tumor, and thus systemic hypertension, tends to be episodic; failure to document systemic hypertension does not rule out pheochromocytoma. Measurement of urinary catecholamine concentrations or their metabolites can strengthen the tentative diagnosis of pheochromocytoma but is not commonly performed in cats. Preliminary studies indicate that plasma normetanephrine levels may be a potential diagnostic test for pheochromocytoma in cats.[55] Because many of the clinical signs and blood pressure alterations are similar for pheochromocytoma and adrenal-dependent hyperadrenocorticism, it is important to rule out adrenal-dependent hyperadrenocorticism before focusing on pheochromocytoma.

SEX HORMONE–SECRETING ADRENAL TUMORS

A functional tumor arising from the adrenal cortex could secrete excessive amounts of adrenal progestagens, androgens, or estrogens. Progesterone-secreting adrenal tumors have been the most common sex hormone secreting adrenal tumor reported in cats.* Clinical signs are similar to those in cats with cortisol-secreting tumors. Excessive progesterone secretion in affected cats causes DM and fragile skin syndrome, which is characterized by progressively worsening dermal and epidermal atrophy, endocrine alopecia, and easily torn skin.

Recently, a male cat that had developed a strong urine odor and aggressive behavior was documented to have a functional adrenal adenoma associated with high circulating concentration of androstenedione and testosterone.[32] After adrenalectomy serum concentrations of the androgens decreased and urine spraying and aggression resolved.

Some adrenocortical tumors, especially carcinomas, may secrete glucocorticoids or sex steroids in addition to mineralocorticoids. In particular, hyperprogesteronism with associated DM has been reported in combination with hyperaldosteronism in two cats.[9,12] The putative mechanism for concurrent hyperprogesteronism and hyperaldosteronism is either increased production of progesterone, as an intermediate in the synthesis of aldosterone, from neoplastic cells of the zona glomerulosa alone, or increased secretion of aldosterone and progesterone from neoplastic cells of the zona glomerulosa and fasciculata/reticularis, respectively.

In most cats with sex steroid–secreting adrenal tumors, results of tests of the pituitary-adrenocortical axis are normal to suppressed, and the contralateral adrenal gland is normal in size and shape on abdominal ultrasound. Diagnosis requires documenting an increased concentration of one or more adrenal sex steroids, ideally measured before and after ACTH stimulation.

HYPERALDOSTERONISM

Etiology and Pathophysiology

Aldosterone is the major mineralocorticoid secreted by the adrenal cortex and, as such, is responsible for regulation of the body's sodium and potassium balance, as well as maintenance of intravascular fluid volume and acid–base status. Hyperaldosteronism, a condition resulting from increased secretion of aldosterone from the adrenal glomerulosa, may be related to either a primary or a secondary cause.

*References 6, 7, 9, 12, 42, 47.

Secondary hyperaldosteronism develops in cats, as in other species, as a physiologic response to stimulation of the renin–angiotensin–aldosterone system. The renin–angiotensin–aldosterone system acts to maintain the volume of extracellular fluid, circulatory pressure, and electrolyte homeostasis through integrated effects of enzymes and hormones, chiefly on the vasculature and kidney. Therefore secondary hyperaldosteronism can develop in any disease that overstimulates the renin–angiotensin–aldosterone system, such as dehydration, hypotension, or reduced renal perfusion secondary to renal disease.

Primary hyperaldosteronism (Conn's syndrome) appears to be a relatively rare disease of older cats characterized by excessive autonomous secretion of aldosterone from one or both adrenal glands, resulting in clinical signs relating to hypertension or hypokalemia or both.* About one half of cats with primary hyperaldosteronism have unilateral aldosterone-secreting adrenal adenomas, and most of the remaining cats have unilateral adrenal carcinomas. Rarely, cats with Conn's syndrome develop bilateral adrenocortical tumors.[42] Finally, bilateral adrenal hyperplasia of the zona glomerulosa can also cause primary hyperaldosteronism in cats, but the prevalence of nontumorous disease is unclear.[22] Until recently, primary hyperaldosteronism in cats was considered a rare disease, but it is now becoming increasingly recognized as a cause of hypokalemia and hypertension in cats.

Clinical Features

Signalment

Primary hyperaldosteronism is a disease of the middle-aged to older cat. There does not appear to be any breed or sex predilection.[44]

Clinical Signs and Physical Examination Findings

The signs associated with hyperaldosteronism are due to sodium retention (which leads to hypertension) and potassium depletion (which leads to weakness). Historical findings are generally nonspecific and can include generalized weakness (sometimes episodic), lethargy, depression, stiffness, muscle pain, blindness, polyuria, and polydipsia.† Physical examination findings might include ventroflexion of the neck, hypertension, blindness, and retinal vessel tortuosity or retinal detachment.

The major clinical signs exhibited by the cat depend, in part, on whether primary hyperaldosteronism results from adrenal adenoma, carcinoma, or bilateral adrenocortical hyperplasia. Although the presenting clinical signs relate directly to the increased circulating aldosterone concentrations, they can be divided broadly into two general subgroups, which include hypokalemic polymyopathy and acute onset of blindness.

*References 1, 9, 12, 16, 22, 42, 44-46.

†References 1, 9, 12, 16, 22, 42, 44-46.

HYPOKALEMIC POLYMYOPATHY

Hypokalemic polymyopathy is the most common presentation for cats with primary hyperaldosteronism caused by adrenal adenoma or carcinoma.* These cats develop generalized muscle dysfunction, and owners may report cervical ventroflexion; hind limb weakness; ataxia; and, less commonly, limb stiffness or collapse. In some cats the muscular features are mild and episodic, whereas in others the signs are severe and acute in onset. This presentation is less common in the subgroup of cats with bilateral adrenal hyperplasia, with only about one quarter developing signs related to hypokalemia.[22]

ACUTE ONSET OF BLINDNESS

Although subclinical hypertension is common in cats with primary hyperaldosteronism caused by adrenal neoplasia, acute blindness secondary to intraocular hemorrhage or retinal detachment is relatively rare in that subgroup of cats. In contrast, hypertensive retinopathy appears to be the most common presenting sign in cats with primary hyperaldosteronism associated with bilateral adrenal hyperplasia. More than one half of cats with bilateral adrenocortical hyperplasia present with retinal detachment or subretinal, intraretinal, and intravitreal hemorrhages associated with severe systemic hypertension.[22]

Routine Laboratory Findings

No specific hematologic abnormalities have been identified in cats with primary hyperaldosteronism. Serum chemistry analysis commonly reveals hypokalemia but its severity is variable. However, because hypokalemia develops in cats for many other reasons, most commonly renal disease, hyperaldosteronism is commonly overlooked as a differential by many veterinarians simply because they do not realize that the condition exists.

Most cats with primary hyperaldosteronism caused by adrenal neoplasia are examined because of clinical signs related to hypokalemia.† Persistence of hypokalemia despite supplementation with potassium should always prompt suspicion of the possibility of hyperaldosteronism in cats.

Although hypokalemia is common in cats with primary hyperaldosteronism, the finding of a normal potassium concentration in a cat with documented hypertension should never exclude the possibility of primary hyperaldosteronism. In fact, in the reported cats with bilateral adrenal hyperplasia, only one half were mildly hypokalemic at initial presentation, but most had

*References 1, 9, 12, 16, 42, 44-46.

†References 1, 9, 12, 16, 42, 44-46.

severe hypertension.[22] The diagnosis of hyperaldosteronism in such cats would be missed if hypokalemia were considered to be a prerequisite before initiation of a diagnostic evaluation for hyperaldosteronism.

Despite the common finding of hypokalemia, serum sodium concentrations usually are normal. Hypernatremia, when present, is generally mild. The lack of marked hypernatremia in cats with primary hyperaldosteronism may be explained by concurrent volume expansion secondary to sodium retention.

High creatine kinase activity is common in cats with hypokalemic myopathy, but the degree of enzyme elevation is highly variable. A metabolic alkalosis may be observed, which is related to aldosterone-mediated urinary excretion of hydrogen ions. Serum urea nitrogen and creatinine may be slightly high at the time of diagnosis, and progression of renal disease may be the cause of death in some cats with primary hyperaldosteronism. The presence of azotemia may hinder the diagnosis in some cases because the presence of hypokalemia or hypertension may simply be considered a consequence of the renal disease itself.

In human beings progressive renal disease is a recognized sequela to Conn's syndrome, with renal damage occurring because of a combination of intraglomerular hypertension, inflammation, and renal fibrosis. This is also thought to occur in cats suffering from primary hyperaldosteronism as a result of bilateral adrenal hyperplasia, in which a progressively worsening azotemia is a common finding.[22]

Diagnostic Imaging

Adrenal masses are rarely visible radiographically. However, if an adrenal mass is seen on radiographs, it is more likely to be an adrenocortical carcinoma than an adenoma. Bilateral adrenocortical hyperplasia, of course, would never be detected on radiographic examination.

In most cats with primary hyperaldosteronism caused by adrenal neoplasia, abdominal ultrasonography is a valuable aid for confirming the presence of an adrenal mass (Figure 24-26). In these cats the contralateral adrenal gland should appear normal in size and shape. It is important that the contralateral gland be assessed to help differentiate a unilateral adrenal tumor from bilateral adrenal hyperplasia. Ultrasonography also should attempt to identify the presence and degree of invasion of the caudal vena cava by the tumor or related thrombus and the presence of metastases to other organs, such as the liver.

Diagnosis

Plasma Aldosterone Concentration

The possibility of primary hyperaldosteronism should be considered in any cat with a history of hypokalemia

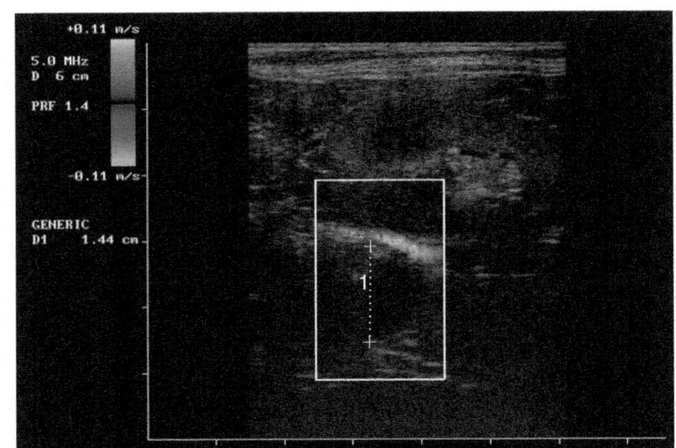

FIGURE 24-26 Ultrasonographic appearance of adrenal gland in a cat with hyperaldosteronism showing proximity of vasculature (shown with color Doppler). Hemorrhage is the major surgical risk associated with adrenalectomy, and ultrasonography can aid in assessing this risk.

or hypertension. Similarly, the finding of an "incidental" adrenal mass by ultrasound should prompt the veterinarian to rule out a functional aldosterone-secreting adrenal tumor.

Confirmation of diagnosis relies mainly on demonstrating a high plasma aldosterone concentration. The assay is widely available at most commercial endocrine laboratories, and requirements for collection and handling of serum or plasma are routine. There is no diagnostic benefit in measuring an ACTH-stimulated aldosterone value over a baseline concentration alone.

Most cats with primary hyperaldosteronism due to adrenal neoplasia have marked elevated circulating aldosterone concentrations.* However, in mild cases of primary hyperaldosteronism, and particularly in cats with bilateral adrenal hyperplasia, it is possible for plasma aldosterone values to be within the upper end of reference range.[22] Finally, there may be wide variation in circulating aldosterone concentrations in cats with secondary hyperaldosteronism, with some also developing very high values, so the results must always be assessed together with the clinical signs and laboratory findings.

Ideally, plasma aldosterone concentrations would be interpreted together with plasma renin activity (discussed later). Plasma renin would be expected to be high in cases of secondary hyperaldosteronism and suppressed in cats with primary hyperaldosteronism. However, there are difficulties in measuring plasma renin activity, and it is usually not possible to do so in a clinical situation.

As a consequence, the finding of an adrenal mass together with a markedly high plasma aldosterone concentration is considered sufficient to make a diagnosis

*References 1, 9, 12, 16, 42, 44-46.

of aldosterone-secreting adrenocortical tumor in cats. This is especially true if the cat has persistent hypokalemia or hypertension, or both. Normalization of the high circulating aldosterone concentrations after medical or surgical treatment helps confirm the diagnosis, as does histopathologic confirmation of adrenal neoplasia.

Primary hyperaldosteronism associated with bilateral adrenal hyperplasia is more difficult to diagnose without assessment of plasma renin activity. In these cats potential causes of secondary hyperaldosteronism must always be excluded with appropriate investigations, including evaluation for renal, liver, and cardiac disease. The fact that both cats with primary renal disease and cats with hyperaldosteronism associated with bilateral adrenal hyperplasia develop progressive azotemia is problematic. Without concurrent determination of both plasma aldosterone and plasma renin activity, it is difficult to differentiate these two groups of cats.

Plasma Renin Activity and the Aldosterone–Renin Ratio

Reliably distinguishing primary from secondary hyperaldosteronism requires assessment of activity of the entire renin–angiotensin system by measurement of plasma renin activity (PRA). This can be problematic, insofar as the plasma renin assay is not generally commercially available, and plasma samples must be processed quickly and kept frozen until assayed for renin activity. Furthermore, drugs (e.g., angiotensin-converting enzyme [ACE] inhibitors and beta blockers) and dietary salt intake also may influence PRA measurement.

PRA determinations in cats with primary hyperaldosteronism caused by adrenal neoplasia are usually low to undetectable but may be within the lower half of the reference range in some cats.[44] Therefore PRA alone cannot be used to diagnose primary hyperaldosteronism, inasmuch as a normal PRA value may be found in cats with primary hyperaldosteronism caused by either an adrenal tumor or bilateral adrenal hyperplasia.[22,44]

The ratio of plasma aldosterone concentration to PRA, known as the aldosterone–renin ratio, is regarded as the most reliable screening test, with a high aldosterone–renin ratio indicating primary hyperaldosteronism in cats. Even if the plasma aldosterone concentration is within reference range limits, a high aldosterone–renin ratio provides evidence for inappropriate (excessive) aldosterone secretion, diagnostic for primary hyperaldosteronism.[22] Cats with secondary hyperaldosteronism, in contrast, have a low aldosterone–renin ratio inasmuch as these cats would be expected to have high PRA values.

Mineralocorticoid Function Tests

In human medicine mineralocorticoid suppression tests are used as confirmatory tests for primary hyperaldosteronism. These suppression tests assess the response to treatments designed to suppress the renin–angiotensin system and thus decrease circulating concentrations of aldosterone. Examples of mineralocorticoid suppression tests include oral sodium loading, saline infusion, fludrocortisone administration with sodium supplementation, and the captopril challenge test.

Mineralocorticoid suppression tests have recently been developed and are being investigated for use in cats. A recent report assessed changes of the urinary aldosterone-to-creatinine ratio in normal cats in response to increased dietary salt or administration of fludrocortisone acetate.[13] In that study normal cats showed a more consistent decrease in the urinary aldosterone-to-creatinine ratio with administration of fludrocortisone acetate than with dietary salt supplementation. One cat with an aldosterone-secreting adrenal carcinoma had a high urinary aldosterone-to-creatinine ratio that did not decrease in response to fludrocortisone acetate administration.

Treatment

Initial treatment of primary hyperaldosteronism is directed at controlling hypokalemia, hypertension, or both. Medical treatment of hypokalemia includes parenteral or oral potassium supplementation, as well as correction of any fluid deficits and acid–base imbalances. For this purpose potassium gluconate is generally given at the dosage of 2 to 6 mEq per day, with the dose adjusted as necessary to maintain normokalemia.*

In cats with hypertension, amlodipine besylate (0.625 to 1.25 mg/cat daily) is the initial treatment of choice. Most hypertensive cats become normotensive with amlodipine treatment, but higher doses may be required and hypertension can become refractory to treatment.

If necessary, the diuretic spironolactone, which acts as an aldosterone receptor antagonist, can also be administered at the dosage of 2 to 4 mg/kg/day, assisting in the control of both hypokalemia and hypertension.†

Surgical adrenalectomy is the treatment of choice in most cats with hyperaldosteronism that do not have evidence of metastatic disease (see Figure 24-25). For cats with documented unilateral adrenal tumors, surgical adrenalectomy is recommended because it is potentially curative. However, the procedure has been associated with high mortality, with about one third of reported cases dying in the intraoperative or postoperative period as a result of severe acute hemorrhage. Because hyperaldosteronism does not suppress pituitary ACTH secretion, postoperative cortisol insufficiency after excision of unilateral aldosterone-secreting tumors in cats would not be expected to develop. However, it is possible that short-term mineralocorticoid replacement might be needed, especially if postoperative hyperkalemia develops.

*References 1, 9, 12, 16, 42, 44-46.

†References 1, 9, 12, 16, 22, 42, 44-46

Patients should be stabilized medically before surgery, and meticulous preoperative planning is required.[46] For those cats that have bilateral adrenal hyperplasia or metastatic disease or cats whose owners have declined surgery, medical management with oral spironolactone and potassium can be continued indefinitely.

HYPOADRENOCORTICISM

In cats, as in other species, hypoadrenocorticism results from deficient adrenocortical secretion of glucocorticoids, either alone or concurrent with reduced secretion of mineralocorticoids. Hypoadrenocorticism can be a naturally occurring disease or iatrogenic and is extremely rare in cats (especially the naturally occurring disorder). The first cat with primary hypoadrenocorticism was described approximately 30 years ago,[23] and since then fewer than 20 well-documented cases of naturally occurring adrenal insufficiency in cats have been reported.

Etiology and Pathophysiology

Primary hypoadrenocorticism results from primary adrenal failure, in which destruction of more than 85% to 90% of both adrenal cortices leads to deficient secretion of glucocorticoids and mineralocorticoids.

Secondary hypoadrenocorticism may result from deficient pituitary ACTH secretion, which leads to atrophy of the adrenal cortex and impaired glucocorticoid secretion. In cats with secondary hypoadrenocorticism, the zona glomerulosa is spared, so adequate mineralocorticoid secretion is maintained.

Primary Hypoadrenocorticism

The cause of the complete destruction or atrophy of both adrenal cortices in cats with naturally occurring primary hypoadrenocorticism is usually unknown (idiopathic atrophy). It is likely that many of these cats have immune-mediated destruction of the adrenal cortices, as in humans and dogs with this disease.[23,37] There are occasional reports of cats with primary hypoadrenocorticism thought to be subsequent to abdominal trauma and adrenal hemorrhage.[5,8] Primary hypoadrenocorticism has also been described secondary to bilateral adrenal gland infiltration by multicentric lymphoma in two cats.[35]

Iatrogenic primary hypoadrenocorticism is a rarely reported but well recognized complication of surgical treatment for pituitary-dependent hyperadrenocorticism (Cushing's disease) by bilateral adrenalectomy.[15]

Clinical signs in all cats with primary hypoadrenocorticism result from the deficiency of both glucocorticoids and mineralocorticoids. Because the primary insult is to the adrenal glands, pituitary production of ACTH continues unhindered. In fact, reduced cortisol production results in decreased negative feedback at the pituitary gland, allowing increased release of ACTH. Therefore cats with primary hypoadrenocorticism usually have greatly increased circulating concentrations of ACTH.[5,37,52]

Secondary Hypoadrenocorticism

Secondary hypoadrenocorticism arises from either (1) an underlying hypothalamic pituitary disorder (such as a pituitary or hypothalamic tumor) resulting in deficient ACTH production or (2) administration of drugs that suppress pituitary ACTH production.[14,31,41] Secondary hypoadrenocorticism has not yet been recognized as a naturally occurring disorder in cats but is likely to develop in some cats with large pituitary tumors.

Iatrogenic hypoadrenocorticism caused by chronic administration of either glucocorticoids or progestagens is the most common type of secondary adrenocortical failure encountered in cats.[14,31,36,41] Although hypophysectomy is an uncommon procedure to treat pituitary-dependent hyperadrenocorticism in cats, iatrogenic secondary hypoadrenocorticism is well recognized as a complication of this procedure.[28]

Deficient ACTH secretion results in a decrease in glucocorticoid production caused by atrophy of the zona fasciculata and zona reticularis. The adrenal zona glomerulosa is preserved because ACTH has little stimulatory effect on mineralocorticoid production. The clinical signs are due to deficiency in glucocorticoid production and so are similar to those observed in cats with primary hypoadrenocorticism. However, the derangements associated with mineralocorticoid deficiency (and subsequent electrolyte disturbances) are absent. Consequently, clinical signs observed are usually less severe than those that develop in cats with primary hypoadrenocorticism.

Clinical Features

Naturally occurring primary hypoadrenocorticism has been well documented in 18 cats.* Of these 18 cats, 14 had idiopathic atrophy of the adrenal cortex, two had traumatically induced hypoadrenocorticism, and two had adrenal lymphoma. The cats documented with idiopathic hypoadrenocorticism were of mixed breed, ranging in age from 1 to 14 years (median age, 4 years), and had no obvious sex predilection.

These 18 reported cats with primary hypoadrenocorticism had clinical signs and physical examination findings similar to those recognized in dogs with the disease. Lethargy, anorexia, and weight loss are the most common presenting signs (Table 24-11). Vomiting, polyuria, and polydipsia are less commonly reported. The clinical manifestations may wax and wane in some cases; this

*References 3, 5, 8, 23, 35, 37, 43, 52, 53.

TABLE 24-11 Clinical Features in 18 Cats with Primary Hypoadrenocorticism

Clinical Features	Number of Cats	% of Cats
HISTORICAL OWNER COMPLAINTS		
Lethargy or depression	18	100%
Anorexia	17	94%
Weight loss	14	78%
Vomiting	10	56%
Waxing and waning course	7	39%
Previous response to therapy	6	33%
Polyuria and polydipsia	5	28%
Dysphagia	1	6%
PHYSICAL EXAMINATION FINDINGS		
Depression	18	100%
Dehydration	16	89%
Weakness	14	78%
Hypothermia	12	67%
Slow capillary refill time	8	44%
Weak pulse	7	39%
Collapse/inability to rise	5	28%
Bradycardia	2	11%
Painful abdomen	1	6%
Constipation	1	6%

temporary remission usually occurs after parenteral fluid and corticosteroid administration.

The most common findings on physical examination are depression, dehydration, weakness, hypothermia, slow capillary refill time, and weak pulse. Collapse, bradycardia, and a painful abdomen are observed less frequently.

Diagnosis

Routine Clinicopathologic Features

HEMATOLOGY

The most noteworthy hematologic findings (if present) in cats with primary hypoadrenocorticism are eosinophilia or lymphocytosis; a mild normocytic, normochromic, nonregenerative anemia is also possible (Table 24-12). The finding of normal or high eosinophil and lymphocyte counts in a sick cat with signs suggestive of hypoadrenocorticism is clinically significant because the expected response to stress is eosinopenia and lymphopenia.

BIOCHEMISTRY

Hyponatremia, hypochloremia, and hyperkalemia are classical electrolyte changes associated with mineralocorticoid deficiency that occur in most cats with primary hypoadrenocorticism (see Table 24-12). Prerenal azotemia and hyperphosphatemia often result from extracellular fluid volume contraction (and subsequent decreased renal perfusion) associated with primary adrenocortical insufficiency (see Table 24-12).

However, most sick cats with altered serum electrolyte changes found on biochemical testing will *not* have primary hypoadrenocorticism. In one study of 49 sick cats with decreased sodium-to-potassium ratios, the final diagnoses included gastrointestinal disease, urinary disease, cardiorespiratory disease, and artefactually decreased Na : K ratios.[4] None of these 49 cats had a final diagnosis of hypoadrenocorticism.

TABLE 24-12 Diagnostic Features in 18 Cats with Primary Hypoadrenocorticism

Diagnostic Features	Number of Cats	% of Cats
HEMATOLOGY		
Anemia	5	28%
Lymphocytosis	4	22%
Eosinophilia	1	6%
BIOCHEMISTRY		
Sodium-to-potassium ratio less than 27:1	18	100%
Hyponatremia	18	100%
Hyperkalemia	17	94%
Azotemia	15	83%
Hyperphosphatemia	13	72%
Hypochloremia	13	72%
Low total CO_2 (metabolic acidosis)	4	22%
Hypercalcemia	3	17%
URINALYSIS		
Specific gravity less than 1.030	10/15	75%
Specific gravity greater than 1.030	5/15	25%
PITUITARY ADRENAL FUNCTION TESTS		
Low basal serum cortisol	17	94%
Subnormal ACTH-stimulated cortisol	17/17	100%
High endogenous ACTH concentration	10/10	100%

ACTH, Adrenocorticotropic hormone.

URINALYSIS

Pretreatment USG varies, but urine may be more dilute than would be expected in a cat with prerenal azotemia. Care must be taken not to misdiagnose primary renal failure in these cases (see Table 24-12). The cause of this apparent loss of renal concentrating ability is poorly understood but may be secondary to renal sodium loss resulting in medullary washout.

Radiography and Electrocardiography

Radiography demonstrated hypoperfusion of the lungs and microcardia in approximately one half of the cats described with primary hypoadrenocorticism.[3,37,43,52,53] Electrocardiography revealed sinus bradycardia in 2 of 18 cats, and atrial premature contractions in one.[37] Interestingly, no cats with primary hypoadrenocorticism showed the other electrocardiographic changes commonly associated with hyperkalemia in dogs and humans, such as peaking of the T wave, reduced or absent P wave, or atrial standstill.

Pituitary Adrenal Function Tests

ADRENOCORTICOTROPIC HORMONE RESPONSE TEST

The ACTH response test is the most accurate screening test for hypoadrenocorticism in cats. Low basal serum cortisol concentration with a subnormal or negligible response to ACTH is diagnostic for adrenocortical insufficiency but does not differentiate between primary and secondary causes of hypoadrenocorticism. It is imperative to compare test results to reference interval values obtained in healthy cats because cats tend to respond to ACTH with a smaller rise in peak serum cortisol concentrations than dogs.[14,40]

One common protocol for ACTH response testing in cats is to collect blood for determination of circulating cortisol concentration before and 60 minutes after intravenous administration of 0.125 mg synthetic ACTH (tetracosactide or cosyntropin).[38,40] It is important to administer ACTH intravenously, especially if the cat is dehydrated. In addition, findings in healthy cats indicate that ACTH given by the intravenous route induces a greater and more prolonged adrenocortical stimulation than does intramuscular administration.[38]

Many glucocorticoid preparations, including hydrocortisone and prednisolone or prednisone, cross-react in most cortisol assays to give a falsely elevated endogenous cortisol determination and therefore should not be administered until the ACTH response test is completed. Dexamethasone, on the other hand, can be administered before the ACTH response test because it has little or no influence on the measurement of endogenous cortisol concentrations.

A subnormal serum cortisol response to ACTH administration accompanied by serum electrolyte findings of hyperkalemia and hyponatremia is consistent with primary hypoadrenocorticism. If serum electrolytes changes are not found, one of the following may be present:

- Early primary hypoadrenocorticism with at least some residual mineralocorticoid secretion
- Secondary hypoadrenocorticism resulting from pituitary or hypothalamic disease
- Most commonly, secondary hypoadrenocorticism resulting from the administration of drugs such as glucocorticoids or progestagens[14,31,36,41]

ENDOGENOUS ADRENOCORTICOTROPIC HORMONE CONCENTRATION

Steroid or progestagen administration (or any other iatrogenic cause of hypoadrenocorticism) should first be excluded; then circulating ACTH concentration should be determined to help distinguish between primary and secondary hypoadrenocorticism. Extremely high plasma ACTH concentrations are found in cats with primary hypoadrenocorticism,[5,37,52] whereas cats with secondary hypoadrenocorticism have inappropriately low plasma ACTH concentrations when compared with circulating cortisol concentrations.[14,41] Samples for plasma ACTH determination must be collected before treatment with glucocorticoids because these drugs will suppress pituitary ACTH secretion and may therefore result in false normal or low plasma ACTH concentrations in cats with primary hypoadrenocorticism. Special handling is required for blood samples intended for determination of endogenous ACTH concentration because ACTH can degrade rapidly after collection. Mishandling of samples potentially results in falsely decreased values, which could erroneously suggest secondary rather than primary hypoadrenocorticism. Ideally, the veterinarian should speak to laboratory personnel before sampling to be sure to meet the laboratory's requirements.

Treatment

Initial Treatment

In cats with acute or life-threatening primary adrenal failure, initial therapy should be aimed at (1) restoring the circulating blood volume; (2) providing an immediate source of glucocorticoid; and (3) correcting serum electrolyte disturbances (i.e., hyperkalemia, hyponatremia).

FLUID THERAPY

An indwelling intravenous catheter should be placed, preferably in the jugular vein, to allow for the administration of large volumes of isotonic fluids. 0.9% saline is the intravenous fluid of choice and should be administered at 40 to 60 mL/kg per hour during the first 1 to 3 hours. The rate of administration may be slowed before the total bolus has been given if the cat begins to improve. The end point of resuscitation is an improvement in tissue perfusion, clinically recognized by an improvement in mucous membrane color, better-quality pulses, a decrease in the heart rate toward normal, and improved mentation.

Once fluid deficits are restored, the rate of fluid administration should be decreased to maintenance rates of 2.5 mL/kg per hour (60 mL/kg per day), given by constant-rate infusion. Fluid administration is further tapered when azotemia resolves, serum electrolyte abnormalities are corrected, and the cat is eating and drinking on its own.

GLUCOCORTICOID THERAPY

Rapid intravenous administration of a glucocorticoid is also extremely important in the initial management of severe adrenocortical insufficiency. Dexamethasone, administered at a dose of 0.5 mg/kg intravenously, is adequate in most cases and will not interfere with concurrent ACTH response testing. Hydrocortisone can be administered (as an alternative) at a dose of 5 to 10 mg/kg intravenously every 6 hours or by constant-rate infusion (0.5 to 0.625 mg/kg per hour) for the first 24 hours. These doses are based on studies in dogs because no feline specific dosages have been evaluated. If hydrocortisone is used as initial glucocorticoid therapy, it should not be administered until the ACTH response test has been completed.

Once the ACTH response test has been completed and the cat is stable, glucocorticoid replacement should then be continued as prednisolone at 0.2 mg/kg per day intramuscularly. Transferring to oral administration of the same daily glucocorticoid dosage can be instituted once the cat can swallow without vomiting. In cats use of prednisolone is preferred over the prodrug prednisone, which must be converted to prednisolone to be metabolically active. In one study of cats, only 21% of orally administered prednisone was absorbed and converted to prednisolone in the circulation.[19]

MINERALOCORTICOID THERAPY

Mineralocorticoid replacement therapy should also be started once the cat is stabilized and can swallow without vomiting; fludrocortisone acetate is administered orally at 0.1 mg/cat per day.[14,37,41,43] Desoxycorticosterone pivalate (DOCP) is a mineralocorticoid that also works well in most cats when administered intramuscularly at an initial dosage of 12.5 mg/cat monthly,[14,37,41,43] although this is not available in most countries other than the United States. The mineralocorticoid effects of either fludrocortisone acetate or DOCP enhance renal potassium excretion and sodium resorption, thereby normalizing serum electrolyte abnormalities.

Signs of weakness, lethargy, and anorexia may persist for 3 to 5 days in cats with acute adrenocortical insufficiency, despite appropriate management. This is in direct contrast to dogs, in which the major clinical signs of primary hypoadrenocorticism usually resolve rapidly within a day or two of treatments.[37,53]

Long-Term Treatment and Prognosis

Once stabilized, maintenance therapy for cats with primary adrenocortical insufficiency consists of lifelong mineralocorticoid and glucocorticoid supplementation. With appropriate replacement therapy, the long-term prognosis of cats with primary (especially idiopathic) hypoadrenocorticism is excellent.

Chronic mineralocorticoid therapy can be either fludrocortisone acetate given orally or injections of DOCP given intramuscularly.* The dosage is adjusted as needed, on the basis of serial serum electrolyte concentrations determined every 1 to 2 weeks during the initial maintenance period. The treatment goal with mineralocorticoid supplementation is normalization of the serum sodium and potassium concentrations.

Glucocorticoid replacement, as needed, is usually accomplished with oral administration of prednisolone, at a total dosage of 1 to 1.25 mg daily. If owners find it difficult to administer oral medication, repositol methylprednisolone acetate can be given intramuscularly, at a total dosage of 10 mg monthly. Adverse effects associated with iatrogenic hyperadrenocorticism (i.e., polyuria, polydipsia, polyphagia, pendulous abdomen, hair loss) rarely, if ever, develop in cats at these low replacement glucocorticoid doses.

References

1. Ash RA, Harvey AM, Tasker S: Primary hyperaldosteronism in the cat: a series of 13 cases, *J Feline Med Surg* 7:173, 2005.
2. Bailey DB, Page RL: Tumors of the endocrine system. In Withrow SJ, Vail DM, editors: *Withrow & MacEwen's small animal clinical oncology*, ed 4, St Louis, 2007, Saunders Elsevier, p 583.
3. Ballmer-Rusca E: [What is your diagnosis? Hypoadrenocorticism in a domestic cat], *Schweiz Arch Tierheilkd* 137:65, 1995.
4. Bell R, Mellor DJ, Ramsey I et al: Decreased sodium:potassium ratios in cats: 49 cases, *Vet Clin Pathol* 34:110, 2005.
5. Berger SL, Reed JR: Traumatically induced hypoadrenocorticism in a cat, *J Am Anim Hosp Assoc Assoc* 29:337, 1993.
6. Boag AK, Neiger R, Church DB: Trilostane treatment of bilateral adrenal enlargement and excessive sex steroid hormone production in a cat, *J Small Anim Pract* 45:263, 2004.
7. Boord M, Griffin C: Progesterone secreting adrenal mass in a cat with clinical signs of hyperadrenocorticism, *J Am Vet Med Assoc* 214:666, 1999.
8. Brain PH: Trauma-induced hypoadrenocorticism in a cat, *Aust Vet Pract* 27:178, 1997.
9. Briscoe K, Barrs VR, Foster DF et al: Hyperaldosteronism and hyperprogesteronism in a cat, *J Feline Med Surg* 11:758, 2009.
10. Daley CA, Zerbe CA, Schick RO et al: Use of metyrapone to treat pituitary-dependent hyperadrenocorticism in a cat with large cutaneous wounds, *J Am Vet Med Assoc* 202:956, 1993.
11. de Lange MS, Galac S, Trip MR et al: High urinary corticoid/creatinine ratios in cats with hyperthyroidism, *J Vet Intern Med* 18:152, 2004.
12. DeClue AE, Breshears LA, Pardo ID et al: Hyperaldosteronism and hyperprogesteronism in a cat with an adrenal cortical carcinoma, *J Vet Intern Med* 19:355, 2005.
13. Djajadiningrat-Laanen SC, Galac S, Cammelbeeck SE et al: Urinary aldosterone to creatinine ratio in cats before and after suppression with salt or fludrocortisone acetate, *J Vet Intern Med* 22:1283, 2008.
14. Duesberg C, Peterson ME: Adrenal disorders in cats, *Vet Clin North Am Small Anim Pract* 27:321, 1997.
15. Duesberg CA, Nelson RW, Feldman EC et al: Adrenalectomy for treatment of hyperadrenocorticism in cats: 10 cases (1988-1992), *J Am Vet Med Assoc* 207:1066, 1995.

*References 5, 14, 37, 41, 43, 52, 53.

16. Eger CE, Robinson WF, Huxtable CRR: Primary aldosteronism (Conn's syndrome) in a cat; a case report and review of comparative aspects, *J Small Anim Pract* 24:293, 1983.
17. Feldman EC, Nelson RW: Hyperadrenocorticism in cats (Cushing's syndrome). In Feldman EC, Nelson RW, editors: *Canine and feline endocrinology and reproduction*, Philadelphia, 2004, Elsevier, p 358.
18. Goossens MM, Meyer HP, Voorhout G et al: Urinary excretion of glucocorticoids in the diagnosis of hyperadrenocorticism in cats, *Domest Anim Endocrinol* 12:355, 1995.
19. Graham-Mize CA, Rosser EJ, Hauptman J: Absorption, bioavailability, and activity of prednisone and prednisolone in cats. In Hiller A, Foster AP, Kwochka KW, editors: *Advances in veterinary dermatology*, Oxford, 2005, Blackwell, p 152.
20. Henry CJ, Clark TP, Young DW et al: Urine cortisol:creatinine ratio in healthy and sick cats, *J Vet Intern Med* 10:123, 1996.
21. Hoenig M: Feline hyperadrenocorticism—where are we now? *J Feline Med Surg* 4:171, 2002.
22. Javadi S, Djajadiningrat-Laanen SC, Kooistra HS et al: Primary hyperaldosteronism, a mediator of progressive renal disease in cats, *Domest Anim Endocrinol* 28:85, 2005.
23. Johnessee JS, Peterson ME, Gilbertson SR: Primary hypoadrenocorticism in a cat, *J Am Vet Med Assoc* 183:881, 1983.
24. Kley S, Alt M, Zimmer C et al: Evaluation of the low-dose dexamethasone suppression test and ultrasonographic measurements of the adrenal glands in cats with diabetes mellitus, *Schweiz Arch Tierheilkd* 149:493, 2007.
25. Lien YH, Huang HP, Chang PH: Iatrogenic hyperadrenocorticism in 12 cats, *J Am Anim Hosp Assoc* 42:414, 2006.
26. Lowe AD, Campbell KL, Barger A et al: Clinical, clinicopathological and histological changes observed in 14 cats treated with glucocorticoids, *Vet Rec* 162:777, 2008.
27. Mayer MN, Greco DS, LaRue SM: Outcomes of pituitary tumor irradiation in cats, *J Vet Intern Med* 20:1151, 2006.
28. Meij BP: Hypophysectomy as a treatment for canine and feline Cushing's disease, *Vet Clin North Am Small Anim Pract* 31:1015, 2001.
29. Meij BP, van der Vlugt-Meijer RH, van den Ingh TS et al: Melanotroph pituitary adenoma in a cat with diabetes mellitus, *Vet Pathol* 42:92, 2005.
30. Meij BP, Voorhout G, Van Den Ingh TS et al: Transsphenoidal hypophysectomy for treatment of pituitary-dependent hyperadrenocorticism in 7 cats, *Vet Surg* 30:72, 2001.
31. Middleton DJ, Watson AD, Howe CJ et al: Suppression of cortisol responses to exogenous adrenocorticotrophic hormone, and the occurrence of side effects attributable to glucocorticoid excess, in cats during therapy with megestrol acetate and prednisolone, *Can J Vet Res* 51:60, 1987.
32. Millard RP, Pickens EH, Wells KL: Excessive production of sex hormones in a cat with an adrenocortical tumor, *J Am Vet Med Assoc* 234:505, 2009.
33. Moore LE, Biller DS, Olsen DE: Hyperadrenocorticism treated with metyrapone followed by bilateral adrenalectomy in a cat, *J Am Vet Med Assoc* 217:691, 2000.
34. Neiger R, Witt AL, Noble A et al: Trilostane therapy for treatment of pituitary-dependent hyperadrenocorticism in 5 cats, *J Vet Intern Med* 18:160, 2004.
35. Parnell NK, Powell LL, Hohenhaus AE et al: Hypoadrenocorticism as the primary manifestation of lymphoma in two cats, *J Am Vet Med Assoc* 214:1208, 1999.
36. Peterson ME: Effects of megestrol acetate on glucose tolerance and growth hormone secretion in the cat, *Res Vet Sci* 42:354, 1987.
37. Peterson ME, Greco DS, Orth DN: Primary hypoadrenocorticism in ten cats, *J Vet Intern Med* 3:55, 1989.
38. Peterson ME, Kemppainen RJ: Comparison of intravenous and intramuscular routes of administering cosyntropin for corticotropin stimulation testing in cats, *Am J Vet Res* 53:1392, 1992.
39. Peterson ME, Kemppainen RJ: Dose-response relation between plasma concentrations of corticotropin and cortisol after administration of incremental doses of cosyntropin for corticotropin stimulation testing in cats, *Am J Vet Res* 54:300, 1993.
40. Peterson ME, Kemppainen RJ, Orth DN: Plasma concentrations of immunoreactive proopiomelanocortin peptides and cortisol in clinically normal cats, *Am J Vet Res* 55:295, 1994.
41. Peterson ME, Randolph JF, Mooney CT: Endocrine diseases. In Sherding RG, editor: *The cat: diseases and clinical management*, ed 2, New York, 1994, Churchill Livingstone, p 1403.
42. Quante S, Sieber-Ruckstuhl N, Wilhelm S et al: [Hyperprogesteronism due to bilateral adrenal carcinomas in a cat with diabetes mellitus], *Schweiz Arch Tierheilkd* 151:437, 2009.
43. Redden B: Feline hypoadrenocorticism, *Compend Contin Educ Pract Vet* 27(9):697, 2005.
44. Refsal KR, Harvey AM: Primary hyperaldosteronism. In August JR, editor: *Consultations in feline internal medicine*, ed 6, St Louis, 2010, Saunders Elsevier, p 254.
45. Rijnberk A, Voorhout G, Kooistra HS et al: Hyperaldosteronism in a cat with metastasised adrenocortical tumour, *Vet Q* 23:38, 2001.
46. Rose SA, Kyles AE, Labelle P et al: Adrenalectomy and caval thrombectomy in a cat with primary hyperaldosteronism, *J Am Anim Hosp Assoc* 43:209, 2007.
47. Rossmeisl JH, Jr., Scott-Moncrieff JC, Siems J et al: Hyperadrenocorticism and hyperprogesteronemia in a cat with an adrenocortical adenocarcinoma, *J Am Anim Hosp Assoc* 36:512, 2000.
48. Schoeman JP, Evans HJ, Childs D et al: Cortisol response to two different doses of intravenous synthetic ACTH (tetracosactrin) in overweight cats, *J Small Anim Pract* 41:552, 2000.
49. Schwedes CS: Mitotane (o,p′-DDD) treatment in a cat with hyperadrenocorticism, *J Small Anim Pract* 38:520, 1997.
50. Sellon RK, Fidel J, Houston R et al: Linear-accelerator-based modified radiosurgical treatment of pituitary tumors in cats: 11 cases (1997-2008), *J Vet Intern Med* 23:1038, 2009.
51. Skelly BJ, Petrus D, Nicholls PK: Use of trilostane for the treatment of pituitary-dependent hyperadrenocorticism in a cat, *J Small Anim Pract* 44:269, 2003.
52. Stonehewer J, Tasker S: Hypoadrenocorticism in a cat, *J Small Anim Pract* 42:186, 2001.
53. Tasker S, MacKay AD, Sparkes AH: A case of feline primary hypoadrenocorticism, *J Feline Med Surg* 1:257, 1999.
54. Watson PJ, Herrtage ME: Hyperadrenocorticism in six cats, *J Small Anim Pract* 39:175, 1998.
55. Wimpole JA, Adagra CFM, Billson MF et al: Plasma free metanephrines in healthy cats, cats with non-adrenal disease and a cat with suspected phaeochromocytoma, *J Feline Med Surg* 12:435, 2010.
56. Zerbe CA, Refsal KR, Peterson ME et al: Effect of nonadrenal illness on adrenal function in the cat, *Am J Vet Res* 48:451, 1987.
57. Zimmer C, Horauf A, Reusch C: Ultrasonographic examination of the adrenal gland and evaluation of the hypophyseal-adrenal axis in 20 cats, *J Small Anim Pract* 41:156, 2000.

PITUITARY DISORDERS

Mark E. Peterson

Disorders of the pituitary gland are rare in the cat. The pituitary disorders that are reported to occur in cats are primarily related to neoplasia (almost exclusively adenomas) of the pars distalis or pars intermedia.[17,33,70,102] Only one case of a pituitary tumor arising from the pars nervosa (pituicytoma) has been reported.[101] Many pituitary tumors appear to be nonfunctional and are incidental findings at necropsy.[17,70] Occasionally, clinical signs related to central nervous system dysfunction and hypopituitarism are observed because of the compressive nature of a large pituitary tumor.[32,91,101,102] With functional pituitary tumors, clinical disorders that have been reported are limited to those diseases related to increased production of ACTH or GH (i.e., Cushing's disease and acromegaly).[6,66,67,74,76]

DI, most commonly caused by deficient vasopressin (ADH) secretion from the pars nervosa, is a rare disorder in the cat, with fewer than 20 cases reported.*

ANATOMY AND PHYSIOLOGY

The feline pituitary gland (hypophysis) is a small, whitish, ovoid body (weighing approximately 35 mg in the adult) that lies at the base of the brain in the sella turcica, a concavity of the sphenoid bone.[25,44,87] Unfortunately, a most confusing terminology has arisen in connection with this gland. The pituitary gland is of dual epithelial and neural origin, with the adenohypophysis (which originates embryologically from an invagination of the buccal cavity) consisting of the pars distalis, pars tuberalis, and pars intermedia and the neurohypophysis (pars nervosa) originating as a direct ventral extension of the diencephalon.[12,20,25] The pituitary can be divided grossly into two parts, usually referred to as the *anterior and posterior lobes,* which are separated by the hypophyseal cleft. On this basis the anterior lobe consists of the pars distalis, whereas the posterior lobe would consist of the pars nervosa and the small strip of cells lying between the pars nervosa and the hypophyseal cleft, the pars intermedia. However, the terms *anterior* and *posterior,* based on the anatomy of the human pituitary, are not totally applicable for the cat, because the feline pars distalis almost completely surrounds the pars nervosa (unlike in humans) and the feline pars nervosa actually lies dorsal, as well as posterior, to the pars distalis.[12,20,25]

Of all the endocrine glands, the pituitary, affectionately referred to as the *master gland,* is probably the most complex, with many different cell types involved in the secretion and control of a wide variety of trophic hormones. The hormones secreted by the pars distalis include TSH; ACTH or corticotrophin and related hormones (e.g., lipotropins, endorphins); GH; and the gonadotrophic hormones, follicle-stimulating hormone (FSH) and luteinizing hormone (LH).[20,76] The pars intermedia is also involved in the secretion of ACTH, endorphins, and melanocyte-stimulating hormones (e.g., alpha-MSH).[20,73,75,76]

The pars nervosa is probably best noted for its function as a storage depot for arginine vasopressin (AVP, also called *ADH*) and oxytocin. Both vasopressin and oxytocin are produced in cell bodies of the supraoptic, paraventricular, and several accessory nuclei of the hypothalamus. The peptides are then transported along the axons of the hypothalamo-neurohypophyseal nerve tract and stored in nerve terminals of the pars nervosa in granules until secreted into the circulation.[20,84]

*References 4, 14-16, 23, 36, 43, 49, 56, 58, 81, 86, 94, 99.

DISEASES OF THE PITUITARY GLAND

Pituitary Dwarfism

Congenital GH deficiency (pituitary dwarfism), which occurs in dogs secondary to cystic distention of the craniopharyngeal duct, has not been well documented in the cat. Most dwarf cats have either congenital hypothyroidism (see the section on Thyroid Gland Disorders) or mucopolysaccharidosis.[24,35,48,89] One hypothyroid kitten with dwarfism[82] was found to have low circulating levels of insulin-like growth factor-1 (IGF-1) levels, a peptide hormone produced by the liver after GH stimulation. However, primary GH deficiency has yet to be documented in cats.

Pituitary Macrotumors

Cats with large pituitary tumors may develop signs related to central nervous system dysfunction alone (inactive pituitary tumors) or associated with secretion of the pituitary hormones (Cushing's or acromegaly). Clinical signs that may develop in cats with large invasive pituitary tumors include marked lethargy, weakness, personality change, incoordination, and blindness.[17,32,91,96]

Because of the large size of these pituitary tumors at the time of diagnosis, surgical removal is generally not feasible.[51,52,55] Radiation therapy may effectively reduce tumor size and help control neurologic signs in cats with large pituitary tumors.[50,91]

Adrenocorticotropic Hormone–Secreting Pituitary Adenomas: Cushing's Disease

As in humans and dogs, hyperfunctioning ACTH-secreting adenomas of the feline pituitary corticotrophs have been reported to cause hyperadrenocorticism (Cushing's disease).* Such tumors may arise from either the pars intermedia or pars distalis corticotroph cells. As in dogs with intermediate lobe adenomas, pars intermedia tumors in the cat can secrete excessive concentrations of endorphins and alpha-MSH, in addition to ACTH.[73,76] See the section on Adrenal Gland Disorders, for more information.

Growth Hormone–Secreting Pituitary Tumors: Acromegaly

In cats, chronic hypersecretion of GH by a functional adenoma of the pituitary gland causes acromegaly, a

*References 17, 29, 32, 52, 54, 77, 102.

syndrome characterized by insulin-resistant DM and progressive overgrowth of soft tissue, membranous bone, and viscera.[30,38,74,76,78]

Published reports of acromegaly in cats are relatively sparse but have been gradually increasing since the disease was first described 30 years ago.* Although thought to be a rare disorder by most veterinarians, recent research suggests that the prevalence underlying acromegaly in cats with diabetes may actually be as high as 25% to 35%.[6,66] This strongly suggests that this disorder is greatly underdiagnosed by practicing veterinarians today.[80]

Once secreted by the pituitary, GH exerts its effects on the body through both direct and indirect actions.[21,57,60] The indirect actions of GH are mediated by IGF-1, a peptide hormone produced by the liver after GH stimulation. IGF-1 has anabolic effects and can induce increased protein synthesis and soft tissue and skeletal growth. By contrast, the direct effects of GH are predominantly catabolic and include lipolysis and restricted cellular glucose transport.

With time, acromegalic cats end up suffering from the catabolic and diabetogenic effects of GH; the anabolic effects of IGF-1; and, in some cases, the space-occupying effect of a pituitary macroadenoma.[38,67,78] Normally, GH is an important modulator of insulin sensitivity.[26] A GH-induced postreceptor defect in insulin action at the level of target tissues leads to concurrent DM, usually associated with severe insulin resistance.[29,38,67,74,76]

Cause of Acromegaly

In the cat, as in man, acromegaly is most often caused by a GH-secreting adenoma of the pituitary gland.† In addition, GH-producing hyperplasia of these cells has also been reported as a rare cause.[66,67] This latter process might represent a pre-adenomatous change or a separate disease process. Further, one cat with a double pituitary adenoma causing both acromegaly and hyperadrenocorticism has been reported.[55]

As in dogs, administration of progestogens to cats can induce expression of the mammary GH gene and thereby stimulate the local production of GH in mammary tissue.[59] Indeed, progestin-induced fibroadenomatous changes in the mammary gland of cats are also associated with locally enhanced GH expression. In cats this mammary gene is identical to the pituitary-expressed gene and is driven by the same promoter.[59] However, this local production of GH has never been shown to result in high circulating GH concentrations or the clinical state of acromegaly in cats.[67,72]

*References 1, 2, 6, 9, 13, 27-29, 34, 37, 46, 47, 53, 55, 61, 68, 74, 85, 93, 95.

†References 2, 27, 29, 34, 38, 46, 47, 55, 74.

Clinical Features of Acromegaly

The earliest clinical signs of feline acromegaly, present in almost all cats reported to date, include progressive polyuria, polydipsia, and polyphagia, all of which are associated with poorly controlled or insulin-resistant DM.* Additional clinical findings that may develop in these cats weeks to months after development of diabetes may include enlargement of one or more organs (i.e., heart, liver, kidneys, spleen, tongue), progressive increase in body size and weight, disproportionate enlargement and thickening of the head and paws, prognathia of the lower jaw, degenerative arthropathy, renal failure, congestive heart failure, and central nervous signs caused by enlargement of the pituitary tumor.

The clinical features of feline acromegaly, listed according to the signs that may develop as the disease progresses when left untreated, are presented in Box 24-3. At the time of diagnosis, many diabetic cats with acromegaly do not exhibit the "classic" physical changes associated with the disease, such as enlargement of the face and extremities.[38,66,67,74] This is one reason that this endocrine disorder has frequently gone undiagnosed or misdiagnosed as "routine" diabetes. It is important to consider acromegaly as a differential diagnosis in all cats with DM, especially if the cat is poorly controlled or develops moderate to severe insulin resistance.

SIGNALMENT

Acromegaly develops in middle-aged to older cats without obvious breed predilection. All reported cases of feline acromegaly have been mixed-breed cats (domestic shorthair). There is a strong male sex predilection, with approximately 90% of cats being male.[38,66,67,74] This is in contrast to humans, wherein acromegaly has no sex predilection, and in dogs, wherein females are affected most commonly.[30,78]

GENERAL APPEARANCE

In humans the earliest recognizable signs of acromegaly are soft tissue swelling and hypertrophy of the face and extremities.[19,57] Overt DM, although it does develop in up to half of human patients with acromegaly, is generally not the initial patient complaint.[7] Similarly, alterations in facial features and body dimensions are observed in some cats with acromegaly, generally at a later stage of the disease (see Box 24-3). GH-induced proliferation of connective tissue results in an increase in body size, most frequently manifested as marked weight gain and enlargement of the abdomen. The increases in body weight may occur despite the presence of the catabolic state of unregulated DM. As the disease progresses, growth and hypertrophy of all organs in the body (e.g., heart, liver, kidneys, tongue) is also a characteristic sign of acromegaly.

*References 1, 2, 6, 9, 13, 27-29, 34, 37, 46, 47, 53, 55, 61, 68, 74, 85, 93, 95.

BOX 24-3

Clinical Features of Cats with Untreated Acromegaly: Progression Over Time*

Initial Clinical Signs

Polyuria and polydipsia
Polyphagia
Diabetes mellitus
Physical appearance generally quite normal

Clinical Signs Noticed After a Few Weeks

Insulin resistance (increasing need for high doses of insulin)
Weight gain/increase in body size
Abdominal enlargement
Organomegaly (e.g., liver, kidneys, heart, tongue)

Clinical Signs That May Be Noticed After a Few Months

Systolic cardiac murmurs
Respiratory stridor
Lameness/degenerative arthropathies
Broad facial features
Prognathia inferior
Increase in paw size

Clinical Signs That May Develop After a Few Years

Renal failure
Congestive heart failure
Central nervous system signs

*Not all acromegalic cats will develop all these clinical features.

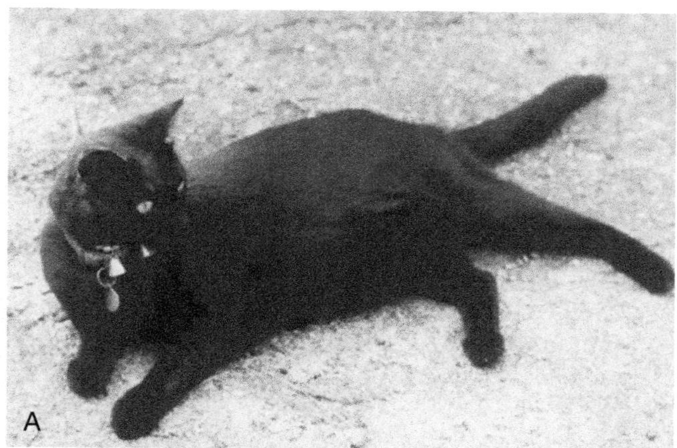

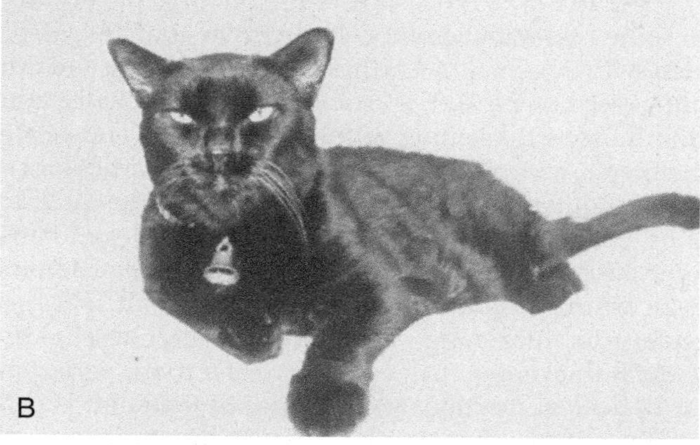

FIGURE 24-27 Photography of a 10-year-old male domestic shorthair before **(A)** and 3 years after **(B)** the diagnosis of insulin-resistant diabetes mellitus. Acromegaly was confirmed 9 months after the onset of the diabetic state. Notice the broad facial features, large head, and club paws development of acromegaly.

Cats with acromegaly may also develop mandibular enlargement resulting in prognathism, widened interdental spaces, thickening of the bony ridges of the skull, large head, large paws, and soft tissue swelling of the head and neck (see Box 24-3).[38,66,67,74] Obviously, not all acromegalic cats will develop all these conformational changes. However, because many of these changes develop and progress gradually, subtle conformational changes might not always be noticeable by owners who see their affected cat every day. Reviewing old photographs of the cat taken years earlier frequently helps determine whether changes in the cat's appearance have indeed occurred (Figure 24-27).

DIABETES MELLITUS

The earliest and most commonly recognized clinical manifestation of acromegaly in most cats is insulin-resistant DM (see Box 24-3). GH, especially in carnivores (and especially in cats and dogs), displays powerful diabetogenic activity and appears to provoke hyperglycemia mainly by inducing peripheral insulin resistance.[8,100] Excessive GH has been shown to decrease insulin receptor numbers, decrease receptor-binding affinity, and induce a postreceptor insulin defect similar to that observed with cortisol-induced insulin antagonism.[26,62]

Most cats with acromegaly exhibit severe, persistent hyperglycemia that is refractory to insulin therapy and can be controlled only with extremely large doses of exogenous insulin. In one recent study[66] the mean insulin requirements of 59 acromegalic diabetic cats (14 units daily; range, 2 to 70 units daily) were markedly higher than in a matched group of diabetic cats without acromegaly (6 units daily). Other cats have been reported in which even higher insulin dosages (up to 130 U daily) were needed to control hyperglycemia.[74] Despite the presence of such uncontrolled DM, the development of ketoacidosis is rare in cats with acromegaly.

Although polyphagia is a well-recognized clinical sign associated with uncontrolled DM, the excess GH itself is also likely to contribute. Some cats with acromegaly will have persistent, and often extreme, polyphagia, despite reasonable control of the DM.

RESPIRATORY SYSTEM

In cats with acromegaly, GH-induced soft tissue proliferation in the oropharyngeal region can lead to upper airway narrowing, resulting in clinical signs of respiratory disease. In accord with this, inspiratory stridor develops in about half of the cats with acromegaly (see Box 24-3).[66-68] Dyspnea may develop in cats with longstanding untreated acromegaly as a result of pulmonary edema or pleural effusion from GH-induced cardiac failure.[68,74,76]

SKELETAL SYSTEM

In some cats with acromegaly, articular changes (associated with degenerative arthritis) may be severe and crippling (see Box 24-3). The articular changes initially result from fibrous thickening of the joint capsule and related ligaments, as well as bony overgrowth and articular cartilage proliferation.[10,22] Later, as a result of the distorted joint architecture, features more typical of degenerative joint disease develop. Radiographic evidence of acromegalic arthropathy includes an increase in joint space secondary to thickening of the articular cartilage (early), cortical thickening, osteophyte proliferation, periarticular periosteal reaction, and collapse of the joint.[10,22,74,76]

Other bony changes that may occur in acromegaly include enlargement of the mandible, leading to prognathism and an overbite by the lower incisors. There also may be increased spacing between the teeth, as commonly occurs in acromegalic dogs.[78] The bones of the calvarium may be thickened (Figure 24-28), with apparent enlargement of the entire head in some cats. Finally, marked spondylosis deformans of the spine may be evident; this may lead to gait abnormalities such as chronic progressive stiffness and rigidity in some cats.[66,74]

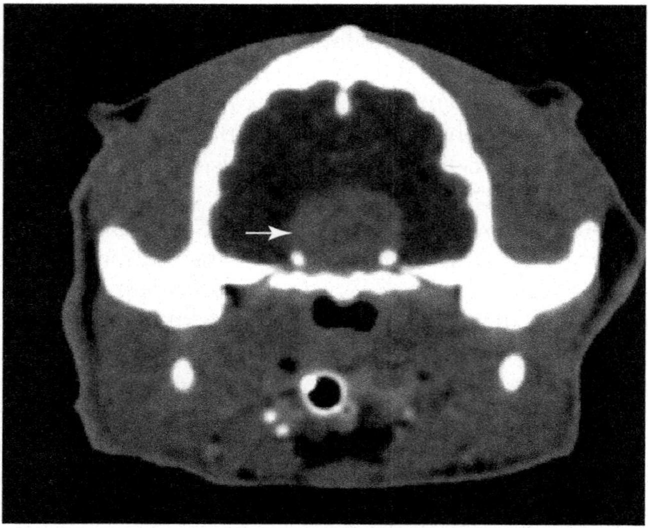

FIGURE 24-28 Computed tomography of the head of a 14-year-old male castrated domestic shorthair with acromegaly. Note the huge pituitary mass, measured at 7.5 mm in height, invading the hypothalamus. Also note the apparent calvarial hyperostosis (thickening of skull).

CARDIOVASCULAR SYSTEM

Another prominent manifestation of chronic acromegaly in some cats is cardiomyopathy. Cardiovascular abnormalities that may be detected on physical examination include the presence of a systolic murmur, gallop rhythm, and, especially late in the course of the disease, signs of congestive heart failure (e.g., dyspnea, muffled heart sounds, ascites) (see Box 24-3). Radiographic findings may include mild to severe cardiomegaly, pleural effusion, and pulmonary edema.[68,74,76] Echocardiography frequently reveals left ventricular and septal hypertrophy but can also be normal; electrocardiographic findings are generally unremarkable. The cause of cardiac disease in acromegaly is not clear but may be related to the general growth-promoting effect of excess GH on tissues.[88]

Hypertension is common in human patients with acromegaly[11,98] and may contribute to cardiac hypertrophy in cats.[38,68] However, in one large case series of acromegalic cats, hypertension was not any more prevalent than would be expected in a group of age-matched control cats.[66] Nevertheless, blood pressure should be determined in all cats with acromegaly, especially if cardiac disease is present, and that treatment is instituted as needed.

NERVOUS SYSTEM

In cats central nervous system signs can develop as a result of expansion of the pituitary tumor beyond the sella turcica. However, central nervous system signs are uncommon because the GH-secreting pituitary tumors tend to be both benign and slow growing, and overt neurologic signs are rare even when a large pituitary tumor is compressing and invading the hypothalamus (see Figure 24-28).[66,74,76] When neurologic signs do develop, they may include stupor, somnolence, and poor appetite.

RENAL SYSTEM

Polyuria and polydipsia are common signs of acromegaly in cats and appear to develop primarily because of the associated diabetic state. However, acromegaly also produces several other alterations in renal function. The kidneys may hypertrophy, and GFR and renal plasma flow may increase. The nephromegaly is also associated with an increase in both secretory and absorptive functions.[5,69] In cats with long-standing acromegaly, however, development of azotemia, proteinuria, and clinical signs of renal failure commonly develop (see Box 24-3). Histologically, the kidneys of acromegalic cats can show mesangial thickening of the glomeruli, changes similar to those described in human patients with diabetic nephropathy. Although the mechanism of impairment of renal function in feline acromegaly is not clear, it may result from the glomerulosclerosis associated with the unregulated DM or GH-mediated glomerular hyperfiltration.

Diagnosis of Acromegaly

Confirming a diagnosis of acromegaly can be difficult because of the disorder's insidious onset, the cost of pituitary imaging procedures, and the frequent lack of a readily available GH assay validated for use in cats.[30,38,67,76] As is the case in many feline endocrinopathies, a combination of suggestive clinical features and multiple diagnostic tests is generally required to make the definitive diagnosis of acromegaly (Box 24-4).

Acromegaly should be suspected in any cat that has severe insulin-resistant DM (persistent hyperglycemia despite daily insulin doses greater than 10 U daily), especially if other characteristic signs of acromegaly (especially arthopathy or cardiomyopathy) are also present. The diagnosis of acromegaly can be established by demonstrating markedly elevated circulating GH or IGF-1 concentrations, especially when combined with the finding of a pituitary mass with brain imaging (see Box 24-4).

ROUTINE LABORATORY TESTING

In addition to findings expected in a poorly controlled diabetic cat (e.g., hyperglycemia and glycosuria), clinicopathologic testing of an acromegalic cat may reveal high serum hepatic enzyme activities, hyperproteinemia, hyperphosphatemia, proteinuria, and mild erythrocytosis.[38,67,68,74]

Mild increases in the activities of serum ALT and ALP appear to develop secondary to the hepatic lipidosis associated with the GH-induced DM. Mild hyperphosphatemia appeared to be caused by a GH-induced increase in the renal tubular reabsorption of phosphate.[39,92] The mechanism of the hyperproteinemia (which is associated with a normal pattern of distribution on serum protein electrophoresis) is unclear but is relatively common, occurring in over half of cats.[66,74] Mild erythrocytosis, which also develops in some cats with acromegaly, probably represents another manifestation of the anabolic effects of excessive GH.

In the latter stages of the disease, routine laboratory tests may reveal high serum concentrations of urea nitrogen and creatinine, as the cat develops renal disease as a complication of the acromegalic state.[68,74]

SERUM GROWTH HORMONE CONCENTRATION

Ideally, the diagnosis of acromegaly is confirmed by demonstrating high serum GH concentrations, the primary hormone responsible for the disease. Overall, use of basal serum GH concentrations appears to be the most accurate diagnostic test for feline acromegaly. All cats with acromegaly thus far reported have had clearly high GH concentrations.* This is in contrast to the normal serum IGF-1 values occasionally reported in some cats with acromegaly (see the discussion later in this chapter on serum insulin-like growth factor-1 concentration).[68,85]

In a recent study a validated feline GH radioimmunoassay proved useful in distinguishing 19 clinically normal cats from 19 acromegalic cats, with no overlap occurring between the two groups.[65] In a separate study using the same feline GH assay, however, 2 out of 34 diabetic cats (without acromegaly) were wrongly classified as being acromegalic using the same diagnostic criteria. Nevertheless, the specificity and sensitivity of this assay were both high at 95% and 84%, respectively.[66]

Although many acromegalic cats have been diagnosed by demonstrating high serum or plasma GH concentrations, this test has never been widely available to the practicing veterinarian; the assay is performed in only a few specialized laboratories around the world. A GH radioimmunoassay validated for both dogs and cats has been available at Utrecht University, The Netherlands, for many years,[53,93] and a validated feline GH assay is now available at the Royal Veterinary College, University of London.[65] But even in the best of circumstances, it remains extremely inconvenient for most practicing veterinarians to ship frozen samples to Europe

*References 28, 34, 46, 65, 66, 74, 93.

BOX 24-4

Diagnosis of Acromegaly in Cats

Supportive Clinical Features

Insulin-resistant diabetes mellitus (daily insulin doses of >2 IU/kg)
Changes in physical appearance (larger head or paws)
Weight gain despite poorly controlled diabetes

Routine Laboratory Findings

Hyperglycemia and glucosuria
Lack of ketonuria
Hyperproteinemia

Specific Tests for Acromegaly

High serum or plasma growth hormone concentrations
High serum insulin-like growth factor-1 concentrations

Pituitary Imaging

Pituitary tumor on computed tomography or magnetic resonance imaging for serum GH analysis. The fact that most veterinarians do not have convenient access to a veterinary laboratory capable of measuring serum GH has greatly hindered the diagnostic evaluation of cats with suspected acromegaly.

Because of this lack of GH assays for cats, the diagnosis of feline acromegaly generally must be based on the characteristic clinical, laboratory, and imaging features (see Boxes 24-3 and 24-4) with demonstration of a high serum IGF-1 concentration alone (discussed in the next section).

SERUM INSULIN-LIKE GROWTH FACTOR-1 CONCENTRATION

In human medicine, determination of circulating concentrations of the polypeptide hormone IGF-1 is a very useful diagnostic test for acromegaly. The basis for use of IGF-1 as a diagnostic test for acromegaly is that circulating GH activates the hepatic and peripheral tissue production of IGF-1, which is responsible for many of the actions normally attributable to GH itself. In fact, other than DM, most of the clinical features of acromegaly are *not* the result of a direct catabolic effect of GH excess, but rather result from an indirect anabolic effect of GH excess mediated through the production of the IGF-1 (e.g., overgrowth of soft tissue, bony enlargement, and organomegaly).[57] Therefore circulating IGF-1 levels serve as a biomarker for assessing the peripheral biological effect of GH hypersecretion, which, at least in human patients, tends to correlate better with the severity of the acromegalic state than does random circulating GH determinations.

In cats with suspected acromegaly, use of IGF-1 measurements is also a very useful diagnostic test, with many studies now demonstrating that serum IGF-1 can differentiate cats with acromegaly from clinically normal cats.[2,6,66,68,85] For the practicing veterinarian, IGF-1 determinations are widely available and are performed by most commercial veterinary laboratories, in contrast to the limited availability of feline GH assays.

As with all diagnostic tests, however, the serum IGF-1 test is not a perfect test for acromegaly. An abnormally high serum IGF-1 concentration strongly suggests acromegaly, but the disease should not be excluded if values are within the high-normal range. Portal insulin is necessary for hepatic IGF-1 production, which means that in an acromegalic diabetic cat before or at the start of insulin therapy, IGF-1 can prove falsely low.[85] However with insulin treatment the IGF-1 level may well eventually increase into the acromegalic range with increasing portal insulin concentrations. In one study the sensitivity of IGF-1 as a diagnostic test for feline acromegaly was calculated to 0.84 (positive diagnostic test in 84% of the acromegalic cats tested)[6]; accordingly, that indicates that 16% of acromegalic cats would be expected to have single IGF-1 values that were within reference range limits (false-negative test result).

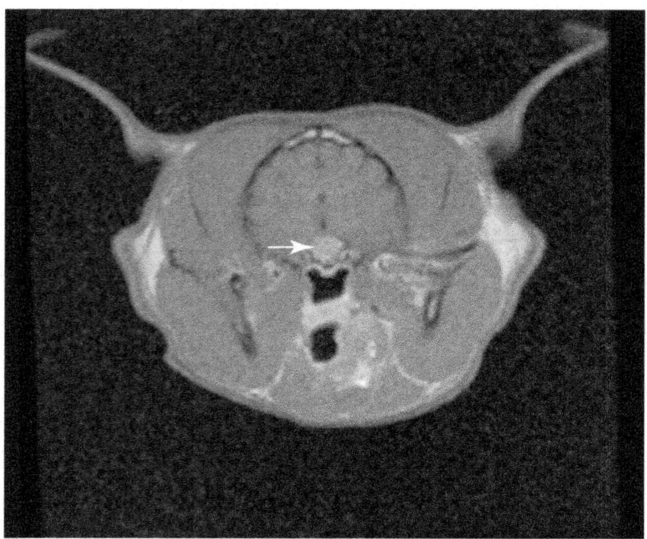

FIGURE 24-29 Magnetic resonance imaging of the brain of a 12-year-old male castrated domestic shorthair with acromegaly. Notice the obvious pituitary mass, measured at 1.9 mm in height.

In addition, high serum IGF-1 concentrations have recently been reported in diabetic cats *without* acromegaly, so false-positive test results can also occur.[45,95] In one study the test specificity of IGF-1 in cats without acromegaly was calculated to be 0.92 (normal test result in 92% of the nonacromegalic cats evaluated)[6]; accordingly, that indicates that 8% of cats without acromegaly would be expected to have a false-positive, high IGF-1 value.

PITUITARY IMAGING PROCEDURES

Documentation of a pituitary mass by CT) or MRI provides further support for the diagnosis (Figures 24-28 and 24-29). It appears that MRI may be a more sensitive diagnostic test for this condition.[29] However, although almost all cats with acromegaly have a clearly visible pituitary tumor on CT or MRI imaging, it should be remembered that normal intracranial imaging (no visible pituitary tumor) does preclude a diagnosis of feline acromegaly.[66,67]

In addition to documenting the presence of a pituitary tumor, determining the size and location of the tumor is helpful in establishing the mode of therapy (i.e., surgery, medical, radiotherapy) and monitoring the tumor response to therapy.[27,47,50,55,91]

Differential Diagnoses for Acromegaly

Any disease causing insulin-resistant diabetes should be considered a differential diagnosis for acromegaly, as should diabetes management issues that can lead one to suspect insulin resistance (e.g., lack of compliance, inappropriate insulin storage, and administration problems).

Hyperadrenocorticism, especially the pituitary-dependent form of the disease, is the major differential for acromegaly for many reasons. First of all, both acromegaly and hyperadrenocorticism commonly cause insulin-resistant DM.[76,90] Both disorders are caused by a hormone-secreting (ACTH or GH) pituitary tumor, and bilateral adrenal enlargement is common in both acromegaly and pituitary-dependent hyperadrenocorticism.[66,74]

Differentiating between the two disorders is sometimes difficult. However, looking at specific clinical signs for each disease is generally quite helpful in making the differentiation. For example, broad facial features, clubbed paws, arthropathy, and prognathia inferior should lead the veterinarian to suspect feline acromegaly, whereas truncal hair loss; pendulous abdomen; and thin, fragile, or tearing skin are associated with hyperadrenocorticism (see the section on Adrenal Gland Disorders). In addition, the insulin resistance associated with acromegaly is usually much more severe than that observed in cats with hyperadrenocorticism, as demonstrated by their much higher insulin requirements. Finally, dexamethasone suppression tests have generally proved useful in differentiating the two disorders because tests of the pituitary–adrenal axis generally remain normal in cats with acromegaly.[30,76]

Treatment of Acromegaly

In acromegalic cats three potential treatment options are available, including external radiation therapy, hypophysectomy, and medical therapy. Of these, radiotherapy is currently considered to be the most effective, although the response can vary in individual cats.

Conservative supportive treatment also represents a genuine alternative option, especially in cats for which definitive treatment is simply not possible (e.g., too costly). It is possible for an acromegalic cat to maintain a reasonable quality of life if it receives high (and generally increasing) daily doses of insulin to treat the insulin-resistant DM.

EXTERNAL RADIATION THERAPY

Currently, radiotherapy is considered by most to be the best treatment option for cats with acromegaly. Although earlier reports suggested that radiotherapy for cats with acromegaly offered only a limited or partial response, more recent studies indicate that most acromegalic cats respond favorably to external radiation therapy.[27,34,50,91] In cats that have a good to excellent response to radiotherapy, pituitary tumors generally decrease in size and high circulating concentrations of GH normalize. In such cats insulin resistance resolves and overall diabetic control improves; some cats may even go into diabetic remission.[27,34]

Despite the fact that external radiation therapy remains the most effective treatment for cats with acromegaly, this treatment modality has many disadvantages. The most important drawbacks to this treatment include the limited availability, the need for frequent hospital visits and multiple anesthetic procedures, and the high cost.[27,34,50,91] In addition, it is not uncommon for cats to relapse months to years after treatment, with recurrence of uncontrolled or insulin-resistant DM.[74]

The final outcome of radiotherapy is not always predictable. Not all cats will respond completely to radiotherapy, with some showing improvement of DM but persistence of other acromegalic signs. In many of these latter cats, serum GH normalizes but serum IGF-1 concentrations remain high (so-called GH–IGF-1 discordance).[65,67] This suggests that radiotherapy may decrease circulating GH concentration to levels such that diabetogenic effects are no longer present but not to a level required to normalize IGF-1 secretion and reverse its associated biological complications.[27,47,67] Because of this GH–IGF-1 discordance, use of serum GH concentrations alone are not recommended as a marker to judge cure of the acromegalic state after treatment.

SURGICAL THERAPY (HYPOPHYSECTOMY)

Hypophysectomy, the therapeutic modality of choice for human patients suffering from acromegaly, may also appear to be a logical choice for cats with GH-secreting tumors. In human patients, however, surgical cure is most likely to result if the pituitary tumor is small and noninvasive. Large, invasive pituitary tumors, similar to those identified in many cats with acromegaly, are only rarely cured by surgery.[19,57]

Experience with transsphenoidal hypophysectomy as a treatment for cats with acromegaly is very limited. It is a highly specialized procedure and is not likely to be available to many clinicians in the near future. This surgical procedure is also associated with relatively high morbidity and mortality rates.[52] However, in cats with small pituitary tumors, hypophysectomy can be curative.[55]

Cryohypophysectomy represents an alternative technique that was successful in treatment of two reported cats with acromegaly. However, this technique also requires further evaluation and longer-term follow-up before it can be strongly recommended.[2,3,9]

MEDICAL THERAPY

Compared with the situation in human patients, only limited information is available on medical treatment of cats with acromegaly. In human patients three types of medication are used in the treatment of acromegaly, all with variable degrees of success.[18,57]

First-line medical treatment for acromegaly included the use of the somatostatin analogs (e.g., octreotide and lanreotide). These analogs are synthetic forms of the hypothalamic hormone, somatostatin, which acts to inhibit GH production. These drugs improve symptoms and signs of acromegaly in the majority of human patients, with normalization of the serum GH and IGF-1 concentrations in 50% to 70%.[18,19,57]

Dopamine agonists (e.g., bromocriptine and selegiline) make up the second medication group. These drugs are not as effective as the other medications at lowering GH or IGF-I levels and also cause more adverse effects.

The third group of drugs for the medical treatment of acromegaly is the use of a GH receptor antagonist (pegvisomant). By blocking the action of the endogenous GH molecules, this compound is able to normalize IGF-I levels and control disease activity in virtually all patients.[18,19,57] The disadvantage of this form of medical therapy is that the drug is not directed at the pituitary tumor itself but at the peripheral GH receptor sites; therefore the pituitary tumor continues to grow, and the circulating GH concentrations remain high.

Although medical treatment for acromegaly would be a very attractive option for many cat owners, neither somatostatin analogs nor dopamine agonists have been successful in lowering serum GH concentrations or improving insulin sensitivity in cats with acromegaly.[1,61,74,76] A recent study did show an acute lowering of serum GH after intravenous octreotide administration, suggesting that perhaps a small subset of cats with acromegaly might be suited to treatment with somatostatin analogs.[93] However, a recent trial with lanreotide, a long-acting somatostatin analog, produced disappointing results in cats with acromegaly.[67] It may be that at least some GH-secreting pituitary adenomas of cats lack the somatostatin receptors possessing high affinity for the somatostatin analogs, thereby explaining the apparent lack of effect of these drugs in cats.

Pegvisomant has not yet been evaluated in cats with acromegaly; however, this drug would be expected to be effective only if there is sufficient homology between feline and human GH receptors. In addition, the drug must be given daily by subcutaneous injection and might be too costly for many cat owners.

Prognosis of Acromegaly

In cats with acromegaly, the severity of clinical signs and clinical course are related to the high circulating GH and IGF-1 concentrations, as well as the duration of the disease. The short-term prognosis for most cats with acromegaly is relatively good. Severe insulin-resistant DM can generally be satisfactorily controlled using large, divided doses of insulin. Mild to moderate cardiac disease responds well to diuretic therapy and ACE inhibitors (i.e., enalapril or benazepril), at least initially.

Definitive treatment with external radiation therapy or hypophysectomy improves long-term prognosis, but complete long-term cure of feline acromegaly is rare. Survival times of both aggressively and conservatively treated cats vary enormously, with some cats not surviving more than a few weeks beyond diagnosis and others living for many years (>5 years) and dying from causes likely unrelated to the disease. If left untreated, most cats eventually die or are euthanized because of the development of severe congestive heart failure, renal failure, respiratory distress, or the neurologic effects of an expanding pituitary tumor.

Diabetes Insipidus

DI is an uncommon condition characterized by marked polyuria and secondary polydipsia. The disorder may be classified as either neurogenic (central) or nephrogenic in origin. Central DI results from a complete or partial failure of the neurohypophysis to secrete vasopressin (also called *ADH*), whereas nephrogenic DI is related to a lack of renal responsiveness to the antidiuretic actions of vasopressin.[31,79]

Cause of Diabetes Insipidus in Cats

DI is an extremely rare disorder in cats, with only 18 reported cases.* All cats have had central DI; a primary nephrogenic form of DI (congenital DI) has not yet been described in cats. As in dogs, cats can develop either partial or complete forms of central DI.[58,86,94]

In most cats the exact cause of the disorder cannot be determined (idiopathic DI) but is thought to be a congenital defect in vasopressin secretion. Head trauma, however, is a relatively common identifiable cause of DI in cats, with about a third of the reported cases having such a history.[4,16,56,86,94] Other less common causes of DI in cats include pituitary macrotumors[31] or pituitary malformation.[99]

Clinical Features of Diabetes Insipidus

All 18 reported cats with DI have been kittens or young adults, with an average age at diagnosis of 16 months (range, 2 months to 5 years).† Of the 18 cats, 12 (67%) have been males. There is no breed predilection.

The major clinical signs of feline DI are marked polydipsia (generally above 100 mL/kg daily; normal, 40 to 70 mL/kg daily) and polyuria, usually of several months' duration.[79] The severity of clinical signs varies because DI may result from a partial to complete defect in either arginine vasopressin secretion or action. Other clinical signs affected cats show less consistently include weight loss (resulting from a preoccupation with drinking) and dehydration (if access to water has been restricted). Physical examination findings are usually unremarkable.

---

*References 4, 14-16, 23, 36, 43, 49, 56, 58, 81, 86, 94, 99.

†References 4, 14-16, 23, 36, 43, 49, 56, 58, 81, 86, 94, 99.

Diagnostic Workup for Polyuria and Polydipsia

The first step for any cat presented with the owner complaint of polyuria and polydipsia is to establish that the problem actually exists, preferably by a combination of history; random USG determinations; and, if necessary, home measurement of water consumption over several days.

The diagnosis of DI requires that it be differentiated from other medical diseases that cause polyuria and polydipsia in cats.[64,79] The most important ones to rule out for polyuria and polydipsia in cats include primary renal disease, DM, and hyperthyroidism, all of which are much more common that DI. Although primary (psychogenic) polydipsia, a rare disorder associated with compulsive water drinking, has not been well-documented in the cat, it may play a role in the polyuria and polydipsia that develops in more than a third of cats with hyperthyroidism.[71,83]

In general, routine hematologic and serum biochemical testing in cats with central DI are either normal or show evidence of mild dehydration (e.g., mild increases in packed cell volume, total protein, and sodium). In contrast, most of the other differential disorders for polyuria and polydipsia result in marked abnormalities in these screening tests (e.g., elevated serum urea nitrogen, creatinine, glucose, or T_4).

In central DI complete urinalysis is unremarkable except for the finding of persistently dilute urine. In cats the finding of USGs consistently below 1.008 is usually associated with either DI or hyperthyroidism.[71,79] Obviously, hyperthyroidism should be ruled out before initiating testing procedures for DI. It is important to realize that the finding of a USG below 1.008 in a cat excludes mild (occult) renal disease, so further workup for renal disease or precautions associated with the water deprivation test are not necessary.

The workup for polyuric cats with USGs about 1.008 is more complicated. Finding a USG of 1.008 to 1.012 or greater (but less than 1.030) can be associated with hyperthyroidism, stage 1 (occult) renal insufficiency, or pyelonephritis, as well as partial forms of central DI.[71,79] The first step in workup of this group of cats is to exclude hyperthyroidism.

If the serum T_4 concentration is normal, pyelonephritis and early renal insufficiency should next be ruled out. The veterinarian should never perform a water deprivation test in a cat until renal disease is excluded, inasmuch as water deprivation could induce overt renal failure or urosepsis in a cat with unsuspected renal insufficiency.[31,79]

For the workup of pyelonephritis and early renal insufficiency, the following stepwise diagnostic approach is recommended. First, the veterinarian should perform a urine culture to help exclude pyelonephritis and associated urinary tract infection. If the urine culture is negative, renal size and architecture are evaluated by abdominal radiography or, preferably, renal ultrasonography.[42,79] If urine culture results are negative and radiographic or ultrasonographic findings are equivocal, determination of GFR[40] or renal biopsy[97] may be indicated. Because the urine culture can sometimes be negative in cats with pyelonephritis, a therapeutic trial with an appropriate antibiotic (e.g., enrofloxacin) should be instituted, especially if clinical or ultrasonographic findings suggest occult pyelonephritis.

Confirming the Diagnosis of Diabetes Insipidus

Several different diagnostic approaches can be used to confirm central DI, nephrogenic DI, and primary (psychogenic) polydipsia. The water deprivation test is generally considered by most authorities to be the best diagnostic test to differentiate these disorders. However, the water deprivation test is labor intensive, is difficult to perform correctly, is unpleasant for the cat, relies heavily on repeated emptying of the bladder, and can lead to untoward complications and misdiagnosis in some cats.[31,64,79]

A simpler and more practical method of diagnosis that can be recommended as an alternative to water deprivation testing is evaluation of the clinical response to a closely monitored therapeutic trial with the vasopressin analog, desmopressin.[31,64,79] This approach is less complicated and time consuming than the water deprivation test and is certainly easier on the cat. The cost of the two approaches varies according to circumstances but is often comparable. Again, before a desmopressin trial is initiated, it is extremely important to rule out all other common causes of polyuria and polydipsia, limiting the differential diagnosis to central DI, primary nephrogenic DI, and primary (psychogenic) polydipsia.

To perform the test, the owner should first measure the cat's 24-hour water intake for 2 to 3 days before desmopressin is initiated, allowing free-choice water intake. The cat is then treated with therapeutic dosages of desmopressin (see the section on the treatment of diabetes insipidus later in this chapter), which ideally are administered subcutaneously at the dosage of 1.0 μg twice daily for a period of 5 to 7 days. If subcutaneous injections cannot be given, administration of desmopressin by the conjunctival (1 drop twice daily) or oral routes (75 mg twice daily) can be used (Tables 24-13 and 24-14). During this treatment period the owner should continue to measure the cat's daily water intake and monitor the degree of urine output.

A dramatic reduction in water intake (more than 50% of pretreatment measurements) and polyuria strongly suggests a diagnosis of central DI, whereas a lack of any reduction in polydipsia and polyuria is most consistent with primary nephrogenic DI. With more prolonged treatment, water consumption and urine output should completely normalize in cats with central DI.

TABLE 24-13 **Desmopressin Formulations Available in the United States**

Formulation	Concentration	How Supplied	Storage	Trade Name	Manufacturer
Nasal solution and sprays	0.1 mg/mL (100 μg/mL)	2.5-mL bottle	Refrigerate	DDAVP Rhinal Tube	Sanofi Aventis
	0.1 mg/mL (100 μg/mL)	5-mL bottle	Room temp	DDAVP Nasal Spray	Sanofi Aventis
	0.1 mg/mL (100 μg/mL)	2.5-mL bottle	Room temp	Minirin (DDAVP) Nasal Spray	Ferring Pharmaceuticals
	1.5 mg/mL (1,500 μg/mL)	2.5-mL bottle	Room temp	Stimate Nasal Spray	CSL Behring
	0.1 mg/mL (100 μg/mL)	5-mL bottle	Refrigerate	Desmopressin Acetate Nasal Soln (generic)	Bausch and Lomb
	0.1 mg/mL (100 μg/mL)	5-mL bottle	Room temp	Desmopressin Acetate Nasal Soln (generic)	Apotex Corporation
Injectable	4 μg/mL	1-mL single-dose vial 10-mL multiuse vial	Refrigerate	DDAVP Injection	Sanofi Aventis
	4 μg/mL	1-mL vial	Refrigerate	Minirin injection	Ferring Pharmaceuticals
	4 μg/mL	1-mL vial	Refrigerate	Desmopressin Acetate Injection (generic)	Hospira
	4 μg/mL	1-mL vial	Refrigerate	DDAVP injection (generic)	Teva Pharmaceuticals
Tablets	0.1 mg; 0.2 mg	Bottle of 100 tabs	Room temp	DDAVP Tablets	Sanofi Aventis
	0.1 mg; 0.2 mg	Bottle of 30 tabs	Room temp	Minirin Tablets	Ferring Pharmaceuticals
	0.1 mg; 0.2 mg	Bottle of 100 tabs	Room temp	DDAVP Tablets (generic)	Teva Pharmaceuticals
	0.1 mg; 0.2 mg	Bottle of 100 tabs	Room temp	Desmopressin Acetate Tablets (generic)	Apotex Corporation
Melt	60 mg; 120 mg; 240 mg	10, 20, or 100 wafers	Refrigerate	Minirin Melt®	Ferring Pharmaceuticals

Company websites for more information:
Sanofi Aventis: http://www.sanofi-aventis.us/live/us/en/layout.jsp?scat=BD0DB735-32D7-41C4-898F-74F67D343145
Ferring Pharmaceuticals: http://www.ferring.com/en/therapeutic/urology/Products.htm
http://www.mims.com/Page.aspx?menuid=mng&name=Minirin+(DDAVP)+nasal+spray&CTRY=TW&brief=false
CSL Behring: http://www.stimate.com/
Bausch and Lomb: http://www.bausch.com/en_us/msds/msds_listing.aspx
Hospira: http://www.hospira.com/default.aspx
Teva Pharmaceuticals: http://www.tevausa.com/
Apotex Corporation: http://www.apotex.com/us/en/
Desmopressin acetate is also available generically (many companies) and may also be known by the following synonyms and internationally registered trade names: *Concentraid, D-Void, Defirin, Desmogalen, Desmospray, Desmotabs, Emosint, Minurin, Nocutil, Octim, Octostim, or Presinex.*

TABLE 24-14 **Treatment with Desmopressin in Cats**

Formulation	Concentration	Route of Administration	Expected Daily Dose	Frequency of Administration	Cost of Generic Product
Nasal spray or solution	0.1 mg/mL (100 μg/mL)	Conjunctival drops	2-4 medium to large drops	Once daily or given every 8 or 12 hours	Intermediate ($1.50-$3.00/day)
Nasal spray or solution	0.1 mg/mL (100 μg/mL)	Subcutaneous	2-4 μg/day	Once daily or given every 12 hours	Cheapest ($0.60-$1.20/day)
Injectable solution	4 μg/mL	Subcutaneous	2-4 μg/day	Once daily or given every 12 hours	Most expensive ($12-$24/day)
Oral tablet	0.1 mg or 0.2 mg (100 μg and 200 μg)	Oral	50-150 μg/day	Given every 8 or 12 hours	Expensive ($3.50-7.50/day)

In any older cat that develops DI, the veterinarian should consider pituitary imaging with CT or MRI to exclude a pituitary mass. This is especially true if the affected cat has associated neurologic signs.

Treatment of Diabetes Insipidus

Treatment with arginine vasopressin (the cat's ADH) or its analogs restores medullary hypertonicity and a normal urinary concentrating ability in cats with central DI. Historically, ADH tannate in oil, an extract of arginine vasopressin prepared from bovine and porcine pituitary glands, was administered every 2 to 3 days as needed to control polyuria and polydipsia. Because this product is no longer available, desmopressin acetate, a synthetic analog of arginine vasopressin with prolonged and enhanced antidiuretic activity, has become the drug of choice for the treatment of central DI in cats.

Desmopressin acetate is available in preparations for intranasal, parenteral (injectable), or oral administration (see Table 24-13).

NASAL SPRAYS OR SOLUTIONS OF DESMOPRESSIN

The nasal formulations are supplied with two different delivery systems: either a spray pump or a rhinal tube delivery system (see Table 24-13) in which the desmopressin is "sprayed" or "blown" into the nose, respectively. Obviously, most cats will not tolerate either of these intranasal delivery methods. Drops placed in the conjunctival sac provide a more suitable alternative for cats.

With the rhinal tube delivery formulation (DDAVP Rhinal Tube, Sanofi Aventis), the desmopressin is packaged with a small, calibrated plastic catheter so that exact amounts of the drug can be measured and administered. The calibrated rhinal tube has four graduation marks that measure amounts of 0.05 mL, 0.1 mL, 0.1 mL, and 0.2 mL and thereby can deliver doses of 5 to 20 μg of desmopressin. Although this system allows for accurate dosing, it is awkward to use. In addition, because this rhinal tube delivery system is not available as a generic product, this formulation is quite expensive.

The most common intranasal formulations of desmopressin are marketed as nasal sprays or solutions equipped with a compression pump that delivers 10 μg of drug with each spray. For use in cats this spray bottle should be opened and the desmopressin solution transferred to a sterile vial; this dispensing vial then allows the user to place the desmopressin drops within the cat's conjunctival sac. These intranasal preparations of desmopressin are generally supplied as a concentration of 100 μg/mL; depending on the size of the drop, 1 drop of nasal solution corresponds to 1.5 to 4 μg of desmopressin. One highly concentrated nasal solution (1.5 mg/mL) is marketed for use in hemophilia (see Table 24-13), but it should not be used to treat cats with DI because of the strong likelihood of overdosage.

In most cats 1 to 2 drops of the intranasal preparation administered once or twice daily are sufficient to control polyuria and polydipsia (see Table 24-14). Use of a tuberculin or insulin syringe allows for more accurate dosing. Application of desmopressin into the conjunctival sac may cause local irritation because the solution is acidic. Some cats may object to the daily eye drops, making this route of administration ineffective.[4,81]

ORAL DESMOPRESSIN TABLETS

The oral preparation of desmopressin is available both as a sublingual dissolve melt tablet (not suitable for treating cats) and as 0.1-mg and 0.2-mg tablets. Each 0.1-mg (100-μg) tablet is roughly comparable to 5 to 10 μg (1 or 2 large drops) of the nasal solution (see Table 24-13). In one report of five cats with DI,[4] all were treated successfully with oral desmopressin. Doses were variable, but most were well-controlled using oral dosages of 50 μg administered twice or three times daily.[4]

The tablet form of desmopressin is a more cost-prohibitive alternative than the conjunctival or subcutaneous routes of administration. The cost of daily oral desmopressin in cats is roughly 2.5 times that of the cost of conjunctival drops and roughly 6 times the cost of subcutaneous injections of desmopressin. For some cat owners, however, the use of a tablet form may prove to be a more convenient, or the only possible, route of administration.

INJECTABLE DESMOPRESSIN SOLUTIONS FOR SUBCUTANEOUS OR INTRAVENOUS USE

An injectable sterile solution of desmopressin acetate (4 μg/mL) marketed for intravenous use is available (see Table 24-13) and can be used in cats with DI. However, the cost of the injectable desmopressin is approximately 7 to 15 times higher per μg than the intranasal preparation, making this formulation cost prohibitive for use in most cats. To circumvent this cost issue, the intranasal form of desmopressin—although not designed for parenteral use—can be given subcutaneously to cats with excellent results.[14,16,43,81] Because the nasal forms of desmopressin are not considered to be sterile, however, it is best to first sterilize the product by passing the nasal solution through a 0.2-micron bacteriostatic syringe filter[31,63] (see www.whatman.com/GDXSyringeFilters.aspx for more information). Clinically the nasal and injectable preparations of desmopressin induce indistinguishable responses when administered subcutaneously.

To make dosing easier, the desmopressin is best administered with an U-100 low-dose insulin syringe. The solution can be diluted in sterile physiologic saline to make dosing easier.

The subcutaneous route of desmopressin administration has many advantages over the other routes of administration. These advantages include the following:

- First, drug appears to be most effective when administered via the subcutaneous route.
- Second, the duration of action is longer after subcutaneous injection than when administered orally or through the conjunctival sac.
- Third, because of the smaller subcutaneous doses required to control signs (about 15% and 40% of the oral and conjunctival doses, respectively), the cost of treatment is greatly reduced.
- Fourth, many cats seem to prefer long-term subcutaneous injections to the chronic use of eye drops or oral medication.

DOSE ADJUSTMENTS FOR DESMOPRESSIN

Recommended initial doses of desmopressin vary depending on the route by which it is being administered. If the conjunctival route is employed, 1 or 2 drops of the intranasal preparation administered once or twice daily is usually sufficient to control polyuria (see Table 24-14). With the subcutaneous route of administration, the initial recommended dose is 1 to 2 μg once or twice daily. If the nasal solution (100 μg/mL) were used for this purpose, the veterinarian would inject only 0.01 to 0.02 mL (or 1 to 2 U with a U-100 insulin syringe). With the oral tablets a starting dose of 0.05 μg to 0.075 μg (50 to 75 μg) once or twice daily is initiated.

In cats with central DI, daily administration of desmopressin may completely eliminate polyuria and polydipsia. However, because of individual differences in absorption and metabolism, the dose required to achieve complete, around-the-clock control varies from patient to patient. The maximal effect of desmopressin occurs from 2 to 8 hours after administration, and the duration of action varies from 8 to 24 hours.[31,63] Larger doses of the drug appear to both increase its antidiuretic effects and prolong its duration of action; however, expense can become a limiting factor for some owners.

No matter what route of administration is used, the daily dose should be gradually adjusted as needed to control signs of polydipsia and polyuria. The morning and evening doses can be adjusted separately if needed.

ADVERSE EFFECTS OF DESMOPRESSIN

Desmopressin is relatively safe for use in cats with central DI. Adverse effects of desmopressin are uncommon, but overdosage can lead to fluid retention, hyponatremia, and decreased plasma osmolality.[31,63] Although extremely rare, fluid intoxication associated with desmopressin overdosage can lead to central nervous system disturbances, including depression, increased salivation, vomiting, ataxia, muscle tremors, coma, and convulsions.[31,41] In such instances furosemide can be given to induce diuresis.

To avoid the potential problem of overdosage, cats should not be allowed free access to water immediately after each dose of desmopressin, especially if severe polydipsia and polyuria have redeveloped. Without such short-term (1 to 2 hours) water restriction, the cat many consume excessive amounts of water that cannot be subsequently excreted, insofar as the desmopressin is absorbed and has its peak antidiuretic effects on the renal tubules.

COST OF DESMOPRESSIN

The principle drawback with the use of any of the desmopressin preparations in the treatment of central DI is the drug's considerable expense. The oral route of administration is the most expensive, and the subcutaneous route of administration (using the sterilized nasal solutions) is generally the most cost-effective.

Prognosis of Diabetes Insipidus

In some cats with DI, the owner may elect not to treat the cat because of financial concerns. Because polyuria and polydipsia do not pose a serious health hazard in these cats (as long as adequate access to water is available), treatment is not essential or mandatory. In cats with untreated DI, however, it is imperative that the water never be restricted because the inability to concentrate urine may lead to dehydration and possibly even death from neurologic complications.

Cats with idiopathic, traumatic, or congenital DI usually respond well to treatment with desmopressin, with near complete resolution of clinical signs of polyuria and polydipsia. With proper care these cats have an excellent prognosis and a normal life expectancy.

In contrast, cats with DI caused by large or aggressive hypothalamic masses or pituitary macrotumors have a grave prognosis. External radiation therapy in combination with desmopressin medical treatment offers the best chance for decreasing tumor size while controlling signs of polyuria in such cats.[50,91] Fortunately, this appears to be an extremely rare cause of DI in cats.

References

1. Abraham LA, Helmond SE, Mitten RW et al: Treatment of an acromegalic cat with the dopamine agonist L-deprenyl, *Aust Vet J* 80:479, 2002.
2. Abrams-Ogg A, Holmberg DL, Stewart WA et al: Acromegaly in a cat: diagnosis by magnetic resonance imaging and treatment by cryohypophysectomy, *Can Vet J* 34:682, 1993.
3. Abrams-Ogg A, Holmberg DL, Quinn RF et al: Blindness now attributed to enrofloxacin therapy in a previously reported case of a cat with acromegaly treated by cryohypophysectomy, *Can Vet J* 43:53, 2002.
4. Aroch I, Mazaki-Tovi M, Shemesh O et al: Central diabetes insipidus in five cats: clinical presentation, diagnosis and oral desmopressin therapy, *J Feline Med Surg* 7:333, 2005.
5. Auriemma RS, Galdiero M, De Martino MC et al: The kidney in acromegaly: renal structure and function in patients with

acromegaly during active disease and 1 year after disease remission, *Eur J Endocrinol* 162:1035, 2010.
6. Berg RI, Nelson RW, Feldman EC et al: Serum insulin-like growth factor-I concentration in cats with diabetes mellitus and acromegaly, *J Vet Intern Med* 21:892, 2007.
7. Biering H, Knappe G, Gerl H et al: [Prevalence of diabetes in acromegaly and Cushing syndrome], *Acta Med Austriaca* 27:27, 2000.
8. Bishop JS, Steele R, Altszuler N et al: Diminished responsiveness to insulin in the growth hormone-treated normal dog, *Amer J Physiol* 212:272, 1967.
9. Blois SL, Holmberg DL: Cryohypophysectomy used in the treatment of a case of feline acromegaly, *J Small Anim Pract* 49:596, 2008.
10. Bluestone R, Bywaters EG, Hartog M et al: Acromegalic arthropathy, *Ann Rheum Dis* 30:243, 1971.
11. Bondanelli M, Ambrosio MR, degli Uberti EC: Pathogenesis and prevalence of hypertension in acromegaly, *Pituitary* 4:239, 2001.
12. Brahms S: The development of the hypophysis of the cat (felis domestica), *Am J Anat* 50:251, 1932.
13. Brearley MJ, Polton GA, Littler RM et al: Coarse fractionated radiation therapy for pituitary tumours in cats: a retrospective study of 12 cases, *Vet Comp Oncol* 4:209, 2006.
14. Brown B, Peterson ME, Robertson GL: Evaluation of the plasma vasopressin, plasma sodium and urine osmolality response to water restriction in normal cats and a cat with diabetes insipidus, *J Vet Intern Med* 7:113, 1993.
15. Burnie AG, Dunn JK: A case of central diabetes insipidus in the cat: Diagnosis and treatment, *J Small Anim Pract* 23:237, 1982.
16. Campbell FE, Bredhauer B: Trauma-induced central diabetes insipidus in a cat, *Aust Vet J* 86:102, 2008.
17. Carpenter JL, Andrews LK, Holzworth J: Tumors and tumor-like lesions. In Holzworth J, editor: *Diseases of the cat: medicine and surgery*, Philadelphia, 1987, Saunders, p 406.
18. Chanson P: Emerging drugs for acromegaly, *Expert Opin Emerg Drugs* 13:273, 2008.
19. Chanson P, Salenave S, Kamenicky P et al: Pituitary tumours: acromegaly, *Best Pract Res Clin Endocrinol Metab* 23:555, 2009.
20. Chastain CB, Ganjam VK: The endocrine brain and clinical tests of its function In: Chastain CB, Ganjam VK, editors, *Clinical endocrinology of companion animals*, Philadelphia, 1986, Lea & Febiger, p 37.
21. Clemmons DR: Roles of insulin-like growth factor-I and growth hormone in mediating insulin resistance in acromegaly, *Pituitary* 5:181, 2002.
22. Colao A, Pivonello R, Scarpa R et al: The acromegalic arthropathy, *J Endocrinol Invest* 28:24, 2005.
23. Court MH, Watson AD: Idiopathic neurogenic diabetes insipidus in a cat, *Aust Vet J* 60:245, 1983.
24. Daminet S: Feline hypothyroidism In Mooney CT, Peterson ME, editors: *BSAVA manual of canine and feline endocrinology*. ed 4, Shurdington, Cheltenham, 2011, British Small Animal Veterinary Association (in press).
25. Dellmann HD: The endocrine system In Dellmann HD, Brown EM, editors: *Textbook of veterinary histology*, Philadelphia, 1976, Lea & Febiger, p 373.
26. Dominici FP, Argentino DP, Munoz MC et al: Influence of the crosstalk between growth hormone and insulin signalling on the modulation of insulin sensitivity, *Growth Horm IGF Res* 15:324, 2005.
27. Dunning MD, Lowrie CS, Bexfield NH et al: Exogenous insulin treatment after hypofractionated radiotherapy in cats with diabetes mellitus and acromegaly, *J Vet Intern Med* 23:243, 2009.
28. Eigenmann JE, Wortman JA, Haskins ME: Elevated growth hormone levels and diabetes mellitus in a cat with acromegalic features, *J Am Anim Hosp Assoc* 20:747, 1984.
29. Elliott DA, Feldman EC, Koblik PD et al: Prevalence of pituitary tumors among diabetic cats with insulin resistance, *J Am Vet Med Assoc* 216:1765, 2000.
30. Feldman EC, Nelson RW: Disorders of growth hormone. In Feldman EC, Nelson RW, editors: *Canine and feline endocrinology and reproduction*, Philadelphia, 2004, Elsevier, p 69.
31. Feldman EC, Nelson RW: Water metabolism and diabetes insipidus In Feldman EC, Nelson RW, editors: *Canine and feline endocrinology and reproduction*, ed 3, Philadelphia, 2004, Saunders, p 2.
32. Fracassi F, Mandrioli L, Diana A et al: Pituitary macroadenoma in a cat with diabetes mellitus, hypercortisolism and neurologicsigns, *J Vet Med A Physiol Pathol Clin Med* 54:359, 2007.
33. Gembardt C, Loppnow H: Pathogenesis of spontaneous diabetes mellitus in the cat. II. Acidophilic adenoma of the pituitary gland and diabetes mellitus in 2 cases, *Berl Munch Tierarztl Wochenschr* 89:336, 1976.
34. Goossens MM, Feldman EC, Nelson RW et al: Cobalt 60 irradiation of pituitary gland tumors in three cats with acromegaly, *J Am Vet Med Assoc* 213:374, 1998.
35. Greco DS: Pediatric endocrinology, *Vet Clin North Am Small Anim Pract* 36:549, 2006.
36. Green RA, Farrow CS: Diabetes insipidus in a cat, *J Am Vet Med Assoc* 164:524, 1974.
37. Heinrichs M, Baumgartner W, Krug-Manntz S: Immunocytochemical demonstration of growth hormone in an acidophilic adenoma of the adenohypophysis in a cat, *Vet Pathol* 26:179, 1989.
38. Hurty CA, Flatland B: Feline acromegaly: a review of the syndrome, *J Am Anim Hosp Assoc* 41:292, 2005.
39. Hurxthal LM: The serum phosphorus level as an index of pituitary growth hormone activity in acromegaly; a preliminary report, *Lahey Clin Bull* 5:194, 1948.
40. Kerl ME, Cook CR: Glomerular filtration rate and renal scintigraphy, *Clin Tech Small Anim Pract* 20:31, 2005.
41. Kim RJ, Malattia C, Allen M et al: Vasopressin and desmopressin in central diabetes insipidus: adverse effects and clinical considerations, *Pediatr Endocrinol Rev* 2(Suppl 1):115, 2004.
42. Konde LJ: Sonography of the kidney, *Vet Clin North Am Small Anim Pract* 15:1149, 1985.
43. Kraus KH: The use of desmopressin in diagnosis and treatment of diabetes insipidus in cats, *Compend Cont Ed Prac Vet* 9:752, 1987.
44. Latimer HB: The weights of the hypophysis, thyroid, and supradrenals in the adult cat, *Growth* 3:435, 1939.
45. Lewitt MS, Hazel SJ, Church DB et al: Regulation of insulin-like growth factor-binding protein-3 ternary complex in feline diabetes mellitus, *J Endocrinol* 166:21, 2000.
46. Lichtensteiger CA, Wortman JA, Eigenmann JE: Functional pituitary acidophil adenoma in a cat with diabetes mellitus and acromegalic features, *Vet Pathol* 23:518, 1986.
47. Littler RM, Polton GA, Brearley MJ: Resolution of diabetes mellitus but not acromegaly in a cat with a pituitary macroadenoma treated with hypofractionated radiation, *J Small Anim Pract* 47:392, 2006.
48. Macri B, Marino F, Mazzullo G et al: Mucopolysaccharidosis VI in a Siamese/short-haired European cat, *J Vet Med A Physiol Pathol Clin Med* 49:438, 2002.
49. Mason KV, Burren VS: Successful management of a case of feline diabetes insipidus with occular instilation of desmoporessin, *Aust Vet Practitioner* 15:156, 1985.
50. Mayer MN, Greco DS, LaRue SM: Outcomes of pituitary tumor irradiation in cats, *J Vet Intern Med* 20:1151, 2006.
51. Meij BP: Hypophysectomy as a treatment for canine and feline Cushing's disease, *Vet Clin North Am Small Anim Pract* 31:1015, 2001.
52. Meij BP, Voorhout G, Van Den Ingh TS et al: Transsphenoidal hypophysectomy for treatment of pituitary-dependent hyperadrenocorticism in 7 cats, *Vet Surg* 30:72, 2001.

53. Meij BP, van der Vlugt-Meijer RH, van den Ingh TS et al: Somatotroph and corticotroph pituitary adenoma (double adenoma) in a cat with diabetes mellitus and hyperadrenocorticism, *J Comp Pathol* 130:209, 2004.
54. Meij BP, van der Vlugt-Meijer RH, van den Ingh TS et al: Melanotroph pituitary adenoma in a cat with diabetes mellitus, *Vet Pathol* 42:92, 2005.
55. Meij BP, Auriemma E, Grinwis G et al: Successful treatment of acromegaly in a diabetic cat with transsphenoidal hypophysectomy, *J Feline Med Surg* 12:406, 2010.
56. Mellanby RJ, Jeffery ND, Gopal MS et al: Secondary hypothyroidism following head trauma in a cat, *J Feline Med Surg* 7:135, 2005.
57. Melmed S: Acromegaly pathogenesis and treatment, *J Clin Invest* 119:3189, 2009.
58. Miller MS: Diagnosis of partial central diabetes insipidus in a kitten, *Pulse* 33:19, 1991.
59. Mol JA, van Garderen E, Rutteman GR et al: New insights in the molecular mechanism of progestin-induced proliferation of mammary epithelium: induction of the local biosynthesis of growth hormone (GH) in the mammary glands of dogs, cats and humans, *J Steroid Biochem Mol Biol* 57:67, 1996.
60. Moller N, Jorgensen JO: Effects of growth hormone on glucose, lipid, and protein metabolism in human subjects, *Endocr Rev* 30:152, 2009.
61. Morrison SA, Randolph J, Lothrop CD, Jr.: Hypersomatotropism and insulin-resistant diabetes mellitus in a cat, *J Am Vet Med Assoc* 194:91, 1989.
62. Muggeo M, Bar RS, Roth J et al: The insulin resistance of acromegaly: evidence for two alterations in the insulin receptor on circulating monocytes, *J Clin Endocrinol Metab* 48:17, 1979.
63. Nichols R, Hohenhaus AE: Use of the vasopressin analogue desmopressin for polyuria and bleeding disorders, *J Am Vet Med Assoc* 205:168, 1994.
64. Nichols R: Polyuria and polydipsia. Diagnostic approach and problems associated with patient evaluation, *Vet Clin North Am Small Anim Pract* 31:833, 2001.
65. Niessen SJ, Khalid M, Petrie G et al: Validation and application of a radioimmunoassay for ovine growth hormone in the diagnosis of acromegaly in cats, *Vet Rec* 160:902, 2007.
66. Niessen SJ, Petrie G, Gaudiano F et al: Feline acromegaly: an underdiagnosed endocrinopathy? *J Vet Intern Med* 21:899, 2007.
67. Niessen SJ: Feline acromegaly: an essential differential diagnosis for the difficult diabetic, *J Feline Med Surg* 12:15, 2010.
68. Norman EJ, Mooney CT: Diagnosis and management of diabetes mellitus in five cats with somatotrophic abnormalities, *J Feline Med Surg* 2:183, 2000.
69. O'Shea MH, Layish DT: Growth hormone and the kidney: a case presentation and review of the literature, *J Am Soc Nephrol* 3:157, 1992.
70. Patnaik AK, Liu SK, Hurvitz AI et al: Nonhematopoietic neoplasms in cats, *J Natl Cancer Inst* 54:855, 1975.
71. Peterson ME, Kintzer PP, Cavanagh PG et al: Feline hyperthyroidism: pretreatment clinical and laboratory evaluation of 131 cases, *J Am Vet Med Assoc* 183:103, 1983.
72. Peterson ME: Effects of megestrol acetate on glucose tolerance and growth hormone secretion in the cat, *Res Vet Sci* 42:354, 1987.
73. Peterson ME, Kemppainen RJ: Pituitary intermediate lobe in cats: active secretion of alpha-MSH and in vivo evidence for dopaminergic and beta-adrenergic regulation. Program of the 72nd Annual Meeting of The Endocrine Society 1990;121 (Abstract).
74. Peterson ME, Taylor RS, Greco DS et al: Acromegaly in 14 cats, *J Vet Intern Med* 4:192, 1990.
75. Peterson ME, Kemppainen RJ, Orth DN: Plasma concentrations of immunoreactive proopiomelanocortin peptides and cortisol in clinically normal cats, *Am J Vet Res* 55:295, 1994.
76. Peterson ME, Randolph JF, Mooney CT: Endocrine diseases. In Sherding RG, editor: *The cat: diagnosis and clinical management*, ed 2, New York, 1994, Churchill Livingstone, p 1404.
77. Peterson ME: Feline hyperadrenocorticism. In Mooney CT, Peterson ME, editors: *BSAVA manual of canine and feline endocrinology*, ed 3, Gloucester, 2004, British Small Animal Veterinary Association, p 205.
78. Peterson ME: Acromegaly. In Mooney CT, Peterson ME, editors: *BSAVA manual of canine and feline endocrinology*, ed 3, Gloucester, 2004, British Small Animal Veterinary Association, p 187.
79. Peterson ME, Nichols R: Investigation of polyuria and polydipsia. In Mooney CT, Peterson ME, editors: *BSAVA manual of canine and feline endocrinology*, ed 3, Gloucester, 2004, British Small Animal Veterinary Association, p 16.
80. Peterson ME: Acromegaly in cats: are we only diagnosing the tip of the iceberg? *J Vet Intern Med* 21:889, 2007.
81. Pittari JM: Central diabetes insipidus in a cat, *Feline Practice* 24:18, 1996.
82. Quante S, Fracassi F, Gorgas D et al: Congenital hypothyroidism in a kitten resulting in decreased IGF-I concentration and abnormal liver function tests, *J Feline Med Surg* 12:487, 2010.
83. Radcliffe CE: Observations on the relationship of the thyroid to the polyuria of experimental diabetes insipidus, *Endocrinology* 415, 1943.
84. Reaves TA, Liu HM, Qasim MM et al: Osmotic regulation of vasopressin in the cat, *Am J Physiol* 240:E108, 1981.
85. Reusch CE, Kley S, Casella M et al: Measurements of growth hormone and insulin-like growth factor 1 in cats with diabetes mellitus, *Vet Rec* 158:195, 2006.
86. Rogers WA, Valdez H, Anderson BC et al: Partial deficiency of antidiuretic hormone in a cat, *J Am Vet Med Assoc* 170:545, 1977.
87. Romeis B: Innersekretorische drüsen II: Hypophyse (Dritter Teil) In: Möllendorff WV, ed. *Handbuch der Mikroskopischen Anatomie des Menschen, Sechster Band, Blutgefäss-Und Lymphgefässappart Innerskretorische Drüsen*, Berlin, 1940, Verlag Von Julius Springer, p 280.
88. Sacca L, Cittadini A, Fazio S: Growth hormone and the heart, *Endocr Rev* 15:555, 1994.
89. Sande RD, Bingel SA: Animal models of dwarfism, *Vet Clin North Am Small Anim Pract* 13:71, 1983.
90. Scott-Moncrieff JC: Insulin resistance in cats, *Vet Clin North Am Small Anim Pract* 40:241, 2010.
91. Sellon RK, Fidel J, Houston R et al: Linear-accelerator-based modified radiosurgical treatment of pituitary tumors in cats: 11 cases (1997-2008), *J Vet Intern Med* 23:1038, 2009.
92. Slatopolsky E, Rutherford WE, Rosenbaum R et al: Hyperphosphatemia, *Clin Nephrol* 7:138, 1977.
93. Slingerland LI, Voorhout G, Rijnberk A et al: Growth hormone excess and the effect of octreotide in cats with diabetes mellitus, *Domest Anim Endocrinol* 35:352, 2008.
94. Smith JR, Elwood CM: Traumatic partial hypopituitarism in a cat, *J Small Anim Pract* 45:405, 2004.
95. Starkey SR, Tan K, Church DB: Investigation of serum IGF-I levels amongst diabetic and non-diabetic cats, *J Feline Med Surg* 6:149, 2004.
96. Troxel MT, Vite CH, Van Winkle TJ et al: Feline intracranial neoplasia: retrospective review of 160 cases (1985-2001), *J Vet Intern Med* 17:850, 2003.
97. Vaden SL: Renal biopsy of dogs and cats, *Clin Tech Small Anim Pract* 20:11, 2005.
98. Vitale G, Pivonello R, Auriemma RS et al: Hypertension in acromegaly and in the normal population: prevalence and determinants, *Clin Endocrinol (Oxf)* 63:470, 2005.
99. Winterbotham J, Mason KV: Congenital diabetes insipidus in a kitten, *J Small Anim Pract* 24:569, 1983.

100. Young FG: Growth hormone and diabetes, *Rec Progr Horm Res* 8:471, 1953.
101. Zaki F, Harris J, Budzilovich G: Cystic pituicytoma of the neurohypophysis in a Siamese cat, *J Comp Path* 85:467, 1975.
102. Zaki FA, Liu SK: Pituitary chromophobe adenoma in a cat, *Vet Pathol* 10:232, 1973.

DISORDERS OF CALCIUM METABOLISM

Randolph M. Baral

CALCIUM HOMEOSTASIS

Calcium plays a key role in many physiologic processes. In addition to skeletal support, these include muscle contractions (skeletal, smooth, and cardiac muscle), transmission of nerve impulses, and blood clotting.[41]

In most cases plasma or serum biochemistry analytes are assessed by determining where the analyte is produced and excreted, as well as taking into account other influences. For example, albumin is produced by the liver and excretion is by way of renal or gastrointestinal routes. This means that in most cases a decrease in albumin is due to decreased production (indicating hepatopathy) or increased loss (due to renal or gastrointestinal causes). A further influence is dehydration, which can increase albumin results. In contrast to albumin, calcium regulation is exceedingly complex. In the first instance routine measurements of plasma or serum calcium are of total calcium (tCa), but calcium exists in three forms[83]:

1. Ionized (free) calcium (iCa), which is the only physiologically active form and makes up 50% to 60% of tCa
2. Protein-bound calcium that accounts for approximately 10% of tCa
3. Complexed calcium (bound to e.g., phosphate, bicarbonate, lactate), which makes up 30% to 40% of tCa

Ionized calcium (iCa) must be measured immediately in-house or collected and separated anaerobically and measured within 2 hours (at room temperature) or 6 hours (if kept refrigerated).[7]

Our measurements of calcium are a reflection of extracellular fluid (ECF) calcium levels. The influences on ECF calcium are shown in Figure 24-30. Not only is ECF calcium increased by absorption from the gastrointestinal tract and decreased by secretion back to the gastrointestinal tract for excretion (90%), but filtration occurs through the kidneys for urinary excretion (10%). The kidneys also reabsorb 99% of this filtered calcium. Further, approximately 99% of total body calcium is stored in bones, which act as reservoirs, releasing calcium when ECF calcium reduces.[41]

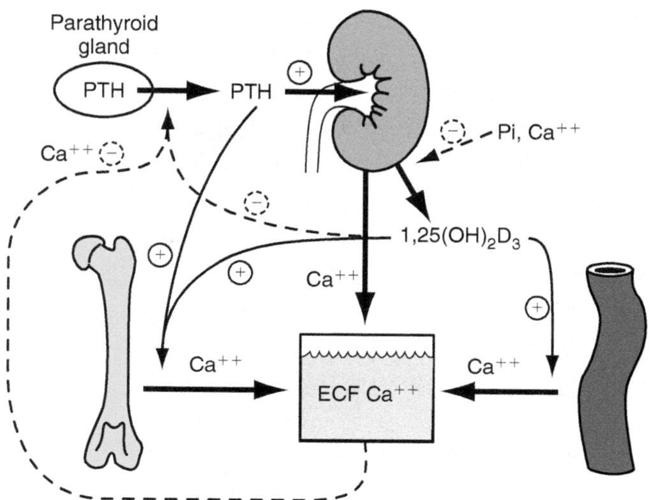

FIGURE 24-30 Influences on calcium concentrations. Extracellular fluid calcium is increased by absorption from the gastrointestinal tract, released from bone (where 99% of body calcium is stored) and reabsorbed by the kidneys. Extracellular fluid calcium reduces by secretion back to the gastrointestinal tract for excretion (90%) and filtration through the kidneys for urinary excretion (10%). These interactions are mediated by parathyroid hormone and calcitriol (activated vitamin D). Parathyroid hormone responds to decreased ionized calcium. Parathyroid hormone release results in increased calcitriol production by the kidneys. *(From Schenck PA, Chew DJ, Behrend EN: Update on hypercalcemic disorders. In August JR, editor:* Consultations in feline internal medicine, *ed 5, St Louis, 2006, Elsevier Saunders, p 157.)*

These interactions between the gastrointestinal tract, kidneys, and bone to maintain ECF calcium within a relatively narrow range are predominantly mediated by the following[41]:

1. Parathyroid hormone (PTH)
   - Produced by "chief cells" within the parathyroid gland
2. Calcitriol, or 1,25-dihydroxycholecalciferol, the most active form of vitamin D
   - The final stage of the conversion of vitamin D to calcitriol occurs within the kidneys
3. Calcitonin
   - Secreted by the thyroid gland
   - Has only a minor role in decreasing plasma calcium concentration

PTH acts to increase ECF calcium, and in a normal cat PTH is secreted in response to decreased levels of ECF calcium (or increased phosphate) and results in the following[41]:

1. Increased calcium (and phosphate) absorption from bone
2. Decreased calcium excretion from the kidneys (and increased phosphate excretion)
3. Increased calcitriol formation by the kidneys

Increased calcitriol levels result in the following[41]:

1. Increased intestinal absorption of calcium (and phosphate)
2. Enhancement of the ability of PTH to resorb bone
3. Decreased renal calcium and phosphate excretion (minor effect)

All these interactions are also influenced by plasma phosphate (PO_4) concentrations.[41]

APPROACH TO THE CAT WITH HYPERCALCEMIA

The clinical signs of hypercalcemia are very nonspecific. Mild hypercalcemia may not result in any signs. More severe clinical signs are usually associated with a concurrent problem (e.g., malignancy). Extreme hypercalcemia can cause depression of the nervous system, polyuria and polydipsia may be seen, and uroliths can form. A list of the clinical signs of hypercalcemia is shown with the pathophysiologic reason in Table 24-15. Mostly, however, hypercalcemia is detected by plasma biochemistry screening of a generally unwell cat with nonspecific signs such as lethargy or inappetence.

The following approaches to a cat with hypercalcemia must take into account physical examination and other laboratory findings as well as the cat's signalment (e.g., neoplasia is much less likely to occur in a kitten) and clinical history (e.g., possible exposure to rodenticide).

The main diagnostic steps are as follows:

1. Confirm finding of elevated tCa.
2. Measure iCa.
3. Measure PTH.
4. Measure parathyroid hormone-related protein (PTHrP) and vitamin D metabolites.
5. Assess results and relationships of tCa, iCa, and PTH concentrations.

Assessment of the results of these tests narrows down the potential causes of hypercalcemia considerably, particularly when the cat's age, clinical history, and physical examination findings are taken into account. Step 4, testing for vitamin D metabolites (calcidiol and calcitriol) and PTHrP should be considered as an optional step. The results of these tests are sometimes helpful, but a diagnosis can often be reached without testing for these. Together with further diagnostics, these will be discussed under the specific conditions where their testing is appropriate.

TABLE 24-15 **Clinical Signs of Hypercalcemia**

Clinical Sign	Pathophysiology
Polyuria and polydipsia	Impaired response of renal tubules to antidiuretic hormone Impaired renal tubular resorption of sodium and chloride Secondary to renal damage
Weakness, depression, mental dullness	Depressed excitability of muscular and nervous tissue
Anorexia, vomiting, constipation	Decreased contractility of the smooth muscle of the gastrointestinal tract
Muscle twitching, shivering, seizures	Direct effect on central nervous system
Cardiac arrhythmias	Direct neurologic effect
Lower urinary tract signs	Presence of uroliths

Modified from Barber PJ: Disorders of calcium homeostasis in small animals, *In Pract* 23:262, 2001

Step 1: Confirm Finding of Elevated Total Calcium

The tCa is usually measured by a colorimetric assessment and so is susceptible to spurious increases caused by lipemia or hemolysis. Additionally, mild hypercalcemia may be transient. A second sample should be taken after a 12-hour fast because food intake can sometimes cause mild hypercalcemia, as well as lipemia. If the finding of hypercalcemia is repeatable, then iCa should be measured. Further, iCa can be increased when tCa is normal. In these cases tCa will be at the high end of the normal reference range, so it is appropriate to test iCa concentrations in those cats with repeatable high normal tCa concentrations.[85] It is prudent to collect a sample with the special handling required for iCa (discussed later) at the time of sampling for confirmation of elevated tCa.

Correction equations that take into account total protein or albumin levels have been devised for people and dogs to improve diagnostic interpretation of tCa values.[55,62] These equations are controversial in these two species. In cats the equations are even less reliable because the relationship between tCa and albumin is too variable.[37]

Step 2: Measure Ionized Calcium

The iCa should be measured in all cases where tCa is elevated or on the high side of the normal reference range. iCa values can be artefactually increased by exposure to air because pH and temperature affect the equilibrium between the three fractions of ionized, protein-bound, and complex-bound calcium.[7,85] Therefore samples should be tested immediately with an in-house analyzer or collected anaerobically and sent chilled (4° C) to a commercial laboratory.

When heparinized whole blood is used for in-house iCa sampling, it results in a lower iCa concentration than serum samples.[40] These differences should be taken into account by using different reference ranges. Commercial laboratories measure iCa from serum. Ethylenediaminetetraacetic acid (EDTA) plasma must never be used for either in-house or commercial laboratory assessment of ionized calcium because EDTA chelates calcium, which falsely reduces the concentration.[85]

Anaerobic collection of serum requires two serum vacutainer tubes, a centrifuge, and a spinal needle. Silicon separator vacutainer tubes should not be used because calcium is released from the silicone gel, falsely elevating the calcium level. The needle of the syringe used to collect the blood sample from the cat should placed directly through the stopper of the first vacutainer tube (without opening the tube) to transfer the sample from syringe to blood tube. The blood should be allowed to clot (approximately 20 minutes), then separated by centrifugation. The spinal needle (attached to a syringe that does not contain air) is used to withdraw serum from this tube without opening it. This serum is then transferred to the second vacutainer tube (again, without opening the tube). The sample is refrigerated and then sent to the reference laboratory with an ice pack.[83]

Step 3: Measure Parathyroid Hormone

PTH is an 84-chain amino acid. The amino acid sequence of PTH is known for the dog, cow, pig, rat, chicken, and human, and most mammals appear to have very similar amino-terminal portions of the molecule.[87] Mature feline PTH is 84% identical to human PTH.[97] At least two PTH assays have been validated for use in the cat. Both are two-site immunoradiometric assays (IRMA) for human intact PTH. *Two-site* means using antibodies that bind with epitopes at the two terminals of the molecule and therefore avoids measuring the PTH fragments that can be present in blood and would otherwise potentially be detected by a one-site assay (rendering it less accurate).[10,77] Serum or plasma can be assayed but should be separated with minimal exposure of samples to room temperature (less than 2 hours). The samples then should be refrigerated or frozen before analysis to prevent degradation.[6,85,87]

The serum sample for iCa requires similar handling. It is therefore practical to use the same serum for both iCa and PTH at a reference laboratory.

Step 4: Measure PTH-Related Protein and Vitamin D Metabolites

PTHrP is secreted by some malignant neoplasms and mimics the action of PTH by binding to PTH receptors. It is elevated in some cases of hypercalcemia of malignancy, but not all. One study of 322 cats with elevated iCa found PTH in the lower half of the normal reference range in 263 cats (81.7%), yet PTHrP was elevated in only 31 cats (9.6%). Clinical records were not available for all cats, and only seven cats had confirmed malignancy.[77] It is highly likely that a large number of cats with normal PTHrP had hypercalcemia caused by malignancy.

Two-site assays for human PTHrP have been validated for cats.[77] PTHrP is best measured from fresh or frozen EDTA plasma.[84]

Vitamin D metabolites are identical in all species, so radioimmunoassays used for humans are appropriate for cats.[84] Human endocrinology laboratories often offer this testing, and developing a relationship with such a laboratory at a local human hospital can be beneficial for practitioners. The different vitamin metabolites should be considered. Calcidiol (25-hydroxyvitamin D) increases with ingestion of cholecalciferol-containing rodenticides. Calcitriol (1,25-dihydroxyvitamin D) increases with ingestion of calcitriol-containing plants (such as *Cestrum diurnum* [day-blooming jessamine]) and granulomatous inflammation. Calcidiol and calcitriol are best measured from chilled serum. Neither analyte is increased with hypercalcemia caused by ingestion of calcipotriene, a vitamin D analog found in psoriasis cream.[84]

Step 5: Assess tCa, iCa, and Parathyroid Hormone Relationships

Table 24-16 outlines common conditions that result in hypercalcemia together with the tCa, iCa, PO_4, and PTH results. Broadly, disorders resulting in hypercalcemia should be classified as those for which PTH is typically increased, those for which PTH is typically reduced, and those for which PTH is normal. Exceptions to these findings do occur, and these are addressed under the specific conditions. The most common causes of hypercalcemia in cats, with the most common iCa and PTH findings, are as follows:

1. Neoplasia:
   - iCa often very high
   - PTH often undetectable, may be in lower half of reference range
2. Renal disease:
   - iCa often normal
   - PTH elevated
3. Idiopathic hypercalcemia
   - iCa often mildly elevated
   - PTH in lower half of normal range

Mnemonics, such as "GOSH DARN IT"[85] for all causes of hypercalcemia and "SHIRT"[24] for common causes of hypercalcemia have been devised. These are listed in Boxes 24-5 and 24-6. Veterinarians are advised to remember the causes of hypercalcemia in terms of PTH results because this gives a better understanding of the underlying processes.

TABLE 24-16 **Common Conditions That Result in Hypercalcemia with Expected Calcium (Total and Ionized), Albumin, Phosphate, Parathyroid Hormone, and Other Calcemic Indices***

	tCa	iCa	Alb	PO_4	PTH	PTHrP	25-OH vit D	$1,25(OH)_2$ vit D
INCREASED PTH								
Primary hyperparathyroidism	↑	↑	N	↓ or N	↑	N	N	N or ↑
Renal secondary hyperparathyroidism	↑	N or ↓	N	↑	↑	N	N or ↓	N or ↓
Tertiary hyperparathyroidism	↑	↑	N	↑	↑	N	N or ↓	↓ or N
REDUCED PTH								
Neoplasia Humoral hypercalcemia	↑	↑	N or ↓	↓ or N	↓ or N	↑ or N	N	↓ or N or ↑
Neoplasia Local osteolytic	↑	↑	N or ↓	N or ↑	↓ or N	N or ↑	N	N
Hypervitaminosis D Calcitriol (including granulomatous inflammation)	↑	↑	N	N or ↑	↓	N	N	↑
Hypervitaminosis D Cholecalciferol (rodenticide)	↑	↑	N	↑ or N	↓	N	↑	N or ↑
NORMAL PTH								
Idiopathic	↑	↑	N	N or ↑	N or ↓	N	N	N or ↓ or ↑
MISCELLANEOUS CAUSES								
Dehydration	↑	N or ↑	↑ or N	N or ↑	N or ↓	N	N	N
Hypoadrenocorticism	↑	↑	N or ↓	↑ or N	↓ or N	N	N	↓ or N
Hyperthyroidism	N or ↑ or ↓	↑ or ↓	N	N or ↑	↑ or N or ↓	N	N	N or ↓

tCa, Total calcium; *iCa,* ionized calcium; *alb,* albumin; *PO_4,* phosphate; *PTH,* parathyroid hormone; *PTHrP,* PTH-related peptide; *25-OH vit D, calcidiol; $1,25(OH)_2$ vit D,* calcitriol; *N,* normal.

*Note that the most common conditions are highlighted yellow. Variations in expected results are indicated with the more common result noted first.

BOX 24-5

"GOSH DARN IT" Mnemonic to Help Remember Causes of Hypercalcemia

Granulomatous disease
Osteolysis
Spurious (e.g., laboratory error; presence of lipemia, hemolysis)
Hyperparathyroidism, **H**ouse plant ingestion, **H**yperthyroidism
D toxicosis (i.e., vitamin D toxicosis), **D**ehydration
Addison's disease (hypoadrenocorticism), **A**luminum toxicity
Renal disease
Neoplasia, **N**utritional
Idiopathic
Temperature (hyperthermia)

Modified from Schenck PA, Chew DJ, Behrend EN: Update on hypercalcemic disorders. In August JR, editor: *Consultations in feline internal medicine,* ed 5, St Louis, 2006, Elsevier Saunders, p 157.

BOX 24-6

"SHIRT" Mnemonic to Help Remember Common Causes of Hypercalcemia

Spurious (lipemia, hemolysis; always verify before proceeding)
Hyperparathyroidism
Idiopathic
Renal disease (mostly normal iCa despite elevated tCa)
Tumors (lymphoma, carcinoma, multiple myeloma)

Modified from Cook AK: Guidelines for evaluating hypercalcemic cats, *Vet Med* 103:392, 2008.

INCREASED PARATHYROID HORMONE WITH HYPERCALCEMIA

Hypercalcemia with increased PTH may be due to primary hyperparathyroidism or renal secondary hyperparathyroidism. Tertiary hyperparathyroidism is a rare consequence of renal secondary hyperparathyroidism. Renal disease is a far more common cause of hypercalcemia than primary hyperparathyroidism. Hypercalcemia from renal disease usually results in increased tCa but normal iCa.

Primary Hyperparathyroidism

Primary hyperparathyroidism is relatively rare in cats. One case series of 71 hypercalcemic cats recognized only four cats with this condition.[82] One small cases series of seven hyperparathyroid cats has been reported,[50] but all other publications have been case reports.* One case was reported in a cat with multiple endocrine neoplasia.[78] Further, nonfunctional parathyroid adenomas were removed from two cats, having been recognized by cervical palpation.[69] The underlying cause is commonly benign, such as adenoma, cystadenoma, or hyperplasia[17,28,50,82,93] but can be malignant adenocarcinoma.[50,57,75]

The age range of affected cats was 8 to 20 years, with no sex predisposition. There are no definitive breed predispositions; five of the seven initial cases were Siamese,[50] most subsequent cases have been mixed-breed cats, but two recent cases were Persian.[2,19]

Presenting clinical signs are generally nonspecific and consistent with hypercalcemia of any cause (see Table 24-15); polydipsia and polyuria do not seem to be commonly reported. Physical examination findings are generally nonspecific; however, a palpable parathyroid (that may be mistaken for an enlarged thyroid gland) may be present in approximately 40% of cases. One cat with probable primary hyperparathyroidism had lytic changes and disruption of normal bone architecture, affecting mainly the femoral diaphyses.[39]

Laboratory results show elevations of tCa and iCa with an inappropriately elevated PTH concentration; phosphate is suppressed by PTH and so should initially be low but may rise with impaired renal function caused by ongoing hypercalcemia. In a physiologically normal cat, hypercalcemia should suppress PTH, so a PTH concentration at the high end of the normal reference range may still suggest primary hyperparathyroidism. Further, PTH concentrations vary with time. In one case five of seven PTH measurements from the same cat were normal; the other two were notably increased.[28]

*References 2, 17, 19, 28, 39, 51, 57, 75, 93.

Ultrasound has been used as a diagnostic aid in some cases.[75,93] In one report parathyroid adenomas in two cats measured greater than 1 cm in diameter and contained hypoechoic regions with distal acoustic enhancement, compared to the hyperechoic homogenous masses.[93] In another case fluid retrieved by fine-needle aspiration from a cystic cervical mass had higher concentrations of PTH than serum from the same cat.[75]

Surgical resection of the abnormal parathyroid tissue is the treatment of choice. Before surgery, it is advisable to use fluid therapy to rehydrate the animal and attempt to reduce the severity of the hypercalcemia. Surgical approaches are as for thyroidectomy (see the section on Thyroid Gland Disorders). During surgery, the ventral and dorsal surfaces of both thyroid and parathyroid complexes should be examined. Any enlarged or discolored parathyroid tissue should be removed. Parathyroid adenomas are usually single nodules, and the remaining normal tissue is typically atrophied and can be difficult to see. However, in some cases, adenomas may be as small as 2 mm in diameter. External parathyroid adenomas are easily removed, but excision of adenomas of internal parathyroid glands may require removal of the entire thyroid and parathyroid complex on that side. It is imperative that at least one parathyroid gland is left intact to prevent permanent hypoparathyroidism. If no abnormal parathyroid gland tissue can be visualized, it is possible that an ectopic parathyroid gland is responsible. A thorough inspection of the ventral neck should be made, although an ectopic gland may be located in the cranial mediastinum. In most cases the abnormal parathyroid gland will be palpated before surgery, making the procedure relatively straightforward.[7]

Because chronic hypercalcemia leads to atrophy of normal parathyroid glands, surgical removal of the autonomously secreting gland will lead to a rapid decline in PTH levels and relative hypoparathyroidism.[6] It is therefore crucial to monitor closely for signs of hypocalcemia. Hypocalcemia that is sufficiently severe to require treatment is likely to develop within 24 to 48 hours, with clinical signs of hypocalcemia occurring 3 to 6 days after surgical removal of a parathyroid gland tumor.[87] Most reported cases have been treated preventively with calcitriol and calcium to reduce this risk, but hypocalcemia has not been a commonly recognized sequela.[28,50,51] Initiating treatment for hypocalcemia before the onset of clinical signs is not recommended because it removes the hypocalcemic stimulus to reverse parathyroid atrophy by actively inhibiting PTH secretion.[6] If hypoparathyroidism does result after surgery, it is usually transient, and treatment can be gradually withdrawn over a few months. In some cases the postoperative stabilization of serum calcium can present a major challenge.[7]

Renal Disease

Chronic renal disease (CRD) is one of the more common underlying causes of hypercalcemia in cats.[82,85] The frequency of hypercalcemia among cats with CRD has been reported from 11.5%[29] to 58%,[9] but the author recognizes far fewer than even this lower number. The degree of hypercalcemia correlates with the severity of renal disease; in one study of 73 cats with CRD, the frequency of hypercalcemia was 8% in cats with compensated renal disease, 18% in those with uremic renal disease, and 32% in cats with end-stage renal disease (that died within 21 days of sampling).[9]

Hypercalcemia caused by CRD often results in normal to low iCa, but occasionally iCa can be elevated.[9,85] Therefore normal to low iCa concentrations make underlying CRD more likely, but an elevated iCa concentration does not rule out CRD.

Insofar as hypercalcemia can *cause* CRD, the presence of both concomitantly creates a diagnostic challenge. Hypercalcemia *caused by* renal failure is usually quite mild. The primary cause is phosphate retention resulting from the failing kidneys' inability to secrete sufficient phosphate, leading to PTH secretion. Other mechanisms are also responsible, including alterations to serum protein binding and decreased GFR.[41] In most cases tCa will be increased but iCa will be normal or low (the increase in tCa being related to altered protein binding)—if this is the case, it is easier to resolve the etiology (renal failure causing the hypercalcemia), and the lack of ionized hypercalcemia means that specific therapy is not required.

Deleterious effects of hypercalcemia occur in patients with CRD only if it is associated with increases in serum iCa concentration. Consequently, clinical signs of hypercalcemia are uncommon in CRD patients, and measurement of serum iCa concentration to assess calcium status in CRD patients is important.

Tertiary hyperparathyroidism has been recognized for some time in humans. The term refers to the emergence of ionized hypercalcemia over months to years as a result of progression from renal secondary hyperparathyroidism. Consequently, the patient has elevated tCa, iCa, and PTH because of an alteration in the calcium set point to stimulate release of PTH (i.e., higher concentrations of iCa are necessary to inhibit PTH secretion).[26] As already noted, elevated iCa is sometimes recognized in cats with hypercalcemia caused by CRD[9]; however, tertiary hyperparathyroidism has not specifically been described in cats.

Prevention of phosphate retention is central to the management of CRD and has been shown to reduce renal secondary hyperparathyroidism.[11] Treatment consists primarily of dietary phosphate restriction using phosphate-restricted diets or intestinal phosphate-binding agents (or a combination of the two, if required).

There is a small chance that phosphate-restricted diets or phosphate binders can actually cause hypercalcemia. In one study 2 of 15 cats with CRD developed hypercalcemia while eating a phosphate-restricted veterinary diet designed for treatment of CRD. Hypercalcemia in these cats was associated with a decrease in serum phosphorus and low or undetectable PTH concentrations. Hypercalcemia resulted in clinical signs for one cat. In this cat the dietary therapy was stopped for 6 months. The phosphate-restricted diet was then reintroduced such that the cat was fed two thirds of its energy intake as phosphate-restricted diet and one third as ordinary commercial canned cat food, which halted the rise in plasma phosphate and PTH. The proportion of phosphate-restricted diet was subsequently increased and this reduced plasma phosphate and PTH concentrations to below pretreatment values without recurrence of the hypercalcemia. The other cat showed no clinical signs of hypercalcemia, and calcium returned to normal on cessation of the phosphate-reduced diet.[11]

Theoretically, the agents in phosphate binders could cause hypercalcemia. The most commonly used phosphate binders for cats with CRD contain aluminum phosphate. Aluminum has been shown to experimentally cause hypercalcemia and renal disease in dogs.[43] Alternative phosphate binders for cats contain calcium carbonate. Calcium carbonate is also an ingredient of many antacids used for humans, and hypercalcemia has been recognized as a result of consumption of large amounts of such antacids.[42] Hypercalcemia as a result of ingestion of aluminum hydroxide or calcium carbonate as phosphate binders has not been described in cats but is theoretically possible.

Therapy with low-dose calcitriol has been recommended as preventive management of renal secondary hyperparathyroidism in textbooks and review articles.[21,67,68] One study of 10 cats showed that PTH concentrations were not significantly different after 14 days of calcitriol administration.[47] It is possible that a longer duration of therapy is required to note benefits. An unpublished 1-year-duration randomized, controlled clinical trial failed to show any benefit in cats with varying severity of CKD; the possibility that calcitriol was of benefit was not excluded by the study.[76] Of course, overdosing a cat with calcitriol used for this purpose can, in itself, result in hypercalcemia.

DECREASED PARATHYROID HORMONE WITH HYPERCALCEMIA

The most common reason for hypercalcemia associated with suppressed levels of PTH is neoplasia. In most cases PTH is suppressed to undetectable or very low concentrations (i.e., zero or approaching zero). On some occasions cats with hypercalcemia of malignancy may have PTH concentrations in the middle of the normal reference range,[77] thus creating overlap with idiopathic hypercalcemic cats and potential diagnostic difficulties. An alternative diagnosis for suppressed PTH concentration is hypervitaminosis D, which can result from vitamin D ingestion or granulomatous inflammation.

In many cases there will be a clinical history of toxic ingestion, or potential neoplasia will be recognized at physical examination (e.g., palpation of an abdominal mass), and these overt signs should be investigated in the first instance. Further investigations of hypercalcemia are appropriate in cases when no such toxin exposure or indicative physical examination findings are present.

Distinctions may be found by measuring PTHrP or vitamin D metabolites. However, malignancy-associated hypercalcemia does not necessarily cause an increase in PTHrP, and the different forms of vitamin D create different responses depending on what the toxic agent is. PTHrP and vitamin D metabolite measurements may be considered relatively specific (false-positive results are unlikely) but not very sensitive (false-negative results are a strong possibility).

Neoplasia

Malignancy-associated hypercalcemia may result from two mechanisms:

1. Humoral hypercalcemia of malignancy (HHM)
   - Neoplastic tissues can elaborate numerous cytokines that act like PTH to stimulate bone resorption, thus elevating serum calcium
   - PTHrP is a principal mediator of this effect, but others are possible
2. Local osteolytic hypercalcemia
   - Subsequent to local invasion and dissolution of bone by the tumor

Numerous types of malignancies have been associated with hypercalcemia of malignancy. Most commonly reported is lymphosarcoma[32,33,82] (in various locations) or squamous cell carcinoma[48,54,82] (e.g., in the mandible or ear canal); hypercalcemia of malignancy has also been recognized with multiple myeloma,[14,44,90] osteosarcoma,[82] fibrosarcoma,[82] bronchogenic carcinoma,[82] leukemia,[60] renal carcinoma, and thyroid carcinoma.[77] The author has recently recognized hypercalcemia in a cat with intestinal small cell lymphoma. In many cases neoplasia will be apparent on physical examination. When hypercalcemia is recognized in a generally unwell cat and iCa is increased and PTH is very low or even unrecordable, investigations for neoplasia should take place. Increased concentrations of PTHrP indicate malignancy is present, but failure to detect increased PTHrP does not rule it out; calcidiol and calcitriol concentrations will be normal in most cases.

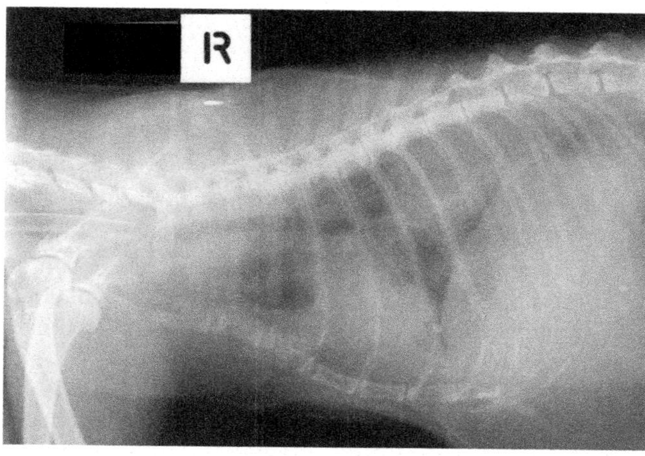

FIGURE 24-31 Lateral thoracic radiograph of a cat with hypercalcemia of malignancy caused by bronchogenic carcinoma. Note that there is not only pleural effusion and a consolidated caudal lung lobe but also osteolysis of the ninth rib. The tumor was also adhered to the diaphragm, so one diaphragmatic crus is farther cranial than the other.

Thoracic radiographs (Figure 24-31), abdominal ultrasonography, and bone marrow aspiration are all appropriate investigations. The order in which these are undertaken will depend on the clinical signs, but sometimes all three are necessary.

Treatment of malignancy-associated hypercalcemia requires treatment of the underlying malignancy; however, therapies to reduce the magnitude of hypercalcemia (discussed later) may be necessary. There are no data in cats to compare survival times of cats with neoplasia with and without hypercalcemia.

Hypervitaminosis D

Hypervitaminosis D is not very common in cats but is an important differential diagnosis for hypercalcemia of malignancy. As with malignancy, hypervitaminosis D results in elevated iCa and suppressed PTH. It is important to obtain a thorough clinical history with potential of ingestion of, or access to, known toxins (discussed later). Presence of an abdominal mass or intrathoracic lesions may indicate that the hypercalcemia is associated with granulomatous inflammation and not neoplasia. Serum calcitriol will be elevated in most cases of hypervitaminosis D (exceptions are noted later).

Granulomatous Inflammation

Hypercalcemia can result from granulomatous inflammation because macrophages can synthesize calcitriol from calcidiol without negative feedback regulation. Hypercalcemia has been recognized in cats with mycobacteriosis,[5,61] nocardiosis,[61] histoplasmosis,[45] toxoplasmosis, pulmonary cryptococcosis, *Actinomyces* rhinitis, and feline infectious peritonitis.[82] A direct association between granulomatous inflammation and hypercalcemia was not made in most reported cases, but elevated calcitriol concentrations were recognized in one cat with both nocardiosis and atypical mycobacterial infection.[61]

In most cases investigations will proceed to diagnose abnormalities found on physical examination and include thoracic radiographs and abdominal ultrasonography. Hypercalcemia may, in such cases, be wrongly considered to be due to neoplasia. An elevated calcitriol concentration can help distinguish such cases as being due to granulomatous inflammation rather than neoplasia. It is, however, theoretically possible for neoplasia to cause a granulomatous response sufficient to cause hypercalcemia; a definitive diagnosis of the cause of hypercalcemia requires cytologic or histologic assessment with culture required to identify the causative agent.

Toxic Exposures

Vitamin D toxicity is not commonly reported in cats because they seem to be resistant to cholecalciferol toxicosis if their diet is otherwise complete and balanced.[91] However, several reports from Japan in the early 1990s documented significant hypercalcemia with clinical signs resulting from hypervitaminosis D associated with commercial diets consisting of fish that contained over 100 times the minimal requirement of cholecalciferol (50 IU/100 g of diet for growing cats).[66,81]

Toxicity can occur from ingestion of vitamin D–containing plants such as *C. diurnum* (known as day-blooming cestrum, or day-blooming jessamine, or day-blooming jasmine).[31] Calcitriol may be used to treat hypoparathyroidism and potentially renal secondary hyperparathyroidism, and overdosing (perhaps after an error by a compounding pharmacist) is another potential source of toxicity.[85] All these toxicities will result in an elevation of calcitriol (1,25-dihydroxyvitamin D) with normal calcidiol (25-hydroxyvitamin D).

Ingestion of cholecalciferol-containing rodenticides such as Quintox or Rampage[65,72] can also cause hypervitaminosis D. In these circumstances calcidiol will be elevated, and calcitriol is often normal but may be elevated. Calcidiol can remain elevated for weeks to months because of lipid storage and slow release.[85]

Calcipotriol or calcipotriene is a calcitriol analog formulated as a topical dermatologic agent to treat psoriasis in people. There are anecdotal reports of cats licking this ointment from their owners' skin[85] and documented cases of toxicity in dogs.[18,34,80,98] With calcipotriol toxicity, calcidiol concentrations remain normal; calcitriol concentrations would be expected to remain normal (or perhaps be suppressed), but this is undetermined.[85]

NORMAL PARATHYROID HORMONE WITH HYPERCALCEMIA

The main consideration for a cat with hypercalcemia and normal PTH concentration is idiopathic hypercalcemia. Because cats with hypercalcemia of malignancy may have PTH levels in the lower half of the normal reference range, there can be considerable overlap with cats with idiopathic hypercalcemia. Cats for which this diagnostic dilemma occurs (but in which occult neoplasia is not detected after thoracic auscultation, abdominal ultrasonography, and bone marrow analysis) should be managed as if they had idiopathic hypercalcemia. These cats also should be serially monitored (every 3 months is appropriate for a stable cat), not only for calcium concentrations but with a thorough examination on each visit with a clinical suspicion of neoplasia. Repeat ancillary testing to look for occult neoplasia is appropriate if clinical signs arise, but after a period of time (1 year can be considered a good yardstick), idiopathic hypercalcemia becomes more likely and the need for repeat diagnostics decreases.

Idiopathic Hypercalcemia

Idiopathic hypercalcemia refers to abnormally elevated serum iCa concentration of unknown cause after extensive medical evaluation to rule out known causes of hypercalcemia.[23] It may now be the most common type of hypercalcemia and has been anecdotally recognized in North America, Europe,[23] and Australia despite being reported only in the United States.[63,88]

With idiopathic hypercalcemia serum calcium concentrations can be increased for months to years without overt clinical signs. Hypercalcemia may initially be recognized as a fortuitous discovery from a blood sample taken in a well cat (e.g., for preanesthetic screening) or a cat with an unrelated condition. One study reported as an abstract assessed 427 cats with idiopathic hypercalcemia recognized at a single diagnostic laboratory; no clinical signs were noted in 46% of cases, 18% had mild weight loss only, chronic constipation was noted in 5% of cats, and inflammatory bowel disease was seen in 6% (although it was not noted how this was diagnosed). Uroliths or renoliths were observed in 15% of cats, and calcium oxalate stones were specifically noted in 10% of cases.[88] Similarly, in an earlier series of 20 cases, 35% of cats had urolithiasis, as well as signs normally attributable to the gastrointestinal tract, such as vomiting and diarrhea.[63] The recognition of intestinal signs is interesting insofar as an association has been made between inflammatory bowel disease and renal urolith formation in humans (possibly because of poor absorption of magnesium and citrate, which are considered stone inhibitors).[59] No such association has been made in cats.

Cats with idiopathic hypercalcemia can be any age; the clinical cases series of 20 cats found an age range of 2 to 13 years (with a mean of 5.8 years)[63] compared with the larger set of 427 cats, which found a mean of 9.8 years (range 0.5 to 20 years).[88] No gender predispositions are recognized, but longhaired cats seem to be overrepresented, including both domestic longhaired cats and purebreds, such as Persians and Himalayans.[63,88]

In most cases elevations of both tCa and iCa concentrations are mild to moderate (10% to 20% above the upper limit of the reference range), but some cats can have markedly high elevations. PTH concentrations are typically normal but at the low end of the reference range, with the mean value equaling 1.1 pmol/L (range 0 to 4) in both series.[63,88] PTHrP was negative in 301 cats tested in one series[88] but increased in 1 of 11 cats in the other. The reason for the abnormally high concentration of PTHrP in this cat could not be determined, but the cat survived more than 3 years after the onset of hypercalcemia, making underlying malignancy an unlikely explanation for the high PTHrP concentration.[63] Calcitriol was normal in 12 cats in one series[88] but increased in one of seven cats in the other. Similar to the cat with increased PTH, this cat lived a further 2 years after the onset of hypercalcemia, and at postmortem examination neither neoplasia nor granulomatous disease was identified.[63]

The relationship between renal disease and idiopathic hypercalcemia is not clear-cut. Renal disease can occur secondary to longstanding idiopathic hypercalcemia (Figure 24-32); some cats with renal disease can have idiopathic hypercalcemia recognized after protracted periods of normocalcemia; in yet other cats, renal disease may be recognized concurrently with recognition of idiopathic hypercalcemia.[85]

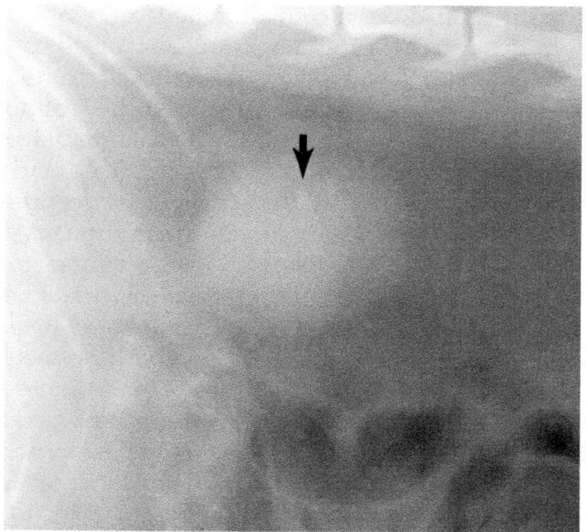

FIGURE 24-32 Small, misshapen kidneys as a consequence of idiopathic hypercalcemia. Note the small urolith (*arrow*). This cat's hypercalcemia with elevated ionized calcium and midrange parathyroid hormone was recognized more than 12 months before the development of azotemia.

Multiple factors have been considered in relation to the underlying cause of idiopathic hypercalcemia. It is unknown whether increased intestinal calcium absorption, increased bone resorption, or decreased renal calcium excretion (or some combination thereof) is the key factor leading to the development of this condition.

Three of five cats in one series[58] and all 14 cats for which diet history was available in another[63] had been fed acidifying diets designed to minimize struvite crystalluria and urolithiasis. Of course, not all cats on acidifying diets develop hypercalcemia, so these patients must have had an additional underlying factor that predisposed them to hypercalcemia. All five cats in that first series[58] had reduced serum calcium when the diet was changed to a high-fiber diet, and two of four cats that could be assessed had a partial response in the second study.[63] Genetics is another consideration, given the overrepresentation of longhaired cats.

Management of idiopathic hypercalcemia is discussed in the following section.

OTHER CAUSES OF HYPERCALCEMIA

Some causes of hypercalcemia are not appropriate for assessment in relation to PTH levels—chiefly, hypercalcemia caused by endocrinopathies. In these cases the underlying condition dictates the clinical investigations and findings, and hypercalcemia is relatively mild and resolves as the underlying disease is managed.

Hyperthyroidism

One study has recognized increased tCa, but normal iCa, in 2 of 26 hyperthyroid cats,[8] and a study of 71 hypercalcemic cats recognized 2 hyperthyroid cats.[82] Conversely, decreased iCa concentrations can be seen, and increased PTH concentration was recognized in 77% of hyperthyroid cats in one of these reports.[8] The reasons for and importance of these changes are not entirely clear. Hypercalcemia almost invariably resolves on treatment of hyperthyroidism.

Hypoadrenocorticism

Naturally occurring primary hypoadrenocorticism has been well documented in 18 cats (see the section on Adrenal Gland Disorders); of these, three cats (17%) were hypercalcemic. Additionally, one cat with iatrogenic hypoadrenocorticism and DM was hypercalcemic,[92] and in a series of 71 hypercalcemic cats, one was hypoadrenocorticoid.[82] The hypercalcemia in these patients is usually mild and has little effect on the outcome of hypoadrenocorticism. The magnitude of hypercalcemia usually parallels the severity of hyperkalemia and hypovolemia. The mechanism of hypercalcemia is unknown and typically resolves with treatment of hypoadrenocorticism.[86]

TREATMENT OF HYPERCALCEMIA

Acute Therapy

The principle treatment aim for a hypercalcemic cat is to identify and *manage the underlying condition*. Treatment to specifically reduce hypercalcemia may be necessary based on the degree of hypercalcemia or severity of clinical signs resulting from hypercalcemia. There is no absolute serum calcium concentration that can be used as a guideline for the decision to treat hypercalcemia aggressively, but a serum calcium concentration of 4 mmol/L (16 mg/dL) or greater has been recommended as a rule of thumb.[87] In practice, hypercalcemia of this magnitude can be expected to be accompanied by clinical signs such as depression, anorexia, vomiting, or dysrhythmia. Concurrent hyperphosphatemia potentiates soft tissue mineralization, and the result of multiplying serum calcium by serum phosphate (calcium × phosphate product) has been used to judge the risk of nephrotoxicity and thus help determine whether immediate treatment is required.[85] When using U.S. units (mg/dL), a calcium × phosphate product of 60 to 80 has been used as the level at which to consider treatment; this correlates to a calcium × phosphate product of approximately 5 to 6.5 when using SI units. The principles of emergency treatment of severe hypercalcemia are summarized in sequential order in Box 24-7.

Intravenous fluid therapy is the first step in symptomatic treatment of hypercalcemia. The initial aim is to correct fluid deficits, but the volume expansion not only dilutes the circulating calcium concentration but also increases renal calcium excretion. Normal (0.9%) saline is the fluid of choice and should be infused at approximately 2 to 3 times the maintenance requirements, which for most cats means 20 to 30 mL per hour. Potassium supplementation is usually required, and maintenance potassium requirements can be calculated as 5 mEq/cat every 24 hours (with additional potassium required if hypokalemia is present).

Diuretic therapy with frusemide (furosemide) can be added after rehydration and after any other electrolyte abnormalities are corrected. Diuretics are appropriate only if intravenous fluid therapy alone is not adequate to correct hypercalcemia. Bolus doses of 1 to 2 mg/kg can be used every 8 to 12 hours, or a constant-rate infusion of 2 to 6 mg/kg every 24 hours can be used. Care must be taken to ensure that the intravenous fluid rates overcome the volume loss induced by diuretic therapy.

> **BOX 24-7**
>
> **Acute Medical Management of Hypercalcemia**
>
> 1. Identify and treat underlying cause.
> 2. Fluid therapy (0.9% saline) at 2-3 times maintenance rates.
>   - Volume expansion to correct dehydration.
>   - Diuresis increases renal calcium excretion.
>   - Potassium supplementation usually required.
> 3. Diuretic therapy with frusemide (furosemide).
>   - Use when fluids alone do not resolve hypercalcemia.
>   - Ensure hydration–electrolyte balance has been corrected and is maintained.
>   - Administer 1-2 mg/kg every 8-12 hours.
> 4. Calcitonin therapy
>   - Use when fluid and diuretic therapy are not successful.
>   - Administer 4-6 IU/kg subcutaneously every 8-12 hours.
>   - May result in anorexia.
> 5. Bisphosphonates
>   - There are few reports of use in cats.
>   - Oral agents can result in esophagitis in humans.
> 6. Glucocorticoids
>   - They should not be used until all diagnostic testing is complete.
>   - They may decrease effectiveness of chemotherapy.

Calcitonin has not been frequently used in cats. It can be tried if fluid diuresis and diuretic treatment do not resolve hypercalcemia. Calcitonin is administered subcutaneously at 4 to 6 IU/kg every 8 to 12 hours. The magnitude and duration of effect are limited, although there is a fast onset of action. Calcitonin causes anorexia in dogs.[85]

Intravenous bisphosphonates have been reported to reduce hypercalcemia in two cats (pamidronate disodium)[46] and have also been used for slowing of tumor growth and pathologic bone turnover associated with oral squamous cell carcinoma (zoledronate).[101] Bisphosphonates reduce the activity and number of osteoclasts after binding to hydroxyapatite. Pamidronate was administered at 1.5 to 2 mg/kg given as a slow (approximately 4-hour) intravenous infusion diluted in normal saline; ionized calcium concentration returned to normal within 48 hours. One cat with idiopathic hypercalcemia remained normocalcemic for 9 weeks; the other cat had nocardiosis, which was successfully treated, and no recurrence was reported.[46] Adequate hydration is required before bisphosphonates should be considered insofar as nephrotoxicity is a potential risk factor.

Glucocorticoids should not be administered to hypercalcemic cats until a diagnosis has been confirmed because they can interfere with the ability to reach a diagnosis, affect chemotherapy efficacy, and reduce immunity against infectious agents (that can cause hypercalcemia associated with granulomatous inflammation). The beneficial effects of glucocorticoids to manage hypercalcemia include reducing bone resorption of calcium, decreasing intestinal calcium absorption, and increasing renal calcium excretion; they are also cytotoxic to neoplastic lymphocytes (and therefore used as part of most chemotherapeutic protocols for these types of neoplasia). The previously noted therapies are rarely unsuccessful in managing hypercalcemia acutely. It is the author's opinion that glucocorticoids should be reserved to manage hypercalcemia in chronic cases when other therapy is unsuccessful.

Chronic Therapy

The key principle for chronic therapy of hypercalcemia is the same for acute management—that is, *manage the underlying cause.* In most cases, management of the underlying cause will be sufficient to reduce hypercalcemia. Consequently, the key condition for which chronic management must be instituted is when the diagnosis is idiopathic hypercalcemia—those instances when thorough investigation fails to uncover an underlying cause. The treatment options for chronic management of hypercalcemia are summarized in Box 24-8.

BOX 24-8

Chronic Medical Management of Hypercalcemia

1. Identify and treat underlying cause.
2. Dietary therapy
   - High-fiber diets
   - Renal disease diets
   - Calcium oxalate–preventive diets
   - Canned diets
3. Subcutaneous fluids (0.9% saline)
   - Not assessed
   - Unlikely to be harmful
4. Low-dose diuretics such as frusemide (furosemide).
   - Not assessed in chronic situation
   - Potential for dehydration
   - Must evaluate for azotemia serially
5. Glucocorticoids
   - Should not be used until all diagnostic testing complete
   - Can decrease efficacy of chemotherapy
   - Prolonged use can increase risk of diabetes mellitus in susceptible cats
6. Bisphosphonates
   - Few reports in cats
   - Oral agents can result in esophagitis in humans

There have been mixed reports of the efficacy of dietary therapy in reducing hypercalcemia. One report noted a return to normocalcemia in all five cats fed a high-fiber diet.[58] In another study three cats were fed a high-fiber diet, three were fed an oxalate urolith–preventive diet, and three were fed a diet for management of CRD; there was minimal response to dietary therapy in any of these cats.[63] An oxalate urolith–preventive diet had no effect on ionized calcium concentrations in three cats with apparent idiopathic hypercalcemia in another study.[56]

High-fiber diets may increase intestinal transit time of calcium; foods designed for cats with renal disease are lower in calcium and phosphorus; oxalate urolith–preventive diets are also calcium restricted; canned diets of any description are generally calcium restricted. There is no firm evidence for the benefits of dietary therapy, but insofar as this management is very unlikely to be harmful and many cats with idiopathic hypercalcemia do not show clinical signs for years, it is appropriate to try dietary therapy in the first instance.

The author recommends starting with canned high-fiber diets (e.g., Hill's Prescription Diet w/d Feline) or adding psyllium fiber (e.g., Metamucil, Procter & Gamble) to a maintenance canned diet and rechecking calcium values at 2- to 4-week intervals. If normocalcemia is not restored after 6 to 8 weeks, alternative diets can be tried similarly. Further therapy is warranted if no benefit is noted from any diet.

Subcutaneous fluid administration at home, as is often recommended for cats with renal insufficiency, is a potential management strategy for hypercalcemic cats. It is important to note that this treatment modality has not been critically assessed for this condition. However, there are few contraindications—namely, congestive heart failure, hypoalbuminemia, and edema or other evidence of fluid overload. Fluid overloading is difficult to achieve with subcutaneous therapy but is a potential issue in a cat with, for example, an unrecognized cardiomyopathy. Certainly, subcutaneous fluid administration is a sensible approach in a hypercalcemic cat that is azotemic because the treatment will, in most cases, manage the two conditions concurrently.

Diuretic therapy with low-dose frusemide (furosemide) has also not been critically assessed as management for chronic hypercalcemia. It is imperative to use extreme caution with diuretics in an already dehydrated (azotemic) cat, including cats with renal disease. Anecdotally, the author has found that cats vary immensely in their sensitivity to frusemide (furosemide). As little as 0.5 mg/kg (or 2.5 mg/cat) frusemide (furosemide) can reduce mild hypercalcemia in many cats and usually does not result in azotemia but can cause severe azotemia in some susceptible individuals. If a low dose is not effective in reducing hypercalcemia and is not causing azotemia, the dose can slowly be titrated upward with weekly rechecks to assess calcium and azotemia. Other potential consequences of chronic diuretic administration are metabolic alkalosis with hypokalemia and reduction of sodium and chloride.

Glucocorticoids, in the form of prednisone (5 to 12.5 mg/cat daily) were effective in resolving hypercalcemia completely in four of six treated cats in one study.[63] Uncited textbook references note that 50% of cats respond to 5 to 10 mg/cat daily of prednisone or prednisolone, but some cats require up to 20 mg/cat daily to restore normocalcemia; some cats escape the effect of glucocorticoid treatment, and hypercalcemia can return despite maximal prednisone doses.[23,85] Glucocorticoid therapy *must not* be initiated until neoplasia and granulomatous inflammation have been conclusively ruled out. In these circumstances, when other therapies have been unsuccessful, prednisone (or prednisolone) can be attempted at 5 mg/cat daily for 1 month before reassessment. If iCa remains increased, the dose can be titrated upward (with reassessments). Chronic administration of corticosteroids can induce DM in susceptible individuals (see Endocrine Pancreatic Disorders). Because of the concern that increased renal excretion of calcium induced by corticosteroids has the potential to aggravate hypercalciuria and calcium oxalate urolithiasis, appropriate monitoring should be instituted.[63]

Bisphosphonates have not been thoroughly assessed but may become a routine alternative for management of hypercalcemia. Intravenous pamidronate was reported to result in normocalcemia for 9 weeks after a single dose of 1.5 to 2 mg/kg in one cat with idiopathic hypercalcemia.[46] The duration of effect is likely to vary from cat to cat and may vary with dose, but it is not unreasonable to suggest that intravenous pamidronate therapy approximately every 2 months may be appropriate management for a cat with idiopathic hypercalcemia. Further, an uncited textbook reference notes that a small number of cats have been treated successfully with 10 mg of alendronate orally once weekly for up to 1 year.[23] Erosive esophagitis is noted as a possibility in humans receiving bisphosphonates, but this risk is most associated with swallowing the medication with little or no water, lying down during or after ingestion of the tablet, continuing to take alendronate after the onset of symptoms, and having preexisting esophageal disorders.[27] These risks may be reduced in cats by following the medication with 5 mL of water syringed into the cat's mouth; dabbing butter on the cat's lips to promote licking and salivation has also been recommended.[23]

HYPOCALCEMIA

Hypocalcemia is not a common clinical finding in cats. When present, signalment and history, with other clinical and routine laboratory findings, usually give an indication of the underlying cause.[7] For example, hypocalcemia in a queen in the first few weeks after delivery is most likely due to eclampsia; low calcium after thyroidectomy is most likely due to iatrogenic hypoparathyroidism; taking a thorough dietary history will help the clinician recognize nutritional secondary hyperparathyroidism. As with hypercalcemia, serum PTH and calcitriol concentrations can help confirm a diagnosis. Calcidiol and PTHrP concentrations are not usually helpful to distinguish causes of hypocalcemia.

Clinical Signs

The clinical signs due to hypocalcemia vary depending on the severity and rate of change of iCa concentrations; mild decreases in iCa concentration may not result in obvious clinical signs.[7] Low plasma iCa increases the excitability of neuromuscular tissue. Typical signs seen are muscle tremors, stiff gait, and even generalized seizures; anorexia and lethargy are noted in cats with primary hypoparathyroidism. In severe cases circulatory effects (hypotension and decreased myocardial contractility) and paralysis of respiratory muscles can result in death.[22,73]

Underlying Causes

Hypocalcemia develops when bone mobilization of calcium is reduced, skeletal calcium accretion is enhanced, urinary losses of calcium are increased, gastrointestinal absorption of calcium is reduced, calcium is translocated intracellularly, or a combination of these mechanisms occurs.[87] Common potential underlying causes of hypocalcemia, with associated biochemistry and calcemic hormone changes, are shown in Table 24-17. It should be noted that renal disease can cause hypocalcemia as well as hypercalcemia. Hypocalcemia has also been recognized in cats with acute pancreatitis and is associated with a poorer prognosis.[53]

Primary Hypoparathyroidism

Primary hypoparathyroidism has been reported in the literature in cats on nine occasions. Aside from one small case series of five cats,[73] other descriptions have been single case reports.[12,38,71,79] This appears to be a disorder of young cats with a mean reported age of 1.8 years (range 0.5 to 6.7 years), with four cats being 1 year old or less. Approximately equal numbers of male and female cases have been reported. All but two cats were domestic shorthairs (one Himalayan and one Siamese). Clinical signs were mostly those expected with prolonged hypocalcemia, such as seizures, tremors, and tetany. Cataracts were noted in five of the nine cases; bilateral protrusion of the nictitating membrane was noted in two cats.

TABLE 24-17 **Anticipated Changes in Calcemic Hormones and Serum Biochemistry Associated with Common Disorders of Hypocalcemia**

	tCa	iCa	Alb	PO_4	PTH	PTHrP	25-OH vit D	$1,25(OH)_2$ vit D
Hypoparathyroidism Idiopathic Iatrogenic	↓	↓	N	↑ or N	↓or N	N	N	N or ↓
Secondary hyperparathyroidism Nutritional Renal	N or ↓	N or ↓	N	N or ↑	↑	N	↓ or N	N or ↓
Eclampsia	↓	↓	N	↓	Mild ↑ or N	N	N	N or ↓
Ethylene glycol toxicity	↓	↓	N	↑ or N	↑	N	N	↓ or N
Phosphate enema	↓	↓	N	↑	↑	N	N	Nor ↓ or ↑
Septic peritonitis	↓ or N	↓	↓ or N	N	↑ or N	N	N	N
Hypoalbuminemia	↓	N	↓	N	N or ↑	N	N	N or ↑

tCa, Total calcium; *iCa*, ionized calcium; *Alb*, albumin; PO_4, phosphate; *PTH*, parathyroid hormone; *PTHrP*, PTH-related peptide; *25-OH vit D*, calcidiol; *1,25(OH)₂ vit D*, calcitriol; *N*, normal.

Eight of nine hypocalcemic cats were also hyperphosphatemic (without azotemia). Some cats had elevated ALT values. PTH concentration was normal in the two cats in which it was measured. In physiologically normal cats, PTH should increase in the face of hypocalcemia. Histopathology of the parathyroid gland was assessed in three cases, and no parathyroid tissue was found in any. In one case a lymphocytic plasmacytic infiltrate was recognized adjacent to the cranial pole of a thyroparathyroid lobe,[38] suggesting an immune-mediated mechanism.

Affected cats may initially require emergency therapy with intravenous calcium gluconate but subsequently require lifelong supplementation with oral calcium and calcitriol supplementation; phosphate binders have been used to reduce high phosphate concentrations. Approaches for therapeutic requirements are the same as for all causes of hypocalcemia and will be covered later in this chapter. When appropriate therapy is instituted, the prognosis is excellent.

Iatrogenic Hypoparathyroidism

Iatrogenic hypoparathyroidism can occur subsequent to parathyroidectomy (as discussed in the section on hyperparathyroidism), bilateral thyroidectomy, sudden correction of chronic hypercalcemia of malignancy, or alkali administration.

The sudden correction of chronic hypercalcemia can lead to hypocalcemia as a result of parathyroid gland atrophy and inadequate ability to synthesize and secrete PTH. This can be a consequence of surgical excision of the affected parathyroid gland on account of primary hyperparathyroidism caused by parathyroid gland adenoma. The degree of parathyroid gland atrophy depends on the magnitude of hypercalcemia and its duration before correction. Rapid correction of hypercalcemia of malignancy after chemotherapy often results in mild hypocalcemia that is usually not associated with clinical signs, but clinical signs of hypocalcemia may occur in some cases.[87]

Postoperative hypocalcemia is reported in 6% to 82% of cats undergoing bilateral thyroidectomy, depending on the surgical method.[15,36] Hypoparathyroidism and associated hypocalcemia result from accidental removal of the external parathyroid glands or disruption of the vascular supply. This consequence becomes transient when parathyroid autotransplantation is used as outlined in the section on Thyroid Gland Disorders; in one study seven of eight cats regained normocalcemia within 20 days of bilateral thyroparathyroidectomy with parathyroid autotransplantation.[70] Hypocalcemia is a rare consequence of unilateral thyroidectomy.

The administration of alkaline agents may result in hypocalcemia. This has been recognized in a cat treated for salicylate intoxication with sodium bicarbonate.[1] Muscle fasciculations increased during treatment with sodium bicarbonate, and serum tCa was low. A single dose of intravenous sodium bicarbonate at 4 mEq/L to cats resulted in a maximal decrease of iCa 10 minutes after infusion; iCa remained below baseline for 3 hours.[20]

Nutritional Secondary Hyperparathyroidism

Nutritional secondary hyperparathyroidism was once a common nutritional disease in small animals,[13] being most frequently encountered in puppies and kittens fed exclusively all-meat diets.[89] More recent reports are sporadic,[95,100] but two very recent papers[30,64] demonstrate the continuing importance of this entity. Theoretically, nutritional secondary hyperparathyroidism may also occur when severe gastrointestinal disease is present (as has been reported in dogs and people), limiting the absorption of calcium and vitamin D.[87]

The two major forms of clinical signs reflect either complications of severe osteopenia or typical signs of hypocalcemia. Typical radiographic findings include an extensive decrease in bone opacity (osteopenia) with decreased contrast between bones and soft tissue. Cortices are thin and diaphyseal, and metaphyseal trabeculation is coarse. Longitudinal limb growth and physeal appearance are normal. Pathologic fractures are a not-uncommon consequence. In contrast, the skull tends to be predominantly affected in osteodystrophy as a result of renal secondary hyperparathyroidism. Hypocalcemia signs can include muscle twitching, excitation, or generalized seizures.[95]

The prognosis for uncomplicated cases is good, and dietary correction alone results in normalized mineralization in 4 to 8 weeks.[30,95] Supplementing diets with additional calcium may accelerate osteoid mineralization but may represent a risk for hypercalcemia when calcitriol levels are markedly increased. Vitamin D administration may also be contraindicated because of its potentiating effect, in concert with PTH, on bone resorption.[95]

Renal Secondary Hyperparathyroidism

The most likely causes of hypocalcemia in renal disease are decreased calcitriol synthesis by diseased kidneys and the response to markedly increased serum phosphorus concentration.[87] One study found that 15% of 74 cats with clinical renal disease were hypocalcemic on the basis of serum tCa.[29] Another found that hypocalcemia was underappreciated when based on results of only tCa measurement (and not iCa), especially with advancing azotemia. In that study 56% of 47 cats with advanced renal disease had ionized hypocalcemia. Only 14% of cats with moderate renal disease had ionized hypocalcemia, and no cats with "compensated" renal disease were hypocalcemic.[8]

Prevention of phosphate retention is central to the management of chronic renal disease, primarily using phosphate-restricted diets. Intestinal phosphate-binding agents can be used for additional phosphate restriction.[7] Low-dose calcitriol therapy has been recommended but is clinically unproven.[47,76]

Eclampsia

Puerperal tetany (eclampsia) is rare in cats but when present typically occurs between 1 and 3 weeks post partum and has been attributed to loss of calcium into milk during lactation.[16,99] Eclampsia was described in four cats in which hypocalcemia developed 3 to 17 days *before* parturition. Signs of depression, weakness, tachypnea, and mild muscle tremors were most common; vomiting and anorexia were less common, and prolapse of the third eyelid occurred in some cats. Hypothermia, instead of hyperthermia as seen in dogs, was observed. All cats responded to parenteral calcium gluconate initially and to oral calcium supplementation throughout gestation and lactation.[35] Calcium supplementation before parturition is not recommended for queens at risk of eclampsia because it may down-regulate PTH secretion and actually increases the risk of eclampsia.[99]

Toxic Exposures

PHOSPHATE ENEMAS

Phosphate enemas (e.g., Fleet enema, Johnson & Johnson) should not be used in cats because the rapid absorption of phosphate results in hyperphosphatemia that can be greater than five times the upper limit of normal. Such significant hyperphosphatemia results in hypocalcemia, with serum tCa decreasing within 45 minutes and persisting for 4 hours.[4,49,96]

ETHYLENE GLYCOL

Ethylene glycol ingestion can result in hypocalcemia. This is due to chelation of calcium by a metabolite and calcium deposition in soft tissues. Hypocalcemia is recognized along with acute renal failure and hyperphosphatemia.[94]

Septic Peritonitis

Hypocalcemia has been recognized with septic peritonitis in 59% of cats (20 of 34) in one study[25] and 89% of cats (49 of 55) in another.[52] No specific signs of hypocalcemia were recognized in any cat in the latter study; although 10 cats in this study received calcium supplementation, no treatment benefit could be demonstrated. Treatment could potentially result in subclinical deleterious effects such as precipitation of calcium in soft tissues or excessive intracellular calcium accumulation, leading to cell death. Therefore routine treatment of hypocalcemia in the septic patient is not recommended. Failure of iCa concentration to normalize during hospitalization may be a negative prognostic indicator.[52]

Hypoalbuminemia

Hypoalbuminemia may result in hypocalcemia because of a decrease in the protein-bound fraction of calcium. Ionized calcium should be evaluated in these circumstances but is usually normal, so clinical signs do not result. Correction formulae based on albumin concentration do not improve the prediction of actual iCa concentration and should not be used.[87]

Treatment of Hypocalcemia

Treatment of hypocalcemia must take into account the underlying cause. Treatment of acute signs of hypocalcemia such as tetany or seizures is identical regardless of cause. However, some causes of hypocalcemia, such as nutritional secondary hyperparathyroidism, eclampsia, and toxicities, will not require supplemental treatment beyond the acute phase. Conversely, conditions such as primary hypoparathyroidism and bilateral thyroparathyroidectomy (without parathyroid autotransplantation) will require lifelong treatment.

Hypocalcemia should be anticipated in cats that undergo bilateral thyroidectomy (even with parathyroid autotransplantation) because transiently lowered serum calcium concentrations can still occur. In humans, assessing PTH as well as calcium concentrations 24 hours after surgery has proved a useful predictor of postoperative hypoparathyroidism.[3] Those cats undergoing parathyroidectomy for primary hyperparathyroidism should be monitored similarly to cats undergoing thyroidectomy. Preemptive therapy to increase serum calcium concentration is appropriate for cats with marked hypocalcemia that do not yet show clinical signs.

Acute Management of Tetany or Seizures

Tetany or seizures caused by hypocalcemia are an indication for an immediate infusion of intravenous calcium gluconate, administered to effect. Ten percent calcium gluconate at a dosage of 10 to 15 mg/kg (1 to 1.5 mL/kg) is slowly infused over a 10- to 20-minute period.[22,74] Calcium gluconate is the calcium salt of choice because it is nonirritating if the solution is inadvertently injected perivascularly.[22] Heart rate and, ideally, electrocardiogram should be monitored during this infusion; bradycardia and shortening of the Q-T interval are indicators of cardiotoxicity and, if recognized, the infusion should be slowed or temporarily discontinued.

Not all clinical signs abate immediately after acute correction of hypocalcemia; there may be a lag of 30 to 60 minutes before signs such as nervousness, panting, and behavioral changes abate, despite attainment of normocalcemia. This may reflect a lag in equilibration between cerebrospinal fluid and extracellular fluid calcium concentrations.[22]

Subacute Management

The initial bolus injection of elemental calcium can be expected to decrease signs of hypocalcemia for as little as 1 hour to as long as 12 hours if the underlying cause of hypocalcemia is still present. Consequently, a constant-rate infusion of calcium gluconate administered with intravenous fluids is required at 60 to 90 mg/kg per day (2.5 to 3.75 mg/kg per hour) of elemental calcium until oral medications provide control of serum calcium concentration. Note that 10 mL of 10% calcium gluconate provides 93 mg of elemental calcium. For a 4-kg cat maintenance fluid rates are approximately 10 mL per hour, so approximately 2.5 mg/kg per hour (or 10 mg/4-kg cat per hour) of calcium is provided by adding 100 mL of calcium gluconate per 1 L fluids (as long as the fluid rate is maintained at 10 mL per hour). Calcium salts should not be added to fluids that contain lactate, acetate, bicarbonate, or phosphates because calcium salt precipitates can occur.[22,86]

Subcutaneous administration of calcium gluconate can result in iatrogenic calcinosis cutis, skin necrosis, and scarring at the injection site[79] and should be avoided. Oral calcium and calcitriol should be started as soon as possible while the cat is receiving intravenous calcium. The intravenous dose of calcium is reduced as oral calcium salts and calcitriol become effective at maintaining serum calcium.[22,74,87]

Chronic Maintenance Therapy

Maintenance therapy is required for conditions (e.g., primary or iatrogenic hypoparathyroidism) for which parathyroid function is lost permanently so that PTH cannot be produced. PTH cannot be supplemented, although supplementing with calcitriol (the secretion of which is stimulated by PTH in a physiologically normal cat) suffices in most cases.

Initially, calcium also must be supplemented. However, in most patients a complete and balanced diet supplies a normal dietary intake of calcium and is sufficient to maintain adequate serum calcium concentrations *as long as calcitriol treatment is continued*. Consequently, oral calcium salt supplementation can be tapered and, for most cats, discontinued after calcitriol reaches adequate levels.[7,87]

Calcium carbonate is the most widely used oral preparation of the calcium salts because it contains the greatest percentage of elemental calcium. Any given volume of calcium carbonate contains 40% of that volume of elemental calcium. Oral calcium is usually administered at 25 to 50 mg/kg per day by way of elemental calcium in divided doses (divided into three or four doses over a day). A 4-kg cat will require 100 to 200 mg daily of elemental calcium, which is equivalent to 250 to 500 mg daily of calcium carbonate. If serum phosphorus concentrations remain increased, oral calcium carbonate can be continued for its intestinal phosphate-binding effects.[74,87]

Calcitriol is the vitamin D metabolite of choice to provide calcemic actions because it has the most rapid onset of maximal action and the shortest biologic half-life. The dose of calcitriol can be adjusted frequently because of its short half-life and rapid effects on serum calcium concentration. If hypercalcemia occurs, it abates quickly after dose reduction. A loading dose of 20 to 30 ng/kg daily has been recommended when more rapid correction of serum calcium concentration is desirable. A maintenance dose of 10 to 20 ng/kg daily divided and given twice daily ensures sustained priming effects on intestinal epithelium for calcium absorption.[87] Dose recommendations should be taken as guidelines, and individual doses should be determined for each cat on the basis of frequent evaluation of calcium concentrations.

Commercially available calcitriol capsules (Rocaltrol, Hoffman-LaRoche) of 0.25- and 0.50-μg (250 and 500 ng) per capsule are not appropriate for cats because the doses are too high to be useful. Furthermore, it is difficult to divide capsules because active calcitriol within the capsule is in a liquid form. Fortunately, there is also a commercial liquid formulation of Rocaltrol with a concentration of 1 μg/mL that can be used to dose cats appropriately. Compounding pharmacists are also able to make up appropriate doses of calcitriol for cats.

Periods of hypocalcemia and hypercalcemia occur sporadically in patients during initial efforts to manage serum calcium concentration. During the stabilization period, serum tCa should be assessed daily. Subsequently, until target serum calcium concentration has been achieved and maintained, serum calcium should be assessed weekly. Measurement of serum tCa concentration is recommended every 3 months thereafter in animals with permanent hypoparathyroidism. Serum calcium concentration should be adjusted to just below the normal reference range. This not only lessens the likelihood that hypercalcemia will develop but also reduces the magnitude of hypercalciuria that occurs in patients with PTH deficiency. Maintaining a mildly decreased serum calcium concentration also ensures a continued stimulus for hypertrophy of the remaining parathyroid tissue in patients with postoperative hypoparathyroidism.[87]

References

1. Abrams KL: Hypocalcemia associated with administration of sodium bicarbonate for salicylate intoxication in a cat, *J Am Vet Med Assoc* 191:235, 1987.
2. Aronson L, Drobatz K: Hypercalcemia following renal transplantation in a cat, *J Am Vet Med Assoc* 217:1034, 2000.
3. Asari R, Passler C, Kaczirek K et al: Hypoparathyroidism after total thyroidectomy: a prospective study, *Arch Surg* 143:132, 2008.
4. Atkins CE, Tyler R, Greenlee P: Clinical, biochemical, acid–base, and electrolyte abnormalities in cats after hypertonic sodium phosphate enema administration, *Am J Vet Res* 46:980, 1985.
5. Baral RM, Metcalfe SS, Krockenberger MB et al: Disseminated *Mycobacterium avium* infection in young cats: overrepresentation of Abyssinian cats, *J Feline Med Surg* 8:23, 2006.
6. Barber PJ: Disorders of the parathyroid glands, *J Feline Med Surg* 6:259, 2004.
7. Barber PJ: Disorders of calcium homeostasis in small animals, *In Pract* 23:262, 2001.
8. Barber PJ, Elliott J: Study of calcium homeostasis in feline hyperthyroidism, *J Small Anim Pract* 37:575, 1996.
9. Barber PJ, Elliott J: Feline chronic renal failure: calcium homeostasis in 80 cases diagnosed between 1992 and 1995, *J Small Anim Pract* 39:108, 1998.
10. Barber PJ, Elliott J, Torrance AG: Measurement of feline intact parathyroid hormone: Assay validation and sample handling studies, *J Small Anim Pract* 34:614, 1993.
11. Barber PJ, Rawlings JM, Markweu PJ et al: Effect of dietary phosphate restriction on renal secondary hyperparathyroidism in the cat, *J Small Anim Pract* 40:62, 1999.
12. Bassett J: Hypocalcemia and hyperphosphatemia due to primary hypoparathyroidism in a six-month-old kitten, *J Am Anim Hosp Assoc* 34:503, 1998.
13. Bennett D: Nutrition and bone disease in the dog and cat, *Vet Rec* 98:313, 1976.
14. Bienzle D, Silverstein D, Chaffin K: Multiple myeloma in cats: variable presentation with different immunoglobulin isotypes in two cats, *Vet Pathol* 37:370, 2000.
15. Birchard SJ, Peterson ME, Jacobson A: Surgical treatment of feline hyperthyroidism: results of 85 cases, *J Am Anim Hosp Assoc* 20:705, 1984.
16. Bjerkas E: Eclampsia in the cat, *J Small Anim Pract* 15:411, 1974.
17. Blunden AS, Wheeler SJ, Davies JV: Hyperparathyroidism in the cat of probable primary origin, *J Small Anim Pract* 27:791, 1986.
18. Campbell A: Calcipotriol poisoning in dogs, *Vet Rec* 141:27, 1997.
19. Cavana P, Vittone V, Capucchio MT et al: Parathyroid adenocarcinoma in a nephropathic Persian cat, *J Feline Med Surg* 8:340, 2006.
20. Chew DJ, Leonard M, Muir W, 3rd: Effect of sodium bicarbonate infusions on ionized calcium and total calcium concentrations in serum of clinically normal cats, *Am J Vet Res* 50:145, 1989.
21. Chew DJ, Nagode LA: Calcitriol in treatment of chronic renal failure. In Kirk RW, Bonagura JD, editors: *Current veterinary therapy XI*, Philadelphia, 1992, Saunders, p 857.
22. Chew DJ, Nagode LA: Treatment of hypoparathyroidism. In Bonagura JD, editor: *Current veterinary therapy XIII small animal practice*, Philadelphia, 2000, Saunders, p 340.
23. Chew DJ, Schenck PA: Idiopathic Feline Hypercalcemia. In Bonagura JD, Twedt DC, editors: *Kirk's current veterinary therapy XIV*, St Louis, 2009, Saunders Elsevier, p 236.
24. Cook AK: Guidelines for evaluating hypercalcemic cats, *Vet Med* 103:392, 2008.
25. Costello MF, Drobatz KJ, Aronson LR et al: Underlying cause, pathophysiologic abnormalities, and response to treatment in cats with septic peritonitis: 51 cases (1990-2001), *J Am Vet Med Assoc* 225:897, 2004.
26. Davies DR, Dent CE, Watson L: Tertiary hyperparathyroidism, *Br Med J* 3:395, 1968.
27. de Groen PC, Lubbe DF, Hirsch LJ et al: Esophagitis associated with the use of alendronate, *N Engl J Med* 335:1016, 1996.
28. den Hertog E, Goossens MM, van der Linde-Sipman JS et al: Primary hyperparathyroidism in two cats, *Vet Q* 19:81, 1997.
29. DiBartola SP, Rutgers HC, Zack PM et al: Clinicopathologic findings associated with chronic renal disease in cats: 74 cases (1973-1984), *J Am Vet Med Assoc* 190:1196, 1987.
30. Dimopoulou M, Kirpensteijn J, Nielsen DH et al: Nutritional secondary hyperparathyroidism in two cats, *Vet Comp Orthop Traumatol* 23:56, 2010.
31. Drazner FH: Hypercalcemia in the dog and cat, *J Am Vet Med Assoc* 178:1252, 1981.
32. Dust A, Norris AM, Valli VE: Cutaneous lymphosarcoma with igg monoclonal gammopathy, serum hyperviscosity and hypercalcemia in a cat, *Can Vet J* 23:235, 1982.
33. Engelman RW, Tyler RD, Good RA et al: Hypercalcemia in cats with feline-leukemia-virus-associated leukemia-lymphoma, *Cancer* 56:777, 1985.
34. Fan TM, Simpson KW, Trasti S et al: Calcipotriol toxicity in a dog, *J Small Anim Pract* 39:581, 1998.
35. Fascetti A, Hickman M: Preparturient hypocalcemia in four cats, *J Am Vet Med Assoc* 215:1127, 1999.
36. Flanders JA, Harvey HJ, Erb HN: Feline thyroidectomy a comparison of postoperative hypocalcemia associated with three different surgical techniques, *Vet Surg* 16:362, 1987.
37. Flanders JA, Scarlett JM, Blue JT et al: Adjustment of total serum calcium concentration for binding to albumin and protein in cats: 291 cases (1986-1987), *J Am Vet Med Assoc* 194:1609, 1989.

38. Forbes S, Nelson RW, Guptill L: Primary hypoparathyroidism in a cat, *J Am Vet Med Assoc* 196:1285, 1990.
39. Gnudi G, Bertoni G, Luppi A et al: Unusual hyperparathyroidism in a cat, *Vet Radiol Ultrasound* 42:250, 2001.
40. Grosenbaugh DA, Gadawski JE, Muir WW: Evaluation of a portable clinical analyzer in a veterinary hospital setting, *J Am Vet Med Assoc* 213:691, 1998.
41. Guyton AC, Hall JE: Parathyroid hormone, calcitonin, calcium and phosphate metabolism, vitamin d, bone, and teeth. In Guyton AC, Hall JE, editors: *Textbook of medical physiology*, ed 11, Philadelphia, 2006, Elsevier-Saunders, p 978.
42. Hakim R, Tolis G, Goltzman D et al: Severe hypercalcemia associated with hydrochlorothiazide and calcium carbonate therapy, *Can Med Assoc J* 121:591, 1979.
43. Henry DA, Goodman WG, Nudelman RK et al: Parenteral aluminum administration in the dog: I. Plasma kinetics, tissue levels, calcium metabolism, and parathyroid hormone, *Kidney Int* 25:362, 1984.
44. Hickford F, Stokol T, vanGessel Y et al: Monoclonal immunoglobulin G cryoglobulinemia and multiple myeloma in a domestic shorthair cat, *J Am Vet Med Assoc* 217:1029, 2000.
45. Hodges R, Legendre A, Adams L et al: Itraconazole for the treatment of histoplasmosis in cats, *J Vet Intern Med* 8:409, 1994.
46. Hostutler R, Chew D, Jaeger J et al: Uses and effectiveness of pamidronate disodium for treatment of dogs and cats with hypercalcemia, *J Vet Intern Med* 19:29, 2005.
47. Hostutler RA, DiBartola SP, Chew DJ et al: Comparison of the effects of daily and intermittent-dose calcitriol on serum parathyroid hormone and ionized calcium concentrations in normal cats and cats with chronic renal failure, *J Vet Intern Med* 20:1307, 2006.
48. Hutson CA, Willauer CC, Walder EJ et al: Treatment of mandibular squamous cell carcinoma in cats by use of mandibulectomy and radiotherapy: seven cases (1987-1989), *J Am Vet Med Assoc* 201:777, 1992.
49. Jorgensen LS, Center SA, Randolph JF et al: Electrolyte abnormalities induced by hypertonic phosphate enemas in two cats, *J Am Vet Med Assoc* 187:1367, 1985.
50. Kallet AJ, Richter KP, Feldman EC et al: Primary hyperparathyroidism in cats: seven cases (1984-1989), *J Am Vet Med Assoc* 199:1767, 1991.
51. Kaplan E: Primary hyperparathyroidism and concurrent hyperthyroidism in a cat, *Can Vet J* 43:117, 2002.
52. Kellett-Gregory LM, Mittleman Boller E, Brown DC et al: Retrospective Study: Ionized calcium concentrations in cats with septic peritonitis: 55 cases (1990-2008), *J Vet Emerg Crit Care* 20:398, 2010.
53. Kimmel S, Washabau R, Drobatz K: Incidence and prognostic value of low plasma ionized calcium concentrations in cats with acute pancreatitis: 46 cases (1996-1998), *J Am Vet Med Assoc* 219:1105, 2001.
54. Klausner JS, Bell FW, Hayden DW et al: Hypercalcemia in two cats with squamous cell carcinomas, *J Am Vet Med Assoc* 196:103, 1990.
55. Labriola L, Wallemacq P, Gulbis B et al: The impact of the assay for measuring albumin on corrected ("adjusted") calcium concentrations, *Nephrol Dial Transplant* 24:1834, 2009.
56. Lulich J, Osborne C, Lekcharoensuk C et al: Effects of diet on urine composition of cats with calcium oxalate urolithiasis, *J Am Anim Hosp Assoc* 40:185, 2004.
57. Marquez GA, Klausner JS, Osborne CA: Calcium oxalate urolithiasis in a cat with a functional parathyroid adenocarcinoma, *J Am Vet Med Assoc* 206:817, 1995.
58. McClain H, Barsanti J, Bartges J: Hypercalcemia and calcium oxalate urolithiasis in cats: a report of five cases, *J Am Anim Hosp Assoc* 35:297, 1999.
59. McConnell N, Campbell S, Gillanders I et al: Risk factors for developing renal stones in inflammatory bowel disease, *BJU International* 89:835, 2002.
60. McMillan FD: Hypercalcemia associated with lymphoid neoplasia in two cats, *Feline Pract* 15:31, 1985.
61. Mealey K, Willard M, Nagode L et al: Hypercalcemia associated with granulomatous disease in a cat, *J Am Vet Med Assoc* 215:959, 1999.
62. Meuten DJ, Chew DJ, Capen CC et al: Relationship of serum total calcium to albumin and total protein in dogs, *J Am Vet Med Assoc* 180:63, 1982.
63. Midkiff AM, Chew DJ, Randolph JF et al: Idiopathic hypercalcemia in cats, *J Vet Intern Med* 14:619, 2000.
64. Moarrabi A, Mosallanejad B, Khadjeh G et al: Nutritional secondary hyperparathyroidism in cats under six-month-old of Ahvaz, *Iranian J Vet Surg* 3:59, 2008.
65. Moore FM, Kudisch M, Richter K et al: Hypercalcemia associated with rodenticide poisoning in three cats, *J Am Vet Med Assoc* 193:1099, 1988.
66. Morita T, Awakura T, Shimada A et al: Vitamin D toxicosis in cats: natural outbreak and experimental study, *J Vet Med Sci* 57:831, 1995.
67. Nagode L, Chew D, Podell M: Benefits of calcitriol therapy and serum phosphorus control in dogs and cats with chronic renal failure: both are essential to prevent or suppress toxic hyperparathyroidism, *Vet Clin North Am Small Anim Pract* 26:1293, 1996.
68. Nagode LA, Chew DJ: Nephrocalcinosis caused by hyperparathyroidism in progression of renal failure: treatment with calcitriol, *Semin Vet Med Surg (Small Anim)* 7:202, 1992.
69. Norsworthy G, Adams V, McElhaney M et al: Palpable thyroid and parathyroid nodules in asymptomatic cats, *J Feline Med Surg* 4:145, 2002.
70. Padgett S, Tobias K, Leathers C et al: Efficacy of parathyroid gland autotransplantation in maintaining serum calcium concentrations after bilateral thyroparathyroidectomy in cats, *J Am Anim Hosp Assoc* 34:219, 1998.
71. Parker JSL: A probable case of hypoparathyroidism in a cat, *J Small Anim Pract* 32:470, 1991.
72. Peterson EN, Kirby R, Sommer M et al: Cholecalciferol rodenticide intoxication in a cat, *J Am Vet Med Assoc* 199:904, 1991.
73. Peterson ME, James KM, Wallace M et al: Idiopathic hypoparathyroidism in five cats, *J Vet Intern Med* 5:47, 1991.
74. Peterson ME, Randolph JF, Mooney CT: Endocrine Diseases. In Sherding RG, editor: *The cat: diseases and clinical management*, ed 2, New York, 1994, Churchill Livingstone, p 1403.
75. Phillips D, Radlinsky M, Fischer J et al: Cystic thyroid and parathyroid lesions in cats, *J Am Anim Hosp Assoc* 39:349, 2003.
76. Polzin DJ, Ross S, Osborne CA: Calcitriol. In Bonagura JD, editor: *Kirk's current veterinary therapy XIV*, Philadelphia, 2008, Saunders Elsevier, p 892.
77. Provencher Bolliger A, Graham PA, Richard V et al: Detection of parathyroid hormone-related protein in cats with humoral hypercalcemia of malignancy, *Vet Clin Pathol* 31:3, 2002.
78. Reimer S, Pelosi A, Frank J et al: Multiple endocrine neoplasia type I in a cat, *J Am Vet Med Assoc* 227:101, 2005.
79. Ruopp J: Primary hypoparathyroidism in a cat complicated by suspect iatrogenic calcinosis cutis, *J Am Anim Hosp Assoc* 37:370, 2001.
80. Saedi N, Horn R, Muffoletto B et al: Death of a dog caused by calcipotriene toxicity, *J Am Acad Dermatol* 56:712, 2007.
81. Sato R, Yamagishi H, Naito Y et al: Feline vitamin D toxicosis caused by a commercially available cat food, *J Japan Vet Med Assoc* 46:577, 1993.
82. Savary K, Price G, Vaden S: Hypercalcemia in cats: a retrospective study of 71 cases (1991-1997), *J Vet Intern Med* 14:184, 2000.
83. Schenck PA, Chew DJ: What's new in assessing calcium disorders Part 1, *Proc 21st ACVIM Forum* 2003;517.

84. Schenck PA, Chew DJ: What's new in assessing calcium disorders Part 2, *Proc 21st ACVIM Forum* 2003;519.
85. Schenck PA, Chew DJ, Behrend EN: Update on hypercalcemic disorders. In August JR, editor: *Consultations in feline internal medicine*, ed 5, St Louis, 2006, Elsevier Saunders, p 157.
86. Schenck PA, Chew DJ, Jaeger JQ. Clinical disorders of hypercalcemia and hypocalcemia in dogs and cats, *Proc 21st ACVIM Forum* 2003, p 521.
87. Schenck PA, Chew DJ, Nagode LA et al: Disorders of calcium: hypercalcemia and hypocalcemia. In DiBartola SP, editor: *Fluid, electrolyte and acid-base disorders in small animal practice*, ed 3, St Louis, 2006, Saunders Elsevier, p 122.
88. Schenck PA, Chew DJ, Refsal K et al: Calcium metabolic hormones in feline idiopathic hypercalcemia [abstract], *J Vet Intern Med* 18:442, 2004.
89. Scott PP: Nutritional secondary hyperparathyroidism in the cat, *Vet Med Small Anim Clin* 62:42, 1967.
90. Sheafor S, Gamblin R, Couto C: Hypercalcemia in two cats with multiple myeloma, *J Am Anim Hosp Assoc* 32:503, 1996.
91. Sih T, Morris J, Hickman M: Chronic ingestion of high concentrations of cholecalciferol in cats, *Am J Vet Res* 62:1500, 2001.
92. Smith S, Freeman L, Bagladi-Swanson M: Hypercalcemia due to iatrogenic secondary hypoadrenocorticism and diabetes mellitus, *J Am Anim Hosp Assoc* 38:41, 2002.
93. Sueda MT, Stefanacci JD: Ultrasound evaluation of the parathyroid glands in two hypercalcemic cats, *Vet Radiol Ultrasound* 41:448, 2000.
94. Thrall MA, Grauer GF, Mero KN: Clinicopathologic findings in dogs and cats with ethylene glycol intoxication, *J Am Vet Med Assoc* 184:37, 1984.
95. Tomsa K, Glaus T, Hauser B et al: Nutritional secondary hyperparathyroidism in six cats, *J Small Anim Pract* 40:533, 1999.
96. Tomsa K, Steffen F, Glaus T: [Life threatening metabolic disorders after application of a sodium phosphate containing enema in the dog and cat], *Schweiz Arch Tierheilkunde* 143:257, 2001.
97. Toribio R, Kohn C, Chew D et al: Cloning and sequence analysis of the complementary DNA for feline preproparathyroid hormone, *Am J Vet Res* 63:194, 2002.
98. Torley D, Drummond A, Bilsland DJ: Calcipotriol toxicity in dogs, *Br J Dermatol* 147:1270, 2002.
99. Waters CB, Scott-Moncrieff JCR: Hypocalcemia in cats, *Comp Contin Educ Vet* 14:497, 1992.
100. Watson ADJ: Treatment of nutritional secondary hyperparathyroidism in the cat, *Can Vet J* 24:107, 1983.
101. Wypij JM, Fan TM, Fredrickson RL et al: In vivo and in vitro efficacy of zoledronate for treating oral squamous cell carcinoma in cats, *J Vet Intern Med* 22:158, 2008.

CHAPTER

25

Hematology and Immune-Related Disorders

Edward Javinsky

OUTLINE

Blood and immune diseases are relatively common in cats and often caused by infectious agents. Many of the presenting signs are nonspecific, requiring a detailed and logical investigation into their cause. Understanding normal physiology is important in recognizing disease. This chapter covers some diagnostic techniques useful in evaluating cats with blood disease. Important, non-neoplastic blood and systemic immune dysfunction is discussed, with an emphasis on diagnosis and treatment. Specific immune disorders of the skin and joints are covered in Chapters 22 and 26, and neoplastic diseases are discussed in Chapter 28.

DIAGNOSTIC TECHNIQUES

Bone Marrow Collection

Bone marrow evaluation is an underutilized technique in veterinary medicine. Any veterinarian with the easily obtained proper supplies can collect bone marrow. For a diagnostic technique so full of potential rewards, the risks are minimal. As with any other diagnostic test, proper patient selection is important to avoid performing an unnecessary procedure.

Indications

Indications for obtaining a sample of bone marrow include the presence of an unexplained nonregenerative anemia, neutropenia, thrombocytopenia, or combination of cytopenias (Box 25-1). Bone marrow collection can be used to stage neoplasia or determine the etiology of hypercalcemia or hypergammaglobulinemia that may be caused by lymphosarcoma or multiple myeloma. Although most healthy cats do not have visible iron stores in the bone marrow, the presence of iron here will eliminate iron deficiency as a cause of anemia.[34] Additional indications for collecting bone marrow include the inappropriate presence of immature hematopoietic cells in the circulation, unexplained leukocytosis or thrombocytosis, and dysplastic changes in the circulating blood cells. Routine evaluation of the bone marrow is not helpful in sorting out the causes of absolute erythrocytosis (polycythemia) because the erythroid morphology of the marrow appears the same in all cases (erythroid hyperplasia).[47]

Contraindications

There are few contraindications for collecting a sample of bone marrow when it is warranted. Most of these relate to the severity of the cat's condition and its ability to tolerate sedation or general anesthesia. Hemorrhage as a result of the bone marrow collection is uncommon even in situations of severe thrombocytopenia. The veterinarian should not hesitate to collect bone marrow when it is indicated.

Equipment and Supplies

Most hospitals will have, or can easily obtain, the supplies required to collect a bone marrow sample. These supplies include a bone marrow biopsy needle, chemical restraint, surgical scrub, sterile fenestrated surgical

BOX 25-1

Indications for Sampling Bone Marrow

Abnormal Peripheral Blood Findings

- Unexplained anemia, leukopenia, or thrombocytopenia
- Unexplained leukocytosis or thrombocytosis
- Myeloproliferative disease
- Lymphoproliferative disease
- Abnormal blood cell morphology
- Rubricytosis (increased nucleated erythrocytes) without polychromasia
- Neutrophilic left shift without inflammatory disease

Historical or Physical Findings

- Fever of unknown origin
- Occult disease
- Unexplained lymphadenopathy
- Drug toxicity
- Neoplasia

Therapeutic Monitoring

- Hematopoietic disorders
- Neoplasia

Abnormal Serum Biochemical Changes

- Unexplained hypercalcemia
- Monoclonal gammopathy
- Polyclonal gammopathy
- Proof of adequate iron stores (normal cats may have no identifiable stored iron)

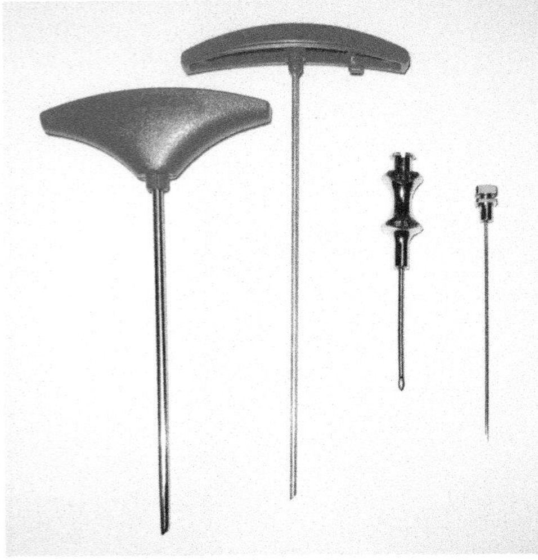

FIGURE 25-1 Bone marrow biopsy needles. *Left to right,* Jamshidi disposable core-aspiration biopsy needle (11-gauge, 4 inches), stylet for the Jamshidi biopsy needle, Rosenthal reusable core-aspiration biopsy needle (16-gauge, $1\frac{5}{16}$ inches), stylet for the Rosenthal needle.

drape, slides, anticoagulant, a 12-mL syringe, a dozen glass microscope slides, sterile gloves, and a scalpel blade. If a core biopsy will be performed, tissue fixative such as 10% formalin will be required. Local anesthesia will be used for patients in which chemical restraint is contraindicated. Other supplies that may be useful, but are not required, include pipettes and microhematocrit tubes.

Several types of bone marrow needles are available (Figure 25-1). An 18-gauge needle is an appropriate size for collecting marrow from a cat. The Jamshidi and Rosenthal needles are made of stainless steel and can be heat sterilized. The Illinois needle contains plastic and requires gas or cold sterilization. The presence of a stylet in the needle keeps the lumen from becoming plugged with a core of cortical bone at the beginning of the procedure. The stylet must be completely in place until the actual sample is collected, or a frustrating obstruction of the needle will occur. For hospitals without a bone marrow needle, an 18-gauge venipuncture needle may be substituted. Because there is no stylet to keep the lumen open, an obstruction of the venipuncture needle is likely. This means a second needle will be needed, and dexterity will be required to find the hole in the cortical bone made by the first needle.

Bone marrow collection is a painful procedure. The struggling of an uncooperative and anxious patient makes collecting a diagnostic sample difficult. It may also be unethical to put a cat through unnecessary pain and anxiety when chemical restraint is available; trauma to assistants can also be avoided. If chemical restraint is not appropriate, a local anesthetic can be used to minimize the pain of passing the needle through the skin to the periosteum. Cortical bone itself has no pain receptors. Unfortunately, the endosteum cannot be anesthetized, and most of the pain of this procedure occurs when the endosteum is torn during sample collection.

Bone marrow clots readily when collected. The use of an anticoagulant is recommended so that there is no rush to process the sample after collection. A 2.5% solution of ethylenediaminetetraacetic acid (EDTA) can be made by injecting 0.35 mL of sterile saline into a 3-mL lavender-top EDTA blood collection tube. The contents are withdrawn and injected into a second EDTA tube.[71] The resulting 0.5 mL volume is placed in a 12-mL syringe and should be adequate for preventing coagulation of the collected marrow sample.

Collection Sites

Bone marrow can be collected from one of three sites: the proximal humerus (Figure 25-2), the iliac crest, or the femur (Figure 25-3). The proximal humerus is easily accessible, has little overlying tissue, and offers a large

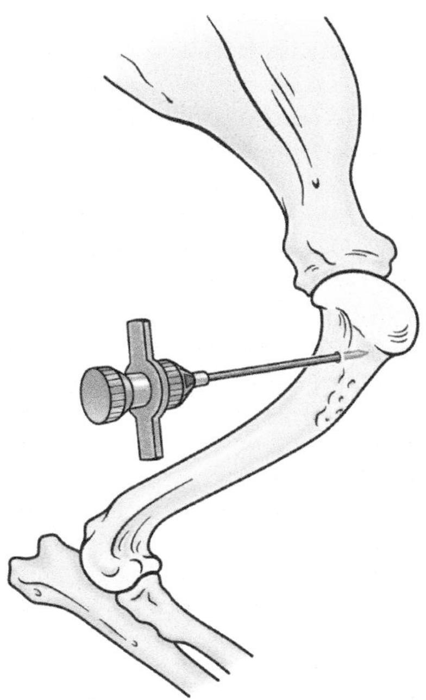

FIGURE 25-2 Bone marrow collection site from the proximal humerus. *(Redrawn from Grindem CB: Bone marrow biopsy and evaluation,* Vet Clin North Am *19:674, 1989.)*

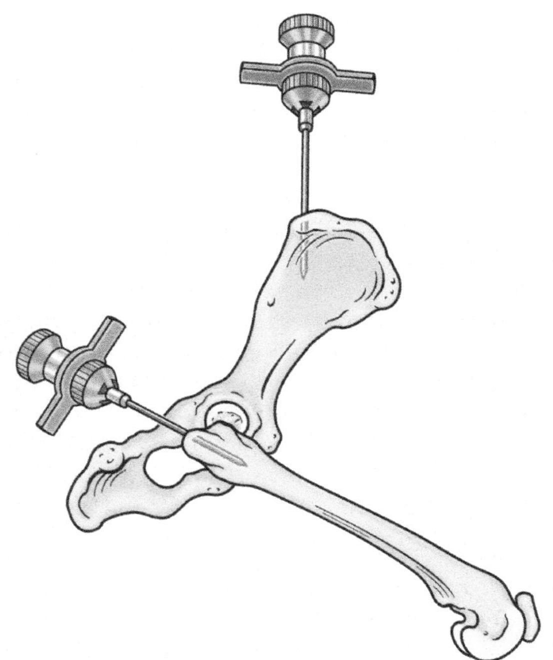

FIGURE 25-3 Bone marrow collection sites from the iliac crest and the proximal femur. *(Redrawn from Grindem CB: Bone marrow biopsy and evaluation,* Vet Clin North Am *19:673, 1989.)*

surface for needle placement. The greater tubercle is palpated, and the needle inserted into the flat surface of the craniolateral humerus just distal to the tubercle. The needle is inserted in a craniomedial direction perpendicular to the long axis of the bone.

The iliac crest may be wide enough only in large cats and is difficult to palpate in obese patients. The needle is directed ventrally and slightly medially into the most dorsally palpable portion of the ilium, where the bone is widest. Occasionally, the needle will come to rest against the opposing cortical wall. If aspirating a sample from the iliac crest is difficult, the clinician should withdraw the needle slightly before concluding that the procedure is a failure.

The proximal femur is an easily accessed site for collecting marrow from cats. The greater trochanter is palpated and the needle inserted into the trochanteric fossa medial to the trochanter. The needle is directed parallel to the long axis of the femur. A potential, but uncommon, complication with using this site is damage to the sciatic nerve running medial and caudal to the greater trochanter. There should be plenty of room, however, to obtain the sample while leaving the nerve untouched.

Aspiration Biopsy

Before preparing the patient, the veterinarian should place all the materials in easy reach. A surgical tray is an excellent choice. Once the cat is anesthetized, it is placed in lateral recumbency with the side to be sampled facing up. The area is shaved, surgically prepared, and draped. While wearing sterile gloves, the veterinarian makes a small incision in the skin and superficial subcutaneous tissue. The incision need only be large enough for the needle to pass through. The veterinarian holds the needle between the thumb and middle finger with the index finger along the shaft for stabilization. The top of the stylet should rest against the palm of the hand so that it does not become displaced during the passage through the cortical bone. The grip is more like holding a screwdriver than a pen and allows for more force to be placed on the needle during the procedure. The veterinarian firmly holds the limb with one hand while advancing the needle through the incision down to the bone.

After ensuring the proper orientation of the needle, the veterinarian begins advancing through the cortical bone with firm clockwise and counterclockwise rotations while maintaining proper orientation. When the needle is properly placed, it will feel solidly seated. For example, if the veterinarian is collecting from the proximal femur, the cat's whole leg should move when the needle is fanned. If the seating does not feel proper or the needle slides down the side of the bone into the soft tissue, the veterinarian should withdraw it to the level of the cortical bone, reposition if necessary, and try again. When the needle is in the soft tissue, it is freely movable.

Once the needle is firmly in the bone, the stylet is removed. If an 18-gauge blood collection needle is being used, it should be removed and a second needle placed in the same hole in the cortical bone. The anticoagulated 12-mL syringe is placed on the end of the needle, and the plunger of the syringe is pulled rigorously to aspirate the marrow. A sample may be obtained with the first aspiration, or several attempts may be required. If no marrow is aspirated, the stylet is replaced. If it does not go all the way in, there may be a bony plug at the end of the needle. If the stylet resumes its normal position, the veterinarian should continue advancing the needle for a short distance and try again.

Once a sample appears in the syringe, no more than 1 or 2 mL of marrow is required. The syringe is removed from the needle and rocked gently to mix the sample with the anticoagulant. The marrow is then expelled onto a glass microscope slide. It should look like blood with small particles in it. The slide is then tilted to allow blood to run off onto a paper towel. What remains on the slide are the whitish to gray bone marrow spicules. These can be collected with a pipette, a microhematocrit tube, or the end of another glass slide. The sample is transferred to a slide and covered with a second slide. The sample is allowed to spread a small amount, and then the two slides are rapidly but gently slid apart. Little, if any, pressure should be applied because this may damage the cells. If a sufficiently large sample is collected, about 12 slides should be made in this manner; if not, as many slides should be made as the sample allows. These slides should be air dried and submitted to the laboratory along with a sample of peripheral blood in a lavender-top tube. The interpretation of a bone marrow sample should always be made in the light of a complete blood cell count (CBC). If the patient suffers from severe thrombocytopenia, direct pressure should be applied to the wound once the needle is removed.

Aspiration of marrow allows for a cytologic evaluation, but architecture cannot be assessed. It is recommended to perform both an aspiration and a core biopsy of the bone marrow so that the procedure does not have to be repeated at a later date. A core biopsy is also recommended if there is a dry tap. Potential causes for a dry tap include myelofibrosis, myelophthisis, marrow necrosis or aplasia, and operator error. The only additional supply required for a core biopsy is tissue fixative. The veterinarian must remember to remove any cytology preparations away from the area when working with formalin. The fumes released when the vial is opened can fix the prepared slides, preventing proper staining of the cells.

Core Biopsy

If an aspiration of the bone marrow has been performed, the needle should still be in place. If not, the veterinarian should follow the instructions for performing an aspiration of bone marrow without aspirating any bone marrow. Collecting a core sample of bone marrow from a separate site may increase the likelihood of identifying metastatic neoplasia.[71]

Once the needle is seated firmly in the bone, or if it is still in place after aspiration, it is advanced another 1 to 1.5 cm, with the stylet removed, using the same rotational pressure as before. This maneuver should cut a core out of the marrow. At this point the needle need no longer be advanced. The core is broken off by several clockwise revolutions of the needle followed by several counterclockwise twists. The needle is withdrawn a short distance and advanced slightly again, this time at an angle slightly off axis. It should be twisted in both directions several times so that the bevel of the needle cuts the core off at the endosteum. The needle is removed by again rotating in both directions. The core sample should be gently pushed out of the top of the needle using the stylet. Bone marrow biopsy needles are tapered at the beveled end, and forcing the core sample through the tip will damage the sample. Once removed, the core can be rolled on a glass microscope slide for cytology if an aspirate has not been obtained. The veterinarian then places the sample into tissue fixative, remembering to remove any cytology preparations from the area before opening a jar of formalin to avoid having the fumes fix the cells on the slide. Direct pressure is placed on the wound to prevent hematoma formation in cats with severe thrombocytopenia.

With a little practice and the proper supplies, which all clinics can obtain easily, the cause of unexplained changes in circulating cells may be elucidated. More specific therapy may then be possible. Other than the risks involved with an anesthetic, there are few, if any, contraindications to the procedure.

Cross-Match

A crossmatch test can identify compatibility or incompatibility between the blood donor and transfusion recipient. It tests for the presence of alloantibodies, induced or naturally occurring, for which blood typing does not test. At the present time, typing for the *Mik* erythrocyte antigen is not readily available. Other, unknown erythrocyte antigens may be present and cause blood incompatibility. Because of the potential presence of unknown alloantibodies in feline blood, a cross-match should be performed before any transfusion, even if both donor and recipient are blood typed and a prior cross-match has indicated compatibility.

The major cross-match tests for alloantibodies in the plasma of the recipient that may hemolyze the donor's red cells. The minor cross-match tests for alloantibodies in the plasma of the donor that may attack the recipient's erythrocytes. Autoagglutination in the major cross-match predicts that antibodies in the recipient's plasma will attack the donor's red cells, likely eliciting a transfusion reaction. A minor cross-match incompatibility suggests that antibodies in the donor's blood will attack the recipient's red cells. Incompatible blood should not be used for transfusions.

A quick means of performing a major cross-match is to mix 2 drops of plasma from the recipient with 1 drop of anticoagulated blood from the donor on a slide at room temperature.[35] The opposite will be a minor cross-match. Development of macroscopic agglutination within a minute suggests the presence of anti-A alloantibodies in the plasma sample of the recipient (major cross-match) or donor (minor cross-match). In either case the blood is incompatible. Autoagglutination can make interpretation of the test difficult. Running a control test using saline instead of plasma may help with interpretation.

For hospitals performing frequent transfusions, a standardized gel agglutination test is available for in-hospital use. Although more time consuming than the previously described method, the gel test is less vulnerable to operator interpretation error. Because it is stable, the test result can be saved and reviewed at a later time if needed.[118] Two commercially available products include the DiaMed-ID cross-match gel (DiaMed, Switzerland) and the Rapid Vet-H companion animal cross-match gel (DMS Laboratories, Flemington, New Jersey). More rigorous and time-consuming methods involving washing, centrifuging, and incubating samples have been published.[25,42]

Slide Agglutination Test

A positive, properly performed slide agglutination test suggests the presence of antibody-coated erythrocytes and negates the need for performing a direct Coombs' test. It is important to differentiate erythrocyte clumping caused by autoagglutination from that caused by rouleaux formation. These types of erythrocyte clumping are differentiated by washing the cells with saline, which will reliably break up clumps formed by rouleaux. A quick method of performing the test is to mix a drop of EDTA anticoagulated blood on a slide with 2 to 5 drops of 0.9% NaCl followed by a gross and microscopic examination of the sample.[54] The "stacked coins" appearance characteristic of rouleaux formation (Figure 25-4) will disperse, whereas the random or rosette clumping of autoagglutination will not (Figure 25-5). If the test is negative, a direct Coombs' test should be requested. An important limitation to this test is its inability to separate primary from secondary immune-mediated disease.

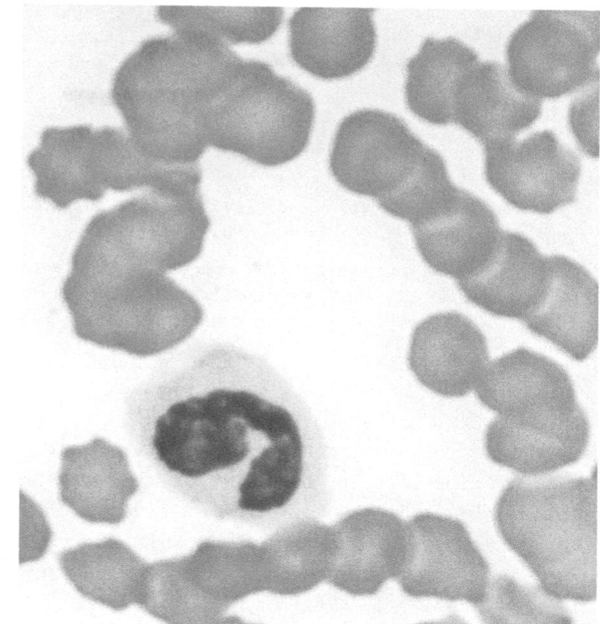

FIGURE 25-4 The "stack of coins" arrangement associated with rouleaux formation. *(Courtesy Rick Cowell.)*

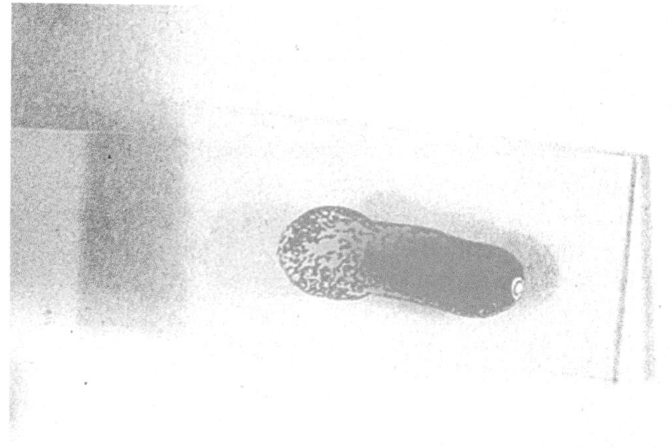

FIGURE 25-5 Macroscopic agglutination is apparent on the slide. If clumping remains after proper washing, autoagglutination would be the conclusion. *(From Fry MM, McGavin MD: Bone marrow, blood cells, and lymphatic system. In McGavin MD, Zachary JF, editors:* Pathologic basis of veterinary disease, *ed 4, St Louis, 2007, Mosby.)*

ERYTHROCYTE PHYSIOLOGY AND DIAGNOSTIC EVALUATION

The erythrocyte is a unique cell with a singular function: to carry oxygen to the tissues. Decreased numbers of red blood cells results in decreased tissue oxygenation; however, an excessive number of erythrocytes make blood more viscous, potentially resulting in less than optimal oxygenation. Changes in the visual appearance of erythrocytes yield clues as to the underlying disease. A change in red blood cell numbers is a sign of disease, not a disease itself. Therefore a change in erythrocyte numbers or appearance requires investigation of the etiology.

The production of erythrocytes by the bone marrow is influenced by the hormone erythropoietin (EPO),

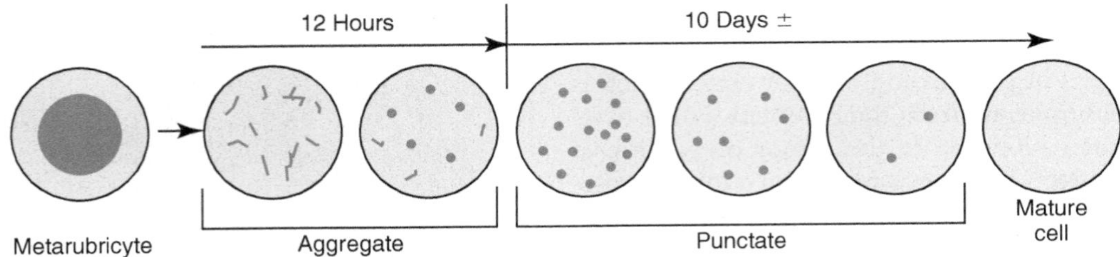

FIGURE 25-6 Diagram depicting the progressive maturation of feline reticulocytes. Aggregate reticulocytes lose their inclusions and mature into punctate reticulocytes in approximately 12 hours. The punctate reticulocytes slowly lose their inclusions over a period of around 10 days. *(From Weiser MG: Disorders of erythrocytes and erythropoiesis. In Sherding RG, editor:* The cat: diseases and clinical management, *ed 2, Philadelphia, 1994, Saunders.)*

which is produced by fibroblasts adjacent to the renal tubules near the corticomedullary junction in response to decreased local oxygen tension.[129] Increased EPO production begins within minutes of onset of hypoxia, with maximal production occurring 24 hours later. Colony-forming-unit erythrocytes in the bone marrow respond to increased concentrations of EPO by increasing production, maturation, and release into circulation of new red cells. Increasing numbers of new circulating erythrocytes will not be apparent for at least 2 or 3 days.

When hypoxia is caused by anemia, immature erythrocytes are released early to the circulation. The immaturity of the released cells is proportional to the severity of the anemia. Reticulocytes are immature erythrocytes that still contain ribosomes, are larger than mature red cells, and have lower concentrations of hemoglobin. The ribosomes stain a bluish color, giving reticulocytes their characteristic blue-gray color. Their presence in circulation is responsible for the variation in cell size and color observed on a blood smear examination in regenerative anemias.

Two types of feline reticulocytes are recognized: aggregate and punctate. Aggregate reticulocytes have long, linear chains of ribosomes; are larger and bluer than mature red cells; and are the less mature of the two types of reticulocytes. The ribosomes appear dark blue after staining with new methylene blue. Most of the ribosomes are removed within 12 hours as the cell matures into a punctate reticulocyte. Punctate reticulocytes have a few small dots representing the remaining ribosomes and are the color of a mature red cell. It takes up to 10 to 14 days for the remaining ribosomes to be removed and the cell to become a mature erythrocyte. Some punctate reticulocytes are present in healthy cats, and punctate reticulocytes may be present in the circulation for up to 1 month after an anemic event.

It is important to realize that these two types of reticulocytes are not different cells but rather a progression in the maturation of the erythrocyte (Figure 25-6). As the anemia becomes more severe, younger reticulocytes are released in an attempt to increase the number of oxygen-carrying red cells. The result is an increase in the number of aggregate reticulocytes in the circulation. Because they mature so quickly to punctate reticulocytes, the presence of increased numbers of circulating aggregate reticulocytes suggests ongoing hypoxia. An important concept regarding feline anemia is that an increase in the numbers of aggregate reticulocytes (above the reference range for the laboratory) is required before a moderate to severe anemia is considered regenerative. Unless the anemia is mild, and the more immature aggregate reticulocytes are not required, the presence of punctate reticulocytes alone is not evidence of regeneration. In cats the absolute number of aggregate reticulocytes is a more reliable indicator of regeneration than the corrected reticulocyte percentage or the reticulocyte production index.[54]

EPO also stimulates hemoglobin synthesis. Feline hemoglobin is unique in that it has less affinity for oxygen than the hemoglobin found in other species; consequently, oxygen is more easily released to the tissues. This may be one explanation for why the packed cell volume (PCV) and hemoglobin concentration in the normal cat are lower than those of normal dogs.[54] In a healthy cat the production and removal of erythrocytes is balanced. The life span of the normal, mature feline erythrocyte is approximately 73 days, after which they are removed from circulation by macrophages in the spleen, and the heme and iron recycled.

Quantitative Erythrocyte Parameters

Erythrocytes can be classified by their size and hemoglobin concentration on the basis of quantitative parameters such as the mean corpuscular volume (MCV, the average cell size), the red cell distribution width (RDW), and the mean corpuscular hemoglobin concentration (MCHC). *Macrocytosis, normocytosis,* and *microcytosis* refer to cell size above, within, or below the reference range, respectively. The RDW is derived from the cell numbers versus cell volume histogram (Figure 25-7); an increase in RDW indicates a greater than normal variation in cell size. The RDW may be artifactually affected by the overlap in size between feline platelets and red cells. *Normochromia* and *hypochromia* refer to MCHC within or below the reference range, respectively. Hemoglobin makes up approximately 33% of the volume of the cell. Erythrocytes cannot carry more hemoglobin in their cytoplasm than normal, so they cannot be hyperchromic. An increased MCHC is usually associated with hemolysis, either a result of disease or of improper venipuncture or sample handling. A change in any of these parameters requires a review of a blood smear for an explanation.[126]

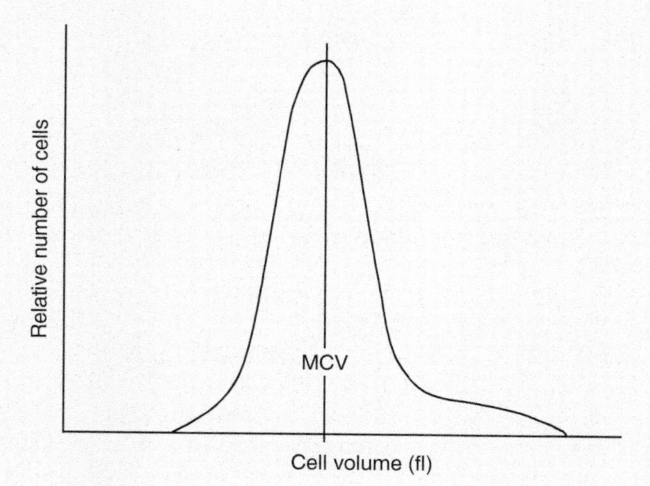

FIGURE 25-7 The erythrocyte volume distribution histogram. The mean cell volume is represented by the *vertical bar.* Increased variation in cell volume (anisocytosis) causes the curve to widen, increasing the red cell distribution width (RDW). *(From Weiser MG: Disorders of erythrocytes and erythropoiesis. In Sherding RG, editor:* The cat: diseases and clinical management, *ed 2, Philadelphia, 1994, Saunders.)*

Qualitative Erythrocyte Parameters

Qualitative erythrocyte parameters are based on a blood smear evaluation. Increased variations in cell size, color, and shape are known as *anisocytosis, polychromasia,* and *poikilocytosis,* respectively. Anisocytosis is present if there is a combination of normal-size cells along with an appreciable number of larger or smaller cells. Anisocytosis may result in an increased RDW. The larger cells are often reticulocytes, although infection with the feline leukemia virus (FeLV) can result in larger cells without increased reticulocyte numbers. Polychromasia is usually due to the presence of increased numbers of aggregate reticulocytes and indicates regeneration.[126] Lack of polychromasia, however, does not rule out regeneration.[18] Variations in cell shape may be artifactual or due to disease (Figure 25-8). Echinocytes are crenated red cells with uniform, often pointy, projections. They are usually artifacts but are important to recognize; when the projections are viewed end on, they may appear as small rings and mimic the ring form of hemoplasmosis (e.g., *Mycoplasma haemofelis).* Acanthocytes are similar to echinocytes but have fewer and more rounded projections. They are frequently present in cats with hepatic disease. Erythrocyte fragments, such as schistocytes or keratocytes, are the result of cell trauma. When there are many fragments, the presence of turbulent blood flow or microangiopathic disorders such as hemangiosarcoma or disseminated intravascular coagulation (DIC) should be considered. Iron deficiency may also cause increased fragmentation.[18] Spherocytes are smaller cells that are

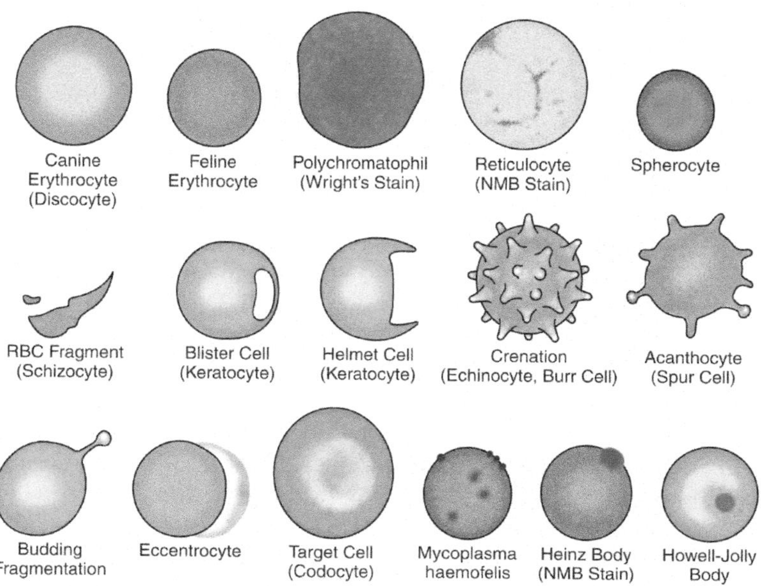

FIGURE 25-8 Some common terms and synonyms are given beneath a drawing of selected morphologic changes in red blood cells. These illustrations are of the cell as it appears on a Wright-stained smear, except for reticulocytes and Heinz bodies, which are preferentially stained with new methylene blue. A canine erythrocyte is included for comparison purposes. *(From Weiss D, Tvedten H: The complete blood cell count and bone marrow examination: general comments and selected techniques. In Willard MD, Tvedten H, editors:* Small animal diagnosis by laboratory methods, *ed 4, St Louis, 2004, Saunders.)*

the product of immune-mediated removal of antibody-coated parts of the erythrocyte membrane, after which the cell is reconfigured into a sphere. Because normal feline erythrocytes are small and lack central pallor, spherocytosis in this species is difficult or impossible to appreciate and identification is best left to an experienced veterinary hemocytologist.

Microagglutination and rouleaux formation may be visible on blood smears. Agglutination appears as a random, disorganized clumping of cells not dispersed by the addition of saline. True autoagglutination indicates an immune-mediated disease affecting the erythrocyte. Rouleaux formation looks similar to a stack of coins (see Figure 25-4) and will disperse after the addition of saline (see Figure 25-5). Circulating monocytes may phagocytose antibody-covered red cells; this is called *erythrophagocytosis.* Although not observed very often, erythrophagocytosis also suggests the presence of immune-mediated red cell damage. Heinz bodies are areas of oxidatively denatured hemoglobin within the cell (discussed later). The altered hemoglobin is pushed off to one side and often seen as a projection off the surface of the cell membrane. Heinz bodies stain dark with new methylene blue stain, somewhat clear with Diff-Quik, and the same as the cytoplasm with Wright's stain[18] (Figures 25-9 and 25-10). Howell–Jolly bodies are intracytoplasmic remnants of nuclear material found in erythrocytes that may mimic red cell parasites. Blood smear examination is an essential part of a CBC, particularly when it comes to evaluating the erythron. There is no other way to identify the morphologic changes in red cells that can yield clues to the etiology of erythrocyte disease. Without a blood smear evaluation, a CBC is incomplete.

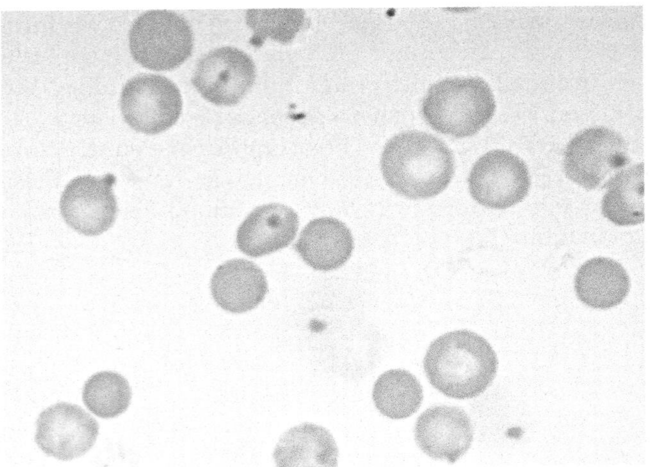

FIGURE 25-9 Heinz bodies appear as dark-stained structures in this new methylene blue–stained smear of feline blood. *(Courtesy Rick Cowell.)*

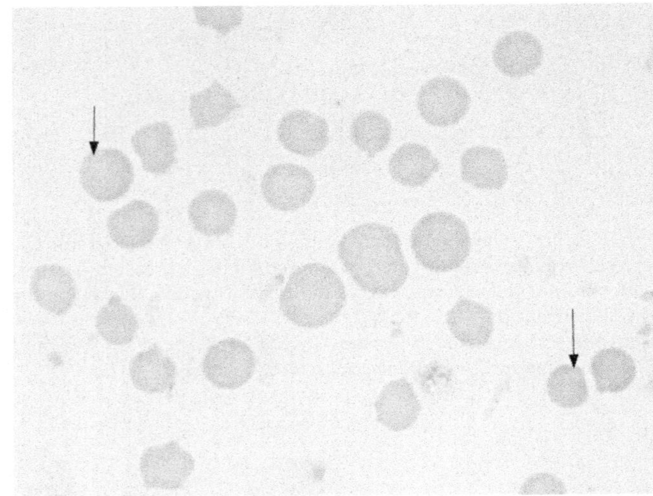

FIGURE 25-10 Heinz bodies stain pale on a Wright-stained feline blood smear. They may be seen projecting from some erythrocytes, whereas others appear as pale areas in the erythrocyte, as shown by the *arrows. (Courtesy Rick Cowell.)*

Blood Types

There are three well-known, clinically important blood groups in cats: A, B, and AB. Another potentially important group called *Mik* has recently been identified.[124] The blood groups are genetically determined erythrocyte surface antigens. The *A*-allele is dominant over the *b*-allele so that cats with genotypes *A/A* and *A/b* will be type A, whereas only the homozygous *b/b* will have the type B phenotype. A third allele, *Ab,* occurs rarely and is said to be recessive to the *A*-allele and dominant to the *b*-allele, although controversy exists regarding the exact inheritance. A and B antigens are produced on the same red cell only in cats with the genotypes *Ab/b* or *Ab/Ab.*[35] A more in-depth discussion of feline blood types has recently been published.[7] Blood typing can be performed by a diagnostic laboratory using various methods or in the hospital with a card typing system (DMS RapidVet-H [feline], DMS Laboratories). If the card-typing system is used, type AB and type B results should be confirmed by a referral laboratory because some cross-reactions have been known to occur.[104] A recently introduced option for patient-side blood typing is the gel column agglutination test (DiaMed-Vet feline typing gel, DiaMed, Switzerland). This test is easier to interpret than the card method, although it requires a specially designed centrifuge that may be cost prohibitive in some settings.[118] An evaluation of various blood typing methods for the cat concluded that the gel column test is reliable compared with the gold standard, the Penn tube assay.[104]

Genetic blood typing using buccal mucosal swabs is available from certain labs and may allow breeders to identify heterozygous type A cats (*A/b*). Breeding two of these cats together would be expected to produce 25% type B kittens (*b/b*) and 50% heterozygous type A kittens (*A/b*). However, genetic typing cannot distinguish between type A and type AB.

Understanding feline blood groups is important because, unlike other mammals, cats produce naturally occurring antibodies, called *alloantibodies,* against the erythrocyte antigens not present on their own cells. The kitten produces these alloantibodies at approximately 2 to 3 months of age, as a result of exposure to antigens on plants, bacteria, or protozoa that are structurally similar to red cell antigens. No alloantibodies are produced against antigens that are similar to self-antigens, and no previous exposure to blood products (transfusions) is necessary to produce the alloantibodies.

Knowledge of this system is important in the prevention of transfusion reactions and neonatal isoerythrolysis. Cats with type B blood have anti-A antibodies with strong hemolytic potential. Even a small volume of type A or AB blood administered to a type B cat can cause potentially life-threatening hemolysis within minutes of the transfusion.[36] Hemolysis of type B blood administered to a type A cat will result in a reduced life span of the transfused erythrocytes, but severe reactions are uncommon.[42] Ingestion of colostrum from a type B queen by a type A newborn results in absorption of anti-A alloantibodies and subsequent rapid hemolysis of the kitten's erythrocytes. This is known as *neonatal isoerythrolysis* and occurs only when type A or AB kittens are born to a type B queen.

The distribution of blood types varies by geographic region and breed (Tables 25-1 and 25-2). Type A is the most common type among cats. There is, however, a geographic variation in the number of type B domestic shorthair cats. More than 10% of the domestic shorthair cats in Australia, France, Greece, India, Italy, Japan, Turkey, and some regions of England are type B. Distribution of blood types among pedigreed breeds does not vary as much by location because of the international exchange of breeding cats. More than 30% of British Shorthair cats, Cornish and Devon Rex cats, and Turkish Angora or Vans have type B blood. In contrast, Siamese and related breeds are almost exclusively type A. Ragdoll cats appear to be unique with regard to blood types. Approximately 3% of Ragdoll cats are discordant when genotyping is compared to serology, necessitating further investigation in this breed.[7] The AB blood type is very rare, and the frequency of the *Mik* blood type is unknown. The presence of erythrocyte antigens in addition to the A and B groups may explain why transfusion compatibility is not guaranteed by blood typing; cross-matching is recommended before any transfusion.[124] Breeding queens, along with blood donors and, if possible, blood recipients, should be blood typed.

TABLE 25-1 **Geographic Distribution of Blood Type Frequencies in Domestic Cats**

Region	Number of Cats	A%	B%	AB%
US (British Virgin Island)	32	100	0	0
US (New England)	69	100	0	0
Finland	61	100	0	0
Hungary (Budapest area)	73	100	0	0
US	432	99.77	0.23	0
US (82% Philadelphia area)	1072	99.72	0.28	0
Switzerland	1014	99.6	0.4	0
Japan	238	89.9	0.9	9.2
US (Northeast)	1450	99.7	0.3	0
US (North Central)	506	99.4	0.4	0.2
US (Southeast)	812	98.5	1.5	0
US (Southwest)	483	97.5	2.5	0
US (West Coast)	812	94.8	4.7	0
Germany (Berlin and Brandenburg area)	372	98.7	1.1	0.3
Denmark (Copenhagen area)	105	98.1	1.9	0
Argentina (Buenos Aires area)	76	96.1	2.6	1.3
Brazil (Rio de Janeiro area)	172	94.8	2.9	2.3
Scotland	70	97.1	2.9	0
Austria	101	97	3	0
England (Manchester)	477	97	3	0
Portugal (North)	147	89.1	4.1	6.8
Netherlands	95	94.8	4.2	0.1
Spain (Barcelona area)	100	94	5	1
Germany (Gieben area)	404	94.1	5.9	0
Gran Canaria	97	88.7	7.2	4.1
Italy (Piedmont region)	122	86.9	7.4	5.7
UK (Edinburgh area)	139	87.1	7.9	5
Italy (Lombardy region)	57	89.5	8.8	1.7
Japan (Tokyo)	207	90	10	0
Italy (Tuscany region)	363	87.1	12.9	0
France (Paris area)	350	85	15	0
Greece	207	78.3	20.3	1.4
Turkey	301	73.1	24.6	2.3
Australia (Brisbane area)	1895	73.3	26.3	0.4
England (Southeast)	105	67.6	30.5	1.9
Australia (Sydney region)	187	62	36	1.6

US, United States; *UK,* United Kingdom.

From Bighignoli B, Owens S, Froenicke L, et al: Blood types of the domestic cat. In August JR: *Consultations in feline internal medicine,* ed 6, St Louis, 2010, Elsevier.

Clinical Evaluation of Cats with Anemia

Anemia is defined as a decrease in the number of circulating red blood cells, the PCV, or the hemoglobin concentration. Because anemia is a sign of disease, making

TABLE 25-2 **Worldwide Frequencies of Blood Types A, B, and AB in Different Breeds**

Breed	Country	Number of Cats	A%	B%	AB%
Abyssinian	US	230	86.5	13.5	0
Abyssinian	US	194	79.9	20.1	0
Birman	US	216	82.4	17.6	0
British Shorthair	UK	121	39.7	58.7	1.6
British Shorthair	US	85	41.2	58.8	0
British Shorthair	Germany	33	54.5	45.5	0
British Shorthair	Germany	35	71.4	28.6	0
British Shorthair	Denmark	30	66.7	33.3	0
Burmese	Australia	30	93	3	3
Burmese	US	25	100	0	0
Chartreux (Kartäuser)	Germany	27	77.8	18.5	3.7
Devon Rex	US	288	50.3	49.7	0
Devon Rex	US	100	57	43	0
Devon Rex*	Australia	71	45	54	1.4
Himalayan	US	35	80	20	0
Maine Coon	Germany	25	96	4	0
Persian	US	230	90.4	9.6	0
Persian	US	170	75.9	24.1	0
Persian	Germany	157	91.7	7.6	0.6
Persian	Denmark	56	96.4	3.6	0
Persian	Italy	38	97.4	2.6	0
Ragdoll	Italy	36	72.2	8.3	19.4
Scottish Fold	US	27	85.2	14.8	0
Siamese	US	99	100	0	0
Siamese	Germany	46	100	0	0
Siamese	Italy	26	96.2	3.8	0
Somali	US	27	77.8	22.2	0
Tonkinese	US	31	100	0	0
Turkish Angora	Turkey	28	53.6	46.4	0
Turkish Van	Turkey	85	40	60	0

US, United States; *UK*, United Kingdom.
*Also includes hybrids.
From Bighignoli B, Owens S, Froenicke L, et al: Blood types of the domestic cat. In August JR: *Consultations in feline internal medicine,* ed 6, St Louis, 2010, Elsevier.

appropriate therapeutic decisions depends on identifying the underlying etiology. As with any disease, the first, most important steps include taking a thorough history and performing a detailed physical examination. The signs associated with anemia are often nonspecific. They are the result of decreased oxygen-carrying capacity of the blood, decreased blood volume, or the underlying disease. The severity of the signs is related to the rate of onset of the disease and the severity of the anemia. Most anemic cats are presented for evaluation of weakness, lethargy, or anorexia. Bleeding may or may not be obvious, depending on its location. The owner should be asked about previous illnesses in addition to the duration and course of the present illness. Exposure to drugs or toxins, such as acetaminophen or onions, as well as the outdoors is important to ascertain. Cats that go outside have a greater risk of trauma and increased exposure to other cats and thus infectious diseases such as retroviral infections. Outdoor cats are also more likely to be exposed to fleas or ticks, possible vectors for important infectious causes of anemia. Discolored urine from hemoglobinuria must be distinguished from hematuria. The geographic location of the cat and its travel history may provide clues as to the cause of the disease. The blood type of a neonate's parents may be critical information if an ill day-old kitten exhibits signs of neonatal isoerythrolysis. Other signs, such as polyuria and polydipsia, can indicate the presence of chronic diseases. Gastrointestinal signs may lead to the consideration of chronic blood loss or inflammatory disease. Recent surgery or trauma may result in blood loss anemia.

Mucous membrane pallor is a common physical finding. If hemolysis is present, the mucous membrane color may be icteric. Decreased peripheral perfusion from causes such as shock or congestive heart failure may also cause pallor, whereas hepatic failure can result in icterus. Evidence of volume contraction, such as tacky mucous membranes or prolonged skin tenting, may be present. Remember that older cats lack skin elasticity and may have a prolonged skin tent even if well hydrated. A moderate decrease in erythrocyte numbers leads to decreased blood viscosity and tissue hypoxia. A soft murmur may be present because turbulent blood flow is directly related to decreased blood viscosity. Hypoxia leads to vasodilation, resulting in an increased heart rate in an attempt to increase cardiac output and oxygen delivery to the tissues. Tachypnea is also a common finding. Fleas or ticks may be found during a detailed examination of the skin, particularly in young animals. Fever may be present in cats with infectious causes of anemia, and splenomegaly is a common finding in cats with hemolysis of any etiology. Small kidneys may be appreciated in a cat with chronic renal disease. Any abdominal mass should be noted for further evaluation. Petechial or ecchymotic hemorrhages indicate bleeding from hemostatic disorders, whereas bleeding wounds may be evidence of recent trauma. Discolored urine may stain the perineum of a longhaired white cat. The severity of the clinical signs shown by anemic cats is more often related to the chronicity than degree of anemia. Chronic anemia allows the cat to adapt physiologically and behaviorally to decreased tissue oxygenation, whereas acute anemia does not allow this adaptation to take place.

When presented with a pale cat, the first diagnostic step is to measure the PCV and total plasma protein concentration. If the PCV is normal, the veterinarian should look for other causes of pallor. If the PCV is low, the next step is to determine if the anemia is regenerative or nonregenerative (Figure 25-11). The single, best indicator of regeneration is an increase in the absolute aggregate reticulocyte count.[126] The severity of anemia should not be assessed until any volume deficits have been corrected. A CBC with a platelet and aggregate reticulocyte count and a blood smear examination will provide evidence of regeneration as long as sufficient time has elapsed since the initial insult. If the protein content is low, acute bleeding should be suspected. Additional tests to consider include a slide agglutination test, a direct Coombs' test, testing for retroviral infection, and a polymerase chain reaction (PCR) test for hemotrophic *Mycoplasma*. Other tests to consider include thoracic and abdominal radiography and abdominal ultrasonography, a serum biochemical profile, urinalysis, and coagulation profile. If the anemia is nonregenerative, evaluation of the bone marrow may be required to make an etiologic diagnosis. An attempt should be made to biopsy any masses identified during the evaluation. Examination and sampling of the gastrointestinal mucosa may be required to diagnose causes of blood loss from this system. To differentiate anemia of inflammatory disease from iron deficiency anemia, serum iron, ferritin, and transferrin (total iron-binding capacity) will have to be measured. By following a logical, ordered diagnostic approach to anemia, the veterinarian can often make an etiologic diagnosis, allowing specific therapy to be instituted.

SUPPORTIVE CARE FOR CATS WITH ANEMIA

Specific treatment for an anemic cat can be attempted only after the cause has been identified. Until that time, supportive care is essential. Bleeding should be controlled to prevent further blood loss. Home care while awaiting test results may be adequate if the anemia is mild. Avoiding stressful situations, such as excessive handling, barking dogs, or fractious cats, will help reduce oxygen requirements. Correction of volume contraction may improve the patient's attitude and appetite. Intravenous fluids may be necessary if volume depletion is significant. Concerns regarding reduction of oxygen-carrying capacity by reducing the PCV with fluid therapy are probably unfounded. The total body hemoglobin and oxygen-carrying ability remains unchanged. However, cats with low plasma protein levels are at risk of edema formation as a result of dilution by aggressive fluid administration. Cats with severe signs related to the anemia, such as respiratory distress or extreme weakness, may require a transfusion. Oxygen administration adds little to the ability to improve tissue hypoxia in anemic patients.[35] The low solubility of oxygen in plasma results in a very small increase in the dissolved oxygen content when 100% oxygen is inhaled. In addition, the stress a cat may experience during oxygen administration may be deleterious.

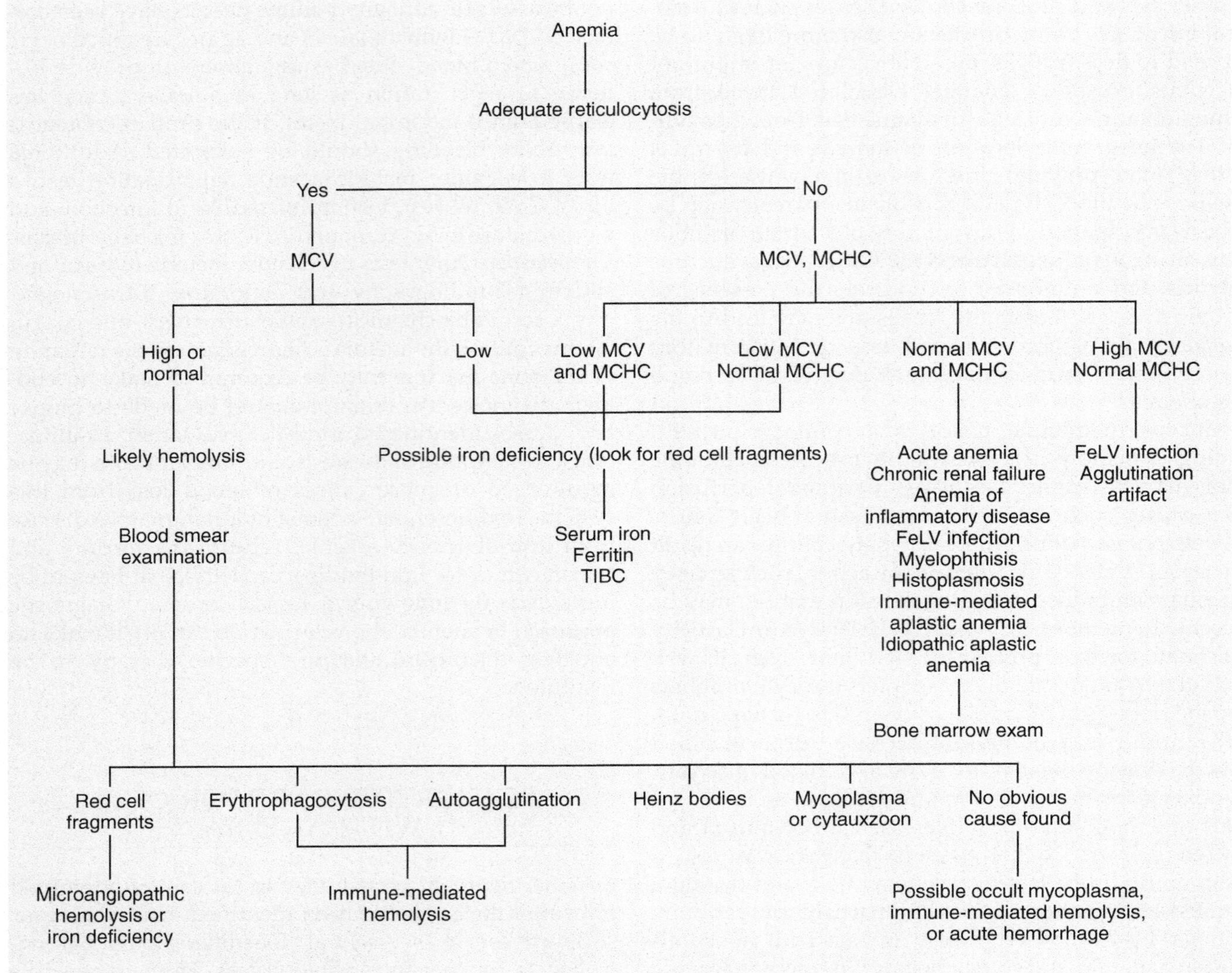

FIGURE 25-11 An algorithm that may be useful in evaluating a cat with anemia. Clinical judgment should be used when following any algorithm because an individual cat may not follow the rules. Further testing should be performed as needed.

Basic Feline Transfusion Medicine

The indications for the use of blood products are many and include hemorrhage, anemia, hemostatic defects, and hypoproteinemia.[42] Many blood products are available or may be prepared, although most veterinary hospitals have hospital cats to use as needed for whole blood donation.

Many blood products are available and have specific uses. Fresh, whole blood contains erythrocytes, platelets, clotting factors, and serum proteins. Storage of whole blood results in the loss of platelets in 2 to 4 hours and clotting factors V and VIII within 24 hours of collection.[42] Packed red cells maintain the oxygen-carrying capacity of whole blood in a smaller volume. This product may be used when volume expansion is unwanted, such as anemic cats with heart disease. Fresh frozen plasma contains albumin and all the clotting factors and is used in cats hemorrhaging from coagulation disorders such as liver failure, DIC, or anticoagulant rodenticide toxicity. The use of plasma products to treat hypoalbuminemia is beneficial only in the short-term because transfused albumin rapidly equilibrates with the extravascular space.[25] The addition of synthetic colloids may prolong the oncotic effects of a plasma transfusion in these cats.[42] Platelet-rich plasma is indicated for cats bleeding from platelet deficiency or dysfunction. Sources for products other than fresh whole blood include a local emergency or referral hospital or a regional veterinary blood bank. Oxyglobin (Biopure, Cambridge, Mass.) is a bovine hemoglobin product containing 130 g/L of hemoglobin that has been licensed for use in dogs. Because no cell membranes are present, there is no antigenicity and the product can be used when compatible blood is unavailable. However, availability of the product has been erratic, and at the time of this writing, it is not available.

Donor cats should be healthy larger cats with a PCV above 35% and fully vaccinated.[42] Donors should be blood typed before blood is collected. No abnormal morphologic cell types should be present, and platelet numbers should be in the reference range. The American College of Veterinary Internal Medicine (ACVIM) consensus statement on screening blood donors recommends testing donor cats for *M. haemofelis; Candidatus* Mycoplasma haemominutum; FeLV antigen; feline immunodeficiency virus (FIV) antibody; and, possibly, *Bartonella* infections.[122] Cats that test positive for FIV antibody should be excluded even if vaccinated against the disease because development of reliable tests to discriminate between antibodies present from a natural infection versus vaccination has been difficult. Heartworm disease cannot be transmitted by blood donation, insofar as the larvae require passage through the mosquito to become infective. Screening for cytauxzoonosis is unnecessary because most cats with the disease are ill. Toxoplasmosis and feline infectious peritonitis have not been documented to be transmitted by transfusion.[122] Donor cats should be kept indoors to reduce the risk of exposure to infectious diseases. Healthy cats can donate 10% to 20% of their total blood volume without adverse effects. A cat's total blood volume is approximately 66 mL/kg. For example, approximately 50 mL of blood (10 mL/kg) can be collected from a 5-kg cat no more often than every 4 to 6 weeks. Subcutaneous fluids should be administered at 2 to 3 times the volume of donated blood. Collection of more than 70 mL of blood from a 5-kg cat can lead to hypovolemia, and the volume should be replaced with intravenous fluids. Many donors resent sitting still long enough to have this volume of blood removed and may require sedation or general anesthesia.

For the treatment of anemia, there are no established levels of PCV below which a cat requires a blood transfusion. The decision to transfuse is instead based on the condition of the patient and assessment of the potential benefits weighed against the risks. Indications that an anemic cat may require a transfusion include respiratory distress, weak pulses, or severe weakness.[126] Both the donor and recipient should be blood typed. Even if the blood types are known, cross-matching should be performed before blood administration to prevent incompatible transfusions caused by untested or unknown erythrocyte antigens such as *Mik*. The half-life of appropriately matched red blood cells in the cat is 29 to 39 days, but for mismatched transfusions the half-life may be a matter of hours. When type B blood is transfused to a type A cat, the life span of transfused red blood cells is only 2 days. When type A blood is transfused to a type B cat, in addition to a potentially severe and fatal reaction, the life span of the transfused cells is only a few hours. A cross-match should be performed again if more than 4 days have elapsed since the last transfusion from the same donor or if another donor is used.

Blood collected for immediate use can be anticoagulated with heparin. Heparin has no preservative properties, and heparinized blood should be used within 8 hours.[42] If blood is to be stored for a longer period, citrated anticoagulants should be used. The required blood volume can be collected into a large syringe. If stored blood is used, it should be warmed to room temperature. Blood is administered through a filter connected to a dedicated intravenous line or a line without the presence of calcium-containing fluids. The transfusion is usually administered using gravity flow, although an infusion pump can be used if the manufacturer has stated that it can be used for this purpose. Bacterial contamination is a potential risk, and aseptic techniques for blood collection should be followed. Blood products can be administered intravenously or intraosseously in small patients.

For severely anemic cats the goal of transfusing whole blood is to ameliorate life-threatening decreases in PCV. This can be accomplished by attempting to raise the PCV to over 20%.[42] The volume of whole blood required to increase the PCV to a desired level can be calculated by using the following formula:

$$\begin{matrix}70 \times \text{recipient's body} \\ \text{weight in kg}\end{matrix} \times \left[\frac{\text{desired PCV} - \text{recipient PCV}}{\text{donor PCV}}\right]$$

The volume to be delivered is equal to 70 times the recipient cat's weight in kilograms times the difference between the desired and the patient's PCV divided by the donor's PCV. Administer 2 to 3 mL of typed and cross-matched blood over 5 minutes and watch for evidence of adverse reaction, such as an increased body temperature, increased heart or respiratory rate, or a prolongation of the capillary refill time. Whole blood can be administered at 10 mL/kg/hour in a normovolemic cat or 2 to 4 mL/kg/hour in a cat with heart disease. The recipient should be constantly monitored for increased heart and respiratory rate, fever, and any signs of adverse reaction (e.g., vomiting) until the transfusion is complete. The transfusion should be completed within 4 hours to avoid bacterial contamination and the PCV measured 1 to 2 hours after completion.

For cats with incompatible cross-matches or in cases when blood products are unavailable, Oxyglobin (Biopure, Cambridge, Mass.) may be administered at a dose of 5 to 15 mL/kg at a rate of 5 mL/kg/h. Because the product contains no red cells, the hemoglobin concentration is measured to assess the effectiveness of the treatment. Oxyglobin has high colloidal properties, and cats are prone to volume overload with its use. Adverse reactions in cats included vomiting, pulmonary edema, and pleural effusion. In one study of cats receiving Oxyglobin, 20% of cats developing respiratory signs required furosemide or supplemental oxygen during or after treatment. Most of these cats had preexisting heart disease.[32] The lower dose should be used cautiously in cats with cardiac disease. The oxygen-carrying effects of Oxyglobin last up to 3 days in circulation.[42]

Adverse effects of blood transfusions can be immunologic reactions to incompatible blood or nonimmune events and may occur within 1 or 2 hours after the transfusion begins. Occasionally, they may be seen up to 48 hours later.[42] In a study of 126 cats that received blood transfusions, 11 cats (8.7%) suffered acute reactions.[53] Multiple red blood cell transfusions (either whole blood or packed red blood cells) are also well tolerated in cats and may be critical for survival of some severely ill patients.[98] Immune-mediated reactions can include hemolysis, allergic reactions, fever, or graft-versus-host reactions. Bacterial contamination of the blood product, hemolysis, hypocalcemia (from citrate toxicity), hypothermia, hyperammonemia, and volume overload are examples of nonimmune adverse reactions. In either case, the life span of the transfused erythrocytes may be shortened. Some reactions are severe enough to cause death. Despite the best efforts to prevent them, transfusion reactions may still occur. Depending on the severity, therapy may include glucocorticoids, epinephrine, crystalloid intravenous fluids, and discontinuation of the transfusion. Fever is usually mild, requiring no treatment. Furosemide should be administered if volume overload occurs. To prevent hypothermia, the blood product can be warmed to no more than 37° C. If the reaction is relatively mild, the transfusion can be restarted at a slower rate. Cross-matching blood is the best means of preventing immune-mediated transfusion reactions even if the blood type is known for both cats. It is also imperative that blood be collected and administered as aseptically as possible and that cats receiving blood products be carefully monitored.

ERYTHROCYTE DISORDERS

Regenerative (Responsive) Anemia

Definition

Regenerative anemia is recognized by a decrease in the PCV, erythrocyte count, and hemoglobin concentration, along with evidence of bone marrow production of new erythrocytes. The presence of polychromasia or increased reticulocyte numbers (or both) is evidence that the bone marrow has increased production of new cells. Regenerative anemia is recognized in a cat with blood loss of longer than 4 to 7 days or with destruction (hemolysis) of erythrocytes faster than they can be replaced. Blood loss anemia can be caused by gastrointestinal bleeding; bleeding secondary to vessel damage from trauma or surgery; bleeding associated with hemostatic defects such as platelet or coagulation disorders; or the early stages of flea or tick infestations. Red cell destruction has myriad potential causes, including primary immune-mediated mechanisms; immune-mediated destruction secondary to infectious disease or drug administration; direct damage from hemoglobin oxidation or blood parasites; congenital defects resulting in erythrocyte membrane fragility; or exposure to alloantibodies from incompatible transfusions or neonatal isoerythrolysis. An anemia is regenerative if there are adequate numbers of circulating aggregate reticulocytes for the degree of anemia. An anemia may not appear regenerative for 4 to 7 days, the time it takes the bone marrow to produce and release new aggregate reticulocytes.

History and Physical Examination

The signs associated with anemia are often nonspecific and have been covered in a previous section of this chapter (Clinical Evaluation of Cats with Anemia).

Diagnostic Plans

A regenerative anemia of greater than 5 days' duration would be expected to show specific changes in a CBC. All cats suspected of being anemic on the basis of the history and clinical signs should have blood drawn for a CBC to include erythrocyte indices, a reticulocyte count, and a blood smear evaluation. The presence of pinpoint hemorrhages (petechiae) should prompt a platelet count. A CBC from a cat with a regenerative anemia should reveal evidence of a reduced erythrocyte mass such as a decreased PCV, red blood cell count, and hemoglobin concentration. The presence of reticulocytes, which are larger and have less hemoglobin than mature erythrocytes, should result in an increased MCV and decreased MCHC. This is why regenerative anemias are classified as macrocytic (increased MCV) and hypochromic (decreased MCHC). Examining a properly made blood smear is very important. The blood smear evaluation may reveal populations of cells of different sizes (anisocytosis) and colors (polychromasia). Morphologic changes may also be present that may give clues as to the cause of the anemia. Blood parasites and Heinz bodies may be seen on a blood smear. Because of the small size of feline erythrocytes, recognizing spherocytes in this species is difficult and is best left to an experienced veterinary cytopathologist. Microscopic agglutination and rouleaux formation can be appreciated when looking at a blood smear. The presence of a population of immature erythrocytes will increase the RDW, and a histogram of cell size versus numbers may contain two peaks representing two populations of cells—mature and immature. If the anemia has not been present long enough, few reticulocytes will be in the circulation and the red cell indices are likely to be within the reference range for the laboratory. It may be necessary to repeat a CBC at a later date to reveal regeneration.

After recognizing a regenerative anemia, the veterinarian must decide if the anemia is due to hemorrhage or to hemolysis. Coagulation parameters and, if not part of the initial CBC, a platelet count may illuminate the cause of unknown bleeding. Endoscopic examination may be required to identify causes of gastrointestinal blood loss. Radiography of the thorax and an abdominal ultrasound examination should be performed to look for the presence of an effusion or mass. Congenital or acquired coagulopathy or trauma may result in a hemorrhagic effusion. A mass lesion may indicate the presence of neoplasia that could result in a secondary immune-mediated event. An abdominal radiograph may reveal the presence of a metallic foreign body in the gastrointestinal tract. Such a foreign body may be a zinc-containing coin, suggesting a possible nonimmune cause for the hemolytic anemia. A slide agglutination test should be performed on a washed or saline diluted EDTA blood sample. If there is no obvious agglutination on gross examination of the slide, a microscopic exam should be performed. Because both test for the presence of antibodies coating the erythrocyte, a direct Coombs' test is unnecessary if the slide agglutination test is positive. If the slide agglutination test is negative, a direct Coombs' test should be performed. Occasionally, FeLV will cause immune-mediated hemolysis. Testing for FeLV antigen is recommended in cats with a regenerative anemia, as is a PCR test for hemotrophic mycoplasma DNA.

Acute Blood Loss

Early in the course of blood loss, before reticulocytes can be produced and released, the anemia may appear nonregenerative. The physiologic response to volume loss is to shunt blood away from the skin and spleen to protect the heart, brain, and viscera.[34] Pallor seen in this situation is not due to anemia but to decreased blood flow to the mucosa. During and immediately after significant blood loss, the PCV may remain normal, insofar as there is loss of both erythrocytes and plasma. A shift of fluid from the interstitial to intravascular space occurs within 12 to 24 hours, diluting the erythrocytes.[129] The result is a decrease in the PCV and total protein concentration. These decreases occur earlier if intravenous fluids have been administered. Erythrocyte morphology at this point will be normal, as will the MCV and MCHC. For 3 to 5 days, the anemia will appear nonregenerative and the diagnosis of a blood loss anemia is made on the basis of suspicion, history, physical findings, and a decreased total protein concentration. Once sufficient time has elapsed, reticulocytes appear and the anemia becomes regenerative. If the bleeding is controlled, the transient increase in aggregate reticulocyte numbers is followed by a rise in the number of punctate reticulocytes as the aggregate ones mature.[34] If clinical signs are sufficiently severe, a whole blood transfusion should be considered.

If the cause of the bleeding is not determined or controlled, loss of iron stores will lead to an iron deficiency anemia. Gastrointestinal bleeding should be considered if a cause for the blood loss is not obvious. Bleeding gastrointestinal tumors, inflammatory bowel disease, gastric ulcers from overzealous use of nonsteroidal anti-inflammatory drugs (NSAIDs), and gastrointestinal parasitism are all potential causes of external blood loss.[34] Urinary blood loss is unlikely to cause depletion of iron stores.[129] Young kittens infested with fleas can experience significant blood loss, insofar as 100 fleas can consume approximately 1 mL of blood daily.[34] This represents about 10% of a 1-kg kitten's blood volume over a 1-week period.

Immune-Mediated Hemolysis

Immune-mediated hemolytic anemia (IMHA) occurs when an immune response is directed against antigens on erythrocytes, leading to their removal by the mononuclear phagocyte system of the spleen (extravascular hemolysis) or complement-mediated lysis (intravascular hemolysis). If the immune-mediated event is associated with another disease, it is a secondary IMHA. Infectious or inflammatory disease may lead to secondary IMHA, as might neoplasia or drug administration. When no underlying cause can be discerned, it is termed *primary IMHA.*

Dysregulation of the immune system results in a loss of self-tolerance. Antibodies may be formed against erythrocyte antigens (type II hypersensitivity), against a non-erythrocyte antigen attached to the red cell surface (type III hypersensitivity), or an antibody may be produced against an unassociated antigen that is similar to an erythrocyte antigen. Alloantibodies present in transfused blood or in colostrum from a type B queen ingested by a type A kitten may lead to immune-mediated hemolysis. Some erythrocyte antigens are hidden and exposed to the immune system only after the cell membrane has been damaged. New antigens that cross-react with red cell antigens or attach to the red cell membrane may be released into circulation by infection or inflammation.[34]

The antibodies involved in the immune process are usually IgG, although IgM can be present alone or with IgG. Macrophages of the mononuclear phagocyte system have receptors for the Fc portion of the IgG antibody but not for IgM. Fc receptors are proteins on the surfaces of cells such as macrophages and neutrophils that contribute to the protective functions of the immune system. Fc receptors bind to the Fc portion of antibodies attached to pathogens or infected cells and stimulate the activity of phagocytic or cytotoxic cells. The antibody-coated cells are removed after antibody binds to the receptor on the macrophage, mostly in the red pulp of the spleen. The result is extravascular hemolysis. Complete phagocytosis may not occur, and only a portion of the membrane may be removed. The cell's volume-to-surface-area ratio is reduced, and the cell becomes spherical. Spherocytes are less able to deform, making passage through the spleen more difficult. Because of the nonsinusoidal nature of the feline spleen (see the section on splenic diseases later in this chapter), less cell deformability is required for cells to pass through, and decreased numbers of spherocytes are trapped and destroyed than in dogs. Splenic macrophages also have receptors for complement. If a sufficient quantity of IgG antibodies coat the cell membrane, complement may also bind to the erythrocyte. The presence of complement on the cell membrane increases the efficiency of erythrocyte removal. If a sufficient number of the antibodies are IgM, complement-mediated lysis can occur, resulting in intravascular hemolysis. However, none of the 19 cats with primary IMHA in one study had intravascular hemolysis despite the presence of IgM in 8 of the cats.[57]

Cats with IMHA, whether primary or secondary, will exhibit signs related to the anemia. These can include anorexia, lethargy, weakness, or respiratory difficulties. Additional signs as a result of the underlying disease may be present in cats with secondary IMHA. Most of the cats with primary IMHA are young adults. In the previously mentioned report of 19 cats with primary disease, six were younger than 2 years old; the median age for all 19 cats was 2 years.[57] Eleven of the cats were male, and eight female. Cats with secondary disease will have a signalment related to the underlying disease. Physical changes that might be present include pale or icteric mucous membranes, tachycardia, tachypnea, or splenomegaly as a consequence of increased processing of damaged erythrocytes. Tachypnea and tachycardia are attempts at compensating for the decreased oxygen-carrying capacity of the anemic patient; pulmonary thromboembolism, so common in dogs with IMHA, is rare in cats.[57] Splenomegaly occurs in many nonimmune disorders causing hemolysis as the organ attempts to deal with the increased numbers of damaged red cells. Body temperature is likely to be normal unless the patient is moribund, in which case hypothermia may be noted. A systolic murmur may be heard during auscultation of the thorax.

Diagnosis of IMHA can be frustrating. There are many mechanisms causing hemolysis that do not involve the immune system. Distinguishing primary from secondary IMHA is important because therapy may be different. With aggressive diagnostic investigation, an underlying cause is often found. Two sources state that primary IMHA is rare in cats.[34,75] However, Kohn and coworkers[57] found that of 23 anemic cats with a positive Coombs' test or persistent erythrocyte agglutination, an underlying cause was identified in only four patients after an extensive workup. Put another way, 19 of the 23 Coombs'-positive cats had primary IMHA.

To make a diagnosis of primary IMHA, other causes of hemolysis must be eliminated. A CBC with reticulocyte and platelet counts, serum biochemical profile, and urinalysis should be performed. The cat's retroviral status should be ascertained and a PCR test for *M. haemofelis* DNA should be run. Thoracic radiography and an abdominal ultrasound examination should be performed to rule out the presence of potential bronchial infections, or thoracic or abdominal masses. A bone marrow evaluation may be useful when a regenerative response to the anemia is equivocal. Specific immunodiagnostic tests such as a slide agglutination test and a direct Coombs' test should be performed.

If the hemolysis is severe enough and the anemia is not peracute, there should be evidence of regeneration in the CBC report. Increased numbers of aggregate reticulocytes should be present. Polychromasia and rubricytosis (nucleated red blood cells) may be present. The hallmark of IMHA in dogs, spherocytosis, is unlikely to be identified. The PCV may be surprisingly low for the condition of the patient; cats seem to tolerate a lower PCV than dogs.[57] The lower the PCV, the higher the aggregate reticulocyte count should be. If the reticulocyte count is not appropriate for the degree of anemia, it may be nonregenerative. In this case an immune response directed at erythrocyte precursors in the bone marrow might be considered. Another difference from dogs is the lack of leukocytosis or neutrophilia with left shift in cats with primary IMHA. In the aforementioned study by Kohn and coworkers[57] 17 of the 19 cats with primary IMHA had a white cell count within the reference range. The platelet count should be within the reference range, too. Evans syndrome, a combination of immune-mediated damage to both erythrocytes and platelets, is rare in cats. Although evidence of DIC is common in dogs with IMHA, it is uncommon in cats. Before convicting a cat with anemia of also having thrombocytopenia on the basis of an automated cell count, a blood smear should be examined to determine whether platelet clumping is present. The smear examination will also allow identification of intraerythrocytic parasites or morphologic changes in the erythrocyte that may suggest causes of anemia other than IMHA.

There are no pathognomic changes for IMHA in the biochemical profile. Anemia may cause hepatic centrilobular hypoxia, hepatocyte injury, and subsequent increases in serum alanine transferase (ALT) activity. Hyperbilirubinemia and hyperproteinemia may be present. Volume contraction may be reflected by azotemia, which is likely prerenal in cats with primary IMHA. Other changes may be present if there is an underlying disease (secondary IMHA). Any thoracic or abdominal masses should be biopsied. An airway wash with cytology and culture might be attempted in cats with peribronchial thickening.

The direct Coombs' test detects the presence of antibodies or complement on the red cell surface. A positive test is consistent with, but not necessarily diagnostic for, IMHA. However, a diagnosis of IMHA should include a positive direct Coombs' test.[34] False-negative tests are unlikely. In the study by Kohn and coworkers, 78 cats with anemia had a direct Coombs' test performed and 55 were negative, all of which had nonimmune etiologies identified as causing the anemia; an additional 14 cats without anemia were also direct Coombs' test negative.[57] The direct Coombs' test may become negative after a patient with IMHA enters remission, although a few days of immunosuppressive therapy is unlikely to cause a negative test.[34] A limitation of the test is the inability to differentiate between primary and secondary IMHA. A properly performed slide agglutination test may detect anti-erythrocyte IgM or large quantities of anti-erythrocyte IgG coating the erythrocytes. Autoagglutination must be distinguished from rouleaux formation by proper washing or dilution of the blood on the slide. A direct Coombs' test is unnecessary if the slide agglutination test is positive because they both test for anti-erythrocyte antibodies; autoagglutination is considered indicative of IMHA.[57] Autoagglutination may artifactually increase the MCV because clumps of cells are counted as one.

Therapy for IMHA depends on the cause and severity of the anemia and must be tailored to the individual. Removal of an underlying cause or trigger will help bring secondary IMHA under control. If an infection, such as *M. haemofelis,* is thought to be contributing to the disorder, use of appropriate antibiotics is required. Surgical drainage of any fight-wound abscesses or removal of potentially neoplastic masses may be necessary. Removal of nonessential drugs, particularly those known to induce an immune response, may eliminate a potential trigger for the immune-mediated process.

Supportive measures should not be forgotten. Volume expansion in a severely ill cat will improve organ perfusion. Concerns regarding exacerbating hypoxia by decreasing the PCV with intravenous fluids are unwarranted. Although the PCV may decrease, the total amount of hemoglobin in the body does not. However, rehydration will reveal the true severity of the anemia. Depending on the cat's condition and PCV, a blood transfusion may be required. A major cross-match before collecting and administering blood is imperative, even if the blood type of the donor and recipient is known. Unfortunately, autoagglutination may make interpretation of the cross-match difficult. Alternatively, a hemoglobin-containing solution, Oxyglobin, may be used to improve oxygen-carrying capacity. Stressful situations while in hospital, such as frequent handling or exposure to barking dogs, should be minimized in severely ill cats.

Reduction of the immune-mediated destruction of erythrocytes is the goal of drug therapy. The optimal drug protocol will decrease phagocytosis of antibody or complement coated red cells, reduce complement activation, and eliminate the production of anti-erythrocyte antibodies (Table 25-3). Glucocorticoids are the initial drug of choice. These drugs are both antiinflammatory and immunosuppressive, although higher doses are required to accomplish the latter. Oral prednisone is the most commonly used glucocorticoid, but it requires conversion by the liver to the active form, prednisolone.[100] There is some evidence that intestinal absorption or hepatic conversion of prednisone to prednisolone may be poor in cats,[119] thus prednisolone is thought by some to be a better initial choice in this species. The pharmacologic effects are due to interference with cellular communication and interaction among cells of the immune system. Glucocorticoids also inhibit production of cytokines used to amplify the immune response.[75] Decreased production of IL-2 leads to decreased T_h1 helper cell proliferation and cytotoxicity.[27] Glucocorticoids stimulate maturation of T-suppressor cells and inhibit antibody-dependent cytotoxicity by natural killer cells,[27] resulting in inhibition of the cellular arm of the immune system. They are beneficial in reducing binding of the Fc component of the attached IgG to the Fc receptors on

TABLE 25-3 **Immunosuppressive Drugs**

Drug	Trade Name	Dose	Preparation
Prednisone/prednisolone		2-4 mg/kg/day	
Dexamethasone		0.25-1 mg/kg/day	
Chlorambucil	Leukeran	0.1-0.2 mg/kg q24h or 2 mg/cat q48-72h	2-mg tablets
Cyclophosphamide	Cytoxan	2-4 mg/kg q24h 4 days/week	25- and 50-mg tablets
Cyclosporine	Atopica, Neoral	1-5 mg/kg q12-24h use ideal body weight for obese cats	10-, 25-, 50-, and 100-mg capsules (Atopica) 25- and 100-mg capsules, 100-mg/mL oral suspension (Neoral)
Leflunomide	Arava	2-4 mg/kg q24h	10- and 20-mg tablets

splenic macrophages. In addition, they may decrease antibody binding to the red cell membrane and complement activation.[34] There are few direct effects on B-lymphocytes, and therefore there is little effect on antibody production.[27,90] Cats have fewer and less sensitive cytoplasmic glucocorticoid receptors than dogs.[16] This may explain why cats typically have less pronounced side effects; for instance, polyuria and polydipsia and steroid hepatopathy are not typical side effects of glucocorticoid use in cats.[27] Cats receiving immunosuppressive doses of glucocorticoids may have difficulty eliminating infections on their own, and some infections may be inapparent because the inflammation associated with the infection may be blunted by the antiinflammatory effect of the glucocorticoid.

An initial immunosuppressive dose of prednisone or prednisolone is 2 to 4 mg/kg orally every 24 hours. The biological duration of action of these drugs is 24 to 36 hours, which is longer than the plasma half-life. Therefore there is little advantage in dividing the daily dose in two other than to reduce the gastric irritation some patients experience at very high doses.[16] If oral medication is contraindicated because of vomiting or severe oral cavity or esophageal disease, injectable dexamethasone may be substituted at 0.25 to 1 mg/kg every 24 hours subcutaneously, intramuscularly, or intravenously. Repository glucocorticoids such as methylprednisolone acetate (Depo-Medrol, Pfizer) prevent accurate titrating of the dose, and their use is not recommended.[16] Response is indicated by a stable or rising PCV and can be expected within a week. Appropriately treated secondary IMHA may respond more quickly. The Coombs' test will remain positive, possibly for months, despite a normal PCV. Once the PCV has reached and remains in the low part of the reference range for at least 1 week, consideration may be given to slowly decreasing the glucocorticoid dose. A rapid response may allow for a more rapid reduction in dose. The dose may be reduced by 25% to 50% every 2 to 4 weeks. Once the dose of prednisolone has reached 0.5 mg/kg, alternate-day therapy may begin. It is imperative to ensure the maintenance of remission before each dose reduction. There is no sense in reducing the dose in a cat that is deteriorating. Once a physiologic dose (0.25 mg/kg) of prednisolone has been reached, an attempt can be made to discontinue the drug. Whether this is possible depends on the individual cat. Relapses are to be expected and should be treated by increasing to the last effective dose.

Additional immunosuppressive drugs may be required if the response to prednisolone is inadequate, if control occurs only at high doses of prednisolone, or if side effects are unacceptable. Chlorambucil is an acceptable additional drug to use in cats. Although not as potent as cyclophosphamide, it is well tolerated by cats and is the preferred first choice when an additional drug is required. Dosages range from 2 mg/cat orally every 48 to 72 hours[119] to 0.1 to 0.2 mg/kg orally every 24 hours.[88] Hemorrhagic cystitis has not been reported in cats, and myelosuppression is uncommon[119]; however, myelotoxicity may result in neutropenia, with a nadir occurring 7 to 14 days after starting the drug. A white blood cell count should be performed at that time. If the neutrophil count is less than $0.5 \times 10^9/L$, the veterinarian should administer prophylactic antibiotics and reduce the dose by 25%.[85]

Other immunosuppressive drugs include cyclophosphamide, cyclosporine, and leflunomide. An alkylating agent similar to chlorambucil, cyclophosphamide may have a more rapid onset of action.[87] Cats seem more resistant to the adverse effects of this medication than dogs[87]; however, gastrointestinal signs such as vomiting, diarrhea, nausea, and anorexia are possible. Although it is metabolized in the liver to active metabolites, production of substances toxic to the bladder epithelium do not seem to be produced as they are in dogs,[87] and sterile hemorrhagic cystitis has not been reported in cats receiving cyclophosphamide. The drug is cytotoxic and decreases the production of white blood cells and antibodies. As with chlorambucil, a white blood cell count should be performed 7 to 14 days after starting the drug. The dose is 2 to 4 mg/kg orally every 24 hours for 4 consecutive days per week.[29] The tablet is not homogeneous and therefore should not be split; compounding may be required to enable accurate dosing.

Cyclosporine acts by suppressing cytokine release from T cells, particularly IL-2.[119] This, in turn, prevents early activation of T_h1 helper cells and cytotoxic T cells. Cyclosporine has little effect on nonstimulated T cells, is not cytotoxic or myelosuppressive,[58] and spares other rapidly dividing cells.[40] Common adverse effects include anorexia and vomiting, which respond to a decrease in the dose. It has a bitter taste that may cause refusal to eat if mixed with food.[87] Hepatotoxicity is not a problem except at extremely high blood levels,[40] but reversible nephrotoxicity, although not as common as in people, can occur in cats at any blood level.[40] Monitoring of renal function in cats receiving cyclosporine is warranted. The gingival lesions seen in dogs receiving cyclosporine have not been reported in cats.[119] Patients receiving cyclosporine may also have an increased risk of developing neoplasia, particularly lymphosarcoma.[40] This effect may be due to decreased surveillance for neoplastic cells by the cellular arm of the immune system. Only the modified formulations of cyclosporine are recommended. A veterinary preparation of the emulsified form, Atopica (Novartis Animal Health), is available in capsules, allowing more accurate dosing in cats. This formulation is administered orally at 1 to 5 mg/kg of ideal body weight every 12 to 24 hours, and routine drug monitoring is generally unnecessary[87] unless the patient is not responding as expected. Measuring 2-hour postadministration cyclosporine concentrations is more closely correlated with the drug's area under the curve than trough blood levels and more accurately predicts clinical response.[87] Because cyclosporine is extensively bound to erythrocytes, whole blood levels are higher than plasma concentrations.[58]

Leflunomide (Arava, Sanofi Aventis) is a prodrug that is metabolized into the active form by the intestinal mucosa.[40] The active form inhibits a lymphocyte growth factor receptor[40] and mitochondrial enzymes, leading to inhibition of T cell proliferation.[40,92] It is particularly effective in inhibiting B cell proliferation and antibody production. The drug is metabolized by the liver and excreted in the urine.[92] The gastrointestinal problems experienced by dogs do not seem to occur in cats,[40] insofar as the metabolite causing the gastrointestinal distress is less toxic to cats.[130] Cats with inadequate renal function may, however, accumulate enough of the metabolite to cause gastrointestinal upset.[130] Leflunomide is administered orally at 2 to 4 mg/kg every 24 hours. Once remission is achieved, the dose can be reduced to once or twice weekly to maintain adequate blood levels.[40] Leflunomide orally at 10 mg per day has been used along with methotrexate to induce remission of refractory rheumatoid arthritis in cats. Once control is achieved, the dose is reduced to 10 mg twice weekly.

Because of the severe myelosuppression that occurs in cats, azathioprine is not recommended. When weaning off treatment using multiple drugs, the veterinarian should start by reducing the cytotoxic drugs. Once they are discontinued, reduction in glucocorticoid doses can begin. In the rare instance that combination therapy is ineffective, splenectomy may be required.

The prognosis for cats with IMHA depends on response to therapy, the prognosis associated with any underlying disease, and the occurrence of complications. The mortality rate for cats with primary IMHA is thought to be much lower than in dogs. Kohn and coworkers[57] reported a mortality rate of 23.5% compared with much higher rates in dogs. Life-threatening complications such as DIC or pulmonary thromboembolism also occur at a much lower rate in cats.

In summary, primary IMHA may be more common in cats than previously thought. Diagnosis remains an exclusionary one; elimination of other disorders by comprehensive investigation is required before making a diagnosis of primary IMHA. Therapy depends on whether an underlying condition exists but usually involves the use of immunosuppressive drugs. Fortunately, the prognosis for cats with primary IMHA is better than for dogs.

Inherited Erythrocyte Abnormalities Causing Hemolysis

The erythrocyte membrane is composed of a lipid bilayer attached to the membrane skeleton. Numerous glycoproteins act as receptors or transporters. The membrane sodium/potassium (Na/K) ATPase is lost during maturation, and, subsequently, the cytoplasmic sodium and potassium concentrations are similar to plasma. Because erythrocytes lack mitochondria, energy generation is exclusively anaerobic. Pyruvate kinase (PK) is involved in the last step in energy production and catalyzes the production of pyruvate from phosphoenolpyruvate, yielding a high-energy ATP molecule.[55] Some of this energy is responsible for maintaining the pliability of the cell membrane, which allows the cell to squeeze through small capillaries. Two inherited defects in the feline erythrocyte occur in the related Abyssinian and Somali breeds of cat. Both defects affect erythrocyte survival time. One involves a PK deficiency; the other an idiopathic increase in red cell osmotic fragility. Both are inherited in an autosomal recessive manner and are identified in young cats with Coombs'-negative hemolytic anemia. Other, more common causes of hemolysis must be eliminated as possible causes of anemia before considering inherited defects. This requires an exhaustive effort to find other causes of regenerative anemia. A CBC, including an aggregate reticulocyte count and measurement of red cell indices, serum biochemical profile, and a urinalysis, should be performed. The patient should be screened for retroviral and hemoplasma infection and have a direct Coombs' test run.

Abyssinian and Somali cats with PK deficiency are usually young adults when presented for evaluation, although cats younger than 1 year old may be affected. These cats exhibit the common signs associated with anemia, including lethargy, weakness, pale mucous membranes, and anorexia. The signs are often intermittent and mild, even in cats with severe anemia. Physical findings are not specific for PK deficiency and may include pallor, lethargy, icterus, or weight loss. Mild to moderate splenomegaly is common. At presentation, most, but not all, cats are anemic, with a PCV between 13% and 29% (median of 25%) reported in one study.[55] The anemia in most is regenerative with macrocytosis, polychromasia, and an aggregate reticulocytosis. Some cats have a lymphocytosis and a polyclonal hyperglobulinemia, possibly as a result of nonspecific immune system stimulation. A genetic test is available for PK deficiency and might be useful in all breeding Abyssinian and Somali cats, particularly those related to cats with anemia. Affected cats are homozygous for the causative mutation and have very low PK activity.[33] Heterozygotes have intermediate PK activity and, because they are asymptomatic carriers, can transmit the defect unknowingly. Therapy is limited for cats with PK deficiency. They are often misdiagnosed with IMHA or hemoplasmosis and receive prednisolone, doxycycline, or both. Prednisolone may be beneficial in reducing the number of hemolytic crises by delaying phagocytosis by macrophages in the spleen. Splenectomy should be considered when recurrent hemolytic episodes occur or if the spleen becomes so large that it restricts expansion of the stomach, leading to anorexia.[55] Stressful events can lead to a life-threatening hemolytic crisis and should be avoided. The prognosis for a cat with PK deficiency is variable. Most cats that die do so during a hemolytic crisis. In contrast to dogs, cats do not develop progressive osteosclerosis.[33] Some cats can live to an older age; according to one source,[34] the oldest PK-deficient cat lived to 13 years of age.

A population of Somali and Abyssinian cats has been identified with increased fragility of the erythrocyte membrane.[56] The cause for the increased fragility has not been elucidated, but an inherited defect in the cell membrane is suspected with a likely autosomal recessive mode of inheritance. The disorder has also been identified in Siamese and domestic shorthair cats.[34] All of the cats had normal PK activity. The age at the initial visit was between 6 months and 5 years (mean of 2 years). The most common presenting complaints included lethargy, anorexia, weight loss, and pale mucous membranes—signs typical of anemia. In some cats the signs were episodic. Physical examination revealed the presence of pallor and splenomegaly. As these cats age, the splenomegaly appears to become more profound. As with PK deficiency, the initial presentation may be misinterpreted for some other cause of hemolysis. Most blood samples were severely hemolyzed after an overnight stay in refrigeration. Although the PCV was most often in the range of 15% to 25%, during a hemolytic crisis it dropped to as low as 5%. The anemia was usually mildly to moderately regenerative with macrocytosis, anisocytosis, polychromasia, and an aggregate reticulocytosis. Macroscopic agglutination was present in 50% of the cats but disappeared after proper washing. The agglutination may have artifactually increased the MCV as aggregates of cells passed through the cell counter. Many cats had a lymphocytosis and polyclonal hyperglobulinemia. Retroviral tests were negative, as was a direct Coombs' test. Microscopic examination for hemoplasma infection was negative; because of the insensitivity of this test in detecting the bacteria, cats were treated with doxycycline anyway. Osmotic fragility testing is performed by placing the patient's red cells in serial dilutions of a saline solution. Because mature erythrocytes have no Na/K ATPase, the amount of water inside the cell rapidly equilibrates with that of the solution and the cell increases in volume. Hemolysis of patient erythrocytes occurs at much higher concentrations of saline than control samples. Affected erythrocytes are osmotically fragile even when there are no clinical signs. Whereas some of the cats responded to glucocorticoid administration, others improved without treatment. Splenectomy was performed in cats that did not respond or had recurrent hemolytic events. This effectively removed the organ responsible for phagocytosis of the damaged erythrocytes.

In summary, cats with PK deficiency and increased erythrocyte fragility have many clinical and hematologic similarities, such as the young age of onset, character and chronicity of the hemolytic anemia, splenomegaly, and treatments available. Because of the similarity of the two diseases, testing for both in a patient in whom the disease is suspected may be wise. A DNA test for PK deficiency is available for Abyssinian and Somali cats. Osmotic fragility testing requires an EDTA blood sample from both the patient and a control. Cats with PK deficiency have relatively normal osmotic fragility, and those with severe osmotic fragility have normal PK activities.

Neonatal Isoerythrolysis

The strong hemolytic characteristics of the anti-A alloantibodies found in the serum of type B cats is responsible for the often fatal hemolysis that occurs in very young kittens. When the pathologic basis for neonatal isoerythrolysis is understood, it is easy to see how it can be prevented. Treatment of the disorder is often unrewarding.

The *A* and *Ab* alleles in cats are dominant to the *b* allele. Type B queens mated to type A or AB toms may have kittens that have expressed type A (or AB) antigens on their erythrocytes. Because the placenta in cats is impermeable to the passage of immunoglobulins, in utero hemolysis does not occur. Once the kitten is born, however, passive absorption of proteins from colostrum, including anti-A antibodies, occurs for the first 12 to 24 hours. Exposure to the strongly hemolyzing anti-A antibodies leads to massive, often fatal erythrocyte destruction in type A and AB kittens. The severity of signs is related to the amount of colostral antibody absorbed before closure of the kitten's intestinal tract to passive immune transfer. Once gut closure occurs, the kitten is no longer at risk for neonatal isoerythrolysis. The time at which this occurs varies among individuals.

Kittens at risk are born healthy and become ill only after consuming anti-A antibodies in the colostrum. Clinical signs appear within the first few hours to days of life and may range in severity from sudden death to development of tail-tip necrosis from vessel obstruction by agglutinating erythrocytes. Some kittens develop dark-colored urine. These kittens may also stop nursing, fail to thrive or gain weight, and develop anemia and icterus; they usually die within the first week after birth. The diagnosis is confirmed by blood typing the queen and affected kittens.

Because of the acute nature of the disease, therapy is usually unsuccessful. The kitten should be removed from the queen for the first 24 hours after birth, and the body temperature should be well controlled. Between 2 and 3 mL of type B blood may be transfused through an intraosseous catheter. Type B blood is used because the only alloantibodies present in the sick newborn kitten are the anti-A antibodies from the queen's colostrum; the kitten has not yet made any of its own alloantibodies. Ideally, the blood would come from the queen because she has no antibodies directed against her own red cells. Kittens start to produce their own anti-B alloantibodies soon after birth. If a further transfusion is necessary 3 days after birth, type A blood should be used.

Preventing the disorder, however, is much more successful than treating it. Blood typing of breeding individuals in breeds known to have a high percentage of type B cats will identify matings at risk of producing neonatal isoerythrolysis (see Tables 25-1 and 25-2). If mating a type B queen with a type A or AB tom is desired, plans should be made to foster the kittens to a type A queen for the first 24 hours of life. Alternatively, these kittens can be fed with kitten milk replacer for the first 24 hours. If there is concern about lack of passive transfer of maternal immunity in kittens fed milk replacer, 5 mL of serum from a type A cat can be administered subcutaneously or intraperitoneally every 8 hours for the first 24 hours.[60] Type B kittens receiving anti-B antibodies from the colostrum of type A queens are not known to be at risk of developing isoerythrolysis.

Because blood typing is readily available, preventing kitten death from neonatal isoerythrolysis is rather easy. It is recommended that cats of breeds with high frequency of type B blood, whether intended for breeding or as pets, have their blood typed at the earliest opportunity in case the information is needed in an urgent situation in the future.

Cytauxzoonosis

Cytauxzoonosis is a tick-borne blood disease of cats caused by the protozoal organism *Cytauxzoon felis*. The reservoir for the organism is the North American bobcat *(Lynx rufus)*. Infection in domestic cats is usually rapidly fatal, insofar as they are a terminal host.[9] The only proven vector for the organism is the tick *Dermacentor variabilis*. Cytauxzoonosis presently has a limited geographic distribution in the central, south-central, southeastern, and mid-Atlantic areas of the United States. This is also the geographical area where *D. variabilis* is encountered.

After the tick ingests parasitized erythrocytes from an infected host, the parasite is released into the gut, undergoes reproduction, and migrates to the salivary glands. When the tick feeds on a domestic cat, the parasite enters the circulation and infects mononuclear phagocytes. Massive replication in the phagocytes (tissue phase) causes the cells to swell and burst. Freed parasites are found in erythrocytes 1 to 3 days later (erythrocyte phase).[39] Interestingly, inoculation of infected red cells results in a chronic erythrocyte parasitemia without the severe illness normally seen in domestic cats. In order for the parasite to cause virulent disease, it must develop in the tick.[9] There is no evidence the parasite can infect humans.

The prepatent period for the disease is between 2 and 3 weeks. The tissue phase is responsible for many of the clinical signs because the swollen macrophages obstruct vessels, resulting in decreased organ perfusion. Damage to the lungs, liver, spleen, bone marrow, and brain account for many of the clinical signs. Erythrocyte infection and destruction occur 2 to 3 days before death, not enough time for the hemolytic anemia to become regenerative. Surviving cats may have a regenerative anemia if a sufficient number of erythrocytes are destroyed. If the hemolysis is severe enough, the resulting hypoxia will exacerbate organ damage. By-products of the parasite may be cytotoxic, pyrogenic, and vasoactive.[39] Once clinical signs are present, death follows in less than 1 week.

There is no age or gender predilection, although younger cats seem to represent many of the cases. Cats that go outside have an increased the risk of tick exposure. Most infections are identified during early spring to early fall, when the ticks are most active. Cats infected with *C. felis* exhibit vague, nonspecific signs such as lethargy, anorexia, pallor, icterus, or respiratory distress. Physical examination of an infected cat may reveal fever, hepatosplenomegaly, tachycardia, tachypnea, and pale or icteric mucous membranes. Alterations in mentation, seizures, and vocalizing may be seen in cats in the later stages of the disease. Recumbency, hypothermia, and coma are seen in terminally ill cats. Death usually occurs a few days after the temperature peaks.

Diagnostic plans entail a CBC, including a platelet and aggregate reticulocyte count and blood smear evaluation; serum biochemical profile, and urinalysis. The cat's retrovirus status should be determined. If hepatosplenomegaly is palpated, an abdominal ultrasound examination is warranted. The goal of testing is to logically eliminate potential causes of the clinical signs. Diagnosing a *C. felis* infection requires an index of suspicion for the disease. Cats in an endemic area with acute onset of vague signs of disease should be considered candidates for this infection. Finding a tick on the cat's body can be an enormous clue. Anemia is not present until later in the course of illness and is usually normocytic and normochromic, with no increase in the number of aggregate reticulocytes. A neutrophilic leukocytosis may be present; however, if parasite-laden macrophages fill up the bone marrow, myelophthisis may lead to neutropenia. Thrombocytopenia may be present as a result of consumption, possibly from DIC. Hepatic infiltration with parasite-loaded macrophages may cause hyperbilirubinemia and increases in liver enzyme activities.

A definitive diagnosis involves identifying the parasite in macrophages or red blood cells. Because erythrocyte infection takes place later in the course of disease, aspiration of liver, spleen, lymph nodes, lung or bone marrow is more likely to produce a diagnosis. Infected monocytes may be identified at the feathered edge of a blood smear. The organism is recognized as a basophilic, possibly lobulated area taking up much of the cytoplasm of the phagocyte (Figure 25-12). The parasite can be demonstrated in the erythrocyte as a characteristic round signet ring form (Figure 25-13). Other forms found in the red cells include small dots and an ovoid safety-pin shape. There is usually only one parasite per red cell, but pairs and tetrads are seen occasionally.[39] Because erythrocyte infection occurs later in the disease, parasitemia may not be present early; a repeated smear examination should reveal the parasite.

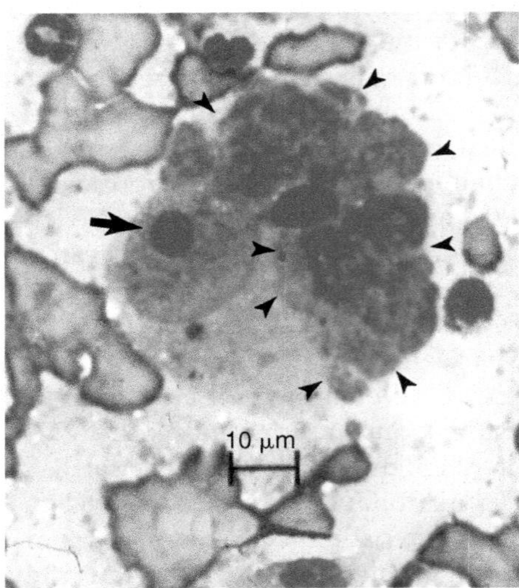

FIGURE 25-12 A macrophage from a feline liver contains a developing *Cytauxzoon* schizont. The early schizont is outlined by *arrowheads* and appears as a lobulated basophilic area within the cytoplasm of the cell. A large prominent nucleolus in the host nucleus is indicated by the *long arrow* (Wright-Giemsa, ×165). *(From Greene CE, Meinkoth J, Kocan A: Cytauxzoonosis. In Greene CE, editor:* Infectious diseases of the dog and cat, *ed 3, St Louis, 2006, Saunders/Elsevier.)*

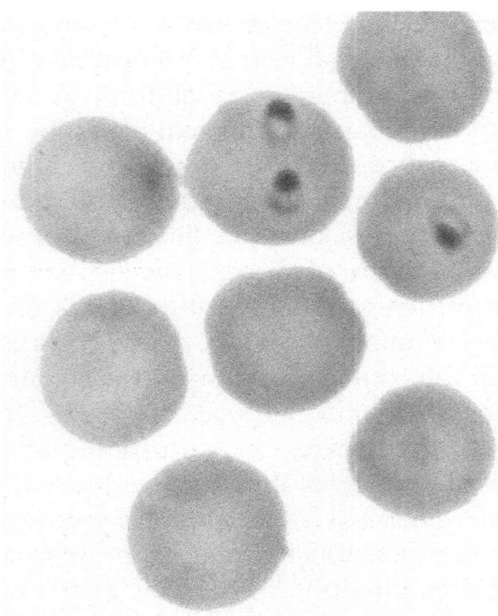

FIGURE 25-13 Feline erythrocytes infected with the characteristic signet-ring shaped *Cytauxzoon* piroplasms. The clear nuclear area in the parasite allows the organism to be differentiated from hemotropic *Mycoplasma* organisms (Wright-Giemsa, ×330). *(From Greene CE, Meinkoth J, Kocan A: Cytauxzoonosis. In Greene CE, editor:* Infectious diseases of the dog and cat, *ed 3, St Louis, 2006, Saunders/Elsevier.)*

Even though infection with *C. felis* is usually fatal, cats have survived, including some that received only aggressive supportive care. A population of 18 cats from the Arkansas–Oklahoma border area survived, suggesting the presence of a less virulent strain of the parasite.[72] Goals of therapy include preventing DIC and bacterial septicemia, promoting perfusion, and improving tissue oxygenation. Aggressive intravenous fluid administration will help preserve intravascular volume, maintain tissue perfusion, and consequently improve tissue oxygenation and help prevent DIC. The prophylactic use of heparin to prevent DIC has been suggested.[9] Even though antibiotics are not able to directly control the protozoa, they have been used in most cats that have survived.[9] Effective drugs able to eradicate *C. felis* are not yet available. In fact, many cats that survived infection did so without the benefit of antiprotozoal drugs.

Therapy is often unrewarding; most cats die despite aggressive treatment. Until effective protocols for treating *C. felis* infections are developed, prevention of the initial infection should be the goal of the veterinarian and owner. Tick control is mandatory in preventing infection, as is confinement indoors during the tick season to minimize exposure to the protozoal parasite. Daily grooming to remove ticks is also helpful. Preliminary data have been published regarding the use of oral atovaquone 15 mg/kg every 8 hours in combination with oral azithromycin 10 mg/kg every 24 hours for 10 days along with aggressive supportive care. The protocol resulted in the survival of 14 of 22 infected cats.[8] It is possible that some of these cats were infected with the less virulent strain of *C. felis*.

Heinz Body Anemia

Heinz bodies are indicative of oxidative injury to the erythrocyte. They are clumps of irreversibly denatured hemoglobin attached to the erythrocyte cell membrane (see Figures 25-9 and 25-10). Feline hemoglobin is quite sensitive to oxidative injury because there are more targets on the molecule to oxidize than in other mammals and cats have reduced capacity for scavenging oxidative substances. Feline hemoglobin also dissociates more readily than other species.[14] Because of the nonsinusoidal nature of the feline spleen, rigid bodies such as erythrocytes with Heinz bodies are not forced to squeeze their way through the red pulp. Therefore the feline spleen is inefficient in removing Heinz bodies, and they accumulate. Still, the result is decreased erythrocyte survival time. Oxidation of the iron in the hemoglobin can occur without denaturing the hemoglobin. The Fe^{+2} is oxidized

BOX 25-2

Substances and Diseases Associated with Oxidative Damage to Erythrocytes

Foods

- Onions
- Propylene glycol
- Broccoli
- Garlic
- Salmon-based food

Drugs

- Acetaminophen
- Benzocaine
- Propofol
- DL-methionine
- Vitamin K_3

Metals

- Zinc
- Copper

Disease

- Diabetes mellitus (especially with ketoacidosis)
- Hyperthyroidism
- Hepatic lipidosis
- Lymphosarcoma

to Fe^{+3}, which is unable to bind oxygen. The result is methemoglobinemia.

Oxidative substances are free radicals that damage cell structures. They may accumulate when there is increased production or decreased detoxification of the free radical, which can be produced spontaneously from oxygen. They may also be the result of drugs, plants, or chemicals with oxidative properties.[14] Many substances or diseases can produce Heinz bodies (Box 25-2).

Heinz bodies are reported as the percentage of red cells containing Heinz bodies. Because of the nature of the feline spleen, up to 10% of erythrocytes in healthy cats may have Heinz bodies.[126] Any amount over this percentage should generate questions for the owner regarding diet and drug exposure. Owners who give their cats homemade diets or meat-based baby food may be inadvertently feeding enough onion powder to cause up to 50% Heinz bodies.[14] Cats ingesting an oxidative diet may be more susceptible to oxidative drugs. Cats with diseases generating increased numbers of Heinz bodies should not be given foods with Heinz body–producing potential insofar as the effects can be additive.

Cats are more susceptible to damage from oxidative drugs than other species. A number of drugs can produce oxidative damage to the red blood cell. In cats acetaminophen is particularly dangerous. Cats cannot metabolize the drug through glucuronidation, and oxidative metabolites are formed that damage the erythrocyte and the hemoglobin. Several diseases can produce substances that cause oxidative injury. Ketoacidotic cats may have up to 70% large Heinz bodies.[14] Diabetic cats without ketosis have a lesser degree of Heinz bodies. Owners should refrain from feeding onion-containing baby food to diabetic cats.

Signs of Heinz body anemia are similar to those found in most anemic cats: lethargy, anorexia, pale mucous membranes, tachycardia, and tachypnea. The addition of the lowered oxygen-carrying capacity of methemoglobin caused by iron oxidation can make the signs of hypoxia appear worse than the lowered PCV would suggest. If over 15% of the hemoglobin is in the form of methemoglobin, the color of the mucosa and blood can be altered to appear darker red or brownish in color. Significant methemoglobin is rarely associated with diet or diseases that produce Heinz bodies.[14]

The development and degree of anemia depends on the size, number, and rate of formation of Heinz bodies. Heinz bodies are produced at a slower rate by diet or disease compared with oxidative drugs and are less likely to be associated with acute hemolysis. Anemia is more likely when the Heinz bodies are large and affect over 30% of the erythrocytes. Heinz bodies appear dark when stained with new methylene blue stain. Ghost cells may appear on the slide if the erythrocytes are seen to be extruding the Heinz body. These cells look like empty circular rims with an attached Heinz body. As opposed to dogs, cats often have single, large Heinz bodies. The presence of many large Heinz bodies can artifactually increase the MCHC and automated leukocyte count. Once Heinz body anemia has been discovered, the veterinarian should carefully evaluate the cat for drug or onion ingestion or diabetes mellitus. It is important to search for an underlying cause for anemia even if Heinz bodies are present; they are a sign of disease, not the disease itself. Thoracic and abdominal radiography and abdominal ultrasonography may help identify any malignancies or metallic foreign bodies. Offending dietary substances may be identified on the food's package label. Owners sometimes unwittingly administer acetaminophen to cats that seem to be in pain.

Therapy for Heinz body anemia should first be directed at removing the cause of the oxidative damage (e.g., eliminating onion-containing foods or treating the underlying disease). As with any anemia-causing disease, supportive care based on the cat's condition is important. Intravenous fluid therapy to correct volume contraction is always important in dehydrated cats. If the clinical signs warrant, a blood transfusion may become necessary. Lastly, antioxidant therapy may be required if the disorder is severe. N-acetylcysteine is used to treat acetaminophen toxicity (see Chapter 31). Methylene blue can be administered intravenously to cats at 1 to 1.5 mg/kg once; however, additional doses may exacerbate the Heinz body anemia. Once the oxidative substance is removed from the cat, the Heinz bodies should disappear over the next 1 to 4 weeks.

Acute Hemolysis Secondary to Severe Hypophosphatemia

Phosphorus exists in the body as organic and inorganic phosphates. Organic phosphate is an important component of many cellular structures and molecules in the cat such as adenosine-5′-triphosphate (ATP), cyclic adenosine monophosphate (cAMP), the electron transport chain, and cell membranes. These, in turn, are important in maintaining the integrity of the cell. Inorganic phosphate is present mostly in the extracellular space and is an important substrate for oxidative phosphorylation and glycogenolysis.[74] Acute hemolysis due to hypophosphatemia has been recognized in cats treated for diabetes mellitus and hepatic lipidosis.[1] Cats with these diseases may already have low serum phosphate concentrations; treatment of the disease may result in a further decrease as exogenous insulin is administered to diabetic patients or endogenous insulin increases when chronically anorexic cats are refed. Insulin results in an intracellular shift of phosphate as it follows glucose into cells. The intraerythrocytic phosphate concentration is dependent on the serum phosphate concentration.

Severe hypophosphatemia leads to decreased erythrocyte phosphate and consequently depletion of ATP. The resultant loss of the high-energy phosphate leads to an inability to maintain the cell's biconcave shape,[1] a reduction in membrane deformability, increased osmotic fragility, and increased susceptibility to oxidative stress.[34] The result is a rigid, oxidatively stressed, fragile cell. The macrophages in the spleen remove these cells, and anemia develops. The presence of Heinz bodies in diabetic cats can exacerbate the anemia caused by hypophosphatemia.

Anemia caused by acute hemolysis develops within 1 to 2 days of documentation of a serum phosphate concentration less than 0.65 mmol/L. Because of the acute nature of the hemolysis, the anemia will be normocytic and normochromic and appear nonregenerative. In one report the PCV dropped between 9 and 18 percentage points.[1] Increased numbers of Heinz bodies may be found when examining a blood film. Cats that survive are expected to develop an aggregate reticulocytosis during recovery.

Supplementation is recommended when the serum phosphate is less than 0.65 mmol/L. Intravenous sodium phosphate or potassium phosphate is administered at 0.01 to 0.06 mmol/kg per hour in calcium-free solutions.[49] Serum calcium and phosphate concentrations should be monitored every 6 hours because hypocalcemia is a common complication (it is treated with intravenous calcium gluconate).[34] Once serum phosphate is over 0.65 mmol/L, the dosage can be decreased by half and discontinued shortly thereafter. Oral supplementation is started at this time.

Hypophosphatemia-associated acute hemolytic anemia is a complication of treating a diabetic cat or can result from refeeding syndrome. It is important to remember to evaluate the serum phosphate levels in these cats because the development of anemia can complicate recovery. Prophylactic use of phosphate supplementation for these patients may be considered if proper monitoring is available.

Feline Hemoplasmosis (Hemobartonellosis)

Feline hemoplasmas are epicellular gram-negative organisms causing anemia and illness in cats around the world. In one study 27% of 310 cats with acute or regenerative anemia tested positive for hemoplasmosis.[109] Another investigation found that 14% of all anemic cats were positive for hemoplasmosis.[83] Four distinct hemoplasmas have been detected in cats by PCR testing: *M. haemofelis, Candidatus* Mycoplasma haemominutum, *Candidatus* Mycoplasma turicensis, and *Candidatus* Mycoplasma haematoparvum. The most common hemoplasma found in cats is *Candidatus* M. haemominutum; mixed infections are not unusual.[109] *M. haemofelis* is the most pathogenic of the hemoplasmas and can cause potentially fatal hemolytic anemia. *Candidatus* M. haemominutum usually causes little to no illness in cats,[31] unless there is FeLV co-infection or co-infection with another hemoplasma. *Candidatus* M. turicensis has caused anemia when inoculated into specific-pathogen free cats.[108] The pathogenicity of *Candidatus* M. haematoparvum is as yet undetermined.

Erythrocyte cell membrane damage occurs as a result of attachment of the organism. Consequently, cell survival time is affected. The damaged membrane can also reveal antigens previously hidden from the immune system. Antibodies directed against these antigens (type II immune reaction) as well as the organism itself (type III immune reaction) can lead to Coombs'-positive immune-mediated hemolysis. The spleen removes these damaged cells, leading to a reduction in the PCV. Macrophages in the spleen may also remove the bacteria from the surface of the red cell and, if it is not too severely damaged, return the erythrocyte back into the circulation.[111] Despite appropriate therapy, cats that recover can remain subclinically infected for a period of time. PCR remains positive in these cats while the bacteria disappears from the erythrocytes and the PCV reaches the reference range. Cats that become carriers have reached a steady state between organism replication and macrophage phagocytosis and removal of erythrocytes. Carriers are more likely to occur after infection with *Candidatus* M. haemominutum than with *M. haemofelis*.[111]

The mode of transmission is poorly understood. Traditionally, it was thought that transmission of hemoplasmas occurred by fleas *(Ctenocephalides felis)*. Although PCR tests have documented the presence of hemoplasma DNA in flea larvae, feces, and eggs, ingestion of these did not result in transmission to cats under experimental conditions.[133] Transmission of infection has been found after fleas infected with hemoplasma fed on cats in an experimental setting. Experimental ingestion of infected blood, but not infected feline saliva,[79] also resulted in transmission of infection. Whether these results translate to the clinical setting is unknown, but this research leads to speculation that aggressive interactions between cats may also play a role in the transmission of the organism.[83]

Cats infected with hemoplasmas can be males or females of any age and are brought to the veterinarian for reasons similar to those of most other cats with anemia. They are often lethargic, pale, not eating well, and losing weight. The course may be waxing and waning as circulating parasite numbers fluctuates. The severity of the clinical signs depends on the species involved, the rate of development, and the degree of anemia. Cats infected with *M. haemofelis* or *Candidatus* M. turicensis are more likely to become anemic than cats infected with *Candidatus* M. haemominutum. The presence of FeLV co-infection results in a more severe illness; however, concurrent infection with FIV is not associated with more severe disease.[108] Physical findings include fever, pale mucous membranes, splenomegaly, and icterus. Cats infected with *Candidatus* M. haemominutum may have no physical abnormalities at all.[108] An ill cat infected with *Candidatus* M. haemominutum and no co-infection should be evaluated for other causes of anemia.

Evaluation of a cat experiencing the aforementioned clinical signs should include a CBC with a blood smear examination, an aggregate reticulocyte, and a platelet count; a Coombs' test; and retroviral testing. The anemia caused by feline hemoplasma infection should be macrocytic, normochromic to hypochromic and regenerative if enough time has elapsed to allow production of new erythrocytes. Increases in aggregate reticulocyte numbers should be present if the anemia is moderate to severe. If the anemia is mild, only punctate reticulocytes may be observed. The Coombs' test is often positive.[111] The cat should be evaluated for other causes of regenerative anemia as warranted by other clinical signs, such as bleeding.

Specific tests for hemoplasmosis include close inspection of erythrocytes on the blood smear for evidence of the organism and PCR tests for organism DNA. Occasionally, the organisms may appear on the blood smear

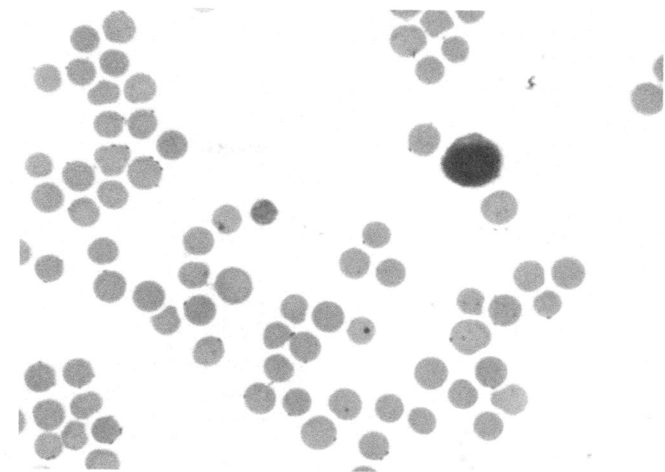

FIGURE 25-14 Giemsa-stained blood smear form a cat with *Mycoplasma haemofelis* infection. The organisms are attached to the surface of the erythrocytes. Anisocytosis (variation in cell size) is present on the slide. *(From Tasker S, Lappin MR: Update on hemoplasmosis. In August JR, editor:* Consultations in feline internal medicine, *ed 5, St Louis, 2006, Elsevier.)*

(Figure 25-14). The likelihood of finding organisms in this manner is affected by the cyclic nature of the parasitemia and, possibly, by sample handling issues. Slides should be made within 1 hour of collection to prevent the unlikely possibility that the organism will dislodge from the red cells.[111] Infected erythrocytes must be differentiated from Howell–Jolly bodies, stain precipitate, and ribosome-containing reticulocytes. PCR is a more sensitive test and is considered the test of choice for the infection. Cats undergoing antibiotic treatment are often PCR negative and should not be tested with this technique. A positive test result indicates the presence of organism DNA and may not correlate with clinical disease. Carriers of the infection are identified with this test.

Traditionally, cats with hemoplasma infections have been treated with tetracycline. Oral doxycycline at 10 mg/kg every 24 hours can be effective in treating the illness caused by hemoplasmosis. Courses longer than 21 days may be required for elimination of the organism. Esophageal strictures are a possible complication of doxycycline administration in tablet or capsule form and can be prevented by ensuring passage of the drug into the stomach by syringing a small amount of food or water after administering the pill to the cat. Doxycycline can also be compounded into a suspension. Applying a small amount of butter or margarine to the nose may accomplish the same thing. Fluoroquinolone antibiotics have been shown to be effective in treating cats with hemoplasma infections. Enrofloxacin (Baytril, Bayer HealthCare) at 5 mg/kg orally every 24 hours was associated with improvement in clinical signs, although elimination of the infection was uncommon.[21] Daily doses higher than this may cause retinal degeneration in cats. Other fluoroquinolones may be effective.

Marbofloxacin (Zeniquin, Pfizer Animal Health) at 2 mg/kg orally every 24 hours is effective at treating illness but may not result in clearance of the infection.[110] Retinal toxicity has not yet been identified in cats receiving marbofloxacin. Pradofloxacin (Veraflox, Bayer AG) at 5 mg/kg orally every 24 hours appears to be safe and effective in treating illness caused by hemoplasma infections. It also appears to be more effective in clearing the organism than doxycycline.[22] Prednisolone, initially dosed at 2 mg/kg orally every 24 hours, before dose tapering has been used to control the immune-mediated component of the disease. However, this drug may be unnecessary because some cats recover without the use of glucocorticoids.[111] If the illness and anemia are severe, a transfusion may be required.

Cats with anemia caused by hemoplasmosis have an excellent prognosis for recovery.[83] The prognosis may not be as good for cats with concurrent disease, such as co-infection with FeLV. Prevention of the disease may include flea control and preventing aggressive interactions with other cats. The efficacy of these tactics is unknown insofar as the mode of transmission of the infection is still not clear. Cats with a positive PCR test should not be used as blood donors.

Nonregenerative (Nonresponsive) Anemia

Definition

Nonregenerative anemia is defined as a decreased erythrocyte mass (decreased PCV, red cell count, and hemoglobin concentration) without evidence of increased bone marrow production of new red blood cells. Lack of regeneration can be caused by decreased EPO production, decreased responsiveness of the bone marrow to EPO, decreased erythroid precursors in the bone marrow, or iron deficiency. Numerous disorders can lead to a nonregenerative anemia, including chronic renal disease, liver disease, inflammatory disease, FeLV infection, immune-mediated destruction of erythrocyte precursors, and primary bone marrow disease such as neoplasia and myelodysplasia. An anemia is nonregenerative if there are inadequate numbers of circulating aggregate reticulocytes for the degree of anemia. It is important to remember that an acute onset of anemia may also appear nonregenerative if there has not been enough time (4 to 7 days) for the bone marrow to produce and release aggregate reticulocytes.

History and Physical Examination

The signs associated with anemia are often nonspecific and have been covered in a previous section of this chapter (Clinical Evaluation of Cats with Anemia).

Diagnostic Plans

A CBC, along with measurement of erythrocyte indices, a blood smear evaluation, and a reticulocyte count, should be performed in all cats in which anemia is a suspected cause of the clinical signs. Nonregenerative anemias are most often normocytic and normochromic. As with regenerative anemias, the PCV, erythrocyte count, and hemoglobin concentration are all decreased. However, because there is no increase in reticulocyte production, the MCV is usually within the reference range. The RDW is also in the reference range because most of the erythrocytes are similar in size. These parameters may lie outside the reference range in disorders such as iron deficiency and infection with FeLV. Most of the erythrocytes will have their normal allotment of hemoglobin, so the MCHC is also in the reference range.

Once a nonregenerative anemia has been identified, the goal of further diagnostic procedures is to identify extramarrow causes of the anemia before pursuing intramarrow disorders. A serum biochemical profile, urinalysis, and retroviral tests should be performed.[18] If the duration of illness is shorter than 5 days, the cat's bone marrow may not have had enough time to increase erythrocyte production. Another CBC and reticulocyte count should be performed to ensure that the anemia is nonregenerative. Other diagnostic procedures that may be useful include thoracic radiographs and abdominal imaging. If these steps have not identified a cause for the anemia, evaluation of the bone marrow should be performed.

Iron Deficiency

Iron exists in the body in the form of hemoglobin, myoglobin, labile iron, tissue iron, and transported iron.[129] Hemoglobin concentrations inside the maturing erythrocyte help determine when cell division stops; erythrocytes undergo extra divisions, resulting in smaller cells when decreased hemoglobin is available. In most species the anemia of iron deficiency is microcytic (decreased MCV) and hypochromic (decreased MCHC), but cats are less likely to develop these changes.[18] Early in the course of iron deficiency, the anemia is likely to be regenerative. Sufficient polychromasia and reticulocytosis may be present.[18] As iron stores are depleted, polychromasia and reticulocytosis decrease and the anemia becomes nonregenerative. The degree of anemia ranges from mild to life threatening.[129] Variations in red cell shape (poikilocytosis)[129] and fragmented erythrocytes (schistocytosis)[18] are commonly observed on the blood smear. Poikilocytosis is also common in cats with liver disease.[126]

Kittens are at risk of developing iron deficiency anemia as a result of endoparasitism or ectoparasitism. Repeated blood sampling from kittens can also lead to iron depletion. Severe flea-bite anemia occurs in young kittens as a result of iron loss.[129] Anemia from total body iron depletion is unusual in adult cats.[129] Chronic blood loss caused by gastrointestinal ulceration or neoplasia may result in an iron deficiency anemia. If the amount of blood lost at any one time is small, there will not be

TABLE 25-4 Anemia of Inflammatory Disease Versus Iron-Deficiency Anemia

	Anemia of Inflammatory Disease	Iron-Deficiency Anemia
Erythrocyte indices	Normocytic, normochromic	Microcytic, hypochromic
Serum iron concentration	Low	Low
Total iron-binding capacity (transferrin)	Often decreased	Often normal
Bone marrow iron	May be increased	Absent (also a finding in normal cats)
Serum ferritin	High	Low
Inflammatory disease	Present	Need not be present

evidence of regeneration; the anemia will be caused by chronic iron loss. Careful evaluation of the gastrointestinal tract may be required insofar as there may be no overt evidence of gastrointestinal disease (e.g., vomiting, melena).[93] Loss through the urinary tract from bleeding transitional cell carcinoma or cystitis is unlikely to lead to iron loss sufficient to cause anemia.[129]

Diagnosis of an iron deficiency anemia can be difficult. The changes in the erythron can be similar to anemia of inflammatory disease (AID; see later discussion). Sometimes the diagnosis can be made on the basis of the history and physical examination because there will be evidence of blood loss or active inflammation. Often, more information is required. Healthy cats typically do not have visible iron stores in their bone marrow. Although the presence of iron in the bone marrow rules out iron deficiency, its absence does not prove it.[34,128] An iron profile can prove useful (Table 25-4). Serum iron concentrations alone are too nonspecific.[128] Assessing the total iron-binding capacity (TIBC) and serum ferritin concentrations can be helpful. The TIBC is a measure of the concentration of transferrin, a plasma protein that functions in iron transport. In an iron-deficient cat, transferrin (and TIBC) would be expected to be normal to slightly increased[34] in an attempt to offer more capacity for transport of iron to the cells. Because serum iron is low, the saturation of transferrin is decreased. Iron sequestration and decreased iron transport are a consequence of inflammatory disease so that transferrin concentrations (and TIBC) are decreased.[126] Ferritin is a cytoplasmic protein that stores iron in a soluble phase inside the cell.[34] In states of iron deficiency, cytoplasmic iron stores are decreased, resulting in decreased ferritin requirements and decreased plasma concentrations. Ferritin also happens to be an acute phase inflammatory protein. In conditions involving inflammation, ferritin concentrations are expected to be elevated.[128] In summary, transferrin (TIBC) is increased and ferritin decreased in iron deficiency, whereas the reverse may be true for AID.

When a cat with iron deficiency is being treated, it is imperative that the cause of blood loss be identified and addressed. If the cat's clinical signs warrant it, a transfusion may be required. Iron replacement therapy involves administering ferrous sulfate at 50 to 100 mg/cat orally every 24 hours. If gastrointestinal upset occurs, the dose may be divided. The dose should be decreased by 50% once the PCV is in the reference range. If intestinal absorption is questionable, iron dextran should be administered intramuscularly at 50 mg every 3 to 4 weeks until the gastrointestinal disease is under control. Occasionally, hypersensitivity reactions will occur with iron dextran injections. Evidence of regeneration, such as polychromasia and reticulocytosis, should be apparent within several days[18] as hemoglobin synthesis and erythropoiesis accelerate.

Anemia of Inflammatory Disease

Inflammatory conditions cause mild to moderate nonregenerative anemia.[43,126] The PCV is often greater than 20% and is generally associated with an inflammatory leukogram[18] and fever.[126] Cytokines released by inflammatory cells in response to infection, cell damage, or malignancy cause iron sequestration by macrophages. Because iron is an essential growth factor for microorganisms,[86] this is thought to be a protective mechanism against infection. It also leaves less iron for erythropoiesis. The inflammatory environment leads to decreased erythrocyte survival, decreased EPO secretion in response to anemia, and decreased bone marrow response to existing EPO.[86] This process has been known as anemia of chronic disease; however, cats in one study had a decreased PCV within 2 days of onset of an inflammatory disease.[86] Many of the cats developed hyperglobulinemia as a result of the inflammation.

The diagnosis of AID is one of exclusion. Other causes of nonregenerative anemia must first be eliminated.[86] Evidence for this mechanism of anemia may be found in the history or physical examination. Decreases in serum iron concentrations may mimic iron deficiency and are not confirmatory for either disease. Measuring serum ferritin concentrations may be helpful. In addition to being an iron-carrying protein, it is also an acute phase protein and may be elevated in inflammatory disorders.[128] Bone marrow cytology is nonspecific because changes such as myeloid hyperplasia and erythroid hypoplasia are common. This results in an increased myeloid to erythroid (M:E) ratio.[18]

Therapy for AID involves treating the underlying disease. When treated successfully, the anemia should resolve within several weeks.[86] Because the anemia is usually mild to moderate, specific therapy, such as blood transfusions, is usually not required. Supplementation with iron products is not recommended because the increased iron may promote the growth of pathogenic bacteria or tumor cells.[86] Occasionally, the anemia is severe, and a blood transfusion is needed. In a retrospective study, only 3 of 21 cats with nonregenerative anemia associated with inflammatory disease required a transfusion.[86]

Chronic Renal Disease

Anemia is an expected consequence of chronic renal disease (CRD) in cats and contributes significantly to their lack of well-being.[91] Marked azotemia and an inappropriate urine specific gravity are usually present by the time CRD causes a significant anemia.[18] The cause of anemia is multifactorial and may be exacerbated by concurrent illness.[93] There are four major causes of the anemia:

1. Uremic toxins may suppress the maturation of erythroid precursors in the bone marrow.
2. Erythrocyte life span may be shortened in animals with CRD.
3. Blood loss is often overlooked as a cause of anemia in CRD patients. Uremia can lead to platelet dysfunction and to gastrointestinal ulceration.[129] Evidence of gastrointestinal blood loss can be difficult to find because melena may not be present.[93]
4. The most important contributing factor to the anemia of CRD is EPO deficiency. EPO is produced in the peritubular fibroblasts deep in the renal cortex in response to hypoxia. Decreasing renal mass results in decreased numbers of EPO-producing cells.

The anemia of CRD is normocytic, normochromic, and hypoproliferative.[97] Poikilocytes may be noted during examination of a blood smear.[93] Initially, the anemia is mild, but as renal disease progresses, the anemia becomes correspondingly more severe.[129] Occasionally, a transfusion becomes necessary. Bone marrow cytology may reveal erythroid hypoplasia and an increased myeloid to erythroid (M:E) ratio.

Specific therapy directed at treating anemia of CRD includes EPO replacement and minimizing blood loss. An overlooked but obvious consideration is minimizing the number and volume of blood samples obtained when a patient is hospitalized. Repeated blood monitoring should be limited to that which is essential to manage the patient.[93] Occult gastrointestinal blood loss can lead to significant anemia in patients that would otherwise have enough EPO to maintain the PCV in an acceptable range. Because of the difficulty in proving gastrointestinal blood loss, empirical use of H_2 receptor blockers along with sucralfate should be considered.[93]

Recombinant human EPO (rhEPO) is a genetically engineered protein used to treat anemia in humans.[19] The structure of EPO is relatively well conserved across species, allowing for biological activity of rhEPO in cats.[128] Hormone replacement using rhEPO is the treatment of choice for anemia associated with erythropoietic failure in cats with chronic renal failure.[93] Consideration for use of rhEPO should be limited to patients with severe anemia that affects quality of life. The initial dose is 100 units/kg subcutaneously three times weekly. This dose may be modified if the anemia is particularly severe without requiring a transfusion. If the PCV is less than 14%, 150 U/kg may be administered subcutaneously three times weekly. Should the patient be hypertensive or if the anemia is not particularly severe (yet still causing clinical signs), a dose of 50 U/kg may be effective in increasing the PCV while preventing a further increase in blood pressure.[93] The initial dose is continued for 8 to 12 weeks until the target PCV of 30% is reached.[19] The PCV should be measured weekly so the dose can be altered when the target is reached.[70] At that point, dosing frequency is reduced to once or twice weekly to maintain the PCV above 30%. The dosage and dosing interval must be individualized for each patient.[128] Changes in dose should be made infrequently because there is a lag between a dosage change and its effect on the PCV. Generally, the dose should not be changed more than once monthly.[93] If iatrogenic erythrocytosis occurs, the dose or dosing interval (or both) should be decreased. A cat that does not respond should be evaluated for iron deficiency, external blood loss, AID, or the development of antibodies directed against rhEPO.[19] Improper storage, handling, or administration by the owner should also be considered.[93] The drug vial should be refrigerated, and care should be taken not to vigorously shake the vial to prevent protein denaturation.

Potential adverse effects of rhEPO administration include iron deficiency, hypertension, erythrocytosis, anaphylaxis, local reactions to the injection,[94] and most important the development of anti-EPO antibodies.[128] The rapid increase in erythropoiesis can lead to the use of large amounts of iron. If iron is not supplemented, iron deficiency will develop. All cats receiving rhEPO should also receive ferrous sulfate at 50 to 100 mg/cat per day orally. Chronic anemia leads to vasodilation[19] to facilitate delivery of blood to the tissues. Once the anemia is corrected by using rhEPO, total peripheral resistance increases, although clinical hypertension is uncommon. In a study of cats receiving recombinant feline EPO (rfEPO), only 2 of 26 cats that responded developed hypertension requiring antihypertensive therapy.[94]

Although the rhEPO molecule is very similar to the cat's endogenous EPO, it is not identical. There is enough structural variation for the immune system of some cats to recognize rhEPO as a foreign protein and mount an immune response against it.[94] Approximately 20% to 50% of cats receiving rhEPO will develop antibodies against the protein.[91,128] These antibodies usually develop in cats receiving rhEPO for longer than 4 weeks.[128] Unfortunately, these antibodies block the biological effects not only of rhEPO but also of the cat's endogenous EPO.[94] This can lead to a life-threatening red cell aplasia as the patient's PCV drops to below pretreatment levels. This condition is reversible with cessation of the drug, but it may be months before the PCV recovers.[70] Until that time transfusions may be necessary to support the cat. After developing antibodies against rhEPO, its use is contraindicated. Because of the development of these antibodies, rhEPO should be reserved for patients most in need. Proper client education and communication are important when making decisions regarding the use of this therapy.

Evaluation of an rfEPO has been reported. Although the product is not available, it seems to be effective in reversing the anemia of chronic renal failure.[94] It also reversed the red cell aplasia caused by antibodies against rhEPO in some cats. Unexpectedly, 8 of the 26 cats receiving rfEPO redeveloped a nonregenerative anemia after an initial response. It was postulated that perhaps there are variations in the endogenous EPO in the cat population, allowing immune response against the molecule. Other possible targets of an immune reaction are the carbohydrate moiety on the molecule or some additive in the rfEPO preparation.[94]

Darbepoietin is a longer acting form of rhEPO. Anecdotally, it seems to have similar efficacy and safety as rhEPO.[97] It can be administered as a weekly injection and may be less immunogenic in animals, but this has not been documented. Darbepoietin acts similarly to EPO by stimulating erythropoiesis in the bone marrow. Adverse effects in animals are unknown but are likely similar to rhEPO because darbepoietin causes increased erythropoiesis and improved oxygen delivery to tissues. This may result in hypertension, erythrocytosis, and iron deficiency. Until proven otherwise, darbepoietin should be considered potentially immunogenic.

With the availability of rhEPO, the ability to control anemia caused by chronic renal failure has improved. Careful patient selection, proper patient monitoring, and constant client communications are crucial to successful management of these patients. Supplementation with ferrous sulfate and control of gastrointestinal bleeding are also essential.

Feline Leukemia Virus Infection

Various hematologic abnormalities are common in cats infected with FeLV. Anemia can be caused by bone marrow suppression, myelodysplasia, myelophthisis due to lymphosarcoma or leukemia, or immune-mediated hemolysis.[129] Most of the anemias caused by FeLV are nonregenerative. The anemia can be normocytic, normochromic, and nonregenerative or macrocytic, normochromic, and nonregenerative. If there is immune-mediated hemolysis, a regenerative anemia may occur.[18] Hemolysis may be a direct result of the virus or due to co-infection with *M. haemofelis*.

The virus causes nonregenerative anemia by infecting erythroid precursors in the bone marrow and the stromal cells supporting the marrow.[59] Integration of proviral DNA into the marrow cell may cause marrow dysfunction by altering regulatory mechanisms or inducing the expression of an unknown antigen on the surface of the erythrocyte precursor or stromal fibroblast, leading to immune-mediated destruction of these cells.[107] The result is depletion and maturation arrest of erythrocyte precursors in the bone marrow.[59] Granulocyte precursors and megakaryocytes may also be affected, causing leukopenia and thrombocytopenia or thrombocytosis.[125] Cats with macrocytic nonregenerative anemias are often FeLV antigen positive.[18] Macrocytosis is thought to result from a skipped mitosis during erythropoiesis; reticulocyte numbers are not increased.[129]

Some FeLV-infected cats will have normocytic nonregenerative anemias with anisocytosis but no polychromasia. Anisocytosis results from a subpopulation of mature cells that are larger than the others but are not reticulocytes.[26] These cats may have an increased RDW reported on a hemogram. If a histogram of red cell size is provided, two peaks may be present, reflecting the two populations of cells: one of normal size and one a bit larger. Macrocytosis without anemia may be seen in some cats with hyperthyroidism.[14] A spurious macrocytosis may result from the agglutination of erythrocytes as they pass through automated cell counters.

A cat with hematologic changes that is negative for circulating FeLV antigen may still be infected with the virus. Latent FeLV infections are defined as circulating antigen negative and bone marrow positive. The provirus is present in a nonreplicating form in myelomonocytic precursors in the marrow.[107] The viral particles may be identified by performing an indirect fluorescent antibody test on marrow smear or by using a PCR test. A study of a population of cats with various types of nonregenerative cytopenias of unknown origin was performed to assess the role of latent FeLV infections. All the cats had a negative test for circulating FeLV antigen. Only 2 of the 37 cats had a positive PCR test for FeLV proviral DNA in the bone marrow. The researchers concluded that FeLV latency does not play an important role in cats with nonregenerative cytopenias.[107]

Any cat with anemia without obvious cause (e.g., trauma, blood loss) should be checked for the presence of FeLV antigen. If the anemia is regenerative, additional testing for blood parasites such as *M. haemofelis* is indicated. Therapy for cats with FeLV-associated anemia is supportive. Concurrent infection with blood parasites should be treated appropriately. Immunosuppressive doses of prednisolone should be used if immune-mediated hemolysis is a factor.[128] Blood transfusions will be useful in ameliorating clinical signs of anemia. Some cats may respond to the administration of rhEPO, although most cats already have high circulating concentrations of EPO.[59]

Pure Red Cell Aplasia

Pure red cell aplasia (PRCA) is characterized by a severe normocytic, normochromic, nonregenerative anemia along with erythroid hypoplasia and increased lymphocyte numbers in the bone marrow.[125] Granulocytes and megakaryocytes are left intact. This is a rare syndrome[129] thought to be caused by immune-mediated response against erythrocyte precursors in the marrow. Infection with FeLV subgroup C has also been implicated in the pathogenesis of the disease. It appears to be a disease of younger cats.[125] A Coombs' test may be positive, and other causes of anemia are absent. The PCV is often lower than 20%.[26] Aggressive combination immunosuppressive therapy with prednisolone and another drug (such as chlorambucil) is often required to control the immune-mediated damage (see the previous section on treating immune-mediated hemolytic anemia). Response to treatment may not be apparent for several weeks.

Acute Blood Loss or Hemolysis

Acute loss of sufficient erythrocytes either by hemorrhage or hemolysis leads to hypoxia and increased production of EPO by the kidneys. If the cat is evaluated before aggregate reticulocytes are released by the bone marrow, the circulating red cell morphology will appear nonregenerative. Immediately upon bleeding, both red cells and plasma are lost and no decrease in PCV is detected. Within 12 to 24 hours of acute hemorrhage, interstitial fluid shifts into the intravascular space. The increase in plasma volume dilutes the red cells and is recognized as anemia. Acute hemolysis will also lead to decreased erythrocyte numbers. In both situations the anemia may be evaluated before the appearance of aggregate reticulocytes in the circulation. A CBC performed at this time will reveal the presence of a normocytic, normochromic, nonregenerative anemia without polychromasia or increased aggregate reticulocyte numbers. The anemia will not be recognized as regenerative until aggregate reticulocytes are released 4 or 5 days after the initial event. A second CBC should be performed 5 days after onset of illness before the conclusion is reached that an anemia is nonregenerative.

Bone Marrow Disease

Numerous types of bone marrow disorders can cause nonregenerative anemia in cats, although they are very uncommon. Disorders include aplastic anemia, myelofibrosis, myelodysplasia, and myelophthisis secondary to inflammatory diseases or neoplasia. Many are associated with FeLV. The etiologic diagnosis of bone marrow disease requires a cytologic or histopathologic evaluation of a bone marrow sample.

Aplastic anemia is defined as the presence of bicytopenia or pancytopenia. Most of the hematopoietic space of the marrow is replaced by adipose tissue. Cats most commonly have a nonregenerative anemia along with leukopenia, thrombocytopenia, or both. Although it may be idiopathic in cats, aplastic anemia is also associated with chronic renal disease, FeLV infections, and methimazole and griseofulvin toxicity.[125] Starvation and emaciation appear to have a role in the pathogenesis of the disorder in association with chronic renal disease and those with idiopathic aplastic anemia.[127] Some cats may survive for prolonged periods despite the presence of hypocellular bone marrow.[127]

Myelofibrosis is defined as proliferation of fibroblasts or collagen in the bone marrow. It can be primary or secondary. Primary or idiopathic myelofibrosis is a disorder of dysplastic megakaryocytes, which produce cytokines that induce proliferation of fibroblasts.[52] Secondary myelofibrosis in cats is associated with immune-mediated anemia, myelodysplasia, acute myelogenous leukemia, CRD,[125] and FeLV infection.[52] Most commonly, a moderate to severe nonregenerative anemia is found in cats.[125] Myelofibrosis should be suspected when repeated bone marrow aspirates are unsuccessful, and definitive diagnosis is based on finding excessive fibroblasts on histopathologic examination of a bone marrow core biopsy.[52]

Myelodysplastic syndrome (MDS) comprises a group of proliferative hematologic disorders originating from a mutation in a hematopoietic stem cell.[125] Most cats are anemic, and many have other cytopenias. The anemia is commonly macrocytic, normochromic, and nonregenerative. Almost 80% of cats with MDS are FeLV positive.[129] MDS is thought to be a preneoplastic condition and may be lethal without progression to leukemia.[129] Therapy for cats with MDS is supportive and may include blood transfusions, antibiotics for those with severe leukopenia, and corticosteroids. Survival time for a cat with MDS is likely to be measured in days to weeks from the time of diagnosis. However, some cats may survive for longer than 1 year.

By definition, *myelophthisis* is the replacement of hematopoietic space of the bone marrow by neoplastic, inflammatory, or collagen-producing cells.[52] Acute and chronic leukemia may infiltrate the bone marrow, leading to a nonregenerative anemia. Acute inflammatory lesions in the marrow have been associated with immune-mediated hemolytic anemia, bacterial sepsis, and infection with the coronavirus responsible for feline infectious peritonitis. Pyogranulomatous inflammation has been observed in cats with disseminated histoplasmosis. The anemia in cats with myelophthisis is often moderate to severe.[125]

Unfortunately, nonregenerative anemia can be a frustrating problem to solve and sometimes unrewarding to treat. A lack of increased numbers of aggregate reticulocytes in the face of a decreased PCV is indicative of this type of anemia. Extensive testing is often required to achieve a diagnosis. Some cats remain a diagnostic dilemma and must be treated symptomatically with blood transfusions, antibiotics, and corticosteroids. Frequent monitoring is often required to detect changes that may affect the cat's well-being.

Feline Erythrocytosis

Definition

Erythrocytosis, also known as *polycythemia,* is defined as an increase in the red blood cell mass as measured by an increase in the PCV, red blood cell count, and hemoglobin concentration. Like anemia, erythrocytosis is a sign of disease, not a disease in itself. Erythrocytosis is an uncommon finding in cats. EPO is a hormone produced by fibroblasts adjacent to proximal convoluted tubules deep in the renal cortex.[47] These cells are subject to negative feedback based on systemic or local oxygen tension. They respond to hypoxia by increasing the production of EPO. Red blood cell precursors in the bone marrow respond to EPO by dividing and maturing into cells capable of carrying oxygen to the tissues. Optimal oxygen delivery in normovolemic cats occurs at a PCV between 35% and 45%.[84] When hypoxia resolves, EPO production decreases, and production of new erythrocytes slows.

Clinical Signs and Physical Findings

The signs associated with erythrocytosis are due to increased blood viscosity. This leads to a decrease in the rate of blood flow in the microcirculation followed by distention and possibly thrombosis of these vessels. Hyperemia, bleeding, and central nervous system signs are the result of these changes. With increased hemoglobin concentration comes a greater chance of exceeding the 50 g/L level of deoxygenated hemoglobin, above which cyanosis becomes evident, making the detection of hyperemia difficult. Bleeding occurs because of rupture of the distended small vessels. Vessel obstruction and bleeding may result in central nervous system hypoxia and subsequent alterations in mentation, seizures, weakness, ataxia, and blindness. Approximately 25% of cats will have splenomegaly.[47] Other clinical signs may be present if there is an underlying disease.

Classification and Pathophysiology

Erythrocytosis can be classified into categories, each with its own unique underlying pathophysiology (Figure 25-15). The disorder can be relative or absolute. Relative erythrocytosis is caused by decreased plasma volume and a "relative" increase in the red blood cell volume as measured by the PCV. Whereas the PCV is mildly increased, the total erythrocyte mass is not. Any disease leading to fluid loss and volume contraction may result in a relative erythrocytosis. Common causes include diarrhea and burns. EPO concentrations and reticulocyte numbers would be expected to be low to normal. Splenic contraction does not significantly elevate erythrocyte numbers in cats.[84]

Absolute erythrocytosis, characterized by an actual increase in the red blood cell mass, is further categorized into primary and secondary absolute erythrocytosis. Primary erythrocytosis is a neoplastic disease seen in young to middle-aged cats in which autonomous erythrocyte precursors in the bone marrow divide and mature in the absence of EPO.[84] The other cell lines in the bone marrow remain unaffected.

Secondary absolute erythrocytosis is associated with increased EPO production and is divided further into physiologically appropriate or inappropriate. Appropriate secondary erythrocytosis occurs as a normal response to systemic hypoxia and is an appropriate, compensatory response. The most common causes include congenital cardiac disease with right-to-left shunting of blood, a high-altitude environment, chronic pulmonary parenchymal disease, and severe obesity (Pickwickian syndrome).[47,84] Serum EPO would be expected to be normal to high.

Inappropriate secondary erythrocytosis is defined as increased erythrocyte mass without evidence of systemic hypoxia. The most common cause in cats is renal disease, including solid tumors or diffusely infiltrative neoplasia, polycystic kidney disease, amyloidosis, or pyelonephritis.[47] Locally reduced renal parenchymal blood flow due to compression or infiltration leads to focal hypoxia in the cortex, resulting in increased production of EPO.[84] Tumors of other body systems may produce EPO or EPO-like substances as a paraneoplastic syndrome. As with appropriate secondary erythrocytosis, EPO levels would be expected to be normal to high.

Diagnostic Plans

A logical approach to the diagnosis of erythrocytosis is important, insofar as treatment depends on the underlying cause. A thorough history and detailed physical examination, along with a CBC with a reticulocyte count, serum biochemical profile, and urinalysis is the recommended minimum database.[84]

Relative erythrocytosis should be evident at this phase of the workup; the history and physical examination should reveal evidence of disease causing volume contraction. Along with an elevated PCV, the reticulocyte count should be low because erythropoiesis is not increased. The total plasma protein concentration should be elevated, along with the presence of azotemia and an appropriate increase in urine specific gravity. A

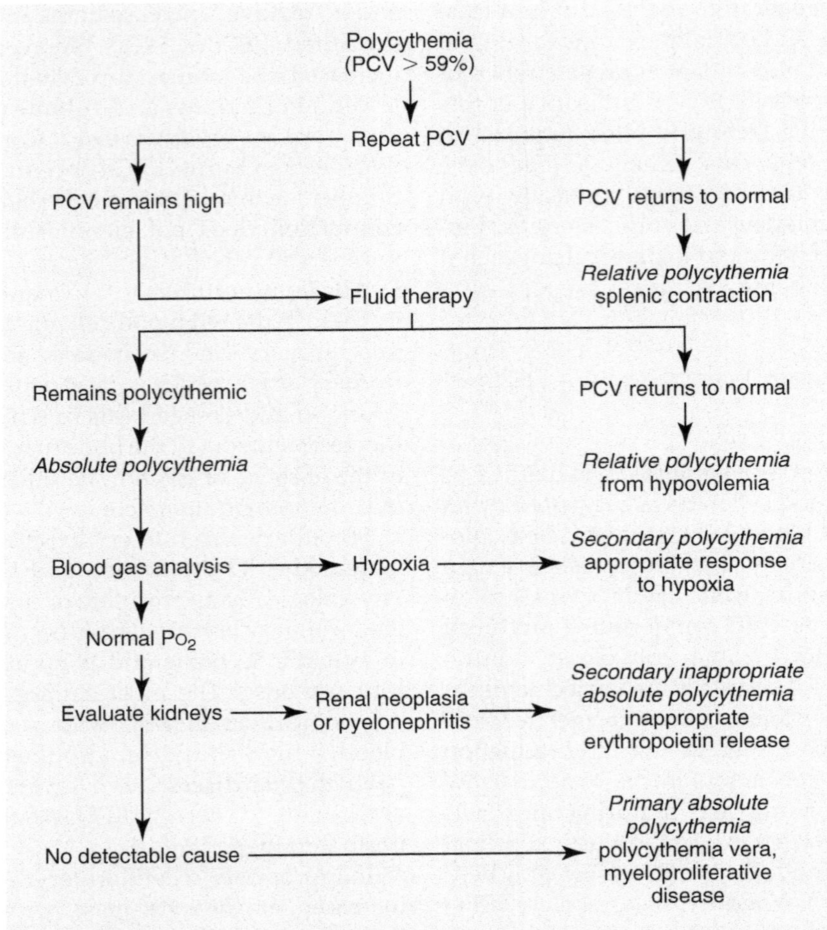

FIGURE 25-15 An algorithm that may be useful in deciding the classification of erythrocytosis. A diagnosis of primary erythrocytosis is made only when all other potential causes have been eliminated. The veterinarian should use clinical judgment when following an algorithm because an individual cat may not follow the rules. *PCV,* Packed cell volume. *(Modified from Figure 3-6; Weiss D, Tvedten H: Erythrocyte disorders. In Willard MD, Tvedten H, editors:* Small animal diagnosis by laboratory methods, *ed 4, St Louis, 2004, Saunders.)*

reduction in PCV after volume expansion confirms the diagnosis.

If the erythrocytosis is not relative, the next step is to look for evidence of hypoxia and accelerated erythropoiesis. An increased reticulocyte count in the face of an increased PCV suggests increased erythropoietic activity.[47] Severe obesity causing decreased pulmonary function may be present.[84] Cats with hypoxia often show evidence of respiratory distress and possibly cyanosis. Pulse oximetry and arterial blood gas assessment should confirm hypoxia. An etiologic diagnosis should be pursued by obtaining thoracic radiographs and performing an echocardiogram. Mild bronchointerstitial changes in the lungs and mild left ventricular hypertrophy may be found in cats with hyperviscosity from any cause.[47] Rarely, methemoglobinemia in cats can lead to erythrocytosis.

If no evidence of hypoxia is found, a diligent search for disorders causing an inappropriate production of EPO should be performed. Because renal neoplasia (both carcinoma and lymphosarcoma) is the most common cause, imaging of the kidneys is prudent.[84] Abdominal radiography, intravenous pyelography, and abdominal ultrasonography may identify structural abnormalities of the kidneys. These procedures may also reveal tumors of other organs that may be producing EPO or EPO-like substances.

Primary erythrocytosis is a diagnosis made by exclusion.[84] Most cats with this disease will have normal laboratory parameters, other than the hemogram, and normal imaging results. EPO concentrations would be expected to be low to normal[84]; if not, the veterinarian should reconsider the likelihood of inappropriate secondary erythrocytosis. Bone marrow examination is not helpful in the diagnosis, insofar as there are no markers for abnormal erythrocyte precursors, and absolute erythrocytosis leads to marrow erythroid hyperplasia, no matter the cause.[47]

Therapeutic Plans

Phlebotomy should be the initial treatment for symptomatic cats with absolute erythrocytosis from any cause. The goal is to maintain the PCV such that clinical signs are alleviated. This is usually in the range of 50% for cats, unless they have hypoxia causing an appropriate secondary erythrocytosis.[47] No more than 10 to 20 mL/kg should be removed daily to reduce the PCV to the target level, and when it is safe to do so, the veterinarian should administer an equal volume of intravenous fluids or re-infuse the patient's removed plasma to further reduce viscosity. This should be repeated as needed to maintain the PCV at that range.

Phlebotomy is a generally safe procedure. However, phlebotomy is more physically demanding for the operator when dealing with erythrocytosis because of the increased viscosity of the blood being removed. Potential unwanted sequelae include hypovolemia and hypoproteinemia.[84] Frequent blood removal may also lead to iron deficiency, and iron supplementation may be required.

Therapy for relative erythrocytosis involves volume expansion with appropriate intravenous fluids or blood products and correction of the underlying cause. Successful treatment of inappropriate secondary erythrocytosis resulting from EPO-secreting tumors involves surgical removal of the offending neoplasm after stabilization of the cat's clinical status and PCV.[84] Presurgical phlebotomy may reduce the risk of bleeding or thrombosis during surgery. Drainage of large cysts and antimicrobial therapy may be useful in cats with polycystic kidney disease or pyelonephritis, respectively.

Appropriate secondary erythrocytosis is a compensatory mechanism to combat hypoxia; therefore removing too much blood by phlebotomy may exacerbate the hypoxia experienced by the cat. Systemic oxygenation declines with a PCV over 60%, so the veterinarian should attempt to maintain a PCV in the range of 55% to 60%.[47,84] Treating the underlying cause is imperative. Severely obese cats should have a proper weight loss program instituted, and cats with heart disease and those with chronic bronchial disease should be treated appropriately. Because cats with cardiac disease may already be volume expanded, crystalloid replacement of the volume of blood removed by phlebotomy may result in volume overload and pulmonary edema.

Cats with primary absolute erythrocytosis will require phlebotomy for the rest of their lives. If the procedure needs to be performed too frequently or is ineffective in maintaining the PCV at an appropriate level, the addition of hydroxyurea should be considered. Hydroxyurea is an alkylating chemotherapeutic agent that suppresses production of erythrocytes. The dose should be individualized to maintain an acceptable PCV. The regimen begins with 10 to 15 mg/kg orally every 12 hours until the target PCV is met, then continues every other day at the lowest dose needed to maintain that PCV. The dose is increased if the PCV starts to climb.[120]

Hydroxyurea may cause reversible myelosuppression,[47] so a CBC with platelet count should be performed periodically to assess white blood cell and platelet numbers. If cell numbers decrease significantly, the medications should be discontinued until cell counts become normal, and the drug is restarted at a lower dose. Other potential side effects include vomiting, anorexia, and methemoglobinemia at high doses.

Prognosis

The prognosis for cats with erythrocytosis depends on the underlying cause. Removal of a renal tumor in a patient with secondary inappropriate erythrocytosis may be curative as long as metastasis has not occurred. Animals with primary erythrocytosis have lived for many years with appropriate treatment.[47]

SELECTED LEUKOCYTE DISORDERS

Evaluation of White Blood Cell Changes

Interpretation of the leukogram seems straightforward, and often it is. As with investigating any other body system, evaluation of white blood cells involves integration of the signalment, history, and physical findings with the numbers reported on the CBC. Abnormal cell numbers in a healthy cat may be normal for that particular cat. A thorough white blood cell evaluation is both quantitative (cell numbers) and qualitative (smear examination). Interpretation of absolute cell numbers for each of the different cell types is essential; relative cell percentages are often inaccurate and should be ignored. It is also important to look at the value reported for each cell, not just those flagged as abnormal. An important aspect of a CBC is examining a well-made smear for changes in cell appearance. White blood cells are short lived in the circulation, and changes can be rapid. It is important to remember a CBC is an evaluation at a set point in time, and repeated CBCs may be necessary to identify important trends.

Neutrophilia

Physiologic Leukogram

This increase in leukocyte count is transient and nonpathologic (Box 25-3). The fear or excitement a cat experiences during a trip to the veterinarian results in an increase in epinephrine secretion with subsequent increases in heart rate, blood pressure, and blood flow. Neutrophils and lymphocytes are mobilized out of the marginated pool next to the vessel wall and into the

BOX 25-3

Some Causes of Neutrophilia in Cats

Physiologic Leukocytosis

- Stress
- Illness
- Glucocorticoid administration

Inflammatory

- Tissue trauma
- Pancreatitis
- Surgery
- Burns
- Immune-mediated tissue injury

Infection

- Pyothorax
- Pyometra
- Abscesses
- Peritonitis
- Mycotic

Metabolic

- Uremia
- Diabetic ketoacidosis

Acute Hemolysis

- Drug induced
- Immune-mediated (uncommon)
- Hemoplasmosis

Neoplasia

- Lymphosarcoma
- Granulocytic leukemia
- Adenocarcinomas
- Ulcerated or necrotic masses

circulating pool. Because many of the neutrophils in cats are in the marginated pool, the increase in neutrophil numbers can be significant, up to three to four times the upper level of the reference range. The same degree of increase may be expected in the lymphocyte count.[10] The changes are immediate and usually last 20 to 30 minutes. A physiologic leukocytosis is, then, mature neutrophilia with lymphocytosis. There should not be an increase in immature neutrophils.

Stress Leukogram

Chronic pain and illness cause secretion of glucocorticoids, leading to a change in the leukocyte count known as a *stress leukogram,* which is also recognized in cats receiving exogenous glucocorticoids for disease management. The increased glucocorticoid concentration results in decreased diapedesis of neutrophils into the tissues, increased mobilization of neutrophils out of the marginated pool and into the circulating pool, and increased production and release of neutrophils by the bone marrow. The stress leukogram is characterized by a mature neutrophilia (no bands), lymphopenia, and eosinopenia. Unlike in dogs, monocytosis is an uncommon finding in cats with a stress leukogram. Resolution of a stress leukogram may take days after cessation of glucocorticoid administration.

Inflammatory Leukogram

The number of neutrophils in the blood represents balances among bone marrow production and release, physiologic changes in blood flow, diapedesis, and tissue demands. Inflammation from many different causes increases demands for neutrophils, and the bone marrow responds through increased release of stored mature neutrophils and accelerated production of new neutrophils. If the bone marrow can supply enough neutrophils to meet the needs of the inflamed tissue, there should be increases in the number of mature and immature neutrophils in the circulation. This is called a *regenerative left shift* and is characterized by a neutrophilia with an increased number of band neutrophils. A left shift should not be thought of as just the result of a bacterial infection, although this is a common cause. Immature neutrophils representing greater than 10% of the neutrophils in a cat with neutropenia is also called a *regenerative left shift.*

When tissue requirements for neutrophils outpaces the bone marrow's ability to replace them, most of the mature neutrophils will be in the tissues and the circulating neutrophils will be composed mostly of immature cells. If the number of bands (or other immature neutrophils) is greater than the number of mature neutrophils, a *degenerative left shift* is present and is often associated with a guarded to poor prognosis.

Severe inflammation can cause changes in the morphology of the maturing neutrophil, leading to the presence of what are known as toxic changes. Döhle bodies are small, retained accumulations of grey-staining cytoplasmic endoplasmic reticulum. They represent mild toxic changes. Retention of ribosomes in the cytoplasm causes basophilia and, along with vacuolization, suggests more severe inflammation. In one study the presence of toxic neutrophils was associated with longer hospitalization.[102] This same study also found that, unlike dogs, toxicity was not associated with increased mortality in cats. Toxic granules represent severe inflammation and, in Birman cats, must be differentiated from the nonpathologic neutrophil granulation anomaly seen in this breed.

Extreme neutrophilic leukocytosis is defined as a white blood cell count over $50 \times 10^9/L$ with more than 50% of the cells identified as neutrophils.[64] This finding is associated with a grave prognosis; 76 of the 104 cats in a study of extreme neutrophilic leukocytosis died as a result of the underlying disease.[64] Surprisingly, only 29 of the cats were febrile. Categories of disease causing this extreme white blood cell count included various types of infections, malignancies, immune-mediated diseases, and severe tissue necrosis. The highest risk of death associated with extreme neutrophilic leukocytosis was in cats with neoplasia.[64]

Neutropenia

A neutrophil count below the reference range for the laboratory may be caused by overwhelming tissue needs, decreased production or abnormal release of neutrophils by the bone marrow, or immune-mediated destruction (Box 25-4). Deficient neutrophil production is caused by infection with FeLV, FIV, or feline parvovirus (panleukopenia); drug administration; or myelophthisis. Because the half-life of circulating neutrophils, at 7 to 10 hours, is shorter than that for erythrocytes or platelets, neutropenia is often the first evidence of bone marrow disease.

Approximately half of cats with FeLV-related disease have neutropenia.[43] Mild neutropenia appears to be the most common change and is associated with mild lymphopenia and normal hematopoiesis. Moderate neutropenia is associated with hypoplastic bone marrow and must be differentiated from infection with feline parvovirus.[43] Severe neutropenia is caused by ineffective maturation and release of neutrophils by the bone marrow and is associated with a paradoxical marrow granulocyte hyperplasia because the cells produced are not released to the circulation effectively. FeLV can also cause a cyclic neutropenia, with the lowest neutrophil count occurring every 8 to 18 days.[43]

Occasionally, a healthy cat will be identified with neutropenia after a CBC is performed as part of wellness or preanesthestic testing. It is often difficult to know how aggressively this finding should be pursued. The history and physical examination should be revisited in a more thorough manner. The veterinarian should ensure that a blood smear has been examined to confirm the neutropenia. A new blood sample of adequate volume should be collected for a repeated CBC to eliminate laboratory or blood collection errors.[13] If the cat is easygoing, the sample may be collected after exposure to a mild stressful event such as running tap water. Epinephrine secretion will mobilize neutrophils from the marginated pool into the circulating pool for sampling. If the neutrophil count is over 2×10^9/L, monitoring the cat's temperature and attitude at home is probably sufficient.[85] Another reason for an apparently healthy cat to have a mild neutropenia is the manner in which laboratory reference ranges are determined. The reference range is designed to catch 90% of normal patients, meaning that 5% of normal cats will fall below the reference range for neutrophil counts and be considered neutropenic despite being normal for that individual. Sometimes the neutrophil count will persist below 1×10^9/L, necessitating further investigation. A serum biochemical profile and urinalysis should be performed if not already done. Urine can also be collected for culture. The cat's retroviral status should be ascertained and imaging of the chest and abdomen performed to look for abnormalities. If the neutropenia persists for more than 1 week, the veterinarian should consider performing a bone marrow examination in an attempt to catch bone marrow disease early.[13]

An afebrile cat with a neutrophil count below 0.5×10^9/L has an increased risk of infection with normal gastrointestinal, nasal cavity, or skin bacteria. Broad-spectrum antibiotics should be administered when

BOX 25-4

Some Causes of Neutropenia in Cats

1. Increased tissue demand or destruction
   a) Severe bacterial infections
   b) Drug induced
   c) Immune mediated
   d) Paraneoplastic
2. Neutrophil shift from circulating to marginated pool
   a) Endotoxic shock
3. Decreased bone marrow production
   a) Myelophthisis
      i. Neoplasia
      ii. Myelofibrosis
   b) Drug-induced (idiosyncratic)
      i. Chloramphenicol
      ii. Trimethoprim–sulfa
      iii. Griseofulvin (especially in FIV-positive cats)
      iv. Methimazole
      v. Propylthiouracil
      vi. Albendazole
      vii. Anticancer drugs
      viii. Immunosuppressive drugs (e.g., azathioprine)
   c) Infectious disease
      i. FeLV
      ii. FIV
      iii. Feline parvovirus (panleukopenia)
      iv. Histoplasmosis
   d) Idiopathic
4. Defects in neutrophil precursor maturation and release from bone marrow
   a) Drug-induced (as above)
   b) FeLV/FIV infection
   c) Myelodysplasia
   d) Cyclic neutropenia

FIV, Feline immunodeficiency virus; *FeLV,* feline leukemia virus.

neutrophil counts drop below 0.5×10^9 cells/L and continued until the neutrophil count is over 2×10^9/L.[85] These cats should be isolated at home to decrease the risk of infection. They should be kept indoors, and the owner should monitor the cat's appetite, attitude, and temperature. The owner should refrain from giving the cat table scraps.[13] Constant communication between the veterinarian and owner is essential.

A cat with a neutrophil count below 0.5×10^9/L, fever, and an unconfirmed bacterial infection should be hospitalized, preferably in isolation, for investigation into the cause of the neutropenia and supportive care. The evaluation would be similar to the workup mentioned previously. Additional tests, depending on physical findings, might include arthrocentesis, cerebrospinal fluid collection, airway wash, echocardiography, and blood cultures.[13] The cat should be closely monitored while hospitalized. Parameters to monitor include temperature, respiratory rate, body weight, urine output, blood pressure, and central venous pressure. Hands should be thoroughly washed and laboratory coats changed before handling these cats. One thermometer should be designated for use in this particular cat. Broad-spectrum bactericidal antibiotics should be administered through an aseptically maintained intravenous catheter. Antibiotic administration should continue for 1 to 7 days past the return of the neutrophil count to above 1×10^9/L *and* resolution of the fever.[85] Cats with confirmed pulmonary, urinary tract, or soft tissue infections require antibiotics for a minimum of 7 days past return of the neutrophil count to above 1×10^9/L *and* resolution of clinical signs *and* radiographic changes.[85] A reduction in fever would be expected 72 hours after appropriate antibiotic administration.[85] Potential causes for apparent treatment failure include infection with something other than bacteria, a bacteria not sensitive to the chosen drug, or poor host defenses.

Changes in the Numbers of Other Leukocytes

A significant eosinophilia may be seen in cats with endoparasitism or ectoparasitism, certain neoplasms such as mast cell tumors, hypersensitivity reactions such as asthma and eosinophilic gastritis, hypereosinophilic syndrome, or hyperthyroidism.[43] An increased eosinophil count by itself should not be used to confirm eosinophilic disease, and the degree of eosinophilia is not helpful in differentiating among the various eosinophilic disorders. Non-neoplastic lymphocytosis in cats can be seen along with a mature neutrophilia in a physiologic leukocytosis or after antigenic stimulation. Lymphopenia is a nonspecific finding in many ill cats. Monocytosis is also a nonspecific finding in cats and has little diagnostic value. A decreased number of monocytes is insignificant. Basophilia is interpreted in a manner similar to eosinophilia.

Hypereosinophilic Syndrome

Hypereosinophilic syndrome is a disease characterized by a mature eosinophilia and eosinophilic infiltration into many organs and is usually fatal. Clonal expansion of type 2 helper T (T_h2) cells secreting eosinopoietic factors such as interleukin-5 (IL-5) result in increased eosinophil survival.[134] The eosinophils infiltrate the liver, spleen, lymph nodes, bone marrow, and the gastrointestinal tract and result in organ failure. Almost three times as many female cats are affected as male cats.[11] Clinical signs depend on the organ affected. Vomiting, diarrhea, anorexia, fever, weight loss, and pruritus have been reported. Diagnosis depends on demonstrating excessive eosinophilic infiltration into numerous organs. Often, a fine-needle aspiration biopsy of the liver, spleen, or an affected lymph node will suffice. Although glucocorticoids have been used, no therapy has proved effective in cats. Imatinib mesylate (Gleevec, Novartis), a signal inhibitor, has been used successfully in humans.[10] Other promising treatments include the use of anti-IL-5 antibodies, IL-5 receptor blockers, and eosinophil chemotaxis inhibitors.[134]

Birman Hypotrichosis and Thymic Atrophy

A severe combined immunodeficiency has been identified in Birman kittens born hairless. These kittens are T cell deficient as a result of thymic atrophy and die within a few days of birth. Necropsy findings include a lack of a thymus and aplastic lymph nodes. The disorder has an autosomal recessive mode of inheritance.[28]

Birman Neutrophil Granulation Anomaly

Birman neutrophil granulation anomaly is a hereditary trait in Birman cats. The trait is transmitted in an autosomal recessive manner. Neutrophil function is unaffected, and no treatment is necessary. The increased granularity of the cytoplasm of the abnormal neutrophils resembles the cytoplasm of immature cells. The main concern is to differentiate the anomaly from toxic granulation found in severely ill cats.[10]

Chédiak–Higashi Syndrome

Although light blue smoke-colored Persian cats with yellow-green eyes may be attractive, they also may have Chédiak–Higashi syndrome (CHS). Homozygous cats affected by CHS are prone to bleeding and infections and usually die at an early age. They also tend to have abnormal brain stem auditory evoked responses.[11] The disease is an autosomal recessive inherited trait. Decreased bone marrow release of neutrophils leads to neutropenia. The neutrophils that do make their way into circulation have defects of intracellular killing and motility.[10] The large granules found in the neutrophils are friable and rupture spontaneously, causing tissue damage such as cataracts noted in cats with this disease.[115] Impaired natural killer (NK) cell and cytotoxic lymphocyte function has also been identified. Abnormal platelet granule release results in impaired platelet aggregation and an increased buccal mucosal bleeding time. Diagnosis is based on signalment, history, and physical findings. A few large, eosinophilic granules can be found in the neutrophils, and comparison of the hair shafts of affected animals to those of normal cats reveals large melanin granules in the affected cat.[10] At present, there is no cure for the disease. Care should be taken to avoid and control hemorrhage in affected cats. Use of drugs known to cause platelet dysfunction is contraindicated. Administration of recombinant canine granulocyte colony-stimulating factor (rcG-CSF) or IL-2 has been shown temporarily to improve neutrophil function. A bone marrow transplant may resolve the neutrophil and platelet dysfunction, but the neurologic and renal changes will remain.[10] Affected cats should not be bred, and their unaffected parents, who are obligate carriers, should be removed from breeding programs.

Pelger–Huët Anomaly

Pelger–Huët anomaly is an uncommon, benign congenital defect of leukocyte development found in domestic shorthair cats that is transmitted in an autosomal dominant manner.[10] Affected cats are heterozygous because the homozygous defect is lethal in utero. The disorder is characterized by hyposegmentation of granulocytes and monocytes. Cell function is normal, and no treatment is necessary. Affected neutrophils resemble immature band cells; affected cells, however, have mature, clumped chromatin. A healthy cat with this anomaly may be reported as having a degenerative left shift without toxic change. It is important to differentiate a true left shift associated with sick cats from healthy cats with this anomaly to avoid unnecessary, potentially expensive, and possibly invasive testing and treatment.

Pseudo Pelger–Huët anomaly is a transient condition caused by various illnesses and administration of drugs such as ibuprofen or anticancer agents.[10] The changes resolve after resolution of the disease or withdrawal of the offending drug. Drug-associated changes are idiosyncratic.

DISORDERS OF HEMOSTASIS

Hemostasis is a complex and coordinated system, with a balance between clot formation and dissolution. Its sole purpose is to seal the defects in vessel walls that occur in health and disease until they can be mended. Disorders of this system can lead to clinically significant bleeding. Fortunately, abnormalities of hemostasis are rare in cats, and spontaneous bleeding is uncommon in patients with these abnormalities. Normal hemostasis comprises primary and secondary hemostasis and fibrinolysis. Primary hemostasis involves interactions among the vessel wall, platelets, and von Willebrand factor (vWf), whereas secondary hemostasis results in the formation of a fibrin mesh. Fibrinolysis is the process of dissolving previously formed clots. It is important to realize that hemostasis (primary and secondary) and fibrinolysis, along with the various inhibitory and amplification steps, are all happening at the site of vascular injury simultaneously, and not in a stepwise fashion.

Primary Hemostasis

Platelets are small anucleate cells formed in the bone marrow by fragmentation of megakaryocytes. A single megakaryocyte may produce thousands of platelets, with thrombopoiesis taking approximately 4 days. The survival time of platelets in circulation is 1 to 2 days, after which they are removed by macrophages of the mononuclear phagocyte system in the spleen.

Vascular damage leads to local vasoconstriction and exposes subendothelial collagen, to which platelets adhere by way of a membrane receptor. Adhesion to collagen is made more efficient by the presence of vWf. After adhesion platelets undergo shape change (to increase their surface area) and activation (release of granular contents), with the subsequent recruitment of more platelets that adhere to the wound and one another. Platelet-to-platelet adhesion is known as *aggregation*. Platelet adhesion to the vessel wall and aggregation to one another form a temporary and unstable plug in the damaged vessel that is sufficient to stem bleeding from the minor defects associated with daily life.

Secondary Hemostasis

Mediators of secondary hemostasis are produced in the liver (clotting factors) and cells in and surrounding the vessel wall (tissue factor). Clotting factors are released into circulation in inactive form and require activation to become functional. For the hepatocyte to produce factors II, VII, IX, and X, vitamin K_1 must be present in adequate quantities.

Vascular damage exposes tissue factor to the circulation, which combines with circulating activated factor VII (VIIa) to activate factor X (Xa), the extrinsic pathway of coagulation. Factor Xa activates and combines with factor V (Va). Factors Xa and Va combine with ionized calcium (Ca^{2+}) and phospholipid on the platelet membrane, which localizes the formation of thrombin from prothrombin to the area of the platelet plug. The formation of thrombin is the beginning of the common pathway. Thrombin catalyzes the conversion of fibrinogen to soluble fibrin and amplifies the coagulation process by activating other procoagulant factors, particularly those of the intrinsic pathway. Finally, after activation by thrombin, factor XIIIa catalyzes the cross-linking of the fibrin strands into an insoluble mesh that stabilizes the platelet plug produced by primary hemostasis.

Classically, the intrinsic and extrinsic pathways were thought to be equally important in initiating the coagulation process. However, in live animals the beginning of the intrinsic pathway, activation of factor XI, is catalyzed by thrombin generated by the extrinsic pathway. Therefore it is more appropriate to consider the extrinsic pathway as the initiator of coagulation and the intrinsic pathway as the sustainer or amplifier of coagulation.[103]

Inhibition of coagulation prevents excessive and uncontrolled clot formation. Antithrombin (AT), previously known as *antithrombin 3,* is produced by the liver and inhibits the actions of thrombin, IXa, Xa, and XIa. The presence of heparin on the surface of the vascular endothelial cell augments the function of AT and helps control clot formation at the edges of the damaged vessel localizing the clot to the damaged area.[103] Like factors II, VII, IX and X, synthesis of protein C and protein S is vitamin K_1 dependent, and they are released in inactive form by the liver. After binding to thrombomodulin on the endothelial cell, thrombin loses its coagulant activity and activates protein C, which combines with protein S to inactivate factors V and VIII.[103]

Fibrinolysis

Clot dissolution is mediated by plasmin produced by the liver as plasminogen. Tissue plasminogen activator (tPA) is produced by endothelial cells and, as its name suggests, activates plasminogen. Plasmin degrades fibrinogen and soluble and insoluble fibrin into fibrin degradation products (FDPs), which also have inhibitory actions on platelets and various clotting factors. Degradation of cross-linked or insoluble fibrin also results in the production of D-dimers. Inhibition of fibrinolysis occurs by way of inhibition of tPA or plasmin by various proteins.

Etiology of Hemostatic Disorders

Primary hemostatic defects result from vasculopathy, thrombocytopenia, platelet dysfunction, or a combination of these (Box 25-5). They may be congenital or acquired. Ehlers–Danlos syndrome is an uncommon inherited defect of collagen. Cats with this condition typically have hyperelastic skin. Because normal subendothelial collagen is required for platelet adhesion to the damaged vessel, cats with Ehlers–Danlos syndrome have a propensity to bleed, similar to cats with platelet dysfunction. Acute, traumatic bleeding may result in thrombocytopenia as the platelets are consumed in an attempt to control the bleeding. However, the decrease is usually mild insofar as thrombopoiesis ramps up quickly and the spleen releases sequestered platelets. Very low platelet counts in bleeding cats are usually the cause of the bleeding, not caused by bleeding.[66]

Reduced activity or concentrations of clotting factors can be congenital or acquired and result in secondary hemostatic disorders (Table 25-5). Factor XII deficiency is the most common congenital coagulopathy in cats.[89] This is an autosomal recessive disorder resulting in prolongation of the partial thromboplastin time (PTT) or activated clotting time (ACT). Because in vivo generation of fibrin does not require activated factor XII, no spontaneous bleeding is associated with this defect. It is most often identified in the course of a preoperative evaluation before an elective surgery or invasive diagnostic procedure such as a liver biopsy.[12] Factor IX deficiency (hemophilia B) also results in prolongation of the PTT and ACT.[38] This is an X-linked recessive disorder that may lead to bleeding in severely affected male cats. As with all bleeding from factor deficiencies, hematomas and cavitary bleeding are most likely. A definitive diagnosis is based on identification of decreased factor IX activity. Once the gene encoding the feline factor IX protein is sequenced, a genetic test may become

TABLE 25-5 **Secondary Hemostatic Defects**

Inherited Factor Deficiency	Comments
Factor I (fibrinogen)	DSH, DLH
Factor VII	DSH
Factor VIII (hemophilia A)	DSH, DLH, Persian, Havana brown, Siamese, Himalayan
Factor IX (hemophilia B)	DSH, DLH, British Shorthair, Siamese
Factor X	DSH
Factor XII	DSH, DLH (does not cause bleeding)
Acquired Factor Deficiency	
Hepatic disease	Factors II, VII, IX, and X
DIC	FDPs also inhibit the function of multiple factors
Vitamin K_1 Antagonism or Deficiency	
Anticoagulant rodenticide	
Severe cholestasis	Decreased bile-associated fat-soluble vitamin absorption
Phenobarbital	Decreased activities of factors II and VII

DSH, Domestic shorthair; *DLH,* domestic longhair; *FDPs,* fibrin degradation products.

BOX 25-5 Selected Primary Hemostatic Disorders

Thrombocytopenia

A—Decreased Bone Marrow Production

Infection
- Retroviral infections
- Systemic mycosis involving the marrow
- Feline infectious peritonitis
- Cytauxzoonosis

Neoplasia

Drugs
- Methimazole
- Propylthiouracil
- Griseofulvin
- Cytotoxic drugs such as chlorambucil
- Chloramphenicol
- Trimethoprim–sulfa
- Albendazole

Myelodysplasia

B—Increased Destruction

Immune mediated

Primary

Secondary
- Drugs
  - Penicillins
  - Cephalosporins
  - Sulfonamides
  - Methimazole
  - Propylthiouracil
- Infection
  - Retroviral infections
  - *Mycoplasma haemofelis*
  - Bacterial
- Neoplasia
- Modified-live vaccines
- Inflammatory disorders such as pancreatitis

C—Increased Use/Consumption

DIC
- Liver disease
- Neoplasia
- Sepsis
- FIP
- Shock

Hemorrhage (mild decrease only)

D—Sequestration in the Spleen

Infiltrative disease

Splenitis

Platelet Functional Defects

A—Inherited

von Willebrand disease

Chédiak–Higashi syndrome

B—Acquired

Drugs
- NSAIDs
- Clopidogrel
- Penicillins
- Diazepam
- Acepromazine
- Ketamine
- Propofol

Uremia

Antiplatelet antibodies from IMTP

Fibrin degradation products from DIC

Liver disease

Myeloproliferative disease

Vessel (Endothelial) Disorders

Ehlers–Danlos syndrome

Vasculitis
- FIP

NSAIDs, Nonsteroidal antiinflammatory drugs; *IMTP*, immune-mediate thrombocytopenia; *DIC*, disseminated intravascular coagulation; *FIP*, feline infectious peritonitis.

available. Cats with less than 1% of the normal activity often die at birth from umbilical bleeding. Cats with greater than 5% activity may have no clinical signs until challenged by trauma or surgery.[38] Clinically affected cats are treated with appropriately typed and cross-matched fresh frozen plasma or, if sufficiently anemic, whole blood transfusions. It must be remembered that hemostatic abnormalities in cats are very uncommon, and spontaneous bleeding associated with them is even more unusual.[89]

A combination of primary and secondary disorders may be found in cats with DIC. In one retrospective study, 21 of 69 cats with hemostatic abnormalities had laboratory evidence of DIC, the most common hemostatic abnormality. Most of these cats did not have clinically significant bleeding. Neoplasia, feline infectious peritonitis, and hepatic disease were the most common causes of DIC in this study.[89] Another study identified neoplasia and pancreatitis as the most common diseases associated with DIC.[24] Only 7 of the 46 cats with DIC in this study had evidence of hemorrhage. DIC consists of excessive thrombin formation combined with the loss of inhibitory control and stimulation of inflammation.[105] Normally kept out of circulation by the vascular endothelium, intravascular production of tissue factor by neoplastic cells or inflammatory cytokine-stimulated monocytes initiates DIC.[105] The initial phase of DIC is hypercoagulable, with inhibitors counterbalancing the formation of thrombin. This is the non-overt or compensated stage of DIC. Although difficult to detect clinically, treatment at this stage may prevent progression to the next stage. When coagulation inhibitors are overwhelmed, widespread microthrombosis occurs, leading to tissue hypoxia and death. This overt or decompensated phase is clinically important in the deterioration of the patient's condition. In the study by Estrin and coworkers,[24] 43 of 46 cats with DIC died or were euthanized. The thrombotic stage is much more common than the hemorrhagic stage of DIC, as demonstrated by the few cats in DIC that bleed.[24] The late stage occurs when there is consumption of clotting factors and platelets. Neoplasms can also cause hemostatic abnormalities by causing thrombocytopenia or platelet dysfunction or by producing procoagulants. Inhibition of clotting factors and intrinsic anticoagulants are also potential mechanisms by which substances produced by neoplasms can affect the clotting system.

A multifactorial clotting factor defect has been identified in Devon Rex cats involving a decrease in the vitamin K_1–dependent activity of the enzyme gamma-glutamyl carboxylase.[62] Without the function of this enzyme, vitamin K_1 is not properly recycled, resulting in decreased activation of clotting factors II, VII, IX, and X. An autosomal recessive mode of inheritance is suspected.[62,67] Affected cats may present for spontaneous intracavitary bleeding or uncontrolled postoperative hemorrhage. There may be a history of similar episodes in related cats. Both the prothrombin and activated partial thromboplastin times are significantly prolonged.[67] Severe liver failure, intestinal malabsorption, and exposure to anticoagulant rodenticide toxins must be ruled out. Treatment involves transfusion with appropriately typed and cross-matched blood because there are many individuals with blood type B in this breed. Intravenous or subcutaneous administration of vitamin K_1 at 5 mg/cat every 24 hours is also required. Long-term normalization of the laboratory and clinical abnormalities is accomplished by using oral vitamin K_1 at 2.5 to 5 mg/cat every 24 hours.[62,67] Treatment may be required for the life of the patient. This disorder should be suspected in any Devon Rex cat presenting with a history of unexpected bleeding.

Clinical Evaluation

Cats with hemostatic abnormalities are often brought to see the veterinarian for reasons other than spontaneous bleeding. Unlike dogs, cats with hemophilia rarely develop detectable spontaneous bleeding; the disease is suspected after prolonged intraoperative bleeding is noted, often during elective surgery such as ovariohysterectomy or castration. Cats tolerate thrombocytopenia and lower concentrations of clotting factors better than dogs do.[66,89] This may be partially due to a cat's more sedentary lifestyle. Many platelet disorders are secondary to other diseases, and the patient may exhibit signs related to that disease. The patient may be volume contracted or have signs of anemia such as weakness, lethargy, pallor, or respiratory distress. Cats with severe hereditary hemostatic disorders may exhibit bleeding at a young age before elective surgery. Owners should be questioned about potential exposure to anticoagulant rodenticides or drugs known to cause platelet dysfunction. Evidence of hemostatic problems such as melena, bruising, or petechiation may not be recognized by the owner as bleeding. Excessive or prolonged bleeding from previous traumatic events, surgery, dental procedures, or nail trims should be queried.

Spontaneous bleeding resulting from severe thrombocytopenia or platelet dysfunction usually arises from small breaks in capillaries that cannot be plugged by platelets. These pinpoint hemorrhages in the skin, mucosa, or conjunctiva are known as *petechiae*. Coalescence of petechiae into a larger area of bruising is known as *ecchymosis*. A cat presenting with either of these two abnormalities likely suffers from severe platelet disease. However, cats with platelet disorders may also have epistaxis, hematemesis, melena, hyphema, or hematuria, signs often associated with clotting factor abnormalities. Cats with congenital factor XII deficiency rarely bleed spontaneously. A palpably enlarged spleen may be present if there is excessive immune-mediated destruction of platelets.[132]

Diagnostic Plans

Most hemostatic abnormalities in cats are identified unexpectedly because they are usually subclinical. Once trauma has been ruled out, diagnostic evaluation of a bleeding cat revolves around deciding if the abnormality is with primary or secondary hemostasis or both. The initial step is to perform a CBC with a platelet count and blood smear examination. Additional tests to consider, depending on clinical signs and results of the CBC, include a serum biochemical profile and urinalysis to identify potential systemic diseases (e.g., hepatic or renal failure) that may result in bleeding diathesis. Retroviral testing is imperative because FeLV is a common cause of thrombocytopenia. Thoracic radiography and abdominal ultrasonography might identify evidence of bacterial bronchitis or abdominal masses or organomegaly that may be responsible for immune-mediated thrombocytopenia or DIC. Sampling the bone marrow may yield clues as to the cause of unidentified thrombocytopenia. Because *M. haemofelis* infection occasionally causes thrombocytopenia, PCR testing for hemoplasmosis is suggested. If anemia is present, a positive Coombs' test may help prove the presence of Evans syndrome (primary immune-mediated anemia and thrombocytopenia).

Laboratory Evaluation of Primary Hemostasis

Primary hemostasis consists of interactions between vascular endothelial cells, platelets, and vWf. A buccal mucosa bleeding time (BMBT), along with a platelet count, is performed before evaluating the levels of vWf. A BMBT should be performed using a standardized stylet rather than a scalpel blade or a hypodermic needle; however, the latter instruments will suffice if the stylet is unavailable. The BMBT is difficult to perform in nonsedated cats and should be less than 4 minutes.[66] Longer times suggest an abnormality in any of the components of primary hemostasis. A normal BMBT eliminates primary hemostatic defects as a cause of the bleeding.[103]

Platelet counting can be performed by an automated cell counter or manually using a hemacytometer, or it can be estimated by examination of the blood smear. The most common cause of thrombocytopenia when reported from a laboratory is artifact caused by platelet clumping. Clumped platelets cannot be counted separately by automated cell counters, which also have difficulty differentiating between the rather large feline platelet and the small feline erythrocyte. The following handling factors are among those that predispose feline platelets to clump:

- Traumatic venipuncture
- Slow sampling from a peripheral vein
- Refrigeration
- Use of EDTA for anticoagulation
- Sampling from a recently used vein or through catheters

A smear made from fresh blood should accompany any sample to the laboratory in case it is needed for estimation of platelet numbers. Smears made by the laboratory will be from blood refrigerated before making the smear. Using sodium citrate as an anticoagulant can reduce, but not eliminate, the amount of clumping. A normal platelet count reported by the laboratory is probably normal and can be trusted. A low platelet count reported by an automated cell counter should always be confirmed by a manual count or by examination of a fresh blood smear. Estimation of platelet numbers is performed by examining the monolayer of a smear (which is an essential part of a CBC anyway) under oil immersion and counting the number of platelets in 5 to 10 fields. The average number of platelets per oil field is multiplied by 20 to get the number of platelets $\times 10^9/L$.[66] Many clumps suggest a normal number of platelets. A smear examination also allows for identification of shift platelets, evidence of increased marrow production of platelets. The presence of shift platelets precludes the necessity for collecting bone marrow. FeLV infection, a common cause of thrombocytopenia, is also associated with increased platelet volume.[44]

Spontaneous bleeding caused by thrombocytopenia in cats usually occurs only when the platelet count is lower than $30 \times 10^9/L$.[51] If bleeding occurs in a cat with a platelet count above this, the veterinarian should consider a concurrent platelet function defect or a secondary hemostatic problem. Because the BMBT evaluates hemostatic abnormalities resulting from platelet disorders in addition to problems with the vascular endothelium, it is unnecessary to perform this test when platelet counts are severely depressed. A prolonged BMBT in a cat with a platelet count over $30 \times 10^9/L$ suggests a vessel problem such as vasculitis or an inherited collagen defect, congenital or acquired platelet dysfunction, or von Willebrand disease. A detailed history should eliminate the possible exposure to drugs that can cause platelet dysfunction. Platelet function testing is usually performed only by special hemostasis laboratories and often requires freshly drawn blood samples.

Laboratory Evaluation of Secondary Hemostasis

Tests evaluating secondary hemostasis include those that test the extrinsic, intrinsic, and common pathways of secondary hemostasis and tests of fibrinolysis. The prothrombin time (PT) evaluates the extrinsic (the initiating pathway) and the common pathway by using tissue factor to activate factor VII and initiate clot formation. The test is rather insensitive insofar as it will be normal until more than 65% of the factor activity is lost[103] and is not affected by thrombocytopenia. The activated partial thromboplastin time (aPTT) evaluates the intrinsic (amplification pathway) and common pathways by activating factor XII to initiate clotting. Prolongation of this test also occurs only when over 65% of factor activity is lost. Thrombocytopenia does not affect the test results. The ACT essentially mimics the aPTT in that it also initiates clotting by activating factor XII. Accuracy is affected by variations in the temperature at which the test is performed and by the experience of the operator in recognizing the endpoint of the test, which is the formation of a clot. The ACT is very insensitive insofar as it is not prolonged until more than 90% of the factor activity is lost. Severe thrombocytopenia will erroneously prolong the test as platelet cell membranes provide the phospholipids required by the test. An abnormal PT in the face of a normal aPTT suggests an abnormality in factor VII activity, because of either an inherited deficiency or early vitamin K_1 antagonism. An abnormal aPTT with a normal PT will occur if there are abnormalities in factors VIII (hemophilia A), IX (hemophilia B), XI, or XII. A patient with a prolonged aPTT is not predisposed to spontaneous bleeding.[103] If both the PT and aPTT are prolonged, a common pathway defect, multiple factor involvement, or late vitamin K_1 antagonism should be considered. Testing for hepatic failure would be appropriate in this situation. Specific factor activities can be assessed depending on the test results. A low platelet count in association with a prolonged PT and aPTT is consistent with DIC, and an evaluation of fibrinolysis is warranted.

Laboratory Evaluation of Fibrinogen and Fibrinolysis

Measurement of the thrombin time evaluates the conversion of fibrinogen to fibrin, and prolongation is suggestive of fibrinogen deficiency, abnormal fibrinogen structure, or inhibition of thrombin by FDPs or heparin. Low fibrinogen concentrations are due to an inherited deficiency, decreased production by the liver, or increased utilization from DIC. FDPs are formed by the plasmin-mediated dissolution of fibrinogen, soluble (not cross-linked) fibrin or insoluble (cross-linked) fibrin. Increased FDPs are indicative only of plasmin activation because they can be produced by breakdown of fibrinogen without the presence of a clot. D-dimers are the result of plasmin dissolution of cross-linked fibrin found in clots, and increases in this substance truly represent active thrombosis and fibrinolysis. Controversy exists regarding the sensitivity of the D-dimers test for the detection of DIC in cats.[105,112] A combination of prolonged PT and aPTT, thrombocytopenia, and elevations in D-dimers is consistent with a diagnosis of consumptive coagulopathy, particularly if there are signs compatible with DIC or a disease known to cause DIC (e.g., neoplasia) is present.

Supportive Care for Cats with Hemostatic Disorders

Although most cats with hemostatic disorders do not present with spontaneous bleeding, supportive care for those that do is important in preventing serious consequences. It is important to identify and control underlying disease; this may remove any triggers for secondary thrombocytopenia, platelet dysfunction, or DIC. Gentle handling is essential in preventing further damage to vessels. Cage rest in the hospital or at home, if possible, is imperative until the cause of the bleeding is isolated and brought under control. Pressure bandages may be required to control bleeding from surgical sites. Fractious cats may require sedation. Offering soft food may prevent gingival bleeding.[132] Unnecessary trauma such as elective surgery or intramuscular injections should be avoided. However, should collection of bone marrow be required, the veterinarian should not hesitate to perform the procedure because bleeding is rarely a problem.

Drugs that affect platelet function, particularly NSAIDs, should be avoided. If the cat is thrombocytopenic, interfering with function of the remaining platelets will make the situation worse. Blood should be collected as atraumatically and infrequently as possible using small bore needles and preferably sampling from the jugular vein. Several minutes of compression after blood collection may be necessary to prevent hematoma formation. Cats requiring additional fluid support should receive fluids intravenously through a small-gauge catheter. Thoracocentesis or abdominocentesis is not recommended unless respiratory distress is present. Cats suspected of ingesting anticoagulant rodenticides should receive vitamin K_1. Cats with bleeding disorders related to biliary obstruction may also benefit from parenteral vitamin K_1.

A blood transfusion using fresh whole blood may supply needed clotting factors; platelets; and, if the patient is anemic, erythrocytes to cats with DIC. Blood administered to patients with DIC is more effective in controlling clotting factor consumption if heparin is used at the same time. Because cats usually tolerate thrombocytopenia without excessive bleeding, platelet transfusion should be considered when the count is less than 5×10^9/L, which is rarely encountered in this species. However, the veterinarian should always use clinical judgment and not base treatment solely on a number. Administration of platelets to cats with destructive or consumptive causes of thrombocytopenia is usually ineffective because the transfused platelets are quickly lost. Platelets administered to cats with bone marrow failure will last a few days, the normal life span of a platelet.

Thrombocytopenia

A genuine decrease in platelet numbers is an uncommon finding in cats. The most common cause of thrombocytopenia is clumping of platelets. If it is determined that the low platelet count is real, a concerted effort should be made to identify the underlying cause. One study of

41 cats with thrombocytopenia identified only one cat with primary immune-mediated platelet destruction.[51] Even in cats with documented presence of platelet-bound antibodies, 17 of the 19 cats had identifiable underlying causes for the immune-mediated disease.[132] The most commonly identified causes of feline thrombocytopenia are infectious. In the previously mentioned study of 41 cats with thrombocytopenia, 19 (46%) had infectious diseases identified as the cause of the thrombocytopenia. Of those 41 cats, 37 were tested for FeLV antigen and 11 (30%) of them were positive. The next most common cause was various types of malignancy, which affected 16 (39%) of the cats.[51]

Immune-mediated thrombocytopenia (IMTP) is caused by the removal of antibody-coated platelets by macrophages in the spleen. Similar to IMHA, these antibodies may be directed against antigens on the surface of the platelet or against antigens similar in structure to platelet antigens. Disease may reveal hidden antigens on the platelet surface. Antigen–antibody complexes may deposit on the platelet membrane and elicit a type 3 hypersensitivity response (innocent bystander destruction). Platelets also have Fc receptors on their surface and may bind the Fc portion of an antibody to these receptors. Antiplatelet antibodies may also contribute to platelet dysfunction.[132] Because primary IMTP is rare in cats, it is important not to immediately administer immunosuppressive doses of glucocorticoids to cats with thrombocytopenia. Laboratory proof of the presence of antiplatelet antibodies is difficult to obtain. Specialized laboratories may be able to perform a flow cytometric assay for platelet-bound antibodies. In most veterinary hospitals the diagnosis of primary IMTP is made by the elimination of secondary etiologies of platelet destruction and response to immunosuppressive therapy.

Once secondary causes of IMTP have been eliminated, primary IMTP may respond well to oral prednisolone at 2 to 4 mg/kg every 24 hours.[66] In a report of four cats with presumed primary IMTP, two of the three survivors required either administration of a different glucocorticoid or the addition of another immunosuppressive drug to control the disease.[6] More information on the use of additional immunosuppressive drugs is found in the section on treating IMHA. The immunosuppressive regime is continued until the platelet count has reached and remains above 75 to 100 × 10^9/L for at least 1 to 2 weeks. Attempts at reducing the dose should not be made unless the platelet count is acceptable and stable. The veterinarian should start by reducing the dose of any drug added to the glucocorticoid. There is no sense in reducing the dose if the patient is not in remission, as defined by a stable platelet count at a reasonable level and a cat that is not bleeding. It may not be possible, and indeed is unnecessary, to have the platelet count reach the reference range for the laboratory. Once the prednisolone dose reaches 0.5 mg/kg every 24 hours, alternate-day dosing may be attempted. If the platelet count starts to decrease at any point, the veterinarian should return to the last effective dose. Frequent monitoring is necessary because relapses are common.[6]

The etiology of hemostatic disorders is often difficult to identify, insofar as hemostasis is complex and difficult to fully understand. Lack of experience in dealing with these disorders contributes to the difficulty. Fortunately, hemostatic diseases in cats are rare, and significant spontaneous bleeding is even more uncommon.

DISORDERS OF THE SPLEEN

The spleen has long been recognized as inessential for life. It is not, however, unimportant; its function in maintaining homeostasis is slowly being recognized. Understanding the microanatomy of the spleen is necessary to understand its function in health and disease. The functions of the spleen include storage of erythrocytes and platelets, extramedullary hematopoiesis, and blood filtration. It is also an important immune organ. Disorders of the feline spleen are uncommonly diagnosed.[20]

Microanatomy and Circulation

The splenic parenchyma is made mostly of white and red pulp. White pulp is composed of lymphoid nodules and loose collections of lymphocytes surrounding small arterioles. Red pulp consists of venous spaces into which arteriolar blood empties along with the macrophage-populated structural framework of the spleen. In addition to the macrophages, there are increased numbers of lymphocytes and megakaryocytes in the red pulp. Blood enters at the hilus and makes its way through small arterioles to capillaries terminating in the lymphoid nodules of the white pulp or to capillaries leading into the red pulp. Some of the arterioles entering the white pulp continue on to the venous side of the circulation. Venous blood exits the spleen at the hilus and enters the portal circulation. The path an erythrocyte takes between the arterioles and the venous circulation varies by species. In dogs the circulation is sinusoidal; to enter the red pulp, cells have to squeeze through splenic cords and vessel endothelial cells. Cats, however, have nonsinusoidal microcirculation.[68] Most erythrocytes pass into the red pulp and flow directly into the venous circulation unimpeded by endothelial cells and unscrutinized by immune cells.[44]

Function

The four major functions of the spleen are storing blood, filtering blood, serving as a site for hematopoiesis, and acting as an organ of immunity. The spleen can store between 10% and 20% of the circulation erythrocyte mass and up to 30% of the platelets.[68,113] There are three patterns of blood flow through the spleen. Under normal conditions most (90%) of the blood enters the rapid pool and flows through the spleen in 30 seconds. The remainder flows through in approximately 8 minutes (the intermediate pool) or 60 minutes (the slow pool). Blood can be shunted in and out of these pools as needed during times of stress. Because of the nonsinusoidal nature of the feline spleen, splenic contraction does not result in the movement of as many erythrocytes into the circulation as it does in dogs.[84] Most of the stored platelets are in the slow pool. Iron from recycled erythrocytes is stored in the spleen while awaiting transport to the bone marrow for use in the production of hemoglobin for incorporation into new erythrocytes.

The spleen functions as an organ of filtration. As erythrocytes squeeze through the parenchyma, they come into contact with macrophages whose function is to remove rigid particulate matter from the cell. These particles include parasites, nuclear remnants (Howell–Jolly bodies), and denatured hemoglobin (Heinz bodies). The high metabolic activity in the spleen results in areas with a slightly anaerobic environment.[113] The decreased oxygen content causes the cell membrane of old, badly damaged, or abnormal erythrocytes to stiffen. This renders them unable to undergo the deformation required to pass through the sinuses, and they are removed from circulation.[113] These cells, and those coated in antibodies, are phagocytosed by nearby macrophages, which process the hemoglobin and recycle the iron. Owing to the nonsinusoidal nature of the feline spleen, the cat is less efficient at removing these cells than is the dog and is one reason that normal cats have higher numbers of Heinz bodies present in the circulation. In addition to obsolete erythrocytes, the spleen also removes bacteria from the blood.[68]

The fetal hematopoietic function of the spleen in cats ceases at birth.[68] In situations of increased need overwhelming the bone marrow, the adult spleen can resume these functions. These conditions can include infiltrative bone marrow disease, immune-mediated hemolysis or thrombocytopenia, inflammatory or infectious diseases, and malignancy. Splenic extramedullary hematopoiesis results in either generalized or nodular splenomegaly and is less common than in dogs.

The spleen serves as a major site for clearing microorganisms and is important in the immune response to circulating antigens.[113] The spleen is the principle site of IgM production and is therefore important in the early immune response. The many macrophages act in the phagocytosis and processing of antigens. Various cytokines are produced in the spleen to both improve neutrophil function and activate complement. Soluble antigens are sent to the lymphoid centers of the white pulp, whereas particulate antigens lodge in the red pulp, where they are phagocytosed and sent by macrophages to the lymphoid follicles in the white pulp for further processing.[113] The spleen also removes antibody-coated erythrocytes (extravascular hemolysis) and platelets during immune-mediated events.

Clinical Signs and Physical Findings

Historical findings in cats with splenic disorders are often vague and usually relate to an underlying disorder. Common complaints include anorexia, vomiting, diarrhea, weight loss, and an enlarged, sometimes painful abdomen. Most of these signs relate to a mass effect in the abdomen with organ displacement. Polyuria and polydipsia may occur; the pathogenesis is unclear, and it resolves after splenectomy.[2] The most reliable physical finding in cats with splenic disease is splenomegaly. The enlargement may be generalized or focal. However, not all enlarged spleens are abnormal, nor are they always palpable. Gentle palpation is important because a diseased spleen is often friable and may rupture with rough handling. Other physical changes may be present depending on the primary disease. Peripheral or abdominal lymph node enlargement may be present. At times, it is difficult to differentiate splenomegaly from enlargement of the liver.

Diagnostic Plans

When splenomegaly is identified in a patient, a search should begin for an underlying cause. Blood should be obtained for a CBC. Splenic disease is a possible cause for the presence of nucleated red blood cells in the face of a normal PCV. Hypercalcemia may be due to lymphosarcoma. If malignancy is suspected, radiographic views of the chest should be obtained to look for evidence of metastasis. Morphologically abnormal cells or a proliferation of normal cells in the circulation may suggest leukemia. A bone marrow biopsy may be required in this situation. All cats with splenic enlargement should also be checked for retroviral infection.

Compiling a list of differentials may be facilitated by classifying the enlargement as generalized or focal. Generalized enlargement (or splenomegaly) can be caused by congestion or by infiltration with neoplastic or inflammatory cells and is the most common type found in cats.[113] Focal enlargement can be caused by neoplastic or non-neoplastic lesions. The nonsinusoidal nature of the feline spleen decreases its susceptibility to the formation of nodular hyperplasia and hematomas.[113]

Visualizing the spleen is important in determining the type of enlargement. Abdominal radiography allows for easy visualization of the spleen, although the location varies owing to its mobility within the abdomen. The head of the spleen is located caudal to the stomach and cranial to the left kidney and appears triangular on a

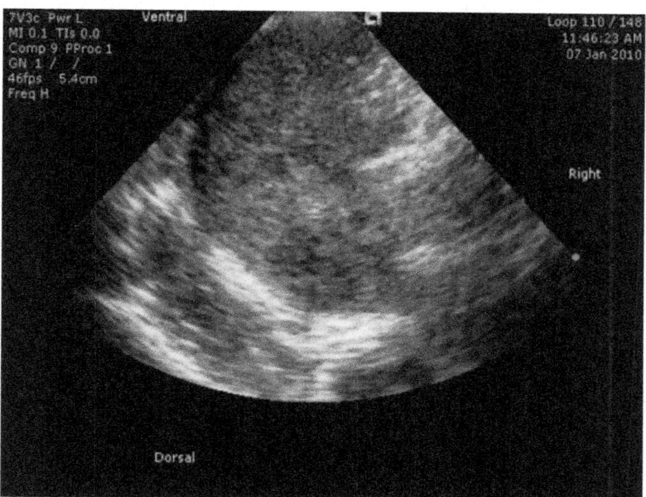

FIGURE 25-16 A transverse sonogram of the spleen of a cat with mast cell infiltration. Note the irregular hypoechoic (darker) area in the middle of the image.

ventrodorsal projection. The tail of the spleen is uncommonly seen in cats,[2] so visualizing the tail on an abdominal radiograph is supportive of splenomegaly. Lesions rarely alter the radiodensity of the spleen. Ultrasonography allows assessment of the parenchymal architecture and the surface contour (Figure 25-16). Ultrasonography is sensitive in detecting splenic lesions, but a definitive diagnosis requires sampling the lesion.[4] Focal changes in the parenchyma and irregularities in the surface are criteria for lesions in the spleen. Nodular changes within the parenchyma are easily identified as hypoechoic or hyperechoic to the rest of the parenchyma. Benign nodules are difficult to differentiate from malignant masses without using contrast ultrasonography or splenic biopsy techniques. Fine-needle aspiration biopsies can be guided by the ultrasound image. Unfortunately, there are no objective criteria for evaluating the size of the organ in cats.

Sampling the splenic parenchyma is crucial in establishing an etiologic diagnosis. A fine-needle aspiration biopsy of a lesion may be sufficient because most diseases of the spleen exfoliate readily.[2] In a study evaluating the correlation of the sonographic appearance of splenic lesions to cytologic and histologic diagnoses in 29 dogs and 3 cats, 19 of the aspirated samples matched the histologic diagnosis.[4] Carefully performed fine-needle biopsies of the spleen are safe in cats with thrombocytopenia or coagulopathy.[2] If ultrasound is unavailable for guidance, an enlarged spleen can be immobilized manually. A 22-gauge needle can be used to obtain cells by moving the needle in and out multiple times. Minimal blood contamination can be achieved by not applying suction with a syringe. The veterinarian must take care not to reposition the needle while it is in the spleen because this may result in laceration of the capsule and potentially catastrophic bleeding. If a mass is palpable in the spleen, fine-needle aspiration should be avoided until an ultrasound examination can verify that the lesion is not cavitated. Cavitated lesions, while uncommon in cats, are best dealt with by splenectomy. Aspiration biopsies may be unnecessary in cats with diffuse homogeneous splenomegaly without clinical signs.[2] Normal cell types collected from a splenic biopsy include medium and large lymphocytes. Neutrophils are rare.

Generalized Splenomegaly

Congestion of the spleen can occur after administration of a sedative or general anesthetic (Box 25-6). The capsule relaxes and allows for an increase in the storage capacity of the parenchyma. Portal venous or caudal vena caval obstruction or congestion from right-sided heart failure will infrequently cause splenic congestion. Infarcts may occur secondary to hepatic or renal disease and may obstruct the efferent blood supply.

Infiltrative lesions of the spleen are the result of neoplasia, hyperplasia of normally occurring cell types, or inflammation. The most common splenic abnormalities in a report of 101 cats with splenic disease were lymphosarcoma (n = 30), mast cell tumor (n = 27), and extramedullary hematopoiesis and/or lymphoid hyperplasia (n = 27).[45] Hyperplasia may occur in response to an increased workload. Massive hemolysis (whether immune mediated or caused by some other mechanism) or the presence of bloodborne antigens increases the number of mononuclear phagocytes and lymphocytes required to do the work. Extramedullary hematopoiesis requires an increase in blood-forming cells in the spleen. Eosinophilic infiltrates may be present in cats with hypereosinophilic syndrome. Different inflammatory cell types are associated with different types of infection. Infectious agents can cause splenomegaly by direct injury or by chronic antigenic stimulation. Potential infectious causes of splenomegaly in cats include retroviral infection, feline infectious peritonitis, hemotrophic *Mycoplasma* infections, ehrlichiosis, and cytauxzoonosis.[2] Patients with peripheral neutrophilia or eosinophilia may have splenic aspirates with increases in those cell types because of the increased numbers in the circulation, not from neutrophilic or eosinophilic inflammatory disease.[2]

Localized Lesions

Focal enlargements in the spleen of cats are less common than generalized splenomegaly.[68] Non-neoplastic lesions are more common than neoplastic lesions, but these types are indistinguishable from each other at the time of surgery. Neoplastic lesions can be malignant, benign, or metastatic. Hematomas, nodular hyperplasia,

BOX 25-6

Causes of Splenomegaly

Focal Enlargement

Infectious Inflammation
Bacterial abscess

Neoplastic
Lymphosarcoma
Hemangiosarcoma
Hemangioma
Sarcomas arising from other splenic cell types
Metastatic lesions

Non-neoplastic
Extramedullary hematopoiesis
Hematoma
Myelolipoma
Hyperplastic lymphoid nodules

Diffuse Enlargement

Infectious Inflammation
Bacterial:
- Mycobacteriosis
- Salmonellosis
- Hemoplasmosis
- Other various organisms

Mycotic:
- Sporotrichosis
- Histoplasmosis

Protozoal:
- Toxoplasmosis

Viral:
- Feline leukemia virus
- Feline immunodeficiency virus
- Feline infectious peritonitis

Neoplastic
Mast cell tumor
Lymphosarcoma
Multiple myeloma
Myelolymphoproliferative disorder
Malignant histiocytosis

Non-neoplastic
Amyloidosis
Extramedullary hematopoiesis
Pyruvate kinase deficiency
Excessive osmotic fragility
Other noninflammatory hemolysis

Noninfectious Inflammation
Plasmacytic–lymphocytic enteritis
Hypereosinophilic syndrome
Immune-mediated hemolytic anemia

Congestive
Portal hypertension
Drug induced (sedation, anesthesia)
Right-sided heart failure

abscesses, and foreign bodies may present as focal lesions.

Therapy

Treatment of generalized splenomegaly is focused on treating the underlying disorder. Splenectomy may be considered in cats with immune-mediated anemia or thrombocytopenia refractory to aggressive immunosuppressive therapy.[2] Splenectomy should be performed in all cats with mass lesions of the spleen because it is difficult to tell neoplastic lesions from non-neoplastic ones. The outcome of this mode of therapy depends on the underlying disease and the patient's preoperative condition. In a report of 19 cats undergoing splenectomy for various reasons, only weight loss had any prognostic significance.[37] The median survival time following splenectomy for the three cats with weight loss was 3 days compared with 293 days for those without. The loss of the filtration function of the spleen can predispose the cat to infections.[2] The loss of the filter may lead to increases in morphologically abnormal erythrocytes such as those with Heinz bodies.[113] Because the spleen plays a major role in the removal of erythrocyte parasites, splenectomized cats may be more susceptible to infections with hemotrophic mycoplasma. Before performing splenectomy to treat cytopenias, it is important to be certain that the bone marrow is functioning properly. If splenic extramedullary hematopoiesis is the primary source of the missing blood cells, its removal could prove fatal.[113]

LYMPHADENOPATHY

Definition

Diseases of lymph nodes are almost always recognized by enlargement. The enlargement may be solitary, regional, or generalized. Solitary lymphadenopathy, as its name suggests, is enlargement of a single lymph node, whereas regional lymphadenopathy is enlargement of lymph nodes draining an anatomic area. *Generalized lymphadenopathy* refers to enlargement of lymph nodes draining multiple anatomic areas. The enlargement is due to infiltration of cells into the node; the cell types may be normal lymph node constituents, inflammatory cells, or neoplastic infiltrates.

Anatomy and Function

Lymph nodes are kidney-shaped structures located throughout the body (Figure 25-17). Afferent and efferent blood vessels enter and exit at the hilus. Afferent lymphatic vessels enter at various points of the periphery. Lymph flows toward the hilus, percolating through cortical, paracortical, and medullary regions of the

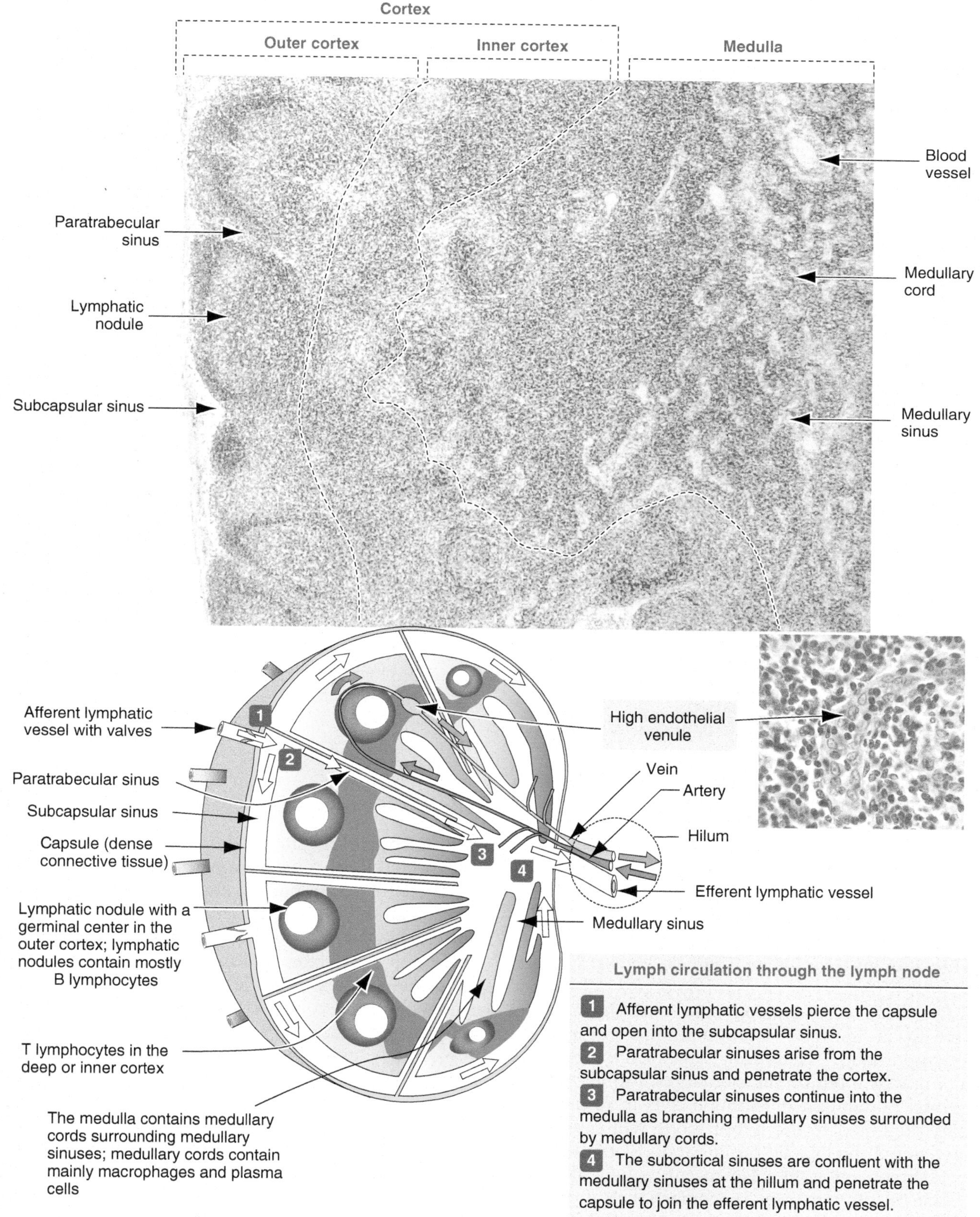

FIGURE 25-17 Anatomic and histologic structure of a lymph node. *(From Kierszenbaum AL:* Histology and cell biology: an introduction to pathology, *St. Louis, 2002, Mosby).*

BOX 25-7

Causes of Generalized Lymphadenopathy

Infectious

Bacterial
Viral:
- Feline leukemia virus
- Feline immunodeficiency virus
- Feline infectious peritonitis
- Postvaccinal

Noninfectious

Immune mediated:
- Chronic progressive polyarthritis

Idiopathic:
- Distinctive lymph node hyperplasia of young cats
- Generalized lymphadenopathy resembling lymphosarcoma

Neoplastic:
- Lymphosarcoma
- Myelolymphoproliferative disease
- Myeloma
- Mast cell tumor

Non-neoplastic:
- Hypereosinophilic syndrome

BOX 25-8

Causes of Single or Regional Lymphadenopathy

Infectious

Bacterial:
- Mycobacteriosis
- Hemoplasmosis
- Various other organisms

Mycotic:
- Histoplasmosis
- Blastomycosis
- Cryptococcosis
- Sporotrichosis
- Phycomycosis

Viral:
- Feline leukemia virus
- Feline immunodeficiency virus
- Feline infectious peritonitis

Noninfectious

Idiopathic:
- Plexiform vascularization
- Distinctive lymph node hyperplasia of young cats

Local inflammation

Neoplastic:
- Hemolymphatic neoplasms
- Metastatic neoplasia

Non-neoplastic:
- Eosinophilic granuloma complex

lymph node, and exits at the hilus through the efferent lymphatic vessel. Lymph then flows to other lymph nodes or into the venous circulation.

The cortex of the lymph node is primarily composed of follicles of B cells surrounded by a rim of T cells. The medullary area is made of cords of macrophages, lymphocytes, and plasma cells. The endothelium in the medulla is discontinuous, allowing for exposure of fluid and particles to the immune cells. Between the cortex and medulla is the paracortical area containing small T cells and macrophages acting as antigen-presenting cells.[46]

The lymph node functions as a filter of interstitial fluid. It retains particles, cells, and antigens brought to it by the afferent lymphatics. The best known function of the lymph node is as an immune organ. All the cell types (B cells, T cells, macrophages, and plasma cells) required for an immune response are brought together in the lymph node.[81] These functions form the basis for explaining why a lymph node enlarges. Proliferation of the normal population of immune cells in response to antigens presented to the lymph node will cause it to enlarge, as will neoplastic proliferation of the resident cells. Enlargement will also occur when there is infiltration by inflammatory or neoplastic cells from processes in the region drained by the lymph node. Etiologies causing lymphadenopathy can be found in Boxes 25-7 and 25-8. Neoplastic enlargement is discussed in Chapter 28.

Clinical Signs and Physical Findings

The discovery of an enlarged lymph node is often unexpected. The owner may be concerned about a lump found while petting the cat or enlarged lymph nodes may be discovered during a physical examination for a vague illness or during a wellness visit. Questions should be directed at identifying potential underlying illness, as well as the duration of the changes. It is also important to find out how fast the lump is growing.

Normally palpable lymph nodes include the mandibular, superficial cervical (prescapular), and popliteal. The ileocecocolic lymph node is sometimes palpable in normal cats. All these nodes are more difficult to palpate in cats than in dogs.[81] The fat surrounding a lymph node in an obese cat may give the impression of increased size; however, with more careful palpation the firmer node can be felt in the middle of the fat. If there is significant inflammation, the enlarged lymph node may be painful and the area warm to the touch. Clinical signs in other areas may be present if the locally enlarged lymph node is acting as a space-occupying lesion:

- Dysphagia may be present if a retropharyngeal node is enlarged.
- Swelling of the head, neck, and cranial sternal areas (precaval syndrome) may be present if a mediastinal or cervical lymph node is enlarged.
- Intrathoracic lymphadenopathy may cause pleural effusion and subsequent respiratory distress.
- Horner's syndrome may be present if there is mediastinal lymphadenopathy.
- The cat may have tenesmus if the sublumbar lymph node is large.

Diagnostic Plans

Numerous diagnostic procedures are available to evaluate a cat with lymphadenopathy. The easiest, fastest, and most noninvasive means of obtaining information about a palpably enlarged lymph node is a fine-needle biopsy. In some cases the results provide an etiologic diagnosis; in others the results lead to the selection of additional tests that may be helpful. Retroviral testing should be performed on all cats with generalized lymphadenopathy. Thoracic radiographs and thoracic and abdominal ultrasound examination may reveal an enlarged lymph node in these areas. An exploratory laparotomy should be considered if a lymph node presents as a large abdominal mass.

The cytologic appearance of the normal lymph node is a heterogeneous population of small lymphocytes. Any enlarged lymph node with normal cytology should be considered reactive (hyperplastic) because normal nodes do not enlarge.[46] Increased numbers of medium and large lymphocytes and plasma cells are also to be expected in a reactive lymph node. Lymphadenitis is either suppurative, pyogranulomatous, or eosinophilic. Suppurative lymph nodes should be cultured. If a fine-needle biopsy is inconclusive (as it often is in cats), an excisional biopsy should be performed. Other tests to contemplate depending on the results of the fine-needle biopsy include a CBC, serum biochemical profile, urinalysis, bone marrow biopsy, and infectious disease serology.[81]

Therapy

Treatment of a cat with lymphadenopathy involves treating any identified underlying disease. If an underlying cause cannot be identified, the temptation to use glucocorticoids in an attempt to shrink the size of the lymph node should be resisted. Idiopathic lymphadenopathies have been reported in cats that either require only patience or can be treated surgically.

Distinctive Lymph Node Hyperplasia of Young Cats

There is a report of 14 cats with peripheral lymphadenopathy with microscopic architecture of the lymph nodes similar to cats with experimental feline leukemia viral infections.[77] The 14 cats were young (5 months to 2 years of age) with no gender predilection. Eight of the 14 cats were healthy aside from the lymphadenopathy. The others had a combination of signs such as lethargy, anorexia, fever, or hepatosplenomegaly. Vaccines had not been administered for at least 4 months and were not considered responsible for the lymph node enlargement. Generalized peripheral lymphadenopathy was present in 13 of the 14 cats; the other had only an enlarged mandibular lymph node. The nodes were judged to be 2 to 3 times the normal size. Some of the cats had abnormalities such as anemia, neutrophilia, and lymphocytosis, and 6 of 9 cats tested were positive for FeLV antibodies. The outcome was known for 10 of the 14 cats. Two were euthanized because of the positive FeLV status; the other eight were followed for 5 years. One cat developed mediastinal lymphosarcoma, and six experienced complete resolution of the lymphadenopathy over a 2- to 28-week period. The remaining cat had episodic lymphadenopathy. The cause of the spontaneous lymph node hyperplasia in these young cats was not determined. The similarities of the lesions to those found in cats with experimental FeLV infections and the exposure to the feline leukemia virus in six of the cats suggest that the virus may be involved in the pathogenesis of the disease.

Generalized Lymphadenopathy Resembling Lymphosarcoma

There is a report of six young cats with generalized lymphadenopathy with lesions similar to those of lymphosarcoma.[76] The cats were 1 to 4 years of age and were either Maine Coons (three) or domestic shorthairs (three). Four of the cats were initially seen for urinary or upper respiratory disease. The other two were from FeLV-positive homes. The only significant physical finding was generalized lymphadenopathy. One cat was euthanized after an initial diagnosis of lymphosarcoma. Of the other five cats, four had a persistent leukocytosis with two of them having atypical lymphocytes or a lymphocytosis. FeLV antigen tests were negative in the five cats. Histopathologic evaluation of the lymph nodes revealed some features consistent with lymphosarcoma; however, some of the findings were not compatible with malignancy, such as a lack of high-grade anaplastic changes, no capsular invasion, a mix of infiltrating cell types, and the presence of normal follicles. None of the cats was treated because the clinical and histopathologic features of their disease were equivocal for neoplasia.

Surprisingly, all went on to experience regression of the lymphadenopathy within 1 to 17 weeks. All the cats were still alive and doing well 1 to 7 years after the initial examination for lymphadenopathy, supporting the diagnosis of nonmalignant lymphadenopathy.

Plexiform Vascularization of Lymph Nodes

An unusual cause of lymphadenopathy in cats has been reported,[81] specifically in adult cats ranging in age from 3 to 14 years. All cats were clinically normal except for one or two enlarged lymph nodes. Two cats with inguinal lymphadenopathy were affected bilaterally. The disease was characterized by replacement of the follicles by a plexiform proliferation of small blood vessels. The cause of this change was unknown, but removal of the affected gland(s) was curative.

Because lymphadenopathy has many potential causes, a cat presenting with generalized lymphadenopathy should not automatically be convicted of having malignant disease. Many cats may prove to have curable diseases when approached with a systematic, logical evaluation.

CYTOKINES

Currently, there is great interest in exploring the use of cytokines in feline medicine. Imbalances in cytokine profiles are associated with a wide range of diseases in cats. Potential uses include use as tools for investigating the underlying pathogenesis of disease and for the diagnosis, monitoring, and therapy of disease. Efforts are hampered by the lack of specifically cloned feline molecules, the complexity of the cytokine regulatory system, and the paucity of cats available for evaluation. Individual cytokines may have actions in cats that are not predicted by their effects in humans and mice.[95]

Definition

Cytokines are small glycoproteins secreted by many different cells, including dendritic cells, lymphocytes, macrophages, monocytes, endothelial cells, and fibroblasts in response to specific stimuli. Interleukins, interferons, lymphokines, tumor necrosis factors, and hematopoietic growth factors such as EPO are examples of cytokines. They act locally in intercellular communication to regulate cell growth and maturation, regulate immune and inflammatory responses, and modify hematopoiesis. They affect multiple cell types and are important enough that the effects often overlap those of other cytokines, acting as a natural backup system. Some cytokines have different effects depending on the concentration; for example, interferon (INF)-alpha has immunostimulating properties at low concentrations but immunoinhibitory properties at high concentrations. Cytokine structure is not well preserved across mammalian species so that administration of a nonfeline cytokine to a cat often elicits an antibody response, resulting in loss of function.[63]

Physiology

Production of cytokines is induced by alteration in gene expression and is usually transient. Cytokines act by binding to specific receptors on the surface of the target cell, with a subsequent modification of gene expression in that cell. This changes cell proliferation, differentiation, or function, often in concert with other mediators. Circulating non–cell-associated receptors for the cytokines may be present to prevent systemic actions if some should reach the circulation.[23]

Normal embryonic development may be affected by alterations in cytokine concentrations, leading to birth defects.[23] Hematopoiesis is modified by the presence or absence of EPO, thrombopoietin (TPO), or colony-stimulating factors (Figure 25-18). Cytokines are active in immunoregulation through a complex interaction among the various cytokines, which activate or suppress helper T cells (T_h cells) (Figure 25-19). The outcome of these interactions is an alteration in the balance of cell-mediated and humoral immunity. Activated macrophages elaborate various cytokines important in the acute inflammatory response by altering vascular permeability, increasing endothelial leukocyte adhesion and leukocyte chemotaxis (Box 25-9). The acute phase inflammatory response is, in part, mediated by cytokines secreted by these macrophages. Nonspecific effects of chronic inflammation such as cachexia and tissue destruction may be due to the presence of cytokines. Growth factors have a role in wound healing by stimulating the migration of fibroblasts into the wound and increasing angiogenesis.

Therapeutic Uses

Manipulation of cytokines for use in treating disease can involve administration of the cytokine itself in one form or another. Presently, cytokines are primarily used to treat hematocytopenias. The best-known example is the use of EPO to treat hypoproliferative anemia. Cytokines may also be used to treat tumors. Intralesional injections of IL-2 may be beneficial as an adjunctive therapy for fibrosarcoma.[23] In the future it may be possible to use cytokines to augment the immune response to disease or alter tissue repair. Inhibiting cytokine activity may modulate the immune response and result in novel methods of treating immune-mediated and allergic disease. Glucocorticoids and cyclosporine are examples of drugs that inhibit production of proinflammatory cytokines such as IL-2. Glucocorticoids also stimulate

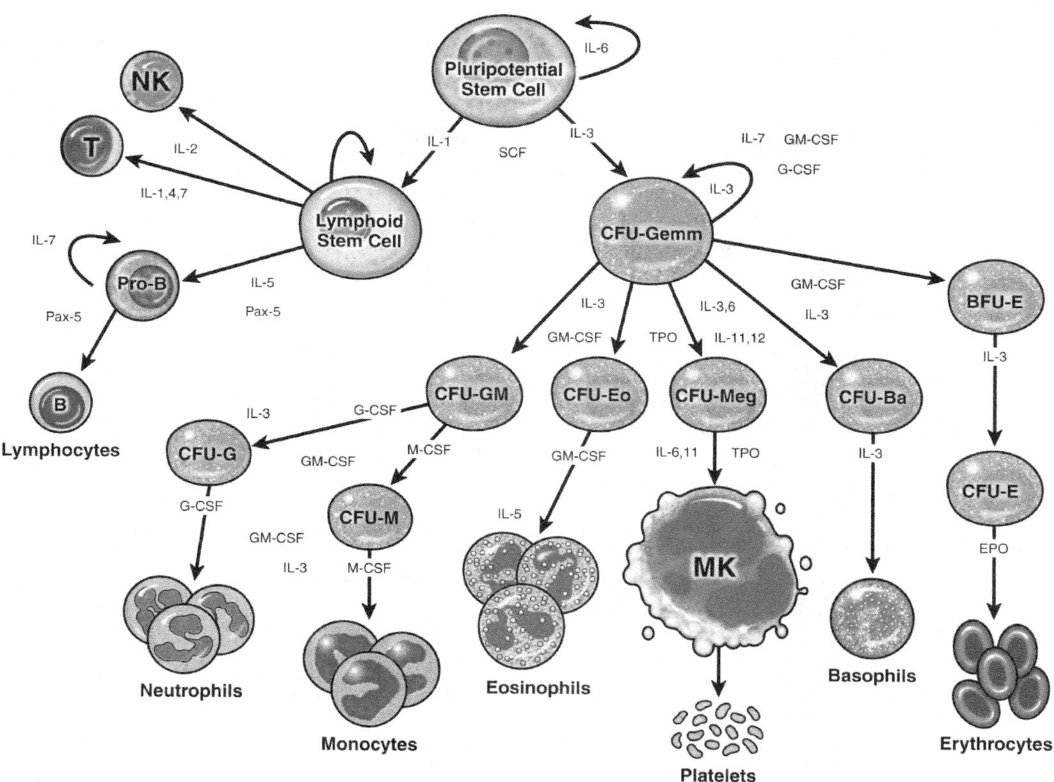

FIGURE 25-18 Cytokines important in proliferation and differentiation of cell types during hematopoiesis. *B*, B-lymphocyte; *BFU-E*, burst-forming unit-erythrocyte; *CFU-Ba*, colony-forming unit-basophil; *CFU-E*, colony-forming unit-erythrocyte; *CFU-Eo*, colony-forming unit-eosinophil; *CFU-G*, colony-forming unit-granulocyte; *CFU-Gemm*, colony-forming unit-granulocyte-erythroid-monocyte-megakaryocyte; *CFU-GM*, colony-forming unit-granulocyte-monocyte; *CFU-M*, colony-forming unit-monocyte; *CFU-Meg*, colony-forming unit-megakaryocyte; *EPO*, erythropoietin; *G-CSF*, granulocyte colony-stimulating factor; *GM-CSF*, granulocyte-monocyte colony-stimulating factor; *IL*, interleukin; *M-CSF*, macrophage-monocyte colony-stimulating factor; *MK*, megakaryocyte; *NK*, natural killer cell; *Pax-5*, transcription factor produced by expression of PX-5 gene in B-lymphocyte development; *T*, T-lymphocyte; *TPO*, thrombopoietin.

BOX 25-9

Important Cytokines Released from Stimulated Macrophages

Interleukin-8

- Induces inflammation by stimulating leukocytes
- Chemotactic for neutrophils
- Serves as principle secondary mediator of inflammation

Interleukin-6

- Stimulates hepatocytes to synthesize acute phase proteins
- Serves as principle growth factor for B cells

Interleukin-1

- Enhances proliferation of helper T cells
- Enhances growth and differentiation of B cells
- Stimulates interleukin-2 production by T_h1 cells
- Stimulates nearby macrophages to produce interleukin-6 and interleukin-8

Tumor Necrosis Factor

- Causes vascular endothelium to become adhesive for leukocytes
- Activates inflammatory leukocytes
- Stimulates nearby macrophages to produce interleukin-1, interleukin-6, and interleukin-8

Interferon-alpha

- Inhibits viral replication in adjacent cells
- Inhibits cell proliferation in adjacent cells
- Increases class I major histocompatibility complex (MHC) expression in adjacent cells
- Increases lytic potential of natural killer (NK) lymphocytes

Interleukin-12

- Enhances interferon-gamma production by T_h1 cells and further activation of macrophages
- Inhibits T_h2 cell proliferation and activation

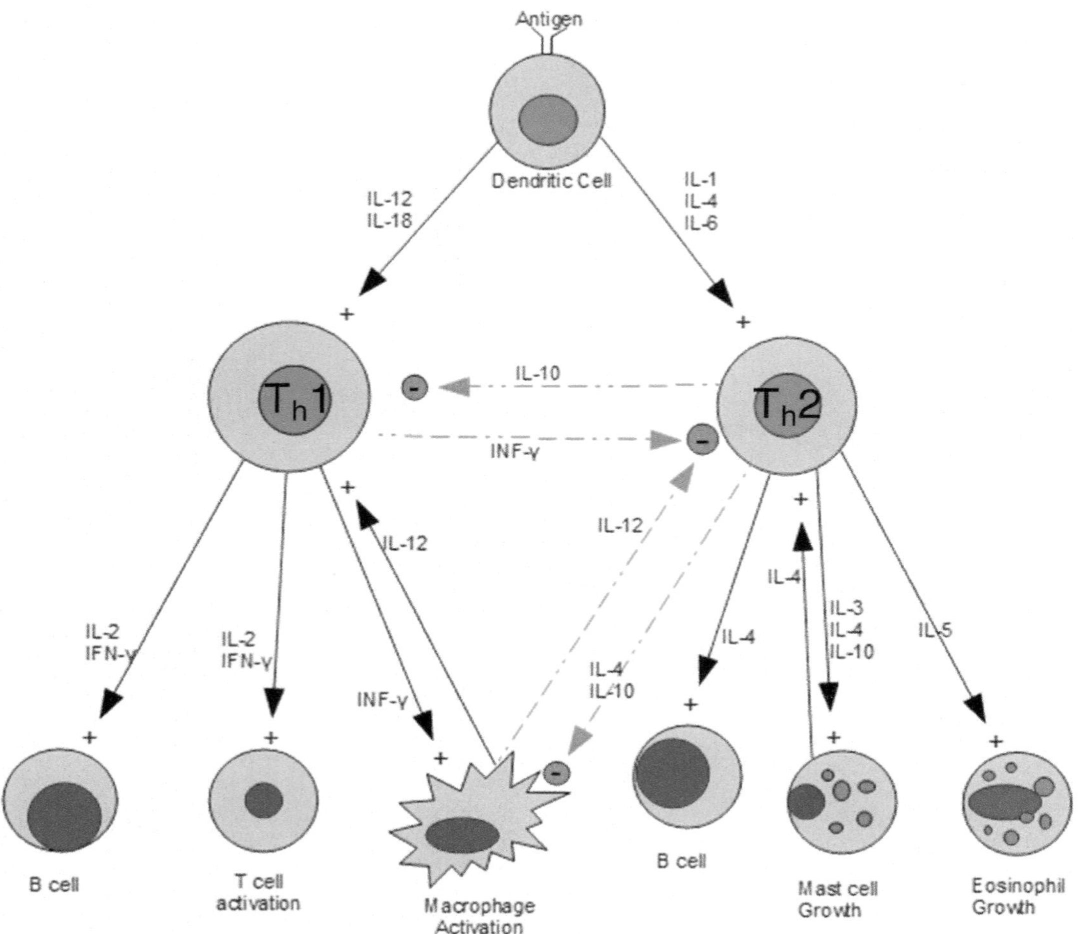

FIGURE 25-19 Regulatory effects of interleukins secreted by macrophages and T_h1 and T_h2 lymphocytes on the cell-mediated and humoral immune response after antigen presentation by dendritic cells. *Red, dashed lines* represent inhibitory effects. *Solid black lines* represent stimulatory effects. *IL,* interleukin; *INF,* interferon.

the production of IL-10, an immunosuppressive cytokine. Antibodies against the cytokine or its receptor may help reduce its activity. Inactivation may also be accomplished by the use of direct cytokine antagonists or administration of their receptors in soluble form. IL-2 receptor antagonist protein (IRAP) has shown promise in reducing the severity of inflammatory bowel disease.[23] Manipulation of a single cytokine may trigger mechanisms that control its activity and neutralize or enhance its effect.[114] No treatment is without potential adverse effects, and cytokine therapy is no exception. Systemic use of cytokines has resulted in fever, anorexia, nausea, pain, anemia, shock, pulmonary edema, coma, or death.

Interleukins

Interleukins are cytokines produced by antigen-activated dendritic cells, lymphocytes, and macrophages (see Figure 25-19). As with all cytokines, they act by binding to specific receptors on the effector cell. In health fewer than 15% of immune cells have interleukin receptors on the surface. This guards against an overzealous immune response.[48] Bacterial and viral infections stimulate T_h1 cells to produce interleukins such as IL-2, interferon (INF)-gamma, and tumor necrosis factor-alpha that are responsible for enhancing cell-mediated immunity. These interleukins activate natural killer (NK) cells, cytotoxic lymphocytes, and macrophages. IL-12 is secreted by activated macrophages with subsequent activation and recruitment of new T_h1 cells, thereby acting as a positive feedback loop to amplify the cell-mediated immune response. IL-12 is also a potent stimulator of NK cell and cytotoxic lymphocytes. Large, extracellular parasites activate T_h2 cells to secrete interleukins that result in augmentation of the humoral arm of the immune system.[48] Increases in B lymphocytes, eosinophils, and mast cells follow. T_h2 cells also release the antiinflammatory interleukins, IL-4 and IL-10. These potent inhibitors of INF-gamma secretion by T_h1 cells act to reduce cell-mediated immune activity. These two interleukins also stimulate activation of B lymphocytes and mast cells.[48] Of course, there is never stimulation or inhibition of only T_h1 or T_h2 cells; a balance must be maintained, or illness ensues.

IL-2, part of cell-mediated immunity, may be useful in the treatment of malignancy. For example, IL-2 activates the tumoricidal effects of pulmonary alveolar cells.[48] Animals with depressed cell-mediated immunity may have derangements in IL-2 production. Dogs with generalized demodicosis have decreased expression of IL-2 and decreased numbers of lymphocytes with IL-2 receptors. Production of IL-2 by feline lymphocytes infected with retroviruses is decreased. IL-8 is a potent neutrophil activator and may be useful in disorders characterized by neutrophil dysfunction. Antagonists of IL-8 may have a role in combating asthma. IL-12 is a potent inhibitor of tumor angiogenesis and has potent antitumor effects that may be used to treat neoplasia. IL-12 may also have a role in the development of autoimmune diseases.

Hematopoietic Growth Factors

Differentiation, proliferation, and maturation of the different types of stem cells in the bone marrow are stimulated by various cytokines. EPO and TPO stimulate increases in production and release of erythrocytes and platelets, respectively. A number of cytokines mediate similar activities on leukocytes. Granulocyte colony-stimulating factor (G-CSF) is produced by bone marrow stroma, neutrophils, and endothelial cells. The receptor for G-CSF is found on both immature and mature neutrophils and stimulates proliferation and maturation of neutrophils. G-CSF also enhances neutrophil chemotaxis and antibody-dependent cell-mediated cytotoxicity and increases the expression of Fc receptors on the neutrophil surface.[63] A neutrophilia reliably occurs 24 hours after administration of recombinant human (rh)-G-CSF to healthy cats and is useful in preventing chemotherapeutic neutropenia. Using G-CSF to reverse an established neutropenia, such as seen in cats with FeLV infection, is unrewarding. The action of rh-G-CSF in cats ends when the patient starts making antibodies against the cytokine. The recombinant canine product, however, retains its efficacy, suggesting that antibodies are not produced.[63]

Granulocyte monocyte (GM)-CSF is made in fibroblasts, endothelial cells, T lymphocytes, and monocytes. The targeted cells are neutrophils, eosinophils, monocytes, and their respective progenitor cells. GM-CSF prolongs the survival of the target cells and enhances their function. GM-CSF–activated macrophages recognize and kill tumor cells and present their antigens to T_h cells as a part of tumor immune surveillance.[63] Macrophage-CSF promotes the survival and functions of macrophages and may be useful in treating fungal infections.[63] Stem cell factor is produced by bone marrow support cells and endothelial cells and may find uses in treating aplastic anemia, myelofibrosis, or bone marrow toxicity.

Investigational Use

Cytokine profiles and individual cytokines are being used by researchers investigating many different disorders in cats. The cytokine profile information can elucidate the extent to which each arm of the immune system is involved in the pathogenesis of the disease. Are the increases or decreases in the various cytokines measured consistent with activation of T_h1 or T_h2 cells? Is the response stimulatory or inhibitory? Assessment of individual cytokines may present opportunities for intervention in the disease process. Many different body systems and individual infectious diseases have been examined with regard to cytokines. Tumor necrosis factor-alpha is produced by cardiac myocytes in response to ventricular pressure overload in cats with cardiomyopathy and has been implicated in the pathogenesis of cardiac cachexia, ventricular dysfunction, and the development of congestive heart failure.[73] Evaluations of the cytokine profiles of the nasal and oral cavities in cats suggest that a T_h1 profile of cytokines is present to protect against bacterial and viral infections of these tissues. An increase in T_h1 cytokines is associated with progression of the signs and histologic changes of nasal cavity disease. Humans with allergic rhinitis have T_h2 profiles.[50] IL-4–producing lymphocytes have been found in lesional and nonlesional skin from cats with allergic dermatitis, but not from the skin of healthy control cats, which suggests a role for IL-4 in allergic skin disease in this species.[96] IL-5, thought to be a major regulator for eosinophils, was not correlated with the number of eosinophils in cats with suspected allergic dermatitis, whereas IL-2 was.[80] This is an example of an investigation with a conclusion that steers therapeutic intervention away from what theory suggests should be effective. Antibodies against IL-5 and IL-5 receptor blockers are under investigation for the treatment of hypereosinophilic syndrome.[134]

Inflammatory disease in other body systems would seem to be reasonable areas of investigation. Indeed, cytokine evaluation in cats with inflammatory bowel disease (IBD) is an ongoing area of interest. Nguyen Van and coworkers found a statistically significant increase in both proinflammatory and regulatory cytokine expression in cats with inflammatory lesions of the intestine compared with those without inflammation. They concluded that the pathogenesis of IBD involves aberrations in both regulatory and inflammatory aspects of the immune system.[82] The ACVIM consensus statement on gastrointestinal inflammation suggests that a role for decreased immunoregulation is predicted in the pathogenesis of IBD in cats based on the cytokine profile from humans and rodents.[123] The pathogenesis and response to treatment of allergic airway disease in cats involves alterations in cytokine profiles. An imbalance in cytokine production favoring T_h2 cell products in response to environmental aeroallergens is thought to be a major part of the pathogenesis of this disease.[101] These T_h2-derived cytokines lead to increased production of allergen-specific IgE. Investigators are evaluating different substances for their efficacy in altering or inhibiting the activity of these cytokines.[101] Even behavior can be affected by cytokines. Increased IL-2 in certain areas of the brain has been found to potentiate defensive rage behavior in cats.[5]

Perhaps the most important area of study of cytokines is in the pathogenesis and treatment of infectious diseases. This area of study may be important in designing prevention and therapies for infections with FIV. Increased IL-10, an immunosuppressive T_h2 cytokine, was found in the early stages of FIV infection corresponding to high viral replication. This was followed by an increase in IFN-gamma levels to bring the ratio back into balance. The increase in IFN-gamma was associated with a decreased tissue viral load.[3] In a challenge study, cats infected with FIV and then challenged with *Toxoplasma gondii* infections produced significantly lower amounts of T_h1 (proinflammatory) cytokines compared with challenged FIV-negative controls. The FIV-positive cats also maintained the elevated levels of IL-10 found before the challenge with *T. gondii.*[61] Imbalances in T_h1 versus T_h2 cytokines were also suggested as a cause for the development of lesions in the neurologic form of FIP. It was also thought that a failure to increase IFN-gamma concentrations in the infected tissues might be an important reason these cats succumbed to the FIP infection.[30] Another example of using a cytokine for the treatment of infectious disease is the use of rhIFN-alpha to treat cats with FeLV infections.[23] Although the use of cytokines holds great promise for feline medicine, much research must still be performed to fully understand the complexity of the system and the implications of manipulating it and to develop new strategies for using cytokines to intervene in the management of sick cats.

SYSTEMIC LUPUS ERYTHEMATOSUS

Definition

Systemic lupus erythematosus (SLE) is a rare disease characterized by autoimmune damage to multiple tissues and organ systems. The most commonly affected tissues in cats include synovial joints, glomeruli, skin, blood cells, and the central nervous system (Box 25-10). The syndrome mimics many other disorders, and diagnosis can be difficult because diseases including infectious and neoplastic causes must first be eliminated.

BOX 25-10

Disorders Consistent with Systemic Lupus Erythematosus

Major Signs

Immune-mediated hematologic disease
- Immune-mediated hemolytic anemia
- Immune-mediated thrombocytopenia
- Immune-mediated leukopenia

Polymyositis
Glomerulonephritis
Non-erosive immune-mediated polyarthritis
Vesicobullous dermatitis

Minor Signs

Oral ulceration
Fever of unknown origin
Central nervous system disturbances
- Seizures
- Dementia
- Coma

Pleuritis
Myocarditis
Pericarditis
Peripheral lymphadenopathy

Signalment

Young to middle-aged cats are most commonly affected,[65] and unlike in humans, there is no gender predilection.[69] Purebred cats are more likely to be affected than domestic cats.[106]

Clinical Signs and Physical Findings

Clinical signs depend on the body system affected. These can include fever; lameness; muscle pain; lymphadenopathy; ulcerative stomatitis; skin lesions such as crusts, erythema, and ulceration; depigmentation around the head and paws; pale mucous membranes; and central nervous system signs ranging from subtle behavioral changes to alterations in mentation and seizures. These signs may be exacerbated by ultraviolet radiation from the sun or concurrent infection.[106]

Pathophysiology

The changes resulting from SLE are due to inflammation of the affected body part. Dysregulation of the immune system (possibly the result of abnormal function of T suppressor cells) leads to an attack against the body's self-antigens and is responsible for the inflammation. Circulating antigen–autoantibody complexes deposit in the vessel walls of the synovium, glomerulus, or choroid plexus (type 3 hypersensitivity). Complement is activated, and neutrophils and macrophages are recruited, resulting in vasculitis and damage to tissues. Less commonly, antibodies against nuclear, cytoplasmic, and membrane antigens (type 2 hypersensitivity) alter cell function. Direct T cell damage of tissues (type 4 hypersensitivity) is also possible.[106]

Diagnostic Plans

Diagnosis of SLE requires an increased index of suspicion for a cat with apparent multisystemic disease. Various criteria have been proposed for the diagnosis of SLE in dogs and cats based on those used for the diagnosis in people. One such proposal requires evidence for autoimmune injury to at least two organ systems, along with a positive antinuclear antibody (ANA) test, or three affected organ systems with a negative ANA titer. A positive ANA titer is neither sufficient nor required for a diagnosis.[106] Most commonly, a combination of the following occurs:

- IMHA
- IMTP
- Immune-mediated skin disease
- Glomerulonephritis
- Central nervous system signs
- Non-erosive immune-mediated polyarthritis[106]

No single test is available to diagnose SLE. A CBC, serum biochemical profile, ANA test, and urinalysis should be performed along with thoracic radiographs to rule out potential bronchial infections. The ANA test is relatively sensitive in identifying anti-self antibodies. The results are reported as a titer along with an immunofluorescence pattern that is clinically insignificant.[106] Many false-positive and false-negative tests occur. False-positive tests may occur in cats with infectious, neoplastic, or chronic inflammatory diseases. About 10% of healthy cats will have a low titer for ANA.[106] Therefore a high ANA titer is more consistent with SLE than is a low titer. A lupus erythematosus (LE) cell preparation identifies neutrophils with phagocytosed nuclei in the cytoplasm. Interpretation depends on the experience of the technician, and many false-negatives occur.[106] Because of the difficulty in performing the test and problems with sensitivity, it has largely been replaced with the ANA test. If there is evidence of a regenerative anemia, the veterinarian should perform a Coombs' test and a PCR test for hemotrophic mycoplasmosis. The cat's retroviral status should also be ascertained. If there is joint pain or effusion, synovial fluid should be obtained for cytology; the synovial neutrophils should be well preserved in a cat with SLE. If the neutrophils are lytic or if bacteria are present, a culture of the fluid should be performed.[69] Cats with azotemia and proteinuria should have the urine protein to creatinine (UPC) ratio measured. A renal biopsy should be performed if the UPC ratio is high because the elevated protein may be due to glomerulonephritis. One cat was identified with coagulation defects because of the presence of a circulating lupus anticoagulant, an antibody against phospholipid that interferes with function of the common coagulation pathway and platelets (see the section on hemostasis). This cat had prolongation of both PT and aPTT. No overt bleeding was reported.[65] Any skin lesions should be biopsied in an appropriate manner.[69,106] To make a diagnosis of SLE, infectious and neoplastic causes must be eliminated as possible explanations for the cat's clinical signs.

Therapeutic Plans

Control of tissue inflammation and addressing organ failure are the goals of therapy for SLE. In situations where there is mild pain, NSAIDs may suffice.[69,106] If not, or if the signs are more severe, immunosuppressive doses of corticosteroids should be started. Prednisolone at 2 to 4 mg/kg daily should be effective. If there is no improvement in 1 week, consideration should be given to a change in therapeutic plans such as the addition of cytotoxic immunosuppressants. Ultraviolet light can be a trigger for some cats with SLE, and they should be kept out of the sun.

Additional immunosuppression can be achieved by adding cytotoxic drugs such as chlorambucil. Chlorambucil is well tolerated, with minimal side effects; however, the dose must be individualized to the particular patient. A good starting point is 0.25 to 0.5 mg/kg orally every 24 to 48 hours.[69] Side effects include anorexia and myelosuppression. Constant communication between owner and veterinarian is essential.

Once remission has been achieved, a reduction in drug dose can begin. Remission is defined as resolution of clinical signs and initial radiographic and laboratory changes.[106] If combination therapy has been used, the chlorambucil should be reduced first. The dose is reduced by 50% for 4 weeks. As long as clinical remission continues, further reductions can take place every month. Usually a minimum of 6 months of therapy is required.[106] If a relapse occurs, the veterinarian should return to the previous effective dosage until remission is accomplished. Further attempts at reducing drug dosages should be made more slowly. Some cats will require lifelong therapy.

Prognosis

Because SLE in cats is rare, the natural course of the disease is unknown. Many cats will achieve remission, and drug doses can be tapered; however, relapses should be expected to occur. Frequent follow-up examinations and laboratory evaluations may be necessary.

SYSTEMIC ANAPHYLAXIS

Systemic anaphylaxis is a life-threatening allergic event resulting in massive, generalized mast cell degranulation. The inflammatory mediators released by mast cells result in grave consequences if not treated promptly. Because time is of the essence, recognizing the signs of anaphylactic shock is essential if the veterinarian is to institute appropriate therapy.

Pathophysiology

An anaphylactic reaction is mediated by interactions among antigens, IgE antibodies, and mast cells. This type I hypersensitivity reaction requires previous exposure to an antigen and production of IgE against that antigen. Many different substances can play the role of antigen, including drugs such as NSAIDs and antibiotics, insect or reptile venom, food, vaccines, and inhaled allergens. Most animals produce IgA or IgG when exposed to an environmental allergen, whereas others have an exaggerated T_h2 response and produce excessive amounts of IgE.[116] Once the cat is re-exposed to the antigen, it can be bound to IgE molecules on the mast cell surface. Cross-linking occurs when the antigen is bound to two IgE molecules at the same time. Once the two antibodies are cross-linked, IgE receptors signal the mast cell to degranulate, produce increased quantities of phospholipase A_2, and begin production of new inflammatory cytokines.

Degranulation of mast cells results in the release of preformed mediators of inflammation. This occurs rapidly, with evidence of their effects appearing within seconds to minutes of exposure to the antigen. These mediators, which include but are not limited to histamine, heparin, kallikrein, and inflammatory cell chemotactic factors, result in physiologic changes responsible for many of the clinical signs recognized as anaphylactic shock. Histamine bound to H_1 receptors causes smooth muscle contraction in the intestinal tract and in the airways and pulmonary vasculature. H_1 activation also results in increased vascular permeability and neutrophil and eosinophil chemotaxis. Binding to the H_2 receptor is followed by increased production of airway mucus and bronchodilation. The balance between H_1 and H_2 stimulation results in hypotension, bronchospasm, airway obstruction, hyperperistalsis, increased vascular permeability, and pruritus.[15] Chemotactic factors amplify the inflammatory reaction by recruiting neutrophils and eosinophils. Consequences of the release of other mast cell mediators include complement activation, enhanced smooth muscle contraction, increased vascular permeability, and stimulation of pain sensors.[121]

Phospholipase A_2 acts on the phospholipids in the cell membranes to form arachidonic acid. Although not as immediate as degranulation, this process still occurs within minutes of exposure to the antigen. Production of secondary inflammatory mediators such as prostaglandins, leukotrienes, thromboxane, and platelet-activating factor augments inflammation, bronchoconstriction, and vascular permeability.

A late-phase inflammatory reaction occurs after newly produced cytokines are released by the mast cell. This occurs between 2 and 24 hours after exposure to the antigen. Cytokines produced by mast cells include IL-4, IL-5, IL-6, IL-13, IL-16, tumor necrosis factor-alpha, and macrophage inflammatory protein 1-alpha. These are either proinflammatory or promote a T_h2 response with increased IgE antibody production.[116] They also augment vasodilation and stimulate the production of cell adhesion proteins on endothelial cell membranes, which increases the ability of circulating inflammatory cells to stick to and then move through the vessel wall into the tissues.[15]

An anaphylactoid reaction is the result of mast cell degranulation without an immune component.[116] IgE is not involved, and previous exposure to the antigen is not required; mast cells are activated directly or, more commonly, indirectly by complement activation. Other than the initial stimulus, the two processes are virtually the same. Anaphylactoid reactions can be caused by drugs such as NSAIDs or opioids, iodinated radiographic contrast materials, or dextrans. Ingestion of certain types of spoiled fish can cause an anaphylactoid reaction. Bacterial contamination of tuna, mackerel, or mahi-mahi converts the abundant histidine in the fish to histamine.[41] Anaphylactic and anaphylactoid reactions have the exact same clinical signs and treatment, so differentiating between the two is immaterial in the emergency situation.

Clinical Evaluation

The major shock organ in the cat is the lung, with the intestinal tract involved to a lesser degree. The signs of anaphylaxis are the result of the actions of all the different inflammatory mediators released by the mast cells. Respiratory distress is the major sign of anaphylactic shock in cats. Increases in respiratory rate and effort are consequences of laryngeal edema, bronchoconstriction, and increased production of airway mucus; open-mouth breathing may be noticed. Pruritus about the face and head may be present, and increased salivation may be noted along with vomiting, pale mucous membranes, poor pulse quality, and a prolonged capillary refill time. Hypovolemia owing to increased vascular permeability and vasodilation leads to decreased tissue oxygenation. Progression to collapse, coma, and death may follow rapidly. Diagnosis of anaphylactic shock is based on recognizing the presenting signs and the acute nature of illness. A cursory initial examination of the cat is often all that time will allow, insofar as many are life-threateningly ill. A detailed history and physical examination of less severely affected cats may yield clues to the cause of the anaphylaxis. An insect stinger in the tongue of a cat with open-mouth breathing is suggestive of an allergic reaction to a bee sting.

Therapy

Once anaphylaxis is recognized, rapid and aggressive treatment may be life saving. Following the precepts of basic emergency medicine gives the veterinarian the best chance at success. The veterinarian must first ensure that the airway is patent and be ready to intubate if laryngeal edema is causing an airway obstruction. Tracheotomy may be necessary if intubation is not possible. If the upper airway is not obstructed and the cat is having respiratory difficulties, administration of oxygen may be required. Cardiovascular and respiratory dysfunction can be addressed with intravenous fluids and drugs.

Intravenous access should be established early on so that volume contraction can be corrected. Intravenous fluids at 50 to 60 mL/kg over the first hour should be administered to cats with severe anaphylaxis. After the first hour the cat should be reassessed and fluids continued. Fluid rates will likely need to be greater than maintenance rates but should be tailored to the individual patient. Monitoring the central venous pressure (CVP) is an excellent means of assessing fluid requirements. Fluids can be administered until the CVP reaches 3 to 5 cm of water. Otherwise, the pulse quality and rate, capillary refill time, and mucous membrane color are used as clinical guides to fluid therapy after the initial shock rates are completed. If DIC is present, blood products may be used to replace clotting factors consumed in the process. The addition of heparin alone to augment the effectiveness of the transfusion is controversial. In humans a combination of antithrombin and heparin has shown promise in reducing mortality, as has administration of activated protein C.[99] Use of these modalities has not yet been reported in cats or dogs.

Many of the pathophysiologic derangements that occur with anaphylactic shock can be ameliorated by the administration of epinephrine (Table 25-6). Stimulation of the alpha-adrenergic receptors results in vasoconstriction, thereby decreasing blood pooling in the splanchnic circulation, increasing venous return to the heart, and improving cardiac contractility. Beta-adrenergic receptor stimulation decreases bronchoconstriction and impedes further mast cell degranulation while also improving cardiac output through positive inotropic and chronotropic effects. Epinephrine is used as a 1:10,000 dilution and administered intravenously at 0.02 mg/kg, which is 0.2 mL/kg or 1 mL for a 5-kg cat. To create 10 mL of a 1:10,000 dilution of epinephrine, 1 mL of the 1:1,000 solution is mixed with 9 mL of sterile saline. If venous access cannot be established, the volume can be doubled and administered through a urinary catheter passed through an endotracheal tube and wedged in a small bronchus.[131] Alternatively, epinephrine can be administered in the sublingual vein. If the patient's condition is not serious, the epinephrine can be administered intramuscularly or subcutaneously. The cat's heart rate and rhythm should be monitored because epinephrine can precipitate cardiac dysrhythmias. Epinephrine should be readministered in 15 to 20 minutes.

A positive response to parenteral fluid and epinephrine administration should be noticed within minutes of

TABLE 25-6 **Drugs Useful for the Treatment of Anaphylaxis**

Drug	Dose	Use
Epinephrine (intravenous)	0.2 mL/kg of a 1:10,000 dilution repeat in 15 minutes	Initial treatment along with intravenous fluids
Epinephrine (intratracheal or intrabronchial)	0.4 mL/kg of a 1:10,000 dilution repeat in 15 minutes	Initial treatment along with intravenous fluids; administer through a urinary catheter
Aminophylline	5 mg/kg IV slowly	Respiratory distress refractory to epinephrine
Atropine	0.02-0.04 mg/kg IV or IM	Bradycardia refractory to epinephrine
Dopamine	4-10 μg/kg/min constant-rate infusion	Refractory hypotension
Dexamethasone sodium phosphate	1-4 mg/kg IV	After correction of volume contraction
Prednisone sodium succinate (Solu-Delta-Cortef)	10-25 mg/kg IV slowly	After correction of volume contraction
Diphenhydramine (Benadryl)	0.5-1 mg/kg IV slowly	H_1 receptor blockade After correction of volume contraction
Tripelennamine	1 mg/kg IV or IM	H_1 receptor blockade After correction of volume contraction

IV, Intravenously; *IM,* intramuscularly.

beginning therapy. If not, additional drugs should be considered. If respiratory distress is still present, aminophylline 5 mg/kg administered slowly and intravenously may help reduce bronchoconstriction and strengthen contraction of the respiratory muscles.[121] If additional cardiovascular support is required, infusions of dopamine or dobutamine may be considered. Atropine at 0.02 to 0.04 mg/kg intravenously or intramuscularly may be used if bradycardia is refractory to epinephrine.

Once the life-threatening crisis is dealt with, glucocorticoids and antihistamines can be administered. They are not useful for the acute treatment of anaphylaxis.[121] Glucocorticoids cause vasodilation and decreased cardiac contractility and are detrimental if administered before correction of hypovolemia with intravenous fluids. Rapid-acting glucocorticoids such as dexamethasone sodium phosphate at 1 to 4 mg/kg intravenously may be beneficial by enhancing beta-receptor sensitivity and decreasing phospholipase A_2 activity. H_1-receptor–blocking antihistamines such as diphenhydramine (Benadryl, McNeil PPC) at 0.5 to 1 mg/kg administered slowly and intravenously or tripelennamine 1 mg/kg intravenously or intramuscularly may reduce the further effects of histamine on the target tissues. This may be of limited benefit insofar as histamine is only one of many mediators released by mast cells. H_2-receptor–blocking antihistamines may be used if gastric ulceration is suspected.

The cat experiencing anaphylactic shock should be monitored closely for the next 24 hours, the time period over which new cytokine synthesis and release occurs. Parameters to follow include respiratory rate and effort, heart rate and rhythm, pulse quality, capillary refill time, the patient's attitude, urine output, systemic blood pressure, and oxygen saturation as measured by pulse oximetry. Bloody diarrhea may signal the presence of DIC. Preparations should be made to act on significant changes in any of these parameters.

Prognosis

The effectiveness of therapeutic interventions in cats with anaphylactic shock depends on timely and aggressive action on the part of the veterinarian and support staff. The prognosis for these patients varies with the individual and the individual's response to initial therapy. The sooner appropriate therapy can begin, the better chance the cat has of surviving. However, some patients will die despite the best efforts of the veterinarian.

Prevention

Once the acute crisis is over, the owner can be questioned regarding recent vaccination and exposure to insects, drugs, reptiles, and new foods. Any intravenous injections in the future should be administered slowly. Avoidance of any triggers is advisable. If this is not possible, as may be the case with vaccinations, pretreatment with antihistamines or glucocorticoids may help minimize the severity of any reaction. Any cat experiencing anaphylaxis after vaccination should remain at the hospital for 20 to 30 minutes after subsequent vaccinations to allow for immediate intervention should anaphylaxis recur. If a severe reaction has not begun within that time frame, it is unlikely to happen.[17] Although they are uncommon, anaphylactic and anaphylactoid reactions can occur at any time. Anticipating the needs of a cat experiencing this frightening reaction is essential to a successful outcome.

Vaccine-Associated Adverse Events

Vaccination represents a common scenario in which cats are exposed to foreign proteins. Fortunately, the chance of a vaccine-associated adverse event (VAAE) occurring, although slightly higher than in dogs, is quite low.[78,117] Vaccine reactions are usually mild and transient.[117] In a report of almost 500,000 vaccinated cats, VAAEs were reported in approximately 0.5% of these cats. The most common adverse event was lethargy followed by localized vaccine-site reactions, vomiting, facial edema, and generalized pruritus.[78] Only four cats died within 48 hours of vaccine administration; two of them fit the description of anaphylaxis. The chances of developing a VAAE increased with the number of agents vaccinated against at one time.[78] A reduction in the number of vaccinations administered at one time might reduce the chances of VAAE development. Localized swellings appear 24 hours after vaccination, may be painful and hot, and usually last about 1 week.[117] These localized swellings occur two to five times more frequently in cats than in dogs.[78] Although this has not been studied in cats, there is limited evidence supporting an association between vaccine administration and the development of immune-mediated disorders in dogs.[117] Vaccination against calicivirus has been associated with polyarthritis and postvaccination lameness in cats.[117] Injection-site sarcomas are covered in Chapter 28.

References

1. Adams LG, Hardy RM, Weiss DJ et al: Hypophosphatemia and hemolytic anemia associated with diabetes mellitus and hepatic lipidosis in cats, *J Vet Intern Med* 7:266, 1993.
2. Autran de Morais H, O'Brien R: Non-neoplastic diseases of the spleen. In Ettinger S, Feldman E, editors: *Textbook of veterinary internal medicine*, ed 6, St Louis, 2005, Elsevier/Saunders, p 1944.
3. Avery PR, Hoover EA: Gamma interferon/interleukin 10 balance in tissue lymphocytes correlates with down modulation of mucosal feline immunodeficiency virus infection, *J Virol* 78:4011, 2004.

4. Ballegeer EA, Forrest LJ, Dickinson RM et al: Correlation of ultrasonographic appearance of lesions and cytologic and histologic diagnoses in splenic aspirates from dogs and cats: 32 cases (2002-2005), *J Am Vet Med Assoc* 230:690, 2007.
5. Bhatt S, Siegel A: Potentiating role of interleukin 2 (IL-2) receptors in the midbrain periaqueductal gray (PAG) upon defensive rage behavior in the cat: role of neurokinin NK(1) receptors, *Behav Brain Res* 167:251, 2006.
6. Bianco D, Armstrong PJ, Washabau RJ: Presumed primary immune-mediated thrombocytopenia in four cats, *J Feline Med Surg* 10:495, 2008.
7. Bighignoli B, Owens S, Froenicke L et al: Blood types of the domestic cat. In August J, editor: *Consultations in feline internal medicine*, ed 6, St Louis, 2010, Elsevier/Saunders, p 628.
8. Birkenheuer A, Cohn L, Levy M et al: Atovaquone and azithromycin for the treatment of *Cytauxzoon felis*, *J Vet Intern Med* 22:703, 2008.
9. Bondy P, Cohn L, Kerl M: Feline cytauxzoonosis, *Compend Contin Educ Pract Vet* 27, 2005.
10. Brockus C: Interpreting the leukogram. In August J, editor: *Consultations in feline internal medicine*, ed 5, St Louis, 2006, Elsevier/Saunders, p 585.
11. Brockus C: Leukocyte disorders. In Ettinger S, Feldman E, editors: *Textbook of veterinary internal medicine*, ed 6, St Louis, 2006, Elsevier/Saunders, p 1937.
12. Brooks M, DeWilde L: Feline factor XII deficiency, *Compend Contin Educ Pract Vet* 28:148, 2006.
13. Brown R, Riogers K: Neutropenia in dogs and cats, *Compend Contin Educ Pract Vet* 23:534, 2001.
14. Christopher M: Disorders of feline red blood cells. In Bonagura J, editor: *Kirk's current veterinary therapy XIII small animal practice*, Philadelphia, 2000, Saunders, p 421.
15. Cohen R: Systemic anaphylaxis. In Bonagura J, editors: *Kirk's current veterinary therapy XII small animal practice*, Philadelphia, 1995, Saunders, p 150.
16. Cohn L: Glucocorticoid therapy. In Ettinger S, Feldman E, editors: *Textbook of veterinary internal medicine*, ed 6, St Louis, 2005, Elsevier/Saunder, p 503.
17. Cowell A, Cowell R: Management of bee and other hymenoptera stings. In Bonagura J, editor: *Kirk's current veterinary therapy XII small animal practice*, Philadelphia, 1995, Saunders, p 226.
18. Cowell R, Tyler R, Meinkoth J: Diagnosis of anemia. In August J, editor: *Consultations in feline internal medicine*, ed 5, St Louis, 2006, Elsevier/Saunders, p 565.
19. Cowgill L: CVT update: use of recombinant human erythropoietin. In Bonagura J, editor: *Kirk's current veterinary therapy XII small animal practice*, Philadelphia, 1995, Saunders, p 961.
20. Culp WT, Aronson LR: Splenic foreign body in a cat, *J Feline Med Surg* 10:380, 2008.
21. Dowers KL, Olver C, Radecki SV et al: Use of enrofloxacin for treatment of large-form *Haemobartonella felis* in experimentally infected cats, *J Am Vet Med Assoc* 221:250, 2002.
22. Dowers KL, Tasker S, Radecki SV et al: Use of pradofloxacin to treat experimentally induced *Mycoplasma hemofelis* infection in cats, *Am J Vet Res* 70:105, 2009.
23. Dunham SP: Cytokines and anti-cytokine therapy: clinical potential for treatment of feline disease, *J Feline Med Surg* 1:7, 1999.
24. Estrin MA, Wehausen CE, Jessen CR et al: Disseminated intravascular coagulation in cats, *J Vet Intern Med* 20:1334, 2006.
25. Feldman B: Blood transfusion guidelines. In Bonagura J, editor: *Kirk's current veterinary therapy XIII small animal practice*, Philadelphia, 2000, Saunders, p 400.
26. Feldman B: Nonregenerative anemia. In Ettinger S, Feldman E, editors: *Textbook of veterinary internal medicine*, ed 6, St Louis, 2005, Elsevier/Saunders, p 1908.
27. Feldman E, Nelson R: *Glucocorticoid therapy: canine and feline endocrinology and reproduction*, ed 3, St Louis, 2004, Saunders, p 464.
28. Felsburg P: Hereditary and acquired immunodeficiency diseases. In Bonagura J, editor: *Kirk's current veterinary therapy XIII small animal practice*, Philadelphia, 2004, Saunders, p 516.
29. Foley J: Feline infectious peritonitis and feline enteric coronavirus. In Ettinger S, Feldman E, editors: *Textbook of veterinary internal medicine*, ed 6, St Louis, 2005, Elsevier/Saunders, p 663.
30. Foley JE, Rand C, Leutenegger C: Inflammation and changes in cytokine levels in neurological feline infectious peritonitis, *J Feline Med Surg* 5:313, 2003.
31. George JW, Rideout BA, Griffey SM et al: Effect of preexisting FeLV infection or FeLV and feline immunodeficiency virus coinfection on pathogenicity of the small variant of *Haemobartonella felis* in cats, *Am J Vet Res* 63:1172, 2002.
32. Gibson GR, Callan MB, Hoffman V et al: Use of a hemoglobin-based oxygen-carrying solution in cats: 72 cases (1998-2000), *J Am Vet Med Assoc* 221:96, 2002.
33. Giger U: Hereditary erythrocyte disorders. In August J, editor: *Consultations in feline veterinary internal medicine*, ed 4, Philadelphia, 2001, Saunders, p 484.
34. Giger U: Regenerative anemias caused by blood loss or hemolysis. In Ettinger S, Feldman E, editors: *Textbook of veterinary internal medicine*, ed 6, St Louis, 2005, Elsevier/Saunders, p 1886.
35. Giger U: Blood-typing and crossmatching. In Bonagura J, Twedt D, editors: *Kirk's current veterinary therapy XIV*, St Louis, 2009, Saunders/Elsevier, p 260.
36. Giger U, Bucheler J: Transfusion of type-A and type-B blood to cats, *J Am Vet Med Assoc* 198:411, 1991.
37. Gordon SS, McClaran JK, Bergman PJ et al: Outcome following splenectomy in cats, *J Feline Med Surg* 12:256, 2010.
38. Goree M, Catalfamo JL, Aber S et al: Characterization of the mutations causing hemophilia B in 2 domestic cats, *J Vet Intern Med* 19:200, 2005.
39. Greene C, Meinkoth J, Kocan A: Cytauxzoonosis. In Greene C, editor: *Infectious diseases of the dog and cat*, ed 3, St Louis, 2006, Saunders, p 716.
40. Gregory C: Immunosuppressive agents. In Bonagura J, Twedt D, editors: *Kirk's current veterinary therapy XIV*, St Louis, 2009, Saunders/Elsevier, p 254.
41. Guilford W: The gastrointestinal tract and adverse reactions to food. In August J, editor: *Consultations in feline internal medicine*, ed 4, Philadelphia, 2001, Saunders, p 113.
42. Haldane S, Roberts J, Marks S et al: Transfusion medicine, *Compend Contin Educ Pract Vet* 26, 2004.
43. Hall R: Interpreting the leukogram. In August J, editor: *Consultations in feline internal medicine*, ed 2, Philadelphia, 1994, Saunders, p 489.
44. Hammer A, Couto C: Disorders of the lymph nodes and spleen. In Sherding R, editor: *The cat: diseases and clinical management*, ed 2, Philadelphia, 1994, Saunders, p 671.
45. Hanson JA, Papageorges M, Girard E et al: Ultrasonographic appearance of splenic disease in 101 cats, *Vet Radiol Ultrasound* 42:441, 2001.
46. Hardie R, Petrus D: Lymphatics and lymph nodes. In Slatter D, editor: *Textbook of small animal surgery*, ed 3, Philadelphia, 2003, Saunders, p 1063.
47. Hasler A: Polycythemia. In Ettinger S, Feldman E, editors: *Textbook of veterinary internal medicine*, ed 6, St Louis, 2005, Elsevier/Saunders, p 215.
48. Helfand S: Hematopoietic cytokines: the interleukin array. In Bonagura J, editor: *Kirk's current veterinary therapy XIII small animal practice*, Philadelphia, 2000, Saunders, p 408.
49. Holan K: Feline hepatic lipidosis. In Bonagura J, Twedt D, editors: *Kirk's current veterinary therapy XIV*, St Louis, 2009, Saunders/Elsevier, p 570.

50. Johnson LR, De Cock HE, Sykes JE et al: Cytokine gene transcription in feline nasal tissue with histologic evidence of inflammation, *Am J Vet Res* 66:996, 2005.
51. Jordan HL, Grindem CB, Breitschwerdt EB: Thrombocytopenia in cats: a retrospective study of 41 cases, *J Vet Intern Med* 7:261, 1993.
52. Kearns S, Ewing P: Causes of canine and feline pancytopenia, *Compend Contin Educ Pract Vet* 28, 2006.
53. Klaser DA, Reine NJ, Hohenhaus AE: Red blood cell transfusions in cats: 126 cases (1999), *J Am Vet Med Assoc* 226:920, 2005.
54. Knottenbelt S, Blackwood L: The blood. In Chandler E, Gaskell C, Gaskell R, editors: *Feline medicine and therapeutics*, ed 3, Oxford, 2004, Blackwell Publishing, p 235.
55. Kohn B, Fumi C: Clinical course of pyruvate kinase deficiency in Abyssinian and Somali cats, *J Feline Med Surg* 10:145, 2008.
56. Kohn B, Goldschmidt MH, Hohenhaus AE et al: Anemia, splenomegaly, and increased osmotic fragility of erythrocytes in Abyssinian and Somali cats, *J Am Vet Med Assoc* 217:1483, 2000.
57. Kohn B, Weingart C, Eckmann V et al: Primary immune-mediated hemolytic anemia in 19 cats: diagnosis, therapy, and outcome (1998-2004), *J Vet Intern Med* 20:159, 2006.
58. Langston C, Ludwig L: Renal transplantation. In Ettinger S, Feldman E, editors: *Textbook of veterinary internal medicine*, ed 6, St Louis, 2005, Elsevier/Saunders, p 1752.
59. Levy J, Crawford P: Feline leukemia virus. In Ettinger S, Feldman E, editors: *Textbook of veterinary internal medicine*, ed 6, St Louis, 2005, Elsevier/Saunders, p 653.
60. Levy JK, Crawford PC, Collante WR et al: Use of adult cat serum to correct failure of passive transfer in kittens, *J Am Vet Med Assoc* 219:1401, 2001.
61. Levy JK, Liang Y, Ritchey JW et al: Failure of FIV-infected cats to control Toxoplasma gondii correlates with reduced IL2, IL6, and IL12 and elevated IL10 expression by lymph node T cells, *Vet Immunol Immunopathol* 98:101, 2004.
62. Littlewood JD, Shaw SC, Coombes LM: Vitamin K-dependent coagulopathy in a British Devon rex cat, *J Small Anim Pract* 36:115, 1995.
63. London C: Hematopoietic cytokines: the myelopoietic factors. In Bonagura J, editor: *Kirk's current veterinary therapy XIII small animal practice*, Philadelphia, 2000, Saunders, p 403.
64. Lucroy MD, Madewell BR: Clinical outcome and diseases associated with extreme neutrophilic leukocytosis in cats: 104 cases (1991-1999), *J Am Vet Med Assoc* 218:736, 2001.
65. Lusson D, Billiemaz B, Chabanne JL: Circulating lupus anticoagulant and probable systemic lupus erythematosus in a cat, *J Feline Med Surg* 1:193, 1999.
66. Mackin A: Platelet disorders. In August J, editor: *Consultations in feline internal medicine*, ed 5, St Louis, 2006, Elsevier/Saunders, p 575.
67. Maddison JE, Watson AD, Eade IG et al: Vitamin K-dependent multifactor coagulopathy in Devon Rex cats, *J Am Vet Med Assoc* 197:1495, 1990.
68. Marino D: Diseases of the spleen. In Bonagura J, editor: *Kirk's current veterinary therapy XIII small animal practice*, Philadelphia, 2000, Saunders, p 520.
69. Marks S, Henry C: CVT update: diagnosis and treatment of systemic lupus erythematosus. In Bonagura J, editor: *Kirk's current veterinary therapy XIII small animal practice*, Philadelphia, 2000, Saunders, p 514.
70. May S, Langston C: Managing chronic renal failure, *Compend Contin Educ Pract Vet* 28, 2006.
71. McSherry L: Techniques for bone marrow aspiration and biopsy. In Ettinger S, Feldman E, editors: *Textbook of veterinary internal medicine*, ed 6, St Louis, 2005, Elsevier/Saunders, p 285.
72. Meinkoth J, Kocan AA, Whitworth L et al: Cats surviving natural infection with *Cytauxzoon felis*: 18 cases (1997-1998), *J Vet Intern Med* 14:521, 2000.
73. Meurs KM, Fox PR, Miller MW et al: Plasma concentrations of tumor necrosis factor-alpha in cats with congestive heart failure, *Am J Vet Res* 63:640, 2002.
74. Miller C, Bartges J: Refeeding syndrome. In Bonagura J, editor: *Kirk's current veterinary therapy XIII small animal practice*, Philadelphia, 2000, Saunders, p 87.
75. Miller E: Immune-mediated hemolytic anemia. In Bonagura J, Twedt D, editors: *Kirk's current veterinary therapy XIV*, St Louis, 2009, Saunders/Elsevier, p 266.
76. Mooney SC, Patnaik AK, Hayes AA et al: Generalized lymphadenopathy resembling lymphoma in cats: six cases (1972-1976), *J Am Vet Med Assoc* 190:897, 1987.
77. Moore FM, Emerson WE, Cotter SM et al: Distinctive peripheral lymph node hyperplasia of young cats, *Vet Pathol* 23:386, 1986.
78. Moore GE, DeSantis-Kerr AC, Guptill LF et al: Adverse events after vaccine administration in cats: 2,560 cases (2002-2005), *J Am Vet Med Assoc* 231:94, 2007.
79. Museux K, Boretti FS, Willi B et al: In vivo transmission studies of '*Candidatus* Mycoplasma turicensis' in the domestic cat, *Vet Res* 40:45, 2009.
80. Nakazato A, Momoi Y, Kadoya M et al: Measurement of feline serum interleukin-5 level, *J Vet Med Sci* 69:843, 2007.
81. Neer T: Splenomegaly and lymphadenopathy. In August J, editor: *Consultations in feline internal medicine*, ed 4, Philadelphia, 2001, Saunders, p 439.
82. Nguyen Van N, Taglinger K, Helps CR et al: Measurement of cytokine mRNA expression in intestinal biopsies of cats with inflammatory enteropathy using quantitative real-time RT-PCR, *Vet Immunol Immunopathol* 113:404, 2006.
83. Nibblett BM, Snead EC, Waldner C et al: Anemia in cats with hemotropic mycoplasma infection: retrospective evaluation of 23 cases (1996-2005), *Can Vet J* 50:1181, 2009.
84. Nitsche E: Erythrocytosis in dogs and cats: diagnosis and management, *Compend Contin Educ Pract Vet* 26, 2004.
85. Ogg A, Kruth S: Antimicrobial therapy for the neutropenic dog and cat. In Bonagura J, editor: *Kirk's current veterinary therapy XIII small animal practice*, Philadelphia, 2000, Saunders, p 267.
86. Ottenjann M, Weingart C, Arndt G et al: Characterization of the anemia of inflammatory disease in cats with abscesses, pyothorax, or fat necrosis, *J Vet Intern Med* 20:1143, 2006.
87. Papich M: Drug therapy in cats: precautions and guidelines. In August J, editor: *Consultations in feline internal medicine*, ed 5, St Louis, 2006, Elsevier/Saunders, p 279.
88. Paterson S: Diagnosis and management of pemphigus foliaceus. In August J, editor: *Consultations in feline internal medicine*, ed 5, St Louis, 2006, Elsevier/Saunders, p 261.
89. Peterson JL, Couto CG, Wellman ML: Hemostatic disorders in cats: a retrospective study and review of the literature, *J Vet Intern Med* 9:298, 1995.
90. Platt S, Abramson C, Garosi L: Administering corticosteroids in neurological disease, *Compend Contin Educ Pract Vet* 27, 2005.
91. Plotnick A: Feline chronic renal failure: long-term medical management, *Compend Contin Educ Pract Vet* 29, 2007.
92. Plumb D: Leflunomide. In *Plumb's veterinary drug handbook*, ed 6, Stockholm, WI, 2008, PharmaVet Inc.
93. Polzin D, Osborne C, Ross S: Chronic kidney disease. In Ettinger S, Feldman E, editors: *Textbook of veterinary internal medicine*, ed 6, St Louis, 2005, Elsevier/Saunders, p 1756.
94. Randolph JE, Scarlett JM, Stokol T et al: Expression, bioactivity, and clinical assessment of recombinant feline erythropoietin, *Am J Vet Res* 65:1355, 2004.
95. Rojko J, Hardy W: Feline leukemia virus and other retroviruses. In Sherding R, editor: *The cat: diseases and clinical management*, ed 2, Philadelphia, 1994, Saunders, p 263.
96. Roosje PJ, Dean GA, Willemse T et al: Interleukin 4-producing CD4+ T cells in the skin of cats with allergic dermatitis, *Vet Pathol* 39:228, 2002.

97. Roudebush P, Polzin DJ, Ross SJ et al: Therapies for feline chronic kidney disease. What is the evidence? *J Feline Med Surg* 11:195, 2009.
98. Roux FA, Deschamps JY, Blais MC et al: Multiple red cell transfusions in 27 cats (2003-2006): indications, complications and outcomes, *J Feline Med Surg* 10:213, 2008.
99. Rudloff E, Kirby R: Disseminated intravascular coagulation: diagnosis and management. In Bonagura J, Twedt D, editors: *Kirk's current veterinary therapy XIV*, St Louis, 2009, Saunders/Elsevier, p 287.
100. Sartor L, Trepanier L: Rational pharmacological therapy of hepatobiliary disease in dogs and cats, *Compend Contin Educ Pract Vet* 25, 2003.
101. Schooley EK, McGee Turner JB, Jiji RD et al: Effects of cyproheptadine and cetirizine on eosinophilic airway inflammation in cats with experimentally induced asthma, *Am J Vet Res* 68:1265, 2007.
102. Segev G, Klement E, Aroch I: Toxic neutrophils in cats: clinical and clinicopathologic features, and disease prevalence and outcome—a retrospective case control study, *J Vet Intern Med* 20:20, 2006.
103. Smith J, Day T, Mackin A: Diagnosing bleeding disorders, *Compend Contin Educ Pract Vet* 27, 2005.
104. Stieger K, Palos H, Giger U: Comparison of various blood-typing methods for the feline AB blood group system, *Am J Vet Res* 66:1393, 2005.
105. Stokol T, Brooks M: Diagnosis of DIC in cats: is it time to go back to the basics? *J Vet Intern Med* 20:1289, 2006.
106. Stone M: Systemic lupus erythematosus. In Ettinger S, Feldman E, editors: *Textbook of veterinary internal medicine*, ed 6, St Louis, 2005, Elsewhere/ Saunders, p 1952.
107. Stutzer B, Muller F, Majzoub M et al: Role of latent feline leukemia virus infection in nonregenerative cytopenias of cats, *J Vet Intern Med* 24:192, 2010.
108. Sykes JE, Drazenovich NL, Ball LM et al: Use of conventional and real-time polymerase chain reaction to determine the epidemiology of hemoplasma infections in anemic and nonanemic cats, *J Vet Intern Med* 21:685, 2007.
109. Sykes JE, Terry JC, Lindsay LL et al: Prevalences of various hemoplasma species among cats in the United States with possible hemoplasmosis, *J Am Vet Med Assoc* 232:372, 2008.
110. Tasker S, Caney SM, Day MJ et al: Effect of chronic FIV infection, and efficacy of marbofloxacin treatment, on *Mycoplasma haemofelis* infection, *Vet Microbiol* 117:169, 2006.
111. Tasker S, Lappin M: Update on hemoplasmosis. In August J, editor: *Consultations in feline internal medicine*, ed 5, St Louis, 2006, Elsevier/Saunders, p 605.
112. Tholen I, Weingart C, Kohn B: Concentration of D-dimers in healthy cats and sick cats with and without disseminated intravascular coagulation (DIC), *J Feline Med Surg* 11:842, 2009.
113. Tillson D: Spleen. In Slatter D, editor: *Textbook of small animal surgery*, ed 3, Philadelphia, 2003, Saunders, p 1046.
114. Tizard I: Drugs and other agents that affect the immune system. In Tizard I, editor: *Veterinary immunology: an introduction*, ed 8, St Louis, 2009, Saunders/Elsevier, p 480.
115. Tizard I: Primary immunodeficiencies. In Tizard I, editor: *Veterinary immunology: an introduction*, ed 8, St Louis, 2009, Saunders/Elsevier, p 448.
116. Tizard I: Type I hypersensitivity. In Tizard I, editor: *Veterinary immunology: an introduction*, ed 8, St Louis, 2009, Saunders/Elsevier, p 329.
117. Tizard I: The use of vaccines. In Tizard I, editor: *Veterinary immunology: an introduction*, ed 8, St Louis, 2009, Saunders/Elsevier, p 270.
118. Tocci LJ, Ewing PJ: Increasing patient safety in veterinary transfusion medicine: an overview of pretransfusion testing, *J Vet Emerg Crit Care (San Antonio)* 19:66, 2009.
119. Trepanier L: Idiopathic inflammatory bowel disease in cats. Rational treatment selection, *J Feline Med Surg* 11:32, 2009.
120. Vail D, Thamm D: Hematopoietic tumors. In Ettinger S, Feldman E, editor: *Textbook of veterinary internal medicine*, ed 6, St Louis, 2005, Elsevier/Saunders, p 732.
121. Waddell L: Systemic anaphylaxis. In Ettinger S, Feldman E, editor: *Textbook of veterinary internal medicine*, ed 6, St Louis, 2005, Elsevier/Saunders, p 458.
122. Wardrop KJ, Reine N, Birkenheuer A et al: Canine and feline blood donor screening for infectious disease, *J Vet Intern Med* 19:135, 2005.
123. Washabau RJ, Day MJ, Willard MD et al: Endoscopic, biopsy, and histopathologic guidelines for the evaluation of gastrointestinal inflammation in companion animals, *J Vet Intern Med* 24:10, 2010.
124. Weinstein NM, Blais MC, Harris K et al: A newly recognized blood group in domestic shorthair cats: the MiK red cell antigen, *J Vet Intern Med* 21:287, 2007.
125. Weiss D: Nonregenerative anemias. In Bonagura J, Twedt D, editors: *Kirk's current veterinary therapy XIV*, St Louis, 2009, Sanders/Elsevier, p 272.
126. Weiss D, Tvedten H: Erythrocyte disorders. In Willard M, Tvedten H, editors: *Small animal clinical diagnosis by laboratory methods*, ed 4, St Louis, 2004, Saunders, p 38.
127. Weiss DJ: Aplastic anemia in cats—clinicopathological features and associated disease conditions 1996-2004, *J Feline Med Surg* 8:203, 2006.
128. White C, Reine N: Feline nonregenerative anemia: diagnosis and treatment, *Compend Contin Educ Pract Vet* 31, 2009.
129. White C, Reine N: Feline nonregenerative anemia: pathophysiology and etiologies, *Compend Contin Educ Pract Vet* 31, 2009.
130. Williams CR, Sykes JE, Mehl M et al: In vitro effects of the active metabolite of leflunomide, A77 1726, on feline herpesvirus-1, *Am J Vet Res* 68:1010, 2007.
131. Wohl J, Murtaugh R: Use of catecholamines in critical care patients. In Bonagura J, editor: *Kirk's current veterinary therapy XII small animal practice*, Philadelphia, 1995, Saunders, p 188.
132. Wondratschek C, Weingart C, Kohn B: Primary immune-mediated thrombocytopenia in cats, *J Am Anim Hosp Assoc* 46:12, 2010.
133. Woods JE, Wisnewski N, Lappin MR: Attempted transmission of *Candidatus* Mycoplasma haemominutum and *Mycoplasma haemofelis* by feeding cats infected *Ctenocephalides felis*, *Am J Vet Res* 67:494, 2006.
134. Young K, Moriello K: Eosinophils and eosinophilic diseases. In August J, editor: *Consultations in feline internal medicine*, ed 5, St Louis, 2006, Elsevier/Saunders, p 239.

CHAPTER

26

Musculoskeletal Diseases

Greg L.G. Harasen and Susan E. Little

OUTLINE

Conditions of the musculoskeletal system in the cat have received comparatively little attention in the literature. Much of what has been published assumes similarities with dogs and humans that may not be accurate. Developmental diseases, especially genetically determined conditions, are much less common in the cat than in the dog. Even those that are seen, including patellar luxation and hip dysplasia, are relatively uncommon. Trauma is the major source of musculoskeletal abnormality in the cat, and thus the entire patient must be evaluated.

The feline patient also presents challenges in examination and observation of abnormal gaits because many cats are uncooperative at best and fractious at worst when exposed to the clinic environment. To appreciate subtle gait disturbances, the clinician must frequently rely on patience when examining the cat, as well as on owner observations or videotapes taken in the home environment.

The cat has a number of anatomic and physiologic differences compared with the dog. Some are mere curiosities, whereas others can be extremely significant from a diagnostic perspective.[96] The presence of a free-floating clavicle in the cranial shoulder region falls into the category of curiosity, but it is sometimes mistaken for a fracture or foreign body (Figure 26-1). The median nerve and brachial artery pass through the supracondylar foramen on the medial side of the distal humerus in the cat, whereas the same structures lie medial to the humerus in the dog (Figure 26-2). The presence of these vital structures within the humeral metaphysis of the cat restricts the placement of orthopedic hardware in this region. In the condylar region of the distal humerus, there is no supratrochlear foramen in the cat as there is in the dog. This is one of the main reasons that humeral condylar fractures are relatively less common in cats.[65] Approximately 40% of cats have a sesamoid bone in the tendon of origin of the supinator muscle on the dorsal surface of the proximal radius (Figure 26-3). This structure may be visible on lateral radiographic projections of the elbow and should not be mistaken for a chip fracture. The round ligament of the femoral head provides significant vascular supply to the femoral head in the cat, which is not the case in the dog. This may be one reason that aseptic necrosis of the femoral head is not described in the cat. The cranial cruciate ligament is larger and thicker than the caudal cruciate ligament in cats, which is the reverse of what is found in the dog. This may be an important factor explaining why rupture of the cruciate ligament is much less common in the cat. The range of motion in the feline shoulder and hip is greater than in the dog, but in the feline carpus and stifle range of motion is less than in the dog. However, supination of the carpus and paw is much greater in the cat and is important in grooming behavior.[13,65,96,103]

FRACTURES

Fractures make up a large percentage of musculoskeletal problems in the cat, with the distribution of fractures being somewhat unique to this species. Although both dogs and cats suffer a majority of their fractures in the hind limb or pelvis, this percentage exceeds 70% of all fractures seen in the cat.[48] When the 11% to 23% of feline

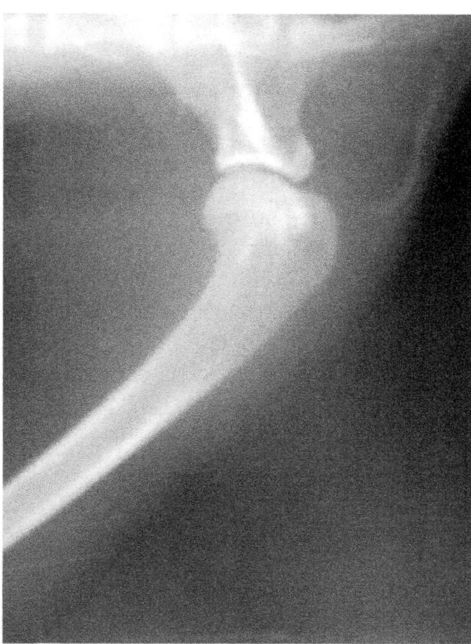

FIGURE 26-1 The clavicle is located cranial to the proximal humerus.

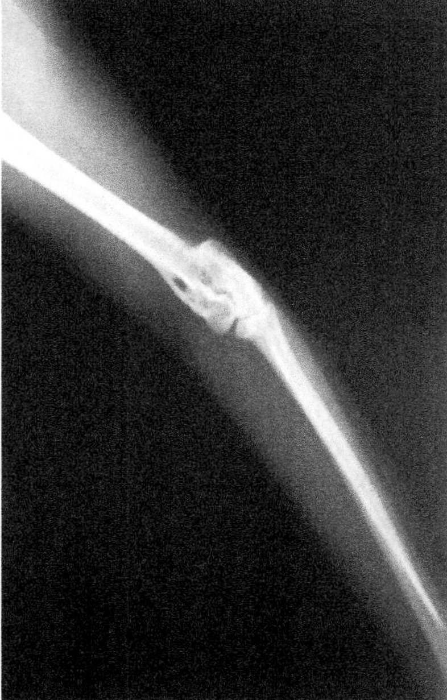

FIGURE 26-2 The supracondylar foramen is a unique anatomic feature of the medial aspect of the distal humerus in the cat through which pass the brachial artery and median nerve.

fractures that involve the maxillae, mandible, or facial bones are included, these two regions account for the overwhelming majority of fractures in the cat.

Because most fractures are associated with significant trauma, a thorough evaluation of the entire cat beyond the fracture is essential. Published estimates suggest that as many as 40% of fracture patients also have thoracic trauma, which may affect not only the treatment plan but also the patient's very survival.[13]

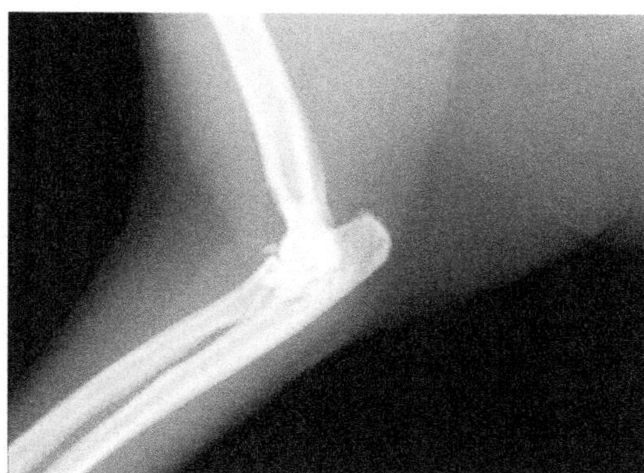

FIGURE 26-3 Approximately 40% of cats have a sesamoid bone located in the origin of the supinator muscle. It can be seen on a lateral radiographic projection of the elbow.

Much commonality exists between dogs and cats in the fractures that are seen and the repair techniques that can be used successfully. Certain fractures with unique considerations in the cat bear special consideration.

Mandibular and Maxillary Fractures

Fractures involving the mandible or maxillae of cats are unique if for no other reason than that they are at least tenfold more common in the cat than in the dog.[86] Vehicular trauma and high-rise syndrome are the most common causes of these fractures, which occur when the cat absorbs a face-first impact. Not surprisingly, such trauma is frequently associated with additional injuries, including broken teeth, thoracic injury, head trauma, and forelimb fractures. Fracture of the mandibular symphysis accounts for nearly three quarters of mandibular and maxillary injuries.[47,86] Circumferential wiring of the symphysis combined with 3 to 4 weeks of a soft diet followed by wire removal is usually successful (Figure 26-4). At the time of wire removal, some residual mobility may still be present at the symphysis, but this is due in part to the fact that the joint is cartilaginous and is not rigid, even in the normal state. Most patients do well clinically, regardless of the mobility.

Midsagittal splits of the hard palate are another common consequence of frontal facial impact trauma in the cat. Minor splits of 1 to 2 mm usually require no specific repair; however, wider splits should be compressed. This can be accomplished by running surgical wire in a figure-of-eight pattern across the split along the oral surface of the hard palate and around the base of a tooth on each side of the maxillae. Alternatively, a Kirschner wire can be driven across the maxillae between teeth so that the ends of the wire are exposed through the gingiva on either side of the maxillae, just dorsal to

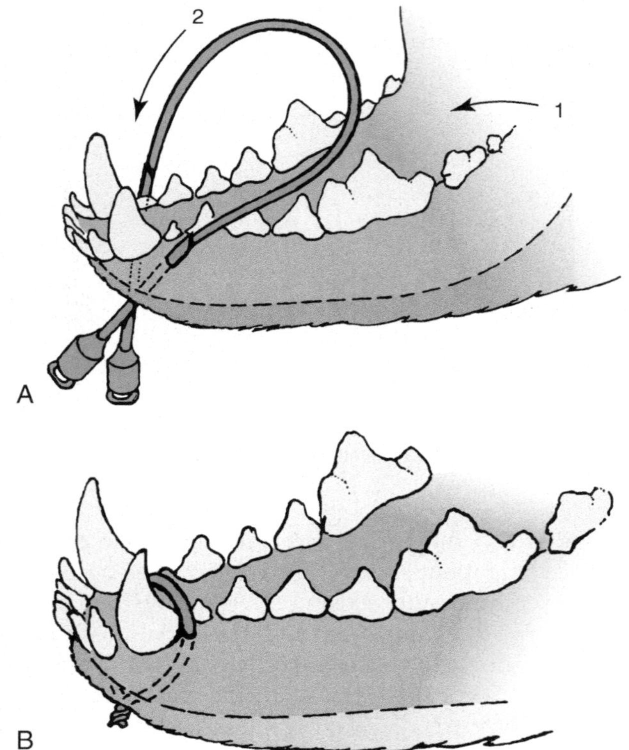

FIGURE 26-4 Mandibular symphyseal fractures can be stabilized with a loop of surgical wire passed around the cranial mandible, caudal to the canine teeth. *(Reprinted with permission from Piermattei D, Flo G, DeCamp C:* Brinker, Piermattei, and Flo's handbook of small animal orthopedics and fracture repair, *ed 4, St Louis, 2006, Saunders Elsevier.)*

the level of the hard palate. A figure-of-eight tension band wire is then placed around each end of the wire and tightened to achieve compression of the palatine split. The Kirschner wire ends can be bent over to prevent trauma to the lips. The hardware is removed after 4 weeks.[47]

Treatment of more complex mandibular or maxillary fractures can involve many of the same techniques used in dogs, including interdental wiring, intraoral splints, bone plates, and external skeletal fixators. Regardless of the technique, the primary goal is to restore perfect dental occlusion. It bears remembering that the most beautiful surgical repair is of little consequence if the teeth do not fit. An adhesive tape muzzle can be used effectively in the cat despite its short, conical muzzle. A length of tape is wrapped around the muzzle with the adhesive side facing out, caudal to the level of the canine teeth. Care is taken to ensure that the canine teeth interdigitate properly but that there is enough space between the incisor teeth to allow the cat to lap liquid diets and water. Performing the procedure under general anesthesia with an endotracheal tube in place usually provides the proper amount of space. A length of tape is then passed behind the ears and stuck to the adhesive surface of the muzzle wrap on the each side of the muzzle. Another wrap of tape is placed around the muzzle to hold the second length of tape in place. A final length of tape is placed from the head strap on both sides and beneath the cat's throat to prevent the head strap from pulling up over the ears.[47,96] In cases in which fracture comminution precludes surgical reconstruction and stabilization, when financial constraints eliminate a surgical option, or in young kittens whose soft bone and erupting teeth make the use of surgical hardware difficult, a tape muzzle permits the maintenance of normal dental occlusion and often produces surprisingly good results.[47,86,96]

Patellar Fractures

Traumatic fractures of the patella can occur in cats. If fracture fragments are sufficiently large, they can be stabilized with a pin and tension band wire. Small fragments may be removed. In either case the integrity of the quadriceps muscle and patellar tendon mechanism must be maintained.[63] Some cats may be born with bipartite patellas. The radiographic appearance reveals smooth edges to the patellar fragments and frequently a similar appearance bilaterally. The condition is usually an incidental finding but can cause diagnostic confusion in a lame cat.

An additional subset of young adult cats develops fractures of one or both patellae with no history or evidence of trauma. Lameness is acute but usually mild to moderate. Although the etiology is unclear, these have been characterized as stress fractures.[62] Evidence for this pathogenesis includes the lack of known trauma in most cases and the presence of radiographic sclerosis of the fracture fragments and often the contralateral patella if it is intact. The fractures are simple transverse, involve the proximal one third of the patella, and are bilateral about half the time. In one survey about half of the contralateral patellae subsequently fractured at a mean time of 3 months.[62] Attempts at surgical repair by pin and tension band wire have met with almost universal failure, characterized by iatrogenic fracture of the remaining fragments; hardware failure; or, most often, nonunion. However, most cats regained reasonable function of the limb, with stiffness or intermittent lameness in about half the cases.[62] Some of the cats were found to have retained deciduous teeth or delayed dental eruption (Figure 26-5, *A*). In humans there is a connection between dentinogenesis imperfecta, which involves a number of dental abnormalities, and osteogenesis imperfecta, a condition involving brittle, easily fractured bones that is also seen in cats (discussed later).

Of 34 cats with apparently atraumatic patellar fractures, 10 also had a history of previous, concurrent, or subsequent fracture of other bones (see Figure 26-5, *B*).[62] It may be that some of these cats with patellar fractures

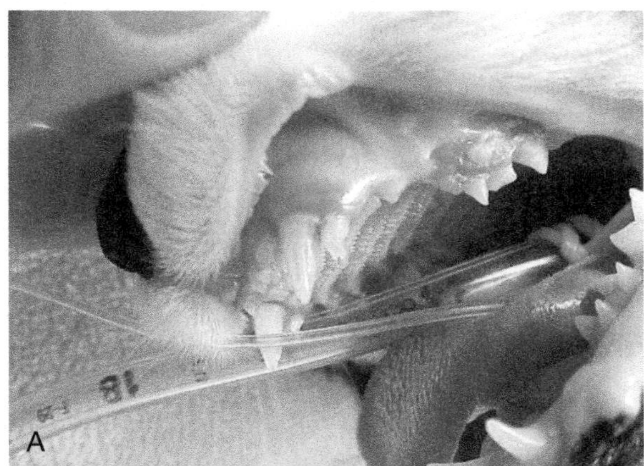

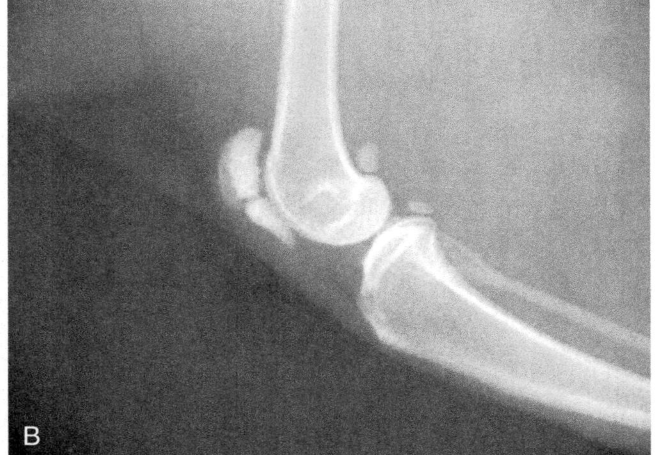

FIGURE 26-5 **A,** Persistent deciduous teeth are evidence of dentinogenesis imperfecta in this cat with a patellar fracture. **B,** A patellar fracture in a cat without history of trauma. *(A courtesy Dr. Steven Bailey.)*

have a form of osteogenesis imperfecta. Conservative treatment of these patellar fractures would appear to be the most prudent course, especially if distraction of fracture fragments is mild to moderate. If fragments are significantly distracted, then a circumferential wire may be preferred over an attempt to pass a pin through sclerotic bone. Alternatively, partial patellectomy may be performed. Complete patellectomy does not usually produce satisfactory function.[62]

Radial and Ulnar Fractures

Fractures of the radius and ulna are relatively uncommon in cats, composing between 5% and 13.8% of feline fractures.[84] Further, surgical repair of these fractures, especially when comminuted or open, is associated with a high complication rate.[103] This would appear to be primarily due to the cat's ability to pronate the front limb and paw to a much greater degree than the dog. This increased mobility between the bones means that the standard surgical approach in the dog of stabilizing only the radius, when both bones are fractured, may not

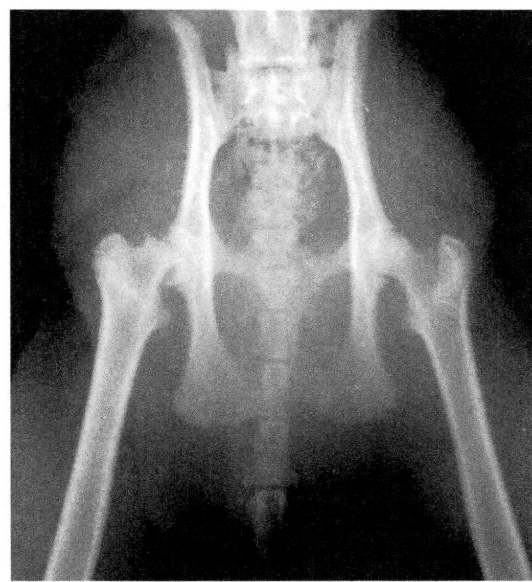

FIGURE 26-6 Unilateral slipped capital femoral epiphysis.

confer enough stability to produce consistently good results in the cat. Adding an intramedullary pin to the ulna in addition to the radial repair has been associated with more reliable surgical outcomes in this species.[103] In addition, the ulna, especially its proximal portion, has been identified as a common site of nonunion in the cat, which may also be a significant contributory factor to surgical complication statistics for these fractures.[84]

Capital Femoral Physeal Fractures

Capital femoral physeal fracture is a common traumatic injury in cats, but it appears as though just as many cases arise without a traumatic episode (Figure 26-6). Affected cats usually present with acute hind limb lameness, although the lameness may be mild and chronic in some instances. Most of these cases are seen in overweight, neutered males between 4 and 24 months of age.[11,19,45,79] One report found a preponderance of domestic shorthairs,[79] whereas another found a large number of Siamese cats.[19]

The first report of this problem described it as metaphyseal osteopathy of the femoral neck, which was thought to result from an aseptic necrosis, not unlike Legg-Calve-Perthes disease in the dog.[88] However, further examination of serial radiography and histopathologic specimens suggests that the changes in the femoral neck are more likely to be resorptive and remodeling changes secondary to the Salter–Harris I physeal fracture rather than a vascular impairment as is seen in Legg-Calve-Perthes disease in the dog (Figure 26-7).[19,45,79] The etiopathogenesis of this condition seems to revolve around abnormalities of the physis. Radiographically and histologically, these cats have abnormally wide physes that remain open long after they would be expected to have closed.

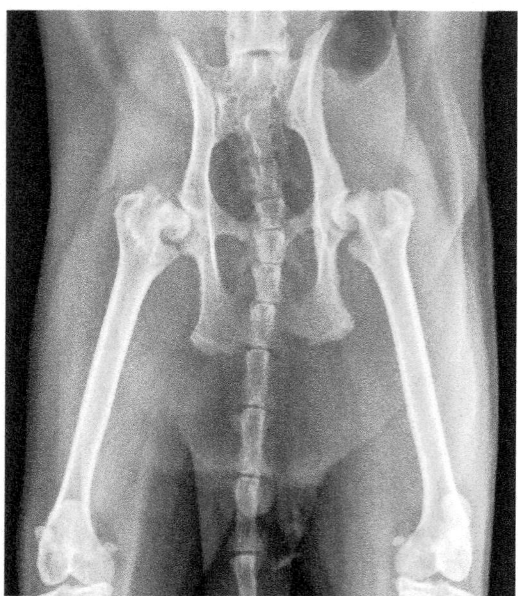

FIGURE 26-7 An acute slipped capital femoral epiphysis on the right side of the figure and a chronic example of the same injury on the left side. Note the resorption of the femoral neck and extensive remodeling.

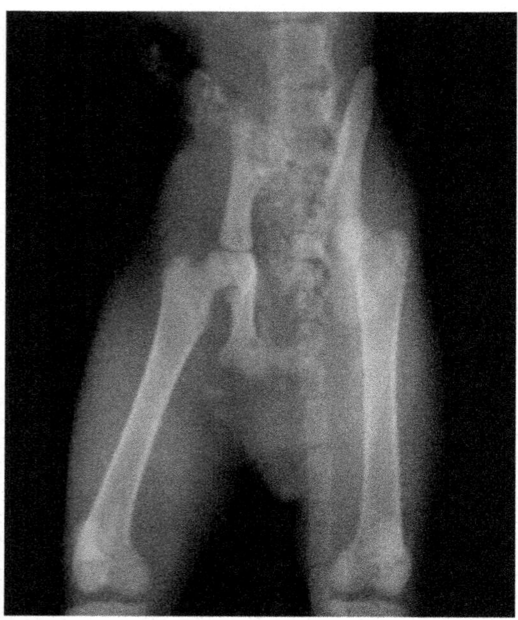

FIGURE 26-8 A kitten with multiple pelvic fractures. Note the significant decrease in pelvic canal diameter.

Histologically, these physes are characterized by an irregular arrangement of chondrocytes rather than the normal columnar appearance, which has resulted in the use of the term *physeal dysplasia* to describe the process.

Although genetic factors may certainly be involved in the development of the physeal dysplasia, endocrine factors may also play a role. Neutering at an early age has been shown to delay physeal closure times in the cat,[53] and it has been suggested that neutering before 6 months of age may be the endocrine factor contributing to the physeal dysplasia and slipped femoral capital physis.[79] A similar syndrome occurs in young, overweight adolescent humans, especially those that are hypothyroid, are receiving growth hormone supplementation, or have hypogonadism.[72] It may be that early neutering is one factor in the development of a physeal dysplasia, a wide physis, and a physis that remains open longer than normal, particularly in individuals that may be predisposed. If the cat becomes overweight, the stresses on the abnormal capital femoral physis may cause it to "slip," producing the characteristic Salter–Harris I fracture. Published reports suggest that between 24% and 38% of affected cats will develop bilateral fractures.[19,45,79,88] The condition is best treated with femoral head and neck excision (FHNE), which will produce a return to normal function in the majority of cases.[45,79] Primary repair with Kirschner wires has been described[20,29] but has much greater potential for complications than FHNE, with few, if any, demonstrated advantages.

Pelvic Fractures

Pelvic fractures are extremely common in the cat, especially after vehicular trauma, and make up at least 22% of all fractures seen (Figure 26-8).[64] Most pelvic fractures are multiple, unstable, and displaced, at least to some degree. Regardless, most will heal with conservative therapy. However, the issue is not whether they will heal but rather the severity and consequences of the malunion that almost invariably results. Although surgery can be considered to hasten pain relief and return to function, in most practical applications there are two primary indications for surgery:

Displaced acetabular fractures: Approximately 17.5% of feline pelvic fractures involve the acetabulum. Any degree of fracture malunion in the coxofemoral joint will lead to degenerative joint disease (DJD) and pain. Such a fracture can be addressed near the time of the initial trauma by primary fixation methods that include plates, screws, and tension band wires.[64] Traditionally, caudal acetabular fractures have often been treated conservatively because this area of the acetabulum was not considered to be weight bearing. However, recent research has suggested that the central and caudal portions of the acetabulum are actually the major weight-bearing regions within the coxofemoral joint of the cat.[4] Alternatively, femoral head and neck ostectomy can be performed several days or weeks later, once the patient's condition has stabilized, and where there is evidence of ongoing disability.

Pelvic canal narrowing: Ilial and acetabular fractures commonly displace axially, producing a narrowing of the pelvic canal. This can have immediate traumatic effects on bladder and bowels, but the greater concern is the prospect of producing obstipation and megacolon in the longer term. These problems are extremely frustrating to treat and are much better prevented. Thus pelvic fractures that produce more than 25% to 30% narrowing of the pelvic canal are best treated surgically. This can be efficiently done, in most cases utilizing bone plates, within 5 days of the initial trauma. After that time it becomes more difficult to break down fibrous tissue and surgically reduce these fractures. Pelvic canal–widening procedures such as pelvic symphyseal osteotomy can be performed if constipation has been present for less than 6 months. If constipation has been present for more than 6 months, the colon is often beyond reclamation and subtotal colectomy should be performed.[17]

BOX 26-1

Clinical Signs Associated with Degenerative Joint Disease in the Cat[3,15,37,50]

1. Pain
2. Reduced activity, difficulty with jumping or stairs
3. Anorexia, weight loss
4. Irritability, aggression
5. Inappropriate urination, constipation
6. Decreased grooming
7. Lameness or stiff gait
8. Alopecia over affected joints

BOX 26-2

Physical Examination Findings Associated with Degenerative Joint Disease in Cats[3]

1. Pain on joint manipulation
2. Soft tissue swelling
3. Periarticular thickening
4. Joint effusion
5. Restricted range of movement
6. Muscle atrophy
7. Crepitus
8. Heat

Nonunion Fractures

Cats may be characterized as the "perfect orthopedic patient" in many ways because their straight bones, lightweight frames, and legendary healing abilities have resulted in many amazing outcomes in fracture cases. However, the old adage that fractured feline bones will heal if placed in the same room is not always true. Feline fracture nonunions do occur, at a rate of 4.3% according to one report.[84] The tibia and proximal ulna were identified as the most common sites for nonunions. Increasing age and body weight, as well as open and comminuted fractures, were identified as risk factors.[84]

ARTHRIDITIES

Degenerative Joint Disease

The slowly progressive degeneration of articular cartilage with osteophyte production, usually associated with acute or chronic joint trauma, is the most common form of joint disease seen in the cat and is variously described as DJD, osteoarthritis, or osteoarthrosis. It is only relatively recently that the common occurrence of DJD has been recognized in the cat. Knowledge about DJD in cats—prevalence, impact on lifestyle, efficacy of therapy—is less well developed than for the dog. Because cats have a small body size and are light and agile, they compensate for orthopedic diseases better than dogs. Cats are also notorious for hiding signs of illness, especially if onset is insidious, and it is more difficult to interpret signs of pain or discomfort in this species.[100]

Twenty-two percent of cats in a general population older than 1 year of age[37] and 90% of cats older 12 years of age[51] were found to have radiographic evidence of DJD. The elbow was the most frequently affected joint in the older population. The coxofemoral joint may also be affected, and most cats have bilateral involvement.[15] Relatively few of these cats had clinical signs associated with the radiographic findings, or, perhaps more accurately, clinical signs were infrequently recognized by owners and veterinarians.[16] This may be because the most common clinical sign associated with DJD in the dog is lameness. Owing to the cat's lightweight frame and behavioral differences, it appears as though there may be other, more significant clinical signs of DJD that need to be recognized (Box 26-1). Physical examination findings for DJD in cats are also different than those for dogs (Box 26-2).

It is assumed that the etiopathogenesis of DJD is the same for cats and dogs, although little evidence currently exists to support this assumption. Suspected causes include primary degeneration (wear and tear), joint dysplasia, joint injury, fractures, luxations and dislocations, congenital malformations, cranial cruciate ligament rupture, infection, and neoplasia. The clinical presentation of DJD in cats is different from dogs, and the radiographic signs differ slightly. Joint injuries are less common in cats than dogs, but hip dysplasia is probably underestimated in cats.

The hallmark of DJD is the progressive and permanent damage of articular cartilage.[82] Injury of the chondrocytes leads to the production of inflammatory mediators such as cytokines (especially interleukin-1 [IL-1]) and tumor necrosis factor-alpha. IL-1 stimulates production of degradative enzymes, inhibits production of proteoglycans, and stimulates fibroplasia of the joint capsule. The thickened joint capsule contributes to stiffness and decreased range of movement.

The degradative enzymes set in motion a process that damages collagen and causes it to swell. The abnormal cartilage cannot bear loads normally, causing increased load on certain areas of the joint and leading to further cartilage damage. The underlying subchondral bone is stressed, and pain receptors are stimulated. Osteophytes are bony proliferations formed at the conjunction of the synovium, perichondrium, and periosteum. They are believed to be caused by mechanical instability of the joint and joint inflammation. They may contribute to joint pain.

Even though the clinical signs of DJD may wax and wane, the changes to the joint are permanent, with limited ability to repair the articular surface or joint capsule. The vicious cycle of inflammation, degeneration, and mechanical dysfunction leads to progressive disease.

The diagnostic approach to joint disease in cats is similar to that in dogs. A medical history, physical examination, and radiographs are most commonly employed. Further diagnostic steps might include joint fluid analysis and culture, arthroscopy, myelography, or advanced imaging such as magnetic resonance imaging (MRI) or computed tomography (CT).

When taking a medical history, especially for senior cats, the veterinarian should focus the questions on changes in activity and behavior rather than solely on lameness. Many signs of chronic pain are not obvious to owners or may be misinterpreted as due to aging.[100] The degree of impairment caused by chronic pain may not be apparent to some owners until improvements occur after treatment.

Unfortunately, gait analysis is rarely helpful in cats, and orthopedic examinations are limited by the lack of data on normal ranges of motion for feline joints and the difficulty of detecting small changes associated with joint disease. In the examination room it may be possible to evaluate gait by allowing the cat to walk around the room. In addition, the cat can be encouraged to jump off a chair or jump up to get into its carrier. Cats with lumbosacral joint disease may be reluctant to jump and may exhibits signs of being in pain when the lower back is petted or examined. Cats with hip dysplasia may have no clinical signs at all, although cats with more advanced disease may have lameness and pain.

Radiographic signs of DJD in cats are variable.[1,16,36] Radiographs are best at demonstrating bony changes, and changes in the cartilage and synovium are not well demonstrated on plain radiographs. Joint effusions and joint capsule thickening are rarely evident. Typical bony changes include osteophyte development, subchondral sclerosis, perichondral bone erosion, and change in congruity of articular surfaces. Soft tissue swelling around the joint may be present. Lumbosacral DJD may be indicated by collapse of the L7-S1 disk space, sclerosis of the L7-S1 endplates, and spondylosis deformans.

Infectious Arthridities

Bacterial

Septic bacterial arthritis is most commonly associated with bite wounds sustained in cat fights. Hematogenous spread of bacteria from other sites in the body appears to be relatively rare in the cat, although it may occasionally be seen in kittens. Septic arthritis may develop secondary to orthopedic surgical procedures. Clinical signs include pain and swelling of the affected joint. Pyrexia and leukocytosis are usual but not invariable.[56] Radiographic signs in the early stages will be confined to joint effusion and soft tissue swelling. As the condition progresses, and depending on the infective organism, there may be evidence of a periosteal reaction, bony sclerosis, and varying degrees of bone lysis at the periosteum and in the subchondral bone. Diagnosis is based on clinical signs and the results of arthrocentesis. Cytology, as well as aerobic and anaerobic culture combined with bacterial sensitivity testing, is essential, although a negative culture result is not uncommon. Therapy with bactericidal antibiotics (based on sensitivity testing) is indicated for 4 to 6 weeks. In the absence of a positive culture, while awaiting results, or where empirical treatment is desired, cephalosporin or amoxicillin–clavulanate antibiotics are reasonable choices, with metronidazole a useful addition in confirmed or suspected anaerobic infections.[56] All of these antibiotic choices, and others besides, commonly cause vomiting or inappetence in cats, which may necessitate changes in therapy. Surgical drainage or flushing of infected joints is rarely necessary except in the most severe cases. Analgesics and other supportive care may be indicated.

Although up to 15% of cats have been found to be seropositive for *Borrelia burgdorferi*, they seem to be resistant to clinical disease, and no reports of arthritis associated with Lyme disease have been documented in this species.[56]

Mycoplasma

Rare cases of polyarthritis and tenosynovitis associated with *Mycoplasma gateae* and *Mycoplasma felis* have been reported in the literature.[56,107] Hematogenous spread from areas of active or latent infection in respiratory mucous membranes or the urogenital tract, most often in otherwise debilitated or immunocompromised individuals, appears to be the pathogenesis of the arthritis. There is potential for diagnostic confusion with immune-mediated arthridities because *Mycoplasma* arthritis may appear similar. Radiographically, there is the potential for erosive lesions. Synovial fluid analysis and a negative aerobic culture may suggest immune-mediated arthritis. The organisms may be detected on a synovial fluid smear stained with Wright, Leishman, or Giemsa stains, or it may be grown on anaerobic culture from synovial fluid or synovium.[56,107] The clinician should have an index of suspicion for *Mycoplasma* arthritis when dealing with debilitated individuals that appear to have immune-mediated arthritis. Tylosin, erythromycin, and gentamicin have traditionally been the most recommended therapies. However, fluoroquinolones represent a more recent, readily available alternative that is effective, convenient, and safe in cats.[107]

Viral

A short-term, self-limiting polyarthritis associated with calicivirus has been described in kittens younger than 6 months of age.[7,21] The arthritis may be caused by infective intraarticular live virus or by the deposition of immune complexes within the synovium. The condition may be seen in association with the typical respiratory infection, or it may be seen 5 to 7 days after vaccination with modified-live calicivirus vaccine. Vaccine-associated arthritis is now uncommon because vaccine manufacturers have for the most part discontinued the use of virus strains associated with the problem. Diagnosis is made largely on the basis of history and clinical signs, and therapy is supportive, including analgesia, because the condition is self-limiting.[7,21]

Autoimmune Arthridities

Autoimmune arthridities are characterized in the first instance by inflammation of the synovium. They may be subdivided as "erosive" when there are deforming, lytic lesions to cartilage and subchondral bone, and "nonerosive" when no such lesions are found and inflammation is confined to the synovium. Arthrocentesis produces similar results in most cases. Increased amounts of a watery, turbid joint fluid with a poor mucin clot are commonly encountered. White cell counts in the joint fluid are increased, and the majority of cells are nondegenerate polymorphonuclear cells. Bacteria are not seen, and culture is negative. All types are similar clinically, presenting with stiffness and swollen, painful joints and typically resulting in an irritable cat. Some cases may have fever and inappetence or anorexia.

Erosive

PERIOSTEAL PROLIFERATIVE POLYARTHRITIS

Periosteal proliferative polyarthritis (PPP) is the most common erosive form of arthritis seen in the cat. It most often affects the hocks and carpi of young adult male cats. Clinical signs begin acutely with fever, depression, stiffness, joint effusion, and pain. Over the course of a few weeks, the disease enters a chronic phase in which extensive periosteal new bone forms around the hocks and carpi and at the attachments of ligaments and tendons. New bone production may be extensive enough to produce ankylosis of joints. Erosive lesions may also be seen in subchondral bone and at tendinous attachments.[21,56] Erosive lesions or periosteal new bone formation at attachment points of ligaments, tendons, or fascia are referred to as *enthesopathies.*[7] The criteria proposed by Bennett and Nash for diagnosing PPP are found in Box 26-3.[7]

BOX 26-3

Criteria Proposed for the Diagnosis of Periosteal Proliferative Polyarthritis[7]

1. Erosive polyarthritis
2. Periosteal new bone formation at affected joints
3. Negative for rheumatoid factor in the blood
4. Enthesopathies
5. Primarily the hocks and carpi are involved

NOTE: The first three criteria must be met to make the diagnosis; however, the last two are variable.

An etiologic link has been proposed between feline syncytium-forming virus (FeSFV) and PPP insofar as all cats with PPP appear to have FeSFV. However, attempts to experimentally induce PPP by inoculating cats with the virus have failed, and FeSFV has been found as a normal inhabitant in the joints of many asymptomatic cats.[21] A role for feline leukemia virus (FeLV) and feline immunodeficiency virus (FIV) has also been proposed in producing immunosuppression that allows proliferation of FeSFV; however, FeLV and FIV are frequently not found in cats with PPP.[5,21] Occasionally symptoms of immune-mediated arthritis may be found in cats immunocompromised for other reasons, including chemotherapy and hyperadrenocorticism.

PPP bears some similarities to Reiter's disease, which is seen most commonly in men. Urethritis and diarrhea can be seen, in addition to the arthritic lesions in humans, and there is at least one report of hematuria associated with polyarthritis in a cat.[5] Conjunctivitis and lesions of skin and mucous membranes, which are common in humans, have been found in some cats. In light of these types of lesions, a link between Reiter's disease and *Chlamydia* infection has been explored, and the organism has been implicated in humans.[7] The prognosis for cats with PPP is guarded to poor. Few will experience anything more than marginal improvement on therapy, and many will end up being euthanized. However, decisions of that sort should be based on assessments of the patient's function and comfort level.

RHEUMATOID ARTHRITIS

By all accounts, rheumatoid arthritis (RA) is much less common in the cat than in the dog. RA is a synovitis

BOX 26-4

Diagnostic Criteria for Establishing a Diagnosis of Rheumatoid Arthritis in the Cat[7]

1. Stiffness after rest
2. Pain on manipulation of at least one joint
3. Swelling of at least one joint
4. Swelling of at least one other joint within a 2-month period
5. Symmetric joint swelling
6. Subcutaneous nodules
7. Erosive radiographic changes
8. Positive rheumatoid factor blood test
9. Abnormal synovial fluid (poor mucin clot, predominance of polymorphonuclear cells)
10. Characteristic histologic changes in the synovium (villous hypertrophy)
11. Characteristic histologic changes in the subcutaneous nodules

NOTE: Criteria 1 to 5 must be present for at least 6 weeks, and at least two of criteria 7, 8, and 10 must be present to establish the diagnosis.

caused by the production of autoantibodies against immunoglobulin G (rheumatoid factor). The deposition of immune complexes within the synovium leads to an erosive, deforming arthritis. As with other immune-mediated arthridities, RA causes generalized stiffness, pain, and swelling of joints. In contrast to PPP and idiopathic immune-mediated arthridities, there is seldom malaise or inappetence, and the course tends to be more gradual in onset. Joint deformity to the point of subluxation and luxation is often a prominent feature. Bennett[7,21] has described 11 diagnostic criteria, patterned after those used in man and the dog, for establishing a diagnosis of RA in the cat (Box 26-4). The criteria recognize the fact that a positive blood test for rheumatoid factor is not always present, and a positive test is not necessarily specific for the disease. The presence of subcutaneous nodules is common in humans but has not been described in the cat.[7]

One report of 12 cases of RA in the cat described an average age of 5.9 years, with Siamese cats overrepresented.[44] With aggressive forms of antirheumatic therapy, discussed at the end of this section, the prognosis for RA seems to be much better than PPP, with 58% showing a marked improvement.[44]

Non-Erosive

SYSTEMIC LUPUS ERYTHEMATOSUS

Systemic lupus erythematosus (SLE) is an uncommon cause of arthritis in cats. It is characterized by multisystemic involvement with polyarthritis and usually one of the following: autoimmune hematologic disease (thrombocytopenia, hemolytic anemia, and leukopenia),

BOX 26-5

Idiopathic Polyarthritis Subgroups[7]

Type I: idiopathic
Type II: idiopathic associated with other infections. These may be found in the respiratory or urogenital tracts, skin, or oral cavity.
Type III: idiopathic associated with gastrointestinal disease
Type IV: idiopathic associated with neoplasia. In the cat this is most often myeloproliferative neoplasia, which may be FeLV or FIV.

dermatitis, glomerulonephritis, or meningitis.[7] There are no destructive or deforming lesions on radiography or gross examination. The disease results from an autoimmune reaction to nucleic acid, which manifests as the hemolytic anemia, leukopenia, or thrombocytopenia. Deposition of the resulting immune complexes produces synovitis, glomerulonephritis, meningitis, dermatitis, or occasionally polymyositis. Onset of symptoms is usually acute and includes pain, especially on handling, and joint swelling.

Clinical pathology is essential to diagnose SLE. Antinuclear antibody (ANA) blood tests are invariably positive at a level of 1:40 or greater in the cat.[7] Although a diagnosis of SLE cannot be established without such a positive ANA value, the test is not specific and may be elevated in the acute phase of other disease conditions, including FeLV, FIV, and feline infectious peritonitis (FIP). Moreover, lower titers of ANA can be found in otherwise healthy cats.[7] Hematologic abnormalities (anemia, thrombocytopenia, and leukopenia) are common, as is proteinuria.[7] The diagnostic criteria to establish SLE are as follows:

1. Multisystem involvement, which most often includes polyarthritis and one other body system
2. ANA titre of 1:40 or greater
3. Presence of antibodies to blood cells or immune complexes in histopathology of affected tissues

Criteria 1 and 2 are essential for the diagnosis, which cannot be made solely on the basis of an elevated ANA titer.[7] Reports of treatment for SLE in cats are rare in the literature, but the prognosis appears to be guarded.

IDIOPATHIC POLYARTHRITIS

Polyarthridities that do not fit into any of the other classifications end up in the idiopathic category. There are four subgroups of idiopathic polyarthritis (Box 26-5).[7]

Idiopathic arthritis may present at any age, but most affected cats are young adults that develop symptoms acutely or subacutely. The pathogenesis is undoubtedly a synovitis arising from the deposition of immune complexes. Clinical signs are acute in all but type IV cases, which have a more chronic course. Most cases of all types exhibit signs of stiffness and pain, with occasional lameness. Joint and soft tissue swelling is usually present. These changes, along with the clinical signs, tend to be bilaterally symmetric. Pyrexia and inappetence are common. Type II idiopathic polyarthritis in the cat is most often associated with respiratory symptoms, including increased lung sounds, congestion, and conjunctivitis. Cats with type III frequently have diarrhea and dysentery, with occasional vomiting.[7] Toxoplasmosis has been identified as one possible cause.[7] Radiography is normal, except for joint effusion in some cases. The prognosis with treatment is generally good, especially in type I cases or in type II and III cases in which the underlying systemic illness can be identified and treated. Relapses, especially in types I and IV, are common.

Scottish Fold Arthropathy

Scottish Fold cats have an autosomal dominant trait that impairs enchondral ossification and produces abnormal cartilage maturation called *Scottish Fold arthropathy* (also known as *osteochondrodysplasia* and *osteodystrophy*). Heterozygotes for this trait have the characteristic "folded ear" appearance for the breed and may have mild signs of arthropathy. Homozygotes develop a progressive ankylosing arthropathy with radiographic lesions evident as early as 7 weeks of age. The condition is characterized by the production of new bone that bridges joints throughout the body but most prominently in the paws, spine, tail, and distal hind limbs (Figure 26-9). Affected individuals have a short, squat appearance that has been described as a form of dwarfism[14] and experience decreased range of motion in affected joints. Clinical signs include stiffness, lameness, and inability to jump. The condition is progressive and can produce dramatic periarticular new bone, most prominently on the plantar aspect of the calcaneal–tarsal–metatarsal articulation. Exostoses in this area can produce ulceration of overlying skin. Surgical excision of the exostoses or radiation therapy have been used as successful palliative therapies for extended periods.[14,54,78] Nonsteroidal anti-inflammatory drugs (NSAIDs), pentosan polysulfate, and oral glycosaminoglycans have been reported to provide symptomatic relief.[14,74] One report has described the use of pantarsal arthrodesis to improve function.[78]

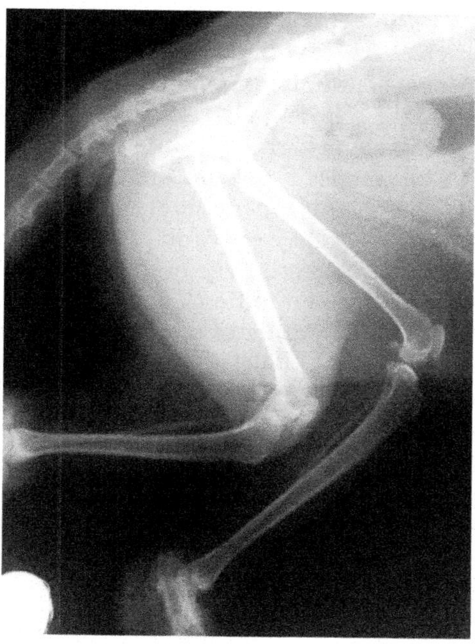

FIGURE 26-9 Scottish Fold arthropathy. Note the ankylosing arthropathy characterized by new bone production in the hock, stifle, and vertebral (especially coccygeal) joints.

Arthritis Therapy

It has been argued that no pharmaceutical therapy has a greater impact on the arthritic patient than weight control in the obese patient. The owner may also be able to make adjustments in the cat's environment, such as placing litter boxes within easy access of the arthritic cat or making it easier for the cat to attain its customary perch in several small steps instead of one big jump.

Therapy for Degenerative Joint Disease

The goals of treatment for cats with DJD include reduction of pain and inflammation, improvement in joint function, and slowing the disease process, if possible. Treatments fall into four broad categories:

1. Weight loss
2. Drug therapy
3. Chondroprotectants
4. Nutraceuticals

Weight loss is indicated if the patient is overweight or obese and will reduce forces on the joint surfaces. Weight loss may also lead to decreased dose or frequency of drug administration.

Drug therapy is indicated to control inflammation, provide pain relief, and improve function. The development of several NSAIDs specifically for the small animal veterinary market is arguably one of the most significant therapeutic advances in veterinary medicine during the last 50 years. Despite this, relatively little information exists regarding the safety and efficacy of these drugs in the cat, and virtually nothing is known about the long-term use of these drugs in this species for chronic pain and inflammation, such as is seen in DJD. What is known is that the cat has a significantly decreased ability to metabolize most of these drugs through hepatic glucuronidation. The result is a much longer half-life for most NSAIDs in the cat and thus a greater potential for accumulation and toxicity. Whereas gastrointestinal upset characterized by vomiting, inappetence, and diarrhea is the most common toxic effect, renal insufficiency is the most serious potential adverse reaction. Both of these adverse reactions arise from the antiprostaglandin effect of NSAIDs, specifically on the cyclooxygenase 1 (COX-1) isomer in the inflammatory pathway. Prostaglandins have a protective effect on gastric mucosa, presumably through increased secretion of mucus in the gastrointestinal tract. Inhibition of this secretion, combined with the acidic nature of most NSAIDs, produces gastric inflammation and ulceration. In the kidney, prostaglandins play a role in maintaining renal blood flow, particularly in the face of dehydration or hypotension. Inhibition of this effect has been associated with catastrophic renal failure in some cats.[13,67,91] The potential for these adverse reactions undoubtedly explains some of the reluctance on the part of pharmaceutical manufacturers to pursue the use of NSAIDs in this species. Nevertheless, limited research has resulted in label recommendations in some parts of the world for feline use of carprofen, ketoprofen, tolfenamic acid, and meloxicam.[13,43,67,80,91] Only meloxicam has a label for extended duration of administration in some countries, but cautious off-label use of various NSAIDs has been successful for much longer periods.[43,91,99a]

Carprofen is labeled for use in the cat in the United Kingdom, Europe, Australia, and New Zealand; however, the indication is for one-time postsurgical subcutaneous administration at a dose of 4 mg/kg.[67,80,91] No information exists on long-term use other than an individual report of toxicity after oral administration.[67] The drug has an extremely variable half-life (9 to 49 hours) in the cat, which increases the likelihood for toxicity with repeated use in some cats. Consequently, carprofen cannot be recommended as a safe option for management of DJD.

Ketoprofen is approved for use in the cat in Europe, Australia, and Canada at a dose of 1 mg/kg orally, once daily for up to 5 days, and 2 mg/kg subcutaneously, once daily for up to 3 days. Although the drug is eliminated by hepatic glucuronidation in the dog, the half-lives in both dogs and cats are similar. This, combined with other evidence, suggests the possibility of another excretory pathway for ketoprofen in the cat, which may imply a higher degree of safety; however, no long-term data corroborate this.[67] The drug is known to have a relatively greater activity against COX-1, which increases its inhibitory effect on platelet aggregation and may be significant in terms of renal or gastrointestinal side effects with long-term use.[67]

Tolfenamic acid is licensed for use in cats in Canada, Australia, New Zealand, and most of Europe. The recommended dose is 4 mg/kg orally or subcutaneously, once daily for 3 to 5 days. The product is labeled for the treatment of fever and upper respiratory disease, although its use as an analgesic and antiinflammatory is established in the literature.[67] Information provided by the manufacturer claimed no significant toxic effects when up to twice the recommended dose of the oral tablet or the injectable solution were given for up to 10 days to two groups of 12 cats. Increases characterized as "mild" were noted in the alanine transaminase (ALT) and aspartate aminotransferase (AST) of treated cats, and a positive test for fecal occult blood was noted in two cats from each group. There are anecdotal reports of DJD treatment in cats with tolfenamic acid for 3 to 5 consecutive days each week for extended periods, but little information in the literature supports this recommendation.

Most of what little information exists regarding the chronic use of NSAIDs for DJD in the cat concerns meloxicam. In contrast to the metabolism of most other NSAIDs in the cat, meloxicam is excreted by oxidative enzymes and thus has a similar half-life in both the cat and dog.[67] One recent study showed a COX-1–sparing effect for meloxicam in cats.[38] Consequently, the drug lends itself more readily to longer-term use in this species. In North America meloxicam is supplied in a 1.5 mg/mL honey-flavored oral formulation that is well tolerated by cats. In many countries it is supplied in a cat-specific formulation of 0.5 mg/mL. The same strength is available in the United States as a small dog formulation. It is labeled for feline use in the United States, Europe, Australia and New Zealand at a dose of 0.3 mg/kg for one-time subcutaneous use. Further, chronic use of the oral solution at 0.05 mg/kg per day is described on the package insert in many countries.[91] Several other recommendations for oral dosing appear in the literature (Box 26-6).

Administration of 1 drop of the 1.5 mg/mL oral liquid preparation on the cat's daily food was tolerated without significant adverse effects compared with controls in 46 cats with a mean age of 12.9 years that were given the drug for a mean duration of 5.8 months.[43] Good to excellent results were reported by at least 80% of the owners and veterinarians surveyed.[43] Palatability was not reported to be a problem with meloxicam. The most commonly encountered side effect appears to be gastrointestinal upset.[91]

The currently available information, although far from overwhelming, would suggest that meloxicam is a viable option for long-term treatment of DJD in cats. Before starting NSAID therapy, a complete blood cell count, serum chemistries, and a urinalysis should be performed. Ideally, NSAIDs should be prescribed only to normotensive, normovolemic adult cats with no history of renal, hepatic, or gastrointestinal disease. However, for some cats the benefits of NSAID therapy outweigh the risks, insofar as the quality of life may be more important than the length of life. NSAIDs are not recommended in patients taking certain medications,

BOX 26-6

Published Doses for Meloxicam in the Cat

Source	Dose
Label: US, Australia, New Zealand, EU	0.3 mg/kg subcutaneously, once
Label: Australia, New Zealand, EU	0.1 mg/kg on day one, followed by 0.05 mg/kg per day, orally
Wallace 2003,[103a] Carroll & Simonson 2005[12a]	0.2 mg/kg on day 1, followed by 0.1 mg/kg/day for 2 days, then 0.025 mg/kg/day or 0.1 mg/cat 2-3 times/week
Lascelles 2007[67]	0.1 mg/kg on day 1, followed by 0.05 mg/kg for 1 to 4 days, then reduction to the lowest effective dose (0.025 mg/kg every 24-48 hours)
Robertson 2008[91]	0.05 mg/kg given once, followed by 0.025 mg/kg or less once daily
Gunew 2008[43]	0.1 mg/kg for four days, followed by 0.1 mg/cat once daily

such as diuretics and corticosteroids. Blood tests should be monitored periodically for cats on long-term therapy, and owners should be cautioned to monitor for vomiting, diarrhea, anorexia, increased thirst, increased urination, and lethargy. One author suggests re-evaluation every 8 to 12 weeks.[90]

Renal values and urine protein levels should be monitored; hepatic sensitivity to NSAIDs seems to be primarily a canine problem.[13,67,91] It may be helpful to recommend that cats taking NSAIDs be fed only or primarily canned foods because this increases water consumption by up to 50% and may help prevent subclinical dehydration in predisposed patients.

Glucocorticoids are controversial drugs for treatment of DJD. These drugs can reduce inflammation through various mechanisms, but chronic use has been found to delay healing and even damage cartilage.[3] Furthermore, the potential adverse effects of glucocorticoids in cats are well known. Use of these drugs should be limited to cases in which all other therapies have failed and for short periods only.

Analgesics can be very useful in the treatment of feline DJD and may be added to other therapies. Commonly used analgesics include buprenorphine (0.01 to 0.03 mg/kg every 8 to 12 hours, by way of buccal mucosa), gabapentin (3 to 5 mg/kg orally, every 8 to 12 hours), and tramadol (2 mg/kg orally, every 12 hours).

Although the use of oral and injectable chondroprotectives is reported for arthritic conditions of various kinds in the cat,[14,74] little objective evidence exists as to their effectiveness. Oral preparations include several combinations in which chondroitin sulfate and either hydrochloride or sulfate salts of glucosamine predominate. Little is known about the differences, if any, among various formulations; what dose rates and durations of therapy are best; and which patients, if any, will benefit. Virtually all of the currently available research has been done in the dog. Injectable chondroprotectants include polysulfated glycosaminoglycan (Adequan, Novartis) and pentosan polysulfate (Cartrophen, Biopharm, Australia or Pentosan, Naturevet, Australia), which are labeled for use in the dog but have been used with apparent benefit and without adverse effect in the cat.[14,78] Pentosan polysulfate is given at a dose of 3 mg/kg subcutaneously, once weekly for four consecutive treatments. Polysulfated glycosaminoglycan is given at a dose of 4 mg/kg intramuscularly, twice weekly for 4 weeks. Both chondroprotectants are given as needed after the first course of therapy. Oral or parenteral chondroprotectants have their beneficial effect in three primary ways:

1. By stimulating and enhancing the metabolism of chondrocytes and synoviocytes, including the provision of substrate for the production of cartilage matrix and synovial fluid
2. By inhibiting degradative enzymes and other entities, including prostaglandins, complement, and free radicals that play a role in the osteoarthritic destruction of the joint
3. By inhibiting the production of thrombi in the microvasculature of the synovium and subchondral bone, which have been shown to play a role in osteoarthritis[46]

Omega-3 fatty acids have been shown to have an inhibitory effect on arachidonic acid, which is a key player in the inflammatory pathway in arthritic joints. Supplements of omega-3 fatty acids or diets containing these compounds have been used with apparent success in dogs. Diets for joint health are relatively new for cats. The first products on the market (Medi-Cal Royal Canin Mobility Support, Hill's Prescription Diet Feline j/d) contain omega-3 fatty acids as well as glucosamine and chondroitin sulfate.

Therapy for Immune-Mediated Arthritis

Prednisolone at immunosuppressive doses is the first-line treatment for immune-mediated arthritis in the cat.

Prednisone and prednisolone are interchangeable in the dog, but many cats are unable to adequately absorb prednisone and convert it to the active metabolite, prednisolone, within the liver.[40] The cat with immune-mediated arthritis should be started on a total daily dose of 2 to 4 mg/kg in two divided doses. This dose is continued for 2 weeks and then gradually tapered over a further 6 to 8 weeks.[7,28,56,80] The short- and long-term side effects of corticosteroid therapy are well known, but most cats seem to be relatively more resistant to these effects compared with dogs or humans.

The determination of when to begin tapering the dose and how quickly that should be done is based on improvement of clinical signs and the results of follow-up joint taps starting at 2 weeks after the initiation of therapy. Most immune-mediated arthridities have synovial fluid profiles with high numbers of nondegenerate polymorphonuclear cells. Follow-up samples should show significant declines in absolute white cell counts (preferably below 4000/μL), but equally important is a shift to a predominantly mononuclear cell population. Results satisfying those criteria would suggest a favorable prognosis and would also be an indication to begin tapering the corticosteroid.[7,56]

If, however, follow-up joint taps do not show favorable changes in cell numbers and populations, then the addition of a cytotoxic drug, most often cyclophosphamide in the cat, should be considered. Similarly, if clinical signs cannot be kept in remission or doses of prednisolone become high and side effects are problematic, cyclophosphamide should be added. Some have advised that both prednisolone and cyclophosphamide should be used together from the outset of therapy, especially in the erosive arthridities, for which the prognosis is much less favorable.[7] Cyclophosphamide is given at a dose of 2.5 mg/kg orally, once daily for 4 consecutive days a week in combination with prednisolone at an antiinflammatory dose of 1 mg/kg orally, divided twice daily. This regimen should be continued for 4 weeks after remission of clinical signs.[7]

The introduction of cytotoxic drugs mandates a higher level of monitoring because of their potential for adverse effects. Hematuria is one such side effect and should be monitored with urinalysis every 2 weeks during therapy. Every 1 to 2 weeks, complete blood counts (CBCs) should also be done to detect any significant decrease in white cell or platelet counts. Neutrophil counts below 1000/μL or platelet counts below 50,000/μL should result in a decrease in cyclophosphamide dose by 25%. If neutropenia (<1000/μL) is found on the next CBC, a further reduction in drug dose is warranted.[32]

Azathioprine, which is a popular cytotoxic drug in the dog, should not be used in cats because they seem particularly sensitive to its myelosuppressive effects. Tapering of medication is unique to every case of feline polyarthritis in that some will rapidly respond and can be quickly tapered without recurrence. At the other end of the spectrum are cats that respond poorly and can be managed only with continuous therapy. Many variations of drug combinations and doses, as well as frequency and duration of treatment, have been used in the cat, so the clinician must find what works best in each case.

An alternative therapy for RA in the cat using methotrexate and leflunomide produced encouraging results in 12 cases.[44] Methotrexate inhibits inflammation and joint destruction through the promotion of adenosine release within the joint. Leflunomide has similar effects through inhibition of T lymphocytes.[44] Methotrexate was given on the same day each week at an oral dose of 2.5 mg at 0, 12, and 24 hours, for a total dose of 7.5 mg during the 24-hour period. Leflunomide was given orally at a dose of 10 mg/cat daily. When clinical signs were deemed to have significantly improved, the dose of methotrexate was reduced to 2.5 mg once weekly, and 10 mg of the leflunomide was given twice weekly.[44] The cats in the test group were treated for periods ranging from 2 to 6 months. Two of the twelve cats were determined to have had no beneficial response, and two were deemed to be in remission. More than 80% of the cats had a moderate or marked beneficial response in clinical signs. Rheumatoid factor was retested in only three cats but was decreased by at least 50% in all. Hepatotoxicity has been encountered with the use of these drugs, especially in humans, but was not encountered in these cats.[44] Severe cases of erosive arthridities may require surgical arthrodesis, especially of carpal and tarsal joints, to improve function and decrease pain in affected individuals.

The results of RA treatment with methotrexate and leflunomide notwithstanding, the expected outcomes with treatment are generally much poorer in erosive versus idiopathic immune-mediated arthridities. Type I idiopathic arthritis has the best prognosis. It is common for response to treatment to be rapid and for the condition to resolve without relapse. Types II and III idiopathic arthritis have a similar expected outcome, provided the mitigating medical factors can be identified and corrected. Type IV idiopathic arthritis obviously carries a much poorer expected response to treatment given the grave nature of most of the myeloproliferative diseases associated with it. For this reason the recommendation has been made that all cats with polyarthritis should have a bone marrow aspirate as well as FeLV and FIV tests included in the diagnostic workup.[7] Euthanasia is a common eventual outcome in cases of erosive immune-mediated feline polyarthridities. Cats with PPP do not go into remission but may be able to maintain a reasonably comfortable lifestyle on treatment. SLE arthritis may be controllable, but disease processes in other organ systems may be more challenging to manage.

CONDITIONS OF THE FRONT LIMB

Dorsal Scapular Luxation

The scapula is attached to the thoracic body wall by the serratus ventralis, rhomboideus, and trapezius muscles. Trauma incurred by falling from a height can cause partial or complete rupture of these muscles, which will displace the scapula, especially during weight-bearing activities. If these cats are presented acutely there will be a non–weight-bearing lameness accompanied by pain and swelling between the dorsal scapula and the body wall. After a few days, this inflammation will subside and the cat will begin bearing weight. This produces an unusual gait because the scapula is dorsally displaced with each step. Most cats will regain a reasonable degree of mobility, and if the cat is not especially active, no further treatment need be undertaken. The cat will, of course, retain the distinctive gait abnormality. If the owner is unsettled by the gait or feels that it represents a disability for the cat, surgical stabilization can be undertaken. This consists of exploration of the dorsal aspect of the scapula and primary suturing of the torn muscles, where possible. In addition, two holes are drilled in the dorsocaudal area of the scapula and the scapula is attached in a normal position to an adjacent rib with nonabsorbable suture or surgical wire. Care must be taken that the thoracic cavity is not entered while passing the wire. The limb is then bandaged against the chest so it cannot be used for 2 weeks.[48]

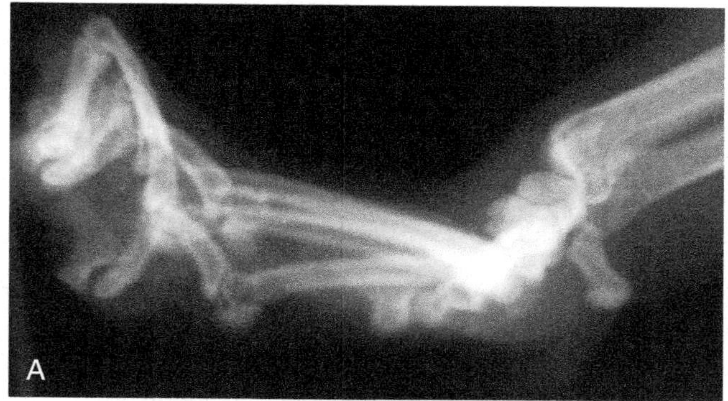

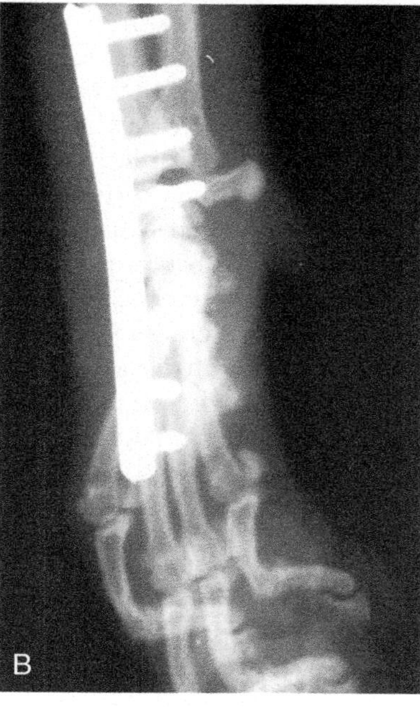

FIGURE 26-10 **A,** Stressed radiographic view demonstrating hyperextension at the carpometacarpal joint level. **B,** Postoperative radiograph from the cat in Figure 26-16 after pancarpal arthrodesis with a length of veterinary cuttable plate and 2-mm screws.

Carpal Hyperextension Injuries

Another injury commonly associated with falling from a height is hyperextension of the carpus. Alternatively, the carpus may become hyperextended on account of the degenerative process of an immune-mediated arthritis. Stress radiography will delineate the level at which the hyperextension has occurred, with antebrachial-carpal and carpometacarpal hyperextensions being most common (Figure 26-10, *A*). In some cases the hyperextension may involve more than one joint level, or it may be unclear which levels are affected.

The most common treatment for carpal hyperextension injuries in the cat is pancarpal arthrodesis (see Figure 26-10, *B*). Although a number of methods have been described, including cross pins, external skeletal fixators, and circular external skeletal fixation, the most commonly used and consistently effective technique involves the dorsal placement of a bone plate. After the articular cartilage is débrided from the joint surfaces and the gaps are packed with cancellous bone graft (usually from the ipsilateral proximal humerus), a plate is placed over the dorsal surface of the distal radius, carpus, and third metacarpal bone. Two types of plates work well in this application. A carpal arthrodesis plate (CAP) is designed to place larger-diameter screws in the distal radius and smaller-diameter screws in the carpal and metacarpal bones. In addition, the CAP is manufactured such that it tapers in thickness from the radial to metacarpal portions and so that it places the arthrodesed carpus into a slightly extended standing angle of about 5 degrees. The plate can be contoured to alter this angle, but that is seldom necessary. CAPs come in an assortment of sizes, with the two smallest sizes being applicable to cats. The majority of cats will do well with the CAP that accommodates 2-mm diameter screws in the radius and 1.5-mm screws in the third metacarpal bone. Some large cats may fit a 2.7/2.0 CAP with 2.7-mm screws proximally and 2-mm screws distally. The average feline third metacarpal bone is 3.15 to 4.13 mm in diameter, so a 1.5-mm screw would occupy less than 50% of the bone's diameter, lessening the chance of iatrogenic fracture, a reasonably common complication. Thus the 2.0/1.5 CAP is the best fit for the average cat.[12] The CAP is also engineered to cover more than 50% of the length of the third metacarpal, which has also been found to decrease the chance of iatrogenic fracture in dogs.

A cost-effective alternative to the CAP is the veterinary cuttable plate (VCP). The plate is sold in 50-hole lengths of two sizes. The screw holes in the small VCP accommodate 1.5-mm or 2-mm screws. The larger VCP accommodates 2-mm and 2.7-mm screws. An 8- or 9-hole length of the 1.5/2.0 VCP is usually the best choice when using VCPs. This allows one 2-mm screw to be placed first in the radial carpal bone, four 2-mm screws to be placed in the distal radius, and three to four 1.5- or 2-mm screws in the distal carpal bones and third metacarpal bone. The biggest advantage of the VCP is its cost. An 8- or 9-hole length of 1.5/2.0 VCP would be approximately 25% to 30% of the cost of a CAP. The plate can be used for many orthopedic applications, making it a versatile addition to a clinic inventory, whereas the CAP has few applications beyond carpal arthrodesis. The disadvantages of the VCP is that it is not as strong as the CAP; however, a second length of VCP can be stacked on top of the first length to increase its bending strength if this is deemed necessary in a very heavy cat. With limited soft tissues to close over the plate, this can sometimes increase tension on the incision but is usually not a significant problem.

The VCP also has only round holes, whereas the CAP has dynamic compression holes. It is common to load the most distal radial and most proximal metacarpal hole in compression; however, the importance of this in the cat is unknown. The principles of carpal arthrodesis have largely been extrapolated from experience with the dog, and data in the cat are scarce.[12] Because the dorsal application of a plate is not on the "tension" side of the bone, it has been deemed to be in a mechanically inferior position to withstand cyclic loading. Thus in dogs it is routine to augment the plate arthrodesis, usually with a cast or splint for at least the first 4 to 6 weeks. Support of the plate has also been attempted with one or two additional Kirschner wires angled across the carpal joint. These have commonly been found to migrate. Good results have been achieved with limited or no additional support for the plate, a fact that leads to speculation as to whether additional support is necessary in the cat.[12]

Complications of pancarpal arthrodesis primarily seem to involve a decrease in jumping and climbing behavior, based on the results of an owner survey.[12] Given the degree to which cats pronate and supinate the antebrachium and given the degree to which this would be affected by carpal arthrodesis, it has always been postulated that pancarpal arthrodesis would dramatically affect behaviors involving pronation and supination, such as grooming and batting of objects with the paw. Owners of cats that underwent pancarpal arthrodesis did not feel that this was a significant issue.[12]

When it can be clearly demonstrated that hyperextension involves the carpometacarpal joint level, partial carpal arthrodesis is an option in the cat.[12] T-plates (1.5 or 2.0 mm) allow fusion of the distal carpal and carpometacarpal joint levels while preserving function at the radial-carpal level. In dogs it has been shown that partial carpal arthrodesis results in the progression of DJD in adjacent joint levels that are not arthrodesed. Whether this also happens in cats and its potential clinical significance is not known.

CONDITIONS OF THE HIND LIMB

Hip Dysplasia

Hip dysplasia is a less common condition in cats than dogs; however, the exact incidence is unclear. One survey identified 6.6% of a population of 684 cats as being radiographically dysplastic.[58] The frequency of clinical signs attributable to hip dysplasia is another matter, however. Although reports of hind limb stiffness, weakness, or pain are few, there is an increasing realization that the signs associated with DJD in the cat are underdiagnosed. There is an increased incidence in female and purebred cats, with the Maine Coon, Siamese, Persian, and Himalayan breeds overrepresented.[58,96] The radiographic signs of hip dysplasia in the cat differ somewhat from those seen in the dog. The primary finding is a shallow acetabulum, even given the fact that the normal acetabulum is shallower in the cat than the dog (Figure 26-11). Hip joint laxity, as measured by distraction index, is greater in dysplastic cats, although coxofemoral subluxation on the hip extended radiographic view is much less commonly seen in the cat than in the dog. Distraction indices have been reported as 0.6 in dysplastic cats and 0.49 or less in normal cats.[61] The mean Norberg angle in a random group of cats was found to be 84 degrees among those considered dysplastic and 92.4 degrees among those considered normal, compared with 103 degrees in normal dogs.[61] Degenerative changes seen in the hips of dysplastic cats also differed from the most common signs seen in dogs in that the craniodorsal acetabulum showed the most changes, whereas the femoral neck was relatively unaffected.[58] Treatment for dysplastic cats seldom seems necessary, but some may benefit from the previously discussed protocol for treating DJD, including weight control, modifications to the cat's environment, and NSAIDs. Conceivably, surgical salvage procedures such as femoral head and neck ostectomy could be used. Surgical prostheses are now available so that total hip replacement can be performed on cats; however, it is currently unclear whether this procedure offers any functional advantages over femoral head and neck ostectomy.[70]

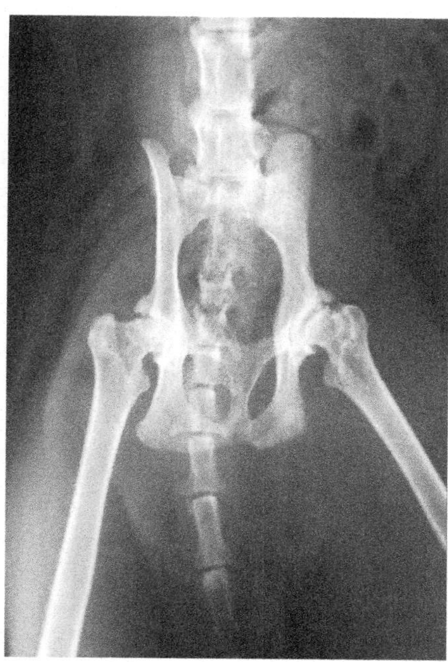

FIGURE 26-11 The primary finding in feline hip dysplasia is a shallow acetabulum; changes associated with degenerative joint disease are also common findings.

Patellar Luxation

Although patellar luxation occurs in the cat, it is much less common than in the dog, at least when it comes to the development of clinical signs. Many cats have some degree of mobility in their patellas. One may even go so far as to say that the classic description of a "grade 1" patellar luxation in the dog, wherein the patella can be luxated with moderate force but immediately returns to its normal position, may be a normal state of affairs for some cats. Certainly, such a state rarely would be associated with any clinical lameness in the cat. Grade 2 luxations are described as being easily achieved, but the patella spends most of its time in the normal position. Grade 3 luxations are characterized by a patella that is usually found luxated but can be reduced manually. Grade 4 luxations involve a continuously luxated patella that cannot be manually reduced. It should be pointed out that the previously described rating system, while useful in communicating what has been detected on physical examination, does not imply prognosis, nor does it correlate well with clinical signs.

As in the dog, most feline patellar luxations are medial, usually congenital, and bilateral. A small percentage of cases are lateral luxations, and a few cats seem to have the curious ability to luxate their patellas in either direction. Traumatic injury, especially malunions of femoral fractures, account for a small number of patellar luxation cases. Devon Rex, Abyssinian, and domestic shorthair cats have been identified as having a high incidence.[60,73,96] Although patellar luxation can be found at any age, most cats that develop clinical signs will do so within the first 1 to 2 years of life. Clinical signs in cats differ somewhat from those seen in dogs in that the "skipping lameness" characteristic of a poodle with medial patellar luxation is uncommon in the cat. A locking of the stifle with extension of the hind limb is a common presentation. Many cat owners will describe an associated painful response from the cat. There may be some degree of lameness or a crouched gait in some cases. The clinical signs may be described as acute in some cases and more intermittent and chronic in others.[73,96]

Although much more is known about the pathogenesis of congenital patellar luxation in dogs, it does appear as though the developmental abnormalities of the hip (coxa vara), femoral bowing, and tibial torsion that are instrumental in the canine condition are not commonly encountered in the cat. More often, the problem arises from a shallow trochlear groove and an underdeveloped medial trochlear ridge. Occasionally, some medial deviation of the tibial tuberosity may be present but this is much less common than in dogs.[60,73,96] An association has been noted between hip dysplasia and medial patellar luxation in that in one study cats were three times more likely to have both conditions together than either alone.[99] The clinical significance of this finding is unknown. The majority of cats with patellar luxation will never need treatment because they will never show clinical signs; some evidence suggests that even cats with clinical signs should initially be treated conservatively.[73] Rest and NSAIDs may be sufficient to manage intermittent episodes of lameness.

Radiographically, signs of DJD are slow to develop in cats with patellar luxation, and attempting to prevent such DJD is not a justification for surgery. Similarly, the decision to go to surgery should not be based on the grade of luxation but rather on the clinical signs and the degree of disability they cause the cat. In cats with more severe signs for which medical management has not been successful, surgery is associated with a high success rate. In dogs tibial tuberosity transposition is the most important procedure linked with a successful outcome. In cats that is usually not the case. If medial (or lateral) deviation of the tibial tuberosity is encountered, then transposition should be done. The keys to successfully performing this procedure are to make a sufficiently large osteotomy that will accommodate at least two Kirschner wires of 0.045 or 0.062 mm diameter. The osteotomy can be performed with a power-driven saw or an osteotome and mallet and should be at least 0.5 cm in thickness and depth and 1 cm in length. The veterinarian should always err on the side of making the osteotomy larger than necessary, for as long as the cut is positioned cranial to the insertion of the cranial cruciate ligament, no harm will arise. However, an inadequately small osteotomy will split when implants are driven into it or will not stand up to weight bearing, resulting in a surgical complication that is very difficult to deal with. The osteotomy should be continued distally only far enough so that the tuberosity can be lateralized (or serialized). There is no need to completely detach the tuberosity. In most cases if a tibial tuberosity transposition is required at all, it will only be necessary to move the tuberosity a very few millimeters, sometimes only one or two. The most frequent complications in tibial tuberosity transposition are fracture of the osteotomized fragment or implant failure if the fragment is too small, lateral (or medial) patellar luxation if transposition is over exuberant or inadequate, and pin migration.

The most common surgical procedures to stabilize a patellar luxation in cats are deepening of the trochlear groove (trochleoplasty) or sulcus (sulcoplasty) and soft tissue procedures involving medial and lateral joint capsule and fascia. Trochleoplasty or sulcoplasty involves deepening the trochlear groove so that the patella will tend to remain in place. Originally, trochlear sulcoplasty simply involved taking a bone rasp to the groove to abrade cartilage and subchondral bone until a sufficient depth was achieved. The procedure destroys the articular cartilage and results in its replacement by fibrocartilage.[59] While many animals have done well with this procedure, many others have developed very extensive and clinically-significant DJD. As a result, the procedure has largely fallen out of favor in the wake of procedures that spare the articular cartilage.

The first of these was the wedge recession trochleoplasty, in which a lengthwise elliptical wedge is cut from the trochlear groove. A second cut is usually performed a millimeter or less from the edge of the original saw cut, and then the wedge is replaced in the deepened sulcus. It is not necessary to fix the wedge in place because the pressure of the patella maintains it in position.[59,96] Usually, the cuts are made with a handsaw because this gives the surgeon more control over what is a reasonably delicate cut. Because the most common problem seen in the cat is an underdeveloped medial trochlear ridge, the surgeon may find it helpful to angle the cuts somewhat steeper medially so that the resulting sulcus will be deeper on the medial side. If the wedge does not sit solidly, the bottom surface can be trimmed with a scalpel blade until it is stable. A variation of the wedge recession is the block recession trochleoplasty in which a rectangular block of articular cartilage and subchondral bone is removed from the trochlear groove utilizing a bone saw and osteotome. Once the block is removed, additional bone is removed from the underlying defect and from the underside of the block. This allows the replaced block to be recessed below the original surface, producing a deepened groove. The advantage of this procedure is that a greater area of the sulcus is involved in the recession, especially in the proximal portion. The proximal aspect of the groove may be the most critical area, especially when the stifle is in extension.[59,96]

Recently, a rotating dome trochleoplasty technique, in which the trochlear groove is osteotomized and rotated medially, has been described. The procedure was performed on feline cadavers but showed some potential advantages over the currently used trochleoplasty techniques, particularly in increasing the size of the medial trochlear ridge. The ultimate utility of the procedure awaits clinical trials.

Soft tissue surgical corrections for patellar luxation include joint capsule and fascial imbrication and desmotomy. Essentially, one tightens the tissues on the side away from the luxation and loosens them on the side of the luxation. In the most usual case of a medial luxation, the surgeon would start with a medial parapatellar arthrotomy. This would allow inspection of the joint and completion of the trochleoplasty, if desired. A corresponding incision in the lateral joint capsule would allow placement of an osteotome to perform a tibial tuberosity transposition if that is deemed necessary. The medial incision can, in some cases, be continued as much as one third of the way up the distal femur if this relieves medial pressure from the patella and lessens the tendency for luxation. At surgical closure there is no need to do anything on the medial side. Joint capsule, muscle, and fascia may all be left open in what can be called a medial desmotomy. On the lateral side, the same incised tissues can be closed in one layer with mattress sutures, vest-over-pants sutures, or simply large bits of tissue in a simple interrupted pattern. The principle is to "gather or tighten up," otherwise referred to as imbricating, the tissues on the lateral side. Although some have described the use of nonabsorbable sutures for this procedure, the author has not found these to be necessary. Most absorbable sutures are present for an adequate period to allow healing of the tissues. Nonabsorbable sutures cannot be expected to hold the tissues in an unaltered state for an indefinite period.

Although soft tissue procedures can be very helpful in surgically stabilizing a luxating patella, they are rarely sufficient by themselves. "Bony procedures," such as trochleoplasty or tibial tuberosity transposition are the key components to surgical success. In those rare cats that luxate their patellas both laterally and medially and have clinical lameness, surgical correction with a wedge or block recession trochleoplasty and bilateral soft tissue imbrication is the most effective course.

Although the majority of cats with patellar luxation will have the problem bilaterally, not all will show clinical signs bilaterally. As previously mentioned, the decision to do surgery must be based on clinical signs, not the finding of the problem on a physical examination. If a cat is clinically affected bilaterally, it will easily tolerate bilateral surgery, and the surgeon need not be afraid to correct both stifles at the same surgery session.

Postoperative care of patellar luxation patients involves nothing more complex than adequate analgesia for a few days and exercise restriction for 4 to 6 weeks.

Stifle Ligamentous Injury

Cats suffer ligamentous injury to the stifle because of either trauma, where there are often multiple injuries to supporting structures, or as the result of a degenerative process that culminates in rupture of the cranial cruciate ligament. In the former case the most common trauma is a "falling" injury which can result in ligamentous and meniscal injury to the extent of complete stifle disruption or luxation. On physical examination, these cats have profound stifle instability in most planes. Radiographically, the most common appearance is of the tibia luxated cranially due to the almost invariable rupture of both the cranial and caudal cruciate ligaments. The medial collateral ligament is the next most likely structure to be compromised, followed by meniscal tearing in 50% of cases, with the lateral meniscus being most common.[18,49] An assessment of the ligamentous injuries can usually be deduced through radiography, stress radiography, and a thorough physical examination, under general anesthesia. Ultimately, surgical exploration of the joint will reveal all.

Stifle disruption can be treated surgically in two potential ways. The initial step in both procedures is exploratory arthrotomy to identify the pathology and to débride any meniscal tears. In many cases, damage to one or both menisci will be severe enough to require complete meniscectomy. Ligamentous damage can be addressed either by reconstruction or by transarticular pinning. Occasionally it may be possible to suture or plicate stretched collateral ligaments with absorbable suture, but in most cases reconstructive techniques will be necessary to replace torn ligaments or reinforce suture repairs.

The most straightforward approach to collateral and cruciate ligament reconstruction in the cat begins with a conventional lateral extracapsular cranial cruciate ligament procedure. Although there are dozens of variations to extracapsular cruciate ligament procedures, most involve the placement of a nonabsorbable suture from behind the fabellae, behind the distal patellar tendon, and through a hole in the proximal tibia. Monofilament nylon leader material of 40 pound test strength is a popular choice in the cat. The ends can be fastened at the starting point with a metal crimp tube or any of several knots. Lateral placement of this extracapsular suture replaces the stability provided by the cranial cruciate and lateral collateral ligaments. Care must be taken not to overtighten the suture if the medial collateral ligament is compromised because a valgus deformity at the stifle can be created. Varus or valgus deformity can alternatively be prevented by the temporary placement of a transarticular pin, which is removed after ligamentous reconstruction.

On the medial side of the stifle, if caudal cruciate or medial collateral ligaments are torn, reconstruction is best accomplished by placing 2.7-mm screws and washers or bone anchors in the distal femur and proximal tibia. In the proximal and distal planes, these anchor points should be placed at the mid-level of the femoral condyle and about 1 cm distal to the level of the tibial plateau. The final femoral anchor point is then slightly caudal to the midcondyle and the tibial anchor point slightly cranial of a line drawn distally from the intercondylar eminences of the tibia. A figure-of-eight suture between the anchor points then provides reconstruction of the medial collateral ligament, but the slightly caudoproximal to craniodistal course also mimics the course of the caudal cruciate ligament and provides stability in the absence of that ligament. Again, monofilament nylon leader material is a popular choice.

Another way to stabilize a disrupted stifle after resection of damaged meniscal tissue is to place a transarticular pin. A 3- to 3.5-mm Steinmann pin can be introduced at the intercondylar eminences on the tibial plateau and driven in a distocranial direction to exit at the distal extent of the tibial tuberosity. The chuck is then attached to the distal extent of the pin, and it is drawn flush to the surface of the tibial plateau. The stifle joint is then placed in a standing angle of approximately 30 to 40 degrees of flexion, and the pin is driven proximally through the intercondylar fossa of the femur until the pin is lodged in the cranial cortex of the distal femur. The joint capsule and remaining soft tissues are then closed routinely.[18,49] Distally, the pin is cut with enough room to allow its removal in 4 weeks. External support, especially in larger cats, in the form of a lateral splint can be helpful because the pin very frequently bends and occasionally breaks. Although stifle range of motion is ultimately reduced to some degree, owners and clinicians are generally amazed at the level of function and the range of motion that returns in these limbs.[18,49] The procedure is relatively simple and requires little in the way of specialized equipment, but it usually allows a very serious situation to be salvaged.

Cats also rupture their cranial cruciate ligaments without any apparent trauma. There is epidemiologic and histologic evidence that they suffer from the same type of degenerative cruciate disease as dogs.[49,95] Histologic disorganization of collagen fibers interspersed with acellular or hypocellular areas, chondroid metaplasia, and mineralization are found in degenerative cruciate ligaments along with granulation tissue formed in an attempt to repair the damage.[49]

Affected cats tend to be older and overweight, with a mean age of 8.5 years and a mean weight of 6.5 kg identified in one survey.[49] They are presented with rear limb lameness, reluctance to jump, and generally decreased activity. Diagnosis of cranial cruciate ligament (CCL) rupture is fairly straightforward on physical examination insofar as cranial drawer motion is usually present and quite easy to demonstrate, even in the nonsedated cat on the examination table. However, in some chronic cases or in the occasional case of early degeneration or partial ligament tear, the detectable stifle instability may be minor. Although the diagnostic challenge of partial CCL tears and mild inflammation of the ligament without grossly detectable stifle instability is commonly encountered in the dog, this seems to be relatively rare in the cat. The author (GH) has encountered some cats with cruciate ligament disease in which little stifle instability is present.

The more common obstacle to accurate diagnosis of CCL rupture in the cat is often the absence of an index of suspicion on the part of the clinician. Radiographically, cats with CCL rupture will usually have some joint effusion, although the amount is seldom as impressive as in the dog. Degenerative osteoarthritic changes are common and increase with chronicity (Figure 26-12). Cats develop a prominent osteoarthritic spur on the distal aspect of the patella in most cases. Distal displacement of the popliteal sesamoid bone is a variable radiographic finding.[49] A unique radiographic feature in the cat that is commonly encountered in CCL rupture is the development of mineralization within the stifle joint. Radiodense mineralized bodies are most often seen in the cranial joint space but can also be seen in the caudal joint space of the stifle. In most cases this mineralization forms as dystrophic calcification at the insertion point of the CCL on the cranial tibial plateau. Occasionally, the mineralization originates in the cranial horn of the medial or lateral meniscus.[89] Although the pathogenesis of calcification at the insertion of the ruptured ligament would seem to involve resolution at a site of inflammation and hemorrhage, the reasons for the development of calcified meniscal cartilages are less clear. Both processes are associated with CCL rupture in the overwhelming majority of cases, and it appears that excision of the calcified tissue, along with extracapsular stabilization of the stifle, is curative.[49,89] Although the presence of a degenerative process partially explains the rupture of many CCLs in the cat, little else is known about the pathogenesis. For example, a clear genetic predisposition has been demonstrated in the dog but remains a subject of speculation in the cat. An increased tibial plateau angle also appears to be an important contributing factor in some dogs and has recently been shown to be of potential importance in the cat.[95] A comparison of 21 cats with CCL rupture to a control group of 34 cats showed that the CCL group had a significantly higher tibial plateau angle (24.7 versus 21.6 degrees).[95] Still, the tibial plateau angle in the CCL group could not be considered "steep," at least by canine standards, in which angles of over 30 or 35 degrees are common, so the significance of this finding is unclear.

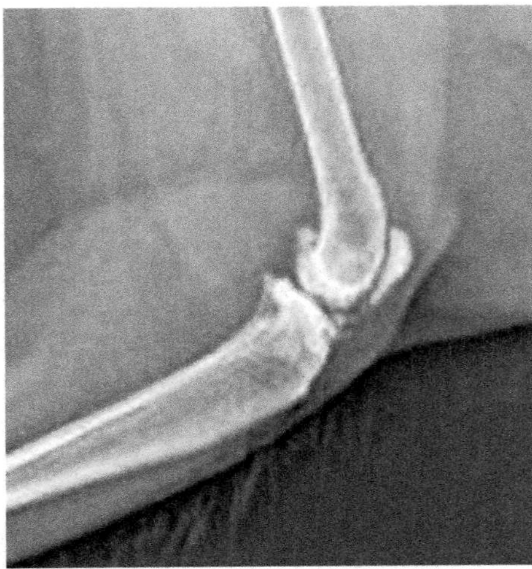

FIGURE 26-12 Dystrophic mineralization in the stifle of a cat with cranial cruciate ligament rupture.

Treatment of CCL rupture remains somewhat controversial. If there can be said to be any dogma on this topic, it would be that isolated unilateral CCL rupture should be treated conservatively with NSAIDs and exercise restriction. However, as is so often the case in veterinary science, this recommendation emanates from one paper that is nearly 25 years old and involves only 18 cats.[94] Although it is true that many cats seemingly do well without surgical repair, the advancement of DJD in these joints is undeniable. In light of the underrecognized clinical signs, prevalence, and lifestyle impact of DJD in the cat, one must wonder whether cats are always best served by conservative management. Some clinicians adopt the approach of starting with conservative management but opting for surgery if lameness persists past 4 weeks. Extracapsular repair techniques reliably return cats to weight bearing, often in less than 1 week; offer an opportunity to débride intraarticular calcification or meniscal pathology; and will provide normal or near-normal function in nearly all cats.[49] This is the approach advocated by the author (GH) in light of seemingly increasing numbers of older, overweight cats that do not seem to do well with conservative therapy.

A curious addition to the limited published information on CCL rupture in the cat proposes a link with hypertrophic cardiomyopathy. In a report of three cats that died shortly after CCL surgery, as a result of apparent heart failure, the presence of hypertrophic cardiomyopathy was confirmed at necropsy in two of the cases.[55] No other reports have been published to corroborate such a connection; however, two of eight cats in another report that underwent CCL surgery were diagnosed with hyperthyroidism within 2 years of their surgeries.[49] Apart from being interesting, this information probably only reinforces the advice to do a thorough diagnostic workup on all cats in which surgery is contemplated, a workup that may include echocardiogram and thoracic radiography in some cases.

Common Calcaneal Tendon Ruptures

The common calcaneal tendon (CCT) consists of the combined tendons of the gracilis, semitendinosus, and bicep femoris muscles that insert on the medial aspect of the calcaneus; the superficial digital flexor muscle that passes over the top of the calcaneus and fans out to insert on the plantar surface of the second phalanges; and the calcaneal tendon, which is the major part of the CCT and ends on the lateral side of the calcaneus as the tendon of insertion of the gastrocnemius and soleus muscles. Equally important is the proximal end of this muscle group, which originates as paired heads of the gastrocnemius muscle on the caudal cortex of the distal femur, just proximal to the femoral condyles. The CCT group acts together with the quadriceps group of the cranial thigh region to flex the stifle and extend the hock.

Cats can be presented with acute or chronic histories of being "down in the hock," or in a plantigrade stance in which the plantar surface of the hock is in contact with the ground (Figure 26-13). Some animals will exhibit a partial plantigrade stance if the CCT tendon components are torn except for the superficial digital flexor tendon. These incomplete ruptures of the CCT are also characterized by hyperflexion of the digits, especially if the stifle is extended and the hock is flexed. This manipulation stretches the superficial digital flexor tendon, which is the sole remaining component of the CCT, thus flexing the digits. Incomplete plantigrade stances may also be related to tibial neuropathies caused by diabetes mellitus, trauma, or degenerative conditions. Complete plantigrade stance presentations may be unilateral or bilateral.

Laceration of the CCT is a common cause, as is calcaneal fracture or tendon avulsion resulting from falling injuries. In dogs tendinopathy of the CCT or degenerative rupture is well known, especially in older animals. There does appear to be a similar degenerative condition in older cats that can lead to CCT rupture, often bilaterally, without any history of trauma. There are also anecdotal reports of degenerative CCT ruptures that may be associated with the administration of fluoroquinolone antibiotics in the cat. Fluoroquinolones have been shown to have an inhibitory effect, in canine and human cell culture, on fibroblast, chondrocyte, and tendon cell proliferation, as well as collagen and proteoglycan synthesis.[69,97,105] These effects have been linked to Achilles tendon ruptures in humans and caused the United States Food and Drug Administration to issue a warning to physicians in July 2008.[87]

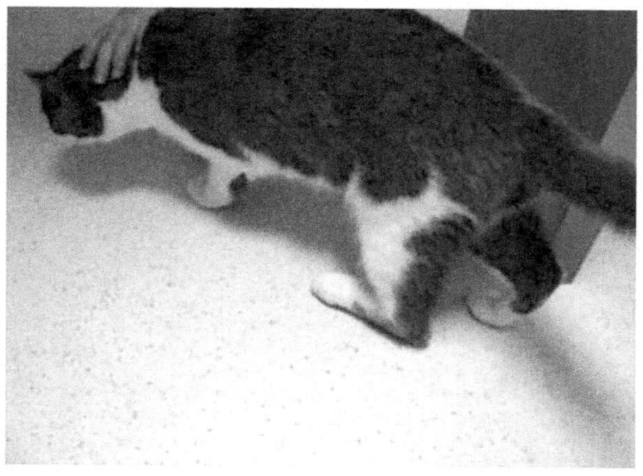

FIGURE 26-13 Cat demonstrating plantigrade stance after rupture of the common calcaneal tendon.

Diagnosis of CCT tendon ruptures are based on the history of plantigrade stance and the findings of a physical examination. In most cases a palpable defect in the distal one third of the tendon is present, but in some cases the gastrocnemius tendon avulses from the calcaneus. A unique presentation of CCT failure that seems to occur mostly in cats involves a plantigrade stance but no detectable defect in the distal tendon. Avulsion of the paired heads of the gastrocnemius muscle at their origin on the caudal cortex of the distal femur will produce the same clinical signs but can be more of a diagnostic challenge. Careful palpation of the area caudal and proximal to the stifle will generate a painful response in the acute phase but will often reveal a defect in the muscle. The integrity of the CCT can also be tested by placing the stifle in extension and flexing the hock joint. In the normal hock joint, it is abnormal to be able to flex the paw much below an angle of 140 degrees. The hock joint in cats with CCT rupture can often be flexed to 90 degrees or less.[81] Geriatric cats may have more range of motion on hock flexion when tested in this manner but may still be normal. This is due to decreased muscle mass, especially in the hind limbs. Comparison should be made to the normal limb so that the test is not misinterpreted.

Treatment of CCT ruptures is usually surgical. Débridement of fibrotic tendon tissue followed by suturing with a three-loop pulley or similar tension-distributing suture is completed. Nonabsorbable sutures such as polydioxanone (2/0 or 0) work well for this purpose because these sutures maintain their integrity for more than the time necessary for healing. The hock should be placed in more extension than the standing angle to relieve tension on the repair, and then the hock joint is immobilized with a splint, cast, or transarticular external skeletal fixator for 4 weeks. Occasionally, if sufficient fibrotic tendon is débrided, the hock may have to be placed in nearly complete extension. This is not associated with any serious consequences for the limited time that the hock is immobilized. If the defect in the tendon is even greater, then the gap can be bridged or the repair can be reinforced with a length of fascia lata harvested from the thigh region of the ipsilateral limb.

Recently, evidence produced in human and canine patients suggests that early controlled flexion of the hock joint may help align fibroblasts in a linear and stronger arrangement, thus making for faster, stronger healing. This can be accomplished with gentle passive range-of-motion exercises beginning 3 weeks after the operation. A bivalved cast or splint that can be removed as needed or an external skeletal fixator with hinges that can be loosened will facilitate this sort of physiotherapy. The prognosis for healing and return to function in isolated traumatic ruptures is good. In older cats with degenerative ruptures, the prognosis is somewhat more guarded. Some cases, especially more chronic ruptures in older, less active cats, have been treated conservatively with an acceptable outcome. The hock is placed in a steeper angle of extension than the normal standing angle, and a splint or cast is placed for 6 weeks, followed by another month of controlled exercise.[81] Although these patients are likely to retain a more plantigrade stance than normal, they will be free of pain and usually have satisfactory function. In cats with bilateral rupture, especially where primary repair procedures have failed, arthrodesis of the tarsocrural joint is a treatment option. The development of a tarsal arthrodesis plate that can be applied to the medial surface of the hock and permits placement of 2.7-mm screws in the tibia and 2-mm screws in the tarsus and metatarsus has greatly simplified tarsocrural arthrodesis in the cat (Figure 26-14). The major potential complication of this procedure, however, is breakdown of the incision over the plate. This complication may require soft tissue care until the plate can be removed, which is at least 4 months postoperatively.

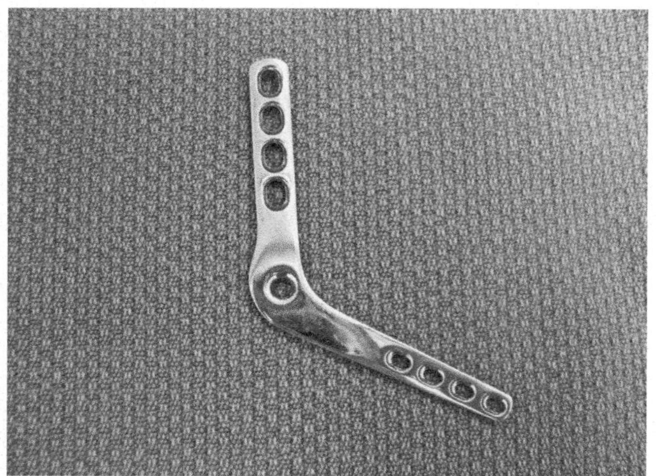

FIGURE 26-14 Tarsal arthrodesis plate that allows placement of 2.7-mm screws in the tibia and 2-mm screws in the tarsal and metatarsal bones.

NEOPLASIA

Primary musculoskeletal neoplasia is uncommon in cats. Although osteosarcoma (OSA) accounts for approximately 80% of primary malignant bone tumors, these cases account for fewer than 1% of all feline malignancies. OSA is a disease of older cats, with most cases being older than 9 years of age. Some reports have described a preponderance of female, domestic shorthair cats, with the hind limbs being involved most commonly. OSA can be divided into cases that involve the appendicular skeleton, primarily the distal femur or proximal tibia, but also the proximal humerus, and the less common axial skeletal cases involving the skull, pelvis, ribs, and vertebrae (Figure 26-15).[8] Clinical signs include lameness and pain, which can be chronically progressive or acute in the case of a pathologic fracture. Local swelling may be noted at the tumor site and in axial OSA of the vertebrae; the initial signs may be neurologic because of swelling or vertebral collapse around spinal cord and nerves. Diagnosis initially requires radiography, which will show a primarily lytic lesion of the affected bone. New bone production may be present but tends to be less prominent than in the dog. Biopsy of the lesion is the only way to confirm a diagnosis. This is best accomplished using a Jamshidi needle. Taking at least three to four samples is the best way to maximize the likelihood of obtaining a definitive diagnosis.

The prognosis with appendicular OSA in the cat is much more positive than in the dog. The tumor seems to be less aggressive in the cat and seldom metastasizes in the early stages. That means that limb amputation may be curative, and adjunctive chemotherapy is seldom

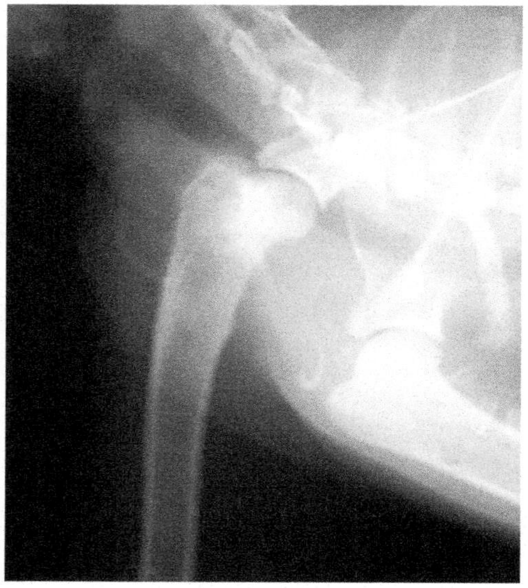

FIGURE 26-15 Osteosarcoma of the proximal humerus. Note the periosteal reaction in the proximal humeral cortices.

necessary. Median survival times after amputation were 49.2 months in one study[8] and 11.8 months in another.[52] Although a curious discrepancy exists between those studies in survival times for appendicular OSA, the authors largely agree on the much graver prognosis for survival with axial OSA, citing 5.5 months in the first study and 6.07 months in the second. Some of the difference in reported survival times for appendicular OSA may be related to histologic grade and mitotic index of specific tumors, which has been directly linked to prognosis.[22]

Chemotherapy of axial OSA using doxorubicin, carboplatin, or both after surgical excision has been described. Radiation therapy may also be of use in axial OSA. Some tumors histologically classified as OSA are "extraskeletal," arising in assorted soft tissues, most often previous injection sites, but also orbital, oral, intestinal, hepatic, or mammary gland–associated sites.[52] One report labeled 38% of feline OSA tumors as being extraskeletal and found affected cats to have a median survival time similar to appendicular cases.[52]

OSTEOMYELITIS

Osteomyelitis occurs uncommonly in the cat under three different circumstances. First, it can arise secondary to deep bite wounds from other cats that involve bone in the septic process. Second, postsurgical osteomyelitis can develop in patients that have undergone surgical repair of traumatic fractures. Third, metaphyseal osteomyelitis can be seen, presumably by way of hematogenous infection, in young kittens. The latter condition seems to be much less common in the cat than in other species. *Staphylococcus* spp. are the most common bacteria involved and will produce mixed lytic and proliferative radiographic lesions in the metaphyseal region of affected long bones; will commonly produce systemic signs such as pain, swelling, pyrexia, and anorexia; and will usually respond to appropriate antibiotic therapy.[10]

Staphylococcus spp. are also the most common bacteria isolated in postsurgical osteomyelitis. Methicillin-resistant *Staphylococcus aureus* does not presently seem to be a common problem in cats; when it is isolated, the source seems to be from humans.[6] Cats with osteomyelitis involving an orthopedic surgery site may show systemic signs, including pain, swelling, and lameness in the affected limb; pyrexia; and anorexia. Radiographically, elements of a proliferative periosteal or lytic reaction may be seen. Occasionally, a sequestrum of necrotic bone may be identified on radiographs. Soft tissue swelling is also prominent, and some cases may have draining fistulous tracts.

Treatment of this problem follows all the rules of managing a soft tissue infection: supportive care of the patient should be provided as needed, bacteriologic samples for culture and antibiotic sensitivity are invaluable, drainage and lavage of areas with purulent exudate must be established, and appropriate bactericidal antibiotic therapy must be initiated. Antibiotic sensitivity testing will guide the selection of an appropriate drug, but pending those results an amoxicillin–clavulanate combination or a cephalosporin antibiotic is a good empirical choice. Both drugs attain good levels in bone and have a broad spectrum of activity against most common bacterial pathogens; however, some cats will become anorexic or will vomit after taking these drugs. Fluoroquinolones and clindamycin are other less desirable choices, in the former case because of poor levels in bone and in the latter case because of increasing instances of bacterial resistance. Orthopedic hardware such as pins and plates should be maintained if the fracture repair is stable, insofar as fractures will heal in the face of osteomyelitis. However, once the fracture is healed, it is often necessary to remove orthopedic hardware to ultimately resolve recurring osteomyelitis episodes. Stainless-steel hardware becomes coated in a protein calyx, which harbors bacteria and shields it from the effects of antimicrobials. Removal of all hardware will usually resolve the problem.

Treatment of osteomyelitis related to bite wounds follows the same principals of drainage, lavage as necessary, and antimicrobial therapy. The propensity for cat bite wounds to become infected is well known, with as many as 80% of cat bites to humans becoming infected, according to some surveys.[31] *Pasteurella multocida* is the most commonly cultured bacterium from these wounds, and surveys have suggested up to 90% of the cat population harbor this organism in their mouths.[31] In excess of 95% of isolates were found to be sensitive to benzylpenicillin, amoxicillin–clavulanate, cefazolin, and erythromycin, which would give some guidance for empirical therapy of affected cats pending specific microbiologic testing results. Osteomyelitis is best treated with antimicrobials for at least 4 to 6 weeks.

DYSOSTOSES

Dysostoses are congenital bone deformities involving individual bones or portions thereof. There are two of clinical significance in the cat.

Polydactyly

Many cats are presented with extra digits, and aside from occasional minor problems caused by lack of attention to regular nail trimming, the condition, known as polydactyly, is primarily a curiosity. It is the result of an autosomal dominant trait with variable expression.[101]

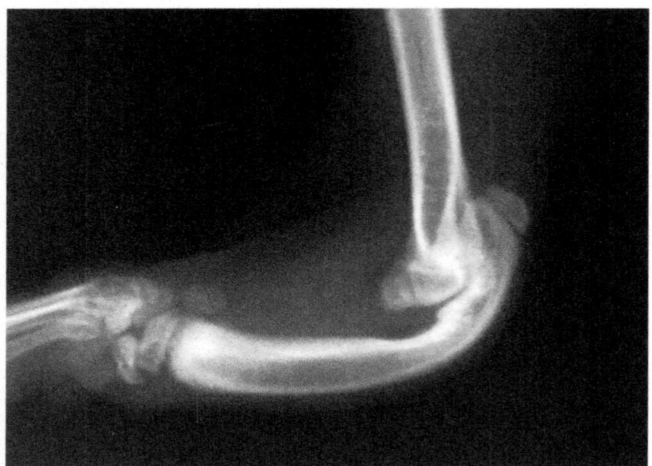

FIGURE 26-16 Forelimb radiograph of a cat with radial hemimelia. The only remnant of a radius in this limb is the small, oval density dorsal to the distal ulnar physis.

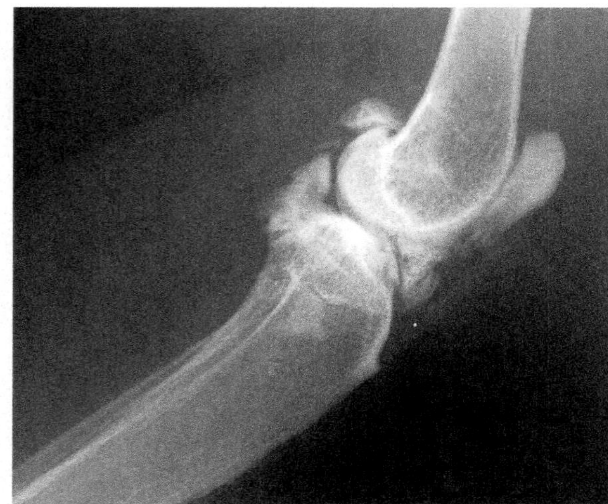

FIGURE 26-17 Synovial osteochondromatosis. This is a benign process, but it can affect joint range of motion.

Radial Hemimelia

Radial hemimelia involves complete or partial absence of the radius (Figure 26-16). As the limb develops without a radius, the action of flexor and extensor tendons deforms the ulna. A varus flexed deformity of the antebrachium produces a "flipperlike" appearance and leaves the front limbs largely nonfunctional. Although the condition can be unilateral and has been described as hereditary in Siamese and domestic shorthair cats, the practical significance of radial hemimelia in the cat is that it is a trait that is selected for by unscrupulous breeders. "Twisty cats" or "kangaroo cats" are marketed as uniquely desirable pets and get their names from the deformity of their front limbs that causes them to hop along on their back legs like rabbits or kangaroos. Occasionally, these cats may be presented to a veterinary clinic as the suspected victims of abuse. Although their deformity is not painful and usually cannot be significantly improved surgically, their lack of mobility may make them prone to attack from dogs or other animals.[71,101]

MISCELLANEOUS MUSCULOSKELETAL CONDITIONS

Extraneous Skeletal Mineralization

The terminology surrounding extraneous mineralization of the cat skeleton is highly confusing. *Osteochondroma, osteochondromatosis, multiple cartilaginous exostoses, synovial osteochondromatosis,* and *synovial chondrometaplasia* are similar terms used to describe sometimes vastly different things. There are two primary syndromes that are seen with some regularity in the cat and must be distinguished. Osteochondromatosis involves the production of exostoses of cartilage and subchondral bone at multiple sites that most often involve the skull, ribs, pelvis, scapula, and vertebrae. The lesions get progressively larger and can become aggressive, transforming to malignant neoplasms typed as OSA or chondrosarcoma. Affected cats are young adults that are nearly always test positive for FeLV. The exostoses may cause clinical signs because they grow by impinging on other structures. In this way neurologic signs are common when vertebrae are involved. Surgical debulking of the masses may be of some temporary benefit, but the progressive nature of the condition and the leukemia virus infection usually results in euthanasia.[22,39,68]

More commonly seen is synovial osteochondromatosis, which is a much more benign condition that has been previously described in dogs (Figure 26-17).[30,41] Cats have a propensity for producing mineralization in and around their joints, especially in the face of chronic inflammation. Radiographically visible mineralization at the CCL insertion or of meniscal cartilage is commonly seen in cats with cruciate ligament rupture. Synovial osteochondromatosis is an excessively exuberant variation of that tendency in which impressive amounts of intraarticular and extraarticular calcification forms. Chronic inflammatory stimulation of synoviocytes results in metaplasia, such that mineralized bodies are produced in association with synovial membranes. These "joint mice" may produce pain and lameness and are frequently large enough to restrict joint range of motion. Affected cats can be of any age but are generally middle-aged or older. There is no connection with FeLV, and although it is chronically progressive, the condition follows a much more benign course and does not necessitate euthanasia. Treatment can involve surgical excision but should also address the source of the chronic

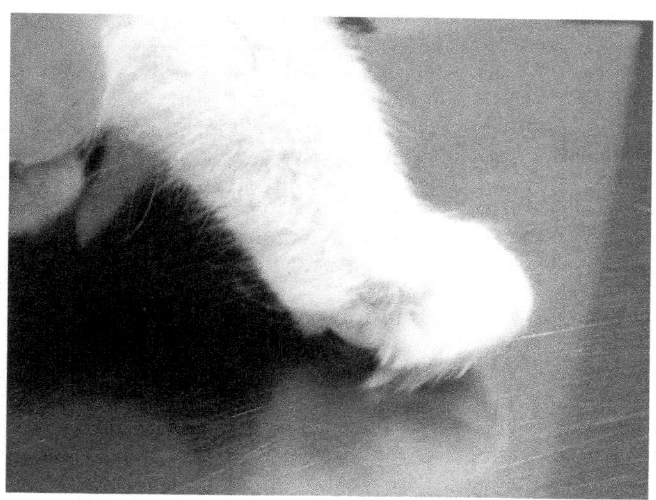

FIGURE 26-18 Tendon contracture involving the digit of an adult cat that had undergone an amputation of P1 and P2 after a traumatic injury.

inflammation (e.g., CCL rupture). Recurrence after surgery is common but does not always result in the return of clinical signs.[22,30,39,41,68]

Tendon Contracture

Cats have a tendency to develop contracture of their tendons in two distinct instances: as newborns and as adults. Newborn kittens can develop a tendon contracture condition that produces deformity of the distal limb and paw, primarily in the hind limbs (see Chapter 41). This condition seems to resolve as the kittens become ambulatory, and the cause is unknown. The significant point to remember is that these kittens may be brought to the veterinarian for euthanasia because of what the owner mistakenly believes is a hopeless congenital deformity.

Adults can develop tendon contracture, which may be associated with trauma. The most common source of such trauma is onychectomy. Remnants of the flexor process on the third phalanx may still have the deep digital flexor tendon attached. As the tissue heals, there may be contraction of the flexor tendon, producing flexion of the toes into a "claw grip" (Figure 26-18). This produces pain and lameness for the cat. Alternatively, cats may develop progressive flexor tendon contracture involving the front limbs without any history of trauma. The flexor carpi radialis and flexor carpi ulnaris tendons are preferentially affected, producing deformity and disability. The cause of the contracture is unknown, but a parallel has been drawn to Dupuytren's contracture in humans, which is a genetic condition. However, Dupuytren's contracture involves the palmar fascia of the hands, whereas the problem in cats seems to involve the tendons. Tendon contracture, of whatever cause, can be treated with stretching exercises and intermittent splinting if the contracture is minor. In advanced cases tendon transection may be required.[48]

Osteogenesis Imperfecta

Osteogenesis imperfecta is a genetic mutation of a gene coding for type I collagen. The result is a syndrome of fragile bones that develop pathologic fractures with minimal trauma. The condition has been described in humans, cattle, and dogs and infrequently in cats.[26] The fractures usually begin to appear between 10 and 18 weeks of age. In addition to the history of multiple fractures with minimal trauma (e.g., jumping from a low height), radiology will reveal "folding fractures," which are typical of pathologic etiology, as well as thin long bone cortices with decreased density, and there may be evidence of other healed fractures. Primary and secondary hyperparathyroidism are differential diagnoses; however, these can usually be ruled out by normal serum chemistry and parathyroid hormone levels. In cats there also appears to be a link between osteogenesis imperfecta and dentinogenesis imperfecta. Because dentin is composed of type I collagen, cats with osteogenesis imperfecta commonly have abnormal dentin development characterized by pink discoloration of the teeth and tooth fractures. Cats with patellar fractures, and often with evidence of other healing fractures, have been noted to have persistent deciduous teeth, which are thought to be another manifestation of the osteogenesis imperfecta–dentinogenesis imperfecta link.

Definitive diagnosis of osteogenesis imperfecta involves analysis of type I collagen cultured from dermal fibroblasts; however, this test is not readily available. Alternatively, bone biopsy, which may be obtained during surgical fracture repair, will reveal decreased cortical and trabecular bone, reduced numbers of osteons with porous lamellar bone interspersed with loose connective tissue.[26] The prognosis for these cats is guarded to poor because even the most patient owner is likely to find it difficult to manage the recurrent fractures. Therapy with vitamin C has been suggested because it plays a role in collagen formation and tissue repair. In addition, bisphosphonate therapy, specifically alendronate at 3 mg/kg orally, every 12 hours, has been suggested, although little information exists regardings its efficacy for this condition in cats. Bisphosphonates act by inhibiting osteoclastic bone resorption and have been credited with reducing pathologic fractures in osteoporotic menopausal women and in children with osteogenesis imperfecta, where these drugs also appear to increase bone density.[26]

Transitional Vertebrae

Transitional vertebrae are defined as abnormal vertebrae that occur in the areas between segments of the vertebral

TABLE 26-1 Congenital Myopathies in the Cat

Disease	Affected Breeds and Geographic Provenance	Mode of Inheritance	Underlying Defect	Clinical Signs	Prognosis
Congenital myotonia	DSH (NZ, US)	Autosomal recessive	Probable defect in chloride channels	Stiff gait; hyperactivity of the selected muscle groups when startled; percussion dimple	Fair to good (nonprogressive condition; cats enjoy normal quality of life)
Devon Rex myopathy	Devon Rex (AUS, GB)	Autosomal recessive	Unknown	Cervical ventroflexion; generalized muscle weakness; abnormal gait; megaloesophagus	Poor (many cats die of asphyxiation)
Dystrophin-deficient myopathy	DSH (US, NL, CH)	X-linked recessive	Dystrophin deficiency	Skeletal muscle hypertrophy with possible complications; sensitivity to stress; stiff gait	Guarded to fair (cats can have almost normal quality of life but may require more frequent veterinary visits)
Glycogen storage disease type IV	Norwegian forest cats (US, Europe)	Autosomal recessive	Glycogen branching enzyme deficiency	Stillbirth; muscle tremor; muscle atrophy; cardiomyopathy	Poor (all cats eventually die)
Hypokalemic myopathy	Burmese (AUS, NZ, GB, NL)	Probably autosomal recessive	Unknown	Transient, paroxysmal clinical signs with generalized muscle weakness, cervical ventroflexion	Good response to potassium supplementation
Malignant hyperthermia	DSH	Unknown	Unknown	Severe hyperthermia during anesthesia (halothane)	Poor (the two reported cats died)
Merosin-deficient myopathy	DSH, Siamese (US)	Unknown	Merosin (laminin alpha$_2$) deficiency	Hindlimb weakness from 6 months old, worsening to muscle atrophy and contractures at 1 year old	Poor (both cats were euthanized before 2 years of age)
Myasthenia gravis (MG)	DSH	Unknown	Lack of acetylcholine receptors	Generalized muscle weakness	Fair, generally good response to therapy
Nemaline myopathy	DSH (US)	Possibly autosomal recessive	Unknown	Progressive weakness (6-18 months); rapid, choppy, hyperthemic gait; tremor, exercise intolerance	Poor (all five reported cats died or were euthanized)

DSH, Domestic shorthair; *NZ,* New Zealand; *US,* United States; *AUS,* Australia; *GB,* Great Britain; *NL,* Netherlands; *CH,* Switzerland.
Gaschen FP, Jones BR: Feline myopathies. In Ettinger SJ, Feldman EC, editors: *Textbook of veterinary internal medicine—diseases of the dog and cat,* ed 6, St Louis, 2005, Elsevier Saunders, p 907.

column. They may be thoracolumbar, lumbosacral or sacrococcygeal transitional vertebrae. Transitional vertebrae may display characteristics of the vertebrae types on either side; they may display abnormalities of length, spinous or transverse process formation; and they may be asymmetrical in shape in either the dorsoventral or left and right planes. For the most part, transitional vertebrae do not produce clinical signs, and their significance is as a unique feature rarely encountered on radiographs. In dogs lumbosacral transitional vertebrae have been linked to an increased incidence of hip dysplasia and lumbosacral stenosis. There may be a similar connection in the cat.[83]

MYOPATHIES

Myopathies are uncommon in the cat, but several congenital (Table 26-1)[35] and acquired diseases (Box 26-7) have been described in the literature. This chapter covers only the most common of a rare group of diseases. For more information on neuromuscular diseases, see Chapter 27. Common clinical signs seen in cats with myopathies include weakness and a stiff, stilted gait. Weak cats often show neck ventroflexion (Figure 26-19). The diagnosis of myopathies in the cat includes a minimum database (CBC, serum chemistries and electrolytes, urinalysis, +/− total T_4) and may also include

BOX 26-7

The Most Common Acquired Myopathies in the Cat

Inflammatory

Infectious: *Toxoplasma, Clostridium,* feline immunodeficiency virus
Idiopathic/immune mediated

Metabolic

Hypokalemia
Hyperthyroidism

Ischemic

Thromboembolic disease associated with congestive heart failure

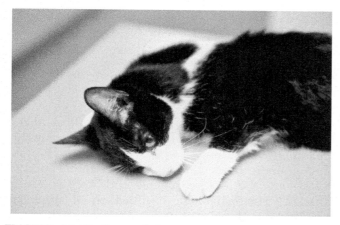

FIGURE 26-19 Cats with hypokalemia may exhibit profound muscle weakness.

infectious disease testing (e.g., *Toxoplasma*, FeLV, FIV) and special investigative techniques (e.g., electromyography, motor nerve conduction studies, muscle biopsy with histologic analysis, and immunohistochemical staining). Clinicians should consult the diagnostic laboratory before performing muscle biopsies for requirements regarding sampling, handling, and shipping. Generally, fresh or flash-frozen samples are preferred.[35] Fixing biopsy samples in formaldehyde does not allow for a comprehensive examination.

Because the half-life of creatine kinase (CK) is thought to be short in the cat, as it is in other species, an elevated serum CK level indicates recent changes. However, many factors other than myopathies can cause an elevated CK level in cats, such as prolonged anorexia.[27] Serum concentrations of AST and ALT may also be increased in cats with myopathic disorders.[35] Referral to a specialized facility may be necessary for diagnosis of some myopathies and neuromuscular diseases.

Infectious Polymyositis

The most common cause of infectious polymyositis in cats is toxoplasmosis. Affected cats are generally young, and clinical signs include weakness, reluctance to move, and muscle hyperesthesia.[24] Systemic signs of infection include anterior uveitis; chorioretinitis; and central nervous system, respiratory tract, and gastrointestinal tract signs. Most cats have fever and weight loss. Hematology and serum chemistry abnormalities include nonregenerative anemia, neutrophilia, lymphocytosis, eosinophilia, hyperglobulinemia, and increases in serum bilirubin and liver enzymes.[93] Serum immunoglobulin G (IgG) and immunoglobulin M (IgM) titers are generally positive, although some cats do not develop IgG titers either in the acute or convalescent stages of infection.[93]

Diagnosis of *Toxoplasma* polymyositis is based on history, clinical signs, minimum laboratory database results, serology, and response to therapy. A definitive diagnosis may be reached with identification of parasites in muscle biopsy samples. The recommended treatment for toxoplasmosis in cats is clindamycin (10 mg/kg orally, every 8 hours for at least 4 weeks).[24]

Burmese Hypokalemic Polymyopathy

Hypokalemia is a well-known cause of muscle weakness in the cat. Hypokalemia may be caused by systemic loss, reduced intake, or a shift of potassium from the extracellular to the intracellular space. The most common cause of hypokalemia, especially in older cats, is chronic kidney disease.[23] Other common causes of hypokalemia include chronic vomiting or diarrhea, hyperthyroidism, and administration of diuretics.

A hereditary disease with a probable autosomal recessive mode of inheritance causing hypokalemia and weakness has been reported in Burmese cats, primarily in the United Kingdom, the Netherlands, Australia, and New Zealand.* Signs are episodic and include acute onset of neck ventroflexion, head nodding, stiff gait, exercise intolerance, and weakness. Severely affected cats are reluctant to move and have myalgia. Exercise and stressors may induce clinical signs. Death resulting from cardiac arrest or respiratory paralysis has been reported.[77] Affected cats are typically from 2 to 12 months of age (mean age, 7.4 months) and are usually normal between episodes. There is no gender predisposition.

The molecular basis of the defect has not been determined but is most likely a channelopathy similar to hypokalemic periodic paralysis in humans.[42] Electromyography and muscle biopsies are normal in affected cats.[42] During episodes of clinical signs, serum potassium is decreased (<3.0 mEq/L) and serum CK is

*References 9, 25, 42, 57, 66, 77.

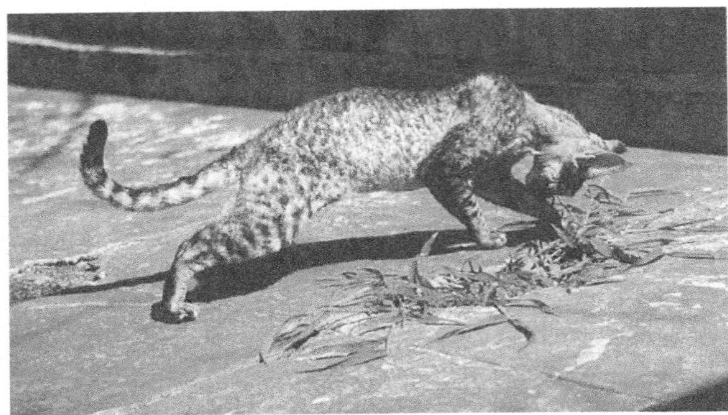

FIGURE 26-20 The prominent shoulder blades and neck ventroflexion characteristic of Devon Rex myopathy.

increased (often >100,000 IU/L). Clinical signs respond to potassium supplementation (potassium gluconate, typically 2 to 4 mmol/cat/day, orally but higher doses are required in some cats). Some affected cats appear to improve spontaneously.

Devon Rex and Sphynx Myopathy

A hereditary myopathy with presumed autosomal recessive inheritance has been reported in Devon Rex and Sphynx cats.[75,76,92,98] The condition came to light in the 1970s and was first called "spasticity." Affected cats have been reported in the United Kingdom, Australia, New Zealand, the United States, and other countries. Clinical signs typically develop between 4 to 7 weeks of age but may not appear until 3 months or later. Signs often fluctuate in severity. The condition does not appear to be painful. Affected kittens have a peculiar high-stepping gait, with the shoulder blades held high and the neck ventroflexed, often with the head tucked into the sternum (Figure 26-20). When resting, the head is laid to one side. Generalized weakness and exercise intolerance are seen in moderately to severely affected cats and may be provoked by exertion, stress, concurrent disease, or excitement. A characteristic "dog-begging" or "chipmunk" position is adopted where the front legs are rested on an object and the head is held erect (Figure 26-21). The head may be rested on elevated objects for support when sitting or lying down. Some cats have difficulty prehending food, because of both oropharyngeal weakness and the abnormal head position. Severely affected cats may develop megaesophagus. The condition eventually stabilizes as the kitten matures and learns to cope with the disability.[75]

Diagnosis is suspected on signalment and history and ruling out of other common causes of weakness, such as hypokalemia. The results of common laboratory tests, including serum CK concentrations, are usually within normal limits. Electrodiagnostic studies may be within normal limits, and examination of the central and

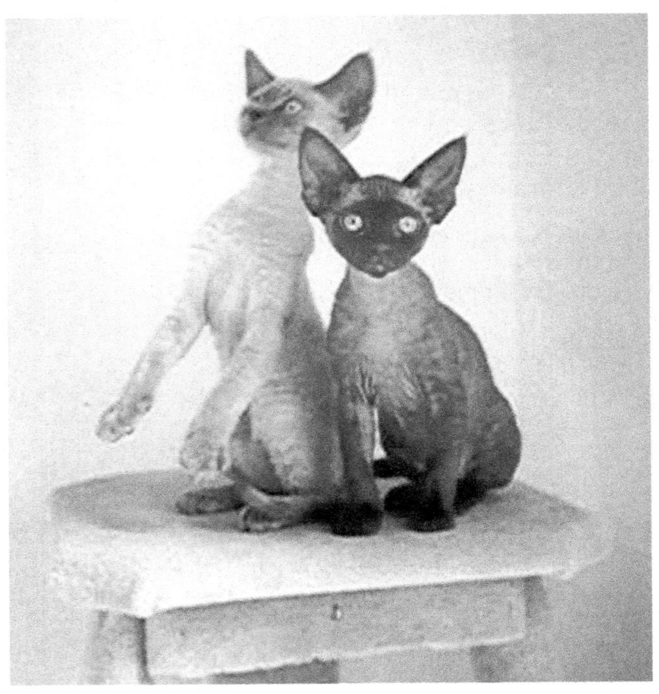

FIGURE 26-21 The characteristic "dog-begging" or "chipmunk" position adopted by Devon Rex cats with myopathy is shown in the cat on the *left*, compared to the normal littermate on the *right*.

peripheral nervous system is normal. Definitive diagnosis is established by examination of muscle biopsies histopathologically and with histochemistry and immunofluorescence staining.[76] Sites recommended for biopsy are the triceps brachii and dorsal cervical muscles.[75] Histopathologic examination of specimens shows changes consistent with a dystrophy (e.g., variation in muscle fiber size, internal nuclei, myofiber degeneration and regeneration, muscle atrophy and hypertrophy, and fibrosis).[75,93] Recent studies have characterized this disease as a novel dystroglycanopathy, with loss of natively glycosylated alpha-dystroglycan.[76] A causative genetic mutation has not yet been identified.

There is no specific treatment for this disease. Feeding affected cats by hand or from an elevated position is recommended because the major cause of death is aspiration pneumonia or obstruction of the pharynx or larynx with food. Environmental modifications and avoidance of stressors and exertion may also be helpful.

Glycogen Storage Disease Type IV in Norwegian Forest Cats

A myopathy was first recognized in Norwegian Forest cats in 1992 and identified as glycogen storage disease (GSD) type IV; it is inherited in an autosomal recessive manner.[33,34,35] There are many types of GSDs reported in the literature, most affecting humans. The disease in

Norwegian Forest cats is due to a deficiency of glycogen branching enzyme (GBE) and characterized by accumulation of abnormal glycogen in several tissues, including skeletal muscle, hepatocytes, and neurons.

The prognosis is very poor for affected cats because there is no effective treatment. Many kittens are stillborn or die within the first few days of life. Those that survive will generally develop clinical signs between 5 and 7 months of age, including persistently elevated body temperature, generalized muscle tremors, intermittent lethargy, and a "bunny hopping" type of movement.[35] Muscle weakness and muscle atrophy progress rapidly, resulting in the inability to chew, contractures of certain joints, and quadriplegia. Death typically occurs before 1 year of age.

Routine laboratory testing is not helpful in diagnosis, although increases in serum CK and ALT are commonly seen. Further diagnostic studies include nerve conduction velocities (typically normal) and electromyography. Samples obtained through biopsy or during necropsy show cytoplasmic inclusions containing periodic acid-Schiff and toluidine blue positive material. Nervous tissue and skeletal and cardiac muscle are most affected. A genetic test is available using buccal swabs or whole blood from PennGen Laboratories, at the University of Pennsylvania.

When an affected kitten is identified, it means that both parents are carriers of the defective gene, which has implications for future breeding. Ideally, carrier cats would be removed from breeding programs. In a recent report, 402 privately owned Norwegian Forest cats were tested, with 58 carriers and four affected cats identified.[34]

Myositis Ossificans

Myositis ossificans (fibrodysplasia ossificans) is a rare disorder generally reported in young cats.[2,85,102,104,106] The disease is characterized by ossification of skeletal muscle–associated connective tissue and adjacent skeletal muscle. Similar disorders are reported in humans and pigs. The disease appears to be inherited in an autosomal dominant manner in those species, but the etiology in cats is unknown. Typically, disease progression is rapid (over a few weeks to a few months), and most affected cats are euthanized. Clinical signs include muscle enlargement and limb stiffness that progresses and becomes painful with decreased range of motion. Fever and lymphadenopathy have also been reported.[102] The results of routine laboratory tests are within normal limits; serum CK may be normal or elevated. Diagnosis is based on clinical signs, radiographic findings (mineralization of skeletal muscles), and histopathologic examination of muscle biopsy specimens (fibrosis, ossification without inflammation). No effective treatment for myositis ossificans in cats has been identified; therapy with vitamin E, selenium, prednisone, and etretinate have all proved ineffective.

References

1. Allan GS: Radiographic features of feline joint diseases, *Vet Clin North Am Small Anim Pract* 30:281, 2000.
2. Asano K, Sakata A, Shibuya H et al: Fibrodysplasia ossificans progressiva-like condition in a cat, *J Vet Med Sci* 68:1003, 2006.
3. Beale BS: Orthopedic problems in geriatric dogs and cats, *Vet Clin North Am Small Anim Pract* 35:655, 2005.
4. Beck AL, Pead MJ, Draper E: Regional load bearing of the feline acetabulum, *J Biomech* 38:427, 2005.
5. Becker K, Brown N, Denardo G: Polyarthropathy in a cat seropositive for feline synctial-forming virus and feline immunodeficiency virus, *J Am Anim Hosp Assoc* 30:225, 1994.
6. Bender JB, Torres SM, Gilbert SM et al: Isolation of methicillin-resistant *Staphylococcus aureus* from a non-healing abscess in a cat, *Vet Rec* 157:388, 2005.
7. Bennett D, Nash AS: Feline immune-based polyarthritis: a study of thirty-one cases, *J Small Anim Pract* 29:501, 1988.
8. Bitetto WV, Patnaik AK, Schrader SC et al: Osteosarcoma in cats: 22 cases (1974-1984), *J Am Vet Med Assoc* 190:91, 1987.
9. Blaxter A, Lievesley P, Gruffydd-Jones T et al: Periodic muscle weakness in Burmese kittens, *Vet Rec* 118:619, 1986.
10. Bradley WA: Metaphyseal osteomyelitis in an immature Abyssinian cat, *Aust Vet J* 81:608, 2003.
11. Burke J: Physeal dysplasia with slipped capital femoral epiphysis in a cat, *Can Vet J* 44:238, 2003.
12. Calvo I, Farrell M, Chase D et al: Carpal arthrodesis in cats. Long-term functional outcome, *Vet Comp Orthop Traumatol* 22:498, 2009.

12a. Carroll GL, Simonson SM: Recent developments in nonsteroidal antiinflammatory drugs in cats, *J Am Anim Hosp Assoc* 41:347, 2005.

13. Chandler JC, Beale BS: Feline orthopedics, *Clin Tech Small Anim Pract* 17:190, 2002.
14. Chang J, Jung J, Oh S et al: Osteochondrodysplasia in three Scottish Fold cats, *J Vet Sci* 8:307, 2007.
15. Clarke SP, Bennett D: Feline osteoarthritis: a prospective study of 28 cases, *J Small Anim Pract* 47:439, 2006.
16. Clarke SP, Mellor D, Clements DN et al: Prevalence of radiographic signs of degenerative joint disease in a hospital population of cats, *Vet Rec* 157:793, 2005.
17. Colopy-Poulsen S, Danova N, Hardie R et al: Managing feline obstipation secondary to pelvic fractures, *Comp Cont Edu Pract Vet* 27:662, 2005.
18. Connery NA, Rackard S: The surgical treatment of traumatic stifle disruption in a cat, *Vet Comp Orthop Traumatol* 13:208, 2000.
19. Craig L: Physeal dysplasia with slipped capital femoral epiphysis in 13 cats, *Vet Pathol* 38:92, 2001.
20. Culvenor JA, Black AP, Lorkin KF et al: Repair of femoral capital physeal injuries in cats: 14 cases, *Vet Comp Orthop Traumatol* 9:182, 1996.
21. Dawson S, Bennett D, Carter SD et al: Acute arthritis of cats associated with feline calicivirus infection, *Res Vet Sci* 56:133, 1994.
22. Dimopoulou M, Kirpensteijn J, Moens H et al: Histologic prognosticators in feline osteosarcoma: a comparison with phenotypically similar canine osteosarcoma, *Vet Surg* 37:466, 2008.
23. Dow S, Fettman M, Curtis C et al: Hypokalemia in cats: 186 cases (1984-1987), *J Am Vet Med Assoc* 194:1604, 1989.
24. Dubey JP, Lappin MR: Toxoplasmosis and neosporosis. In Greene CE, editor: *Infectious diseases of the dog and cat*, ed 3, St Louis, 2006, Saunders Elsevier, p 754.
25. Edwards CM, Belford CJ: Hypokalemic polymyopathy in Burmese cats, *Aust Vet Pract* 25:58, 1995.

26. Evason MD, Taylor SM, Bebchuk TN: Suspect osteogenesis imperfecta in a male kitten, *Can Vet J* 48:296, 2007.
27. Fascetti A, Mauldin G, Mauldin G: Correlation between serum creatinine kinase activities and anorexia in cats, *J Vet Intern Med* 11:9, 1997.
28. Feldman D: Glucocorticoid-responsive, idiopathic, nonerosive polyarthritis in a cat, *J Am Anim Hosp Assoc* 30:42, 1994.
29. Fischer HR, Norton J, Kobluk CN et al: Surgical reduction and stabilization for repair of femoral capital physeal fractures in cats: 13 cases (1998-2002), *J Am Vet Med Assoc* 224:1478, 2004.
30. Flo GL, Stickle RL, Dunstan RW: Synovial chondrometaplasia in five dogs, *J Am Vet Med Assoc* 191:1417, 1987.
31. Freshwater A: Why your housecat's trite little bite could cause you quite a fright: a study of domestic felines on the occurrence and antibiotic susceptibility of *Pasteurella multocida*, *Zoonoses Public Health* 55:507, 2008.
32. Frimberger A: Principles of chemotherapy. In Ettinger S, Feldman EC, editors: *Textbook of veterinary internal medicine*, ed 6, St Louis, 2005, Saunders Elsevier, p 708.
33. Fyfe JC, Giger U, Van Winkle TJ et al: Glycogen storage disease type IV: inherited deficiency of branching enzyme activity in cats, *Pediatr Res* 32:719, 1992.
34. Fyfe JC, Kurzhals RL, Hawkins MG et al: A complex rearrangement in GBE1 causes both perinatal hypoglycemic collapse and late-juvenile-onset neuromuscular degeneration in glycogen storage disease type IV of Norwegian forest cats, *Mol Genet Metab* 90:383, 2007.
35. Gaschen F, Jaggy A, Jones B: Congenital diseases of feline muscle and neuromuscular junction, *J Feline Med Surg* 6:355, 2004.
36. Godfrey DR: Osteoarthritis (OA) in cats: a retrospective series of 31 cases, *J Small Anim Pract* 43:260, 2002.
37. Godfrey DR: Osteoarthritis in cats: a retrospective series of 31 cases, *J Small Anim Pract* 43:260, 2002.
38. Goodman LA, et al: In vivo effects of firocoxib, meloxicam and tepoxalin administration on eicosanoid production in target tissues of normal cats (abstract), *J Vet Intern Med* 23:767, 2009.
39. Gradner G, Weissenbock H, Kneissl S et al: Use of latissimus dorsi and abdominal external oblique muscle for reconstruction of a thoracic wall defect in a cat with feline osteochondromatosis, *J Feline Med Surg* 10:88, 2008.
40. Graham-Mize CA, Rosser EJ, Hauptman J: Absorption, bioavailability and activity of prednisone and prednisolone in cats. In Hillier A, Foster A, Bertola G, editors: *Advances in veterinary dermatology*, Ames, Iowa, 2005, Blackwell Publishing, p 152.
41. Gregory SP, Pearson GR: Synovial osteochondromatosis in a Labrador retriever bitch, *J Small Anim Pract* 31:580, 1990.
42. Gruffydd-Jones T, Sparkes AH, Caney SA et al: Hypokalaemic episodic weakness in Burmese kittens (abstract), *J Vet Intern Med* 10:175, 1996.
43. Gunew MN, Menrath VH, Marshall RD: Long-term safety, efficacy and palatability of oral meloxicam at 0.01-0.03 mg/kg for treatment of osteoarthritic pain in cats, *J Feline Med Surg* 10:235, 2008.
44. Hanna FY: Disease modifying treatment for feline rheumatoid arthritis, *Vet Comp Orthop Traumatol* 18:94, 2005.
45. Harasen G: Atraumatic proximal femoral physeal fractures in cats, *Can Vet J* 45:359, 2004.
46. Harasen G: Good stuff for joints!, *Can Vet J* 46:933, 2005.
47. Harasen G: Maxillary and mandibular fractures, *Can Vet J* 49:819, 2008.
48. Harasen G: Feline orthopedics, *Can Vet J* 50:669, 2009.
49. Harasen GL: Feline cranial cruciate rupture: 17 cases and a review of the literature, *Vet Comp Orthop Traumatol* 18:254, 2005.
50. Hardie EM: Management of osteoarthritis in cats, *Vet Clin North Am Small Anim Pract* 27:945, 1997.
51. Hardie EM, Roe SC, Martin FR: Radiographic evidence of degenerative joint disease in geriatric cats: 100 cases (1994-1997), *J Am Vet Med Assoc* 220:628, 2002.
52. Heldmann E, Anderson M, Wagner-Mann C: Feline osteosarcoma: 145 cases (1990-1995), *J Am Anim Hosp Assoc* 36:518, 2000.
53. Houlton J, McGlennon N: Castration and physeal closure in the cat, *Vet Rec* 131:466, 1992.
54. Hubler M, Volkert M, Kaser-Hotz B et al: Palliative irradiation of Scottish Fold osteochondrodysplasia, *Vet Radiol Ultrasound* 45:582, 2004.
55. Janssens LAA, Janssens GO, Janssens DL: Anterior cruciate ligament rupture associated with cardiomyopathy in three cats, *Vet Comp Orthop Traumatol* 4:35, 1991.
56. Johnson KA, Watson ADJ: Skeletal diseases. In Ettinger S, editor: *Textbook of veterinary internal medicine*, ed 6, St Louis, 2005, Saunders Elsevier, p 1958.
57. Jones BR, Swinney GW, Alley MR: Hypokalaemic myopathy in Burmese kittens, *NZ Vet J* 36:150, 1988.
58. Keller GG, Reed AL, Lattimer JC et al: Hip dysplasia: a feline population study, *Vet Radiol Ultrasound* 40:460, 1999.
59. L'Eplattenier H, Montavon P: Patellar luxation in dogs and cats: management and prevention, *Comp Contin Edu Pract Vet* 24:292, 2002.
60. L'Eplattenier H, Montavon P: Patellar luxation in dogs and cats: pathogenesis and diagnosis, *Comp Contin Edu Pract Vet* 24:234, 2002.
61. Langenbach A, Giger U, Green P et al: Relationship between degenerative joint disease and hip joint laxity by use of distraction index and Norberg angle measurement in a group of cats, *J Am Vet Med Assoc* 213:1439, 1998.
62. Langley-Hobbs SJ: Survey of 52 fractures of the patella in 34 cats, *Vet Rec* 164:80, 2009.
63. Langley-Hobbs SJ, Brown G, Matis U: Traumatic fracture of the patella in 11 cats, *Vet Comp Orthop Traumatol* 21:427, 2008.
64. Langley-Hobbs SJ, Sissener TR, Shales CJ: Tension band stabilisation of acetabular physeal fractures in four kittens, *J Feline Med Surg* 9:177, 2007.
65. Langley-Hobbs SJ, Straw M: The feline humerus: an anatomical study with relevance to external skeletal fixator and intramedullary pin placement, *Vet Comp Orthop Traumatol* 18:1, 2005.
66. Lantinga E, Kooistra HS, van Nes JJ: [Periodic muscle weakness and cervical ventroflexion caused by hypokalemia in a Burmese cat], *Tijdschr Diergeneeskd* 123:435, 1998.
67. Lascelles BD, Court MH, Hardie EM et al: Nonsteroidal anti-inflammatory drugs in cats: a review, *Vet Anaesth Analg* 34:228, 2007.
68. Levitin B, Aroch I, Aizenberg I et al: Linear osteochondromatosis in a cat, *Vet Radiol Ultrasound* 44:660, 2003.
69. Lim S, Hossain MA, Park J et al: The effects of enrofloxacin on canine tendon cells and chondrocytes proliferation in vitro, *Vet Res Commun* 32:243, 2008.
70. Liska WD, Doyle N, Marcellin-Little DJ et al: Total hip replacement in three cats: surgical technique, short-term outcome and comparison to femoral head ostectomy, *Vet Comp Orthop Traumatol* 22:505, 2009.
71. Lockwood A, Montgomery R, McEwen V: Bilateral radial hemimelia, polydactyly and cardiomegaly in two cats, *Vet Comp Orthop Traumatol* 22:511, 2009.
72. Loder RT, Aronsson DD, Dobbs MB et al: Slipped capital femoral epiphysis, *J Bone Joint Surg Am* 82:1170, 2000.
73. Loughlin C, Kerwin S, Hosgood G et al: Clinical signs and results of treatment in cats with patellar luxation: 42 cases (1992-2002), *J Am Vet Med Assoc* 228:1370, 2006.
74. Malik R, Allan G, Howlett C et al: Osteochondrodysplasia in Scottish Fold cats, *Aust Vet J* 77:85, 1999.
75. Malik R, Mepstead K, Yang F et al: Hereditary myopathy of Devon Rex cats, *J Sm Anim Pract* 34:539, 1993.

76. Martin PT, Shelton GD, Dickinson PJ et al: Muscular dystrophy associated with [alpha]-dystroglycan deficiency in Sphynx and Devon Rex cats, *Neuromuscular Disord* 18:942, 2008.
77. Mason K: A hereditary disease in Burmese cats manifested as an episodic weakness with head nodding and neck ventroflexion, *J Am Anim Hosp Assoc* 24:147, 1988.
78. Mathews KG, Koblik PD, Knoeckel MJ et al: Resolution of lameness associated with Scottish fold osteodystrophy following bilateral ostectomies and pantarsal arthrodeses: a case report, *J Am Anim Hosp Assoc* 31:280, 1995.
79. McNicholas WT, Jr, Wilkens BE, Blevins WE et al: Spontaneous femoral capital physeal fractures in adult cats: 26 cases (1996-2001), *J Am Vet Med Assoc* 221:1731, 2002.
80. Mollenhoff A, Nolte I, Kramer S: Anti-nociceptive efficacy of carprofen, levomethadone and buprenorphine for pain relief in cats following major orthopedic surgery, *J Vet Med Series A* 52:186, 2005.
81. Mughannam A, Reinke J: Avulsion of the gastrocnemius tendon in three cats, *J Am Anim Hosp Assoc* 30:550, 1994.
82. Neil K, Caron J, Orth M: The role of glucosamine and chondroitin sulfate in treatment for and prevention of osteoarthritis in animals, *J Am Vet Med Assoc* 226:1079, 2005.
83. Newitt ALM, German AJ, Barr FJ: Lumbosacral transitional vertebrae in cats and their effects on morphology of adjacent joints, *J Feline Med Surg* 11:941, 2009.
84. Nolte D, Fusco J, Peterson M: Incidence of and predisposing factors for nonunion of fractures involving the appendicular skeleton in cats: 18 cases (1998-2002), *J Am Vet Med Assoc* 226:77, 2005.
85. Norris A, Pallett L, Wilcock B: Generalized myositis ossificans in a cat, *J Amer Anim Hosp Assoc* 16:659, 1980.
86. Owen MR, Langley-Hobbs SJ, Moores AP et al: Mandibular fracture repair in dogs and cats using epoxy resin and acrylic external skeletal fixation, *Vet Comp Orthop Traumatol* 17:189, 2004.
87. Ozaras R, Mert A, Tahan V et al: Ciprofloxacin and Achilles' tendon rupture: a causal relationship, *Clin Rheumatol* 22:500, 2003.
88. Queen J, Bennett D, Carmichael S et al: Femoral neck metaphyseal osteopathy in the cat, *Vet Rec* 142:159, 1998.
89. Reinke J, Muqhannam A: Meniscal calcification and ossification in six cats and two dogs, *J Am Anim Hosp Assoc* 30:145, 1994.
90. Robertson S, Taylor P: Pain management in cats—past, present and future. Part 2. Treatment of pain—clinical pharmacology, *J Fel Med Surg* 6:321, 2004.
91. Robertson SA: Managing pain in feline patients, *Vet Clin North Am Sm Anim Pract* 38:1267, 2008.
92. Robinson R: "Spasticity" in the Devon rex cat, *Vet Rec* 130:302, 1992.
93. Ruehlman D: Myopathic disorders. In August J, editor: *Consultations in feline internal medicine*, ed 6, St Louis, 2010, Saunders Elsevier, p 602.
94. Scavelli T, Schrader S: Nonsurgical management of rupture of the cranial cruciate ligament in 18 cats, *J Am Anim Hosp Assoc* 23:337, 1987.
95. Schnabl E, Reese S, Lorinson K et al: Measurement of the tibial plateau angle in cats with and without cranial cruciate ligament rupture, *Vet Comp Orthop Traumatol* 22:83, 2009.
96. Scott H, McLaughlin R: *Feline orthopedics*, London, 2007, Manson Publishing Ltd.
97. Shakibaei M, de Souza P, van Sickle D et al: Biochemical changes in Achilles tendon from juvenile dogs after treatment with ciprofloxacin or feeding a magnesium-deficient diet, *Arch Toxicol* 75:369, 2001.
98. Shelton DG, Sturges BK, Lyons LA et al: Myopathy with tubulin-reactive inclusions in two cats, *Acta Neuropathol* 114:537, 2007.
99. Smith G, Langenbach A, Green P et al: Evaluation of the association between medial patellar luxation and hip dysplasia in cats, *J Am Vet Med Assoc* 215:40, 1999.
99a. Sparkes AH, Heiene R, Lascelles BDX et al: ISFM and AAFP consensus guidelines: long-term use of NSAIDs in cats, *J Feline Med Surg* 12:521, 2010.
100. Taylor P, Robertson S: Pain management in cats—past, present and future. Part 1. The cat is unique, *J Fel Med Surg* 6:313, 2004.
101. Towle H, Breur G: Dysostoses of the canine and feline appendicular skeleton, *J Am Vet Med Assoc* 225:1685, 2004.
102. Valentine B, George C, Randolph J et al: Fibrodysplasia ossificans progressive in the cat: a case report, *J Vet Intern Med* 6:335, 1992.
103. Wallace AM, De La Puerta B, Trayhorn D et al: Feline combined diaphyseal radial and ulnar fractures. A retrospective study of 28 cases, *Vet Comp Orthop Traumatol* 22:38, 2009.
103a. Wallace J: Meloxicam, *Comp Contin Edu Pract Vet* 25:64, 2003.
104. Warren H, Carpenter J: Fibrodysplasia ossificans in three cats, *Vet Pathol* 21:495, 1984.
105. Williams RJ 3rd, Attia E, Wickiewicz TL et al: The effect of ciprofloxacin on tendon, paratenon, and capsular fibroblast metabolism, *Am J Sports Med* 28:364, 2000.
106. Yabuzoe A, Yokoi S, Sekiguchi M et al: Fibrodysplasia ossificans progressiva in a Maine Coon cat with prominent ossification in dorsal muscle, *J Vet Med Sci* 71:1649, 2009.
107. Zeugswetter F, Hittmair KM, de Arespacochaga AG et al: Erosive polyarthritis associated with Mycoplasma gateae in a cat, *J Feline Med Surg* 9:226, 2007.

CHAPTER

27

Neurology

Georgina Barone

OUTLINE

Neurologic diseases in cats present a unique challenge to the feline practitioner because of the inherent difficulties of examining feline patients. Cats are not prone to the same diseases as dogs, and often clinical signs in cats may be atypical, further complicating the veterinarian's ability to develop a neuroanatomic diagnosis. The neurologic exam may be markedly altered in cats as a result of their high sympathetic overdrive and their physiologic responses to stress; therefore, in many instances, unless the patient is extremely obtunded or unusually compliant, a complete examination may not be possible. Because the examiner may have difficulty even eliciting the most basic reflexes and postural responses in an apprehensive cat, minimal restraint, a quiet environment, and extreme patience are imperative. Although a complete neurologic assessment may not always be possible in a fractious cat, a thorough history, physical examination, and observation of the cat in most cases will allow the practitioner to develop a neuroanatomic diagnosis. On the basis of this diagnosis, the veterinarian can generate a reasonable list of differentials and determine appropriate ancillary testing. Detailed descriptions of individual disorders and abnormalities on the neurologic exam are discussed in the following sections. For a detailed description of the neurologic exam, the reader is referred to *Veterinary Neuroanatomy and Clinical Neurology*, by Dr. A. DeLahunta and Dr. R. Glass (Box 27-1).

INTRACRANIAL DISEASES

Seizure Disorders

Seizure disorders in cats present a significant diagnostic challenge and may result from primary intracranial disease or extracranial disease. Seizures can be classified as focal, partial, or generalized.[34] A *focal* seizure is one in which there is spontaneous discharge of neurons of the prosencephalon in the absence of clinical signs and that may be present in the interictal period but is detectable only with use of an electroencephalogram (EEG). A *partial* seizure is a focal seizure that may be observed clinically and consists of varying degrees of motor or sensory abnormalities in the absence of loss of consciousness. A *simple partial* seizure results in abnormal motor activity such as twitching, tremors, limb flexion, ptyalism, facial twitching, and mydriasis with no alteration in sensorium. A *complex partial* seizure may resemble the simple partial seizure, but changes in the mental status are evident, including maniacal running, staring into space, aggression, and self-inflicted trauma.[34] *Generalized seizures* (grand mal) are more easily recognized by pet owners and result in loss of consciousness, recumbency, tonic–clonic muscle activity in the limbs, chewing movements, ptyalism, mydriasis, and loss of stool and urine.[34] The seizure type does not necessarily reflect underlying etiology,[114] although seizure pattern in cats is reportedly different from that of dogs, with complex partial seizures being more common than generalized seizures.[109] Cluster seizures are defined as more than two seizures in a 24-hour period, whereas status epilepticus (SE) is a seizure lasting more than 5 minutes or multiple seizures between which there is no recovery.[34] Structural brain disease has been identified as the most common cause of seizures in cats and includes meningoencephalitis, feline ischemic encephalopathy, neoplasia, trauma, abscess, and vascular disorders.[4,109] However, *idiopathic epilepsy* (defined as recurrent seizures in the absence of an underlying cause) is an important and often

BOX 27-1
Additional Resources

DeLahunta A, Glass R: *Veterinary neuroanatomy and clinical neurology*, St Louis, 2009, Saunders.
Brain tumors in dogs and cats, North Carolina State College of Veterinary Medicine: http://cvm.ncsu.edu/vth/clinical_services/neuro/brain_tumor.html
Comparative neuromuscular laboratory, University of California, San Diego: http://vetneuromuscular.ucsd.edu/

overlooked cause of seizures in cats, accounting for 25% of cases in one report of 91 cats.[114] Cats with idiopathic epilepsy tended to be younger than those with structural brain disease, with a mean age of 3.5 years in two publications.[114,126] Feline hippocampal necrosis should also be considered in the differential diagnosis for a seizuring cat. It is characterized by acute onset seizures and behavioral changes in young to middle-aged cats with poor response to conventional anticonvulsant therapy and progressively worsening signs.[40] Histopathologic findings include severe, diffuse, bilateral necrosis of neurons in the hippocampus and piriform lobes.[40] Prognosis is guarded.

Diagnosis

Evaluation of affected cats requires a thorough history and neurologic exam, as well as consideration of the breed, age, and vaccine history of the patient. A thorough description of the seizure as well as duration, frequency, and the presence or absence of interictal abnormalities are vital to formulate a diagnostic plan. An initial minimum database should include a complete blood count, chemistry panel, blood pressure measurement, urinalysis, and testing for feline leukemia virus (FeLV) and feline immunodeficiency virus (FIV). Thoracic radiographs, abdominal ultrasonography, echocardiography, bile acid assessment, and thyroid testing may all be part of the workup, depending on the results of the physical examination, history, and preliminary testing. If a metabolic or systemic cause is ruled out through the preliminary workup, advanced imaging and cerebrospinal fluid (CSF) analysis is indicated. Magnetic resonance imaging (MRI) is the most reliable imaging modality for the diagnosis of structural diseases of the brain on account of its superior anatomic detail.[4,34]

CSF analysis is an invaluable resource in the diagnosis of many primary encephalopathies, but findings are rarely specific and results must be interpreted in light of clinical and MRI findings. CSF analysis infrequently provides a definitive diagnosis, unless infectious agents such as *Cryptococcus* (Figure 27-1) or neoplastic cells are identified. In one report, despite extensive evaluation, a definitive diagnosis could not be made after CSF analysis in 37% of cats.[17]

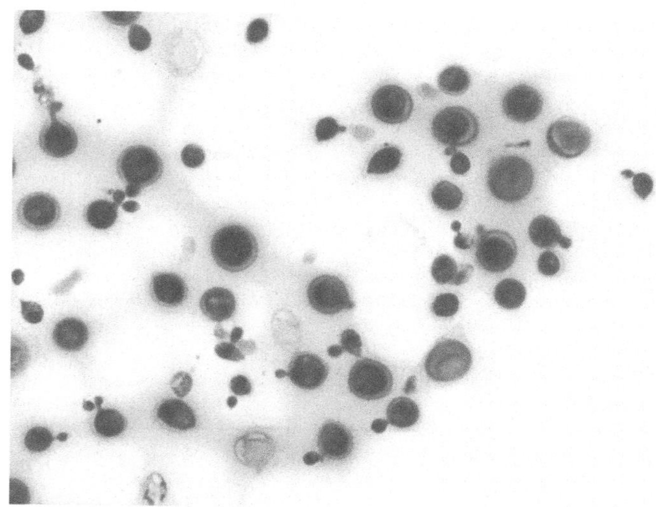

FIGURE 27-1 Cryptococcus organisms found in cerebrospinal fluid. (Wright's stain.) *(From Cowell RL, Tyler RD, Meinkoth JH et al, editors:* Diagnostic cytology and hematology of the dog and cat, *ed 3, St Louis, 2008, Mosby Elsevier.)*

Processing of CSF is typically done by a clinical pathologist and may include evaluation of the following parameters: color, turbidity, specific gravity, protein concentration, red blood cell count, nucleated cell count and differential analysis, and glucose concentration. In cases of specific infectious diseases, culture and sensitivity, gram stain, infectious disease titers, or polymerase chain reaction (PCR) assays may be indicated. Cytologic analysis should be performed using a hemocytometer after concentration of the sample because of the typically low number of cells present in CSF, even in the face of inflammatory disease.

Collection techniques require a thorough understanding of neuroanatomy as well as application of the proper technique.[17] In most cats the cerebellomedullary cistern is the site of choice, although lumbar collection may be preferable in cats with a thoracolumbar myelopathy.

A 22-g, 1.5-inch spinal needle with a stylet is appropriate for most cats. General anesthesia is induced, and the desired site of collection is clipped and aseptically prepped. For collection from the cerebellomedullary cistern, the cat is placed in right lateral recumbency for a right-handed clinician with the neck flexed. The wings of the atlas and occipital protuberance are palpated and an imaginary line drawn between the wings of the atlas and the point where this line transects midline. The spinal needle is inserted slowly, with frequent removal of the stylet to evaluate CSF flow. When the subarachnoid space is entered, the CSF (at least 1 mL) can be allowed to passively drip into a sterile glass tube.[17]

Collection from the lumbar cistern can be performed with the patient in sternal or right or left lateral recumbency. In cats fluid is typically collected from the L6-7

TABLE 27-1 **Drugs Used for Control of Seizures in Cats**

Drug	Dose	Adverse effects	Comments
Phenobarbital	2.5 mg/kg, PO, every 12 hours	Thrombocytopenia, facial pruritus, neutropenia, swelling of the feet, hepatotoxicity	Monitor drug levels 10 days after starting therapy or change in dose; monitor drug levels, CBC, chemistries, bile acids every 4 months
Zonisamide	5 mg/kg, PO, once daily	Anorexia, vomiting, diarrhea, somnolence, ataxia	Recommended for cats refractory to phenobarbital
Levetiracetam	20 mg/kg, PO, every 8 hours	Not reported	No hepatic metabolism
Potassium bromide		Eosinophilic pneumonitis	Not recommended
Diazepam		Hepatic necrosis	Not recommended

PO, By mouth; *CBC*, complete blood count.

intervertebral space. With the patient positioned such that the spine is flexed, L7 is palpated and the spinal needle inserted perpendicularly along the cranial border of the dorsal spinous process of L7. A twitch of the tail or limb can be felt once the needle is advanced into the canal. It is best to attempt to collect from the dorsal subarachnoid space instead of passing the needle through the nervous structures to the floor of the canal. Once CSF flow is evident, fluid can be collected passively into a glass tube or extracted with a 3-mL syringe and T-connector.

Although CSF collection is usually a safe and rapid diagnostic procedure, it may be contraindicated in some instances. For example, cats with known or suspected increased intracranial pressure may be at high risk of brain herniation, either of the cerebrum under the tentorium cerebelli or of the brain stem and cerebellum through the foramen magnum. Many patients with neurologic disease are poor anesthetic candidates, and clinicians should carefully consider the risk-to-benefit ratio, as well as take special precautions in anesthetizing these cases. Ketamine is considered relatively unsafe in patients with disorders of the brain because of its potential to increase intracranial pressure, whereas propofol is relatively safe as an induction agent. An adequate plane of anesthesia is vital to prevent movement of the patient during the spinal tap. Intubation and supplemental oxygen are indicated in most cases to maintain the airway and provide inhalant anesthesia if necessary.

Specific testing and descriptions for most primary diseases of the brain are described in further detail later in this chapter, in the section that deals with disorders of the brain.

Treatment

Treatment is directed at the underlying disease and pharmacologic management of the seizures (Table 27-1). Phenobarbital (PB) is the drug of choice for most feline seizure disorders because of its efficacy, relative safety, ease of administration, and bioavailability.[34,133] A starting dose of 2.5 mg/kg, administered orally every 12 hours, is recommended,[133] but serum PB concentrations vary greatly among individuals on the same dosage, which suggests that there are differences in elimination kinetics among populations of cats.[23] These differences emphasize the need for individual monitoring of cats receiving PB,[23] and researchers recommend more frequent monitoring of PB levels in cats compared with dogs.[108] Elimination of PB may be accelerated in cats receiving steroids and in kittens, which suggests a probable need for higher dosing in these individuals.[108] Toxicity is extremely unusual in cats receiving therapeutic doses but may include thrombocytopenia, facial pruritus, neutropenia, or swelling of the feet.[108] Hepatotoxicity is equally rare. The author suggests checking PB levels approximately 10 days after initiation of therapy or after a change in dose, as well as every 4 months along with a complete blood count, chemistry panel, and assessment of bile acids. Samples can be drawn at any time during the day.

Potassium bromide (KBr) is commonly used in dogs as an add on to PB or in patients with hepatic disease. Although relatively effective for seizure control (seizures were eradicated in 7 of 15 cats in one report), KBr has fallen out of favor for cats because of the high incidence of drug-induced eosinophilic pneumonitis associated with its use.[13] Similarly, diazepam, once considered the second line of therapy for controlling seizures in cats, is not recommended owing to the risk of fatal hepatic necrosis associated with oral administration.[18] Zonisamide, a newer anticonvulsant medication, has been used by the author in cats refractory to PB with promising results. Toxicity is reportedly low, but approximately half the cats in one study developed adverse reactions such as anorexia, vomiting, diarrhea, somnolence, and ataxia.[52] Further studies are needed regarding efficacy and pharmacokinetics of this drug, but anecdotally, a starting dose of 5 mg/kg, administered orally once daily, has proved effective in a number of cases.

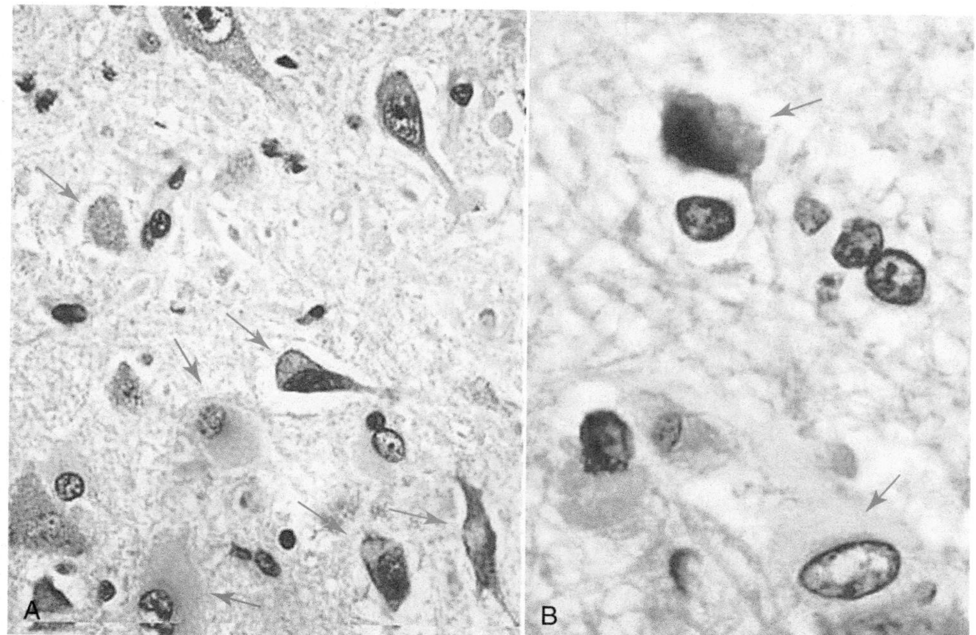

FIGURE 27-2 **A,** Storage vacuoles in neurons of an animal with Niemann–Pick disease. **B,** Cytoplasmic pallor of choroid plexus epithelium due to accumulation of storage material. *(Reprinted with permission from DeLahunta A: Degenerative diseases of the central nervous system. In Summers BA, Cummings JF, DeLahunta A, editors:* Veterinary neuropathology, *St Louis, 1995, Mosby.)*

Levetiracetam, another relatively new drug, has been shown to be an effective and safe drug when used as an adjunct to PB therapy in cats with idiopathic epilepsy.[3] Adverse effects were not reported, and 7 of 10 cats treated experienced a greater than 50% reduction in seizure frequency and none of the cats experienced SE after beginning the drug.[3] It is noteworthy that there appears to be no hepatic metabolism. The suggested starting dose is 20 mg/kg, administered orally every 8 hours.

Prognosis for seizure disorders depends on the underlying cause and is discussed for individual diseases in detail in the following section. It is important to note that severity of seizures does not predict prognosis,[108] and cats without other neurologic abnormalities may have excellent outcomes with aggressive management.[4,108]

Degenerative Disorders

Lysosomal storage diseases are genetic disorders resulting in accumulation of large cytoplasmic inclusions containing undigested products of cellular metabolism (Figure 27-2).[30] Most are inherited as an autosomal recessive trait and result in a deficiency or malfunction of key enzymes within the lysosomal catabolic pathway.[125] Storage diseases are highly diverse and have been organized into subgroups (on the basis of the deranged metabolic pathway), including the glycoproteinoses, the oligosaccaridoses, the sphingolipidoses, the mucopolysaccharidoses (MPS), and the proteinoses.[125] Features common to the storage diseases include equal distribution between males and females, a slowly progressive clinical course (with the cat being normal at birth and in the first few months of life), and in some cases a history of neonatal deaths within the litter.[30] The neurologic signs can be highly diverse depending on the specific disease; multiple organ systems and all levels of the nervous system may be affected. However, the predominant clinical signs usually begin with cerebellar or cerebellovestibular impairment.[125] In some disorders, such as Niemann–Pick disease type A or globoid cell leukodystrophy (GCL), signs of a peripheral neuropathy may predominate. Similarly, ceroid lipofuscinosis, reported rarely in Siamese cats, may present with primarily prosencephalic signs, including seizures and blindness.[125]

Diagnosis

Diagnosis of a storage disease can be challenging, and an index of suspicion may be raised if an at-risk breed is involved or if there is a history of prior progeny of the same parents being similarly affected.[30] Results of routine hematologic and biochemical testing is usually normal in these patients, although careful examination of blood smears may alert the clinician to the presence of storage vacuoles within leukocytes.[125] Biopsy of lymphoid tissue, including the spleen, or liver may reveal evidence of vacuolation.[125] In some subgroups, such as MPS, connective tissue abnormalities are common and radiography may reveal skeletal abnormalities, particularly of the spine. Muscle biopsies may reveal pathologic changes, particularly with glycogen storage diseases, and peripheral nerve biopsies are advocated in the diagnosis of GCL.[125] Urine metabolic screening is available (Josephine Deubler Genetic Disease Testing Laboratory, University of Pennsylvania) to identify the presence of urinary excretory products, with characteristic excretory profiles being described for specific diseases.[125] A definitive means of diagnosing a storage disease is through the use of lysosomal enzyme analysis, in which activity of select lysosomal enzymes in the affected cat are measured against an age-matched control. Affected animals typically have 0% to 5% of the normal activity of the enzyme in question, whereas carrier animals have approximately 50% of normal activity.[125] Molecular genetic testing will become increasingly available in the coming years as another means of diagnosing this group of disorders; currently, DNA testing is available only for MPS 6 in cats.[125]

Anomalous and Congenital Disorders

Malformations of the brain are not uncommon in veterinary patients, with the majority resulting from hereditary causes and in utero exposure to toxins or infectious agents.[34] Infectious agents lead to both hypoplasia after destruction of progenitor cells and atrophy secondary to destruction of differentiated actively growing tissue.[34]

Hydrocephalus

Hydrocephalus is one of the more commonly recognized congenital central nervous system (CNS) disorders in young cats, with clinical signs becoming apparent in kittens as young as 2 to 3 months of age.[22] It is characterized by an increase in volume of CSF caused by compensatory or obstructive mechanisms leading to varying degrees of dilation of the ventricular system.[34] Enlargement of the cranium, small stature, an open fontanelle, calvarial distortion, divergent strabismus, abnormal behavior, ataxia, seizures, visual deficits, head pressing, and stupor may all be sequelae to hydrocephalus, depending on the severity of the pathologic changes in the brain.[22] Advanced imaging is necessary to confirm the diagnosis and rule out other causes of intracranial disease. Typical findings on MRI (Figure 27-3) include varying degrees of ventricular dilation, reduction of periventricular white matter, expansion of the cranial cavity, and loss of cortical bone.

Treatment of congenital hydrocephalus may include medical management with the aim of reducing CSF volume and production through the use of diuretics and corticosteroids.[22] Furosemide at a dose of 0.5 to 4.4 mg/kg PO, IV, IM, every 12 to 24 hours, may be used to decrease CSF production through inhibition of the sodium–potassium cotransport system.[22] Acetazolamide (Diamox) may be used in a similar fashion at 10 mg/kg PO, every 8 hours; it acts to decrease CSF production through inhibition of carbonic anhydrase.[22] Prednisone

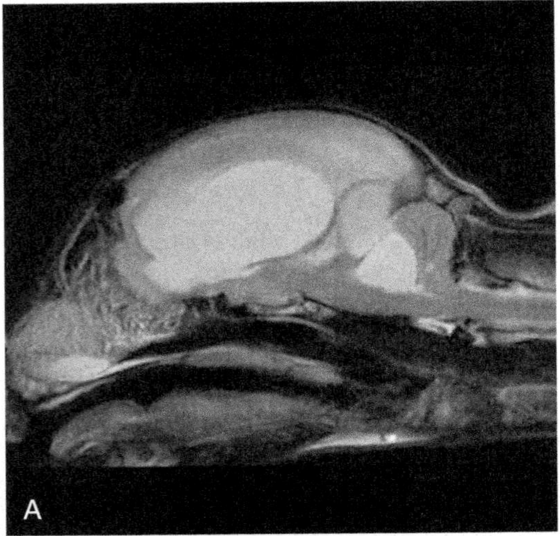

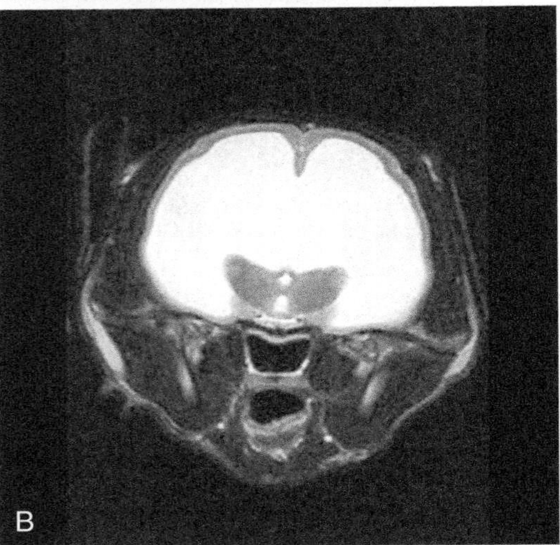

FIGURE 27-3 **A,** Sagittal T2-weighted image of a 1-year-old cat with blindness, seizures, and lethargy. Note the massive dilation of the lateral ventricles, in which fluid appears hyperintense (bright). **B,** Axial T2-weighted view of the same cat with hydrocephalus. Note the small and misshapen diencephalon.

may also be administered to reduce production of CSF, but medical management usually provides only temporary relief of clinical signs.[22] Surgical intervention requires placement of a ventriculoperitoneal or ventriculoatrial shunt, with prognosis dependent on the severity of the underlying disease.[22]

Cerebellar Hypoplasia

Cerebellar hypoplasia is a well-recognized syndrome in cats resulting from in utero or perinatal exposure to feline panleukopenia virus.[34] The virus has a predilection for rapidly dividing cells and targets the external germinal layer of the cerebellum. As such, hypoplasia of the granule layer and disorganization of the Purkinje cells results (Figure 27-4), leading to varying degrees of impairment.[34] Clinical signs become evident as soon as the animal is able to walk and include a base-wide

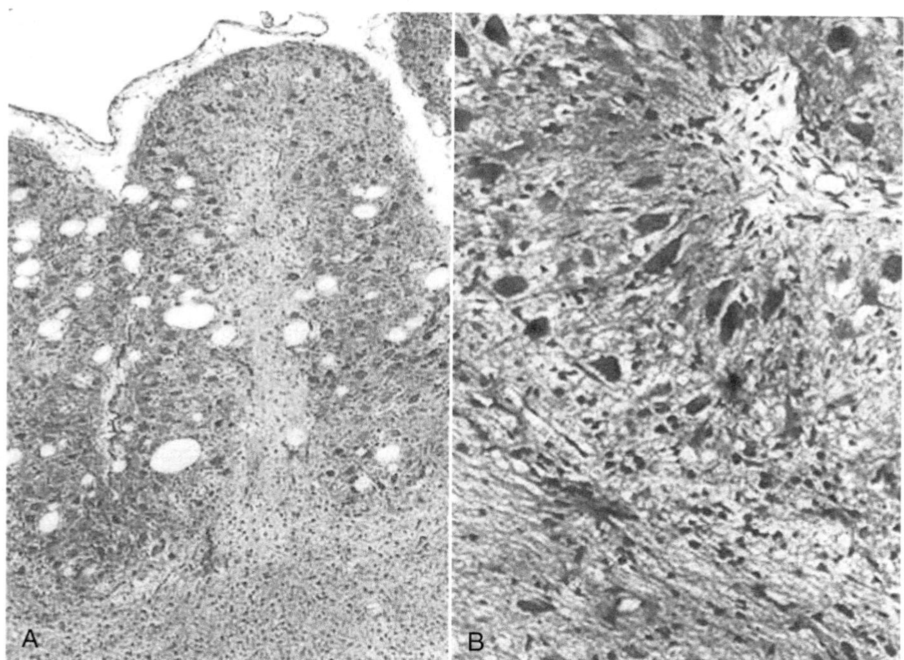

FIGURE 27-4 Cerebellar hypoplasia in a kitten. The Purkinje neurons are disorganized, and the granular layer is absent. *(Reprinted with permission from DeLahunta A, Glass R:* Veterinary neuroanatomy and clinical neurology, *St Louis, 2009, Saunders.)*

stance, coarse whole body tremors, intention tremors, cerebellar quality ataxia, and hypermetria. Neurologic deficits are symmetric and nonprogressive in nature.[34] Depending on severity of disease, an affected kitten can have a good quality of life, provided adequate measures are taken to prevent injury from falling and to keep it indoors. This disorder is best prevented by vaccinating queens before pregnancy.[34] Although similar clinical signs are seen in cats with cerebellar abiotrophy, the two disorders can be readily distinguished given that signs resulting from abiotrophy usually do not become apparent until several months to years of age and are progressive in nature.[6]

Miscellaneous Anomalies

Other congenital anomalies are less well recognized and occur sporadically from genetic, toxic, or infectious causes. Meningoencephalocele has been well recognized in Burmese kittens as part of an inherited craniofacial malformation and has also been associated with in utero exposure to griseofulvin.[34] Intracranial arachnoid cysts have been reported to arise in the quadrigeminal cistern in Persian cats, with clinical signs including obtundation and collapse.[80,110] Lissencephaly with microencephaly in Korat cats has been reported and is associated with signs of abnormal behavior and self-mutilation.

Metabolic and Nutritional Encephalopathies

Numerous metabolic diseases result in neurologic signs in cats through effects on the metabolism of neurons in the CNS.[34] Hypoglycemia is a well-recognized cause of seizures in pediatric patients and has also been reported infrequently in older cats with insulinoma or other insulin-secreting tumors.[50,67] Additional causes include hepatic disease, sepsis, lysosomal storage diseases, inadvertent overdose of insulin, and hypoadrenocorticism.[67] Clinical signs associated with neuroglycopenia in addition to seizures may include lethargy, weakness, disorientation, ataxia, and visual deficits. Chronic hypoglycemia may cause irreversible nerve damage in cats,[67] and thus prompt treatment aimed at correcting the underlying problem is essential.

Hepatic encephalopathy is most often seen in young cats with portosystemic shunts (PSSs) and has also been recognized in other hepatic disorders (e.g., lipidosis, damage caused by hepatotoxic drugs). Toxic products that are released from the gut normally are detoxified by the liver, but in affected cats increased levels of ammonia, benzodiazepine-like substances, and other metabolites circulate to the brain.[34] Resultant clinical signs include seizures (often postprandial), circling, depression, ptyalism, blindness, head pressing, disorientation, and poor growth.[145] Gastrointestinal and urinary signs as well as poor growth often accompany neurologic deficits. A complete description of diagnosis and treatment of PSS and other hepatopathies can be found in Chapter 23.

Various endocrinopathies and electrolyte abnormalities have also been associated with intracranial signs. Diabetic ketoacidosis and diabetic hyperosmolar nonketotic syndrome may produce neurologic dysfunction leading to signs of lethargy, depression, anorexia, and stupor.[138] Coma may result from dehydration of brain cells secondary to chronic hypovolemia, osmotic diuresis, and shifts in fluid balance between the intracellular and extracellular compartments.[138]

Hyperthyroidism has been reported to cause restlessness, hyperexcitability, pacing, circling, anxiety, and mental confusion.[61] Seizures may also be seen, either as a direct result of thyroid hormones decreasing the electric threshold of cerebral tissue or related to a vascular accident secondary to hypertension.

Naturally occurring hypoparathyroidism results in severe hypocalcemia and results in focal or generalized muscle tremors, seizures, ataxia, disorientation, stilted gait, lethargy, anorexia, and elevated nictitans. Other causes of hypocalcemia include renal disease, ethylene glycol toxicity, pancreatitis, eclampsia, phosphate-containing enemas, and iatrogenic causes related to thyroidectomy.[41]

Hypercalcemia can cause disturbances of the CNS such as depression and seizures and is most often associated with hypercalcemia of malignancy or renal failure, although there are rare reports of primary hyperparathyroidism in cats.[41]

Hypernatremia, defined as a serum sodium concentration above 165 mEq/L in cats, results in clinical signs of weakness, ataxia, seizures, and coma.[86] The severity of clinical signs is related directly to the acuteness of onset and degree of hypernatremia[86] and is attributed to rapid shifts of water from the intracellular to the extracellular space.[48] Rapid correction with inappropriate fluid therapy can lead to severe complications, including cerebral edema and death.[48]

Thiamine-deficiency encephalopathy is well recognized in cats and is characterized by vestibular-quality ataxia, mydriasis, cervical ventroflexion, and seizures.[30] Affected cats often have a history of eating a raw-fish diet, which is rich in thiaminase.[30] The author has observed a number of cats with presumed thiamine deficiency in which clinical signs were preceded by prolonged anorexia, such as with hepatic lipidosis. Administration of thiamine (10 to 25 mg administered intramuscularly and followed by oral supplementation) will result in complete resolution of clinical signs. If the condition is left untreated, signs progress to prostration, opisthotonos and spasticity, coma, and death.[30] On postmortem examination, petechial hemorrhages are found bilaterally in the brain stem, with degenerative lesions found in the caudal colliculi, lateral geniculate, vestibular, oculomotor, and habenular nuclei.[30]

Neoplasia

Brain tumors occur in cats with an overall incidence of 3.5 cases per 100,000 cats and account for 2.2% of all tumors.[76] Primary brain tumors include meningioma, glioma (astrocytoma, oligodendroglioma), ependymoma, choroid plexus tumor, and rare embryonal tumors (e.g., neuroblastoma, primitive neurectodermal tumors, medulloblastoma).[139] Secondary tumors include pituitary tumors, tumors that invade by direct extension into the brain (e.g., nasal tumors, otic tumors, ocular tumors), and metastatic tumors (e.g., mammary adenocarcinoma).[76] In a retrospective study of 160 cats with intracranial neoplasia,[141] tumor prevalence was determined to be as follows: 58.1% meningioma, 14.4% lymphoma, 8.8% pituitary, 7.5% glioma, 5% neuroepithelial, 5.6% metastatic, and 3.8% direct extension. There is no reported breed predisposition in cats, and the median age for developing a brain tumor is 11 years.[139]

Intracranial tumors infiltrate the parenchyma of the brain, leading to disruption of blood flow, cerebral edema, local necrosis, disruption of CSF flow leading to obstructive hydrocephalus, and increased intracranial pressure (which can result in herniation).[99] Primary intracranial tumors rarely metastasize, but in some cases they may spread to the lungs by drainage through the venous sinus plexuses in the cranial vault.[99] Clinical signs can include behavioral changes, circling, seizures, visual deficits, ataxia, and paresis[115]; however, signs can be nonspecific, and in one report 21% of cats presented only for anorexia and lethargy.[136] Signs are often slowly progressive and asymmetric in nature; however, in some asymptomatic patients tumors may be found as incidental findings at necropsy.[141]

Meningiomas

Meningiomas are the most common primary brain tumor in cats and are mesenchymal in origin, arising from the arachnoid layer of the meninges. The majority of cases involve older patients[34,93] with males slightly overrepresented at a ratio of 3:2.[33] Their topography is similar to that of dogs, with most being supratentorial and frequently involving the third ventricle.[33,140] There is a tendency in cats for these tumors to be multiple, and in one report 19% of cats had more than one meningioma.[148] In another report three cats had two meningiomas, and another cat had four meningiomas.[43] The presence of multiple lesions may result in multifocal signs, confounding the clinical picture and differential diagnosis. However, despite multiple lesions, 75% of cats in one study presented with signs suggestive of a focal lesion.[43]

Microscopically, most feline meningiomas are meningotheliomatous or psammomatous, and many have cholesterol deposits.[33] Clinical signs depend on the location and rate of growth of the tumor but are usually insidious in onset because of their slow growth rate.[115] The median duration of clinical signs before presentation was 1.25 months in a retrospective of 42 cats and included mentation changes (100%), visual deficits (93%), paresis (83%), and seizures (19%).[49]

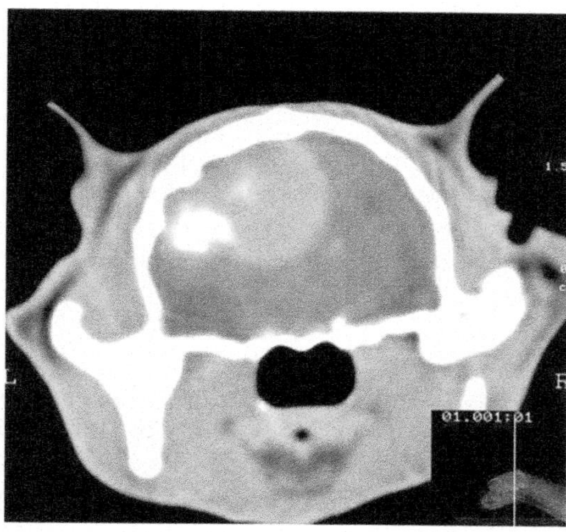

FIGURE 27-5 Computed tomography scan of a cat with confirmed meningioma. Note the hyperdense area of calcification ventrally and the hyperostosis in the overlying calvaria. *(Courtesy Dr. Kerry Bailey, Oradell Animal Hospital.)*

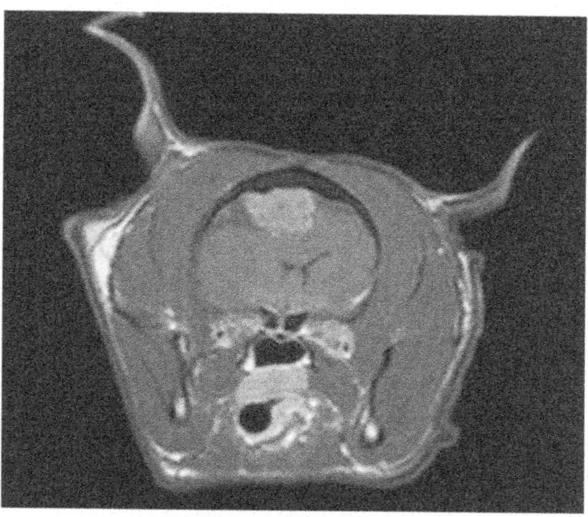

FIGURE 27-6 Magnetic resonance imaging of a cat with a confirmed meningioma. Note the extraaxial location and mass effect typical for this tumor type. *(Courtesy Dr. Mark Troxel, In Town Veterinary Group.)*

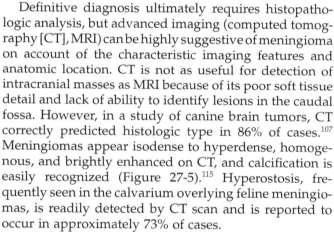

Definitive diagnosis ultimately requires histopathologic analysis, but advanced imaging (computed tomography [CT], MRI) can be highly suggestive of meningioma on account of the characteristic imaging features and anatomic location. CT is not as useful for detection of intracranial masses as MRI because of its poor soft tissue detail and lack of ability to identify lesions in the caudal fossa. However, in a study of canine brain tumors, CT correctly predicted histologic type in 86% of cases.[107] Meningiomas appear isodense to hyperdense, homogenous, and brightly enhanced on CT, and calcification is easily recognized (Figure 27-5).[115] Hyperostosis, frequently seen in the calvarium overlying feline meningiomas, is readily detected by CT scan and is reported to occur in approximately 73% of cases.

MRI is considered the superior modality for detecting these tumors and correctly identified meningioma on the basis of MRI features alone in 96% of cases in 33 cats.[140] Imaging features are variable but include an extraaxial location, distinct margins, mild peritumoral edema, mass effect, dural tail, and broad base (Figure 27-6).[140] In one report enlargement of the lateral ventricle was present in 64% of cases, and herniation under the tentorium or cerebellum was evident in 63% of cases.[140] Results of CSF analysis in cats with meningioma have not been reported, but in dogs they are nonspecific and unlikely to be of diagnostic benefit.

The mainstay of treatment for feline meningioma is surgical removal. Surgery is often successful owing to the superficial location over the cerebral convexities and frontal lobes, the lack of invasion of underlying parenchyma (unlike dogs), and the well-circumscribed nature of these generally benign tumors. Postoperative mortality rates have been reported to be as high as 19%,[49] but in the author's experience and that of other experienced clinicians,[115] the mortality rate is typically lower. The most common postoperative complication after meningioma excision is anemia, which occurs in as many as one third of cats.[49] Overall, median survival time (MST) in a study of 42 cats was 26 months, with a 1-year survival rate of 66% and a 2-year survival rate of 50%.[49] In the same report 30% of cats developed a recurrence of neurologic signs, with a median time of 30.75 months. In another report of 34 cats with surgically treated meningioma, MST was 685 days, with 20% of cats experiencing a recurrence of clinical signs (285 days). Data regarding treatment of feline meningioma with radiation or chemotherapy are lacking, probably because of the high success and long survival times after surgery.

Pituitary Tumors

Pituitary tumors are rarely diagnosed in cats and often exert their clinical effects through excessive secretion of growth hormone. Clinical signs include acromegaly, characterized by enlargement of the head, lameness, dyspnea resulting from cardiomegaly, protrusion of the mandible, respiratory stridor caused by hypertrophy of oropharyngeal soft tissues, and widening of the interdental space.[128] Severe insulin-resistant diabetes is often evident. However, neurologic signs (e.g., seizures, behavioral changes, blindness) may occur in the absence of an endocrinopathy.[62,88] Middle-aged to older male cats are overrepresented.[88,128]

Definitive diagnosis requires advanced imaging of the brain (CT or MRI) and usually reveals a mass lesion in the sella with dorsal expansion into the overlying diencephalon (Figure 27-7). The majority of macroadenomas are contrast enhancing and may have areas of necrosis, hemorrhage, or calcification.

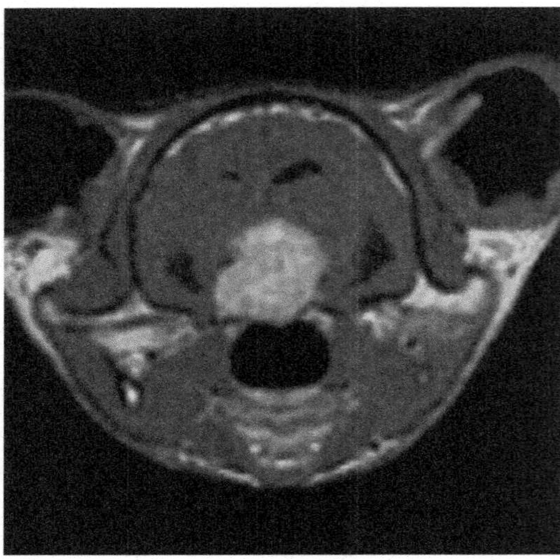

FIGURE 27-7 T1-weighted magnetic resonance imaging after contrast administration in a cat with a confirmed pituitary macroadenoma. Note the strong contrast uptake and obliteration of the diencephalon. *(Reprinted with permission from DeLahunta A, Glass R: Veterinary neuroanatomy and clinical neurology, St Louis, 2009, Saunders.)*

Medical management of these tumors is largely unrewarding, and more definitive treatment requires surgical intervention or radiation. In seven cats treated with transphenoidal hypophysectomy, surgery was well tolerated in most cases, with clinical signs resolving in five cats and two cats surviving 28 and 46 months after surgery.[89] However, surgeons competent in this procedure are lacking, and complications, including chronic oronasal fistula, can have a significant impact on quality of life.[89] Treatment with radiation therapy has been shown to ameliorate or resolve clinical signs and has been associated with prolonged survival times in numerous studies.[62,88] Median survival time in a report of eight cats treated with radiation was 17.4 months (range, 8.4 to 63.1 months).[62]

Lymphoma

Lymphoma of the brain can be primary or secondary or may be an aspect of multicentric disease.[76] It is seen uncommonly, accounting for only 14.4% of cases in a series of 160 cats with intracranial tumors.[141] In a retrospective of 18 cats with CNS lymphoma, 14 had intracranial involvement and 10 presented with a chief complaint of seizures.[98] Most important, the prevalence of involvement of bone marrow and other organs was extremely high, suggesting that perhaps the most reliable means of diagnosing lymphoma in the CNS is through confirming its presence in other body systems.[98]

There are no pathognomonic findings on MRI of cats with intracranial lymphoma, and in some cases imaging features are similar to those of meningioma.[140] CSF analysis may be highly useful, and malignant cells were seen in the CSF of 5 of 11 cats in one report[98] and 6 of 17 in another.[72]

Although lymphoma is considered chemotherapy sensitive, prognosis in affected cats is guarded, with a MST of approximately 21 days in patients treated with prednisone alone.[141] Chemotherapy alone has not proved to substantially prolong survival times, but when combined with radiation, the MST was found to be 125 days (range 40 to 210 days).[98]

Other Tumors

The incidence of other tumors of the brain in cats is not known, but they are seen only rarely in clinical practice. Of 160 cats with intracranial tumors, astrocytoma, oligodendroglioma, olfactory neuroblastoma, and ependymoma accounted for only 7.6% of cases. Because of the rarity of these tumors, there is a paucity of information regarding treatment and prognosis. However, gliomas typically appear to carry a grave prognosis, and in a cat with an astrocytoma treated with surgery and radiation, the survival time was only 179 days.[141] Ependymomas carry a more favorable prognosis and seem to respond well to surgical intervention, with survival times as long as 2 years reported.[124,141]

Inflammatory Disorders

Feline Infectious Peritonitis

Feline infectious peritonitis (FIP) is the most common and clinically significant inflammatory disorder in the CNS, accounting for 48% of cases of infectious neurologic diseases reported in cats.[14] The causative agent, a highly pathogenic variant of feline enteric corona virus (FIPV), produces immune-mediated disease through infection of macrophages, with severity of signs determined by host susceptibility, host-specific immune response, and virus strain.[42] The majority of cases are younger than 2 years of age and come from multicat households, with males and purebreds being overrepresented.[35,42]

Neurologic signs can be seen with both the effusive ("wet") and the noneffusive ("dry") form of this disease, but the dry form appears more commonly to involve the CNS.[35] Signs referable to cerebellomedullary involvement are most common,[32] but seizures may also be evident and have been reported in up to 25% of cats with histopathologically confirmed FIP.[135] Ataxia, spastic paresis, head tilt, nystagmus, hyperesthesia, proprioceptive deficits, blindness, and behavioral changes have all been reported.[35,42] Non-neurologic signs frequently accompany the CNS signs and include uveitis, chorioretinitis, respiratory infections, mesenteric lymphadenopathy, dehydration, weight loss, lethargy, fever, and pica.[42]

Antemortem diagnosis of FIP can be extremely challenging and requires a high index of suspicion, especially in those patients with no obvious systemic

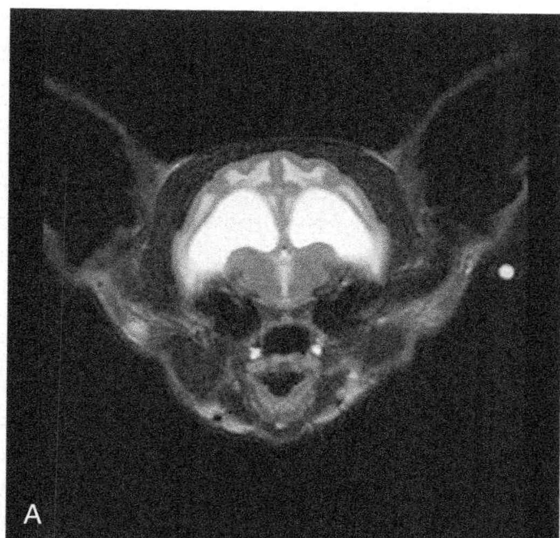

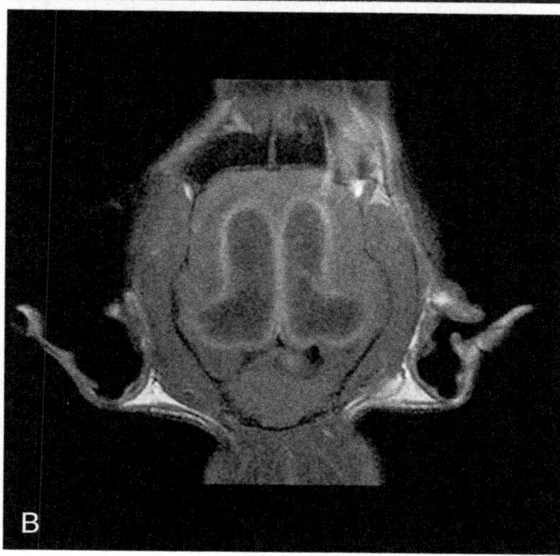

FIGURE 27-8 **A,** T2-axial magnetic resonance imaging of a cat with progressive ataxia and seizures. Polymerase chain reaction for feline infectious peritonitis virus was positive in the cerebrospinal fluid. Note the massive ventricular dilation and edema in the corona radiata. **B,** T1 postcontrast magnetic resonance imaging of same cat in **A.** Note the strong uptake of contrast in the ependymal lining of the lateral ventricles.

involvement (see Chapter 33). Complete blood count findings are nonspecific, but serum protein concentration is often elevated, specifically the alpha-2, beta, and gamma-globulins.[35] CSF analysis in cats with FIP is characterized by increased cellularity (which may be predominantly neutrophilic or mononuclear), as well as increased protein levels as high as 2 g/L. The presence of anti-coronavirus antibodies in either serum or CSF proves only that the cat has been exposed to a coronavirus and is not a means of definitively diagnosing FIP. In a prospective study of 67 cats, detection of anti-coronavirus antibodies in CSF had a sensitivity of 60% and a specificity of 90%.[11]

MRI is a useful adjunctive tool in cases of suspected intracranial FIP, both to help confirm the diagnosis and rule out other causes of neurologic signs (Figure 27-8). Typical findings include ventricular dilation, ependymitis, choroid plexitis, meningitis (most evident on the ventrocaudal surfaces of the brain), cervical syringomyelia, and periventricular inflammation.[42,100] However, there are no pathognomonic imaging findings, and results must be considered in light of clinical and clinicopathologic findings. PCR can be performed on CSF and other fluids (e.g., abdominal effusion) or tissues, but its sensitivity is relatively low, and a negative test does not necessarily rule out FIP.[42]

Postmortem examination of the brain often reveals gross lesions, including meningeal opacity around the medulla and choroid plexus of the fourth ventricle and coating of the choroid plexuses with a white tenacious exudate.[32] Ependymal cells may be coated by fibrin and may lead to hydrocephalus rostral to the obstruction. Histologically, there is a severe pyogranulomatous leptomeningitis, choroiditis, ependymitis, and encephalomyelitis, with lesions predominantly surface oriented.[32] Prognosis is extremely grim, and despite claims of effective treatments for FIP, it appears that the disease is uniformly fatal, even with supportive care and immunomodulatory therapies.

Toxoplasmosis

Toxoplasma gondii is a protozoal parasite for which the cat can serve as both the intermediate and definitive host.[32,79] Infection occurs by direct ingestion of tissue cysts in meat or sporulated oocysts from cats feces, as well as transplacentally.[32] After infection bradyzoite organisms will become encysted in various tissues, including muscle and CNS, but often the infection remains latent and the patient will be asymptomatic.[32] Clinical disease occurs with a variety of immunocompromising factors, including steroid administration, concurrent infection with FIV or FeLV, stress, a large infective dose in very young animals, and neoplasia.[32,79]

Clinical findings include fever, pneumonia, icterus, abdominal discomfort, dyspnea, pericardial effusion, ascites, pancreatitis, and mesenteric lymphadenopathy.[79,134] Lesions in the CNS are uncommon, accounting for only 7 of 100 cats with histologically confirmed toxoplasmosis.[36a] Clinical signs of CNS involvement are often multifocal and include seizures, blindness, ataxia, abnormal behavior, depression, anisocoria, head tilt, and nystagmus.[36a,79]

Antemortem diagnosis can be challenging and use of an IgG-based test (e.g., enzyme-linked immunosorbent assay [ELISA], latex agglutination test) requires demonstration of a fourfold increase in IgG over 2 to 3 weeks.[79] CSF can be used to determine intrathecal antibody production, but results must be interpreted cautiously because *T. gondii*–specific IgG has been found in the CSF of normal cats.[79] PCR has also been used to detect *T. gondii* in CSF, and results were found to be positive in seven of seven cats with immunohistochemical or

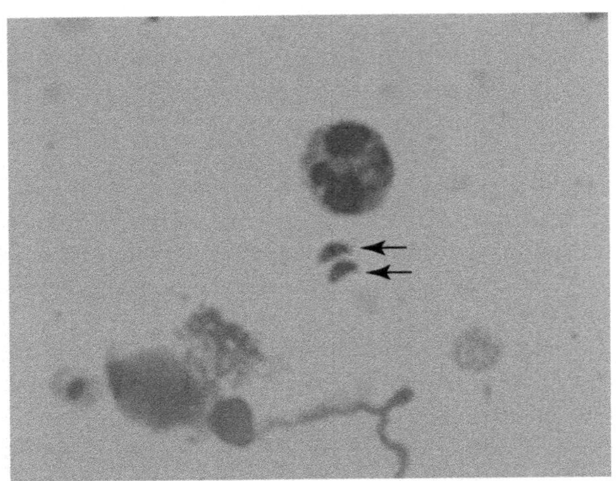

FIGURE 27-9 Cerebrospinal fluid of a cat infected with *Toxoplasma gondii (arrows).*

serologic evidence of toxoplasmosis.[113] In rare cases organisms may be seen directly in CSF (Figure 27-9) or other biologic material, such as fluid obtained through bronchial lavage.

Histologically, nonsuppurative meningoencephalitis affecting gray and white matter is seen with occasional periventricular involvement.[32] Necrosis may be severe, especially in congenital infections, and organisms may be visualized at the margins of lesions, within macrophages, and in tissue cysts.[32] Treatment may yield a favorable response, and clindamycin (10 to 12 mg/kg, administered orally every 12 hours for 4 weeks) is considered the drug of choice.[79] Alternatively, trimethoprim sulfa (15 mg/kg, administered orally every 12 hours for 4 weeks) can be used.

Fungal Infections

Fungal infections are occasionally identified in the CNS in cats, with *Cryptococcus neoformans* being the most commonly reported. Because cats with cryptococcosis frequently are infected through inhalation of unencapsulated organisms, it is not unusual for the cat to have concurrent upper respiratory signs as well as swelling of the nose.[74] Clinical signs usually reflect a multifocal process, but forebrain signs may predominate because of the proposed route of entry. Ocular involvement often accompanies lesions in the CNS, with organisms being found between the choroid and the retina.[32] There is no significant age or sex predilection, and both indoor and outdoor cats can become infected.

Definitive diagnosis can be obtained with the latex agglutination (LA) test for capsular antigen, a test that is both highly sensitive and specific. LA may also be performed on CSF and may be preferable in cats without obvious systemic involvement. The organism may also be directly visualized in CSF, nasal exudates, skin lesions, urine, and lymph node aspirates.[74] In cases in which the organism is not seen in CSF, it is generally still abnormal and may yield neutrophilic, eosinophilic, mononuclear, or mixed pleocytosis with elevated protein.[74] MRI of affected cats is variable and may include a solitary granuloma, multifocal masses, meningeal inflammation, and enhancement of the ependyma and choroid plexuses.[130] Microscopic findings include the presence of numerous, tightly packed organisms filling the subarachnoid space and expanding the sulci with a mild nonsuppurative inflammatory response in the meninges and parenchyma (Figure 27-10).[32]

The treatment of choice is currently fluconazole (25 to 50 mg orally every 12 hours) because of its ability to cross the blood–brain barrier, its relative safety margin, and its reported efficacy.[74] However, prognosis is considered extremely guarded in cats with CNS involvement and relapses are common. Other fungal infections, such as *Blastomyces dermatitidis*, *Histoplasma capsulatum*, and *Cladophialophora* spp., are sporadically reported in endemic areas and are typically associated with a grave prognosis.[74,127]

Borna Disease

Borna disease virus (BDV) is the cause of a severe nonsuppurative encephalomyelitis reported in many parts of the world, particularly Europe and Australia. It is most often seen in rural cats prone to hunting birds and rodents and is characterized by pelvic limb ataxia followed by mentation changes, visual deficits, photophobia, circling, and seizures.[9] Clinical signs last from 1 to 4 weeks and usually result in progressive impairment and death, although in some cases recovery is possible. Cats that have recovered have permanent ataxia, behavioral changes, and polyphagia.[9]

Definitive diagnosis can be difficult, and other causes of multifocal CNS disturbances, such as FIP, must be ruled out. Fewer than half of affected cats test positive for BDV-specific antibodies, and PCR has not proved to be a reliable test in this species.[9] The disease can be definitively diagnosed only through postmortem examination. Findings include inflammatory changes, mostly in gray matter, perivascular cuffing, neuronophagia, and detection of BDV antigen in the CNS parenchyma.[9] Prognosis is grave, and there is no known treatment. Many other infectious encephalitides in cats have been reported uncommonly, including rabies, FIV, rickettsial disease, pseudorabies, and feline spongiform encephalopathy.

Toxic Disorders

Toxin ingestion should be considered in any cat presenting with acute neurologic signs, particularly in those cats with a history of indiscriminate ingestion of foreign materials or those that have had access to the outdoors with no supervision. Because many toxins can produce effects similar to naturally occurring diseases on the CNS, a thorough history, as well as a complete

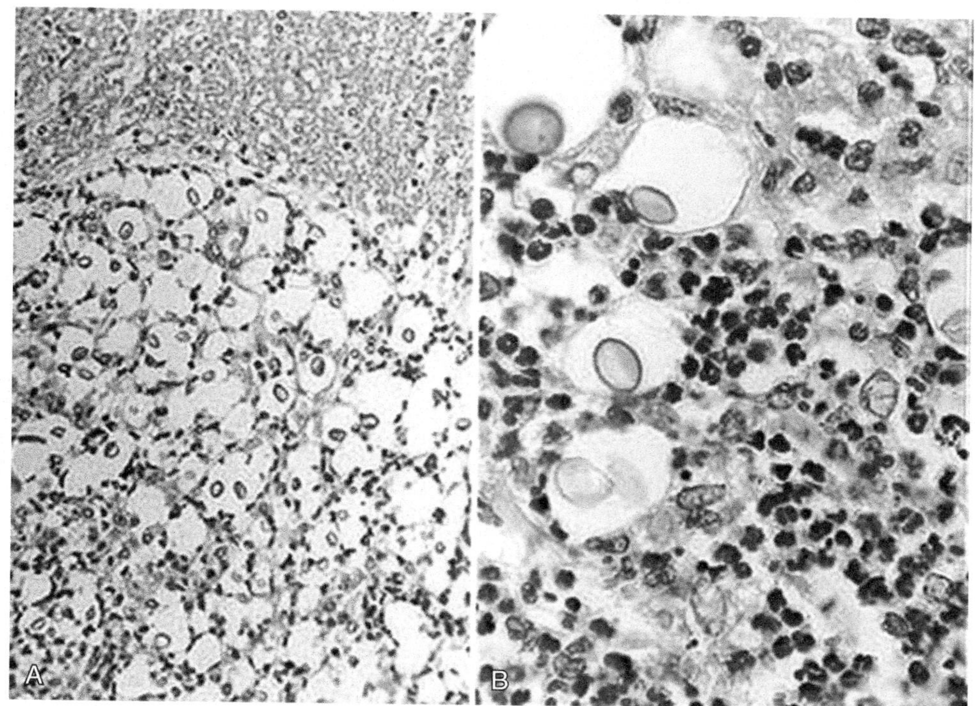

FIGURE 27-10 Hippocampus of a cat infected with *Cryptococcus neoformans* (H & E, ×140). Cavities representing perivascular spaces distended with organisms are readily seen. *(Reprinted with permission from DeLahunta A: Inflammatory diseases of the nervous system. In Summers BA, Cummings JF, DeLahunta A, editors:* Veterinary neuropathology, *St Louis, 1995, Mosby.)*

neurologic examination, is essential. Although the list of potential neurotoxins is endless, this section addresses only the most common and clinically relevant ones seen by feline practitioners (see also Chapter 31).[25]

Topical pesticides represent a significant source of toxicity in cats and usually result from inappropriate administration of flea and tick products. Clinical signs of permethrin toxicity include tremors and muscle fasciculations, twitching, hyperesthesia, seizures, ataxia, mydriasis, and central blindness. Severe clinical signs require intensive treatment, and left unchecked, death from aspiration pneumonia, respiratory arrest, or electrolyte abnormalities may result. However, the majority of cats will have a good outcome with no long-term complications.[12,37] Organophosphate and carbamate insecticides act by inhibiting acetylcholinesterase, resulting in signs consistent with a "cholinergic crisis" marked by muscarinic, nicotinic, and mixed signs.[36] Tremors, depression, seizures, miosis, abnormal behavior, and cervical ventroflexion all have been reported in affected cats within minutes to hours after exposure.[36]

A number of drugs have been reported to cause neurologic signs in cats, the most well described being metronidazole.[16,112] Neurologic signs include disorientation, ataxia, central blindness, and seizures. All reported cases have been on doses greater than 30 mg/kg per day. Withdrawal of the medication and institution of supportive care result in rapid resolution of clinical signs within several days.[16,112] Ivermectin is also reported to cause seizures, as well as ataxia, blindness, mydriasis, coma, disorientation, and death.

Plant toxicities account for approximately 10% of reported exposures to poison control centers, with more than 50% of cases being less than 1 year of age.[58] These are often particularly challenging to the clinician because many pet owners do not know the names of the plants the cat may have ingested, and in some cases it is unclear whether the animal did in fact ingest the plant material. Tobacco, marijuana, and other hallucinogenic plants have all been reported to cause a multitude of signs, from depression to ataxia, seizures, and death.[58]

Ingestion of lead continues to be an important toxicologic problem in cats, particularly in those living in homes constructed before 1977. Owners of cats with suspected lead poisoning should be questioned carefully to determine whether remodeling is taking place because the grooming habits of cats put them at risk for ingesting lead-containing particles.[36] Neurologic signs, including behavioral changes, seizures, blindness, and ataxia usually develop after acute, high-level lead exposure.[36] In cats gastrointestinal signs (e.g., vomiting, anorexia, abdominal pain, constipation, and megaesophagus) are more common than neurologic signs. The diagnosis of lead poisoning can be confirmed by measuring a blood lead level greater than 0.22 ppm.[36]

Although numerous other toxins have the potential to affect the nervous system in cats, a complete discussion is beyond the scope of this chapter; the reader is referred elsewhere for an excellent review of veterinary toxicology.[103]

Vascular Encephalopathies

Cerebrovascular Accidents

Cerebrovascular accidents (CVAs) are becoming recognized in veterinary medicine with increasing frequency because of the greater availability of MRI. CVAs can be divided into two broad categories: ischemic stroke, in which a vessel is occluded by thrombus or vasospasm, and hemorrhagic stroke, which arises from rupture of blood vessels into CNS parenchyma or subarachnoid space.[45] The incidence of CVA in cats is unknown, insofar as the majority of reports in the veterinary literature are based on canine studies. Risk factors include hyperfibrinogenemia, polycythemia, coagulopathies, neoplasia (e.g., intravascular lymphoma), hypertension, multiple myeloma, cardiac disease, infectious diseases (e.g., FIP), renal disease, vasculitis, and others.[45,53,55] Postanesthetic cerebellar ischemia has been reported in Persian cats after anesthesia with ketamine.[116]

Clinical signs reflect the location and extent of the affected area and are usually acute in onset and asymmetric, with minimal progression after the first 24 hours. The cerebellum is the most common site for vascular accidents to occur,[19,34] but the cerebral hemispheres and thalamus are also frequently affected. A minimum database in any cat with suspected brain infarction should include a complete blood count, chemistry panel, FeLV and FIV testing, urinalysis, thyroid panel if applicable, coagulation profile if applicable, multiple blood pressure measurements, electrocardiogram, and possible thoracic radiographs and abdominal ultrasound. If cardiomyopathy is suspected, echocardiography should also be performed. Definitive diagnosis requires advanced imaging of the brain, with MRI considered the superior modality for detecting intracranial infarction (Figure 27-11). Findings may vary depending on the amount of time that has elapsed between the onset of the stroke and performance of imaging. Typical abnormalities noted on MRI include a focal, sharply demarcated lesion that is hyperintense on T2 and FLAIR images, hypointense on T1, with a discrete cutoff between normal and abnormal tissue. Mass effect or midline shifting is usually not seen, and there is minimal, if any, contrast enhancement.

There is no specific treatment for vascular accidents in most feline patients, and care must be taken to try to identify and correct an underlying cause. Acutely, supportive care, especially when signs are severe, is aimed at maintaining perfusion to the brain through judicious use of intravenous fluids and administration of oxygen. Mannitol (0.5 to 1 g/kg administered intravenously) may be indicated in the acute phase if cerebral edema is a concern, provided the cat is hemodynamically stable and electrolytes are normal. Corticosteroids have not been shown to play a role in the treatment of stroke and in fact may exacerbate oxidative damage to the brain. Prognosis depends on a number of factors, including underlying cause, severity of clinical signs, and the extent of the lesion, but the majority of patients will improve over a period of days to weeks.

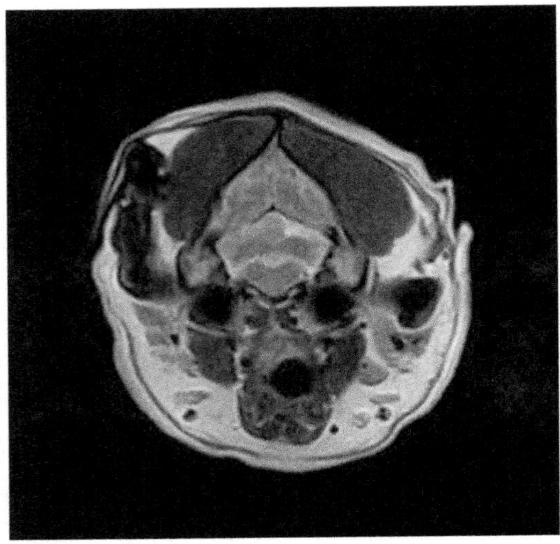

FIGURE 27-11 T2-axial magnetic resonance imaging of a brain infarct. Note the sharply delineated borders and wedge shape. *(Courtesy Dr. Boaz Levitin, NYC Veterinary Specialists.)*

Feline Ischemic Encephalopathy

A unique vascular disorder of the CNS, feline ischemic encephalopathy is well described in cats and thought to be related to *Cuterebra* larvae myasis.[34,47] Affected cats typically have access to the outdoors and present in summer and early fall with unilateral prosencephalic signs, including progressive seizures, behavioral changes (often aggression), blindness, and depression. In some cases neurologic signs are preceded by signs of upper respiratory disease, including sneezing.[47] Abnormal rectal temperatures, either hyperthermia or hypothermia, were noted.[47]

Neither routine hematology nor CSF analysis is specific for this disorder. MRI of the brain (Figure 27-12) may show parasitic track lesions, as well as cerebrocortical degeneration caused by toxin release by the parasite.[34] Grossly, marked atrophy of the affected cerebral hemisphere can be apparent (Figure 27-13). Vasospasm secondary to release of toxin produced by the parasite results in infarction in the region perfused by the middle cerebral artery or its branches.[34]

Histologic findings include parasitic track lesions, superficial laminar cerebrocortical necrosis, cerebral infarction, subependymal rarefaction, and subpial astrogliosis.[146] Larvae are most commonly found in the olfactory bulbs and peduncles, optic nerves, and cribriform plate, suggesting entry from the nasal cavity.[146]

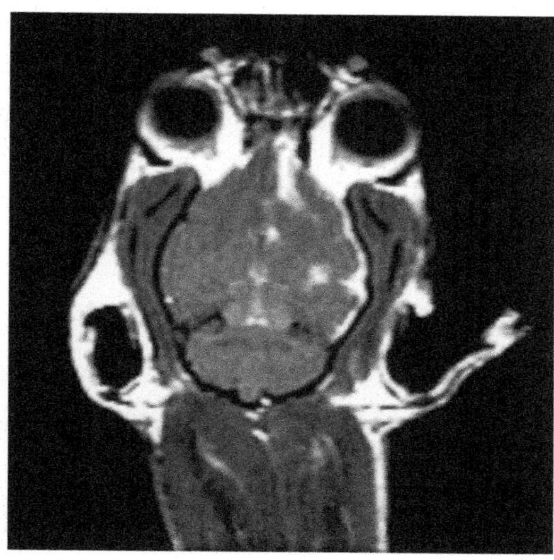

FIGURE 27-12 T1 postcontrast magnetic resonance imaging (coronal) of a cat with feline ischemic encephalopathy. Contrast uptake associated with necrosis caused by the parasite is seen in the olfactory and prefrontal lobe on the right. *(Reprinted with permission from DeLahunta A, Glass R:* Veterinary neuroanatomy and clinical neurology, *St Louis, 2009, Saunders.)*

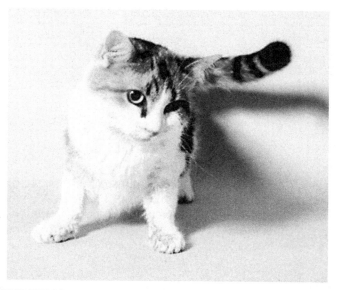

FIGURE 27-14 Kitten with left head tilt secondary to otitis media-interna. *(Reprinted with permission from DeLahunta A, Glass R:* Veterinary neuroanatomy and clinical neurology, *St Louis, 2009, Saunders.)*

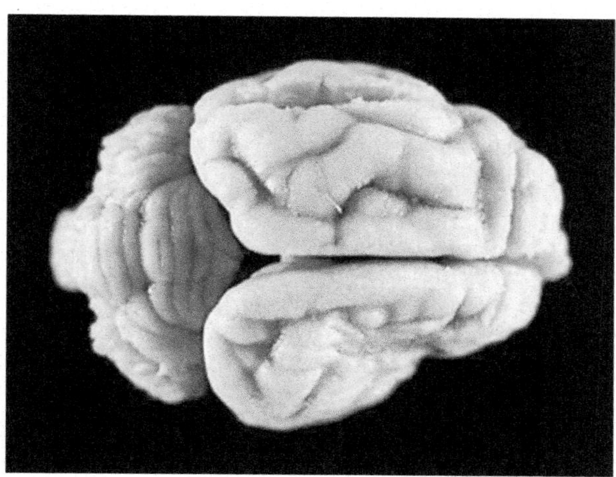

FIGURE 27-13 Gross specimen of a cat with feline ischemic encephalopathy. Atrophy is evident in the affected hemisphere *(left)* in the distribution of the middle cerebral artery. *(Reprinted with permission from DeLahunta A, Glass R:* Veterinary neuroanatomy and clinical neurology, *St Louis, 2009, Saunders.)*

Treatment options are extremely limited, and most cats are euthanized because of severe neurologic impairment and aggression.

PERIPHERAL VESTIBULAR DISEASES

The vestibular system is responsible for maintaining the position of the eyes, neck, trunk, and limbs relative to the position of the head in space.[34] Dysfunction of the vestibular system results in dramatic clinical presentations, including head tilt (Figure 27-14), nystagmus, falling, vomiting, rolling, wide-based stance, loss of equilibrium, and vestibular quality ataxia.[34] It is of key importance that the clinician recognizes whether the signs are due to peripheral or central disturbances of the vestibular system; this is primarily ascertained with a thorough neurologic examination and history (Table 27-2). The presence of a head tilt and vestibular-quality ataxia can be seen with either peripheral or central disease; however, paresis, spasticity, hypermetria, or postural deficits are suggestive of a central lesion. Likewise, horizontal or rotary nystagmus with the fast phase opposite the side of the lesion can be seen in both central and peripheral disease, but vertical nystagmus is typically seen with central disease. Nystagmus with a fast phase directed toward the side of the lesion or that changes with changing position of the head is consistent with a central lesion.[34] The presence of cranial nerve abnormalities (other than VII) is also more common with central lesions, whereas Horner's syndrome is more often seen with peripheral dysfunction. Bilateral peripheral vestibular disease is characterized by a crouched gait, wide head excursions, absent oculocephalic reflex, and a wide-based stance.[34] It should be noted that blue-eyed cats often have a resting pendular nystagmus because of the larger portions of axons of the optic nerve crossing in the chiasm compared with normal animals. This is of no clinical significance and occurs in the absence of other vestibular signs.[34]

There are myriad causes of vestibular signs in cats, but this section covers only those affecting the peripheral vestibular system. Common causes of peripheral disease in cats include feline idiopathic peripheral vestibular disease, otitis media-interna (OMI), nasopharyngeal

TABLE 27-2 **Clinical Signs Associated with Central Versus Peripheral Vestibular Disease**

Central	Peripheral	Bilateral peripheral	Both central and vestibular
Paresis, spasticity, hypermetria, postural deficits, vertical nystagmus, nystagmus with a fast phase directed toward the side of the lesion or that changes with changing position of the head, cranial nerve abnormalities (other than VII)	Horner's syndrome Facial paralysis	Crouched gait, wide head excursions, absent oculocephalic reflex, wide-base stance	Head tilt, vestibular quality ataxia; horizontal or rotary nystagmus with the fast phase opposite the side of the lesion

polyps, neoplasia (e.g., ceruminous gland adenocarcinoma, squamous cell carcinoma), and toxicity. A review of disorders affecting the central vestibular system can be found in the preceding section on intracranial diseases.

Idiopathic Vestibular Disease

Idiopathic vestibular disease is the most common cause of peripheral signs in cats, accounting for 43% of cases of peripheral vestibular disease in one report.[96] Clinical signs are often severe, with rolling and rapid nystagmus quite evident. There is no sex or breed predilection, and the average age of affected cats is 4 years, although it may be seen in any age. Interestingly, there is a higher incidence of this disorder in summer and fall, suggesting an environmental or infectious cause. Prevalence is higher in certain regions of the United States, especially the Northeast.

Although usually acute and nonprogressive in nature, there have been some reports of clinical signs progressing for up to 3 weeks.[96] Signs resolve rapidly without definitive treatment, usually in the first week, although some patients may have a persistent head tilt.[96] Diagnosis is through excluding other known causes of peripheral vestibular disease; there is no definitive diagnostic testing, nor is there definitive treatment. Some cats may require fluid and antiemetic therapy if vomiting does not resolve the first day.

Nasopharyngeal Polyps

Nasopharyngeal polyps are non-neoplastic, inflammatory growths originating in the middle ear or auditory tube and may potentially lead to peripheral vestibular signs.[70] They are primarily seen in cats younger than 2 years of age, but reported cases range in age from 2 months to 15 years. In addition to head tilt, ataxia, and abnormal nystagmus, respiratory signs such as stertorous breathing, sneezing, nasal discharge, and upper airway obstruction may be evident. The cause is unknown, but chronic respiratory tract infection, chronic OMI, ascending infection from the nasopharynx, and congenital causes have all been proposed.[70] Drainage of middle ear secretions through the auditory tube may be blocked by the polyp, leading to otorrhea and a misdiagnosis of otitis externa.

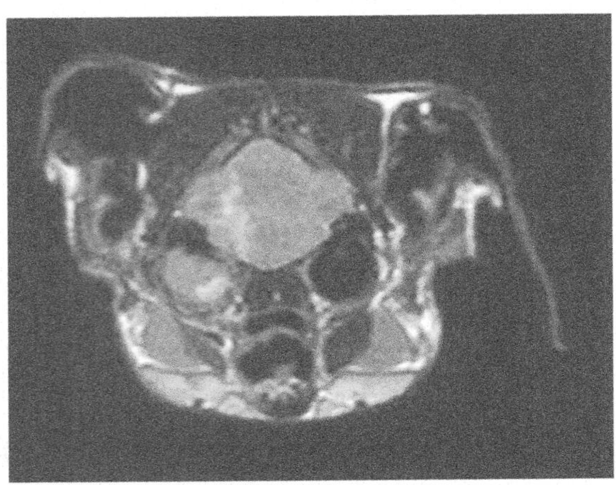

FIGURE 27-15 T1 postcontrast axial magnetic resonance imaging of cat with otogenic encephalopathy. Note the rim of contrast around the abscess in the left brain stem and cerebellum, as well as the mild contrast uptake and soft tissue density within the left bulla.

Otitis Media-Interna

OMI is one of the primary rule outs for cats with suspected nasopharyngeal polyps as the clinical signs may be identical. OMI may be associated with Horner's syndrome as well as facial nerve paralysis ipsilateral to the affected ear and can be accompanied by pain and signs of otitis externa. Remember that while a thorough otoscopic exam is indicated in all patients presenting with suspected peripheral vestibular dysfunction, the presence of an intact tympanic membrane does not exclude middle ear infection. While the most common etiologic agents in cats are bacterial (e.g., *Pseudomonas* spp., *Staphylococcus pseudointermedius*), *Cryptococcus* infection has also been implicated in a number cats with OMI and an index of suspicion should be raised in cats living in endemic areas.[8] Intracranial complications of OMI are well recognized and result from extension of organisms from the inner ear to the brainstem along the nerves and vessels of the internal acoustic meatus (Figure 27-15). This can result in severe, life-threatening disease requiring rapid surgical intervention and aggressive, long

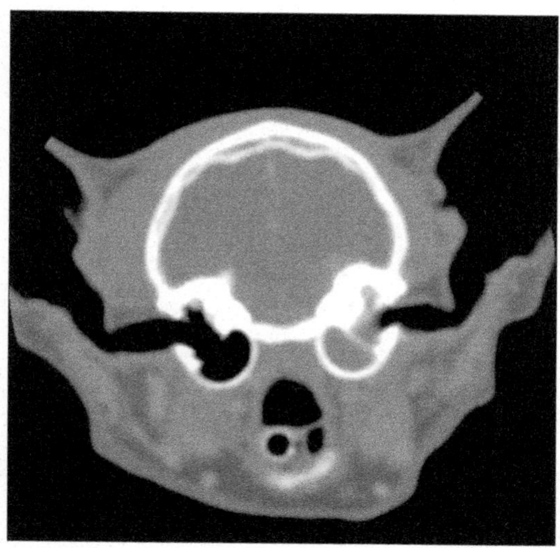

FIGURE 27-16 Computed tomography scan of a cat with unilateral otitis media-interna. There is mild sclerosis of the bony structures around the right bulla.

term medical management based on cultures obtained at the time of surgery.[131]

Malignant Tumors

Malignant tumors of the middle and inner ear occur uncommonly but also must be considered on the differential list of patients with peripheral vestibular signs, particularly in geriatric cats. Ceruminous gland adenocarcinoma and squamous cell carcinoma occur with equal frequency in cats and may be accompanied by obvious mass effect, aural discharge, pain, and pruritus.[147]

Diagnosis and Treatment of Peripheral Vestibular Disease

Definitive diagnosis of disease of the middle and inner ear may require advanced imaging in the form of CT or MRI (Figures 27-16, 27-17, and 27-18), insofar as plain radiography often results in false-negative results or underestimation of the extent of disease.[10] Imaging of the ear provides vital information about the extent of involvement, the possibility of bilateral disease, and integrity of adjacent structures and assists in ruling out concurrent lesions in the CNS. MRI can provide excellent detail of the structures of the cochlea and semicircular canals as well as the adjacent brain stem and is the imaging modality of choice at the author's institution. CT scanning may be preferable in cases in which the abnormality primarily involves bony structures.

Treatment depends on diagnosis, and in cases of nasopharyngeal polyps, ventral bulla osteotomy (VBO) combined with traction removal of the polyp is recommended.[70] Prognosis is excellent, although recurrence is possible.

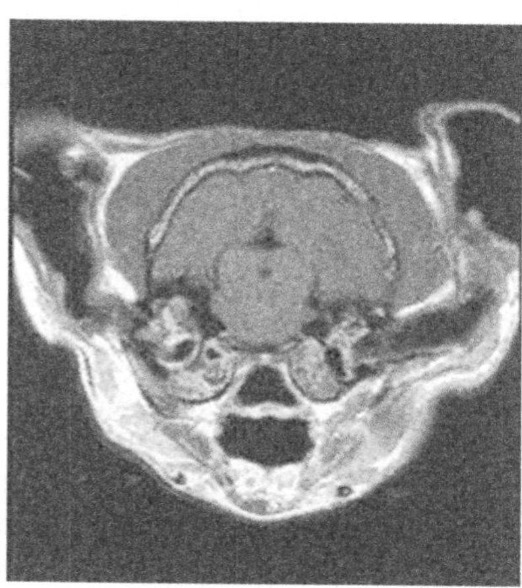

FIGURE 27-17 T1 postcontrast axial magnetic resonance imaging of cat with bilateral otitis media-interna. The bullae are expanded, and there is mild contrast uptake within the homogenous material in both bullae.

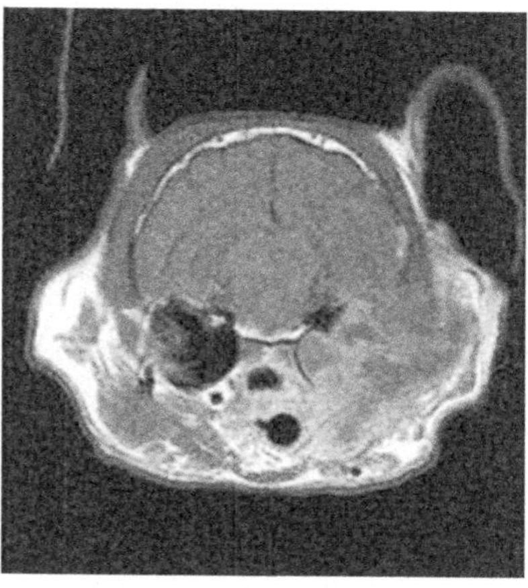

FIGURE 27-18 T1 postcontrast axial magnetic resonance imaging of cat with severe vestibular ataxia, head tilt, and facial paralysis. A mass obliterating the affected bulla and surrounding soft tissue structures is evident. Histopathology was consistent with ceruminous gland adenocarcinoma.

Newly diagnosed cases of OMI require antimicrobial therapy for a minimum of 4 to 6 weeks. Failure to respond to medical therapy or recurrence of OMI warrants surgical intervention (i.e., VBO and antimicrobials based on cultures obtained intraoperatively). Prognosis for malignancies of the ear is fair for ceruminous gland adenocarcinoma and guarded for squamous cell carcinoma after aggressive ear ablation and bulla osteotomy, provided there is no intracranial involvement or lymphatic or vascular invasion.[147]

MYELOPATHIES

Feline myelopathies encompass a wide range of diseases and often present a challenge to the clinician, both with respect to attaining a neuroanatomic diagnosis as well as creating a reasonable list of differential diagnoses. Common cardiovascular and orthopedic conditions can mimic disorders of the spine, making decisions regarding appropriate diagnostic testing particularly taxing. A thorough neurologic assessment is necessary to determine lesion location, with careful attention paid to gait, postural responses, and segmental reflexes. Although many feline patients are reluctant to walk in the clinical setting, the provision of adequate space, a quiet setting, and nonslippery flooring may facilitate the examination. The unique temperament of many cats, difficulty with gait evaluation in this species, and the fact that many live outdoors and thus are less closely observed than other species further impede the assessment of feline patients. Additionally, most of the literature regarding feline myelopathies is based on single cases or small group case reports. Although a description of all spinal disorders is beyond the scope of this chapter, a brief overview of some of the most clinically relevant disorders is presented.

Typically, if the cervical spine is affected, tetraparesis and ataxia are evident, with delayed postural responses in all four limbs. Cats with lesions located between C1 and C5 will show an upper motor neuron/general proprioceptive (UMN/GP) ataxia in all four limbs, whereas those with a C6-T2 myelopathy may have a short-strided gait with decreased tone and segmental reflexes in the thoracic limbs. Those with a lesion between T3 and L3 will have normal thoracic limbs with paraparesis or paraplegia and, if ambulatory, UMN/GP ataxia in the pelvic limbs. Reflexes in the pelvic limbs will be normal to increased, and postural responses may be delayed. Lesions located between L4 and S3 will result in paraparesis/paraplegia, a short-strided gait, postural deficits, decreased tone and reflexes, decreased perineal reflexes, fecal or urinary incontinence (or both), and poor tail tone.

Degenerative Myelopathies

Intervertebral Disk Disease

Although extremely well documented in the veterinary literature in dogs, intervertebral disk disease (IVDD) in cats has been reported only sporadically, with the incidence ranging from 0.02% to 0.12%, compared with dogs, in which the incidence is as high as 2.3%.[56,92] Although IVDD is clearly less common in the clinical setting in cats than in dogs, necropsy evaluations have revealed that disk extrusion, protrusion, and rupture are commonly found, generally in middle-aged to older cats in all segments of the spine. When clinically significant IVDD is found in cats, it typically affects the thoracolumbar spine, with one study showing a peak incidence at L4-5 (Figure 27-19).[92] Any age, breed, or sex may be affected, although purebreds appear to be overrepresented and account for approximately 38% of reported cases.

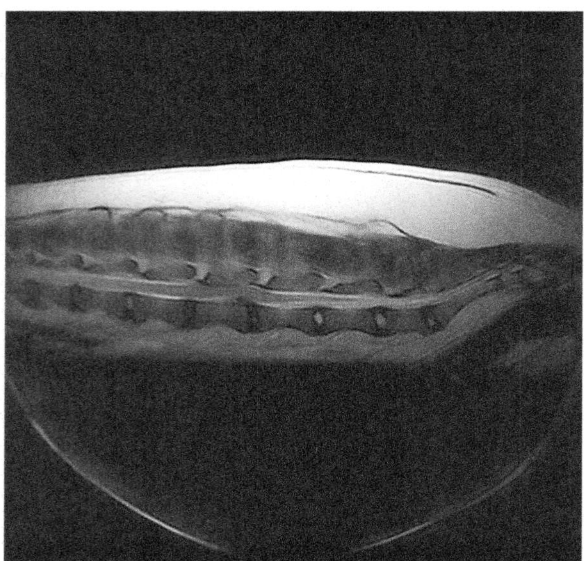

FIGURE 27-19 Sagittal magnetic resonance imaging of the lumbar spine of an acutely paraparetic cat. A degenerate disk with moderate compression of the overlying spinal cord is seen at L4-5.

BOX 27-2

Grading Clinical Signs Caused by Spinal Cord Lesions

- Grade 5: Normal strength and coordination
- Grade 4: Readily stands and walks with minimal paraparesis and ataxia
- Grade 3: Able to stand to walk unassisted but with difficulty; often stumbles and falls but can walk; mild to moderate paraparesis and ataxia
- Grade 2: Unable to stand unassisted; when assisted, able to move the pelvic limbs but constantly stumbles and often falls; moderate to severe paraparesis and ataxia
- Grade 1: Unable to stand unassisted; when assisted, only slight pelvic limb movements; severe paraparesis and ataxia
- Grade 0: Unable to stand unassisted; when assisted, complete absence of any pelvic limb movements, paraplegia

From DeLahunta A, Glass R: *Veterinary neuroanatomy and clinical neurology*, St Louis, 2009, Saunders.

Clinical signs are variable and can include spinal hyperesthesia alone, mild paraparesis, ataxia, paraplegia, urinary or fecal incontinence (or both), and loss of tail or anal tone (Box 27-2). The thoracolumbar spine is typically affected. Involvement of the cervical spinal cord is extremely rare, and to the author's knowledge there is only one case of a surgically treated cervical disk

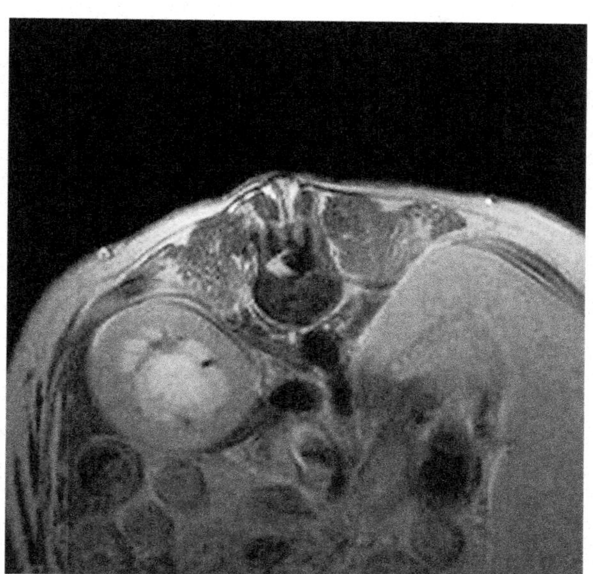

FIGURE 27-20 Axial MRI of a traumatic disc rupture. Note the compression and deviation of the spinal cord by calcified disc material.

in a cat, which succumbed to respiratory arrest several days after a ventral slot at C2-3.[85]

Diagnostic testing can include CT scan or MRI, and most frequently will reveal a single extradural compressive lesion (Figure 27-20). MRI may also reveal loss of the normal signal from the nucleus pulposus of the intervertebral disk, narrowing of the ventral subarachnoid space, and displacement of the spinal cord or epidural fat. With increasing availability of advanced imaging modalities, myelography is becoming less commonly used, but it still remains a viable means of diagnosing this disorder. Plain radiographs are of little value in definitively diagnosing IVDD but may help rule out other causes of myelopathy, such as fracture or osteosarcoma.

As with dogs, treatment options can be tailored to the individual patient depending on clinical signs and owner preference. Conservative management in the form of strict rest, corticosteroids, pain management, and bladder care can be a viable treatment option, especially in patients still able to ambulate. However, recurrence rates with conservative care alone are significantly higher than with surgical management, and gait, bladder, and bowel deficits may persist. Surgical treatment includes hemilaminectomy, dorsal laminectomy, and fenestration, with the majority of reports limited to cases of thoracolumbar IVDD. In a study of thoracolumbar IVDD in 10 cats, all patients undergoing surgical intervention were judged to have an excellent outcome,[92] whereas in another study five of six cats undergoing hemilaminectomy responded favorably, having good to excellent postoperative recovery.[66]

Other Degenerative Myelopathies

Other degenerative diseases of the spine are extremely rare in cats but include degenerative myelopathy, lysosomal storage diseases, and other inborn errors of metabolism. Degenerative myelopathy, typically seen in large-breed dogs such as the German Shepherd, has been reported in cats and follows a similar clinical course as that seen in canines. Signs are usually slowly progressive and limited to the pelvic limbs, with nonpainful UMN/GP ataxia and paraparesis evident. Bowel and bladder dysfunction may occur late in the course of the disease. The cause is unknown, but feline leukemia virus antigen has been isolated in the spinal cord lesions from some affected cats.[15] Inborn errors of metabolism, such as Niemann–Pick disease, neuroaxonal dystrophy, mucopolysaccharidosis, and other storage diseases, typically have a genetic basis and clinical signs become apparent at a young age.[30] Many of these disorders cause skeletal abnormalities, resulting in compressive spinal lesions, whereas others lead to vacuolation within neurons and glial cells with concomitant demyelination. There is no known treatment for these disorders.

Congenital and Developmental Anomalies

Anomalies of the spinal column are infrequently seen in cats and may go undiagnosed or be discovered only incidentally because many cause no clinical abnormalities. Because the embryologic development of the spine is closely related to development of other body systems, a thorough examination of the patient should be performed to assess viability. Although many spinal anomalies occur sporadically, the possibility of a genetic basis in potential breeding animals should be carefully considered. Animals with anomalies of the spinal cord will have clinical signs present from birth, whereas those with vertebral anomalies may not show evidence of a myelopathy until skeletally mature.

The Manx cat has been the subject of numerous reports of spinal anomalies because of its caudal vertebral aplasia specifically selected for in breeding programs. The trait is inherited as an autosomal dominant gene and in the homozygous state is lethal, whereas variable expression is seen in heterozygotes.[34] Associated with this anomaly is a high incidence of sacrocaudal spina bifida and meningoceles; meningomyeloceles; and myelodysplasia of the caudal lumbar, sacral, and caudal segments.[30] Specifically, spina bifida involves failure of the dorsal elements of the vertebrae to form during development and may occur alone in the absence of other clinical signs (spina bifida occulta). Spina bifida may occur in conjunction with meningocele (protrusion of meninges and CSF outside the vertebral canal) or meningomyelocele (protrusion of meninges, CSF, and neural tissue outside the vertebral canal) (Figure 27-21).

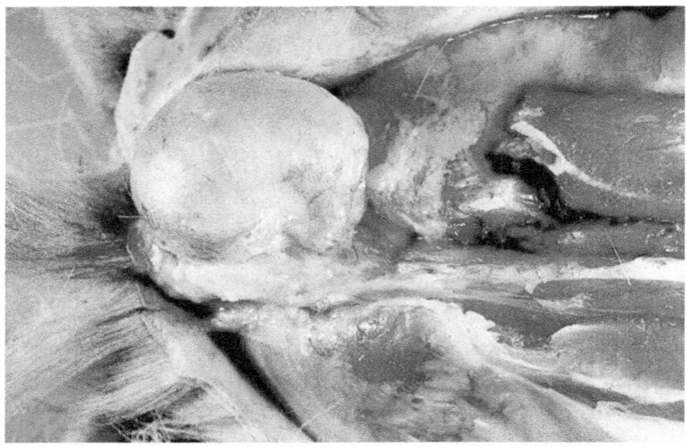

FIGURE 27-21 Necropsy of Manx cat, showing cerebrospinal fluid–distended meningomyelocele. *(Reprinted with permission from DeLahunta A, Glass R:* Veterinary neuroanatomy and clinical neurology, *St Louis, 2009, Saunders.)*

These are often associated with myelodysplasia, including hydromyelia, syringomyelia, and abnormal gray matter differentiation.[34] All these abnormalities could easily be avoided by selecting for Manx cats with normally developed tails. For humane reasons Manx breeders should be strongly encouraged by veterinarians to stop such unethical practices with known deleterious effects.

Clinical findings in Manx and similarly affected cats include abnormal hair growth or dimpling of the skin over the affected spinal segment, an open tract draining CSF, urinary or fecal incontinence (or both), depressed or absent tone and reflexes in the anus and perineum, a "bunny-hopping" gait, and paresis or paralysis. Severely affected animals are usually euthanized, and less severely affected animals may succumb to infections or pyelonephritis. Treatment options are extremely limited and focus on palliative care and bladder management.

Multiple cartilaginous exostosis occurs in younger cats and originates from the perichondrium of flat bones such as ribs, skull, scapulae, and vertebrae.[59] The nodules are composed of cartilaginous tissue with a bony component and arise from the growth plates. Malignant transformation has been documented. Clinical signs reflect the affected spinal segment, but involvement of the thoracic spine is most common. Radiographically, lesions within the canal may be difficult to visualize, but those on the projecting processes or lamina can be identified with conventional radiography.[2] Myelography, CT scanning, or MRI is necessary to assess the extent of the lesion (or lesions) and for surgical planning. Prognosis after surgery depends on the severity of clinical signs and whether multiple sites are affected.

Other less common anomalies are sporadically reported, usually as single cases. A retrospective study of 200 cats revealed abnormalities in 46 patients, including block vertebrae, transitional vertebrae, and extra ribs.[97] Syringomyelia has also been described and was seen in one kitten in conjunction with hydrocephalus after parvoviral infection. Spinal arachnoid cyst, spinal dermoid sinus, atlantoaxial malformation, hemivertebrae, inborn errors of skeletal growth, and others have also been documented in the veterinary literature.

Metabolic and Nutritional Myelopathies

Metabolic and nutritional myelopathies are rarely reported in cats, with hypervitaminosis A perhaps being the most well described. Cats fed a diet with high levels of vitamin A, such as raw liver, are at risk, and clinical signs result from bony proliferation related to synovial joints.[34,106] Lesions are often confined to the cervical spine and lead to spinal hyperpathia, tetraparesis, cervical rigidity, Horner's syndrome, palpable bony masses over the cervical region, lethargy, and weight loss. Lesions can be seen on plain radiographs and consist of multiple exostosis and possible fusion of the spine. Prognosis is extremely guarded, but dietary adjustments may slow disease progression. Other osteodystrophies of suspected nutritional etiology have been reported, as have lesions in the gray matter of the cervical cord in a cat with an extrahepatic shunt.[84]

Inflammatory and Infectious Myelopathies

Infectious meningomyelitis has been identified as an important cause of myelopathy in feline patients, representing 32% of cases of spinal cord disease in 208 specimens submitted for histopathologic evaluation.[84] The majority of cases will occur in cats younger than 2 years of age with clinical signs present for less than 30 days.[84] Unlike other myelopathies, infectious and inflammatory disease most often affects the cervical spinal cord, perhaps because of extension of inflammatory disease in the brain, insofar as they are often seen in conjunction with intracranial lesions. Although many infectious diseases have the potential to affect the spine, FIP is at the top of the differential list.

Lesions of FIP consist of pyogranulomatous inflammation of the meninges and ependymal cells, spongy degeneration, malacia, and syringomyelia.[132] Concurrent intracranial signs (e.g., ataxia, seizures) and weight loss, fever, chorioretinitis, and anorexia often accompany the signs of spinal cord dysfunction (e.g., paraparesis, tetraparesis, spinal hyperesthesia). Prognosis is extremely grave. A more comprehensive discussion of FIP is available in the section on encephalopathies.

Other infectious diseases of the spine are seen sporadically and agents include *Cryptococcus, Toxoplasma,* bacterial meningomyelitis, *Coccidioides, Histoplasma,* FIV, rabies, BDV, and others. A FeLV-associated myelopathy was reported in 16 cats with signs consisting of abnormal vocalization, hyperesthesia, and paresis progressing to paralysis.[15] The clinical course involved gradually progressive neurologic dysfunction resulting in euthanasia. Microscopically, white-matter degeneration with dilation of myelin sheaths and swollen axons was identified in the spinal cord and brain stem of affected animals. Neither neoplastic nor hematologic diseases commonly associated with FeLV infection were present.[15]

Noninfectious inflammatory conditions of the spine include idiopathic poliomyelitis and eosinophilic meningomyelitis and can be difficult to distinguish from other forms of myelitis in the absence of additional clinical signs. Because history, clinical signs, and neurologic examination findings can be virtually identical in all of these disorders, the clinician must rely on concurrent systemic signs, potential exposure to an infectious agent, serology, and risk of exposure (e.g., geographical location).

Advanced imaging such as CT scan or MRI should be recommended when attempting to distinguish inflammatory myelopathies from other spinal disorders. However, although these tests are highly sensitive, they are not specific to the etiologic agent responsible for any inflammatory changes that may be evident.

Treatment is aimed at the underlying cause and may include antibiotics, antifungal agents, bladder management, pain control, and corticosteroids. Although the use of corticosteroids in treating infectious diseases may raise concerns for immunosuppression, adjunctive corticosteroid administration in children and adults with bacterial meningitis reduces both morbidity and mortality, and studies suggest that results are best when corticosteroids are administered immediately before the onset of antibiotics. Surgical decompression may be indicated if a discrete compression of the spinal cord is present, such as may be seen with a fungal granuloma.[44] Prognosis is dictated by specific cause, response to medical management, and neurologic status but in general is extremely guarded.

Spinal Neoplasia

Tumors of the spine represent a wide variety of cancers and are classified as extradural, intradural-extramedullary, or intramedullary. Extradural tumors account for approximately 50% of cases, intradural-extramedullary tumors represent 35%, and intramedullary tumors represent 15%. They may arise from the vertebrae and surrounding soft tissues, meninges, or neuroparenchyma. In a retrospective study of 205 cats affected by spinal disease, 27% were affected by neoplasia, the majority (36%) being diagnosed with lymphosarcoma.[84] Clinical signs will reflect the segment of spinal cord affected, and care must be taken to do a complete examination to rule out involvement of the brain or other body systems.

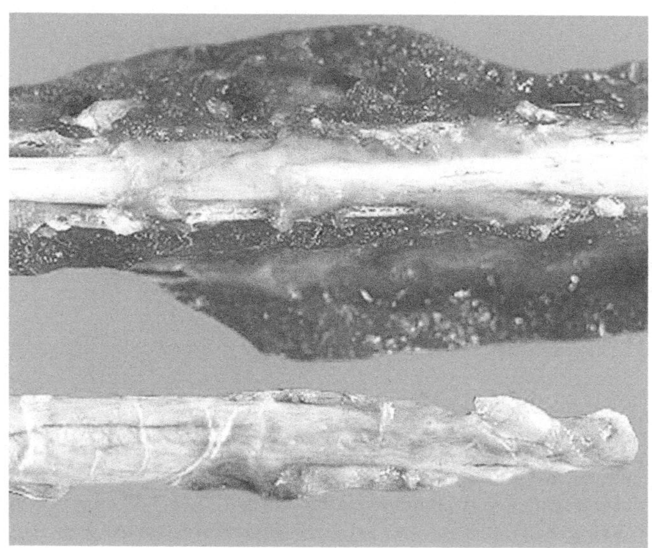

FIGURE 27-22 Feline epidural lymphoma. In the top specimen soft, gray-white neoplastic tissue invests the spinal cord. The bottom specimen depicts a similar lesion associated with portion of the spinal cord fixed and removed from the vertebral canal. *(Reprinted with permission from DeLahunta A: Degenerative diseases of the central nervous system. In Summers BA, Cummings JF, DeLahunta A, editors:* Veterinary neuropathology, *St Louis, 1995, Mosby, p 208.)*

Lymphoma, as previously mentioned, is the most common tumor affecting the spine of cats and is typically seen in a younger subset of patients (median age, 24 months) with a short duration of clinical signs (less than 7 days). Reported neurologic signs include spinal hyperesthesia, asymmetric postural deficits, paraparesis and paraplegia, ataxia, tetraparesis, lower motor neuron tail and/or bladder, upper motor neuron bladder, and lack of deep pain.[83] Nonspecific abnormalities, such as anorexia, lethargy, weight loss, renomegaly, chorioretinitis, and lymphadenopathy may also be found. There is an association with spinal lymphoma and FeLV infection, and in one report results of FeLV testing were positive in 84.2% (16 of 19) of cases with necropsy confirmation of spinal lymphoma.[129] Spinal lymphoma has also been found to be associated with FIV.[7] Extraneural lymphoma is commonly found in affected patients, with the most common locations being bone marrow and kidneys followed by liver, skeletal muscle, spleen, lymph nodes, vertebrae, and heart.[83,142] The majority of clinical cases are located in the thoracolumbar spine and are most frequently reported to be extradural (Figure 27-22). However, histopathologic examination of 33 cats revealed 87.9% to have both intradural and extradural components, with 42.9% of cats examined having concurrent lymphoma in the brain.[83]

Diagnosis of spinal lymphoma requires a high index of suspicion and careful attention to involvement of other body systems. Hematologic abnormalities are frequently found and include anemia, leukopenia,

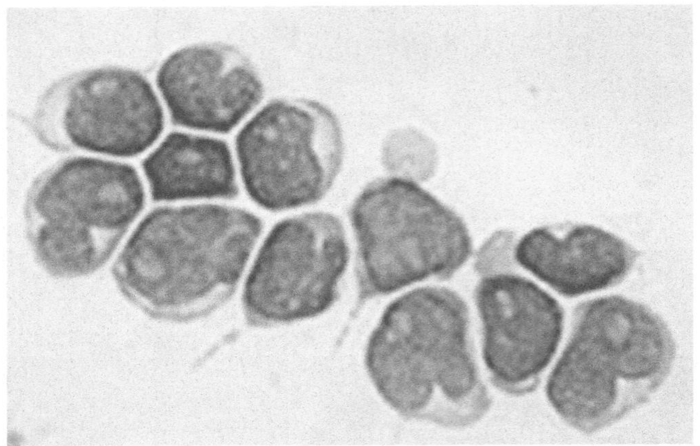

FIGURE 27-23 Large lymphoid cells with dispersed chromatin, prominent nucleoli, and scant cytoplasm in the cerebrospinal fluid of a cat with spinal lymphoma.

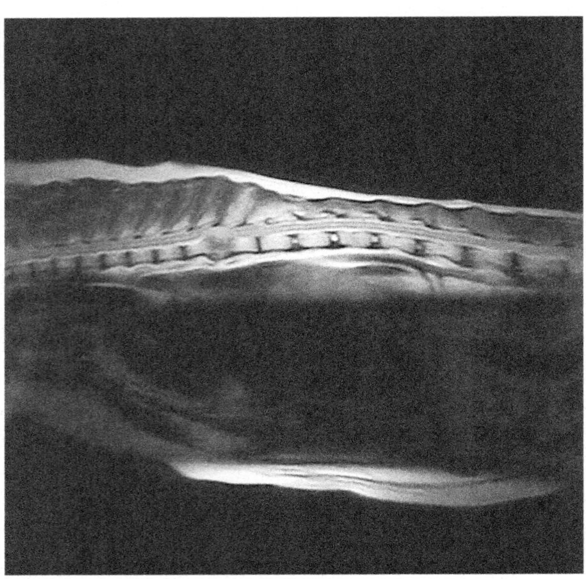

FIGURE 27-24 Magnetic resonance imaging of the spine showing an extraaxial mass lesion in a cat with progressive paraparesis and spinal hyperesthesia.

thrombocytopenia, and circulating lymphoblasts. Bone marrow involvement is also seen in more than 68% of cases, with the lymphoma being high-grade lymphoblastic or immunoblastic in all cats.[129] A careful fundic examination, three-view thoracic radiographs, lymph node aspirates if lymphadenopathy is evident, and abdominal ultrasonography are all warranted.

A positive FeLV test raises the index of suspicion for spinal lymphoma, but confirmatory neurodiagnostics are warranted and may include myelography, CT scan, MRI, and CSF analysis. Myelography generally is abnormal, but lesion location (e.g., intramedullary versus extramedullary) may not always be delineated on the basis of this modality alone, and the presence of an extradural lesion does not distinguish lymphoma from other tumor types. CT in combination with myelography is likely to provide greater detail regarding the extent and location of the lesion, whereas MRI increases the ability to visualize the spinal cord and surrounding structures in a less invasive manner. Plain radiographs of the vertebral column are of little value in attaining a diagnosis, with bony lysis being detected very infrequently.[83]

CSF collected from the lumbar spine may show elevated protein and white blood cells, predominantly lymphocytes, although abnormal CSF is seen more commonly in dogs because of their higher incidence of leptomeningeal involvement. Occasionally, lymphoblasts (Figure 27-23) can be seen, and in one report neoplastic lymphocytes were identified on CSF analysis in 6 of 17 cats evaluated.[72]

Treatment options depend on tumor location, histologic grade, extent of CNS involvement, and whether multicentric disease is present. Chemotherapy, either alone or in combination with other modalities, has been shown to be beneficial. In one study of cats treated with cyclophosphamide, vincristine, and prednisone, complete remission was attained in 50% of cases, with a median duration of remission of 14 weeks.[129] Surgery in the form of hemilaminectomy or dorsal laminectomy may allow complete removal or cytoreduction of the tumor in some cases, alleviating pain and paresis and providing samples for histologic analysis. When this is combined with chemotherapy, prolonged remission of up to 62 weeks after surgery has been reported.[129] However, it may not be advisable if intramedullary lesions are present or multiple levels of the spinal cord are involved. Radiation can be used in combination with chemotherapy or surgery (or both) because the spinal cord seems to be relatively resistant to the acute effects of radiation. Long-term prognosis is extremely guarded, despite the greater availability of treatment options and advanced neurosurgical techniques.

Other neoplasms of the spine are rare but include meningioma, osteosarcoma, glioma, malignant nerve sheath neoplasm, meningeal sarcoma, and lipoma (Figure 27-24).[78,84,111] Median age is typically much higher than in cats with lymphoma (median 12 years), and the clinical course is more protracted because of the slow-growing nature of many of these tumors. Osteosarcoma and meningioma appear to be the most common malignant and benign tumors, respectively,[111] and accounted for 24% of cases reported in a large retrospective study.[83] As with lymphoma, clinical signs reflect the neuroanatomic location, with the most common clinical signs being pain and paraparesis or paraplegia. Unlike lymphoma, conventional radiography can be a useful initial diagnostic tool. Eight of nine cats with confirmed osteosarcoma had bony lysis, and lytic lesions were detected in 14 of 18 cats with other nonlymphoid spinal neoplasms.[83] Vertebral bodies and dorsal lamina are more frequently affected than the dorsal or transverse processes. Additional radiographic signs that may help with antemortem diagnosis include widening of the intervertebral foramen, expansion of the vertebral canal, thinning of the bone, or pathologic fractures. Advanced imaging is indicated even when a lesion is identified on radiography for the purpose of further defining the extent of the lesion and for surgical planning. MRI is considered the superior modality for its excellent anatomic detail and three-dimensional capabilities.

Only a few reports in the veterinary literature address treatment and long-term prognosis in cats with nonlymphoid spinal tumors.[78,111] Resectability and severity of clinical signs dictate treatment plan, with the primary goal to relieve spinal cord compression, either through surgical management or the use of glucocorticoids. Although surgical intervention may not always achieve complete resection of the mass, cytoreduction will alleviate clinical signs and allow for histopathologic confirmation of tumor type. In a retrospective study of 26 cats undergoing surgery alone for nonlymphoid vertebral and spinal cord neoplasms, the median survival times for malignant (e.g., osteosarcoma) and benign (e.g., meningioma) tumors were 110.5 and 518 days, respectively.[111] In another report one cat with meningioma was alive 1400 days postoperatively, and another was alive 2190 days after resection of a nerve sheath neoplasm.[78] Overall, it appears that surgical treatment, even when complete resection is not possible, will palliate clinical signs and may result in sustained quality of life. Data regarding radiation and chemotherapy are lacking in these feline patients, but studies in dogs suggest that one or both of these modalities may prolong MST in some cases.

Spinal Trauma

Many feline patients have access to the outdoors, and thus vehicular accidents and other forms of external trauma to the spine are a common occurrence. Fractures, traumatic disk rupture (discussed previously), luxation, nerve root avulsion, and contusion to the spinal cord are not uncommon. Secondary effects include ischemia, hemorrhage, decreased perfusion, and edema and may have greater potential to damage nervous tissue than the inciting injury.[73] The craniocervical, cervicothoracic, thoracolumbar, and lumbosacral junctions appear particularly susceptible to the effects of external trauma,[73] but in one report the thoracic and lumbosacral regions were overrepresented.[84] Careful physical examination is warranted before any neurodiagnostic testing because many of these patients have sustained injuries of the thoracic, abdominal, or pelvic viscera and require immediate stabilization. Concurrent orthopedic injuries are also quite common.

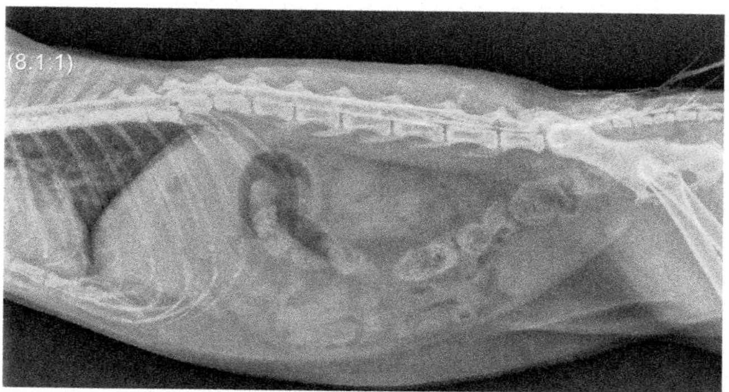

FIGURE 27-25 Myelogram of a cat after being hit by a car. Note the luxation and attenuation of contrast medium at T12-13.

Confirmatory testing begins with conventional radiography and may require sedation, anesthesia, or both. However, the potential for iatrogenic potentiation of spinal trauma exists during handling and positioning of the anesthetized patient, and extreme care must be exercised as such. Complete vertebral radiographs should be taken because a second fracture of the spine is seen in up to 20% of cases.[73] Advanced imaging in the form of myelography (Figure 27-25), CT scan, or MRI provides additional information regarding the extent of the injury and may assist in surgical planning and for prognostic purposes.

There is considerable controversy regarding the appropriate treatment of spinal fractures in veterinary medicine, but most practitioners agree that the therapeutic plan must be dictated by the patient's neurologic status. Cats with mild signs such as minor pain, ambulatory paresis, motor deficits, and stable fractures are good candidates for attempting medical management. However, early decompressive surgery may be associated with a more favorable outcome and is considered the best option for animals with unstable fractures, unrelenting pain, severe paresis or paraplegia, or progressive signs. In human studies early surgical intervention reduced complications, length of hospital stay, and cost of care in patients with traumatic spinal injury.[69] Additionally, early decompression alleviates the compression and thus decreases the cascade of secondary events.[69]

Routine use of corticosteroids has fallen out of favor in recent years for a number of reasons. Dexamethasone, once considered the drug of choice for initial treatment in spinal injuries, has not been shown to inhibit the secondary detrimental effects of trauma on the CNS and is associated with a greater incidence of adverse effects in veterinary patients. Experimental studies in animals suggest that only soluble glucocorticoids (e.g., methylprednisolone sodium succinate) given within 8 hours of injury are of benefit,[102] but adverse effects are common and include gastrointestinal hemorrhage, vomiting, diarrhea, anorexia, and hypotension.

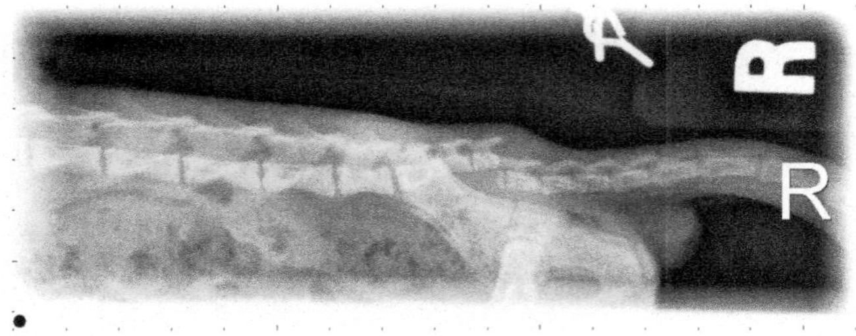

FIGURE 27-26 Radiograph of a kitten with coccygeal separation after having its tail caught in a door.

Supportive care in the form of pain control, bladder expression, physical therapy, appropriate bedding and housing, and management of concurrent injuries may be required in varying degrees. Clinicians and pet owners must be advised of the potentially significant financial and time investment necessary in caring for these patients. Prognosis depends on neurologic status but is considered extremely grave in animals that are paraplegic with loss of deep pain perception.

A unique clinical syndrome in cats results from sacrococcygeal or coccygeal separation (Figure 27-26), a sequela to abrupt pulling of the tail away from the body.[71] Laceration or avulsion of the nerves in the cauda equine leads to varying degrees of compromise to the tail, perineum, pelvic viscera, and pelvic limbs. Clinical signs can range from diminished motor function in the tail alone to signs as severe as complete loss of bowel, bladder, and tail function. Hyperesthesia at the base of the tail is common.[71] Treatment consists of pain control, prevention of urine scald, stool softeners, and bladder management.

The bladder may require manual evacuation if the patient is unable to empty it or if urethral spasm is occurring. Pharmacologic bladder care may include the use of bethanechol, a parasympathomimetic, at 1 to 2 mg/kg, administered orally every 8 hours, to facilitate bladder contraction, or phenoxybenzamine, an alpha-agonist, at 1 mg/kg, administered orally every 8 hours, to relieve urethral spasm. The use of bethanechol alone is strictly contraindicated if increased urethral tone is present because of the risk of bladder rupture.

Tail amputation may be necessary if ischemic necrosis, frequent soiling, or chronic pain is evident.[71] Prognosis may be quite good, especially in those cases with mild signs, but clients must be advised that if no improvement is seen within the first month, the outcome is less favorable.

Vascular Myelopathies

Spinal cord infarction (SCI) is becoming increasingly recognized in veterinary medicine as an important cause of acute myelopathy. Clinical signs are peracute in onset and typically nonprogressive, and the patient may be monoparetic/monoplegic, tetraparetic/tetraplegic, or paraparetic/paraplegic. Hyperesthesia is not common, although some reports suggest pain at the immediate onset of the infarction. The most well-documented type of SCI in veterinary medicine is fibrocartilaginous embolic myelopathy, in which fibrocartilaginous material derived from the nucleus pulposus gains access to the spinal vasculature.[34] The mechanism of action remains controversial, but intervertebral disk degeneration adjacent to the fibrocartilaginous embolic myelopathy is often seen.

Myelographic findings are typically normal, although mild swelling of the spinal cord at the affected site may be appreciated. MRI reveals an intramedullary lesion that is hyperintense on T2 weighting and isointense on T1 weighting with no contrast uptake.[90] Neutrophilic pleocytosis or cytoalbuminologic dissociation is reported in cases in which spinal fluid was analyzed.[1] Prognosis depends largely on severity of clinical signs, which reflect the degree of ischemic injury and necrosis of the spinal cord. Involvement of the gray matter in the cervical or lumbar intumescence is often associated with a less favorable outcome.[34] Many patients recover spontaneously, and those in which improvement is seen within the first week often will go on to make significant improvement.

Other causes of SCI include thromboembolism, hypercoagulable states, vasculopathy, and septic emboli.[95] An underlying cause should be thoroughly investigated whenever SCI is suspected. Diagnostic workup should include complete blood count, chemistry panel, urinalysis, FeLV and FIV serology, three-view thoracic radiographs, and thyroid panel if indicated. Hypertension has been seen secondary to renal disease in a cat with a cervical infarct,[34] so a careful retinal exam for evidence of hemorrhage, as well as blood pressure monitoring, is necessary in some cats. In a series of 13 cats with a diagnosis of SCI, 6 of 13 were found to be hypertensive and seven cats were found to have hypertrophic cardiomyopathy.[3a] Depending on physical examination and historical abnormalities, coagulation panel, abdominal ultrasound, CSF analysis, or echocardiography may be warranted. MRI is warranted to attain a definitive diagnosis and for prognostic purposes, insofar as the extent of the lesion as seen on MRI, as well as gray matter involvement, may influence outcome (Figure 27-27).

A syndrome of ischemic poliomyelomalacia has been described in cats after abdominal trauma or prolonged vasospasm or embolization of the lumbar arteries.[34] Cats typically present with severe neurologic deficits, including paraplegia, absent nociception in the pelvic limbs, absent tail and anal tone, and inability to void. A recent history of abdominal trauma or abdominal surgery is often reported, and clinical signs are acute in nature. Spinal fractures or evidence of external spinal trauma is

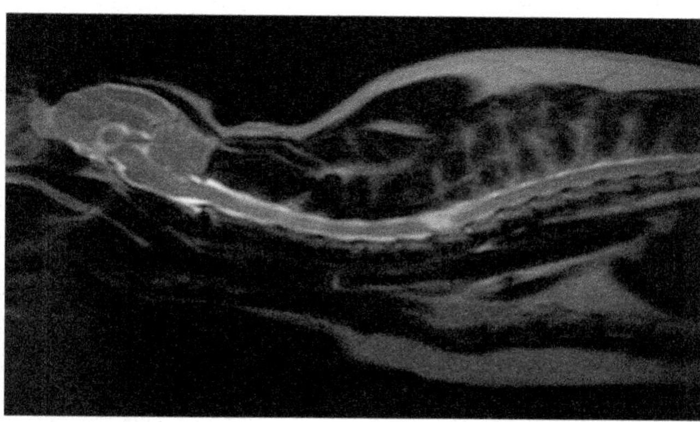

FIGURE 27-27 Sagittal magnetic resonance imaging of a cat with an infarction in the caudal cervical spine. Note the well-defined margins of the lesion, as well as the lack of mass effect. *(Courtesy Dr. Kerry Bailey, Oradell Animal Hospital.)*

lacking. Evidence of retroperitoneal hemorrhage and, in one cat, an avulsed kidney has been reported. Microscopically, the lesions consist of complete ischemic necrosis of both gray matter and white matter, and such findings have been reproduced experimentally by ligating the aorta at or cranial to the level of the renal arteries.[34] There is no known treatment, and prognosis is grave.

NEUROMUSCULAR DISEASES

Disorders of the motor unit are rare in cats and affect skeletal muscle, the neuromuscular junction, or the lower motor neuron. Weakness is the most salient clinical sign common to all these disorders and may vary considerably in severity and distribution, with signs including exercise intolerance, dysphagia, regurgitation, dysphonia, and difficulty jumping.[120] In addition to weakness, a striking sign often seen in cats is cervical ventroflexion (Figure 27-28), in which the patient is unable to lift the head and the chin rests at the level of the thoracic inlet.[75]

Diagnosis of neuromuscular disorders can be challenging, and a thorough neurologic examination, along with an accurate history, is imperative. A minimum database should include a complete blood count, chemistry panel (including creatine kinase levels), urinalysis, abdominal ultrasound, and possibly thyroid levels. Advanced neurodiagnostics may be indicated as well, including electrophysiologic testing (e.g., electromyogram [EMG], nerve conduction velocities) and nerve and muscle biopsy. This discussion focuses on some of the more common disorders of the motor unit, the diagnostic techniques necessary for making a diagnosis, and therapeutic approaches available for some of these diseases.

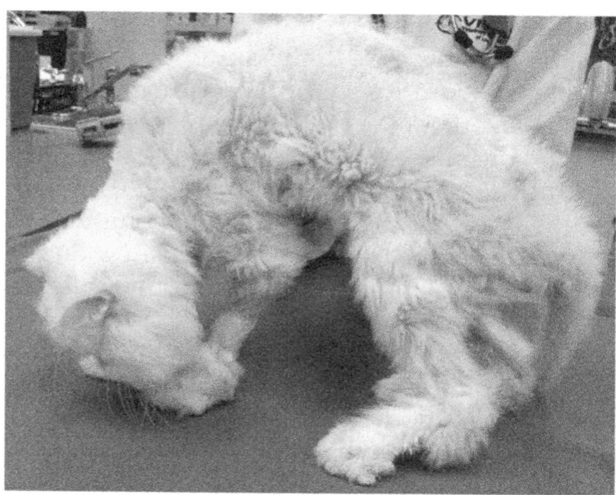

FIGURE 27-28 Severe weakness and cervical ventroflexion in a cat with end-stage renal disease and hypokalemia.

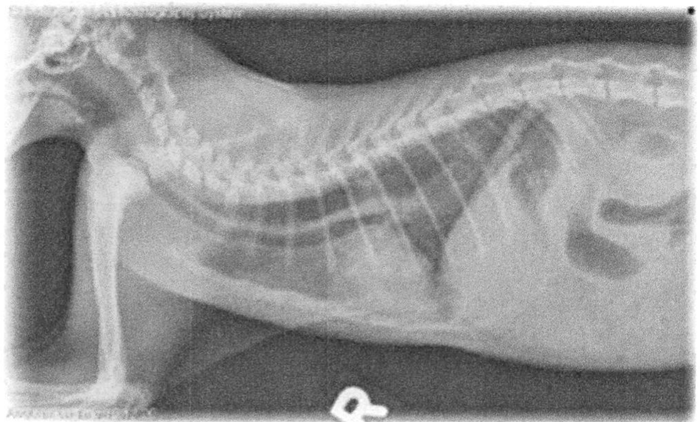

FIGURE 27-29 Thoracic radiograph of a myasthenic cat with megaesophagus and regurgitation.

Disorders of the Neuromuscular Junction

Myasthenia Gravis

Myasthenia gravis (MG) is a disorder of neuromuscular transmission resulting from a reduction in the number of acetylcholine receptors at the level of the neuromuscular junction. Acquired MG occurs when antibodies are produced against the acetylcholine receptors, leading to their destruction. Clinical signs may be difficult to distinguish from other neuromuscular disorders and may include generalized weakness and exercise intolerance, collapse, a short-strided gait, and weak palpebral reflexes. Focal signs, including megaesophagus (Figure 27-29) and dysphagia without signs of generalized weakness, may also be seen.[117] Abyssinians and the related Somalis are at the highest relative risk for MG, suggesting a genetic basis for this autoimmune disorder.[117] A form of acquired MG in cats has been associated with administration of methimazole,[119] with clinical signs developing 2 to 4 months after beginning treatment for hyperthyroidism. Congenital MG is extremely rare and can be diagnosed only through electrophysiologic testing and response to therapy.

The gold standard for confirming a diagnosis of MG is by documentation of antibodies against acetylcholine receptors by precipitation radioimmunoassay (available through the Comparative Neuromuscular Laboratory, University of California; http://vetneuromuscular.ucsd.edu). This assay is both highly sensitive and specific. Intravenous administration of edrophonium chloride may temporarily ameliorate clinical signs, but the response of cats to this drug is less reliable than that in dogs.[26] In addition to acetylcholine receptor antibody levels, the diagnostic workup should include thoracic radiographs, even in the absence of respiratory signs, on account of the high incidence of thymomas diagnosed in myasthenic cats as well as the potential for megaesophagus. In a retrospective report of 105 cases of acquired MG in cats, 27 of 105 (25.7%) were identified with thymoma. The incidence of megaesophagus is typically lower in cats with MG than it is in dogs because of the different distribution of skeletal muscle in the esophagus of the two species, but megaesophagus was still identified in 14.3% of myasthenic cats in the same study.[117]

The first line of therapy includes anticholinesterase drugs (pyridostigmine bromide starting at 0.5 mg/kg, administered orally every 12 hours), which help alleviate weakness by prolonging the action of acetylcholine at the neuromuscular junction. Cats may have a greater sensitivity than dogs to the side effects of this drug and may develop ptyalism, tremors, respiratory distress, vomiting, and diarrhea, especially at higher doses. If an optimal response to therapy is not seen or unacceptable side effects are observed, corticosteroids may be indicated but should be used with great caution, particularly in cats with megaesophagus. Immunosuppressive doses are not recommended because of the risk of aspiration pneumonia and the potential for corticosteroids to worsen muscle weakness.[122] Many cats will go into remission spontaneously after months of therapy, and monitoring acetylcholine receptor antibody levels every 3 months is useful in guiding medical management.

Disorders of Muscle

Muscle disorders are uncommonly identified in cats and can be divided into inflammatory and noninflammatory causes.[120] Noninflammatory myopathies are grouped into those that are primary and those that are secondary to diverse systemic illnesses. Inflammatory myopathies are divided into infectious and noninfectious causes and can appear similar to MG in presentation. The muscle biopsy is the most important diagnostic test for evaluation of muscle diseases[122] and must be performed before the institution of medical therapy (e.g., corticosteroids).

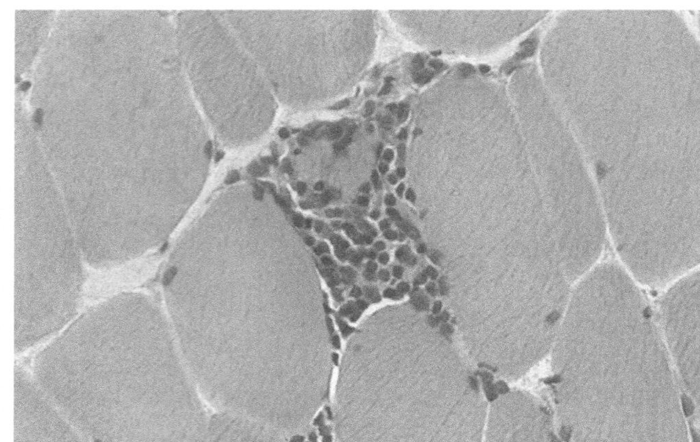

FIGURE 27-30 Muscle biopsy from a cat with polymyositis. Multifocal areas of lymphocytic infiltration are seen. No organisms were present within the biopsies. *(Courtesy Dr. Diane Shelton, Comparative Neuromuscular Laboratory, University of California.)*

Inflammatory Myopathies

Polymyositis is characterized by myalgia, exercise intolerance, myocarditis, dysphagia, muscle swelling or atrophy, and elevations in serum creatine kinase levels. The degree of elevation of creatine kinase is highly variable, however, and ultimately, a diagnosis of myositis depends on evaluation of muscle biopsy (Figure 27-30).[120] Additionally, serum CK levels can be significantly elevated in anorectic cats,[39] so blood results must be interpreted cautiously in light of the patient's recent nutritional history. Polymyositis can be further divided into either infectious or noninfectious causes (i.e., immune mediated or paraneoplastic). Immune-mediated polymyositis occurs sporadically in cats, but in a review of feline muscle biopsy specimens evaluated at the Comparative Neuromuscular Laboratory, University of California (http://vetneuromuscular.ucsd.edu), polymyositis in cats was most often secondary to infectious (FeLV, FIV) or paraneoplastic (prelymphoma, thymoma) disorders.

INFECTIOUS MYOPATHIES

Although not common, *Toxoplasma* infection may manifest as a primary myopathy or can be seen in conjunction with systemic disease, including pneumonia, uveitis, chorioretinitis, intracranial signs, hepatomegaly, vomiting, and diarrhea.[134] Clinical confirmation requires documentation of cysts on muscle biopsy or through serologic testing. A fourfold rise in IgG over a few weeks or a high IgM titer is suggestive of disease, but many cats can remain positive for IgM over years. Similarly, IgG titers suggest only that the cat has been exposed to *Toxoplasma* and is not a reliable means of diagnosis. PCR can allow for identification of *T. gondii* on tissue, blood, or aqueous humor samples.[134] Immunosuppression is often a factor in the development of clinically relevant toxoplasmosis in cats, so FeLV and FIV testing should be performed.

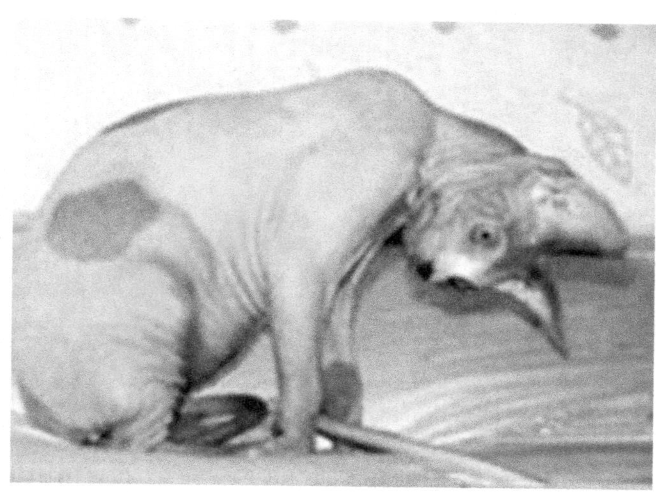

FIGURE 27-31 Devon Rex cat with inherited myopathy. Note the typical posture with passive ventroflexion of the head and neck and dorsal protrusion of the scapulae. *(Courtesy Dr. Diane Shelton, Comparative Neuromuscular Laboratory, University of California.)*

The treatment of choice is clindamycin (25 mg/kg administered orally every 8 to 12 hours) for 2 to 4 weeks, with resolution of clinical signs typically beginning within 1 week after starting therapy.

Other infectious agents reported to cause myositis in cats include *Neospora*, *Clostridium* spp., and *Sarcocystis*. An inflammatory myopathy associated with FIV has been reported and is characterized by elevated creatine kinase levels, abnormalities in EMG testing, mononuclear cellular infiltrates in multiple muscle groups, and myonecrosis.[104] Interestingly, clinical signs associated with these abnormalities have not been reported.

Primary Noninflammatory Myopathies

Primary noninflammatory myopathies are usually associated with abnormalities of the intrinsic metabolic machinery of the muscle or abnormalities in muscle membranes or ion channels.[120] Many are inherited disorders and have been reported exclusively in certain breeds (e.g., hypokalemic myopathy of Burmese cats, type IV glycogen storage disease in Norwegian Forest cats, and Devon Rex myopathy) (Figure 27-31).

MYOTONIA CONGENITA

Myotonia congenita is characterized by prolonged muscle contraction after cessation of voluntary effort.[120] This is believed to be due to a chloride channel abnormality inherited as an autosomal recessive trait in some species.[144] Clinical signs include difficulty opening the mouth, muscle hypertrophy, and a stiff gait, with the stiffness decreasing during exercise. Startling of the animal may lead to hyperextension of the limbs and falling to lateral recumbency or spasm of the orbicularis oculi muscle, prolonged prolapse of the nictitating membranes, and flattening of the ears. Endotracheal intubation may be difficult on account of the inability to open the mouth to a wide angle and narrowing of the glottis caused by muscle spasm.[54]

The diagnosis is supported by characteristic changes on EMG, in which the classic myotonic discharges and "dive-bomber"-like sounds are noted. Further support for the diagnosis is the presence of a sustained contraction of the tongue muscle when tapped, or a "myotonic dimple." Long-term prognosis is guarded, although affected cats may be able to enjoy some quality of life provided that aspiration pneumonia is avoided.

MUSCULAR DYSTROPHIES

Muscular dystrophies (MDs) are a diverse group of inherited, noninflammatory, degenerative muscle disorders leading to muscle atrophy, hypertrophy of select muscles (e.g., tongue, diaphragm), stiff gait, joint contracture, weakness, exercise intolerance, regurgitation, and dysphagia.[121] The most well-characterized MD in feline medicine is X-linked muscular dystrophy, also called *hypertrophic feline muscular dystrophy (HFMD)*, which is associated with an absence of dystrophin and mutations of the dystrophin gene. Other apparently autosomal forms of MD have recently been described, including merosin (laminin alpha-2) deficiency and a unique MD in Sphynx and Devon Rex cats.[87]

Muscle biopsy is characterized by extensive muscle necrosis with large accumulations of macrophages, fibrosis, lipid accumulation, and satellite cells in regenerating muscle.[34] Affected cats are typically male, with clinical signs beginning at several months of age. Although cats have been reported to live as long as 5 years, overall prognosis is grave and dysphagia, regurgitation, and dyspnea from hypertrophy of the lingual, pharyngeal, and esophageal musculature as well as the diaphragm will lead to poor nutritional intake and death from aspiration pneumonia.[121]

FIBRODYSPLASIA OSSIFICANS PROGRESSIVA

Fibrodysplasia ossificans progressiva is a disorder affecting the epimysium, tendons, and fascia with marked proliferation of fibrovascular connective tissue and associated chondroid and osseous metaplasia.[143] Clinical signs are characterized by progressive stiffness in the gait, enlargement of the proximal limb musculature, pruritus, and joint pain and are typically seen in young to middle-aged cats of both sexes. Radiographically, multiple mineralized densities (Figure 27-32) can be seen. Muscle biopsy shows collagen proliferation, focal areas of lymphocytic infiltration, and areas of cartilage and ectopic bone formation within the muscle tissue, with the pathologic abnormalities appearing to have originated from the fascial connective tissue. The clinical course progresses rapidly, and there is no known treatment. Prognosis is grave.

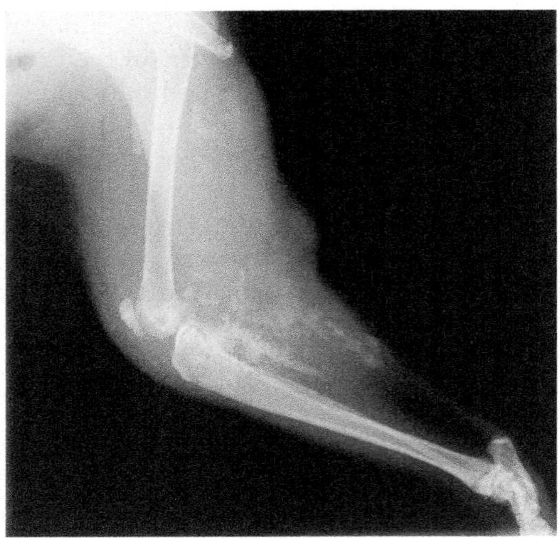

FIGURE 27-32 Lateral radiograph of the pelvic limb showing multifocal mineralized densities in the adjacent musculature in a cat with fibrodysplasia ossificans progressiva. *(Courtesy Dr. Diane Shelton, Comparative Neuromuscular Laboratory, University of California.)*

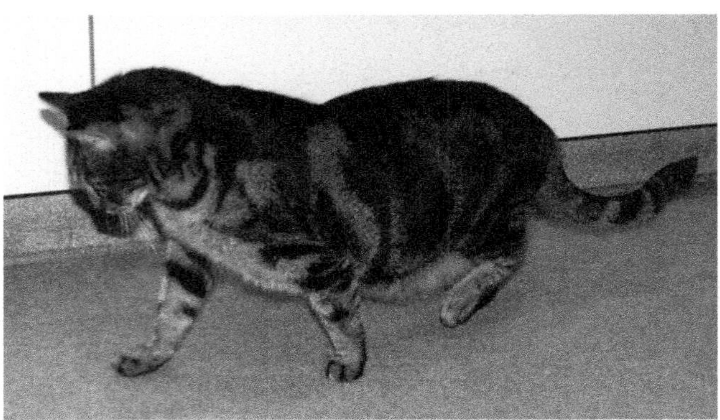

FIGURE 27-33 Cat with hypokalemia resulting from postobstructive dieresis. Note the typical posture of cervical ventroflexion.

Secondary Noninflammatory Myopathies

Secondary noninflammatory myopathies result from nutritional, metabolic, and toxic etiologies. Perhaps the most well recognized of these is hypokalemic polymyopathy, a generalized muscle disorder resulting from low serum potassium levels (1.5 to 3.5 mEq/L), which leads to signs of weakness, cervical ventroflexion (Figure 27-33), myalgia, stiff gait, and a broad-based stance of the pelvic limbs. Reduced potassium intake or increases in the fractional excretion of potassium in the urine secondary to renal disease often precipitate clinical signs. In addition to decreased intake, cats with increased potassium loss through the gastrointestinal tract secondary to vomiting and diarrhea are also at risk.

Other disorders that may give rise to potassium-depletion myopathy include hyperaldosteronism, postobstructive diuresis, diuretic administration, inappropriate fluid therapy, diabetic ketoacidosis, and others. Differential diagnoses include thiamine deficiency, hyperthyroidism, myasthenia gravis, polymyositis, polyneuropathy, hypocalcemic myopathy, and hypernatremic myopathy.[75] Treatment is aimed at reestablishing normal serum potassium levels and correcting the underlying disorder.

When first examining an adult cat with acute onset of lower motor neuron signs, the clinician should be sure to ascertain whether there has been any recent drug or toxin exposure. Most notably, pyrethrins and organophosphates have been known to result in severe cervical ventroflexion and tremors, as well as seizures. The mechanism of action for these agents is believed to be through the reduction of acetylcholinesterase activity in both the central and peripheral nervous system. Clinical signs can begin within a few hours of exposure, and cats with suspected exposure should be bathed to remove any residual insecticide. Supportive care in the form of muscle relaxants and, if necessary, anticonvulsants, will lead to resolution of signs in 48 hours. Other reported toxins include acrylamide, thallium, chlorpyrifos, vincristine, salinomycin, and others.

Disorders of the Lower Motor Neuron

Polyneuropathies of cats can affect sensory, motor, and autonomic neurons with a variety of clinical presentations. Those with involvement of motor fibers will have weakness and muscle atrophy, whereas those with sensory neuropathy may present with ataxia, anesthesia, or paraesthesia.[20] Involvement of autonomic neurons may result in ptyalism, excessive lacrimation, regurgitation secondary to megaesophagus, urine retention, constipation, and mydriasis. Both inherited and acquired disorders have been reported, and signalment plays a key role in guiding the clinician in differentiating between the two. Definitive diagnosis of polyneuropathy requires electrophysiologic (EMG, NCV, F-waves) testing to confirm the diagnosis and determine the location of the lesion, and nerve biopsy further defines the type of pathology present.[20] The ensuing discussion focuses on the more clinically relevant neuropathies seen in feline patients.

Congenital Polyneuropathies

Congenital polyneuropathies are typically seen in cats younger than 1 year of age, with most being progressive and ultimately fatal.[20] Clinical signs usually include progressive tremors, paraparesis or tetraparesis, generalized weakness, sensory deficits, and depressed segmental reflexes.[20] Concurrent clinical signs, as well as signalment, are critical in helping the clinician arrive at a definitive diagnosis. For example, cats with an inherited primary hyperchylomicronemia develop multifocal neuropathies secondary to lipid deposition and compression of nerves, especially at the level of the intervertebral

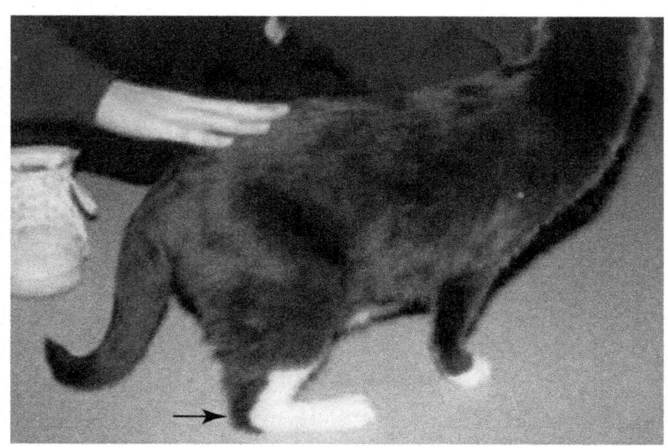

FIGURE 27-34 Diabetic cat with polyneuropathy and plantigrade stance. *(Courtesy Dr. Diane Shelton, Comparative Neuromuscular Laboratory, University of California.)*

foramina. Severe fasting hyperlipidemia and lipemia retinalis are present. Dietary management in the form of a restricted-fat diet results in resolution of clinical signs.[60]

Primary hyperoxaluria is seen in kittens between 5 and 8 months of age, with a rapid course of severe generalized weakness, anorexia, and dehydration.[20] This is reportedly an autosomal recessive disorder leading to renal failure from oxalate deposition in renal tubules. The pathogenesis is unclear, but all patients described thus far succumbed to the disease before the age of 12 months.

Other inherited neuropathies include hypertrophic polyneuropathy, glycogen storage disorders in Norwegian Forest cats, and distal axonopathy of Birman cats.[20]

Acquired Polyneuropathies and Neuronopathies

DIABETIC NEUROPATHY

Neuropathy associated with poorly controlled diabetes mellitus has been well described in the veterinary literature. Symmetric weakness may develop with progressive paraparesis, plantigrade stance (excessive hock flexion), patellar hyporeflexia, and poor postural responses (Figure 27-34).[68] Clinical signs may progress to involve the thoracic limbs. Functional, structural, and biochemical defects of motor and sensory nerves in both thoracic and pelvic limbs have been identified with Schwann cell injury, leading to demyelination and axonal damage.[91] Strict glycemic control reverses the clinical signs of neuropathy in some cats, although many cats continue to show degrees of clinical weakness even with specific therapy that includes oral hypoglycemic agents or insulin. Acetyl-l-carnitine appears to be of benefit in the treatment of diabetic peripheral neuropathy in humans and has been used in a few cats with persistent clinical signs of neuropathy with subjectively good results.[27,38,123]

IDIOPATHIC POLYNEUROPATHY

Idiopathic polyneuropathy results in acute onset of generalized weakness; tetraparesis or tetraplegia; decreased segmental reflexes; and, in severe cases, respiratory depression.[46] Age of onset varies from 3 months to several years, with animals of both sexes affected. The underlying cause is poorly understood, but an immune-mediated basis is suspected. In some cases a toxin (e.g., snake envenomation) or infectious agent may be an inciting factor, and kittens vaccinated against *Microsporum canis* infection have reportedly shown acute flaccid tetraparesis.[20] Definitive diagnosis can be attained only by obtaining a representative nerve biopsy; demyelination, axonal loss, and mononuclear inflammation have been reported.[46] Complete recovery is possible, and treatment with a tapering dose of prednisone over several weeks is recommended. Relapses are not uncommon, however, and cats may ultimately become refractory to treatment with corticosteroids.

FELINE ISCHEMIC NEUROMYOPATHY

Occlusion of the aorta or iliac arteries ("saddle thrombus") is a well-recognized disorder in cats, occurring most often in cats with hypertrophic cardiomyopathy. Clinical signs include acute onset of paraparesis or paraplegia, dysuria, and apparent pain.[81] Occasionally, a thoracic limb lameness of monoplegia may be seen with a thrombus in the brachial artery. Physical examination findings include poor or absent femoral pulses; foot beds and nail beds that are cyanotic and cool; hypothermia; severe weakness distal to the stifle; depressed patellar reflexes; inability to flex or extend the hock; and, in some cases, loss of nociception. Histopathologically, peripheral nerve changes begin at the level of the midthigh and include ischemic degeneration of axons and paranodal and segmental demyelination of the sciatic nerve.[31] In the cranial tibial muscles, rhabdomyolysis can be noted.[31] Treatment is aimed at treating the underlying cardiac disorder (see Chapter 20), but prognosis is extremely guarded.

FACIAL PARALYSIS

Facial paralysis affecting one or both facial nerves is commonly seen either alone or in association with myriad disorders. Idiopathic facial paralysis is much less common in cats than in dogs, accounting for only 25% of cases in one report.[64] Clinical signs include drooling from one side of the mouth, inability to blink on the affected side, and halitosis caused by accumulation of food in the affected oral commissure. A facial droop is not as apparent in cats as it is in dogs. Corneal ulceration may be evident as a result of damage to the parasympathetic fibers responsible for tear production or exposure keratitis resulting from the inability to blink.[5] On physical examination both the menace response and the palpebral reflex are absent, but sensation to the face remains intact. When it is a result of disease in the middle ear, facial paralysis may be accompanied by concurrent Horner's syndrome or vestibular signs. A minimum database should include a complete blood count, chemistry panel, otic exam, corneal fluorescein staining, and Schirmer tear test. Advanced imaging (CT or MRI) may be necessary for evaluation of the bullae and brain stem.[5]

ADULT-ONSET MOTOR NEURON DISEASE

Adult-onset motor neuron disease has been seen in cats with slowly progressive signs of generalized weakness, cervical ventroflexion, dysphagia, and muscle atrophy.[118] Clinical signs are progressive, and in the end stage spinal reflexes became undetectable. Evidence of denervation can be seen in muscle biopsies, and electrodiagnostics will reveal abnormalities consistent with a neuronopathy. Necropsy examination of the spinal cord in affected cats reveals a decrease in the number of cell bodies in the ventral horn, astrocytosis, and wallerian degeneration in the ventral roots.[118] The cause is unknown, but viral, hereditary, immune-mediated, nutritional, and toxic etiologies have all been proposed. Prognosis is grave, but some cats can live many years with mild clinical signs. A similar inherited disorder has been reported in young Maine Coon cats.

DYSAUTONOMIA

Feline dysautonomia (Key–Gaskell syndrome) is a polyneuropathy affecting primarily the autonomic nervous system. Clinical signs include mydriatic pupils that are unresponsive to light, elevation of the third eyelid, dry oral and nasal mucosae, dysphagia, megaesophagus, vomiting, constipation, bradycardia, and incontinence or urine retention (Figure 27-35).[34,65] Signs are usually acute but may progress over the course of several days or more. The cause is unknown, but a neurotoxin is highly suspected. The disorder was first recognized in cats in the United Kingdom but has been sporadically reported elsewhere, including the midwestern United States. Primarily young domestic shorthair cats of either sex are susceptible.

Confirmation of a suspected diagnosis based on clinical signs can be confirmed through administration of 1% pilocarpine drops in both eyes, which will produce constriction of the pupils in affected cats but not normal cats. Alternatively, assays of plasma and urine may reveal reduced amounts of noradrenaline and adrenaline.[51] Histopathologic evaluation of affected animals reveals lesions in both sympathetic and parasympathetic ganglia, with neuronal loss, satellite cell proliferation, and light fibrosis.[31] Prognosis is extremely poor, and there is no known treatment.[65]

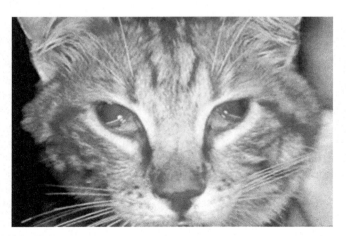

FIGURE 27-35 Cat with dysautonomia. Note the elevated third eyelids and dilated pupils. *(Courtesy Dr. D. O'Brien, College of Veterinary Medicine, University of Missouri.)*

MISCELLANEOUS NEUROLOGIC CONDITIONS

Horner's Syndrome

Horner's syndrome results from loss of sympathetic innervation to the eye and is characterized by miosis, ptosis, enophthalmos, and protrusion of the third eyelid (Figure 27-36).[28] Other rare signs of Horner's syndrome include alterations in iris color and change in coat color of Siamese cats secondary to peripheral vasodilation of blood vessels in the skin.[94] It is helpful to consider that the sympathetic pathway is a three-neuron system, and as such Horner's syndrome can be classified as first, second, or third order.

First-order Horner's syndrome, or upper motor neuron Horner's syndrome, may originate anywhere along the pathway from its origin in the hypothalamus through the lateral tectotegmentospinal system in the cervical spinal cord to its termination in the lateral gray column from T1-3.[28] Typically, first-order Horner's syndrome is accompanied by significant neurologic deficits

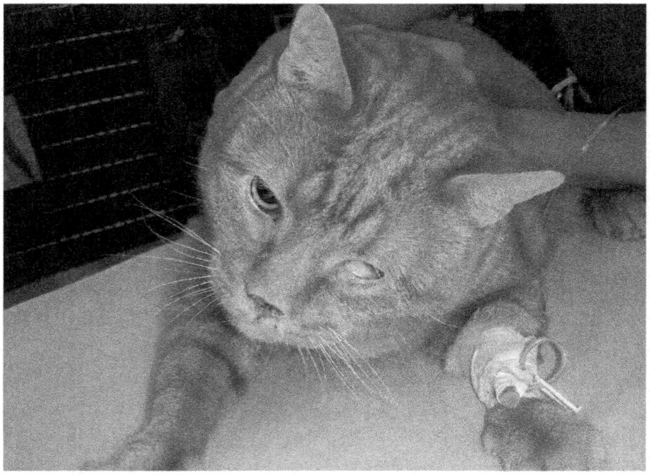

FIGURE 27-36 Cat with classic signs of Horner's syndrome.

and has reportedly been associated with neoplasia, trauma, infarctions, and meningoencephalomyelitis.[28,63]

Second-order Horner's syndrome (preganglionic) results from a lesion in the pathway beginning from T1-3, through the associated spinal roots and ramus communicans, and up the cranial thoracic and cervical parts of the sympathetic trunk. This trunk travels with the vagus nerve, forming the vagosympathetic trunk, located in the carotid sheath.[28] Trauma, aggressive jugular venipuncture, bite wounds, mediastinal lymphoma, and brachial plexus avulsion have all reportedly been the cause of second-order Horner's syndrome.[28,63]

Third-order Horner's syndrome is most commonly recognized associated with otitis media (Figure 27-37) and results from lesions rostral to the termination of the preganglionic axons in the cranial cervical ganglion, located at the level of the tympanic bulla. In some cases a cause may not be determined, and in a review of 26 cats with Horner's syndrome, a definitive diagnosis could not be attained in 42.3% of cases.[63]

An initial database should include a thorough otic exam as well as three-view thoracic radiographs to evaluate the mediastinum and other associated structures. A complete neurologic examination can help guide the clinician in determining neuroanatomic diagnosis and whether advanced imaging is necessary. Denervation hypersensitivity of the iris to subpharmacologic concentrations of sympathomimetic drugs is a consequence of Horner's syndrome in dogs and cats and can be used to help predict the site of the lesion in affected patients.[63] Instillation of 10% phenylephrine topically will result in mydriasis in less than 20 minutes in cats with third-order Horner's syndrome. In cats with second-order Horner's syndrome, mydriasis will take 20 to 45 minutes to develop, and in those with first-order Horner's syndrome it will take greater than 45 minutes. However, the sensitivity and specificity of this test have not been determined, and the results should be interpreted cautiously, with the history and examination findings being the most useful means of predicting underlying cause. Treatment of Horner's syndrome is unnecessary, and therapeutic efforts should instead be directed at the primary etiology.

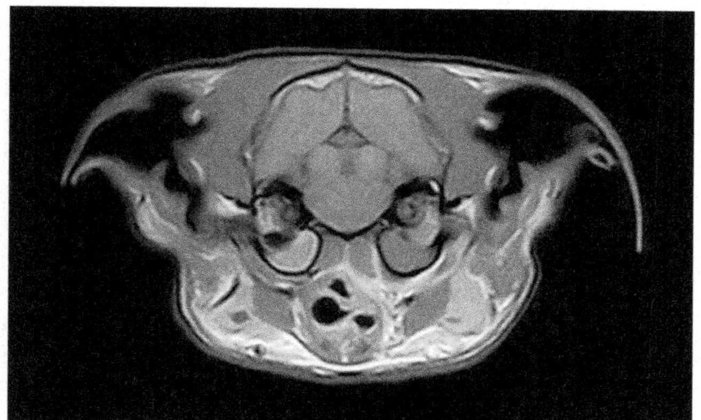

FIGURE 27-37 Magnetic resonance imaging of the cat from Figure 27-36. Note the fluid-filled tympanic bullae bilaterally.

Feline Hyperesthesia Syndrome

Feline hyperesthesia syndrome (FHS) is a poorly understood disorder characterized by myriad clinical signs, including rippling of the skin over the lumbar muscles, excessive grooming, tail chasing, mydriasis, self-mutilation, aggression, frantic biting at the feet and tail base, and vocalization.[21,101] Palpation of the lumbar musculature may elicit signs of pain. Affected cats commonly stare at their tail, then attack the tail or flanks.[21] Although all breeds can be affected, Siamese, Burmese, Persian, and Abyssinian cats are more commonly afflicted.[57] The behavior may be induced by petting or stroking the cat's fur and most commonly occurs in the morning or later in the evening.

Differential diagnoses relate to disorders of the skin, nervous system, musculoskeletal system, and behavioral disorders.[21] Dermatologic disorders such as flea allergy dermatitis and atopy must be ruled out as possible triggers. Likewise, diseases of the spine, such as IVDD, should be considered and ruled out as a potential source of lumbar pain. Numerous theories point to a compulsive disorder resulting in self-injurious behavior.[21] Others propose that it is a seizure disorder and best treated with anticonvulsant medication. However, results of EMG and muscle biopsy in five cats with signs of FHS were consistent with an inclusion body myositis/myopathy, suggesting myalgia as a trigger.[82]

There have been no controlled studies comparing the efficacy of various treatments for FHS, and cat owners must be made aware that a significant trial-and-error period may be necessary before the desired clinical response is attained. The most common treatments used for FHS are flea medications, corticosteroids, anticonvulsants, and anti-anxiety drugs (Table 27-3). The author has not had success with steroids and usually will instead begin treatment with PB (2 mg/kg, administered orally every 12 hours) and increase the dose according to clinical response and drug levels (discussed previously). Alternatively, gabapentin at 10 mg/kg, administered orally every 8 to 12 hours, has both anticonvulsant as well as pain-relieving properties and is considered safe for use in cats. The clinician must be aware that gabapentin pediatric suspension contains xylitol; if a suspension must be used, a xylitol-free product must be obtained from a compounding pharmacy.

Selective serotonin reuptake inhibitors (SSRIs) such as fluoxetine (0.5 to 2 mg/kg administered orally every 24 hours) are occasionally recommended when anticonvulsants do not prove effective.[21] The adverse effects of SSRIs include sedation, anorexia, irritability, vomiting,

TABLE 27-3 **Drugs Used for Treatment of Feline Hyperesthesia Syndrome**

Drug	Dose	Comments
Phenobarbital	2 mg/kg, PO, every 12 hours	Increase dose according to response and drug levels; for monitoring, see Table 27-1
Gabapentin	10 mg/kg, PO, every 8 to 12 hours	Ensure suspensions are xylitol free
Fluoxetine	0.5 to 2 mg/kg, PO, every 24 hours	Adverse effects include sedation, anorexia, irritability, vomiting, and diarrhea; inhibition of hepatic cytochrome P450 enzymes
Clomipramine	0.5 to 1 mg/kg, PO, every 24 hours	Adverse effects include sedation, anticholinergic effects, potentiation of arrhythmias, lowering of the seizure threshold

PO, By mouth.

and diarrhea. In addition, SSRIs inhibit the function of the liver cytochrome P450 enzymes, and care should be taken when prescribing concurrent medications that rely on these enzymes for their metabolism (e.g., PB, carbamazepine, benzodiazepines). Tricyclic antidepressants, such as clomipramine (0.5 to 1 mg/kg, administered orally every 24 hours)[21] can also be used to treat FHS. Adverse effects associated with this drug include sedation, anticholinergic effects, potentiation of arrhythmias in predisposed patients, and lowering of the seizure threshold in patients with seizure disorders.[21] Long-term medical and behavioral management may be necessary, and cats with FHS often require ongoing adjustments in type or dosage of medication (or both).

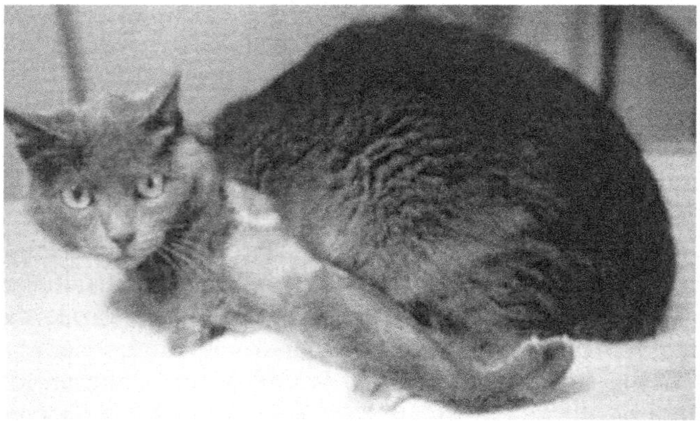

FIGURE 27-38 A cat with focal tetanus after suffering a wound to the affected limb. *(Courtesy www.felipedia.org.)*

Tetanus

Tetanus is a result of sustained muscle contraction without relaxation that is most commonly caused by infection with the anaerobic, ubiquitous organism *Clostridium tetani.*[24,29] Under certain conditions (e.g., penetrating wound) neurotoxin produced by the bacterium is transported up axons in a retrograde fashion to the level of the spinal cord or brain.[24] Ultimately, tetanus toxin (called *tetanospasmin)* acts on inhibitory interneurons, preventing the release of glycine in the spinal cord and gamma-aminobutyric acid in brain stem motor nuclei.[29] Tetanospasmin may remain bound for up to 3 weeks.[29] The main binding site is inhibitory interneurons that act on motor neurons innervating the antigravity extensor muscles.[29] Species susceptibility is highly variable, but cats are generally regarded as quite resistant.[24,29] Nonetheless, there are sporadic reports of this disease in cats,[77,105,137] and the author has witnessed a handful of cases over the past 10 or more years.

Clinical signs usually are seen 5 to 10 days after wound infection or surgical procedure,[24,29,77] but can be delayed by up to 21 days.[77,137] The site where clinical signs first are noted will usually reflect the site of entry of the toxin into the CNS. For example, cats that have developed tetanus after castration will typically develop signs first in the pelvic limbs, after which there will be rapid and diffuse spread of the toxin throughout the CNS.[29] However, tetanus may remain focal (Figure 27-38), with signs remaining confined to a single extremity where the toxin first entered the CNS.[29] In the generalized form the gait is stiff, there is increased muscle tone, and there may be excessive contraction of the facial muscles, known as the classic *risus sardonicus.* Prolapse of the third eyelid, wrinkling of the forehead, and trismus (lockjaw) may also be evident.[24,29] In the most severe form, the patient is recumbent, with opisthotonos and extensor rigidity in all four limbs, and seizures or respiratory arrest may ensue.[24,29]

Diagnosis is largely based on history and the classical physical examination findings, and in some cases a recent wound or surgical procedure may not always be evident.[24] Treatment is largely supportive, although if a wound is present, débridement and antibiotics to kill any remaining *C. tetani* organisms are indicated. Penicillin G is considered the drug of choice, but amoxicillin–clavulanic acid and metronidazole have also been reportedly effective.[137] The benefit of tetanus antitoxin in cats remains uncertain insofar as there is too little information in the literature regarding its safety and efficacy. Supportive care depends on severity of signs, and cats severely affected may require muscle relaxants, physical therapy, bladder management, and nutritional assistance. Recovery can be prolonged, and periods lasting from several weeks to up to 5 months have been reported in affected cats before clinical resolution.[105,137]

References

1. Abramson C, Platt S, Stedman N: Tetraparesis in a cat with fibrocartilaginous emboli, *J Am Anim Hosp Assoc* 38:153, 2002.
2. Bailey CS, Morgan JP: Congenital spinal malformations, *Vet Clin North Am Small Anim Pract* 22:985, 1992.
3. Bailey KS, Dewey CW, Boothe DM et al: Levetiracetam as an adjunct to phenobarbital treatment in cats with suspected idiopathic epilepsy, *J Am Vet Med Assoc* 232:867, 2008.

3a. Bailey K: Personal communication, July 2010.

4. Barnes H, Chrisman C, Mariani C et al: Clinical signs, underlying cause, and outcome in cats with seizures: 17 cases (1997-2002), *J Am Vet Med Assoc* 225:1723, 2004.
5. Barone G, Dewey CW: Facial paralysis, idiopathic. In Cote E, editor: *Clinical veterinary advisor*, St Louis, 2007, Mosby Elsevier, p 374.
6. Barone G, Foureman P, deLahunta A: Adult-onset cerebellar abiotrophy and retinal degeneration in a domestic shorthair cat, *J Am Anim Hosp Assoc* 38:51, 2002.
7. Barr MC, Butt MT, Anderson KL et al: Spinal lymphosarcoma and disseminated mastocytoma associated with feline immunodeficiency virus infection in a cat, *J Am Vet Med Assoc* 202:1978, 1993.
8. Beatty JA, Barrs VR, Swinney GR et al: Peripheral vestibular disease associated with cryptococcosis in three cats, *J Feline Med Surg* 2:29, 2000.
9. Berg A: Borna disease in cats. In Bonagura JD, editor: *Current veterinary therapy small animal practice*, ed 13, Philadelphia, 2000, Saunders, p 976.
10. Bischoff MG, Kneller SK: Diagnostic imaging of the canine and feline ear, *Vet Clin North Am Small Anim Pract* 34:437, 2004.
11. Boettcher IC, Steinberg T, Matiasek K et al: Use of anti-coronavirus antibody testing of cerebrospinal fluid for diagnosis of feline infectious peritonitis involving the central nervous system in cats, *J Am Vet Med Assoc* 230:199, 2007.
12. Boland LA, Angles JM: Feline permethrin toxicity: retrospective study of 42 cases, *J Feline Med Surg* 12:61, 2010.
13. Boothe DM, George KL, Couch P: Disposition and clinical use of bromide in cats, *J Am Vet Med Assoc* 221:1131, 2002.
14. Bradshaw J, Pearson G, Gruffydd-Jones T: A retrospective study of 286 cases of neurological disorders of the cat, *J Comp Pathol* 131:112, 2004.
15. Carmichael K, Bienzle D, McDonnell J: Feline leukemia virus–associated myelopathy in cats, *Vet Pathol* 39:536, 2002.
16. Caylor K, Cassimatis M: Metronidazole neurotoxicosis in two cats, *J Am Anim Hosp Assoc* 37:258, 2001.
17. Cellio B: Collecting, processing, and preparing cerebrospinal fluid in dogs and cats, *Comp Contin Edu Pract Vet* 23:786, 2001.
18. Center SA, Elston TH, Rowland PH et al: Fulminant hepatic failure associated with oral administration of diazepam in 11 cats, *J Am Vet Med Assoc* 209:618, 1996.
19. Cherubini GB, Rusbridge C, Singh BP et al: Rostral cerebellar arterial infarct in two cats, *J Feline Med Surg* 9:246, 2007.
20. Chrisman CL: Polyneuropathies of cats, *J Small Anim Pract* 41:384, 2000.
21. Ciribassi J: Understanding behavior: feline hyperesthesia syndrome, *Compend Contin Educ Pract Vet* 31:116, 2009.
22. Coates J, Axlund T, Dewey C et al: Hydrocephalus in dogs and cats, *Comp Contin Edu Pract Vet* 28:136, 2006.
23. Cochrane SM, Parent JM, Black WD et al: Pharmacokinetics of phenobarbital in the cat following multiple oral administration, *Can J Vet Res* 54:309, 1990.
24. Coleman E: Clostridial neurotoxins: tetanus and botulism, *Comp Contin Edu Pract Vet* 20:1089, 1998.
25. Cote E, Khan SA: Intoxication versus acute, non-toxicological illness: differentiating the two. In Ettinger SJ, Feldman EC, editors: *Textbook of veterinary internal medicine*, ed 6, Philadelphia, 2005, Saunders, p 242.
26. Cuddon PA: Feline neuromuscular disease. In Kirk RW, Bonagura JD, editors: *Current veterinary therapy VI*, Philadelphia, 1992, Saunders, p 1024.
27. De Grandis D, Minardi C: Acetyl-L-carnitine (levacecarnine) in the treatment of diabetic neuropathy. A long-term, randomised, double-blind, placebo-controlled study, *Drugs R D* 3:223, 2002.
28. De Lahunta A, Glass EN: *Lower motor neuron: general visceral efferent system.* In De Lahunta A, Glass R, editors: *Veterinary neuroanatomy and clinical neurology*, St Louis, 2009, Saunders, p 169.
29. De Lahunta A, Glass EN: *Upper motor neuron.* In De Lahunta A, Glass R, editors: *Veterinary neuroanatomy and clinical neurology*, St Louis, 2009, Saunders, p 193.
30. DeLahunta A: Degenerative diseases of the central nervous system. In Summers BA, Cummings JF, DeLahunta A, editors: *Veterinary neuropathology*, St Louis, 1995, Mosby, p 208.
31. DeLahunta A: Diseases of the peripheral nervous system. In Summers BA, Cummings JF, De Lahunta A, editors: *Veterinary neuropathology*, St Louis, 1995, Mosby, p 469.
32. DeLahunta A: Inflammatory diseases of the nervous system. In Summers BA, Cummings JF, DeLahunta A, editors: *Veterinary neuropathology*, St Louis, 1995, Mosby, p 95.
33. DeLahunta A: Tumors of the central nervous system. In Summers BA, Cummings JF, DeLahunta A, editors: *Veterinary neuropathology*, St Louis, 1995, Mosby, p 351.
34. DeLahunta A, Glass R: *Veterinary neuroanatomy and clinical neurology*, St Louis, 2009, Saunders.
35. Diaz JV, Poma R: Diagnosis and clinical signs of feline infectious peritonitis in the central nervous system, *Can Vet J* 50:1091, 2009.
36. Dorman DC, Dye JA: Chemical toxicities. In Ettinger SJ, Feldman EC editors: *Textbook of veterinary internal medicine*, ed 6, St Louis, 2005, Saunders, p 256.

36a. Dubey JP, Carpenter JL: Histologically confirmed clinical toxoplasmosis in cats: 100 cases (1952-1990), *J Am Vet Med Assoc* 203:1556, 1993.

37. Dymond NL, Swift IM: Permethrin toxicity in cats: a retrospective study of 20 cases, *Aust Vet J* 86:219, 2008.
38. Evans JD, Jacobs TF, Evans EW: Role of acetyl-L-carnitine in the treatment of diabetic peripheral neuropathy, *Ann Pharmacother* 42:1686, 2008.
39. Fascetti A, Mauldin G, Mauldin G: Correlation between serum creatinine kinase activities and anorexia in cats, *J Vet Intern Med* 11:9, 1997.
40. Fatzer R, Gandini G, Jaggy A et al: Necrosis of hippocampus and piriform lobe in 38 domestic cats with seizures: a retrospective study on clinical and pathologic findings, *J Vet Intern Med* 14:100, 2000.
41. Feldman EC: Disorders of the parathyroid glands. In Ettinger SJ, Feldman EC, editors: *Textbook of veterinary internal medicine*, ed 6, St Louis, 2005, Saunders, p 1508.
42. Foley J, Lapointe J, Koblik P et al: Diagnostic features of clinical neurologic feline infectious peritonitis, *J Vet Intern Med* 12:415, 1998.
43. Forterre F, Tomek A, Konar M et al: Multiple meningiomas: clinical, radiological, surgical, and pathological findings with outcome in four cats, *J Feline Med Surg* 9:36, 2007.
44. Foureman P, Longshore R, Plummer S: Spinal cord granuloma due to *Coccidioides immitis* in a cat, *J Vet Intern Med* 19:373, 2005.

45. Garosi LS: Cerebrovascular disease in dogs and cats, *Vet Clin North Am Small Anim Pract* 40:65, 2010.
46. Gerritsen RJ, van Nes JJ, van Niel MH et al: Acute idiopathic polyneuropathy in nine cats, *Vet Q* 18:63, 1996.
47. Glass E, Cornetta A, De Lahunta A et al: Clinical and clinicopathologic features in 11 cats with Cuterebra larvae myiasis of the central nervous system, *J Vet Intern Med* 12:365, 1998.
48. Goldkamp C, Schaer M: Hypernatremia in dogs, *Compend Contin Educ Vet* 29:148, 2007.
49. Gordon LE, Thacher C, Matthiesen DT et al: Results of craniotomy for the treatment of cerebral meningioma in 42 cats, *Vet Surg* 23:94, 1994.
50. Greene SN, Bright RM: Insulinoma in a cat, *J Small Anim Pract* 49:38, 2008.
51. Guilford WG, O'Brien DP, Allert A et al: Diagnosis of dysautonomia in a cat by autonomic nervous system function testing, *J Am Vet Med Assoc* 193:823, 1988.
52. Hasegawa D, Kobayashi M, Kuwabara T et al: Pharmacokinetics and toxicity of zonisamide in cats, *J Feline Med Surg* 10:418, 2008.
53. Henrich M, Huisinga M, Bauer N et al: A case of intravascular lymphoma with mixed lineage antigen expression in a cat, *J Vet Med A Physiol Pathol Clin Med* 54:575, 2007.
54. Hickford FH, Jones BR, Gething MA et al: Congenital myotonia in related kittens, *J Small Anim Pract* 39:281, 1998.
55. Hillock SM, Dewey CW, Stefanacci JD et al: Vascular encephalopathies in dogs: incidence, risk factors, pathophysiology, and clinical signs, *Comp Contin Edu* 28:196, 2006.
56. Hoerlein BF: Intervertebral disk disease. In Oliver J, Hoerlein B, Mayhew I, editors: *Veterinary neurology*, Philadelphia, 1987, Saunders, p 321.
57. Horwitz DF, Neilson JC: Psychogenic alopecia/overgrooming: feline: *Blackwell's five-minute veterinary consult—clinical companion—canine and feline behavior*, Ames, Iowa, 2007, Blackwell, p 425.
58. Hovda LR: Plant toxicities. In Ettinger SJ, Feldman EC, editors: *Textbook of veterinary internal medicine*, ed 6, St Louis, 2005, Saunders, p 250.
59. Hubler M, Johnson KA, Burling RT et al: Lesions resembling osteochondromatosis in two cats, *J Small Anim Pract* 27:181, 1986.
60. Jones B, Johnstone A, Cahill J et al: Peripheral neuropathy in cats with inherited primary hyperchylomicronaemia, *Vet Rec* 119:268, 1986.
61. Joseph RJ, Peterson ME: Review and comparison of neuromuscular and central nervous system manifestations of hyperthyroidism in cats and humans, *Prog Vet Neurol* 3:114, 1993.
62. Kaser-Hotz B, Rohrer CR, Stankeova S et al: Radiotherapy of pituitary tumours in five cats, *J Small Anim Pract* 43:303, 2002.
63. Kern TJ, Aromando MC, Erb HN: Horner's syndrome in dogs and cats: 100 cases (1975-1985), *J Am Vet Med Assoc* 195:369, 1989.
64. Kern TJ, Erb HN: Facial neuropathy in dogs and cats: 95 cases (1975-1985), *J Am Vet Med Assoc* 191:1604, 1987.
65. Kidder AC, Johannes C, O'Brien DP et al: Feline dysautonomia in the Midwestern United States: a retrospective study of nine cases, *J Feline Med Surg* 10:130, 2008.
66. Knipe M, Vernau K, Hornof W et al: Intervertebral disc extrusion in six cats, *J Feline Med Surg* 3:161, 2001.
67. Kraje A: Hypoglycemia and irreversible neurologic complications in a cat with insulinoma, *J Am Vet Med Assoc* 223:812, 2003.
68. Kramek BA, Moise NS, Cooper B et al: Neuropathy associated with diabetes mellitus in the cat, *J Am Vet Med Assoc* 184:42, 1984.
69. Kube SA, Olby NJ: Managing acute spinal cord injuries, *Compend Contin Educ Pract Vet* 30:496, 2008.
70. Kudnig ST: Nasopharyngeal polyps in cats, *Clin Tech Small Anim Pract* 17:174, 2002.
71. Kuntz CA: Sacral fractures and sacrococcygeal injuries in dogs and cats. In Bonagura JD, editor: *Current veterinary therapy XIII*, Philadelphia, 2000, Saunders, p 1023.
72. Lane S, Kornegay J, Duncan J et al: Feline spinal lymphosarcoma: a retrospective evaluation of 23 cats, *J Vet Intern Med* 8:99, 1994.
73. Lauer SK: Fractures of the spine/luxations of the spine. In Cote E, Harari J, editors: *Clinical veterinary advisor*, St Louis, 2007, Mosby Elsevier, p 419.
74. Lavely J, Lipsitz D: Fungal infections of the central nervous system in the dog and cat, *Clin Tech Small Anim Pract* 20:212, 2005.
75. LeCouteur RA: Feline neuromuscular disorders, *Proceedings North Am Vet Conf*, Orlando, Fla, 2006, p 709.
76. LeCouteur RA, Withrow SJ: Tumors of the nervous system. In Withrow SJ, Vail DM, editors: *Small animal clinical oncology*, St Louis, 2007, Saunders, p 659.
77. Lee EA, Jones BR: Localised tetanus in two cats after ovariohysterectomy, *N Z Vet J* 44:105, 1996.
78. Levy MS, Mauldin G, Kapatkin AS et al: Nonlymphoid vertebral canal tumors in cats: 11 cases (1987-1995), *J Am Vet Med Assoc* 210:663, 1997.
79. Lindsay D, Blagburn B, Dubey J: Feline toxoplasmosis and the importance of the *Toxoplasma gondii* oocyst, *Comp Contin Edu* 19:448, 1997.
80. Lowrie M, Wessmann A, Gunn-Moore D et al: Quadrigeminal cyst management by cystoperitoneal shunt in a 4-year-old Persian cat, *J Feline Med Surg* 11:711, 2009.
81. MacDonald K, Cote E: Hypertrophic cardiomyopathy. In Cote E, editor: *Clinical veterinary advisor*, St Louis, 2007, Mosby Elsevier, p 554.
82. March PA, Fisher JR: Electromyographic and histologic abnormalities in epaxial muscles of cats with feline hyperesthesia syndrome (abstract), *J Vet Intern Med* 13:238, 1999.
83. Marioni-Henry K, Van Winkle TJ, Smith SH et al: Tumors affecting the spinal cord of cats: 85 cases (1980-2005), *J Am Vet Med Assoc* 232:237, 2008.
84. Marioni-Henry K, Vite CH, Newton AL et al: Prevalence of diseases of the spinal cord of cats, *J Vet Intern Med* 18:851, 2004.
85. Maritato KC, Colon JA, Mauterer JV: Acute non-ambulatory tetraparesis attributable to cranial cervical intervertebral disc disease in a cat, *J Feline Med Surg* 9:494, 2007.
86. Marshall M, Manning A: Hypernatremia. In Cote E, editor: *Clinical veterinary advisor*, St Louis, 2007, Mosby Elsevier.
87. Martin PT, Shelton GD, Dickinson PJ et al: Muscular dystrophy associated with [alpha]-dystroglycan deficiency in Sphynx and Devon Rex cats, *Neuromuscul Disord* 18:942, 2008.
88. Mayer MN, Greco DS, LaRue SM: Outcomes of pituitary tumor irradiation in cats, *J Vet Intern Med* 20:1151, 2006.
89. Meij BP, Voorhout G, Van Den Ingh TS et al: Transsphenoidal hypophysectomy for treatment of pituitary-dependent hyperadrenocorticism in 7 cats, *Vet Surg* 30:72, 2001.
90. Mikszewski JS, Van Winkle TJ, Troxel MT: Fibrocartilaginous embolic myelopathy in five cats, *J Am Anim Hosp Assoc* 42:226, 2006.
91. Mizisin AP, Shelton GD, Burgers ML et al: Neurological complications associated with spontaneously occurring feline diabetes mellitus, *J Neuropathol Exp Neurol* 61:872, 2002.
92. Munana K, Olby N, Sharp N et al: Intervertebral disk disease in 10 cats, *J Am Anim Hosp Assoc* 37:384, 2001.
93. Nafe LA: Meningiomas in cats: a retrospective clinical study of 36 cases, *J Am Vet Med Assoc* 174:1224, 1979.
94. Neer TM: Horner's syndrome: anatomy, diagnosis, and causes, *Comp Contin Edu Pract Vet* 6:740, 1984.
95. Neer TM: Fibrocartilaginous emboli, *Vet Clin North Am Small Anim Pract* 22:1017, 1992.
96. Negrin A, Cherubini GB, Lamb C et al: Clinical signs, magnetic resonance imaging findings and outcome in 77 cats with vestibular disease: a retrospective study, *J Feline Med Surg* 12:291, 2010.
97. Newitt A, German AJ, Barr FJ: Congenital abnormalities of the feline vertebral column, *Vet Radiol Ultrasound* 49:35, 2008.

98. Noonan M, Kline K, Meleo K: Lymphoma of the central nervous system: a retrospective study of 18 cats, *Comp Contin Educ Pract Vet* 19:497, 1997.
99. O'Brien DP, Axlund TW: Brain disease. In Ettinger SJ, Feldman EC, editors: *Textbook of veterinary internal medicine*, ed 6, St Louis, 2005, Saunders, p 803.
100. Okada M, Kitagawa M, Ito D et al: MRI of secondary cervical syringomyelia in four cats, *J Vet Med Sci* 71:1069, 2009.
101. Overall KL: Fears, anxieties, and sterotypies: *Clinical behavioral medicine for small animals*, St Louis, 1997, Mosby, p 209.
102. Platt SR: Recommendations for corticosteroid use in neurological diseases, *Proceedings 20th Annual Am Coll Vet Intern Med Forum*, Dallas, Tex, 2002, p 370.
103. Plumlee KH: *Veterinary clinical toxicology*, St Louis, 2004, Mosby.
104. Podell M, Chen E, Shelton GD: Feline immunodeficiency virus associated myopathy in the adult cat, *Muscle Nerve* 21:1680, 1998.
105. Polizopoulou Z, Kazakos G, Georgiadis G et al: Presumed localized tetanus in two cats, *J Feline Med Surg* 4:209, 2002.
106. Polizopoulou Z, Kazakos G, Patsikas M et al: Hypervitaminosis A in the cat: a case report and review of the literature, *J Feline Med Surg* 7:363, 2005.
107. Polizopoulou ZS, Koutinas AF, Souftas VD et al: Diagnostic correlation of CT-MRI and histopathology in 10 dogs with brain neoplasms, *J Vet Med A Physiol Pathol Clin Med* 51:226, 2004.
108. Quesnel A, Parent J, McDonell W: Clinical management and outcome of cats with seizure disorders: 30 cases (1991-1993), *J Am Vet Med Assoc* 210:72, 1997.
109. Quesnel A, Parent J, McDonell W et al: Diagnostic evaluation of cats with seizure disorders: 30 cases (1991-1993), *J Am Vet Med Assoc* 210:65, 1997.
110. Reed S, Cho DY, Paulsen D: Quadrigeminal arachnoid cysts in a kitten and a dog, *J Vet Diagn Invest* 21:707, 2009.
111. Rossmeisl JH, Jr., Lanz OI, Waldron DR et al: Surgical cytoreduction for the treatment of non-lymphoid vertebral and spinal cord neoplasms in cats: retrospective evaluation of 26 cases (1990-2005), *Vet Comp Oncol* 4:41, 2006.
112. Saxon B, Magne MI: Reversible central nervous system toxicosis associated with metronidazole therapy in three cats, *Prog Vet Neurol* 4:25, 1993.
113. Schatzberg S, Haley N, Barr S et al: Use of a multiplex polymerase chain reaction assay in the antemortem diagnosis of toxoplasmosis and neosporosis in the central nervous system of cats and dogs, *Am J Vet Res* 64:1507, 2003.
114. Schriefl S, Steinberg TA, Matiasek K et al: Etiologic classification of seizures, signalment, clinical signs, and outcome in cats with seizure disorders: 91 cases (2000-2004), *J Am Vet Med Assoc* 233:1591, 2008.
115. Sessums K, Mariani C: Intracranial meningioma in dogs and cats: a comparative review, *Compend Contin Educ Vet* 31:330, 2009.
116. Shamir M, Goelman G, Chai O: Postanesthetic cerebellar dysfunction in cats, *J Vet Intern Med* 18:368, 2004.
117. Shelton G, Ho M, Kass P: Risk factors for acquired myasthenia gravis in cats: 105 cases (198601998), *J Am Vet Med Assoc* 216:55, 2000.
118. Shelton G, Hopkins A, Ginn P et al: Adult-onset motor neuron disease in three cats, *J Am Vet Med Assoc* 212:1271, 1998.
119. Shelton G, Joseph R, Richter K et al: Acquired myasthenia gravis in hyperthyroid cats on Tapazole therapy (abstract), *J Vet Intern Med* 11:120, 1997.
120. Shelton GD: Differential diagnosis of muscle diseases in companion animals, *Prog Vet Neurol* 2:27, 1991.
121. Shelton GD: Inherited neuromuscular disease. *Proceedings 20th Annual Am Coll Vet Intern Med Forum*, Dallas, Tex, 2002, p 334.
122. Shelton GD: Practical approach to the diagnosis and treatment of neuromuscular disorders. *Proceedings 20th Annual Am Coll Vet Intern Med Forum*, Dallas, Tex, 2002, p 325.
123. Sima AA, Ristic H, Merry A et al: Primary preventive and secondary interventionary effects of acetyl-L-carnitine on diabetic neuropathy in the bio-breeding Worcester rat, *J Clin Invest* 97:1900, 1996.
124. Simpson DJ, Hunt GB, Tisdall PL et al: Surgical removal of an ependymoma from the third ventricle of a cat, *Aust Vet J* 77:645, 1999.
125. Skelly B, Franklin R: Recognition and diagnosis of lysosomal storage diseases in the cat and dog, *J Vet Intern Med* 16:133, 2002.
126. Smith Bailey K, Dewey CW: The seizuring cat. Diagnostic work-up and therapy, *J Feline Med Surg* 11:385, 2009.
127. Smith JR, Legendre AM, Thomas WB et al: Cerebral *Blastomyces dermatitidis* infection in a cat, *J Am Vet Med Assoc* 231:1210, 2007.
128. Snead E: Acromegaly. In Cote E, editor: *Clinical veterinary advisor*, St Louis, 2007, Mosby Elsevier, p 25.
129. Spodnick GJ, Berg J, Moore FM et al: Spinal lymphoma in cats: 21 cases (1976-1989), *J Am Vet Med Assoc* 200:373, 1992.
130. Stevenson TL, Dickinson PJ, Struges BK et al: Magnetic resonance imaging of intracranial Cryptococcosis in dogs and cats. *Proceedings Am Coll Vet Intern Med Forum*. Minneapolis, 2004.
131. Sturges BK, Dickinson PJ, Kortz GD et al: Clinical signs, magnetic resonance imaging features, and outcome after surgical and medical treatment of otogenic intracranial infection in 11 cats and 4 dogs, *J Vet Intern Med* 20:648, 2006.
132. Tamke P, Petersen M, Dietze A et al: Acquired hydrocephalus and hydromelia in a cat with feline infectious peritonitis: a case report and brief review, *Can Vet J* 29:997, 1988.
133. Thomas WB: Seizures and narcolepsy. In Dewey CW, editor: *A practical guide to canine and feline neurology*, Ames, Iowa, 2003, Iowa State Press, p 193.
134. Tieber Nielson LM, Macintire DK: Toxoplasmosis/neosporosis. In Cote E, editor: *Clinical veterinary advisor*, St Louis, 2007, Mosby Elsevier, p 1093.
135. Timmann D, Cizinauskas S, Tomek A et al: Retrospective analysis of seizures associated with feline infectious peritonitis in cats, *J Feline Med Surg* 10:9, 2008.
136. Tomek A, Cizinauskas S, Doherr M et al: Intracranial neoplasia in 61 cats: localisation, tumour types and seizure patterns, *J Feline Med Surg* 8:243, 2006.
137. Tomek A, Kathmann I, Faissler D et al: [Tetanus in cats: 3 case descriptions], *Schweiz Arch Tierheilkd* 146:295, 2004.
138. Towell T, Shell L: Endocrinopathies that affect the central nervous system of cats and dogs, *Comp Contin Edu Pract Vet* 16:1461, 1994.
139. Troxel M, Dewey CW: Brain neoplasia. In Cote E, editor: *Clinical veterinary advisor*, St Louis, 2007, Mosby Elsevier, p 151.
140. Troxel M, Vite C, Massicotte C et al: Magnetic resonance imaging features of feline intracranial neoplasia: retrospective analysis of 46 cats, *J Vet Intern Med* 18:176, 2004.
141. Troxel M, Vite C, Van Winkle T et al: Feline intracranial neoplasia: retrospective review of 160 cases (1985-2001), *J Vet Intern Med* 17:850, 2003.
142. Vail DM, MacEwen EG: Feline lymphoma and leukemias. In Withrow SJ, MacEwen EG, editors: *Small animal clinical oncology*, ed 3, Philadelphia, 2001, Saunders, p 590.
143. Valentine B, George C, Randolph J et al: Fibrodysplasia ossificans progressive in the cat: a case report, *J Vet Intern Med* 6:335, 1992.
144. Vite CH: Myotonia and disorders of altered muscle cell membrane excitability, *Vet Clin North Am Sm Anim Pract* 32:169, 2002.
145. Webster CRL: Hepatic encephalopathy. In Cote E, editor: *Clinical veterinary advisor*, St Louis, 2007, Mosby Elsevier, p 489.
146. Williams KJ, Summers BA, De Lahunta A: Cerebrospinal cuterebriasis in cats and its association with feline ischemic encephalopathy, *Vet Pathol* 35:330, 1998.
147. Withrow SJ, Vail DM: *Small animal clinical oncology*, St Louis, 2007, Saunders.
148. Zaki FA, Hurvitz AI: Spontaneous neoplasms of the central nervous system of the cat, *J Small Anim Pract* 17:773, 1976.

CHAPTER

28

Oncology

OUTLINE

BASIC APPROACH TO THE FELINE CANCER PATIENT

Brooke Fowler

SIGNS OF CANCER

All too commonly, the veterinarian sees a feline patient after clinical signs have exceeded the client's perception of health. Subtle behavioral changes may occur long before overt clinical signs appear. These changes vary depending on the type of malignancy and which body systems are most affected. General changes in activity, appetite, and litter box use are perhaps the most common first indications that a disease process is under way (see Box 37-3).

SCREENING DIAGNOSTICS

General health screening is the first step for the ill cat or a cat whose clinical signs designate the location of the disease. A complete blood count (CBC) can reveal hematologic malignancies and bone marrow–infiltrating diseases. The CBC is also an excellent way to primitively assess the innate immune system. Biochemistry data aid in the evaluation of general organ function as well as screening for hepatic lipidosis, the most common secondary disease.[1] General body cavity imaging is necessary because not all malignancies lead to biochemical alterations. Complete staging generally includes both abdominal and thoracic radiographs and potentially abdominal ultrasound, computed tomography (CT), and magnetic resonance imaging (MRI).

GENERAL STAGING TECHNIQUES

Each cancer type has its own predilection for sites of metastasis, and therefore staging is tailored to individual type. However, general assumptions can be made. By knowing the cell type of origin, the veterinarian can predict the route by which cancer will metastasize. Round cell tumors tend to metastasize by way of the lymphatics. Therefore examination of the draining lymph nodes surrounding round cell tumors is part of any thorough cancer workup. Mesenchymal cell tumors tend to metastasize hematogenously. Therefore thoracic radiographs are always indicated. Lastly, epithelial tumors tend to metastasize by way of either lymphatics or blood. Lymph node imaging and aspiration, as well as thoracic radiographs, are warranted to assess the metastatic status of a patient with a carcinoma. Aberrant metastatic patterns can suggest aggressive behavior. Sarcomas spreading by lymphatics or round cell tumors metastatic to pulmonary parenchyma may suggest a worse-than-typical prognosis for that patient. CT scans and MRI can be used to diagnose disease in closed cavities such as the skull, spine, and thoracic cavity. CT and MRI scans can be used to better plan for surgery. Another commonly used diagnostic modality is nuclear scintigraphy. Radioactive isotopes can be tagged to target certain body tissues. These radioisotopes can be used to locate bony lysis or even to elucidate the biological activity of a thyroid mass.

Fine-Needle Aspiration and Cytology

Most palpable masses can be aspirated with a needle. Fine-needle aspiration is the least invasive diagnostic approach that still offers high yield to define the malignancy.

Technique

The veterinarian should use the smallest needle necessary to safely and adequately collect cells for diagnosis. Needles of 22 to 25 gauge are typically sufficient, even for masses present in bone. Two methods exist for a fine-needle aspirate. The first method uses a needle without an attached syringe or with a syringe containing 6 mL of air. In an oscillating motion, the clinician inserts the needle into the lesion multiple times to collect sufficient cells for a smear. Using 6 mL of air, the clinician forcefully expels the contents of the needle onto a slide. The expelled material is gently spread on a blank slide to create a monolayer of cells. One slide is stained to ensure that cells were obtained and adequately prepared. The rest of the sample is sent unstained to a clinical pathologist. The second technique involves placing the needle into the lesion and aspirating with the syringe. The clinician removes the needle, fills the syringe with 6 mL of air, reattaches the needle, and then forcefully expels the contents of the needle onto a slide and prepares as previously described.

Advantages

Fine-needle aspiration is minimally invasive and rarely requires sedation or anesthesia. A diagnosis often can be made rapidly and at little cost to the patient and the client. This technique can be performed for skin, bone, and internal organ lesions.

Disadvantages

This approach collects a small sample that is assumed to be representative of the entire tumor population. The heterogenous nature of tumors with varied oxygenation and inflammatory components can confound this assumption. This test may yield nondiagnostic results and delay the diagnosis. Cytologic diagnosis often depends on the type of tumor. Round and epithelial cells may exfoliate more completely than tumors of mesenchymal origin.

BIOPSY TECHNIQUES

Biopsy samples should be taken along the periphery of a lesion, as a general rule. This will ensure that the necrotic center of a mass will not be sampled instead of the viable portion. This also facilitates skin closure. Neoplastic tissue has poor healing capabilities. The one exception to this rule is a tumor of bone. When a biopsy of bony tumors is performed, the track should include the center of the lesion. Aspirates or biopsies performed at the periphery of a bone lesion will likely yield reactive bone.

Punch Biopsy and Needle Biopsy

Punch biopsy and needle biopsy are the least invasive of the biopsy techniques. A punch biopsy is more suitable for external skin lesions. A Tru-Cut biopsy is more suitable for sampling internal organ lesions with imaging guidance.

Technique

When a biopsy punch is used, cutaneous and subcutaneous samples can be acquired transdermally or through a small skin incision. The biopsy punch is twisted, always in the same direction, into the lesion to the desired depth within the mass. With Metzenbaum scissors the sample is cut away from adherent underlying tissues. The sample is placed in formalin at a ratio of 1:10 (tumor:formalin) and submitted to a pathologist, who will provide a complete microscopic description, diagnosis, grade, margin description, and mitotic index as indicated. For a needle biopsy, a Tru-Cut biopsy needle is required. A Tru-Cut biopsy requires a special tool. This needle biopsy tool is inserted into the lesion. The core of the needle biopsy device is extended into the tissue mass. The sheath of the needle biopsy device is then advanced, and a portion of tissue is cut free within the notch of the core. Multiple specimens should be collected. Automatic firing devices can speed the collection of each sample. However, these automated, spring-loaded devices can be too vigorous for internal organs, causing organ damage in smaller patients.[3]

Advantages

These techniques require either a short anesthetic experience or sedation and a local block. These techniques require minimal surgical closure, resulting in less risk of dehiscence or infection compared with a major surgery. These techniques may allow a pathologist to identify the neoplastic process with description of the tumor's architecture. These samples may also allow for immunohistochemical stains and further prediction of the biological behavior of the tumor.

Disadvantages

These procedures may result in a nondiagnostic sample. Crush artifact is a common occurrence with these techniques. Surgical dehiscence is also a potential complication, as well as the aforementioned risk of organ damage associated with automated devices.

Wedge Biopsy

Removing a small but representative sample of the tumor facilitates identification of tissue architecture, allowing the pathologist to make a diagnosis and identify potential lymphatic or vascular invasion. A wedge of tissue is incised into the lesion along the edges. This wedge should have the smallest side along the center of the lesion and the longest side along the lateral margins.

Advantages

This technique allows a larger sample to be obtained. Sample architecture can be examined by a pathologist. Further information may be gained, including biological behavior and immunohistochemical staining. Because the portion of tissue that is being sampled is larger, the likelihood of obtaining a diagnosis is higher.

Disadvantages

This technique involves general anesthesia and all its associated risks. This procedure also carries a greater risk of dehiscence. Tumors do not heal as well as normal tissue does. This procedure carries some risk of spreading the tumor within normal tissue and requires careful planning to keep cells and hemorrhage contained within the ideal excisional surgical field.

Excisional Biopsy

Complete excision of the tumor can be at once diagnostic and therapeutic. Failure of complete excision functionally spreads the tumor farther inside the patient, potentially worsening the prognosis.[2]

Technique

Excision of a mass should be attempted only with careful prior planning to ensure a complete excision. Lateral margins must be at least 2 to 3 cm wide, and one complete fascial plane must be resected deep to the mass for the excision to be considered complete. Given the small size of the feline patient, this may not be feasible. Such margins can be particularly difficult to achieve with injection-site sarcomas, making preoperative imaging necessary for surgical planning. If complete excision is not considered highly likely, the veterinarian should consider an incisional biopsy for diagnosis before a major surgical procedure.

Advantages

This technique provides a potentially curative sampling diagnostic.

Disadvantages

This is the most aggressive biopsy technique. It may not be advisable if the surgery is a potential threat to patient function. This technique also requires general anesthesia.

References

1. Armstrong PJ, Blanchard G: Hepatic lipidosis in cats, *Vet Clin North Am Small Anim Pract* 39: 599, 2009.
2. Hershey AE, Sorenmo KU, Hendrick MJ et al: Prognosis for presumed feline vaccine-associated sarcoma after excision: 61 cases (1986-1996), *J Am Vet Med Assoc* 216: 58-61, 2000.
3. Proot SJ, Rothuizen J: High complication rate of an automatic Tru-Cut biopsy gun device for liver biopsy in cats, *J Vet Intern Med* 20: 1327, 2006.

CHEMOTHERAPY FOR THE FELINE CANCER PATIENT

Jenna H. Burton

Chemotherapy is primarily effective against tumors of minimal bulk with a high mitotic proportion. Some cancers, such as lymphoma, are treated primarily with chemotherapy. For other tumor types, chemotherapy is used in an adjuvant setting after radiation therapy or surgery (or both) or a neoadjuvant setting before radiation or surgery (or both). Treating cats with chemotherapy is no more technically challenging than many veterinary procedures. However, the decision to administer chemotherapy must include an assessment of risk to staff and cats that is unique to this modality, as well as the expense and practicalities of safely storing, preparing, and administering chemotherapeutic agents.

Treating cancer in cats is similar to managing any chronic disease in this species; the veterinarian's goals should be to treat the underlying disease while maintaining or improving the pet's quality of life throughout treatment. To ensure that chemotherapy is both safe and appropriate for the cat, an accurate cytologic or histologic diagnosis must be reached, and any concurrent health problems must be identified to assess the risk of toxicity to the individual cat. Staging tests, such as CBC, serum chemistry profile, urinalysis, thoracic radiographs, abdominal ultrasound, CT scan, MRI, and bone marrow aspirate cytology, are often needed to determine if the cancer is localized to one area or if it has metastasized. Advanced-stage cancers generally carry a poorer prognosis and increased risk of toxicosis as a result of treatment. This may alter the owner's willingness to pursue treatment. The owner should understand the expected prognosis for the cat as well as the possible risks, cost, and time commitment associated with therapy.

The aim of this section is to provide information regarding the safe handling and administration of chemotherapy as well as information regarding dosing and potential toxicoses of some of the chemotherapy agents commonly administered to cats. Additional resources are found in Box 28-1.

BOX 28-1

Additional Resources

ASHP guidelines on handling hazardous drugs, *Am J Health Syst Pharm* 63:1172-1191, 2006. http://www.ashp.org/DocLibrary/BestPractices/PrepGdlHazDrugs.aspx.

Burroughs GE, Connor TH, McDiarmid MA et al: Preventing occupational exposure to antineoplastic and other hazardous drugs in health care settings, National Institute for Occupational Safety and Health, 2004. http://www.cdc.gov/niosh/docs/2004-165/.

Chemotherapy and managing oncologic emergencies. In Henry CJ, Higginbotham ML: *Cancer management in small animal practice*, St. Louis, 2010, Saunders Elsevier, pp 101-135.

Chun R, Garrett LD, Vail DM: Cancer chemotherapy. In Withrow SJ, Vail DM: *Withrow and MacEwen's small animal clinical oncology*, ed 4, St. Louis, 2007, Saunders Elsevier, pp 163-192.

Thamm DH, Vail DM: Aftershocks of cancer chemotherapy: managing adverse effects, *J Am Anim Hosp Assoc* 43:1, 2007.

CHEMOTHERAPY PREPARATION

The risk of exposure of personnel to chemotherapy drugs is greatest during preparation and administration. These cytotoxic drugs may have mutagenic and carcinogenic effects. All staff members should be aware of the risks of exposure to these drugs and follow protocols to minimize these risks. Clinics that administer chemotherapy should have a written set of guidelines for the safe handling of chemotherapy drugs and plans for managing chemotherapy spills or other exposures.[1,6] Areas where chemotherapy is prepared and administered should be clearly marked, and traffic through those areas should be limited. Storage or consumption of food and beverages, including gum chewing, should be prohibited in these areas to prevent accidental ingestion. Cytotoxic drugs should be stored separately from other medications and their location clearly identified.

Facilities where injectable chemotherapy agents are prepared ideally should have a class II biologic safety cabinet that is vented to the outside and located in a space designated for chemotherapy preparation. The area should be free of clutter, and workroom surfaces should be disinfected with bleach. The work surface should be covered with an absorbent pad with a nonporous backing to help contain any spills that do occur. Compounding pharmacies can be used to prepare drugs for administration if space and proper equipment are cost prohibitive for the clinic. Items required for preparation of antineoplastic drugs are listed in Box 28-2. Personal protective equipment (PPE), including gloves, gown, protective eyewear, shoe covers, and a respirator or heavy-duty mask, should be worn when preparing cytotoxic drugs. Gowns should be made of a low-permeability fabric and have a closed front and long sleeves with elastic cuffs. Chemotherapy gloves or two pairs of latex, nitrile, or neoprene gloves are recommended, and gloves should be worn over the cuffs of the gown. Powder-free gloves should be used because the powder may absorb contaminants and increase the risk of exposure. A chemotherapy spill kit should be easily accessible in all areas where chemotherapy is handled. Box 28-3 lists the items necessary for a chemotherapy spill kit; alternatively, ready-made spill kits can also be purchased.

Reconstitution of chemotherapy drugs may cause aerosolization of the agent. For this reason devices designed to prevent aerosolization should be used. Chemotherapy dispensing pins are venting devices with a 0.22-micron filter that reduce pressure in the chemotherapy vial when reconstituting and dispensing chemotherapy drugs, thereby decreasing the risk of spraying or spillage. Optimally, a closed-system drug delivery device such as PhaSeal (Carmel Pharma, Columbus, Ohio) or a contained medication system such as

BOX 28-2

Requirements for Chemotherapy Preparation and Administration

Chemotherapy Preparation

- Personal protective equipment
- Absorbent pad with nonporous backing to cover preparation surface
- Needles, Luer-Lok syringes, syringe caps
- Drug-containment devices such as PhaSeal or ONGUARD
- Appropriate diluent, as indicated on the drug package insert
- Sealable plastic bag for transporting chemotherapy
- Hazardous waste container
- Dedicated chemotherapy sharps container
- Labels

Chemotherapy Administration

- Personal protective equipment
- Properly labeled chemotherapy drug
- Disposable, absorbent pad with nonporous backing
- Catheter setup: Surgical prep, butterfly or over-the-needle catheter, tape, T-port adapter
- PhaSeal adapter (if appropriate)
- Two syringes of nonheparinized saline flush
- Bandage for catheter site (after removal)

BOX 28-3

Chemotherapy Spill Kit Requirements

- Two pairs powder-free latex or nitrile gloves or chemotherapy gloves
- Disposable closed-front gown with elastic cuffs
- Disposable shoe covers
- Protective eyewear
- Respirator or heavy-duty mask
- Absorbable pads (disposable diapers, Chemosorb pad)
- Several large, sealable plastic bags for chemo waste

ONGUARD (B Braun, Bethlehem, Penn.) can be used. Closed-system devices prevent aerosolization of drugs and provide leak-free (dry) connection between the vial, syringe, infusion set, and the cat; they have been demonstrated to decrease surface contamination and personnel exposure.[43,44] Regardless of the venting or delivery device used, the use of Luer-Lok syringes is essential when reconstituting or drawing up chemotherapy drugs to prevent accidental disconnection of the syringe from the delivery system. Intravenous fluid lines should be primed before the addition of the chemotherapy agent to the infusion bag to prevent contamination when

BOX 28-4

Suppliers of Chemotherapy Safety Equipment

Biological Safety Cabinets

- Esco Technologies
- NuAire Laboratory Equipment Supply
- Terra Universal
- Thermo Fisher Scientific

Chemotherapy Delivery Devices

- Chemotherapy dispensing pins
  - B Braun Medical
  - Specialty Medical Group
- PhaSeal; Carmel Pharma
- ONGUARD; B Braun Medical

priming the line. Once chemotherapy preparation is complete, the drug should be placed in a sealable plastic bag for transport to the administration area to contain any leaks or spills that may occur during transportation. Suppliers of chemotherapy equipment are listed in Box 28-4.

All materials that have been in contact with chemotherapy agents during preparation and administration should be disposed of in a designated chemotherapy waste container. This includes gloves, gowns, absorbent pads, catheter materials, syringes, fluid bags, and intravenous lines that that have been used for chemotherapy administration. Sharps should be disposed of in a designated chemotherapy sharps container. To prevent accidental inoculation, needles should never be recapped. Waste that has been identified as chemotherapy waste should be handled separately from other hospital waste. Regulations regarding proper disposal of hazardous waste vary among municipalities; local and state officials should be consulted to ensure that disposal meets with Environmental Protection Agency standards in the United States and with the standards of the respective authorities in other countries.

CHEMOTHERAPY DOSING AND ADMINISTRATION

Obtaining a thorough history at each visit will help the practitioner identify any toxicosis that the cat may have experienced during prior chemotherapy, as well as guide treatment delays and dose reductions if the owner decides that the cat's quality of life is adversely affected by treatment. At each appointment cats should have their body weight, temperature, heart rate, and respiratory rate recorded and receive a complete physical examination. A CBC should be performed before each dose of chemotherapy. A biochemical panel should be performed as needed depending on the toxicity profile of the drug to be administered. Cats that appear to be feeling unwell at the time of the chemotherapy appointment should not be administered chemotherapy that day, and appropriate diagnostic tests should be performed to identify any new problems or complications from therapy. If the cat is determined to be ill secondary to its cancer, it should be treated with the goal of obtaining remission and improving the cat's quality of life.

The cat's chemotherapy dose should be calculated from the current body weight. The clinician should pay particular attention to whether the drug is to be dosed on the basis of body weight (kilograms) or body surface area (m^2). A chart converting body weight into body surface area should be easily accessible when calculating the chemotherapy dose. A system by which a second person double-checks drug type, dosage, and calculation of dose is important to prevent dosing errors. The cat's name, drug type, and drug dose should be double-checked again against the label on the drug, the patient chart, and patient identification tag or collar before administration to ensure that the cat receives the correct type and amount of drug. Additionally, a record documenting the drug given, dose and route administered, vein used for chemotherapy administration, initials of person administering the drug, and any adverse reactions should be maintained in the cat's chart. The various routes of chemotherapy administration are discussed in greater detail in subsequent sections.

Personnel should be instructed in the proper handling and disposal of waste from chemotherapy patients. Owners should be given written instructions regarding these as well. Depending on the drug administered, urine, feces, saliva, and vomitus may contain small amounts of chemotherapy agents and their metabolites for as long as 72 hours after administration; chemotherapy drugs that undergo substantial protein binding may not be fully excreted for as long as 21 days after treatment.[26] While the cat is in the hospital, cage cards identifying chemotherapy patients should be used to alert staff members responsible for cleaning soiled cages. Soiled linens should be washed separately, and disposable gloves should be worn when cleaning up urine, feces, or vomitus during this time. Litter boxes should be changed daily for several days after treatment, and use of litter-box liners may help prevent aerosolizing chemotherapy metabolites. Cats in multicat households do not need to be separated because there is no reported risk associated with sharing litter boxes or food dishes.

Oral Administration

Numerous oral antineoplastic drugs are commonly used in veterinary oncology. Although these are often perceived by pet owners to be safer and easier to administer than intravenous agents, clients must be counseled regarding the proper handling of these medications. Tablets should never be split or crushed, and capsules should not be opened; doing so may lead to the owner's exposure through inhalation, skin contact, or ingestion. Similarly, liquid medications should never be compounded. Owners should be given disposable, latex, powder-free gloves to wear when handling oral chemotherapy agents, and hands should be washed after administration. Cats should be encouraged to eat a small amount of food or carefully syringed several milliliters of water after administration of the drug to ensure passage of the tablet or capsule into the stomach. Some owners will request that the oral chemotherapy agent be administered while the pet is at the hospital. This can be problematic if the cat is prone to motion sickness and vomits the medication during the car ride home. If the owner is capable, administration of the drug once the pet is at home is preferable.

Intravenous Administration

It is recommended that the jugular veins be used for blood collection to preserve peripheral veins for chemotherapy administration. An atraumatically placed indwelling intravenous catheter should be used for administration of chemotherapy volumes greater than several milliliters. This step is critical in prevention of extravasation because many chemotherapy drugs are potent vesicants. If the catheter is not placed cleanly on the first attempt, the clinician should remove the catheter and attempt placement in a different peripheral vein. Sedation should be considered for fractious cats to ensure that the intravenous catheter remains in place throughout infusion of the chemotherapy agent. If possible, the catheter site should not be bandaged to allow the clinician to observe any signs of extravasation during administration.

Box 28-2 lists the equipment necessary for intravenous administration of cytotoxic drugs. PPE, as previously described, should be worn by the individual administering the drug and any personnel involved in restraint of the cat. An absorbent pad with a plastic backing should be placed underneath the limb into which the drug is to be delivered. A butterfly catheter can be used for cooperative cats receiving small chemotherapy volumes (<3 mL). For larger volumes an indwelling catheter should be placed and the cat closely monitored throughout the infusion. The catheter should be flushed thoroughly with nonheparinized saline before administration to ensure its patency. Chemotherapy agents should not be infused with an intravenous fluid pump. Chemotherapy drugs should be administered by slow gravity drip or manual syringe infusion over the recommended time of administration. The fluid bag should be lowered beneath the cat every few minutes to ensure that blood is able to flow back in the catheter. If the drug is administered through a syringe, the plunger should be aspirated back several times during administration of the drug to ensure that blood still appears in the hub of the catheter. The catheter site should be monitored throughout administration and administration discontinued if any swelling at the catheter site is observed. Once the chemotherapy infusion is complete, the catheter should be flushed again with nonheparinized saline before removal. A light bandage should be placed over the catheter site after removal.

Intramuscular, Subcutaneous, and Intralesional Administration

Intramuscular or subcutaneous injections are administered in the same manner as any other intramuscular or subcutaneous injection, but disposable gloves should always be worn. Because L-asparaginase is more likely to cause an anaphylactic reaction when administered intravenously, aspiration of the syringe should be performed before intramuscular or subcutaneous administration to ensure that a blood vessel has not been inadvertently entered. Chemotherapy drugs that are administered intralesionally are always suspended in oil or another vehicle to help prevent the drug from leaking out of the tumor tissues into the bloodstream. Disposable gloves and a protective gown and eyewear should be worn during administration, and a disposable, absorbent pad should be placed underneath the part of the body to receive the intralesional chemotherapy. All materials used in intramuscular, subcutaneous, or intralesional chemotherapy administration should be disposed of in the same manner as for intravenous administration. Urinary and fecal waste should be handled as previously described in the hospital and at home after intralesional injection.

Intracavitary Administration

Chemotherapy agents such as carboplatin and mitoxantrone may be administered in the pleural or peritoneal space to mitigate malignant effusions. The intracavitary dose of chemotherapy is generally the same as that administered intravenously and can be administered into a single body cavity or divided between the thorax and the abdomen. The chemotherapy drug should be diluted with the appropriate diluent to a maximal volume of 60 mL for intrathoracic administration and 250 mL for intraabdominal administration.[34] As appropriate, effusions should be drained from the cavity before instillation of the chemotherapy agent.

For intrathoracic chemotherapy administration, the cat can be positioned in sternal or lateral recumbency and the thoracic wall overlying the seventh to ninth ribs aseptically prepared. Proper PPE should be worn in a similar fashion as for intravenous administration. An 18-gauge catheter is then inserted between the ribs, the stylet removed, and the catheter flushed with 2 to 5 mL of warmed saline to ensure patency. If the cat is uncomfortable or begins to cough, or the catheter does not flush easily, the catheter should be removed and a new one inserted. If the cat tolerates the flush well, the drug can then be administered while the catheter site is monitored continuously to ensure that the drug is not inadvertently administered subcutaneously. The catheter insertion site can be blocked with a small amount of buffered lidocaine before the procedure to minimize discomfort.

For intraperitoneal administration the cat should be placed in dorsal recumbency, and a site on the abdomen just caudal to the umbilicus should be aseptically prepared. The urinary bladder should be identified with palpation to prevent accidental puncture. The 18-gauge catheter can then be placed and the chemotherapy administered as previously described. After administration of intracavitary chemotherapy, some authorities recommend allowing the cat to move around for several minutes to ensure distribution of the drug throughout the body cavity.

GENERAL ADVERSE EFFECTS OF CHEMOTHERAPY

Gastrointestinal

Chemotherapy agents can be directly cytotoxic to the intestinal epithelial crypt cells resulting in gastrointestinal side effects about 2 to 5 days after administration. Less commonly, some chemotherapy agents may cause release of 5-HT from enterochromaffin cells in the gastrointestinal tract, which binds to 5-HT_3 receptors on peripherally vagal nerves or centrally in the chemoreceptor trigger zone. 5-HT_3–mediated nausea and vomiting tend to occur within 24 hours of chemotherapy administration. These side effects may include mild to severe inappetence, nausea, vomiting, and diarrhea. For the majority of cats, gastrointestinal side effects secondary to chemotherapy are mild and self-limiting and often can be easily managed by owners at home with the administration of oral antinausea and antidiarrheal drugs on an as-needed basis. Oral antiemetics such as metoclopramide, ondansetron, and maropitant (see Table 28-5) can be dispensed at the time of the first chemotherapy appointment, whereupon owners should be instructed when to give the medications. Medications such as tylosin and metronidazole can be dispensed in a similar manner for owners to administer in the case of soft stools or diarrhea. Probiotics can also be administered throughout the duration of chemotherapy and have been anecdotally reported to decrease the frequency and severity of chemotherapy-induced diarrhea.

Cats that are unwilling to eat for several days or that have intractable vomiting should be hospitalized for supportive care with intravenous fluids to correct any hydration deficits and electrolyte abnormalities. Injectable antiemetics should be administered until the cat is eating readily on its own. Dosage of the particular chemotherapy agent should be reduced by 20% for cats that require hospitalization for significant gastrointestinal toxicosis.

Hematologic

Myelosuppression, particularly neutropenia, is a common sequela of chemotherapy administration. Most affected cats remain asymptomatic, but a small number may develop serious, life-threatening complications as a result of neutropenia and subsequent development of sepsis. The neutrophil nadir occurs approximately 7 to 10 days after chemotherapy administration, with exceptions to this noted in subsequent sections. To monitor for myelosuppression, a CBC should be checked before each chemotherapy administration to ensure that neutrophil and platelet counts are adequate. Treatment with chemotherapy should be delayed if the neutrophil count is less than 2000 to 3000 cells/uL or if the platelet count is less than 75,000 to 100,000 cells/uL. These ranges are merely guidelines, and CBC values should be assessed in conjunction with the overall health of the cat in mind. If neutropenia or thrombocytopenia occurs, a treatment delay of 5 to 7 days is generally recommended, at which time a CBC should be rechecked to ensure that cell counts have normalized. For chemotherapy agents that are administered every 2 to 3 weeks, a CBC should be checked 7 to 10 days after the first treatment with that drug. If neutrophil counts are greater than 1000 to 1500 cells/uL and the cat is afebrile and clinically well, reduction in subsequent doses is not needed.

Cats with neutrophil counts greater than 1000 cells/uL have a low risk of systemic infection. Most cats with significant neutropenia (≤1000 neutrophils/uL) can be managed on an outpatient basis, provided they are feeling well and afebrile. A broad-spectrum oral antimicrobial that is sparing to the normal gastrointestinal flora, such as trimethoprim–sulfa or enrofloxacin, can be administered for 5 to 7 days prophylactically. Cats that are febrile or systemically unwell with a concurrent neutropenia should be hospitalized for supportive therapy with intravenous fluids and antimicrobials to correct any hydration deficits or electrolyte abnormalities. In addition to a CBC, a biochemical profile and urinalysis should be obtained at admission. Treatment with intravenous broad-spectrum antimicrobials should be instituted until the cat is eating well and able to receive oral medications. Cats generally recover from febrile neutropenic episodes in 1 or 2 days. Cats that are slow to recover or are declining in the face of appropriate therapy should have thoracic radiographs, urine culture, and blood cultures performed to determine whether a resistant source of infection exists. Neutrophil counts need not be normal before the cat is released from the hospital as long as it is afebrile, eating, and tolerating oral medications.

Alopecia

Alopecia is a common concern for pet owners whose cat may require chemotherapy as part of its cancer treatment. Cats rarely develop diffuse alopecia, but this can happen with chronic administration of high-dose chemotherapy. Owners should be cautioned that most cats undergoing treatment with chemotherapy may lose their whiskers and other guard hairs, and previously shaved areas may be slow to regrow. Generally, hair will grow back once chemotherapy is discontinued.

Extravasation

Many intravenously administered chemotherapy agents are vesicants and can cause local tissue irritation or necrosis if administered outside of the vein. Of the more common chemotherapy drugs used in cats, doxorubicin, vincristine, and vinblastine are all vesicants. If there is any doubt as to whether a drug is a vesicant, it should be administered as though it is.

Signs of extravasation may include pain, erythema, moist dermatitis, and necrosis and may appear 1 to 10 days after extravasation of the drug.[28] If extravasation is suspected at the time of administration, the infusion should be stopped immediately. An attempt should be made to aspirate the drug with up to 5 mL of blood back into the syringe. The catheter is removed once this has been accomplished. Recommendations regarding additional treatment are generally extrapolated from experiences in human oncology and are based on the type of drug that was extravasated. In the case of vinca alkaloid extravasation, warm, dry compresses can be applied for several hours and hyaluronidase injected into the local site.[10] The volume of hyaluronidase injected should equal the volume of drug extravasated. Administration of dexrazoxane (Zinecard), a free-radical scavenger marketed to prevent doxorubicin-associated cardiotoxicity in humans, is indicated in the case of doxorubicin extravasation. The recommended dose is 1:10 of vesicant to dexrazoxane, and this should be administered intravenously through a separate catheter within 6 hours of extravasation.[10,30] Dexrazoxane is expensive and may be too costly for practitioners to stock. Availability at a local human hospital should be investigated because timely administration (within 3 to 6 hours) after extravasation may help mitigate tissue necrosis. Alternatively, topically applied dimethyl sulfoxide (DMSO) to the site of extravasation may help minimize tissue damage as well.[51] Aggressive surgical débridement may be required to manage severe cases of perivascular necrosis.

Hypersensitivity Reactions

L-asparaginase and doxorubicin are drugs that may cause hypersensitivity reactions in cats. Cats receiving doxorubicin should be monitored for pruritus, head shaking, erythema of the skin and mucous membranes, facial edema, wheezing, and dyspnea during the doxorubicin infusion. If any of these signs are noted, the infusion should be stopped and the cat administered diphenhydramine (2 to 4 mg/kg intramuscularly) and dexamethasone SP (0.2 to 0.4 mg/kg intravenously). Once the reaction has subsided, then infusion can be restarted at a slower rate of administration. Treatment with L-asparaginase may result in anaphylaxis. This generally occurs within 60 minutes of administration and is more likely to occur with subsequent doses than the first dose. Cats that have been treated with L-asparaginase should be closely monitored for 60 minutes after treatment for respiratory difficulty, vomiting, diarrhea, and collapse. Aggressive supportive care may be required if anaphylaxis occurs. Cats that have previously experienced hypersensitivity reactions should be premedicated with diphenhydramine and dexamethasone SP before every subsequent dose of the drug to which they had the reaction. Reactions that are severe warrant discontinuation of the drug. Subsequent hypersensitivity reactions can be more severe or even life-threatening.

COMMONLY USED CHEMOTHERAPY DRUGS

This section deals with chemotherapy agents commonly used for treating cats with cancer, as well as some newer agents about which limited information is known. Table 28-1 summarizes these chemotherapy drugs, common indications, dosages, and associated toxicities.

Alkylating Agents

Chlorambucil (Leukeran)

Chlorambucil is an orally administered DNA alkylating agent that is used to treat low-grade lymphoma, chronic lymphocytic leukemia, and, less commonly, multiple myeloma. Reported dosages include 2 mg orally every 2 or 3 days, 2 to 4 mg/m^2 orally every other day, 15 mg/m^2 orally every day for 4 consecutive days once every 3 weeks, and 20 mg/m^2 orally once every 2 weeks.[13,23,49]

Chlorambucil is generally well tolerated, and gastrointestinal signs are uncommon. Myelosuppression may occur after prolonged used. Rare toxicities may include neurotoxicity, which has been reported in a single cat, and there may be an increased risk of developing a second malignancy with prolonged therapy.[4,49]

Cyclophosphamide (Cytoxan)

Cyclophosphamide is a prodrug that requires hepatic activation and is excreted primarily by the kidneys. It is most commonly combined with other chemotherapy drugs to treat lymphoma or various sarcomas. It can be administered either orally or intravenously, and dosages range from 200 to 300 mg/m^2 or 10 mg/kg, as dictated by the protocol used. Cyclophosphamide may be administered as a single bolus, or the oral dose may be divided over 3 to 4 days. For example, if the cat's total dose is 75 mg, then the cat may be administered a 25-mg tablet orally once daily for 3 days. Tablets should never be divided, and it may be necessary to compound cyclophosphamide for smaller cats. Alternatively, the injectable form is relatively inexpensive, and dosing is very flexible.

Common side effects include myelosuppression and gastrointestinal toxicity. Less commonly, sterile hemorrhagic cystitis may develop secondary to cyclophosphamide administration.[8] If signs of hematuria, pollakiuria, or stranguria are observed in a cat that has been recently treated with cyclophosphamide, a urinalysis and urine culture should be performed. If the urine culture is negative, a presumptive diagnosis of sterile hemorrhagic cystitis can be made, and cyclophosphamide therapy should be discontinued permanently.

Lomustine (CCNU, CeeNU)

Lomustine is an oral DNA alkylating agent that is most frequently used against mast cell tumors and lymphoma.[11,41,42] Because of its ability to cross the blood–brain barrier, it is also used to treat brain tumors, but efficacy against these tumor types is not documented in cats. It may be efficacious against fibrosarcoma and multiple myeloma.[11] Lomustine is administered at 50 to 60 mg/m^2 or 10 mg/cat orally once every 3 to 6 weeks.[11,41,42] It may be necessary to compound capsules to smaller sizes for more accurate dosing because the 10 mg/cat dose may underdose or overdose some cats.

Myelosuppression, particularly neutropenia, is the dose-limiting toxicity for lomustine. Severe and persistent thrombocytopenia can occur that warrants discontinuation of the drug if platelet numbers do not return to normal levels in 6 weeks. Gastrointestinal signs can occur with this drug as well. Hepatotoxicity has not been reported in cats to date, but routine monitoring of liver enzymes is still recommended. Pulmonary fibrosis can occur in people treated with CCNU, and a report of pulmonary fibrosis developing after chronic CCNU therapy exists for a single cat.[46] Renal toxicity is an uncommon side effect in humans and has not been reported in cats, but routine monitoring of kidney values

TABLE 28-1 **Commonly Used Chemotherapy Drugs**

Drug	Main Indications	Toxicities	Dosage
ALKYLATING AGENTS			
Cyclophosphamide	LSA, leukemia, sarcoma	Myelosuppression, GI, sterile hemorrhagic cystitis	200 to 300 mg/m^2 PO or IV or 10 mg/kg IV, depending on protocol used
Chlorambucil	Low-grade LSA, CLL, MM	GI and myelosuppression (uncommon)	2 mg PO every 2-3 days; 2-3 mg/m^2 PO every other day; 15 mg/m^2 PO × 4 days every 3 weeks; 20 mg/m^2 PO every 2 weeks
Lomustine	MCT, LSA	Myelosuppression, GI, pulmonary fibrosis (rare)	50 to 60 mg /m^2 PO or 10 mg/cat every 3 to 6 weeks
Melphalan	MM, LSA	Myelosuppression (thrombocytopenia)	0.1 mg/kg/day PO; 0.1 mg/kg PO every 24 hours for 14 days, then 0.1 mg/kg PO every other day
ANTHRACYCLINES			
Doxorubicin	LSA, various sarcomas and carcinomas	Myelosuppression, GI, nephrotoxicity, perivascular vesicant, hypersensitivity reaction	1 mg/kg or 25 mg/m^2 IV every 2-3 weeks
Liposome-encapsulated doxorubicin (Doxil)	ISS	GI, nephrotoxicity, perivascular vesicant, cutaneous, hypersensitivity	1 mg/kg IV every 3 weeks
Mitoxantrone	LSA, various sarcomas and carcinomas	GI, myelosuppression	6 to 6.5 mg/m^2 IV every 3 weeks
ANTIMETABOLITES			
Cytosine arabinoside	LSA, leukemia	Mild myelosuppression, GI	600 mg/m^2 SC, divided into 4 doses given every 12 hours for 2 days
Gemcitabine	SCC, other carcinomas	May cause increase hematologic and local tissue toxicity when used as a radiosensitizer	Not assessed as single agent in cats
Methotrexate	LSA	GI, myelosuppression	0.8 mg/kg PO or IV as directed by protocol
ANTITUBULIN AGENTS			
Vinblastine	MCT, LSA	GI, myelosuppression	Unknown, 2 mg/m^2 IV weekly or every other week
Vincristine	LSA, leukemia	GI, myelosuppression, peripheral neuropathy	0.5 to 0.75 mg/m^2 IV weekly
Vinorelbine	Not assessed	Not assessed	Not assessed
TYROSINE KINASE INHIBITORS			
Imatinib (Gleevec)	MCT, ISS	Mild GI	10 mg/kg PO daily
Masitinib (Kinavet)	Not assessed	Not assessed	Not assessed
Toceranib (Palladia)	Not assessed	GI	2.8 mg/kg PO every other day or Monday, Wednesday, Friday
MISCELLANEOUS			
L-asparaginase	LSA	Hypersensitivity	400 IU/kg or 10,000 IU/m^2 SC or IM
Carboplatin	Carcinoma or sarcoma	Myelosuppression; GI	240 mg/m^2 IV every 3-4 weeks
Imiquimod 5% cream (Aldara)	Cutaneous SCC *in situ* or actinic SCC	Localized erythema	Topical
Prednisone/ prednisolone	LSA, MM, MCT	GI, polyuria, polydipsia, polyphagia, diabetes mellitus	2 mg/kg PO once daily; taper according to protocol
Hydroxyurea	Polycythemia vera, chronic myelogenous leukemia	GI, myelosuppression	10 mg/kg PO daily

LSA, Lymphosarcoma; *GI,* gastrointestinal; *PO,* orally; *IV,* intravenously; *CLL,* chronic lymphocytic leukemia; *MM,* multiple myeloma; *MCT,* mast cell tumor; *ISS,* injection-site sarcoma; *SCC,* squamous cell carcinoma; *SC,* subcutaneously; *IM,* intramuscularly.

should be performed for cats with documented renal insufficiency that are receiving CCNU.

Melphalan

Melphalan is an oral DNA alkylating agent that is most commonly used in treatment of multiple myeloma and occasionally lymphoma. Melphalan can be administered at 0.1 mg/kg orally once daily or 0.1 mg/kg orally daily for 14 days followed by 0.1 mg/kg orally every other day.[5,7] Tablets may need to be compounded for more accurate dosing because they should not be split.

Myelosuppression, in particular thrombocytopenia, is the most common toxicity and generally occurs with chronic administration. A CBC should be monitored once weekly for the first month and then every 4 to 8 weeks during melphalan therapy.

Anthracyclines

Doxorubicin (Adriamycin)

Doxorubicin is an anthracycline that exerts its antineoplastic effects by way of a number of mechanisms, including topoisomerase II inhibition, intercalation of DNA, and generation of free radicals. Doxorubicin is commonly used in multidrug protocols for lymphoma, injection-site and other soft tissue sarcomas, and feline mammary carcinomas. Doxorubicin is diluted in 30 to 50 mL 0.9% NaCl and administered at 1 mg/kg or 25 mg/m^2 intravenously over 20 to 60 minutes every 2 to 3 weeks.

More common side effects of doxorubicin administration include gastrointestinal signs and myelosuppression. Doxorubicin is a potent vesicant, and utmost caution should be used to ensure that extravasation does not occur during administration. Cumulative nephrotoxicity may occur with doxorubicin administration, and this drug should not be used in cats with renal insufficiency.[36] Renal values and urine specific gravity should be monitored routinely in cats receiving doxorubicin and the drug discontinued if isosthenuria or azotemia occur. Cats can also have an acute hypersensitivity reaction with doxorubicin, and some practitioners routinely premedicate cats receiving doxorubicin with diphenhydramine or dexamethasone SP (or both). Regardless of whether premedication with antihistamines or corticosteroids is performed, the cat should be closely monitored during the infusion for any indications of a hypersensitivity reaction, such as head shaking, erythema of the pinna or mucous membranes, facial swelling, dyspnea, and agitation. Cumulative cardiotoxicity with doxorubicin administration is well documented in humans and dogs but is infrequent in cats.[36] Administration of doxorubicin to cats with underlying cardiac disease is discouraged, and some practitioners recommend not exceeding cumulative doses of 180 to 240 mg/m^2 in cats with normal cardiac function.

Liposmal-Encapsulated Doxorubicin (Doxil)

Liposomal-encapsulated doxorubicin was formulated to avoid the significant cardiotoxicity in humans that limits doxorubicin administration. This drug may have efficacy against similar tumor types as doxorubicin, including injection-site sarcomas, and is dosed at 1 mg/kg intravenously every 3 weeks.[40]

Liposomal-encapsulated doxorubicin has a similar toxicity profile in cats as native doxorubicin. Gastrointestinal side effects are generally mild and self-limiting. Liposomal-encapsulated doxorubicin is associated with nephrotoxicity, and renal function should be closely monitored after administration of the drug.[40] It is a vesicant and should be administered only through a cleanly placed intravenous catheter. Cats may also develop a nonpainful alopecia and erythema with hyperpigmentation around their mouths and distal limbs.[40] Cats may experience a hypersensitivity reaction characterized by salivation and bradycardia during their first treatment with liposomal-encapsulated doxorubicin; this can be managed with administration of diphenhydramine and dexamethasone SP.[40] Intracavitary administration of liposomal-encapsulated doxorubicin has been reported in dogs but has not been evaluated in cats.

Mitoxantrone

Mitoxantrone is an anthracycline derivative that exerts its cytotoxic effects by inhibiting topoisomerase II. This drug likely has a similar antitumor profile to doxorubicin and may be efficacious against lymphoma and various carcinomas and sarcomas.[35] The mitoxantrone dosage is 6 to 6.5 mg/m^2 intravenously every 3 weeks. The drug is diluted in 20 to 50 mL 0.9% NaCl before intravenous administration over 10 to 15 minutes. Mitoxantrone can be administered in the pleural or peritoneal space to help alleviate malignant effusions.

The most common adverse effects observed with mitoxantrone are mild, self-limiting gastrointestinal signs and myelosuppression. Unlike doxorubicin, mitoxantrone does not induce hypersensitivity reactions and is not as potent a vesicant if extravasated. Owners should be cautioned that urine and sclera may be blue-tinged after administration.[7]

Antimetabolites

Cytosine Arabinoside (Cytarabine, Cytosar-U, ara-C)

Cytosine arabinoside is a deoxycytidine analog that interferes with DNA synthesis through DNA polymerase inhibition. Because this drug is cell cycle specific with an extremely short plasma half-life, it is most efficacious when administered by constant-rate infusion or with the dose divided into twice-daily subcutaneous injections over several days. Cytosine arabinoside is used in cats primarily to treat lymphoma or leukemia, particularly when there is central nervous system (CNS) involvement, because of the ability of the drug to cross the blood–brain barrier. Cytosine arabinoside is often substituted for cyclophosphamide for treatment of renal lymphoma because CNS involvement occurs in approximately 40% of these cases.[33] The dosage of cytosine arabinoside is 600 mg/m^2 divided into four doses administered subcutaneously twice daily for 2 days or administered as a constant-rate infusion at 300 mg/m^2 per day for 2 days.[7]

Cytosine arabinoside is generally well tolerated, with myelosuppression being most common and gastrointestinal signs occurring rarely.

Gemcitabine

Gemcitabine is an analog of deoxycytidine that is activated intracellularly, resulting in DNA synthesis inhibition. There is limited information on the use of gemcitabine as a single agent in cats. It has been used as a radiation sensitizer in the treatment of oral squamous cell carcinoma (SCC) and also in combination with carboplatin as therapy for various carcinomas.[22,29,31] This drug is expensive compared with other chemotherapy drugs, and optimal dosing in cats is not known at this time.

Adverse effects when administered intravenously at 2 mg/kg weekly in conjunction with carboplatin included moderate gastrointestinal toxicity and myelosuppression.[31] When administered intravenously at 25 mg/m^2 twice weekly as a radiation sensitizer, significant hematologic and local tissue toxicity occurred.[29] Additional research investigating efficacy, dosage, and toxicity of gemcitabine as a single agent drug is necessary before it can be used routinely in cats with cancer.

Methotrexate

Methotrexate is an antifolate that inhibits dihydrofolate reductase, thereby blocking DNA synthesis. It has been used primarily in combination chemotherapy protocols for lymphoma at a dosage of 0.8 mg/kg weekly, either intravenously or orally.[32,33,45]

Adverse effects of methotrexate administration are most commonly gastrointestinal signs, with myelosuppression occurring less commonly.

5-Fluorouracil (5-FU)

5-Fluorouracil (5-FU) is available in injectable and topical formulations. Because this drug has been documented to cause fatal neurotoxicity in cats, it should not be administered, even topically, to this species.[17,18,52]

Antitubulin Agents

Vinblastine and vincristine are naturally occurring vinca alkaloids derived from the periwinkle plant, and vinorelbine is a second-generation synthetic vinca alkaloid. These drugs disrupt cell division by binding to the microtubular proteins in the mitotic spindle. Metabolism of this class of drugs occurs in the liver, and dosage adjustments should be made for liver dysfunction. The antitubulin agents share a similar toxicity profile, with exceptions for each drug noted in subsequent sections. They are generally well tolerated, but mild gastrointestinal toxicosis and myelosuppression may occur. The antitubulin agents are all vesicants and should be administered using a cleanly placed catheter.

Vinblastine

Vinblastine is used as a treatment for mast cell tumor or substituted for vincristine in lymphoma protocols when vincristine is not tolerated by the cat or the disease has become refractory to vincristine in a rescue setting. Anecdotally, cats can tolerate intravenous dosages of 2 mg/m^2 weekly to every other week, but published data are lacking.

Vincristine

Vincristine is used commonly to treat lymphoma and leukemia; reported dosages range from 0.5 to 0.75 mg/m^2 given as an intravenous bolus once weekly. Peripheral neuropathy, which may present as constipation in cats, is uncommon but may occur with prolonged administration.[7]

Vinorelbine (Navelbine)

There is no published information regarding vinorelbine and its possible antitumor spectrum, dosage, or toxicity profile in tumor-bearing cats.

Platinum Drugs

Carboplatin

Carboplatin is a platinum-derived alkylating agent that may have efficacy against various carcinomas and sarcomas.[7,24] The most common route of administration is intravenous, but carboplatin can also be administered intracavitarily, in the thorax or abdomen, and intralesionally. Carboplatin is administered intravenously at 240 mg/m^2 every 3 to 4 weeks. Dosing of carboplatin on the basis of glomerular filtration rate has been investigated and may allow for more appropriate dosing in cats, but this is clinically impractical for most practitioners.[2,3] Carboplatin can also be used intralesionally for facial SCC. General anesthesia is required for treatment, and carboplatin is administered at 1.5 mg/cm^3 in purified sesame oil emulsion injected every 0.5 cm in the tumor and adjacent tissues weekly for up to four treatments.[53] Carboplatin has been reported to be administered intracavitarily at 180 to 200 mg/m^2 to help alleviate malignant effusions; however, information regarding efficacy is limited.[47,48]

Myelosuppression is the dose-limiting toxicity of carboplatin. Neutrophil and platelet nadirs generally occur 2 to 3 weeks after administration.[24] Gastrointestinal signs occur less commonly with carboplatin. Because carboplatin is excreted by the kidneys, it is important to assess renal function (blood urea nitrogen, creatinine, and urine specific gravity) before each treatment. Carboplatin is not commonly directly nephrotoxic, but decreased excretion occurs with decreased renal function, thereby increasing the likelihood of toxicity.

Cisplatin

Administration of cisplatin to cats induces a fatal pulmonary edema. It should not be administered to cats at any dosage.[25]

Tyrosine Kinase Inhibitors

Tyrosine kinases are proteins expressed on cell surfaces that are integral to regulation of cell growth and differentiation. These kinases, such as KIT, epithelial growth factor receptor (EGFR), vascular endothelial growth factor receptor (VEGFR), and platelet-derived growth factor receptor (PDGFR), bind their specific growth factor, leading to downstream intracellular signaling and regulation of cell growth, differentiation, and survival. Tyrosine kinases can become constitutively activated with some types of cancer, thereby leading to unregulated cell growth. Tyrosine kinase inhibitors are a newer class of antineoplastic agents that inhibit these kinases by binding to the ATP-binding pocket, resulting in downregulation of cellular growth. Tyrosine kinase inhibitors used in veterinary oncology include imatibinib (Gleevec; Novartis), toceranib (Palladia; Pfizer), and masitinib (Kinavet CA-1; AB Science). Both toceranib and masitinib have recently been approved by the Food and Drug Administration for the treatment of canine mast cell tumors. Gastrointestinal side effects are common in dogs, and it is recommended that patients have a "drug holiday" until gastrointestinal signs resolve. Use of these drugs for cats remains off-label, and there is limited information regarding dosage, tumor specificity, efficacy, and toxicity of tyrosine kinase inhibitors in this species.

Imatinib (Gleevec)

Imatinib has been used to treat feline cutaneous, splenic, and disseminated mast cell tumors at doses at 10 to 15 mg/kg orally once daily. The most common side effects noted are mild gastrointestinal upset.[20,21,27]

Toceranib (Palladia)

Information regarding use of toceranib in cats is limited. Preliminary results suggest that dosage of 2.8 mg/kg orally every other day or on a Monday/Wednesday/Friday schedule may have some efficacy against oral SCC and injection-site sarcomas.[19] Most common side effects are gastrointestinal, particularly anorexia with weight loss and vomiting.[19]

Masitinib (Kinavet CA-1)

Masitinib has been administered to healthy cats at a dosage of 50 mg/cat orally every 24 to 48 hours and was well tolerated over a 4-week period.[9] Gastrointestinal toxicosis was most common, with neutropenia and proteinuria occurring less frequently.[9] There is no information at this time regarding dosage, safety, and efficacy for masitinib in cats with cancer.

Miscellaneous

L-asparaginase

L-asparaginase is an enzyme derived from *Escherichia coli* that depletes cells of asparagine, an essential amino acid for protein synthesis. Lymphoreticular cells are particularly sensitive to the effects of L-asparaginase because they lack asparagine synthetase and cannot produce asparagine. For this reason L-asparaginase is primarily used in treatment of lymphoma and leukemia. It is administered at 400 mg/kg or 10,000 IU/m^2 intramuscularly or subcutaneously as part of a multidrug protocol.

The most common toxicity associated with L-asparaginase administration is anaphylaxis, which may be characterized by dyspnea, pruritus, edema, vomiting, diarrhea, hypotension, and collapse. Additional rare side effects may include myelosuppression, particularly when administered simultaneously with vincristine, or pancreatitis.

Hydroxyurea

Hydroxyurea is an oral chemotherapy agent that suppresses proliferation of myeloid, erythroid, and platelet precursors by inhibiting DNA synthesis.[37] The main indications for hydroxyurea are treatment of polycythemia vera and chronic myelogenous leukemia. The recommended dosage is 10 mg/kg orally once daily.[7]

Side effects associated with hydroxyurea therapy in cats may include myelosuppression and gastrointestinal toxicity.[7]

Imiquimod (Aldara)

Imiquimod 5% cream (Aldara) is a topical immune response modifier that has been shown to have antitumor effects by enhancement of both innate and cell-mediated immunity. Data are limited at this time, but imiquimod 5% cream may be effective in treating multifocal, cutaneous SCC *in situ* or actinic (solar-induced) SCC in cats.[14,38] Reported topical application schedules range from once daily to three times a week on affected areas.

Adverse events that have been reported include mild erythema at the site of application.[14,38] Potential systemic toxicities have been reported as well, and these are likely secondary to ingestion of imiquimod 5% cream by the cat because the drug should not have systemic effects when applied topically. These side effects include mild gastrointestinal upset, neutropenia, and elevated liver enzymes.[14] It is recommended that routine monitoring of CBC and biochemistry panel be performed every 4 to 8 weeks in cats treated with imiquimod 5% until more information is known about this drug in cats.

Prednisone and Prednisolone

Prednisolone and its prodrug prednisone are glucocorticoids frequently used in veterinary oncology. In most species prednisone is converted to prednisolone in the liver, but there is some concern that this step does not occur efficiently in some cats. Therefore use of prednisolone rather than prednisone is recommended in this species.[39] Prednisolone is commonly used in multidrug chemotherapy protocols, and there is evidence that prednisolone has activity against lymphoma, plasma cell tumors, and mast cell tumors.* The antitumor dose of prednisolone is 2 mg/kg orally once daily. This dose is tapered over approximately 1 month and then generally discontinued when used in combination chemotherapy protocols. Other common uses for prednisolone include decreasing edema associated with tumors of the CNS and as an antiinflammatory for pain control in cats that cannot tolerate administration of nonsteroidal antiinflammatory drugs. For these indications, prednisolone is generally administered at antiinflammatory dosages (0.5 to 1 mg/kg orally once daily).

Prednisolone is generally well tolerated in cats. Adverse effects may include polyphagia, polydipsia, polyuria, and gastrointestinal irritation. Rarely, chronic high-dose prednisolone therapy may lead to development of diabetes mellitus in cats.[12]

References

1. ASHP guidelines on handling hazardous drugs, *Am J Health Syst Pharm* 63:1172, 2006.
2. Bailey DB, Rassnick KM, Dykes NL et al: Phase I evaluation of carboplatin by use of a dosing strategy based on a targeted area under the platinum concentration-versus-time curve and individual glomerular filtration rate in cats with tumors, *Am J Vet Res* 70:770, 2009.
3. Bailey DB, Rassnick KM, Erb HN et al: Effect of glomerular filtration rate on clearance and myelotoxicity of carboplatin in cats with tumors, *Am J Vet Res* 65:1502, 2004.
4. Benitah N, de Lorimier L-P, Gaspar M et al: Chlorambucil-induced myoclonus in a cat with lymphoma, *J Am Anim Hosp Assoc* 39:283, 2003.
5. Betts GJ, Clarke SL, Richards HE et al: Regulating the immune response to tumours, *Adv Drug Del Rev* 58:948, 2006.

*References 7, 15, 16, 45, 49, 50.

6. Burroughs GE, Connor TH, McDiarmid MA et al: *Preventing occupational exposure to antineoplastic and other hazardous drugs in health care settings in Cincinnati, OH*, National Institute for Occupational Safety and Health, 2004.
7. Chun R, Garrett LD, Vail DM: Cancer chemotherapy. In Withrow SJ, Vail DM, editors: *Withrow & MacEwen's small animal clinical oncology*, ed 4, St Louis, 2007, Saunders Elsevier, pp 163-192.
8. Crow SE, Theilen GH, Madewell BR et al: Cyclophosphamide-induced cystitis in the dog and cat, *J Am Vet Med Assoc* 171:259, 1977.
9. Daly M, Sheppard S, Cohen N et al: Safety of masitinib mesylate in healthy cats, *J Vet Intern Med* 25:297, 2011.
10. Dhaliwal RS: Managing oncologic emergencies. In Henry CJ, Higginbotham ML, editors: *Cancer managment in small animal practice*, St Louis, Mo, 2010, Saunders Elsevier, pp 122-135.
11. Fan TM, Kitchell BE, Dhaliwal RS et al: Hematological toxicity and therapeutic efficacy of lomustine in 20 tumor-bearing cats: critical assessment of a practical dosing regimen, *J Am Anim Hosp Assoc* 38:357, 2002.
12. Feldman EC, Nelson RW: Feline diabetes mellitus. In Feldman EC, Nelson RW, editors: *Canine and feline endocrinology and reproduction*, ed 3, St Louis, 2004, Saunders, pp 539-579.
13. Fondacaro J, Ritcher K, Carpenter J et al: Feline gastrointestinal lymphoma: 67 cases (1988-1996), *Eur J Comp Gastroenterol* 4:5, 1999.
14. Gill VL, Bergman PJ, Baer KE et al: Use of imiquimod 5% cream (Aldara™) in cats with multicentric squamous cell carcinoma in situ: 12 cases (2002-2005), *Vet Comp Oncol* 6:55, 2008.
15. Hadden AG, Cotter SM, Rand W et al: Efficacy and toxicosis of velcap-c treatment of lymphoma in cats, *J Vet Intern Med* 22:153, 2008.
16. Hanna F: Multiple myelomas in cats, *J Feline Med Surg* 7:275, 2005.
17. Harvey HJ, MacEwen EG, Hayes AA: Neurotoxicosis associated with use of 5-fluorouracil in five dogs and one cat, *J Am Vet Med Assoc* 171:277, 1977.
18. Henness AM, Theilen GH, Madewell BR et al: Neurotoxicosis associated with use of 5-florouracil, *J Am Vet Med Assoc* 171:692, 1977.
19. Hohenhaus AE: Biological activity and adverse event profile in cats treated with toceranib phosphate. Annual Conference of the Veterinary Cancer Society, San Diego, Calif, 2010, p 64.
20. Isotani M, Tamura K, Yagihara H et al: Identification of a c-kit exon 8 internal tandem duplication in a feline mast cell tumor case and its favorable response to the tyrosine kinase inhibitor imatinib mesylate, *Vet Immunol Immunopathol* 114:168, 2006.
21. Isotani M, Yamada O, Lachowicz JL et al: Mutations in the fifth immunoglobulin-like domain of kit are common and potentially sensitive to imatinib mesylate in feline mast cell tumours, *Br J Haematol* 148:144, 2010.
22. Jones PD, de Lorimier L-P, Kitchell BE et al: Gemcitabine as a radiosensitizer for nonresectable feline oral squamous cell carcinoma, *J Am Anim Hosp Assoc* 39:463, 2003.
23. Kiselow MA, Rassnick KM, McDonough SP et al: Outcome of cats with low-grade lymphocytic lymphoma: 41 cases (1995-2005), *J Am Vet Med Assoc* 232:405, 2008.
24. Kisseberth WC, Vail DM, Yaissle J et al: Phase I clinical evaluation of carboplatin in tumor-bearing cats: a veterinary cooperative oncology group study, *J Vet Intern Med* 22:83, 2008.
25. Knapp DW, Richardson RC, DeNicola DB et al: Cisplatin toxicity in cats, *J Vet Intern Med* 1:29, 1987.
26. Knobloch A, Mohring SAI, Eberle N et al: Drug residues in serum of dogs receiving anticancer chemotherapy, *J Vet Intern Med* 24:379, 2010.
27. Lachowicz JL, Post GS, Brodsky E: A phase I clinical trial evaluating imatinib mesylate (Gleevec) in tumor-bearing cats, *J Vet Intern Med* 19:860, 2005.
28. Lana SE, Dobson JM: Principles of chemotherapy. In Dobson JM, Lascelles BDX, editors: *BSAVA manual of canine and feline oncology*,

ed 3, Gloucester, UK, 2011, British Small Animal Veterinary Association, pp 60-79.
29. LeBlanc AK, LaDue TA, Turrel JM et al: Unexpected toxicity following use of gemcitabine as a radiosensitizer in head and neck carcinomas: a veterinary radiation therapy oncology group pilot study, *Vet Radiol Ultrasound* 45:466, 2004.
30. Mahoney JA, Bergman PJ, Camps-Palau MA et al: Treatment of doxorubicin extravasation with intravenous dexrazoxane in a cat, *J Vet Intern Med* 21:872, 2007.
31. Martinez-Ruzafa I, Dominguez PA, Dervisis NG et al: Tolerability of gemcitabine and carboplatin doublet therapy in cats with carcinomas, *J Vet Intern Med* 23:570, 2009.
32. Mooney S, Hayes AA, MacEwen EG et al: Treatment and prognostic factors in lymphoma in cats: 103 cases (1977-1981), *J Am Vet Med Assoc* 194:696, 1989.
33. Mooney S, Hayes AA, Matus RE et al: Renal lymphoma in cats: 28 cases (1977-1884). *J Am Vet Med Assoc* 191:1473, 1987.
34. Ogilvie GK, Moore AS: Drug handling and adminsitration. In Ogilvie GK, Moore AS, editors: *Feline oncology: a comprehensive guide to compassionate care*, Trenton, NJ, 2001, Veterinary Learning Systems, pp 53-61.
35. Ogilvie GK, Moore AS, Obradovich JE et al: Toxicoses and efficacy associated with administration of mitoxantrone to cats with malignant tumors, *J Am Vet Med Assoc* 202:1839, 1993.
36. O'Keefe DA, Sisson DD, Gelberg HB et al: Systemic toxicity associated with doxorubicin administration in cats, *J Vet Intern Med* 7:309, 1993.
37. Paz-Ares L, Donehower RC, Chabner BA: Hydoxyurea. In Chabner BA, Longo DL, editors: *Cancer chemotherapy and biotherapy*, ed 4, Philadelphia, 2006, Lippincott Williams & Wilkins, pp 229-236.
38. Peters-Kennedy J, Scott DW, Miller Jr WH: Apparent clinical resolution of pinnal actinic keratoses and squamous cell carcinoma in a cat using topical imiquimod 5% cream, *J Feline Med Surg* 10:593, 2008.
39. Plumb DC: *Plumb's veterinary drug handbook*, ed 6, Stockholm, Wisconsin, 2008, PharmaVet.
40. Poirier VJ, Thamm DH, Kurzman ID et al: Liposome-encapsulated doxorubicin (Doxil) and doxorubicin in the treatment of vaccine-associated sarcoma in cats, *J Vet Intern Med* 16:726, 2002.
41. Rassnick KM, Gieger TL, Williams LE et al: Phase I evaluation of CCNU (Lomustine) in tumor-bearing cats, *J Vet Intern Med* 15:196, 2001.
42. Rassnick KM, Williams LE, Kristal O et al: Lomustine for treatment of mast cell tumors in cats: 38 cases (1999-2005), *J Am Vet Med Assoc* 232:1200, 2008.
43. Sessink PJ, Connor TH, Jorgenson JA et al: Reduction in surface contamination with antineoplastic drugs in 22 hospital pharmacies in the US following implementation of a closed-system drug transfer device, *J Oncol Pharm Pract* 17:39, 2011.
44. Siderov J, Kirsa S, McLauchlan R: Reducing workplace cytotoxic surface contamination using a closed-system drug transfer device, *J Oncol Pharm Pract* 16:19, 2010.
45. Simon D, Eberle N, Laacke-Singer L et al: Combination chemotherapy in feline lymphoma: treatment outcome, tolerability, and duration in 23 cats, *J Vet Intern Med* 22:394, 2008.
46. Skorupski KA, Durham AC, Duda L et al: Pulmonary fibrosis after high cumulative dose nitrosourea chemotherapy in a cat, *Vet Comp Oncol* 6:120, 2008.
47. Sparkes A, Murphy S, McConnell F et al: Palliative intracavitary carboplatin therapy in a cat with suspected pleural mesothelioma, *J Feline Med Surg* 7:313, 2005.
48. Spugnini EP, Crispi S, Scarabello A et al: Piroxicam and intracavitary platinum-based chemotherapy for the treatment of advanced mesothelioma in pets: preliminary observations, *J Exp Clin Cancer Res* 27:6, 2008.
49. Stein TJ, Pellin M, Steinberg H et al: Treatment of feline gastrointestinal small-cell lymphoma with chlorambucil and glucocorticoids, *J Am Anim Hosp Assoc* 46:413, 2010.
50. Teske E, van Straten G, van Noort R et al: Chemotherapy with cyclophosphamide, vincristine, and prednisolone (COP) in cats with malignant lymphoma: new results with an old protocol, *J Vet Intern Med* 16:179, 2002.
51. Thamm DH, Vail DM: Aftershocks of cancer chemotherapy: managing adverse effects. *J Am Anim Hosp Assoc* 43:1, 2007.
52. Theilen G: Adverse effect from use of 5% fluorouracil, *J Am Vet Med Assoc* 191:276, 1987.
53. Theon AP, VanVechten MK, Madewell BR: Intratumoral administration of carboplatin for treatment of squamous cell carcinomas of the nasal plane in cats, *Am J Vet Res* 57:205, 1996.

SELECTED FELINE CANCERS

Cats are affected by a wide variety of cancers and a complete discussion is beyond the scope of this chapter. In general, information on the most common cancers will be found elsewhere in this book with the relevant body system. Presented here is an overview of three important cancers that deserve more in-depth discussion—lymphoma, injection-site sarcoma, and mammary tumors. For more detailed information on feline oncology, the reader is referred to a current textbook, such as *Cancer Management in Small Animal Practice*, edited by Carolyn Henry and Mary Lynn Higginbotham (St. Louis, 2010, Saunders).

LYMPHOMA

Kevin Choy and Jeffrey N. Bryan

INCIDENCE, ETIOLOGY, AND RISK FACTORS

Lymphoma (also termed *malignant lymphoma* and *lymphosarcoma)* is the most common feline neoplasm, comprising more than half of all hemolymphatic tumors.[29,39,54] Lymphoma can be found in cats of any age, breed, or sex, although purebred cats such as the Manx, Burmese, and Siamese may have an increased risk.[16,25,29,39,54] The precise etiology of feline lymphoma in many cases is unknown; however, viral causes of feline lymphoma are well defined, with both feline leukemia virus (FeLV) and feline immunodeficiency virus (FIV) infections implicated. Before the widespread use of FeLV testing and control regimens that began in the 1980s, up to 70% of diagnosed feline lymphoma was caused by FeLV infection. Over the following decades a shift away from FeLV-associated tumors has been seen, with only 14% to 25% of cats with lymphoma having documented FeLV infection despite an overall increase in diagnosed cases of feline lymphoma.* Although FeLV has a direct role in tumorigenesis, FIV is thought to indirectly contribute to an increased risk of feline lymphoma by immunosuppression.[2,17] This association with immune compromise is further supported by a report describing 95 feline renal transplant patients receiving immunosuppressive therapy, in which 9.5% of cats developed *de novo* malignant neoplasia, predominantly lymphoma.[55] FeLV infection in one study increased the risk of lymphoma 62-fold, FIV infection sixfold, and concurrent FeLV and FIV infection 77-fold.[44] Exposure to second-hand cigarette tobacco smoke is also reported to increase the risk of developing lymphoma 2.4- to 3.2-fold over background, depending on duration of exposure.[3] Chronic inflammation may also play a role in the development of feline lymphoma, as seen in other tumors, such as injection-site sarcomas.[26] An association has been suggested between inflammatory bowel disease and intestinal lymphoma in which one progresses to the other, although supporting evidence is not well developed.[6,26,34,41,42]

CLINICAL FEATURES

Cats with lymphoma exhibit a bimodal pattern of clinical presentation. The first group comprises cats approximately 2 years of age (although cats as young as 6 months have been reported) with FeLV-associated disease, typically with mediastinal lymph node involvement and pleural effusion resulting in dyspnea.[16] The second group comprises mature cats 6 to 12 years of age that are serologically FeLV negative and present with alimentary (particularly intestinal) lymphoma or lymphoma in a multicentric or extranodal pattern.[8,25] Clinical signs of alimentary lymphoma commonly include vomiting, diarrhea, anorexia, and weight loss. A palpable abdominal mass or thickening of the intestinal tract is often appreciated. Nonalimentary locations for lymphoma are quite varied and can include virtually every tissue in the body; renal, mediastinal, respiratory (particularly nasal), CNS (brain and spinal), multicentric (lymph node), skeletal muscle, cutaneous, conjunctival, and cardiac lymphoma have been reported, with clinical signs referable to the respective organ system dysfunction.† Hypercalcemia may also be a feature of lymphoma, but this is seen less commonly than in canine lymphoma.[4] Prevalence, presenting clinical signs, and biological behavior of feline lymphoma vary significantly with geographical location and may reflect regional differences in feline populations as well as differences in retroviral strains and prevalence.‡

*References 1, 5, 7, 13-16, 25, 27, 29, 48, 50, 54.

†References 1-3, 5-8, 16, 17, 25, 26, 29, 30, 34, 41, 42, 44, 52.

‡References 7, 13-16, 27, 48, 50.

DIAGNOSIS AND STAGING

Because feline lymphoma is a neoplasm of the lymphoid system that generally affects multiple locations, a thorough diagnostic evaluation is recommended to confirm diagnosis and anatomic localization(s) and establish baseline data points to evaluate response to subsequent therapy. Feline lymphoma is usually classified on the basis of anatomic location rather than the traditional World Health Organization (WHO) staging scheme commonly used in dogs. Anatomic site of origin is important insofar as each type of lymphoma appears to have different specific clinical behavior, therapy considerations, and prognosis.[5,8,29,34,54]

Diagnosis of most anatomic forms of lymphoma in the cat can be made from cytologic examination of fine-needle aspirates of an enlarged lymph node, affected tissues, or cavitary fluids (e.g., pleural effusions in mediastinal lymphoma). When cytologic findings are equivocal, histopathology and immunohistochemistry are recommended. Histopathology is particularly important in alimentary lymphoma in which endoscopic (partial thickness) or surgical (full thickness) biopsies of the gastrointestinal tract are generally required for a diagnosis to differentiate between severe lymphoplasmacytic intestinal inflammation and malignant lymphoma. Inclusion of the intestinal muscularis is necessary for a definitive diagnosis of lymphoma. If histopathology is inconclusive, molecular analysis techniques such as polymerase chain reaction for antigen receptor rearrangement (PARR) test for T and B cell receptor gene clonality assessment can provide further support for malignancy, but this is not yet established as a gold standard for diagnosis. Nasal lymphoma also commonly requires a biopsy using a blind or rhinoscopic approach to confirm diagnosis, with advanced imaging such as CT helpful in assessing the extent of disease.[49]

After the diagnosis of lymphoma, complete staging should include a detailed physical examination, with particular attention to lymph node size (including tonsils), abdominal palpation (masses, thickened intestinal loops, organomegaly), cranial thoracic compression (mediastinal mass), and ophthalmic examination. Peripheral lymphadenopathy is less common in cats than in dogs. Laboratory evaluation should include a CBC, serum biochemistry profile, urinalysis with culture and sensitivity (to assess for preexisting urinary tract infections that may represent a nidus for sepsis during immunosuppressive chemotherapy), and FIV and FeLV serology. Three-view thoracic radiographs (right lateral, left lateral, and ventrodorsal views) should be made to assess lymph node, pulmonary, mediastinal, and pleural structures. Abdominal ultrasound examination is useful to assess gastrointestinal wall thickness, mesenteric lymph node size, and organ size and echotexture (liver, spleen, kidney). Ultrasound-guided fine-needle aspirates should be performed where appropriate. Bone marrow aspirates should be performed to evaluate this compartment for disease infiltration. Complete staging with anatomic classification will guide appropriate therapy selection, minimize toxicity, and reduce therapy-associated complications.

BIOLOGICAL BEHAVIOR

As with dogs, most anatomical classifications of feline lymphoma are non-Hodgkin–like disease that tends to progress to systemic involvement during the course of disease.[19,51] Because of the anatomic syndromic nature of lymphoma in cats, the clinical signs associated with the site of origin are most important for prognostication. Immunophenotype for B- or T-lymphocytes varies by location and etiology but has not been shown to be significantly prognostic for outcome.[1,5,30,37,54] Age, weight, sex, FIV status, and stage (based on WHO criteria) also do not appear to be prognostic in cats.[30,32] FeLV infection has been shown by some studies to be a negative prognostic factor because of a more rapid emergence of drug resistance, but other studies have not found a similar association.[1,11,50] The most important prognostic factor for feline lymphoma is response to therapy and anatomic localization of disease.

TREATMENT AND PROGNOSIS

Systemic chemotherapy is the primary treatment modality for feline lymphoma. Without medical therapy mortality rates in cats with lymphoma are approximately 40% and 75% at 4 and 8 weeks after diagnosis, respectively.[20] For aggressive high-grade lymphoblastic lymphoma, multi-agent chemotherapy is considered the standard of care, with a variety of protocols and response rates reported. There is a general lack of consensus regarding the gold-standard protocol. Consequently, many treatment regimens are specific to a particular institution or practice.

The combination protocol COP (cyclophosphamide, vincristine, and prednisone) has been reported to result in complete remission in 50% to 75% of cats, with a median survival time (MST) ranging from 2 to 9 months.[32,47,48] Single-agent doxorubicin chemotherapy has been less successful, with a response rate of 42% and median duration of response of 64 days in cats.[23,38] However, when doxorubicin is included into multi-agent protocols either as part of a CHOP (H = doxorubicin) protocol or as maintenance therapy (COP followed by doxorubicin), significantly longer durations of remission have been reported in cats that responded compared with cats that received only COP therapy.[32,47] These reports suggest that a subset of cats may benefit from the addition of doxorubicin. Doxorubicin should be used with caution in cats because it is potentially nephrotoxic and cardiotoxic; thus a COP-based protocol may be preferable for cats with preexisting renal or cardiac disease.[35] The doxorubicin-containing CHOP protocol that is used at Washington State University is provided (Table 28-2), but consultation with a veterinary oncologist is recommended before starting induction therapy. The most reliable prognostic indicator is response to therapy; individuals achieving complete remission typically enjoy the best outcomes, with MST approaching 1 year, and longer-term survival reported. Conversely, failure to achieve complete remission is generally associated with MST of a few months.[6,11,30,42,47] Single-agent therapy with prednisolone at 2 mg/kg

TABLE 28-2 **Modified Madison-Wisconsin (Short) Protocol for Feline Lymphoma at Washington State University**

Week	1	2	3	4	5	6	7	8	9	10	11	12	13	14	15	16	17	18	19	20	21	22	23	24	25
Vincristine	•		•			•		•			•				•				•				•		
Cyclophosphamide		•					•						•								•				
Doxorubicin				•					•								•								•
Prednisone	•	•	•	•	•	•	•	•	•	•	•	•	•	•	•	•	•	•	•	•	•	•	•	•	•

Complete blood counts are performed before and weekly after each dose of chemotherapy. If the total segmented neutrophil count is below 2500, treatment is delayed for 1 week or until count increases above 2500. Watch for sterile hemorrhagic cystitis resulting from cyclophosphamide therapy. Serum biochemistry profiles and urinalysis should be checked once monthly to monitor for potential nephrotoxicity associated with doxorubicin therapy.
Vincristine: 0.5 mg/m^2 intravenously (do not exceed 0.12 mg/dose); *vesicant.*
Cyclophosphamide: 200 mg/m^2 intravenously or orally; *wear gloves if given orally.*
Doxorubicin: 25 mg/m^2 intravenously. Dilute into 50 mL of saline and administer intravenously over 40 to 60 minutes; *severe vesicant.*
Prednisone: 2 mg/kg orally daily for the first 2 weeks, then 1 mg/kg orally daily for the next 2 weeks, then 1 mg/kg orally every other day thereafter for long-term use.

orally once daily for 2 weeks and then tapered to 1 mg/kg thereafter may provide varying degrees of palliation, with reported MST of approximately 60 days.[1,47] Rescue protocols are not well defined in cats. Single-agent lomustine (CCNU) has been used in cats as primary therapy or in a rescue setting at reported dosages of 50 to 65 mg/m^2 orally every 3 to 6 weeks depending on degree and duration of myelosuppression. The advantages are simplicity and relative inexpensiveness, but response rates are variable, with generally shorter MSTs reported. Chronic administration of lomustine has been associated with severe thrombocytopenia and pulmonary fibrosis in cats.[1,5,21,40,45] Cats with renal lymphoma have been shown to have a reduced risk of CNS metastasis with the addition of cytosine arabinoside to a standard COP protocol (COAP).[5,31]

Malignant lymphocytes are radiosensitive, and radiation therapy has been reported for treatment of localized lymphoma.* Although radiation is effective for control of local disease, particularly nasal lymphoma, adjunctive systemic chemotherapy is generally advised to target residual tumor cells and delay systemic progression. Survival times of cats treated by localized radiation therapy with or without chemotherapy for nasal lymphoma often exceed 1 year, with durable MSTs approaching 3 years reported.[9,10,12,18,43] Whole-abdomen irradiation has also been used as adjunctive or rescue therapy for gastrointestinal lymphoma. In one pilot study eight cats with gastrointestinal or abdominal lymphoma that achieved remission during an abbreviated 6-week CHOP chemotherapy protocol received abdominal radiation therapy 2 weeks later. Five cats remained in remission for at least 266 days after starting therapy, with a range from 266 to 1332 days.[53] In another study a rapid abdominal radiation protocol delivered over 2 days for cats with relapsed or chemotherapy-resistant gastrointestinal lymphoma resulted in a response in 10 of 11 cats, with a postirradiation MST of 214 days.[36]

Large granular lymphoma is an uncommon, morphologically distinct variant of lymphoma in cats that carries a poor prognosis. Response to chemotherapy is generally poor, and an MST of 57 days after diagnosis has been reported.[22]

Feline alimentary lymphoma presents a therapeutic challenge. MSTs for cats experiencing complete remission can exceed 11 months.[24,42,45,56] High-grade lymphoblastic forms of alimentary lymphoma should be treated with combination chemotherapy (COP, CHOP). Low-grade small-cell gastrointestinal lymphoma (also termed *lymphocytic intestinal lymphoma)* is considered an indolent neoplasm that can be successfully treated with a combination of daily prednisone or prednisolone (2 to 3 mg/kg orally daily tapering to 1 mg/kg orally every 48 hours) and chlorambucil therapy (20 mg/m^2 orally every 2 weeks or 15 mg/m^2 orally every 24 hours for 4 consecutive days every 3 weeks). Prognosis was reported to be good, with overall response rates of up to 96%, up to 76% of cats achieving complete remission, and median clinical remission durations of approximately 19 to 26 months reported.[24,42,46,56] Please refer to Chapter 23 for further information on the management of gastrointestinal lymphoma.

Regardless of the anatomic form, most cats with lymphoma benefit from supportive care, particularly cats that are anorexic, vomiting, or severely debilitated because of chronic disease progression. Nutritional and fluid support is critical for cats that are inappetent because of either the malignancy or the chemotherapy. The placement of an esophageal, gastric, or jejunal feeding tube (bypassing the affected tissues) is often quite helpful to allow adequate nutrition, hydration, and administration of oral medication, particularly during early stages of treatment. Appetite stimulants, antiemetics, and thorough nursing care may also be necessary to improve body condition and tolerance to therapy.[34,54]

*References 9, 10, 12, 18, 19, 28, 36, 43, 53.

References

1. Argyle DJ, Brearly MJ, Turek MM: *Decision making in small animal oncology—feline lymphoma and leukemia*, Ames, Iowa, 2008, Wiley-Blackwell, pp 197-209.
2. Beatty JA, Lawrence CE, Callanan JJ et al: Feline immunodeficiency virus (FIV)–associated lymphoma: a potential role for immune dysfunction in tumorigenesis, *Vet Immunol Immunopathol* 23:309, 1998.
3. Bertone ER, Snyder LA, Moore AS: Environmental tobacco smoke and risk of malignant lymphoma in pet cats, *Am J Epidemiol* 156:268, 2002.
4. Bolliger AP, Graham PA, Richard V et al: Detection of parathyroid hormone–related protein in cats with humoral hypercalcemia of malignancy, *Vet Clin Pathol* 31:3, 2002.
5. Bryan JN: Feline lymphoma. In Henry CJ, Higginbotham ML, editors: *Cancer management in small animal practice*, ed 1, St Louis, 2010, Saunders Elsevier, pp 348-351.
6. Carreras JK, Goldschmidt M, Lamb M et al: Feline epitheliotropic intestinal malignant lymphoma: 10 cases (1997-2000), *J Vet Intern Med* 17:326, 2003.
7. Court EA, Watson AD, Peaston AE: Retrospective study of 60 cases of feline lymphosarcoma, *Aust Vet J* 75:424, 1997.
8. Couto CG, Nelson RW: *Small animal internal medicine*, ed 4, St Louis, 2009, Mosby/Elsevier, pp 1174-1186.
9. de Lorimier LP, Fan TM, Haney S et al: Feline sinonasal neoplasia: CT staging and prognosis with mega voltage radiation therapy, *Vet Comp Oncol* 3:39, 2005.
10. Elmslie RE, Ogilvie GK, Gillette EL et al: Radiotherapy with and without chemotherapy for localized lymphoma in cats, *Vet Radiol Ultrasound* 32:277, 1991.
11. Ettinger SN: Principles of treatment for feline lymphoma, *Clin Tech Small Anim Pract* 18:98, 2003.
12. Evans SM, Hendrick M: Radiotherapy of feline nasal tumors: a retrospective study of nine cases, *Vet Radiol Ultrasound* 30:128, 1989.

13. Gabor LJ, Canfield PJ, Malik R: Haematological and biochemical findings in cats in Australia with lymphosarcoma, *Aust Vet J* 78:456, 2000.
14. Gabor LJ, Jackson ML, Trask B et al: Feline leukaemia virus status of Australian cats with lymphosarcoma, *Aust Vet J* 79:476, 2001.
15. Gabor LJ, Love DN, Malik R et al: Feline immunodeficiency virus status of Australian cats with lymphosarcoma, *Aust Vet J* 79:540, 2001.
16. Gabor LJ, Malik R, Canfield PJ: Clinical and anatomical features of lymphosarcoma in 118 cats, *Aust Vet J* 76:725, 1998.
17. Gregory CR, Madewell BR, Griffey SM et al: Feline leukemia virus–associated lymphosarcoma following renal transplantation in a cat, *Transplantation* 52:1097, 1991.
18. Haney SM, Beaver J, Turrel CA et al: Survival analysis of 97 cats with nasal lymphoma: a multi-institutional retrospective study (1986-2006), *J Vet Intern Med* 23:287, 2009.
19. Holt E, Goldschmidt MH, Skorupski K: Extranodal conjunctival Hodgkin's-like lymphoma in a cat, *Vet Ophthalmol* 9:141, 2006.
20. Jarrett WF, Crighton GW, Dalton RG: Leukaemia and lymphosarcoma in animals and man. I: Lymphosarcoma or leukaemia in domestic animals, *Vet Rec* 79:693, 1966.
21. Komori S, Nakamura S, Takahashi K et al: Use of lomustine to treat cutaneous nonepitheliotropic lymphoma in a cat, *J Am Vet Med Assoc* 226:237, 2005.
22. Krick EL, Little L, Patel R et al: Description of clinical and pathological findings, treatment and outcome of feline large granular lymphocyte lymphoma (1996-2004), *Vet Comp Oncol* 6(2):102, 2008.
23. Kristal O, Lana SE, Ogilvie GK, et al: Single agent chemotherapy with doxorubicin for feline lymphoma: a retrospective study of 19 cases (1994-1997), *J Vet Intern Med* 15:125, 2001.
24. Lingard AE, Briscoe K, Beatty JA et al: Low-grade alimentary lymphoma: clinicopathological findings and response to treatment in 17 cases, *J Fel Med Surg* 11:692, 2009.
25. Louwerens M, London CA, Pedersen NC et al: Feline lymphoma in the post-feline leukemia virus era, *J Vet Intern Med* 19:329, 2005.
26. Madewell BR, Gieger TL, Pesavento PA et al: Vaccine site–associated sarcoma and malignant lymphoma in cats: a report of six cases (1997-2002), *J Am Anim Hosp Assoc* 40:47, 2004.
27. Malik R, Gabor LJ, Foster SF, et al: Therapy for Australian cats with lymphosarcoma, *Aust Vet J* 79:808, 2001.
28. Mansfield CM, Hartman GV, Reddy EK: A review of the role of radiation therapy in the treatment of non-Hodgkin's lymphomas, *J Natl Med Assoc* 70(2):103, 1978.
29. Meuten DJ: *Tumors in domestic animals*, ed 4, Ames, Iowa, 2002, Blackwell, pp 144-151.
30. Milner RJ, Peyton J, Cooke K et al: Response rates and survival times for cats with lymphoma treated with the University of Wisconsin-Madison chemotherapy protocol: 38 cases (1996-2003), *J Am Vet Med Assoc* 227:1118, 2005.
31. Mooney SC, Hayes AA, Matus RE et al: Renal lymphoma in cats: 28 cases (1977-1984), *J Am Vet Med Assoc* 191:1473, 1987.
32. Moore AS, Cotter SM, Frimberger AE et al: A comparison of doxorubicin and COP for maintenance of remission in cats with lymphoma, *J Vet Intern Med* 10:372, 1996.
33. Moore PF, Woo JC, Vernau W, et al: Characterization of feline T cell receptor gamma (TCRG) variable region genes for the molecular diagnosis of feline intestinal T cell lymphoma, *Vet Immunol Immunopathol* 106:167, 2005.
34. Ogilvie GK, Moore AS. *Feline oncology—feline lymphoma and leukemia*, Trenton, NJ, 2001, Veterinary Learning Systems, pp 191-219.
35. O'Keefe DA, Sisson DD, Gelberg HB et al: Systemic toxicity associated with doxorubicin administration in cats, *J Vet Intern Med* 7:309, 1993.
36. Parshley DL, LaRue SM, Kitchell B et al: Abdominal irradiation as rescue therapy for feline gastrointestinal lymphoma: a retrospective study of 11 cats (2001-2008), *J Fel Med Surg* 13:63, 2011.
37. Patterson-Kane JC, Kugler BP, Francis K: The possible prognostic significance of immunophenotype in feline alimentary lymphoma: a pilot study, *J Comp Pathol* 130:220, 2004.
38. Peaston AE, Maddison JE: Efficacy of doxorubicin as an induction agent for cats with lymphosarcoma, *Aust Vet J* 77:442, 1999.
39. Preister WA, McKay FW: The occurrence of tumors in domestic animals. In Zeigler JL, editor: National Cancer Institute Monographs, Bethesda, 1980, U.S. Dept of Health and Human Services.
40. Rassnick KM, Gieger TL, Williams LE et al: Phase I evaluation of CCNU (lomustine) in tumor-bearing cats, *J Vet Intern Med* 15:196, 2001.
41. Richter KP: Feline gastrointestinal lymphoma. In Bonagura JR, Twedt DC, editors: *Kirk's current veterinary therapy XIV*, St Louis, 2009, Saunders, pp 340-342.
42. Richter KP: Feline gastrointestinal lymphoma, *Vet Clin North Am Small Anim Pract* 33:1083, vii, 2003.
43. Sfiligoi G, Theon AP, Kent MS: Response of nineteen cats with nasal lymphoma to radiation therapy and chemotherapy, *Vet Radiol Ultrasound* 48(4):388, 2007.
44. Shelton GH, Grant CK, Cotter SM et al: Feline immunodeficiency virus and feline leukemia virus infections and their relationships to lymphoid malignancies in cats: a retrospective study (1968-1988), *J Acquir Immune Defic Syndr* 3:623, 1990.
45. Skorupski KA, Durman AC, Duda L et al: Pulmonary fibrosis after high cumulative dose nitrosourea chemotherapy in a cat, *Vet Comp Oncol* 6(2):120, 2008.
46. Stein TJ, Pellin M, Steinberg H et al: Treatment of feline gastrointestinal small-cell lymphoma with chlorambucil and glucocorticoids, *J Am Anim Hosp Assoc* 46:413, 2010.
47. Taylor SS, Goodfellow MR, Browne WJ et al: Feline extranodal lymphoma: response to chemotherapy and survival in 110 cats, *J Small Anim Pract* 50:584, 2009.
48. Teske E, van Straten G, van Noort R, Rutteman GR: Chemotherapy with cyclophosphamide, vincristine, and prednisolone (COP) in cats with malignant lymphoma: new results with an old protocol, *J Vet Intern Med* 16:179, 2002.
49. Tromblee TC, Jones JC, Etue AE et al: Association between clinical characteristics, computed tomography characteristics, and histologic diagnosis for cats with sinonasal disease, *Vet Radiol Ultrasound* 47:241, 2006.
50. Vail DM, Moore AS, Ogilvie GK, et al: Feline lymphoma (145 cases): proliferation indices, cluster of differentiation 3 immunoreactivity, and their association with prognosis in 90 cats, *J Vet Intern Med* 12:349, 1998.
51. Walton RM, Hendrick MJ: Feline Hodgkin's-like lymphoma: 20 cases (1992-1999), *Vet Pathol* 38:504, 2001.
52. Waly NE, Gruffydd-Jones TJ, Stokes CR et al: Immunohistochemical diagnosis of alimentary lymphomas and severe intestinal inflammation in cats, *J Comp Pathol* 133:253, 2005.
53. Williams LE, Pruitt AF, Thrall DE: Chemotherapy followed by abdominal cavity irradiation for feline lymphoblastic lymphoma, *Vet Radiol Ultrasound* 51:681, 2010.
54. Withrow SJ, Vail DM: *Withrow and MacEwen's small animal clinical oncology: feline lymphoma and leukemia*, St Louis, 2007, Saunders, pp 733-756.
55. Wooldridge JD, Gregory CR, Mathews KG et al: The prevalence of malignant neoplasia in feline renal-transplant recipients, *Vet Surg* 31:94, 2002.
56. Zwahlen CH, Lucroy MD, Kraegel SA et al: Results of chemotherapy for cats with alimentary malignant lymphoma: 21 cases (1993-1997), *J Am Vet Med Assoc* 213:1144, 1998.

INJECTION-SITE SARCOMA

William C. Kisseberth

INCIDENCE, ETIOLOGY, AND RISK FACTORS

Injection-site sarcomas, also referred to as vaccine-associated sarcomas, were first recognized as a distinct histopathologic and clinical entity 20 years ago, when an increase in the number of feline fibrosarcoma biopsy accessions was first observed.[13] The increased number of fibrosarcomas in cats could largely be explained by an increase in the number of tumors occurring at anatomic sites commonly used for vaccination (e.g., hindlimb, dorsal neck/interscapular, dorsal lumbar, flank, and dorsolateral thorax). It also was observed that the increase in tumor incidence coincided with significant changes in routine vaccination practices used in cats, notably the introduction of FeLV vaccines and legally mandated rabies vaccination of cats.[13] Often, sarcomas occurring at these locations were surrounded by lymphocytes and macrophages containing foreign material identical to that previously described in postvaccinal inflammatory injection site reactions.[13,14] Furthermore, the foreign material was found to contain aluminum, which is commonly used in vaccine adjuvants.[13] Although aluminum-adjuvanted rabies vaccines were the first to be associated with sarcoma formation in cats, subsequent epidemiologic studies identified an increased risk for sarcoma formation associated with other vaccines and other types of injections in cats, including adjuvanted and nonadjuvanted rabies, FeLV, and feline viral rhinotracheitis/calicivirus/panleukopenia vaccines, long-acting penicillins, and methylprednisolone acetate injections.[14,17,18] However, no specific manufacturer's product has ever been identified as being of greater risk.[18] Apparently, not all injectable products are associated with the same risk. For example, diabetic cats receiving frequent insulin injections (and probably other injections associated with hospitalizations) were not found to be at increased risk for sarcoma formation.[17]

The hypothesized pathogenesis of sarcoma formation in cats induced by injections is that inflammatory and immunologic reactions associated with the presence of foreign material in injection sites predisposes the cat to a derangement of its fibrous connective tissue repair response, eventually leading to neoplasia in some cases.[13] In fact, in some tumors transitional areas can be identified, where microscopic foci of sarcoma are found in areas of granulomatous inflammation. It has been pointed out that there is precedent for this type of oncogenesis in the cat.[13] Sarcomas have been reported to develop in the eyes of cats after persistent or previous trauma.[7] The pathogenesis of ocular sarcomas could be similar to that proposed for injection-site sarcomas. Although the histologic, epidemiologic, and clinical evidence supports an important role for injections in sarcoma formation in cats, other host and environmental factors also must be of critical importance because only a very small proportion of injections result in sarcoma formation. Although there is a feline sarcoma virus, it does not have a role in the pathogenesis of these tumors. Similarly, FeLV, FIV, papillomavirus, and polyomavirus viruses have all been undetectable in feline injection-site sarcomas and do not appear to have a role in pathogenesis.[8,19-21] The expression of a variety of oncogenes, tumor suppressor genes, and growth factors has been investigated in feline injection-site sarcomas, including p53, PDGF-R, KIT, TGF-alpha, FGFb, and STAT3.[15,25,27,30] A variable proportion of injection-site sarcomas exhibit dysregulated expression of each of these proteins; however, their role, if any, in pathogenesis is unclear at this time. In a recent study both injection-site sarcomas and spontaneous sarcomas in cats exhibited an extensive range of genomic imbalances, some of which were highly recurrent. Interestingly, deletions of two specific regions were significantly associated with the non–injection-site sarcoma (spontaneous) phenotype.[31]

The true incidence of injection-site sarcomas is unknown. The most common estimate given is between 1 of 1000 and 1 of 10,000 vaccines administered; however, a more recent epidemiologic study estimated the incidence of vaccine-associated sarcoma to be 0.63 sarcoma in 10,000 cats vaccinated and 0.32 sarcoma in 10,000 doses of all vaccines administered.[4,12,26] Thus the incidence is now believed to be one case for every 10,000 to 30,000 cats vaccinated.

CLINICAL FEATURES

The clinical presentation of injection-site sarcoma is that of a subcutaneous or intramuscular mass occurring at the site of a previous injection (although an injection history may not be known) (Figure 28-1). Injection-site sarcomas are most commonly located in the dorsal thoracic region between the shoulder blades, a common location for vaccination and other injections in cats. Other affected areas include the femoral, flank, lumbar, and gluteal regions; however, there is some evidence for a changing anatomic distribution of these tumors, presumably related to current vaccine administration recommendations made in response to this disease.[18,29] In the case of vaccine-associated sarcomas, tumors have been reported to form 4 weeks to 10 years after vaccination, although most appear to develop within 3 years.[12,24] Masses are typically nonpainful and firm to fluctuant and may contain cystic areas. Occasionally, large masses are ulcerated. Usually, affected cats show no systemic signs of illness, except in advanced disease. Feline

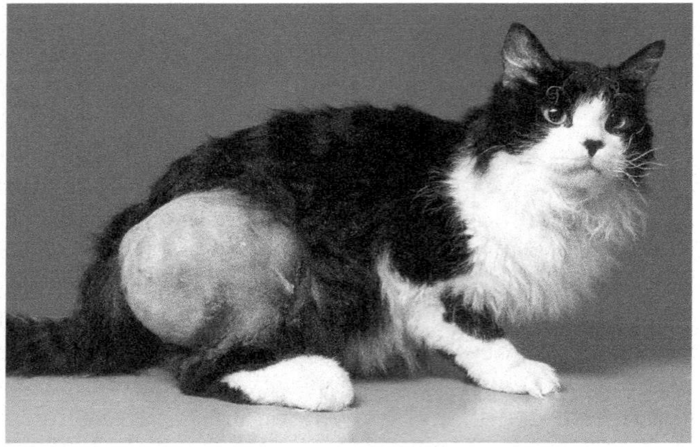

FIGURE 28-1 Injection-site sarcoma arising from the caudal thigh of a cat. *(Courtesy C. Guillermo Couto.)*

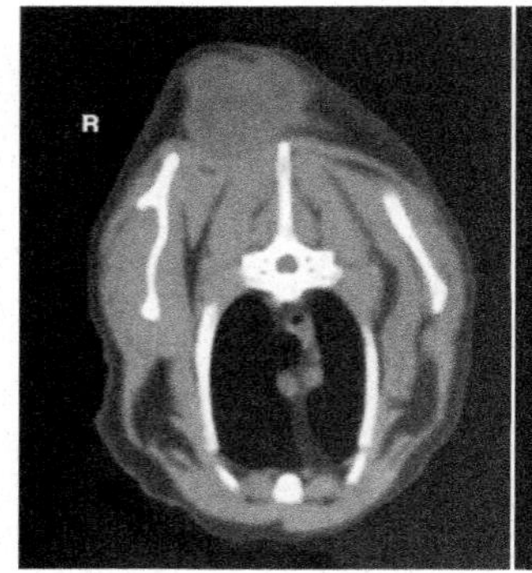

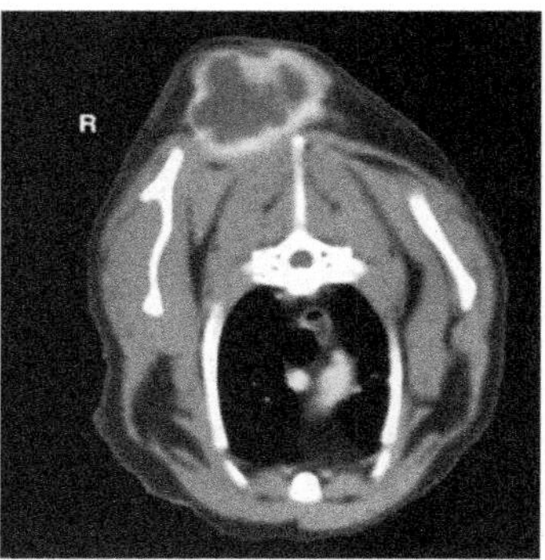

FIGURE 28-2 Computed tomography image of a contrast rim enhancing interscapular injection-site sarcoma in a cat. *(Courtesy Eric Green.)*

injection-site sarcomas are highly aggressive and locally invasive, making them challenging to treat. They are more likely to recur after surgical excision than spontaneous sarcomas at other sites.[14] Histologic subtypes of soft tissue sarcomas reported at the site of vaccination include fibrosarcoma, malignant fibrous histiocytoma, osteosarcoma, rhabdomyosarcoma, undifferentiated sarcoma, liposarcoma, and chondrosarcoma.[15]

Although injection-site sarcoma is the primary differential diagnosis in most cases, differential diagnoses may include other tumors (e.g., lymphoma), abscess, foreign body, and postvaccine reaction. Local vaccine or injection reactions in particular must be distinguished from sarcoma. In response to the recognition of injection-site sarcoma as a significant and iatrogenically caused health problem in cats, the Vaccine-Associated Feline Sarcoma Task Force (VAFSTF) was created.[32] VAFSTF concluded that owner education is imperative and cat owners should be warned of the risk of vaccine- and injection-associated sarcomas and the occurrence of local vaccine and injection reactions. Furthermore, owners should be taught how to examine the injection site and seek veterinary assistance if any of the three following scenarios occur (i.e., the "3-2-1" recommendation):

- A mass persists at the injection site for more than 3 months after injection.
- A mass is present and is larger than 2 cm, regardless of time since injection.
- A mass is still increasing in size 1 month after injection.[32,33]

DIAGNOSIS AND STAGING

A presumptive diagnosis of injection-site sarcoma can often be made on the basis of history, anatomic location, and fine-needle aspiration cytology; however, a biopsy should be performed to confirm the diagnosis. Tru-Cut needle biopsy, punch biopsy, or wedge biopsy is recommended, and the practitioner should strictly follow standard biopsy techniques and principles. Staging of injection-site sarcoma includes a minimum database consisting of a CBC and differential, serum chemistry profile, urinalysis, and FeLV and FIV serology. If regional lymph nodes are accessible for fine-needle aspiration cytology, they should be aspirated. Thoracic radiographs are made to assess for lung metastasis. CT or MRI imaging is extremely useful for assessing tumor invasiveness into surrounding structures and for surgical and radiation therapy planning (Figure 28-2).

BIOLOGICAL BEHAVIOR

Injection-site sarcomas are aggressive, locally invasive tumors with a moderate metastatic potential. Primary tumors grow at a variable rate, invading surrounding and underlying tissues and making surgical resection difficult. Metastasis occurs primarily in the lungs but also can occur at other sites, such as regional lymph nodes, mediastinum, pericardium, liver, pelvis, and eye.[9,10,28] Lung metastases are radiographically visible in 10% to 24% of the cases at the time of diagnosis.[5,16]

TREATMENT AND PREVENTION

Although injection-site sarcomas have the potential for metastasis, treatment is focused on local control of the primary tumor, at least initially. Because injection-site sarcomas are aggressive and locally invasive, establishing control of the primary tumor is often challenging. Treatment generally begins with wide and sometimes radical surgical excision of the primary tumor, provided the mass is determined to be surgically resectable using multiplanar imaging. Aggressive resection should include at least 3-cm lateral surgical margins and be one

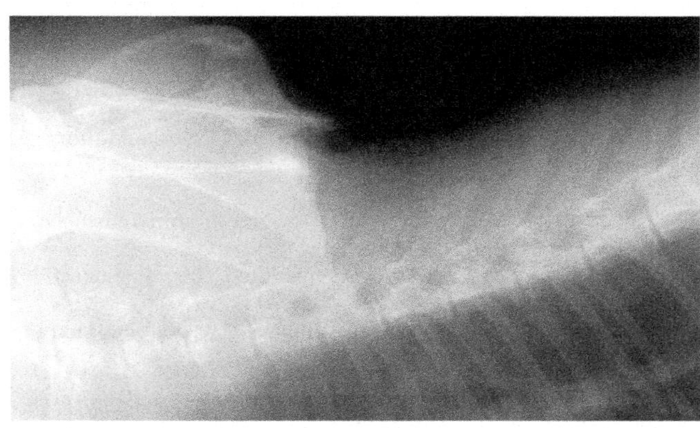

FIGURE 28-3 Postsurgical lateral radiograph of a cat with an interscapular injection-site sarcoma. Removal of vertebral dorsal processes was required to achieve complete resection. *(Courtesy Stephen J. Birchard.)*

uninvolved fascial layer deep. Because of the invasive nature of these tumors, depending on the anatomic location it may also be necessary to resect bony structures. Partial scapulectomy and removal of dorsal processes of vertebrae may be necessary with interscapular masses (Figure 28-3) and rib resections, and body wall reconstructions may be required to adequately resect masses affecting the body wall and flanks.[22] Masses occurring in the pelvic limb are often best managed by limb amputation or hemipelvectomy, provided the mass is distal enough to obtain a clean surgical margin. Surgical staples should be placed in the tumor bed to define the margins of the surgical field if radiation therapy will potentially be included in the postsurgical treatment plan. The margins of the excised mass should be clearly marked with surgical ink or suture before fixing and submitting for histopathology.[11] The best surgical outcomes are associated with aggressive surgeries performed by specialist surgeons.[16] The median recurrence-free interval for injection-site sarcomas excised at a referral institution was 274 days, significantly longer than a median of 66 days in those cats whose tumors were excised by referring veterinarians.[16] Even with aggressive wide excision, surgical margins are often infiltrated with neoplastic cells.[11] Overall, the local recurrence rate is 30% to 70%, and even when no evidence of tumor cells is detected histopathologically at the surgical margins, there may be a 50% local recurrence rate.[3,24] For this reason the decision to incorporate postoperative radiation therapy in the treatment plan of these patients should not unduly rely on whether tumor-free surgical margins are achieved. Cats treated with aggressive excision at first attempt have longer tumor-free intervals than those treated with marginal excision (325 days versus 79 days), and cats with complete excision have a longer tumor-free interval (>16 months versus 4 months) and survival time (>16 months versus 9 months) than those whose excisions were incomplete.[6,16]

Although surgical excision is the primary treatment modality for most cats with injection-site sarcomas, a multimodality treatment approach may provide better outcomes for cats with incomplete surgical excisions (whether or not the surgical margins are assessed to be "clean"). Radiation therapy can be incorporated into the treatment plan either preoperatively or postoperatively. There is no clear evidence as to whether preoperative or postoperative irradiation is better for injection-site sarcoma. In one study evaluating the effectiveness of preoperative radiation and surgery in 33 cats, the median disease-free interval was 398 days and the median overall survival time was 600 days.[5] Local recurrence of the tumor was noted in 45%. In another study 76 cats received postoperative radiation. The median disease-free interval was 405 days, and the median overall survival time was 469 days. The local recurrence rate was 41%.[3] Because these are different studies, with different confounding factors, results are not directly comparable. No clinical study has ever directly compared the two treatment approaches. When used, radiation treatment is typically performed in conjunction with surgery, except in the palliative setting.

The role of chemotherapy in the treatment of injection-site sarcoma is poorly defined. There are no studies that support its use as the primary, or sole, form of treatment in the gross disease setting and little evidence for its use in the adjuvant (after surgery or radiation) setting either. Nonetheless, chemotherapy is commonly used in an attempt to palliate nonresectable tumors; in the neoadjuvant setting to cytoreduce large tumors before surgery; and in the adjuvant setting, especially for histologically high-grade tumors. It has also been used as a radiation sensitizer. Chemotherapy drugs that have been used clinically include doxorubicin, cyclophosphamide, carboplatin, mitoxantrone, and vincristine.[24] In general, use of these drugs has resulted in some partial responses and infrequent complete responses. Usually, responses are not durable. Of these drugs doxorubicin has received the most attention, both as a single agent and in combination with cyclophosphamide. In one study evaluating the use of combined doxorubicin and cyclophosphamide in cats with nonresectable tumors, the overall response rate was 50%, with 17% having resolution of all clinically detectable tumor.[1] Unfortunately, the responses were not durable, with a median response duration of 125 days. In another study 69 cats were treated with four cycles of doxorubicin combined with surgical excision 10 days after the second chemotherapy cycle. No differences in the rates of recurrence or overall survival were found between the groups.[23] Several studies have investigated multimodality treatment, combining preoperative or postoperative radiation, surgery, and/or chemotherapy. One study compared surgery and radiation therapy with or without doxorubicin, and the other compared surgery and radiation therapy with or without doxorubicin and cyclophosphamide.[2,3] No significant differences between the group receiving adjuvant chemotherapy and the group that did not were found in either study for overall survival or median time to recurrence.

In conclusion, aggressive wide surgical excision performed by an experienced specialist surgeon that includes advanced imaging in the treatment planning is recommended for most cats with injection-site sarcomas. There is evidence that some cats may benefit from preoperative or postoperative radiation therapy. The role for chemotherapy in a multimodality approach for this disease remains to be defined; however, its continued empiric use is reasonable in light of the lack of definitive studies addressing its efficacy and the potential benefits some drugs might provide.

Based on what is known and suspected regarding the pathogenesis of injection-site sarcomas in cats, prevention strategies are likely to have the greatest impact in decreasing the morbidity and mortality rates associated with injection-site sarcoma in the pet cat population. The VAFSTF and others have suggested strategies and guidelines that may help decrease the incidence of injection-site sarcoma and decrease morbidity and mortality rates. In addition to the 3-2-1 recommendations for management of vaccine reactions, it is recommended that rabies vaccines be administered as far distally as possible in the right rear limb; FeLV vaccines (unless containing rabies antigen as well) be given as distally as possible in the left rear limb; and vaccines containing any other antigens except rabies or FeLV be given on the right shoulder, with care taken to avoid the midline or interscapular space.[32] The location of the injection should be in an area that is amenable for possible surgical removal. The vaccination site, dose, manufacturer, and lot number should be accurately recorded.[33] The recommended vaccination protocols for cats are critically important, with the understanding that these protocols should be tailored to the individual needs of the patient.[26] Additionally, discussion with cat owners regarding vaccination practices and sarcoma risk should be part of routine client education by veterinarians.

References

1. Barber LG, Sorenmo KU, Cronin KL et al: Combined doxorubicin and cyclophosphamide chemotherapyfor nonresectable feline fibrosarcoma, *J Am Anim Hosp Assoc* 36:416, 2000.
2. Bregazzi VS, LaRue SM, McNiel E et al: Treatment with combination of doxorubicin, surgery, and radiation versus surgery and radiation alone for cats with vaccine-associated sarcomas: 25 cases (1995-2000), *J Am Vet Med Assoc* 218:547, 2001.
3. Cohen M, Wright JC, Brawner WR et al: Use of surgery and electron beam irradiation, with or without chemotherapy, for treatment of vaccine-associated sarcomas in cats: 78 cases (1996-2000), *J Am Vet Med Assoc* 219:1582, 2001.
4. Coyne MJ, Reeves NC, Rosen DK: Estimated prevalence of injection-site sarcomas in cats during 1992, *J Am Vet Med Assoc* 210:249, 1997.
5. Cronin K, Page RL, Sponick G et al: Radiation therapy and surgery for fibrosarcoma in 33 cats, *Vet Radiol Ultrasound* 39:51, 1998.
6. Davidson EB, Gregory CR, Kass PH: Surgical excision of soft tissue sarcomas in cats, *Vet Surg* 26:265, 1997.
7. Dubielzig RR, Everitt J, Shadduck JA, et al: Clinical and morphologic features of post-traumatic ocular sarcomas in cats, *Vet Pathol* 27:62, 1990.
8. Ellis JA, Jackson ML, Barfsch RC et al: Use of immunohistochemistry and polymerase chain reaction for detection of oncornaviruses in formalin-fixed, paraffin-embedded fibrosarcomas from cats, *J Am Vet Med Assoc* 209:767, 1996.
9. Esplin DG, Campbell R: Widespread metastasis of a fibrosarcoma associated with vaccination site in a cat, *Feline Pract* 23:13, 1995.
10. Esplin DG, Jaffe MH, McGill LD: Metastasizing liposarcoma associated with a vaccination site in a cat, *Feline Pract* 24:20, 1996.
11. Giudice C, Stefanello D, Sala M et al: Feline injection-site sarcoma: recurrence, tumour grading and surgical margin status evaluated using the three-dimensional histological technique, *Vet J* 186:84, 2010.
12. Gobar GM, Kass PH: World Wide Web–based survey of vaccination practices, postvaccinal reactions, and vaccine site-associated sarcomas in cats, *J Am Vet Med Assoc* 220:1477, 2002.
13. Hendrick MJ, Goldschmidt MH, Shofer FS et al: Postvaccinal sarcomas in the cat: epidemiology and electron probe microanalytical identification of aluminum, *Cancer Res* 52:5391, 1992.
14. Hendrick MJ, Shofer FS, Goldschmidt MH et al: Comparison of fibrosarcomas that developed at vaccination sites and at nonvaccination sites in cats: 239 cases (1991-1992), *J Am Vet Med Assoc* 205:7425, 1994.
15. Hendrick MJ, Brooks JJ: Postvaccinal sarcomas in the cat: histology and immunohistochemistry, *Vet Pathol* 31:126, 1994.
16. Hershey AE, Sorenmo KU, Hendrick MJ et al: Prognosis for presumed feline vaccine-associated sarcoma after excision: 61 cases (1986-1996), *J Am Vet Med Assoc* 216:58, 2000.
17. Kass PH, Barnes WG, Spangler WL et al: Epidemiologic evidence for a causal relation between vaccination and fibrosarcoma tumorigenesis in cats, *J Am Vet Med Assoc* 203:396, 1993.
18. Kass PH, Spangler WL, Hendrick MJ et al: Multicenter case-control study of risk factors associated with development of vaccine-associated sarcomas in cats, *J Am Vet Med Assoc* 223:1283, 2003.
19. Kidney BA, Ellis JA, Haines DM et al: Evaluation of formalin-fixed paraffin-embedded tissues obtained from vaccine site-associated sarcomas of cats for DNA of feline immunodeficiency virus, *Am J Vet Res* 61:1037, 2000.
20. Kidney BA, Haines DM, Ellis JA et al: Evaluation of formalin-fixed paraffin-embedded tissues from vaccine site-associated sarcomas of cats for polyomavirus DNA and antigen, *Am J Vet Res* 62:828, 2001.
21. Kidney BA, Haines DM, Ellis JA et al: Evaluation of formalin-fixed paraffin-embedded tissues from vaccine site-associated sarcomas of cats for papillomavirus DNA and antigen, *Am J Vet Res* 62:833, 2001.
22. Lidbetter DA, Williams FA, Krahwinkel DJ et al: Radical lateral body wall resection with reconstruction using polypropylene mesh and a caudal superficial epigastric axial pattern flap: a retrospective clinical study of the technique and results in 6 cats, *Vet Surg* 31:57, 2002.
23. Martano M, Morello E, Ughetto M et al: Surgery alone versus surgery and doxorubicin for the treatment of feline injection site sarcomas: a report on 69 cases, *Vet J* 170:84, 2005.
24. McEntee MC, Page RL: Feline vaccine-associated sarcomas, *J Vet Intern Med* 15:176, 2001.
25. Nieto A, Sanchez MA, Martinez E et al: Immunohistochemical expression of p53, fibroblast growth factor-b, and transforming growth factor-alpha in feline vaccine-associated sarcomas, *Vet Pathol* 40:651, 2003.

26. O'Rourke K: Controversy, confusion continue to surround vaccine guidelines, *J Am Vet Med Assoc* 225:814, 2004.
27. Petterino C, Martano M, Cascio P et al: Immunohistochemical study of STAT3 expression in feline injection-site fibrosarcomas, *J Comp Path* 134:91, 2006.
28. Rudmann DG, Van Alstine WG, Doddy F et al: Pulmonary metastasis of a feline vaccine-site fibrosarcoma, *J Vet Diagn Invest* 10:79, 1998.
29. Shaw SC, Kent MS, Gordon IK et al: Temporal changes in characteristics of injection-site sarcomas in cats: 392 cases (1990-2006), *J Am Vet Med Assoc* 234:376, 2009.
30. Smith AJ, Njaa BL, Lamm CG: Immunohistochemical expression of c-KIT protein in feline soft tissue fibrosarcomas, *Vet Pathol* 46:934, 2009.
31. Thomas R, Valli VE, Ellis P et al: Microarray-based cytogenetic profiling reveals recurrent and subtype-associated genomic copy number aberrations in feline sarcomas, *Chromosome Research* 17:987, 2009.
32. Vaccine-Associated Feline Sarcoma Task Force: Diagnosis and treatment of suspected sarcomas, *J Am Vet Med Assoc* 214:1745, 1999.
33. Vaccine-Associated Feline Sarcoma Task Force: The current understanding and management of vaccine-associated sarcomas in cats, *J Am Vet Med Assoc* 226:1821, 2005.

MAMMARY TUMORS

Kevin Choy

INCIDENCE, ETIOLOGY, AND PATHOGENESIS

Mammary tumors are the third most common feline tumor, accounting for up to 17% of all neoplasms in female cats.[6,10,19,24] Male cats can also be affected by mammary tumors, although much less often, with reported incidence of up to 5% compared with females.[9,31] Domestic short hair and Siamese breeds appear to have an elevated risk for mammary tumors.[9,24] Mammary neoplasia is generally seen in older cats with a median age of 10.8 years (mean 10 to 12 years), although cats as young as 9 months have been reported to be affected.* The precise etiology of feline mammary tumors is uncertain, but hormones, particularly estrogen and progesterone, are thought to play a significant role in tumorigenesis.[22] In a case control study, cats that underwent ovariohysterectomy before 6 months and 1 year of age had a 91% and 86% reduction in risk, respectively, of developing mammary carcinoma compared with intact cats.[22] Parity was not found to significantly affect risk for tumor development.[22] Both female and male cats regularly exposed to exogenous progestins or estrogen–progestin combinations such as medroxyprogesterone acetate have been identified to be at increased risk of developing mammary carcinoma.[15,17,22,28]

*References 9, 10, 18, 23, 24, 27, 31.

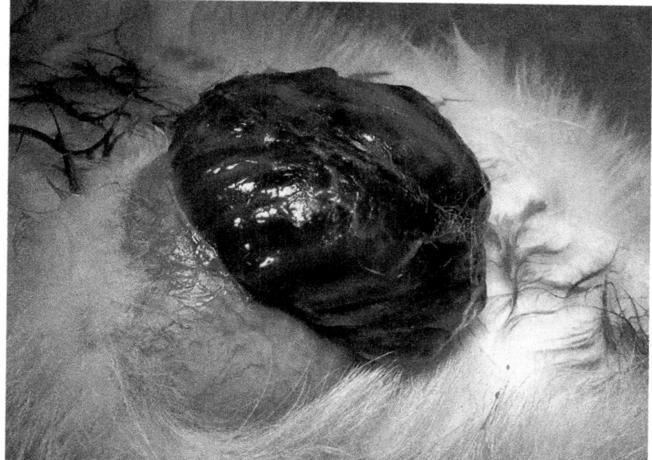

FIGURE 28-4 Gross appearance of a solitary ulcerated mammary tumor in an adult cat diagnosed by histopathology as an adenocarcinoma.

CLINICAL FEATURES

In contrast to canine mammary tumors, the vast majority (80% to 96%) of feline mammary masses are malignant, with most diagnosed as adenocarcinomas (tubular, papillary, and solid types). Less common malignant lesions include SCCs, soft tissue sarcomas, mucinous carcinomas, complex and mixed carcinomas, and inflammatory mammary carcinomas.* Cats are typically presented for palpable nodules of single or multiple mammary glands detected by the owner or found incidentally during routine physical examination. More than half of affected cats have multiple gland involvement.[34] Mammary tumors in cats may remain undetected until they become large, fixed, and ulcerated and involve multiple mammary glands or local lymph nodes (Figure 28-4).[11,12] Thus mammary carcinomas are often in an advanced state at the time of examination. If pulmonary metastatic disease is present, cats may present with acute dyspnea as a result of malignant pleural effusion, often containing exfoliating malignant cells.[27,34]

Feline fibroepithelial hyperplasia, a benign hypertrophy of the mammary glands, should not be confused with malignant mammary neoplasms. Other terms for this condition include *mammary fibroadenomatosis, pericanalicular fibroadenoma, benign mammary hypertrophy,* and *mammary adenomatosis.* Unlikely mammary carcinomas, which are less common in males, fibroepithelial hyperplasia is seen in both sexes. The condition is seen most typically in young cats shortly after a silent estrus or after chronic exogenous progestins. One or more glands may be enlarged, with occasional severe bilateral

*References 1-3, 10-12, 21, 24, 27, 29, 34.

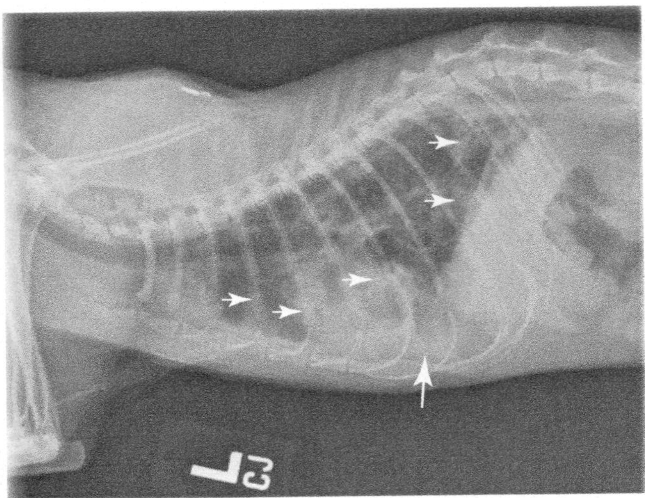

FIGURE 28-5 Left lateral thoracic radiograph from a 12-year-old domestic shorthair with metastatic mammary carcinoma. Note the diffuse interstitial to nodular metastatic pattern *(small arrows)* along with malignant pleural effusion *(large arrow)*.

TABLE 28-3 Modified World Health Organization (WHO) Staging System for Classification of Feline Mammary Tumors

T = PRIMARY TUMOR SIZE			
T_1	<2 cm maximum diameter		
T_2	2-3 cm maximum diameter		
T_3	>3 cm maximum diameter		
N = REGIONAL LYMPH NODE INVOLVEMENT			
N_0	No histologic/cytologic evidence of metastasis		
N_1	Histologic / cytologic evidence of metastasis		
M = DISTAL METASTASIS			
M_0	No evidence of metastasis		
M_1	Evidence of metastasis		
STAGES			
I	T_1	N_0	M_0
II	T_2	N_0	M_0
III	T_{1-2} T_3	N_1 N_{0-1}	M_0 M_0
IV	Any T	Any N	M_1

enlargement noted. The affected glands are often traumatized, leading to secondary ulceration, necrosis, and discomfort. Benign feline fibroepithelial hyperplasia is treated by removing hormonal exposures of exogenous progestin therapy or performing ovariohysterectomy. It may take several months for mammary lesions to resolve.[1,12,27,34] More information on treatment of this condition is found in Chapter 40.

DIAGNOSIS AND STAGING

Because feline mammary tumors are often malignant, thorough evaluation of cats with mammary tumors is prudent to confirm diagnosis and, if malignancy is confirmed, to establish clinical stage for prognostication. Evaluation should include CBC, serum biochemistry profile and urinalysis, and evaluation of the primary tumor, regional lymph nodes, and distant metastatic sites (particularly the thoracic cavity). The primary tumor(s) should be assessed for number, site, size, consistency, ulceration, fixation to skin or abdominal wall, and nipple discharge if present. Local lymph nodes should be carefully palpated with any identified nodes aspirated or biopsied. Three-view thoracic radiographs (right lateral, left lateral, and ventrodorsal views) are vital to assess for pulmonary, lymph node, and pleural metastatic disease. Mammary tumor pulmonary metastases appear as interstitial densities ranging from small and indistinct to large and discrete nodules and may be accompanied by miliary pleural lesions with or without pleural effusion (Figure 28-5).

Reported metastatic rates for feline mammary carcinomas range from 25% to 100%, with the most common sites being lungs and draining lymph nodes (axillary, inguinal, sternal).[11,12,33] Metastasis to other organs or body tissues is less common, with involvement of the liver, spleen, kidney, adrenal gland, peritoneal surface, heart, and bone reported.[3,27] A literature review of 799 cats with malignant mammary tumors found extraskeletal metastases in 338 cases. Skeletal metastasis was rare in cats compared with breast cancer in humans and mammary carcinoma in dogs.[33]

Biopsy of the mammary lesion is required for histopathologic confirmation of malignancy. Samples may be obtained before surgery by incisional biopsy or at the time of definitive surgery by excisional biopsy. Cytologic examination using fine-needle aspiration of mammary lesions in cats may confirm an epithelial neoplasm but will not distinguish reliably between benign and malignant tumors. Cytology may be helpful in ruling out nonmammary cutaneous or subcutaneous neoplasms such as mast cell tumors. Cytology is also indicated to assess suspected lymph node metastasis or malignant pleural effusions.[11,12]

Staging of feline mammary tumors is based on the modified WHO scheme first established in 1980 that assesses primary tumor size, lymph node involvement, and evidence of distant metastasis (Table 28-3).[12,34]

TREATMENT

Surgery

Surgery remains the most widely accepted primary treatment modality for feline mammary carcinomas; however, it is usually not curative. Surgery can be considered alone or, more commonly, in combination with adjuvant chemotherapy. Unilateral or bilateral (staged 2 weeks apart) radical chain mastectomies are generally recommended. Complete mastectomies are associated with decreased rate of local recurrence but do not have a significant effect on overall survival rates. The cat, unlike the dog, has four pairs of mammary glands: two cranial (thoracic) and two caudal (abdominal). The cranial glands drain to axillary and sternal lymph nodes, whereas the caudal glands drain to the inguinal nodes. The inguinal node should always be removed if the caudal mammary gland is affected. Excision of the axillary lymph node should be attempted only if enlarged and tumor involvement is confirmed on cytology because prophylactic removal of axillary lymph nodes can create significant subcutaneous dead space and is unlikely to have a therapeutic benefit.[7,11,12,25,34] Malignant mammary tumors in the cat often have lymphatic or vascular invasion, and therefore principles of surgical oncology must be observed, including early vessel ligation, gentle tumor tissue handling, *en bloc* resection of tumor, and copious flushing of the resulting surgical bed to help remove neoplastic cells.[7] The entire mammary chain should be submitted for histologic examination for tissue grading and assessment of margins. The role of ovariohysterectomy in the management of malignant mammary tumors is controversial. No impact of concurrent ovariohysterectomy with mastectomy has been demonstrated on survival rates, but some authors continue to recommend the practice to remove hormonal stimulation of the tumor.[3,9,30]

Chemotherapy

Chemotherapy is generally recommended as adjuvant therapy; however, there are no well-controlled large-scale studies documenting its role in the management of feline mammary gland tumors. Doxorubicin-based protocols are the most frequently reported, but protocols and efficacy vary among studies. Doxorubicin and cyclophosphamide combination therapy has been described, with short-term measurable responses observed in approximately half of cats with metastatic or nonresectable local disease (stage III or IV).[16,20] Retrospective analysis of single-agent doxorubicin in 67 cats (1 mg/kg intravenously every 21 days for five planned treatments) given postoperatively starting at the time of suture removal resulted in a MST of 448 days, with 1-, 2-, and 5-year survival rates at 58.9%, 37.2%, and 16.7%, respectively.[26] Doxorubicin should be used with care in cats because of the risk of nephrotoxicity. Mitoxantrone may be a suitable alternative for cats with compromised renal function. In an unpublished randomized prospective trial comparing mitoxantrone (6 mg/m^2 intravenously every 21 days for four doses) to doxorubicin (20 mg/m^2 intravenously every 21 days for four doses) for adjuvant therapy of feline mammary tumors after unilateral or bilateral radical mastectomy, no significant difference in MST or metastasis-free interval was observed between the two groups (Carolyn Henry, personal communication). MST was 747 days for mitoxantrone-treated cats and 484 days for doxorubicin-treated cats.[11-13]

Radiation

The role of radiation therapy is not well established for feline mammary tumors and is not used routinely as primary therapy. There is no evidence in current published literature supporting its efficacy or influence on survival for cats with mammary tumors. Anecdotally, according to the author's experience, hypofractionated radiation therapy in conjunction with concurrent chemotherapy may play a palliative role in inoperable local disease, with clinical responses observed.

PROGNOSIS

Average survival time between detection of primary tumor and death in untreated cats is 10 to 12 months.[8] Prognosis for malignant mammary tumors in male cats is comparable to that for female cats.[1]

Tumor size is the single most important and reliable prognostic factor in feline mammary cancer. In one study of 39 cats with mammary adenocarcinoma, a MST of 12 months for tumors larger than 3 cm was reported, compared with a MST of 21 months for tumors smaller than 3 cm after surgical excision only.[32] Prognosis for cats treated with combination surgery and adjuvant chemotherapy was discussed earlier. Other negative prognostic factors include increased WHO stage (lymph node or distant metastasis), lymphatic invasion, or immunohistochemical markers such as high AgNOR count or Ki-67 index greater than 25.2.* Histologic diagnosis is also prognostic; cats with complex carcinomas have a more favorable prognosis, with a reported MST of 32.6 months compared with 15.5 months for other mammary carcinomas. Inflammatory mammary carcinomas in cats, as in dogs, carry a poor prognosis, with rapid onset of clinical signs and euthanasia between 10 and 45 days after diagnosis.[29]

*References 4, 5, 13, 14, 27, 32.

References

1. Argyle DJ, Brearly MJ, Turek MM: *Decision making in small animal oncology—feline mammary tumors*, Ames, Iowa, 2008, Wiley-Blackwell, pp 332-335.
2. Bostock DE: Canine and feline mammary neoplasms, *Br Vet J* 142:506-515, 1986.
3. Carpenter JL, Andrews LK, Holzworth J et al: Tumors and tumor-like lesions. In Holzworth J, editor: *Diseases of the cat: medicine and surgery*, Philadelphia, 1987, Saunders.
4. Castagnaro M, Casalone C, Ru G et al: Argyrophilic nucleolar organizer regions (AgNORs) coindicator of post-surgical prognosis in feline mammary carcinomas, *Res Vet Sci* 64:97, 1998.
5. Castagnaro M, de Maria R, Bozetta E et al: Ki-67 index as indicator of the post-surgical prognosis in feline mammary carcinomas, *Res Vet Sci* 65:223, 1998.
6. Dorn CR, Taylor DON, Schneider R et al: Survey of animal neoplasms in Alameda and Contra Costa Counties, California. II. Cancer morbidity in dogs and cats from Alameda County, *J Natl Cancer Inst* 40:307, 1968.
7. Gimenez F, Hecht S, Craig LE et al: Early detection, aggressive therapy: optimizing the management of feline mammary masses, *J Feline Med Surg* 12(3):214, 2010.
8. Hahn KA, Adams WH: Feline mammary neoplasia: biological behavior, diagnosis and treatment alternatives, *J Feline Pract*, 25:5, 1997.
9. Hayes HM Jr, Milne KL, Mandell CP: Epidemiological features of feline mammary carcinomas, *Vet Rec* 108:476, 1981.
10. Hays AA, Mooney S: Feline mammary tumors, *Vet Clin North Am* 15:513-520, 1985.
11. Henry CJ: Feline mammary cancer. In Bonagura JR, Twedt DC, editors: *Kirk's current veterinary therapy XIV*, St Louis, 2009, Saunders, pp 366-368.
12. Henry CJ, Higginbotham ML: *Cancer management in small animal practice—feline mammary cancer*, St Louis, 2010, Saunders Elsevier, pp 280-282.
13. Henry CJ, Higginbotham ML, Rodriguez C et al: Prospective evaluation of doxorubicin versus mitoxantrone for adjuvant therapy of feline mammary carcinoma, *Proceedings of the 2006 Veterinary Cancer Society*, Callaway Gardens, Oct 19-22, 2006, p 54.
14. Ito T, Kadosawa T, Mochizuki M et al: Prognosis of malignant mammary tumors in 53 cats, *J Vet Med Sci* 58(8):723, 1996.
15. Jacobs TM, Hoppe BR et al: Mammary adenocarcinomas in three male cats exposed to medroxyprogesterone acetate (1990-2006), *J Feline Med Surg* 12:169, 2010.
16. Jeglum KA, DeGuzman E, Young K: Chemotherapy of advanced mammary adenocarcinoma in 14 cats, *J Am Vet Med Assoc* 187: 157, 1985.
17. Keskin A, Yilmazbas G et al: Pathological abnormlaities after long-term administration of medroxyprogesterone acetate in a queen, *J Feline Med Surg* 11:518, 2009.
18. Kessler M, Vonbomhard D: Mammary tumors in cats: epidemiologic and histologic features in 2,386 cases (1990-1995), *Kleinterpraxis* 42:459, 1997.
19. MacEwen EG, Hayes AA, Harvey JK et al: prognostic factors for feline mammary tumors, *J Am Vet Med Assoc* 185:201, 1984.
20. Mauldin GN, Matus RE, Patnaik AK et al: Efficacy and toxicity of doxorubicin and cyclophosphamide used in the treatment of selected malignant tumors in 23 cats, *J Vet Intern Med* 23:60, 1988.
21. Meuten DJ: *Tumors in domestic animals*, ed 4, Ames, Iowa, 2010, Blackwell, pp 575-606.
22. Misdorp W: Progestagens and mammary tumors in dogs and cats, *Acta Endocrinol (Cophnh)125 Suppl* 1:27-31, 1991.
23. Morrison WB: *Cancer in dogs and cats*, ed 2, Jackson Hole, Wyo, 2002, Teton NewMedia, pp 570-571.
24. Moulton JE: *Tumors in domestic animals*, ed 2, Berkeley, 1978, University of California Press, pp 367.
25. Novosad CA: Principles of treatment for mammary gland tumors, *Clin Tech Small Anim SA Pract* 18(2): 107-109, 2003.
26. Novosad CA, Bergman PJ, O'Brien MG et al: Retrospective evaluation of adjunctive doxorubicin for the treatment of feline mammary gland adenocarcinoma: 67 cases, *J Am Anim Hosp Assoc* 42:110, 2006.
27. Ogilvie GK, Moore AS. *Feline oncology—mammary tumors*, Trenton, NJ, 2001, Veterinary Learning Systems, pp 355-365.
28. Overley B, Shofer FS, Goldschmidt MH: Association between ovariohysterectomy and feline mammary carcinoma, *J Vet Intern Med* 19:560, 2005
29. Perez-Alenza MD, Jimenez A, Nieto AL: First description of feline inflammatory mammary carcinoma: clinicopathological and immunohistochemical characteristics of three cases, *Breast Cancer Res* 6(4):R300, 2004.
30. Rutteman GR, Misdorp W: Hormonal background of canine and feline mammary tumors, *J Reprod Fertil Suppl* 47:483-487, 1993.
31. Skorupski KA, Overly B, Shoter FS et al: Clinical characteristics of mammary carcinoma in male cats, *J Vet Intern Med* 19:52, 2005.
32. Viste JR, Myers SL, Singh B et al: Feline mammary adenocarcinoma: tumor size as a prognostic indicator, *Can Vet J* 43:33, 2002
33. Waters DJ, Honeckman A, Cooley DM et al: Skeletal metastasis in feline mammary carcinoma: case report and literature review, *J Am Anim Hosp Assoc* 34:103, 1998.
34. Withrow SJ, Vail DM: *Withrow and MacEwen's small animal clinical oncology*, St Louis, 2007, Saunders, pp 628-633.

PARANEOPLASTIC SYNDROMES

Chamisa Herrera

A paraneoplastic syndrome (PNS) is a phenomenon by which cancer cells cause a disease that is not due to the physical presence of the tumor or its metastasis. This is most often by secretion of cytokines or hormones that have some effect on body systems distant to the tumor. In cats there are a unique set of PNSs of which the veterinary clinician should be aware, including the dermatologic syndromes associated with pancreatic and thymic tumors. There are also PNSs shared among species, such as hypercalcemia and anemia. Early detection of a PNS can alert the clinician to the need for a cancer workup, including a CBC, biochemical profile, urinalysis, FeLV and FIV serology, thoracic radiographs, and abdominal imaging.

It is important to recognize that PNSs may occur before any other signs of cancer, and they may also serve as a sentinel for return of cancer in patients believed to be in remission. For this reason, if a PNS is suspected, the cat should be thoroughly screened for cancer and should be closely monitored for return of the syndrome once the cancer is in remission. Some PNSs are related to only one or a few types of neoplasia, and their presence can help narrow the differential list. PNSs can also serve as the main source of morbidity in the feline patient. When responsible for decreasing quality of life, a PNS may necessitate prioritizing symptomatic treatment before the cancer itself can be addressed.

Documented feline PNSs, their differentials, and their treatments are discussed in the subsequent sections. The reader is directed to a veterinary oncology textbook for documented canine PNSs. There is crossover in the syndromes associated with cancer in both dogs and cats. As yet undocumented PNSs in cats could recapitulate those syndromes documented in dogs.

DERMATOLOGIC MANIFESTATIONS

Feline Paraneoplastic Alopecia

Feline paraneoplastic alopecia (FPA) is a syndrome that is unique to the cat and has been associated with pancreatic, bile duct, and hepatocellular carcinomas.[32,55,69] Cats with FPA present with a nonpruritic bilaterally symmetric progressive alopecia of the ventral thorax and abdomen, limbs, and perineum.[92] The foot pads can also be involved and appear dry and crusted.[98] FPA is unique in that the skin appears thin and glistening, devoid of elasticity, and the hairs are easily epilated (Figure 28-6).[69] On histopathologic examination, findings consistent with FPA include a nonscarring alopecia with follicular telogenization, miniaturization, and atrophy.[97] The exact mechanism of alopecia is unknown, although it has been proposed that hypoproteinemia or deficiencies in biotin, zinc, or fatty acids may be responsible for the skin lesions.[32] Resolution of the alopecia has been reported with surgical removal of the tumor,[92] but FPA usually appears late in the course of malignancy. If surgical resection of the primary tumor is not possible, the prognosis is usually poor. Noncancerous differentials for alopecia include dermatophytosis, ectoparasites, demodecosis, hyperthyroidism, and hyperadrenocorticism.

It is important to note that in the workup of a cat with alopecia, the finding of pruritus or *Malassezia* infection does not rule out FPA alopecia. In fact, a retrospective study of feline skin biopsies with *Malassezia*-associated dermatitis found that 7 out of 15 cases had dermatopathologic findings consistent with FPA.[58]

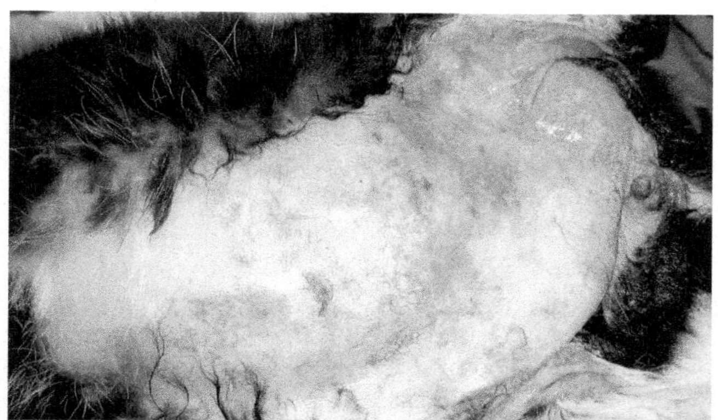

FIGURE 28-6 Abdomen of a cat with feline paraneoplastic alopecia. The entire abdomen is alopecic and the underlying skin is thin and glistening, which is typical of this syndrome. *(From Hnilica KA, editor:* Small animal dermatology, a color atlas and therapeutic guide, *ed 3, St Louis, 2011, Saunders.)*

Thymoma-Associated Exfoliative Dermatitis

Thymoma-associated exfoliative dermatitis is a rare PNS that has been described in cats diagnosed with mediastinal thymoma. The disease is characterized by a mild erythema of the head and pinnae that progresses to a nonpruritic generalized exfoliative dermatitis.[97] Most cats demonstrate generalized desquamation, alopecia on the body, and multifocal crusts, particularly on the head.[77] Differentials for this form of dermatitis include systemic lupus erythematosus, drug eruptions, epitheliotropic T-cell lymphoma, erythema multiforme, cheyletiellosis, demodecosis, *Malassezia* dermatitis, dermatophytosis, FeLV/FIV dermatitis, parapsoriasis, and sebaceous adenitis.[77] Histopathology of full-thickness skin lesions is helpful for diagnosis and shows perkeratotic hyperkeratosis with lymphocytic interface dermatitis.[86,88] The pathophysiology of thymoma-associated exfoliative dermatitis has not been completely elucidated; however, one theory is that an immune-mediated process directed against the tumor is occurring. This hypothesis is supported by the fact that the interface dermatitis is composed predominately of CD3+ lymphocytes.[77] The prognosis for feline thymoma and associated dermatitis is good with excision of the primary tumor, with a 1-year survival rate approaching 90%.[109]

Another PNS that has been documented in cats with thymoma is myasthenia gravis, which in a recent report occurred along with thymoma-associated dermatitis in a single cat.[86]

Cutaneous Necrosis of the Hindfeet

Symmetric cutaneous necrosis of the hindfeet has been described in a single cat with multicentric lymphoma as a presumed PNS. In this case the cat had necrosis of the hindfeet, but there were no neoplastic cells present on histopathology of this lesion, which is suggestive of a PNS.[1] Paraneoplastic digital necrosis has been described in humans with multiple malignancies, and there may be crossover between species. One hypothesis for the pathogenesis of this lesion is local or systemic vasculitis secondary to circulating tumor antigens.[11,39,72]

HEMATOLOGIC ALTERATIONS

Hyperglobulinemia

A hyperglobulinemia is an increase in serum proteins other than albumin. In cats PNSs resulting in hyperglobulinemia are rare and include multiple myeloma, plasmacytoma, and lymphoma.[6,23,93] The primary mechanism of paraneoplastic hyperglobulinemia is production of excess gammaglobulin(s) by the tumor. Serum protein electrophoresis can be used to differentiate polyclonal from monoclonal gammopathies.[93] Monoclonal gammopathies are rare and, when observed in cats, are most often associated with neoplasia.[50,93] Other differentials for hyperglobulinemia include chronic infectious diseases such as feline infectious peritonitis, FeLV, FIV, inflammatory bowel disease, fungal disease, tick-borne disease, and immune-mediated disease (e.g., rhinitis and immune-mediated hemolytic anemia).[93]

Cats with hyperglobulinemia can develop a host of secondary complications, including infection, bleeding, and end-organ damage. Infections are common because of the decreased production of normal immunoglobulins, and antimicrobial treatment should be considered even when signs of infection are absent.[34,104] As hyperglobulinemia worsens, serum viscosity increases and leads to hyperviscosity syndrome. In humans hypergammaglobulinemia is the most common cause of hyperviscosity syndrome.[62] Increased blood viscosity results in decreased perfusion, ultimately leading to multiorgan damage. Patients with hyperviscosity syndrome present with or develop renal, retinal, or cardiac disease or neurologic abnormalities.[6,27,34] They may also have spontaneous hemorrhage with a normal platelet count, although the mechanism for this is unknown.[34] The treatment of choice for hyperglobulinemia is control of the underlying neoplasm. When immediate relief from hyperviscosity syndrome is needed, plasmapheresis can be used, including for immediate relief from congestive heart failure secondary to hyperviscosity syndrome.[9,27] Prognosis is poor if end-organ damage has occurred or the underlying neoplasm cannot be controlled.

Anemia

The causes of anemia in the feline cancer patient are numerous, including hemorrhage, immune-mediated destruction of red blood cells, and decreased red blood cell production. If a minimum database including a CBC with a manual differential, a biochemical profile, and FeLV/FIV serology do not reveal the etiology of the anemia, cancer should be considered on the differential list. The first step in differentiating causes of anemia is to determine if the anemia is regenerative (corrected reticulocyte count >60,000) or nonregenerative. A regenerative anemia is likely due to hemorrhage or hemolysis, although a hemorrhage identified early will not always be accompanied by regeneration. A common cause of a nonregenerative anemia is inflammatory disease, but such an anemia can also be attributed to decreased erythropoietin (EPO) production or bone marrow pathology. Immune-mediated destruction of red blood cells can result in either a regenerative or nonregenerative anemia.[105] In cats retroviral infection commonly causes cytopenias of various cell lines, including red blood cells, neutrophils, and platelets. A negative FeLV antigen test is a reliable means for ruling out FeLV infection as a cause of cytopenias, with only approximately 5% of cats harboring latent infections testing negative on antigen tests and positive on bone marrow polymerase chain reaction.[91]

Anemia associated with cancer can be secondary to most of the aforementioned mechanisms, making anemia difficult to definitively pinpoint as a PNS. For example, hemorrhage can occur secondary to a bleeding tumor in the gastrointestinal tract, the nasal cavity, or the thoracic or abdominal cavities. Although hemoperitoneum in cats is rare, almost half of cats with that diagnosis in one study had intraabdominal neoplasia, most often hemangiosarcoma.[19] Hemolysis of red blood cells with cancer is secondary to production of anti-erythrocyte antibodies. This has been documented in lymphoma in the cat.[44,52] Renal failure, and therefore decreased EPO production, can be secondary to a primary renal tumor or a tumor that is metastatic to the renal parenchyma or caused by renal hypoxia secondary to a neoplastic embolism. Cancer itself can serve as a chronic source of inflammation and lead to anemia of inflammatory disease (AID). The mechanisms of AID are multifactorial and include decreased red blood cell survival, iron sequestration, and insufficient EPO production or bone marrow response (or both).[68] One of the main mediators of AID is believed to be hepcidin, which is a hormone responsible for iron homeostasis that is upregulated in inflammatory conditions in response to interleukin-6. This upregulation of hepcidin is thought to deprive infectious agents of iron but also reduces iron stores necessary for erythropoiesis.[17,61,87,106]

A unique mechanism that can contribute to anemia in cancer is erythrophagocytosis of red blood cells by the tumor. This has been documented in an extranodal T-cell lymphoma, histiocytic sarcoma, mast cell tumors, and multiple myeloma in the cat.[13,40,54,103]

The prognosis for anemia associated with cancer depends on the underlying mechanism, the degree of anemia, and the animal's response to symptomatic treatment of the anemia or treatment of the underlying neoplasia.

Polycythemia

Polycythemia is another neoplastic syndrome that is more commonly described in cats than dogs, but it is rare in veterinary medicine. Diagnosis of polycythemia is uncomplicated and easily diagnosed by performing packed cell volume and total protein measurements. It is important to rule out non-neoplastic causes of polycythemia. A relative polycythemia results from dehydration or hypovolemia, is often accompanied by high serum total protein, and will resolve with fluid therapy. An absolute polycythemia can be primary, as in polycythemia vera, or secondary to conditions such as chronic hypoxia, excessive EPO production, and cancer. Serum EPO concentrations have been used for differentiating polycythemia vera from secondary polycythemia; however, there is overlap between the two groups, and testing is not readily available.[35]

Secondary polycythemia in feline cancer patients has been documented in primary renal tumors.[37,43] Similar to hyperglobulinemia, polycythemia can result in hyperviscosity syndrome. The most common clinical signs are neurologic and include seizures and ataxia.[43,75] Paraneoplastic polycythemia is thought to arise from renal hypoxia, production of EPO by the tumor, or both.[22] In patients with an absolute secondary polycythemia and a hematocrit greater than 65%, symptomatic treatment is achieved by therapeutic phlebotomy.[28] Leeching as an initial treatment for feline patients for whom phlebotomy proves impossible has also been documented.[66]

Prognosis is variable. Resolution of polycythemia has been achieved with nephrectomy of the affected kidney, although this requires unilateral disease and adequate function of the contralateral kidney.[43]

Thrombocytopenia and Disseminated Intravascular Coagulation

Thrombocytopenia is conservatively defined as a platelet count of less than 200,000/μL and frequently occurs in various disease states. One of the most common reasons for this finding is laboratory error because of the tendency of feline platelets to aggregate and be misread by automated systems.[67] The first step when thrombocytopenia is suspected in a cat is to have a manual platelet count performed to rule out platelet aggregation as a cause.

Differentials for a true thrombocytopenia include infectious disease (e.g., FeLV, FIV, feline infectious peritonitis, other infectious and inflammatory causes), neoplasia (e.g., leukemia, lymphoma, hemangiosarcoma), cardiac disease, and primary immune-mediated disease, with infectious disease and neoplasia within the bone marrow being the most common causes.[41] The pathophysiologic mechanisms of thrombocytopenia include destruction, decreased production, consumption, and sequestration within the spleen. Many of these mechanisms may also play a role in thrombocytopenia associated with cancer. For example, platelet-bound antibodies have been demonstrated in cats with immune-mediated thrombocytopenia secondary to lymphoma.[44] Cancer can also cause thrombocytopenia as a result of decreased production secondary to bone marrow invasion, sequestration of platelets within the spleen, and consumption resulting from disseminated intravascular coagulation (DIC). When DIC occurs in cats, neoplasia is often an underlying etiology and survival rates are poor.[25]

Thrombocytopenia can result in spontaneous hemorrhage when platelet numbers fall below 30,000/μL. Prognosis for thrombocytopenia secondary to a malignancy is variable and depends on the underlying mechanism leading to thrombocytopenia, the degree of thrombocytopenia, and the responsiveness of the tumor to antineoplastic therapies.

Eosinophilia

Dramatic increases in peripheral eosinophil counts can occur for a variety of reasons in the cat, including parasitism, allergic diseases, hypereosinophilic syndrome, and eosinophilic leukemia.[16,18,108] Eosinophilia can also occur as a PNS and in cats has been documented in lymphoma, mast cell tumors, and transitional cell carcinoma.[4,71,82] Lymphoma and various other sarcomas and carcinomas have also been documented as causes of paraneoplastic eosinophilia in dogs and humans.[26,49,89,99,100]

The mechanism of eosinophilia is believed to be production of cytokines important in eosinophil proliferation, particularly interleukin-3, interleukin-5, granulocyte macrophage colony-stimulating factor, and potentially some other eosinophilotactic factors produced by the tumor.[3,82,94,102] Diagnosis of paraneoplastic eosinophilia relies on ruling out other causes of eosinophilia, including hypereosinophilic syndrome and eosinophilic leukemia, or seeing resolution of the eosinophilia with treatment of the underlying neoplasia. Prognosis for paraneoplastic eosinophilia in cats is not well studied. In humans peripheral eosinophilia in association with a tumor usually carries a poor prognosis—not because of the eosinophils themselves but because this is associated with widespread metastasis of the underlying malignancy.[53]

ENDOCRINOLOGIC MANIFESTATIONS

Hypercalcemia of Malignancy

Hypercalcemia of malignancy (HM) is one of the most recognized paraneoplastic syndromes in veterinary medicine; however, it is less commonly reported in the cat than in the dog.[24] In cats the most common tumors resulting in HM are lymphoma and SCC.[78] Other tumors reported to cause HM in cats include leukemia, fibrosarcoma, osteosarcoma, multiple myeloma, and various carcinomas, particularly bronchogenic adenocarcinoma.[8,15,70,78,80] The distribution of clinical signs in the cat is unique, with the most common being anorexia and lethargy followed by gastrointestinal signs, polyuria and polydipsia, urinary signs, and neurologic signs.[78] Hypercalcemia commonly causes significant morbidity when elevations are profound, including renal failure, arrhythmias, seizures, and coma. The most common mechanism of HM is thought to be production of parathyroid hormone–related peptide (PTH-rp) by the tumor; however, other mechanisms of HM include skeletal metastasis and diffuse osteolysis caused by production of humoral products produced by the tumor.[78] The most common non-neoplastic cause of hypercalcemia is renal failure.[78] Other causes include idiopathic hypercalcemia, vitamin D toxicosis, and granulomatous disease.[38,60,63,73] Primary hyperparathyroidism has been reported in cats and, although extremely rare, also results in hypercalcemia.[20]

In general, hypercalcemia is more profound when related to a malignant process than hypercalcemia associated with non-neoplastic diseases, and may be indicative of, although not definitive for, the underlying process.[78] Diagnosis relies on ruling out other causes of hypercalcemia. In the past a PTH-rp assay could be performed to look for production of parathyroid hormone–related peptide production by the tumor,[8] but this diagnostic tool recently became unavailable. The best treatment option for HM is to treat the underlying neoplasia. When this is not possible or when the hypercalcemia itself is causing significant morbidity (e.g., renal failure, arrhythmias, seizures), symptomatic treatment should be aggressive and immediate. Initial treatment is fluid diuresis with a calcium-poor solution (0.9% NaCl).[79] Furosemide, prednisone, salmon calcitonin, and bisphosphonates can also be used to decrease serum calcium.[64,79,107] Use of furosemide should be limited to patients that are well hydrated. In the patient with hypercalcemia of unknown origin, treatment with prednisone can make diagnosis of lymphoma difficult by inducing remission and can also cause chemotherapeutic resistance. For this reason steroid treatment of hypercalcemia should not be instituted until lymphoma has been ruled out. In cases of severe hypercalcemia that require management without a cancer diagnosis, administration of bisphosphonates is preferred. Prognosis for patients with HM is considered poor, regardless of the underlying neoplasia.

Hypoglycemia

Hypoglycemia, defined as a blood glucose below 70 mg/dL, has been documented to occur as a PNS in both cats and dogs suffering from cancer. The mechanisms of paraneoplastic hypoglycemia are variable, but production of insulin by an insulinoma is probably the most common.[46] Other mechanisms of cancer-associated hypoglycemia include liver failure secondary to metastasis and production of insulin-like growth factor II by the tumor.[76] In the cat tumor types that have been shown to cause hypoglycemia include insulinoma, lymphoma, and hepatoma.[30,36,45,95] In dogs tumors associated with hypoglycemia include hepatocellular carcinoma, leiomyosarcoma, hemangiosarcoma, melanoma, and various carcinomas[5,51,76] and could theoretically also cause hypoglycemia in a similarly affected cat. Clinical signs associated with hypoglycemia include weakness, lethargy, muscle twitching, and seizures. Neurologic complications might become irreversible with chronic hypoglycemia secondary to insulinoma, even after treatment and normalization of glucose levels.[45] A diagnosis of paraneoplastic hypoglycemia should be considered when an adult cat presents with a persistent hypoglycemia and other causes have been ruled out. Non-neoplastic differentials include sepsis, hepatic disease, hypoadrenocorticism, portosystemic shunt, and insulin overdose. Diagnosis of an insulinoma can be made when a persistent hypoglycemia with concurrent normal to increased serum insulin concentrations are present. Diagnosis of other causes of paraneoplastic hypoglycemia is likely to be presumptive or require biopsy and immunohistochemical staining to demonstrate the underlying mechanism. Alternatively, documenting glycemic control with treatment of the tumor supports the diagnosis of this PNS. Prognosis for an insulinoma in cats is guarded because of the metastatic nature of the disease; however, prolonged survival times have been documented with surgical excision when no metastases were present.[33] Prognosis with other causes of paraneoplastic hypoglycemia varies depending on the tumor type and mechanism by which the tumor induces glucose dysregulation.

NEUROMUSCULAR MANIFESTATIONS

Peripheral Neuropathy

The characteristic physical examination findings associated with a peripheral neuropathy include hyporeflexia, motor or sensory involvement (or both), and occasionally autonomic dysfunction. There are numerous etiologies of peripheral neuropathies in cats, including inherited disorders, endocrine diseases (e.g., diabetes mellitus, hyperthyroidism), infectious disease (FeLV, FIV), nutritional disorders (e.g., phenylalanine deficiency, tyrosine deficiency), toxins (e.g., organophosphates, carbamates, heavy metals), drugs (e.g., aminoglycosides, vincristine), neoplastic invasion of a tumor into a nerve, and paraneoplastic peripheral neuropathies (PPNs).[14] In cats a single case report of PPN has been described in a cat with renal lymphoma.[14] Muscle and nerve sections from the cat showed demyelination, axonal degeneration, and muscle denervation.[14] No neoplastic cells were observed in the affected muscle or nerve biopsies, which is consistent with a PPN.[14] Although this is the first described case in a cat, several tumors have been implicated in PPN in dogs, including insulinoma, lymphoma, primary lung tumors, multiple myeloma, mammary adenocarcinoma, and melanoma.[10,56,74,101] Polyneuropathy has been reported in various neoplasms in human-medicine literature as well.[31] The underlying cause is thought to be autoimmunity through the production of onconeural antibodies by the tumor.[59,90] These antibodies can be directed at any part of the peripheral nerve, including the cell body, axon, myelin sheath, and presynaptic region. Treatment of PPN is removal or treatment of the underlying neoplasm and supportive care; however, given the presumed immune-mediated component, immunosuppressive medications may be another treatment modality to consider.

Myasthenia Gravis

Acquired myasthenia gravis is an immune-mediated neuromuscular disorder by which antibodies alter, block, or destroy acetylcholine receptors (AChRs), resulting in muscle weakness and fatigue. In cats myasthenia gravis usually results in generalized weakness, although focal signs such as dysphagia and megaesophagus can also be seen.[84] Other clinical signs may include gait abnormalities, voice change, neck ventroflexion, and regurgitation.[42] Approximately 25% of cats in a study of risk factors for myasthenia gravis had a cranial mediastinal mass, most of which were thymomas.[84] This is very different from myasthenia in dogs, in which only about 3% of cases have a mediastinal mass.[85] Production of onconeural antibodies by the tumor is the likely mechanism of AChR blockade and is by definition a type of PNS. Definitive diagnosis of myasthenia gravis can be achieved by demonstrating AChR antibodies by immunoprecipitation radioimmunoassay. A feline-specific immunoprecipitation radioimmunoassay should be used, although there is some cross-reactivity between species.[83] Treatment for paraneoplastic myasthenia gravis in cats is not well described, although removal of the tumor has been shown to cause complete resolution of focal myasthenia gravis in a dog.[48] Acetylcholine esterase inhibitors and antiinflammatory doses of corticosteroids may also be useful in the absence of aspiration pneumonia.[81]

CANCER CACHEXIA AND ANOREXIA

Some cancer patients experience anorexia or weight loss secondary to treatment or because of the location of the tumor (gastrointestinal), which is beyond the scope of this discussion and occurs by a mechanism likely to be different from that of cancer cachexia. Those patients who involuntarily lose weight before diagnosis or independent of treatment of their disease have the PNS termed *cancer cachexia*. Cancer cachexia can occur with or without anorexia, although weight loss is often seen despite normal caloric intake.[7] The mechanisms of this disease are multifactorial and poorly understood but result in weight loss through the depletion of lean muscle mass and adipose tissue, which differentiates it from malnutrition.[65] The true prevalence of cachexia in human cancer patients is unknown, and the literature reveals huge variability, ranging from less than 3% to 87% of cancer patients, depending on the definition, type of cancer, and stage of disease used in each study.[21,29] One well-recognized phenomenon in human oncology patients is that cancer cachexia is associated with a higher incidence of treatment failure and reduced survival.[21,57] Production of cytokines and hormones by the tumor or host immune system are thought to contribute to cachexia and anorexia by altering appetite, increasing resting energy expenditure, increasing lipolysis, altering fat metabolism, increasing protein catabolism, and depressing protein synthesis.[96] Excessive glucose use by tumor cells may also play a role in weight loss.[12] A single study investigating the prevalence and prognostic significance of weight loss and body condition score (BCS) has been reported in cats. This study evaluated cats with various tumor types and found that 60% had reduced fat mass and 91% had reduced muscle mass. They also found that patients with a BCS below 5 (on a 9-point scale) had an MST of 3.3 months compared with 16.7 months for cats with a BCS of 5 or above.[2] Based on this information, physical examination monitoring (including estimates of muscle and fat mass), as well as recording of BCS and trends in weight, should occur in all cats with cancer. This information may provide prognostic data and serve as a guide for attempted intervention. Because cancer cachexia is not solely caused by inadequate caloric intake, treatment aimed at increasing caloric intake may not be effective. Studies in humans have investigated various drugs for treatment of cancer cachexia and anorexia, including appetite stimulants, 5-HT_3 antagonists, and cyclooxygenase-2 inhibitors, none of which have proved successful.[47] With continued research and understanding of the mechanisms involved in cancer cachexia and anorexia, new pharmacologic interventions may become available.

References

1. Ashley PF, Bowman LA: Symmetric cutaneous necrosis of the hind feet and multicentric follicular lymphoma in a cat, *J Am Vet Med Assoc* 214(2):211, 1999.
2. Baez JL, Michel KE, Sorenmo K et al: A prospective investigation of the prevalence and prognostic significance of weight loss and changes in body condition in feline cancer patients, *J Feline Med Surg* 9(5):411, 2007.
3. Bain BJ: Review: eosinophils and eosinophilic leukemia, *Clin Adv Hematol Oncol* 8(12):901, 2010.
4. Barrs VR, Beatty JA, McCandlish IA et al: Hypereosinophilic paraneoplastic syndrome in a cat with intestinal T cell lymphosarcoma, *J Small Anim Pract* 43(9):401, 2002.

5. Battaglia L, Petterino C, Zappulli V et al: Hypoglycaemia as a paraneoplastic syndrome associated with renal adenocarcinoma in a dog, *Vet Res Commun* 29(8):671, 2005.
6. Bienzle D, Silverstein DC, Chaffin K: Multiple myeloma in cats: variable presentation with different immunoglobulin isotypes in two cats, *Vet Pathol Online* 37(4):364, 2000.
7. Blum D, Omlin A, Baracos VE et al: Cancer cachexia: a systematic literature review of items and domains associated with involuntary weight loss in cancer, *Crit Rev Oncol Hematol*, 2011. Accessed March 26, 2011 at http://www.ncbi.nlm.nih.gov/pubmed/21216616.
8. Bolliger AP, Graham PA, Richard V et al: Detection of parathyroid hormone-related protein in cats with humoral hypercalcemia of malignancy, *Vet Clin Pathol* 31(1):3, 2002.
9. Boyle TE, Holowaychuk MK, Adams AK et al: Treatment of three cats with hyperviscosity syndrome and congestive heart failure using plasmapheresis, *J Am Anim Hosp Assoc* 47(1):50, 2011.
10. Braund KG, McGuire JA, Amling KA et al: Peripheral neuropathy associated with malignant neoplasms in dogs, *Vet Pathol* 24(1):16, 1987.
11. Burnouf M, Mahé E, Verpillat P et al: [Cutaneous necrosis is predictive of cancer in adult dermatomyositis], *Ann Dermatol Venereol* 130(3):313, 2003.
12. Burt BM, Humm JL, Kooby DA et al: Using positron emission tomography with [(18)F]FDG to predict tumor behavior in experimental colorectal cancer, *Neoplasia* 3(3):189, 2001.
13. Carter JE, Tarigo JL, Vernau W et al: Erythrophagocytic low-grade extranodal T-cell lymphoma in a cat, *Vet Clin Pathol* 37(4):416, 2008.
14. Cavana P, Sammartano F, Capucchio MT et al: Peripheral neuropathy in a cat with renal lymphoma, *J Feline Med Surg* 11(10):869, 2009.
15. Cavana P, Vittone V, Capucchio MT et al: Parathyroid adenocarcinoma in a nephropathic persian cat, *J Feline Med Surg* 8(5):340, 2006.
16. Center SA, Randolph JF, Erb HN et al: Eosinophilia in the cat: a retrospective study of 312 cases (1975 to 1986), *J Am Anim Hosp Assoc* 26(4):349, 1990.
17. Cheng P, Jiao X, Wang X et al: Hepcidin expression in anemia of chronic disease and concomitant iron-deficiency anemia, *Clin Exp Med* 11(1):33, 2011.
18. Craig LE, Hardam EE, Hertzke DM et al: Feline gastrointestinal eosinophilic sclerosing fibroplasia, *Vet Pathol* 46(1):63, 2009.
19. Culp WTN, Weisse C, Kellogg ME et al: Spontaneous hemoperitoneum in cats: 65 cases (1994-2006), *J Am Vet Med Assoc* 236(9):978, 2010.
20. den Hertog E, Goossens MM, van der Linde-Sipman JS et al: Primary hyperparathyroidism in two cats, *Vet Q* 19(2):81, 1997.
21. Dewys WD, Begg C, Lavin PT et al: Prognostic effect of weight loss prior to chemotherapy in cancer patients. Eastern Cooperative Oncology Group, *Am J Med* 69(4):491, 1980.
22. Durno AS, Webb JA, Gauthier MJ et al: Polycythemia and inappropriate erythropoietin concentrations in two dogs with renal T-cell lymphoma, *J Am Anim Hosp Assoc* 47(2):122, 2011.
23. Dust A, Norris AM, Valli VE: Cutaneous lymphosarcoma with IgG monoclonal gammopathy, serum hyperviscosity and hypercalcemia in a cat, *Can Vet J* 23(8):235, 1982.
24. Engelman RW, Tyler RD, Good RA et al: Hypercalcemia in cats with feline-leukemia-virus-associated leukemia-lymphoma, *Cancer* 56(4):777, 1985.
25. Estrin MA, Wehausen CE, Jessen CR et al: Disseminated intravascular coagulation in cats, *J Vet Intern Med* 20(6):1334, 2006.
26. Fews D, Scase TJ, Battersby IA: Leiomyosarcoma of the pericardium, with epicardial metastases and peripheral eosinophilia in a dog, *J Comp Pathol* 138(4):224, 2008.
27. Forrester SD, Greco DS, Relford RL: Serum hyperviscosity syndrome associated with multiple myeloma in two cats, *J Am Vet Med Assoc* 200(1):79, 1992.
28. Foster ES, Lothrop CD: Polycythemia vera in a cat with cardiac hypertrophy, *J Am Vet Med Assoc* 192(12):1736, 1988.
29. Fox KM, Brooks JM, Gandra SR et al: Estimation of cachexia among cancer patients based on four definitions, *J Oncol* 2009:1, 2009.
30. Gabor LJ, Canfield PJ, Malik R: Haematological and biochemical findings in cats in Australia with lymphosarcoma, *Aust Vet J* 78(7):456, 2000.
31. Giglio P, Gilbert MR: Neurologic complications of cancer and its treatment, *Curr Oncol Rep* 12(1):50, 2010.
32. Godfrey DR: A case of feline paraneoplastic alopecia with secondary *Malassezia*-associated dermatitis, *J Small Anim Pract* 39(8):394, 1998.
33. Greene SN, Bright RM: Insulinoma in a cat, *J Small Anim Pract* 49(1):38, 2008.
34. Hanna F: Multiple myelomas in cats, *J Feline Med Surg* 7(5):275, 2005.
35. Hasler AH, Giger U: Serum erythropoietin values in polycythemic cats, *J Am Anim Hosp Assoc* 32(4):294, 1996.
36. Hawks D, Peterson ME, Hawkins KL et al: Insulin-secreting pancreatic (islet cell) carcinoma in a cat, *J Vet Intern Med* 6(3):193, 1992.
37. Henry CJ, Turnquist SE, Smith A et al: Primary renal tumours in cats: 19 cases (1992-1998), *J Feline Med Surg* 1(3):165, 1999.
38. Hodges RD, Legendre AM, Adams LG et al: Itraconazole for the treatment of histoplasmosis in cats, *J Vet Intern Med* 8(6):409, 1994.
39. Iamandi C, Dietemann A, Grosshans E et al: Unusual presentations of lung cancer: case 3. Paraneoplastic digital necrosis in a patient with small-cell lung cancer, *J Clin Oncol* 20(23):4600, 2002.
40. Ide K, Setoguchi-Mukai A, Nakagawa T et al: Disseminated histiocytic sarcoma with excessive hemophagocytosis in a cat, *J Vet Med Sci* 71(6):817, 2009.
41. Jordan HL, Grindem CB, Breitschwerdt EB: Thrombocytopenia in cats: a retrospective study of 41 cases, *J Vet Intern Med* 7(5):261, 1993.
42. Joseph RJ, Carrillo JM, Lennon VA: Myasthenia gravis in the cat, *J Vet Intern Med* 2(2):75, 1988.
43. Klainbart S, Segev G, Loeb E et al: Resolution of renal adenocarcinoma-induced secondary inappropriate polycythaemia after nephrectomy in two cats, *J Feline Med Surg* 10(3):264, 2008.
44. Kohn B, Weingart C, Eckmann V et al: Primary immune-mediated hemolytic anemia in 19 cats: diagnosis, therapy, and outcome (1998-2004), *J Vet Intern Med* 20(1):159, 2006.
45. Kraje AC: Hypoglycemia and irreversible neurologic complications in a cat with insulinoma, *J Am Vet Med Assoc* 223(6):812-814, 2003.
46. Kruth SA, Carter RF: Laboratory abnormalities in patients with cancer, *Vet Clin North Am Small Anim Pract* 20(4):897, 1990.
47. Kumar NB, Kazi A, Smith T et al: Cancer cachexia: traditional therapies and novel molecular mechanism-based approaches to treatment, *Curr Treat Options Oncol* 11(3-4):107, 2010.
48. Lainesse M, Taylor S, Myers S et al: Focal myasthenia gravis as a paraneoplastic syndrome of canine thymoma: improvement following thymectomy, *J Am Anim Hosp Assoc* 32(2):111, 1996.
49. Laingo Andrianarison JF, Ranoharison D, Rakotoarivelo RA et al: [A misleading case of hypereosinophilia revealing colonic adenocarcinoma in a patient from a tropical area], *Med Trop (Mars)* 69(5):517, 2009.
50. Larsen AE, Carpenter JL: Hepatic plasmacytoma and biclonal gammopathy in a cat, *J Am Vet Med Assoc* 205(5):708, 1994.
51. Leifer CE, Peterson ME, Matus RE et al: Hypoglycemia associated with nonislet cell tumor in 13 dogs, *J Am Vet Med Assoc* 186(1):53, 1985.

52. Lenard ZM, Foster SF, Tebb AJ et al: Lymphangiosarcoma in two cats, *J Feline Med Surg* 9(2):161, 2007.
53. Lowe D, Jorizzo J, Hutt MS: Tumour-associated eosinophilia: a review, *J Clin Pathol* 34(12):1343, 1981.
54. Madewell BR, Gunn C, Gribble DH: Mast cell phagocytosis of red blood cells in a cat, *Vet Pathol* 20(5):638, 1983.
55. Marconato L, Albanese F, Viacava P et al: Paraneoplastic alopecia associated with hepatocellular carcinoma in a cat, *Vet Dermatol* 18(4):267, 2007.
56. Mariani CL, Shelton SB, Alsup JC: Paraneoplastic polyneuropathy and subsequent recovery following tumor removal in a dog, *J Am Anim Hosp Assoc* 35(4):302, 1999.
57. Mariani L, Lo Vullo S, Bozzetti F: Weight loss in cancer patients: a plea for a better awareness of the issue (on behalf of the SCRINIO Working Group), *Support Care Cancer* 2011. Accessed March 25, 2011 at http://www.springerlink.com/content/7n59570606038676/.
58. Mauldin EA, Morris DO, Goldschmidt MH: Retrospective study: the presence of *Malassezia* in feline skin biopsies. A clinicopathological study, *Vet Dermatol* 13(1):7, 2002.
59. Maverakis E, Goodarzi H, Wehrli LN et al: The etiology of paraneoplastic autoimmunity, *Clinic Rev Allerg Immunol* 2011. Accessed March 18, 2011, at http://www.springerlink.com/content/k9540n712385517v/.
60. Mealey KL, Willard MD, Nagode LA et al: Hypercalcemia associated with granulomatous disease in a cat, *J Am Vet Med Assoc* 215(7):959, 1999.
61. Means RT: Hepcidin and anaemia, *Blood Rev* 18(4):219, 2004.
62. Mehta J, Singhal S: Hyperviscosity syndrome in plasma cell dyscrasias, *Semin Thromb Hemost* 29(5):467, 2003.
63. Midkiff AM, Chew DJ, Randolph JF et al: Idiopathic hypercalcemia in cats, *J Vet Intern Med* 14(6):619, 2000.
64. Milner RJ, Farese J, Henry CJ et al: Bisphosphonates and cancer, *J Vet Intern Med* 18(5):597, 2004.
65. Moley JF, Aamodt R, Rumble W et al: Body cell mass in cancer-bearing and anorexic patients, *JPEN J Parenter Enteral Nutr*, 11(3):219, 1987.
66. Nett CS, Arnold P, Glaus TM: Leeching as initial treatment in a cat with polycythaemia vera, *J Small Anim Pract* 42(11):554, 2001.
67. Norman EJ, Barron RCJ, Nash AS et al: Prevalence of low automated platelet counts in cats: comparison with prevalence of thrombocytopenia based on blood smear estimation, *Vet Clin Pathol* 30(3):137, 2001
68. Ottenjann M, Weingart C, Arndt G et al: Characterization of the anemia of inflammatory disease in cats with abscesses, pyothorax, or fat necrosis, *J Vet Intern Med* 20(5):1143, 2006.
69. Pascal-Tenorio A, Olivry T, Gross TL et al: Paraneoplastic alopecia associated with internal malignancies in the cat, *Vet Dermatol* 8(1):47, 1997
70. Patel RT, Caceres A, French AF et al: Multiple myeloma in 16 cats: a retrospective study, *Vet Clin Pathol* 34(4):341, 2005.
71. Peaston AE, Griffey SM: Visceral mast cell tumour with eosinophilia and eosinophilic peritoneal and pleural effusions in a cat, *Aust Vet J* 71(7):215, 1994.
72. Peschken CA, Walker SL, El-Gabalawy HS et al: Digital necrosis as a paraneoplastic syndrome, *J Clin Rheumatol* 3(6):339, 1997.
73. Peterson EN, Kirby R, Sommer M et al: Cholecalciferol rodenticide intoxication in a cat, *J Am Vet Med Assoc* 199(7):904, 1991.
74. Presthus J, Teige J: Peripheral neuropathy associated with lymphosarcoma in a dog, *J Small Animal Practice* 27(7):463, 1986.
75. Quesnel AD, Parent JM, McDonell W et al: Diagnostic evaluation of cats with seizure disorders: 30 cases (1991-1993), *J Am Vet Med Assoc* 210(1):65, 1997.
76. Rossi G, Errico G, Perez P et al: Paraneoplastic hypoglycemia in a diabetic dog with an insulin growth factor-2-producing mammary carcinoma, *Vet Clin Pathol* 39(4):480, 2010.
77. Rottenberg S, von Tscharner C, Roosje PJ: Thymoma-associated exfoliative dermatitis in cats, *Vet Pathol* 41(4):429, 2004.
78. Savary KC, Price GS, Vaden SL: Hypercalcemia in cats: a retrospective study of 71 cases (1991-1997), *J Vet Intern Med* 14(2):184, 2000.
79. Schaer M: Therapeutic approach to electrolyte emergencies, *Vet Clin North Am Small Anim Pract* 38(3):513, 2008.
80. Schoen K, Block G, Newell SM et al: Hypercalcemia of malignancy in a cat with bronchogenic adenocarcinoma, *J Am Anim Hosp Assoc* 46(4):265, 2010.
81. Scott-Moncrieff JC, Cook JR, Lantz GC: Acquired myasthenia gravis in a cat with thymoma, *J Am Vet Med Assoc* 196(8):1291, 1990.
82. Sellon RK, Rottman JB, Jordan HL et al: Hypereosinophilia associated with transitional cell carcinoma in a cat, *J Am Vet Med Assoc* 201(4):591, 1992.
83. Shelton GD: Routine and specialized laboratory testing for the diagnosis of neuromuscular diseases in dogs and cats, *Vet Clin Pathol* 39(3):278, 2010.
84. Shelton GD, Ho M, Kass PH: Risk factors for acquired myasthenia gravis in cats: 105 cases (1986-1998), *J Am Vet Med Assoc* 216(1):55, 2000.
85. Shelton GD, Schule A, Kass PH: Risk factors for acquired myasthenia gravis in dogs: 1,154 cases (1991-1995), *J Am Vet Med Assoc* 211(11):1428, 1997.
86. Singh A, Boston SE, Poma R: Thymoma-associated exfoliative dermatitis with post-thymectomy myasthenia gravis in a cat, *Can Vet J* 51(7):757, 2010.
87. Smirnov OA: [Anemia during inflammatory processes: pathogenesis and clinical and morphological manifestations], *Arkh Patol* 72(2):56, 2010.
88. Smits B, Reid MM: Feline paraneoplastic syndrome associated with thymoma, *N Z Vet J* 51(5):244, 2003.
89. Snyder MC, Lauter CB: Eosinophilic and neutrophilic leukemoid reaction in a woman with spindle cell sarcoma: a case report, *J Med Case Reports* 4:335, 2010.
90. Storstein A, Monstad SE, Haugen M et al: Onconeural antibodies: improved detection and clinical correlations, *J Neuroimmunol* 232(1-2):166, 2011.
91. Stützer B, Müller F, Majzoub M et al: Role of latent feline leukemia virus infection in nonregenerative cytopenias of cats, *J Vet Intern Med* 24(1):192, 2010.
92. Tasker S, Griffon DJ, Nuttall TJ et al: Resolution of paraneoplastic alopecia following surgical removal of a pancreatic carcinoma in a cat, *J Small Anim Pract* 40(1):16, 1999.
93. Taylor SS, Tappin SW, Dodkin SJ et al: Serum protein electrophoresis in 155 cats, *J Feline Med Surg* 12(8):643, 2010.
94. Tefferi A, Patnaik MM, Pardanani A: Eosinophilia: secondary, clonal and idiopathic, *Br J Haematol* 133(5):468, 2006.
95. Thompson JC, Hickson PC, Johnstone AC et al: Observations on hypoglycaemia associated with a hepatoma in a cat, *N Z Vet J* 43(5):186, 1995.
96. Tisdale MJ: Mechanisms of cancer cachexia, *Physiol Rev* 89(2):381, 2009.
97. Turek MM: Cutaneous paraneoplastic syndromes in dogs and cats: a review of the literature, *Vet Dermatol* 14(6):279, 2003.
98. van der Luer R, van den Ingh T, van Hoe N: [Feline paraneoplastic alopecia], *Tijdschr Diergeneeskd* 133(5):182, 2008.
99. Van Mens SP, Buist MR, Walter AW et al: [Eosinophilia and a solid tumour: ovarian sarcoma], *Ned Tijdschr Geneeskd* 154(8):A1031, 2010.
100. Vassilatou E, Fisfis M, Morphopoulos G et al: Papillary thyroid carcinoma producing granulocyte-macrophage colony-stimulating factor is associated with neutrophilia and eosinophilia, *Hormones (Athens)* 5(4):303, 2006.

101. Villiers E, Dobson J: Multiple myeloma with associated polyneuropathy in a German shepherd dog, *J Small Anim Pract* 39(5):249, 1998.
102. Wasserman SI, Goetzl EJ, Ellman L et al: Tumor-associated eosinophilotactic factor, *N Engl J Med* 290(8):420, 1974.
103. Webb J, Chary P, Northrup N et al: Erythrophagocytic multiple myeloma in a cat, *Vet Clin Pathol* 37(3):302, 2008.
104. Weber NA, Tebeau CS: An unusual presentation of multiple myeloma in two cats, *J Am Anim Hosp Assoc* 34(6):477, 1998.
105. Weiss DJ: Bone marrow pathology in dogs and cats with non-regenerative immune-mediated haemolytic anaemia and pure red cell aplasia, *J Comp Pathol* 138(1):46, 2008.
106. White C, Reine N: Feline nonregenerative anemia, *Compend Contin Educ Vet* 31(7):E1-E19, 2009.
107. Whitney JL, Barrs VRD, Wilkinson MR et al: Use of bisphosphonates to treat severe idiopathic hypercalcaemia in a young Ragdoll cat, *J Feline Med Surg* 13(2):129, 2011.
108. Wilson SC, Thomson-Kerr K, Houston DM: Hypereosinophilic syndrome in a cat, *Can Vet J* 37(11):679, 1996.
109. Zitz JC, Birchard SJ, Couto GC et al: Results of excision of thymoma in cats and dogs: 20 cases (1984-2005), *J Am Vet Med Assoc* 232(8):1186, 2008.

PALLIATIVE CARE

Jackie M. Wypij

The term *palliative care* refers to medical therapy primarily administered to treat the symptoms of cancer, as opposed to directly treating the cancer itself. The ultimate goal is to maintain or improve quality of life. Palliative care is commonly used for advanced stage and terminal cancer alone or in combination with standard cancer therapies. Palliative care is *not* synonymous with giving up. Unfortunately, in very advanced-stage disease traditional cancer therapy may in fact worsen the pet's quality of life and offer little chance of providing significant benefit to the patient. Conversely, palliative care still improves patient comfort levels, even when prolongation of life is not possible. Compassionate and humane palliative treatment for the pet also contributes to client satisfaction.

The primary clinical signs associated with advanced feline cancer include physical and mechanical dysfunction (e.g., dysphagia, cramping, obstipation, dyspnea) and concerns secondary to metabolic or paraneoplastic processes (e.g., anorexia, nausea, fever, anemia, cachexia, and electrolyte imbalances). These problems may be exhibited as overt pain, discomfort, lack of social interaction, or anxiety, in addition to physical dysfunction.

QUALITY OF LIFE SCORE SYSTEMS

Although many feline cancers are not curable, palliation of clinical signs will improve the quality of life in most cats with cancer. This is a major concern for pet owners; quality of life is often more important than the length of life. Assessing quality of life in feline patients can be very difficult and depends on the individual cat's behavior as well as owners' perceptions. Several quality of life score systems have been proposed for cats.[3,4] Dr. Villalobos's quality of life scoring system, "HHHHHMM," incorporates measures of "*h*urt, *h*unger, *h*ygiene, *h*ydration, *h*appiness, *m*obility, and *m*ore good days than bad" and attempts to provide a more objective means for the caregiving team (client and veterinary staff) to determine appropriate intervention or euthanasia (Table 28-4).[3] The key is open communication between veterinarian and pet owner about factors that contribute to decreased quality of life, as well as monitoring relatively feline-specific behaviors such as hiding, lack of grooming, and lack of social interaction.

TABLE 28-4 **The HHHHHMM Quality of Life Scale***

Score	Criterion
Hurt: 0-10	Is pain successfully managed?
Hunger: 0-10	Is the cat eating enough? Is a feeding tube required?
Hydration: 0-10	Is the cat dehydrated? Is subcutaneous fluid therapy necessary?
Hygiene: 0-10	The cat should be groomed and cleaned regularly; avoid pressure sores and keep all wounds clean.
Happiness: 0-10	Does the cat express interest in its environment? Is it responsive to family, toys, other pets, and so forth?
Mobility: 0-10	Can the cat move without assistance? Are neurologic signs or pain impairing mobility?
More good days than bad: 0-10	When bad days outnumber good days, quality of life may be compromised. When a healthy human-animal bond is no longer possible, the owner should be aware that the end is near. Euthanasia may be necessary to prevent further pain and suffering.
Total =	A total of 35 points or more is acceptable for good quality of life.

*Score patients on a scale of 1 (poor) to 10 (best).
Adapted from Myers F: Palliative care: end of life "pawspice" care. In Villalobos A, Kaplan L, editors: *Canine and feline geriatric oncology: honoring the human-animal bond*, Ames, Iowa, 2007, Wiley-Blackwell.

ANALGESIA

Pain control is an important aspect of cancer care in feline patients. Pain may be visceral (e.g., gastrointestinal lymphoma), somatic (e.g., jaw pain with oral tumor), or neuropathic (e.g., extension of a soft tissue sarcoma along nerve fibers). If pain is suspected despite a lack of apparent clinical signs, analgesic intervention may function as a diagnostic test for pain as well as a directed therapy. To address cancer-related pain in cats, the veterinarian should consider several strategies,[2] including the following:

1. Direct treatment of painful site: Bulky tumors or those involving bone may be amenable to direct therapy such as cytoreductive surgery or palliative (coarse fraction) radiation therapy. Intravenous aminobisphosphonates (e.g., pamidronate, zoledronate) may also be useful for malignant bone lysis, such as a primary bone tumor (e.g., osteosarcoma), metastatic bone tumor (e.g., digital metastasis of primary lung tumor), and local tissue invasion (e.g., oral SCC, injection-site sarcoma). These drugs are potentially nephrotoxic and should be used with caution, especially in conjunction with other analgesics and chemotherapeutics. In some cases systemic chemotherapy may also be effective to palliate clinical signs. The treatment goals may focus on reduction of inflammation or pain, reduction in tumor volume, or slowing of growth to improve clinical signs rather than cure of the disease.
2. Remove or reduce contributing environmental factors: Care should be taken to modify the cat's home environment for maximal comfort. Cats with intranasal tumors may benefit from a room humidifier. To help cats with limited mobility, items such as litter boxes, food, and water bowls should be easily accessible (e.g., at floor level). The owner should minimize the necessity of high jumps and stairs and provide safe, comfortable, and accessible private resting areas away from other household pets that might contribute to patient stress. For cats with oral tumors, moistened or canned food and soft toys should be used.
3. Local analgesic techniques: Although rarely practical for long-term use, local analgesic options (e.g., nerve blocks, topical analgesics, local analgesic patches) may be considered in certain cases.
4. Systemic analgesia: This is the most common form of clinical pain management in cats and often includes nonsteroidal antiinflammatory drugs and opioids. Patients with cancer may be at increased risk of organ toxicity as a sequela of the tumor, primary treatment, or supportive medications. Cats are more sensitive than dogs to the toxic side effects of many analgesics, and most feline cancer patients are also geriatric. Contraindications and interactions with other medications should be taken into consideration, particularly with drugs that are potentially nephrotoxic or hepatotoxic. Some chemotherapy agents may potentiate organ toxicity. For example, doxorubicin and carboplatin are commonly used chemotherapy agents that are potentially nephrotoxic. Sedation and anesthesia should be minimized but may be necessary for procedures such as radiation therapy or feeding tube placement; this may place additional stress on kidneys and other organs.
5. Complementary therapies: Physical therapy and rehabilitation techniques such as physical manipulation are poorly tolerated by most cats but could be considered in certain cases. Options include range-of-motion exercises, massage therapy, acupuncture, acupressure, and chiropractic care. Client instruction for home care may be more feasible than in-hospital physical therapy.

For more complete information on feline analgesia, please refer to Chapter 6.

NUTRITIONAL CARE

Nutritional care of feline cancer patients should address route of administration, optimal nutritional content, palatability, appetite stimulation, nutritional supplementation, supportive care of gastrointestinal upset, and recognition of the effects of cancer cachexia. Cancer-bearing cats are often underweight, with most exhibiting reduced fat stores and muscle mass. BCS is prognostic in cats, with average or obese cats living significantly longer than thin cats.[1]

Cancer cachexia is a poorly understood paraneoplastic process in veterinary patients. In human oncology cancer cachexia is recognized as a complex metabolic syndrome that manifests as severe weight loss, muscle wasting, and inappetence. Contributing factors include maldigestion and malabsorption as well as functional abnormalities leading to decreased nutritional intake. Examples include painful oral tumors, obstructive or malabsorptive gastrointestinal tumors, and systemic cancers that induce nausea, vomiting, and diarrhea. Metabolic and physiologic alterations are more subtle contributing factors to cachexia and may include altered nutrient metabolism (carbohydrates, protein, and fats), altered insulin response, and cytokine abnormalities. These derangements can result in severe weight loss even in the face of normal or apparent increased food intake.

Enteral feeding is always preferred because it maintains gastrointestinal epithelial health and offers safety and convenience. For short-term care of hospitalized patients, a nasogastric tube is easily managed. Esophagostomy tubes (E-tubes) are ideal for both short- and longer-term home care for patients with oral tumors or nonspecific inappetence that are not actively vomiting. E-tubes are easily placed during a short anesthesia procedure and are extremely well-tolerated by cats (see Chapter 18). Newer feline-specific E-tubes are commercially available and are appropriately sized, flexible, and radio-opaque to optimize placement. Cats are able to eat on their own with E-tubes in place, and this provides a low-stress option for owners to administer both nutrition and medication. Another less commonly used long-term home option is a gastrostomy tube. In select cases partial parenteral or total parenteral nutrition is used in the intensive care unit for short-term support of hospitalized patients, such as after an invasive surgical procedure. Hand feeding may also encourage food intake, although assisted feeding in the form of force feeding or syringe feeding is often poorly tolerated and may lead to food aversion and bite injuries to pet owners.

The ideal diet for the feline cancer patient has yet to be determined. Given the metabolic alterations of cancer cachexia, a diet low in simple carbohydrates with moderate lipids and easily digestible protein sources is ideal. Many adult commercial cat foods meet these criteria. Because many cats may be geriatric or have chronic renal insufficiency, these medical concerns should also be taken into consideration when selecting an appropriate diet. In addition to adequate nutritional composition, palatability is a major concern. The best answer to the question, "What should I feed my cat with cancer?" is usually, "Whatever he or she will eat." Standard methods to improve palatability include trying different brands of cat food, canned cat food, or human food, such as tuna, deli meats, and cheese. Warming up the food or adding cooking liquids or milk may also improve palatability for some cats. The role of specific nutritional supplements is poorly understood in clinical feline patients. However, supplementation should be instituted as clinically indicated (e.g., vitamin B_{12} supplementation in cats with intestinal lymphoma). Specific recommendations for nutritional care of feline cancer patients can be found in Chapter 18.

Appetite stimulants are most effective in mildly affected cats or in temporary situations such as when the cat is recovering from anesthesia or surgery. Appetite stimulants may not adequately improve food intake and may have inconsistent results. Mirtazapine is a newer appetite stimulant with good efficacy in cats. Cyproheptadine may also be effective, although cyproheptadine and mirtazapine should not be used concurrently because their actions are antagonistic. In a hospital or short-term situation, oral diazepam could be administered if other oral medications are ineffective. Side effects and toxicity may occur with all these medications, and they should be prescribed with appropriate monitoring. For example, mirtazapine dose should be reduced in the presence of renal insufficiency.

Other supportive gastrointestinal medications include histamine receptor (H_2) antagonists (e.g., famotidine), coating agents such as sucralfate, and proton pump inhibitors (e.g., omeprazole) (Table 28-5). Fiber supplementation or lactulose may alleviate constipation in predisposed cats or in cases complicated by abdominal, pelvic, or intestinal discomfort. Antiemetics may be effective for nonobstructive gastrointestinal cancer or nonspecific/systemic cancers that contribute to nausea or vomiting. Some options include metoclopramide (a prokinetic and centrally acting antiemetic); 5-HT_3 receptor antagonists (ondansetron, dolasetron); and, more recently, the neurokinin-1 receptor antagonist maropitant citrate (Cerenia). Although routinely used in small animal patients, metoclopramide is less effective in cats than in dogs because of differences in CNS neurotransmitter receptors at the chemoreceptor trigger zone. Options for management of acute and chronic diarrhea in feline cancer patients include dietary modification, addition of dietary prebiotics and feline-specific probiotics, and direct medical therapy. Metronidazole is most commonly used and should be prescribed at the lowest effective dose.

Outpatient or at-home subcutaneous fluid therapy should be instituted for cats with inadequate fluid intake and those with increased risk of renal toxicity. Cats with preexisting renal insufficiency or those receiving nephrotoxic medications (e.g., nonsteroidal antiinflammatory drugs, chemotherapy agents such as doxorubicin and carboplatin) and geriatric animals undergoing procedures requiring sedation should be supported with appropriate fluid therapy.

For further information on drug therapy and fluid therapy, please refer to Chapters 4 and 5.

MISCELLANEOUS CARE

Sick cats and those with oral tumors often stop grooming, necessitating additional home care by the pet owner. Oral health concerns such as bacterial infections and malocclusion should be assessed and treated as needed. Cats undergoing systemic chemotherapy may be at increased risk of myelosuppression and susceptibility to secondary bacterial infections. Common routes of entry include the oral cavity, colon and intestinal tract, lower urinary tract, skin, and ears. Pleural effusion secondary to mediastinal lymphoma, primary or metastatic lung tumors, or carcinomatosis (microscopic tumor seeding of pleura) may decrease the cat's quality of life, and thoracocentesis can be performed as an acute palliative measure, although effusion often progresses quickly. Abdominal effusion is less likely to reduce the patient's quality of life, and therapeutic abdominocentesis should be performed only if clinically necessary to reduce losses of protein and electrolytes and minimize patient stress.

In summary, a variety of supportive and medical therapies can be instituted for feline cancer patients. The goal of palliative care is to maintain and maximize the pet's quality of life and should incorporate a whole-health approach.

TABLE 28-5 **Selected Supportive Gastrointestinal Medications in Feline Cancer Patients**

Drug	Action	Mechanism	Site of Action	Feline Dose
Famotidine (Pepcid AC)	Gastric acid reduction	Histamine H_2-receptor antagonist	Peripheral	0.5-1 mg/kg PO, SC, IV every 12 to 24 hours
Ranitidine (Zantac)	Gastric acid reduction Prokinetic	Histamine H_2-receptor antagonist	Peripheral	1-2 mg/kg PO, SC, IV every 12 hours
Omeprazole (Prilosec)	Gastric acid reduction	Proton pump inhibitor	Peripheral	0.5-1 mg/kg PO every 24 hours
Maropitant (Cerenia)	Antiemetic	NK-1 antagonist	Central Peripheral	Empirical 0.5-1 mg/kg short-term
Metoclopramide (Reglan)	Antiemetic	Dopaminergic antagonist Suspected acetylcholine sensitization?	Peripheral Central	Empirical 0.2-0.4 mg/kg PO, SC every 6-8 hours
Ondanestron (Zofran)	Antiemetic	5-HT3 serotonin antagonist	Central Peripheral	Empirical 0.1-0.5 mg/kg every 12 hours
Mirtazapine	Appetite stimulant	Noradrenergic agonist Serotonin agonist	Central	3.75 mg PO/cat every 72 hours or 1 mg/cat per day, compounded
Metronidazole (Flagyl)	Anticolitis Antidiarrheal	Antibiotic Other	Peripheral	10-15 mg/kg PO every 12 hours, short-term (3-5 days)

PO, Orally; *SC*, subcutaneously; *IV*, intravenously.

References

1. Baez JL, Michel KE, Sorenmo K et al: A prospective investigation of the prevalence and prognostic significance of weight loss and changes in body condition in feline cancer patients, *J Feline Med Surg* 9:411, 2007.
2. Looney A: Oncology pain in veterinary patients, *Top Companion Anim Med* 25:32, 2010.
3. Myers F: Palliative care: end of life "pawspice" care. In Villalobos A, Kaplan L, editors: *Canine and feline geriatric oncology: honoring the human-animal bond*, Ames, Iowa, 2007, Wiley-Blackwell.
4. Tzannes S, Hammond MF, Murphy S et al: Owners perception of their cats' quality of life during COP chemotherapy for lymphoma, *J Fel Med Surg* 10:73, 2008.

CHAPTER

29

Ophthalmology

Christine C. Lim and David J. Maggs

OUTLINE

Feline ophthalmology is a vast and important field in which feline practitioners need to be reasonably adept, given the frequency with which clients note ocular disease in their cats and the importance they place on good vision from a pain-free globe. In this chapter we have attempted to highlight conditions that are unique to cats and emphasize feline-specific considerations for more common ocular diseases. Less attention has been paid to those conditions for which management strategies differ little from those employed in dogs, insofar as these topics have been amply covered in standard veterinary ophthalmology texts.

OPHTHALMIC EXAMINATION AND DIAGNOSTIC TECHNIQUES

History

A great deal of information can be gleaned from a complete history and thorough ophthalmic examination. A detailed history does much to narrow the list of differential considerations. Important background information includes the chief complaint, duration of clinical signs, concurrent ocular or systemic medical conditions, previous therapies, and current ophthalmic or systemically administered medications.

Examination Techniques and Order

Basic necessities for a complete ophthalmic examination include a consistent, systematic approach to the examination; a bright, focal light source; magnification; and a darkened room. Diagnostic tests such as the Schirmer tear test (STT), tonometry (assessment of intraocular pressure), fluorescein staining, and funduscopic examination are important components of the examination and need to be done at prescribed times. The following is a recommended order for the ophthalmic examination.

Whereas assessment of dogs begins by observing while the patient navigates into the examination room, most cats are carried in and refuse to participate in any obstacle courses set up by the examiner. Cats also seem to mask vision loss much more effectively than dogs; therefore clinical assessment of vision tends to be much more difficult in the cat than in the dog. For this the examiner may need to rely more heavily on historical information and other examination findings.

The examiner should begin at eye level with the cat. The cat's head should first be observed from a distance, avoiding excessive manipulation of the face by the restrainer. This allows for detection of nonocular abnormalities that may be related to the ocular disease, such as facial asymmetry, oral or nasal discharge, and the presence of a head tilt. The examiner should then perform the neuro-ophthalmic examination (Table 29-1). The neuro-ophthalmic assessment for cats can yield very different results than that for the dog. For example, the menace response (Figure 29-1) tends to be inconsistently elicited in cats, with many normal cats failing to blink in response to a menacing gesture. Likewise, stressed cats with higher sympathetic tone often have resting mydriasis and diminished pupillary light reflexes (PLRs).

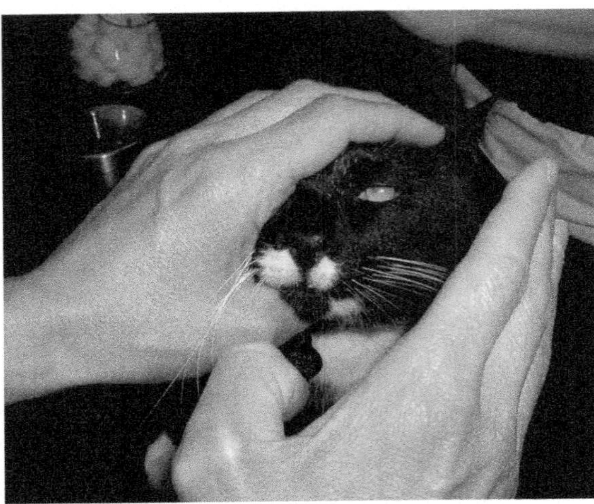

FIGURE 29-1 Proper technique for eliciting the menace response. The contralateral eye must be covered with one hand to prevent it from viewing the menacing gesture. Care should be taken to keep from generating wind currents or directly touching the highly sensitive vibrissae when performing the menacing gesture.

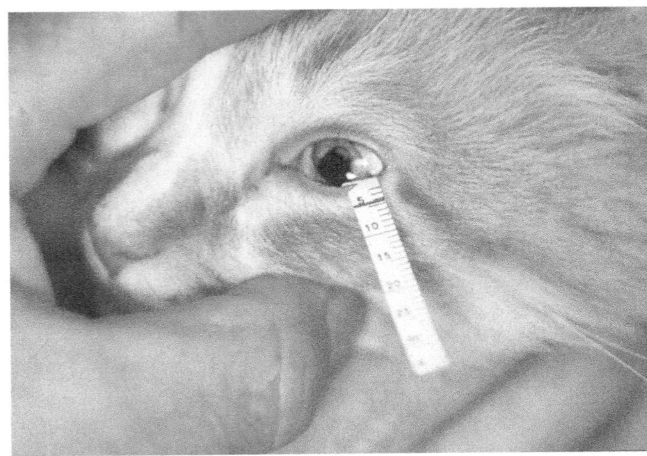

FIGURE 29-2 The Schirmer tear test in a cat. The test strip should be folded at the notch and placed in the ventrolateral conjunctival fornix and left in place for 60 seconds. Care should be taken not to touch the lower part of the strip with the hands because oil on the skin can affect the capillary action of the strip and test result. *(From Maggs D: Slatter's fundamentals of veterinary ophthalmology, ed 4, St Louis, 2007, Saunders.)*

TABLE 29-1 **Components of the Neuro-Ophthalmic Examination**

Test	Tested Structures
Menace response	CN II and VII, visual cortex, and cerebellum
Palpebral reflex	CN V and VII
Oculocephalic reflex	CN III, IV, and VI
Direct and consensual pupillary light reflexes	CN II and III and central visual pathways excluding the visual cortex
Dazzle reflex	CN II and VII and subcortical visual pathways

If a STT is to be performed, it must be done before any eye drops are applied to the eye. It is performed in the same manner as in the dog (Figure 29-2); however, normal STT measurements vary widely in cats.[194] For example, the authors have recorded STT values less than 5 mm/min in cats without detectable ocular disease. Conversely, cats with significant keratoconjunctival disease may have STT results within the normal reference range.[106] Such discrepancies emphasize the importance of interpreting the STT in context with the overall clinical examination and comparing them between the affected and unaffected eyes in cats with unilateral or asymmetric ocular disease. After the STT, intraocular pressure (IOP) should be assessed. Although there is some variability, normal feline IOP tends to be between 10 and 25 mm Hg.[140] Both the Schiotz and TonoPen tonometers require application of a topical anesthetic agent before obtaining an IOP measurement, whereas the TonoVet does not (Figure 29-3). Although retropulsion can be useful in detecting space-occupying lesions of the orbit, it is not considered an acceptable technique for measurement of IOP. If the IOP is within normal limits, a single drop of 0.5% or 1% tropicamide should then be applied to each eye to achieve pupillary dilation, which is essential for examination of the lens, vitreous, and ocular fundus. In cats tropicamide induces mydriasis within 15 minutes, for 8 to 9 hours.[87] Pharmacologic mydriasis is not recommended if the IOP is elevated because dilation may further increase the IOP.

The remainder of the ophthalmic examination may be performed during and after pupillary dilation, and the techniques used in cats differ little from those used in other species. Sequential examination of all structures moving from peripheral to axial and from superficial to deep ensures a complete and orderly examination. The examiner should begin with retroillumination of the tapetal reflection from arm's length (Figure 29-4) to identify opacities in the visual axis. Magnification, in the form of head loupes (Figure 29-5), should then be employed throughout the entire ophthalmic examination, except for the fundic examination. The examiner should employ focal illumination and transillumination (Figure 29-6) from various angles when assessing the ocular surface. Depth and spatial relationships are best assessed using the slit beam of the direct ophthalmoscope. The detection of aqueous flare (plasma protein in the anterior chamber) is a pathognomonic change in anterior uveitis, and therefore its detection forms a critical part of the ophthalmic examination in all cats. Aqueous flare is best detected when the room has been darkened completely and the smallest, most focal white light beam on the direct ophthalmoscope head is used

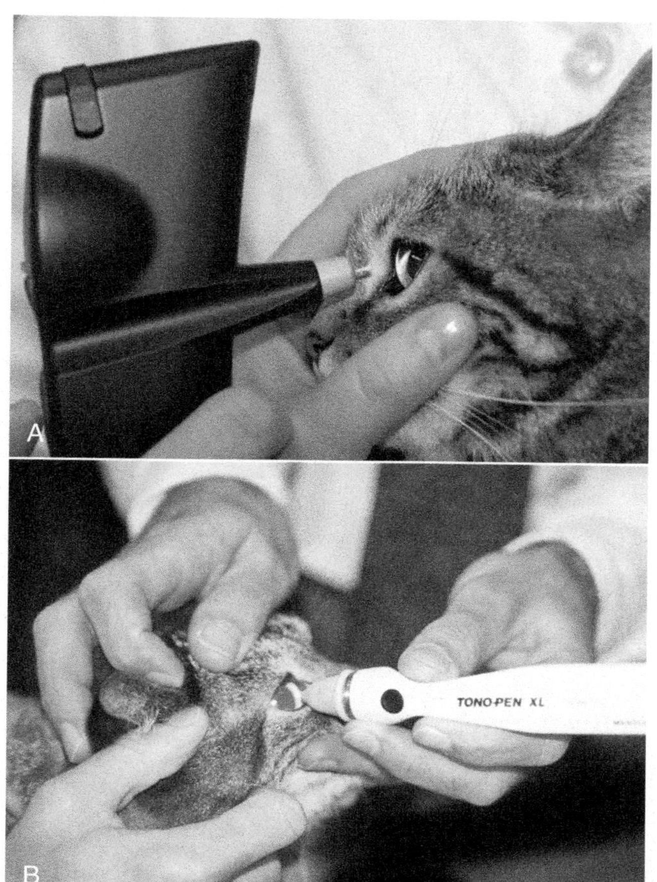

FIGURE 29-3 The TonoVet **(A)** and TonoPen **(B)** being used to measure intraocular pressure in cats. The tips of both instruments should be directed toward the central cornea according to the manufacturer's directions. The operator should take care to ensure that excessive pressure is not placed directly on the globe when holding the eyelids open or on the jugular veins as the animal is restrained because both can elevate intraocular pressure readings.

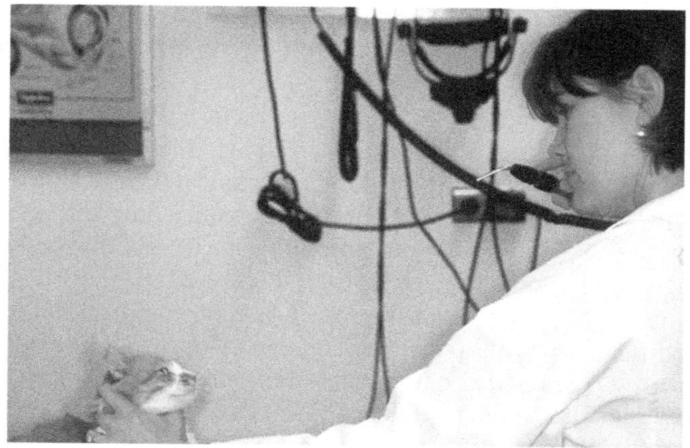

FIGURE 29-4 Correct technique for performing retroillumination. The light source is held next to the examiner's eye and the patient examined at arm's length in a darkened room. The examiner should alter his or her viewing angle until the fundic reflection is elicited. This can be used to assess pupil symmetry and any opacities within the tear film, cornea, anterior chamber, lens, and vitreous.

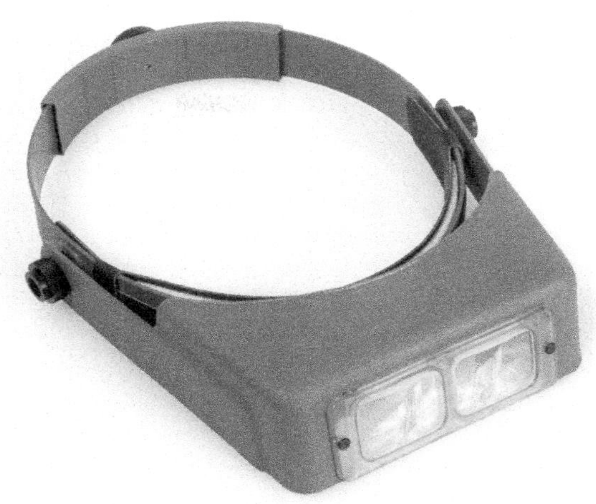

FIGURE 29-5 Magnification is an essential component of the entire ophthalmic examination, with the exception of the fundic examination. It is especially important for assessment of aqueous flare and after application of fluorescein stain. The Optivisor is inexpensive and extremely useful for the ophthalmic examination, as well as surgery and suture removal in general practice.

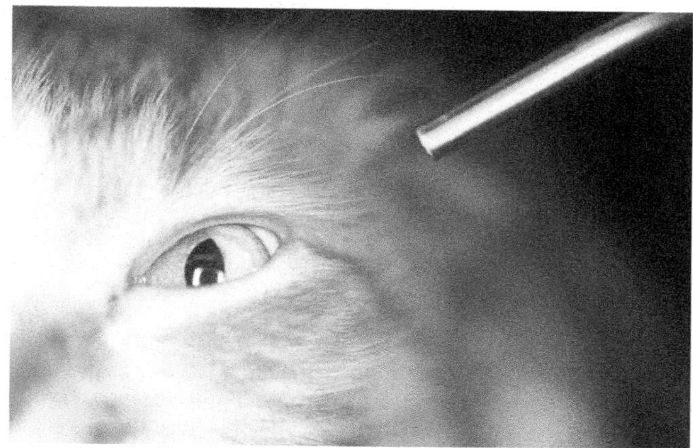

FIGURE 29-6 Technique for transillumination. The light source and examiner should move around the animal such that multiple highly variable combinations of viewing and illumination angles are achieved throughout the ophthalmic examination. This will greatly increase the chance that lesions will be found. In particular, this technique improves or facilitates depth perception within the eye, assessment of topography, and evaluation of reflections from transparent surfaces. *(From Maggs D:* Slatter's fundamentals of veterinary ophthalmology, *ed 4, St Louis, 2007, Saunders.)*

very close to the cat's eye to examine the clarity of the anterior chamber. Any "smokiness" detected as the beam traverses the anterior chamber between the cornea and the lens should prompt consideration of and further investigation for anterior uveitis. The iris face is a frequent site of pathology in cats and must be evaluated before dilation. By contrast, thorough assessment of the lens, vitreous, and fundus can be performed only after full dilation has been achieved. Also, aqueous flare may be more easily detected after full mydriasis has been

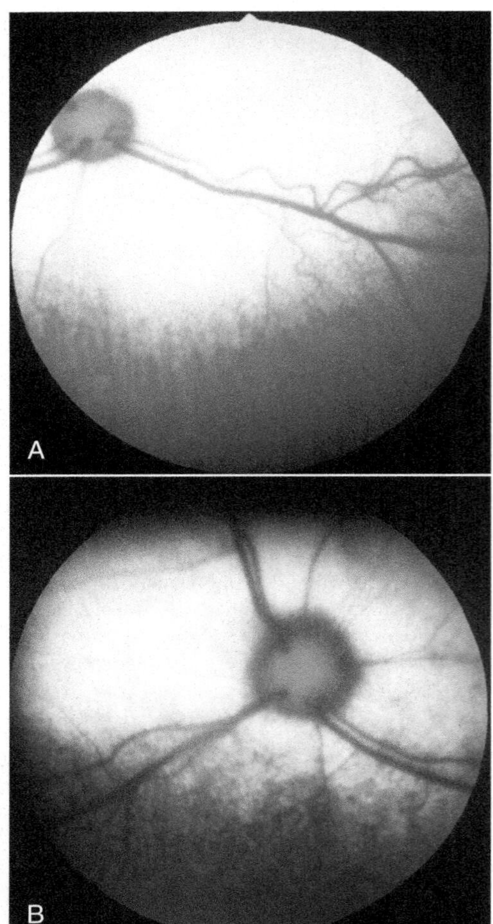

FIGURE 29-7 Two variations of the normal feline fundus. **A,** A subalbinotic fundus is a normal variation typically seen in pigment-dilute individuals. The relative lack of melanin in the retina and choroid allows visualization of the choroidal vessels in the nontapetal fundus. In some subalbinotic fundi, the tapetum is absent. **B,** Normal feline fundus. Melanin in the retina and choroid prevents visualization of the choroidal vessels seen in image **A**. The optic disc appears circular and gray because of the lack of myelin and is located immediately dorsal to the tapetal–nontapetal junction. Three or four larger retinal venules extend from the edges of the optic disc to the periphery of the retina. The tapetum is usually green or yellow.

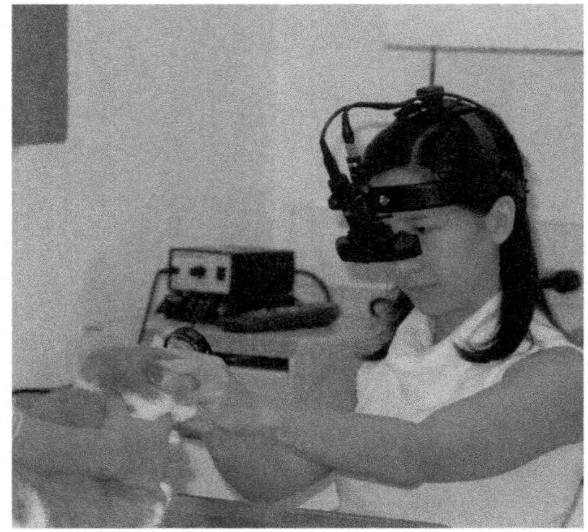

FIGURE 29-8 The binocular headset improves depth perception and frees one hand for manipulation of the patient's eyelids and head.

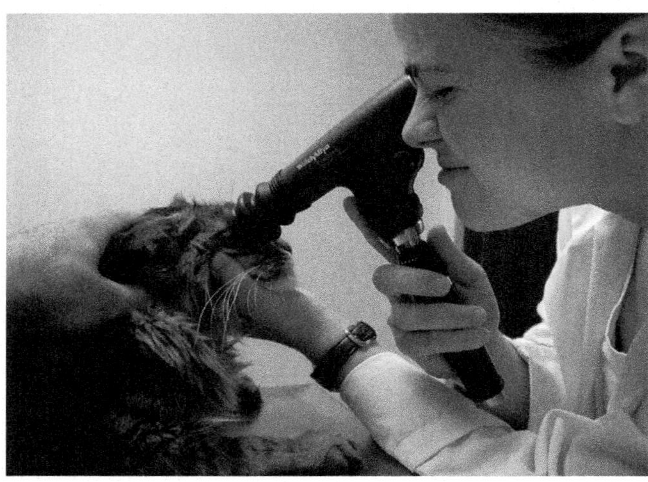

FIGURE 29-9 Technique for fundic examination using the Panoptic. After the instrument is focused for the examiner's eye, the fundic reflection is identified while looking through the Panoptic from approximately 10 to 15 centimeters away from the patient. The examiner then moves toward the patient until the eyecup of the ophthalmoscope contacts the patient's face. If this causes eyelid closure, the eyecup can be removed.

achieved, insofar as the black background of the pupil provides contrast with which to view the gray beam of light traversing the anterior chamber. Direct and indirect ophthalmoscopy are the two traditional methods for examining the fundus (Figure 29-7). Direct ophthalmoscopy is relatively easy to learn and provides the examiner with an upright image of the retina but is not a good method for examination of the fundus. The main disadvantage of direct ophthalmoscopy is the limited field of view, a result of extreme magnification. This makes complete retinal examination difficult, and peripheral regions and smaller lesions are often missed. Indirect ophthalmoscopy is considered to be the best method for viewing the fundus, despite the steeper learning curve. The image produced is an inverted representation of the fundus. When the binocular headset (Figure 29-8) is used, indirect ophthalmoscopy provides superior depth perception. The larger field of view obtained by indirect ophthalmoscopy makes complete fundic examination easier and allows the practitioner to view a larger portion of the fundus in less time, which is extremely valuable for uncooperative patients. The direct ophthalmoscope can then be used for more detailed examination of any focal lesions identified. A newer ophthalmoscope, the Panoptic offers a field of view and level of magnification intermediate to the traditional ophthalmoscopes (Figure 29-9). Although it is unable to provide much depth perception, its ease of use and moderate field of view make the Panoptic a reasonable compromise between direct and indirect ophthalmoscopy.

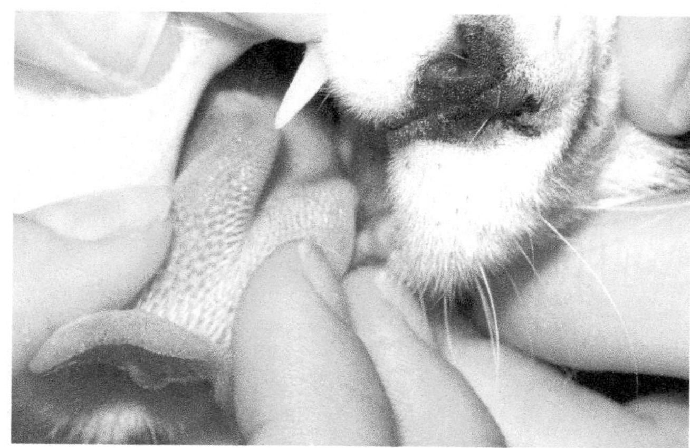

FIGURE 29-10 The Jones test. Appearance of fluorescein dye at the nares or in the mouth within a few minutes after application to the ocular surface indicates patency of the nasolacrimal ducts, or a positive Jones test. In many cats, especially those with brachycephalic conformation, the nasolacrimal duct opens sufficiently caudally within the nose that fluorescein is noted on the tongue rather than at the naris. This highlights the importance of testing the side of interest first, because laterality cannot be determined when fluorescein is detected in the mouth. *(Image courtesy UC Davis Veterinary Ophthalmology Service.)*

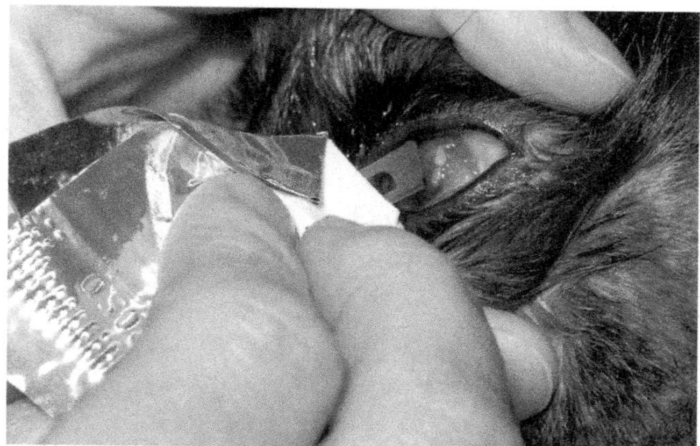

FIGURE 29-11 Technique for collection of corneal or conjunctival samples for diagnostic testing. After application of topical anesthetic, the blunt end of a scalpel blade is used to carefully scrape surface cells from the cornea or conjunctiva. These can then be gently blotted onto a microscope slides for cytologic or immunologic assessment or can be inoculated onto a swab or directly into agar plates for microbiologic assessment.

Application of fluorescein dye may be used to detect corneal ulceration and corneal perforation and may be used to assess tear film stability and patency of the nasolacrimal drainage system. It should be performed only after all other parts of the examination are complete because it will affect results of microbial testing, the STT, and the appearance of many ocular structures.

The Jones test is an assessment of nasolacrimal duct patency (Figure 29-10). A minimum of 2 minutes after placing fluorescein dye into the conjunctival sacs, the nares and mouth are examined for evidence of fluorescein. Presence of fluorescein (positive Jones test) confirms patency of the nasolacrimal duct, whereas absence of fluorescein (negative Jones test) is suggestive of obstruction and should be followed with nasolacrimal flushing.

The tear film break-up time (TFBUT) evaluates stability of the precorneal tear film. It is the time between eyelid opening and the first spot of evaporation within the precorneal tear film. The examiner first places fluorescein dye into the conjunctival sac, then closes the eyelids. Timing begins when the eyelids are opened. Using magnification, the examiner observes one area of the cornea, usually the dorsolateral aspect. Timing ends when the first black spot, signifying evaporation, appears within the green tear film. The normal TFBUT in a cat is 16.7+/−4.5 seconds,[36] whereas more rapid TFBUTs suggest tear film instability.

Ancillary Tests

Techniques for ancillary diagnostic tests such as corneal scrapings (Figure 29-11), conjunctival swabs, and conjunctival biopsies (Figure 29-12) are identical to those for the dog. However, the effect of topical anesthetics required to obtain these samples is shorter in cats than it is in dogs. Whereas a single drop of 0.5% proparacaine provides up to 45 minutes of corneal anesthesia in the dog, the same dose achieves only 25 minutes of corneal anesthesia for the cat, with maximal effect 5 minutes after application.[16,88] This time difference should be taken into account if the practitioner is unable to obtain samples shortly after administering topical anesthesia. Cannulation of the nasolacrimal puncta is more challenging in cats than dogs because of the tight fit of the eyelids to the globe. Also, in cats more often than in dogs, the nasal opening of the nasolacrimal duct is located more

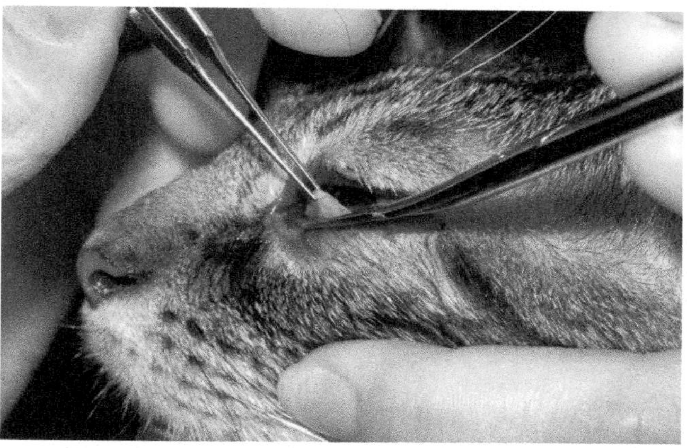

FIGURE 29-12 A biopsy of the conjunctiva can be easily obtained in almost all cats without sedation or general anesthesia. After application of topical anesthetic, forceps are used to tent the conjunctiva, which is then incised with small scissors. The conjunctival defect will heal by second intention. *(From Maggs D:* Slatter's fundamentals of veterinary ophthalmology, *ed 4, St Louis, 2007, Saunders.)*

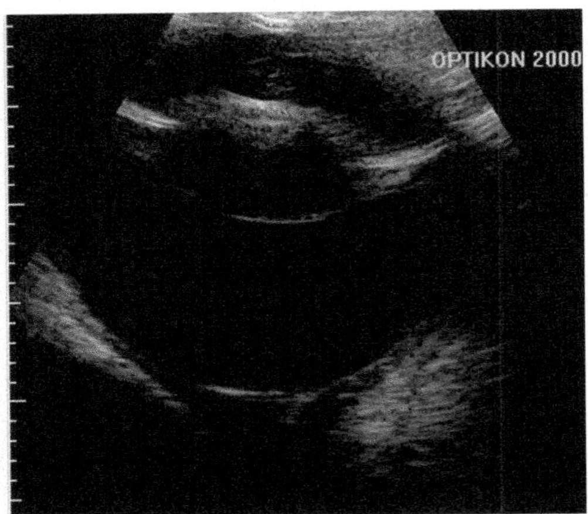

FIGURE 29-13 Ultrasonographic appearance of the normal feline globe. This technique is particularly useful for assessing intraocular structures, especially retinal detachment, in globes with anterior segment pathology that prevent direct visualization. Normal features include the highly echoic convex anterior lens capsule and concave posterior lens capsule; the anechoic anterior chamber, lens, and vitreous cavity; and the echoic concave monolayer of the posterior globe representing sclera, choroid, and retina in close apposition with one another. Orbital structures such as the optic nerve and extraocular muscle cone are sometimes seen. Because of the close proximity of the ultrasound probe to the anterior structures, the anteriormost ocular structures are less well defined than those posterior to them. In the example shown, the anterior chamber and anterior lens appear artifactually hyperechoic. *(Image courtesy UC Davis Veterinary Ophthalmology Service.)*

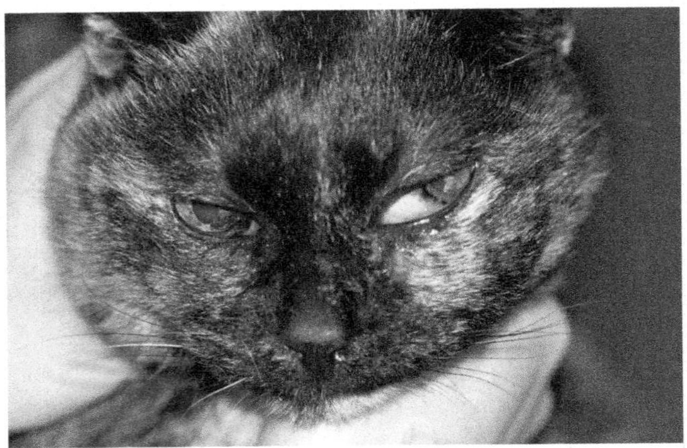

FIGURE 29-14 Left-sided orbital disease in a cat. Comparison of the palpebral fissures shows distortion of the left palpebral fissure, as well as dorsal and lateral displacement of the left globe and elevation of the left nictitans, all of which are highly supportive of orbital, rather than ocular, disease. *(Image courtesy WCVM Veterinary Ophthalmology Service.)*

caudally, such that fluid will be flushed into the oral cavity rather than out the nares (as with fluorescein in Figure 29-10).

Advanced imaging is required when opaque ocular media prevent complete examination of the globe or when orbital or neurologic disease is suspected. Ocular ultrasound is very useful for characterizing lesions within the globe but may not allow full evaluation of orbital lesions[156] (Figure 29-13). Skull radiography and computed tomography (CT) also may not clearly show borders of a lesion, but they will detect bony changes.[156] Magnetic resonance imaging (MRI) is of limited value for bony lesions but offers excellent resolution of soft tissues, including the globe, orbit, and optic nerves.[73]

ORBITAL DISEASE

In cats the most common clinical sign accompanying orbital disease is exophthalmos.[66] Epiphora, enophthalmos, strabismus, elevation of the third eyelid, and decreased retropulsion are other possible examination findings (Figure 29-14). If eyelid movement has been compromised, exposure keratitis or corneal ulceration may also be found (Figure 29-15). Inflammatory and neoplastic conditions make up the bulk of feline orbital disease; orbital vascular anomalies and cystic lesions

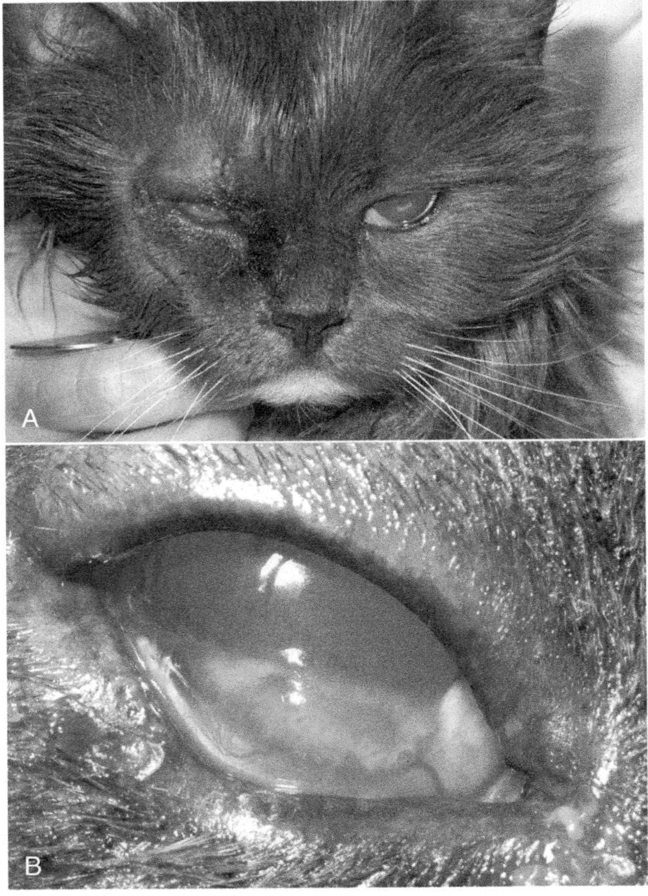

FIGURE 29-15 Right-sided orbital disease caused by squamous cell carcinoma. The globe is enophthalmic. In this patient tumor-induced facial nerve paralysis resulted in exposure keratitis and ulceration of the central cornea. *(Image courtesy UC Davis Veterinary Ophthalmology Service.)*

have not been reported in cats. Identification of the underlying disease process is important because of significant differences in treatment and prognosis. At minimum, a complete blood count (CBC), serum biochemical profile, urinalysis, and fine-needle aspirate or biopsy of the orbital lesion are recommended. Based on the results of these tests, CT or MRI may be warranted to determine the extent of the lesion.

Infectious and Neoplastic Orbital Disease

Orbital cellulitis and abscess formation in the cat are diagnosed and treated in a similar manner as in dogs. As in dogs, orbital extension of dental disease is responsible for many of these cases, but foreign body migration, fungal infections, and iatrogenic trauma (mainly during dental procedures) are also documented causes.[110,157] However, these conditions occur much less frequently in cats than in dogs, and neoplasia should always be considered when a cat presents with orbital disease.[157] In cats the majority of orbital neoplasia is secondary, with direct extension from adjacent structures accounting for 71% of cases.[66] Squamous cell carcinoma (SCC) is the most common orbital neoplastic process in cats,[66] but many other neoplasms may occur.* Regardless of type, 90% of orbital neoplasms are malignant, with mean postdiagnosis survival times less than 2 months.[8,66]

Ocular Proptosis

Ocular proptosis is seen less commonly in cats than in dogs, likely because of cats' deep orbits and relatively tightly fitting adnexa. For this reason the amount of force required to displace the globe from the feline orbit is large, and cats with ocular proptosis usually present with severe intraocular trauma, as well as concurrent cranial or systemic injuries that require more immediate attention. Ocular proptosis in cats often occurs in conjunction with skull fractures and trauma to the globe.[65] As with dogs, enucleation or emergency replacement of the globe followed by temporary tarsorrhaphy is required. However, the prognosis after traumatic ocular proptosis in cats is worse than in dogs. In one retrospective review, all proptosed feline eyes were permanently blind, and 12 of 18 required enucleation.[65]

Feline Orbital Pseudotumor

Feline orbital pseudotumor (FOP) is currently described as a progressive inflammatory disease with similarities to idiopathic orbital inflammation in humans. However, only eight feline cases have been described, and the definition is still evolving.[15,127] All affected cats were middle-aged to older.[15,127] The majority of cats presented with unilateral disease that later became bilateral. In all cases onset of clinical signs was insidious, ultimately characterized by exophthalmos, lagophthalmos, exposure keratitis, and restriction of ocular movements.[15,127] Resistance to retropulsion was also found in the majority of cases.[15,127]

No specific changes are seen on blood work, and fine-needle aspirates tend to be nondiagnostic. Orbital ultrasound may show increased echogenicity of orbital tissues.[15] CT appears to be the most useful imaging modality, often revealing physical compression of the globe. Biopsy of orbital tissues (often obtained during enucleation or exenteration) is essential, with histopathology being characterized by proliferating fibrous tissue with lymphocytic–plasmacytic inflammation.[15]

As for its human counterpart,[20] prognosis for FOP is poor and specific therapeutic guidelines do not exist. Immunosuppressive doses of systemic corticosteroids, oral antibiotics, and radiation therapy have all been attempted with little success.[15,127,192] One author reports having managed FOP for a period of 1.5 years with immunosuppressive corticosteroid therapy before clinical disease returned.[192] This author also reports clinical improvement in one cat after radiation therapy, but this case has not been described nor followed up in the literature.[192] Enucleation or exenteration followed medical therapy in all published cases,[15,127] and in one case series, all seven cats were eventually euthanized because of either recurrence of disease or appearance of the disease in the contralateral orbit.[15]

A viral etiology has been suggested for FOP, perhaps in part because of the suggestion that herpes simplex virus (HSV-1) is a proposed cause of human idiopathic orbital inflammation.[189] In the case series of seven cats, three exhibited signs suggestive of feline herpesvirus (FHV-1) infection, including upper respiratory disease before or after development of clinical signs of orbital disease, followed by development of gingival hyperplasia.[15] However, the authors were unable to establish FHV-1 infection in these cats. More recently, FOP has been suggested to be a neoplastic disease, with spindle cell sarcoma identified in the orbital tissue of one cat and the suggestion that FOP be renamed *feline restrictive orbital sarcoma*.[48]

EYELID AND ADNEXAL DISEASE

Eyelid Agenesis

Eyelid agenesis, or eyelid coloboma, is the most common congenital eyelid disease of cats.[133] It has been documented to occur in the Persian, Burmese, and domestic shorthair, as well as snow leopards and a Texas cougar.[11,40,100,124,205] Affected cats have bilateral, incomplete development of the upper lateral eyelids (Figures

*References 8, 44, 66, 73, 94, 161, 197, 206.

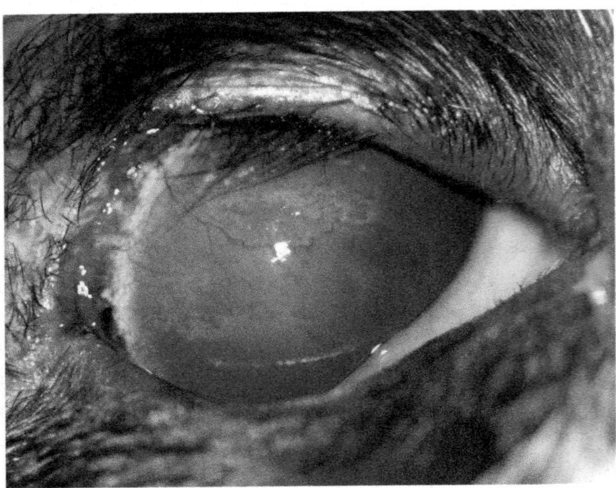

FIGURE 29-16 Right eye of a cat with agenesis of approximately 30% of the upper lateral eyelid margin. The result is trichiasis, incomplete eyelid closure (lagophthalmos), and exposure keratitis. *(Image courtesy WCVM Ophthalmology Service.)*

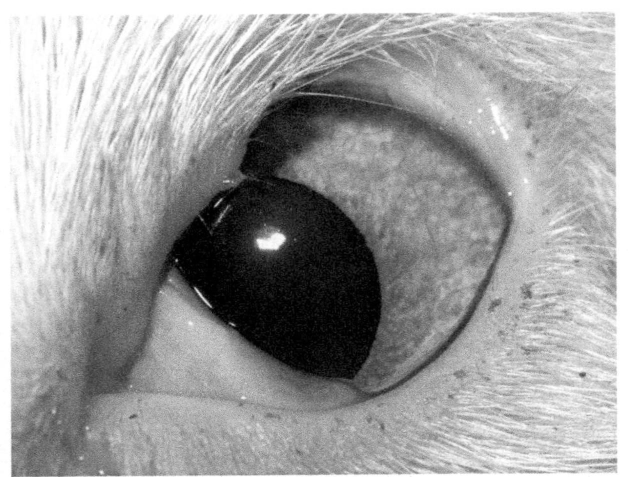

FIGURE 29-17 Agenesis of almost 50% of the left upper eyelid. Although the eyelid defect in this patient is larger than the defect in Figure 29-16, the degree of keratitis is less. *(Image courtesy UC Davis Veterinary Ophthalmology Service.)*

29-16 and 29-17). The extent of the defect ranges widely, from a barely perceptible absence of the eyelid margin at the lateral extent of the eyelid to complete absence of the upper eyelid margin. The cause is unknown; viral etiologies, intrauterine events, and genetic mutations are proposed mechanisms, although there is no clear evidence supporting any of these theories.[124]

Most owners do not notice abnormalities until kittens are a few months of age, probably because of the small eye size of young kittens. On occasion, eyelid agenesis has been mistaken for upper eyelid entropion; however, close inspection reveals absence of the eyelid margin rather than an inward roll. Varying degrees of chronic keratitis resulting from trichiasis and lagophthalmos almost always accompany the eyelid defect (see Figure

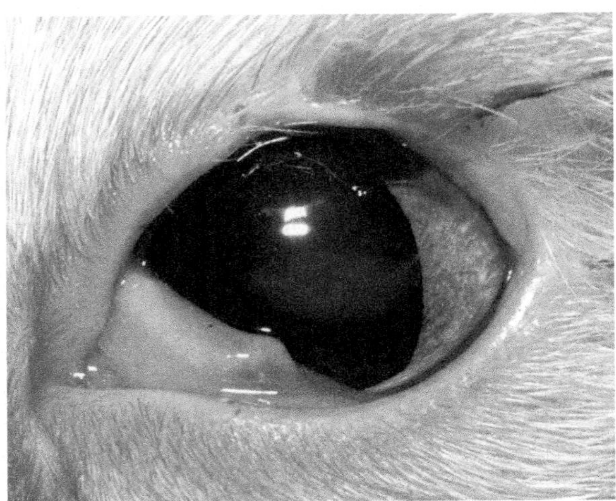

FIGURE 29-18 Patient in Figure 29-17 after completion of a rotating skin flap and subsequent cryoepilation of resulting trichiasis. Although the eyelids are not completely normal, there is improved coverage of the globe during normal blinking and the trichiasis is decreased from before surgery. *(Image courtesy UC Davis Veterinary Ophthalmology Service.)*

29-16). The conjunctival fornix at the site of the malformed eyelid also tends to be shallow or replaced by a thin band of conjunctiva directly connecting the globe to the eyelid. Other ocular abnormalities may accompany eyelid agenesis—most commonly, persistent pupillary membranes, which are remnants of dysplastic uveal tissue visible as thin sheets of pigmented tissue usually extending from the iris to the cornea. Colobomas of the iris, choroid, or optic nerve; retinal dysplasia; and keratoconjunctivitis sicca may also accompany eyelid agenesis.[71,124] Like the eyelid defect itself, the associated developmental abnormalities range in severity, sometimes even among kittens from the same litter.[124]

Treatment varies with the extent of the eyelid malformation. Very small defects may require cryoepilation or primary closure for resolution of trichiasis; however, most defects of clinical significance require more extensive blepharoplasty. Surgical reconstruction usually involves two separate surgeries, the first to correct the defect and the second to correct residual trichiasis. The most common procedure is rotation of a flap of skin from the lower eyelid with a functional outcome (Figure 29-18). Subsequent cryoepilation or a Holtz–Celsus procedure can be employed to address trichiasis from the skin flap.

Entropion

In the authors' experience, feline breed-related entropion differs greatly from the same condition in dogs. In cats the majority of breed-related entropion is mild and located at the medial aspect of the lower eyelid in brachycephalic cats (Figure 29-19). The clinical significance is often minimal but may be associated with

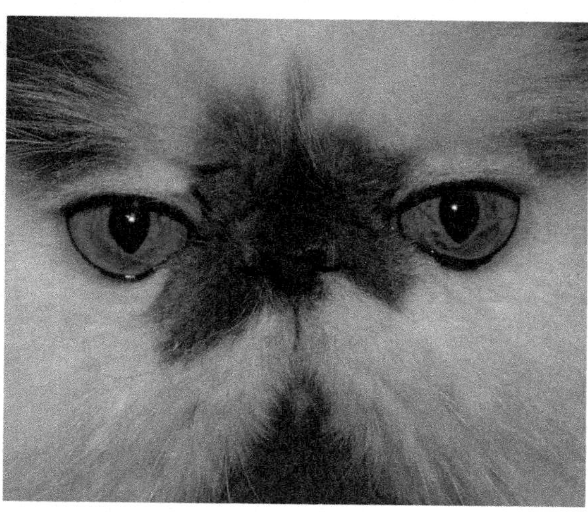

FIGURE 29-19 Ventromedial entropion is present in all brachycephalic cats and usually does not require treatment. Surgical correction is required when entropion causes excessive frictional irritation with corneal ulcer or sequestrum formation or epiphora with moist dermatitis and tear staining. *(Image courtesy Dr. Kathleen Doyle.)*

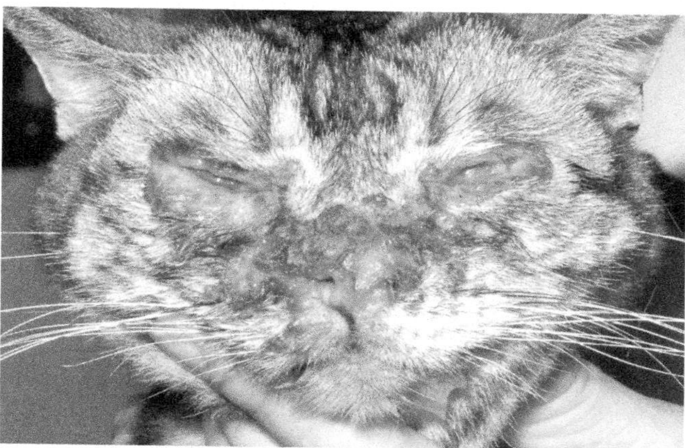

FIGURE 29-20 Herpetic dermatitis causing a chronic ulcerative dermatitis of the periocular skin, nasal planum, and muzzle. Histology revealed extensive eosinophilic infiltration and viral inclusion bodies and polymerase chain reaction confirmed presence of feline herpesvirus-1 DNA. This patient responded very well to famciclovir administration. *(Image courtesy UC Davis Veterinary Ophthalmology Service.)*

epiphora and tear staining caused by wicking of the tears by trichiasis, kinking of the nasolacrimal canaliculi, and frictional irritation of the cornea. However, these cats frequently have other abnormalities, such as exophthalmos, poor corneal sensitivity, unstable tear film, low blink rates, and lagophthalmos, that predispose them to chronic keratitis, including sequestrum formation. In these patients medial canthoplasty may be necessary to correct the entropion, lagophthalmos, and macropalpebral fissure. Breed-related entropion is believed to be more clinically significant in intact male Maine Coon cats, where it may be related to excessive skin around the face.[202]

Unlike breed-related entropion, acquired entropion in cats is often associated with clinically significant keratitis. Acquired entropion occurs in response to a primary pathologic process, typically as a result of blepharospasm or symblepharon formation caused by keratoconjunctivitis, or because of changes in globe position or size owing to enophthalmos or phthisis–microphthalmos, respectively. Enophthalmos may be seen in older cats or cachexic cats because of the loss of orbital fat. Surgical correction of feline entropion uses similar techniques as for the dog, which are published elsewhere. However, treatment (and preferably resolution) of any underlying cause before surgery is essential, and some authors have suggested that although the surgical technique is the same, cats require excision of a larger amount of tissue than do dogs.[202]

Herpetic Dermatitis

Periodically, FHV-1 has been identified as a cause of dermatologic lesions, particularly those surrounding the

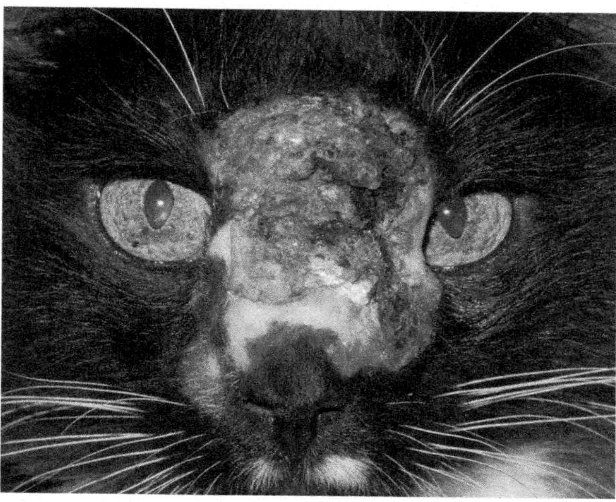

FIGURE 29-21 In contrast to Figure 29-20, in this cat the herpetic dermatitis manifests as dry, proliferative crusts over the nasal planum. *(Image courtesy UC Davis Veterinary Dermatology Service.)*

eyes and involving nasal skin of domestic and wild felidae* (Figures 29-20 and 29-21). This is not surprising given the marked epithelial tropism of this virus and the reliability with which HSV-1 causes dermal lesions.[115] Herpetic dermatitis typically presents with raised, thickened plaques and chronic, nonhealing cutaneous ulcers. Most commonly, the periocular skin, nasal planum, and the skin around the muzzle are affected; however, lesions may also occur on forelimbs and other sites in contact with oral and ocular secretions.[80,97] Oral ulcers and rhinitis may accompany dermal lesions.[80,132,184] Most published cases had concurrent immune compromise, in the form of recent glucocorticoid administration or systemic

*References 79, 80, 93, 97, 132, 184.

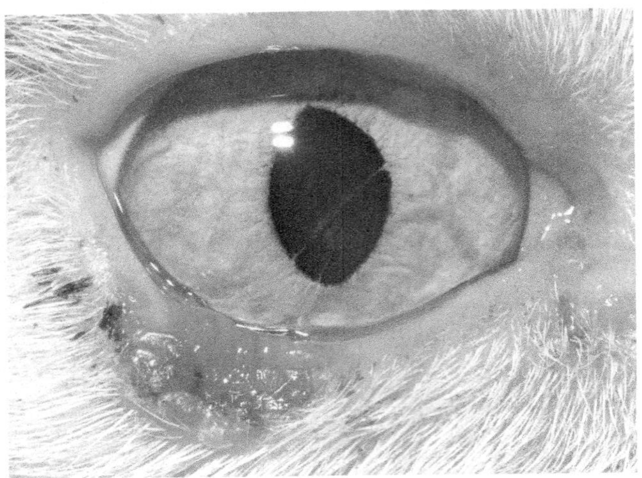

FIGURE 29-22 An alopecic, hyperemic ulcerative lesion is characteristic of eyelid squamous cell carcinoma in cats. Usually, the adjacent skin and conjunctiva are inflamed to some degree. Cats with lightly pigmented skin are more often affected. These tumors tend to be locally invasive and can require extensive blepharoplasty procedures. *(Image courtesy UC Davis Veterinary Ophthalmology Service.)*

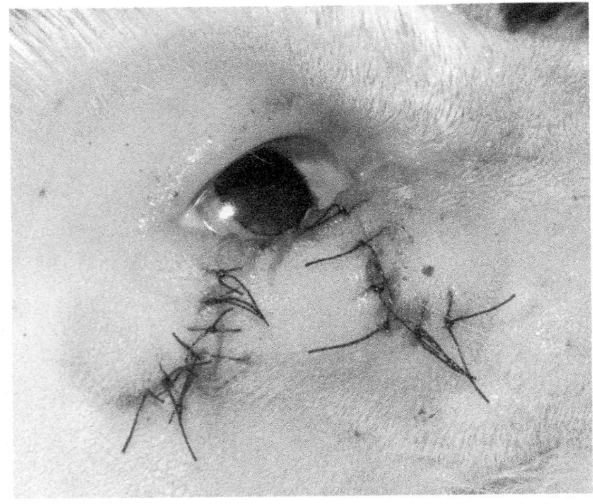

FIGURE 29-23 Immediate postoperative photograph of the cat in Figure 29-22. An advancement flap was performed to close the large defect created by excision of the eyelid tumor with adequate surgical margins. *(Image courtesy UC Davis Veterinary Ophthalmology Service.)*

disease.[80,184] Histologic changes are often diagnostic; however, because of the eosinophilic infiltration, misinterpretation of lesions as eosinophilic granuloma may occur.[80] Unlike herpetic corneal or conjunctival disease, which is not reliably diagnosed using the polymerase chain reaction (PCR), this assay seems diagnostically useful for herpetic dermatitis. When results of histologic examination were used as the gold standard in one study of cats with dermatitis, sensitivity and specificity of the PCR assay were 100% and 95%, respectively.[93] Although prospective controlled studies are lacking, this disease seems responsive to systemic administration of famciclovir (see the section on corneoconjunctival disease later in this chapter).

Eyelid Neoplasia

In contrast to dogs, most feline eyelid neoplasms are malignant, and many tumors are locally invasive.[125,138,204] SCC is the most common feline eyelid tumor, although a variety of neoplasms have been reported (Figure 29-22).* Eyelid neoplasia tends to occur in cats older than 10 years of age.[125,138] However, one study found SCC affected slightly older cats (12.4 years), whereas mast cell tumors were more common in younger cats (6.5 years).[138] This same study also underscored the systemic significance of eyelid tumors. Cats with eyelid or third eyelid lymphoma, adenocarcinoma, SCC, and peripheral nerve sheath tumors frequently experienced tumor recurrence or died as a result of tumor-related causes.[138] Conversely, the literature suggests that recurrence is unlikely after excision of hemangiosarcoma or mast cell tumor.[83,138,149]

*References 83, 92, 125, 138, 204, 206.

Regardless, presurgical diagnosis through incisional biopsy or aspirate, diagnostic assessment for systemic metastases, and tumor resection with wide surgical margins are recommended for all eyelid tumors of cats. Given the essential role that eyelids play in ocular, especially corneoconjunctival, health, extensive blepharoplasty procedures are often required to guarantee postoperative eyelid function when surgical margins result in loss of more than 25% of the eyelid length (Figure 29-23). In some cases sufficiently wide margins cannot be achieved without enucleation or exenteration of a normal globe, and even then these procedures are often accompanied by extensive axial pattern flaps to cover the defect created (Figure 29-24).

Apocrine hidrocystoma is an unusual and relatively uncommon neoplasm affecting feline eyelids and, as one of the few benign neoplasms affecting the eyelid of cats, warrants separate discussion. It represents a proliferative lesion of the apocrine glands within the eyelid. Although histologic confirmation is necessary for definitive diagnosis, the typical appearance of the lesion is a smooth-surfaced, hairless, often pigmented, slightly translucent eyelid mass (Figure 29-25). Apocrine hidrocystomas may occur singly, or there may be multiple lesions on the same eyelid.[69] Persian cats are predisposed.[25,69,208] Isolated masses may be removed with simple excision, although recurrence is common and cryosurgery is recommended as an adjunctive therapy.[25,28] There is one report of ablation using trichloroacetic acid (TCA).[208] In this case the hidrocystomas were eliminated without adverse effects, and no recurrence was noted 1 year after treatment.[208] This treatment should be used with caution because TCA has the ability to cause painful blisters and burns to normal skin.[208]

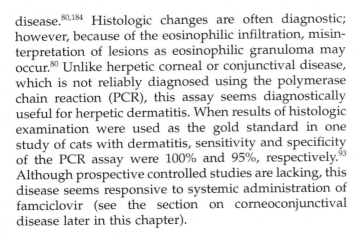

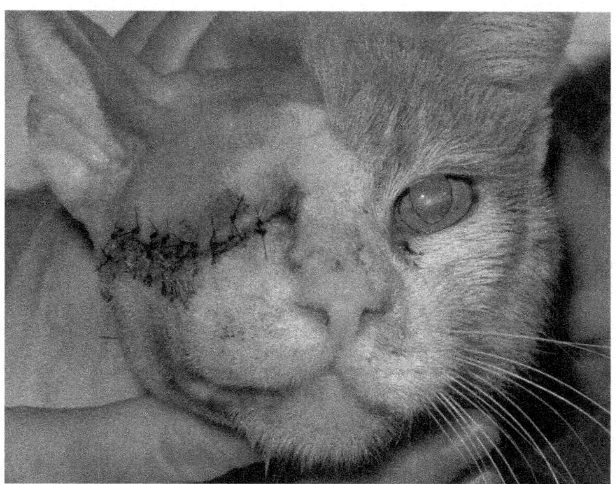

FIGURE 29-24 Immediate postoperative photograph after exenteration of the globe and orbital contents for removal of a large, infiltrative eyelid squamous cell carcinoma. Previous surgeries in this patient failed to completely remove the eyelid tumor, and exenteration was necessary to obtain adequate surgical margins. An advancement flap was required to close the surgical defect. *(Image courtesy UC Davis Veterinary Ophthalmology Service.)*

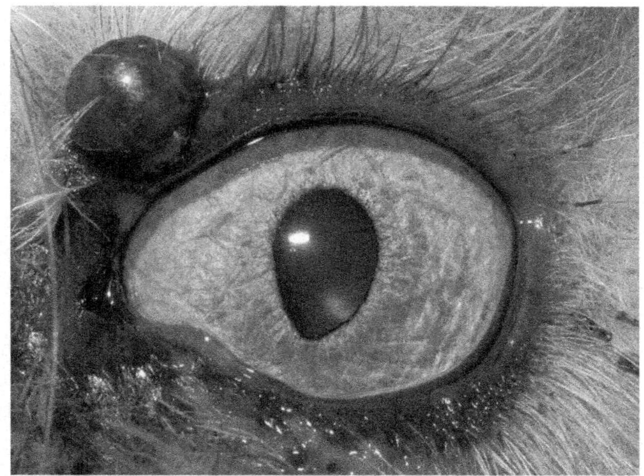

FIGURE 29-25 The typical appearance of an apocrine hidrocystoma is a smooth, hairless, darkly pigmented round mass on the eyelid of a cat. *(Image courtesy UC Davis Veterinary Ophthalmology Service.)*

Third Eyelid Disease

Disease affecting only the third eyelid in cats appears to be uncommon; however, the third eyelid is occasionally the site of primary neoplasia.[138,149] Prolapse of the gland of the third eyelid ("cherry eye") has been reported in the cat, and it has been suggested that the Burmese may be predisposed.[100] As in the dog, surgical replacement of the gland is required, with specific techniques being published elsewhere.[7] Elevation of the third eyelid, without gland prolapse, may be a sign of Horner's syndrome if accompanied by signs such as miosis and ptosis. Pharmacologic testing and other diagnostic

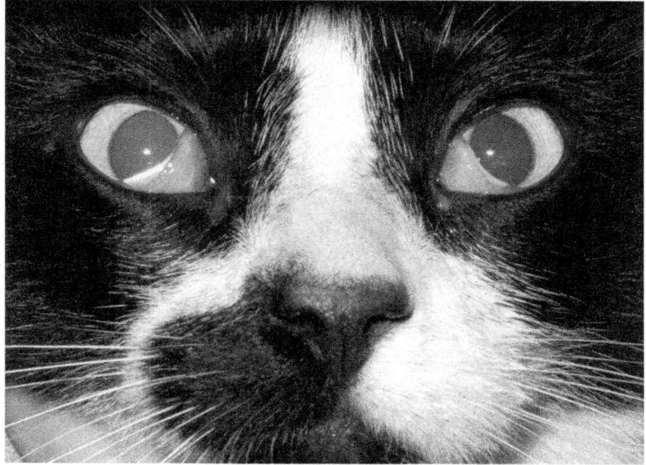

FIGURE 29-26 Haw's syndrome is characterized by bilateral elevation of the nictitans. This condition is idiopathic and self-limiting, usually within days. *(Image courtesy UC Davis Veterinary Ophthalmology Service.)*

investigations are similar to those used for dogs. Cats also occasionally have bilateral elevation of the third eyelids without other ocular abnormalities (Haw's syndrome) (Figure 29-26). Infectious etiologies have been proposed for this syndrome when it occurs in conjunction with diarrhea,[123,131] but the condition is thought to be self-limiting when no other abnormalities are found.

Nasolacrimal System Disease

Primary disease of the nasolacrimal duct occurs infrequently in the cat. However, its physical characteristics make it prone to involvement when adjacent structures are diseased. For example, the lack of osseous protection of the distal lacrimal sac leaves it susceptible to inflammation from adjacent respiratory mucosa.[139] In addition, a portion of the nasolacrimal duct lies in very close proximity to the root of the canine tooth, which is a common site of dental disease in cats.[122,139] Because of ventromedial entropion, the puncta are often in poor apposition with the globes of brachycephalic cats. This, combined with the fact that the nasolacrimal ducts of brachycephalic cats undergo sharper turns, increases the chances of impaired tear drainage and epiphora[21] (Figure 29-27).

CORNEAL AND CONJUNCTIVAL DISEASE

Surface ocular disease is common in cats and, in contrast to dogs, is almost always infectious in origin. The most commonly implicated agents are FHV-1—a primary conjunctival and, to a lesser extent, corneal pathogen—and *Chlamydophila felis* (previously *Chlamydia psittaci*)—a pathogen of the conjunctiva but not the cornea.

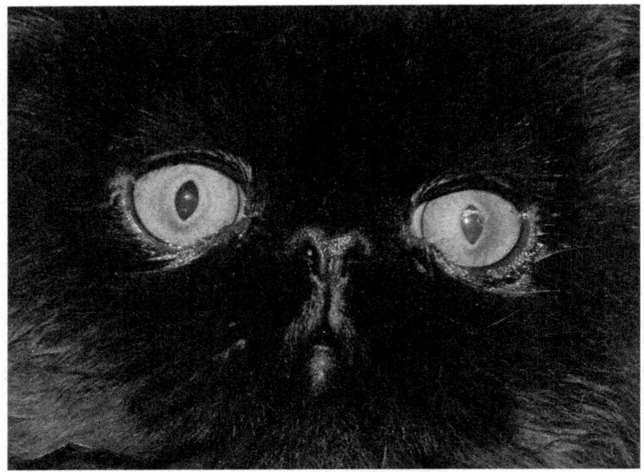

FIGURE 29-27 Brachycephalic cats often exhibit chronic epiphora as a result of ventromedial entropion and sharper turns in the course of the path of the nasolacrimal ducts. *(Image courtesy Dr. Kathleen Doyle.)*

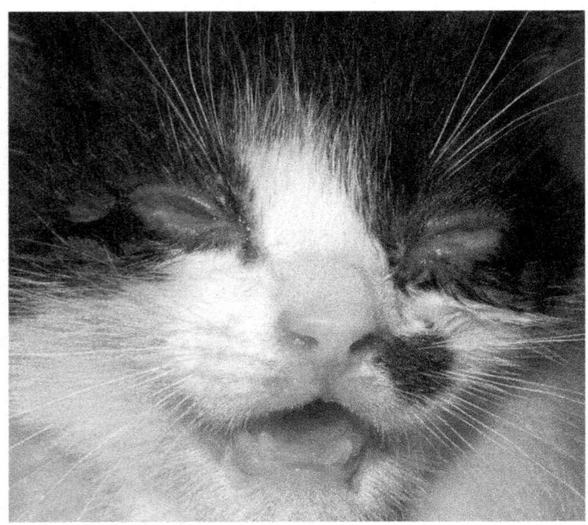

FIGURE 29-28 Primary infection with feline herpesvirus-1 is characterized by upper respiratory disease in addition to bilateral ocular disease. The mucopurulent and serosanguineous ocular and nasal discharge seen in this photo is typical. *(Image courtesy UC Davis Veterinary Ophthalmology Service.)*

Mycoplasma species and *Bordetella bronchiseptica* are also conjunctival, but not corneal, pathogens. Although feline calicivirus is often included in lists of differential considerations for feline conjunctivitis, patients infected with calicivirus are presented to veterinarians with severe upper respiratory disease and glossitis, although close examination can sometimes reveal mild conjunctivitis. This knowledge leads to a basic philosophical approach to feline surface ocular disease that can be helpful: Corneal disease should be presumed infectious and likely caused by FHV-1, and conjunctivitis should be assumed to be caused by *C. felis* or FHV-1 until proven otherwise. Because therapy for these two organisms differs so markedly, the obvious question is how to make a definitive etiologic diagnosis. Because both FHV-1 and *C. felis* can be detected in normal cats, diagnostic tests are unable to differentiate vaccine from wild-type organism, and false-positive and false-negative test results are common, laboratory testing is usually unhelpful. For these reasons the mainstay of diagnosis in cats with surface ocular disease is critical observation of clinical signs and judgment of response to therapy. This requires understanding of the biologic behavior of both organisms and the mode of action and expected effect of common antichlamydial and antiviral therapies. This will be the major focus of the subsequent sections.

Feline Herpesvirus

As a typical alphaherpesvirus, FHV-1 is highly host-specific; replicates rapidly in epithelial cells, where it causes cytolysis; establishes lifelong latency within ganglia; periodically reactivates from latency, especially during periods of stress; and during reactivation can either cause cell lysis again or activate immune-mediated pathology. Although the virus typically persists for life in the ganglia of latently infected cats, it is extremely labile in the environment and is susceptible to most disinfectants and to desiccation. For example, FHV-1 is relatively rapidly killed in fluorescein stain and proparacaine; however, it can survive in eyewash for 5 days.[181] Assuming that adequate hygiene is practiced in veterinary clinics, this short environmental survival time means that cats, rather than fomites, are the major source of viral persistence. Infection results from direct mucosal (oral, nasal, conjunctival) transfer of viral-laden macrodroplets, generated during sneezing but not normal respiratory movements. Up to 97% of cats are seropositive, and the virus is considered to be responsible for 45% of all upper respiratory infections.[58,118,182] All studies to date suggest little variation in pathogenicity between viral strains, found worldwide.[95,111-112,166]

After initial infection of a naïve cat, the incubation period is 2 to 10 days; however, this and disease severity are likely dose dependent. Viral shedding in ocular, oropharyngeal, and nasal secretions begins as early as 24 hours after inoculation and can persist for 1 to 3 weeks. Subsequent intermittent shedding is characteristic of the lifelong carrier state. The virus causes disease through a number of theorized mechanisms, each of which requires a different therapeutic approach. The initial period of rapid intraepithelial replication and associated cytolysis manifests clinically as erosion and ulceration of the ocular, oropharyngeal, and nasal mucosa, often with a serosanguineous discharge (Figure 29-28). The pathognomonic dendritic ulcerative pattern is sometimes seen in the cornea (Figure 29-29); however, their absence should not be used to rule out FHV-1 as a causative agent.

Primary disease is usually self-limiting within 10 to 20 days. Viremia occurs during this phase of infection,

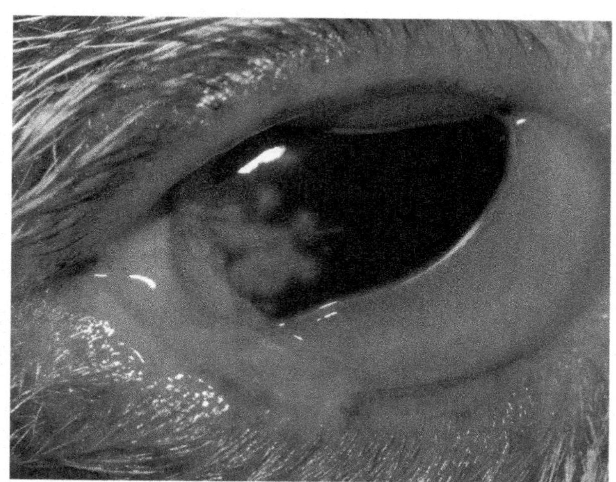

FIGURE 29-29 Dendritic corneal ulcers are considered pathognomonic for disease resulting from feline herpesvirus-1 infection. These can be very small and reinforce the need for examination with a cobalt blue light and a source of magnification after application of fluorescein dye. *(Image courtesy UC Davis Veterinary Ophthalmology Service.)*

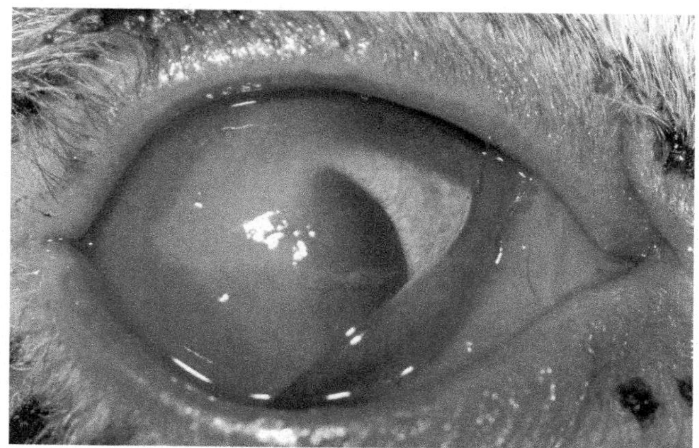

FIGURE 29-30 Stromal keratitis is characterized by vascularization, fibrosis, edema, and white blood cell infiltration of a nonulcerated cornea. It is believed to be due to persistence of feline herpesvirus-1 antigen within the corneal stroma. *(Image courtesy UC Davis Veterinary Ophthalmology Service.)*

but because systemic FHV-1-related syndromes are poorly defined, its significance is unknown. Also during this period, viral latency is established in the majority of cats, often as early as 4 days after infection, presumably by way of the ascent of the sensory axons of the trigeminal nerve. Latency is a period of viral quiescence during which there is no clinical evidence of disease, no histologically detectable inflammation within nerves or ganglia, no detectable virus using standard culture techniques, and limited viral transcriptional activity. In some animals intermittent episodes of viral reactivation from the latent state may be followed by centrifugal spread of virus along the sensory axons to peripheral epithelia. Viral recrudescence occurs when this results in clinically evident disease at peripheral epithelial sites. Recrudescent disease may be of the same ulcerative character as primary disease or may cause disease through recruitment of host immunologic mechanisms. It is often unilateral and typically not associated with generalized malaise or severe respiratory signs. The severity and extent of recrudescent disease range widely among individuals and even between episodes, making diagnosis more challenging. However, as a rule, conjunctivitis is milder and less ulcerative than seen in the primary infection, sometimes instead with substantial conjunctival thickening and hyperemia secondary to inflammatory cell infiltration. Corneal recrudescence may involve only the epithelial tissues, in which case dendritic and later geographic corneal ulceration may be seen; however, stromal keratitis is also common. This is characterized by vascularization, fibrosis, edema, and white blood cell infiltration of a nonulcerated cornea (Figure 29-30) and is believed to be due to FHV-1 antigen persistence within these tissues. Predicting which animals within a population are going to suffer recrudescent disease is currently not possible. The important concept is that although the majority of cats appear to become latently infected, only a minor percentage of them experience chronic or recurrent herpetic disease (Box 29-1). The pathogenesis of FHV-1 is summarized in Figure 29-31.

Chlamydophila felis

Although *C. felis* has some unique biological features, it shares a number of them with FHV-1: It is an obligate intracellular organism spread by macrodroplets and direct contact, it replicates within epithelial cells, it persists within the host but poorly in the environment, and it is highly host adapted. The recent reclassification of the feline chlamydial organism from *Chlamydia psittaci var. felis* to its own distinct species reflects this host specificity and low zoonotic potential.[108] Although there is little evidence of zoonotic transmission,[84] owners, especially the immunosuppressed, should be advised to practice adequate hygiene when handling cats with suspect chlamydial conjunctivitis. Like FHV-1, *C. felis* prefers to replicate in epithelial cells; however, it appears to do so in a more diverse range of tissues than does FHV-1, including rectal and vaginal epithelia, as well as lung, spleen, liver, peritoneum, and kidneys.[185] This knowledge helps explain why systemic therapy is now recommended for cats with chlamydial conjunctivitis, even if no extraocular signs are noted.

After an incubation period of approximately 3 to 5 days, cats develop conjunctivitis, mild fever, and sometimes submandibular lymphadenopathy. In contrast to FHV-1, respiratory signs are mild to absent, and the clinical disease course tends to be more insidious and persistent but not lifelong. The typical clinical

BOX 29-1

Important Virologic Considerations for Cats Infected with Feline Herpesvirus-1

1. Feline populations themselves, not the environment, act as the major reservoir of feline herpesvirus-1 (FHV-1).
2. FHV-1 infection (but not necessarily disease) is common in individual cats.
3. FHV-1 establishes lifelong latency within neural tissues in approximately 80% of infected individuals.
4. FHV-1 reactivates from latency commonly with or without obvious cause and with or without clinical evidence of reactivation.
5. FHV-1 reactivation is associated with recrudescent disease in only a small percentage of cats.
6. FHV-1 induces disease by way of (at least) two distinct mechanisms, with important therapeutic implications:
   - Cytolysis (cell-rupturing) due to viral replication. An antiviral agent may be needed; immunomodulation is contraindicated.
   - Immunopathology (immune-mediated injury); however, the antigen is not proven, and the immune-mediated disease may involve no or low-grade viral replication. Antiviral agents may not be effective as sole therapeutic agents. In these cases, antiinflammatory therapy may be indicated, usually in addition to antiviral agents.

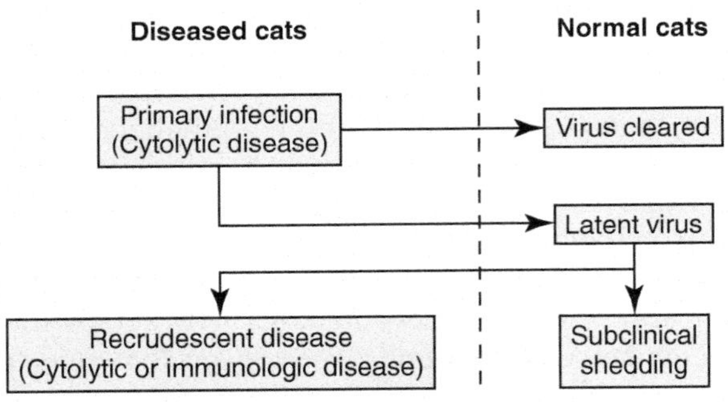

FIGURE 29-31 Summary of the pathogenesis of feline herpesvirus-1. Although most cats are exposed to the virus, become infected, and may even shed virus later in life, only a minority of these cats are expected to experience recrudescent disease. This figure also highlights why diagnostic tests can produce false-positive results.

presentation is periods of chronic mild conjunctivitis alternating with quiescent phases. Many cats shed chlamydial organisms for at least 60 days. Although the organisms may be spontaneously cleared, many cats require appropriate therapy for complete elimination. This helps explain why treatment of in-contact cats is often recommended for individual cats with chlamydial conjunctivitis. Co-infection with FHV-1 and *C. felis* appears to be very uncommon.[24,109,155,195,196]

TABLE 29-2 Comparison of the Biological Behavior of *Chlamydophila felis* and Feline Herpesvirus-1

	Feline herpesvirus-1	*Chlamydophila felis*
Organism	Obligate intracellular alphaherpesvirus	Obligate intracellular gram-negative bacterium
Strains	Few; biologically similar	Multiple; variable virulence
Environmental stability	12-18 hours	A few days
Preferred replication site	Conjunctival epithelium	Conjunctival epithelium
Infection	Macrodroplets	Macrodroplets
Carrier state	Lifelong latency within trigeminal ganglia	Persistent (6-9 months) ocular and nonocular infections
Reinfection	Unlikely	Common
Subclinical shedding	More likely	Less likely

Diagnosis

A major paradox exists with respect to the diagnosis of FHV-1.[118] Cats experiencing primary FHV-1 infection shed virus in sufficient quantities that viral detection is relatively easy. However, clinical signs during this phase of infection tend to be characteristic and self-limiting, making definitive diagnosis less necessary. By contrast, the diversity and ambiguity of clinical signs in more chronic FHV-1–associated syndromes makes viral identification more desirable, but the elusive nature of the virus in these syndromes makes this difficult. Indeed, the diagnosis of FHV-1 in individual cats represents one of the greatest challenges in the management of chronic FHV-1–related diseases. The situation is equally challenging for *C. felis*. Culture is the gold-standard method of diagnosis; however, this requires special transport media and conditions and rigorous culture techniques and is expensive. The increased sensitivity and ease of organism detection using PCR have made it a preferred technique; however, it appears that many chlamydial organisms may not be detected by standard PCR assay.[196] For these reasons clinical judgment using assessment of a number of helpful, but not pathognomonic, characteristics (Table 29-2) followed by response to appropriate therapeutic trials may be preferred.

Antiviral Treatment

Several antiviral drugs have been studied for their efficacy against FHV-1 and their safety in cats. However, it is critical to realize that because they were developed for use against human herpesviruses, they are not approved for use in cats, many are toxic to cats, some have

BOX 29-2

General Principles Regarding Antiviral Drugs

Virostatic
- Apply frequently
- Do not taper

Not antibacterial or antifungal
- Use an adjunctive antimicrobial when indicated

Generally more toxic than antibacterial drugs
- Use only when necessary

Monitor for systemic or topical toxicity

dramatically reduced efficacy against FHV-1, and the pharmacokinetics and metabolism are often notably different in cats compared with humans. Provided that these limitations are understood and antiviral drugs are chosen in an evidence-based manner, response to therapy is an excellent way to support or refute the clinical diagnosis of FHV-1. Naturally, this must be tempered by an appreciation that both chlamydial and herpetic disease can wax and wane without therapy. The more commonly used and available antiviral drugs will be individually discussed in subsequent sections; however, some general comments regarding antiherpetic drugs are possible (Box 29-2).

First and perhaps most important is the fact that all antiviral drugs are virostatic and therefore merely reduce viral replication, permitting host immune response to overcome the virus. An appreciation that inappropriate immune response is likely what allows viral reactivation and disease recrudescence helps moderate clinical expectations for antiviral drugs in FHV-1–infected cats. It also reinforces the critical importance of administering these drugs at an appropriately high frequency. Next, the fact that no antiviral drugs have antibacterial or antifungal properties necessitates that the clinician consider adjunctive antimicrobial therapy for primary or secondary nonviral organisms. This is most relevant when treating a herpetic corneal ulcer, when a topical antibiotic is also required. Finally, these drugs typically target enzymes or replicative mechanisms that are shared between viruses and their eukaryotic hosts, creating a much narrower margin of safety than for most antibacterial agents. This is most important when antiviral agents are administered systemically but may also be evident after topical use, especially if therapy is protracted. Signs of topical toxicity include conjunctivitis and punctate corneal erosions, which closely mimic the signs of viral infection; it is therefore particularly important that the clinician remain alert to this potential and discontinue or change topical antiviral agents if there is worsening of disease during therapy or after prolonged therapy. One reasonable approach is to discontinue topical antiviral therapy after 4 to 6 weeks of therapy, even if clinical signs have not resolved, and to wait 1 to 2 weeks before restarting or changing the topical antiviral. Corneal toxicity can also be avoided through use of systemic, rather than topical, antiviral medication.

In vitro efficacy data permit us to concentrate in vivo attention on the more efficacious agents and to ignore, for example, foscarnet. Clinical application requires at a minimum that consideration be given to cost, frequency of application, adverse effects, toxicity, pharmacokinetics, and route of therapy. This often means that some of the more potent drugs are not widely used clinically. Idoxuridine is a nonspecific inhibitor of DNA synthesis. Therefore host cells are affected, systemic therapy is not possible, and corneal toxicity can occur. It was commercially available in Canada and the United States as a 0.1% ophthalmic solution or 0.5% ointment but now must be compounded. It should be applied to the affected eye a minimum of 5 to 6 times daily. This drug is reasonably tolerated by most cats and seems efficacious in many. Vidarabine is believed to reduce viral DNA synthesis by interfering with DNA polymerase. Like idoxuridine, vidarabine is well tolerated when applied topically but because it is nonselective in its effect, it is associated with notable host toxicity if administered systemically. Vidarabine may be effective in patients whose disease seems resistant to idoxuridine because it affects a viral replication step different from that targeted by idoxuridine. Vidarabine is also commercially unavailable in Canada and the United States but can be compounded as a 3% ophthalmic ointment, which should be applied at least 5 to 6 times daily. Trifluridine is a nucleoside analog of thymidine that is too toxic to be administered systemically and often produces unacceptable signs of toxicity (keratoconjunctivitis and apparent stinging on application), even when applied topically. This is unfortunate because it is the most potent drug against FHV-1 in vitro and it has excellent corneal epithelial penetration. It is commercially available in both Canada and the United States as a 1% ophthalmic solution that should be applied to the affected eye at least 5 to 6 times daily.

Acyclovir has relatively low potency, poor bioavailability, and potential bone marrow toxicity when systemically administered to cats.[142] In the authors' opinion, the availability of safer and more effective drugs makes systemic administration of acyclovir difficult to justify. However, in countries where acyclovir is available as an ophthalmic ointment and can be applied very frequently, this may be effective and should circumvent systemic toxicity.[203] In vitro data suggest that interferon exerts a synergistic effect with acyclovir that could permit an approximately eightfold reduction in acyclovir dose,[198] but in vivo validation of these data is needed. Valacyclovir is a prodrug of acyclovir that is more efficiently absorbed from the feline gastrointestinal tract and is converted to acyclovir within the liver. Unfortunately, valacyclovir administration is associated with plasma acyclovir concentrations that are elevated to a point of causing fatal myelosuppression and renal and hepatic necrosis,[135] and valacyclovir should never be used in cats. Penciclovir has a similar mechanism of action as acyclovir but with much more potent antiviral activity against FHV-1. Like acyclovir, its relatively poor bioavailability can probably be overcome by oral administration of the prodrug famciclovir. Pharmacokinetic, safety, and efficacy studies in cats reveal that famciclovir is remarkably effective and apparently safe in cats when administered at 90 mg/kg orally, thrice daily.[121,187,188] Although clinical efficacy at lower doses has been reported,[121] because of the nonlinear pharmacokinetics of famciclovir in the cat, further research is needed to establish the appropriate dose.

Cidofovir is a relatively new antiviral with good efficacy against FHV-1. When compounded with methylcarboxycellulose into a 0.5% ophthalmic solution and administered twice daily to experimentally infected cats, cidofovir was associated with reduced viral shedding and clinical disease.[62] Although twice-daily dosing offers a clear advantage over all other topical antiherpetic drugs, cidofovir is not yet commercially available in Canada or the United States, and there are reports of its topical use in humans being associated with stenosis or cicatrization of the nasolacrimal drainage system components. As cidofovir becomes used more widely in cats, this potential side-effect should be monitored.

Lysine is an adjunctive therapy for FHV-1, but there are contradictory research data regarding its efficacy. In vitro data suggest that lysine exerts its antiviral effect by antagonism of arginine.[116] In vivo studies demonstrated that administration of 500 mg lysine orally, twice daily, was associated with less severe conjunctivitis during primary infection[179] and that 400 mg lysine orally, once daily, reduced viral shedding during latent infections.[119] However, other clinical studies failed to show a positive effect or even demonstrated worsening of disease and increased viral shedding[47,120,158] in two studies in which lysine was administered as a dietary supplement rather than in bolus form.[47,120] For that reason cat owners should be advised to administer lysine as a twice-daily 500-mg bolus rather than by sprinkling it on food. Because lysine appears to be most effective when initiated before clinical disease, it may be most useful when administered indefinitely to cats experiencing repeated recrudescent disease,[179] rather than being administered only during periods of active disease.

The interferons are a group of cytokines that have diverse immunologic and antiviral functions largely through limiting cell-to-cell viral spread. Although interferons may play important physiologic roles in the control of viral infections, data regarding potential therapeutic applications are conflicting. In vitro, interferon significantly reduced FHV-1 titer or cytopathic effect (or both) without detectable cytotoxic changes in the host cell lines[162,170] and was associated with a nearly eightfold reduction in the required dose of acyclovir, especially when introduced to the viral culture before infection.[198] However, there are relatively few peer-reviewed, placebo-controlled, prospective clinical trials of interferon administration in cats. Those that exist show minimal or no beneficial effects.[76] Further research is necessary to determine dosage, timing, and efficacy (if any) of this group of compounds, especially in the more chronic or recrudescent infections.

Antichlamydial Treatment

Traditionally, feline chlamydial conjunctivitis has been treated with topical tetracycline ointment. However, because cats harbor and shed *C. felis* from nonocular sites and apparently normal cats can shed organisms, systemic drugs should also be used and consideration should be given to treating all cats in contact with the affected cat.[141,172,185] The preferred systemic drug is doxycycline at 5 to 10 mg/kg orally once to twice daily for at least 3 to 4 weeks. Azithromycin has good efficacy against chlamydial (and mycoplasmal) organisms and shows reasonably rapid absorption, adequate bioavailability, and useful concentrations in ocular tissues for at least 3 days after a single oral dose of 5 mg/kg. However, doxycycline has superior capacity to reduce organism shedding. A topical tetracycline or erythromycin ointment should be considered in addition to systemic doxycycline if conjunctivitis is severe so as to guarantee high drug concentrations at the ocular surface and provide some surface ocular lubrication.

Contraindicated Therapies

Because triple antibiotic is ineffective against *C. felis* and FHV-1, it should not be used to treat primary conjunctivitis in cats. It is useful for prevention of infection of a superficial corneal ulcer. Topically or systemically administered corticosteroids may sometimes produce symptomatic improvement in infectious corneoconjunctival disease but do not reduce, and may actually increase, organism load. This is presumably why they are often associated with rebound worsening of disease once they are discontinued. Ironically, this can falsely lead the clinician to reinstitute the steroid therapy, further exacerbating the underlying disease. Topically administered corticosteroids induce deeper and more persistent corneal disease and protracted viral shedding.[137] Systemic administration of corticosteroids is contraindicated and is a well-established, reliable means of inducing viral reactivation.[91] Although steroids may be used in select cases that are suspected to be due to immunopathologic mechanisms, the potential for dramatic clinical decompensation warrants extreme caution, close monitoring, and concurrent use of antiviral medication. The potential complications from using corticosteroids have prompted interest in the use of nonsteroidal antiinflammatory drugs (NSAIDs) for managing the inflammatory effects of ocular FHV-1 infection. Although there are no studies of their effects in cats infected with FHV-1, they have similar negative effects to corticosteroids in humans infected with HSV-1. Use of cyclosporine in chronic feline herpetic disease has been inadequately studied. Cyclosporine is capable of suppressing inflammatory events operative in viral stromal and eosinophilic keratitis but also impairs viral clearance from the eye and suppresses some beneficial immune responses. The authors are unaware of any studies examining the effects of tacrolimus on ocular herpetic infections in any species. This suggests that use of these agents should, as a minimum, be restricted by the same principles that govern the use of corticosteroids in humans with HSV-1.

Conjunctivitis

Conjunctivitis is an extremely common finding in the cat. However, when reaching this clinical diagnosis, clinicians must always first determine if the cat is affected by conjunctivitis only and then must determine the cause of the conjunctivitis. The first consideration is crucial because many diseases, including blepharitis, keratitis, uveitis, glaucoma, orbital disease, and scleritis all produce conjunctival hyperemia (Figure 29-32). However, these diverse diseases often have completely different causes, require completely different diagnostic investigations, have different ramifications for vision or even patient survival, and necessitate completely different treatments. This emphasizes why a complete ophthalmic examination should always be performed, even if the clinical presentation looks like simple conjunctivitis. If ocular examination fails to reveal further pathology, then it is justifiable to diagnose conjunctivitis and begin searching for the cause. Fortunately, in contrast to dogs, there are few likely causes of feline conjunctivitis. As discussed previously, FHV-1 and *C. felis* are the top two etiologic diagnoses with *Mycoplasma* spp., *Bordetella,* and possibly *Bartonella* lower on the list. Once clinical judgment has identified the most likely cause (see Table 29-2), specific and evidence-based treatment should be initiated because response to therapy is the next "diagnostic test." These therapies are described earlier in this chapter and should include systemic doxycycline with or without topical tetracycline or erythromycin ointment if *C. felis* is suspected, or a topical or systemic antiviral with or without lysine if FHV-1 is suspected. Antichlamydial treatment is required for 3 to 4 weeks, whereas antiviral drugs should be continued for approximately 1 week after clinical resolution is noted.

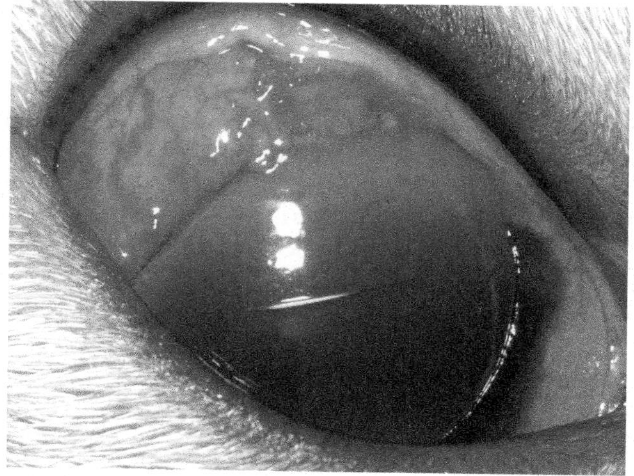

FIGURE 29-32 Conjunctival and episcleral vascular congestion and mild corneal edema in a cat with uveitis. Although the conjunctival hyperemia suggests "simple" conjunctivitis, the larger episcleral vascular engorgement along with the corneal edema make this diagnosis untenable and instead make glaucoma or uveitis most likely. This underscores the importance of always performing a complete ophthalmic examination, including assessment of aqueous flare and intraocular pressure. *(Image courtesy UC Davis Veterinary Ophthalmology Service.)*

Mucinomimetic therapy is a safe and important component of the treatment of conjunctivitis. Chronic conjunctivitis is associated with conjunctival goblet cell atrophy and an associated mucin-deficient qualitative tear film abnormality characterized by premature evaporation of the tear film and corneal drying. This, in turn, worsens conjunctivitis, leading to a perpetually exacerbating cycle unless remedied with topical mucin replacement.[38] Although this is likely true for many causes of conjunctivitis, FHV-1 has specifically been proved to induce a drastic decline of conjunctival goblet cell density to normalize for at least 1 month after FHV-1 infection.[106] Mucinomimetic tear replacement agents break this cycle by increasing stability of the precorneal tear film. Numerous formulations exist; however, sodium hyaluronate demonstrates superior corneal retention time compared with other tear substitutes.[171] Unlike most medications, artificial tear substitutes have the added advantage of being available in single-dose packaging, bypassing corneal cytotoxicity that is a feature of preservatives in ophthalmic medications[23,30] (Figure 29-33).

Symblepharon

Symblepharon is a term that describes adhesions between conjunctiva and adjacent conjunctiva or cornea, and is expected after marked or chronic ulceration and exposure of subepithelial connective tissue. Its clinical appearance is characteristic, but significance varies greatly depending on the extent and location of adhesions (Figure 29-34). Corneal involvement is associated with reduced vision, and conjunctival adhesions may obstruct lacrimal drainage, prohibit normal globe or

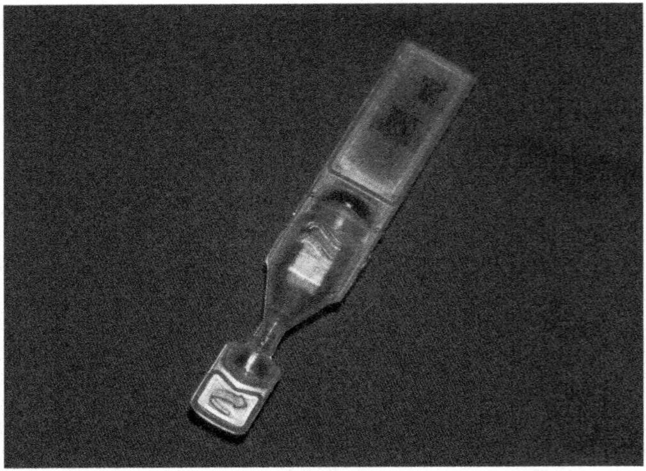

FIGURE 29-33 Artificial tear formulations are often available in single-dose containers. Single-dose medications are advantageous because they are free of preservatives, which are toxic to the corneal epithelium. This is especially important when medications are administered 4 or more times daily, multiple medications are being administered, or there is known hypersensitivity.

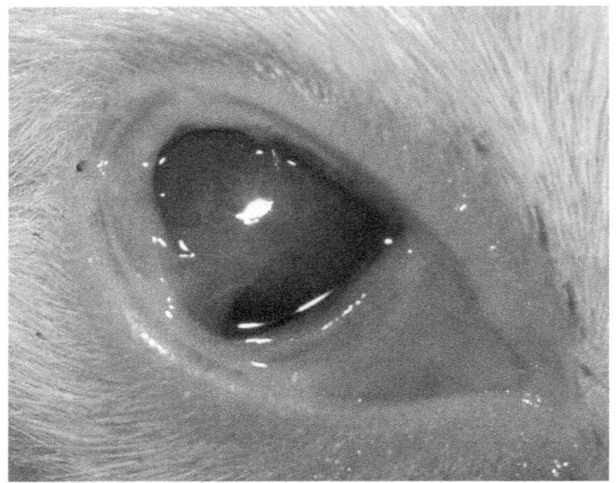

FIGURE 29-34 Symblepharon between the conjunctiva and the cornea following primary infection with feline herpesvirus-1. Because of the central location of the adhesions in this cat, reduced vision is probable. *(Image courtesy UC Davis Veterinary Ophthalmology Service.)*

eyelid movements and position, or cause nictitans protrusion (Figure 29-35). Feline herpesvirus is most frequently blamed, presumably because it is so common in cats. Because medications cannot break down adhesions, surgical resection is the only possible therapy. However, recurrence is common because surgery involves a combination of conjunctivectomy and superficial lamellar keratectomy, which re-expose subepithelial connective tissue. Minor adhesions are therefore best left untreated. When surgical management is elected, preoperative and postoperative control of active herpetic recrudescence is essential. In addition, various mechanical devices to separate the exposed surfaces during healing, often accompanied by a staged approach, have been used. Referral for these procedures is recommended.

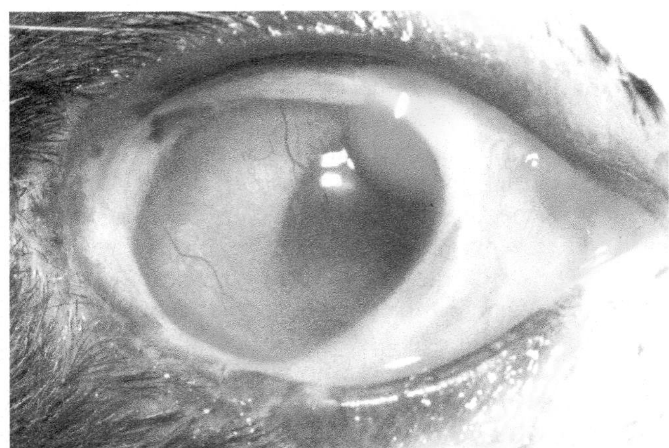

FIGURE 29-35 Symblepharon involving the bulbar and palpebral conjunctiva, nictitans, and cornea. The adhesions in this cat prevent normal movement of the third eyelid. Epiphora is caused by adhesions over the nasolacrimal puncta. *(Image courtesy UC Davis Veterinary Ophthalmology Service.)*

Corneal Ulceration

As in dogs, there are three main principles for treating corneal ulceration in cats:

1. Find and treat the primary cause.
2. Prevent secondary infection.
3. Provide specific supportive care if stromal involvement or chronicity are present.

The major difference between feline and canine ulcers is that infectious causes of ulcers are rare in dogs, whereas feline ulcers are considered to be due to FHV-1 until proved otherwise. If thorough clinical examination fails to reveal evidence of a foreign body, ectropion, entropion, distichia, ectopic cilia, trichiasis, lagophthalmos, blepharitis with an abrasive eyelid margin (all of which are very uncommon in cats), or periocular or intraocular trauma, then the ulcer should be assumed to be herpetic in origin. Herpetic ulcers have either a pathognomonic dendritic pattern or a highly suggestive appearance—superficial, epithelial loss, sometimes with a nonadherent lip. Herpetic ulcers do not involve stromal loss unless there is secondary bacterial infection. If FHV-1 is believed to be the originating cause, then a decision must be made regarding antiviral therapy. If the ulcer is acute, unilateral, and in an otherwise healthy cat without previous recrudescent herpetic disease, then allowing the patient's own immunity the chance to overcome the herpetic reactivation is justifiable. Otherwise, the clinician must initiate topical or systemic antiviral medication. Antiviral therapy should be continued until ulcer resolution and should not be tapered.

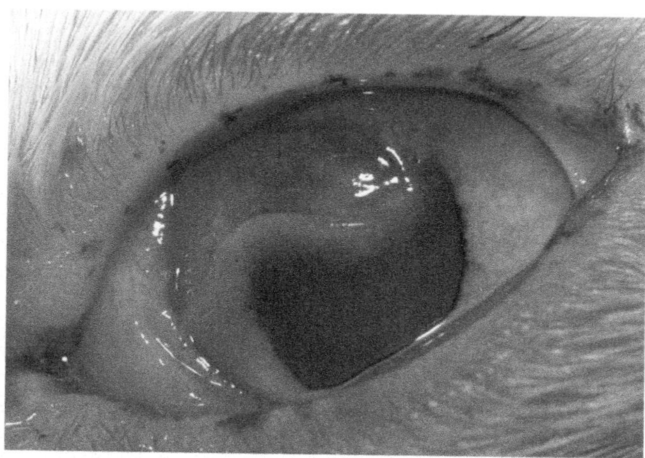

FIGURE 29-36 Deep corneal ulcer secondary to feline herpesvirus-1. Note the loss of corneal stroma; the thickened, hyperemic conjunctiva; mild corneal edema; and deep corneal vessels. *(Image courtesy UC Davis Veterinary Ophthalmology Service.)*

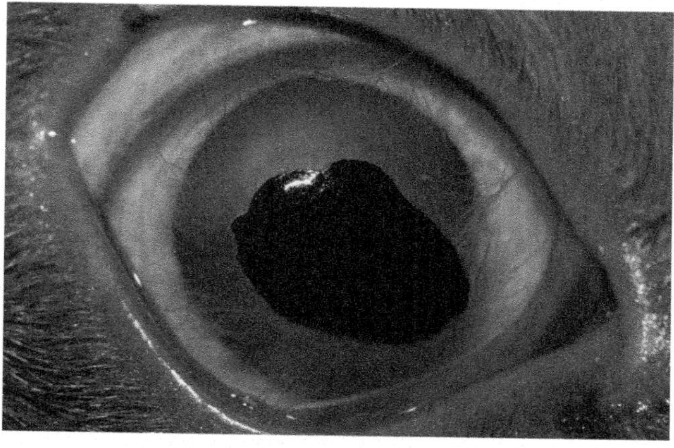

FIGURE 29-37 Corneal sequestrum with chronic, superficial keratitis. Superficial corneal vessels span the entire visible cornea, and a lip of granulation tissue is seen at the ventral edge of the sequestrum. *(Image courtesy UC Davis Veterinary Ophthalmology Service.)*

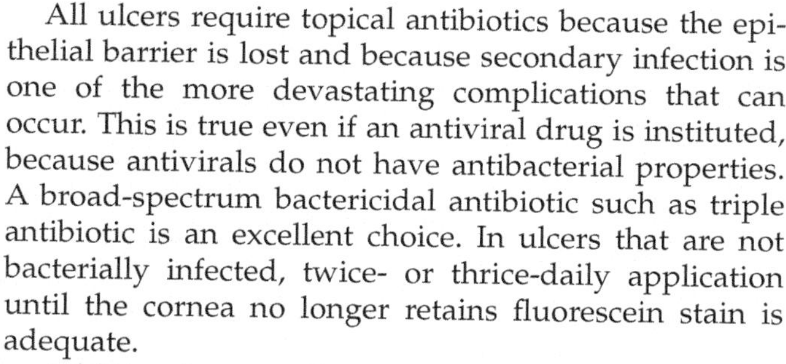

All ulcers require topical antibiotics because the epithelial barrier is lost and because secondary infection is one of the more devastating complications that can occur. This is true even if an antiviral drug is instituted, because antivirals do not have antibacterial properties. A broad-spectrum bactericidal antibiotic such as triple antibiotic is an excellent choice. In ulcers that are not bacterially infected, twice- or thrice-daily application until the cornea no longer retains fluorescein stain is adequate.

Additional supportive treatment is required for any ulcer with stromal involvement (stromal loss, malacia, or white blood cell infiltration) (Figure 29-36). These changes typically indicate secondary bacterial infection, and as in other species, cytology and culture and sensitivity are recommended. Unlike in dogs, *Mycoplasma* spp. can cause rapidly progressive stromal ulcers in cats; this should be considered when requesting culture at the laboratory. A broad-spectrum bactericidal ophthalmic antibiotic solution such as fluoroquinolone should be administered as often as 6 times daily until culture results are available. If *Mycoplasma* is suspected, then tetracycline ointment should be considered. In all deep ulcers, adjunctive therapy with serum should be considered to provide anticollagenases, which reduce stromal melting, and growth factors, which speed healing. Typically, serum is administered at the same frequency as the topical antibiotic. If there is danger of rupture or healing is delayed, referral for placement of a conjunctival graft is recommended. Third eyelid flaps are not recommended because they prohibit the two things the ulcer needs most: medication and observation.

Ulcers are also classified as complicated when they persist beyond 7 days, even if they remain superficial. A particular type of chronic nonhealing superficial ulcer occurs in cats and shares some features with the indolent ulcer of dogs; it involves epithelium only (no stromal loss) and has a lip of nonadherent epithelium that is easily débrided with a cotton-tipped applicator. However, indolent ulcers of dogs are caused by an anatomical defect preventing adhesion between the corneal epithelium and stroma and are treated by grid keratotomy. No such syndrome has been proved to occur in cats. In fact, if nonhealing ulcers in cats are treated by grid keratotomy, they are particularly likely to form corneal sequestra (discussed later in this chapter). These chronic, superficial ulcers, which débride easily in cats, may be due to FHV-1. One treatment protocol involves use of a topical antiviral and antibacterial agent following corneal débridement. If this is unsuccessful, referral is wise.

Corneal Sequestration

Corneal sequestration is an entity unique to the cat. It is an area of ulcerated, necrotic cornea characterized clinically by gradual progression of a dark (amber, brown, or black) discoloration usually involving the central cornea (Figure 29-37). Prior, and usually chronic, corneal ulceration is common but not always reported. Blood vessels often extend to the lesion and are deep or superficial, depending on depth of the sequestrum. The necrotic corneal stroma may be surrounded by zones of variably intense corneal stromal edema, inflammatory cell infiltration, or both. Sequestra are usually unilateral but may occur bilaterally. Frequently, the eye appears to be causing the cat pain, but some cats display only minor signs of discomfort. Histologically, the plaque consists of a sequestered, desiccated region of necrotic corneal stroma surrounded by a variable "foreign body–type" inflammatory cell response with extensive granulation tissue development. The characteristic

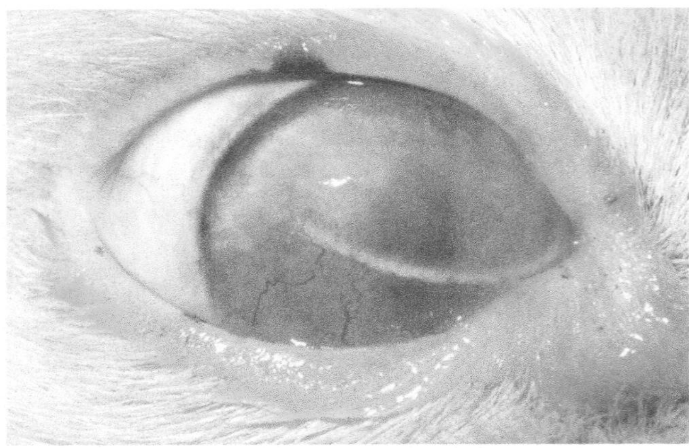

FIGURE 29-38 Postoperative photo after excision of a corneal sequestrum. In this case excision of the sequestrum resulted in a deep corneal defect that required grafting. A corneoconjunctival transposition was performed to maintain a relatively clear visual axis in the central cornea. *(Image courtesy UC Davis Veterinary Ophthalmology Service.)*

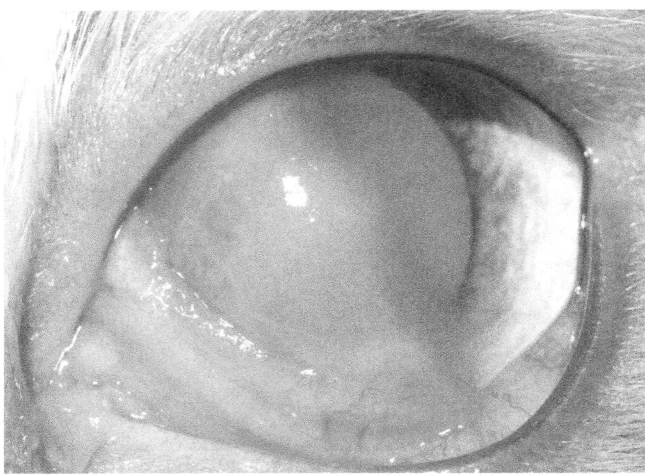

FIGURE 29-39 The characteristic appearance of feline eosinophilic keratitis includes thickened and hyperemic conjunctiva, corneal vascularization, and white corneal plaques. Cytologic assessment of the corneal plaques revealed eosinophils and mast cells. *(Image courtesy UC Davis Veterinary Ophthalmology Service.)*

clinical appearance is considered diagnostic; however, differential diagnoses should include corneal foreign body; dermoid, anterior synechia–staphyloma; or limbal melanoma. Feline herpesvirus may be involved in approximately 50% of cases.[136] Other causes of chronic corneal irritation such as entropion, distichiasis, tear film deficiencies, and lagophthalmos appear also to predispose to sequestrum formation. This may explain the predilection for Persian, Himalayan, and Siamese cats to develop corneal sequestra. Identification and correction of any underlying causes are important whenever possible. Lamellar keratectomy with a sliding corneal or conjunctival graft is the treatment of choice, especially if the cat appears to be in pain or the lesion is deep or chronic (Figure 29-38). Unfortunately, approximately 33% of cases experience recurrence. Medical management is generally not recommended because of the potential for corneal perforation and the degree of discomfort usually present. However, if the cat appears comfortable, it may be attempted because sequestra can spontaneously slough over a period of weeks to months. Medical management includes prophylactic topical antibiotics, as for corneal ulceration and treatment of reflex uveitis, if evident. Many recommend using antiviral medications and mucinomimetic tear-replacement formulations because altered tear film quality or evaporation or both have been blamed for these lesions. Surgical procedures to reduce corneal exposure and irritation such as temporary or permanent partial tarsorrhaphy and correction of entropion should be considered to reduce recurrences.

Eosinophilic Keratoconjunctivitis

Feline eosinophilic keratitis (FEK) is an enigmatic disease of cats. Clinically, FEK appears as a focal, raised, yellow to pink corneal plaque resembling granulation tissue (Figure 29-39). Typically, only the lateral cornea is affected initially, but in advanced cases the entire cornea may be involved. Adjacent areas of corneal ulceration are often present. Eyelid or conjunctival involvement (including third eyelids) is seen relatively commonly with keratitis but occasionally occurs alone. Cytologic evaluation of scrapings from affected cornea or conjunctiva reveals neutrophils, eosinophils, and mast cells, along with hyperplastic or dysplastic epithelial cells. Histology may reveal lymphocytes and plasma cells. Diagnosis is suggested by clinical appearance and confirmed using cytology. The cause is undetermined; however, the condition appears to be due to an aberrant immune response. In many cases the antigenic stimulus is unrecognized; however, FHV-1 DNA can be detected in corneal samples from approximately 75% of cats with FEK.[136] Given the inability to identify the inciting antigen, this disease has traditionally been treated with topical corticosteroids. Potential involvement of FHV-1 presents clinicians with a dilemma, because use of immunomodulatory drugs, especially topical corticosteroids, for treatment of an eye that is potentially infected with FHV-1 warrants caution. Given the likely involvement of FHV-1, it is prudent to simultaneously administer an antiviral agent and recheck frequently. If there is improvement and the owners are compliant, continuation of this regimen may be all that is necessary. The use of 1.5% cyclosporine has recently been described, with promising results.[173] Antiviral treatment should be continued for as long as there is evidence of active viral replication and certainly while ulceration is present, and corticosteroids are tapered judiciously as clinical signs improve. Early diagnosis and treatment of recurrences will limit the need for protracted therapy.

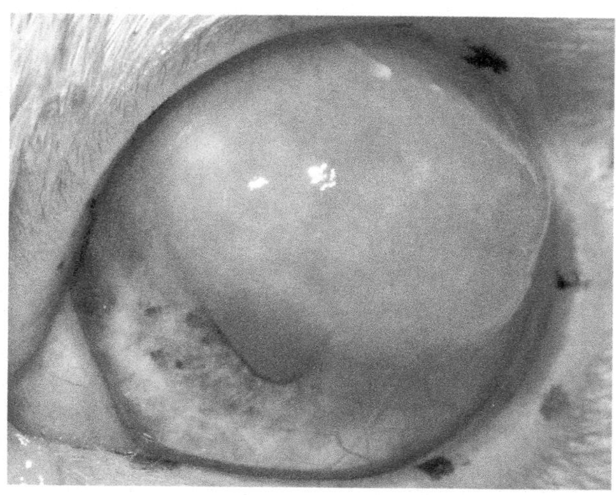

FIGURE 29-40 Acute bullous keratopathy is characterized by rapid onset of massive corneal edema, with bulla formation and keratoconus. Superficial corneal vessels are also visible in this cat, suggesting a previous keratitis. This is not a necessary feature. Urgent surgical intervention is required to stabilize the cornea. *(Image courtesy UC Davis Veterinary Ophthalmology Service.)*

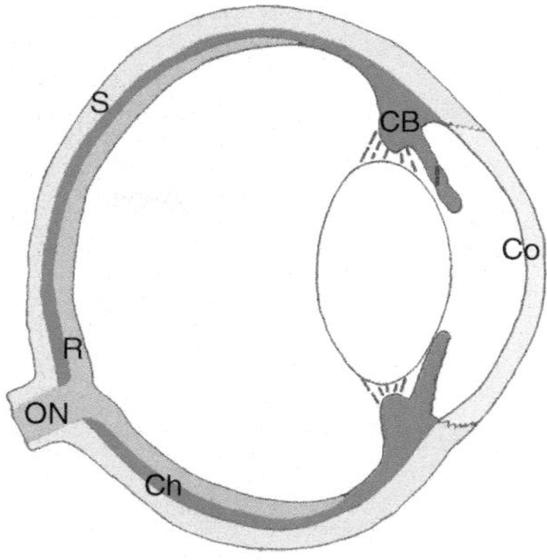

FIGURE 29-41 Basic anatomy of the globe. The anterior uvea is composed of the iris and ciliary body, and the posterior uvea is composed of the choroid. *Co*, Cornea; *I*, iris; *CB*, ciliary body; *R*, retina; *Ch*, choroid; *S*, sclera; *ON*, optic nerve. *(From Maggs D:* Slatter's fundamentals of veterinary ophthalmology, *ed 4, St Louis, 2007, Saunders.)*

Acute Bullous Keratopathy

Although acute bullous keratopathy (ABK) is a rare condition, feline clinicians should be aware of it because it is seen only in cats, has a characteristic clinical appearance, and requires emergency management to avoid globe rupture.

As its name suggests, ABK involves the cornea only and is extremely rapid in onset, occurring within minutes to hours. Profound edema and bullae formation within the corneal stroma are the predominant features[72] (Figure 29-40). There is usually marked epiphora and blepharospasm, as well as some conjunctival hyperemia and chemosis, as is expected with all cases of keratitis. With this clinical appearance, the major differential considerations are a peracute progressive stromal ulcer or a corneal laceration; however, the bullous nature of the corneal distention and the typical lack of stromal inflammatory cells are characteristic of ABK. The condition can present in one or both eyes. Cats of any age may be affected, but the few cases reported in the literature suggest that the syndrome is more common in younger cats. To date, no predisposing cause or history is recognized, although an association with systemic antiinflammatory and immunosuppressive medication has been suggested.[147a] Unlike other causes of corneal edema, which result from defects in the corneal epithelium or endothelium, the defect in ABK is proposed to involve the corneal stroma itself. Bacterial, viral, protozoal, and fungal organisms have not been detected when tested for by cytology, culture, or serology.

Some cases have been reported to improve without treatment; however, most require referral for emergency conjunctival grafting and sometimes thermokeratoplasty. In the latter technique, the cornea is treated with multiple, very carefully applied, highly focal applications of heat. A scar forms in the treated area, and associated tissue contraction expels fluid from the corneal stroma, limiting further corneal distention. Application of a bandage in the form of a temporary tarsorrhaphy has also been reported to reduce edema. Although third-eyelid flaps may provide some support to the cornea, they are not recommended because they prevent medication and observation of the cornea, which are critical to proper management. If aggressive treatment is initiated promptly, the prognosis for vision and for the globe is good; however, extensive bullous keratopathy, especially with globe perforation, carries a poorer prognosis.

DISEASES OF THE UVEAL TRACT

Uveitis

The uvea or vascular layer of the eye is composed of the iris and ciliary body (anterior uvea), and choroid (posterior uvea) (Figure 29-41). Uveal inflammation may involve the iris and ciliary body alone (anterior uveitis), the choroid and adjacent retina (posterior uveitis or chorioretinitis), or the entire uveal tract (panuveitis). Recognition of this common, painful condition is vital, as the consequences of untreated uveitis can be blinding and underlying causes of uveitis can be fatal.

Unlike dogs, cats with uveitis less commonly present with sudden, overt clinical signs. Instead, feline uveitis is insidious, with subtle changes that may easily be dismissed, often as "conjunctivitis," unless a thorough ophthalmic examination is performed. Therefore all reddened eyes in cats should be assessed for signs considered pathognomonic or at least highly suggestive of

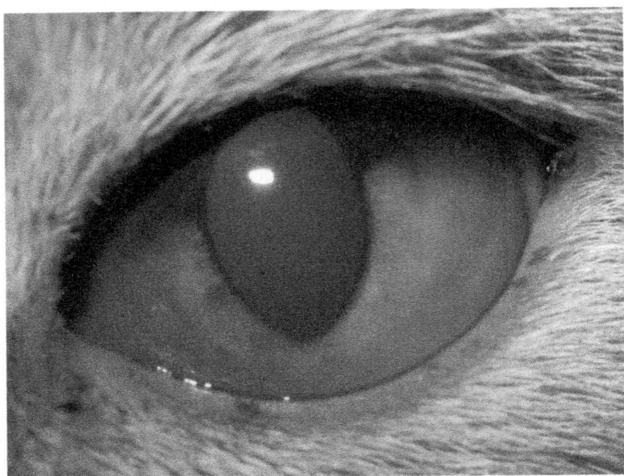

FIGURE 29-42 Examination findings typical of uveitis include corneal edema, rubeosis iridis, a thickened or "muddy" iris, and keratic precipitates on the ventral corneal endothelium. *(Image courtesy of the WCVM Ophthalmology Service.)*

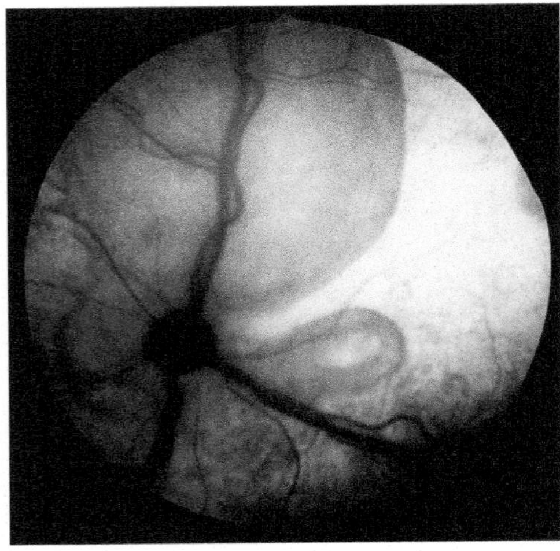

FIGURE 29-43 Multiple focal bullous retinal detachments around the optic nerve of a cat that also demonstrated neurologic abnormalities. A diagnostic workup failed to reveal an underlying cause; however, the owner reported that the cat regained normal mentation, neurologic status, and vision. This case reinforces the importance of a fundic examination in patients demonstrating neurologic signs. *(Image courtesy UC Davis Veterinary Ophthalmology Service.)*

anterior uveitis (or at the very least incompatible with a diagnosis of conjunctivitis), such as aqueous flare; hypopyon; hyphema; anterior chamber fibrin; keratic precipitates; episcleral congestion; corneal edema; rubeosis iridis; a thickened, swollen, or "muddy"-looking iris; miosis (or a delayed response to mydriatic agents); anterior or posterior synechiae; and altered IOP (Figure 29-42). The IOP in eyes with anterior uveitis is generally low; however, with secondary glaucoma, it may also be normal or elevated. Posterior uveitis is not always accompanied by outward clinical signs or anterior segment changes, which emphasizes the importance of performing a fundic examination with each ophthalmic examination. Clinical findings indicative of posterior uveitis include vitreous debris, hyporeflective areas within the tapetum, chorioretinal infiltration with white blood cells, retinal vascular tortuosity, retinal or vitreous hemorrhage (or both), or retinal detachment (Figure 29-43).

Once uveitis has been diagnosed, the next important step is to search for an underlying cause, even if this is expected to be unrewarding (Table 29-3). Causes of uveitis are generally referred to as *exogenous* or *endogenous*. Exogenous causes are usually easily diagnosed by clinical examination, tend to result from trauma or surgery, and include corneal ulceration and blunt or penetrating ocular trauma. Endogenous causes require further testing to achieve a diagnosis, and include infectious, neoplastic, and immune-mediated factors. Although examination findings are nonspecific with regard to etiology, some clinical findings are more suggestive of certain etiologies. For example, large, cellular keratic precipitates (often described as resembling mutton fat) usually reflect diseases causing granulomatous inflammation, such as systemic mycoses or feline infectious peritonitis (FIP) (Figure 29-44). Presence of a mature or hypermature cataract may be suggestive of lens-induced uveitis; however, unlike dogs, cats tend to develop cataracts secondary to uveitis, and the cataract should not be assumed to be the original cause of intraocular inflammation. Idiopathic uveitis occurs more often in male cats older than 9 years and is more likely to be unilateral, whereas uveitis secondary to systemic disease is more often bilateral.[43]

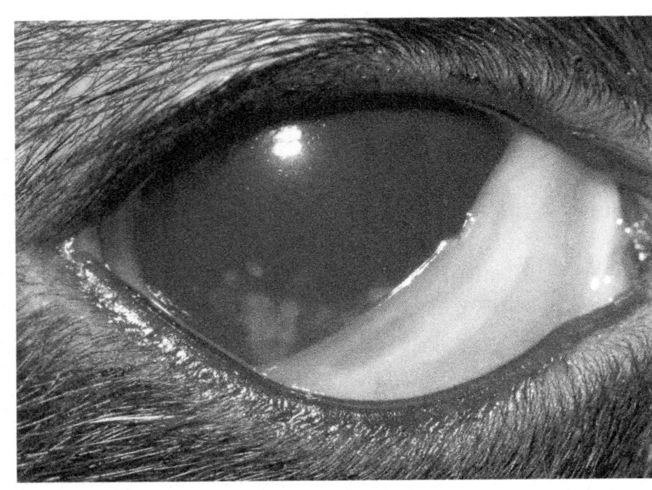

FIGURE 29-44 Mild corneal edema and granulomatous keratic precipitates in a cat with uveitis caused by feline infectious peritonitis. *(Image courtesy UC Davis Veterinary Ophthalmology Service.)*

Because many systemic diseases have been implicated as being able to cause uveitis in cats, the list of differential considerations is long (Box 29-3). Feline immunodeficiency virus (FIV) and FIP directly cause

TABLE 29-3 **Suggestive Clinical Examination Findings for Several Common Causes of Uveitis in the Cat**

Cause	Clinical Course	Typical Location	Suggestive Signs*
Trauma	Acute	Anterior uveitis	Hyphema; AC fibrin; miosis; aqueous flare; hypotony
Reflex uveitis (due to ulcerative keratitis)	Acute	Anterior uveitis	Miosis; aqueous flare; hypopyon (if ulcer is infected); hypotony
FIP	Subacute	Panuveitis (anterior uveitis may dominate)	KPs; aqueous flare; AC fibrin; hypopyon; retinal vascular engorgement and increased tortuosity; perivascular chorioretinal granulomas; retinal detachment
Lymphoma	Subacute	Anterior uveitis	Hypopyon; hyphema; AC fibrin; aqueous flare; iridal thickening; iridal nodules; rubeosis iridis; iris bombé; secondary glaucoma
Systemic mycoses	Subacute	Panuveitis (posterior uveitis dominates)	Hypopyon; hyphema; AC fibrin; aqueous flare; iridal thickening; rubeosis iridis; iris bombé; vitreal debris/infiltrates; secondary glaucoma; chorioretinal granulomas; retinal detachment
Lens-induced uveitis	Phacoclastic (acute)	Anterior uveitis	Hypopyon; hyphema; AC fibrin; aqueous flare; iridal thickening; posterior synechiae; ocular hypertension; miosis
	Phacolytic (chronic)		Aqueous flare; iridal thinning/atrophy; rubeosis iridis; posterior synechiae; mature/hypermature cataract; secondary glaucoma
Idiopathic	Chronic or recurrent	Anterior or intermediate uveitis	Iridal thinning/atrophy; iridal nodules; rubeosis iridis; aqueous flare; KPs; snow banking; vitreous debris/infiltrates; posterior synechiae; cortical cataract; secondary glaucoma
Primary uveal neoplasia	Chronic	Anterior uveitis or chorioretinitis depending on site of tumor	**Anteriorly located** Hypopyon; hyphema; AC fibrin; aqueous flare; anterior iridal displacement; rubeosis iridis; vitreous debris/infiltrates; secondary glaucoma **Posteriorly located** Retinal detachment; subretinal neoplasm; vitreous debris/infiltrates
FIV	Chronic	Intermediate uveitis	Vitreous debris/infiltrates; snow banking; iridal thinning/atrophy; rubeosis iridis; aqueous flare; posterior synechiae; cortical cataract; secondary glaucoma

AC, Anterior chamber; *FIP*, feline infectious peritonitis; *KPs*, keratic precipitates; *FIV*, feline immunodeficiency virus.
*Note the considerable overlap of signs. No sign is pathognomonic for a given cause, and absence of one or more of the signs listed does not allow a cause to be eliminated. Rather, these features can be used to rank the likelihood of potential causes for further diagnostic testing.
From Maggs DJ: Feline uveitis: an "intraocular lymphadenopathy," *J Feline Med Surg* 11:167-182, 2009.

BOX 29-3

Infectious Causes of Uveitis in Cats

Viral	Bacterial	Fungal/algal	Parasitic	Protozoal
FIP	*Bartonella* species	*Cryptococcus neoformans*†	*Cuterebra*	*Toxoplasma gondii*
FeLV*	*Mycobacterium* species	*Histoplasma capsulatum*†		*Leishmania* species
FIV*	*Ehrlichia* species‡	*Blastomyces dermatitidis*†		
FHV	*Borrelia burgdorferi*‡	*Candida albicans*		
		Coccidioides immitis†		
		Aspergillus species		

FIP, Feline infectious peritonitis; *FeLV*, feline leukemia virus; *FIV*, feline immunodeficiency virus; *FHV*, feline herpesvirus.
*Via immunosuppression or oncogenesis.
†Chorioretinitis predominates.
‡Seroprevalence data only (no clinical evidence).
From Maggs DJ: Feline uveitis: an "intraocular lymphadenopathy," *J Feline Med Surg* 11:167-182, 2009.

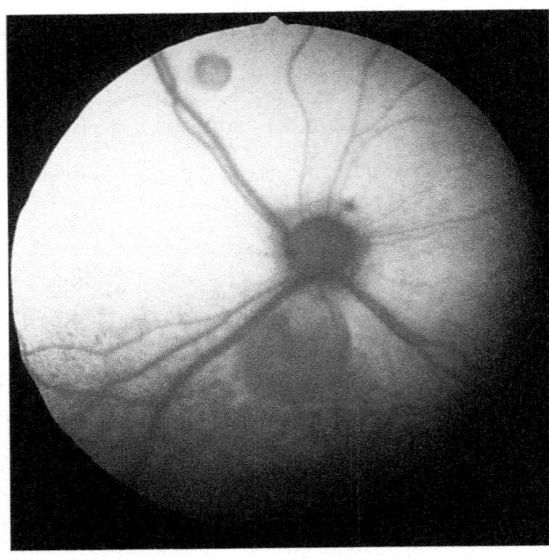

FIGURE 29-45 Multiple focal bullous retinal detachments and chorioretinal hemorrhage in a cat with systemic cryptococcosis. *(Image courtesy UC Davis Veterinary Ophthalmology Service.)*

uveitis in cats.[59,114] Lymphoma or superinfection resulting from immunosuppression and anemia induced by feline leukemia virus (FeLV) also cause uveitis; however, FeLV itself does not seem to directly result in ocular disease.[22] There is also evidence suggesting that intraocular presence of FHV-1 may be associated with feline uveitis.[117] Bacteremia or septicemia may also manifest as uveitis. Although *Bartonella* species have been implicated by some authors,[103] other controlled studies have revealed that many normal animals are seropositive[61] and can even have organism DNA demonstrated in their aqueous humor.[103] These facts confound diagnosis of these and many other organisms. By contrast, *Toxoplasma gondii* and *Leishmania* species are well established as a cause of feline uveitis.* Intraocular migration of nematodes such as *Cuterebra* species may cause uveitis.[82,177,207] Dematiaceous fungi, as well as systemic infections of *Cryptococcus* species, *Histoplasma capsulatum, Blastomyces dermatitidis,* and *Coccidioides immitis,* may also cause uveitis in cats† (Figure 29-45). Primary and metastatic neoplasia also causes uveitis. In cats, iris melanoma is the most common primary ocular tumor, whereas lymphoma is the most common metastatic tumor associated with feline uveitis.[43,147]

Although a large number of systemic diseases are capable of causing uveitis, uveitis remains idiopathic in approximately 70% of cats undergoing a thorough diagnostic investigation.[43,147] Regardless, thorough diagnostic investigation is indicated because many causes are treatable, have human health implications, or affect management of cats. In particular, failure to identify a cause means that corticosteroids may be used at sufficiently high doses to be effective without concern regarding their safety in systemically infected animals or animals with neoplasia in which a more complete chemotherapeutic protocol might be chosen. Therefore a diagnosis of uveitis without obvious exogenous cause should always be followed by a complete physical examination, CBC, serum biochemical profile, urinalysis, and testing for FIV and FeLV. Further diagnostics, such as chest or abdominal radiography and ultrasonography or fine-needle aspirates of lymph nodes, may be indicated depending on clinical suspicion.

Serology for infectious disease is variably useful for obtaining a diagnosis. Serology is unable to differentiate between vaccine-associated virus and wild-type virus, and titers against some infectious diseases may remain elevated long after infection has occurred. For example, immunoglobulin G titers to *T. gondii* remain elevated for years after initial exposure in healthy cats.[104] With *Bartonella* there appears to be no correlation between titers and uveitis.[61] It may be of more value to use negative titers to rule out disease than to use positive titers to rule in infectious disease; however, care must be taken not to falsely interpret negative titers in acutely affected animals. Aqueous humor may also be submitted for infectious disease titers. However, similar pitfalls exist for interpretation of aqueous titers as for serum titers. In addition, intraocular antibody production can persist or recur in response to nonspecific antigenic stimuli and may occur in the absence of uveitis. Cytology of aqueous humor also tends to be of low-yield except for lymphoma. Culture is of benefit only with endophthalmitis, typically after a penetrating injury. However, evaluation of aqueous may be of some value when uveitis is unresponsive to treatment and other diagnostics have been unrewarding. When an eye has become blind and painful despite treatment, enucleation is indicated and histopathologic evaluation of the globe is essential.

Treatment for uveitis should be aggressive and prompt given the high potential for blinding sequelae. The main goals of treatment are to address any underlying etiology, control intraocular inflammation, provide analgesia, and minimize secondary complications. Anterior uveitis may be treated with topical medications alone; however, the presence of posterior uveitis requires systemic administration of medications because of the inability of eye drops to achieve therapeutic drug concentrations posterior to the lens. Treatment of an identified underlying etiology is essential. Failure to address an underlying cause will almost certainly lead to failure to control uveitis. In addition, specific treatment often does more to reduce inflammation than nonspecific antiinflammatory medications and can result in lower doses of and shorter treatment periods with antiinflammatory medications.

*References 42, 89, 90, 105, 151, 152.

†References 6, 13, 19, 67, 75, 144, 147.

Corticosteroids or NSAIDs are used to control intraocular inflammation. In the absence of corneal ulceration, topical 1% prednisolone or 0.1% dexamethasone ophthalmic suspensions may be used up to 4 times daily to treat anterior uveitis. Hydrocortisone, found in combination antibiotic–corticosteroid preparations, is a weak steroid that does not penetrate an intact corneal epithelium and should not be used to treat uveitis. Because systemic absorption from topically applied medications is generally minimal, especially acutely, and because control of inflammation is essential (irrespective of cause), topical steroids are usually safe for use when infectious systemic disease is present. However, when treating posterior uveitis, the clinician should refrain from using systemic steroids until infectious etiologies have been ruled out or when results of diagnostic tests may be affected by the use of corticosteroids. Topical 0.1% diclofenac, 0.03% flurbiprofen, and 0.1% nepafenac are NSAIDs that may all be used up to 4 times daily to control uveitis. Because they tend to be more expensive and less potent than steroids, they are usually reserved for situations in which when corticosteroids are contraindicated. Because of the potential for platelet inhibition, these medications should be avoided if hyphema is present. Likewise, systemic NSAID therapy is used when systemic corticosteroids are contraindicated or while awaiting results of diagnostic testing but should be avoided if a bleeding disorder is suspected.

The pain associated with anterior uveitis results from spasm of the ciliary body muscle. Although this cannot be assessed directly, it can be assumed to be present if the pupil is miotic. Administration of cycloplegic medication such as 1% atropine will provide analgesia by preventing ciliary muscle spasm. Clinicians should use the presence of a dilated pupil to infer that paralysis of the ciliary muscle has also occurred. Initially, atropine may be required up to 3 times daily to achieve mydriasis. After the pupil has dilated, atropine is administered only as often as is required to maintain dilation, which may be as infrequently as every other day or every few days. The bitter taste of atropine may result in profuse salivation after administration in cats; use of the ointment form rather than the solution may minimize this side effect. In addition to its analgesic effects, atropine also stabilizes the blood–ocular barrier, and the resulting mydriasis decreases the chance of posterior synechia formation. The IOP should be checked frequently in patients receiving atropine treatment because the dilated pupil may potentiate peripheral anterior synechia, which obstruct the iridocorneal angle, and cycloplegia can also reduce aqueous outflow, thereby increasing IOP.

Initial uveitis treatment should be aggressive, with judicious tapering of antiinflammatory and cycloplegic agents based on clinical improvement. Recheck examinations should be frequent and at increasing intervals as signs abate. Initial rechecks may need to be as frequent as twice weekly to manage complications should they arise. Patients should also be rechecked beyond the time that all medications are completely discontinued on account of the potential for recurrence. Owners should also be warned that patients who have experienced past bouts of uveitis are at risk of future episodes. Some patients, particularly those diagnosed with idiopathic uveitis, may require lifelong low-dose-antiinflammatory medications to control clinical signs, reduce complications, and minimize recurrence of disease.

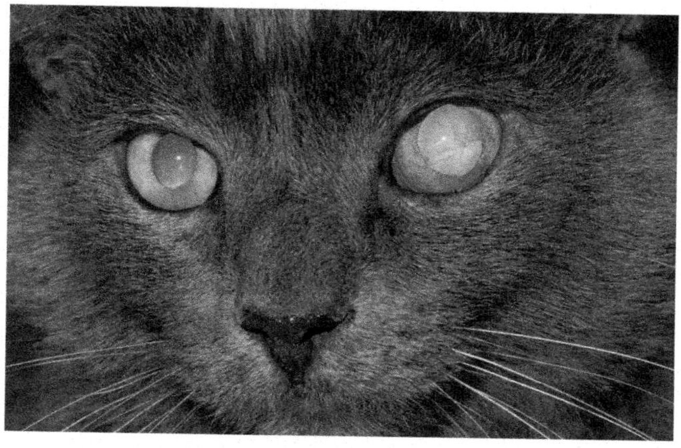

FIGURE 29-46 Bilateral uveitis in a cat. Rubeosis iridis and keratic precipitates are visible in the right eye. Mydriasis and buphthalmos of the left eye are due to glaucoma, which has developed secondary to uveitis. There is also a cataract in the left eye, likely caused by the uveitis. This case reinforces the need for early and aggressive therapy of uveitis in cats, with slow tapering of therapy based only on reduction of clinical evidence of uveitis. Unrecognized or inadequately treated uveitis is associated with severe and blinding sequelae. *(Image courtesy UC Davis Veterinary Ophthalmology Service.)*

In some cases uveitis may prove intractable. Secondary complications in these patients are common. The most important sequelae of chronic uveitis in cats are glaucoma, lens luxation, cataract, and retinal detachment[43,147] (Figure 29-46). Should glaucoma arise, treatment with the carbonic anhydrase inhibitor dorzolamide, twice or thrice daily, should be instituted. Unfortunately, glaucoma can be challenging to treat and may ultimately necessitate enucleation of the affected eye. Cataract formation and lens luxation are other common complications of uveitis that may be difficult to treat. An advanced cataract may exacerbate ocular disease by inciting phacolytic uveitis; however, most cats are not candidates for phacoemulsification because of the severity of ocular pathology. Similarly, surgical removal of a luxated lens carries a poor prognosis if uveitis is ongoing. In many patients with these sequelae to uveitis, a blind and painful globe eventuates, and enucleation is necessary

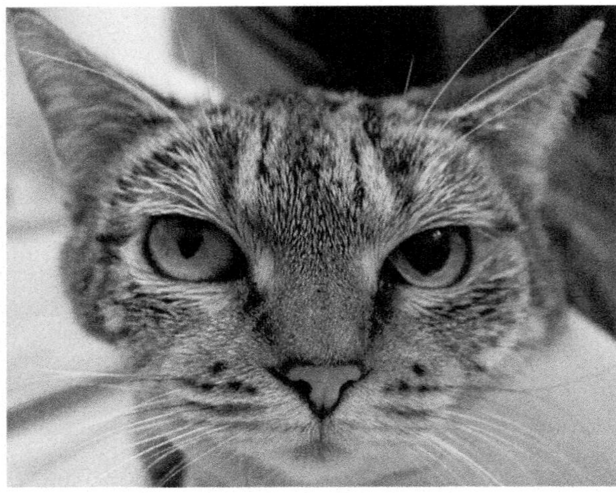

FIGURE 29-47 Note the anisocoria in this patient. Pupillary light reflexes were also abnormal, and the degree of anisocoria changed over time. These features are suggestive of feline spastic pupil syndrome, which is thought to be due to neuritis of cranial nerve 3, induced by feline leukemia virus. *(Image courtesy UC Davis Veterinary Ophthalmology Service.)*

to reduce pain, permit cessation of medical therapy and frequent recheck examinations, minimize risk of intraocular sarcoma development (discussed later in this chapter), and allow a histologic diagnosis that may permit more appropriate treatment of the opposite eye.

Spastic Pupil Syndrome

Spastic pupil syndrome (SPS) is a condition unique to cats in which clients report anisocoria, which may sometimes be transient and independent of ambient light levels (Figure 29-47). Clinically, cats with SPS appear to be healthy, are visual, and have no ocular abnormalities besides unusual behavior of the pupils. Clinical examination reveals anisocoria, failure to achieve complete mydriasis in dark conditions, and sluggish PLRs; however, examination findings can be normal because signs may be transient. It is claimed that all cats with SPS test positive for FeLV, although this is not always the case at the initial examination. The lesion is proposed to result from virally induced neuritis involving cranial nerve 3. No treatment is possible, and the prognosis for long-term survival is poor.[174]

Uveal Neoplasia

Few primary intraocular tumors have been documented in cats. These include iridociliary epithelial tumors,[145] melanoma,[143] feline ocular sarcoma (FOS),[49] and perhaps extramedullary plasmacytoma.[126] Ultimately, an eye with a suspected primary neoplastic process should be removed after a thorough physical examination and diagnostic workup are performed to rule out obvious systemic metastasis. However, both diffuse iris melanoma (DIM) and FOS have special considerations that warrant specific discussion. They are considered to be the two most common and most significant primary intraocular tumors in cats. FOS is discussed in the upcoming section on diseases of the lens.

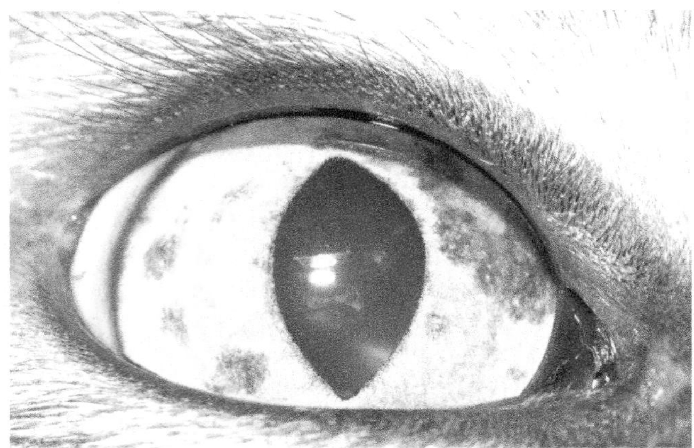

FIGURE 29-48 Multiple, diffuse to coalescing areas of iridal hyperpigmentation, highly suggestive of diffuse iris melanoma. At this stage, where the only ocular change is iridal hyperpigmentation, determining if these lesions are due to benign melanosis or malignant melanoma is highly challenging. Referral is recommended. *(Image courtesy UC Davis Veterinary Ophthalmology Service.)*

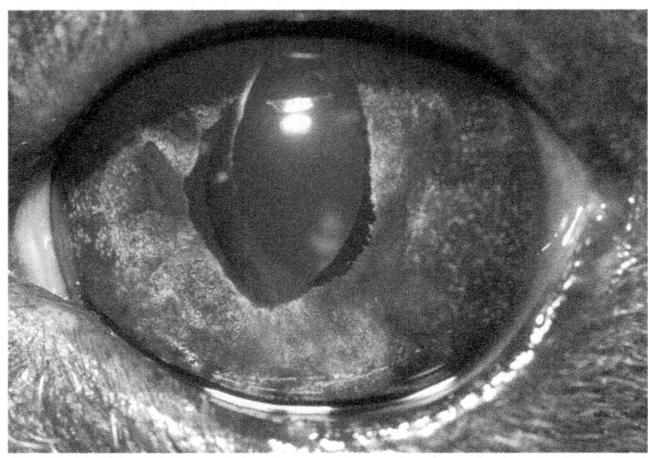

FIGURE 29-49 Diffuse iris melanoma. Although histology is ultimately required to confirm a diagnosis, the raised nature of the melanotic lesions and the dyscoria are highly suggestive of a malignant process. *(Image courtesy UC Davis Veterinary Ophthalmology Service.)*

Iris Melanoma

DIM is the most common primary intraocular tumor in cats.[130] Unlike dogs with intraocular melanoma, which typically develop a discrete raised mass on their anterior iris face, cats most commonly demonstrate diffuse and insidious iridal melanosis with little or no projection above the iris surface (Figures 29-48 and 29-49). Clinical recognition in the early stages of disease can be difficult because of the similar appearance of benign iris melanosis, a common aging change in cats.[50] Definitive diagnosis is further complicated by the difficulty of obtaining an iris biopsy, as well as the potential for benign areas of melanosis to later undergo transformation into malignant melanoma.[56,130] Until better methods to differentiate these syndromes are discovered, practitioners and owners must sometimes elect to remove an eye that potentially has only benign melanosis or risk metastatic disease by delaying removal of an eye containing neoplastic cells.

No breed or gender predilection exists, but the average affected cat is middle-aged to older, presenting at an average age of 11 years.[12,143] DIM usually first appears as a focal area of brown iridal hyperpigmentation.[1,50,53,130] In the early stages distinguishing between DIM and benign iris melanosis is sometimes impossible.[50] The appearance of early DIM may remain static for months or years, but it is ultimately progressive, resulting in visible enlargement of iridal discoloration.[1,56] Although DIM has no pathognomonic clinical features, thickening of the iris, hyperpigmentation extending beyond the anterior iris surface, and alterations of pupillary function increase the suspicion for melanoma.[12,130] Without treatment, there is progressive infiltration of the anterior uvea and ocular drainage pathways, eventually resulting in uveitis and secondary glaucoma.[53,130,200]

Diode laser photocoagulation, as reported for the treatment of focal areas of iridal hyperpigmentation in dogs,[33] has not been recommended for cats because of incomplete destruction and potentially dispersal of neoplastic cells and tissue. One reasonable management approach is to monitor areas of iris color change over time. Photographic documentation of such lesions is extremely helpful. However, because of the risk of metastatic disease, enucleation is ultimately the recommended treatment for enlarging iridal hyperpigmentation.[53,56,98,130]

Latency times of up to a few years have been reported for metastatic disease, with documented metastatic rates as high as 62.5%.[143] The liver is the most common site for metastatic disease; however, lungs, regional lymph nodes, and other sites may also be affected.[14,56,130,143] A thorough diagnostic workup is therefore recommended before surgery. Enucleation should be performed early in the disease course.[98] Although this may risk removal of eyes with subsequent histologically diagnosed benign iridal melanosis, this risk should be weighed against treatment delay, given the fact that survival time decreases with progressive tumor infiltration into the uvea.[98] Compared with a control group, equivalent survival times were achieved when enucleation was performed while the melanoma was confined to the iris stroma.[56,98] In contrast, tumor infiltration into the ciliary body or drainage pathways, especially with development of glaucoma, strongly correlates with markedly decreased survival time.[56,98] Although increased metastatic rate is associated with high mitotic index and evidence of scleral invasion,[56,98] cellular characteristics such as cell shape, nucleus to cytoplasm ratio, number of nucleoli, and melanin content do not appear to be of value for determining prognosis.[56]

Amelanotic DIM has been described and presents similarly to the classical DIM except that the discoloration appears gray rather than brown.[17] Clinical progression and potential for metastasis should be considered to be the same as for classical DIM. A second variant, atypical ocular melanoma, has also been reported. Unlike DIM, atypical ocular melanoma originates from multiple areas within the uveal tract and may have a more aggressive clinical course.[81] Cats with atypical ocular melanoma had neoplastic infiltration of the entire uveal tract and sclera at the time of initial presentation,[81] whereas in DIM neoplastic cells remain in the anterior uvea. At this time it is not clear if the advanced nature of disease at presentation was due to more aggressive behavior at the cellular level or a result of tumor arising from the posterior, rather than anterior, uvea.

Iris melanoma can be experimentally induced after anterior chamber inoculation with FeLV and feline sarcoma virus (FeSV), leading to speculation that these viruses may play a role in the development of DIM.[4,5] An association has been documented between naturally arising DIM and FeLV/FeSV; however, this was seen in a minority of cases of one study only.[175] At this time there is no evidence that FeLV or FeSV is involved in the pathogenesis of DIM.[37]

Secondary Intraocular Neoplasia

Any systemic neoplastic process has the potential to metastasize to the eye. Intraocular metastases secondary to SCC, pulmonary adenocarcinoma, hemangiosarcoma, and lymphosarcoma have been documented.[32,34,68,99] Of these, lymphosarcoma is by far the most common[204] (Figure 29-50). Because hematogenous spread appears to be the main route into the eye, metastatic intraocular neoplasia first affects the uvea.[27,54,68] In cats choroidal metastases may occur more often than metastases to the anterior uvea.[54] A discrete uveal mass is possible; however, more diffuse metastases with signs of uveitis are more common.[34,54] In fact, uveitis may be the first clinical sign of underlying systemic neoplasia.[34] For this reason systemic neoplasia should always be considered when evaluating a patient presenting with uveitis. Thorough physical examination and diagnostic investigation are essential, as for all other cases of uveitis. Ocular ultrasound is useful when intraocular structures are not easily seen on clinical examination. Although rare, intraocular metastasis of pulmonary adenocarcinoma warrants special mention because of its unique presentation in cats. In addition to the nonspecific signs of uveitis,

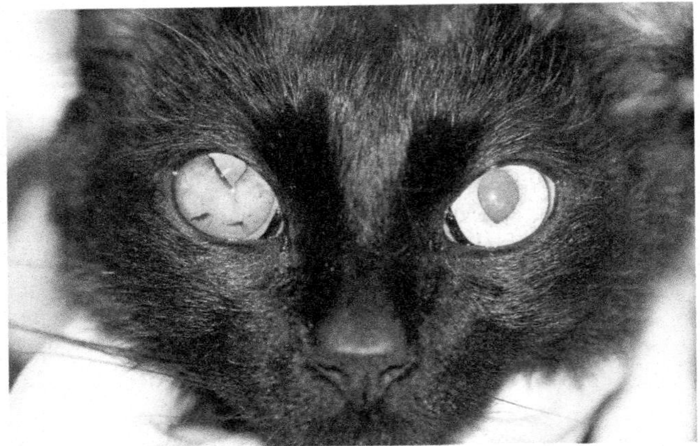

FIGURE 29-50 Dyscoria due to an iridal mass in the right eye of a cat. The histopathologic diagnosis was lymphosarcoma. *(Image courtesy WCVM Ophthalmology service.)*

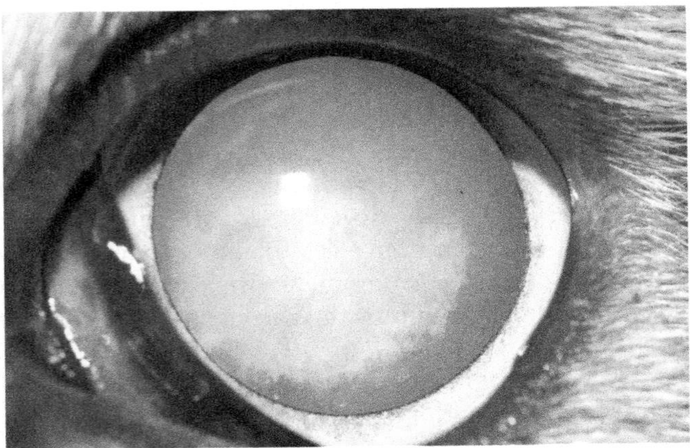

FIGURE 29-51 Incomplete cataract involving the lens nucleus. *(Image courtesy UC Davis Veterinary Ophthalmology Service).*

this tumor causes characteristic wedge-shaped areas of fundic discoloration resulting from ischemic chorioretinopathy.[27]

Treatment for metastatic intraocular neoplasia should include both nonspecific treatment for uveitis as well as treatment of the underlying neoplastic process. With tumors that are responsive to chemotherapy (in particular, lymphosarcoma), the reduction in uveitis tends to correlate well with response of the tumor at extraocular sites and is often dramatic. By contrast, ocular tissues do not tolerate irradiation, and so radiation-responsive intraocular tumors often necessitate enucleation as a palliative measure.

DISEASES OF THE LENS

Cataract and Lens Luxation

The most common diseases of the feline lens are cataract and lens luxation, both of which occur as primary syndromes much less frequently in cats than in dogs[70] (Figure 29-51). Rather, in cats both diseases tend to occur as a result of chronic uveitis; therefore patients should be thoroughly examined for signs of uveitis and its causes. Diabetic cats rarely develop cataracts, presumably because of decreased aldose reductase centrations in the feline lens compared with the canine lens.[159] Congenital cataracts have been reported in conjunction with such ocular abnormalities as eyelid agenesis, microphakia, and Chédiak–Higashi syndrome but are also considered to be uncommon.[2,31,128] Primary lens luxation is believed to occur in cats, but peer-reviewed descriptions do not exist and a breed predilection has not been reported. Instead, lens dislocations in the cat occur secondary to other ocular disease, such as uveitis, glaucoma, and senile zonular degeneration[165] (Figure 29-52). Treatments for cataracts and lens luxation are similar to those for dogs and require referral to a veterinary ophthalmologist.

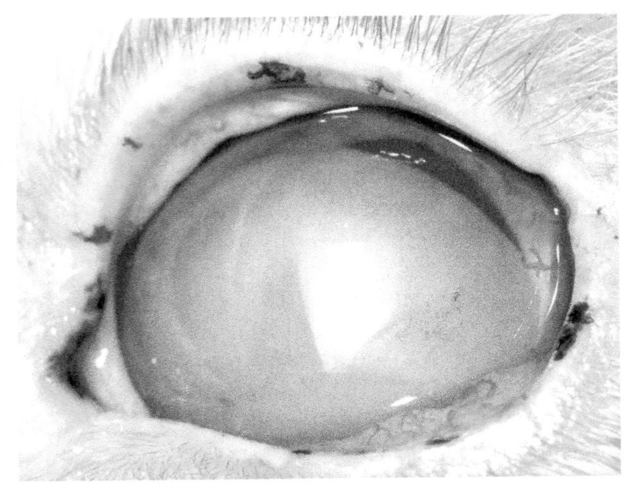

FIGURE 29-52 Complete cataract and anterior lens luxation in the left eye of a cat. The lens is seen anterior to the iris. Note the superficial corneal vessels, which are commonly seen with lens luxation. Serology indicated that this cat was positive for feline immunodeficiency virus. Lens luxation in cats is associated with uveitis, cataract, and glaucoma and should initiate referral. If the eye is irreversibly blind, enucleation with histopathology should be performed. *(Image courtesy UC Davis Veterinary Ophthalmology Service.)*

Feline Ocular Sarcoma

FOS is an aggressive ocular tumor resulting in tumor-related death of the majority of affected cats. Because of this, many ophthalmologists strongly recommend enucleation of blind and painful feline globes, regardless of cause, to prevent subsequent malignant transformation to FOS. For these reasons, this tumor warrants special mention here.

Most cats diagnosed with primary ocular sarcoma have a known history of trauma to the affected eye

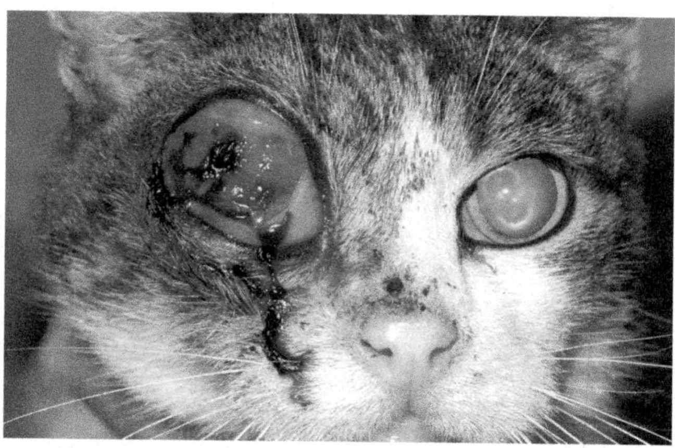

FIGURE 29-53 An intraocular mass has caused glaucoma, buphthalmos, and rupture of the right eye of this cat. Histopathology identified this tumor to be feline ocular sarcoma that had migrated into the orbit. The orbit was exenterated as a palliative measure, but the owner was warned to expect tumor recurrence and death as a result of local invasion and recurrence. *(Image courtesy UC Davis Veterinary Ophthalmology Service.)*

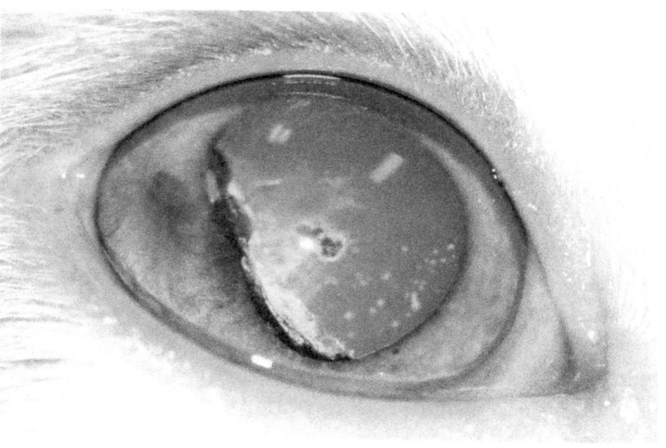

FIGURE 29-54 Clinical signs of globe perforation. Note the anterior synechiae at the 9 o'clock position, indicating corneal perforation. Dyscoria is a result of posterior synechiae along the lateral pupillary margin, consistent with uveitis. The presence of melanin on the anterior lens capsule and within the lens as well as early cataract are highly suggestive of lens capsule perforation. This cat is at risk of developing of developing feline ocular sarcoma. *(Image courtesy WCVM Ophthalmology Service.)*

several years prior.* For this reason FOS is sometimes referred to as *posttraumatic intraocular sarcoma*. Chronic uveitis and intraocular injections have also been reported as precursors to the development of FOS.[180] Quite often, the affected eye has been blind for several years, and the reason for presentation is a change in the appearance of the eye.[52,77] Cats rarely show overt signs of discomfort at the time of presentation.[49,51] Clinical examination often shows an opaque cornea.[49,52,77] An anterior chamber mass can sometimes be appreciated, but intraocular structures are often difficult to discern[52,77,180] (Figure 29-53). Ultrasound may be useful for confirmation of an intraocular mass when clinical examination is limited. The affected globe may also have an abnormal shape; quite frequently, the globe is phthisical or buphthalmic.[9,52]

Histologically, there is obliteration of normal architecture of globes from cats with FOS.† Neoplastic cells tend invade the sclera, preferentially exiting the globe at the posterior pole/optic nerve and the limbus.[49,52,146] Severe pathology of the lens, particularly lens rupture, has been found in almost all cases.[49,52,146] Although the origin of FOS was unknown for years, it is now accepted that the tumor arises from lens epithelial cells.[26,55,209] It is believed that the anterior epithelium of the lens undergoes a malignant transformation in response to trauma in a manner similar to the development of fibrosarcoma at sites of vaccination.[209] FeLV and FeSV are not believed to play a role in the pathogenesis of FOS.[37]

Given the relationship between FOS and lens rupture, cats with perforating lens injury should be referred for treatment immediately and followed up rigorously for life. Treatment options include medical management, phacoemulsification, or enucleation. A small lens capsule perforation may self-seal and respond to medical management for the associated uveitis; however, the liberation of lens material into the eye necessitates long-term follow-up for these patients. Larger lens capsule ruptures require either phacoemulsification to remove free lens material from the eye or enucleation (Figure 29-54). Development of FOS has been reported in cats that previously underwent surgical lens extraction.[55] Although development of FOS has not been reported after phacoemulsification specifically, its development is theoretically possible, thus necessitating long-term follow-up.

Likewise, cats with a known history of ocular trauma should also be monitored closely because of the potential for FOS. Clinical suspicion of an intraocular mass or observation of a phthisical globe in a cat, especially one known to have undergone ocular trauma, should prompt the clinician to recommend enucleation after diagnostic investigation for metastatic disease. Although it is not known if early enucleation decreases the mortality rate, treatment should not be delayed because of the aggressive nature of the disease. In the vast majority of reported cases, patients died from tumor-related disease within months of enucleation as a result of local invasion of the orbit, extension along the optic nerve into the central nervous system, or metastatic disease.[9,49,52,77,146] At this time, there are no reports of adjunctive treatments, such as radiation or chemotherapy, for the management of FOS.

*References 9, 49, 52, 55, 77, 146.

†References 9, 52, 53, 77, 146, 180.

GLAUCOMA

It is essential to measure IOP during every ophthalmic examination to avoid overlooking a diagnosis of glaucoma, especially because glaucoma can be a very subtle and insidious disease in cats. In contrast to dogs, glaucoma occurs infrequently in the cat, and secondary glaucoma is far more common than primary glaucoma.[18,160,200] In addition, the rare aqueous humor misdirection syndrome (AHMS) arises naturally in cats but has not yet been reported in dogs. Although any animal can be affected, the typical feline patient with glaucoma is middle-aged or older.[18,41,78,160,190]

Because clinical signs of feline glaucoma tend to develop gradually rather than acutely, irreversible blindness is frequently present by the time of presentation for ophthalmic evaluation.[18,160] Cats often do not develop obvious corneal edema or overtly red eyes in the same manner that dogs do. Instead, the most common findings on initial presentation include absent menace response, absent PLR, and buphthalmos.[18]

A diagnosis of glaucoma is made on the basis of IOP measurements greater than 25 to 30 mm Hg combined with evidence of ocular abnormalities (Figure 29-55). A single elevated IOP reading, in the absence of clinical signs, should not be used to make a diagnosis of glaucoma. Tonometry technique, excessive neck pressure, diurnal variation, and fractious patients can all contribute to elevated readings.[45,102] Eyes should be re-evaluated if IOP is greater than 25 mm Hg or there is a greater than 12 mm Hg difference between eyes.[102] As mentioned previously in this chapter, the neuro-ophthalmic examination will be abnormal. Retinal degeneration may be present if disease is advanced. Optic disc cupping, a feature of canine glaucoma, is often difficult to appreciate in the cat because of the unmyelinated nature of the feline optic disc. Because the vast majority of feline glaucoma is secondary to anterior uveitis and intraocular neoplasia,[18,200] abnormalities such as aqueous flare, cataract, intraocular mass, or iris discoloration are often also present. Primary glaucoma is possible if such clinical findings are absent, although this condition is rare.[18,96,200] Referral for gonioscopy is necessary to make the diagnosis of primary glaucoma.

AHMS is a rare condition arising from misdirection of aqueous humor into the vitreous cavity instead of into the posterior then anterior chambers and out through the iridocorneal angle. The pathogenesis for this condition is not well understood. It is hypothesized that a defect of the anterior hyaloid membrane acts as a one-way valve, allowing aqueous humor to enter, but not exit, the vitreous cavity. As pressure builds up within the vitreous, the lens and anterior uvea are anteriorly displaced. As a consequence of this shift, there is increased iris–lens contact, producing mydriasis and reduced flow of aqueous humor to the anterior chamber as a result of "pupillary block," which further exacerbates ocular hypertension. Patients with AHMS present with similar neuro-ophthalmic examination abnormalities as cats with other forms of glaucoma.[41] Ophthalmic findings required for diagnosis of AHMS include intact lens zonules, juxtaposition of the ciliary body, consolidated anterior vitreous face, narrow approach to the iridocorneal angle, and a uniformly shallow anterior chamber.[41] Compared with the other examination findings, a uniformly narrow anterior chamber is more easily recognized in a general practice setting and is the characteristic sign of AHMS[41] (Figure 29-56). The uniform narrowing helps differentiate between AHMS and glaucoma due to other causes. In other forms of glaucoma,

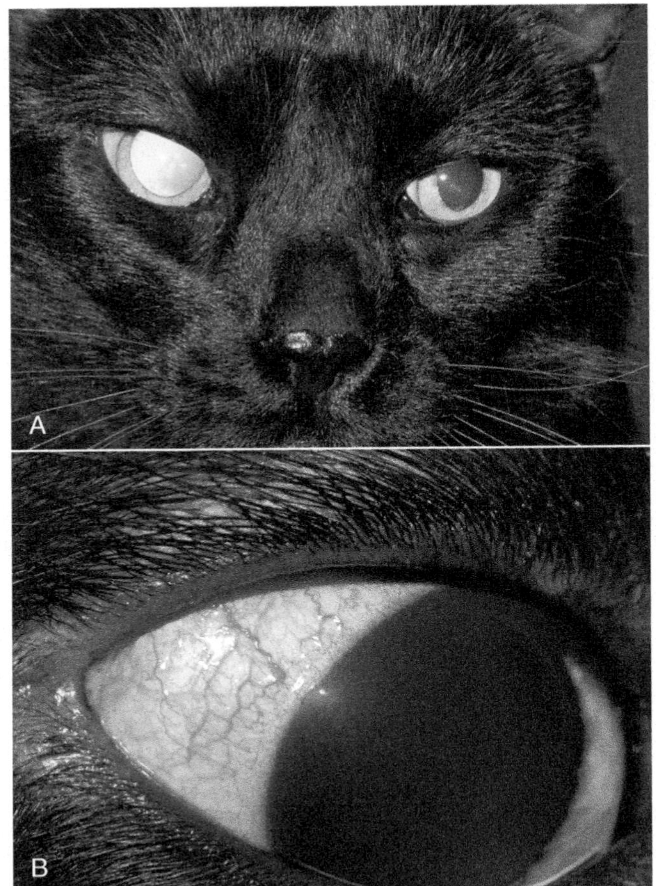

FIGURE 29-55 **A,** Uveitis and marked secondary glaucoma in the right eye of a cat. Despite the intraocular pressure in the right eye being 73 mm Hg, the signs of discomfort, mydriasis, and visible ophthalmic abnormalities are minimal. Signs to look for in this cat are mydriasis, subtle corneal edema, and episcleral injection, none of which can be associated with conjunctivitis alone. Note too that buphthalmos is evident only when the entire head is viewed and symmetry of the globes is assessed. **B,** Finally, note the difference in tapetal reflection between the eyes. This subtle change is sometimes the most obvious sign of ophthalmic disease, usually indicates serious intraocular disease, and should therefore never be ignored. *(Image courtesy UC Davis Veterinary Ophthalmology Service.)*

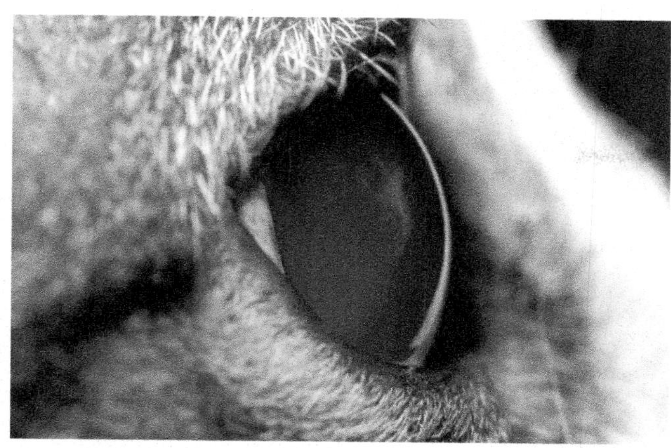

FIGURE 29-56 A narrow anterior chamber is characteristic of aqueous humor misdirection syndrome. The slit beam of the direct ophthalmoscope helps identify the narrowed distance between the bright reflections off the cornea and the anterior lens capsule. In this cat the presence of an anterior cortical cataract also helps demonstrate forward displacement of the lens. This cat's intraocular pressure was 40 mm Hg but responded well to phacoemulsification and anterior vitrectomy. *(Image courtesy UC Davis Veterinary Ophthalmology Service.)*

buphthalmos causes deepening of the anterior chamber. With iris bombé, the peripheral anterior chamber narrows but the central anterior chamber remains deep. The IOP in patients with AHMS is elevated, sometimes markedly so. However, unlike most other forms of glaucoma wherein pharmacologic mydriasis causes a further elevation in IOP, the IOP of some patients with AHMS may be reduced by pupil dilation because of a reduction in pupillary block. AHMS may occur unilaterally at first but often becomes bilateral.

Regardless of cause, treatment of glaucoma should always address the underlying disease if identified. Because many of these primary conditions are intractable, feline glaucoma is usually advanced at presentation, and few antiglaucoma medications are effective in the cat, feline glaucoma is particularly challenging to treat. Medical control of IOP is achieved in 21% to 58% of treated eyes.[18,160] The carbonic anhydrase inhibitor dorzolamide appears to be one of the most useful antiglaucoma drugs for cats. Topical carbonic anhydrase inhibitor therapy is preferred over systemic therapy because of the susceptibility of cats to adverse systemic effects. Dorzolamide is effective for lowering IOP when applied twice daily; however, 4 or 5 days of therapy are needed to reach a reliable decrease.[154] Dorzolamide may also be administered in combination with timolol twice daily, although the additional benefit of timolol appears to be marginal.[46] The carbonic anhydrase inhibitor brinzolamide is ineffective in cats,[74] as are the prostaglandin analogs bimatoprost, unoprostone, and latanoprost, which are quite successful in dogs.[10,183] The hypotensive effect of travoprost in cats is not known. Although prostaglandin analogs do not effectively decrease IOP, they do induce miosis in cats as they do in dogs. Pilocarpine also has hypotensive effects in cats[201]; however, on account of its propensity to induce uveitis,[101] as well as systemic side effects, its use is generally discouraged.[41]

Mydriatics are generally contraindicated in glaucoma. Although atropine therapy is a vital component of the treatment of aqueous misdirection in humans, beneficial effects of mydriatic therapy for AHMS have not been demonstrated. In one study application of tropicamide was followed by an increase in IOP.[41] Use of miotics such as pilocarpine and timolol may worsen glaucoma associated with AHMS and should therefore be avoided.

Unfortunately, cyclodestructive procedures appear to provide limited benefit in cats, perhaps because they exacerbate or fail to address the underlying inflammation present in most cases.[78,160] A combination of lensectomy by phacoemulsification in association with posterior capsulotomy and anterior vitrectomy appears to permit redirection of aqueous from the vitreous and correct pupillary block and narrowing of the anterior chamber and holds promise for the control of IOP in AHMS.[41] When medical and surgical interventions fail to control IOP, enucleation should be performed for all blind globes that appear to be causing pain.

CHORIORETINAL DISEASE

Hypertensive Chorioretinopathy

Because it is an end organ, the eye is susceptible to damage resulting from systemic hypertension. Specifically, persistently elevated blood pressure causes pathology to the retina, choroid, and optic nerve. *Hypertensive retinopathy* is a blanket term used to describe all the ocular lesions arising from damage to these structures. Incidence of ophthalmic lesions in hypertensive cats has been estimated to be as high as 60% to 77%.[57,176]

A short review of anatomy may assist in understanding pathogenesis (Figure 29-57). Briefly, vessels are located in only the innermost layers of the feline retina. The outermost retina is highly metabolically active but avascular. The choriocapillaris is a network of capillaries supplying choroidal blood to the outer retina. Although the choroidal vasculature is permeable to most substances, the blood–ocular barrier prevents entry of solutes and fluid into the retina from the choroid and systemic circulation. Exclusion of substances from the retina assists in maintaining retinal attachment.

Hypertensive ocular lesions ultimately arise from ischemic injury to vessel walls. In the face of chronically elevated blood pressure, autoregulatory mechanisms within the retina become deranged and there is leakage of angiotensin II into both the extracellular choroidal space and optic nerve. Consequently, there is vasoconstriction of the retinal vessels, choriocapillaris, and

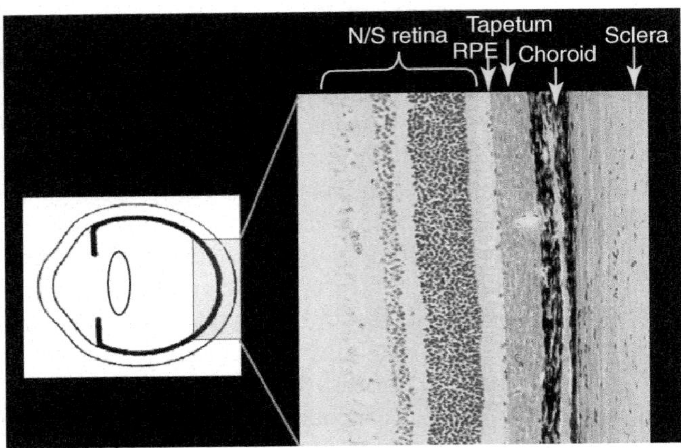

FIGURE 29-57 Normal anatomy of the feline fundus, including the sclera, choroid proper, tapetum (which is actually part of the choroid), retinal pigment epithelium, and neurosensory retina. The blood–retinal barrier normally prevents solutes and fluid from entering the potential space between the retinal pigmented epithelium and the neurosensory retina. Leakage of substances from the choroidal vasculature into this potential space results in retinal detachment.

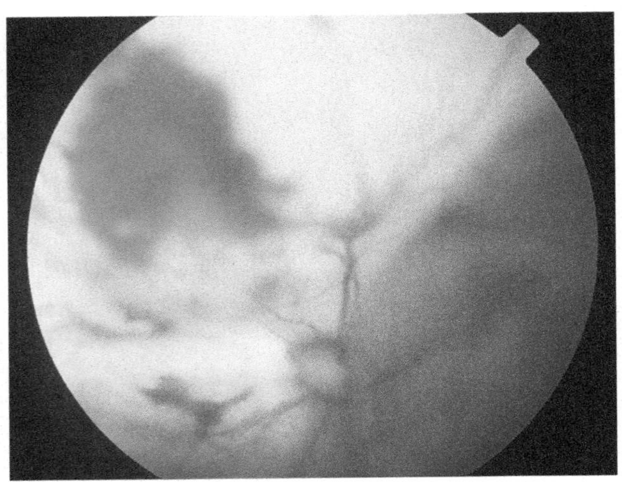

FIGURE 29-59 Complete retinal detachment and multiple retinal hemorrhages are characteristic findings in cats with systemic hypertension, with vision loss being the most frequent reason for presentation to a veterinarian. *(Image courtesy UC Davis Veterinary Ophthalmology Service.)*

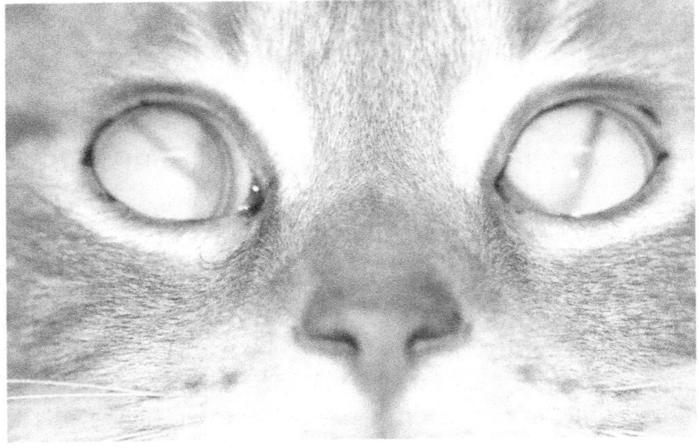

FIGURE 29-58 Evidence of retinal detachment can often be seen during retroillumination, before performing the fundic examination. In this patient complete, bilateral retinal detachment has resulted in mydriasis, and the retinal vessels can be seen in focus immediately posterior to the lens. *(Image courtesy WCVM Ophthalmology Service.)*

vessels supplying the optic nerve. The ischemic damage resulting from prolonged vasoconstriction causes vessel wall necrosis and leakage of fluid from these vessels. Clinically, these changes are manifested as retinal edema, retinal hemorrhage, and serous retinal detachment (Figures 29-58 and 29-59). Papilledema, seen in other species, has not been reported in cats.[35]

The magnitude and duration of blood pressure elevation required to induce ocular lesions is not known. In one study hypertensive ocular lesions were associated with systolic blood pressure measurements above 168 mm Hg[164]; however, the majority of studies show the systolic blood pressure in most cats with hypertension-induced ocular lesions to be above 200 mm Hg.[107,129,163,191]

Ocular lesions may be more likely to develop after pronounced hypertension of prolonged duration, and hypertensive cats with ocular lesions have significantly higher blood pressure than hypertensive cats without ocular lesions.[29,129] For cats with ocular lesions, no significant difference was found between systolic blood pressure of cats presenting with retinal detachment (and acute blindness) compared with that of cats that did not present with acute blindness.[57] Hypertensive cats with ocular lesions are likely to have more severe cardiac pathology than hypertensive cats without ocular lesions.[29]

The typical cat with systemic hypertension is older than 10 years of age.[107,129,164,176] Gender predilections have been suggested but not confirmed.[107,164] The most common reason for presentation is acute blindness.[57,107,163] In fact, in many patients ocular disease is the first indicator of systemic disease.[186] Serous retinal detachment, usually accompanied by retinal hemorrhage, is the most common examination finding, supporting the notion that choroidal pathology accounts for the majority of ocular lesions in cats.[113] Other common examination findings include resting mydriasis, slow to absent PLRs, hyphema, iris hemorrhage, retinal edema, and retinal vessel tortuosity (see Figure 29-59).

Systemic hypertension should be considered in all cats presenting with intraocular hemorrhage or retinal detachment. A thorough diagnostic work up is essential. Diagnosis of hypertensive retinopathy is confirmed when systolic blood pressure measurements exceed 160 to 170 mm Hg and potential causes of posterior uveitis have been excluded. Chronic renal failure is the most common underlying disease associated with systemic hypertension.[107,113,129,176] Primary hypertension and hypertension associated with hyperthyroidism, diabetes mellitus, and hyperaldosteronism should also be considered, but these occur less frequently.[113,176,193]

Antiinflammatory treatment should be considered in cats with anterior segment disease. Corticosteroids are preferred over NSAIDs, which can exacerbate bleeding. To prevent potential systemic effects of corticosteroid therapy, these should be administered topically.[150] Ultimately, the most important components of treating hypertensive retinopathy are control of blood pressure and treatment of any underlying disease. Medical control of blood pressure will allow for improvement of hypertensive ocular lesions in the majority of patients.[57,107,113,129,191] In recent years the calcium channel blocker amlodipine besylate has emerged as a successful treatment for systemic hypertension and related ocular lesions. At doses ranging from 0.625 to 1.25 mg orally, every 12 to 24 hours, amlodipine may be more effective than other classes of drugs for reduction of intraocular hemorrhage and retinal edema and reattachment of serous retinal detachments.[113] For further discussion about the treatment of systemic hypertension, please see Chapter 20.

Prognosis for return to vision depends on both duration and severity of ocular lesions. Mild retinal edema and hemorrhage, without retinal detachment, may completely resolve with successful control of blood pressure.[113] Prognosis becomes guarded if retinal detachment is present. Histologically, retinal degeneration is visible within 1 hour of detachment, and extensive photoreceptor damage occurs within 2 weeks.[60] Therefore, although retinal reattachment is possible with medical management, many cats remain blind or visually impaired due to the retina becoming irreversibly degenerated while detached.[113,129] Prognosis is also guarded in cats with intraocular hemorrhage, particularly hyphema, because of the increased potential of secondary glaucoma.[163]

Enrofloxacin Toxicity

Accounts of blindness in association with enrofloxacin administration in cats were rare until almost a decade after Baytril was first approved by the Food and Drug Administration for use in dogs and cats; these reports appeared to coincide with a labeling change that allowed higher doses to be given to cats. Subsequent toxicologic studies have confirmed that retinal degeneration is dose related rather than idiosyncratic and led to a maximum recommended oral dose of 5 mg/kg per day for cats. Blindness of rapid onset, sometimes as soon as 4 days into treatment, and mydriasis are the typical signs noted by owners. Clinical findings included absent menace responses, sluggish to absent PLRs, variable degrees of tapetal hyperreflectivity, and retinal vascular attenuation[64] (Figure 29-60). Electroretinography has confirmed reduction in retinal function as early as 24 hours after initiation of therapy at 50 mg/kg per day.[63] No common signalment, duration of therapy, or underlying medical condition for which enrofloxacin was prescribed has been noted.[64] In one study oral enrofloxacin doses ranged from 4.6 mg/kg once daily to 27 mg/kg twice daily.[64] After cessation of treatment, a limited amount of vision was preserved or regained in four cats. At higher doses (50 mg/kg daily), some cats also demonstrate neurologic signs.[63] Although the exact mechanism by which enrofloxacin exerts its effects is not known, hypertensive retinopathy does not appear to be a contributing cause.[63]

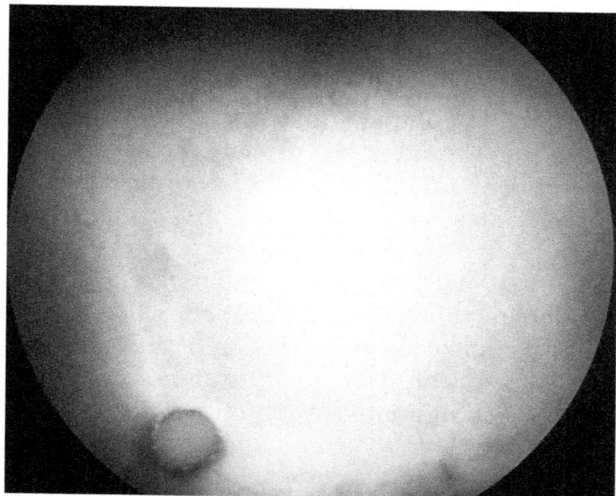

FIGURE 29-60 Tapetal hyperreflectivity and marked retinal vascular attenuation are indicators of advanced retinal degeneration in this cat. Although these signs are pathognomonic for retinal degeneration, they do not permit definitive diagnosis of a cause, which may include taurine deficiency, progressive retinal atrophy, enrofloxacin toxicity, glaucoma, and severe and prolonged previous retinal detachment from any cause. Reaching an etiologic diagnosis requires a complete history and ophthalmic and general physical examination. *(Image courtesy UC Davis Veterinary Ophthalmology Service.)*

Although a dose of 5 mg/kg daily is in accordance with the manufacturer's recommendations, retinal degeneration may still be possible at this dose.[64] Several factors, such as large drug doses or plasma drug concentrations, rapid intravenous infusion, prolonged treatment, and advanced patient age, may increase the risk of toxicity.[199] In particular, cats older than 12 years are more likely to experience adverse effects than are cats younger than 9 years, perhaps because of a higher incidence of hepatic or renal disease causing impaired drug clearance.[199] Exposure to ultraviolet A light during treatment, drug interactions, and drug accumulation (secondary to impaired metabolism or clearance) may also increase the likelihood of retinal degeneration.[199]

A study conducted in 2- to 8-week-old kittens found that oral administration of enrofloxacin at a dose of 5 mg/kg daily failed to achieve therapeutic plasma concentrations but that parenteral administration was successful in achieving target plasma concentrations.[169] This study also suggested that doses higher than 5 mg/kg per day were necessary. This was attributed to the differences in volume of distribution and drug clearance in kittens compared with adult cats. No ocular lesions were found in this study. It is worth noting, however, that at this time the manufacturer's label indicates that enrofloxacin should not be used in kittens younger than 12 weeks of age and that parenteral administration is not licensed in cats.

Because there is no treatment for enrofloxacin toxicity and the vast majority of cats remain permanently blind, practitioners must exercise caution when dispensing fluoroquinolones to cats. Selection of a fluoroquinolone should be made only after culture and sensitivity testing confirms that alternative antibiotics are not suitable. A complete ophthalmic examination, including a fundic examination, should be performed before and after treatment. Owners should be warned of the potential for adverse effects. Should signs of mydriasis, altered PLRs, or visual impairment be noted, treatment should be stopped immediately and the cat brought in for evaluation. Enrofloxacin oral doses in cats should never exceed a maximum of 5 mg/kg per day, and duration should not exceed the manufacturer's recommendation of 2 to 3 days beyond cessation of clinical signs. Caution is especially warranted in patients of advanced age or those with concurrent medical conditions that may impair drug metabolism or elimination. Enrofloxacin is not approved for parenteral use in cats; therefore off-label use of injectable enrofloxacin should be avoided.

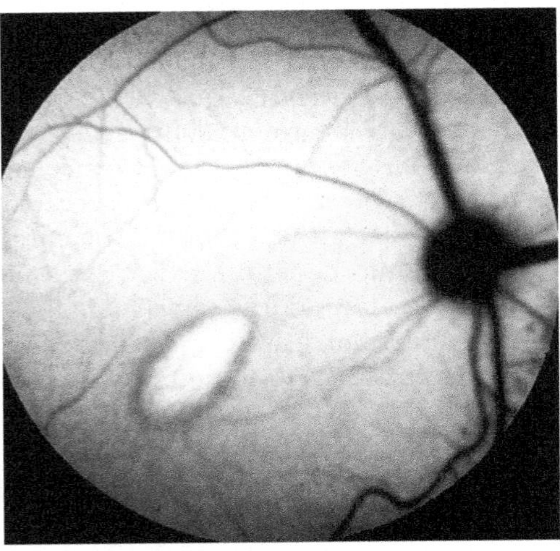

FIGURE 29-61 A focal, elliptical area of tapetal hyperreflectivity dorsolateral to the optic disc is one of the early signs of taurine-deficient retinopathy. This would be considered stage 2 degeneration in a 5-stage scaling system. *(Image courtesy UC Davis Veterinary Ophthalmology Service.)*

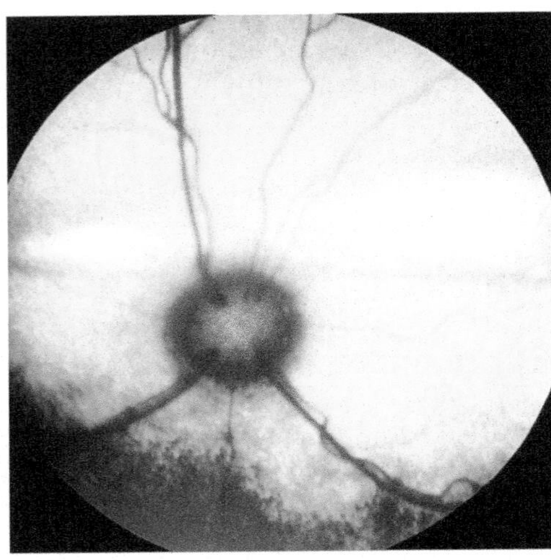

FIGURE 29-62 Prolonged taurine deficiency has led to stage 3 retinal degeneration with hyperreflective regions dorsolateral and dorsomedial to the optic disc. Continued dietary deficiency will lead to complete retinal degeneration (stage 5). *(Image courtesy UC Davis Veterinary Ophthalmology Service.)*

Taurine-Deficient Retinopathy

In the 1970s several authors demonstrated that cats fed taurine-deficient diets showed funduscopic evidence of retinal degeneration and decreased retinal function. In the following years, naturally arising cases of taurine-deficient retinopathy were documented. In particular, this syndrome was recognized in cats fed dog food, which tends to have minimal taurine concentrations.[3] Since then, the practice of feeding dog food to cats has largely stopped, and because most cat foods contain adequate levels of taurine,[178] retinopathy secondary to dietary taurine deficiency is relatively rare. However, with the increased interest in homemade pet diets, the potential for resurgence of this condition remains. Recognition of this condition is important not only for prevention of blindness but also for prevention of dilated cardiomyopathy; another disease associated with taurine deficiency.[148]

Because the half-life of retinal taurine is protracted, it may take several months of dietary deficiency for retinal degeneration to occur.[167,168] Early signs of taurine-deficient retinopathy are similar to those of early progressive retinal atrophy. The first abnormality is a granular appearance to the area centralis, followed by the development of hyperreflectivity[167] (Figures 29-61 and 29-62). If taurine deficiency is corrected, this is the limit of the fundic changes; however, with continued dietary deficiency, extension of degeneration to the midperipheral retina is possible. Should the clinician suspect dietary taurine deficiency in a cat with retinal degeneration, confirmation of low plasma taurine is warranted. If plasma taurine is demonstrated to be low, dietary supplementation is required. With supplementation partial reversal of retinal degeneration is possible in cats with mild to moderate stages of disease, but prevention of further progression is the major therapeutic goal.[85,86]

Progressive Retinal Atrophy

Inherited retinal degeneration or dysplasia (often grouped together as progressive retinal atrophy) occurs in cats, particularly the Abyssinian and Persian breeds.[39,134,153] An autosomal recessive, early onset retinal photoreceptor dysplasia is seen in Persian cats and as an autosomal dominant condition in Abyssinian cats as early as 2 to 3 weeks of age.[39,153] In the Persian the earliest ocular abnormalities are subtly diminished PLRs at 2 weeks of age, progressing to minimal PLRs and resting mydriasis by 17 weeks of age. Funduscopic signs of retinal degeneration, such as retinal vascular attenuation, tapetal hyperreflectivity, and optic nerve head darkening, are minimal at 4 to 5 weeks but marked by 17 weeks of age. In the Abyssinian early onset retinal degeneration is a result of an autosomal dominant photoreceptor dysplasia.[39] As with the Persian, abnormal PLRs are first noted at approximately 2 to 3 weeks of age, but the terminal stage of disease is not reached until approximately 1 year of age.[39] Nystagmus accompanies this form of retinal degeneration.[39] A later onset autosomal recessive retinal degeneration also occurs in the Abyssinian. Early ophthalmoscopic evidence of retinal degeneration is visible at approximately 1.5 to 2 years of age, in the form of a gray discoloration of the peripapillary fundus and the area centralis in particular.[134] Disease progression is much slower than for early onset disease, with terminal stages being reached at approximately 3.5 to 4 years of age.[134] No treatment is possible for any of these conditions. Affected animals should not be bred.

Resources for Cat Owners

http://www.petplace.com/cats/living-with-a-blind-cat/page1.aspx

References

1. Acland GM, McLean IW, Aguirre GD et al: Diffuse iris melanoma in cats, *J Am Vet Med Assoc* 176:52, 1980.
2. Aguirre G, Bistner S: Microphakia with lenticular luxation and subluxation in cats, *Vet Med Small Anim Clin* 68:498, 1973.
3. Aguirre GD: Retinal degeneration associated with the feeding of dog foods to cats, *J Am Anim Hosp Assoc* 172:791, 1978.
4. Albert DM, Shadduck JA, Craft JL et al: Feline uveal melanoma model induced with feline sarcoma virus, *Invest Ophthalmol Vis Sci* 20:606, 1981.
5. Albert DM, Shadduck JA, Liu H-S et al: Animal models for the study of uveal melanoma, *Int Ophthalmol Clin* 20:143, 1979.
6. Angell J, Shively J, Merideth R et al: Ocular coccidioidomycosis in a cat, *J Am Vet Med Assoc* 187:167, 1985.
7. Aquino SM: Management of eyelid neoplasms in the dog and cat, *Clin Tech Small Anim Pract* 22:46, 2007.
8. Attali-Soussay K, Jegou J-P, Clerc B: Retrobulbar tumors in dogs and cats: 25 cases, *Vet Ophthalmol* 4:19, 2001.
9. Barrett PM, Meredith RE, Alarcon FL: Central amaurosis induced by an intraocular, posttraumatic fibrosarcoma in a cat, *J Am Anim Hosp Assoc* 31:242, 1995.
10. Bartoe JT, Davidson H, Horton MT et al: The effects of bimatoprost and unoprostone isopropyl on the intraocular pressure of normal cats, *Vet Ophthalmol* 8:247, 2005.
11. Bellhorn R, Barnett K, Henkind P: Ocular colobomas in domestic cats, *J Am Vet Med Assoc* 159:1015, 1971.
12. Bellhorn R, Henkind P: Intraocular malignant melanoma in domestic cats, *J Small Anim Pract* 10:631, 1970.
13. Bernays ME, Peiffer RL: Ocular infections with dematiaceous fungi in two cats and a dog, *J Am Vet Med Assoc* 213:507, 1998.
14. Bertoy RW, Brightman AH, Regan K: Intraocular melanoma with multiple metastases in a cat, *J Am Vet Med Assoc* 192:87, 1988.
15. Billson FM, Miller-Michau T, Mould JR et al: Idiopathic sclerosing orbital pseudotumor in seven cats, *Vet Ophthalmol* 9:45, 2006.
16. Binder DR, Herring IP: Duration of corneal anesthesia following topical administration of 0.5% proparacaine hydrochloride solution in clinically normal cats, *Am J Vet Res* 67:1780, 2006.
17. Bjerkas E, Arnesen K, Peiffer RL: Diffuse amelanotic iris melanoma in a cat, *Vet Comp Ophthalmol* 7:190, 1997.
18. Blocker T, Van der Woerdt A: The feline glaucomas: 82 cases (1995-1999), *Vet Ophthalmol* 4:81, 2001.
19. Blouin P, Cello R: Experimental ocular cryptococcosis. Preliminary studies in cats and mice, *Invest Ophthalmol Vis Sci* 19:21, 1980.
20. Brannan PA: A review of sclerosing idiopathic orbital inflammation, *Curr Opin Ophthalmol* 18:402, 2007.
21. Breit S, Kunzel W, Oppel M: The course of the nasolacrimal duct in brachycephalic cats, *Anat Histol Embryol* 32:224, 2003.
22. Brightman AH, Ogilvie GK, Tompkins MB: Ocular disease in FeLV-positive cats: 11 cases (1981-1986), *J Am Vet Med Assoc* 198:1049, 1991.
23. Burstein N: Preservative cytotoxic threshold for benzalkonium chloride and chlorhexidine digluconate in cat and rabbit corneas, *Invest Ophthalmol Vis Sci* 19:308, 1980.
24. Cai Y, Fukushi H, Koyasu S et al: An etiological investigation of domestic cats with conjunctivitis and upper respiratory tract disease in Japan, *J Vet Med Sci* 64:215, 2002.
25. Cantaloube B, Raymond-Letron I, Regnier A: Multiple eyelid apocrine hidrocystomas in two Persian cats, *Vet Ophthalmol* 7:121, 2004.
26. Cassotis N, Dubielzig R, Davidson M: Immunohistochemical analysis of primary ocular sarcomas in cats: 38 cases, *Proceedings of the American College of Veterinary Ophthalmologists*, 22, 1999.
27. Cassotis N, Dubielzig R, Gilger B et al: Angioinvasive pulmonary carcinoma with posterior segment metastasis in four cats, *Vet Ophthalmol* 2:125, 1999.
28. Chaitman J, van der Woerdt A, Bartick T: Multiple eyelid cysts resembling apocrine hidrocystomas in three Persian cats and one Himalayan cat, *Vet Pathol* 36:474, 1999.
29. Chetboul V, Lefebvre HP, Pinhas C et al: Spontaneous feline hypertension: clinical and echocardiographic abnormalities, and survival rate, *J Vet Intern Med* 17:89, 2003.
30. Chung S-H, Lee SK, Cristol SM et al: Impact of short-term exposure of commercial eyedrops preserved with benzalkonium chloride on precorneal mucin, *Mol Vis* 12:415, 2006.
31. Collier L, Bryan G, Prieur D: Ocular manifestations of the Chédiak-Higashi syndrome in four species of animals, *J Am Vet Med Assoc* 175:587, 1979.
32. Cook C, Peiffer R, Stine P: Metastatic ocular squamous cell carcinoma in a cat, *J Am Vet Med Assoc* 185:1547, 1984.
33. Cook CS, Wilkie DA: Treatment of presumed iris melanoma in dogs by diode laser photocoagulation: 23 cases, *Vet Ophthalmol* 2:217, 1999.
34. Corcoran KA, Peiffer RL, Koch SA: Histopathological features of feline ocular lymphosarcoma: 49 cases (1978-1992), *Vet Comp Ophthalmol* 5:35, 1995.
35. Crispin S, Mould J: Systemic hypertensive disease and the feline fundus, *Vet Ophthalmol* 4:131, 2001.
36. Cullen C, Lim C, Sykes J: Tear film breakup times in young healthy cats before and after anesthesia, *Vet Ophthalmol* 8:159, 2005.

37. Cullen CL, Haines DM, Jackson ML et al: Lack of detection of feline leukemia and feline sarcoma viruses in diffuse iris melanomas of cats by immunohistochemistry and polymerase chain reaction, *J Vet Diagn Invest* 14:340, 2002.
38. Cullen CL, Njaa BL, Grahn BH: Ulcerative keratitis associated with qualitative tear film abnormalities, *Vet Ophthalmol* 2:197, 1999.
39. Curtis R, Barnett KC, Leon A: An early-onset retinal dystrophy with dominant inheritance in the Abyssinian cat, *Invest Ophthalmol Vis Sci* 28:131, 1987.
40. Cutler TJ: Bilateral eyelid agensis repair in a captive Texas cougar, *Vet Ophthalmol* 5:143, 2002.
41. Czederpiltz JM, La Croix NC, Van der Woerdt A et al: Putative aqueous humor misdirection syndrome as a cause of glaucoma in cats: 32 cases (1997-2003), *J Am Vet Med Assoc* 227:1434, 2005.
42. Davidson MG, Lappin MR, English RV et al: A feline model of ocular toxoplasmosis, *Invest Ophthalmol Vis Sci* 34:3653, 1993.
43. Davidson MG, Nasisse MP, English RV et al: Feline anterior uveitis: a study of 53 cases, *J Am Anim Hosp Assoc* 27:77, 1991.
44. de Lormier L-P: Primary orbital melanoma without ocular involvement in a Balinese cat, *Can Vet J* 47:225, 2006.
45. Del Sole MJ, Sande PH, Bernades JM et al: Circadian rhythm of intraocular pressure in cats, *Vet Ophthalmol* 10:155, 2007.
46. Dietrich U, Chandler M, Cooper T et al: Effects of topical 2% dorzolamide hydrochloride alone and in combination with 0.5% timolol maleate on intraocular pressure in normal feline eyes, *Vet Ophthalmol* 10:95, 2007.
47. Drazenovich T, Fascetti A, Westermeyer H et al: Effects of dietary lysine supplementation on upper respiratory and ocular disease and detection of infectious organisms in cats within an animal shelter, *Am J Vet Res* 70:1391, 2009.
48. Dubielzig R, Bell C, Schobert C: *Feline orbital pseudotumor: a morphologic review of 14 cases, ACVO Annual Conference*, Boston, 2008.
49. Dubielzig R, Everitt J, Shadduck J et al: Clinical and morphological features of post-traumatic ocular sarcomas in cats, *Vet Pathol* 27:62, 1990.
50. Dubielzig R, Lindley D: The relationship between pigmented spots on the feline iris and diffuse iris melanoma, *Vet Pathol* 30:451, 1993.
51. Dubielzig RR: Feline ocular sarcomas. In Peiffer RL, Simons KB, editors: *Ocular tumors in animals and humans*, Ames, Iowa, 2001, Iowa State Press.
52. Dubielzig RR: Ocular sarcoma following trauma in three cats, *J Am Vet Med Assoc* 184:578, 1984.
53. Dubielzig RR, Everitt J, Shadduck JA et al: Feline ocular melanoma and post traumatic sarcoma, *Proceedings of the American College of Veterinary Ophthalmologists* 441, 1986.
54. Dubielzig RR, Grendahl RL, Orcutt JC et al: Metastases. In Peiffer RL, Simons KB, editors: *Ocular tumors in animals and humans*, Ames, Iowa, 2001, Iowa State Press, p 337.
55. Dubielzig RR, Hawkins KL, Toy KA et al: Morphologic features of feline ocular sarcomas in 10 cats: light microscopy, ultrastructure, and immunohistochemistry, *Vet Comp Ophthalmol* 4:7, 1994.
56. Duncan D, Peiffer R: Morphology and prognostic indicators of anterior uveal melanomas in cats, *Prog Vet Comp Ophthalmol* 1:25, 1991.
57. Elliott L, Barber P, Syme H et al: Feline hypertension: clinical findings and response to antihypertensive treatment in 30 cases, *J Small Anim Pract* 42:122, 2001.
58. Ellis T: Feline respiratory virus carriers in clinically healthy cats, *Aust Vet J* 57:115, 1981.
59. English RV, Davidson MG, Nasisse MP et al: Intraocular disease associated with feline immunodeficiency virus infection in cats, *J Am Vet Med Assoc* 196:1116, 1990.
60. Erickson PA, Fisher SK, Anderson DH et al: Retinal detachment in the cat: the outer nuclear and out plexiform layers, *Invest Ophthalmol Vis Sci* 24:927, 1983.
61. Fontenelle JP, Powell CC, Hill AE et al: Prevalence of serum antibodies against *Bartonella* species in the serum of cats with or without uveitis, *J Feline Med Surg* 10:41, 2008.
62. Fontenelle JP, Powell CC, Veir JK et al: Effect of topical ophthalmic application of cidofovir on experimentally induced primary ocular feline herpesvirus-1 infection in cats, *Am J Vet Res* 69:289, 2008.
63. Ford MM, Dubielzig RR, Giuliano EA et al: Ocular and systemic manifestations after oral administration of a high dose of enrofloxacin in cats, *Am J Vet Res* 68:190, 2007.
64. Gelatt KN, van der Woerdt A, Ketring KL et al: Enrofloxacin-associated retinal degeneration in cats, *Vet Ophthalmol* 4:99, 2001.
65. Gilger BC, Hamilton HL, Wilkie DA et al: Traumatic ocular proptosis in dogs and cats: 84 cases (1980-1993), *J Am Vet Med Assoc* 206:1186, 1995.
66. Gilger BC, McLaughlin SA, Whitley RD et al: Orbital neoplasms in cats: 21 cases (1974-1990), *J Am Vet Med Assoc* 201:1083, 1992.
67. Gionfriddo J: Feline systemic fungal infections, *Vet Clin N Am Small Anim Pract* 30:1029, 2000.
68. Gionfriddo JR, Fix AS, Niyo Y et al: Ocular manifestations of a metastatic pulmonary adenocarcinoma in a cat, *J Am Vet Med Assoc* 197:372, 1990.
69. Giudice C, Muscolo MC, Rondena M et al: Eyelid multiple cysts of the apocrine gland of Moll in Persian cats, *J Feline Med Surg* 11:487, 2009.
70. Glaze MB: Congenital and hereditary ocular abnormalities in cats, *Clin Tech Small Anim Pract* 20:74, 2005.
71. Glaze MB, Gelatt KN: Feline ophthalmology. In Gelatt KN, editor: *Veterinary ophthalmology*, ed 3, Baltimore, 1999, Lippincott Williams & Wilkins, p 997.
72. Glover T, Nasisse M, Davidson M: Acute bullous keratopathy in the cat, *Vet Comp Ophthalmol* 4:66, 1994.
73. Grahn BH, Stewart WA, Towner RA et al: Magnetic resonance imaging of the canine and feline eye, orbit, and optic nerves and its clinical application, *Can Vet J* 34:418, 1993.
74. Gray H, Willis A, Morgan R: Effects of topical administration of 1% brinzolamide on normal cat eyes, *Vet Ophthalmol* 6:285, 2003.
75. Greene RT, Troy GC: Coccidioidomycosis in 48 cats: a retrospective study (1984-1993), *J Vet Intern Med* 9:86, 1995.
76. Haid C, Kaps S, Gonczi E et al: Pretreatment with feline interferon omega and the course of subsequent infection with feline herpesvirus in cats, *Vet Ophthalmol* 10:278, 2007.
77. Hakanson N, Shively JN, Reed RE et al: Intraocular spindle cell sarcoma following ocular trauma in a cat: case report and literature review, *J Am Anim Hosp Assoc* 26:63, 1990.
78. Hampson E, Smith R, Bernays M: Primary glaucoma in Burmese cats, *Aust Vet J* 80:672, 2002.
79. Hargis AM, Ginn PE: Feline herpesvirus 1-associated facial and nasal dermatitis and stomatitis in domestic cats, *Vet Clin N Am Small Anim Pract* 29:1281, 1999.
80. Hargis AM, Ginn PE, Mansell JE et al: Ulcerative facial and nasal dermatitis and stomatitis in cats associated with feline herpesvirus 1, *Vet Dermatol* 10:267, 1999.
81. Harris BP, Dubielzig RR: Atypical primary ocular melanoma in cats, *Vet Ophthalmol* 2:121, 1999.
82. Harris BP, Miller PE, Bloss JR et al: Ophthalmomyiasis interna anterior associated with *Cuterebra* spp in a cat, *J Am Vet Med Assoc* 216:352, 2000.
83. Hartley C, Ladlow J, Smith KC: Cutaneous haemangiosarcoma of the lower eyelid in an elderly white cat, *J Feline Med Surg* 9:78, 2007.
84. Hartley J, Stevenson S, Robinson A et al: Conjunctivitis due to *Chlamydophila felis (Chlamydia psittaci* feline pneumonitis agent) acquired from a cat: case report with molecular characterization of isolates from the patient and cat, *J Infect* 43:7, 2001.
85. Hayes K, Carey RE: Retinal degeneration associated with taurine deficiency in the cat, *Science* 88:949, 1975.

86. Hayes K, Rabin AR, Berson EL: An ultrastructural study of nutritionally induced and reversed retinal degeneration in cats, *Am J Pathol* 78:504, 1975.
87. Herring IP: Clinical pharmacology and therapeutics Part 1: Mydriatics/cycloplegics, anesthetics, ophthalmic dyes, tear substitutes and stimulators, intraocular irrigating fluids, topical disinfectants, viscoelastics, fibrinolytics amd antifibrinolytics, antifibrotic agents, tissue adhesives, and anticollagenase agents. In Gelatt KN, editor: *Veterinary ophthalmology*, ed 4, Ames, Iowa, 2007, Blackwell, p 332.
88. Herring IP, Bobofchak MA, Landry MP et al: Duration of effect and effect of multiple doses of topical ophthalmic 0.5% proparacaine hydrochloride in clinically normal dogs, *Am J Vet Res* 66:77, 2005.
89. Hervás J, Chacón-M De Lara F, Sánchez-Isarria M et al: Two cases of feline visceral and cutaneous leishmaniosis in Spain, *J Feline Med Surg* 1:101, 1999.
90. Hervás J, Chacon-Manrique de Lara F, Lopez J et al: Granulomatous (pseudotumoral) iridociclitis associated with leishmaniasis in a cat, *Vet Rec* 149:624, 2001.
91. Hickman M, Reubel G, Hoffman D et al: An epizootic of feline herpesvirus, type 1 in a large specific pathogen-free cat colony and attempts to eradicate the infection by identification and culling of carriers, *Lab Animal* 28:320, 1994.
92. Hoffmann A, Blocker T, Dubielzig R et al: Feline periocular peripheral nerve sheath tumor: a case series, *Vet Ophthalmol* 8:153, 2005.
93. Holland JL, Outerbridge CA, Affolter VK et al: Detection of feline herpesvirus 1 DNA in skin biopsy specimens from cats with or without dermatitis, *J Am Vet Med Assoc* 229:1441, 2006.
94. Holt E, Goldschmidt MH, Skorupski K: Extranodal conjunctival Hodgkin's-like lymphoma in a cat, *Vet Ophthalmol* 9:141, 2006.
95. Horimoto T, Limcumpao J, Xuan X et al: Heterogeneity of feline herpesvirus type 1 strains, *Arch Virol* 126:283, 1992.
96. Jacobi S, Dubielzig RR: Feline primary open angle glaucoma, *Vet Ophthalmol* 11:162, 2008.
97. Junge R, Miller R, Boever W et al: Persistent cutaneous ulcers associated with feline herpesvirus type 1 infection in a cheetah, *J Am Vet Med Assoc* 198:1057, 1991.
98. Kalishman JB, Chappell R, Flood LA et al: A matched observational study of survival in cats wtih enucleation due to diffuse iris melanoma, *Vet Ophthalmol* 1:25, 1998.
99. Kirschner S, Niyo Y, Betts D: Intraocular hemangiosarcoma in three dogs and a cat, *Proceedings of the American College of Veterinary Ophthalmologists*, 1986.
100. Koch SA: Congenital ophthalmic abnormalities in the Burmese cat, *J Am Vet Med Assoc* 174:90, 1979.
101. Krohne SG: Effect of topically applied 2% pilocarpine and 0.25% demecarium bromide on blood-aqueous barrier permeability in dogs, *Am J Vet Res* 55:1729, 1994.
102. Kroll MM, Miller PE, Rodan I: Intraocular pressure measurements obtained as part of a comprehensive geriatric health examination from cats seven years of age or older, *J Am Vet Med Assoc* 219:1406, 2001.
103. Lappin M, Kordick D, Breitschwerdt E: *Bartonella* spp antibodies and DNA in aqueous humour of cats, *J Feline Med Surg* 2:61, 2000.
104. Lappin MR, Burney DP, Hill SA et al: Detection of *Toxoplasma gondii*-specific IgA in the aqueous humor of cats, *Am J Vet Res* 56:774, 1995.
105. Leiva M, Lloret A, Pena T et al: Therapy of ocular and visceral leishmaniasis in a cat, *Vet Ophthalmol* 8:71, 2005.
106. Lim CC, Reilly CM, Thomasy SM et al: Effects of feline herpesvirus type 1 on tear film break-up time, Schirmer tear test results, and conjunctival goblet cell density in experimentally infected cats, *Am J Vet Res* 70:394, 2009.
107. Littman MP: Spontaneous systemic hypertension in 24 cats, *J Vet Intern Med* 8:79, 1994.
108. Longbottom D, Coulter L: Animal chlamydioses and zoonotic implications, *J Comp Pathol* 128:217, 2003.
109. Low HC, Powell CC, Veir JK et al: Prevalence of feline herpesvirus 1, *Chlamydophila felis*, and *Mycoplasma* spp DNA in conjunctival cells collected from cats with and without conjunctivitis, *Am J Vet Res* 68:643, 2007.
110. Lybaert P, Delbecke I, Cohen-Solal A: Diagnosis and management of a wooden foreign body in the orbit of a cat, *J Feline Med Surg* 11:219, 2009.
111. Maeda K, Kawaguchi Y, Ono M et al: Restriction endonuclease analysis of field isolates of feline herpesvirus type 1 and identification of heterogeneous regions, *J Clin Microbiol* 33:217, 1995.
112. Maeda K, Kawaguchi Y, Ono M et al: Comparisons among feline herpesvirus type 1 isolates by immunoblot analysis, *J Vet Med Sci* 57:147, 1995.
113. Maggio F, DeFrancesco TC, Atkins CE et al: Ocular lesions associated with systemic hypertension in cats: 69 cases (1985-1998), *J Am Vet Med Assoc* 217:695, 2000.
114. Maggs DJ: Feline uveitis: an "intraocular lymphadenopathy," *J Feline Med Surg* 11:167, 2009.
115. Maggs DJ, Chang E, Nasisse MP et al: Persistence of herpes simplex virus type 1 DNA in chronic conjunctival and eyelid lesions of mice, *J Virol* 71:9166, 1998.
116. Maggs DJ, Collins BK, Thorne JG et al: Effects of L-lysine and L-arginine on in vitro replication of feline herpesvirus type-1, *Am J Vet Res* 61:1474, 2000.
117. Maggs DJ, Lappin MR, Nasisse MP: Detection of feline herpesvirus-specific antibodies and DNA in aqueous humor from cats with or without uveitis, *Am J Vet Res* 60:932, 1999.
118. Maggs DJ, Lappin MR, Reif JS et al: Evaluation of serologic and viral detection methods for diagnosing feline herpesvirus-1 infection in cats with acute respiratory tract or chronic ocular disease, *J Am Vet Med Assoc* 214:502, 1999.
119. Maggs DJ, Nasisse MP, Kass PH: Efficacy of oral supplementation with L-lysine in cats latently infected with feline herpesvirus, *Am J Vet Res* 64:37, 2003.
120. Maggs DJ, Sykes JE, Clarke H et al: Effects of dietary lysine supplementation in cats with enzootic upper respiratory disease, *J Feline Med Surg* 9:97, 2007.
121. Malik R, Lessels N, Webb S et al: Treatment of feline herpesvirus-1 associated disease in cats with famciclovir and related drugs, *J Feline Med Surg* 11:40, 2009.
122. Manfra Marretta S: Feline dental problems: diagnosis and treatment, *Feline Pract* 20:16, 1992.
123. Muir, P, Jones T, Howard P: A clinical and microbiological study of cats with protruding nictitating membranes and diarrhoea: isolation of a novel virus, *Vet Research* 127:324-330, 1990.
124. Martin CL, Stiles J, Willis M: Feline colobomatous syndrome, *Vet Comp Ophthalmol* 7:39, 1997.
125. McLaughlin SA, Whitley RD, Gilger BC et al: Eyelid neoplasms in cats: a review of demographic data, *J Am Anim Hosp Assoc* 29:63, 1993.
126. Miller Michau T, Proulx DR, Rushton SD et al: Introcular extramedullary plasmacytoma in a cat, *Vet Ophthalmol* 6:177, 2003.
127. Miller SA, Van der Woerdt A, Bartick TE: Retrobulbar pseudotumor of the orbit in a cat, *J Am Vet Med Assoc* 216:356, 2000.
128. Molleda J, Martin E, Ginel P et al: Microphakia associated with lens luxation in the cat, *J Am Anim Hosp Assoc* 31:209, 1995.
129. Morgan RM: Systemic hypertension in four cats: ocular and medical findings, *J Am Anim Hosp Assoc* 22:615, 1986.
130. Mould JR, Petersen-Jones SM, Peruccio C et al: Uveal melanocytic tumors. In Peiffer RL, Simons KB, editors: *Ocular tumors in animals and humans*, Ames, Iowa, 2001, Iowa State Press.
131. Muir P, Harbour D, Gruffydd-Jones T et al: A clinical and microbiological study of cats with protruding nictitating membranes and diarrhoea: isolation of a novel virus, *Vet Rec* 127:324, 1990.

132. Munson L, Wack R, Duncan M et al: Chronic eosinophilic dermatitis associated with persistent feline herpes virus infection in cheetahs *(Acinonyx jubatus)*, *Vet Pathol* 41:170, 2004.
133. Narfstrom K: Hereditary and congenital ocular disease in the cat, *J Feline Med Surg* 1:135, 1999.
134. Narfstrom K: Progressive retinal atrophy in the Abyssinian cat, *Invest Ophthalmol Vis Sci* 26:193, 1985.
135. Nasisse M, Dorman D, Jamison K et al: Effects of valacyclovir in cats infected with feline herpesvirus 1, *Am J Vet Res* 58:1141, 1997.
136. Nasisse MP, Glover TL, Moore CP et al: Detection of feline herpesvirus 1 DNA in corneas of cats with eosinophilic keratitis or corneal sequestration, *Am J Vet Res* 59:856, 1998.
137. Nasisse MP, Guy JS, Davidson MG et al: Experimental ocular herpesvirus infection in the cat, *Invest Ophthalmol Vis Sci* 30:1758, 1989.
138. Newkirk K, Rohrbach B: A retrospective study of eyelid tumors from 43 cats, *Vet Pathol* 46:916, 2009.
139. Noller C, Henninger W, Gronemeyer DH et al: Computed tomography-anatomy of the normal feline nasolacrimal drainage system, *Vet Radiol Ultrasound* 47:53, 2006.
140. Ollivier FJ, Plummer CE, Barrie KP: Ophthalmic examination and diagnostics: the eye examination and diagnostic procedures. In Gelatt KN, editor: *Veterinary ophthalmology*, ed 4, Ames, Iowa, 2007, Blackwell, p 438.
141. Owen W, Sturgess C, Harbour D et al: Efficacy of azithromycin for the treatment of feline chlamydophilosis, *J Feline Med Surg* 5:305, 2003.
142. Owens J, Nasisse M, Tadepalli S et al: Pharmacokinetics of acyclovir in the cat, *J Vet Pharmacol Ther* 19:488, 1996.
143. Patnaik A, Mooney S: Feline melanoma: a comparative study of ocular, oral, and dermal neoplasms, *Vet Pathol* 25:105, 1988.
144. Pearce J, Giuliano E, Galle L et al: Management of bilateral uveitis in a *Toxoplasma gondii*-seropositive cat with histopathologic evidence of fungal panuveitis, *Vet Ophthalmol* 10:216, 2007.
145. Peiffer R: Ciliary body epithelial tumors in the dog and cat: a report of 13 cases, *J Small Anim Pract* 24:347, 1983.
146. Peiffer RL, Monticello T, Bouldin TW: Primary ocular sarcomas in the cat, *J Small Anim Pract* 29:105, 1988.
147. Peiffer RL, Wilcock BP: Histopathologic study of uveitis in cats: 139 cases (1978-1988), *J Am Vet Med Assoc* 198:135, 1991.
147a. Pierce KE, Bartoe JT, Wilkie DA et al: An association between acute bullous keratopathy and administration of systemic anti-inflammatory/immunosuppressive therapy in cats, *Proceedings of the American College of Veterinary Ophthalmologists*, 2010, p 50.
148. Pion P, Kittleson M, Thomas W et al: Clinical findings in cats with dilated cardiomyopathy and relationship of findings to taurine deficiency, *J Am Vet Med Assoc* 201:267, 1992.
149. Pirie CG, Dubielzig RR: Feline conjunctival hemangioma and hemangiosarcoma: a retrospective evaluation of eight cases (1993-2004), *Vet Ophthalmol* 9:227, 2006.
150. Ployngam T, Tobias A, Smith S et al: Hemodynamic effects of methylprednisolone acetate administration in cats, *J Am Vet Med Assoc* 67:583, 2006.
151. Powell CC, Lappin MR: Causes of feline uveitis, *Compendium* 23:128, 2001.
152. Powell CC, Lappin MR: Clinical ocular toxoplasmosis in neonatal kittens, *Vet Ophthalmol* 4:87, 2001.
153. Rah H, Maggs DJ, Blankenship TN et al: Early-onset, autosomal recessive, progressive retinal atrophy in Persian cats, *Invest Ophthalmol Vis Sci* 46:1742, 2005.
154. Rainbow ME, Dziezyc J: Effects of twice daily application of 2% dorzolamide on intraocular pressure in normal cats, *Vet Ophthalmol* 6:147, 2003.
155. Rampazzo A, Appino S, Pregel P et al: Prevelance of *Chlamydophila felis* and feline herpesvirus 1 in cats with conjunctivitis in Northern Italy, *J Vet Intern Med* 17:799, 2003.
156. Ramsey DT, Gerding PA, Losonsky JM et al: Comparative value of diagnostic imaging techniques in a cat with exophthalmos, *Vet Comp Ophthalmol* 4:198, 1994.
157. Ramsey DT, Marretta SM, Harmor RE et al: Ophthalmic manifestations and complications of dental disease in dogs and cats, *J Am Anim Hosp Assoc* 32:215, 1996.
158. Rees T, Lubinski J: Oral supplementation with L-lysine did not prevent upper respiratory infection in a shelter population of cats, *J Feline Med Surg* 10:510, 2008.
159. Richter M, Guscetti F, Speiss B: Aldose reductase activity and glucose-related opacities in incubated lenses from dogs and cats, *Am J Vet Res* 63:1591, 2002.
160. Ridgway MD, Brightman AH: Feline glaucoma: a retrospective study of 29 clinical cases, *J Am Anim Hosp Assoc* 25:485, 1989.
161. Ruhli MB, Speiss B: Retrobulbare raumforderungen bei hund und katze: symptome und diagnostik, *Tierarztl Prax* 23:306, 1995.
162. Sandmeyer LS, Keller CBB, Bienzle, D: Effects of interferon-alpha on cytopathic changes and titers for feline herpesvirus-1 in primary cultures of feline corneal epithelial cells, *Am J Vet Res* 66:210, 2005.
163. Sansom J, Barnett K, Dunn K et al: Ocular disease associated with hypertension in 16 cats, *J Small Anim Pract* 35:604, 1994.
164. Sansom J, Rogers K, Wood JL: Blood pressure assessment in healthy cats and cats with hypertensive retinopathy, *Am J Vet Res* 65:245, 2004.
165. Sapienza JS: Feline lens disorders, *Clin Tech Small Anim Pract* 20:102, 2005.
166. Scherba G, Hajjar A, Pernikoff D et al: Comparison of a cheetah herpesvirus isolate to feline herpesvirus type 1, *Arch Virol* 100:89, 1988.
167. Schmidt SY, Berson EL, Hayes K: Retinal degeneration in cats fed casein. I Taurine deficiency, *Invest Ophthalmol* 15:47, 1976.
168. Schmidt SY, Berson EL, Watson G et al: Retinal degeneration in cats fed casein III. Taurine deficiency and ERG amplitudes, *Invest Ophthalmol Vis Sci* 16:673, 1977.
169. Seguin MA, Papich MG, Sigle KJ et al: Pharmacokinetics of enrofloxacin in neonatal kittens, *Am J Vet Res* 65:350, 2004.
170. Siebeck N, Hurley DJ, Garcia M et al: Effects of human recombinant alpha-2b interferon and feline recombinant omega interferon on in vitro replication of feline herpesvirus-1, *Am J Vet Res* 67:1406, 2006.
171. Snibson G, Greaves J, Soper N et al: Ocular surface residence times of artificial tear solutions, *Cornea* 11:288, 1992.
172. Sparkes A, Caney S, Sturgess C et al: The clinical efficacy of topical and systemic therapy for the treatment of feline ocular chlamydiosis, *J Feline Med Surg* 1:31, 1999.
173. Spiess AK, Sapienza JS, Mayordomo A: Treatment of proliferative feline eosinophilic keratitis with topical 1.5% cyclosporine: 35 cases, *Vet Ophthalmol* 12:132, 2009.
174. Stiles J: Ophthalmic manifestations of systemic disease part 2: the cat. In Gelatt KN, editor: *Veterinary ophthalmology*, ed 3, Baltimore, 1999, Lippincott Williams & Wilkins, p 1448.
175. Stiles J, Bienzle D, Render J et al: Use of nested polymerase chain reaction (PCR) for detection of retroviruses from formalin-fixed, paraffin-embedded uveal melanomas in cats, *Vet Ophthalmol* 2:113, 1999.
176. Stiles J, Polzin DJ, Bistner SI: The prevalence of retinopathy in cats with systemic hypertension and chronic renal failure or hyperthyroidism, *J Am Anim Hosp Assoc* 30:564, 1994.
177. Stiles J, Rankin A: Ophthalmomyiasis interna anterior in a cat: surgical resolution, *Vet Ophthalmol* 9:165, 2006.
178. Stiles J, Townsend WM: Feline ophthalmology. In Gelatt KN, editor: *Veterinary ophthalmology*, ed 4, Ames, Iowa, 2007, Blackwell, p 1095.
179. Stiles J, Townsend WM, Rogers QR et al: Effect of oral administration of L-lysine on conjunctivitis caused by feline herpesvirus in cats, *Am J Vet Res* 63:99, 2002.

180. Stoltz J, Carpenter J, Albert D et al: Histologic, immunohistochemical, and ultrastructural features of an intraocular sarcoma of a cat, *J Vet Diagn Invest* 6:114, 1994.
181. Storey ES, Gerding PA, Scherba G et al: Survival of equine herpesvirus-4, feline herpesvirus-1, and feline calicivirus in multidose ophthalmic solutions, *Vet Ophthalmol* 5:263, 2002.
182. Studdert M, Martin M: Virus diseases of the respiratory tract of cats. 1. Isolation of feline rhinotracheitis virus, *Aust Vet J* 46:99, 1970.
183. Studer ME, Martin CL, Stiles J: Effects of 0.005% latanoprost solution on intraocular pressure in healthy dogs and cats, *Am J Vet Res* 51:1220, 2000.
184. Suchy A, Bauder B, Gelbmann W et al: Diagnosis of feline herpesvirus infection by immunohistochemistry, polymerase chain reaction, and in situ hybridization, *J Vet Diagn Invest* 12:186, 2000.
185. Sykes J, Studdert V, Browning G: Comparison of the polymerase chain reaction and culture for the detection of feline *Chlamydia psittaci* in untreated and doxycycline-treated experimentally infected cats, *J Vet Intern Med* 13:146, 1999.
186. Syme HM, Barber PJ, Markwell PJ et al: Prevalence of systolic hypertension in cats with chronic renal failure at initial evaluation, *J Am Vet Med Assoc* 220:1799, 2002.
187. Thomasy SM, Lim CC, Reilly CM et al: Safety and efficacy of orally administered famciclovir in cats experimentally infected with feline herpesvirus 1, *Am J Vet Res* 72:85, 2011.
188. Thomasy SM, Maggs DJ, Moulin NK et al: Pharmacokinetics and safety of penciclovir following oral administration of famciclovir to cats, *Am J Vet Res* 68:1252, 2007.
189. Tornerup NR, Fomsgaard A, Nielsen NV: HSV-1-induced acute retinal necrosis syndrome presenting with severe inflammatory orbitopathy, proptosis, and optic nerve involvement, *Ophthalmology* 107:397, 2000.
190. Trost K, Peiffer RL, Nell B: Goniodysgenesis associated with primary glaucoma in an adult European Short-haired cat, *Vet Ophthalmol* 10:3, 2007.
191. Turner JL, Brogdon JD, Lees GE et al: Idiopathic hypertension in a cat with secondary hypertensive retinopathy associated with a high-salt diet, *J Am Anim Hosp Assoc* 26:647, 1990.
192. van der Woerdt A: Orbital inflammatory disease and pseudotumor in dogs and cats, *Vet Clin N Am Small Anim Pract* 38:389, 2008.
193. Van der Woerdt A, Peterson ME: Prevalence of ocular abnormalities in cats with hyperthyroidism, *J Vet Intern Med* 14:202, 2000.
194. Veith LA, Cure TH, Gelatt KN: The Schirmer tear test—in cats, *Mod Vet Pract* 51:48, 1970.
195. Volopich S, Benetka V, Schwendenwein I et al: Cytologic findings, and feline herpesvirus DNA and *Chlamydophila felis* antigen detection rates in normal cats and cats with conjunctival and corneal lesions, *Vet Ophthalmol* 8:25, 2005.
196. von Bomhard W, Polkinghorne A, Lu ZH et al: Detection of novel chlamydiae in cats with ocular disease, *Am J Vet Res* 64:1421, 2003.
197. Ward D, McEntee M, Weddle D: Orbital plasmocytoma in a cat, *J Small Anim Pract* 38:576, 1997.
198. Weiss R: Synergistic antiviral activities of acyclovir and recombinant human leukocyte (alpha) interferon on feline herpesvirus replication, *Am J Vet Res* 50:1672, 1989.
199. Wiebe V, Hamilton P: Fluoroquinolone-induced retinal degeneration in cats, *J Am Vet Med Assoc* 221:1568, 2002.
200. Wilcock B, Peiffer R, Davidson M: The causes of glaucoma in cats, *Vet Pathol* 27:35, 1990.
201. Wilkie D, Latimer C: Effects of topical administration of 2.0% pilocarpine on intraocular pressure and pupil size in cats, *Am J Vet Res* 52:441, 1991.
202. Williams D, Kim J: Feline entropion: a case series of 50 affected animals (2003-2008), *Vet Ophthalmol* 12:221, 2009.
203. Williams D, Robinson J, Lay E et al: Efficacy of topical aciclovir for the treatment of feline herpetic keratitis: results of a prospective clinical trial and data from in vitro investigations, *Vet Rec* 157:254, 2005.
204. Williams LW, Gelatt KN, Gwin RM: Ophthalmic neoplasms in the cat, *J Am Anim Hosp Assoc* 17:999, 1981.
205. Wolfer J: Correction of eyelid coloboma in four cats using subdermal collagen and a modified Stades technique, *Vet Ophthalmol* 5:269, 2002.
206. Wray JD, Doust RT, McConnell F et al: Retrobulbar teratoma causing exophthalmos in a cat, *J Feline Med Surg* 10:175, 2008.
207. Wyman M, Starkey R, Weisbrode S et al: Ophthalmomyiasis (interna posterior) of the posterior segment and central nervous system myiasis: *Cuterebra* spp. in a cat, *Vet Ophthalmol* 8:77, 2005.
208. Yang S-H, Liu C-H, Hsu C-D et al: Use of chemical ablation with trichloroacetic acid to treat eyelid apocrine hidrocystomas in a cat, *J Am Vet Med Assoc* 230:1170, 2007.
209. Zeiss C, Johnson E, Dubielzig R: Feline intraocular tumors may arise from transformation of lens epithelium, *Vet Pathol* 40:355, 2003.

CHAPTER

30

Respiratory and Thoracic Medicine

OUTLINE

THE UPPER RESPIRATORY TRACT

Jessica Quimby and Michael R. Lappin

Clinical signs of upper respiratory tract disease, including sneezing and nasal discharge, are common in cats (Box 30-1). Some diseases are associated with sneezing, and others are more commonly associated with stertorous breathing, with or without gagging. Coughing can sometimes be present, as well as epiphora, halitosis, dysphagia, and nonspecific signs such as lethargy, inappetence, and weight loss.[1,12,33] Laryngeal disease is rare in the cat but may present as acute or chronic dyspnea, stridor, dysphagia, and signs of upper airway obstruction.[84] Common causes of upper respiratory disorders in cats include trauma, foreign bodies, infectious agents, brachycephalic syndrome, inflammatory polyps, tooth root infections or other oral disease, nasopharyngeal stenosis, chronic rhinosinusitis, and neoplasia.[1,12,33] The most common causes of laryngeal disease in the cat are laryngeal paralysis and laryngeal neoplasia.[92] A complete diagnostic workup is important to determine the etiology so that the treatment regimen can be appropriately directed and maximal response to therapy is obtained.[76,77]

CLINICAL SIGNS

Nasal Disease

Nasal discharge is the most common clinical sign associated with nasal disease and can be serous, mucopurulent, or hemorrhagic[1,12,33] (see Box 30-1). Serous nasal discharge is characteristic of most acute diseases of the nasal cavity and may precede mucopurulent nasal discharge. If the serous nasal discharge is chronic, viral and allergic etiologies are most common. Mucopurulent nasal discharge implies inflammation and occurs in association with fungal disease, primary bacterial disease, or overgrowth of normal bacterial flora secondary to any chronic nasal disease, including neoplasia, chronic rhinosinusitis, oronasal fistula, foreign body, inflammatory polyp, fungal disease, and viral disease. In addition, cats with vomiting or regurgitation can develop sneezing or nasal discharge by aspirating gastrointestinal content into the nose through the nasopharynx.

Epistaxis alone is most common with trauma, acute foreign body, hypertension, and coagulopathy. Epistaxis that develops in conjunction with or after mucopurulent discharge is most common with fungal disease,

BOX 30-1

Differential Diagnoses for Nasal Discharge in Cats

Serous

Viral infection
Precursor to disease with mucopurulent discharge
Normal

Mucopurulent

Associated with oral disease
- Tooth root abscess
- Oronasal fistula

Nasopharyngeal polyp
Foreign body
Bacterial infection
- Primary or secondary

Viral infection
- Feline herpesvirus-1
- Feline calicivirus

Fungal infection
- *Cryptococcus* spp.
- *Aspergillus* spp.

Chronic rhinosinusitis
Neoplasia
- Lymphoma
- Squamous cell carcinoma
- Adenocarcinoma

Hemorrhagic

Nasal disease
- Trauma
- Foreign body
- Chronic rhinosinusitis
- Neoplasia
- Fungal disease

Systemic disease
- Hypertension
- Polycythemia
- Coagulopathy
- Hyperviscosity syndrome

neoplasia, oronasal fistula, and occasionally chronic foreign bodies. Vasculitis occurs in dogs with diseases such as ehrlichiosis and bartonellosis but is rare in cats. Unilateral nasal discharge is more likely with foreign bodies, oronasal fistula, and neoplasia, although the latter can become bilateral as it progresses. Bilateral discharge is nonspecific and can be found with almost any etiology.[33]

Sneezing is a superficial reflex that originates in the mucous membranes lining the nasal cavity and is easily induced by chemical or mechanical stimuli. The sneeze results in forceful expulsion of air that passes through the airways with great velocity to clear the respiratory passageways. Sneezing is a common manifestation of nasal disease but is relatively nonspecific.

Stertor is a harsh, audible snoring sound associated with inspiratory breathing. Cats that experience stertor while awake are also likely to snore when sleeping. Stertor indicates airway obstruction and is most common with such conditions as nasopharyngeal polyps, nasopharyngeal stenosis, and neoplastic masses that occlude the airway. It may also occur as a result of airway occlusion caused by turbinate inflammation. Facial deformity is relatively uncommon but is usually associated with neoplastic processes and fungal infections, particularly *Cryptococcus* spp.[1]

Laryngeal Disease

Laryngeal disease is rare in the cat but may present as acute or chronic dyspnea, signs of upper airway obstruction, stridor (a harsh, high-pitched sound heard on inspiration), and dysphagia. Coughing or gagging may also be appreciated, and aphonia (loss of voice) or a change in voice has been reported.[84]

GENERAL DIAGNOSTICS

Signalment and lifestyle will often help refine the differential list and direct a diagnostic workup. Brachycephalic breeds may be predisposed to nasal disorders because of their physical conformation.[85,112] Neoplasia is more likely in older cats,[33] and nasopharyngeal polyps are more common in younger cats.[40] Cats with outdoor access are more likely to develop foreign bodies, trauma, or infectious etiologies.[33] Cats in crowded housing conditions such as catteries, shelters, and multicat households are more likely to develop acute or chronic viral or bacterial rhinitis.[32] Obtaining a complete history is important for determining the duration of the clinical signs. Acute onset of clinical signs is common with viral agents, foreign bodies, and trauma. The diagnostic workup of sneezing and nasal discharge is commonly completed in three phases (Box 30-2).

Phase 1: Noninvasive Tests

Most cats with acute disease are generally evaluated with noninvasive tests and therapeutic trials. A complete physical examination with careful attention to the head and neck should be performed, including ocular retropulsion. Firm resistance to retropulsion of the orbit or a painful reaction could be indicative of a retrobulbar lesion. Otic examination should be completed to evaluate for bulging or discoloration of the tympanum; these changes commonly occur with nasopharyngeal polyps. Deformation of the nose or face, exophthalmia, or pain

BOX 30-2

Staged Workup of Upper Respiratory Disease

Phase 1 (Noninvasive)

History
Physical exam
CBC, chemistry, urinalysis
Thoracic +/− cervical radiographs
Cytology of nasal discharge
Cryptococcus antigen titer
Feline leukemia/feline immunodeficiency virus serology

Phase 2 (Sedation or Anesthesia Required)

Oral, pharyngeal, and laryngeal exam
Computed tomography
Nasal radiography
Nasal biopsy and histopathology
Tissue fungal and bacterial culture

Phase 3

Exploratory rhinotomy
Repetition of earlier phases

on palpation of the nasal or facial bones is most consistent with fungal disease or neoplasia.[1] Oral examination should be performed to assess for dental disease that could be causing an oronasal fistula, gingivostomatitis that could be consistent with feline herpesvirus (FHV-1) or feline calicivirus (FCV) infections, and defects in the hard or soft palate. External ocular examination may reveal conjunctivitis that could indicate FHV-1, FCV, *Mycoplasma* spp., or *Chlamydophila felis* infections. Fundic examination is performed to evaluate for lesions consistent with lymphoma or *Cryptococcus neoformans* infection. A cold microscope slide can be placed in front of the nose to assess airflow and may aid in determining if disease is unilateral or bilateral, although this should not limit diagnostic investigation to the obstructive side of the nose because bilateral disease may be present.

Although fungal organisms are uncommonly identified, cytology of nasal discharge should be performed on all cats with mucoid to mucopurulent nasal discharge to evaluate for the presence of *C. neoformans, Sporothrix schenckii,* or hyphae consistent with *Aspergillus* spp. or *Penicillium* spp. Neutrophils and bacteria are commonly detected if mucopurulent disease is present but do not prove primary bacterial disease. Hyphae also do not confirm primary fungal disease; they may represent contamination or infection secondary to another underlying cause. Secondary infections result in the same discharge as primary infections.

If lymph nodes draining the head are enlarged, they should be aspirated to evaluate for the presence of lymphoma, metastatic neoplasia, and fungal agents. Bacterial culture and antimicrobial susceptibility testing on nasal discharges are generally not recommended because results are difficult to interpret in that they typically yield normal intranasal bacterial flora.[43] However, in respiratory outbreaks in catteries, pet stores, shelters, and multicat households, culture may be indicated to determine whether a pathogenic *Bordetella bronchiseptica* isolate is present.

Molecular diagnostic assays are now available for many respiratory agents, including FHV-1, FCV, *C. felis, Mycoplasma* spp., and *B. bronchiseptica.* However, cats can be asymptomatic carriers of these agents, and the FHV-1, FCV, *B. bronchiseptica,* and *C. felis* assays also amplify vaccine strains of the organisms, which means that positive results do not prove a disease association. This is especially true for FHV-1 and FCV, which may have a relatively high prevalence in the healthy cat population.[52,78,98] Recently, a study failed to link *Bartonella* spp. infection to rhinitis in cats; therefore at this time recommendations to perform *Bartonella* spp. serology, culture, or polymerase chain reaction (PCR) assays in cats with upper respiratory tract signs are controversial.[6] If a clinician chooses to test for evidence of *Bartonella* spp. infection, the cat should be evaluated by serology and PCR or culture because serology alone has been shown to yield false-negative results in up to 15% of infected cats.[8] In addition, because only approximately 40% of seropositive cats are currently infected, a positive serologic test result does not prove bartonellosis.[8] See Chapter 33 and the subsequent sections in this chapter about individual agents for a further discussion of molecular assays.

A complete blood cell count (CBC), serum biochemical panel, and urinalysis is recommended to rule out other systemic disease processes in cats with chronic disease. In general, results of the CBC are of low yield but may reveal eosinophilia in some cats with fungal or allergic disease, thrombocytopenia in some cats with epistaxis, or other cytopenias that might accompany feline leukemia (FeLV) or feline immunodeficiency virus (FIV) infections. FeLV and FIV do not cause sneezing and nasal discharge primarily, but they have been associated with lymphoma and may induce immunodeficiency that predisposes to other infections; therefore testing for these agents is indicated. A *Cryptococcus* antigen test is also recommended as a preliminary test for any cat with chronic nasal discharge, but particularly for those with nasal deformation, lymphadenopathy, or retinal lesions.[59] Although thoracic radiographs are generally normal, they are still indicated to rule out pulmonary involvement of fungal disease and metastatic neoplasia. In cats with epistaxis, blood pressure measurement, coagulation profile, and buccal mucosal bleeding test are recommended, and thromboelastography may also be useful.

During phase 1, therapeutic trials are commonly attempted in cats with mild disease and usually consist of antibiotics, antiviral drugs, immunomodulators, or antihistamines (see the discussions of specific diseases that follow).

Phase 2: Imaging, Biopsy, Deep Cultures

If the physical examination indicates further diagnostic workup, a definitive diagnosis is not made during phase 1, or routine therapeutic trials fail, more aggressive diagnostic testing is indicated (typically requiring general anesthesia). Phase 2 diagnostics usually consist of pharyngeal and laryngeal examination, computed tomography (CT) scan or skull and dental radiographs, rhinoscopy, bacterial and fungal cultures, and biopsy to obtain samples for histology. In preparation for biopsies, a platelet estimate and an activated clotting time or other coagulation function test should be performed before anesthesia.

General anesthesia is induced by administering approximately one third of an induction dose of propofol (4 to 6 mg/kg intravenously), a short-acting thiobarbiturate, or ketamine combined with diazepam (ketamine 5 mg/kg intravenously and valium 0.3 mg/kg intravenously). The arytenoids are examined before intubation to make sure both are abducting normally on inspiration. Dopram can be used to stimulate respiration and increase intrinsic laryngeal motion at a dose of 2.2 mg/kg, administered intravenously. Oropharyngeal examination is performed to evaluate thoroughly for masses, foreign bodies, or palate defects. A spay hook and dental mirror can be used to help manipulate the soft palate to a position allowing visualization of the nasopharynx so that polyps, other masses, foreign material, or nasopharyngeal stenosis can be checked (Figure 30-1). A thorough dental examination should be performed and all teeth probed for evidence of oronasal fistula.

If a definitive diagnosis is not made, a CT scan or nasal, sinus, and dental radiographs are performed. If radiographs are performed, anesthesia is required for accurate positioning and should include a lateral view, ventrodorsal view, and intraoral and open-mouth bullae views. Nasal imaging can reveal increased density in the nasal cavity or bony lysis that could be consistent with a mass, turbinate destruction consistent with chronic rhinosinusitis or fungal disease, as well as radio-opaque foreign objects or tooth root abscessation.[44,69] Although more expensive and not widely available, a CT scan has the added advantage of better visualization of the sinuses and tympanic bullae and better assessment of bony lysis; it also allows assessment of the cribriform plate and brain so that the extent of a lesion can be evaluated[86] (Figure 30-2). It is also faster to perform than a full series of skull radiographs and allows for radiotherapy treatment planning if indicated. It is the preferred imaging

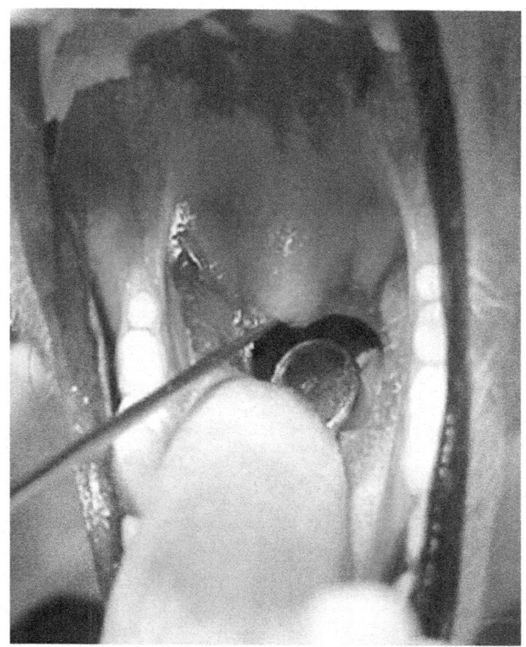

FIGURE 30-1 A spay hook and mirror can be used to assess the nasopharyngeal area.

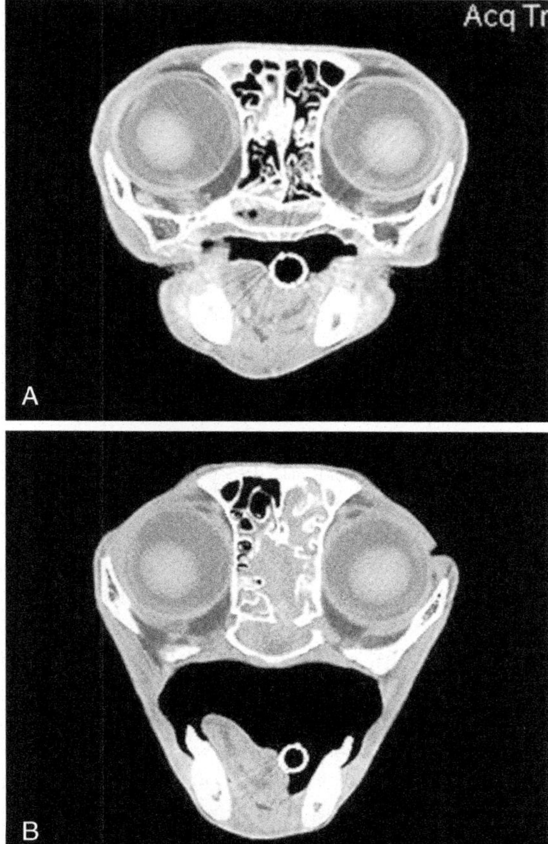

FIGURE 30-2 CT appearance of chronic rhinitis **(A)** versus nasal tumor **(B)**. A mass effect and bony lysis is noted in the nasal cavity.

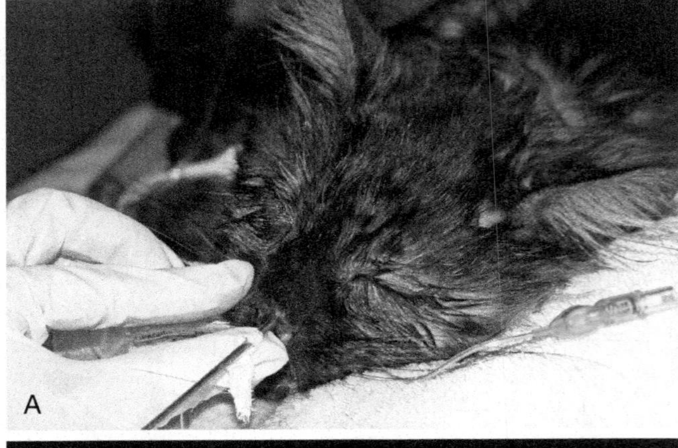

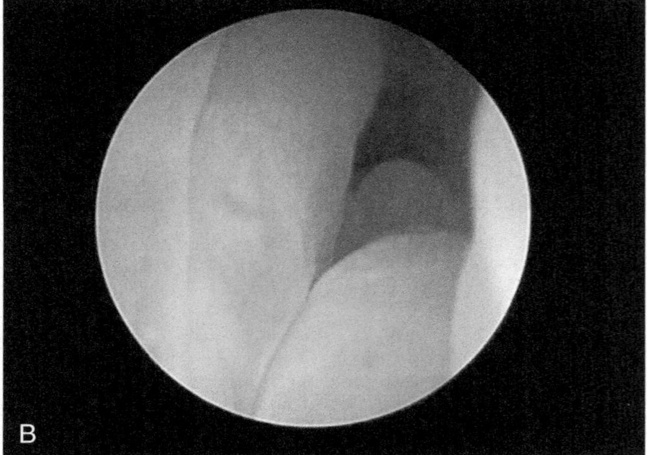

FIGURE 30-3 **A,** Rhinoscopy allows visualization of the nasal mucosa as well as sample collection. **B,** Erythematous and irregular nasal mucosa.

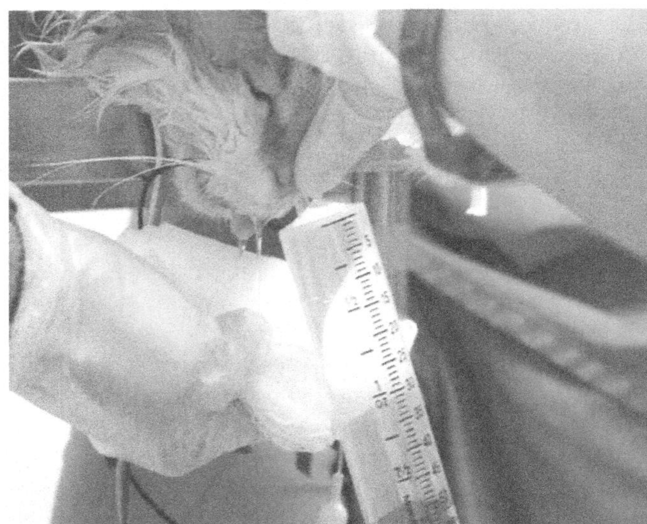

FIGURE 30-4 Nasal flush can be performed for diagnostic and therapeutic purposes.

modality, especially if a mass is suspected. Imaging should be performed before rhinoscopy and biopsy to prevent hemorrhage from obscuring details in the nasal passages.

Depending on imaging findings, the nasopharynx is examined with a flexible rhinoscope, and rigid rhinoscopy of the anterior nasal cavity is then performed (Figure 30-3). Rhinoscopy allows direct visualization of the nasal cavity, detection and removal of foreign objects, detection and débridement of fungal plaques, as well as assessment for inflammation, turbinate destruction, and masses. However, should a mass be present, rhinoscopy does not allow assessment of the extent of bony lysis (hence the importance of additional imaging). In addition, because gross appearance of the nasal mucosa on rhinoscopy does not always correlate with histopathologic diagnosis, biopsies should always be performed.[37]

If no foreign material is visualized on rhinoscopy, the nasal cavity is flushed with sterile saline to evaluate for the presence of hidden material. The cuff of the endotracheal tube should be checked for full inflation before performing nasal lavage with saline administered under pressure. In cats lavaging should be performed from the anterior nares caudally. Gauze should be placed in the oropharyngeal area and then a 20-, 35-, or 60-mL syringe can be used to forcefully flush saline through the nose while the nares are being pinched off to create pressure (Figure 30-4). Material flushed from the nose (or oropharynx) should be caught on the gauze and examined for foreign objects. If no foreign material is located, biopsies are then made using a bone curette or the largest biopsy instrument that can be passed through the nares. Most rigid endoscopes are too large for the biopsy sleeve to be used in many cats; a gastroscopic biopsy instrument can often be passed next to the camera of a rigid scope to perform directed biopsies. Alternatively, the biopsy site can be directed by the results of diagnostic imaging or by rhinoscopy. If indicated, bacterial and fungal cultures are made using material from flush or biopsied tissues.[39]

Phase 3: Exploratory Rhinotomy

Exploratory rhinotomy allows for direct visualization of the nasal cavity to identify foreign objects, masses, or fungal plaques and is occasionally performed to aid in the diagnostic workup and the treatment of some diseases. However, in cats it is rarely performed, except for cases requiring removal of chronically embedded foreign bodies or cases of *Aspergillus* spp. or other infections in the sinus in which endoscopic débridement was not sufficient or the condition was refractory to treatment. Surgical debulking is rarely required for cats with nasal cryptococcosis. In general, there is also no added benefit to debulking nasal tumors before chemotherapy (e.g., lymphoma) or radiation therapy. Although turbinate tissue can be removed to increase airflow through the nasal cavities, bacterial osteomyelitis is often present as well as nasal discharge, so this procedure is generally not recommended for cats with chronic inflammatory rhinitis.

DISEASE-SPECIFIC RECOMMENDATIONS: THE NASAL CAVITY

Anatomic and Functional Disorders

Nasopharyngeal Polyps

Nasopharyngeal polyps are non-neoplastic, inflammatory nodules that occur most commonly in young cats. They originate in the middle ear or auditory canal and can grow out through the nasopharynx or, alternatively, the tympanum.[34,40] Why the growths occur is unknown, but because they tend to occur when the cat is young, a congenital etiology has been postulated.[2] The possible association of polyps with infectious agents has also been explored, including FHV-1, FCV, *C. felis, Mycoplasma* spp., and *Bartonella* spp.,[41,108] but to date no organism has definitely been proven to be a cause. Large polyps can be detected by palpation through the soft palate, and otic examination may reveal discoloration or bulging of the tympanum. When extending into the nasopharynx, polyps disrupt the normal flow of secretions, resulting in secondary bacterial infections, mucopurulent nasal discharge, stertorous breathing, and gagging. Signs of middle ear involvement, such as Horner's syndrome and head tilt, can also be seen. Diagnosis can be confirmed with examination of the nasopharynx under sedation with a dental mirror and spay hook or rhinoscope, as previously described. A bulla radiography series or CT scan should be performed to determine whether there is bulla involvement. However, if there is no evidence of middle ear–associated clinical disease and the polyp can be removed by way of the mouth, many clinicians will perform removal using traction and wait for a recurrence before performing a bulla osteotomy on account of the high incidence of morbidity associated with bulla osteotomy[40,108] (Figure 30-5). Complications of this procedure include Horner's syndrome, facial nerve paralysis, and discomfort, and the recovery period is similar to that for a relatively invasive surgery. Without bulla osteotomy approximately 30% will be recurrent.[108] However, combining removal by traction with a tapering course of glucocorticoids (1 to 2 mg/kg per day, by mouth, for 14 days followed by a taper dosage over the next 2 weeks) may improve the success rate.[64] Bulla osteotomy is an effective surgical treatment, and when it is performed at initial presentation or at recurrence, most cases generally experience complete resolution.[40,103,108]

Brachycephalic Syndrome

Cats with brachycephalic conformation may experience difficulty with airflow due to the severe malformation of their nasal passages and nares, and potentially could be predisposed to nasal disease. A recent CT study of brachycephalic cats documented some of the abnormalities associated with this condition. It was found that the greater the degree of brachycephalia, measured by the amount of dorsal rotation of the maxillary canine tooth, the narrower the nasal cavity, nasal passages and nares.[85] Stenotic nares also serve to limit inspired airflow. This condition may be improved by alar fold excision, performed with a laser or scalpel technique or alternatively a punch resection alaplasty.[104] Nasopharyngeal turbinates have also been documented in brachycephalic cats and may serve to further reduce airflow through the nasopharyngeal area.[25] Little information is available regarding surgical options for nasopharyngeal turbinates.

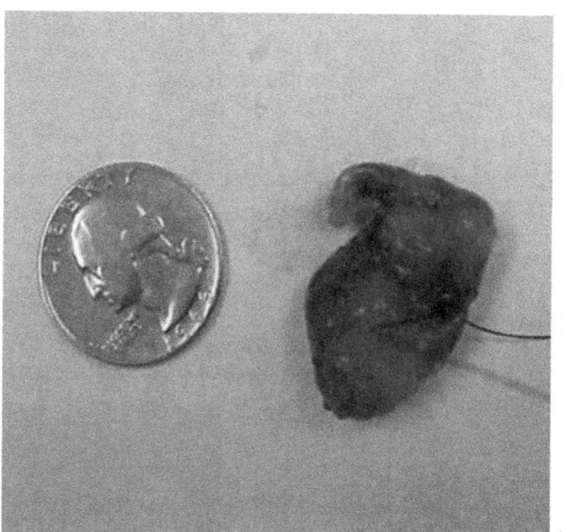

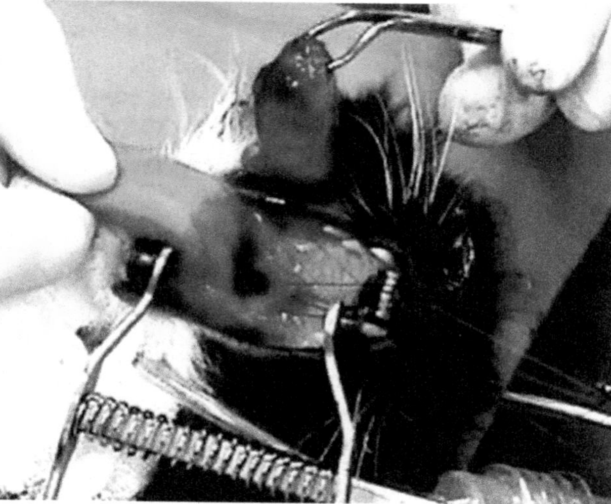

FIGURE 30-5 Manual removal of nasopharyngeal polyp.

Nasopharyngeal Stenosis

Nasopharyngeal stenosis is a rare condition that involves narrowing of the choanae to the extent that little air is able to pass. This can occur as a result of chronic infections, aspiration rhinitis, or congenital defect.[33,96] Clinical signs typically include stertorous, labored breathing and, less typically, nasal discharge. Diagnosis is determined by retroflex rhinoscopic assessment of the nasopharynx. In the past manual dilation and advanced surgical procedures combined with steroid therapy were the only therapeutic options, and recurrence was common.[33] More recently, stenting of the nasopharynx has been described as a successful palliative measure.[5]

Infectious Disorders

Bacterial Agents

DIAGNOSIS

Almost all cats with mucopurulent or purulent nasal discharge have a bacterial component to their disease. The bacterial agents that have been described as primary respiratory pathogens in cats include *B. bronchiseptica, C. felis, Streptococcus canis,* and *Mycoplasma* spp. However, *Corynebacterium* spp., *Escherichia coli, Pasteurella multocida, Pseudomonas aeruginosa, Streptococcus viridans,* and *Staphylococcus intermedius* are also commonly detected but generally thought to be secondary invaders.* Culture of either nasal flush samples or tissue biopsy samples yields similar species results, but aerobic and anaerobic cultures of nasal flushes were positive significantly more often in one study.[39] Culture of nasal biopsies may be more representative for deep mucosal infections,[38] but this has not been definitively shown. In another study different organisms were isolated from each collection technique, so it may be most complete to culture both nasal flush and biopsy samples.[38] However, it should be remembered that positive culture results may not correlate with the cause of the disease on account of the presence of normal flora and other superficial bacteria.

Although *B. bronchiseptica* is a well-defined primary pathogen in dogs, the organism can be isolated from many clinically normal cats.[32] Thus the positive predictive value (PPV) of serologic test results, culture, and PCR assay is low in cats. Many cats have antibodies against *B. bronchiseptica,* the organism is commonly cultured from cats in crowded environments, and there are sporadic reports of severe lower respiratory disease caused by bordetellosis in kittens and cats in crowded environments or other stressful situations.[7,110] The organism was cultured on necropsy from the lower airways of several cats from shelters in Colorado, and in one shelter the organism was cultured from 19 of 40 cats (47.5%) with upper respiratory disease.[91] However, the significance of infection in otherwise healthy pet cats appears to be minimal. For example, in client-owned cats in north central Colorado, the organism was rarely cultured from cats with rhinitis or lower respiratory disease (approximately 3%).[109] *B. bronchiseptica* is easily grown, and culture is superior to PCR for this agent because antimicrobial susceptibility testing can be performed on isolates. Because the organism is not usually eliminated by treatment, follow-up culture or PCR assay after treatment has minimal benefit.[9]

C. felis is a common differential diagnosis for cats with clinical evidence of conjunctivitis and rhinitis; it is not a common cause of lower airway disease. The organism is difficult to culture, so PCR detection of microbial DNA from conjunctival swabs can be useful clinically. Because of the intracellular nature of the organism, adequate cellular material must be obtained from the conjunctival swab for analysis.[28] PCR assay results can be used to prove a cattery has been cleared of the infection after treatment.[95] Most, but not all, PCR-positive cats are clinically ill (e.g., 3.3% if healthy cats were positive in one study).[13]

Mycoplasma spp. are normal commensal organisms of the mucous membranes of multiple species, including cats. *M. felis* has been associated primarily with conjunctivitis but is suspected as a primary cause of rhinitis in cats as well.[31,38,39] There are multiple *Mycoplasma* spp. of cats, and the pathogenic potential for most is unknown. If other primary diseases are present, even nonpathogenic *Mycoplasma* spp. may be associated with the disease process. *Mycoplasma* spp. culture can be difficult and takes longer than routine culture, and antimicrobial susceptibility is not provided by most laboratories. Culture of nasal biopsy samples rather than nasal flush samples may increase yield.[39] *Mycoplasma* spp. PCR assays have at least some clinical utility, with some assays allowing for speciation, which is helpful in assessing the pathogenic potential of the organism. However, because *Mycoplasma* spp. are common flora, the PPV of the assays is likely to be low. Because the organism is not usually eliminated by treatment, follow-up culture or PCR assay after treatment has minimal benefit.

TREATMENT

If primary bacterial infections are suspected, doxycycline 10 mg/kg, administered orally once daily for cats with rhinitis with or without conjunctivitis, is usually effective (Table 30-1). Doxycycline is the treatment of choice for *B. bronchiseptica, Mycoplasma* spp., and *C. felis* infections,[19,28] and in the last has been shown to be superior to topical administration of tetracycline.[90] Side-effects in young kittens are less of a concern with doxycycline than tetracycline but should still be taken into consideration. Amoxicillin–clavulanate is a good choice in young animals and is effective for most organisms, with the exception of *Mycoplasma* spp. because these organisms lack a cell wall. Pradofloxacin has been

*References 7, 9, 16, 31, 83, 88, 91, 109, 110.

TABLE 30-1 **Pharmacologic Treatment of Upper Respiratory Tract Disease**

Class	Drug	Dosage
Antibiotics	Amoxicillin	10-22 mg/kg, PO, every 12 hours
	Amoxicillin-clavulanate	13.75 mg/kg, PO, every 12 hours
	Azithromycin	15 mg/kg, PO, every 24 hours
	Cefadroxil	22 mg/kg, PO, every 12 hours
	Cephalexin	22 mg/kg, PO, every 8 hours
	Chloramphenicol	10-15 mg/kg, PO, every 12 hours
	Clindamycin	10-12 mg/kg, PO, every 24 hours
	Doxycycline	10 mg/kg, PO, every 24 hours
	Enrofloxacin	2.5-5 mg/kg, PO, every 24 hours
	Marbofloxacin	2.5-5 mg/kg, PO, every 24 hours
	Metronidazole	10-15 mg/kg, PO, every 12 hours
	Orbifloxacin	2.5-5 mg/kg, PO, every 24 hours
	Pradofloxacin	5-10 mg/kg, PO, every 24 hours
	Trimethoprim-sulfonamide	15 mg/kg, PO, every 12 hours
Antihistamines	Cetirizine	2.5-5 mg/cat, PO, every 24 hours
	Chlorpheniramine	2 mg/cat, PO, every 12 hours
	Clemastine	0.68 mg/cat, PO, every 12 hours
	Fexofenadine	5-10 mg/cat, PO, every 12 to 24 hours
	Hydroxyzine	5-10 mg/cat, PO, every 8 to 12 hours
	Loratadine	5 mg/cat, PO, every 24 hours
Antifungals	Deoxycholate amphotericin B	1) IV: 0.1-0.5 mg/kg: M, W, F; to 16 mg/kg total cumulative dose 2) SC: 0.5-0.8 mg/kg in 400 mL of 0.45% saline/2.5% dextrose; M, W, F; to 16 mg/kg total cumulative dose
	Fluconazole	50 mg/cat, PO, every 12 to 24 hours
	Itraconazole	10 mg/kg, PO, every 24 hours
	Liposomal amphotericin B	1 mg/kg IV; Mon, Wed, Fri; to 12 mg/kg total cumulative dose
Antivirals	Cidofovir topical (0.5%)	1 drop OU, every 12 hours
	Famciclovir	62.5 mg/cat, PO, every 12 hours, 14 days
	Interferon-alpha	10 U PO, every 24 hours (chronic); 10,000 U SC, every 24 hours, 21 days (acute)
	Lysine	500 mg/cat, PO, every 12 hours
NSAIDs	Meloxicam	0.025-0.1 mg/kg, PO, every 2 to 3 days
	Piroxicam	0.3 mg/kg, PO, every 2 days
Glucocorticoids	Beclomethasone (inhaled)	1-2 puffs, every 12 to 24 hours
	Fluticasone (inhaled)	1-2 puffs, every 12 to 24 hours
	Methylprednisolone acetate	5-15 mg IM, every 3 to 4 weeks, as needed
	Prednisolone	2.5-5 mg/cat, PO, every 1 to 2 days

PO, By mouth; *IV*, intravenously; *SC*, subcutaneously; *OU*, each eye; *NSAIDs*, nonsteroidal antiinflammatory drugs; *IM*, intramuscularly.

shown to have efficacy against *Mycoplasma* spp.[16,31] Enrofloxacin has also been shown to be effective for *C. felis*[23] but should be used with caution in young cats because of possible adverse effects on cartilage. Although the drug has not been shown to damage chondrocytes in cats, this does occur in several other species. Clindamycin penetrates bone and tissues well and has an excellent anaerobic spectrum. Administering the liquid form of this drug is generally well tolerated if given cold. Azithromycin therapy (15 mg/kg, administered orally once daily) can be tried for cats with suspected resistant bacterial infections.*

Doxycycline and clindamycin have been associated with esophagitis and esophageal strictures in cats[4,24,61] because of the poor secondary esophageal contractions in this species. The authors recommend never administering dry pills or capsules to cats. Drugs should be compounded into a liquid, administered, and then followed with a 3- to 6-mL liquid bolus or food, administered coated with butter or a product such as Nutri-Cal, or administered in a pill-delivery treat.[27,50,111] Cats with acute disease are treated for 7 to 10 days, except for *C. felis*, in which 28 days of therapy is needed to eliminate infection.[31,95] Chronic bacterial disease may require treatment for 6 to 8 weeks to adequately clear the infection if osteomyelitis exists. Pulse therapy may help some chronically affected cats but may induce antimicrobial resistant bacteria in other cats. Most cases of bacterial rhinitis are secondary to other diseases, including trauma, neoplasia, inflammation induced by viral

*References 16, 31, 83, 91, 94, 95.

infection, foreign bodies, inflammatory polyps, chronic rhinosinusitis, and tooth root abscessation. Thus if routine antibiotic therapy fails, a diagnostic workup should be performed.

PREVENTION

The currently available *B. bronchiseptica* vaccine for intranasal administration can be administered as early as 4 weeks of age, has an onset of immunity as early as 72 hours, and has a minimum duration of immunity of 1 year.[81] The American Association of Feline Practitioners (AAFP) Feline Vaccine Advisory Panel, and the European Advisory Board on Cat Diseases (ABCD) recommendations suggest that *Bordetella* vaccination should be considered primarily for use in cats at high risk for exposure and disease, such as those with a history of respiratory problems and living in humane shelters with culture-proven outbreaks.[19,81] However, because the vaccine is administered by the intranasal route, mild sneezing and coughing can result, which may influence case management of kittens housed in shelters or humane societies. Because the disease is apparently not life-threatening in adult cats, is uncommon in pet cats, responds to a variety of antibiotics, and is considered minimally zoonotic,[18] routine use of this vaccine in the majority of client-owned cats seems unnecessary.

Killed and modified live *C. felis*–containing vaccines are available. In recent studies *C. felis* was amplified from conjunctival swabs of 3.2% of cats with conjunctivitis[49] but 0% of nasal discharges from cats housed in a humane society.[91] FVRCP vaccines that also contained *C. felis* were associated with more vaccine reactions in cats when compared to other products.[63] Because infection of cats by *C. felis* generally results only in mild conjunctivitis, is easily treated with antibiotics, has variable prevalence rates, and is of minimal zoonotic risk to humans, some researchers have questioned whether *C. felis* vaccination is ever necessary in the United States.[14] Duration of immunity for *Chlamydophila* vaccines may be short-lived, so high-risk cats, such as those in multicat environments or where there is a history of chlamydial infection, should be immunized before a potential exposure.

Viral Agents

DIAGNOSIS

The most common viruses associated with feline respiratory disease are FCV and FHV-1. Both viruses are extremely common in cats, particularly those from crowded environments such as pet stores, catteries, and shelters.[14,32] There are many strains of FCV, and mutations resulting in new strains are common. This organism is a common differential diagnosis for cats with clinical evidence of rhinitis, stomatitis, oral ulceration, and conjunctivitis (Figure 30-6). Less commonly, FCV is associated with polyarthritis, lower airway disease in kittens, and virulent systemic disease.[78] Some variants of FCV are thought to induce systemic vasculitis in cats (virulent systemic calicivirus [VS-FCV]), and clinical signs can be severe even in cats previously vaccinated with FVRCP vaccines.[10,36,72,87,105] VS-FCV strains arise spontaneously from endogenous FCV strains, and outbreaks have resolved quickly after the initial cases were recognized. Currently, it is unknown how often these outbreaks occur and whether the number of outbreaks is increasing. The VS-FCV strains evaluated to date have been genetically and antigenically diverse.[42,71]

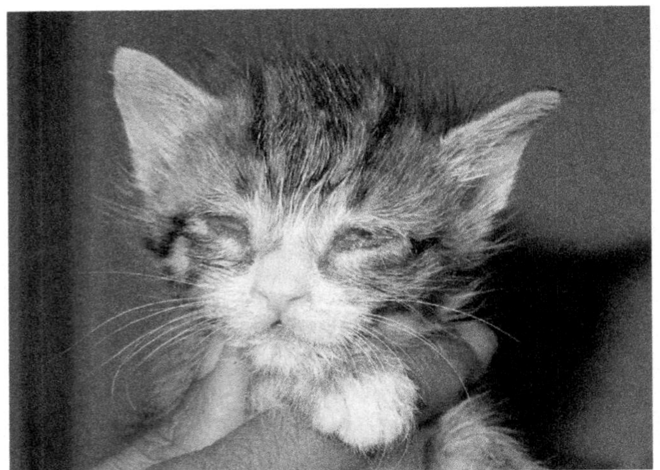

FIGURE 30-6 Clinical appearance of a kitten with herpesvirus infection.

Virus isolation can be used to document current infection but takes at least several days for results and is not performed by all laboratories. Because of widespread exposure and vaccination, the PPV of serologic tests is poor. Reverse transcriptase (RT) PCR assays can be used to amplify the RNA of calicivirus, and results can be made available quickly. However, these assays also amplify vaccine strains of FCV (Lappin MR: unpublished data, 2010). FCV RNA can be amplified from samples collected from normal carrier cats as well as clinically ill cats, and PCR assays therefore have poor PPV. In addition, amplification of FCV RNA cannot be used to prove virulent systemic calicivirus infection.[78] False-negative results of FCV RT-PCR can also occur if inadequate RNA is present on the submitted swab or if the organism has been cleared to levels below the sensitivity limits of the assay by specific immune responses. Because treatment does not eliminate FCV infection, there is no benefit to follow-up culture or RT-PCR testing.

FHV-1 is a common differential diagnosis for cats with clinical evidence of rhinitis, stomatitis, conjunctivitis, keratitis, and facial dermatitis. Because of widespread exposure and vaccination, the PPV of serologic tests is poor. FHV-1 infection can be documented by direct fluorescence staining of conjunctival scrapings, virus isolation, or PCR.[98] FHV-1 DNA can be amplified from conjunctival cells of approximately 20% of healthy cats; therefore the PPV of PCR assays for this agent is low.[79] Currently used PCR assays also detect vaccine strains of FHV-1, further lessening the PPV.[52] Quantitative PCR may ultimately prove to correlate with the presence or absence of disease but failed to correlate to presence of conjunctivitis in one small study in the authors' laboratory.[49] The negative predictive value of the FHV-1 PCR assays is also in question because many cats that are likely to have FHV-1–associated disease are PCR negative. This may relate to clearance of FHV-1 DNA from tissues by the immune reaction. Tissue biopsies have greater sensitivity than conjunctival swabs but do not necessarily have greater predictive value.[93] FHV-1 DNA can be amplified from the aqueous humor of some cats, but whether this indicates FHV-1–associated uveitis is unknown.[54] Because treatment does not eliminate FHV-1 infection, there is no benefit to follow-up culture or PCR testing.

TREATMENT

Therapy for FCV consists mainly of supportive care, which is often needed for cats with VS-FCV infections, and may consist of intravenous fluids, antibiotics for concurrent bacterial infections, and interferon. Interferon may augment immune responses to viral infections by upregulating key cytokines.[101] Feline interferon omega (1 to 2.5 million IU/kg, intravenously or subcutaneously, every 24 to 48 hours for up to 5 doses, then reduce to twice weekly and eventually to once weekly, depending on clinical response) (Virbagen Omega, Virbac Animal Health) inhibits FCV replication in vitro, but results of controlled studies evaluating efficacy in clinically affected cats with respiratory disease are not available. If human alpha interferon is used systemically for cats with life-threatening FCV or FHV-1 infections, 10,000 U/kg, administered subcutaneously, can be administered safely once daily, but controlled data concerning efficacy are not available. Recently, use of feline interferon therapy has been used to improve quality of life in cats with FeLV and FIV infections.[11] In one study low-dose oral interferon therapy (10 U/kg, orally, daily alternating 7 days on, 7 days off, for 6 months) improved quality of life in cats with FIV infections.[73] The effect of oral interferon is thought to be from mediation of inflammatory cytokines. There may also be effects against chronic FHV-1 or FCV infections, but controlled data are not available. Topical administration of alpha interferon in saline to the eyes of cats with conjunctivitis or the nose has been recommended by some veterinarians as an aid in the management of some cats with acute or chronic FHV-1 or FCV infections.

Recently, antiviral drugs have become more popular in the management of cats with acute or chronic FHV-1 infections. Currently available antiviral medications are efficacious only for DNA viral infections such as FHV-1, and not RNA viruses such as FCV, because they interfere with viral DNA synthesis and thus viral replication. Acyclovir and valacyclovir have been administered to some cats but can induce bone marrow suppression and are minimally effective for FHV-1; therefore they should no longer be used.[51,66] Famciclovir is safe and effective and is used for both acute and long-term therapy for cats with FHV-1 infections. One dose that has been used with apparent clinical efficacy is 62.5 mg, orally, every 12 hours for 14 days.[58] However, recent pharmacokinetic studies indicate that higher doses may be needed for activity against FHV-1.[99]

Idoxuridine and trifluridine have been used topically in cats with conjunctivitis or keratitis resulting from FHV-1 infection, but these must be administered multiple times per day and are irritating. Recently, cidofovir was used in a small experimental FHV-1 conjunctivitis study and was shown to lessen clinical signs and FHV-1 shedding.[21] Lysine at 250 to 500 mg, orally, every 12 hours may be helpful in some cats with acute or chronic rhinosinusitis caused by FHV-1 infection (not FCV).[53] However, in several controlled studies of cats fed a lysine-fortified diet, a significant positive effect was not noted.[17,55,80]

Intranasal administration of modified live FHV-1 and FCV vaccines may lessen disease in some chronically infected cats, but controlled data are lacking. If there is a positive response to intranasal vaccination in a cat with chronic disease, this form of immunotherapy can be administered up to three times per year. Intranasal vaccination has been shown to potentiate cell-mediated immunity to FHV-1 better than parenteral vaccination.[48] Chronic administration of one commercially available probiotic (FortiFlora, Purina Veterinary Diets) was shown to enhance T-helper lymphocyte numbers in cats.[106] When this probiotic was administered to cats with chronic FHV-1 infections that were then subjected to mild stress, improved conjunctivitis scores were noted in some of the cats in the treatment group.[47] See the section on chronic rhinosinusitis for a discussion of other nonspecific therapies.

PREVENTION

Specific pathogen-free (SPF) cats inoculated with one dose of intranasal modified live FVRCP vaccine had significantly less clinical signs than control cats as soon as 4 days when challenged with virulent FHV-1 in one study.[45] Administration of the intranasal FVRCP vaccine was also shown to induce FCV antibody responses in SPF kittens more quickly than a modified live FVRCP vaccine administered parenterally.[46] Thus the intranasal route of administration may be preferred for the primary or booster immunization of kittens housed in environments at high risk for exposure to FHV-1 or FCV, such as shelters, humane societies, catteries, boarding facilities, and multicat households. However, because administration of intranasal FHV-1 and FCV vaccines can induce transient mild sneezing or coughing, the owners should be informed of these potential side effects. Additionally, these vaccine side effects may influence case management of kittens housed in shelters or humane societies. Subcutaneous vaccines are recommended if concerns about the respiratory side effects of intranasal vaccines exist. Currently, yearly revaccination for cats in high-risk environments (e.g., shelters, catteries, multicat household) and a 3-year revaccination interval for cats in low-risk environments (indoor-only with no contact with other cats) are recommended.[78,81,98]

Inactivated vaccines containing VS-FCV are now available (Calicivax, Boehringer Ingelheim Vetmedica). The product contains a traditional FCV vaccine strain as well as a VS-FCV strain. Cross-neutralization studies show that cats inoculated with more than one FCV strain inactivate more FCV strains in vitro than cats inoculated with one FCV strain.[74,75] In addition, a recent challenge study illustrated that kittens vaccinated with the dual-strain product were protected from clinical signs of VS-FCV.[35]

Fungal Agents

C. neoformans and *Aspergillus* spp. are the most common causes of respiratory tract fungal infection in cats.[3,57,68] Cryptococcosis is most common and should be considered a differential diagnosis for cats with respiratory tract disease, subcutaneous nodules, lymphadenopathy, intraocular inflammation, fever, and central nervous system disease.[57] Infected cats range from 6 months to 16 years of age, and male cats are overrepresented in some studies.[67] Infection of the nasal cavity is reported most frequently and commonly results in sneezing and nasal discharge. The nasal discharge can be unilateral or bilateral, ranges from serous to mucopurulent, and often contains blood. Granulomatous lesions extruding from the external nares, facial deformity over the bridge of the nose, and ulcerative lesions on the nasal planum are common (Figure 30-7). Submandibular lymphadenopathy is detected in most cats with rhinitis. Definitive diagnosis of cryptococcosis is based on antigen testing or cytologic, histopathologic, or culture demonstration of the organism.

Cats with cryptococcosis have been treated with amphotericin B, ketoconazole, itraconazole, fluconazole, and 5-flucytosine alone and in varying combinations. Responses have varied among studies, but good to excellent treatment responses are often achieved in cats administered fluconazole or itraconazole.[60,67] Because of toxicity and the availability of more efficacious drugs, ketoconazole is no longer recommended by these authors. Fluconazole at 50 mg per cat, orally, once or twice daily is recommended because it results in the fewest side effects, has the best penetration across the blood–brain and blood–ocular barriers of the azoles, and has been shown to have good efficacy.[60,67] If life-threatening infection is occurring or the cat is failing to respond to an azole drug, amphotericin B should be used.[67] A typical amphotericin protocol involves intravenous infusions on a Monday–Wednesday–Friday schedule until a cumulative dose of 16 mg/kg has been reached. Nephrotoxicity is the most serious side effect, and an initial infusion dose of 0.1 mg/kg is used as a test dose. The dose can be slowly increased to 0.5 mg/kg if it is well tolerated clinically and if renal values remain stable.[26,56] A successful subcutaneous protocol has also been described in which 0.5 to 0.8 mg/kg is added to 0.45% saline/2.5% dextrose, and the total volume is given two to three times weekly to a cumulative dose of 8 to 26 mg/kg.[56,67]

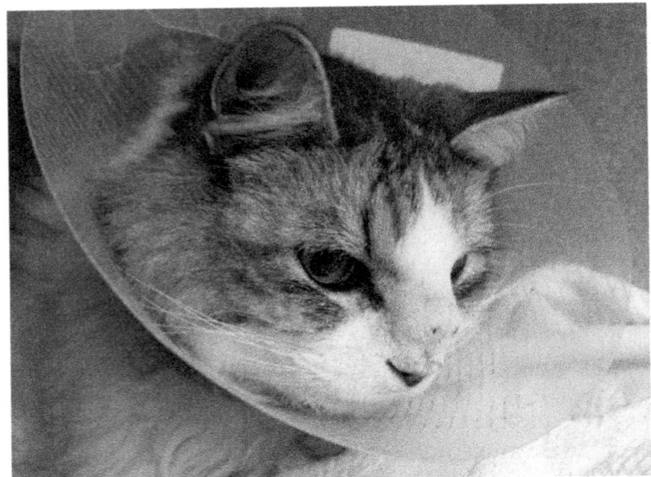

FIGURE 30-7 Although *Cryptococcus* and *Aspergillus* are the most common upper respiratory fungal infections in cats, nasal deformity may also be associated with *Sporothrix* spp. infection.

In addition to the deoxycholate form of amphotericin B, a liposomal formulation is also available. It is thought that less nephrotoxicity is seen with the liposomal product, and a recommended dose regimen is 1 mg/kg, intravenously, on a Monday–Wednesday–Friday schedule until a cumulative dose of 12 mg/kg has been reached.[26] Focal nasal and cutaneous cryptococcosis generally resolves with treatment; central nervous system, ocular, and disseminated diseases are less likely to respond to treatment.[60,67] Treatment should be continued for at least 1 to 2 months past resolution of clinical disease, or until antigen titers are negative.[20,67] People and animals can have the same environmental exposure to *Cryptococcus* spp., but zoonotic transfer from contact with infected animals is unlikely.

Aspergillosis is less common than cryptococcosis but can be equally devastating.[3,102,112] Clinical signs of mild disease are similar to those of nasal cryptococcosis. Sino-orbital aspergillosis was recently described in cats and appears to be more aggressive than canine aspergillosis, involving invasion into surrounding structures.[3] Ocular involvement, such as exophthalmos and ocular discharge, can be seen in addition to nasal signs. Diagnosis of aspergillosis is based on visualization of fungal plaques on rhinoscopy or fungal hyphae on cytology or biopsy. Infection can be caused by either *Aspergillus* spp. or *Penicillium* spp., which can be difficult to differentiate cytologically. Fungal culture seems less sensitive and specific than visualization on rhinoscopy or biopsy.[112] Therapy with oral itraconazole and fluconazole has been documented as 50% to 60% efficacious,[102,112] and better efficacy with nasal clotrimazole therapy has been reported in a few cases.[102]

Chronic Inflammatory Disorders

Chronic Rhinosinusitis

Lymphocytic–plasmacytic, eosinophilic, and idiopathic rhinosinusitis are a constellation of diagnoses obtained by way of histopathology that are collectively referred to as *chronic rhinosinusitis.* In many cases this is a diagnosis of exclusion when other etiologies have been ruled out. This syndrome is one of the most significant causes of sneezing and nasal discharge in the cat.[33] The nasal discharge is generally serous, but secondary bacterial infections can result in the development of mucopurulent nasal discharge (Figure 30-8), and inflammation can be severe enough to cause intermittent hemorrhage.[33] The clinical signs can persist for years. Cats with relatively stable disease that encounter a sudden change in severity should be re-evaluated for the presence of a more severe secondary disease, such as fungal rhinitis or neoplasia.

There is a subset of chronic rhinosinusitis cats that have a history of acute FHV-1 or FCV upper respiratory infections at a younger age, and it is postulated that an early severe viral infection may trigger chronic disease.[38] In addition, it is estimated that approximately 80% of cats are latently infected with FHV-1,[22] and so another possible scenario for chronic viral rhinosinusitis is the presence of latent FHV-1 viral infections that are triggered into recrudescence by stressful events. In such cats with a prior history of viral infection, therapies such as lysine, antivirals, and immunomodulators are often tried, as previously discussed. Subjective improvement in clinical signs has been noted in response to cationic liposome DNA complexes (CLDC) immunomodulatory therapy in a small pilot study currently under way at Colorado State University, as well as in a previously published study.[107] Stress is thought to play a role in the clinical severity and potential for recurrence of chronic viral rhinosinusitis, particularly if FHV-1 latency or chronic FCV infections are involved. Environmental measures to decrease stress, allocate resources in multicat households, and provide antianxiety therapies such as feline facial pheromone use (Feliway, Ceva Animal Health) may also provide some benefit. Controversy surrounds the use of immunosuppressive therapy in these patients: It may not be beneficial and runs the risk of exacerbating viral and bacterial components of the disease syndrome.

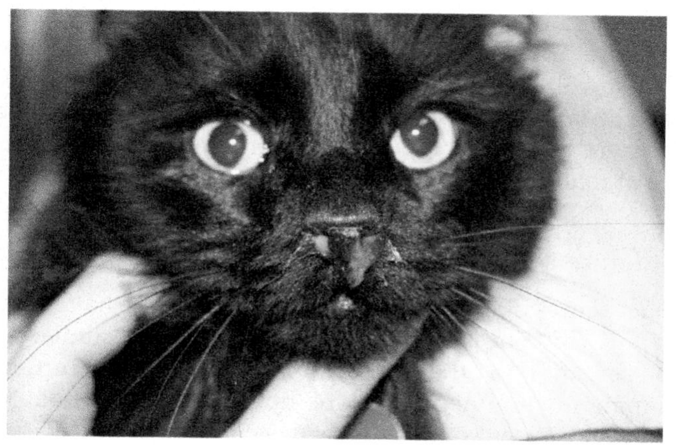

FIGURE 30-8 Mucopurulent nasal discharge is common with chronic rhinosinusitis.

In many cases there is no history of viral infection or any other predisposing cause. Generally, idiopathic chronic rhinosinusitis is somewhat refractory to treatment, and palliation of clinical signs, rather than cure, is the goal of medical management. Broad-spectrum antibiotics are often prescribed to manage secondary infections. Administration of antihistamines such as chlorpheniramine at 1 to 2 mg, orally, every 12 hours may lessen clinical signs of disease in some cats. Several newer antihistamines are now available (see Table 30-1), and because response to therapy is variable from patient to patient, an alternative drug should be tried if no improvement is seen with the initial choice. Moistening therapies such as nebulization and saline nasal drops can help loosen secretions and soothe mucosa, particularly in drier climates.

The role of immunosuppressive drugs as therapeutic agents in the treatment of chronic idiopathic rhinosinusitis is poorly understood, likely because of the multifactorial nature of this condition. Individual patients will respond variably to this approach. Prednisolone may be used at a maximum dose of 1 to 2 mg/kg, orally, every 12 hours. If a positive response is noted, the lowest dose and the longest dosing interval that is effective should be determined by adjusting the dose over time. Inhaled glucocorticoids can be used as an alternative to decrease the systemic side effects of oral glucocorticoid use and have the benefit of directly affecting the nasal mucosa. Beclomethasone or fluticasone can be administered by metered dose inhaler (MDI) with an inhalation chamber at 1 to 2 puffs once to twice daily. Resistant cases may respond to administration of cyclosporine at up to 7.5 mg/kg, orally, daily or every other day, but controlled data are lacking. Trough blood levels should be checked 2 weeks after initiation of therapy to ensure that excessive blood levels are not achieved; this may activate latent infectious diseases.

Neoplasia

Neoplasia of the nasal cavity is relatively rare in the cat compared with the dog; lymphoma is the most common tumor type, followed by adenocarcinoma and squamous cell carcinoma.[12,33,65] Lymphoma is treated with chemotherapy, often in conjunction with radiation therapy, and has potential for a good long-term prognosis.[89] Palliative radiation therapy is indicated for other nasal neoplasms, and surgical debulking is generally not required.[62] Prognosis depends on the aggressiveness and extent of the tumor, which is best determined by CT scan. Piroxicam administered at 0.3 mg/kg, orally, every 48 to 72 hours can control inflammation and clinical signs of disease in some cats with nonlymphoproliferative nasal neoplasia. Meloxicam (0.1 mg/kg, orally, every other day) may be another efficacious alternative. However, neither drug may result in antitumor effects against squamous cell carcinoma because it has been shown that there is minimal expression of cyclooxygenase-2 in this cancer type in the cat.[15] If nonsteroidal antiinflammatory therapy is used, the cat should be monitored for renal and gastrointestinal side effects (e.g., PCV to assess for gastrointestinal hemorrhage and renal values) because these are potential side effects of this drug family.

Spontaneous Disorders

Trauma

Trauma to the nasal cavity most commonly results in massive hemorrhage, and thus initial evaluation should include assessment and treatment for hypovolemic shock. Nasal tissue may be easily damaged because of its fragile structure. Placement of a nasal cannula may aid in airflow and allowing healing that maintains a nasal passage. It may take 2 to 3 weeks for healing to occur. Generally, surgical correction of fractures in the nasal cavity is not necessary, although solitary bone fragments should be removed to prevent the formation of sequestra. Trauma may also lead to chronic complications as a result of damage to the nasal passage.[33]

Foreign Bodies

Nasal foreign bodies are more common in cats than generally realized.[33,82] In dogs the foreign material is usually inspired into the anterior nares and is found in the ventral meatus just caudal to the nares. Most nasal foreign bodies in cats are plant material that lodges above the soft palate after coughing or vomiting. Clinical signs may include sneezing, reverse sneezing, gagging, and repeated attempts at swallowing. Retroflex rhinoscopic examination of the nasopharynx can sometimes confirm diagnosis and aid in removal of the object. Nasal lavage under general anesthesia is often more effective. The cuff of the endotracheal tube should be checked for full inflation before performing nasal lavage with saline administered under pressure. In cats lavaging from the anterior nares caudally is recommended. Gauze should be placed in the oropharyngeal area, and then a 20-, 35-, or 60-mL syringe can be used to forcefully flush saline through the nose while the nares are being pinched off to create pressure. Material flushed from the nose (or oropharynx) should be caught on the gauze and examined for foreign material.

DISEASE-SPECIFIC RECOMMENDATIONS: THE LARYNX

Laryngeal Paralysis

Laryngeal paralysis is a relatively rare condition in the cat compared with the dog, but it may occur as a result of a variety of etiologies.[84] Clinical signs include respiratory distress, inspiratory stridor, change in vocalization, coughing, dysphagia, and nonspecific signs such as weight loss and anorexia. Continuous positive airway pressure may be helpful in managing acute cases when intubation is not possible.[100] When possible, depending on the stability of the patient, cervical and thoracic radiographs are helpful for ruling out other causes of dyspnea. In a recent study 60% of cats with laryngeal paralysis had evidence of upper airway obstruction on radiographs. Findings included lung hyperinflation; caudal displacement of the larynx; and air in the larynx, pharynx, esophagus, and stomach.[84] Insofar as laryngeal paralysis is a functional disease, laryngeal examination provides a definitive diagnosis. In one study 75% of cats examined had bilateral disease.[84] In this study medical management was instituted for cats with unilateral disease with good outcome. Surgical management with arytenoid lateralization is reported to be variably successful (50% to 70%) for cats with laryngeal paralysis and is more commonly recommended in cats with bilateral disease. Aspiration pneumonia (with bilateral lateralization procedures), temporary tracheotomy necessitated by laryngeal swelling, and repetition of the surgery have been reported as possible sequelae of surgical management.[30]

Inflammatory Laryngitis

A few cases of inflammatory laryngeal disease have been reported.[97] These are clinically and grossly similar in presentation to other causes of laryngeal disease but are apparently non-neoplastic and noninfectious in etiology. Thus a biopsy should always be performed to distinguish inflammatory disease from a neoplastic process. Histopathology of this condition appears to be either granulomatous or lymphocytic-plasmacytic and neutrophilic. A temporary tracheostomy may be necessary while treatment is initiated, and surgical resection of inflamed tissue may be necessary. Favorable response to glucocorticoids has been reported, with good long-term prognosis in some cases.[97]

Laryngeal Neoplasia

Laryngeal neoplasia most commonly presents with clinical signs similar to those of other laryngeal disorders. A physical examination with special attention to the cervical area may identify a mass originating from tissues adjacent to the larynx. Laryngeal examination may reveal a mass, swelling, or irregularity in the appearance of the larynx. A biopsy is necessary to confirm the diagnosis and differentiate the condition from inflammatory laryngeal disease. The most common laryngeal neoplasms are lymphoma, squamous cell carcinoma, and adenocarcinoma.[70] Lymphoma may respond to chemotherapy. Complete surgical excision is usually not possible in this anatomic area, but it can be performed as a palliative measure. The long-term prognosis is poor. Permanent tracheostomy can be performed, but complications are common.[29,92]

References

1. Allen HS, Broussard J, Noone K: Nasopharyngeal diseases in cats: a retrospective study of 53 cases (1991-1998), *J Am Anim Hosp Assoc* 35:457, 1999.
2. Baker G: Nasopharyngeal polyps in cats, *Vet Rec* 111:43, 1982.
3. Barrs VR, Beatty JA, Lingard AE et al: Feline sino-orbital aspergillosis:an emerging clinical syndrome, *Aust Vet J* 85:N23, 2007.
4. Beatty JA, Swift N, Foster DJ et al: Suspected clindamycin-associated oesophageal injury in cats: five cases, *J Feline Med Surg* 8:412, 2006.
5. Berent AC, Weisse C, Todd K et al: Use of a balloon-expandable metallic stent for treatment of nasopharyngeal stenosis in dogs and cats: six cases (2005-2007), *J Am Vet Med Assoc* 233:1432, 2008.
6. Berryessa NA, Johnson LR, Kasten RW et al: Microbial culture of blood samples and serologic testing for bartonellosis in cats with chronic rhinosinusitis, *J Am Vet Med Assoc* 233:1084, 2008.
7. Binns SH, Dawson S, Speakman AJ et al: Prevalence and risk factors for feline *Bordetella bronchiseptica* infection, *Vet Rec* 144:575, 1999.
8. Brunt J, Guptill L, Kordick DL et al: American Association of Feline Practitioners 2006 Panel report on diagnosis, treatment, and prevention of *Bartonella* spp. infections, *J Feline Med Surg* 8:213, 2006.
9. Coutts AJ, Dawson S, Binns S et al: Studies on natural transmission of *Bordetella bronchiseptica* in cats, *Vet Microbiol* 48:19, 1996.
10. Coyne KP, Jones BR, Kipar A et al: Lethal outbreak of disease associated with feline calicivirus infection in cats, *Vet Rec* 158:544, 2006.
11. de Mari K, Maynard L, Sanquer A et al: Therapeutic effects of recombinant feline interferon-omega on feline leukemia virus (FeLV)-infected and FeLV/feline immunodeficiency virus (FIV)-coinfected symptomatic cats, *J Vet Intern Med* 18:477, 2004.
12. Demko JL, Cohn LA: Chronic nasal discharge in cats: 75 cases (1993-2004), *J Am Vet Med Assoc* 230:1032, 2007.
13. Di Francesco A, Piva S, Baldelli R: Prevalence of *Chlamydophila felis* by PCR among healthy pet cats in Italy, *New Microbiol* 27:199, 2004.
14. Di Martino B, Di Francesco CE, Meridiani I et al: Etiological investigation of multiple respiratory infections in cats, *New Microbiol* 30:455, 2007.
15. DiBernardi L, Dore M, Davis JA et al: Study of feline oral squamous cell carcinoma: potential target for cyclooxygenase inhibitor treatment, *Prostaglandins Leukot Essent Fatty Acids* 76:245, 2007.
16. Dossin O, Gruet P, Thomas E: Comparative field evaluation of marbofloxacin tablets in the treatment of feline upper respiratory infections, *J Small Anim Pract* 39:286, 1998.
17. Drazenovich TL, Fascetti AJ, Westermeyer HD et al: Effects of dietary lysine supplementation on upper respiratory and ocular disease and detection of infectious organisms in cats within an animal shelter, *Am J Vet Res* 70:1391, 2009.
18. Dworkin MS, Sullivan PS, Buskin SE et al: *Bordetella bronchiseptica* infection in human immunodeficiency virus–infected patients, *Clin Infect Dis* 28:1095, 1999.
19. Egberink H, Addie D, Belak S et al: *Bordetella bronchiseptica* infection in cats. ABCD guidelines on prevention and management, *J Feline Med Surg* 11:610, 2009.
20. Flatland B, Greene RT, Lappin MR: Clinical and serologic evaluation of cats with cryptococcosis, *J Am Vet Med Assoc* 209:1110, 1996.
21. Fontenelle JP, Powell CC, Veir JK et al: Effect of topical ophthalmic application of cidofovir on experimentally induced primary ocular feline herpesvirus-1 infection in cats, *Am J Vet Res* 69:289, 2008.
22. Gaskell RM, Povey RC: Experimental induction of feline viral rhinotracheitis virus re-excretion in FVR-recovered cats, *Vet Rec* 100:128, 1977.
23. Gerhardt N, Schulz BS, Werckenthin C et al: Pharmacokinetics of enrofloxacin and its efficacy in comparison with doxycycline in the treatment of *Chlamydophila felis* infection in cats with conjunctivitis, *Vet Rec* 159:591, 2006.
24. German AJ, Cannon MJ, Dye C et al: Oesophageal strictures in cats associated with doxycycline therapy, *J Feline Med Surg* 7:33, 2005.
25. Ginn JA, Kumar MS, McKiernan BC et al: Nasopharyngeal turbinates in brachycephalic dogs and cats, *J Am Anim Hosp Assoc* 44:243, 2008.
26. Greene CE, Hartmann K, Calpin J: Antimicrobial Drug Formulary. In Greene CE, editor: *Infectious diseases of the dog and cat*, ed 3, St Louis, 2006, Elsevier, p 1200.
27. Griffin B, Beard DM, Klopfenstein KA: Use of butter to facilitate the passage of tablets through the esophagus of cats, *J Vet Intern Med* 17:445, 2003.
28. Gruffydd-Jones T, Addie D, Belak S et al: *Chlamydophila felis* infection. ABCD guidelines on prevention and management, *J Feline Med Surg* 11:605, 2009.
29. Guenther-Yenke CL, Rozanski EA: Tracheostomy in cats: 23 cases (1998-2006), *J Feline Med Surg* 9:451, 2007.
30. Hardie RJ, Gunby J, Bjorling DE: Arytenoid lateralization for treatment of laryngeal paralysis in 10 cats, *Vet Surg* 38:445, 2009.
31. Hartmann AD, Helps CR, Lappin MR et al: Efficacy of pradofloxacin in cats with feline upper respiratory tract disease due to *Chlamydophila felis* or *Mycoplasma* infections, *J Vet Intern Med* 22:44, 2008.
32. Helps CR, Lait P, Damhuis A et al: Factors associated with upper respiratory tract disease caused by feline herpesvirus, feline calicivirus, *Chlamydophila felis* and *Bordetella bronchiseptica* in cats: experience from 218 European catteries, *Vet Rec* 156:669, 2005.

33. Henderson SM, Bradley K, Day MJ et al: Investigation of nasal disease in the cat—a retrospective study of 77 cases, *J Feline Med Surg* 6:245, 2004.
34. Holt DE: Nasopharyngeal polyps. In King L, editor: *Textbook of respiratory disease in dogs and cats*, Philadelphia, 2004, Saunders, p 328.
35. Huang C, Hess J, Gill M et al: A dual-strain feline calicivirus vaccine stimulates broader cross-neutralization antibodies than a single-strain vaccine and lessens clinical signs in vaccinated cats when challenged with a homologous feline calicivirus strain associated with virulent systemic disease, *J Feline Med Surg* 12:129, 2010.
36. Hurley KE, Pesavento PA, Pedersen NC et al: An outbreak of virulent systemic feline calicivirus disease, *J Am Vet Med Assoc* 224:241, 2004.
37. Johnson LR, Clarke HE, Bannasch MJ et al: Correlation of rhinoscopic signs of inflammation with histologic findings in nasal biopsy specimens of cats with or without upper respiratory tract disease, *J Am Vet Med Assoc* 225:395, 2004.
38. Johnson LR, Foley JE, De Cock HE et al: Assessment of infectious organisms associated with chronic rhinosinusitis in cats, *J Am Vet Med Assoc* 227:579, 2005.
39. Johnson LR, Kass PH: Effect of sample collection methodology on nasal culture results in cats, *J Feline Med Surg* 11:645, 2009.
40. Kapatkin AS, Matthiesen DT, Noone KE et al: Results of surgery and long-term follow-up in 31 cats with nasopharyngeal polyps, *J Am Anim Hosp Assoc* 26:387, 1990.
41. Klose TC, Rosychuk RA, MacPhail CM et al: Association between upper respiratory tract infections and inflammatory aural and nasopharyngeal polyps in cats, *J Vet Intern Med* 21:628, 2007.
42. Kreutz LC, Johnson RP, Seal BS: Phenotypic and genotypic variation of feline calicivirus during persistent infection of cats, *Vet Microbiol* 59:229, 1998.
43. Kuehn NF: Chronic rhinitis in cats, *Clin Tech Small Anim Pract* 21:69, 2006.
44. Lamb CR, Richbell S, Mantis P: Radiographic signs in cats with nasal disease, *J Feline Med Surg* 5:227, 2003.
45. Lappin MR, Sebring RW, Porter M et al: Effects of a single dose of an intranasal feline herpesvirus 1, calicivirus, and panleukopenia vaccine on clinical signs and virus shedding after challenge with virulent feline herpesvirus 1, *J Feline Med Surg* 8:158, 2006.
46. Lappin MR, Veir J, Hawley J: Feline panleukopenia virus, feline herpesvirus-1, and feline calicivirus antibody responses in seronegative specific pathogen-free cats after a single administration of two different modified live FVRCP vaccines, *J Feline Med Surg* 11:159, 2009.
47. Lappin MR, Veir JK, Satyaraj E et al: Pilot study to evaluate the effect of oral supplementation of Enterococcus faecium SF68 on cats with latent feline herpesvirus 1, *J Feline Med Surg* 11:650, 2009.
48. Lappin MR, Veir JK, Sebring RW et al: Feline lymphocyte blastogenesis in response to feline herpesvirus-1 antigens and concanavalin A after vaccination with five FVRCP vaccines, *J Vet Intern Med* 19:467, 2005.
49. Low HC, Powell CC, Veir JK et al: Prevalence of feline herpesvirus 1, *Chlamydophila felis,* and *Mycoplasma* spp DNA in conjunctival cells collected from cats with and without conjunctivitis, *Am J Vet Res* 68:643, 2007.
50. MacPhail CM, Bennet AD, Gibbons DS et al: The esophageal transit time of tablets or capsules following administration with FlavorRx pill glide or pill delivery treats, *J Vet Intern Med* 23:736, 2009.
51. Maggs DJ, Clarke HE: In vitro efficacy of ganciclovir, cidofovir, penciclovir, foscarnet, idoxuridine, and acyclovir against feline herpesvirus type-1, *Am J Vet Res* 65:399, 2004.
52. Maggs DJ, Clarke HE: Relative sensitivity of polymerase chain reaction assays used for detection of feline herpesvirus type 1 DNA in clinical samples and commercial vaccines, *Am J Vet Res* 66:1550, 2005.
53. Maggs DJ, Collins BK, Thorne JG et al: Effects of L-lysine and L-arginine on in vitro replication of feline herpesvirus type-1, *Am J Vet Res* 61:1474, 2000.
54. Maggs DJ, Lappin MR, Nasisse MP: Detection of feline herpesvirus–specific antibodies and DNA in aqueous humor from cats with or without uveitis, *Am J Vet Res* 60:932, 1999.
55. Maggs DJ, Nasisse MP, Kass PH: Efficacy of oral supplementation with L-lysine in cats latently infected with feline herpesvirus, *Am J Vet Res* 64:37, 2003.
56. Malik R, Craig AJ, Wigney DI et al: Combination chemotherapy of canine and feline cryptococcosis using subcutaneously administered amphotericin B, *Aust Vet J* 73:124, 1996.
57. Malik R, Krockenberger MB, O'Brien CR et al: Cryptococcus. In Greene CE, editor: *Infectious diseases of the dog and cat*, ed 3, St Louis, 2006, Elsevier, p 584.
58. Malik R, Lessels NS, Webb S et al: Treatment of feline herpesvirus-1 associated disease in cats with famciclovir and related drugs, *J Feline Med Surg* 11:40, 2009.
59. Malik R, McPetrie R, Wigney DI et al: A latex cryptococcal antigen agglutination test for diagnosis and monitoring of therapy for cryptococcosis, *Aust Vet J* 74:358, 1996.
60. Malik R, Wigney DI, Muir DB et al: Cryptococcosis in cats: clinical and mycological assessment of 29 cases and evaluation of treatment using orally administered fluconazole, *J Med Vet Mycol* 30:133, 1992.
61. Melendez LD, Twedt DC, Wright M: Suspected doxycycline-induced esophagitis and esophageal stricture formation in three cats, *Feline Pract* 28:10, 2000.
62. Mellanby RJ, Herrtage ME, Dobson JM: Long-term outcome of eight cats with non-lymphoproliferative nasal tumours treated by megavoltage radiotherapy, *J Feline Med Surg* 4:77, 2002.
63. Moore GE, DeSantis-Kerr AC, Guptill LF et al: Adverse events after vaccine administration in cats: 2,560 cases (2002-2005), *J Am Vet Med Assoc* 231:94, 2007.
64. Muilenburg RK, Fry TR: Feline nasopharyngeal polyps, *Vet Clin North Am Small Anim Pract* 32:839, 2002.
65. Mukaratirwa S, van der Linde-Sipman JS, Gruys E: Feline nasal and paranasal sinus tumours: clinicopathological study, histomorphological description and diagnostic immunohistochemistry of 123 cases, *J Feline Med Surg* 3:235, 2001.
66. Nasisse MP, Dorman DC, Jamison KC et al: Effects of valacyclovir in cats infected with feline herpesvirus 1, *Am J Vet Res* 58:1141, 1997.
67. O'Brien CR, Krockenberger MB, Martin P et al: Long-term outcome of therapy for 59 cats and 11 dogs with cryptococcosis, *Aust Vet J* 84:384, 2006.
68. O'Brien CR, Krockenberger MB, Wigney DI et al: Retrospective study of feline and canine cryptococcosis in Australia from 1981 to 2001: 195 cases, *Med Mycol* 42:449, 2004.
69. O'Brien RT, Evans SM, Wortman JA et al: Radiographic findings in cats with intranasal neoplasia or chronic rhinitis: 29 cases (1982-1988), *J Am Vet Med Assoc* 208:385, 1996.
70. Ogilvie GK, Moore AS: Laryngeal tumors. In: Ogilvie GK, Moore AS, editors: *Feline oncology*, Trenton, NJ, 2000, Veterinary Learning Systems, p 375.
71. Ossiboff RJ, Sheh A, Shotton J et al: Feline caliciviruses (FCVs) isolated from cats with virulent systemic disease possess in vitro phenotypes distinct from those of other FCV isolates, *J Gen Virol* 88:506, 2007.
72. Pedersen NC, Elliott JB, Glasgow A et al: An isolated epizootic of hemorrhagic-like fever in cats caused by a novel and highly virulent strain of feline calicivirus, *Vet Microbiol* 73:281, 2000.
73. Pedretti E, Passeri B, Amadori M et al: Low-dose interferon-alpha treatment for feline immunodeficiency virus infection, *Vet Immunol Immunopathol* 109:245, 2006.

74. Porter CJ, Radford AD, Gaskell RM et al: Comparison of the ability of feline calicivirus (FCV) vaccines to neutralise a panel of current UK FCV isolates, *J Feline Med Surg* 10:32, 2008.
75. Poulet H, Brunet S, Leroy V et al: Immunisation with a combination of two complementary feline calicivirus strains induces a broad cross-protection against heterologous challenges, *Vet Microbiol* 106:17, 2005.
76. Quimby JM, Lappin MR: Update on feline upper respiratory diseases: introduction and diagnostics, *Compend Cont Ed Pract Vet* 31, 2009.
77. Quimby JM, Lappin MR: Update on feline upper respiratory diseases: condition-specific recommendations, *Compend Cont Ed Pract Vet* 32, 2010.
78. Radford AD, Addie D, Belak S et al: Feline calicivirus infection. ABCD guidelines on prevention and management, *J Feline Med Surg* 11:556, 2009.
79. Rampazzo A, Appino S, Pregel P et al: Prevalence of *Chlamydophila felis* and feline herpesvirus 1 in cats with conjunctivitis in northern Italy, *J Vet Intern Med* 17:799, 2003.
80. Rees TM, Lubinski JL: Oral supplementation with L-lysine did not prevent upper respiratory infection in a shelter population of cats, *J Feline Med Surg* 10:510, 2008.
81. Richards JR, Elston TH, Ford RB et al: The 2006 American Association of Feline Practitioners Feline Vaccine Advisory Panel report, *J Am Vet Med Assoc* 229:1405, 2006.
82. Riley P: Nasopharyngeal grass foreign body in eight cats, *J Am Vet Med Assoc* 202:299, 1993.
83. Ruch-Gallie RA, Veir JK, Spindel ME et al: Efficacy of amoxycillin and azithromycin for the empirical treatment of shelter cats with suspected bacterial upper respiratory infections, *J Feline Med Surg* 10:542, 2008.
84. Schachter S, Norris CR: Laryngeal paralysis in cats: 16 cases (1990-1999), *J Am Vet Med Assoc* 216:1100, 2000.
85. Schlueter C, Budras KD, Ludewig E et al: Brachycephalic feline noses: CT and anatomical study of the relationship between head conformation and the nasolacrimal drainage system, *J Feline Med Surg* 11:891, 2009.
86. Schoenborn WC, Wisner ER, Kass PP et al: Retrospective assessment of computed tomographic imaging of feline sinonasal disease in 62 cats, *Vet Radiol Ultrasound* 44:185, 2003.
87. Schorr-Evans EM, Poland A, Johnson WE et al: An epizootic of highly virulent feline calicivirus disease in a hospital setting in New England, *J Feline Med Surg* 5:217, 2003.
88. Schulz BS, Wolf G, Hartmann K: Bacteriological and antibiotic sensitivity test results in 271 cats with respiratory tract infections, *Vet Rec* 158:269, 2006.
89. Sfiligoi G, Theon AP, Kent MS: Response of nineteen cats with nasal lymphoma to radiation therapy and chemotherapy, *Vet Radiol Ultrasound* 48:388, 2007.
90. Sparkes AH, Caney SM, Sturgess CP et al: The clinical efficacy of topical and systemic therapy for the treatment of feline ocular chlamydiosis, *J Feline Med Surg* 1:31, 1999.
91. Spindel ME, Veir JK, Radecki SV et al: Evaluation of pradofloxacin for the treatment of feline rhinitis, *J Feline Med Surg* 10:472, 2008.
92. Stepnik MW, Mehl ML, Hardie EM et al: Outcome of permanent tracheostomy for treatment of upper airway obstruction in cats: 21 cases (1990-2007), *J Am Vet Med Assoc* 234:638, 2009.
93. Stiles J, McDermott M, Bigsby D et al: Use of nested polymerase chain reaction to identify feline herpesvirus in ocular tissue from clinically normal cats and cats with corneal sequestra or conjunctivitis, *Am J Vet Res* 58:338, 1997.
94. Sturgess CP, Gruffydd-Jones TJ, Harbour DA et al: Controlled study of the efficacy of clavulanic acid–potentiated amoxycillin in the treatment of *Chlamydia psittaci* in cats, *Vet Rec* 149:73, 2001.
95. Sykes JE, Studdert VP, Browning GF: Comparison of the polymerase chain reaction and culture for the detection of feline *Chlamydia psittaci* in untreated and doxycycline-treated experimentally infected cats, *J Vet Intern Med* 13:146, 1999.
96. Talavera Lopez J, Josefa Fernandez Del Palacio MA, Cano FG et al: Nasopharyngeal stenosis secondary to soft palate dysgenesis in a cat, *Vet J* 181:200, 2009.
97. Tasker S, Foster DJ, Corcoran BM et al: Obstructive inflammatory laryngeal disease in three cats, *J Feline Med Surg* 1:53, 1999.
98. Thiry E, Addie D, Belak S et al: Feline herpesvirus infection. ABCD guidelines on prevention and management, *J Feline Med Surg* 11:547, 2009.
99. Thomasy SM, Lim CC, Reilly CM et al: Safety and efficacy of orally administered famciclovir in cats experimentally infected with feline herpesvirus-1, *Am J Vet Res* 72:85, 2011.
100. Ticehurst K, Zaki S, Hunt GB et al: Use of continuous positive airway pressure in the acute management of laryngeal paralysis in a cat, *Aust Vet J* 86:395, 2008.
101. Tompkins WA: Immunomodulation and therapeutic effects of the oral use of interferon-alpha: mechanism of action, *J Interferon Cytokine Res* 19:817, 1999.
102. Tomsa K, Glaus TM, Zimmer C et al: Fungal rhinitis and sinusitis in three cats, *J Am Vet Med Assoc* 222:1380, 2003.
103. Trevor PB, Martin RA: Tympanic bulla osteotomy for treatment of middle-ear disease in cats: 19 cases (1984-1991), *J Am Vet Med Assoc* 202:123, 1993.
104. Trostel CT, Frankel DJ: Punch resection alaplasty technique in dogs and cats with stenotic nares: 14 cases, *J Am Anim Hosp Assoc* 46:5, 2009.
105. Turnquist SE, Ostlund E: Calicivirus outbreak with high mortality in a Missouri feline colony, *J Vet Diagn Invest* 9:195, 1997.
106. Veir JK, Knorr R, Cavadini C et al: Effect of supplementation with *Enterococcus faecium* (SF68) on immune functions in cats, *Vet Ther* 8:229, 2007.
107. Veir JK, Lappin MR, Dow SW: Evaluation of a novel immunotherapy for treatment of chronic rhinitis in cats, *J Feline Med Surg* 8:400, 2006.
108. Veir JK, Lappin MR, Foley JE et al: Feline inflammatory polyps: historical, clinical, and PCR findings for feline calici virus and feline herpes virus-1 in 28 cases, *J Feline Med Surg* 4:195, 2002.
109. Veir JK, Ruch-Gallie R, Spindel ME et al: Prevalence of selected infectious organisms and comparison of two anatomic sampling sites in shelter cats with upper respiratory tract disease, *J Feline Med Surg* 10:551, 2008.
110. Welsh RD: *Bordetella bronchiseptica* infections in cats, *J Am Anim Hosp Assoc* 32:153, 1996.
111. Westfall DS, Twedt DC, Steyn PF et al: Evaluation of esophageal transit of tablets and capsules in 30 cats, *J Vet Intern Med* 15:467, 2001.
112. Whitney BL, Broussard J, Stefanacci JD: Four cats with fungal rhinitis, *J Feline Med Surg* 7:53, 2005.

LOWER RESPIRATORY TRACT DISEASES

Randolph M. Baral

Lower respiratory tract (LRT) diseases include the following:

1. Bronchial disease (i.e., pathology affecting the airways distal to the tracheal bifurcation)
2. Pulmonary interstitial disease, which is predominantly pneumonia or neoplasia (but also pulmonary edema and pulmonary fibrosis)

These distinctions are important to make for management purposes, but the clinician should not lose sight of the fact that combinations of these can occur, such as in bronchopulmonary pneumonia. Severe cases of LRT disease usually present for dyspnea or tachypnea. In milder cases cats may present for coughing, wheezing, or "loud breathing."

The diagnostic processes must not only distinguish bronchial from interstitial disease but also LRT diseases from upper respiratory tract (URT) or cardiac disease and other intrathoracic diseases (e.g., those causing pleural effusion or intrathoracic masses). LRT diseases can be classified as infectious or noninfectious, and noninfectious causes can be considered as neoplastic or non-neoplastic. The most common LRT conditions encountered are idiopathic bronchial diseases, commonly described as asthma or chronic bronchitis.

CLINICAL SIGNS

The most common presenting signs for cats with LRT disorders are dyspnea, coughing, or other abnormal respiratory sounds or patterns; some cats can present for general malaise, and respiratory signs are first recognized by the clinician rather than the owner. Signs can be intermittent or constant. The clinician must, in the first instance, distinguish LRT signs from those caused by URT, cardiac, or pleural disorders. A recent study of 90 dyspneic cats divided the underlying causes (and proportions) as cardiac (38%), non-neoplastic URT and LRT disease (32%), and neoplasia of the URT, LRT, or pleural cavity (20%).[263]

Typically, louder (or harsher) *expiratory* sounds are auscultated with LRT disease compared with the harsher *inspiratory* sounds auscultated with URT disorders. Disease confined to the pleural space or pulmonary parenchyma does not result in auscultatory change when the airways are not affected. Rapid breathing with decreased depth indicates restrictive disease which can result from alveolar or interstitial infiltrates or masses (LRT) or pleural diseases such as effusion, mediastinal masses, diaphragmatic herniation, or pneumothorax. Auscultation of a murmur usually points toward cardiac disease, but cardiomyopathies do not necessarily result in a murmur.

Coughing and wheezing are considered typical signs of LRT disorders such as bronchial diseases or pneumonia and do not typically occur with congestive heart failure (CHF) in cats.

Palpably decreased chest wall compliance is considered typical of pleural diseases such as effusion or masses but is certainly recognized with bronchopulmonary disease as well.

DIAGNOSTICS

Radiology

Radiology is the hallmark modality to diagnose LRT diseases and distinguish them from pleural and cardiac diseases. In acute cases screening images to determine the anatomic location of pathology should be taken in the most comfortable position for the cat; many cats are comfortable sitting sternally, with their elbows stabilizing themselves, which can allow a dorsoventral image. Multiple views of good-quality images are important for precise diagnostics but only after respiratory distress has been relieved. When radiographs are taken for more precise diagnostics, three views should be taken: (1) left lateral, (2) right lateral, and (3) dorsoventral or ventrodorsal.

Typically, bronchopulmonary disease is interpreted radiographically by a pattern-based approach of assessment[28] (Table 30-2).

Bronchial patterns result from fluid or cellular infiltrate within the bronchial walls and peribronchial and perivascular connective tissue of the lung. This leads to increased radiodensity of bronchial walls. When these prominent bronchi are viewed longitudinally, they appear as paired, parallel lines that branch and have been compared to train tracks. In cross-section they appear as tissue-dense circles with radiolucent centers that have been described as resembling "doughnuts" (Figure 30-9).

Vascular patterns result from an increase (or decrease) in prominence (i.e., size, shape, number) of pulmonary arteries and veins. Vessels appear as radiodense linear structures running parallel to the main lobar airways that taper. Vascular patterns are more common in cardiovascular disease than LRT disease.

Alveolar patterns result from alveolar collapse or flooding of pulmonary acini with fluid. The acini are those parts of the lung distal to each terminal bronchiole. As each acinus becomes flooded, the fluid spreads to the adjoining acinus, resulting in a "fluffy" density. As these "fluffy" densities spread, they coalesce. Any bronchial structures within the density appear as radiolucent lines (known as "air bronchograms"). Alveolar patterns indicate that the disease process is within the end-air spaces and not the lung interstitium (or pleural space or mediastinum) (Figure 30-10).

Interstitial patterns result from fluid or cellular accumulation within the lung interstitium (i.e., not airways). The consequence is generally a haze or "veil" over the lung fields that obscures the vascular outlines. Distinct linear densities or nodules are also possible (Figure 30-11).

In most cases a combination of patterns (mixed pattern) will result. For example, bronchopneumonia may result in alveolar and bronchial patterns. In all cases

TABLE 30-2 Radiographic Features of Pulmonary Patterns in Dyspneic Cats

Pattern Name	Radiographic Features	Comments	Disease Examples (Not All Inclusive)
Alveolar	Lobar sign; uniform soft tissue opacity; air bronchograms; will not see pulmonary vessels or airways; border effacement of heart or diaphragm	Location is important for formulating a differential list; is the easiest pulmonary pattern to recognize	Aspiration pneumonia; bronchopneumonia; cardiogenic and noncardiogenic pulmonary edema; neoplasia; hemorrhage; smoke inhalation; etc.
Bronchial	Rings and lines are noted within the pulmonary parenchyma; visible in the periphery and away from the pulmonary hilum	Usually generalized; be sure to evaluate in the peripheral lung fields and in the thin areas of lung	Chronic bronchitis; pulmonary infiltrates with eosinophilia; heartworm disease; allergic lung disease; feline asthma
Vascular	Increased in size of the pulmonary arteries, veins or both (left-to-right shunting lesions)	Added lung opacity secondary to enlargement of the pulmonary vessels	Pulmonary arteries—heartworm disease or cor pulmonale; pulmonary veins—left-sided heart failure; both—left-to-right PDA, VSD, ASD, or overcirculation secondary to volume overload
Interstitial—nodules or miliary pattern (structured)	Multiple "millet seeds" or small miliary nodules noted throughout the lung fields; variably sized pulmonary nodules	Usually needs to be at least 5 mm in size to be seen as a distinct nodule; "fake-outs" include nipples, end-on vessels, and pulmonary osteomas	Lymphoma, disseminated neoplasia (carcinoma), and fungal disease; parasitic, eosinophilic, or pyogranulomatous pneumonias; nodules can be cavitated
Unstructured interstitial	Increased opacity to the lung fields with decreased visualization of the pulmonary vessels, aorta, and caudal vena cava	Typically generalized and never mild!	Check exposure factors, expiration, lymphoma, fibrosis, fungal infection, edema, hemorrhage, infectious etiologies

PDA, Patent ductus arteriosus; *VSD,* ventricular septal defect; *ASD,* atrial septal defect.
From Berry CR: Small animal thoracic radiology: the dyspneic cat, in *Proceedings,* Western Veterinary Conference, 2010.

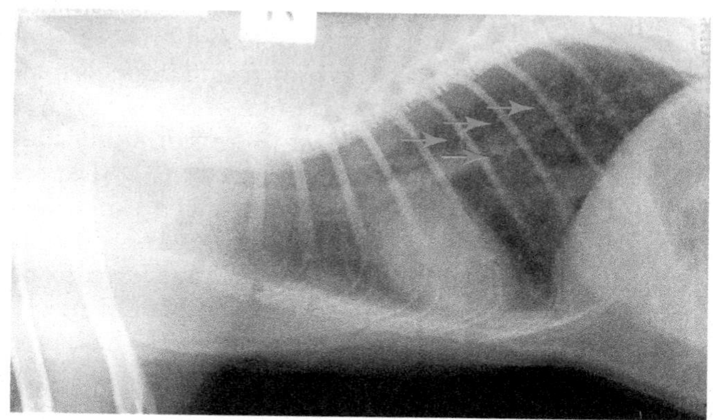

FIGURE 30-9 Thoracic radiograph (right lateral projection) demonstrating bronchial pattern. Note the increased radiodensity of bronchial walls resulting in "tram tracks" (two, marked with *green arrows)* and "doughnuts" (one, marked with a *red arrow).*

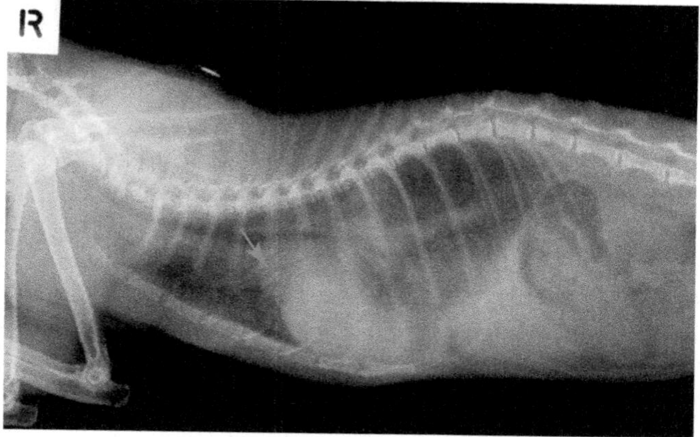

FIGURE 30-10 Thoracic radiograph (right lateral projection) demonstrating alveolar pattern. This cat has pulmonary edema subsequent to congestive heart failure. Note the bronchial structure ("air bronchogram") within the density caused by flooded alveoli appearing as a radiolucent line (marked with *green arrow).* There is also cardiomegaly, and the stomach is filled with air, as is often the case with dyspneic cats.

the clinician must determine the dominant pattern to help decide the most appropriate next diagnostic step.

Although radiography narrows down the possible diagnoses, a precise diagnosis cannot be made without a cytologic assessment. The radiographic pattern can help decide which sampling technique is likely to produce a higher cellular yield. Sampling from airways (bronchoalveolar washing) is more likely to be successful when bronchial or alveolar patterns are present. Aspiration directly from lung tissue is more likely to aid diagnosis when an interstitial pattern predominates or discrete nodules are present.

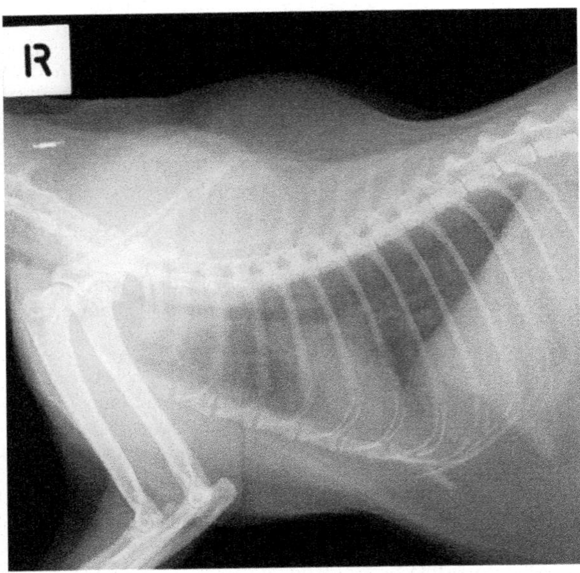

FIGURE 30-11 Thoracic radiograph (right lateral projection) demonstrating interstitial pattern. Note that the radiodensity of the lung fields is increased with a "veil-like" quality. The radiodensity of normal lung fields should approach that of the air surrounding the cat.

Computed Tomography

CT is being used more frequently in referral practice. CT eliminates superimposition of overlying structures and offers superior contrast resolution compared with conventional radiography. Most reports of CT, often with CT-guided fine-needle aspiration (FNA), for diagnosis of feline LRT disorders have been for neoplastic disease.[106,292] CT is also useful for assessment of airway wall thickening, mucus obstruction, emphysematous changes, secondary bronchiectasis, mucus accumulation in small airways, and air trapping.[120,121]

Bronchoscopy

Bronchoscopy is not yet widely available in general practice but is becoming more so. Bronchoscopy allows examination of patency, color, and character of mucosa; presence and character of secretions; and presence and location of masses or foreign bodies. A major limitation of feline bronchoscopy is the requirement for very narrow bronchoscopes (2.5 to 3.8 mm outer diameter). Even with such narrow scopes, the airways are mostly occluded, requiring intravenous anesthesia for maintenance as well as induction. Oxygen can be supplied through jet ventilation or an oxygen cannula passed adjacent to the scope. In one study of bronchoscopy in 68 cats, complications resulted in approximately one third of cases (26 of 68 cats). In most cases the complications were mild, but in six cases they were serious, with death resulting in four cats. The deaths were considered to be associated with the severity of the underlying pulmonary disease. Complications were predominantly associated with oxygen desaturation of hemoglobin. Pretreatment with terbutaline (0.01 mg/kg subcutaneously) and preoxygenation appear to reduce complication rates.[122,132]

When bronchial disease is recognized radiographically or suspected despite no radiographic evidence, airway fluid should be collected for analysis by blind or transoral bronchial lavage or by bronchoscopy. Pretreatment with terbutaline (0.01 mg/kg subcutaneously) is recommended for blind sampling as well as with bronchoscopic evaluation.

Bronchoalveolar Lavage

Bronchoscopic bronchoalveolar lavage (BAL) samples are taken after visual inspection. The bronchoscope is removed from the airway and the biopsy channel rinsed and the outer surface wiped. The bronchoscope is then reintroduced and wedged in the smallest bronchus that accommodates it. Three 10-mL aliquots of warmed, sterile saline are introduced and then retrieved.[121] The technique for blind bronchial lavage[170,222] is described in Box 30-3 (Figure 30-12). Samples collected should be assessed cytologically and submitted for culture and sensitivity testing. Samples should be evaluated promptly because storage for 48 hours may alter cytologic evaluation.[193] Table 30-3 summarizes normal bronchial lavage cytologic findings from several studies.

BAL findings are dependent on cell recovery and yield, which is influenced by the distribution and location of lesions in the lung. One study found poor correlation between BAL cytology findings and histology[199]; however, this is in direct contrast to a prior study that found good correlation.[91] A retrospective of 88 BAL specimens from 80 cats with broad-ranging lower respiratory diseases found inconclusive results in 28 cases.[79] Series of cats with bronchial disease have mostly shown consistent BAL cytologic findings. Moise and colleagues[188] recognized exudates in 58 of 65 bronchial washes. Dye and colleagues[63] showed that severely affected cats with bronchial disease had significantly higher percentages of eosinophils or neutrophils (or both) than moderately affected cats compared with normal cats. Corcoran and coworkers[45] found that 16 of 24 had BAL cytologic findings consistent with bronchial disease, and the other eight cats had milder radiographic changes. Foster and coworkers[75] found no association between BAL cytology or radiographic severity and disease severity, but no direct comparison of cytology to radiologic changes were made. These findings can be summarized as follows: BAL will give helpful clinical information in most (but not all) cases with diffuse bronchial disease. Generalized interstitial disease or focal lesions are less likely to lend themselves to cytologic diagnosis from BAL.

BOX 30-3

Blind Bronchoalveolar Lavage Technique

Equipment

1. Two sterile 10-mL red-top blood collection tubes to submit samples for cytology and culture
2. Sterile endotracheal (ET) tube (usually 4 mm)
3. Two or three sterile 10-mL syringes filled with 5-mL aliquots of warmed sterile 0.9% saline
4. Sterile red rubber feeding tube or polypropylene catheter (usually 8 French). The end of the red rubber feeding tube should be cut off and smoothed so that the sterile saline will flow more easily than through the side holes. The proximal end of the feeding tube may also need to be trimmed so that the syringe will fit.
5. Laryngoscope and topical lidocaine

Procedure

1. Premedicate with an injectable bronchodilator such as terbutaline.
2. Administer a short-acting intravenous anesthetic agent (e.g., propofol, ketamine, midazolam). The entire procedure will only take a few minutes if all the equipment is organized in advance.
3. Desensitize the larynx with topical lidocaine, and use the laryngoscope to insert the sterile endotracheal tube, trying to avoid contamination of the tip of the tube in the oral cavity.
4. Provide a few minutes of supplemental oxygen before the procedure.
5. With the cat in lateral recumbency, the sterile red rubber feeding tube or polypropylene catheter is inserted into the lumen of the endotracheal tube and advanced until resistance is felt when the tip is lodged in a small airway. Do not force the catheter too far into the airway, or trauma may result.
6. A syringe with warmed saline is attached to the end of the red rubber feeding tube or catheter and a 5-mL aliquot is instilled. With gentle suction the fluid is aspirated back from the airways. When negative pressure is felt on the syringe, suction should be decreased, the catheter backed out slightly, and aspiration continued. The hindquarters of the cat can be elevated to facilitate aspiration, and gentle coupage of the chest wall may also be helpful. The presence of foam in the aspirated fluid indicates surfactant and a successful deep alveolar lavage. The volume of saline retrieved is typically less than half of what was instilled. If an inadequate volume is retrieved, a second aliquot can be instilled and the procedure repeated. Typically a total volume of 5 to 10 mL sterile saline is required to retrieve adequate samples, although total volumes of up to 60 mL have been described in cats.
7. The red rubber feeding tube or catheter is removed from the endotracheal tube, and supplemental oxygen is provided until the cat is ready for extubation. Elevating the hindquarters and providing gentle coupage can assist in clearance of remaining fluid from the airways. Once the endotracheal tube is removed, the cat should be closely observed for respiratory distress for the next 15 to 30 minutes.
8. Samples collected should be divided into sterile red-top blood collection tubes and submitted for cytology as well as culture.

Adapted from McCarthy G, Quinn PJ: The development of lavage procedures for the upper and lower respiratory tract of the cat, *Irish Vet J* 40:6, 1986; Reinero CR: Bronchoalveolar lavage fluid collection using a blind technique, *Clinician's Brief* 8:58, 2010.

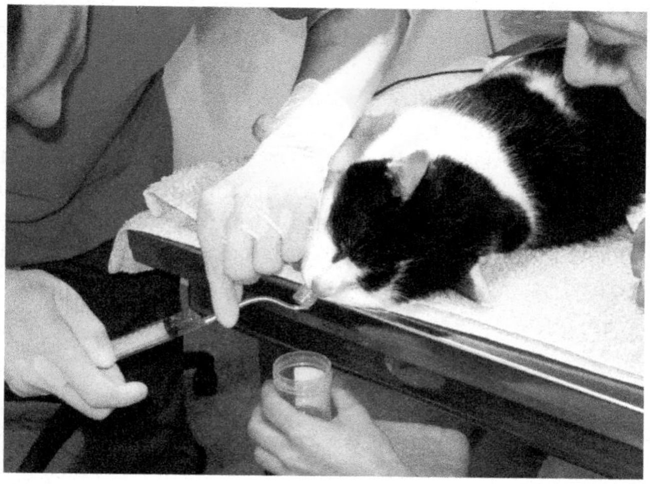

FIGURE 30-12 Blind bronchoalveolar lavage. Note that the 8F feeding tube is within the endotracheal tube.

Fine-Needle Aspiration

Focal lesions can be assessed by FNA. Although *aspiration* is the commonly used term for this technique, it is a misnomer because, when tissue samples are obtained by ultrasound guidance, the needle tip (with attached syringe) should be moved back and forth gently within the lesion 5 to 10 times, instead of using negative pressure to obtain lung tissue. This technique has been described as "woodpeckering"; it decreases sample volume but improves the cellularity of the sample because there is less hemodilution.[180] The reported accuracy of samples obtained by FNA compared with histopathology ranges from 83% to 89%.[52,266,290]

Lung Parenchymal Biopsy

Lung parenchymal biopsy may be warranted when a diagnosis cannot be reached and empiric treatment has

TABLE 30-3 **Bronchial Lavage Cytologic Findings of Normal Cats: Cell Counts and Percentage of Major Cell Types Found**

Authors (year)	Total Nucleated Cell Counts (/μL ± SEM)	Alveolar Macrophages (%)	Eosinophils (%)	Neutrophils (%)
McCarthy, Quinn (1986)[170]	300	90.5	7.5	0.7
Hawkins et al (1990)[102]	241 ± 101	70.6	16.1	6.7
Padrid et al (1991)[211]	301 ± 126	*	25	*
Lecuyer et al (1995)[144]	280 ± 270	60	11	24
Mills et al (2006)[184]	185	71	7	6
Dehard et al (2008)[54]	567 ± 74	89	3.1	7.4

SEM, Standard error of the mean.
*Unreported. Alveolar macrophages are noted as "cell type most frequently encountered."

not been successful. A surgical technique of obtaining lung biopsies by a "keyhole" approach has been described. Smaller incisions result in less tissue trauma.[200] Nevertheless, the decision to obtain lung biopsy samples should be weighed against the potential additional morbidity that may be created by thoracotomy in a cat with respiratory disease.

LOWER RESPIRATORY TRACT DISEASES

LRT diseases may be defined as noninfectious or infectious. Noninfectious LRT disease can be considered as non-neoplastic or neoplastic. By far the most common LRT disorders encountered are idiopathic bronchopulmonary diseases,[79] commonly referred to as *feline asthma* and *chronic bronchitis*.

ASTHMA AND CHRONIC BRONCHITIS

Definition

There are no formal definitions of feline idiopathic, inflammatory airway diseases, highlighting the fact that these diseases are still poorly understood. The terms *asthma, bronchial asthma, allergic bronchitis, acute bronchitis,* and *chronic bronchitis* have all been borrowed from human medical literature. The cat is the only animal species that commonly develops a syndrome of asthma similar to that experienced by humans, with eosinophilic airway inflammation, spontaneous bronchoconstriction, and airway remodeling.[208,227] Despite these similarities, direct comparison between human and feline lower airway disease is difficult because pulmonary function testing is used to help classify bronchial diseases in humans, and this testing is not readily available for cats.[188,227]

Essentially, *asthma* is defined as reversible bronchoconstriction, and *chronic bronchitis* results from airway remodeling, leading to fixed airway obstruction. Clinically, reversible bronchoconstriction (the defining feature of asthma) can be recognized by the rapid response to treatment with a bronchodilator such as terbutaline, and chronic bronchitis requires the presence of a daily cough (which may be intermittent with asthma).[207] Asthma is characterized by predominantly eosinophilic airway inflammation and chronic bronchitis by nondegenerate neutrophilic inflammation.[135,192,278]

Because the diagnosis, prognosis, and management overlap considerably, these conditions will be considered concurrently.

Epidemiology

One study recognized 128 cases of feline bronchial disease compared to 13,831 hospital admissions over the same period, giving a disease prevalence of approximately 1%.[188] Cats with idiopathic bronchial disease can present between 4 months and 15 years of age, with a mean age of 4.9 years in one study[63] and medians of 5, 5.5, 6, and 9 years reported in others.[2,45,75,260] Sex predisposition findings have been inconsistent, with two studies finding two thirds of cases to be female,[2,188] another two studies finding two thirds to be male,[63,260] and two others finding no sex predispositions.[45,75] Two North American studies found Siamese to be overrepresented, accounting for between 16% and 17% of cases, with one of these studies compared to a hospital population of 0.6% Siamese cats over the duration of the study[63,188]; one European study reported 12 of 22 cats (55%) to be Siamese, compared with a hospital prevalence of 30%.[2]

Etiopathogenesis

The clinical signs of feline bronchial disease can result from bronchoconstriction caused by increased airway reactivity or increased mucus production (or both) and smooth muscle hypertrophy arising from inflammation of the bronchial wall.[121,207,208,278] The underlying cause of airway inflammation is believed to be instigated by antigenic or allergic stimulation causing activation of a T-Helper 2 (T_h2) response. A T_h2 response instigates secretion of interleukins (IL) 4, 5, and 13, and this cascade results in recruitment of and subsequent degranulation of eosinophils. Degranulation of eosinophils results in damage and destruction of the epithelial lining of the airways.[73,201] Cats with predominantly neutrophilic inflammation may have similar toxic damage with subsequent repair processes.[121]

The consequences of these responses are metaplasia and proliferation of airway epithelium, hyperplasia of mucous glands with production of excess mucus, hypertrophy and hyperplasia of airway smooth muscle, and distal emphysematous changes in the pulmonary parenchyma. Hyperresponsiveness of airway smooth muscle results in airway constriction in response to nonspecific stimuli such as airway irritants, allergens, parasites, and viral particles.[121]

Experimental models in which cats are first sensitized and then challenged with Bermuda grass antigen, house dust mite antigen, or pig roundworm *(Ascaris suum)* have been developed. These models have resulted in not only the clinical signs but also the airway hyperreactivity, typical airway cytology, and histologic lesions that are recognized in cats with naturally occurring bronchial disease.[133,201]

Clinical Signs

Cats with bronchial diseases typically present for coughing, wheezing, loud breathing, and rapid or labored respiration. Exercise intolerance can be seen, and some cats present for general lethargy without the owner realizing that the signs are attributable to respiratory disease. Because coughing can be such an active process involving considerable abdominal effort, owners sometimes confuse it with regurgitation or vomiting and may mention gastrointestinal signs to the veterinarian at presentation. The frequency of clinical signs can vary from intermittent (with cats apparently entirely normal between episodes) to daily.

Physical examination findings vary markedly. Cats presenting with severe respiratory distress should have only a cursory initial examination, during which the clinician's aim is to determine if the clinical signs are from LRT disease or pleural effusion. Radiographs in the position most comfortable for the cat may be required to help make this distinction. Oxygen therapy should be instituted as soon as practicable, and a bronchodilator such as terbutaline (0.01 mg/kg subcutaneously) administered if bronchial disease is suspected. At the other extreme, some cats have no specific abnormalities present. In all but emergency situations, it is ideal to observe the cat before handling to watch for tachypnea and any signs of increased or prolonged expiratory effort. Auscultation often reveals increased expiratory sounds, which can sound harsh or wheezy. Chronic disease can result in a barrel-chested appearance and decreased thoracic compliance.

Diagnosis

Idiopathic, inflammatory bronchial disease is the most common cause of coughing and wheezing in cats. There is no single diagnostic test that is pathognomonic for this diagnosis. Diagnosis is made on the basis of collection of diagnostic clues, the results of which can sometimes be inconsistent, and the exclusion of other known causes of lower respiratory disease, mainly parasitic (e.g., lungworm, heartworm) or other infectious causes. Other causes of respiratory signs, such as pleural effusion, cardiomyopathies, and neoplasia, are mostly distinguished on the basis of radiographic findings.

In most cases radiography and bronchial wash analysis, together with clinical history and physical examination findings, will give enough information for a working diagnosis. Response to therapy is also a useful indication; most cats with asthma will respond to corticosteroid therapy within 1 week.[207] Lungworm and heartworm can be difficult to rule out definitively; these parasites are considered in subsequent sections.

Radiography

Radiography is a vital aspect in diagnosis of lower airway disease but cannot provide a definitive diagnosis of the cause of bronchial disease. The radiographic finding of a bronchial pattern helps guide the clinician to determine the cause; however, the absence of such a pattern does not rule out bronchial diseases. Cats with bronchial diseases can have a variety of radiographic findings, including no abnormalities.[45]

One recent study assessed the radiographic findings of 40 cats with bronchial disease; 37 of 40 cats (92.5%) had a bronchial pattern, but a large number of these cats also had an unstructured interstitial pattern (30 of 40 cats). Nonspecific respiratory signs were also prominent, with lung hyperinflation (31 of 40), hyperlucency (21 of 40), and aerophagia (19 of 40) recognized. Further, lung soft tissue opacities were seen in 11 of 40 cats. This study also found variation in interobserver interpretation; however, there was disagreement in only 2 of 24 cases with severe bronchial disease.[83]

These findings are similar to one other study in which Foster and coworkers[75] found a bronchial or mixed bronchial pattern in 20 of 22 cats (91%). Adamama-Moraitou and coworkers[2] recognized a bronchial pattern in 16 of 22 cats (73%), whereas Corcoran and coworkers[45] found a bronchial or mixed bronchial–interstitial pattern to be less consistent, occurring in only 17 of 29 cats (59%). Moise and coworkers[188] used a bronchial pattern as part of the inclusion criteria but found that 46% also had an interstitial pattern and 37% also had a patchy alveolar pattern. The other consistent radiographic finding in cats with bronchial disease is collapsed lung lobes, occurring in 4% to 11% of cases*; the right middle lung lobe is most frequently collapsed because this lobe's main bronchus has a dorsal-ventral orientation within the bronchial tree, so the accumulated mucus is subject to the effects of gravity.[208] With chronicity, miliary broncholithiasis can develop that appears radiographically as a generalized nodular pattern with multiple mineral opacities.[264]

Figures 30-13 and 30-14 show the progression of radiographic appearance of a cat with bronchial disease over a 9-year period.

In summary, a bronchial or bronchointerstitial pattern has a high correlation with idiopathic bronchial diseases, but other findings, including normal radiographs, still allow the possibility of this diagnosis.

Airway Cytology and Culture

Airway cytology and culture are important in the diagnosis of idiopathic bronchial disease, as well as to rule out specific causes of LRT disease, such as infection. As noted previously, samples can be obtained bronchoscopically (after bronchoscopic examination) or by blind BAL. There are no definitive guidelines for assessment of tracheobronchial wash cytology; contamination of samples is hard to avoid, and up to 75% of cases will result in light growth of bacteria that are not clinically relevant.[63,75] Studies of healthy cats have found highly variable nucleated cell counts in BAL fluid, as well as a variation in the proportion of cell types; eosinophils have been reported to make up as much as 25% of the cells retrieved in normal cats (see Table 30-3).[184,211] However, comparisons of bronchial wash cytology of cats with bronchial diseases, when directly compared with that of healthy cats, have shown higher cell counts in those cats with airway inflammation.[54,63,187] Cell counts from normal cats are typically in the order of 200 to 300 nucleated cells/μL; however, counts as a high as 600/μL can occur. In contrast, cell counts can exceed 1500/μL with airway inflammation.[54,102] The predominant cell type in bronchial wash fluid is alveolar macrophages, which can make up as much as 90% of the population of cells retrieved from healthy cats.[54,170,171] For asthma and chronic bronchitis, the predominant cell type can be eosinophils or neutrophils.[45,63,75,188] It has been suggested that asthma (reversible bronchoconstriction) can be characterized by eosinophilic inflammation, and chronic bronchitis (permanently remodeled airways) may have neutrophils as the predominant inflammatory cell present.[278] Although this has not been confirmed clinically, experimental models in which cats are sensitized to an antigen such as Bermuda grass or house dust mites have shown substantial increases in BAL eosinophil proportions from less than 10% to 35% to 45%.[145,201] The proportions of inflammatory cells found in wash cytology are not always mentioned in clinical reports, but in one study all eosinophilic exudates comprised more than 60% eosinophils,[75] and another noted that mixed cell exudates contained 30% to 50% eosinophils.[188] Although a mean of 25% eosinophils was found in one population of healthy cats,[211] it could be expected that 25% eosinophils from a wash of 1500 to 3000 nucleated cells/μL would have greater significance than the same proportion found in a wash of only 200 to 300 cells/μL. A large proportion of eosinophils may also reflect other conditions, such as parasitism, which must be ruled out. When the neutrophil population is elevated, the distinction of inflammatory disease from infection must be made. As well as the expectation of a positive culture result (from bacterial infection), the neutrophils associated with infection can be expected to show toxic, degenerative changes, whereas nondegenerate neutrophils resembling those of normal peripheral blood would be expected with inflammatory, noninfectious disease.

Not only is culture of *Mycoplasma* spp. important to rule out pneumonia, but this organism may have an interaction with idiopathic bronchial diseases.[35,76,78,273] *Mycoplasma* spp. infections will be considered with infectious bronchial diseases.

*References 2, 45, 75, 83, 188, 260.

Less Routine Diagnostic Interventions

BRONCHOSCOPY

Bronchoscopy requires specific training and experience because the procedure carries the risks of bronchospasm and pneumothorax. The consequences of these risks are increased because the patient cannot be intubated. In competent hands bronchoscopy allows direct visualization of airways and a means of guided BAL. However, in most cases, bronchoscopy is not required to make an accurate diagnosis of asthma or bronchitis.

COMPUTED TOMOGRAPHY

CT provides more precise imaging information than radiography. Specifically for lower airway diseases, CT can provide precise information about airway thickening, mucus accumulation, and lung lobe consolidation.

EXHALED BREATH CONDENSATE ANALYSIS

Exhaled breath condensate (EBC) analysis has been assessed experimentally in cats.[136,253] Essentially, increased concentrations of particular biomarkers are recognized in the exhaled air of people, and this technique has been applied to cats to measure exhaled hydrogen peroxide (H_2O_2). This noninvasive technique involves cats being placed in a chamber similar to an oxygen chamber; the exhaled air is passed through a steel tube that runs through an ice bath for condensation of the exhaled air. The steel tube is disconnected and shaken vigorously to collect the condensate droplets, which are then assessed

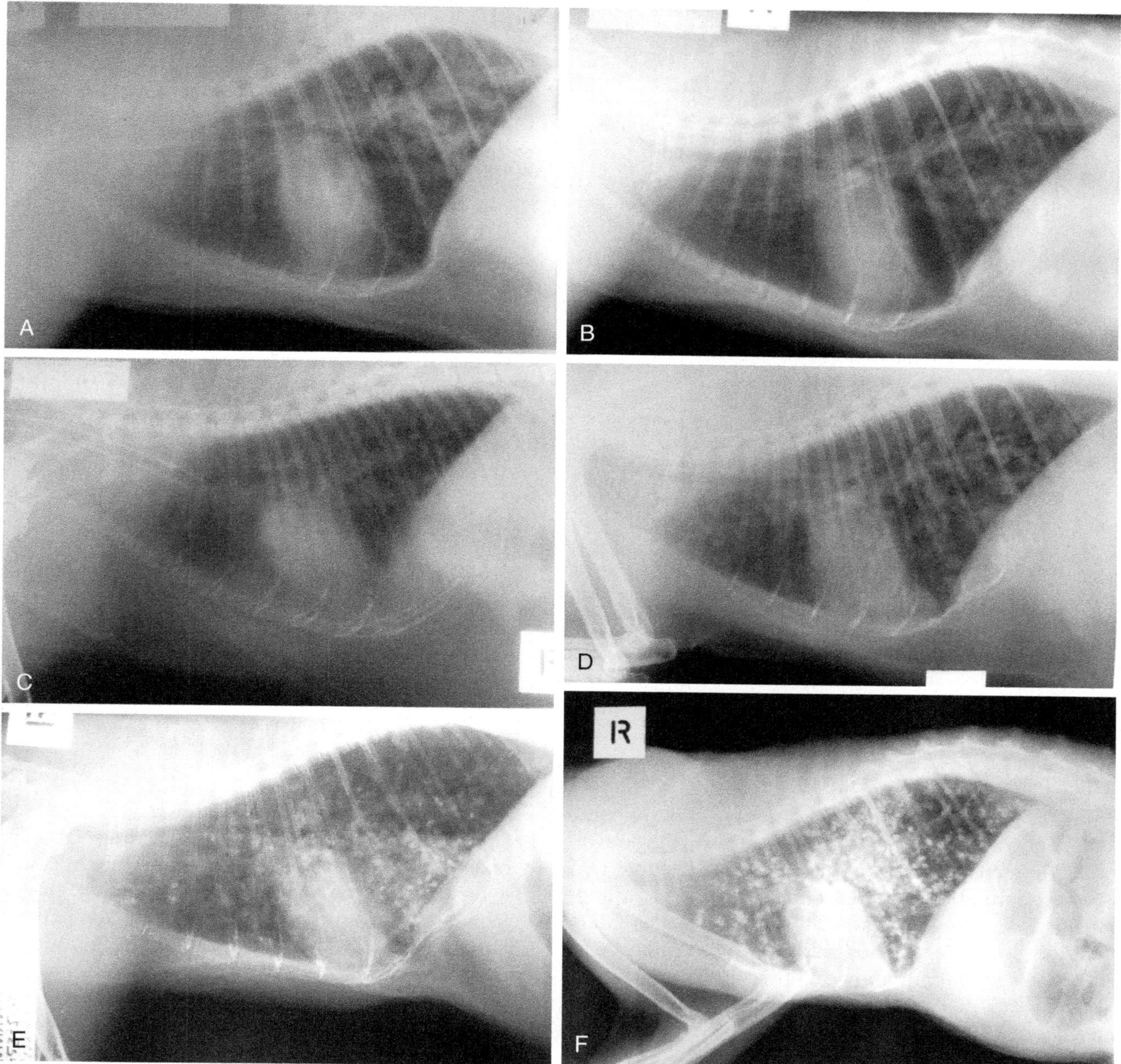

FIGURE 30-13 Progression of radiographic appearance (right lateral views) of a cat with bronchial disease over 9 years. **A,** A bronchointerstitial pattern, with the interstitial change focused about the bronchial tree. Hyperinflation of the lungs is evident. Initially, the cat was diagnosed with *Mycoplasma* infection. **B,** Six weeks after the prior radiograph, after treatment with doxycyline during that time. Note improvement in the interstitial pattern, with a bronchial pattern predominating. Bronchoalveolar lavage at this stage showed eosinophils predominating. **C,** Three years after the initial radiographs. Although the bronchial pattern is less intense, there is evidence of early stage mineralization about the airways. **D,** Five years after the initial radiographs. Mineralization is more obvious and beginning to organize into nodules. **E,** Seven years after the initial diagnosis. Note an organized nodular pattern with multiple mineral opacities, typical of broncholithiasis. A collapsed lung lobe is also visible caudoventrally; this is more evident on the dorsoventral view (see Figure 30-14). **F,** Nine years after the initial diagnosis. Note further broncholithiasias; where lung is visible caudally, a bronchial pattern can be seen. After the initial course of doxycyline, this cat remained on prednisolone and terbutaline, which (for the most part) managed this cat's clinical signs for the duration of this series.

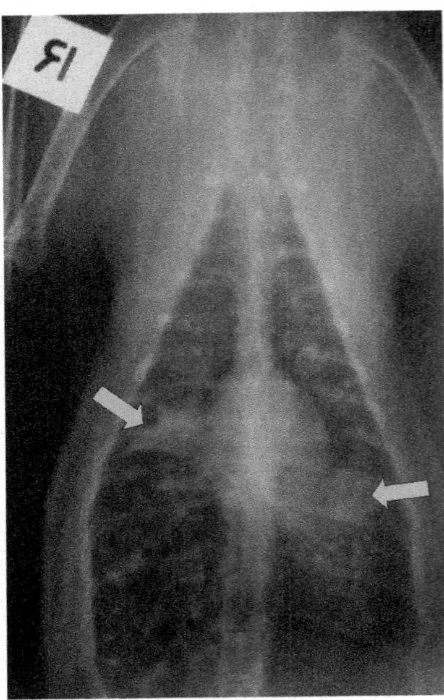

FIGURE 30-14 Dorsoventral view of cat with chronic bronchial disease in prior figures. Note that the collapsed lung lobes (marked with *green arrows*) are dependent lobes. There is also marked broncholithiasis.

to measure H_2O_2, considered to be a marker of lower airway inflammation.[136,253]

PULMONARY FUNCTION TESTING

Pulmonary function testing is commonly used in people to determine airway resistance associated with reduced airway diameter caused by bronchoconstriction and mucus accumulation. There are descriptions of pulmonary function testing in cats, but this testing is not widely available.[63,111,134] Plethysmography allows pulmonary function testing in conscious cats by calculating expiratory time and peak inspiratory and expiratory flows from a cat in a sealed (and calibrated) Plexiglas box.[111,134]

IDENTIFICATION OF ALLERGENS

Identification of allergens has been performed for cats with bronchial diseases in both clinical[190] and experimental[145,198] settings with both intradermal skin testing(IDT)[145,190] and IgE serology.[145,190,198] These studies show promise, and if specific allergens can be identified, immunotherapy is conceivable as a treatment option. The remaining obstacles for allergy testing of cats with lower respiratory disease are that positive allergen reactions reflect only exposure and may not be clinically relevant. Further, IDT in cats is regarded as problematic to interpret because subtle positive reactions occur and repeatability of both serum IgE and IDT testing cannot always be demonstrated.[190] Interestingly, one study found case recruitment difficult because numerous cats had concurrent allergic skin disease (an exclusion criteria for this study); concurrent allergic skin disease and lower airway disease had not previously been reported.[190]

Treatment

Aims

Treatment aims are as follows:

1. To reduce airway smooth muscle contraction (bronchodilators)
2. To decrease underlying inflammation (corticosteroids)

Use of bronchodilators is the primary method of treatment when acute signs develop but are not appropriate as sole therapy. It is important to recognize that human (and most likely feline) airways show evidence of chronic, ongoing inflammation whether the patient is showing clinical signs or not; thus many cats require long-term treatment with corticosteroids.[208] Asthma is a chronic disorder without a cure, and even well-controlled patients may experience occasional exacerbations of clinical signs. Although the prognosis for most patients receiving appropriate diagnostic evaluation and treatment is good for control of disease, owners should have realistic expectations about the need for long-term therapy.

Emergency Treatment

Cats presenting with acute respiratory distress such as open-mouth breathing or abdominal breathing should be handled minimally (to reduce further stress). The clinician's primary aim should be to distinguish LRT disease from pleural effusion or pulmonary edema; to this end, survey radiographs should be taken in the position most comfortable for the cat (usually dorsoventrally, with the cat supported by its elbows) after the patient has been stabilized as much as possible. It is appropriate to provide the cat with an oxygen-rich environment; details of supplementary oxygen–delivery techniques can be found in Box 30-5 later in the chapter. A bronchodilator such as terbutaline should be administered at 0.01 mg/kg parenterally. A response is usually seen in 10 to 30 minutes. The response to terbutaline alone can aid in the diagnosis of bronchoconstriction as the cause of respiratory distress. Terbutaline can be readministered 30 minutes later at the same dose if minimal effect has been noted. An alternative is to administer salbutamol–albuterol using an MDI (discussed later). The typical dose is 2 actuations every 30 minutes as needed. The drug takes effect rapidly with improvement in clinical signs seen in less than 5 minutes. If oxygen therapy and bronchodilation do not substantially reduce respiratory rate and effort, corticosteroids such as dexamethasone sodium phosphate (0.2 to 1 mg/kg, intravenously or intramuscularly) can be administered. Failure to respond to these therapeutic measures should alert the clinician to other causes of respiratory distress.

Long-Term Treatment Corticosteroids

Corticosteroids are the mainstay for treatment of inflammatory airway disease, having demonstrated success in several clinical studies.[45,75] Corticosteroids reduce inflammation and migration of inflammatory cells into the airway. However, there have been few studies to determine efficacy or optimal dosing routines for systemic corticosteroids in cats with asthma. One study has shown that prednisolone administered at 5 mg/cat every 12 hours orally for 2 weeks resulted in a significantly lower percentage of eosinophils (mean = 5%) in BAL cytology compared with a control substance (mean eosinophils = 33.7%).[226] Typical recommendations are for prednisolone to be administered at 1 to 2 mg/kg every 12 hours for 5 to 10 days before tapering the dose over at least 2 months (e.g., reducing at weekly intervals until 0.5 mg/kg every second day).[121,208]

Treatment with injectable long-acting corticosteroids (e.g., methylprednisolone acetate, 10 to 20 mg/cat, intramuscularly every 4 to 8 weeks) is the least desirable approach and should be reserved for patients for which no other method of drug administration is possible. Chronic use of these formulations often results in serious side effects, such as weight gain, diabetes mellitus, and an impaired immune response. Owners should be fully informed of the significant risks of this form of therapy.

Inhaled corticosteroids have been used to manage feline bronchial diseases for over a decade.[204] In veterinary medicine human MDIs containing a propellant rather than dry powder inhalers (e.g., Diskus inhalers) are used. Inhalational delivery of corticosteroids by use of MDI allows for local antiinflammatory activity while minimizing systemic absorption and the potential adverse effects that may arise. Systemic absorption of inhaled medications still occurs with some drugs; one study demonstrated hypothalamic–pituitary–adrenal axis (HPAA) suppression in healthy cats receiving 250 μg flunisolide every 12 hours,[223] but another study of cats receiving 220 μg fluticasone every 12 hours showed no suppression.[40] Research using nebulized radiopharmaceutical agents has demonstrated that inhaled medications delivered using a face mask and spacer can be distributed throughout the lung fields of cats.[242] The most commonly used inhaled corticosteroid is fluticasone, although others are sometimes available (e.g., beclomethasone) and may be less expensive (but potentially less effective). Fluticasone has the longest half-life of the available inhalant corticosteroids, is the most potent, and is the least likely to be absorbed systemically.[205] The drug is available in three strengths per actuation, with the labeling varying by country: 44 or 50 μg, 110 or 125 μg, and 220 or 250 μg. In the United States, MDIs are labeled by the amount of drug delivered at the mouthpiece, whereas in other countries, they are labeled by the amount of drug delivered from the valve, which accounts for what appears to be different strengths of the same product. Inhaled fluticasone at doses of 44 μg every 12 hours and 110 μg every 12 hours was found to be effective in ameliorating signs and reducing inflammation in experimentally induced eosinophilic airway inflammation.[40] Further, 220 μg of inhaled fluticasone every 24 hours reduced the inflammatory response in cats with neutrophilic airway inflammation (but no clinical signs).[135]

Each MDI delivers a set dose per actuation (a "puff"), and each container has a fixed number of doses. For MDIs that do not include a dose-counting mechanism, the owner must keep track of the doses used so that an empty container is not used. MDIs require slow, deep inhalation on the part of the patient. This type of inspiration is not possible for animals and infants, so a spacer and face mask must be used. Spacers decrease the amount of drug deposited in the oropharynx. A spacer and face mask of appropriate size for cats should be used (e.g., AeroKat, Trudell Medical International). To administer the medication, the MDI is shaken to open an internal valve in the canister and is then attached to the spacer. If the spacer does not contain a valve, the spacer and mask should be applied to the cat's face before the MDI is actuated. The MDI is then actuated to deliver the drug into the spacer and the owner should observe the cat take 7 to 10 breaths to ensure that the drug has been inhaled. The AeroKat system has an indicator valve that makes it easier for the owner to tell when the cat takes a breath. If a patient is receiving both an inhaled bronchodilator and corticosteroid, the bronchodilator should be administered first and the corticosteroid 5 to 10 minutes later. The owner should follow the manufacturer's instructions for cleaning and maintenance of the mask and spacer system.

It has been stated that the most effective long-term treatment of asthma is systemically administered corticosteroids,[208] and it is prudent to start severely affected cats with oral prednisolone with a view to maintenance with inhaled fluticasone when the severity of signs has decreased. It is appropriate to start therapy with inhaled fluticasone in mildly to moderately affected cases. Anecdotal responses indicate that 44/50 μg fluticasone is not always effective clinically but that 110/125 μg every 12 hours is effective in managing most cases of mild to moderate disease and cats with more serious disease require 220/250 μg every 12 hours; it has been suggested that once-daily dosing is occasionally effective and dosing less often is not helpful.[208] Inhaled corticosteroid therapy is considerably more expensive than oral therapy, and cost will be a barrier for some owners.

The author's approach to corticosteroid use in severe cases has been to use oral prednisolone, starting at 10 mg/cat every 24 hours or 5 mg/cat every 12 hours and tapering weekly until 5 mg/cat every second day is reached. At this point inhaled therapy with fluticasone can be started on the days prednisolone is not given; it should be given daily when the cat has been weaned from prednisolone entirely. It may take 1 to 2 weeks for fluticasone to take effect, so weaning from oral prednisolone should take place over a 2- to 3-week period. Mild to moderately affected cats can be started with inhaled fluticasone (without use of systemic corticosteroids). The author uses an MDI product containing 250 μg fluticasone combined with 25 μg salmeterol and has found that most cats can be managed at dosages between one puff every second day and two puffs twice a day. MDIs containing fluticasone combined with salmeterol are not available in all countries, although they may be available as separate products. Salmeterol is available as 25 μg/actuation in some countries and as 21 μg/actuation in others. Management appears to be most successful when the dose is started higher and reduced at 1- to 2-week intervals to the lowest effective dose.

Avoidance of oral corticosteroids may be important for certain patients with concurrent diseases, such as diabetes mellitus or herpesvirus infection. In one series of 300 cases,[206] 80% of 246 cats with mild to moderate disease were weaned from oral corticosteroids and maintained on inhaled fluticasone alone. Of 54 cats with severe disease, 63% were weaned from oral corticosteroids and maintained on inhaled fluticasone. The remaining cats were maintained on a combination of oral and inhaled corticosteroids, but in most cases with a lower oral dose than if inhaled medication was not used. About 85% of owners were able to use a mask and spacer system effectively, and the rate of adverse effects was low, such as 5% of cats with ocular irritation.

Box 30-4 provides details of guidelines for the use of inhaled medications in cats (Figures 30-15 and 30-16).

BRONCHODILATORS

Because bronchoconstriction is considered a major aspect of inflammatory airway disease, bronchodilators can be

BOX 30-4

Guidelines for Use of Inhaled Medications in Cats

Inhaled medications have been successfully used to manage bronchial diseases in cats for more than a decade. Successful therapy depends on habituating the cat (and the owner) to receiving (and giving) medication in this way. There are several commercially available spacers designed for both veterinary and human pediatric use. The clinician should explore available options and become familiar with the equipment.

Choices of chamber and mask should be made based on the basis of the following factors:

1. Size of chamber: Ideally, the size of the chamber should be appropriate for a cat's tidal volume (10 to 20 mL/kg). Veterinary brands and those designed for human neonates that are approximately 10 to 12 cm long and 3 to 4 cm in diameter are appropriate.
2. Is there a valve present? Presence of a valve between the chamber and the mask allows preloading of the chamber. This reduces the potential stress of the noise of actuating the metered dose inhaler. When using a chamber without such a valve, the owner may need to habituate the cat to the sound of the actuation.
3. Does the mask fit snugly over the cat's muzzle? Commercial spacers usually have a specially shaped opening that allows only their brand of mask to be fitted. Veterinary systems often include more than one size of mask. Sometimes masks can be cut down to fit better.

Habituation:

1. Some cats dislike the mask being placed over their muzzle. These cats can be introduced to the mask slowly by offering food from the mask (just a few kibbles) without the chamber attached for approximately 1 week and then allowing the cat to breathe air through the mask before attaching the chamber. After a few weeks, medications can be introduced to the chamber. Cats may need oral medication during the period of habituation.
2. When using a chamber without a valve, the owner may need to habituate the cat to the sound of the actuation.

Dosing:

1. Anecdotal information indicates that 44 to 50 μg fluticasone is not effective clinically but that 110 to 125 μg every 12 hours is effective in managing most cases of mild to moderate disease and that cats with more serious disease require 220 to 250 μg every 12 hours; it has been suggested that once-daily dosing is occasionally effective and dosing less often is not helpful.
2. The author uses an MDI with 250 μg fluticasone/25 μg salmeterol and has found that most cats can be managed between one puff every second day and two puffs twice day. Management appears to be most successful when the dose is started higher and reduced at 1- to 2-week intervals to the lowest effective dose.
3. Albuterol/salbutamol 90 to 100 μg per actuation can be used before administering fluticasone or, in emergencies, every 30 minutes for up to 4 to 6 hours. Chronic use of albuterol/salbutamol is not recommended.
4. It may take 1 to 2 weeks for fluticasone to take full effect, so some patients may benefit from concurrent administration of oral prednisolone in tapering doses over 2 to 3 weeks.

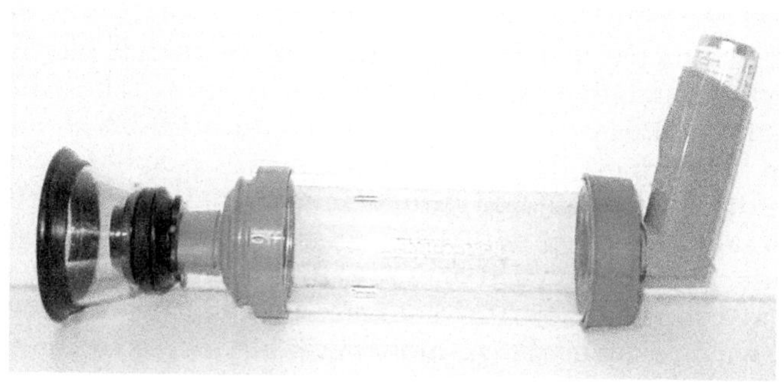

FIGURE 30-15 Metered dose inhaler connected to chamber and mask ready for delivery of inhaled medication. The mask should fit snugly and comfortably over the cat's muzzle. The ideal chamber size should approximate the cat's tidal volume.

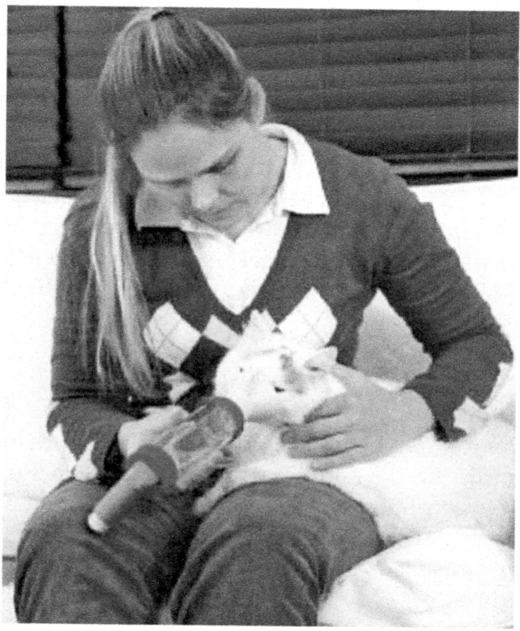

FIGURE 30-16 Administration of inhaled medications should be in a relaxed setting where the cat feels comfortable.

expected to be beneficial. Reductions in airway obstruction have been demonstrated with the beta$_2$-receptor agonists, terbutaline (intravenously)[63] and a combination of inhaled salbutamol (albuterol) and ipratropium.[132] The bronchodilatory effects of inhaled salbutamol, salmeterol, and ipratropium have also been demonstrated against induced bronchoconstriction in healthy cats.[148]

There are three major classes of bronchodilators: beta$_2$-receptor agonists, methylxanthines, and anticholinergics.

BETA$_2$-RECEPTOR AGONISTS The most commonly used beta$_2$-receptor agonists are terbutaline (mostly used through injectable routes or orally) and salbutamol/albuterol (mostly used as an inhaled medication but available in oral preparations). Beta$_2$-receptor specificity should reduce cardiovascular side effects, but tachycardia has been recognized with terbutaline.[63] Terbutaline can be given parenterally (subcutaneously, intramuscularly, or intravenously) at 0.01 mg/kg[63,64,175] for emergency care and is recommended to be given before bronchoscopy or blind BAL. Oral dosing has been determined to be 0.625 mg every 12 hours.[64,175] Terbutaline should be used with care in patients with preexisting cardiac disease, hyperthyroidism, hypertension, or seizures.

Salbutamol (International Nonproprietary Name) and albuterol (United States Adopted Name) are different names for the same drug. The drug is available in an MDI as salbutamol (100 µg/actuation) in most of the world and as albuterol (90 µg/actuation) in the United States. In humans salbutamol or albuterol results in significant bronchodilation within 5 to 15 minutes and lasts for 3 to 4 hours.[65] Similar results have been found in cats; the longer acting beta$_2$-receptor agonist salmeterol had less effect but lasted for 24 hours.[148] There are two forms (enantiomers) of salbutamol or albuterol, the pharmacologically active R-salbutamol or albuterol and inactive S-salbutamol or albuterol; most formulations available are combinations of the two forms, with the proportion of active form varying from 16% to 50%.[4,100,117,202,228] Chronic use of the inactive form can result in worsening airway inflammation in humans[100,117,202] and in cats.[228] Where available, single enantiomer R-salbutamol or albuterol should be used. It is used once daily when needed and is administered before fluticasone. Salbutamol or albuterol should be used with care in patients with preexisting cardiac disease, hyperthyroidism, hypertension, or seizures.

The addition of inhaled long acting beta$_2$-agonists to corticosteroids is believed to increase the efficacy of inhaled corticosteroid effects in moderate to severe asthma and chronic obstructive pulmonary disease in humans.[36] The author uses 100 µg salbutamol or albuterol as emergency treatment and 25 µg salmeterol (combined with fluticasone) as maintenance therapy for cats with stable disease.

METHYLXANTHINES Theophylline and aminophylline are not recommended for routine use; however, propentofylline may show promise. Drugs of this class are generally considered less potent bronchodilators than beta$_2$-agonists[209] and remain controversial in human respiratory medicine, with some authors considering these drugs obsolete for airway disease.[141] The recommended dose of standard-preparation theophylline is 4 mg/kg orally every 8 to 12 hours; the sustained release preparation dose has been reported at 10 mg/kg orally every 24 hours[121] and 25 mg/kg orally every 24 hours.[208] However, sustained-release formulations known to have acceptable pharmacokinetics in cats, such as Theo-Dur, were discontinued more than 10 years ago. Extended-release formulations from various manufacturers do not have the same pharmacokinetics, preventing extrapolation of doses from brand to brand and making routine use of these products impractical. In addition, there are several known drug interactions with theophylline that the clinician must consider. The dose rate for aminophylline is reported to be 5 to 6 mg/kg orally every 12 hours.[208] A recent clinical study indicated that cats treated with propentofylline (a methylxanthine derivative marketed for dementia in dogs) improved more on owner and clinician scoring as well as radiographic features than those treated with prednisolone alone.[260] This drug's usefulness could be assessed further by a crossover study (which is not usually practical for a clinical study as was undertaken).

ANTICHOLINERGICS Anticholinergics are not widely used in veterinary medicine. Several recent papers have indicated synergistic benefit of inhaled ipratropium bromide when used with salbutamol in healthy cats[148] and experimentally allergen-sensitized cats.[132] These drugs may prove useful in cats with severe disease in which more routinely used bronchodilators are not sufficiently helpful.

Other Therapies

ANTIBIOTICS

Antibiotic use is not warranted in a great majority of cases of feline idiopathic airway disease. Antimicrobial therapy should be instituted only on the basis of culture and sensitivity findings from bronchial wash fluid. However, a positive culture result does not always indicate a lower respiratory infection and must be interpreted on the basis of cytologic findings, whether there is pure or mixed growth, and how heavy the growth is. Generally, greater than 10^5 organisms/mL is consistent with infection.[208] LRT infections with *Mycoplasma* spp. have the strongest association with idiopathic airway disease. *Mycoplasma* spp. have not been isolated from airways of healthy cats,[221] and associations have been made with human asthma and mycoplasma infection.[76,78] Treatment with doxycycline 5 mg/kg orally every 12 hours for 3 weeks is effective to clear infection in most cases. More information about mycoplasma infections appears later in this chapter in the section about LRT infections.

CYCLOSPORIN-A

An initial study indicated that cyclosporin-A (CsA) inhibits late phase asthmatic responses in experimentally induced allergic airway disease in cats,[210] but a subsequent study by the same investigators showed that CsA treatment does not inhibit the early phase asthmatic response or mast cell degranulation.[185] No further work appears to have been done, and no recommendations to use CsA for idiopathic lower airway disease can be made as of this writing.

ANTIHISTAMINES

One study has demonstrated that cyproheptadine blocks airway smooth muscle contraction in vitro,[212] but the author of this paper has stated that clinical observations do not support these in vitro findings.[208] A subsequent study showed minimal reduction in BAL eosinophil percentage compared with a control substance and far less reduction than inhaled or orally administered corticosteroids; however, two of six cats did indicate reduced airway resistance.[226] A more recent paper confirmed minimal reduction in BAL eosinophil percentage for both cyproheptadine and another antihistamine, cetirizine, compared with a placebo in experimentally induced allergic airway disease.[240] No recommendations to use antihistamines for idiopathic lower airway disease can be made as of this writing.

ANTILEUKOTRIENES

Antileukotrienes such as zafirlukast or montelukast have been advocated for the treatment of feline bronchial diseases.[165] However, one study failed to show any significant reduction in BAL eosinophil percentage for zafirlukast compared with a placebo in experimentally induced allergic airway disease.[226] There is no evidence to support the use of this class of drug for feline bronchial diseases.

OMEGA-3 POLYUNSATURATED FATTY ACIDS

A recent study has indicated a significant modulation in the development of allergen-induced airway disease in cats administered a combination of lipid extract of New Zealand green-lipped mussel (providing omega-3 polyunsaturated fatty acids) and lutolein.[147] This treatment shows promise as a therapeutic option for feline allergic airway disease.

IMMUNOTHERAPY

The identification of allergens responsible for lower airway disease allows the possibility of allergen-specific immune therapy. Several studies from the same investigative group have demonstrated the success of immune therapy in experimentally induced allergic lower airway disease.[146,224,225] Because disease was experimentally induced in these cases, the inciting allergen (Bermuda grass allergen) was known; the challenge remains to demonstrate efficacy in natural cases where the inciting allergen (or allergens) must be determined from intradermal skin testing (notoriously difficult in cats) or IgE serology. Nevertheless, immunotherapy holds great promise not only to manage allergic airway disease (as other treatments do) but actually to *cure* the underlying disease so that ongoing therapy is no longer required.

Long-Term Management

In the great majority of cases, cats with lower airway disease require chronic, mostly lifelong, treatment.

Cats undergoing long-term therapy (for any condition) should be assessed at regular intervals. Follow-up visits should be scheduled approximately 2 weeks after instituting therapy, 1 month later, and subsequently every 3 to 6 months. The schedules are not fixed and cats should be seen ahead of schedule if the cat fails to respond to treatment. The initial visits are important to assess not only the cat's response to therapy but also the owner's ability to administer medication, whether inhaled or oral. As well as the cat's clinical signs at home at examination, doses and frequency of medication should be assessed and confirmed. Home control measures should be discussed with the clients, such as avoidance of aerosol triggers such as cigarette smoke, fireplace smoke, and dusty cat litters; use of air filters can also help control signs. Cats on long-term systemic glucocorticoid treatment should also have periodic blood glucose assessment. Repeat thoracic radiographs or other investigations may be warranted if a cat's clinical signs persist, recur, or are not controlled entirely.

OTHER NONINFECTIOUS LOWER RESPIRATORY TRACT DISEASE

The diagnosis of noninfectious, non-neoplastic causes of LRT disease in cats is often aided by clinical history. For example, a history of blunt trauma, exposure to smoke inhalation, lipid aspiration from owner administration of mineral oil, or electric shock is often known at the time of admission; likewise, aspiration pneumonia is usually associated with an esophageal disorder and chronic vomiting if not associated with anesthesia. The major exception to this generalization is idiopathic pulmonary fibrosis.

Idiopathic Pulmonary Fibrosis

Despite few reports, idiopathic pulmonary fibrosis has been well characterized in one case series of 23 cats[41] that included 16 cats from an earlier study,[286] which detailed the histologic findings and compared the condition to that in people. Most cats in this study were middle-aged or older, with a median age of 8.3 years (range 1.9 to 15 years). Most cases present for respiratory signs—predominantly labored or rapid respiration but also coughing. Lethargy, anorexia, and weight loss are also prominent (but not always present). Respiratory distress is often recognized at presentation and is often inspiratory or mixed inspiratory and expiratory compared with bronchial disease, in which expiratory signs predominate. Respiratory sounds auscultated were described as harsh or loud in numerous cases and wheezes or crackles, or both were recognized in approximately half of the cases.[41]

Radiographic changes affecting the parenchyma resulting in an interstitial or bronchointerstitial pattern are usually marked with diffuse involvement (Figure 30-17), but patchy distribution with greater severity in some regions (particularly caudal lung lobes) was recognized in 10 of 18 cats. BAL findings may show a mild increase in nondegenerate neutrophils or be normal. FNA, when performed, is either nondiagnostic or misleading. Diagnosis depends on histopathologic examination of affected lung tissue; either performed ante mortem by thoracotomy or thorascopic biopsy but usually at necropsy. The characteristic histopathologic finding is interstitial fibrosis with fibroblast or myofibroblast foci, honeycombing with alveolar interstitial smooth muscle metaplasia. Interstitial inflammation is not a prominent feature. As in people, coincident neoplasia may be present.[41,286] CT has been used to diagnose idiopathic pulmonary fibrosis presumptively in people with an accuracy of approximately 90%; the key feature is cystic dilation of air spaces leading to peripheral honeycombing. Although this has not been described in cats, it may serve as a useful diagnostic aid.[130]

There is no known effective treatment. Corticosteroids (e.g., prednisolone at 10 mg/cat, orally every 24 hours) and bronchodilators (e.g., terbutaline) appear to help some cats but have no beneficial effect in many. Cyclophosphamide (12.5 mg orally, on 4 days out of 7) was used for several weeks in the only cat that was alive at the time the report was written. With no definitive cause or known pathogenesis, there can be no definitive treatment. Therapeutic approaches in human patients are aimed at interactions between fibroblasts and other pulmonary cells.[41]

Aspiration Pneumonia

Aspiration pneumonia results from the aspiration of endogenous secretions or exogenous substances into the LRT. The extent of damage depends on the frequency, volume, and character of the aspirated material, as well as the effectiveness of host defense mechanisms. Defense mechanisms include airway closure during swallowing; cough reflex; mucociliary transport apparatus; and pulmonary cellular defenses, which minimize the degree of damage when minimal amounts of material are aspirated.[265]

Aspiration pneumonia is a potential consequence in cats with esophageal or swallowing disorders, including those that are anesthetized, comatose, or otherwise debilitated. Gastric contents are acidic and therefore result in chemical pneumonitis that can cause necrosis of bronchial and alveolar epithelium, as well as pulmonary edema. Supportive care with oxygen therapy is appropriate, and treatment for pulmonary edema may be required.[265]

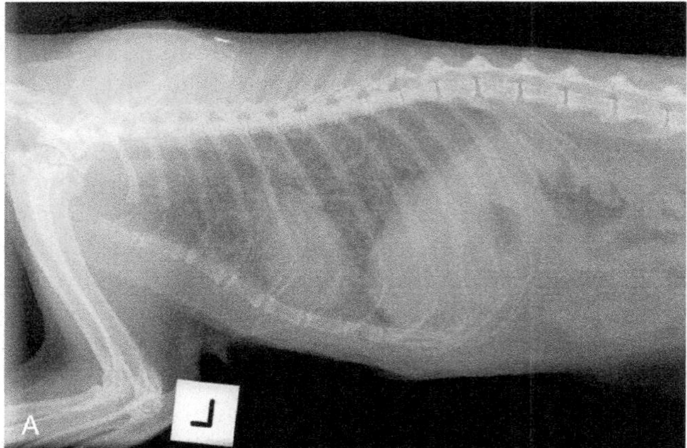

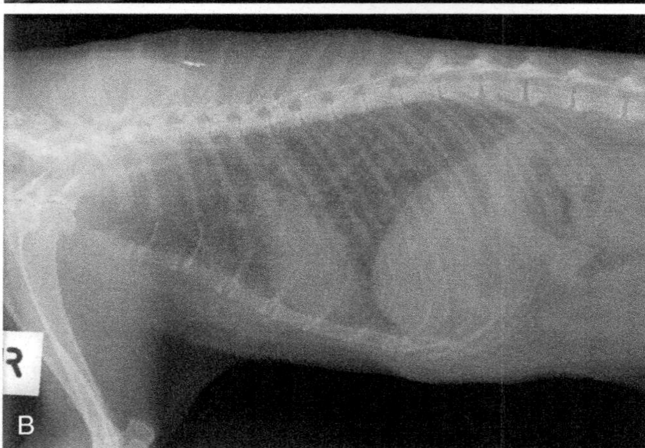

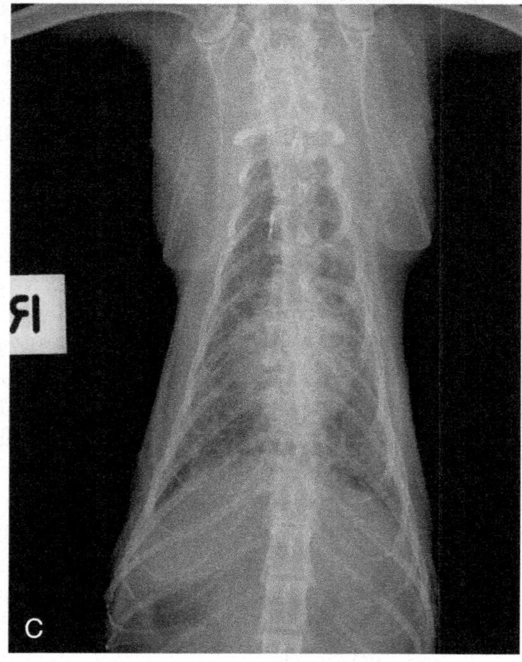

FIGURE 30-17 Left lateral **(A)**, right lateral **(B)**, and dorsoventral **(C)** radiographic views of cat with idiopathic pulmonary fibrosis. Note the diffuse reticular interstitial pattern present throughout all lung lobes. The left caudal lung lobe has consolidation caudally.

Aspiration of small amounts of inert substances such as water or barium (or less acidic gastric material) usually results in transient, self-limiting hypoxia. Larger volumes aspirated can result in asphyxia, and solid material aspirated may result in a more severe reaction than gastric fluid alone. Solid material, such as food particles, should be removed by suction or bronchoscopy and must be removed as soon as possible to prevent death from asphyxiation. Oxygen therapy and other supportive care should also be instituted.[265] Bacterial pneumonia is a longer-term consequence, and preemptive antibiotics are appropriate.

Overnight fasting before anesthesia reduces the risk of aspiration pneumonia as an anesthetic complication.

Lipid aspiration pneumonia may result if mineral or paraffin oil is inhaled during oral administration for management of hairballs.[34] Because such oils are nonirritating, they do not cause reflex inhibition of aspiration. The resultant pneumonia elicits an extensive macrophage response with fibrosis. A mixed alveolar–interstitial infiltrate is often seen in the middle lung lobe, but diffuse nodular densities that may be confused with metastatic lesions can also be seen.[34,265] This condition can be fatal; bronchodilators and corticosteroids may help some cats, but effective treatment may require lobectomy.

Endogenous lipid pneumonia can result when underlying obstructive pulmonary disease damages pneumocytes, allowing release of lipid from degenerating cells, which acts as a direct irritant to the lung and triggers an inflammatory response. This condition does not normally result in death, and the underlying condition should be managed.[125]

Trauma

Thoracic trauma subsequent to automobile accidents or high-rise falls can result in pulmonary contusion (accumulation of blood and other fluids) or bullae (acutely formed pockets of air). Contused lung appears in a patchy alveolar pattern, similar to pulmonary edema; lung cysts appear as isolated air-fluid levels with poorly delineated margins within lung parenchyma and, if they rupture, can result in pneumothorax. Lung cysts and contusions are more obvious radiographically 24 to 48 hours after trauma. These lesions usually resolve with cage rest as other traumatic injuries are managed. Lung cysts sometimes require lobectomy of the affected lobe.[6]

Smoke Inhalation

Both carbon monoxide intoxication and direct bronchopulmonary injury result from smoke inhalation. Compromise to surfactant activity causes atelectasis, resulting in necrotizing bronchiolitis and intraalveolar hemorrhage. Radiographic changes include diffuse peribronchial densities or patchy, interstitial infiltration and, as with trauma, may not be apparent for 24 hours. Cats should be placed in an oxygen chambers (see Box 30-5), and bronchodilators are indicated. Prognosis depends on the degree of damage caused, which is associated with the amount of smoke inhaled.[265]

NEOPLASIA

Primary pulmonary neoplasia is rare in cats[179,182,267]; no recent prevalence data are available, but the annual incidence was estimated at 2.2 per 100,000 cats approximately 30 years ago.[267] Older cats are more likely to be affected, with a mean age of 10 to 14 years reported.[13,179] Most tumors are adenocarcinomas of bronchial or bronchoalveolar origin.[94] Presenting signs are most commonly referable to the respiratory tract and can include coughing, exercise intolerance, tachypnea, and dyspnea[94]; however, cats can present for nonrespiratory signs such as lethargy, inappetence, and lameness associated with metastasis to digits; this is also known as "lung–digit syndrome" and carries an extremely poor prognosis.[87,189] Metastasis to other locations such as skin,[217] skeletal muscle,[142,181] and the eye[32] has also been reported. Hypercalcemia of malignancy is possible,[5,22,238] and hypertrophic osteodystrophy has been reported in 5% to 25% of cases.[13,94]

In many cases all lung lobes are affected when assessed radiographically, and pleural effusion is present in 35% to 65% of cases. Typical radiographic findings are a mixed bronchoalveolar pattern, an ill-defined alveolar mass, or a mass with cavitation. Some form of bronchial disease is often present and may represent local airway metastasis (Figure 30-18).[10,13,179,182]

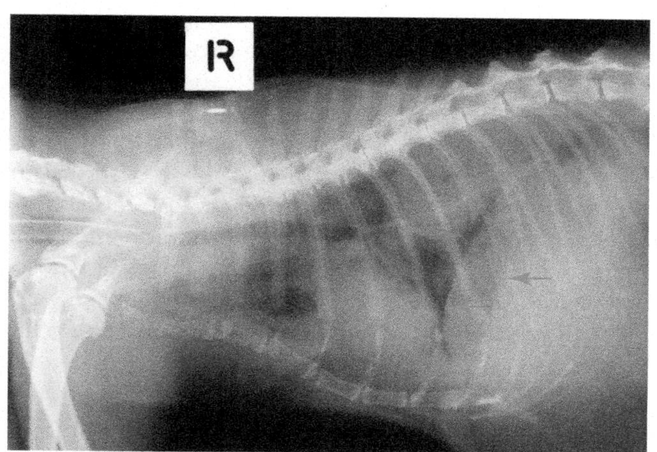

FIGURE 30-18 Right lateral radiographic view of a cat with primary pulmonary adenocarcinoma. As well as the overt lung lobe consolidation and pleural effusion, local osteolysis of the ninth rib *(red arrow)* is evident and the two crurae of the diaphragm *(green arrows)* are not aligned. The tumor was adhered to the rib and one diaphragmatic crus.

In comparison, pulmonary metastasis from other locations appears radiographically as interstitial nodules (either well or ill defined) or a diffuse pulmonary pattern. The latter often consists of an alveolar pattern with or without ill-defined pulmonary nodules or pleural effusion. The most commonly represented primary tumor is mammary gland adenocarcinoma.[74]

Definitive diagnosis depends on cytologic or histologic assessment. Ultrasound-guided FNA of discrete masses or pleural fluid can provide a cytologic diagnosis in many cases but can lead to missed diagnoses because of poor cell recovery as a result of small sample size, poor exfoliation of certain cell types and minimal exfoliation of certain cell types (e.g., mesenchymal cells), necrosis, or failure to obtain a representative sample.[52] Histology of lung biopsy samples may be required for definitive diagnosis.[52,199,200]

The prognosis for long-term survival with pulmonary adenocarcinoma has been reported to be poor.[13] The degree of differentiation of the tumor is the only recognized prognostic factor associated with survival in cats with primary pulmonary neoplasia; cats with moderately differentiated tumors survived a median 698 days (19 to 1526 days) compared with cats that had poorly differentiated tumors at 75 days (13 to 634 days), although all cats eventually died of metastatic disease. The overall median survival time is 115 days.[95] Long-term individual treatment success is possible: A recent paper reported that a cat remained well, with no radiographic evidence of disease at 34 months after left-sided pneumonectomy and adjuvant chemotherapy with mitoxantrone, administered every 3 to 5 weeks, for 10 doses after surgery.[38]

LOWER RESPIRATORY TRACT INFECTIONS

In most cases LRT infection results in pneumonia (inflammation of the lung parenchyma) in cats, although occasionally pathology is limited to the airways.[17,78,161] Pneumonia is uncommon in cats, which is demonstrated by the scarcity of case series that have been published, including only 39 cases over 10 years[161] and 21 cases over 5 years,[78] each from teaching hospitals. The potentially serious nature of infectious pneumonia is highlighted by two[17,161] of only three case series being postmortem studies; however, early recognition and intervention can lead to successful treatment, as noted in 18 of 20 cats in the only clinical cases series.[78] Successful treatment has also been noted in numerous case reports.[76,80]

Isolation of organisms from BAL fluid or tissue obtained from focal lesions by way of FNA or fuller biopsy forms the basis for diagnosis of infectious pneumonia.[78,161] Isolation of bacteria may represent contamination or commensal organisms, although culture of a single organism ("pure" culture) implies infection.[207] Diagnosis of LRT infection, therefore, is based on identification of an organism with supportive historical, clinical, radiographic, and cytologic findings; further, diagnosis is confirmed only with an unambiguous response to appropriate therapy.[78]

Clinical signs may not relate directly to the respiratory tract. In one study 14 of 39 cats (36%) did not have respiratory signs,[161] although in another, 18 of 20 cats (90%) had coughing (15 of 20) or dyspnea (3 of 20).[78] Anorexia, lethargy, and fever were absent in 14 of 39 cats (41%) in one study,[161] and pyrexia was noted in only 25% in another.[78] Hematologic indication of infection (neutrophilia with or without a left shift) is helpful diagnostically if present but can also be absent.[161] Infectious pneumonia is most often associated with an alveolar radiographic pattern, but any pattern is possible; one study found predominantly interstitial patterns (with normal radiographs in 3 of 13 cats),[161] and another, although finding 67% with an alveolar pattern, also found 81% with a bronchial pattern.[78] Neutrophils with toxic changes can be expected to predominate in bronchial wash fluid.

Treatment requires appropriate antibiosis, ideally based on culture and sensitivity findings, as well as supportive care to maintain hydration and electrolyte balance. In some cases of focal pneumonia, pulmonary lobectomy may be required to effect a cure by removing the nidus of infection.[191]

Viral

Until recently, most, if not all, viral causes of LRT infection were diagnosed with lung histopathology and specific viral detection techniques, such as virus isolation by culture, immunofluorescent antibody testing, electron microscopy, or PCR of pulmonary parenchyma obtained, in most cases, post mortem* but in one case ante mortem.[124] In one recent paper, influenza A (H_1N_1), commonly known as "swine flu," was identified by PCR of BAL fluid.[255] Perhaps the increasing availability of PCR testing will allow more ante mortem diagnoses of viral pneumonia in such a manner. Most reported cases of viral pneumonia have been in kittens, but virulent strain calicivirus[115,216] and influenza virus† have also been regularly described in adult cats. Additionally, a case series of nine cats with herpesvirus pneumonia included two adult cats.[37]

Herpesvirus

Herpesvirus infections most often result in URT and ocular clinical signs. Necrotizing pneumonia arises in rare cases in kittens or otherwise immune-debilitated cats.* In a recent study, three of nine kittens were also FeLV positive.[37] In all but one[124] reported case, herpesvirus pneumonia has been fatal. The airways, as well as lung parenchyma, are affected either diffusely or in multifocal distribution with fibrinonecrotic pneumonia. Concurrent infections such as *B. bronchiseptica* or *E. coli* may be recognized, and these most likely represent secondary infection. In many cases typical signs of herpesvirus URT infections may be recognized before lower respiratory signs. There may be an overrepresentation of male cats for herpesvirus pneumonia[37] (although not for herpesvirus causing only URT signs), but with so few cases recognized, this may be a statistical anomaly. The one reported case of survival from herpesvirus pneumonia also had orthopoxvirus demonstrated by immunohistochemistry and electron microscopy on a sample of lung tissue obtained by Tru-Cut biopsy. The cat was 5 years old, and herpesvirus infection was thought to be as a result of recrudescence. The cat required approximately 2 weeks of hospitalization with supportive care of intravenous fluids and parenteral broad-spectrum antibiotics.[124]

Calicivirus

Pneumonia as a result of calicivirus infection was first described in the 1940s.[9] Then, as now, most cases of calicivirus infection resulted in URT signs, often with glossal ulceration. Pneumonia usually cannot be demonstrated ante mortem, but necropsies often reveal grayish, densely consolidated areas in the anterior lobes. The disease is rarely fatal. These findings were confirmed with experimental infection studies in the 1970s that indicated pneumonia was transient and resolved with an appropriate immune response.[112,220] Occasional reports of kittens dying with calicivirus pneumonia after natural infection[160] were most likely associated with either an inability to mount an appropriate immune response or the pathogenicity of the strain of virus.

Outbreaks of virulent strains of calicivirus (named *FCV-Ari* and *FCV-Kaos*) in the late 1990s and early 2000s led to new cases of calicivirus pneumonia.[115,215,216] Signs referable to pneumonia were not a clinical feature of cats affected with these virulent strains of calicivirus, but severe pneumonia, often with secondary infection, such as with *Aspergillus* spp., was demonstrated postmortem. Distinctive clinical signs included facial and limb edema in febrile, anorexic, dehydrated cats, with hair loss and ulcerative dermatitis of the face and feet, and sudden death.[115,215] In these outbreaks 33% to 50% of infected cats died. Cats need intensive supportive care of intravenous fluids and parenteral antibiotics. Phosphorodiamidate morpholino oligomers (PMOs) are compounds that enter cells to target viral-specific sequences and block viral replication. Use of an

*References 17, 37, 115, 137, 157, 160, 161, 216.

†References 55, 137, 139, 157, 252, 255, 268, 291.

*References 17, 37, 69, 82, 113, 159, 247, 256.

anticalicivirus-specific PMO appeared to improve survival in cats affected with virulent calicivirus.[249] The virus transmits readily, including by way of fomite dissemination, and sodium hypochlorite solution should be used for disinfection whenever contamination is suspected.[115] These outbreaks of virulent calicivirus appeared to be self-limiting, but others may occur in the future given the nature of these organisms to mutate readily. More information on virulent calicivirus infections is found in Chapter 33.

Influenza

Until this century, clinical signs resulting from influenza viruses were not recognized in cats despite the recognition that cats mount an immunologic response and develop antibodies against experimental infection.[110,213,232]

The H_5N_1 avian influenza pandemic in southeast Asia from the early 2000s resulted in sporadic deaths from natural infection in domestic cats. Infection results from ingestion of the carcass of infected birds,[139,252] and horizontal transmission to other cats by respiratory and gastrointestinal routes has been demonstrated after experimental infections.[139] Infected cats can develop clinical signs, including significant pyrexia, in 1 to 5 days after infection, and virus attachment in the LRT can result in pneumonic signs in only 1 more day.[139,230,274] The disease can be fatal, but some cats are asymptomatic, and this wide range of severity of clinical signs is thought to be dose dependent.[149] Supportive care with intravenous fluids and parenteral, broad-spectrum antibiotics to treat secondary infection is warranted. There have been no reports of humans contracting the infection from diseased cats.[101]

The pandemic (H_1N_1) 2009 influenza virus (swine flu) was first reported in pigs in Canada in May of 2009[281] and has subsequently been recognized in multiple species, including humans, on multiple continents. Natural infection has been reported in three domestic cats between the ages of 8 and 13 years; in each case the cats are believed to have been infected by aerosol transmission from their owners.[157,255] Pneumonia was recognized radiographically between 1 and 4 days after the onset of clinical signs of inappetence, lethargy, and dyspnea. In one case four other cats in the household had less severe respiratory signs that resolved without any intervention. Two cats died, and H_1N_1 was diagnosed by PCR of postmortem samples (one of lung tissue and the other of a nasal swab).[157] The other cat was diagnosed by PCR of BAL fluid. The BAL fluid comprised 65% macrophages, 25% nondegenerate neutrophils, and 10% small lymphocytes, and radiographs demonstrated opacity of right and left caudal lung lobes. The cat was essentially managed as an outpatient with at-home administration of subcutaneous fluids and oral, broad-spectrum antibiotics.[255]

Experimental infection of cats with H_1N_1 influenza resulted in lesions confined to the lungs compared with experimental infection with H_5N_1 influenza, which also results in extrarespiratory lesions.[275]

A seroprevalence survey across several states in the United States during the 2009 to 2010 influenza season found that 17 of 78 (21.8%) cats sampled had appreciable antibody titers against the novel H_1N_1 strain. The high seroprevalence and infrequent reporting of confirmed disease suggest that most infections are clinically inapparent, because there was no increase in pneumonia of undiagnosed cause over the same duration.[174]

Poxvirus

Cowpox, of the genus *Orthopoxvirus,* is found only in Eurasia, and the reservoir hosts are voles or wood mice.[19] Poxvirus-associated pneumonia is rare in cats. This virus typically causes focal cutaneous lesions, with few to no systemic signs.[18,218] Experimental infection of domestic cats has been shown to induce fatal pulmonary disease,[293] and occasional fatal pneumonia has been reported in natural cases.[109,239,243] A recent report described the diagnosis and successful treatment of a 5-year-old cat with cowpox virus and herpesvirus pneumonia. Radiographs demonstrated a consolidated caudal right lung lobe. Neutrophils predominated on BAL cytology. Bacterial culture of the BAL fluid yielded a negative result. Tru-Cut biopsy of the consolidated lung lobe demonstrated severe, acute, necrotizing bronchopneumonia with necrosis affected both the bronchiolar and the alveolar epithelium. Cowpox virus and herpesvirus were demonstrated by immunohistochemistry and electron microscopy. Interestingly, the cat had skin lesions additional to the respiratory signs. The cat improved after nearly 2 weeks of hospitalization with intravenous fluid therapy and parenteral antibiotics. The reason for the prolonged hospitalization was that the owner was concerned about the zoonotic potential.[124] The potential of poxvirus infection to veterinary staff and owners should be considered when treating affected cats because cat-to-human transmission has been reported.[103,243]

Coronavirus

In one study feline infectious peritonitis (FIP) was the cause of pneumonia in 9 of 11 cats with viral pneumonia.[161] FIP is unlikely to cause pneumonia in cats without pleural effusion, and there are usually other indicators of infection, such as fever. FIP is covered in detail in Chapter 33.

Bacterial

Bacteria represent the most common cause of LRT infections, with postmortem studies recognizing bacterial pneumonia in approximately 50% of infectious pneumonia cases[17,161] and a clinical study recognizing 18 of 21

(86%) LRT infections to be bacterial.[78] A postmortem study noted 12 of 20 cases (60%) of pneumonia to be due to hematogenous spread.[161] A clinical study used BAL as the major mode to retrieve samples, also finding a bronchial radiographic pattern in 81% of cases[78]; these findings indicate airway involvement and may suggest inhalation as the primary route of infection. These disparate findings may represent the difference between an antemortem and a postmortem study.

Important causes of bacterial pneumonia in cats include *Mycoplasma* spp.,* *Neisseria animaloris* (previously described as Eugonic Fermenter 4a or EF-4a),† *Pasteurella* spp.,[17,78,161,186,257] *B. bronchiseptica*,‡ *Streptococcus* spp.,[17,161,261] *Mycobacterium* spp.,[12,46,80,93,126] *E. coli*,[17,37,108,262] *Salmonella* spp.,[16,72,78,231,258] and *Yersinia pestis*.[67,127]

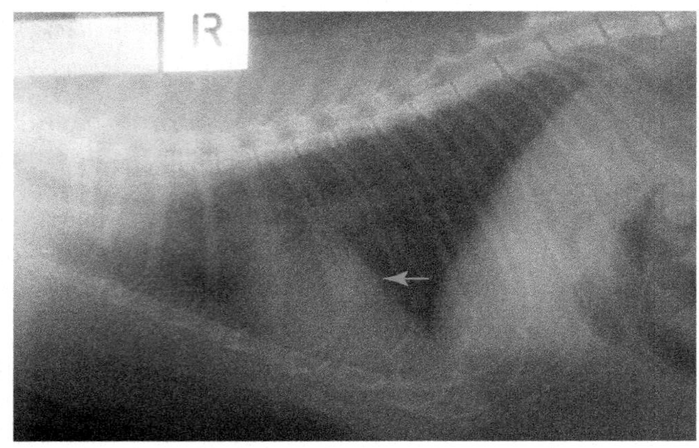

FIGURE 30-19 Right lateral radiographic view of pulmonary abscess *(green arrow)* caused by *Mycoplasma* infection. Note that because the abscess is over the cardiac silhouette, the abscess could not be seen in a left lateral projection.

Mycoplasma

Mycoplasma spp. deserve special mention in relation to feline LRT infections. In case series, two postmortem studies reported *Mycoplasma* pneumonia prevalence of 0%[161] and 15%,[17] respectively, yet a clinical paper found 13 of 17 (76%) of bacterial LRT infections to have mycoplasma infection (and 11 of 13 had purely mycoplasma infection).[78] Further, *Mycoplasma* spp. feature prominently in other reports of feline LRT infections.[35,48,76,163,273] This discrepancy between antemortem and postmortem findings may be because *Mycoplasma* spp. lends itself to more ready diagnosis and successful treatment can be achieved in most cases. *Mycoplasma* spp. have not been isolated from airways of healthy cats,[221] yet mycoplasma LRT infections are often considered to be a consequence of preexisting pulmonary disease, mostly asthma or chronic bronchitis. In human asthma it is recognized that mycoplasma infection can exacerbate asthma and that asthma is induced subsequent to mycoplasma infection; similar associations may apply in feline medicine.[76,78] In most cases infection is associated with the airways, but pulmonary parenchymal involvement also may be present (see Figure 30-13).[35,76,78,221,273] In some cases pulmonary abscessation may be seen (Figure 30-19).[48,78]

In most cases treatment with doxycycline 5 mg/kg orally every 12 hours for 3 weeks is often effective to clear infection, but if a cat has underlying airway disease (asthma or chronic bronchitis), management of the concurrent disease is required.[78]

Neisseria animaloris

One of the most frequently reported causes of feline pneumonia is *Neisseria animaloris*,† which was not formally classified until 2006[276] despite reports in cats dating back to 1973.[118] *N. animaloris* is considered to be part of the normal oral flora of the dog and cat and has been recovered from the oral cavity of 30% to 82% of normal dogs[8,234]; no specific studies appear to have been done in cats, but they are thought to be normal flora in this species also.[279] The organism causes fatal necrotizing pneumonia with a multifocal distribution, which suggests hematogenous dissemination. The precise pathogenesis of *N. animaloris* infection in cats is not well understood. All previous cases have appeared acute clinically, with death occurring within 1 week of onset of clinical signs and often within 2 days, although necropsy and histologic findings were indicative of chronicity. *N. animaloris* has been shown to have inherently low virulence because experimental inoculation of guinea pigs with low numbers of bacteria did not result in any discernible change, but inoculation with larger numbers resulted in death within 18 hours.[156] It has been postulated that prolonged infection overwhelms the host's defenses, resulting in periodic subclinical bacteremia with hematogenous dissemination to the lungs and an eventual acute on chronic terminal exacerbation.[70] Thus the eventual outcome for the patient most likely depends on whether the organism spreads to locations that favor its survival and replication. Because of its small size and Gram stain reaction, the organism is difficult to visualize in cytologic and histologic preparations, necessitating culture of specimens to recognize infection. The organism is susceptible to a broad range of antibiotics, but no successful treatment has been recorded on account of the severity of signs at time of presentation.[11]

Pasteurella *spp.*

Pasteurella spp. represent approximately one quarter of all LRT infections in two studies[17,161] and 32 of 68 (47%) of positive bacterial lower airway cultures in another.[257]

*References 17, 35, 48, 76, 78, 163, 273.

†References 33, 43, 44, 58, 92, 118, 161, 176, 284.

‡References 17, 66, 116, 167, 282, 287.

The organism is recognized as indigenous microflora of the nasopharynx and large airways of dogs and cats.[89] Prior respiratory disease such as viral infection[89] or potassium bromide–induced airway disease[78] contributes to proliferation and then migration to lower airways. Reduced defense mechanisms lead to impaired bacterial clearance from the lung and resultant pneumonia. *Pasteurella* spp. are usually susceptible to a broad range of antibiotics; however, the pneumonia may be slow to resolve, and abscesses or pleuritis may develop.[89]

Bordetella

Pneumonia as a result of *B. bronchiseptica* infection has been recognized both experimentally[47,116] and as a result of natural infection,[282,287] although in most cases disease will be confined to the URT. It is likely that in cases of natural infection other factors may be involved in disease, including environmental factors such as stress or overcrowding or, in some cases, preexisting viral infection.[37,66] Multiple cases of LRT disease associated with *Bordetella* have been reported in breeding catteries, boarding catteries, and in veterinary clinics with boarding facilities. Dogs with *Bordetella* may spread the infection to cats.[21,105,154] Most cases of *Bordetella* pneumonia are in kittens; a postmortem study of pneumonia in which 65% of cases were kittens younger than 12 weeks of age found 30% of confirmed bacterial infections to be *B. bronchiseptica*,[17] whereas only 1 of 68 (1.5%) of positive lower airway cultures from cats of unspecified age were recognized in another study.[257]

Antibiotic choice should be based on sensitivity findings; however, almost all isolates of *B. bronchiseptica* from cats are sensitive to tetracyclines, and doxycycline dosed at 5 mg/kg orally every 12 hours for 21 days is the antimicrobial of choice. Feline isolates of *B. bronchiseptica* are less susceptible to clavulanate-potentiated amoxicillin, and a high level of resistance has been detected to ampicillin and trimethoprim.[254] Supportive care is almost always required initially. Feline vaccines against *B. bronchiseptica* are available in many countries. Although pneumonia is a severe consequence of this organism, in most cases bordetellosis is a mild disease of low prevalence in the small populations typical of most pet cats, so routine vaccinations are not recommended. Use of this vaccine should be limited to those cats living in or moving into high-density populations of cats with a history of bordetellosis.[66] *B. bronchiseptica* is a zoonosis, and disease has been reported in immunecompromised humans in association with living with cats.[283]

Others

Other bacteria have been recognized as causative agents of pneumonia in cats. Some, such as *E. coli*,[17] *Salmonella* spp.,[72,258] or *Streptococcus* spp.[261] may be recognized in cases of disseminated septicemia. However, these same organisms have been recognized in cases of apparent primary respiratory infection[17,108,231,262] or in association with viral pneumonia.[37] Interestingly, *Salmonella* pneumonia has been recognized on two occasions with the lungworm *Aelurostrongylus abstrusus*, and it has been suggested that migrating lungworm larvae may act as carriers for intestinal bacteria.[16,78] The pneumonic form of plague, caused by *Y. pestis*, was found in 10% of cats with this disease in one study.[67] The overall mortality of plague in cats is 33%, with pneumonic cases posing the greatest risk.[67,127] Various forms of mycobacterial species have been recognized to cause pneumonia both as part of disseminated[12,93,126] and localized disease.[46,80] In all cases logical approaches to diagnosis by defining organisms from cultures from BAL fluid or FNA or fuller biopsy samples and treatment by antibiotics determined from sensitivity studies with appropriate supportive care should be used.

Fungal

Fungal pneumonia is rare in cats, representing 0.8%,[17] 5%,[78] and 15%[161] of pneumonia cases in case series. The incidence of fungal infections, generally, depends on whether organisms are endemic to particular regions. Even in endemic areas, fungal pneumonia is not a common consequence of infection, as demonstrated by the fact that there was only one case *(Cryptococcus neoformans)* among 20 cats with pneumonia in Sydney, Australia,[78] where this organism is considered endemic. A diagnosis of fungal pneumonia, therefore, should lead to a high degree of suspicion of immune suppression. Reported causes of fungal pneumonia in cats include *Cryptococcus neoformans*,* *Histoplasma capsulatum*,† *Aspergillus* spp.,‡ *Sporothrix schenkii*,§ *Blastomycosis dermatitides*,¶ *Coccidioides immitis*,[90] and *Mucor* spp.,[17,203] and *Candida* spp.[161,172,203] In many cases pneumonia is one manifestation of systemic, disseminated disease.

Parasitic

Parasitic infections of the feline LRT include the metastrongyloid *A. abstrusus*; the capillarid *Eucoleus aerophilus*; and, in endemic areas, the trematode *Paragonimus kellicotti*. Collectively, *A. abstrusus* and *E. aerophilus* are known as lungworm; *P. kellicotti* is known as lung fluke. Additionally, the filarioid, *Dirofilaria immitis*, or heartworm, although a resident of the pulmonary artery in cats, causes predominantly respiratory disease, and the

*References 51, 78, 85, 99, 161, 164, 178.

†References 39, 51, 123, 162, 166, 288, 289.

‡References 17, 29, 51, 81, 104, 172, 203, 236.

§References 49, 51, 62, 129, 241, 251.

¶References 3, 24, 25, 51, 86, 119, 183, 194, 233, 245, 246, 251, 290.

protozoan *Toxoplasma gondii* can lead to pulmonary involvement in systemic disease.

Lungworm

A. abstrusus has worldwide distribution.[42] Adult *A. abstrusus* lungworms live in the respiratory bronchioles and alveolar ducts of cats. After mating, the females produce eggs that hatch in this same location. The first stage larvae (L1) then ascend the bronchial tree to the pharynx, from where they are swallowed and subsequently excreted in the feces and into the environment. L1s are then ingested by slugs and snails that act as intermediate hosts, with rodents, frogs, lizards, snakes, or birds acting as paratenic hosts. Cats become infected by ingesting a mollusk or a paratenic host (or both).[272]

Most infections are subclinical[96,244]; however, heavy infections can result in clinical signs as a result of damage to the lung parenchyma induced by eggs and larvae. Severe disease can be fatal. Severe clinical disease was reproduced experimentally after kittens were infected with 800 L3 larvae; coughing developed 6 weeks after exposure.[97] *A. abstrusus* infection can mimic allergic respiratory disease because radiographs often demonstrate a bronchointerstitial pattern (although an alveolar pattern predominates during the period of heaviest larval shedding at 5 to 15 weeks post infection) and BAL fluids comprise predominantly eosinophils; further, cats can show an initial positive response to administration of corticosteroids and bronchodilators.[88,271]

Diagnosis depends on recognition of the organism in feces, BAL fluid, or pleural fluid.[140,272] In one study standard fecal examination recognized *A. abstrusus* in only 21.7% of infected cats.[128] Using the Baermann technique to examine feces is considered the most sensitive method for larval detection; however, sensitivity is less than 90%.[140,285] A PCR assay for *A. abstrusus* has recently been validated for use on Baermann sediment, feces, and pharyngeal swabs. This shows great promise to aid in diagnosis, with a reported specificity of 100% and sensitivity of 96.6%.[272]

Many parasiticides have proved to be effective in treating cats with *A. abstrusus* infection. Fenbendazole has been used at 20 mg/kg orally every 24 hours for 5 days or 50 mg/kg orally every 24 hours for 15 days.[16,88,98] Ivermectin (0.4 mg/kg subcutaneously, repeated 2 weeks later) has been reported to be effective in some reported cases.[27,131] Abamectin (0.3 mg/kg subcutaneously, repeated 2 weeks later) was effective in the treatment of one cat.[78] A single topical application of imidacloprid/moxidectin reduced larval counts by 100% in one study,[269a] and topical application of emodopside/praziquental reduced larval counts by 99.4% in another.[272a] Two applications of selamectin (6 mg/kg, topical) were effective in the treatment of only one of three cats.[88]

Eucoleus aerophilus (formerly *Capillaria aerophilus)* has been recognized worldwide.[15,197,270] The life cycle is considered direct. There is, however, some speculation that earthworms may serve as a paratenic or intermediate host. Infection may not result in clinical signs; alternatively, a chronic cough and weight loss may develop. Infection is rarely fatal.[42] Definitive diagnosis is by detection of eggs on sugar and zinc sulfate solution fecal flotation[270]; eggs may also be detected in BAL samples.[15] Radiographs typically show a diffuse interstitial lung pattern, and BAL cytology shows an eosinophilic inflammatory response.[42] Abamectin (0.3 mg/kg subcutaneously, repeated 2 weeks later) has been reported as effective treatment in one cat.[15] Other anthelmintics, such as ivermectin or milbemycin oxime, may also be effective in cats.[42]

Lung Fluke

P. kellicotti is a trematode that can infect the lungs of cats and dogs in the Eastern United States, mainly in areas surrounding the Mississippi River. Other species of *Paragonimus* can affect cats across eastern Asia and Central and South America. The disease in man is endemic in southeast Asia and portions of central Africa.[214] Adult flukes live within cysts inside the lung parenchyma and are about 6 mm long. Eggs are deposited into the lung tissue, where they are coughed up, swallowed, and then passed in the feces. If the eggs enter fresh water, they begin to develop and produce a ciliated miracidium, which hatches and seeks out a young snail host. After asexual multiplication in the snail, the cercarial stage is produced, which penetrates the shell of a crayfish and encysts in an area near the heart of the crustacean. Within the crayfish the cercaria forms a cyst wall and becomes a metacercaria. When the crayfish is ingested by a cat (or dog), the excised metacercariae penetrate the intestinal tract and enter the peritoneal cavity, within which they migrate for 7 to 10 days before entering the pleural cavity through the diaphragm. The lungs are entered approximately 2 weeks after infection.[259] Dogs and cats typically become infected by eating metacercariae in crayfish, but rats can serve as paratenic hosts and transmammary or transplacental transmission is also thought to be possible.[23] Clinical signs such as occasional coughing are usually mild, although pneumothorax can result from migrating flukes. Early lesions appear radiographically as indistinct nodular densities containing small air cavities and having irregular, sharply defined margins; older cysts are usually air-filled pneumatocysts, but ill-defined interstitial nodular densities may also be seen.[229,280] Successful treatment has been reported with praziquantel (25 mg/kg orally every 8 hours for a total dose of 150 mg/kg) and albendazole (25 mg/kg orally every 12 hours for 11 to 24 days).[23,61,114]

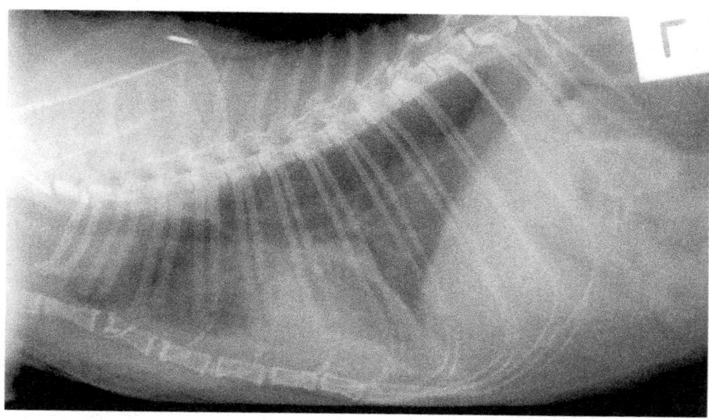

FIGURE 30-20 Left lateral radiographic view of cat with *Toxoplasma* pneumonia. There is a mixed pattern with consolidated ventral lung lobe and pleural effusion.

Toxoplasma

Toxoplasma gondii may cause self-limiting small bowel diarrhea but typically causes no disease in cats. However, transplacentally or lactationally infected kittens and immune-suppressed older cats can show severe systemic signs.[60] In a study of 100 cases with histologically confirmed toxoplasmosis, 76.7% of 86 lung tissue samples assessed had organisms present, and in the 36 cats considered to have generalized toxoplasmosis, 26 had predominantly pulmonary lesions.[59] Retrospective studies of feline LRT infection have found *T. gondii* in 1 of 20 cats (5%)[78] and 6 of 245 cases (2.4%).[17] Diagnosis is achieved by recognition of *Toxoplasma* tachyzoites, which can be found in BAL fluid[14] or FNA of affected lung tissue.[219,235] Diffuse interstitial to alveolar patterns are typically described,[14,219,235] but a bronchial influence is also possible[14] (Figure 30-20). Serology can aid diagnosis.[60] Recognition of *Toxoplasma* in an adult cat should instigate investigations to determine a cause of immune suppression, which is often FIV related[50,78] but can be iatrogenic (e.g., due to administration of corticosteroids or cyclosporin).[14,77] Treatment is covered in detail in Chapter 23 but is typically with clindamycin at 12.5 to 25 mg/kg orally every 12 hours for 2 weeks[60]; combination therapy with pyrimethamine at 0.25 to 0.5 mg/kg orally every 12 hours may help the prognosis.[14] Supportive care such as oxygen therapy maintenance of fluid and electrolyte balance is also important. Successful treatment of clinical feline toxoplasmosis has been described infrequently.[14,59,143]

Heartworm

Despite prevalence studies demonstrating a worldwide distribution and recognizing heartworm infection in up to 18% of cats tested,* the prevalence rate being approximately 5% to 10% of that found in dogs,[84,150,153] and the prevalence being found similar to that of FIV and FeLV infection,[150,151,158] feline heartworm disease remains underdiagnosed in general practice.[30,195] This is likely because clinical signs vary dramatically from no signs to sudden death and definitive diagnosis can be difficult.[20,30,153,196]

Heartworm disease is caused by the filarioid nematode *Dirofilaria immitis,* which is transmitted by mosquitos and for which dogs are the usual definitive host. Therefore a prerequisite for heartworm infection is a climate with adequate temperature and humidity to support a viable mosquito population and allow maturation of larvae within the intermediate host. The sexually dimorphic adult heartworm mate within an infected dog's pulmonary artery, producing immature forms called *microfilariae.* Circulating microfilariae are ingested by mosquitoes feeding on infected dogs. Within mosquitoes, microfilariae transform into larval stages. There are five larval stages (L1 to L5); L1 to L3 transformations occur within the mosquito, and L3 is the form that is transmitted from mosquitos to dogs and cats. Maturation from L3 to other larval stages occurs in subcutaneous tissues and peripheral veins of mammalian hosts; immature worms in peripheral veins are carried in the bloodstream to and through the heart, with adult heartworms ultimately residing at the caudal pulmonary arteries.[1]

There are significant differences between feline and canine heartworm disease because the parasite is only partially adapted to the cat. The cat is susceptible to heartworm infection but more resistant than the dog. The cat represents a dead-end host because it cannot act as a reservoir for infection. The prepatent period in the cat is 7 to 8 months (1 to 2 months longer than in dogs).[169] In dogs, most juvenile worms mature into adults that can live for 5 to 7 years, whereas in cats most juvenile worms die shortly after arriving in the pulmonary arteries, instigating a severe vascular and parenchymal inflammatory response. Pulmonary lesions may be long lasting. The clinical response in the cat has been termed *heartworm-associated respiratory disease (HARD).* In a small percentage of cats, a few worms develop to mature adults that can live for 2 to 3 years.[195]

Cats with adult heartworms develop pulmonary changes characterized by intimal proliferation, eosinophilic endarteritis, intimal fibrosis, and disruption of the internal elastic lamina. Arterial wall changes can lead to pulmonary hypertension with resultant pulmonary arterial distention.[173] Damage can be caused by juvenile heartworms without development to the adult stage, resulting in increase in thickness of the pulmonary arterial wall that in turn causes occlusion.[26,56] There have been suggestions that *Wolbachia pipientis*, a symbiotic gram-negative intracellular bacterium harbored by *D. immitis* induces further pulmonary pathology.[57] A strong antibody response against *Wolbachia* surface protein has

*References 31, 71, 84, 107, 138, 150, 151, 155, 158, 197, 269, 285.

been demonstrated in heartworm-infected cats. Further research is required to define the exact relationship between *Wolbachia* and HARD in cats. Upon death of heartworms, it has been hypothesized that degenerating parasites may cause an acute anaphylactic reaction and thromboembolism, which can result in fulminant pulmonary failure and sudden death of the cat.[152] Even the death of one adult heartworm can be lethal. Adult heartworms are able to suppress pulmonary intravascular macrophage activity and therefore induce little inflammation until they die.

Clinical signs can vary from no clinical signs, reported in 28% to 79% of cases,[7,84] to acute or chronic respiratory tract signs. Sudden death has been reported in 7% to 47% of naturally infected cats with mature adult heartworm infections.[7,68,84,277] Additional signs that may be seen include neurologic signs or vomiting.[7,277]

On most occasions cats will present clinically with respiratory tract signs mimicking asthma or chronic bronchitis, such as coughing or dyspnea.[7,84,277] Physical examination findings are nonspecific. Investigations should follow those for any cats with respiratory signs, but the diagnosis of heartworm disease is sometimes reached only when a high degree of suspicion of this disease is maintained. Cats are rarely microfilaremic, so filtration or immunofluorescent assay for microfilaria is not recommended. No single diagnostic test can detect feline heartworm at all life stages of the worm (Table 30-4). Serologic testing, if positive, is the most straightforward for demonstration of infection, but false-negative results occur frequently. According to the American Heartworm Society, the primary reasons for heartworm testing in cats are as follows:

1. To establish a diagnosis in cats that, on the basis of other clinical evidence, are suspected of infection
2. To monitor the clinical course of cats diagnosed with heartworm disease
3. To establish a baseline reference prior to starting prophylaxis

Heartworm antigen testing detects mature female heartworm genital parts, so sensitivity increases when more female worms are present. Because heartworm antigen testing is regarded as highly specific, false-positive results are very rare. One study found 36% sensitivity with only one female heartworm and increasing to 93% sensitivity with seven females present. Cats with only male heartworms test as negative.[177] A more recent study comparing antigen tests detected 79.3% to 86.2% of necropsy confirmed heartworm infections. Most cats with false-negative antigen tests had a single male worm.[20] On the basis of this study, it can be assumed that antigen testing will detect at least three quarters of cats infected with adult heartworm. However, as previously noted, clinical signs can result from larval infections that do not progress to adult stage heartworms.

Antibody tests will help determine exposure, but up to 79% cats with exposure do not become symptomatic.[84] A negative antibody test does not rule out infection. The different antibody tests available vary in sensitivity and specificity, insofar as each brand may detect a different stage of larval development. Also, up to 30% of cats on

TABLE 30-4 **Interpretation of Heartworm Diagnostic Procedures Tests in the Cat**

Test	Description	Result	Interpretation	Limitation
Antibody test	Detects antibodies produced in response to heartworm larvae; may detect infection as early as 8 weeks after transmission	Negative Positive	Lowers index of suspicion Increases index of suspicion, confirms cat is at risk of disease; 50% or more of cats will have pulmonary arterial disease	Antibodies confirm infection with heartworm larvae but do not confirm disease causality
Antigen test	Detects antigen produced by adult female heartworms or from >5 dying male or female heartworms	Negative Positive	Lowers index of suspicion Confirms presence of heartworms	Immature or male-only heartworm infections are rarely detected
Thoracic radiography	Detects vascular enlargement, pulmonary parenchymal inflammation, edema	Normal Signs consistent with heartworm disease	Lowers index of suspicion Enlarged arteries greatly increases index of suspicion	Radiographic signs are subjective, affected by clinical interpretation
Echocardiography	Detects echogenic walls of immature or mature heartworms in the lumen of the pulmonary arterial tree	No heartworms seen Heartworms seen	Does not change index of suspicion Confirms presence of heartworms	Experience of ultrasonographer influences accuracy

Note: In the cat no single test will detect all heartworm cases. Although the antigen tests are highly specific for detecting adult heartworm antigen, they will not detect infections with only live male worms. The clinician must use a combination of test results to determine the likelihood of heartworm disease as the etiology of the cat's clinical signs.
Adapted and reprinted with permission from the American Heartworm Society (www.heartwormsociety.org/veterinary-resources/feline-guidelines.html).

heartworm prophylaxis may become antibody positive, although they are not at risk for HARD. Combining antigen and antibody testing achieves higher sensitivity than either test alone but may generate more false-positive results.[250]

Radiographic findings may add to a clinician's index of suspicion for heartworm disease, but results are inconsistent. Significant enlargement of the central and peripheral caudal lobar pulmonary arteries (greater than 1.6 times the width of the ninth rib) in the ventrodorsal view has been considered a typical radiographic sign of heartworm infection in cats. However, this was recognized in only 53% of cases in one study[237] and only 1 of 11 cats in another.[277] The latter study found diffuse or focal bronchointerstitial patterns to be most common, with focal changes supporting a better prognosis.[277]

Echocardiography, in experienced hands, can also aid diagnosis. Adult heartworms typically appear as two echodense parallel lines within the pulmonary artery, one of its branches, or the right ventricle. One study found heartworms in 17 of 43 cats with echocardiography but, it is important to note, allowed a definitive diagnosis to be made in five cats in which antigen test results were negative; four of these five cats had positive antibody test results.[53]

There is no definitive treatment for heartworm disease in cats. Most cats with infection are asymptomatic, and it is appropriate to start prophylactic treatment in these cats. Heartworm prophylactic treatments have been demonstrated to be slowly adulticidal in dogs,[168] and there is no reason to assume that this would not also be the case in cats. Ivermectin has the most potent adulticidal activity, milbemycin the least, with selamectin and moxidectin in between.[168] More rapid kill of adult heartworm with arsenical agents such as thiacetarsemide or melarsomine is *not* recommended. These agents are believed to be less potent in cats and have significant toxicity, and death of heartworms may result in fatal pulmonary embolism.[153] Successful surgical removal of heartworms has been reported, although there are substantial risks associated with the procedure. In particular, crushing or transecting the adult heartworms can induce a fatal shock reaction. Trauma to the jugular vein during multiple heartworm retrievals may result in transection of the vein.[248]

In most cases, in addition to heartworm prophylaxis, it is appropriate to manage the clinical signs of infected cats with corticosteroids and bronchodilators. Prednisolone has been used at 2 mg/kg orally every 24 hours and then tapered at remission of clinical signs.[84] If *W. pipientis* is demonstrated to be relevant to clinical disease, a 3-week course of doxycycline (5 mg/kg orally every 12 hours) would be appropriate.[57] Monitoring of heartworm-infected cats with radiographic evidence of disease may include repeat thoracic radiographs at 6- to 12-month intervals. Infected cats can also be monitored with repeat serologic testing. Recovery is indicated by an improvement in radiographic signs and seroconversion of a positive antigen test to negative.

In areas where heartworm is endemic for dogs, all serologic evidence points to the appropriateness of cats (including those confined to indoors) receiving regular prophylactic treatment. There are several macrocytic lactone drugs registered for feline heartworm prophylaxis: ivermectin (Heartguard FX chewables, Merial), milbemycin oxide (Milbemax, Novartis), moxidectin (Advocate/Advantage Multi, Bayer; NB also contains imidacloprid), and selamectin (Revolution or Stronghold, Pfizer).

References

1. Abraham D: Biology of *Dirofilaria immitis*. In Boreham PFL, Atwell RB, editors: *Dirofilariasis*, Boca Raton, Fla, 1988, CRC Press, p 29.
2. Adamama-Moraitou KK, Patsikas MN, Koutinas AF: Feline lower airway disease: a retrospective study of 22 naturally occurring cases from Greece, *J Feline Med Surg* 6:227, 2004.
3. Alden CL, Mohan R: Ocular blastomycosis in a cat, *J Am Vet Med Assoc* 164:527, 1974.
4. Ameredes BT, Calhoun WJ: (R)-albuterol for asthma: pro [a.k.a. (s)-albuterol for asthma: con], *Am J Resp Crit Care Med* 174:965, 2006.
5. Anderson T, Legendre A, McEntee M: Probable hypercalcemia of malignancy in a cat with bronchogenic adenocarcinoma, *J Am Anim Hosp Assoc* 36:52, 2000.
6. Aron DN, Kornegay JN: The clinical significance of traumatic lung cysts and associated pulmonary abnormalities in the dog and cat, *J Am Anim Hosp Assoc* 19:903, 1983.
7. Atkins CE, DeFrancesco TC, Coats JR et al: Heartworm infection in cats: 50 cases (1985-1997), *J Am Vet Med Assoc* 217:355, 2000.
8. Bailie WE, Stowe EC, Schmitt AM: Aerobic bacterial flora of oral and nasal fluids of canines with reference to bacteria associated with bites, *J Clin Microbiol* 7:223, 1978.
9. Baker JA: A virus causing pneumonia in cats and producing elementary bodies, *J Exp Med* 79:159, 1944.
10. Ballegeer EA, Forrest LJ, Stepien RL: Radiographic appearance of bronchoalveolar carcinoma in nine cats, *Vet Radiol Ultrasound* 43:267, 2002.
11. Baral RM, Catt MJ, Soon L et al: Successful treatment of a localised CDC Group EF-4a infection in a cat, *J Feline Med Surg* 9:67, 2007.
12. Baral RM, Metcalfe SS, Krockenberger MB et al: Disseminated *Mycobacterium avium* infection in young cats: overrepresentation of Abyssinian cats, *J Feline Med Surg* 8:23, 2006.
13. Barr F, Gruffydd-Jones TJ, Brown PJ et al: Primary lung tumours in the cat, *J Small Anim Pract* 28:1115, 1987.
14. Barrs VR, Martin P, Beatty JA: Antemortem diagnosis and treatment of toxoplasmosis in two cats on cyclosporin therapy, *Aust Vet J* 84:30, 2006.
15. Barrs VR, Martin P, Nicoll RG et al: Pulmonary cryptococcosis and Capillaria aerophila infection in an FIV-positive cat, *Aust Vet J* 78:154, 2000.
16. Barrs VR, Swinney GR, Martin P et al: Concurrent *Aelurostrongylus abstrusus* infection and salmonellosis in a kitten, *Aust Vet J* 77:229, 1999.
17. Bart M, Guscetti F, Zurbriggen A et al: Feline infectious pneumonia: a short literature review and a retrospective immunohistological study on the involvement of *Chlamydia* spp. and distemper virus, *Vet J* 159:220, 2000.

18. Bennett M, Gaskell CJ, Baxby D et al: Feline cowpox virus infection, *J Small Anim Pract* 31:167, 1990.
19. Bennett M, Gaskell RF, Baxby D: Poxvirus infection. In Greene CE, editor: *Infectious diseases of the dog and cat*, ed 3, St Louis, 2006, Saunders Elsevier, p 158.
20. Berdoulay P, Levy JK, Snyder PS et al: Comparison of serological tests for the detection of natural heartworm infection in cats, *J Am Anim Hosp Assoc* 40:376, 2004.
21. Binns S, Dawson S, Speakman A et al: Prevalence and risk factors for feline *Bordetella* bronchiseptica infection, *Vet Rec* 144:575, 1999.
22. Bolliger AP, Graham PA, Richard V et al: Detection of parathyroid hormone—related protein in cats with humoral hypercalcemia of malignancy, *Vet Clin Pathol* 31:3, 2002.
23. Bowman DD, Frongillo MK, Johnson RC et al: Evaluation of praziquantel for treatment of experimentally induced paragonimiasis in dogs and cats, *Am J Vet Res* 52:68, 1991.
24. Breider MA, Walker TL, Legendre AM et al: Blastomycosis in cats: five cases (1979-1986), *J Am Vet Med Assoc* 193:570, 1988.
25. Breshears DE: What is your diagnosis? *J Am Vet Med Assoc* 152:1555, 1968.
26. Browne LE, Carter TD, Levy JK et al: Pulmonary arterial disease in cats seropositive for Dirofilaria immitis but lacking adult heartworms in the heart and lungs, *Am J Vet Res* 66:1544, 2005.
27. Burgu A, Sarimehmetoglu O: *Aelurostrongylus abstrusus* infection in two cats, *Vet Rec* 154:602, 2004.
28. Burk RL, Feeney DA: *The thorax: small animal radiology and ultrasonography: a diagnostic atlas and text*, St Louis, 2003, Saunders Elsevier, p 25.
29. Burk RL, Joseph R, Baer K: Systemic aspergillosis in a cat, *Vet Radiol* 31:26, 1990.
30. Buzhardt L, Blagburn BL, Cousins M et al: Feline heartworm disease, *Compendium* 30:1, 2008.
31. Carleton RE, Tolbert MK: Prevalence of *Dirofilaria immitis* and gastrointestinal helminths in cats euthanized at animal control agencies in northwest Georgia, *Vet Parasitol* 119:319, 2004.
32. Cassotis NJ, Dubielzig RR, Gilger BC et al: Angioinvasive pulmonary carcinoma with posterior segment metastasis in four cats, *Vet Ophthalmol* 2:125, 1999.
33. Ceyssens K, Devriese LA, Maenhout T: Necrotizing pneumonia in cats associated with infection by EF-4a bacteria, *Zentralbl Veterinarmed B* 36:314, 1989.
34. Chalifoux A, Morin M, Lemieux R: Lipid pneumonia and severe pulmonary emphysema in a Persian cat, *Feline Pract* 17:6, 1987.
35. Chandler JC, Lappin MR: Mycoplasmal respiratory infections in small animals: 17 Cases (1988-1999), *J Am Anim Hosp Assoc* 38:111, 2002.
36. Chung K, Caramori G, Adcock I: Inhaled corticosteroids as combination therapy with β adrenergic agonists in airways disease: present and future, *Eur J Clin Pharmacol* 65:853, 2009.
37. Chvala-Mannsberger S, Bagó Z, Weissenböck H: Occurrence, morphological characterization and antigen localization of felid herpesvirus–induced pneumonia in cats: a retrospective study (2000-2006), *J Comp Pathol* 141:163, 2009.
38. Clements DN, Hogan AM, Cave TA: Treatment of a well differentiated pulmonary adenocarcinoma in a cat by pneumonectomy and adjuvant mitoxantrone chemotherapy, *J Feline Med Surg* 6:199, 2004.
39. Clinkenbeard KD, Cowell RL, Tyler RD: Disseminated histoplasmosis in cats: 12 cases (1981-1986), *J Am Vet Med Assoc* 190:1445, 1987.
40. Cohn LA, DeClue AE, Cohen RL et al: Effects of fluticasone propionate dosage in an experimental model of feline asthma, *J Feline Med Surg* 12:91, 2010.
41. Cohn LA, Norris CR, Hawkins EC et al: Identification and characterization of an idiopathic pulmonary fibrosis-like condition in cats, *J Vet Intern Med* 18:632, 2004.
42. Conboy G: Helminth parasites of the canine and feline respiratory tract, *Vet Clin North Am Small Anim Pract* 39:1109, 2009.
43. Corboz L, Ossent P, Gruber H: Isolation and characterization of group EF-4 bacteria from various lesions in cat, dog and badger, *Zentralbl Bakteriol* 279:140, 1993.
44. Corboz L, Ossent P, Gruber H: [Local and systemic infections with bacteria of group EF-4 in dogs, cats and in a badger: bacteriologic and pathologico-anatomic results], *Schweizer Archiv fur Tierheilkunde* 135:96, 1993.
45. Corcoran BM, Foster DJ, Fuentes VL: Feline asthma syndrome: a retrospective study of the clinical presentation in 29 cats, *J Small Anim Pract* 36:481, 1995.
46. Couto SS, Artacho CA: *Mycobacterium fortuitum* pneumonia in a cat and the role of lipid in the pathogenesis of atypical mycobacterial infections, *Vet Pathol* 44:543, 2007.
47. Coutts AJ, Dawson S, Binns S et al: Studies on natural transmission of *Bordetella* bronchiseptica in cats, *Vet Microbiol* 48:19, 1996.
48. Crisp MS, Birchard SJ, Lawrence AE et al: Pulmonary abscess caused by a Mycoplasma sp in a cat, *J Am Vet Med Assoc* 191:340, 1987.
49. Crothers SL, White SD, Ihrke PJ et al: Sporotrichosis: a retrospective evaluation of 23 cases seen in northern California (1987-2007), *Vet Dermatol* 20:249, 2009.
50. Davidson MG, Rottman JB, English RV et al: Feline immunodeficiency virus predisposes cats to acute generalized toxoplasmosis, *Am J Pathol* 143:1486, 1993.
51. Davies C, Troy G: Deep mycotic infections in cats, *J Am Anim Hosp Assoc* 32:380, 1996.
52. DeBerry JD, Norris CR, Samii VF et al: Correlation between fine-needle aspiration cytopathology and histopathology of the lung in dogs and cats, *J Am Anim Hosp Assoc* 38:327, 2002.
53. DeFrancesco TC, Atkins CE, Miller MW et al: Use of echocardiography for the diagnosis of heartworm disease in cats: 43 cases (1985-1997), *J Am Vet Med Assoc* 218:66, 2001.
54. Dehard S, Bernaerts F, Peeters D et al: Comparison of bronchoalveolar lavage cytospins and smears in dogs and cats, *J Am Anim Hosp Assoc* 44:285, 2008.
55. Desvaux S, Marx N, Ong S et al: Highly pathogenic avian influenza virus (H5N1) outbreak in captive wild birds and cats, Cambodia, *Emerg Infect Dis* 15:475, 2009.
56. Dillon AR, Blagburn BL, Tillson DM et al: Immature heartworm infection produces pulmonary parenchyma, airway, and vascular disease in cats [abstract], *J Vet Intern Med* 21:608, 2007.
57. Dingman P, Levy JK, Kramer LH et al: Association of *Wolbachia* with heartworm disease in cats and dogs, *Vet Parasitol* 170:50, 2010.
58. Drolet R, Kenefick KB, Hakomaki MR et al: Isolation of group eugonic fermenter-4 bacteria from a cat with multifocal suppurative pneumonia, *J Am Vet Med Assoc* 189:311, 1986.
59. Dubey JP, Carpenter JL: Histologically confirmed clinical toxoplasmosis in cats: 100 cases (1952-1990), *J Am Vet Med Assoc* 203:1556, 1993.
60. Dubey JP, Lappin MR: Toxoplasmosis and neosporosis. In Greene CE, editor: *Infectious diseases of the dog and cat*, ed 3, St Louis, 2006, Saunders Elsevier, p 754.
61. Dubey JP, Stromberg PC, Toussant MJ et al: Induced paragonimiasis in cats: clinical signs and diagnosis, *J Am Vet Med Assoc* 173:734, 1978.
62. Dunstan RW, Reimann KA, Langham RF: Feline sporotrichosis, *J Am Vet Med Assoc* 189:880, 1986.
63. Dye JA, McKiernan BC, Rozanski EA et al: Bronchopulmonary disease in the cat: historical, physical, radiographic, clinicopathologic, and pulmonary functional evaluation of 24 affected and 15 healthy cats, *J Vet Intern Med* 10:385, 1996.
64. Dye JA, McKiernan BC, Rozanski EA et al: Pharmacokinetics of terbutaline in two cats [abstract], *J Vet Intern Med* 4:118, 1990.

65. Easton PA, Jadue C, Dhingra S et al: A Comparison of the bronchodilating effects of a beta-2 adrenergic agent (albuterol) and an anticholinergic agent (ipratropium bromide), given by aerosol alone or in sequence, *New Engl J Med* 315:735, 1986.
66. Egberink H, Addie D, Belák S et al: *Bordetella bronchiseptica* infection in cats. ABCD guidelines on prevention and management, *J Feline Med Surg* 11:610, 2009.
67. Eidson M, Thilsted JP, Rollag OJ: Clinical, clinicopathologic, and pathologic features of plague in cats: 119 cases (1977-1988), *J Am Vet Med Assoc* 199:1191, 1991.
68. Evans EA, Litster AL, Gunew MNM et al: Forty-five cases of feline heartworm in Australia 1990-1998, *Aust Vet Pract* 30:11, 2000.
69. Feinstein L, Miller GF, Penney BE: Diagnostic exercise: lethal pneumonia in neonatal kittens, *Lab Anim Sci* 48:190, 1998.
70. Fenwick BW, Jang SS, Gillespie DS: Pneumonia caused by a eugonic fermenting bacterium in an African lion, *J Am Vet Med Assoc* 183:1315, 1983.
71. Fernandez C, Chikweto A, Mofya S et al: A serological study of *Dirofilaria immitis* in feral cats in Grenada, West Indies, *J Helminthol* 84:390, 2010.
72. Foley JE, Orgad U, Hirsh DC et al: Outbreak of fatal salmonellosis in cats following use of a high-titer modified-live panleukopenia virus vaccine, *J Am Vet Med Assoc* 214:67, 1999.
73. Fondati A, Carreras E, Fondevila MD et al: Characterization of biological activities of feline eosinophil granule proteins, *Am J Vet Res* 65:957, 2004.
74. Forrest LJ, Graybush CA: Radiographic patterns of pulmonary metastasis in 25 cats, *Vet Radiol Ultrasound* 39:4, 1998.
75. Foster SF, Allan GS, Martin P et al: Twenty-five cases of feline bronchial disease (1995-2000), *J Feline Med Surg* 6:181, 2004.
76. Foster SF, Barrs VR, Martin P et al: Pneumonia associated with *Mycoplasma* spp in three cats, *Aust Vet J* 76:460, 1998.
77. Foster SF, Charles JA, Canfield PJ et al: Reactivated toxoplasmosis in a FIV-positive cat, *Aust Vet Pract* 28:159, 1998.
78. Foster SF, Martin P, Allan GS et al: Lower respiratory tract infections in cats: 21 cases (1995-2000), *J Feline Med Surg* 6:167, 2004.
79. Foster SF, Martin P, Braddock JA et al: A retrospective analysis of feline bronchoalveolar lavage cytology and microbiology (1995-2000), *J Feline Med Surg* 6:189, 2004.
80. Foster SF, Martin P, Davis W et al: Chronic pneumonia caused by *Mycobacterium thermoresistibile* in a cat, *J Small AnimPract* 40:433, 1999.
81. Fox JG, Murphy JC, Shalev M: Systemic fungal infections in cats, *J Am Vet Med Assoc* 173:1191, 1978.
82. Fulton RW, Cho DY, Downing M et al: Isolation of feline herpesvirus 1 from a young kitten, *Vet Rec* 106:479, 1980.
83. Gadbois J, d'Anjou MA, Dunn M et al: Radiographic abnormalities in cats with feline bronchial disease and intra- and interobserver variability in radiographic interpretation: 40 cases (1999-2006), *J Am Vet Med Assoc* 234:367, 2009.
84. Genchi C, Venco L, Ferrari N et al: Feline heartworm *(Dirofilaria immitis)* infection: a statistical elaboration of the duration of the infection and life expectancy in asymptomatic cats, *Vet Parasitol* 158:177, 2008.
85. Gerds-Grogan S, Dayrell-Hart B: Feline cryptococcosis: a retrospective evaluation, *J Am Anim Hosp Assoc* 33:118, 1997.
86. Gilor C, Graves TK, Barger AM et al: Clinical aspects of natural infection with Blastomyces dermatitidis in cats: 8 cases (1991-2005), *J Am Vet Med Assoc* 229:96, 2006.
87. Gottfried S, Popovitch C, Goldschmidt M et al: Metastatic digital carcinoma in the cat: a retrospective study of 36 cats (1992-1998), *J Am Anim Hosp Assoc* 36:501, 2000.
88. Grandi G, Calvi LE, Venco L et al: *Aelurostrongylus abstrusus* (cat lungworm) infection in five cats from Italy, *Vet Parasitol* 134:177, 2005.
89. Greene CE, Norris-Reinero C: Bacterial respiratory infections. In Greene CE, editor: *Infectious diseases of the dog and cat*, ed 3, St Louis, 2006, Saunders Elsevier, p 866.
90. Greene RT, Troy GC: Coccidioidomycosis in 48 cats: a retrospective study (1984-1993), *J Vet Intern Med* 9:86, 1995.
91. Greenlee PG, Roszel JF: Feline bronchial cytology: histologic/cytologic correlation in 22 cats, *Vet Pathol* 21:308, 1984.
92. Guérin-Faublée V, Thollot I, Fournel C et al: The isolation of Group EF-4 bacteria from a case of septic pleural effusion in a cat. [French], *Revue de Medecine Veterinaire* 146:821, 1995.
93. Gunn-Moore DA, Jenkins PA, Lucke VM: Feline tuberculosis: a literature review and discussion of 19 cases caused by an unusual mycobacterial variant, *Vet Rec* 138:53, 1996.
94. Hahn KA, McEntee MF: Primary lung tumors in cats: 86 cases (1979-1994), *J Am Vet Med Assoc* 211:1257, 1997.
95. Hahn KA, McEntee MF: Prognosis factors for survival in cats after removal of a primary lung tumor: 21 cases (1979-1994), *Vet Surg* 27:307, 1998.
96. Hamilton JM: *Aelurostrongylus abstrusus* infestation of the cat, *Vet Rec* 75:417, 1963.
97. Hamilton JM: The number of *Aelurostrongylus abstrusus* larvae required to produce pulmonary disease in the cat, *J Comp Pathol* 77:343, 1967.
98. Hamilton JM, Weatherley A, Chapman AJ: Treatment of lungworm disease in the cat with fenbendazole, *Vet Rec* 114:40, 1984.
99. Hamilton TA, Hawkins EC, DeNicola DB: Bronchoalveolar lavage and tracheal wash to determine lung involvement in a cat with cryptococcosis, *J Am Vet Med Assoc* 198:655, 1991.
100. Handley D: The asthma-like pharmacology and toxicology of (S)-isomers of beta agonists, *J Allergy Clin Immunol* 104:S69, 1999.
101. Harder TC, Vahlenkamp TW: Influenza virus infections in dogs and cats, *Vet Immunol Immunopathol* 134:54, 2010.
102. Hawkins EC, DeNicola DB, Kuehn NF: Bronchoalveolar lavage in the evaluation of pulmonary disease in the dog and cat, *J Vet Intern Med* 4:267, 1990.
103. Hawranek T, Tritscher M, Muss WH et al: Feline orthopoxvirus infection transmitted from cat to human, *J Am Acad Dermatol* 49:513, 2003.
104. Hazell K, Swift I, Sullivan N: Successful treatment of pulmonary aspergillosis in a cat, *Aust Vet J* 89:101, 2011.
105. Helps C, Lait P, Damhuis A et al: Factors associated with URT disease caused by feline herpesvirus, feline calicivirus, *Chlamydophila felis* and *Bordetella bronchiseptica* in cats: experience from 218 European catteries, *Vet Rec* 156:669, 2005.
106. Henninger W: Use of computed tomography in the diseased feline thorax, *J Small Anim Pract* 44:56, 2003.
107. Hermesmeyer M, Limberg-Child RK, Murphy AJ et al: Prevalence of *Dirofilaria immitis* infection among shelter cats, *J Am Vet Med Assocn* 217:211, 2000.
108. Highland MA, Byrne BA, DebRoy C et al: Extraintestinal pathogenic *Escherichia coli*–induced pneumonia in three kittens and fecal prevalence in a clinically healthy cohort population, *J Vet Diagn Invest* 21:609, 2009.
109. Hinrichs U, van de Poel H, van den Ingh TSGAM: Necrotizing pneumonia in a cat caused by an orthopox virus, *J Comp Pathol* 121:191, 1999.
110. Hinshaw VS, Webster RG, Easterday BC et al: Replication of avian influenza A viruses in mammals, *Infect Immun* 34:354, 1981.
111. Hoffman AM, Dhupa N, Cimetti L: Airway reactivity measured by barometric whole-body plethysmography in healthy cats, *Am J Vet Res* 60:1487, 1999.
112. Hoover EA, Kahn DE: Experimentally induced feline calicivirus infection: clinical signs and lesions, *J Am Vet Med Assoc* 166:463, 1975.
113. Hoover EA, Rohovsky MW, Griesemer RA: Experimental feline viral rhinotracheitis in the germfree cat, *Am J Pathol* 58:269, 1970.

114. Hoskins JD, Malone JB, Root CR: Albendazole therapy in naturally-occurring feline paragonimiasis, *J Am Anim Hosp Assoc* 17:265, 1981.
115. Hurley KF, Pesavento PA, Pedersen NC et al: An outbreak of virulent systemic feline calicivirus disease, *J Am Vet Med Assoc* 224:241, 2004.
116. Jacobs AA, Chalmers WS, Pasman J et al: Feline bordetellosis: challenge and vaccine studies, *Vet Rec* 133:260, 1993.
117. Jacobson GA, Chong FV, Wood-Baker R: (R,S)-salbutamol plasma concentrations in severe asthma, *J Clin Pharm Ther* 28:235, 2003.
118. Jang SS, Demartini JC, Henrickson RV et al: Focal necrotizing pneumonia in cats associated with a gram negative eugonic fermenting bacterium, *Cornell Vet* 63:446, 1973.
119. Jasmin AM, Carroll JM, Baucom JN et al: Systemic blastomycosis in siamese cats, *Vet Med Small Anim Clin* 64:33, 1969.
120. Johnson EG, Wisner ER: Advances in respiratory imaging, *Vet Clin North Am Small Anim Pract* 37:879, 2007.
121. Johnson LR: Bronchial disease. In August JR, editor: *Consultations in feline internal medicine*, ed 5, St Louis, 2006, Elsevier Saunders, p 361.
122. Johnson LR, Drazenovich TL: Flexible bronchoscopy and bronchoalveolar lavage in 68 cats (2001-2006), *J Vet Intern Med* 21:219, 2007.
123. Johnson LR, Fry MM, Anez KL et al: Histoplasmosis infection in two cats from California, *J Am Anim Hosp Assoc* 40:165, 2004.
124. Johnson MS, Martin M, Stone B et al: Survival of a cat with pneumonia due to cowpox virus and feline herpesvirus infection, *J Small Anim Pract* 50:498, 2009.
125. Jones DJ, Norris CR, Samii VF et al: Endogenous lipid pneumonia in cats: 24 cases (1985-1998), *J Am Vet Med Assoc* 216:1437, 2000.
126. Jordan HL, Cohn LA, Armstrong PJ: Disseminated *Mycobacterium avium* complex infection in three Siamese cats, *J Am Vet Med Assoc* 204:90, 1994.
127. Kaufmann AF, Mann JM, Gardiner TM et al: Public health implications of plague in domestic cats, *J Am Vet Med Assoc* 179:875, 1981.
128. Kelly JD, Ng BKY, Whitlock HV: Helminth parasites of dogs and cats, *Aust Vet Pract* 6:89, 1976.
129. Kier AB, Mann PC, Wagner JE: Disseminated sporotrichosis in a cat, *J Am Vet Med Assoc* 175:202, 1979.
130. King TE, Costabel U, Cordier J-F et al: Idiopathic pulmonary fibrosis: diagnosis and treatment. international consensus statement, *Am J Resp Crit Care Med* 161:646, 2000.
131. Kirkpatrick CE, Megella C: Use of ivermectin in treatment of *Aelurostrongylus abstrusus* and *Toxocara cati* infection in a cat, *J Am Vet Med Assoc* 190:1309, 1987.
132. Kirschvink N, Leemans J, Delvaux F et al: Bronchodilators in bronchoscopy-induced airflow limitation in allergen-sensitized cats, *J Vet Intern Med* 19:161, 2005.
133. Kirschvink N, Leemans J, Delvaux F et al: Functional, inflammatory and morphological characterisation of a cat model of allergic airway inflammation, *Vet J* 174:541, 2007.
134. Kirschvink N, Leemans J, Delvaux F et al: Non-invasive assessment of airway responsiveness in healthy and allergen-sensitised cats by use of barometric whole body plethysmography, *Vet J* 173:343, 2007.
135. Kirschvink N, Leemans J, Delvaux F et al: Inhaled fluticasone reduces bronchial responsiveness and airway inflammation in cats with mild chronic bronchitis, *J Feline Med Surg* 8:45, 2006.
136. Kirschvink N, Marlin D, Delvaux F et al: Collection of exhaled breath condensate and analysis of hydrogen peroxide as a potential marker of lower airway inflammation in cats, *Vet J* 169:385, 2005.
137. Klopfleisch R, Wolf PU, Uhl W et al: Distribution of lesions and antigen of highly pathogenic avian influenza virus A/Swan/Germany/R65/06 (H5N1) in domestic cats after presumptive infection by wild birds, *Vet Pathol* 44:261, 2007.
138. Kramer L, Genchi C: Feline heartworm infection: serological survey of asymptomatic cats living in northern Italy, *Vet Parasitol* 104:43, 2002.
139. Kuiken T, Rimmelzwaan G, van Riel D et al: Avian H5N1 influenza in cats, *Science* 306:241, 2004.
140. Lacorcia L, Gasser RB, Anderson GA et al: Comparison of bronchoalveolar lavage fluid examination and other diagnostic techniques with the Baermann technique for detection of naturally occurring *Aelurostrongylus abstrusus* infection in cats, *J Am Vet Med Assoc* 235:43, 2009.
141. Lam A, Newhouse MT: Management of asthma and chronic airflow limitation. Are methylxanthines obsolete? *Chest* 98:44, 1990.
142. Langlais LM, Gibson J, Taylor JA et al: Pulmonary adenocarcinoma with metastasis to skeletal muscle in a cat, *Can Vet J* 47:1122, 2006.
143. Lappin MR, Greene CE, Winston S et al: Clinical feline toxoplasmosis. Serologic diagnosis and therapeutic management of 15 cases, *J Vet Intern Med* 3:139, 1989.
144. Lecuyer M, Dube PG, DiFruscia R et al: Bronchoalveolar lavage in normal cats, *Can Vet J* 36:771, 1995.
145. Lee-Fowler TM, Cohn LA, DeClue AE et al: Comparison of intradermal skin testing (IDST) and serum allergen-specific IgE determination in an experimental model of feline asthma, *Vet Immunol Immunopathol* 132:46, 2009.
146. Lee-Fowler TM, Cohn LA, DeClue AE et al: Evaluation of subcutaneous versus mucosal (intranasal) allergen-specific rush immunotherapy in experimental feline asthma, *Vet Immunol Immunopathol* 129:49, 2009.
147. Leemans J, Cambier C, Chandler T et al: Prophylactic effects of omega-3 polyunsaturated fatty acids and luteolin on airway hyperresponsiveness and inflammation in cats with experimentally-induced asthma, *Vet J* 184:111, 2010.
148. Leemans J, Kirschvink N, Bernaerts F et al: A pilot study comparing the antispasmodic effects of inhaled salmeterol, salbutamol and ipratropium bromide using different aerosol devices on muscarinic bronchoconstriction in healthy cats, *Vet J* 180:236, 2009.
149. Leschnik M, Weikel J, Mostl K et al: Subclinical infection with avian influenza A (H5N1) virus in cats, *Emerg Infect Dis* 13:243, 2007.
150. Levy JK, Edinboro CH, Glotfelty C-S et al: Seroprevalence of *Dirofilaria immitis*, feline leukemia virus, and feline immunodeficiency virus infection among dogs and cats exported from the 2005 Gulf Coast hurricane disaster area, *J Am Vet Med Assoc* 231:218, 2007.
151. Levy JK, Snyder PS, Taveres LM et al: Prevalence and risk factors for heartworm infection in cats from northern Florida, *J Am Anim Hosp Assoc* 39:533, 2003.
152. Litster A, Atkins C, Atwell R: Acute death in heartworm-infected cats: unraveling the puzzle, *Vet Parasitol* 158:196, 2008.
153. Litster AL, Atwell RB: Feline heartworm disease: a clinical review, *J Feline Med Surg* 10:137, 2008.
154. Little S: *Bordetella bronchiseptica* infection in a cat, *Feline Pract* 28:12, 2000.
155. Liu J, Song KH, Lee SE et al: Serological and molecular survey of *Dirofilaria immitis* infection in stray cats in Gyunggi province, South Korea, *Vet Parasity* 130:125, 2005.
156. Lloyd J, Allen JG: The isolation of group EF-4 bacteria from a case of granulomatous pneumonia in a tiger cub, *Aust Vet J* 56:399, 1980.
157. Lohr CV, DeBess EE, Baker RJ et al: Pathology and viral antigen distribution of lethal pneumonia in domestic cats due to pandemic (H1N1) 2009 influenza A virus, *Vet Pathol* 47:378, 2010.

158. Lorentzen L, Caola AE: Incidence of positive heartworm antibody and antigen tests at IDEXX Laboratories: trends and potential impact on feline heartworm awareness and prevention, *Vet Parasitol* 158:183, 2008.
159. Love DN: Feline herpesvirus associated with interstitial pneumonia in a kitten, *Vet Rec* 89:178, 1971.
160. Love DN: Pathogenicity of a strain of feline calicivirus for domestic kittens, *Aust Vet J* 51:541, 1975.
161. Macdonald ES, Norris CR, Berghaus RB et al: Clinicopathologic and radiographic features and etiologic agents in cats with histologically confirmed infectious pneumonia: 39 cases (1991-2000), *J Am Vet Med Assoc* 223:1142, 2003.
162. Mahaffey E, Gabbert N, Johnson D et al: Disseminated histoplasmosis in three cats, *J Am Anim Hosp Assoc* 13:46, 1977.
163. Malik R, Love DN, Hunt GB et al: Pyothorax associated with a *Mycoplasma* species in a kitten, *J Small AnimPract* 32:31, 1991.
164. Malik R, Wigney DI, Muir DB et al: Cryptococcosis in cats: clinical and mycological assessment of 29 cases and evaluation of treatment using orally administered fluconazole, *Med Mycol* 30:133, 1992.
165. Mandelker L: Experimental drug therapy for respiratory disorders in dogs and cats, *Vet Clin North Am Small Anim Pract* 30:1357, 2000.
166. Mavropoulou A, Grandi G, Calvi L et al: Disseminated histoplasmosis in a cat in Europe, *J Small Anim Pract* 51:176, 2010.
167. McArdle HC, Dawson S, Coutts AJ et al: Seroprevalence and isolation rate of *Bordetella bronchiseptica* in cats in the UK, *Vet Rec* 135:506, 1994.
168. McCall JW: The safety-net story about macrocyclic lactone heartworm preventives: a review, an update, and recommendations, *Vet Parasitol* 133:197, 2005.
169. McCall JW, Calvert CA, Rawlings CA: Heartworm infection in cats: a life-threatening disease, *Vet Med* 89:639, 1994.
170. McCarthy G, Quinn PJ: The development of lavage procedures for the upper and lower respiratory tract of the cat, *Ir Vet J* 40:6, 1986.
171. McCarthy GM, Quinn PJ: Bronchoalveolar lavage in the cat: cytological findings, *Can J Vet Res* 53:259, 1989.
172. McCausland IP: Systemic mycoses of two cats, *N Z Vet J* 20:10, 1972.
173. McCracken MD, Patton S: Pulmonary arterial changes in feline dirofilariasis, *Vet Pathol* 30:64, 1993.
174. McCullers JA, Van De Velde LA, Schultz RD et al: Seroprevalence of seasonal and pandemic influenza A viruses in domestic cats, *Arch Virol* 156(1):117, 2011.
175. McKiernan BC, Dye JA, Powell M et al: Terbutaline pharmacokinetics in cats [abstract], *J Vet Intern Med* 5:122, 1991.
176. McParland PJ, O'Hagan J, Pearson GR et al: Pathological changes associated with group EF-4 bacteria in the lungs of a dog and a cat, *Vet Rec* 111:336, 1982.
177. McTier TL, Supakorndej N, McCall JW et al: Evaluation of ELISA-based adult heartworm antigen test kits using well-defined sera from experimentally and naturally infected cats, *Proceedings of the American Association of Veterinary Parasitologists* 38:37, 1993.
178. Medleau L, Jacobs GJ, Marks MA: Itraconazole for the treatment of cryptococcosis in cats, *J Vet Intern Med* 9:39, 1995.
179. Mehlhaff CJ, Mooney S: Primary pulmonary neoplasia in the dog and cat, *Vet Clin North Am Small AnimPract* 15:1061, 1985.
180. Menard M, Papageorges M: Technique for ultrasound-guided fine needle biopsies, *Vet Radiol Ultrasound* 36:137, 1995.
181. Meyer A, Hauser B: [Lung tumor with unusual metastasis in a cat—a case report], *Schweizer Archiv fur Tierheilkunde* 137:54, 1995.
182. Miles KG: A review of primary lung tumors in the dog and cat, *Vet Radiol* 29:122, 1988.
183. Miller PE, Miller LM, Schoster JV: Feline blastomycosis: a report of three cases and literature review:(1961-1988), *J Am Anim Hosp Assoc* 26:417, 1990.
184. Mills PC, Litster A: Using urea dilution to standardise cellular and non-cellular components of pleural and bronchoalveolar lavage (BAL) fluids in the cat, *J Feline Med Surg* 8:105, 2006.
185. Mitchell RW, Cozzi P, Maurice Ndukwu I et al: Differential effects of cyclosporine A after acute antigen challenge in sensitized cats in vivo and ex vivo, *Br J Pharmacol* 123:1198, 1998.
186. Mohan K, Kelly PJ, Hill FWG et al: Phenotype and serotype of *Pasteurella multocida* isolates from diseases of dogs and cats in Zimbabwe, *Comp Immunol Microbiol Infect Dis* 20:29, 1997.
187. Moise NS, Blue JT: Bronchial washings in the cat: procedure and cytology evaluation, *Comp Cont Ed Pract Vet* 5:621, 1983.
188. Moise NS, Wiedenkeller D, Yeager AE et al: Clinical, radiographic, and bronchial cytologic features of cats with bronchial disease: 65 cases (1980-1986), *J Am Vet Med Assoc* 194:1467, 1989.
189. Moore AS, Middleton DJ: Pulmonary adenocarcinoma in three cats with nonrespiratory signs only, *J Small Anim Pract* 23:501, 1982.
190. Moriello KA, Stepien RL, Henik RA et al: Pilot study: prevalence of positive aeroallergen reactions in 10 cats with small-airway disease without concurrent skin disease, *Vet Derm* 18:94, 2007.
191. Murphy ST, Mathews KG, Ellison GW et al: Pulmonary lobectomy in the management of pneumonia in five cats, *J Small Anim Pract* 38:159, 1997.
192. Nafe LA, DeClue AE, Lee-Fowler TM et al: Evaluation of biomarkers in bronchoalveolar lavage fluid for discrimination between asthma and chronic bronchitis in cats, *Am J Vet Res* 71:583, 2010.
193. Nafe LA, DeClue AE, Reinero CR: Storage alters feline bronchoalveolar lavage fluid cytological analysis, *J Feline Med Surg* 13:94, 2011.
194. Nasisse MP, van Ee RT, Wright B: Ocular changes in a cat with disseminated blastomycosis, *J Am Vet Med Assoc* 187:629, 1985.
195. Nelson CT: *Dirofilaria immitis* in cats: anatomy of a disease, *Compendium* 30:382, 2008.
196. Nelson CT: *Dirofilaria immitis* in cats: diagnosis and management, *Compendium* 30:393, 2008.
197. Nolan TJ, Smith G: Time series analysis of the prevalence of endoparasitic infections in cats and dogs presented to a veterinary teaching hospital, *Vet Parasitol* 59:87, 1995.
198. Norris CR, Decile KC, Byerly JR et al: Production of polyclonal antisera against feline immunoglobulin E and its use in an ELISA in cats with experimentally induced asthma, *Vet Immunol Immunopathol* 96:149, 2003.
199. Norris CR, Griffey SM, Samii VF et al: Thoracic radiography, bronchoalveolar lavage cytopathology, and pulmonary parenchymal histopathology: a comparison of diagnostic results in 11 cats, *J Am Anim Hosp Assoc* 38:337, 2002.
200. Norris CR, Griffey SM, Walsh P: Use of keyhole lung biopsy for diagnosis of interstitial lung diseases in dogs and cats: 13 cases (1998-2001), *J Am Vet Med Assoc* 221:1453, 2002.
201. Norris Reinero CR, Decile KC, Berghaus RD et al: An experimental model of allergic asthma in cats sensitized to house dust mite or Bermuda grass allergen, *Int Arch Allergy Immunol* 135:117, 2004.
202. Nowak R, Emerman C, Hanrahan JP et al: A comparison of levalbuterol with racemic albuterol in the treatment of acute severe asthma exacerbations in adults, *Am J Emerg Med* 24:259, 2006.
203. Ossent P: Systemic aspergillus and mucormycosis in 23 cats, *Vet Rec* 120:330, 1987.
204. Padrid P: Feline asthma. Diagnosis and treatment, *Vet Clin North Am Small Anim Pract* 30:1279, 2000.
205. Padrid P: Use of inhaled medications to treat respiratory diseases in dogs and cats, *J Am Anim Hosp Assoc* 42:165, 2006.

206. Padrid P: Inhaled steroids to treat feline lower airway disease: 300 cases 1995-2007, *Proceedings of the American College of Veterinary Internal Medicine Forum* 456, 2008.
207. Padrid P: Chronic bronchitis and asthma in cats. In Bonagura JD, Twedt DC, editors: *Current veterinary therapy XIV*, Philadelphia, 2009, Saunders Elsevier, p 650.
208. Padrid P: Asthma. In August JR, editor: *Consultations in feline internal medicine*, ed 6, St Louis, 2010, Elsevier Saunders, p 447.
209. Padrid P, Church DB: Drugs used in the management of respiratory diseases. In Maddison JE, Page SW,Church DB, editors: *Small animal clinical pharmacology*, ed 2, Philadelphia, 2008, Saunders Elsevier, p 458.
210. Padrid PA, Cozzi P, Leff AR: Cyclosporine A inhibits airway reactivity and remodeling after chronic antigen challenge in cats, *Am J Resp Crit Care Med* 154:1812, 1996.
211. Padrid PA, Feldman BF, Funk K et al: Cytologic, microbiologic, and biochemical analysis of bronchoalveolar lavage fluid obtained from 24 healthy cats, *Am J Vet Res* 52:1300, 1991.
212. Padrid PA, Mitchell RW, Ndukwu IM et al: Cyproheptadine-induced attenuation of type-I immediate-hypersensitivity reactions of airway smooth muscle from immune-sensitized cats, *Am J Vet Res* 56:109, 1995.
213. Paniker CK, Nair CM: Infection with A2 Hong Kong influenza virus in domestic cats, *Bull World Health Org* 43:859, 1970.
214. Pechman RD Jr: Pulmonary paragonimiasis in dogs and cats: a review, *J Small AnimPract* 21:87, 1980.
215. Pedersen NC, Elliott JB, Glasgow A et al: An isolated epizootic of hemorrhagic-like fever in cats caused by a novel and highly virulent strain of feline calicivirus, *Vet Microbiol* 73:281, 2000.
216. Pesavento PA, Maclachlan NJ, Dillard-Telm L et al: Pathologic, immunohistochemical, and electron microscopic findings in naturally occurring virulent systemic feline calicivirus infection in cats, *Vet Pathol* 41:257, 2004.
217. Petterino C, Guazzi P, Ferro S et al: Bronchogenic adenocarcinoma in a cat: an unusual case of metastasis to the skin, *Vet Clin Pathol* 34:401, 2005.
218. Pfeffer M, Kaaden OR, Pfleghaar S et al: Retrospective investigation of feline cowpox in Germany, *Vet Rec* 150:50, 2002.
219. Poitout F, Weiss DJ, Dubey JP: Lung aspirate from a cat with respiratory distress, *Vet Clin Pathol* 27:10, 1998.
220. Povey RC, Hale CJ: Experimental infections with feline caliciviruses (picornaviruses) in specific-pathogen-free kittens, *J Comp Pathol* 84:245, 1974.
221. Randolph JF, Moise NS, Scarlett JM et al: Prevalence of mycoplasmal and ureaplasmal recovery from tracheobronchial lavages and of mycoplasmal recovery from pharyngeal swab specimens in cats with or without pulmonary disease, *Am J Vet Res* 54:897, 1993.
222. Reinero CR: Bronchoalveolar lavage fluid collection using a blind technique, *Clinician's Brief* 8:58, 2010.
223. Reinero CR, Brownlee L, Decile KC et al: Inhaled flunisolide suppresses the hypothalamic-pituitary-adrenocortical axis, but has minimal systemic immune effects in healthy cats, *J Vet Intern Med* 20:57, 2006.
224. Reinero CR, Byerly JR, Berghaus RD et al: Rush immunotherapy in an experimental model of feline allergic asthma, *Vet Immunol Immunopathol* 110:141, 2006.
225. Reinero CR, Cohn LA, Delgado C et al: Adjuvanted rush immunotherapy using CpG oligodeoxynucleotides in experimental feline allergic asthma, *Vet Immunol Immunopathol* 121:241, 2008.
226. Reinero CR, Decile KC, Byerly JR et al: Effects of drug treatment on inflammation and hyperreactivity of airways and on immune variables in cats with experimentally induced asthma, *Am J Vet Res* 66:1121, 2005.
227. Reinero CR, DeClue AE, Rabinowitz P: Asthma in humans and cats: Is there a common sensitivity to aeroallegens in shared environments? *Environ Res* 109:634, 2009.
228. Reinero CR, Delgado C, Spinka C et al: Enantiomer-specific effects of albuterol on airway inflammation in healthy and asthmatic cats, *Int Arch Allergy Immunoly* 150:43, 2009.
229. Rendano VT: Paragonimiasis in the cat: a review of five cases, *J Small Anim Pract* 15:637, 1974.
230. Rimmelzwaan GF, van Riel D, Baars M et al: Influenza A virus (H5N1) infection in cats causes systemic disease with potential novel routes of virus spread within and between hosts, *Am J Pathol* 168:176, 2006.
231. Rodriguez CO, Jr., Moon ML, Leib MS: Salmonella choleraesuis pneumonia in a cat without signs of gastrointestinal tract disease, *J Am Vet Med Assoc* 202:953, 1993.
232. Romvary J, Rozsa J, Farkas E: Infection of dogs and cats with the Hong Kong influenza A (H3N2) virus during an epidemic period in Hungary, *Acta Vet Acad Sci Hung* 25:255, 1975.
233. Roomiany PL, Axtell RC, Scalarone GM: Comparison of seven *Blastomyces dermatitidis* antigens for the detection of antibodies in humans with occupationally acquired blastomycosis, *Mycoses* 45:282, 2002.
234. Saphir DA, Carter GR: Gingival flora of the dog with special reference to bacteria associated with bites, *J Clin Microbiol* 3:344, 1976.
235. Sardinas JC, Chastain CB, Collins BK et al: Toxoplasma pneumonia in a cat with incongruous serological test results, *J Small Anim Pract* 35:104, 1994.
236. Sauter JH, Steelte DS, Henry JE: Aspergillosis in a cat, *J Am Vet Med Ass* 127:518, 1955.
237. Schafer M, Berry CR: Cardiac and pulmonary artery mensuration in feline heartworm disease, *Vet Radiol Ultrasound* 36:499, 1995.
238. Schoen K, Block G, Newell SM et al: Hypercalcemia of malignancy in a cat with bronchogenic adenocarcinoma, *J Am Anim Hosp Assoc* 46:265, 2010.
239. Schöniger S, Chan DL, Hollinshead M et al: Cowpox virus pneumonia in a domestic cat in Great Britain, *Vet Rec* 160:522, 2007.
240. Schooley EK, McGee Turner JB, JiJi RD et al: Effects of cyproheptadine and cetirizine on eosinophilic airway inflammation in cats with experimentally induced asthma, *Am J Vet Res* 68:1265, 2007.
241. Schubach TM, Schubach A, Okamoto T et al: Haematogenous spread of Sporothrix schenckii in cats with naturally acquired sporotrichosis, *J Small Anim Pract* 44:395, 2003.
242. Schulman RL, Crochik SS, Kneller SK et al: Investigation of pulmonary deposition of a nebulized radiopharmaceutical agent in awake cats, *Am J Vet Res* 65:806, 2004.
243. Schulze C, Alex M, Schirrmeier H et al: Generalized fatal cowpox virus infection in a cat with transmission to a human contact case, *Zoonoses Public Health* 54:31, 2007.
244. Scott DW: Current knowledge of aelurostrongylosis in the cat, *Cornell Vet* 63:483, 1973.
245. Sekhon AS, Bogorus MS, Sims HV: Blastomycosis: report of three cases from Alberta with a review of Canadian cases, *Mycopathologia* 68:53, 1979.
246. Sheldon WG: Pulmonary blastomycosis in a cat, *Lab Anim Care* 16:280, 1966.
247. Shields RP, Gaskin JM: Fatal generalized feline viral rhinotracheitis in a young adult cat, *J Am Vet Med Assoc* 170:439, 1977.
248. Small MT, Atkins CE, Gordon SG et al: Use of a nitinol gooseneck snare catheter for removal of adult *Dirofilaria immitis* in two cats, *J Am Vet Med Assoc* 233:1441, 2008.
249. Smith AW, Iversen PL, O'Hanley PD et al: Virus-specific antiviral treatment for controlling severe and fatal outbreaks of feline calicivirus infection, *Am J Vet Res* 69:23, 2008.
250. Snyder PS, Levy JK, Salute ME et al: Performance of serologic tests used to detect heartworm infection in cats, *J Am Vet Med Assoc* 216:693, 2000.
251. Soltys MA, Sumner-Smith G: Systemic mycoses in dogs and cats, *Can Vet J* 12:191, 1971.

252. Songserm T, Amonsin A, Jam-on R et al: Avian influenza H5N1 in naturally infected domestic cat, *Emerg Infect Dis* 12:681, 2006.
253. Sparkes AH, Mardell EJ, Deaton C et al: Exhaled breath condensate (EBC) collection in cats—description of a non-invasive technique to investigate airway disease, *J Feline Med Surg* 6:335, 2004.
254. Speakman AJ, Dawson S, Binns SH et al: *Bordetella bronchiseptica* infection in the cat, *J Small Anim Pract* 40:252, 1999.
255. Sponseller BA, Strait E, Jergens A et al: Influenza A pandemic (H1N1) 2009 virus infection in domestic cat, *Emerg Infect Dis* 16:534, 2010.
256. Spradbrow PB, Carlisle C, Watt DA: The association of a herpesvirus with generalised disease in a kitten, *Vet Rec* 89:542, 1971.
257. Stein JE, Lappin MR: Bacterial culture results in cats with upper and lower airway disease: 255 cases (1995-1999) [abstract], *J Vet Intern Med* 15:320, 2001.
258. Stiver SL, Frazier KS, Mauel MJ et al: Septicemic salmonellosis in two cats fed a raw-meat diet, *J Am Anim Hosp Assoc* 39:538, 2003.
259. Stromberg PC, Dubey JP: The life cycle of *Paragonimus kellicotti* in cats, *J Parasitol* 64:998, 1978.
260. Stursberg U, Zenker I, Hecht S et al: Use of propentofylline in feline bronchial disease: prospective, randomized, positive-controlled study, *J Am Anim Hosp Assoc* 46:318, 2010.
261. Sura R, Hinckley LS, Risatti GR et al: Fatal necrotising fasciitis and myositis in a cat associated with *Streptococcus canis*, *Vet Rec* 162:450, 2008.
262. Sura R, Van Kruiningen HJ, DebRoy C et al: Extraintestinal pathogenic *Escherichia coli*–induced acute necrotizing pneumonia in cats, *Zoonoses Public Health* 54:307, 2007.
263. Swift S, Dukes-McEwan J, Fonfara S et al: Aetiology and outcome in 90 cats presenting with dyspnoea in a referral population, *J Small Anim Pract* 50:466, 2009.
264. Talavera J, del Palacio MJF, Bayon A et al: Broncholithiasis in a cat: clinical findings, long-term evolution and histopathological features, *J Feline Med Surg* 10:95, 2008.
265. Tams TR: Aspiration pneumonia and complications of inhalation of smoke and toxic gases, *Vet Clin North Am Small Animal Pract* 15:971, 1985.
266. Teske E, Stokhof A, van den Ingh T et al: Transthoracic needle aspiration biopsy of the lung in dogs and cats with pulmonic disease, *J Am Anim Hosp Assoc* 27:289, 1991.
267. Theilen GH, Madewell BR: Tumours of the respiratory tract and thorax. In Theilen GH, Madewell BR, editors: *Veterinary cancer medicine*, ed 1, Philadelphia, 1979, Lea & Febiger, p 341.
268. Thiry E, Zicola A, Addie D et al: Highly pathogenic avian influenza H5N1 virus in cats and other carnivores, *Vet Microbiol* 122:25, 2007.
269. Traversa D, Di Cesare A, Conboy G: Canine and feline cardiopulmonary parasitic nematodes in Europe: emerging and underestimated, *Parasit Vectors* 3:62, 2010.
269a. Traversa D, Di Cesare A, Milillo P et al: Efficacy and safety of imidacloprid 10%/moxidectin 1% spot-on formulation in the treatment of feline aelurostrongylosis, *Parasitol Res* 105:S55, 2009.
270. Traversa D, Di Cesare A, Milillo P et al: Infection by *Eucoleus aerophilus* in dogs and cats: is another extra-intestinal parasitic nematode of pets emerging in Italy? *Res Vet Sci* 87:270, 2009.
271. Traversa D, Guglielmini C: Feline aelurostrongylosis and canine angiostrongylosis: a challenging diagnosis for two emerging verminous pneumonia infections, *Vet Parasitol* 157:163, 2008.
272. Traversa D, Iorio R, Otranto D: Diagnostic and clinical implications of a nested PCR specific for the ribosomal DNA of feline lungworm Aelurostrongylus abstrusus (Nematoda, Strongylida), *J Clin Microbiol* 46:1811, 2008.
272a. Traversa D, Milillo P, Di Cesare A et al: Efficacy and safety of emodepside 2.1%/praziquantel 8.6% spot-on formulation in the treatment of feline aelurostrongylosis, *Parasitol Res* 105:S83, 2009.
273. Trow AV, Rozanski EA, Tidwell AS: Primary mycoplasma pneumonia associated with reversible respiratory failure in a cat, *J Feline Med Surg* 10:398, 2008.
274. Vahlenkamp TW, Harder TC, Giese M et al: Protection of cats against lethal influenza H5N1 challenge infection, *J Gen Virol* 89:968, 2008.
275. van den Brand JM, Stittelaar KJ, van Amerongen G et al: Experimental pandemic (H1N1) 2009 virus infection of cats, *Emerg Infect Dis* 16:1745, 2010.
276. Vandamme P, Holmes B, Bercovier H et al: Classification of Centers for Disease Control Group Eugonic Fermenter (EF)-4a and EF-4b as *Neisseria animaloris* sp. nov. and *Neisseria zoodegmatis* sp. nov., respectively, *Int J Syst Evol Microbiol* 56:1801, 2006.
277. Venco L, Genchi C, Genchi M et al: Clinical evolution and radiographic findings of feline heartworm infection in asymptomatic cats, *Vet Parasitol* 158:232, 2008.
278. Venema CM, Patterson CC: Feline asthma: What's new and where might clinical practice be heading? *J Feline Med Surg* 12:681, 2010.
279. Weaver RE, Hollis DG, Bottone EJ: Gram-negative fermentative bacteria and *Francisella tularensis*. In Lennette EH, Balows A, Hausle Jr WJ et al, editors: *Manual of clinical microbiology*, Washington DC, 1985, American Society for Microbiology, p 309.
280. Weina PJ, England DM: The American lung fluke, *Paragonimus kellicotti*, in a cat model, *J Parasitol* 76:568, 1990.
281. Weingartl HM, Berhane Y, Hisanaga T et al: Genetic and pathobiologic characterization of pandemic H1N1 2009 influenza viruses from a naturally infected swine herd, *J Virol* 84:2245, 2010.
282. Welsh R: *Bordetella bronchiseptica* infections in cats, *J Am Anim Hosp Assoc* 32:153, 1996.
283. Wernli D, Emonet S, Schrenzel J et al: Evaluation of eight cases of confirmed *Bordetella bronchiseptica* infection and colonization over a 15-year period, *Clin Microbiol Infect* 17:201, 2011.
284. Weyant RS, Burris JA, Nichols DK et al: Epizootic feline pneumonia associated with Centers for Disease Control group EF-4a bacteria, *Lab Anim Sci* 44:180, 1994.
285. Willard MD, Roberts RE, Allison N et al: Diagnosis of *Aelurostrongylus abstrusus* and *Dirofilaria immitis* infections in cats from a human shelter, *J Am Vet Med Assoc* 192:913, 1988.
286. Williams K, Malarkey D, Cohn L et al: Identification of spontaneous feline idiopathic pulmonary fibrosis, *Chest* 125:2278, 2004.
287. Willoughby K, Dawson S, Jones RC et al: Isolation of *B. bronchiseptica* from kittens with pneumonia in a breeding cattery, *Vet Rec* 129:407, 1991.
288. Wolf AM, Belden MN: Feline histoplasmosis: a literature review and retrospective study of 20 new cases, *J Am Anim Hosp Assoc* 20:995, 1984.
289. Wolf AM, Green RW: The radiographic appearance of pulmonary histoplasmosis in the cat, *Vet Radiol* 28:34, 1987.
290. Wood EF, O'Brien RT, Young KM: Ultrasound-guided fine-needle aspiration of focal parenchymal lesions of the lung in dogs and cats, *J Vet Intern Med* 12:338, 1998.
291. Yingst SL, Saad MD, Felt SA: Qinghai-like H5N1 from domestic cats, northern Iraq, *Emerg Infect Dis* 12:1295, 2006.
292. Zekas LJ, Crawford JT, O'Brien RT: Computed tomography-guided fine-needle aspirate and tissue-core biopsy of intrathoracic lesions in thirty dogs and cats, *Vet Radiol Ultrasound* 46:200, 2005.
293. Zhukova OA, Tsanava SA, Marennikova SS: Experimental infection of domestic cats by cowpox virus, *Acta Virol* 36:329, 1992.

THE THORACIC CAVITY

Randolph M. Baral

GENERAL CONSIDERATIONS

The thoracic cavity is contained within the thoracic wall and the diaphragm caudally. It encloses the lungs and the mediastinum, the potential space located between the right and left pleural cavities. The mediastinum contains numerous vital structures, including the heart, trachea, esophagus, thymus, and great vessels. The pleural space is lined by the visceral and parietal pleura, with visceral pleura covering the surface of the lungs and parietal pleura covering the diaphragm, costal surface, and mediastinum.

Diseases affecting the thoracic cavity most commonly result in the following:

1. Fluid accumulation within the pleural space (pleural effusion)
2. Air accumulation within the pleural space (pneumothorax)
3. Solid tissue within the pleural space; such tissue may arise from within the thoracic cavity, such as neoplastic masses, or be introduced, such as abdominal viscera with diaphragmatic herniation

In most cases cats with pathology affecting the thoracic cavity will present with dyspnea, but in early stages signs may be so mild that no obvious effect on respiration is evident. Recognition of a disorder affecting the thoracic cavity usually requires radiographic recognition of fluid, air, or masses within the chest or disruption of the diaphragm or chest wall.

CLINICAL SIGNS

The presence of fluid, air, or masses within the pleural cavity restricts lung expansion, resulting in rapid, shallow breaths with increased inspiratory effort. Lung volume and expansion are also affected with pathology of the pulmonary parenchyma (e.g., pneumonia, pulmonary edema), so a similar breathing pattern may result. In early stages, signs may be subtle, and cats may simply reduce activity levels. Cats may prefer a sitting or crouched sternal posture with elbows abducted from the thorax, perhaps with head or neck extended to maximize air intake. Coughing is not considered a typical sign with pleural space disease but may result from tracheal compression (e.g., from neoplasia) or pulmonary parenchymal involvement or pleuritis.[11,105] Coughing was recognized in 30 of 37 cats with chylothorax in one series.[39] Other clinical signs depend on the underlying cause of intrathoracic disease but may include weight loss, anorexia, or fever.

PHYSICAL EXAMINATION

Cats presenting in severe respiratory distress should have minimal initial handling and only a cursory examination on presentation because further stress can lead to decompensation. Cats in this situation often need supplemental oxygen (see Box 30-5 later in this chapter). In some circumstances, survey radiographs in the position most comfortable for the cat (often dorsoventral with the cat resting on its elbows) should be taken in lieu of a physical examination. Some authors advocate thoracocentesis (see Box 30-6 later in this chapter) ahead of thoracic radiography when pleural effusion is strongly suspected.[42,77]

On auscultation, heart and lung sounds may be reduced or absent, particularly ventrally. These signs are obvious in severe cases but may be subtle or absent with milder disease. Thoracic percussion is difficult to perform in cats; tapping against an intercostal space can result in dull, hyporesonant sounds in the case of pleural effusion or pulmonary consolidation; a "drumlike," resonant sound may be recognized with pneumothorax.

Other physical examination findings can be helpful to determine the underlying cause. For example, the presence of a heart murmur, tachycardia, or jugular distention or pulsation can point toward primary cardiac disease (but absence of these signs does not preclude an underlying cardiopathy); hyperthyroidism can result in cardiac disease, so palpation for a thyroid nodule is important in older cats; signs of neoplasia may be present in other locations around the body; abdominal palpation may reveal displaced organs in cats with diaphragmatic hernia. In many cases the signalment of the cat and clinical history will direct the approach. For example, an older cat with a poor body condition score may have neoplasia or hyperthyroidism-associated CHF; a young cat with a fever may have FIP; a cat with known trauma may have diaphragmatic herniation, pneumothorax, or hemothorax.

PLEURAL EFFUSION

In normal cats the pleural space contains a tiny amount of fluid (approximately 0.25 mL/kg in dogs) that enables lubrication of intrathoracic organs during respiration. The control of volume and composition of the pleural liquid is affected by a number of mechanisms, including Starling forces (the balance of interstitial and capillary hydrostatic and oncotic pressures), lymphatic drainage through the parietal pleura stomata, as well as the activity of mesothelial cells.[90,91,140] Pleural effusions arise when one or more of these factors are altered—that is, fluid formation or accumulation is increased, absorption is decreased, or both. Multiple underlying processes can result in pleural effusion, but in most cases the underlying cause is FIP, CHF, neoplasia, pyothorax, or idiopathic chylothorax. A recent review accumulated results from five prior studies ascertaining that of 265 cats with a definitive diagnosis of pleural effusion, 88% to 100% of cases had one of these first four diagnoses[11]; idiopathic chylothorax is a diagnosis of exclusion and represents 10% to 15% of cats with pleural effusion.[23,129,141]

Because clinical signs of pleural effusion are essentially the same as for other diseases affecting the pleural space, radiography (or ultrasonography) is required to confirm the presence of pleural fluid.

Radiography

Radiography should only be used to confirm the presence or absence of pleural effusion in a dyspneic cat *but cannot determine the nature or etiology of the effusion.* Multiple radiographic views for precise diagnostics should be attempted only in stable cats. In severe cases, the stress from handling can result in decompensation and death, so some authors advocate thoracocentesis (discussed later and in Box 30-6) *before* radiography when pleural effusion is suspected.[42,77] In many circumstances, cats with pleural effusion present very similarly to cats with pulmonary edema or bronchial disease, and radiography is required to confirm the presence of pleural fluid. Handling should be minimal, and initially only a single radiograph in the position most comfortable for the cat should be taken, with no additional handling to improve symmetry, for example. In most cases dyspneic cats are most comfortable sitting sternally and resting on their elbows, so a dorsoventral view is most appropriate. Supplementary oxygen should be provided by mask or flow-by ventilation if this is not stressful to the cat (see Box 30-5). Horizontal beam radiographs can be used to document fluid lines or distinguish masses from free-flowing fluid; in one study, however, this view did not contribute additional information to that gained from plain radiographs in eight of nine cats.[23]

Small volumes of pleural effusion are not visible radiographically. It has been shown that 50 mL of effusion is required before radiographic signs are visible in 15-kg dogs,[73] but no similar studies appear to have been performed in cats. The first radiographic signs in small volume effusions are interlobar fissure lines, rounding of lung margins at costophrenic angles, separation of lung borders from the thoracic wall, scalloping of lung margins dorsal to the sternum, blurring to absence of the cardiac silhouette, and widening of the mediastinum. With larger volume effusions the visibility of the heart and mediastinum reduces, lung lobes may collapse, the trachea can be elevated dorsally, and the diaphragm and liver may be displaced dorsally[42,94,97] (Figures 30-21, 30-22, 30-23, and 30-24).

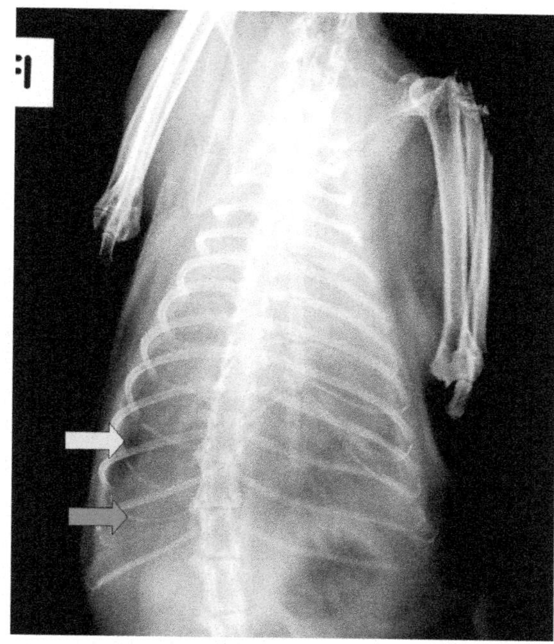

FIGURE 30-21 For dyspneic cats it is appropriate to take a single radiographic view in the position most comfortable for the cat, even if the radiograph is imperfect. In this poorly aligned dorsoventral radiograph, the lung is separated from the thoracic wall *(yellow arrow)* and the lung margins are rounded *(red arrow)*. The cardiac silhouette is barely visible. Additionally, pulmonary edema can be seen as patchy opacities in lung lobes on the left side. In this case pleural effusion is more obvious in the lateral view (see Figure 30-22). This cat was subsequently diagnosed with congestive heart failure secondary to hypertrophic cardiomyopathy.

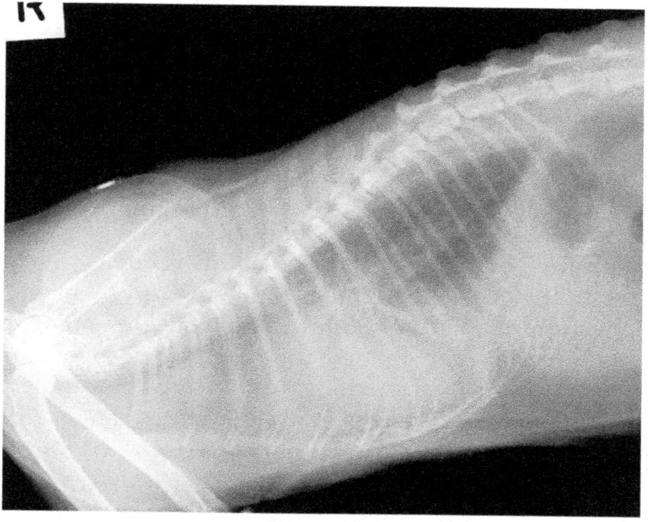

FIGURE 30-22 Right lateral radiographic view of cat from Figure 30-21. Pleural effusion is recognized by interlobar fissure lines, rounding of lung margins at costophrenic angles, separation of lung borders from the thoracic wall, scalloping of lung margins dorsal to the sternum, blurring of the cardiac silhouette, and dorsal elevation of the trachea. This cat was subsequently diagnosed with congestive heart failure secondary to hypertrophic cardiomyopathy.

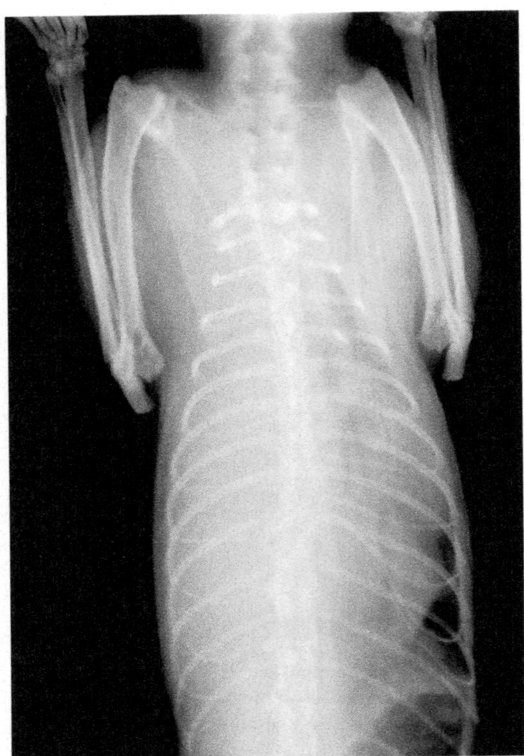

FIGURE 30-23 Dorsoventral radiographic view of severe pleural effusion. This cat had pyothorax.

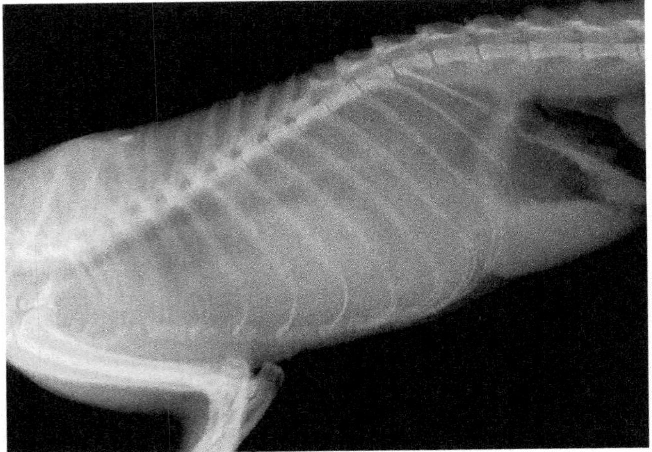

FIGURE 30-24 Right lateral radiographic view of severe pleural effusion. Note the distention of the thoracic cavity resulting in extreme dorsal displacement of the diaphragm and liver. This cat had pyothorax.

Ultrasonography can be used to detect the presence of small volumes of pleural effusion when radiographic findings are equivocal.[72,101] In one study in humans, pleural fluid was recognized by ultrasonography in 93% of cases, compared with only 83% by radiology.[53] Ultrasonography can also provide gross estimations of effusion volume and assess effusion characteristics on the basis of echogenicity.[72,101]

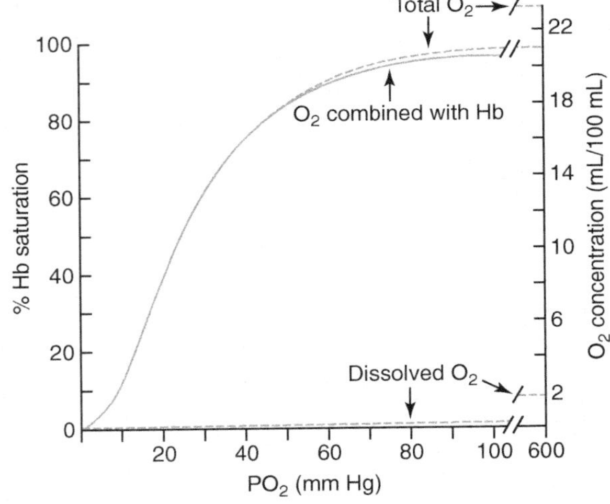

FIGURE 30-25 Oxygen–hemoglobin dissociation curve demonstrating that as oxygen partial pressure (PO_2) decreases below 60 mm Hg, the hemoglobin saturation percentage drops rapidly. *(From West JB:* Respiratory physiology: the essentials, *ed 5, Philadelphia, 1995, Williams & Wilkins.)*

Stabilization

Cats (and other animals) with respiratory disease decompensate easily because although the oxygen saturation of hemoglobin is relatively stable, this is only provided the arterial partial pressure of oxygen (PO_2) remains above approximately 60 mm Hg. Below this point the amount of oxygen carried by hemoglobin drops dramatically, so for an already respiratory-compromised cat, very small reductions in oxygen intake can result in extreme clinical effects. This is demonstrated by the oxygen–hemoglobin dissociation curve (Figure 30-25), where it can be seen that on the flat (right-hand side) part of the curve, decreases in PO_2 from 100 to 60 mm Hg result in only small drops in oxygen hemoglobin saturation. As PO_2 decreases below approximately 60 mm Hg, the curve drops to the left steeply, demonstrating the large decrease in the amount of oxyhemoglobin that results from only small drops in PO_2; PO_2 less than 60 mm Hg is defined as hypoxemic respiratory failure. If a cat is underventilating for any reason, the arterial carbon dioxide (PCO_2) will rise; therefore, if the patient is inspiring room air, hypoxia will worsen; PCO_2 greater than 45 mm Hg is defined as hypercapnic (ventilatory) respiratory failure.[55,77] A patient can have both hypercapnic and hypoxemic respiratory failure occurring to differing degrees simultaneously.

Stabilization requires an increase in the patient's arterial oxygen pressure to enable increased oxygen saturation of hemoglobin—that is, a shift to the right of the oxygen–hemoglobin dissociation curve. The two key components of stabilization are as follows:

1. Oxygen therapy
2. Pleurocentesis

Administration of an oxygen-enriched inspired gas mixture will at least partially correct hypoxemia depending on severity of hypoventilation, atmospheric pressure, flow rates, underlying pathology, hemoglobin concentration, cardiac output, and method of administration. The administration of an oxygen-enriched inspired gas mixture improves oxygenation for most respiratory causes of hypoxia.

Provision of pure oxygen provides higher concentrations of oxygen than normal air, so a greater amount of oxygen is moved to the alveoli with each breath. Oxygen therapy can be provided in the short term by flow-by delivery (Figure 30-26) or face mask delivery (Figure 30-27). More prolonged oxygen delivery can be achieved with the use of an Elizabethan collar canopy (Figure 30-28) or nasal catheter (Figure 30-29). Oxygen cages are widely used but can be problematic. Many commercially available cages do not permit manipulation of the temperature and humidity within the cage (Figure 30-30); the increasing heat and humidity caused by the presence of the cat in the sealed cage increases the cat's oxygen demands, thus further reducing the oxygen saturation of hemoglobin. Moreover, each time the cage door is opened to access the patient, the oxygen-rich environment not only is lost (which can lead to decompensation) but takes time to reach the desired oxygen concentration again. Human neonatal incubators (humidicribs) are most appropriate because they do allow manipulation of temperature and humidity, as well as having smaller openings (Figure 30-31). In severe cases intratracheal catheterization may be necessary, and those cats that cannot sustain PO_2 greater than 60 mm Hg through their own efforts despite conventional oxygen supplementation will require mechanical ventilation. Further details about oxygen therapy are contained in Box 30-5.

Drainage of pleural fluid by pleurocentesis (puncture and aspiration from the pleural cavity) allows improved lung expansion, thereby enabling further oxygen saturation of hemoglobin. Some authors advocate thoracocentesis (puncture and aspiration from the thorax and not necessarily from the pleural space) *before* imaging when pleural effusion is strongly suspected because it can result in life-saving improvement for the patient.[42,77] In experienced hands thoracocentesis is a safe procedure and very well tolerated by cats. The major complications are pneumothorax, hemothorax, pneumohemothorax, or organ laceration, and these risks may be greater in cases when there is a small volume effusion (including no effusion), uncooperative patients, use of a large needle, and the need for multiple needle passes.[103] Thoracocentesis is usually performed at the 6th, 7th, or 8th intercostal space, just ventral to the costochondral junction; this site should be clipped and surgically prepared. The positioning of the cat will vary from case to case. Sternal recumbency is ideal for maximal drainage of fluid, but access ventrally can be difficult when the cat is in this position; having the cat stand is appropriate, but this requires too much effort for many cats with respiratory distress; lateral recumbency results in the best access but may be too stressful for the cat. Butterfly catheter needles of 19 to 23G are appropriate to use and ideally should be mounted to a three-way stopcock and a 10-mL to 20-mL syringe.[42,103] It is important that fluid be collected for assessment as well as drained for therapeutic purposes. Further details about pleurocentesis are contained in Box 30-6 and Figure 30-32.

Pleural Effusion Analysis

Assessment of pleural effusion fluid is the key step to determining the underlying cause. Assessments are based initially on the gross appearance (color, turbidity, presence of fibrin), then the protein concentration and cytology. The findings should always take into account the signalment of the cat and clinical findings.

Opaque effusion fluid can be milky white or milky pink (chyle), red (hemorrhage, although blood contamination can give a similar appearance); pyothorax often results in green or yellow opaque, malodorous fluid with flocculent material (but this can vary). Translucent effusions can be clear, yellow, or pink tinged and are initially distinguished by protein concentration, with lower protein effusions most typically arising from CHF and higher protein effusions most typically arising from FIP. Neoplasia can result in chylous, hemorrhagic, or translucent effusions of high or low protein concentration; cytology is often, but not always, helpful for diagnosis. More details about pleural fluid analysis can be found in Table 30-5.

CAUSES OF PLEURAL EFFUSION

Congestive Heart Failure

Effusion Characteristics

Effusion fluid from cats with CHF may be translucent (often clear to pale yellow, but blood contamination during pleurocentesis can result in pink or reddish tinge) or chylous (white or pink if blood contamination). The fluid is often a modified transudate (with protein concentrations of 25 to 50 g/L), but transudative or chylous effusion is also possible. Left-sided CHF typically results in pleural effusion in cats associated with increased ventricular diastolic pressure resulting in increased capillary hydrostatic pressure. Right-sided CHF can also cause pleural effusion, and chylothorax is often seen in this circumstance[41,68] (Figure 30-33).

BOX 30-5
Supplemental Oxygen Delivery

The fraction of inspired oxygen (FiO_2) in normal room air is 0.21 (21%). Providing dyspneic cats with supplemental oxygen (O_2) aims to increase FiO_2 and thus help increase the patient's arterial oxygen pressure; this, in turn, enables an increase in the oxygen saturation of hemoglobin—that is, a shift to the right of the oxygen–hemoglobin dissociation curve (see Figure 30-25). Different modes of O_2 supplementation provide differing FiO_2s and require differing O_2 flow rates.

Flow-by oxygen (Figure 30-26)

- O_2 line held 1 to 3 cm in front of the cat's nose and mouth
- O_2 flow rate of 6 to 8 L/min used
- FiO_2 of 0.25 to 0.45 typically achieved
- Minimal stress to patient
- Requires physical presence of caregiver to hold O_2 line in place
- High O_2 flow rates
- Appropriate at initial presentation while carrying out other procedures (e.g., thoracocentesis)

Face mask (Figure 30-27)

- Well-fitted mask held over cat's muzzle
- O_2 flow rate of 6 to 8 L/min used
- FiO_2 of 0.35 to 0.55 typically achieved (reservoir bag may increase to as high as 0.8)
- Poor elimination of carbon dioxide
- Stressful for many cats (stress further increases O_2 requirements)
- Only to be used if tolerated

Elizabethan collar canopy (Figure 30-28)

- Elizabethan collar placed snugly around the neck
- O_2 line placed inside the collar from caudal direction (tip may be taped inside collar)
- Front of the collar then covered in plastic wrap with vent holes created or portion left uncovered (to eliminate expired air)
- FiO_2 of 0.30 to 0.40
- O_2 flow rate of 2 to 5 L/min
- Mostly well tolerated
- Stable patient can be left in cage, affording full accessibility for examination, treatment
- Potential heat and humidity, CO_2 retention within canopy if vents inadequate
- Variability in O_2 concentration within the hood, depending on the size of the vent, minute ventilation, exact placement of the oxygen hose within hood

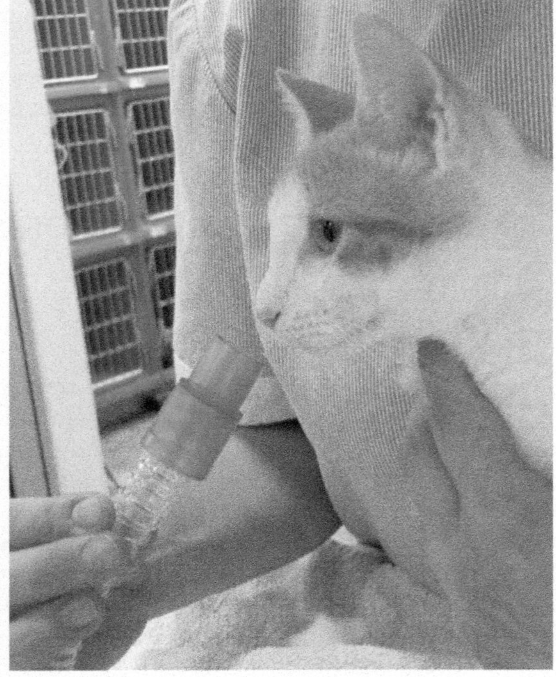

FIGURE 30-26 "Flow-by" oxygen delivery.

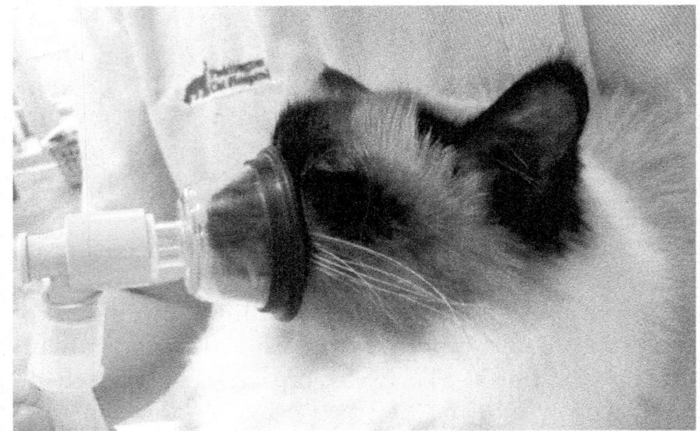

FIGURE 30-27 Face mask oxygen delivery.

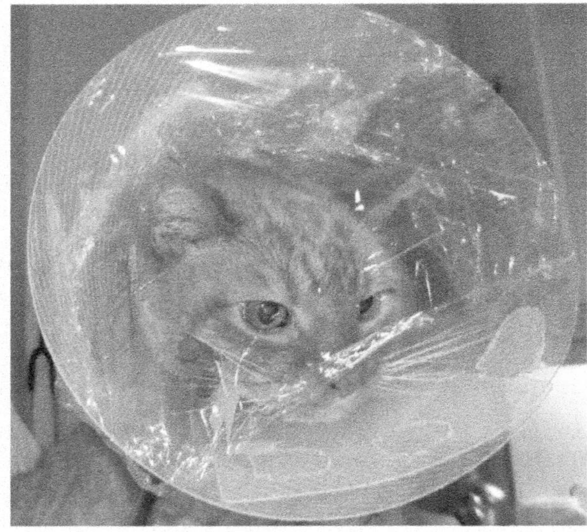

FIGURE 30-28 Elizabethan collar canopy.

BOX 30-5—cont'd

Supplemental Oxygen Delivery

Nasal catheter (Figure 30-29)

- Topical anesthetic (e.g., 2% lidocaine, proparacaine) instilled into one nostril
- 5 Fr lubricated, soft rubber catheter (with multiple fenestrations distally) introduced through nostril to the level of the medial canthus then secured to the skin at the nostril with adhesive glue or suture (usually least irritant long term)
- Remainder of catheter attached to dorsolateral aspect of nose and head with further sutures or adhesive, then attached to the O_2 source
- Ideal for in-line bubble humidifier
- FiO_2 of 0.3 to 0.5
- O_2 flow rates of 100 to 150 mL/kg/min
- Stable patient can be left in cage, affording full accessibility for examination, treatment
- Can be stressful for the patient, so severe respiratory distress may preclude safe placement

Oxygen chamber (Figures 30-30 and 30-31)

- Most commercially available oxygen chambers/cages inappropriate
- Must be able to regulate O_2 concentration, eliminate expired CO_2, as well as ambient temperature and humidity
- Without temperature and humidity regulation, overheating of patient almost inevitable (leading to increased O_2 demand)
- Human neonatal incubators (humidicribs) most appropriate (see Figure 30-31)
- FiO_2 of 0.4 to 0.5
- Flow rates variable, determined by unit
- Temperature to be maintained ~22°C (~70°F), humidity 40-50%
- Inability to conduct physical examination while animal in O_2-rich environment
- Loss of O_2-rich environment when cage door opened, several minutes to refill with O_2

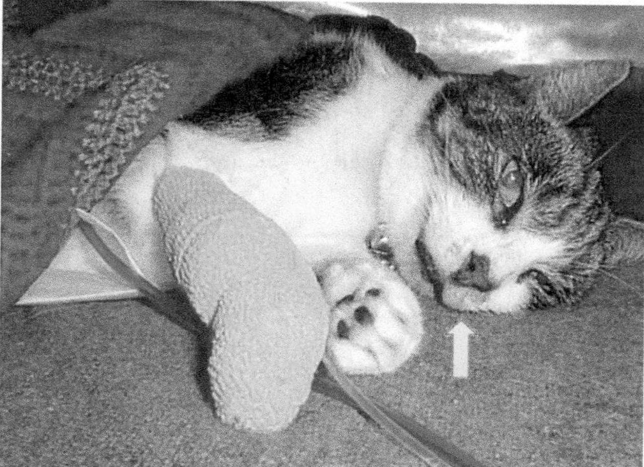

FIGURE 30-29 Nasal catheter oxygen delivery to a recumbent cat. The catheter is marked with a yellow arrow and is glued to the cat's zygomatic arch. *(Courtesy Dr. Peter Best, South Tamworth Animal Hospital, Tamworth, Australia.)*

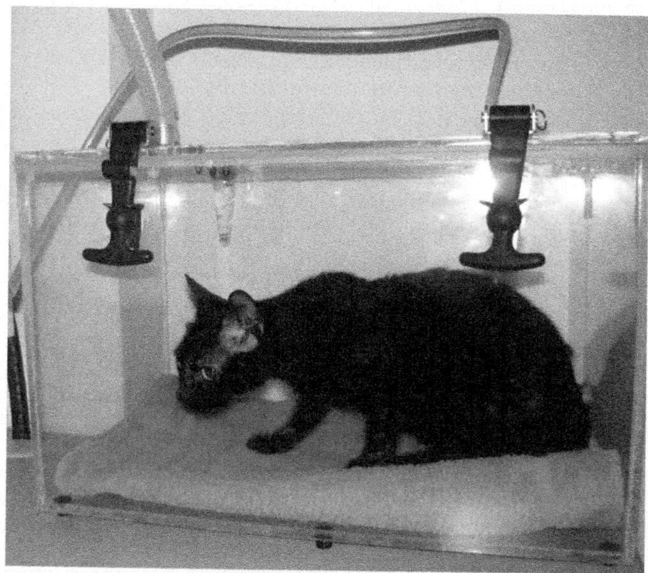

FIGURE 30-30 Cat in an inappropriate oxygen cage with no temperature, humidity, or fraction of inspired oxygen control.

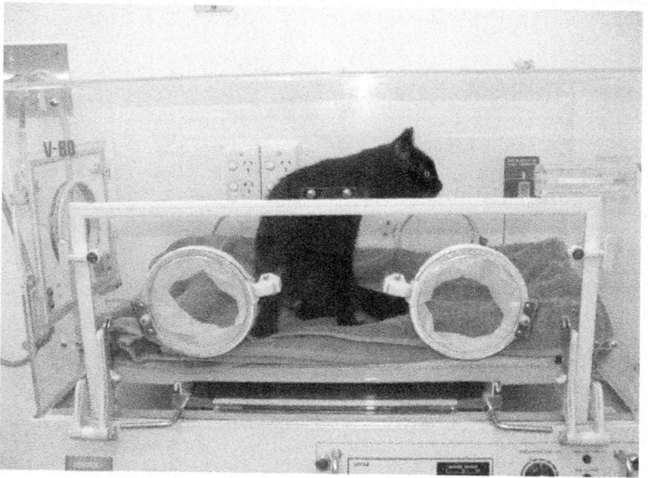

FIGURE 30-31 Cat in a human neonatal incubator (humidicrib). *(Courtesy Dr. Peter Best, South Tamworth Animal Hospital, Tamworth, Australia.)*

Adapted from Camps-Palau MA, Marks SL, Cornick JL: Small animal oxygen therapy, *Compend Contin Educ Pract Vet* 21:587, 1999; Drobatz KJ, Hackner S, Powell S: Oxygen supplementation. In Bonagura JD, Kirk RW, editors: *Kirk's current veterinary therapy XII*, Philadelphia, 1995, Saunders, p 175; Manning AM: Oxygen therapy and toxicity, *Vet Clin North Am Small Anim Pract* 32:1005, 2002; Tseng LW, Drobatz KJ: Oxygen supplementation and humidification. In King LG, editor: *Textbook of respiratory disease in dogs and cats*, St Louis, 2004, Saunders, p 205.

BOX 30-6

Thoracocentesis

- Thoracocentesis should be considered both a therapeutic and diagnostic procedure.
- Ultrasound guidance is helpful but rarely necessary for large volume effusions.
- Equipment required:
  - 19- to 23-gauge butterfly needle; larger bore appropriate for thicker secretions such as pyothorax, does not seem more painful to cats
  - Alternatively, an IV catheter can be used (up to 18 gauge); in this case, the skin is punctured, but the thorax is not penetrated until after tunneling along 1 rib space. The needle is then withdrawn, leaving the catheter in place. This technique may allow further penetration into the thoracic cavity with minimal increased risk of trauma
  - Three-way stopcock; so only one placement of needle
  - 10- to 20-mL syringe; 10-mL syringe provides more manual control and can generate more negative pressure but requires more draws

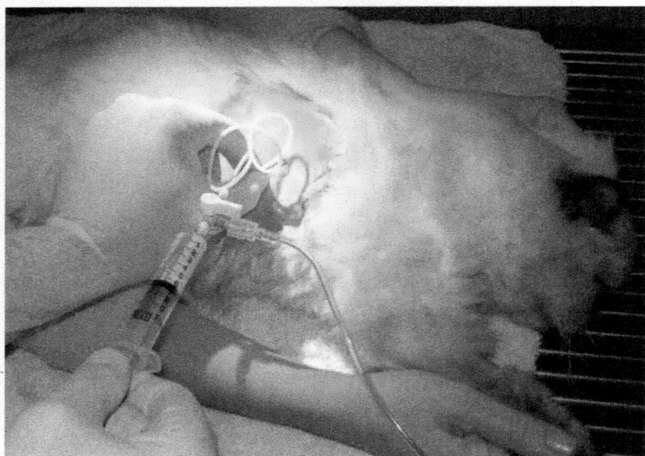

FIGURE 30-32 Thoracocentesis. Note the milky appearance of the effusion. This chylous effusion was subsequent to right-sided congestive heart failure.

  - Extension tubing attached for drainage away from cat
- Positioning of cat: Different positions have different advantages and disadvantages.
  - Sternal recumbency ideal for maximal drainage of fluid, but ventral access can be difficult when the cat is in this position
  - Cat standing appropriate but too much effort for many cats with respiratory distress
  - Best access in lateral recumbency, but too much respiratory stress for some cats
- Location for needle insertion:
  - 6th, 7th, or 8th intercostal space
  - Ventral to the costochondral junction
  - Care taken to avoid intercostal vessels and nerves near the caudal rib margin
  - Necessary to clip and surgically prepare the site
- Anesthetics/sedation:
  - Usually not necessary since tolerated well by most cats
  - Local anesthetic instillation recommended by some; appears to hurt as much (or more) than placement of butterfly needle
- Samples of pleural fluid (first aliquot) to be collected:
  - EDTA tube for cell counts and cytology
  - Plain serum tube for biochemical analysis
  - Sterile container for aerobic *and* anaerobic culture (e.g., pediatric BACTEC bottle that will grow both aerobes and anaerobes); must be inoculated without letting air in
  - Slides with smears should be prepared and subsequently assessed
- Drainage:
  - After collection of diagnostic specimens
  - Stay in one location but continue removing fluid
  - Three-way stopcock adjusted for syringe filling and emptying
  - Sometimes slight repositioning of needle necessary to keep fluid flowing because the lungs move in relation to the pleura as fluid drains
  - After no more fluid retrieved at initial site, repeat on contralateral side

Further Diagnostics

The underlying cardiac disease can be determined only by echocardiography; cardiomyopathies such as hypertrophic or unclassified cardiomyopathy are most common. Auscultable changes such as a murmur or gallop rhythm are not necessarily present, and cardiac disease may be secondary to another problem, such as hyperthyroidism. CHF is covered in more detail in Chapter 20.

Feline Infectious Peritonitis

In one survey of 390 cats with effusive FIP, 17% had thoracic effusions, 62% had ascites, and 21% had effusions in both body cavities[57] (Figure 30-34).

Effusion Characteristics

The effusion fluid found with FIP is typically straw colored to golden yellow (although the shade can vary

TABLE 30-5 **Guidelines for Categorization of Feline Pleural Effusions**

	Translucent Effusions			*Opaque Effusions*		
	Transudate	**Modified Transudate**	**Nonseptic Exudate**	**Septic exudate**	**Chylous Effusion**	**Hemorrhage**
Color	Colorless to pale yellow	Yellow or pink	Yellow or pink	Yellow or pink	Milky white	Red
Turbidity	Clear	Clear to cloudy	Clear to cloudy	Cloudy to opaque; flocculent	Opaque	Opaque
Protein (g/L)	<25	25-50	30-60 (FIP: 35-85)	30-70	25-60	>30
Fibrin	Absent	Absent	Present	Present	Variable	Present
Triglyceride	Absent	Absent	Absent	Absent	Present	Absent
Bacteria	Absent	Absent	Absent	Present	Absent	Absent
Nucleated cells/UL	<1000	1000-7,000 (LSA: 1000-100,000)	5000-20,000 (LSA: 5,000-100,000)	7000-300,000	1000-20,000	Similar to that of peripheral blood
Cytologic features	Mostly mesothelial cells	Mostly macrophages and mesothelial cells; few nondegenerative neutrophils; may be neoplastic cells (LSA, carcinoma) in some cases	Mostly nondegenerate neutrophils and macrophages; neoplastic cells (LSA, carcinoma) in some cases	Mostly degenerate neutrophils, bacteria, also macrophages	Small lymphocytes, neutrophils, and macrophages in variable proportions	Mostly erythrocytes; macrophages with erythrocytosis
Disease associations	Hypoalbuminemia (glomerulopathy, hepatopathy, protein-losing enteropathy); early CHF (rare); hyperthyroid has been reported	CHF; neoplasia (LSA, carcinoma); diaphragmatic hernia	FIP; neoplasia; diaphragmatic hernia; lung lobe torsion; pancreatitis	Pyothorax	Chylothorax; obstructed thoracic duct or cranial vena cava (lymphangectasia, central venous thrombosis); ruptured thoracic duct, CHF, heartworm, neoplasia, idiopathic	Hemothorax Trauma Coagulopathies Lung lobe Torsion Neoplasia
Further diagnostics to differentiate causes	Blood biochemistry (perhaps T_4), urinalysis with UPC; If primary hepatic: abdominal U/S and FNA, or fuller hepatic biopsy. If primary cardiac, echocardiography	Echocardiography NB hernia may not be seen on radiographs	May need biopsy sample to differentiate neoplasia and FIP (although signalment often helpful); FIP: unresponsive pyrexia, hyperglobulinemia, nonregen erative anemia, lymphopenia (perhaps serology), coronavirus IFA of effusion fluid may help diagnose; neoplasia: LSA may be noted from cytology; pancreatitis may require laparotomy and biopsy	Culture and sensitivity required for appropriate antibiosis	Echocardiography; neoplasia may require FNA or biopsy; idiopathic by rule outs	Must distinguish between blood contamination of effusion; haemothorax fluid as haematocrit of 25-50% of that of peripheral blood History, presentation (mainly for trauma, exposure to rodenticides) Clotting factors. Neoplasia by U/S and FNA or biopsy (clotting factors first!)

FIP, Feline infectious peritonitis; *LSA,* lymphosarcoma; *CHF,* congestive heart failure; *U/S,* ultrasound; *UPC,* urine protein:creatinine ratio; *FNA,* fine-needle aspirate; *IFA,* immunofluorescent assay; *NB,* nota bene.
Repeat radiography after pleurocentesis of effusion is often helpful diagnostically.

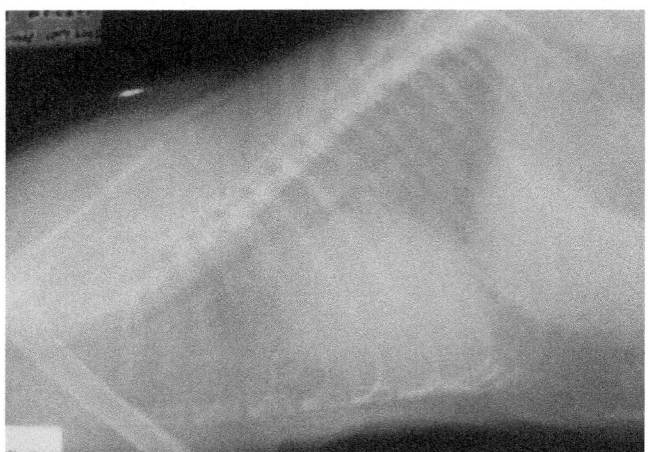

FIGURE 30-33 Right lateral thoracic radiograph showing pleural effusion and pulmonary edema caused by congestive heart failure. Note the significant cardiomegaly.

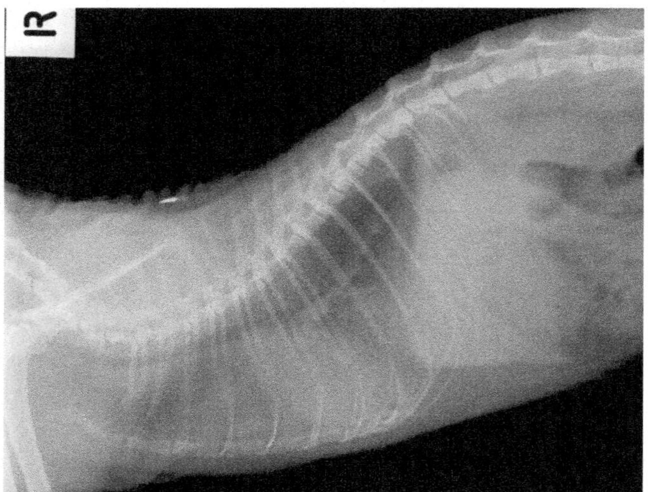

FIGURE 30-34 Right lateral thoracic radiograph showing pleural effusion caused by feline infectious peritonitis (FIP); there is no distinguishing radiological feature to discern FIP. The color of the fluid and the high protein content in a young, febrile cat were clinical clues of the diagnosis.

quite a bit), often contains fibrin clots, and has a high protein concentration. The total protein content is greater than 35 g/L, and often greater than 45 g/L, with globulins making up 50% or more.[114] One study described an effusion with total protein greater than 80 g/L as 90% specific, 55% sensitive, and having a 0.78 PPV for the diagnosis of FIP.

Further Diagnostics

The Rivalta test recognizes high-protein content, as well as high concentrations of fibrinogen and inflammatory mediators in effusion fluid. It has been found to be very sensitive but only 80% specific; this test is performed by adding one drop of acetic acid (98%) to 5 mL of distilled water. This fluid is mixed thoroughly, and then one drop of effusion is gently placed on the surface of the mixture. If the drop stays at the top of the fluid or slowly floats to the bottom, the test is considered to be positive. This test can give inaccurate results if inappropriate technique is used or if there is a significant temperature difference between the fluid sample and the acetic acid solution. A positive Rivalta test can also result from lymphosarcoma or septic effusions (these can be distinguished from FIP by cytology and culture). Immunofluorescence staining of effusion fluid for coronavirus antigen in macrophages has a PPV of 1.00 but a negative predictive value of 0.57.[58]

The potential clinical presentations, diagnostics, and management of FIP are covered in greater detail in Chapter 33.

Neoplasia

Effusion Characteristics

Effusion fluid resulting from neoplasia can vary greatly depending on the mechanism responsible for fluid production. For example, exudates are more likely to occur when large numbers of neoplastic cells are exfoliated, and modified transudates are associated with less exfoliation. However, inflammation associated with neoplasia can result in an exudate with poorly exfoliating neoplasia. Chylous effusions can result when there is obstruction of intrathoracic lymph flow. Occasionally, hemorrhagic effusions may result from hemorrhagic neoplasia or vessel rupture from neoplastic invasion.

Further Diagnostics

Cytologic analysis is often useful to recognize neoplasia. One study showed that cytology had a sensitivity of 61% and a specificity of 100% in detecting neoplasia in body cavity effusions.[62] Direct smears are often of adequate cellularity for assessment, but samples should be concentrated before examination in cases of low cellularity. In cases when cytology is not diagnostic, repeat radiography after drainage of pleural fluid often reveals a mass, commonly in the mediastinum, cranial to the cardiac silhouette. Care should be taken when interpreting radiographs because atelectatic lung lobes may mimic the appearance of a mass. Ultrasound-guided FNA can usually be used to confirm the diagnosis in these cases; in some cases, thoracotomy (or thoracoscopy) is required for an adequate biopsy sample.[70]

Specific Causes

Most studies cite mediastinal lymphosarcoma (Figure 30-35) as the most common neoplastic cause of pleural effusion in cats, representing approximately two thirds to three quarters of cases.[21,23,52,62] One study indicated that pleural effusion occurred in 90% of cats (55 of 61) with mediastinal lymphosarcoma.[21] In a more recent study, however, only one of five cases (20%) of cats with pleural effusion associated with neoplasia was

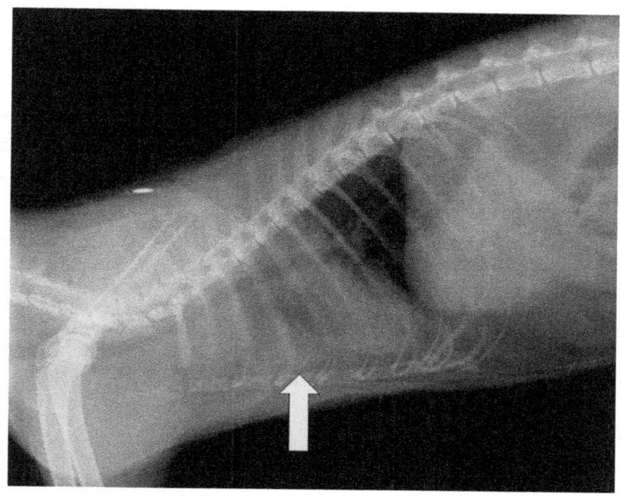

FIGURE 30-35 Right lateral thoracic radiograph showing mediastinal mass (marked with *yellow arrow*). Fine-needle aspiration allowed a cytologic diagnosis of lymphosarcoma.

diagnosed with lymphosarcoma, with the remaining four cases associated with carcinoma.[141] Most cats, particularly young cats, with mediastinal lymphosarcoma seem to respond well to routine lymphosarcoma treatment protocols.[76,119,124]

Primary pulmonary neoplasia is rare in cats.[84,86,120] In many cases all lung lobes are affected when assessed radiographically, and pleural effusion is present in between 35% and 65% of cases. Other radiographic findings can include a mixed bronchoalveolar pattern, an ill-defined alveolar mass, or a mass with cavitation. Some form of bronchial disease is often present and may represent local airway metastasis.[5,6,84,86] Pulmonary metastasis from other locations appears radiographically as interstitial nodules (which may be well or ill defined) or a diffuse alveolar patter with or without ill-defined pulmonary nodules or pleural effusion (or both). Mammary gland adenocarcinoma is the most commonly represented primary tumor.[32] Digital metastasis of bronchial carcinomas is also recognized as an uncommon cause of lameness in older cats; it is also known as *lung–digit syndrome* and carries an extremely poor prognosis.[48] The prognosis for long-term survival with pulmonary adenocarcinoma is generally poor, with an overall median survival time of 115 days reported.[56]

Differential Diagnoses

Other mediastinal pathology can result in mediastinal masses; most cases are thymoma, which does not typically (but can) result in pleural effusion; thymic hyperplasia; idiopathic mediastinal and thymic hemorrhage; cystic thymus[24]; and thymolipoma.[125] Thymic masses can be associated with paraneoplastic processes such as exfoliative dermatitis and myasthenia gravis.*

*References 19, 24, 34, 47, 100, 107, 111, 113, 123.

Thymectomy typically results in resolution of all clinical signs (including paraneoplastic signs) and results in prolonged survival,* with one study noting median survival of 1825 days.[139] Occasional reports have recognized the development of myasthenia gravis after a thymectomy.[47,107]

Pyothorax

Effusion Characteristics

Septic exudates are usually turbid to opaque because of a large cell count and often contain flocculent material. They are usually cream or pale yellow in color but can be pink, green tinged, or red tinged. Greater than 80% of cases of pyothorax are caused by mixed anaerobic infections; consequently the effusion is typically malodorous (like cat-fight abscesses, which are also largely due to anaerobic bacterial infection). A lack of odor does not rule out pyothorax but makes aerobic or yeast infection probable in an effusion predominated by neutrophils. Typical of exudates, the protein content is greater than 30 g/L because of a high nucleated cell count (at least 7,000/μL), which often comprises more than 85% degenerate neutrophils; bacteria may be recognized intracellularly or extracellularly.[8]

Other Findings

Cats with pyothorax are not necessarily dyspneic on presentation and may present with nonspecific systemic signs of inappetence or lethargy. Pyothorax is typically a disease of young cats, with a mean age of 4 to 6 years reported, but cats of any age can be affected.[7,23,25,128,130] Pyrexia is not necessarily present; hypothermia and bradycardia can be present as indicators of severe sepsis.[128] Hematology may reflect sepsis with a left shift neutrophilia, and neutropenia with a degenerative left shift can occur with advanced sepsis. Plasma biochemistry may demonstrate hyperglobulinemia with hypoalbuminemia, and hyperglycemia or hypoglycemia are potential consequences of sepsis.

Treatment

Treatment of pyothorax should be considered in terms of treatment of a cat-fight abscess—that is, drainage, appropriate antibiotic therapy, and any required supportive care.

DRAINAGE AND LAVAGE

Drainage is best achieved by placement of bilateral thoracostomy tubes, which generally remain in place for 5 to 6 days to enable repeated thoracic lavage. Placement of thoracostomy tubes is covered in Box 30-7.

One study reported shorter total duration of tube placement for patients treated with lavage than those

*References 34, 47, 75, 100, 107, 111, 113, 123, 139.

BOX 30-7

Placement of Thoracostomy Tubes

- Thoracostomy tubes should be placed after stabilization of respiratory compromise (by thoracocentesis and oxygen therapy) as well as any fluid and electrolyte imbalances.
- Tubes should be placed bilaterally:
  - Helps effective drainage if loculation of fluid or mediastinum intact
  - Drainage still provided if single side tube failure (obstruction or kinking)
- Commercially available veterinary thoracic trocar catheters are available; generally 14 to 16 Fr are the most appropriate size.
- General anesthesia is required with intubation.
  - Intermittent positive pressure ventilation (IPPV) required; ~10-12 breaths per minute, with a tidal volume of about 20 mL per kg.
- The chest tube enters the skin two or more intercostal spaces (ICSs) caudal to where the tube enters the thoracic cavity (Figure 30-36).
  - Surgical site prepared
  - Small stab incision (just large enough to accommodate the size of the thoracic drain but no larger) for entry of catheter at approximately 10th to 12th ICS (dorsally).
  - Subcutaneous tunnel made cranioventrally with trocar as far as 7th to 8th ICS
  - Helpful if assistant pulls the thoracic skin approximately 5 cm cranially and ventrally just before driving trocar through thoracic wall; enables the trocar to enter thoracic wall perpendicularly
  - Trocar advanced through subcutaneous tunnel, and then driven into the pleural space at 7th to 8th ICS
  - Tube pushed off the trocar and advanced ~12 to 18 cm cranially and ventrally within the thoracic cavity (assistant releases the skin)
  - End of tube clamped to prevent pneumothorax
- Alternative technique:
  - Direct dissection of the subcutaneous tunnel using Mayo scissors or hemostat
  - Red rubber catheter grasped and clamped in the tips of a hemostat, to drive into the pleural space.
- Tube is secured to the thoracic wall with purse-string suture, and a Chinese finger trap suture is placed to prevent the tube from slipping (Figure 30-37).
- Three-way stopcock is placed at the end of the tube, and any remaining exudate or air that entered during the procedure is evacuated
- After bilateral tubes are placed, each tube should be used to lavage the thorax on two or three occasions, with about 100 mL of warmed lactated Ringer's solution (Figure 30-38).
  - The thorax should be lavaged multiple times in the first 24 to 48 hours.
  - Subsequently, two to three times daily lavage is appropriate.
- A light two-layer bandage should be applied *without* excessive pressure (not so tight that it interferes with the cat's breathing) (Figure 30-39).
- Hygienic precautions such as wearing gloves should be adhered to at all times when changing bandage dressing or performing manual aspiration of the tube.

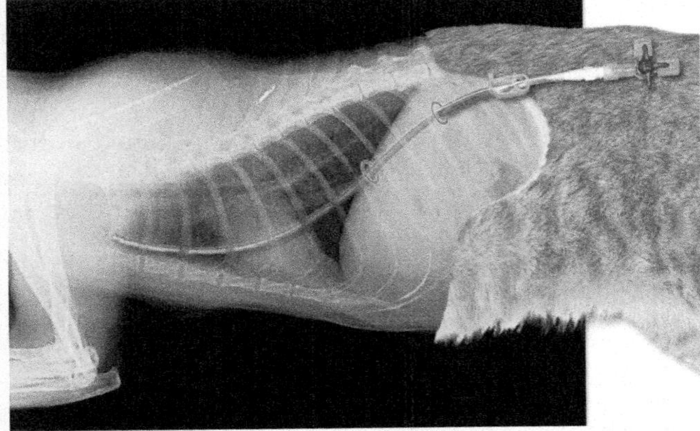

FIGURE 30-36 Positioning of a thoracostomy tube within the pleural space. *(From Barrs VR, Beatty JA: Feline pyothorax: new insights into an old problem. Part 2: Treatment recommendations and prophylaxis,* Vet J *179:171, 2009.)*

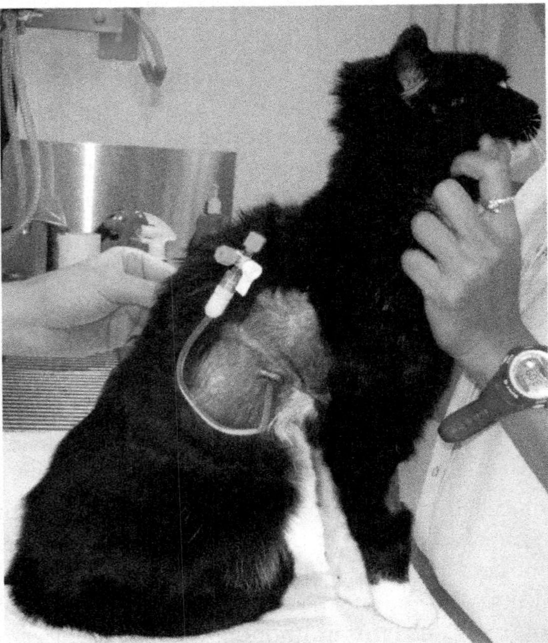

FIGURE 30-37 Thoracostomy tube *in situ,* secured to the thoracic wall with purse-string suture and a Chinese finger trap suture (which cannot easily be seen).

BOX 30-7—cont'd

Placement of Thoracostomy Tubes

- Tubes are generally removed after 4 to 6 days on the basis of the following factors:
  - Reduction of pleural effusion to approximately 2 mL/kg per day
  - Resolution of pleural effusion on thoracic radiographs
  - Cytologically:
    - Absence of microorganisms
    - Reduction of neutrophil numbers with loss of degenerative appearance
- Appearance of macrophages

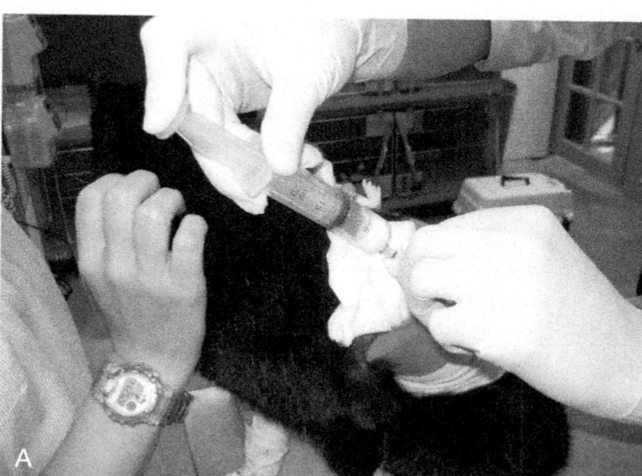

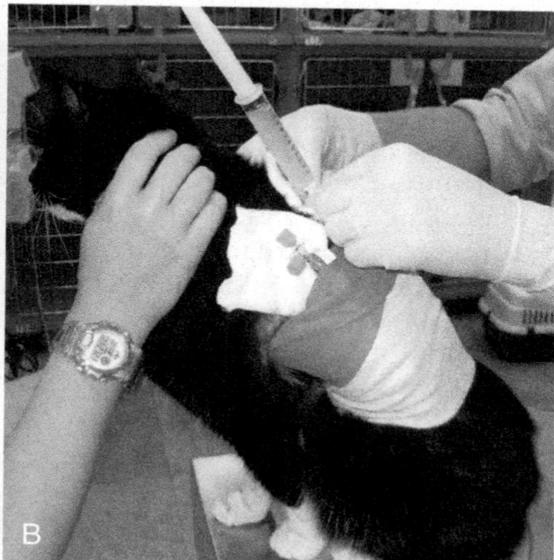

FIGURE 30-38 **A,** Warmed lactated Ringer's solution is used to lavage the pleural space. The author uses multiple 20-mL syringes for this. **B,** Introduced fluid is removed. Note the discoloration of the fluid compared with that in the prior image.

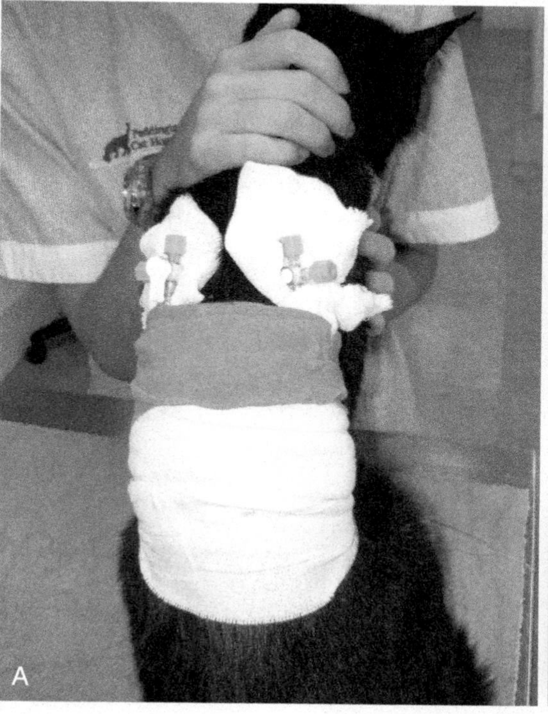

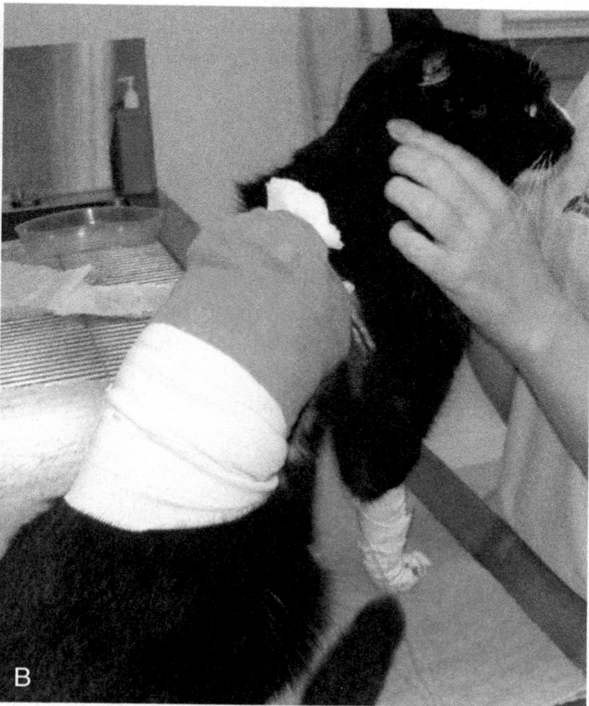

FIGURE 30-39 **A,** Thoracoscopy tubes covered by a light two-layer bandage should be applied without excessive pressure. In this view the three-way stopcocks are exposed (as when lavage and drainage are performed) to show gauze used as padding under the stopcocks. **B,** The three-way stopcocks should be covered over for when the cat is returned to its hospital cage.

managed with drainage only; however, the authors note that few cases were treated without lavage.[25] Repeated thoracic lavage allows drainage and assessment of exudates but also débrides the pleura, including breaking down adhesions and diluting bacterial and inflammatory mediator concentrations; further, the chance of thoracostomy tube obstruction with thick exudates is reduced. Before lavage, suction should be attempted to determine the volume and nature of pleural effusion. Warmed (to body temperature) compound sodium lactate is used for lavage (use of 0.9% sodium chloride can result in hypokalemia[7]) with volumes from 10 to 25 mL/kg per lavage. The volume of fluid introduced and aspirated should be recorded for each side, with expected recovery of 75% or more of lavage fluid. Recovery of smaller volumes should prompt investigations (usually with imaging) for thoracostomy tube complications or loculation of pockets of fluid as a result of adhesions. There are no definitive guidelines for frequency of lavage; every 4 hours for the first 24 to 48 hours and subsequently two to three times daily has been recommended.[9] Removal of thoracostomy tubes is indicated when the volume of pleural effusion has reduced to approximately 2 mL/kg per day; pleural effusion has resolved radiographically; and infection has resolved, as indicated by absence of organisms, reduction of neutrophil numbers, and loss of their degenerative appearance and appearance of macrophages. Recent studies have reported a median duration of thoracic drainage of 5 to 6 days.[7,25,128]

Continuous water seal suction has also been used[59] but offers no real advantage over intermittent suction and lavage as described. Continuous suction offers the advantage of maximal drainage but does not decrease the time needed to manage pyothorax. Further, water-seal chest drainage units require continuous monitoring because leakage between the pleural cavity and the water seal can be fatal.[59]

Needle thoracocentesis (on one occasion or multiple times) is the alternative to thoracoscopy tube placement but is associated with higher mortality and should be reserved for cases with low volume effusion or when thoracostomy tube placement is declined by the owner (e.g., because of financial concerns).

ANTIBIOTIC THERAPY

Antibiotic therapy should be governed by culture and sensitivity findings; however, therapy should be instigated as soon as practical after diagnosis, and, further, sensitivity results for anaerobic bacteria are not routinely available (another consideration is that samples should be collected anaerobically). The bacteria most commonly responsible for pyothorax are anaerobes, typical of oral flora; the most commonly isolated aerobes, *Pasteurella* spp., have been recognized in 12.5% to 20% of cases, in many cases in addition to anaerobes.[7,74,130] Empiric therapy with penicillin-based antibiotics (including aminopenicillins or potentiated penicillins), therefore, should be effective against these bacteria. It is important to use parenteral antibiotics initially because affected cats are debilitated and unlikely to be eating. Most intravenous antibiotics require dosing at 6- to 8-hour intervals; in some cases antibiotics can be added to the intravenous fluids and provided as constant-rate infusion. Antibiotic therapy should be continued for an extended duration, typically 6 to 8 weeks.[7,25] Amoxicillin–clavulanate at 15-20 mg/kg twice daily is an appropriate empiric antibiotic choice in most cases; cefovecin has an appropriate in vitro spectrum,[116] and the author has successfully used this antibiotic in cases when the owner has had difficulty administering oral antibiotics; however, the revisits for repeat injections at 10- to 14-day intervals are vital, and the owner should be reminded of appointments in the preceding days.

SUPPORTIVE CARE

Fluid therapy should be provided for supportive care at approximately twice maintenance rates until the cat is rehydrated and continued at maintenance rates thereafter. Electrolyte status should be evaluated and taken into account with fluid therapy. Most cats are inappetent or anorexic and will require nutritional support.

Idiopathic Chylothorax

Differential Diagnoses and Effusion Characteristics

There are no distinctive radiographic features of idiopathic chylothorax (Figure 30-40).

The recognition of milky white or pink pleural effusion (see Figure 30-32) does not constitute a diagnosis of idiopathic chylothorax because thoracic chylous effusions can result from multiple causes, including CHF,[12,39,41,60,122] neoplasia,[19,33,61] trauma,[50,85] infections (including heartworm),[26,27,83] and potentially FIP. The color of chylous effusions varies depending on dietary

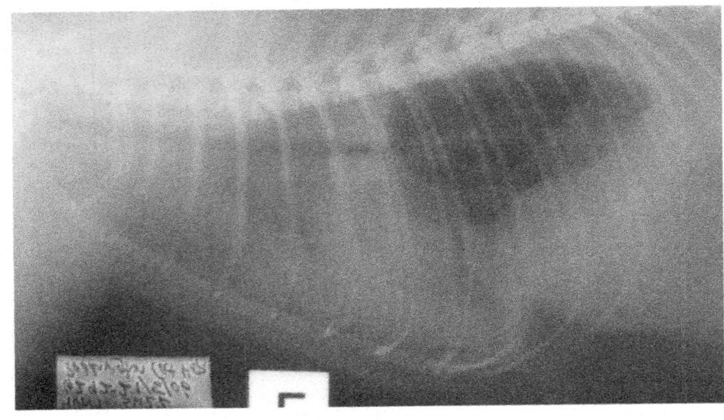

FIGURE 30-40 Left lateral radiograph of pleural effusion caused by idiopathic chylothorax. There are no distinguishing radiologic features to determine the nature of this effusion.

fat content and whether there is concurrent hemorrhage. The protein concentration is variable and often raised artefactually by the high lipid content of the fluid. The total nucleated cell count is often less than 10,000/µL, consisting of predominantly small lymphocytes or neutrophils as well as lipid-laden macrophages.[37] Pleural effusions with triglyceride concentrations greater than 1.12 mmol/L (100 mg/dL) are always chylous; chylous effusions have a greater pleural fluid triglyceride concentration but a lower or equal cholesterol concentration compared with serum.[129] Pseudochylous effusions are rare; these effusions grossly resemble chyle but are distinguished by having a greater cholesterol concentration than serum.[37] Despite multiple possible causes, in the majority of cases, no specific etiology for the chylous effusion is found, leaving the diagnosis as idiopathic.[39,66] However, because the management of these disparate causes varies so greatly, thorough investigations should be undertaken.

Further Diagnostics

The two major modes of investigating chylous effusions are to repeat thoracic radiographs subsequent to drainage of effusion fluid and echocardiography. Mediastinal masses can be difficult to appreciate radiographically when there is a large volume pleural effusion; masses recognized to result in chylothorax include mediastinal lymphosarcoma,[33,61] thymoma,[19] and one case of a cryptococcal granuloma.[83] Ultrasound-guided FNA is required to distinguish these (or other) conditions. Echocardiography should be performed on all cats with chylothorax; cardiac diseases recognized to result in chylous effusion include cardiomyopathies,[12,41] congenital disorders,[41] cardiac neoplasia,[41] pericardial disease,[41] paroxysmal heart block,[31] and heartworm disease.[27,45,108] Additional investigations for heartworm disease, such as antigen and antibody testing, are also appropriate.

Medical Management

There is no definitive medical treatment for idiopathic chylothorax, and surgery should be considered if attempts at medical management are unsuccessful. If the effusion recurs despite dietary and drug therapy (as is often the case), then intermittent repeat thoracocentesis is required. Cats should be managed with low-fat diets containing 6% or less fat on a dry matter basis.[37] Rutin is a benzopyrone plant extract available from health food stores that has been reported to improve and occasionally successfully resolve idiopathic chylothorax; recommended doses are 50 to 100 mg/kg (or 250 to 500 mg/cat) orally, three times daily.[49,69,121] Octreotide is a somatostatin analog that has been anecdotally reported to resolve idiopathic chylothorax when administered at 10 µg/kg subcutaneously, three times daily for 2 to 3 weeks; prolonged administration has been associated with gallstone formation in people. The condition does occasionally resolve spontaneously after several weeks to months.[37] Persistent chylothorax resulting from incomplete treatment can lead to fibrosing pleuritis as a complication; this condition appears to develop subsequent to any prolonged exudative or blood-stained effusion. The fibrosis restricts normal pulmonary expansion and carries a very guarded prognosis.[38]

Surgical Treatment

If medical management fails to resolve or alleviate the clinical signs of chylothorax, surgical intervention becomes the only therapeutic option. Thoracic duct ligation (TDL) in conjunction with pericardiectomy (PC) is the most widely accepted technique; one study reported an 80% success rate for resolving idiopathic chylothorax in cats.[40] These procedures have been performed successfully with thoracoscopy in dogs.[2] Pleural omentalization has been performed in addition to TDL and PC but does not appear to improve results.[15] The techniques for these procedures have been recently reviewed.[37]

Other Causes of Pleural Effusion

Beyond CHF, FIP, neoplasia, pyothorax, and idiopathic chylothorax, clinicians will be directed toward most other causes of pleural effusion from clinical history (e.g., known trauma), physical examination findings, and routine investigations. Trauma can result in hemothorax (Figure 30-41), chylothorax (from thoracic duct rupture), or effusion associated with diaphragmatic hernia; urinothorax subsequent to diaphragmatic herniation and kidney prolapse has been reported in one cat.[117] Other reported underlying conditions include pancreatitis,[102] congenital thoracic duct abnormalities,[28]

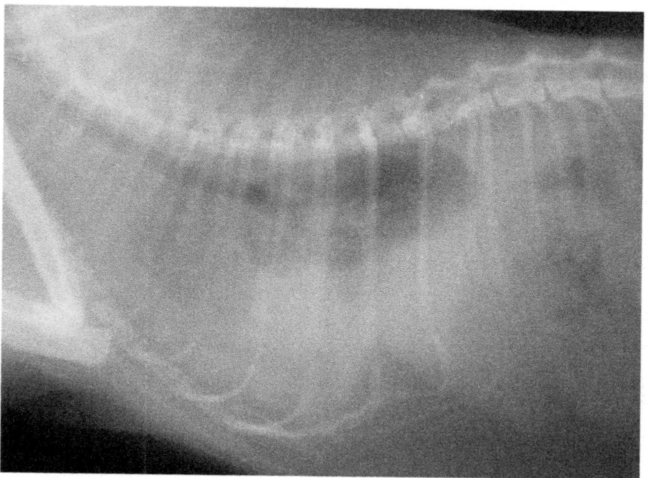

FIGURE 30-41 Right lateral radiograph demonstrating hemothorax associated with trauma. Note that the lung mass is greatly compressed by effusion, pulmonary contusions are evident, and the increased radiodensity over the cardiac silhouette is associated with clot formation. The diaphragm can be followed and is intact. *(Courtesy Dr. Susan Little.)*

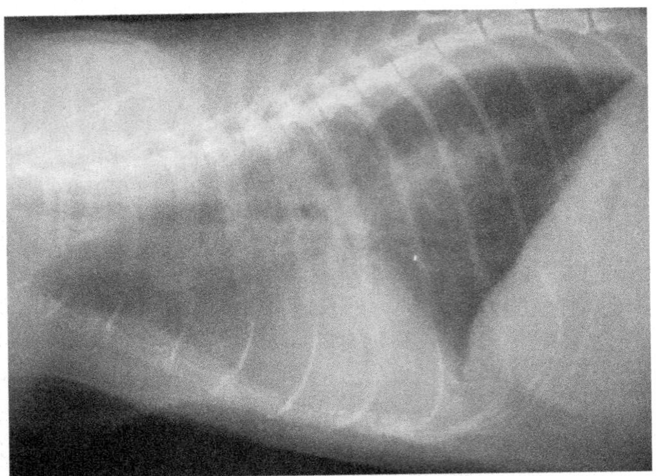

FIGURE 30-42 Right lateral radiograph demonstrating pleural effusion associated with hypoalbuminemia. Note that there is also pulmonary edema. This cat's plasma albumin concentration was 15 g/L and was associated with severe intestinal disease. A total of 115 mL of effusion was removed using bilateral thoracocentesis. *(Courtesy Dr. Susan Little.)*

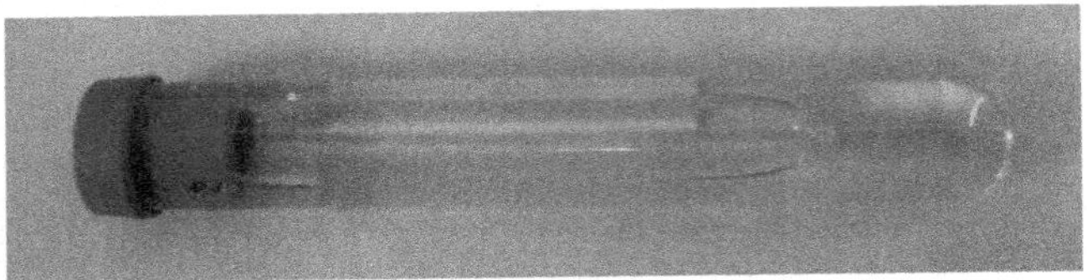

FIGURE 30-43 Effusion fluid drained from hypoalbuminemic cat (radiograph shown in Figure 30-42); note that the fluid is clear, with no evidence of cellularity. *(Courtesy Dr. Susan Little.)*

aelurostronglylosis,[87] cardioperitoneal and pleuroperitoneal hernias, and lung lobe torsion.[67,81] Low-protein pleural transudates (Figures 30-42 and 30-43) are rarely recognized and have been described in one cat with a preexisting perinephric pseudocyst in direct communication with the pleural space[98] and another with a severe protein-losing glomerulopathy.[4]

Pleural Access Ports

Recent studies[13,16] have documented the use of pleural access ports for cats with chronic pleural effusions. These devices are inserted during thoracotomy; they allow drainage of chronic thoracic effusion in circumstances such as neoplasia when effusion is profuse in a patient undergoing chemotherapy.

PNEUMOTHORAX

The normal pressure of the pleural cavity remains below normal atmospheric air pressure, varying from −5 cm of water at beginning of inspiration (equal to the amount of suction required to hold the lungs open to their resting level) to −7.5 cm of water as inspiration creates more negative pressure.[54] Pneumothorax results from the accumulation of free air or gas of atmospheric pressure within the thoracic cavity[95]; this loss of negative intrapleural pressure causes the lungs to collapse as a result of elastic recoil.[71] When the lungs collapse, the tidal volume is reduced, prompting tachypnea in an attempt to maintain the minute ventilation. Local hypoxia induces vasoconstriction of pulmonary vessels, diverting blood flow to ventilated areas. Vasoconstriction, combined with collapse of blood vessels caused by atelectasis, eventually leads to pulmonary hypertension and increased work for the right side of the heart.[79]

Causes and Classification

Pneumothorax most commonly results from trauma in cats[64]; spontaneous pneumothorax is occasionally reported.[10,20,88,110,132] Iatrogenic pneumothorax can result from anesthetic complications in association with intubation, positive pressure ventilation, and failure to reopen anesthetic machine pop-up valves,* subsequent to endoscopic retrieval of foreign bodies from the trachea or esophagus[17,138] or subsequent to thoracic FNA.[79]

There are two basic classes of pneumothorax: open and closed. Open pneumothorax is associated with a body wall wound that allows entry of free air. Depending on the wound size, pressure within the pleural space is less than or equal to atmospheric pressure. Closed pneumothorax occurs when the air within the pleural space has entered through a wound of the lung parenchyma or trachea. Open pneumothorax is further divided into simple and tension forms. Simple closed pneumothorax occurs when a puncture of the lung allows air to enter the pleural space during inspiration and exit during expiration. This allows the pressure within the pleural space to equilibrate with atmospheric pressure. In tension pneumothorax, the wound in the lung acts as a flap valve, allowing air to enter the pleural space during inspiration but not allowing it to escape during expiration. This results in a gradual increase in pleural space pressure and progressive pulmonary atelectasis. With large wounds pleural pressure can eventually exceed atmospheric pressure. Untreated tension pneumothorax therefore results in progressively worsening dyspnea, subsequent cardiovascular dysfunction, and ultimately death.[71]

Diagnosis and Radiography

Cats with pneumothorax typically present with dyspnea; in most cases there is a history of trauma or, in iatrogenic cases, a procedure that could potentially cause pneumothorax. Radiography readily confirms the diagnosis

*References 14, 30, 78, 82, 92, 96.

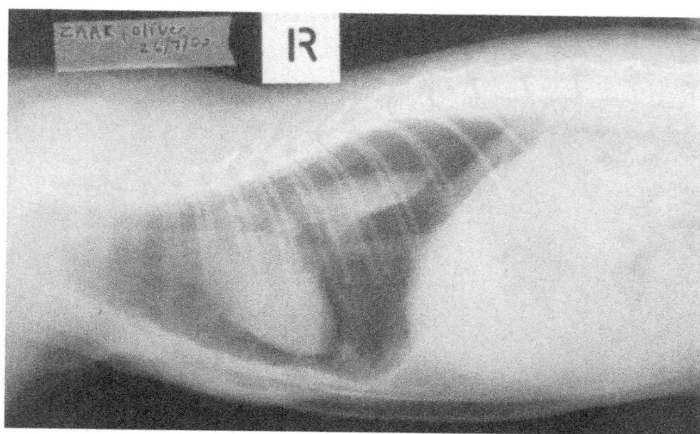

FIGURE 30-44 Right lateral radiograph of cat with pneumothorax. This cat fell onto a kitchen knife that was held upright in a kitchen strainer. Note the greatly increased width of the air-filled pleural space. Because the lung is decreased in size and air content, it appears radiopaque compared with the surrounding air-filled pleural space. Subcutaneous emphysema can be seen ventrally.

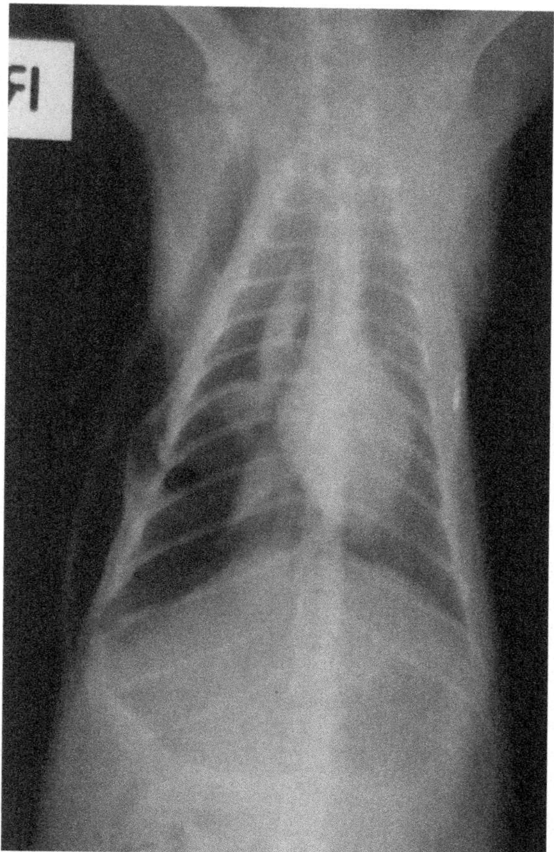

FIGURE 30-45 Dorsoventral view of the same cat in Figure 30-44. The chest wall emphysema is in the position where the knife entered the thoracic cavity. Subcutaneous emphysema surrounds this position.

(Figures 30-44 and 30-45). Spontaneous pneumothorax is typically recognized after thoracic radiography and, in many cases, unknown trauma is assumed.

Pneumothorax is recognized radiographically by the increased width of the air-filled pleural space with accompanying partial pulmonary atelectasis and retraction of the lung margins. This results in the absence of vascular shadows in the peripheral portions of the thorax. Because the lung is decreased in size and air content, it appears relatively radiopaque compared with the air-filled pleural space. The heart is typically displaced dorsally from the sternum in recumbent lateral views. Minimal pneumothorax can be difficult to visualize and requires recognition of retracted lobar edges. Tension pneumothorax is best recognized by sequential radiographs demonstrating the accumulation of progressively larger amounts of pleural air.[93]

Diagnosis of spontaneous pneumothorax requires recognition of a potential underlying cause or resolution of pneumothorax after appropriate treatment of a potential cause such as bronchial disease.[10,20,132] CT was used to recognized a pulmonary bulla in a recent report.[88]

Treatment

The treatment of pneumothorax varies greatly depending on severity, cause, and class of pneumothorax. In all cases large volumes of pleural air should be drained by thoracocentesis using a three-way stopcock (see Box 30-6). Subsequently, many cases with simple closed pneumothorax can be managed successfully with cage rest; the air leak usually seals itself within hours, and the residual pleural air is resorbed over a few days.[64] Oxygen therapy (see Box 30-5) maintains a dissolved gas pressure gradient between pulmonary vessels and the pleural cavity and can aid resorption of pleural air.

Open pneumothorax requires surgical correction; open wounds should be covered immediately with any available material. Intermittent positive pressure ventilation is required through anesthesia until the wound is repaired and air evacuated.

Worsening dyspnea, with reaccumulation of pleural air, in cats with closed pneumothorax (no overt penetrating injury) suggests tension pneumothorax. Thoracostomy tubes (see Box 30-7) are not often indicated in cats but may be required in some cases to facilitate drainage, and closed suction systems may be indicated for continuous drainage of air. Water-seal chest drainage units require continuous monitoring because failure of the system can result in acute respiratory distress or death.[59] In severe cases of massive air reaccumulation, surgical thoracotomy is required to identify and correct the underlying cause.

DIAPHRAGMATIC HERNIA

Diaphragmatic hernia refers to the entry of abdominal contents into the thoracic cavity caused by a defect of the diaphragm. *Peritoneopericardial hernia (PPDH)* refers to entry of abdominal contents into the pericardial sac owing to a congenital communication from the abdomen[36]; PPDH is addressed in Chapter 20. The more commonly encountered pleuroperitoneal hernias are predominantly the result of trauma, with motor vehicle accidents the most common cause of trauma in these cases[44,89,104,135,136]; interestingly, high-rise trauma does not commonly result in diaphragmatic herniation.[126,134] Abdominal pressure at impact is dissipated cranially, causing the diaphragm to tear, with the location and size of the tear depending on the position of the animal at the time of the impact.[36] Occasional cases of congenital diaphragmatic hernia have been described, including so called "true herniation," in which the serosa remains intact.[18,46,65,127]

Clinical Signs

The severity of clinical signs varies greatly depending on the size of the tear and the organ that has herniated. Respiratory signs such as dyspnea or tachypnea are often, but not always, present. Lack of respiratory signs can result in the diagnosis being missed; in one study 50 of 116 cases of diaphragmatic hernia (of cats and dogs) were not diagnosed within 30 days,[135] and in some cats the condition may remain unrecognized for years. Muffled heart or lung sounds are a common clinical finding; some cats will refuse to lie in particular positions because of the resultant dyspnea; the abdomen may have an empty or "tucked-up" appearance; and gastrointestinal signs may be present, including gastric dilation.* Because the most common cause is trauma, there are often other injuries present; mortality rates appear to be more correlated with concurrent injuries than the degree of diaphragmatic damage or chronicity.[104]

Diagnosis

Radiography is the most reliable means of diagnosis; typical radiographic signs include loss of continuity of the diaphragmatic outline and readily identifiable abdominal organs within the thorax such as gas-filled loops of intestine (Figure 30-46).[43,118,135] In more subtle cases a soft tissue density may be recognized in the caudal thorax (Figures 30-47 and 30-48).[18,133] Pleural effusion is present in 20% to 25% of cases (see Figure 30-47).[43,118,135] Ultrasonography can be used to confirm the diagnosis if radiographic findings are equivocal; one study correctly diagnosed diaphragmatic hernia by ultrasonography in 20 of 21 cats (95%), with the only false-negative result being due to adhesions imitating the appearance of an intact diaphragm.[115]

*References 43, 64, 89, 104, 135, 136.

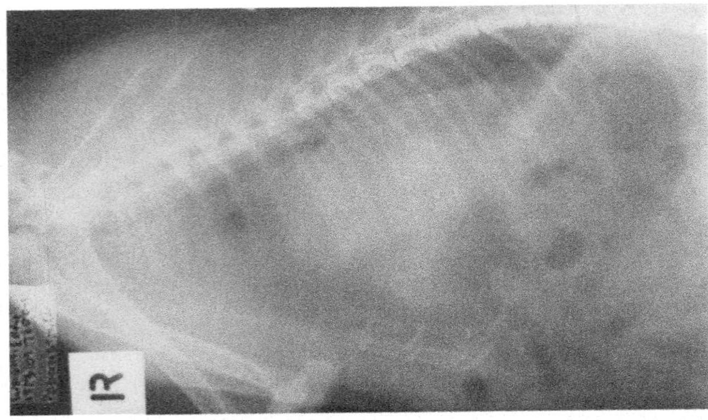

FIGURE 30-46 Right lateral radiograph showing severe diaphragmatic hernia. As well as the overt abdominal contents within the thoracic cavity resulting in dorsal elevation of the heart, there is loss of continuity of the diaphragm and pleural effusion.

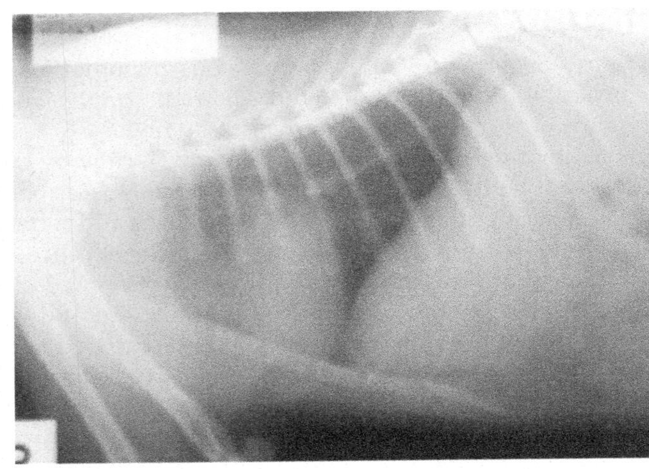

FIGURE 30-47 Right lateral radiograph showing more subtle diaphragmatic hernia than prior image. The herniation looks like a mass ventrally, just caudal to the heart. There is also pleural effusion present.

Treatment

Diaphragmatic herniation requires surgical repair (Figure 30-49). However, in many cases surgery should be delayed until other consequences of trauma, such as shock, have been stabilized; gastric dilation warrants immediate surgical attention.[36] Intermittent positive pressure ventilation must be provided throughout anesthesia, and residual air must be evacuated from the thorax when surgical repair is complete; the clinician must be aware of the possibility of postsurgical pneumothorax, which can usually be managed by thoracocentesis. In most cases hernias may be repaired by primary closure, but in some chronic or congenital cases, the defect may be too large; in one such case a commercial small intestinal submucosal graft was used.[3] Recent studies report an excellent prognosis. In one study 28 of

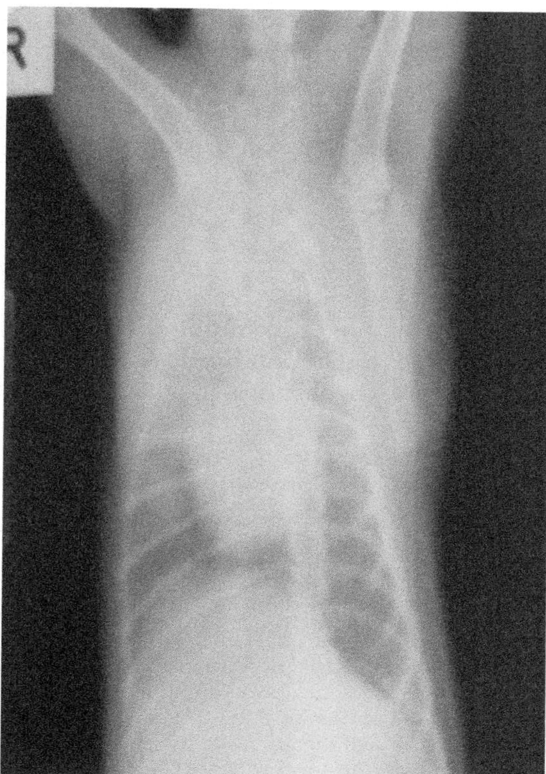

FIGURE 30-48 Ventrodorsal view of the same cat in Figure 30-47. The discontinuity of the diaphragm is evident on *left* of the image (cat's right).

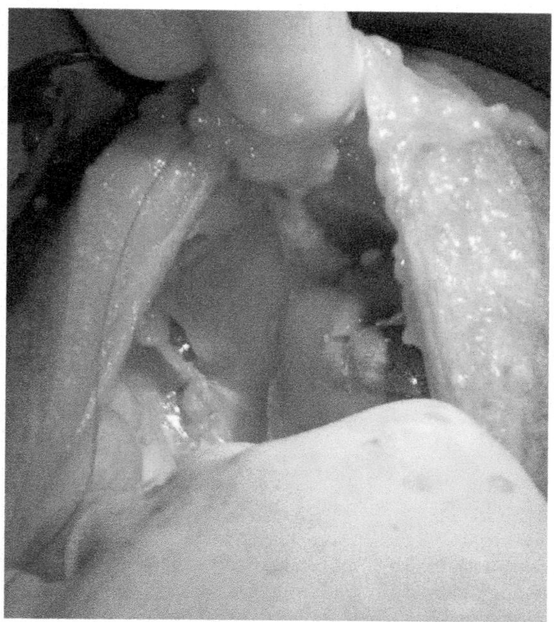

FIGURE 30-49 Gross appearance of diaphragmatic hernia during laparotomy for repair.

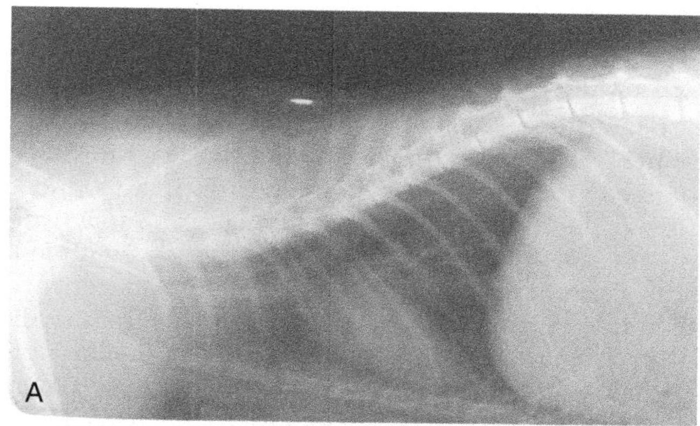

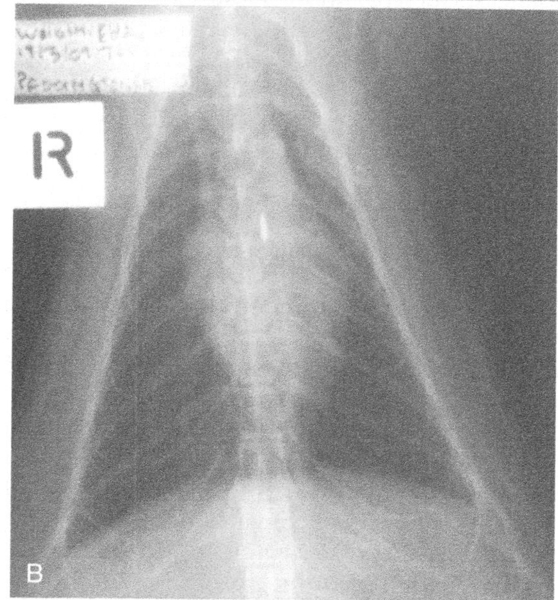

FIGURE 30-50 Postsurgical radiographs (right lateral **[A]** and ventrodorsal **[B]** views) of the cat depicted in Figure 30-43 demonstrating continuity of diaphragm. There is a small amount of residual pleural effusion.

34 cats (82%) survived, with concurrent injuries being recognized as the most common contributing factor for failure to survive[104]; another study reported survival in 16 of 16 (100%) of chronic cases with duration of herniation greater than 2 weeks[89] (Figure 30-50).

CHEST WALL PATHOLOGY

Chest wall pathology is not common in cats, and many cases produce no clinical signs. Awareness of these conditions is important for completeness of differential diagnoses of thoracic conditions and to rule out inconsequential change.

Trauma

Trauma is the most common chest wall abnormality. Blunt trauma may result in rib fractures, but these typically occur with other injuries, such as pulmonary contusions, pneumothorax, and hemothorax.[1] Subcutaneous emphysema may also result but is usually of little significance in itself, often requiring no specific treatment as long as the underlying cause is addressed.[36] Rib fractures also rarely contribute to morbidity in themselves. In one study 11 of 17 (65%) of cats with traumatic rib fractures survived, with all deaths (including euthanasia) attributable to concurrent injuries.[1] Similarly, the damage to the chest wall sustained by penetrating trauma is rarely of itself of major consequence but may be the only clue to other consequences, such as thoracic soft tissue trauma or pneumothorax.[36] Cases should be managed on a case-by-case basis, addressing basic wound management principles and taking into account thoracic cavity physiology—primarily, that intrathoracic pressure is lower than atmospheric pressure.

Nontraumatic Rib Fractures

In a recent study approximately half of rib fractures recognized (16 of 33, or 48%) had no known associated trauma. Pathologic fractures associated with neoplasia were one recognized cause, but in many cases (11 of 16, or 69%) the fractures were associated with chronic respiratory disorders such as bronchial diseases, pleural effusion, and URT disorders; the authors postulate these to be stress fractures associated with repetitive mechanical stress and chronic microtrauma caused by increased or more forceful respirations. In no case were the rib fractures deemed to specifically affect any cat's clinical course, but recognition of such fractures without trauma should prompt attention to determine the underlying cause or provide an additional measure of the severity of known underlying pathology.[1]

Pectus Excavatum

Pectus excavatum has been sporadically reported in cats.* It is a congenital condition resulting in dorsal deviation of the caudal part of the sternum or a dorsoventral flattening of the entire thorax that is thought to be associated with shortening of the central tendon of the diaphragm (see Figure 41-8). Many cats show respiratory signs, but the abnormality is recognized visually or by palpation by their owner. When respiratory signs do occur, they are present at birth or not long afterward; such signs may include reduced exercise tolerance, dyspnea, recurrent respiratory infections, and cyanosis; additionally, gastrointestinal signs such as vomiting may occur. Diagnosis is usually made by visual recognition and is confirmed radiographically. Surgical correction techniques using either temporary external splints[35,80,112,137] or internal stabilization[22,99,106] have been described as successful. The reader is directed to these sources for details of these techniques.

*References 22, 35, 51, 63, 80, 99, 106, 109, 112, 137.

Neoplasia

Neoplasia affecting the ribs of cats is rare. Occasional cases of plasma cell tumors or multiple myeloma have been recognized to result in rib fractures[1] or rib osteolysis.[131] One case series of chondrosarcoma mentions only 2 of 67 (3%) cases involving the ribs.[29] Rare occurrences such as this must be managed on a case-by-case basis using general oncologic principles; no overall recommendations can be made.

References

1. Adams C, Streeter EM, King R et al: Retrospective study: cause and clinical characteristics of rib fractures in cats: 33 cases (2000-2009), *J Vet Emerg Crit Care* 20:436, 2010.
2. Allman DA, Radlinsky MG, Ralph AG et al: Thoracoscopic thoracic duct ligation and thoracoscopic pericardectomy for treatment of chylothorax in dogs, *Vet Surg* 39:21, 2010.
3. Andreoni AA, Voss K: Reconstruction of a large diaphragmatic defect in a kitten using small intestinal submucosa (SIS), *J Feline Med Surg* 11:1019, 2009.
4. Asano T, Tsukamoto A, Ohno K et al: Membranoproliferative glomerulonephritis in a young cat, *J Vet Med Sci* 70:1373, 2008.
5. Ballegeer EA, Forrest LJ, Stepien RL: Radiographic appearance of bronchoalveolar carcinoma in nine cats, *Vet Radiol Ultrasound* 43:267, 2002.
6. Barr F, Gruffydd-Jones TJ, Brown PJ et al: Primary lung tumours in the cat, *J Small Anim Pract* 28:1115, 1987.
7. Barrs VR, Allan GS, Martin P et al: Feline pyothorax: a retrospective study of 27 cases in Australia, *J Feline Med Surg* 7:211, 2005.
8. Barrs VR, Beatty JA: Feline pyothorax: new insights into an old problem. Part 1: Aetiopathogenesis and diagnostic investigation, *Vet J* 179:163, 2009.
9. Barrs VR, Beatty JA: Feline pyothorax: new insights into an old problem. Part 2: Treatment recommendations and prophylaxis, *Vet J* 179:171, 2009.
10. Barrs VR, Swinney GR, Martin P et al: Concurrent *Aelurostrongylus abstrusus* infection and salmonellosis in a kitten, *Aust Vet J* 77:229, 1999.
11. Beatty J, Barrs V: Pleural effusion in the cat: a practical approach to determining aetiology, *J Feline Med Surg* 12:693, 2010.
12. Birchard SJ, Ware WA, Fossum TW et al: Chylothorax associated with congestive cardiomyopathy in a cat, *J Am Vet Med Assoc* 189:1462, 1986.
13. Brooks AC, Hardie R: Use of the subcutaneous pleuralport device for management of chronic pleural effusions in the dog and cat [abstract], *Vet Surg* 38:E27, 2009.
14. Brown DC, Holt D: Subcutaneous emphysema, pneumothorax, pneumomediastinum, and pneumopericardium associated with positive-pressure ventilation in a cat, *J Am Vet Med Assoc* 206:997, 1995.
15. Bussadori R, Provera A, Martano M et al: Pleural omentalisation with en bloc ligation of the thoracic duct and pericardiectomy for idiopathic chylothorax in nine dogs and four cats, *Vet J* 188:234-236, 2011.

16. Cahalane AK, Flanders JA, Steffey MA et al: Use of vascular access ports with intrathoracic drains for treatment of pleural effusion in three dogs, *J Am Vet Med Assoc* 230:527, 2007.
17. Cariou MP, Lipscomb VJ: Successful surgical management of a perforating oesophageal foreign body in a cat, *J Feline Med Surg* 13:50, 2011.
18. Cariou MPL, Shihab N, Kenny P et al: Surgical management of an incidentally diagnosed true pleuroperitoneal hernia in a cat, *J Feline Med Surg* 11:873, 2009.
19. Carpenter JL, Holzworth J: Thymoma in 11 cats, *J Am Vet Med Assoc* 181:248, 1982.
20. Cooper ES, Syring RS, King LG: Pneumothorax in cats with a clinical diagnosis of feline asthma: 5 cases (1990-2000), *J Vet Emerg Crit Care* 13:95, 2003.
21. Creighton SR, Wilkins RJ: Thoracic effusions in the cat. Etiology and diagnostic features, *J Am Anim Hosp Assoc* 11:66, 1975.
22. Crigel M: Pectus excavatum surgically repaired using sternum realignment and splint techniques in a young cat, *J Small Anim Pract* 46:352, 2005.
23. Davies C, Forrester SD: Pleural effusion in cats: 82 cases (1987 to 1995), *J Small Anim Pract* 37:217, 1996.
24. Day MJ: Review of thymic pathology in 30 cats and 36 dogs, *J Small Anim Pract* 38:393, 1997.
25. Demetriou JL, Foale RD, Ladlow J et al: Canine and feline pyothorax: a retrospective study of 50 cases in the UK and Ireland, *J Small Anim Pract* 43:388, 2002.
26. Donahoe JM: Experimental infection of cats with *Dirofilaria immitis*, *J Parasitol* 61:599, 1975.
27. Donahoe JM, Kneller SK, Thompson PE: Chylothorax subsequent to infection of cats with Dirofilaria immitis, *J Am Vet Med Assoc* 164:1107, 1974.
28. Duncan NM: Chylothorax in a kitten, *J S Afr Vet Assoc* 62:75, 1991.
29. Durham AC, Popovitch CA, Goldschmidt MH: Feline chondrosarcoma: a retrospective study of 67 cats (1987-2005), *J Am Anim Hosp Assoc* 44:124, 2008.
30. Evans AT: Anesthesia case of the month. Pneumothorax, pneumomediastinum and subcutaneous emphysema in a cat due to barotrauma after equipment failure during anesthesia, *J Am Vet Med Assoc* 212:30, 1998.
31. Ferasin L, vande Stadt M, Rudorf H et al: Syncope associated with paroxysmal atrioventricular block and ventricular standstill in a cat, *J Small Anim Pract* 43:124, 2002.
32. Forrest LJ, Graybush CA: Radiographic patterns of pulmonary metastasis in 25 cats, *Vet Radiol Ultrasound* 39:4, 1998.
33. Forrester SD, Fossum TW, Rogers KS: Diagnosis and treatment of chylothorax associated with lymphoblastic lymphosarcoma in four cats, *J Am Vet Med Assoc* 198:291, 1991.
34. Forster-Van Hijfte MA, Curtis CF, White RN: Resolution of exfoliative dermatitis and Malassezia pachydermatis overgrowth in a cat after surgical thymoma resection, *J Small Anim Pract* 38:451, 1997.
35. Fossum T, Boudrieau R, Hobson H: Pectus excavatum in eight dogs and six cats, *J Am Anim Hosp Assoc*, 1989.
36. Fossum TW: Pleural and extrapleural diseases. In Ettinger SJ, Feldman EC, editors: *Textbook of veterinary internal medicine*, Philadelphia, 2000, Saunders, p 1098.
37. Fossum TW: Chylothorax. In August JR, editor: *Consultations in feline internal medicine*, ed 5, St Louis, 2006, Elsevier Saunders, p 369.
38. Fossum TW, Evering WN, Miller MW et al: Severe bilateral fibrosing pleuritis associated with chronic chylothorax in five cats and two dogs, *J Am Vet Med Assoc* 201:317, 1992.
39. Fossum TW, Forrester SD, Swenson CL et al: Chylothorax in cats: 37 cases (1969-1989), *J Am Vet Med Assoc* 198:672, 1991.
40. Fossum TW, Mertens MM, Miller MW et al: Thoracic duct ligation and pericardectomy for treatment of idiopathic chylothorax, *J Vet Intern Med* 18:307, 2004.
41. Fossum TW, Miller MW, Rogers KS et al: Chylothorax associated with right-sided heart failure in five cats, *J Am Vet Med Assoc* 204:84, 1994.
42. Fossum TW, Relford RL: Pleural effusion: physical, biochemical, and cytologic characteristics. In August JR, editor: *Consultations in feline internal medicine 2*, Philadelphia, 1994, Saunders, p 287.
43. Garson HL, Dodman NH, Baker GJ: Diaphragmatic hernia. Analysis of fifty-six cases in dogs and cats, *J Small Anim Pract* 21:469, 1980.
44. Gibson TWG, Brisson BA, Sears W: Perioperative survival rates after surgery for diaphragmatic hernia in dogs and cats: 92 cases (1990-2002), *J Am Vet Med Assoc* 227:105, 2005.
45. Glaus TM, Jacobs GJ, Rawlings CA et al: Surgical removal of heartworms from a cat with caval syndrome, *J Am Vet Med Assoc* 206:663, 1995.
46. Gombač M, Vrecl M, Svara T: Congenital diaphragmatic eventration in two closely related British Shorthair cats, *J Feline Med Surg* 13:276-279, 2011.
47. Gores BR, Berg J, Carpenter JL et al: Surgical treatment of thymoma in cats: 12 cases (1987-1992), *J Am Vet Med Assoc* 204:1782, 1994.
48. Gottfried SD, Popovitch CA, Goldschmidt MH et al: Metastatic digital carcinoma in the cat: a retrospective study of 36 cats (1992-1998), *J Am Anim Hosp Assoc* 36:501, 2000.
49. Gould L: The medical management of idiopathic chylothorax in a domestic long-haired cat, *Can Vet J* 45:51, 2004.
50. Graber ER: Diagnosis and treatment of ruptured thoracic duct in the cat, *J Am Vet Med Assoc* 146:242, 1965.
51. Grenn H, Lindo D: Case report. Pectus excavatum (funnel chest) in a feline, *Can Vet J* 9:279, 1968.
52. Gruffydd–Jones TJ, Flecknell PA: The prognosis and treatment related to the gross appearance and laboratory characteristics of pathological thoracic fluids in the cat, *J Small Anim Pract* 19:315, 1978.
53. Gryminski J, Krakówka P, Lypacewicz G: The diagnosis of pleural effusion by ultrasonic and radiologic techniques, *Chest* 70:33, 1976.
54. Guyton AC, Hall JE: Pulmonary ventilation. In Hall JE, editor: *Textbook of medical physiology*, ed 11, Philadelphia, 2006, Elsevier Saunders, p 471.
55. Guyton AC, Hall JE: Transport of oxygen and carbon dioxide in blood and tissue fluids. In Hall JE, editor: *Textbook of medical physiology*, ed 11, Philadelphia, 2006, Elsevier Saunders, p 502.
56. Hahn KA, McEntee MF: Prognosis factors for survival in cats after removal of a primary lung tumor: 21 cases (1979-1994), *Vet Surg* 27:307, 1998.
57. Hartmann K: Feline infectious peritonitis, *Vet Clin North Am Small Anim Pract* 35:39, 2005.
58. Hartmann K, Binder C, Hirschberger J et al: Comparison of different tests to diagnose feline infectious peritonitis, *J Vet Intern Med* 17:781, 2003.
59. Hawkins EC, Fossum TW: Medical and surgical management of pleural effusion. In Bonagura JD, editor: *Kirk's current veterinary therapy XIII small animal practice*, Philadelphia, 2000, Saunders, p 819.
60. Hayes G: Chylothorax and fibrosing pleuritis secondary to thyrotoxic cardiomyopathy, *J Small Anim Pract* 46:203, 2005.
61. Hinrichs U, Puhl S, Rutteman GR et al: Lymphangiosarcomas in cats: a retrospective study of 12 cases, *Vet Pathol* 36:164, 1999.
62. Hirschberger J, DeNicola DB, Hermanns W et al: Sensitivity and specificity of cytologic evaluation in the diagnosis of neoplasia in body fluids from dogs and cats, *Vet Clin Pathol* 28:142, 1999.
63. Johnston S, Moon M, Atkinson R et al: Pectus excavatum and left to right intracardiac shunt in a kitten, *J Small Anim Pract* 34:577, 1993.
64. Kagan KG: Thoracic trauma, *Vet Clin North Am Small Anim Pract* 10:641, 1980.

65. Keep JM: Congenital diaphragmatic hernia in a cat, *Aust Vet J* 26:193, 1950.
66. Kerpsack SJ, McLoughlin MA, Birchard SJ et al: Evaluation of mesenteric lymphangiography and thoracic duct ligation in cats with chylothorax: 19 cases (1987-1992), *J Am Vet Med Assoc* 205:711, 1994.
67. Kerpsack SJ, McLoughlin MA, Graves TK et al: Chylothorax associated with lung lobe torsion and a peritoneopericardial diaphragmatic hernia in a cat, *J Am Anim Hosp Assoc* 30:351, 1994.
68. Kittleson MD: Pathophysiology of heart failure. In Kittleson MD, Kienle RD, editors: *Small animal cardiovascular medicine*, St Louis, 1998, Mosby, p 136.
69. Kopko SH: The use of rutin in a cat with idiopathic chylothorax, *Can Vet J* 46:729, 2005.
70. Kovak JR, Ludwig LL, Bergman PJ et al: Use of thoracoscopy to determine the etiology of pleural effusion in dogs and cats: 18 cases (1998-2001), *J Am Vet Med Assoc* 221:990, 2002.
71. Kramek BA, Caywood DD: Pneumothorax, *Vet Clin North Am Small Anim Pract* 17:285, 1987.
72. Larson MM: Ultrasound of the thorax (noncardiac), *Vet Clin North Am Small Anim Pract* 39:733, 2009.
73. Lord PF, Suter PF, Chan KF et al: Pleural, extrapleural and pulmonary lesions in small animals: a radiographic approach to differential diagnosis, *Vet Radiol* 13:4, 1972.
74. Love DN, Jones RF, Bailey M et al: Isolation and characterisation of bacteria from pyothorax (empyaemia) in cats, *Vet Microbiol* 7:455, 1982.
75. Malik R, Gabor L, Hunt GB et al: Benign cranial mediastinal lesions in three cats, *Aust Vet J* 75:183, 1997.
76. Malik R, Gabor LJ, Foster SF et al: Therapy for Australian cats with lymphosarcoma, *Aust Vet J* 79:808, 2001.
77. Mandell DC: Respiratory distress in cats. In Lesley GK, editor: *Textbook of respiratory disease in dogs and cats*, St Louis, 2004, Saunders, p 12.
78. Manning MM, Brunson DB: Barotrauma in a cat, *J Am Vet Med Assoc* 205:62, 1994.
79. Maritato KC, Colon JA, Kergosien DH: Pneumothorax, *Compend Contin Educ Vet* 31:232, 2009.
80. McAnulty J, Harvey C: Repair of pectus excavatum by percutaneous suturing and temporary external coaptation in a kitten, *J Am Vet Med Assoc* 194:1065, 1989.
81. McLane MJ, Buote NJ: Lung lobe torsion associated with chylothorax in a cat, *J Feline Med Surg* 13:135, 2011.
82. McMurphy RM, Hodgson DS, Cribb PH: Modification of a nonrebreathing circuit adapter to prevent barotrauma in anesthetized patients, *Vet Surg* 24:352, 1995.
83. Meadows RL, MacWilliams PS, Dzata G et al: Chylothorax associated with cryptococcal mediastinal granuloma in a cat, *Vet Clin Pathol* 22:109, 1993.
84. Mehlhaff CJ, Mooney S: Primary pulmonary neoplasia in the dog and cat, *Vet Clin North Am Small Anim Pract* 15:1061, 1985.
85. Meincke JE, Hobbie WV, Jr., Barto LR: Traumatic chylothorax with associated diaphragmatic hernias in the cat, *J Am Vet Med Assoc* 155:15, 1969.
86. Miles KG: A review of primary lung tumors in the dog and cat, *Vet Radiol* 29:122, 1988.
87. Miller BH, Roudebush P, Ward HG: Pleural effusion as a sequela to aelurostrongylosis in a cat, *J Am Vet Med Assoc* 185:556, 1984.
88. Milne ME, McCowan C, Landon BP: Spontaneous feline pneumothorax caused by ruptured pulmonary bullae associated with possible bronchopulmonary dysplasia, *J Am Anim Hosp Assoc* 46:138, 2010.
89. Minihan AC, Berg J, Evans KL: Chronic diaphragmatic hernia in 34 dogs and 16 cats, *J Am Anim Hosp Assoc* 40:51, 2004.
90. Miserocchi G: Physiology and pathophysiology of pleural fluid turnover, *Eur Respir J* 10:219, 1997.
91. Miserocchi G, Agostoni E: Contents of the pleural space, *J Appl Physiol* 30:208, 1971.
92. Mitchell SL, McCarthy R, Rudloff E et al: Tracheal rupture associated with intubation in cats: 20 cases (1996-1998), *J Am Vet Med Assoc* 216:1592, 2000.
93. Myer W: Pneumothorax: a radiography review, *Vet Radiol* 19:12, 1978.
94. Myer W: Radiography review: pleural effusion, *Vet Radiol* 19:75, 1978.
95. Pawloski DR, Broaddus KD: Pneumothorax: a review, *J Am Anim Hosp Assoc* 46:385, 2010.
96. Pawloski DR, Brunker JD, Singh K et al: Pulmonary *Paecilomyces lilacinus* infection in a cat, *J Am Anim Hosp Assoc* 46:197, 2010.
97. Prittie J, Barton L: Hemothorax and sanguineous effusions. In Lesley GK, editor: *Textbook of respiratory disease in dogs and cats*, St Louis, 2004, Saunders, p 610.
98. Rishniw M, Weidman J, Hornof WJ: Hydrothorax secondary to a perinephric pseudocyst in a cat, *Vet Radiol Ultrasound* 39:193, 1998.
99. Risselada M, De Rooster H, Liuti T et al: Use of internal splinting to realign a noncompliant sternum in a cat with pectus excavatum, *J Am Vet Med Assoc* 228:1047, 2006.
100. Rottenberg S, von Tscharner C, Roosje PJ: Thymoma-associated exfoliative dermatitis in cats, *Vet Pathol* 41:429, 2004.
101. Saunders HM, Keith D: Thoracic imaging. In Lesley GK, editor: *Textbook of respiratory disease in dogs and cats*, St Louis, 2004, Saunders, p 72.
102. Saunders HM, VanWinkle TJ, Drobatz K et al: Ultrasonographic findings in cats with clinical, gross pathologic, and histologic evidence of acute pancreatic necrosis: 20 cases (1994-2001), *J Am Vet Med Assoc* 221:1724, 2002.
103. Sauvé V: Thoracocentesis. In Lesley GK, editor: *Textbook of respiratory disease in dogs and cats*, St Louis, 2004, Saunders, p 137.
104. Schmiedt CW, Tobias KM, Stevenson MAM: Traumatic diaphragmatic hernia in cats: 34 cases (1991-2001), *J Am Vet Med Assoc* 222:1237, 2003.
105. Sherding RG: Diseases of the pleural cavity. In Sherding RG, editor: *The cat: diseases and clinical management*, New York, 1994, Churchill Livingstone, p 1053.
106. Shires P, Waldron D, Payne J: Pectus excavatum in three kittens, *J Am Anim Hosp Assoc* 24:203, 1988.
107. Singh A, Boston SE, Poma R: Thymoma-associated exfoliative dermatitis with postthymectomy myasthenia gravis in a cat, *Can Vet J* 51:757, 2010.
108. Small MT, Atkins CE, Gordon SG et al: Use of a nitinol gooseneck snare catheter for removal of adult Dirofilaria immitis in two cats, *J Am Vet Med Assoc* 233:1441, 2008.
109. Smallwood J, Beaver B: Congenital chondrosternal depression (pectus excavatum) in the cat, *Vet Radiol Ultrasound* 18:141, 1977.
110. Smith JW, Scott-Moncrieff JC, Rivers BJ: Pneumothorax secondary to *Dirofilaria immitis* infection in two cats, *J Am Vet Med Assoc* 213:91, 1998.
111. Smits B, Reid MM: Feline paraneoplastic syndrome associated with thymoma, *N Z Vet J* 51:244, 2003.
112. Soderstrom MJ, Gilson SD, Gulbas N: Fatal reexpansion pulmonary edema in a kitten following surgical correction of pectus excavatum, *J Am Anim Hosp Assoc* 31:133, 1995.
113. Spadavecchia C, Jaggy A: Thymectomy in a cat with myasthenia gravis: a case report focusing on perianaesthetic management, *Schweiz Arch Tierheilkd* 150:515, 2008.
114. Sparkes A, Gruffydd-Jones T, Harbour D: Feline infectious peritonitis: a review of clinicopathological changes in 65 cases, and a critical assessment of their diagnostic value, *Vet Rec* 129:209, 1991.

115. Spattini G, Rossi F, Vignoli M et al: Use of ultrasound to diagnose diaphragmatic rupture in dogs and cats, *Vet Radiol Ultrasound* 44:226, 2003.
116. Stegemann MR, Passmore CA, Sherington J et al: Antimicrobial activity and spectrum of cefovecin, a new extended-spectrum cephalosporin, against pathogens collected from dogs and cats in Europe and North America, *Antimicrob Agents Chemother* 50:2286, 2006.
117. Störk CK, Hamaide AJ, Schwedes C et al: Hemiurothorax following diaphragmatic hernia and kidney prolapse in a cat, *J Feline Med Surg* 5:91, 2003.
118. Sullivan M, Lee R: Radiological features of 80 cases of diaphragmatic rupture, *J Small Anim Pract* 30:561, 1989.
119. Teske E, van Straten G, van Noort R et al: Chemotherapy with cyclophosphamide, vincristine, and prednisolone (cop) in cats with malignant lymphoma: new results with an old protocol, *J Vet Intern Med* 16:179, 2002.
120. Theilen GH, Madewell BR: Tumours of the respiratory tract and thorax. In Theilen GH, Madewell BR, editors: *Veterinary cancer medicine*, ed 1, Philadelphia, 1979, Lea & Febiger, p 341.
121. Thompson MS, Cohn LA, Jordan RC: Use of rutin for medical management of idiopathic chylothorax in four cats, *J Am Vet Med Assoc* 215:345, 1999.
122. Trumpa M, Stephan I, Baumgartner W et al: [Case report. Restrictive cardiomyopathy with chylothorax in a cat: the pathogenesis], *Dtsch Tierarztl Wochenschr* 111:438, 2004.
123. Turek MM: Cutaneous paraneoplastic syndromes in dogs and cats: a review of the literature, *Vet Dermatol* 14:279, 2003.
124. Vail DM, Moore AS, Ogilvie GK et al: Feline lymphoma (145 cases): proliferation indices, cluster of differentiation 3 immunoreactivity, and their association with prognosis in 90 cats, *J Vet Intern Med* 12:349, 1998.
125. Vilafranca M, Font A: Thymolipoma in a cat, *J Feline Med Surg* 7:125, 2005.
126. Vnuk D, Pirkic B, Maticic D et al: Feline high-rise syndrome: 119 cases (1998-2001), *J Feline Med Surg* 6:305, 2004.
127. Voges AK, Bertrand S, Hill RC et al: True diaphragmatic hernia in a cat, *Vet Radiol Ultrasound* 38:116, 1997.
128. Waddell LS, Brady CA, Drobatz KJ: Risk factors, prognostic indicators, and outcome of pyothorax in cats: 80 cases (1986-1999), *J Am Vet Med Assoc* 221:819, 2002.
129. Waddle JR, Giger U: Lipoprotein electrophoresis differentiation of chylous and nonchylous pleural effusions in dogs and cats and its correlation with pleural effusion triglyceride concentration, *Vet Clin Path* 19:80, 1990.
130. Walker AL, Jang SS, Hirsh DC: Bacteria associated with pyothorax of dogs and cats: 98 cases (1989-1998), *J Am Vet Med Assoc* 216:359, 2000.
131. Webb J, Chary P, Northrup N et al: Erythrophagocytic multiple myeloma in a cat, *Vet Clin Path* 37:302, 2008.
132. White HL, Rozanski EA, Tidwell AS et al: Spontaneous pneumothorax in two cats with small airway disease, *J Am Vet Med Assoc* 222:1573, 2003.
133. White JD, Tisdall PLC, Norris JM et al: Diaphragmatic hernia in a cat mimicking a pulmonary mass, *J Feline Med Surg* 5:197, 2003.
134. Whitney WO, Mehlhaff CJ: High-rise syndrome in cats, *J Am Vet Med Assoc* 191:1399, 1987.
135. Wilson GP, 3rd, Newton CD, Burt JK: A review of 116 diaphragmatic hernias in dogs and cats, *J Am Vet Med Assoc* 159:1142, 1971.
136. Worth AJ, Machon R: Traumatic diaphragmatic herniation: pathophysiology and management, *Compend Contin Educ Pract Vet* 27:178, 2005.
137. Yoon HY, Mann F, Jeong S: Surgical correction of pectus excavatum in two cats, *J Vet Sci* 9:335, 2008.
138. Zambelli AB: Pneumomediastinum, pneumothorax and pneumoretroperitoneum following endoscopic retrieval of a tracheal foreign body from a cat, *J S Afr Vet Assoc* 77:45, 2006.
139. Zitz JC, Birchard SJ, Couto GC et al: Results of excision of thymoma in cats and dogs: 20 cases (1984-2005), *J Am Vet Med Assoc* 232:1186, 2008.
140. Zocchi L: Physiology and pathophysiology of pleural fluid turnover, *Eur Resp J* 20:1545, 2002.
141. Zoia A, Slater LA, Heller J et al: A new approach to pleural effusion in cats: markers for distinguishing transudates from exudates, *J Feline Med Surg* 11:847, 2009.

CHAPTER

31

Toxicology

Jill A. Richardson and Susan E. Little

OUTLINE

According to the old saying, "curiosity killed the cat." Usually, this is just a metaphor used to describe the ill effects of being nosy. But in many cases, it can actually be true. One of the instances when this phrase is true occurs when curious cats are exposed to poisons. Exposure may occur by way of the oral, cutaneous, or inhalation routes, although most feline toxicoses result from ingestion. Cats may chew on poisonous plants, ingest chemicals spilled on their fur, or swallow poisons in food or water. Sometimes cats are exposed to poisons through inappropriate administration by their owners. Many of these situations have the potential of being fatal without proper and prompt treatment.

Although toxicoses are not as common in cats as in dogs, they still accounted for 10% of the calls to a pet poison helpline.[19] Most veterinarians report that pyrethrin–permethrin and plant intoxications are the most common toxicoses seen in cats.[17] Cats are deficient in their ability to metabolize certain compounds, leading to poor detoxification and excretion of many chemicals and drugs. Cats are more sensitive to adverse drug reactions than most companion animals for several reasons. Cats are deficient in glucuronyl transferase activity, an enzyme that conjugates many chemicals. Moreover, the feline red blood cell is more susceptible to oxidative damage than that of other species, resulting in Heinz body formation and methemoglobinemia.

According to Paracelsus, the father of toxicology, everything is toxic—the dose makes the poison. That is especially true with cats. Although there are thousands of potential poisons for cats, the ones that are of special note include permethrin topical spot-ons, members of the *Lilium* and *Hemerocallis* genera of plants, acetaminophen, and ethylene glycol (EG). This chapter focuses on these toxicants and several others that can be dangerous for cats. A list of online resources for toxicology information is provided in Box 31-1.

PESTICIDES

Cats may have exposure to pesticides either through accidental ingestion of inappropriately stored products or through malicious poisonings.

Snail and Slug Baits

Metaldehyde is a polymer of acetaldehyde and is often used as snail and slug bait. Commercial products are available in various forms, such as granules, pellets, and liquids, and are designed to be used in and around gardens (Figure 31-1). Toxicosis is more common in dogs, which are more likely to ingest bait in a garden or from an improperly stored container. The minimum lethal dose of metaldehyde in cats is not known; however, in dogs it is 100 mg/kg.[42] Serious adverse effects occur at much lower doses. Although the mechanism of action of metaldehyde is not known, its effects are well established. Both metaldehyde and its metabolite, acetaldehyde, will distribute widely in the body and cross the blood–brain barrier.

After ingestion affected animals have signs of tachycardia, nervousness, sensitivity to light and noise, panting, drooling, ataxia, hyperthermia, tremors, and

BOX 31-1

Online Resources for Toxicology Information

American Association for the Prevention of Cruelty to Animals, Animal Poison Control Center: http://www.aspca.org/apcc
Pet Poison Helpline: http://www.petpoisonhelpline.com
American Board of Veterinary Toxicology: http://www.abvt.org
National Pesticide Information Center: http://npic.orst.edu
Environmental Protection Agency: http://www.epa.gov
American Association of Poison Control Centers: http://www.aapcc.org

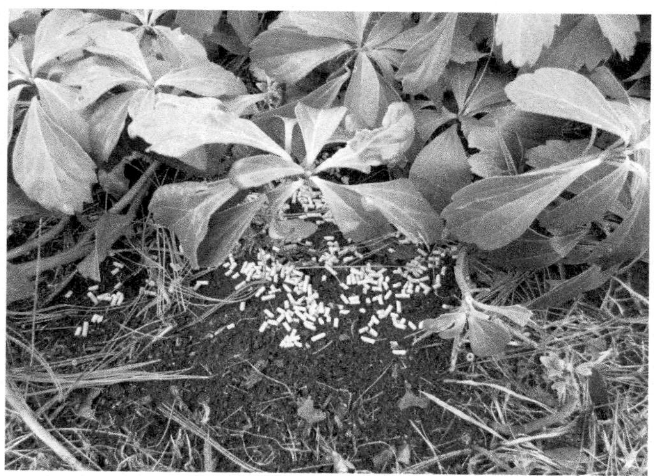

FIGURE 31-1 Pelleted slug and snail bait is often placed under plant foliage in gardens, either scattered loosely or in small traps. Nontoxic slug and snail bait containing ferric phosphate is readily available.

seizures.[42] Onset of clinical signs in dogs generally occurs within 3 to 5 hours of ingestion but can occur in as soon as 30 minutes. Clinical signs can last for up to 5 days but will lessen over 12 to 72 hours with appropriate treatment.[51] Metabolic acidosis often occurs with toxicity, and in some cases hepatic failure may occur within 2 or 3 days after exposure.[42]

The diagnosis of metaldehyde toxicosis is based on history of exposure and associated clinical signs. If necessary, serum and urine can be assayed for acetaldehyde. Lesions on necropsy are generally nonspecific.

Treatment includes early decontamination, supportive care, and seizure control. Emesis can be induced in appropriate patients, or gastric lavage may be used under sedation or anesthesia. Activated charcoal may help inhibit metaldehyde absorption. Methocarbamol has been used successfully to control tremors and seizures from metaldehyde toxicosis in dogs (Table 31-1).[42] Other options for seizure control include diazepam, barbiturates, and inhalant anesthesia. Affected animals should be monitored for metabolic acidosis and hyperthermia. Intravenous fluid therapy is indicated to combat hyperthermia and dehydration. Metabolic acidosis may be treated with bicarbonate if necessary. A warm, quiet, comfortable environment helps lessen anxiety and nervousness. Treatment should continue until clinical signs are resolved, which may take several days.

Fly Bait

Methomyl is an extremely toxic carbamate insecticide that is found in certain fly baits. The mechanism of action of carbamates is through the inhibition of both acetylcholinesterases and pseudocholinesterases.[3] Almost immediately after ingestion, seizures and pulmonary edema occur. The signs occur rapidly and are so severe that most cases are fatal.[3] Atropine, a cholinergic agent, is antidotal for methomyl toxicity.[3] In addition, seizure control is recommended. Because the clinical signs occur so quickly, decontamination is usually not an option.

RODENTICIDES

Rodenticides are designed to kill rats, mice, gophers, and other rodents. Cats may be exposed to rodenticides either through accidental ingestion of the bait or through eating poisoned rodents. Sometimes people mix rodenticides with foods such as tuna or peanut butter, inadvertently luring pets as well as rodents to the bait. The most commonly reported toxicoses are caused by anticoagulant rodenticides, bromethalin, cholecalciferol, strychnine, and zinc phosphide.[31] In many cases diagnosis is based on a history of exposure and compatible clinical signs. In some cases laboratory testing is necessary to establish the diagnosis, especially when an accurate history is not available. Response to treatment may also be a valuable indicator. Although antidotes are not available for all rodenticides, decontamination and symptomatic and supportive treatments are important.

Emetics may be administered to appropriate patients (e.g., those without seizures, depression, or coma) if exposure occurred within the previous 1 to 2 hours. Activated charcoal is administered as an adsorbent and may be combined with a cathartic.

Anticoagulant Rodenticides

Anticoagulant rodenticides include the short-acting warfarin and long-acting chemicals such as pindone, diphacinone, difethialone, chlorophacinone, brodifacoum, and bromadiolone. They are readily available in many formats, including pellets and powders, from several sources, including feed stores and home and

TABLE 31-1 **Selected Drugs Useful in the Treatment of Toxicoses in the Cat**

Drug	Indication	Dose
Acetylcysteine	Acetaminophen toxicity	140 mg/kg PO for initial dose, then 70 mg/kg PO every 4 hours for 3-5 treatments
Activated charcoal	Adsorbent for ingested toxicants	2-5 g/kg PO; slurry made with 1 g per 5-10 mL water
Ascorbic acid	Acetaminophen toxicity	20-30 mg/kg, PO, every 6 hours
Atropine	OP, carbamate toxicity	0.2-0.5 mg/kg; ¼ given IV, remainder IM or SC; every 4-8 hours as needed
Cimetidine	Acetaminophen toxicity	5-10 mg/kg PO or IV, every 6 to 8 hours
Dapsone	Brown recluse spider envenomation	1 mg/kg PO, once daily for 14 days
Diazepam	Control of seizures	0.25-0.5 mg/kg IV or rectally; repeat as needed
Ethanol (20%): add 250 mL 100% ethanol to 1 L crystalloid fluids	Ethylene glycol toxicity	5 mL/kg, CRI over 1 hour; every 6 hours for 5 treatments, then every 8 hours for 4 treatments
Kaolin/pectin	Gastrointestinal protectant	1-2 mL/kg PO, every 6 hours
Methocarbamol	Control of tremors, muscle fasciculations	55-200 mg/kg IV or PO, every 8 hours; maximum 330 mg/kg/day
Misoprostol	Gastric protectant, NSAID toxicity	1-3 μg/kg PO, every 12 hours
Pamidronate	Cholecalciferol toxicity	1.3-2 mg/kg IV, diluted with saline and given over 2 hours
Phenobarbital	Control of seizures	2-6 mg/kg IV bolus, repeat up to 2 times at 20-minute intervals
Pralidoxime chloride (2-PAM)	OP toxicity (not for carbamate toxicity)	10-15 mg/kg IM or SC, every 8-12 hours
Sodium sulfate	Cathartic	250 mg/kg PO
Sorbitol (70% solution)	Cathartic	1-2 mL/kg PO
Sucralfate	Oral, esophageal, gastric, duodenal ulceration	0.25-0.5 g/cat PO, every 8 to 12 hours
Vitamin K_1	Anticoagulant rodenticide toxicity	3-5 mg/kg PO or SC, every 8 to 12 hours with food
For Induction of Emesis*	**Comments**	**Dose**
Apomorphine	Dissolve 6 mg tablet in water or saline; flush conjunctival sac after emesis; antagonized with yohimbine (0.1 mg/kg, IV or 0.5 mg/kg SC or IM)	0.04 mg/kg IV or 0.25 mg/kg, conjunctival sac
Hydrogen peroxide (3%)	Take care to avoid aspiration	2 mL/kg PO; maximum 10 mL/cat
Xylazine	May cause respiratory depression, reversed with yohimbine (0.1 mg/kg IV or 0.5 mg/kg SC or IM)	0.44-1.1 mg/kg IM

PO, By mouth; *OP,* organophosphate; *IV,* intravenously; *IM,* intramuscularly; *SC,* subcutaneously; *CRI,* constant-rate infusion; *NSAID,* nonsteroidal antiinflammatory drug.

*Emesis should not be induced in patients that have ingested corrosive or caustic substances or substances that may cause aspiration pneumonia. In addition, induction of emesis is contraindicated in animals with decreased consciousness or those that have or are likely to have seizures.

garden stores. One of the first rodenticides marketed was warfarin, but resistance rapidly developed in target species, so newer generation compounds have been developed. Anticoagulants act by blocking the recycling of vitamin K_1 in the liver, which results in a coagulopathy. Dysfunctional forms of clotting factors II, VII, IX, and X are released into circulation.[31]

Clinical signs of an anticoagulant toxicity include ecchymoses, petechiae, frank hemorrhage, pale mucous membranes, weakness, exercise intolerance, lameness, dyspnea, coughing, and swollen joints. Early signs may be vague, such as lethargy and anorexia.[21] The most common clinical presentation is acute onset of dyspnea caused by bleeding into the thoracic cavity.[24] Other presentations include otic bleeding, hematoma, melena, and hematochezia.[21] Sudden death without preceding clinical signs is also possible. Clinical signs are seen several days after the bait is ingested because of the time needed to completely block the coagulation pathways. The duration of action, and thus the length of treatment required, is highly variable, ranging from 14 days to several weeks, depending on the chemical involved.[24]

Commonly used coagulation tests include bleeding time, activated clotting time (ACT), prothrombin time (PT), and activated partial thromboplastin time (APTT). ACT and APTT measure the intrinsic clotting cascade. PT measures the extrinsic coagulation pathway. Anticoagulant rodenticides affect both the extrinsic and intrinsic pathways. When vitamin K is depleted, the first clotting factor to be affected is factor VII of the extrinsic coagulation pathway. In early cases of toxicoses (36 to 72 hours after ingestion), the PT will be prolonged, but the animal will still appear clinically normal because the other pathways are functioning.[30] However, after 72 hours factor IX becomes depleted and shuts down the intrinsic pathway, prolonging other coagulation tests, at which time hemorrhage is possible.

The PIVKA (protein induced in vitamin K antagonism) test (Thrombotest; Axis-Shield PoC, Oslo, Norway) is a newer diagnostic tool for anticoagulant rodenticide toxicosis. It evaluates the extrinsic and common pathways.[22] However, if the PT is prolonged, the PIVKA test adds no further information. PIVKA times are also prolonged in any vitamin K_1–responsive coagulopathy.

Decontamination is helpful only with early recognition of ingestion. Vomiting may be induced if ingestion occurred within the previous 4 hours.[24] Activated charcoal may be useful if a significant amount of chemical has been ingested. Other treatment is aimed at providing functional clotting factors. PT and PIVKA are monitored at baseline and 48 and 73 hours later.[24] Because PT elevates before clinical signs occur, it is a useful indicator of when vitamin K_1 therapy is indicated. Testing for both PT and PIVKA must be performed before vitamin K_1 is administered to prevent false-negative results.

In some cases initial treatment may require transfusion of fresh frozen plasma or whole blood to supply clotting factors.[21] Oral vitamin K_1 (phytonadione) therapy is antidotal for anticoagulant rodenticides. Injectable vitamin K_1 is not recommended because of the risk of anaphylactic reactions. Vitamin K_3 is contraindicated because it is not effective and may induce hemolytic anemia.[30] Treatment should continue as long as necessary, depending on the type of rodenticide (e.g., 14 days for warfarin, 21 days for bromadiolone, 30 days for other compounds). Confirming a normal PT 48 to 72 hours after the last dose of vitamin K_1 can ensure that it is not needed further. The prognosis is generally good if the toxicity is recognized and treated early.

Bromethalin

Bromethalin has been sold since the 1980s and is typically available in grain-based pellet form. Bromethalin is an uncoupler of oxidative phosphorylation and causes a reduction of adenosine-5′-triphosphate (ATP), decreasing nerve impulse conduction.[12] After ingestion absorption is rapid and peak plasma levels are reached in a few hours.[30] Clinical signs can occur at any time from 24 hours after ingestion to 2 weeks later and include muscle tremors, seizures, hyperexcitability, forelimb extensor rigidity, ataxia, depression, loss of vocalization, paresis, paralysis, and death.[11,12,30] Low-dose exposure causes slow development of clinical signs, starting with hindlimb ataxia and paresis, with hindlimb paralysis following.[11] Affected animals also show decreased conscious proprioception, loss of deep pain, and upper motor neuron bladder paralysis.[11] The most common postmortem lesions include cerebral and spinal cord edema and a spongy appearance to the cerebellum.[12]

Diagnosis is based on history of exposure and compatible clinical signs. Because there is no antidote to this rodenticide and the clinical effects can be extremely severe, early aggressive decontamination is critical. If ingestion occurred recently (within 2 hours of presentation), emetics, activated charcoal, and a cathartic should be administered.[11] Activated charcoal may be required every 4 to 8 hours for at least 3 days. Cats with cerebral edema may be treated with mannitol (250 mg/kg intravenously, every 6 hours) and dexamethasone (2 mg/kg intravenously, every 6 hours).[11] Seizures may be managed with diazepam or phenobarbital. Unfortunately, treatment of such severely affected animals is often futile. Mildly affected animals may recover in 1 to 2 weeks. More severely affected animals may require prolonged nutritional support and nursing care.

Cholecalciferol

Cholecalciferol (vitamin D_3) is metabolized in the liver to calcifediol (25-hydroxycholecalciferol). Calcifediol is then metabolized by the kidney to calcitriol (1,25-dihyd roxycholecalciferol). Cholecalciferol increases intestinal absorption of calcium, stimulates bone resorption, and enhances renal tubular reabsorption of calcium. Toxic ingestion results in hypercalcemia, which can lead to renal failure, cardiovascular abnormalities, and tissue mineralization. Plasma phosphorus and calcium increase within 72 hours of ingestion. The (calcium × phosphorus) product may exceed 130 mg^2/dL^2 (10.5 $mmol^2/L^2$), well above the level at which soft tissue mineralization occurs.[29] Other laboratory abnormalities include increased blood urea nitrogen (BUN) and creatinine, hyperkalemia, acidosis, and decreased urine specific gravity.[30]

Clinical signs usually occur 18 to 36 hours after ingestion and include vomiting, diarrhea, inappetence, depression, polyuria, polydipsia, and cardiac arrhythmia.[29,30] With high doses renal failure results from the deposition of calcium in the kidney and occurs in 24 to 48 hours.[29] Death is often due to acute renal failure, and animals that survive may have permanent loss of renal function and other abnormalities. Cholecalciferol is highly lipid soluble and is eliminated slowly from the body.[29] Clinical signs, and therefore duration of treatment, may last for weeks.

Diagnosis is based on a history of exposure and compatible clinical signs. Other causes of hypercalcemia must be ruled out. Assessment of serum parathyroid hormone, parathyroid hormone–related polypeptide, and 25-hydroxycholecalciferol levels may be helpful in the differential diagnosis.

Decontamination is recommended with early exposures. Emesis may be induced in appropriate patients. Activated charcoal should be administered concurrently with a cathartic. Baseline and serial monitoring of serum BUN, creatinine, phosphorus, and calcium is necessary. In cats that develop clinical signs or changes in laboratory parameters, diuresis with intravenous 0.9% saline is indicated. Furosemide is added to the therapy once the cat is hydrated to increase renal calcium excretion.[29] Oral prednisone may be used to decrease serum calcium by decreasing bone resorption, decreasing intestinal absorption, and increasing renal excretion.

Severely affected cats or those that relapse after initial therapy may require treatment with a bisphosphonate. Pamidronate (see Table 31-1) inhibits osteoclastic bone resorption and has been used successfully to treat exposures in combination with fluid therapy and supportive care.[29] Once calcium levels are normal, they should be monitored daily for 4 days. Retreatment may be required.

Strychnine

Strychnine is an alkaloid derived from the nux vomica tree that is used to kill rodents and also other pests, including coyotes.[30] Strychnine is considered a restricted pesticide in many states. It is often, but not always, found as red-colored grain-based pellets. Cats are less commonly affected than dogs but may be poisoned by accidental or malicious exposure. Strychnine is a glycine antagonist in the central nervous system (CNS) and results in excessive neuronal activity, causing muscle spasms and severe convulsions.[52] The lethal dose in cats is 2 mg/kg.[52] Early signs of toxicity (within minutes) include apprehension and stiffness, progressing to tonic extensor rigidity, especially in response to stimulation (light, sound, touch).[30] Clinical signs affect the face, neck, and limb muscles first.[52] Convulsions with opisthotonos can appear quickly. Death may occur as a result of hypoxia from impaired respiration as soon as 10 minutes after ingestion or up to 24 to 48 hours later.[52] The differential diagnosis includes a wide variety of possibilities, including rabies and other intoxications.

Diagnosis is based on a history of exposure, compatible clinical signs, and strychnine testing (on urine, tissues, or stomach contents). If exposure is recent and the patient's status is stable, activated charcoal may be administered to reduce further absorption. Emetics should be used with care insofar as they may precipitate violent muscle or convulsive activity.[52] It may be safer to perform gastric lavage on a sedated or anesthetized patient. Seizure control in most cases is difficult but may include the use of methocarbamol, propofol, or barbiturates. Diazepam is usually not recommended because its efficacy for strychnine-induced seizures is variable.[30]

Respiration should be monitored closely and mechanical ventilation initiated if severe respiratory depression occurs. Supportive care includes intravenous fluid therapy and provision of a quiet, dark environment. Most poisoned animals require hospitalization for 24 to 72 hours. Patients presented late in the progression of the disease are at higher risk of death.

Zinc Phosphide

Zinc phosphide is commonly found in mole and gopher baits at concentrations up to 5% and is highly toxic.[1] It is used for vermin control in areas where rodents have become resistant to other chemical control methods and is usually a restricted-use pesticide. Dogs and cats are the species most likely to suffer accidental ingestion and toxicosis. Cats that eat very recently poisoned rodents may also be at risk of toxicity from zinc phosphide still in the gastrointestinal tract of the target animal.[1] For most species a lethal dose is 20 to 40 mg/kg.[1]

After ingestion, phosphide is converted to phosphine gas by stomach acid.[1] Released phosphine gas causes severe irritation to the pulmonary tissues, which results in respiratory distress and death occurring secondary to respiratory failure. Clinical signs are typically seen in 15 minutes to 4 hours, depending on when the animal last ingested a meal.[1] Early signs of toxicosis include anorexia and depression, followed by rapid and deep respirations.[1] Vomiting is common and often contains blood.

Treatment includes early decontamination (induction of emesis or gastric lavage, activated charcoal with a cathartic) and supportive care for the associated clinical effects (e.g., acidosis, respiratory compromise, depression). Some animals suffer liver failure.[1] There is no specific antidote for zinc phosphide. Because the conversion of zinc phosphide to phosphine gas is enhanced with gastric acidity, treatment with antacids is highly recommended.

The phosphine gas emitted from the affected animal is a human health hazard and can be dangerous to hospital personnel even at levels that cannot be detected by smell. Therefore precautions such as adequate ventilation should be taken to protect staff members.[1]

INSECTICIDES

Insecticides are primarily used in and around cats for flea control. They can be used as sprays, powders, flea collars, dips, and spot-on treatments. When used according to the label directions, most insecticides can be used safely around cats. In the United States these products are regulated as pesticides by the Environmental Protection Agency (EPA). Most incidents reported to the EPA are minor, but major incidents, including death, have occurred. Serious adverse effects are most likely to occur when products labeled for dogs—often bearing a name similar to that of a product labeled for cats—are inappropriately or mistakenly applied to cats, especially products containing permethrin. Problems may also occur when products are not applied according to label directions, or are applied to ill cats. In addition, cats have been affected by exposure to treated dogs. It may be prudent to keep cats away from dogs immediately after treatment with spot-on products. Adverse effects should be reported to the product manufacturer. In the United States veterinarians should also report incidents to the National Pesticide Information Center and the EPA (see Box 31-1).

Pyrethrins and Pyrethroids

Pyrethrins are naturally derived from chrysanthemum flowers, whereas pyrethroids are synthetic analogs. These compounds modify the sodium channels in nervous tissue and muscle cell membranes, causing repetitive discharging of the cell and clinical signs of neurotoxicity. Most insecticidal products labeled for use in cats contain low levels of pyrethrin and, if used appropriately, are relatively safe for cats.[37]

Permethrin is derived from a combination of esters that are extracted from dried chrysanthemum flowers and is further classified as a type I pyrethroid.[37] This insecticide is used in spot-on flea treatments for dogs but is contraindicated in cats because of the high risk of toxicity. Cautionary labeling on canine products may not be visible enough or adequate to prevent inappropriate use, and risk awareness among pet owners may be low. Cats are highly sensitive to the effects of permethrin, probably because of their deficiency of hepatic glucuronidase transferase.[6] Permethrin toxicity is one of the most commonly reported feline toxicities.[28,50]

Cats are most commonly exposed to concentrated permethrin compounds inappropriately or accidentally through exposure to topical flea products intended for canine use only. These spot-on products can contain 45% to 65% permethrin or more. The most commonly seen clinical signs include tremors, muscle fasciculations, ear twitching, facial twitching, hyperesthesia, ataxia, ptyalism, pyrexia, mydriasis, and seizures.[6] Clinical signs may occur with exposure to only a few drops of the concentrated solution and may occur within a few hours or several days. In general, clinical signs will continue for 24 to 72 hours but may last up to 7 days.[37,50] Death occurs in about 10% of cases.[50]

Diagnosis of permethrin toxicity is based on a history of recent exposure and typical clinical signs. Differential diagnoses include other causes of seizures and tremors. Treatment should focus on seizure control, decontamination, and supportive care (Box 31-2). With recent exposures to permethrin, the cat should be bathed completely using lukewarm water and mild hand dishwashing detergent or shampoo to remove any residual product. Hot water should not be used because it may increase dermal perfusion and uptake of permethrin. Seizures and tremors typically respond to methocarbamol (see Table 31-1).[37] Other options for seizure control include propofol, barbiturates, diazepam, and inhalant anesthetics. In addition, supportive care, including maintaining normal body temperature, supplying intravenous fluids, and providing nutritional support, is needed.

Cholinesterase Inhibitors

Cholinesterase inhibitors include carbamates and organophosphates. These compounds have been widely used in agricultural and veterinary medicine for decades. Cats may be exposed accidentally or by inappropriate use of products. Organophosphates are very toxic to cats and not recommended in this species. Carbamates (e.g., carbaryl) are less toxic and are found in several insecticides marketed for use in cats in various formulations (e.g., shampoos, powders, collars). These compounds bind to and inhibit cholinesterases, causing excess accumulation of acetylcholine and resulting in cholinergic excitation and muscarinic and nicotinic signs.[27] Organophosphates have higher binding affinity than carbamates and are often called *irreversible inhibitors.*

Clinical signs result from overstimulation of the cholinergic nervous system, as well as skeletal muscle and the CNS, and appear within minutes to hours after exposure.[53] Clinical signs of toxicity include classic muscarinic signs often referred to as *SLUDGE signs:* salivation, *l*acrimation, *u*rination, *d*efecation, *g*astrointestinal upset, and *e*mesis.[27] Nicotinic signs include ataxia, weakness, tremors, and muscle fasciculations. Cholinesterase inhibitors can also cause seizures, increased bronchial secretions, pulmonary edema, and bradycardia.[27]

Diagnosis is based on history of exposure and compatible clinical signs. To confirm exposure to a

BOX 31-2

Recommendations for Treatment of Permethrin Toxicosis* in the Cat

Veterinary Treatment Plan:

1. **Seizure control**
   - Diazepam: 0.25-0.5 mg/kg IV (can also be given rectally), repeat as needed every 3-5 min
   - Midazolam: 0.3 mg/kg IV/IM, repeat as needed every 3-5 min

If ongoing seizures after benzodiazepine bolus × 2, then consider:
   - Propofol: 4-6 mg/kg slow IV as a bolus, then 0.05-0.3 mg/kg per min IV as a CRI
   - Alfaxalone CD: 2-3 mg/kg slow IV bolus
   - Phenobarbitone: 2-4 mg/kg slow IV, diluted 1:10 with 0.9% NaCl. Repeat as needed every 2 h, total dose should not exceed 20 mg/kg/day
2. **Muscle fasciculation control.** Note that the aim is not to completely anaesthetize the patient but to decrease the severity of clinical signs.
   - Methocarbamol (if available): 55-200 mg/kg IV/PO every 8 hours, up to a maximum dose of 330 mg/kg per day
   - Midazolam: 0.2 mg/kg/hour IV as a CRI
   - Propofol: 0.05-0.3 mg/kg per min IV as a CRI
3. **Ensure patent airway.** Swab/suction pharynx if patient is hypersalivating. Provide oxygen support if needed (maintain SpO_2 >95%).
4. **Skin decontamination.** Warm bath with mild detergent, towel, warm blow dry.
5. **Temperature monitoring and control.** Maintain body temperature 38°-39° C.
6. **IV crystalloids.** Aim for 1.5 × maintenance rates. Monitor packed cell volume/total plasma protein, electrolytes every 12 hours; check urine specific gravity when available.
7. **Ocular lubrication.** Every 4 h (e.g., Lacrilube/Opticin)
8. **Bladder expression or urethral catheterization:** Every 6-8 h (lower motor neuron [LMN] bladder).
9. **Quiet, darkened environment.**
10. **Maintain sterna recumbency,** head slightly elevated, turn hind legs every 6 h.
11. **Prevent self-grooming.** Apply Elizabethan collar once mobility begins to improve.

IV, Intravenously; *IM,* intramuscularly; *CRI,* constant-rate infusion; *PO,* by mouth.

**Source: Protocols, Animal Referral Hospital, Sydney, NSW, Australia.*

From: Boland LA, Angles JM: Feline permethrin toxicity: retrospective study of 42 cases, *J Feline Med Surg* 12:61, 2010.

cholinesterase inhibitor, whole blood, serum, or plasma cholinesterase enzyme activity (ACHE test) can be evaluated through an accredited veterinary laboratory. The diagnosis is confirmed if the cholinesterase activity is less than 25% of normal. In addition, the insecticide can be detected in stomach contents and tissues. Changes on complete blood cell count, serum chemistry panel, and urinalysis are generally nonspecific.[53]

Patients affected by organophosphate or carbamate toxicity may deteriorate quickly so treatment must be initiated as soon as possible. Respiratory failure is the main cause of death, so artificial respiration may be required. Treatment also includes control of seizures. The specific antidote for organophosphate toxicity is pralidoxime chloride (2-PAM; Protopam, Ayerst Laboratories), which releases cholinesterase from the organophosphate. 2-PAM will control nicotinic signs and is most effective when given as soon as possible after exposure (preferably within 24 to 48 hours). Clinical improvement should occur within 3 to 4 days, and treatment is continued as long as needed. This drug is usually not recommended for carbamate toxicity.[53]

Although atropine is often considered an antidote to cholinesterase inhibitors insofar as it blocks the effects of the excess acetylcholine at the neuromuscular junction, it should be used with caution. If muscarinic signs are present, a test dose (0.02 mg/kg intravenously) can be given to determine if the signs are due to organophosphate or carbamate toxicity versus other causes. If the heart rate increases and the pupils dilate in response to the test dose, the clinical signs are probably not due to organophosphate or carbamate toxicity. This is because the atropine dose required to resolve clinical signs caused by insecticide toxicity is about 10 times the preanesthetic dose of the drug. If insecticide toxicity is confirmed, atropine can be administered to control muscarinic signs (see Table 31-1). The dose is adjusted by monitoring response, especially heart rate and secretion production.

Activated charcoal may be used to bind insecticide in the gastrointestinal tract, and bathing with soap and water can be used for cats with dermal exposure to prevent further absorption. Additional treatments may include methocarbamol, diazepam, or phenobarbital to control seizures and muscle tremors.[53] Good supportive and nursing care, including intravenous fluid therapy and nutritional management, is essential.

Other Topical Spot-On Products

There is limited published information regarding adverse effects of most topical spot-on products approved for use in cats, although they appear to be generally safe.[39] Most products are applied to the area between the shoulder blades and are intended for use every 30 days. Oral exposure to topical products may result in excessive drooling and gastrointestinal upset owing to the bitter taste. Hypersensitivity skin reactions may occur with any topical product, and signs are expected to resolve with bathing and supportive care (e.g., topical corticosteroids, antihistamines).

Imidacloprid

Imidacloprid is a chloronicotinyl nitroguanide insecticidal agent that is used as a spot-on product labeled to kill fleas (but not ticks) in dogs and cats. It is marketed as Advantage Topical Solution (Bayer HealthCare, Shawnee Mission, Kansas). In combination with moxidectin, it is marketed as Advantage Multi and Advocate (Bayer HealthCare). When applied topically, it spreads rapidly over the cat's skin by translocation but is not absorbed systemically. Imidacloprid acts by blocking the nicotinergic pathways, which results in a buildup of acetylcholine at the neuromuscular junction, causing impairment of normal nerve function and death of the insect.[20] Imidacloprid is also found in combination with permethrin in dog-only products (K9 Advantix, Bayer HealthCare), which can be dangerous if used accidentally or inappropriately on a cat because of the permethrin.

Imidacloprid products formulated for use on cats have a low order of toxicity. The manufacturer recommends caution when used in debilitated, elderly, pregnant, or nursing animals and kittens younger than 4 months of age. There is one report of a cat with a thymoma that developed dermatosis (erythema multiforme) and systemic signs shortly after being treated with imidacloprid.[14] A combination of paraneoplastic syndrome and drug reaction may have caused the cat's clinical signs.

Oral exposure to imidacloprid through grooming may cause mild and self-limiting drooling or retching as a result of the bitter taste of the product.[20,39] Imidacloprid poisoning would be expected to produce nicotinic signs.[39] Dermal hypersensitivity reactions from topical application should be treated by bathing with a non-insecticidal shampoo and symptomatic care (e.g., antihistamines, hydrocortisone). Ocular exposure is treated with lavage.

Fipronil

Fipronil is a phenylpyrazole antiparasitic agent introduced in the United States in 1996 as a flea and tick control product. It is marketed for veterinary use as Frontline Top Spot and Frontline Spray (Merial; Duluth, Georgia). It may be found in combination with methoprene, an insect growth regulator (Frontline Plus, Merial). Fipronil is classified as a gamma-aminobutyric acid (GABA) agonist, and it causes its effects on insects by disrupting CNS activity.[20] After topical application the product spreads over the skin by translocation and collects in skin oils and hair follicles.

Fipronil products for veterinary use have a low order of toxicity by dermal, oral, and inhalation exposure.[20] Oral exposure may cause mild and self-limiting drooling and vomiting. A dermal hypersensitivity reaction may occur within hours of application of topically applied products.[58] Affected cats should be bathed in a non-insecticidal shampoo and treated symptomatically (e.g., antihistamines, hydrocortisone). Ocular exposure causes mild reactions that are treated with lavage.

Selamectin

Selamectin is a semisynthetic avermectin developed specifically for broad-spectrum use in dogs and cats and was introduced in the United States in 2000. It is marketed as the spot-on product Revolution (Pfizer Animal Health). Selamectin causes parasite death through neuromuscular paralysis by increasing permeability in neuronal chloride channels.[20] Mammals have less sensitive chloride channels and so are less affected.

Topical selamectin is labeled for use in cats against fleas *(Ctenocephalides felis)*, ear mites *(Otodectes cynotis)*, hookworm *(Ancylostoma tubaeforme)*, and roundworm *(Toxocara cati)*. It is also approved as a preventive for heartworm disease. Although it is applied topically, it is absorbed systemically, with peak plasma levels occurring approximately 15 hours after application in cats.[34] Selamectin is distributed selectively to the sebaceous glands, where it acts against external parasites. According to studies, adverse effects of selamectin are rare.[20] The most common adverse effect is minor skin irritation (redness, irritation) or transient alopecia at the site of application.[58] Other possible adverse effects include diarrhea, vomiting, muscle tremors, anorexia, pruritus/urticaria, erythema, lethargy, salivation, and tachypnea. Accidental oral ingestion through grooming causes self-limiting salivation and intermittent vomiting in cats. There is no specific antidote, and treatment is symptomatic and supportive.

POISONOUS PLANTS

Lilies

Several species of the *Lilium* genus, including Easter lily *(Lilium longiflorum)*, tiger lily *(Lilium lancifolium,* formerly *tigrinum)*, Asian lily *(Lilium asiatica)*, Stargazer lily *(Lilium auratum)*, and others have been shown to cause acute kidney failure in cats, characterized by acute tubular necrosis.[40,48,54] Also, some species of daylily *(Hemerocallis* genus) are potentially dangerous for cats.[15] These flowering plants are common in gardens, as potted houseplants, and as cut flowers (Figures 31-2, 31-3, and 31-4).

Exposure to any part of the plant, including the pollen, can lead to toxicosis. Even consuming less than one leaf can lead to severe consequences.[23] Cats appear to be the only species in which this poisoning occurs, and the mechanism of action and toxic ingredient is not known, although it appears to be water soluble and most concentrated in the flowers.[23] The case fatality rate is often high, and surviving cats may suffer permanent renal damage.[48]

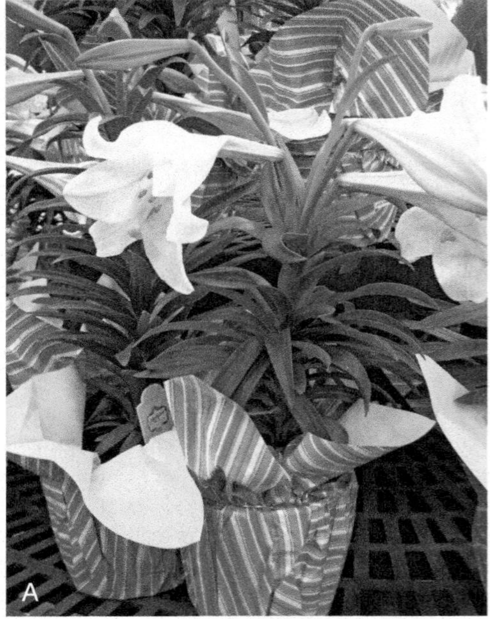

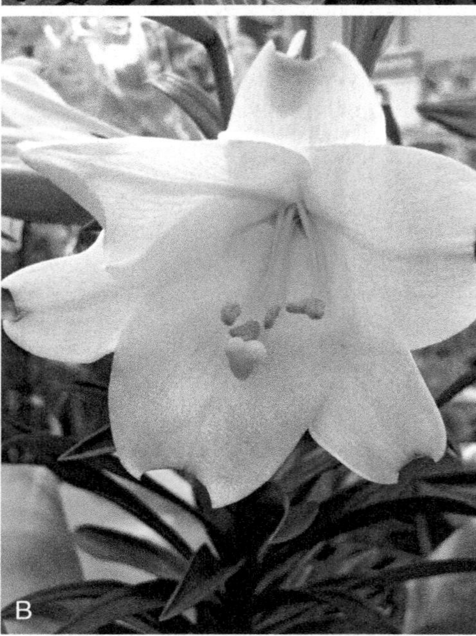

FIGURE 31-2 **A,** Easter lilies *(Lilium longiflorum)* are popular houseplants in the spring. **B,** All parts of the plant are highly toxic. *(Courtesy Dr. Vicki Thayer.)*

Clinical signs typically develop within 12 hours of ingestion (but may be delayed for up to 5 days) and include vomiting, anorexia, depression, polyuria, and polydipsia (Table 31-2).[16] Less frequent signs include disorientation, ataxia, face and paw edema, head pressing, and seizures.[5] The initial vomiting often subsides in 4 to 6 hours, leading to a false impression that the cat is recovering from an innocuous problem.[16] Renal failure develops within 24 to 96 hours of ingestion.[54] Laboratory abnormalities include azotemia (with creatinine disproportionately increased compared with BUN), glycosuria,

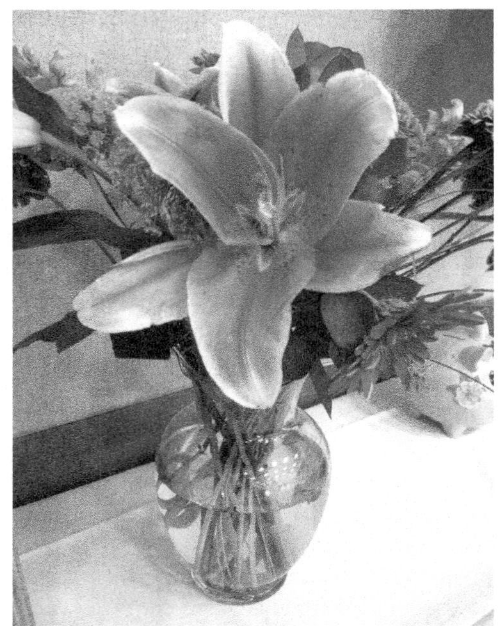

FIGURE 31-3 Stargazer lilies *(Lilium auratum)* are also highly toxic to cats and are found as garden plants and as cut flowers. *(Courtesy Dr. Edward Javinsky.)*

TABLE 31-2 **Onset and Duration of Common Clinical Signs and Changes with Lily Toxicosis in Cats**

Clinical Sign/ Parameter	Onset	Duration from Onset
Vomiting	0-3 h	4-6 h
Salivation	0-3 h	4-6 h
Anorexia	0-3 h	Throughout syndrome
Depression	0-3 h	Throughout syndrome
Proteinuria	12-24 h	Until anuria develops
Urinary casts	12-24 h	Until anuria develops
Glucosuria	12-24 h	Until anuria develops
Isosthenuria	12-24 h	Until anuria develops
Polyuria	12-30 h	12-24 h
Dehydration	18-30 h	Until corrected
Serum chemistry changes	>24 h	Until corrected
Vomiting reoccurs	30-72 h	Through remainder of syndrome
Anuria	24-48 h	Through remainder of syndrome
Weakness	36-72 h	Through remainder of syndrome
Recmbency	48-72 h	Through remainder of syndrome
Death	3-7 days	

From Hall J: Lily. In Plumlee KH, editor: *Clinical veterinary toxicology,* St Louis, 2004, Mosby, p 434.

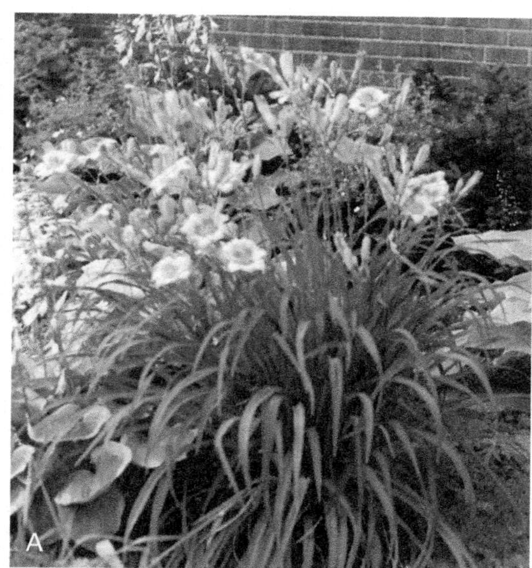

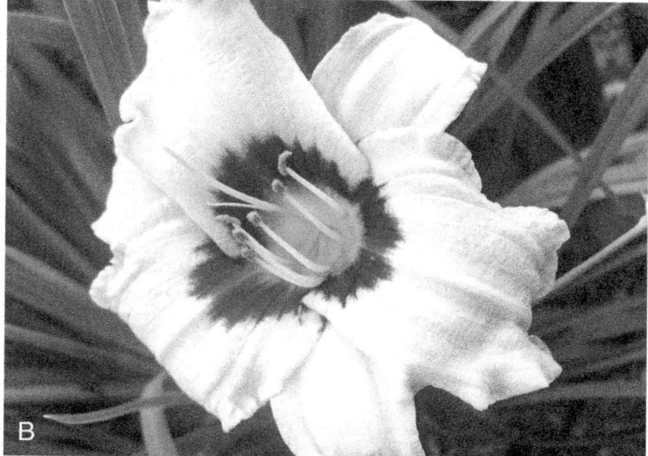

FIGURE 31-4 **A** and **B,** Day lilies (*Hemerocallis* spp.) are common garden plants available in thousands of varieties that are toxic to cats. *(A courtesy Tori-Rose Javinsky).*

proteinuria, isosthenuria, and tubular epithelial urinary casts.[16,23,54] No crystalluria occurs with lily toxicity.[16] Increases in liver enzymes may occur late in the course of illness.[16] The differential diagnosis includes EG toxicity, nonsteroidal antiinflammatory drug (NSAID) toxicity, and chronic renal disease.

With recent exposures decontamination followed by fluid diuresis at twice the maintenance rate with lactated Ringer's solution for a minimum of 48 hours is recommended.[40] If ingestion occurred less than 2 hours before presentation and no clinical signs have appeared, emesis can be induced (even if the cat has already vomited), followed by activated charcoal with a cathartic.[23] Dehydration is an important component in the development of renal damage, so initiation of fluid therapy is necessary to prevent permanent damage. Ideally, a central venous catheter and closed urine collection system should be placed. Referral to a 24-hour treatment facility

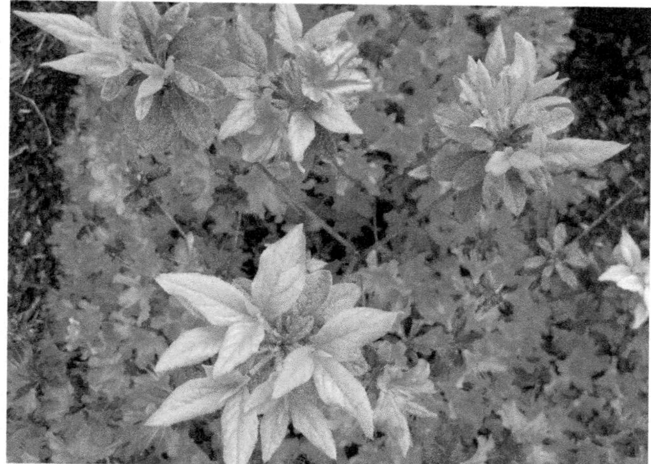

FIGURE 31-5 Azalea is an ornamental shrub that contains highly toxic grayanotoxins. *(Courtesy Dr. Vicki Thayer.)*

may be necessary. Baseline laboratory data (particularly serum chemistries and urinalysis) should be obtained. Renal function should be monitored for 2 to 3 days or more. Delayed treatment, even by 18 hours, can result in irreversible renal failure, leading to death or euthanasia.[54] Cats that receive prompt and aggressive treatment have a good prognosis. Cats that become oliguric or anuric have a poor prognosis but may respond to peritoneal dialysis. Cats that do not receive treatment will die in 3 to 7 days.[54]

Rhododendron Species

Rhododendron species (azalea, rhododendron, rosebay) contain grayanotoxin glycosides, which affect sodium channels in cell membranes, leading to neurologic, gastrointestinal, and cardiovascular dysfunction (Figures 31-5 and 31-6).[18] Grayanotoxins are found in all parts of the plant, including the flowers and nectar, and as few as two leaves may cause serious poisonings. Clinical signs include vomiting, diarrhea, abdominal pain, weakness, depression, cardiac arrhythmias, hypotension, shock, cardiopulmonary arrest, pulmonary edema, dyspnea, lethargy, seizures, and death.[18]

Decontamination and cardiovascular support are recommended after exposure. There is no specific antidote. Early induction of emesis followed by activated charcoal with a cathartic is important. Electrocardiography should be used to monitor heart rate and rhythm, and blood pressure should also be monitored. Cardiovascular support may require aggressive intravenous fluid therapy and sodium channel-blocking drugs (e.g., quinidine, procainamide, atropine) may be useful for some patients.[18]

Plants Containing Cardiac Glycosides

Hundreds of cardiac glycosides have been identified in plants; the most commonly known is digitalis, which has

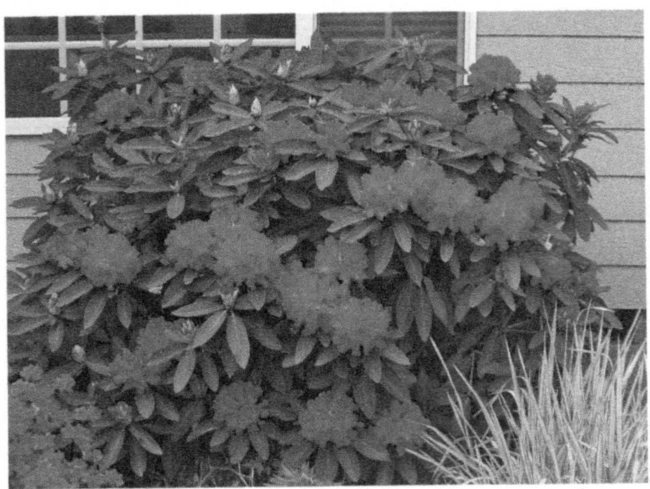

FIGURE 31-6 Rhododendrons are popular ornamental shrubs. Grayanotoxins are found in every part of the plant. *(Courtesy Dr. Vicki Thayer.)*

been used medicinally in human and veterinary medicine for many years. All parts of cardiac glycoside–containing plants are toxic, and even small amounts can cause significant clinical signs, including death. Examples of cardiac glycoside–containing plants include oleander *(Nerium oleander)*, lily-of-the-valley *(Convallaria majalis)*, foxglove *(Digitalis purpurea)*, certain milkweeds *(Asclepias* spp.), and squill *(Urginea maritima)*.[18]

Cardiac glycosides inhibit the sodium–potassium ATPase pump and slow cardiac electrical conductivity.[18] Onset of clinical signs varies with the species of plant ingested but may occur within hours of ingestion and last for several days. Clinical signs are related to the cardiovascular system and the gastrointestinal tract and include vomiting, abdominal pain, bradycardia, ventricular arrhythmias, and even sudden death.[18] Diagnosis is based on identification of the plant ingested.

Treatment includes early induction of emesis, followed by activated charcoal with a cathartic.[13,18] Monitoring with electrocardiography is recommended for at least 24 hours. Further treatment varies with the specific cardiac abnormalities detected. Prognosis is poor without early and aggressive intervention.[18]

Castor Bean Plant

The castor bean plant *(Ricinus communis)* is used as a decorative plant, and oil extracted from the seeds is used in industry and medicine. The toxic principle is ricin,[2] which is one of the most potent toxins known, and it is often linked to bioterrorism. All parts of the castor bean plant are toxic, but the seeds contain the highest concentration of ricin and are most commonly associated with poisoning.[2] Damage to the seed coat (usually by chewing) is required to allow the ricin to be available for absorption. Castor bean oil should not contain ricin if it is properly manufactured.[2] Another decorative plant containing a similar phytotoxin (abrin) is the rosary pea or jequirity bean *(Albrus precatorius)*.[18] It is used in Latin America to make jewelry for tourists and is also grown in Florida and Hawaii.

Clinical signs appear within hours of ingestion and may last for up to 5 days. Ricin is a cellular toxin, and its major effects are on the intestinal mucosa.[2] Initial clinical signs include vomiting, diarrhea, and abdominal pain, progressing to hemorrhagic gastroenteritis, seizures, and cerebral edema.[18] There is no specific antidote, and treatment consists of decontamination and supportive care. Prognosis is poor once clinical signs appear.[18]

Cycad Palms (Cycas, Zamia Species)

Cycad palms and similar ornamental plants are generally found in tropical to subtropical climates but may also be grown as houseplants in more temperate climates. Cycasin is considered to be the toxic principle that is responsible for the hepatoxicity and gastrointestinal signs generally seen with toxicosis.[18,59] Most parts of the plant are toxic, but the seeds contain a higher concentration of cycasin. Clinical signs include vomiting and diarrhea, lethargy, depression, liver failure, coagulopathy, and death. Neurologic signs, such as weakness, ataxia, seizures, and coma, may also be seen.[18] There is no specific antidote. Treatment includes early decontamination and supportive care.

Plants Containing Insoluble Calcium Oxalates

Many plants, including peace lily (*Spathiphyllum* spp.), calla lily (*Zantedeschia* spp.) (Figure 31-7), *Philodendron* spp. (Figure 31-8), and *Dieffenbachia* spp. (Figure 31-9) contain insoluble calcium oxalate crystals.[26] These crystals can cause mechanical irritation of the oral cavity. The clinical signs seen with ingestion of these plants include oral pain, difficulty swallowing, hypersalivation, swelling of the oral cavity, vomiting, depression, and inappetence.[26] Clinical signs are temporary and rarely severe and usually respond to supportive care, such as rinsing the mouth with water and offering a small quantity of milk or yogurt. Oral swelling can be treated with an antihistamine, and a protectant such as kaolin/pectin can reduce gastrointestinal irritation.[26]

HOUSEHOLD HAZARDS

Ant and Roach Baits

Ant and roach baits are common objects found in households. They are also referred to as hotels, traps, or stations. The insecticides used most commonly in these

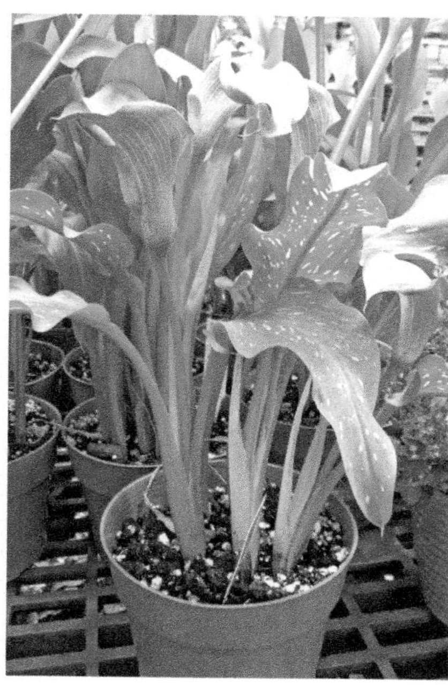

FIGURE 31-7 The calla lily (*Zantedeschia* spp.) is not a true lily but is toxic to cats on account of the presence of calcium oxalates found in all parts of the plant.

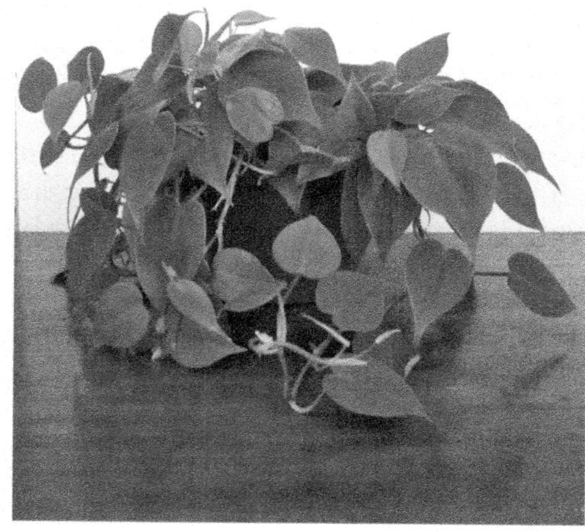

FIGURE 31-8 Philodendrons are tropicals that are common ornamental houseplants. The leaves contain insoluble calcium oxalates, which can cause oral irritation.

baits are present only in small amounts and include chlorpyrifos, sulfluramid, fipronil, avermectin, boric acid, and hydramethylnon. The baits usually contain inert ingredients such as peanut butter, breadcrumbs, sugars, and fats, which could be attractive to pets. Exposures to these types of baits usually do not require decontamination or treatment. Most often, if signs are seen at all, they are mild in nature and self-limiting and are usually attributed to the inert ingredients instead of the active ingredient. However, cats that ingest baits containing chlorpyrifos, an organophosphate, may require decontamination and treatment (as discussed previously).

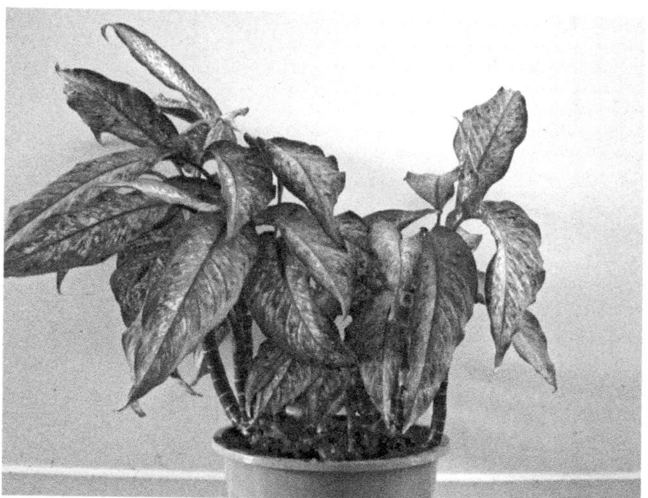

FIGURE 31-9 Dieffenbachia (dumb cane) belongs to the tropical *Araceae* family and also contains insoluble calcium oxalates.

Silica Gel Packets

Silica gel is used as a desiccant and often comes in paper packets or plastic cylinders. These products are used to absorb moisture with leather, medication, and some food packaging. Silica is considered to be chemically inert if ingested. However, if large amounts are ingested, it is possible to see signs of gastrointestinal upset, such as nausea, vomiting, and inappetence. Additional problems could occur if the silica gel was used as a desiccant in medication packaging because the silica may have absorbed qualities of the medication.

Liquid Potpourri and Essential Oils

Liquid potpourri is used as a fragrance, often heated over a candle or other heat source (Figure 31-10). Cats may be exposed by ingesting the oil directly from the container or licking oil from fur or feet. Liquid potpourri is made with essential oils, sometimes in combination with cationic detergents, both of which can be harmful.[35] Essential oils can cause mucous membrane and gastrointestinal irritation, CNS depression, and dermal hypersensitivity and irritation. Severe clinical signs can be seen with potpourri products that contain cationic detergents, which can be corrosive to the skin and mucous membranes. Dermal exposure to cationic detergents can result in erythema, edema, intense pain, and ulceration. Ingestion of cationic detergents can lead to tissue necrosis and inflammation of the mouth, esophagus, and

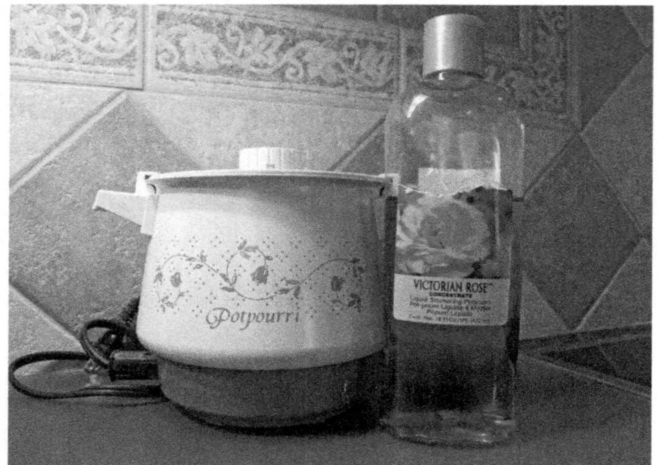

FIGURE 31-10 Liquid potpourri is heated in an electric appliance or over a candle as a room fragrance. It contains essential oils and cationic detergents that are highly toxic to cats if ingested. *(Courtesy Dr. Vicki Thayer.)*

stomach.[35,49] Additional clinical signs include hyperthermia, tachypnea, ptyalism, and lethargy.[49] Cationic detergents can also be found in some household cleaners, disinfectants, sanitizers, and fabric softeners.

If the exposure is detected promptly, dilution of the chemicals with milk or water may be attempted.[28] Induction of emesis is avoided, as is the use of activated charcoal.[28] Sulcralfate as a slurry can be used to coat and protect oral lesions. Pain management is indicated for cats with ulcerations. Supportive care, including nutritional support (sometimes through a nasogastric or esophageal feeding tube) and intravenous fluids, may be required for several days.

Melaleuca oil is another essential oil derived from the leaves of the Australian tea tree *(Melaleuca alternifolia)*. Melaleuca oil products are sold as topical treatments for skin problems, as insect repellants, and for many other uses. Unfortunately, it is a myth that melaleuca oil is nontoxic for dogs and cats; toxicities are not uncommon, especially when 100% oil is used topically for parasite control. The toxic components are cyclic hydrocarbons and terpenes.[7]

Melaleuca oil is rapidly absorbed from the skin and gastrointestinal tract.[7] Cats are probably at higher risk of toxicity than dogs because they have a limited ability to perform hepatic glucuronidation of terpenes.[7] Clinical signs of toxicity include weakness, ataxia, muscle tremors, depression, vomiting, diarrhea, and hypothermia.[25,53] Elevation in liver enzymes and even liver failure may occur.[25] Onset of clinical signs is 2 to 8 hours, and duration is 1 to 2 days.[7,53]

There is no antidote for tea tree oil toxicity, and treatment consists of decontamination and supportive care (e.g., intravenous fluids, maintenance of body temperature). Removal of the oil from the skin can be accomplished by bathing in a mild shampoo or detergent. If ingestion has occurred as a result of grooming, activated charcoal and a cathartic may be used. Induction of emesis is contraindicated.[25] Most affected cats recover over a 2- to 3-day period.[53]

Pennies

United States pennies minted after 1982 are composed of copper plating around a zinc core.[38] One penny contains approximately 2440 mg of zinc, and poisoning has been reported as a result of ingesting just one coin.[38] Zinc can affect the renal, hepatic, and the hematopoietic tissues. Zinc can also cause hemolytic anemia, which could lead to hemoglobinemia, hemoglobinuria, or both.[38] Surgical removal of the penny is recommended over chelation therapy.[38] Supportive care, including gastrointestinal protectants, fluid diuresis, and blood transfusions, may be needed.[38]

Ethylene Glycol

EG is a hydrocarbon derivative.[41] Most commercial antifreeze preparations contain between 95% to 97% EG and are usually mixed 50:50 when used in automobile radiators. Cats may be exposed accidentally through ingestion of radiator leaks or product spills. Unfortunately, the taste appears to be attractive to cats. EG may also be added to toilets in winter months to prevent pipe freezing, and cats that drink water out of the toilets may be exposed. The minimum lethal dose of undiluted EG is approximately 1.4 mL/kg in cats, so even small ingestions can be dangerous.[41,47]

EG is rapidly absorbed and can be measured in the blood within 30 minutes. EG is metabolized in the liver to more toxic compounds—to glycoaldehyde by alcohol dehydrogenase, and then glycoaldehyde is oxidized to glycolic acid and glyoxylic acid.[41] Glyoxylic acid is primarily converted to oxalic acid; calcium is bound to oxalic acid, resulting in calcium oxalate crystal formation, which is deposited in the kidneys. A wide range of tissue toxicities is seen with EG toxicity (gastric irritation, CNS dysfunction, metabolic acidosis, and renal failure).[55]

In most cases of EG poisonings, the animal begins vomiting within the first few hours. In 1 to 6 hours, signs of depression, ataxia and knuckling, weakness, tachypnea, hypothermia, polyuria, and polydipsia are seen.[47,55] Cats are less likely to exhibit polydipsia than dogs.[55] By 18 to 36 hours, acute oliguric renal failure occurs. The kidneys may be swollen and painful.[55] Other signs seen with EG toxicosis include seizures, coma, and death.[41,47]

Common laboratory changes include increased anion gap, hyperosmolality, increased BUN and creatinine, hypocalcemia, isosthenuria, and calcium oxalate crystalluria.[22,47] Quantitative EG tests can be run through human diagnostic laboratories on an urgent basis for diagnosis as early as 30 minutes after ingestion.[41] Insofar as the minimum toxic blood level is not known in cats, any detection of EG would necessitate treatment.

In some cases it is helpful to examine the cat's oral cavity, face, paws, vomitus, and urine with a Wood's lamp for fluorescence.[55] This is because many (but not all) antifreeze solutions contain sodium fluorescein. Detection of fluorescence in a cat with compatible clinical signs may help confirm the diagnosis, but failure to detect fluorescence does not eliminate the possibility of EG toxicity.

In most cases of feline exposure to EG, decontamination steps are not helpful because it is absorbed too quickly. Emesis may be helpful only if it occurs within 30 minutes of exposure, and activated charcoal may be helpful only if given within 1 hour of ingestion.[41] Activated charcoal should not be administered if ethanol treatment is planned because it will inhibit absorption.[55]

The drug 4-methylpyrazole (4-MP) is an alcohol dehydrogenase inhibitor that inhibits conversion of EG to its more toxic metabolites. However, 4-MP has poor efficacy in cats when used at the canine dose and currently is not recommended,[10,47] although further research to identify the optimal dose may improve outcomes.[9] Intravenous ethanol is the treatment of choice in cats (see Table 31-1), despite its drawbacks (CNS depression, short-half life). Ethanol is the preferred substrate for alcohol dehydrogenase and is used to inhibit EG metabolism. Ethanol is most effective if started within 12 hours of ingestion.[47] Intravenous ethanol may have to be continued for up to 72 hours to ensure complete EG elimination. Supportive treatment, including intravenous fluid therapy, control of hyperkalemia and acidosis, diuresis, and nutritional support, is an important part of therapy. Prognosis is poor to guarded with most cases of EG poisoning in cats because most patients are presented for treatment too late in the course of the disease. The earlier treatment is initiated (preferably within 3 hours of ingestion), the better the chance of recovery.

ANIMAL HAZARDS

Bufo Toad

Cane or marine toads *(Bufo marinus)* are native to Central and South America and have been introduced throughout Oceania (including Australia) and the Caribbean. Colorado River toads *(Bufo alvarius)* are found in several U.S. states, including Florida, Texas, and Colorado. These toads are highly toxic. The skin of the Bufo toads contains a potent neurotoxin and cardiotoxin called *bufotoxin.*[45] When a cat has oral contact with this toad, the bitter taste initially causes hypersalivation and vomiting, which may help in self-decontamination. With ingestion of bufotoxin, clinical signs can include weakness, cardiac arrhythmias, seizures, nystagmus, coma, and death.[45]

Diagnosis is based on a history of exposure and compatible clinical signs. The mouth of a cat suspected of oral exposure to Bufo toads should be flushed thoroughly with water to remove any residue and the patient treated supportively for neurologic and cardiac abnormalities. Seizures may be treated with diazepam, and marked bradycardia with atropine. Most animals recover if treated early.

Poisonous Snakes

There are two types of poisonous snakes in North America: those that produce myotoxins, and those that produce neurotoxins. Pit vipers (crotalids) include rattlesnakes, copperheads, and water moccasins. Pit vipers are widespread in the United States and account for 99% of all snakebites.[32] Crotalid venom causes a disseminated intravascular coagulopathy–like syndrome but also has effects on many body systems because of the complex mix of toxins produced by the various snakes.[8,32] Clinical signs include severe localized pain at the site of the bite wound, salivation, weakness, hypotension, and bleeding. Onset of clinical signs may occur several hours after the bite occurred.

Coral snakes (elapids) are less commonly involved in envenomation because they must chew on their victim to inject venom, and their venom potency is low.[32] Elapid venom affects the CNS, and clinical signs do not occur for more than 10 hours after contact.[8] It may take up to 2 weeks for the venom to be cleared.[32] In cats clinical signs include ascending flaccid quadriplegia, loss of cutaneous nociception, depression, and hypothermia. Death is typically caused by respiratory collapse.

According to studies, specific antivenins can increase the chances of a full recovery but only if they are used before moderate to severe signs are seen.[32] Unfortunately, most snake bites in cats are not witnessed, and most envenomation may not be identified until the cat becomes symptomatic. In addition to antivenins, cases of snake bites should be treated symptomatically and supportively according to the clinical signs and affected body systems. Prognosis is poor with severe clinical signs.

Poisonous Spiders

There are two types of poisonous spiders in North America. Just as with snake bites, most spider bites are not witnessed, and until clinical signs are seen or the bite wound is visualized, the spider bite may not be known. The venom of the widow spiders (*Latrodectus* spp.) contains potent neurotoxins including alpha-latrotoxin, which causes a massive release of neurotransmitters, including acetylcholine, norepinephrine, and dopamine.[44] Unlike the brown recluse bite, there is minimal tissue reaction at the site of the bite of the widow spiders. Diagnosis usually depends on onset of systemic clinical signs, which begin within 8 hours of envenomation.[8] The bite causes severe generalized pain, which results in the cat becoming extremely vocal and agitated. Hypersalivation, vomiting, diarrhea, and tremors are also commonly seen. Later stages result in muscle paralysis and death caused by cardiopulmonary collapse.[44] Supportive and symptomatic therapy is required for stabilization, including pain management.[8,44] The most effective treatment is the slow intravenous administration of antivenin (*Latrodectus* antivenin). The product acts rapidly, with resolution of clinical signs within 30 minutes.[8]

Because most bites by the brown recluse or violin spider (*Loxosceles* spp.) go unnoticed, the cat is usually presented with a severe wound that is several days old. *Loxosceles* venom contains necrotizing enzymes, and the lesions produced by them can persist for months.[8] One portion of the venom, the enzyme sphingomyelinase, may cause systemic effects, including hemolysis, hyperthermia, and nausea.[8] Although there is no specific antivenin for this spider bite, dapsone has been recommended to inhibit the influx of neutrophils and thus vasculitis at the site of the bite (see Table 31-1).[8,44] Dapsone should be administered within 36 hours of the envenomation.[44]

DRUGS

Cats may be exposed to dangerous medications either through accidental exposure or through inappropriate use by uninformed owners.

Acetaminophen

Acetaminophen (also known as paracetamol) is a derivative of P-aminophenol that has analgesic and antipyretic activity. Acetaminophen inhibits the effects of pyrogens by blocking prostaglandin synthesis and also by inhibiting cyclooxygenase (COX), which results in an increased pain threshold.[36] It is a common ingredient found in many human pain-relief products and cold and flu remedies and is available in more than 200 prescription and nonprescription formulations.[36] Cats are typically exposed when well-intentioned but uninformed owners administer the drug without consulting a veterinarian.

Although acetaminophen can be used safely in canine patients at a dose of 10 mg/kg every 12 hours, there is no safe dose for cats.[36] In fact, a single dose of 10 mg/kg has produced signs of poisoning in cats.[36] The reason for feline sensitivity to acetaminophen is based on the limited glucuronyl transferase activity in this species. Glucuronidation and sulfation pathways become saturated, and cellular glutathione stores are depleted. This results in the production of a highly reactive metabolite, *N*-acetyl-parabenzequinoneimine (NAPQI), which causes hepatocyte damage and also oxidative stress to red blood cells that leads to hemolysis and methemoglobinemia.[36]

The major adverse effects of acetaminophen toxicosis are related to methemoglobin and hemolysis. Clinical signs of acetaminophen poisoning in cats include vomiting, lethargy, facial and paw edema, brown-colored mucous membranes, dyspnea, and death.[43] Centrilobular or diffuse hepatic necrosis is also a possible complication but less common in cats than in dogs.[36,43]

With recent exposures to acetaminophen, decontamination through emesis and activated charcoal should take place. However, before administering activated charcoal, a preliminary dose of N-acetyl cysteine (NAC) should be given (see Table 31-1). NAC binds reactive toxic metabolites and is a glutathione precursor.[43] Treatment is most effective if started within 8 hours of ingestion.[43] Activated charcoal can then be given 2 hours later to help prevent the adsorption of NAC. NAC therapy and supportive care are indicated with any exposure. Cimetidine or ranitidine may be included as part of the treatment to reduce the metabolism of acetaminophen.[43] There is also some evidence that silymarin[4] and s-adenosylmethionine[57] may protect liver tissue against oxidative damage in cats with acetaminophen toxicity.

Ibuprofen and Other Nonsteroidal Antiinflammatory Drugs

The NSAIDs reduce inflammation by inhibiting the COX enzyme system. NSAID toxicity affects the gastrointestinal, renal, hepatic, and CNS through a variety of effects on COX enzymes. Most cats are poisoned through inappropriate administration by owners.

Ibuprofen is a substituted phenylalkanoic acid with nonsteroidal antiinflammatory, antipyretic, and analgesic properties. According to studies of acute ingestion of ibuprofen in dogs, vomiting, diarrhea, nausea, anorexia, gastric ulceration, and abdominal pain can be seen with doses of 50 to 125 mg/kg. These signs in combination with renal damage can be seen at doses at or above 175 mg/kg. At doses at or above 400 mg/kg, CNS effects such as seizure, ataxia, and coma may occur.[36] Cats are considered to be twice as sensitive as dogs because they have a limited glucuronyl-conjugating capacity.[36] Other NSAIDs may have similar toxicity, but limited published data are available.

The most common signs of NSAID toxicoses include anorexia, nausea, vomiting, lethargy, diarrhea, melena, ataxia, polyuria, and polydipsia. Postmortem lesions associated with NSAID toxicoses include perforations, erosion, ulceration, and hemorrhage of the gastrointestinal tract.[36]

The primary goal of treatment is to prevent or treat gastric ulceration, renal failure, CNS effects, and possibly hepatic effects. There is no specific antidote available. Prognosis is good if the animal is treated promptly and appropriately. Delay in treatment can decrease survival potential with large exposures. Fluid diuresis for 24 to 48 hours is recommended when ibuprofen doses approach or exceed approximately 75 mg/kg in cats.[36] Peritoneal dialysis may be necessary if unresponsive oliguric or anuric renal failure develops.

Misoprostol (Cytotec, Pfizer) may be helpful for treating or preventing gastric ulceration caused by ibuprofen.[36] Sucralfate can be used to bind to erosions and ulcers and protect them from exposure to gastric acid, bile acids, and pepsin.[36] H_2 blockers or proton pump inhibitors may also be helpful.

Gastric protection is recommended for at least 5 to 7 days. When renal failure is possible, BUN, creatinine, and urine specific gravity should be monitored closely. A baseline level and then rechecks at 36, 48, and 72 hours are recommended.[36] The animal should also be monitored for acidosis and electrolyte shifts during treatment. Symptomatic treatment for gastric signs and renal failure should be provided until the animal fully recovers.

Aspirin

Aspirin (acetylsalicylic acid) is the salicylate ester of acetic acid and is derived from phenol. Salicylates are commonly used as analgesics, and they also have antipyretic and antiinflammatory properties. In addition to its antiprostaglandin effect, aspirin uncouples oxidative phosphorylation and can cause an increase in oxygen consumption and carbon dioxide production. Aspirin can also inhibit platelet aggregation. Unlike ibuprofen, renal injury is uncommon in acute aspirin toxicosis, although hepatic injury has occasionally been reported.

The therapeutic dose in cats is 10 to 20 mg/kg every 48 hours.[34] Cats are deficient in glucuronyl transferase and therefore have a prolonged excretion rate and are more susceptible to toxicity.[43] For example, a dose of 25 mg/kg in a cat has an elimination half-life of almost 45 hours.[34] Caution is necessary for doses of more than 30 mg/kg, especially in geriatric cats, kittens, and cats with preexisting renal or hepatic disease.

Signs of aspirin toxicosis may include fever, hyperpnea, vomiting, melena, abdominal pain, seizures, and coma.[43] Clinical laboratory abnormalities may include elevations in liver enzymes, respiratory alkalosis, metabolic acidosis, and increased bleeding time.[43] There is no specific antidote, so treatment is symptomatic and supportive, including decontamination, intravenous fluid therapy to maintain renal function, and management of acidosis. Gastrointestinal protection with sucralfate or cimetidine may prevent further damage to the mucosa but may be required for up to 2 weeks.[43]

5-Fluorouracil

5-Fluorouracil (5-FU) is a fluorinated pyrimidine antagonist, which acts as an antineoplastic antimetabolite.[7] It is used in human patients to treat solar and actinic keratoses and some superficial skin tumors. Topical fluorouracil is available as 1% or 5% cream (Efudex, Valeant Pharmaceuticals). 5-FU can inhibit RNA processing and functioning as well as DNA synthesis and repair. The toxicity effects of 5-FU, as with other antineoplastic agents, occur mainly through destruction of rapidly dividing cell lines such as bone marrow stem cells and the epithelial layer of the intestinal crypts.[7] The drug is no longer recommended for topical treatment of squamous cell carcinoma in cats because it can cause severe toxicity and death. Cats are very sensitive to the effects of 5-FU, and even a few licks may cause life-threatening toxicity.[7]

Early effects seen with 5-FU include generalized grand mal seizures, tremors, vomiting, and ataxia.[7] Cardiac arrhythmia, respiratory distress, and hemorrhagic gastroenteritis are also seen. Clinical signs develop within 1 hour and are usually life threatening. Death often occurs within 6 to 16 hours after exposure. Induction of emesis is usually not recommended, given the rapid onset of toxicity. Thorough gastric lavage may be the preferred method of decontamination, followed by activated charcoal.[7] Seizures and tremors are often poorly responsive to treatment with diazepam, and other options, such as barbiturates, propofol, or gas anesthesia, must be used. Further treatment may include blood transfusion, intravenous fluid therapy, gastrointestinal protectants, analgesics, and broad-spectrum antibiotics. In those cats that survive the initial effects, bone marrow suppression may take 2 to 3 weeks to resolve.[7]

Isoniazid

Isoniazid (INH) is a medication used to treat tuberculosis and has a very narrow margin of safety.[56] The LD_{50} is estimated to be about 50 mg/kg in dogs. Isoniazid is available as an elixir, injection, syrup, and tablets (in strengths of 50, 100, and 300 mg). INH causes a decreased level of gamma-aminobutyric acid in the brain, and it also depletes the CNS of pyridoxine, the precursor of the coenzyme pyridoxal phosphate, which is necessary for the activity of the enzyme glutamic acid decarboxylase.[56] Overdoses produce life-threatening signs, including seizures, acidosis, and coma. Pyridoxine (vitamin B_6) is a direct agonist of INH.[56]

PRINCIPLES OF TREATMENT

When facing a potential poisoning exposure, the veterinarian must first evaluate the situation. It is very important to obtain as much information as possible about the exposure. *Who, what, when,* and *how* are key questions to ask your client. First, who was exposed? Second, what is the patient's signalment? Next, to what was the animal exposed? Finally, when did the exposure occur, and how? Obtaining the medical history and the exposure history is very important and can affect the way the patient is treated. Important elements of the toxicologic history are found in Box 31-3.

The initial examination of the patient should be performed quickly, with as little stress as possible, and should include assessment of the respiratory rate, capillary refill time, mucous membrane color, heart rate, and body temperature. Examination of a cat that is unconscious, in shock, seizing, or in distress must be conducted simultaneously with stabilization measures. If the cat is stable, a full history of the cat and the exposure should be taken, followed by a systematic physical examination. Patterns of clinical signs may be suggestive for certain drugs or toxins (Table 31-3).

In cases of contact with chemicals or medicines, the veterinarian should ask the pet owner to bring in the packaging information to confirm product contents. For example, a pet owner may say that the cat was given a "baby aspirin" when in fact it was actually an aspirin-free formulation containing acetaminophen. The treatment and prognosis for acetaminophen are quite different than those for aspirin.

BOX 31-3

Important Elements in Taking a Toxicologic History

1. Listen to the client, avoiding bias or preconceptions.
2. Observe the animal.
3. Identify and treat immediate life-threatening problems (e.g., seizures, arrhythmias); do not wait for confirmation of poisoning to initiate supportive therapy.
4. Identify the animal's home environment; determine whether other animals or children could be involved.
5. Identify any current medications, preexisting disease conditions, or pertinent previous medical history.
6. Investigate the history of the exposure: how long ago, what toxin, what concentration, how much? What toxins/poisons could be in the home environment?
7. Identify the poison if possible: Estimate the mg/kg dose, and determine the worst-case scenario.
8. Establish a timeline for the exposure and onset of clinical signs: Is the animal getting better, deteriorating, or showing no clinical signs?
9. Establish a minimum database.
10. Always treat the patient, not the poison.

Modified from Fitzgerald K: Taking a toxicological history. In Peterson M, Talcott P, editors: *Small animal toxicology,* ed 2, St Louis, 2006, Saunders Elsevier, pp 39-46.

Stabilization of Vital Functions

Stabilizing the cat is always a priority, and the ABCs should always be followed (i.e., airway, breathing, circulation). A patent airway should be established and artificial respiration given if the animal is dyspneic. The cardiovascular system should be monitored closely, preferably with an electrocardiographic monitor, and any cardiovascular abnormality should be corrected. If cardiac arrest occurs, cardiopulmonary resuscitation should be attempted. The placement of an indwelling intravenous catheter may be necessary for the administration of medications and intravenous fluids. Anticonvulsant therapy should be given if the animal has tremors or seizures (see Table 31-1), and attention should be paid to hypothermia or hyperthermia.

Once the cat is stable, metabolic derangements should be assessed and a management plan formulated. The minimum database for a suspected toxicosis includes a complete blood cell count, serum electrolytes, serum chemistries (especially glucose, BUN, creatinine, calcium), and urinalysis. Depending on the presenting signs and the suspected toxin, other laboratory tests may be necessary, such as coagulation testing, electrocardiography, blood gases, and radiographs of the chest and abdomen.

Decontamination

Preventing absorption of the toxicant through decontamination is important for treating a toxicosis. It is also important that the members of the veterinary staff protect themselves from exposure while treating affected animals by using protective gear such as gloves, safety glasses, and aprons. After dermal exposure to a toxicant, the cat should be bathed with a mild liquid hand dish detergent or a non-insecticidal shampoo, then thoroughly rinsed and dried. It may be necessary to repeat the procedure. Care should be taken when bathing debilitated or unstable animals. Oily substances can be removed with commercial hand-cleaning degreasers (avoiding those containing citrus), but care should be taken to wash the animal afterward with warm water and soap to remove the degreasing product. It may help to clip the hair coat of longhaired cats. The veterinarian

TABLE 31-3 **Clinical Signs Associated with Selected Toxins in Cats**

Toxin	Vital Signs	Mentation	Clinical Signs and Findings
Acetaminophen	Normal in early stages	Normal	Anorexia, vomiting, facial and paw edema, brown mucous membranes, dyspnea
Ethylene glycol	Tachypnea	Lethargy to coma	Vomiting, depression, ataxia, seizures, hypothermia
Metaldehyde	Hyperthermia, tachypnea, tachycardia	Lethargy to coma	Salivation, ataxia, tremors, seizures
Organophosphates and carbamates	Changes in blood pressure, heart rate, respiration	Lethargy to coma	Vomiting, diarrhea, salivation, tremors, seizures, ataxia
Pyrethrins/pyrethroids	Variable	Lethargy to coma	Vomiting, diarrhea, salivation, tremors, ataxia, seizures, mydriasis
Salicylates (aspirin)	Hyperthermia, tachycardia	Agitation, then lethargy to coma	Anorexia, vomiting, melena, abdominal pain, seizures

Modified from Fitzgerald K: Establishing a minimum database in small animal poisonings. In Peterson M, Talcott P, editors: *Small animal toxicology,* ed 2, St Louis, 2006, Saunders Elsevier, pp 61-73.

should monitor the skin for redness, swelling, or pain. Skin exposed to caustic substances should be flushed thoroughly with tepid water and handled gently to avoid mechanical injury. It is important to note that most dermal exposures in cats also lead to oral exposure through grooming.

For ocular exposures a minimum of 20 to 30 minutes of irrigation with tepid tap water, lactated Ringer's solution, or physiologic saline is recommended.[46] Fractious animals or those experiencing pain may require sedation. If the substance is corrosive, the veterinarian should examine the eyes for evidence of corneal ulceration. In cases involving corneal damage, the cat may require follow-up examinations or consultations with a veterinary ophthalmologist.

Inducing emesis can help remove toxicants from recent ingestions. Cats do have the ability to vomit; however, the length of time since ingestion, the cat's age, its previous medical history, and the type of poison can affect the decision to attempt emesis. Any cat with a history of cardiovascular abnormalities, epilepsy, recent abdominal surgery, or severe debilitation is not a candidate for emesis induction.[46] Emesis should not be induced in an animal that is severely depressed or in a coma because doing so could lead to aspiration. On the other hand, inducing vomiting in a hyperactive animal could trigger a seizure. Moreover, inducing vomiting in a cat that has already vomited is usually not recommended.

Another factor affecting the decision to induce emesis is the nature of the substance ingested. Emesis is contraindicated for corrosive materials such as cationic detergents, acids, and alkali. Induction of vomiting is not recommended with corrosives because of re-exposure of the esophageal tissues to the corrosive material. Instead, dilution with milk or water is the recommended initial treatment. Emesis is also contraindicated when a hydrocarbon has been ingested, with the main concern being aspiration. Some examples of hydrocarbon-containing products are tar, lubrication oils, fuel oil, kerosene, mineral spirits, and gasoline.

Establishing the time of exposure is important because emesis will be useful only if induced soon after the exposure (typically within 4 hours) and if food or liquid is present in the stomach. Several substances have been used as emetics but are generally unreliable and not recommended (e.g., dry salt, salt water, liquid dishwashing soap).[46] Other substances, such as syrup of ipecac, have been used, but the safest and most reliable emetics are hydrogen peroxide and apomorphine (see Table 31-1).

Hydrogen peroxide solution (3%), which can be purchased over the counter, has been shown to be an effective emetic for cats. Hydrogen peroxide can be administered with an eyedropper or a syringe by owners at home, under the direction of a veterinarian. Hydrogen peroxide causes mild gastric mucosal irritation, resulting in emesis. Typically, vomiting occurs within 15 minutes. If not, 3% hydrogen peroxide can be repeated one additional time at the same dose. Apomorphine can be used in cats to induce emesis; however, caution should be exercised because some cats will experience a paradoxical hyperactivity reaction with opioids. It is also not as reliable an emetic in cats as in dogs.

In cases when emesis is contraindicated but emptying stomach contents is essential, a gastric lavage under general anesthesia and using a cuffed endotracheal tube may be considered. A stomach tube is passed no further than the xiphoid process, and the patient is positioned with the head lower than the chest at approximately a 20-degree angle. Warm saline (10 mL/kg) is instilled, and manual agitation of the stomach is performed while the fluid is allowed to drain by gravity or is aspirated.[33] The procedure is repeated (often 10 to 20 times) until the lavage fluid is clear. The veterinarian should avoid overdistention of the stomach and occlude the end of the tube before removal. Complications of gastric lavage include aspiration pneumonia, laryngospasm, hypoxia, mechanical injury, and fluid and electrolyte imbalances.[33] Careful technique and patient selection can help minimize these risks.

Activated charcoal is a nonspecific adsorbent that binds to many substances through weak chemical forces and prevents their absorption. It is ineffective for corrosive substances; hydrocarbons; and most heavy metals, such as iron, lead, mercury, and arsenic.[46] Activated charcoal is available commercially in liquid, powder, and granular forms. The granular or powder form of activated charcoal can be mixed with water to facilitate administration. Activated charcoal can be administered orally with a syringe or by gastric tube (see Table 31-1). It is advisable to wait 1 to 2 hours after attempting emesis before administering activated charcoal to minimize the risk of aspiration through vomiting. However, waiting for more than 2 hours after most exposures will reduce the benefit. For toxins that undergo enterohepatic circulation, repeated doses of activated charcoal every 6 to 8 hours over several days may be beneficial.[46]

When gastric lavage is performed, activated charcoal may be administered before the lavage to slow absorption of the toxin and administered again after the lavage has been completed.[33] Contraindications to the use of activated charcoal include significant risk of aspiration, severe vomiting, and gastrointestinal perforation.[46]

Cathartics increase the clearing of intestinal contents. Two types are readily available: saline solutions (e.g., sodium sulfate [Glauber's salt], magnesium sulfate [Epsom salt]) and saccharide solutions (e.g., sorbitol). Mineral oil should never be used as a cathartic because of the high risk of aspiration and interference with charcoal adsorption.[46] Cathartics are used to enhance the elimination of activated charcoal and adsorbed toxicant. Premixed products that contain both activated charcoal and a cathartic (usually sorbitol) are available as commercial preparations, or cathartics can be added to solutions of activated charcoal. Veterinarians are advised to administer activated charcoal with a cathartic to facilitate removal of the charcoal-bound substance, unless the cat already has diarrhea or is dehydrated. Increasing the transit time of the activated charcoal through the gastrointestinal system will decrease the chances that the bonds between the charcoal and poison can weaken and allow the poison to be released. If activated charcoal is administered in multiple doses, the cathartic should be included only with the first dose to prevent fluid and electrolyte imbalances. Contraindications to the use of cathartics include ingestion of a corrosive substance, hypotension, dehydration, electrolyte abnormalities, abdominal trauma, and intestinal damage such as obstruction or perforation.[33]

Supportive Care

The cat's clinical signs should be managed with symptomatic and supportive care. The appropriate antidote or antagonist should be administered, if one exists. Monitoring of the acid–base balance, serum chemistry profile, hydration, or electrolytes may be necessary, depending on the potential effects of the toxicant involved. Some toxicants, such as iron, copper, acetaminophen, and arsenic, are hepatotoxic, whereas others, such as estrogen, lead, and antineoplastic medications, can cause anemia.

Diuresis may be beneficial with exposures to nephrotoxic agents or to enhance elimination of the poison. Examples of nephrotoxic agents that could benefit from diuresis include EG, zinc, mercury, oxalic acids, NSAIDs, diquat herbicide, and aminoglycoside antibiotics. Adverse effects associated with diuresis include pulmonary edema, cerebral edema, metabolic acidosis or alkalosis, and water intoxication; therefore close monitoring is necessary.

Supportive care should continue until the patient fully recovers. When the cat is released to the owner, the veterinary staff should take the time to explain what signs should be monitored for and how medication or treatment should be given and schedule follow-up visits as needed.

References

1. Albretsen J: Zinc phosphide. In Plumlee KH, editor: *Clinical veterinary toxicology*, St Louis, 2004, Mosby, p 456.
2. Albretsen JC: Lectins. In Plumlee KH, editor: *Clinical veterinary toxicology*, St Louis, 2004, Mosby, p 406.
3. Arnett D, Richardson J, Gwaltney-Brant SM et al: Clinical signs associated with methomyl toxicoses in dogs (January 1998-December 2001) (abstract), *J Vet Intern Med* 17:431, 2003.
4. Avizeh R, Najafzadeh H, Razijalali M et al: Evaluation of prophylactic and therapeutic effects of silymarin and N-acetylcysteine in acetaminophen-induced hepatotoxicity in cats, *J Vet Pharmacol Ther* 33:95, 2010.
5. Berg RI, Francey T, Segev G: Resolution of acute kidney injury in a cat after lily *(Lilium lancifolium)* intoxication, *J Vet Intern Med* 21:857, 2007.
6. Boland LA, Angles JM: Feline permethrin toxicity: retrospective study of 42 cases, *J Feline Med Surg* 12:61, 2010.
7. Brutlag A: Topical toxins. In Ettinger S,Feldman E, editors: *Textbook of veterinary internal medicine: diseases of the dog and cat*, ed 7, St Louis, 2010, Saunders Elsevier, p 565.
8. Burns P: Venomous bites and stings. In Ettinger S, Feldman E, editors: *Textbook of veterinary internal medicine: diseases of the dog and cat*, ed 7, St Louis, 2010, Saunders Elsevier, p 556.
9. Connally H, Hamar D, Thrall M: Inhibition of canine and feline alcohol dehydrogenase activity by fomepizole, *Am J Vet Res* 61:450, 2000.

10. Dial S, Thrall M, Hamar D: Comparison of ethanol and 4-methylpyrazole as treatments for ethylene glycol intoxication in cats, *Am J Vet Res* 55:1771, 1994.
11. Dorman D: Bromethalin. In Plumlee KH, editor: *Clinical veterinary toxicology*, St Louis, 2004, Mosby, p 446.
12. Dunayer E: Bromethalin: the other rodenticide, *Vet Med* 98:732, 2003.
13. Galey F: Cardiac glycosides. In Plumlee KH, editor: *Clinical veterinary toxicology*, St Louis, 2004, Mosby, p 386.
14. Godfrey DR: Dermatosis and associated systemic signs in a cat with thymoma and recently treated with an imidacloprid preparation, *J Small Anim Pract* 40:333, 1999.
15. Hadley R, Richardson J, Gwaltney-Brant S: A retrospective study of daylily toxicosis in cats, *Vet Hum Toxicol* 45:38, 2003.
16. Hall J: Lily. In Plumlee KH, editor: *Clinical veterinary toxicology*, St Louis, 2004, Mosby, p 433.
17. Hall K: Toxin exposures and treatments: a survery of practicing veterinarians. In Bonagura J,Twedt D, editors: *Kirk's current veterinary therapy XIV*, St Louis, 2009, Saunders Elsevier, p 95.
18. Hovda L: Plant toxicities. In Ettinger S, Feldman E, editors: *Textbook of veterinary internal medicine: diseases of the dog and cat*, ed 7, St Louis, 2010, Saunders Elsevier, p 561.
19. Hovda LR: Toxin exposures in small animals. In Bonagura J,Twedt D, editors: *Kirk's current veterinary therapy XIV*, St Louis, 2009, Saunders Elsevier, p 92.
20. Hovda LR, Hooser SB: Toxicology of newer pesticides for use in dogs and cats, *Vet Clin North Am Small Anim Pract* 32:455, 2002.
21. Kohn B, Weingart C, Giger U: Haemorrhage in seven cats with suspected anticoagulant rodenticide intoxication, *J Fel Med Surg* 5:295, 2003.
22. Luiz JA, Heseltine J: Five common toxins ingested by dogs and cats, *Compend Contin Educ Vet* 30:578, 2008.
23. Mason J, Khan S, Gwaltney-Brant SM: Recently recognized animal toxicants. In Bonagura J, Twedt D, editors: *Kirk's current veterinary therapy XIV*, St Louis, 2009, Saunders Elsevier, p 138.
24. Means C: Anticoagulant rodenticides. In Plumlee KH, editor: *Clinical veterinary toxicology*, St Louis, 2004, Mosby, p 444.
25. Means C: Essential oils. In Plumlee KH, editor: *Clinical veterinary toxicology*, St Louis, 2004, Mosby, p 149.
26. Means C: Insoluble calcium oxalates. In Plumlee KH, editor: *Clinical veterinary toxicology*, St Louis, 2004, Mosby, p 340.
27. Meerdink G: Anticholinesterase insecticides. In Plumlee KH, editor: *Clinical veterinary toxicology*, ed 1, St. Louis, 2004, Mosby, p 178.
28. Merola V, Dunayer E: The 10 most common toxicoses in cats, *Vet Med* 101:339, 2006.
29. Morrow C, Volmer P: Cholecalciferol. In Plumlee KH, editor: *Clinical veterinary toxicology*, St Louis, 2004, Mosby, p 448.
30. Murphy M: Rodenticides, *Vet Clin North Am Sm Anim Pract* 32:469, 2002.
31. Murphy M: Rodenticide toxicoses. In Bonagura J,Twedt D, editors: *Kirk's current veterinary therapy XIV*, St Louis, 2009, Saunders Elsevier, p 117.
32. Peterson M: Reptiles. In Plumlee KH, editor: *Clinical veterinary toxicology*, St Louis, 2004, Mosby, p 103.
33. Peterson M: Toxicological decontamination. In Peterson M, Talcott P, editors: *Small animal toxicology*, ed 2, St Louis, 2006, Saunders Elsevier, p 128.
34. Plumb D: *Veterinary drug handbook*, ed 5, Ames, Iowa, 2005, Iowa State Press.
35. Richardson J: Potpourri hazards in cats, *Vet Med* 94:1010, 1999.
36. Richardson J: Management of acetaminophen and ibuprofen toxicoses in dogs and cats, *J Vet Emerg Crit Care* 10:285, 2000.
37. Richardson J: Permethrin spot on toxicoses in cats, *J Vet Emerg Crit Care* 10:103, 2000.
38. Richardson J: Zinc toxicosis from penny ingestion in dogs, *Vet Med* 97:96, 2002.
39. Richardson J: Atypical topical spot-on products. In Peterson M,Talcott P, editors: *Small animal toxicology*, ed 2, St Louis, 2006, Saunders Elsevier, p 978.
40. Richardson J, Gwaltney-Brant SM: Lily toxicoses in cats, *Stand Care Emerg Crit Care Med* 4:5, 2002.
41. Richardson J, Gwaltney-Brant SM: Ethylene glycol toxicosis in dogs and cats, *Clinicians Brief* 1:13, 2003.
42. Richardson J, Welch S, Gwaltney-Brant SM et al.: Metaldehyde toxicoses in dogs, *Comp Contin Edu Pract Vet* 25:376, 2003.
43. Roder J: Analgesics. In Plumlee KH, editor: *Clinical veterinary toxicology*, St Louis, 2004, Mosby, p 282.
44. Roder J: Spiders. In Plumlee KH, editor: *Clinical veterinary toxicology*, St Louis, 2004, Mosby, p 111.
45. Roder J: Toads. In Plumlee KH, editor: *Clinical veterinary toxicology*, St Louis, 2004, Mosby, p 113.
46. Rosendale ME: Decontamination strategies, *Vet Clin North Am Small Anim Pract* 32:311, 2002.
47. Rumbeiha W, Murphy M: Nephrotoxicants. In Bonagura J, Twedt D, editors: *Kirk's current veterinary therapy XIV*, St Louis, 2009, Saunders Elsevier, p 159.
48. Rumbeiha WK, Francis JA, Fitzgerald SD et al: A comprehensive study of Easter lily poisoning in cats, *J Vet Diagn Invest* 16:527, 2004.
49. Schildt JC, Jutkowitz LA, Beal MW: Potpourri oil toxicity in cats: 6 cases (2000-2007), *J Vet Emerg Crit Care* 18:511, 2008.
50. Sutton NM, Bates N, Campbell A: Clinical effects and outcome of feline permethrin spot-on poisonings reported to the Veterinary Poisons Information Service (VPIS), London, *J Feline Med Surg* 9:335, 2007.
51. Talcott P: Metaldehyde. In Plumlee KH, editor: *Clinical veterinary toxicology*, St Louis, 2004, Mosby, p 182.
52. Talcott P: Strychnine. In Plumlee KH, editor: *Clinical veterinary toxicology*, St Louis, 2004, Mosby, p 454.
53. Talcott P: Insecticide toxicoses. In Bonagura J, Twedt D, editors: *Kirk's current veterinary therapy XIV*, St Louis, 2009, Saunders Elsevier, p 119.
54. Tefft K: Lily nephrotoxicity in cats, *Comp Contin Edu Pract Vet* 26:149, 2004.
55. Thrall M, Connally H, Grauer G et al.: Ethylene glycol. In Peterson M, Talcott P, editors: *Small animal toxicology*, ed 2, St Louis, 2006, Saunders Elsevier, p 703.
56. Villar D, Knight MK, Holding J et al: Treatment of acute isoniazid overdose in dogs, *Vet Hum Toxicol* 37:473, 1995.
57. Webb C, Twedt D, Fettman M et al: S-adenosylmethionine (SAMe) in a feline acetaminophen model of oxidative injury, *J Fel Med Surg* 5:69, 2003.
58. Wismer T: Novel insecticides. In Plumlee KH, editor: *Clinical veterinary toxicology*, St Louis, 2004, Mosby, p 183.
59. Youssef H: Cycad toxicoses in dogs, *Vet Med* 103:242, 2008.

CHAPTER

32

Urinary Tract Disorders

OUTLINE

THE UPPER URINARY TRACT

Margie Scherk

The recognition and management of renal disease are important in small animal practice: Cats are popular companions, and the average life expectancy has increased. The purpose of this chapter is not only to explore renal disease in depth but also to remind veterinarians that although the clinical signs may look the same, they should strive to identify specific etiologies insofar as these may have specific treatments.

DIAGNOSTIC METHODS

Various diagnostic methods are available for evaluation of the upper urinary tract, including imaging, renal function tests, urinalysis, urine culture, urine protein: creatinine ratio, and renal biopsy. Table 32-1 describes how diagnostic tests can be used to localize disorders.

Renal Size

Renal size is measured radiographically relative to the length of the second lumbar (L2) vertebra. Although there is no difference between the sexes in this parameter, there is an effect of gonadectomy on kidney size. A significant size difference was determined between intact and neutered cats, with intact cats having larger kidneys. Normal feline renal length ratios range from 1.9 to 2.6 for neutered cats and 2.1 to 3.2 for intact cats, which suggests that reproductive status should be taken into consideration when interpreting renal size.[202] Box 32-1 lists the causes of renomegaly in the cat.

Renal Function Tests

Assessment of renal function using the standard measures of urine specific gravity (USG), creatinine (Cr), and blood urea nitrogen (BUN) is extremely crude because these parameters are not altered until significant renal function has been lost (approximately 75%) and because they also reflect nonrenal factors. BUN can be especially

TABLE 32-1 Use of Diagnostic Tests to Localize Lesions within the Urinary Tract

Diagnostic Test	Renal Function Assessed	Localized to Kidneys?	Localized Distal to Kidneys?
Blood urea nitrogen	GFR	Not necessarily*	No
Serum creatinine	GFR	Not necessarily*	No
Iohexol clearance	GFR	No	No
IV urography	GFR and crude estimate of renal blood flow	Yes	Yes
Urine specific gravity	Tubular reabsorption	Not necessarily*	No
Urine osmolality	Tubular reabsorption	Not necessarily*	No
Water deprivation and vasopressin response tests	Tubular reabsorption	Not necessarily*	No
Ultrasound	No	Yes	Yes
Renal biopsy	No	Yes	N/A
Renal tubular epithelial cells	No	No, unless in casts	No
Hematuria	No	No, unless in casts	Yes, if sample not contaminated by blood
Proteinuria	No	Not necessarily†	Not necessarily
Pyuria	No	No, unless in casts	Yes, if sample not contaminated by genital tract
Significant bacteriuria	No	No	Yes, if sample not contaminated by genital tract or coat
Urinary casts	No	Yes	N/A

GFR, Glomerular filtration rate; *IV*, intravenous.
*Changes to renal parameters may occur secondary to other nonrenal diseases.
†The presence of large quantities of protein in the absence of red blood cells and white blood cells is suggestive of glomerular disease, and a urine protein:creatinine ratio should be calculated.
Adapted from Osborne CA, Stevens JB: Table 2-3. In *Urinalysis: a clinical guide to compassionate patient care*, 1999, Bayer Corporation.

BOX 32-1
Causes of Renomegaly in the Cat

- Polycystic kidneys
- Perinephric pseudocyst
- Hydronephrosis
- Obstructive nephrosis
- Pyonephrosis
- Pyelonephritis
- Feline infectious peritonitis
- Neoplasia (most common is lymphoma)

difficult to interpret because it reflects ammonia intake, production, and excretion. Urea is a by-product of ammonia metabolism that is excreted in bile, reabsorbed by way of enterohepatic recirculation, and also is eliminated by the kidney. The majority of the ammonia produced in the body is by bacterial fermentation in the gut, with lesser amounts produced by catabolism of endogenous protein and other molecules such as heme and some of the cytochromes that are rich in nitrogen. Because dietary factors can be important—there have been reports of animals fed organ meats as treats that produced spuriously high urea readings—everything the patient is ingesting must be taken into consideration. Bleeding into the gastrointestinal tract is one of the most common pathologic causes because of the large amount of nitrogen in blood, which is broken down by the bacteria. Other potential causes include factors that could change the amount of ammonia being produced by the bacteria in the gut, such as shifts in bacterial populations and changes in motility and gastrointestinal transit of food. Any metabolic derangement that causes excessive catabolism of protein in the body as an energy substrate has the potential to increase urea levels. Increases in urea (independent of Cr) are common in diabetes mellitus (DM) and hyperthyroidism. Interestingly, urea can be elevated in renal disease when Cr is normal, especially in neonates or animals with muscle wasting insofar as these patients have decreased muscle mass compared with the normal population and therefore correspondingly lower Cr levels. In this situation urea may be more sensitive than Cr for predicting renal disease. In most cases, a diagnosis of renal insufficiency will be made based on elevations in BUN and/or Cr along with a dilute USG.

Numerous tests have been evaluated for the assessment of glomerular filtration rate (GFR) or renal function. The standard 24-hour Cr clearance test is unwieldy, and renal scintigraphy is not widely available.[121] One group evaluated a single injection of either inulin or Cr in normal cats and then compared plasma inulin and Cr clearances. The results showed that inulin may be a better indicator of GFR than Cr.[166] The same researchers subsequently assessed iohexol and found that plasma clearance of this marker not only is a sensitive test for the detection of diminished renal function before changes in either BUN or Cr but also can be performed noninvasively in conscious cats.[167] Another single-injection inulin clearance study compared inulin and iohexol clearance and showed excellent correlation between the two methods in their ability to detect alterations in GFR. The investigators concluded that an "inulin excretion test" sampling blood 3 hours after the administration of 3000 mg/m^2 body surface area can be used for the assessment of renal function in daily practice.[100] Excretory urography is another method to determine GFR; one study compared iohexol with amidotrizoate and concluded that iohexol was safer and produced better-quality urograms.[6]

Renal hemodynamics (resistance and pulsatility index) of intrarenal arteries has been studied using pulsed-wave Doppler; quantitative scintigraphy (^{99m}Tc-MAG3) was used to study relative renal function and relative renal blood flow. Of clinical relevance is that significant differences were found between awake and isoflurane-anesthetized cats for all pulsed-wave Doppler and quantitative renal scintigraphic measurements.[165] Recently, a group evaluated an enzyme-linked immunosorbent assay (ELISA) test for gadolinium diethylenetriamine pentaacetic acid as a means to determine GFR. This test did not offer a sufficiently accurate estimation of GFR in cats when compared with plasma clearance of iohexol and plasma concentrations of BUN and Cr.[203] Box 32-2 lists additional tests for renal function.

BOX 32-2

Diagnostic Tests for Evaluation of Renal Function

Tubular concentration capacity:
- Water deprivation test
- Pitressin concentration test

Glomerular filtration rate measurement:
- Plasma iohexol clearance
- Plasma inulin clearance
- Renal scintigraphy
- Phenolsuphonphthalein (PSP) clearance

Markers:
- Blood urea nitrogen (BUN)
- Serum creatinine
- Amylase, lipase

Excretory urography

Urinalysis

A complete urinalysis is indicated when disease of the urinary tract is suspected. These include the following:

- Chronic renal insufficiency
- Acute renal failure (ARF)
- Urinary tract infection (kidneys, ureters, bladder, urethra—the last only if urine sample is voided)
- Urolithiasis or crystalluria
- Neoplasia: occasionally exfoliation of neoplastic cells occurs from urinary tract neoplasia

In addition, a voided sample evaluates the urethra, prostate, and vagina.

A urinalysis is indicated as part of a minimum database in any ill cat. For example, pyelonephritis is an occult condition without necessarily any clinical signs referable to the urinary tract. Urinalysis results reflect the health and function of many body systems because urine is, in essence, filtered blood. Examples of some of the non–urinary tract conditions with significant changes detected through urine evaluation include DM (glucosuria) and ketoacidosis (ketonuria), diabetes insipidus (hyposthenuria), hepatic disease and hemolytic disease (bilirubinuria), prerenal azotemia (concentrated urine), and severe inflammation or multiple myeloma (proteinuria).

Throughout this chapter the term *urinalysis* refers to a complete urinalysis consisting of macroscopic evaluation (e.g., appearance, concentration, semiquantitative urine biochemical dip strip tests for pH and urine constituents: protein, glucose, blood) a USG assessment, and microscopic evaluation of spun urine sediment (e.g., cells, crystals, bacteria).

As with any laboratory test, it is possible to generate invalid and misleading results. The usefulness of a urine specimen is significantly affected by the timing of collection and the way it is collected, handled, stored, and examined. Additionally, the veterinarian should note all the drugs that a patient is receiving because many therapeutic agents affect the results of urinalysis (Box 32-3).[177]

Timing of Sample Collection

Samples collected after fasting or in the early morning may show highest concentrating ability and highest yield of sediment. The exception to this is the cat with access at all times to a litter box. This sample is also least likely to show glucosuria. Cytologic quality of the cells will be altered by prolonged exposure to waste products, osmolality, and pH variations.

Recently formed urine provides better cytologic detail, and bacteria are more easily identified. If the sample is dilute, tubular concentrating ability cannot be evaluated. Dilute samples also may distort cells.

BOX 32-3

Effects of Drugs on Urine Sample

1. Parenteral and oral fluids and diuretics
   a. Alter urine specific gravity (USG) and osmolality
   b. Furosemide may acidify urine
   c. Increased urine volume may dilute biochemical parameters, resulting in false-negative results
   d. Dilute urine affects cell integrity and promotes lysis
   e. Glucose-containing fluids may result in iatrogenic glucosuria
2. Antimicrobial agents
   a. Ideally samples for microbiologic culture should be collected before starting antimicrobial therapy. However, culture of urine while on this class of agent will reflect organisms not susceptible to the antimicrobial being used. To evaluate efficacy of therapy, the patient should be off that treatment for a minimum of 3 days.
3. Acidifying and alkalinizing agents (therapeutic, dietary, or added to urine sample)
   a. Alter crystal composition of the sample
   b. Extreme alkalinity may cause false-positive protein reactions on urine strips
   c. Vitamin C (ascorbic acid) causes false-negative glucose reactions on urine strips, as well as red cells, hemoglobin, and myoglobin
4. Iodinated radiopaque contrast materials
   a. Given intravenously will increase USG if preadministration USG was <1.040, but will decrease the USG if the preadministration USG was >1.040
   b. Given by catheter into the lower urinary tract will increase the USG
   c. Affect cell structure and survival of bacteria in the sample

Collection Technique

The most reliable method for collecting urine from cats is by cystocentesis. Cystocentesis samples reflect prerenal, renal, ureteral, and bladder health. Voided samples reflect the aforementioned, as well as the urethra, prostate, vagina, and perineal fur. Further, voided samples reflect where the cat has urinated (e.g., the litter box, consultation table, or floor). The yield of the sediment must also be interpreted in light of collection technique. The bladder contracts circumferentially; however, sediment depends on gravity. Thus, for a cystocentesis-collected sample, the sediment yield may be improved by gently shaking the bladder just before inserting the needle.[178] Voided samples also do not reflect sediment proportionately because of sediment remaining in the bladder as it contracts; thus samples collected in this manner may underestimate the degree of inflammation, crystalluria, and so on.

Cystocentesis: The bladder must contain a sufficiently large volume of urine for the veterinarian to be able to identify it by palpation and immobilize it manually. The two approaches used are either through the lateral abdominal wall with the cat on its side or ventrally with the cat in dorsal recumbency. Ideally, the hair is shaved and the skin disinfected; however, as this adds to stress for the patient, it is often not performed. After the bladder is agitated, the needle should be inserted in the caudoventral direction on an angle so that the layers of the bladder wall seal the puncture better. By using a smaller-gauge needle (e.g., 23 to 25 G) and not applying pressure to the bladder with the mobilizing hand, the veterinarian can reduce the risk of urine leakage.

If a swirl of blood is seen to enter the hub of the syringe, collection should be discontinued and the blood (an iatrogenic cause for hematuria) should be noted in the medical record. This bleeding is extremely unlikely to result in postcollection complications, however. Iatrogenic hematuria is commonly seen in cystocentesis samples and may be differentiated from true hematuria by comparison with a free catch–voided sample collected by the client at home 24 to 48 hours later. Clients can use a long-handled spoon such as a soup ladle or put clean aquarium gravel or Nosorb in a clean, empty litter box to collect the sample. Penetration of a bowel loop during cystocentesis is unlikely to cause problems other than in the interpretation of bacteriuria (discussed later). The most disconcerting postprocedural complication is the rare occurrence of vomiting and hypotensive collapse. Although the mechanism is unclear, it is believed to be a vasovagal response. With standard fluid therapy (to support volume and systemic blood pressure [BP]) and quiet, patients recover within 30 minutes to 1 hour.

Voided sample: Midstream collection reduces the chance of collecting debris (particulate material including feces and bacteria) from the perineal region; however, a voided sample is never completely free from risk of contamination. Veterinarians often make do with samples collected from the examination table, examination room floor, cage, litter box, or carrier base. These may also be used as long as the veterinarian is aware that the sample is likely to include artifacts (and know which types are most likely).

Catheter collection is another possibility; however, it requires sedation in both sexes to ensure humane treatment and minimize potential trauma to the urethra. In the very young kitten (younger than 3 or 4 weeks of age), a urine sample may be obtained by stimulating the anogenital region with a warm moist cotton ball.

Handling the Urine Specimen

In an ideal world urine should be kept at room temperature and evaluated within 30 minutes of collection. Storage time and temperature alter and affect pH, USG, and crystal formation.[7] If it cannot be examined in this time frame, the following suggestions will help preserve the integrity of the specimen.

1. Refrigerate at 41° F (5° C) for 2 to 3 hours or possibly overnight. The sample should be warmed to room temperature before analysis for accuracy of USG and for glucose assessment. Do not freeze the sample.
2. Protect the sample from light. Bilirubin becomes undetectable within 1 hour of exposure to sunlight.
3. Casts and cellular material deteriorate in alkaline urine. Over time, more crystals will develop depending on the pH of the sample; therefore the pH should be determined promptly.
4. Although preservatives for urine are available, each type alters the characteristics of the sample; specific information has been published elsewhere.[178]

Examination of the Sample

To minimize interassay variation, a standardized protocol should be used for every sample. Refrigerated samples should be rewarmed to room temperature before evaluation. Urine strips and other reagents should be kept cool but not refrigerated. These and the urine should not be exposed to sunlight or other light for significant amounts of time. It is important to read and interpret the test results at the times designated by the test manufacturer. Centrifugation of urine sediment should be at 1000 to 1500 rpm for 3 to 5 minutes. Most important, the timing and method of collection should be taken into consideration when interpreting the significance of the results relative to the patient.

Urinalysis Interpretation[177,190]

Volume: The normal 24-hour urine volume production for an adult cat is 20 to 40 mL/kg per day. When the USG is greater than 1.040, polyuria is unlikely. Occasionally, cats with renal insufficiency may paradoxically concentrate their urine above 1.040.

Color: Clarity and color are affected by many things, which, in turn, affect the USG value perceived with an optical refractometer. Conversely, urine color should also be interpreted in light of the USG. The color of the sample may be important insofar as it can affect interpretation of the colorimetric dry chemistries (urine strips). Color comparisons are subjective and are affected by colored urine constituents. Color should be assessed by a trained professional, in a consistently well-lit area and using fresh urine (Figure 32-1). Urine color may provide valuable information, including the following:

- Urine that is colorless is very dilute.
- Normal urine color ranges from transparent to light yellow, medium yellow, and amber. Normally, highly concentrated urine is amber as a result of increased urochrome or urobilin. Urochrome levels are also high in states of fever or starvation. Nitrofurantoin and riboflavin (vitamin B_2) will cause urine to appear deep yellow.
- Orange-yellow color reflects high concentration, or excessive urobilin, bilirubin, or fluorescein (e.g., when used to identify a cat that is urinating inappropriately).
- Red, pink, red-brown, red-orange, or orange color suggests hematuria, the presence of hemoglobin, myoglobin, porphyrin, or warfarin. In humans ingestion of rhubarb, beets, phenothiazines, and other substances may cause this discoloration.
- A brown tint suggests methemoglobin; melanin; and, in humans, several drugs, including bismuth, mercury, and sulfasalazine.
- Yellow- or green-brown discoloration signifies the presence of bile pigment.
- Brown to black discoloration is actually brown or red-brown if evaluated as a thinner layer.
- Milky white urine is a result of chyle, pus, or phosphate crystals.

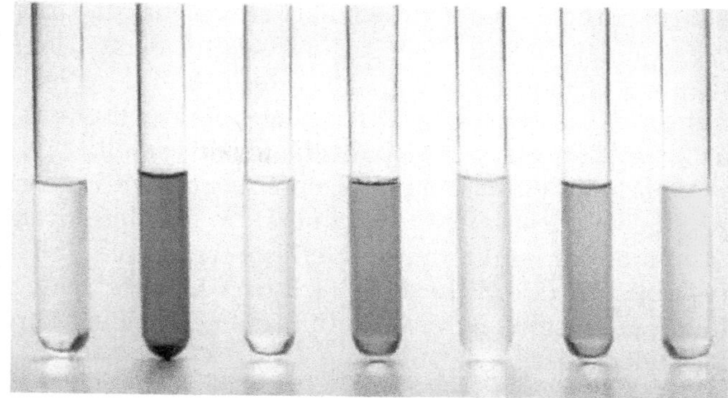

FIGURE 32-1 Urine color is best assessed in good lighting against a white background.

Turbidity: Transparency is assessed by holding a clear glass tube against a printed page and assessing the legibility of the print. Concentrated urine is more likely to be turbid than dilute urine. Refrigeration changes clarity, as do substances affecting pH. Most commonly, turbidity is caused by sediment—namely, crystals, cells (red blood cells, white blood cells, epithelial cells), bacteria, yeast, semen, or contaminants from the collection container (as well as litter box, carrier, table top, floor) or feces. If there is lipid (from pericystic fat) in the urine, it will rise to the surface of the sample.

Crystal formation is affected by temperature; these may form as urine cools from body temperature to room or refrigerator temperature. Hematuria results in brownish to reddish (rarely black) turbid urine. Myoglobin and hemoglobin create a similarly colored, but clear, urine.

Odor: Cat urine has a characteristic odor that is stronger when the urine is concentrated. Tomcat urine has an almost pathognomonic smell that helps identify an intact cat or a cat that has been incompletely castrated (e.g., retained testicle) or a cat with a testosterone-secreting tumor. It has been speculated that felinine, the amino acid unique to cats, is responsible for this smell.

Abnormal odors may indicate infection with urease-producing bacteria. Warm temperature facilitates transformation of ammonium [NH_4] to ammonia [NH_3], resulting in odor. The odor of urine ketones may be detected by some humans. A putrid smell suggests bacterial degradation of protein.

USG: USG is a measure of the density of the urine relative to the density of water measured at the same temperature. The density of water is 1.000 under set circumstances of temperature and pressure. Temperature affects USG inversely (i.e., increasing urine temperature causes a decrease in its USG, whereas decreasing the urine temperature increases the USG). Solutes affect the density of urine, and each solute may affect it to a different degree, even when each one is present in equal amounts.

The accepted method for determining USG in cats is by using a refractometer. This tool assesses refractive index (ratio of velocity of light in air to the velocity of light in a solution). The refractive index is affected by the type and quantity of solutes present. Although refractometers are calibrated to a reference temperature, they compensate to a certain degree. They should be stored at room temperature. Veterinary refractometers measure a wider range of specific gravity and are therefore best suited for cat urine that may have USG in excess of 1.080. Human refractometers read only to 1.050. Digital refractometers appear to correlate with optical refractometers and have the advantage of less subjectivity.[22] Some reagent strips include a pad for USG. Because these are developed for human urine, the highest value they detect is 1.030, which is inadequate for feline urine. Urinometers, devices that float in urine to measure USG, are imprecise. Osmometers assess osmolality rather than specific gravity. Regardless of the method used, all factors that affect refraction still should be taken into consideration.

The normal USG for a cat depends on hydration status and age. By the time a kitten is 4 weeks of age, USG is 1.020 to 1.038; full concentrating ability (up to 1.080) is reached by 8 weeks of age. In a dehydrated cat normal renal function (specifically, concentrating ability), is suggested by USG of 1.040 or above, depending on the diet fed. In cats fed exclusively canned food, a "normal" USG may be 1.025 or greater, whereas in cats fed exclusively dry food, USG should be 1.035 to 1.040 or higher.[52] In a well-hydrated cat, it may fall between 1.035 and 1.060. *Specific gravity varies within the same individual throughout the day; therefore a single urine sample with a low USG is not reliable evidence of a decline in renal function.*

When nephrons are no longer able to modify glomerular filtrate, a fixed USG of 1.008 to 1.012 develops. USG of 1.007 to 1.039 in a dehydrated cat with or without azotemia is highly suggestive of renal insufficiency (or renal failure, depending on the degree of azotemia once the patient is rehydrated).[176] Hypoadrenocorticism and hyperaldosteronemia are less common causes of such a drop in urine concentration. There is a subgroup of cats with impaired renal function that paradoxically remain able to concentrate urine to greater than 1.045, such that renal azotemia precedes a decline in USG.[177] Because these patients are uncommonly identified, veterinarians must rely on finding USG of 1.045 or greater in the face of azotemia as indicating a prerenal cause for the azotemia.

Urine pH: Urine pH can be used as an index of body acid–base balance; however, this parameter changes so rapidly to provide homeostatic balance to the body that it is a rough guide at best. Obligate carnivores create a great deal of acidic metabolic waste. They regulate their acid–base balance by excreting hydrogen (H^+), ammonium ion (NH_4^+), and phosphates (PO_4^+) in urine (metabolic route) and by exhaling CO_2 (respiratory route). pH is one of the factors affecting crystal formation and may be manipulated to encourage dissolution of some crystal types. Acidic urine inhibits bacterial growth.

Stress affects urine pH. In one study it was reported that the urine pH of a cat increased by 1.4 U when the cat was transported from home to a veterinary clinic. The authors concluded that the most likely cause was anxiety-induced hyperventilation (excessive panting).[43] Another study suggested the opposite—namely, that increasing activity of the sympathetic nerves and the adrenal glands will most likely lead to increased metabolism, including catabolic conversion of proteins, which in turn increases sulfuric acid production and lowers urinary pH. This effect can also be seen in the fasted, inappetent, or anorectic cat.[60]

Eating affects urine pH. Postprandial alkaline tide (alkaline urine) is believed to be a result of increased hydrochloride acid secretion after a meal. In their feral state cats eat many (8 to 15) small meals per day rather than two, as are fed in many homes, making the effect of this pH swing much smaller. Frequency of feeding along with quality of food ingested and the composition of the meal will affect urine pH. Higher-protein, meat- and fish-based diets create more acidic urine; lower-protein, grain- and vegetable-based diets create more alkaline urine.

The pH of urine in the healthy "normal" cat generally ranges between 6.0 and 7.5. The pH of urine least likely to result in crystal formation is 6.2 to 6.4. The method used to measure urine pH is critical; pH meters are inexpensive and are most accurate. Hydrogen paper (pH 5.5 to 9.0) is satisfactory. The urine reagent strips most commonly used in clinics are extremely unreliable. pH values measured with reagent strips are accurate only to within 0.5 units, meaning that the color subjectively translated into a pH value may vary by +/− 0.5, resulting in one whole unit variability.

Acidic urine may be a result of an acidifying diet, respiratory or metabolic acidosis, diabetic ketoacidosis, renal failure, starvation or anorexia, pyrexia, protein catabolism, hypoxia, or severe diarrhea. Severe vomiting resulting in chloride depletion may cause paradoxical acidosis.

Alkaline urine is associated with an alkalinizing diet; drug therapy; respiratory or metabolic alkalosis; vomiting; renal tubular acidosis; chronic metabolic acidosis resulting in ammonium ion (NH_4^+) secretion; and infection with urease-producing bacteria, such as *Proteus* and *Staphylococcus*, organisms seen infrequently in the urinary tract of cats.

Drugs may alter urine pH. Acidifiers include DL-methionine, furosemide, ammonium chloride (NH_4Cl), ascorbic acid at supertherapeutic doses, and phosphate salts. Alkalinizing agents include sodium bicarbonate ($NaHCO_3$), potassium citrate, sodium lactate, and chlorothiazide.

Artifacts affecting urine pH include containers contaminated with detergents or disinfecting agents, CO_2 loss resulting from storing urine at room temperature, and contamination of the sample by urease-producing bacteria from the environment or the distal urethra.

Glucose: The glucose pad on a urine strip is a colorimetric test based on glucose oxidase activity. Although it is easy to use, several points are worth noting. Because the test involves multiple enzymatic steps, it must be performed according to label instructions. The colorimetric indicators can react with substances other than glucose, and some substances may inhibit the test; this means that false-positive and false-negative results are possible. Glucose oxidase is labile, so the expiration date of the strips should be respected. The reaction is also pH dependent. Because the test is temperature dependent, the urine has to be tested at room or body temperature.

Glucose is filtered by the glomerulus and reabsorbed by the proximal tubules. Physiologic or stress glucosuria occurs when serum glucose exceeds the renal threshold for glucose of greater than 260 mg/dL (14 mmol/L). Pharmacologic agents that can result in transient glucosuria include epinephrine, phenothiazines, glucagon, adrenocorticotropic hormone (ACTH) and morphine. Persistent glucosuria may be a result of DM, hyperprogesteronemia, acromegaly, hyperadrenocorticism, and pheochromocytoma. Renal glucosuria may be caused by acute tubular injury.

Urine glucose monitoring for insulin dose titration in the diabetic cat should not be used because the relationship between serum glucose concentration and that in the urine is variable.[177]

Ketones: Ketones (ketone bodies) are produced when metabolism shifts to using stored fat as a source of energy, such as in cellular starvation (unregulated DM or lack of eating) or when excessive fat is ingested. In other species it also occurs with insufficient carbohydrate metabolism. The three ketones produced are acetoacetic acid, acetone, and beta-hydroxybutyric acid. The first two are detectable in urine using the reagents in urine strips; beta-hydroxybutyric acid is not. All three types can be measured in blood. Another colorimetric reaction on urine strips, ketone pad color interpretation, is subjective and is affected by colored urine constituents.

Bilirubin: Bilirubin is a by-product of heme (from hemoglobin) catabolism. The portion that is bound to albumin (unconjugated/indirect bilirubin) is removed from circulation by the liver where it is conjugated. Once conjugated, it is water soluble. The majority of the conjugated portion is transported in bile to the intestinal tract, where bacteria convert it into urobilinogen. It is oxidized to urobilin, the pigment that provides the brown color to feces. A small amount of the urobilinogen is reabsorbed into circulation and is excreted into urine. The small quantity of conjugated bilirubin that evades the bile is excreted into glomerular filtrate.

An increase in urinary bilirubin is associated with increased destruction of red blood cells (hemolytic disease), hepatocellular disease preventing normal elimination of this product, or bile duct obstruction (cholestatic disease). Altered selective permeability of glomerular capillaries in glomerulonephropathy can also potentially cause bilirubinuria by changing the renal threshold of affected nephrons. Bilirubinuria may precede clinically recognizable icterus and even bilirubinemia. Unlike in dogs, bilirubinuria is not found in normal cats, even in highly concentrated urine samples, presumably because of a higher renal threshold for bilirubin in this species.[177]

Bilirubin is an unstable compound, especially when exposed to room air or light. The degradation products formed under those circumstances (including biliverdin) do not react with the test, causing false-negative test results. To avoid this, urine should be evaluated within 30 minutes of collection or be refrigerated, kept dark, and (for other tests) brought to room temperature just before analysis. This test should also be run before centrifugation (or filtration) because precipitates in the centrifuged (or filtered) sample may absorb bilirubin.

Urobilinogen: The reagent strip test detects normal and increased amounts but not the absence of urobilinogen. Because of this, it cannot be used to detect complete bile duct obstruction. Increased concentration is suggestive of hemolytic disease or decreased hepatic function. For results to be meaningful, a fresh urine specimen is required.

Occult blood, hemoglobin, and myoglobin: Hemoglobinuria (red to brown urine) is suggestive of intravascular hemolysis; a serum sample from the patient collected concurrently should have a reddish discoloration. Myoglobinuria (brownish urine) is suggestive of muscle disease; the serum from the patient may be clear.

Free hemoglobin and myoglobin, but not intact red blood cells, cause a positive reaction. This urine strip chemical reaction augments and complements the microscopic findings of red cells on urine sediment evaluation. This test must be interpreted in concert with the USG as well as the microscopic sediment evaluation. Very dilute or very alkaline urine may lyse red cells. Serum creatinine kinase should be assessed when a positive reaction occurs and hemoglobinemia has been ruled out to differentiate between myoglobinuria and hemoglobinuria.

Lack of red cells in the sediment with a positive test reaction implies hemoglobinuria, myoglobinuria, low urine concentration, low pH causing red cell lysis, or misidentification of red cells in the sediment. When red blood cells are seen on microscopic examination but the urine test pad is negative, it suggests that the strips are outdated, the sample was improperly mixed or centrifuged, there are too few red cells in the sediment to hemolyze, or red cells have been misidentified in the sediment.

Hematuria indicates blood loss into any part of the urinary tract. Identification of the site of bleeding is the next step. Idiopathic renal hematuria has been recognized in cats and dogs. It is not known whether it is due to a vascular bed abnormality or to an abnormality in podocyte attachment, as occurs in humans.[220]

Protein: Numerous types of protein (as many as 40 kinds) may be found in the urine of cats. Hemoglobin and myoglobin have already been mentioned. Protein detected in urine may be prerenal, glomerular, or postglomerular in origin. Small amounts of protein are routinely found in the urine of healthy individuals, but under normal circumstances plasma proteins included in urine are restricted by size and are 66,000 daltons or lower. Because protein loss may be transient, it is essential to verify that proteinuria is persistent before considering appropriate diagnostics and therapeutics. Sample-to-sample variation may be considerable. Centrifugation removes cells that may be causing positive reactions; therefore if protein is detected on an uncentrifuged sample, the test should be repeated on the supernatant after centrifugation.

The aspects of the glomeruli that determine whether protein leaves the glomerular capillaries are size, electrical charge, and hemodynamics. In general, proteins at or below 45,000 daltons with a positive charge are most likely to pass through. Albumin is 66,000 daltons and has a negative charge, which is why there are negligible amounts of albumin in the urine of a cat with normally functioning glomeruli despite high plasma concentrations (Table 32-2). Plasma hemoglobin is normally bound to haptoglobin, making it too large to cross the glomeruli. When this binding capacity is exceeded, as may occur in hemolysis, then unbound hemoglobin can enter urine.

TABLE 32-2 **Examples of Proteins Found in Urine, Their Relative Size, and Implied Reason for Presence**

Protein	Approximate Molecular Weight (Daltons)	Implication When Found in Urine
Smaller proteins (e.g., beta$_2$-microglobulin, muramidase)	11,800-14,400	Unknown
Myoglobin	17,600	Ischemic or traumatic injury to muscles (heat stroke, electrocution, severe muscular exertion, snake bite, crush injury)
Bence Jones proteins	22,000-44,000	Multiple myeloma
Alpha$_1$-microglobulin	27,000	Unknown
Alpha$_1$-acid glycoprotein	40,000	Unknown
Hemoglobin (unbound to haptoglobin)	64,500	Low urine specific gravity, alkaline urine, intravascular hemolysis
Albumin	66,000	Significant glomerular disease

Adapted from Osborne C, Stevens J, Lulich J et al: A clinician's analysis of urinalysis. In Osborne C, Finco D, editors: *Canine and feline nephrology and urology*, ed 1, Baltimore, 1995, Williams & Wilkins.

Because tubules reabsorb filtered protein, a great deal of protein has to be lost through the glomeruli, exceeding the capacity of the functional or impaired tubules to reabsorb it, for it to be present in the ultrafiltrate. Some proteins originate from the urinary tract. The distal tubules and collecting ducts secrete Tamm–Horsfall mucoprotein. The urothelium secretes immunoglobulins as necessary (e.g., to protect against ascending infection).

Interpretation of the significance of protein in urine depends on the USG. For example, mild 1+ proteinuria with USG of 1.010 implies greater protein loss than 1+ protein in a sample with USG of 1.040. Localization of the protein source requires knowledge of collection technique and the urine sediment constituents (Table 32-3).

Numerous test methods exist to detect urine protein, each having a different specificity and sensitivity. It should be noted that small amounts of protein normally found in urine are not detected by routine methods. When 4+ (approximately 1000 mg/dL) protein is found in the supernatant of a centrifuged specimen, a urine protein:Cr ratio (UPC) should be performed. The UPC should be repeated two to three times at 2-week

TABLE 32-3 **Localization, Causes, and Findings in Proteinuria**

Urinary Protein Source	Findings
Hemorrhage into urinary tract (trauma, inflammation, neoplasia)	Occult blood test +, TNTC red blood cells + white blood cells in sediment, high protein
Inflammation in urinary tract	Variable number of white blood cells in sediment, protein rarely >2+ unless concurrent hemorrhage
Infection in urinary tract	Many white blood cells and bacteria in sediment, protein rarely >2+ unless concurrent hemorrhage
Glomerular and/or tubular disease	No occult blood, no significant sediment findings, +/− casts, protein higher in glomerular than tubular disease
Functional extrarenal causes for transient glomerular changes (e.g., fever, stress, extreme environmental temperatures, seizures, venous congestion of kidneys, exercise)	No occult blood, lack of significant sediment findings, +/− casts, high protein, transient
Hemoglobinuria, myoglobinuria	Variable amounts protein, no significant sediment findings

TNTC, Too numerous to count.
Adapted from: Osborne C, Stevens J, Lulich J et al: A clinician's analysis of urinalysis. In Osborne C, Finco D editors: *Canine and feline nephrology and urology*, ed 1, Baltimore, 1995, Williams & Wilkins.

intervals to verify the persistence of the problem before pursuing additional diagnostics (e.g., biopsy) or therapeutics.

The reader is referred to the ACVIM Consensus Statement[143] for a comprehensive discussion of causes, significance, identification, and management of proteinuria in dogs and cats. This topic is discussed in greater detail later in this chapter.

Nitrite: In humans this test is used to screen for certain bacterial pathogens. This test is *not* valid in cats (or dogs).

Leukocytes: In humans this test is used to detect the presence of leukocyte esterase and is a semiquantitative assessment for leukocytes in urine. This test is *not* valid in cats (or dogs).

Urine sediment: Microscopic examination of urine sediment is akin to exfoliative cytology of the urinary tract. It is critically important in the interpretation of color, specific gravity, turbidity, protein, pH, occult blood, and so forth. Without this procedure it is not possible to differentiate, for example, proteinuria caused by glomerular disease from that of inflammatory response to bacterial insult at any level of the urinary tract or the genital tract. Conversely, the sediment cannot be interpreted without knowledge of the physical and biochemical characteristics of the sample.

To minimize interassay variation, a standardized procedure should be followed. Centrifugation speed for urine sediment is slow: 1000 to 1,500 rpm for 3 to 5 minutes. Faster or longer centrifugation will lead to artifacts. Normal constituents in urine sediment include a few epithelial cells, red and white blood cells, hyaline casts, some fat, mucus, sperm, and some struvite or oxalate crystals. Yeast bodies are contaminants. Abnormal constituents in urine sediment include more than a few red or white blood cells; hyperplastic or neoplastic epithelial cells; more than a few hyaline or granular, cellular, hemoglobin, fatty, or waxy casts; a large number of crystals; any parasite ova; bacteria in a properly collected, transported, and prepared sample; or many yeast organisms.

Storage of urine can alter crystalluria dramatically and therefore the clinician's diagnosis and treatment planning. A study performed to look at the effects of storage on the diagnosis of crystalluria and casts in cats with no history of urinary tract disease was performed. Crystalluria was detected in at least one aliquot in 92% of stored samples as opposed to only 24% of samples examined fresh. Regardless of whether the sample was stored or fresh, urine from cats fed an exclusively canned diet did not have crystals.[208]

Pitfalls of interpretation may be avoided by examining unstained sediment using a reduced microscope light intensity. This can be achieved by either lowering the condenser or closing the iris diaphragm. Stain artifact may include bacteria growing in the stain and foreign material. Stain should be filtered weekly or monthly (depending on the number of samples being examined) and should be kept in the refrigerator. Additionally, staining procedures that require washing and counterstaining may result in loss of sediment in the process. Ideally, some of the sediment should be examined unstained, and if there is enough, some of it should be saved for staining. A lack of bacteria on examination does not mean that bacteria are not present.

Urine Culture and Sensitivity

In cats with chronic kidney disease (CKD), the prevalence of urinary tract infections (UTIs) is 22%; in cats with uncontrolled DM and in cats with hyperthyroidism, it is 12%. Many cats with UTIs have no clinical

BOX 32-4

Factors that May Explain Lack of Growth on Urine Culture when Bacteria Were Identified in the Sediment

1. Bacteria nonviable in the urine at time of collection (e.g., antimicrobial therapy, immunologic defenses)
2. Urine sample improperly handled or preserved, causing death of bacteria
3. Organisms fastidious, did not survive time between collection and culture outside of the body
4. Improper culture technique (e.g., anaerobic organism processed as an aerobe)
5. Bacteria misidentified in sediment (look-alikes)

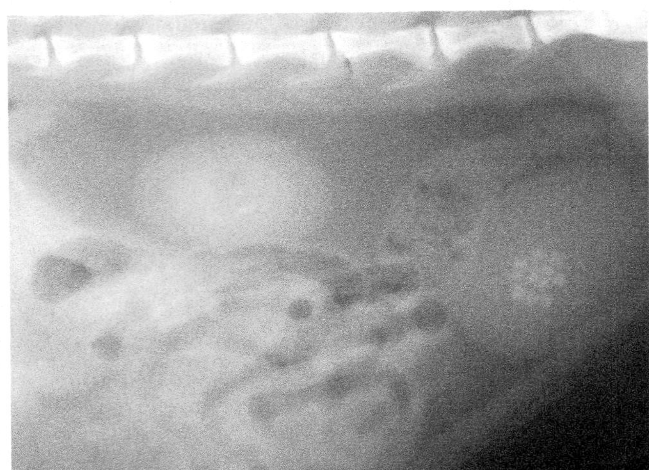

FIGURE 32-2 This radiograph shows a cluster of radio-opaque calculi in the bladder lumen as well as five smaller densities in the kidney. On ultrasound two calculi were also seen in the ipsilateral ureter.

signs of lower urinary tract disease or changes in their laboratory values indicative of infection.[156] Because UTI is so common in cats with hyperthyroidism, DM, and CKD, urine culture and sensitivity is recommended as part of the minimum database for cats with these conditions, especially if the USG is 1.030 or lower regardless of sediment and, in more concentrated samples, if significant numbers of white blood cells or bacteria are seen. Box 32-4 shows causes of negative growth on urine culture in the face of the detection of bacteria in the sediment.

Urine Protein : Creatinine Ratio

Renal proteinuria occurs by one of two mechanisms. The first is a loss of integrity of the glomerular filtration barrier in excess of tubular reabsorption capacity; this may cause mild to marked proteinuria. The second occurs when the tubules fail to reabsorb normal proteins; this may cause mild to moderate proteinuria. Cr is excreted by the kidneys exclusively by glomerular filtration. Comparing these two urine components gives a measure of protein loss relative to renal function. The equation is simple:

Urine protein (mg/dL or mmol/L) divided by urine Cr (mg/dL or mmol/L)

In cats a UPC below 0.2 is considered nonproteinuric. Values between 0.2 and 0.4 reflect borderline proteinuria and should be reassessed within 2 months and reclassified as appropriate. A UPC above 0.4 is considered clinically significant proteinuria.

Microalbuminuria

In humans microalbuminuria is predictive of future renal health. In cats the predictive significance of microalbuminuria is not understood at present. The recommendation of the International Renal Interest Society (IRIS; http://www.iris-kidney.com/) is to continue to monitor this level of proteinuria.[96]

The reader is referred to the ACVIM Consensus Statement[143] for a comprehensive discussion of the causes, significance, identification, and management of proteinuria in dogs and cats. (This topic is also discussed later in this chapter.)

Imaging of the Kidney and the Ureters

Imaging studies commonly used in the assessment of the upper urinary tract of cats include survey radiography, contrast excretory studies, and ultrasound. The normal signal intensities have been determined for magnetic resonance imaging (MRI) of the normal feline cranial abdomen.[173] Each test has a role to play in patient diagnostics. Plain radiographs allow assessment of the number, size, location, and density of the kidneys. The limitations of survey radiography include an inability to visualize kidneys in the thin cat lacking retroperitoneal fat or if retroperitoneal fluid is present. Moreover, survey radiography cannot delineate problems of the renal pelvis or of the ureters unless there is radio-opaque material present (e.g., renoliths or ureteroliths, dystrophic mineralization) (Figure 32-2). Fecal material may obscure the outflow tract. Abdominal compression (e.g., using a wooden spoon over the organ of interest or a general abdominal wrap) may help enhance the image of a specific area by eliminating some of the superimposition encountered with survey radiographs.[11]

Excretory urography is the technique of choice when the renal parenchyma, renal pelvis, or ureters are of concern. This study may be useful to establish the relationship between a renal mass and the pelvis or ureter, to locate an avulsed or congenitally displaced kidney, to identify and possibly distinguish between acute and chronic pyelonephritis, to detect a nonfunctional kidney, to diagnose hydronephrosis, and to outline radiolucent uroliths.[119]

Ultrasound has the advantage of being noninvasive and quick. It is safer for the patient because no contrast material is needed and safer for the patient and owner because there is no exposure to ionizing radiation. It can be used to guide renal biopsy should this be indicated. This modality is useful for evaluating renal masses, cysts, diseases of the renal pelvis (calculi, hydronephrosis, pyonephrosis[53]) and adjacent abdominal structures. Although it is difficult to visualize the normal feline ureters ultrasonographically, various abnormalities associated with ureteral dilation may be revealed, including ectopic ureter, ureterocele, and certain causes of ureteral obstruction. Ultrasonographic evidence of hypoechoic subcapsular thickening in feline kidneys is associated with renal lymphosarcoma.[215] Ultrasound guidance facilitates certain interventional diagnostic procedures for the ureters.[135] Its limitations include the inability to visualize structures through abdominal air or bone (i.e., pelvic structures occlude the urethra).

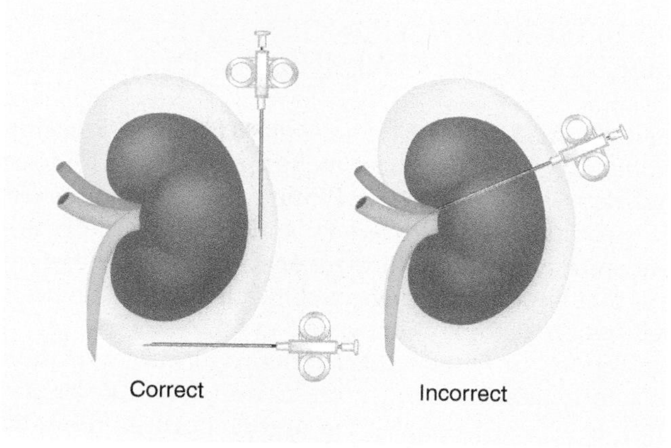

FIGURE 32-3 This drawing depicts the correct way to direct the renal biopsy needle. The needle should remain in the renal cortex and not cross the corticomedullary junction or enter the medulla or the renal pelvis. *(From Vaden SL: Renal biopsy: methods and interpretation,* Vet Clin North Am Small Anim Pract *34:887, 2004.)*

Renal Biopsy

Histopathology of a kidney biopsy sample can provide information by revealing a pathologic process other than chronic interstitial nephritis. Patient selection is important. This procedure should be recommended in those individuals whose treatment will change because of information the results provide. Thus those with proteinuria believed to be of glomerular origin, those with ultrasound evidence of infiltrative disease, or those in ARF are appropriate candidates. The benefits of biopsy in patients with renomegaly outweigh risks; in general, however, for patients with small, scarred kidneys, it is unlikely to be of use. To obtain the best possible results, the veterinarian must be well prepared and understand the laboratory's sample-handling requirements.[214] The laboratory should ideally be able to perform not just light microscopy but also electron microscopy (EM). The latter requires a specific transport medium, gluteraldehyde, which is available through the laboratory.

Two centers that provide this comprehensive service are the Texas Veterinary Renal Pathology Service (Texas A&M University, College Station, Tex) and the Veterinary Pathology Diagnostic Centre (Utrecht University, Utrecht, The Netherlands). They encourage submission as part of the World Small Animal Veterinary Association (WSAVA) Renal Standardization study in order to increase understanding of glomerular diseases of dogs and cats. EM is needed for complete histologic examinations, especially to define early stages of kidney diseases (minimal changes disease, epithelial tubular pathologies, and tubular basement membrane and glomerular basement membrane changes). Along with clinical, histologic, histochemical, and immunologic examinations, it is an essential method for diagnosis and prognosis of renal disease.[198] Because complications after renal biopsy are usually minor, provided the biopsy is performed properly, this tool for diagnostic evaluation should be encouraged.[164,214]

A sample may be collected by tissue-core biopsy (e.g., Tru-Cut) percutaneously with ultrasound guidance or surgically by laparotomy or keyhole approach. The first technique requires only very good sedation and local analgesia, whereas the latter requires general anesthesia. Regardless of technique, monitoring for postprocedural bleeding is critical. This and other possible complications (e.g., peritonitis, local infection, neoplastic seeding) still occur in fewer than 2% of patients undergoing percutaneous sampling. Unless the procedure inadvertently interferes with significant vasculature, GFR is not substantially affected.[74] By guiding the biopsy needle through cortex only from pole to pole, the veterinarian is able to avoid the medulla and the medullary-cortical junction and significant vascular supply (Figure 32-3). The patient should be monitored to ensure that adequate analgesia is being used; palpation over and around the biopsy site will be a good guide. Renal biopsy is contraindicated in patients with coagulopathy, those receiving drugs affecting bleeding, and those with cavitated lesions (e.g., vascular lesion, cyst, abscess, hydronephrosis) to avoid leakage of contents or bleeding.[26] More information on performing renal biopsy can be found later in this chapter.

INHERITED, CONGENITAL, AND DEVELOPMENTAL RENAL DISEASES

Renal anomalies are rare in cats. The most common familial disorders in cats include renal amyloidosis, renal dysplasia, polycystic kidney disease, glomerular basement membrane disorders, and tubular dysfunction (Fanconi's syndrome).[98] Errors of embryologic development that have been recognized in cats include agenesis, renal fusion, ectopic kidney, and cysts.

In reports of renal agenesis, the right kidney is more likely to be absent along with its ureter (*in toto* or partially). In affected females the uterine horn on the same side is also partially or completely missing. The ovary, having a different cellular origin, is present. In affected males the vas deferens and epididymis may be lacking, but the ipsilateral testicle will be normal.[81]

In the recent literature, two cases with urogenital abnormalities have been reported. The first, a 9-month-old female domestic shorthair, was lacking the right kidney and ureter and a segment of the uterine horn on the same side. The cat was brought in because of acute vomiting, depression, and shivering caused by hydrometra of the right uterine horn segment.[51] The second case described was of a 1.5-year-old female Persian with azotemia and inappetence. Like the earlier case, the cat also had renal and ureteral agenesis with segmental aplasia of the uterine horn on the right side; however, in this cat the affected uterine segment was caudal, resulting in cranial uterine horn distention.[91] In a study in which 257 Ragdoll cats were screened for polycystic kidney disease, 0.8% were identified with renal agenesis/aplasia.[179] In a large study of more than 53,000 cats presented for ovariohysterectomy, uterine anomalies were detected in 0.09% of cats (n = 49). The kidneys were also evaluated in 34 of the affected cats, and ipsilateral renal agenesis was found in 29% (10 of 34).[158]

Crossed renal ectopia with fusion was identified in an adult neutered male cat that was presented for polyuria and polydipsia and shown to have renal disease and hypertension. Imaging revealed an ectopic left kidney fused with an orthotopic right kidney.[8] Bilateral renal dysplasia was found in a 5-month-old Norwegian Forest Cat; histopathology revealed primary tubular disorganization and changes in the glomeruli.[10]

Membranoproliferative glomerulonephritis (GN) was reported in a 9-month-old domestic shorthair cat in Japan.[15] In another report a series of 8 young, related Abyssinian cats of both sexes presented with hematuria and were found to have varying degrees of proteinuria. Six of the eight developed nephrotic syndrome with peripheral edema. Histopathology revealed mild glomerular changes, including mesangial hypercellularity with adhesions between Bowman's capsule and the glomerular tuft consistent with focal proliferative glomerulopathy. Genetic analysis was not available in this report.[222]

In Norway, 11 Ragdoll cats were evaluated after two unrelated queens were found suddenly dead as a result of oxalate nephrosis with chronic or acute-on-chronic underlying renal disease.[105] Renal abnormalities were found on ultrasound of five cats. Although investigated as an inherited condition, the etiology and mode of inheritance were not elucidated. Primary hyperoxaluria was ruled out by urine oxalate and liver enzyme analysis.

Cystic Diseases

Polycystic Kidney Disease

Polycystic kidney disease (PKD) is found in Persian, Himalayan, and Exotic Shorthair cats around the world and is reported extensively in the United States,[58] United Kingdom,[46] Australia,[17,20] France,[18] Italy,[31] and Slovenia.[69] The prevalence rates in these studies are between 40% and 50%. Many young Persian cats are asymptomatic, and renal function may not begin to decline until the cat is 7 or 8 years of age. Other breeds of cats manifest this condition rarely; a case report describing a Chartreux cat was recently published.[217] It has been shown to have an autosomal dominant mode of inheritance in all of these breeds.[27,153] All affected individuals are heterozygous for the causative mutation; homozygous individuals die in utero. Concurrent with the renal cysts, unilocular or multilocular cysts may be seen in the liver with or without congenital hepatic fibrosis,[33] as well as other abdominal organs (Figure 32-4).[69]

Cats may exhibit no clinical disease, slowly progressive renal insufficiency as adults, or significant disease as young cats, with marked renomegaly. Because of the variable clinical picture and because of the autosomal dominant inheritance in a pedigreed population,

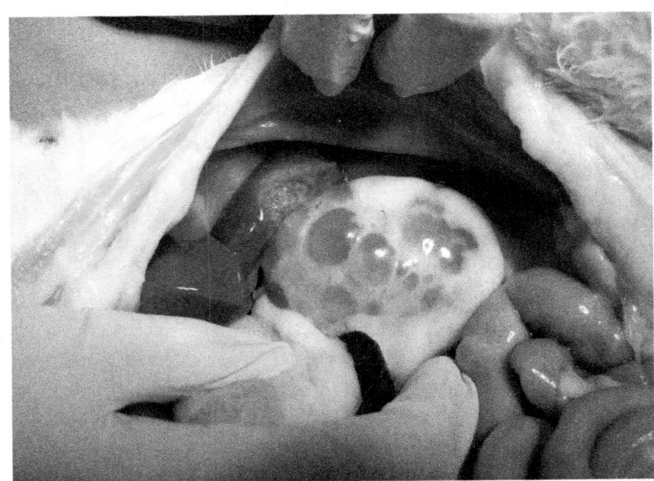

FIGURE 32-4 This necropsy image shows the typical appearance of a polycystic kidney in a Persian cat. *(Courtesy Dr. Susan Little.)*

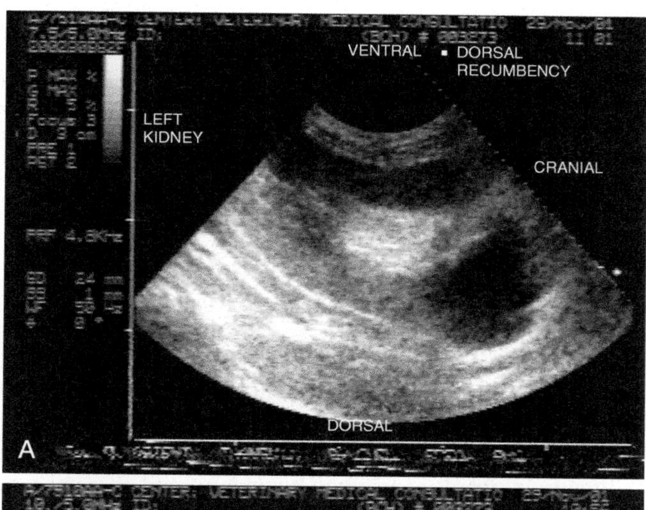

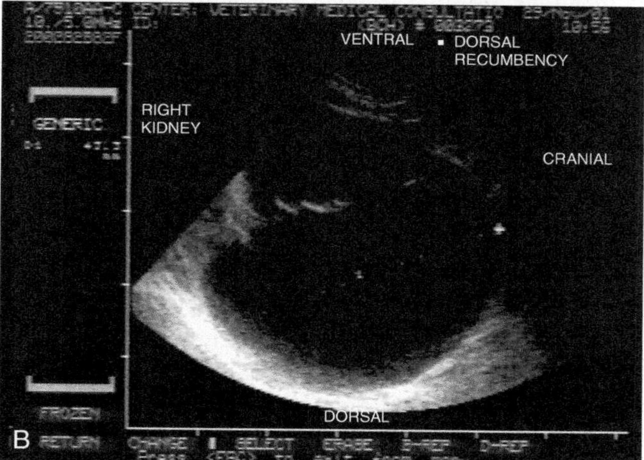

FIGURE 32-5 **A,** Ultrasound of the left kidney of a cat with polycystic kidney disease. Note the anechogenicity of the cyst. **B,** This ultrasound is of the right kidney and shows that cysts are of variable sizes within the same cat. *(Courtesy Dr. Edward Javinsky.)*

screening to identify affected individuals is essential. The condition may be unilateral or bilateral with irregular, enlarged kidney (or kidneys) on palpation. Radiographically, the affected kidney will be irregularly enlarged; on excretory urogram multiple radiolucent areas will be seen. Ultrasound is readily available and may help identify affected cats long before they show clinical signs. Thus sonographic screening is recommended in kittens older than 13 weeks of age; a skilled ultrasonographer can detect cysts in affected kittens as young as 6 to 8 weeks of age. Absence of cysts at a young age does not predict that the kitten will not develop them at a later age. Conversely, a cat with cysts may never show clinical disease. Cysts are located in the medulla or cortex (or both) and are anechoic to hypoechoic, round to irregularly shaped structures of variable size that may grow over time (Figure 32-5). Affected kidneys have indistinct corticomedullary junctions and may have mineralized foci. Further evaluation using intravenous contrast medium allows more definitive identification of cysts with computed tomography (CT), as well as identification of distortion of the renal pelves by cysts.[189]

Genetic testing has been developed to detect a C→A transversion at position 3284 on exon 29 of the *PKD1* gene, resulting in a stop mutation. A real-time polymerase chain reaction (PCR) assay using fluorescent hybridization probes and melting curve analysis has recently (2009) been developed that may be as reliable but faster than previous methods.[63] It is, however, recommended to use both ultrasound as well as genetic testing to improve sensitivity and specificity[32] to decrease the prevalence of the disease in the Persian population.[58] PKD is the leading cause of renal disease in Persian and Persian-related breeds.

Therapy for hepatic and renal cysts is warranted when there is significant compression of adjacent tissue or pain from capsular stretch. Drainage may be performed using ultrasound guidance. In one study of dogs and cats, the drained cysts were infused with alcohol for two periods of 3 minutes. Short-term discomfort was noted in all the patients, with anorexia, lethargy, or vomiting occurring in some.[229]

Interestingly, although dogs with renal cysts and humans with PKD have hypertension, cats with PKD are normotensive. One study that looked at the effects of the angiotensin-converting enzyme inhibitor (ACE-I) enalapril on BP, renal function, and the renin-angiotensin-aldosterone system (RAAS) in affected cats compared with healthy controls found that the ACE-I reduced BP in all and resulted in changes in RAAS enzyme activities and hormone concentrations with minimal effects on renal function.[163]

Perinephric Pseudocysts

Much less common than PKD, perinephric pseudocysts (PNPs) surround one or both kidneys, which may be normal or subnormal in size. Not a true cyst, the fibrous sac lacks an epithelial lining; thus the fluid it contains is extravasated rather than secreted. There is no single etiology, and this condition may follow renal trauma (urine leakage resulting in scarification) or perirenal fat necrosis (resulting in inflammation), may be associated with neoplasia (e.g., transitional cell carcinoma[186]), or may be categorized as idiopathic. Regardless of the initiating cause, anechoic fluid accumulates between the renal capsule and the parenchyma. The sac is often at a pole, but the fluid dissects between the kidney and its capsule or is extracapsular. Fluid cytology reveals a transudate with urea nitrogen close to that of serum. Because the structure does not communicate with renal parenchyma, contrast does not fill it, and on ultrasound it is seen to envelop the kidney rather than exist within it. One report describes a case in which the pseudocyst communicated with the pleural space, resulting in hydrothorax.

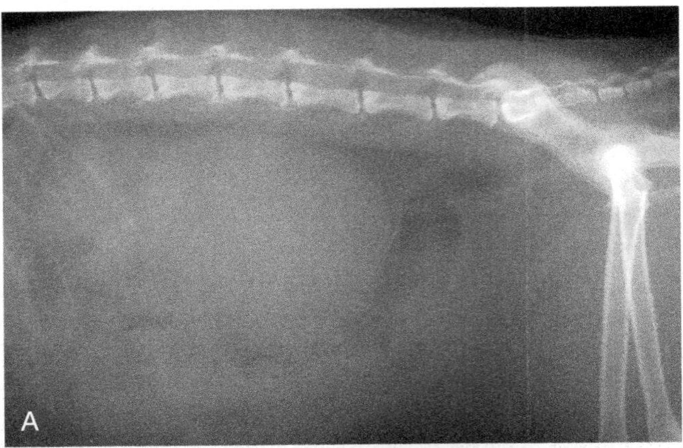

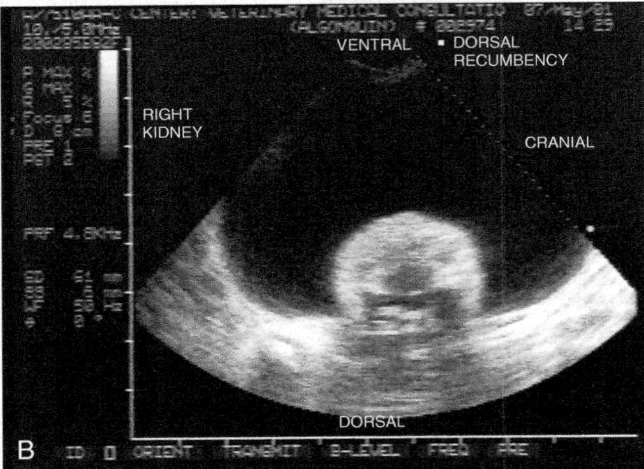

FIGURE 32-6 **A,** This lateral radiograph shows a soft tissue density in the region of the kidney. **B,** This ultrasound of the same patient reveals that the mass is a classic perinephric pseudocyst. *(Courtesy Dr. Edward Javinsky.)*

Unilateral nephrectomy of the affected kidney resulted in resolution of the hydrothorax.[191]

Affected cats are generally older (older than 8 years of age); there is no sex or breed predisposition.[21,175] The lesion is initially detected on palpation; renal insufficiency may be diagnosed on the basis of serum biochemistries and urinalysis, either due to associated interstitial fibrosis or the effect of compression. Imaging reveals the nature of the lesion (Figure 32-6).

Surgical resection of cyst walls is recommended, although reduction by drainage may provide temporary relief. There is one report of cyst wall omentalization with good long-term outcome.[108] Another case report describes laparoscopic fenestration of the capsule wall with resulting improvement in GFR of the affected kidney; no relapse was seen.[157] In other cases renal disease progresses, with the outcome being related to the severity of the renal disease.

Acquired Cysts

Cysts may also be acquired as a result of intraluminal obstruction of renal tubules by inflammatory debris or exudate or because of extraluminal compression associated with interstitial inflammation or fibrosis. Cysts may be unilateral but are more commonly bilateral. Regardless of cause, if cysts enlarge or become more numerous, resulting damage (compression) to parenchyma occurs, function is compromised, and azotemia develops.

RENAL AMYLOIDOSIS

Amyloidosis involves the deposition of insoluble proteins that have a specific pleated conformation. In cats, the condition occurs in the pancreas, where an islet-associated polypeptide form of amyloid is frequently found and is co-secreted with insulin.[118,152] Another form of localized amyloidosis has been reported in a cat with a plasmacytoma.[47]

Systemic amyloidosis with amyloid deposition primarily in the kidney is seen in Abyssinian cats; however, other breeds may also be affected (e.g., Siamese and other Oriental breeds, in which deposition is primarily in the liver). In the former it appears to be a result of a reactive inflammatory response, as reflected by the presence of amyloid protein AA and identification of concurrent inflammatory lesions in the tissues of approximately half of the examined cats.[67] Amyloid is deposited in the kidneys between 9 and 24 months of age. Renal insufficiency can progress rapidly, resulting in renal failure within 1 year, or deposits may be so mild that the effect may remain clinically undetected, allowing affected cats to live into old age. The condition affects females to males in a 1.4:1 ratio.[35] It is inherited in an autosomal dominant fashion but has a wide spectrum of disease expression because of variable penetrance.

In non-Abyssinian cats, the inflammatory aspect is lacking; a few cases have been associated with hypervitaminosis A.[55,56] The mean age is 7 years and the male:female ratio favors males 2:1.

Clinical illness reflects renal impairment, with the degree of involvement and location of the amyloid deposits playing a role. If glomeruli are involved, proteinuria will be present, whereas if lesions are restricted to the interstitium, azotemia with decreased urine-concentrating ability will be evoked. Affected cats will be in various degrees of renal insufficiency (uremic ulcers, inappetence, weight loss, dehydration, polyuria, polydipsia, lethargy). Metabolic acidosis, azotemia, hyperphosphatemia, hypokalemia, stress hyperglycemia/glucosuria, nonregenerative anemia, and low USG may all be components.

Definitive diagnosis requires renal biopsy; if the deposits are restricted to the medulla, they will be missed by needle biopsy because the procedure is limited to sampling the cortex (discussed previously).[184] In addition to routine hematoxylin and eosin (H&E) staining, when Congo red is applied to the section and it is viewed with polarized light, birefringence and an apple-green color specifically represent amyloid. Thioflavine T stain results in a yellow-green stain when visualized with ultraviolet light. Typically, papillary necrosis, chronic tubulointerstitial nephritis characterized by a lymphoplasmacytic infiltrate, and fibrosis with variable degrees of glomerular deposits are present.

In addition to the kidneys, amyloid is found in other organs of affected Abyssinian and non-Abyssinian cats. These may include the tongue, stomach, small and large intestines, liver, pancreas, spleen, heart, and adrenal and thyroid glands.

Treatment goals include supportive care for renal disease, identification and treatment of underlying inflammatory disease if identified, and attempts to mobilize the offending amyloid. Dimethyl sulfoxide (DMSO), by reducing serum amyloid protein A concentrations and through its antiinflammatory effects, could be considered were it tolerated therapeutically by cats. Colchicine is used in dogs and humans with amyloidosis to prevent formation of the amyloid; however, a safe and effective dose has *not* been established in cats.

POLYARTERITIS NODOSA

Polyarteritis nodosa is an extremely rare abnormality in which small and medium arteries undergo segmental inflammation and necrosis. The lesions may be restricted to the kidneys or affect multiple organs. When the kidney is involved, regions supplied by affected vessels become infarcted. There are only a handful of feline cases reported in the literature. Histologic changes were described as fibrinoid necrosis of the tunica media of implicated arteries with concurrent mononuclear cell infiltration. Glomerular lesions are noteworthy. Diagnosis requires biopsy, and therapy centers on supportive care and immunosuppression once cultures prove negative for bacterial infection. Prognosis has been poor in the few documented cases.

FELINE INFECTIOUS PERITONITIS

The dry or noneffusive form of feline infectious peritonitis (FIP) often involves the kidneys, along with other organs (liver, central nervous system [CNS], mesenteric lymph nodes, and eyes). Bilateral, asymmetric renomegaly is common. As might be expected with this disease, vague, nonspecific clinical signs are noted: inappetence, lethargy, muscle wasting, weight loss, and dehydration. Fever may be noted; however, it is also easily missed because of its intermittent nature. Only if, or once, renal involvement is marked, will polyuria and polydipsia become evident. In addition to hyperglobulinemia, a serum albumin:globulin ratio below 0.4; an inflammatory leukogram; an inappropriate USG of less than 1.040, with or without proteinuria; and cytology of the enlarged kidneys revealing pyogranulomatous inflammation suggest a diagnosis of FIP.[103] Pyogranulomas (neutrophils, macrophages, lymphocytes, and plasma cells) are generally limited to the renal cortex and may result in lumpy, irregularly enlarged kidneys. Thanks to better diagnostic sensitivity of both biopsy and fine-needle aspirate (FNA) of the liver compared with the kidney, it is advisable to sample both tissues concurrently. Additionally, because false-negative results are not uncommon, use of both Tru-Cut biopsy and FNA together improves diagnostic value.[88] Lymphoma may manifest in a similar clinical fashion; cytology may be expected to differentiate between the two conditions insofar as cytology will reveal a monomorphic population of lymphocytes in the neoplastic condition. FIP is covered in greater detail in Chapter 33.

RENAL NEOPLASIA

Lymphoma is the most common type of neoplasia affecting feline kidneys; however, primary renal neoplasms that are not hemolymphatic in origin are reported infrequently. Carcinoma and nephroblastoma are less frequent, and mesenchymal tumors (hemangiosarcoma, fibrosarcoma, chondrosarcoma, and leiomyosarcoma) are rare. Metastatic tumors are common in this organ because of the large blood supply.[216] Evaluation of the records and tissues from four veterinary colleges and one private referral practice over a 6-year period revealed only 19 cases of renal tumors. The majority of these (13 of 19) were renal carcinomas (11 tubular and 2 tubulopapillary), with three transitional cell carcinomas, one malignant nephroblastoma, one hemangiosarcoma, and one adenoma.[106] In addition, the recent literature includes a cat with a renal cystadenoma,[169] one with a transitional cell carcinoma forming a perirenal cyst,[186] and two with renal adenocarcinoma–induced polycythemia.[126] Lymphoma, in contrast, is very common, with 31% of 118 cats with multicentric lymphoma in one report having renal involvement,[85] or as high a percentage as 45% according to another source.[216]

Diagnosis of lymphoma is made by FNA or renal biopsy. Cancer staging (I-V) is recommended because treatment planning will be affected. This involves palpation, hematology, serum biochemistry, survey abdominal radiographs or ultrasonography, and bone marrow aspiration (see Chapter 28). The presence of ultrasonographic evidence of hypoechoic subcapsular thickening in feline kidneys is associated with renal lymphosarcoma. In one study the positive predictive value of this finding was 80.9%, and the negative predictive value was 66.7%. This resulted in a sensitivity of 60.7% and a specificity of 84.6%.[215]

Surgical management is generally not recommended for lymphoma. In cats with renal or multicentric lymphoma, chemotherapy is recommended. Numerous induction and maintenance protocols using multiple chemotherapeutic drugs have been described. These agents include vincristine, cyclophosphamide, L-asparaginase, doxorubicin, methotrexate, and prednisolone. One study evaluated the response to chemotherapy in 110 cats with extranodal lymphoma, of which 35 had renal lymphoma. The conclusions of this retrospective study were that cats with extranodal lymphoma respond to chemotherapy and achieve survival times comparable to those with disease in other locations. Corticosteroid pretreatment reduced survival time in cats achieving complete remission.[212] The prognosis for a cat with renal lymphoma depends on the stage of the tumor, existing renal function, responsiveness to chemotherapy, and retrovirus status.[216] More information about lymphoma can be found in Chapter 28.

PYELONEPHRITIS

Pyelonephritis refers to bacterial infection of one or both kidneys. Resulting inflammation may be centered in the pelvic region and adjacent medulla, which suggests ascending infection. Alternately, if the route of infection is hematogenous, a more generalized distribution of lesions may be expected (Figure 32-7). The clinical presentation in either case may be vague (lethargy, inappetence, anorexia, and dehydration) or may include more marked but still poorly specific signs of weight loss, vomiting, polyuria, and polydipsia. Fever may remain undetected because of its tendency to wax and wane. Clinical signs may be brief with self-resolution or may persist over time.

Because of the infrequent use of biopsy as a diagnostic tool in feline medicine and the less common prevalence of infection of the urinary tract in cats compared with dogs, it is unclear how often infection by either route (ascending versus hematogenous) occurs. In humans ureteral obstruction by casts or ureteronephroliths contributes to risk of infection; this occurs at least experimentally in cats. Pyelonephritis potentially predisposes to ongoing inflammation and may contribute to chronic interstitial nephritis. However, it is unlikely that this is the originating cause of chronic interstitial nephritis, the most common histopathologic form of chronic renal disease in the majority of cats.

Urine culture and renal imaging are required for definitive diagnosis. Minimum database tests (hematology, biochemistries, urinalysis, and BP assessment) yield results that point to renal infection. Neutrophilia with a left shift may be present in acute disease. A stress leukogram may reflect inflammation and chronicity along with a nonregenerative anemia. Biochemistry findings

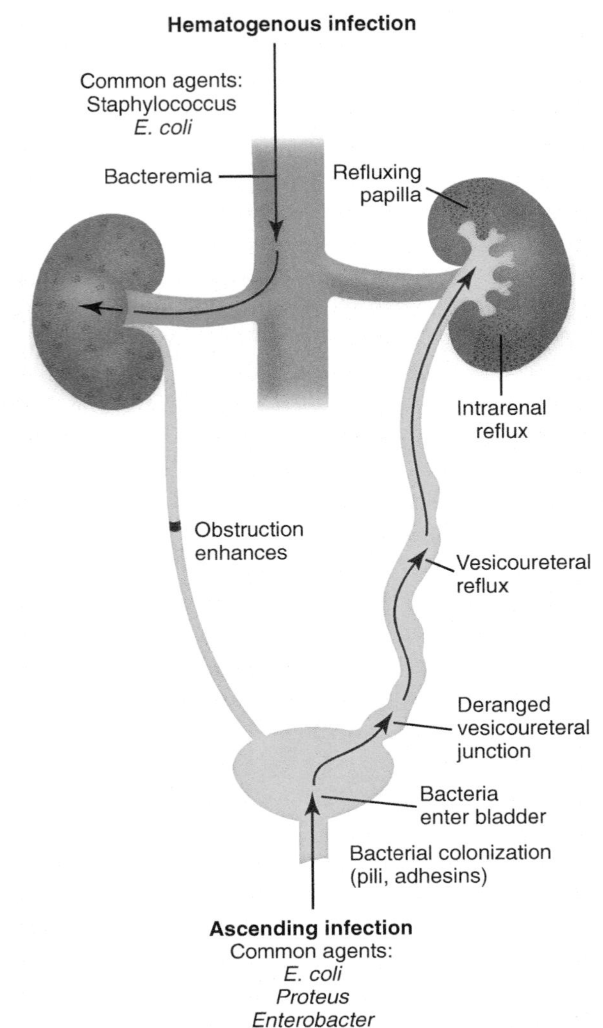

FIGURE 32-7 Infection of the kidney resulting in pyelonephritis may occur by either the hematogenous spread of bacteria or from ascending infection. *(Adapted from Cotran RS, Kumar V, Robbins SL: The kidney. In Cotran RS, Kumar V, Robbins SL, editors:* Robbins pathologic basis of disease, *ed 5, Philadelphia, 1994, Saunders.)*

include azotemia, hyperphosphatemia, and metabolic acidosis. Urinalysis shows proteinuria, bacteriuria with pyuria, and hematuria indicative of infection, but imaging (ultrasound or a contrast radiographic study) is needed to determine what part of the urinary tract is affected. Although it might be expected that concurrent typical signs of stranguria and pollakiuria, with or without periuria (inappropriate urination), indicate lower urinary tract involvement, a remarkable 29% (38 of 132) of cats with positive urine cultures lacked these clinical signs in one study. There was a significant predisposition to being female among these patients, and *Enterococcus faecalis* was the most commonly isolated bacteria, ahead of *Escherichia coli* phylogenetic group B2.[151] Finding leukocyte casts in the urine localizes the disorder to the kidneys; however, because casts are infrequently reported, a diagnosis of pyelonephritis should not rely on this finding.

Either ultrasound or an excretory urogram may be used to suggest a diagnosis of pyelonephritis. Ultrasound findings suggestive of this condition include a dilated renal pelvis with hyperechoic, edematous mesentery and peritoneal or retroperitoneal effusion reflecting inflammation of these tissues. In contrast, the far more common hydronephrosis may be characterized by a similarly dilated renal pelvis, but with anechoic contents and no findings indicative of peritonitis.[53]

Older cats with low USG associated with CKD or glucosuria caused by poorly controlled DM are more prone to upper or lower UTI. A study was performed to ascertain whether antibiotic sensitivity profiles can be used to distinguish between relapsing (or persisting) UTIs from reinfection by different clones of uropathogenic *E. coli*. Results showed that they cannot be relied on for this purpose in the cat.[84]

Similar to lower UTI, antimicrobial therapy should be continued for 4 to 5 weeks for an initial episode of pyelonephritis; subsequent occurrences require a 5- to 8-week course of antibiotic therapy, as determined by sensitivity spectrum. Follow-up urine culture after and possibly during therapy is required to document eradication of infection. Culture during therapy may be considered with the intention of verifying that no additional organisms have become apparent as a result of treatment. Given the potential for infection-instigated inflammation favoring chronic renal insufficiency and interstitial nephritis, complete and thorough treatment with documentation of cure is extremely important.

GLOMERULONEPHRITIS

GN occurs as a sequela to one of two instigating pathways for immune-mediated damage of the glomeruli. In the autoimmune form antibodies react with glomerular basement membrane antigen; in the other form soluble circulating immune complexes become entrapped in the glomerular capillary wall. Any infectious, inflammatory, neoplastic, or degenerative processes capable of sustained antigenic stimulation can induce immune-mediated glomerular injury.[174] It is this latter form that is seen in cats. Because the underlying cause for antigen production is so varied and generally not associated directly with the kidney itself, it is important to try to identify and treat the underlying cause. Most cases are deemed to be idiopathic in cats because the cause is not usually apparent.[93,94] Box 32-5 lists causes of GN in cats.

Cats with GN tend to be young adults (mean age 4 years, range up to 12 years) and male (intact or altered). They present with either classic nephrotic syndrome (subcutaneous edema, ascites, muscle wasting) or variable degrees of clinical signs associated with chronic renal insufficiency. These may include inappetence; anorexia; weight loss; lethargy; polyuria; polydipsia; vomiting; pale mucous membranes; and small, firm kidneys.

BOX 32-5

Causes of Glomerulonephritis in Cats

Idiopathic: most common
Infectious: e.g., feline infectious peritonitis, bacterial, feline leukemia virus, *Mycoplasma gatae*
Inflammatory: e.g., systemic lupus erythematosus?, chronic progressive polyarthritis
Neoplastic: e.g., lymphoma, myeloproliferative disorders
Toxicity: e.g., hydrocarbons?[188], mercury?
Familial: Abyssinians[222]

Proteinuria is certainly a hallmark finding for glomerular disease. It must, however, be remembered that proteinuria may also be a result of prerenal inflammation or tubular or interstitial disease, as well as originating in the urinary tract distal to the kidney. Thus proteinuria itself is not pathognomonic for GN. In the cat with nephrotic syndrome, proteinuria, hypercholesterolemia, and hypoalbuminemia with mild azotemia may be expected and the USG may remain between 1.030 and 1.050. In the cat with clinical signs of renal insufficiency, the azotemia is more moderate to severe in degree, the USG is lower, and a nonregenerative anemia may be present. The other laboratory findings reflect CKD. In addition to a complete blood count (CBC), serum biochemistries, urinalysis, and BP evaluation, retroviral serology is indicated. If joints are affected, joint fluid analysis should be considered. Antinuclear antibody titer and lupus erythematosus cell preparations may also be considered. Urine or blood culture (or both) may be warranted.

On the basis of light microscopy, immunofluorescence, transmission electron microscopy, and scanning electron microscopy, there are a number of types of GN that have been reported in cats. The following definitions or descriptions are in order:

- Membranous GN has a thickened glomerular basement membrane.
- Proliferative GN (mesangioproliferative GN) is characterized by glomerular hypercellularity with accumulation of mesangial matrix.
- Membranoproliferative GN has a thickened glomerular basement membrane but also is hypercellular.
- Glomerulosclerosis is characterized by both an increase in mesangial matrix and glomerular scarring.

- "Minimal change disease" is characterized by minimal increases in mesangial cell proliferation, abnormal podocyte foot processes, and a lack of immunoglobulin deposition when stained with immunofluorescent preparations.

Eleven cases of membranous nephropathy,[225] two types of membranoproliferative,[15,113] nonamyloidotic fibrillary glomerulonephritis,[49] and glomerular fibrosis ("collagenofibrotic glomerulonephropathy")[170] have been reported in cats. The GN of six related Abyssinians was not characterized beyond light microscopic evaluation.[222] Experimentally, immune-complex proliferative GN (more similar to the disease in humans than other feline forms) has been induced using intravenous injections of cationic bovine or human serum albumin.[28,29,30,171] In this model cats develop hypoalbuminemia before signs of clinical disease occur. However, the appearance of proteinuria may be misleading insofar as it occurred in some of the control cats without GN as well.[29] In a study evaluating histopathology of renal biopsies with clinical data in dogs and cats, higher Cr values were suggestive of (and correlated with) changes of interstitial nephritis. High urinary protein values correlated with glomerular disease. Although no relationship between different types of nephropathy and age were found, in general, cats (and dogs) with chronic tubulointerstitial nephritis were, on average, older than animals with glomerulopathies.[164]

In another study of naturally occurring renal disease in dogs and cats, myofibroblast induction was studied. Immunohistochemical expression of myofibroblast markers, alpha-smooth muscle actin (alpha-SMA) and vimentin were evaluated quantitatively. In cats, Cr concentrations correlated with fibrosis, alpha-SMA expression correlated with Cr and fibrosis, tubular vimentin expression correlated with fibrosis, and interstitial vimentin expression correlated with Cr.[227] The relevance is that the correlations found in dogs were different, indicating that the severity of CKD is mediated by different pathways associated with myofibroblast expression in dogs compared with cats.

In a patient with persistent proteinuria of renal origin, a biopsy of the kidney is indicated. Indeed, it is necessary for the accurate diagnosis of GN and may help guide therapy. Indications for renal biopsy are summarized in Box 32-6. When performed correctly (i.e., in a carefully monitored, sedated, or anesthetized cat with no history of a bleeding disorder, using ultrasound guidance and a Tru-Cut biopsy needle or by a surgical keyhole approach, harvesting only cortex [pole to pole] and monitoring for postprocedural bleeding), there is minimal risk even in the face of renal dysfunction. The sample must be handled carefully and submitted in the correct medium to a laboratory able to perform not just light microscopy (standard histopathology and immunofluorescent staining) but also EM for ultrastructural examination (Box 32-7).

BOX 32-6
Indications for Renal Biopsy

Acute nephritis: Yes, if injury is recent, active, and ongoing
Acute nephrosis: Maybe; it may help assess severity and reversibility, but it will not direct therapy
Glomerulopathy: Yes, can establish diagnosis and aid in directing therapy
Renal proteinuria: Yes, if higher UPC and lower creatinine; maybe if borderline but not responding to therapy
Chronic kidney disease, IRIS late stage 3 or stage 4: No, generally will not provide clinically useful information

UPC, Urine protein: creatinine ratio.
Adapted from Lees GE, Berridge BR: Renal biopsy—when & why, *NAVC Clinician's Brief* 7:26, 2009.

BOX 32-7
Centers that Perform Comprehensive Renal Biopsy Evaluations*

Texas A&M University—Texas Veterinary Renal Pathology Service
- Dr. George E. Lees: glees@cvm.tamu.edu; telephone 1-888-778-5523 (toll free) or 1-979-845-2351

Utrecht University—Dept. of Clinical Sciences of Companion Animals, Yalelaan 108, NL 3584 CM Utrecht; mailing address: P.O. Box 80.154, NL 3508 TD Utrecht
- Dr. Astrid M. van Dongen: A.M.vanDongen@uu.nl; telephone +31 (0)30 2537767, fax +31 (0)30 2518126

*At the time of this writing.

The centers that perform full assessment of renal biopsies provide kits containing detailed instructions along with the materials necessary to collect, properly preserve, and submit the samples to their laboratories. The veterinarian should speak with the person who will be evaluating the tissue sample to obtain complete instructions and ensure that he or she feels comfortable with the technique before proceeding.

Renal biopsy samples should be processed in several ways[146,147]:

1. Using light microscopy, samples are stained with H&E, periodic acid-Schiff (PAS), Masson's

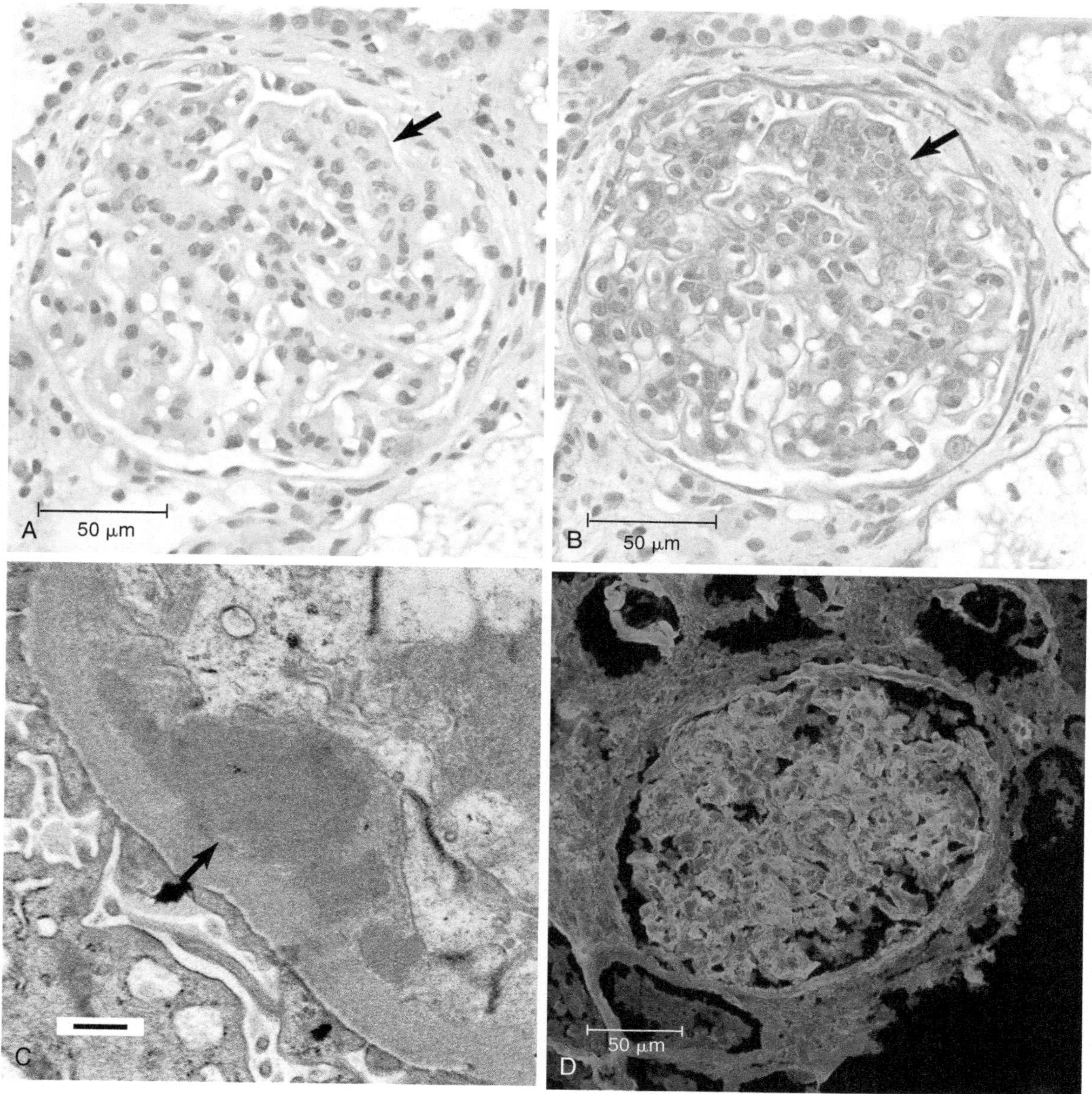

FIGURE 32-8 Pathologic findings in a renal biopsy obtained from a 5-year-old neutered male domestic shorthair cat with glomerular disease. **A** (H&E stain) and **B** (PAS stain), Photomicrographs of a glomerulus that exhibits histologic changes consistent with membranoproliferative glomerulonephritis. The capillary lumens are effaced by mesangial and endocapillary hypercellularity in the marked glomerular lobule *(arrows)*. **C**, Transmission electron photomicrograph of subendothelial electron-dense deposits *(arrows)* in a glomerular capillary wall (bar = 500 nm). **D**, Immunofluorescence photomicrograph of a glomerulus labeled for immunoglobulin G. *(A, B, and D courtesy Dr. George E. Lees, Texas A&M University; C courtesy Dr. Fred J. Clubb, Jr., Texas A&M University.)*

trichrome, Jones' methenamine silver (JMS), and Congo red to fully characterize lesions.
2. Immunohistochemical stains are applied to evaluate sections with immunofluorescence.
3. Lastly, transmission electron microscopy is performed on glutaraldehyde-preserved samples to examine ultrastructural detail.

Figure 32-8 shows renal biopsy samples from a patient with glomerular disease.

Renal biopsies can be performed in two ways[145]:

1. Using an automated needle biopsy device and ultrasound guidance
2. By a surgical approach: keyhole needle or wedge biopsies or using laparotomy

All techniques require that the patient be anesthetized rather than sedated for comfort and immobilization. Ultrasound-guided needle biopsy is appropriate when the expected lesions are diffusely distributed in the cortex (e.g., ARF, GN). When the clinician is experienced, this approach is less traumatic for the patient than the surgical options and can yield adequate to excellent samples. Extensive practice in aspiration and biopsy of other organs is recommended before attempting this procedure because there is little room for error. An automated device, such as a Tru-Cut or similar biopsy needle, is used. The needle throw should be short (e.g., 11 mm, 7 mm specimen notch); an 18G diameter needle is appropriate for cats of most sizes. Patient positioning will depend to some degree on the preference of the ultrasonographer or radiologist. The goal is to present as much of the cortex as possible while minimizing inadvertent damage of hilar blood vessels that could result in bleeding and subsequent infarction or outright fatal hemorrhage. Assuming that both kidneys are affected, the advantage of sampling the right kidney is that it is less mobile than the left. The left kidney, on the other hand, is more superficial and more caudally placed than the right.

The veterinarian should position the cat for an optimal view of the cortex: Ventrodorsal recumbency reveals the lateral cortex, and lateral recumbency exposes the dorsal cortex. Both these positions place the hilus in a less vulnerable, more distal location. An ultrasound guide may be used to position the needle biopsy device alongside the probe once the optimal view is achieved; alternately, the probe and the needle device can be used independently (freehand) of each other. The latter requires excellent hand–eye coordination. Once the direction of the needle placement has been selected, the veterinarian makes a small stab incision with a scalpel blade through the skin and then advances the biopsy needle through the body wall up to and just through the capsule before activating the biopsy device (see Figure 32-3).

Next, the veterinarian harvests a minimum of two cortical core samples. Ideal samples are 10 mm in length or longer. If they are shorter than this, a third tissue core should be collected. The veterinarian should use a gentle flow of sterile saline through a 25G needle to flush the tissue from the biopsy needle onto a glass slide to keep the biopsy needle sterile for the next sample and keep from traumatizing the sample. The veterinarian flushes the biopsy needle with more saline and greater force (away from the sample) to dislodge any debris remaining in the cutting channel. This is repeated until two or three good cores have been collected. It is important to check that the samples contain glomeruli using the 10× to 40× lens on a microscope, a handheld magnifying lens, or an ocular loupe.

Should a surgical approach be preferred over ultrasound guidance, a keyhole incision may be made over the kidney or a celiotomy or laparotomy may be performed. Because it is very easy to penetrate too deeply without the benefit of ultrasound to visualize the difference between the cortical and medullary echos, a wedge biopsy is preferable to using the automated needle biopsy device. The sample is taken by incising the cortex with a small elliptical incision, and the sample is excised by cutting it off with a flat bottom before the medulla is penetrated. The wedge can then be subdivided into samples, as recommended by the appropriate staff member at the renal pathology center.

It is important to keep the tissue cores moist on saline-soaked swabs. They should never be handled with toothed forceps. They should be placed in the appropriate preservative and fixatives promptly according to the directions provided by the renal pathology service.

On the basis of ultrastructural studies, as well as the type and distribution pattern of the immunoglobulins or complement, clues to the pathogenesis of GN in the individual patient may be determined, thereby allowing a rational and specific treatment plan to be made. Additionally, the clinical problems should be addressed. For the nephrotic, edematous, or ascitic patient with minimal or no azotemia, diuretic therapy is indicated. The patient should be closely monitored to ensure adequate but not excessive diuresis because dehydration and hypovolemia are detrimental to tissue perfusion, including that of the kidneys. An ACE-I is of value in reducing glomerular loss of protein by reducing glomerular pressure and GFR. GFR reduction (and the potential for increased azotemia) is mild and will stabilize. The urine protein:creatinine ratio (UPC) should be monitored for improvement; in patients in which no reduction of proteinuria is noted, the ACE-I should be discontinued. Corticosteroids may be considered to reduce the inflammatory response and production of antibodies for antigen-antibody complexes. Increasing dietary protein by using a growth diet or adding hard-boiled eggs or cooked egg white to the cat's food may be beneficial by countering the hypoalbuminemia caused by the glomerular protein loss. Sodium restriction should be considered if sodium retention is apparent.

For those GN patients with moderate to severe azotemia, corticosteroids and furosemide are not recommended. Instead, treatment is as for the cat with interstitial nephritis (CKD) but with additional dietary protein to offset their urinary losses. In both clinical presentations hypertension should be addressed (discussed later). If urine culture has revealed bacterial involvement, a prolonged course (minimally 5 to 8 weeks) of the appropriate antimicrobial is indicated, with reculture after discontinuation of the antibiotic.

The prognosis is extremely variable and depends on the instigating cause of the immune mechanism. If it is bacterial in origin and the infection is successfully eliminated, cure may occur. If the underlying disease is FIP, the course will be short and the prognosis grim. With nephrotic syndrome or less severe azotemia, good control may be achieved for several years. If azotemia is advanced and multiple components of renal disease are present, such as hyperphosphatemia, hypertension, nonregenerative anemia, and muscle wasting, the prognosis is poor.

URETERONEPHROLITHIASIS

Renal calculi are a significant cause of CKD and hydronephrosis, although urolithiasis occurs less frequently in the cat than the dog. Concomitant UTI is also much less common with feline struvite urolithiasis than it is in dogs.

The first of the two largest retrospective studies of feline and canine ureteronephroliths was published in 1998 (71 cats with *renal* calculi from 1981 to 1993) and reported that 38 of the renal calculi were from female cats and 33 were from male cats. Pedigreed cats were predisposed to renal calculus formation compared with random bred cats. Increased age was identified as a predisposing factor. Somewhat surprisingly, more than 50% of renal calculi were identified in the first known episode of urolithiasis, justifying radiography as part of the minimum database in affected patients (Figures 32-2 and 32-9). Additionally, the risk of forming renal calculi was found to be higher in cats than in dogs compared with other sites of stone formation (approximately 4.95 per 100 stone-forming cats versus 2.88 per 100 dogs). Unilateral disease favors the left kidney; approximately 9% of cats with renal stones had bilateral involvement. Stone composition analysis in this study showed oxalate and apatite as the main contenders, and there was no sex predisposition for stone composition or for concurrent/causative bacterial infection.[150] Struvite stones are more commonly induced by diet in cats; however infection-based stones may occasionally occur as well in cats with conditions predisposing to UTI (e.g., DM, perineal urethrostomy).

The second large study,[131] reported in 2005, reviewed the records of 163 cats with *ureteral* calculi evaluated from 1984 to 2002. Of note was that the number of cats in which ureterolithiasis was diagnosed each year increased progressively during the study period, notably after the year 2000. The median age of affected cats was 7 years, with a range of 8 months to 16 years. Clinical signs recorded included inappetence and anorexia in 45% of cats, vomiting in 42%, lethargy in 31%, weight loss in 27%, polyuria and polydipsia in only 18%, and the remaining signs (stranguria and pollakiuria, hematuria, pain on abdominal palpation, inappropriate urination, ptyalism, urethral obstruction, and obtundation) in fewer than 9%. On laboratory evaluation a surprising 48% of 150 cats tested were anemic. Either renal or prerenal azotemia (elevation of either BUN or Cr) was found in 83% of the total cats tested (76% of those with unilateral and 96% with bilateral calculi), 54% had hyperphosphatemia (43% if unilateral), 35% were hyperkalemic, and 14% were hypercalcemic. This implies that the function of the contralateral kidney was impaired, the cats were dehydrated, or both. UTI was found in 8% of the cats; crystalluria was reported in 36 of 124 (29%) urine samples.

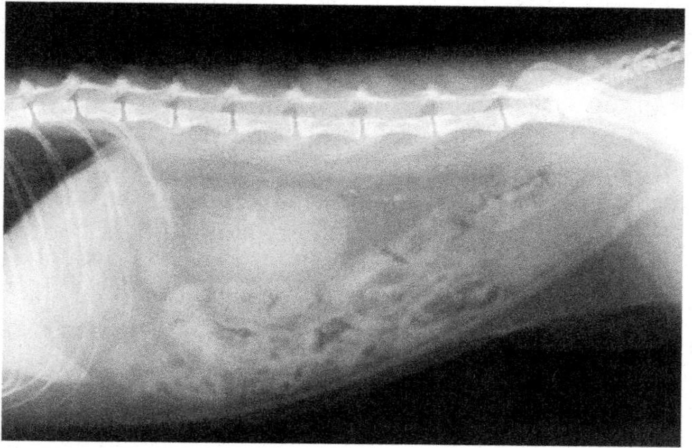

FIGURE 32-9 This lateral radiograph shows numerous radioopacities in the region of the kidney and ureter. A ventrodorsal view or an abdominal ultrasound is required to localize these lesions to the kidney and ureter; however, this is suggestive of urolithiasis.

The sensitivity of ultrasound in identifying ureteral calculi was 77%. Radiography on its own identified 81% of ureteroliths. When ultrasound and radiography were combined, the detection sensitivity rose to 90%. Based on the finding of a dilated renal pelvis or proximal ureter, ureteral obstruction was identified in 143 (92%) of 155 cats that underwent abdominal ultrasound. Interestingly, 73 of the cats had surgical or necropsy confirmation of the diagnosis, yet a combination of radiography and ultrasound revealed only 66 (90%) of those cases. Therefore it seems prudent to pursue both imaging modalities when investigating the possibility of ureteral calculi. In fact, in seven cats the calculi were an incidental finding during ultrasound of the abdomen for another problem. Of additional note is that in this ureterolith population, 101 cats had concurrent renal calculi (62%) and 14 had cystic calculi (<1%). Other imaging modalities that may be considered (and were used in some of these patients) are intravenous urography, antegrade pyelography, nuclear scintigraphy, and CT.[132]

Clinical signs of renal or ureteral stones may be vague to nonexistent. Cats may present with apparently painless hematuria or with ill thrift associated with infection or azotemia. Excessive grooming over the dorsolumbar region or abdomen has been noted by the author in a few cases. Thus, because clinical signs are so variable and ureteronephroliths are so common, screening radiographs can be justified as part of the workup of an older cat with or without renal insufficiency. In a patient with clinical illness, abdominal ultrasound as well as radiography may well be justified.

Ureteral stones were analyzed in 93 cats in the second study; calcium oxalate (CaOx) was identified in 81 cats, mixed CaOx and calcium phosphate ($CaPO_4$) in seven cats, $CaPO_4$ in two cats, and mixed CaOx and urate in two cats, the last being mixed CaOx and amorphous calcium.[131] One paper from Norway reports an oxalate-like nephrosis in Ragdoll cats.[105] The diagnosis of primary hyperoxaluria types 1 and 2 was excluded in 11 cats tested; both etiology and inheritance remain unknown.

Therapy may initially include IV fluids and diuretics (the goals being to increase urine production and voiding and supportive care for underlying renal insufficiency), but some cats will need additional surgical assistance. Because bilateral chronic interstitial fibrosis is common in cats with ureteroliths or nephroliths, nephrectomy should not be considered unless it has been established that the contralateral kidney has adequate function to support the patient. Renal transplantation may be a feasible option.

In a study of 153 cats with ureteral calculi,[132] management and outcome were evaluated. After medical therapy for all cats, 66% of the patients received additional treatments. Nephrostomy tubes were placed in a few of these cats to improve urine drainage, and a few patients received hemodialysis. Possible surgical solutions depended on the location of the ureteronephrolith. For proximal ureteral stones, ureterotomy was used; for more distal stones partial ureterectomy and ureteroneocystostomy were the treatment of choice. Postoperative complication rates were 31% in those patients proceeding to surgery (e.g., urine leakage resulting in uroabdomen, persistent ureteral obstruction). The postoperative mortality rate was 18%. Yet the 24-month survival rate of those that received only medical treatment was 66%, and when cats were euthanized, it occurred within 1 month of diagnosis. In the surgical (after medical stabilization) group, 12- and 24-month survival rates were 91% and 88%, respectively.[132]

Any stones removed surgically or passed during medical treatment should be submitted for quantitative analysis to allow institution of appropriate preventive therapy, when it exists. Similarly, if bacterial infection is identified, antimicrobial therapy based on sensitivity profiles and overall health should be followed for a minimum of 5 to 8 weeks. Subsequent medical care should focus on achieving a moderate urine pH of 6 to 6.5 and USG of approximately 1.035 (should the cat have a higher USG) to reduce the likelihood of recurrence of stones. Recurrence was found in 14 of 35 cats (40%) that were monitored serially with abdominal radiography after medical or surgical therapy.[132]

A very small case-control study attempted to evaluate whether the presence of nephroliths negatively affected progression of renal disease in cats with IRIS stage II or III disease. It was found that in the 14 cats (7 with nephroliths) there was neither an increase in the rate of progression nor increased mortality from renal disease.[194]

Lithotripsy has been evaluated in cats. Compared to canine CaOx stones, feline CaOx uroliths are less susceptible to fragmentation by shock wave lithotripsy. Studies have concluded that the high numbers of shock waves required for adequate fragmentation of the CaOx nephroliths may cause renal or ureteral injury in some cats.[3,90] Ureteroliths are often not fixed in location and are capable of spontaneous retrograde movement. In contrast, laser lithotripsy may be more suitable for fragmentation of bladder uroliths—in essence, any urolith that can be accessed using a flexible or rigid cystoscope. A few caveats apply, however. Even when the stones are broken into sandlike fragments, ureteral or possibly urethral obstruction may still occur. Given the anatomic challenges of the narrower male urethra, this technique should be considered in female cats only.

HYDRONEPHROSIS

Hydronephrosis is defined as the distention of the renal pelvis and calices with urine as a result of obstruction of the urinary outflow tract. Obstruction can occur at various places in the urinary tract (Figure 32-10). It usually occurs as a result of ureterolithiasis or urethral obstruction; however, neoplasia, pregnancy, infection, and strictures may also be causes of this condition. Rarely, hydronephrosis may be congenital because of a deformity of, or affecting, the ureter. The condition has been seen in cats of any age and all breeds; a literature search does not reveal a sex predilection.

Depending on the cause, as well as the speed, of treatment, hydronephrosis may be reversible. The condition may be unilateral or bilateral. When it is unilateral, the relative size difference between the affected enlarged kidney and the unaffected normal or fibrosed contralateral organ can be very marked. The patient with unilateral disease may be expected to have a much more gradual onset of illness because the unaffected kidney compensates for the decreased function of its partner. Less commonly, both kidneys are distended concurrently, and these patients will present more acutely in crisis before extensive destruction and remodeling have occurred. If obstruction becomes complicated by infection, pyonephrosis may develop, resulting in lethargy, anorexia, fever, leukocytosis, bacteriuria, and pyuria.

In the case of unilateral hydronephrosis, diagnosis is suggested on finding unilateral renomegaly and verified through imaging. Intravenous urography will show a decreased uptake of contrast material by the kidney, which often has become merely a thin rim of cortical tissue. Ultrasound shows a dilated renal pelvis filled with anechoic fluid and a loss of renal parenchyma.[53] Depending on the structural cause, the obstruction may or may not be seen with either form of imaging. Because the fluid is urine, the cytology of a sample will reflect the character of the urine in that patient; it may be unremarkable or may contain renal tubular cells, red blood cells, or white blood cells. Over time it becomes more quiescent. Serum biochemistries and urinalysis results will reflect the patient's disease status (e.g., unilateral,

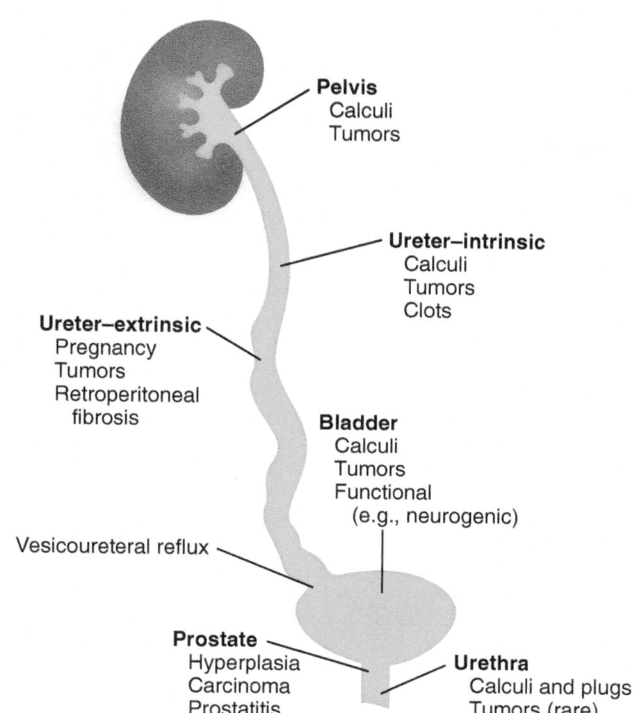

FIGURE 32-10 Although urethral obstruction is frequently recognized, obstruction to the urinary tract may occur at other locations. Calculi are underrecognized. *(Adapted from Cotran RS, Kumar V, Robbins SL: The kidney. In Cotran RS, Kumar V, Robbins SL, editors:* Robbins pathologic basis of disease, *ed 5, Philadelphia, 1994, Saunders.)*

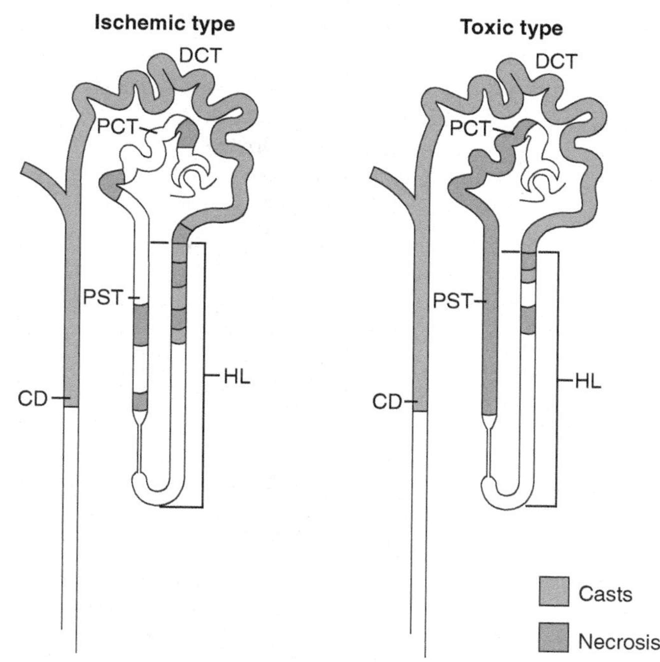

FIGURE 32-11 Acute tubular necrosis (ATN) is the most common cause of acute renal failure. This drawing depicts the two mechanisms by which ATN occurs. With ischemic damage tubular necrosis is patchy, affecting short segments of the proximal straight tubule (PST) and the loop of Henle (HL). When the insult is toxic, the damage is extensive along both the PST and proximal convoluted tubule (PCT), with some damage to the HL as well. Both forms of tubular necrosis result in accumulation of debris in the distal convoluted tubule (DCT) and the collecting duct (CD), resulting in urine casts. *(From Cotran RS, Kumar V, Robbins SL: The kidney. In Cotran RS, Kumar V, Robbins SL, editors:* Robbins pathologic basis of disease, *ed 5, Philadelphia, 1994, Saunders.)*

bilateral, duration, concurrent infection). Histopathology of the affected kidney shows a cystic structure with remnants of renal parenchyma, insofar as the kidney is, in essence, an innocent bystander to obstruction.

Treatment, including dialysis and supportive fluid therapy, is aimed at relief of obstruction and optimal restoration of renal function. The longer the obstruction, the poorer the chance of return to function. In some cases renal transplantation may be warranted.

ACUTE RENAL FAILURE

ARF may be a result of ischemia, infectious agents, or toxicity. What appears to be ARF may in fact be an acute decompensation of chronic renal disease. In this case one would expect a long-standing history of polyuria, polydipsia, and weight loss and a finding of anemia, whereas in the case of "true" ARF, exposure to a nephrotoxin or to a potential cause of ischemia (trauma, surgery, and thromboembolism) may precede the onset of acute disease in a previously unaffected individual. Recovery from ARF (but not from CKD) is potentially possible, depending on the type and degree of pathology induced, its location, and the rapidity with which adequate treatment is initiated. The lesions in ARF may be glomerular or tubular.

In general, *ischemic* damage results in focal tubular necrosis at multiple points in the nephron with unaffected regions in between. Where affected, the basement membrane may be ruptured and the tubules may be occluded by casts. Epithelial regeneration occurs such that, if treated promptly, over time no residual evidence of damage remains.[59] *Toxic* insults, on the other hand, tend to predominantly affect the proximal tubules with extensive necrosis, but because the basement membrane often remains intact, tubular regeneration may build on this scaffold.[64] In the case of ethylene glycol poisoning, in addition to casts, CaOx crystals may plug the lumen (Figure 32-11).[59]

From a therapeutic perspective, it is helpful to think of ARF in three phases:

1. The latent phase describes the period between exposure to insult and onset of renal dysfunction.
2. During the second (maintenance) phase, azotemia and reduction in urine production progress.
3. The final possible phase is that of recovery of as much function as is possible owing to innate mechanisms as well as therapy.

Prerenal ARF is a result of hypovolemia, hypotension, inadequate cardiac output, shock, or hypoxia. Reduced renal perfusion results in local ischemia, which, if sufficiently severe and long in duration, results in renal failure. Hypotension occurring during anesthesia is a common prerenal cause of ARF and may be preventable through careful monitoring. Likewise, hypovolemia can be easily addressed at any time. Hypothermia, another anesthetic risk, should also be avoided and, if noted, treated.

ARF originating from causes directed at the kidney includes ischemia and nephrotoxins. These toxins will be discussed to a limited degree later; the reader should refer to Chapter 31 for more detailed information.

Postrenal causes for ARF may be related to obstruction of urine outflow. Examples of luminal obstruction include plugs, calculi, and sludge in the urethra; however, external compression of the urethra by a mass (e.g., in the prostate, colon, lymph node) or urethral wall thickening from scarring or neoplasia will have the same end effect. Renal failure may occur within 48 to 72 hours of complete obstruction. If the obstruction has been relieved promptly and the cat is supported with fluid therapy, ARF associated with this cause is generally reversible. Uroperitoneum is another potential cause for postrenal ARF.

Although cats may react serologically to *Leptospira* species, they seem remarkably resistant to clinical disease. Cats may become infected and develop bacteremia after 5 to 10 days. The infection localizes in the kidney tubules, where it may cause impairment of renal function, but the clinical significance in this species is questionable. Experimentally infected cats are not usually clinically affected but may have mild to severe nephritis on histology, resulting in gradual chronic renal insufficiency over 1 to 3 years.

There are numerous toxic causes for ARF, however. These may be divided into plant, drug, or chemical toxicities. Cats may be especially predisposed to exposure to topical toxins because of their fastidious grooming behavior; if a toxic material is found on the hair coat or feet, it will be ingested.[207]

Lilies of many types can cause acute nephrotoxicosis. Easter lilies are not only nephrotoxic but also pancreotoxic.[197] The dose and species of plant ingested, the part of the plant eaten, and the stage of its life cycle may play a role, as may the efficiency of the cat's gastrointestinal absorption, the preexistence of renal disease (or lack thereof), and the cat's overall health. Not all lilies are toxic and not all plants called lilies are, in fact, lilies. Table 32-4 lists lilies known to be nephrotoxic to cats.[9]

Clinical signs of lily intoxication include peracute gastrointestinal signs (vomiting, ptyalism), neurologic signs (ataxia, tremors, depression, head pressing, and seizures), and ARF. Swelling of face and paws has been reported.[23] The gastrointestinal and neurologic signs occur within hours of ingestion, but the renal failure develops within 3 to 5 days. Oliguria, anuria, renomegaly, and even renal pain may occur. Azotemia is severe. Urinalysis reveals tubular damage (i.e., casts, glucosuria, and proteinuria). Changes wrought by the as yet unidentified toxic principal consist of acute tubular necrosis with development of polarized crystals in the collecting tubules. Additionally, in the case of the Easter lily, degeneration of pancreatic acinar cells also occurs.

TABLE 32-4 Nephrotoxic Lilies

Common Name	Latin Name
Asiatic Lily (Asian lily)	*Lilium asiatica*
Day Lilies (many varieties)	*Hemerocallis* spp.
Easter Lily	*Lilium longiflorum*
Gloriosa Lily (Glory Lily, Climbing Lily, Superb Lily)	*Gloriosa superba*
Japanese Show Lily	*Lilium speciosum*
Red Lily	*Lilium umbellatum*
Rubrum Lily	*Lilium speciosum cultivar*
Stargazer Lily	*Lilium orientalis*
Tiger Lily	*Lilium tigrinum*
Wood Lily	*Lilium umbellatum*

Source: American Society for the Prevention of Cruelty to Animals: *Toxic and non-toxic plants* (website): http://www.aspca.org/pet-care/poison-control/plants/. Accessed July 23, 2010.

Therapy involves gastrointestinal decontamination, fluid diuresis +/− dialysis. Cats treated within 6 hours of ingestion may be spared from developing ARF; those not treated until after 18 hours are expected to develop ARF. Cats developing anuria or oliguria have a poorer prognosis[136,224] but may still recover.[23] Cats that survive ARF may have residual damage resulting in chronic renal insufficiency.[136,207]

In a retrospective evaluation of 32 cases of ARF seen at one institution, the authors reported that the causes included nephrotoxins in 18 cats (56%) (nine from lilies; four from nonsteroidal antiinflammatory drugs [NSAIDs]; two from ethylene glycol; and one each from tulips, tar, and plant food), ischemia in four cats, and 10 cases from other causes. There were 18 oliguric cats. Prognostically, initial BUN and Cr levels were *not* predictive; however, low serum albumin or bicarbonate was negatively correlated to survival. Most significantly, potassium level increases on presentation equated with decreased chance of survival regardless of cause; for every 1 mEq/L increase, chance of survival decreased by 57%. All the nonoliguric cats survived, and all cats that died were oliguric or anuric. There were 17 (53%) cats that survived; azotemia resolved in eight cats, and the other nine were discharged with persistent azotemia.[224]

Raisins and grapes have recently been recognized as being nephrotoxic in dogs and cats. The literature includes reports in dogs; cases in cats are reported only anecdotally. The toxic principal is unknown, and the lowest dose known to be toxic in dogs is 0.7 oz/2.2 lb (19.8 g/kg) body weight for grapes and 0.11 oz/2.2 lb (3 g/kg) for raisins. Initial signs are gastrointestinal (vomiting, diarrhea, anorexia, abdominal pain) and lethargy. ARF may develop as soon as 24 hours after ingestion. As with lilies, oliguria and anuria are associated with a poor prognosis. Histopathologic changes in dogs with grape- and raisin-induced ARF include an intact basement membrane; thus with aggressive therapy (diuresis, dialysis), some affected individuals will recover.

Aminoglycoside antibiotics are well known to have a dose- and frequency-dependent potential to be both nephrotoxic and ototoxic in cats. The renal insult occurs in the proximal tubules. Gentamicin has been toxic when administered by the topical,[160] intravenous,[117] and intramuscular routes.[102] Orally administered paromomycin, used in the treatment of enteritis from tritrichomoniasis or cryptosporidiosis, has also resulted in ARF.[92]

With the growing awareness of pain and increased concern about analgesia in cats, NSAIDs have a significant role to play. A great deal of concern exists regarding the renal safety of NSAIDs both for acute, short-term use as well as longer periods in the patient with an ongoing problem, such as degenerative joint disease. It is certainly possible to cause ARF in the young, renally competent cat when an accidental overdose is administered. However, it is in the older cat, more likely to require long-term analgesia, that the concern regarding preexisting renal disease and the effect of NSAIDs becomes most pertinent. Selective cyclooxygenase (COX)-2 inhibitors spare housekeeping prostaglandins required for renal health. In excessive doses, even this subtype of NSAID may result in COX-1 inhibition and renal damage. Thus dose and frequency, as well as type of NSAID used, play a role in toxicity. Volume depletion or dehydration precipitates renal failure by reducing renal perfusion. Similarly, hypotension, most commonly associated with anesthesia, has adverse effects by itself. In combination with an inappropriate type, dose, or frequency of NSAID, ARF may arise. Nevertheless, there are numerous studies in older cats showing safe use, particularly of meloxicam, over long periods. An extensive review of the subject may be found in the ISFM and AAFP Consensus Guidelines for Long-Term Use of NSAIDs in Cats.[204]

Vitamin D (as cholecalciferol, vitamin D_3) is well known in rodenticide preparations. Cats can also ingest it by grooming the hair coat or feet if they are exposed to vitamin D–containing human medications (for parathyroid or hypophosphatemic disorders, osteomalacia or osteoporosis, renal failure, and psoriasis) or by eating a diet with excessive levels of vitamin D. In 2006 a prescription diet manufacturer caused an inadvertent overdose in vitamin D_3 levels in specific feline (and canine) products because of an error originating with the vitamin–mineral premix supplier. In addition to managing the tubular necrosis–based ARF, hypercalcemia must be addressed. Corticosteroids, saline diuresis, furosemide, bisphosphonates, and calcitonin are possible therapies to attempt to keep the calcium × phosphorus product below 60 mg/dL (4.85 mmol/L) in order to prevent soft tissue mineralization.

In 2004 and 2007 there were two outbreaks of ARF in dogs and cats associated with melamine and cyanuric acid contamination of pet food. The site of injury is the distal tubule, with unique polarizable striated crystals found there as well as in the collecting ducts.[37] These fan-shaped birefringent crystals are light green to slightly basophilic in color. Additional perivascular and intravascular lesions may also be seen.[54] In addition to the acute and marked azotemia and crystalluria, severe hyperphosphatemia occurs. Neither melamine nor cyanuric acid on its own was found to cause ARF.[68,185]

Ethylene glycol may be ingested directly or by the cat grooming the toxic product from the hair coat or feet. There is a well-recognized seasonality in ethylene glycol toxicity cases, with the majority occurring during the fall and winter; however, this agent is found not only in automotive radiator antifreeze but also in lock de-icer, windshield-wiper fluid, some gasoline additives, and film-processing chemicals. The site of damage is the renal tubule. Ethylene glycol is metabolized to several toxic compounds (glycoaldehyde, glycolic acid, glyoxylic acid, and oxalic acid) that cause marked metabolic acidosis and ARF. Characteristic clinicopathologic findings include an increased anion gap, increased osmolal gap, metabolic acidosis, and CaOx crystalluria. If cats are presented in the latent phase (30 minutes to 12 hours after exposure), ataxia, stupor, and muscle fasciculations may be seen, along with relatively nonspecific signs such as anorexia, lethargy, vomiting, dehydration, hypothermia, and oral ulceration. Once the patient becomes oliguric (12 to 72 hours after ingestion), the likelihood of recovery is dramatically decreased. Thus an index of suspicion warrants checking serum or urine (or both) ethylene glycol levels in the clinic. CaOx crystalluria (monohydrates predominate over other forms) may be seen in cats as soon as 3 hours after ingestion. Serum ethylene glycol levels peak 1 to 6 hours after exposure but are no longer detectable after 48 hours.[213]

The goal of treatment is to block alcohol dehydrogenase (ADH), in order to prevent metabolism of the ethylene glycol into the aforementioned toxic compounds. Ethanol competes with ethylene glycol and has a higher affinity for ADH. It must be given by constant-rate infusion or every 4 hours because of its short half-life. The adverse effects of intravenous ethanol are CNS depression, as well as a worsening of the metabolic acidosis, osmotic diuresis, and serum hyperosmolality. Whereas fomepizole (4-methyl-pyrazole [4-MP]) is the treatment of choice in dogs, it has only recently been shown to be effective in cats and superior to ethanol only if given within 3 hours of ingestion of ethylene glycol.[57] The dose used in this prospective study was 125 mg/kg, intravenously as an initial dose, followed by 31.25 mg/kg at 12, 24, and 36 hours; this is higher than doses recommended for dogs. If treatment is delayed until 4 hours after ingestion, mortality rates are high regardless of whether ethanol or 4-MP is used. Intensive physiologic monitoring and aggressive use of intravenous fluids and sodium bicarbonate will be required because electrolyte and fluid shifts are dramatic. The reader should refer to Chapter 31 for more information. Many patients that are already in oliguric renal failure at presentation will require hemodialysis or peritoneal dialysis to survive.[86,87]

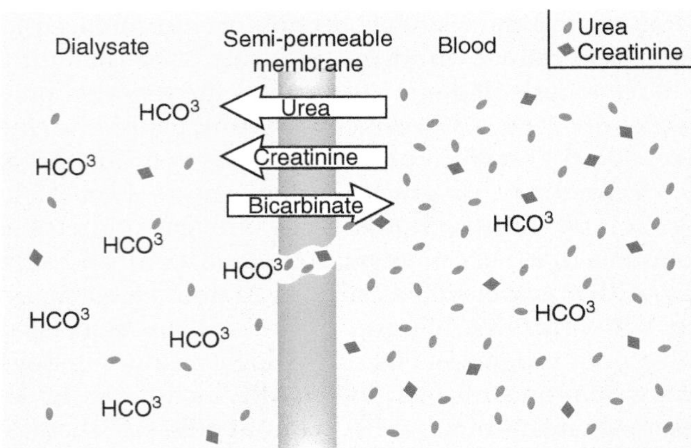

FIGURE 32-12 Blood flows past a semipermeable membrane (the peritoneal lining or the dialyzer in peritoneal dialysis and hemodialysis, respectively), and a dialysate–dialysis fluid flows by or resides on the opposite side of the membrane. (*From Fischer JR, Pantaleo V, Francey T et al: Veterinary hemodialysis: advances in management and technology, Vet Clin North Am Small Anim Pract 34:935, 2004.*)

INTENSIVE MANAGEMENT OF RENAL DISEASES

Dialysis

Treatment for all patients with ARF, regardless of the inciting cause, may require peritoneal dialysis or hemodialysis. Although these procedures are not common in feline medicine, they are becoming more readily available, and it is useful to understand the basic indications and contraindications to help with treatment planning and client education. Additionally, as clients become more aware of these treatment options through their own research on the Internet or elsewhere, it is helpful to understand some basic concepts.

Dialysis may be used to reduce azotemia and correct severe electrolyte abnormalities, acid–base imbalances, or overhydration. It is useful for the treatment of ARF associated with intoxication (drug or toxin) or urinary tract outflow obstruction or in the treatment of end-stage chronic renal failure that is nonresponsive to medical therapy and as part of stabilizing the patient in preparation for renal transplantation. Both hemodialysis and peritoneal dialysis have been used for more than 10 years in veterinary medicine and are becoming more widely available and affordable.

The principle underlying dialysis is that solutes diffuse across a semipermeable membrane depending on their concentration, the relative pressure on either side of the membrane (i.e., gradient), and the size of the molecule relative to the pores in the membrane. Solutes move from an area of high concentration or pressure to an area of low concentration or pressure; smaller molecules (e.g., electrolytes, urea, and albumin) move more readily than larger molecules (e.g., blood cells, Cr, and globulins). Applying this clinically, blood flows past a semipermeable membrane (the peritoneal lining or the dialyzer in peritoneal dialysis and hemodialysis, respectively), and a dialysate–dialysis fluid flows by or resides on the opposite side of the membrane (Figure 32-12).

In hemodialysis a dedicated, double-lumen hemodialysis catheter is placed in the jugular vein. Blood is run through an extracorporeal filter (dialyzer) in the opposite direction to the dialysate, resulting in a countercurrent flow pattern. Because the blood is continuously exposed to fresh dialysate, the diffusion occurs more rapidly than in peritoneal dialysis. In peritoneal dialysis the dialysate is infused into the peritoneal cavity and left there for variable amounts of time ("dwell time") before it is drained from the abdomen. Dialysis may be continuous (continuous renal replacement therapy by hemodialysis), or intermittent (hemodialysis or peritoneal dialysis).

Standard dialysate is a solution that mimics normal serum composition. Variations of sodium, potassium, magnesium, phosphorus, and bicarbonate concentrations may be made to adjust the patient's levels as necessary. *Sodium profiling* refers to regular adjustments of sodium concentration during dialysis to reduce the likelihood of complications. The prescription for an individual patient will change as the patient's status changes. To increase water loss in the overhydrated patient, mannitol may be added or the dextrose concentration may be increased. In the hypoalbuminemic patient that is receiving adequate dietary protein, an amino acid dialysate may be considered.

The complication rate for peritoneal dialysis is high but not insurmountable. Peritoneal dialysis requires intensive monitoring of the drain (for obstruction) and the stoma (for subcutaneous leakage, infection), as well as the patient; however, this procedure is more accessible to veterinarians because of the relatively lower cost of equipment compared with that needed for hemodialysis. Rapid solute removal and electrolyte shifts can result in hypovolemia, hypotension, cramping, nausea, vomiting, and dialysis disequilibrium syndrome.[83] In both peritoneal dialysis and hemodialysis, catheters may become obstructed, and prevention of catheter infection requires diligence. The interested reader is referred to the listed references, in particular Dzyban et al and Dorval et al (for peritoneal dialysis) and Fischer (for hemodialysis).*

Another possible method of treatment, diuretic renal scintigraphy using ^{99m}Tc-DTPA plus furosemide, has been evaluated to date as a diagnostic test. This procedure is noninvasive and fast to perform and may have application in patients with significantly impaired renal function and obstructive uropathies.[104]

Renal Transplantation

The first successful feline renal transplant was performed in 1987 at the University of California, Davis, by Dr. Clare Gregory. Since that time, the procedure has been performed at numerous centers around the world for cats in chronic renal failure. Clients must understand that this is not a cure; the goal is to provide good quality of life for a cat that otherwise would not survive. Indications are early chronic renal disease (ideally before decompensation) or irreversible ARF. It cannot be a last-ditch effort because the patient must not be too debilitated nor have concurrent conditions. Additionally, the veterinarian cannot ethically justify removing a healthy kidney from a donor cat unless there is a good chance of success for the recipient. Careful screening and early referral of stable cats for renal transplantation improves the likelihood of a successful outcome.[4,24]

Exclusion criteria include significant cardiac disease, feline leukemia virus infection, active feline immunodeficiency virus infection, UTI, uncontrolled hyperthyroidism, neoplasia, DM, a poor starting body condition score, and a fractious temperament. Some centers will perform transplants on cats with CaOx uroliths.[14] Screening tests that determine suitability as a recipient include a CBC, serum biochemistries including total T_4, urinalysis and urine culture, UPC, thoracic radiographs and echocardiogram, electrocardiogram, abdominal radiographs, heartworm antigen test, and *Toxoplasma* titers. If the cat has positive *Toxoplasma* immunoglobulin IgM or IgG titers, it will be started on clindamycin or trimethoprim sulfa preoperatively and likely kept on the antibiotic for the rest of its life. A renal biopsy for crossmatching and a 2-week cyclosporine challenge will be required, the latter to see if subclinical UTIs or upper respiratory tract infections surface.[128]

Preparation of the successful transplant candidate includes correction of electrolyte and acid–base imbalances, anemia (with appropriate blood products and darbepoietin), and azotemia (may require dialysis) and improvement of nutritional status (may require a feeding tube). Alleviation of preoperative azotemia is essential insofar as this results in a decreased risk of CNS disorders after surgery.[5]

Donors are healthy young adult cats in good body condition with normal CBCs, serum chemistries, and urinalyses. They should also test negative for retrovirus and *Toxoplasma* infections, with no abnormalities found on renal ultrasound. They are blood typed and crossmatched to potential recipients, and renal tissue compatibility is assessed. The kidney size must be relatively similar (not too much larger) to that of the recipient. Computed tomography renal angiography is used in some centers because it is superior to intravenous urography to evaluate the vascular architecture of potential donors.[34] Transplantation will not be considered if the client is unwilling to care for the donor and provide it with a home.

The donor's left kidney is harvested because of its greater vein length. The kidney is flushed and then preserved in a solution that can store the organ for 3 to 4 days, allowing a matched donor and recipient to reside in different parts of the world. Several techniques (e.g., renal arterial end-to-end anastomosis to the external iliac artery or end-to-side anastomosis to the aorta) may be employed to anastomose the new kidney to the recipient's renal vessels and ureter.[25] The technique used for ureteral attachment is ureteroneocystostomy. Several different techniques have been evaluated; an extravesical technique using a simple interrupted pattern has been found to be most favorable.[161]

Postoperative care is intensive because several risks exist. Routine care consists of close intensive care unit monitoring and treatment with intravenous fluids, analgesics, antibiotics, gastric protectants, blood products as needed, and enteral nutrition. Ionized (but not total) serum magnesium concentrations are decreased in feline renal transplant recipients in the perioperative period. In addition, ionized serum calcium and potassium concentrations are below normal in many cats as well, although a case of hypercalcemia has been published.[13] Hence electrolyte monitoring is required. Profound weakness and depression commonly seen in feline renal transplant recipients in the immediate postoperative period may, in part, be a result of these electrolyte disturbances.[223] Interestingly, in a study of 86 cats with post-transplant hypophosphatemia, survival was unaffected regardless of whether this abnormality was treated.[180]

Postoperative malignant hypertension with systolic pressures in excess of 300 mm Hg can result in seizures and neurologic complications, including death. Uncontrolled uremia is believed to cause increased endothelial

*References 70, 75, 76, 83, 137, 138, 149.

catecholamine sensitivity. Additional possible instigating causes include anesthesia and pain. Treatment with subcutaneous hydralazine has been shown to be effective in correcting hypertension and minimizing or preventing neurologic complications.[134]

Other possible postoperative complications directly related to the graft may include torsion, thrombosis, or hemorrhage of the pedicle; this possibility is greatly reduced through pexy of the new kidney to the body wall. Retroperitoneal fibrosis has also been reported.[12] The most likely complication is ischemic injury and ureteral obstruction resulting in delayed graft function.[162] Delayed graft function may be identified through ultrasonographic monitoring of renal blood flow and may occur as late as 21 days postoperatively.[172]

The recipient will require lifelong immunosuppressive therapy (microemulsified cyclosporine or potentially tacrolimus) to prevent graft rejection.[130] This calls for a dedicated caregiver. Acute allograft rejection initially has minimal clinical signs: a 1° F (<1° C) increase in temperature at 21 days after transplant. Markers of oxidative stress from venous blood were not found to be helpful in one experimental study.[101] Cr levels should be monitored routinely in patients as an increase in this parameter is suspicious for allograft rejection; a biopsy of the renal allograft is needed for definitive diagnosis.[133] Rejection is a result of a lack of adequate plasma cyclosporine levels. Treatment with intravenous cyclosporine and prednisolone will reverse 60% of rejection cases.

Approximately 20% of the cats undergoing a renal transplant procedure die at the time of surgery or during the first week after surgery. Older cats and cats with severe azotemia, hypertension, and cardiovascular disease may have an increased mortality risk after renal transplantation. For cats that are successfully discharged from hospital, survival rates are approximately 80% for 6-month and 45% for 3-year survival.[201] Causes of mortality include the following:

- Poor client compliance in giving oral cyclosporine and failure to have cyclosporine trough levels checked routinely
- Infection: In a retrospective study of 169 recipients, infections developed in 25% of the cases, with bacterial causes being most common, viral next most common, and fungal or protozoal least common. Infection was the second most common cause of death after acute rejection of the transplant, accounting for 14% of deaths overall in this study group. Cats with diabetes had a significantly greater risk of developing this complication.[120]
- Acute rejection of the kidney
- Development of cardiac disease, hepatopathy, pancreatitis, neoplasia, diabetes, and other conditions
- Uncommonly, post-transplantation malignant neoplasia may occur, resulting in a shorter survival time. Lymphoma is the most common form; however, a variety of tumor types are reported.[200,223]

The longest survival time attained after feline renal transplantation was 14 years, as of the autumn of 2009.[99] The average life expectancy after transplantation is approximately 3 to 6 years, depending on the age of the cat at the time of surgery. All recipients should be considered to have renal insufficiency regardless of how well they do; therefore ongoing monitoring is necessary, just as with any other cat with CKD. In addition, because of the cyclosporine therapy, urine cultures must be performed regularly. Hypertension should be diligently treated.

CHRONIC KIDNEY DISEASES

Despite the tendency to use the terms "chronic kidney disease" and "chronic renal insufficiency" (CKD/CRI) as a single entity, it is helpful to bear in mind that these terms refer to a cluster of clinical signs that may be a result of a number of different etiologies and pathologic entities. Box 32-8 lists recognized causes of CKD in cats. Another term, "chronic renal failure," may also be misleading and should be used judiciously; many patients are far from failure given the wide variability in renal impairment despite the Cr value at initial presentation.[38,78] Using this potentially inappropriate terminology may distress clients who might believe that the condition is more advanced than it is and may choose not to begin treatment at all (i.e., euthanize) or to discontinue therapy earlier than is warranted.

The most common histopathologic form of chronic disease in the kidneys of cats is tubulointerstitial nephritis characterized by the infiltration of lymphocytes and

BOX 32-8

Causes of Chronic Kidney Disease in Cats

Chronic tubulointerstitial nephritis of unknown etiology
Hydronephrosis secondary to ureteronephroliths
Hypokalemic nephropathy
Polycystic renal disease
Neoplasia (primarily lymphoma)
Hypercalcemia resulting from hypervitaminosis D
Nephrotoxicoses
Chronic glomerulonephritis
Chronic pyelonephritis
Amyloidosis
Dry feline infectious peritonitis: pyogranulomatous interstitial nephritis
Polyarteritis nodosa

plasma cells with concurrent and variable degrees of fibrosis. Retrospective studies evaluating the prevalence of type of renal disease resulting in chronic changes are sparse. A study undertaken in 1987 classified the morphologic category of CKD in 74 cats. 53% were chronic tubulointerstitial nephritis.[66] The other causes listed in Box 32-8 are less prevalent. What initiates this lymphoplasmacytic inflammatory response is unclear and may not be the same in all individuals. Several studies have been undertaken to investigate the role of antigenic stimulation through routine vaccination. The antigen source that has been evaluated is Crandell–Rees feline kidney (CRFK) cell lysate because this cell line was used to grow many vaccine viruses. Although antibodies to CRFK have been identified in all tissues tested, the only cats in which significant inflammation was detected were those given doses of CRFK cell lysate far in excess of that which any cat could receive in its lifetime.[140,141] Thus this aspect of routine vaccination does not appear to be a cause of tubulointerstitial nephritis.

An interesting theory is that tubulointerstitial nephritis might, in fact, be a mortality antagonist, meaning that it provides an evolutionary survival benefit. A study evaluated the histopathologic findings from the necropsies of nearly 700 adult cats that were maintained for life as residents of the same colony, over a period of 22 years. The surprising finding was that the cats that died or were euthanized because of renal disease lived longer than those cats dying from other causes. It was also noted that they had higher, but uniform, mean renal histologic scores across ages, compared with cats that had other causes of death. A decline in body condition was a negative prognostic indicator in all cats.[142]

Clinical Findings

Regardless of cause, the clinical presentation of a cat with any CKD is similar. On physical examination a dull, often spiky coat with a delay in skin elasticity and muscle wasting are very common findings. Oral ulcers may be seen; mucous membrane pallor is variable. Although one or both kidneys may be smaller and firmer than normal, renal size cannot be relied on because some cats retain normal size, others have renomegaly, and yet others have small kidneys surrounded by sufficient perirenal fat to obscure the real size. Cats may present in a lethargic or depressed state, with poor or no appetite and concurrent weight loss. Nausea or vomiting is common. Polyuria may go unnoticed unless the cat lives indoors only, without feline housemates, and uses clumping litter and the client pays attention to the size and number of urine clumps in the litter. Polydipsia may likewise be overlooked in this species because, as a result of their desert origin, cats tend to dehydrate and become constipated before they start to drink more.

International Renal Interest Society Classification

Chronic renal insufficiency refers to a gradual decline in renal function and is extremely common in cats. In one retrospective study clinical and laboratory evidence of renal insufficiency from renal disease were present in 7% (11 of 153) of dogs and 20% (27 of 137) of cats.[219] As in human medicine, this syndrome of chronic renal insufficiency has been divided into stages. The International Renal Interest Society (IRIS; http://www.iris-kidney.com/) bases the categories on serum Cr levels once the cat is rehydrated as well as the patient's clinical signs. Substaging is based on the presence or absence of hypertension as well as of proteinuria insofar as both of these parameters are critical in treatment, disease progression, and prognosis for the individual. There are numerous benefits to assigning a stage to an individual patient. Staging ensures that the veterinarian evaluates all the appropriate parameters. The veterinarian then has the information required to focus on cure when possible (e.g., pyelonephritis, early stages 1 and 2), alleviation of factors that affect progression of disease (e.g., hypertension and proteinuria), treatment of clinical uremia, or provision of palliative care. These tools also direct the practitioner to logical monitoring (parameters and frequency) and also provide more information on which to base a prognosis. Having distinctly defined categories allows practitioners to communicate clearly about patients. Table 32-5 and Boxes 32-9 and 32-10 summarize the IRIS definitions. Figures 32-13 to 32-15 are algorithms for staging and substaging patients with CKD.

Patients are classified on the basis of their serum Cr value *once rehydrated* and then substaged on the basis of the presence or absence of hypertension or proteinuria. Thus stage 1 reflects the earliest stage of renal disease with an inappropriate USG for the hydration state of the cat. The Cr is still within normal reference intervals, but proteinuria or hypertension may be present. These cats will not have clinical signs of illness at this time unless significant proteinuria or hypertension are present; this stage is detected by screening cats in an age category at risk (>7 to 8 years of age) and verifying abnormalities as found.

Azotemia may be misleading if a cat is dehydrated. It is not possible to stage, prognosticate, or plan appropriate therapy until the individual has been *re*hydrated. Using the IRIS staging system, stage 1 cats are not azotemic but are classified according to whether they have inadequate renal concentrating ability (a USG ≤1.035) in a *de*hydrated state. The diuretic effect of diet (e.g., high sodium, canned versus dry) or drugs will make assessment of USG difficult. Collecting urine after a period of sleep may help counter this effect somewhat.

TABLE 32-5 **IRIS Definitions for Classification of Renal Disease**

Stage	1. Nonazotemic Renal Disease	2. Mild Renal Azotemia	3. Moderate Renal Azotemia	4. Severe Renal Azotemia/ "Chronic Renal Failure"
Creatinine: mg/dL (mmol/L)	<1.6 mg/dL (<140 mmol/L)	1.6-2.8 mg/dL (140-249 mmol/L)	2.9-5.0 mg/dL (250-439 mmol/L)	>5.0 mg/dL (>440 mmol/L)
Clinical signs	None	+/− inappetence, weight loss, PU/PD	Usually inappetence, weight loss, PU/PD	Uremia, clinically ill
Progression	Stable for long periods of time	Stable for long periods of time	May progress	Fragile
Therapeutic goals	Identify and treat specific primary kidney disease (e.g., acute pyelonephritis, nephrolithiasis)	Identify and treat specific primary kidney disease (e.g., acute pyelonephritis, nephrolithiasis)	Modify progression: phosphorus restriction, omega 3 fatty acids?	Ameliorate uremic signs: protein restriction, antiemetics, erythropoietin, fluid therapy, appetite stimulation, dialysis, etc.
Proteinuria	Classify	Classify	Classify	Classify
Blood pressure	Classify	Classify	Classify	Classify

PU/PD, Polyuria/polydipsia.
Comments: Stage 1: Some other renal abnormality present e.g. inadequate concentrating ability without identifiable non-renal cause; abnormal renal palpation and/or abnormal renal imaging findings; persistent proteinuria of renal origin; abnormal renal biopsy results, progressively elevating creatinine levels. Stage 2: Lower end of the range lies within the reference range for many labs but the insensitivity of creatinine as a screening test means that animals with creatinine values close to the upper limit of normality often have excretory failure.
Adapted from International Renal Interest Society: (website): http://www.iris-kidney.com/. Accessed November 28, 2010.

BOX 32-9
IRIS Definitions Regarding Proteinuria

Proteinuria (determined by evaluating sequential urine protein:creatinine ratios)

Nonproteinuric = UPC < 0.25
Borderline proteinuria = UPC 0.25-0.5 Re-evaluate after 2 months
Proteinuria = UPC > 0.4

Adapted from International Renal Interest Society (website): http://www.iris-kidney.com/. Accessed November 28, 2010.

BOX 32-10
IRIS Definitions Regarding Classification of Blood Pressure

NH = nonhypertensive = <150 mm Hg with no complications
BP = borderline hypertensive = 150-160 mm Hg with no complications
Hnc = hypertension no complications = consistent systolic blood pressure values >160 mm Hg
Hc = hypertension with extra-renal complications = signs + > 150 mm Hg

Adapted from International Renal Interest Society (website): http://www.iris-kidney.com/. Accessed November 28, 2010.

Stages 2 to 4 are based on elevation of Cr levels. Again, as with USG, numerous nonrenal factors may affect this parameter. When inadequate protein is available for ongoing needs, cats, being obligate carnivores, catabolize protein stores (e.g., muscle) to fuel metabolic pathways, resulting in an artificially low serum Cr value. Prerenal azotemia associated with dehydration will have the opposite effect. BUN can be especially difficult to interpret insofar as it reflects ammonia intake, production, and excretion (discussed previously).

Regardless of serum Cr concentration, evaluation of BP and urinary protein is required for complete IRIS staging. Hypotension is detrimental to renal perfusion; hypertension, to cardiac output and potentially to renal function. Hypertension increases the risk of vascular damage to target organs (brain, kidneys, and eyes). A persistent UPC higher than 0.4 has been shown to be associated with increased mortality,[129] as well as progression of renal insufficiency.

Diagnosis

Standard diagnostics for renal disease include the minimum database of CBC and differential, serum biochemistries, BP, and urinalysis with, if significant urinary protein is present, a UPC. It can be argued that radiographs should also be included. Earlier diagnosis could help to blunt pathologic processes and stop progression of CKD.[96,144]

Azotemia (an increase in either or both BUN and serum Cr) is present and commonly has a prerenal as

History and/or physical examination suggest chronic kidney disease (CKD)
Measure blood creatinine
Creatinine <130 µmol/L <1.6 mg/dL
Creatinine 140-249 µmol/L 1.6-2.8 mg/dL
Creatinine >250 µmol/L >2.8 mg/dL
Firm evidence of CKD absent
Firm evidence of CKD present
Re-evaluate in 2-3 months, then every 3 months if creatinine rising; every 3-6 months if creatinine stable
Stage 1 Substage by UP/C & BP
Radiographs and ultrasound, UP/C, BP, and urine culture
Institute management plan for Stage 1 patients
Measure urine specific gravity
<1.030
≥1.030
Radiographs and ultrasound, UP/C, BP, and urine culture
Normal: re-evaluate within 2 months Abnormal: Stage 2 Substage by UP/C & BP
Institute treatment
Clinical evaluation
If underlying extra-renal abnormalities, correct and re-evaluate within 6 months
Clinical evaluation
Pre- or post-renal azotemia
Renal azotemia
Correct underlying abnormalities and re-evaluate immediately
Stage 3 or 4 Substage by UP/C & BP
Institute treatment

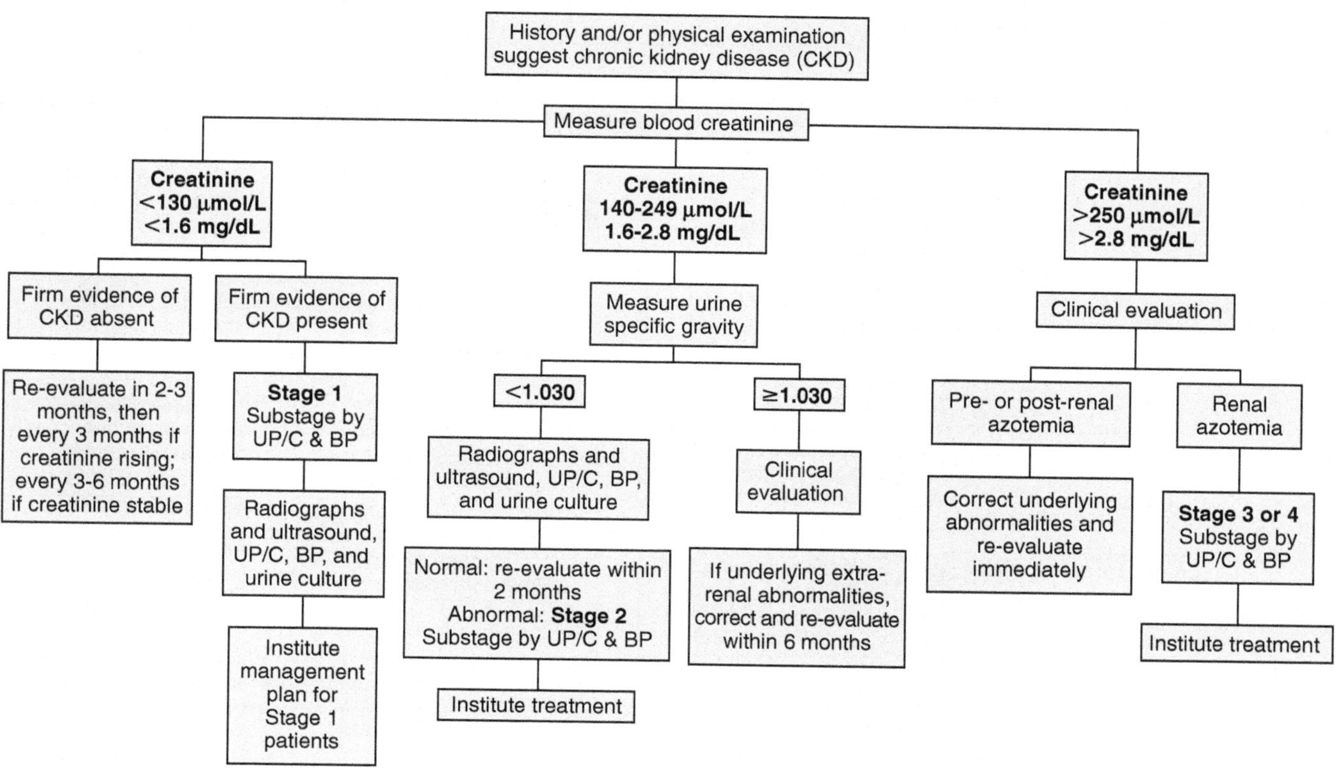

FIGURE 32-13 Algorithm for staging chronic kidney disease. *(Adapted from Bonagura JD, Twedt DC:* Kirk's current veterinary therapy, *ed 14, St Louis, 2008, Saunders/Elsevier.)*

CKD diagnosed & staged 1-4 Urine dipstick examination
+
−
Questionable proteinuria; Urinalysis with sediment examination
Non-proteinuric (NP)
Sediment abnormal/"active"
Sediment "inactive"/unremarkable/hyaline casts
Conduct further work-up, e.g., rule out lower urinary tract disease
Determine UP/C
Cat
UP/C <0.2 Non-proteinuric NP
UP/C >0.4* Proteinuric (P)
UP/C 0.2-0.4* Borderline proteinuric (BP) Re-evaluate within 2 months
*Demonstrate persistence by re-evaluating:
if borderline proteinuric in 2 weeks to 2 months
if proteinuric in 2-4 weeks
if UPC >2 no need to demonstrate persistence prior to initiating therapy (severe proteinuria)

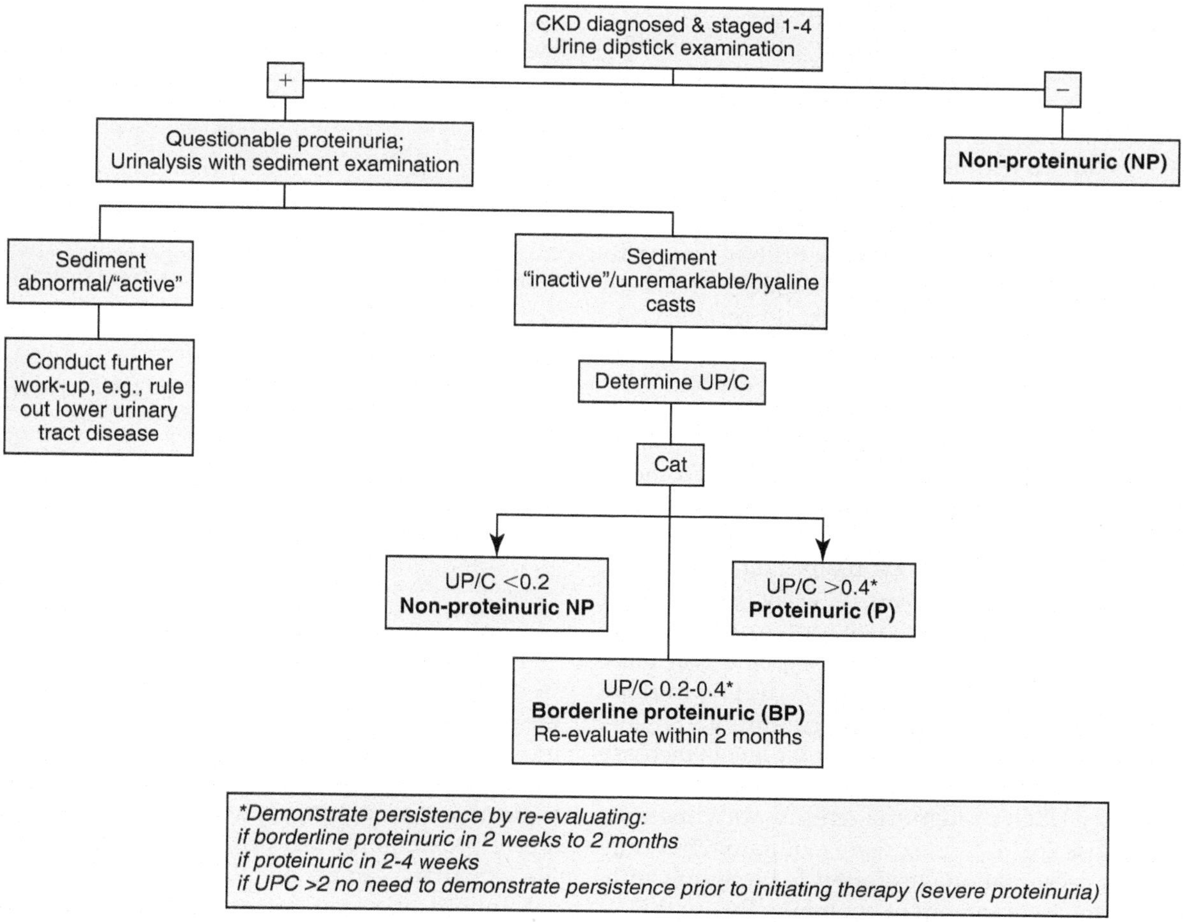

FIGURE 32-14 Algorithm for substaging chronic kidney disease by proteinuria. *(Adapted from Bonagura JD, Twedt DC:* Kirk's current veterinary therapy, *ed 14, St Louis, 2008, Saunders/Elsevier.)*

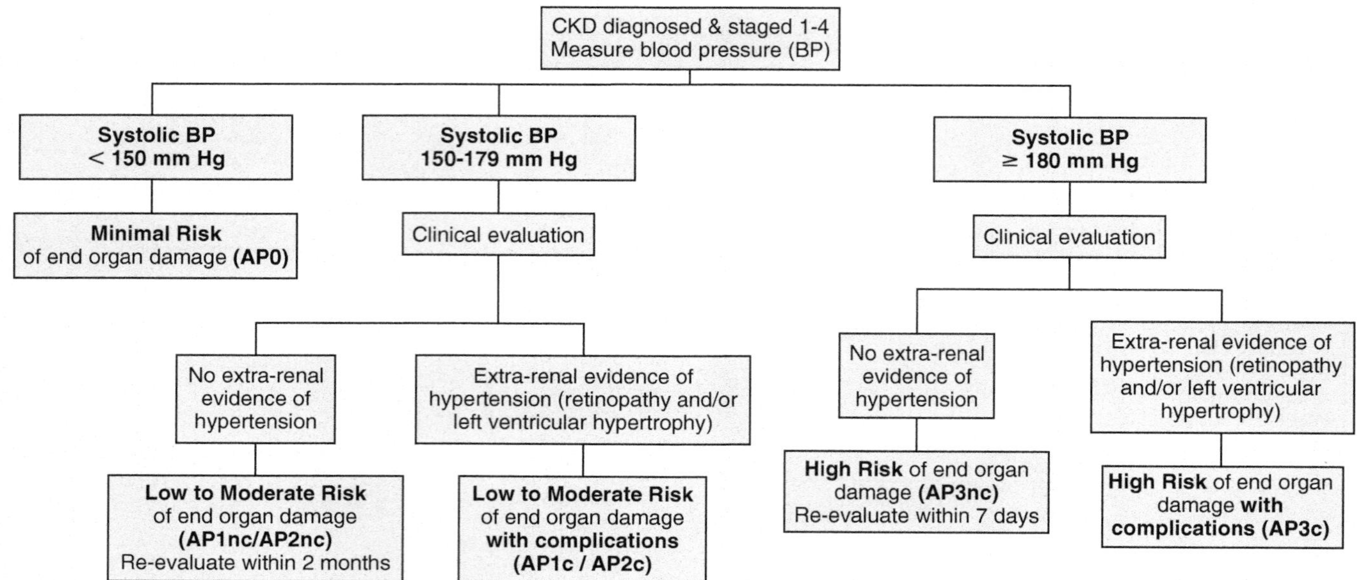

FIGURE 32-15 Algorithm for substaging chronic kidney disease by blood pressure. This is based on the risk of target organ damage due to hypertension. *(Adapted from Bonagura JD, Twedt DC:* Kirk's current veterinary therapy, *ed 14, St Louis, 2008, Saunders/Elsevier.)*

well as the defining renal component; variable acid–base and electrolyte changes occur. These are most notably a metabolic acidosis with variable potassium, phosphorus, and calcium levels depending on the mechanism as well as the duration of the problem. A urinalysis reveals a subnormal specific gravity in the face of dehydration (i.e., ≤1.035) with or without cellular, bacterial, and cast components. Systolic BP is commonly elevated and has been reported to occur in as many as 60% of cats with CKD.[127,206] More recently, in a study of 103 cats with CKD, 20 (19.4%) were found to have systolic BP in excess of 175 mm Hg.[209] Serum T_4 levels are suppressed in cats with CKD. In a study of 128 cats with CKD, 48% of cats with CKD had low total serum T_4. Total T_4 levels were 12.3 +/− 8.4 nmol/L (0.96 +/− 0.65 μg/dL) compared with healthy, age-matched cats in which the total T_4 range was 27.0 +/− 10.4 nmol/L (2.1 +/− 0.81 mcg/dL).[159] Only a small proportion of cats with CKD have significant proteinuria.

In human medicine numerous biomarkers have been evaluated (Table 32-6) to identify early ischemic or nephrotoxic kidney injury. To date, only a few studies have been published in veterinary medicine that have attempted to find markers that detect a decline in renal function before urine-concentrating ability is lost (approximately 66% nephrons lost) or Cr levels increase (approximately 75% nephrons lost).

In one study USG, proteinuria, and N-acetyl-beta-D-glucosaminidase (NAG) index were evaluated, but only proteinuria at presentation was found to be significantly associated with development of azotemia. Evaluation of NAG index offered no additional benefit.[115] The same group attempted to assess the correlation between NAG index, plasma Cr concentration, and proteinuria. They concluded that the NAG index in cats with CKD may be indicative of ongoing lysosomal activity rather than active proximal tubular cell damage. Also, although the NAG activity can be quantified in feline urine using a colorimetric technique, results should be interpreted cautiously because of high interassay variation.[116]

TABLE 32-6 **Protein Biomarkers Used in Human Medicine for the Early Detection of Acute Renal Injury**

Biomarker	Associated Renal Injury
Cystin C	Proximal tubule injury
KIM-1	Ischemia and nephrotoxins
NGAL (lipocalin)	Ischemia and nephrotoxins
Cytokines (IL-6, IL-8, IL-18)	Ischemia, prerenal, postrenal acute kidney injury
Actin-actin depolymerizing F	Toxic, delayed graft function
a-GST	Ischemia and delayed graft function
p-GST	Proximal tubule injury, acute rejection
L-FABP	Ischemia and nephrotoxins
Netrin-1	Ischemia and nephrotoxins, sepsis
Keratin-derived chemokine	Ischemia and delayed graft function

Adapted from Ronco C, Haapio M, House AA et al: Cardiorenal syndrome, *J Am Coll Cardiol* 52:1527, 2008.

Another study looked at whether urine NAG might be a predictor for the development of CKD in hyperthyroid cats. Unfortunately, baseline NAG did not differentiate azotemic from nonazotemic treated hyperthyroid cats. It was speculated that it might be of help when combined with USG in adjusting methimazole therapy.[139]

As a matter of interest, although it is specific for myocardial damage or necrosis, cardiac troponin I (cTnI) concentration can be elevated in azotemic renal failure, suggesting that stage 4 renal disease may result in clinically inapparent myocardial injury or possibly altered elimination of cTnI.[183]

In stages 1 and 2 veterinarians have the best chance to identify treatable causes of renal disease. Hence, in addition to the aforementioned basic measures, urine culture, radiographs, abdominal ultrasound, and possibly renal biopsy should ideally be pursued. Urine cultures are worth performing when USG is 1.030 or lower regardless of sediment characteristics and, in more concentrated samples, if significant numbers of white blood cells or bacteria are seen. If a hematogenous source of infection is suspected, blood culture may be considered. Abdominal ultrasound is useful to assess gross renal pathology, guide in collection of intrarenal urine samples, and help with the performance of renal biopsies if indicated. Determination of the cause of CKD should be encouraged in stable patients because this knowledge provides the only chance for accurate treatment of potentially reversible renal disease. When there is concern for primary or secondary cardiac pathology, an echocardiogram and thoracic radiographs should be evaluated. Contributing systemic disease (including electrolyte imbalances) should be identified and stabilized if possible.

Regardless of stage, diagnostics are directed at finding treatable and potentially reversible problems. Thus it is appropriate to try to identify and remove any cause that has compromised renal function, such as a nephrotoxic drug, diet, or plant; prerenal causes of ischemia (hypotension, hypoxia, hypovolemia, hypothermia); postrenal causes of obstruction of urine flow (intraluminal uroliths or sludge, mural or extramural); and UTI (lower tract or upper tract). The veterinarian should evaluate for hypertension and proteinuria.

Therapy

Treatment of CKD in cats consists of etiology-specific and etiology-nonspecific therapy. Specific entities to address include pyelonephritis, nephrotoxicoses, ureteronephroliths, and neoplasia. Problems resulting from these and other causes of CKD requiring therapeutic attention include metabolic acidosis, proteinuria, hypertension, dehydration, electrolyte abnormalities (hyperphosphatemia, hypokalemia, hyperkalemia), renal secondary hyperparathyroidism, inappetence and anorexia, nausea and vomition, protein:calorie malnutrition, and anemia.

One paper has recently reviewed the literature regarding treatment modalities for CKD and assessed the quality of the evidence behind each one using evidence-based medicine (EBM) definitions.[195] The grading scheme used was as follows:

Grade I: Evidence based on properly designed, randomized, controlled clinical trials performed in clinical feline patients

Grade II: Evidence from properly designed, randomized, controlled clinical trials of cats with spontaneous disease in a research setting

Grade III: Evidence from appropriately controlled studies without randomization, cohort, or case-control studies; studies using models of disease or simulations in cats; case series; or dramatic results from uncontrolled studies

Grade IV: Evidence from studies in other species, reports of expert committees, descriptive studies, case reports, pathophysiologic justification, and opinions of recognized experts

This comprehensive review elegantly categorizes the studies in the literature using the evidence-based medicine criteria. The therapies evaluated were fluid therapy, calcitriol, antihypertensives, ACE-I, erythropoietin, supplementation with potassium or antioxidants, alkalinization, dietary phosphorus restriction and intestinal phosphate binders, therapeutic renal diets, assisted feeding, dialysis, and renal transplantation. The authors concluded that, with the exception of renal diets, the quality of the evidence is weak for other therapies (Table 32-7). One could argue that it is not possible to design a double-blind, randomized, controlled clinical trial for some of these treatments; for example, not treating hypertension when identified would be unethical and constitute malpractice despite the lack of grade 1 (highest level) evidence. Similarly, it could be argued that if the patient will not take the recommended treatment or the patient–caregiver relationship is negatively affected, the practitioner must adapt the treatment plan accordingly.

Management of Specific Diseases

PYELONEPHRITIS

Antimicrobial therapy must be based on urine culture and sensitivity results. When urine culture and sensitivity is negative despite evidence of bacteria on urinalysis, several possible explanations exist (see Box 32-4). It may be necessary to harvest the urine specimen directly from the renal pelvis using ultrasound guidance to obtain a representative sample.

Antimicrobial therapy should continue for 3 to 5 weeks for the initial episode and for 5 to 8 weeks should

TABLE 32-7 **Summary of Evidence Grades Supporting Recommendations for Therapy of Chronic Kidney Disease**

Evidence Grade	Therapy
Grade I	Some therapeutic diets ACE inhibitors to reduce proteinuria, increase appetite in cats with UPC > 1
Grade III	Some therapeutic diets Antihypertensive therapy with amlodipine Recombinant human/feline erythropoietin Potassium supplementation for cats with hypokalemia Dietary phosphorus restriction for cats in IRIS stages 3 and 4
Grade IV	Long-term SC fluid therapy Potassium supplement for all cats with CKD Intestinal phosphate binders Alkalinizing therapy Assisted feeding ACE inhibitors for nonproteinuric cats

ACE, Angiotensin-converting enzyme; *UPC*, urine protein:creatinine ratio; *IRIS*, International Renal Interest Society; *SC*, subcutaneous; *CKD*, chronic kidney disease.

Adapted from: Roudebush P, Polzin DJ, Ross SJ et al: Therapies for feline chronic kidney disease. What is the evidence?, *J Feline Med Surg* 11:195, 2009.

re-infection or relapse occur. Urine may be cultured during therapy to verify antimicrobial efficacy and should be repeated 1 week after the end of treatment to ensure that infection has been eradicated.

VITAMIN D NEPHROTOXICOSIS

Nephrotoxicoses generally result in ARF; however, accumulation of vitamin D or overexuberant calcitriol therapy and subsequent hypercalcemia or hyperphosphatemia-induced hypercalcemia cause gradual onset of mineralization. Treatment for hypervitaminosis D may be required in addition to reducing calcitriol dose or addressing hyperphosphatemia. In 2006 an inadvertent error resulted in excess vitamin D addition to several diet formulations.

Appropriate diagnostics are serum ionized calcium and serum 25-hydroxyvitamin D, a marker for vitamin D_3 levels. The half-life of cholecalciferol (vitamin D_3) in the body is about 6 months, and as it is slowly released from the fat stores, it can potentially cause ongoing toxicity. These patients need to be monitored for at least 6 months.

Acute therapy consists of intravenous fluids, corticosteroids, furosemide, and calcitonin. Chronic monitoring and ongoing treatment is necessary because the hypercalcemia can last for months. The use of intravenous bisphosphonates is recommended and has been shown to control hypercalcemia in most cases for at least 3 to 4 weeks after a single dose. Some patients will require repeated doses; others require only a single dose. A single dose may provide enough time for the hypercalcemia to lessen when the drug wears off. Pamidronate, a second-generation bisphosphonate, has been used intravenously at 1.3 to 2 mg/kg diluted in saline, with intravenous fluid administration before, during, and after the pamidronate infusion. Serum calcium concentration is usually normal within 48 hours.[110]

HYPOKALEMIC NEPHROPATHY

Hypokalemia is a condition that is known to cause clinical muscle weakness, especially of the cervical muscles. Hypokalemic myopathy is truly a functional disorder insofar as that although electromyographic measurements are abnormal and serum creatine kinase (CK) levels are elevated, on histologic examination the muscle is normal. The feline potassium requirement is related to the dietary protein level; the higher the protein, the more potassium is needed.[109] Potassium depletion results in weight loss and poor hair coat because this electrolyte is required for protein synthesis. In 1993 a paper reported on the development of nephropathy in cats fed a commercial diet that was potassium depleted.[65] Additionally, acidification of the diet plays a role. Diets that are more extremely acidified may result in metabolic acidosis, and over time this can lead to urinary potassium loss.[71-73]

Cats with hypokalemia-induced nephropathy may or may not have an increased fractional excretion of potassium (FE_K). Serum potassium levels of less than 3.1 mEq/L, increased CK levels, azotemia, hyperchloremic metabolic acidosis, and isosthenuria with possible hyperphosphatemia are noted. On histopathology morphologic changes in the kidneys include interstitial fibrosis, lymphocytic–plasmacytic interstitial infiltration, tubular dilation, and atrophy with varying glomerular sclerosis.[65,72]

Treatment of this condition differs from that of chronic tubulointerstitial nephrosis in that diligent attention must be paid to establishing eukalemia by intravenous and oral potassium therapy. It is not unusual for serum potassium levels to decrease initially, despite potassium-supplemented fluid therapy as a result of dilution, increased tubular flow as GFR improves, and cellular uptake of potassium. Clinical improvement should be noticed within 3 to 4 days. Intravenous fluids should not contain more than 40 mEq potassium/L because this can cause vascular pain and damage; the delivery rate of potassium should not exceed 0.5 mEq/kg body weight/hour. Chronic oral potassium gluconate therapy will be required, adjusting the oral dose as needed to achieve normal serum levels. Renal function will stabilize or improve in some cases. Should the hypokalemia be refractory to treatment, serum magnesium should be evaluated, and, if normal, the possibility of hyperaldosteronism should be investigated, especially in the patient with hypertension.

Treatment of ureteronephroliths and renal neoplasia is discussed in an earlier section.

Nonspecific Management Strategies

SLOWING THE INHERENT PROGRESSION OF CHRONIC KIDNEY DISEASE

The IRIS categorization focuses in its staging system on factors that, when managed, slow the rate of inherent progression. These are azotemia, proteinuria, hyperphosphatemia, hypertension, and metabolic acidosis (Box 32-11).

Because azotemia, metabolic acidosis, and (to some degree) hyperphosphatemia are affected by hydration, optimizing hydration by using canned diets, adding water to food, encouraging drinking by use of flavored liquids or a fountain, and administering subcutaneous fluids daily are beneficial to the well-being of the patient. Similarly, for well-being the patient should enjoy the diet offered, regardless of the specific illness. It is always more important that the cat eat, rather than what the cat eats. The amount consumed must be monitored; this requires calculating the caloric requirements for each individual. A reasonable goal is 50 kcal/kg ideal body weight daily. The client should be advised how much food this is equivalent to so that if the cat does not eat that amount, the veterinarian can be notified. It also prevents confusion in that weight loss associated with progressing disease and weight loss associated with inadequate nutrient intake can be more easily distinguished. Inadequate intake results in a negative nitrogen balance; protein: calorie malnutrition; and deterioration of protective mechanisms that affect immunity, red cell hemoglobin content, and muscle mass, as well as tissue healing ability.

HYDRATION

Undoubtedly, rehydration is of critical and key importance to perfuse tissues with oxygen and support nutrient-carrying and waste-scavenging mechanisms.[95] Rehydration aids in acid–base homeostasis and helps improve renal blood flow, tissue perfusion, and GFR. With an impaired ability to concentrate urine, despite polydipsia, exogenous fluids (isotonic, polyionic fluids administered intravenously or subcutaneously) are required. Plenty of fresh water should be available at all times. Increasing oral intake of water can be encouraged by provision of a circulating water fountain, flavored water (broth) or ice cubes, milk, and canned foods. Supplementation with water-soluble vitamins should be considered.

In cats with IRIS stage 1 disease, home fluid therapy is generally not yet required; however, in-clinic rehydration as needed may be advisable. See Box 32-12 for an example of how to calculate fluid volume and rate. It is not too early in the progression of chronic renal insufficiency to mention this helpful treatment that the client may consider providing at home in the future, when the disease advances. Many clients are willing to give daily or less frequent subcutaneous fluids at home once they understand how it is done and see the improvement in demeanor that rehydration offers. They can assess the cat's state of hydration by evaluating the character of the feces; feces should be moist and shaped like logs rather than pellets or pieces. Once rehydrated, the goal is to maintain this state; in other words, the skin should not become less elastic, the feces should not become more firm, and so on.

METABOLIC ACIDOSIS

Metabolic acidosis is common in cats with CKD. In one study it was reported in 52.6% of cats with severe renal

BOX 32-11

Factors That Can Be Managed to Affect Progression of Feline Renal Insufficiency

Azotemia
Metabolic acidosis
Hyperphosphatemia
Proteinuria
Hypertension

BOX 32-12

Example of Subcutaneous Fluid Calculation for a Dehydrated Cat

Ideal healthy hydrated weight: 4 kg
Ill, dehydrated inappetent weight: 3.2 kg
Estimated deficit (firm feces, delay in skin elasticity, slightly dry oral mucous membranes, normal eye position): 8%

Deficit 8% × 4 kg	= 320 mL
Maintenance 60 mL (6%) × 4 kg/day	= 240 mL
Ongoing losses unknown at present	= ? mL
Fluids needed in first 24 hours	= 560 mL

The 560 mL can be given intravenously at 23 mL/hour **or**, were this to be given subcutaneously, for some reason, as 3 boluses of 185 mL over the 24-hour period.

Once rehydrated, the cat should receive maintenance dose of 60 mL/kg ideal weight/day = 240 mL/day. If the cat has not completely absorbed the subcutaneous fluids (e.g., fluid retention in axilla, lower limb), then reduce the dose but not the frequency. If the fluids are completely absorbed and the feces is still passed in firm pieces rather than moist logs, then increase the volume.

After the patient is rehydrated, then a dose of 60 mL/kg per day (6% ideal weight) = 240 mL is needed daily to maintain hydration.

failure (Cr >400 mmol/L).[80] It is important because it promotes severe catabolism of endogenous proteins, exacerbates azotemia regardless of diet, promotes wasting (degradation of protein), inhibits protein synthesis, causes a negative nitrogen balance, and enhances hypokalemia. In most cats, however, it is generally mild in degree and readily treated with subcutaneous fluid therapy. When it is persistent, sodium bicarbonate therapy may be required: 160 to 320 mg orally every 8 hours, to be titrated on the basis of serum bicarbonate/tCO_2 response. Baking soda contains 5 g $NaHCO_3$/tsp. Urine pH will be affected, and this treatment may result in struvite crystal formation in a predisposed individual.

HYPERTENSION

What role, if any, *systemic* hypertension plays in the progression of renal disease in the feline species is unknown. However, at any IRIS stage, if a persistent systolic BP higher than 160 mm Hg is detected, treatment for hypertension should be instituted to minimize the risk to target organs (CNS, retina, heart). Should target organ damage already be present, treatment is warranted without re-evaluation for persistence if another cause for this damage is not identified. The suggested schedule for re-evaluation of a questionable systolic BP elevation is as follows:

- A systolic BP of 160 to 179 mm Hg constitutes a moderate risk for target organ damage; BP should be re-evaluated after 2 months.
- A systolic BP of 180 mm Hg or higher constitutes a severe risk for target organ damage; BP should be re-evaluated after 1 to 2 weeks.

The 2007 American College of Veterinary Internal Medicine (ACVIM) Consensus Statement on identifying, evaluating, and managing systemic hypertension is an excellent guide on hypertension in general.[39]

Reduction of systemic hypertension should be gradual to avoid hypotension and inadvertent activation of the RAAS. Recent publications have looked at the role of dietary sodium in lower urinary tract disease, renal disease, and BP in cats. Increasing dietary sodium has been evaluated as a way to increase urine output and reduce specific gravity, thereby not only increasing frequency of voiding but also reducing the relative supersaturation of solutes to reduce risk of urolith formation.[50]

As far as renal disease goes, there is much conflict in reported results. In one study cats eating a higher-sodium diet had an increase in serum Cr, BUN, and phosphorus compared with cats on a lower-sodium diet.[125] Another study showed that a low-sodium diet resulted in a reduced GFR, increased urinary potassium loss, and activation of the RAAS.[44] A third study showed that feeding higher levels of sodium, along with magnesium, protein, and dietary fiber, resulted in a lower risk for development of chronic renal failure.[112] In a different study, feeding a classic restricted-protein, -phosphorus, and -sodium diet to cats in renal insufficiency resulted in fewer renal-related deaths.[193] Finally, in a study evaluating the effects of increased salt intake on renal function or any other health parameter, no adverse effects were seen.[226]

There is no strong evidence that increased dietary sodium increases the risk of hypertension in dogs and cats, and the current recommendation for hypertensive animals is to avoid high dietary salt intake without making a specific effort to restrict it, insofar as restriction may, in fact, activate the RAAS.[50] Reduction of sodium has not been shown to have an effect on blood pressure (systolic, diastolic, or mean)[44,125] and may, in fact, result in hypotension in cats, especially if these cats are on an ACE-I.[148]

It is important to recognize that these studies vary with respect to diet composition and the definition of what constituted high versus low sodium levels. The studies reported in these six papers are designed differently, so drawing conclusions relative to the other papers is not really possible.

Medical reduction of hypertension is most effectively achieved using the calcium channel blocker amlodipine.[155] After an initial dose of 0.625 mg/cat orally once daily, the BP should be assessed after 3 to 5 days. If this dose is inadequate in controlling the systolic BP at below 160 mm Hg, it may be titrated upwards as needed to as much as 0.5 mg/kg/day, rechecking its effect on systolic BP after 3 to 5 days each time. If this is insufficient, the cat may, in fact, not be receiving the medication *or* may be hyperaldosteronemic, and serum aldosterone levels should be measured. ACE-I have minimal, if any, effect in reducing systemic hypertension in cats and do not reduce RAAS activation in this species.[205] However, they are indicated for cats with proteinuria of glomerular origin. More information on treatment of hypertension is found in Chapter 20.

PROTEINURIA

Several studies have shown that plasma Cr concentration and proteinuria are highly related to survival in cats with naturally occurring renal insufficiency.[124,211] Preliminary studies also suggest that proteinuria may predict the development of azotemia in normal geriatric cats. It is unclear whether proteinuria is a marker or a mediator of renal injury in the cat, and the pathologic mechanisms remain unclear.[210] As with Cr, the source of the proteinuria must be determined before attributing significance to the value. Additionally, persistence of proteinuria must be confirmed because transient physiologic events (e.g., fever, excessive physical activity) may cause nonrenal proteins to spill into the urine. Other prerenal causes of proteinuria include increases in normal inflammatory proteins (e.g., from chronic inflammation or infection) or abnormal protein (e.g., from myeloma). Postrenal protein increases are most typically the result of UTI or inflammation. Once persistence and renal origin have been verified, localizing the protein as being glomerular, interstitial, or tubular remains difficult. However, because the latter two are less likely to cause significant proteinuria, the veterinarian can assume that UPC elevations are associated with alterations in glomerular integrity or hyperfiltration associated with a decline in the number of functional nephrons.[143] Because the significance of microalbuminuria in cats is unclear, UPC remains the test of choice.[97]

Glomerular hypertension promotes urinary protein loss because of a pressure gradient between the preglomerular blood and postglomerular ultrafiltrate. The mechanism of action of ACE-I is a selective dilation of glomerular efferent arterioles. Benazepril has undergone a large, multi-institutional study to assess its effects on CKD in cats. Results of this and other smaller studies show that using benazepril or placebo did not make any significant difference in survival time for all CKD cats unless proteinuria was present.[123,124,168] However, for cats with urinary protein loss based on UPC, benazepril-treated cats had longer survival times and better appetite than placebo-treated urinary protein–losing cats. Cats with an increased UPC (>0.4) that are started on this medication should be rechecked within 3 to 7 days and have renal parameters, hydration, body weight, appetite, and overall health monitored. Thereafter, re-evaluation should occur every 2 to 4 months in a stable patient. If there is no decrease in UPC, the medication should be discontinued because the possibility of adverse effects on renal function should not be completely discounted.[148]

NUTRITION AND DIETARY PROTEIN

There is only one certainty regarding feeding the cat with CKD, and that is that each patient's response to the disease and to nutritional intervention varies dramatically, requiring individualized therapy. The patient must be re-evaluated for response to nutritional therapy.[42,45,77,182]

In ARF and mild to moderate CKD, restriction of dietary protein may limit the kidney's compensatory response to injury. Protein restriction may lead to protein malnutrition, which impairs immunologic response, decreases hemoglobin production and thus promotes anemia, decreases plasma protein levels, and promotes muscle wasting. Inadequate protein intake also decreases urinary excretion of magnesium; this may result in $CaPO_4$ precipitation in the kidneys. It is more important for cats with mild to moderate CKD (IRIS stages 1 and 2) to maintain adequate caloric intake and thereby avoid protein-calorie malnutrition. Monitoring for evidence of protein-calorie malnutrition should include monitoring for weight loss, hypoalbuminemia, poor hair coat quality, and muscle wasting.

Dietary therapy for patients in IRIS stages 3 and 4 (Cr >2.9 mg/dL [>250 μmol/L]) is not controversial; restriction of both protein and phosphorous is required to prevent uremic complications. Benefits of protein restriction are related to *non*renal effects (toxins affect organs other than kidneys). Being obligate carnivores, cats require more of their dietary calories from protein than omnivores do. The minimum daily requirement for cats is 4.5 to 5 g/kg body weight. However, not all proteins are equivalent in bioavailability. Using protein sources of high biological value is important. In addition, should there be concurrent intestinal disease (e.g., inflammation associated with uremic gastritis), there may be alterations in nutrient absorption. Table 32-8 illustrates the differences in protein source as well as quantity of protein in a variety of protein-restricted diets.

Protein restriction may actually be harmful in renal patients that are inappetent, insofar as sustained calorie deficit causes body proteins to be catabolized to supply calories, and the nitrogenous end products of this process will further accentuate uremic signs. Unlike omnivores and herbivores, adult cats are often unwilling to eat a very-low-protein diet. Thus inappetence may be an indication for avoiding protein-restricted diets. Uremia is associated with variable dietary intake, intestinal malabsorption, metabolic acidosis, and comorbid conditions, which independently influence nitrogen balance.

Despite numerous experimental studies[1,2,82] and clinical trials,[79,181,193] questions about feeding protein to the cat with renal disease still remain. These include the following:

1. What is the optimal amount of protein for the cat with renal disease?
2. When should protein restriction be implemented?
3. Does the type of protein make a difference?
4. How much restriction is necessary?
5. Will a cat in IRIS stage 3 or 4 benefit if phosphorus is restricted by other means?

The answer to question 2 is that protein restriction should be considered when moderate azotemia persists in the well-hydrated state (IRIS stage 3). If the cat is unwilling to eat adequate quantities of food, it will have inadequate intake of all nutrients and be receiving even less protein than was intended. Thus it must always be remembered that anorexia and the catabolic state is as or more deleterious to the patient than the higher-protein diet the cat will eat willingly. Increasing fat content provides additional nonprotein calories and may increase palatability.

One of the most recent clinical trials[193] states that the "renal diet evaluated in this study was superior to an adult maintenance diet in minimizing uremic episodes and renal related deaths in cats with spontaneous stage

TABLE 32-8 Comparison of North American Therapeutic Renal Diets (as of July, 2011)

Feline (US & Canada) July 2011	Eukanuba Multi-stage Renal	Hill's k/d Feline Renal Health*	Hill's g/d Feline Early Cardiac-Healthy Aging	Purina NF Kidney Function	Royal Canin†	Royal Canin‡
CANNED						
Energy kcal/can	199 kcal/can	183 kcal/can	165 kcal/can	193 kcal/can	219 kcal/6 oz can	84 kcal/2.5 oz can
Moisture g/100 g as fed	74.9%	73.7%	74.9%	71.0%	78%	80%
Protein g/100 kcal ME	7.2	6.5	8.2	6.7	5.2	5.6
Source	Beef liver, chicken, beef by-products, corn meal, chicken fat, corn starch, dried egg product, fish oil	Pork liver, chicken, pork by-products, rice, oats, chicken fat	Turkey, pork liver, corn flour, barley, fish oil	Poultry by-products, beef, rice, meat by-products, chicken, fish oil	Pork by-products, chicken, chicken liver, chicken fat, pork, fish oil, rice, rice flour, mackerel	Pork by-products, chicken liver, chicken by-products, corn flour, chicken, fish oil, vegetable oil, dried egg white
Fat g/100 kcal ME	5.1	6.1	4.6	6.4	7.3	6.7
Carbohydrate g/100 kcal ME	7.1	7.9	9.2	6.3	3.0	4.3
Phosphorus mg/100 kcal ME	128	85	123	120	95	80
Potassium mg/100 kcal ME	217	264	171	320	189	200
Sodium mg/100 kcal ME	82	68	76	50	81	50
DRY						
Energy kcal/cup	514 kcal/cup	492 kcal/cup	297 kcal/cup	398 kcal/cup	358 kcal/cup	428 kcal/cup
Moisture g/100 g as fed	7.9%	7.5%	7.5%	7.4%	8.0%	8.0%
Protein g/100 kcal ME	7.1	6.8	7.9	7.2	5.7	6.2
Source	Corn grits, chicken, corn gluten meal, chicken fat, soy protein isolate, fish oil	Rice, corn gluten meal, pork fat, chicken by-product meal, dried egg, dried chicken, fish meal	Rice, corn gluten meal, pork fat, chicken by-product meal, soybean mill run, pork protein isolate, fish meal	Rice, corn, corn gluten meal, soybean meal, animal fat, fish meal, fish oil	Rice, ground corn, chicken fat wheat, corn gluten meal, soy protein isolate, fish oil	Pork meal, ground corn, chicken fat, rice, wheat, corn gluten meal, fish oil
Fat g/100 kcal ME	5.6	5.3	4.5	3.0	4.3	5.1
Carbohydrate g/100 kcal ME	7.8	9.9	9.8	11.9	10.9	8.5
Phosphorus mg/100 kcal ME	94	109	128	100	120	80
Potassium mg/100 kcal ME	143	175	181	210	240	220
Sodium mg/100 kcal ME	87	56	77	50	80	70

*Hill's k/d canned with chicken.
†Renal LP Modified pate (canned); LP Modified-C (dry).
‡Renal LP Modified in gravy (canned); LP Modified-P (dry).
Note: Manufacturers change diet compositions from time to time, and diets differ in different parts of the world.

II or III CKD" but goes on to acknowledge that "these findings emphasize the value of considering individual dietary components in the overall assessment of the benefits of dietary therapy. Individually or in combination, similar dietary modifications in the present study may have minimized the number of uremic crises and mortality rate." This underscores the difficulties in trying to isolate single factors as being of greatest importance in treating CKD.

Several other studies have attempted to identify what role different dietary components play. Based on natural occurrence as well as experimental study it is known that insufficient dietary potassium in an acidifying diet precipitates the development of renal insufficiency in normal cats and exacerbates pre-existing interstitial nephritis and fibrosis.[65] Some Burmese cats, primarily in the UK, Australia, and Europe, have been found to be predisposed to hypokalemic nephropathy/myopathy due to a presumed autosomal recessive genetic mutation.[154]

Another avenue of research has evaluated the role of oxidative stress in the progression of chronic renal insufficiency in cats.[41] Dietary supplementation of a dry food with the antioxidants vitamins E and C and beta-carotene resulted in significantly reduced oxidative damage to DNA in cats with spontaneous renal insufficiency.[228] This effect may also have been part of the difference noted in the diet effect seen in the Plantinga et al study.[181]

A survey of cats with CKD was conducted in 2002 to evaluate risk factors for the development of CKD using diet and lifestyle variables. It found that increased levels of dietary protein, sodium, magnesium, and fiber were associated with lower odds of developing CKD, whereas *ad libitum* feeding and increased ash intake were associated with an increased risk of developing CKD.[112]

In addition to paying attention to specific nutrients, ultimately with a goal to improve the quality and length of life, the veterinarian must ensure that the patient is receiving an adequate amount of energy (including protein). Uremic gastritis is a common cause of anorexia, nausea, or vomiting in cats with renal disease. This is a result of excessive gastric acid secretion caused by increased plasma gastrin levels. Given that gastrin is metabolized by the kidneys, a decline in renal function may also contribute to increased levels of this hormone.[89] Histamine-2 (H_2) receptor antagonists and proton pump inhibitors are important therapies for the reduction of gastric acid secretion. Cats may show only signs of partial anorexia or nausea rather than outright vomiting. The H_2 receptor antagonist famotidine (0.5 to 1 mg/kg orally every 24 to 48 hours) or ranitidine (2 to 3 mg/kg orally every 12 hours) may be tried if inappetence is apparent. The proton pump inhibitor omeprazole may be dosed at 0.7 to 1.5 mg/kg orally every 12 to 24 hours.

Appetite stimulants should be needed as a short-term measure only. Antiemetics can be administered to treat nausea (Table 32-9). If a cat is not eating enough calories on its own or if muscle wasting and nausea have been addressed, then a feeding tube should be considered proactively to enhance quality of life, rather than considered only as a salvage measure. Box 32-13 lists criteria for the consideration of feeding tube placement.

TABLE 32-9 **Antiemetics for Use in the Cat**

Generic Name	Brand Name	Dose
Chlorpromazine	Thorazine, Largactil	0.5 mg/kg q8h IM
Prochlorpromazine	Compazine	0.1 mg/kg q6h IM
Diphenhydramine	Benadryl	2.0-4.0 mg/kg q8h PO 2.0 mg/kg q8h IM
Dimenhydrinate	Dramamine, Gravol	8.0 mg/kg q8h PO
Metoclopramide	Reglan	1-2 mg/kg constant rate infusion over 24 hours
Ondansentron	Zofran	0.1-0.15 mg/kg slow push IV q6-12 hours prn
Dolasetron	Anzemet	0.6 mg/kg IV, SC q24h
Mirtazapine	Remeron	1.88-3.75 mg/cat PO q72h
Maropitant	Cerenia	0.5-1 mg/kg SC, IV, or PO q24 hr ≤5 days

IM, Intramuscular; *PO*, by mouth; *IV*, intravenous; *prn*, as needed; *SC*, subcutaneous.

BOX 32-13

When to Consider a Feeding Tube

Nutritional support should be considered for the following:

- The severely malnourished cat (e.g., 20% weight loss, body condition score 1-2/9)
- The moderately malnourished cat (e.g., 10% weight loss, body condition score 3-4/9) that also has catabolic disease
- Some cats will benefit from early intervention even at normal weight and condition if they suffer from advanced renal disease, hepatopathy, protein-losing gastrointestinal or glomerular disease, pancreatitis, or bile duct obstruction.

HYPERPHOSPHATEMIA

It is important to restrict phosphorus in moderately azotemic patients; this is more important than protein restriction to survival in remnant kidney model dogs and has been shown to produce less severe renal lesions in remnant kidney model cats. Suggested serum phosphorus targets are listed in Table 32-10. In an experimental study (using a reduced renal mass model) comparing the effect of dietary phosphorus restriction to a normal

TABLE 32-10 **Suggested Serum Phosphorus Targets**

Iris Stage	Creatinine	Target Serum Phosphorus	Method: Adjust on the Basis of Individual Response
2	1.6-2.8 mg/dL (141.44-247.52 μmol/L)	2.5-4.5 mg/dL (0.81-1.45 mmol/L)	Dietary restriction or normal diet + intestinal phosphate binder
3	2.9-4.9 mg/dL (256.36-433.16 μmol/L)	2.5-5 mg/dL (0.81-1.61 mmol/L)	Dietary restriction ± intestinal phosphate binder
4	≥5 mg/dL (>442 μmol/L)	2.5-6 mg/dL (0.81-1.94 mmol/L)	Dietary restriction ± intestinal phosphate binder

Adapted from Elliott J, Brown S, Cowgill L et al: Phosphatemia management in the treatment of chronic kidney disease: a roundtable discussion: Vetoquinol, 2006.

phosphorus diet, no difference in renal function was found; however, histopathologic changes (mineralization, mononuclear inflammation, and interstitial fibrosis) were more severe in the cats on the normal phosphorus diet.[192]

When a cat refuses to eat a restricted-protein diet but requires phosphorus restriction, intestinal phosphate binders are an option. To be effective, they must be given within 2 hours of a meal because they act by binding the phosphorus in the lumen of the gastrointestinal tract, preventing absorption of the phosphorus and facilitating its excretion in feces. Aluminum hydroxide, aluminum carbonate, and calcium carbonate are traditional choices. They are dosed at 90 mg/kg per day, divided and given with meals. Many cats object to being given these agents.[122] Epakitin (Vétoquinol, Lavaltrie, Quebec) is designed as an alternative to feeding renal diets as a method to reduce serum phosphorus. It is composed of chitosan and calcium carbonate. There are two published clinical studies of this agent. Serum urea and phosphorus levels were significantly reduced during the treatment period with minimal increase in serum calcium.[40,218]

Renalzin (lanthanum carbonate with kaolin and vitamin E, Bayer AG) is another option recently introduced in some European countries that has been shown to increase fecal phosphorus excretion in cats with surgically reduced renal mass.[199]

HYPERPARATHYROIDISM

Hyperparathyroidism is a common complication of chronic renal disease in cats. As parathyroid hormone (PTH) levels increase as a result of a decrease in calcitriol production and serum ionized calcium levels, intracellular calcium concentrations increase, which can result in cell death. High PTH concentration also affects the cardiovascular system, glucose and lipid metabolism, nerve and brain function, and the gastrointestinal tract.[16] Because phosphorus is retained in CKD, sufficient increases in serum Ca can result in a serum calcium × phosphorus product sufficiently high that soft tissue mineralization occurs.

Along with phosphorus restriction, oral calcitriol therapy has been suggested to enhance gastrointestinal absorption of calcium, providing feedback to the parathyroid glands to reduce PTH secretion. It must not be used until hyperphosphatemia is corrected. Its use is still controversial.[111,195]

Advocates suggest that it should be started at 2.5 to 3.5 ng/kg daily in early renal insufficiency when Cr is 2 to 3 mg/dL (175 to 265 mmol/L), USG is compatible with CKD as cause of azotemia, and phosphorus is below 6 mg/dL (<1.94 mmol/L). In these patients the PTH levels are often normal and the calcitriol is used to prevent PTH increase to slow progression of the CKD and prevent symptoms related to PTH toxicity. In patients with a serum Cr higher than 3 mg/dL (>265 mmol/L) and serum phosphorous lower than 6 mg/dL (<1.94 mmol/L) the dose is 3.5 ng/kg per day, administered orally. Good client compliance is critical for ongoing monitoring of ionized calcium and PTH.

ANEMIA

Cats with CKD may develop anemia by several mechanisms, including the following:

- "Anemia of chronic disease" (believed to be associated with iron sequestration)
- Anemia from protein malnutrition (from inappetence or being fed a diet not meeting protein requirements)
- Blood loss (associated with uremic gastritis–induced gastrointestinal bleeding)
- Erythropoietin (EPO) deficiency

EPO is produced in the mesangial cells of the glomerulus in response to hypoxia. When administered parenterally, EPO can cause a rapid correction of anemia by stimulating marrow progenitor cells. In 1994 the first report of the use of human recombinant EPO (r-HuEPO) (Eprex) to treat anemia associated with CKD was published.[107] Subsequently, a multicenter study evaluated the safety and efficacy of using r-HuEPO (Epogen) in cats with anemia caused by CKD. The benefits reported include increased appetite, energy, weight gain, alertness, strength, and playfulness to varying degrees but also that anemia, anti-r-HuEPO antibody production, seizures, systemic hypertension, and iron deficiency occurred, albeit inconsistently, in some of the study subjects.[62] In 2000 a study reported the development of a recombinant adeno-associated virus vector containing the feline erythropoietin gene (rAAV/feEpo). When normal healthy cats were given an intramuscular injection, a dose-related increase in hematocrit over a 7-week period was seen.[19] An attempt was made to create recombinant feline EPO (rfEPO) in 2004; unexpectedly, 8 of 26 cats developed anemia that was refractory to additional rfEPO treatments.[187]

Despite these setbacks, r-HuEPO therapy should still be considered in the anemic cat with CKD. As with any agent, some patients may experience adverse effects, but no patients can benefit if it is not used.[61] The veterinarian should consider using EPO when the packed cell volume is below 20%; 100 U/kg should be administered subcutaneously three times weekly until the packed cell volume is in the low-normal range (35%), then the dose and frequency should be reduced to 50 to 75 U/kg subcutaneously twice a week. It is important to monitor the packed cell volume every 2 weeks for the first 60 to 90 days to check for development of anti-EPO antibodies (Ab). If they occur, EPO must be ceased immediately. The cat may be transfusion dependent for 2 to 4 months until Ab levels decrease. The veterinarian should administer iron at the start of the treatment regimen and continue until the appetite is good. Iron dextran may be administered at 50 mg intramuscularly every 3 to 4 weeks or ferrous gluconate at 50 to 100 mg per cat orally per day. Although there is a risk of Ab development, the majority of cats will enjoy the benefits of an improved hemogram. Darbepoietin (Aranesp) may be less antigenic than EPO and is administered less frequently at 0.45 μg/kg weekly.

With or without EPO therapy, cats with renal disease may require a transfusion; in one review from a university teaching hospital, 20% of the cats needing blood products had CKD.[48] With diligent and proper preparation and monitoring, it has been shown that multiple red cell transfusions are well tolerated by cats regardless of underlying disease.[196]

HYPOKALEMIA

Hypokalemia is a common problem in renal insufficiency. It is a result of inappetence, muscle wasting, and polyuria. Dietary acidification in cats with or without renal function deficiencies contributes to acidosis, which shifts potassium out of cells, falsely elevating serum potassium. Because 94% of body potassium is intracellular, even small changes in serum potassium concentrations reflect significant intracellular events. Thus even serum potassium levels at the low end of the reference interval should be considered to possibly reflect subnormal cellular potassium levels. Acidosis should be corrected. Intravenous potassium chloride is used therapeutically until the patient is eating; after this, oral supplementation with potassium gluconate should be instituted. The starting dose for potassium gluconate is 2 to 4 mEq orally twice daily; it should be titrated to effect on the basis of serum electrolyte levels.

Some cats have persistently low potassium levels despite therapy. In these patients hypomagnesemia and hyperaldosteronemia should be considered. It has been suggested that in the latter, a neoplastic or non-neoplastic endocrine condition may be implicated in the progression of kidney disease.[114]

Prognosis

Chronic renal disease caused by tubulointerstitial nephritis will progress to eventual renal failure. The prognosis is variable because progression occurs at widely differing times in different individuals. Because amelioration of metabolic acidosis, azotemia, hyperphosphatemia, hypertension, and proteinuria have all been shown to halt or slow this progression, the earlier these are identified and treated, the better. Three studies have profiled cats with naturally occurring chronic renal disease. The first showed the following in a group of 184 cats with CKD[221]:

- Male cats with CKD were significantly younger than female cats with CKD.
- Younger cats were more likely to be diagnosed at an advanced stage of disease than older cats.
- The age at which cats were diagnosed with CKD was influenced by the veterinary clinic where the cats were treated.
- Breed did not appear to play a significant role in the development of CKD in this survey.

The second, a retrospective review, evaluated the duration of survival of 211 cats with naturally occurring CKD.[36] IRIS stage of CKD based on serum Cr at the time of diagnosis was found to be strongly predictive of survival. Median survival for cats in IRIS stage 2b at the time of diagnosis was 1151 days (range 2 to 3107) and was longer than survival in stage 3 (median 778, range 22 to 2100) or stage 4 (median 103, range 1 to 1920).

The third study evaluated 190 cats with stage 2 or higher CKD, half of which were treated with benazepril and half with placebo. Cats were followed for up to 3 years. Compared with cats in the treatment group, increased Cr, increased UPC, and increased blood leukocyte count were significantly ($P < 0.01$) associated with a shorter renal survival time and were independent risk factors. Increased concentrations of plasma phosphate or urea and lower blood hemoglobin concentration or hematocrit were significantly ($P < 0.01$) associated with a shorter renal survival time, but they correlated with plasma Cr concentration at the beginning of the study. Blood pressure was not routinely measured; thus this study was unable to include the effects of hypertension on outcome.[124]

These three studies underscore the need to diagnose this condition early and to treat and correct the aforementioned factors. Cats with CKD have widely variable and often lengthy survival times depending on when they are identified and how they are treated.

References

1. Adams LG, Polzin DJ, Osborne CA et al: Effects of dietary protein and calorie restriction in clinically normal cats and in cats with surgically induced chronic renal failure, *Am J Vet Res* 54:1653, 1993.
2. Adams LG, Polzin DJ, Osborne CA et al: Influence of dietary protein/calorie intake on renal morphology and function in cats with 5/6 nephrectomy, *Lab Invest* 70:347, 1994.
3. Adams LG, Williams JC, Jr., McAteer JA et al: In vitro evaluation of canine and feline calcium oxalate urolith fragility via shock wave lithotripsy, *Am J Vet Res* 66:1651, 2005.
4. Adin CA: Screening criteria for feline renal transplant recipients and donors, *Clin Tech Small Anim Pract* 17:184, 2002.
5. Adin CA, Gregory CR, Kyles AE et al: Diagnostic predictors of complications and survival after renal transplantation in cats, *Vet Surg* 30:515, 2001.
6. Agut A, Murciano J, Sanchez-Valverde MA et al: Comparison of different doses of iohexol with amidotrizoate for excretory urography in cats, *Res Vet Sci* 67:73, 1999.
7. Albasan H, Lulich JP, Osborne CA et al: Effects of storage time and temperature on pH, specific gravity, and crystal formation in urine samples from dogs and cats, *J Am Vet Med Assoc* 222:176, 2003.
8. Allworth MS, Hoffmann KL: Crossed renal ectopia with fusion in a cat, *Vet Radiol Ultrasound* 40:357, 1999.
9. American Society for the Prevention of Cruelty to Animals: Toxic and non-toxic plants (website): http://www.aspca.org/pet-care/poison-control/plants/. Accessed July 23, 2010.
10. Aresu L, Zanatta R, Pregel P et al: Bilateral juvenile renal dysplasia in a Norwegian Forest Cat, *J Feline Med Surg* 11:326, 2009.
11. Armbrust L, Biller D, Hoskinson J: Compression radiography: an old technique revisited, *J Am Anim Hosp Assoc* 36:537, 2000.
12. Aronson L: Retroperitoneal fibrosis in four cats following renal transplantation, *J Am Vet Med Assoc* 221:984, 2002.
13. Aronson L, Drobatz K: Hypercalcemia following renal transplantation in a cat, *J Am Vet Med Assoc* 217:1034, 2000.
14. Aronson LR, Kyles AE, Preston A et al: Renal transplantation in cats with calcium oxalate urolithiasis: 19 cases (1997-2004), *J Am Vet Med Assoc* 228:743, 2006.
15. Asano T, Tsukamoto A, Ohno K et al: Membranoproliferative glomerulonephritis in a young cat, *J Vet Med Sci* 70:1373, 2008.
16. Barber PJ, Rawlings JM, Markweu PJ et al: Effect of dietary phosphate restriction on renal secondary hyperparathyroidism in the cat, *J Small Anim Pract* 40:62, 1999.
17. Barrs V, Gunew M, Foster S et al: Prevalence of autosomal dominant polycystic kidney disease in Persian cats and related-breeds in Sydney and Brisbane, *Aust Vet J* 79:257, 2001.
18. Barthez P, Rivier P, Begon D: Prevalence of polycystic kidney disease in Persian and Persian related cats in France, *J Feline Med Surg* 5:345, 2003.
19. Beall CJ, Phipps AJ, Mathes LE et al: Transfer of the feline erythropoietin gene to cats using a recombinant adeno-associated virus vector, *Gene Ther* 7:534, 2000.
20. Beck C, Lavelle R: Feline polycystic kidney disease in Persian and other cats: a prospective study using ultrasonography, *Aust Vet J* 79:181, 2001.
21. Beck J, Bellenger C, Lamb W et al: Perirenal pseudocysts in 26 cats, *Aust Vet J* 78:166, 2000.
22. Bennett A, Gunn-Moore D: Comparison of digital and optical handheld refractometers for the measurement of feline urine specific gravity, *J Feline Med Surg* 13:152, 2011.
23. Berg RI, Francey T, Segev G: Resolution of acute kidney injury in a cat after lily *(Lilium lancifolium)* intoxication, *J Vet Intern Med* 21:857, 2007.
24. Bernsteen L, Gregory CR, Kyles AE et al: Renal transplantation in cats, *Clin Tech Small Anim Pract* 15:40, 2000.
25. Bernsteen L, Gregory CR, Pollard RE et al: Comparison of two surgical techniques for renal transplantation in cats, *Vet Surg* 28:417, 1999.
26. Bigge L, Brown D, Penninck D: Correlation between coagulation profile findings and bleeding complications after ultrasound-guided biopsies: 434 cases (1993-1996), *J Am Anim Hosp Assoc* 37:228, 2001.
27. Biller D, DiBartola S, Eaton K et al: Inheritance of polycystic kidney disease in Persian cats, *J Hered* 87:1, 1996.
28. Bishop SA, Bailey M, Lucke VM et al: Antibody response and antibody affinity maturation in cats with experimental proliferative immune complex glomerulonephritis, *J Comp Pathol* 107:91, 1992.
29. Bishop SA, Lucke VM, Stokes CR et al: Plasma and urine biochemical changes in cats with experimental immune complex glomerulonephritis, *J Comp Pathol* 104:65, 1991.
30. Bishop SA, Stokes CR, Lucke VM: Experimental proliferative glomerulonephritis in the cat, *J Comp Pathol* 106:49, 1992.
31. Bonazzi M, Volta A, Gnudi G et al: Prevalence of the polycystic kidney disease and renal and urinary bladder ultrasonographic abnormalities in Persian and Exotic Shorthair cats in Italy, *J Feline Med Surg* 9:387, 2007.
32. Bonazzi M, Volta A, Gnudi G et al: Comparison between ultrasound and genetic testing for the early diagnosis of polycystic kidney disease in Persian and Exotic Shorthair cats, *J Feline Med Surg* 11:430, 2009.
33. Bosje JT, van den Ingh TS, van der Linde-Sipman JS: Polycystic kidney and liver disease in cats, *Vet Q* 20:136, 1998.
34. Bouma JL, Aronson LR, Keith DG et al: Use of computed tomography renal angiography for screening feline renal transplant donors, *Vet Radiol Ultrasound* 44:636, 2003.
35. Boyce J, BiBartola S, Chew D et al: Familial renal amyloidosis in Abyssinian cats, *Vet Pathol* 21:33, 1984.
36. Boyd LM, Langston C, Thompson K et al: Survival in cats with naturally occurring chronic kidney disease (2000-2002), *J Vet Intern Med* 22:1111, 2008.
37. Brown CA, Jeong KS, Poppenga RH et al: Outbreaks of renal failure associated with melamine and cyanuric acid in dogs and cats in 2004 and 2007, *J Vet Diagn Invest* 19:525, 2007.
38. Brown S: Evaluation of chronic renal disease: a staged approach, *Compend Contin Educ Pract Vet* 21:752, 1999.
39. Brown S, Atkins C, Bagley R et al: Guidelines for the identification, evaluation, and management of systemic hypertension in dogs and cats, *J Vet Intern Med* 21:542, 2007.
40. Brown S, Rickertsen M, Sheldon S: Effects of an intestinal phosphate binder on serum phosphorus and parathyroid hormone concentration in cats with reduced renal function, *Int J Appl Res Vet Med* 6:155, 2008.
41. Brown SA: Oxidative stress and chronic kidney disease, *Vet Clin North Am Small Anim Pract* 38:157, 2008.
42. Brown SA, Finco DR, Bartges JW et al: Interventional nutrition for renal disease, *Clin Tech Small Anim Pract* 13:217, 1998.
43. Buffington C, Chew D: Intermittent alkaline urine in a cat fed an acidifying diet, *J Am Vet Med Assoc* 209:103, 1996.
44. Buranakarl C, Mathur S, Brown S: Effects of dietary sodium chloride intake on renal function and blood pressure in cats with normal and reduced renal function, *Am J Vet Res* 65:620, 2004.
45. Burkholder W: Dietary considerations for dogs and cats with renal disease, *J Am Vet Med Assoc* 216:1730, 2000.
46. Cannon M, MacKay A, et al: Prevalence of polycystic kidney disease in Persian cats in the United Kingdom, *Vet Rec* 149:409, 2001.

47. Carothers M, Johnson G, DiBartola S et al: Extramedullary plasmacytoma and immunoglobulin-associated amyloidosis in a cat, *J Am Vet Med Assoc* 195:1593, 1989.
48. Castellanos I, Couto C, Gray T: Clinical use of blood products in cats: a retrospective study (1997-2000), *J Vet Intern Med* 18:529, 2004.
49. Cavana P, Capucchio MT, Bovero A et al: Noncongophilic fibrillary glomerulonephritis in a cat, *Vet Pathol* 45:347, 2008.
50. Chandler ML: Pet food safety: sodium in pet foods, *Top Companion Anim Med* 23:148, 2008.
51. Chang J, Jung JH, Yoon J et al: Segmental aplasia of the uterine horn with ipsilateral renal agenesis in a cat, *J Vet Med Sci* 70:641, 2008.
52. Chew D: Personal communication, Jan 24, 2010.
53. Choi J, Jang J, Choi H et al: Ultrasonographic features of pyonephrosis in dogs, *Vet Radiol Ultrasound* 51:548, 2010.
54. Cianciolo RE, Bischoff K, Ebel JG et al: Clinicopathologic, histologic, and toxicologic findings in 70 cats inadvertently exposed to pet food contaminated with melamine and cyanuric acid, *J Am Vet Med Assoc* 233:729, 2008.
55. Clark L, Seawright AA: Amyloidosis associated with chronic hypervitaminosis A in cats, *Aust Vet J* 44:584, 1968.
56. Clark L, Seawright AA: Generalised amyloidosis in seven cats, *Pathol Vet* 6:117, 1969.
57. Connally HE, Thrall MA, Hamar DW: Safety and efficacy of high-dose fomepizole compared with ethanol as therapy for ethylene glycol intoxication in cats, *J Vet Emerg Crit Care* 20:191, 2010.
58. Cooper B, Piveral P: Autosomal dominant polycystic kidney disease in Persian cats, *Feline Pract* 28:20, 2000.
59. Cotran R, Kumar V, Robbins S: The kidney. In Cotran R, Kumar V, Robbins S, editors: *Robbins pathologic basis of disease*, ed 5, Philadelphia, 1994, Saunders.
60. Cottam YH, Caley P, Wamberg S et al: Feline reference values for urine composition, *J Nutr* 132:1754S, 2002.
61. Cowgill L: Advanced therapeutic approaches for the management of uraemia—"the met and unmet needs," *J Feline Med Surg* 5:57, 2003.
62. Cowgill L, James K, Levy J et al: Use of recombinant human erythropoietin for management of anemia in dogs and cats with renal failure, *J Am Vet Med Assoc* 212:521, 1998.
63. Criado-Fornelio A, Buling A, Barba-Carretero JC: Identification of feline polycystic kidney disease mutation using fret probes and melting curve analysis, *Res Vet Sci* 86:88, 2009.
64. DiBartola SP: *Selected diseases of the feline kidney*, Lakewood, Colo, 1992, American Animal Hospital Association.
65. DiBartola SP, Buffington CA, Chew DJ et al: Development of chronic renal disease in cats fed a commercial diet, *J Am Vet Med Assoc* 202:744, 1993.
66. DiBartola SP, Rutgers HC, Zack PM et al: Clinicopathologic findings associated with chronic renal disease in cats: 74 cases (1973-1984), *J Am Vet Med Assoc* 190:1196, 1987.
67. DiBartola SP, Tarr MJ, Benson MD: Tissue distribution of amyloid deposits in Abyssinian cats with familial amyloidosis, *J Comp Pathol* 96:387, 1986.
68. Dobson RL, Motlagh S, Quijano M et al: Identification and characterization of toxicity of contaminants in pet food leading to an outbreak of renal toxicity in cats and dogs, *Toxicol Sci* 106:251, 2008.
69. Domanjko-Petric A, Cernec D, Cotman M: Polycystic kidney disease: a review and occurrence in Slovenia with comparison between ultrasound and genetic testing, *J Feline Med Surg* 10:115, 2008.
70. Dorval P, Boysen SR: Management of acute renal failure in cats using peritoneal dialysis: a retrospective study of six cases (2003-2007), *J Feline Med Surg* 11:107, 2009.
71. Dow S, Fettman M, Curtis C et al: Hypokalemia in cats: 186 cases (1984-1987), *J Am Vet Med Assoc* 194:1604, 1989.
72. Dow SW, Fettman MJ, LeCouteur RA et al: Potassium depletion in cats: renal and dietary influences, *J Am Vet Med Assoc* 191:1569, 1987.
73. Dow SW, Fettman MJ, Smith KR et al: Effects of dietary acidification and potassium depletion on acid-base balance, mineral metabolism and renal function in adult cats, *J Nutr* 120:569, 1990.
74. Drost WT, Henry GA, Meinkoth JH et al: The effects of a unilateral ultrasound-guided renal biopsy on renal function in healthy sedated cats, *Vet Radiol Ultrasound* 41:57, 2000.
75. Dzyban LA, Labato MA, Ross LA et al: Peritoneal dialysis: a tool in veterinary critical care, *J Vet Emerg Crit Care* 10:91, 2000.
76. Elliott DA: Hemodialysis, *Clin Tech Small Anim Pract* 15:136, 2000.
77. Elliott DA: Nutritional management of chronic renal disease in dogs and cats, *Vet Clin North Am Small Anim Pract* 36:1377, 2006.
78. Elliott J, Barber PJ: Feline chronic renal failure: clinical findings in 80 cases diagnosed between 1992 and 1995, *J Small Anim Pract* 39:78, 1998.
79. Elliott J, Rawlings JM, Markwell PJ et al: Survival of cats with naturally occurring chronic renal failure: effect of dietary management, *J Small Anim Pract* 41:235, 2000.
80. Elliott J, Syme HM, Markwell PJ: Acid-base balance of cats with chronic renal failure: effect of deterioration in renal function, *J Small Anim Pract* 44:261, 2003.
81. Finco D: Congenital, inherited, and familial renal diseases. In Osborne CA, Finco D, editors: *Canine and feline nephrology and urology*, ed 1, Baltimore, 1995, Williams & Wilkins.
82. Finco D, Brown S, Brown C et al: Protein and calorie effects on progression of induced chronic renal failure in cats, *Am J Vet Res* 59:575, 1998.
83. Fischer JR, Pantaleo V, Francey T et al: Veterinary hemodialysis: advances in management and technology, *Vet Clin North Am Small Anim Pract* 34:935, 2004.
84. Freitag T, Squires RA, Schmid J et al: Antibiotic sensitivity profiles do not reliably distinguish relapsing or persisting infections from reinfections in cats with chronic renal failure and multiple diagnoses of Escherichia coli urinary tract infection, *J Vet Intern Med* 20:245, 2006.
85. Gabor LJ, Malik R, Canfield PJ: Clinical and anatomical features of lymphosarcoma in 118 cats, *Aust Vet J* 76:725, 1998.
86. Gaynor A, Dhupa N: Acute ethylene glycol intoxication. Part I. Pathophysiology and clinical stages, *Compend Contin Educ Pract Vet* 21:1014, 1999.
87. Gaynor A, Dhupa N: Acute ethylene glycol intoxication. Part II. Diagnosis, treatment, prognosis, and prevention, *Compend Contin Educ Pract Vet* 21:1124, 1999.
88. Giordano A, Paltrinieri S, Bertazzolo W et al: Sensitivity of Tru-cut and fine needle aspiration biopsies of liver and kidney for diagnosis of feline infectious peritonitis, *Vet Clin Pathol* 34:368, 2005.
89. Goldstein R, Marks S, Kass P et al: Gastrin concentrations in plasma of cats with chronic renal failure, *J Am Vet Med Assoc* 213:826, 1998.
90. Gonzalez A: Evaluation of the safety of extracorporeal shock-wave lithotripsy in cats (abstract), *J Vet Intern Med* 16:376, 2002.
91. Goo M-J, Williams BH, Hong I-H et al: Multiple urogenital abnormalities in a Persian cat, *J Feline Med Surg* 11:153, 2009.
92. Gookin J, Riviere J, Gilger B et al: Acute renal failure in four cats treated with paromomycin, *J Am Vet Med Assoc* 215:1821, 1999.
93. Grant D, Forrester S: Glomerulonephritis in dogs and cats: diagnosis and treatment, *Compend Contin Educ Pract Vet* 23:798, 2001.
94. Grant D, Forrester S: Glomerulonephritis in dogs and cats: glomerular function, pathophysiology, and clinical signs, *Compend Contin Educ Pract Vet* 23:739, 2001.
95. Grauer GF: Fluid therapy in acute and chronic renal failure, *Vet Clin North Am Small Anim Pract* 28:609, 1998.
96. Grauer GF: Early detection of renal damage and disease in dogs and cats, *Vet Clin North Am Small Anim Pract* 35:581, 2005.

97. Grauer GF: Measurement, interpretation, and implications of proteinuria and albuminuria, *Vet Clin North Am Small Anim Pract* 37:283, 2007.
98. Greco D: Congenital and inherited renal disease of small animals, *Vet Clin North Am Small Anim Pract* 31:393, 2001.
99. Gregory C: Personal communication, January 2010.
100. Haller M, Rohner K, Muller W et al: Single-injection inulin clearance for routine measurement of glomerular filtration rate in cats, *J Feline Med Surg* 5:175, 2003.
101. Halling KB, Ellison GW, Armstrong D et al: Evaluation of oxidative stress markers for the early diagnosis of allograft rejection in feline renal allotransplant recipients with normal renal function, *Can Vet J* 45:831, 2004.
102. Hardy ML, Hsu RC, Short CR: The nephrotoxic potential of gentamicin in the cat: enzymuria and alterations in urine concentrating capability, *J Vet Pharmacol Ther* 8:382, 1985.
103. Hartmann K, Binder C, Hirschberger J et al: Comparison of different tests to diagnose feline infectious peritonitis, *J Vet Intern Med* 17:781, 2003.
104. Hecht S, Lane IF, Daniel GB et al: Diuretic renal scintigraphy in normal cats, *Vet Radiol Ultrasound* 49:589, 2008.
105. Heiene R, Rumsby G, Ziener M et al: Chronic kidney disease with three cases of oxalate-like nephrosis in Ragdoll cats, *J Feline Med Surg* 11:474, 2009.
106. Henry C, Turnquist S, Smith A et al: Primary renal tumours in cats: 19 cases (1992-1998), *J Feline Med Surg* 1:165, 1999.
107. Henry P: Human recombinant erythropoetin used to treat a cat with anemia caused by chronic renal failure, *Can Vet J* 35:375, 1994.
108. Hill TP, Odesnik BJ: Omentalisation of perinephric pseudocysts in a cat, *J Small Anim Pract* 41:115, 2000.
109. Hills DL, Morris JG, Rogers QR: Potassium requirement of kittens as affected by dietary protein, *J Nutr* 112:216, 1982.
110. Hostutler RA, Chew DJ, Jaeger JQ et al: Uses and effectiveness of pamidronate disodium for treatment of dogs and cats with hypercalcemia, *J Vet Intern Med* 19:29, 2005.
111. Hostutler RA, DiBartola SP, Chew DJ et al: Comparison of the effects of daily and Intermittent-dose calcitriol on serum parathyroid hormone and ionized calcium concentrations in normal cats and cats with chronic renal failure, *J Vet Intern Med* 20:1307, 2006.
112. Hughes KL, Slater MR, Geller S et al: Diet and lifestyle variables as risk factors for chronic renal failure in pet cats, *Prev Vet Med* 55:1, 2002.
113. Inoue K, Kami-ie J, Ohtake S et al: Atypical membranoproliferative glomerulonephritis in a cat, *Vet Pathol* 38:468, 2001.
114. Javadi S, Djajadiningrat-Laanen SC, Kooistra HS et al: Primary hyperaldosteronism, a mediator of progressive renal disease in cats, *Domest Anim Endocrinol* 28:85, 2005.
115. Jepson RE, Brodbelt D, Vallance C et al: Evaluation of predictors of the development of azotemia in cats, *J Vet Intern Med* 23:806, 2009.
116. Jepson RE, Vallance C, Syme HM et al: Assessment of urinary N-acetyl-beta-D-glucosaminidase activity in geriatric cats with variable plasma creatinine concentrations with and without azotemia, *J Am Vet Med Assoc* 71:241, 2010.
117. Jernigan AD, Hatch RC, Wilson RC et al: Pathologic changes and tissue gentamicin concentrations after intravenous gentamicin administration in clinically normal and endotoxemic cats, *Am J Vet Res* 49:613, 1988.
118. Johnson KH, O'Brien TD, Jordan K et al: Impaired glucose tolerance is associated with increased islet amyloid polypeptide (IAPP) immunoreactivity in pancreatic beta cells, *Am J Pathol* 135:245, 1989.
119. Johnston G, Walter P, Feeney D: Diagnostic imaging of the urinary tract. In Osborne CA, Finco D, editors: *Canine and feline nephrology and urology*, ed 1, Baltimore, 1995, Williams & Wilkins.
120. Kadar E, Sykes JE, Kass PH et al: Evaluation of the prevalence of infections in cats after renal transplantation: 169 cases (1987-2003), *J Am Vet Med Assoc* 227:948, 2005.
121. Kerl ME, Cook CR: Glomerular filtration rate and renal scintigraphy, *Clin Tech Small Anim Pract* 20:31, 2005.
122. Kidder AC, Chew D: Treatment options for hyperphosphatemia in feline CKD: What's out there? *J Feline Med Surg* 11:913, 2009.
123. King JN, Gunn-Moore DA, Tasker S et al: Tolerability and efficacy of benazepril in cats with chronic kidney disease, *J Vet Intern Med* 20:1054, 2006.
124. King JN, Tasker S, Gunn-Moore DA et al: Prognostic factors in cats with chronic kidney disease, *J Vet Intern Med* 21:906, 2007.
125. Kirk CA, Jewell DE, Lowry SR: Effects of sodium chloride on selected parameters in cats, *Vet Ther* 7:333, 2006.
126. Klainbart S, Segev G, Loeb E et al: Resolution of renal adenocarcinoma-induced secondary inappropriate polycythaemia after nephrectomy in two cats, *J Feline Med Surg* 10:264, 2008.
127. Kobayashi DL, Peterson ME, Graves TK et al: Hypertension in cats with chronic renal failure or hyperthyroidism, *J Vet Intern Med* 4:58, 1990.
128. Kuwahara Y, Kobayashi R, Iwata J et al: Method of lymphocytotoxic crossmatch test for feline renal transplantation, *J Vet Med Sci* 61:481, 1999.
129. Kuwahara Y, Ohba Y, Kitoh K et al: Association of laboratory data and death within one month in cats with chronic renal failure, *J Small Anim Pract* 47:446, 2006.
130. Kyles A, Gregory C, Craigmill A et al: Pharmacokinetics of tacrolimus after multidose oral administration and efficacy in the prevention of allograft rejection in cats with renal transplants, *Am J Vet Res* 64:926, 2003.
131. Kyles A, Hardie E, Wooden B et al: Clinical, clinicopathologic, radiographic, and ultrasonographic abnormalities in cats with ureteral calculi: 163 cases (1984-2002), *J Am Vet Med Assoc* 226:932, 2005.
132. Kyles A, Hardie E, Wooden B et al: Management and outcome of cats with ureteral calculi: 153 cases (1984-2002), *J Am Vet Med Assoc* 226:937, 2005.
133. Kyles AE, Gregory CR, Griffey SM et al: Evaluation of the clinical and histologic features of renal allograft rejection in cats, *Vet Surg* 31:49, 2002.
134. Kyles AE, Gregory CR, Wooldridge JD et al: Management of hypertension controls postoperative neurologic disorders after renal transplantation in cats, *Vet Surg* 28:436, 1999.
135. Lamb CR: Ultrasonography of the ureters, *Vet Clin North Am Small Anim Pract* 28:823, 1998.
136. Langston C: Acute renal failure caused by lily ingestion in six cats, *J Am Vet Med Assoc* 220:49, 2002.
137. Langston C: Hemodialysis in dogs and cats, *Compend Contin Educ Pract Vet* 24:540, 2002.
138. Langston C: Advanced renal therapies: options when standard treatments are not enough, *Vet Med* 98:999, 2003.
139. Lapointe C, Bélanger MC, Dunn M et al: N-Acetyl-beta-d-Glucosaminidase index as an early biomarker for chronic kidney disease in cats with hyperthyroidism, *J Vet Intern Med* 22:1103, 2008.
140. Lappin M, Jensen W, Jensen T et al: Investigation of the induction of antibodies against Crandall-Rees feline kidney cell lysates and feline renal cell lysates after parenteral administration of vaccines against feline viral rhinotracheitis, calicivirus, and panleukopenia in cats, *Am J Vet Res* 66:506, 2005.
141. Lappin MR, Basaraba RJ, Jensen WA: Interstitial nephritis in cats inoculated with Crandell Rees feline kidney cell lysates, *J Feline Med Surg* 8:353, 2006.
142. Lawler DF, Evans RH, Chase K et al: The aging feline kidney: a model mortality antagonist? *J Feline Med Surg* 8:363, 2006.

143. Lees G, Brown S, Elliott J et al: Assessment and management of proteinuria in dogs and cats: 2004 ACVIM Forum consensus statement (small animal), *J Vet Intern Med* 19:377, 2005.
144. Lees GE: Early diagnosis of renal disease and renal failure, *Vet Clin North Am Small Anim Pract* 34:867, 2004.
145. Lees GE, Bahr A, Sanders MH: Performing renal biopsy, *NAVC Clinician's Brief* 8(4):67, 2010.
146. Lees GE, Berridge BR, Cianciolo RE: Renal biopsy stains, *NAVC Clinician's Brief* 8:27, 2010.
147. Lees GE, Berridge BR, Clubb FJ: Evaluation of renal biopsy samples, *NAVC Clinician's Brief* 7:67, 2009.
148. Lefebvre HP, Toutain PL: Angiotensin-converting enzyme inhibitors in the therapy of renal diseases, *J Vet Pharmacol Ther* 27:265, 2004.
149. Lew S, Kuleta Z, Pomianowski A: Peritoneal dialysis in dogs and cats, *Pol J Vet Sci* 8:323, 2005.
150. Ling G, Ruby A, Johnson D et al: Renal calculi in dogs and cats: prevalence, mineral type, breed, age, and gender interrelationships (1981-1993), *J Vet Intern Med* 12:11, 1998.
151. Litster A, Moss S, Platell J et al: Occult bacterial lower urinary tract infections in cats-urinalysis and culture findings, *Vet Microbiol* 136:130, 2009.
152. Lutz TA, Rand JS: Detection of amyloid deposition in various regions of the feline pancreas by different staining techniques, *J Comp Pathol* 116:157, 1997.
153. Lyons LA, Biller DS, Erdman CA et al: Feline polycystic kidney disease mutation identified in PKD1, *J Am Soc Nephrol* 15:2548, 2004.
154. Mason K: A hereditary disease in Burmese cats manifested as an episodic weakness with head nodding and neck ventroflexion, *J Am Anim Hosp Assoc* 24:147, 1988.
155. Mathur S, Syme H, Brown C et al: Effects of the calcium channel antagonist amlodipine in cats with surgically induced hypertensive renal insufficiency, *Am J Vet Res* 63:833, 2002.
156. Mayer-Roenne B, Goldstein RE, Erb HN: Urinary tract infections in cats with hyperthyroidism, diabetes mellitus and chronic kidney disease, *J Feline Med Surg* 9:124, 2007.
157. McCord K, Steyn PF, Lunn KF: Unilateral improvement in glomerular filtration rate after permanent drainage of a perinephric pseudocyst in a cat, *J Feline Med Surg* 10:280, 2008.
158. McIntyre RL, Levy JK, Roberts JF et al: Developmental uterine anomalies in cats and dogs undergoing elective ovariohysterectomy, *J Am Vet Med Assoc* 237:542, 2010.
159. McLoughlin M, DiBartola SP, Birchard S et al: Influence of systemic nonthyroidal illness on serum concentration of thyroxine in hyperthyroid cats, *J Am Anim Hosp Assoc* 29:227, 1993.
160. Mealey K, Boothe D: Nephrotoxicosis associated with topical administration of gentamicin in a cat, *J Am Vet Med Assoc* 204:1919, 1994.
161. Mehl ML, Kyles AE, Pollard R et al: Comparison of 3 techniques for ureteroneocystostomy in cats, *Vet Surg* 34:114, 2005.
162. Mehl ML, Kyles AE, Reimer SB et al: Evaluation of the effects of ischemic injury and ureteral obstruction on delayed graft function in cats after renal autotransplantation, *Vet Surg* 35:341, 2006.
163. Miller R, Lehmkuhl L, Smeak D et al: Effect of enalapril on blood pressure, renal function, and the renin-angiotensin-aldosterone system in cats with autosomal dominant polycystic kidney disease, *Am J Vet Res* 60:1516, 1999.
164. Minkus G, Reusch C, Hörauf A et al: Evaluation of renal biopsies in cats and dogs—histopathology in comparison with clinical data, *J Small Anim Pract* 35:465, 1994.
165. Mitchell S, Toal R, Daniel G et al: Evaluation of renal hemodynamics in awake and isoflurane-anesthetized cats with pulsed-wave Doppler and quantitative renal scintigraphy, *Vet Radiol Ultrasound* 39:451, 1998.
166. Miyamoto K: Evaluation of single-injection method of inulin and creatinine as a renal function test in normal cats, *J Vet Med Sci* 60:327, 1998.
167. Miyamoto K: Clinical application of plasma clearance of iohexol on feline patients, *J Feline Med Surg* 3:143, 2001.
168. Mizutani H, Koyama H, Watanabe T et al: Evaluation of the clinical efficacy of benazepril in the treatment of chronic renal insufficiency in cats, *J Vet Intern Med* 20:1074, 2006.
169. Mosenco AS, Culp WT, Johnson V et al: Renal cystadenoma in a domestic shorthair, *J Feline Med Surg* 10:102, 2008.
170. Nakamura S, Shibata S, Shirota K et al: Renal glomerular fibrosis in a cat, *Vet Pathol* 33:696, 1996.
171. Nash AS, Mohammed NA, Wright NG: Experimental immune complex glomerulonephritis and the nephrotic syndrome in cats immunised with cationised bovine serum albumin, *Res Vet Sci* 49:370, 1990.
172. Newell S, Ellison G, Graham J et al: Scintigraphic, sonographic, and histologic evaluation of renal autotransplantation in cats, *Am J Vet Res* 60:775, 1999.
173. Newell SM, Graham JP, Roberts GD et al: Quantitative magnetic resonance imaging of the normal feline cranial abdomen, *Vet Radiol Ultrasound* 41:27, 2000.
174. Nichols R: Allergic- and immune-associated diseases of the urinary tract, *Vet Clin North Am Small Anim Pract* 24:749, 1994.
175. Ochoa V, DiBartola S, Chew D et al: Perinephric pseudocysts in the cat: a retrospective study and review of the literature, *J Vet Intern Med* 13:47, 1999.
176. Osborne C, Stevens J: *Urinalysis: a clinical guide to compassionate patient care*, Shawnee Mission, Kan, 1999, Bayer.
177. Osborne C, Stevens J, Lulich J et al: A clinician's analysis of urinalysis. In Osborne C,Finco D editors: *Canine and feline nephrology and urology*, ed 1, Baltimore, 1995, Williams & Wilkins, p 136.
178. Osborne CA: Techniques of urine collection and preservation. In Osborne CA,Finco DR editors: *Canine and feline nephrology and urology*, ed 1, Baltimore, 1995, Williams & Wilkins, p 100.
179. Paepe D, Saunders JH, Bavegems V et al: Screening of Ragdoll cats for kidney disease: a retrospective evaluation (abstract), *J Vet Intern Med* 24:677, 2010.
180. Paster ER, Mehl ML, Kass PH et al: Hypophosphatemia in cats after renal transplantation, *Vet Surg* 38:983, 2009.
181. Plantinga E, Everts H, Kastelein A et al: Retrospective study of the survival of cats with acquired chronic renal insufficiency offered different commercial diets, *Vet Rec* 157:185, 2005.
182. Polzin D, Osborne C, Ross S et al: Dietary management of feline chronic renal failure: where are we now? in what direction are we headed? *J Feline Med Surg* 2:75, 2000.
183. Porciello F, Rishniw M, Herndon WE et al: Cardiac troponin I is elevated in dogs and cats with azotaemia renal failure and in dogs with non-cardiac systemic disease, *Aust Vet J* 86:390, 2008.
184. Pressler B, Vaden S: Managing renal amyloidosis in dogs and cats, *Vet Med* 98:320, 2003.
185. Puschner B, Poppenga RH, Lowenstine LJ et al: Assessment of melamine and cyanuric acid toxicity in cats, *J Vet Diagn Invest* 19:616, 2007.
186. Raffan E, Kipar A, Barber PJ et al: Transitional cell carcinoma forming a perirenal cyst in a cat, *J Small Anim Pract* 49:144, 2008.
187. Randolph J, Scarlett J, Stokol T et al: Expression, bioavailability, and clinical assessment of recombinant feline erythropoietin, *Am J Vet Res* 65:1355, 2004.
188. Ravnskov U: Hydrocarbon exposure may cause glomerulonephritis and worsen renal function: evidence based on Hill's criteria for causality, *QJM* 93:551, 2000.
189. Reichle JK, DiBartola SP, Leveille R: Renal ultrasonographic and computed tomographic appearance, volume, and function of cats with autosomal dominant polycystic kidney disease, *Vet Radiol Ultrasound* 43:368, 2002.

190. Reine NJ, Langston CE: Urinalysis interpretation: how to squeeze out the maximum information from a small sample, *Clin Tech Small Anim Pract* 20:2, 2005.
191. Rishniw M, Weidman J, Hornof WJ: Hydrothorax secondary to a perinephric pseudocyst in a cat, *Vet Radiol Ultrasound* 39:193, 1998.
192. Ross LA, Finco DR, Crowell WA: Effect of dietary phosphorus restriction on the kidneys of cats with reduced renal mass, *Am J Vet Res* 43:1023, 1982.
193. Ross SJ, Osborne CA, Kirk CA et al: Clinical evaluation of dietary modification for treatment of spontaneous chronic kidney disease in cats, *J Am Vet Med Assoc* 229:949, 2006.
194. Ross SJ, Osborne CA, Lekcharoensuk C et al: A case-control study of the effects of nephrolithiasis in cats with chronic kidney disease, *J Am Vet Med Assoc* 230:1854, 2007.
195. Roudebush P, Polzin DJ, Ross SJ et al: Therapies for feline chronic kidney disease. What is the evidence? *J Feline Med Surg* 11:195, 2009.
196. Roux FA, Deschamps J-Y, Blais M-C et al: Multiple red cell transfusions in 27 cats (2003-2006): indications, complications and outcomes, *J Feline Med Surg* 10:213, 2008.
197. Rumbeiha WK, Francis JA, Fitzgerald SD et al: A comprehensive study of Easter lily poisoning in cats, *J Vet Diagn Invest* 16:527, 2004.
198. Scaglione FE, Catalano D, Bestonso R et al: Comparison between light and electron microscopy in canine and feline renal pathology: a preliminary study, *J Microsc* 232:387, 2008.
199. Schmidt B, Delport P, Spiecker-Hauser U: G07 Bay 78-1887, a novel lanthanum-based phosphate binder, decreases intestinal phosphorus absorption in cats, *J Vet Pharmacol Ther* 29:206, 2006.
200. Schmiedt CW, Grimes JA, Holzman G et al: Incidence and risk factors for development of malignant neoplasia after feline renal transplantation and cyclosporine-based immunosuppression, *Vet Comp Oncol* 7:45, 2009.
201. Schmiedt CW, Holzman G, Schwarz T et al: Survival, complications, and analysis of risk factors after renal transplantation in cats, *Vet Surg* 37:683, 2008.
202. Shiroma J, Gabriel J, Carter R et al: Effect of reproductive status on feline renal size, *Vet Radiol Ultrasound* 40:242, 1999.
203. Sox EM, Chiotti R, Goldstein RE: Use of gadolinium diethylene triamine penta-acetic acid, as measured by ELISA, in the determination of glomerular filtration rates in cats, *J Feline Med Surg* 12:738, 2010.
204. Sparkes AH, Heiene R, Lascelles BDX et al: ISFM and AAFP consensus guidelines: Long-term use of NSAIDs in cats, *J Feline Med Surg* 12:521, 2010.
205. Steele JL, Henik RA, Stepien RL: Effects of angiotensin-converting enzyme inhibition on plasma aldosterone concentration, plasma renin activity, and blood pressure in spontaneously hypertensive cats with chronic renal disease, *Vet Ther* 3:157, 2002.
206. Stiles J, Polzin D, Bistner S: The prevalence of retinopathy in cats with systemic hypertension and chronic renal failure or hyperthyroidism, *J Am Anim Hosp Assoc* 30:564, 1994.
207. Stokes JE, Forrester SD: New and unusual causes of acute renal failure in dogs and cats, *Vet Clin North Am Small Anim Pract* 34:909, 2004.
208. Sturgess C, Hesford A, Owen H et al: An investigation into the effects of storage on the diagnosis of crystalluria in cats, *J Feline Med Surg* 3:81, 2001.
209. Syme H, Barber P, Markwell P et al: Prevalence of systolic hypertension in cats with chronic renal failure at initial evaluation, *J Am Vet Med Assoc* 220:1799, 2002.
210. Syme HM: Proteinuria in cats. Prognostic marker or mediator? *J Feline Med Surg* 11:211, 2009.
211. Syme HM, Markwell PJ, Pfeiffer D et al: Survival of cats with naturally occurring chronic renal failure is related to severity of proteinuria, *J Vet Intern Med* 20:528, 2006.
212. Taylor SS, Goodfellow MR, Browne WJ et al: Feline extranodal lymphoma: response to chemotherapy and survival in 110 cats, *J Small Anim Pract* 50:584, 2009.
213. Thrall M, Connally H, Dial S et al: Advances in therapy for antifreeze poisoning, *California Veterinarian* 52:18, 1998.
214. Vaden R, Levine J, Lees G et al: Renal biopsy: a retrospective study of methods and complications in 283 dogs and 65 cats, *J Vet Intern Med* 19:794, 2005.
215. Valdes-Martinez A, Cianciolo R, Mai W: Association between renal hypoechoic subcapsular thickening and lymphosarcoma in cats, *Vet Radiol Ultrasound* 48:357, 2007.
216. Veterinary Society of Surgical Oncologists: Renal tumors (website): http://www.vsso.org/Renal_Tumors_-_Feline.html. Accessed September 11, 2010.
217. Volta A, Manfredi S, Gnudi G et al: Polycystic kidney disease in a Chartreux cat, *J Feline Med Surg* 12:138, 2010.
218. Wagner E, Schwendenwein I, Zentek J: Effects of a dietary chitosan and calcium supplement on Ca and P metabolism in cats, *Berl Munch Tierarztl Wochenschr* 117:310, 2004.
219. Watson A: Indicators of renal insufficiency in dogs and cats presented at a veterinary teaching hospital, *Aust Vet Pract* 31:54, 2001.
220. Westropp J: Personal communication, April 2010.
221. White JD, Norris JM, Baral RM et al: Naturally-occurring chronic renal disease in Australian cats: a prospective study of 184 cases, *Aust Vet J* 84:188, 2006.
222. White JD, Norris JM, Bosward KL et al: Persistent haematuria and proteinuria due to glomerular disease in related Abyssinian cats, *J Feline Med Surg* 10:219, 2008.
223. Wooldridge JD, Gregory CR, Mathews KG et al: The prevalence of malignant neoplasia in feline renal-transplant recipients, *Vet Surg* 31:94, 2002.
224. Worwag S, Langston CE: Acute intrinsic renal failure in cats: 32 cases (1997-2004), *J Am Vet Med Assoc* 232:728, 2008.
225. Wright NG, Nash AS, Thompson H et al: Membranous nephropathy in the cat and dog: a renal biopsy and follow-up study of sixteen cases, *Lab Invest* 45:269, 1981.
226. Xu H, Laflamme DPL, Long GL: Effects of dietary sodium chloride on health parameters in mature cats, *J Feline Med Surg* 11:435, 2009.
227. Yabuki A, Mitani S, Fujiki M et al: Comparative study of chronic kidney disease in dogs and cats: induction of myofibroblasts, *Res Vet Sci* 88:294, 2010.
228. Yu S, Paetau-Robinson I: Dietary supplements of vitamins E and C and beta-carotene reduce oxidative stress in cats with renal insufficiency, *Vet Res Commun* 30:403, 2006.
229. Zatelli A, D'Ippolito P, Bonfanti U et al: Ultrasound-assisted drainage and alcoholization of hepatic and renal cysts: 22 cases, *J Am Anim Hosp Assoc* 43:112, 2007.

THE LOWER URINARY TRACT

Susan E. Little

Feline lower urinary tract disease (FLUTD) was described as early as 1925 and remains one of the most common problems encountered in feline medicine. A 1999 survey reported that FLUTD affected 1.5% of cats evaluated in private practice.[117] In a 2001 study 8% of cats presented to veterinary teaching hospitals were presented for FLUTD.[101] Because inappropriate elimination, often seen in cats with FLUTD, is an important risk factor for relinquishment to a shelter, accurate diagnosis and management are welfare as well as medical issues.[143]

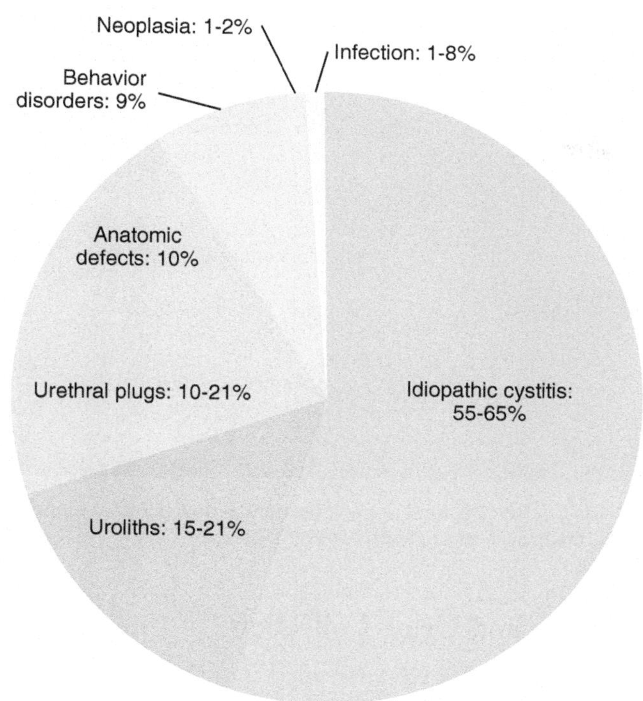

FIGURE 32-16 Prevalence of the causes of feline lower urinary tract disease. *(Adapted from Gerber B, Boretti FS, Kley S et al: Evaluation of clinical signs and causes of lower urinary tract disease in European cats,* J Small Anim Pract *46:571, 2005; Kruger JM, Osborne CA, Goyal SM et al: Clinical evaluation of cats with lower urinary tract disease,* J Am Vet Med Assoc *199:211, 1991; Buffington CA, Chew DJ, Kendall MS et al: Clinical evaluation of cats with nonobstructive urinary tract diseases,* J Am Vet Med Assoc *210:46, 1997.)*

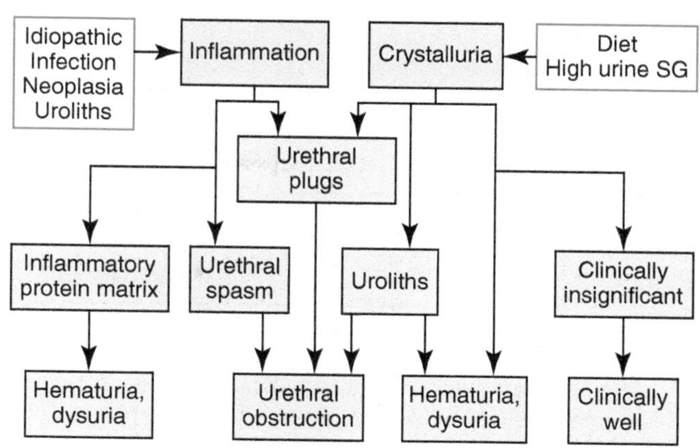

FIGURE 32-17 Interactions between urinary tract inflammation and crystalluria to produce common clinical presentations of feline lower urinary tract disease. *(Adapted from Gunn-Moore D: Feline lower urinary tract disease,* J Feline Med Surg *5:133, 2003.)*

Over the years various terms such as "feline urologic syndrome" (dating to 1970) and FLUTD (dating to the 1980s) have been used to describe the group of clinical signs related to problems voiding urine.[131] However, these umbrella terms do not identify the underlying etiology. The clinician is encouraged to determine the specific cause for lower urinary tract signs in cats in order to recommend appropriate treatment because FLUTD is not a diagnosis in itself.

A variety of disorders have been implicated as causes of FLUTD, including feline idiopathic cystitis (FIC), urolithiasis, urethral plugs, anatomic defects, neoplasia, infection, and behavioral problems (Figure 32-16). Published studies show general agreement on the relative prevalence of these causes.[27,60,91] The most common cause is FIC (55% to 65% of cases). Urolithiasis affects about 15% to 20% of cats presenting with FLUTD. Behavioral problems and anatomic defects may account for about 10% of cases. Neoplasia (1% to 2%) and UTIs (1% to 8%) are the least common causes.

Antibiotics are overprescribed for cats with FLUTD, given that bacterial infection is one of the least common diagnoses. In one survey of 301 veterinary practices in the United Kingdom, 47% of practices reported providing treatment for cats presenting for the first time with clinical signs of FLUTD without any investigation.[46] In addition, 68% of practices reported prescribing antibiotics in combination with other options on first presentation. FIC is the most common form of FLUTD and is typically self-limiting. Many cats appear to respond to antibiotic therapy because they have self-limiting disease. This may explain why antibiotics continue to be prescribed in clinical practice despite evidence that they are useless in the majority of FLUTD cases.

Many of the components of FLUTD are not independent factors but instead may be related in a type of unifying hypothesis, leading to the major clinical presentations of FLUTD. In particular, inflammation and crystalluria may be the necessary elements for urolith formation, urethral obstruction, and cystitis (Figure 32-17). This concept was first introduced in the early 1990s by Osborne and colleagues and has since been refined.[69,136]

Various factors have been associated with risk of FLUTD. In particular, an indoor lifestyle and feeding a diet consisting exclusively of dry food have been implicated.[84] However, because a great many cats worldwide are confined indoors and fed dry diets but do not have clinical signs of FLUTD, it seems reasonable that some underlying predisposition to FLUTD, as yet uncharacterized, may exist in affected cats.

DIAGNOSTIC METHODS

The underlying causes for FLUTD are varied, and a focused diagnostic plan will help the clinician reach a diagnosis and target treatment (Figure 32-18). A diagnostic evaluation should always include a complete medical and dietary history, physical examination, and urinalysis. Depending on the patient, investigation may

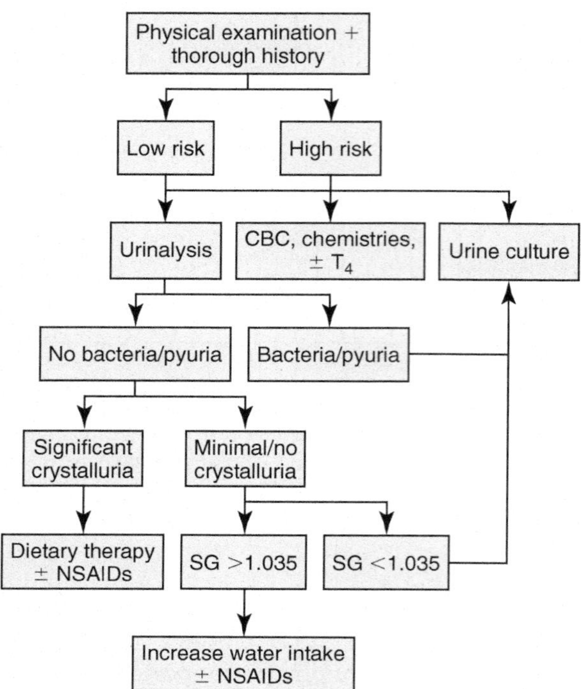

FIGURE 32-18 Decision tree for the initial diagnostic plan for the first occurrence of lower urinary tract signs in a cat without urethral obstruction. Low risk: young to middle-aged cat (<10 years) with no concurrent disease; high risk: older cat (>10 years), with or without concurrent diseases. *SG,* Urine specific gravity; *NSAIDs,* nonsteroidal antiinflammatory drugs.

also include urine culture and sensitivity testing, bladder imaging (e.g., plain and contrast radiography, ultrasound, cystoscopy), and other laboratory investigations (e.g., CBC, chemistry profile, total T_4, retroviral serology). Cats that present with only periuria (urinating outside the litter box) or urine spraying as clinical signs may have a purely behavioral problem or a medical problem with a behavioral component. A behavioral approach to periuria and urine spraying is found in Chapter 13.

Physical Exam and Clinical Signs

It is not possible to determine the cause of FLUTD on the basis of clinical signs alone. Common clinical signs regardless of underlying cause include pollakiuria, dysuria, stranguria, vocalizing during attempts to urinate, hematuria, and periuria. Bilateral ventral abdominal and inguinal alopecia is occasionally seen in cats with bladder pain (Figure 32-19). One of the first steps when evaluating a male cat with FLUTD is to determine urethral patency. Cats with urethral obstruction present with dysuria, stranguria, increased grooming of the penis and perineum, pain, and variable signs of systemic involvement. The bladder may be markedly distended.

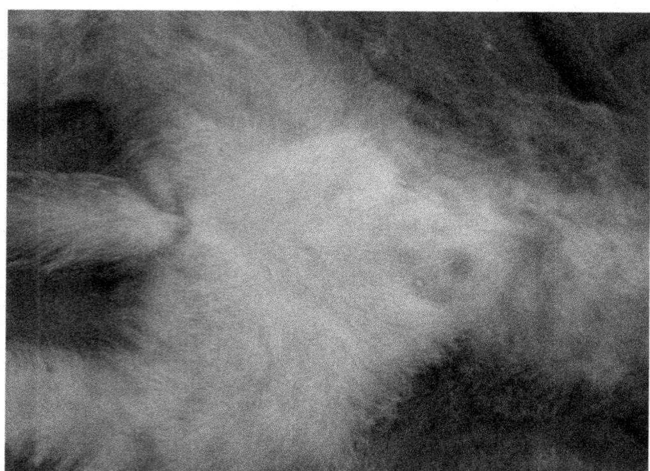

FIGURE 32-19 Bilateral ventral abdominal and inguinal alopecia is occasionally seen in cats with bladder pain.

Urinalysis and Urine Collection

A urinalysis should be performed for all cats presenting with signs of FLUTD. Urine samples should be evaluated within 30 to 60 minutes of collection, which means that ideally samples should be analyzed in-house rather than at a referral laboratory. It also means that samples collected at home by the owner and brought to the veterinary clinic for analysis have limited usefulness. Storage for periods of time longer than 60 minutes, especially with refrigeration, may cause in vitro formation of struvite or CaOx crystals.[2,173] In vitro formation of struvite crystals is especially a risk in stored urine samples from cats fed dry food diets.[173] Use of a urinalysis preservative tube (BD Vacutainer Plus Urinalysis Preservative Tube; Becton, Dickinson & Co.) may decrease the risk of in vitro crystal formation in stored urine samples.[82] Urine pH and specific gravity are not significantly affected by storage.[2] More information on urinalysis is contained in the section on upper urinary tract diseases in this chapter. Although not always a first-line diagnostic test, a urine culture should be performed for any cat with recurrent FLUTD or an identified risk factor. More information on bacterial lower UTI and urine culture is found later in this chapter.

Although urine may be collected in various ways, cystocentesis has become the standard of practice in most situations (Table 32-11).[108] It may be performed blindly using palpation or with ultrasound guidance, especially in obese patients. The benefits of cystocentesis include ease of performance, tolerance by patients, and the collection of samples that are not contaminated by the distal urogenital tract. However, care must be taken with technique to avoid iatrogenic bladder trauma. Because cystocentesis is performed in the veterinary practice, it is helpful if the patient arrives with a full urinary bladder. Owners can be advised to place the cat

TABLE 32-11 Assessment of Urine Collection Methods Based on Patient Safety and Sample Diagnostic Quality

	Collection Method			
Purpose of Sample Collection	**Cystocentesis**	**Voided Midstream**	**Catheterization**	**Manual Expression**
Screening test	P	A	N	N
Diagnostic urine culture	P	A	N	N
FLUTD	P	A	N	N
Urolithiasis	P	A	N	N
Bladder neoplasia	N	P	N	N
Disease distal to the bladder	N	P	N	N

P, Preferred; *A,* acceptable; *N,* not advised, *FLUTD,* feline lower urinary tract disease.
Adapted from: Lulich J, Osborne C: Cystocentesis: lessons from thirty years of clinical experience, *Clin Brief* 2:11, 2004.

in its carrier or in a room without a litter box for several hours before the veterinary visit. Some cats with FLUTD are pollakiuric as a result of bladder pain; providing analgesia (e.g., buprenorphine, or meloxicam in a well-hydrated patient) can reduce stranguria and may facilitate urine collection. More information on cystocentesis and other methods of urine collection is contained in the section on upper urinary tract diseases in this chapter.

Urethral catheterization is most often performed for diagnostic procedures (e.g., contrast cystography) and for relief of urethral obstruction rather than for collection of urine samples. The procedure for the male cat is described later in this chapter, in the section about the management of cats with urethral obstruction. The procedure for female cats is very similar to that for the female dog and is usually performed under sedation or general anesthesia. Catheterization should always be performed aseptically. The cat is placed in sternal recumbency with the hind legs hanging off the end of the examination table. It is important to keep the body position straight. A 3.5 to 5 French soft catheter with a stylet or a more rigid polypropylene catheter should be used. Because the vaginal vault of the female cat is small, visualization of the urethral opening is not usually possible. Wearing sterile gloves, the veterinarian palpates the urethral papilla on the floor of the vagina with the index finger.[154] The lubricated urinary catheter is then passed under the index finger and directed down and into the urethra. If resistance is felt, the catheter has likely encountered the cervix and must be repositioned.

BOX 32-14

Common Indications for Contrast Cystography

- Suspected bladder rupture
- Bladder tumor
- Chronic cystitis
- Radiolucent calculi
- Bladder diverticuli
- Incontinence
- Congenital anomalies

Adapted from Essman SC: Contrast cystography, *Clin Tech Small Anim Pract* 20:46, 2005.

Imaging

Imaging is recommended for cats with recurrent or persistent FLUTD signs, palpation of a bladder mass, or a history of urolithiasis. Survey radiographs are most useful for detection of radiodense uroliths at least 3 mm in size. The entire urinary tract, including the urethra, should be radiographed. Both lateral and dorsoventral views should be obtained, and ideally the colon should be emptied with an enema before the procedure to improve visualization of the bladder.

Contrast cystography is relatively easy to perform in clinical practice. The indications are described in Box 32-14. All procedures are performed under general anesthesia and require urethral catheterization. Multiple radiographic views (right and left lateral, ventrodorsal and dorsoventral) have been recommended.[54] A brief discussion of the techniques follows; more detailed information has been published.[54] Risks of contrast cystography are few but include urethral trauma or perforation during catheterization, overdistention of the bladder (potentially leading to ischemia, hemorrhage, or rupture), and fatal air embolism.[54]

The simplest technique is negative contrast cystography (pneumocystogram), performed with approximately 10 mL/kg of a negative contrast agent (room air, carbon dioxide, or nitrous oxide) (Figure 32-20). This technique is best for demonstrating the location and size of the bladder and bladder wall thickness but does not provide good mucosal detail, and small bladder tears may be overlooked. When the bladder is distended, normal wall thickness is 1 to 2 mm.

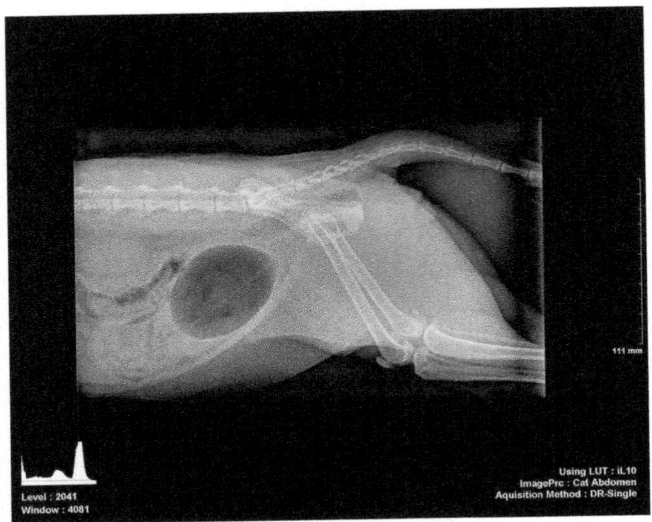

FIGURE 32-20 Negative contrast cystogram with no abnormal findings performed on a 5-year-old neutered male domestic shorthair cat with recurrent signs of feline lower urinary tract disease. *(Courtesy Dr. Janet Cohn, Veterinary Information Network.)*

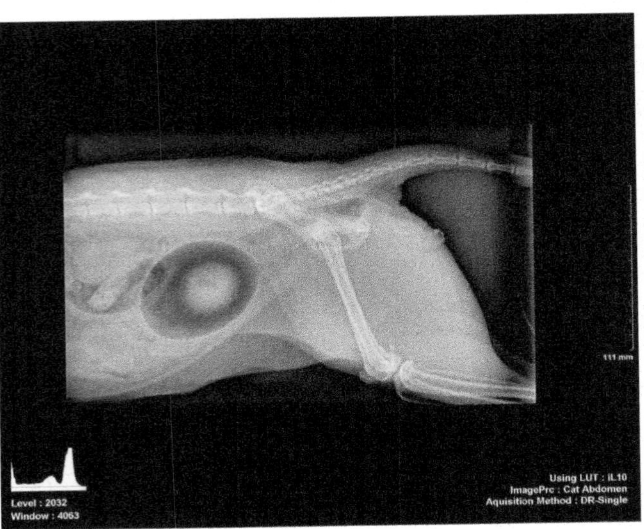

FIGURE 32-21 Double contrast cystogram with no abnormal findings performed on the same cat in Figure 32-20. *(Courtesy Dr. Janet Cohn, Veterinary Information Network.)*

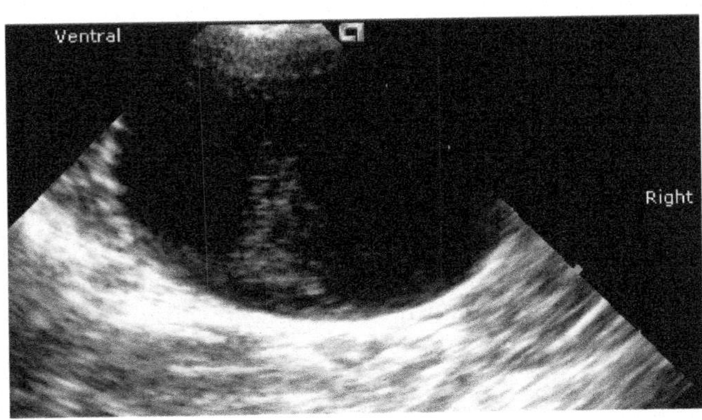

FIGURE 32-22 Ultrasound examination of the bladder of an 11-year-old spayed female domestic shorthair cat with clinical signs of feline lower urinary tract disease. Echogenic debris (cells, debris, +/− crystals), sometimes seen in cats with idiopathic cystitis, is present. *(Courtesy Dr. Edward Javinsky.)*

Positive contrast cystography is used for determining bladder size and shape, detecting bladder tears through leakage of contrast, assessment of wall thickness, and identification of small filling defects. It is poor for assessing mucosal detail. It is performed with approximately 10 mL/kg of an organic iodinated contrast medium; barium and sodium iodide are never used.

Double contrast cystography is more involved but is the best technique for detection of most common feline diseases, such as bladder wall abnormalities, mucosal changes, and calculi. First 0.5 to 1 mL of contrast medium is infused into the bladder, followed by approximately 10 mL/kg of a negative contrast agent such as room air. The contrast medium forms a pool in the dependent portion of the bladder; calculi appear as radiolucent objects in the pool (Figure 32-21).

Ultrasonographic equipment is less expensive than in the past, and image quality has improved, making the procedure affordable and accessible. It has the benefit of being a rapid noninvasive imaging technique that also allows for evaluation of other abdominal organs without sedation or anesthesia in many patients. Another benefit is that veterinary staff is not exposed to radiation. Ultrasonographic examination of the distended bladder may be used to evaluate bladder wall thickness, mass lesions, calculi, blood clots, echogenic debris, diverticula, and ectopic ureters (Figure 32-22). Although ultrasonography has become a popular diagnostic tool for FLUTD, it is important to understand that it does not replace survey radiography but instead should be considered complementary, particularly for patients with uroliths.[113]

One in vitro study concluded that ultrasonography was more sensitive than survey and contrast radiography for detection of canine uroliths.[180] The false-negative detection rate (i.e., the chance of missing the lesion) for CaOx uroliths was lowest with ultrasonography (2%) and highest with double contrast radiography (7%). The false-negative detection rate for struvite uroliths was 0% with ultrasonography, double contrast radiography, and pneumocystography and 2% with survey radiography.

However, ultrasonography does not provide information that may be useful in determining urolith composition. As well as providing an indication of mineral composition (Table 32-12), radiographs also provide information about urolith number, size, and location.

Cystoscopy

Transurethral cystoscopy, available at some referral centers, is performed under general anesthesia with a rigid endoscope and a balanced electrolyte solution for

TABLE 32-12 Predicting Mineral Composition of Feline Uroliths on the Basis of Radiographic Appearance

Mineral	Radiographic Opacity Compared with Soft Tssue	Surface Contour	Shape	Usual Number	Appropriate Size
CaOx monohydrate	+++ to ++++	Smooth, but occasionally bosselated	Commonly round, but also rosette	>5	1 mm-5 mm
CaOx dihydrate	+++ to ++++	Rough to smooth	Rosettes	>3	1 mm-7 mm
Sterile MAP	++ to +++	Slightly rough	Round or discoid	Usually 1-3, occasionally many	3 mm-10 mm
Infection MAP	+ to +++	Smooth to slightly rough	Round to faceted	Few to many	2 to >7 mm
Urate	– to ++	Smooth	Round to ovoid	Usually 1, but up to 5	2 mm to 10 mm
CaP	+++ to ++++	Rough	Too rare to comment	Too rare to comment	1 mm-4 mm
Cystine	– to +++	Rough	Round	Many, but some with few	1 mm-4 mm
Silica	++ to ++++	Too rare to comment	Too rare to comment	Too rare to comment	1 mm-4 mm
Xanthine	– to +	Smooth	Round to ovoid	1-3	1 mm-5 mm

CaOx, Calcium oxalate; *MAP,* magnesium ammonium phosphate; *CaP,* calcium phosphate.
From Lulich JP, Osborne CA: Changing paradigms in the diagnosis of urolithiasis, *Vet Clin North Am Small Anim Pract* 39:79, 2009.

flushing and distention of the bladder. Because of the narrowness of the feline urethra, it is most commonly performed in female cats (or male cats with a perineal urethrostomy), typically using a 1.9-mm diameter, 18-cm long instrument.[34] Cystoscopy may be used for diagnosis of bladder diseases through visualization of abnormalities (e.g., ectopic ureters, masses, uroliths, glomerulations) as well as biopsy of masses and calculi removal. In skilled hands the procedure is quick and minimally invasive. Risks include urethral or bladder trauma or perforation as well as overdistention of the bladder.[151]

IDIOPATHIC CYSTITIS

FIC is a chronic, sterile, inflammatory process causing signs of lower urinary tract disease. The etiology is incompletely understood, and treatment is often frustrating for both clinician and owner. It is the most common diagnosis for young cats with FLUTD (the second most common being urolithiasis). FIC is important not only because of the pain and distress it causes patients, but also because it is highly associated with house soiling, an important cause of relinquishment of cats to shelters.[143]

Terminology can be confusing with this disease. *Interstitial cystitis* is a term best reserved for that subset of FIC patients with chronic or frequent signs and cystoscopic findings consistent with the National Institutes of Health criteria for humans.[73] *Idiopathic cystitis* is a more generic, umbrella term for those cats with acute or chronic signs of FLUTD in which cystoscopy has not been performed or has not revealed changes associated with interstitial cystitis.

Prevalence

FIC appears to be a modern disease, having first been mentioned in the early 1990s when it was discovered that no specific diagnosis could be made in most cats with FLUTD signs.[91] Currently, approximately 55% to 65% of cats younger than 10 years of age with signs of FLUTD have no specific cause identified for their clinical signs and are classified as having FIC.

Patient Signalment and Risk Factors

Most patients are 2 to 6 years of age at diagnosis; FIC is uncommon in cats younger than 1 year of age or older than 10 years of age. FIC is less likely as a new diagnosis in geriatric cats, and other causes of FLUTD should be pursued aggressively in this age group. In one questionnaire-based study of 31 cats with FIC compared with 24 normal housemates and 125 other normal cats, certain risk factors were identified: male sex, being overweight, pedigreed breed, and stress factors, especially conflict with another cat in the home.[33] Other studies have found male and female cats equally affected. Additional risk factors variably reported as associated with FLUTD include an indoor lifestyle, no access to outdoors for elimination (exclusive litter box use), and a predominantly dry-food diet.[84,187] Outdoor cats may be affected, particularly if the neighborhood cat population is dense. It is important to note that not all studies agree on all risk factors. Studies have been conducted in various locations using different criteria and sample sizes. In addition, concentrating on single risk factors rather than the interplay of factors may be too simplistic an approach. For example, in a study of 238 healthy indoor-housed cats, 157 cats with FLUTD, and 70 cats with other diseases, few differences in lifestyle, environment, or diet were detected among the groups.[29] Instead, the authors of this study postulate that an internal predisposition exists in some cats rather than that environmental factors directly cause disease.

An indoor lifestyle protects cats against hazards, such as predation, trauma, and many infectious diseases. However, in some cats the indoor lifestyle may bring unintended health consequences, such as obesity and FLUTD. Undoubtedly, many cats have adapted to indoor living without health problems. A successful adaptation to the indoor lifestyle may depend on the quality of the indoor environment and the ability of the cat itself to adapt.

Some individual cats may be unusually sensitive to features of an indoor lifestyle.[24] This is understandable insofar as cats are a less socially interactive species than dogs or humans and free-roaming cats often live in low-density populations. If the home ranges of free-roaming cats overlap, they avoid meeting by using a time-sharing schedule. These natural behaviors are inhibited to greater or lesser degrees with indoor housing. In addition, many indoor environments are boring and predictable, factors considered stressful. Lack of control in an environment and perceptions of threat are also important triggers of stress responses.

The behavioral stress response is accompanied by immunologic, neurologic, endocrinologic, and vascular responses. Comorbid conditions with FLUTD and FIC include obesity, separation anxiety, gastrointestinal tract problems, and hypertrophic cardiomyopathy.[29,156,160] In one study owners of cats with lower urinary tract disease were more likely to describe their cats as fearful, nervous, or aggressive than healthy cats or cats with other diseases.[29] These findings suggest that FIC is a disease process that affects more than the urinary bladder. Even healthy cats may exhibit temporary signs of illness affecting multiple body systems (e.g., anorexia, inappropriate elimination, vomiting, or diarrhea) in response to stressful events.[169] The reader is referred to an excellent review of the stress response and its role in certain feline diseases for more information.[24]

Clinical Signs

The most common clinical signs in cats with FIC are periuria, pollakiuria, dysuria, vocalizing during attempts to urinate, and hematuria. These clinical signs are not specific to FIC and may also occur in cats with other causes of FLUTD. The clinical signs typically wax and wane and often follow or are exacerbated by stressful events. The episodes are usually self-limiting and of short duration (3 to 7 days). About 50% of cats will have recurrent signs within 1 to 2 years. It appears that recurrent episodes decrease in frequency and severity as the cat becomes older.[90,92]

Some cats (fewer than 15%) will have more frequent recurrences or chronic persistent clinical signs.[41,85,92] Whether this represents an extreme on the spectrum of cats with FIC or is an indication that FIC is not a single disease entity remains unknown. Some male cats with FIC will suffer a urethral blockage caused by mucus plugs that include proteins, cells, and debris with or without crystals.

Pathophysiology

Over the years, many theories as to the cause of FLUTD and FIC have been advanced and discarded. In the 1960s and 1970s, bacterial infection was considered to be the main cause of lower urinary tract signs. Many factors contributed to this erroneous theory, such as a high rate of false-positive results on urinalysis and urine culture and extrapolation of information from other species. Various viruses, such as calicivirus, have been associated with FLUTD, but convincing evidence for a causative role is lacking despite decades of investigation. In the 1970s and 1980s, it was thought that vesicourachal diverticula played a role in FLUTD, and surgical correction of the defect was often recommended. However, one case series determined that diverticula resolved within 2 to 3 weeks with medical management to resolve FLUTD signs without surgical intervention and did not recur.[134]

The pathophysiology of FIC is not well understood, although advances have been made in recent years. It seems likely that FIC is a syndrome that may have several underlying causes that may act separately or may be interrelated.[92] FIC is thought to involve complex interactions among the CNS, bladder, and endocrine system. Cats with FIC are described by Buffington and colleagues as "sensitive cats in a provocative environment." These cats may be unusually sensitive to stressors, such as changes in their environment and diet, weather changes, moving to a new home, holiday activities, and intercat conflict.[24,29,33,84] FIC has many similarities to nonulcerative interstitial cystitis in humans, although the ulcerative form (Hunner's ulcer) has also rarely been reported in cats.[42]

Cats with FIC have been shown to have enhanced activation of stress responses, particularly in the sympathetic nervous system (SNS). Stress and pain stimulate increased SNS activity—the "fight or flight" response—that results in release of catecholamines. Tyrosine hydroxylase is the rate-limiting enzyme of catecholamine synthesis and is produced in response to acute or chronic stress. Cats with FIC have increased tyrosine hydroxylase activity in the brain stem and hypothalamus and an increased release of norepinephrine and other catecholamine metabolites during stress compared with normal cats.[153,182] Moreover, cats with FIC have functional desensitization of central $alpha_2$ adrenoceptors, probably as a result of chronic stimulation from elevated catecholamine levels.[183]

Activation of the SNS may increase epithelial permeability and permit noxious agents in the urine to access sensory afferent neurons, resulting in pain and inflammation. In support of this hypothesis, cats with FIC are known to have significantly higher bladder permeability than healthy cats, as well as epithelial damage and dysfunction.[58,97] Biopsies of the bladder of cats with FIC often show submucosal edema, hemorrhage, and vasodilation, sometimes with large numbers of mast cells.[30,168] Products of activated mast cells could play a role in the pain and inflammation associated with FIC. The exact role of mast cells is difficult to determine insofar as mastocytosis also occurs in the bladders of cats with urolithiasis.[167] In addition, the other histopathologic abnormalities are not specific for FIC and may not correlate well with the presence of clinical signs. It is also unknown if the changes represent primary dysfunction of the urothelium or appear secondary to injury.

Other abnormalities have been found in the bladders of cats with FIC. Neurogenic inflammation is initiated by excitation of C-fiber sensory afferent neurons and mediated by neuropeptides such as substance P. The bladder afferent neurons in cats with FIC show increased excitability to stimuli compared with those of healthy cats.[162] In addition, substance P receptors are increased in the bladder of cats with FIC.[31] The interaction of neuropeptides with tissue receptors results in many changes, such as vasodilation, increased vascular permeability, and mast cell activation. The combined effects of neuropeptides and mast cell mediators may result in pain, inflammation, tissue injury, and fibrosis.[92]

A thin layer of glycosaminoglycan (GAG) covers and protects the bladder urothelium. Similar to humans with interstitial cystitis, urinary GAG excretion is decreased in some cats with FIC compared with healthy cats.[26,144] It has been hypothesized that the low GAG levels in urine reflect qualitative and quantitative changes in the GAG layer and may be associated with increased bladder permeability. The cause of the alterations to the GAG layer is not understood, nor is it known if the changes are a cause of disease or appear secondary to other mechanisms.

Abnormalities are also found in the hypothalamic–pituitary–adrenal axis, which, unlike the SNS, does not appear to be activated. One of the roles of glucocorticoids such as cortisol is to restrain catecholamine synthesis and metabolism, thus balancing the stress response. Cats with FIC have significantly decreased serum cortisol responses compared with normal cats and have smaller adrenal glands with reduced size of the zona fasciculata and zona reticularis.[186] Despite the subnormal cortisol responses in cats with FIC, treatment with prednisolone has not been effective.[135]

Thus the response of the hypothalamic–pituitary–adrenal axis appears to be dissociated from the response of the SNS to stress in cats with chronic FIC. Essentially, FIC is an exaggerated SNS response to stress with an inadequate adrenocortical response, although the cause of these abnormalities is not understood. The complex involvement of the CNS may explain why therapies directed only at the bladder have a high failure rate. In effect, according to this theory, the bladder is an innocent bystander.

An interesting question is why the bladder appears to be the primary target for cats with FIC, although given the presence of comorbid diseases, it is probably not the only target. The SNS is involved in both micturition and sensory arousal, and it is well known that involuntary urination is a response to severe stress. Overlap between micturition and fear pathways may put the bladder at risk during stress responses.[25]

Diagnosis

There is no gold-standard test for diagnosis of FIC; it is essentially a diagnosis of exclusion. Physical examination of cats with FIC may be unrewarding, or it may reveal a painful thickened bladder. Some cats have bilateral ventral abdominal and inguinal alopecia as a result of chronic overgrooming of the area over the bladder. The minimum initial workup at first presentation calls for a complete history, including environmental and diet history, thorough physical examination, and urinalysis (see Figure 32-18).

A variety of abnormal findings may be revealed on urinalysis, none of which is specific for any particular bladder disease. Hematuria is commonly found, although it may be present in one sample and not in another from the same cat. Hematuria may also be induced by the sample-collection method (i.e., manual expression, cystocentesis, or catheterization). Proteinuria and crystalluria may also be found in some cats. Because mild crystalluria may be found in normal cats, it is important not to overinterpret this finding. Crystals do not damage a healthy urothelium. In fact, it appears likely that crystals form secondary to bladder inflammation rather than being the cause. Neurogenic inflammation of the bladder mucosa leads to leakage of plasma proteins into urine, thereby increasing the urine pH and allowing struvite crystals to form. USG is often very high with FIC, especially in cats fed exclusively dry foods. A low USG (under 1.035) should prompt investigation for systemic disease. Some normal cats fed only a canned diet may have USG as low as 1.025.

Urine culture is a low-yield test on account of the low prevalence of bacterial UTIs in cats younger than 10 years of age. Urine culture should be performed in cats older than 10 years, cats with recurrent clinical signs (two or more episodes), cats with low USG, cats with concurrent diseases, cats that have undergone perineal urethrostomy, and cats in which a urethral catheter was recently placed.

A survey radiograph of the urinary tract (including the entire urethra) may provide clinically relevant information because 15% to 20% of cats with lower urinary tract signs have urinary calculi. Together urinalysis and survey radiographs are the most commonly used diagnostic tests for cats with lower urinary tract signs. In young cats negative findings on both tests warrant a presumptive diagnosis of FIC and initiation of a treatment plan.

Further imaging studies are indicated in cats with recurrent signs that do not respond to initial treatment as well as in senior cats. Contrast cystography may detect radiolucent calculi and other lesions, such as masses. Double contrast cystography may be useful insofar as certain findings have been associated with FIC in approximately 15% of cases.[161] These include focal or diffuse bladder wall thickening and irregularities of the bladder mucosa. Ultrasonography may also be used to evaluate cats for cystic calculi, mass lesions, bladder wall characteristics, and other abnormalities, such as blood clots.

Cystoscopy should be considered for cats with recurrent bouts of FLUTD when available and when other diagnostics have failed to find a cause. Because of the narrowness of the feline urethra, cystoscopy is limited to evaluation of female cats weighing at least 3 kg (6.6 lb) or male cats with a perineal urethrostomy. Cystoscopy allows for visualization of the bladder wall and evaluation for abnormalities associated with FIC, such as increased blood vessel density and tortuosity, edema, and submucosal petechial hemorrhages (glomerulations) (Figure 32-23). However, because these abnormalities have also been seen in otherwise healthy cats, cystoscopy is best performed to rule out other causes for the clinical signs, such as small cystic calculi and ectopic ureters and masses.

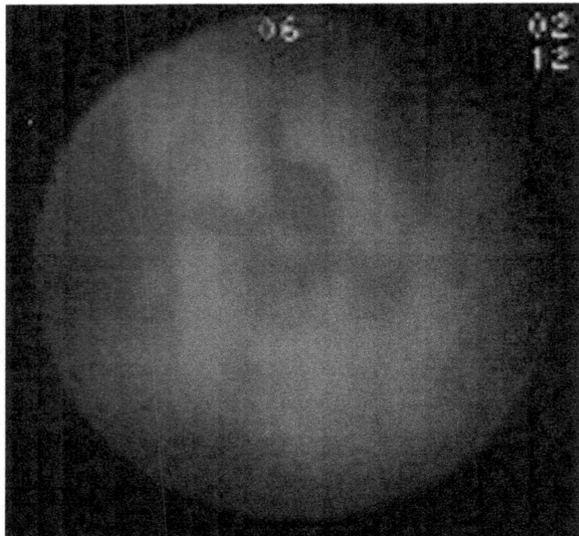

FIGURE 32-23 Cystoscopic appearance of the bladder of a female cat with idiopathic cystitis showing submucosal petechial hemorrhages (glomerulations). *(Courtesy Dr. Joseph Bartges.)*

Management

Environmental Modification

Given that the etiology of FIC is still unknown, current treatment recommendations are directed at decreasing the severity and frequency of clinical signs rather being curative. Perhaps the most important part of the treatment plan is ensuring that the owner understands FIC and is willing to make the recommended changes. FIC is a frustrating disease, one that often requires long-term management, and a strategy that provides owners with ongoing support and information is essential.

Because increased activity of the SNS stress response seems to maintain the chronic inflammatory response, therapy is directed at reducing stressors. Another goal of therapy is to reduce the noxious properties of urine that irritate the bladder mucosa. The recommended standard of care to achieve these goals includes environmental enrichment and stress reduction, increased water intake, litter box management, management of interactions in multiple cat homes, and potentially drug therapy.[185]

Environmental enrichment is a tool to help decrease sympathetic overdrive, reduce stress, and prolong time between episodes of FIC. The goal is to increase choices to provide the cat with a sense of control over the environment and allow it to behave in a species-appropriate way. Provisional recommendations have been published that focus on identifying key resources, as well as feeding and litter box management.[24] Indoor and high-density cat populations are risk factors for FIC.[24] Indoor cats need places to climb, scratch, sleep, perch on high, and hide, in addition to food and water. Many cats find it stressful to compete for these resources daily. Owners often do not understand the importance of resources other than food, water, and a litter box. Box 32-15 is a resource checklist designed to help owners identify and correct problems. In addition, owners are often unfamiliar with the signs of intercat conflict and stress, given

BOX 32-15

A Resource Checklist for Cat Owners

Enhanced stress response system activity seems to be central in exacerbating clinical signs in cats with feline idiopathic cystitis. Any treatment strategy to decrease sympathetic nervous system outflow may be important in reducing these signs. By altering the environment of a cat that has had previous episodes of feline idiopathic cystitis, the veterinarian can decrease clinical signs and increase the interepisode intervals. The authors provide this list to clients and tailor these resources on a case-by-case basis. Although most cats do not require all suggestions from this list, a detailed history obtained from the owner will dictate which areas seem to be most relevant for each patient. If drug therapy is necessary in the patient, it should be used in conjunction with appropriate environmental strategies listed in the following.

Litter Box Management	Yes	No
Boxes are located on more than one level in multilevel houses.	–	–
Boxes are located so that another animal cannot sneak up on the cat while it uses it.	–	–
Boxes are located away from appliances or air ducts that could come on unexpectedly while the cat uses them.	–	–
The litter is kept clean, scooped as soon after use as possible (at least daily).	–	–
Boxes are washed regularly (at least weekly) with a mild detergent (e.g., dishwashing liquid), rather than strongly scented cleaners.	–	–
Unscented clumping litter is used.	–	–
The brand or type of litter purchased is changed infrequently (less than monthly).	–	–
If a type of litter is offered, it is put in a separate box so that the cat can choose to use it if it wants to.	–	–
Each cat has its own litter box in a convenient, well-ventilated location that still gives the cat some privacy while using it.	–	–

Food and Water	Yes	No
Each cat has its own food and water bowl in a convenient location that provides some privacy while eating or drinking.	–	–
Bowls are located such that another animal cannot sneak up on the cat while it eats.	–	–
Bowls are located away from appliances or air ducts that could come on unexpectedly while the cat eats or drinks.	–	–
Food and water is kept fresh (daily).	–	–
Bowls are washed regularly (at least weekly) with a mild detergent.	–	–
The brand or type of food purchased is changed infrequently (less than monthly).	–	–
If a new food is offered, it is put in a separate dish next to the familiar food so that the cat can choose to eat it if it wants to do so.	–	–

Environmental Considerations	Yes	No
Scratching posts are provided.	–	–
Toys are provided, rotated, or replaced regularly.	–	–
Each cat has the opportunity to move to a warmer or cooler area if it chooses to do so.	–	–
Each cat has a hiding area where it can get away from threats if it chooses to do so.	–	–
Each cat has its own space that it can use if it chooses to do so.	–	–

Rest	Yes	No
Each cat has its own resting area in a convenient location that still provides some privacy.	–	–
Resting areas are located such that another animal cannot sneak up on the cat while it rests.	–	–
Resting areas are located away from appliances or air ducts that could come on unexpectedly while the cat rests.	–	–
If a new bed is provided, it is placed next to the familiar bed so that the cat can choose to use it if it wants to do so.	–	–
Movement—each cat has the opportunity to move about freely, explore, climb, stretch, and play if it chooses to do so.	–	–
Social contact—each cat has the opportunity to engage in play with other animals or the owner if it chooses to do so.	–	–

From Westropp JL, Buffington CA, Chew DJ: Feline lower urinary tract diseases. In Ettinger SJ, Feldman EC, editors: *Textbook of veterinary internal medicine: diseases of the dog and cat*, ed 6, St Louis, 2005, Elsevier Saunders, p 1839.

BOX 32-16
Recommended Reading and Resources

Techniques

Essman SC: Contrast cystography, *Clin Tech Small Anim Pract* 20:46, 2005.
Lulich J, Osborne C: Cystocentesis: lessons from thirty years of clinical experience, *Clin Brief* 2:11, 2004.
Reine NJ, Langston CE: Urinalysis interpretation: how to squeeze out the maximum information from a small sample, *Clin Tech Small Anim Pract* 20:2, 2005.
Sabino C, Boudreau A, Mathews K: Emergency management of urethral obstruction in male cats, *Clin Brief*:57, 2010.

Behavior and Environmental Enrichment

Ellis SLH: Environmental enrichment: Practical strategies for improving feline welfare, *J Feline Med Surg* 11:901, 2009.
Herron ME, Buffington CA: Environmental enrichment for indoor cats, *Compend Contin Educ Vet* 32, 2010.
Indoor pet initiative, Ohio State University: http://indoorpet.osu.edu/
Overall K, Rodan I, Beaver B et al: Feline behavior guidelines from the American Association of Feline Practitioners, *J Am Vet Med Assoc* 227:70, 2005.

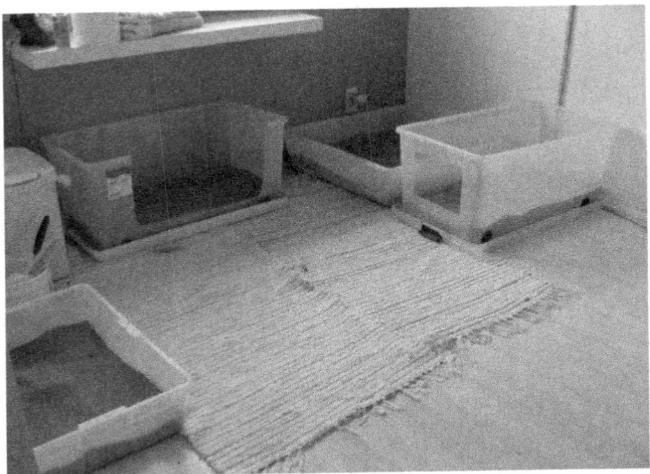

FIGURE 32-24 Large litter boxes can be made by modifying plastic storage bins. *(Courtesy Dr. Margie Scherk.)*

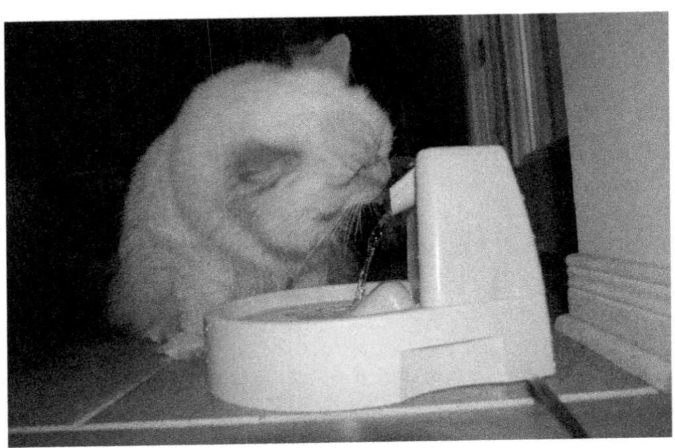

FIGURE 32-25 Water can be provided in a way that stimulates interest, such as a water fountain. *(Courtesy Dr. Emma Thom.)*

that the signs are typically subtle to the uninformed observer and usually stop short of actual fighting. Cats typically prefer to avoid others rather than engage in fighting, so that sufficient three-dimensional space must be available in multicat homes. Enrichment should also provide mental stimulation through the use of toys, food puzzles, window perches, and so on. The reader is referred to further resources that provide more information on environmental enrichment for cats (Box 32-16). More information is also found in Chapter 14.

Litter boxes should be in a quiet and easily accessible area and should be scooped daily and cleaned weekly. Clumping, unscented litters and those containing activated carbon are preferred by most cats.[128] Citrus-scented litters should be avoided. It is commonly recommended that owners provide a minimum of one more litter box than the number of cats in the household, although supportive evidence is lacking. Boxes should be located in at least two easily accessible but quiet areas. Cats also seem to prefer large or jumbo-size boxes; commercial cat litter boxes are often too small. Plastic storage bins (e.g., sweater or under-bed storage boxes) or dog litter boxes are good alternatives (Figure 32-24). Further discussion of litter box management is found in Chapter 13.

Feeding is not a social function for cats as it is for humans. In a multicat household, there should be enough food and water stations for each cat to eat and drink alone. Some cats may benefit from being fed in a separate room. Food puzzles are mentally stimulating, and hiding food throughout the home allows cats to engage in normal hunting behavior. Water should be provided in large bowls (e.g., dog bowls) or in a more interesting way that stimulates investigation (e.g., pet water fountain) (Figure 32-25).

Unfortunately, published trials that have evaluated the usefulness of the various components of environmental enrichment for cats with FIC are scarce. A recent case report detailed successful management of FIC in an indoor cat living with five other cats using environmental modification.[163] In an uncontrolled study of 46 client-owned cats, multimodal environmental modification (MEMO) was instituted, and the cats were followed for 10 months.[28] The components of MEMO are available for owners and veterinarians on the website of the Indoor Pet Initiative (see Box 32-16). Significant decreases were documented in signs of FLUTD, fearfulness, nervousness, and aggressive behavior. Moreover, owners reported a reduction in clinical signs referable to the respiratory and gastrointestinal tracts. The results of the study remain difficult to interpret, however, because no controls were included and dietary or drug interventions were used concurrently with MEMO.

Pheromones are fatty acids that induce changes in the limbic system and hypothalamus and appear to alter emotional states in cats.[67] Feliway (Ceva) is a synthetic analog of a feline facial pheromone, available as both a spray and a plug-in room diffuser. Facial pheromones are deposited on prominent objects (e.g., furniture) by facial rubbing when cats feel comfortable and safe. Use of Feliway has been associated with increased grooming and food intake in hospitalized cats,[67] decreased urine spraying,[126] and decreased scratching.[140] Little data are available to evaluate the efficacy of Feliway for cats with FIC. In one pilot study nine cats with FIC completed a randomized, double-blind, placebo-controlled crossover study of the efficacy of Feliway.[70] Although there were no statistical differences between the treatment groups, there was a trend for cats exposed to Feliway to show fewer days with clinical signs. Current recommendations are that Feliway should be used in conjunction with other management strategies. Further investigation into the use of pheromones in the management of FIC is warranted.

Increasing Water Intake

There is no evidence to suggest that diets designed to prevent urolithiasis or promote "urinary tract health" should be recommended for cats with FIC. Indeed, dietary change is a stress in itself. However, increasing water intake appears to be important in the management of FIC. Increased water intake may dilute noxious components in urine that irritate the bladder mucosa, thereby decreasing pain and inflammation. The treatment goal should be to decrease the cat's USG until it is below 1.040 and even below 1.030 if possible by feeding canned foods containing at least 60% moisture.[40] Although cats fed a dry diet drink more water than cats fed canned diets, the total daily water volume ingested is greater in cats fed canned food because of the high water content of canned foods. In addition, feeding the daily food allowance divided into at least two or three meals has been shown to increase water intake in healthy cats.[88]

In a nonrandom prospective study, 54 client-owned cats with FIC were monitored for 1 year.[118] The cats were fed either a dry or canned formulation of a diet designed for management of lower urinary tract disease. Signs of FIC recurred in only 11% of cats on the canned diet and in 39% cats fed the dry diet. Cats fed the dry formulation had an average USG of 1.050 compared with 1.030 for cats fed the canned formulation.

To reduce the stress of change, owners should be instructed to offer old and new foods side by side in similar dishes, allowing the cat to become accustomed to the new diet before withdrawing the old diet. Other suggestions for changing diets are found in Box 18-5. If the FIC patient will not change to a canned diet, increased water intake can be accomplished by various other means (see Box 18-16).

A common recommendation to increase water consumption is to use a pet water fountain. One study of 12 healthy cats found that water intake was slightly greater from a fountain than a bowl.[64] However, urine osmolality was not reduced, which suggests that measurement of water intake from the fountain was falsely elevated. The lowest urine osmolality and specific gravity achieved was only 1901 mOsm/L and 1.044, respectively. One problem encountered during this study was the tendency for cats to play with water in the fountain, thus splashing water out and making assessment of actual intake difficult.

Drug and Nutraceutical Therapy

Many drug therapies have been recommended for FIC, but few controlled studies have been performed. Because FIC is a painful disease, analgesics may be prescribed for acute episodes. It is important to break the pain–inflammation–pain cycle. A common choice is transmucosal buprenorphine (0.02 to 0.03 mg/kg, every 6 to 12 hours) for 3 to 5 days.[40] Other analgesics that have been recommended include fentanyl transdermal patch, butorphanol (0.1 to 0.2 mg/kg, orally, every 8 to 12 hours), oxymorphone, and NSAIDs. Ease of use is important to decrease the stress associated with administration of the medication.

Dysuric male cats with FIC may benefit from antispasmodics to relax the urethra. Recommended medications include phenoxybenzamine, prazosin, and dantrolene (Table 32-13). Many of these drugs also have sedative properties, which may be beneficial in the short term.

Amitriptyline is a tricyclic antidepressant with anticholinergic, antihistaminic, sympatholytic, antiinflammatory, and analgesic properties and has been recommended for severe FIC cases in which environmental enrichment and diet change have not provided relief. In an uncontrolled study 15 cats with severe recurrent FIC were treated with 10 mg/cat, orally once daily in the evening.[41] Clinical signs were eliminated in 73% of cats for the first 6 months of the study and in 60% of cats for the full 12 months of the study. However, cystoscopic abnormalities persisted despite clinical remission. Side effects noted included weight gain, lethargy, and decreased grooming. Cystic calculi were noted in four cats and resolved spontaneously in three of the cats. Amitriptyline is not effective in the short term and therefore is not useful for acute treatment of FIC insofar as

TABLE 32-13 **Drugs Used in the Management of Cats with Urethral Obstruction and Other Lower Urinary Tract Disorders**

Drug	Class	Indication	Dose	Adverse Effects
Acepromazine	Phenothiazine	Sedation, antispasmodic (smooth muscle)	0.02-0.05 mg/kg, SC, q6-8h	Hypotension
Bethanecol	Parasympathomimetic	Detrusor atony	1.25-5.0 mg/cat, PO, q12h	Vomiting, diarrhea, salivation
Buprenorphine	Opiate	Analgesia	0.01-0.02 mg/kg, SC, q8-12h	Sedation
Butorphanol	Opiate	Analgesia	0.2-0.4 mg/kg, PO/SC, q8-12h	Sedation
Dantrolene	Skeletal muscle relaxant	Antispasmodic (striated muscle)	0.5-2.0 mg/kg, PO, q8h	Hepatotoxicity
Diazepam	Benzodiazepine	Antispasmodic (striated muscle)	2.5-5.0 mg/cat, PO, q8h	Sedation, appetite stimulation
Fentanyl	Opiate	Analgesia	25 μg/hour transdermal patch	Respiratory depression, bradycardia
Hydromorphone	Opiate	Analgesia, sedation	0.02-0.05 mg/kg, IV/IM/SC, q4h	Respiratory depression, hyperthermia, vomiting
Phenoxybenazmine	Alpha$_1$-adrenergic antagonist	Antispasmodic (smooth muscle)	2.5-7.5 mg/cat, PO, q12h	Sedation, hypotension
Prazosin	Alpha$_1$-adrenergic antagonist	Antispasmodic (smooth muscle)	0.25-0.5 mg/cat, PO, q12h	Sedation, hypotension

SC, Subcutaneous; *PO*, by mouth; *IM*, intramuscular.

the drug takes several weeks to exert maximal effect.[89,90] It appears to be a safe drug, having been prescribed by behaviorists for many years, and may be effective at a lower dose (2.5 to 5 mg/cat daily). Transdermal formulations of amitriptyline have poor systemic absorption and cannot be recommended.[122] Other drugs have been used for cats with FIC (e.g., clomipramine, fluoxetine, buspirone), but no clinical studies evaluating efficacy have been published. Appropriate monitoring of CBC and serum chemistry profile should be performed before starting any psychotropic medication and repeated periodically during treatment.

GAG therapy is used with short-term success in some human patients with interstitial cystitis. The rationale is to help repair the defective urothelium to decrease permeability, as well as provide analgesic and antiinflammatory effects. There is one case report in the veterinary literature on the apparent successful use of sodium pentosan polysulfate in a cat with biopsy-diagnosed interstitial cystitis,[42] although two other clinical studies failed to show any difference between cats receiving placebo and cats receiving treatment.[38,179]

Glucosamine is a natural substrate for the biosynthesis of GAG and is available combined with chondroitin sulfate as Cosequin (Nutramax). In a recent study oral glucosamine was compared to placebo in a randomized, double-blind, placebo-controlled study of 40 patients with FIC over 6 months.[71] Owners kept a diary of FIC-related events and graded the severity of the cat's clinical signs at the start and at the end of the trial. There was no significant difference between the two groups when considering the owners' assessment of mean health score, the average monthly clinical score, or the average number of days with clinical signs. Most cats in the study did improve clinically, but this was attributed to a change to a canned food diet in 90% of the cats. The mean USG at the beginning of the study was 1.050; 1 month into the trial, it decreased significantly to 1.036. Despite this, clinical signs recurred in 65% of the cats, so dietary therapy alone was not sufficient. It is difficult to recommend GAG therapy given the lack of any veterinary studies demonstrating efficacy in FIC.

UROLITHIASIS AND URETHRAL PLUGS

Prevalence

Uroliths are organized concretions containing primarily crystalloids with a small amount of organic matrix. The most common components of uroliths are struvite and CaOx,[35,77] but recently uroliths composed of dried solidified blood have been reported.[184] Urine is commonly supersaturated with crystalloids, so crystalluria itself is not a disease and does not need to be treated unless it is associated with clinical signs. It is important to understand that finding crystalluria in cats with signs of

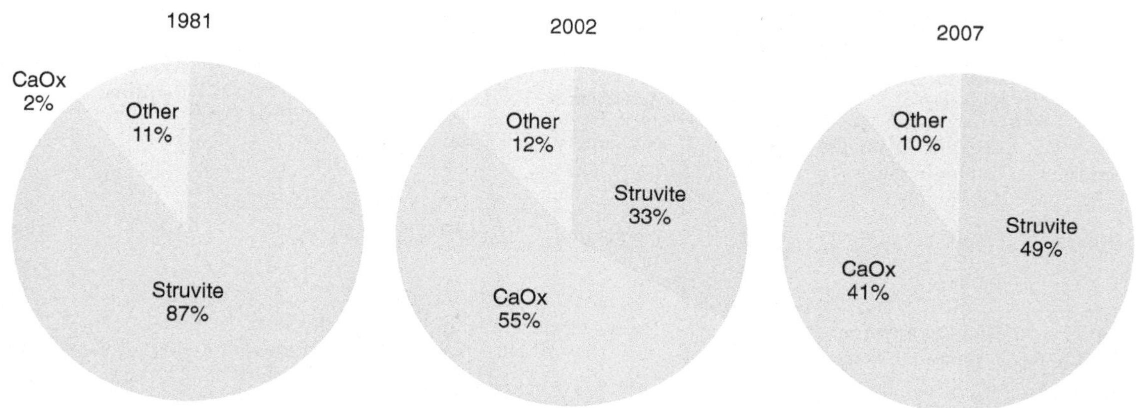

FIGURE 32-26 Composite of changes in feline urolith composition over time (1981-2007) reported by American and Canadian urolith analysis centers. *(Adapted from Cannon AB, Westropp JL, Ruby AL et al: Evaluation of trends in urolith composition in cats: 5,230 cases (1985-2004),* J Am Vet Med Assoc *231:570, 2007; Houston DM, Moore AEP: Canine and feline urolithiasis: examination of over 50,000 urolith submissions to the Canadian Veterinary Urolith Centre from 1998 to 2008,* Can Vet J *50:1263, 2009; Osborne CA, Lulich JP, Kruger JM et al: Analysis of 451,891 canine uroliths, feline uroliths, and feline urethral plugs from 1981 to 2007: perspectives from the Minnesota Urolith Center,* Vet Clin North Am Small Anim Pract *39:183, 2009.)*

FLUTD does not guarantee that the crystals are actually the cause of the clinical signs.

In the last 25 years, dramatic change in the prevalence of different urolith types has occurred (Figure 32-26). Until the mid-1980s, struvite uroliths made up 78% of submissions to the Minnesota Urolith Center (MUC).[139] Starting in the mid-1980s, a dramatic increase in the frequency of CaOx uroliths, along with a decrease in struvite uroliths, was noted. By 2002 55% of uroliths submitted to the MUC were CaOx, whereas only 33% were struvite. However, in recent years the prevalence of urolith types has changed again. In 2007 49% of uroliths submitted to the MUC were struvite and 41% were CaOx. The ratio of CaOx to struvite uroliths also increased significantly in submissions to the Gerald V. Ling Urinary Stone Analysis Laboratory from 1985 to 2004.[35] But as with the MUC study, by 2002-2004, 44% of uroliths were struvite and 40% were CaOx.

The prevalence of struvite uroliths presented to the Canadian Veterinary Urolith Centre (CVUC) decreased in the 10-year period from 1998 to 2008, whereas that of CaOx uroliths remained constant.[78] In 2008 49% of uroliths submitted to the CVUC were CaOx and 42% were struvite. In Europe the prevalence of CaOx uroliths also increased from 1994 to 2004.[147] In 1994 77% of uroliths were struvite and 12% were CaOx. By 2003 61% of uroliths were CaOx and 32% were struvite.

Despite these comprehensive data sets, it is important to note that they may not truly reflect the prevalence of urolith types for several reasons. For example, not all cats with uroliths are diagnosed or treated, and not all uroliths are submitted for analysis. It is also possible that CaOx uroliths are more likely to be removed and submitted for analysis than struvite uroliths because there is no medical dissolution option for this type of urolith.

It seems likely that the increase in CaOx uroliths seen in the 1980s was driven by changes in feline diets. The widespread use of diets designed to dissolve struvite uroliths meant that fewer were surgically removed and submitted for analysis. At the same time, the modification of maintenance diets to prevent struvite uroliths may have caused an increase in CaOx uroliths. Some dietary factors that decrease the risk of struvite uroliths can increase the risk of CaOx uroliths. The more recent changes in prevalence of urolith type may be associated with further modification of maintenance diets to minimize the risk of CaOx uroliths and improvements in and increased use of therapeutic diets designed to reduce risk factors for CaOx uroliths.

Methods for Urolith Removal

Various methods for urolith removal are available for cats: surgical removal, basket retrieval by way of cystoscopy, voiding urohydropropulsion (VU), and lithotripsy. Dietary dissolution is available only for struvite uroliths (see Chapter 18). The choice of method will be dictated by patient factors and stone type, as well as the equipment and expertise available (Table 32-14). Regardless of the method used, imaging should be used to confirm complete removal.

Cystotomy is the most commonly used method to retrieve bladder uroliths. The procedure is well known, surgery times are short, and complications are rare.[188] Suture nidus uroliths have been reported to form after cystotomy (discussed later).[5] Incomplete surgical removal of uroliths occurs in approximately 15% to 20% of patients.[116] Several precautions can be taken to reduce this risk.[112] If time has elapsed since the original diagnosis, imaging studies should be repeated the day of surgery to confirm the number and location of the

TABLE 32-14 **Comparison of Bladder Urolith Treatment Methods**

Technique	Urolith Size/ Number	Urolith Type	Advantages	Disadvantages	Anesthesia Required?	Equipment Required
Voiding urohydropropulsion	<3-5 mm in females <1 mm in males Any number	All	No surgery	Urethral obstruction	Yes	Catheter
Cystoscopic retrieval	Small, any number	All	No surgery	Limited to small uroliths	Yes	Rigid cystoscope, stone basket
Laser lithotripsy	Small to medium, moderate number	All	No surgery	Limited availability, long procedure times, not well evaluated in cats, limited to females or males with perineal urethrostomy	Yes	Cystoscope, laser lithotripter
Cystotomy	Any	All	Rapid, readily available	Invasive, longer recovery time	Yes	Surgical instruments
Medical dissolution	Any size, number	Struvite only	Noninvasive	Limited to struvite stones, takes several weeks	No	Prescription diet

Adapted from Langston C, Gisselman K, Palma D et al: Methods of urolith removal, *Compend Contin Educ Vet* 32, 2010.

uroliths. Urethroliths can be flushed retrograde into the bladder before surgery. The urethral catheter can be left in place during surgery to prevent migration of uroliths into the urethra during the procedure. Finally, the urethra can be flushed before closing the incision in the bladder. The catheter tip is inserted just inside the distal urethra. The urethra is occluded by pinching it around the catheter during retrograde flushing. Postoperative imaging should always be performed to ensure that all uroliths have been removed. Laparoscopy-assisted cystotomy for the removal of bladder uroliths has been described in dogs but has also been used clinically in cats.[152]

VU can be used successfully for removal of uroliths with a diameter smaller than the urethral lumen; in cats this means uroliths smaller than 3 to 5 mm in females and 1 mm in males.[17,95] Smooth uroliths are more likely to be successfully removed than irregular uroliths or ones with sharp edges. The patient is anesthetized, and a urinary catheter is placed and attached to a three-way stopcock. The bladder is filled with sterile saline until distended. Overdistention is discouraged; the typical volume used is 4 to 6 mL/kg. The patient is then held in a fully upright position with the spine perpendicular to the table. The bladder is gently agitated to loosen any uroliths adhered to the mucosa, and the urinary catheter is removed. The bladder is expressed manually to void the saline and uroliths. The bladder is compressed dorsally and cranially during expression; the bladder should not be compressed into the pelvic canal. The steps are repeated as needed until imaging confirms that all uroliths have been removed. The clinician should be prepared for surgical removal of any uroliths that cannot be removed by VU. Hematuria and dysuria may be expected for 1 to 2 days after the procedure.[115] It has been recommended that antibiotics be administered for up to 5 days to prevent UTI.

Cystoscopic retrieval using a urolith basket is possible in female cats and male cats that have undergone a perineal urethrostomy. It is useful only for uroliths small enough to be withdrawn through the distended urethra (<5 mm). It is a desirable approach for patients with bladders that are too fragile for manual expression, such as patients that have recently undergone cystotomy. Only one urolith is removed at a time, and a large urolith should never be forced through the urethra.

Lithotripsy has been evaluated for stone fragmentation and removal in dogs and cats. Extracorporeal shock wave lithotripsy is best suited for fragmentation of uroliths that are fixed in one location, such as nephroliths. Laser lithotripsy (holmium:YAG) is used for intracorporeal fragmentation of bladder calculi in humans. In veterinary medicine transurethral laser lithotripsy can be performed through small-diameter flexible endoscopes. In cats the small diameter of the male urethra is a limitation, so the procedure is feasible only in females or males that have had a perineal urethrostomy. After lithotripsy the fragments are removed through VU or cystoscopy.

One in vitro study found that holmium laser energy was able to fragment various types of canine uroliths into fragments smaller than 3.5 mm in diameter.[192] Three in vivo studies that evaluated laser lithotripsy in dogs reported bladder urolith removal rates of 83% to 96% in females and 68% to 81% in males.[1,65,114] Reported complications included bladder and urethral perforation, urethral swelling causing obstruction, and hemorrhage. Most complications were short-lived. Laser lithotripsy has been compared with surgical removal for bladder uroliths in dogs.[21] The procedures were equally successful. Laser lithotripsy procedures were on average 23 minutes longer than surgical procedures, but lithotripsy patients were discharged from the hospital about 12 hours sooner. To date, no published studies have evaluated the use of laser lithotripsy for treatment of bladder uroliths in cats.

Struvite Uroliths

Risk Factors

Struvite uroliths have also been called *triple phosphate* or *magnesium ammonium phosphate* uroliths. They most commonly occur in the bladder and usually form in sterile urine in the cat. Infection-induced uroliths may occur in young cats (younger than 1 year of age) and senior cats (older than 10 years of age).[175] Cats with struvite uroliths are generally younger (peak age, 4 to 7 years) than cats with CaOx uroliths. No clear sex predisposition exists. Other risk factors include an indoor sedentary lifestyle, obesity, low water intake, and alkaline urine. Certain breeds appear to be predisposed (e.g., Persian, Himalayan, Ragdoll, Chartreux, Oriental Shorthair), whereas other breeds appear to be at low risk (Rex, Abyssinian, Burmese, Russian Blue, Birman, Siamese).[175]

Formation of struvite uroliths is influenced by urine pH, urine concentration, and the presence of calculogenic materials. Early research demonstrated that struvite urolithiasis could be induced in cats by feeding a diet very high in magnesium (3 to 10 times the level found in commercial diets). This led to the erroneous assumption that magnesium was the main cause of struvite urolithiasis in cats. Subsequent research showed that urine pH influences the formation of struvite uroliths and that these uroliths can be dissolved when the urine pH is reduced to less than 6.4. In a study evaluating the association between dietary factors and struvite formation, diets with the highest magnesium, phosphorus, calcium, chloride, or fiber content; moderate protein content; and low fat content were associated with increased risk.[102] However, struvite formation is likely a complex process in which individual dietary factors cannot be considered in isolation but instead interact with one another and with factors such as breed, age, sex, and environment.

Clinical Signs and Diagnosis

Cats with struvite uroliths have the generic signs of lower urinary tract disease: hematuria, pollakiuria, periuria and dysuria. Struvite uroliths are typically round, ellipsoid, or tetrahedral in shape and may be present singly or in large numbers. Survey abdominal radiographs are often sufficient for detection of radiopaque uroliths that are 3 mm or more in diameter. Detection of small uroliths or nonradiopaque uroliths may be improved with double contrast cystography or ultrasonography (Figure 32-27). Urinalysis typically shows an alkaline pH; struvite crystals may be present but are not always associated with urolith formation. The index of suspicion for struvite uroliths in patients with lower urinary tract signs is increased in cats younger than 7 years old, those with a prior history, and those with struvite crystalluria and alkaline urine. Definitive diagnosis requires removal and chemical analysis.

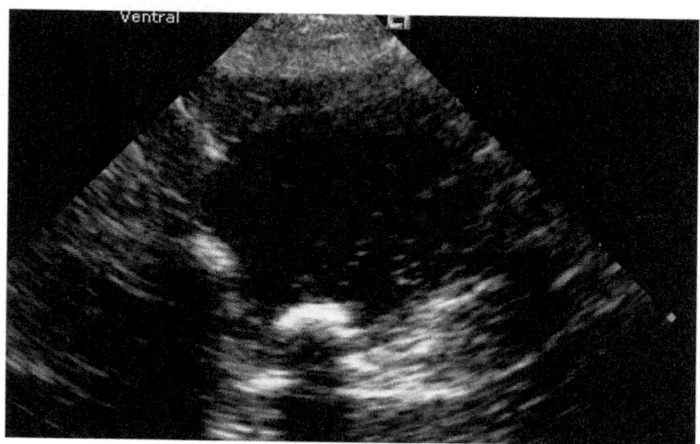

FIGURE 32-27 Ultrasound examination of the bladder of a 2-year-old neutered male domestic shorthair cat with hematuria. A urolith is seen as an echogenic object (6.2 × 3.7 mm) with an acoustic shadow adjacent to the dorsal bladder wall. Some echogenic debris is present in the bladder lumen. *(Courtesy Dr. Edward Javinsky.)*

Treatment

Both stone dissolution by way of dietary therapy and stone removal are options for cats with struvite uroliths (see Table 32-14). Dissolution therapy is noninvasive but dependent on owner and patient compliance. Treatment failure may occur if the urolith type is misidentified or if the uroliths have a complex composition. Therapeutic diets that reduce urine pH to below 6.4 and contain restricted magnesium levels are used. Dietary therapy is effective; in one study dissolution of sterile struvite uroliths occurred in a mean of 36 days (compared with 44 days for infected uroliths).[138] In another study using a different diet, struvite uroliths dissolved completely in 31 of 39 cats in an average of 30 days.[79]

Once a dissolution diet is prescribed, owners should feed this diet exclusively and be cautioned against feeding treats, table food, milk, and similar substances. Radiographs should be reassessed once monthly, and the diet should be fed for 2 to 4 weeks after radiographic disappearance to ensure that the smallest uroliths that are not radiographically detectable have resolved.[141] If urine culture indicates the presence of a bacterial UTI, antibiotics must be administered or dissolution therapy may not be effective. Antibiotic therapy should be continued for 1 month after radiographic dissolution because bacteria may be released from uroliths as they dissolve.[138]

Struvite dissolution diets should not be used in growing cats, cats with acidemia, or pregnant cats. Some authorities do not recommend use of dissolution diets in male cats because of the risk of urethral obstruction as the uroliths decrease in size.[141] However, there is no published evidence to support this concern.

After medical dissolution or stone removal, measures should be taken to minimize urolith recurrence. In one study of 1821 cats with struvite uroliths, 2.7% had a first recurrence and 0.2% had a second recurrence.[3] In the past urinary acidifiers (such as DL-methionine and ammonium chloride) were commonly used to reduce urine pH, but they are rarely indicated today. Several struvite-preventive diets are commercially available that acidify urine and avoid excessive magnesium, phosphorus, calcium, and chloride. However, no randomized, controlled studies have evaluated their efficacy. *Ad libitum* feeding may decrease the postprandial alkaline tide, but care must be taken to avoid obesity. Water intake should be increased to encourage diuresis and reduce urine concentration of mineral precursors for urolith formation. This is best accomplished by feeding a canned diet; other methods to increase water intake are listed in Box 18-16. Recommendations on how to change a cat's diet are found in Box 18-5.

Routine monitoring (e.g., urinalysis, radiographs) is recommended for early detection of recurrence. Initially, reassessment should occur every 3 months. Urinalysis should be monitored for crystalluria, pH, and specific gravity. Urine pH should be maintained at less than 6.5 and USG should be less than 1.030. A pH meter is preferable to urine dipsticks for monitoring because meters provide more precise measurement of pH and are not affected by pigments in urine.

Calcium Oxalate Uroliths

Risk Factors

Risk factors for development of CaOx urolithiasis include age (mean age, 7 years) and breed (Persian, Himalayan, British Shorthair, Exotic Shorthair, Havana Brown, Foreign Shorthair, Ragdoll, Scottish Fold).[35,78,86,100,147] Some studies suggest male cats are at higher risk than females.[35,78,100] Diets low in sodium or potassium and those formulated to increase urine acidity increase the risk of CaOx uroliths.[102] The source of drinking water is thought to be an unlikely contributor to the development of CaOx uroliths.[86]

Altered systemic calcium metabolism may play a role in the formation of CaOx uroliths in some cats. Mild hypercalcemia (11.5 to 13.5 mg/dL [2.88-3.38 mmol/L]) was documented in more than one third of cats with CaOx urolithiasis in one study.[132] Other studies have also reported hypercalcemia in cats with CaOx urolithiasis.[120,125,158] Many of the cats in these studies had a history of being fed a urine-acidifying diet. Chronic dietary acidification can cause metabolic acidosis, increased serum ionized calcium concentrations, hypercalcemia, and increased bone turnover of calcium. Dietary acidification therefore predisposes cats to hypercalciuria and CaOx urolithiasis. It is important to assess dietary needs throughout all life stages in cats and avoid continuation of a urine-acidifying diet prescribed early in life into the later years. Other factors, such as increased absorption of calcium or oxalate from the gastrointestinal tract or renal tubular dysfunction leading to hypercalciuria or hyperoxaluria, may also be involved but have not been well investigated in cats.[125]

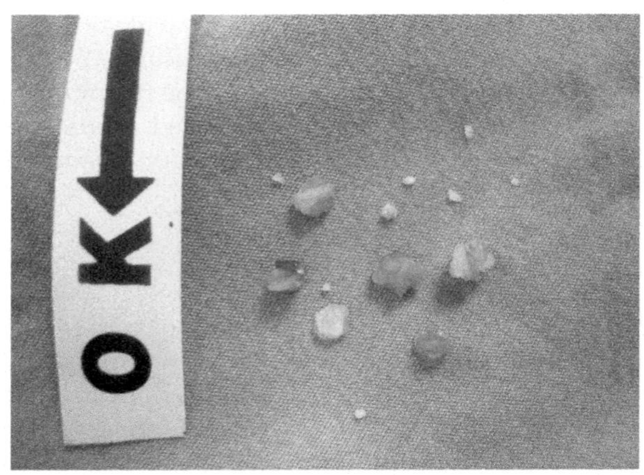

FIGURE 32-28 Multiple calcium oxalate uroliths surgically removed from the bladder of a 12-year-old spayed female domestic longhair cat with hematuria.

Clinical Signs and Diagnosis

When CaOx uroliths form in the lower urinary tract, clinical signs include stranguria, hematuria, pollakiuria, periuria, and urethral obstruction. CaOx uroliths are radiopaque and usually white and hard, with either an irregular or smooth surface (Figure 32-28). They may be present as either single or multiple stones. Survey abdominal radiographs are often sufficient for detection of CaOx uroliths (Figure 32-29). Detection of small uroliths or nonradiopaque uroliths may be improved with double contrast cystography or ultrasonography, both of which have a false-negative rate of less than 5%.[94] The index of suspicion for CaOx versus struvite uroliths in the bladder would be higher in male cats, cats over 7 years of age, and in susceptible breeds. Definitive diagnosis of CaOx uroliths requires removal and chemical analysis.

Ruling out concurrent diseases and evaluating for hypercalcemia is important in cats suspected or known to have CaOx uroliths. Cats with CaOx uroliths should have a CBC and serum biochemistry profile performed, as well as a urinalysis and urine culture. Evaluation of hypercalcemia includes assessment of total serum calcium, ionized calcium, and PTH. Because the

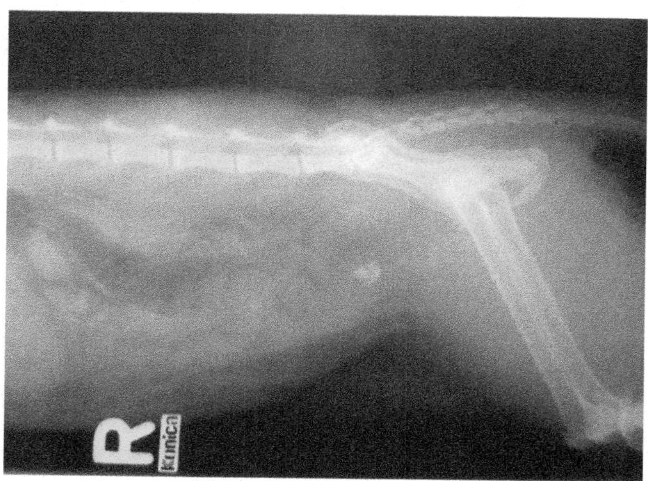

FIGURE 32-29 Radiographic appearance of the bladder uroliths pictured in Figure 32-28.

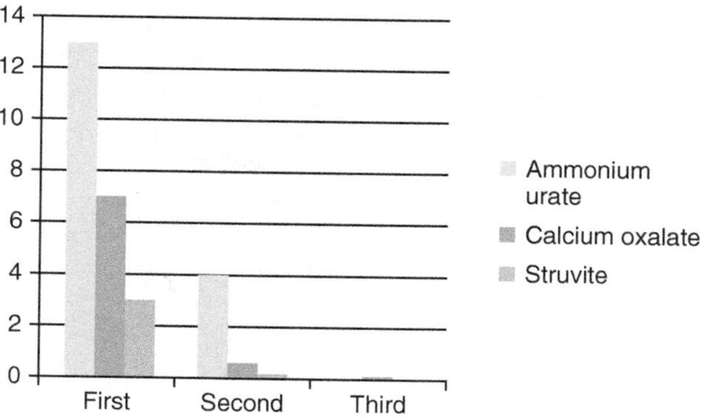

FIGURE 32-30 Percentage of cats with recurrence of uroliths. Recurrence was usually, but not always, with the same urolith type. *(Adapted from Albasan H, Osborne C, Lulich J et al: Rate and frequency of recurrence of uroliths after an initial ammonium urate, calcium oxalate, or struvite urolith in cats,* J Am Vet Med Assoc *235:1450, 2009.)*

hypercalcemia is usually idiopathic, the total serum calcium and ionized calcium are increased but the PTH concentration is normal or low.

Urinalysis typically shows an acidic pH in cats with CaOx uroliths. These uroliths are not usually associated with infection, although secondary bacterial infections, especially with *E. coli*, may be present in some patients.[17] Although CaOx crystals may be seen on urinalysis, they are not a reliable indicator of whether uroliths are present or of urolith composition. Some cats with uroliths do not have crystalluria, and uncommonly those with uroliths may have urinary crystals that are different from the type in the stone.[23]

Treatment

To date, no calculolytic diets for CaOx uroliths exist. The only effective treatment is physical removal of the stones, usually by way of surgery or VU. Lithotripsy is available at some referral centers. Cystotomy must be performed for larger uroliths, but care must be taken to remove all the stones. Uroliths causing urethral obstruction should be retropulsed into the bladder.[17]

Recurrence of CaOx uroliths in cats after treatment is common (Figure 32-30). In a study of 2393 cats with CaOx uroliths, 7% had one recurrence, 0.6% had a second recurrence, and 0.1% had a third recurrence (usually, but not always, of the same urolith type).[3] Recommendations for the management and prevention of CaOx uroliths include the following (see also Box 18-14):

1. Feed a protein-restricted, high-moisture, alkalinizing diet designed to prevent CaOx uroliths[109]; avoid foods high in oxalates, and avoid supplements of ascorbic acid and vitamin D.[137]
2. Reduce the USG to less than 1.025 by feeding canned food (other suggestions for increasing water consumption are found in Box 18-16)
3. Maintain a urine pH of 7 to 7.5 by using a therapeutic diet or supplementing with potassium citrate (50 to 75 mg/kg with food, every 12 hours)
4. Other strategies include supplementing with vitamin B_6 (2 to 4 mg/kg, daily to every other day, orally) and administration of hydrochlorothiazide to promote calcium reabsorption (2 to 4 mg/kg, orally, every 12 hours)[75]
5. If hypercalcemia is present, use a high-fiber diet and potassium citrate; other options include glucocorticoids (start prednisolone at 5 mg/cat daily orally for 1 month and reassess) and once weekly oral alendronate (10 mg/cat)[39]

The appropriate dietary sodium content for prevention of CaOx uroliths is currently a matter of controversy, and guidelines are lacking. For more information, see Chapter 18.

After urolith removal, cats should be re-evaluated within 1 month and then again at 3 months and 6 months. In addition to a physical examination and medical history, a urinalysis should be performed as well as bladder imaging (radiography, ultrasonography, or both). Ideally, bladder imaging should be performed every 6 months. Some cats will require monitoring of total and ionized calcium, and cats receiving diuretics will require monitoring of electrolytes.

Other Urolith Types

Although struvite and CaOx are the most common urolith types in cats, many other mineral types have been identified, including urates (Figure 32-31), apatite, cystine, potassium magnesium pyrophosphate, calcium phosphate, xanthine, and silica.[35,77,139] Mixed, compound, and matrix uroliths have also been identified.

Uroliths not composed of mineral salts may also form. In one report 49 of 21,784 (0.2%) feline uroliths were

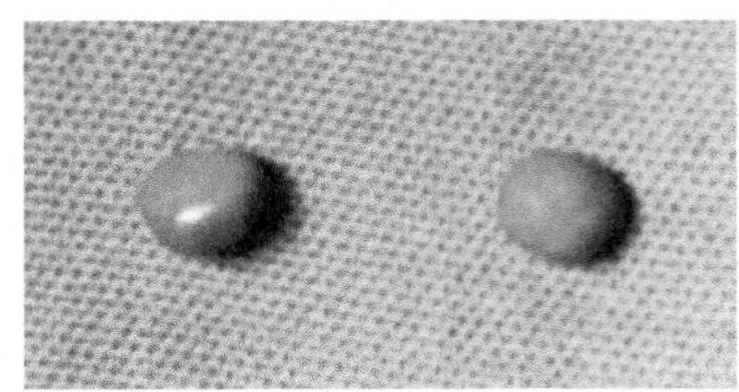

FIGURE 32-31 Uroliths composed of ammonium urate (95%) and calcium oxalate (5%) surgically removed from the bladder of a 5-year-old spayed female Egyptian Mau with pollakiuria, hematuria, and inappropriate elimination.

composed of dried solidified blood (DSB).[184] These uroliths were firm and stonelike and did not resemble blood clots. Almost half had been submitted after 2001. The mean age of affected cats was 9 years. Although they were found throughout the urinary tract, most of these uroliths (57%) were removed from the bladder or urethra. DSB calculi do not appear to be radiodense and may not be detected on ultrasound examination. In another report 60 of 5230 (1.1%) uroliths were determined to be composed of DSB.[35] The majority had been submitted in 1999 or later, and male cats were found to be overrepresented.

Foreign objects, such as sutures placed in the bladder during cystotomy, may act as a nidus for urolith formation. From 1999 to 2006, 0.17% of feline bladder uroliths submitted to the CVUC contained a suture nidus.[5] The most common mineral composition of the uroliths was CaOx, but struvite and compound minerals were also identified. It seems to take an extended period of time, approximately 1 year, for a clinically apparent urolith to form around a suture nidus. The authors of the study recommended certain precautions when closing the bladder after cystotomy, such as avoiding full-thickness bites, long-lasting absorbable sutures, and nonabsorbable sutures.

Urethral Plugs

Most urethral plugs are composed primarily of a proteinaceous matrix (mucoprotein and inflammatory debris) with trapped crystals. They are typically found at the tip of the penis where the urethral diameter is smallest or in other areas of the urethra where a narrowing occurs (i.e., caudal to the bulbourethral gland or between the bladder and prostate gland). Although CaOx uroliths are now at least as common as struvite uroliths, the mineral composition of urethral plugs continues to be predominantly struvite.[53,77,139] Other urethral plugs are composed almost totally of matrix or sloughed tissue and blood. It is currently not known what causes urethral plugs to form. One theory suggests that urethral plugs form in cats with underlying inflammation.[181] Plasma proteins may enter the urine from suburothelial vascular leakage and may trap crystals in the lumen of the urethra, resulting in obstruction. Oozing of plasma proteins into urine combined with active inflammation may increase the urine pH, thus contributing to the precipitation of struvite crystals.

MANAGEMENT OF URETHRAL OBSTRUCTION

Urethral obstruction is a common feline medical condition, although data on prevalence in the general cat population is lacking. It was diagnosed in 18% of more than 22,000 cats with FLUTD presented to veterinary teaching hospitals[101] and in 10% of cats presented to a large urban emergency service.[99] Little information is available regarding risk factors. In a recent study of 82 cats with urethral obstruction compared with sex- and time-matched controls, the majority of affected cats were between 1 and 7 years old.[164] The proportion of cats consuming exclusively dry food was significantly higher in the cats with urethral obstruction. Increased body weight, which may be a marker for decreased activity, was also associated with increased risk. Cats with access to outdoors were at decreased risk. In another study risk was greatest for cats between 4 and 10 years of age.[101]

Fortunately, the frequency of urethral obstruction has been declining in recent decades. In veterinary teaching hospitals in Canada and the United States, the hospital proportional morbidity rate for urethral obstruction declined from 19 cases per 1000 cats evaluated in 1980 to 7 cases per 1000 cats in 1999.[103] This coincides with, and is likely due to, at least in part, the widespread availability of diets designed to minimize struvite crystalluria.

Obstructive uropathy is most common in males because of the small diameter of the male urethra compared with that of female cats. The age at time of castration does not affect the diameter of the urethra and so does not affect risk of urethral obstruction.[155] Typical clinical signs include dysuria, hematuria, frequent attempts to urinate, vocalizing in the litter box, and licking of the penis or prepuce. Owners may not notice that the cat has not voided urine recently, and some cats will be erroneously presented for constipation or for difficulty walking. Some cats will have signs of systemic illness, such as lethargy, anorexia, weakness, and vomiting. Cats suffering from prolonged obstruction may present moribund or dead.

Diagnosis is relatively simple and is accomplished by palpating a large, firm bladder, which seems to be painful for the cat. Palpation of a distended bladder should be performed gently to avoid tears or ruptures. In some cases owners present cats relatively soon after obstruction has occurred, in which case the bladder may not be overdistended but it will not be possible to express urine. Urethral obstruction should be considered as a differential diagnosis for any young to middle-aged sick male cat.

Obstruction may be caused by an intraluminal object, mural thickening, or compression by an extraurethral mass. Urethral plugs and urethroliths have been identified as the most common causes of obstruction in male cats,[60,91] although more than 50% of cases were classified as idiopathic in a recent study.[61] Other potential causes include urethrospasm, trauma, congenital defects, stricture, and neoplasia.

Stabilization

Cats with urethral obstruction should be treated as emergencies when presented. Although most patients are stable at presentation, 10% or more have significant physiologic compromise. In particular, cats that have been obstructed 48 hours or more may be severely ill and require crisis management. The initial approach to management should be adapted to the cat's condition because it can make a life-or-death difference to the most severely compromised patients. The most common immediately life-threatening issue is not the obstruction itself but the resulting cardiovascular compromise.

A thorough assessment of the cat's condition should be made before attempting to relieve the obstruction as specific stabilization measures may be necessary, particularly before sedation is provided or anesthesia is induced. Physical evaluation should include mucous membrane color, capillary refill time, pulse quality and rate, cardiac auscultation, and rectal temperature. Hypothermia may occur secondary to circulatory shock. Cats with urethral obstruction would be expected to have a high heart rate on account of stress and pain. The presence of an inappropriately slow heart rate may be associated with hyperkalemia; an electrocardiogram should be performed and serum potassium concentration measured. Supplemental oxygen may be provided by face mask or flow-by delivery.

An intravenous catheter should be placed promptly to administer fluids and medication and obtain blood samples. Blood is collected for a CBC, serum chemistries, and electrolytes. For critically ill cats an emergency database would be packed cell volume, total protein (TP), electrolytes, ionized calcium, blood glucose, BUN, and Cr. Venous blood gases are also useful if available. Analgesia should be provided at the earliest opportunity. Appropriate agents include butorphanol, buprenorphine, hydromorphone, and other opioids. NSAIDs are inappropriate in this clinical setting.

Obstructed cats may have moderate to severe dehydration and varying degrees of electrolyte disturbances and azotemia, so the prompt initiation of fluid therapy is extremely important. In one study 85% of cats with urethral obstruction were azotemic.[164] A balanced electrolyte solution is recommended for rehydration and stabilization. In two studies metabolic acidosis resolved more slowly in critically ill cats with urethral obstruction treated with 0.9% NaCl than in those treated with balanced electrolyte solutions, but there was no difference in the final outcome between the two treatments.[45,48] In severely dehydrated or moribund cats, 20 to 30 mL/kg may be administered as an initial intravenous bolus, adjusting the subsequent fluid rate on the basis of initial response.[47] More information on fluid therapy for cats with postrenal azotemia due to urethral obstruction is found in Chapter 5.

Common electrolyte abnormalities in cats with urethral obstruction that may require correction include hyperkalemia, metabolic acidosis, and hypocalcemia. The measures outlined in subsequent paragraphs have temporary effects but will help stabilize the patient as fluid therapy is instituted and until the inciting cause is corrected. In one study approximately 24% of 199 obstructed cats had mild to severe hyperkalemia (≥6.0 mEq/L).[99] About 12% of the cats in the same study had multiple, life-threatening metabolic derangements (particularly hyperkalemia and concurrent hypocalcemia). In another study hyperkalemia (48%), ionized hypocalcemia (56%), and hyponatremia (55%) were common findings.[164]

In most cases metabolic abnormalities resolve with administration of fluids and relief of the obstruction. However, in some cases specific treatment should be considered. Severe metabolic acidosis ($pH < 7.1$) has profound effects on the cardiac system, respiratory system, and CNS. Treatment with sodium bicarbonate may be required in unstable cats with severe metabolic acidosis. If it is not possible to evaluate blood gases, severely ill cats can be treated with 1 to 2 mEq/kg sodium bicarbonate given slowly and intravenously. It is important to monitor serum calcium because sodium bicarbonate lowers the ionized portion of plasma calcium and some patients are already hypocalcemic at presentation; therefore the hypocalcemia should be corrected first. More information on treatment of metabolic acidosis with sodium bicarbonate is found in Chapter 5.

Potassium is involved in cellular function and neuromuscular transmission. Hyperkalemia may have profound cardiac effects, with characteristic electrocardiographic changes that include bradycardia, peaking and narrowing of the T wave, a shortened QT interval, widening of the QRS complex, and decreased amplitude or loss of the P wave. It is not possible to correlate the electrocardiographic changes with the severity of the hyperkalemia. Some cats have significant hyperkalemia without electrocardiographic changes. The effect of hyperkalemia in cats with severe electrocardiographic disturbances can be countered with calcium gluconate, which directly antagonizes potassium at the cell membrane level. The veterinarian should administer 50 to 100 mg/kg intravenously over 2 to 3 minutes while monitoring the electrocardiogram for calcium-induced arrhythmias. The effects are almost immediate and will last about 30 minutes.

Plasma potassium can be further decreased if necessary by driving it intracellularly using regular insulin (0.1 to 0.25 U/kg intravenously). The insulin should be followed with an IV bolus of 50% dextrose (0.5 g/kg, diluted) to prevent hypoglycemia. Serum potassium will decrease within 1 hour. Blood glucose should be monitored for several hours after administration of insulin, and intravenous fluids can be supplemented with 2% to 5% dextrose to maintain normoglycemia.

In one study, ionized hypocalcemia (<2.4 mEq/L) was identified in 75% of 24 obstructed male cats, usually associated with high serum phosphorus (caused by decreased renal excretion).[49] Cats with severe ionized hypocalcemia (<1.6 mEq/L) may have impaired cardiac electrical and mechanical dysfunction, requiring administration of intravenous calcium (as detailed previously).

Cystocentesis is useful to decompress the bladder before attempting to catheterize the urethra.[181] This helps relieve pain and distention and makes subsequent attempts to flush the urethra easier by reducing back pressure. The procedure may be performed with a 22- or 23-gauge butterfly needle or a 22-gauge needle attached to an extension set, stopcock, and 20-mL syringe. The veterinarian inserts the needle into the bladder halfway between the apex and the neck of the ventral or ventrolateral wall while the bladder is stabilized manually. The needle should enter the bladder at an oblique angle and should be directed caudally.[108] The veterinarian should be careful not to apply excessive pressure to the bladder during the procedure to minimize the risk of urine leakage. As much of the urine as possible should be removed, and the samples should be saved for urinalysis and urine culture. The most important complication is damage to the bladder wall or bladder rupture and would be most likely to occur in cats with friable, compromised bladder walls. Bladder rupture could also occur in these patients during attempts to relieve urethral obstruction without prior cystocentesis. Although rupture is an uncommon event, the veterinarian should be prepared for surgical intervention should it occur.

Urinalysis findings in cats with urethral obstruction may include hematuria, proteinuria, pyuria (usually caused by inflammation), alkaluria, crystalluria, and glucosuria (stress induced). In one study 12% of cats also had bilirubinuria, although the cause was unclear.[164]

Finally, radiographs provide useful information to direct treatment, such as the presence, location, and number of uroliths. The entire urethra should be radiographed to detect urethroliths that may be lodged distally.

BOX 32-17

Supplies for Urethral Catheterization and Relief of Obstruction

- Sterile lidocaine gel
- Open-end urethral catheter to relieve urethral obstruction
- Intravenous extension set
- Sterile lubricant
- Sterile saline flush
- Sterile gloves
- Several 10-mL syringes
- Indwelling urethral catheter
- Empty intravenous fluid bag and sterile intravenous line

Establishing Urethral Patency

Establishing urethral patency is begun *after* the patient is stable. In particular, severe hyperkalemia and cardiac dysrhythmias should be corrected before anesthesia is induced. The choice of sedation versus anesthesia and the drug protocols employed will vary depending on the condition of the patient and the experience of the clinician. Drugs that require renal excretion should be used with caution. A commonly used combination is ketamine (2 to 5 mg/kg) with diazepam (0.2 to 0.5 mg/kg) or midazolam (0.2 to 0.5 mg/kg) administered intravenously to effect; lower doses may also be adequate. Ketamine should be avoided in cats with cardiac arrhythmia or cardiac disease. Hydromorphone and midazolam is another common choice. Mask induction with isoflurane or intravenous propofol may be used if additional time for procedures is needed. Obtunded patients may not require sedation for urethral catheterization.

The supplies required for urethral catheterization and relieving obstruction are found in Box 32-17. The patient is placed in dorsal or lateral recumbency, and the hair is clipped around the perineal area, especially in longhair cats. Surgical scrub is used to gently cleanse the prepuce and tip of the penis. Wearing sterile gloves, the veterinarian should extrude the penis from the sheath and gently massage it to expel very small calculi and urethral plugs lodged at the tip of the penis. In some cases massaging the urethra through the rectum may dislodge an obstruction. Extrusion of the penis can be difficult in obese cats. Drawing the hind limbs forward may provide better exposure.

Catheters useful for relief of urethral obstruction include the standard open-ended tomcat catheter (3.5 Fr polypropylene, 4.5 to 5.5 inches) or Minnesota olive-tipped urethral catheters (22-G, ½ to 1½ inch) (Figure 32-32), which is the author's first choice for obstructions in the distal urethra. The tip of the catheter is lubricated

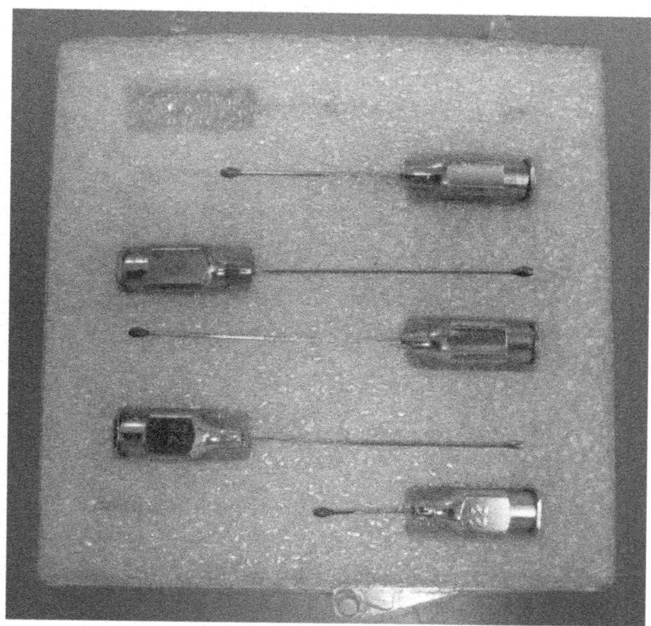

FIGURE 32-32 A set of 22-G Minnesota olive-tip catheters ranging in length from 0.5 to 1.5 inches (1.2 to 3.8 cm).

with lidocaine gel and inserted into the external urethral orifice. The tip of the penis can be allowed to retract into the prepuce once the catheter has been inserted. Extending the penis until it is parallel to the cat's spine by pulling the prepuce caudally and dorsally will help straighten the urethra as much as possible and facilitate catheter placement. Alternately, an assistant can apply pressure ventrally through the rectum to help guide the catheter over the pelvic brim. The catheter is gently advanced until the obstruction is reached. Then an intravenous extension set is attached, and a 10-mL syringe filled with saline is used to liberally flush the urethral lumen. It may be helpful to add a small amount of sterile lubricant to the saline flush (shake to form an emulsion). Walpole's solution should never be used because it has an acidic pH and is highly irritating to the already traumatized mucosa; use may result in serious inflammation of the urethra and bladder and even urethral stricture.

It may take several attempts at gentle advancement and flushing to relieve the obstruction. If resistance is felt when saline is injected into the catheter, the catheter should be backed out slightly until the saline can be flushed more easily. Gently massaging the penis during flushing may help dislodge the obstructing material. Occlusion of the urethra may also help distend the urethral lumen and dislodge plugs or uroliths. This can be accomplished in two ways. The urethra can be compressed through the rectum during hydropropulsion. Alternatively, the tip of the penis can be pinched to occlude the urethral lumen and increase pressure by preventing flush from exiting the external urethral orifice. It is important to watch carefully for expulsion of urethral plugs or calculi during flushing so that the material can be saved for analysis.

Any procedures involving the urethra should be carried out as gently as possible to avoid inflammation and long-term damage. The catheter itself should never be used to push obstructing material into the bladder. One series of 15 cats requiring perineal urethrostomy had sustained urethral trauma during catheterization using inappropriate technique or equipment.[44] Physical examination abnormalities included perineal hematoma, deviation of the penis, and scrotal swelling. Contrast radiography was performed in 10 cats; urethral stricture (one cat) and urethral rupture (five cats) were found. The other four cats had a stricture at the external urethral orifice.

Once the obstruction has been relieved, any urine remaining in the bladder should be aspirated. The bladder is then flushed and drained repeatedly with saline until the harvested solution appears relatively clear of blood and debris. The catheter used to relieve the obstruction is withdrawn slowly while continuing to flush saline. An indwelling urinary catheter (3.5 to 5 Fr) is not required for all obstructed patients. Factors such as ease of establishing urethral patency, quality of urine stream, size of bladder at presentation, and the presence of systemic illness must all be considered. Marked hematuria is another indication for an indwelling catheter because it represents risk of re-obstruction with blood clots and indicates severe bladder distention, which may impair detrusor contractility. If an indwelling urinary catheter is not used, the bladder should be palpated after natural voiding to assess completeness of emptying. If the cat without a urinary catheter is not voiding regularly or not fully emptying the bladder, the bladder should be expressed manually 3 or 4 times daily.

The best choices for indwelling catheters are made of soft material, such as a polyvinyl red-rubber feeding tube, a silicone tomcat urethral catheter, a polyurethane E-Z-GO urinary catheter (Mila International, Inc.), or a polytetrafluoroethylene Slippery Sam tomcat urethral catheter. These catheters are more flexible than polypropylene catheters and reduce urethral irritation and trauma. Softer catheters are sometimes too flexible to insert easily, especially if a stylet is not included; storing the catheters in the freezer is helpful because they become stiff when cold. The tip of the catheter should be advanced only a short distance into the bladder lumen. Inserting the catheter too far can cause irritation and straining. If the catheter tip lies in the proximal urethra, this will also cause irritation and discomfort. The position of the catheter can be checked radiographically. The catheter should be sutured to the cat's prepuce near the external urethral orifice using a tape "butterfly"; some catheters come with "wings" for this purpose.

Indwelling catheters should be attached to closed collection systems to reduce the risk of ascending bacterial contamination. A urine collection bag or an empty intravenous fluid bag and intravenous administration set can be used to construct a collection system. After flushing the bladder, the veterinarian should leave 10 to 20 mL of lavage fluid in the bladder lumen. This provides fluid to fill the tubing and immediately indicates that the system is working properly. It is important to check that the intravenous administration line is not clamped closed. The collection bag should be positioned below the level of the cat to provide a siphon effect and prevent retrograde flow of urine. An Elizabethan collar should be used to prevent the cat from biting the catheter or tubing.

Indwelling catheters are generally left in place from 1 to 3 days. Clinical judgment is used to determine the optimal time to remove the catheter. Indications for catheter removal include resolution of clinical signs such as lethargy, weakness, anorexia and vomiting, diminishing hematuria, and resolution of metabolic derangements and postobstructive diuresis. A recovered bladder will feel small and firmly contracted around the tip of the catheter on palpation. When the catheter is removed, risk of postcatheterization voiding problems may be assessed by evaluating the functional status of the urethra. Between 20 and 30 mL of sterile saline may be instilled into the bladder just before catheter removal. As soon as the catheter is removed, the bladder is expressed, and the quality of the urine stream is evaluated.

Whenever possible, antibiotic therapy should not be instituted while an indwelling catheter is in place. Although antibiotics may reduce the risk of postcatheter bacterial infection with short-term catheter placement, infections that do occur may be highly resistant. In addition, prophylactic antibiotic use cannot prevent infection when catheters remain in place for longer than 3 days. Antibiotic use with an indwelling catheter is reserved for cats with evidence of urinary tract or systemic infection at the time of diagnosis. Antibiotics may be required once the catheter is removed. In one study of 13 cats with indwelling urethral catheters, 69% developed bacteriuria.[80] In a study in dogs, culture of the tip of the catheter at removal had poor predictive value.[166] Urine should be cultured on the day of catheter removal or within 24 hours. To culture urine on the day of removal, the clinician should clamp the collection system to allow urine to accumulate in the bladder about 1 to 2 hours before the catheter is removed. Then the collection system is removed, and a midstream urine sample is collected through the catheter; this sample is submitted for culture and sensitivity testing. If an infection is diagnosed, an appropriate antibiotic should be administered for a minimum of 10 days and the urine recultured 1 week after the end of therapy.

Corticosteroids should not be administered to cats with indwelling urinary catheters, insofar as this increases the risk of lower UTI. Furthermore, corticosteroids predispose these patients to bacterial pyelonephritis and fail to lessen inflammation.[14] In patients with normal renal function and hydration status, NSAIDs may be considered to reduce inflammation.

Reobstruction after catheter removal may be due to various causes, such as incomplete removal of obstructing material (urethral plug or urethrolith) or urethrospasm caused by inflammation. Other causes of reobstruction include obstruction of the proximal urethral opening by a urolith or mass in the bladder or external compression of the urethra by a mass. Additional investigation with imaging should be considered in these cases.

Although the standard of care for cats with urethral obstruction is relief of the obstruction by way of urethral catheterization, treatment often involves extended hospitalization and may be too costly for some owners. Euthanasia or relinquishment is usually the only alternative in such circumstances. Recently, a protocol for managing urethral obstruction without catheterization using medication (acepromazine, buprenorphine, medetomidine); repeated decompressive cystocentesis; subcutaneous fluid therapy as needed; and a quiet, dark, low-stress environment has been described. In one report 15 cats were treated with this protocol.[43] Cats with serious metabolic or physiologic derangements were excluded from treatment, and a lateral abdominal radiograph was obtained to rule out cystic or urethral calculi. Treatment was successful in 11 of 15 cats, defined as spontaneous urination within 72 hours and discharge from hospital. Of the 11 cats, 9 urinated spontaneously within 48 hours. In the remaining four cats, uroabdomen or hemoabdomen developed. Necropsy was performed in three cats, but none had evidence of bladder tear or rupture.

Ongoing Medical Management

After stabilization ongoing monitoring should include assessment of hydration, temperature, mentation, and urine output. Any abnormalities on initial assessment should be re-evaluated as needed (e.g., electrolytes, ionized calcium, blood glucose, BUN, Cr, acid–base status).

Cats that were obstructed for longer than 48 hours or that were severely azotemic may experience significant postobstructive diuresis (urine output greater than 2 mL/kg per hour) for a period of 2 to 5 days. In one retrospective study postobstructive diuresis occurred in 13 of 28 cats (46%) within the first 6 hours of treatment.[55] Cats with acidemia (venous pH less than 7.35) on admission were at greatest risk. Urine output should be monitored and fluid therapy carefully titrated to prevent dehydration. The cat should be carefully monitored for hypokalemia. After azotemia resolves, fluid therapy may be gradually tapered. More information on fluid therapy for cats with postobstructive diuresis is found in Chapter 5.

In addition to analgesics, other drugs may be used in the management of urethral obstruction (see Table 32-13). Urethral spasms are a common cause for reobstruction once the catheter has been removed, so preemptive therapy with an antispasmodic is warranted starting while the catheter is still in place and once the patient is stable. The proximal (preprostatic) portion of the feline urethra is primarily controlled by smooth muscle, whereas the distal (postprostatic and penile) portion is primarily controlled by striated muscle. Acepromazine may be useful for its antispasmodic effects on urethral smooth muscle. Alternative drugs to decrease urethral smooth muscle tone are the $alpha_1$ antagonists such as phenoxybenzamine and prazosin. The penile portion of the urethra is the principle portion contributing to excessive outflow resistance in recently obstructed cats. Diazepam may be used to relax the striated muscle component of the urethra, although its clinical efficacy is unclear. Dantrolene may be more effective than diazepam, based on studies in healthy cats.[171,172] This drug can cause hepatotoxicity and should not be used in patients with preexisting hepatic disease and should be used used with caution in patients with severe cardiac or pulmonary disease (e.g., asthma). Some clinicians also find judicious use of NSAIDs (e.g., meloxicam) helpful for management of postobstructive urethral spasms as long as the patient is well hydrated and is not azotemic.

Prolonged distention of the bladder may induce detrusor atony by causing separation of the tight junctions of the detrusor muscle, resulting in weak and ineffective muscle contractions. Patients with detrusor atony may require prolonged urethral catheterization (7 days or more) because the bladder must be kept as small as possible to re-establish tight junction connections. With prolonged catheterization the risk of bacterial infection increases. Frequent urinalyses should be performed and antibiotics prescribed if necessary on the basis of culture and sensitivity testing. The cholinergic drug bethanecol may be used in conjunction with prazosin or phenoxybenzamine to stimulate detrusor contractions once the patient is stabilized and there is no outflow resistance.

The survival rate to discharge from the hospital for cats with obstructive uropathy is over 90%.[22,61,99,164] However, recurrence rates may be high (22% to 36%), particularly if the underlying cause is not identified and corrected or successfully managed.[22,61,164] Therefore every attempt should be made to identify and treat the etiology while relieving the obstruction. Cats with urethral plugs should be managed the same way as idiopathic cystitis patients. Between 15% and 20% of cats with FLUTD have radiographic evidence of cystic calculi, so bladder imaging is important, especially for cats with recurrent FLUTD.[27] Dietary therapy should be appropriate for the urolith or crystal type. In general, cats with obstruction from urethral plugs or urethroliths should be changed to canned diets to decrease urine concentration and supersaturation with calculogenic precursors.

Surgical Management

Perineal urethrostomy is a salvage procedure that may be indicated for the occasional patient with urethral obstruction (Figure 32-33). Ideally, a decision to perform the surgery should not be based on the number of times the cat has experienced urethral obstruction. Rather, the functional state of the urethra should be the basis of the decision. Indications would include urethral stricture, urethral or penile trauma, and priapism. However, in some cases the frequency and severity of recurrent obstructions, the owner's perception of the cat's quality of life, and the ongoing costs may influence the decision to perform surgery. The procedure, which is described elsewhere, requires thorough knowledge of anatomy and good surgical technique.[188]

Data on the frequency with which perineal urethrostomy is performed in cats with urethral obstruction is scarce. In two recent studies perineal urethrostomy was performed in 10% of 82 cats in Israel[164] and 22% of 45 cats in Switzerland.[61] The frequency of perineal urethrostomy performed at veterinary teaching hospitals in North America has been sharply declining. The proportional morbidity rate was reported as 13 cases

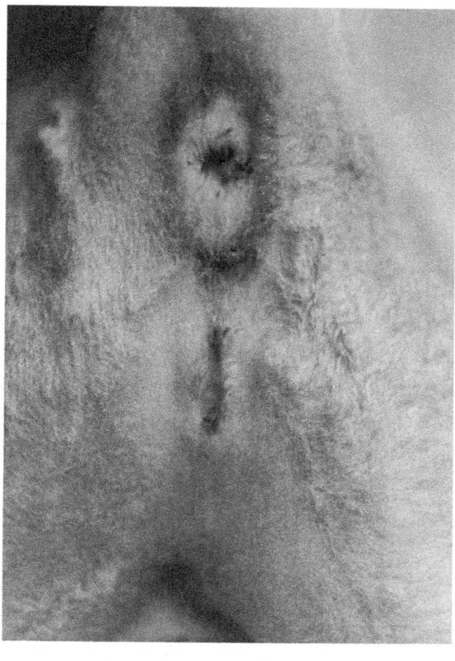

FIGURE 32-33 The 2-week postoperative appearance of a perineal urethrostomy site that is healing normally.

per 1000 cats evaluated in 1980 compared with four cases per 1000 cats in 1999.[103]

Complications of perineal urethrostomy are common and include stricture of the stoma necessitating surgical revision, wound dehiscence, urine scalding, urine leakage into perineal tissue, perineal hernia, and urinary incontinence.[18,61,130,146] The most common complication is recurrent bacterial UTI, which occurs in 17% to 58% of cases.[18,44,61,66] However, long-term disease-free outcomes may be achieved with good quality of life.[18,44,61,164] Clients should be aware that the surgery does not always correct the underlying problem, and recurrent episodes of idiopathic cystitis or uroliths may still occur.

Prepubic urethrostomy is a salvage procedure for cats with failed perineal urethrostomy or stenosis or rupture of the intrapelvic urethra. The complication rate may be high. In one study of 16 cats, six were eventually euthanized because of urinary incontinence, skin necrosis, and unresolved idiopathic lower urinary tract disease.[11] Alternate salvage techniques include subpubic or transpelvic urethrostomy. In a study of 11 cats, the postoperative complication rate for transpelvic urethrostomy was low.[20] The authors suggested that this surgical technique could be considered as an alternative for perineal urethrostomy.

LOWER URINARY TRACT INFECTION

Prevalence and Risk Factors

The normal feline lower urinary tract has a number of defense mechanisms against infection. These include normal micturition (e.g., frequent and complete voiding), normal anatomy (e.g., length of urethra), uroepithelial mucosal barriers, antimicrobial properties of normal urine (e.g., high specific gravity and osmolality), and a normal immune system.[16] The lower urogenital tract and the perineal area have a resident population of normal flora, a ready source of pathogens for ascending infections in susceptible individuals.

Information on the prevalence of bacterial lower UTI varies with the population of cats studied. Prospective studies of young cats with FLUTD identified bacterial UTIs in fewer than 2% of cases.[27,91] Higher rates of UTI in cats with FLUTD have been documented (8% to 33%), although the data reported are often not stratified by age or other factors.* Bacterial UTI can also occur in cats without clinical signs. A study of 132 urine specimens from cats without signs of FLUTD collected for routine screening or other diagnostic evaluation found 29% with bacterial infection.[106] Older female cats were at highest risk. Some of the differences in study results may be due to differences between cats seen as first-opinion cases versus those seen as referral cases.

Persian breed, female sex, increasing age, and decreasing body weight are typically found to be risk factors for UTI.[9,10,87,101] Urethral catheterization and perineal urethrostomy also increase the risk of bacterial UTI.[66] Bacterial UTI can develop in healthy male cats with indwelling urinary catheters; risk of infection increases with duration of catheterization.[16] The risk of infection also increases with open indwelling systems, corticosteroid administration, diuresis, and preexisting lower urinary tract disease. The practice of administering antimicrobials while an indwelling urinary catheter is in place is tempting, but this should be discouraged because it may promote the development of multidrug-resistant infections.[16]

UTI is an important problem of senior cats (older than 10 years).[101,106] It is assumed that the decline in immune competence with aging is responsible in part, as well as the increased prevalence of concurrent diseases in this age group. Cats with hyperthyroidism (12% to 22% prevalence of UTI), DM (10% to 13%), and CKD (13% to 22%) are at increased risk.[8,9,10,87,119] Interestingly, decreasing USG was not associated with a positive urine culture in cats with CKD, DM and hyperthyroidism in one study[9] although other studies have reported significantly lower USG in cats with UTI.[106]

Rarely, lower UTI with fungal organisms has been documented in cats, particularly *Candida* spp.[83,110,149] In addition to signs of lower urinary tract disease, affected cats may also show systemic signs of illness (e.g., lethargy, anorexia, dehydration, weight loss, pyrexia, and weakness).[83] Most affected cats have concurrent problems causing local or systemic immune compromise, such as perineal urethrostomy, lower urinary tract disease (e.g., chronic bacterial cystitis, atonic bladder), DM, neoplasia, and chronic renal disease or have a history of prolonged treatment with antibiotics or glucocorticoids. Treatment options include fluconazole and itraconazole, although resolution of predisposing factors is important for success.

Clinical Signs and Diagnosis

Cats with infections of the lower urinary tract have typical nonspecific signs of FLUTD, including pollakiuria, dysuria, stranguria, hematuria, and periuria. However, asymptomatic infections are also possible.[8,106,119] Differential diagnosis includes other lower urinary tract diseases, such as idiopathic cystitis, urolithiasis, neoplasia, and behavioral disorders. A full urinalysis (USG, urine chemistries, and microscopic sediment examination) should be performed on all cats with signs of FLUTD and should be part of the routine minimum database for older cats or ill cats. Changes on urinalysis consistently associated with bacterial UTI

*References 51, 60, 89, 101, 142, 176.

include bacteriuria, pyuria (>5 white blood cells/high power field), and hematuria. Proteinuria may also be present. In a dilute urine sample, the magnitude of these changes may be masked. Conversely, there may be no changes on urinalysis or routine laboratory data to indicate UTI.[119]

Urine culture and sensitivity testing is recommended for cats at increased risk of UTI because of concurrent disease or with recurrent episodes of lower urinary tract disease. Samples for culture should be collected before any therapy is initiated, preferably by cystocentesis.[176] Voided samples or samples collected by catheterization are often contaminated, making interpretation difficult and risking overdiagnosis. Urine samples for culture should be processed as soon as possible. If processing will be delayed for more than 30 minutes, the sample should be refrigerated in a sterile container. A sample collected by cystocentesis may be stored in this way for 6 to 12 hours without additional bacterial growth.[111] Commercially available urine culture collection tubes containing preservative may be used to refrigerate urine specimens for up to 72 hours.[15] The most commonly isolated organisms are *E. coli* and *Enterococcus*.[8,10,107,119] Other organisms that have been isolated include *Staphylococcus* spp., *Streptococcus* spp., *Klebsiella* spp., and *Enterobacter* spp. *Corynebacterium* spp. have been identified as a cause of UTI in cats with preexisting lower urinary tract abnormalities and a history of previous UTI with other organisms.[7,37,150]

Treatment

Administration of appropriate antimicrobials is the main treatment for bacterial UTI. The choice of drug is based on susceptibility testing, but other considerations are important, such as ease of administration, risk of adverse effects, availability, and cost. Most *E. coli* isolates associated with UTI in cats are sensitive to commonly used antimicrobials (e.g., amoxicillin or amoxicillin–clavulanate), and *Enterococcus* is also sensitive to amoxicillin–clavulanate.[8,68,106,189] Therefore cats with bacteriuria may be started on amoxicillin–clavulanate pending the results of urine culture and sensitivity testing. Uncomplicated bacterial UTIs occur in cats with no underlying structural or functional abnormality. These infections are usually treated with an appropriate antimicrobial for at least 14 days. Clinical signs can be expected to abate within 48 hours.[16] Ideally, a urine culture is performed 1 week after the end of therapy.

Unfortunately, many cats with bacterial UTI have complicated infections with identifiable predisposing factors (e.g., CKD, DM, or hyperthyroidism). These cats should be treated with an appropriate antimicrobial for 4 to 6 weeks. Urine should be recultured 3 to 5 days after the start of therapy, again just before therapy is discontinued, and 1 week after completion of treatment.

Pradofloxacin (Veraflox, Bayer AG) is a third-generation fluoroquinolone antibiotic that is active against a range of feline urinary pathogens, including *E. coli* and *Staphylococcus* spp. It is available as a palatable 2.5% oral suspension that is administered at 0.2 mL/kg once daily. In a recent study 27 cats treated with pradofloxacin all had negative posttreatment urine cultures.[105] Pradofloxacin appears to have no retinal toxic effects in cats.[124] Cefovecin (Convenia, Pfizer Animal Health) is an extended spectrum semisynthetic cephalosporin with a 14-day dosing interval after a single subcutaneous injection. A recent study of posttreatment urine cultures showed that cefovecin eliminated 76% of *E. coli* infections compared with 62% for cephalexin. However, this is lower than the efficacy of cefovecin for treatment of canine UTI.[142] These newer antimicrobial agents should not be used as first-line therapy but should be reserved for bacterial organisms that are resistant to other drugs on the basis of culture and sensitivity testing or for cats that cannot be treated using other medications.

Relapses are recurrent infections with the same organism that occur for a variety of reasons, such as failure to eradicate the original infection, inappropriate antimicrobial choice (or dose, dose frequency, or length of treatment), or other complicating factors. Re-infections are recurrences caused by a different pathogen than the original infection and typically occur weeks to months after the first infection. Re-infection, as well as persistent and relapsing infection with *E. coli*, has been documented in older cats with chronic renal disease.[56] Cats with concurrent diseases and other risk factors such as perineal urethrostomy are also likely at risk. Prophylactic antimicrobial treatment for frequent re-infections has not been evaluated in cats.

One strategy employed in human medicine to prevent recurrent bacterial UTIs in women is the use of cranberry products.[81] Cranberry contains proanthocyanidins, which inhibit adherence of *E. coli* to the bladder epithelium.[72] To date, no data on safety or efficacy of cranberry products for prevention or treatment of UTI in cats has been published.

OTHER LOWER URINARY TRACT PROBLEMS

Neoplasia

Although tumors can occur anywhere in the lower urinary tract of cats, the bladder is the most common location, possibly because the bladder epithelium has prolonged exposure to carcinogenic substances contained in urine. Cats seem to be less susceptible to bladder tumors than dogs and humans. Overall, neoplasia of the lower urinary tract is rare, although data on prevalence is scarce. The most commonly reported bladder tumor in cats is transitional cell carcinoma (TCC); other tumor types reported include squamous cell carcinoma, adenocarcinoma, leiomyosarcoma, hemangiosarcoma, and lymphoma.* Most feline bladder tumors are malignant and locally invasive. Urethral tumors are very rarely reported; most cases have been TCC.[12,174]

The mean age of cats with lower urinary tract neoplasia ranges from 9 to 13 years. Compared with cats younger than 10 years old, cats 10 to 15 years old were 6 times more likely and cats older than 15 years were 19 times more likely to have neoplasia of the lower urinary tract in one study.[101] The same study showed a slightly increased risk in spayed females (2 times greater) and neutered males (2.5 times greater) than in intact cats. In a study of 25 cats with TCC, neutered males were most commonly affected.[190]

Clinical signs of lower urinary tract neoplasia may be general (e.g., lethargy, anorexia, weight loss) or specific to the lower urinary tract (e.g., hematuria, stranguria, dysuria, pollakiuria). Most urinary tract tumors are locally invasive and will eventually interfere with normal function. Inflammation and disruption of the urethral and bladder mucosa cause signs of cystitis. Masses in the urethra or the trigone of the bladder may cause urinary obstruction, as well as abnormalities in the kidneys (hydroureter, hydronephrosis). Metastasis to distant sites (abdominal organs, lungs) is common. Physical examination may be normal, or a palpably thickened urinary bladder may be appreciated.

The differential diagnosis includes other causes of lower urinary tract signs, such as urolithiasis. A thorough diagnostic evaluation including imaging should be performed in cats older than 10 years of age with lower urinary tract signs. Common findings on routine laboratory testing include azotemia, anemia, and hematuria. Hypereosinophilia as a paraneoplastic syndrome was associated with TCC in one reported case.[165] Neoplastic cells may be present on examination of urine sediment, although a definitive diagnosis should not be based solely on these findings.[59,190] Neoplastic cells often do not exfoliate into urine. Because UTI is common in these patients, urine culture and sensitivity testing should be part of the diagnostic evaluation.

Ultrasonography is a noninvasive, rapidly performed diagnostic tool that is very useful in evaluation of older cats with signs of lower urinary tract disease (Figures 32-34 and 32-35). When available, abdominal ultrasound should be part of the initial evaluation for these patients. In addition to finding bladder masses, ultrasound examination may detect other abdominal abnormalities, such as lymphadenopathy, abdominal effusion, hydroureter, or hydronephrosis.

*References 19, 59, 145, 157, 178, 190, 191.

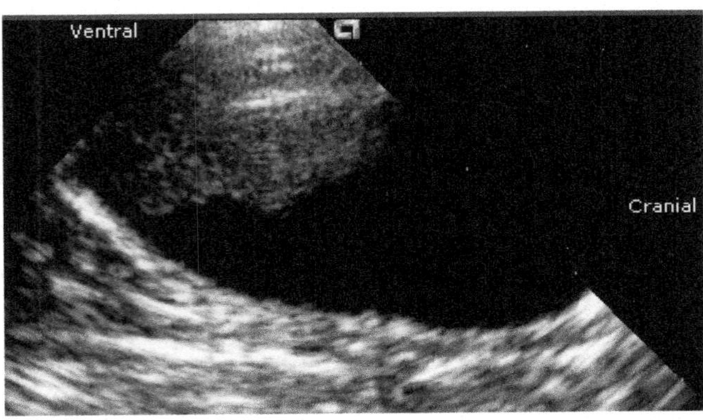

FIGURE 32-34 Ultrasound examination of the bladder of a 12-year-old spayed female domestic shorthair cat with weight loss, anorexia, and azotemia. A 1.5 × 1.0 cm (0.6 × 0.4 in) mass with an irregular surface is present on the caudal ventral bladder wall. Unilateral renomegaly was also found on ultrasonographic examination. *(Courtesy Dr. Edward Javinsky.)*

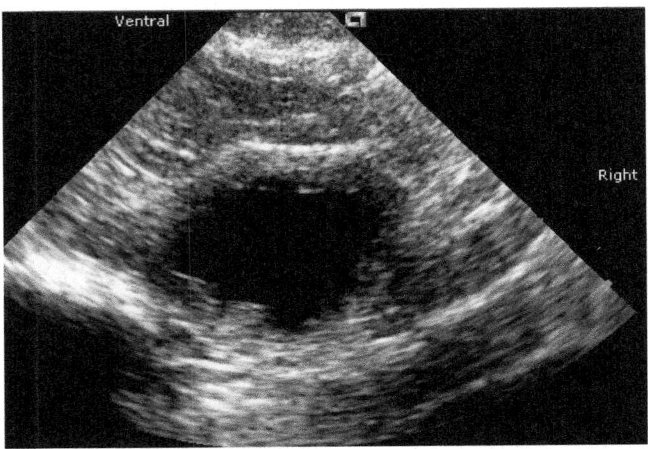

FIGURE 32-35 Ultrasound examination of the bladder of a 15-year-old spayed female domestic shorthair cat with clinical signs of feline lower urinary tract disease. The bladder wall is thickened and irregular. At the thickest point the bladder wall measures 3.9 mm (normal <2 mm). *(Courtesy Dr. Edward Javinsky.)*

Survey radiographs may detect bladder masses as well as evidence of metastasis. If survey radiographs are unrewarding and ultrasonography is not available, contrast cystography may reveal masses or bladder wall thickening. Other findings associated with neoplasia include decreased bladder distensibility and mineralization of the bladder wall. Contrast urethrography has been used for diagnosis of urethral TCC.[174] Other options for diagnostic imaging include CT, MRI, and cystoscopy.

Definitive diagnosis requires histopathologic examination of biopsy specimens. Biopsies may be collected by way of percutaneous aspiration, traumatic catheterization, cystoscopy, or laparotomy. Ultrasound-guided percutaneous fine-needle aspiration is relatively easy to perform with minimal complications.[104] Tumor seeding of the needle tract has been reported.[63,129,177,190]

Clinical staging is important to guide treatment decisions. Imaging of the chest and abdomen should be performed to evaluate for metastasis. The best treatment for tumors of the lower urinary tract is not known and is complicated by the fact that disease is often advanced at the time of diagnosis and many affected patients may have concurrent diseases. Tumors in the apex or body of the bladder can be surgically resected, although risk of recurrence and metastasis is high. TCC is often found in the trigone, where it is not amenable to surgery. In a case report of a cat with urethral TCC, treatment with surgery and radiation produced a survival time of 386 days.[174] Although piroxicam has been associated with clinical improvement in dogs with TCC, no data on safety and efficacy exists for cats. In a series of 25 cats with TCC of the bladder, various treatments were attempted, including surgery, chemotherapy (carboplatin, doxorubicin, cyclophosphamide), and piroxicam.[190] The rate of metastasis at time of diagnosis was 20%. Median survival time regardless of treatment modality was 261 days, and almost all deaths were attributed to advancement of the tumor.

Trauma

The most common lower urinary tract injury is bladder rupture, although urethral rupture can also occur. Causes of lower urinary tract injury include blunt or penetrating abdominal trauma, pelvic trauma, neoplasia, excessive pressure applied to a distended and compromised bladder during palpation or manual expression, repeated cystocentesis of a compromised bladder, urethral calculi, and improper urethral catheterization technique.[4,6,57] With bladder rupture urine will accumulate in the abdomen or in the tissues of the perineal area. With a urethral rupture urine may accumulate in the perineal subcutaneous tissues, causing swelling and hemorrhage. Physical examination of the cat with lower urinary tract injury may also show evidence of trauma such as bruising, as well as pain and lack of a discrete bladder on abdominal palpation. However, in one report of cats with uroabdomen, the bladder was palpable in some cats with bladder rupture.[6] Depending on the amount of urine accumulation, cats with uroabdomen may have abdominal distention. Anuria may be present, but the ability to urinate does not exclude a diagnosis of lower urinary tract rupture. As uremia develops, clinical signs appear and worsen, such as vomiting, anorexia, depression, and dehydration. Pain may be caused by inflammation from urine in subcutaneous tissues or chemical peritonitis from uroabdomen. Preexisting UTIs may cause septic peritonitis in cats with uroabdomen.

Diagnosis is based on physical examination findings, evaluation of a minimum database (CBC, serum chemistries and electrolytes, urinalysis) and radiography. Azotemia and electrolyte disturbances similar to those of cats with urethral obstruction will develop secondary to urinary tract rupture. Uroabdomen can result in third spacing, with volume depletion and hemodynamic compromise. Hematuria is a common finding on urinalysis. Survey radiography may show abdominal fluid, ileus (induced by chemical peritonitis), and loss of the normal bladder shadow. The presence of pelvic fractures in a trauma patient should always prompt investigation of the condition of the bladder and urethra. If abdominal fluid is present, a sample is collected using sterile technique through abdominocentesis, and the Cr and potassium content of the fluid is compared with the serum Cr and potassium. A serum Cr:abdominal fluid ratio of 1:2 (range 1.1:1 to 4:1) and a serum potassium:abdominal fluid ratio of 1.9:1 (range 1.2:1 to 2.4:1) is diagnostic for urine.[6] A retrograde positive contrast urethrogram or cystogram is used to confirm rupture of the urethra or bladder and determine the location of the lesion. Contrast studies should be performed only once the patient is stable and metabolic disturbances have been corrected.

Initial management and stabilization for cats with lower urinary tract rupture are the same as for cats with urethral obstruction. Trauma patients may require further stabilization measures depending on the type and severity of other injuries. For cats with bladder rupture, percutaneous placement of a peritoneal drainage catheter can be used for drainage of urine from the abdomen to assist in stabilization of the patient. Peritoneal dialysis catheters can be used if available; alternatives include trocar chest tubes and balloon-tip catheters. The reader is referred to other resources for description of peritoneal catheter placement.[50,57] Placement of a urethral catheter is recommended to keep the bladder decompressed. Bladder wall defects must be repaired surgically once the patient is stable. Small iatrogenic bladder tears may be treated conservatively with good outcomes by placement of an indwelling urethral catheter for continuous bladder decompression during healing in carefully selected cases.[133]

Treatment options for urethral trauma include surgical repair of the defect and use of a catheter as a stent during healing. In cases not amenable to surgical repair or stenting, urethrostomy is the best option. An important complication of urethral trauma is stricture formation, partly from exposure of the injured tissue to the irritating qualities of urine. Prompt placement of a urethral catheter using appropriate technique protects the tissues from urine. If the urethra is too traumatized to be catheterized, urine can be diverted with a tube cystostomy. The technique for placement of a prepubic cystostomy tube is described elsewhere.[121,170] In one retrospective case series of 37 dogs and 39 cats with cystostomy tubes, 49% had complications (e.g., inadvertent

BOX 32-18

Some Causes of Urinary Incontinence in Cats

Spinal cord lesions: upper motor neuron, lower motor neuron, Manx syndrome
Detrusor atony: prolonged urethral obstruction, dysautonomia
Generalized weakness: neuromuscular disorders
Congenital defects: ectopic ureters
Associated with feline leukemia virus

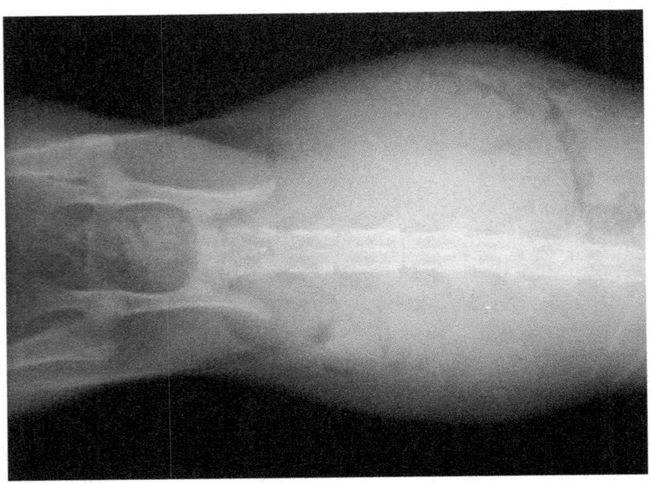

FIGURE 32-36 Ventrodorsal radiographic view of a stray cat with overflow incontinence. The cat has a Manx phenotype with a shortened tail. Note the severely distended bladder.

tube removal, UTI, inflammation around the exit site, urine leakage around the tube), although most were easily resolved.

Indwelling urethral catheters can also be used to align the urethra during healing. In one study of 11 cats with urethral rupture, placement of a urethral catheter was possible in 10 cats.[123] Catheterization was performed retrograde in five cats and normograde by cystotomy in the other five cats. The catheter was left in place for 5 to 14 days. A positive outcome was achieved in 8 of the 10 cats; two cats developed urethral strictures. Primary surgical repair of the urethra may also be performed; in one study risk of stricture formation was reduced in dogs by use of an indwelling urethral catheter during healing.[98]

In a retrospective study of 29 cats with urethral trauma, the outcome was generally good, regardless of the method of treatment. The only poor prognostic factor was the presence of multiple traumatic injuries.[4]

Incontinence

Urinary incontinence is far less common in cats than dogs. The most common causes are neurologic disorders or congenital abnormalities (Box 32-18). Urethral sphincter incompetence is the most common cause in dogs, reported to affect 5% to 10% of spayed females, but is rarely reported in spayed cats.

Micturition disorders are characterized as neurogenic or non-neurogenic. Lesions cranial to the sacral spinal cord cause upper motor neuron dysfunction. Sensory and motor function to the bladder is lost, but urethral resistance is maintained or increased. The coordination of detrusor contraction with urethral relaxation may be disrupted, leading to reflex dyssynergia. Lumbosacral invertebral disk disease affecting L7 to S1 has been associated with urinary incontinence.[74] One report describes intermittent urinary incontinence in a cat with a spinal arachnoid cyst at T11-12.[159]

Lesions of the sacral spinal cord, cauda equina, or peripheral nerves may result in lower motor neuron dysfunction. In this situation sensory and motor input to the bladder is lost, as well as urethral tone, leading to overflow incontinence. This type of micturition disorder may be seen in cats with pelvic or sacral fractures. Manx cats or cats with congenital sacral lesions may also be affected with this type of incontinence (Figure 32-36).

Non-neurogenic causes are classified according to whether the bladder is distended. A common non-neurogenic micturition disorder presenting with a distended bladder is detrusor atony, which may be seen after prolonged urethral obstruction and is discussed elsewhere in this chapter. A rare cause of detrusor atony is dysautonomia (see Chapter 27). Non-neurogenic causes of incontinence presenting with a nondistended bladder include congenital defects. Ectopic ureter has been reported in cats and results in dysfunction during the storage phase of micturition.* One or both ureters enter the lower urogenital tract at an abnormal location. Affected cats display intermittent or persistent incontinence from a young age and are at increased risk for UTI. Other urinary tract abnormalities, such as renal hypoplasia, hydronephrosis, and hydroureter may be associated with ectopic ureter. Urinary incontinence with normal bladder size has been reported in cats infected with FeLV.[13,36,96]

A thorough history is important to determine whether the problem is truly incontinence or another problem (e.g., urine spraying, inappropriate urination, polyuria, pollakiuria). Owners are often unable to distinguish among these various urinary tract signs. Urinary incontinence is characterized by intermittent or constant leakage of urine, usually small volumes. Questions to ask the owner should help establish when the problem occurs, when it was first noticed, if there is a history of trauma, whether the urine appears normal, and whether the cat urinates normally at times. Age at onset is

*References 32, 52, 62, 76, 93, 148.

important because incontinence that manifests during kittenhood is likely to be the result of a congenital defect such as ectopic ureter. Physical examination should include palpation of the bladder and an attempt to manually express urine. Ideally, the cat should be observed while voiding urine. Owners can make a video at home for the clinician to review. The residual volume of urine after voiding should not exceed 0.2 to 0.4 mL/kg.[127] If the bladder cannot be expressed manually, the urethra should be catheterized to determine if an anatomic abnormality is causing obstruction. A neurologic examination should be performed because neurogenic micturition disorders are accompanied by other neurologic deficits.

A minimum database for the diagnosis of incontinence includes CBC, serum chemistries and electrolytes, complete urinalysis, and retroviral serology. A urine culture should be performed if dictated by findings on examination of the urine sediment. Survey radiography may detect evidence of pelvic or spinal trauma. Contrast radiography (e.g., intravenous urography, positive contrast urethrography) or cystoscopy is useful for diagnosis of congenital defects such as ectopic ureter. Advanced imaging of the spinal cord (e.g., myelography, CT, MRI) may be indicated in some patients. Various procedures for urodynamic and electrodiagnostic testing of bladder and urethral function (e.g., cystometry, urethral pressure profilometry, urethral electromyography) have been described in cats and may be available at referral institutions.

Treatment for urinary incontinence relies on correction of underlying causes whenever possible, as well as pharmacologic therapy. Treatment choices for an ectopic ureter include ureter reimplantation and ureterovesicular anastomosis. Nephrectomy or ureterectomy may be required when hydronephrosis or hydroureter are present. Few drugs have been evaluated for micturition disorders in cats (see Table 32-13). Bethanecol, a parasympathomimetic drug, is indicated for detrusor atony as long as the bladder is easily expressed and no physical or functional urethral obstruction is present. Relaxation of the urethra may be accomplished with phenoxybenzamine, prazosin, diazepam, or dantrolene. Other management options include frequent manual expression and intermittent urinary catheterization. Cats with lack of urethral tone are at increased risk of UTIs, so urinalysis and urine culture should be performed periodically. Urine scalding of the perineum is common; the affected skin should be kept clean and dry and a nonzinc barrier cream applied.

References

1. Adams LG, Berent AC, Moore GE et al: Use of laser lithotripsy for fragmentation of uroliths in dogs: 73 cases (2005-2006), *J Am Vet Med Assoc* 232:1680, 2008.
2. Albasan H, Lulich JP, Osborne CA et al: Effects of storage time and temperature on pH, specific gravity, and crystal formation in urine samples from dogs and cats, *J Am Vet Med Assoc* 222:176, 2003.
3. Albasan H, Osborne C, Lulich J et al: Rate and frequency of recurrence of uroliths after an initial ammonium urate, calcium oxalate, or struvite urolith in cats, *J Am Vet Med Assoc* 235:1450, 2009.
4. Anderson RB, Aronson LR, Drobatz KJ et al: Prognostic factors for successful outcome following urethral rupture in dogs and cats, *J Am Anim Hosp Assoc* 42:136, 2006.
5. Appel SL, Lefebvre SL, Houston DM et al: Evaluation of risk factors associated with suture-nidus cystoliths in dogs and cats: 176 cases (1999-2006), *J Am Vet Med Assoc* 233:1889, 2008.
6. Aumann M, Worth LT, Drobatz KJ: Uroperitoneum in cats: 26 cases (1986-1995), *J Am Anim Hosp Assoc* 34:315, 1998.
7. Bailiff N, Westropp J, Jang S et al: Corynebacterium urealyticum urinary tract infection in dogs and cats: 7 cases (1996-2003), *J Am Vet Med Assoc* 226:1676, 2005.
8. Bailiff NL, Nelson RW, Feldman EC et al: Frequency and risk factors for urinary tract infection in cats with diabetes mellitus, *J Vet Intern Med* 20:850, 2006.
9. Bailiff NL, Westropp JL, Nelson RW et al: Evaluation of urine specific gravity and urine sediment as risk factors for urinary tract infections in cats, *Vet Clin Pathol* 37:317, 2008.
10. Bailiff NL, Westropp JL, Sykes JE et al: Comparison of urinary tract infections in cats presenting with lower urinary tract signs and cats with chronic kidney disease, hyperthyroidism, and diabetes mellitus (abstract), *J Vet Intern Med* 21:649, 2007.
11. Baines SJ, Rennie S, White RS: Prepubic urethrostomy: a long-term study in 16 cats, *Vet Surg* 30:107, 2001.
12. Barrett RE, Nobel TA: Transitional cell carcinoma of the urethra in a cat, *Cornell Vet* 66:14, 1976.
13. Barsanti JA, Downey R: Urinary incontinence in cats, *J Am Anim Hosp Assoc* 20:979, 1984.
14. Barsanti JA, Shotts EB, Crowell WA et al: Effect of therapy on susceptibility to urinary tract infection in male cats with indwelling urethral catheters, *J Vet Intern Med* 6:64, 1992.
15. Bartges J: Diagnosis of urinary tract infections, *Vet Clin North Am Small Anim Pract* 34:923, 2004.
16. Bartges JW: Revisiting bacterial urinary tract infection. In August J, editor: *Consultations in feline internal medicine*, ed 5, St Louis, 2006, Elsevier Saunders, p 439.
17. Bartges JW, Kirk C, Lane IF: Update: management of calcium oxalate uroliths in dogs and cats, *Vet Clin North Am Small Anim Pract* 34:969, 2004.
18. Bass M, Howard J, Gerber B et al: Retrospective study of indications for and outcome of perineal urethrostomy in cats, *J Small Anim Pract* 46:227, 2005.
19. Benigni L, Lamb CR, Corzo-Menendez N et al: Lymphoma affecting the urinary bladder in three dogs and a cat, *Vet Radiol Ultrasound* 47:592, 2006.
20. Bernarde A, Viguier E: Transpelvic urethrostomy in 11 cats using an ischial ostectomy, *Vet Surg* 33:246, 2004.
21. Bevan JM, Lulich JP, Albasan H et al: Comparison of laser lithotripsy and cystotomy for the management of dogs with urolithiasis, *J Am Vet Med Assoc* 234:1286, 2009.
22. Bovee KC, Reif JS, Maguire TG et al: Recurrence of feline urethral obstruction, *J Am Vet Med Assoc* 174:93, 1979.
23. Buffington C, Chew D: Diet therapy in cats with lower urinary tract disorders, *Vet Med* 94:626, 1999.
24. Buffington CA: External and internal influences on disease risk in cats, *J Am Vet Med Assoc* 220:994, 2002.
25. Buffington CA: Comorbidity of interstitial cystitis with other unexplained clinical conditions, *J Urol* 172:1242, 2004.
26. Buffington CA, Blaisdell JL, Binns SP, Jr., et al: Decreased urine glycosaminoglycan excretion in cats with interstitial cystitis, *J Urol* 155:1801, 1996.

27. Buffington CA, Chew DJ, Kendall MS et al: Clinical evaluation of cats with nonobstructive urinary tract diseases, *J Am Vet Med Assoc* 210:46, 1997.
28. Buffington CA, Westropp JL, Chew DJ et al: Clinical evaluation of multimodal environmental modification (MEMO) in the management of cats with idiopathic cystitis, *J Feline Med Surg* 8:261, 2006.
29. Buffington CA, Westropp JL, Chew DJ et al: Risk factors associated with clinical signs of lower urinary tract disease in indoor-housed cats, *J Am Vet Med Assoc* 228:722, 2006.
30. Buffington CAT, Chew DJ, Woodworth BE: Animal model of human disease—feline interstitial cystitis, *Comp Pathol Bull* 29:3, 1997.
31. Buffington CAT, Wolfe SA: High affinity binding sites for [(3) H] substance P in urinary bladders of cats with interstitial cystitis, *J Urol* 160:605, 1998.
32. Burbridge HM, Jones BR, Mora MT: Ectopic ureter in a male cat, *N Z Vet J* 37:123, 1989.
33. Cameron ME, Casey RA, Bradshaw JW et al: A study of environmental and behavioural factors that may be associated with feline idiopathic cystitis, *J Small Anim Pract* 45:144, 2004.
34. Cannizzo KL, McLoughlin MA, Chew DJ et al: Uroendoscopy. Evaluation of the lower urinary tract, *Vet Clin North Am Small Anim Pract* 31:789, 2001.
35. Cannon AB, Westropp JL, Ruby AL et al: Evaluation of trends in urolith composition in cats: 5,230 cases (1985-2004), *J Am Vet Med Assoc* 231:570, 2007.
36. Carmichael KP, Bienzle D, McDonnell JJ: Feline leukemia virus–associated myelopathy in cats, *Vet Pathol* 39:536, 2002.
37. Cavana P, Zanatta R, Nebbia P et al: *Corynebacterium urealyticum* urinary tract infection in a cat with urethral obstruction, *J Feline Med Surg* 10:269, 2008.
38. Chew D, Bartges JW, Adams LG et al: Randomized, placebo-controlled clinical trial of pentosan polysulfate sodium for treatment of feline interstitial (idiopathic) cystitis (abstract), *J Vet Intern Med* 23:690, 2009.
39. Chew D, Schenck P, Hardy B: Management of idiopathic hypercalcemia in cats with calcium oxalate stones, in *Proceedings. Am Coll Vet Int Med Forum* 2009.
40. Chew DJ, Buffington CA: Managing cats with nonobstructive idiopathic interstitial cystitis, *Vet Med* 104:568, 2009.
41. Chew DJ, Buffington CA, Kendall MS et al: Amitriptyline treatment for severe recurrent idiopathic cystitis in cats, *J Am Vet Med Assoc* 213:1282, 1998.
42. Clasper M: A case of interstitial cystitis and Hunner's ulcer in a domestic shorthaired cat, *N Z Vet J* 38:158, 1990.
43. Cooper ES, Owens TJ, Chew DJ et al: A protocol for managing urethral obstruction in male cats without urethral catheterization, *J Am Vet Med Assoc* 237:1261, 2010.
44. Corgozinho KB, de Souza HJ, Pereira AN et al: Catheter-induced urethral trauma in cats with urethral obstruction, *J Feline Med Surg* 9:481, 2007.
45. Cunha MGMCM, Freitas GC, Carregaro AB et al: Renal and cardiorespiratory effects of treatment with lactated Ringer's solution or physiologic saline (0.9% NaCl) solution in cats with experimentally induced urethral obstruction, *Am J Vet Res* 71:840, 2010.
46. Dean RS, Adams V. Managing feline lower urinary tract disease in first opinion practice—a survey of 431 practices, in *Proceedings. Br Small Anim Vet Assoc* 2009.
47. Drobatz KJ: Urethral obstruction in cats. In Bonagura JD, Twedt DC, editors: *Kirk's current veterinary therapy XIV*, St Louis, 2008, Saunders Elsevier, p 951.
48. Drobatz KJ, Cole SG: The influence of crystalloid type on acid–base and electrolyte status of cats with urethral obstruction, *J Vet Emerg Crit Care* 18:355, 2008.
49. Drobatz KJ, Hughes D: Concentration of ionized calcium in plasma from cats with urethral obstruction, *J Am Vet Med Assoc* 211:1392, 1997.
50. Dzyban LA, Labato MA, Ross LA et al: Peritoneal dialysis: a tool in veterinary critical care, *J Vet Emerg Crit Care* 10:91, 2000.
51. Eggertsdottir AV, Lund HS, Krontveit R et al: Bacteriuria in cats with feline lower urinary tract disease: a clinical study of 134 cases in Norway, *J Feline Med Surg* 9:458, 2007.
52. Eisele JG, Jackson J, Hager D: Ectopic ureterocele in a cat, *J Am Anim Hosp Assoc* 41:332, 2005.
53. Escolar E, Bellanato J: Analysis of feline urinary calculi and urethral plugs by infrared spectroscopy and scanning electron microscopy, *Vet Rec* 152:625, 2003.
54. Essman SC: Contrast cystography, *Clin Tech Small Anim Pract* 20:46, 2005.
55. Francis BJ, Wells RJ, Rao S et al: Retrospective study to characterize post-obstructive diuresis in cats with urethral obstruction, *J Feline Med Surg* 12:606, 2010.
56. Freitag T, Squires RA, Schmid J et al: Antibiotic sensitivity profiles do not reliably distinguish relapsing or persisting infections from reinfections in cats with chronic renal failure and multiple diagnoses of Escherichia coli urinary tract infection, *J Vet Intern Med* 20:245, 2006.
57. Gannon K, Moses L: Uroabdomen in dogs and cats, *Comp Contin Edu Pract Vet* 24:604, 2002.
58. Gao X, Buffington CA, Au JL: Effect of interstitial cystitis on drug absorption from urinary bladder, *J Pharmacol Exp Ther* 271:818, 1994.
59. Geigy CA, Dandrieux J, Miclard J et al: Extranodal B-cell lymphoma in the urinary bladder with cytological evidence of concurrent involvement of the gall bladder in a cat, *J Small Anim Pract* 51:280, 2010.
60. Gerber B, Boretti FS, Kley S et al: Evaluation of clinical signs and causes of lower urinary tract disease in European cats, *J Small Anim Pract* 46:571, 2005.
61. Gerber B, Eichenberger S, Reusch CE: Guarded long-term prognosis in male cats with urethral obstruction, *J Feline Med Surg* 10:16, 2008.
62. Ghantous SN, Crawford J: Double ureters with ureteral ectopia in a domestic shorthair cat, *J Am Anim Hosp Assoc* 42:462, 2006.
63. Gilson SD, Stone EA: Surgically induced tumor seeding in eight dogs and two cats, *J Am Vet Med Assoc* 196:1811, 1990.
64. Grant DC: Effect of water source on intake and urine concentration in healthy cats, *J Feline Med Surg* 12:431, 2010.
65. Grant DC, Werre SR, Gevedon ML: Holmium: YAG laser lithotripsy for urolithiasis in dogs, *J Vet Intern Med* 22:534, 2008.
66. Griffin DW, Gregory CR: Prevalence of bacterial urinary tract infection after perineal urethrostomy in cats, *J Am Vet Med Assoc* 200:681, 1992.
67. Griffith C, Steigerwald E, Buffington C: Effects of a synthetic facial pheromone on behavior of cats, *J Am Vet Med Assoc* 217:1154, 2000.
68. Guidi G, Cerri D, Ebani VV et al: Survey on bacterial isolates from cats with urinary tract infections and their in vitro sensitivity in Italy, *Rev Med Vet* 154:27, 2003.
69. Gunn-Moore D: Feline lower urinary tract disease, *J Feline Med Surg* 5:133, 2003.
70. Gunn-Moore D, Cameron M: A pilot study using synthetic feline facial pheromone for the management of feline idiopathic cystitis, *J Feline Med Surg* 6:133, 2004.
71. Gunn-Moore D, Shenoy C: Oral glucosamine and the management of feline idiopathic cystitis, *J Feline Med Surg* 6:219, 2004.
72. Gupta K, Chou MY, Howell A et al: Cranberry products inhibit adherence of p-fimbriated Escherichia coli to primary cultured bladder and vaginal epithelial cells, *J Urol* 177:2357, 2007.
73. Hanno PM: Interstitial cystitis—epidemiology, diagnostic criteria, clinical markers, *Rev Urol* 4 Suppl 1:S3, 2002.

74. Harris JE, Dhupa S: Lumbosacral intervertebral disk disease in six cats, *J Am Anim Hosp Assoc* 44:109, 2008.
75. Hezel A, Bartges JW, Kirk CA et al: Influence of hydrochlorothiazide on urinary calcium oxalate relative supersaturation in healthy young adult female domestic shorthaired cats, *Vet Ther* 8:247, 2007.
76. Holt P, Gibbs C: Congenital urinary incontinence in cats: a review of 19 cases, *Vet Rec* 130:437, 1992.
77. Houston D, Moore A, Favrin M et al: Feline urethral plugs and bladder uroliths: a review of 5484 submissions 1998-2003, *Can Vet J* 44:974, 2003.
78. Houston DM, Moore AEP: Canine and feline urolithiasis: examination of over 50,000 urolith submissions to the Canadian Veterinary Urolith Centre from 1998 to 2008, *Can Vet J* 50:1263, 2009.
79. Houston DM, Rinkardt NE, Hilton J: Evaluation of the efficacy of a commercial diet in the dissolution of feline struvite bladder uroliths, *Vet Ther* 5:187, 2004.
80. Hugonnard M, Dernis J, Vialard J et al: Evaluation of catheter-induced urinary tract infections in feline obstructive lower urinary tract disease (LUTD): a prospective study of 13 cats (abstract), *J Vet Intern Med* 22:1464, 2008.
81. Jepson RG, Craig JC: Cranberries for preventing urinary tract infection, *Cochrane database Syst Rev* Jan 23:CD001321, 2008.
82. Jillings E, O'Connell A, Forsyth S et al: Comparative clinical evaluation of BD Vacutainer Plus Urinalysis Preservative Tube and plastic tube for urinalysis in dogs and cats (abstract), *J Vet Intern Med* 24:769, 2010.
83. Jin Y, Lin D: Fungal urinary tract infections in the dog and cat: a retrospective study (2001-2004), *J Am Anim Hosp Assoc* 41:373, 2005.
84. Jones BR, Sanson RL, Morris RS: Elucidating the risk factors of feline lower urinary tract disease, *N Z Vet J* 45:100, 1997.
85. Kalkstein T, Kruger J, Osborne C: Feline idiopathic lower urinary tract disease. Part 1. Clinical manifestations, *Comp Contin Educ Pract Vet* 21:15, 1999.
86. Kirk C, Ling G, Franti C et al: Evaluation of factors associated with development of calcium oxalate urolithiasis in cats, *J Am Vet Med Assoc* 207:1429, 1995.
87. Kirsch M: Incidence of bacterial cystitis in recently diagnosed diabetic dogs and cats. Retrospective study 1990-1996, *Tierarztl Prax Ausg K Klientiere Heimtiere* 26:32, 1998.
88. Kirschvink N, Lhoest E, Leemans J et al: Effects of feeding frequency on water intake in cats (abstract), *J Vet Intern Med* 19:476, 2005.
89. Kraijer M, Fink-Gremmels J, Nickel R: The short-term clinical efficacy of amitriptyline in the management of idiopathic feline lower urinary tract disease: a controlled clinical study, *J Feline Med Surg* 5:191, 2003.
90. Kruger J, Conway T, Kaneene J et al: Randomized controlled trial of the efficacy of short-term amitriptyline administration for treatment of acute-nonobstructive, idiopathic lower urinary tract disease in cats, *J Am Vet Med Assoc* 222:749, 2003.
91. Kruger JM, Osborne CA, Goyal SM et al: Clinical evaluation of cats with lower urinary tract disease, *J Am Vet Med Assoc* 199:211, 1991.
92. Kruger JM, Osborne CA, Lulich JP: Changing paradigms of feline idiopathic cystitis, *Vet Clin North Am Small Anim Pract* 39:15, 2009.
93. Kuzma AB, Holmberg DL: Ectopic ureter in a cat, *Can Vet J* 29:59, 1988.
94. Langston C, Gisselman K, Palma D et al: Diagnosis of urolithiasis, *Comp Contin Educ Pract Vet* 30:447, 2008.
95. Langston C, Gisselman K, Palma D et al: Methods of urolith removal, *Compend Contin Educ Vet* 32, 2010.
96. Lappin MR, Barsanti JA: Urinary incontinence secondary to idiopathic detrusor instability: cystometrographic diagnosis and pharmacologic management in two dogs and a cat, *J Am Vet Med Assoc* 191:1439, 1987.
97. Lavelle JP, Meyers SA, Ruiz WG et al: Urothelial pathophysiological changes in feline interstitial cystitis: a human model, *Am J Physiol Renal Physiol* 278:F540, 2000.
98. Layton CE, Ferguson HR, Cook JE et al: Intrapelvic urethral anastomosis. A comparison of three techniques, *Vet Surg* 16:175, 1987.
99. Lee JA, Drobatz KJ: Characterization of the clinical characteristics, electrolytes, acid-base, and renal parameters in male cats with urethral obstruction, *J Vet Emerg Crit Care* 13:227, 2003.
100. Lekcharoensuk C, Lulich J, Osborne C et al: Association between patient-related factors and risk of calcium oxalate and magnesium ammonium phosphate urolithiasis in cats, *J Am Vet Med Assoc* 217:520, 2000.
101. Lekcharoensuk C, Osborne C, Lulich J: Epidemiologic study of risk factors for lower urinary tract diseases in cats, *J Am Vet Med Assoc* 218:1429, 2001.
102. Lekcharoensuk C, Osborne C, Lulich J et al: Association between dietary factors and calcium oxalate and magnesium ammonium phosphate urolithiasis in cats, *J Am Vet Med Assoc* 219:1238, 2001.
103. Lekcharoensuk C, Osborne CA, Lulich JP: Evaluation of trends in frequency of urethrostomy for treatment of urethral obstruction in cats, *J Am Vet Med Assoc* 221:502, 2002.
104. Leveille R: Ultrasonography of urinary bladder disorders, *Vet Clin North Am Small Anim Pract* 28:799, 1998.
105. Litster A, Moss S, Honnery M et al: Clinical efficacy and palatability of pradofloxacin 2.5% oral suspension for the treatment of bacterial lower urinary tract infections in cats, *J Vet Intern Med* 21:990, 2007.
106. Litster A, Moss S, Platell J et al: Occult bacterial lower urinary tract infections in cats—urinalysis and culture findings, *Vet Microbiol* 136:130, 2009.
107. Litster A, Moss SM, Honnery M et al: Prevalence of bacterial species in cats with clinical signs of lower urinary tract disease: recognition of *Staphylococcus felis* as a possible feline urinary tract pathogen, *Vet Microbiol* 121:182, 2007.
108. Lulich J, Osborne C: Cystocentesis: lessons from thirty years of clinical experience, *Clin Brief* 2:11, 2004.
109. Lulich J, Osborne C, Lekcharoensuk C et al: Effects of diet on urine composition of cats with calcium oxalate urolithiasis, *J Am Anim Hosp Assoc* 40:185, 2004.
110. Lulich JP, Osborne CA: Fungal infections of the feline lower urinary tract, *Vet Clin North Am Small Anim Pract* 26:309, 1996.
111. Lulich JP, Osborne CA: Urine culture as a test for cure: why, when, and how? *Vet Clin North Am Small Anim Pract* 34:1027, 2004.
112. Lulich JP, Osborne CA: Incomplete urolith removal: prevention, detection, and correction. In Bonagura JD, Twedt DC, editors: *Kirk's current veterinary therapy XIV*, St Louis, 2008, Saunders Elsevier, p 936.
113. Lulich JP, Osborne CA: Changing paradigms in the diagnosis of urolithiasis, *Vet Clin North Am Small Anim Pract* 39:79, 2009.
114. Lulich JP, Osborne CA, Albasan H et al: Efficacy and safety of laser lithotripsy in fragmentation of urocystoliths and urethroliths for removal in dogs, *J Am Vet Med Assoc* 234:1279, 2009.
115. Lulich JP, Osborne CA, Carlson M et al: Nonsurgical removal of urocystoliths in dogs and cats by voiding urohydropropulsion, *J Am Vet Med Assoc* 203:660, 1993.
116. Lulich JP, Osborne CA, Sanderson SL et al: Voiding urohydropropulsion. Lessons from 5 years of experience, *Vet Clin North Am Small Anim Pract* 29:283, 1999.
117. Lund E, Armstrong P, Kirk C et al: Health status and population characteristics of dogs and cats examined at private veterinary practices in the United States, *J Am Vet Med Assoc* 214:1336, 1999.
118. Markwell PJ, Buffington CA, Chew DJ et al: Clinical evaluation of commercially available urinary acidification diets in the

management of idiopathic cystitis in cats, *J Am Vet Med Assoc* 214:361, 1999.

119. Mayer-Roenne B, Goldstein RE, Erb HN: Urinary tract infections in cats with hyperthyroidism, diabetes mellitus and chronic kidney disease, *J Feline Med Surg* 9:124, 2007.
120. McClain H, Barsanti J, Bartges J: Hypercalcemia and calcium oxalate urolithiasis in cats: a report of five cases, *J Am Anim Hosp Assoc* 35:297, 1999.
121. McLoughlin MA: Surgical emergencies of the urinary tract, *Vet Clin North Am Small Anim Pract* 30:581, 2000.
122. Mealey KL, Peck KE, Bennett BS et al: Systemic absorption of amitriptyline and buspirone after oral and transdermal administration to healthy cats, *J Vet Intern Med* 18:43, 2004.
123. Meige F, Sarrau S, Autefage A: Management of traumatic urethral rupture in 11 cats using primary alignment with a urethral catheter, *Vet Comp Orthop Traumatol* 21:76, 2008.
124. Messias A, Gekeler F, Wegener A et al: Retinal safety of a new fluoroquinolone, pradofloxacin, in cats: assessment with electroretinography, *Doc Ophthalmol* 116:177, 2008.
125. Midkiff A, Chew D, Randolph J et al: Idiopathic hypercalcemia in cats, *J Vet Intern Med* 14:619, 2000.
126. Mills DS, White JC: Long-term follow up of the effect of a pheromone therapy on feline spraying behaviour, *Vet Rec* 147:746, 2000.
127. Moreau P: Neurogenic disorders of micturition in the dog and cat, *Comp Contin Educ Pract Vet* 4:12, 1982.
128. Neilson JC: The latest scoop on litter, *Vet Med* 104:140, 2009.
129. Nyland TG, Wallack ST, Wisner ER: Needle-tract implantation following us-guided fine-needle aspiration biopsy of transitional cell carcinoma of the bladder, urethra, and prostate, *Vet Radiol Ultrasound* 43:50, 2002.
130. Osborne C, Caywood D, Johnston G et al: Feline perineal urethrostomy: a potential cause of feline lower urinary tract disease, *Vet Clin North Am Small Anim Pract* 26:535, 1996.
131. Osborne C, Kruger J, Lulich J et al: Feline urologic syndrome, feline lower urinary tract disease, feline interstitial cystitis: what's in a name? *J Am Vet Med Assoc* 214:1470, 1999.
132. Osborne C, Lulich J, Thumchai R et al: Feline urolithiasis: etiology and pathophysiology, *Vet Clin North Am Small Anim Pract* 26:217, 1996.
133. Osborne C, Sanderson S, Lulich J et al: Medical management of iatrogenic rents in the wall of the urinary bladder, *Vet Clin North Am Small Anim Pract* 26:551, 1996.
134. Osborne CA, Kroll RA, Lulich JP et al: Medical management of vesicourachal diverticula in 15 cats with lower urinary tract disease, *J Small Anim Pract* 30:608, 1989.
135. Osborne CA, Kruger JM, Lulich JP et al: Prednisolone therapy of idiopathic feline lower urinary tract disease: a double-blind clinical study, *Vet Clin North Am Small Anim Pract* 26:563, 1996.
136. Osborne CA, Kruger JP, Lulich JP et al: Feline matrix-crystalline urethral plugs: a unifying hypothesis of causes, *J Small Anim Pract* 33:172, 1992.
137. Osborne CA, Lulich JP, Forrester D et al: Paradigm changes in the role of nutrition for the management of canine and feline urolithiasis, *Vet Clin North Am Small Anim Pract* 39:127, 2009.
138. Osborne CA, Lulich JP, Kruger JM et al: Medical dissolution of feline struvite urocystoliths, *J Am Vet Med Assoc* 196:1053, 1990.
139. Osborne CA, Lulich JP, Kruger JM et al: Analysis of 451,891 canine uroliths, feline uroliths, and feline urethral plugs from 1981 to 2007: perspectives from the Minnesota Urolith Center, *Vet Clin North Am Small Anim Pract* 39:183, 2009.
140. Pageat P, Gaultier E: Current research in canine and feline pheromones, *Vet Clin North Am Small Anim Pract* 33:187, 2003.
141. Palma D, Langston C, Gisselman K et al: Feline struvite urolithiasis, *Compend Contin Educ Vet* 31, 2009.
142. Passmore CA, Sherington J, Stegemann MR: Efficacy and safety of cefovecin for the treatment of urinary tract infections in cats, *J Small Anim Pract* 49:295, 2008.
143. Patronek G, Glickman L, Beck A et al: Risk factors for relinquishment of cats to an animal shelter, *J Am Vet Med Assoc* 209:582, 1996.
144. Pereira DA, Aguiar JA, Hagiwara MK et al: Changes in cat urinary glycosaminoglycans with age and in feline urologic syndrome, *Biochim Biophys Acta* 1672:1, 2004.
145. Phillips B: Bladder tumors in dogs and cats, *Comp Contin Educ Pract Vet* 21:540, 1999.
146. Phillips H, Holt DE: Surgical revision of the urethral stoma following perineal urethrostomy in 11 cats: (1998-2004), *J Am Anim Hosp Assoc* 42:218, 2006.
147. Picavet P, Detilleux J, Verschuren S et al: Analysis of 4495 canine and feline uroliths in the Benelux. A retrospective study: 1994-2004, *J Anim Physiol Anim Nutr (Berl)* 91:247, 2007.
148. Popp JP, Trebel B, Schimke E et al: [Bilateral ectopic ureter in a Persian cat—a possible cause of urinary incontinence], *Tierarztl Prax* 19:530, 1991.
149. Pressler BM, Vaden SL, Lane IF et al: *Candida* spp. urinary tract infections in 13 dogs and seven cats: predisposing factors, treatment, and outcome, *J Am Anim Hosp Assoc* 39:263, 2003.
150. Puskar M, Lemons C, Papich MG et al: Antibiotic-resistant Corynebacterium jeikeium urinary tract infection in a cat, *J Am Anim Hosp Assoc* 43:61, 2007.
151. Rawlings CA: Diagnostic rigid endoscopy: otoscopy, rhinoscopy, and cystoscopy, *Vet Clin North Am Small Anim Pract* 39:849, 2009.
152. Rawlings CA, Mahaffey MB, Barsanti JA et al: Use of laparoscopic-assisted cystoscopy for removal of urinary calculi in dogs, *J Am Vet Med Assoc* 222:759, 2003.
153. Reche Junior A, Buffington CA: Increased tyrosine hydroxylase immunoreactivity in the locus coeruleus of cats with interstitial cystitis, *J Urol* 159:1045, 1998.
154. Reine NJ, Langston CE: Urinalysis interpretation: how to squeeze out the maximum information from a small sample, *Clin Tech Small Anim Pract* 20:2, 2005.
155. Root MV, Johnston SD, Johnston GR et al: The effect of prepuberal and postpuberal gonadectomy on penile extrusion and urethral diameter in the domestic cat, *Vet Radiol Ultrasound* 37:363, 1996.
156. Rush J, Freeman L, Fenollosa N et al: Population and survival characteristics of cats with hypertrophic cardiomyopathy: 260 cases (1990-1999), *J Am Vet Med Assoc* 220:202, 2002.
157. Sapierzynski R, Malicka E, Bielecki W et al: Tumors of the urogenital system in dogs and cats. Retrospective review of 138 cases, *Pol J Vet Sci* 10:97, 2007.
158. Savary K, Price G, Vaden S: Hypercalcemia in cats: a retrospective study of 71 cases (1991-1997), *J Vet Intern Med* 14:184, 2000.
159. Schmidt MJ, Schachenmayr W, Thiel C et al: Recurrent spinal arachnoid cyst in a cat, *J Feline Med Surg* 9:509, 2007.
160. Schwartz S: Separation anxiety syndrome in cats: 136 cases (1991-2000), *J Am Vet Med Assoc* 220:1028, 2002.
161. Scrivani PV, Chew DJ, Buffington CA et al: Results of double-contrast cystography in cats with idiopathic cystitis: 45 cases (1993-1995), *J Am Vet Med Assoc* 212:1907, 1998.
162. Sculptoreanu A, de Groat WC, Tony Buffington CA et al: Abnormal excitability in capsaicin-responsive DRG neurons from cats with feline interstitial cystitis, *Exp Neurol* 193:437, 2005.
163. Seawright A, Casey R, Kiddie J et al: A case of recurrent feline idiopathic cystitis: the control of clinical signs with behavior therapy, *J Vet Behav* 3:32, 2008.
164. Segev G, Livne H, Ranen E et al: Urethral obstruction in cats: predisposing factors, clinical, clinicopathological characteristics and prognosis, *J Feline Med Surg* 13:101, 2011.
165. Sellon RK, Rottman JB, Jordan HL et al: Hypereosinophilia associated with transitional cell carcinoma in a cat, *J Am Vet Med Assoc* 201:591, 1992.

166. Smarick SD, Haskins SC, Aldrich J et al: Incidence of catheter-associated urinary tract infection among dogs in a small animal intensive care unit, *J Am Vet Med Assoc* 224:1936, 2004.
167. Specht A, Kruger JM, Fitzgerald SD et al: Histochemical and immunohistochemical light microscopic features of chronic feline idiopathic cystitis (abstract), *J Vet Intern Med* 18:416, 2004.
168. Specht AJ, Kruger JM, Fitzgerlad SD et al: Light microscopic features of chronic feline idiopathic cystitis (abstract), *J Vet Intern Med* 17:436, 2003.
169. Stella JL, Lord LK, Buffington CAT: Sickness behaviors in response to unusual external events in healthy cats and cats with feline interstitial cystitis, *J Am Vet Med Assoc* 238:67, 2011.
170. Stiffler K, Stevenson M, Cornell K et al: Clinical use of low-profile cystostomy tubes in four dogs and a cat, *J Am Vet Med Assoc* 223:325, 2003.
171. Straeter-Knowlen IM, Marks SL, Rishniw M et al: Urethral pressure response to smooth and skeletal muscle relaxants in anesthetized, adult male cats with naturally acquired urethral obstruction, *Am J Vet Res* 56:919, 1995.
172. Straeter-Knowlen IM, Marks SL, Speth RC et al: Effect of succinylcholine, diazepam, and dantrolene on the urethral pressure profile of anesthetized, healthy, sexually intact male cats, *Am J Vet Res* 55:1739, 1994.
173. Sturgess C, Hesford A, Owen H et al: An investigation into the effects of storage on the diagnosis of crystalluria in cats, *J Feline Med Surg* 3:81, 2001.
174. Takagi S, Kadosawa T, Ishiguro T et al: Urethral transitional cell carcinoma in a cat, *J Small Anim Pract* 46:504, 2005.
175. Thumchai R, Lulich J, Osborne C et al: Epizootiologic evaluation of urolithiasis in cats: 3,498 cases (1982-1992), *J Am Vet Med Assoc* 208:547, 1996.
176. Van Duijkeren E, Van Laar P, Houwers DJ: Cystocentesis is essential for reliable diagnosis of urinary tract infections in cats, *Tijdschr Diergeneeskd* 129:394, 2004.
177. Vignoli M, Rossi F, Chierici C et al: Needle tract implantation after fine needle aspiration biopsy (FNAB) of transitional cell carcinoma of the urinary bladder and adenocarcinoma of the lung, *Schweiz Arch Tierheilkd* 149:314, 2007.
178. Walker DB, Cowell RL, Clinkenbeard KD et al: Carcinoma in the urinary bladder of a cat: cytologic findings and a review of the literature, *Vet Clin Pathol* 22:103, 1993.
179. Wallius BM, Tidholm AE: Use of pentosan polysulphate in cats with idiopathic, non-obstructive lower urinary tract disease: a double-blind, randomised, placebo-controlled trial, *J Feline Med Surg* 11:409, 2009.
180. Weichselbaum RC, Feeney DA, Jessen CR et al: Urocystolith detection: comparison of survey, contrast radiographic and ultrasonographic techniques in an in vitro bladder phantom, *Vet Radiol Ultrasound* 40:386, 1999.
181. Westropp JL, Buffington CA, Chew DJ: Feline lower urinary tract diseases. In Ettinger SJ, Feldman EC, editors: *Textbook of veterinary internal medicine: diseases of the dog and cat*, ed 6, St Louis, 2005, Elsevier Saunders, p 1828.
182. Westropp JL, Kass PH, Buffington CA: Evaluation of the effects of stress in cats with idiopathic cystitis, *Am J Vet Res* 67:731, 2006.
183. Westropp JL, Kass PH, Buffington CA: In vivo evaluation of alpha(2)-adrenoceptors in cats with idiopathic cystitis, *Am J Vet Res* 68:203, 2007.
184. Westropp JL, Ruby AL, Bailiff NL et al: Dried solidified blood calculi in the urinary tract of cats, *J Vet Intern Med* 20:828, 2006.
185. Westropp JL, Tony Buffington CA: Feline idiopathic cystitis: current understanding of pathophysiology and management, *Vet Clin North Am Small Anim Pract* 34:1043, 2004.
186. Westropp JL, Welk KA, Buffington CA: Small adrenal glands in cats with feline interstitial cystitis, *J Urol* 170:2494, 2003.
187. Willeberg P: Epidemiology of naturally occurring feline urologic syndrome, *Vet Clin North Am Small Anim Pract* 14:455, 1984.
188. Williams J: Surgical management of blocked cats. Which approach and when? *J Feline Med Surg* 11:14, 2009.
189. Wilson BJ, Norris JM, Malik R et al: Susceptibility of bacteria from feline and canine urinary tract infections to doxycycline and tetracycline concentrations attained in urine four hours after oral dosage, *Aust Vet J* 84:8, 2006.
190. Wilson HM, Chun R, Larson VS et al: Clinical signs, treatments, and outcome in cats with transitional cell carcinoma of the urinary bladder: 20 cases (1990-2004), *J Am Vet Med Assoc* 231:101, 2007.
191. Wimberly HC, Lewis RM: Transitional cell carcinoma in the domestic cat, *Vet Pathol* 16:223, 1979.
192. Wynn VM, Davidson EB, Higbee RG et al: In vitro effects of pulsed holmium laser energy on canine uroliths and porcine cadaveric urethra, *Lasers Surg Med* 33:243, 2003.

SECTION V

INFECTIOUS DISEASES AND ZOONOSES

Editor: Melissa Kennedy

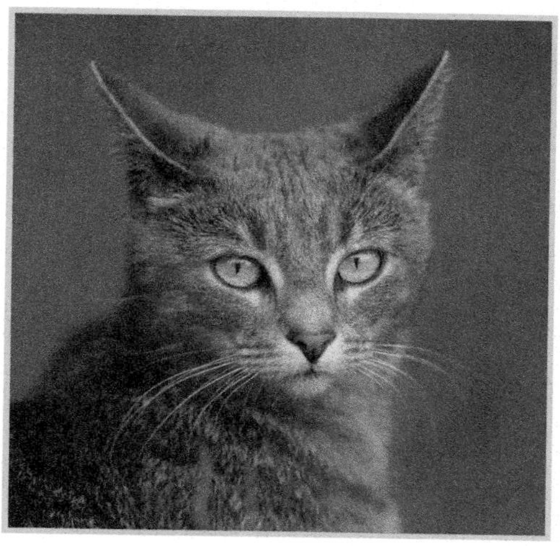

CHAPTER

33

Infectious Diseases

OUTLINE

FUNGAL AND RICKETTSIAL DISEASES

Jennifer Stokes

FUNGAL DISEASES

Systemic fungal infections are rarely documented in cats. Approximately 7 per 10,000 of the total population of animals presenting to veterinary teaching hospitals in North America are diagnosed with a systemic mycosis.[10] In most cases, dogs are the more susceptible species; the exception is cryptococcosis, which is 5 to 6 times more likely to be diagnosed in cats.[42] Cryptococcosis, histoplasmosis, coccidioidomycosis, blastomycosis, and sporotrichosis will be discussed separately, and recommendations for treatment will be described at the end of the section.

Cryptococcosis

Of the organisms causing systemic mycosis in cats, *Cryptococcus* is most commonly diagnosed. In the largest retrospective study evaluating deep mycotic infections in 571 cats, 46.1% of the infections were due to *Cryptococcus*.[10] The organism is round to ovoid in shape, thin walled with diameter of 2.5 to 8 μm (Figure 33-1).[17,20] In tissues, it is surrounded by a heteropolysaccharide capsule that varies in thickness depending on the strain and environment. The capsule provides resistance to desiccation and virulence.[20] *Cryptococcus* multiplies asexually with narrow-based budding. The infectious particle, the basidiospore, is adapted to be dispersed by air and has properties that allow it to adhere to and penetrate respiratory epithelium and cause infection.[20]

Typically, cryptococcosis in people and domestic animals is caused by one of two species: *Cryptococcus neoformans* (var. *neoformans* or var. *grubii*) or *C. gattii*.[20] Globally, *C. neoformans* var. *grubii* is the most common isolate associated with disease in people and animals. *C. neoformans* causes almost all cases in the United States and Europe.[20,31] Within the United States, the highest incidence of cryptococcosis in cats is reported in California, Florida, Virginia, and Iowa.[10] *C. gattii* most commonly causes disease in tropical and subtropical areas, including Australia, Papua New Guinea, Southeast Asia, and Central Africa; it has also been documented to cause infection in the temperate climate of the Pacific northwest, including Vancouver, Canada.[37] *C. albidus* was confirmed to cause one case of systemic disease in a cat in Japan but has not been recognized as a significant pathogen in cats.[31]

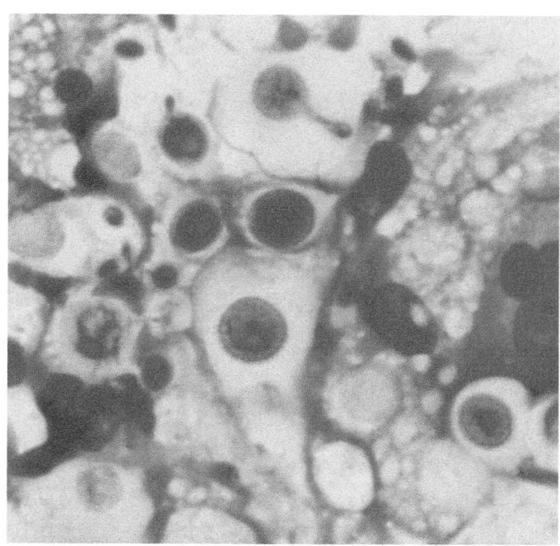

FIGURE 33-1 Cytologic diagnosis of *Cryptococcus* showing encapsulated yeast forms in a Diff Quik-stained smear. *(Courtesy Richard Malik. [Figure 61-2, B in Greene CE, editor:* Infectious diseases of the dog and cat, *ed 3, St Louis, 2006, Elsevier.])*

Cryptococcus can be isolated from a variety of substances, depending on the geographic location of the organism as well as the species.[42] *C. neoformans* is consistently found in pigeon feces and soil enriched by avian feces and less often in milk, fermenting fruit juices, air, dust, wasp nests, grass, and insects.[20,42] *C. gattii* is found in hollows of *Eucalyptus* and fig trees in Australia and some fir trees in western Canada.[20,42] Risk factors for *C. gattii* infection in pets in Vancouver include proximity to logging sites or other areas of commercial soil disruption and owners hiking or visiting a botanical garden.[14] It is viable in feces for up to 2 years in moist environments.[20] Ultraviolet light and dry conditions can decrease viability.

The exact mode of transmission is unknown, but most likely occurs by inhalation of yeast cells or basidospores.[13,20] Once inhaled, *Cryptococcus* lodges in the nasal passages and causes mycotic rhinitis; lower respiratory infection is uncommon because most organisms are larger than the alveolar diameter of 2 μm.[17] Some strains are particularly virulent and will destroy adjacent facial bones and spread locally.[20] Rarely, cryptococcosis occurs secondary to a penetrating skin wound, causing localized infection.[37]

Clinical signs depend upon location of infection. Infection usually involves the nasal cavity, skin, subcutis, central nervous system (CNS), and regional lymph nodes. Dissemination has been documented (Figure 33-2). As mycotic rhinitis of the rostral nasal cavity occurs most often, sneezing, wheezing, and unilateral or bilateral nasal discharge are common presenting complaints. Respiratory signs have been reported in 26% to 83% of cats with cryptococcosis.[12,39] In another study, 63% of 263 cats had nasal discharge, and 12.5% had cough or dyspnea.[10] Thickening and inflammation of nasal mucosa or nasal granulomas may be visible. Osteomyelitis may occur, leading to facial deformity, including broadening of the nose or swelling of adjacent tissue (Figure 33-3). If the nasopharynx is affected, clinical signs may be absent until the infection spreads through cribriform plate and causes meningitis.[38] Alternatively, cats may present dyspneic or with stertorous breathing because of obstruction by fungal granulomas. Lymph node involvement was present in 39% of 263 cats.[10] Mycotic pneumonia and hilar lymphadenomegaly because of *Cryptococcus* is rare in cats.

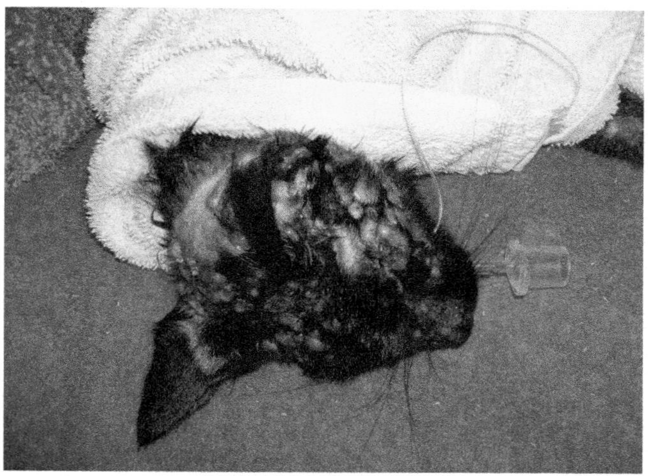

FIGURE 33-2 Disseminated *Cryptococcus* infection. *(Courtesy Richard Malik.)*

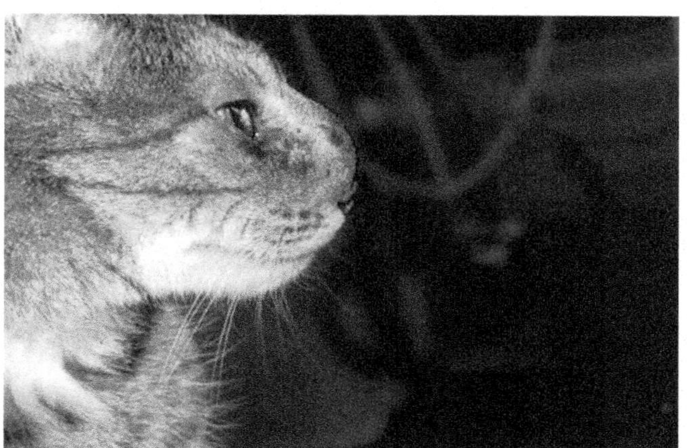

FIGURE 33-3 Cryptococcal osteomyelitis may lead to facial deformity. *(Courtesy Richard Malik.)*

Cutaneous nodules were documented in 41% of 263 cats with cryptococcosis (Figures 33-4 and 33-5).[10] Oral lesions occasionally occur in cats with *Cryptococcus* infection and may appear as diffuse ulceration of the oral mucosa of the tongue, gingiva, or palate, or as proliferative lesions.[43] Central nervous system involvement also occurs, either because of erosion of nasal infection through the cribriform plate or possibly by

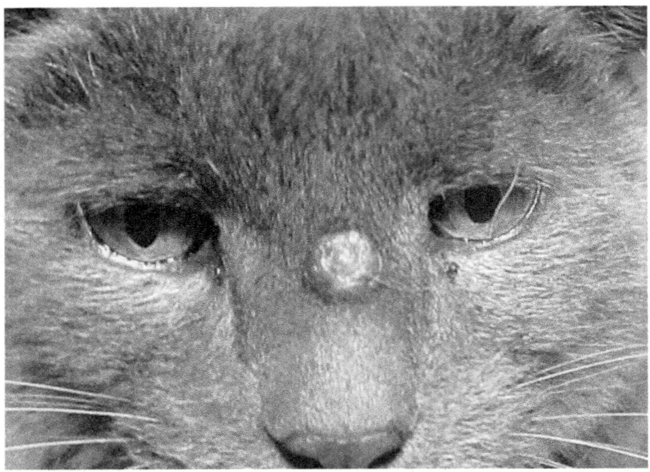

FIGURE 33-4 Cutaneous *Cryptococcus* nodule on the nasal planum. *(Courtesy Jessica Baron.)*

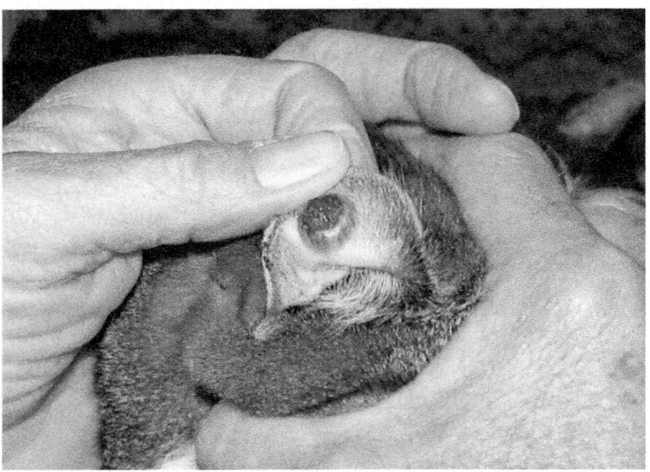

FIGURE 33-5 Cutaneous *Cryptococcus* nodule on the inside of the pinna. *(Courtesy Paige May.)*

hematogenous spread. Neurologic signs occur in 8% to 26% of cats with cryptococcosis and may manifest as blindness, pupil changes, ataxia, depression, and temperament changes.[10,12,41]

Cryptococcosis has been diagnosed in cats less than 1 month of age and in those greater than 15 years of age. The mean age at diagnosis is about 6 years, with 58% of cats being between 2 to 7 years of age.[10,17] Some, but not all studies, have shown breed predisposition, with Abyssinian, Siamese, Birman, and Ragdoll cats being overrepresented compared with domestic shorthairs.[10,17,42] Indoor as well as outdoor cats are susceptible to infection. A gender predisposition for cryptococcosis in male cats is inconsistently reported. Cryptococcosis occurs most commonly in immunocompromised people, but most studies of the infection in cats do not show an association with retrovirus infection or other causes of immunosuppression.[20]

BOX 33-1

Methods for Diagnosis of Cryptococcosis in Cats

1. Fungal culture
2. Cytology
   a. Nasal swab or wash
   b. Biopsy or aspiration samples
   c. Vitreous or subretinal fluid
3. Serology: antigen latex agglutination
   a. Serum
   b. Cerebrospinal fluid
   c. Vitreous fluid

A definitive diagnosis of cryptococcosis requires culturing the organism from infected tissue (Box 33-1). Both *C. neoformans* and *C. gattii* can be cultured from the nasal cavity of asymptomatic patients. Culture of most systemic fungal infections is laborious and poses a zoonotic hazard to laboratory staff. Culture of *Cryptococcus* on Abouraud dextrose agar may take up to 6 weeks to be evident.[17] In most cases, a presumptive diagnosis is made by cytologic evaluation. The organism may be detected from nasal swab samples, nasal washing, and nasal tissue biopsy imprint or from aspiration of other infected tissues. Rhinoscopy or advanced imaging may aid in diagnosis. If ocular involvement is present without evidence of disease elsewhere, vitreous or subretinal fluid may be aspirated for cytologic evaluation. Quik-Dip (Mercedes Medical, Sarasota, Fla.), Wright Giemsa, or new methylene blue stains enhance visualization of the thickly encapsulated, broad-based budding yeast cells. If cryptococcosis cannot be confirmed cytologically or histopathologically, then serology can be performed. The antigen latex agglutination test is highly specific and sensitive in detecting *Cryptococcus* capsular antigen in dogs. It can be performed on serum, cerebral spinal fluid, or vitreous fluid. The specificity and sensitivity has not been described in cats, but infected cats can have extremely high titers (>1:65,536).[37] Serial serologic testing can be used to assess response to treatment, and a favorable prognosis often accompanies a decrease in titer.

Overall, the prognosis for cats with cryptococcosis is good, if the disease is not severe, there is no CNS involvement, and treatment is of appropriate duration. Animals presenting with or progressing to CNS disease are 4 times more likely to die than those without CNS signs.[12] In one retrospective study of 59 cats from Sydney, Australia with cryptococcosis, 76% were successfully treated.[41] Determining the ideal duration for treatment can be difficult. It is typically recommended to treat for at least 1 month past clinical resolution, and sometimes therapy is needed for 9 months or longer. If fungal granulomas are present in the nasal cavity or nasopharynx, debulking the abnormal tissue may aid in treatment. Itraconazole is the drug most commonly used for treatment of feline cryptococcosis, but other azoles as well as amphotericin B have been used successfully.[37]

There is no evidence that cryptococcosis is either contagious or zoonotic, but pets may act as sentinels for people.

Histoplasmosis

The second most common cause of systemic mycosis in cats is due to *Histoplasma*; 16.7% of 571 cats diagnosed with systemic fungal disease had histoplasmosis in one study.[10] *Histoplasma* has a global distribution. Pathogenic species include *H. capsulatum, H. duboisii*, and *H. farciminosum*. *H. capsulatum* causes infection in the continental United States, and *H. duboisii* is the causative agent in Africa. The organism thrives in warm (22° C to 29° C) and moist environments, particularly in temperate and subtropical areas.[22] *H. capsulatum* is most commonly isolated from moist, nitrogen-rich soil containing bird or bat feces.[20,32] In the environment, the organism exists as a mycelial form and within a host as a yeast.

H. capsulatum is most commonly diagnosed in North and South America, India, and southeastern Asia, although it has been documented in every continent with the exception of Antarctica.[22] *H. capsulatum* is endemic in the U.S. Midwest, South and areas along the Ohio, Mississippi, and Missouri rivers. It is sporadically reported elsewhere, including California, Ontario, Canada, and Australia.[7] Although reported in 31 states within the United States, the highest incidence is in Oklahoma, Texas, Virginia, and Louisianna.[10,22]

The life cycle of *H. capsulatum* is similar to other dimorphic fungi. The mycelial stage living in soil is resistant to environmental damage. It sporulates at temperatures around 22° C, and the spores are known as microconidia or macroconidia.[22] Lower respiratory infection most likely occurs because of inhalation of infective microconidia. Some cases of histoplasmosis are isolated to the gastrointestinal (GI) system, but an oral route of infection has not been confirmed.[22] At body temperature (37° C), the inhaled organism transforms into the yeast phase within the lungs, is phagocytized, and replicates intracellularly. Infection may be limited to the lower respiratory system and regional lymph nodes, or yeast-laden macrophages may disseminate the organism via lymphatics or hematogenously. In most patients, cell-mediated immunity is effective in controlling the infection; however, if a large number of organisms are inhaled or if immune compromise exists, severe disease may occur.[22] In patients with an effective immune system, dormant infections may be reactivated because of immunocompromise.

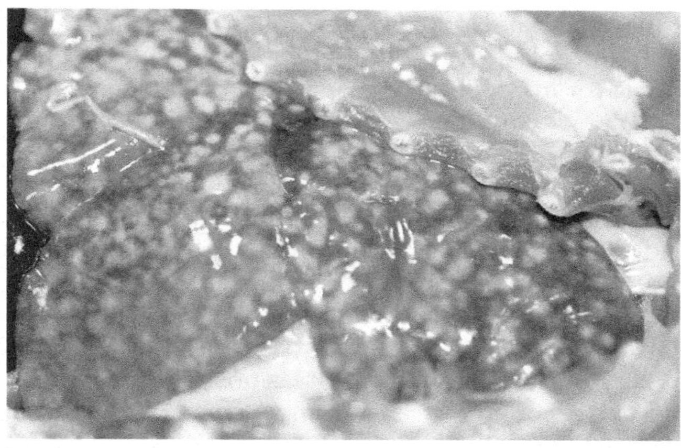

FIGURE 33-6 Histoplasmosis pneumonia in a cat. *(Courtesy Eric Snook.)*

Unlike other systemic fungal infections, histoplasmosis occurs equally in dogs and cats.[32] Histoplasmosis has been diagnosed in cats less than 8 weeks of age to more than 15 years, and it occurs most commonly in cats less than 4 years of age.[10,32] The mean age at time of diagnosis is 3.9 years.[7] Both outdoor and exclusively indoor cats are at risk of infection.[10,30] No consistent gender bias is reported. Breed predilection is not consistently described, but Persian cats were predisposed in one report.[10] Although one retrospective study found that concurrent infection with feline leukemia virus (FeLV) was present in 15% of 96 cats with histoplasmosis, in most reports co-infection with feline retroviruses is uncommon.[10,29,30,32]

Although infection with *H. capsulatum* may be asymptomatic and self-limiting, dissemination is common in cats and may occur in up to 95% of cases, despite a lack of systemic clinical signs.[10] The organs most commonly affected include the lungs (Figure 33-6), GI tract, lymph nodes, spleen, liver, bone marrow, eyes, and adrenal glands. The incubation period is approximately 12 to 16 days in people and dogs and is likely the same for cats.[10,22] Clinical signs are often present for 2 to 3 months prior to presentation.[29] In 96 cats with histoplasmosis, the most common clinical signs, which occurred in 67% of infected cats, were nonspecific and included lethargy, weakness, and fever.[10] Respiratory signs were present in 39% of the cats and ocular in 24%. When pulmonary involvement is present, clinical signs may include abnormal lung sounds, tachypnea, or dyspnea. Ocular abnormalities included blepharitis, conjunctivitis, anterior uveitis, chorioretinitis, optic neuritis, and retinal detachment.[10,22] Lymphadenopathy and hepatosplenomegaly can occur with dissemination. If present, bone marrow involvement may lead to cytopathies.[32] Uncommon sites for infection include skin, bone, CNS, and oral cavity.[33,53] Specific GI signs occur less commonly in cats than in dogs. Oral infection may manifest as ulcerated tissue or proliferative lesions on the gingiva or palate.[33]

Routine laboratory tests are often abnormal in cats with histoplasmosis, but findings are not pathognomonic for infection. Anemia, thrombocytopenia, leukopenia, or pancytopenia may be present. The most common hematologic abnormality is normocytic, normochromic, nonregenerative anemia, which may be due to chronic inflammation, bone marrow involvement, and GI blood loss. Neutrophilic leukocytosis with monocytosis can also be diagnosed, or the leukogram may be normal. The organism can be seen in phagocytic cells on blood smears, and in a study of 56 cases, it was evident in 20% of the cats with histoplasmosis.[10] Other abnormalities reported include thrombocytopenia and severe pancytopenia.[22] Biochemical abnormalities have included hypoalbuminemia, hyperglobulinemia, elevated liver enzyme activity, hyperbilirubinemia, and hypercalcemia.[32] In one report, radiographic abnormalities were present in over 87% of cats with histoplasmosis, and the most common finding was a diffuse or nodular interstitial pattern in the lungs.[10] Hilar lymphadenomegaly was rare. Abdominal fluid, hepatomegaly, or splenomegaly may be present.

Definitive diagnosis of histoplasmosis requires identification of the organism cytologically or histologically. *Histoplasma* is usually present in clusters within cells of the mononuclear phagocyte system in the infected organs. When stained with Wright or Giemsa, *H. capsulatum* appears as a small (2 to 4 μm) round body with a basophilic center and lighter halo caused by shrinkage of the yeast during the staining process.[22] Diff-Quik can also be used to stain cytologic preparations. In cats, the organism is most commonly found by fine-needle aspirate cytology of infected organs, including lung, lymph node, dermal lesions, spleen, liver, or bone marrow. Organisms may be seen on evaluation of fluid collected by endotracheal wash, bronchoalveolar lavage, thoracocentesis, or cerebrospinal tap. Histopathologic abnormalities include granulomatous inflammation, but *H. capsulatum* may be difficult to see with routine staining. If fungal disease is suspected then special stains, such as periodic acid–Schiff (PAS), Gomoris methenamine silver, or Gidley fungal stain, should be requested. Immunostaining has been used to diagnose histoplasmosis in skin biopsy samples.[22]

Diagnosis of histoplasmosis by culture of the organism is rarely performed because of the zoonotic risk for laboratory personnel; it can also take up to 4 weeks for results to be available. Serologic testing is unreliable and false negatives are common in animals with clinical disease, and false-positive results may occur in previously infected patients with residual antibodies.[22] MiraVista Diagnostics (Indianapolis, Ind., www.miravistalabs.com) has developed a test that can detect *H. capsulatum* antigens in urine, serum, or cerebrospinal fluid (CSF); this has been used to diagnose histoplasmosis in people. Sensitivity is increased if both urine and serum is tested. The test can be used to monitor response to treatment; titers decrease with effective therapy and increase with disease relapse. In people, cross reactivity occurs with blastomycosis, coccidioidomycosis, and penicilliosis. At the author's institution, the urine antigen test has been used for monitoring purposes in dogs confirmed to have histoplasmosis, based on cytologic diagnosis. The test is likely applicable in cats, but more research needs to be performed to determine sensitivity and specificity.

Although histoplasmosis may be self-limiting when isolated to the lungs, treatment is recommended to avoid dissemination. As with most systemic fungal diseases diagnosed in cats, itraconazole is the medication of choice. Prognosis varies depending on the extent of disease. Of 56 cats in which the outcome was known in one study, 68% died or were euthanized.[10]

Prevention consists of avoiding exposure to soils likely to harbor *H. capsulatum*, including those contaminated by bird or bat feces. Histoplasmosis is not zoonotic.

Coccidioidomycosis

Coccidioidomycosis was diagnosed in 9.2% of cats with systemic fungal disease in one study.[10] *Coccidioides* is a dimorphic fungus that grows in soil as a mycelium. Mycelia germinate to form thick-walled, barrel-shaped, rectangular, multinucleate arthroconidia that are 2 to 4 μm wide and 3 to 10 μm in length.[24] Mycelium can persist in soil indefinitely and arthroconidia are environmentally resistant. When soil containing *Coccidioides* is disturbed, arthroconidia are released and dispersed.[24] They can germinate and produce new hyphae or serve as a source of infection.

Coccidioides is found in a specific ecologic location, known as the Lower Sonoran life zone.[24] This area includes the southwestern United States, Mexico, and Central and South America.[21] It is also known as valley fever. These regions have sandy, alkaline soil, and high temperatures, with the summer mean greater than 26.6° C and the winter mean 4° C to 12° C.[24] In addition, elevation and annual rainfall are low. During prolonged periods of dry, hot weather, *Coccidioides* survives below the soil as deep as 20 cm.[24] After rainfall, the organism replicates near the soil surface and releases large numbers of infective arthroconidia that disseminate.[24]

Infection is most common when the soil is dry and is disturbed, such as by dust storms, earthquakes, or crop harvesting, or following the rainy season.[21] *C. immitis* is the species found in California in the San Joaquin Valley, while *C. posadasii* is found in all other endemic areas.[24] Disease is most common in California, Arizona, and southwestern Texas and less commonly diagnosed in New Mexico, Nevada, and Utah. Infections outside of endemic areas are sporadic. In such cases, the individual may have traveled to an endemic area and then had activation of dormant organisms years later.[24] In people, most infections are asymptomatic, with only 40% of people developing clinical signs.[24] This may be true in other species.

Coccidioidomycosis occurs primarily following inhalation of infective arthrospores, and less than 10 organisms can cause infection.[21] Uncommonly, infection will occur following inoculation of the organism into the skin. There is one case report of a veterinary assistant developing coccidioidomycosis after being bitten by an infected cat.[16] Rarely, there have been suspect cases of dogs becoming infected after contacting fomites contaminated with arthrospheres.[21]

Once inhaled and spread to the alveoli, arthroconidia convert to spherules because of the higher temperature and increased carbon dioxide level.[21,24] Once the spherule matures, it eventually ruptures, releasing up to 300 endospores.[24] After inhalation, it takes approximately 3 days for the endospores to form, but clinical signs usually do not occur for 2 weeks.[21] It is thought that endospores are able to disseminate through blood and lymphatics to distant sites, and cats with disseminated disease may have no infection in the respiratory system.[49] When skin inoculation occurs, infection may be limited to the dermis or subcutis.

As is typical of fungal disease, cell-mediated immunity is much more effective in resolving infection with *Coccidioides* than is humoral immunity. Antibody formation typically occurs but is more useful as a diagnostic aid than in fighting the infection. Although people who recover from coccidioidomycosis are considered immune to reinfection, recurrence in dogs and cats is common. It is not known if this is due to premature discontinuation of treatment or to a lack of long-term immunity to *Coccidioides*.[21]

Clinical disease varies from subclinical to fatal; it is not known why some infected animals have self-limiting disease and others die despite treatment. Evaluation of necropsy reports from 1995 to 2005 from the Arizona Veterinary Diagnostic Laboratory found that in fatal coccidioidomycosis cases, 25% of the animals involved were cats. It is unclear if this finding is due to more severe disease in cats or if coccidioidomycosis is underdiagnosed antemortem in cats. Infection is most commonly reported in middle-aged cats, with no breed predisposition. There is also no correlation between coccidioidomycosis and feline retrovirus infection.[21]

Specific clinical manifestations depend on the site of infection and are extremely varied, making early diagnosis a challenge. *Coccidioides* appears to be able to infect most tissues. Fever is commonly present at diagnosis, as well as nonspecific signs, including lethargy, anorexia, and weight loss. Respiratory signs are uncommonly recognized, and lung and bone involvement occurs less frequently in cats than in dogs. Ocular lesions, including chorioretinitis and anterior uveitis, occur with similar frequency among cats and dogs.[24] In cats, approximately 50% of cases are disseminated.[21] Subclinical infection may occur in up to 70% of dogs; it is unknown if this is true in cats.[21]

Coughing is uncommon, but 25% of cats may present dyspneic. The CNS can be infected, and granulomatous mass lesions in the brain are more common than fungal meningitis. Ocular signs may include anterior uveitis, subretinal granulomas, retinal detachment, and blindness. There is also a report of cats that presented for periocular swellings with systemic signs, including weight loss, unkempt hair coat, and lethargy. Clinical ophthalmologic abnormalities were bilateral in each cat and included hyperemia, conjunctival masses, fluid-filled periorbital swellings, granulomatous chorioretinitis, nonhematogenous retinal detachments, and anterior uveitis.[51] Cats were diagnosed with coccidioidomycosis using a combination of clinical findings, serology, and, in two cases, visualization of *Coccidioides* spherules by either aspiration cytology or biopsy. Active anterior uveitis and periocular swelling resolved with treatment. Chorioretinal granulomas, although persistent, significantly decreased in size.[51]

Infection is often limited to the lungs and perihilar lymph nodes, although dissemination of the organism through the blood and lymphatics can occur.[21] When dissemination occurs, the skin is the most frequent site of infection. In 15 cats with coccidioidomycosis that underwent post-mortem evaluation, all had multiorgan involvement.[21] Nonhealing cutaneous lesions, including abscesses, dermatitis, chronic draining tracts, and ulcerations are the most common clinical manifestations.[21] Cutaneous and subcutaneous lesions were reported in 56% of cats in one series of 48 cases.[49]

In infected cats, laboratory abnormalities have included nonregenerative anemia, neutrophilic leukocytosis with left shift, monocytosis, eosinophilia, hypoalbuminemia, and hyperglobulinemia. Sensitivity and specificity of serology in cats is unknown. In the report of 48 cats with coccidioidomycosis, of the 39 cats undergoing testing, all were seropositive at some point during their illness.

Cytologic confirmation may be made by evaluation of aspirates of affected lymph nodes, skin lesions, or lungs. The organism can be seen on unstained slides and appears as a large (10 to 80 μm) round, double-walled structure containing endospores.[24] Multiple biopsy samples may need to be collected and evaluated in order to see the organism histologically. Although spherules can be detected with routine hematoxylin and eosin stain (H&E), they are easier to see when PAS or Grocott-Gomoris methenamine silver stain is used. Commercial laboratories that practice biosafety precautions can isolate *Coccidioides* on culture. The mycelia that grow on culture media are highly infectious. Serologic testing using tube precipitin and complement fixation techniques were useful in 48 cats with coccidioidomycosis.[24]

Itraconazole is typically used for treatment of feline coccidioidomycosis. Of 53 cats diagnosed with coccidioidomycosis, 67% survived with treatment.[10]

Blastomycosis

Blastomyces dermatitidis is the saprophytic dimorphic fungus that causes blastomycosis. It exists in a mycelial form and reproduces sexually, producing infective spores. At body temperature, the spores transform into yeast and replicate asexually. Budding yeasts are 5 to 20 μm in diameter and have a thick, refractile, double-contoured cell wall.[36] Dogs and people are the species infected most commonly, but blastomycosis has been reported in other animals, including bats, horses, sea lions, wolves, ferrets, and nondomestic cats.[19,36] It is rarely reported in domestic cats.

The most likely reservoir for *Blastomyces* is soil. Because normal soil organisms destroy most *Blastomyces* organisms, specific environmental conditions are needed for *Blastomyces* to survive. *Blastomyces* thrives in a sandy, acidic soil near water. It has also been isolated from decaying wood and vegetation, animal excrement, a beaver dam, and animal waste.[19,36] Even in endemic areas, blastomycosis occurs in geographically restricted foci. Living near water is a risk factor for blastomycosis in dogs. In people, disturbing soil is associated with infection, and precipitation may facilitate the release of infective spores. Most people and dogs are likely exposed to *Blastomyces* on their own property, because there has been documentation of repeated cases occurring at the same location despite occupation by multiple families.[3] The source of infection in cats is unclear. Many reported cases of feline blastomycosis have occurred in strictly indoor cats. One study analyzed 60 environmental samples obtained from four homes in which blastomycosis was diagnosed in cats, and all were negative for *B. dermatitidis*.[3,19]

During a 10-year period, eight cases of blastomycosis were diagnosed in cats at the veterinary teaching hospital (VTH) in Illinois, while during a span of 11 years, 5 cats were diagnosed with blastomycosis at the VTH in Tennessee.[3,19] The prevalence of canine blastomycosis in Tennessee between 1979 and 1989 was 1.2%, compared with less than 0.1% in cats.[4] Of 571 cats diagnosed with systemic mycosis, 41 (7.1%) were infected with *B. dermatitidis*.[10] *B dermatitidis* mainly causes disease in the United States and Canada, but is endemic in Africa and India and has been documented in Europe and South America.[6] Within North America, endemic areas include the Mississippi, Missouri, and Ohio river valleys; the mid-Atlantic states; and the Canadian provinces of Manitoba, Ontario, and Quebec.[36] Blastomycosis has also been diagnosed in New York, Wyoming, South Dakota, Colorado, and Saskatchewan.[6,27,36] In a retrospective review of 41 cats diagnosed with blastomycosis, most cases occurred in Oklahoma, Tennessee, and Wisconsin.[10] Risk factors and the epidemiology of blastomycosis are unknown in cats because of its rarity.

Infection occurs most commonly by inhalation of infective spores, which establish infection within the lungs. Direct inoculation of the organism through skin puncture may occur. Blastomycosis is thought to disseminate through lymphatics and hematogenously. There is great variation in host response to infection, because dogs are 10 times more likely to develop blastomycosis than people; blastomycosis is rarer in cats. No seasonality has been reported in infected cats.

There are so few cases described in the literature that it is not possible to determine predisposing factors. Many reports provide conflicting data. Most cases described in the literature were diagnosed at necropsy.[19] Males may be slightly predisposed; one study reported that 69% of 36 infected cats were male.[3] Breeds described as being predisposed include Siamese, Abyssinian, and the Havana Brown, but this is not supported in all reports.[10,19] Affected cats have ranged in age from 6 months to 18 years.[4] The typical age of infected cats varies among publications: In three studies, 75% were less than 4 years of age, 42% were less than 4 years, and 87% of cats were greater than 7 years.[19] Duration of clinical signs prior to diagnosis has ranged from 3 days to 7 months.[10,19] A history of immunosuppression is rarely present; 10% of 41 cats with blastomycosis were FeLV positive, none were FIV positive, and one was positive for feline infectious peritonitis (FIP).[10]

Based on thoracic radiographs and necropsy data, infection in cats occurs most commonly in the lung, even though respiratory signs may be absent (Figure 33-7).[19] *B. dermatitidis* has been documented in lymph node, kidney, eye, CNS, skin, GI tract, pleura, peritoneum,

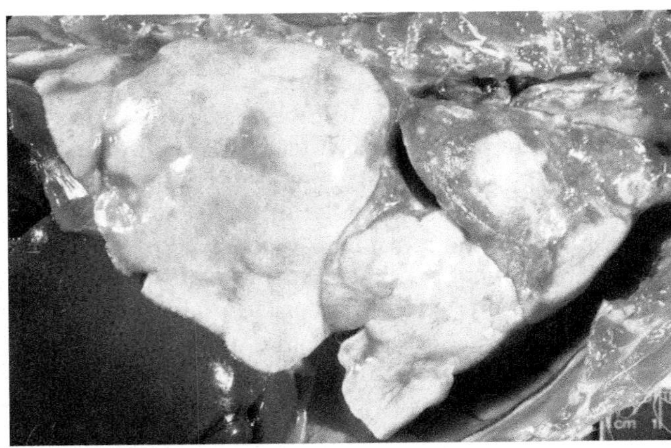

FIGURE 33-7 Pulmonary blastomycosis in a cat. *(Courtesy Jennifer Stokes.)*

heart, liver spleen, trachea, and adrenal glands.[19,36] Infection is frequently disseminated. Clinical signs vary depending on the site of infection. The most commonly reported clinical signs in cats with blastomycosis vary among publications, but dyspnea, lethargy, weight loss, and fever are frequently present.[19] Other reported respiratory signs have included cough, tachypnea, sneezing, and increased bronchovesicular signs.[19] Central nervous system, ocular, and dermatologic involvement may manifest clinically as well. Ocular changes described include retinal granulomas and detachment, chemosis, corneal edema, and uveititis.[6,7,19] Skin lesions may be draining tracts or nonulcerated dermal masses and range from a few millimeters to a few centimeters in diameter.[19]

Diagnosis of blastomycosis can be difficult in cats, particularly because there are no pathognomonic clinical manifestations. Hematologic and biochemical changes are neither specific nor consistent among infected cats but may include anemia, leukopenia or leukocytosis, monocytosis, hyperglobulinemia, hypoalbuminemia, and hypercalcemia.[19] Radiographic changes may include poorly defined soft tissue opacities with nodules or masses or alveolar lung consolidation and pleural effusion.[10,19]

Definitive diagnosis is made by cytologic or histologic identification of *B. dermatitidis*. Pyogranulomatous inflammation is commonly seen associated with large numbers of broad-based budding yeasts. Diagnosis has occurred by cytologic exam of fine-needle aspirate samples of infected skin, draining tracts, lymph nodes, and lung. Bronchoalveolar lavage can also be performed to diagnose pulmonary blastomycosis.[19] In dogs, the sensitivity and specificity of the agar-gel immunodiffusion test (AGID) was reported as 91% and 96%, respectively. The usefulness of AGID testing for blastomycosis in cats is unknown. Of three cats with blastomycosis tested using AGID, one was positive.[10] MiraVista Diagnostics offers an antigen test for *B. dermatitidis* that has been validated in dogs and has the greatest sensitivity when urine is tested.[50] It is unknown if this test is sensitive or specific in cats.

Currently, treatment with itraconazole is recommended.[6] The prognosis is guarded to poor. Of four cats treated for blastomycosis, three died within 12 days of diagnosis.[3]

Sporotrichosis

Sporotrichosis is a mycotic disease of humans and many animal species caused by the dimorphic fungus *Sporothrix schenckii,* which is endemic worldwide. Zoonotic transmission of *S. schenckii* between cats and people has been documented and is considered an emerging zoonosis.[11,45,48,54,55] *S. schenckii* survives in the environment, typically in decaying vegetation, and people and animals are infected by wound contamination or penetrating foreign bodies. The organism becomes pathogenic because of its dimorphic abilities. After entering the skin through a puncture, bite, or scratch, the fungus converts to a yeast phase. The organism has also been isolated from the nails and oral cavity of cats and presumably can be inoculated into bites, scratches, or puncture wounds.[47,48] Three clinical syndromes of sporotrichosis are known in cats:

1. Localized cutaneous
2. Lymphocutaneous
3. Multifocal disseminated

The localized and lymphocutaneous forms are the most common. Cutaneous lesions are most commonly found on the face, nasal planum (Figure 33-8), tail base, and legs and may be solitary or multiple. Lesions appear after an incubation period of about 1 month and first appear as draining puncture wounds mimicking bacterial fight-wound abscesses or cellulitis. Treatment with antibiotics does not result in resolution. The lesions may then become ulcerated and form large, crusted areas. The localized form may progress to the lymphocutaneous form, especially if not treated. In the lymphocutaneous form, cutaneous nodules may progress to draining ulcers of the skin, subcutis, and lymph nodes. The disseminated form is primarily found in the liver and lungs, but involvement of other organs has been documented.

Outbreaks of sporotrichosis are thought to be rare. In a large series of 347 cats with naturally acquired sporotrichosis in an epidemic in Rio de Janeiro, the median age was 2 years, and cats of male gender predominated.[46] Most cats were infected through fight wounds, and multiple skin lesions were common. Most lesions were on the head. The skin lesions were varied and included small crusted lesions, subcutaneous nodules that progressed to draining lesions and ulcers, extensive

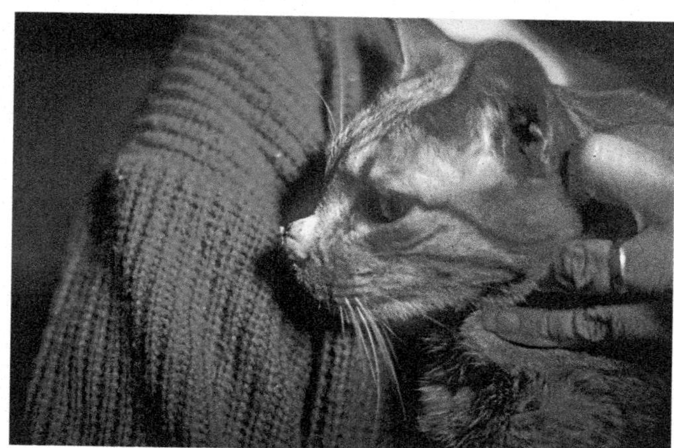

FIGURE 33-8 Sporotrichosis nodule on the nasal planum of a cat. *(Courtesy Vic Menrath.)*

exudative ulcers, and extensive zones of necrosis that exposed muscle and bone. More than 25% of cats had lymphangitis and regional lymphadenitis. The most common extracutaneous signs were respiratory signs, such as sneezing and dyspnea. Subclinical infections were also documented.

It does not appear that infection with FeLV or feline immunodeficiency virus (FIV) is a predisposing factor for sporotrichosis in cats.[46,54] Concurrent infection with FIV does not affect clinical outcome.[46]

Diagnosis of sporotrichosis in cats is most often by cytologic examination of exudates and aspirates from abscesses or nodules or impression smears from skin lesions. Smears stained with a Romanowsky-type stain typically contain large numbers of yeastlike organisms that are often cigar shaped but may appear as round budding shapes. Histopathology is not a reliable method of diagnosis; in two published case series, the organism was not present in more than 1 of 3 affected cats.[9,46] Failure to find the organism in biopsy specimens may be due to sampling early in infection or individual variation in immune response. Definitive diagnosis is by fungal culture of exudate from deep within a draining tract and/or macerated tissue samples.

The drug of choice for sporotrichosis in cats is oral itraconazole. Ketoconazole and sodium iodide have also been reported as effective treatments, but the rate of adverse effects is high.[46,54] Successful treatment of localized disease with a combination of oral itraconazole and intralesional amphotericin B has been described.[25] Secondary bacterial infections should be treated according to culture and sensitivity results for 4 to 8 weeks. Antifungal treatment should be continued for 1 month past resolution of clinical signs to prevent recurrence. Treatment may be required for months to over 1 year; therefore client compliance may be an obstacle to achieving cure even though the prognosis is good. People handling cats suspected or confirmed with sporotrichosis should wear gloves as well as wash their hands and arms with a disinfectant scrub.

Antifungal Therapy

The best therapy for management of systemic fungal disease in cats is ultimately dependent on the individual patient. Preexisting medical conditions, site of fungal infection, and cost of therapy are factors to consider when choosing treatment (Table 33-1).

Amphotericin B is fungicidal and causes cell death by binding to ergosterol in the fungal cell membrane and disrupting membrane stability. It has a broad spectrum of efficacy against many fungal species and was initially the treatment of choice for systemic mycosis in people and animals. It has been proven to eliminate fungal meningitis.[37] Its potential for nephrotoxicity limits the total dose that may safely be administered to a patient, and its use in patients with compromised renal function is not recommended. Newer formulations are safer but more expensive. The three types of newer formulations of amphotericin B include a lipid mixture (Abelcet), a colloidal suspension (Amphotec), and a liposome-encapsulated form (AmBisome). The lipid complex is the least expensive and has been used the most in veterinary medicine.[26] It is 8 to 10 times less nephrotoxic than the original amphotericin B, when administered to healthy dogs.[26] The new formulations are taken up rapidly by the reticuloendothelial system, leading to the high drug levels in infected organs, including the liver, spleen, and lungs.[26] A higher cumulative dose of the new formulations may be administered without increasing risk of drug uptake by the kidneys and nephrotoxicity. The lipid-complexed amphotericin B has been used successfully in veterinary patients for treatment of cryptococcal meningitis, histoplasmosis, coccidioidomycosis, blastomycosis, and other systemic mycoses.

Indications for use of lipid complexed amphotericin B include cryptococcosis with CNS involvement, in mycotic infections that are severe or progressive and in cats that cannot tolerate oral administration of antifungal agents. An appropriate dose of Abelcet in cats is 1 mg/kg intravenously spanning 2 hours. Therapy is

TABLE 33-1 **Drugs for Treatment of Systemic Fungal Infections in Cats**

Drug	Dose	Comments
Amphotericin B	Original formulation: 0.5 mg/kg, IV, 3 times/week Lipid mixture (Abelcet): 1 mg/kg, IV for 2 hours, 3 times/week	Cumulative dose in cats should not exceed 4 to 6 mg/kg for the original formulation, and 12 mg/kg for the lipid mixture
Flucytosine (Ancobon)	50 mg/kg, PO, q8h	Used in combination with amphotericin B
Itraconazole (Sporanox)	10 mg/kg, PO, q24h	Administer capsules with food; administer liquid on empty stomach
Fluconazole (Diflucan)	30-50 mg/cat PO q12h 75 mg/cat PO q12-24h	

Note: Duration of treatment is difficult to determine but should be at least 1 month past clinical resolution.

administered 3 times weekly for an accumulative dose of 12 mg/kg.[26] If the original formulation of amphotericin B is used, a dose of 0.5 mg/kg IV 3 times weekly has been recommended.[37] Monitoring for changes in renal function, such as creatinine, blood urea nitrogen (BUN), and glucosuria, is indicated. Amphotericin B may also be effective as a fungicide by causing immunomodulation and activating macrophage uptake and killing of fungal organisms.[26] Amphotericin B combined with flucytosine may provide the greatest efficacy when treating cats with disseminated disease and/or CNS involvement. This combination is considered by some as the treatment of choice for feline cryptococcosis.[37]

Flucytosine is rarely used as sole therapy, but is combined with other antifungals to increase efficacy. It is synergistic when combined with amphotericin B and penetrates the blood–brain barrier. It has been associated with drug reactions in dogs, and its use may be limited to the first 10 to 14 days of treatment.[37]

Azole antifungals inhibit ergosterol biosynthesis, interfering with fungal membrane function.[26] One benefit of azole drugs is that they allow for treatment of patients without hospitalization. Itraconazole is considered the drug of choice for treatment of most cases of systemic mycoses that are not immediately life threatening in cats.[26,37] It does not easily cross the blood–brain, blood–eye, or blood–prostate barriers. Although it does not penetrate these organs well, it has been used successfully to treat fungal meningitis in cats. Such success may be due to a decrease in the blood–brain barrier associated with inflammation. It is more effective than ketoconazole and has fewer side effects. Side effects can include GI upset, hepatic disease with elevations in alanine aminotransferase activity, and rarely, cutaneous lesions resulting from vasculitis. The capsule formulation of itraconazole should be administered with food to increase absorption, while the liquid formulation should be given after a fast. It should not be administered with antacids. Itraconazole is typically dosed at 10 mg/kg PO q24h for treatment of cryptococcosis, histoplasmosis, coccidioidomycosis, and blastomycosis.[6,22,37]

Fluconazole is effective in treatment of systemic mycoses, particularly when there is involvement of the CNS, eye, or urinary system. It may be the most effective antifungal for treatment of feline cryptococcosis.[37] It has also been used in cats that cannot tolerate itraconazole or in which itraconazole is ineffective. Published doses include 30 to 50 mg/cat PO q12h and 75 mg/cat PO q12-24h.[37] Ketoconazole is not considered a drug of choice for management of feline fungal disease but has been used successfully in treatment of *C. gattii*. It has a higher rate of side effects and is less efficacious than itraconazole.

Newer azoles are on the market and are being used in veterinary medicine. Voriconazole is a derivative of fluconazole but has greater potency and a broader spectrum of activity. It is highly bioavailable when administered orally and also comes in an IV formulation.[26] Posaconazole is an itraconazole analog. It has been used successfully in animal models for the treatment of systemic histoplasmosis and coccidioidomycosis, as well as cryptococcal meningitis.[26] There is little published data describing use of these newer azoles in cats.

In summary, itraconazole can be considered the first choice for treatment of systemic fungal disease in cats. Cats with severe, progressive, or immediately life-threatening disease may need amphotericin B therapy. When cats are suspected to have CNS involvement, flucytosine combined with amphotericin B may be the best treatment. Patients should be monitored regularly for drug toxicity and side effects. The ideal duration of treatment is unknown, but treatment for at least 1 month past clinical resolution is recommended; if the patient's owner can afford to treat for an additional month or two, that is recommended in order to decrease risk of recurrence. A decrease in antibody titers is often associated with effective treatment but does not always indicate cure. In the future, with newer diagnostic tests available, including the fungal antigen tests offered by MiraVista Diagnostics, we may be able to serially monitor antigen levels in infected cats and determine an appropriate time to discontinue antifungal therapy.

RICKETTSIAL DISEASES

Rickettsia are obligate intracellular gram-negative bacteria that are transmitted by an arthropod vector, typically a tick. Their pathogenicity in people and dogs is well understood; in cats little is known currently. *Ehrlichia* organisms primarily infect leukocytes, while *Anaplasma* species typically infect erythrocytes, endothelial cells, platelets, as well as leukocytes. Reclassification of several rickettsial organisms within the families Rickettsiaceae and Anaplasmataceae (order Rickettsiales) occurred in 2001.[40] The genera *Ehrlichia* was moved from the family Rickettsiaceae to the family Anaplasmataceae, while the genera *Rickettsia* remains in the family Rickettsiaceae.[40] Within the genera *Ehrlichia*, *E. phagocytophila*, *E. equi*, and *E. platys* were moved to the genus *Anaplasma*, while *E. risticii* and *E. sennetsu* now belong to the genus *Neorickettsia*.[40]

Specific information about ehrlichiosis, anaplasmosis, and *Rickettsia felis* will be described subsequently. Cats appear less susceptible than dogs to common vector-borne diseases, including ehrlichiosis and anaplasmosis. There are several reports of ill cats presenting with clinical signs that are similar to the ones caused by rickettsial disease in dogs. Presumptive diagnosis of clinical rickettsial disease in cats has been based on appropriate clinical signs combined with the presence of morulae (intracellular clusters of organisms), positive serology, positive polymerase chain reaction (PCR) analysis, and/or response to treatment with doxycycline.

Confirmation of rickettsial organisms as the causative agent of disease in cats is difficult. *Rickettsia* are difficult to culture, and morulae are infrequently present.[35] In addition, the presence of morulae that are *E. canis*-like, for example, does not confirm infection with the specific *Ehrlichia* species because the morulae may belong to another species or genera. Serology has been used to diagnose rickettsial infections, but there are limitations. Serologic techniques among diagnostic laboratories are not standardized. Because there may be yet undiscovered rickettsial species targeting cats, serology results may be negative despite clinical disease. There is serologic cross reactivity among some rickettsial organisms, making diagnosis of infection with a specific species difficult.

The use of molecular techniques including real-time PCR may increase detection of rickettsial pathogens in cats. PCR is sensitive and specific, particularly in the early phase of disease prior to antibody formation. It can be used to detect rickettsial DNA in blood, body fluids, bone marrow, and tissue samples. However, positive PCR results do not confirm an infection in the absence of clinical disease. Although PCR is highly sensitive, false-negative results can occur. If a rickettsial organism is harbored within a tissue, then PCR of blood samples would likely be negative. In addition, in infections with intermittent or brief bacteremia, negative results from testing of blood cannot rule out infection.

At this point, it is recommended that both PCR and serology be used to diagnose suspect rickettsial infections in cats. In addition, measurement of convalescent titers and serial examination of blood or tissue samples by PCR are likely to increase diagnostic efficiency. It is also important to recognize that one arthropod host may transmit multiple pathogens, leading to co-infection. This may explain the variation in clinical signs and response to therapy of cats suspected of having rickettsial disease. It is recommended that samples be screened for multiple organisms simultaneously in areas in which vectors for rickettsial disease are endemic.

Although the most effective therapy for treatment of feline rickettsial diseases is unknown, the American College of Veterinary Internal Medicine recommends that suspect ehrlichial cases be managed with doxycycline at a dose of 10 mg/kg/day for 28 days.[35] Treatment of other rickettsial infections with doxycycline is also appropriate.

Ehrlichiosis

Vectors for *E. canis* include the ticks *Rhipicephalus sanguineus* and *Dermacentor variabilis,* and clinical ehrlichiosis in dogs has been well recognized and understood for decades.[40] Although the first evidence of naturally transmitted ehrlichiosis occurring in cats was described in 1986, our understanding of the disease in cats and which *Ehrlichia* species are infective to cats is incomplete.[35] Evidence for feline ehrlichiosis includes cytologic identification of *E. canis*-like morulae on blood smears, positive *E. canis* serology, and PCR evidence of ehrlichial organism DNA in blood.[35]

Feline ehrlichiosis has been recognized globally, because blood from five cats in North America and France was positive for DNA most consistent with *E. canis*.[35] In addition, *Ehrlichia*-like morulae have been detected in peripheral leukocytes of cats in the United States, Kenya, France, Brazil, Sweden, and Thailand.[5,35] Serology has been used as a diagnostic tool for evaluation of feline ehrlichiosis; however, a limitation is that seropositivity does not equate with active infection. There is a lack of standardization in available methodologies, and variable serologic cross reactivity occurs among species of *Ehrlichia*, *Neorickettsia*, and *Anaplasma*.[35] Some cats with presumed ehrlichiosis test negative for *E. canis* antibodies but positive for *N. risticii*. Antibodies for *N. risticii* and *Ehrlichia* have been detected cats from Maryland, Virginia, California, and Colorado.

The pathogenesis of feline ehrlichiosis is thought to be similar to that of ehrlichiosis in dogs.[35] Clinical disease has been described in 55 cats with probable *E. canis*-morulae in mononuclear cells, *E. canis*-like DNA in blood, or seropositivity for *E. canis* +/− *N. risticii*.[35] Affected cats ranged from 1 to 14 years of age with no gender predisposition; most cats were domestic shorthairs[5,35] Some cats had a history of tick infestation. Clinical signs included fever, anorexia, lethargy, weight loss, pallor, splenomegaly, lymphadenopathy, and anemia.[35] Clinicopathologic abnormalities included anemia (both regenerative and nonregenerative), hyperglobulinemia, hypoalbuminemia, and positive antinuclear antibody titers. Both leukocytosis and leukopenia were documented.[35] Some cats had radiographic evidence of interstitial lung disease.[35] Concurrent infection with *Mycoplasma haemofelis*, *M. haemominutum*, *Cryptococcus neoformans,* feline immunodeficiency virus, or feline leukemia virus were documented.[35]

Cats with suspect ehrlichiosis have been treated with doxycycline, tetracycline, or imidocarb.[35] In three cats, clinical resolution occurred with doxycycline therapy: 5 mg/kg PO q12h for 21 days. Five cats seropositive for *N. risticii* initially had clinical relapse after doxycycline therapy, but clinical resolution occurred after treatment with a higher dose: 10 mg/kg PO q12h for 21 days. Imidocarb dosed at 5 mg/kg IM administered as two injections 14 days apart was successful in treating two cats in Kenya.

The modes of transmission of feline ehrlichiosis are unknown, although vector transmission and spread through blood transfusion have been documented. Prevention may be managed by minimizing a cat's exposure to vectors, administering monthly flea and tick preventatives, as well as by screening potential blood donors for rickettsial species.

Although people, dogs, and cats may develop ehrlichiosis, there is no evidence that the disease can be transmitted directly from cats to other species.

Anaplasmosis

Anaplasma phagocytophilum is the causative agent of anaplasmosis in dogs and people, and there is evidence that cats can develop the disease after experimental inoculation as well as natural transmission. *Ixodes* tick species are vectors for transmission of *A. phagocytophilum* to dogs and are likely vectors for cats.[2,34] At this point, it is not known if other modes of transmission, such as the ingestion of or contact with *A. phagocytophilum*–infected rodents, occurs in cats.[34] In initial research studies, cats inoculated with *A. phagocytophilum* were found to have morulae in eosinophils but were asymptomatic.[34] In a subsequent study, when cats with and without FIV infection were inoculated, they developed clinical disease.[34]

Other evidence for the susceptibility of cats to anaplasmosis includes the detection of *A. phagocytophilum* DNA in the blood of naturally infected cats in Sweden, Denmark, Ireland, and the United States. Additionally *A. phagocytophilum*–like morulae have been detected in neutrophils of infected cats in, Brazil, Kenya, and Italy.[34] *A. phagocytophilum* morulae have been confirmed in the neutrophils of Swedish cats.[34] Prevalence of *A. phagocytophilum* antibodies in 416 cats from six states in the United States was 4.3%, but blood samples were PCR negative for DNA from *Anaplasma* and *Ehrlichia* species.[2] In Florida, 553 cats were tested for *A. phagocytophilum* by PCR and all were negative.[2] At this time, it is not known if the prevalence of anaplasmosis is rare in cats or underdiagnosed because of limitations of current diagnostic tests.

The pathogenesis of feline anaplasmosis is likely similar to that in other species. The clinical manifestations of anaplasmosis in six cats diagnosed with infection, based on PCR documentation of *A. phagocytophilum* DNA with or without serologic evidence have been described.[34] Cats were 9 to 14 months of age, and both castrated males and spayed females were infected.[34] Cases occurred in Massachusetts, Connecticut, and Sweden.[34] Clinical abnormalities were most often mild and included fever, lethargy, anorexia, tachypnea, and the presence of *Ixodes* tick.[34]

Clinicopathologic abnormalities included thrombocytopenia, neutrophilia with left shift, lymphopenia, and mild hyperglycemia. All cats were FIV and FeLV negative. Morulae were detected in only one cat; 24% of its neutrophils were affected. Of the three cats in which *A. phagocytophilum* serology was performed at presentation, two were seronegative and the third had a titer of greater than 1:640. Subsequently, the seronegative cats seroconverted, illustrating that negative serology at the time of initial clinical illness does not rule out anaplasmosis in cats. Titers for *A. phagocytophilum* increased, decreased, or fluctuated over time, so use of serology to confirm resolution of infection is not recommended. With treatment, five of the six cats became PCR negative within 15 to 139 days after diagnosis.[34] All cats were seronegative for *E. canis*.[34] Clinical disease in these 6 cats was milder than anaplasmosis in dogs; data from one study of cats experimentally co-infected with FIV and *A. phagocytophilum* suggests that immunocompromised cats may have more severe clinical disease.[15]

Although initial microbial therapy varied among the six affected cats, all were ultimately treated with tetracycline or doxycycline for 20 to 28 days. The dose of doxycycline administered was 5 to 10 mg/kg PO q12h and 22 mg/kg PO q8h for tetracycline. All cats had clinical improvement within 48 hours after administration of tetracycline or doxycycline.

Rickettsia felis

The cat flea, *Ctenocephalides felis* is a reservoir and vector for *R. felis*, which is widely disseminated within tissues of the cat flea.[1,44] Naturally infected *C. felis* fleas have been found worldwide, although prevalence of infection based on detection of *R. felis* DNA using PCR varies.[8,28,44,52] In Italy, prevalence of *R. felis* in 320 cat fleas from 117 animals was 11.9%, while the prevalence was 9% in Germany.[8,18] In one study in the United States, the prevalence of *R. felis* DNA in 226 cat fleas from 103 animals was 9%, while in another study 67% of cat fleas collected from cats from Alabama, Maryland, and Texas were positive for *R. felis*.[1,28] *R. felis*–infected fleas have also been found in California, Florida, Georgia, Louisiana, New York, North Carolina, Oklahoma, and Tennessee. *Rickettsia felis* DNA has been found in two research cats exposed to fleas infected with *R. felis*.[28] Most cats exposed to *R. felis*–infected fleas do not develop antibodies. This data suggest that *R. felis* may not cause clinical disease in cats, bacteremia may be brief or intermittent, or the organism is harbored in tissues so that blood samples tested by PCR are negative.

Cats may be potential reservoirs for *Rickettsia felis* and a source of infection in people. The pathogenicity of *Rickettsia felis* in cats is poorly understood. Cats experimentally infected remained asymptomatic but seroconverted between 2 to 4 months.[23]

References

1. Bayliss DB, Morris AK, Horta MC et al: Prevalence of *Rickettsia* species antibodies and *Rickettsia* species DNA in the blood of cats with and without fever, *J Feline Med Surg* 11:266, 2009.

2. Billeter SA, Spencer JA, Griffin B et al: Prevalence of *Anaplasma phagocytophilum* in domestic felines in the United States, *Vet Parasitol* 147:194, 2007.
3. Blondin N, Baumgardner DJ, Moore GE et al: Blastomycosis in indoor cats: suburban Chicago, Illinois, USA, *Mycopathologia* 163:59, 2007.
4. Breider MA, Walker TL, Legendre AM et al: Blastomycosis in cats: five cases (1979-1986), *J Am Vet Med Assoc* 193:570, 1988.
5. Breitschwerdt EB, Abrams-Ogg AC, Lappin MR et al: Molecular evidence supporting *Ehrlichia canis*-like infection in cats, *J Vet Intern Med* 16:642, 2002.
6. Bromel C, Sykes JE: Epidemiology, diagnosis, and treatment of blastomycosis in dogs and cats, *Clin Tech Small Anim Pract* 20:233, 2005.
7. Bromel C, Sykes JE: Histoplasmosis in dogs and cats, *Clin Tech Small Anim Pract* 20:227, 2005.
8. Capelli G, Montarsi F, Porcellato E et al: Occurrence of *Rickettsia felis* in dog and cat fleas *(Ctenocephalides felis)* from Italy, *Parasit Vectors* 2(Suppl 1):S8, 2009.
9. Crothers SL, White SD, Ihrke PJ et al: Sporotrichosis: a retrospective evaluation of 23 cases seen in northern California (1987-2007), *Vet Dermatol* 20:249, 2009.
10. Davies C, Troy GC: Deep mycotic infections in cats, *J Am Anim Hosp Assoc* 32:380, 1996.
11. de Lima Barros MB, Schubach TM, Galhardo MC et al: Sporotrichosis: an emergent zoonosis in Rio de Janeiro, *Mem Inst Oswaldo Cruz* 96:777, 2001.
12. Duncan C, Stephen C, Campbell J: Clinical characteristics and predictors of mortality for *Cryptococcus gattii* infection in dogs and cats of southwestern British Columbia, *Can Vet J* 47:993, 2006.
13. Duncan C, Stephen C, Lester S et al: Follow-up study of dogs and cats with asymptomatic *Cryptococcus gattii* infection or nasal colonization, *Med Mycol* 43:663, 2005.
14. Duncan CG, Stephen C, Campbell J: Evaluation of risk factors for *Cryptococcus gattii* infection in dogs and cats, *J Am Vet Med Assoc* 228:377, 2006.
15. Foley JE, Leutenegger CM, Dumler JS et al: Evidence for modulated immune response to *Anaplasma phagocytophila* sensu lato in cats with FIV-induced immunosuppression, *Comp Immunol Microbiol Infect Dis* 26:103, 2003.
16. Gaidici A, Saubolle MA: Transmission of coccidioidomycosis to a human via a cat bite, *J Clin Microbiol* 47:505, 2009.
17. Gerds-Grogan S, Dayrell-Hart B: Feline cryptococcosis: a retrospective evaluation, *J Am Anim Hosp Assoc* 33:118, 1997.
18. Gilles J, Just FT, Silaghi C et al: *Rickettsia felis* in fleas, Germany, *Emerg Infect Dis* 14:1294, 2008.
19. Gilor C, Graves TK, Barger AM et al: Clinical aspects of natural infection with *Blastomyces dermatitidis* in cats: 8 cases (1991-2005), *J Am Vet Med Assoc* 229:96, 2006.
20. Gionfriddo JR: Feline systemic fungal infections, *Vet Clin North Am Small Anim Pract* 30:1029, 2000.
21. Graupmann-Kuzma A, Valentine BA, Shubitz LF et al: Coccidioidomycosis in dogs and cats: a review, *J Am Anim Hosp Assoc* 44:226, 2008.
22. Greene C: Histoplasmosis. In Greene C, editor: *Infectious diseases of the dog and cat*, ed 3, St Louis, 2006, Elsevier, p 577.
23. Greene CG, Breitschwerdt, EB: Cat-flea typhuslike illness (*Rickettsia felis* infection). In Greene C, editor: *Infectious diseases of the dog and cat*, ed 3, St Louis, 2006, Elsevier, p 242.
24. Greene RT: Coccioidomycosis and paracoccidioidomycosis. In Greene C, editor: *Infectious diseases of the dog and cat*, ed 3, St Louis, 2006, Elsevier, p 598.
25. Gremião IDF, Schubach TMP, Pereira SA et al: Intralesional amphotericin B in a cat with refractory localised sporotrichosis, *J Feline Med Surg* 11:720, 2009.
26. Grooters AM, Taboada J: Update on antifungal therapy, *Vet Clin North Am Small Anim Pract* 33:749, 2003.
27. Harasen GL, Randall JW: Canine blastomycosis in southern Saskatchewan, *Can Vet J* 27:375, 1986.
28. Hawley JR, Shaw SE, Lappin MR: Prevalence of *Rickettsia felis* DNA in the blood of cats and their fleas in the United States, *J Feline Med Surg* 9:258, 2007.
29. Hodges RD, Legendre AM, Adams LG et al: Itraconazole for the treatment of histoplasmosis in cats, *J Vet Intern Med* 8:409, 1994.
30. Johnson LR, Fry MM, Anez KL et al: Histoplasmosis infection in two cats from California, *J Am Anim Hosp Assoc* 40:165, 2004.
31. Kano R, Kitagawat M, Oota S et al: First case of feline systemic *Cryptococcus albidus* infection, *Med Mycol* 46:75, 2008.
32. Kerl ME: Update on canine and feline fungal diseases, *Vet Clin North Am Small Anim Pract* 33:721, 2003.
33. Lamm CG, Rizzi TE, Campbell GA et al: Pathology in practice. *Histoplasma capsulatum* infections, *J Am Vet Med Assoc* 235:155, 2009.
34. Lappin MR, Bjoersdorff A, Breitschwerdt EB: Feline granulocytotropic anaplasmosis. In Greene CG, editor: *Infectious diseases of the dog and cat*, ed 3, St Louis, 2006, Elsevier, p 227.
35. Lappin MR, Breitschwerdt, EB: Feline mononuclear ehrlichiosis. In Greene C, editor: *Infectious diseases of the dog and cat*, ed 3, St Louis, 2006, Elsevier, p 224.
36. Legendre AM: Blastomycosis. In Greene C, editor: *Infectious diseases of the dog and cat*, ed 3, St Louis, 2006, Elsevier, p 569.
37. Malik R, Krockenberger M, O'Brien CR, et al: Cryptococcosis. In Greene C, editor: *Infectious diseases of the dog and cat*, ed 3, St Louis, 2006, Elsevier, p 584.
38. Malik R, Martin P, Wigney DI et al: Nasopharyngeal cryptococcosis, *Aust Vet J* 75:483, 1997.
39. Malik R, Wigney DI, Muir DB et al: Cryptococcosis in cats: clinical and mycological assessment of 29 cases and evaluation of treatment using orally administered fluconazole, *J Med Vet Mycol* 30:133, 1992.
40. Neer MT, Harrus S: Canine monocytotropic ehrlichiosis and neoricketsisos (*E. canis, E. chaffeensis, E. ruminatium, N. sennetsu*, and *N. risticii* infections). In Greene C, editor: *Infectious diseases of the dog and cat*, ed 3, St Louis, 2006, Elsevier, p 203.
41. O'Brien CR, Krockenberger MB, Martin P et al: Long-term outcome of therapy for 59 cats and 11 dogs with cryptococcosis, *Aust Vet J* 84:384, 2006.
42. O'Brien CR, Krockenberger MB, Wigney DI et al: Retrospective study of feline and canine cryptococcosis in Australia from 1981 to 2001: 195 cases, *Med Mycol* 42:449, 2004.
43. Odom T, Anderson JG: Proliferative gingival lesion in a cat with disseminated cryptococcosis, *J Vet Dent* 17:177, 2000.
44. Reif KE, Macaluso KR: Ecology of *Rickettsia felis:* a review, *J Med Entomol* 46:723, 2009.
45. Reis RS, Almeida-Paes R, Muniz Mde M et al: Molecular characterisation of *Sporothrix schenckii* isolates from humans and cats involved in the sporotrichosis epidemic in Rio de Janeiro, Brazil, *Mem Inst Oswaldo Cruz* 104:769, 2009.
46. Schubach T, Schubach A, Okamoto T et al: Evaluation of an epidemic of sporotrichosis in cats: 347 cases (1998-2001), *J Am Vet Med Assoc* 224:1623, 2004.
47. Schubach TM, de Oliveira Schubach A, dos Reis RS et al: *Sporothrix schenckii* isolated from domestic cats with and without sporotrichosis in Rio de Janeiro, Brazil, *Mycopathologia* 153:83, 2002.
48. Schubach TM, Valle AC, Gutierrez-Galhardo MC et al: Isolation of *Sporothrix schenckii* from the nails of domestic cats *(Felis catus)*, *Med Mycol* 39:147, 2001.
49. Shubitz LF, Dial SM: Coccidioidomycosis: a diagnostic challenge, *Clin Tech Small Anim Pract* 20:220, 2005.
50. Spector D, Legendre AM, Wheat J et al: Antigen and antibody testing for the diagnosis of blastomycosis in dogs, *J Vet Intern Med* 22:839, 2008.

51. Tofflemire K, Betbeze C: Three cases of feline ocular coccidioidomycosis: presentation, clinical features, diagnosis, and treatment, *Vet Ophthalmol* 13:166, 2010.
52. Tsai KH, Lu HY, Huang JH et al: *Rickettsia felis* in cat fleas in Taiwan, *Vector Borne Zoonotic Dis* 9:561, 2009.
53. Vinayak A, Kerwin SC, Pool RR: Treatment of thoracolumbar spinal cord compression associated with *Histoplasma capsulatum* infection in a cat, *J Am Vet Med Assoc* 230:1018, 2007.
54. Welsh R: Sporotrichosis, *J Am Vet Med Assoc* 223:1123, 2003.
55. Yegneswaran PP, Sripathi H, Bairy I et al: Zoonotic sporotrichosis of lymphocutaneous type in a man acquired from a domesticated feline source: report of a first case in southern Karnataka, India, *Int J Dermatol* 48:1198, 2009.

VIRAL DISEASES

Melissa Kennedy and Susan E. Little

Viral infections of cats are common, especially in the young. Many of the viral agents affecting cats can cause serious, even lethal disease. Several cause lifelong infections and affected cats are important sources in multicat settings. Most of the agents are very contagious, spreading easily from cat to cat. Additionally, some such as feline parvovirus and calicivirus, are quite hardy and may persist in the environment for weeks or months. Identification of the infecting agent is critical in these multicat settings in order to aid control and prevention. Vaccines to protect against several of these agents have been developed, some of which are considered core vaccine components. Like viral diseases in other species, very few antiviral chemotherapeutics are available for treatment. However, the repertoire of efficacious drugs is increasing as more research is performed. This chapter describes the most common viral agents of concern in cats.

FELINE HERPESVIRUS-1

Feline herpesvirus-1 (FHV-1) is the agent of viral rhinotracheitis and is a common respiratory pathogen of cats. An Alphaherpesvirinae subfamily member of the Herpesviridae family, the virus is a double-stranded DNA virus with an icosahedral protein capsid and a lipid envelope containing several viral glycoproteins. As a DNA virus, the mutation rate of herpesviruses is relatively low; thus antigenic variation among FHV-1 strains is not a major concern. The lipid membrane encasing the virion is derived from the infected cell, and contributes to the virus' ability to survive desiccation, making it an efficient respiratory pathogen. However, it also contributes to the virus' lability in the environment; it survives up to 18 hours in a damp environment (less in dry conditions) after shedding onto inanimate objects and is unstable as an aerosol.[87] In addition, it is easily inactivated by any detergent or soap.

Transmission and Pathogenesis

Most cats become infected with feline herpesvirus as kittens. Direct contact with an infected cat is the most efficient mode of transmission, but spread by aerosolized droplets over short distances or by indirect contact with contaminated objects is also important. Unlike herpesviruses of other animal species, feline herpesvirus primarily targets epithelia of the upper respiratory tract and conjunctiva and only rarely spreads beyond these tissues to cause systemic disease. Virus replication in these cells results in cell death (cytolysis) and loss. This may manifest as ulceration, necrosis, and inflammation in the oronasal and pharyngeal tissue. In the conjunctiva, epithelial necrosis may also occur, with serosanguinous to purulent discharge, which may be profuse. In severe cases, erosion to the bone may occur in the nasal cavity from rhinitis, and the resultant distortion of bone and cartilage may lead to chronic rhinosinusitis (cats known as "snufflers").

In a manner similar to all herpesviruses, FHV-1 enters a latent state in innervating sensory nerves after acute infection. In cats, this most commonly occurs in the trigeminal ganglion, and is estimated to occur in about 80% of infections.[88] From this latent state, the virus can be reactivated, especially during stressful episodes, leading to replication in the epithelia, virus shedding, and in a minority of cats, disease. Termed recrudescence, it can be stimulated by any stressor, including trauma, concurrent disease, parturition, boarding, or changes in social hierarchy. Recrudescent episodes are often asymptomatic, and may be an important mechanism of maintaining the virus in a population. As new, immunologically naïve kittens are introduced, whether by birth (e.g., breeding cattery) or intake (e.g., shelter setting), asymptomatic shedders may expose them to the virus.

Clinical Signs

The typical presentation of FHV infection is that of upper respiratory tract disease (see also Chapter 30): sneezing, nasal and/or ocular discharge, fever, depression, and decreased appetite following an incubation period of 2 to 6 days.[13] Conjunctivitis is not uncommon, and can progress to severe hyperemia and chemosis, with mucopurulent ocular discharge (see also Chapter 29). Infection may lead to corneal ulceration because of the viral damage of the corneal epithelium. In fact, FHV-1 is believed to be the most common cause of feline ocular disease, and corneal ulceration in a cat should be assumed to be a consequence of FHV-1 infection until proven otherwise.[110] This may manifest as a typical dendritic ulcer or may progress to involve the stroma, leading to a desmetocele.[110] Occasionally, cats may manifest with stromal keratitis; this uncommon manifestation is a consequence of the immune response to herpesvirus

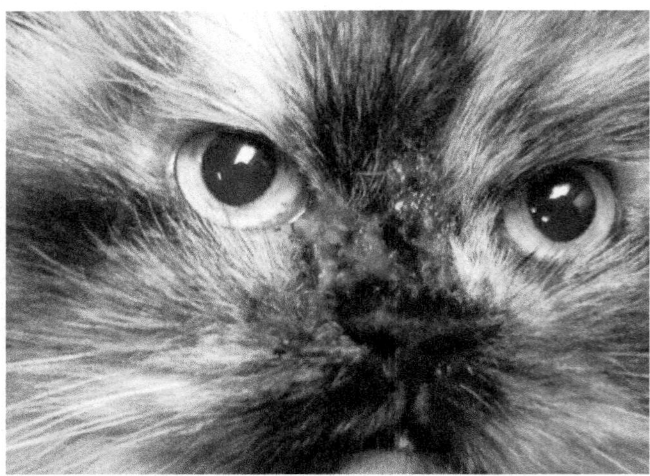

FIGURE 33-9 Herpesvirus may cause an ulcerative dermatitis that may be multifocal, often involving the face or planum nasale.

antigen rather than direct destruction by the virus itself. The corneal stroma becomes infiltrated with mononuclear white blood cells, primarily lymphocytes, which may lead to blindness.[110]

Less common manifestations of FHV-1 are ulcerative dermatitis and stomatitis. Ulcerative dermatitis may be multifocal, often involving the face or planum nasale, but may involve other areas of the skin (Figure 33-9). Affected cats may not have concurrent or historical evidence of respiratory infection.[161] Because lesions may involve eosinophils in addition to neutrophils, and intranuclear viral inclusions may not always be found, misdiagnosis as eosinophilic granuloma complex is a concern.[161] Cases of stomatitis are also relatively uncommon and may involve the soft palate and tongue.[109,161] An association with chronic gingivostomatitis has not been found.[238]

Diagnosis

Diagnostic testing for FHV-1 infection primarily involves virus detection, because most cats are seropositive from either natural exposure or vaccination. Prevalence rates for seropositive status may be as high as 97%.[180] In addition, studies have shown that the magnitude of the FHV-1-specific antibody levels does not necessarily correlate with presence of either acute or chronic FHV-1 infection.[180]

Diagnosis of the classic presentation of upper respiratory tract disease in kittenhood is relatively straightforward. Methods for viral detection include virus isolation, viral antigen detection, and detection of viral genetic material. With ocular involvement, conjunctival and/or corneal swabs, scrapings, or brushings are collected for testing. In addition, pharyngeal and/or nasal swabs should be collected from cats with upper respiratory tract disease.[299]

Virus isolation is the gold standard because it identifies actively replicating virus, but may have a turnaround time of several days to a week. Samples should be shipped chilled and preferably overnight to the testing laboratory. Virus isolation may be falsely negative with chronic herpesviral-induced disease. This is due to the presence of locally produced neutralizing antibodies on the mucosal surface, preventing viral replication in cell culture. In addition, virus may be isolated from clinically normal cats.[277] Viral antigen detection using immunofluorescence is fast and inexpensive; however, sensitivity is relatively low, especially in chronic infections. This testing is done on corneal, conjunctival, or oropharyngeal scrapings, and samples must be collected prior to fluorescein administration to avoid test interference.

Genetic detection using polymerase chain reaction (PCR) has become the most commonly used assay for virus detection. This assay, done on similar samples as those described above, amplifies viral genetic material through repeated rounds of DNA synthesis. The amplified viral material is generally identified using a probe (e.g., TaqMan real-time PCR). This technology has very high sensitivity and specificity, and does not require viable virus, unlike virus isolation. The exquisite sensitivity of PCR is a double-edged sword, however, because it may detect subclinical, recrudescent, and even latent infections; thus positive results must be interpreted carefully.[110,284,291] Studies have shown that, using PCR, FHV-1 may be detected in many clinically normal cats,[178,276,291] as well as in normal corneas.[277] In addition, it appears possible that PCR assays may detect vaccine virus as well as field strains.[178] Therefore an increase in test sensitivity does not necessarily equate with diagnostic sensitivity. Genetic detection by PCR may also be used to identify virus in skin lesions of ulcerative dermatitis resulting from FHV-1.[161] In addition, histopathology may identify viral inclusions, and immunohistochemistry can be used for viral detection in biopsy samples.[109,161]

Treatment

Advancements have been made in the treatment of FHV infection in cats, and in fact, this is one agent for which specific antiviral medications are available. Although none are approved for veterinary use in the United States, some success has been achieved with their use. It is critical to remember, however, that human antiviral medications should not be used unless safety and efficacy have been proven in cats because some have proven to be highly toxic, even fatal to cats. Topical antivirals used in cases of FHV-1 ocular disease include trifluridine, vidaribine, and idoxuridine. These drugs are virostatic, and must be given often; thus owner compliance may be a challenge. Typically, recommendations are to apply these as many times as possible throughout the day, usually every 4 to 6 hours being the maximum. Recently, topical instillation of a 0.5% cidofovir solution every 12 hours led to clinical improvement and decreased viral shedding in experimental FHV-1 infection.[80] Its usefulness in natural infection is being evaluated. The advantage to this medication is its less frequent administration.

Systemic nucleoside analogs developed for human herpesvirus infections have shown some efficacy against feline herpesvirus, at least in vitro. Toxic side effects have been reported with some, such as acyclovir, but others, such as ganciclovir, may prove to be useful clinically. Famciclovir has been shown to be effective for FHV-1–associated ocular disease, rhinosinusitis, and dermatitis in at least one study.[184] Clinical trials are required to optimize the dose and schedule.

Interferon (IFN; both human IFN-alpha and recombinant feline IFN-omega) has been used with some success, and has been shown to be efficacious in vitro.[267] To date, recombinant feline interferon omega (rFeIFN) is not available in North America. Effectiveness of rFeIFN in vivo for dermatitis associated with FHV-1 has been shown in at least one case report.[105]

L-lysine given orally inhibits herpesviral protein synthesis and restricts virus replication by antagonizing the growth promoting effect of arginine. In vitro, FHV-1 replication was significantly reduced when lysine was present in the growth medium.[179] It is optimal when used early in infection, or as a means to prevent recrudescence during stress, where it has been shown to reduce viral shedding in latently infected cats.[181] However, studies evaluating its usefulness in preventing upper respiratory tract disease (URTD) in multicat settings, such as shelters, have shown no positive effect from daily lysine supplementation.[243] In fact, one study actually found increased viral shedding and severity of signs of URTD in shelter cats fed lysine supplements.[62] In another study evaluating the effectiveness of dietary lysine supplementation in shelter cats with enzootic upper respiratory disease, mean disease scores were higher for cats fed the lysine-supplemented diet.[183] However, food intake (and therefore lysine intake) decreased when lysine was added to the diet. In addition, cats in the study were group housed and group fed so that individual lysine intake could not be monitored. Despite this, oral administration as a bolus (250 to 500 mg/cat/day) for acute infections and as a supplement for prophylaxis in cats with recurrent signs has been recommended.[182] Lysine administration to cats appears to be safe, though the effects of long-term administration on plasma arginine concentrations are not known.[183] In one study, plasma arginine concentrations declined in lysine-supplemented cats during a 52-day monitoring period, leading the authors to recommend monitoring of plasma arginine in cats receiving long-term lysine supplementation.[183]

In experiments, bovine lactoferrin has been shown to inhibit virus attachment and entry, and may eventually be available as an antiviral treatment for FHV-1.[17] An immune-enhancing probiotic, *Enterococcus faecium* SF68, used as a dietary supplement has been shown to reduce evidence of clinical disease associated with chronic infection.[160] Although the study size was small (12 cats), the findings warrant further clinical evaluation. At least one study has shown improvement in adult cats with chronic rhinitis by administration of liposomal complexes containing interleukin-2 (IL-2) DNA as an immunotherapeutic.[298] Another approach under investigation is the use of ribonucleic acid interference to inhibit FHV-1 replication.[305]

Prevention and Control

Protection following recovery is not long-lived, and reinfections may occur. Antigenic variation is not a significant problem with feline herpesvirus; thus the antigenic coverage of available vaccines is adequate. Vaccines do not prevent infection or production of the carrier state. They do offer protection from disease, however, and FHV-1 is considered a core component of feline vaccines.[50,249,284] The nonadjuvanted modified live vaccines that contain FHV-1 in combination with other agents have been shown to be both efficacious and safe when administered as directed. In multicat situations where FHV-1 infection is endemic, intranasal vaccination may be used in kittens for early protection from clinical disease and decreased viral shedding.[159] In addition, response to intranasal vaccination is not affected by the presence of maternal antibody. More information on FHV-1 vaccination is found in Chapter 8.

FELINE CALICIVIRUS

Feline calicivirus (FCV) is a highly contagious respiratory pathogen of cats. In addition to the classic respiratory disease, FCV is associated with several other disease syndromes, including polyarthritis, gingivostomatitis, and systemic vasculitis. The virus is classified as a *Vesivirus* in the family *Caliciviridae*. It is a small nonenveloped virus, making it very hardy in the environment, and it is easily spread by fomites, including pet owners and hospital staff.[133] The viral genome is single-stranded RNA, giving it a significant mutation rate, much higher than that of FHV-1. This may lead to changes in antigenicity (many strains that vary antigenically exist) as well as virulence.

The gene encoding the capsomer protein, the major structural protein, has variable regions that distinguish strains of FCV. These regions also contain important immunologic epitopes; thus antigenic variability among strains is common, and has an impact on vaccine

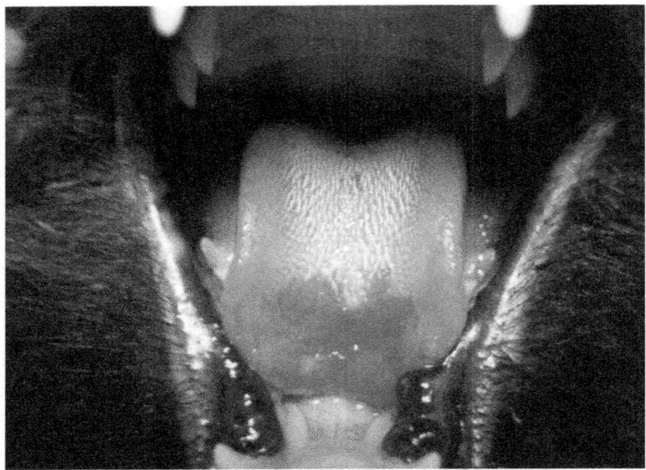

FIGURE 33-10 The most common lesion associated with feline calicivirus infection is oral ulceration, commonly on the margins of the tongue.

efficacy. For most vaccines, there is sufficient antigenic overlap to allow cross protection to heterologous strains following immunization with one strain of FCV, but protection against all field strains may not be equal. Genetic variability may also have an impact on disease phenotype, but does not segregate with antigenicity; that is, differences in disease manifestations do not correlate with differences in antigenicity. This, too, has an impact on vaccine design and development.

Transmission and Pathogenesis

FCV is shed in secretions from the oropharynx, conjunctiva, and nose. Transmission is most efficient by direct cat-to-cat contact and by fomites. Aerosol transmission is less important, because sneezed macrodroplets do not travel far (less than 4 feet). A major source of infection is asymptomatic carrier cats that shed virus continuously. Unlike FHV-1, FCV shedding is not influenced by stress. There is a high prevalence of FCV in healthy cats (up to 24%, depending on the assay). Carrier cats may shed for months to years (even lifelong),[302] although one study showed that 50% of infected cats ceased shedding within 75 days.[86] Long-term analysis of FCV shedding patterns in five naturally infected colonies revealed three distinct patterns of shedding in individuals: cats that shed virus consistently, cats that shed virus intermittently, and cats that never shed virus.[45] Re-infection after recovery is possible.

Feline calicivirus primarily targets epithelia of the upper respiratory tract, oral cavity, and conjunctiva. Unlike FHV-1, it is not associated with corneal infection and ulceration. The most common lesion associated with FCV infection is oral ulceration. In general, clinical signs begin as vesicular lesions in the mouth, and are commonly seen on margins of the tongue (Figure 33-10).[239]

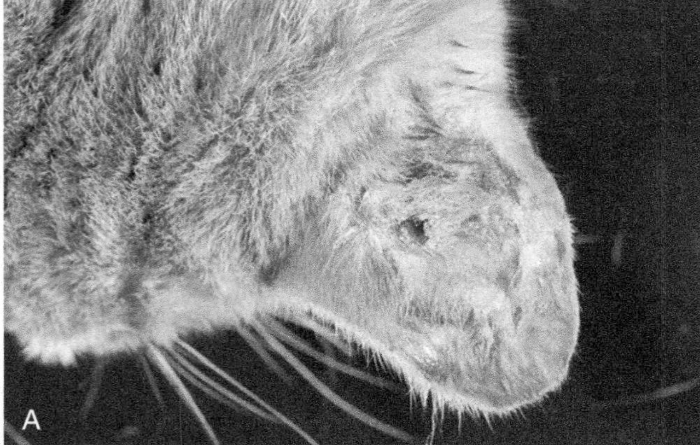

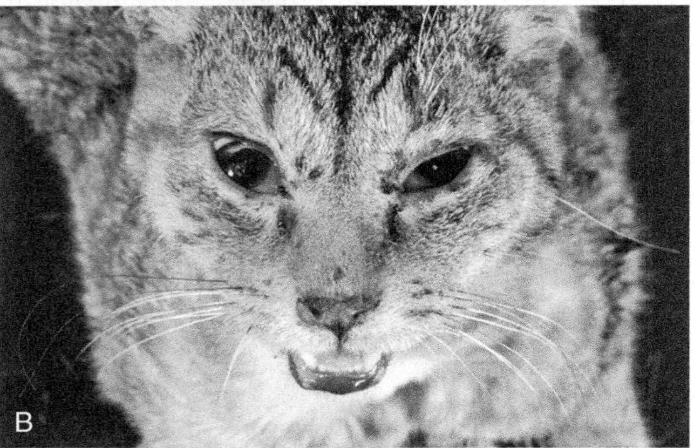

FIGURE 33-11 Epithelial necrosis associated with virulent systemic calicivirus infection occurs in skin as well as mucous membranes, leading to ulceration that often involves the ears **(A)**, face **(B)**, and paws. *(Courtesy Dr. Patricia Pesavento, University of California, Davis, Calif.)*

As the overlying epithelia necroses, the lesions ulcerate and become inflamed. Feline calicivirus may also target alveolar epithelia of the lower respiratory tract. Some strains appear to be quite pneumotropic, leading to severe interstitial pneumonia.

Infection with FCV also produces a transient viremia, leading to widespread distribution of the virus.[239] In most cases, this dissemination does not manifest clinically. Uncommonly, disease beyond the respiratory tract may occur. Lameness associated with acute synovitis may occur, and although the precise mechanism of disease remains unclear, viral antigen associated with joint macrophages has been identified.[239]

Rarely, a virulent systemic (VS-FCV) manifestation may occur, and may appear as an outbreak within a population.[132,223,247,260] This syndrome involves widespread vasculitis and multiorgan failure and has occurred in vaccinated animals.[223] Epithelial infection and necrosis occurs in skin as well as mucous membranes, leading to ulceration that often involves the ears, face, and paws (Figures 33-11).[239] The mortality rate of this syndrome is quite high.

The underlying pathogenesis of this virulent clinical manifestation appears to involve viral mutations leading to hypervirulence, though the precise mutation remains unknown. In each documented outbreak where data is available, the virulent strain seems to have appeared spontaneously by mutation from caliciviruses already present in the group. Each isolate has been genetically unique. VS-FCV isolates are not members of a single clade.[212] Instead, these mutant viruses are emerging from several different lineages intermixed with other field strain FCVs. In addition, the emergence of these variants seems to involve host and environmental conditions as well. Thus far, no common mutation has been identified; however, at least one report describes point mutations leading to an additional glycosylation site in the capsomer protein of some hemorrhagic isolates.[2] Interestingly, most of the outbreaks associated with this form of FCV have arisen in shelter or rescue situations. One theory is that in these settings, FCV infection may be endemic in the population; in these situations, rapidly replicating virus that can attain high titers in a relatively short period of time is selected for because of the immunity of the endemically infected population.[239] When introduced into a population, this rapidly replicating, "hot" variant may lead to systemic dissemination and disease.

Host parameters have also been speculated to play a role in VS-FCV cases. In particular, immunopathologic mechanisms may contribute to the disease production.[74] Local modulation of cytokine levels have been found associated with lesions, and may contribute to the vasculitis and increased vascular permeability seen.

Clinical Signs

Clinical presentations with FCV infection can vary from mild upper respiratory tract disease to viral pneumonia to lethal systemic disease. The typical presentation is similar to FHV infection; though the ocular discharge generally remains serous, corneal ulcers do not occur and oral ulcers are common. Typically, cats present with vesicular and ulcerative lesions of the oral cavity that may also involve the lips, nares, and even paronychial skin. Sneezing, hypersalivation, serous ocular and nasal discharge, and fever are seen. Ocular lesions include conjunctival hyperemia, chemosis, and blepharospasm.[133] The majority of infections are mild and self-limiting. Acute lameness with joint and muscle pain may be seen in kittens associated with either FCV vaccine strains or field virus.[219] Affected cats may be febrile, and about 25% have oral ulceration. Clinical signs resolve quickly, usually within 72 to 96 hours.[239] Feline calicivirus has also been associated with chronic lymphoplasmacytic gingivostomatitis.[61] However, other pathogens and host factors likely also play a role in this syndrome.[239]

For virulent systemic FCV (VS-FCV) infection, disease is typically more severe in adults than kittens. Clinicopathologic abnormalities associated with VS-FCV are generally nonspecific, such as neutrophilia, hyperglobulinemia, and elevated liver enzymes. Characteristic clinical signs that have been described include subcutaneous edema, particularly of the head and limbs, ulceration of pinna and footpads, and crusting lesions of the face, ears, and limbs.[133,239] In addition, signs such as jaundice, dyspnea, vomiting, and diarrhea, may be observed. However, mild or subclinical infections may also occur, and asymptomatic cats are able to transmit fatal disease.[133] Mortality rates have been reported as high as 60%.[228] On necropsy, affected cats commonly have hepatocellular necrosis, interstitial pneumonia, and fluid in body cavities.[133,228]

Persistent infections following recovery from acute disease are not uncommon. Unlike FHV, persistent FCV infections are not latent and shedding is continuous. These asymptomatic shedders are important sources of the virus in a population and may be the source of new variants. Infected cats may continue to shed the virus throughout their lifetime, but most shed for periods of weeks to a few months.

Diagnosis

The presence of severe oral ulcerations is an important clinical indicator of FCV infection, even in cases of VS-FCV. Confirmation of a diagnosis of FCV, as with FHV, relies primarily on detection of the virus, because the majority of cats are seropositive for FCV. Viral identification is particularly important in multicat settings. Virus isolation is the gold standard, because it detects replicating virus. Virus can be isolated from conjunctival and nasals swabs, but the highest success rate is achieved with oropharyngeal swabs. Samples should be shipped cooled (e.g., with ice packs) overnight to the testing laboratory. Antigen detection on slides made from swabs of the same sites, as for virus isolation, can also be done but is generally of lower sensitivity. As with FHV, detection of FCV nucleic acid by PCR is being used more frequently for diagnosis and is done on the same samples as for virus isolation.[3] The drawback of PCR testing for FCV not observed with FHV is the genetic variation of FCV, potentially leading to false-negative results. At least one report has identified a highly conserved genetic region of the virus that can be targeted for detection of the majority of field strains.[3,4] However, it is possible that PCR assays may also detect vaccine virus in addition to field strains.[157] It is recommended that samples submitted for PCR NOT be frozen; refrigeration and shipment on an ice pack is suggested.[157]

None of the assays described can distinguish the virus of virulent systemic disease from those causing more classic disease; this classification is currently based on clinical presentation. In cases of suspected VS-FCV, samples from the same sites as for typical presentations should be collected. In addition, tissue samples from those animals that die should be submitted for histopathology and immunohistochemistry or PCR. These samples should include parenchymal organs and ulcerated lesions (e.g., skin, foot pads, lingual areas).

Interpretation of positive results for each of these ante mortem assays must be done in light of the fact that asymptomatic carrier states are not uncommon; thus finding the virus in an ill cat does not necessarily prove causation of the current disease.

Treatment

Treatment of FCV infection primarily involves symptomatic and supportive care. Fluids and nutritional support (e.g., esophagostomy or gastrostomy tube feeding) are important for anorectic cats, and oxygen therapy for dyspneic cats is critical. Broad-spectrum antibiotics should be used if bacterial infection is suspected. Recombinant feline interferon has demonstrated antiviral activity in vitro, but in vivo effectiveness is unclear.[209] Currently, no specific antiviral medication for FCV exists. A recent study showed efficacy of virus-specific compounds in blocking FCV replication in vivo.[270] This technology, which is referred to as phosphorodiamidate morpholino oligomer (PMO), uses virus-specific nucleic acid sequences that bind to viral RNA, preventing translation of viral proteins. In at least one study, it was safe and reduced disease development, virus shedding, and mortality.[270] As this technology is developed, a commercially produced medication may become available. For cats with VS-FCV, intensive care using parameters described above are needed, and corticosteroids for the immunopathologic component may be beneficial.[133,239] Oral interferon-alpha has also been used in these cases, though it is not clear if it contributed to survival.[133]

Prevention and Control

Vaccination is the main means of control, and, as with FHV, prevents disease but not infection nor the carrier state. Calicivirus is considered a core component of feline vaccines.[50,239,249] Most vaccines contain a single strain, typically strain F9 or strain 225, and these strains have been shown to be broadly cross-reactive based on neutralization studies.[234] Traditional calicivirus vaccines, however, do not appear to be protective against virulent systemic disease. Manufacturers are investigating the utility and inclusion of additional strains in vaccines to increase the spectrum of protection. Newer vaccine strains appear to induce neutralizing antibodies against a higher proportion of calicivirus field strains.[129,235] A vaccine containing a virulent systemic strain is available, although the ability of this vaccine to protect against future outbreaks of VS-FCV disease is unknown. A bivalent vaccine containing two strains with broad cross-antigenicity based on in vitro cross-neutralization evaluation was found to provide protection against heterologous strains.[235] This study validated the use of cross-neutralization tests to evaluate cross-protection of vaccine strains. It is important to bear in mind that inclusion of two or more strains isolated from different disease manifestations does not necessarily insure broad protection against the varied pathogenic phenotypes. Rather, neutralization assays are critical for assessing the protective spectrum of any new vaccine. It will be difficult to achieve a vaccine that provides protection against all strains in circulation because of the antigenic variability of FCV, and continued evaluation of prevalent strains and their antigenic relatedness to vaccine strains will be critical. In a clinical setting, if vaccine breakthroughs are occurring within a cat population, boosting with a different strain of FCV may enhance the protection of the population. More information on calicivirus vaccines is found in Chapter 8.

Environmental decontamination is also important for control in multicat situations, including veterinary clinics. Because of the environmental hardiness of the virus, detergent alone will not inactivate FCV. The virus can persist for days to weeks in the environment, and disinfection requires products with oxidizing activity, such as 5% sodium hypochlorite diluted 1:32 and potassium peroxymonosulfate.[239] Quaternary ammonium products are not effective against FCV.[69] Thus decontamination following examination or housing of any cat with URT infection should include cleaning with a detergent to remove organic matter, followed by disinfection.[133] During outbreaks of virulent disease because of FCV, stringent quarantine measures and barrier nursing are required to prevent the spread of the virus. All affected and exposed cats should be strictly isolated, and if possible, treatment away from the veterinary hospital is ideal.[239] Additional and more detailed control measures can be found elsewhere.[133,239]

INFLUENZA VIRUS

Influenza virus is an uncommon pathogen of cats, but several occurrences have been documented. The virus known as highly pathogenic avian influenza H5N1 (HPAI H5N1) was found to infect cats in 2004 in Southeast Asia, while the human pandemic strain of 2009 (H1N1) was transmitted from a human to a cat in 2009. Because of these occurrences, it is important that veterinarians understand the virus and its pathogenesis not only for patient care but, perhaps, even more importantly for communication with the public.

Influenza viruses are members of the Orthomyxoviridae family. These viruses are enveloped viruses with a genome of single-stranded RNA. The majority of influenza viruses are classified antigenically as type A (based on internal viral proteins). Subtypes of the virus are based on antigenicity of the two viral glycoproteins embedded in the viral envelope, the hemagglutinin (H) and neuraminidase (N) proteins, and are designated by numbers (H1-16; N1-9). In addition to antigenicity, the hemagglutinin also affects virulence of the virus, and certain subtypes are associated with more pathogenic strains, notably H5 and H7. Another important characteristic of this family is the segmentation of the genome, with each virus containing seven to eight separate genetic segments encoding individual viral proteins. This allows for a unique form of viral mutation called reassortment. As with all RNA viruses, the mutation rate of the genome is quite high, and generally manifests as small point mutations, which lead to relatively minor amino acid changes in the viral proteins. Reassortment involves the exchange of entire gene segments when one or more distinct influenza viruses infect the same cell. This is often the mechanism of significant changes in antigenicity, virulence, or host/tissue tropism of influenza viruses. For example, the 2009 pandemic H1N1 influenza is a quadruple reassortant, having gene segments from four distinct influenza viruses, two mammalian and two avian in origin.[24] Reassortment is often referred to as "antigenic shift," reflecting the relatively large change in the viral genome, while "antigenic drift" refers to the smaller point mutations observed from season to season within a single strain.

The natural reservoirs of influenza viruses are birds, primarily waterfowl. The most common mammalian species affected are pigs, horses, and humans; more recently, dogs have experienced infection with a variant derived from equine influenza virus H3N8. Cats are only rarely infected with influenza virus.

In 1997, outbreaks of the HPAI H5N1 occurred in poultry in Southeast Asia. Subsequent spread of H5N1 strains in birds has occurred in Europe, the Middle East, and Africa. Sporadic cases of H5N1 in humans have also occurred with relatively high mortality. In 2004, the first report of H5N1 in domestic cats in Thailand was made by the World Health Organization.[287] Subsequent occurrences in domestic cats, as well as tigers and leopards, have been documented in Turkey, Iraq, China, Germany, and Austria.[18] In the majority of cases, exposures occurred from contact with infected poultry. HPAI H5N1 has not occurred in North or South America in either birds or mammals, to date.

In 2009, a new strain of H1N1 spread to humans causing a worldwide pandemic. This virus is a reassortant that has infected a number of species, including turkeys, ferrets, and swine. Infection of a domestic cat in the United States was documented in 2009, with infection occurring from an infected person to the pet cat in the household.[274]

Transmission and Pathogenesis

Oral infection of cats, particularly with avian influenza (e.g., by consumption of infected bird carcasses) can occur. In addition, aerosol and direct contact may be a means of transmission (i.e., spread of human H1N1 to cats by contact with infected owners). Finally, indirect contact, for example, with feces from birds infected with HPAI H5N1, may occur. Infections may be subclinical or may manifest with mild to severe disease ending in death. Factors such as dose of virus, strain virulence, and host factors may have an impact on the severity of disease. Prevalence of influenza infection in cats is very low, including in areas where HPAI H5N1 occurs, and cats are not believed to be important in maintenance or transmission of influenza virus for humans.[187] In fact, transmission of the virus from cats to humans has never been documented.[186,187] It is currently not known how well HPAI H5N1 can spread from cat to cat under natural conditions, although it has been shown to occur in experimental settings.[152,296]

Natural and experimental infections with HPAI H5N1 lead to viral replication in the upper respiratory and gastrointestinal tracts.[285] Spread to the lower respiratory tract with viral replication in type II pneumocytes may occur leading to alveolar damage.[286] This may manifest as severe pneumonia.[186,286] With HPAI H5N1, viremia may also occur, leading to spread to other tissues. In fact, in addition to pneumonia, hepatic necrosis is a common finding and contributes to the pathogenesis of this virus in cats.[150] In addition, neurologic disease associated with a nonsuppurative encephalitis has been found in natural infection with HPAI H5N1.[285] Infected cats may shed the virus in respiratory secretions and feces.[186]

Clinical Signs

In general, the incubation period for influenza in cats is quite short, usually 2 to 3 days. Typical signs, whether HPAI H5N1 or human pandemic H1N1, are fever, decreased appetite and activity, and respiratory signs such as dyspnea.[18,285] Conjunctivitis may also be observed.[285] With HPAI H5N1, signs of systemic spread may include icterus, hemorrhagic lesions, and neurologic signs such as seizures and ataxia.[285]

Diagnosis

Diagnosis may be established by virus detection or serology for virus-specific antibodies. For the former, virus isolation as well as genetic detection by PCR may be performed on oropharyngeal swabs or tissues post mortem.[186,285] In addition, immunohistochemistry for viral antigen may be performed on tissues post mortem.[285]

Treatment and Control

Treatment using human antiviral medication, such as oseltamivir (Tamiflu, Genentech, South San Francisco, Calif.) has not been clinically evaluated and is not recommended.[18] Supportive treatment, including oxygen therapy as needed, is generally all that is recommended. No vaccine is currently commercially available for any influenza of cats, although experimental vaccines have been designed. Control is by and large aimed at preventing exposure, including avoiding access to uncooked poultry.[18,186] Additional recommendations may be found elsewhere.[18,186]

FELINE PANLEUKOPENIA

Feline panleukopenia is caused by feline parvovirus (FPV), and remains a significant disease of cats. In addition to FPV, the newer canine variants of canine parvovirus (CPV), specifically CPV-2a, CPV-2b, and CPV-2c reacquired the ability to replicate and cause disease in cats. All of these variants are closely related, sharing approximately 99% DNA homology. Parvoviruses are small nonenveloped viruses with a single-stranded DNA genome. A notorious property of the parvoviruses is their extreme hardiness in the environment. They are shed in feces of infected animals and may remain infectious in the environment for months, or even years, when protected by organic matter.[101]

Parvoviruses are unique among most DNA viruses in that they have a significant mutation rate, more similar to that of RNA viruses; thus mutations occur in circulating field virus. Feline parvovirus is in evolutionary stasis as compared with CPV.[55] Canine parvovirus-2 is believed to be ancestrally related to FPV. It emerged in 1978, and as it adapted to dogs, additional variants arose with relatively minor amino acid changes in the capsomer protein genes. The original CPV-2 is now believed to be extinct, and CPV-2b is the most prevalent variant in circulation. In recent years, additional variants have emerged, and differ from CPV-2b by just a few amino acid residues, with some leading to antigenic differences. The nomenclature of these variants is confusing and has led to the reporting of several distinct CPV-2c isolates. These variants have been identified in Asia, Europe, South America, and most recently, the United States.[55,124,134] One of these variants contains a mutation at amino acid residue 426 of the major capsid protein, an important antigenic epitope of CPV, leading to substitution of an aspartic acid residue with glutamic acid.[56] This mutant has been reported to be replacing CPV-2b in Italy and is present in dogs in the United States. The disease associated with these newer variants appears to be similar to that seen with earlier strains, including vomiting, diarrhea that may be hemorrhagic, and leukopenia. The mortality rate thus far does not seem to be significantly different from that of previous isolates. Interestingly, the new canine variants that emerged from the original variant, CPV-2 (which lacked the ability to infect cats), have all reacquired the ability to infect and cause disease in cats.[54,85,134] This includes both CPV-2b and CPV-2c, which are currently the most prevalent variants in circulation. Thus when we discuss feline panleukopenia, it is important to bear in mind that the infecting agent may be either feline or canine in origin.

Transmission and Pathogenesis

FPV is shed from all body secretions during active disease but is most consistently found in feces. Replication of the virus in intestinal epithelia leads to fecal shedding of the virus, which is at very high levels in the acute phase of disease ($\geq 10^9$ $TCID_{50}/g$). The period of viral shedding is usually only a few days, but recovered cats can shed virus in urine and feces for as long as 6 weeks.[49] Infection with FPV occurs through the oral cavity, where the virus initially replicates in local lymphoid tissue. From there, the virus disseminates via lymphatics and blood to many tissues. As discussed below, successful viral replication leading to cell lysis occurs only in those cells that are actively replicating. Destruction of intestinal crypt cells leads to blunting or complete loss of intestinal villi, while bone marrow infection leads to profound leukopenia. In addition, destruction of lymphoid tissues can contribute to the virus-induced immunodeficiency.

All parvoviruses share a tropism for cells of high mitotic index; that is, these viruses can only complete their replication cycle in cells that are rapidly dividing. With its small genomic coding capacity, much of the replication machinery for the virus must be provided by the infected cell. Parvoviruses, unlike larger DNA viruses, such as adenoviruses, have no ability to "push" cells into the cell cycle; thus cells must be actively dividing to support parvovirus replication. In kittens and adult cats, this includes cells of lymphoid tissue, blood cell precursors in the bone marrow, and intestinal crypt epithelia. In the neonate, this also includes tissues such as the cerebellum and myocardium. The virus may also target a wide variety of cells in the developing embryo or fetus, causing reproductive loss. The virus causes a lytic infection in target cells, leading to their destruction. The typical clinical presentation in kittens reflects the bone marrow and intestinal epithelia involvement. For the former, because of the shorter half-life of white blood cells compared with red blood cells, this destruction generally manifests as a severe leukopenia, though anemia can occur. Anemia can also occur as a consequence of blood loss in the intestines.

Clinical Signs

The clinical presentation of FPV infection includes profound depression, a consequence of the bone marrow depletion, anorexia, and fever. Signs referable to the intestinal infection may not be evident initially or may only include vomiting, but diarrhea that may be hemorrhagic is a hallmark sign in most infections.[42,293] Kittens quickly become dehydrated and may be moribund with subnormal body temperatures. The classic disease presentation is most common in kittens at the time that maternal immunity wanes and mortality is high. A study of kitten mortality in the United Kingdom revealed 25% of kitten deaths were due to FPV.[37]

Infection of kittens in late gestation or in the neonatal period may result in myocardial or cerebellar destruction. The latter syndrome manifests as permanent ataxia and intention tremors.[293] Myocardial infection has been postulated to contribute to cardiomyopathy development, but a causal association has not been proven.[193]

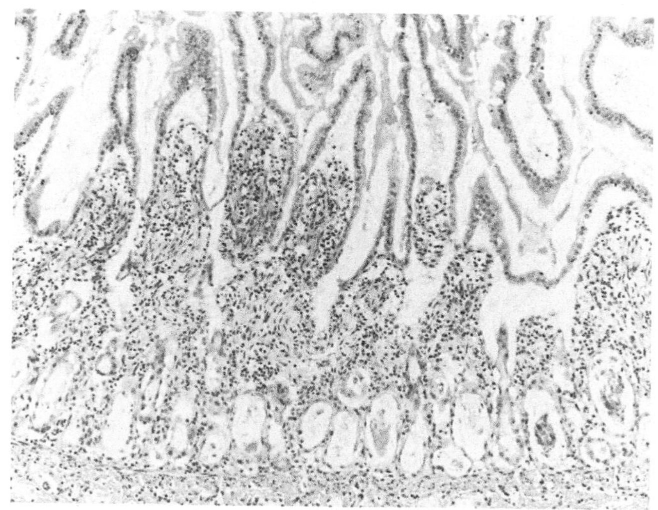

FIGURE 33-12 Feline panleukopenia virus infection in the small intestine. Photomicrograph of small intestine with radiomimetic type injury of cryptal necrosis. Crypts are dilated and lined by a reduced number of attenuated epithelial cells (H&E stain, 200×). *(Courtesy Dr. Robert Foster, Ontario Veterinary College and Yager-Best Histovet, Guelph, Ontario, Canada.)*

Diagnosis

Diagnosis of feline panleukopenia is generally based on clinical presentation, the presence of severe leukopenia (often <2000 cells/μL), and virus detection, which is often done in-house at veterinary clinics using commercial fecal enzyme-linked immunosorbent assay (ELISA) kits. Most kits use monoclonal antibodies, specific for a single epitope of the virus, to detect the virus in fecal samples. Typically, fecal ELISA test kits designed to detect CPV-2 variants of dogs will also detect FPV.[1,203] Evaluation of ELISA results must be interpreted in light of vaccination history, especially in shelter situations. It has been shown that some ELISA kits may detect vaccine virus for as long as 2 weeks postvaccination.[218] Commercial ELISA kits currently available have shown good sensitivity and specificity for detection of virus shedding in the unvaccinated animal.

Other diagnostic options include electron microscopy to visualize the virus in fecal samples, which is typically only available at laboratories affiliated with academic institutions, and PCR for genetic detection of the virus. Electron microscopy offers the advantage of being nonspecific—that is, it is an assay for any virus that may be causing enteritis, and it can detect agents such as coronavirus, rotavirus, or other viral enteric pathogens. The PCR assay is very sensitive and may detect vaccine virus or subclinical parvovirus infections; thus positive results by PCR must be interpreted in light of other relevant clinical data. Virus isolation, as well as histopathology and immunohistochemistry, can also be performed on tissues collected postmortem.[156] Histopathologic examination reveals crypt necrosis with villus blunting in the small intestines and cellular depletion in bone marrow and lymphoid tissues (Figure 33-12).[156]

Treatment

Treatment of panleukopenia is directed at supportive care. Strict isolation and barrier nursing must be used when treating affected cats in a clinic setting. Fluids to combat dehydration, and restoration of electrolyte and acid–base balance are critical in the treatment of panleukopenia.[293] Colloids, plasma, or whole blood transfusion may be required in hypoproteinemic cats (protein <5 g/dL). B-vitamin supplementation should be given parenterally because of decreased food intake and loss in diuresis. A platelet count and activated coagulation time should be evaluated for signs of disseminated intravascular coagulopathy (DIC). Initially, oral intake of food should be avoided to lessen vomiting and slow the bowel mitotic activity necessary for viral replication. Antiemetics may be necessary to control persistent vomiting. In addition to dehydration, a major concern is secondary bacterial septicemia resulting from the leukopenia and intestinal epithelial necrosis; thus parenteral broad-spectrum antibiotics with activity against gram-negative and anaerobic bacteria (e.g., amoxicillin/clavulanic acid with an aminoglycoside, fluoroquinolone, or cephalosporin) are an important management tool. Return to enteral nutrition is vital once vomiting ceases.[293] Feline recombinant interferon-omega has been shown to inhibit viral replication in vitro, and may be beneficial clinically.[293] Its administration has also been recommended in pregnant queens and neonatal kittens prior to introduction to a potentially contaminated environment in order to enhance antibody production.[215]

The antiviral medication oseltamivir (Tamiflu) has been proposed as part of the treatment regimen for CPV infection in dogs.[258] This drug, designed to combat influenza virus, inhibits neuraminidase enzyme activity. Parvovirus encodes no neuraminidase function; therefore this medication has no direct effect on the virus. Proponents of its use indicate it is beneficial because of its effect on bacterial neuraminidase enzymes. The efficacy and, more importantly, the safety of this medication in cats have not been evaluated, and its use is not recommended for panleukopenia cases.

Prevention and Control

Panleukopenia is most common in kittens and is uncommon in adults. Despite the ability of CPV-2a, CPV-2b, and CPV-2c to infect cats, FPV remains the most common cause of panleukopenia in cats.[55] Panleukopenia is a major concern in shelter and rescue situations where it may accumulate and survive disinfection. Thorough cleaning with a detergent to remove all organic matter, followed by disinfection with an appropriate product with oxidizing activity (e.g., 6% sodium hypochlorite, potassium peroxymonosulfate), is needed to inactivate the virus.[69] The virus survives disinfection with 70% alcohol and quaternary ammonium compounds.[69,101] Contaminated fomites and caretakers can be an important mode of transmission, and stringent precautions to prevent spread must be taken.

Passive immunization with serum from vaccinated or recovered cats is very effective, even after exposure, as long as clinical signs are not present. Serum donors should be selected with the same care as blood donors (see Chapter 25). Products containing immunoglobulins against parvovirus are available in some European countries for cats and are marketed for prophylactic and therapeutic use. Cats cannot be vaccinated with a modified live virus (MLV) product for 3 weeks after administration of immunoglobulin to avoid neutralization of vaccine virus. Repeated treatment should be avoided or anaphylactic reactions may occur.[293]

Immunity after recovery is likely lifelong.[42] Vaccination is recommended for every cat, given the severity of disease and the ability of the virus to persist in the environment.[50,249,293] The modified live vaccine is recommended as early as 6 weeks of age and continuing through 16 weeks to ensure that maternally derived immunity has not interfered with vaccine response.[249] In the face of an outbreak, kittens can be vaccinated as early as 4 weeks with a MLV vaccine to provide rapid onset of immunity. Current guidelines recommend re-vaccination at 1 year of age followed by vaccination every 3 years. Vaccination of pregnant queens or neonates (<4 weeks) with a MLV vaccine is not recommended, because the live attenuated virus may infect and produce lesions in the fetus or neonate.

FELINE CORONAVIRUS

Appearing for the first time in the 1950s, feline infectious peritonitis (FIP) continues to be a significant disease in domestic cats. Approximately 1 out of every 200 new feline cases seen at veterinary medical teaching hospitals are cats diagnosed with FIP.[252] The pathogenesis of FIP is complex, involving feline coronavirus (FCoV) and an inappropriate humoral response to the virus. A minority of FCoV-infected cats develops the lethal disease, and both host and virus genetic factors are believed to play a role.

Feline coronavirus is a member of the Coronaviridae, and is antigenically related to canine enteric coronavirus as well as transmissible gastroenteritis virus of swine. It is an enveloped virus, which is unusual for an enteric pathogen. There is a relatively large amount of glycoprotein embedded in the envelope in the form of peplomers, such as the spike protein, and this may contribute to the virus' stability. The virus may survive in the environment for up to 7 weeks under dry conditions[264] but is readily inactivated by common detergents and disinfectants.

The spike protein is used for cellular attachment and may play a role in cellular tropism of the virus as well as the pathogenesis of FIP. The genome of FCoV is single-stranded RNA and is one of the largest RNA genomes of the animal viruses. The coronaviruses have a high mutation rate, including point mutations, deletions, and recombination with heterologous coronaviruses. For example, FCoV serotype 2 is a recombinant between FCoV and canine enteric coronavirus, specifically, in the gene encoding the spike protein. Thus this serotype of FCoV is more antigenically related to canine coronavirus than to FCoV serotype 1.[195,300]

As alluded to above, there are two antigenically distinct serotypes of FCoV, based primarily on the antigenicity of the viral spike protein. Viruses capable of causing FIP may be of either serotype; however, the majority of field strains are serotype 1.[19] Feline coronaviruses are also characterized according to virulence, referred to as virus biotype. The most common biotype is that of mild or no disease associated with enteric infection by the virus, and it is often referred to as feline enteric coronavirus (FECV). This is actually a misnomer, because even in asymptomatic infections, the virus can spread systemically, albeit at relatively low levels. The biotype associated with FIP (FIPV) occurs in only a small percentage of infected cats. The viral properties responsible for the difference in biotype are the subject of intense research.

Virus factors are important to disease development, because virus strains vary in virulence. It has been theorized that a viral mutation is responsible for the change in biotype of the virus, leading to disease production. Speculation on the genomic locale of this mutation has involved the gene encoding the spike protein, as well as genes encoding several nonstructural proteins including 3c, 7a, and 7b. However, no consistent genetic difference between virulent and avirulent biotypes has been found. In fact, one study found 100% homology in the 3-prime one third of the genome when comparing the enteric and nonenteric forms of the virus from a cat with FIP.[65] Recently, genetic analysis of 56 isolates from cases of FIP (n=8) and asymptomatic FCoV infection (n=48) revealed biotype-specific genotypes in the gene encoding the membrane (M) protein.[30] In addition, phylogenetic clustering of virulent isolates was observed when based upon the genes encoding the spike structural protein and 7b nonstructural protein. These researchers concluded that based on their analyses, cases of FIP arise from infection with a distinct strain rather than in vivo mutation.

Other studies have shown that the product of the nonstructural 3c gene may also play a role in pathogenesis.[38,225] One research group found deletions within this gene occurring in the majority of FIPV isolates examined (n=28) but intact in all FECV isolates (n=27).[38] They speculate that these deletions lead to poor replication of the virus in the intestines of cats and may explain, at least in part, why FIP outbreaks are uncommon. Another research group had similar findings when analyzing the virus in eight cats that died of FIP, in that extraintestinal virus from FIP lesions in the majority of cases (74%) had deletional mutations in the 3c gene, leading to truncation of the protein, while fecal virus in all cats had an intact 3c gene and presumably functional 3c gene product.[225]

One phenotypic change in the virus associated with FIP disease production appears to be efficiency of replication in monocytes and macrophages, in that viruses causing FIP have acquired significant tropism for macrophages. Although FECV may spread beyond the intestines, it does so at relatively low levels, probably because of a poor ability to replicate in monocytes and macrophages.[144,192,269] The virus of FIP, on the other hand, replicates at high levels in macrophages and may disseminate throughout the body. Macrophage tropism appears to reside in a region of the spike protein.[254] Quantitative differences in viral RNA levels in the blood of cats with and without FIP have been found.[143] Rising amounts of viral RNA in the blood seen in end-stage disease may indicate enhanced viral replication and disease progression. This increased viral replicative capacity may be a key element of FIP pathogenesis. It is likely that the viral properties responsible for development of FIP do not lie in a single or, even necessarily, the same mutation in all cases, but instead lie in the high mutability of the virus and multiple genetic changes. It is also likely that each virulent isolate arises individually.

Transmission and Pathogenesis

Feline enteric coronavirus is spread by the fecal–oral route because the virus is primarily shed in feces and rarely in saliva or other body fluids. Virus may infect intestinal epithelial cells from the lumen after ingestion. From there, systemic spread by infection of monocytes/macrophages may occur. In multicat environments, kittens are infected at a young age, typically at 4 to 6 weeks as maternally derived antibodies wane.[8] However, infection as young as 2 weeks of age has been documented.[176] Fecal shedding occurs within 1 week following infection and may continue for weeks, months, or even lifelong. Two types of shedding patterns are observed: cats that shed virus almost continuously and cats that shed virus only intermittently.[77] In addition, a small number of cats are seropositive for FCoV, but never shed virus in feces, apparently having a high degree of immunity.[77] Chronic carriers are an important source of the virus for other cats within the household. Virus persists primarily in the colon; it may also persist in tissue macrophages, giving rise to recurrent viremia.[147] It is important to note that although FECV (the benign biotype) is highly infectious, FIPV (the virulent biotype) is infrequently spread in a horizontal manner.[221] FIPVs are strongly cell-associated and tissue-associated so that shedding into feces would not normally be possible.

Enzootic disease is common in multicat environments, such as catteries, where losses are sporadic and unpredictable. Overall mortality during a period of years is usually less than 5%.[221] Very occasionally, epizootics with high mortality have been reported that generally last less than 12 months. Epizootics are probably multifactorial, involving factors such as population stresses, overcrowding, high kitten birth rates, and genetically predisposed breeding cats. Risk factors for FIP in catteries include individual cat age, individual cat coronavirus titer, overall frequency of fecal coronavirus shedding, and the proportion of cats in the cattery that are chronic shedders.[78]

In addition to changes in viral properties causing the shift from a benign to virulent biotype, the pathogenesis of FIP also involves host factors. Genetic predisposition along familial lines has been observed, and breeds in certain countries or areas appear to have a predisposition for FIP development.[75,206,229] However, the incidence of FIP in cat breeds can vary greatly among countries, suggesting that susceptibility to disease is more related to bloodlines than the breed itself.[221] These host factors may manifest in the immune response of the cat to systemic spread of FCoV. In cats that develop FIP, a strong humoral response to infection occurs, with inadequate cell-mediated response by cytotoxic T lymphocytes.[220]

The antibody production is ineffective in clearing the virus and contributes to the immune-mediated disease.[138] The factors responsible for this unsuccessful immune response are unknown, but various mechanisms appear to be at work. As stated above, they seem to involve the immune response to FCoV infection, in particular, a shift from a T-helper lymphocyte type I (Th1) to a T-helper lymphocyte type 2 (Th2) response to the infection. The former is important in coordinating cell-mediated immunity, which is protective against FIP, while the latter is important in humoral response. This shift results in an exaggerated humoral response that is not protective, and, in fact, actually enhances the disease progression as the virus-specific antibody opsonizes the virus for phagocytosis by monocytes and macrophages.

Another finding in cats with FIP is lymphocyte depletion, particularly T lymphocytes,[106] through apoptosis. The resultant depletion of T lymphocytes contributes to enhanced viral replication, because these cells are important in cell-mediated immunity. At least one group of investigators propose that the virus-driven T-lymphocyte depletion occurring in infected cats that do not mount a quick and effective cell-mediated immune response leads to loss of immune control and unchecked viral replication.[51] The virus does not replicate in lymphocytes; so, some other mechanism must be responsible for this process.

Because lymphocytes are not target cells of FCoV, it is theorized that secreted factors, including cytokines, are critical to these lymphocyte effects, including the Th2 response and T-lymphocyte depletion. In fact, the T-lymphocyte response appears to be the decisive factor in disease progression. Monocytes and macrophages are major cytokine producers and are the target of FIPV infection. The cytokine secretion patterns from these cells thus determine the magnitude and direction of the immune response. Cytokines associated with cell-mediated immunity, such as IL-10, IL-12, and IFN-gamma have been found to decrease in cats that develop FIP. Elevations in cytokines IL-1beta and IL-6 have also been found in affected cats, which may contribute to the humoral response.[79] An increase in tumor necrosis factor-alpha (TNF-alpha) has been observed in some studies, and may contribute to the T-lymphocyte apoptosis.[282] A recent study has shown that FCoV-infected macrophages produce factors that promote B-lymphocyte differentiation into plasma cells.[281] This may contribute to the exaggerated humoral response.

Much focus has been placed on interferon-gamma, because of its role in enhancing the cell-mediated immune response. Although serum interferon-gamma concentrations were not found to differ between cats with FIP and healthy cats with feline coronavirus in catteries with a low incidence of FIP, higher serum concentrations were seen in healthy cats with feline coronavirus compared with cats with FIP in catteries with a high prevalence of FIP.[91] In addition, higher interferon-gamma concentrations were associated with FIP lesions, indicating that, at least at the tissue level, cell-mediated immunity may contribute to lesion development.[91] In particular, it indicates that local activation of macrophages by interferon-gamma may be occurring, leading to enhanced viral replication.[22] In contrast, a systemic increase in interferon-gamma concentrations, as indicated by elevated expression in blood, may protect infected cats from disease.[89,91]

Clinical Signs

The disease of FIP is predominantly immune mediated. Lesions are distributed along the vasculature, particularly along veins.[146] Vasculitis is the hallmark lesion of FIP, whether the effusive or noneffusive form. Emigration of infected monocytes/macrophages from blood vessels into perivascular regions incites local inflammatory responses. Type II and type III hypersensitivity responses occur with complement activation and cellular destruction. This may occur widely throughout an infected cat's tissues, leading to increased vascular permeability, extensive pyogranulomatous lesions, and the classic signs of the effusive, or wet, form of FIP. Alternatively, focal lesions may be confined to one or more organ systems in the noneffusive, or dry, form of FIP. The cells involved in the inflammatory process are primarily macrophages and neutrophils; however, B lymphocytes play a critical role in producing disease.[145]

The incubation period for FIP is unknown, but is probably weeks or months, in some cases, even years.[221] The cat with FIP generally presents with weight loss, fever, and inappetence. The fever may wax and wane and is not responsive to antibiotics. Kittens are often underweight and unthrifty compared with normal littermates (Figure 33-13). Icterus may be seen with both effusive and noneffusive forms (Figure 33-14). Abdominal palpation of affected cats may reveal thickened bowel loops, mesenteric lymphadenopathy, or irregular serosal surfaces of abdominal organs. Cats with the effusive form characteristically present with significant abdominal ascites. In fact, FIP is the leading cause of ascites in young cats, proving a more common cause than cardiac disease, neoplasia, and hepatic or renal disease.[307] The enlarged abdomen can contain a surprising amount of fluid and may be mistaken for pregnancy by owners of female cats. Typically, the abdominal distension is nonpainful, and a fluid wave can be palpated. Effusion in the thorax and/or pericardial sac may also occur. If pleural effusion occurs, the primary clinical signs may include dyspnea, tachypnea, open-mouth breathing, and cyanotic mucous membranes. Heart sounds will be muffled on thoracic auscultation.

With the noneffusive form, signs may be referable to virtually any organ, singly or in combination (Table

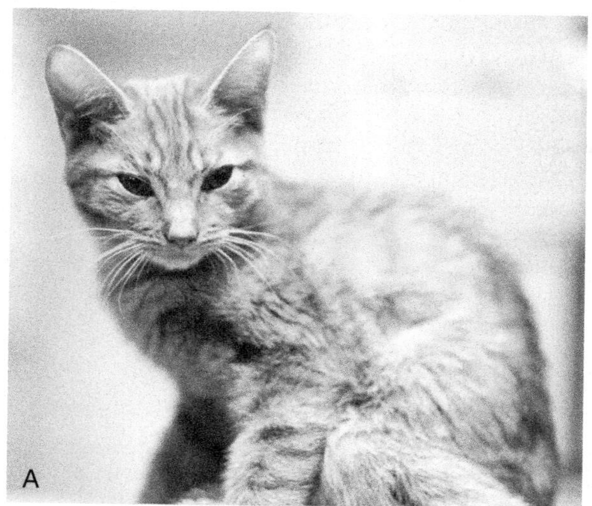

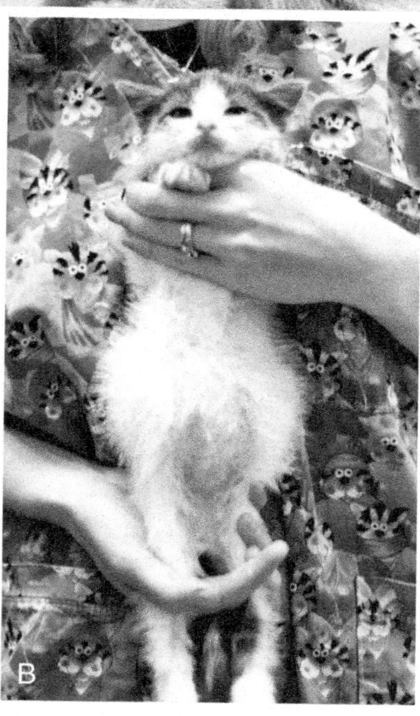

FIGURE 33-13 Kittens with FIP are often underweight and unthrifty compared with normal littermates. Pleural effusion may cause dyspnea **(A)**, and ascites may cause abdominal enlargement **(B)**.

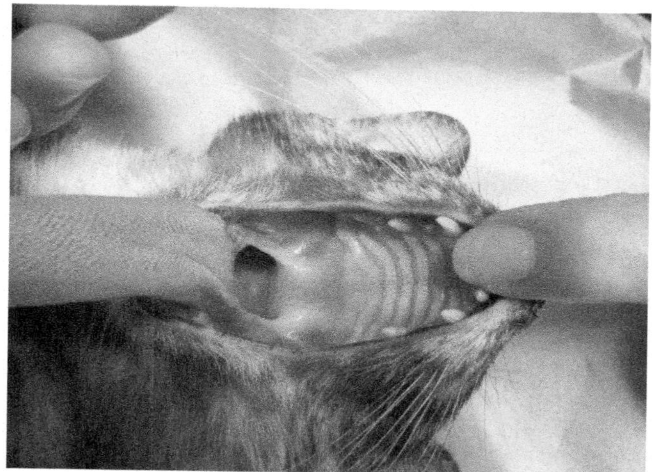

FIGURE 33-14 A Burmese kitten with noneffusive FIP. Icterus may be seen with both effusive and noneffusive forms of FIP.

TABLE 33-2 **Variability in Clinical Signs of Noneffusive Feline Infectious Peritonitis**

Clinical Signs Referable to Involvement of:	% of Affected Cats
Peritoneal cavity	32.0
CNS	23.0
Eyes	15.0
CNS and eyes	8.5
Peritoneal cavity and eyes	7.4
Peritoneal and pleural cavities	4.3
Peritoneal and pleural cavities, CNS	3.2
Peritoneal and pleural cavities, eyes	2.1
Peritoneal cavity, CNS, eyes	2.1
Pleural cavity	1.1
Pleural cavity, CNS, eyes	1.1

Adapted from Table 2 in Pedersen NC: A review of feline infectious peritonitis virus infection: 1963-2008, *J Feline Med Surg* 11:225, 2009.

33-2). Thoracic or abdominal effusions are either absent or too scant to be appreciated clinically. Granulomatous lesions may occur in the eye, including retinal changes, iritis, an irregular pupil, and uveitis with hyphema, hypopyon, aqueous flare, miosis, and keratic precipitates.[58] Ocular disease may be the sole manifestation of FIP in affected cats, or it may be combined with CNS or abdominal involvement. CNS lesions may be single or multifocal and may involve the spinal cord, cranial nerves, or meninges, causing seizures, ataxia, nystagmus, tremors, depression, behavior or personality changes, paralysis or paresis, circling, head tilt, hyperesthesia, or urinary incontinence.[149] FIP is the most common inflammatory disease of the CNS in cats[28] and is a leading cause of spinal disease.[185] Affected cats are typically young (less than 2 years old) and come from multicat environments.[76] In one study of 24 cats with FIP and neurologic involvement, 75% had hydrocephalus at necropsy.[149] The occurrence of seizures indicates extensive brain damage and is an unfavorable prognostic sign.[288]

Abdominal involvement with FIP may include granulomas in mesenteric lymph nodes, kidneys or liver, as well as adhesions throughout the omentum and mesentery that may be palpable as masses and visible with ultrasonography (Figure 33-15). With intramural intestinal involvement, diarrhea and vomiting may be observed. Focal granulomas may be found in the ileum, ileocecocolic junction, or colon. Involvement of the cecum and colon produces a distinct form of FIP with signs of colitis (soft stools containing blood and mucus).[116]

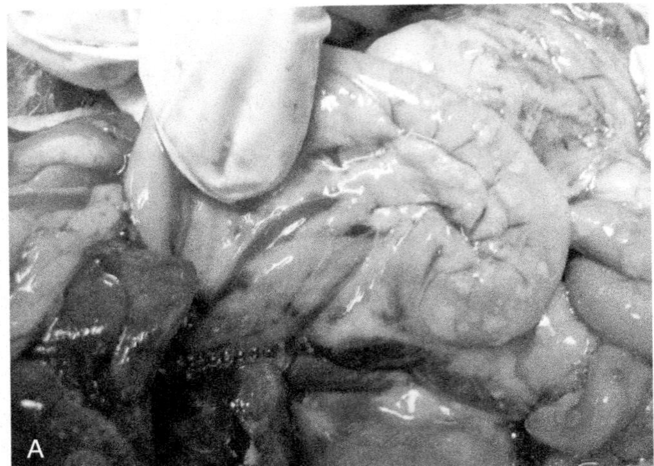

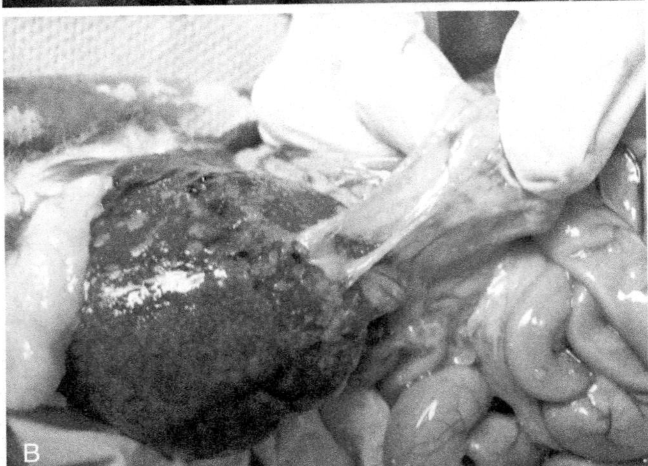

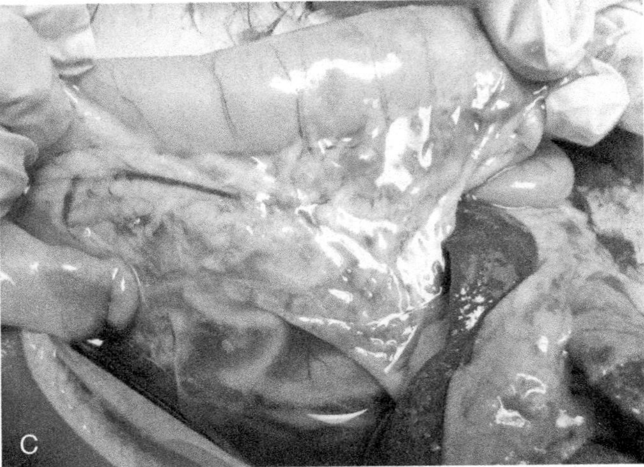

FIGURE 33-15 Abdominal involvement with FIP may include granulomas on the serosal surface of the intestines **(A)**; in mesenteric lymph nodes, kidneys, or liver **(B)**; as well as adhesions throughout the omentum and mesentery **(B)** and accumulation of straw-colored fluid **(C)**.

Uncommon manifestations of noneffusive FIP include cutaneous lesions, such as intradermal papules.[57] Skin lesions resulting from coronavirus-induced vasculitis have been reported in a cat with FIP and concurrent feline immunodeficiency virus infection.[33] Scrotal enlargement may occur because of extension of the peritonitis to the tunics surrounding the testes or because of chronic fibrinous necrotizing orchitis (Figure 33-16).[81,268]

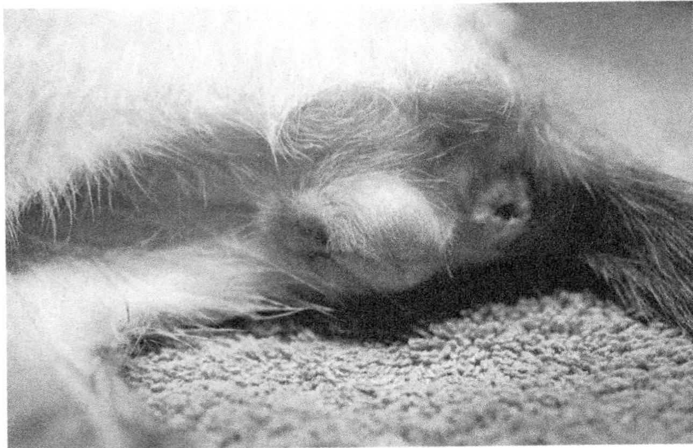

FIGURE 33-16 A Siamese kitten with FIP. Scrotal enlargement may occur because of extension of the peritonitis to the tunics surrounding the testes or because of chronic fibrinous necrotizing orchitis.

In addition, a combination of effusive and noneffusive forms may occur, and transition between the two can occur in any given cat with FIP. The onset of FIP may be acute or insidious. For the former, rapid development of effusion may occur, and the disease course may be short. For the latter, a subclinical state may exist for sometime or may be preceded by months or even years of vague illness and poor growth.[221]

Diagnosis

Diagnosis of FIP can be challenging, especially for the noneffusive form. Clinical signs of FIP, particularly the noneffusive form, are often vague; in addition, changes in clinical parameters are not pathognomonic for FIP. The effusive form of FIP is the easiest to diagnose, but only about 50% of cats that present with effusions will have FIP. The most common diseases that produce effusions similar to FIP include lymphocytic cholangitis and malignancies.[273] Feline coronavirus infection is common, thus evidence of infection is not diagnostic for FIP. Though diagnosis of FIP is critical, given the poor prognosis, ante mortem diagnosis of FIP can be a challenge, requiring a combination of evidence gathered from patient signalment, medical history, physical examination, imaging, and laboratory findings. There is no single test, other than histopathology and immunohistochemistry, that will confirm a diagnosis of FIP.

Diagnosing FIP starts with obtaining an animal's history and noting its signalment. Most cases occur in young cats (usually <1 year of age); it occurs more frequently in purebred than it does in mixed-breed cats; and affected cats usually originate from or are currently housed in multicat situations.[9] In breeding catteries, examination of records may reveal a genetic connection

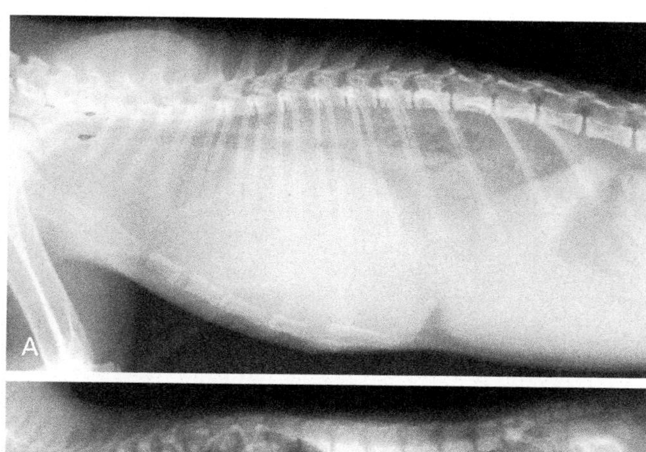

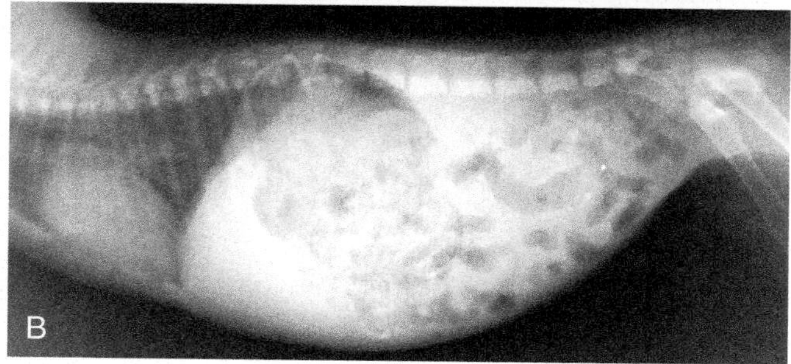

FIGURE 33-17 **A,** A thoracic radiograph of the kitten with pleural effusion shown in Figure 33-13, A. **B,** An abdominal radiograph of the kitten with ascites shown in Figure 33-13, B.

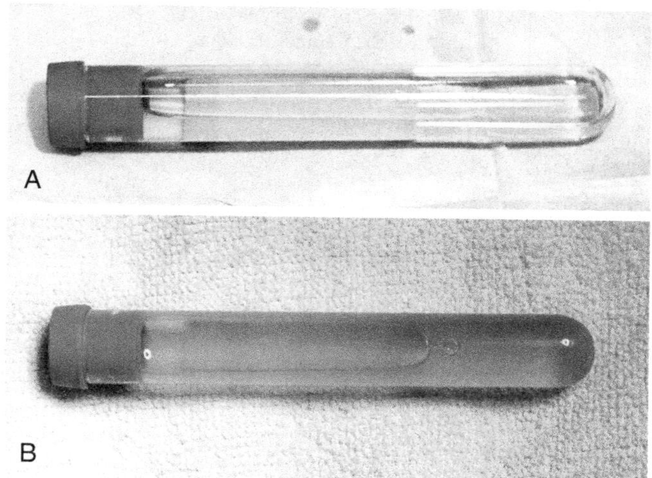

FIGURE 33-18 The effusion characteristic of FIP is straw to golden yellow in color, viscous, clear **(A)** to slightly cloudy **(B),** depending on cell count, often frothy when shaken.

BOX 33-2

Characteristics of the Effusion Found in Feline Infectious Peritonitis[217]

- Nonseptic exudate
- Straw to golden yellow color, viscous, clear to slightly cloudy, frothy when shaken
- High specific gravity (1.017 to 1.047)
- High protein (typically >3.5 g/dL, often 5 to 12 g/dL)
- Albumin:globulin ratio less than 0.45
- Low to moderate cellularity (<5000 cells/μL)

among cases. A history of a stressful event, such as spay or neuter, adoption from a shelter, or trauma, may precede the onset of signs by several weeks. An event that qualifies as a stressor may also be more subtle, such as a change of social hierarchy within the population.

Imaging, such as radiography and ultrasonography are useful to rule out other diseases and identify effusions, especially in cats with abdominal enlargement or dyspnea. A recent study of abdominal ultrasonographic findings in 16 cats with FIP identified a variety of nonspecific changes, such as renomegaly, irregular renal contour and hypoechoic subcapsular echogenicity, abdominal lymphadenopathy, peritoneal or retroperitoneal effusion, and diffuse changes within the intestines.[171] However, a normal abdominal ultrasonograph does not exclude a diagnosis of FIP.

For cats with effusion, evaluation of this fluid can be informative. Tests on effusions have greater diagnostic reliability than tests on blood or serum. Therefore the first step should be evaluation of the patient for evidence of effusion using radiographs and/or ultrasonography if necessary (Figure 33-17). The fluid has been described as straw-colored (Figure 33-18) and is usually viscous because of the high-protein content (Box 33-2). It usually has a relatively low cellular content that is pyogranulomatous (macrophages and neutrophils—usually no toxic changes in the latter) in nature. Detection of feline coronavirus antigen by immunofluorescence within inflammatory cells (macrophages) in effusive fluid correlates with a diagnosis of FIP.[112,217] Viral antigen detection by immunofluorescence is offered by many diagnostic laboratories and can be performed on sediment from submitted abdominal fluid. RT-PCR has been shown to differentiate FIP effusions from effusions because of other causes.[112] High levels of protein and a low albumin to globulin ratio in the fluid are also indicative of FIP.[112,217]

The Rivalta test is a simple and inexpensive supportive test on effusions in the diagnosis of FIP. It distinguishes between exudates and transudates. A test tube is filled with distilled water and one drop of 98% acetic acid is added, followed by one drop of effusion sample. If the effusion drop dissipates in the solution, the test is negative and not supportive of FIP. If the drop retains its shape, the test is positive and supportive of FIP. In one large retrospective study, the positive predictive value of the Rivalta test was 86%, and the negative predictive value was 97%.[112]

Serum chemistry profiles reveal that many cats with FIP have elevated serum total protein concentrations, because of the high globulin concentrations; however, even with normal total protein concentrations, a decreased albumin to globulin ratio may be evident. As

TABLE 33-3 **Specificity, Sensitivity, Positive Predictive Value, Negative Predictive Value, and Optimum Cutoff Value of Different Total Protein Concentrations, Gamma-Globulin Concentrations, and Albumin to Globulin Ratios in Effusions**

Total Protein					*Gamma-Globulin*					*Albumin to Globulin Ratio*				
Total Protein (g/dL)	**SP**	**SE**	**PPV**	**NPV**	**Gamma-Globulin (g/dL)**	**SP**	**SE**	**PPV**	**NPV**	**Albumin to Globulin Ratio**	**SP**	**SE**	**PPV**	**NPV**
5.0	0.10	1.00	0.56	1.00	0.5	0.47	0.94	0.67	0.87	0.5	0.89	0.62	0.86	0.76
6.0	0.33	0.88	0.60	0.71	0.1*	0.83	0.82	0.84	0.80	0.6	0.85	0.67	0.83	0.70
7.0	0.53	0.82	0.66	0.72	1.5	0.93	0.65	0.91	0.70	0.7	0.82	0.69	0.81	0.71
8.0*	0.90	0.55	0.78	0.62	2.0	0.97	0.44	0.94	0.61	0.8	0.79	0.78	0.80	0.68
9.0	0.93	0.32	0.84	0.55	2.5	0.99	0.35	0.98	0.57	0.9*	0.74	0.86	0.79	0.82
10.0	0.95	0.23	0.85	0.52	3.0	1.00	0.26	1.00	0.55	1.0	0.65	0.94	0.75	0.91
11.0	0.98	0.12	0.87	0.50										
12.0	0.99	0.07	0.89	0.49										

SP, Specificity; *SE*, sensitivity; *PPV*, positive predictive value; *NPV*, negative predictive value.
*Optimum cutoff value as determined by differential positive rate analysis.
Adapted from Table 3 in Hartmann K, Binder C, Hirschberger J et al: Comparison of different tests to diagnose feline infectious peritonitis, *J Vet Intern Med* 17:781, 2003.

this ratio approaches 0.5, a diagnosis of FIP becomes more likely (Table 33-3).[112] Other abnormalities may be evident depending on the tissues involved (e.g., elevated hepatic enzyme activities, azotemia, hyperbilirubinemia, hyperbilirubinuria).[271,273]

Complete blood count (CBC) results are variable and nonspecific but may include neutrophilia with a mild left shift, lymphopenia (<1500/μl), and anemia of chronic disease.[214,271,273] Lymphopenia may be present in the face of an elevated total white blood cell count. Immunophenotyping shows that the T lymphocytes, in particular, are depleted; in fact, a normal T-lymphocyte count has a significant negative predictive value for FIP. Immunophenotyping or flow cytometry is often offered by laboratories associated with academic institutions.[51] Results of serum chemistries and CBC may also be normal in cats with FIP.

In addition to high serum globulin concentrations, elevation in acute phase proteins also occurs. Elevations in alpha-1 acid glycoprotein (AGP) in serum have been noted in cats with FIP and may aid diagnosis. In one study that evaluated the usefulness of measuring AGP to diagnose FIP, it was found that high AGP concentrations (>1.5 g/L) in serum, plasma, or effusion samples are a discriminating marker for FIP.[64,216] Measurement of AGP can be specifically requested from some but not all commercial labs and is more commonly available in Europe than North America. However, it must be remembered that many other inflammatory conditions, such as lymphoma and FIV, can lead to an increase in serum AGP; so, it is not diagnostic for FIP by itself.

FIP is one of the most frequent causes of neurologic disease in the cat, especially in cases with multifocal clinical signs. Examination of cerebrospinal fluid from cats with neurologic FIP reveals a marked pleocytosis (>100 cells/mL) primarily consisting of neutrophils, high protein content (>200 mg/dL), and coronavirus antibody titer greater than 1:25.[241] Magnetic resonance imaging (MRI) is useful to confirm the presence of inflammatory disease and demonstrate abnormalities consistent with FIP, such as periventricular contrast enhancement, ventricular dilatation, and hydrocephalus.[76,202]

Serum Antibody and Virus Detection Assays

Feline coronavirus-specific assays can generally be categorized as FCoV-specific antibody measurement or virus detection assays. Because of the inability to identify a consistent viral mutation correlating with FIP, no FIP virus-specific test exists. Serologic analysis detects only antibody to the coronavirus and does not reflect the virus' biotype. Unfortunately, some commercial diagnostic laboratories use the misnomer "FIP test" for coronavirus antibody titer. Although a high antibody titer is consistent with a diagnosis of FIP, it is not confirmatory; in addition, some cats with FIP have low antibody titers or are seronegative.[9] This latter situation may occur in fulminant cases or may be due to high virus levels that bind antibody, making it undetectable in the serologic assay. Therefore serology should only be used as an aid to rule in or rule out the possibility of FIP, and a diagnosis of FIP should never be made on antibody titers alone.

Serologic assays for antibody to a single virus-specific protein (as opposed to antibody to multiple virus proteins) have been developed. In particular, a serologic test for antibody to the 7b protein has been offered as a diagnostic aid to FIP. This protein is a viral nonstructural protein whose function is unknown, but, as described above, it may play a role in disease development. It has been theorized that this protein is not expressed in all feline coronavirus infections; when expression does occur, perhaps because of a viral mutation allowing 7b expression, FIP may develop. Cats with high concentrations of antibody to the 7b protein would, by definition, be infected with the FIP viral biotype. However, subsequent studies have shown that 7b expression occurs in most infections; 7b-specific antibodies, although consistently present at high concentrations in cats with FIP, are also present in healthy cats with feline coronavirus.[142] Thus, although 7b seronegative status would lessen the likelihood of a diagnosis of FIP, this test cannot be used to confirm FIP.

Because of the problems associated with serology, it is difficult to use FCoV antibody testing to control or eliminate FIP from catteries.[221] In most cases, it is not possible to interpret the results of FCoV testing cats in catteries. Most catteries with an active breeding program, and having at least six cats, will have endemic FECV, and 50% or more of the cats will have FCoV titers of 1:100 or greater at any given time.[221] Unfortunately, antibody titers do not provide the type of information the breeder requires, such as whether any cats have FIP, whether a particular cat will develop FIP, and which cats are shedding FECV.

Virus detection assays also suffer from a lack of specificity for FIP virus. That is, finding the virus by antigen detection (e.g., immunofluorescent staining of ascitic macrophages) or genetic detection (e.g., real-time polymerase chain reaction testing of whole blood) is consistent with a diagnosis of FIP but is not necessarily confirmatory. At least one commercial laboratory (Auburn University College of Veterinary Medicine) offers a RT-PCR assay that quantitates the level of viral messenger RNA (mRNA) in the monocytes of cats. Although it is not known precisely how the cutoff levels were determined, high levels of viral mRNA do reflect efficient viral replication in circulating monocytes.[269] However, in a recent study, FCoV mRNA was detected in 14 of 26 blood samples, yet only one of these cats had clinical signs compatible with FIP.[32] As stated above, high viral loads in the blood are consistent with FIP, especially in the end stage; however, high viral loads in the blood are also found in healthy cats in endemically infected populations.[148,192] In addition, absence of circulating virus detectable by PCR has been observed in noneffusive, localized forms of FIP (Dr. Alfred Legendre, personal communication). Virus detection and quantitation is thus not confirmatory for FIP but does offer diagnostic information. In general, results of any single assay claiming specificity for the virus of FIP must be interpreted with great caution.

The gold standard for FIP diagnosis remains histopathology and immunohistochemistry for feline coronavirus antigen.[221,283] Granulomatous lesions are vascular and perivascular, primarily involving small and medium veins. Cellular composition is mainly monocytes and macrophages with a minority of neutrophils. B lymphocytes and plasma cells may be found at the periphery of lesions, while T lymphocytes are few. Detection of viral antigen (immunohistochemistry) or nucleic acid (in situ hybridization) in infected cells within lesions is found and is confirmatory; this testing is offered by some pathology laboratories.

Treatment

In the past, treatment has focused on two areas: suppressing the immune response or modulating the immune response. The former generally involves administering immunosuppressive drugs to inhibit the immune response, while the latter attempts to enhance the cell-mediated response through the administration of cytokines such as interferon. Immunosuppression by using prednisolone or cyclophosphamide will sometimes slow disease progression but will not provide a cure.[114] Antibiotics are not justified unless neutropenia occurs as a result of cytotoxic drug therapy. Good nutritional support and avoidance of stressors are also recommended.

Although human and feline recombinant interferon has been shown to inhibit feline coronavirus replication in vitro, in vivo studies have shown no effect on survival time or quality of life. Recombinant feline interferon-omega (Virbagen Omega, Virbac, Carros, France) had showed some initial promise in a small, uncontrolled clinical trial.[135] However, a larger placebo-controlled double-blind trial found no statistically significant difference in the survival time of cats treated with recombinant feline interferon-omega versus a placebo.[250]

Recently, a new drug tested in three cats with the dry form of FIP demonstrated efficacy in prolonging life and alleviating signs.[162] The drug, a polyprenyl immunostimulant, is an investigatory veterinary biologic and acts by upregulating mRNA expression of T-helper lymphocytes responsible for effective cell-mediated immunity. In this study, two cats with FIP were still alive 2 years after diagnosis, while one cat survived 14 months. As of this writing, further studies are underway to assess its potential for FIP treatment.

Finally, it is rarely necessary to isolate a cat with FIP from other cats in the home, particularly if the other cats are healthy adults. Transmission of FIP directly from cat to cat is the exception, not the rule. Isolation of an already sick kitten or young cat simply provides another stressor that may further impair the immune response.

Prevention and Control

Preventing FIP is challenging, because the only effective means of control is preventing infection with feline coronavirus. The widespread nature of the virus and its ease of transmission, as well as the existence of persistent infections, make this difficult in a multicat situation. If one cat in a multicat population dies of FIP, the other members are likely already infected with the circulating virus. The likelihood that other cats in the population will develop FIP is not high, but it can occur, especially if there are genetic links to the affected cat. There may be some risk to introducing a new cat to this population, but generally, outbreaks of FIP are not observed. In most pet cat homes, where the number of cats is small, there should be little risk to introduction of a new cat after a resident cat has died of FIP. To decrease the risk, owners should consider adopting older (greater than 16 weeks) rather than younger kittens, or even a young adult cat.

Various strategies have been used to eliminate or prevent feline coronavirus infection in a cat population (Box 33-3). In breeding catteries, isolating pregnant queens nearing parturition and queens and kittens after parturition, as well as early weaning at 5 to 6 weeks of age, has been advocated (Table 33-4).[5,6] This prevention method, which requires strict quarantine measures and low (<5) numbers of cats in the population, is designed to delay infection until the kitten is older and can more easily eliminate the virus after exposure. One of the most important measures that can be used in a breeding cattery is to maintain complete breeding records. Heritability of FIP susceptibility is known to exist; thus continued breeding of parents, particularly sires that have produced kittens that developed FIP, is not recommended.

Other means of control involve removing chronic shedders from the population. Detection of virus in the feces by using PCR testing is the optimal method for identifying viral shedding in multicat environments. PCR testing without quantitation is offered at many commercial laboratories. Testing multiple samples from an animal over time can identify chronic shedding.[120] Because these animals may shed the virus intermittently, at least two fecal samples (preferably more), collected at weekly to monthly intervals should be tested. An example regimen would be three samples collected daily, followed by three samples daily 1 month later. Some laboratories may offer pooling of samples to reduce costs. Serology may also be helpful, because cats that maintain high antibody levels are likely shedding high levels of virus.[10] However, it may be almost impossible to maintain a group of cats free of FCoV without strict quarantine measures and barrier nursing techniques that are typically beyond the capabilities of most breeding catteries.

BOX 33-3

Methods for Control of Feline Infectious Peritonitis in Multicat Environments[221]

1. Eliminate overcrowding: maintain no more than six breeding cats, keep cats in stable small groups
2. Maintain cats 3 years and older as a larger proportion of the population
3. Manage litter boxes properly: have adequate numbers of litter boxes, limit spread of litter and dust, scoop boxes regularly, empty and disinfect boxes at least weekly
4. Have a selective breeding program: produce the least number of kittens necessary, do not use any tom cat in a breeding program that has produced kittens that have developed feline infectious peritonitis, preferably do not use such queens either

TABLE 33-4 **Protocol for Early Weaning and Isolation to Prevent Coronavirus Infection of Kittens**

Step	Description
Prepare kitten room	1. Remove all cats and kittens 1 week before introducing new queen. 2. Disinfect room using 1:32 dilution of sodium hypochlorite (bleach). 3. Dedicate separate litter trays and food and water bowls to this room, and disinfect with sodium hypochlorite. 4. Introduce single queen 1-2 weeks before parturition.
Practice barrier nursing	1. Work in the kitten room before tending other cats. 2. Clean hands with disinfectant before going into kitten room. 3. Have shoes and coveralls dedicated to the kitten room.
Wean and isolate kittens early	1. Test queen for FCoV antibodies either before or after she gives birth. 2. If queen is seropositive, she should be removed from the kitten room when the kittens are 5-6 weeks old. 3. If the queen is seronegative, she can remain with the kittens until they are older.
Test kittens	1. Test kittens for FCoV antibodies after 10 weeks of age.

Adapted from Table 11-5 in Addie DD, Jarrett O: Feline coronavirus infections. In Greene CE, editor: *Infectious diseases of the dog and cat*, ed 3, St Louis, 2006, Saunders Elsevier, p 101.

At least one commercially available vaccine for feline coronavirus exists. It is an intranasal vaccine containing a temperature-sensitive mutant of feline coronavirus allowing replication in the upper respiratory tract but not systemically. The vaccine is given as two doses, 3 or more weeks apart, but is not started until 16 weeks of age or older. Although this vaccine appears to be safe, its efficacy has been questioned. A small reduction in the number of FIP cases was noted in one study when the vaccine was given to seronegative cats.[244] However, in cats with preexisting antibody, the vaccine showed no protection. In another field study, the vaccine failed to prevent FIP in kittens with preexisting FCoV antibodies in a cattery.[72]

In households in which feline coronavirus is endemic or in which FIP has occurred, most cats are seropositive and thus not aided by vaccination. Kittens at highest risk for FIP are those born into colonies in which the virus is endemic, where infection often occurs by 4 to 6 weeks of age. However, the vaccine is not given until 16 weeks of age; thus the vaccine is of dubious usefulness in those situations in which the risk is greatest. It may provide some protection for seronegative cats entering an infected population, but currently, this vaccine is not recommended as part of core vaccines for routine use.[5,50,249]

RABIES

Rabies is a member of the Rhabdoviridae family and belongs to the *Lyssavirus* genus along with European bat lyssaviruses 1 and 2. Rabies virus particles (rhabdovirions) are a characteristic bullet shape because of the cylindrical form of the nucleocapsid core. Rabies is an enveloped single-stranded RNA virus. Although all warm-blooded animals are susceptible to infection with rabies, mammals are the only known vectors and reservoirs. Species susceptibility varies considerably; for example, cats, foxes, and raccoons are highly susceptible while domestic dogs, horses, and goats are moderately susceptible, and birds have low susceptibility. Younger animals are generally more susceptible than older animals. Rabies virus is neurotrophic, traveling quickly to the CNS after infection. Salivary glands have high concentrations of virus, thus allowing efficient transmission through bites or saliva-contaminated scratches. An infected cat will be able to transmit the disease in saliva about 3 days before clinical signs appear. Environmental transmission by fomites is rare and infected animals are not viremic, so blood is not infectious. As an enveloped virus, rabies is inactivated by many disinfectants and labile when exposed to ultraviolet light and heat. The virus can remain viable in a carcass for several days or longer, depending on temperature.

Large parts of Europe are now rabies-free because of wildlife vaccination programs. Strict quarantines have kept several countries free of rabies, such as Japan and the United Kingdom. Worldwide, the majority of human rabies cases are due to dog bites, because dog rabies is endemic in many developing countries. In Canada and the United States, domestic dogs have been effectively eliminated as a reservoir. However, rabies virus continues to be a concern for cat owners; in 2008, 294 cases of rabies in cats were reported in the United States and Puerto Rico compared with 75 cases in dogs.[27] The risk of exposure to outdoor cats from infected wildlife is significant. Raccoons, skunks, and bats are the main reservoirs in the United States, but other species such as foxes, coyotes, and bobcats may also be infected. In addition, importation of rabies infected animals from areas of endemic infection, such as Africa, poses a risk and requires practitioners to be aware of potential cases, even in rabies-free areas.

Following exposure an incubation period of weeks to months may follow, but once symptoms appear, death occurs within days. The typical incubation period in cats is 2 to 24 weeks (average 4 to 6 weeks) before CNS signs appear.[102] Once rabies virus enters the CNS, damage to lower motor neurons (LMN) causes the typical ascending paralysis. After replicating in the CNS, the virus spreads via peripheral, sensory, and motor nerves. Virus reaches the salivary glands via cranial nerves. Virtually any tissue may be infected, but spread outside the CNS does not occur in every case.

Classically, rabies has been divided into two clinical presentations—furious and paralytic. However, rabies is variable in its presentation and atypical signs are common. Usually the initial history includes a bite wound. The prodromal phase in cats lasts up to 2 days and is characterized by behavior changes, erratic behavior, and fever spikes. In the furious form, cats show erratic and unusual behavior, aggression, restlessness, muscle tremors, and weakness or incoordination. The paralytic phase typically follows as LMN paralysis progresses. Mandibular and laryngeal paralysis is less common in cats than dogs. However, increased frequency of vocalization and a change in voice pitch are common in cats.[73] Ascending paralysis terminates in coma and death, usually after as little as 3 to 4 days.[255] There is no effective therapy for animals with rabies, and supportive care is not recommended. Clinically normal cats with suspected exposure to rabies should be quarantined as recommended by local authorities. Postexposure vaccination is forbidden in most countries.

Rabies should be considered as a differential diagnosis in any cat with profound behavior changes and/or LMN paralysis, particularly if there is a history of contact with wildlife. The definitive diagnostic test is demonstration of rabies virus antigen by direct fluorescent antibody testing of brain tissue. No ante mortem tests are considered sensitive enough for rabies diagnosis. Handling live cats suspected of rabies must be done with extreme care, using heavy protective gloves, cages, catchpoles, and other equipment. The animal must be humanely euthanized and the head removed and refrigerated until the brain can be examined. Specimens should be transported according to the specifications of the individual laboratory and should always be identified as hazardous.

Rabies titer testing may be required to export a pet to a rabies-free country. Although no "protective" titer is known in animals, a titer of less than or equal to 0.5 IU/mL detected by the fluorescent antibody virus neutralization (FAVN) method is accepted by most countries. Depending on the country, other requirements must be fulfilled, such as identification with microchip or tattoo.

Virus neutralizing antibody is critical for protection against rabies following exposure. Rabies is considered a core vaccination in countries where the disease is endemic.[50,82,249] Current vaccines provide excellent protection; the presence of neutralizing antibody at the time of exposure eliminates the virus prior to neuronal infection. In the unvaccinated cat, this immune response occurs too late to prevent neuronal spread. Rarely, rabies can occur in vaccinated animals; thus any animal exhibiting signs compatible with rabies should be handled as such, regardless of vaccination history.[199] Any cat dying from neurologic disease for which antemortem diagnosis was not obtained should be submitted for rabies testing.

FELINE RETROVIRUSES

The feline retroviruses, feline leukemia virus (FeLV) and feline immunodeficiency virus (FIV), are members of the Retroviridae and are among the most common and important infectious diseases of cats. FeLV and FIV are found worldwide, with variable seroprevalence depending on geography and risk factors (Table 33-5). Although infected cats may remain clinically well for prolonged periods (especially with FIV infection), retroviruses are associated with a wide variety of clinical problems, such as anemia, lymphoma, chronic inflammatory diseases, and secondary and opportunistic infections. Testing for FeLV and FIV should be part of the minimum database for all sick cats, even if previously tested negative.

Certain risk factors for infection are common to both FeLV and FIV worldwide. Sick cats are more likely to be seropositive than healthy cats, with sick feral cats having the highest risk. Other risk factors include age (>6 months), male gender, and access to outdoors. Low-risk groups include juvenile cats (<6 months) and spayed or neutered cats.[94,170,172,196] However, in one large study in the United States, seroprevalence in healthy feral cats was similar to that of healthy outdoor pet cats.[170] An important risk factor is bite wounds. In a study of over 900 cats with bite wounds or abscesses, 19.3% of cats

TABLE 33-5 **Seroprevalence of FeLV and FIV in Selected Areas and Populations of Cats**

Location	FeLV%	FIV%	Population
Japan[137]	N/A	28.9	3,323 cats
Belgium[59]	3.8	11.3	346 stray cats
Istanbul[308]	5.8	22.3	103 owned, outdoor cats
United Kingdom[196]	3.5	10.4	517 stray cats
Finland[278]	1.0	6.6	196 stray cats
Germany[92,94]	3.7	3.2	17,462 cats
South Africa[259]	12.3	22.2	454 sick cats; 3.5% co-infected
Australia[205]	N/A	8	340 owned/feral cats
United States[170]	2.3	2.5	18,038 cats; 0.3% co-infected
Canada[172]	3.4	4.3	11,144 cats; 0.5% co-infected

FeLV, Feline leukemia virus; *FIV,* feline immunodeficiency virus; *N/A,* not available.

were seropositive for one or both viruses (FeLV 8.8%, FIV 12.7%, co-infected 2.2%) at the time of treatment.[95]

FeLV and FIV share several important properties. They are single-stranded diploid RNA viruses with a cone-shaped capsid made up of the core protein. They possess a lipid envelope in which the glycoproteins needed for attachment and entry into the host cell are embedded. Outside of the host animal, these viruses are very labile, lasting only minutes in the environment; thus direct contact between animals is the most efficient mode of spread.

During replication of the retroviruses, the RNA genome is converted into double-stranded DNA (provirus) by the viral enzyme reverse transcriptase. This enzyme has no proofreading ability and is mistake-prone. As a result, the retroviruses have a high mutation rate, and even within a host, the population is heterologous, differing slightly from one another; thus each animal is infected with a cloud of variants, rather than a single genotype. These mutations may lead to changes in phenotype, which will be discussed with the individual viruses, as well as antigenicity. After conversion to DNA, the viral genome becomes incorporated into the host cell DNA. This integration is permanent; thus for total elimination of the virus, all infected cells must be removed. This viral DNA then serves as the template for new viral RNA genomes, which are ultimately packaged and released from the infected cell.

Feline Leukemia Virus

Feline leukemia virus was first described in 1964 in a cat with lymphoma and was formerly classified in the subfamily Oncovirinae, referring to its oncogenic ability. The subfamilies of the Retroviridae were renamed, and FeLV is now classified as a gammaretrovirus. Within the gammaretroviruses, FeLV is classified into A, B, C, and T subgroups based on antigenicity and host cell target (Table 33-6). Subgroup A viruses are generally mildly pathogenic and are the forms horizontally transmitted. Subgroups B, C, and T arise by point mutations of subgroup A members, and in the case of subgroup B, by recombination with endogenous retroviruses. All cats have endogenous retroviral genetic material that is normally present in the genome and is inherited. These pieces of endogenous DNA are not pathogenic themselves and do not produce infectious virus particles. However, they can recombine with exogenous retroviruses, such as FeLV-A, and increase the pathogenicity of the infecting virus.

Although FeLV was only "discovered" in 1964, genomic analysis has determined that it evolved from a virus in an ancestor of the rat.[21] This event likely took place up to 10 million years ago in the North African desert, an area where both cats and rats lived.

Transmission and Pathogenesis

Viremic FeLV-infected cats shed virus in many body fluids, including saliva, feces, milk, and urine. FeLV transmission occurs through sustained close contact among cats. Behaviors such as mutual grooming, sharing of food and water bowls and litter boxes, and fighting can contribute to transmission, primarily through saliva. Resistance to persistent infections increases with age, although the degree of natural resistance is unknown. Kittens less than 16 weeks of age are most likely to remain persistently infected after exposure. However, adult cats may be susceptible to FeLV infection after long-term exposure.[100]

FeLV can be transmitted to kittens by various routes from infected queens. Infected pregnant queens may suffer reproductive loss; kittens that survive to term are generally born viremic and fade quickly. Up to 20% of vertically infected kittens may survive to become persistently infected adults.[111] Transmission to kittens may also occur through the milk from an infected queen or through saliva when the queen cleans the kittens.[111]

FeLV subgroups are associated with distinct pathologies: Subgroup B is associated with lymphomas, C with nonregenerative anemia, and T with immunosuppression. This reflects the distinct syndromes that may be seen with FeLV infection—proliferative (cancer), degenerative (blood cell line depletion), and immunosuppression. The pathogenesis of FeLV infection can be thought of as occurring in six stages:

1. Virus enters through the oral cavity (e.g., by mutual grooming), where it infects and replicates in mononuclear white blood cells in the tonsils.
2. Transient cell-associated lymphatic and viremic spread of the virus to regional lymphatics occurs.
3. Spread of the virus to systemic lymphoid tissue occurs.
4. Infection of the blood cell precursors in the bone marrow occurs.
5. Secondary viremia disseminates the virus.
6. Virus replicates in many epithelial cells, including those of salivary glands, intestines, and conjunctiva.

In the past, it was thought that about one third of cats would become persistently viremic and two thirds would eventually clear infection.[125] Depending upon several factors, including immune status, age, dose, and strain of the virus, infection may be eliminated in the first three stages. Once bone marrow infection occurs, it becomes much less likely that the cat will clear the virus.

TABLE 33-6 **Classification of FeLV Subgroups**

Viral Subgroups	Frequency of Isolation in FeLV-Positive Cats	Associated Disease	Comparison by Species of In Vitro Replication
A	100% viremic cats, mildly pathogenic but highly contagious, mildly cytopathogenic	Hematopoietic neoplasia, experimentally may cause hemolysis	Cat, rabbit, pig, mink, human
B	Occurs with subgroup A in 50% or more of cats with neoplastic disease (lymphoma)	Not pathogenic alone, virulent in recombination with subgroup A, noncontagious	Cat, dog, cow, hamster, pig, human
C	Rarely isolated, arises by mutation from FeLV subgroup A	Nonregenerative anemia and erythremic myelosis, nonreplicating and noncontagious	Cat, dog, guinea pig, human
T*	Highly cytopathic, T-cell tropic virus; affinity for two host cell proteins: Pit1 and FeLIX; evolved from FeLV subgroup A	Lymphopenia, neutropenia, fever, diarrhea	Cat

*Subgroup T is a variant of subgroup A. Changes in the envelope protein result in increased cytopathogenicity of T strains.

Adapted from Table 13-2 in Hartmann K: Feline leukemia virus infection. In Greene CE, editor: *Infectious diseases of the dog and cat*, ed 3, St Louis, 2006, Saunders Elsevier, p 107. Modified from Jarrett O: Feline leukemia virus subgroups. In Hardy WD, Essex M, McClelland AJ, editors: *Feline leukemia virus*, New York, 1990, Elsevier; and Nakata R, Myiazawa T, Shin YS, et al: Reevaluation of host ranges of feline leukemia virus subgroups, *Microbes Infect* 5:947-950, 2003.

TABLE 33-7 Outcomes of Feline Leukemia Virus Infection

Outcome of FeLV Exposure	FeLV p27 Antigen in Blood	Viral Blood Culture	Viral Tissue Culture	Viral RNA in Blood	Proviral DNA in Blood	Viral Shedding	FeLV-Associated Disease
Progressive infection	Positive	Positive	Positive	Positive	Positive	Positive	Likely
Regressive infection	Negative or transiently positive	Negative or transiently positive	Negative or transiently positive	Transiently or persistently positive	Positive	Negative	Unlikely
Abortive exposure	Negative	Negative	Negative	Not tested	Negative	Negative	Unlikely
Focal infection	Negative	Negative	Positive	Not tested	Not tested	Variable	Unlikely

Adapted from Table 1 in Levy J, Crawford C, Hartmann K et al: 2008 American Association of Feline Practitioners' feline retrovirus management guidelines, *J Feline Med Surg* 10:300, 2008.

Evaluation of the FeLV-host relationship has been evaluated using real-time PCR, which provided new insight and evolving ideas on infection with FeLV.[289] This technology detects viral genetic material and can be designed to detect viral RNA or DNA (provirus—the DNA-integrated form of the virus). Researchers examined FeLV infection in vaccinated and unvaccinated cats and were able to define four separate classes of infection: abortive, regressive, latent, and progressive (Table 33-7):

1. Abortive infections are those in which the exposed cat produces an effective and early immune response preventing viral replication and eliminating virus-infected cells. These cats are negative for circulating viral antigen (core protein) and viral genetic material.
2. Regressive infections are those in which viral replication is limited, and a small population of virus-infected cells remain. These cats are also antigen negative, but viral genetic material can be detected in a small percentage of blood cells by PCR. These cats may go on to eliminate the virus completely. Regressively infected cats are not viremic (and therefore not contagious), but proviral DNA may be infectious through blood transfusion.[39]
3. Latent infection refers to those in which a moderate amount of proviral-infected cells remain. These cats are antigen negative but PCR positive. These latently infected cells have the potential for reactivation of virus replication but are not contagious as long as the infection remains latent.
4. Progressive infections are those in which virus replication is not eliminated; both viral antigen and genetic material can be detected in the blood of these cats, and they are actively shedding virus primarily in saliva and feces.[96,98] These cats are likely to become ill with FeLV-related disease.

In this study, these classifications were attained in the exposed cats within 4 to 8 weeks post-infection; however, these classifications are likely dynamic, especially in the intermediate stages. Interestingly, vaccination was not found to prevent provirus integration; thus vaccinated cats that are exposed to FeLV may become latently infected. Finally, focal infections were reported in early studies, describing FeLV infection restricted to certain tissues.[117]

These and other results suggest that many cats may remain infected with FeLV for life following exposure but may revert to a regressive state.[97,122,227] One study of 597 Swiss cats found that 10% of cats negative on ELISA for p27 antigen were positive for FeLV provirus by PCR.[122] The provirus is integrated into the cat's genome, and so, it may not be possible to clear infection.[36] The clinical significance of antigen-negative, PCR-positive cats is unclear. One study evaluated 152 necropsied cats, with various disorders, that were negative for viral antigen but positive for FeLV provirus in bone marrow. A significant association with anemia, panleukopenia, and purulent inflammation, but not lymphosarcoma, was found.[280]

Clinical Signs

Following exposure, cats may exhibit mild clinical signs, such as fever and malaise, or may remain asymptomatic. For cats that remain persistently infected, this acute phase is followed by a period of asymptomatic infection that may last months or years. Ultimately, persistently infected cats develop one of several FeLV-associated disorders (Box 33-4).

The B subgroup variants, which as stated above, arise in about 50% of infected cats by recombinational mutation between the infecting A subgroup with endogenous retroviruses, are oncogenic primarily by insertional mutagenesis. The provirus integration into the host cell genome activates a cellular oncogene or disrupts a tumor suppressor gene.[84] Some of these genomic loci for cellular integration have been identified, such as those for lymphomas,[84] the most common tumor of cats. The most common malignancies associated with FeLV are lymphomas and leukemias, but nonhematopoietic

BOX 33-4

Retrovirus-Associated Illnesses in Cats

- Common illnesses associated with feline leukemia virus (FeLV) infection
  - Hematologic disease: anemia (most commonly nonregenerative), neutropenia, thrombocytopenia
  - Lymphoma: common sites include mediastinum, eye, and multicentric forms
  - Myelopathy: gradually progressive neurologic dysfunction; abnormal vocalization and behavior, hyperesthesia, paresis progressing to paralysis
- Common illnesses associated with FIV infection
  - Stomatitis: variable severity, often refractory to conservative treatment
  - Neoplasia: most commonly lymphoma, but also other tumor types, including sarcomas and carcinomas
  - Ocular disease: most commonly uveitis and chorioretinitis
  - Central and peripheral neurologic disease: abnormal behavior, nystagmus, ataxia, seizures, paresis, and paralysis
  - Hematologic disease: anemia and leukopenia; often more than one cell line involved
  - Renal disease: similar to nephropathy in human immunodeficiency virus (HIV) patients
- Common secondary diseases in retrovirus-infected cats
  - Systemic infections: *Toxoplasma*, *Cryptococcus*, *Mycoplasma haemofelis*, feline infectious peritonitis
  - Gastrointestinal: stomatitis/gingivitis, parasitism (*Giardia*, coccidia, *Cryptosporidia*), bacterial infection (*Salmonella*, *Campylobacter*), chronic diarrhea
  - Dermatologic: *Demodex*, ringworm
  - Respiratory/ocular: herpesvirus keratitis, chronic upper respiratory infections/sinusitis, uveitis, chorioretinitis, spastic pupil syndrome (FeLV associated)
  - Urinary tract: pyelonephritis, bacterial cystitis

malignancies are occasionally seen. Prior to the 1980s, about 80% of feline lymphomas were FeLV-related. A dramatic shift has occurred, where now only a small percentage of cats with these malignancies are FeLV-positive. For example, only 8% of cats with lymphoma treated at the Animal Medical Center in New York between 1988 and 1994 were FeLV positive.[44] PCR detection of proviral DNA in tumor tissue may uncover more cases than FeLV antigen testing alone.[111,303a] Lymphomas are classified based on anatomic locale as mediastinal (thymic; Figure 33-19), alimentary, multicentric (lymph nodes), or extranodal (kidneys, CNS, skin). Leukemias are generally classified as to the cellular origin (e.g., erythroid, granulocytic, myelocytic).

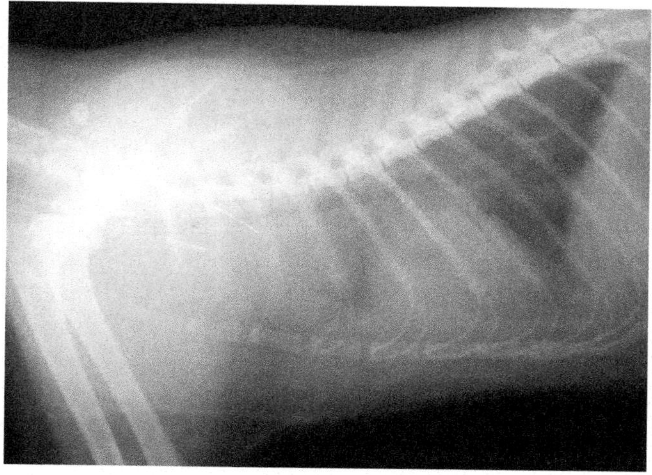

FIGURE 33-19 Radiograph of a mediastinal mass in a young cat with FeLV.

Anemias, mainly nonregenerative, are one of the most common clinical problems in FeLV-infected cats. Occasionally, regenerative anemia associated with *M. haemofelis* or immune-mediated destruction is seen. FeLV-infected cats may also develop anemia of chronic disease. The C subgroup variants are rare and are associated with fatal red cell aplasia. These variants arise from mutations in the envelope glycoprotein gene of the infecting subgroup A virus. This mutation leads to a change in cell receptors used by the virus from the thiamine transporter to the heme exporter.[265] This switch in host receptors is believed to disrupt early erythropoiesis, leading to a nonregenerative anemia, typically with a hematocrit less than 15%, that is resistant to therapy.

Immunosuppression is one of the most common manifestations of FeLV infection, and is very complex. Some viral proteins, particularly the transmembrane protein p15e, are directly immunosuppressive. The p15e protein affects the interleukin 2 signaling pathway.[155,191] In addition, FeLV infection may lead to lymphopenia, especially a decrease in CD8+ cytotoxic T lymphocytes, which are critical for viral immunity. Granulocytopenia may also occur, as well as effects on neutrophil function. The result is recurrent or chronic infections with other pathogens (e.g., poxvirus, *M. haemofelis*, *Cryptococcus*, *Toxoplasma gondii*), including agents that are usually of little clinical significance, such as *Salmonella* or *Listeria*.[175,240] Concurrent infection with feline coronavirus may lead to FIP development. Other infections, such as abscesses, rhinitis, and stomatitis, may be slow to resolve.[175]

FeLV may be neuropathogenic.[60] Neurologic disease not associated with malignancy has been described and manifests clinically as anisocoria (Figure 33-20) and mydriasis, Horner syndrome, urinary incontinence, abnormal vocalization, hyperesthesia, as well as paresis and paralysis.[29,34]

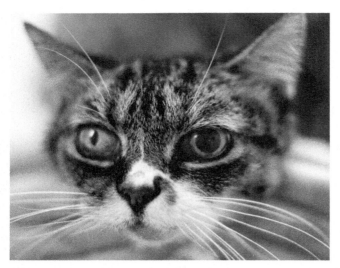

FIGURE 33-20 FeLV may cause neurologic disease not associated with malignancy that may manifest as anisocoria.

Diagnosis

Diagnosis of FeLV-related disorders is multifaceted. Clearly, confirmation of FeLV infection is of primary importance, but since FeLV-infected cats may be concurrently infected with other pathogens that are treatable, such as *M. haemofelis*, identification of any concomitant pathogen is critical as well. A minimum database (CBC, serum chemistry panel, urinalysis) is important for the investigation of any sick cat, including cats that may have retroviral infections. Low neutrophil and thrombocyte levels are commonly seen in FeLV-infected cats, as well as anemia.[92,93] No consistent abnormalities are seen in serum chemistry panels from FeLV-infected cats.

Confirmation of FeLV infection relies on detection of the virus. There are several in-clinic screening ELISA-based kits available that detect the core protein of the virus (p27). These tests vary in sensitivity and specificity, but most have high negative and positive predictive values.[113,256] In-clinic kits may be used with anticoagulated whole blood, serum, or plasma, although the test kit should be checked for the manufacturer's recommendations. Most cats will test positive for soluble FeLV antigen with ELISA early in primary viremia, within 30 days of exposure. The exception is those ELISA tests using saliva and/or tears; these tests do not detect viral antigen until the epithelial cells are infected, at stage 6, and are thus not ideal for routine screening. As well, they are known to have a high rate of false results.[165]

Because ELISA tests for FeLV detect viral antigen, and not antibody to the virus, maternal immunity will not interfere with testing. Vaccination generally does not interfere with testing; however, blood samples drawn immediately following vaccination may contain detectable FeLV vaccine antigen.[166] It is unknown how long this type of test interference lasts; FeLV testing should always be performed before vaccination. Confirmation of a positive result obtained by ELISA is recommended, particularly in healthy cats. False-positive results are possible, and may be due to a number of factors, including improper testing or kit storage and hemolyzed samples. A false-negative test result can occur if the cat is tested too early in the course of infection for detection of soluble antigen (less than 4 weeks). In addition, because ELISA testing on serum can detect early infection, it does not distinguish transient from persistent infection. The confirmatory test recommended is the immunofluorescence assay (IFA), which detects virus infected cells, primarily neutrophils. It is best performed on a smear prepared from fresh whole blood, because anticoagulants can interfere with results.[15] This assay can detect infection only after the blood cell precursors in the bone marrow have been infected (stage 4), 6 to 8 weeks after exposure. Thus an IFA positive result indicates that the cat is likely persistently infected. False-negative IFA results may occur in leukopenic cats. False-positive results may occur if the smear is too thick, if background fluorescence is high, or if the test is performed and interpreted by inexperienced personnel.[166]

Early in infection a cat may be ELISA positive and IFA negative; these cats should be rechecked with ELISA in 1 to 3 months to determine their status. If the ELISA result remains positive, a second IFA test should be performed to confirm. Uncommonly, a cat may remain discordant (ELISA positive, IFA negative); the reason for this is unclear but may be seen in a latently infected cat that is periodically antigenemic. In these cases, PCR may be used to detect proviral DNA. PCR can also be used to detect provirus DNA in antigen-negative cats that are regressively or latently infected. PCR is recommended only for cats that are to be used as blood donors, cats with persistently discordant ELISA/IFA results, or antigen-negative cats that are believed to have a FeLV-related disorder, like lymphoma.

Recently, a novel PCR for detection of FeLV viral RNA in saliva has been described.[97] The diagnostic sensitivity and specificity, as well as positive and negative predictive values for the PCR, were very high when compared with conventional ELISA. In situations where the cost of testing is a barrier, such as shelters and multicat households, it is possible that pooled saliva samples could be used for screening. The method is sensitive enough to detect one infected cat in a pool of up to 30 samples.[98]

Treatment

Illness in the FeLV-infected cat requires prompt attention for accurate diagnosis and institution of appropriate treatment. Because of the immunosuppression associated with FeLV, identification of secondary infections and treatment, which may be prolonged compared with noninfected cats, is required. Immunosuppressive drugs, such as corticosteroids, should be avoided unless specifically indicated.[175] For FeLV-associated anemias, transfusions may be necessary. Treatment of FeLV-associated neoplasia should follow established regimens. Symptomatic and supportive treatment may also be required for FeLV-associated diseases.

Immunomodulatory treatment has been investigated for the FeLV-infected cat. *Staphylococcus* protein A (SPA), a cell wall component of the bacterium with immunoenhancing activity has been evaluated in FeLV-infected cats. In at least one study, although subjective assessment of owners indicated improvement with SPA treatment, objective parameters did not differ from those in cats given the saline control.[190] Several other treatments, such as acemannan and *Proprionibacterium acnes*, have been evaluated and either failed to demonstrate efficacy or suffer from poorly-designed studies.

Interferon, an important antiviral cytokine has also been evaluated in FeLV-infected cats. The effects on the virus in cell culture were induction of apoptosis in infected but not uninfected cells, decreasing the amount of viral replication overall.[41] In vivo studies have had conflicting results; at least one study showed no improvement.[190] However, this study used human recombinant interferon. Treatment with feline recombinant interferon (Virbagen Omega, Virbac) has shown evidence of improved clinical picture and survival, but evaluation of virologic parameters was not performed in these studies.[52,189] A suggested treatment protocol is 1 million U/kg, SC, every 24 hours for 5 consecutive days.

Lymphocyte T-cell immunomodulator (LTCI; ProLabs, St. Joseph, Mo.) is a product of the thymic stromal epithelial cells that is now commercially available for feline retrovirus-infected cats. It enhances interleukin-2 and interferon production by T-helper lymphocytes, which, in turn, enhances cytotoxic T-lymphocyte activity.[90] LTCI is supplied in 1-mL single dose vials for SC injection, and the recommended protocol is an initial three-dose regimen given at weekly intervals, with further treatments as necessary. LTCI is reported to improve clinical and hematologic parameters. However, controlled clinical trials have not been published.

The antiretroviral drug 3′-azido-2′3′-dideoxythymidine (AZT) has shown some positive effects but can have serious side effects at higher dosages (recommended dose is 5 to 10 mg/kg, PO, every 12 hours).[175] Careful monitoring of the patient's CBC is necessary, because AZT can cause bone marrow suppression, especially anemia. Many other antiretroviral drugs are too toxic for use in the cat or are not effective against FeLV or FIV.

FeLV-infected cats that are otherwise healthy can be maintained, sometimes for years, without problems. Data on survival of retroviral infected cats indicate that the lifespan of FeLV-infected cats is generally shorter than that of uninfected cats. In one study conducted in the United States, records of 67,963 cats that were tested for FeLV and FIV in 2000, and that had outcome information available 6 years later, were analyzed.[169] Survival of infected cats was compared with age-matched and sex-matched uninfected cats. The 6-year survival rates were 90% for uninfected cats, 65% for FIV-positive cats, and 51% for FeLV-positive cats. Most deaths in cats with FeLV or FIV occurred in the first year after diagnosis, probably because of the illness that prompted the original veterinary visit or because of euthanasia for purposes of infection control. A study of 17,289 cats in Germany tested for FeLV and FIV from 1993 to 2002 included survival data on 100 randomly selected cats: 19 FIV positive, 18 FeLV positive, and 63 uninfected.[94] The mean survival time of FeLV-positive cats (312 days) was significantly shorter than that of FeLV-negative cats (732 days).

Owners should be advised that certain precautions should be instituted with FeLV-infected cats, including isolation from uninfected cats (Box 33-5). This protects not only the uninfected cats from FeLV, but it also serves to limit the risk of exposure of the FeLV-infected cat to other feline pathogens.[175] Given that many

BOX 33-5

Client Education for Owners of Retrovirus-Infected Cats

- Confine retrovirus-infected cats indoors to prevent disease transmission to other cats and to protect the infected cat from trauma and infectious disease.
- Spay and neuter intact cats.
- Whenever possible, isolate infected cats from uninfected cats to prevent disease transmission.
  - Feline leukemia virus (FeLV) is primarily spread by close, intimate contact (i.e., between friendly cats); vaccination of any FeLV-negative in-contact cats is recommended.
  - Feline immunosuppressive virus (FIV) is primarily spread by bite wounds (i.e., between unfriendly cats); transmission is unlikely in socially stable households, and a decision to vaccinate any FIV-negative in-contact cats should be taken with care because of vaccine interference with testing.
- Feed a high-quality commercial diet.
- Avoid raw meat and eggs, and unpasteurized milk as potential sources of bacterial or parasitic infections.
- Monitor infected cats closely for potential signs of illness, such as
  - Changes in social interactions with people or other pets.
  - Changes in activity level and sleeping habits.
  - Changes in food or water consumption.
  - Unexpected weight loss or weight gain.
  - Bad breath odor.
- Consult a veterinarian promptly at the earliest sign of illness.

BOX 33-6

Wellness Examination Procedures for Retrovirus-Infected Cats

- Obtain a detailed medical, dietary and behavior history.
- Perform a thorough physical examination, with special attention to the lymph nodes, skin, eyes, and oral cavity.
- Weigh the patient accurately.
- Perform a complete blood cell count, serum chemistries, and urinalysis (cystocentesis collection) at least once yearly.
- Feline leukemia virus (FeLV)-infected cats should have a complete blood cell count at least every 6 months.
- Perform fecal examinations if the patient is at risk of intestinal parasite infection or has signs of gastrointestinal disease.

BOX 33-7

Prevention of Retrovirus Transmission in Veterinary Hospitals

- Feline leukemia virus (FeLV) and feline immunosuppressive virus (FIV) are fragile viruses that do not persist in the environment and are susceptible to all common detergents and disinfectants.
- Ensure routine infection-control measures are in place.
  - Ensure routine handwashing.
  - Disinfect equipment, cages, instruments, food/water bowls, litter boxes, and so forth.
  - Do not re-use dental or surgical instruments without sterilization.
  - Do not re-use needles/syringes or share bags of intravenous fluids among patients.
  - Avoid multidose vials of medication and vaccines.
  - Feed all cats individually; do not share dishes of food.
  - Carefully handle/dispose of infected body fluids (blood, urine, saliva, feces).
- House infected cats individually but not in special isolation or contagious disease areas.
- Screen blood donors appropriately for blood type and infectious diseases.

retrovirus-infected cats will survive for years after diagnosis, veterinarians should be familiar with guidelines for management of infected cats.[166,175] Wellness exams should be performed every 6 to 12 months to detect problems early (Box 33-6). Otherwise healthy retrovirus-infected cats require routine veterinary care, including surgical sterilization and dental prophylaxis. Simple precautions in the veterinary hospital will enable these patients to receive appropriate care safely (Box 33-7). FeLV is not considered a zoonotic disease; one study of 204 veterinarians and others with potential exposure to retroviruses, including needle sticks, failed to detect retrovirus infection using serologic and molecular methods.[31]

The necessity of vaccination of healthy FeLV-infected cats with core vaccines should be evaluated on an individual basis. Inactivated vaccines are often recommended because modified live virus vaccines have a theoretical risk of reversion to virulence in an immunosuppressed animal. However, definitive clinical evidence to support this recommendation is not available. FeLV vaccination is of no benefit and should not be administered to FeLV-infected cats.

Prevention and Control

FeLV testing may be performed for a variety of reasons (Box 33-8). The American Association of Feline Practitioners (AAFP) has stated that the retrovirus status of all cats should be known because the consequences of infection are important to the patient and any in-contact cats.[166] Preventing exposure of healthy cats to FeLV-infected cats by test and removal or isolation is an important way to prevent spread of the disease and is not replaced by vaccination as a control method.[253]

Kittens can be tested for FeLV at any age, because passively acquired maternal antibody does not interfere with testing for viral antigen. Newborn kittens infected from FeLV-positive queens may not test positive for weeks to months after birth. Although it may be tempting to test only a queen and not her kittens in an attempt to conserve resources in shelter or rescue settings, it is inappropriate to test one cat as a representative for others. Even young kittens may be exposed to cats other than the dam; for example, feral queens often share mothering of kittens. If a queen or any one of her kittens tests FeLV positive, all should be considered potentially infected and isolated, with follow-up testing to resolve status.[111] If a queen or one kitten in a litter tests negative, it cannot be guaranteed that the others are also negative. Shelters or rescue groups sometimes test pooled blood samples from litters of kittens in order to save money; the reliability of this method is unknown and cannot be recommended.

Certain populations of cats require tailored recommendations for control of retrovirus infections. Retrovirus testing and management for multicat environments such as shelters is discussed in Chapter 46. Breeding catteries have a low prevalence of FeLV infections, since the advent of test and removal programs over 30 years ago. However, these multicat environments require

BOX 33-8

Summary of Feline Leukemia (FeLV) and Feline Immunosuppressive Virus (FIV) Testing Recommendations

1. Cats that should be tested for FeLV and FIV include
   a. At-risk cats: sick cats, cats with bite wounds or oral disease, cats with known exposure to a retrovirus-infected cat, cats in multicat environments where the status of all cats is not known, cats entering shelters or rescue organizations
      - Sick cats should be tested regardless of a negative FeLV or FIV test result in the past
   b. Newly acquired cats and kittens
   c. Cats about to be vaccinated for FeLV or FIV
2. Test for FeLV antigen and FIV antibody at presentation with in-clinic or referral laboratory enzyme-linked immunosorbent assay (ELISA)
   a. Cats that test positive for FeLV and/or FIV
      - If FeLV positive, confirm with immunofluorescence assay (IFA)
      - If FIV positive and greater than 6 months of age
        i. If not FIV vaccinated, confirm with Western blot
        ii. If known or possibly FIV vaccinated, confirm with an alternative test methodology, such as a validated polymerase chain reaction (PCR) test

        If FIV positive and less than 6 months of age, re-test at intervals of 30 days until the kitten tests negative or is greater than or equal to 6 months of age
   b. Cats that test negative for FeLV and FIV
      - Ideally, all cats should have confirmatory testing performed to ensure negative status; however, it is most important for sick cats and cats with bite wounds
        i. Although FeLV retesting alone can be performed in a minimum of 30 days, it is may be more practical and cost effective to re-test for both viruses in a minimum of 60 days with in-clinic or referral laboratory ELISA
3. Cats at ongoing risk of infection (e.g., cats with access to outdoors) should be tested annually for FeLV and for FIV, if not FIV vaccinated, with in-clinic or referral laboratory ELISA
4. Cats used for blood or tissue donation in practice or in shelters should have negative screening tests for FIV antibody, as well as FeLV antigen and FeLV provirus by serology and real-time PCR, respectively

ongoing disease surveillance because factors such as group living and introduction of new cats favor transmission of infectious diseases. The retrovirus status of all cats in a breeding cattery should be known, and ideally negative test results should be confirmed.

BOX 33-9

Retrovirus Infection Prevention Recommendations for Breeding Catteries

- Any newly acquired cats should be isolated and tested before introduction into the population.
- Queens sent outside the cattery for breeding should only be mated to toms known to be retrovirus negative. Upon return, the queen should be isolated and tested in 60 days.
- Cats that have left the cattery for a cat show do not need to be re-tested, because cat shows are very low-risk environments for retrovirus transmission.
- Catteries that maintain retrovirus-negative status do not require vaccination of cats against feline leukemia virus (FeLV) or feline immunodeficiency virus (FIV), as long as no cats have access to outdoors.
- Catteries that rely heavily on sending queens to an outside stud service should consider FeLV vaccination of queens in addition to testing.
- Vaccination against FIV is not recommended because FIV is uncommon in catteries and vaccination interferes with common testing methods.

Adapted from Levy J, Crawford C, Hartmann K et al: 2008 American Association of Feline Practitioners' feline retrovirus management guidelines, *J Feline Med Surg* 10:300, 2008.

Infected cats should be removed from the cattery. Additional recommendations for breeding catteries are found in Box 33-9.

Vaccination against FeLV is not considered a core vaccine but is recommended for cats at risk of exposure[50,175,249] (e.g., cats with access to outdoors, cats living with known FeLV-infected cats, multicat environments where the status of all cats is not known). In addition, vaccination of all kittens has been recommended,[249] because a kitten's status (indoor vs. outdoor; low risk vs. high risk) may change, and susceptibility to persistent infection is highest in kittenhood. Several vaccines are available, including whole inactivated virus, subunit, and recombinant canarypox vector vaccines (which may be administered subcutaneously or intradermally). Testing of cats prior to vaccination is recommended to ensure negative status. Inadvertent use of FeLV vaccine in a cat infected with FeLV is not harmful, but it is also of no benefit. However, vaccination of a cat that is unknowingly retrovirus-infected gives false expectations to the owner and will give rise to unnecessary questions of vaccine efficacy when the infection is eventually discovered.

The efficacy of the available vaccines is controversial.[272] Many of the published efficacy trials have been conducted or supported by the vaccine manufacturer, and most studies do not evaluate more than one vaccine.

Other factors hamper interpretation of vaccine efficacy, such as lack of standard challenge and testing protocols, and the difficulty of infecting adult cats for a trial. Generally, inactivated whole virus vaccines have been recommended. In addition, a recombinant FeLV vaccine provided protection against persistent antigenemia equivalent to an efficacious inactivated whole virus vaccine.[104] One study using whole inactivated virus vaccines found that, after challenge, vaccinated cats had no detectable viral antigen, RNA, proviral DNA, or infectious virus.[290] Other studies have shown that vaccines do not prevent the persistence of proviral DNA following exposure.[123] Despite these findings, several current vaccines are efficacious at preventing persistent virus persistence and replication, as well as FeLV-associated disease.[121]

Feline Immunodeficiency Virus

Feline immunodeficiency virus (FIV) was discovered in 1986 in a California cattery where cats had immunodeficiency-like illnesses.[224] FIV is a member of the Retroviridae, along with FeLV, but is classified in a different subfamily, Lentivirinae, along with HIV, equine infectious anemia virus, and ovine progressive pneumonia/caprine arthritis encephalitis viruses. The immunodeficiency viruses of domestic cats are classified into several subtypes or clades, designated A to E, based on the antigenicity of the envelope glycoprotein, gp120. Some authorities also recognize a sixth clade (F) that is found predominantly in Texas. Prevalence of the various clades varies geographically, although most field isolates belong to clades A or B. In the United States, clades A, B, C, and F have been identified, with clade B being predominant.[303] In Canada, clades A, B and C have been identified.[246] In the United Kingdom, only clade A is found, and in Japan, all clades have been identified. In general, clade A is thought to be less pathogenic than clades B and C. Within a clade, variations in genotype as well as phenotype may occur, including emergence of more pathogenic subtypes.[53,230] Recombination between two distinct isolates may also occur with co-infection, leading to new strains as well.[118]

Infection with lentiviruses related to FIV has also been documented in many nondomestic cat species around the world, such as the lion, puma, and Florida panther. In general, the isolates from nondomestic cats are less pathogenic than domestic cat FIV. This suggests that nondomestic cats have been living with the virus for a long time and that infection of domestic cats is more recent. Domestic cats can be infected with isolates from nondomestic felids, but do not develop the same clinical and immunologic abnormalities found in FIV-infected cats.[292,297]

Variations in the envelope glycoprotein affect cross-reactivity and cross-protection among virus strains. The virus structure, stability, genomic characteristics, and replication at the cellular level are similar to FeLV. One of the main target cells of FIV is the CD4+ T-helper lymphocyte, which is essential for both cell-mediated and humoral immunity. Dysfunction and destruction of these cells are critical to the pathogenesis of disease. But FIV has a relatively broad cell tropism, and it is not restricted to cells expressing CD4; it may also use chemokine receptors for cellular attachment and entry. The virus also replicates in B lymphocytes, monocytes and macrophages, salivary gland epithelia, and fibroblast and neural cell lines.

FIV has a high mutation rate because of an error-prone reverse transcriptase enzyme, leading to the circulation of many heterologous strains, even within a single host. Some of these mutations may lead to changes in virulence or antigenicity.[53,230] This tremendous variation has an impact on diagnostics, therapeutics, and vaccine development.

Transmission and Pathogenesis

The virus is present in saliva of infected cats, and FIV infection is most likely to occur in male cats and free-roaming cats, reflecting the efficient transmission by bite wounds. Queens may be infected during mating if bitten by an infected tom cat. However, transmission through sustained contact among infected and uninfected cats, as with FeLV, may occur.[7] In addition, *in utero* and lactogenic transmission to kittens from queens may occur, especially if the queen is experiencing high levels of viremia.[12,208] *In utero* transmission may lead to fetal resorption, abortion, or stillbirth and is likely due to placental inflammation.[40] However, experimental evidence suggests that not all kittens in a litter will acquire infection *in utero* from an FIV-infected queen.[207,208,251] When the pregnant queen is acutely infected and has a high viral load, most of the kittens will become infected. However, when the pregnant queen is chronically infected and healthy, with low a viral load, few kittens will become infected. Complicating the picture is the fact that some kittens born to FIV-infected queens have FIV provirus detected in tissues, but not blood, and are negative for FIV antibody in blood.[11] In experiments, queens can be infected through semen, but it is unknown how important this mode of transmission is in nature.[139]

After inoculation of FIV, the virus replicates in T-helper (CD4+) lymphocytes, which are critical cells for appropriate and adequate immune responses to infecting pathogens. The virus binds through CD134 molecules and may also use a chemokine receptor (CXCR4) for attachment on the cell surface.[68] CD134 protein is upregulated on activated T lymphocytes, thus making these cells the primary target of FIV. Viral infection of these cells leads to disruption of normal function, as well as cell death. In addition, during the acute phase of infection, infection of a subset of T-helper cells, the

T-regulatory lymphocytes, contributes to the disease process. These cells have an immunosuppressor function. It has been shown that infection of these cells with FIV leads to activation, and, by definition, immunosuppression. This may contribute to the ineffective FIV clearance with resultant chronic infection, as well as immunodeficiency.[194] In addition to T lymphocytes, the virus infects macrophages and dendritic cells.

Following cellular infection, as part of the replication cycle, viral RNA is transcribed to double-stranded DNA by the viral enzyme reverse transcriptase. The DNA product then integrates into the cellular DNA as a provirus. In activated lymphocytes, viral RNA is transcribed using the DNA template by the cellular RNA polymerase. This is followed by viral protein synthesis, assembly of the virion, and release of the infectious virus. In nonactivated cells, the replication cycle may stop at the provirus stage; this is referred to as a latent infection, which may be reactivated with activation of the lymphocyte, allowing completion of the viral replication cycle.[126] This ability of the virus to persist integrated into the cellular genome makes treatment as well as prevention through vaccination challenging.

Most infected cats will mount an immune response to the virus, which leads to decreased virus replication and viral load in infected cats, but not elimination of infection. This generally occurs within 1 to 3 months postinfection, and the cat will then enter an asymptomatic phase. Virus replication continues, but at very low levels. This phase may last for months or years. Initially, levels of both CD4+ and CD8+ lymphocytes decline. As the cat mounts an immune response, a rebound of CD8+ lymphocytes above preinfection levels occurs. This causes an inversion of the CD4+:CD8+ lymphocyte ratio (the normal ratio is 2:1) that is persistent. Over time, the level of both CD4+ and CD8+ lymphocytes may gradually decline, ultimately leading to immunodeficiency in the infected cat.

Clinical Signs

FIV infection can be categorized into clinical stages similar to HIV infection, and various schemes for staging cats have been devised.[99,136,222] A simplified and useful categorization for the practicing clinician is as follows, bearing in mind there may not be clear distinction between phases and not all cats will demonstrate each phase:

1. Acute phase: Clinically, cats may present in the acute phase of infection with signs such as depression, anorexia, fever, and lymphadenopathy. Some cats, however, remain asymptomatic immediately following infection.
2. Clinically latent phase: A significant period of asymptomatic infection follows that may last for months or years. During this asymptomatic stage, however, changes in blood cell values may occur. Although hematologic abnormalities are less common than in FeLV-infected cats, FIV infection of bone marrow cells may lead to peripheral cytopenia of one or more cell lines.[83,93] In addition, FIV-infected cats have higher serum total protein and globulin concentrations than uninfected cats. In one study, FIV-infected cats also had lower serum aspartate transaminase (AST) and glutamate dehydrogenase than uninfected cats.[93]
3. Acquired immunodeficiency syndrome (AIDS)-related complex (ARC) phase: As the cat progresses to the immunodeficient state, secondary infections may occur. In addition, immune-mediated diseases resulting from immune cell activation may also occur. These manifestations generally occur later in life, perhaps years after initial FIV infection. Cats may present with single or combinations of infectious agents, including viral, bacterial, fungal, protozoal, and parasitic, and clinical signs may involve any system. Infections may be chronic or intermittent/recurring in nature.
4. Acquired immunodeficiency syndrome (AIDS) phase: This terminal phase of infection is characterized by neurologic disorders, neoplasia, multiple concurrent infections, and serious opportunistic infections. Survival time is no more than a few months.

The clinical signs and illnesses associated with FIV are varied and nonspecific (see Box 33-4) and are usually not a direct effect of the virus but resulting from secondary infections that may be treatable, such as *Demodex*-associated skin disease (Figure 33-21). One of the most common clinical presentations is chronic gingivostomatitis (Figure 33-22),[126] though the precise pathogenic mechanisms at work are unclear. Histologic findings include lymphocytes, plasma cells, and variable neutrophilic and eosinophilic infiltrates. Ocular disease has been well characterized in cats with FIV, with abnormalities in both the anterior (uveitis [Figure 33-23], glaucoma) and posterior (pars planitis, retinal degeneration, retinal hemorrhage) segments.[70,158,306] Neoplasia is also common in cats with FIV and includes various tumors, such as lymphomas (primarily B lymphocyte) and leukemias. FIV may infect neural tissue, causing neurologic disease, affecting central or peripheral nerves. Clinical signs reported include seizures, behavior changes, cognitive difficulties, and paresis.[126] Renal disease has also been associated with FIV infection and may be similar to HIV-associated nephropathy. Affected cats have glomerular and tubulointerstitial lesions, elevations in BUN and creatinine, and proteinuria.[232,233] In one group of 155 cats with FIV, azotemia and proteinuria were more common than in age-matched uninfected cats.[164] In an Australian case-control study of 73 cats with chronic

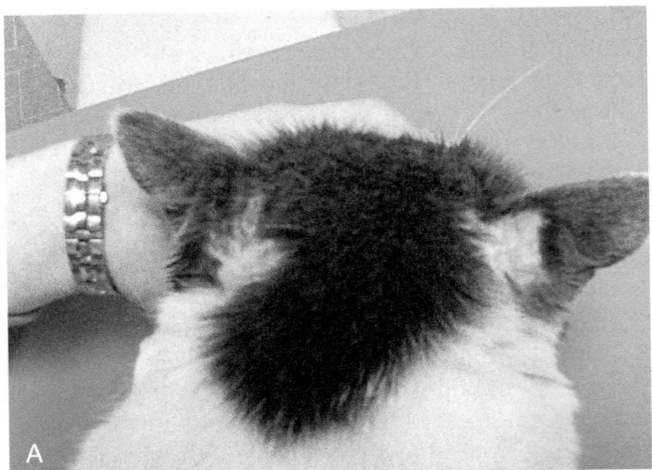

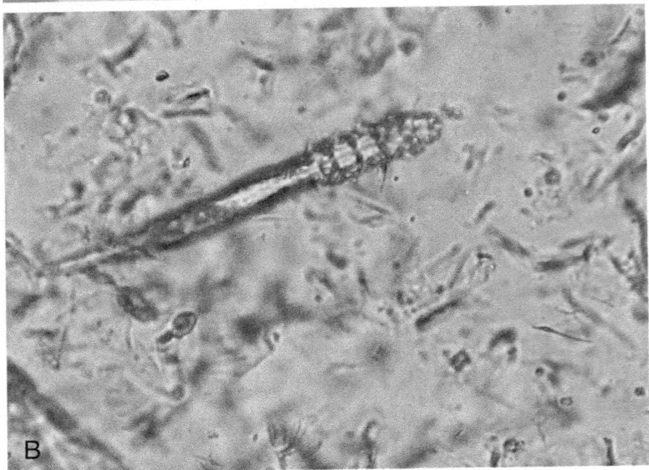

FIGURE 33-21 Secondary causes of disease are common in FIV-infected cats, such as this cat with alopecia and pruritus **(A)**. Skin scrapings revealed infection with *Demodex cati* **(B)**.

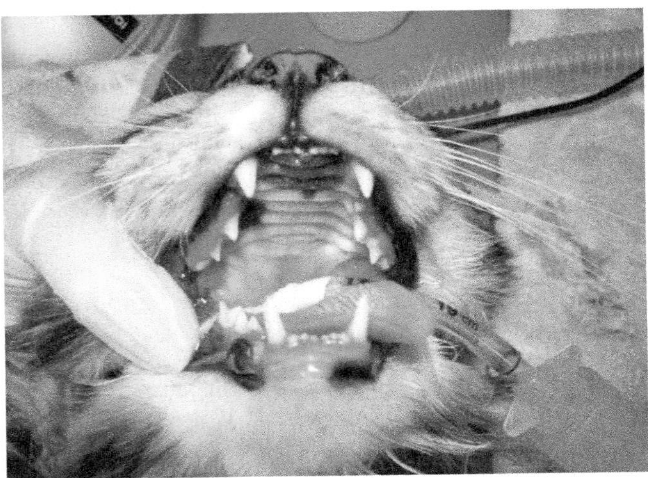

FIGURE 33-22 One of the most common clinical presentations in cats with FIV is chronic gingivostomatitis.

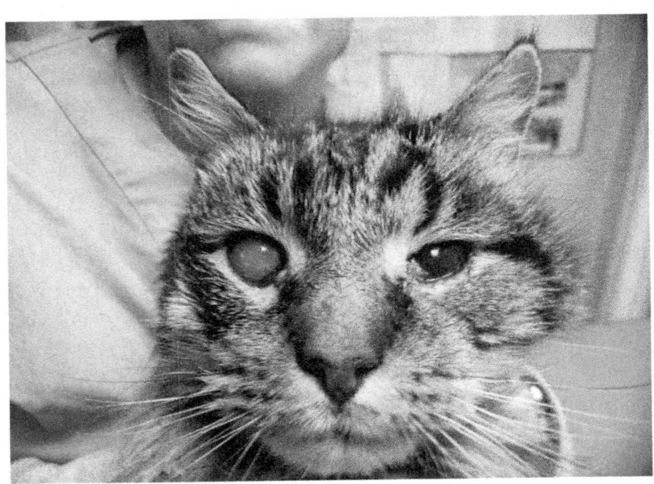

FIGURE 33-23 Ocular disease has been well characterized in cats with FIV, such as the anterior uveitis seen in this cat.

kidney disease (CKD) and 69 control cats, cats less than 11 years of age with CKD were significantly more likely to be FIV positive than cats of similar age without CKD.[304]

Diagnosis

Routine diagnosis of FIV infection currently relies on detection of virus-specific antibody. Rapid screening for viral antigen is not possible, because the amount of circulating virus is low after the acute stage of infection. FIV produces a persistent, lifelong infection so that the detection of antibodies is sufficient for diagnosis as long as the cat has not been vaccinated for FIV. Detection of FIV-specific antibodies is initially performed using a point-of-care ELISA or immunochromatography kits. Using these kits, most cats will have detectable FIV antibody within 60 days of infection, but some cats take up to 4 months to seroconvert.[15] Comparison of several diagnostic kits that are commercially available indicate a high sensitivity and specificity and significant (>90%) negative and positive predictive values in cats with no history of FIV vaccination.[113,168] Despite these results, confirmation of positive ELISA results when screening a healthy cat is recommended. Although virus culture is considered the gold standard for FIV infection, it is not readily available in many countries, and it is time-consuming and labor-intensive. A different soluble antibody test has been recommended as a confirmatory test,[166] but to date, only one FIV antibody test is commercially available in Canada and the United States. Western blot and immunofluorescent antibody assays are available in many countries. These assays detect antibodies against an increased number of viral antigens and are suggested as confirmatory tests in seropositive cats with no history of FIV vaccination.

Kittens born to infected or FIV-vaccinated queens may acquire FIV antibodies in colostrum. In a study of such kittens, FIV antibodies persisted past 8 weeks of age in more than 50% of kittens (n=55) born to FIV-vaccinated queens (n=12), but were no longer detectable at 12 weeks of age.[177] In another study, passively acquired antibodies in five kittens from infected queens declined to undetectable levels only by 17 weeks of age.[237] None of the routine testing methods can distinguish passively acquired maternal antibodies from antibodies produced by infected kittens; thus kittens less than 6 months of age testing positive using these assays should be retested when maternal antibodies wane. For example, kittens can be rested at intervals of 30 days until negative for FIV antibody. Though infection of kittens, even those born to infected queens, is uncommon, one must assume a kitten testing positive is contagious until a negative result is achieved. Kittens greater than 6 months of age with FIV antibodies are more likely to be infected. Because of concerns regarding detection of passively acquired FIV antibodies, it is tempting to delay testing kittens for FIV until after 6 months of age. Because they are a low-risk group, most kittens test negative and can reliably be considered clear of infection. However, infected kittens could be a source of infection for other cats if they are not identified and isolated. Compliance of both owners and veterinarians with retroviral testing recommendations was low in one published study so that delaying testing of newly acquired kittens until 6 months of age would potentially result in many cats that never undergo FIV testing at all.[95]

The recent development of a vaccine for FIV has complicated testing in countries where it is available (e.g., Canada, United States, Australia, New Zealand, and Japan, but not Europe), because the current technology used for screening tests cannot distinguish natural infection from vaccination.[168] Antibodies derived from vaccination persist for more than 1 year, and possibly for more than 4 years.[166,168] In some cats, it may be difficult to determine if a positive FIV antibody test means the cat is truly infected with FIV, is vaccinated against FIV but not infected, or is vaccinated against FIV and also infected. Detection of viral nucleic acid by PCR has been proposed as an alternative testing method for vaccinated cats. However, both false-negative and false-positive results may occur.[25,46] For the former, the most common cause is the inherent genetic variability of FIV strains, making development of a genetic assay that can detect all strains challenging. False-positive results have been observed in vaccinated cats.[46] In one study, the sensitivity and specificity of PCR testing for FIV varied tremendously among laboratories. The most accurate test was the real-time PCR, but it had a sensitivity of only 76%.[46] Newer PCR technologies, such dual-emission fluorescence resonance energy transfer (FRET) real-time PCR, may prove more reliable for discrimination of FIV-vaccinated from FIV-infected cats.[301]

Because of the limited sensitivity of currently available assays, PCR is not useful as a screening tool for FIV and will not replace in-clinic or referral laboratory ELISA tests. Rather, PCR testing should be reserved for FIV antibody–positive cats that have an unknown vaccination history or that have been vaccinated against FIV but where infection is still suspected. PCR test results must be interpreted with caution. A positive FIV PCR result from a laboratory with stringent quality control should confirm FIV infection and should not be affected by FIV vaccination. However, a negative FIV PCR result does not rule out infection, but may reflect a level of viral nucleic acid below the limit of detection, or a strain of FIV that is not detected by the test.

Recently, a study has shown that cats vaccinated for but not infected with FIV may not produce antibodies to all FIV epitopes. The process of inactivation of the virus for vaccine production leads to alteration of the native structure of some virus proteins.[154] This alteration leads to loss of certain viral epitopes. As a result, cats infected with FIV would have antibody able to recognize these epitopes, while vaccinated cats would not, which has been shown in one study.[167] Use of these viral proteins to distinguish vaccine response from FIV infection may become commercially available.

Treatment

As for FeLV infection, sick FIV-infected cats require prompt attention to diagnosis and appropriate treatment. Retrovirus-infected cats may respond to treatment as well as uninfected cats, although in some cases, longer or more intensive courses of therapy may be needed. It is important for both the veterinarian and owner to allow enough time for response to treatment and not become discouraged too quickly. Treatment of the ill FIV cat requires a full health evaluation, including a minimum database (CBC, chemistry panel, urinalysis) and identification of any secondary infecting agent. When secondary infections are identified, institution of appropriate treatment (e.g., doxycycline for *M. haemofelis* infection) may resolve the clinical problem. Supportive treatment may also be indicated depending on the severity of the illness. Treatment of chronic stomatitis with corticosteroids is controversial because of adverse effects with long-term use. Griseofulvin should never be used in FIV-infected cats, because it causes bone marrow suppression[266]; newer azole drugs are safe and effective for treatment of fungal infections.

Treatment of the FIV infection itself has focused primarily on drugs developed against HIV. Reverse transcriptase (RTase) inhibitors, such as AZT (zidovudine; Retrovir, GlaxoSmithKline), have been used in cats, both alone and in combination with other drugs. Reduced viral load and improved clinical status have been observed with AZT treatment (5 mg/kg, PO, every 12 hours).[126] Side effects are possible, including nonregenerative anemia, and cats should be monitored carefully during treatment, including complete blood cell counts. One study has shown that AZT alone or in combination with another inhibitor of RTase was effective in preventing infection after exposure (treated cats that were exposed to the virus did not become infected), but did not have therapeutic value in chronically infected cats.[14] Another study showed in vitro viral replication was inhibited by AZT in combination with other nucleoside analogs.[26] AZT is best reserved for treatment of severe stomatitis/gingivitis or neurologic disease.[166] Another RTase inhibitor, stampidine, has shown antiretroviral activity in FIV-infected cats and is well tolerated.[294,295]

Other drugs that may potentially be valuable for FIV treatment but have not yet been tested in cats include other reverse transcriptase inhibitors, as well as inhibitors of viral protease, integrase, and envelope fusion.[47,210,257] A selective antagonist (AMD3100) to the cellular co-receptor for FIV (chemokine receptor CXCR4) has shown in vitro and in vivo activity against the virus, leading to reduced viral load.[115] In addition, side effects were not observed. A protease inhibitor that showed in vitro activity against FIV (TL-3) was shown to prevent and even counteract changes in the CNS from FIV.[131] As research continues, additional medications may become available and useful for FIV treatment.

Immune modulation has also been attempted for the FIV-infected cat. Cytokines, such as granulocyte colony–stimulating factor (G-CSF) and erythropoietin have been used to stimulate blood cell production in cases of neutropenia and anemia, respectively. As they are human in origin, antibodies to these cytokines are produced in treated cats, reducing the drugs' effectiveness within a few weeks.[231] Interferons, both human and feline origin, have also been used in FIV-infected cats. To date, only one study has been published on the use of recombinant feline interferon (rFeIFN; Virbagen Omega, Virbac) for FIV, and the study population consisted of 24 cats co-infected with FeLV.[52] In this multicenter, double-blind, placebo-controlled trial, rFeIFN-treated cats (1 million U/kg/day SC for 5 days in three courses: days 0 to 4, days 14 to 18, days 60 to 64) had improved clinical scores in the first 4 months, minor improvement in hematologic parameters, and lower rates of mortality. However, evaluation of virologic parameters was not performed and the study is difficult to interpret, because the data was not broken down by infection type (FeLV-infected only versus FeLV/FIV-infected). Ironically, one study evaluating human interferon (10 IU/kg, PO, once daily using a 7-day on, 7-day off treatment schedule) in 24 FIV-infected cats did show clinical improvement and improved survival in infected cats compared with six placebo-treated cats despite no change in viral loads.[226] However, the control group was small, and all cats were treated with antiparasitic drugs and antibiotics as needed.

To modulate the lymphocyte activation and proliferation, which may play a role in chronic inflammation associated with FIV (e.g., stomatitis), the antiinflammatory product bovine lactoferrin may affect lymphocyte proliferation and cytokine production, and may provide clinical improvement.[151] Investigation of in vivo effects is ongoing.

As for FeLV, lymphocyte T-cell immunomodulator (LTCI; ProLabs) has been evaluated in cats with FIV. Limited data from placebo-controlled trials in small groups of cats has been published, reporting increased lymphocyte counts, more rapid recovery from respiratory infections, and reduced viral load in LTCI-treated cats.[90]

Data on survival of retroviral infected cats indicate that the lifespan of FIV-infected cats appears similar to that of uninfected cats. FIV-infected cats may have a long disease-free period, especially if wellness care is provided and exposure to other infectious diseases is limited. In one study conducted in the United States, records of 67,963 cats that were tested for FeLV and FIV in 2000, and that had outcome information available 6 years later, were analyzed.[169] The 6-year survival rates were 90% for uninfected cats and 65% for FIV-positive cats. Most deaths in cats with FIV occurred in the first year after diagnosis, probably because of the illness that prompted the original veterinary visit or because of euthanasia for purposes of infection control. A study of 17,289 cats in Germany tested for FeLV and FIV from 1993 to 2002 included survival data on 100 randomly selected cats, including 19 FIV-positive cats. There was no statistically significant difference in the mean survival time of FIV-positive cats (785 days) compared with FIV-negative cats (625 days).[94] In a study of 1,205 cats tested for FeLV and FIV in western Canada, FIV-positive/FeLV-negative cats were compared with randomly selected, age-matched and sex-matched FIV/FeLV-negative cats. The median survival time for FIV-positive cats (n=39, 3.9 years) was not significantly different from that of FIV-negative cats (n=22, 5.9 years).[242]

Management of the FIV-infected cat is similar to the FeLV-infected cat, including client education about isolation (again, not only to prevent spread of FIV, but to protect the FIV-infected cat from infectious agents carried by other cats) and other management issues (see Box 33-5). Guidelines for management of retrovirus-infected cats have been published.[126,166] Wellness exams should be performed every 6 to 12 months to allow early detection, diagnosis, and treatment of health problems (see Box 33-6). FIV-infected cats will require hospitalization both for treatment of illness and for routine wellness care (e.g., surgical sterilization, dental prophylaxis); simple infection control precautions should be instituted (see Box 33-7). Administration of perioperative broad-spectrum antibiotics should be considered for surgical and dental procedures. As for FeLV, FIV is not considered a zoonotic disease, and one study of 204 veterinarians and others with potential exposure to retroviruses failed to detect infection using serologic and molecular methods.[31]

Vaccination of healthy FIV-infected cats against core diseases should be evaluated on a case-by-case basis, taking into account individual risk factors. As for FeLV, inactivated vaccines are often recommended but no data exist to support the recommendation. Healthy cats with FIV have adequate immune responses to vaccination.[48,163] Concern exists that activation of infected lymphocytes by vaccinations may increase viral replication[48]; however, the clinical significance is unclear.[126] FIV vaccination is of no benefit and should not be administered to FIV-infected cats.

Prevention and Control

Control of FIV is aimed primarily at preventing infection. FIV testing may be performed for a variety of reasons (see Box 33-8), including identification of infected cats to prevent disease transmission. It has been recommended that the retrovirus status of all cats should be known.[166] Neutering may limit aggressive behavior, thus limiting spread by fighting and bite wounds. Restricting contact with cats outside the household, especially feral cats that are at risk for FIV infection, is the ideal method of prevention.

A vaccination for FIV is commercially available, and contains inactivated whole virus isolates from clades A and D with an adjuvant. It has been found to induce antibodies as well as cell-mediated responses.[211] Studies of the currently available vaccine (Fel-O-Vax FIV; Boehringer Ingelheim Vetmedica, Inc.) conducted by the inventor or manufacturer have demonstrated efficacy when vaccinated cats were challenged with subtypes A and B.[127,128,153,236] One independent study showed that the vaccine was not able to protect cats when they were challenged by a subtype A field strain from the United Kingdom.[63] Although it offers some protection to some cats at high risk, its use remains controversial, and it is listed as noncore or not recommended by the major vaccine advisory groups.[50,126,249] An informed decision to use the vaccine requires local knowledge about prevalent FIV subtypes, which is typically not available to the practitioner, as well as better evaluation of vaccine efficacy against FIV field strains. Another important concern is that current screening/testing methods cannot distinguish naturally infected from vaccinated cats. In addition, because high-risk cats are those that are free roaming, these animals may be more likely to be seized by animal control authorities. Without identification and access to vaccination records, these cats may be inappropriately euthanized if tested FIV positive at the receiving facility.

Cats should be tested for FIV infection prior to vaccination. The AAFP guidelines recommend clients be informed of the difficulties interpreting FIV test results in vaccinated cats, the lack of knowledge about vaccine efficacy, and that vaccinated cats should be permanently identified, such as with a microchip, tattoo, and/or collar.[166] Microchip databases can be used to record FIV vaccination histories.

As for FeLV, certain populations of cats require tailored recommendations for control of FIV. Retrovirus testing and management for multicat environments is discussed in Chapter 46. Although FIV is uncommon in breeding catteries, the retrovirus status of all breeding cats should be known. Vaccination against FIV is generally not required in catteries. Additional recommendations for control of retrovirus infections in breeding catteries are found in Box 33-9.

MISCELLANEOUS VIRUSES

Other Viral Enteritis Agents

Agents of viral enteritis in cats other than coronavirus include astrovirus, rotavirus, reovirus, enterovirus, and calicivirus/norovirus.* These agents, all nonenveloped RNA viruses, may survive for extended periods in contaminated environments. They are transmitted orally, and unlike parvoviruses, infect the intestinal epithelia from the lumen. They target mature epithelia at the villus tips, leading to intestinal villus atrophy. Disease, which manifests as diarrhea without blood, is typically only seen in very young animals, where turnover/replacement of intestinal epithelia is slower than in adults. The most serious consequence of disease in affected kittens is dehydration. Because these are not systemic infections, changes in leukocyte levels and other signs of systemic disease, such as depression and fever, may not be seen. Diagnosis can generally only be accomplished using electron microscopy. Treatment is supportive, with fluids being the key component. Environmental decontamination involves cleaning with a detergent to remove all organic matter followed by disinfection with an appropriate product with oxidizing activity (e.g., 6% sodium hypochlorite, potassium peroxymonosulfate). Zoonotic transmission of rotavirus and perhaps norovirus is possible; thus owners should take appropriate precautions when handling affected cats.[43,263]

Bornavirus

Borna disease was named after a town in Saxony, Germany where, in 1895, an outbreak of fatal neurologic disease occurred in horses. The causative virus was identified in 1925 and named Bornavirus. Since that report, Bornavirus has been identified in a number of species, including cattle, donkeys, dogs, wild birds, and ostriches, and occurs virtually worldwide.[140] It is a cause of encephalomyelitis in many species. In the mid-1990s,

*References 42, 43, 188, 248, 263, 275.

Bornavirus was isolated from cats experiencing a neurologic disease in Sweden called "staggering disease."[174] Since that report, evidence of potential Bornavirus-associated disease has been described in cats in Australia, the United Kingdom, and Japan.[141,201,213,245] Evidence of infection with Bornavirus, but not necessarily disease, has been found in several countries. FIV-infected cats may have a higher prevalence of infection.[119,130]

Bornavirus is a single-stranded RNA virus in the family Bornaviridae with a helical capsid and a lipid envelope. Its genome is nonsegmented and approximately 9000 bases in length. Interestingly, the virus does not appear to be cytolytic. In affected animals, the disease is a nonsuppurative meningoencephalitis, and pathology includes an inflammatory response in the CNS and demyelinating lesions.[103] Asymptomatic infection has also been documented.[204]

The most characteristic clinical sign is hindlimb paraparesis and ataxia (staggering); other clinical signs include behavioral changes, lumbosacral pain, anorexia, hypersalivation, hypersensitivity to light and sound, visual impairment, seizures, and inability to retract the claws.[103] The clinical signs progress over 1 to 4 weeks until the patient either deteriorates to the point of death or euthanasia, or stabilizes. Recovered cats may be permanently affected with motor dysfunction or personality changes.[103]

The mode of transmission of Bornavirus is unclear, though vectorborne transmission has been postulated because of its seasonality, with most cases occurring in spring and summer.[103] Transmission by bodily fluids has also been proposed, and rodents and birds have been postulated to be reservoirs.[103] The virus is believed to reach the CNS from its site of entry by axonal migration. The immune response is believed to play a role in disease development and is primarily mediated by CD8+ T lymphocytes.[23]

Diagnosis is problematic and controversial, because the presence of antibody is not confirmatory and virus is present at low levels, even in affected tissue. Ante mortem, it is a diagnosis by elimination of other causes. As well as postmortem examination, histopathology, and immunohistochemistry of CNS gray matter for Bornavirus antigen may be required for diagnosis. Treatment is largely supportive; however, given the immunopathologic component, corticosteroids may be beneficial.

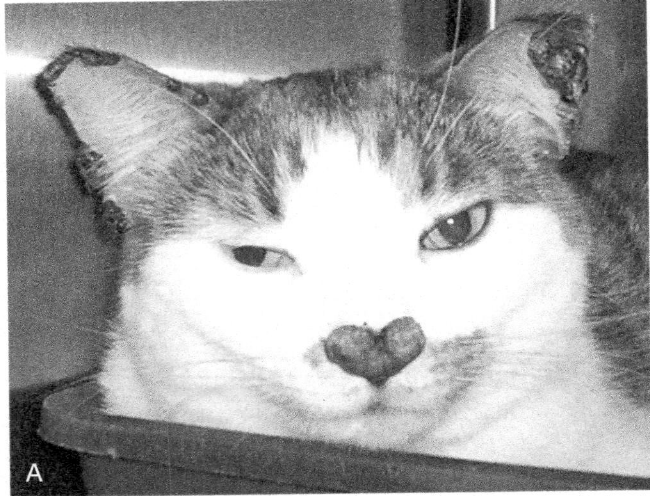

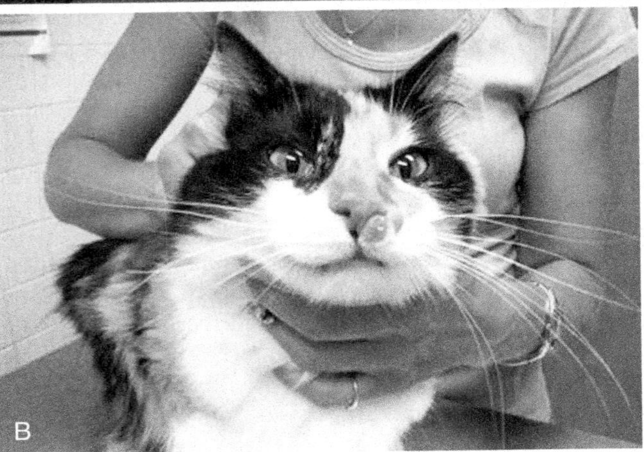

FIGURE 33-24 Papillomavirus lesions in cats appear distinct from those in other species and are locally extensive, often multiple, and can appear on the skin or in the oral cavity. Cutaneous papillomas may be rough, raised, pigmented **(A)** or nonpigmented **(B)**, scaly plaques. (**A** courtesy Kelly St. Denis. **B** courtesy Lisa Henderson, Veterinary Information Network.)

Papillomavirus

Papillomaviruses are members of the Papovaviridae family and cause cutaneous warts in a number of animal species, including domestic and nondomestic cats. They are small, nonenveloped DNA viruses that are highly species specific, although there is one report in the literature of a feline papilloma associated with human papillomavirus type 9.[198] In cats, though infection appears to be infrequent, papillomaviruses have been associated with papillomas, fibropapillomas, and squamous cell carcinomas.* Papillomavirus skin lesions have also been reported in a cat with FIV infection.[66]

Papillomas most likely develop after introduction of the virus through skin lesions or abrasions. The papillomaviruses have a specific tropism for squamous epithelial cells. Lesions in cats appear distinct from those in other species and are locally extensive, often multiple, and can appear on the skin or in the oral cavity.[279] Oral papillomas are small, soft, light pink, oval, slightly raised, flat, and appear on the ventral lingual surface.[279] Cutaneous papillomas may be rough, raised, pigmented or nonpigmented, scaly plaques (Figure 33-24).[279] Histologic examination reveals pigmented, hyperplastic

*References 35, 67, 108, 173, 197, 261.

epidermal plaques without evidence of inflammation.[67] Papillomavirus DNA has been identified in plaques and invasive squamous cell carcinomas. The virus causes hyperplasia of epithelia and contributes to epithelial proliferation in cutaneous neoplasms.[197]

The histology of feline fibropapillomas is very similar to equine sarcoid, and in one report, 17 of 19 tumors were positive for a papillomavirus most similar to bovine papillomavirus type 1.[108,261] Fibropapillomas appear to be most common in outdoor cats living in rural areas and cats with known exposure to cattle. Like equine sarcoids, local recurrence after excision is common and metastasis has not been reported.

Definitive diagnosis of feline papillomatosis is by immunohistochemical staining of tissue obtained during biopsy or surgical resection. PCR can also be used to demonstrate viral DNA in lesions. No specific treatment has been identified; surgical excision is rarely warranted. Spontaneous regression has occurred in other species, such as dogs.

Poxvirus

Cats are most commonly infected with cowpox,[200] an orthopoxvirus in the Poxviridae family that is only found in Europe and Asia. Orthopoxviruses are enveloped DNA viruses that are relatively stable in the environment, surviving under dry conditions for months to years. They are readily inactivated by common disinfectants. The reservoir hosts are small rodents, such as voles and wood mice. Cowpox infection is seen primarily in rural cats that hunt rodents, and cases are typically seasonal, occurring in the summer and fall.[20]

The virus is probably inoculated under the skin through a bite wound. The virus replicates locally, producing a skin lesion, and then spreads systemically, causing more widespread skin lesions within 1 to 3 weeks. The skin lesions are small nodules at first, but form well-circumscribed ulcers that become scabbed.[20] The lesions gradually exfoliate after 4 to 5 weeks, and new hair growth occurs, although some lesions may result in permanent bald patches. Signs of systemic illness occur early in infection in some cats; they are generally mild and include pyrexia, anorexia, and depression. Severe or fatal disease is rare and is typically associated with immunosuppression, such as from retrovirus infection or administration of immunosuppressive drugs.[20,262]

Feline cowpox virus infection is diagnosed by culturing dried scab material, electron microscopy, or PCR. Serum antibodies can also be detected. Histologic examination of lesions reveals epithelial hyperplasia, vesicle formation and ulceration. Infected cells may contain intracytoplasmic eosinophilic inclusion bodies. No specific treatment has been identified; therapy is primarily supportive, such as broad-spectrum antibiotics for secondary bacterial infections. Corticosteroids should be avoided.

Cat-to-cat and cat-to-human transmission has been documented.[16,71,107,262] Human cowpox infection is rare in the United Kingdom, but more than half of cases are due to transmission from cats.[16] Cowpox causes skin lesions in humans, as well as systemic infections. Basic hygiene precautions will help prevent transmission from infected cats to humans, and euthanasia of infected cats is not warranted.

References

1. Abd-Eldaim M, Beall M, Kennedy M: Detection of feline panleukopenia virus using a commercial ELISA for canine parvovirus, *Vet Ther* 10:E1, 2009.
2. Abd-Eldaim M, Potgieter L, Kennedy M: Genetic analysis of feline caliciviruses associated with a hemorrhagic-like disease, *J Vet Diagn Invest* 17:420, 2005.
3. Abd-Eldaim MM, Wilkes RP, Thomas K et al: Development and validation of a TaqMan real-time reverse transcription-PCR for rapid detection of feline calicivirus, *Arch Virol* 154:555, 2009.
4. Reference deleted in pages.
5. Addie D, Belak S, Boucraut-Baralon C et al: Feline infectious peritonitis ABCD guidelines on prevention and management, *J Feline Med Surg* 11:594, 2009.
6. Addie D, Jarrett O: Control of feline coronavirus infections in breeding catteries by serotesting, isolation, and early weaning, *Feline Pract* 23:92, 1995.
7. Addie DD, Dennis JM, Toth S et al: Long-term impact on a closed household of pet cats of natural infection with feline coronavirus, feline leukaemia virus and feline immunodeficiency virus, *Vet Rec* 146:419, 2000.
8. Addie DD, Jarrett O: A study of naturally occurring feline coronavirus infections in kittens, *Vet Rec* 130:133, 1992.
9. Addie DD, Jarrett O: Feline coronavirus infections. In Greene CE, editor: *Infectious diseases of the dog and cat*, ed 3, St Louis, 2006, Saunders Elsevier, p 88.
10. Addie DD, Paltrinieri S, Pedersen NC: Recommendations from workshops of the second international feline coronavirus/feline infectious peritonitis symposium, *J Feline Med Surg* 6:125, 2004.
11. Allison RW, Hoover EA: Covert vertical transmission of feline immunodeficiency virus, *AIDS Res Hum Retroviruses* 19:421, 2003.
12. Allison RW, Hoover EA: Feline immunodeficiency virus is concentrated in milk early in lactation, *AIDS Res Hum Retroviruses* 19:245, 2003.
13. Andrew SE: Immune-mediated canine and feline keratitis, *Vet Clin North Am Sm Anim Pract* 38:269, 2008.
14. Arai M, Earl DD, Yamamoto JK: Is AZT/3TC therapy effective against FIV infection or immunopathogenesis? *Vet Immunol Immunopathol* 85:189, 2002.
15. Barr MC: FIV, FeLV, and FIPV: interpretation and misinterpretation of serological test results, *Semin Vet Med Surg (Small Anim)* 11:144, 1996.
16. Baxby D, Bennett M, Getty B: Human cowpox 1969-93: a review based on 54 cases, *Br J Dermatol* 131:598, 1994.
17. Beaumont SL, Maggs DJ, Clarke HE: Effects of bovine lactoferrin on in vitro replication of feline herpesvirus, *Vet Ophthalmol* 6:245, 2003.
18. Beeler E: Influenza in dogs and cats, *Vet Clin North Am Small Anim Pract* 39:251, 2009.
19. Benetka V, Kubber-Heiss A, Kolodziejek J et al: Prevalence of feline coronavirus types I and II in cats with histopathologically verified feline infectious peritonitis, *Vet Microbiol* 99:31, 2004.

20. Bennett M, Gaskell CJ, Baxbyt D et al: Feline cowpox virus infection, *J Small Anim Pract* 31:167, 1990.
21. Benveniste R, Sherr C, Todaro G: Evolution of type C viral genes: origin of feline leukemia virus, *Science* 190:886, 1975.
22. Berg AL, Ekman K, Belak S et al: Cellular composition and interferon-gamma expression of the local inflammatory response in feline infectious peritonitis (FIP), *Vet Microbiol* 111:15, 2005.
23. Berg AL, Johannisson A, Johansson M et al: Peripheral and intracerebral T cell immune response in cats naturally infected with Borna disease virus, *Vet Immunol Immunopathol* 68:241, 1999.
24. Bi Y, Fu G, Chen J et al: Novel swine influenze virus reassortants in pigs, China, *Emerg Inf Dis* 16:1162, 2010.
25. Bienzle D, Reggeti F, Wen X et al: The variability of serological and molecular diagnosis of feline immunodeficiency virus infection, *Can Vet J* 45:753, 2004.
26. Bisset LR, Lutz H, Boni J et al: Combined effect of zidovudine (ZDV), lamivudine (3TC) and abacavir (ABC) antiretroviral therapy in suppressing in vitro FIV replication, *Antiviral Res* 53:35, 2002.
27. Blanton JD, Robertson K, Palmer D et al: Rabies surveillance in the United States during 2008, *J Am Vet Med Assoc* 235:676, 2009.
28. Bradshaw J, Pearson G, Gruffydd-Jones T: A retrospective study of 286 cases of neurological disorders of the cat, *J Comp Pathol* 131:112, 2004.
29. Brightman AH 2nd, Ogilvie GK, Tompkins M: Ocular disease in FeLV-positive cats: 11 cases (1981-1986), *J Am Vet Med Assoc* 198:1049, 1991.
30. Brown MA, Troyer JL, Pecon-Slattery J et al: Genetics and pathogenesis of feline infectious peritonitis virus, *Emerg Infect Dis* 15:1445, 2009.
31. Butera ST, Brown J, Callahan ME et al: Survey of veterinary conference attendees for evidence of zoonotic infection by feline retroviruses, *J Am Vet Med Assoc* 217:1475, 2000.
32. Can-Sahna K, Soydal Ataseven V, Pinar D et al: The detection of feline coronaviruses in blood samples from cats by mRNA RT-PCR, *J Feline Med Surg* 9:369, 2007.
33. Cannon MJ, Silkstone MA, Kipar AM: Cutaneous lesions associated with coronavirus-induced vasculitis in a cat with feline infectious peritonitis and concurrent feline immunodeficiency virus infection, *J Feline Med Surg* 7:233, 2005.
34. Carmichael KP, Bienzle D, McDonnell JJ: Feline leukemia virus-associated myelopathy in cats, *Vet Pathol* 39:536, 2002.
35. Carney HC, England JJ, Hodgin EC et al: Papillomavirus infection of aged Persian cats, *J Vet Diagn Invest* 2:294, 1990.
36. Cattori V, Tandon R, Pepin A et al: Rapid detection of feline leukemia virus provirus integration into feline genomic DNA, *Mol Cell Probes* 20:172, 2006.
37. Cave T, Thompson H, Reid S et al: Kitten mortality in the United Kingdom: a retrospective analysis of 274 histopathological examinations (1986 to 2000), *Vet Rec* 151:497, 2002.
38. Chang HW, de Groot RJ, Egberink HF et al: Feline infectious peritonitis: insights into feline coronavirus pathobiogenesis and epidemiology based on genetic analysis of the viral 3c gene, *J Gen Virol* 91:415, 2010.
39. Chen H, Bechtel MK, Shi Y et al: Pathogenicity induced by feline leukemia virus, Rickard strain, subgroup A plasmid DNA (pFRA), *J Virol* 72:7048, 1998.
40. Coats KS: The feline immunodeficiency virus-infected cat: a model for lentivirus-induced placental immunopathology and reproductive failure [mini-review], *Am J Reprod Immunol* 54:169, 2005.
41. Collado VM, Gomez-Lucia E, Tejerizo G et al: Effect of type I interferons on the expression of feline leukaemia virus, *Vet Microbiol* 123:180, 2007.
42. Cook AK: Feline infectious diarrhea, *Top Companion Anim Med* 23:169, 2008.
43. Cook N, Bridger J, Kendall K et al: The zoonotic potential of rotavirus, *J Infect* 48:289, 2004.
44. Cotter SM: Feline viral neoplasia. In Greene CE, editor: *Infectious diseases of the dog and cat*, ed 2, Philadelphia, 1998, Saunders, p 71.
45. Coyne KP, Dawson S, Radford AD et al: Long-term analysis of feline calicivirus prevalence and viral shedding patterns in naturally infected colonies of domestic cats, *Vet Microbiol* 118:12, 2006.
46. Crawford PC, Slater MR, Levy JK: Accuracy of polymerase chain reaction assays for diagnosis of feline immunodeficiency virus infection in cats, *J Am Vet Med Assoc* 226:1503, 2005.
47. D'Ursi AM, Giannecchini S, Esposito C et al: Development of antiviral fusion inhibitors: short modified peptides derived from the transmembrane glycoprotein of feline immunodeficiency virus, *Chembiochem* 7:774, 2006.
48. Dawson S, Smyth NR, Bennett M et al: Effect of primary-stage feline immunodeficiency virus infection on subsequent feline calicivirus vaccination and challenge in cats, *AIDS* 5:747, 1991.
49. Dawson S, Willoughby K, Gaskell RM et al: A field trial to assess the effect of vaccination against feline herpesvirus, feline calicivirus and feline panleucopenia virus in 6-week-old kittens, *J Feline Med Surg* 3:17, 2001.
50. Day MJ, Horzinek MC, Schultz RD: WSAVA guidelines for the vaccination of dogs and dats, *J Small Anim Pract* 51:338, 2010.
51. de Groot-Mijnes JD, van Dun JM, van der Most RG et al: Natural history of a recurrent feline coronavirus infection and the role of cellular immunity in survival and disease, *J Virol* 79:1036, 2005.
52. de Mari K, Maynard L, Sanquer A et al: Therapeutic effects of recombinant feline interferon-omega on feline leukemia virus (FeLV)-infected and FeLV/feline immunodeficiency virus (FIV)-coinfected symptomatic cats, *J Vet Intern Med* 18:477, 2004.
53. de Rozieres S, Mathiason CK, Rolston MR et al: Characterization of a highly pathogenic molecular clone of feline immunodeficiency virus clade C, *J Virol* 78:8971, 2004.
54. Decaro N, Buonavoglia D, Desario C et al: Characterisation of canine parvovirus strains isolated from cats with feline panleukopenia, *Res Vet Sci* 89:275, 2010.
55. Decaro N, Desario C, Miccolupo A et al: Genetic analysis of feline panleukopenia viruses from cats with gastroenteritis, *J Gen Virol* 89:2290, 2008.
56. Decaro N, Desario C, Parisi A et al: Genetic analysis of canine parvovirus type 2c, *Virology* 385:5, 2009.
57. Declercq J, De Bosschere H, Schwarzkopf I et al: Papular cutaneous lesions in a cat associated with feline infectious peritonitis, *Vet Dermatol* 19:255, 2008.
58. Doherty MJ: Ocular manifestations of feline infectious peritonitis, *J Am Vet Med Assoc* 159:417, 1971.
59. Dorny P, Speybroeck N, Verstraete S et al: Serological survey of *Toxoplasma gondii*, feline immunodeficiency virus and feline leukaemia virus in urban stray cats in Belgium, *Vet Rec* 151:626, 2002.
60. Dow SW, Hoover EA: Neurologic disease associated with feline retroviral infection. In Kirk R, Bonagura J, editors: *Current veterinary therapy*, Philadelphia, 1992, Saunders, p 1010.
61. Dowers KL, Hawley JR, Brewer MM et al: Association of *Bartonella* species, feline calicivirus, and feline herpesvirus 1 infection with gingivostomatitis in cats, *J Feline Med Surg* 12:314, 2010.
62. Drazenovich TL, Fascetti AJ, Westermeyer HD et al: Effects of dietary lysine supplementation on upper respiratory and ocular disease and detection of infectious organisms in cats within an animal shelter, *Am J Vet Res* 70:1391, 2009.
63. Dunham SP, Bruce J, MacKay S et al: Limited efficacy of an inactivated feline immunodeficiency virus vaccine, *Vet Rec* 158:561, 2006.
64. Duthie S, Eckersall PD, Addie DD et al: Value of alpha 1-acid glycoprotein in the diagnosis of feline infectious peritonitis, *Vet Rec* 141:299, 1997.
65. Dye C, Siddell SG: Genomic RNA sequence of feline coronavirus strain FCoV C1Je, *J Feline Med Surg* 9:202, 2007.

66. Egberink HF, Berrocal A, Bax HA et al: Papillomavirus associated skin lesions in a cat seropositive for feline immunodeficiency virus, *Vet Microbiol* 31:117, 1992.
67. Egberink HF, Horzinek MC: Feline viral papillomatosis. In Greene C, editor: *Infectious diseases of the dog and cat*, ed 3, St Louis, 2006, Saunders Elsevier, p 160.
68. Elder JH, Sundstrom M, de Rozieres S et al: Molecular mechanisms of FIV infection, *Vet Immunol Immunopathol* 123:3, 2008.
69. Eleraky N, Potgieter L, Kennedy M: Virucidal efficacy of four new disinfectants, *J Am Anim Hosp Assoc* 38:231, 2002.
70. English RV, Davidson MG, Nasisse MP et al: Intraocular disease associated with feline immunodeficiency virus infection in cats, *J Am Vet Med Assoc* 196:1116, 1990.
71. Essbauer S, Pfeffer M, Meyer H: Zoonotic poxviruses, *Vet Microbiol* 140:229, 2010.
72. Fehr D, Holznagel E, Bolla S et al: Placebo-controlled evaluation of a modified life virus vaccine against feline infectious peritonitis: safety and efficacy under field conditions, *Vaccine* 15:1101, 1997.
73. Fogelman V, Fischman H, Horman J et al: Epidemiologic and clinical characteristics of rabies in cats, *J Am Vet Med Assoc* 202:1829, 1993.
74. Foley J, Hurley K, Pesavento P et al: Virulent systemic feline calicivirus infection: local cytokine modulation and contribution of viral mutants, *J Feline Med Surg* 8:55, 2006.
75. Foley J, Pedersen N: The inheritance of susceptibility to feline infectious peritonitis in purebred catteries, *Feline Pract* 24:14, 1996.
76. Foley JE, Lapointe JM, Koblik P et al: Diagnostic features of clinical neurologic feline infectious peritonitis, *J Vet Intern Med* 12:415, 1998.
77. Foley JE, Poland A, Carlson J et al: Patterns of feline coronavirus infection and fecal shedding from cats in multiple-cat environments, *J Am Vet Med Assoc* 210:1307, 1997.
78. Foley JE, Poland A, Carlson J et al: Risk factors for feline infectious peritonitis among cats in multiple-cat environments with endemic feline enteric coronavirus, *J Am Vet Med Assoc* 210:1313, 1997.
79. Foley JE, Rand C, Leutenegger C: Inflammation and changes in cytokine levels in neurological feline infectious peritonitis, *J Feline Med Surg* 5:313, 2003.
80. Fontenelle JP, Powell CC, Veir JK et al: Effect of topical ophthalmic application of cidofovir on experimentally induced primary ocular feline herpesvirus-1 infection in cats, *Am J Vet Res* 69:289, 2008.
81. Foster R, Caswell J, Rinkardt N: Chronic fibrinous and necrotic orchitis in a cat, *Can Vet J* 37:681, 1996.
82. Frymus T, Addie D, Belak S et al: Feline rabies ABCD guidelines on prevention and management, *J Feline Med Surg* 11:585, 2009.
83. Fujino Y, Horiuchi H, Mizukoshi F et al: Prevalence of hematological abnormalities and detection of infected bone marrow cells in asymptomatic cats with feline immunodeficiency virus infection, *Vet Microbiol* 136:217, 2009.
84. Fujino Y, Ohno K, Tsujimoto H: Molecular pathogenesis of feline leukemia virus-induced malignancies: insertional mutagenesis, *Vet Immunol Immunopathol* 123:138, 2008.
85. Gamoh K, Shimazaki Y, Makie H et al: The pathogenicity of canine parvovirus type-2b, FP84 strain isolated from a domestic cat, in domestic cats, *J Vet Med Sci* 65:1027, 2003.
86. Gaskell CJ, Gaskell RM, Dennis PE et al: Efficacy of an inactivated feline calicivirus (FCV) vaccine against challenge with United Kingdom field strains and its interaction with the FCV carrier state, *Res Vet Sci* 32:23, 1982.
87. Gaskell R, Dawson S, Radford A et al: Feline herpesvirus, *Vet Res* 38:337, 2007.
88. Gaskell RM, Povey RC: Experimental induction of feline viral rhinotracheitis virus re-excretion in FVR-recovered cats, *Vet Rec* 100:128, 1977.
89. Gelain ME, Meli M, Paltrinieri S: Whole blood cytokine profiles in cats infected by feline coronavirus and healthy non-FCoV infected specific pathogen-free cats, *J Feline Med Surg* 8:389, 2006.
90. Gingerich D: Lymphocyte T-cell immunomodulator (LTCI): review of the immunopharmacology of a new veterinary biologic, *Intern J Appl Res Vet Med* 6:61, 2008.
91. Giordano A, Paltrinieri S: Interferon-gamma in the serum and effusions of cats with feline coronavirus infection, *Vet J* 180:396, 2009.
92. Gleich S, Hartmann K: Feline immunodeficiency virus and feline leukemia virus—a retrospective study in 17462 cases, *J Vet Intern Med* 21:578, 2007.
93. Gleich S, Hartmann K: Hematology and serum biochemistry of feline immunodeficiency virus-infected and feline leukemia virus-infected cats, *J Vet Intern Med* 23:552, 2009.
94. Gleich SE, Krieger S, Hartmann K: Prevalence of feline immunodeficiency virus and feline leukaemia virus among client-owned cats and risk factors for infection in Germany, *J Feline Med Surg* 11:985, 2009.
95. Goldkamp CE, Levy JK, Edinboro CH et al: Seroprevalences of feline leukemia virus and feline immunodeficiency virus in cats with abscesses or bite wounds and rate of veterinarian compliance with current guidelines for retrovirus testing, *J Am Vet Med Assoc* 232:1152, 2008.
96. Gomes-Keller MA, Gonczi E, Grenacher B et al: Fecal shedding of infectious feline leukemia virus and its nucleic acids: a transmission potential, *Vet Microbiol* 134:208, 2009.
97. Gomes-Keller MA, Gonczi E, Tandon R et al: Detection of feline leukemia virus RNA in saliva from naturally infected cats and correlation of PCR results with those of current diagnostic methods, *J Clin Microbiol* 44:916, 2006.
98. Gomes-Keller MA, Tandon R, Gonczi E et al: Shedding of feline leukemia virus RNA in saliva is a consistent feature in viremic cats, *Vet Microbiol* 112:11, 2006.
99. Goto Y, Nishimura Y, Mizuno T et al: Quantification of viral ribonucleic acid in plasma of cats naturally infected with feline immunodeficiency virus, *Am J Vet Res* 61:1609, 2000.
100. Grant CK, Essex M, Gardner MB et al: Natural feline leukemia virus infection and the immune response of cats of different ages, *Cancer Res* 40:823, 1980.
101. Greene C, Addie D: Feline parvovirus infections. In Greene C, editor: *Infectious diseases of the dog and cat*, ed 3, St Louis, 2006, Saunders Elsevier, p 78.
102. Greene C, Rupprecht C: Rabies and other Lyssavirus infections. In Greene C, editor: *Infectious diseases of the dog and cat*, ed 3, St Louis, 2006, Saunders Elsevier, p 167.
103. Greene CE, Berg AL, Chomel BB: Miscellaneous viral infections. In Greene C, editor: *Infectious diseases of the dog and cat*, ed 3, St Louis, 2006, Saunders Elsevier, p 162.
104. Grosenbaugh DA, Leard T, Pardo MC et al: Comparison of the safety and efficacy of a recombinant feline leukemia virus (FeLV) vaccine delivered transdermally and an inactivated FeLV vaccine delivered subcutaneously, *Vet Ther* 5:258, 2004.
105. Gutzwiller ME, Brachelente C, Taglinger K et al: Feline herpes dermatitis treated with interferon omega, *Vet Dermatol* 18:50, 2007.
106. Haagmans BL, Egberink HF, Horzinek MC: Apoptosis and T-cell depletion during feline infectious peritonitis, *J Virol* 70:8977, 1996.
107. Haenssle HA, Kiessling J, Kempf VA et al: Orthopoxvirus infection transmitted by a domestic cat, *J Am Acad Dermatol* 54:S1, 2006.
108. Hanna PE, Dunn D: Cutaneous fibropapilloma in a cat (feline sarcoid), *Can Vet J* 44:601, 2003.

109. Hargis A, Ginn P, Mansell J et al: Ulcerative facial and nasal dermatitis and stomatitis in cats associated with feline herpesvirus 1, *Vet Dermatol* 10:267, 1999.
110. Hartley C: Aetiology of corneal ulcers: assume FHV-1 unless proven otherwise, *J Feline Med Surg* 12:24, 2010.
111. Hartmann K: Feline leukemia virus infection. In Greene C, editor: *Infectious diseases of the dog and cat*, ed 3, St Louis, 2006, Saunders Elsevier, p 105.
112. Hartmann K, Binder C, Hirschberger J et al: Comparison of different tests to diagnose feline infectious peritonitis, *J Vet Intern Med* 17:781, 2003.
113. Hartmann K, Griessmayr P, Schulz B et al: Quality of different in-clinic test systems for feline immunodeficiency virus and feline leukaemia virus infection, *J Feline Med Surg* 9:439, 2007.
114. Hartmann K, Ritz S: Treatment of cats with feline infectious peritonitis, *Vet Immunol Immunopathol* 123:172, 2008.
115. Hartmann K, Stengel S, Klein D et al: Efficacy of the chemokine receptor inhibitor 1,1′-bis-1,4,8,11-tetraazacyclotetradekan against feline immunodeficiency virus infection [abstract], *Sixth International Feline Retrovirus Research Symposium*, Amelia Island, Fla, 2002, p 26.
116. Harvey CJ, Lopez JW, Hendrick MJ: An uncommon intestinal manifestation of feline infectious peritonitis: 26 cases (1986-1993), *J Am Vet Med Assoc* 209:1117, 1996.
117. Hayes KA, Rojko JL, Tarr MJ et al: Atypical localised viral expression in a cat with feline leukaemia, *Vet Rec* 124:344, 1989.
118. Hayward JJ, Rodrigo AG: Recombination in feline immunodeficiency virus from feral and companion domestic cats, *Virol J* 5:76, 2008.
119. Helps CR, Turan N, Bilal T et al: Detection of antibodies to Borna disease virus in Turkish cats by using recombinant p40, *Vet Rec* 149:647, 2001.
120. Herrewegh AA, de Groot RJ, Cepica A et al: Detection of feline coronavirus RNA in feces, tissues, and body fluids of naturally infected cats by reverse transcriptase PCR, *J Clin Microbiol* 33:684, 1995.
121. Hofmann-Lehmann R, Cattori V, Tandon R et al: How molecular methods change our views of FeLV infection and vaccination, *Vet Immunol Immunopathol* 123:119, 2008.
122. Hofmann-Lehmann R, Huder JB, Gruber S et al: Feline leukaemia provirus load during the course of experimental infection and in naturally infected cats, *J Gen Virol* 82:1589, 2001.
123. Hofmann-Lehmann R, Tandon R, Boretti FS et al: Reassessment of feline leukaemia virus (FeLV) vaccines with novel sensitive molecular assays, *Vaccine* 24:1087, 2006.
124. Hong C, Decaro N, Desario C et al: Occurrence of canine parvovirus type 2c in the United States, *J Vet Diagn Invest* 19:535, 2007.
125. Hoover EA, Mullins JI: Feline leukemia virus infection and diseases, *J Am Vet Med Assoc* 199:1287, 1991.
126. Hosie MJ, Addie D, Belak S et al: Feline immunodeficiency ABCD guidelines on prevention and management, *J Feline Med Surg* 11:575, 2009.
127. Huang C, Conlee D, Gill M et al: Dual-subtype feline immunodeficiency virus vaccine provides 12 months of protective immunity against heterologous challenge, *J Feline Med Surg* 12:451, 2010.
128. Huang C, Conlee D, Loop J et al: Efficacy and safety of a feline immunodeficiency virus vaccine, *Anim Health Res Rev* 5:295, 2004.
129. Huang C, Hess J, Gill M et al: A dual-strain feline calicivirus vaccine stimulates broader cross-neutralization antibodies than a single-strain vaccine and lessens clinical signs in vaccinated cats when challenged with a homologous feline calicivirus strain associated with virulent systemic disease, *J Feline Med Surg* 12:129, 2010.
130. Huebner J, Bode L, Ludwig H: Borna disease virus infection in FIV-positive cats in Germany, *Vet Rec* 149:152, 2001.
131. Huitron-Resendiz S, De Rozieres S, Sanchez-Alavez M et al: Resolution and prevention of feline immunodeficiency virus-induced neurological deficits by treatment with the protease inhibitor TL-3, *J Virol* 78:4525, 2004.
132. Hurley K, Pesavento P, Pedersen N et al: An outbreak of virulent systemic feline calicivirus disease, *J Am Vet Med Assoc* 224:241, 2004.
133. Hurley K, Sykes J: Update on feline calicivirus: new trends, *Vet Clin North Am Sm Anim Pract* 33:759, 2003.
134. Ikeda Y, Nakamura K, Miyazawa T et al: Feline host range of canine parvovirus: recent emergence of new antigenic types in cats, *Emerg Infect Dis* 8:341, 2002.
135. Ishida T, Shibanai A, Tanaka S et al: Use of recombinant feline interferon and glucocorticoid in the treatment of feline infectious peritonitis, *J Feline Med Surg* 6:107, 2004.
136. Ishida T, Tomoda I: Clinical staging of feline immunodeficiency virus infection, *Nippon Juigaku Zasshi* 52:645, 1990.
137. Ishida T, Washizu T, Toriyabe K et al: Feline immunodeficiency virus infection in cats of Japan, *J Am Vet Med Assoc* 194:221, 1989.
138. Jacobse-Geels HE, Daha MR, Horzinek MC: Isolation and characterization of feline C3 and evidence for the immune complex pathogenesis of feline infectious peritonitis, *J Immunol* 125:1606, 1980.
139. Jordan HL, Howard JG, Bucci JG et al: Horizontal transmission of feline immunodeficiency virus with semen from seropositive cats, *J Reprod Immunol* 41:341, 1998.
140. Kamhieh S, Flower RL: Borna disease virus (BDV) infection in cats. A concise review based on current knowledge, *Vet Q* 28:66, 2006.
141. Kamhieh S, Hodgson JL, Bode L et al: Borna disease virus: evidence of naturally-occurring infection in cats in Australia, *APMIS Suppl* 50, 2008.
142. Kennedy MA, Abd-Eldaim M, Zika SE et al: Evaluation of antibodies against feline coronavirus 7b protein for diagnosis of feline infectious peritonitis in cats, *Am J Vet Res* 69:1179, 2008.
143. Kipar A, Baptiste K, Barth A et al: Natural FCoV infection: cats with FIP exhibit significantly higher viral loads than healthy infected cats, *J Feline Med Surg* 8:69, 2006.
144. Kipar A, Bellmann S, Gunn-Moore DA et al: Histopathological alterations of lymphatic tissues in cats without feline infectious peritonitis after long-term exposure to FIP virus, *Vet Microbiol* 69:131, 1999.
145. Kipar A, Bellmann S, Kremendahl J et al: Cellular composition, coronavirus antigen expression and production of specific antibodies in lesions in feline infectious peritonitis, *Vet Immunol Immunopathol* 65:243, 1998.
146. Kipar A, May H, Menger S et al: Morphologic features and development of granulomatous vasculitis in feline infectious peritonitis, *Vet Pathol* 42:321, 2005.
147. Kipar A, Meli ML, Baptiste KE et al: Sites of feline coronavirus persistence in healthy cats, *J Gen Virol* 91:1698, 2010.
148. Kiss I, Kecskemeti S, Tanyi J et al: Preliminary studies on feline coronavirus distribution in naturally and experimentally infected cats, *Res Vet Sci* 68:237, 2000.
149. Kline K, Joseph R, Averill D: Feline infectious peritonitis with neurological involvement: clinical and pathological findings in 24 cats, *J Am Anim Hosp Assoc* 30:111, 1994.
150. Klopfleisch R, Wolf PU, Uhl W et al: Distribution of lesions and antigen of highly pathogenic avian influenza virus A/Swan/Germany/R65/06 (H5N1) in domestic cats after presumptive infection by wild birds, *Vet Pathol* 44:261, 2007.
151. Kobayashi S, Sato R, Aoki T et al: Effect of bovine lactoferrin on functions of activated feline peripheral blood mononuclear cells during chronic feline immunodeficiency virus infection, *J Vet Med Sci* 70:429, 2008.
152. Kuiken T, Rimmelzwaan G, van Riel D et al: Avian H5N1 influenza in cats, *Science* 306:241, 2004.

153. Kusuhara H, Hohdatsu T, Okumura M et al: Dual-subtype vaccine (Fel-O-Vax FIV) protects cats against contact challenge with heterologous subtype B FIV infected cats, *Vet Microbiol* 108:155, 2005.
154. Kusuhara H, Hohdatsu T, Seta T et al: Serological differentiation of FIV-infected cats from dual-subtype feline immunodeficiency virus vaccine (Fel-O-Vax FIV) inoculated cats, *Vet Microbiol* 120:217, 2007.
155. Lafrado LJ, Lewis MG, Mathes LE et al: Suppression of in vitro neutrophil function by feline leukaemia virus (FeLV) and purified FeLV-p15E, *J Gen Virol* 68(Pt 2):507, 1987.
156. Lamm CG, Rezabek GB: Parvovirus infection in domestic companion animals, *Vet Clin North Am Small Anim Pract* 38:837, 2008.
157. Lappin MR: Infectious disease diagnostic assays, *Top Companion Anim Med* 24:199, 2009.
158. Lappin MR, Marks A, Greene CE et al: Serologic prevalence of selected infectious diseases in cats with uveitis, *J Am Vet Med Assoc* 201:1005, 1992.
159. Lappin MR, Sebring RW, Porter M et al: Effects of a single dose of an intranasal feline herpesvirus 1, calicivirus, and panleukopenia vaccine on clinical signs and virus shedding after challenge with virulent feline herpesvirus 1, *J Feline Med Surg* 8:158, 2006.
160. Lappin MR, Veir JK, Satyaraj E et al: Pilot study to evaluate the effect of oral supplementation of *Enterococcus faecium* SF68 on cats with latent feline herpesvirus 1, *J Feline Med Surg* 11:650, 2009.
161. Lee M, Bosward KL, Norris JM: Immunohistological evaluation of feline herpesvirus-1 infection in feline eosinophilic dermatoses or stomatitis, *J Feline Med Surg* 12:72, 2010.
162. Legendre AM, Bartges JW: Effect of polyprenyl immunostimulant on the survival times of three cats with the dry form of feline infectious peritonitis, *J Feline Med Surg* 11:624, 2009.
163. Lehmann R, Franchini M, Aubert A et al: Vaccination of cats experimentally infected with feline immunodeficiency virus, using a recombinant feline leukemia virus vaccine, *J Am Vet Med Assoc* 199:1446, 1991.
164. Levy J: CVT Update: feline immunodeficiency virus. In Bonagura J, editor: *Kirk's current veterinary therapy XIII: small animal practice*, Philadelphia, 2000, Saunders, p 291.
165. Levy J: FeLV and non-neoplastic FeLV-related disease. In Ettinger S, Feldman E, editors: *Textbook of veterinary internal medicine*, ed 5, Philadelphia, 2000, Saunders, p 424.
166. Levy J, Crawford C, Hartmann K et al: 2008 American Association of Feline Practitioners' feline retrovirus management guidelines, *J Feline Med Surg* 10:300, 2008.
167. Levy JK, Crawford PC, Kusuhara H et al: Differentiation of feline immunodeficiency virus vaccination, infection, or vaccination and infection in cats, *J Vet Intern Med* 22:330, 2008.
168. Levy JK, Crawford PC, Slater MR: Effect of vaccination against feline immunodeficiency virus on results of serologic testing in cats, *J Am Vet Med Assoc* 225:1558, 2004.
169. Levy JK, Lorentzen L: Long-term outcome of cats with natural FeLV and FIV infection [abstract], *8th International Feline Retrovirus Research Symposium*, Washington, DC, 2006.
170. Levy JK, Scott HM, Lachtara JL et al: Seroprevalence of feline leukemia virus and feline immunodeficiency virus infection among cats in North America and risk factors for seropositivity, *J Am Vet Med Assoc* 228:371, 2006.
171. Lewis KM, O'Brien RT: Abdominal ultrasonographic findings associated with feline infectious peritonitis: a retrospective review of 16 cases, *J Am Anim Hosp Assoc* 46:152, 2010.
172. Little S, Sears W, Lachtara J et al: Seroprevalence of feline leukemia virus and feline immunodeficiency virus infection among cats in Canada, *Can Vet J* 50:644, 2009.
173. Lozano-Alarcon F, Lewis TP 2nd, Clark EG et al: Persistent papillomavirus infection in a cat, *J Am Anim Hosp Assoc* 32:392, 1996.
174. Lundgren A-L, Zimmermann W, Bode L et al: Staggering disease in cats: isolation and characterization of the feline Borna disease virus, *J Gen Virol* 76:2215, 1995.
175. Lutz H, Addie D, Belak S et al: Feline leukaemia ABCD guidelines on prevention and management, *J Feline Med Surg* 11:565, 2009.
176. Lutz H, Gut M, Leutenegger C et al: Kinetics of FCoV infection in kittens born in catteries of high risk for FIP under different rearing conditions, *Proceedings of the Second International Feline Coronavirus/Feline Infectious Peritonitis Symposium*, Glasgow, Scotland, 2002.
177. MacDonald K, Levy JK, Tucker SJ et al: Effects of passive transfer of immunity on results of diagnostic tests for antibodies against feline immunodeficiency virus in kittens born to vaccinated queens, *J Am Vet Med Assoc* 225:1554, 2004.
178. Maggs D, Clarke H: Relative sensitivity of polymerase chain reaction assays used for detection of feline herpesvirus type 1 DNA in clinical samples and commercial vaccines, *Am J Vet Res* 66:1550, 2005.
179. Maggs D, Collins B, Thorne J et al: Effects of l-lysine and l-arginine on in vitro replication of feline herpesvirus type-1, *Am J Vet Res* 61:1474, 2000.
180. Maggs D, Lappin M, Reif J et al: Evaluation of serologic and viral detection methods for diagnosing feline herpesvirus-1 infection in cats with acute respiratory tract or chronic ocular disease, *J Am Vet Med Assoc* 214:502, 1999.
181. Maggs D, Nasisse M, Kass P: Efficacy of oral supplementation with l-lysine in cats latently infected with feline herpesvirus, *Am J Vet Res* 64:37, 2003.
182. Maggs DJ: Update on pathogenesis, diagnosis, and treatment of feline herpesvirus type 1, *Clin Tech Small Anim Pract* 20:94, 2005.
183. Maggs DJ, Sykes JE, Clarke HE et al: Effects of dietary lysine supplementation in cats with enzootic upper respiratory disease, *J Feline Med Surg* 9:97, 2007.
184. Malik R, Lessels NS, Webb S et al: Treatment of feline herpesvirus-1 associated disease in cats with famciclovir and related drugs, *J Feline Med Surg* 11:40, 2009.
185. Marioni-Henry K, Vite CH, Newton AL et al: Prevalence of diseases of the spinal cord of cats, *J Vet Intern Med* 18:851, 2004.
186. Marschall J, Hartmann K: Avian influenza A H5N1 infections in cats, *J Feline Med Surg* 10:359, 2008.
187. Marschall J, Schulz B, Harder Priv-Doz TC et al: Prevalence of influenza A H5N1 virus in cats from areas with occurrence of highly pathogenic avian influenza in birds, *J Feline Med Surg* 10:355, 2008.
188. Martella V, Campolo M, Lorusso E et al: Norovirus in captive lion cub *(Panthera leo)*, *Emerg Infect Dis* 13:1071, 2007.
189. Maynard L, De Mari K, Lebreux B: Efficacy of a recombinant feline omega interferon in the treatment of symptomatic FeLV- or FeLV- and FIV-positive cats, *Proceedings of the 10th Congress of the European Society of Veterinary Internal Medicine*, Neuchatel, Switzerland, 2000, p 122a.
190. McCaw DL, Boon GD, Jergens AE et al: Immunomodulation therapy for feline leukemia virus infection, *J Am Anim Hosp Assoc* 37:356, 2001.
191. Mehrotra S, Mishra KP, Yadav VS et al: Immunomodulation by peptide analogs of retroviral envelope protein, *Peptides* 24:979, 2003.
192. Meli M, Kipar A, Muller C et al: High viral loads despite absence of clinical and pathological findings in cats experimentally infected with feline coronavirus (FCoV) type I and in naturally FCoV-infected cats, *J Feline Med Surg* 6:69, 2004.
193. Meurs K, Fox P, Magnon A et al: Molecular screening by polymerase chain reaction detects panleukopenia virus DNA in formalin-fixed hearts from cats with idiopathic cardiomyopathy and myocarditis, *Cardiovasc Pathol* 9:119, 2000.

194. Mexas AM, Fogle JE, Tompkins WA et al: CD4+CD25+ regulatory T cells are infected and activated during acute FIV infection, *Vet Immunol Immunopathol* 126:263, 2008.
195. Motokawa K, Hohdatsu T, Aizawa C et al: Molecular cloning and sequence determination of the peplomer protein gene of feline infectious peritonitis virus type I, *Arch Virol* 140:469, 1995.
196. Muirden A: Prevalence of feline leukaemia virus and antibodies to feline immunodeficiency virus and feline coronavirus in stray cats sent to an RSPCA hospital, *Vet Rec* 150:621, 2002.
197. Munday JS, Dunowska M, De Grey S: Detection of two different papillomaviruses within a feline cutaneous squamous cell carcinoma: case report and review of the literature, *N Z Vet J* 57:248, 2009.
198. Munday JS, Hanlon EM, Howe L et al: Feline cutaneous viral papilloma associated with human papillomavirus type 9, *Vet Pathol* 44:924, 2007.
199. Murray KO, Holmes KC, Hanlon CA: Rabies in vaccinated dogs and cats in the United States, 1997-2001, *J Am Vet Med Assoc* 235:691, 2009.
200. Naidoo J, Baxby D, Bennett M et al: Characterization of orthopoxviruses isolated from feline infections in Britain, *Arch Virol* 125:261, 1992.
201. Nakamura Y, Watanabe M, Kamitani W et al: High prevalence of Borna disease virus in domestic cats with neurological disorders in Japan, *Vet Microbiol* 70:153, 1999.
202. Negrin A, Lamb CR, Cappello R et al: Results of magnetic resonance imaging in 14 cats with meningoencephalitis, *J Feline Med Surg* 9:109, 2007.
203. Neuerer FF, Horlacher K, Truyen U et al: Comparison of different in-house test systems to detect parvovirus in faeces of cats, *J Feline Med Surg* 10:247, 2008.
204. Nishino Y, Funaba M, Fukushima R et al: Borna disease virus infection in domestic cats: evaluation by RNA and antibody detection, *J Vet Med Sci* 61:1167, 1999.
205. Norris JM, Bell ET, Hales L et al: Prevalence of feline immunodeficiency virus infection in domesticated and feral cats in eastern Australia, *J Feline Med Surg* 9:300, 2007.
206. Norris JM, Bosward KL, White JD et al: Clinicopathological findings associated with feline infectious peritonitis in Sydney, Australia: 42 cases (1990-2002), *Aust Vet J* 83:666, 2005.
207. O'Neil LL, Burkhard MJ, Diehl LJ et al: Vertical transmission of feline immunodeficiency virus, *Semin Vet Med Surg (Small Anim)* 10:266, 1995.
208. O'Neil LL, Burkhard MJ, Hoover EA: Frequent perinatal transmission of feline immunodeficiency virus by chronically infected cats, *J Virol* 70:2894, 1996.
209. Ohe K, Takahashi T, Hara D et al: Sensitivity of FCV to recombinant feline interferon (rFeIFN), *Vet Res Commun* 32:167, 2008.
210. Oishi S, Kodera Y, Nishikawa H et al: Design and synthesis of membrane fusion inhibitors against the feline immunodeficiency virus, *Bioorg Med Chem* 17:4916, 2009.
211. Omori M, Pu R, Tanabe T et al: Cellular immune responses to feline immunodeficiency virus (FIV) induced by dual-subtype FIV vaccine, *Vaccine* 23:386, 2004.
212. Ossiboff RJ, Sheh A, Shotton J et al: Feline caliciviruses (FCVs) isolated from cats with virulent systemic disease possess in vitro phenotypes distinct from those of other FCV isolates, *J Gen Virol* 88:506, 2007.
213. Ouchi A, Kishi M, Kobayashi T et al: Prevalence of circulating antibodies to p10, a non-structural protein of the Borna disease virus in cats with ataxia, *J Vet Med Sci* 63:1279, 2001.
214. Paltrinieri S, Cammarata MP, Cammarata G et al: Some aspects of humoral and cellular immunity in naturally occuring feline infectious peritonitis, *Vet Immunol Immunopathol* 65:205, 1998.
215. Paltrinieri S, Crippa A, Comerio T et al: Evaluation of inflammation and immunity in cats with spontaneous parvovirus infection: consequences of recombinant feline interferon-omega administration, *Vet Immunol Immunopathol* 118:68, 2007.
216. Paltrinieri S, Giordano A, Tranquillo V et al: Critical assessment of the diagnostic value of feline alpha1-acid glycoprotein for feline infectious peritonitis using the likelihood ratios approach, *J Vet Diagn Invest* 19:266, 2007.
217. Paltrinieri S, Parodi MC, Cammarata G: In vivo diagnosis of feline infectious peritonitis by comparison of protein content, cytology, and direct immunofluorescence test on peritoneal and pleural effusions, *J Vet Diagn Invest* 11:358, 1999.
218. Patterson EV, Reese MJ, Tucker SJ et al: Effect of vaccination on parvovirus antigen testing in kittens, *J Am Vet Med Assoc* 230:359, 2007.
219. Pedersen N, Laliberte L, Ekman S: A transient febrile "limping" syndrome of kittens caused by two different strains of feline calicivirus, *Feline Pract* 13:26, 1983.
220. Pedersen NC: Virologic and immunologic aspects of feline infectious peritonitis virus infection, *Adv Exp Med Biol* 218:529, 1987.
221. Pedersen NC: A review of feline infectious peritonitis virus infection: 1963-2008, *J Feline Med Surg* 11:225, 2009.
222. Pedersen NC, Barlough JE: Clinical overview of feline immunodeficiency virus, *J Am Vet Med Assoc* 199:1298, 1991.
223. Pedersen NC, Elliott JB, Glasgow A et al: An isolated epizootic of hemorrhagic-like fever in cats caused by a novel and highly virulent strain of feline calicivirus, *Vet Microbiol* 73:281, 2000.
224. Pedersen NC, Ho EW, Brown ML et al: Isolation of a T-lymphotropic virus from domestic cats with an immunodeficiency-like syndrome, *Science* 235:790, 1987.
225. Pedersen NC, Liu H, Dodd K et al: Significance of coronavirus mutants in feces and diseased tissues of cats suffering from feline infectious peritonitis, *Viruses* 1:166, 2009.
226. Pedretti E, Passeri B, Amadori M et al: Low-dose interferon-alpha treatment for feline immunodeficiency virus infection, *Vet Immunol Immunopathol* 109:245, 2006.
227. Pepin AC, Tandon R, Cattori V et al: Cellular segregation of feline leukemia provirus and viral RNA in leukocyte subsets of long-term experimentally infected cats, *Virus Res* 127:9, 2007.
228. Pesavento PA, MacLachlan NJ, Dillard-Telm L et al: Pathologic, immunohistochemical, and electron microscopic findings in naturally occurring virulent systemic feline calicivirus infection in cats, *Vet Pathol* 41:257, 2004.
229. Pesteanu-Somogyi L, Radzai C, Pressler B: Prevalence of feline infectious peritonitis in specific cat breeds, *J Feline Med Surg* 8:1, 2006.
230. Phadke AP, de la Concha-Bermejillo A, Wolf AM et al: Pathogenesis of a Texas feline immunodeficiency virus isolate: an emerging subtype of clade B, *Vet Microbiol* 115:64, 2006.
231. Phillips K, Arai M, Tanabe T et al: FIV-infected cats respond to short-term rHuG-CSF treatment which results in anti-G-CSF neutralizing antibody production that inactivates drug activity, *Vet Immunol Immunopathol* 108:357, 2005.
232. Poli A, Abramo F, Matteucci D et al: Renal involvement in feline immunodeficiency virus infection: p24 antigen detection, virus isolation and PCR analysis, *Vet Immunol Immunopathol* 46:13, 1995.
233. Poli A, Abramo F, Taccini E et al: Renal involvement in feline immunodeficiency virus infection: a clinicopathological study, *Nephron* 64:282, 1993.
234. Porter CJ, Radford AD, Gaskell RM et al: Comparison of the ability of feline calicivirus (FCV) vaccines to neutralise a panel of current UK FCV isolates, *J Feline Med Surg* 10:32, 2008.
235. Poulet H, Jas D, Lemeter C et al: Efficacy of a bivalent inactivated non-adjuvanted feline calicivirus vaccine: relation between in vitro cross-neutralization and heterologous protection in vivo, *Vaccine* 26:3647, 2008.

236. Pu R, Coleman J, Coisman J et al: Dual-subtype FIV vaccine (Fel-O-Vax FIV) protection against a heterologous subtype B FIV isolate, *J Feline Med Surg* 7:65, 2005.
237. Pu R, Okada S, Little ER et al: Protection of neonatal kittens against feline immunodeficiency virus infection with passive maternal antiviral antibodies, *AIDS* 9:235, 1995.
238. Quimby JM, Elston T, Hawley J et al: Evaluation of the association of *Bartonella* species, feline herpesvirus 1, feline calicivirus, feline leukemia virus and feline immunodeficiency virus with chronic feline gingivostomatitis, *J Feline Med Surg* 10:66, 2008.
239. Radford AD, Addie D, Belak S et al: Feline calicivirus infection ABCD guidelines on prevention and management, *J Feline Med Surg* 11:556, 2009.
240. Raith K, Müntener T, Vandevelde M et al: Encephalomyelitis resembling human and ruminant rhombencephalitis caused by *Listeria monocytogenes* in a feline leukemia virus-infected cat, *J Vet Intern Med* 24:983, 2010.
241. Rand J, Parent J, Percy D et al: Clinical, cerebrospinal fluid, and histological data from twenty-seven cats with primary inflammatory disease of the central nervous system, *Can Vet J* 35:103, 1994.
242. Ravi M, Wobeser GA, Taylor SM et al: Naturally acquired feline immunodeficiency virus (FIV) infection in cats from western Canada: prevalence, disease associations, and survival analysis, *Can Vet J* 51:271, 2010.
243. Rees TM, Lubinski JL: Oral supplementation with L-lysine did not prevent upper respiratory infection in a shelter population of cats, *J Feline Med Surg* 10:510, 2008.
244. Reeves N, Pollock R, Thurber E: Long-term follow-up study of cats vaccinated with a temperature-sensitive feline infectious peritonitis vaccine, *Cornell Vet* 82:117, 1992.
245. Reeves NA, Helps CR, Gunn-Moore DA et al: Natural Borna disease virus infection in cats in the United Kingdom, *Vet Rec* 143:523, 1998.
246. Reggeti F, Bienzle D: Feline immunodeficiency virus subtypes A, B and C and intersubtype recombinants in Ontario, Canada, *J Gen Virol* 85:1843, 2004.
247. Reynolds BS, Poulet H, Pingret J-L et al: A nosocomial outbreak of feline calicivirus associated virulent systemic disease in France, *J Feline Med Surg* 11:633, 2009.
248. Rice M, Wilks CR, Jones BR et al: Detection of astrovirus in the faeces of cats with diarrhoea, *N Z Vet J* 41:96, 1993.
249. Richards JR, Elston TH, Ford RB et al: The 2006 American Association of Feline Practitioners Feline Vaccine Advisory Panel report, *J Am Vet Med Assoc* 229:1405, 2006.
250. Ritz S, Egberink H, Hartmann K: Effect of feline interferon-omega on the survival time and quality of life of cats with feline infectious peritonitis, *J Vet Intern Med* 21:1193, 2007.
251. Rogers A, Hoover E: Fetal feline immunodeficiency virus infection is prevalent and occult, *J Infect Dis* 186:895, 2002.
252. Rohrbach BW, Legendre AM, Baldwin CA et al: Epidemiology of feline infectious peritonitis among cats examined at veterinary medical teaching hospitals, *J Am Vet Med Assoc* 218:1111, 2001.
253. Romatowski J, Lubkin S: Use of an epidemiologic model to evaluate feline leukemia virus control measures, *Feline Pract* 25:6, 1997.
254. Rottier PJ, Nakamura K, Schellen P et al: Acquisition of macrophage tropism during the pathogenesis of feline infectious peritonitis is determined by mutations in the feline coronavirus spike protein, *J Virol* 79:14122, 2005.
255. Rupprecht CE, Childs J: Feline rabies, *Feline Pract* 24:15, 1996.
256. Sand C, Englert T, Egberink H et al: Evaluation of a new in-clinic test system to detect feline immunodeficiency virus and feline leukemia virus infection, *Vet Clin Pathol* 39:210, 2009.
257. Savarino A, Pistello M, D'Ostilio D et al: Human immunodeficiency virus integrase inhibitors efficiently suppress feline immunodeficiency virus replication in vitro and provide a rationale to redesign antiretroviral treatment for feline AIDS, *Retrovirology* 4:79, 2007.
258. Savigny MR, Macintire DK: Use of oseltamivir in the treatment of canine parvoviral enteritis, *J Vet Emerg Crit Care (San Antonio)* 20:132, 2010.
259. Schoeman J, Kahn R, Meers J et al: Seroprevalence of FIV and FeLV infection and determination of FIV subtypes in sick domestic cats in South Africa (abstract), *J Vet Intern Med* 19:950, 2005.
260. Schorr-Evans E, Poland A, Johnson W et al: An epizootic of highly virulent feline calicivirus disease in a hospital setting in New England, *J Feline Med Surg* 5:217, 2003.
261. Schulman FY, Krafft AE, Janczewski T: Feline cutaneous fibropapillomas: clinicopathologic findings and association with papillomavirus infection, *Vet Pathol* 38:291, 2001.
262. Schulze C, Alex M, Schirrmeier H et al: Generalized fatal Cowpox virus infection in a cat with transmission to a human contact case, *Zoonoses Public Health* 54:31, 2007.
263. Scipioni A, Mauroy A, Vinje J et al: Animal noroviruses, *Vet J* 178:32, 2008.
264. Scott F: Update on FIP, *Proceedings of the 12th Kal Kan Symposium*, 1988, p 43.
265. Shalev Z, Duffy SP, Adema KW et al: Identification of a feline leukemia virus variant that can use THTR1, FLVCR1, and FLVCR2 for infection, *J Virol* 83:6706, 2009.
266. Shelton GH, Grant CK, Linenberger ML et al: Severe neutropenia associated with griseofulvin therapy in cats with feline immunodeficiency virus infection, *J Vet Intern Med* 4:317, 1990.
267. Siebeck N, Hurley DJ, Garcia M et al: Effects of human recombinant alpha-2b interferon and feline recombinant omega interferon on in vitro replication of feline herpesvirus-1, *Am J Vet Res* 67:1406, 2006.
268. Sigurdardottir OG, Kolbjornsen O, Lutz H: Orchitis in a cat associated with coronavirus infection, *J Comp Pathol* 124:219, 2001.
269. Simons FA, Vennema H, Rofina JE et al: A mRNA PCR for the diagnosis of feline infectious peritonitis, *J Virol Methods* 124:111, 2005.
270. Smith AW, Iversen PL, O'Hanley PD et al: Virus-specific antiviral treatment for controlling severe and fatal outbreaks of feline calicivirus infection, *Am J Vet Res* 69:23, 2008.
271. Sparkes A, Gruffydd-Jones T, Harbour D: An appraisal of the value of laboratory tests in the diagnosis of feline infectious peritonitis, *J Am Anim Hosp Assoc* 30:345, 1994.
272. Sparkes AH: Feline leukaemia virus and vaccination, *J Feline Med Surg* 5:97, 2003.
273. Sparkes AH, Gruffydd-Jones TJ, Harbour DA: Feline infectious peritonitis: a review of clinicopathological changes in 65 cases, and a critical assessment of their diagnostic value, *Vet Rec* 129:209, 1991.
274. Sponseller BA, Strait E, Jergens A et al: Influenza A pandemic (H1N1) 2009 virus infection in domestic cat, *Emerg Infect Dis* 16:534, 2010.
275. Squires RA: An update on aspects of viral gastrointestinal diseases of dogs and cats, *N Z Vet J* 51:252, 2003.
276. Stiles J, McDermott M, Bigsby D et al: Use of nested polymerase chain reaction to identify feline herpesvirus in ocular tissue from clinically normal cats and cats with corneal sequestra or conjunctivitis, *Am J Vet Res* 58:338, 1997.
277. Stiles J, Pogranichniy R: Detection of virulent feline herpesvirus-1 in the corneas of clinically normal cats, *J Feline Med Surg* 10:154, 2008.
278. Sukura A, Salminen T, Lindberg LA: A survey of FIV antibodies and FeLV antigens in free-roaming cats in the capital area of Finland, *Acta Vet Scand* 33:9, 1992.
279. Sundberg JP, Van Ranst M, Montali R et al: Feline papillomas and papillomaviruses, *Vet Pathol* 37:1, 2000.
280. Suntz M, Failing K, Hecht W et al: High prevalence of non-productive FeLV infection in necropsied cats and significant

association with pathological findings, *Vet Immunol Immunopathol* 136:71, 2010.
281. Takano T, Azuma N, Hashida Y et al: B-cell activation in cats with feline infectious peritonitis (FIP) by FIP-virus-induced B-cell differentiation/survival factors, *Arch Virol* 154:27, 2009.
282. Takano T, Hohdatsu T, Hashida Y et al: A "possible" involvement of TNF-alpha in apoptosis induction in peripheral blood lymphocytes of cats with feline infectious peritonitis, *Vet Microbiol* 119:121, 2006.
283. Tammer R, Evensen O, Lutz H et al: Immunohistological demonstration of feline infectious peritonitis virus antigen in paraffin-embedded tissues using feline ascites or murine monoclonal antibodies, *Vet Immunol Immunopathol* 49:177, 1995.
284. Thiry E, Addie D, Belak S et al: Feline herpesvirus infection ABCD guidelines on prevention and management, *J Feline Med Surg* 11:547, 2009.
285. Thiry E, Addie D, Belak S et al: H5N1 avian influenza in cats ABCD guidelines on prevention and management, *J Feline Med Surg* 11:615, 2009.
286. Thiry E, Zicola A, Addie D et al: Highly pathogenic avian influenza H5N1 virus in cats and other carnivores, *Vet Microbiol* 122:25, 2007.
287. Tiensin T, Chaitaweesub P, Songserm T et al: Highly pathogenic avian influenza H5N1, Thailand, 2004, *Emerg Inf Dis* 11:1664, 2005.
288. Timmann D, Cizinauskas S, Tomek A et al: Retrospective analysis of seizures associated with feline infectious peritonitis in cats, *J Feline Med Surg* 10:9, 2008.
289. Torres AN, Mathiason CK, Hoover EA: Re-examination of feline leukemia virus: host relationships using real-time PCR, *Virology* 332:272, 2005.
290. Torres AN, O'Halloran KP, Larson LJ et al: Feline leukemia virus immunity induced by whole inactivated virus vaccination, *Vet Immunol Immunopathol* 134:122, 2010.
291. Townsend WM, Stiles J, Guptill-Yoran L et al: Development of a reverse transcriptase-polymerase chain reaction assay to detect feline herpesvirus-1 latency-associated transcripts in the trigeminal ganglia and corneas of cats that did not have clinical signs of ocular disease, *Am J Vet Res* 65:314, 2004.
292. Troyer JL, Vandewoude S, Pecon-Slattery J et al: FIV cross-species transmission: an evolutionary prospective, *Vet Immunol Immunopathol* 123:159, 2008.
293. Truyen U, Addie D, Belak S et al: Feline panleukopenia ABCD guidelines on prevention and management, *J Feline Med Surg* 11:538, 2009.
294. Uckun FM, Chen CL, Samuel P et al: In vivo antiretroviral activity of stampidine in chronically feline immunodeficiency virus-infected cats, *Antimicrob Agents Chemother* 47:1233, 2003.
295. Uckun FM, Waurzyniak B, Tibbles H et al: In vivo pharmacokinetics and toxicity profile of the anti-HIV agent stampidine in dogs and feline immunodeficiency virus-infected cats, *Arzneimittelforschung* 56:176, 2006.
296. Vahlenkamp TW, Harder TC, Giese M et al: Protection of cats against lethal influenza H5N1 challenge infection, *J Gen Virol* 89:968, 2008.
297. VandeWoude S, O'Brien SJ, Langelier K et al: Growth of lion and puma lentiviruses in domestic cat cells and comparisons with FIV, *Virology* 233:185, 1997.
298. Veir JK, Lappin MR, Dow SW: Evaluation of a novel immunotherapy for treatment of chronic rhinitis in cats, *J Feline Med Surg* 8:400, 2006.
299. Veir JK, Ruch-Gallie R, Spindel ME et al: Prevalence of selected infectious organisms and comparison of two anatomic sampling sites in shelter cats with upper respiratory tract disease, *J Feline Med Surg* 10:551, 2008.
300. Vennema H, Poland A, Hawkins K et al: A comparison of the genomes of FECVs and FIPVs and what they tell us about the relationships between feline coronaviruses and their evolution, *Feline Pract* 23:40, 1995.
301. Wang C, Johnson C, Ahluwalia S et al: Dual-emission FRET real-time PCR differentiates feline immunodeficiency virus and separates infected from vaccinated cats, *J Clin Microbiol* 48:1667, 2010.
302. Wardley RC, Povey RC: The clinical disease and patterns of excretion associated with three different strains of feline caliciviruses, *Res Vet Sci* 23:7, 1977.
303. Weaver EA: A detailed phylogenetic analysis of FIV in the United States, *PLoS One* 5, 2010.
303a. Weiss ATA, Klopfleisch R, Gruber AD: Prevalence of feline leukaemia provirus DNA in feline lymphomas, *J Feline Med Surg* 12:929, 2010.
304. White JD, Malik R, Norris JM et al: Association between naturally occurring chronic kidney disease and feline immunodeficiency virus infection status in cats, *J Am Vet Med Assoc* 236:424, 2010.
305. Wilkes RP, Kania SA: Evaluation of the effects of small interfering RNAs on in vitro replication of feline herpesvirus-1, *Am J Vet Res* 71:655, 2010.
306. Willis AM: Feline leukemia virus and feline immunodeficiency virus, *Vet Clin North Am Small Anim Pract* 30:971, 2000.
307. Wright KN, Gompf RE, DeNovo RC Jr: Peritoneal effusion in cats: 65 cases (1981-1997), *J Am Vet Med Assoc* 214:375, 1999.
308. Yilmaz H, Ilgaz A, Harbour DA: Prevalence of FIV and FeLV infections in cats in Istanbul, *J Feline Med Surg* 2:69, 2000.

BACTERIAL INFECTIONS

Melissa Kennedy, Susan E. Little, and Randolph M. Baral

Primary bacterial diseases are less common in cats compared with other domestic species and humans. Important canine bacterial diseases, such as leptospirosis and Lyme disease (borreliosis), are not clinically important in cats even though seroconversion after exposure has been documented. Secondary bacterial infections, however, are common complications of many conditions, such as viral diseases, trauma, and surgery. The most common bacterial diseases are discussed elsewhere in this book along with the relevant body system. This chapter addresses bartonellosis, mycobacterial infections, and nocardiosis. A summary of less common bacterial diseases is found in Table 33-8.

BARTONELLOSIS

Bartonella spp. are receiving increasing attention both in veterinary and human medicine. Historically, their role in feline disease has been unclear and without consensus. As more is learned about these bacteria, their function as disease-causing agents will become clarified. The current understanding of *Bartonella* in cats is discussed here.

Bartonella spp. are very small gram-negative bacteria that can survive and replicate intracellularly in their mammalian hosts, not unlike rickettsial organisms. Their primary targets are vascular endothelial cells and red blood cells, and spread to various tissues is facilitated through infection of macrophages.[11] There are many

TABLE 33-8 Less Common Bacterial Diseases of Cats

Disease	Agent	Clinical Signs	Diagnosis	Treatment	Comments
Tetanus[5,7,30]	*Clostridium tetani* Motile, gram-positive, anaerobic, spore-forming bacillus	Appear within 5 to 21 days; localized and generalized forms; limb stiffness, stiff gait, dorsally curved tail, muscle rigidity, hyperthermia, cranial nerve signs, facial and masticatory muscle spasms, reflex muscle spasms/tonic contraction, seizures, death from respiratory compromise	History of a recent wound, clinical signs; serum antibody titers to tetanus toxin	Tetanus antitoxin, penicillin G or metronidazole; chlorpromazine, barbiturates, benzodiazepines; muscle relaxants, such as methocarbamol; nursing care	Transmission by environmentally resistant spores introduced into wounds; disease caused by neurotoxin formed during vegetative growth; localized forms have better prognosis, mortality from complications in generalized disease is high
Tularemia[4,28,70,73]	*Francisella tularensis* Gram-negative, non–spore-forming bacillus	Fever, depression, generalized lymphadenomegaly, hepatomegaly, splenomegaly, oral ulcers, icterus, draining abscesses, panleukopenia	Serology for microscopic agglutinating antibody	No validated treatment; suggested antibiotics include aminoglycosides, tetracyclines, fluoroquinolones	Zoonotic; type A and B strains isolated from cats in United States; transmission through contact with wildlife reservoirs (rodents, rabbits), tick vectors or contaminated environment
Plague[24,61]	*Yersinia pestis* Gram-negative, non–spore-forming, facultative anaerobe coccobacillus	Bubonic form: fever, dehydration, lymphadenomegaly, cervical/submandibular abscesses, hyperesthesia; septicemic form: septic shock, rapidly fatal; pneumonic form can develop by hematogenous or lymphogenous spread; 50% die acutely	Clinical signs, epidemiologic information; contact public health laboratory for guidance on submission of samples for culture (fluids, tissues, aspirates, blood), direct fluorescent antibody testing, serology	Strict barrier nursing techniques required; eliminate fleas; recommended antimicrobials include aminoglycosides, penicillins	Zoonotic; transmitted by ingestion of infected rodents or rabbits, bites from infected fleas on prey

species of *Bartonella*, and many of them can infect humans. Various species of mammalian hosts are adapted to the various *Bartonella* spp. and maintain a bacteremia for long periods without any effects. The organisms are spread by a variety of vectors, including sand flies, lice, and fleas; ticks may be a vector, but this has not been definitively proven.[11]

Several *Bartonella* species have been identified in cats. *B. clarridgeiae* causes asymptomatic bacteremia of cats. Other species have been found in isolated cases, but the primary species of concern in cats is *B. henselae*, the agent of cat scratch disease.[35]

Epidemiology

Bartonella-infected cats have been found throughout the world, but prevalence appears to be highest in warm, humid climates.[35] In the United States, prevalence studies have shown rates from 5% to 40%. In addition to transmission by biting insect vectors, cats may become infected by a bite or scratch from another infected animal.[10] Infection of domestic and nondomestic felids with *B. henselae* has been documented. Interestingly, the genetic variation among *B. henselae* isolates is significant, which may account for the bacteria's ability to persist in an infected animal as well as the fact that infected cats may be reinfected with heterologous strains.[35]

B. henselae is naturally transmitted among cats by cat fleas (*Ctenocephalides felis felis*), specifically by flea excrement. Cat-to-cat transmission, even by transplacental exposure, is rare to nonexistent.[35] The resultant bacteremia is often chronic in nature though it may be intermittent.

Pathogenesis and Clinical Signs

After infection, the bacteria enter red blood cells and endothelial cells where they are protected from the immune response. In experiments, infection of bone marrow progenitor cells has been documented and may be the mechanism for red blood cell infection.[10] The intraerythrocyte locale facilitates transmission throughout the host tissues, as well as vector transmission. Transient fever has been associated with primary infection as well as recurrence of bacteremia in chronically infected cats following a stressor, such as surgery.[10] Lethargy, anorexia, and lymphadenomegaly have been reported following experimental infection, and less commonly, transient mild neurologic manifestations, such as nystagmus and tremors, have been noted.[35] In natural infection, however, clinical signs are uncommon. *Bartonella* infection has been associated with gingivostomatitis, but causation has not been shown.[67] In fact, a lack of association of *Bartonella* infection and chronic gingivostomatitis has also been documented.[23] No association with other disease syndromes, including kidney, pancreatic, neurologic, nasal, or ocular diseases, has been proven. More severe disease has been seen in immunocompromised humans infected with *Bartonella*, but no such enhancement of disease has been found with concurrent FIV or FeLV infection in cats. However, an association between FeLV and *B. henselae* co-infection has been observed, indicating that infection with the former may predispose to infection with the latter.[14] Large epidemiologic studies are needed to determine what role, if any, *B. henselae* plays in feline disease.

Diagnosis

Veterinarians may be asked to test pet cats because of a diagnosis of *Bartonella*-associated disease in the cat owner. Diagnosis of active infection is difficult, and will likely rely on multiple assays. Finding the organism in red blood cells on smears is notoriously insensitive and is not considered a viable method for diagnosis.[35] Serology alone is also difficult, because both false-negative and false-positive results occur. Antibody levels may remain elevated for prolonged periods, even if the organism is cleared; in addition, the latter is difficult to document. Antigen preparations vary among the different serologic assays, affecting results. Having said this, although the positive predictive value of a positive test is low, the negative predictive value of a seronegative result is much higher.[35]

Definitive diagnosis of infection should be performed with culture and/or PCR on blood samples. Generally, multiple samples must be tested because of the intermittent nature of bacteremia. Culture is done by sterile blood collection in ethylenediaminetetraacetic acid (EDTA)-containing tubes. Tubes should be kept chilled until reaching the diagnostic laboratory. Because special conditions and enriched media are required, labs having experience with this organism should be selected and consulted for optimal collection and transport methods.[35]

Nucleic acid detection by PCR is much more rapid, but is no more sensitive than culture, and reveals nothing about organism viability. The same care as required for sample collection for culture is required for PCR.

Treatment

The efficacy of treatment is difficult to assess because of the intermittent nature of the bacteremia. Because of concern over antibiotic resistance, only treatment of clinically ill cats is recommended.[34] Optimal treatment regimens have not been determined. Currently, recommendations are that doxycycline or amoxicillin-clavulanate should be used initially; if no response is seen in 7 days, and other diagnoses are ruled out, treatment with azithromycin or fluoroquinolones may be needed.[13] In addition, prolonged treatment (at least 4 weeks) is recommended. Owners should be made aware of the limitations of diagnostics as well as the caveats of positive results.

Prevention

The emphasis for control of *Bartonella* infections should focus on year-round flea control.[13] Cats that are seropositive for *Bartonella* should not be used as blood donors.[35] No vaccine is available.

MYCOBACTERIAL INFECTIONS

Mycobacterium is a genus of aerobic, non–spore-forming, nonmotile, gram-positive, pleomorphic bacterial rods with wide variations in host affinity and pathogenic potential. Traditionally, mycobacteria are classified by their growth in culture (slow, difficult to cultivate, rapid), whether they produce tubercles or lepromatous or granulomatous disease, and whether or not there is dissemination (Table 33-9). More recently, DNA sequencing of various genomic regions has provided more insight into taxonomy and discovered three new fastidious mycobacterial species. In cats, this diverse class of bacteria produces various, seemingly unrelated syndromes that this chapter will address as

1. Slow-growing organisms that do or do not produce tubercles
   a. Tuberculous mycobacteria
   b. *Mycobacterium avium* complex (MAC) and other slow-growing saprophytes
2. Leproid granuloma-producing organisms that cannot be cultured using standard methods
   a. Feline leprosy
3. Rapidly growing mycobacteria that are easily cultivated

Mycobacterium tuberculosis Complex

Feline tuberculosis is caused by the *Mycobacterium tuberculosis* complex, primarily *M. microti* and *M. bovis*. Tuberculous mycobacteria survive within mammalian hosts. The only reservoir hosts for *M. tuberculosis* are humans, cattle are the predominant host for *M. bovis*, and *M. microti* is prevalent in small rodents, such as voles, shrews and field mice in the United Kingdom. Cats are naturally more resistant to *M. tuberculosis* than to *M. bovis* or *M. microti*.

Epidemiology

Feline infections with *M. tuberculosis* are considered an anthropozoonosis; the direction of transmission is from human to animal. Spread of infection back from cats to people has not been reported. In general, the tubercle bacilli are not as transmissible as other bacterial pathogens, requiring frequent exposure or exposure to a large dose of pathogen to produce disease.

The primary mode of transmission of *M. tuberculosis* is by inhalation of aerosolized droplets of about 3 to 5 μm diameter that are able to reach the alveoli. The prevalence of human and animal *M. tuberculosis* infections has been decreasing in developed countries because of effective infection control measures in people, although unanticipated increases in prevalence have occurred in certain human populations because of many factors, such as immunosuppression from HIV infection and illicit drug use. Multidrug-resistant tuberculosis has thus emerged in these populations because of poor compliance with drug therapy. This may increase the risk of infection in cats in contact with these human populations.

M. bovis infects many species of animals as well as people, and is found worldwide, although bovine tuberculosis has been eradicated in most industrialized countries. The most common route of infection for *M. bovis* is via the gastrointestinal tract through the consumption of contaminated milk or meat from cattle. Bovine tuberculosis has become established in wildlife hosts in many countries (e.g., white-tailed deer in Michigan,[45] badgers in the United Kingdom,[21] and brushtail possums in New Zealand[15]) so that cats may continue to become infected even in areas where infection of domestic animals is uncommon. In this situation, cats are most likely to be infected by eating secondarily infected small wild mammals.[20,22]

Cats are more commonly infected with *M. bovis* than dogs, and can excrete the organism in feces and thus disseminate and maintain infection on farms. In the United States, cats are rarely responsible for transmission of infection to humans.[71] However, in some areas of the world, such as Buenos Aires, *M. bovis* infection of cats may be a significant human health hazard.[75]

M. microti infection is most commonly seen in rural cats in Great Britain. Infection is most likely transmitted by hunting and ingesting prey species, such as mice and voles.[33,41]

Pathogenesis

Tubercle bacilli enter the body through either the respiratory or alimentary tract or by skin penetration. In cats, *M. bovis* infection is more common than *M. tuberculosis* infection so that tonsils, mandibular lymph nodes, and ileocecal lymph nodes are often infected. The ileocecal nodes are the most common sites for localization and shedding of *M. bovis* organisms.

Cats with mucocutaneous infections caused by *M. tuberculosis* or *M. avium*-complex organisms develop a pyogranulomatous infiltrate with variable amounts of necrosis, presence of multinucleated giant cells, and degrees of lymphoid infiltration.[47] *M. tuberculosis* organisms are frequently extracellular, whereas *M. avium* complex organisms are usually intracellular.

TABLE 33-9 Species of *Mycobacterium* Infecting Cats

Organism	Environmental Factors	Clinical Features	Drug Susceptibility or Reported Successful Therapy*
SLOW-GROWING TUBERCULOUS: TUBERCLES AND LYMPHADENITIS, OCCASIONAL DISSEMINATION			
M. tuberculosis	Urban, close contact with affected person	Usually respiratory, pulmonary localization, can disseminate systemically	Isoniazid, rifampin, ethambutol, pyrazinamide
M. bovis	Rural cats, ingest raw beef or dairy products or infected wildlife	Usually alimentary disorders; may get respiratory, cutaneous, or lymphatic involvement, sometimes systemic dissemination	Rifampin, clarithromycin, fluoroquinolones, ethambutol, isoniazid, surgical excision of skin lesions
M. microti	Rural, suburban, hunter, bite wounds, prey exposure, ingestion of rodents	Nodular cutaneous lesions draining, ulceration, peripheral lymphadenomegaly, local myositis, arthritis, osteomyelitis, sometimes pneumonia, peritoneal infection, or systemic dissemination	Clarithromycin/azithromycin, fluoroquinolones + rifampin; rifampin, isoniazid, ethambutol
LEPROMATOUS: CUTANEOUS NODULAR DERMATOSIS			
M. lepraemurium	Cooler wet climates, winter months, cats less than 3 years of age exposed to infected rodent prey	Single to multiple cutaneous and subcutaneous dermal nodules on head and extremities, ulcers, fistulas, abscesses regional spread only	Clarithromycin, clofazimine, doxycycline or minocycline, rifampin, surgical removal
Feline leprosy, *Mycobacterium* sp. strain Tarwin	Central coast New South Wales, Australia, New Zealand, older cats greater than 10 years of age, feline immunodeficiency virus predisposes	Multiple subcutaneous dermal nodules, no ulceration, sometimes dissemination	Clarithromycin, clofazimine, rifampin
"Candidatus *M. visibile*"	Western Canada and United States, environmental exposure?	Cutaneous and disseminated	Clofazimine
NONTUBERCULOUS: PYOGRANULOMATOUS			
Saprophytic Slow Growing: Cutaneous Lesions, Lymphadenitis, Dissemination in Immunocompromised Hosts			
M. avium complex	Exposure to infected soil, water or dust; acidic soils contaminated with bird feces or carcasses, most prevalent in Siamese and Abyssinian cats	Dermal and regional lymph node granulomas, alimentary infiltration, corneal granulomas, systemic dissemination	Clarithromycin, clofazimine, doxycycline or minocycline, rifabutin, ethambutol; rifampin preferred for better penetration if central nervous system involvement
M. genavense	Environmental exposure in immunocompromised host	Disseminated lymphadenitis	Clarithromycin, ethambutol, fluoroquinolones, clofazimine
M. terrae complex	Environmental exposure	Cutaneous lesions	Clarithromycin, fluoroquinolones, rifampin
M. simiae	Environmental exposure	Cutaneous and disseminated	Clarithromycin, fluoroquinolones, rifampin?
M. ulcerans	Environmental exposure	Cutaneous	Surgical removal, clarithromycin
Saprophytic Rapidly Growing Mycobacteria (RGM): Cutaneous and Subcutaneous Pyogranulomatous Infections			
Mycobacterial panniculitis: *M. smegmatis* (Australia), *M. fortuitum* (United States)	Soil and water exposure; bite and puncture wounds; immunocompromised host	Cutaneous and subcutaneous granulomas, especially inguinal region, ulcers, drainage, with regional spread only; secondary wound infections	Surgical removal, wide excision, variable susceptibility to fluoroquinolones, doxycycline, aminoglycosides, clofazimine, clarithromycin, trimethoprim-sulfonamide

*A minimum of two and often three drugs should always be used in combination.
Adapted from Table 50-2 in Greene CE, editor: *Infectious diseases of the dog and cat*, ed 3, St Louis, 2006, Elsevier.

Clinical Signs

Feline tuberculosis is frequently a subclinical disease, often acquired through contact with *M. tuberculosis* or *M. bovis*-infected people.[69] When clinical signs are present, they are similar whether infection is by *M. tuberculosis*, *M. microti*, or *M. bovis* and typically reflect the site of granuloma formation. Cats may develop localized cutaneous infections with *M. bovis* and *M. microti* seen as dermal nodules and nonhealing, draining ulcers at the site of a bite or scratch wound or a penetrating injury. Regional lymphadenomegaly may develop.[33] Pulmonary infection causes dyspnea and cough.[33] Dysphagia, retching, hypersalivation, and tonsillar enlargement may result from ulcerated and chronically draining oropharyngeal lesions. Localized intestinal lesions may cause weight loss, anemia, vomiting, and diarrhea, as well as enlarged mesenteric lymph nodes and abdominal effusion.

Disseminated disease resulting from *M. bovis* or *M. microti* may develop from cutaneous lesions and cause respiratory dysfunction.[33] Other signs of disseminated disease include abdominal masses, organ enlargement, generalized lymphadenomegaly, anorexia, weight loss, and fever. *M. bovis* may be associated with tuberculous choroiditis and retinal detachment.[25] Sudden death can also occur.

Mycobacterium avium Complex

The *M. avium* complex (MAC) organisms are opportunistic mycobacteria that survive in soil and water (i.e., are saprophytic). Other slow-growing saprophytic mycobacteria, such as *M. genavense*, *M. simiae*, *M. xenopi*, *M. terrae*, and *M. kansasii*, have a similar environmental niche and can cause similar clinical disease in cats and thus should be considered in the same context. Clinical infection with these organisms results in granulomas but not true tubercles. In cats, localized lymphadenitis can occur, but disease can disseminate if the cat does not mount an appropriate immune response. Disseminated MAC infection occurs, therefore, in immunocompromised animals, such as cats receiving immunosuppressive therapy after renal transplantation[31] and cats with retroviral infections;[40] congenital immune deficiencies are also considered to be a possible predisposing factor.[6]

Epidemiology

MAC and other slow-growing saprophytic mycobacteria are ubiquitous worldwide in soil and water when conditions are acidic (pH 5.0 to 5.5) and soils are high in organic matter, such as swamps, coastal plains, and brackish coastal waters.[48] MAC is found in large numbers in the feces of infected birds. Infection of cats occurs by ingestion of infected meat or contact with infected soil or contaminated fomites. Despite the widespread nature of MAC organisms in the environment, infections in cats have been uncommon because of natural resistance. No evidence has been found for spread of MAC organisms from animals to people.

Pathogenesis

Infection with MAC organisms begins with ingestion of contaminated food or contact with the organism in the environment. MAC infections in cats are often disseminated through many tissues and are due to organisms closely related to the *M. avium* subspecies *paratuberculosis* that causes chronic granulomatous enteritis in ruminants (Johne's disease). It is thought that animals with Johne's disease acquire the infection as neonates, although it initially becomes quiescent. Stress or immunosuppression later in life allows the organisms to replicate and produce disease. A similar scenario may occur in predisposed cat breeds (Siamese, Abyssinian) in which disseminated infections typically develop while cats are young, possibly because of defects in cell-mediated immunity.[6,44]

Clinical Signs

Localized infections often follow bite or scratch wounds so that clinical signs include enlarged regional lymph nodes and subcutaneous swellings, especially around the head and face. Other signs include weight loss, anorexia, and fever. Disseminated infection can occur with clinical signs reflecting the areas involved.[6,8] Clinical findings may include thickened intestinal loops, hepatomegaly, splenomegaly, and lymphadenomegaly; in one series of 12 cats, 10 of 12 cats had enlarged mesenteric lymph nodes, and 6 of 12 had enlarged popliteal lymph nodes.[6] Pulmonary nodular interstitial infiltration is commonly recognized radiographically but does not necessarily result in respiratory signs (Figures 33-25

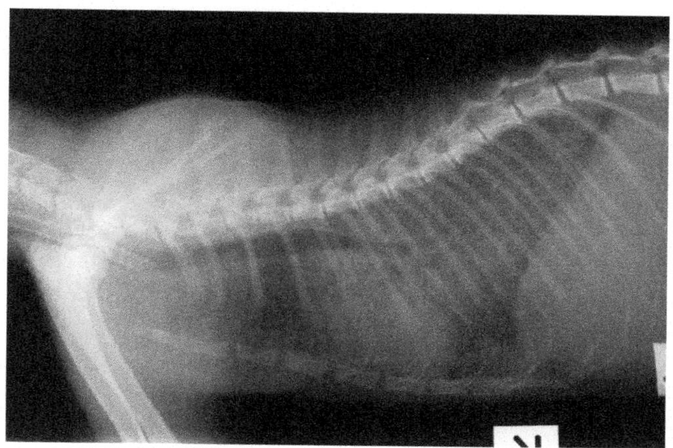

FIGURE 33-25 Lateral radiograph of a 1-year-old neutered male Abyssinian. The diffuse pulmonary interstitial pattern was caused by disseminated MAC infection. *(From Baral RM, Metcalfe SS, Krockenberger MB et al: Disseminated* Mycobacterium avium *infection in young cats: overrepresentation of Abyssinian cats,* J Feline Med Surg *8:23, 2006.)*

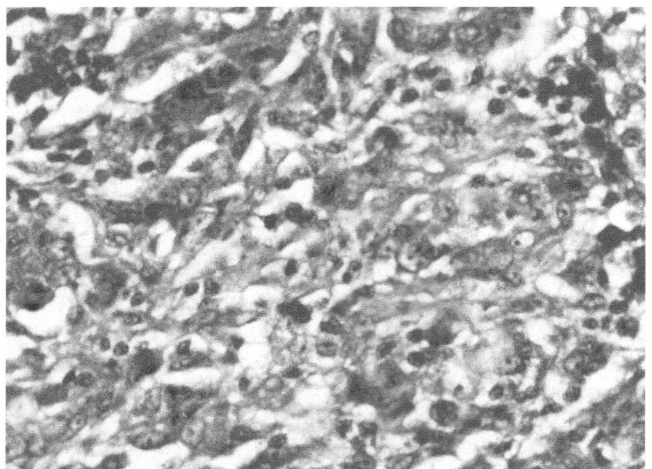

FIGURE 33-26 A high-power photomicrograph of a lymph node from the cat shown in Figure 33-25. The Ziehl-Neelsen stain shows intracellular acid-fast bacilli (staining pink with the carbol fuchsin) in macrophages. *(Courtesy Dr. Randolph Baral.)*

and 33-26). Disseminated infection is particularly noted in Abyssinians, where signs of illness develop before 5 years of age.[6,66]

Diagnosis of M. tuberculosis *Complex and MAC Infections*

Clinical laboratory findings in mycobacterial infections are typically nonspecific. Non-regenerative anemia may be seen, and has been reported to be macrocytic in some cats with intestinal infections.[44] Other findings include neutrophilic leukocytosis, hyperglobulinemia, and hypercalcemia.[1,6,59] Imaging studies may reveal masses in various organ systems. Tracheobronchial lymphadenomegaly, interstitial pulmonary infiltrates, calcified pulmonary lesions, and pleural or pericardial fluid may be seen with thoracic radiography. Hepatomegaly, splenomegaly, solitary abdominal masses, and ascites may be seen on abdominal radiography or ultrasonography.

Specific diagnostic methods include acid-fast staining, mycobacterial culture, biopsy with histopathologic examination and direct detection of organisms. Intradermal tuberculin testing is not reliable in cats, unlike other species, including dogs.

Acid-fast (Ziehl-Neelsen) staining of cytologic specimens obtained by tissue aspirates or impressions smears from biopsy samples is a widely available and useful method of diagnosis. Acid-fast organisms may also be demonstrated within lesions on histopathologic examination of tissue biopsy samples or in direct smears of exudates or fluids. Intracellular tubercle bacilli have a clubbed shape and beaded appearance. *M. tuberculosis* bacilli may be found in extracellular locations.[47] MAC organisms are generally smaller and present in high numbers within infected cells. When biopsy samples are obtained from lesions where mycobacterial infection is suspected, the sample should be divided into three pieces. One piece is fixed in formalin for histopathology and acid-fast staining, and one is sent for routine bacterial culture. A third piece is placed in a sterile container and frozen. If the first sample is acid-fast positive, the frozen sample can be submitted for mycobacterial culture. PCR testing can be performed on formalin-fixed samples.

Finding acid-fast staining organisms confirms mycobacterial infection, but culture is required to determine the species in order to evaluate zoonotic risk, sources of infection, and treatment options. Unfortunately, mycobacterial organisms are very slow-growing and may fail to culture. A specialized laboratory should be consulted for advice on specimen preparation and transport media.

Specific detection methods for mycobacterial organisms in body fluids and tissue specimens include enzyme-linked immunosorbent assay, radioimmunoassay and PCR. PCR appears to be highly sensitive when organisms are abundant in the specimen, but false-negative results are possible when organisms are few because the nucleic acid is difficult to extract and purify. Therefore methods based on detection of nucleic acid should not replace conventional mycobacterial isolation methods but may be complementary, such as to identify organisms found in culture of clinical specimens.

At necropsy, generalized emaciation is a common finding. Multifocal granulomas appear in many organs as grayish-white to yellow, circumscribed, nodular lesions. The primary lesion sites in cats are ileocecal and mesenteric lymph nodes. Disseminated infection may lead to lesions in the mesenteric lymph nodes, spleen, and skin. Uncommon sites for lesions include bones, joints, genitals, and conjunctiva. Histologically, granulomas consist of focal necrosis surrounded by plasma cells and macrophages in a connective tissue capsule.

Precautions should always be taken whenever handling potentially tuberculous material to prevent human infection. In many countries, specific laws govern the diagnosis and reporting of suspected tuberculosis cases.

Therapy of M. tuberculosis *Complex and MAC Infections*

Treatment of tuberculous mycobacterial infections should be considered separate from treatment of disseminated infections with slow-growing saprophytic mycobacteria. This is because of the zoonotic potential of *M. tuberculosis; M. bovis*–infected cats do not appear to be a major risk for their owners,[18,19] and reports of *M. microti* infections in people appear to be associated with direct contact with rodents.[60] Additional considerations are the need for long-term (sometimes indefinite) drug administration that is expensive and can make patient compliance uncertain; and whether immunosuppressed people may be exposed. Also, increasing antimicrobial resistance to drugs used to treat human tuberculosis must be considered, because the routine treatment of animal infections might contribute to the development of resistance. Infections with saprophytic mycobacteria, such as MAC and *M. microti,* are the appropriate mycobacterial infections to consider treating.

When a decision to treat a cat has been made, treatment should be started based on cytologic or histopathologic diagnosis, because results of mycobacterial culture and species identification typically take several weeks if the organism grows in culture at all. Treatment of mycobacterial disease poses several difficulties. To be effective, antimicrobials must reach therapeutic concentrations within phagocytes in various tissues but with minimal toxicity to the host. Importantly, there is a propensity for mycobacteria species, in general, and MAC organisms, in particular, to spontaneously and rapidly develop antibiotic-resistant mutants.[58] Multiple agents should therefore be used to reduce the chance of resistant clones developing. Using several agents concurrently, however, increases the likelihood of adverse drug reactions, because each agent has a potential toxicity profile. Furthermore, some of these toxicity profiles overlap.[58]

M. bovis and *M. microti* infections in cats have been successfully treated with a combination of rifampin, plus enrofloxacin or marbofloxacin, plus clarithromycin or azithromycin.[18,33] It is appropriate to treat localized MAC infections (or other slow-growing saprophytes) with surgical excision followed by combination antibiotic therapy with clarithromycin and doxycycline.[46] Disseminated MAC infections (or other slow-growing saprophyte) are best treated with clarithromycin in combination with at least one other agent, such as clofazimine or rifampin.[6] There is widespread resistance of MAC strains to the traditional fluoroquinolones,[2] but newer agents, such as moxifloxacin, may have some role in treating these organisms. More details about these drugs including dosages are included in Table 33-10.

Prevention of Mycobacterium tuberculosis *Complex and MAC Infections and Public Health Considerations*

Cats (and dogs) should be evaluated as temporary sources for dissemination of infection when *M. tuberculosis* is identified in people and when outbreaks of *M. bovis* in cattle occur on farms. Prevention of infection in cats involves discouraging the hunting of prey and avoiding the feeding of potentially infected meat and milk. MAC organisms may be acquired from the environment by both cats and people.

Mycobacteria are more resistant to heat, pH changes, ultraviolet light, and routine disinfection than are other pathogenic bacteria. Contaminated equipment should always be manually cleaned with a neutral detergent before disinfection. Mycobacteria are killed by 5% household bleach within 15 minutes and 2% glutaraldehyde for 10 minutes at room temperature. Ethyl and isopropyl alcohols can be used as a terminal rinse.

Feline Leprosy

Feline leprosy was first described in the 1960s and consists of solitary or multiple, well-circumscribed, nodular granulomas in the skin and/or subcutis, resulting from mycobacterial infection. Unfortunately, the causative species are fastidious and typically cannot be grown using routine mycobacteriologic techniques, even in specialist laboratories. Recent studies incorporating PCR methodologies have led to the recognition that there are numerous agents associated with feline leprosy, including *M. lepraemurium* as well as at least three novel mycobacterial agents.[4,7,27] In Australia and New Zealand, feline leprosy has typically been considered to be composed of two syndromes: one caused by *M. lepraemurium* (affecting younger, mostly immunocompetent cats) and one caused by a novel mycobacterial species currently described as *Mycobacterium* sp. cat (affecting older, immunocompromised cats).[52] However, a recent study has recognized another organism from a specific regional area, described as *Mycobacterium* sp. strain Tarwin, with no obvious age or sex predisposition in affected cats.[27] In a study of 26 cases in New Zealand and British Columbia, Canada, various species were identified, such as *M. lepraemurium, M. intracellulare, M. mucogenicum, M. septicum,* as well as one case of *Mycobacterium* sp. cat.[17] Three cats from the northwestern United States and western Canada have been diagnosed with diffuse cutaneous and disseminated disease similar to diffuse lepromatous leprosy in people caused by *M. visibile.*[7]

Feline leprosy has been reported from many areas of the world, including New Zealand, Australia, the United Kingdom, the Netherlands, the United States, Canada, and Italy. Many cases originate in temperate coastal areas, suggesting that the route of infection may be rodent or insect bites or contamination of cat fight wounds with soilborne organisms.[56]

Feline leprosy is characterized by single or multiple nodules of the skin and/or subcutis, often on the head, face, limbs or trunk. The nodules are painless, well circumscribed, moveable, and firm or soft on palpation. Overlying skin may be intact or may ulcerate if lesions are large. In advanced disease, regional lymph nodes and local tissues may become involved as well as the liver or spleen.

Diagnosis is similar to that for other mycobacterial infections; an index of suspicion on the part of the clinician is essential. Other causes of cutaneous and subcutaneous nodular lesions must be ruled out (see Chapter 22). Samples obtained for cytology and histopathology by fine-needle aspiration or biopsy can be stained with Ziehl-Neelsen to demonstrate acid-fast organisms surrounded by granulomatous to pyogranulomatous

TABLE 33-10 **Antimicrobial Drug Therapy for Slow-Growing Mycobacterial Infections**

Drug	Dose (mg/kg)[a]	Route	Interval (Hour)	Toxicities
***TUBERCULOUS MYCOBACTERIA:* M. TUBERCULOSIS, M. BOVIS, M. MICROTI**				
Treatment (minimum of two, and preferably three, of different classes of the following drugs in combination)[b]				
Isoniazid	10-20[c]	PO	24	Hepatotoxic, seizures, acute renal failure, peripheral neuritis
Rifampi(ci)n	10-20[d]	PO	24	Hepatotoxic; discolors mucosae, tears, and urine
Ethambutol	10-25	PO	24	Optic neuritis
Dihydrostreptomycin	15	IM	24	Ototoxic
Pyrazinamide[e]	15-40	PO	24	Hepatotoxic, GI signs, arthralgia
Clarithromycin	5-15 62.5 total	PO PO	12 12	GI signs, hepatotoxic, cutaneous erythema, allergic reactions
Azithromycin	7-15	PO	24	GI signs?
Enrofloxacin	5	PO	24	Vomiting, retinal toxicity
Marbofloxacin	2	PO	24	Retinal toxicity?
***SLOW-GROWING SAPROPHYTIC MYCOBACTERIA:* M. AVIUM COMPLEX, M. TERRAE, M. SIMIAE, M. ULCERANS**				
Clarithromycin	7.5-15	PO	12	Cutaneous erythema, hepatotoxicity
Clofazimine[f]	8-10 25 mg total[g]	PO PO	24 24	Orange staining body fluids, hepatotoxic, GI signs, photosensitization
Rifampi(ci)n	10-20 75 mg total	PO PO	24 24	Hepatotoxic, cutaneous erythema, discolors body fluids
Doxycycline	5-10[h]	PO	12	Vomiting, esophagitis

[a]Dose per administration at specified interval. After daily dosing for weeks to months, switch to twice weekly administration for 6 to 9 months.
[b]Treatment for 2 months minimum with three drugs in combination (e.g., rifampin with a fluoroquinolone [e.g., marbofloxacin] and with either clarithromycin or azithromycin). Maintenance therapy for 4 months thereafter consists of the same dosages of any two of the three drugs.
[c]Maximum 300 mg daily.
[d]Maximum 600 mg daily.
[e]Ineffective for *M. bovis* strains.
[f]Only available from a compounding pharmacist in most countries.
[g]Alternatively, 50 mg total can be given every 48 hours.
[h]Can increase dosage up to 10 mg/kg for improved efficacy, but only if this level is tolerated; give with food or administer water to avoid esophageal injury; if possible, use monohydrate salt to minimize gastrointestinal irritation.
GI, Gastrointestinal; *IM*, intramuscular; *PO*, by mouth.
Adapted from Table 50-4 in Greene CE, editor: *Infectious diseases of the dog and cat*, ed 3, St Louis, 2006, Elsevier.

inflammation. With Romanowski stains, mycobacterial rods are "negatively" stained and are typically located within macrophages and giant cells. Culturing these organisms is usually unsuccessful, but they are readily detected using PCR methodologies in laboratories with mycobacterial expertise.

Feline leprosy is divided into two forms: lepromatous and tuberculoid, which correspond to the host's immune response to infection.[65] The lepromatous form corresponds with a poor cell-mediated immune response. Histopathologic findings are primarily pyogranulomatous, and lymphocytes and plasma cells are absent. Large numbers of mycobacterial organisms are present. The tuberculoid form is associated with a more effective cell-mediated immune response and is characterized by pyogranulomatous dermatitis and panniculitis. Histopathologic findings are primarily epitheloid histiocytes with moderate numbers of lymphocytes and plasma cells but moderate to few mycobacterial organisms. The tuberculoid form accounts for about two-thirds of cases in Canada,[17] most cases in New Zealand and the Netherlands, but few cases in Australia.[52] Invasion of peripheral nerves, a feature of human leprosy, is not usually found in feline patients.

Because the organisms responsible for feline leprosy cannot be grown in culture, therapy cannot be guided by susceptibility testing, and no firm guidelines exist to direct therapy. Aggressive surgical resection of lesions with wound reconstruction when required is often recommended, especially when the disease is diagnosed early and lesions are localized.[50,62,72] Adjunctive antibiotic therapy is recommended to prevent local recurrence and should be continued for at least 2 months.[24,52] The most commonly recommended drugs are a combination of clarithromycin, rifampicin, and/or clofazimine.[52] Monotherapy is avoided to prevent development of resistance.

Human leprosy is acquired from the environment and is caused by *M. leprae. M. lepraemurium* has no zoonotic potential.

Rapidly Growing Mycobacteria

Rapidly growing mycobacteria (RGM) were formerly called Runyon group IV or atypical mycobacteria and are characterized by the ability to form colonies in solid media culture within 1 week. These mycobacteria are ubiquitous in the environment, including soil and water sources. The taxonomy of RGM has been redefined based on molecular methods and now includes the *Mycobacterium chelonae-abscessus, Mycobacterium fortuitum*, and *Mycobacterium smegmatis* groups among others. RGM are not known to be transmissible among animals.

RGM cause opportunistic disease in both healthy and immunocompromised cats. Disseminated disease typically occurs only in cats with underlying immunosuppression. The most common presentation is localized infection in healthy cats, most typically chronic panniculitis[72]; there have been occasional reports of pneumonia caused by RGM.[16,26] Many individual case reports are in the veterinary literature as well as a case series of 29 affected cats in Australia.[17] Other countries with reported cases include the United States,[49] Canada,[17,74] New Zealand,[17] France,[68] Finland,[1] the Netherlands,[43] and Switzerland.[3] In Australia, organisms from the *M. smegmatis* group account for most feline cases,[53,57] while in the United States, most cases are caused by members of the *M. fortuitum* group.[39,42]

Infection typically starts in the inguinal fat pad, possibly after a cat-fight wound has become contaminated,[56] and it may spread to the abdominal wall, perineum, and tail base. Other penetrations of the integument (such as through bite wounds, penetrating foreign bodies, injections, surgical wounds) may also allow RGM infections to become established in subcutaneous tissues, especially in fat. RGM organisms appear to prefer tissues rich in lipid so that certain areas of the body are more likely to be affected, and overweight or obese cats are at most risk. Initial lesions are circumscribed plaques or nodules at the site of injury, although trauma to the skin is not always reported.[39] Many patients are initially treated for a cat fight abscess with surgical drainage and antibiotics, although the lesions do not have a fetid odor or the typical bacterial discharge. Wound breakdown and development of a nonhealing suppurating tract then occurs. Later, the subcutaneous tissue becomes thickened, and the overlying skin becomes adherent and alopecic, with watery exudate discharging from fistulas. Gradually, the affected area may involve the entire ventral abdomen, adjacent flank areas, and limbs. Lesions typically remain localized, and most cats have few signs of systemic illness. In severe cases, depression, fever, inappetence, weight loss, and reluctance to move may be noted. Hypercalcemia of granulomatous disease develops only occasionally.

Diagnosis of mycobacterial panniculitis is similar to other mycobacterial infections; an index of suspicion on the part of the clinician is essential. Specimens for cytology (acid-fast staining) and culture are best obtained by fine-needle aspiration of pockets of purulent material through intact skin that has been disinfected with 70% ethanol (to eliminate skin-dwelling mycobacterial species).[55] Material from draining tracts is usually unsuitable, because of the high numbers of contaminating secondary bacteria. Tissue homogenates from surgically collected samples can also be used for cytology and culture. The diagnostic laboratory should be consulted in advance for advice on sample submission and supplies.

The medical and surgical management of mycobacterial panniculitis is well described.[55] However, recommendations continue to evolve as new drugs, such as fourth-generation fluoroquinolones and tetracycline derivatives, become available.[29] The use of appropriate antimicrobial agents based on susceptibility data and aggressive surgical resection, when warranted, improves outcome. However, some cases, especially those caused by *M. fortuitum* in the United States remain frustrating to treat.[39] Initial treatment should be with one or two oral antimicrobials chosen empirically, then adjusted based on susceptibility data. In Australia, doxycycline and/or a fluoroquinolone (such as pradofloxacin or moxifloxacin) are appropriate choices for first-line therapy, whereas in the United States, clarithromycin is the drug of choice for empiric therapy. Treatment durations are typically 3 to 12 months, and agents should be administered for at least 1 to 2 months after affected tissues look and feel completely normal. Surgical resection of persistently nonhealing tissue may be necessary.[63] In human medicine, RGM infections may develop resistance to quinolones (but not doxycycline or clarithromycin) during therapy.[12] For this reason, many veterinary dermatologists in Australia routinely use combination therapy with doxycycline and a fluoroquinolone from the outset. Although some RGM strains show in vitro susceptibility to amoxicillin-clavulanate, this drug combination has no efficacy in vivo.

Once susceptibility data is obtained, drug therapy may be refined. The highest possible doses are used because of the poor perfusion of affected tissues. Patients should be reassessed every 3 to 4 weeks to determine response to treatment and whether surgical resection is required. If surgery is required, it is most important to remove as much abnormal subcutaneous tissue as possible. Some cases require removal of large portions of infected tissue followed by reconstruction to close the wound without tension. Latex or closed suction drains must be used in large areas of dead space. Vacuum-assisted wound closure has been used in some challenging cases.[32]

NOCARDIOSIS

Nocardiosis is caused by several species of gram-positive aerobic actinomycetes that are ubiquitous soil saprophytes. These facultative intracellular pathogens with a propensity to erode blood vessels grow in branching filaments, often in tangles, and fragment into rods and cocci. They are somewhat acid fast. The most commonly isolated species are the *Nocardia asteroides* complex (including *N. farcinica, N. nova*), but infections in cats have also been reported to be caused by *N. brasiliensis, N. otitidiscaviarum, N. elegans, N. tenerifensis,* and *N. africana.*[9,36-38,51,54,64] Infections are opportunistic and are introduced primarily through scratches and bite wounds. Males are overrepresented in the published cases. The most common clinical scenario is infection of the skin and subcutis following penetrating wounds, with lesions typically located in regions subjected to cat bite or scratch injuries, including limbs, body wall, inguinal panniculus, and the nasal bridge (Figure 33-27). Pneumonia and pyothorax, possibly following aspiration of plant material, such as grass awns, and disseminated disease associated with immunodeficiency have also been documented.

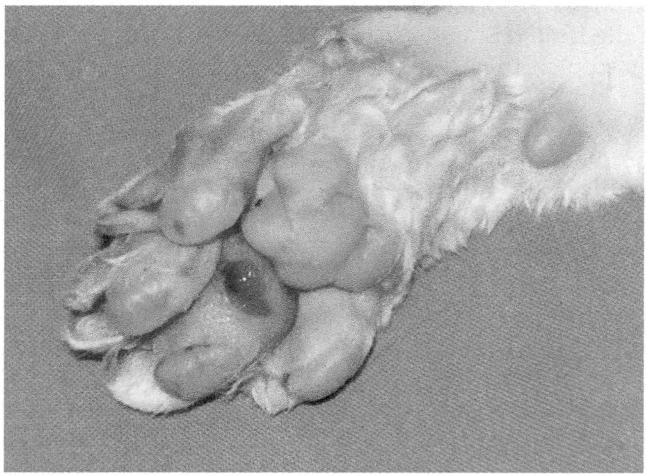

FIGURE 33-27 Lesion on the paw of a 13-year-old neutered male Devon Rex. Tangles of gram-positive branching filaments were seen on cytologic examination, and pyogranulomatous inflammation was seen on histopathologic examination. *Nocardia nova* infection was confirmed on culture. Treatment with clarithromycin (62.5 mg/cat, PO, every 12 hours) for 1 month resolved the lesion. *(Courtesy Dr. Randolph Baral.)*

Chronic nonhealing wounds often start as an abscess but spread circumferentially as well as by development of satellite lesions. The clinical appearance may be very similar to those caused by rapidly growing mycobacteria. In a series of 17 cases from eastern Australia, the majority of cats presented with spreading lesions of the skin and subcutis associated with draining tracts.[54] Most of the cats were male (14 of 17) and random bred (14 of 17). About half (9 of 17) were 10 years old or older. The majority of infections were due to *N. nova*. Several of the cats had conditions predisposing to immunosuppression, such as renal transplantation, chronic corticosteroid administration, postsurgical status, and FIV infection. The prognosis was considered to be guarded, and factors predisposing to treatment failure included delayed treatment resulting from misdiagnosis and insufficient duration of treatment.

Differential diagnoses include other infections associated with pyogranulomatous inflammation, such as mycobacterial panniculitis, *Rhodococcus* spp., *Corynebacterium* spp., and sporotrichosis. Clinical laboratory findings are nonspecific, such as nonregenerative anemia, neutrophilic leukocytosis with a left shift, monocytosis, and hyperproteinemia. Hypercalcemia associated with granulomatous disease has been reported,[59] but localized infections may show no clinical laboratory changes. Analysis of fluids and aspirates of abscesses demonstrates a suppurative to pyogranulomatous inflammation. The causative agent may be observed as a gram-positive, partially or weakly acid-fast, branching filamentous organism, either individually or in groups. Sulfur granules are not common. Diagnosis is confirmed by culture, usually within a few days, although 2 to 4 weeks of incubation may be necessary if samples have a high bacterial load or the patient was receiving antibiotics. Species identification is important for determining optimal antimicrobial treatment. Although traditionally species have been identified by phenotypic features, DNA-based techniques provide more rapid and reliable detection methods.

The primary drugs for treatment of nocardiosis are sulfonamides, such as trimethoprim-sulfamethoxazole (15 to 30 mg/kg, PO, every 12 hours). Prolonged courses of treatment, such as 3 to 6 months, are required to prevent recurrence. Sulfonamides may not be well tolerated for such long treatment durations because of drug reactions (anemia, leukopenia) and gastrointestinal side effects. *N. nova* infections are often susceptible to ampicillin, sulfonamides, clarithromycin, tetracyclines, amikacin, and imipenem but resistant to fluoroquinolones and amoxicillin clavulanate.[38,54] One recommended treatment regime for *N. nova* infections is amoxicillin (20 mg/kg, PO, every 12 hours) and/or erythromycin (10 mg/kg, PO, every 8 hours) or clarithromycin (62.5 mg/cat, PO, every 12 hours). Extensive débridement of skin lesions may be necessary in some cases.

References

1. Alander-Damsten Y, Brander E, Paulin L: Panniculitis, due to *Mycobacterium smegmatis*, in two Finnish cats, *J Feline Med Surg* 5:19, 2003.
2. Alangaden GJ, Lerner SA: The clinical use of fluoroquinolones for the treatment of mycobacterial diseases, *Clin Infect Dis* 25:1213, 1997.
3. Albini S, Mueller S, Bornand V et al: [Cutaneous atypical mycobacteriosis due to Mycobacterium massiliense in a cat], *Schweiz Arch Tierheilkd* 149:553, 2007.
4. Baldwin CJ, Panciera RJ, Morton RJ et al: Acute tularemia in three domestic cats, *J Am Vet Med Assoc* 199:1602, 1991.
5. Baral R, Catt M, Malik R: Localised tetanus in a cat, *J Feline Med Surg* 4:221, 2002.
6. Baral RM, Metcalfe SS, Krockenberger MB et al: Disseminated *Mycobacterium avium* infection in young cats: overrepresentation of Abyssinian cats, *J Feline Med Surg* 8:23, 2006.
7. Baral RM, Norris JM, Malik R: Localized and generalized tetanus in cats. In August J, editor: *Consultations in feline internal medicine*, Philadelphia, 2006, Saunders, p 57.
8. Barry M, Taylor J, Woods JP: Disseminated *Mycobacterium avium* infection in a cat, *Can Vet J* 43:369, 2002.
9. Beaman BL, Sugar AM: *Nocardia* in naturally acquired and experimental infections in animals, *J Hyg (Lond)* 91:393, 1983.
10. Breitschwerdt EB: Feline bartonellosis and cat scratch disease, *Vet Immunol Immunopathol* 123:167, 2008.
11. Breitschwerdt EB, Maggi RG, Chomel BB et al: Bartonellosis: an emerging infectious disease of zoonotic importance to animals and human beings, *J Vet Emerg Crit Care* 20:8, 2010.
12. Brown-Elliott BA, Wallace RJ Jr: Clinical and taxonomic status of pathogenic nonpigmented or late-pigmenting rapidly growing mycobacteria, *Clin Microbiol Rev* 15:716, 2002.
13. Brunt J, Guptill L, Kordick DL et al: American Association of Feline Practitioners 2006 Panel report on diagnosis, treatment, and prevention of *Bartonella* spp. infections, *J Feline Med Surg* 8:213, 2006.
14. Buchmann AU, Kershaw O, Kempf VAJ et al: Does a feline leukemia virus infection pave the way for *Bartonella henselae* infection in cats? *J Clin Microbiol* 48:3295, 2010.
15. Caley P, Hickling GJ, Cowan PE et al: Effects of sustained control of brushtail possums on levels of *Mycobacterium bovis* infection in cattle and brushtail possum populations from Hohotaka, New Zealand, *N Z Vet J* 47:133, 1999.
16. Couto SS, Artacho CA: *Mycobacterium fortuitum* pneumonia in a cat and the role of lipid in the pathogenesis of atypical mycobacterial infections, *Vet Pathol* 44:543, 2007.
17. Davies JL, Sibley JA, Myers S et al: Histological and genotypical characterization of feline cutaneous mycobacteriosis: a retrospective study of formalin-fixed paraffin-embedded tissues, *Vet Dermatol* 17:155, 2006.
18. de Lisle GW, Collins DM, Loveday AS et al: A report of tuberculosis in cats in New Zealand, and the examination of strains of *Mycobacterium bovis* by DNA restriction endonuclease analysis, *N Z Vet J* 38:10, 1990.
19. Dean R, Gunn-Moore D, Shaw S et al: Bovine tuberculosis in cats, *Vet Rec* 158:419, 2006.
20. Delahay RJ, Cheeseman CL, Clifton-Hadley RS: Wildlife disease reservoirs: the epidemiology of *Mycobacterium bovis* infection in the European badger (*Meles meles*) and other British mammals, *Tuberculosis (Edinb)* 81:43, 2001.
21. Delahay RJ, De Leeuw AN, Barlow AM et al: The status of *Mycobacterium bovis* infection in UK wild mammals: a review, *Vet J* 164:90, 2002.
22. Delahay RJ, Smith GC, Barlow AM et al: Bovine tuberculosis infection in wild mammals in the South-West region of England: a survey of prevalence and a semi-quantitative assessment of the relative risks to cattle, *Vet J* 173:287, 2007.
23. Dowers KL, Hawley JR, Brewer MM et al: Association of *Bartonella* species, feline calicivirus, and feline herpesvirus 1 infection with gingivostomatitis in cats, *J Feline Med Surg* 12:314, 2010.
24. Eidson M, Tierney LA, Rollag OJ et al: Feline plague in New Mexico: risk factors and transmission to humans, *Am J Public Health* 78:1333, 1988.
25. Formston C: Retinal detachment and bovine tuberculosis in cats, *J Small Anim Pract* 35:5, 1994.
26. Foster SF, Martin P, Davis W et al: Chronic pneumonia caused by *Mycobacterium thermoresistibile* in a cat, *J Small Anim Pract* 40:433, 1999.
27. Fyfe JA, McCowan C, O'Brien CR et al: Molecular characterization of a novel fastidious mycobacterium causing lepromatous lesions of the skin, subcutis, cornea, and conjunctiva of cats living in Victoria, Australia, *J Clin Microbiol* 46:618, 2008.
28. Gliatto JM, Rae JF, McDonough PL et al: Feline tularemia on Nantucket Island, Massachusetts, *J Vet Diagn Invest* 6:102, 1994.
29. Govendir M, Hansen T, Kimble B et al: Susceptibility of rapidly growing mycobacteria isolated from cats and dogs, to ciprofloxacin, enrofloxacin and moxifloxacin, *Vet Microbiol* 147:113, 2011.
30. Greene CE: Tetanus. In Greene CE, editor: *Infectious diseases of the dog and cat*, ed 3, St Louis, 2006, Saunders Elsevier, p 395.
31. Griffin A, Newton A, Aronson L et al: Disseminated *Mycobacterium avium* complex infection following renal transplantation in a cat, *J Am Vet Med Assoc* 222:1097, 2003.
32. Guille AE, Tseng LW, Orsher RJ: Use of vacuum-assisted closure for management of a large skin wound in a cat, *J Am Vet Med Assoc* 230:1669, 2007.
33. Gunn-Moore DA, Jenkins PA, Lucke VM: Feline tuberculosis: a literature review and discussion of 19 cases caused by an unusual mycobacterial variant, *Vet Rec* 138:53, 1996.
34. Guptill L: Bartonellosis, *Vet Microbiol* 140:347, 2010.
35. Guptill L: Feline bartonellosis, *Vet Clin North Am Small Anim Pract* 40:1073, 2010.
36. Harada H, Endo Y, Sekiguchi M et al: Cutaneous nocardiosis in a cat, *J Vet Med Sci* 71:785, 2009.
37. Hattori Y, Kano R, Kunitani Y et al: *Nocardia africana* isolated from a feline mycetoma, *J Clin Microbiol* 41:908, 2003.
38. Hirsh DC, Jang SS: Antimicrobial susceptibility of *Nocardia nova* isolated from five cats with nocardiosis, *J Am Vet Med Assoc* 215:815, 1999.
39. Horne KS, Kunkle GA: Clinical outcome of cutaneous rapidly growing mycobacterial infections in cats in the southeastern United States: a review of 10 cases (1996-2006), *J Feline Med Surg* 11:627, 2009.
40. Hughes M, Ball N, Love D et al: Disseminated *Mycobacterium genavense* infection in a FIV-positive cat, *J Feline Med Surg* 1:23, 1999.
41. Huitema H, Jaartsveld FH: *Mycobacterium microti* infection in a cat and some pigs, *Antonie Van Leeuwenhoek* 33:209, 1967.
42. Jang S, Hirsh D: Rapidly growing members of the genus *Mycobacterium* affecting dogs and cats, *J Am Anim Hosp Assoc* 38:217, 2002.
43. Jassies-van der Lee A, Houwers DJ, Meertens N et al: Localised pyogranulomatous dermatitis due to *Mycobacterium abscessus* in a cat: a case report, *Vet J* 179:304, 2009.
44. Jordan HL, Cohn LA, Armstrong PJ: Disseminated *Mycobacterium avium* complex infection in three Siamese cats, *J Am Vet Med Assoc* 204:90, 1994.
45. Kaneene JB, Bruning-Fann CS, Dunn J et al: Epidemiologic investigation of *Mycobacterium bovis* in a population of cats, *Am J Vet Res* 63:1507, 2002.
46. Kaufman A, Greene C, Rakich P et al: Treatment of localized *Mycobacterium avium* complex infection with clofazimine and doxycycline in a cat, *J Am Vet Med Assoc* 207:457, 1995.

47. Kipar A, Schiller I, Baumgartner W: Immunopathological studies on feline cutaneous and (muco)cutaneous mycobacteriosis, *Vet Immunol Immunopathol* 91:169, 2003.
48. Kirschner R, Parker B, Falkinham J: Epidemiology of infection by nontuberculosis mycobacteria, *Am Rev Respir Dis* 145:271, 1992.
49. Kunkle GA, KGulbas NK, Fadok V et al: Rapidly growing mycobacteria as a cause of cutaneous granulomas: report of five cases, *J Am Anim Hosp Assoc* 19:513, 1983.
50. Lewis DT, Kunkle GA: Feline leprosy. In Greene CE, editor: *Infectious diseases of the dog and cat*, ed 2, Philadelphia, 1998, Saunders, p 321.
51. Luque I, Astorga R, Tarradas C et al: *Nocardia otitidiscaviarum* infection in a cat, *Vet Rec* 151:488, 2002.
52. Malik R, Hughes M, James G et al: Feline leprosy: two different clinical syndromes, *J Feline Med Surg* 4:43, 2002.
53. Malik R, Hunt GB, Goldsmid SE et al: Diagnosis and treatment of pyogranulomatous panniculitis due to *Mycobacterium smegmatis* in cats, *J Small Anim Pract* 35:524, 1994.
54. Malik R, Krockenberger MB, O'Brien CR et al: *Nocardia* infections in cats: a retrospective multi-institutional study of 17 cases, *Aust Vet J* 84:235, 2006.
55. Malik R, Martin P, Wigney D et al: Infections caused by rapidly growing mycobacteria. In Greene CE, editor: *Infectious diseases of the dog and cat*, ed 3, St Louis, 2006, Elsevier, p 482.
56. Malik R, Norris J, White J et al: "Wound cat," *J Fel Med Surg* 8:135, 2006.
57. Malik R, Wigney DI, Dawson D et al: Infection of the subcutis and skin of cats with rapidly growing mycobacteria: a review of microbiological and clinical findings, *J Feline Med Surg* 2:35, 2000.
58. Masur H: Recommendations on prophylaxis and therapy for disseminated *Mycobacterium avium* complex disease in patients infected with the human immunodeficiency virus. Public Health Service Task Force on Prophylaxis and Therapy for *Mycobacterium avium* Complex, *N Engl J Med* 329:898, 1993.
59. Mealey K, Willard M, Nagode L et al: Hypercalcemia associated with granulomatous disease in a cat, *J Am Vet Med Assoc* 215:959, 1999.
60. Niemann S, Richter E, Dalugge-Tamm H et al: Two cases of *Mycobacterium microti* derived tuberculosis in HIV-negative immunocompetent patients, *Emerg Infect Dis* 6:539, 2000.
61. Orloski K, Lathrop S: Plague: a veterinary perspective, *J Am Vet Med Assoc* 222:444, 2003.
62. Pedersen NC: Atypical mycobacteriosis. In Pedersen NC, editor: *Feline infectious diseases*, Goleta, Calif, 1988, American Veterinary Publications, p 197.
63. Plaus WJ, Hermann G: The surgical management of superficial infections caused by atypical mycobacteria, *Surgery* 110:99, 1991.
64. Ramos-Vara JA, Wu CC, Lin TL et al: *Nocardia tenerifensis* genome identification in a cutaneous granuloma of a cat, *J Vet Diagn Invest* 19:577, 2007.
65. Schiefer HB, Middleton DM: Experimental transmission of a feline mycobacterial skin disease (feline leprosy), *Vet Pathol* 20:460, 1983.
66. Sieber-Ruckstuhl NS, Sessions JK, Sanchez S et al: Long-term cure of disseminated *Mycobacterium avium* infection in a cat, *Vet Rec* 160:131, 2007.
67. Sykes JE, Westropp JL, Kasten RW et al: Association between *Bartonella* species infection and disease in pet cats as determined using serology and culture, *J Feline Med Surg* 12:631, 2010.
68. Thorel MF, Boisvert H: Abscess due to *Mycobacterium chelonei* in a cat, *Bull Acad Vet France* 47:415, 1974.
69. Une Y, Mori T: Tuberculosis as a zoonosis from a veterinary perspective, *Comp Immun Microbiol Infect Dis* 30:415, 2007.
70. Valentine BA, DeBey BM, Sonn RJ et al: Localized cutaneous infection with *Francisella tularensis* resembling ulceroglandular tularemia in a cat, *J Vet Diagn Invest* 16:83, 2004.
71. Wilkins MJ, Bartlett PC, Berry DE et al: Absence of *Mycobacterium bovis* infection in dogs and cats residing on infected cattle farms: Michigan, 2002, *Epidemiol Infect* 136:1617, 2008.
72. Wilkinson GT, Mason KV: Clinical aspects of mycobacterial infections of the skin. In August JR, editor: *Consultations in feline internal medicine*, Philadelphia, 1991, Saunders, p 129.
73. Woods J, Crystal M, Morton R et al: Tularemia in two cats, *J Am Vet Med Assoc* 212:81, 1998.
74. Youssef S, Archambault M, Parker W et al: Pyogranulomatous panniculitis in a cat associated with infection by the *Mycobacterium fortuitum/peregrinum* group, *Can Vet J* 43:285, 2002.
75. Zumarraga MJ, Vivot MM, Marticorena D et al: *Mycobacterium bovis* in Argentina: isolates from cats typified by spoligotyping, *Rev Argent Microbiol* 41:215, 2009.

MOLECULAR ASSAYS USED FOR THE DIAGNOSIS OF FELINE INFECTIOUS DISEASES

Julia Veir and Michael R. Lappin

Infectious agents of cats are associated with many clinical disease syndromes evaluated by practicing veterinarians. A definitive diagnosis is best made by documenting current infection, which can be achieved with a variety of techniques that vary by the body system; these include fecal flotation, cytology, histopathology, immunohistochemistry, culture, antigen tests, and molecular diagnostic assays. For some agents, antibody test results are also used to help make a clinical diagnosis. However, presence of antibodies may only document prior exposure, not current infection.

Sensitivity is the ability of an assay to detect a positive sample; specificity is the ability of an assay to detect a negative sample. Sensitivity and specificity vary with each assay. Positive predictive value (PPV) is the ability of a test result to predict presence of disease; negative predictive value (NPV) is the ability of a test result to predict absence of disease. Many of the infectious agents encountered in feline practice infect a large percentage of the population, resulting in positive organism detection techniques or serum antibody production. However, they only induce disease in a small number of cats in the infected group. Classic examples include coronaviruses, *Toxoplasma gondii*, and *Bartonella* spp. For these agents, even though assays with good sensitivity and specificity are available, the predictive value of a positive test is actually very low.

MOLECULAR ASSAYS

Types of molecular assays used in cats were recently reviewed.[33] Molecular assays rely upon detection of the nucleic acids deoxyribonucleic (DNA) and ribonucleic (RNA) acid. Nucleic acids are part of the genetic makeup of the organism and consist of four nucleotides in varying sequences. Many portions of DNA and RNA are highly conserved among organisms, while others are specific to the organism on a family, genus, species, or even strain level. The sequence specificity is used to detect the organisms within clinical samples using some form of complementary sequence and sometimes a signaling molecule. Signaling molecules are often some form of a fluorescent molecule in order to improve sensitivity.

Detection of Pathogens Without Amplification

The simplest application of molecular tools for detection of infectious organisms is to apply a complementary nucleic acid sequence, termed a probe, which has been tagged with a fluorescent molecule. This probe is then applied directly to a clinical sample and hybridizes to a target sequence in an organism if present. Probes with different fluorescent tags can be applied to a single sample, allowing for detection of several organisms. However, sensitivity is poor compared with other molecular techniques, because the target DNA is not amplified. When probes are designed for use with tissues, it is termed in situ hybridization. Use of this technique can allow for detection of the organisms of interest in association with inflammatory lesions or specific areas of tissue. Fluorescent molecules are the most common signaling mechanism used with this technique, which is abbreviated FISH (fluorescent in situ hybridization).

Detection of Pathogens with Amplification: Polymerase Chain Reaction

The polymerase chain reaction (PCR) was first described in 1985.[28] This technique results in the cyclic amplification of a single strand of DNA to produce an exponential number of identical copies that then can be easily detected, usually on a gel (conventional or end-point PCR), to determine if it is the predicted size for the reaction (Figure 33-28). PCR is superior in sensitivity to probe hybridization techniques because of this amplification step. The great sensitivity of these assays requires strict adherence to good laboratory practice to avoid false-positive results from contamination within the laboratory.

Detection of microbial nucleic acids in a feline sample does not prove the organism is alive, capable of replication, or actually causing clinical signs in the host. Correlation with clinical signs of a known syndrome associated with the organism and/or a response to therapy must be used in conjunction with results of PCR. False-negative reactions can occur with PCR on some tissues or fluids that may have PCR inhibitors present.

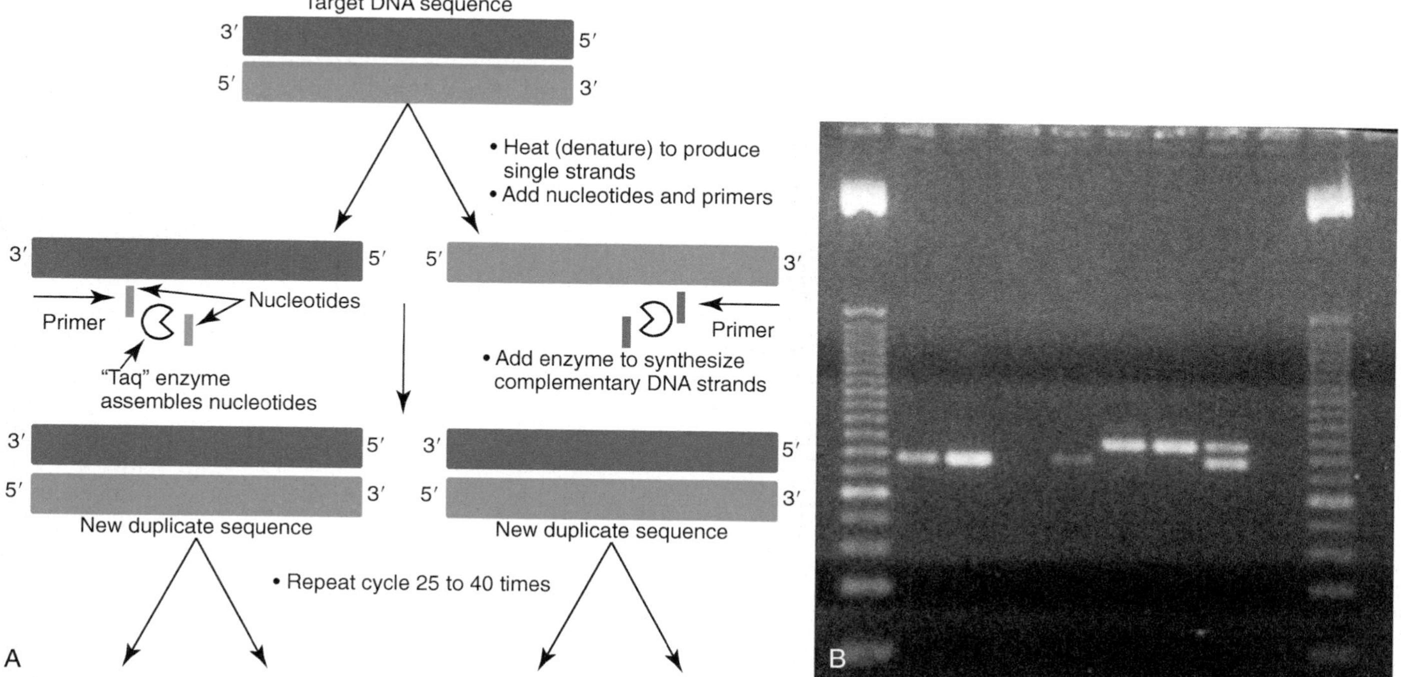

FIGURE 33-28 Traditional polymerase chain reaction. **A,** Short sequences of nucleotides called primers are annealed to the target DNA after the separation of the double strands. A proprietary enzyme is used to produce complementary strands of DNA during the synthesis step. Denaturation is repeated, and replication of the newly formed DNA strands, as well as the original target DNA, is repeated. **B,** The DNA produced in the reaction is then visualized using gel electrophoresis. The size of the product is compared with a standard to confirm that the predicted product has been obtained. *(From Veir JK, Lappin MR: Molecular diagnostic assays for infectious diseases in cats,* Vet Clin North Am Small Anim Pract *40:1189, 2010.)*

This problem varies by the syndrome as well as the assay and should be considered in each case. Finally, in order to prevent false negatives, samples tested should be obtained prior to treatment, which may decrease organism load below the level of detection of the assay even though the organism is still present in the host.

The enzyme used in PCR can only duplicate strands of DNA, and so, to detect RNA, the sample must first have a reverse transcription (RT) step to create a complementary strand of DNA from the target RNA. Amplification of the complementary DNA by polymerase chain reaction is then performed; this method is commonly known as RT-PCR.

PCR is used most commonly in veterinary medicine to detect infectious disease agents: The primers used in PCR can be designed to amplify the nucleic acids only of members of a certain genus, species, or even strain of organism. When a single organism is targeted in an assay, it is termed a singleplex PCR. If multiple targets can be detected in a single assay, it is termed a multiplex assay. It is clearly most attractive to investigate the presence of multiple organisms in a single assay. However, each target sequence competes with the others for the common building blocks in the PCR assay: the enzyme, nucleotide, and various buffers and ions that allow the reaction to proceed. Therefore multiplex reactions can be less sensitive than singleplex assays.

The use of broad-range or degenerate primers amplifying members of an entire genus or even kingdom can be used, targeting highly conserved regions of the nucleic acids. The most common application of this is for rapid detection and identification of eubacteria or fungi in clinical samples.[18,29] Subsequent analysis of the PCR product may then be used to identify the infecting organism much more rapidly than traditional microbiologic techniques and may be more sensitive for detection of fastidious organisms. It must be noted that antimicrobial sensitivity is not available using this technique; therefore it is complementary to traditional culture techniques. However, the use of PCR for detection of certain genes that encode for antimicrobial resistance genes is starting to gain clinical use as well and may provide additional rapid information prior to sensitivity results being available.[23]

It is difficult to acquire quantification information using traditional end-point PCR. Real-time PCR or quantitative PCR (qPCR) is the most recent application of PCR.[12] In this technique, production of DNA is monitored during each amplification cycle so that the original starting quantity could be extrapolated by identification of the logarithmic amplification phase of each individual reaction. This technique uses fluorescent dyes or probes that produce a signal after formation of the product (Figure 33-29). During each amplification cycle, a detector records the amount of fluorescence in the sample. Pathogen detection and load are one of the many applications of this technology. This assay has all the advantages of traditional end-point PCR (good sensitivity, specificity) but also offers a more rapid result and the ability to quantify microbial DNA or RNA load and so can be used to monitor therapy in some cases (see the following sections of the chapter). Because qPCR is very sensitive, strict quality control must be maintained. In addition, accuracy of quantification is reliant upon the availability of a reproducible, high-quality, standard curve. Although minimum laboratory standards have been proposed and are generally met for published protocols,[4] many diagnostic laboratories use proprietary reactions that are not subject to peer review. Thus all laboratories providing PCR assays may not be equivalent, and so, use of laboratories that have published results of their assays may be prudent.

CURRENT CLINICAL APPLICATIONS OF MOLECULAR ASSAYS IN FELINE MEDICINE

In the following subsections, a brief review of the benefits and problems associated with PCR assays currently used in feline medicine is presented.

Respiratory Agents

Feline calicivirus (FCV) is a common differential diagnosis for cats with clinical evidence of rhinitis and stomatitis. Less commonly, FCV is associated with conjunctivitis, polyarthritis, and lower airway disease in kittens. Virus isolation can be used to document current infection but takes at least several days for results to return. Because of widespread exposure and vaccination, the positive predictive value of serologic tests is poor. Reverse transcriptase (RT)-PCR assays can be used to amplify the RNA of FCV, and results can be returned quickly. However, these assays also amplify vaccine strains of FCV.[27] FCV RNA can be amplified from samples collected from normal carrier cats as well as clinically ill cats and so have poor positive predictive value.[24] For example, in one study in our laboratory, presence of FCV RNA failed to correlate with the presence or absence of stomatitis in cats.[26] In addition, amplification of FCV RNA cannot be used to prove virulent systemic calicivirus infection. The negative predictive value for FCV RT-PCR assays is currently unknown. Feline caliciviruses, as RNA viruses, have genetic variability among the different strains. Depending on the viral genetic region targeted by the assay, the degree of genetic variation among strains at that site will vary. Most laboratories design their assays to target conserved regions of the viral genome, but even this cannot guarantee that all strains are detectable by any individual assay.

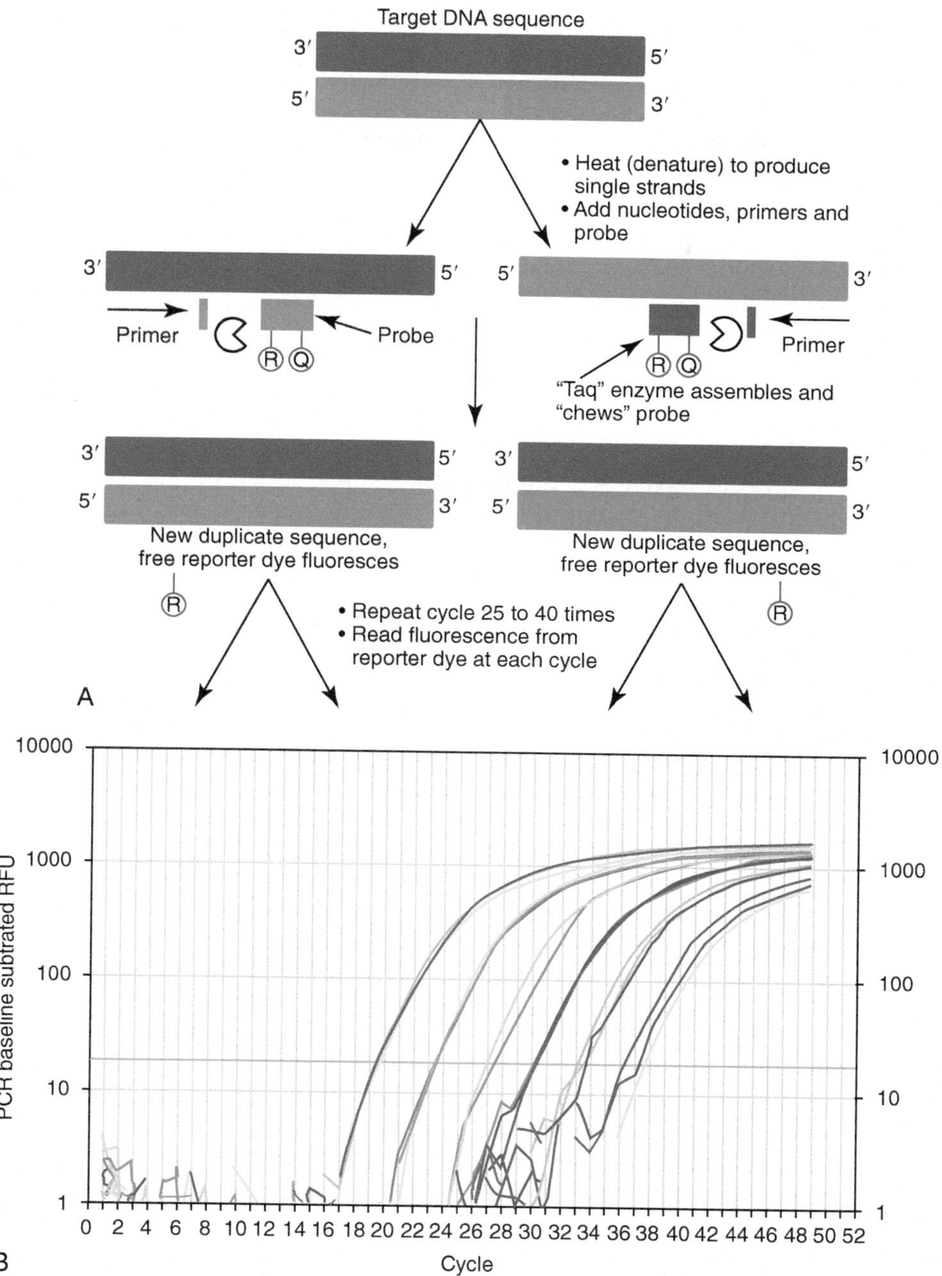

FIGURE 33-29 Quantitative polymerase chain reaction. **A,** The standard PCR assay is enhanced by using a fluorescent probe that fluoresces only after the removal of a quencher dye in close proximity to the reporter dye. The quencher dye is removed by the enzyme that synthesizes new strands of DNA as in traditional PCR. At each step, fluorescence is measured, allowing for the extrapolation of the amount of product present during each replication phase. **B,** The change in fluorescence is then plotted against time (number of cycles), and a starting quantity can be calculated by the extrapolation of the signal produced during the exponential replication phase. *(From Veir JK, Lappin MR: Molecular diagnostic assays for infectious diseases in cats,* Vet Clin North Am Small Anim Pract *40:1189, 2010.)*

FHV-1 is a common differential diagnosis for cats with clinical evidence of rhinitis, stomatitis, conjunctivitis, keratitis, and facial dermatitis. Because of widespread exposure and vaccination, the positive predictive value of serologic tests is poor. FHV-1 can be documented by direct fluorescent staining of conjunctival scrapings, virus isolation, or PCR. FHV-1 DNA can be amplified from conjunctiva, nasal discharges, and pharynx of healthy cats, and so, the positive predictive value of conventional PCR assays is low.[34] Currently used PCR assays also detect vaccine strains of FHV-1, further lessening the positive predictive value of the assays.[21] In one study in our laboratory, presence of FHV-1 DNA failed to correlate with the presence or absence of stomatitis in cats.[26] Quantitative PCR may ultimately prove to correlate with the presence or absence of disease, but it failed to correlate with the presence of conjunctivitis in one study.[20] The negative predictive value of FHV-1 PCR assays is also in question, because many cats that are likely to have FHV-1 associated disease are negative. This may relate to clearance of FHV-1 DNA from tissues by a hypersensitivity reaction. Tissue biopsies have greater sensitivity than conjunctival swabs but do not necessarily have greater predictive value. FHV-1 DNA can be amplified from aqueous humor of some cats, but whether this indicates FHV-1 associated uveitis is unknown.[22]

Mycoplasma spp., *Chlamydophila felis*, and *Bordetella bronchiseptica* are other common respiratory pathogens in cats. As for FHV-1 and FCV, PCR-positive test results for these organisms cannot be used to distinguish a carrier from a clinically ill cat. However, in one recent study, *Mycoplasma* spp. DNA was amplified from conjunctival swabs from more kittens with conjunctivitis than control cats in the same shelters, suggesting the organism can be pathogenic in some cats.[36] In addition, PCR assays do not provide antimicrobial drug susceptibility testing, and so, for cats with potential bordetellosis, culture and sensitivity is the optimal diagnostic technique, especially if an outbreak is occurring. *Toxoplasma gondii* DNA has been amplified from airway washings of some cats with lower respiratory tract disease, and so, PCR is an option for evaluation of samples from diseased animals from which the organism is not identified cytologically.

Gastrointestinal Agents

The diagnosis of *Giardia* spp. infection is generally made with the combination of fecal flotation techniques and wet mount examination. Fecal antigen tests are also accurate, and there are several assays available for point-of-care use, including one labeled for veterinary use. Fecal PCR assays are often falsely negative because of PCR inhibitors in stool, and so, PCR should not be used as a screening procedure for this agent. However, *Giardia* spp. PCR can be used to determine whether the infective species is a zoonotic assemblage, which is the primary indication for this technique. However, it now appears that assemblage determination should be performed on more than one gene for most accurate results.[30]

Although *Cryptosporidium* spp. infection is common, it is unusual to find *C. felis* oocysts after fecal flotation in cats. Acid-fast staining of a thin fecal smear is cumbersome and insensitive. Antigen assays titrated for use with human feces are inaccurate when used with cat feces. Thus PCR may be aid in the diagnosis of cryptosporidiosis in dogs and cats and has been shown to be more sensitive than immunofluorescence assay (IFA) in cats.[31] *Cryptosporidium* spp. PCR assays are indicated in IFA-negative cats with unexplained small bowel diarrhea and when the genotype of *Cryptosporidium* is to be determined. However, *C. felis* infection in cats is common, and so, positive tests results do not always prove that the agent is the cause of the clinical disease. No drug is known to eliminate *Cryptosporidium* spp. infections, and small animal strains are not considered significant zoonotic agents; so, PCR is never indicated in healthy animals.

PCR assays are also available for detection of DNA of *Tritrichomonas foetus*, *Salmonella* spp., *Campylobacter* spp., *Clostridium* spp., parvoviruses, and *T. gondii*, and a RT-PCR assay is available for coronaviruses. Trophozoites of *T. foetus* can often be detected on wet mount examination of fresh feces, which can be completed as an in-clinic test. PCR for *T. foetus* DNA is indicated if wet mount examination is negative and results return more quickly than culture. However, DNA of *T. foetus* can be detected in healthy carrier cats, and so, positive results do not always prove illness from the organism.[8] Cases with suspected salmonellosis or campylobacteriosis should be cultured rather than assessed by PCR to determine the anti-microbial susceptibility patterns. In dogs, the PPV of *Clostridium* spp. PCR assays on feces is low and, if used, should be combined with enterotoxin assays. Information in cats is currently lacking. There is no current evidence that parvovirus PCR on feces is superior to currently available antigen assays. It was recently shown that cats vaccinated with modified live panleukopenia–containing vaccines shed parvovirus DNA in feces within several hours.[7] Thus parvovirus PCR testing should not be used to diagnose panleukopenia virus outbreaks in recently vaccinated cats. *Toxoplasma gondii* is only shed for about 7 to 10 days, and millions of oocysts are generally shed during this time, making the organism very easy to identify. Thus PCR assays are usually not needed to diagnosis this infection. Because virus isolation is not practical clinically, RT-PCR is used most frequently to detect coronavirus RNA in feces. However, positive test results do not differentiate FIP-inducing strains from enteric coronaviruses. Additionally, in one study, presence of coronavirus RNA did not correlate to the presence of diarrhea in shelter cats.[7]

Bloodborne Agents

Mycoplasma haemofelis (Mhf), "*Candidatus* Mycoplasma haemominutum" (Mhm), and "*Candidatus* M. turicensis" (Mtc) all can be found in cats. In experimentally infected cats, Mhf is apparently more pathogenic than Mhm. It appears that Mtc has intermediate pathogenicity. Diagnosis is based on demonstration of the organism on the surface of erythrocytes on examination of a thin blood film or PCR assay. Organism numbers fluctuate, and so, blood film examination can be falsely negative up to 50% of the time. The organism may be difficult to find cytologically, particularly in the chronic phase. Thus PCR assays are the tests of choice because of sensitivity.[13] Primers are available that can amplify all three hemoplasmas. Real-time PCR assays can be used to monitor copy numbers during and after treatment but do not have greater sensitivity, specificity, or predictive value than conventional PCR assays.[32] PCR assays should be considered in the evaluation of cats with unexplained fever or anemia that are cytologically negative. In addition, the American College of Veterinary Internal Medicine (ACVIM) recommends screening cats for use as blood donors by PCR assays for hemoplasmas.[35] Many cats (approximately 15%) are carriers of the relatively nonpathogenic *Candidatus* M. haemominutum, and so, positive test results may not always correlate with the presence of disease (poor PPV).

Cats can be infected by *E. canis*-like organism[2] and *Anaplasma phagocytophilum*.[15] Little is known about the other agents in these genera regarding cats. Because the organisms are in different genera, serologic cross reactivity is variable. Thus although the clinical syndromes can be similar, there is no one serologic test to document infection, and there is currently no standardized serology for cats. In addition, some cats with *E. canis* infection do not seroconvert, and so, PCR assay is superior to serology in cats. PCR assays can be designed to amplify each organism. Alternatively, primers are available to amplify all of the organisms in a single reaction, and then sequencing can be used to determine the infective species. However, positive test results do not always correlate with the presence of disease. *Anaplasma phagocytophilum* DNA has been amplified from the blood of healthy cats for more than 10 weeks after experimental infection by exposure to *Ixodes* ticks (MR Lappin, unpublished data, 2011).

Cats can be infected by *Rickettsia felis* and have been shown to have antibodies against *R. rickettsii*. Fever, headache, myalgia, and macular rash in humans have been attributed to *R. felis* infection in several countries around the world. In recent study in our laboratory, we assayed 92 pairs of cat blood and flea extracts from Alabama, Maryland, and Texas, using PCR assays that amplify a region of the citrate synthase gene *(gltA)* and the outer membrane protein B gene *(ompB)*. Of the 92 pairs, 62 of 92 (67.4%) flea extracts and none of the cat blood samples were positive for *R. felis* DNA.[11] In another study, we showed *R. felis* and *R. rickettsii* antibody prevalence rates in cats with fever to be 5.6% and 6.6%, respectively, but neither organism was amplified from blood.[1] These results prove that cats are sometimes exposed, but further data are needed to determine the significance of disease associations. Whether *Rickettsia* spp. PCR assays are indicated for use in cats at this time is unknown.

Blood culture, PCR assay on blood, and serologic testing can be used to assess individual cats for *Bartonella* spp. infection.[3] Cats that are culture negative or PCR negative and antibody negative, and cats that are culture negative or PCR negative and antibody positive, are probably not a source of flea, cat, or human infection. However, bacteremia can be intermittent, and false-negative culture or PCR results can occur, limiting the predictive value of a single battery of tests.[17] Although serologic testing can be used to determine whether an individual cat has been exposed, both seropositive and seronegative cats can be bacteremic, limiting the diagnostic utility of serologic testing. Thus testing healthy cats for *Bartonella* species infection is not currently recommended.[3,14] Testing should be reserved for cats with suspected clinical bartonellosis. Because *Bartonella* spp. infection is so common in healthy cats, even culture-positive or PCR-positive results do not prove clinical bartonellosis. For example, although we detected *Bartonella* spp. DNA in more cats with fever than in pair-matched cats without fever, the healthy cats were still commonly positive.[16] Combined serology with PCR in evaluation of cats with suspected bartonellosis is likely to give the best predictive value.

Cytauxzoon felis is usually easily identified on cytologic examination of blood smears or splenic aspirates during evaluation of clinically ill cats. Serologic testing is not commercially available at this time. PCR can be used to amplify organism DNA from blood from cats that are cytologically negative.[9]

Antibodies against feline immunodeficiency virus (FIV) are detected in serum in clinical practice most frequently by enzyme-linked immunosorbent assay (ELISA). Comparisons among different tests have shown the results of most assays are comparable.[10] Results of virus isolation or RT-PCR on blood are positive in some antibody-negative cats. False-positive reactions can occur using ELISA; hence, positive ELISA results in healthy or low-risk cats should be confirmed using Western blot immunoassay. Kittens can have detectable, colostrum-derived antibodies for several months. If antibodies persist at 6 months of age, the kitten is likely infected. Virus isolation or RT-PCR on blood can also be performed to confirm infection. However, FIV is not present in the blood at high levels, and so, false-negative results are common. In addition, there are variable results among laboratories.[6]

Most cats with feline leukemia virus infection are viremic, and so, molecular diagnostic assays are not usually needed in clinical practice. However, use of newer sensitive real-time PCR assays has been used to accurately characterize the stages of infection.[19] However, these assays are not commonly available commercially.

RNA of both FIPV and FECV can be amplified from the blood of cats, and so, positive test results do not always correlate with the development of FIP. Amplification of the mRNA of the *M* gene by RT-PCR had mixed results in two studies performed to date. In the one study, 13 of 26 apparently normal cats were positive for FECV mRNA in blood, suggesting that the positive predictive value of this assay for the diagnosis of FIP was low.[5]

Ocular Agents

Toxoplasma gondii, *Bartonella* spp., FHV-1 and coronavirus are the organisms for which DNA or RNA has been amplified most frequently from the aqueous humor of cats with endogenous uveitis.[22,25] Although little is known about the predictive value of these assays when used with aqueous humor, the combination of molecular assays with local antibody production indices may aid in the diagnosis of some cases.

References

1. Bayliss DB, Morris AK, Horta MC et al: Prevalence of *Rickettsia* species antibodies and *Rickettsia* species DNA in the blood of cats with and without fever, *J Feline Med Surg* 11:266, 2009.
2. Breitschwerdt EB, Abrams-Ogg ACG, Lappin MR et al: Molecular evidence supporting *Ehrlichia canis*-like infection in cats, *J Vet Intern Med* 16:642, 2002.
3. Brunt J, Guptill L, Kordick DL et al: American Association of Feline Practitioners 2006 Panel report on diagnosis, treatment, and prevention of *Bartonella* spp. infections, *J Feline Med Surg* 8:213, 2006.
4. Bustin SA, Benes V, Garson JA et al: The MIQE guidelines: minimum information for publication of quantitative real-time PCR experiments, *Clin Chem* 55:611, 2009.
5. Can-Sahna K, Soydal Ataseven V, Pinar D et al: The detection of feline coronaviruses in blood samples from cats by mRNA RT-PCR, *J Feline Med Surg* 9:369, 2007.
6. Crawford P, Slater M, Levy J: Accuracy of polymerase chain reaction assays for diagnosis of feline immunodeficiency virus infection in cats, *J Am Vet Med Assoc* 226:1503, 2005.
7. Gingrich E, Scorza A, Leutenegger C et al: Common enteric pathogens in cats before and after placement in an animal shelter [poster], *J Vet Intern Med* 24:766, 2010.
8. Gookin JL, Stebbins ME, Hunt E et al: Prevalence of and risk factors for feline *Tritrichomonas foetus* and *Giardia* infection, *J Clin Microbiol* 42:2707, 2004.
9. Haber MD, Tucker MD, Marr HS et al: The detection of *Cytauxzoon felis* in apparently healthy free-roaming cats in the USA, *Vet parasitol* 146:316, 2007.
10. Hartmann K, Griessmayr P, Schulz B et al: Quality of different in-clinic test systems for feline immunodeficiency virus and feline leukaemia virus infection, *J Feline Med Surg* 9:439, 2007.
11. Hawley JR, Shaw SE, Lappin MR: Prevalence of *Rickettsia felis* DNA in the blood of cats and their fleas in the United States, *J Feline Med Surg* 9:258, 2007.
12. Higuchi R, Dollinger G, Walsh PS et al: Simultaneous amplification and detection of specific DNA sequences, *Biotechnology (N Y)* 10:413, 1992.
13. Jensen W, Lappin M, Kamkar S et al: Use of a polymerase chain reaction assay to detect and differentiate two strains of *Haemobartonella felis* in naturally infected cats, *Am J Vet Res* 62:604, 2001.
14. Kaplan JE, Benson C, Holmes KK et al: Guidelines for prevention and treatment of opportunistic infections in HIV-infected adults and adolescents, *MMWR Recomm Rep* 58:1, 2009.
15. Lappin M, Breitschwerdt E, Jensen W et al: Molecular and serologic evidence of *Anaplasma phagocytophilum* infection in cats in North America, *J Am Vet Med Assoc* 225:893, 2004.
16. Lappin MR, Breitschwerdt EB, Brewer M et al: Prevalence of *Bartonella* species antibodies and *Bartonella* species DNA in the blood of cats with and without fever, *J Feline Med Surg* 11:141, 2009.
17. Lappin MR, Hawley J: Presence of *Bartonella* species and *Rickettsia* species DNA in the blood, oral cavity, skin and claw beds of cats in the United States, *Vet Dermatol* 20:509, 2009.
18. Lau A, Chen S, Sorrell T et al: Development and clinical application of a panfungal PCR assay to detect and identify fungal DNA in tissue specimens, *J Clin Microbiol* 45:380, 2007.
19. Levy J, Crawford C, Hartmann K et al: 2008 American Association of Feline Practitioners' feline retrovirus management guidelines, *J Feline Med Surg* 10:300, 2008.
20. Low HC, Powell CC, Veir JK et al: Prevalence of feline herpesvirus 1, *Chlamydophila felis*, and *Mycoplasma* spp DNA in conjunctival cells collected from cats with and without conjunctivitis, *Am J Vet Res* 68:643, 2007.
21. Maggs D, Clarke H: Relative sensitivity of polymerase chain reaction assays used for detection of feline herpesvirus type 1 DNA in clinical samples and commercial vaccines, *Am J Vet Res* 66:1550, 2005.
22. Maggs D, Lappin M, Nasisse M: Detection of feline herpesvirus-specific antibodies and DNA in aqueous humor from cats with or without uveitis, *Am J Vet Res* 60:932, 1999.
23. Mapes S, Rhodes DM, Wilson WD et al: Comparison of five real-time PCR assays for detecting virulence genes in isolates of *Escherichia coli* from septicaemic neonatal foals, *Vet Rec* 161:716, 2007.
24. Pedersen N, Sato R, Foley J et al: Common virus infections in cats, before and after being placed in shelters, with emphasis on feline enteric coronavirus, *J Feline Med Surg* 6:83, 2004.
25. Powell CC, McInnis CL, Fontenelle JP et al: *Bartonella* species, feline herpesvirus-1, and *Toxoplasma gondii* PCR assay results from blood and aqueous humor samples from 104 cats with naturally occurring endogenous uveitis, *J Feline Med Surg* 12:923, 2010.
26. Quimby JM, Elston T, Hawley J et al: Evaluation of the association of *Bartonella* species, feline herpesvirus 1, feline calicivirus, feline leukemia virus and feline immunodeficiency virus with chronic feline gingivostomatitis, *J Feline Med Surg* 10:66, 2008.
27. Ruch-Gallie RA, Veir JK, Hawley JR et al: Results of molecular diagnostic assays targeting feline herpesvirus-1 and feline calicivirus in adult cats administered modified live vaccines, *J Feline Med Surg*, in press. Epub March 23, 2011.
28. Saiki RK, Scharf S, Faloona F et al: Enzymatic amplification of beta-globin genomic sequences and restriction site analysis for diagnosis of sickle cell anemia, *Science* 230:1350, 1985.
29. Schabereiter-Gurtner C, Nehr M, Apfalter P et al: Evaluation of a protocol for molecular broad-range diagnosis of culture-negative bacterial infections in clinical routine diagnosis, *J Appl Microbiol* 104:1228, 2008.
30. Scorza A, Lappin M, Ballweber L: Genotyping of *Giardia duodenalis* isolates of mammals (dogs, cats, bobcats and cattle) by the β-giardin, glutamate dehydrogenase and triose phosphate isomerase genes [poster], *Third International Giardia and Cryptosporidium Conference*, Orvieto, Italy, 2009.
31. Scorza AV, Brewer MM, Lappin MR: Polymerase chain reaction for the detection of *Cryptosporidium* spp. in cat feces, *J Parasitol* 89:423, 2003.
32. Tasker S, Helps CR, Day MJ et al: Use of a Taqman PCR to determine the response of *Mycoplasma haemofelis* infection to antibiotic treatment, *J Microbiol Methods* 56:63, 2004.
33. Veir JK, Lappin MR: Molecular diagnostic assays for infectious diseases in cats, *Vet Clin North Am Small Anim Pract* 40:1189, 2010.

34. Veir JK, Ruch-Gallie R, Spindel ME et al: Prevalence of selected infectious organisms and comparison of two anatomic sampling sites in shelter cats with upper respiratory tract disease, *J Feline Med Surg* 10:551, 2008.
35. Wardrop K, Reine N, Birkenheuer A et al: Canine and feline blood donor screening for infectious diseases, *J Vet Intern Med* 19:135, 2005.
36. Zirofsky D, Powell CC, Reckers W et al: Feline herpesvirus-1 and *Mycoplasma* spp. infections in cats with acute conjunctivitis in an animal shelter (abstract), *J Vet Intern Med* 24:705, 2010.

CHAPTER

34

Feline Zoonotic Diseases and Prevention of Transmission

Marcy J. Souza and John C. New, Jr.

OUTLINE

Zoonoses are estimated to make up approximately 75% of today's emerging infectious diseases. These infectious agents can be transmitted by many different animals, including wildlife, exotic pets, and even traditional pets, such as dogs and cats. Recent studies have shown that cats, both healthy and with diarrhea, can shed zoonotic organisms in their feces. Between 13% and 40% of the cats examined were shedding at least one zoonotic, enteric pathogen.[18,36] Although the prevalence of shedding was variable for the specific pathogens, numerous organisms, including *Toxocara cati, Giardia, Cryptosporidium, Salmonella,* and *Campylobacter* were identified. This chapter will highlight transmission routes of zoonotic diseases that are commonly associated with domestic cats and what steps can be taken to reduce exposure and transmission (Box 34-1). Additional zoonotic infections are rarely associated with cats (Table 34-1), and more information on these can be found in the American Association of Feline Practitioners 2003 Report on Feline Zoonoses.[6]

CAT BITES

Although dog bites account for approximately 80% of reported animal bites, cats are the second most common animal reported to cause bites.[32] Because cats typically cause puncture wounds when biting, introduction of bacteria deeply into the tissues of the wound is common. Infection rates for cat bites have been reported to range from 30% to 50%, while infection of wounds resulting from dog bites is reportedly lower, 2% to 4%. *Pasteurella multocida* is the most common bacteria isolated from wounds resulting from cat bites and can cause sepsis, meningitis, and septic arthritis among other complications. Cat bites to the hands often require extensive treatment and are more likely than dog bites to result in complications, such as cellulitis, osteomyelitis, and tenosynovitis.[32]

Prevention of cat bites can often be achieved by understanding feline behavior, using sedation in fractious cats when appropriate, and wearing thick gloves, such as those worn by welders, to prevent penetration of teeth into hands or forearms. Despite these efforts, cat bites will still occur and should be treated as soon as possible. Delaying treatment is a risk factor for infection and other complications. Pain, swelling, erythema, and swelling of local lymph nodes can occur within 1 to 2 hours of a cat bite. Wound care is essential, and the use of prophylactic antibiotics is still controversial. However, one study that examined a small number of humans who had been bitten by cats found that 67% of those not treated with antibiotics developed infection, while 0% of those treated with antibiotics developed infection.[14] Additionally, postexposure prophylaxis for rabies virus may be indicated, depending on the vaccination history

BOX 34-1

Precautions to Reduce the Risk of Contracting a Zoonotic Disease from a Domestic Cat[12]

- Wash hands after handling cats and before eating.
- Annual checkups and fecal exams should be performed for all cats.
- Rabies vaccinations should be kept current.
- Flea and tick control should be performed.
- Do not allow a cat to lick your face, food utensils, or plate.
- Keep cats indoors.
- Seek medical attention for cat bites.
- Cats should be fed cooked or commercially processed food.
- Fecal material should be removed from litter boxes daily.
- Dispose of fecal material in a location where water supplies will not be contaminated.
- Clean litter boxes periodically with scalding water and detergent.
- Avoid handling unfamiliar cats, especially those that appear sick.
- Do not allow cats to drink from the toilet.
- Have the cat's claws trimmed frequently, or consider the use of soft nail caps.
- Never tease or provoke cats.

of the cat and the circumstances of the bite. The victim's history of tetanus prophylaxis should also be reviewed. Treatment for cat bites will vary from case to case, but all should include aggressive and careful wound care (e.g., cleaning, irrigation and débridement when necessary) and measures to prevent infection with bacteria, such as *Pasteurella multocida* or rabies virus.

BACTERIAL ZOONOSES

Bartonella henselae is the most common etiologic agent of cat scratch disease (CSD), but other *Bartonella* spp. have been found in cats, including *B. clarridgeiae, B. koehlerae*, and *B. weissii*.[6] Seroprevalence among domestic cats in the United States can vary but has been reported to be as high as 81%.[6] Young cats are more commonly bacteremic, and most human cases are associated with kitten exposure. Fleas will feed on bacteremic cats, and the bacteria can then replicate in the gut of fleas and survive in flea feces for days. Human infection occurs after the bite or scratch of a cat, which allows introduction of the bacteria into the skin and subcutaneous tissue (Figure 34-1).[11] The bacteria are typically found in flea feces located on the cat (under the claws, in the mouth). Cat scratch disease is usually self-limiting in immune-competent individuals but can

TABLE 34-1 Other Less Common Zoonoses Associated with Cats

Organism	Feline Clinical Signs	Human Symptoms	Route of Infection for Human	Relative Risk of Infection for Humans
Bordetella spp.	Subclinical, upper respiratory, pneumonia (rare)	Pneumonia in immunosuppressed patients	Aerosolization	Extremely rare
Capnocytophaga canimorsus	Subclinical	Bacteremia, keratitis	Bite wounds, possibly scratches	Extremely rare
Cheyletiella	Pruritic skin disease	Pruritic skin disease	Direct contact	Occasional
Coxiella burnetii (agent of Q fever)	Subclinical, abortion, stillbirth	Fever, pneumonitis, myalgia, lymphadenopathy, arthritis, hepatitis, endocarditis	Contact with infected tissues (placenta, birthing fluids)	Extremely rare
Francisella tularensis (agent of tularemia or rabbit fever)	Septicemia, pneumonia	Ulceroglandular, glandular, oculoglandular, pneumonic, typhoidal depending on route of exposure	Bite wounds	Rare
Mycoplasma felis	Chronic draining tracts, polyarthritis	Cellulitis, polyarthritis	Bite wound	Extremely rare
Sporothrix schenckii	Chronic draining of cutaneous tracts	Chronic draining of cutaneous tracts	Potentially contact with exudates from feline wounds	Rare

Modified from Table 1, p. 938 in Brown RR, Elston TH, Evans L et al: American Association of Feline Practitioners 2003 report on feline zoonoses, *Comp Contin Edu Pract Vet* 25:936, 2003.

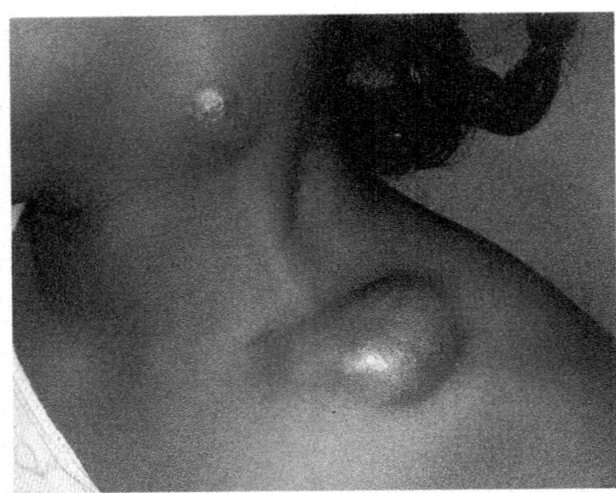

FIGURE 34-1 Bartonellosis. Papular lesion and enlarged lymph node in the supraclavicular area and neck of a girl that frequently cuddled her kitten over her chest and shoulder. *(From Rabinowitz P, Conti L: Human-animal medicine: clinical approaches to zoonoses, St Louis, 2010, Saunders Elsevier.)*

lead to atypical and serious consequences in immune-suppressed individuals, including bacillary angiomatosis and bacillary peliosis.[16] CSD can most effectively be prevented by maintaining good flea and tick prevention in cats and encouraging gentle play that does not involve the owner's hands or feet to reduce biting and scratching, especially with kittens. Nails can also be kept trimmed to reduce the likelihood of skin penetration. Additionally, immune-compromised individuals who want to obtain a cat should be encouraged to adopt an adult cat, because they are less likely to be bacteremic.

Yersinia pestis causes plague and can lead to different forms of clinical disease in humans and cats, including bubonic, bacteremic, and pneumonic plague. Plague must be treated with antibiotics or the infection can be rapidly fatal. Human plague is typically associated with exposure to wild rodent fleas; however, exposure to domestic cats can also be a risk factor.[11,17] A study that examined human cases of plague in the western United States found that approximately 8% of the reported cases were attributable to contact with domestic cats.[17] Exposure occurred through bites, scratches, or other contact with infected cats. Feline and human exposure to *Y. pestis*, especially in the western United States where plague is endemic, can be reduced by maintaining good flea and tick prevention, keeping cats indoors to reduce exposure to prey species, such as rodents (and associated fleas), and encouraging gentle play.

Methicillin-resistant *Staphylococcus aureus* (MRSA) is an increasing problem and concern in human medicine, and the role of domestic animals in transmission is increasingly being examined.[30] Many studies have focused on canine carriage of or infection with MRSA,[24,28] but studies have also identified MRSA in domestic cats.[29,33,37,38] Although no definitive evidence of transmission of MRSA from a cat to a human is available, reports of identical isolates in humans and their pets suggest that transmission between species is likely.[15,33] Cats likely acquire MRSA from interactions with humans, and a recent study examined risk factors associated with MRSA infections in dogs and cats.[34] Dogs and cats with methicillin-sensitive *Staphylococcus aureus* (MSSA) infections were used as unmatched controls for the MRSA cases. The study found that risk factors associated with MRSA infections included number of courses of antibiotics received, number of days admitted to a veterinary clinic, and having received a surgical implant. Of the 197 animals in the study, only 64 were cats (29 MRSA cases, 34 MSSA controls), and data from dogs and cats were combined for analysis. Further research is needed to determine what risk factors might specifically be associated with MRSA infection in cats. Cats can potentially spread MRSA to humans in home or nursing care settings, although the risk is still likely much less than obtaining infection from other humans. Disposable gloves should be worn when possible, but thorough hand washing has been shown to be the most effective method to prevent the spread of MRSA.[3] Fomites and environmental surfaces are not typically associated with the transmission of MRSA and routine cleaning and decontamination is sufficient. Additionally, appropriate screening (culture and sensitivity) of clinical patients, both feline and human, can reduce the transmission of MRSA.

Historically, numerous texts have cited *Chlamydophila felis* as a zoonotic pathogen. Little evidence has been published to support this claim. A recent review of the literature found only seven cases of human disease associated with *C. felis*.[7] Of those seven cases, only one was definitively diagnosed to be caused by *C. felis*. The human patient had chronic conjunctivitis and was immune-suppressed. Based on the prevalence of *C. felis* infections in cats, particularly kittens, risk of disease in humans is low. Precautions to limit exposure to cats with respiratory and ocular infections should be taken for individuals that are immune-compromised.

Although group A *Streptococcus* has been implicated as zoonoses transmitted from a dog, no literature is available confirming the spread of this bacteria from a cat to a human.[27] Transmission of group A *Streptococcus* from a cat to a human is likely extremely rare.[6] Exposure to other, less common zoonotic bacteria, such as *Salmonella* spp., *Yersinia enterocolitica*, *Helicobacter* spp., and *Campylobacter* spp. can be reduced by

1. Using general hygiene precautions when dealing with feces
2. Wearing disposable gloves when handling feces or litter
3. Washing hands thoroughly with soap and water after handling substances (e.g., litter, newspapers, carriers) that are contaminated with feces

These bacteria are most commonly associated with gastrointestinal illness in humans.[6,11]

VIRAL ZOONOSES

Rabies virus causes invariably fatal encephalitis in mammals when left untreated. Although human rabies exposure in the United States is most commonly associated with bats, domestic cats were the most common nonwildlife species identified with rabies in 2007 and 2008.[4,5] This increased frequency of infection in cats versus other domestic animals is likely caused by spillover of raccoon variant rabies, a lack of enforcement of vaccination and leash laws in cats, and the presence of free-roaming cats. The virus is present in saliva and neural tissue of infected animals, and exposure occurs after an infected animal bites another mammal. Prevention of human rabies exposure from cats can be achieved by vaccinating all cats according to guidelines developed by the National Association of State Public Health Veterinarians,[31] keeping cats indoors to reduce exposure to free-roaming cats and wildlife, and by following appropriate post-exposure procedures as outlined by the Centers for Disease Control (CDC).[26] Briefly, individuals who have received vaccination prior to being bitten should receive two vaccinations on days 0 and 3, but NOT receive rabies immunoglobulin (RIG). Individuals who have not received vaccination prior to being bitten should receive vaccinations on days 0, 3, 7, and 14 and should receive RIG.[9] In addition, all bite wounds should be treated appropriately to prevent bacterial infections.

Felids are considered fairly resistant to influenza type A viruses, but infection with both the avian influenza virus (H5N1) and the pandemic influenza virus (H1N1) have been reported.[2,20,22,35] One study showed that infected cats could transmit the H5N1 virus to other cats.[22] Cats infected with the H5N1 virus likely contracted it from eating infected birds or contact with other infected cats. Cats infected with the H1N1 virus likely contracted it from humans. The ability of either influenza virus to be transmitted from cats to humans is unclear at this time. To prevent cross-species transmission, any human or cat with respiratory disease should be examined by medical personnel and have appropriate diagnostic tests performed. In addition, limiting exposure to infected cats and thorough washing of hands after handling will reduce the spread of the virus. The same precautions that will reduce the risk of spread of human strains from one human to another are also appropriate for preventing cross-species transmission.

Other viral infections of cats, such as feline leukemia virus (FeLV) and feline immunodeficiency virus (FIV), are not zoonotic. In one study of 204 veterinarians and other occupationally exposed individuals, no serologic or molecular evidence of zoonosis with FeLV or FIV was detected.[8] However, cats infected with either of these viruses may be more likely to be infected with and spread other zoonotic pathogens.

PARASITIC ZOONOSES

Toxoplasma gondii is estimated to infect approximately 60 million people in the United States, but most humans have few to no clinical symptoms related to infection.[11] Immune-compromised individuals are more likely to have clinical problems, including central neurologic and ophthalmic lesions, from infection. In addition, approximately 3,000 cases of congenital toxoplasmosis occur annually and can lead to hydrocephalus, mental retardation, convulsions, deafness, blindness, and cerebral palsy.[11] Felids are the definitive host for *Toxoplasma gondii* and *only* felids will shed oocysts in their feces.[19] All vertebrate animals can become infected by ingesting sporulated oocysts from the environment or by ingesting bradyzoites contained in raw or undercooked tissue from an infected animal. Most infections in adult humans occur after ingesting infected, improperly cooked meat. In addition, if a human or animal becomes infected while pregnant, the organism can cross the placenta and infect the fetus, leading to abortion or congenital toxoplasmosis. Pregnant women should not necessarily be advised to get rid of a pet cat. Numerous factors need to be considered, including the infection status of the woman, whether a cat is likely shedding oocysts, and the ability of the woman to avoid potential exposure by not cleaning the litter box. Fecal exams can be performed on felids to determine if oocysts are being shed; however, felids will typically only shed oocysts for approximately 1 to 3 weeks after initial infection.

Human infection can be prevented by

1. Making sure all meat products are cooked to the proper temperature
2. Drinking water from clean sources
3. Scooping cat litter boxes daily to prevent sporulation of oocysts shed in the feces (should not be done by pregnant women)
4. Disposing of cat feces in garbage that will go to landfills designed to not contaminate ground water (do not dispose of feces in toilet)
5. NOT composting cat feces, because oocysts can persist in the environment for extended periods of time and then persist in soil where compost is spread
6. Thoroughly washing hands after cleaning litter boxes
7. Keeping cats indoors to reduce the likelihood of becoming infected (if not already infected)

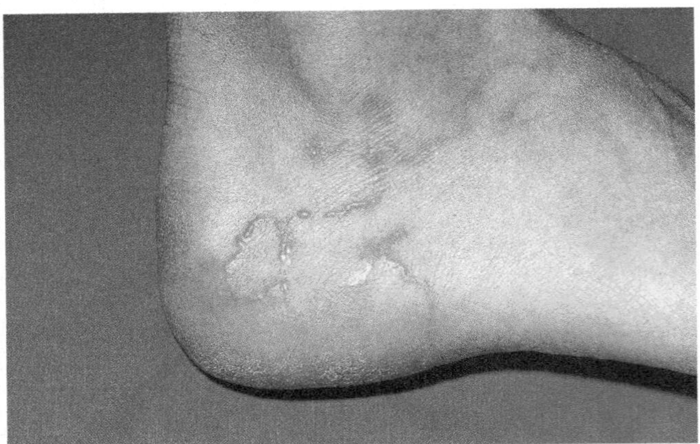

FIGURE 34-2 Cutaneous larval migrans on the foot. *(From Goldman L, Ausiello DA, editors:* Cecil textbook of medicine, *ed 23, Philadelphia, 2008, Saunders, Elsevier.)*

8. Feeding cats only cooked diets or commercially produced diets
9. Determining the infection status of a woman before she becomes pregnant[13]

Ascarids and hookworms commonly infect cats and can lead to visceral and cutaneous larval migrans in humans, respectively (Figure 34-2). *Toxocara cati* is the most common ascarid of cats. Large numbers of eggs are shed in the feces and can inadvertently be ingested by humans. After ingestion by a person, these eggs develop into larvae that can migrate anywhere in the body. Organs commonly affected include the eye, brain, liver, and lung.[10] Cats can also carry numerous types of hookworms, including *Ancylostoma braziliense* and *Ancylostoma tubaeforme*.[6] Larvated eggs of these worms are shed in the feces of infected cats and become free-living larvae in the environment. These larvae can then penetrate the skin of humans, leading to cutaneous larval migrans.[10] Zoonotic ascarid and hookworm infections can be prevented by

1. Administering anthelmintic treatment to cats in accordance with recommendations of the Companion Animal Parasite Council (http://www.capcvet.org)
2. Keeping cats indoors so they are less likely to become infected or shed eggs into the environment
3. Properly disposing of cat feces where they will not contaminate soil or water
4. Washing hands thoroughly after handling cats or cleaning litter boxes
5. Keeping children's sandboxes covered when not in use
6. Wearing shoes while walking outside, especially on beaches

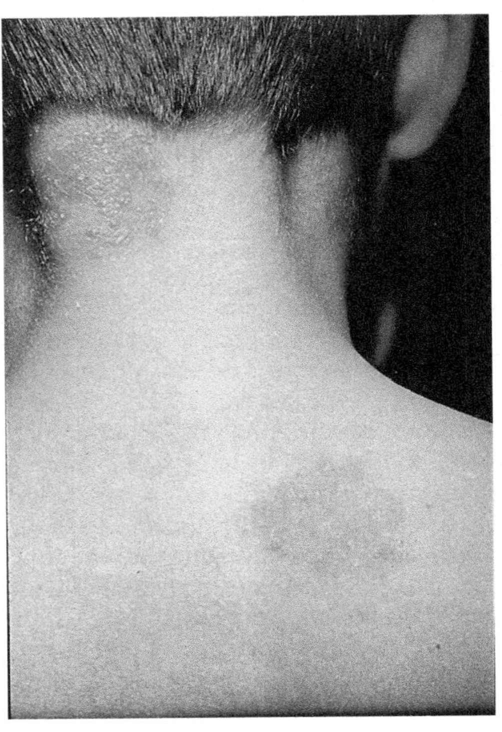

FIGURE 34-3 Tinea corporis caused by *Trichophyton mentagrophytes*. *(From Rabinowitz P, Conti L:* Human-animal medicine: clinical approaches to zoonoses, *St Louis, 2010, Saunders Elsevier.)*

Fleas are the most common ectoparasite of cats, and although fleas are unlikely to live on humans, they can bite, cause pruritus, as well as potentially transmit some serious infectious agents. In addition, fleas carry the tapeworm *Dipylidium caninum*, which has been reported to infect children.[6] Cats can also carry *Sarcoptes scabiei*, which leads to a self-limiting pruritus in humans.[11] Humans can become infected by either of these parasites by coming in contact with infected cats or a contaminated environment. Infection can be prevented by keeping cats indoors and maintaining appropriate flea and tick prevention.

Other parasites, including *Giardia* and *Cryptosporidium*, can be found in cat feces. Recent studies have found that 2% to 7% of cats surveyed were shedding *Giardia* or *Cryptosporidium*.[18,36] The prevalence of shedding is low, and when coupled with appropriate handling of feces, the risk of zoonotic infection should be limited.

FUNGAL ZOONOSES

Numerous dermatophytes can cause cutaneous lesions in both cats and humans, and *Microsporum canis* is likely the most common.[6] In most infected persons, infection typically manifests as red, pruritic, circular lesions at the site of infection; these infections are typically self-limiting (Figure 34-3).[6,11] Immunocompromised individuals may develop more severe infections. Exposure occurs after handling a cat that is carrying the organism on its fur or skin. Some cats may show typical lesions, including broken hair, alopecia, crusting, and scales, while other cats may be asymptomatic carriers (see Chapter 22). Risk factors for human infection include exposure to a kitten recently obtained from a shelter and a known history of infection, or exposure to pet cats that have extensive contact with other animals. In addition, children are more likely to become infected than adults.[6] The risk of infection can be reduced by appropriately treating infected cats, limiting contact with potentially infected cats, wearing gloves when handling potentially infected cats, and thoroughly washing hands after handling cats.

CAT OWNERSHIP FOR IMMUNE-COMPROMISED PERSONS

Interactions with animals can provide positive physical and psychological benefits whether they are pets, outreach animals, or residents of assisted care facilities. Any animal that will be in contact with elderly or immune-compromised individuals should be under the care of a veterinarian. A wellness program for the animal should be designed that takes into account the age, species, and risk factors for disease. The safety of both the animal and human must be taken into account. Wellness recommendations for animals in outreach programs or residents in assisted care facilities have been published and are also available from the American Veterinary Medical Association.[1,23] Cats should be at least six months of age before participating in outreach programs or living in assisted care facilities. Preventive medicine for these cats should include regular wellness exams, appropriate vaccinations, and parasite control. In addition, any animals displaying signs of illness, such as diarrhea, nasal discharge, or conjunctivitis, should not be allowed to interact with elderly or immune-compromised individuals.

Because elderly and immune-compromised individuals are particularly susceptible to zoonotic diseases, including toxoplasmosis and bartonellosis, specific precautions as outlined in Box 8-1 should be closely followed. If possible, litter boxes should not be scooped or cleaned by immune-compromised individuals. However, if cleaning the litter box is unavoidable, individuals should wear disposable gloves and thoroughly wash hands afterward. In addition, immune-compromised individuals should avoid contact with diarrhea from any animal and stool from stray animals or dogs and cats less than 6 months of age.[21] Pets that have diarrhea should be taken to a veterinarian and examined for *Cryptosporidium*, *Salmonella*, *Campylobacter*, and Shiga toxin–producing *E. coli*.[21] Hands should be thoroughly washed after handling any animal feces or any objects or surfaces contaminated by feces.

Elderly and immune-compromised individuals should not necessarily be advised to give up their cats.[21] If considering adoption, elderly and immune-compromised individuals should adopt healthy adult cats (more than 1 year of age) as determined by a veterinarian. Animals should not be adopted from facilities with unsanitary conditions, and cats should be treated for fleas before being adopted. Rough play with cats should be discouraged to decrease the risk of bites or transmission of *Bartonella* spp. In addition, keeping cats indoors will not only prevent exposure of the cat to zoonotic and other infectious diseases, but it will limit human exposure to zoonoses commonly carried by prey species, such as hantavirus and leptospirosis.

PUBLIC HEALTH CONSIDERATIONS

As described above, the role of cats as carriers of numerous zoonotic diseases is documented. Precautions for the individual cat owner have been described; however, the effect of free-roaming cat populations on public health is unclear. Parasitism is the most common infectious problem of free-roaming cats.[25] The deposition of feces into the environment leads to dissemination of infectious agents, including *Toxoplasma* and ascarids, which can potentially infect humans. Humans should avoid contact with free-roaming cats to reduce the risk of bites and exposure to zoonotic diseases, such as rabies and bartonellosis.

Veterinarians must play an active role in the reduction of free-roaming cat populations and disease prevalence in those populations.[39] Methods of population control can be controversial and include trap-neuter-return programs, capture and euthanasia programs, and capture and re-homing programs. Regardless of what program is used in a particular community, veterinarians should encourage owners to neuter their cats and keep them indoors. Additionally, persons should not feed free-roaming cat populations in order to reduce numbers, as well as to reduce the likelihood of humans being exposed to other animals that potentially carry zoonotic diseases. Raccoons, which can transmit rabies and *Baylisascaris procyonis* (the roundworm of raccoons), to humans, will readily eat cat food that is left outside. Although the impact of free-roaming cats on human health is unclear, efforts must be made to reduce populations in order to reduce the spread of infectious diseases to humans and cats, as well as to reduce predation on native wildlife species.

References

1. American Veterinary Medical Association: Wellness guidelines for animals in animal-assisted activity, animal-assisted therapy, and resident animal programs. Available at http://www.avma.org/products/hab/wellness.asp. Accessed May 1, 2010.

2. American Veterinary Medical Association: 2009 H1N1 flu virus outbreak. Available at http://www.avma.org/public_health/influenza/new_virus/default.asp. Accessed May 1, 2010.
3. Association for Professionals in Infection Control and Epidemiology Inc: Guidelines for the control of MRSA. Available http://goapic.org/mrsa.htm. Accessed May 1, 2010.
4. Blanton JD, Palmer D, Christian KA et al: Rabies surveillance in the United States during 2007, *J Am Vet Med Assoc* 233:884, 2008.
5. Blanton JD, Robertson K, Palmer D et al: Rabies surveillance in the United States during 2008, *J Am Vet Med Assoc* 235:676, 2009.
6. Brown RR, Elston TH, Evans L et al: American Association of Feline Practitioners 2003 report on feline zoonoses, *Comp Contin Edu Pract Vet* 25:936, 2003. Available at (http://www.catvets.com/professionals/guidelines/publications/?Id=181; Accessed May 1, 2010.
7. Browning GF: Is *Chlamydophila felis* a significant zoonotic pathogen? *Aust Vet J* 82:695, 2004.
8. Butera S, Brown J, Callahan M et al: Survey of veterinary conference attendees for evidence of zoonotic infection by feline retroviruses, *J Am Vet Med Assoc* 217:1475, 2000.
9. Centers for Disease Control: ACIP provisional recommendations for the prevention of human rabies. Available at http://www.cdc.gov/vaccines/recs/provisional/downloads/rabies-July2009-508.pdf. Accessed May 1, 2010.
10. Centers for Disease Control: Guidelines for veterinarians: prevention of zoonotic transmission of ascarids and hookworms of dogs and cats. Available at http://www.cdc.gov/ncidod/dpd/parasites/ascaris/prevention.htm. Accessed May 1, 2010.
11. Colville J, Berryhill D: *Handbook of zoonoses identification and prevention*, St Louis, 2007, Mosby Elsevier.
12. Cornell Feline Health Center: Zoonotic disease: what can I catch from my cat? Available at http://www.vet.cornell.edu/fhc/brochures/ZoonoticDisease.html. Accessed May 1, 2010.
13. Dabritz HA, Conrad PA: Cats and Toxoplasma: implications for public health, *Zoonoses Public Health* 57:34, 2010.
14. Elenbaas RM, McNabney WK, Robinson WA: Evaluation of prophylactic oxacillin in cat bite wounds, *Ann Emerg Med* 13:155, 1984.
15. Faires MC, Tater KC, Weese JS: An investigation of methicillin-resistant *Staphylococcus aureus* colonization in people and pets in the same household with an infected person or infected pet, *J Am Vet Med Assoc* 235:540, 2009.
16. Florin TA, Zaoutis TE, Zaoutis LB: Beyond cat scratch disease: widening spectrum of *Bartonella henselae* infection, *Pediatrics* 121:e1413, 2008.
17. Gage KL, Dennis DT, Orloski KA et al: Cases of cat-associated human plague in the Western US, 1977-1998, *Clin Infect Dis* 30:893, 2000.
18. Hill S, Cheney J, Taton-Allen G et al: Prevalence of enteric zoonotic organisms in cats, *J Amer Vet Med Assoc* 216:687, 2000.
19. Innes EA: A brief history and overview of *Toxoplasma gondii*, *Zoonoses Public Health* 57:1, 2010.
20. Iowa Department of Public Health: Protecting pets from illness. Available at http://www.idph.state.ia.us/IdphNews/Reader.aspx?id=8FBE90B3-4667-4960-9AF5-1B9B477A3805. Accessed May 1, 2010.
21. Kaplan JE, Benson C, Holmes KK et al: Guidelines for prevention and treatment of opportunistic infections in HIV-infected adults and adolescents, *MMWR Recomm Rep* 58:1, 2009.
22. Kuiken T, Rimmelzwaan G, van Riel D et al: Avian H5N1 influenza in cats, *Science* 306:241, 2004.
23. Lefebvre SL, Peregrine AS, Golab GC et al: A veterinary perspective on the recently published guidelines for animal-assisted interventions in health-care facilities, *J Am Vet Med Assoc* 233:394, 2008.
24. Lefebvre SL, Reid-Smith RJ, Waltner-Toews D et al: Incidence of acquisition of methicillin-resistant *Staphylococcus aureus*, *Clostridium difficile*, and other health-care-associated pathogens by dogs that participate in animal-assisted interventions, *J Am Vet Med Assoc* 234:1404, 2009.
25. Levy J, Crawford P: Humane strategies for controlling feral cat populations, *J Am Vet Med Assoc* 225:1354, 2004.
26. Manning SE, Rupprecht CE, Fishbein D et al: Human rabies prevention–United States, 2008: recommendations of the Advisory Committee on Immunization Practices, *MMWR Recomm Rep* 57:1, 2008.
27. Mayer G, Van Ore S: Recurrent pharyngitis in family of four. Household pet as reservoir of group A streptococci, *Postgrad Med* 74:277, 1983.
28. McLean CL, Ness MG: Meticillin-resistant *Staphylococcus aureus* in a veterinary orthopaedic referral hospital: staff nasal colonisation and incidence of clinical cases, *J Small Anim Pract* 49:170, 2008.
29. Middleton JR, Fales WH, Luby CD et al: Surveillance of *Staphylococcus aureus* in veterinary teaching hospitals, *J Clin Microbiol* 43:2916, 2005.
30. Morgan M: Methicillin-resistant *Staphylococcus aureus* and animals: zoonosis or humanosis? *J Antimicrob Chemother* 62:1181, 2008.
31. National Association of State Publich Health Veterinarians: Compendium of animal rabies prevention and control, 2008. Available at http://www.nasphv.org/Documents/Rabies Compendium.pdf. Accessed May 1, 2010.
32. Patronek GJ, Slavinski SA: Animal bites, *J Am Vet Med Assoc* 234:336, 2009.
33. Sing A, Tuschak C, Hormansdorfer S: Methicillin-resistant *Staphylococcus aureus* in a family and its pet cat, *N Engl J Med* 358:1200, 2008.
34. Soares Magalhaes RJ, Loeffler A, Lindsay J et al: Risk factors for methicillin-resistant *Staphylococcus aureas* (MRSA) infection in dogs and cats: a case-control study, *Vet Res* 41:55, 2010.
35. Songserm T, Amonsin A, Jam-on R et al: Avian influenza H5N1 in naturally infected domestic cat, *Emerg Infect Dis* 12:681, 2006.
36. Spain C, Scarlett J, Wade S et al: Prevalence of enteric zoonotic agents in cats less than 1 year old in central New York state, *J Vet Intern Med* 15:33, 2001.
37. Walther B, Wieler LH, Friedrich AW et al: Methicillin-resistant *Staphylococcus aureus* (MRSA) isolated from small and exotic animals at a university hospital during routine microbiological examinations, *Vet Microbiol* 127:171, 2008.
38. Weese JS, Faires M, Rousseau J et al: Cluster of methicillin-resistant *Staphylococcus aureus* colonization in a small animal intensive care unit, *J Am Vet Med Assoc* 231:1361, 2007.
39. Winter L: Trap-neuter-release programs: the reality and the impacts, *J Am Vet Med Assoc* 225:1369, 2004.

SECTION VI

MANAGING THE CAT WITH CONCURRENT AND CHRONIC DISEASES

Editor: Margie Scherk

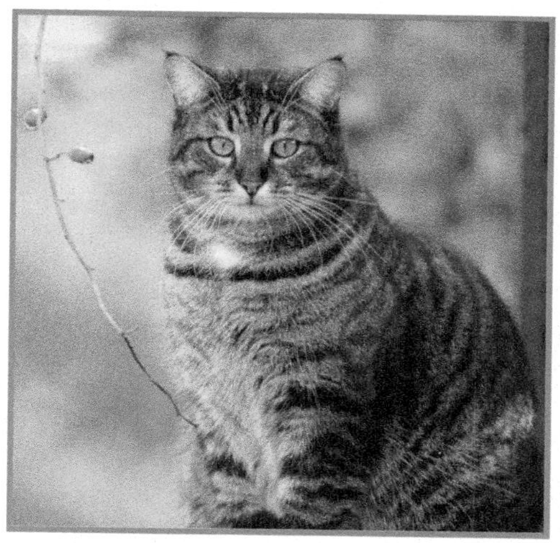

CHAPTER

35

Concurrent Disease Management

OUTLINE

HYPERTHYROIDISM AND CHRONIC KIDNEY DISEASE

Sarah Caney

The most common concurrent illness seen in association with hyperthyroidism is chronic kidney disease (CKD). Both illnesses are common in the older cat and the presence of CKD not only affects diagnosis of hyperthyroidism but also treatment and prognosis. Accurate assessment of patients is required to identify the concurrent problem and any associated complications that may require additional treatment. A more cautious approach to treatment is required to prevent destabilization of a vulnerable patient. With care, it is usually possible to manage both conditions successfully and provide the patient with a good quality and length of life.

Authors of a recent study reported that 14% of hyperthyroid cats had preexisting CKD on first assessment of thyroid disease.[167] Whether there is a causal relationship between hyperthyroidism and CKD or whether both conditions simply occur in concert is not known because they are both common conditions in the older individual. The relationship between these two conditions is complex. It has been postulated that hyperthyroidism causes damage to the kidneys, which may contribute toward long-term development of CKD through several mechanisms. These include tubulointerstitial damage, ultimately fibrosis, and chronic interstitial nephritis caused by an increase in angiotensin II. In addition, systemic hypertension present in a proportion of hyperthyroid cats may contribute to renal damage through microinfarction and subsequent fibrosis. This last effect is recognized in the micropuncture studies on the remnant kidney cat model.[157] Whether this occurs in hypertensive cats with naturally occurring CKD is unknown. However, it is also speculated that hyperthyroidism, in fact, merely masks a preexisting decline in renal function by increasing renal blood flow and hence glomerular filtration rate (GFR).

DIAGNOSTIC CHALLENGES

Evaluation of blood and urine samples is important in the assessment of both hyperthyroid and CKD patients. It not only is valuable in diagnosing these conditions but also in assessing severity and looking for the presence of additional illnesses. Unfortunately, in the case of cats with concurrent hyperthyroidism and CKD, interpretation of laboratory tests becomes especially challenging.

The presence of CKD can make diagnosis of hyperthyroidism problematic because of suppression of thyroid hormones—the so-called sick euthyroid syndrome. Therefore in cats with clinical signs compatible with hyperthyroidism, a normal total thyroxine (total T_4) should not be taken as evidence that the cat does not have this condition. Cats having both creatinine and total T_4 concentrations in the upper normal reference range are likely to have both hyperthyroidism and CKD.[238]

If a normal T_4 result is obtained in a cat suspected of being hyperthyroid, there are several options for further diagnosis. Repeating the same test on another occasion (for example, a few weeks later) can be helpful in those cases where the hyperthyroidism is mild, since fluctuation in levels of thyroxine can result in the total T_4 being intermittently within the reference range. Measurement of free T_4 by equilibrium dialysis is another option. This test is more sensitive in identifying hyperthyroid cats but carries a slightly higher risk of false-positive results (i.e., over diagnosing hyperthyroidism) so is not generally recommended as a screening test for hyperthyroidism.[182] A total T_4 greater than 30 nmol/L (greater than 2.33 μg/dL) in addition to a high free T_4 is supportive of a diagnosis of hyperthyroidism; conversely, if the total T_4 is less than 30 nmol/L (less than 2.33 μg/dL) the cat is extremely unlikely to have hyperthyroidism.[238] Where available, analysis of endogenous thyroid-stimulating hormone (TSH) can be helpful, with hyperthyroid cats having low levels.[238] Thyroid scintigraphy, triiodothyronine (T_3) suppression, and thyrotropin-releasing hormone (TRH) stimulation tests[226] can also be helpful in discriminating hyperthyroid from sick euthyroid patients. Unfortunately, all of these tests are affected by severity of concurrent disease, which can make interpretation of results difficult.

The presence of CKD can affect serum biochemistry and hematology results. Laboratory consequences of hyperthyroidism, such as erythrocytosis, occasionally seen in hyperthyroid cats, may be masked by anemia associated with CKD.

Identifying the presence and quantifying the severity of renal disease in a hyperthyroid cat is difficult. Assessment of kidney function currently depends upon measurement of blood urea and creatinine levels in association with urine specific gravity. Azotemia (elevated blood urea and/or blood creatinine) along with a reduced urine specific gravity are used to diagnose reduced renal function. However, concentrations of urea and creatinine can be affected by hyperthyroidism, and this complicates interpretation of serum chemistry results. Urea tends to be high in hyperthyroid cats as a consequence of polyphagia (and hence increased protein intake), and this may falsely increase the concern that a hyperthyroid cat has CKD. Conversely, creatinine concentrations tend to be misleadingly low, because hyperthyroid cats are thin and have very little muscle mass (creatinine being derived from muscle turnover). The increased GFR present in hyperthyroid cats also tends to reduce blood levels of both urea and creatinine.

Assessment of urine specific gravity is usually helpful to define renal function, but this too can be affected by hyperthyroidism. A healthy urine specific gravity (USG) is generally considered to be greater than 1.040, with concentrations less than 1.035 taken as one of the indications of kidney disease. However, in hyperthyroid cats, the ability to produce concentrated urine is compromised, and a USG less than this figure can be obtained from cats that have healthy kidneys. Additionally, this healthy value varies with the type of diet fed. Cats fed strictly dry food should concentrate urine to greater than 1.045, whereas a USG of greater than 1.025 may be appropriate in cats fed exclusively canned/moist food.[45]

Mild proteinuria is a common finding in hyperthyroid cats.[222] It is thought that the proteinuria may be present as a consequence of glomerular hypertension and hyperfiltration that is known to occur in the hyperthyroid state. The prognostic significance of proteinuria in hyperthyroidism is currently unknown, but it does tend to resolve with treatment, even in cats that develop azotemia.[222,224]

Both hyperthyroidism and CKD are conditions associated with a higher incidence of urinary tract infections. For example, one study showed that 12% of hyperthyroid cats suffered from urinary tract infections.[158] Unfortunately, most of these cats suffer from clinically silent urinary infections and may only show vague clinical signs, such as weight loss and lethargy. It is important to be suspicious of infection and culture the urine to identify and treat any of these additional problems, because it will benefit the cat's current and long-term prognosis.

TREATING CATS WITH CONCURRENT HYPERTHYROIDISM AND CHRONIC KIDNEY DISEASE

All treatments for hyperthyroidism have the potential to worsen kidney function.[58] This is because the hyperthyroid condition increases renal blood flow and GFR. When the hyperthyroidism is treated, the increased cardiac output and renal blood flow to the kidneys decreases. This results in a decrease in GFR by up to 50% of the pretreatment level.[11,16,83] For many hyperthyroid cats, this return to normality is not associated with kidney problems. However, in a proportion of patients, this reduction in blood flow has the potential to unmask kidney disease that was not previously recognized, allowing the preexisting kidney disease to manifest itself clinically. In those cats in which renal disease has been documented before treatment is started, treatment has the potential to worsen renal function and may precipitate a crisis. The reported frequency of this complication has varied in publications. In one report, one third of patients developed this complication following treatment with radioiodine, while other reports have found even higher numbers of cats experiencing a crisis after treatment.[58,212] Affected cats become azotemic and may start to show clinical signs of renal disease. Significant decreases in renal function are generally evident by 4 weeks posttreatment, after which time GFR stabilizes with very little deterioration, depending on the degree or stage of renal disease.[16,233,234]

A number of studies have shown that it is not possible to predict accurately which patients will reveal CKD following treatment of hyperthyroidism. These studies have evaluated pretreatment laboratory variables, such as serum biochemistry, USG, proteinuria, and hematology.[16,192,222,234] In general, no significant differences have been seen when comparing the pretreatment parameters in cats that did develop a posttreatment renal azotemia with those that did not. Although USG is reduced in cats with CKD, it also can be reduced as a consequence of hyperthyroidism, so analysis of this parameter alone is not sufficient to be helpful. Equally, although a pretreatment USG of greater than 1.035 is often reassuring, it cannot be viewed as a guarantee that the cat will not develop a posttreatment renal azotemia.[192] The fact that some cats with primary renal azotemia remain able to concentrate urine to 1.045 or greater complicates the interpretation further.[174]

GFR is reported to be of some value in predicting posttreatment renal azotemia.[2,234] One study reported some value in using a combination of pretreatment GFR, USG, and total T_4 in predicting which patients developed a posttreatment renal azotemia.[234] In the same study, there was a significant difference in pretreatment GFR and USG in those cats that eventually developed posttreatment renal azotemia. Unfortunately, assessment of GFR is not readily available in clinical practice, limiting its usefulness. Iohexol clearance has been evaluated and could be a clinically feasible tool; however, it has not become part of mainstream diagnostics.[11] The usefulness of other markers of renal function, such as the NAG index (urinary N-acetyl-beta-D-glucosaminidase to urinary creatinine ratio) and urinary retinol binding protein, are still being evaluated.[144,232]

For these reasons, most clinicians prefer to treat all hyperthyroid cats with medical management in the first instance. The main advantage of this approach is that it is reversible; in other words, if renal function deteriorates, the treatment for hyperthyroidism can be reduced or discontinued to help stabilize the patient. Medical treatment of hyperthyroidism induces euthyroidism more gradually than surgical thyroidectomy or radioiodine therapy, both of which may result in an acute destabilization of a patient. In cats in which renal function remains stable on medical treatment, permanent treatment of the hyperthyroidism can be considered with a greater degree of confidence. Although no definite guidelines exist, it is probably advisable to monitor patients on medical treatment for at least a few months, possibly as long as 6 months, before making a decision to elect for more permanent, curative treatments.

If a cat is known to have CKD before medical treatment for hyperthyroidism is started, it is probably advisable to start treatment with a lower dose of medication initially while monitoring the renal values closely. For example, if using methimazole, a starting dose of 1.25 to 5 mg every 24 hours should be considered. If any problems are seen, then the methimazole dose can be lowered or the treatment may be discontinued. If, conversely, medication is not associated with renal or other adverse effects, the dose can be titrated to induce and maintain euthyroidism. Frequent and regular re-evaluations are essential to facilitate optimal management of both CKD and hyperthyroidism. The author recommends initial assessment of renal parameters at 3 and 6 weeks following the start of treatment.[39]

Ongoing management of patients with both CKD and hyperthyroidism requires attention to both conditions. International Renal Interest Society (IRIS) guidelines (http://www.iris-kidney.com) should be followed with respect to staging and management of CKD and any complications present as a result of this. Where possible, attempts should be made to induce and maintain euthyroidism as discussed above. In those patients where euthyroidism is associated with a clinical and biochemical worsening of renal disease, it may be necessary to titrate therapy to achieve the best balance possible. The individual priorities of each patient need to be considered to determine which therapy and approach is most appropriate. For example, in some patients, suboptimal control of the hyperthyroidism may be tolerated clinically, whereas euthyroidism may be associated with severe renal dysfunction and a clinical crisis. Success of treatment should be gauged on clinical response to treatment as well as assessment of laboratory parameters. Accurate assessment of body weight and body condition score is vital in addition to a thorough history, general clinical examination, and blood pressure measurement. Fortunately, in many cats, it is possible to achieve a balance between these two conditions and gain a good treatment outcome.

HYPERTHYROIDISM AND DIABETES MELLITUS

Margarethe Hoenig

PREVALENCE

Hyperthyroidism in cats was virtually unknown until the late 1970s and is now the most common endocrine disease of cats and one of the most common diseases in older cats. Diabetes mellitus (DM) is also a commonly encountered endocrine problem in older cats, and its prevalence also has increased dramatically in the last three decades because of a large increase in the prevalence of obesity. According to Joslin (writing in 1934),[128] in people, "the subject of hyperthyroidism and diabetes, as a combination of diseases, is such a small one that it permits but little to be said about," even though diabetes not infrequently co-exists with hypothyroidism and hyperthyroidism in human patients. It is not known how frequently the two diseases co-exist in cats, but anecdotally, it is well known that they can occur concomitantly. There are, however, no epidemiologic or pathophysiologic data linking hyperthyroidism with diabetes, nor is an increase in fasting blood glucose a common feature of the hyperthyroid cat.

PATIENT SIGNALMENT AND RISK FACTORS

Although the increase in both diseases has occurred during the same time span, that is, the last 3 decades, it does not appear that identical factors are involved in the pathogenesis except for the fact that hyperthyroidism and DM occur primarily in older cats, and most patients are more than 10 years old. Hyperthyroidism and DM in young cats are extremely rare, with the exception of DM in Burmese cats in Australia. Other risk factors for DM are body condition (obesity), sex, and reproductive status.[205] At highest risk would be an old, obese, neutered male cat. A genetic predisposition appears to occur in Australian Burmese cats. The marked increase in DM in cats can be traced to the increase in feline obesity.

Several investigators from different continents have evaluated the risk factors for hyperthyroidism and have presented very similar results despite their geographic differences.[64,173,237] As stated, older domestic short- and long-haired cats were more likely to develop the disease than young or purebred cats. The risk increased with increasing age. There was no difference in the risk for males versus females in one study, whereas female cats were identified at higher risk in the others. Hyperthyroid cats were more likely to have used a litter box, to be fed wet cat food from a pop-top can, or were fed all categories of table food, including high-fat dairy products. The plasticizer compounds bisphenol A and phthalates have been suspected, without proof, as a causative agent for obesity and diabetes in man and for hyperthyroidism in cats, but no linkage has been ascertained to date. Environmental factors appear to play an important role, because hyperthyroid cats were more likely to have been exposed to smokers in their environment and to household insecticide treatments. Other risk factors include sleeping on the floor, exposure to organic fertilizers, and dental disease. Interestingly, hyperthyroidism was less likely in multicat households compared with single-cat households.

CLINICAL SIGNS

It is impossible to clearly distinguish hyperthyroidism from DM based on the clinical presentation. The most frequently seen clinical signs for hyperthyroidism and DM are the same, are also similar to other chronic diseases of cats, and will worsen over time. As a result, the early recognition of hyperthyroidism in a diabetic cat and vice versa is difficult because of the shared clinical signs:

- Weight loss
- Excess appetite or inappetence
- Polyuria and polydipsia

Less predictably, both conditions may present with muscle weakness, vomiting, and diarrhea. In addition, cats with extreme hyperthyroidism may show agitation. The diabetic cat with acromegaly may gain, rather than lose weight.[15]

PATHOPHYSIOLOGY

Hyperthyroidism and diabetes are both catabolic states. Hyperthyroidism is caused by excessive secretion of thyroid hormones (triiodothyronine [T_3] and thyroxine [T_4]) by hyperplastic or adenomatous thyroid glands, rarely by malignant thyroid carcinomas.[106,181] Hyperthyroidism in cats is most similar to hyperthyroidism in people caused by toxic nodular goiter. Abnormalities of the G protein and 3′-5′-cyclic adenosine monophosphate (cAMP)-signaling pathway have been implicated in the pathogenesis in both species.[95,178] Although in people antibodies against islet antigens are found with autoimmune thyroid disease, there is no evidence that a similar connection exists in hyperthyroid cats. Autoimmune processes have not been shown to play a role in either disease, and islet antigens have not been detected in diabetic cats.[110]

Thyroid hormones (TH) affect many aspects of metabolism and energy homeostasis, and in general terms, can be viewed as antagonists to insulin. The metabolic alterations during thyrotoxicosis represent direct effects of TH on the expression of TH-responsive genes and are mediated by binding of T_3 to TH receptors in peripheral organs.[10,253] Thyrotoxic human patients exhibit insulin resistance, that is, the effectiveness of insulin in muscle, fat, and liver is hampered.[15,128,136,178,179] Because one of the main roles of insulin is the control of glucose homeostasis, increased insulin resistance is seen as a decrease in glucose tolerance. In a study comparing healthy with hyperthyroid cats, glucose clearance was decreased in hyperthyroid cats, and insulin secretion was increased during an intravenous glucose tolerance test.[105] This pattern is characteristic for peripheral insulin resistance, which causes decreased uptake of glucose into muscle and fat tissue. However, fasting blood glucose concentrations were still normal, suggesting that hepatic glucose output was still normal.

It is known that hyperthyroidism by itself causes increased hepatic glucose production and a dramatic increase in Krebs cycle flux.[59,131,137] One might therefore expect excess glucose production in thyrotoxicosis. However, we have shown in cats that pyruvate cycling flux, a futile cycle, is also stimulated by thyroid hormone, thereby negating an effect on gluconeogenesis.[136] It is conceivable that in hyperthyroid cats, gluconeogenesis is kept low, and fasting blood glucose is kept in the normal range through enhancement of this futile cycle. It has been shown in hyperthyroid rats that gluconeogenesis was only increased 20%, because pyruvate cycling decreased gluconeogenesis by more than two thirds compared with what would be seen were pyruvate cycling not operative, suggesting that pyruvate cycling plays a functional role in protecting against overproduction of glucose in liver.[126] Hyperglycemia is therefore not a feature of hyperthyroidism. Contrary to popular belief, there is no evidence that hyperthyroidism increases intestinal glucose absorption in cats, and data from other species are highly controversial.[165,189]

In contrast to the effect of hyperthyroidism on hepatic glucose regulation, the diabetic cat has lost the ability to regulate glucose output from the liver and shows high fasting blood glucose concentrations. Although it is possible that hyperthyroidism beneficially affects gluconeogenesis in diabetic cats to some degree, it does not overcome the detrimental effects of absolute or relative insulin deficiency that are seen with diabetes. It is certainly conceivable that hyperthyroidism long term could lead to diabetes, because it causes insulin resistance, and insulin resistance is a risk factor for diabetes, but this needs to be investigated in a well-controlled study. To date, there is no evidence for such a link. The deciding factor would be beta-cell mass. As long as a cat has a relatively large beta-cell mass, it will be able to withstand the insult of insulin resistance.

DIAGNOSIS

The diagnosis of hyperthyroidism may be more difficult in a diabetic cat than in a cat with hyperthyroidism alone, because of several confounding factors.

Serum Total Thyroxine (TT_4) Concentration

It has been well documented that nonthyroidal diseases suppress circulating TT_4 concentrations in cats. In fact, diabetes mellitus has one of the most profound effects to reduce TT_4.[182] If TT_4 is normal in a diabetic cat suspected of hyperthyroidism, other tests are indicated, such as circulating free T_4 concentration by dialysis (FT_4D), nuclear scintigraphy, T_3 suppression test, or thyrotropin-releasing hormone (TRH) stimulation. However, normal, and occasionally high, TT_4 and high free T_4 has also been described in obese cats as well (see below). The functional tests (TRH stimulation, T_3 suppression, scintigraphy) have not been systematically studied in obesity, but none of these tests have shown high diagnostic specificity in cases of hyperthyroidism with concomitant nonthyroidal illness.[180,182,226]

Serum Free T_4 Concentration by Dialysis (FT_4D)

Free T_4 concentrations are high in hyperthyroidism and usually normal in cats with diabetes. When cats become obese, FT_4D increases for that animal because of increasing concentrations of non-esterified fatty acids that displace the hormone from its serum binding sites. However, at least in experimentally induced obesity, the FT_4D concentrations usually remain within the normal range.

Fructosamine

In unregulated diabetic cats, serum fructosamine concentrations are high, whereas in hyperthyroid cats, concentration of serum fructosamine may be low because of accelerated protein turnover.[191] Therefore fructosamine concentrations should not be used solely as an indicator of glycemic control in the diabetic cat with concurrent hyperthyroidism.

TREATMENT

If cats develop both diseases, in most instances one occurs before the other. In the case of the cat that is hyperthyroid first and develops diabetes later, the hyperthyroid condition usually has already been well controlled before diabetes occurs and the hyperthyroidism does not affect diabetes treatment.

If a well-controlled diabetic cat develops hyperthyroidism, the glucose control usually deteriorates and the insulin dose needs to be increased to avoid hyperglycemia. Once treatment for hyperthyroidism has begun and hyperthyroidism-induced insulin resistance is reduced, the insulin dose needs to be decreased to avoid hypoglycemia. Diabetes has not been shown to have any influence on the efficacy of drugs used for the treatment of hyperthyroidism, and no dose adjustment of those drugs is needed.

DIABETES MELLITUS AND OBESITY

Margarethe Hoenig

Obesity is the most common nutritional disorder, and diabetes mellitus (DM) is one of the most common endocrine diseases in cats. The prevalence for both has increased dramatically in the last 3 decades. Obesity is now thought to occur in about 40% and DM in about 0.5% to 1% of the cat population. Environmental factors, such as unrestricted food intake and reduced physical activity, are largely responsible for the modern epidemic of obesity. Obesity and DM are tightly linked to each other in cats, as they are in people. It is thought that feline obesity increases the risk to develop diabetes threefold to fivefold. Other risk factors for diabetes are gonadectomy and sex. Obese male neutered cats have the highest risk to develop the disease.[205]

DEFINITION OF DIABETES MELLITUS

Unlike in people, a diagnosis of DM in cats is usually only made when the animal exhibits obvious clinical signs of hyperglycemia. In people, an oral glucose tolerance test (OGTT) is a frequently used test to document diabetes but is rarely applied in pets. In asymptomatic people, a diagnosis of impaired glucose tolerance or diabetes is usually made based on fasting glucose concentrations and the response to a 75-g glucose load. Strict criteria have been established for the interpretation of the results to separate healthy people from people at risk of developing diabetes or already having diabetes. Oral glucose tolerance testing has recently been described in cats.[108] However, as in dogs, the OGTT in cats is associated with high variability of results and is not recommended as a routine clinical diagnostic test. The intravenous glucose tolerance test, although associated with less variability, is labor intensive and not suited for use in clinical practice. Therefore early recognition of cats at risk of developing diabetes is difficult, and no clear pattern of easily measurable parameters has emerged yet that would indicate development or progression of the disease process.

DEFINITION OF OBESITY

Obesity occurs when energy intake exceeds energy output. There are subjective as well as objective methods to measure increases in body mass. One of two (5- or 9-point scales) condition scoring systems are frequently used in practice.[142] Although subjective, they can be easily performed by one person. Longitudinal assessment (i.e., repeated over time) of animals should preferably be performed by the same person to decrease the variability of results. A score of 3/5 or 5/9 indicates that the cat is well proportioned, that is, of normal weight, while a body condition score of 5/5 or 9/9 indicates that the cat is obese and has heavy deposits of fat. Values in between indicate the increase in fat deposits as the numbers rise. Girth circumference may be measured behind the last rib and is a good objective indicator of obesity. Similar to body condition scoring, it can also be performed by one person. Its results correlate very well with fat measurements using more sophisticated methods, such as dual-energy x-ray absorptiometry (DEXA).[109] Because normal girth values are not available for different cat breeds, at this time, this method should only be used to follow the body condition in a given individual animal over time. Plain radiographs may also be helpful in assessing condition by evaluating falciform and paralumbar fat deposits. Other objective methods, such as body mass index, DEXA scanning, or magnetic resonance imaging have also been performed in cats, but not usually in clinical practice. Because normal ranges for those techniques are not available for different breeds, these tests are also valuable only when performed over time in the same cat.

THE LINK BETWEEN OBESITY AND DIABETES

Obesity, in many regards, can be seen as a precursor state to diabetes in humans and cats. It is thought that obese cats develop a form of diabetes that is similar to type 2 diabetes in humans, a disease that is characterized by insulin resistance often caused by obesity, abnormal secretion of insulin and other hormones, and amyloid deposition in the islets of Langerhans. Although many of the pathophysiologic changes are similar in obese and diabetic people and cats, there are also some differences.

It is known that obese cats are insulin resistant. Insulin resistance is the condition in which normal amounts of insulin do not produce a normal insulin response from cells. Insulin resistance is usually measured with a method called the euglycemic hyperinsulinemic clamp. Simply explained, this is a technique in which a constant amount of insulin is infused. Glucose is also infused in the amount necessary to keep blood glucose concentrations in the euglycemic range. The more sensitive a cat is to the effect of insulin, the more glucose needs to be infused. It has been shown in cats that every kilogram in weight gain leads to a 30% loss in the sensitivity to insulin.[111,112] Insulin resistance is seen in muscle, fat, and liver in obese people. In obese cats, the response to insulin is tissue dependent, and even in long-term obese cats, insulin resistance is only seen in adipose and fat tissue. In muscle and fat, the following changes are seen with obesity-induced insulin resistance:

- The expression of the insulin-sensitive, high-Km (i.e., requires a large amount of glucose to achieve maximum reaction velocity) glucose transporter type 4 (GLUT4) is decreased.
- The expression of GLUT1, the insulin-insensitive low-Km (i.e., requires only a small amount of substrate to become saturated and reach maximum velocity) glucose transporter type 1, is unchanged.

This leads to a decrease in glucose clearance when cats are challenged with a high glucose load. These cats do not show a change in glycosylated hemoglobin, and baseline glucose concentrations remain normal even in the long-term obese cat.[20]

An interesting phenomenon, and one that explains the normal baseline blood glucose in obese cats, is the fact that the liver remains responsive to insulin. In a recent study, using nuclear magnetic resonance spectroscopy, we were able to show that insulin suppresses hepatic endogenous glucose production (EGP) by reducing glycogenolysis and gluconeogenesis in obese cats. These cats were hyperinsulinemic, indicated by approximately doubled baseline peripheral insulin concentrations and yet had no difference in glucose concentrations compared with lean cats. This suggests that hepatic autoregulation is intact in obese cats despite peripheral insulin resistance and impaired glucose clearance.[136] The decreased EGP in obese cats might be a compensatory mechanism to ensure normal fasting glucose concentration. It appears therefore that a loss of hepatic autoregulation is an important step in the pathogenesis of diabetes in cats.

Obesity and diabetes are characterized by quantitative and qualitative alterations of insulin secretion. Insulin normally is secreted from beta cells in a biphasic manner in response to high glucose during an intravenous glucose tolerance test. In the cat as in people, other fuels such as amino acids potentiate the secretion of insulin in the presence of glucose. Characteristic changes that are seen in obese cats are a marked increase in the second or maintenance phase of insulin release. The amount of insulin secreted during the second phase is primarily an indicator of glucose uptake into peripheral tissues. Because of the change in glucose transport and the delayed clearance of glucose in obese insulin resistant cats, insulin secretion is increased to overcome the resistance. Over time, the persistent oversecretion leads to a decrease in total insulin secretory capacity, and the animal becomes diabetic when insulin no longer leads to a normal response.[60,107] It is not known when in the course of the development of diabetes hepatic insulin resistance develops and when increased hepatic glucose output contributes to increasing glucose concentrations (known as glucose toxicity) even in the basal state, thereby worsening the demand on beta cells and

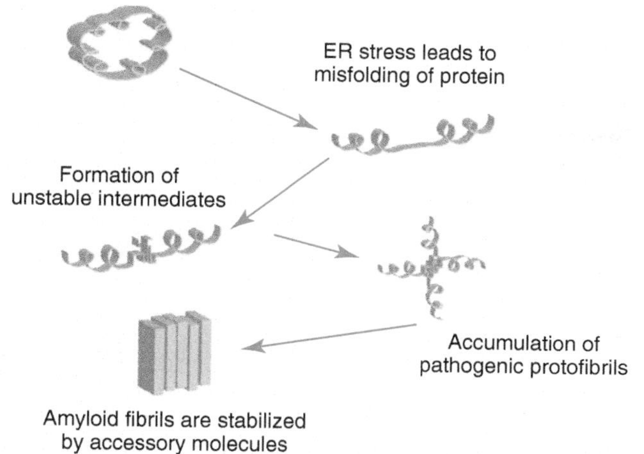

FIGURE 35-1 The effect of stress on endoplasmic reticulum amyloid formation. *(From Hayden MR, Tyagi SC, Kerklo MM, Nicolls MR: Type 2 Diabetes mellitus as a conformational disease,* JOP *6:287, 2005.)*

accelerating their exhaustion.[114] Eventually, beta cells will undergo apoptosis (programmed cell death).[60,195]

Islet amyloid is one of the characteristic features of feline diabetes and of human type 2 diabetes and is associated with a loss of beta cells. The precursor protein of islet amyloid is the hormone islet amyloid polypeptide (IAPP), which is co-localized in secretory granules of beta cells with insulin and is co-secreted with insulin.[129] It is not known why amyloid is formed in the diabetic cat. It is currently believed that the loss of beta cells associated with islet amyloidosis is actually caused by membrane permeable cytotoxic oligomers of IAPP rather than the final product, amyloid, and protective mechanisms in beta cells keeping IAPP in a soluble form must fail to allow these cytotoxic products to form.[93] Because the endoplasmic reticulum is responsible for the proper folding of proteins, including amyloid, it appears that any process that disturbs its function will lead to oligomer formation (Figure 35-1). There are no data about the occurrence of islet amyloid in obese cats compared with age-matched lean cats; however, we have shown that obese cats hypersecrete IAPP as well as insulin, which, long-term, might lead to disruption of regular secretory pathways.

Other hormones likely play a role in the progression from obesity to diabetes in cats (Table 35-1). Leptin is a hormone that is secreted from adipocytes. In lean animals, it leads to satiety and increases energy expenditure. It is known that obese cats have leptin resistance. Similar to the definition for insulin resistance, leptin resistance is the condition where normal amounts of leptin do not cause a normal response. Leptin concentrations are high in obese cats; yet, there is no decrease in food intake or increase in energy expenditure as would be expected in a cat that would respond normally.[6,112] The concentration of adiponectin, a hormone secreted from adipose tissue, which modulates glucose and lipid metabolism, is low in obese cats and correlates with insulin sensitivity.[112]

TABLE 35-1 **Hormonal and Metabolic Changes in Obese Cats Compared with Lean Cats**

Hormone	Concentration in Obese Cats	Effect
Adiponectin	Low	Decreased glucose and fat metabolism
Glucagon-like peptide-1	Low	Decreased hepatic glucose production Decreased gastric emptying Decreased satiety? Lower glucose-dependent insulin release
Insulin	High insulin resistance	Exhaustion of beta cells
Leptin	High leptin resistance	Decreased energy expenditure Decreased satiety?
Thyroid hormone	Higher but usually still within the normal range—thyroid hormone resistance?	Decreased energy expenditure

Thyroid hormone changes contribute to the metabolic alterations of obesity. The energy expenditure is lower in obese cats than lean cats but increases with administration of triiodothyronine (T_3), indicating that thyroid hormone is involved in the low heat production. It has also been shown that free T_4 has the strongest positive correlation with indices of obesity and increases with increases in body mass index, girth, leptin, and fatty acids. This suggests that obesity leads to a form of thyroid hormone resistance.[103,104]

Glucagon-like peptide 1 (GLP-1) has recently been examined in obese cats and was lower than in lean control cats.[108] Changes in GLP-1 concentrations have been associated with changes in glucose control in obese people and people with diabetes. It increases insulin secretion through activation of GLP-1 receptors on beta cells and increases the transcription of the proinsulin gene. It also inhibits glucagon secretion and regulates glucose homeostasis through decreasing glucose production by the liver, decreasing the rate of gastric emptying, and decreasing central effects on satiety.

Obese cats show a marked change in lipid metabolism. We found that obesity does have a significant effect on both plasma lipids and lipoprotein concentrations. Plasma triglycerides were found to be increased with obesity as was the very-low-density lipoprotein fraction (VLDL), the main carrier of triglycerides, whereas the low-density lipoprotein fraction (LDL) was unchanged, and the high-density lipoprotein (HDL) fraction was decreased in long-term but not short-term obese cats compared with lean cats. Using nuclear magnetic resonance spectroscopy, we measured particle size and concentration within each of the lipoprotein fractions and found that obese cats have very similar changes to obese people who are at risk of developing atherosclerosis and cardiovascular disease. Those changes include more large VLDL particles, more medium- and small-sized LDL particles, and more small HDL particles.[127] Despite these changes, atherosclerosis and cardiovascular disease have not been described in obese cats, and only one study has suggested that there might be an increase in cardiovascular disease in diabetic cats; however, this needs to be confirmed in a well-controlled study. Not surprisingly, obese cats have a lower expression of peroxisome proliferator-activated receptors (PPARs), which are transcription factors that play a major role in the regulation of lipid, carbohydrate, and protein metabolism.[104]

Both high plasma glucose and fatty acid concentrations are involved in the mediation of oxidative stress through the generation of reactive oxygen species (primarily oxygen and nitrogen). Oxidative stress may play a role in the progression from obesity to diabetes, but so far this has not been studied in cats. Antibodies to islet antigens do not seem to play a role in the pathogenesis of diabetes in cats.[110] Interestingly, the metabolic sequelae of obesity are not at all, or only to a very limited degree, influenced by dietary components.

In conclusion, obesity is a major risk factor for the development of diabetes. It appears that loss of hepatic autoregulation may be the switch between obesity and diabetes in cats. Once the animal shows hyperglycemia, the toxic effects of glucose become evident as already shown in cats in 1948[60] and, in beta cells, lead to exaggerated apoptosis and further loss of beta-cell mass. It is important to know that the changes described above for obese cats can be reversed with a simple treatment, weight loss. This is one more reason to make sure feline obesity is recorded and treated before the path to diabetes becomes a one-way street.

DIABETES MELLITUS AND FELINE LOWER URINARY TRACT DISORDERS

Deborah S. Greco

Type 2 diabetes mellitus (DM) is characterized by an impaired ability to secrete insulin following a glucose stimulus and is caused by both a defect in pancreatic beta cells and by peripheral insulin resistance. Feline lower urinary tract disease (FLUTD) is a term that describes a constellation of disorders including feline idiopathic cystitis (FIC), which accounts for the majority of cases of FLUTD, urolithiasis, urethral plugs or other causes of obstruction, bacterial cystitis, and, rarely, neoplasia. The purpose of this chapter is to describe the etiology, prevalence, clinical signs, pathogenesis, diagnosis, and treatment of cats with concurrent DM and FLUTD.

ETIOLOGY AND PREVALENCE

Diabetes mellitus is one of the most common feline endocrine diseases. The etiology of type 2 DM is multifactorial, with obesity, genetics, diet, and islet amyloidosis involved in the development of this form of DM in humans and cats.[172,190,255] FLUTD occurs in approximately 1% to 3% of cats seen at general veterinary practices; the etiology is multifactorial, and a cat may be predisposed to the condition because of genetic, dietary, and environmental factors.[31,32,34,118,149]

Concurrent DM and FLUTD may result from two different scenarios. Cats with preexisting DM may experience signs of FLUTD, most often as a result of bacterial cystitis. Although bacterial infections are a rare (<1%) cause of FLUTD in nondiabetic cats, diabetic cats are predisposed to urinary tract infection (UTI) because of impaired local immunity and the presence of glucose (bacterial substrate) in the urine. If the cat has impaired renal function, decreased urine specific gravity (USG) may also contribute to a predisposition to UTI. On the other hand, cats presenting with signs of FLUTD or cats susceptible to repeated episodes of FIC may develop diabetes as a result of the stress of their disease (increased endogenous corticosteroids), inflammation associated with chronicity resulting in insulin resistance, or as a result of therapy for signs of FLUTD (if exogenous steroids have been used).

PATIENT SIGNALMENT AND RISK FACTORS

Risk factors for the development of diabetes mellitus in cats include increased body weight (>6.8 kg), older age (>10 years) and neutering.[176,185] Neutered males (NM) are 1.5 times more likely than females to develop diabetes mellitus. FLUTD is seen most commonly in cats that are young to middle aged, overweight, kept indoors, fed dry food *ad libitum* and live in a multianimal household.[31,32,34,38] Neutered cats are more susceptible, and the risk of urinary tract obstruction is greatest in males.[149] Concurrent FLUTD and DM is most likely to occur in obese middle-aged NM cats kept indoors.

CLINICAL SIGNS

Obesity combined with fasting or postprandial hyperglycemia may be the only clinical sign of early type 2 DM. Owners of diabetic cats may report gait abnormalities, weakness, inappropriate elimination (particularly if the litter box is large or placed in a remote location), and problems with jumping prior to the onset of polydipsia and polyuria.[85] Late signs of DM in cats include polydipsia, polyuria, anorexia, lethargy, and weight loss. The most common physical examination findings in cats suffering from DM are lethargy and depression (70%), dehydration (63%), unkempt hair coat (35%), and muscle wasting (47%).[85,185] Plantigrade rear limb stance resulting from diabetic neuropathy is observed in approximately 8% of diabetic cats.[185]

Cats with lower urinary tract disease can present with signs of dysuria, hematuria, pollakiuria, inappropriate urination, and/or urethral obstruction.[91,118] Nonobstructive cases are self-limiting, usually resolving within 5 to 10 days.

Clinical signs of concurrent diabetes mellitus and FLUTD may include polydipsia, polyuria, pollakiuria, dysuria, hematuria, and inappropriate elimination. In the author's experience, urethral obstruction is rare in a diabetic cat. However, there is considerable overlap in the clinical signs of DM and FLUTD; therefore careful assessment of the history and minimum database, including urine culture and serum fructosamine, may be necessary to make an accurate diagnosis.

PATHOPHYSIOLOGY

To summarize the current hypothesis of the pathogenesis of type 2 DM, peripheral insulin resistance (resulting from obesity, elevated plasma islet amyloid polypeptide [IAPP], or both) causes chronic stimulation of insulin production in the pancreatic beta cells.[190] Amylin is co-synthesized with insulin; therefore abnormal insulin secretion causes IAPP to accumulate in the beta cells.[172] The high local concentration of IAPP causes polymerization of IAPP to form insular amyloid. Eventually a vicious cycle of increased amyloid production and chronic hyperglycemia leads to beta-cell failure and apoptosis (programmed cell death).

Stress plays an important role in the pathogenesis of feline idiopathic cystitis. Recent studies indicate that FIC, the most common cause of FLUTD, may be caused by placing a "susceptible" cat into a "provocative" environment."[244,246,247,249] Activation of an abnormal pituitary-adrenal axis caused by genetic or epigenetic abnormalities, coupled with catecholamine excess caused by environmental stressors, leads to local bladder inflammation. Most cats with signs of FLUTD are obese, and the role of obesity in these diseases is poorly defined. Increased visceral fat causes inflammation[46,166] and predisposes to diseases, such as type 2 DM in both cats and humans. In fact, in the author's experience, many cats that eventually develop DM have had episodes of FLUTD prior to presentation with signs of diabetes.

DIAGNOSIS

Common clinicopathologic features of diabetes mellitus in cats include fasting hyperglycemia, hypercholesterolemia, increased liver enzymes (ALP, ALT), neutrophilic leukocytosis, possible proteinuria, variable urine specific gravity, bacteriuria, and glucosuria.[48] Many cats are susceptible to stress-induced hyperglycemia. In addition, renal glucosuria may be found in animals with renal tubular disease and with stress-induced hyperglycemia. Serum fructosamine evaluation may be beneficial in differentiating early or subclinical diabetes mellitus from stress-induced hyperglycemia in the cat. Serum fructosamine is formed by glycosylation of serum protein, such as albumin, and the concentration of fructosamine in serum is directly related to blood glucose concentration. One study of 17 normal cats showed that transient glucose administration (1 g/kg 50% glucose solution, intravenously) did not cause increased serum fructosamine concentrations.[153]

Cats with FLUTD typically have unremarkable serum biochemistry and hematology values unless urethral obstruction occurs. Urethral obstruction is associated with postrenal azotemia and electrolyte disturbances, particularly hyperkalemia, and a stress leukogram may be present. Urine should be assessed for physical appearance, routine biochemical analysis (including pH and specific gravity), microscopic examination of sediment, and bacterial culture and sensitivity. Although bacterial urinary tract infections are a rare (<1%) cause of uncomplicated FLUTD, signs of FLUTD in a diabetic cat are much more likely to be caused by bacterial cystitis. Repeated culture and sensitivity of urine may be necessary in diabetic cats suffering from lower urinary tract signs, particularly because pyuria is often not observed in these cats partly because of the dilute nature of the urine. Uroliths may be ruled out by the use of ultrasonography or contrast radiography. A diagnosis of feline idiopathic cystitis is one of exclusion; however, in the author's experience, diabetic cats are not often afflicted with idiopathic feline cystitis, perhaps because of frequent voiding caused by osmotic diuresis.

ENVIRONMENTAL AND DIETARY THERAPY

A lower-carbohydrate, higher-protein diet may ameliorate some of the abnormalities associated with diabetes mellitus in the cat. Initial studies using a canned high-protein/low-carbohydrate diet and the starch blocker acarbose have shown that 58% of cats discontinue insulin injections, and those with continued insulin requirements could be regulated on a much lower dosage (1 to 2 U every 12 hours).[159] Comparison of canned high-fiber versus low-carbohydrate diets showed that cats fed low-carbohydrate diets were 3 to 4 times more likely to discontinue insulin injections.[13] The diet formulation is critical in that most dry cat food formulations contain excessive carbohydrates; therefore canned cat foods and preferably higher protein foods should be used for initial treatment of diabetic cats. Caution should be used when initially changing from dry to canned foods as insulin requirements may decrease and a reduction in insulin dosage may be required.

The aim of dietary therapy of FLUTD is to create less concentrated urine (ideally, specific gravity ≤1.035), encourage more frequent urination, and make urolith, crystal, or urethral plug formation less likely. Rather than altering the content of a dry diet, it is preferable to feed a canned diet. Diets designed with a higher protein content that promote weight loss may also be beneficial, because both diabetes mellitus and FLUTD are most often seen in obese cats. Food should be measured and fed to attain an optimal body condition score (4 to 5 on the 9-point scale or 2.5 to 3 on the 5-point scale). For cats with concurrent diabetes and lower urinary tract disease, canned food is recommended both because it contains water and because it is low in carbohydrate content.

Recent evidence suggests that signs of FIC can be reduced by the use of a multimodal environmental modification program.[33] An appropriate number and positioning of the litter boxes should allow the cats to have free access. Although covered litter boxes may be thought to provide a safe and private place to eliminate, many cats will not use them. Daily scooping of urine and feces is essential, and full cleaning of the box and replacement of the litter should take place at least once a week. This is particularly important in diabetic cats with FLUTD because of the presence of polyuria as well as possible odors. The use of Feliway (Ceva Animal Health, Buckinghamshire, England) diffusers during this process is recommended, because it has been shown to reduce signs of defensive aggression and passive withdrawal.[90]

DRUG THERAPY

Cats with diabetes mellitus should be treated with diet and insulin or possibly diet and oral hypoglycemic agents[71,190]; however, the presence of concurrent DM and FLUTD often requires intensive control of hyperglycemia. The presence of FLUTD in a diabetic cat is not necessarily an indication that the cat will not go into diabetic remission. One recent paper showed that when an appropriate ultralow carbohydrate canned diet is used in conjunction with long-acting insulin, most newly diagnosed diabetic cats have a 70% to 90% chance of remission.[156] The reader should refer to Chapters 24 and 32 for an in-depth discussion about treatment of DM and of FLUTD, respectively.

Tricyclic antidepressants have been found to be beneficial in the treatment of some humans with interstitial cystitis, and anecdotally, in a number of cats with FIC because of anticholinergic (including increasing bladder capacity), antiinflammatory (including preventing histamine release from mast cells), antiadrenergic, analgesic, and mood-altering effects.[141] Potential side effects include somnolence, urinary retention, and increased liver enzymes. Liver function should be assessed prior to starting therapy, reassessed 1 month later, and then every 6 to 12 months while the cat is on treatment. It may be difficult to determine if liver enzyme elevations are caused by the diabetes or the tricyclic antidepressant; therefore control of the DM with gradual withdrawal of the agent may be required to determine whether the liver enzyme elevation is drug induced or not.

HEART FAILURE AND CHRONIC KIDNEY DISEASE

Marie-Claude Bélanger

Myocardial disease and chronic kidney disease (CKD) are common disorders of the geriatric cat. The coexistence of heart failure (HF) and CKD is often associated with an adverse outcome, since combined cardiac and renal dysfunctions amplify progression of failure of the individual organ through a complex combination of neurohormonal feedback mechanisms.[197]

In humans, the term cardiorenal syndrome (CRS) has generally been reserved for declining renal function in the setting of advanced congestive heart failure, but recently, a more specific classification of CRS has been published.[198] In this classification, CRS is divided into five subtypes that reflect the pathophysiology, time frame, and nature of concomitant cardiac and renal dysfunction (Box 35-1). The true existence of the negative spiral of primary CKD causing cardiac dysfunction is still unknown in small animals. Except for the consequences of hypertension, CRS subtypes 3 and 4 are probably uncommon in cats. For the purpose of this chapter, CRS will refer to subtype 2, assuming that relatively normal kidneys become dysfunctional because of concomitant HF. A special focus on the therapeutic strategies of concomitant CKD and HF will be presented.

PREVALENCE

Co-morbid dysfunction of the heart and kidney has been reported to be as high as 30% to 50% in hospitalized humans.[100,161,196,209] A lower prevalence of 15% to 30% has

BOX 35-1

Classification of Cardiorenal Syndrome in Humans

Type 1: Abrupt worsening of cardiac function (e.g., acute cardiogenic shock or decompensated congestive heart failure) leading to acute kidney injury

Type 2: Chronic abnormalities in cardiac function (e.g., chronic congestive heart failure) causing progressive and permanent chronic kidney disease

Type 3: Abrupt worsening of renal function (e.g., acute kidney ischemia or glomerulonephritis) causing acute cardiac disorder (e.g., heart failure, arrhythmia, ischemia)

Type 4: State of chronic kidney disease (e.g., chronic glomerular disease) contributing to decreased cardiac function, cardiac hypertrophy and/or increased risk of adverse cardiovascular events

Type 5: Systemic condition (e.g., diabetes mellitus, sepsis) causing both cardiac and renal dysfunction

Adapted from Ronco F, Ronco C: Cardiorenal syndrome, current understanding, *Recent Prog Med* 100:202, 2009.

been found in dogs with mitral valve disease.[170,187] The true incidence of CRS in cats is unknown but also appears common. A study performed on 102 cats with hypertrophic cardiomyopathy reported 59% prevalence for azotemia as compared with 25% in an age-matched control population.[80]

PATHOPHYSIOLOGY

The pathophysiology of CRS is complex and not completely understood. CRS occurs when worsening renal function limits diuresis despite a clinical volume overload associated with HF. The etiology of CRS is multifactorial and involves bidirectional interactions, effects, and reactions between the heart and kidneys. It includes activation of the renin angiotensin aldosterone (RAAS) and sympathetic systems, potentiation of oxidative stress, endothelial dysfunction, and defective nitric oxide metabolism (Figure 35-2). In chronic HF, long-term reduced renal perfusion is responsible for worsening renal function. However, hypoperfusion alone cannot explain progressive renal dysfunction as the cause of

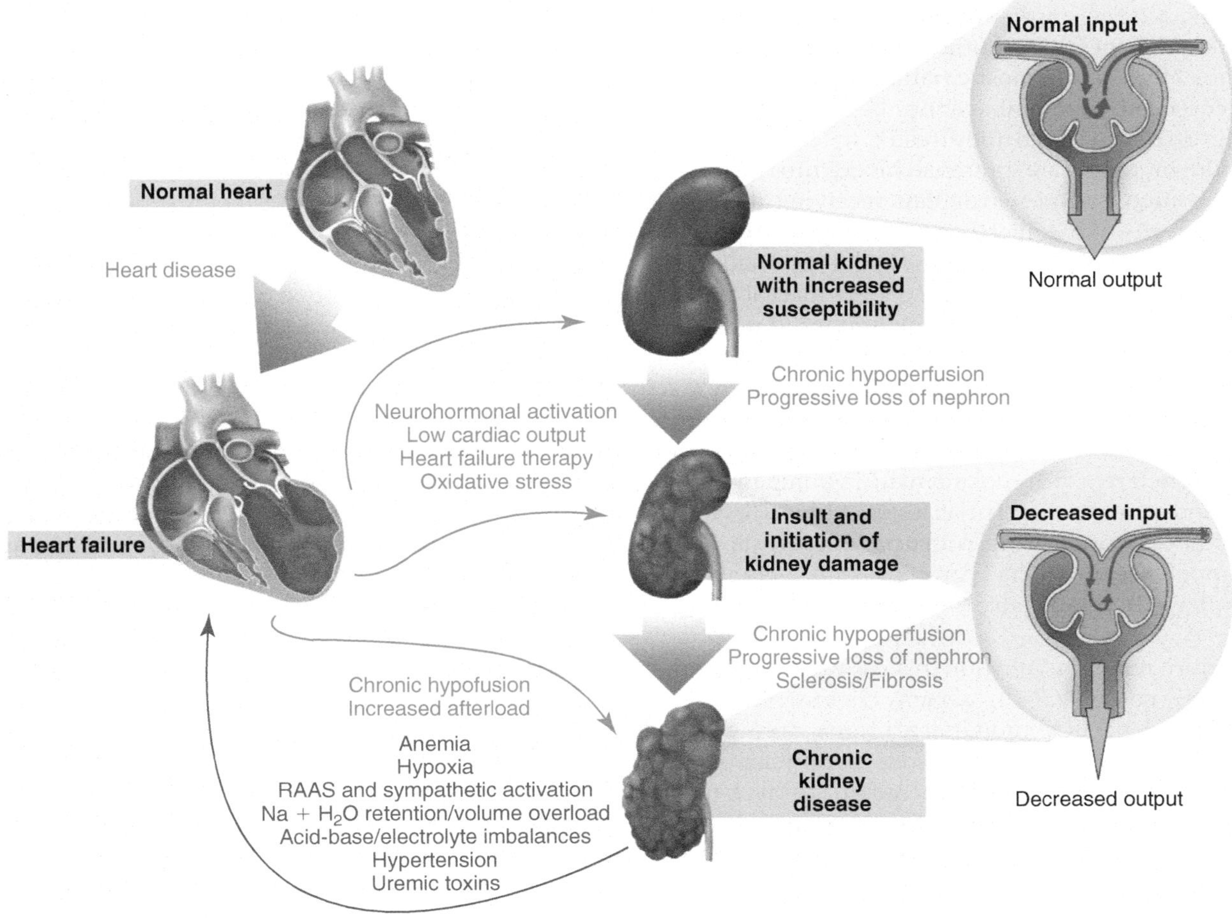

FIGURE 35-2 Pathophysiology of cardiorenal syndrome. *(Drawing by Maxim Moreau.)*

CKD. Numerous neurohormonal mechanisms are implicated and include vasoconstrictive (epinephrine, angiotensin II, endothelin), vasodilatory (BNP, nitric oxide), and inflammatory (C-reactive protein) mediators.[4] Other contributing factors include the deleterious effects of uremia and acidemia on cardiac inotropy, the hypotensive effects of diuresis-associated hypovolemia, and RAAS blockade.[164,171] Whether these mechanisms are responsible for CRS in cats remains speculative.

DIAGNOSIS

While managing a cat for chronic HF, the veterinarian should monitor for and anticipate CRS. This syndrome is suspected when worsening of renal function as determined by a decline in creatinine clearance (eventually leading to azotemia) is observed in cats treated for HF. For both medical planning and prognostic purposes, the glomerular filtration rate (GFR) should be estimated and included in the initial database. In a clinical setting, creatinine concentration can be used as an indirect, albeit insensitive, estimate of GFR. Numerous nonrenal factors affect serum creatinine levels, most notably a decline in muscle mass causes a reduction in this parameter, possibly giving a false sense of improvement in GFR.

The diagnosis of CKD is difficult in cats already being treated for HF. The diagnostic hallmark of isosthenuria in the presence of azotemia cannot be used in patients receiving diuretics, since they result in a lower USG. Also, mild or moderate prerenal blood urea nitrogen (BUN) elevation is expected in cats receiving diuretics, and a mild creatinine increase is also possible.[17,170,187] However, a progressive rise of BUN, and especially creatinine with or without a decreasing USG, in a cat treated for chronic HF should alert the practitioner to potential development of CRS. Longitudinal assessment of serum creatinine is therefore important, and a progressive rise can indicate declining renal function even when values remain in the normal range. Other indices of CKD are hyperphosphatemia, hypokalemia, nonregenerative anemia, and proteinuria. The classical clinical signs of feline CKD (e.g., increasing polyuria/polydipsia [PU/PD], inappetence/anorexia, vomiting, and weight loss; see Chapter 32) should also be considered suspicious for CRS.

To identify renal dysfunction in a cat with HF, a complete blood count (CBC), serum chemistry profile, urinalysis, and urinary protein:creatinine ratio should be determined. Abdominal ultrasonography should be performed to recognize the typical architectural changes of CKD (small kidneys with altered surface contour and poor corticomedullary distinction) and to identify underlying causes of CKD (e.g., pyelonephritis, nephrolithiasis, neoplasia, polycystic kidney disease) that may have specific treatments. Potential aortic thromboembolism resulting in renal infarction and acute decline in renal function should be considered when a cat with HF presents with acute renal failure. Urine culture should be performed to identify and treat possible urinary tract infection. Systemic blood pressure should be evaluated in cats with CRS, since the presence of hypotension will worsen renal perfusion, whereas hypertension will negatively affect cardiac output and renal function. In calm, conscious cats, a systolic blood pressure greater than 160 to 180 mm Hg should be regarded as suspect for hypertension. A complete echocardiogram is usually indicated to optimize treatment of the primary cardiomyopathy and to assess the risk for potential embolic events. Finally, thoracic radiographs should be performed to evaluate the level of control of the HF and to adjust the medical plan accordingly.

A promising tool in the diagnosis of CRS in cats is the measurement of serum amino-terminal probrain natriuretic peptide (Nt-proBNP). Indeed, this biomarker has been shown to offer powerful diagnostic and prognostic information in humans suffering from CRS.[3,235] A commercial Nt-proBNP assay is now available in cats and could eventually prove useful in the diagnosis and management of CRS in this species.

THERAPY

Treatment of CRS in cats is largely empiric, because no clinical trials have been completed. Box 35-2 summarizes the general approach to the cat presented with CRS. The goal is to recognize the syndrome, reverse it as much as possible, and deal with the renal consequences of chronic HF.

The main challenge in the treatment of co-morbid HF and CKD is trying to balance two organs with antagonistic volume needs.[47] The goal is to find a balance between the tendency to "dry-out" HF while hydrating CKD. Unfortunately, HF control is often favored to the detriment of renal support, leading to adverse long-term consequences on the kidneys. Therefore management of cats with CRS should focus on therapeutic strategies aimed at controlling signs of one organ failing while avoiding iatrogenic decompensation of the other organ. Since the degree of compromise of each organ is variable, Table 35-2 describes specific treatment plans in different CRS situations.

Optimizing Heart Failure Therapy

Angiotensin-Converting Enzyme (ACE) Inhibitors

Because of RAAS activation, angiotensin-converting enzyme (ACE) inhibitors are the mainstay of therapy for concomitant HF and CKD, especially in the presence of hypertension and/or proteinuria. Although activation of RAAS is beneficial in the early stages of renal disease,

BOX 35-2

Approach to the Cat with Cardiorenal Syndrome

1. Recognize and anticipate CRS
   - Record baseline BUN/Cr/USG/UPC ratio
   - Monitor for temporal Cr rise
2. Optimize HF therapy
   - Lowest effective dose of furosemide
     - Consider dual-diuretic therapy
     - Consider torsemide if diuretic resistance
   - ACE inhibitors
   - Other cardiac drugs
   - Thoracocentesis/abdominocentesis
3. Evaluate and monitor renal function
   - CBC/serum chemistry profile/urinalysis ± UPC ratio
     - q1-3 months or when changing treatment plan
   - Urine culture
   - Abdominal ultrasonography
4. Control hypertension
   - Assess systolic blood pressure (SBP)
   - Treat when SBP > 160 mm Hg
     - Amlodipine
5. Avoid hypotension
   - If SBP < 100 mm Hg
     - Reassess hypotensive drugs
     - Consider positive inotropes
6. Improve renal therapy
   - Omega-3 fatty acid supplementation
   - Feed renal diet if in ≥ IRIS stage 2 + sodium restriction
   - Phosphate binders
   - K^+ supplementation
   - H_2-blockers if GI signs
   - Consider long-term SC fluids
   - Consider renal replacement therapy
7. Improve cardiac output
   - Consider positive inotropes
     - Dobutamine unconvincing
     - Pimobendan promising
8. Correct anemia of CKD
   - When Hct < 18% to 20%
     - EPO administration
9. Review and modify drug dosages
   - Extend dosage interval of renally excreted drugs
   - Check for drug interactions

ACE, Angiotensin-converting enzyme; *BUN,* blood urea nitrogen; *CBC,* complete blood count; *CKD,* chronic kidney disease; *Cr,* creatinine; *CRS,* cardiorenal syndrome; *EPO,* erythropoietin; *HF,* heart failure; *Hct,* hematocrit; *IRIS,* International Renal Interest Society; *SBP,* systolic blood pressure; *SC,* subcutaneous fluids; *UPC,* urine protein to creatinine ratio; *USG,* urine specific gravity.

TABLE 35-2 **Therapeutic Strategies in Different Cardiorenal Syndrome Situations**

	Renal Dysfunction	
	Normal Cr	**Increased Cr**
HEART FAILURE		
Resolved	Find lowest effective diuretic dose Optimize follow-up	Reduce furosemide dose Reassess ACEI dosage Consider positive inotropes Stimulate water consumption Consider SC fluids
Unresolved Progressive or Severe	Increase furosemide dose Consider dual-diuretic tx Consider furosemide CRI Consider torsemide Control arrhythmias Increase ACEI dosage/frequency Consider pimobendan Consider afterload reduction: arteriodilator/amlodipine	Optimize positive inotrope Consider dual-diuretic tx Control signs of uremia Maintenance SC fluids Increase arteriodilator Control hypertension Avoid iatrogenic hypotension Consider renal replacement tx

ACEI, Angiotensin-converting enzyme inhibitors; *Cr,* creatinine; *CRI,* constant rate infusion; *CRS,* cardiorenal syndrome; *SC,* subcutaneous; *tx,* treatment.

prolonged renal ischemia exacerbates renal injury and may ultimately generate fibrosis in cats as it does in other species.[21] In CKD, ACE inhibitors limit systemic and glomerular capillary hypertension, have an antiproteinuric effect, and retard the development of glomerulosclerosis and tubulointerstitial lesions.[148] In proteinuric dogs, enalapril has been shown to counteract proteinuria and delay the onset or progression of azotemia.[82,147] ACE inhibitors have also shown to be beneficial in cats with proteinuric CKD.[26,133] Historically, some concerns have been expressed regarding the long-term effects of ACE inhibitors on renal function. However, chronic enalapril administration does not adversely affect kidney function in dogs with mitral valve disease.[5]

Cats with CRS should be volume-repleted before being started on low-dose ACE inhibitors (benazepril or enalapril, 0.25 mg/kg, PO, every 24 hours). This dose can eventually be increased (0.5 mg/kg, PO, every 12 to 24 hours) for better control of HF. Benazepril is metabolized in the liver, whereas enalapril is metabolized by liver and kidneys. Consequently, cats with CRS might need a lower dose of enalapril than benazepril. Initiation of ACE inhibition therapy is associated with a transient decrease in GFR and increase in BUN and creatinine concentrations. Cats showing an increased creatinine or those already on an ACE inhibitor while developing renal failure, can remain on therapy. In CRS, ACE inhibitors are beneficial long-term and are generally not responsible for worsening renal function. Lowering the dosage of the ACE inhibitor is usually sufficient in this situation.

Diuretics

As a general rule, if increasing azotemia becomes a concern in cats with CRS, decreasing the furosemide dosage should be the first approach. Diuretics lower cardiac output and renal blood flow, which will tend to increase BUN and creatinine. Elevation of BUN concentration in cats treated with furosemide is mostly prerenal and generally necessary to control HF; therefore it is prudent to use the lowest effective dose of furosemide that controls the HF. The dose has to be continuously reassessed, depending on the type and progression of heart disease, dietary salt intake, and renal adaptation to the diuretic. Conversely, a very important principle when determining the ideal furosemide dosage for an individual HF patient is that the threshold rate of drug excretion must be achieved for optimal efficacy.[75] In other words, the practitioner must find the single effective dose resulting in adequate natriuresis; a cat that is nonresponsive to 5 mg of furosemide will need 10 mg (every 8, 12, or 24 hours) rather than giving 5 mg every 12 hours. Adequate natriuresis can be grossly assessed in a clinical setting by observation of increased urine volume and decreased urine specific gravity. Another important principle with regard to diuretics in CRS cats is to periodically drain pleural effusion or ascites in order to avoid excessive diuretic use.

Diuretic resistance is a phenomenon that can be seen in animals with chronic HF. It is defined as a clinical state in which diuretic response is diminished or lost before the therapeutic goal of relief from edema has been reached. Multiple factors account for diuretic resistance, including insufficient diuretic dose, excessive sodium intake, inappropriate intestinal absorption of oral drugs, increased sodium reabsorption at diuretic-insensitive sites in the nephrons, decreased renal perfusion, and urinary diuretic excretion.[199] When diuretic resistance occurs in cats with CRS, a furosemide constant rate infusion (0.3 to 0.6 mg/kg/h IV) helps to achieve effective natriuresis, since it inhibits sodium reabsorption more consistently and safely than oral or IV boluses do.[204] Once the volume-overloaded state has resolved, most cats will once again respond to oral therapy. Another strategy to consider when diuretic resistance is suspected is to switch to a different oral loop diuretic. Torsemide (Demadex) is useful in CRS patients because of its excellent bioavailability, superior diuretic action, and long half-life. A recent study on eight healthy dogs showed that diuretic resistance developed after 14 days of furosemide, but not torsemide, administration.[115] Torsemide (0.3 mg/kg, PO, every 24 hours) has been evaluated in cats with experimentally induced left ventricular hypertrophy and appears to be 10 times more potent than furosemide.[229] The diuretic effects peak at 4 hours after oral administration and persist for 12 hours. Further studies are needed to establish the dosage range in cats.

Dual-diuretic therapy can be considered when furosemide dosage needs to be decreased. Combination therapy potentiates diuretic effects by acting at multiple sites within the nephron. Spironolactone (1 to 2 mg/kg, PO, every 12 hours) should be used with caution in cats, since it may occasionally cause reversible facial dermititis.[154] Also, in the author's hands, use of aldosterone in patients with renal dysfunction sometimes causes significant hyperkalemia. Thiazide diuretics, such as hydrochlorothiazide (1 to 2 mg/kg, PO, every 12 hours), can also be used but are notably less effective than loop diuretics, especially when creatinine clearance is abnormal.

Normalizing Blood Pressure

Systemic hypertension is common in feline CKD. It complicates management of HF by increasing the afterload, consequently reducing forward cardiac output. In fact, hypertension is known to worsen both CKD and HF and should be aggressively controlled in cats with CRS. ACE inhibitors are not effective as an antihypertensive monotherapy in cats with CKD.[216] Amlodipine (0.625 mg/cat, PO, every 24 hours) should be added to the therapeutic plan as discussed elsewhere in this text. Subsequent blood pressure monitoring should be performed regularly to avoid deleterious iatrogenic hypotension, especially in a patient receiving other drugs with hypotensive effects for control of HF. Systolic blood pressure should ideally be maintained between 100 and 150 mm Hg in cats with CRS.

Improving Cardiac Output

The role of positive inotropes in feline CRS is still to be defined. Indeed, most feline HF patients are primarily affected by hypertrophic cardiomyopathy, which is mainly a diastolic dysfunction. Nevertheless, in advanced stages of HF and CKD, use of a positive inotrope is sometimes helpful in improving renal blood flow and azotemia. Although unapproved in this species, the author has used pimobendan (Vetmedin) on several cats with end-stage CRS, resulting in improved azotemia, demeanor, and appetite. Use of pimobendan may allow a reduction in the diuretic dose. Further study is needed in this area, since a small but significant increase in BUN has been reported in dogs with HF treated with pimobendan.[78] Dobutamine (2 μg/kg/min IV) is another positive inotrope that can be used in hospitalized CRS cats, but its real benefit is still unproven.

Improving Renal Function

Management of feline CKD is discussed in detail in Chapter 32. Specific strategies to optimize renal function in CRS will be discussed in this section.

Dietary Therapy

Appropriate diet therapy is essential in the management of CRS, and nutritional needs of both cardiac and renal dysfunction should be taken into consideration. In HF, high sodium intake can prevent net fluid loss even when adequate diuresis is achieved. Therefore cats with CRS should eat a diet with a maximum sodium content of 0.25% to 0.33% (e.g., Hill's Prescription Diet k/d Feline). More stringent sodium restriction is sometimes needed in CRS cats with severe or progressive HF (e.g., Purina Veterinary Diets NF Feline Formula, Royal Canin Veterinary Diet Renal LP). Distilled or low-sodium bottled water can also be offered for drinking. Owners should be advised to avoid feeding treats with high-sodium content. Examples of low-sodium treats for cats include Purina Whisker Lickin's brands and Stewart Fiber Formula cat treats.

In CKD, dietary modification is recommended for cats in International Renal Interest Society (IRIS) stages 2 to 4. In addition to protein and phosphorus reduction, diets designed for feline CKD usually differ from maintenance diets in several ways that are also beneficial in HF: reduced sodium content, increased B-vitamin content, increased caloric density, neutral effect on acid–base balance, supplementation of omega-3 polyunsaturated fatty acids and potassium. Protein restriction should be tailored on an individual basis in cats with CRS. High-quality, biologically available proteins are important in HF to avoid loss of lean body mass. Protein should be given to the highest level tolerated by the renal dysfunction, that is, without increasing azotemia. A good option for cats with CRS is to have a homemade diet formulated to respond to individual patient needs (see Chapter 18).

Omega-3 Polyunsaturated Fatty Acids

Omega-3 polyunsaturated fatty acids (omega-3 PUFAs) have many beneficial effects on both the heart and the kidney. Dietary supplementation with omega-3 PUFAs is considered renoprotective early in the course of renal insufficiency.[25] In a study of induced renal failure, dogs receiving omega-3 PUFAs supplementation had fewer structural renal lesions, less proteinuria, and preservation of GFR when compared with dogs fed a control, low-PUFA-content diet.[24] A retrospective study on the effects of several renal diets found that survival was greatest among CKD cats fed diets with the highest omega-3 fatty acids content.[184]

Omega-3 PUFAs are also beneficial in animals with cardiac disease. In one study of dogs with HF, fish oil supplementation decreased cytokine production and improved cachexia and appetite.[74] Antiarrhythmic effects of fish oil have also been reported.[130,213] Although these effects have not been studied in cats with CRS, omega-3 PUFAs can be given at the following dosages:

- Eicosapentaenoic acid (EPA): 40 mg/kg, PO, every 24 hours
- Docosahexaenoic acid (DHA): 25 mg/kg, PO, every 24 hours

Fluid Therapy

In volume-depleted CRS patients, administration of IV fluids may be essential to reduce uremia. Increasing extracellular volume with IV fluids will improve renal flow and promote fluid diuresis but may precipitate congestive heart failure. Therefore the main focus will be to determine when the euvolemic status is reached to avoid excessive fluid administration. A good strategy is to use replacement-type fluids (e.g., Plasmalyte-148, lactated Ringer solution) to slowly correct dehydration and then change to maintenance low-sodium crystalloid fluids (e.g., NaCl 0.45% with 2.5% dextrose, Plasmalyte-56 with 5% dextrose) to further improve azotemia. The rate and amount of fluids to administer must be determined on a case-by-case basis. Recording patient weight is easy and important in deciding how to adjust fluid rates. Onset of a new gallop sound, or progressive increase in the respiratory, and/or heart rate in a cat with preexisting heart disease may indicate impending congestive HF and justify fluid rate reduction. Central venous pressure monitoring and echocardiography (monitoring for left atrial dilation) are two useful diagnostic tools that can also be used to guide fluid adjustment. Although controversial, concomitant low-dose constant rate infusion (CRI) of furosemide is sometimes needed in cats with end-stage CRS.

Although there are no scientific studies to support this claim, many cardiologists consider subcutaneous fluids less likely than IV fluids to worsen signs of congestive heart failure.[56] As discussed in Chapter 32, subcutaneous fluid administration can improve dehydration and signs of uremia in cats with CKD. This strategy is also helpful in CRS cats with worsening azotemia. Typically, a balanced electrolyte solution (e.g., lactated Ringer solution) is administered subcutaneously every 24 to 48 hours. Again, the frequency and the amount of fluids to administer should be determined on a case-by-case basis, and close monitoring for volume overload must be done. In fragile patients, it is recommended to start with a small volume, such as 30 mL every 48 hours. If the expected effect on uremia is suboptimal, the volume can cautiously be increased to 50 mL once daily. Serial assessment of hydration, uremic signs, and renal function should be done to adjust fluid therapy accordingly. Sodium-containing fluids given subcutaneously do not provide electrolyte-free water. Therefore providing water through a feeding tube is another option. This approach may be easier for the owner and can also be used to feed some anorectic CRS cats until uremia has improved.

Electrolytes should be monitored closely in CRS animals, especially potassium, because hypokalemia can trigger ventricular tachyarrhythmias and refractoriness to some antiarrhythmics. Hypokalemia can be corrected through fluid therapy (KCl 0.05 to 0.5 mEq/kg/h depending on the level of hypokalemia) or by use of oral supplementation (potassium citrate or gluconate; 1 to 4 mEq/cat, every 12 hours).

Finally, renal replacement therapy, such as hemodialysis or ultrafiltration, can improve survival and quality of life in cats with end-stage CRS. Unfortunately, availability, feasibility, and costs of renal replacement therapy are still a concern for most cat owners.

Correcting Anemia

Anemia is relatively common in cats with CKD. Several mechanisms exist: anemia of chronic disease (iron sequestration), anemia due to decreased erythropoietin (EPO) production, and anemia from inadequate protein intake for normal hemoglobin production. In humans with HF, anemia can also occur secondary to defective erythropoiesis and represents an independent risk factor for poorer outcomes.[56,116] Dogs with HF have been shown to have lower hematocrits than healthy controls.[67] Recently, in human studies, there has been a growing interest in the pathogenic link between EPO deficiency and progression of CRS. Cardiac EPO receptor activation may protect the cardiomyocytes from apoptosis, inflammation, and fibrosis.[193] Clinical studies suggest that EPO supplementation in anemic patients with CRS improves cardiac function.[175] In cats with CRS, significant anemia can be corrected with use of EPO or darbepoetin administration (see Chapter 32). Caution is advised when blood transfusions are given to normovolemic anemic cats with CRS, since it can precipitate congestive HF. Chronic gastrointestinal blood loss of CKD should also be considered and treated in anemic cats with CRS with gastrointestinal protectants such as proton pump inhibitors (e.g., omeprazole), H_2 antagonists (e.g., famotidine), or barrier protectants (e.g., sucralfate).

Reviewing and Modifying Drug Dosages

Since cats with CRS receive many drugs, it is important to review and adjust their dosage at each visit. Special care should be taken to check for drug interactions and to prolong the dosing interval of renally excreted drugs, such as atenolol, propranolol, and enalapril, since higher serum levels should be expected when renal function has decreased. However, dosage adjustments may not be appropriate for drugs that are administered to effect such as amlodipine. Hepatic biotransformation of drugs (e.g., diltiazem) can also be altered in some cats with heart failure. More information on drug dosage adjustment for certain disease states can be found in Chapter 4.

PROGNOSIS

In humans with HF, renal dysfunction is strongly linked to increased morbidity and mortality.[214] Moreover, in HF, relative to a decline in ejection fraction, a fall in GFR is a more important factor for worsening prognosis.[101] Negative predictors for development of renal failure in people with HF include old age, low cardiac output, elevated baseline creatinine concentration, progressive rise in creatinine concentration, hypertension, and diuretic and calcium channel blocker therapy.[79,138,208] In a study of cats with hypertrophic cardiomyopathy, azotemia was correlated to older age, lower body weight, and higher systolic blood pressure.[80] Although renal function may remain stable for months in cats with HF, when CRS occurs, it leads to frequent hospitalization, difficulty maintaining good quality of life, and eventually, euthanasia. The therapeutic strategies discussed above are mainly directed at improving the quality of life for cats with CRS. Whether they also contribute to prolonged survival is unknown.

MANAGEMENT OF CONCURRENT PANCREATITIS AND INFLAMMATORY BOWEL DISEASE

Debra L. Zoran

Feline inflammatory bowel disease (IBD) is a term that is applied to a number of poorly understood chronic enteropathies characterized by infiltration of the gastrointestinal (GI) mucosa with inflammatory cells.

The cellular infiltrate in the mucosa of affected cats is composed of variable populations of lymphocytes, plasma cells, eosinophils, and neutrophils that can be distributed throughout the length of the GI tract as well as all layers of the gut wall.[57,97,125,135,252] In severely affected cats, this infiltrate may be accompanied by changes in the mucosal architecture, including villus atrophy and fusion, fibrosis, and lymphangiectasia.[52,239] Although IBD is a common clinical diagnosis in cats, this is often because the term is used as a catch-all to describe all chronic GI diseases, in some cases without biopsy confirmation or an attempt to truly rule out identifiable causes of intestinal inflammation. Nevertheless, our understanding of the etiopathogenesis of feline IBD, or the local and systemic consequences of the disease, including inflammation of surrounding structures, such as the pancreas or common bile duct, is only in early stages of study.

There is increasing evidence that feline IBD is a consequence of alterations in the GI microflora and concurrent increases in proinflammatory cytokines that together result in a persistent, and ultimately aberrant, mucosal immune response.[121,123,236] To further complicate the clinical picture, an increasing number of cats with IBD are recognized (by GI function testing, ultrasound [US], and biopsy) to have concurrent inflammation (nonsuppurative or lymphoplasmacytic) extending to the pancreas, biliary tract, or both (a condition termed triaditis).[55,228,241,242] Thus although IBD is beginning to be characterized beyond the visible changes in gross histopathology, it is also clear that the idea that IBD is a chronic enteropathy with no relationship to the other two common inflammatory diseases of the feline abdomen (cholangitis and pancreatitis) is not consistent with current evidence. This paper will briefly review the key studies that have furthered our understanding of these diseases, and then focus on the current best recommendations for therapy of cats with concurrent IBD and pancreatitis.

UNDERSTANDING WHY INFLAMMATORY BOWEL DISEASE AND PANCREATITIS OCCUR TOGETHER

One of the most important areas of investigation in current IBD research is seeking to understand the role of enteric microflora in the pathogenesis and immune dysfunction of the disease. In recent work by Janeczko and coworkers, intestinal biopsies were collected from 17 cats undergoing diagnostic investigation of signs of GI disease and from 10 healthy controls.[123] Subjective duodenal histopathology ranged from normal (n = 10) to mild (n = 6), moderate (n = 8), or severe (n = 3) IBD. The number and spatial distribution of mucosal bacteria were determined by fluorescent in situ hybridization (FISH) with probes to 16S rDNA. The mucosal response was evaluated by objective histopathology and cytokine mRNA levels in duodenal biopsies. The number of mucosa-associated Enterobacteriaceae was higher in cats with signs of GI disease than in healthy cats.[123] These pathogens, including *Escherichia coli* and *Clostridium* species, were associated with significant changes in mucosal architecture, principally atrophy and fusion; upregulation of cytokines, particularly interleukin-8 (IL-8); and the number of clinical signs exhibited by affected cats.[123] The study findings indicated that an abnormal mucosa-associated flora is associated with the presence and severity of duodenal inflammation and clinical disease activity in cats.[123]

Additional evidence that bacteria are a key component of IBD in cats is shown in an earlier study by Inness and coworkers, who characterized the gut microflora of both healthy cats and cats with colonic IBD using FISH techniques.[121] In this study, cats with colonic IBD were found to have significantly higher populations of *Desulfovibrio* (a genus of bacteria that produce toxic sulfides) compared with normal cats, which had higher populations of bifidobacteria and bacteroides (normal flora).[121] These authors proposed that modulation of intestinal flora with probiotics and dietary intervention to decrease the production of pathogenic bacteria were likely important in treating cats with IBD. These early studies corroborate the findings in numerous human and rodent studies on IBD that the intestinal microbiome is a key factor in maintenance of the health of the GI tract and can be the focal point of inducing an inflammatory response that results in development of IBD and gut dysfunction.[1,63,73] The importance of these findings for clinical management of cats with IBD is to develop a better understanding of intestinal dysbiosis (imbalance of the intestinal microflora) and its potential role in IBD.

One of the major risk factors for development of any form of pancreatitis in cats is concurrent GI disease and particularly IBD.[240-242] In a recent study, approximately 20% of cats with biopsy confirmed pancreatitis had concurrent IBD.[241] In addition, a recent retrospective of feline necropsies revealed evidence of chronic lymphocytic plasmacytic (LP) pancreatitis in 60% to 65% of the specimens—whether or not they had been previously diagnosed with pancreatic disease.[55] This study revealed that many cats have histopathologic evidence of pancreatitis even in the absence of a clinical diagnosis, thus pointing out that an awareness of this often subclinical problem is paramount to looking for it in cats with IBD.

There are certain factors that may contribute to the increased risk of concurrent pancreatitis in cats with IBD: (1) IBD is a common cause of GI disease in cats and the signs of GI disease and pancreatic disease can overlap, so, differentiation of the two can be difficult and (2) the pancreatic and biliary duct anatomy of the cat allows ready access of duodenal fluid that may be refluxed during vomiting or abnormal duodenal motility. Unlike the dog, the feline pancreaticobiliary sphincter is a common anatomic channel at the duodenal papilla. As a result, reflux either from the biliary tree or the duodenum will affect the pancreatic ductal system.[240] In the case of concurrent IBD, the fluid entering the ductal system likely contains a higher number of pathogenic bacteria (or at least an imbalance), bile salts, and activated pancreatic enzymes that when allowed to perfuse the pancreas and biliary tree results in varying degrees of tissue damage, infection, and inflammation.[240,250] In addition to reflux from vomiting, abnormal GI motility and immune dysregulation are likely important in both the reflux of intestinal contents into the pancreatic ducts and development of the inflammation.[240] In summary, although more studies are required to better understand the pathogenesis of concurrent IBD and LP pancreatitis, it is clear that this phenomenon presents an important clinical problem that feline practitioners must try to identify and manage.

MANAGEMENT OF CONCURRENT INFLAMMATORY BOWEL DISEASE AND PANCREATITIS IN CATS: START WITH INFLAMMATORY BOWEL DISEASE THERAPY

Treatment of cats with IBD has not changed significantly for years: antiinflammatory or immune-suppressive therapy with corticosteroids or drugs such as chlorambucil or cyclosporine (if the cat is corticosteroid intolerant or has severe disease not controlled by the corticosteroids), use of antimicrobials with immune-modulating characteristics (e.g., metronidazole or tylosin), and dietary modification aimed at improving the digestibility and reducing the food-related antigens or factors that may induce intolerance.[227] In humans, IBD therapy has also included the use of antibiotics with immune-modulating capacity, prebiotics, probiotics, and immunosuppression, as well as other drugs that modify cytokine release.[1] Unfortunately, studies assessing therapeutic modulation of enteric flora (using probiotics, prebiotics, or other specific therapy for cytokines) in cats with IBD have not yet been reported. Nevertheless, management of IBD in cats will continue to evolve as more studies reveal the importance of therapy that is focused on the normalization of the intestinal microbiome and more specific suppression of cytokines (e.g., dietary therapy, prebiotics, probiotics, and antiinflammatory drugs that are targeted to the GI tract). For detailed, specific information on the management of IBD in cats, please see Chapter 23. Finally, no matter what approach is used, because the disease is so variable and many causative factors are involved, a staged approach to therapy (when possible) is suggested. Sequential clinical treatment trials with antiparasiticides, dietary therapy, and antibacterials (including prebiotics and probiotics) should be tried before initiating immunosuppressive therapy if possible.

GASTROINTESTINAL FUNCTION TESTING IN PLANNING THERAPY

The important role of cobalamin in normal function of the GI tract and in many other aspects of metabolism is well documented.[201,202] In addition, the diagnostic and therapeutic utility of measuring serum concentrations of cobalamin and folate in cats with suspected intestinal disease is also well established.[201,211] However, in cats with IBD that may also have pancreatitis, specific testing for pancreatic leakage and function should be included in the evaluation: feline pancreatic lipase immunoreactivity (fPLI) and feline trypsin-like immunoreactivity (fTLI) are two important tests to perform. Although there are a number of issues associated with the diagnosis of feline pancreatitis and many limitations of fPLI (see Chapter 23), it remains the test of choice for documenting the presence of enzyme leakage from the pancreas and should be measured in all cats with IBD.[72,250,257]

The fTLI test is the diagnostic test of choice for exocrine pancreatic insufficiency (EPI), and although EPI is currently not commonly recognized in cats, it does occur secondary to chronic pancreatitis and results in weight loss (the most common sign), diarrhea, and poor thrift in affected cats.[217,225] This is a relevant problem, because each of those clinical signs can be confused with uncontrolled or recurrent IBD. The repeated monitoring of fTLI, in addition to cobalamin and folate, are important in the management of cats with concurrent IBD and pancreatitis, because cats without deficiencies at the time of diagnosis may develop them later. Comprehensive therapy of concurrent IBD and pancreatitis requires both recognition and correction of these potential enzyme and vitamin deficiencies.

THE ROLE OF DIETARY MANAGEMENT: FOCUS ON THE GASTROINTESTINAL TRACT

The use of diet in the management of GI or pancreatic disease is not a new concept, but the question of which type of diet to use has become an increasingly complex issue. Additionally, there is no evidence in cats with pancreatitis (as there is in dogs) to suggest that dietary fat levels (or any other dietary component) are involved in the pathogenesis of the disease. Thus two key points must be made at the outset: (1) Cats with pancreatitis should not be held NPO, because this increases the risk of development of hepatic lipidosis and is detrimental to GI health and function, and (2) current recommendations for cats with pancreatitis are to focus on finding an appropriate diet for management of the IBD, because control of this disease may result in an improvement in the pancreas as well.[240,250,257]

Although there are few dietary recommendations for cats with pancreatitis, there have been a number of studies and reviews discussing the role of diet in the development and management of IBD.[89,143,227,254] However, the influence of diet type and composition occurs first in healthy, normal cats, because the diet fed is a major determinant of the intestinal microbiome and specifically determines both the numbers and species of bacteria that populate the intestinal tract.[7,66,194,230] Further, the influence on the microflora that occurs because of diet changes can be profound when a major change occurs (e.g., high carbohydrate to high protein, dry to canned food). Thus changes in diet should be done slowly (over days or longer), with careful assessment of progress (especially monitoring for clinical deterioration). Ideally, probiotic therapy should be added to reduce the probability that major shifts in the microbiome will occur as a result of overgrowth of pathogens.[155] Finally, although diet changes have a significant influence on the microflora of healthy cats, this effect can be even more profound in cats with an abnormal flora (such as occurs in cats with IBD). Thus when planning dietary therapy in cats with IBD, there are three critical areas where, because diet may be the inciting cause of the inflammation, correction can influence therapy: (1) diet effects on microbiome (e.g., dysbiosis, or disruption of the microflora), (2) dietary intolerance (nonimmunologic effects on gut function and microbiome), and (3) true dietary allergy. To address these possible causes of diet-induced GI inflammation requires food trials (of varying lengths) using diets aimed at correcting the possible problem. Unfortunately, there is no single diet, or series of diets, or even family of diets that can address each of these potential problems across all cats; it is a process of elimination for the individual patient. The interested reader is referred to Chapter 17 for a review of the approaches that can be used to make a diagnosis of food allergy.

The remainder of this section will focus on the issues of diet intolerance and dysbiosis—difficult to identify but believed to be the most common reasons for diet-induced inflammation in cats.[89,123,143] In many, if not most, cats with mild IBD, especially those with a mild to moderate infiltrate of inflammatory cells and without significant weight loss, the initial approach should be to feed a highly digestible diet (this could include novel or hydrolyzed diets) with single-source meat protein, low amounts of highly digestible carbohydrates, and fewer additives, flavorings, or other substances that may be associated with poor digestibility or food intolerance.[256] Although diets with a high digestibility are not defined in a regulatory sense, this is generally a product with protein digestibility of greater than 87% (typical diets are 78% to 81%) and fat digestibility of greater than 90% (typical diets are 77% to 85%).[256]

The protein digestibility of a diet is one of the key factors that can determine its success in cats with IBD, primarily because undigested protein is a recognized food source for pathogenic bacteria, and can be associated with toxic products in the GI tract that can increase disruption of the microbiome. As a general rule, meat-source proteins (including meat meals) are more digestible than plant-source proteins (there are some exceptions, such as soy), and animal proteins are more digestible than meat byproducts. Further, in cats with IBD, the type and amount of carbohydrates added to the diet must also be considered, since malabsorption of carbohydrates can occur without causing clinical signs.[54,230] To address this, diets with a single carbohydrate source are preferable to foods with many different sources, and highly digestible carbohydrate sources are better than complex grain source carbohydrates (e.g., wheat or corn).[256]

It is important to recognize that when one diet from this category is not accepted by the cat or does not improve the clinical signs, it cannot be assumed that all diets in this category will not be accepted by the patient or will be ineffective. Many different brands fall under the category of "highly digestible," but they are not all alike and will not necessarily have the same effect in all cats. The formulation of highly digestible diets from different pet food manufacturers is quite variable, with different protein and carbohydrate sources and amounts and different amounts of fat; also some of the diets may contain various additives designed to promote intestinal health (e.g., fructo-oligosaccharides [FOS], mannosoligosaccharides [MOS], omega-3 fatty acids, antioxidant vitamins, and soluble fiber). If one type of highly digestible diet has been fed for at least 2 weeks with minimal response, then it is entirely reasonable to try another diet from the same category, but from a different manufacturer or try an entirely different dietary strategy (e.g., high-protein/low-carbohydrate novel antigen, hydrolyzed diet). As previously mentioned, because changes in diet type and source can result in significant changes in the intestinal microbiota, the addition of probiotics or prebiotics as part of the therapy is reasonable to help prevent further disruption of the microflora.[155]

NORMALIZING THE MICROBIOME: ANTIBIOTICS AND PROBIOTICS

Although correction of the diet is a key step in normalizing the intestinal microbiome, it may not be sufficient to suppress the pathogenic species that have overpopulated the intestinal lumen. As a result, antibiotic therapy with metronidazole has been effectively used for a

TABLE 35-3 **Table of Dosages for Drugs Commonly Used in Feline Pancreatitis and Inflammatory Bowel Disease***

Drug Name	Role	Dosage
Prednisolone/Methylprednisolone 5- or 20-mg tabs/2- or 4-mg tabs	Antiinflammatory and immunosuppressive	1-2 mg/kg, PO, q12-24h
Budesonide (3-mg capsules)	Antiinflammatory: high first-pass metabolism	0.125 mg/kg, PO, q8-12h
Buprenorphine (0.3 mg/mL injectable)	Opioid pain reliever	0.005-0.01 mg/kg, SC, q8h 0.01-0.02 mg/kg, PO, q12h (buccal)
Metronidazole (250-mg tabs, 50 mg/mL suspension)	Antibiotic Immunomodulator	5-15 mg/kg, PO, q12h
Tylosin (2.5-2.7 g/tsp)	Antibiotic	7-15 mg/kg, PO, q12-24h
Chlorambucil (2-mg tabs)	Immunosuppressive	0.1-0.2 mg/kg, PO, q24h once then q48h (monitor CBC)
Cyclosporine (10-, 25-, 50-mg capsules, 100 mg/mL solution)	Immunosuppressive	5 mg/kg, PO, q12h, can reduce to q24h or q48h as clinically indicated
Cyproheptadine (4-mg tabs)	Appetite stimulant	2-4 mg/cat (½ or 1 tablet), PO, q12h
Mirtazapine (15-mg tabs)	Appetite stimulant	⅛ tablet, PO, q3d
Ursodiol (250-mg tabs)	Tertiary bile acid Antiinflammatory	5-15 mg/kg, PO, q24h
S-Adenosylmethionine (SAMe) alone or with Marin (milk thistle) (90-mg tabs)	Antioxidant Antiinflammatory nutraceutical	90 mg/cat, PO, q24h

*Doses from: Papich MG: *Saunders handbook of veterinary drugs*, ed 2, St Louis, 2007, Elsevier.
CBC, Complete blood count.

number of years and continues to be recommended in the therapy of IBD (Table 35-3).[227] A number of other antibiotics have been used empirically in management of feline intestinal disease, but there is no current evidence to indicate the use of other antibiotics that are directed at gram-negative or other bacteria. In fact, frequent use of broad-spectrum antibiotics will result in a further disruption of the microbiome that may contribute to worsening of the inflammation and dysbiosis, rather than improving the situation.

In cats with LP pancreatitis concurrent with IBD, any infection that occurs in the pancreas will be an extension of the flora in the small intestine and thus should be treated with antibiotics appropriate for IBD. At this time, the only form of IBD that is known to be caused by a specific bacterial species is Boxer colitis, which is caused by an enterotoxigenic form of *E. coli*.[210] In that disease, specific antibiotic regimens are suggested based on targeting therapy toward controlling that specific bacterial infection, and in Boxer dogs, complete resolution of the disease is expected by appropriate antibiotic therapy. In feline IBD, however, multiple and different bacterial pathogens have been identified in affected cats[121,194]; so, although bacterial disruption is still believed to be the trigger for the inflammatory disease process, specific antibiotic therapy is currently not recommended, and the therapeutic approach must be aimed at normalizing the intestinal microbiome by other means.

One of the reasons that metronidazole is effective in cats with IBD is likely not only because of its antibacterial properties but also because of its immune-modulating properties.[231] However, because metronidazole may be poorly tolerated and has significant potential for serious adverse effects, including neurotoxicity and reversible DNA damage in intestinal cells, it should not be given indefinitely.[206] The current recommendation is to use metronidazole for no longer than 2 to 3 weeks at a time, then stop therapy for at least several weeks to prevent accumulated DNA damage.[206] An alternative to metronidazole therapy in cats with IBD is tylosin; however, less is known about the effects of tylosin in cats with IBD or if it also has immune-modulating effects in cats, as it appears to have in dogs.[219]

Interest in the role of probiotics in prevention or treatment of gastrointestinal disease in humans and animals has been the most widely known aspect of their long history. Human and experimental studies with probiotics have targeted specific health benefits associated with three functional areas of the gut microbiota: metabolic effects, protective effects, and trophic effects.[155] The *metabolic* effects of probiotics refer to their effects on digestion, particularly in digestion of lactose and other disaccharides, and in the production of intestinal gas, a significant problem in patients with irritable bowel syndrome (IBS). Some microbial species produce large amounts of gas, and other species consume gas particularly hydrogen; however, it is this balance that reflects the amount, frequency, and odor of intestinal gas production. To date, it appears that bifidobacterial species have the highest rates of therapeutic benefit in adult humans with IBS.[73] However, in a study in colicky infants, a *Lactobacillus* strain resulted in the greatest reduction in intestinal bloating and gas.[73] These different responses highlight the complexity of interactions among the microflora in each unique ecological habitat and emphasize the need to be cautious in predicting specific responses in individual subjects.

The *protective* effects of probiotics on the gastrointestinal tract include the prevention and treatment of acute diarrhea due to antibiotics or infectious enteritis and prevention of systemic infections (septicemia) from bacterial translocation.[73,88] There have been a plethora of clinical trials studying the efficacy of probiotics in the treatment of acute diarrhea in adults (e.g., infectious diarrhea, traveler's diarrhea); however, the evidence is most compelling for the administration of probiotics to decrease morbidity in people with antibiotic-associated diarrhea.

The third important area of probiotic influence in the gastrointestinal tract is their *trophic* effects on mucosal immunity and epithelial cell growth. Three specific conditions fall under this umbrella: inflammatory bowel disease (IBD), food allergy, and colon cancer. It is well known that certain bacteria activate proinflammatory mucosal responses, while others downregulate intestinal inflammation. Thus creating a favorable local microecology has been hypothesized to restore homeostasis of the local immune response and would lead to resolution of the intestinal inflammation.[73,88] Although evidence in humans with IBD supports the use of probiotics, there are no similar studies in cats with IBD or other chronic enteropathies.[155] Thus, although probiotic therapy in cats with IBD would be a reasonable therapeutic option, there have been no studies reported to date that identify the best probiotic species or combination of species to use or that show benefit from adding probiotics to the therapeutic plan.

CONTROL OF INFLAMMATION IN PANCREATITIS AND INFLAMMATORY BOWEL DISEASE

Both IBD and pancreatitis are inflammatory diseases for which interruption of the inflammatory process is an important part of the clinical management.[227] However, that being said, there are no studies that have carefully assessed the effectiveness of corticosteroid therapy in treatment of LP pancreatitis in cats. Thus recommendations to use corticosteroid therapy in the treatment of chronic pancreatitis in cats are anecdotal. The most effective antiinflammatory or immunosuppressive drugs for IBD (and presumably pancreatitis) are corticosteroids (i.e., prednisolone or methylprednisolone) or other drugs that interrupt the proinflammatory pathways that are active in the gut (e.g., cytotoxic drugs, such as chlorambucil or cyclosporine).[81,227] Prednisolone is more reliably metabolized than prednisone in cats; therefore the former should be chosen for therapy.[81] Dexamethasone is also effective, but is associated with a much higher incidence of severe adverse events, including intestinal ulceration; so, routine use is not recommended.

However, as is well known, chronic therapy with corticosteroids can result in development of significant insulin resistance, the major precursor to diabetes in obese cats or cats with pancreatitis. Thus alternatives to prednisolone, such as budesonide may also be a reasonable choice. There are no studies showing efficacy of this agent in cats; anecdotal reports suggest variability in clinical response. Alternatively, in cats in which corticosteroids are not effective or are causing additional morbidity, other immunosuppressive drugs may be necessary. The two drugs most commonly recommended and effective for cats in this setting are chlorambucil and cyclosporine. Chlorambucil is the best first choice based on its long record of use in IBD, and although adverse effects such as bone marrow suppression are possible, they are unlikely due to the low frequency of administration (once every 2 to 3 days, PO), also making it attractive for patient management and client compliance.[227] Cyclosporine therapy for cats with IBD has not been studied extensively, but it must be given every 12 hours, is much more expensive, and drug levels must be measured to prevent toxicity and ensure therapeutic dosing levels. Thus cyclosporine is not recommended unless the IBD is severe and unresponsive to other therapy. Whatever therapeutic options are chosen, it is important to use antiinflammatory or immune suppressive therapy judiciously (but long enough) and at the lowest doses necessary to achieve clinical control.

OTHER CONSIDERATIONS IN THERAPY OF PANCREATITIS AND INFLAMMATORY BOWEL DISEASE

In addition to antiinflammatory therapy, modulation of bacteria and dietary therapy for management of cats with concurrent IBD and pancreatitis, there are several other adjunctive therapeutic options that may be important and/or even essential. The first is careful consideration of adding pain therapy into the treatment regimen. It is well known that acute pancreatitis is a painful disease[218]; opioid analgesics are the most appropriate drugs used to control this pain.[240,250] However, because LP pancreatitis is a chronic disease, and may have only focal or low-grade inflammation, this low-grade pain may be difficult to detect.[240,250] In humans with chronic pancreatitis, a disease with a similar presentation and clinical course, low-grade upper quadrant pain is common, and results in lack of appetite and general malaise.[218] Pain in people with pancreatitis that does not resolve with antiinflammatory therapy is frequently managed with either opioid medications or biliary stenting.[218] The key point is that cats may have low-grade pain that is manifested by hiding, decreased appetite, or even occasional vomiting, and thus use of opioid pain medications is indicated (see Table 35-2).

In addition to symptomatic therapy for pain in cats with pancreatitis, use of ursodeoxycholic acid (ursodiol) therapy can be beneficial by improving bile flow, preventing sludging, and reducing inflammation of the biliary tree and pancreas.[183,250] Further, in cats that are intolerant of steroid therapy for control of inflammation, addition of antioxidant and antiinflammatory nutraceuticals into the therapeutic plan can be potentially beneficial. Although no controlled studies evaluating the effectiveness of S-adenosylmethionine (SAMe) therapy in feline pancreatitis or IBD have been performed, studies in cats with liver disease reveal significant increases in liver glutathione concentrations and improvement in liver enzyme levels.[41] This antioxidant nutraceutical is commonly used in humans with chronic pancreatitis and IBD, and thus may also be a reasonable adjunctive therapy in cats.

Finally, because many cats with chronic pancreatitis have bouts of inappetence or decreased appetite, appetite stimulants may be indicated to encourage eating and prevent the need for placement of a feeding tube (see Table 35-2). Mirtazapine therapy in cats is very convenient, because dosing is only needed every 3 to 4 days because of its long half-life. One note of caution about use of mirtazapine in cats is advised, because some cats display significant mood changes or even hyperactivity; so, starting with the lowest possible dose is strongly suggested. Regardless of the appetite stimulant used, calculation of the daily nutritional requirements should be undertaken as well as monitoring the actual amount of food eaten.

CONCLUSION

Management of concurrent IBD and pancreatitis in cats can be a challenge, especially in cats that become diabetic or intolerant of steroid therapy. As in all chronic disease management, the goal of therapy is improving the cat's quality of life by controlling the severity of the disease while aiming for clinical remission. Control of both of these conditions is best achieved by using a combination of dietary therapy, drug therapy as needed, and frequent monitoring of progress. However, each cat will present individual challenges that require the clinician to make adjustments in the therapeutic approach. Also, because cats with chronic pancreatitis can develop diabetes or EPI as a result of progressive loss of functional pancreatic tissue, frequent re-evaluation of GI function testing and clinical response is essential to long-term success.

CHRONIC KIDNEY DISEASE AND HYPERTENSION

Scott A. Brown

PREVALENCE

Chronic kidney disease (CKD) is common in cats, particularly those greater than 10 years of age.[140] Approximately 20% of cats with CKD exhibit elevations of systemic arterial blood pressure (AP),[221] which may contribute to clinical signs, damage tissues and organs, and enhance the rate of progression of CKD.

THE KIDNEY: CAUSE OF HYPERTENSION OR A TARGET ORGAN?

The cause of systemic hypertension in a cat with CKD is usually unknown, although altered handling of fluids and electrolytes by the kidney, as well as alteration in the renin-angiotensin-aldosterone axis (RAAA) and sympathetic nervous system overactivity are potential contributory factors.

Chronically sustained elevations of AP produce injury to tissues; the rationale for treatment of hypertension is to minimize or prevent this injury, which occurs in the kidney, eyes, brain, and/or cardiovascular system.[22] Damage that results from the presence of sustained high AP is commonly referred to as end-organ or target-organ damage (TOD), and the presence of TOD is generally a strong indication favoring antihypertensive therapy. In CKD, the renal microcirculation is more susceptible to barotrauma from elevated AP because of the afferent arteriolar vasodilation that occurs in cats with renal azotemia.[23] In the kidney, TOD is generally manifest as an enhanced rate of decline of renal function, proteinuria, and/or increased mortality rate.[18,27,65,186] Proteinuria is directly related to degree of elevation of AP and rate of decline of kidney function, while inversely related to efficacy and benefit of antihypertensive therapy.[70,186]

RELATIONSHIP OF SYSTEMIC ARTERIAL PRESSURE TO RISK AND INTERNATIONAL RENAL INTEREST SOCIETY CLASSIFICATION

The International Renal Interest Society (IRIS) has proposed that a staging system be used to facilitate the management of feline patients with CKD (see Chapter

32).[65] This classification scheme is based on a three-step process:

- Establish a diagnosis of CKD
- Establish the stage of the disease[168]
- Establish the substages of the disease based on assessment of AP and proteinuria as systemic hypertension and proteinuria may be observed in any stage of CKD

Thus for all cats with CKD, AP measurement and quantification of urinary protein excretion should be performed. This allows the veterinarian to stage the disease properly, linking to prognosis[18] and diagnostic as well as treatment recommendations.[65]

SUBSTAGING CHRONIC KIDNEY DISEASE ON BASIS OF SYSTEMIC ARTERIAL BLOOD PRESSURE

Cats with CKD frequently exhibit elevations of AP.[221] The American College of Veterinary Internal Medicine (ACVIM) Consensus Statement[22] and IRIS[65] have proposed that the risk of TOD is directly related to the degree of AP elevation and have defined systemic hypertension as any elevation of AP that leads to TOD and proposed blood pressure ranges associated with minimal (AP0), low (AP1), moderate (AP2), and severe (AP3) risk of TOD (Table 35-4). A "c" is added to the AP stage if complications (TOD) are present. A notation of "nc" would indicate no complications (TOD) are present. However, kidney disease is generally presumed to be evidence of TOD in cats so that all hypertensive cats with CKD should be denoted as "c". A (T) is added to the substage if the AP measurement was obtained while the cat was receiving antihypertensive therapy.

The IRIS recommends that AP be measured using a device and method individualized for each clinical practice in every cat with CKD and that all target organs be carefully evaluated for the presence of TOD complications.[65] Although some devices provide both systolic and diastolic AP, staging is most often done on the basis of systolic AP measurements, because recent evidence suggests that systolic hypertension is the most important determinant of TOD in other species.[22] Although it is critical for the veterinarian to fully appreciate the subtleties of AP measurement, it is generally preferred to have these measurements obtained by a skilled animal health technician who has been suitably trained. The AP may be affected by stress or anxiety associated with the measurement process, the so-called white-coat effect.[12] It is important for the room in which the measurement is performed to be quiet and for the patient to have 5 to 10 minutes to acclimate to the room prior to evaluation to reduce the likelihood of this anxiety-induced hypertension.

TABLE 35-4 **Arterial Blood Pressure (AP) Substaging of Feline Chronic Kidney Disease**

	Substage			
	AP0 (Minimal or no risk)	**AP1 (Low risk)**	**AP2 (Moderate risk)**	**AP3 (High risk)**
BLOOD PRESSURE (MM HG)				
Systolic	<150	150-159	160-179	≥180
Diastolic	<95	95-99	100-119	≥120

If blood pressure is not measured, the patient is classified as risk not determined (RND).
If complications of high AP are present, a "c" is appended to the substage. If absent then "nc" indicates no complications have been observed. Complications include any evidence of target organ damage in eyes (e.g., intraocular hemorrhage or retinal detachment), central nervous system (e.g., seizures or profound otherwise unexplained depression), cardiovascular system (e.g., congestive heart failure), or kidneys (e.g., azotemia or proteinuria).
If antihypertensive therapy is instituted, subsequent staging of hypertension should be based on the current actual blood pressure, with (T) appended to indicate that this level reflects the effects of therapy.
For example, if a cat with chronic kidney disease (CKD) that presented with a systolic AP of 185 mm Hg (AP substage of AP3c) was treated with the calcium channel blocker amlodipine, and is now being re-evaluated and the systolic AP is 145 mm Hg, the cat's new AP substage is AP0c (T). Here the "c" reflects the presence of complications (i.e., chronic kidney disease, which is always presumed to represent a complication of hypertension), and the (T) indicates that the second set of AP measurements was taken while the cat was on antihypertensive therapy.

The choice of device depends upon operator experience and preference. For indirect devices, the cuff width should be 30% to 40% of the circumference at the chosen measurement site.[22] Measurements may be taken on the antebrachium, brachium, tarsus, or tail. The position of the patient and cuff should be one that is well tolerated with the cuff at, or close to, the level of the right atrium. At least five consecutive, consistent indirect values should be obtained with adequate time between each arterial occlusion. The highest and lowest values are then discarded and the remaining values averaged to produce the actual measurement. Because hypertension in cats with CKD is often a silent condition requiring vigilance and lifelong therapy, it is important to be absolutely certain about the diagnosis: a single high AP measurement may represent true hypertension or white-coat (anxiety-induced) hypertension. Except in the case of rapidly progressive hypertensive crises, multiple measurements should be obtained, preferably separated by at least 24 hours, and always accompanied by a thorough search for TOD before a diagnosis of systemic hypertension is established.

SUBSTAGING CHRONIC KIDNEY DISEASE ON BASIS OF PROTEINURIA

Recent findings have suggested that renal protein leak is not only a marker of severity of renal disease but also of prognostic value in animals treated with

TABLE 35-5 **Proteinuria Substaging of Feline Chronic Kidney Disease**

	Substage		
	Nonproteinuric (NP)	**Borderline Proteinuric (BP)**	**Proteinuric (P)**
Urine protein-to-creatinine ratio (UP/C)	<0.2	0.2-0.4	>0.4

If antihypertensive or antiproteinuric (e.g., restricted protein diet) therapy is instituted, subsequent staging of proteinuria should be based on the current actual UP/C, with (T) appended to indicate that this level reflects the effects of therapy.
For example, suppose a cat with chronic kidney disease (CKD) has a systolic AP of 140 mm Hg (AP0, no antihypertensive therapy indicated). However, the UP/C was 0.8, and thus the proteinuria substage was P. You decided to try to reduce the magnitude of the proteinuria by feeding the cat a protein-restricted diet that is supplemented with fish oil and to administer the angiotensin-converting enzyme inhibitor, benazepril. It is now being re-evaluated and UP/C is 0.3. The proteinuria substage is now BP (T) for borderline proteinuric while on therapy.

antihypertensives.[27,124,223] Proteinuria is associated with increased risk of developing end-stage CKD in cats,[223] and there is an increased risk of mortality in aged cats when proteinuria is present. Further, studies have shown that therapies that reduce the magnitude of proteinuria are often beneficial to the patient and may slow progression of CKD.

According to IRIS recommendations, proteinuria should be assessed in all cats with CKD (or systemic hypertension). A positive finding of proteinuria in a urinalysis with routine dipstick evaluation is the first step, which should lead the veterinarian to carefully evaluate the urine sediment findings to determine if inflammation or infection may be the cause. Because of frequent false positives with routine urine dipsticks in cats, a positive result should be confirmed by a more specific test for proteinuria that provides information on the magnitude of proteinuria, such as measurement of the urine protein/creatinine ratio (UP/C) or quantitative assessment of albuminuria. When monitoring a feline patient with renal proteinuria, it is important to determine if the proteinuria is transient or persistent (at least two tests at 2-week intervals) because only the latter justifies the institution of therapy.

Substaging of renal proteinuria should be performed in all cats with CKD (Table 35-5).[65,147] A (T) is added to the substage if the measurement was obtained when the cat was receiving antihypertensive or antiproteinuric (e.g., restricted protein diet) therapy. If persistent renal proteinuria is present in a patient with CKD and hypertension, further management is generally based on the UP/C and AP measurements.

Complete IRIS staging of a cat with CKD should reflect the IRIS stage and as well as substage for both AP and proteinuria. For example, if a cat with IRIS stage III CKD that is being treated with antihypertensive agents

TABLE 35-6 **Oral Agents for Chronic Antihypertensive Therapy in Cats with Chronic Kidney Disease**

Class	**Drug (Examples of Trade Name)**	**Usual Oral Dosage**
Angiotensin-converting enzyme inhibitor	Benazepril (Lotensin, Fortekor)	0.5-1.0 mg/kg q24h
	Enalapril (Vasotec, Enacard)	0.5-1.0 mg/kg q24h
Calcium channel blocker	Amlodipine (Norvasc)	0.1-0.5 mg/kg q24h
Aldosterone antagonist	Spironolactone (Aldactone)	1.0-2.0 mg/kg q12h
Direct vasodilator	Hydralazine (Apresoline)	2.5 mg/cat q12-24h
Alpha$_1$ blocker	Prazosin (Minipress)	0.25-0.5 mg/cat q24h
	Phenoxybenazime (Dibenzyline)	2.5 mg per cat q8-12h or 0.5 mg/cat q24h
	Acepromazine (PromAce)	0.5-2 mg/kg q8h
Beta blocker	Propranolol (Inderal)	2.5-5 mg/cat q8h
	Atenolol (Tenormin)	6.25-12.5 mg/cat q12h

is re-evaluated and retinal hemorrhages are observed, the systolic AP is 165 mm Hg and the UP/C is 0.5, then the cat is IRIS stage III AP2c P (T). Here the "c" reflects the presence of complications of hypertension (i.e., proteinuria, azotemia, and retinopathy), and the (T) indicates that the measurements have been taken while the cat is on antihypertensive therapy.

EMERGENCY THERAPY: HYPERTENSIVE CRISES

Hypertension generally damages tissues by a slow, insidious process and is rarely an urgent situation. This is always the case for renal injury in cats with CKD. However, emergency antihypertensive therapy may be indicated when a cat is AP2c or AP3c and there is ocular or neurologic TOD that is likely to produce significant permanent abnormalities without rapid lowering of AP (e.g., seizures or retinal detachment where either is attributed to the high AP). If a decision is made to treat a cat with what is judged to be a hypertensive crisis, therapeutic intervention will generally be with a parenteral agent, such as 0.2 mg/kg hydralazine IV or IM, repeated q2h as needed, or an oral calcium channel blocker (CCB) (Table 35-6). If parenteral medications are used, frequent repeated (at least every 30 minutes) AP monitoring is recommended. As an alternative, many veterinarians prefer oral CCBs (e.g., 0.25 to 0.5 mg amlodipine, PO, every 24 hours) because they generally decrease AP regardless of the underlying primary

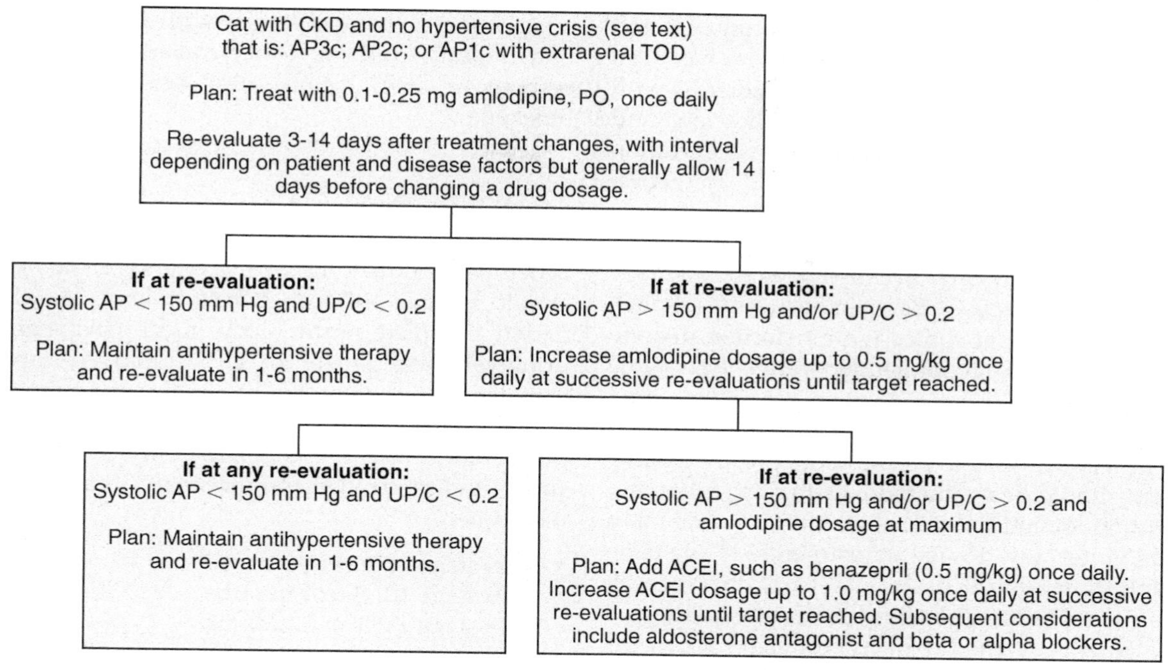

FIGURE 35-3 Approach to treatment of concurrent chronic kidney disease (CKD) and hypertension.

disease. Amlodipine generally reduces BP by 25 to 50 mm Hg in hypertensive cats within 4 hours of oral administration and poses limited risk of causing hypotension. If an oral CCB is used, it may be appropriate to send the animal home to reduce the stress associated with hospitalization and re-evaluate AP and TOD in 24 to 72 hours.

CHRONIC THERAPY: DOSAGES AND MONITORING

Decisions to use antihypertensive drugs should be based on integration of all clinically available information; a decision to treat, which may effectively mandate lifelong drug therapy, warrants periodic, judicious re-evaluation. Antihypertensive therapy must be individualized to the patient and its concurrent conditions. Regardless of the initial level of AP, the ideal goal of therapy should be to maximally reduce the risk of TOD, which generally means stage AP0 (systolic AP < 150 and diastolic AP < 95 mm Hg) and UP/C less than 0.2. Often, a more realistic goal of therapy is to achieve a UP/C less than 0.4 and a reduction by at least one AP stage, which generally equates to a drop in AP greater than 20 mm Hg. Except in hypertensive crises (see above), this can be achieved with a gradual, persistent reduction of AP. Although frequently recommended as an initial step in the management of high AP, restriction of dietary salt is controversial,[35,134] and available evidence suggests significant sodium restriction alone generally does not reduce AP and in fact, in dogs, activates the RAAA with a resulting elevation of AP in certain settings.[84,96] On the other hand, high salt intake may produce adverse consequences,[134] particularly in animals with chronic kidney disease. Until more data are available, the selection of appropriate diet should be based on other patient-specific factors, such as underlying or concurrent diseases and palatability.

In cats with CKD and either an AP in the moderate- or high-risk substage (AP2 and AP3; see Table 35-4) or extrarenal TOD (e.g., hypertensive retinopathy) in substage AP1, antihypertensive therapy is appropriate (Figure 35-3). Once a decision is made to treat a cat with high AP, therapeutic intervention will almost always include a pharmacologic agent.

IMPORTANCE OF SUSTAINING RENAL FUNCTION DURING ANTIHYPERTENSIVE THERAPY

In human beings with essential hypertension, azotemia is absent and diuretics and beta blockers are commonly used as first-line therapy. However, these agents can produce dehydration (diuretics) and activate the renin-angiotensin-aldosterone system (diuretics and beta blockers), which is undesirable in cats with CKD. As a result, antihypertensives whose mode of action is vasodilation are most commonly used in hypertensive cats with CKD. These agents include CCBs and angiotensin-converting enzyme inhibitors (ACEIs), because they tend to sustain renal function while reducing AP and UP/C (see Table 35-6 and Figure 35-3). There has been some concern about acute exacerbation of azotemia with ACEIs, though this is an unusual complication, and modest increases in serum creatinine concentration (<0.5 mg/dL [44.2 μmol/L]) may occur and are generally tolerable.

The ACEIs and CCBs are the most widely used antihypertensive agents in cats. Because of their dramatic antihypertensive efficacy, CCBs, specifically amlodipine, are the treatment of first choice with a starting dose in the lower half of the recommended range (see Table 35-6). Often a 2.5-mg (or 5-mg) tablet is carefully halved or quartered for dosing. This medication may be compounded by a pharmacist to permit more precise dosing.

A patient should be evaluated 3 to 14 days following the institution of antihypertensive therapy and at a similar time after any dosage adjustments. In unstable patients and those with IRIS stage IV CKD, this recheck should be conducted in a shorter time frame, perhaps 3 to 7 days. Patients deemed to be hypertensive emergencies (see above) and hospitalized patients, particularly those receiving fluid therapy or pharmacologic agents with cardiovascular effects, should be assessed daily. The purpose of these short-term assessments is to determine if there are any unexpected (e.g., new or worsening TOD) or adverse findings (e.g., marked worsening of azotemia or development of systemic hypotension). An AP less than 120/60 mm Hg combined with clinical findings of weakness, syncope, and/or marked tachycardia indicates systemic hypotension, and therapy should be adjusted accordingly.

The ideal target is to adjust therapy to achieve an AP with minimal risk of further TOD (i.e., systolic AP < 150 mm Hg) and to eliminate proteinuria (i.e., UP/C < 0.2). In most hypertensive cats with CKD, treatment with a CCB alone or with a CCB plus an ACEI will provide acceptable control of AP and proteinuria. It will be impossible to achieve both targets in many patients, making it important to individualize care using clinical judgment. If adequate antihypertensive effect is observed and the patient remains stable, subsequent re-evaluation may be performed 3 to 6 weeks later. If additional lowering of AP is desired, the CCB dose may be increased (generally by doubling dosage up to the maximum dosage of 0.5 mg/kg, PO, every 24 hours). Amlodipine has a 30-hour duration of effect on AP in cats; so, twice daily dosing is not helpful. If a patient remains proteinuric and/or hypertensive on a CCB, the addition of an ACEI without lowering the CCB dosage is appropriate. If the combination of a CCB plus an ACEI is incompletely effective, an aldosterone antagonist (e.g., spironolactone) or a beta blocker (e.g., atenolol) may be added. The former is of theoretical value, since cats with CKD seem to be prone to hyperaldosteronism. Atenolol or another beta blocker may be more efficacious as supplemental therapy in cats with CKD, hypertension, and hyperthyroidism. Other considerations for poorly responsive cases include oral hydralazine and alpha blockers.

ADDITIONAL PATIENT EVALUATIONS

Scheduled evaluations of hypertensive cats with CKD should include a thorough history and physical examination, complete serum biochemical panel, hematology, urinalysis, assessment of UP/C and AP, ophthalmic examination, and aerobic bacterial urine culture. Evaluations should be done every 1 to 4 months in cats with poorly controlled AP and UP/C. If AP and UP/C are stable and controlled, approximate intervisit intervals would be

- IRIS stages I and II: 6 months
- IRIS stage III: 3 to 4 months
- IRIS stage IV: 1 to 2 months

As noted above, cats with concurrent CKD and hypertension with unstable renal function, extrarenal complications of hypertension, or cats that are undergoing adjustments to therapy should also be seen more frequently, often every 3 to 14 days.

CONCLUSION

The proper management of a cat with concurrent CKD and systemic hypertension requires a clear understanding of the interaction between these two entities, an appreciation of the role of judicious use of antihypertensive agents, and frequent re-evaluations of AP, UP/C, and serum creatinine.

IMMUNE DEFICIENCY, STRESS, AND INFECTION

Lisa M. Singer and Leah A. Cohn

IMMUNODEFICIENCY

A cat is protected from potential pathogens by physical (e.g., epithelial surfaces) and mechanical (e.g., cough reflex) barriers as well as the innate and adaptive immune responses. Generic responses to potential pathogens form the innate immune system. These responses include phagocytosis, attack by natural killer cells, and complement-mediated destruction, among others. For those pathogens that evade physical barriers and innate responses, a more specific, targeted set of responses is evoked. These adaptive responses are particular to a given pathogen, and once they have been stimulated, memory of that response is retained such that subsequent responses to that pathogen are improved in quantity and quality. Both cell-mediated immunity (CMI) and humoral immunity are branches of this adaptive immune response. Both intimately involve the actions of lymphocytes and are guided in part by helper T-lymphocytes (CD4+). In CMI, pathogens are destroyed largely through the actions of cytotoxic T lymphocytes (CD8+), while humoral immunity relies on antibody secreted from activated B lymphocytes (i.e., plasma cells).

Immunodeficiency occurs when one or more components of the immune system are compromised, and cats suffering from immunodeficiency are said to be immunocompromised. These cats are more susceptible to infection than healthy cats, and established infections can be a challenge to cure. In addition, some immunodeficiencies of the adaptive immune system predispose the patient to cancer, especially lymphoproliferative and skin cancers.[50,94,215] Primary immunodeficiency results from an inherited or congenital defect in innate, CMI, and/or humoral immunity. Secondary immunodeficiency occurs when acquired disease or therapy damages immune protections. Although the immune system offers redundant and overlapping protective mechanisms, innate phagocytic, CMI, and humoral immunity are each particularly adept at providing protection from certain types of pathogens (Figure 35-4).

Primary hereditary immunodeficiencies are extremely rare in cats. They are suspected when several related kittens die in utero, fail to thrive after birth, or succumb to early infection. Other clues to the presence of primary immunodeficiency are persistent or recurrent infections in young animals, atypical infections, failure to respond to vaccination, hypoglobulinemia, persistent leukopenia, or morphologic abnormalities in white blood cells. Some hereditary abnormalities of the immune system are benign, while others increase susceptibility to infection to varying degrees. Only a handful of primary immunodeficiencies are recognized in cats (Table 35-7), but it is quite likely that additional abnormalities are as yet unrecognized.

The vast majority of immunocompromised cats have an acquired immunodeficiency state. The causes are varied (Box 35-3) and may impact a single aspect of immunity (e.g., immune mediated neutropenia affects only innate phagocytic immunity) or several components of immunity (e.g., malnutrition affects innate, CMI, and humoral immunity).[132] Some causes of acquired immunodeficiency are reversible, for instance, withdrawal of immunosuppressive drug therapy. Others can be addressed directly, for instance, administration of plasma to kittens with failure of passive transfer.[151] Unfortunately, for many causes of immunodeficiency,

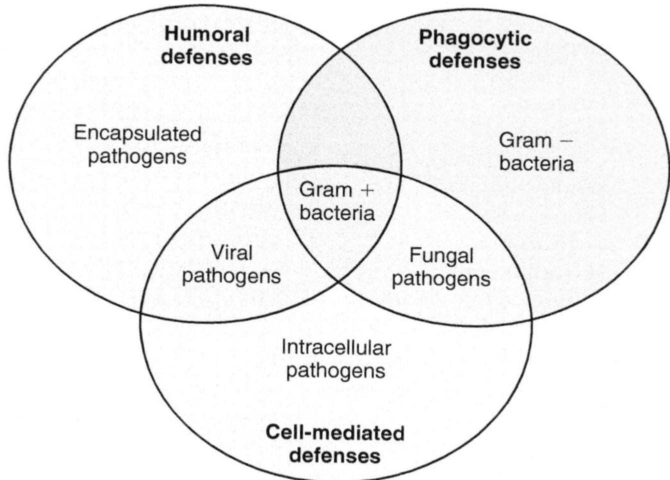

FIGURE 35-4 Although protections from various aspects of the immune system are redundant and overlapping, each is particularly adept at providing protection from certain types of insult. The types of infections that occur offer clues to the type of immunodeficiency present. For instance, defects of phagocytic immunity leave the host particularly susceptible to bacterial and fungal infections without much impact on susceptibility to viral infection.

TABLE 35-7 **Primary Immunodeficiency Syndromes of Cats**

Immunodeficiency	Defect	Effect	Diagnosis
Pelger-Huet anomaly (various cat breeds)[49,145]	Granulocyte nuclear hyposegmentation	Little if any impact on disease susceptibility	Morphologic examination of stained blood smears
Chediak-Higashi Syndrome (blue smoke Persians)[139]	Impaired phagocyte, platelet, and melanin granule membrane fusion	Minimal compromise of innate phagocytic immunity; color dilution; bleeding caused by defective platelet granules	Morphologic examination of stained blood smears
Neutrophil granule anomaly (Birman cats)[102]	Eosinophilic granules in the cytoplasm of neutrophils	Little if any impact on disease susceptibility	Morphologic exam of stained blood smears
Hypotrichosis with thymic atrophy (Birman cats)[40]	Kittens are born hairless and without a thymus, the site of T-lymphocyte development	Stillbirth, early euthanasia, or death because of infections in first 3 months	Suspected in hairless Birman kittens; thoracic imaging; lymphocyte blastogenesis; necropsy

BOX 35-3
Causes of Secondary Immunodeficiency in Cats

- **Infectious disease**
  Feline leukemia virus
  Feline immunodeficiency virus
  Panleukopenia
- **Endocrinopathy**
  Diabetes mellitus
  Hyperadrenocorticism
- **Neoplastic disease**
  Lymphoma
  Leukemia
  Multiple myeloma
- **Immune-mediated disease**
  Immune-mediated neutropenia
- **Metabolic disease**
  Renal failure
  Hepatic failure
  Malnutrition
- **Iatrogenic**
  Splenectomy
  Chemotherapy
  Whole body radiation
  Glucocorticoids
  Cyclosporine
- **Miscellaneous**
  Failure of passive transfer
  Extremes of age
  Pregnancy
  Neutropenia of any cause
  Stress?

while the secondary infections can be treated, the underlying immunodeficiency state cannot be corrected.

The most common causes of immunodeficiency in cats are infection with the retroviruses: feline immunodeficiency virus (FIV) and feline leukemia virus (FeLV). Cats infected with FeLV may develop blood dyscrasias or neoplasia, but often succumb to secondary infections within 1 to 3 years of diagnosis. Cats with FIV infection have a more protracted course and often live for many years before developing complications such as secondary infection. Both viruses affect several aspects of immune responsiveness but are especially damaging to CMI.[117,150,251] Both the American Association of Feline Practitioners and the European Advisory Board on Cat Diseases have recently developed documents that review the pathophysiology, epidemiology, diagnosis, and treatment of cats with retroviral infection.[117,150,152]

Although antiviral drugs have dramatically altered the outcome of retroviral immunodeficiency in people, toxicity and costs make these drugs less useful in cats, and to date, there is no published evidence that antiviral drugs reduce the incidence of secondary infection in this species. Only a few studies have evaluated the potential benefit of immunomodulatory drugs in cats with retroviral infection, with little benefit demonstrated in the way of efficacy.[117,150,152,160] A study of recombinant feline interferon omega suggested an improved survival, but further studies are clearly warranted.[53,92] A new product, Lymphocyte T-Cell Immunomodulator (LTCI; Imulan BioTherapeutics, Prescott, Ariz.), has recently gained conditional approval by the United States Department of Agriculture (USDA) as a treatment aid for FeLV- or FIV-infected cats with opportunistic infection and other retroviral complications. No peer reviewed, controlled studies demonstrating efficacy of this protein in recovery from secondary infection or improved survival in retroviral infected cats have been published to date.

STRESS AND DISEASE

In the 1930s, the endocrinologist Hans Selye coined the term "stress." He postulated that a stressor stimulus could result in a state of stress wherein an organism would respond in a physiologically inappropriate way that could contribute to the development of disease.[207] The stressor could be either physical (e.g., thermal) or psychological (e.g., fear) and could be either real or perceived. In cats, the introduction of a new pet or family member, changes in the familiar environment (e.g., moving to a new home, an outdoor cat becoming an indoor cat, changes in litter box management), changes in food or feeding, and many other seemingly innocuous stimuli might act as stressors. Acute and chronic stress invoke different chemical mediators and different physical effects. Acute stress results in excessive production of sympathetic hormones, such as norepinephrine, while chronic stress results in stimulation of the hypothalamic-pituitary-adrenal axis and excessive cortisol production. Biological stress can have profound effects on not only the nervous and endocrine systems but on the immune systems as well, and stress can play a role in increased susceptibility to infection as well as provoking other physical and behavioral aberrations.[37,43,162,203]

Chronic stress is believed to result in an increased susceptibility to infection, perhaps in part as a result of cortisol excess.[36,200] Unfortunately, the specific effects that stress has on susceptibility to infection are difficult to evaluate except in very homogenous experimental settings. For instance, the prevalence of feline herpes virus (FHV-1) viral shedding in apparently healthy cats surrendered to a shelter for adoption was only 4%, but after 1 week in the stressful shelter environment, 52% of cats were shedding FHV-1.[177] It is essentially impossible to determine if this increase is due to stress-related acquisition of new infection, stress-related recrudescence of latent infections, simple proximity to infected cats, poor sanitation or air quality, or a combination of these and other factors. Exogenous corticosteroids can increase the rate of shedding of FHV-1, and endogenous corticosteroid release is an important component of chronic stress.[99] No treatment to date, including L-lysine, has been found to reduce the rate of FHV-1 shedding in stressed cats.[62]

The role of stress in other disease states, especially interstitial cystitis, is under investigation in cats. Lower urinary tract signs unassociated with urinary infection, urolithiasis, or neoplasia are common in cats. Often identified as interstitial cystitis (IC) or idiopathic feline lower urinary tract disease, this condition has recently been postulated to have a neuroendocrine basis.[28,243,246,248] The psychological stress associated with an indoor-only environment may help account for the increased risk of IC in indoor cats.[30] If IC is largely caused by stress, the ideal treatment is to reduce stress. This includes measures aimed at enriching the environment of the indoor cat; such multimodal environmental modifications are described in the literature and are accessible to veterinarians and owners alike via the Internet (The Indoor Pet Initiative; http://indoorpet.osu.edu).[29] When stress cannot be eliminated, drugs with sympatholytic activity, such as amitriptyline, have been used to treat IC in cats, but these drugs can have serious adverse effects in some cats.[44]

MANAGEMENT OF THE IMMUNOCOMPROMISED CAT

Cats with immunocompromise and no symptomatic infection nonetheless require special considerations, which vary with the cause and type of immunodeficiency. The most common examples include "healthy" cats with retroviral infection or cats receiving immunosuppressive drug therapy. Ideally, immunocompromised cats should be housed indoors-only, and new pets should be introduced to the home only after a complete health screening of both pets. Raw meat diets should be avoided because of the risk of salmonellosis. Ideally, cats with chronic immunocompromise should be examined twice yearly, paying particular attention to oral and ocular evaluation. Veterinarians should address both ectoparasite and endoparasite control.

Depending on the type and severity of immunocompromise, even cats with abnormalities of the adaptive immune system can often mount an effective vaccination response. Therefore these cats should receive vaccinations; however, modified live vaccines are best avoided when adaptive immunity is compromised. Twice yearly screening with CBC, serum biochemistries, and urinalysis are suggested. Owners of immunocompromised cats must be instructed that even seemingly mild illness should prompt veterinary care, because early recognition of infection and appropriate treatment can be life saving. Prophylactic antimicrobial therapy is not indicated in healthy cats with immunocompromise, except prior to dental procedures or in the face of severe ($<1,000 \times 10^3/\mu l$) neutropenia. The role for immunostimulatory drugs (e.g., feline interferon omega, acemannan, granulocyte colony-stimulating factor [G-CSF], *Staphylococcus* protein A) has yet to be defined for most causes of immunodeficiency in cats.[117,150,152,160]

Opportunistic infections are important in animals with immunocompromise. These infections are not always readily apparent, since the clinical signs of infection may be similar to the signs of the underlying cause of immunodeficiency, or because the cause of immunodeficiency may mask clinical signs of infection (e.g., glucocorticoids suppress fever). Although there are a myriad of potential opportunistic pathogens, a few warrant mention. Demodicosis can occur in any cat, but it seems to be a greater problem in cats with immunodeficiency associated with conditions such as FeLV, FIV (see Figure 33-21), diabetes mellitus, and neoplasia.[169] Candidiasis, a major problem in immunocompromised people, is very rare in healthy cats. However, urinary, ocular, and systemic candidiasis has been identified in immunocompromised cats.[76,188] The vast majority of cats infected with *Toxoplasma gondii* remain healthy; cats that develop an immunodeficiency disease or undergo iatrogenic immunosuppression are more likely to develop clinical illness as a result of previously subclinical infection.[8,14,51,76] Immunosuppressive drug therapy has been associated with feline mycobacteriosis.[87,119,163] Retroviral infections are risk factors for several other types of infections, including *Cryptococcus neoformans*, *Mycoplasma haemofelis*, feline infectious peritonitis, and coccidiosis, among others.[9,98,122,220] Immunodeficiency apparently does not increase the risk of feline bartonellosis, but may increase pathogenicity.[19,77]

Active infection in immunocompromised cats requires aggressive treatment. Outpatient treatment reduces the potential for nosocomial infection. If hospitalization is necessary, caretakers should wash their hands before and after handling the cat and should wear gloves. If feasible, the cat should be isolated from other animals and especially other cats. Aseptic technique should be used whenever protective barriers are disrupted (e.g., catheter placement).

Aggressive antimicrobial treatment of infections can be life saving in immunocompromised cats, and even cats with chronic immunosuppressive conditions may be cured of secondary infections. Because bacteriostatic antimicrobials slow bacterial growth but rely on a functional immune system to clear an infection, bactericidal drugs should be used in immunocompromised cats. Empiric antimicrobial choices are best guided by the source, site, and likely pathogens involved in infection, along with cytology and Gram stain results from the infected site. Antimicrobial therapy is instituted pending culture results, but appropriate samples (e.g., cavity effusions, blood, urine,) should be collected. When sepsis is suspected, the ideal is to collect three blood cultures of 10-mL volume but this volume is excessive for many cats.[146] Even in healthy cats, no more than 10 mL/kg of blood should be collected.[120] Cats with severe illness are often anemic and dehydrated, and blood is usually also collected for CBC, serum chemistries, and other diagnostic tests. When the volume of blood for culture is limited, the authors prefer to collect two cultures each with at least 7-mL volume as opposed to more cultures with lower volumes.

Fever in an immunocompromised cat, especially with neutropenia or neutrophilia, is a medical emergency. Bacteremia or sepsis occurs more often in patients with an impaired immune system but can be difficult to recognize in cats.[61] Although hyperglycemia is common in cats with sepsis, this finding is common in cats with many types of illness or stress and thus cannot be relied on as a sign of sepsis.[42,86] When sepsis is suspected, broad-spectrum, parenteral antibiotics are recommended (e.g., a combination of a beta lactam plus either an aminoglycoside or fluoroquinolone; use caution: enrofloxacin can cause blindness at doses exceeding 5 mg/kg/day). If there is no clinical improvement after 48 hours of empiric therapy, a change in antimicrobial agents should be considered. Treatment is continued for at least 1 week beyond resolution of clinical signs.

References

1. Abraham C, Cho JH: Inflammatory bowel disease, *N Eng J Med* 361:2066, 2009.
2. Adams WH, Daniel GB, Legendre AM et al: Changes in renal function in cats following treatment of hyperthyroidism using 131I, *Vet Radiol Ultrasound* 38:231, 1997.
3. Anwaruddin S, Lloyd-Jones DM, Baggish A et al: Renal function, congestive heart failure, and amino-terminal pro-brain natriuretic peptide measurement: results from the ProBNP Investigation of Dyspnea in the Emergency Department (PRIDE) Study, *J Am Coll Cardiol* 47:91, 2006.
4. Arici M, Walls J: End-stage renal disease, atherosclerosis, and cardiovascular mortality: is C-reactive protein the missing link? *Kidney Int* 59:407, 2001.
5. Atkins A, Brown W, Crawford M: Effects of long-term administration of enalapril on clinical indicators of renal function in dogs with compensated mitral regurgitation, *J Am Vet Med Assoc* 221:654, 2002.
6. Backus RC, Havel PJ, Gingerich JL et al: Relationship between serum leptin immunoreactivity and body fat mass as estimated by use of a novel gas-phase Fourier transform infrared spectroscopy deuterium dilution method in cats, *Am J Vet Res* 61:796, 2000.
7. Backus RC, Puryear LM, Crouse BA et al: Breath hydrogen concentrations of cats given commercial canned and extruded diets indicate GI microflora vary with diet, *J Nutr* 132:1763, 2002.
8. Barrs VR, Martin P, Beatty JA: Antemortem diagnosis and treatment of toxoplasmosis in two cats on cyclosporin therapy, *Aust Vet J* 84:30, 2006.
9. Barrs VR, Martin P, Nicoll RG et al: Pulmonary cryptococcosis and *Capillaria aerophila* infection in an FIV-positive cat, *Aust Vet J* 78:154, 2000.
10. Bassett JH, Harvey CB, Williams GR: Mechanisms of thyroid hormone receptor-specific nuclear and extra nuclear actions, *Mol Cell Endocrinol* 213:111, 2002.
11. Becker TJ, Graves TK, Kruger JM et al: Effects of methimazole on renal function in cats with hyperthyroidism, *J Am Anim Hosp Assoc* 36:215, 2000.
12. Belew AM, Barlett T, Brown SA: Evaluation of the white-coat effect in cats, *J Vet Intern Med* 13:134, 1999.
13. Bennett N, Greco DS, Peterson ME et al: Comparison of a low carbohydrate vs high fiber canned diet for the treatment of diabetes mellitus in cats, *J Feline Med Surg* 8:73, 2006.
14. Bernsteen L, Gregory CR, Aronson LR et al: Acute toxoplasmosis following renal transplantation in three cats and a dog, *J Am Vet Med Assoc* 215:1123, 1999.
15. Blois SL, Holmberg DL: Cryohypophysectomy used in the treatment of a case of feline acromegaly, *J Small Anim Pract* 49:596, 2008.
16. Boag AK, Neiger R, Slater L et al: Changes in the glomerular filtration rate of 27 cats with hyperthyroidism after treatment with radioactive iodine, *Vet Rec* 161:711, 2007.
17. Boswood A, Murphy A: The effect of heart disease, heart failure and diuresis on selected laboratory and electrocardiographic parameters in dogs, *J Vet Cardiol* 8:1, 2006.
18. Boyd LM, Langston C, Thompson K et al: Survival in cats with naturally occurring chronic kidney disease, *J Vet Int Med* 22:1111, 2008.
19. Breitschwerdt EB: Feline bartonellosis and cat scratch disease, *Vet Immunol Immunopathol* 123:167, 2008.
20. Brennan CL, Hoenig M, Ferguson DC: GLUT4 but not GLUT1 expression decreases early in the development of feline obesity, *Domest Anim Endocrinol* 26:291, 2004.
21. Brewster UC, Setaro JF, Perazella MA: The renin-angiotensin-aldosterone system: cardiorenal effects and implications for renal and cardiovascular disease states, *Am J Med Sci* 326:15, 2003.
22. Brown S, Atkins C, Bagley R et al: Guidelines for the identification, evaluation, and management of systemic hypertension in dogs and cats: 2007 ACVIM Forum Consensus Statement, *J Vet Intern Med* 21:542, 2007.
23. Brown S, Finco D, Navar LG et al: Impaired renal autoregulatory ability in dogs with reduced renal mass, *J Am Soc Nephr* 5:1768, 1995.
24. Brown SA, Brown CA, Crowell WA et al: Beneficial effects of chronic administration of dietary omega-3 polyunsaturated fatty acids in dogs with renal insufficiency, *J Lab Clin Med* 131:447, 1998.
25. Brown SA, Brown CA, Crowell WA et al: Effects of dietary polyunsaturated fatty acid supplementation in early renal insufficiency in dogs, *J Lab Clin Med* 135:275, 2000.
26. Brown SA, Brown CA, Jacobs G et al: Effects of the angiotensin converting enzyme inhibitor benazepril in cats with induced renal insufficiency, *Am J Vet Res* 62:375, 2001.
27. Brown SA, Finco DR, Boudinot D et al: Evaluation of a single injection method, using iohexol, for estimating glomerular filtration rate in cats and dogs, *Am J Vet Res* 57:105, 1996.
28. Buffington CA, Teng B, Somogyi GT: Norepinephrine content and adrenoceptor function in the bladder of cats with feline interstitial cystitis, *J Urol* 167:1876, 2002.
29. Buffington CA, Westropp JL, Chew DJ et al: Clinical evaluation of multimodal environmental modification (MEMO) in the management of cats with idiopathic cystitis, *J Feline Med Surg* 8:261, 2006.
30. Buffington CA, Westropp JL, Chew DJ et al: Risk factors associated with clinical signs of lower urinary tract disease in indoor-housed cats, *J Am Vet Med Assoc* 228:722, 2006.
31. Buffington CAT, Chew DJ, DiBartola SP: Lower urinary tract disease in cats: is diet still a cause? *J Am Vet Med Assoc* 205:1524, 1994.

32. Buffington CAT, Chew DJ, Woodworth BE: Feline interstitial cystitis, *J Am Vet Med Assoc* 215:682, 1999.
33. Buffington CAT, Westropp JL, Chew DJ et al: Clinical evaluation of multimodal environmental modification (MEMO) in the management of cats with idiopathic cystitis, *J Feline Med Surg* 8:241, 2006.
34. Buffington CAT, Westropp JL, Chew DJ et al: Risk factors associated with clinical signs of lower urinary tract disease in indoor-housed cats, *J Am Vet Med Assoc* 228:722, 2006.
35. Buranakarl C, Mathur S, Brown SA et al: Effects of dietary sodium chloride intake on renal function and blood pressure in cats with normal and reduced renal function, *Am J Vet Res* 65:620, 2004.
36. Buynitsky T, Mostofsky DI: Restraint stress in biobehavioral research: recent developments, *Neurosci Biobehav Rev* 33:1089, 2009.
37. Calcagni E, Elenkov I, Calcagni E et al: Stress system activity, innate and T helper cytokines, and susceptibility to immune-related diseases, *Ann N Y Acad Sci* 1069:62, 2006.
38. Cameron E, Casey RA, Bradshaw JWS et al: A study of the environmental and behavioural factors that may be associated with feline idiopathic cystitis, *J Small Anim Pract* 45:144, 2004.
39. Caney SMA: *Caring for a cat with hyperthyroidism*, Edinburgh, 2009, Cat Professional.
40. Casal ML, Straumann U, Sugg C et al: Congenital hypotrichosis with thymic aplasia in nine Birman kittens, *J Am Anim Hosp Assoc* 30:600, 1994.
41. Center SA, Warner KL, Erb HN et al: Liver glutathione concentration in dogs and cats with naturally occurring liver disease, *Am J Vet Res* 63:1187, 2002.
42. Chan DL, Freeman LM, Rozanski EA et al: Alterations in carbohydrate metabolism in critically ill cats, *J Vet Emerg Crit Care* 16:S7, 2006.
43. Charmandari E, Tsigos C, Chrousos G et al: Endocrinology of the stress response, *Annu Rev Physiol* 67:259, 2005.
44. Chew DJ, Buffington CA, Kendall MS et al: Amitriptyline treatment for severe recurrent idiopathic cystitis in cats, *J Am Vet Med Assoc* 213:1282, 1998.
45. Chew D: Personal communication, January 2010.
46. Coppack SW: Pro-inflammatory cytokines and adipose tissue, *Proc Nutr Soc* 60:349, 2001.
47. Côté E: Seeking the perfect balance: management of concurrent cardiac and renal disease, *Proc Am Coll Intern Med–Medicine Meeting*, 2009.
48. Crenshaw KL, Peterson ME: Pretreatment clinical and laboratory evaluation of cats with diabetes mellitus: 104 cases (1992-1994), *J Am Vet Med Assoc* 209:943, 1996.
49. Cunningham JM, Patnaik MM, Hammerschmidt DE et al: Historical perspective and clinical implications of the Pelger-Huet cell, *Am J Hematol* 84:116, 2009.
50. Dantal J, Soulillou J-P: Immunosuppressive drugs and the risk of cancer after organ transplantation, *N Engl J Med* 352:1371, 2005.
51. Davidson MG, Rottman JB, English RV et al: Feline immunodeficiency virus predisposes cats to acute generalized toxoplasmosis, *Am J Pathol* 143:1486, 1993.
52. Day MJ, Bilzer T, Mansell J et al: Histopathological standards for the diagnosis of gastrointestinal inflammation in endoscopic biopsy samples of the dog and cat: a report from the World Small Animal Veterinary Association Gastrointestinal Standardization Group, *J Comp Pathol* 138:1, 2008.
53. de Mari K, Maynard L, Sanquer A et al: Therapeutic effects of recombinant feline interferon-omega on feline leukemia virus (FeLV)-infected and FeLV/feline immunodeficiency virus (FIV)-coinfected symptomatic cats, *J Vet Intern Med* 18:477, 2004.
54. De'Oliviera LD, Carciolti AC, Oliviera MC et al: Effects of six carbohydrate sources on diet digestibility and post prandial glycemia and insulin response, *J Anim Sci* 86:2237, 2008.
55. DeCock HEV, Forman MA, Farver TB et al: Prevalence and histopathologic characteristics of pancreatitis in cats, *Vet Pathol* 44:39, 2007.
56. DeFrancesco TC: Maintaining fluid and electrolyte balance in heart failure, *Vet Clin Small Anim* 38:727, 2008.
57. Dennis JS, Kruger JM, Mullaney TP: Lymphocytic plasmacytic gastroenteritis in cats: 14 cases (1985-1990), *J Am Vet Med Assoc* 200:1712, 1992.
58. DiBartola SP, Broome MR, Stein BS et al: Effect of treatment of hyperthyroidism on renal function in cats, *J Am Vet Med Assoc,* 208:875,1996.
59. Dimitriadis GD, Raptis SA: Thyroid hormone excess and glucose intolerance, *Exp Clin Endocrinol Diabetes* 109(Suppl2):S225, 2001.
60. Dohan FC, Lukens FDW: Experimental diabetes produced by the administration of glucose, *Endocrinology* 42:244-262, 1948.
61. Dow SW, Jones RL: Bacteremia: pathogenesis and diagnosis, *Compend Contin Educ Prac Vet* 11:432, 1989.
62. Drazenovich TL, Fascetti AJ, Westermeyer HD et al: Effects of dietary lysine supplementation on upper respiratory and ocular disease and detection of infectious organisms in cats within an animal shelter, *Am J Vet Res* 70:1391, 2009.
63. Eckburg PB, Relman DA: The role of microbes in Crohn's disease, *Clin Infect Dis* 44:256, 2007.
64. Edinboro CH, Scott-Moncrieff JC, Janovitz E et al: Epidemiologic study of relationships between consumption of commercial canned food and risk of hyperthyroidism in cats, *J Am Vet Med Assoc* 15:879, 2004.
65. Elliott J, Watson ADJ: Chronic kidney disease: staging and management. In Bonagura JD, Twedt DC, editors: *Current veterinary therapy XIV*, St Louis, 2009, Elsevier Saunders, p 883.
66. Fahey GC, Barry KA, Swanson KS: Age-related changes in nutrient utilization by companion animals, *Ann Rev Nutr* 28:425, 2008.
67. Farabaugh AE, Freeman LM, Rush JE et al: Lymphocyte subpopulations and hematologic variables in dogs with congestive heart failure, *J Vet Intern Med* 18:505, 2004.
68. Ferguson DC, Caffall Z, Hoenig M: Obesity increases free thyroxine proportionally to nonesterified fatty acid concentrations in adult neutered female cats, *J Endocrinol* 194:267, 2007.
69. Reference deleted in pages.
70. Finco D, Braselton W, Cooper T: Relationship between plasma iohexol clearance and urinary exogenous creatinine clearance in dogs, *J Vet Int Med* 215:368, 2001.
71. Ford S: NIDDM in the cat: treatment with the oral hypoglycemic medication, glipizide, *Vet Clin North Am Small Anim Pract* 25:599, 1995.
72. Forman MA, Marks SL, DeCock HE et al: Evaluation of feline pancreatic lipase immunoreactivity and helical computed tomography versus conventional testing for the diagnosis of feline pancreatitis, *J Vet Intern Med* 18:807, 2004.
73. Frank DA, St Amand AL, Feldman RA et al: Molecular-phylogenetic characterization of microbial community imbalances in human inflammatory bowel diseases, *Proc Natl Acad Sci USA* 104:13780, 2007.
74. Freeman LM, Rush JE, Kehayias JJ et al: Nutritional alterations and the effect of fish oil supplementation in dogs with heart failure, *J Vet Intern Med* 12:440, 1998.
75. Geisberg C, Butler J: Addressing the challenges of cardiorenal syndrome, *Cleve Clin J Med* 73:485, 2006.
76. Gerding PA, Morton LD, Dye JA: Ocular and disseminated candidiasis in an immunosuppressed cat, *J Am Vet Med Assoc* 204:1635, 1994.
77. Glaus T, Hofmann-Lehmann R, Greene C et al: Seroprevalence of *Bartonella henselae* infection and correlation with disease status in cats in Switzerland, *J Clin Microbiol* 35:2883, 1997.
78. Gordon S, Miller M, Saunders A: Pimobendan in heart failure therapy—a silver bullet? *J Am Anim Hosp Assoc* 42:90, 2006.

79. Gottlieb SS, Abraham W, Butler J et al: The prognostic importance of different definitions of worsening renal function in congestive heart failure, *J Cardiac Failure* 8:136, 2002.
80. Gouni V, Chetboul V, Pouchelon JL et al: Azotemia in cats with feline hypertrophic cardiomyopathy: prevalence and relationships with echocardiographic variables, *J Vet Cardiol* 10:117, 2008.
81. Graham-Mize CA, Rosser EJ: Bioavailability and activity of prednisone and prednisolone in the feline patient, *Vet Derm* 15(S1):1, 2004.
82. Grauer GF, Greco DS, Getzy DM et al: Effects of enalapril versus placebo as a treatment for canine idiopathic glomerulonephritis, *J Vet Intern Med* 14:526, 2000.
83. Graves TK, Olivier NB, Nachreiner RF et al: Changes in renal function associated with treatment of hyperthyroidism in cats, *Am J Vet Res* 55:1745, 1994.
84. Greco DS, Lees GE, Dzendzel G et al: Effects of dietary sodium intake on blood pressure measurements in partially nephrectomized dogs, *Am J Vet Res* 55:160, 1994.
85. Greco DS: Diagnosis of diabetes mellitus in dogs and cats, *Vet Clin North Am Small Anim Pract* 31:845, 2001.
86. Greiner M, Wolf G, Hartmann K: A retrospective study of the clinical presentation of 140 dogs and 39 cats with bacteraemia, *J Small Anim Pract* 49:378, 2008.
87. Griffin A, Newton AL, Aronson LR et al: Disseminated *Mycobacterium avium* complex infection following renal transplantation in a cat, *J Am Vet Med Assoc* 222:1097, 2003.
88. Guarner F: Probiotics in gastrointestinal diseases. In Versalovic J, Wilson M, editors: *Therapeutic microbiology: probiotics and related strategies*, Washington, DC, 2008, ASM Press, p 255.
89. Guilford WG, Strombeck DR, Rogers Q et al: Food sensitivity in cats with chronic idiopathic gastrointestinal problems, *J Vet Intern Med* 15:7, 2001.
90. Gunn-Moore DA, Cameron ME: A pilot study using synthetic feline facial pheromone for the management of feline idiopathic cystitis, *J Feline Med Surg* 6:133, 2004.
91. Gunn-Moore DA: Feline lower urinary tract disease, *J Feline Med Surg* 5:134, 2003.
92. Gutzwiller ME, Brachelente C, Taglinger K et al: Feline herpes dermatitis treated with interferon omega, *Vet Dermatol* 18:50, 2007.
93. Haataja L, Gurlo T, Huang CJ et al: Islet amyloid in type 2 diabetes, and the toxic oligomer, *Endocr Rev* 29:303, 2008.
94. Hadden JW: Immunodeficiency and cancer: prospects for correction, *Int Immunopharmacol* 3:1061, 2003.
95. Hammer KB, Holt DE, Ward CR: Altered expression of G proteins in thyroid gland adenomas obtained from hyperthyroid cats, *Am J Vet Res* 61:874, 2000.
96. Hansen B, DiBartola SP, Chew DJ et al: Clinical and metabolic findings in dogs with chronic renal failure fed two diets, *Am J Vet Res* 53:326, 1992.
97. Hart JR, Shaker E, Patnaik AK et al: Lymphocytic plasmacytic enterocolitis in cats: 60 cases (1988-1990), *J Am Anim Hosp Assoc* 30:505, 1994.
98. Hartmann K: Feline leukemia virus infection. In Greene C, editor: *Infectious diseases of the dog and the cat*, ed 3, St Louis, 2006, Elsevier Saunders, p 120.
99. Hickman MA, Reubel GH, Hoffman DE et al: An epizootic of feline herpesvirus, type 1 in a large specific pathogen-free cat colony and attempts to eradicate the infection by identification and culling of carriers, *Lab Anim* 28:320, 1994.
100. Hillege H, Nitsch D, Pfeffer M et al: Renal function as a predictor of outcome in a broad spectrum of patients with heart failure, *Circulation* 113:671, 2006.
101. Hillege HL, Girbes AR, de Kam PJ et al: Renal function, neurohormonal activation, and survival in patients with chronic heart failure, *Circulation* 102:203, 2000.
102. Hirsch VM, Cunningham TA: Hereditary anomaly of neutrophil granulation in Birman cats, *Am J Vet Res* 45:2170, 1984.
103. Hoenig M, Caffall Z, Ferguson DC: Obesity increases free thyroxine proportionally to nonesterified fatty acid concentrations in adult neutered female cats, *J Endocrinol* 194:267, 2007.
104. Hoenig M, Caffall Z, Ferguson DC: Triiodothyronine differentially regulates key metabolic factors in lean and obese cats, *Domest Anim Endocrinol* 34:229, 2008.
105. Hoenig M, Ferguson DC: Impairment of glucose tolerance in hyperthyroid cats, *J. Endocrinol* 121:249, 1989.
106. Hoenig M, Goldschmidt MH, Ferguson DC et al: Toxic nodular goitre in the cat, *J Small Anim Pract* 23:1, 1982.
107. Hoenig M, Hall G, Ferguson D et al: A feline model of experimentally induced islet amyloidosis, *Am J Pathol* 157:2143, 2000.
108. Hoenig M, Jordan ET, Ferguson DC et al: Oral glucose leads to a differential response in glucose, insulin, and GLP-1 in lean versus obese cats, *Domest Anim Endocrinol* 38:95, 2009.
109. Hoenig M, Rand JS: Feline obesity. In August JR, editor: *Consultations in feline internal medicine*, ed 5, Philadelphia, 2006, Saunders, p 175.
110. Hoenig M, Reusch C, Peterson ME: Beta cell and insulin antibodies in treated and untreated diabetic cats, *Vet Immunol Immunopathol* 77:93, 2000.
111. Hoenig M, Thomaseth K, Brandao J et al: Assessment and mathematical modeling of glucose turnover and insulin sensitivity in lean and obese cats, *Domest Anim Endocrinol* 31:573, 2006.
112. Hoenig M, Thomaseth K, Waldron M et al: Insulin sensitivity, fat distribution and adipocytokine response to different diets in lean, and obese cats before and after weight loss, *Am J Physiol* 292:R227, 2007.
113. Reference deleted in pages.
114. Hoenig M, MacGregor L, Matschinsky FM: Mechanisms of in vitro exhaustion of pancreatic beta cells, *Am J Physiol* 250:502, 1986.
115. Hori Y, Takusagawa F, Ikadai H et al: Effects of oral administration of furosemide and torsemide in healthy dogs, *Am J Vet Res* 68:1058, 2007.
116. Horwich TB, Fonarow GC, Hamilton MA et al: Anemia is associated with worse symptoms, greater impairment in functional capacity and a significant increase in mortality in patients with advanced heart failure, *J Am Coll Cardiol* 39:1780, 2002.
117. Hosie MJ, Addie D, Belák S et al: Feline immunodeficiency. ABCD guidelines on prevention and management, *J Feline Med Surg* 11:575, 2009.
118. Hostutler RA, Chew DJ, DiBartola SP: Recent concepts in feline lower urinary tract disease. *Vet Clin North Am Small Anim Pract* 35:147, 2005.
119. Hughes MS, Ball NW, Love DN et al: Disseminated *Mycobacterium genavense* infection in a FIV-positive cat, *J Feline Med Surg* 1:23, 1999.
120. Iazbik MC, Ochoa PG, Westendorf N et al: Effects of blood collection for transfusion on arterial blood pressure, heart rate, and PCV in cats, *J Vet Intern Med* 21:1181, 2007.
121. Inness VL, McCartney AL, Khoo C et al: Molecular characterisation of the gut microflora of healthy and inflammatory bowel disease cats using fluorescenece *in situ* hybridisation with special reference to *Desulfovibrio* spp., *J Anim Phys Anim Nutr* 91:48, 2006.
122. Jacobs GJ, Medleau L, Calvert C et al: Cryptococcal infection in cats: factors influencing treatment outcome, and results of sequential serum antigen titers in 35 cats, *J Vet Intern Med* 11:1, 1997.
123. Janeczko S, Atwater D, Bogel E et al: The relationship of mucosal bacteria to duodenal histopathology, cytokine mRNA, and clinical disease activity in cats with inflammatory bowel disease, *Vet Microbiol* 128:178, 2008.

124. Jepson RE, Brodbelt D, Vallance C et al: Evaluation of predictors of the development of azotemia in cats, *J Vet Intern Med* 23:806, 2009.
125. Jergens AE, Moore FM, Hayness JS et al: Idiopathic inflammatory bowel disease in dogs and cats: 84 cases (1987-1990), *J Am Vet Med Assoc* 200:1603, 1992.
126. Jin ES, Burgess SC, Merritt ME et al: Differing mechanisms of hepatic glucose overproduction in triiodothyronine-treated rats vs. Zucker diabetic fatty rats by NMR analysis of plasma glucose. Considerations for diabetics, *Am J Physiol Endocrinol Metab* 288:E654, 2005.
127. Jordan E, Kley S, Le N-A et al: Dyslipidemia in obese cats, *Domest Anim Endocrinol* 35:290, 2008.
128. Joslin EP, Lahey FH: Diabetes and hyperthyroidism, *Ann Surg* 100:629, 1934.
129. Kahn SE, D'Alessio DA, Schwartz MW et al: Evidence of cosecretion of islet amyloid polypeptide and insulin by beta-cells, *Diabetes* 39:634, 1990.
130. Kang JX, Leaf A: Antiarrhythmic effects of polyunsaturated fatty acids: recent studies, *Circulation* 94:1774, 1996.
131. Karlander SG, Khan A, Wajngot AI: Glucose turnover in hyperthyroid patients with normal glucose tolerance, *J Clin Endocrinol Metab* 68:780, 1989.
132. Katona P, Katona-Apte J: The interaction between nutrition and infection, *Clin Infect Dis* 46:1582, 2008.
133. King JN, Gunn-Moore DA, Tasker S et al: Tolerability and efficacy of benazepril in cats with chronic kidney disease, *J Vet Intern Med* 20:1054, 2006.
134. Kirk CA, Jewell DE, Lowry S: Effects of sodium chloride on selected parameters in cats, *Vet Ther* 7:333, 2006.
135. Kleinschmidt S, Harder J, Nolte I et al: Inflammatory and non-inflammatory diseases of the gastrointestinal tract in cats. Diagnostic advantage of full thickness intestinal and extra intestinal biopsies, *J Feline Med Surg* 12:97, 2010.
136. Kley S, Hoenig M, Glushka J et al: The impact of obesity, sex, and diet on hepatic glucose production in cats, *Am J Physiol Regul Integr Comp Physiol* 296:R936, 2009.
137. Klieverik LP, Sauerwein HP, Ackermanns MT et al: Effects of thyrotoxicosis and selective hepatic autonomic denervation on hepatic glucose metabolism in rats, *Am J Physiol Endocrinol Metab* 294:E513, 2008.
138. Knight EL, Glynn RJ, McIntyre KM et al: Predictors of decreased renal function in patients with heart failure during angiotensin-converting enzyme inhibitor therapy: results from the studies of left ventricular dysfunction (SOLVD), *Am Heart J* 138:849, 1999.
139. Kramer JW, Davis WC, Prieur DJ: The Chediak-Higashi syndrome of cats, *Lab Invest* 36:554, 1977.
140. Krawiec D, Gelberg H: Chronic renal disease in cats. In Kirk RW, editor: *Current veterinary therapy X*, Philadelphia, 1989, Saunders, p 1170.
141. Kruger JM, Conway TS, Kaneene JB et al: Randomized controlled trial of the efficacy of short-term amitriptyline administration for treatment of acute, nonobstructive, idiopathic lower urinary tract disease in cats, *J Am Vet Med Assoc* 222:749, 2003.
142. Laflamme D: Development and validation of a body condition score system for cats: a clinical tool, *Feline Pract* 25:13, 1997.
143. Laflamme DP, Xu H, Long G: Evaluation of two diets in the nutritional management of cats with naturally occurring chronic diarrhea, *Vet Therap* 3:43, 2004.
144. Lapointe C, Belanger M-C, Dunn M et al: N-acetyl-beta-D-glucosaminidase index as an early biomarker for chronic kidney disease in cats with hyperthyroidism, *J Vet Intern Med* 22:1103, 2008.
145. Latimer KS, Rakich PM, Thompson DF: Pelger-Huet anomaly in cats, *Vet Pathol* 22:370, 1985.
146. Lee A, Mirrett S, Reller LB et al: Detection of bloodstream infections in adults: how many blood cultures are needed? *J Clin Microbiol* 45:3546, 2007.
147. Lees GE, Brown SA, Elliott J et al: Assessment and management of proteinuria in dogs and cats: 2004 ACVIM Forum Consensus Statement (small animal), *J Vet Intern Med* 19:377, 2005.
148. Lefebvre HP, Toutain PL: Angiotensin-converting enzyme inhibitors in the therapy of renal diseases, *J Vet Pharmacol Therap* 27:265, 2004.
149. Lekcharoensuk C, Osborne CA, Lulich JP: Epidemiological study of risk factors for lower urinary tract diseases in cats, *J Am Vet Med Assoc* 218:1429, 2001.
150. Levy J, Crawford C, Hartmann K et al: 2008 American Association of Feline Practitioners' feline retrovirus management guidelines, *J Fel Med Surg* 10:300, 2008.
151. Levy JK, Crawford PC, Collante WR et al: Use of adult cat serum to correct failure of passive transfer in kittens, *J Am Vet Med Assoc* 219:1401, 2001.
152. Lutz H, Addie D, Belák S et al: Feline leukaemia. ABCD guidelines on prevention and management, *J Fel Med Surg* 11:565, 2009.
153. Lutz TA, Rand JS: A review of new developments in type 2 diabetes mellitus in human beings and cats, *Br Vet J* 149:527, 1993.
154. MacDonald K, Kass P, Kittleson M: Effect of spironolactone on diastolic function and left ventricular mass in Maine Coon cats with familial hypertrophic cardiomyopathy, *J Vet Intern Med* 21:611, 2007.
155. Marks SL, Zoran DL: Probiotics in feline medicine. In August JR, editor: *Consultations in feline internal medicine*, ed 6, St Louis, 2009, Elsevier, p 104.
156. Marshall RD, Rand JS, Morton JM: Treatment of newly diagnosed diabetic cats with glargine insulin improves glycaemic control and results in higher probability of remission than protamine zinc and lente insulins, *J Feline Med Surg* 11:683, 2009.
157. Mathur S, Brown CA, Dietrich UM et al: Evaluation of a technique of inducing hypertensive renal insufficiency in cats, *Am J Vet Res*, 65:1006, 2004.
158. Mayer-Roenne B, Goldstein RE, Erb HN: Urinary tract infections in cats with hyperthyroidism, diabetes mellitus and chronic kidney disease, *J Feline Med Surg* 9:124, 2007.
159. Mazzaferro EM, Greco DS, Turner AS et al: Treatment of feline diabetes mellitus with a high protein diet and acarbose, *J Feline Med Surg* 5:183, 2003.
160. McCaw DL, Boon GD, Jergens AE et al: Immunomodulation therapy for feline leukemia virus infection, *J Am Anim Hosp Assoc* 37:356, 2001.
161. McClellan V, Langston R, Prestley R: Medicare patients with cardiovascular disease have a high prevalence of chronic kidney disease and a high rate of progression to end-stage renal disease, *J Am Soc Nephrol* 15:1912, 2004.
162. McEwen BS, McEwen BS: Physiology and neurobiology of stress and adaptation: central role of the brain, *Physiol Rev* 87:873, 2007.
163. Meeks C, Levy JK, Crawford PC et al: Chronic disseminated *Mycobacterium xenopi* infection in a cat with idiopathic CD4+ T lymphocytopenia, *J Vet Intern Med* 22:1043, 2008.
164. Meyer TW, Hostetter TH: Uremia, *N Engl J Med* 357:1316, 2007.
165. Middleton WR: Thyroid hormones and the gut, *Gut* 12:172, 1971.
166. Miller D, Bartges J, Cornelius L, et al. Tumor necrosis factor-alpha levels in adipose tissue of lean and obese cats, *J Nutr* 128:2751S, 1998.
167. Milner RJ, Channell CD, Levy JK et al: Survival times for cats with hyperthyroidism treated with iodine 131, methimazole, or both: 167 cases (1996-2003), *J Am Vet Med Assoc* 228:559, 2006.
168. Moe L, Heiene R: Estimation of glomerular filtration rate in dogs with 99M-Tc-DTPA and iohexol, *Res Vet Sci* 58:138, 1995.
169. Neel JA, Tarigo J, Tater KC et al: Deep and superficial skin scrapings from a feline immunodeficiency virus-positive cat, *Vet Clin Pathol* 36:101, 2007.

170. Nicolle A, Chetboul V, Allerheiligen T et al: Azotemia and glomerular filtration rate in dogs with chronic valvular disease, *J Vet Intern Med* 21:943, 2007.
171. Nohria A, Hasselblad V, Stebbins A et al: Cardiorenal interactions: insights from the ESCAPE trial, *J Am Coll Cardiol* 51:1268, 2008.
172. O'Brien TD, Butler PC, Westermark P et al: Islet amyloid polypeptide: a review of its biology and potential roles in the pathogenesis of diabetes mellitus, *Vet Pathol* 30:317, 1993.
173. Olczak J, Jones BR, Pfeiffer DU, et al: Multivariate analysis of risk factors for feline hyperthyroidism in New Zealand, *N Z Vet J* 53:53, 2005.
174. Osborne CA, Stevens JB, Lulich JP et al: A clinician's analysis of urinalysis. In Osborne CA, Finco DR, editor: *Canine and feline nephrology and urology*, ed 1, Baltimore, 1995, Williams & Wilkins, p 141.
175. Palazzuoli A, Silverberg DS, Iovine F et al: Effects of beta-erythropoietin treatment on left ventricular remodeling, systolic function, and B-type natriuretic peptide levels in patients with the cardiorenal anemia syndrome, *Am Heart J* 154:645.e9, 2007.
176. Panciera DL, Thomas CB, Eicker SW et al: Epizootiologic patterns of diabetes mellitus in cats, *J Am Vet Med Assoc* 197:1504, 1990.
177. Pedersen NC, Sato R, Foley JE et al: Common virus infections in cats, before and after being placed in shelters, with emphasis on feline enteric coronavirus, *J Feline Med Surg* 6:83, 2004.
178. Peeters ME, Timmermans-Sprang EP, Mol JA: Feline thyroid adenomas are in part associated with mutations in the G(s alpha) gene and not with polymorphisms found in the thyrotropin receptor, *Thyroid* 12:571, 2002.
179. Pestell R, Alford F, Ramos R et al: Insulin secretion, insulin sensitivity and glucose-mediated glucose disposal in thyrotoxicosis: a minimal model analysis, *Clin Endocrinol* 33:481, 1990.
180. Peterson ME, Gamble DA: Effect of nonthyroidal illness on serum thyroxine concentrations in cats: 494 cases (1988), *J Am Vet Med Assoc* 197:1203, 1990.
181. Peterson ME, Kintzer PP, Cavanaugh PG et al: Feline hyperthyroidism: treatment, clinical and laboratory evaluation of 131 cases, *J Am Vet Med Assoc* 183:103, 1983.
182. Peterson ME, Melian C, Nichols R: Measurement of serum concentrations of free thyroxine, total thyroxine, and total triiodothyronine in cats with hyperthyroidism and cats with nonthyroidal disease, *J Am Vet Med Assoc* 218:529, 2001.
183. Piazza F, Montagnani M, Russo C et al: Competition in liver transport between chenodeoxycholic acid and ursodeoxycholic acid as a mechanism for ursodeoxycholic acid and its protection of liver damage, *Dig Liver Dis* 32:318, 2000.
184. Plantinga EA, Everts H, Kastelein AM et al: Retrospective study of the survival of cats with acquired chronic renal insufficiency offered different commercial diets, *Vet Rec* 157:185, 2005.
185. Plotnick AN, Greco DS: Clinical signs of diabetes mellitus in cats and dogs: contrasts and comparisons, *Vet Clin North Am Small Anim Pract* 25:563, 1995.
186. Polzin DJ, Osborne CA: Update—conservative medical management of chronic renal failure. In Kirk RW, editor: *Current veterinary therapy IX*, Philadelphia, 1986, Saunders, p 1167.
187. Pouchelon J, King J, Martignoni L et al: Long-term tolerability of benazepril in dogs with congestive heart failure, *J Vet Cardiol* 6:7, 2004.
188. Pressler BM, Vaden SL, Lane IF et al: *Candida* spp. urinary tract infections in 13 dogs and seven cats: predisposing factors, treatment, and outcome, *J Am Anim Hosp Assoc* 39:263, 2003.
189. Raboudi N, Arem R, Jones RH et al: Fasting and postabsorptive hepatic glucose and insulin metabolism in hyperthyroidism, *Am J Physiol* 256:E159, 1989.
190. Rand JS, Marshall RD: Diabetes mellitus in cats, *Vet Clin North Am Small Anim Pract* 35:211, 2005.
191. Reusch C, Tomsa K: Serum fructosamine concentration in cats with overt hyperthyroidism, *J Am Vet Med Assoc* 215:1297, 1999.
192. Riensche MR, Graves TK, Schaeffer DJ: An investigation of predictors of renal insufficiency following treatment of hyperthyroidism in cats, *J Feline Med Surg* 10:160, 2008.
193. Riksen NP, Hausenloy DJ, Yellon DM: Erythropoietin: ready for prime-time cardioprotection, *Trends Pharmacol Sci* 29:258, 2008.
194. Ritchie L: *Molecular characterization of intestinal bacteria in healthy cats and cats with IBD. MS dissertation*. Texas A&M University, 2008.
195. Robertson RP, Harmon J, Tran PO et al. Glucose toxicity in β-cells: type 2 diabetes, good radicals gone bad, and the glutathione connection, *Diabetes* 52:581, 2003.
196. Ronco C, Cruz DN, Ronco F: Cardiorenal syndromes, *Curr Opin Crit Care* 15:384, 2009.
197. Ronco C, Haapio M, House AA et al: Cardiorenal syndrome, *J Am Coll Cardiol* 52:1527, 2008.
198. Ronco C, House AA, Haapio M: Cardiorenal syndrome: refining the definition of a complex symbiosis gone wrong, *Intensive Care Med* 34:957, 2008.
199. Rose BD: Diuretics, *Kidney Int* 39:336, 1991.
200. Rostagno MH, Rostagno MH: Can stress in farm animals increase food safety risk? *Foodborne Pathog Dis* 6:767, 2009.
201. Ruaux CG, Steiner JM, Williams DA: Early biochemical and clinical responses to cobalamin supplementation in cats with signs of gastrointestinal disease and severe hypocobalaminemia, *J Vet Intern Med* 19:155, 2005.
202. Ruaux CG, Steiner JM, Williams DA: Metabolism of amino acids in cats with severe cobalamin deficiency, *Am J Vet Res* 62:1852, 2001.
203. Salak-Johnson JL, McGlone JJ: Making sense of apparently conflicting data: stress and immunity in swine and cattle, *J Anim Sci* 85:E81, 2007.
204. Salvador D, Rey N, Ramos G: Continuous infusion versus bolus infusion of loop diuretics in congestive heart failure, *Cochrane Database Sys Rev* (3):CD003178, 2005.
205. Scarlett JM, Donoghue S: Association between body condition and disease in cats, *J Am Vet Med Assoc* 212:1725, 1998.
206. Sekis I, Ramstead K, Rishniw M et al: Single dose pharmacokinetics and genotoxicity of metronidazole in cats, *J Feline Med Surg* 11:60, 2009.
207. Selye H: A syndrome produced by diverse nocuous agents, *Nature* 138:32, 1936.
208. Shah MR, O'Connor CM, Sopko G et al: Evaluation study of congestive heart failure and pulmonary artery catheterization effectiveness (ESCAPE): design and rationale, *Am Heart J* 141:528, 2001.
209. Shlipak MG: Pharmacotherapy for heart failure in patients with renal insufficiency, *Ann Intern Med* 138:917, 2003.
210. Simpson KW, Dogan B, Rishniw M et al: Adherent and invasive *E. coli* is associated with granulomatous colitis in Boxer dogs, *Infect Immunol* 74:4778, 2006.
211. Simpson KW, Fyfe J, Cornetta A et al: Subnormal concentrations of serum cobalamin (vitamin B12) in cats with gastrointestinal disease, *J Vet Intern Med* 15:26, 2001.
212. Slater MR, Geller S, Rogers K: Long-term health and predictors of survival for hyperthyroid cats treated with iodine 131, *J Vet Intern Med* 15:47, 2001.
213. Smith CE, Freeman LM, Rush JE et al: Omega-3 fatty acids in Boxer dogs with arrhythmogenic right ventricular cardiomyopathy, *J Vet Intern Med* 21:265, 2007.
214. Smith G, Lichtman J, Bracken M: Renal impairment and outcomes in heart failure: systematic review and meta-analysis, *J Am Coll Cardiol* 47:1987, 2006.
215. Stebbing J, Duru O, Bower M: Non-AIDS-defining cancers, *Curr Opin Infec Dis* 22:7, 2009.

216. Steele JL, Henik RA, Stepien RL: Effects of angiotensin-converting enzyme inhibition on plasma aldosterone concentration, plasma renin activity, and blood pressure in spontaneously hypertensive cats with chronic renal disease, *Vet Ther* 3:157, 2002.
217. Steiner JM, Williams DA: Feline exocrine pancreatic disorders, *Vet Clin North Am Sm Anim Pract* 29:551, 1999.
218. Stevens T, Conwell DL, Zuccaro G et al: Pathogenesis of chronic pancreatitis: evidence based review of past theories and recent developments, *Am J Gastro* 99:907, 2004.
219. Sucholdolski JS, Dowd SE, Westermarck E et al: The effect of the macrolide antibiotic tylosin on microbial diversity in the canine small intestinal tract, *BMC Microbiol* 9:210, 2009.
220. Sykes JE, Terry JC, Lindsay LL et al: Prevalences of various hemoplasma species among cats in the United States with possible hemoplasmosis, *J Am Vet Med Assoc* 232:372, 2008.
221. Syme HM, Barer PJ, Markwell PJ et al: Prevalence of systolic hypertension in cats with chronic renal failure at initial evaluation, *J Am Vet Med Assoc* 220:1799, 2002.
222. Syme HM, Elliott J: Evaluation of proteinuria in hyperthyroid cats, *J Vet Intern Med* 15:299, 2001.
223. Syme HM, Markwell PJ, Pfeiffer D et al: Survival of cats with naturally occurring chronic renal failure is related to severity of proteinuria, *J Vet Int Med* 20:528, 2006.
224. Syme HM: Proteinuria in cats. Prognostic marker or mediator? *J Feline Med Surg* 11:211, 2009.
225. Thompson KA, Parnell NK, Hohenhaus AE et al: Feline exocrine pancreatic insufficiency: 16 cases. (1992-2007), *J Feline Med Surg* 11:935, 2009.
226. Tomsa K, Glaus TM, Kacl GM et al: Thyrotropin-releasing hormone stimulation test to assess thyroid function in severely sick cats, *J Vet Intern Med* 15:89, 2001.
227. Trepanier L: Inflammatory bowel disease in cats: rational treatment selection, *J Feline Med Surg* 11:32, 2009.
228. Twedt DC, Janeczko S, McCord KW et al: Culture independent detection of bacteria in feline inflammatory liver disease, *J Vet Intern Med Abst* 23:673, 2009.
229. Uechi M, Matsuoka M, Kuwajima E et al: The effects of the loop diuretics furosemide and torsemide on diuresis in dogs and cats, *J Vet Med Sci* 65:1057, 2003.
230. Ugarte C, Guilford WG, Markwell P et al: Carbohydrate malabsorption is a feature of feline inflammatory bowel disease but does not increase clinical gastrointestinal signs, *J Nutr* 134:2068, 2004.
231. Van der Auwera P: Immunomodulating effects of antibiotics, *Curr Opin Inf Dis* 1:363, 1988.
232. Van Hoek I, Daminet S, Notebaert S et al: Immunoassay of urinary retinol binding protein as a putative renal marker in cats, *J Immunol Methods* 329:208, 2008.
233. Van Hoek I, Lefebvre HP, Kooistra HS et al: Plasma clearance of exogenous creatinine, exo-iohexol, and endo-iohexol in hyperthyroid cats before and after treatment with radioiodine, *J Vet Intern Med* 22:879, 2008.
234. Van Hoek I, Lefebvre HP, Peremans K et al: Short- and long-term follow-up of glomerular and tubular renal markers of kidney function in hyperthyroid cats after treatment with radioiodine, *Domest Anim Endocrinol* 36:45, 2009.
235. Van Kimmenade RR, Januzzi JL, Jr., Baggish AL et al: Amino-terminal pro-brain natriuretic peptide, renal function, and outcomes in acute heart failure: redefining the cardiorenal interaction? *J Am Coll Cardiol* 48:1621, 2006.
236. Van Nguyen N, Tagliner K, Helps CR et al: Measurement of cytokine mRNA expression in intestinal biopsies of cats with inflammatory enteropathy using quantitative real-time RT-PCR, *Vet Immunol Immunopathol* 113:404, 2006.
237. Wakeling J, Everard A, Brodbelt D et al: Risk factors for feline hyperthyroidism in the UK, *J Small Anim Pract* 50:406, 2009.
238. Wakeling J, Moore K, Elliott J et al: Diagnosis of hyperthyroidism in cats with mild chronic kidney disease, *J Small Anim Pract* 49:287, 2008.
239. Washabau RJ: Endoscopic, biopsy, and histopathologic guidelines for evaluation of gastrointestinal inflammation in companion animals, *J Vet Intern Med* 24:10, 2010.
240. Washabau RJ: Feline pancreatic disease. In Ettinger SJ, Feldman EC, editors: *Textbook of veterinary internal medicine*, ed 7, St Louis, 2010, Elsevier, p 1704.
241. Webb CB, Trott C: Laprascopic diagnosis of pancreatic disease in dogs and cats, *J Vet Intern Med* 22:1263, 2008.
242. Weiss DJ, Gagne JM, Armstrong PJ: Relationship between inflammatory hepatic disease and inflammatory bowel disease, pancreatitis and nephritis in cats, *J Am Vet Med Assoc* 209:114, 1996.
243. Westropp JL, Buffington CA: In vivo models of interstitial cystitis, *J Urol* 167:694, 2002.
244. Westropp JL, Buffington CA: Feline idiopathic cystitis: current understanding of pathophysiology and management, *Vet Clin North Am Small Anim Pract* 34:1043, 2004.
245. Reference deleted in pages.
246. Westropp JL, Kass PH, Buffington CA: Evaluation of the effects of stress in cats with idiopathic cystitis, *Am J Vet Res* 67:731, 2006.
247. Westropp JL, Kass PH, Buffington CA: In vivo evaluation of alpha 2-adrenoceptors in cats with idiopathic cystitis, *Am J Vet Res* 68:203, 2007.
248. Westropp JL, Buffington CA: Feline idiopathic cystitis: current understanding of pathophysiology and management, *Vet Clin North Am Small Anim Pract* 34:1043, 2004.
249. Westropp JL, Welk KA, Buffington CA: Small adrenal glands in cats with feline interstitial cystitis, *J Urol* 170:2494, 2003.
250. Xenoulis PG, Suchodolski JS, Steiner JM: Chronic pancreatitis in dogs and cats, *Comp Cont Ed* 30:166, 2009.
251. Yamamoto JK, Pu R, Sato E et al: Feline immunodeficiency virus pathogenesis and development of a dual-subtype feline-immunodeficiency-virus vaccine, *AIDS* 21:547, 2007.
252. Yamasaki K, Suematsu H, Takahashi T: Comparison of gastric and duodenal biopsy lesions in dogs and cats with and without lymphoplasmacytic enteritis, *J Am Vet Med Assoc* 209:95, 1996.
253. Yen PM: Physiological and molecular basis of thyroid hormone action, *Physiol Rev* 81:1097, 2001.
254. Zentek J, Hellweg P, Khol-Parisini A: Clinical applications of nutritional advances in gastroenterology, *Comp Cont Ed* 29:39, 2007.
255. Zini E, Osto M, Franchini M et al: Hyperglycaemia but not hyperlipidaemia causes beta cell dysfunction and beta cell loss in the domestic cat, *Diabetologia* 52:336, 2009.
256. Zoran DL: Nutritional management of GI disease. In Ettinger SJ, Feldman EC, editors: *Textbook of veterinary internal medicine*, ed 7, St Louis, 2010, Elsevier, p 17.
257. Zoran DL: Pancreatitis in cats: diagnosis and management of a challenging disease, *J Am Anim Hosp Assoc* 42:1, 2006.

CHAPTER

36

Chronic Disease Management

OUTLINE

IMMUNOSUPPRESSIVE DRUG THERAPY

Kristin M. Lewis and Leah A. Cohn

Cats, like other animals, are protected from microbial pathogens through a combination of physical barriers, innate immune effectors (e.g., phagocytic cells, complement system) and acquired immunity (e.g., cell-mediated and humoral effectors). Although these systems do a magnificent job in protection from pathogens, the immune systems occasionally cause or worsen disease when either misdirected against self-tissues or through an overexuberant reaction to exogenous stimuli. In such cases, it is medically advisable to suppress the inflammatory or immune responses.

In an ideal world, only those components of the immune response that cause harm would be suppressed. In reality, therapeutic immune suppression usually suppresses beneficial as well as harmful components of the immune response. Therefore all immunosuppressive therapies have the potential to make manifest quiescent infections (e.g., toxoplasmosis) or increase susceptibility to newly acquired infection.

Immunosuppressive drugs can be divided into several categories, including glucocorticoids (GCs); cytostatic drugs, including alkylating agents (e.g., chlorambucil) and antimetabolites (e.g., azathioprine); immunophilin ligands (e.g., cyclosporine); antibodies (e.g., intravenous immunoglobulin, monoclonal antibodies); and miscellaneous drugs (e.g., cytokine agonists or antagonists, integrin inhibitors). This chapter will focus on those drugs that have been used therapeutically in cats. It is important to note that most immunosuppressive drugs used in feline medicine are used in an off-label fashion. Dose regimens, duration of therapy, and adverse effects are often either anecdotal, or at best, based on small published case series.

GLUCOCORTICOIDS

Glucocorticoids are by far the most commonly used immunosuppressive drugs. They affect nearly every tissue in the body to alter metabolism and suppress inflammation and immune responses in a dose-dependent fashion. Genomic transcription patterns and subsequent protein expression are altered, resulting in impaired cell-mediated immunity, and to a lesser extent, impaired phagocytic and humoral immunity.[8] A multitude of GCs are available that vary in potency and route of administration. Based on data largely derived from other species, these drugs are described as short-, intermediate-, or long-acting based on duration of suppression of the hypothalamic-pituitary-adrenal axis (HPAA; Table 36-1). Duration of action depends upon both the base compound and modifications, such as esterification, that alter GC absorption. For instance, although methylprednisolone is an intermediate-acting compound, it is a very long-acting compound as the repositol formulation methylprednisolone acetate. When used to achieve chronic immunosuppression, intermediate-acting preparations, such as prednisolone, offer the advantage of a practical dose regimen, which allows the dose to be tailored to produce efficacy while minimizing HPAA suppression and adverse effects. The most commonly prescribed GCs are prednisone or its active metabolite prednisolone. In cats, prednisolone is strongly preferred versus prednisone, because of a superior pharmacokinetic profile.[12] The mechanism behind the disparity is not entirely clear, but decreased gastrointestinal (GI) absorption of prednisone or diminished hepatic conversion of prednisone to prednisolone are suspected.

Surprisingly, there is no scientific evidence of exactly what constitutes an immunosuppressive dose of prednisolone (or any other GC) in cats. In dogs, 2 to 4 mg/kg/day has been accepted as an initial immunosuppressive dose. Recommendations for initial immunosuppression in cats range from 2 to 8 mg/kg, while antiinflammatory dosages range from 0.5 to 2 mg/kg/day of prednisolone. Compared with dogs, cats are relatively resistant to many of the effects of GC, perhaps because of lesser numbers of intracytoplasmic GC receptors.[37] However, in the authors' opinion, dosages greater than 4 mg/kg/day are not required; higher dosages recommended in years past may have been based on clinical experience using less biologically available prednisone instead of prednisolone. The initial dose is continued for several days past clinical remission and then gradually tapered over months. In general, the dose may be reduced approximately 25% every 3 to 4 weeks as long as disease remains controlled. In some cases, GCs are continued at the lowest effective dose for an indefinite (even lifelong) period. Disease control should be monitored during dose reduction, a task more easily accomplished for diseases in which there is a measurable end point (e.g., hematocrit in cats with immune-mediated anemia). Although it is tempting to reduce dosages rapidly, early withdrawal may predispose to relapse. Biologically equivalent dosages of other GCs can be used in place of prednisolone (e.g., dexamethasone at 0.3 to 0.55 mg/kg/day). Long-acting repositol formulations of GCs (e.g., methylprednisolone acetate) can be used when owners are unable to administer daily oral medications, but fine adjustments become impossible and adverse effects may be more likely.

TABLE 36-1 **Comparison of Various Glucocorticoid Base Compounds**

	Relative Antiinflammatory Potency	Equivalent Pharmacologic Dose (mg)	Relative Mineralocorticoid Potency	Plasma Half-Life Dogs/People (hours)	Biologic Half-Life in People (hours)
SHORT-ACTING GLUCOCORTICOIDS					
Hydrocortisone	1	20	2	1/1.5	8-12
Cortisone	0.8	25	2	?/1.5	8-12
INTERMEDIATE-ACTING GLUCOCORTICOIDS					
Prednisone	4	5	1	?/1	12-36
Prednisolone	4	5	1	1-3/2-3	12-36
Methylprednisolone	5	4	0	1.5/3	12-36
Triamcinolone	5	4	0	?/4 or more	24-48
LONG-ACTING GLUCOCORTICOIDS					
Dexamethasone	30	0.75	0	2/5 or more	35-54
Betamethasone	30	0.6	0	?/5 or more	>48

From Cohn LA: Glucocorticoid therapy. In Ettinger SJ, Feldman EC, editors: *Textbook of veterinary internal medicine disease of the dog and the cat*, ed 7, vol 1, St. Louis, 2010, Saunders Elsevier.

Adverse reactions of GCs are usually associated with high-dose regimens, and extended administration protocols, such as those used in chronic immune suppression. Although cats are relatively resistant to GC, adverse effects can develop. Polyuria, polydipsia, and polyphagia are less common in cats than in dogs but do occur, while a variety of other adverse effects of GCs have been documented or suggested (e.g., alopecia, pancreatitis).[8] In addition to a stress leukogram, hyperglycemia, hyperalbuminemia, and hyperlipidemia were noted in healthy cats given prednisolone (4.4 mg/kg/day) or dexamethasone (0.55 mg/kg/day) for 56 days.[18] These same cats developed hepatic glycogen deposition as well.[18] The metabolic actions of GCs on glucose balance result in hyperglycemia in healthy cats, and some cats treated with GC develop either temporary or permanent diabetes mellitus.[19,22] The diabetogenic effects of dexamethasone may be more pronounced than those of prednisolone.[18,19] The use of high-dose, long-term systemic GC should be avoided whenever possible in diabetic cats. Cardiac disease and especially congestive heart failure are also relative contraindications to GC use, since GC-associated water retention may exacerbate congestive failure.[35] As with any immunosuppressive therapy, an additional relative contraindication is infection.

Adverse effects of GCs can be minimized by limiting systemic exposure. In addition to using the lowest effective dose of an intermediate-acting GC, this can be achieved by local application of GC whenever possible. In some cases, GCs are formulated in such a way that systemic absorption is limited after local application, and/or absorbed GC is rapidly inactivated through first-pass hepatic metabolism. For example, application of the GCs fluticasone or flunisolide by nebulization or metered dose inhaler to the airway epithelium of cats with feline reactive airway disease (e.g., asthma) delivers the drug directly to the disease site, preserving efficacy while limiting systemic GC exposure.[9,28,29] Similarly, oral budesonide has been used to treat inflammatory bowel disease in dogs, because it delivers GC to the GI epithelium but limits systemic exposure as a result of limited intestinal absorption and first-pass hepatic metabolism.[36] There are no studies showing efficacy of this agent in cats; anecdotal reports suggest variability in clinical response. When adverse effects of GC are pronounced or when GC alone fails to control disease, alternative immunosuppressive drugs may allow a decrease in GC dose or may even permit discontinuation of GC therapy.

IMMUNOPHILIN LIGANDS

The most commonly used immunosuppressive drug in this class is cyclosporine. Cyclosporine inhibits T-lymphocyte activation and inhibits synthesis of cytokines, such as interleukin-2 (IL-2) and gamma interferon, while also reducing activation of antigen-presenting cells and phagocytes.[13,30] Used extensively to prevent rejection of transplanted kidneys, cyclosporine has also been used to treat immune-mediated blood disorders in cats, including immune hemolytic anemia, pure red cell and megakaryocytic aplasia, and immune thrombocytopenia.[6,15,33,34] Cyclosporine has also been used successfully to treat a variety of feline skin diseases, including atopic dermatitis, feline eosinophilic granuloma complex, feline urticaria pigmentosa, pemphigus erythematosus, feline pruritus, atopic dermatitis, granulomatous folliculitis, and furunculosis as well as sebaceous adenitis.[24,25,38,40] Anecdotally, cyclosporine has been used to treat inflammatory bowel disease as well.[1] Cyclosporine has been explored as an additional therapy for feline asthma, with conflicting results. One experimental study suggested cyclosporine inhibited airway remodeling and inflammation, while a second study found no change in initial asthmatic response or mast cell degranulation of experimentally sensitized animals.[23,26]

Cyclosporine is poorly soluble in water. Microemulsified formulations (e.g., Neoral, Atopica) are preferred rather than the original nonaqueous suspension. An initial dose of 5 mg/kg, PO, every 12 hours is reasonable, but there is enough individual variation in absorption that dosage must be adjusted based upon measured drug concentration.[21]Fortunately, the small size of cats makes the cost of treatment reasonable.

Compared with other immunosuppressive therapies, cats tolerate cyclosporine well. Unlike cytostatic drugs, cyclosporine is not myelosuppressive. The most common adverse effect associated with cyclosporine is GI irritation. Hepatotoxicosis or nephrotoxicosis, although rare, is more serious.[24,30] Because there are multiple case reports of cats developing systemic toxoplasmosis during treatment with cyclosporine, the authors recommend that toxoplasma titers be determined prior to initiation of therapy.[2,5,17] Risk must be weighed against benefit for any cat with positive titers. Cats treated with cyclosporine should be monitored with a complete blood count (CBC) and serum chemistry profile at least 3 times per year. In a group of feline renal transplant patients treated with cyclosporine and prednisolone, malignant neoplasias occurred at more than 6 times the expected rate.[32]

Tacrolimus is an immunophilin ligand immunosuppressive agent that is available in both oral and topical formulations, and it has a mechanism of action similar to cyclosporine. It is used in humans to prevent graft rejection and has also been evaluated for prevention of renal allograft rejection in cats.[16] Tacrolimus provided marked improvement in the a small series of cats with proliferative and necrotizing otitis externa refractory to GC, antibiotic, and antifungal therapy.[20]

CYTOSTATIC DRUGS

Alkylating agents act by causing cross-linkage and strand breaks in DNA and RNA. They are commonly used as chemotherapeutic drugs, but they also act on lymphocyte populations impairing both cell-mediated and humoral immunity. Because these agents require at least several weeks to become effective, they are begun along with GC and continued after the GC is tapered or discontinued. The two alkylating agents used most often as immunosuppressant therapies in cats are chlorambucil and cyclophosphamide. Both have been used as adjunctive or alternative therapies to GC in cats with inflammatory bowel disease (IBD).[1] Occasionally, alkylating agents have been used to treat hematologic disorders as well.[34]

Many feline practitioners prefer chlorambucil to cyclophosphamide, because it seems to be better tolerated, but there is little to document an advantage of one versus the other. Chlorambucil is available in a 2-mg tablet form convenient for use in cats. Most cats can be given 2 mg, PO, every 48 hours initially. The dose frequency may be adjusted from every 24 to every 96 hours, depending on the response of the cat to treatment. Both chlorambucil and cyclophosphamide can induce myelosuppression; so, a CBC must be monitored on a regular basis. Initially a CBC should be checked 7 to 10 days after beginning therapy, and even during chronic therapy, a CBC should be monitored at least every 60 days. Additional adverse effects include GI upset and myoclonus (muscle twitching) for chlorambucil or hemorrhagic cystitis for cyclophosphamide.[4,10]

Cytostatic antimetabolite drugs mimic molecules that participate in cellular biochemical reactions but differ enough from the natural molecule to interfere with normal cell division and function. They include nucleic acid analogues as well as antifolate drugs. Most have a more profound effect on T lymphocytes (and therefore on cell-mediated immunity) than on B-lymphocytes. Azathioprine is an antimetabolite commonly used to induce and maintain immunosuppression in dogs and humans. The drug is metabolized to 6-mercaptopurine (6-MP), which interferes with de novo purine synthesis. Unfortunately, a profound and potentially fatal myelosuppression occurs more commonly in cats treated with azathioprine than in dogs or humans, preventing its routine use in felines.[3,27] This difference in the response of cats compared with other species is likely the result of a relative deficiency in the enzyme that catalyzes the conversion of 6-MP to inactive metabolites.[11,31]

Methotrexate is an antimetabolite used to treat rheumatoid arthritis in humans and is occasionally used for chemotherapy or as an immunosuppressive drug in cats. The drug has been used in combination with another antimetabolite drug, leflunomide (Arava), in a small number of cats with spontaneous erosive rheumatoid arthritis.[14] Leflunomide has been used to treat dogs with a wide variety of immune-mediated diseases, but experience in cats is more limited. Leflunomide is converted to an active metabolite that inhibits an enzyme crucial for de novo pyrimidine synthesis. There has been some interest in the use of leflunomide for immunosuppression in feline renal transplantation, since the drug also possesses antiherpesvirus activity.[39]

ANTIBODIES

Antibodies can be used to cause therapeutic immunomodulation. For instance, humanized murine monoclonal antibodies directed against the CD3 molecule on T-lymphocyte receptors are quite effective in the prevention of organ rejection in people. However, human or humanized antibodies may not be effective or safe in cats. To the author's knowledge, the single drug in this class that has been used in feline medicine is human intravenous immunoglobulin (IV-Ig). Derived from a pooled human donor population, IV-Ig contains human polyvalent antibody consisting of predominantly IgG antibodies. Originally developed to treat antibody deficiency syndromes, it has become well accepted for the acute treatment of immune-mediated disease in humans. Although the mechanisms of action are poorly understood, competitive blockade of Fc receptors on macrophages, inhibition of complement activity, and alterations in T-lymphocyte and B-lymphocyte function may each play a role.[7] In cats, IV-Ig has been used to treat severe erythema multiforme and immune-mediated erythroid and megakaryocytic aplasia with a good outcome.[7,41] Although adverse effects were not reported in the few published case reports, it is reasonable to assume that a human-derived protein may lead to anaphylactic reactions, especially with repeated use. Although IV-Ig may eventually be shown to have some utility in initial stabilization of cats with life-threatening immune-mediated disease, this expensive therapy is unlikely to have a role in chronic immunosuppression.

References

1. Allen H: Therapeutic approach to cats with chronic diarrhea. In August J, editor: *Consultations in feline internal medicine*, ed 6, St Louis, 2010, Elsevier, p 244.
2. Barrs VR, Martin P, Beatty JA: Antemortem diagnosis and treatment of toxoplasmosis in two cats on cyclosporin therapy, *Aust Vet J* 84:30, 2006.
3. Beale KM, Altman D, Clemmons RR et al: Systemic toxicosis associated with azathioprine administration in domestic cats, *Am J Vet Res* 53:1236, 1992.
4. Benitah N, de Lorimier LP, Gaspar M et al: Chlorambucil-induced myoclonus in a cat with lymphoma, *J Am Anim Hosp Assoc* 39:283, 2003.

5. Bernsteen L, Gregory CR, Aronson LR et al: Acute toxoplasmosis following renal transplantation in three cats and a dog, *J Am Vet Med Assoc* 215:1123, 1999.
6. Bianco D, Armstrong PJ, Washabau RJ: Presumed primary immune-mediated thrombocytopenia in four cats, *J Feline Med Surg* 10:495, 2008.
7. Byrne KP, Giger U: Use of human immunoglobulin for treatment of severe erythema multiforme in a cat, *J Am Vet Med Assoc* 220:197, 2002.
8. Cohn LA: Glucocorticoid therapy. In Ettinger SJ, Feldman EC, editors: *Textbook of veterinary internal medicine: diseases of the dog and the cat*, ed 7, St Louis, 2010, Elsevier, p 503.
9. Cohn LA, Declue AE, Cohen RL et al: Effects of fluticasone propionate dosage in an experimental model of feline asthma, *J Feline Med Surg* 12:91, 2009.
10. Crow SE, Theilen GH, Madewell BR et al: Cyclophosphamide-induced cystitis in the dog and cat, *J Am Vet Medical Assoc* 171:259, 1977.
11. Foster AP, Shaw SE, Duley JA et al: Demonstration of thiopurine methyltransferase activity in the erythrocytes of cats, *J Vet Intern Med* 14:552, 2000.
12. Graham-Mize CA, Rosser EJ, Hauptman J: Absorption, bioavailability and activity of prednisone and prednisolone in cats. In Hillier A, Foster A, Bertola G et al, editors: *Advances in veterinary dermatology*, ed 5, Ames, Iowa, 2005, Blackwell Publishing, p 152.
13. Guaguere E, Steffan J, Olivry T: Cyclosporin A: a new drug in the field of canine dermatology, *Vet Dermatol* 15:61, 2004.
14. Hanna FY: Disease modifying treatment for feline rheumatoid arthritis, *Vet Comp Orthop Traumatol* 18:94, 2005.
15. Husbands B, Smith SA, Weiss DJ: Idiopathic immune mediated hemolytic anemia (IMHA) in 25 cats [abstract], *J Vet Intern Med* 16:350, 2002.
16. Kyles AE, Gregory CR, Craigmill AL et al: Pharmacokinetics of tacrolimus after multidose oral administration and efficacy in the prevention of allograft rejection in cats with renal transplants, *Am J Vet Res* 64:926, 2003.
17. Last RD, Suzuki Y, Manning T et al: A case of fatal systemic toxoplasmosis in a cat being treated with cyclosporin A for feline atopy, *Vet Dermatol* 15:194, 2004.
18. Lowe AD, Campbell KL, Barger A et al: Clinical, clinicopathological and histological changes observed in 14 cats treated with glucocorticoids, *Vet Rec* 162:777, 2008.
19. Lowe AD, Graves TK, Campbell KL et al: A pilot study comparing the diabetogenic effects of dexamethasone and prednisolone in cats, *J Am Anim Hosp Assoc* 45:215, 2009.
20. Mauldin EA, Ness TA, Goldschmidt MH: Proliferative and necrotizing otitis externa in four cats, *Vet Dermatol* 18:370, 2007.
21. Mehl ML, Kyles AE, Craigmill AL et al: Disposition of cyclosporine after intravenous and multi-dose oral administration in cats, *J Vet Pharmacol Ther* 26:349, 2003.
22. Middleton DJ, Watson AD: Glucose intolerance in cats given short-term therapies of prednisolone and megestrol acetate, *Am J Vet Res* 46:2623, 1985.
23. Mitchell RW, Cozzi P, Ndukwu IM et al: Differential effects of cyclosporine A after acute antigen challenge in sensitized cats in vivo and ex vivo, *Br J Pharmacol* 123:1198, 1998.
24. Noli C, Scarampella F: Prospective open pilot study on the use of ciclosporin for feline allergic skin disease, *J Small Anim Pract* 47:434, 2006.
25. Noli C, Toma S: Three cases of immune-mediated adnexal skin disease treated with cyclosporin, *Vet Dermatol* 17:85, 2006.
26. Padrid PA, Cozzi P, Leff AR: Cyclosporine A inhibits airway reactivity and remodeling after chronic antigen challenge in cats, *Am J Respir Crit Care Med* 154:1812, 1996.
27. Paul AL, Shaw SP, Bandt C: Aplastic anemia in two kittens following a prescription error, *J Am Anim Hosp Assoc* 44:25, 2008.
28. Reinero CR, Brownlee L, Decile KC et al: Inhaled flunisolide suppresses the hypothalamic-pituitary-adrenocortical axis, but has minimal systemic immune effects in healthy cats, *J Vet Intern Med* 20:57, 2006.
29. Reinero CR, Decile KC, Byerly JR et al: Effects of drug treatment on inflammation and hyperreactivity of airways and on immune variables in cats with experimentally induced asthma, *Am J Vet Res* 66:1121, 2005.
30. Robson D: Review of the pharmacokinetics, interactions and adverse reactions of cyclosporine in people, dogs and cats, *Vet Rec* 152:739, 2003.
31. Rodriguez DB, Mackin A, Easley R et al: Relationship between red blood cell thiopurine methyltransferase activity and myelotoxicity in dogs receiving azathioprine, *J Vet Intern Med* 18:339, 2004.
32. Schmiedt CW, Grimes JA, Holzman G et al: Incidence and risk factors for development of malignant neoplasia after feline renal transplantation and cyclosporine-based immunosuppression, *Vet Comp Oncol* 7:45, 2009.
33. Schmiedt CW, Holzman G, Schwarz T et al: Survival, complications, and analysis of risk factors after renal transplantation in cats, *Vet Surg* 37:683, 2008.
34. Stokol T, Blue JT: Pure red cell aplasia in cats: 9 cases (1989-1997), *J Am Vet Med Assoc* 214:75, 1999.
35. Trasida P, Tobias AH, Smith SA, et al: Hemodynamic effects of methylprednisolone acetate administration in cats, *Am J Vet Res* 67:583, 2006.
36. Tumulty JW, Broussard JD, Steiner JM et al: Clinical effects of short-term oral budesonide on the hypothalamic-pituitary-adrenal axis in dogs with inflammatory bowel disease, *J Am Anim Hosp Assoc* 40:120, 2004.
37. Van den Broek AH, Stafford WL: Epidermal and hepatic glucocorticoid receptors in cats and dogs. *Res Vet Sci* 52:312, 1992.
38. Vercelli A, Raviri G, Cornegliani L: The use of oral cyclosporin to treat feline dermatoses: a retrospective analysis of 23 cases, *Vet Dermatol* 17:201, 2006.
39. Williams CR, Sykes JE, Mehl M et al: In vitro effects of the active metabolite of leflunomide, A77 1726, on feline herpesvirus-1, *Am J Vet Res* 68:1010, 2007.
40. Wisselink MA, Willemse T: The efficacy of cyclosporine A in cats with presumed atopic dermatitis: a double blind, randomised prednisolone-controlled study, *Vet J* 180:55, 2009.
41. Zini E, Hauser B, Meli ML et al: Immune-mediated erythroid and megakaryocytic aplasia in a cat, *J Am Vet Med Assoc* 230:1024, 2007.

MONITORING LONG-TERM THERAPY

Melissa Clark and Duncan C. Ferguson

Monitoring drug therapy consists of assessing both the efficacy and the safety of a medication in an individual patient. Monitoring is necessary because the safety of a particular drug may vary among patients, or in the same patient over time, resulting from differences in major organ function (e.g., age-related, breed-related, or disease-related), hydration, body condition, concurrent therapy, and susceptibility to idiosyncratic adverse drug reactions. Likewise, efficacy may be affected by individual patient physiology and disease states as well as by drug interactions, formulation, and delivery. Recognizing early signs of therapeutic failure or unacceptable drug side effects is essential to ensuring appropriate individualized treatment.

CLINICAL MONITORING

Repeated evaluation of a patient's clinical status is the cornerstone of ensuring efficacy and safety. Particularly in cats, client observations are important in making decisions about the benefits and safety of therapy. For example, because cats are often reluctant to ambulate in an exam room, monitoring the efficacy of treatments for osteoarthritis may be impossible without information about the cat's behavior at home. Suggestions for improving clinical monitoring of efficacy and safety include

1. Educating both oneself and the client about adverse effects and indicators of efficacy associated with a particular drug
2. Making follow-up calls to detect adverse effects, since clients will not necessarily report this information without prompting
3. Accurately recording physical examination findings at each recheck visit
4. Having clients keep a treatment log in order to note changes in their pets over time

Monitoring issues associated with some feline drugs for which efficacy assessment is primarily based on clinical observation are listed in Table 36-2.

TABLE 36-2 **Summary of Monitoring Recommendations for Long-Term Drugs That Have Primarily Clinical Efficacy Indices in the Cat***

Drug or Drug Class	Potential Adverse Effects	Monitoring Recommendations
Antifungals (G = griseofulvin, I = itraconazole, T = terbinafine)	Bone marrow suppression; hepatotoxicity; ataxia (G)[18,26,42]; dose-dependent anorexia and vomiting (I)[27]; increased ALT(I)[57,58]; alter therapy if severe or symptomatic; rare hepatotoxicity in humans (T)[11]	CBC +/− liver enzymes before and every 1 to 4 weeks during therapy (G); liver enzymes every 2 to 4 weeks (I); consider baseline and periodic liver enzyme assessment (T)
Antihistamines (e.g., chlorpheniramine)	Transient sedation[31]	Data limited; safety monitoring is primarily clinical at this time
Antivirals	Anemia with zidovudine (AZT) in cats with FeLV[17] and FIV[16]; mild diarrhea and fatigue with feline IFN omega[10]; transient anorexia and weight loss with high-dose human IFN alpha[59]	PCV periodically (AZT); if <20%, discontinue temporarily and restart at lower dose[16]
Appetite stimulants (mirtazapine, cyproheptadine)	Anecdotally, hyperexcitability and vocalization with mirtazapine (possible serotonin syndrome)[1,40]; may respond to dose reduction or treatment with cyproheptadine[28,56]; vomiting, vocalization, and sedation with cyproheptadine (infrequent)[47]	Data limited; safety monitoring is primarily clinical at this time
Cobalamin	None documented in cats; clinical effect measured by improved appetite, weight gain, decreased GI signs[43]	Serum levels can be measured; however, dosing is usually empirical
Fluoroquinolones (long-term use not ideal)	Retinal toxicity at doses as low as 4.6 mg/kg/day (see Chapter 29 for further details)	Monitor for mydriasis or vision loss; discontinue drug if noted
Metronidazole	Neurotoxicosis at chronic doses >58 mg/kg/day[3,33]; reversible DNA disruption after 7 days of treatment (clinical significance unclear)[49]	Monitor for neurologic abnormalities; consider alternative medications for chronic therapy
Meloxicam (chronic use off label in some countries)	Renal and GI toxicity class effect; discontinue if GI upset[15]	Manufacturer recommends CBC and chemistry panel before and periodically during treatment in dogs
Serotonin selective reuptake inhibitors (e.g., fluoxetine)	Intermittent inappetence[39]; shortened REM sleep in laboratory cats at doses of 2.5 mg/kg[51]; increased liver enzymes in humans	Monitor appetite and body weight; consider baseline liver enzyme assessment
Tricyclic antidepressants (e.g., amitriptyline, clomipramine)	Lethargy[4,22,50] and diminished coat quality[4]; anticholinergic effects (urine retention)[37]; cardiac conductivity disturbances in humans (seen in healthy cats only with overdose)[13]; hepatopathy in humans	Consider baseline CBC, chemistry panel, and cardiac evaluation; consider periodic liver enzyme assessment; monitor urine and fecal output
Tramadol	Dysphoria[54]	Data limited; safety monitoring is primarily clinical at this time

*Monitoring therapy with glucocorticoids, chlorambucil, and chemotherapeutic agents is discussed above and in Chapter 28, respectively.
ALT, Alanine transaminase; *AZT,* azidothymidine; *CBC,* complete blood count; *FeLV,* feline leukemia virus; *FIV,* feline immunodeficiency disease; *IFN,* interferon; *PCV,* packed cell volume; *REM,* rapid eye movement.

PHARMACODYNAMIC MONITORING

Specific physiologic end points (pharmacodynamic measures) are helpful in assessing success of therapy for certain drugs. In cats, these drugs include amlodipine, erythropoietin, methimazole, phosphate binders, and potassium supplements. Efficacy and safety monitoring for these drugs is discussed below, and recommendations are summarized in Table 36-3.

Amlodipine

The main objective of efficacy measure for amlodipine, a commonly used antihypertensive in the cat, is blood pressure measurement. Preferred methods for measuring blood pressure in cats, target ranges for blood pressure after treatment, and blood pressure reduction in special situations are discussed in the American College of Veterinary Internal Medicine (ACVIM) Consensus Statement on systemic hypertension[2] and in Chapter 20.

In humans, the effects of amlodipine increase gradually in conjunction with plasma levels during 7 to10 days of dosing.[30] Unfortunately, no specific information is available regarding the pharmacokinetics of amlodipine in cats. Rechecking blood pressure and making dosage adjustments after 7 days of treatment is probably appropriate based on published studies, although anecdotal reports[23] suggest that a clinically significant effect of amlodipine on blood pressure may be seen much sooner (24 to 48 hours). Timing of blood pressure measurement after administration does not appear to be an important factor in evaluating efficacy.[53]

Side effects reported from three studies of amlodipine in cats[8,19,53] included weakness and hypotension (in a patient also receiving propanolol), pruritus, a mild decrease in serum potassium of more than 1 to 2 months following the start of treatment, and need for initiation of potassium supplementation or increase in the dose during the treatment period. Many of the cats in these studies also had some degree of renal dysfunction. Average values for blood urea nitrogen (BUN) and creatinine did not change significantly during the first 1 to 2 months of amlodipine therapy; however, 1 of 10 cats with elevated creatinine in one study became uremic and hypokalemic while on amlodipine.[19] Hence, monitoring of serum potassium concentrations and renal values in cats receiving amlodipine is prudent, particularly if chronic renal disease (CRD) has been diagnosed. Owner monitoring for signs of hypotension may be important in cats taking multiple agents expected to lower blood pressure.[8]

TABLE 36-3 **Summary of Monitoring Recommendations for Drugs with Measurable Pharmacodynamic Parameters***

Drug or Drug Class	Efficacy Monitoring	Safety Monitoring
Amlodipine	Measure blood pressure 7 days after treatment initiation or dose changes; timing of BP measurement with respect to medication not important	Measure serum K periodically during treatment, especially if concurrent CKD Monitor for clinical signs of hypotension (weakness) if cat is taking multiple agents expected to lower BP
Erythropoietin (recombinant human); darbepoetin	Measure PCV every 7-14 days until normalized (25%-30%), then monthly if patient is clinically stable	Monitor for development of anemia (due to anti-rHuEPO antibodies) every 14 days for first 60-90 days Monitor blood pressure periodically Monitor for vomiting, uveitis, or cutaneous/mucocutaneous lesions
Methimazole	Measure serum total T_4 2-4 weeks after initiating therapy or making dose adjustments, then every 6 months	Measure ALT, ALP, bilirubin, BUN, Cr, and USG periodically throughout treatment (example: every 4-6 months after initial control) Monitor CBC periodically, particularly within first 3 months of treatment, and platelet count before surgery Monitor for vomiting or facial excoriation
Phosphate binders (aluminum salts, calcium salts, chitosan/calcium carbonate, lanthanum carbonate)	Measure serum P concentration monthly until within desired range, then every 2-4 months	Monitor for signs of encephalopathy; monitor CBC periodically for microcytosis (aluminum-containing binders) Measure serum Ca periodically to detect hypercalcemia (calcium-containing products) Monitor for constipation (all)
Potassium supplements	Measure serum K 7-14 days after oral supplementation is initiated or dose changes are made	Discontinue supplementation in oliguric/anuric states (acute-on-chronic renal failure, urinary obstruction) to avoid hyperkalemia

*Monitoring insulin therapy is discussed in depth in Chapter 24.
ALP, Alkaline phosphatase; *ALT,* alanine transaminase; *BP,* blood pressure; *BUN,* blood urea nitrogen; *Ca,* calcium; *CBC,* complete blood count; *CKD,* chronic kidney disease; *Cr,* creatinine; *K,* potassium; *PCV,* packed cell volume; *rHuEPO,* recombinant human erythropoietin; *T_4,* thyroxine; *USG,* urine specific gravity.

Erythropoietin

Efficacy of therapy with recombinant human erythropoietin (rHuEPO) is documented by measuring the hematocrit (packed cell volume, PCV). This should be done every 1 to 2 weeks during initial therapy. Once PCV has reached 25% to 30% (often by week 4), the frequency of dosing can be reduced.[6,24] Thereafter, PCV should be monitored periodically (one author suggests monthly[24]) in animals receiving erythropoietin, to avoid creating polycythemia and to detect the severe anemia that can result from development of anti-rHuEPO antibodies.

Anemia secondary to antibody development occurred in of five of seven cats treated for more than 180 days in one study,[6] 4 to 16 weeks after therapy was begun. Darbepoetin, a chemically modified rHuEPO, has not been associated with antibody-positive anemia in human patients to date.[5] No data is available on the likelihood of antibody formation with this form of rHuEPO in cats.

Vomiting, uveitis, seizures, and cutaneous hypersensitivity were reported side effects in a group of 11 cats receiving rHuEPO; both cats with seizures were moderately or severely azotemic, and at least one was hypertensive at the time the seizures were noted.[6] Hypertension can result from use of erythropoietin, possibly due to increased blood viscosity.[24] Erythropoietin treatment increases the demand for iron, and iron deficiency may develop if stores are inadequate. Therefore serum iron should be measured before and during therapy with erythropoietin; supplementation with ferrous gluconate or sulfate may be indicated.

Methimazole

Methimazole therapy is usually monitored by measurement of total thyroxine (T_4) concentrations. Normalization of T_4 levels in treated hyperthyroid cats typically takes 2 to 4 weeks,[55] because the drug inhibits T_4 production but does not affect thyroid hormone that has already been synthesized and is either stored in the gland or in circulation. Timing of sampling during the day does not appear to affect results.[45] Dosage adjustments may be necessary over time, resulting from growth of the thyroid tumor. Thyroid stimulating hormone (TSH) measurement is also possible, because feline TSH shows cross-reactivity in the canine assay.[41] TSH levels are normal to low in cats with adequate thyroid function; elevated TSH levels can indicate overtreatment with antithyroid medication.

Cats with hyperthyroidism and high-normal creatinine levels may progress to mild to moderate azotemia following treatment, regardless of the treatment modality (i.e., medical, surgical, or radioiodine). Development of azotemia typically occurs within the first 30 days following initiation of therapy. Although BUN and creatinine may increase significantly, azotemia is often stable and nonprogressive.[25] It is not clear whether careful dose titration to avoid subnormal T_4 concentrations affects the development of azotemia, but such titration is possible with methimazole therapy (as opposed to radioiodine or surgery). Indicators of renal function, such as urine specific gravity (USG), urine protein:creatinine (UPC) ratio, glomerular filtration rate (GFR) (measured by exogenous creatinine or iohexol clearance), and the urinary enzyme *N*-acetyl-beta-D-glucosaminidase have been investigated as monitoring tools. Their ability to predict propensity for renal decompensation has been poor in most studies.[20] In particular, USG, although simple and noninvasive to measure, is not necessarily predictive, because some cats with renal insufficiency paradoxically retain the ability to concentrate urine to 1.045 or higher.[34]

Other reported side effects of methimazole include vomiting and anorexia (11% to 23% of cats), facial and/or cervical excoriation (2% to 15% of cats, depending on study), agranulocytosis, thrombocytopenia (epistaxis, oral hemorrhage), hepatopathy (anorexia, vomiting, icterus), lymphadenopathy, or acquired myasthenia gravis (all in < 3% of cats). The ideal time frame for monitoring blood values to detect bone marrow suppression and hepatopathy is not known, but in one large study[36] that documented these effects, bone marrow suppression occurred during the first 3 months of therapy.

Alternatives for cats that develop gastrointestinal (GI) side effects include discontinuing the drug and reintroducing it gradually, changing to propylthiouracil, or using transdermal formulations of methimazole. Transdermal methimazole has been reported to cause fewer GI side effects; however, all other adverse reactions may still occur. When a cat develops allergic side effects to methimazole, such as facial pruritus and excoriation, treatment with radiocontrast agents (e.g., iopanoic acid) may be considered. These iodinated compounds inhibit the enzymes that convert T_4 to T_3 (triiodothyronine) but do not alter thyroidal secretion of T_4. Therefore the effect of these drugs is monitored by measuring T_3, not T_4, concentrations. Owners of cats with adverse reactions to methimazole should also be reminded of the options for radioiodine therapy and surgery.

Carbimazole, a prodrug for methimazole, is widely used in Europe, and is being considered for approval in the United States. A sustained-release product, Vidalta (Intervet/Schering-Plough Animal Health, Summit, NJ), allowing once-daily dosing at 10 to 15 mg/cat/day, PO, has been approved in Europe.[14] Monitoring recommendations for carbimazole are similar to those for methimazole; however, more rapid normalization of serum T_4 (mean, 5.7 days after the start of treatment) may be achieved with carbimazole at a dosage of 5 mg/cat, PO, every 8 hours.[32]

Phosphate Binders

Phosphate binders used in cats include aluminum or calcium salts, chitosan/calcium carbonate, sevelamer hydrochloride, and lanthanum carbonate. For most of these compounds, the measurable efficacy indicator is serum phosphate concentration. To date, there are no controlled studies demonstrating the most appropriate values for serum phosphate in cats with renal disease. Suggestions for target values (derived from human medicine) can be found in a recent roundtable discussion on the management of hyperphosphatemia in dogs and cats.[9] After initial achievement of target phosphate levels through dose titration, periodic reassessment is necessary because progression of renal disease or changes in diet may alter serum phosphate concentrations with time. One author recommends measuring serum phosphate concentration monthly after starting therapy until phosphate is in the lower portion of the reference range, then every 2 to 4 months.[21]

A chitosan/calcium carbonate product labeled for veterinary use as a food additive (Epakitin;Vétoquinol, Fort Worth, Tex.) has been shown to lower plasma parathyroid hormone (PTH) concentrations in cats with chronic renal disease. Titrating dose to normalize PTH levels has been recommended,[21] although a dose-response relationship of phosphate binders on PTH has not been established.

There are few studies evaluating the safety of phosphate binders in animals. In humans, all phosphate binders can cause gastrointestinal side effects (e.g., constipation, GI upset). In addition, aluminum-containing phosphate binders are no longer used in human medicine because of occurrences of aluminum toxicity. This complication has also been reported in two dogs with renal disease, after 2 to 6 weeks on doses of 126 to 200 mg/kg/day of aluminum hydroxide. Both dogs had elevated serum aluminum levels; signs of toxicity included lethargy progressing to obtundation and recumbency, with decreased reflexes.[48] Progressive microcytosis preceded the development of neurologic signs in these dogs. For this reason, and because microcytic anemia is also associated with aluminum toxicity in humans, one clinician has advocated serial evaluation of red blood cell (RBC) indices in all animals receiving aluminum-containing phosphate binders.[12]

Hypercalcemia is a concern with calcium-containing phosphate binders and has been observed in cats taking Epakitin.[21] Sevelamer or lanthanum salts may be alternatives in cats with hypercalcemia, although sevelamer has not been used extensively in cats. No adverse effects were observed with administration of a liquid formulation of lanthanum carbonate to 10 cats with renal disease during a 6-month period.[46]

Potassium Supplements

Therapy with oral potassium supplements (potassium gluconate, potassium citrate) is very safe and can be monitored by sequential measurement of serum potassium concentration. One author[38] suggests rechecking potassium concentrations every 7 to 14 days during initial therapy. Once potassium concentration has normalized, frequency of rechecks depends on the severity of concurrent disease. The development of hyperkalemia in cats on potassium supplements is reportedly rare as long as urine production (and, therefore, urinary potassium excretion) is adequate.[7]

PHARMACOKINETIC MONITORING

Measurement of plasma drug concentration is indicated for those drugs that

1. Exhibit inconsistent absorption, elimination, or interaction characteristics, leading to variation in plasma concentration among individuals
2. Show a correlation between drug concentration and toxicity and/or efficacy
3. Have a commercially available assay, validated for veterinary patients, through which results can be obtained in a timely manner[52]

Among drugs used in cats, aminoglycosides, cyclosporine, theophylline, and anticonvulsants satisfy these criteria.

Aminoglycosides are not commonly used long term in the cat. However, assays for measuring serum concentrations are available, and may be useful in certain situations (e.g., treatment of sepsis during protracted hospitalization of a patient with panleukopenia). Aminoglycosides are associated with dose-dependent nephrotoxicity. Monitoring of serum drug concentrations, along with frequent in-hospital testing (e.g., BUN, creatinine, examination of urine sediment for casts) may aid in avoiding this complication.

Cyclosporine is gaining popularity as a treatment for allergic and immune-mediated diseases. As in other species, cyclosporine absorption is unpredictable in the cat.[29] Theophylline has been a recommended treatment for feline bronchitis. For both cyclosporine and theophylline, measurement of plasma drug concentrations may be indicated when lack of efficacy or toxicity is suspected, despite an adequate dose, or when the formulation of the drug is changed.

The main utility of therapeutic drug monitoring in cats at this time is in monitoring therapy with anticonvulsants, particularly phenobarbital. Monitoring of anticonvulsant therapy is discussed in depth in Chapter 27. Recommendations for measurement of aminoglycoside,

TABLE 36-4 **Therapeutic Drug Monitoring in Cats**

Drug	Sample Preparation and Timing[35]*	Target Plasma Concentrations[35]
Aminoglycosides	0.5 mL serum or plasma, shipped on ice; sample at 1, 2, and 4 hours after dose for clearance measurements	Amikacin: peak 40 μg/mL; trough <0.8 μg/mL Gentamicin: peak 20 μg/mL; trough <0.27 μg/mL
Cyclosporine	1 mL whole blood in EDTA tube, shipped on ice; sample at least 48 hours after beginning or altering therapy; trough or peak (2 hours after dosing) samples may be appropriate	Depends on disease; in general, trough should be 300-600 ng/mL
Phenobarbital	0.5 mL serum or plasma; sample at steady state (7-14 days after first dose), any time during dosing interval	15-40 μg/mL (extrapolated from dogs); one author recommends 20-30 μg/mL for cats[44]
Theophylline	0.5 mL serum, shipped on ice; sample at trough; add peak sample for assessment of clearance (timing of peak varies with formulation)	5-20 μg/mL expected to be therapeutic (extrapolated from humans)

*Verify specific instructions for sample handling with laboratory.
EDTA, Ethylenediaminetetraacetic acid.

cyclosporine, phenobarbital, and theophylline levels are found in Table 36-4.

References

1. Adams LG: Updates in management of chronic kidney disease, Western Veterinary Conference 2009 [proceedings online]. Available at http://www.vin.com/Members/Proceedings/Proceedings.plx?CID=wvc2009&PID=pr50998&O=VIN. Accessed February 11, 2009.
2. Brown S, Atkins C, Bagley R et al: Guidelines for the identification, evaluation, and management of systemic hypertension in dogs and cats, *J Vet Intern Med* 21:542, 2007.
3. Caylor KB, Cassimatis MK: Metronidazole neurotoxicosis in two cats, *J Am Anim Hosp Assoc* 37:258, 2001.
4. Chew DJ, Buffington CA, Kendall MS et al: Amitriptyline treatment for severe recurrent idiopathic cystitis in cats, *J Am Vet Med Assoc* 213:1282, 1998.
5. Cournoyer D, Toffelmir EB, Wells GA: Anti-erythropoietin antibody-mediated pure red cell aplasia after treatment with recombinant erythropoietin products: recommendations for minimization of risk, *J Am Soc Nephrol* 15:2728, 2004.
6. Cowgill LD, James KM, Levy JK et al: Use of recombinant human erythropoietin for management of anemia in dogs and cats with renal failure, *J Am Vet Med Assoc* 212:521, 1998.
7. Dow SW, Fettman MJ: Chronic renal disease and potassium depletion in cats, *Sem Vet Med Surg* 7:198, 1992.
8. Elliott J, Barber PJ, Syme HM et al: Feline hypertension: clinical findings and response to antihypertensive treatment in 30 cases, *J Sm An Pract* 42:122, 2001.
9. Elliot J, Brown SA, Cowgill LD et al: Phosphatemia management in the treatment of chronic kidney disease, a roundtable discussion, January 10, 2006. Available at http://www.vetoquinol.ca/documents/Quoi%20de%20neuf/Articles/Round%20table%20discussion.pdf. Accessed January 15, 2010.
10. European Medicines Agency, Veterinary Medicines: European Public Assessment Report, Virbagen Omega. Available at http://www.ema.europa.eu/vetdocs/PDFs/EPAR/virbagenomega/V-061-en1.pdf. Accessed January 15, 2010.
11. Fernandes NF, Geller SA, Fong T: Terbinafine hepatotoxicity: case report and review of the literature, *Am J Gastroenterol* 93:459, 1998.
12. Fischer J: Dealing with renal hyperphosphatemia: the good, the bound, and the ugly, Veterinary Information Network Rounds transcript, June 22, 2008 [website]. Available at http://www.vin.com/Members/CMS/Rounds/default.aspx?id=887. Accessed February 1, 2010.
13. Follmer CH, Lum BK: Protective action of diazepam and of sympathomimetic amines against amitriptyline-induced toxicity, *J Pharm Exp Ther* 222:424, 1982.
14. Frenais R, Rosenberg D, Burgaud S et al: Clinical efficacy and safety of a once-daily formulation of carbimazole in cats with hyperthyroidism, *J Small Anim Pract* 50:510, 2009.
15. Gunew MN, Menrath VH, Marshall RD: Long-term safety, efficacy, and palatability of oral meloxicam at 0.01-0.03 mg/kg for treatment of osteoarthritic pain in cats, *J Feline Med Surg* 10:235, 2008.
16. Hartmann K, Donath A, Kraft W: AZT in the treatment of feline immunodeficiency virus infection, part 2, *Feline Pract*, 23:13, 1995.
17. Haschek WM, Weigel RM, Scherba G et al: Zidovudine toxicity to cats infected with feline leukemia virus, *Fund Appl Toxicol* 14:764, 1990.
18. Helton KA, Nesbitt GH, Caciolo PL: Griseofulvin toxicity in cats: literature review and report of seven cases, *J Am Anim Hosp Assoc* 22:453, 1986.
19. Henik RA, Snyder PS, Volk LM: Treatment of systemic hypertension in cats with amlodipine besylate, *J Am Anim Hosp Assoc* 33:226, 1997.
20. Jepson RE, Brodbelt D, Vallance C et al: Evaluation of predictors of the development of azotemia in cats, *J Vet Intern Med* 23:806, 2009.
21. Kidder A, Chew D: Treatment options for hyperphosphatemia in feline CKD: what's out there? *J Feline Med Surg* 11:913, 2009.
22. King JN, Steffan J, Heath S et al: Determination of the dosage of clomipramine for the treatment of urine spraying in cats, *J Am Vet Med Assoc* 225:881, 2004.
23. Kittleson MD, Kienle RD, editors: *Small animal cardiovascular medicine*, ed 1, St Louis, 1998, Mosby, p 445.
24. Langston CE, Reine NJ, Kittrell D: The use of erythropoietin, *Vet Clin North Am Small Anim Pract* 33:1245, 2003.
25. Langston CE, Reine NJ: Hyperthyroidism and the kidney, *Clin Tech Sm Anim Pract* 21:17, 2006.
26. Levy JK: Ataxia in a kitten treated with griseofulvin, *J Am Vet Med Assoc* 198:105, 1991.
27. Mancianti F, Pedonese F, Zullino C: Efficacy of oral administration of itraconazole to cats with dermatophytosis caused by *Microsporum canis*, *J Am Vet Med Assoc* 213:993, 1998.
28. McDaniel WW: Serotonin syndrome: early management with cyproheptadine, *Ann Pharmacother* 35:1672, 2001.
29. Mehl ML, Kyles AE, Craigmill AL et al: Disposition of cyclosporine after intravenous and multi-dose oral administration in cats, *J Vet Pharmacol Therap* 26:349, 2003.
30. Michel T: Treatment of myocardial ischemia. In Brunton LL, editor: *Goodman and Gilman's the pharmacological basis of therapeutics*, ed 11, Chicago, 2006, McGraw-Hill, p 823.

31. Miller WH, Scott DW: Efficacy of chlorpheniramine maleate for management of pruritus in cats, *J Am Vet Med Assoc* 197:67, 1990.
32. Mooney CT, Thoday KL, Doxey DL: Carbimazole therapy of feline hyperthyroidism, *J Sm Anim Pract* 33:228, 1992.
33. Olson EJ, Morales SC, McVey AS et al: Putative metronidazole toxicosis in a cat, *Vet Pathol* 42:665, 2005.
34. Osborne CA, Stevens JB, Lulich JP et al: A clinician's analysis of urinalysis. In Osborne CA, Finco DR, editors: *Canine and feline nephrology and urology*, ed 1, Baltimore, 1995, Williams & Wilkins, p 141.
35. Papich MG: Therapeutic drug monitoring. In Papich MG, Riviere JE, editors: *Veterinary pharmacology and therapeutics*, ed 9, Ames, Iowa, 2009, Wiley-Blackwell, p 1323.
36. Peterson ME, Kintzer P, Hurvitz AI: Methimazole treatment of 262 cats with hyperthyroidism, *J Vet Intern Med* 2:150, 1988.
37. Pfeiffer E, Guy N, Cribb A: Clomipramine-induced urinary retention in a cat, *Can Vet J* 40:265, 1999.
38. Plotnick A: Feline chronic renal failure: long-term medical management, *Compend Contin Educ Pract Vet* 29:342, 2007.
39. Pryor PA, Hart BL, Cliff KD et al: Effects of a selective serotonin reuptake inhibitor on urine spraying behavior in cats, *J Am Vet Med Assoc* 219:1557, 2001.
40. Quimby JM, Gustafson DL, Samber BJ et al: The pharmacokinetics of mirtazapine in healthy cats [abstract], *J Vet Intern Med* 23:767, 2009.
41. Rayalam S, Eizenstat LD, Davis RR et al: Expression and purification of feline thyrotropin (fTSH): immunological detection and bioactivity of heterodimeric and yoked glycoproteins, *Dom Anim Endocrin* 30:185, 2006.
42. Rottman JB, English RV, Breitschwerdt EB et al: Bone marrow hypoplasia in a cat treated with griseofulvin, *J Am Vet Med Assoc* 198:429, 1991.
43. Ruaux CG, Steiner JM, Williams DA: Early biochemical and clinical responses to cobalamin supplementation in cats with signs of gastrointestinal disease and severe hypocobalaminemia, *J Vet Intern Med* 19:155, 2005.
44. Rusbridge C: Diagnosis and control of epilepsy in the cat, *In Practice* 27:208, 2005.
45. Rutland BE, Nachreiner RF, Kruger JM: Optimal testing for thyroid hormone concentration after treatment with methimazole in healthy and hyperthyroid cats, *J Vet Intern Med* 23:1025, 2009.
46. Schmidt BH, Murphy M: A study on the long-term efficacy of Renalzin™ (Lantharenol® suspension 20%) in cats with experimentally induced chronic kidney disease [poster], *Proc 19th Eur Coll Vet Intern Med Congress*, 2009.
47. Scott DW, Rothstein E, Beningo KE et al: Observations on the use of cyproheptadine hydrochloride as an antipruritic agent in allergic cats, *Can Vet J* 39:634, 1998.
48. Segev G, Bandt C, Francey T et al: Aluminum toxicity following administration of aluminum-based phosphate binders in 2 dogs with renal failure, *J Vet Intern Med* 22:1432, 2008.
49. Sekis I, Ramstead K, Rishniw M et al: Single-dose pharmacokinetics and genotoxicity of metronidazole in cats, *J Feline Med Surg* 11:60, 2009.
50. Seksel K, Lindeman MJ: Use of clomipramine in the treatment of anxiety-related and obsessive-compulsive disorders in cats, *Aust Vet J* 76:317, 1998.
51. Slater IH, Jones GT, Moore RA: Inhibition of REM sleep by fluoxetine, a specific inhibitor of serotonin uptake, *Neuropharmacology* 17:383, 1978.
52. Smith JA: What is the role of therapeutic drug monitoring in antifungal therapy? *Curr Infect Dis Rep* 11:439, 2009.
53. Snyder PS: Amlodipine: a randomized, blinded clinical trial in 9 cats with systemic hypertension, *J Vet Intern Med* 12:157, 1998.
54. Steagall PV, Taylor PM, Brondani JT et al: Antinociceptive effects of tramadol and acepromazine in cats, *J Feline Med Surg*, 10:24, 2008.
55. Trepanier LA: Pharmacologic management of feline hyperthyroidism, *Vet Clin North Am Small Anim Pract* 37:775, 2007.
56. Veterinary Information Network discussion: mirtazapine toxicity? September 14, 2009 [website]. Available at http://www.vin.com/Members/boards/discussionviewer.aspx?DocumentId=4113030. Accessed January 15, 2010.
57. Vlaminck KM, Engelen MA: An overview of pharmacokinetic and pharmacodynamic studies in the development of itraconazole for feline *Microsporum canis* dermatophytosis. In Hillier A, Foster AP, Kwochka K, editors: *Advances in veterinary dermatology*, vol 5, Ames, Iowa, 2005, Blackwell Publishing, p 130.
58. Whitney BL, Broussard J, Stefanacci JD: Four cats with fungal rhinitis, *J Feline Med Surg* 7:53, 2005.
59. Zeidner NS, Myles MH, Mathiason-DuBard CK: Alpha interferon (2b) in combination with zidovudine for the treatment of presymptomatic feline leukemia virus-induced immunodeficiency syndrome, *Antimicrob Agents Chemother* 34:1749, 1990.

MANAGING ADVERSE DRUG REACTIONS

Sidonie Lavergne

Adverse drug reactions (ADR) are a common collateral damage of practicing medicine. They are responsible for high morbidity and even mortality in both human and veterinary medicine every year. The previous chapters and sections have already described numerous adverse drug reactions, well characterized or not, that could be associated with prescribing the therapy options available for the discussed diseases. This chapter section will focus on the general principles and specific aspects that were not already presented earlier.

INCIDENCE OF ADVERSE DRUG REACTIONS

There is no fully established estimate of ADR in veterinary medicine.[3,4,6] Cats, however, appear to have a similar overall incidence of ADR as dogs and humans. The most commonly reported are dose-dependent ADR related to the properties of the drugs (type A). Drugs that are most often associated with adverse events are those that are also the most commonly prescribed: antiparasitic agents, antiinflammatory drugs, antimicrobials, and finally, drugs acting on the neurologic system.

CLASSIFICATION OF ADVERSE DRUG REACTIONS

Type A

Type A adverse drug reactions are dose-dependent and are secondary to the drug characteristics. They will occur in any cat beyond a certain dose. These reactions are predictable and therefore avoidable. There are three different subtypes of type A reactions:

1. Those related to the pharmacologic interaction of the drug with a cell receptor
   a. On-target: for instance, barbiturate- and benzodiazepine-induced sedation, loperamide-associated constipation, immunosuppression from immunosuppressive therapy associated with risks of sepsis
   b. Off-target: for instance, nonsteroidal antiinflammatory drug (NSAID)–associated gastrotoxicity and nephrotoxicity; beta-lactam–induced seizures at high concentrations, erythromycin-induced vomiting, morphine-induced central nervous system stimulation at high doses (greater than 5 mg/kg), xylazine-induced emesis, reversible and dose-dependent bone marrow suppression in cats treated with chloramphenicol
2. Those related to the chemical and/or physical properties of the drug (e.g., most nausea and vomiting reactions, esophageal lesions secondary to tablets or capsules, especially doxycycline and clindamycin)
3. Those related to the toxic properties of a drug metabolite: for instance, metabolite-associated methemoglobinemia and hepatotoxicity with acetaminophen (see Chapter 31), azathioprine-associated bone marrow toxicity (potentially exacerbated in cats by a much lower thiopurine methyltransferase activity compared with humans and dogs); bone marrow toxicity with high doses of griseofulvin in cats infected with feline immunodeficiency virus[8]

The risk of type A ADR increases with the dose and the duration of the treatment, because they are dose-dependent. In addition, drugs can become toxic when used in combination, despite each agent being used at the recommended dosage regimen. Drug interactions are of three types:

1. Pharmaceutical interactions when drugs are not compatible on a chemical or physical level (e.g., diazepam precipitation in lactated Ringer solution or adsorption to plastic, complexation of tetracycline with calcium or magnesium)
2. Pharmacokinetic interactions (e.g., bicarbonates in IV fluids decrease the renal elimination of weak bases; ketoconazole inhibits the metabolism of cyclosporine)
3. Pharmacodynamic interactions during which drugs can synergize their toxic effects (e.g., nephrotoxicity from NSAIDs and aminoglycosides, bleeding risk from aspirin and heparin) or antagonize their therapeutic effects (e.g., immunosuppressive agents with antimicrobials, antiemetic agents with emetic drugs)

Some intrinsic factors may also increase the risk for type A adverse drug reactions, such as age (neonate vs. kitten vs. elderly), percentage of body fat (cachectic vs. normal weight vs. obese), hydration status; and any underlying diseases (especially renal and severe liver dysfunction or meningitis). These factors should always be taken into consideration before deciding on a dosage regimen for any given cat. See type A and type B adverse drug reactions algorithm on page 1164.

Type B

Type B adverse drug reactions are not usually dose-dependent and are secondary to features of the patient rather than the drug. They will not be seen in all cats, even at very high doses, and are sometimes called "idiosyncratic." They are therefore neither predictable nor avoidable (at least before the first episode).

Many type B reactions are thought to be immune mediated and are called "drug allergies" or "drug hypersensitivity reactions." The reaction can be immediate and usually quite severe in cases of anaphylactic or anaphylactoid reactions. Anaphylactic reactions are truly immune mediated, involving immunoglobulin E (type I hypersensitivity), and require a previous exposure. Anaphylactoid reactions, on the other hand, result from the release of powerful inflammatory mediators and can occur at the first exposure. Delayed reactions can be antibody mediated, involving IgG and IgM (type II hypersensitivity) or immune complexes and/or the complement cascade (type III hypersensitivity), or can be cell-mediated, involving T-lymphocytes (type IV). No data have been generated in feline patients, with the exception of propylthiouracil-associated blood dyscrasias, that were shown to involve several antibody markers (antinuclear, anti–red blood cells, and anti-neutrophil).[1,7,9]

Involvement of the immune system has not been confirmed for all type B reactions. The nature of these uncharacterized reactions remains unknown. This was the case for "ivermectin hypersensitivity" in Collies until the *MDR1* genetic mutation was identified in these dogs. It was also the case with fluoroquinolone-induced retinal degeneration until it was shown to be a dose-dependent phenomenon that can happen in all cats with high enough dosages and might involve a drug metabolite (see Chapter 29). It remains the case for carprofen-associated hepatotoxicity in dogs and for diazepam- and glipizide-associated hepatotoxicity in cats.[2,5]

PREVENTING ADVERSE DRUG REACTIONS

Type B reactions are by definition unpredictable, at least until the first episode. Any suspected episode of drug allergy needs to be carefully recorded in the medical record to prevent re-exposure. Type A reactions are, on the other hand, predictable and therefore avoidable. Preventing them, however, requires being aware of their existence. This awareness should be reflected in multiple steps of daily practice through the following protocols:

- Choose drugs with the lowest possible toxicity profile.
- Adjust the dose according to the life stage and health of the patient (especially in very young and old cats, or in cats with renal or severe liver insufficiency).
- Use drugs approved for cats in the disease of interest whenever possible, or research off-label dosage regimen information carefully in the literature before use.
- Try to limit polypharmacy (to decrease the risk of negative drug interactions).
- Realize that most drugs can induce side effects and ALL drugs can be associated with allergic reactions; therefore always warn owners about potential side effects of drugs and nutraceuticals (e.g., SAMe, *N*-acetylcysteine, vitamin C).
- Never prescribe a drug without being perfectly aware of its potentially toxic effects in cats, but also in other species (in case it has not been reported in cats yet), and always use appropriate monitoring tools (e.g., physical examination, CBC, serum chemistry panels, and, when available, drug plasma concentrations).
- Try to limit the use of drugs in sensitive populations, such as kittens, older cats, or pregnant queens.

There is a very limited amount of information on the carcinogenic and/or teratogenic effects of drugs in cats. Metronidazole is thought to be potentially teratogenic in laboratory animals and was shown to be genotoxic in cats. It is recommended, however, to always assume that potential teratogenicity and/or genotoxicity or carcinogenicity demonstrated in other species could occur in cats too. Furthermore, any highly liposoluble drug (e.g., phenobarbital) that will most likely reach the fetus and be excreted in milk, as well as any drug interacting with hormones (e.g., methimazole) or developmental signaling pathway (e.g., cyclooxygenase 2 and kidney development) should not be used in pregnant queens or neonatal kittens, unless strictly necessary and no other treatment alternatives are available.

DIAGNOSING ADVERSE DRUG REACTIONS

A key component of managing an ADR is first to recognize it. This seems like an obvious statement, but most clinicians forget to include ADR in their differential list. Adverse drug events can mimic most diseases, with rare exceptions such as bone fractures, abscesses, or tooth resorption lesions.

Diagnostic Steps for All Adverse Drug Reaction Types

The diagnosis of any ADR involves the following steps:

1. Collection of a complete medical history (previous and present drug exposure and timing); a thorough physical examination; a CBC and serum chemistry panel; +/− a tissue aspirate/biopsy, which should show some specific signs of drug or chemical toxicity but is more important in severe cases.
2. Discontinuation of the drug suspected (a "de-challenge"). If the drug was responsible for the clinical signs, they should resolve when administration of the drug is ceased and the drug has been cleared. Re-challenges are considered unethical, especially in cases of drug allergy, because the next exposure could be associated with much more severe clinical signs.
3. It is critically important to contact and consult with the pharmaceutical company and/or the American Society for the Prevention of Cruelty to Animals (ASPCA) Animal Poison Control Center if necessary (1-888-426-4435; http://www.aspca.org/pet-care/poison-control/).

ADR diagnosis is rendered very challenging by the fact that these drug reactions can mimic miscellaneous non–drug-related diseases. Only the combination of drug exposure and the right timing of events with a given set of clinical signs will allow a clinician to conclude that the patient suffered from a probable adverse drug reaction. Beyond that, there are a very limited number of laboratory tests that a clinician can use to confirm the diagnosis.

Diagnostic Steps for Type A Reactions

Because Type A drug reactions are dose-dependent, and secondary to known features of the drug, getting the following information is useful:

- History: doses and intervals prescribed, but also those that were actually given to the cat by the owner
- Drug plasma concentration, although these tests are not always readily available for the drug of interest (see Table 36-4)
- Specific organ function monitoring depending on the toxicity profile of the suspected drugs, for instance, liver enzymes for diazepam toxicity (see Table 36-2)

Diagnostic Steps for Type B Reactions

Confirming a diagnosis of drug allergy can be difficult. Because they are usually not dose-related, and are often thought to involve a drug metabolite rather than the parent drug, the drug plasma concentration will not be useful. The hematopoietic system, the liver, and the skin are the most common targets of immune-mediated drug reactions, but reports have been published involving miscellaneous organs, such as the lungs, the kidneys, the pancreas, and even the central nervous system. A diagnosis of immune-mediated drug reaction can be suggested by

- The timing of the reaction: occurring immediately after the initial exposure (anaphylactoid reaction), immediately after previous exposure(s) (anaphylaxis), or delayed (usually after at least 5 days of drug administration for the first course); this requires that the clinician inquire about drugs that the cat has been taking within the past month, even if the cat has stopped receiving them at the time of the reactions.
- Clinical signs that may include skin lesions (such as pruritic urticaria-angioedema, maculopapular dermatitis, erythema multiforme, pemphigus foliaceus, vasculitis, and toxic epidermal necrosis), as well as purpura, pale mucosa, jaundice, fever, or polyarthropathy.
- Typical findings from complementary clinical tests that may include blood cytopenia involving one or several cell lines or increased liver enzymes.

When a clinician suspects a drug-induced immune-mediated reaction, some tests specific to the organ targeted by the reaction can be useful: for instance, skin biopsy, liver biopsy, bone marrow aspirate, antinuclear antibody test, and Coombs' test. Some veterinary schools also offer research tests (often free of charge) to help confirm the diagnosis by looking for specific anti-drug antibodies, antitissue antibodies, or drug-specific lymphocytes (lymphocytes recognizing the drug as their target and as their stimulating antigen).

MANAGING ADVERSE DRUG REACTIONS

Fortunately, most adverse drug reactions involve mild clinical signs, and most animals will recover without requiring any specific treatment other than drug discontinuation. The clinical management of some ADR will, however, be more challenging.

Managing Type A Reactions

Because type A reactions are dose-dependent and related to the drug features, the clinician will have to consider either modifying the dosage regimen or discontinuing the drug all together. There is no specific rule in making that decision, but severe clinical signs should probably lead to discontinuing any drug or nutraceutical the cat could be receiving at the time of the reaction. Non–life-threatening reactions can probably be managed by decreasing the dose or increasing the dosing interval.

Type A reactions result from a negative characteristic of the drug that can sometimes be counteracted by antidotes (e.g., folic acid or folinic acid for bone marrow suppression secondary to high doses and long-term trimethoprim/ormetoprim, atipamezole for medetomidine reversal, protamine for heparin overdose, antioxidants when oxidative stress has been proved to be part of the pathogenesis). Some dose-dependent ADR will require complementary organ support (e.g., fluid therapy for hypotension or nephrotoxicity, erythropoietin for anemia, gastroprotectants for NSAID-induced ulcers, antiemetics for vomiting).

Pharmaceutical companies and the ASPCA Animal Poison Control Center (see above) will provide information regarding the treatment of specific dose-dependent ADR.

Managing Type B Reactions

When an idiosyncratic drug reaction is suspected, all drugs and nutraceuticals should be withdrawn, since even a minute amount of drug could elicit an allergic reaction. Most cases of drug allergy are mild, but some allergic reactions can be life threatening, and their clinical management should start as soon as possible and be aggressive. This is the case for anaphylaxis and anaphylactoid drug reactions, blood dyscrasias, liver toxicity, or severe skin reactions, such as Stevens-Johnson syndrome and erythema multiforme majus (approximately 50% survival in humans), and toxic epidermal necrolysis (less than 30% survival in humans).

Anaphylaxis and anaphylactoid reactions are the only true emergency in ADR. Their treatment includes the following steps:

- Ensure patent airway and IV access (central venous access is ideal)
- IV fluids (monitor the rate carefully to avoid pulmonary edema)
- Epinephrine: slow IV if possible (0.1 mL of a 1:1,000 solution per cat, or 1 mL/10 kg of a 1:10,000 dilution or 0.01 mg/kg); or 0.02 mg/kg endotracheal when the cat is intubated or 0.01 mg/kg, SC or IM, in less severe cases, to be repeated as needed every 5 to 15 minutes
- +/− Short-acting water-soluble corticosteroids (prednisolone 50 to 100 μg/cat, IV)

TABLE 36-5 **Examples of Regulatory Agencies Recording Adverse Drug Reaction Reports**

Country	Agency	Website
United States	Federal Drug Administration: Center for Veterinary Medicine (FDA-CVM)	http://www.fda.gov/AnimalVeterinary/SafetyHealth/ReportaProblem/ucm055305.htm
United Kingdom	Veterinary Medicine Directorate: Suspected Adverse Reaction Surveillance Scheme (VMD-SARSS)	http://www.vmd.gov.uk/General/Adverse/adverse.htm
Canada	Health Canada: Veterinary Pharmacovigilance	http://www.hc-sc.gc.ca/dhp-mps/vet/advers-react-neg/index-eng.php

- +/− Antihistamines: anti-H1 receptors (e.g., diphenhydramine 2 mg /kg, IM, every 12 hours) alone or in combination with anti-H2 receptors (e.g., ranitidine 1 to 3.5 mg/kg, IV or SC or PO, every 12 hours; there are reports of hemolytic anemia with famotidine given IV)

It is important to remember that some type I hypersensitivity reactions involve the mucocutaneous system (urticaria and angioedema) without the respiratory and cardiovascular system. These reactions are less severe and can probably be managed with corticosteroids and/or antihistamines alone, under careful surveillance until complete resolution.

Discontinuing any drug and implementing aggressive organ support are the cornerstones of treating all drug allergies. Immunosuppressive therapy (e.g., corticosteroids, human intravenous IgG, cyclosporine) is sometimes included in the management of drug allergies. There is no strong evidence in human medicine, however, and none in feline drug allergies, that they improve the outcome.

If the idiosyncratic reaction is thought to be immune mediated, the cat should never receive the culprit drug again, because the clinical signs could be much more severe at the next exposure. Sometimes, another member of the same drug class may be substituted (e.g., midazolam in cats with a history of diazepam-associated hepatotoxicity, propyluracil in propylthiouracil-sensitive cats). In cases of drug allergies, some clinicians will prefer to use a different drug class to avoid any risk of cross-reactivity (e.g., avoiding all penicillins after amoxicillin allergy). If some of the drugs that were discontinued when the episode started were essential to the cat's survival or quality of life, the clinician should use the following precautions:

- Reintroduce each drug one-by-one, starting with those that are the least likely to have caused the incident.
- Start at a low dose (lower than the therapeutic dose) and increase it very gradually, with strict clinical surveillance and with all the emergency supplies and drugs ready in case of an allergic reaction.

REPORTING ADVERSE DRUG REACTIONS

Reporting an ADR is part of managing the event, even if the clinical signs were only mild, predictable, and/or could have been avoided. The reactions should be reported to the pharmaceutical company (using the phone number on the drug package). The manufacturer is required by law to pass this information on to the necessary governmental agency (Table 36-5). Only cases involving human drugs should be reported directly to a regulatory agency by the veterinarian. The clinician needs to report the adverse drug event as soon as possible, to avoid forgetting important details and to potentially receive key information about managing the reaction and helping the patient.

CONCLUSION

It is important to recognize that ADRs are not uncommon in cats, even though they are less often the subject of publications on ADR than are dogs or humans. The management of an ADR requires being aware of the risks, recognizing reactions promptly, and reporting them.

References

1. Aucoin DP, Peterson ME, Hurvitz AI et al: Propylthiouracil-induced immune-mediated disease in the cat, *J Pharmacol Exp Ther* 234:13, 1985.
2. Center SA, Elston TH, Rowland PH et al: Fulminant hepatic failure associated with oral administration of diazepam in 11 cats, *J Am Vet Med Assoc* 209:618, 1996.
3. Dyer F, Mulugeta R, Spagnuolo-Weaver M et al: Suspected adverse reactions, 2004, *Vet Rec* 156:561, 2005.
4. Hampshire VA, Doddy FM, Post LO et al: Adverse drug event reports at the United States Food and Drug Administration Center for Veterinary Medicine, *J Am Vet Med Assoc* 225:533, 2004.
5. Levy JK, Cullen JM, Bunch SE et al: Adverse reaction to diazepam in cats, *J Am Vet Med Assoc* 205:156, 1994.
6. Maddison JE: Adverse drug reactions: report of the Australian Veterinary Association Adverse Drug Reaction Subcommittee, 1994, *Aust Vet J* 73:132, 1996.
7. Peterson ME, Hurvitz AI, Leib MS et al: Propylthiouracil-associated hemolytic anemia, thrombocytopenia, and antinuclear antibodies in cats with hyperthyroidism, *J Am Vet Med Assoc* 184:806, 1984.

8. Shelton GH, Grant CK, Linenberger ML et al: Severe neutropenia associated with griseofulvin therapy in cats with feline immunodeficiency virus infection, *J Vet Intern Med* 4:317, 1990.
9. Waldhauser L, Uetrecht J: Antibodies to myeloperoxidase in propylthiouracil-induced autoimmune disease in the cat, *Toxicology* 114:155, 1996.

PALLIATIVE MEDICINE: PAIN ASSESSMENT AND MANAGEMENT

Sheilah Robertson

Pain is a component of many chronic diseases and is an important welfare issue. However, it is often overlooked and therefore undertreated. Recognizing long-standing pain and its impact on quality of life is challenging. Some of the behavior changes associated with pain may be mistaken for normal aging. The prevalence of chronic pain in the cat population is unknown, but in one study, 33.9% of cats between 6 months and 16.4 years of age had degenerative joint disease.[9] There is very little scientific evidence on the subject of chronic pain in cats, including treatment options and outcomes, in the veterinary literature.

POTENTIAL CAUSES OF LONG-TERM PAIN AND DISCOMFORT

Clinical conditions likely to result in long-term pain and discomfort in cats include interstitial cystitis, neoplasia, dermatologic diseases, dental and oral diseases, gastrointestinal disease, degenerative joint disease, slow-healing wounds, and diabetic neuropathy. Other causes include treatment-related pain, for example, radiation damage or chemotherapy-induced neuropathy. These conditions can afflict cats of any age, breed, or sex. In these patients, both the disease itself and the pain that is associated with it must be addressed. For example, it is important to regulate blood glucose in a diabetic cat, but the associated pain from neuropathy must also be addressed and often by different methods. In some cases, such as degenerative joint disease, there is little that can be done to halt the disease process, so the focus is to relieve pain.

PATHOPHYSIOLOGY

Defining pain is not a simple matter. It is a multifactorial experience with sensory (how much does it hurt), affective or emotional (how does it make the cat feel), and functional (can the cat still perform normal daily activities) components. Pain can result from obvious causes (e.g., trauma) and last an expected time period, but sometimes pain persists after the original injury or wound appears to be healed. In diseases such as interstitial cystitis, the underlying mechanisms that cause pain are poorly understood, and classical analgesics, such as opioids and anti-inflammatory agents, do not consistently relieve the cat's pain.

In some cases, pain has no obvious cause and is sometimes classified as "idiopathic" or dysfunctional.[10] Dysfunctional pain serves no purpose—it is neither protective nor does it support healing. Historically, pain has been labeled as acute or chronic based solely on its duration; however, this is not a helpful classification. It has been suggested that the terms adaptive and maladaptive be adopted. The term adaptive infers a normal response to tissue damage and involves an inflammatory component (for example, a surgical incision) that is reversible and disappears over a predictable and relatively short time period. Maladaptive pain results from changes in the spinal cord and brain that result in abnormal sensory processing and is usually persistent. Nerve damage results in neuropathic pain that is maladaptive and often persistent, for example after limb amputation. Maladaptive pain can develop if adaptive pain is not quickly and aggressively treated, emphasizing the importance of good pain management for all painful procedures.

Ideally, pain should be classified by the underlying mechanism[31]; for example, inflammatory or neuropathic. Knowing and understanding the underlying cause guides the practitioner in the choice of treatment; otherwise treatment will be empirical. A diagnosis of "cancer" pain is not very helpful, since the cause could be mechanical compression of a nerve, inflammation from tissue necrosis, or mechanical distension of an organ. The underlying cause may be complex, and some mechanisms of pain can co-exist, requiring several different treatment strategies. This approach is discussed in the American Animal Hospital Association (AAHA)/American Association of Feline Practitioners (AAFP) pain management guidelines.[14]

Another challenge to the practitioner is that even if the underlying cause or mechanism is identified, the disease process and associated pain may not be static; "good" days and "bad" days are common in cats with long-term disease. A cat that has good pain management for a tumor can have acute exacerbations if the tumor grows rapidly or becomes necrotic. A concurrent disease condition, such as inflammatory bowel disease, may also change the processing of noxious signals and the pain that the cat perceives.

CLINICAL SIGNS AND DIAGNOSIS

Because of the nature of long-term pain, which is sometimes slow and insidious in onset, the accompanying behavioral changes can be subtle and easily missed. Asking the owner the correct questions about changes in behavior (loss of normal behaviors [e.g., grooming] or appearance of new behaviors [e.g., seeking solitude, aversion to being stroked]) and changes in lifestyle are key to establishing a suspicion of underlying pain. Mobility, activity, grooming, and temperament improve with analgesic intervention in cats with degenerative joint disease.[2,19] It is likely that these four major behavior domains are also altered in other chronic pain states. Keeping track of these questions and answers is also important for evaluating response to therapy. In addition, it can be useful if the owner keeps a diary, noting things such as appetite, playing, hiding, socialization, or interaction with other pets, and to compare current to previous entries. Having a written account can show the owner which therapies appear to help and show when bad days are outnumbering the good days, helping them make decisions on whether or not to continue treatment.

Painful diabetic neuropathy occurs in some but not all human diabetics and can be seen at different times after diagnosis and can resolve as nerves degenerate, but when present is distressing and has a significant impact on quality of life.[30] This component of the disease is less well described in cats; however "irritability, especially when touching the feet" is reported in the literature[21] and by many owners and veterinarians. In humans, sensory changes start in the feet and hands. Unlike humans, changes in sensation to thermal and tactile stimuli have not yet been documented in cats[6]; however, only a very small number of cats have been tested, and only at one time point in the disease process. Clues as to whether diabetic cats are painful include reports by the owner that the cat has recently started to dislike being touched, especially around the distal extremities. Licking of the feet leading to discoloration of the fur can sometimes be seen in light colored cats and suggests tingling or other sensory changes.

Clinical examination by the veterinarian is also an important part of the assessment process.[25] Questioning the owner and performing a comprehensive examination will take time and so should be planned outside of a busy schedule.

TREATMENT

At the outset, some clear treatment goals should be established. In many cases, we are not dealing with curable diseases; quality of life, not quantity of life is the focus of treatment. The aim of treatment is to normalize pain sensitivity.[31] Our goals are to make cats comfortable so that they can perform normal daily activities and to prevent any marked changes in their normal behavior or personality.

The level of treatment must be matched to the level and complexity of the pain present. However, some cats are difficult to medicate, and compliance with a recommended treatment is often poor; therefore the route of administration, number of drugs, and dosing schedules should be carefully evaluated for feasibility in each patient. As previously discussed, chronic diseases are not static and neither is the pain associated with them; therefore frequent modification of the treatment plan may be needed to maintain a constant level of comfort.

Because treatment will often be for a prolonged period of time, it is important to have a discussion with the owner at the outset about the financial, time, and emotional commitment involved and to point out that treatment may require considerable trial and error, with associated disappointment and frustration. It is important to be realistic about what can be achieved and not give false hope or allow the owner to embark on treatment pathways with no scientific basis and with little chance of success.

Drug Therapy

Sometimes it can be difficult to be certain a cat is in pain based on a clinical assessment, or an owner may be convinced that some of the behavioral changes seen are just part of "slowing down and getting old." In these cases, an analgesic trial can be helpful and often results in the owner claiming they did see a change in behavior and the cat is now "like its old self."[2]

Most drugs used for the alleviation of maladaptive pain are used "off label" for the feline species, and doses and dosing intervals are not well established (Table 36-6).

Psychoactive Drugs

Drugs in this category include the selective serotonin reuptake inhibitors (SSRIs [e.g., fluoxetine]), monoamine oxidase inhibitors (MAOIs [e.g., selegiline]), and tricyclic antidepressants (TCAs [e.g., amitriptyline]). These drugs act to alter reuptake, release, and deactivation of catecholamines and serotonin, neurotransmitters known to be involved in pain transmission in the spinal cord. Psychoactive drugs, in particular the TCAs, are used in people for the treatment of chronic and neuropathic pain, often at doses lower than those used to treat depression. Amitriptyline has been used successfully for interstitial cystitis in some cats.[8] The TCAs should not be used concurrently with drugs that also modify the serotonergic system, such as tramadol (also see Drug Interactions below).

Antiepileptics

Gabapentin and pregabalin have been effective in various neuropathic pain states in people. Information on the kinetics of gabapentin in cats is available[27] but there are no scientific publications demonstrating its efficacy for alleviation of long-term pain in this species. However, this author finds gabapentin a particularly useful drug for so-called neuropathic or neurogenic

TABLE 36-6 Suggested Doses of Analgesics That May Be Used for the Alleviation of Long-Standing Pain in the Cat*

Drug and Class	Dose (mg/kg)	Comments
Amantadine (NMDA antagonist)	3.0-5.0 mg/kg, PO, q24h	This drug has not been evaluated for toxicity in the cat. It may be a useful adjunct to NSAIDs in the treatment of cancer-related pain and degenerative joint disease.
Amitriptyline (TCA)	0.5-2.0 mg/kg, PO, q24h	This drug appears to be well tolerated in cats. It has been used for interstitial cystitis. Somnolence (<10% of cats), weight gain, decreased grooming, and transient cystic calculi were observed during treatment in some cats.[8]
Buprenorphine (opioid)	0.01-0.02 mg/kg, oral transmucosal, q8h, or "as needed"	The oral transmucosal route is well tolerated by most cats.
Gabapentin (antiepileptic)	5-10 mg/kg, PO, q12h	Appears to be effective in cats where the underlying cause of pain is neuropathic.
Meloxicam (NSAID)	Oral formulation: Approval was gained in Europe (June 2007) for long-term (unlimited) use of meloxicam in the cat at 0.1 mg/kg, PO, on day 1, followed by 0.05 mg/kg, PO, every 24 hours Lower doses and "every other day" dosing can also be effective Injectable formulation available	This drug is particularly well received by cats, because of its formulation as a liquid. The formulation makes it very easy to gradually and accurately decrease the dose. Meloxicam should be dosed accurately using syringes. Careful titration and monitoring allows the "lowest effective dose" to be reached, thereby avoiding potential side effects. Give with food. Labeled for acute perioperative pain.
Tramadol (mixed analgesic)	1-2 mg/kg, PO, every 12 to 24 hours	Published data suggests the metabolism of tramadol is slower in the cat than in the dog, and the production of the M1 metabolite is very much greater, leading to a greater tendency to see "opioid"-like side effects (pupil dilation euphoria).[24] Very unpalatable even when compounded. Do not use in cats receiving psychoactive drugs.
Transdermal fentanyl patch (opioid)	25 µg/hour patch	A 25 µg/hour patch can be applied to an "average" cat (3.5-5.0 kg, 7.7-11 lb). Uptake is highly variable. Time to onset of action is 6-12 hours. The patches may provide 3-5 days of analgesia in some cases. Following removal at 3 days, the decay in plasma levels following patch removal is slow. Liability issues should be considered when these are used in a home setting. Do not use in cats receiving psychoactive drugs. Do not use in combination with tramadol.
	12.5 µg/hour patch	Smaller cats.

*See text for details. In most cases these drugs are used "off label" for cats, and doses are not well established.
M1 metabolite, O-desmethyl-tramadol; *NMDA,* N-methyl-D-aspartate; *NSAID,* nonsteroidal antiinflammatory drug, *TCA,* tricyclic antidepressant.

pain, at starting doses of 10 mg/kg, PO, every 12 hours. Sedation and ataxia are the main side effects seen in cats.

Sodium Channel Blockade

Although not a convenient mode of delivery for most patients with neuropathic pain, intravenous lidocaine has proven effective for neuropathic pain in humans with single treatments, sometimes offering long-term relief.[7] However, the intravenous administration of lidocaine to cats is associated with cardiovascular depression and is not recommended.[23] There is increasing interest in transdermal lidocaine patches, and a recent study reported on the absorption and kinetics of lidocaine from transdermal patches in cats; plasma lidocaine concentrations remained well below systemically toxic concentrations, and skin concentrations of lidocaine were high.[15] The transdermal technique may prove useful for alleviating pain originating from long-standing wounds and scar tissue.

N-Methyl-D-Aspartate (NMDA) Inhibitors

Preclinical evidence indicates that hyperalgesia (an exaggerated and prolonged response to a noxious stimulus) and allodynia (pain that can be elicited by normally innocuous stimuli) following peripheral tissue or nerve injury depends on NMDA receptor–mediated central changes in synaptic excitability, and also shows quite clearly that NMDA antagonists can attenuate hyperalgesia and allodynia in animal models of neuropathic pain. The NMDA antagonist amantadine (3 to 5 mg/kg, PO, every 24 hours), as an adjunct to NSAID use, is effective in dogs with osteoarthritis.[18] There are no pharmacokinetic studies of amantadine in the cat, and although there are anecdotal reports of use for chronic pain, there are no well-controlled published studies.

In some cats with maladaptive pain, the author has observed improvement after they have been sedated with ketamine for diagnostic tests. Ketamine, as a bolus (2 mg/kg, IV), or as a constant rate infusion (2 to 5 µg/kg/minute) for several hours, may have a role to play in "resetting" the central nervous system in some pain states.

Mixed Analgesics

Although not classified as a true opioid, tramadol has weak binding affinity at OP3 (mu) opioid receptors but also acts at serotonin and adrenergic receptors. There has been considerable interest in evaluating tramadol in cats. Pharmacokinetic evaluation of intravenous and oral tramadol found a relatively long half-life and rapid and significant formation of the M1 metabolite (*O*-desmethyl-tramadol) when compared with use in dogs.[24] The M1 metabolite is considered to be the active metabolite, responsible for analgesia. Tramadol can provide analgesia in the cat, at least in the acute setting (see Chapter 6). As yet, there is no work evaluating the analgesic action of tramadol in chronic or maladaptive scenarios. One of the biggest drawbacks with oral tramadol is its bitter taste, and even with flavoring, this drug can be difficult to administer to cats. The development of palatable formulations that allow high compliance will be essential to future studies. Tramadol should not be given to cats receiving psychoactive drugs (see above, Adverse Drug Reactions).

Opioids

Opioids have variable efficacy in the treatment of maladaptive pain in humans, and their role in this setting is not well defined in cats. Transdermal fentanyl can be an effective way of providing perioperative analgesia in the cat (see Chapter 6). Buprenorphine, given by the oral transmucosal route (OTM), is highly bioavailable, easy to administer, and is antinociceptive in the cat.[26] The major physical side effect of continuous opioid use for weeks or months in humans is constipation, but there are no similar reports in cats. There are anecdotal reports of appetite loss in cats after several days of opioid use, which usually resolves when the dose is lowered or its use is discontinued. Opioid-related euphoria can occur and is undesirable to some owners.

There is no information on dependence or withdrawal with long-term use of opioids in cats. Opioids may have a role to play in controlling "break-through" pain, for example, when a cat whose pain is well controlled with amitriptyline or meloxicam has a "bad day." In this author's experience, OTM buprenorphine can be helpful given in the evening to ensure overnight sleep; the restorative powers of sleep should not be underestimated. In addition, a restless cat can be upsetting and disruptive to the owner. Opioids may also be used in "end-of-life" situations. As discussed below, amitriptyline and fentanyl should not be used concurrently. The liability issues surrounding the use of transdermal patches are discussed in Chapter 6.

Nonsteroidal Antiinflammatory Drugs

Nonsteroidal antiinflammatory drugs (NSAIDs) are the foundation of a treatment plan for many long-term pain patients. The mode of action and use of NSAIDs in cats has been comprehensively reviewed.[17] Meloxicam is approved in Europe and other countries, including Australia, for the treatment of chronic musculoskeletal pain. This approval is for an unlimited time at a dose of 0.05 mg/kg, PO, every 24 hours. A study of 40 cats with degenerative joint disease (DJD)–associated pain suggested that a dose of 0.01 to 0.03 mg/kg, PO, every 24 hours, with mean treatment duration of 5.8 months, was well tolerated.[12] Gastrointestinal upset in 4% of cats was the only adverse effect noted. The first drug in the coxib class of NSAIDs, robenacoxib (Onsior),[11] has been granted approval in Europe for use in cats. In cats with musculoskeletal pain, the indication is for as many as 6 days of therapy at a dose of 1 mg/kg, PO, every 24 hours. Oral NSAIDs should be administered with food.

Adverse Drug Interactions

There is potential for adverse drug interactions when patients with behavioral problems are prescribed psychoactive drugs and require treatment for pain. The main concern is precipitation of serotonin toxicity, sometimes referred to as "serotonin syndrome." This is well recognized in humans[4] and is now reported in animals.[22] Serotonin toxicity results from overdose with one serotonergic drug or by the use of a combination of drugs that influence serotonin levels. Serotonin toxicity resulting from multidrug therapy is not well documented in the veterinary literature but is an increasing concern as treatment strategies become more complex.

Mirtazapine, often used as an appetite stimulant and antiemetic, may cause serotonin syndrome in susceptible individuals. Because of this, other agents may be better choices, should a patient require one of the following drugs with similar serotonin effects. Some opioids, including meperidine, methadone, pentazocine and fentanyl, and tramadol impair reuptake of serotonin, and tramadol may also increase serotonin release. These drugs have precipitated serotonin toxicity when given to humans taking SSRIs, MAOIs, and TCAs. Buspirone is a partial serotonin agonist and could lead to problems when combined with these analgesics.

Before designing a plan for treating long-term pain in a patient, it is important to know which drugs have been prescribed but also what is being given by the owner. Herbal supplements, such as *Hypericum perforatum*, or St. John's Wort, and ginseng have been linked to serotonergic intoxication in humans and dogs.[22] Transdermal fentanyl patches and tramadol should not be used in cats receiving behavior-modification drugs. Buprenorphine does not cause serotonin reuptake inhibition and so can be used as previously described.

Nonpharmacologic Therapies

Environmental Enrichment

Environmental enrichment is important for all cats, especially those confined indoors; however, it may be a critical component of treatment for cats with long-standing disease. Cats with degenerative joint disease (DJD)–associated pain will benefit from exercise, which can be increased by a complex environment, for example, by using cat towers/climbing trees, toys, and hiding food to encourage foraging and hunting behavior. In people, a stimulating environment or being engaged in activities distracts the patient from focusing on their pain, and these techniques could be applied to animals. Environmental enrichment strategies are discussed in detail in Chapter 46.

Physical Therapies

Physical rehabilitation techniques, including controlled exercise, passive range-of-motion (ROM) exercises, and massage can all be incorporated into a treatment plan. The benefits of these treatment strategies are just beginning to be defined in canine medicine but have not yet been evaluated in feline medicine. However, it is likely the same basic principles and benefits will apply to feline patients. ROM and massage techniques can be taught to owners, and these techniques can both help to alleviate muscle pain and also contribute to "environmental" enrichment for the cat; there is more interaction between the owner and cat, and this can use up otherwise empty "time budgets." It also empowers the owner by involving them in treatment. When used as an adjunct to conventional therapy, massage improved pain, discomfort, mood, tension, and stress in human pediatric patients with chronic pain.[29] Similar to massage and ROM exercises, other modalities, such as shock wave therapy, laser therapy, and heat and cold therapy, may well be of benefit in certain circumstances in feline patients, but no well-controlled scientific studies of these modalities in cats have been published.

Gingivostomatitis is challenging to treat in cats and may require several approaches, including multiple tooth extractions, corticosteroids, NSAIDs, antiviral and immunomodulatory drugs, and laser resection.[20] Pain and a poor quality of life are major features of this disease in many cats. Although lasers are widely used for oral surgery, they may also have a potential role in healing and analgesia. In humans with recurrent stomatitis, carbon dioxide (CO_2) laser irradiation provided excellent and rapid pain relief.[32] In cancer patients with mucositis, specific laser phototherapy protocols had a positive effect on pain and healing.[16,28] Once again, clinical studies are lacking in feline medicine.

Complementary Therapies

In recent years, the popularity of more "holistic" or "natural" approaches to medicine for both people and pets has increased. The legitimacy of acupuncture has been questioned because of a lack of well-controlled scientific and clinical trials, and although this is still largely true, in a review of the animal specific acupuncture literature, Habacher[13] stated that there were enough promising results to support pursuing acupuncture as a viable treatment in veterinary patients. However, none of these studies have involved cats.

FUTURE DIRECTIONS IN LONG-TERM PAIN MANAGEMENT

Regenerative Medicine

Regenerative medicine is an emerging area of research as diseases of aging that involve the loss or dysfunction of specific cells become more common. One approach to preventing or treating these diseases is to use autologous adult stem cells, which differentiate into several tissue types and supply trophic factors concurrently. Currently, autologous adipose-derived mesenchymal stem cell therapy is available in the United States (Vet-Stem, Poway, Calif.) for use in animals, primarily for the treatment of osteoarthritis (OA) and tendon injuries. Adipose tissue is surgically harvested from the patient, sent for processing, and several days later, the stem cells are injected into the affected tissue or joints, although intravenous injection is also reported. There are encouraging published results in dogs with OA.[3] Although this treatment modality has been used in cats with osteoarthritis, with anecdotal reports of improvement, there are currently no published studies.

Neurotrophic Agents

ProsaptideTX14 (A) is an exogenous neurotrophic agent given by subcutaneous injection that prevents and reverses neuronal damage and sensory changes in rat models of diabetes. Clinical trials with ProsaptideTX14 (A) have been conducted in cats with naturally occurring diabetes mellitus. Cats that were enrolled underwent a full clinical examination, nerve conduction testing, and collection of a nerve, muscle, and skin biopsy prior to and following 6 months of treatment with either a placebo or Prosaptide injection; results of this study are expected in the near future.[6]

Neurotoxins

Resiniferatoxin, a capsaicin analog, has been injected intrathecally in dogs with severe pain related to osteosarcoma and provided good analgesia.[5] The proposed mechanism of action is a selective effect at the vanilloid receptors in nociceptive neurons, primarily C-fiber afferents of the dorsal horn; motor function and normal nociception are left intact. Other agents, such as substance P-saporin combinations, have been investigated in dogs as potential selective neuroablative agents for managing severe pain.[1] No reports of use of these agents in cats currently exist.

CONCLUSION

There is a growing awareness and concern among practitioners about long-term pain and its impact on quality of life in cats. We are in need of more evidence on the prevalence, recognition of, etiology, treatment protocols, and treatment outcomes of long-term pain issues in cats. The strong desire to help these cats will hopefully pave the way for formulating well-conducted research and clinical trials.

References

1. Allen JW, Mantyh PW, Horais K et al: Safety evaluation of intrathecal substance P-saporin, a targeted neurotoxin, in dogs, *Toxicol Sci* 91:286, 2006.
2. Bennett D, Morton C: A study of owner observed behavioural and lifestyle changes in cats with musculoskeletal disease before and after analgesic therapy, *J Feline Med Surg* 11:997, 2009.
3. Black LL, Gaynor J, Adams C et al: Effect of intraarticular injection of autologous adipose-derived mesenchymal stem and regenerative cells on clinical signs of chronic osteoarthritis of the elbow joint in dogs, *Vet Ther* 9:192, 2008.
4. Boyer EW, Shannon M: The serotonin syndrome, *N Engl J Med* 352:1112, 2005.
5. Brown DC, Iadarola MJ, Perkowski SZ et al: Physiologic and antinociceptive effects of intrathecal resiniferatoxin in a canine bone cancer model, *Anesthesiology* 103:1052, 2005.
6. Calcutt NA, Mizisin AP, Shelton GD: The diabetic cat as a model for diabetic neuropathy—developing therapeutics for neuropathy in companion animals, IASP Special Interest Group: measuring nociception and pain in non-human species: beyond the hot plate and paw pressure test. From the 12th World Congress on Pain, August 2008, Glasgow, Scotland, p 60.
7. Challapalli V, Tremont-Lukats IW, McNicol ED et al: Systemic administration of local anesthetic agents to relieve neuropathic pain, *Cochrane Database Syst Rev* (4):CD003345, 2005.
8. Chew DJ, Buffington CA, Kendall MS et al: Amitriptyline treatment for severe recurrent idiopathic cystitis in cats, *J Am Vet Med Assoc* 213:1282, 1998.
9. Clarke SP, Mellor D, Clements DN et al: Prevalence of radiographic signs of degenerative joint disease in a hospital population of cats, *Vet Rec* 157:793, 2005.
10. Costigan M, Scholz J, Woolf CJ: Neuropathic pain: a maladaptive response of the nervous system to damage, *Annu Rev Neurosci* 32:1, 2009.
11. Giraudel JM, King JN, Jeunesse EC et al: Use of a pharmacokinetic/pharmacodynamic approach in the cat to determine a dosage regimen for the COX-2 selective drug robenacoxib, *J Vet Pharmacol Ther* 32:18, 2009.
12. Gunew MN, Menrath VH, Marshall RD: Long-term safety, efficacy and palatability of oral meloxicam at 0.01-0.03 mg/kg for treatment of osteoarthritic pain in cats, *J Feline Med Surg* 10:235, 2008.
13. Habacher G, Pittler MH, Ernst E: Effectiveness of acupuncture in veterinary medicine: systematic review, *J Vet Intern Med* 20:480, 2006.
14. Hellyer P, Rodan I, Brunt J et al: AAHA/AAFP pain management guidelines for dogs and cats, *J Feline Med Surg* 9:466, 2007.
15. Ko JC, Maxwell LK, Abbo LA et al: Pharmacokinetics of lidocaine following the application of 5% lidocaine patches to cats, *J Vet Pharmacol Ther* 31:359, 2008.
16. Kuhn A, Porto FA, Miraglia P et al: Low-level infrared laser therapy in chemotherapy-induced oral mucositis: a randomized placebo-controlled trial in children, *J Pediatr Hematol Oncol* 31:33, 2009.
17. Lascelles BD, Court MH, Hardie EM et al: Nonsteroidal anti-inflammatory drugs in cats: a review, *Vet Anaesth Analg* 34:228, 2007.
18. Lascelles BD, Gaynor JS, Smith ES et al: Amantadine in a multimodal analgesic regimen for alleviation of refractory osteoarthritis pain in dogs, *J Vet Intern Med* 22:53, 2008.
19. Lascelles BD, Hansen BD, Roe S et al: Evaluation of client-specific outcome measures and activity monitoring to measure pain relief in cats with osteoarthritis, *J Vet Intern Med* 21:410, 2007.
20. Lyon KF: Gingivostomatitis, *Vet Clin North Am Small Anim Pract* 35:89, 2005.
21. Mizisin AP, Nelson RW, Sturges BK et al: Comparable myelinated nerve pathology in feline and human diabetes mellitus, *Acta Neuropathol* 113:431, 2007.
22. Mohammad-Zadeh LF, Moses L, Gwaltney-Brant SM: Serotonin: a review, *J Vet Pharmacol Ther* 3:187, 2008.
23. Pypendop BH, Ilkiw JE: Assessment of the hemodynamic effects of lidocaine administered IV in isoflurane-anesthetized cats, *Am J Vet Res* 66:661, 2005.
24. Pypendop BH, Ilkiw JE: Pharmacokinetics of tramadol, and its metabolite O-desmethyl-tramadol, in cats, *J Vet Pharmacol Ther* 31:52, 2008.
25. Robertson S, Lascelles D: Long-term pain in cats: what do we know about this important welfare issue? *J Feline Med Surg* 12:188, 2010.
26. Robertson SA, Lascelles BD, Taylor P M et al: PK-PD modeling of buprenorphine in cats: intravenous and oral transmucosal administration, *J Vet Pharmacol Ther* 28:453, 2005.
27. Siao KT, Pypendop BH, Ilkiw JE: Pharmacokinetics of gabapentin in cats, *Am J Vet Res* 71:817, 2010.
28. Simoes A, Eduardo FP, Luiz AC et al: Laser phototherapy as topical prophylaxis against head and neck cancer radiotherapy-induced oral mucositis: comparison between low and high/low power lasers, *Lasers Surg Med* 41:264, 2009.
29. Suresh S, Wang S, Porfyris S et al: Massage therapy in outpatient pediatric chronic pain patients: do they facilitate significant reductions in levels of distress, pain, tension, discomfort, and mood alterations? *Paediatr Anaesth* 18:884, 2008.
30. Veves A, Backonja M, Malik RA: Painful diabetic neuropathy: epidemiology, natural history, early diagnosis, and treatment options, *Pain Med* 9:660, 2008.

31. Woolf CJ: Pain: moving from symptom control toward mechanism-specific pharmacologic management, *Ann Intern Med* 140:441, 2004.
32. Zand N, Ataie-Fashtami L, Djavid GE et al: Relieving pain in minor aphthous stomatitis by a single session of non-thermal carbon dioxide laser irradiation, *Lasers Med Sci* 24:515, 2009.

PALLIATIVE MEDICINE, QUALITY OF LIFE, AND EUTHANASIA DECISIONS

Margie Scherk and Bernard E. Rollin

"The death we fear most is dying in pain, unnoticed, and isolated from loved ones. Concern about such an undignified and difficult death has engendered the debate over authorizing voluntary active euthanasia and physician-assisted suicide. Death is fundamental to the nature of being human."
—*Anonymous*

It is the rare adult who does not have an emotional response to thoughts of dying. Once we reach our mid-thirties, we are all inherently aware of our mortality and that of those around us. No different from our clients, despite being veterinary health care providers, we fear the pain and suffering of friends and companions, human or nonhuman, too. Nor do we become elated when considering the probabilities of terminal illness and long-term nursing care.

What is aging? To paraphrase from Robbins[5]: Aging begins at the moment of conception, involves differentiation and maturation and, at some point, leads to the progressive loss of functional capacity characteristic of senescence, ending in death. This occurs at an organismal level as well as at a cellular level. The former may be affected by genetics, social environment, nutrition, and the occurrence of age-related diseases. Cellular aging, on the other hand, includes progressive accumulation of sublethal injury (e.g., from free radical damage), resulting in either cell death or diminished capacity of the cell to repair itself.

Why should we consider this? Home care and end-of-life issues inherently encompass matters of age-related and age-appropriate illnesses. In cats, these include, most significantly, renal insufficiency progressing to failure, hyperthyroidism, diabetes mellitus, degenerative joint disorders, neoplasia, and chronic digestive disorders, including inflammatory bowel disease, pancreatitis, and cholangiohepatitis. In some cases, by addressing organ and cell function, we can have an impact on well-being.

Just as we match nutritional and preventative medical recommendations to life stage, so too can we match stages and types of care to the final stages of life. These roles include providing supportive care; alleviating pain, discomfort, and distress; preparing the animal and client for the end, while ensuring death with dignity intact; and caring for the caregivers.

PROVIDING SUPPORT FOR THE FUNCTION OF CELLS AND ORGANS

Hydration

Hydration is of utmost importance and should be included in any home care program. Most clients are able to give fluids subcutaneously at home if the care team believes in their importance and knows that the client is capable of doing so. Fluids improve well being. Dehydration at a cellular level results in headaches, nausea, sluggishness, inappetence, lethargy, malaise, and constipation. When cells are not getting enough fluid, they take it from urine and feces. In fact, this change is more reliably evaluated than changes in skin elasticity in the early stages of dehydration, and is one that clients can easily monitor. Dehydration results in hard fecal balls rather than the normal log-shaped feces. Inadequately hydrated cells are not able to function adequately, cannot transport toxins or nutrients well, and are not well oxygenated, thereby suffering further damage and lethal changes.

Daily subcutaneous fluid requirements should be calculated in the same manner that intravenous requirements are calculated, namely deficit (as a percentage of ideal body weight in kg) plus maintenance (60 mL/kg [ideal weight]/day) plus ongoing losses sustained by diarrhea or vomiting (Box 36-1).

If this volume is too large for administration at a single time, it may be divided into multiple treatments

BOX 36-1

Example of Subcutaneous Fluid Calculation for a Dehydrated Cat

Ideal, healthy, hydrated weight: 4 kg
Ill, dehydrated, inappetent weight: 3.2 kg
Estimated deficit (assessed by firm feces, delay in skin elasticity, slightly dry oral mucous membranes, normal eye position): 8%

Deficit 8% × 4 kg = 320 mL
Maintenance (60 mL/kg/day) × 4 kg = 240 mL
Ongoing losses unknown at present = ? mL
Fluid requirement in first 24 hours = 560 mL

The 560 mL can be given IV at 23 mL/hour, or, were this to be given SC for some reason, as three boluses of 185 mL during the 24-hour period. After the patient is rehydrated, a dose of 60 mL/kg/day (based on ideal weight) = 240 mL is needed daily to maintain hydration.

BOX 36-2

Sample Client Handout Instructions on Subcutaneous Fluid Administration

To Connect a New Line to a Bag

1. Prepare the line by rolling the wheel to a closed position.
2. Take the sterile cap off the line and place it somewhere where it will stay clean.
3. Remove the white/blue end from the bag of fluids.
4. Insert the white/blue end of the IV line into the bag firmly; squeeze the bulb of the IV line to fill the bulb half full.
5. Open the line by rolling the wheel to the open position and fill the line with fluids.

To Give a Kitty Fluids

1. Wrap your kitty in a towel so his/her shoulder area is exposed.
2. Place an unused needle on the IV line.
3. Make a tent in kitty's skin over his/her shoulders.
4. Holding the needle parallel to your cat's backbone, insert the needle into the tent of skin.
5. Open the IV line and administer the volume of fluids directed by the doctor.
6. Close the IV line by rolling the wheel to the closed position, remove and discard the used needle; place the sterile cap back on the IV line.
CONGRATULATIONS! You've done it!

Notes

1. Your kitty will look like s(he) is wearing shoulder pads. The fluid will droop to one side and down a leg so that it looks like a water wing and then a fat foot. This is normal and will resolve as the fluids are absorbed during 12 to 24 hours.
2. If some of the fluids, or even a bit of blood, leak out of the injection site, there is no need to worry.
3. Warming the fluid bag before giving the fluids may help your kitty be more comfortable. Invert the fluid bag in a warm water bath, being careful to keep the connection between the bulb and the line out of the water. Leave in for 5 minutes, massaging the bag to distribute the warmer portions before you start.
4. Please call us at any time. We are happy to demonstrate again and guide you through this process. We know you CAN do it. Your cat will feel a lot better because of your persistence.

during the day. Warming the fluids may make the experience more pleasant for some cats. Some people prefer to administer the fluids as rapidly as possible using gravity feed and an 18-gauge needle; others prefer a slower delivery rate (resulting in less rapid skin stretch) using a 20-gauge needle. Teflon-coated needles are another available option. A sample client handout for subcutaneous fluid administration is shown in Box 36-2.

Two surgically placed administration options exist. The fenestrated tube implant has been anecdotally reported to have problems, including infection, resulting from movement of the tube at the stoma site. The second option, a skin button or port, shows promise.

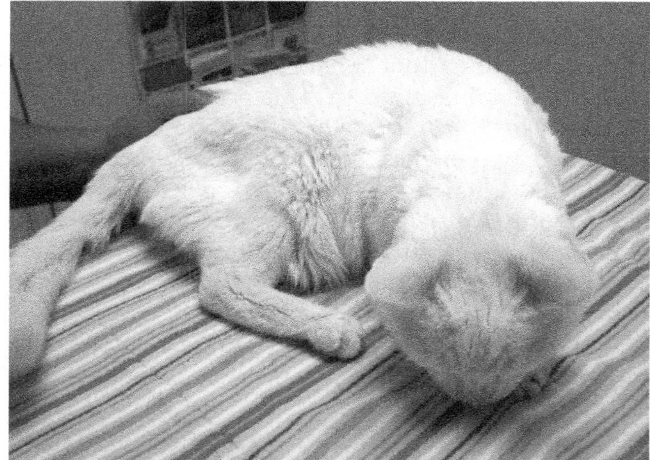

FIGURE 36-1 As cats get older, they may become cachectic. Careful consideration for muscle wasting and weight loss starts with determining whether the cat has a good appetite or a poor appetite. This patient is manifesting protein:calorie malnutrition caused by inadequate protein in the diet.

Nutrition

Attention to nutrition is of paramount importance in order to provide calories from fat and protein and to supply antioxidants and other micronutrients (Figure 36-1). Carbohydrates are less essential for cats as obligate carnivores; however, they can be a good source of energy. The goal is to have a cat eat 50 kcal/kg (ideal weight)/day on its own. When illness interferes with meeting this goal, we have to assist. It is always important to monitor that the amount of food being eaten is adequate, even when appetite stimulants are being used. Aversion to a new diet is readily developed when a therapeutic or other new diet is offered in a clinic setting or when an individual feels ill. Thus it may be advisable to find a food appealing to the patient rather than to insist on a particular dietary formulation.

Pharmacologic agents such as cyproheptadine (Periactin) at 1 mg/cat, PO, q12h or mirtazapine (Remeron) at 2 to 3 mg/cat, PO, q72h can be used. Discontinue cyproheptadine if it is ineffective after four doses. Mirtazapine has the added benefit of being an antiemetic as well as an appetite stimulant. Should disorientation or mania occur with mirtazapine ("serotonin syndrome"), time and a dose of cyproheptadine will resolve the adverse reaction. Although some clinicians view diazepam as an option for appetite stimulation, because of the unnecessary sedative action and the possibility of inducing irreversible, life-threatening toxic hepatopathy, it is contraindicated.

Feeding tubes save lives by making the administration of nutrients and medications less stressful for the client and for the patient. Nasoesophageal tubes can be used short term and require a liquid diet, such as Clinicare Feline or Rebound (1.0 kcal/mL). Human enteral diets are too low in protein for long-term use and have a high osmolarity, resulting in diarrhea. Oral syringe feeding can be performed with minimal stress if several tips are considered. Face the cat away from you and use small volume syringes to ensure that the oral capacity of a cat (approximately 1 mL) is not exceeded. Place the tip of the syringe at the back of the mouth to make it more difficult for the cat to spit out the food. Room- or body-temperature food is less unpleasant. A cat's stomach can hold up to 100 mL when healthy; so, starting with 6 mL and increasing in 6 mL increments to 48 mL total per feeding is realistic with most cats.

Use of large-bore (14- to 16-Fr) feeding tubes is preferable, because a wider variety of diets can be used. Placement of esophagostomy tubes requires only brief anesthesia and eliminates the postoperative risk of peritonitis that a gastrotomy tube (G-tube) might entail (Figure 36-2). These tubes allow for the use of specially formulated, calorically dense, syringeable diets. If the client wants to dilute the diet for ease of syringing, Clinicare or Rebound should be used as the diluent rather than water to prevent loss of caloric density. G-tubes must be aspirated before infusing food to determine residual gastric volume. Either type of tube must be flushed with water following feeding to prevent clogging. Regardless of the method used for assisted feeding, including pharmacologic approaches, the daily caloric needs must be met; this is easily determined by converting to milliliters using the data in Table 36-7.

Pain may interfere with eating. There may be oral pain from periodontal disease, from a tooth resorption lesion, or from a mass (Figure 36-3). Dental health should be optimized wherever possible. Musculoskeletal pain makes crouching or bending the neck uncomfortable. Shape and placement of bowls should be taken into consideration in the ill or older individual, especially if joint pain is present. Nausea associated with uremic gastritis or renal disease may be lessened with famotidine (Pepcid) 5 mg, PO, q24h or another H2 antagonist.

Declining senses (hearing, vision, smell) may result in lack of awareness of food. Warming food to the temperature of freshly killed prey increases its palatability. Small, more frequent meals may suit the older patient better than two meals a day. The texture of the food may play an important role. Canned foods are preferable, should the cat like them, because they contain significantly more water. Practitioners often recommend feeding a prescription diet for a specific ailment. However, cats being the selective creatures they are, as mentioned earlier, it is more important that they eat, than what they eat, and that they eat enough of it.

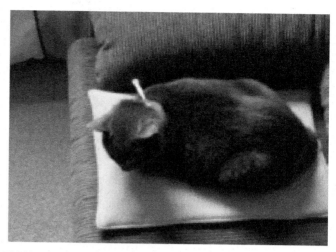

FIGURE 36-2 Supportive feeding helps provide adequate nutrition to slow and possibly reverse catabolic changes. Large-bore feeding tubes, such as the esophageal tube shown here, allow for easy administration of many medications and water for hydration, reducing stress on both the cat and its caregiver.

TABLE 36-7 **Caloric Densities of Convalescent Diets, for Calculating Feeding Volumes**

Product Name	Caloric Density
Rebound	1 kcal/mL
Clinicare	1 kcal/mL
Royal Canin/MediCal Recovery RS	1.23 kcal/mL
Hill's Prescription Diet a/d Canine/Feline	1.3 kcal/mL
Eukanuba Maximum Calorie	2.1 kcal/mL
Purina Veterinary Diets CV	1.3 kcal/mL when one can is blended with 170 mL Rebound/Clinicare 0.7 kcal/mL when one can is blended with 170 mL water

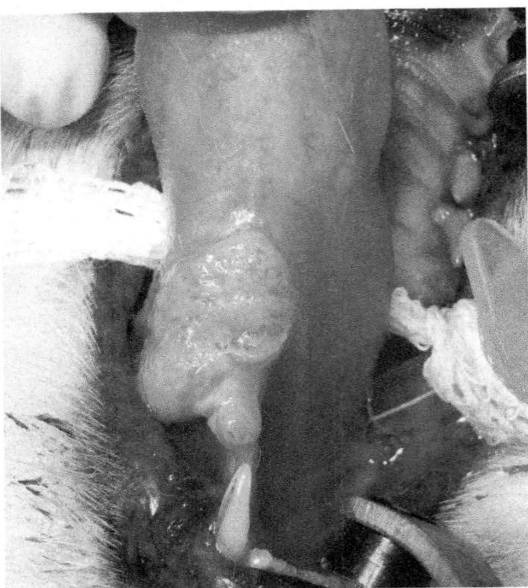

FIGURE 36-3 Working up a patient with a decrease in appetite or weight loss must include evaluation of the dentition and the mouth. Oral lesions, such as this squamous cell carcinoma, may hide under the tongue.

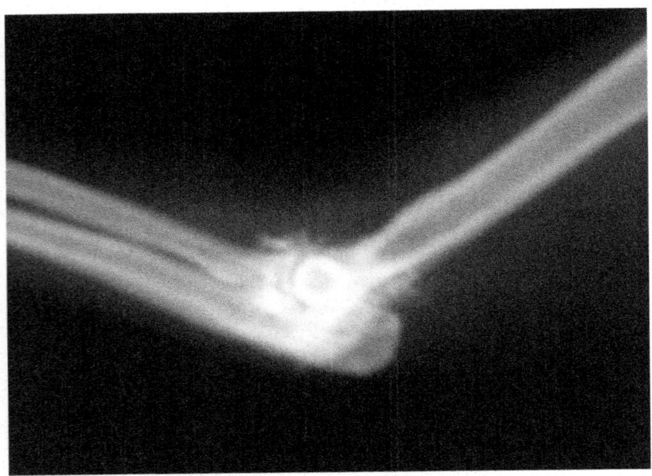

FIGURE 36-4 Proliferative changes of the elbow in a cat with degenerative joint disease. This cat will have difficulty jumping up and climbing down. Appropriate analgesia and environmental modification will allow this patient to have a more comfortable existence. Dietary changes and disease-modifying agents may also be of benefit long term.

Mobility

Mobility often declines in older or ill cats. During the past several years, numerous papers have been published regarding arthritis and degenerative joint disease in our feline patients (Figure 36-4).[9,12] Although estimates vary regarding the frequency of joint disorders, all experts agree that older cats have a greater incidence of joint problems that are clinically underdiagnosed, either because cats are not an exercised species or because they hide their discomfort well. In one paper,[12] a startling 90% of cats over 12 years of age were found to have radiographic evidence of degenerative joint disease, regardless of the reason for which they were presented to the veterinary hospital. Lameness is rarely noted; cats are seen to be "just slowing down" when they jump shorter heights and move less/rest more. If specific questions are asked about movement, one can often determine that there is stiffness or discomfort. "Have you noticed a change in how he jumps/climbs up? Jumps down? Walks?" A useful mobility questionnaire is found in Box 37-4. A recently published study includes another list of useful client evaluation questions suitable for clinic or home use.[3] Care of the older cat must include attention to mobility.

Manifestations of mobility problems include retention constipation, defecating outside of the litter box, falling when jumping onto or off of furniture, inability to climb stairs, and inability to crouch to eat, resulting in weight loss. Regular nail trimming helps by maintaining proper joint relationships. Ramps and steps onto favorite sleeping spots are thoughtful aids. Numerous websites feature ideas for steps and ramps for cats. Warm, soft, padded sleeping places for stiff, painful, possibly bony joints should be considered. Adding another litter box so that the cat does not have to walk as far may reduce inappropriate elimination as well as encourage regular voiding and defecation. Making sure that the rim of the box is not too high, and the opening into the box is not too small is helpful for older cats. Scooping the litter several times a day and making sure that the litter is not too deep or too sparse will encourage regular use.

ALLEVIATING DISCOMFORT AND OPTIMIZING COMFORT

Optimizing cellular function may require medications and supplements. Compliance is best achieved through helping the client understand the cat's illness and how the medication helps. In *Feline Oncology: a Comprehensive Guide to Compassionate Care,*[15] there are excellent handouts for clients that explain cancer terminology, treatment, and help clients to make difficult decisions.

Grooming may be neglected by the cat that has stiffness or one that is simply elderly and less attentive, possibly because of cognitive dysfunction. Diligent patient grooming by the owner may be necessary to help keep a cat's coat clean and healthy. Massage of stiff muscles may be appreciated, and if not, warm soft padded places on which to lie may be.

Cat owners may ask about nighttime yowling. Differential diagnoses include loss of special senses, hypertension, hyperthyroid agitation, pain, and cognitive dysfunction. The first may be discerned and alleviated by simply calling out to the cat so that it is able to locate the client. Hypertension and hyperthyroidism are readily

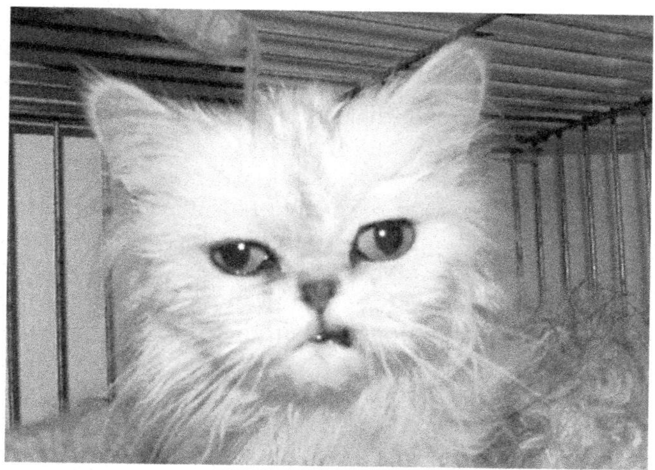

FIGURE 36-5 This cat appears to be in pain, as evidenced by the strained expression around the eyes. The spiky coat suggests dehydration as well as decreased attention to grooming. Dehydration, along with metabolic acidosis, a very common finding in ill cats, results in what humans experience as a "hangover."

diagnosed and controlled medically. Pain may be difficult to assess (see above, Palliative Medicine: Pain Assessment and Management). Often the best way to determine if pain is present is to administer analgesia and see if behavior normalizes. Cognitive dysfunction becomes a diagnosis by exclusion; it has been found that cats with cognitive dysfunction have brain changes similar to humans with dementia.[10]

The American Veterinary Medical Association (AVMA) Veterinarian's Oath states: "I solemnly swear to use my scientific knowledge and skills for … the relief of animal suffering …" Above all else, owners have the right to expect that our focus is going to be on alleviating (and preventing) pain (Figure 36-5). Fortunately, during the past decade, cats have received more attention than they did previously in this regard so that we now have a slightly wider menu from which to create our analgesic protocols. Use of a multimodal approach is often preferable in order to minimize the potential adverse effects of a single agent by using lower doses of several agents. Often a narcotic, such as buprenorphine, hydromorphone, butorphanol or fentanyl, is combined with a nonsteroidal antiinflammatory (NSAID), such as meloxicam or aspirin, or, for a single dose, ketoprofen or carprofen. Topical and local analgesia may also be provided either with EMLA cream (emulsion of lidocaine and prilocaine), a local nerve block, or acupuncture. Corticosteroids should not be combined with NSAIDs but can be used in conjunction with the other drugs.

Because of concern about possible effects on renal function, the general recommendation is to avoid NSAIDs in patients with renal disease. Having said this, at the final stages of life, as long as the owner has been fully informed about the risk, quality of life without arthritic pain may well be preferable to a painful, risk-free existence. As mentioned above, the clinical signs of arthritis include weight loss, anorexia, depression, elimination outside the litter box, poor grooming, and lameness. Meloxicam is licensed in some countries for long-term use for the alleviation of inflammation and pain in chronic musculoskeletal disorders. The registered dose in the European Union is 0.1 mg/kg on the first day, followed by 0.05 mg/kg, PO, every 24 hours, for as long as necessary. In patients with concurrent renal insufficiency, the use of an NSAID is an added reason to recommend daily home subcutaneous fluid therapy. In addition to analgesics, nutraceuticals, and chondroprotectants (such as glucosamine and chondroitin sulfate), may play a role in the management of degenerative joint disease.[2,11] Although efficacy has been shown for acupuncture in a few conditions in people, there is no solid scientific evidence at the time of writing that points to efficacy in cats.[19] For more information on analgesia, refer to the International Veterinary Academy of Pain Management website at http://www.cvmbs.colostate.edu/ivapm/.

Many patients in the later stages of life require numerous medications. The number and frequency of administration is a source of stress for both the patient and the owner. Thus, whenever possible, the importance of the particular agents should be prioritized to ensure that the most important ones are given diligently. If the less critical ones cannot be avoided, perhaps they can be administered in a different, less psychologically distressing manner. Feeding tubes are a tool that allows most oral medications to be given with minimal patient handling. Many clients are comfortable giving subcutaneous injections of agents that can be administered by this route.

PREPARING FOR AN ENDING: DYING WITH DIGNITY

Cats are living longer because of better health care, nutrition, dental care, and immunization to prevent many infectious diseases. We have the wonderful opportunity to know our patients from cradle to grave, often knowing their owners for even more years through numerous companion animals. As a preemptive measure, as a cat reaches its middle to older years, it may help to encourage owners to give consideration to introducing another companion, not only for themselves, but also for other animals that will be left alone. Should they want a kitten, adopting a pair is better for the older cat in order to avoid some of the indignities of kitten behavior. If they are considering adopting another single cat, then a young adult that has learned manners is more suitable than a kitten.

It is tempting as a clinician to treat illnesses as bodily malfunctions requiring politely caring and competent applied scientists. In human medicine, a great deal has been written about the tendency of physicians to forget that patients are persons and to designate patients by such locutions as "the kidney in room 422," "the osteosarcoma," or "the brain-dead." We may also forget that the neutered male, black and white domestic shorthair cat with renal insufficiency has his own experience of the world and the things we are doing to and for him. Although this is an issue affecting all aspects of medicine, it is especially important when we provide palliative care.

Palliative care must not be forgotten in the zeal to preserve life. In 1972, psychiatrists Marks and Sacher were called into the Sloan-Kettering Cancer Center to consult on an outbreak of "insanity," characterized by patients engaging in extreme and emotional behavior.[14] They soon realized that the issue was not madness but, rather, patient response to extreme and untreated cancer pain. Even in human medicine, as recently as 1991, it was reported that although 90% of cancer pain was manageable with available modalities, 80% was not controlled.[7] If pain was ignored as scientifically unreal, what hope was there for other negative sequelae to be treated, such as loss of dignity? Many, if not most, patients fear pain, and the suffering and degradation that extreme pain inflicts on patients and families, more than they fear death; this has resulted in a worldwide movement in favor of voluntary euthanasia and assisted suicide.

Although there are still many instances of animal patients being viewed as disposable property, there are also many in which the cat is viewed as a beloved family member. This has lead to a paradigm shift within veterinary medicine, whereby the practitioner, previously pleading for the chance to treat, may now need to advise discontinuation of treatment. There are several societal reasons for this. In many countries, more than half of marriages end in divorce. People are more separated from extended family, and making friends, particularly in urban areas, is notoriously difficult. Thus the companion animal assumes greater prominence in people's emotional lives, with upwards of 85% of the United States public affirming that their animals are "members of the family."[13] There has been an explosion of veterinary specialty practices, making treatment options previously available only through the limited number of academic institutions much more accessible, even mainstream. As early as 1980, the *Wall Street Journal* reported that clients were spending more than six figures to treat their animals at the Colorado State University Cancer Center (S. Withrow, personal communication to BR, June 2008). Many clients with companion animals will fight their pet's cancer or other terminal illness as aggressively as they would fight their own. For such people, euthanasia is a last resort option. Given this mindset, the cost of treatment is far less of a deterrent to treating animal disease than it once was; many animals that would historically have been euthanized now regain extended and good quality lives.

There is, however, a negative aspect to this for some veterinary patients. Some individuals that should receive the grace of euthanasia are denied it for too long, sometimes resulting in extended unnecessary suffering. With new modalities readily available and a sincere desire on the part of veterinarians to help their patients, it is easy to fall into the trap of doing more. The practitioner may have to guard against overzealous diagnostic and treatment plans to avoid losing sight of the well-being of the individual patient in question. *"Just because we can, doesn't mean we should."*

Similarly, the owner may struggle with assessing their companion's quality of life. When someone is in denial over the need to euthanize their "best friend" or "family member," their despair and hope may result in willingness to "try anything" to save the animal, however deteriorated or suffering it may be. They may reach out to try evidentially baseless, unproven "complementary and alternative medicine."[16] Access to the Internet assures that desperate owners can find an inexhaustible number of allegedly therapeutic modalities to pursue.

One other aspect of veterinary care and caring for animals that risks abuse is animal hospice, sometimes known as "pawspice." In some cases, when an owner wishes to pursue palliative care and legitimate treatment for the cancer patient, and has money but no time to provide care, pet hospice can fulfill a valuable function. But just as often, the hospice can allow the owner to dodge the issue of euthanasia for termination of suffering while endless new treatments are pursued. Catering to an owner's unwillingness to let go can occur in general veterinary practice as well when the needs of the individual animal are not maintained as priority. This occurs as a result of sympathy and empathy for the owner rather than empathy for the patient, along with a belief that one must cater to the desires of the person who is paying the bill. Thus, paradoxically, the rise of love for companion animals can cause new sources of uncontrolled suffering, buttressing the dictum that loving something is neither necessary nor sufficient for ensuring that one provides the beloved with good care. The question to bear in mind is, "At what cost additional life?" It is essential that veterinary medicine learn from the mistakes of human medicine and not sacrifice quality of life to quantity of life.[8]

Aesculapian authority is the unique authority possessed by physicians and veterinarians by virtue of being medical professionals.[18] To deploy such authority on behalf of the animal to end suffering is not only permissible but obligatory. When owners ask, "What would you do if it were your cat, Doctor?", they are appealing to our Aesculapian authority. Part of a veterinarian's job as an animal advocate is to respond to such a cry for exoneration under difficult circumstances, providing the sincere guidance that our training, knowledge, and experience enable us to offer.

This means that we have an obligation to explain to owners some fundamental differences between human and animal mental life that have major and radically distinct implications for quality of life in people versus companion animals. These authors do not deny the richness and moral relevance of animal mental life. There are, however, striking differences between humans and animals facing life-threatening illnesses, even as the tools of medicine dealing with such crises converge in the two areas. Human cognition is such that it can value long-term future goals and endure short-term negative experiences for the sake of achieving them. As humans, we can therefore, rationalize and endure the excruciating pain of cosmetic surgery in order to look better. And we similarly endure chemotherapy, radiation, dialysis, physical therapy, and organ transplants to achieve longer life and a better quality of life than we would have without it, or, in some cases, merely to prolong the length of life to see our children graduate, to complete an opus, or fulfill some other goal.

In the case of animals, however, there is no evidence, either empirical or conceptual, that they have the capability to weigh future benefits or possibilities against current misery. They live in the present moment. To treat our patients morally and with respect, we need to keep in mind their mentational limits. To the animal mind, in a real sense, there is only quality of life, that is, whether experiential content is pleasant or unpleasant in all of the modes it is capable of—bored or occupied, fearful or not fearful, lonely or enjoying companionship, painful or not, hungry or not, thirsty or not, and so forth, at this time. We have no reason to believe that an animal can grasp the notion of extended life, let alone choose to trade current suffering for it.

This, in turn, demands that we realistically assess, as far as possible, what animals are experiencing. An animal cannot weigh being treated for cancer against the suffering that entails. An animal cannot affirm or even conceive of a desire to endure current suffering for the sake of future life, cannot choose to lose a leg to preclude metastasis. We must remember that an animal *is* its pain, and is incapable of anticipating or even *hoping* for cessation of that pain. Thus when we are confronted with life-threatening illnesses that afflict our animals, it is not axiomatic that they be treated at whatever qualitative, experiential cost that may entail. The owner may consider the suffering a treatment modality entails a small price for extra life, but the animal neither values nor comprehends "extra life," let alone the trade-off this entails. Treatment for minor illnesses or injuries can be justified by the virtual certainty of a long pleasant life thereafter. The owner, in turn, may ignore the difference between the human and animal mind and choose the *possibility* of life prolongation at any qualitative cost. It is at this point that the morally responsible veterinarian is thrust into his or her role as animal advocate, speaking for what matters to the animal.

The best way to accomplish this sort of advocacy is to set up the type of relationship with an owner from the outset that has both the owner and the veterinarian agreeing to keep the best interests of the animal in view as the paramount goal of treatment. In this way, the clinician can educate the owner on the nature of animal mentation, suffering, and what matters to the animal. Such education should begin along with treatment, as should the veterinarian's claim for advocacy for animal quality of life. Quality-of-life considerations should be introduced at the beginning of a veterinarian–owner relationship, not suddenly sprung on an owner when treatment is over. In particular, it is useful to recall Plato's dictum that, when dealing with ethics and adults, it far better to *remind* than to teach. For this reason, the owner, who after all knows the animal better than the veterinarian, should be encouraged from the beginning to help define quality of life for that animal.

One of the most troubling things for owners is wondering how they will know "when it is the right time." As veterinary doctors, we try to not take time away from an individual's life or from the time that that cat and its people can spend together and balance that with trying to avoid going beyond the point that the cat has enjoyment of life.

One author (MS) encourages the caregivers to imagine being inside their cat's skin and try to imagine what it is experiencing. Some people are very clear in their assessment of how a cat is doing, others less so. Using a scale of 1 to 10, with 10 being the best day of their life and 1 being equivalent to agony and hopelessness, most of us live at around a 6 or 7. If clients use this as a means to score a given day or part of a day, it allows them an objectivity that is an emotional buffer from the roller coaster of emotions they are living in. (Or, for those who are hiding or numb, it adds content to their cat's experience.) When the scores are mostly 2s and 3s, that is the time to consider helping the cat pass on. This is very helpful when a person is afraid that they allowed their last companion to suffer too long and also encourages the person who cannot let their friend go that it is the right time.

The other author (BR) recommends advising an owner to write a list, that is as long as possible, of the things their cat enjoys doing while the cat is still well or at the beginning of treatment, as might be the case in cancer. This list is then kept in a drawer at home as well as becoming part of the medical record. As the cat becomes more debilitated, the owner can review their reflective and personal criteria and see what changes have occurred despite wishful thinking and potential selfish desires. This objective reality check provides a gauge of progression and reassurance that the decision to euthanize is appropriate while, conversely, also helping the individual who is considering further treatment out of hope and denial.

To help reduce the emotional effects of this period of uncertainty, it is often helpful for owners to feel that they have some control should their cat's condition deteriorate quickly. Things that support this include

- Making sure that they have appropriate emergency care phone numbers and knowing where the emergency facility is.
- Giving them a photocopy of the most recent medical record and laboratory data to keep by their car keys in case they need to go to the emergency clinic. Owners often forget the names of medications and doses that they are giving when they are upset.

Let people know what euthanasia entails beforehand. In a report published in 2001, the AVMA states that "The term euthanasia is derived from two Greek words—*eu*, which means good, and *thanatos*, which means death." They define this "good death" as follows: "Euthanasia is the act of inducing humane death in an animal. It is our responsibility as veterinarians and human beings to ensure that if an animal's life is to be taken, it is done with the highest degree of respect, and with an emphasis on making the death as painless and distress-free as possible."[1]

Communication is critical. Reassure the owner that the dose of barbiturate is painless. One author (MS) places the patient on a thick towel on the owner's lap, informing them that cats generally keep their eyes open and that because muscles relax, the cat may empty its bladder or bowels. Also let them know that some cats may still make breathing movements as death occurs. Although intravenous administration is the most common route for euthanasia agents, unless a cat is agonal, an alternative option, preferred by MS, is to administer a euthanasia solution intraperitoneally (IP), just caudal to a kidney. This avoids restraint and the accompanying fear for the patient. Additionally, the transition from life to death is less sudden: It may take 2 minutes or 20. As soon as the cat is anaesthetized, should the owner want to "hasten the end," a vein can be readily accessed for an additional dose. The time of waiting gives them a good opportunity to remember and cry and laugh. This helps the clinician know that they are working through their grieving normally and are going to be okay. In this author's (MS) experience, owners who have witnessed intravenous euthanasia have said that they prefer the more "natural" passing with the IP route.

CARING FOR THE CAREGIVERS

Most people are able to cope with a loss if they know it is imminent and if they have a support network. Too often, in our modern life, the veterinary team may be the only support the owner has. This is especially sad when friends and family do not appreciate the attachment the person has for their cat. Along with sending a personal card, it is usually greatly appreciated when we check in on the person after a few days. If there is any concern about the owner's emotional security and you are concerned that they might be suicidal, be sure to get help from the human health care system.

In general, however, it helps people to know that they may go through a whole range of emotions, from grief to guilt to anger to uncertainty and emptiness. This is normal and healthy. The practitioner may help an owner understand with an explanation such as, "It is even normal for these feelings to overwhelm you days or weeks after the death of a beloved companion. This reflects the unconscious mind working through things and letting go a little bit at a time. What is NOT normal or healthy is when you get stuck in one emotion." There are also instances in which the death of a cat companion is a reminder of unfinished grieving for another person or pet. There are numerous grief support networks available through veterinary school telephone hotlines, such as Cornell University: http://www.vet.cornell.edu/Org/Petloss/. Some may prefer the electronic support group found at the Rainbow Bridge (http://www.petloss.com).

If owners have not already adopted a new pet, they should give thought to that. Everyone recognizes that the new cat is not a replacement for the one that has died, but by adopting, the newcomer receives a wonderful home and a heart to fill, to ease grief, and bring joy. When the time is right, that new cat will show up.

Finally there is the "cost of caring."[17] We, the care team, experience dying and recovering from it approximately 5 times as often as our human health care equivalents. "Compassion fatigue" goes beyond just normal burnout. Compassion fatigue is a type of physical, emotional, and spiritual exhaustion that comes with frequent exposure to death and having to offer support to owners in highly emotional situations during long periods of time.[6] This is a matter of such importance that there exists a prominent group, The Compassion Fatigue Awareness Project (http://www.compassionfatigue.org). They espouse a series of recommendations, the so-called Eight Laws, regarding healthy caregiving, healthy change, self-care, and a healthy workspace.

Some of the issues that have been associated with compassion fatigue in veterinary medicine include[8]

- Difficulty accepting that the patient's physical problems cannot always be controlled

- Frustration at having invested large amounts of energy in caring for a patient that then dies, taking this investment with them
- Disappointment if expectations for patients to die a "good death," however this may be defined, are not met
- Difficulty ending a life you once saved
- Difficulty establishing realistic boundaries and expectations on veterinary care
- Caring for an animal more than the owner does
- Guilt arising from a cat's death

Without risking the tragedy of arms-length detachment, it is possible to take care of yourself. Suggestions for dealing with and protecting yourself proactively from compassion fatigue include[6]

- Allow yourself to be human
- Acknowledge and honor your own grief and emotions
- Embrace your personal life away from work
- Allow time to debrief and support other team members
- Say your own private "good-bye" to your patients
- Believe in your ability to provide comfort and love to your patients
- Redefine death not as a failure but as an inevitable part of the life cycle
- After euthanasia, know that the individual is no longer suffering
- Think of euthanasia as a gift that owners want and appreciate
- With euthanasia, realize that you are providing a loving and caring time for your patients and owners

CONCLUSION

The end of life is, without a doubt, filled with losses. Although one cannot prevent the loss of function and abilities, their decline can be tempered by addressing cellular needs to some degree, as well as focusing on comfort, prevention, and alleviation of pain and ensuring dignity. When these are no longer possible, we can provide the grace of a good death. This final act holds an inherent responsibility that we do not abuse it or dispense it without the best interests of the patient at heart. So used, it is a gift that provides release for the cat and peace for all remaining.

References

1. AVMA Panel on Euthanasia: 2000 Report of the AVMA panel on euthanasia, *J Am Vet Med Assoc* 218:669, 2001.
2. Beale BS: Use of nutraceuticals and chondroprotectants in osteoarthritic dogs and cats, *Vet Clin North Am Small Anim Pract* 34:271, 2004.
3. Bennett D, Morton C: A study of owner observed behavioural and lifestyle changes in cats with musculoskeletal disease before and after analgesic therapy, *J Feline Med Surg* 11:997, 2009.
4. Clarke SP, Mellor D, Clements DN et al: Prevalence of radiographic signs of degenerative joint disease in a hospital population of cats, *Vet Rec* 157:793, 2005.
5. Cotran RS, Kumar V, Robbins SL: Cellular injury and cellular death. In Cotran RS, Kumar V, Robbins SL, editors: *Robbins' pathologic basis of disease*, ed 5, Philadelphia, 1994, Saunders, p 32.
6. Durrance D: Compassion fatigue, *Proceedings of the 2005 Western Veterinary Conference*, February 20-24, 2005, Las Vegas, Nev.
7. Ferrell BR, Rhiner M: High-tech comfort: ethereal issues in cancer pain management for the 1990s, *J Clin Ethics* 2:108, 1991.
8. Folger W, Addleman R, Rodan I et al: AAFP position statement: end of life issues in feline medicine, *J Feline Med Surg* 12:421, 2010.
9. Godfrey DR: Osteoarthritis in cats: a retrospective radiological study, *J Small Anim Pract* 46:425, 2005.
10. Gunn-Moore DA, McVee J, Bradshaw JM et al: Ageing changes in cat brains demonstrated by beta-amyloid and AT8-immunoreactive phosphorylated tau deposits, *J Feline Med Surg* 8:234, 2006.
11. Hardie EM: Management of osteoarthritis in cats, *Vet Clin North Am Small Anim Pract* 27:945, 1997.
12. Hardie EM, Roe SC, Martin FR: Radiographic evidence of degenerative joint disease in geriatric cats: 100 cases (1994-1997), *J Am Vet Med Assoc* 220:628, 2002.
13. Harris Poll #120: Pets are members of the family, and two-thirds of pet owner buy their pets holiday presents, December 4, 2007. Available at http://www.harrisinteractive.com/harris_poll/index.asp?PID=840. Accessed January 14, 2010.
14. Marks RM, Sacher EJ: Undertreatment of medical inpatients with narcotic analgesics, *Ann Intern Med* 78:173, 1973.
15. Ogilvie GK, Moore AS, editors: *Feline oncology: a comprehensive guide to compassionate care*, Trenton, NJ, 2001, *Veterinary Learning Systems*.
16. Ramey DW, Rollin BE, editors: *Complementary and alternative medicine considered*, Ames, Iowa, 2004, Blackwell.
17. Rollin BE: Euthanasia and moral stress, *Loss Grief Care* 1:115, 1987.
18. Rollin BE: The use and abuse of Aesculapian authority in veterinary medicine, *J Am Vet Med Assoc* 220:1144, 2002.
19. The National Institutes of Health (NIH) Consensus Development Program: Acupuncture. Available at http://consensus.nih.gov/1997/1997Acupuncture107html.htm. Accessed January 8, 2010.

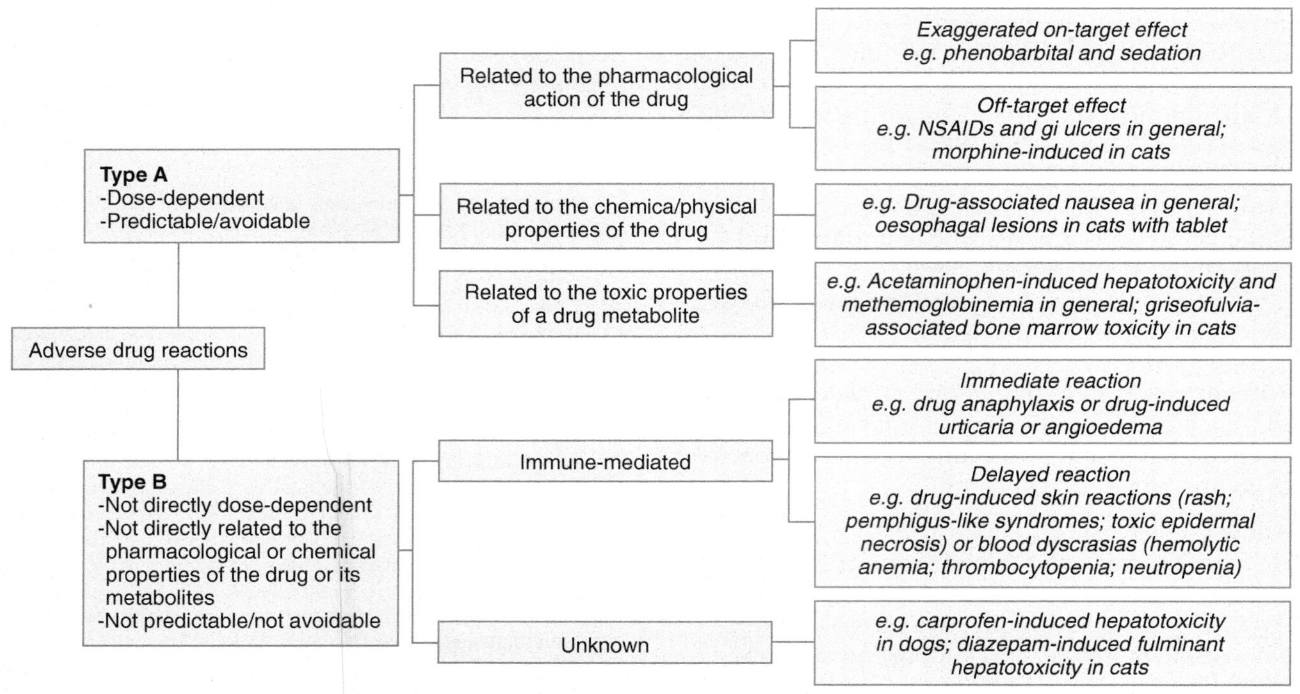

Type A and Type B Adverse Drug Reactions

SECTION VII

SPECIAL CONSIDERATIONS FOR THE SENIOR CAT

Editor: Susan E. Little

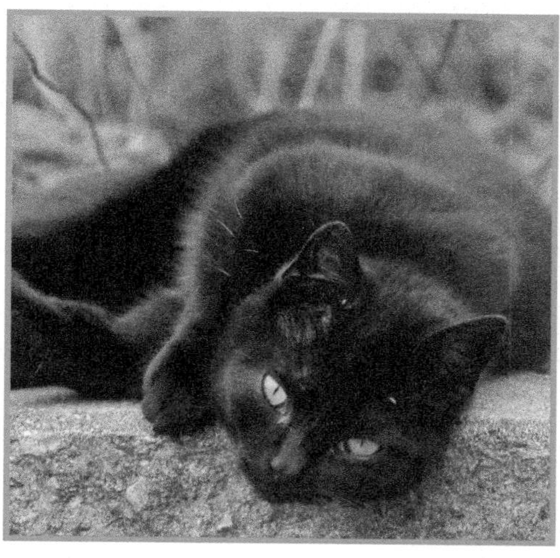

CHAPTER

37

Managing the Senior Cat

Susan E. Little

OUTLINE

Aging, or senescence, is a complex biological process that is not always easy to define. Essentially, aging involves increasing damage and loss of function that occurs over time at both the cellular level and at the level of the entire animal or organism. Many age-related changes are manageable in order to maintain quality of life, and age-related diseases may be manageable or curable. In human medicine, the disciplines of geriatrics (the study of diseases of the elderly) and gerontology (the study of the social, psychological, and biological aspects of aging) are well established. This focus on the unique needs of aging individuals is becoming more important in veterinary medicine as well.

According to the most recently published figures, about one third of American and Canadian households own at least one cat.[40,44] As most veterinarians appreciate, many of these are older cats. For example, a 2008 Canadian survey found that 35% of owned cats are greater than 8 years of age.[40] In the United States and the United Kingdom, senior cats also likely account for at least 30% of the owned cat population. Veterinarians should be familiar not only with normal aging, but also with the common medical problems in this age group and should be able to provide owners with educational support. Unfortunately, the American Animal Hospital Association (AAHA) estimates that only 14% of senior pets receive regular health screenings recommended by veterinarians.[14] The main obstacle is lack of clear recommendations from the veterinary health care team.

The American Association of Feline Practitioners (AAFP)/AAHA feline life stage guidelines define a senior cat as 11 to 14 years old and a geriatric cat as 15 years and older.[48] The term "senior" is often used to refer to all cats greater than about 10 years and will be used as such in this chapter. Owners often ask veterinarians about the human equivalent age of cats. In general, senior cats are approximately equivalent to human ages 60 to 72 and geriatric cats are approximately equivalent to human ages 76 to 100 years. Although these age comparisons are helpful, it is important to remember that the process and speed of aging varies among individuals and may be influenced by genetics, nutrition, environment, and other factors. A cat's chronologic age is not a good indicator of functional age, and even within an individual, different organs may age at different rates.

Of course, old age is not a disease, and both veterinarians and owners must resist the temptation to ascribe signs of illness to aging. For example, pain, dehydration, or hypokalemia might lead to clinical signs that owners attribute to the "slowing down" of old age. Although knowledge of the changes in physiology and disease prevalence resulting from aging is an important part of health care for senior cats, decisions on disease management should never be made on the basis of age alone. In particular, making a diagnosis and formulating a treatment plan should never be avoided simply because of the age of the patient. Many problems of senior cats are chronic and progressive so that early diagnosis and treatment is important for pain management and preservation of quality of life.

IMPACT OF AGING

Unfortunately, little investigation into the physiology of aging has been conducted in cats, and most information is extrapolated from other species or learned through observation of disease states. The impact of aging may be obvious (e.g., white hairs, dulling of senses) or may consist of physiologic changes that are more difficult to appreciate. Aging also brings changes in the sleep/wake cycle and a reduced ability to tolerate stressors and changes in routine and environment. Changes known to occur with aging in some body systems include

1. Immune system: Decreased phagocytic function and neutrophil chemotaxis lead to decreased immune competence. Other changes in cats greater than 10 years of age compared with younger cats include lower total leukocyte counts, as well as reduced numbers of CD4+ and CD8+ T-lymphocytes and an overall reduction in the CD4/CD8 ratio.[9] However, the ability to mount humoral immune responses appears to be preserved even though the cell-mediated response is affected. Immune function may be further affected by the presence of chronic disease states and immunosuppressive drug therapy, leading to increased risk of infection.
2. Skin: Collagen and elastin content is reduced, leading to thinner, less elastic skin. Blood flow to the skin is also reduced. These changes may make assessment of hydration using skin turgor difficult and predispose to infection. Senior cats groom less efficiently than younger cats, leading to hair matting and dermatitis. Nails may be overgrown, thick, and brittle and require more care.
3. Special senses: Reduced vision and hearing may make older cats more easily startled. Lenticular sclerosis is a normal aging change that owners may misinterpret as a cataract. Pupillary light responses are slower, resulting in part from iris atrophy, and retinal changes may occur secondary to hypertension. Decreased olfactory function and taste sensation may impair appetite.
4. Kidney: Aging causes decrease in kidney size, blood flow, and glomerular filtration rate. Mineralization of the renal pelvis is not uncommon, although the significance is unknown, and it should not be confused with nephrolithiasis. Potassium homeostasis is impaired and hypokalemia may be common.
5. Musculoskeletal: Changes in cartilage composition and physiology are associated with degenerative joint disease. Mineralization of some areas of the skeleton, such as costochondral junctions, may be detected on radiographs, but the clinical significance is unknown. Muscle mass may decrease because of weight loss, and muscle atrophy may occur because of inactivity, leading to weakness.
6. Oral cavity: Periodontal disease, tooth resorption, tooth loss, and oral cancer occur more commonly in senior cats, and associated pain can contribute to inappetence and weight loss.

TABLE 37-1 **American Society of Anesthesiologists Physical Status Classification System**

Class	Definition
1	Normal, healthy patient
2	Patient with mild systemic disease
3	Patient with severe systemic disease
4	Patient with severe systemic disease that is a constant threat to life
5	Moribund patient not expected to survive without the procedure

Drug Disposition

An important aspect of aging in cats is that responses to drug therapy change in association with alterations in renal and hepatic function, body composition, and other physiologic responses. These changes can affect the absorption, distribution, metabolism and elimination of drugs. Of these changes, renal insufficiency is probably the most important and common, leading to decreased elimination and increased toxicity of drugs cleared through the kidney. Adjustments in dose and/or frequency of dosing may be necessary in patients with chronic kidney disease (CKD) or hepatic disease. Senior cats may be administered multiple medications and supplements, making monitoring of potential drug interactions critical. More information on drug therapy in senior and geriatric cats is found in Chapter 4.

Veterinarians and owners are often reluctant to administer anesthesia to senior cats, resulting in an impaired ability to make a diagnosis or incomplete treatment. For example, senior cats may require anesthesia for assessment and treatment of oral and dental diseases on multiple occasions. Untreated dental disease is a significant cause of chronic pain and impaired quality of life. As in human medicine, age in itself is not a reason to avoid anesthesia, but changes in physiology and the presence of disease may increase risk and must be considered in formulation of the anesthetic plan (Table 37-1). Aging causes decreased lung compliance and respiratory muscles that fatigue more easily. Heart function may be affected by primary diseases, such as hypertrophic cardiomyopathy, or by changes induced by hyperthyroidism or hypertension. Anesthetic risks also increase with age in cats, independent of the American Society of Anesthesiologists (ASA) physical status grade.[6] Senior cats may be more susceptible to the depressant effects of sedatives and anesthetic agents. As well, senior patients may be more susceptible to hypothermia because of impaired thermoregulation and to prolonged recovery because of reduced metabolic function and hypothermia. Increased anesthetic risk is also associated with decreasing body size in cats.[7] Smaller

TABLE 37-2 **Changes in Various Body Condition and Nutrition Parameters in Different Feline Life Stages**

Age (Years)	Body Weight	Fat Mass	Lean Mass	Fat Digestibility	Protein Digestibility	Urine Volume
1-7	No change or ↑	No change or ↑	No change	>90%	>85%	No change
7-12	↑↑	↑↑	↑	↓	↑	?
12+	↓↓	↓↓	↓↓	↓↓	↓	↑↑

↑, Increase; ↑↑, larger increase; ↓, decrease; ↓↓, larger decrease.
Adapted from Perez-Camargo G: Cat nutrition: what is new in the old? *Comp Contin Educ Pract Vet* 26:5, 2004.

patients may be more at risk of drug overdose (especially if an accurate weight is not used to calculate drug doses), more prone to hypothermia, and more prone to perioperative management difficulties (e.g., intravenous catheter placement, endotracheal intubation).[5] Safety can be improved by thorough preanesthetic patient assessment, stabilization of chronic diseases when possible, appropriate selection of pre-anesthetic and anesthetic drugs, and proper monitoring (e.g., pulse quality and rate, oxygen saturation). More information on anesthetic considerations for senior patients is found in Chapter 7.

Nutritional Requirements

Interestingly, changes in maintenance energy requirements with aging in cats are unlike those in humans and dogs. Short-term studies concluded that cats do not experience a decrease in maintenance energy requirements (MERs) with aging.[8,36,46] However, longer-term studies refined the state of knowledge and concluded that MERs decrease with age by about 3% per year in cats up to about 11 years old.[13,26] However, from about 12 years of age, the MERs of cats actually increase, and this may partly explain the tendency of older cats to be underweight.[13] In contrast, humans and dogs experience a decline of about 20% in maintenance energy requirements with aging. This difference may be because humans and dogs tend to be more active in their younger years, whereas the activity level of most cats, especially those that live indoors, is constant throughout their lives. For most senior cats (the exception being those that are obese), energy provision should not be reduced, because they are susceptible to weight loss. Other reasons for this susceptibility to weight loss may include changing physiology, presence of diseases, and decreased appetite. Older cats are also less efficient at digesting food, particularly fats and proteins, and may need to increase their daily food intake to compensate.[20] Table 37-2 summarizes various body condition and nutrition parameters at different life stages.

Many senior cats, especially those 12 years of age and older, will benefit from being fed a palatable food that is highly digestible and energy dense and that can be offered in small amounts frequently.[25] Specific protein requirements for senior cats compared with younger cats are not known. However, there is no known benefit of protein restriction in healthy senior cats. If there is no specific requirement for a restricted protein diet (e.g., late-stage CKD), current recommendations are to feed a high-quality protein in an amount that meets adult requirements (at least 2 g/lb [5 g/kg] ideal body weight). More information on nutrition for senior and geriatric cats is found in Chapter 16.

WELLNESS CARE FOR SENIOR CATS

Components of wellness care by life stage are found in Table 8-2. Comprehensive wellness examinations, history assessment, and minimum database wellness testing are recommended every 6 months for senior cats.[14,48] This frequency is warranted because an individual's health status may change rapidly in this age group and because early detection and treatment of problems is important to preserve quality of life. As well, the signs of illness in cats are often subtle and may go unnoticed by owners until the problem is well advanced (see the 10 subtle signs of sickness in Chapter 8 and http://www.healthycatsforlife.com). In addition, senior cats with chronic diseases may require more frequent evaluation and laboratory testing.

The minimum database for evaluation of senior cats includes a complete blood count (CBC), full serum chemistry panel (especially total protein, albumin, globulin, alkaline phosphatase [ALP], alanine transaminase [ALT], glucose, blood urea nitrogen [BUN], creatinine, potassium, phosphorus, sodium, and calcium), full urinalysis including microscopic sediment examination, and total thyroxine (T_4). Depending on risk factors and clinical signs, fecal examination and retrovirus testing may also be included in wellness testing. It is important to recognize that serum creatinine may be within the normal reference range in cats with CKD if the patient is thin with reduced muscle mass. In one study, serum calcium, hematocrit, hemoglobin, red blood cells, albumin, and albumin/globulin ratio were significantly lower in older cats (average age 15 years) compared with young cats (average age 2.75 years).[13a] In the same study, total serum protein, albumin, and hematocrit were significantly lower in otherwise healthy senior cats with low body condition scores compared with senior cats of normal weight.

Blood pressure should be measured in cats with known hypertension, cats with predisposing diseases (e.g., CKD, hyperthyroidism) or cats with compatible clinical signs. Experts vary on the utility of routine blood pressure measurement in senior cats with no clinical signs or predisposing diseases because of inherent problems with the procedure, which may lead to overdiagnosis and unnecessary treatment.

It is unknown if senior cats respond to primary vaccination or revaccination in the same way as younger cats. In one study of greater than 2,000 cats receiving a primary course of vaccination against rabies virus, older cats had a significantly greater chance of failing to achieve the titer of 0.5 IU/mL required for international travel.[31] Until more is known about vaccinal responses in aging cats, the AAFP Feline Vaccine Advisory Panel recommends that healthy senior cats and those with stable chronic diseases receive vaccinations according to the same principles as younger cats.[42]

The home environment is critically important for feline wellness, and veterinary staff should be trained to ask questions that uncover pertinent information and counsel clients about enriched environments. This is especially true for senior cats, because they are more likely to live totally indoors than younger cats. An indoor-only life style decreases the risks of trauma and infectious diseases, but welfare may be compromised and illness induced by a stressful or sterile environment. Recent research has shown that stressors (e.g., lack of sufficient resources, presence of visitors, changes in diet, changes in routine, conflict with other cats) can induce physical signs of illness in otherwise healthy cats, including anorexia, vomiting, or diarrhea.[45a] Indoor cats need adequate numbers of "resources"—hiding places, accessible elevated resting places, food and water stations, scratching posts, litter boxes, and stimulating toys.

Senior cats may benefit from environmental modifications, as long as they are made gradually. Examples include a sleeping area that is in a warm place (e.g., on a hot-water radiator) or that has supplemental heat (e.g., covered hot-water bottle), and resting/hiding areas that are in quiet locations away from the main activity of the household and, ideally, that are not accessible by other pets. Modifications may be necessary to allow the cat to reach a favored resting area, such as moving a chair next to a window ledge for easier access. Litter boxes should be large and shallow with low sides and should be placed in easily accessible yet quiet locations, preferably on each floor of the home. Plastic under-bed storage boxes are often better choices than commercially available cat litter boxes, which tend to be too small. Owners may need to clean the litter box more frequently, especially for the cat with polyuria. Placing a night-light near litter boxes and in other places in the home is helpful for senior cats with declining vision.

DISEASES AND HEALTH PROBLEMS OF SENIOR CATS

Several diseases and conditions are more common in senior cats (e.g., hyperthyroidism, chronic kidney disease, neoplasia, dental, and oral diseases), and the practitioner should be aware of these issues and practice active surveillance to detect them. A brief discussion of selected diseases and health problems follows; more complete information on each topic is found elsewhere in this book.

Weight Loss and Dehydration

One of the easiest problems to detect is weight loss and decline in body condition. The body weight, body condition score, and percentage weight change should be determined and recorded at every opportunity, even if a cat has been presented for a nonmedical procedure, such as trimming nails. The prevalence of obesity decreases with age in cats; in fact, senior cats have a tendency to be underweight, especially those greater than the age of 10 to 12 years.[21,39,43] However, this knowledge must not prevent assessment for causes of weight loss. For more on diagnosis and management of weight loss in senior cats, see Chapter 38.

Evaluation of muscle mass is also important, particularly in cats with chronic diseases. Identification of early muscle wasting may be important for the success of diagnostics and therapeutics. Evaluation of muscle mass includes visual examination and palpation over the temporal bones, scapulae, lumbar vertebrae, and pelvic bones. A muscle condition scoring system has been introduced for cats and is undergoing validation (Figure 37-1).[2,33] Table 37-3 is a modified fat and muscle mass scoring system adapted for assessment of weight loss and body condition in feline cancer patients.

Another important aging change in cats is reduced sensitivity to thirst (Figure 37-2), resulting in an increased risk of dehydration even in cats with seemingly normal renal function. Even healthy young cats do not drink large amounts of water, a behavior influenced by the fact that the domestic cat originated in arid environments. The problem is exacerbated in cats with diseases causing polydipsia/polyuria, such as diabetes mellitus and CKD, as well as in cats under the stress of hospitalization or boarding. Healthy geriatric cats have higher water losses than younger cats possibly because of reduced urine concentrating ability even without obvious signs of CKD.[39] A common sequel to chronic dehydration is constipation, which is exacerbated by reduced colonic motility or reluctance to use the litter box because of

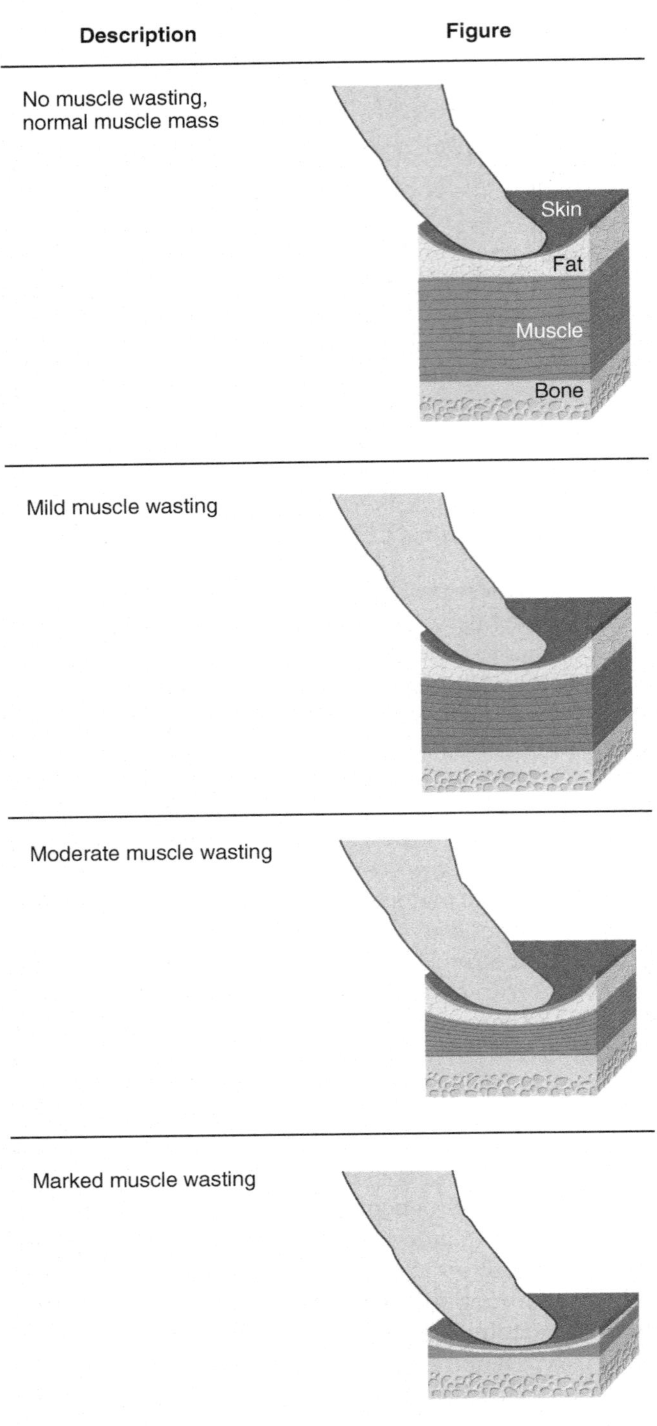

FIGURE 37-1 A muscle condition scoring system includes visual examination and palpation over the scapulae, skull, ribs, lumbar vertebrae, and pelvic bones. *(Adapted from Baldwin K, Bartges J, Buffington T et al: AAHA Nutritional assessment guidelines for dogs and cats,* J Am Anim Hosp Assoc *46:285, 2010.)*

TABLE 37-3 Fat and Muscle Mass Scoring for Cats

Score	Fat Mass	Muscle Mass
0	Absence of palpable subcutaneous fat over the ribs or abdomen	Severe muscle wasting palpable over the scapulae, skull, or wings of the ilia
1	Decreased amounts of palpable subcutaneous fat over the ribs or abdomen	Moderate muscle wasting palpable over the scapulae, skull, or wings of the ilia
2	Normal amounts of palpable subcutaneous fat over the ribs or abdomen	Mild muscle wasting palpable over the scapulae, skull, or wings of the ilia
3	Increased amounts of palpable subcutaneous fat over the ribs or abdomen	Normal muscle mass palpable over the scapulae, skull, or wings of the ilia

Adapted from Baez JL, Michel KE, Sorenmo K et al: A prospective investigation of the prevalence and prognostic significance of weight loss and changes in body condition in feline cancer patients, *J Feline Med Surg* 9:411, 2007.

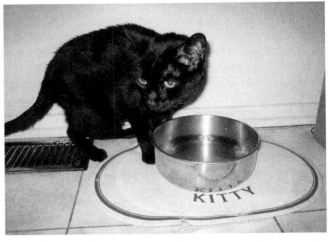

FIGURE 37-2 An important aging change in cats is reduced sensitivity to thirst, resulting in an increased risk of dehydration even in cats with seemingly normal renal function. One way to encourage increased water consumption is to provide large water bowls, such as ones designed for dogs, to prevent the cat's whiskers from touching the sides when drinking.

painful conditions, such as degenerative joint disease. Senior cats may benefit from increased water content through feeding canned foods, ensuring access to fresh water, flavoring water with chicken broth, and so forth. Methods for increasing water consumption are found in Box 18-16. Since older cats do not cope well with changes in daily routine, any changes to food and water should be made gradually.

Cognitive Dysfunction

Increasingly, older cats are being presented to veterinarians because of behavior problems, such as house soiling.[3] However, owners will not always voluntarily mention changes in behavior during veterinary visits; so, it is important for the clinician to obtain a behavioral

BOX 37-1

Behavioral History Questions for Owners of Senior Cats

1. How much does your cat play? Has the way in which your cat plays changed recently?
2. Approximately how many hours does your cat sleep in each 24-hour period? Does your cat sleep well at night? Have there been any recent changes in your cat's sleeping behavior?
3. Does your cat yowl or vocalize at inappropriate times (e.g., at night or in a room when no one is present)?
4. Have there been changes in how your cat interacts with family members or other pets in the home?
5. Does your cat ever pace or wander aimlessly, or appear to be staring into space?
6. Does your cat ever eliminate outside the litter box? Have there been recent changes in your cat's elimination behavior?

Adapted from Crowell-Davis SL: Cognitive dysfunction in senior pets, *Comp Contin Edu Pract Vet* 30:106, 2008.

BOX 37-2

Causes of Nighttime Yowling

1. Hypertension
2. Hyperthyroidism
3. Pain
4. Decreased vision or hearing
5. Cognitive dysfunction

history for all senior cats and ask pertinent questions (Box 37-1). Research suggests that 28% of cats 11 to 14 years old and at least 50% of cats 15 years and older develop behavior problems.[29] The most commonly reported problem in cats age 11 to 14 years was alteration in social interactions, and the most commonly reported problems in cats 15 years and older were alterations in activity and excessive vocalization. Behavior problems, such as nighttime yowling (Box 37-2), can be the result of many different causes in senior cats, particularly medical conditions, such as

1. Hyperthyroidism: anxiety, restlessness, yowling at night
2. Hypertension: yowling at night
3. Diabetes mellitus: decreased social interactions, decreased grooming, inappropriate elimination
4. Feline lower urinary tract disease (FLUTD): inappropriate elimination
5. Conditions causing pain (e.g., degenerative joint disease, oral/dental disease): irritability, decreased social interactions, inappropriate elimination, poor appetite, decreased mobility, yowling at night
6. Conditions causing polyuria (e.g., CKD): inappropriate elimination

Diagnosis of the cause of behavioral problems should be approached as for any medical problem, with a complete medical history, thorough physical examination, blood pressure measurement, and appropriate laboratory testing. Primary behavioral problems affecting senior cats should also be considered.[28] Many conditions found in senior cats cause pain, such as degenerative joint disease, neoplasia, chronic pancreatitis, and chronic oral disease. Pain is associated with impaired recovery from injury or illness as well as behavioral changes. Selection of the most appropriate treatment modality for pain in senior cats must include assessment of major organ function, especially kidney and liver. Information on pain management for chronic conditions is found in Chapter 36.

Cognitive function involves processes such as perception, memory, reasoning, and judgment. In humans and dogs, complex types of learning and memory, such as spatial learning and spatial memory, are affected by age. Very little investigation into cognitive function and aging has been performed in cats, but the available evidence suggests that the same may not be true in this species. In one study, cats age 11 to 16 years performed better on tests of spatial learning than younger cats.[30] Another study found that cats did not undergo age-related declines in spatial memory function or motor function.[32]

In senior cats, cognitive dysfunction (CD) is now recognized as an important problem, although formal diagnostic criteria have not been established. The most common signs of CD in cats are disorientation in time or space, altered learning and memory, house soiling, altered interactions (e.g., attention seeking, aggression, irritability, anxiety), changes in activity (including wandering or pacing), changes in sleep patterns, decreased appetite, decreased grooming, and increased vocalization (especially yowling at night). In dogs, the signs of CD are referred to by the mnemonic DISHA (**D**isorientation, **I**nteractions, **S**leep–wake, **H**ouse-training, **A**ctivity) and this format may be useful for diagnosis of CD in cats as well.

Currently, there are no specific diagnostic tests for feline CD; it is a diagnosis of exclusion after medical and primary behavioral causes are ruled out. Various protocols have been validated using standardized apparatus for assessment of canine cognitive dysfunction, but similar equipment and protocols for assessment of cats have been lacking. Protocols and equipment are being developed for cats based on those used in dogs and horses; validation of neuropsychological testing may eventually improve diagnosis of CD in cats.[29,34] Given that senior cats often have multiple health issues, clinicians should be aware that diagnosis of a medical problem in a cat with behavioral signs does not rule out the possibility of concurrent CD.

The cause of feline CD is unknown, but pathologic brain aging with changes in cerebral blood flow and chronic free radical damage is suspected to play a role. Imaging studies have identified cerebral atrophy and other changes in the brains of elderly cats.[29] Neuron loss and decreased numbers of dendrites associated with Purkinje cells have been found in the cerebellum of old cats, which may affect motor function.[49] Decline in the activity of the cholinergic system in the locus coeruleus has been documented, which may cause cognitive dysfunction and alterations in rapid eye movement (REM) sleep.[49,50] Inconsistent evidence suggests that Alzheimer-type changes, such as vascular and perivascular accumulation of amyloid-beta and microhemorrhage or infarcts, may also contribute to the clinical signs of CD in cats; further investigation is needed to clarify the relationship.[4,12,18] Finally, concurrent medical conditions in senior cats may affect brain blood flow and oxygen supply, such as hypertension, anemia, and cardiac disease. Neurons are particularly sensitive to hypoxia.

Published studies on the efficacy of treatments for feline CD are lacking. Therapies extrapolated from humans and dogs include antioxidant-enriched diets and supplements combined with environmental enrichment. For example, a 3-year study of a canine senior diet containing antioxidants, L-carnitine, alpha-lipoic acid, and omega-3 fatty acids (b/d Canine, Hill's Pet Nutrition) along with environmental enrichment improved clinical signs and slowed cognitive dysfunction.[22,35] Another study of a canine diet containing medium-chain triglycerides to provide an alternate source of energy in the brain (Purina One Vibrant Maturity 7+) improved cognitive function in senior dogs.[38] As of this writing, no diet has been designed to treat CD in cats although therapeutic diets supplemented with antioxidants and essential fatty acids are available for other conditions (e.g., degenerative joint disease).

Dietary supplements containing phosphatidylserine (Senilife, CEVA Animal Health, St. Louis, Mo.) have been associated with clinical improvement in dogs with CD.[1,37] Although this product is also labeled for use in cats, no feline studies have been conducted. Another supplement containing phosphatidylserine, omega-3 fatty acids, vitamins E and C, L-carnitine, alpha-lipoic acid, and other ingredients (Aktivait; VetPlus, Lytham, United Kingdom) improved signs of disorientation, social interaction, and house soiling in dogs.[23] Alpha-lipoic acid is toxic for cats, and although a feline version of the supplement is available without this ingredient, no trials have been published to determine efficacy in cats. S-adenosyl-L-methionine (SAMe) improved activity and awareness in a placebo-controlled trial in dogs with CD.[41] SAMe is commonly used in cats for treatment of hepatic disease, but no trials for treatment of CD have been published.

TABLE 37-4 **Drugs Used for the Treatment of Cognitive Dysfunction in Cats**

Drug	Dose*
Selegiline (Anipryl, Pfizer Animal Health)	0.25-1.0 mg/kg, every 24 hours
Nicergoline (Fitergol, Merial)	1.25 mg/cat, every 24 hours
Propentofylline (Vivitonin, Intervet/Schering-Plough Animal Health)	12.5 mg/cat, every 24 hours
Oxazepam	0.2-0.5 mg/kg, every 12 hours
Lorazepam	0.02-0.1 mg/kg, every 12 hours
Clonazepam	0.1-0.2 mg/kg, every 12 to 24 hours
Buspirone	2.5-5.0 mg/cat, every 12 hours
Fluoxetine	0.5-1.0 mg/kg, every 24 hours

*All drugs are given orally.

Although no drugs are licensed for the treatment of CD in cats, several have been used anecdotally (Table 37-4). Selegiline, also known as L-deprenyl, is a selective monoamine oxidase B inhibitor licensed for the treatment of CD in dogs (Anipryl; Pfizer Animal Health, Overland Park, Kansas). The exact mechanism of action is unclear, although it may enhance the effects of dopamine and have antioxidant effects. In dogs, it has been shown to improve disorientation, sleep patterns, and social interactions in numerous studies. Selegiline has anecdotally been reported to improve signs of disorientation, vocalization, decreased interaction, and repetitive activity in cats with CD.[27] Onset of efficacy may take several weeks. Certain drugs should not be administered at the same time as selegiline, such as selective serotonin reuptake inhibitors (SSRIs) and tricyclic antidepressants (TCAs).

Propentofylline (Vivitonin; Intervet/Schering-Plough Animal Health, Summit, NJ) is a xanthine derivative licensed in some countries for treatment of clinical signs, such as dullness and lethargy, in older dogs, supposedly through improvement in cerebral blood flow and other effects. The drug has anecdotally been reported as useful in cats at a dose of 12.5 mg/cat/day, PO.[17] Another drug available in some countries for canine CD is nicergoline (Fitergol; Merial, Duluth, Ga.). This drug is an ergoline derivative that increases cerebral blood flow and may act as a free radical scavenger. It has been anecdotally used to treat cats with CD at a dose of 1.25 mg/cat/day, PO.[17]

Other drugs may be useful for treatment of specific clinical signs. Antidepressants and anxiolytics may be useful for cats that are yowling and active at night, once medical causes have been ruled out (see Box 37-2). There is evidence of cholinergic decline in senior cats[50] so that drugs with anticholinergic activity (e.g., some SSRIs, such as paroxetine and TCAs) should be avoided. In addition, SSRIs and TCAs should not be combined with selegiline. Drugs that could be considered in senior cats with CD include fluoxetine, buspirone, and the benzodiazepines (see Table 37-4).[29] Selegiline, SSRIs, and TCAs all have long half-lives, so switching from one drug to another requires a prolonged washout period. Changing from selegiline to a TCA or SSRI requires a minimum 2-week washout period, and changing from a TCA or SSRI to selegiline requires a 5-week washout period.[11]

In dogs with CD, dietary therapy is combined with environmental enrichment. No studies have evaluated the use of environmental enrichment for cats with CD. Once signs of CD are apparent, attempting to manipulate the cat's environment may actually have a negative effect because of the stress of change. Therefore change should be kept to a minimum for cats with CD, and when it is necessary, it should be done slowly and patiently. Regular and predictable daily routines are important. Some cats may benefit from restriction of their resources and living space to one room to provide a quiet and controlled environment. Use of Feliway (CEVA Animal Health) is often recommended, but no studies have evaluated efficacy in cats with CD.

Neoplasia

A major component of feline medicine in this era of aging pets is diagnosis and treatment of cancer. Fortunately, recent advances in feline oncology have led to improved treatments and survival times (see Chapter 28). As well, components of palliative care, including nutritional support and pain management, are now better understood in feline oncology patients. The American Association of Feline Practitioners has published a position statement on hospice (palliative) care as an alternative to premature euthanasia for terminally ill cats.[47]

However, many owners are still unaware of the signs of cancer in cats (Box 37-3), the benefits of early detection and the improvements in diagnostics and therapeutics. Accurate diagnosis using cytology or histopathology and disease staging are critical for treatment planning. Owners should be apprised of the prognosis, risks and benefits of treatment, and costs before starting therapy. When possible, an oncologist should be consulted. Discussion of euthanasia is also appropriate, both when treatment is pursued and when treatment is not desirable in a given patient (see Chapter 36).

BOX 37-3

Ten Common Signs of Cancer in Small Animals

1. Abnormal swellings that persist or grow
2. Sores or skin lesions that do not heal
3. Weight loss
4. Loss of appetite
5. Bleeding or discharge from any body opening
6. Offensive odor
7. Difficulty eating or swallowing
8. Decreased activity
9. Persistent lameness or stiffness
10. Difficulty breathing, urinating, or defecating

Adapted from the Veterinary Cancer Society (http://www.vetcancersociety.org).

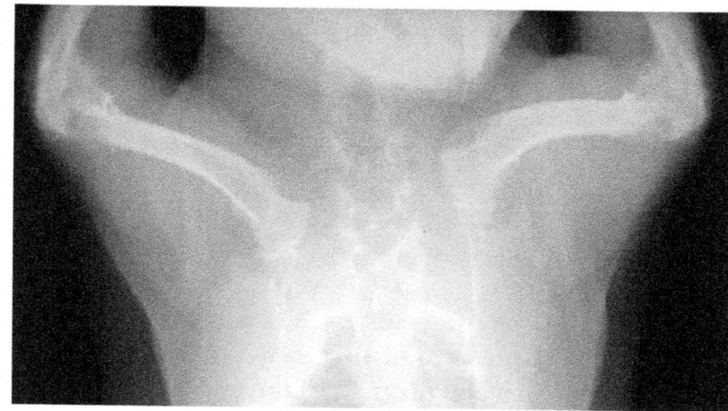

FIGURE 37-3 Bilateral degenerative joint disease of the elbow in a 10-year-old spayed female cat. The lesions were found incidentally when the cat was radiographed because of clinical signs referable to the lower respiratory tract.

Degenerative Joint Disease

Degenerative joint disease (DJD), or osteoarthritis, is a progressive disease where the articular cartilage is slowly destroyed and the underlying bone reacts with remodeling and production of osteophytes. The most commonly affected joints are the shoulder, elbow, and hip (Figure 37-3).[10] Most affected cats are greater than 10 years of age.[10,15,16,19] DJD is an important and under-recognized cause of chronic pain in cats. Clinical signs associated with feline DJD include reduced activity, anorexia and weight loss, irritability and aggression, inappropriate elimination and constipation, decreased grooming, lameness, and alopecia over affected joints. Decreased mobility is less likely to be noticed by cat owners than dog owners, because they are less likely to walk or interact physically with their pet. Some of the clinical signs of DJD overlap with those of cognitive dysfunction. A mobility questionnaire is helpful for early detection of musculoskeletal problems and to increase owner awareness (Box 37-4).

The prevalence of DJD in cats varies with the age of the population studied. In one study, radiographic evidence of DJD was found in 90% of cats greater than 12

BOX 37-4

Mobility Questionnaire for Owners of Senior Cats

Owners should be encouraged to determine whether the answer to each question is "all of the time," "some of the time," or "none of the time."

1. Does your cat sleep more and/or is less active?
2. Is your cat less willing to jump up or down?
3. Will your cat jump up or down only from heights closer to the ground?
4. Is your cat reluctant to use stairs?
5. Does your cat show signs of stiffness, lameness, or limping?
6. Is your cat less likely to greet you or interact with you?
7. Does your cat play with other pets or toys less?
8. Does your cat spend less time grooming and/or have a matted hair coat?
9. Does your cat urinate or defecate outside the litter box?
10. Does your cat have difficulty getting in or out of the cat flap?

Adapted from WellCat for Life, Feline Advisory Bureau (http://www.fabcats.org).

years old.[19] The diagnosis of DJD is achieved through assessment of the medical history, physical examination, and radiography. Many signs of chronic pain are not obvious to owners, or may be misinterpreted as resulting from aging. The goals of treatment for cats with DJD include reduction of pain and inflammation, improvement in joint function and mobility, and slowing the disease process if possible. Treatment options include weight loss if indicated, drug therapy (primary nonsteroidal antiinflammatory drugs [NSAIDs], such as meloxicam, and analgesics), chondroprotectants, nutraceuticals, and dietary therapy. Management of pain has evolved dramatically in the last 10 years, and guidelines have been published by the AAFP/AAHA.[24,45] More information on the treatment of DJD is found in Chapter 26.

Concurrent Disease Management

Senior cats have an increased likelihood of suffering from more than one disease, making management a complex process. The clinician should always have an index of suspicion that another disease may be present in a senior cat, especially if the patient is not responding to treatment as expected. It is most important to remember that as the number of medications administered or the number of interventions (e.g., subcutaneous fluid administration) increases, the human–animal bond and the patient's quality of life may suffer. Prioritizing treatments may mitigate this stress. Treating senior cats may require investigation of novel routes of drug administration and simplified treatment schedules. In addition, the effect of polypharmacy must be monitored, because the administration of some drugs may cause confounding clinical signs (e.g., anorexia, nausea). Age-related changes may also affect the absorption, distribution, and metabolism of drugs, making dose adjustments necessary in some cases. Treatment of concurrent diseases is discussed in Chapter 35.

CONCLUSION

Although both diagnostic and therapeutic tools to help senior pets are more readily available than ever, common sense must be used to assess the quality of life for these patients. Senior cats are less tolerant of change, of interventional treatments, and of hospitalization than younger cats. The degree of tolerance will vary from cat to cat, and in some cases, plans will have to be changed to accommodate the temperament of the individual. It is also important to be proactive in discussing end-of-life issues with owners of senior cats, so that decisions about palliative care and euthanasia can be made at a time that is less stressful than in a life-threatening crisis. For more on palliative care, quality of life and euthanasia decisions, see Chapter 36.

References

1. Araujo JA, Landsberg GM, Milgram NW et al: Improvement of short-term memory performance in aged beagles by a nutraceutical supplement containing phosphatidylserine, *Ginkgo biloba*, vitamin E, and pyridoxine, *Can Vet J* 49:379, 2008.
2. Baldwin K, Bartges J, Buffington T et al: AAHA Nutritional assessment guidelines for dogs and cats, *J Am Anim Hosp Assoc* 46:285, 2010.
3. Bamberger M, Houpt KA: Signalment factors, comorbidity, and trends in behavior diagnoses in cats: 736 cases (1991-2001), *J Am Vet Med Assoc* 229:1602, 2006.
4. Brellou G, Vlemmas I, Lekkas S et al: Immunohistochemical investigation of amyloid beta-protein (Abeta) in the brain of aged cats, *Histol Histopathol* 20:725, 2005.
5. Brodbelt D: Feline anesthetic deaths in veterinary practice, *Top Companion Anim Med* 25:189, 2010.
6. Brodbelt DC, Blissitt KJ, Hammond RA et al: The risk of death: the confidential enquiry into perioperative small animal fatalities, *Vet Anaesth Analg* 35:365, 2008.
7. Brodbelt DC, Pfeiffer DU, Young LE et al: Risk factors for anaesthetic-related death in cats: results from the confidential enquiry into perioperative small animal fatalities (CEPSAF), *Br J Anaesth* 99:617, 2007.
8. Burger IH: Energy needs of companion animals: matching food intakes to requirements throughout the life cycle, *J Nutr* 124:2584S, 1994.
9. Campbell DJ, Rawlings JM, Koelsch S et al: Age-related differences in parameters of feline immune status, *Vet Immunol Immunopathol* 100:73, 2004.
10. Clarke SP, Bennett D: Feline osteoarthritis: a prospective study of 28 cases, *J Small Anim Pract* 47:439, 2006.

11. Crowell-Davis SL: Cognitive dysfunction in senior pets, *Comp Contin Edu Pract Vet* 30:106, 2008.
12. Cummings BJ, Satou T, Head E et al: Diffuse plaques contain C-terminal A beta 42 and not A beta 40: evidence from cats and dogs, *Neurobiol Aging* 17:653, 1996.
13. Cupp C, Perez-Camargo G, Patil A et al: Long-term food consumption and body weight changes in a controlled population of geriatric cats [abstract], *Comp Contin Educ Pract Vet* 26:60, 2004.
13a. Czarnecki-Maulden G, Cupp CJ, Patil AR et al: Effect of aging on blood metabolites in the cat (abstract), *Comp Contin Educ Pract Vet* 26:74, 2004.
14. Epstein M, Kuehn NF, Landsberg G et al: AAHA senior care guidelines for dogs and cats, *J Am Anim Hosp Assoc* 41:81, 2005.
15. Godfrey DR: Osteoarthritis in cats: a retrospective series of 31 cases, *J Small Anim Pract* 43:260, 2002.
16. Godfrey DR: Osteoarthritis in cats: a retrospective radiological study, *J Small Anim Pract* 46:425, 2005.
17. Gunn-Moore D, Moffat K, Christie LA et al: Cognitive dysfunction and the neurobiology of ageing in cats, *J Small Anim Pract* 48:546, 2007.
18. Gunn-Moore DA, McVee J, Bradshaw JM et al: Ageing changes in cat brains demonstrated by beta-amyloid and AT8-immunoreactive phosphorylated tau deposits, *J Feline Med Surg* 8:234, 2006.
19. Hardie EM, Roe SC, Martin FR: Radiographic evidence of degenerative joint disease in geriatric cats: 100 cases (1994-1997), *J Am Vet Med Assoc* 220:628, 2002.
20. Harper EJ: Changing perspectives on aging and energy requirements: aging and digestive function in humans, dogs and cats, *J Nutr* 128:2632S, 1998.
21. Harper EJ: Changing perspectives on aging and energy requirements: aging, body weight and body composition in humans, dogs and cats, *J Nutr* 128:2627S, 1998.
22. Head E: Combining an antioxidant-fortified diet with behavioral enrichment leads to cognitive improvement and reduced brain pathology in aging canines: strategies for healthy aging, *Ann N Y Acad Sci* 1114:398, 2007.
23. Heath SE, Barabas S, Craze PG: Nutritional supplementation in cases of canine cognitive dysfunction—a clinical trial, *Appl Anim Behav Sci* 105:284, 2007.
24. Hellyer P, Rodan I, Brunt J et al: AAHA/AAFP pain management guidelines for dogs and cats, *J Feline Med Surg* 9:466, 2007.
25. Laflamme DP: Nutrition for aging cats and dogs and the importance of body condition, *Vet Clin North Am Small Anim Pract* 35:713, 2005.
26. Laflamme DP, Ballam JM: Effect of age on maintenance energy requirements of adult cats, *Comp Contin Educ Pract Vet* 24:82, 2002.
27. Landsberg G: Therapeutic options for cognitive decline in senior pets, *J Am Anim Hosp Assoc* 42:407, 2006.
28. Landsberg G, Araujo JA: Behavior problems in geriatric pets, *Vet Clin North Am Small Anim Pract* 35:675, 2005.
29. Landsberg GM, Denenberg S, Araujo JA: Cognitive dysfunction in cats: a syndrome we used to dismiss as "old age," *J Feline Med Surg* 12:837, 2010.
30. Levine MS, Lloyd RL, Fisher RS et al: Sensory, motor and cognitive alterations in aged cats, *Neurobiol Aging* 8:253, 1987.
31. Mansfield K, Burr P, Snodgrass D et al: Factors affecting the serological response of dogs and cats to rabies vaccination, *Vet Rec* 154:423, 2004.
32. McCune S, Stevenson J, Fretwell L et al: Ageing does not significantly affect performance in a spatial learning task in the domestic cat (Felis silvestris catus), *Appl Anim Behav Sci* 112:345, 2008.
33. Michel KE, Anderson WI, Cupp C et al: Validation of a subjective muscle mass scoring system for cats, *J Anim Physiol Anim Nutr (Berl)* 93:806, 2009.
34. Milgram NW: Neuropsychological function and aging in cats. *15th Annual Conference on Canine Cognition and Aging*, Laguna Beach, CA, November 2010.
35. Milgram NW, Head E, Zicker SC et al: Long-term treatment with antioxidants and a program of behavioral enrichment reduces age-dependent impairment in discrimination and reversal learning in beagle dogs, *Exp Gerontol* 39:753, 2004.
36. Munday HS, Earle KE, Anderson P: Changes in the body composition of the domestic shorthaired cat during growth and development, *J Nutr* 124:2622S, 1994.
37. Osella MC, Re G, Odore R et al: Canine cognitive dysfunction syndrome: prevalence, clinical signs and treatment with a neuroprotective nutraceutical, *Appl Anim Behav Sci* 105:297, 2007.
38. Pan Y, Larson B, Araujo JA et al: Dietary supplementation with medium-chain TAG has long-lasting cognition-enhancing effects in aged dogs, *Br J Nutr* 103:1746, 2010.
39. Perez-Camargo G: Cat nutrition: what is new in the old? *Comp Contin Educ Pract Vet* 26:5, 2004.
40. Perrin T: The Business Of Urban Animals Survey: the facts and statistics on companion animals in Canada, *Can Vet J* 50:48, 2009.
41. Reme CA, Dramard V, Kern L et al: Effect of S-adenosylmethionine tablets on the reduction of age-related mental decline in dogs: a double-blinded, placebo-controlled trial, *Vet Ther* 9:69, 2008.
42. Richards JR, Elston TH, Ford RB et al: The 2006 American Association of Feline Practitioners Feline Vaccine Advisory Panel report, *J Am Vet Med Assoc* 229:1405, 2006.
43. Scarlett JM, Donoghue S, Saidla J et al: Overweight cats: prevalence and risk factors, *Int J Obes Relat Metab Disord* 18 Suppl 1:S22, 1994.
44. Shepherd AJ: Results of the 2006 AVMA survey of companion animal ownership in US pet-owning households, *J Am Vet Med Assoc* 232:695, 2008.
45. Sparkes AH, Heiene R, Lascelles BDX et al: ISFM and AAFP consensus guidelines: long-term use of NSAIDs in cats, *J Feline Med Surg* 12:521, 2010.
45a. Stella JL, Lord LK, Buffington CAT: Sickness behaviors in response to unusual external events in healthy cats and cats with feline interstitial cystitis, *J Am Vet Med Assoc* 238:67, 2011.
46. Taylor EJ, Adams C, Neville R: Some nutritional aspects of ageing in dogs and cats, *Proc Nutr Soc* 54:645, 1995.
47. Thayer V, Monroe P, Smith R et al: AAFP position statement: veterinary hospice care for cats, *J Feline Med Surg* 12:728, 2010.
48. Vogt AH, Rodan I, Brown M et al: AAFP-AAHA: feline life stage guidelines, *J Feline Med Surg* 12:43, 2010.
49. Zhang C, Hua T, Zhu Z et al: Age-related changes of structures in cerebellar cortex of cat, *J Biosci* 31:55, 2006.
50. Zhang JH, Sampogna S, Morales FR et al: Age-related changes in cholinergic neurons in the laterodorsal and the pedunculo-pontine tegmental nuclei of cats: a combined light and electron microscopic study, *Brain Res* 1052:47, 2005.

CHAPTER

38

Evaluation of the Senior Cat with Weight Loss

Susan E. Little

OUTLINE

PREVALENCE OF WEIGHT LOSS

The easiest problems to detect in senior cats are weight loss and decline in body condition, but they are also problems that may challenge the clinician's diagnostic and therapeutic skills. The American Association of Feline Practitioners (AAFP)/American Animal Hospital Association (AAHA) feline life stage guidelines define a senior cat as 11 to 14 years old and a geriatric cat as 15 years and older.[20] The term "senior" is often used to refer to all cats more than about 10 years of age and will be used as such in this chapter.

The prevalence of obesity decreases with age in cats; in fact, senior cats have a tendency to be underweight (Figure 38-1).[6,10,13,18] In a report of 191 cats at the Waltham Centre for Pet Nutrition (Melton Mowbray, United Kingdom), ranging in age from 1 to 13 years, the heaviest cats were neutered males aged 5 to 8 years, while cats greater than 11 years had a tendency to exhibit lower body weights than younger cats.[6] In a survey of more than 2,000 cats presented to veterinary hospitals in the Northeastern United States, the proportion of overweight cats increased until 7 years of age, after which it declined, especially in cats more than 10 years of age.[18] Similar patterns were found in another study, where the proportion of overweight cats peaked at 7 years of age, and the proportion of underweight cats increased sharply at 11 years of age.[1] Longitudinal data collected on 53 healthy cats more than 11 years of age at the Waltham Centre indicates that for most cats weight loss or weight maintenance, rather than weight gain, is a feature of old age.[6] After 8 years of age, 50% of cats in that report maintained weight and 30% lost weight. It appears that a significant proportion of obese middle-aged cats die before reaching old age (e.g., from diseases such as diabetes mellitus or hepatic lipidosis), and a similar proportion lose weight into their senior years. Those senior cats that are obese have probably been obese for most of their lives.

CAUSES OF WEIGHT LOSS

The reasons for a tendency to weight loss with aging in cats are probably complex and interrelated. As discussed in Chapter 37, maintenance energy requirements (MERs) in cats decrease by about 3% per year until about 11 years of age.[3,9] After 11 years of age, MERs actually increase and may contribute to the tendency of senior cats to be underweight if their energy needs are not met. An investigation of changes in body composition with aging found that lean body mass drops dramatically after 12 years of age, and that by age 15, cats may have a mean lean tissue mass less than 2 kg (4.4 lb), one third less than cats aged 1 to 7 years of age (mean, 3 kg [6.6 lb]).[13] Mean percentage body fat also decreases progressively after 12 years of age so that the lean body mass to fat ratio does not show significant changes with aging. The combination of reduced lean mass and body fat contributes to the frail look of many elderly cats (Figure 38-2).

Changes in digestive efficiency occur with age and may contribute to weight loss. Older cats are less efficient at digesting fats and proteins.[7] In one study, 22%

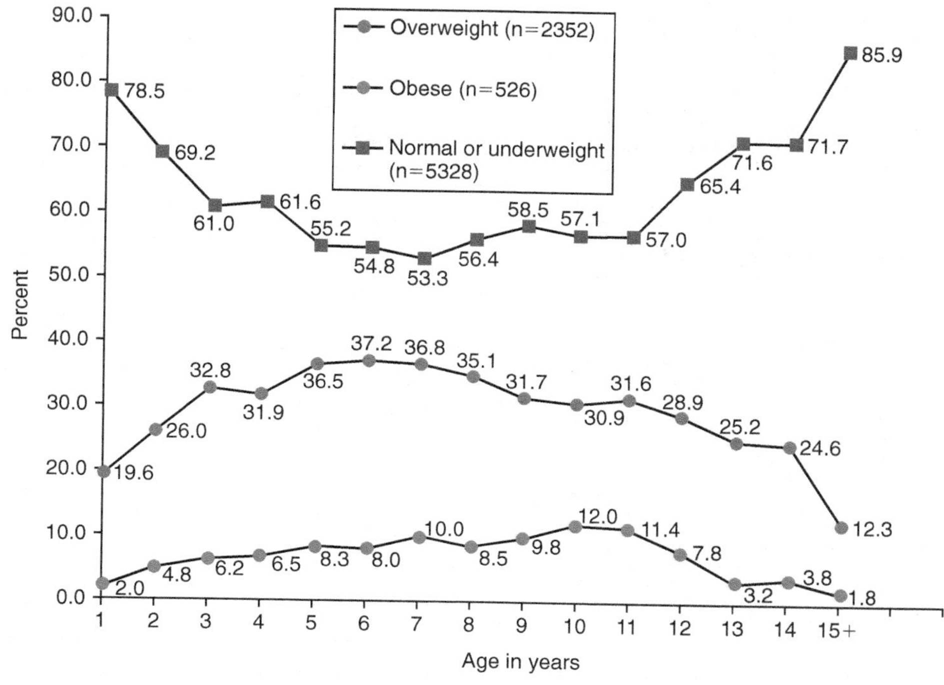

FIGURE 38-1 Prevalence of obesity, overweight, normal, or underweight by age for 8,206 cats examined by veterinarians in the United States. *(Adapted from Lund EM, Armstrong PJ, Kirk CA et al: Prevalence and risk factors for obesity in adult cats from private US veterinary practices,* Intern J Appl Res Vet Med *3:88, 2005.)*

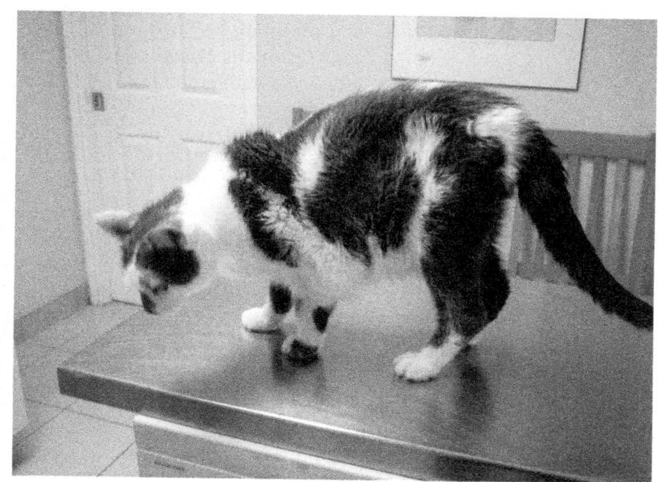

FIGURE 38-2 Many elderly cats have reduced lean body mass and fat mass as well as muscle wasting.

of cats more than 14 years old had protein digestibility of less than 77%, and 33% of cats more than 12 years old had fat digestibility of less than 80%.[11] To compensate, senior cats may need to increase their daily food intake by as much as 25%.[19] In a study of 85 senior cats on a long-term feeding study (spanning 7 years), there was a significant increase in total kcal/kg body weight ingested and total daily food consumption in cats from 10 to 15 years of age.[3,4] Despite the increase in caloric intake, body weight decreased with age, particularly after age 13.

Unfortunately, there are very little data available on changes in gastrointestinal tract function with aging in cats to explain this decline in digestive efficiency. In humans, reduced secretion and activity of pancreatic lipase and reduced capacity for the production, transport, and secretion of bile acids has been documented with aging. It is tempting to speculate that similar mechanisms might be at play in cats.

Although changes in feeding patterns occur with age in some species and may contribute to weight loss, this does not seem to be the case in cats. One study evaluated the effect of age on feeding patterns and determined there was no difference between feeding patterns of younger cats (average age, 3 years) and older cats (average age, 11.6 years).[12] Cats of all ages consumed regular small meals during both day and night. However, owners tend to feed senior cats differently than younger cats. In a telephone survey evaluating feeding of non-therapeutic diets to 429 adult cats, those cats 12 years of age and older were more likely to be fed canned foods and table scraps compared with younger cats.[8]

The dogma that all older cats should be fed reduced energy "senior" diets must be re-evaluated as more is learned about nutritional needs of older cats at various ages. A feeding plan must be tailored to body condition and the presence of diseases as well as life stage. Considering the available data on metabolism and body weight in aging cats, it seems likely that many elderly cats, particularly those more than 12 years of age that are not overweight, would benefit from frequent small meals of energy-dense, highly digestible diets to maintain body weight and lean tissue mass and avoid protein:calorie malnutrition. Protein:calorie malnutrition is associated with important detrimental effects, such as anemia, hypoproteinemia, delayed healing, decreased immune function, and compromised function of major organ systems (gastrointestinal, pulmonary, cardiovascular).[15] Despite the numerous advantages of feeding canned diets to senior cats (e.g., increased water content, higher proportion of animal source protein), most canned diets have a lower caloric density based on volume fed than dry diets. Therefore attention must be paid to ensure the caloric intake of cats on canned diets is appropriate.

Other reasons for the susceptibility of senior cats to lose weight may include the presence of diseases (including those causing pain) and decreased appetite because of dulling senses of taste and smell. Early detection of weight loss is important, because it may lead to early detection of disease. A study of 258 cats in a Nestle Purina colony that died of cancer, renal failure, and hyperthyroidism determined weight loss started about 2.5 years before death.[3] Cats dying from other causes started losing body weight even earlier, about 3.75 years before death. Body weight loss two years prior to death was greater than 6% in cats with cancer, renal failure, and hyperthyroidism. During the last year of life, the average weight loss was greater than 10% for cats dying of all causes. Gradual weight loss is often overlooked by owners. Therefore the body weight and body condition score (see Chapter 3) should be determined and recorded at every opportunity, because weight loss may be the earliest sign of disease. Percentage weight change is an easily performed calculation ([previous weight – current weight]/previous weight) that detects subtle trends. Muscle condition scoring is also useful in senior cats for early detection of loss of body condition (see Chapter 37). It is important to note that diseases causing weight loss in senior cats are not always associated with inappetence. Because weight loss can occur with either an increased or decreased appetite, it is important to encourage owners to report any *change* in appetite.

DIAGNOSIS OF WEIGHT LOSS

Diagnosis of weight loss in senior cats is dependent on thorough data gathering, because there are many potential causes. In human geriatric medicine, a mnemonic consisting of ten "Ds" has been suggested to determine the cause of involuntary weight loss (Box 38-1),[16,21] and many of these categories are useful considerations for senior cats as well. In elderly humans, the most common causes of weight loss are depression, cancer, and benign gastrointestinal disease.

BOX 38-1

The Ten Ds for Weight Loss in Elderly Human Patients

1. Dentition
2. Dysgeusia (an altered ability to taste)
3. Dysphagia
4. Diarrhea
5. Disease (chronic)
6. Depression
7. Dementia
8. Dysfunction
9. Drugs
10. Do not know

Adapted from Robbins LJ: Evaluation of weight loss in the elderly, *Geriatrics* 44:31, 1989. Wise GR, Craig D: Evaluation of involuntary weight loss. Where do you start? *Postgrad Med* 95:143, 1994.

TABLE 38-1 **Signs Suggestive of Pain in Cats**

General Signs	Specific Signs
Changes in normal behavior	Decreased mobility or activity, lethargy, inappetence, decreased grooming
Abnormal behaviors	Inappropriate elimination, inappropriate vocalization, aggression, decreased social interactions, altered facial expression and posture, restlessness, hiding
Reactions to touch	Increased body tension, flinching when painful areas are palpated
Changes in physiologic parameters	Elevated heart rate, elevated respiratory rate, elevated or decreased body temperature, elevated or decreased blood pressure, pupillary dilation

Adapted from Hellyer P, Rodan I, Brunt J et al: AAHA/AAFP pain management guidelines for dogs and cats, *J Feline Med Surg* 9:466, 2007.

A complete history, including a nutritional history, is the first step in diagnosis. Diet quality should be investigated to ensure the patient is receiving an adequate amount of energy and protein. Attention should be paid to trends in food and water consumption and questions should be asked about signs of pain (Table 38-1), behavior changes (see Box 37-1), changes in elimination patterns, and changes in mobility (see Box 37-4), as well as presence of vomiting or diarrhea. Senior cats often have more than one health problem and may be receiving multiple medications, many of which cause gastrointestinal distress, including anorexia, such as nonsteroidal antiinflammatory drugs (NSAIDs), antibiotics, and cardiac medications. A thorough physical examination should include assessment of weight and body condition, an orthopedic examination, and blood pressure

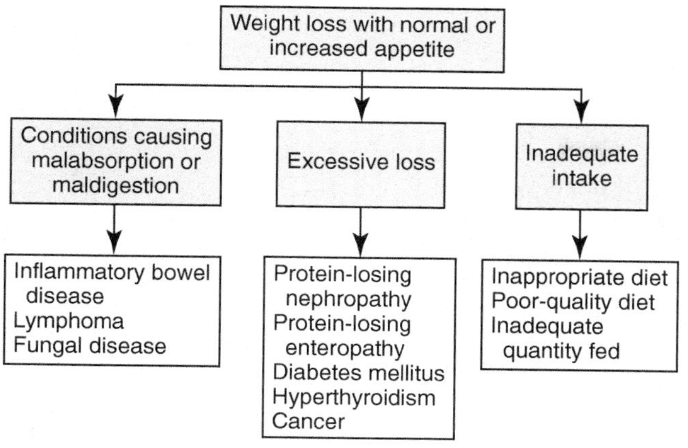

FIGURE 38-3 Diagnostic algorithm for weight loss in senior cats with normal or increased appetite. *(Adapted from Laflamme DP: Nutrition for aging cats and dogs and the importance of body condition,* Vet Clin North Am Small Anim Pract *35:713, 2005.)*

measurement. Specific areas that may yield valuable clues include

1. Oral cavity: Dental and oral diseases (e.g., periodontal disease, tooth resorption, tumors) are common in older cats and may be associated with pain and decreased appetite; feline orofacial pain syndrome is a neuropathic disorder most commonly found in the Burmese breed in the United Kingdom.[17]
2. Eye: An ocular examination, including the retina, may provide evidence consistent with systemic hypertension as well as conditions such as glaucoma, neoplasia, and infectious diseases (e.g., toxoplasmosis, cryptococcosis).
3. Neck and thorax: Thyroid nodules associated with hyperthyroidism may be palpable, and cardiac changes associated with hyperthyroidism or hypertension (e.g., tachycardia, arrhythmia, heart murmur) may be appreciated; decreased thoracic compressibility may be associated with masses or effusions.
4. Abdomen: Thickening of the intestinal wall and mesenteric lymphadenopathy may be associated with inflammatory bowel disease or neoplasia; abdominal masses associated with neoplasia may be found; cranial abdominal pain may be associated with pancreatitis; changes in kidney size and shape may be associated with chronic kidney disease (CKD), polycystic kidney disease, feline infectious peritonitis, hydronephrosis secondary to a ureterolith, pyelonephritis, or neoplasia.
5. Musculoskeletal system: Muscle wasting may be evident especially over the lumbar area; swelling, pain, and stiffness in joints may be associated with degenerative joint disease.

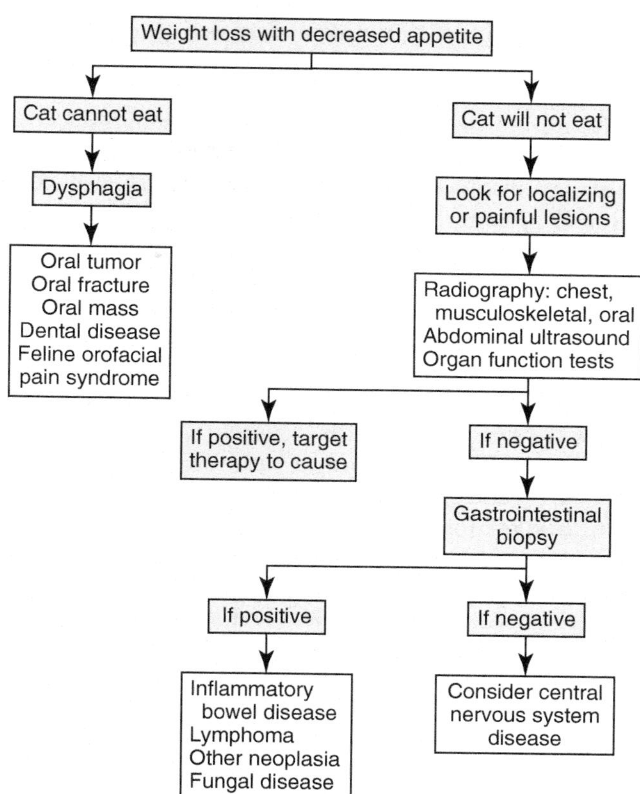

FIGURE 38-4 Diagnostic algorithm for weight loss in senior cats with decreased appetite. *(Adapted from Laflamme DP: Nutrition for aging cats and dogs and the importance of body condition,* Vet Clin North Am Small Anim Pract *35:713, 2005.)*

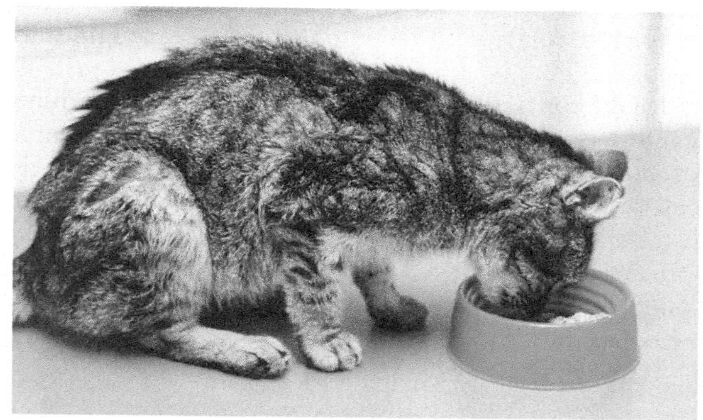

FIGURE 38-5 Weight loss may occur despite a normal or increased appetite in cats with diseases such as hyperthyroidism.

Causes of weight loss in senior cats may be categorized by quality of appetite (Figures 38-3 and 38-4). With a normal or increased appetite, diseases causing malabsorption or maldigestion (e.g., inflammatory bowel disease, gastrointestinal lymphoma) or excessive protein loss (e.g., protein-losing nephropathy or enteropathy, diabetes mellitus, hyperthyroidism) must be considered (Figure 38-5). With a diminished appetite, investigations must focus on oral cavity diseases, systemic diseases (e.g., neoplasia, CKD, liver disease, gastrointestinal disease, retroviral infection), and diseases causing pain (e.g., degenerative joint disease).

The minimum laboratory database for investigation of weight loss in senior cats includes a complete blood count, serum biochemistries and electrolytes, total thyroxine (T_4), complete urinalysis including microscopic examination of sediment, and retroviral testing. Most common causes of weight loss in this age group will be quickly diagnosed or eliminated with this minimum database. Cats with protein:calorie malnutrition may have lymphopenia, anemia, lower than expected blood urea nitrogen (BUN) and creatinine, and increased liver enzymes and bilirubin. In severely protein-deficient animals, serum total protein and albumin may be reduced. Serum creatinine kinase (CK) activity may be a useful marker for assessment and monitoring of nutritional status in cats. In one study, serum CK was significantly increased in hospitalized anorectic cats compared with nonanorectic cats, and was significantly lower after 48 hours of nutritional support through a nasoesophageal tube.[5]

Depending on the physical examination findings and results of initial testing, further laboratory investigations may include bile acid testing and extended thyroid hormone testing. Pancreatic (e.g., chronic pancreatitis) and gastrointestinal disease (e.g., inflammatory bowel disease, lymphoma) are common causes for weight loss that may not be readily apparent from the history, physical examination, and initial laboratory testing. Blood tests for pancreatic and gastrointestinal disease include cobalamin, folate, and feline pancreatic lipase immunoreactivity. Finally, more advanced diagnostics will be indicated for a subset of patients, such as abdominal imaging or endoscopy. Exploratory laparotomy or laparoscopy should be considered when the cause of weight loss remains undiagnosed. During surgery, samples for histopathology should be collected even if the tissue appears grossly normal. Sites to sample include liver, pancreas, lymph nodes, stomach, and multiple areas of the small intestine.

NONSPECIFIC MANAGEMENT OF WEIGHT LOSS

The best chance to reverse weight loss is to diagnose and treat underlying diseases. However, nonspecific measures for nutritional support are often part of the treatment plan. Encouraging increased food intake can be accomplished by feeding an energy-dense, nutrient-dense diet that is palatable to the cat; some cats prefer diets with high moisture content while others prefer dry diets. Examples of appropriate diets include diets designed for growth and recovery or critical care. Box 38-2 discusses ways to encourage senior cats to eat. Even if a therapeutic diet is recommended, initially it is best to feed familiar foods, because learned aversions may be induced by feeding novel foods to sick or hospitalized cats. It is better for a sick cat to eat any food rather than no food at all. Slow introduction of the recommended diet can be made once the cat's condition and appetite have improved and it has been discharged from hospital.

BOX 38-2
Ways to Encourage Senior Cats to Eat

1. Offer fresh favorite and familiar foods to avoid learned aversions
2. Use wide, shallow food and water bowls
3. Warm the food to body temperature
4. Moisten the food
5. Feed in a quiet, stress-free environment
6. Use encouragement (e.g., petting) and praise during feeding

Short-term use of appetite stimulants may be helpful in some anorexic cats. In addition to the drugs listed in Table 18-1, midazolam (2 to 5 µg/kg, IV) has been reported to stimulate appetite within 2 minutes without sedation or other side effects.[14] If adequate food intake cannot be achieved, nutritional support through tube feeding should be considered (see Chapter 18). Nutritional support should be considered earlier rather than later for moderately to severely malnourished cats. Some anorectic patients with diseases such as advanced renal disease, hepatopathy, protein-losing gastrointestinal disease, or protein-losing glomerular disease will benefit from early nutritional support before significant weight loss occurs. This may be especially true for cats with neoplasia. In one study of 57 feline cancer patients, median survival time of cats with a body condition score less than 5/9 was 3.3 months compared with a mean survival time of 16.7 months for cats with a body condition score of 5/9 or greater.[2]

Cats are solitary feeders by nature, and elderly cats often do not cope well with competition and stressors. Therefore many older cats in multicat homes would benefit from being fed separately or being offered supplemental meals. Owners should be educated to monitor the daily food intake of senior cats carefully. One way to do this when cats are fed individually is to weigh food bowls before and after feeding. Many owners are willing to measure the amount fed and record the amount the cat has eaten; this can be valuable information for the clinician.

References

1. Armstrong PJ, Lund EM: Changes in body composition and energy balance with aging, *Vet Clin Nutr* 3:83, 1996.

2. Baez JL, Michel KE, Sorenmo K et al: A prospective investigation of the prevalence and prognostic significance of weight loss and changes in body condition in feline cancer patients, *J Feline Med Surg* 9:411, 2007.
3. Cupp C, Perez-Camargo G, Patil A et al: Long-term food consumption and body weight changes in a controlled population of geriatric cats [abstract], *Comp Contin Educ Pract Vet* 26:60, 2004.
4. Cupp CJ, Jean-Philippe C, Kerr WW et al: Effect of nutritional interventions on longevity of senior cats, *Intern J Appl Res Vet Med* 5:133, 2007.
5. Fascetti AJ, Mauldin GE, Mauldin GN: Correlation between serum creatinine kinase activities and anorexia in cats, *J Vet Intern Med* 11:9, 1997.
6. Harper E: Changing perspectives on aging and energy requirements: aging, body weight and body composition in humans, dogs and cats, *J Nutr* 128:2627S, 1998.
7. Harper J: Changing perspectives on aging and energy requirements: aging and digestive function in humans, dogs and cats, *J Nutr* 128:2632S, 1998.
8. Laflamme DP, Abood S, Fascetti A et al: The effect of age on how cats are fed, *Proceedings 33rd World Small Animal Veterinary Association World Congress,* Dublin, Ireland, August 20-24, 2008.
9. Laflamme DP, Ballam JM: Effect of age on maintenance energy requirements of adult cats, *Comp Contin Educ Pract Vet* 24:82, 2002.
10. Lund EM, Armstrong PJ, Kirk CA et al: Prevalence and risk factors for obesity in adult cats from private US veterinary practices, *Intern J Appl Res Vet Med* 3:88, 2005.
11. Patil AR, Cupp C, Perez-Camargo G: Incidence of impaired nutrient digestibility in aging cats [abstract], *Comp Contin Educ Pract Vet* 26:60, 2004.
12. Peachey SE, Harper EJ: Aging does not influence feeding behavior in cats, *J Nutr* 132:1735S, 2002.
13. Perez-Camargo G: Cat nutrition: what is new in the old? *Comp Contin Educ Pract Vet* 26:5, 2004.
14. Rangel-Captillo A, Avendano-Carillo H, Reyes-Delgado F et al: Immediate appetite stimulation of anorexic cats with midazolam [abstract], *Comp Contin Educ Pract Vet* 26:61, 2004.
15. Remillard RL: Nutritional support in critical care patients, *Vet Clin North Am Small Anim Pract* 32:1145, 2002.
16. Robbins LJ: Evaluation of weight loss in the elderly, *Geriatrics* 44:31, 1989.
17. Rusbridge C, Heath S, Gunn-Moore DA et al: Feline orofacial pain syndrome (FOPS): a retrospective study of 113 cases, *J Feline Med Surg* 12:498, 2010.
18. Scarlett JM, Donoghue S, Saidla J et al: Overweight cats: prevalence and risk factors, *Int J Obes Relat Metab Disord* 18(Suppl 1):S22, 1994.
19. Taylor EJ, Adams C, Neville R: Some nutritional aspects of ageing in dogs and cats, *Proc Nutr Soc* 54:645, 1995.
20. Vogt AH, Rodan I, Brown M et al: AAFP-AAHA: Feline life stage guidelines, *J Feline Med Surg* 12:43, 2010.
21. Wise GR, Craig D: Evaluation of involuntary weight loss. Where do you start? *Postgrad Med* 95:143, 1994.

SECTION VIII

FELINE REPRODUCTION AND PEDIATRICS

Editor: Susan E. Little

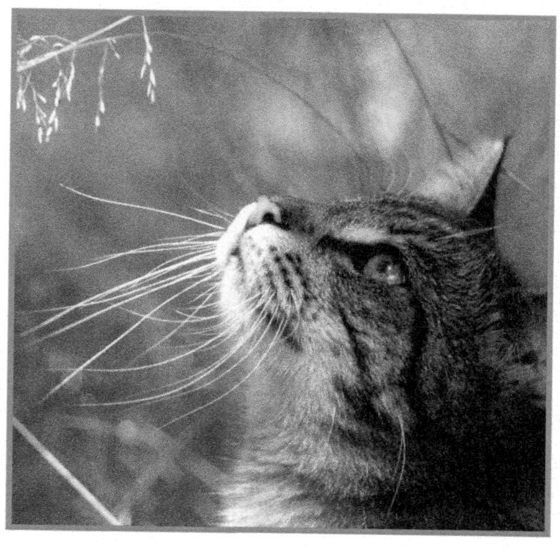

CHAPTER

39

Male Reproduction

Susan E. Little

OUTLINE

MALE ANATOMY

The reproductive tract of the male or tom cat consists of the penis, testes, scrotum, prostate and bulbourethral glands, and the ductus deferens (also called the vas deferens) (Figure 39-1). The fetal testes are inside the abdomen; they descend through the inguinal ring into the scrotum at birth or shortly afterward. By 6 to 8 weeks of age, testes should be palpable in the scrotum. The hair-covered scrotum is divided by a thin wall into two cavities; each cavity contains a testis, epididymis, and the end of the spermatic cord. The testes may not stay in the scrotum permanently until 4 to 6 months of age. The structure of the feline testis is similar to most domestic animals.[9] There are three major cell types in the testes:

1. Interstitial (Leydig) cells: secrete testosterone in response to luteinizing hormone (LH)
2. Sertoli cells: line the seminiferous tubules and secrete estrogen and inhibin to support the developing spermatozoa in response to follicle-stimulating hormone (FSH)
3. Germ cells: spermatozoa in various stages of development present within the seminiferous tubules

Production of spermatozoa occurs in seminiferous tubules; spermatozoa are then transported into the epididymis, where maturation and storage takes place. The seminiferous tubules are closely packed and convoluted and are surrounded by interstitial cells. The tail of the epididymis becomes the ductus deferens, which carries sperm to the penis after passing through the inguinal canal with the rest of the spermatic cord. The spermatic cord consists of the ductus deferens, the testicular artery and vein, lymphatics, and nerve plexus.

The prostate of the cat is approximately 1 cm in length and covers the urethra near the neck of the urinary bladder. The prostate is androgen-dependent and atrophies after castration. Prostatic disease is very rare in the cat, with only a few cases reports of tumors published.[38,39] The bulbourethral glands are two small pea-shaped structures near the bulb of the penis. During ejaculation, spermatozoa from the epididymis are mixed with secretions from the prostate and bulbourethral glands. It is normal for a small proportion of spermatozoa to travel retrograde through the urethra into the bladder (Figure 39-2). The urethra in the male cat is very narrow and shorter than in the dog.

The penis of the cat contains a vestigial os penis (5 mm in length). When not erect, the penis is completely enclosed within the prepuce. The glans of the penis of a mature tom cat is covered with 120 to 150 penile spines that are directed caudally. The spines are testosterone-dependent and start to appear at about 12 weeks of age, are fully developed at puberty, and are absent in neutered males, disappearing by about 6 weeks after castration (Figure 39-3).

In addition to testosterone, important hormones in the male cat include LH and FSH, both produced in the anterior pituitary gland in response to gonadotropin-releasing hormone (GnRH), produced by the hypothalamus. Resting plasma testosterone levels vary widely, because secretion is episodic. Testosterone is not only essential for development of secondary sexual characteristics (e.g., heavy jowls, thick skin) and breeding behavior but also for production of spermatozoa.

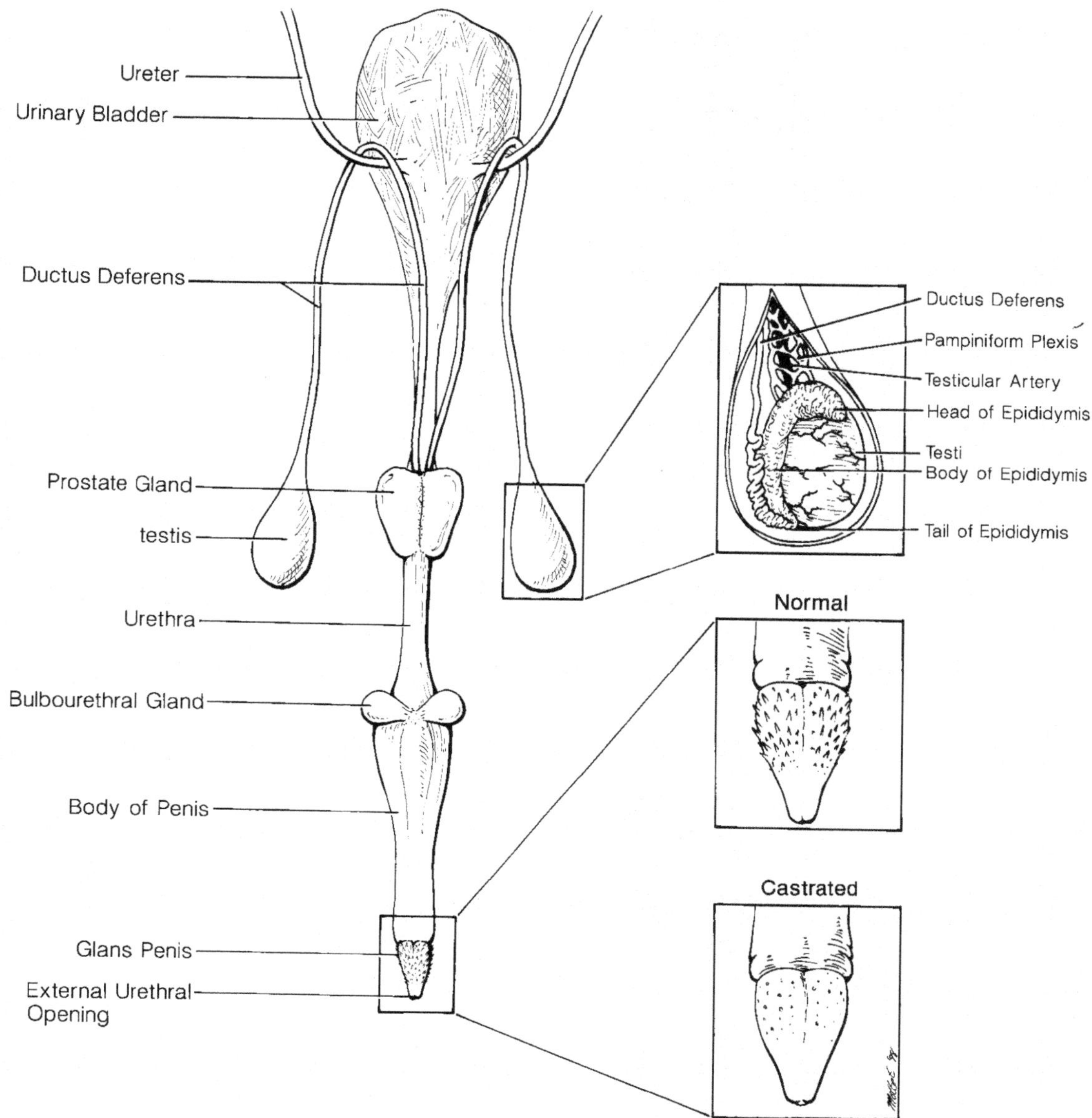

FIGURE 39-1 Anatomy of the reproductive tract of the male cat. *(From Johnston S, Root Kustritz M, Olson P: Sexual differentiation and normal anatomy of the tom cat. In Johnston S, Root Kustritz M, Olson P, editors:* Canine and feline theriogenology, *Philadelphia, 2001, Saunders.)*

Castration causes an immediate drop in blood testosterone, but viable sperm may still be present for up to 7 weeks after surgery.

MATING BEHAVIOR

Spermatozoa are present in the testes by the age of 5 to 9 months, and full maturity of spermatogenesis occurs at 8 to 10 months of age.[37] However, the actual age at which mating begins varies with physical condition, body size, and season. The onset of puberty is typically at 8 to 10 months of age and at a body weight of 2.5 kg or more. However, significant variation among breeds is seen with longhair breeds, such as the Persian, maturing more slowly than shorthair breeds, such as the Siamese. Tom cats probably have a normal breeding lifespan of 10 years or more.

Tom cats are attracted to estrous queens by vocalizing, odors, and behavior. A tom cat will approach a queen in estrus, touch noses, and then investigate her perineum. A flehmen reaction may be exhibited, that is, sampling of the queen's pheromones by the vomeronasal organ. The tom cat grasps the skin on the back of the queen's neck and attempts to mount her. The tom cat then treads on his back feet and slides down over the back of the queen, attempting to position for intromission. The tom cat starts a series of pelvic thrusts, and ejaculation follows within 20 to 30 seconds. Semen is deposited in the posterior vagina. The tom cat then

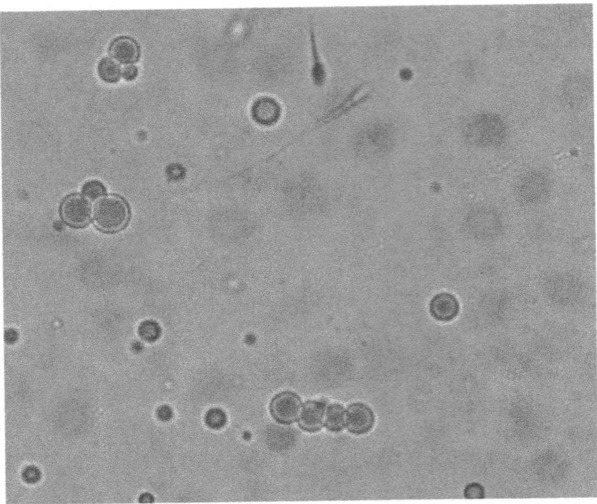

FIGURE 39-2 Because a degree of retrograde ejaculation is normal in the tom cat, collection of a urine sample after ejaculation allows for detection of sperm.

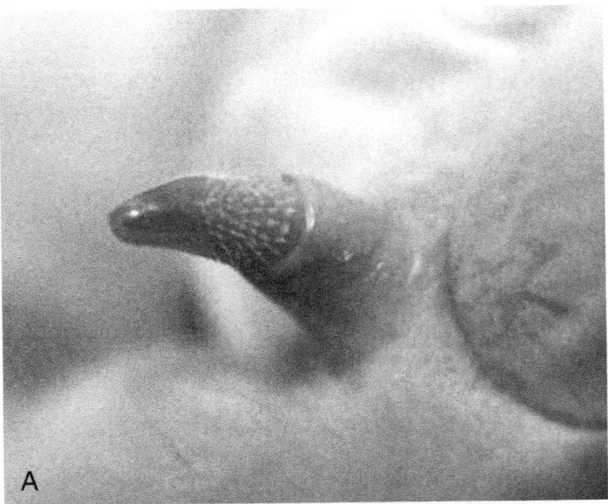

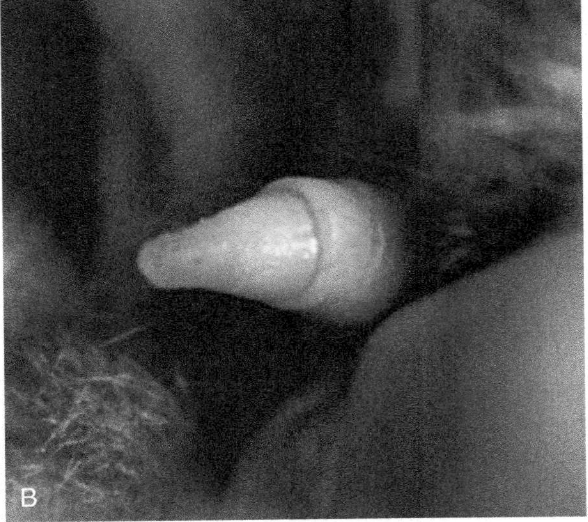

FIGURE 39-3 **A,** Glans of the penis of an intact tom cat with penile spines. **B,** Glans of the penis of a castrated cat without penile spines.

quickly jumps away to avoid being swatted by the queen. Once the queen's postcoital behavior settles down (typically in 10 to 60 minutes), the tom cat will often try to grasp and mount again. A pair may breed several times until the tom cat is exhausted. Breeding usually occurs at night under natural circumstances.

After castration, mating behavior typically ceases, but may persist for years in some mature and experienced tom cats. The behavior may include mounting of other cats or kittens, the owner's legs, or soft inanimate objects. It is important to ensure the cat is not cryptorchid (see below). A rare cause of breeding behaviors in castrated male cats is a testosterone-secreting adrenal tumor.[25] The behavior may be attention seeking or because of a stimulus-poor environment. Ensuring adequate environmental enrichment and interactive time with the owner is often helpful. The behavior should not be rewarded, even inadvertently, by attempts at punishment. Interruption and distraction with another activity is likely to be more effective. Urine spraying may also persist after castration, although typically it resolves in 80% or more of cats. There is one report in the literature on the use of cyproheptadine (2 mg/cat, PO, every 12 hours) for the successful treatment of masturbation and urine spraying in a cryptorchid cat.[32] For more on urine spraying, see Chapter 13.

CONTROL OF REPRODUCTION

Surgical Castration

Castration is the most common procedure used to control fertility in male cats. The surgery is easy to perform, requires simple equipment, is effective and irreversible, and eliminates most of the undesirable traits of an intact male (e.g., aggression, roaming, urine marking).[12] Cats may be castrated using either an open or closed approach. The spermatic cord may be ligated with suture material or the cord may be knotted on itself. Castration may be performed as early as 6 weeks of age (see Chapter 41). Prepuberal castration is more effective at preventing unwanted sexual behaviors than castration after sexual maturity.[13] Complications associated with castration in the tom cat are few but include scrotal swelling, hemorrhage, bruising, and infection.

Vasectomy

Vasectomy involves the bilateral removal or occlusion of a portion of the ductus deferens, causing infertility by preventing ejaculation of sperm during copulation. Vasectomy does not remove or prevent undesirable sexual behaviors, because testosterone is still produced. Therefore it is infrequently used for control of reproduction in male cats. However, "teaser tom cats" (infertile

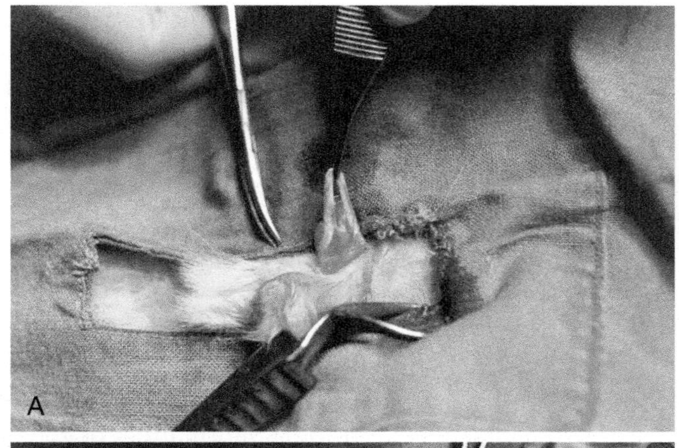

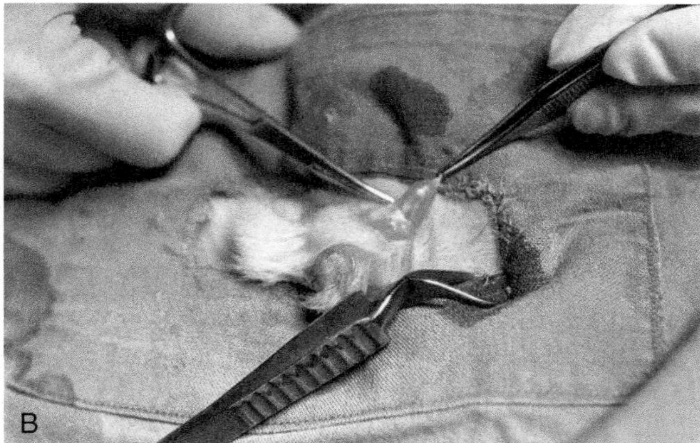

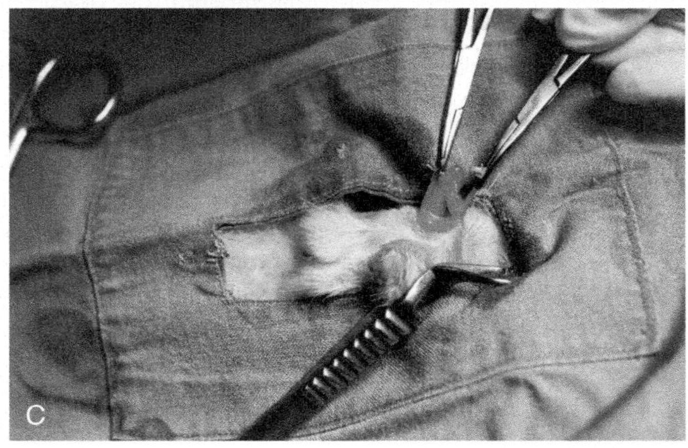

FIGURE 39-4 Vasectomy. **A,** After incision of the skin and subcutaneous tissue, the spermatic cord is identified. **B,** The spermatic cord is exteriorized from the tunica vaginalis using blunt and sharp dissection. **C,** Once the ductus deferens is isolated, a small segment is removed and the severed ends are ligated.

males with good libido) may be used in catteries to bring queens out of heat when pregnancy is not desired. Mating with a teaser tom cat induces a pseudopregnancy in the queen and delays return to estrus. Vasectomy does not alter libido or mating ability in adult tom cats. Live sperm may be present for up to 7 weeks after surgery, however.[30]

Vasectomy is a relatively simple surgical procedure performed through a 1- to 2-cm incision cranial to the scrotum (Figure 39-4).[14] After incision of the skin and subcutaneous tissue, the spermatic cords are identified and exteriorized from the tunica vaginalis using blunt and sharp dissection. Gentle manipulation of the testicle is helpful for identification of the spermatic cord. Once the ductus deferens is isolated, a small segment is removed and the severed ends are ligated. The subcutaneous tissue and skin are closely routinely.

Chemical Castration

An injectable sterilant, zinc gluconate neutralized by arginine (Neutersol, Addison Biological Laboratory, Fayette, Mo.), was licensed for use in puppies (3 to 10 months of age) in the United States from 2003 to 2005 and is currently not available in that country. The product was licensed in Mexico in 2008 (EsterilSol, Ark Sciences, Baltimore, Md.) for use in dogs. A product with the same active ingredient, but at a different concentration and with dimethylsulfoxide (DMSO) as a carrier, was licensed in Brazil in 2009 (Infertile; Rhobifarma, Hortolândia, Brazil), also for use in dogs. The intratesticular injection causes sclerosis of the testes and permanent sterility. In one study comparing intratesticular injection of zinc gluconate with surgical castration in dogs, the product was judged to be valuable for large-scale use, particularly in remote locations or where facilities and expertise for surgical castration are not available.[21] Necrotizing injection site reactions were reported in 4 of 103 treated dogs. Neutersol is reported to be effective in cats, but has not yet been licensed in this species.[19] In one study, 115 cats were injected with EsterilSol (0.3 to 0.4 mL/testis, under sedation) at 6 months of age.[20] Cats were monitored for 12 months, and testicular atrophy, reduced testosterone levels, and absence of sperm were documented.

DISEASES AND CONDITIONS OF THE PENIS

Few problems affect the penis of cats; conditions found more commonly in other species, such as hypospadias and persistent penile frenulum, are rare in the cat. One case report of hypospadias in a 1-year-old Himalayan cat was associated with chronic cystitis.[17] The hypospadias was surgically corrected and the cat recovered fully. A 1-year-old Persian cat presented for infertility was found to have dorsal deviation of the penis resulting from a persistent frenulum.[1]

A small number of cases of phimosis have been reported in the cat.[4,10,22] Phimosis is due to constriction of the preputial opening that prevents protrusion of the penis. Phimosis may be congenital or acquired secondary to trauma, inflammation, or neoplasia. The most common clinical signs are stranguria, pollakiuria, and vocalizing during urination[22]; other clinical signs include dribbling urine, urinating outside the litter box, and inability to mate. The severity of clinical signs varies with the degree of narrowing. Diagnosis is made on physical examination. In many cases, surgical correction of the defect is necessary.

The records of 10 cats diagnosed with phimosis at Michigan State University Veterinary Teaching Hospital have been reviewed.[22] The mean age at presentation was 18.6 weeks (range, 8 weeks to 2.4 years). Two of the cats had other congenital defects (cryptorchidism, penile hypoplasia). Eight of the 10 cats underwent surgical correction of the condition by a full thickness incision in the ventral aspect of the prepuce, with or without resection of a wedge of prepuce. A satisfactory outcome was achieved in seven cats, where long-term follow-up was available. Congenital phimosis has been reported in an 8-week-old domestic shorthair cat presented for hematuria, pollakiuria, and polydipsia.[4] Urine culture was positive for *E. coli*. Surgical correction of the phimosis was accomplished by resection of a small wedge of the dorsal prepuce, and along with antibiotic treatment, led to resolution of clinical signs.

Priapism is persistent abnormal erection of the penis in the absence of sexual stimulation, and may be caused by a variety of factors, such as spinal cord injury, trauma, neoplasia, and inflammation. It is rarely reported in the cat. Priapism may be confused with paraphimosis; however, paraphimosis is associated with a narrow preputial orifice or other preputial abnormalities. Without intervention, the penis may become dry and edematous, and even necrotic. Most cases in the cat require surgical management. In a series of seven cases of priapism, six cases were in Siamese cats.[11] In four of the cases, priapism developed after unsuccessful attempts at mating, despite the fact that three of the cats were castrated. Five of the cats were successfully treated with perineal urethrostomy, and histologic examination revealed thrombosis of the corpus cavernosum.

Priapism was reported in a 1.5-year-old domestic shorthair cat after routine castration.[36] Two days after surgery, the cat developed pollakiuria and stranguria, as well as protrusion of the penis. The cat was successfully treated with perineal urethrostomy. Histology of the resected tissue revealed severe congestion of the corpus cavernosum, with organized thrombi and areas of necrosis. Another case of priapism was reported in a 2-year-old castrated cat with feline infectious peritonitis (FIP).[31a] At necropsy histologic examination of the penis revealed severe pyogranulomatous inflammation and fibrinoid necrosis of the corpus cavernosum.

DISEASES AND CONDITIONS OF THE TESTES

Few conditions of the testes of the cat come to the attention of clinicians, with the exception of cryptorchidism. Other problems that are occasionally encountered include orchitis, neoplasia, and abnormalities of gonadal sex or chromosomal sex.

Orchitis is rare in the cat, although occasionally bacterial orchitis has been reported. Clinical signs include scrotal swelling, pain, and redness. Bacterial orchitis is treated with a broad-spectrum antibiotic for 2 to 3 weeks. Orchitis has also been reported as an uncommon manifestation of FIP[8]; one case report was a cat concurrently infected with FIV.[34] Scrotal swelling may be the only sign associated with FIP in affected cats, at least initially (see Figure 33-16). The vaginal cavity around each testis is confluent with the peritoneal cavity so that fluid accumulated in the abdomen may also appear in the scrotum. Lesions in the testes are consistent with a chronic necrotic and fibrinous orchitis and fibrinous periorchitis with vasculitis.

Testicular neoplasia is uncommon in the cat. Examples of both Sertoli and interstitial cell tumors have been reported.[2,26,29,38] Neoplasia of testicular origin developing after castration has been reported in five cats.[6] All cases involved interstitial cell tumors within the scrotal skin or the spermatic cord. All cats were castrated at 1 year of age or younger, and the mean age at diagnosis of the neoplasia was 9.6 years. Affected cats demonstrated sexual behaviors associated with intact males, such as urine spraying and aggression. Two cats had penile spines. The study authors suggest that care be taken during castration to avoid incising the tunica albuginea to avoid transplantation of small amounts of testicular tissue, and the subsequent development of tumors.

Testicular hypoplasia and infertility may be seen in male tortoiseshell or calico cats. It has been estimated that about 1 in every 3,000 tortoiseshell or calico cats is male.[15] A survey of over 4,500 male cats in the United Kingdom determined that 0.43% were tortoiseshell.[18] Orange is a sex-limited coat color in cats, controlled by a single gene on the X chromosome. Black and orange color may occur together in the female, but normally would not occur together in the male. Males exhibiting black and orange coat color may have various chromosomal abnormalities, such as 39/XXY, mosaicism (two populations of cells with different genotypes from one fertilized egg), or chimerism (two or more populations

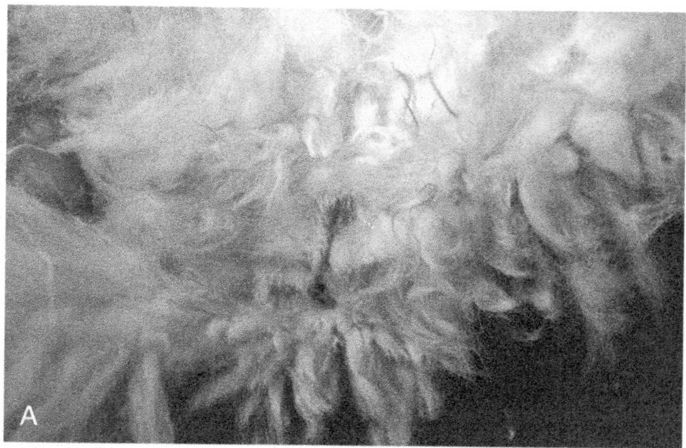

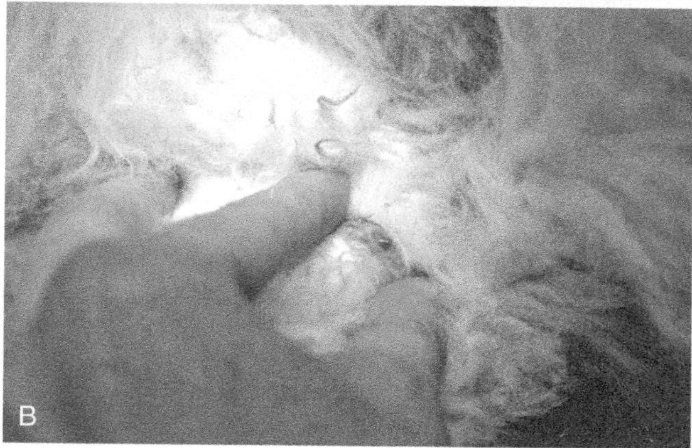

FIGURE 39-5 **A,** External genitalia of an intersex cat presented for ovariohysterectomy that was subsequently found to have one testis next to the vulva. **B,** A small penis-like structure was present in the vulva, and one testis was found subcutaneously near the vulva.

of cells from the fusion of different embryos). Mosaics or chimeras are often fertile.

Both true hermaphroditism and pseudohermaphroditism are very uncommon in the cat. Many cases are unreported, because karyotyping is not widely available for cats. Affected individuals may be discovered at the time of surgical sterilization. For example, the author has examined a blue tabby intersex cat (Figure 39-5). The cat was presented as a female and was spayed without incident. Several months later, the owners complained of a strong smell to the urine, and on examination, a small penis-like structure was present in the vulva and one testis was found subcutaneously near the vulva. The cat's specific condition was not determined, because karyotyping and gonadal histopathology was not performed.

Cryptorchidism

The testes are normally descended into the scrotum by birth or shortly afterward. However, testes may move freely up and down in the inguinal canal prior to puberty. Cryptorchidism is failure of one or both testes to descend into the scrotum and remain there by 7 to 8 months of age. It is the most common congenital defect of the feline urogenital system. The term "monorchid" refers to total absence of one testis. Unilateral testicular agenesis has been reported, with the finding of a rudimentary spermatic cord and no associated testis.[31] The term "anorchid" refers to total absence of both testes (an exceedingly rare event). It is uncertain if cryptorchidism is linked with other congenital defects in cats.

TABLE 39-1 **Data from 4,140 Cats Presented for Castration during a 10-Year Period in Ottawa, Canada**

	No. Presented for Castration	No. Cryptorchid (%)
ALL CATS	4,140	72 (1.7)
BREEDS WITH AT LEAST 10 CATS		
Abyssinian/Somali	15	1 (6.7)
Balinese	10	0
British Shorthair	19	0
Burmese	19	2 (10.5)
Maine Coon	16	2 (12.5)
Persian/Himalayan	135	14 (10.4)
Ragdoll	16	3 (18.75)
Siamese	158	4 (2.5)

The prevalence of cryptorchidism in cats has been reported as 1.3% to 3.8%.[28,31,42] In one study of more than 100,000 feral cats admitted to trap-neuter-return programs, 1.3% of male cats were cryptorchid.[41] In another study of more than 5,000 free-roaming cats admitted to a trap-neuter-return program, 1.9% of the males were cryptorchid.[33] Persian cats are overrepresented in some studies.[28,31] In the author's practice, records of 4,140 cats presented for castration during a 10-year period were reviewed (Table 39-1). Seventy-two cats (1.7%) were identified as cryptorchid. Three cats were identified as monorchid. Of the cats presented for castration, 10.5% were of a pedigreed breed, with a total of 22 breeds represented. Among the pedigreed cats, 6.2% were identified as cryptorchid. The highest incidence was in the Ragdoll breed (>18%).

Cryptorchidism is typically unilateral, with left and right sides equally affected. In one study where the location of the retained testis was recorded, 49% were inguinal, 33% were abdominal, and 14% were within the inguinal ring.[31] In the author's practice, 87% of 72 cats had unilateral cryptorchidism, and the most common configuration was the unilateral, inguinal cryptorchid (51.6% of cases) (Table 39-2). Cats with bilateral cryptorchidism are likely to have abdominally retained testes. If one testis is in the scrotum, it may be difficult to determine if it is on the left or right side. Pushing the scrotal

TABLE 39-2 Location of 124 Testes in 62 Cryptorchid Cats Presented for Castration during a 10-Year Period in Ottawa, Canada

	Abdominal	Inguinal	Inguinal Ring	Scrotal
Right side	11	21	4	26
Left side	11	16	6	29
Totals	22 (17.7%)	37 (29.8%)	10 (8%)	55 (44.3%)

testis dorsally and cranially toward the inguinal canal can help determine its location.[3] It may be difficult to palpate inguinal testes if the cat has large inguinal fat pads, unless the testis is located caudal to the fat pad. The inguinal lymph node and fat pad are commonly confused with inguinal testes on palpation.

Abdominally retained testes have been examined histologically, and typically, no spermatozoa are found. The higher temperature inside the body probably suppresses development of sperm. Cats with retained testes located outside the abdomen, however, may be fertile. Cryptorchid testes produce testosterone; so, affected cats have the typical male phenotype (e.g., thick skin on neck and shoulders, broad face) and behaviors (e.g., libido, aggression, urine marking).

In one study, only 22% of cat owners were aware their pet was cryptorchid.[42] All male cats should be examined for cryptorchidism during initial wellness visits. If a retained testis is suspected, there are two ways to confirm the condition. The simplest is to check for testosterone-dependent penile spines. Gonadotropin stimulation testing has also been used to detect retained testes. Testosterone levels fluctuate in the cat; so, resting samples are not very informative and provocative testing must be used. Various protocols have been described (Box 39-1).

The mode of inheritance for cryptorchidism is suggested to be recessive in cats, as in other species, and cryptorchid males should not be used for breeding.[31] Cryptorchidism is an example of a sex-limited trait. The trait is physically expressed only in the male even though it can be carried by females. Both the sire and dam of an affected cat should be considered to be carriers of the trait. Some full siblings of an affected cat will also be carriers. A reduction in the number of cryptorchid cats in a pedigreed breeding program can be achieved by removing affected males and carrier parents from breeding. If the problem is widespread in a family line, full siblings of an affected cat should also be eliminated from the breeding program.

There is no treatment proven to cause a retained testis to descend into the scrotum. Treatment with gonadotropins has not been successful. In other species, surgical removal of the retained testis is routinely recommended, because the retained testis is at risk for neoplasia or torsion. Torsion of the spermatic cord has not been documented in the cat, and only a few case reports of testicular tumors have been published. Cryptorchid cats that have only the scrotal testis removed will display all the normal behaviors of an intact male. Most studies report cryptorchid cats that have had the scrotal testis removed, with unsuccessful attempts to locate the undescended testis. Owners subsequently seek veterinary care because of odoriferous urine and unwanted behaviors (e.g., urine spraying, aggression, seeking females). Therefore it is important that both testes be removed to avoid unwanted behaviors that may provoke abandonment or relinquishment to a shelter.

Testes that are palpable in the inguinal subcutaneous tissue can be removed through a simple incision. In other cases, a caudal midline incision and dissection deep to the inguinal fat pad is required. The external inguinal ring should be examined, but care should be taken not to damage structures in the femoral triangle. For abdominally retained testes, laparotomy through a midline approach is required, although laparoscopic-assisted cryptorchidectomy has also been described.[23,27,40] Advantages of a laparoscopic technique include minimal invasiveness, reduced tissue trauma, and potentially reduced postoperative pain and fewer complications than laparotomy. The principle disadvantage is the need for specialized equipment with the associated costs and expertise required. Initially, the laparoscopic approach may take longer to perform than a traditional laparotomy until the practitioner gains experience with the technique.

Surgical techniques for removal of abdominal testes have been described elsewhere.[3] Use of a spay hook to retrieve the vas deferens is not recommended because of the risk of damage to the ureters.[31] Abdominal testes are often near the bladder (Figure 39-6) but can be located caudal to the kidney, in the internal inguinal ring or in

BOX 39-1

Hormonal Methods for Diagnosis of Cryptorchidism in the Cat

After collection of a baseline serum testosterone sample:

1. Administer 25 μg gonadotropin-releasing hormone (GnRH) (Cystorelin; Merial, Duluth, Ga.), IM; take second serum testosterone sample 1 hour later[15]
2. Administer 250 IU human chorionic gonadotropin (HCG), IM; take second serum testosterone sample 4 hours later[15]
3. Administer 500 IU HCG, IV; take second serum testosterone sample 2 hours later[24]

Resting testosterone levels in intact male cats are usually less than 3.0 ng/mL, although considerable variation occurs. Provocative testing will induce a marked elevation of serum testosterone in the cryptorchid male.

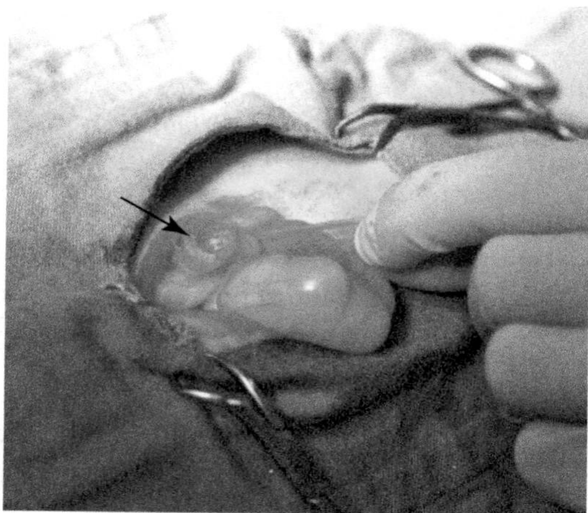

FIGURE 39-6 The testes *(arrow)* in cats with abdominal cryptorchidism are often found near the bladder.

the inguinal canal.[31] The best procedure is to find the vas deferens and follow it caudally to the testis. Applying gentle traction to the vas deferens may facilitate location of the testis by detecting its movement. Although it can be frustrating to locate the retained testis in some cases, it is not appropriate to simply ligate the vas deferens and testicular vessels in the hope the testis will atrophy. It is possible for the blood supply to re-establish and for the testis to remain functional.

INFERTILITY

Causes of infertility are not well studied in the tom cat, partly because of the difficulty in obtaining semen for analysis compared with other species, such as the dog. Regardless, a systematic approach can be taken when the clinician is presented with a potentially infertile tom cat. A thorough evaluation of the queens involved must also be performed (see Chapter 40). Breeders should be encouraged to keep complete records on each breeding male in a cattery (Box 39-2).

Owners of breeding cats may request administration of antimicrobials to prevent transmission of bacterial infections from the queen to the tom cat and vice versa, especially if cases of infertility have occurred in the cattery. However, both the vagina of the queen and the preputial mucosa of the male have normal resident bacterial populations. In one study, bacterial cultures from the preputial mucosa of 29 tom cats (age range, 0.5 to 2.5 years) were all positive for both aerobic and anaerobic bacterial species.[35] The most common aerobic bacteria were *Pasteurella multocida*, unidentified gram-negative rods, and *E. coli*. The most common anaerobic bacteria were *Bacteroides* spp., *Fusobacterium* spp., and *Streptococcus* spp. The type of bacterial populations found in queens differed from that found in the tom cats, suggesting that mating does not lead to a permanent transfer of bacteria. These bacterial populations may play a role in host defense against pathogenic bacteria. Therefore treatment of normal queens or tom cats with antimicrobials may affect the protective bacterial flora and actually increase the risk of infection with pathogenic bacteria.

Successful breeding tom cats must be physically, socially, and sexually mature. Ideally, a young inexperienced tom cat should be paired with a calm, mature, and experienced queen. Tom cats are very territorial, and breeding is most successful if the tom cat is in his home environment and the queen is brought to him. Breeding problems in the tom cat are associated with a wide variety of factors (Box 39-3).

BOX 39-2
Reproductive Data Collection for Breeding Tom Cats

1. Age at puberty
2. Details about libido: interest in estrous queens, willingness to breed
3. Details for each mating
   a. Dates of breeding
   b. Number of copulations
   c. Problems during breeding, for instance, prolonged thrusting, failure to elicit postcoital reaction in queen
   d. Age and parity of each queen bred
   e. Outcome of breeding: pregnancy or date of queen's return to estrus
4. Details of each litter: date born, litter size, sexes, birth weights, stillbirths, congenital defects (if present), illnesses, necropsy findings, and so forth

BOX 39-3
Causes of Breeding Problems in Tom Cats

1. Inexperience or immaturity
2. Nervousness or anxiety
3. New environment or changes to existing environment
4. Inadequate housing
5. Improper breeding management
6. Malpositioning during copulation
7. Medical conditions, both reproductive and nonreproductive
8. Hair rings around the shaft of penis preventing intromission
9. Poor libido
10. Stressors (e.g., showing, travel, social conflicts)

BOX 39-4

Investigation of Infertility in the Tom Cat

1. Normal libido?

If Yes

Investigate breeding management
Investigate queen's fertility
If possible, perform semen evaluation

If No

Ensure queen is in estrus
Investigate behavior problems in tom cat (e.g., shyness, nervousness)
Evaluate general health of tom cat for reproductive and nonreproductive problems
Consider effect of age on libido

2. Normal mating ability?

If Yes

Same as above

If No

Investigate orthopedic or neurologic problems
Check penis for hair ring or other abnormalities that prevent intromission

The first step in investigation of infertility in the tom cat is collection of the reproductive history and a thorough physical examination. Various reproductive disorders causing infertility have been described in the tom cat, such as testicular hypoplasia and persistent penile frenulum.[1] Nonreproductive disease, such as oral cavity disease or degenerative joint disease, may influence willingness or ability to mate. Chronic illness, such as upper respiratory tract infection or diarrhea, may lead to poor body condition and diminished libido. Particular attention should be paid to examination of the penis (position, size, ability to extrude from the prepuce, presence of spines) and testes (size, symmetry, consistency). Ultrasonography may be a useful tool for investigation of testicular abnormalities, although it is performed less frequently in the tom cat than in the male dog.[5] Collection of a minimum database (complete blood count [CBC], serum chemistries, complete urinalysis, feline leukemia virus [FeLV] and FIV testing) is recommended. Information should also be obtained on the cat's housing, diet (including nutritional supplements), and medications (both prescription and nonprescription).

Whether or not the cat has a normal libido determines the next diagnostic steps (Box 39-4). In late-maturing breeds, libido cannot be assessed properly until about 3 years of age. Poor libido is often caused by management problems or underlying medical conditions. The tom cat's environment is very important for breeding success. In pedigreed catteries, tom cats are often housed in cages or enclosures because of urine marking behavior. Tom cats often dislike changes to their territory, even changes in odor, such as when scented cleaners are used. The enclosure for a breeding tom cat must provide enough space to allow for normal exercise. Cats value vertical space; so, provision of areas to climb or shelving is very important. It also provides a way for the tom cat to retreat from the postcoital reaction of the queen to avoid being swatted. Inadequate housing may inhibit the breeding behavior of normal tom cats. For more on breeding management, see Chapter 40. Measurement of baseline testosterone in tom cats with poor libido is not informative; provocative testing must be used, as discussed above in diagnosis of cryptorchidism. Administration of supplemental testosterone in an attempt to correct poor libido is ineffective and inappropriate. Exogenous testosterone may suppress release of GnRH and LH, thereby interrupting testosterone synthesis by the interstitial cells of the testes.

If the male has normal libido, the breeder should attempt to witness matings (either in person or by video camera/web camera) to ensure that normal events are taking place. For example, if no postcoital reaction is seen from the queen, intromission was likely unsuccessful. If prolonged pelvic thrusting occurs in long-haired cats, the base of the penis should be checked for a ring of hair. Observing the breeding pair will also help determine if the tom cat is shy or inhibited, especially by an aggressive queen.

Semen evaluation may be a valuable diagnostic tool for tom cats with normal libido, where other causes of infertility have been ruled out. Semen collection can be performed either by electroejaculation under general anesthesia or by training the tom cat to an artificial vagina; both techniques were first reported in the 1970s and are well described in the literature.[43] Electroejaculation requires specialized equipment that is not widely available, as well as expertise in the technique. Training a tom cat to an artificial vagina is time consuming, requires a "teaser" queen, and will not be successful in all cases. In addition, few clinicians have experience examining semen in cats. These barriers make semen evaluation in the tom cat an uncommon procedure in general clinical practice.

Recently, a novel technique for semen collection in the cat that may be useful in clinical practice has been described.[7,44] In this technique, the tom cat is sedated with medetomidine alone (130 to 140 μg/kg, IM) or medetomidine (100 μg/kg IM) plus ketamine (5 mg/kg, IM). Alpha$_2$-adrenergic agonists are known to stimulate erection and ejaculation in other species. A 3-Fr tom cat catheter is modified by cutting off about 1 cm of the tip with a scalpel blade. The catheter is inserted into the urethra once, to a distance of approximately 9 cm (to the level of the prostatic urethra), and is then withdrawn to collect released semen. It is important to avoid entering the bladder with the catheter so that inadvertent collection of urine does not occur. After collection, the semen is placed in a warmed Eppendorf tube and diluted with semen extender or in vitro fertilization (IVF) medium.

Collected semen should be evaluated macroscopically (appearance, volume) and microscopically (motility, morphology, concentration, viability). Eosin-nigrosin stain can be used to differentiate live and dead spermatozoa. Characteristics of normal cat semen collected by the various techniques have been reported.[7,16,43,44] The volume of semen collected ranges from approximately 30 to 100 μL (collection through artificial vagina) to 200 to 300 μL (collection by electroejaculation). Semen samples collected by urethra catheterization after administration of medetomidine are too small in volume (about 10 μL) and too concentrated to allow evaluation of sperm motility and morphology as is, and so the sample must be diluted before analysis.[44] A variety of morphologic defects have been described for cat sperm. Normal cat semen has less than 30% morphologically abnormal sperm.[43] Teratospermia is characterized by greater than 60% abnormal sperm forms and is associated with decreased genetic variation and low circulating testosterone concentrations.[43] The small volumes of semen collected from cats are challenging to handle and analyze, especially if the clinician performs the procedure infrequently.

When it is not possible to collect a semen sample, vaginal lavage with 1 mL sterile saline of a queen immediately after breeding may allow determination of whether sperm are present. Because a degree of retrograde ejaculation is normal in the tom cat, collection of a urine sample after ejaculation also allows for detection of sperm (see Figure 39-2). Sperm motility and morphology cannot be examined in samples collected from the bladder or by vaginal flush.

References

1. Axner E, Strom B, Linde-Forsberg C et al: Reproductive disorders in 10 domestic male cats, *J Small Anim Pract* 37:394, 1996.
2. Benazzi C, Sarli G, Brunetti B: Sertoli cell tumour in a cat, *J Vet Med A Physiol Pathol Clin Med* 51:124, 2004.
3. Birchard SJ, Nappier M: Cryptorchidism, *Comp Contin Edu Pract* 30:325, 2008.
4. Bright SR, Mellanby RJ: Congenital phimosis in a cat, *J Feline Med Surg* 6:367, 2004.
5. Davidson AP, Baker TW: Reproductive ultrasound of the dog and tom, *Top Companion Anim Med* 24:64, 2009.
6. Doxsee AL, Yager JA, Best SJ et al: Extratesticular interstitial and Sertoli cell tumors in previously neutered dogs and cats: a report of 17 cases, *Can Vet J* 47:763, 2006.
7. Filliers M, Rijsselaere T, Bossaert P et al: In vitro evaluation of fresh sperm quality in tomcats: a comparison of two collection techniques, *Theriogenology* 74:31, 2010.
8. Foster RA, Caswell JL, Rinkardt N: Chronic fibrinous and necrotic orchitis in a cat, *Can Vet J* 37:681, 1996.
9. Franca L, Godinho C: Testis morphology, seminiferous epithelium cycle length, and daily sperm production in domestic cats *(Felis catus)*, *Biol Reprod* 68:1554, 2002.
10. Ghantous SN, Crawford J: Double ureters with ureteral ectopia in a domestic shorthair cat, *J Am Anim Hosp Assoc* 42:462, 2006.
11. Gunn-Moore DA, Brown PJ, Holt PE et al: Priapism in seven cats, *J Small Anim Pract* 36:262, 1995.
12. Hart BL, Barrett RE: Effects of castration on fighting, roaming, and urine spraying in adult male cats, *J Am Vet Med Assoc* 163:290, 1973.
13. Hart BL, Cooper L: Factors relating to urine spraying and fighting in prepubertally gonadectomized cats, *J Am Vet Med Assoc* 184:1255, 1984.
14. Howe LM: Surgical methods of contraception and sterilization, *Theriogenology* 66:500, 2006.
15. Johnston S, Root Kustritz M, Olson P: Disorders of the feline testes and epididymides. In Johnston S, Root Kustritz M,Olson P, editors: *Canine and feline theriogenology*, Philadelphia, 2001, Saunders, p 525.
16. Johnston S, Root Kustritz M, Olson P: Semen collection and evaluation in the cat. In Johnston S, Root Kustritz M, Olson P, editors: *Canine and feline theriogenology*, Philadelphia, 2001, Saunders, p 508.
17. King GJ, Johnson EH: Hypospadias in a Himalayan cat, *J Small Anim Pract* 41:508, 2000.
18. Leaman T, Rowland R, Long S: Male tortoiseshell cats in the United Kingdom, *Vet Rec* 144:9, 1999.
19. Levy J: Non-surgical methods of sterilization: what's new? *World Small Animal Veterinary Association Congress* Sao Paulo, Brazil, 2009.
20. Levy J: Overview of current contraceptive approaches for feral cats. *4th International Symposium on Non-Surgical Contraceptive Methods of Pet Population Control* Dallas, Tex, 2010.
21. Levy JK, Crawford PC, Appel LD et al: Comparison of intratesticular injection of zinc gluconate versus surgical castration to sterilize male dogs, *Am J Vet Res* 69:140, 2008.
22. May LR, Hauptman JG: Phimosis in cats: 10 cases (2000-2008), *J Am Anim Hosp Assoc* 45:277, 2009.
23. Mayhew P: Surgical views: laparoscopic and laparoscopic-assisted cryptorchidectomy in dogs and cats, *Compend Contin Educ Vet* 31:274, 2009.
24. Memon MA, Ganjam VK, Pavletic MM et al: Use of human chorionic gonadotropin stimulation test to detect a retained testis in a cat, *J Am Vet Med Assoc* 201:1602, 1992.
25. Millard RP, Pickens EH, Wells KL: Excessive production of sex hormones in a cat with an adrenocortical tumor, *J Am Vet Med Assoc* 234:505, 2009.
26. Miller MA, Hartnett SE, Ramos-Vara JA: Interstitial cell tumor and Sertoli cell tumor in the testis of a cat, *Vet Pathol* 44:394, 2007.
27. Miller NA, Van Lue SJ, Rawlings CA: Use of laparoscopic-assisted cryptorchidectomy in dogs and cats, *J Am Vet Med Assoc* 224:875, 2004.
28. Millis D, Hauptman J, Johnson C: Cryptorchidism and monorchism in cats: 25 cases (1980-1989), *J Am Vet Med Assoc* 200:1128, 1992.
29. Miyoshi N, Yasuda N, Kamimura Y et al: Teratoma in a feline unilateral cryptorchid testis, *Vet Pathol* 38:729, 2001.
30. Pineda MH, Dooley MP: Surgical and chemical vasectomy in the cat, *Am J Vet Res* 45:291, 1984.
31. Richardson E, Mullen H: Cryptorchidism in cats, *Comp Contin Edu Pract Vet* 15:1342, 1993.

31a. Rota A, Paltrinieri S, Jussich S et al: Priapism in a castrated cat associated with feline infectious peritonitis, *J Feline Med Surg* 10:181, 2008.

32. Schwartz S: Use of cyproheptadine to control urine spraying and masturbation in a cat, *J Am Vet Med Assoc* 214:369, 1999.

33. Scott KC, Levy JK, Crawford PC: Characteristics of free-roaming cats evaluated in a trap-neuter-return program, *J Am Vet Med Assoc* 221:1136, 2002.
34. Sigurdardottir OG, Kolbjornsen O, Lutz H: Orchitis in a cat associated with coronavirus infection, *J Comp Pathol* 124:219, 2001.
35. Strom Holst B, Bergstrom A, Lagerstedt AS et al: Characterization of the bacterial population of the genital tract of adult cats, *Am J Vet Res* 64:963, 2003.
36. Swalec KM, Smeak DD: Priapism after castration in a cat, *J Am Vet Med Assoc* 195:963, 1989.
37. Tsutsui T, Kuwabara S, Kuwabara K et al: Development of spermatogenic function in the sex maturation process in male cats, *J Vet Med Sci* 66:1125, 2004.
38. Tucker AR, Smith JR: Prostatic squamous metaplasia in a cat with interstitial cell neoplasia in a retained testis, *Vet Pathol* 45:905, 2008.
39. Tursi M, Costa T, Valenza F et al: Adenocarcinoma of the disseminated prostate in a cat, *J Feline Med Surg* 10:600, 2008.
40. Vannozzi I, Benetti C, Rota A: Laparoscopic cryptorchidectomy in a cat, *J Feline Med Surg* 4:201, 2002.
41. Wallace JL, Levy JK: Population characteristics of feral cats admitted to seven trap-neuter-return programs in the United States, *J Feline Med Surg* 8:279, 2006.
42. Yates D, Hayes G, Heffernan M et al: Incidence of cryptorchidism in dogs and cats, *Vet Rec* 152:502, 2003.
43. Zambelli D, Cunto M: Semen collection in cats: techniques and analysis, *Theriogenology* 66:159, 2006.
44. Zambelli D, Prati F, Cunto M et al: Quality and in vitro fertilizing ability of cryopreserved cat spermatozoa obtained by urethral catheterization after medetomidine administration, *Theriogenology* 69:485, 2008.

CHAPTER

40

Female Reproduction

Susan E. Little

OUTLINE

NORMAL REPRODUCTION

The pedigreed cat fancy has developed and grown in popularity in North America and around the world during the last 100 years. The widespread appeal of pedigreed cats and cat breeding means that veterinarians need to be familiar with the unique characteristics of feline reproduction and breeding management. In the past 25 years, considerable progress has been made in understanding the behavioral, gonadal, and endocrine factors involved in successful feline reproduction.

Seasonality

The cat is described as being seasonally polyestrous and a long-day breeder. Queens undergo estrous cycles repeatedly during a breeding season unless interrupted by pregnancy, pseudopregnancy, or illness. Estrous cycles will occur at variable intervals but most typically every 14 to 21 days. Cats housed indoors, but largely under the influence of seasonal light, will cycle according to the season. The mechanism of photoperiod influence on estrous cycles through the hypothalamic-hypophysial-gonadal axis and the hormone melatonin has been partly elucidated in the cat. A shorter duration of photoperiod is associated with increased concentrations of melatonin and prolactin and reduction in ovarian activity.

In the northern hemisphere, increasing daylight length in January and February promotes the onset of estrous activity. Peak estrous activity is usually seen in the northern hemisphere from February to April. Regular estrous activity will continue until as late as October or November, depending on the geographic distance from the equator (and therefore the length of daylight). Most cats housed indoors in North America will experience winter anestrus because of the short length of daylight. The effect of seasonality diminishes or disappears near the equator.[12]

Queens housed together may have synchronized estrous cycles. Longhair breeds seem to be more sensitive to the amount of daylight than shorthair breeds. Although many longhair queens (such as the Persian breed) will not exhibit regular estrous cycles even during periods of long daylight, many shorthair queens (such as Siamese and related breeds) exhibit estrous cycles year-round, regardless of daylight length. Inadequate intensity or duration of light is an important cause of infrequent estrous cycles in cats housed indoors. Breeding catteries should provide 12 to 14 hours of daylight or artificial light per day to encourage regular estrous cycles.

Puberty

The first estrus typically occurs in queens between 5 and 9 months of age, but age at onset may be highly variable (3.5 to 18 months).[37] The time of the first estrus is influenced by a number of factors: breed (shorthair breeds reach puberty earlier than longhair breeds), season (which determines the length of daylight), and the queen's body condition. Persian and related breeds may not have their first estrus until 18 months of age or older and may not be sexually mature until 2 to 3 years of age. The average body weight at puberty is 5 to 7 lb (2.3 to 3.2 kg) or 80% of adult body weight.[25] Shorthair breeds,

BOX 40-1

Feline Reproduction Data

Length of estrus: Average 5.8 ± 3.3 days
Length of interestrus: Average 7 days, range 2-19 days
Length of pseudopregnancy: 40-50 days
Length of gestation: 66.9 ± 2.9 days (research colony); 65.1 ± 2.2 days (pedigreed)
Pregnancy rate: 73.9% (research colony)
Queening rate: 65.2% (research colony)
Kittens per litter: Average 3.7, range 1-5 (research colony); 4.6 ± 1.7 (pedigreed)
Number of litters/year: Average 2-2.5; range 1-3
Age at puberty—male: 7-18 months
Age at puberty—female: 4-18 months

Data from Feldman E, Nelson R: Feline reproduction. In Feldman E, Nelson R, editors: *Canine and feline endocrinology and reproduction*, ed 3, St Louis, 2004, Saunders, p 1016; Root MV, Johnston SD, Olson PN: Estrous length, pregnancy rate, gestation and parturition lengths, litter size, and juvenile mortality in the domestic cat, *J Am Anim Hosp Assoc* 31:429, 1995; Sparkes AH, Rogers K, Henley WE, et al: A questionnaire-based study of gestation, parturition and neonatal mortality in pedigree breeding cats in the UK, *J Feline Med Surg* 8:145, 2006; Verstegen J: Physiology and endocrinology of reproduction in female cats. In Simpson G, England G, Harvey M, editors: *Manual of small animal reproduction and neonatology*, Cheltenham, UK, 1998, British Small Animal Veterinary Association, p 11.

such as the Siamese and Burmese, are more precocious and may reach puberty at a lower body weight.

The Feline Estrous Cycle

The feline estrous cycle may be divided into proestrus, estrus, interestrus, anestrus, and luteal (diestrus) phases. See Box 40-1 for feline reproduction data. Proestrus is considerably more difficult to detect in the queen than in the bitch. This part of the estrous cycle may last only one day or so, and the signs may be subtle; so, it is often not detected. In proestrus, many queens rub their head and neck against convenient objects and display affectionate behavior. Occasionally, queens in proestrus have a slight mucoid vulvar discharge and pollakiuria. During proestrus, tom cats may be attracted to the queen, but the queen will not be receptive to breeding.

Estrus is defined as behavioral receptivity to mating. This stage may last from as little as 2 days to as long as 19 days, with the average duration being 5.8 ± 3.3 days.[90] Mating may shorten the length of estrus, although conflicting evidence exists. A queen in estrus will crouch with the front legs pressed to the ground, the back in a position of lordosis, and the tail turned to one side to present the vulva (Figure 40-1). The queen may roll or thrash about on the floor. Queens in estrus often call or vocalize to attract the attention of males. They may be restless, have a poor appetite, and show increased affection to their caretakers. It is not uncommon for

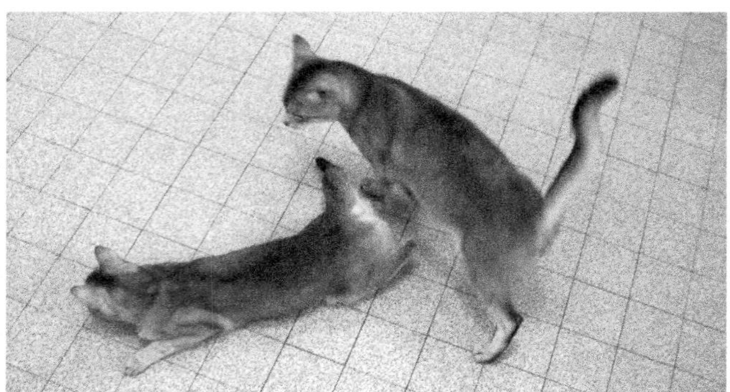

FIGURE 40-1 During estrus, the queen assumes a characteristic body posture of lordosis, with the body positioned low to the ground and the tail turned to one side. *(Courtesy Elise Malandain.)*

inexperienced owners to interpret estrus behavior as a sign of injury or illness.

Occasionally, queens have prolonged estrus (lasting more than 7 days). In some cases, this may be due to the maturation of overlapping waves of follicles with prolonged high estradiol levels.[25] This type of prolonged estrus is most commonly seen in Siamese and related breeds. Other queens with prolonged behavioral estrus, however, have normal distinct patterns of follicular growth.[25] Why these queens show prolonged estrus rather than distinct estrus periods is not understood.

Prolonged estrus can also be associated with cystic ovarian follicles. Functional cystic follicles can produce persistent increases in plasma estradiol levels (>20 pg/mL [>73.4 pmol/L]).[25] Cystic ovarian structures may be identified with abdominal ultrasonography. Another infrequent variation is the split heat, most often associated with young queens. The proestrus signs occur but then subside, only to be followed a few days later by a normal proestrus and estrus. This phenomenon tends to disappear with maturity.

The period between one estrus and the next in queens that have not ovulated is the interestrus. During this time, the plasma estradiol level is low (<15 pg/mL [<55.1 pmol/L]) and no sexual behaviors are seen. The duration of interestrus can range from 2 to 19 days but on average is 7 days.

Anestrus is the absence of cycling activity that may occur naturally in periods of short daylight. In the northern hemisphere, this is between October and December. The effect of season on duration of anestrus diminishes with proximity to the equator.[12] Individual variation is common. During this time, progesterone and estrogen are at baseline concentrations (progesterone <1 ng/mL [<3.2 nmol/L], estrogen 8 to 12 pg/mL [29.4 to 44.0 pmol/L]).[53]

The luteal (diestrus) phase of the queen's estrous cycle is the period after ovulation when the dominant hormone is progesterone. Unlike the bitch, the queen does not experience a pre-ovulatory rise in progesterone. After ovulation, fertilization of oocytes occurs in the oviducts, and the embryos enter a uterine horn 4 to 5 days after ovulation.[101] The embryos then space out along the uterine horns and may even migrate from one horn to another before implantation. Some embryos may be lost in this process. Implantation occurs about 12 to 13 days after breeding, and the implantation rate is estimated to be about 84%.[106] The feline placenta is endotheliochorial in structure and zonary in shape. Pregnancy length varies from 62 to 74 days in queens, with the average length being 65 to 67 days.[90,97]

If the oocytes are not fertilized after ovulation, a pseudopregnancy will occur that lasts about 40 to 50 days. Pseudopregnancy may also result if early embryonic loss occurs. Pseudopregnancy in cats is not usually associated with maternal behaviors or lactation.

Estrus may resume about 10 days after the end of the luteal phase, but nursing queens often experience a lactational anestrus that can last for up to 8 weeks after weaning. Most queens will return to estrus about 4 weeks after weaning their kittens if it is still the breeding season. However, it is entirely possible for a queen to return to estrus while still nursing. Very often the first estrus after a pregnancy is shorter and less fertile. Estrus behavior during gestation has also been reported in the queen, although serum estradiol is not increased and no luteinizing hormone (LH) surge occurs, even if the queen allows copulation.[37,107] Superfetation—kittens of different gestational ages in one litter—has never been proven to occur in the cat. The presence of poorly developed fetuses along with kittens of normal gestational age in a litter is most likely a problem of arrested development.

Hormonal Events of Estrus and Pregnancy

Although little data about follicle stimulating hormone (FSH) concentrations or activity in the queen exist, it is believed to be similar to that in other species. FSH, produced by the pituitary gland, initiates the development of ovarian follicles. Three to seven follicles develop and start producing estradiol-17β. As the follicular activity peaks, plasma estradiol levels increase and also vary widely but usually are greater than 20 pg/mL (greater than 73.4 pmol/L).[32] Estradiol levels stay high for 3 or 4 days during estrus and then abruptly fall. The high estradiol levels produce two important effects: overt estrous behavior and priming of the gonadotropin surge necessary to cause ovulation. Estradiol concentrations rise again about day 58 of gestation and then decline just before parturition.[55]

Ovulation requires the release of luteinizing hormone from the anterior pituitary gland. During intromission, the penis probably causes distention of the posterior vagina[115] and induces release of gonadotropin-releasing hormone (GnRH) from the medioventral hypothalamus resulting from neuroendocrine reflexes. Sufficient stimulus, either copulatory or noncopulatory, is required to provoke the release of GnRH. A surge of LH occurs within minutes of breeding. With multiple copulations, the LH surge is higher in amplitude and lasts longer than when only one breeding occurs, thus increasing the chances that ovulation will occur.

Several days of estradiol priming are required before LH release sufficient to cause ovulation occurs. This is typically reached by the third or fourth day of estrus. There also appears to be a stimulus threshold individual to each queen that must be exceeded in order for adequate LH release to occur. Unlike the rabbit, in which a single mating is sufficient to induce ovulation, queens vary considerably in the number of copulations required to induce sufficient LH release and ovulation. Most queens will ovulate after four or more copulations.[25]

Ovulation occurs 48 hours or more following the LH surge.[95] All oocytes are released at the same time. The remaining granulosa cells of the ovarian follicles undergo luteinization and begin to produce progesterone almost immediately. Progesterone concentrations rise within 24 hours, and may reach highs of 60 to 90 ng/mL (190.8 to 286.2 nmol/L) by 15 to 25 days post-ovulation.[113] Peak progesterone concentrations are highly variable from queen to queen. Throughout pregnancy, progesterone is maintained at high concentrations until the last few days of gestation, when the level falls to about 2 ng/mL (6.4 nmol/L) and to less than 1 ng/mL (3.2 nmol/L) immediately following parturition.[113] A minimum progesterone concentration of 1 ng/mL (3.2 nmol/L) appears to be necessary to sustain pregnancy in the queen.[109] Although progesterone declines at term, baseline concentrations are not required for onset of parturition in the queen, as in the bitch.[55] Progesterone test kits designed for ovulation timing in the bitch have been validated for use in the queen.[6]

As for other induced ovulators, recent research suggests the corpus luteum (CL) may be the primary source of progesterone throughout pregnancy in the cat.[113] Conflicting evidence from earlier research showed maintenance of pregnancy despite ovariectomy at 45 to 50 days of gestation and demonstrated the ability of the feline placenta to synthesize progesterone.

Two other hormones are important in feline pregnancy. Relaxin is produced primarily by the placenta in carnivores, and facilitates delivery by softening the connective tissue of the pelvis, softening the cervix and relaxing uterine musculature. Relaxin concentrations increase as early as day 20 of gestation and are the basis of a commercially available pregnancy test (see below).[107] Prolactin is produced by the anterior pituitary and has various effects, including regulation of lactation. Prolactin concentrations increase from about day 35 of gestation, plateau at about day 50, and then increase abruptly just before parturition.[107] Prolactin appears to be necessary for maintenance of pregnancy by supporting the CL, as the suppression of prolactin with a dopamine agonist results in abortion.

Pseudopregnancy may result if a mating is infertile. High progesterone concentrations are maintained by a centrally mediated blockage of GnRH secretion during both pregnancy and pseudopregnancy.[109] This prevents the queen from returning to estrus until the luteal phase is ended. During pseudopregnancy, progesterone concentrations start to decline by about day 25 to 30 and are less than 1 to 2 ng/mL (<3.2 to 6.4 nmol/L) by day 40 to 50.[113] The feline CL may be preprogrammed to atrophy after 25 to 30 days unless luteotrophic factors are present. These luteotrophic factors may originate from the fetoplacental unit and/or from the pituitary. The two most likely luteotrophic factors in the queen are relaxin and prolactin.[109]

Spontaneous Ovulation

Traditionally, queens are described as reflex-mediated induced ovulators. Ovulation should not occur unless mating or a similar stimulus induces it. However, reports of ovulation without breeding are found in the veterinary literature. Pyometra and mucometra are not uncommon in middle-aged intact virgin queens. Recent studies have found more evidence that spontaneous ovulation not only occurs in cats but occurs with some frequency.

A study of 44 female cats with uterine disease classified them on the basis of ovarian status (active or cystic follicles versus luteal phase ovaries).[65] Of the 44 queens, 35 had no recent exposure to male cats. However, 20 of these 35 queens had luteal phase ovaries, established by histologic examination. In another study, 20 domestic shorthair queens ranging from 2.5 to 11 years old were evaluated.[66] These cats were housed individually, but they could see and hear other cats, including males. Seven of the 20 queens had evidence for spontaneous ovulation, and some queens experienced it repeatedly in the study period. Spontaneous ovulation was most prevalent in older queens (although the study group had a preponderance of older queens, mean age 7.4 years), and it may be that these queens have altered hormonal function.

A study designed to approximate conditions in multicat homes and catteries group housed 15 female cats.[41] The queens were all young and nulliparous. After 3 months, a male cat was housed in the same room but caged separately so that there was no physical contact with the queens. Of the 15 queens, 87% showed evidence of at least one instance of ovulation and pseudopregnancy without mating during the 4.5 months of the study. As well, 67% of the queens had evidence of spontaneous ovulation during the 3 months before the male cat entered the room.

These studies indicate that noncopulatory ovulation may be possible in response to a variety of tactile, visual, auditory, or olfactory cues in queens. Unrecognized spontaneous ovulation and subsequent pseudopregnancy is one important cause for infrequent estrous cycles that must be ruled out in cases of apparent infertility. It is more appropriate to consider the queen to be both an induced and spontaneous ovulator, particularly when investigating cases of infertility or pyometra in a breeding cattery.

Fertility and Breeding Management

The ancient Egyptian goddess of fertility, Bastet, was portrayed as a cat for good reason. Queens are most fertile between the ages of about 18 months to 8 years, although examples of successful production of kittens in aged queens have been reported.[37] Queens more than 8 years of age tend to have more irregular estrous cycles, smaller litters, and more spontaneous abortions and kittens with congenital defects.

The average litter size ranges from 3.7 to 4.6 kittens, but there is wide variability, especially among pedigreed cat breeds.[90,97,106] Given a breeding life of about 10 years and no human interference with breeding, a queen can easily bear up to 100 kittens in a lifetime.[37] Queens are not monogamous and may accept several toms during an estrous cycle, allowing some litters to have multiple sires (superfecundity). Multiple paternity litters may occur more than 70% of the time in free-roaming cats in population-dense urban environments compared with less than 22% of the time in sparsely populated rural environments.[91] Also, queens may use partner selection to control inbreeding. One study of eight queens in a feral colony concluded that queens avoid breeding with closely related toms but not distant relatives.[48]

Breeders of pedigreed cats attempt to exert control over reproduction and plan pairings based on many factors, such as the qualities (e.g., health, color, conformation) desired in the offspring. Breeders also control the timing of litters based on the health of the queen, demand for kittens, show schedules, and lifestyle factors. Breeders should be educated about maintaining proper breeding records for queens (Box 40-2) as part of a sound cattery management plan.

Under optimum conditions, many pedigreed queens can successfully rear two litters per year or three litters during 2 years. Litters may be born anytime in the year, although most studies show there are slightly more litters born to pedigreed cats in the spring. Queens should be fully mature and in good body condition before they are first bred, both to ensure a successful breeding and to ensure a healthy pregnancy and good postpartum care of the kittens. Queens younger than 1 year of age may have irregular estrous cycles and may not display mature maternal behavior.

BOX 40-2

Reproductive Data Collection for Breeding Queens

1. Age at first estrus
2. Dates of each estrous cycle
3. Length of each estrous cycle
4. Details of behavior during proestrus and estrus
5. Details of behavior during breeding
6. Dates of breedings and number of times bred
7. Outcome of each breeding—pregnancy or date of return to estrus
8. Details of each pregnancy—length of gestation, problems with labor or delivery
9. Details of each litter—litter size, sexes, birth weights, stillbirths, congenital defects if present, illnesses, necropsy findings, and so forth
10. Documentation of problems such as vulvar discharges, pyometra, abortions, mastitis, metritis, and so forth

Queens selected for a breeding program should also meet certain health criteria. Breeding queens should be healthy and up to date with vaccinations. They should be free of common problems, such as upper respiratory tract infection, diarrhea, skin disease, and so forth. Ideally, all cats in a cattery should be tested negative for feline leukemia virus (FeLV) and feline immunodeficiency virus (FIV) and any incoming cats should be tested and confirmed free of infection before joining the cattery population. Before breeding, queens should be free of internal and external parasites. In addition, testing for inherited diseases (e.g., polycystic kidney disease, hip dysplasia, and hypertrophic cardiomyopathy) may be desirable for certain breeds and should be accomplished, where possible, before a queen or tom has reproduced. Queens of breeds with a high prevalence of blood type B should be blood typed before breeding to prevent neonatal isoerythrolysis (see Chapter 41).

Introducing young or inexperienced cats into a breeding program can sometimes result in shyness or a refusal to mate. Ideally, two inexperienced cats should not be matched. A shy cat is best exposed to an experienced mate gradually, preferably on a daily basis for short periods (e.g., about 15 minutes), before mating is required. Inexperienced queens should be placed with experienced, but calm and nonaggressive males.

It is preferable to bring the queen to the tom cat, as many tom cats will not breed successfully when outside their own territory. Environmental factors can interrupt mating behavior, especially in tom cats. Tom cats spend considerable time marking their territory. If the area is cleaned too thoroughly, especially if a scented cleaner is used, some tom cats will ignore or even attack a visiting queen until the territory has been re-marked. It may take up to 14 days before the tom cat is comfortable again. Travel stress can adversely affect the female, temporarily upsetting pituitary and ovarian function. It is best to transport the queen to the tom cat several weeks in advance to allow adaptation to the new surroundings and to the tom cat before attempting breeding.

The queen in estrus will signal willingness to breed by displaying interest in the tom cat, and vocalizing or purring. The queen will assume a lordosis position low to the ground with the tail to one side (see Figure 40-1). The tom cat mounts the queen, grasps the skin on the back of the queen's neck and positions the queen for breeding. Intromission and ejaculation occur in a matter of seconds. Immediately after a successful breeding, the queen will vocalize (the "coital cry") and leap away from and often swat at the tom cat. The tom cat should have an avenue of escape; the breeding area should be roomy or should have usable vertical space. For the next several minutes the queen will roll and thrash on the ground, stretching and licking at the perineum. Most pairs will mate several times in a day. On average, the male cat makes 2 to 6 times more attempts at breeding than the female accepts.

Cats may have partner preferences so that a queen that accepts one tom cat may not accept another. Interestingly, some cats appear to dislike cats of other breeds. A queen may have had a previous adverse experience that makes it reluctant to accept a tom cat. Although it is possible to physically restrain a reluctant queen for a tom cat to breed, this is not without considerable risk to the handler.

In rare circumstances, it may be necessary to tranquilize a queen to facilitate breeding. Care must be used in selection of a tranquilizer because the effect of many drugs on reproductive hormones is not well understood. Phenothiazine tranquilizers, such as acepromazine maleate are contraindicated, because they may interfere with release of LH. Benzodiazepine tranquilizers, such as alprazolam, may be used in moderate doses but some adverse effects of these drugs (e.g., paradoxical aggression, ataxia) may be unpredictable and undesirable. Buspirone hydrochloride has some short-term antiaggressive and anxiolytic effects, but it probably affects secretion of pituitary hormones. If the queen's temperament is undesirable, she may not be a good candidate for a breeding program.

One efficient breeding protocol involves breeding the queen 3 times daily (at 4-hour intervals) on the second and third days of estrus. It has been shown to induce ovulation in greater than 90% of queens.[101] Another successful breeding scheme allows the pair of cats to breed *ad libitum* for short periods during the first 3 days of estrus. However, ovulation and pregnancy rates quoted in the literature are derived from random-bred or colony-bred cats and may not always be achieved with pedigreed cats. This is especially true of the Persian and

TABLE 40-1 **Drugs Used for Control of Estrus and Reproduction in the Queen**

Drug	Dose	Effect	Comments
hCG	250-500 IU/cat, IM	Induce ovulation and pseudopregnancy	Effect lasts about 45 days
GnRH	25 μg/cat, IM	Induce ovulation and pseudopregnancy	Effect lasts about 45 days
Megestrol acetate (Ovaban, Megace, others)	(a) 2.5 mg/cat, PO, 5 days, then once/week (b) 2 mg/cat, PO, once	Induce pharmacologic pseudopregnancy Mismating	Progestin; significant adverse effects
Proligestone (Delvosteron)	100 mg/cat, SC	Estrus suppression	Progestin; effect lasts about 6.5 months
Chlormadinone	2 mg/cat, PO, once/week	Estrus suppression	Progestin; not widely used
Melatonin	30 mg/cat/day, PO	Estrus suppression	Takes 30 days to achieve effect, must be given continuously
Deslorelin (Suprelorin)	6 mg, SC implant	Estrus suppression	GnRH analogue; duration of effect variable
PGF_{2alpha}	(a) After day 33: 2 mg/cat/day for 5 days, IM or SC (b) After day 40: 0.5-1.0 mg/kg, twice 24 hours apart, IM or SC	Pregnancy termination after day 33 of gestation	Short-term adverse effects common: vomiting, diarrhea, panting, restlessness
Cabergoline (Galastop)	(a) 1.65 μg/kg/day for 5 days, SC (b) 5-15 μg/kg/day, to effect, PO (c) 5 μg/kg/day, PO with cloprostenol 5 μg/kg every 2 days, to effect, SC (d) 15 μg/kg/day, PO with alfaprostol 10 μg/kg every 2 days, to effect, SC	Pregnancy termination after day 25-30 of gestation	Prolactin inhibitor; abortion occurs within 7-10 days; occasional vomiting reported
Aglepristone (Alizin)	15 mg/kg, twice 24 hours apart, SC	Pregnancy termination after day 25 of gestation	Progesterone antagonist; abortion occurs within 5-9 days; occasional depression and anorexia reported

GnRH, Gonadotropin releasing hormone; *hCG*, human chorionic gonadotropin; *IM*, intramuscular; *PGF_{2alpha}*, prostaglandin F_{2alpha}; *PO*, by mouth; *SC*, subcutaneous.

related breeds that appear to have reduced fertility. Simply housing queen and tom cat together for the duration of the queen's estrus can also result in pregnancy, but it may deplete sperm reserves in tom cats that are frequently used for breeding.

Control of Estrus and Reproduction

Contraception for the cat must be safe, reliable, convenient, and affordable. Surgical methods (ovariohysterectomy and orchidectomy, as well as ovariectomy and, less commonly, vasectomy) are well described, although not without risk.[47] However, there are various reasons why surgery may not be available, affordable, or appropriate for every cat. Even if a cat is not intended for breeding, owners may have negative attitudes toward surgical sterilization. For these reasons, safe and effective methods of nonsurgical contraception are necessary. A list of drugs for control of estrus and reproduction in the queen can be found in Table 40-1.

The simplest method of estrus control is to induce ovulation, which delays return to estrus by causing a luteal phase (pseudopregnancy) that lasts, on average, about 40 to 50 days. Mechanical stimulation of the vagina using an instrument, such as a glass rod or cotton tip swab, will induce ovulation in a queen in estrus. A teaser tom cat (a vasectomized male or a castrated male with intact libido) can also be used to induce ovulation in queens in estrus. Pharmacologic options for induction of ovulation during estrus include human chorionic gonadotropin (hCG) (250 IU/cat, IM) and gonadotropin releasing hormone (Cystorelin, Merial [Duluth, Ga.]; 25 μg/cat, IM).[57] Induction of ovulation will not shorten the length of that estrus period, however. Repeated induction of pseudopregnancy may predispose queens to cystic endometrial hyperplasia-pyometra complex.

Available pharmacologic methods for longer term control of estrus include progestins, androgens and gonadotropin-releasing hormone analogues.[63] Progestins are the oldest class of drugs used to control reproduction in cats. Megestrol acetate (Ovaban, Intervet/Schering-Plough Animal Health [Summit, NJ] and others) is effective for suppressing estrus in queens when given orally, starting in anestrus (2.5 to 5 mg/cat once daily for 5 days, then once weekly). Medroxyprogesterone acetate (Depo-Provera, Pfizer [New York, NY], and other brands) is a long-acting injectable progestin that is also effective at suppressing estrus when given every 6 to 12 months (25 to 100 mg/cat IM). If the queen is intended for breeding, it should be planned for the second estrus after cessation of therapy.

Proligestone (Delvosteron and Covinan, Intervet/Schering-Plough Animal Health) is a long-acting injectable progestin with weaker progestational activity than the other available drugs.[10] It is licensed in Europe for temporary and permanent suppression of estrus in the queen. At the licensed dose of 100 mg/cat given subcutaneously, the effect on estrus suppression lasts about 6.5 months.[63] Although it appears to be safer than other progestins, there are reports of adverse effects, such as hair loss and calcinosis circumscripta at the injection site.[80]

Another progestin, chlormadinone acetate has been reported as safe and effective for prevention of estrus in queens when given by SC or IM injection, orally or by SC implantation. The drug is not widely available. One study reported that long-term oral dosing for up to 4.6 years at 2 mg/cat once weekly was not associated with adverse effects other than weight gain.[103] When treatment was continued for longer periods of time, mammary and uterine disorders similar to those seen with other progestins were noted.

Adverse effects of progestins are well known and include diabetes mellitus, uterine disease and infertility, adrenocortical suppression, mammary hyperplasia, and mammary neoplasia.[10,61,63,67] Progestins are not approved for use in the queen in all countries (the most notable are the United States and Canada) because of the potentially serious adverse effects. Prolonged use should be avoided, and consideration should be given to alternate forms of contraception for valuable breeding queens.

Mibolerone is an androgen that has been used successfully for contraception in the bitch and queen. However, the dose necessary to suppress estrus in the queen is near the drug's toxic dose, and so, its use cannot be recommended, nor is the drug licensed for use in the cat. Adverse effects include hepatotoxicity, skin thickening, and clitoral hypertrophy.[63]

Melatonin is a hormone produced by the pineal gland with secretion controlled by photoperiod. Higher concentrations are produced during times of shorter photoperiod and will suppress ovarian activity. Exogenous melatonin (30 mg/cat, PO, once daily in the evening) was found to be effective at estrus suppression after 30 days of treatment.[34] The effect was reversible, with normal ovarian activity returning 21 to 40 days after melatonin was withdrawn.

Although daily oral administration of a drug may be impractical, subcutaneous melatonin implants have also been investigated in the queen. In one study, SC implants of 12 mg and 60 mg melatonin were evaluated.[38] Queens were monitored for 6 months, and then ovariohysterectomies were performed. No changes in body weight or hematology and serum biochemistries were noted. Estrus was suppressed in two of four cats given 12 mg melatonin and in three of four cats given 60 mg melatonin. The mean time from implantation to estrus suppression was 20 days, and the mean duration of estrus suppression was 75 days. However, histopathology of the ovaries and uterus of all eight treated queens revealed pathologic changes consistent with cystic endometrial hyperplasia.

In another study, a single SC implant containing 18 mg melatonin effectively and reversibly suppressed estrus in nine treated queens for 2 to 4 months without adverse effects.[30] Although ovariohysterectomy and histopathology were not performed on these queens, six of eight treated queens that were bred after return to estrus had normal pregnancies. The implants used in these two studies were manufactured by different companies, so that differences in formulation may account for some of the variability in study outcomes.

Gonadotropin-releasing hormone is the master reproductive hormone, controlling release of LH and FSH from the pituitary gland. Sustained exposure to GnRH analogues causes downregulation of GnRH receptors and decreased release of LH and FSH, thereby suppressing fertility. GnRH analogues are under investigation primarily for control of reproduction in male and female dogs, while few studies have been published for cats. In one placebo-controlled study, a 6-mg deslorelin (Suprelorin; Peptech Animal Health, North Ryde, Australia) implant was administered subcutaneously to 10 queens.[76] A placebo implant was used for 10 control queens. All cats were followed for 14 months, with daily observation for estrus and frequent monitoring of fecal estradiol levels. The deslorelin implant was effective in inducing reversible suppression of estrus, but the duration of suppression varied widely from cat to cat (range, 5 to 14 months or longer). No adverse effects on the health of treated cats were noted.

Nonsurgical pregnancy termination is not often requested for the queen, but several pharmacologic options are described. The traditional mismating treatment has been estrogen (diethylstilbestrol 2 mg/cat, IM or estradiol cypionate 0.25 mg/cat, IM) given 2 to 3 days after breeding. The mechanism of action is thought to be interference with tubal transport of fertilized eggs. However, estrogens will prolong estrus in the queen and are associated with potentially serious adverse effects, such as pyometra and aplastic anemia, and so cannot be recommended. A single oral dose of megestrol acetate (2 mg/cat) is reported to prevent implantation of fertilized eggs.[25]

There are several protocols for induction of midpregnancy abortion in the queen. Prostaglandin F_{2alpha} (Lutalyse, Pfizer Animal Health) may be given daily for 5 days after day 33 of pregnancy (2 mg/cat, IM).[57] After day 40 of pregnancy, the drug may be given twice,

24 hours apart (0.5 or 1.0 mg/kg, SC).[57] Abortion will occur within 1 week. At higher doses, side effects of prostaglandin are well known and include nausea, vomiting, diarrhea, and restlessness. The effects are seen within 10 to 15 minutes of administration and last 1 to 3 hours. Administration of prostaglandin appears to be luteolytic during pregnancy (but not pseudopregnancy), causing a rapid decline in plasma progesterone.

The prolactin inhibitor cabergoline (Galastop; Ceva Animal Health, St. Louis, Mo.) has been studied in Europe for induction of abortion in the queen. Cabergoline (1.65 μg/kg, divided twice daily, SC, for 5 days) given on day 30 of gestation induced abortion in four of five queens 7 to 10 days later.[112] The mechanism of action is luteolysis by inhibition of prolactin release, a luteotrophic hormone in the queen. In a feral cat colony, oral cabergoline (5 to 15 μgkg/day, to effect [typically 5 days]) was successful in inducing abortion when started after day 36 of pregnancy.[49] Cabergoline may also be used with a prostaglandin F_{2alpha} analogue. In one study, cabergoline (5 μg/kg/day, PO, to effect) was combined with cloprostenol (Estrumate, Intervet/Schering-Plough Animal Health; 5 μg/kg, SC, every 2 days, to effect) in five queens after 30 days of pregnancy. All queens aborted in 8 to 10 days with no adverse effects, and no compromise of subsequent fertility.[82] In another study, cabergoline (15 μg/kg/day, PO, to effect) combined with alfaprostol (10 μg/kg, SC, every 2 days, to effect) was effective in inducing abortion when started on days 25 to 42 of pregnancy.[23] The average duration of treatment was 5.6 days (range, 3 to 8 days). Vomiting was reported in 5.5% of treated queens. If treatment is given late in pregnancy, premature birth is induced with early death of kittens.

Aglepristone (Alizin; Virbac, Carros, France) is licensed for pregnancy termination in the bitch in many countries and is also used in the queen. It has the advantage of infrequent administration when compared with other pharmacologic methods. The mechanism of action is by blocking progesterone receptors, which leads to placental detachment.[29] One large study evaluated the efficacy of aglepristone (15 mg/kg, SC, repeated 24 hours later) after 33 days of pregnancy in 61 queens.[27] Termination of pregnancy was achieved in 88.5% of the queens, with 50% of pregnancies terminated within 3 days. Mild depression and anorexia were seen in less than 10% of queens. Termination of pregnancy occurred despite high plasma progesterone concentrations. Another study achieved 87% success in 23 queens when aglepristone (10 mg/kg, SC) was administered on days 25 and 26 of pregnancy.[28] Pregnancy termination occurred within 5 to 9 days.

The majority of the methods described above for control of estrus and reproduction are not suitable for large scale use. Overpopulation of cats in North America and other countries around the world leads to euthanasia and suffering. There is an urgent need for development of safe, effective, inexpensive contraceptives that would be easy to administer to large groups of cats, especially free-roaming or feral cats. One such approach may be immunocontraception—the use of the immune system to block fertility. This concept is under investigation for various reproductive tissues and hormones and may result in a vaccine-type product in the future.[88]

CLINICAL PROBLEMS

Even the practitioner that does not have pedigreed cat breeders as clients will be presented with certain common problems of the reproductive system in cats. Knowledge of the clinical appearance, diagnosis and treatment options for these common conditions is an essential part of feline practice.

Ovarian Remnant Syndrome

Ovarian remnant syndrome (ORS) is the presence of functional ovarian tissue with signs of estrus after ovariohysterectomy (OHE) or ovariectomy. Neoplasia in ovarian remnants, such as granulosa cell tumor, is a rare cause of ORS. Signs of estrus may occur weeks to many years after surgery[74] and include lordosis, vocalizing, rolling on the ground, and receptivity to intact males. Age at time of surgery and breed of cat do not appear to influence risk of ORS, although one report did not find any cases in queens spayed before 4 months of age.[74] The most common causes of ORS are failure to remove all or part of an ovary at surgery, accessory ovarian tissue[74] and revascularization of ovarian tissue inadvertently dropped into the abdomen during OHE.[19]

Diagnosis is most commonly made by observing signs of estrus in a spayed cat and concurrent vaginal cytology consistent with estrus (cornified epithelial cells, absence of red or white blood cells, clear background). Documentation of serum estradiol levels greater than 20 pg/mL (greater than 73.4 pmol/L) while signs of estrus are occurring is also consistent with ORS, although the diagnosis cannot be ruled out if estradiol levels are low. Caution must be exercised with interpretation of baseline estradiol and progesterone concentrations; however, as there is considerable fluctuation with time. The diagnosis may also be established by inducing ovulation of mature ovarian follicles during estrus with GnRH (Cystorelin; Merial; 25 μg, IM) and documentation of elevated serum progesterone (>2 ng/mL [6.4 nmol/L]) 1 to 3 weeks later.[51]

A protocol has also been described to detect ovarian activity when a queen is not in estrus by administering the GnRH analogue buserelin (Receptal; Intervet/Schering-Plough Animal Health; 0.4 μg/kg, IM) with measurement of serum estradiol 2 hours later.[5]

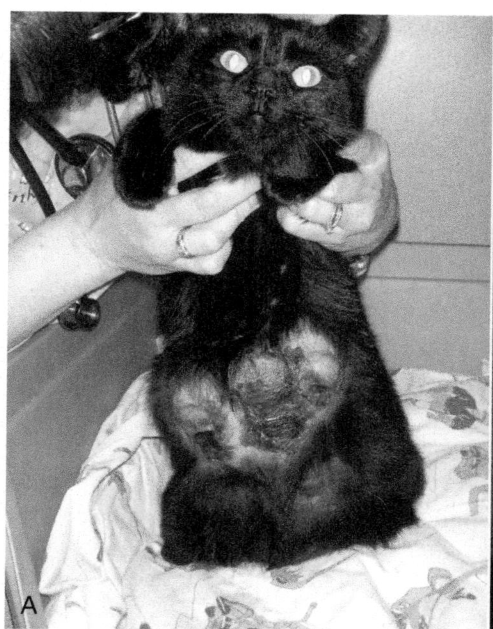

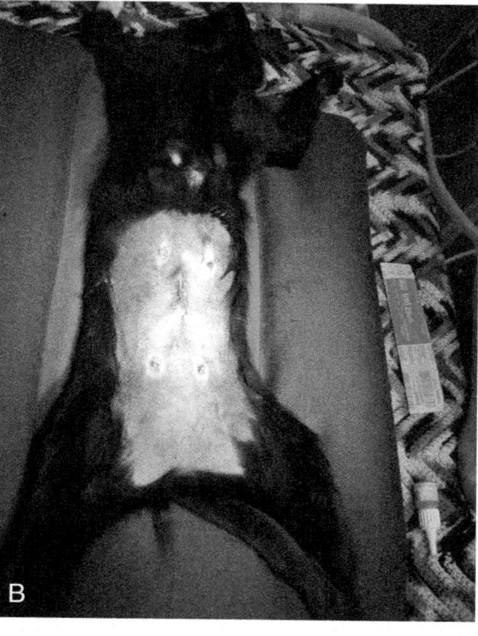

FIGURE 40-2 **A,** Mammary hyperplasia in a young late gestation pregnant queen. A litter of kittens was born 12 days later. The queen was treated with cabergoline, broad-spectrum antibiotics, and analgesics. The kittens were hand raised. **B,** The same queen approximately 2 months later, after ovariohysterectomy. *(Courtesy Shelagh Morrison.)*

Serum estradiol concentrations greater than 3 pg/mL (>11 pmol/L) were consistent with presence of ovarian tissue. No adverse effects from administration of buserelin were noted.

Although evaluation of luteinizing hormone concentrations has been used successfully to determine if a female cat has been spayed or is intact, this assay has not been evaluated in queens with ORS and so should be used with caution.

Once ORS is confirmed, the ovarian tissue should be surgically removed. Queens with ovarian remnants may be at increased risk of mammary and ovarian neoplasia. Many owners will not be tolerant of the estrus behavior. Exploratory laparotomy is required to remove the ovarian remnant. A thorough search of the peritoneal cavity is necessary, starting at the most common location for remnants, the ovarian pedicles. Other common sites for ovarian remnants are the omentum and the peritoneal walls. Remnants may be unilateral or bilateral. Surgery is most rewarding if performed when the cat is in diestrus or has been induced to ovulate. The corpora lutea are visible as yellow-orange structures against the red background of ovarian tissue. Excised tissue should be submitted for histopathology to confirm ovarian tissue has been removed.

Mammary Hyperplasia

Approximately 80% of feline mammary masses are neoplastic, most commonly adenocarcinomas. The remaining 20% are benign and are predominately mammary hyperplasia (also called fibroepithelial hyperplasia and mammary fibroadenomatous hyperplasia). Mammary hyperplasia (MH) is most commonly seen in young cycling queens but may also be seen in pregnant queens and in male or female cats treated with progestins (e.g., megestrol acetate, medroxyprogesterone acetate).[67,69] Typically, most or all of the glands are affected. The hyperplasia can be severe, leading to tissue necrosis, ulceration, and infection. It is often mistaken for neoplasia on gross appearance (Figure 40-2). Histologically, the lesions consist of benign, unencapsulated, fibroglandular proliferation. Progesterone receptors have been commonly found in MH samples, while estrogen receptors have been found in only 50% of cases.[71] The etiology is suspected to be an exaggerated response to natural progesterone or synthetic progestins, but the disease is also rarely reported in sterilized male or female cats with no history of progestin therapy. In spayed queens, ovarian remnant syndrome should be ruled out.

The diagnosis is made by clinical signs, patient signalment and history. Biopsy of affected tissue and histopathology will confirm the diagnosis of MH. However, surgical biopsy of markedly swollen mammary glands may create incisions that are difficult to heal due to wound tension. Treatment varies with the underlying cause. Intact queens should be spayed, and a flank approach is most appropriate (Figure 40-3). If the cat is being treated with progestins, treatment should be stopped. The drug of choice for treatment of MH is the progesterone receptor blocker aglepristone (Alizine, Virbac; 10 to 15 mg/kg/day, SC, days 1, 2, and 7).[33,78] One long-term study monitored 14 queens with MH for 12 months following treatment with aglepristone.[58] Remission of clinical signs occurred in an average of 4 weeks. Cats that had been treated with long-acting

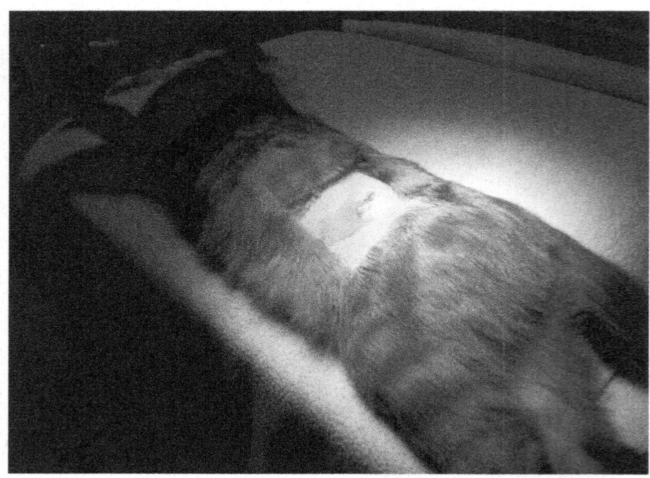

FIGURE 40-3 The flank approach for ovariohysterectomy is useful in situations such as mammary hyperplasia.

medroxyprogesterone acetate required treatment for 5 weeks. Six of the queens were subsequently bred, and four delivered normal litters. Aglepristone may not be available or licensed for cats in every country. For cats that have not received exogenous progestins, other choices include dopamine agonists that reduce prolactin levels, such as cabergoline (5 µg/kg/day, PO, 5 to 7 days)[70a] or bromocriptine (0.25 mg/cat/day, PO, 5 to 7 days).[25,70a] In most countries, these drugs are not licensed in the cat and must be obtained from a compounding pharmacist. Infections should be treated with broad-spectrum antibiotics. Occasionally, MH will resolve spontaneously, but it typically takes several weeks to several months to resolve even with treatment.

Determining Reproductive Status

It may be difficult to determine if an adult queen with unknown history has been previously spayed. Traditional methods to determine reproductive status include observing for signs of estrus and examining the ventral abdomen (or flank) for a surgical scar. Recently, it has been demonstrated that serum luteinizing hormone (LH) can be used to determine reproductive status. LH is released from the anterior pituitary gland in response to copulation. LH stimulates ovulation and luteinization of mature ovarian follicles. In intact queens, serum LH is maintained at basal levels through the negative feedback provided by ovarian estradiol secretion. Following OHE or ovariectomy, this negative feedback is lost and serum LH levels elevate persistently.

A rapid, semiquantitative colorimetric assay is available that shows a positive result when serum LH level is greater than 1 ng/mL (Witness-LH; Synbiotics Corporation, Kansas City, Mo.). The test was developed for canine ovulation timing and has been validated in the queen. Test sensitivity for determination of reproductive status was determined to be 100% and specificity to be 92%.[92] A single negative test is highly likely to indicate a sexually intact queen. A single positive test suggests a spayed queen, although false positives may occur if an episodic LH surge is sampled or the queen is in estrus. The manufacturer recommends that positive tests be confirmed with a second sample taken 2 hours later. Anecdotally, equivocal test results have been reported in some spayed cats.

Some commercial laboratories offer LH testing to veterinarians, but these assays may not have been validated for the dog or cat, so investigation to determine validity is recommended.

Congenital Anomalies

Congenital anomalies of the queen's reproductive tract are not common and are poorly described in the literature. Segmental aplasia/hypoplasia/agenesis of the uterine horn, often called uterus unicornis, may be encountered occasionally and can present difficulties for veterinarians when found incidentally during ovariohysterectomy. Anecdotally, this condition appears to be more common in Ragdoll cats than other breeds or nonpedigreed cats. The abnormality may also be discovered during investigation of infertility in breeding queens.[73] One uterine horn may be missing or reduced to a thread-like remnant, and the ipsilateral kidney is often absent.[7,31,52,70] However, both ovaries are typically present and the surgeon must ensure the ipsilateral ovary is found and removed during ovariohysterectomy (Figure 40-4). Failure to remove the ipsilateral ovary is likely to result in ovarian remnant syndrome and necessitate an exploratory laparotomy at a later date.When one normal uterine horn and ovary are present, the queen may have normal estrous cycles and may even become pregnant. However, segmental aplasia may cause failure to conceive associated with fluid accumulation in the uterine lumen, depending on the location of the occlusion.[70,73]

NORMAL GESTATION AND PARTURITION

Occasionally, practitioners may be called upon to evaluate a pregnant queen or a queen in the midst of labor and delivery. Although many pedigreed cat breeders are knowledgeable about these aspects of feline reproduction, the general public often is not. Accurate evaluation of these patients depends on understanding the normal processes of gestation and parturition.

Pregnancy Diagnosis

The failure of a queen to come back into heat after breeding is one of the most obvious signs of pregnancy, but

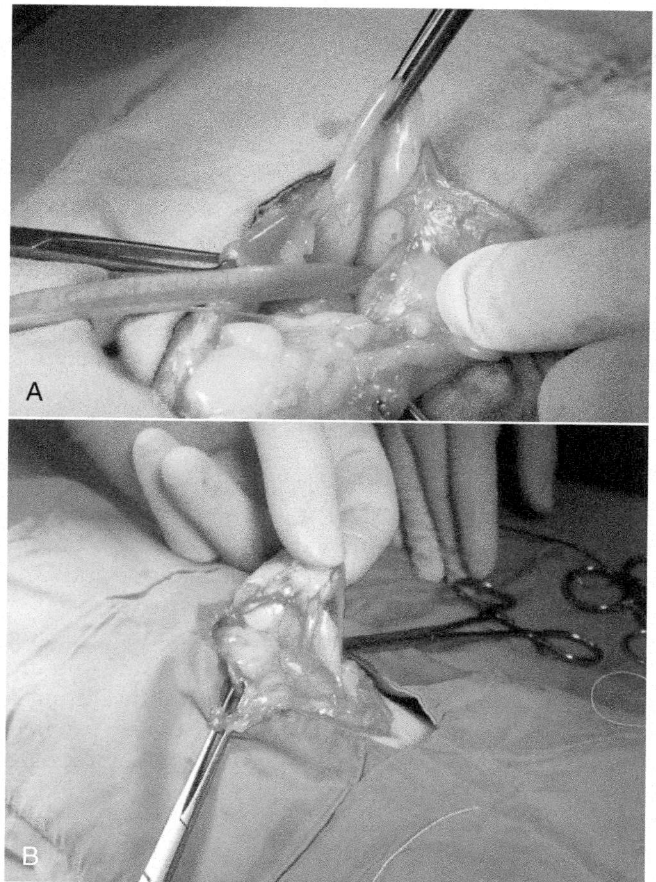

FIGURE 40-4 **A,** Uterus unicornis discovered in a young queen at ovariohysterectomy. **B,** Although one uterine horn may be hypoplastic or missing, the ipsilateral ovary is almost always present. *(Courtesy Jim Sweetman.)*

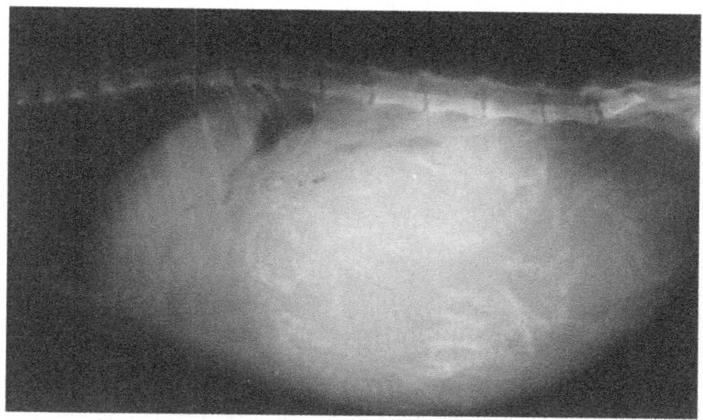

FIGURE 40-5 Radiographic image of a pregnant queen at term. Radiography is useful for determining the number of fetuses by counting the number of skulls present.

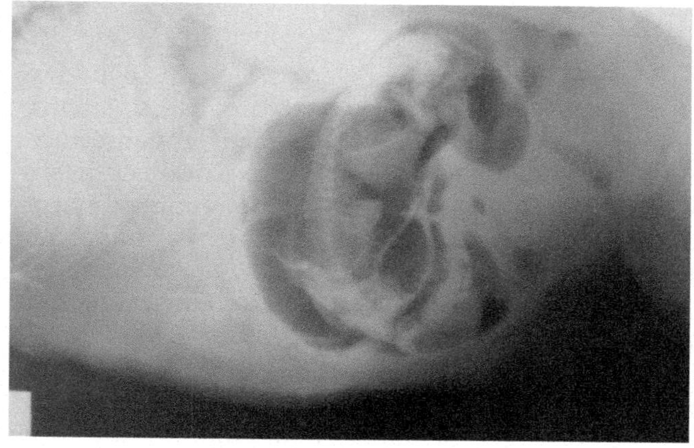

FIGURE 40-6 Radiographic changes associated with fetal death include a hyperextended or hyperflexed body position, collapse of the skull bones, and intrafetal or intrauterine gas.

pseudopregnancy will produce the same effect. However, queens experiencing a pseudopregnancy will usually return to heat within 40 to 50 days after the last estrus. One of the first physical indications of pregnancy is "pinking" of the nipples, which occurs around day 15 to 18 after ovulation. This change in the nipples, which become noticeably pinker and easier to see as the hair around them recedes somewhat and the nipples increase in size, is most obvious in maiden queens. It can be recognized with experience in queens that have had several litters as well.

The developing fetuses can be palpated in the abdomen as early as 14 to 15 days, but most easily at about 21 to 25 days after breeding. They remain distinctly palpable up to about 35 days, when the fetuses and placentas become large enough that they cannot easily be distinguished individually. Toward the end of pregnancy, the heads of fetuses may be very easy to palpate.

Radiography may be used to detect pregnancy once fetal bones begin to mineralize, typically by day 36 to day 45 of gestation.[72] Until this time, only uterine enlargement may be detected, which could be consistent with either pregnancy or uterine disease, such as pyometra. Radiography is useful for determining the number of fetuses by counting the number of skulls present (Figure 40-5). Although fetal death is detected earlier by ultrasonography, radiographic changes include a hyperextended or hyperflexed position, collapse of the skull bones, and intrafetal or intrauterine gas (Figure 40-6).

Ultrasonography is a more sensitive test for pregnancy than radiography. The gestational sac, a spherical anechoic structure slightly compressed at the pole, can be detected at 11 to 14 days and the embryo at 15 to 17 days postbreeding.[17] From day 30, it is possible to identify fetal organs. Details on the time of ultrasound appearance of various fetal and extrafetal structures in the cat have been published.[118,120]

A benefit of ultrasonography is the ability to determine fetal viability by detecting a beating heart (as early as 16 days) and fetal movement (as early as 32 days). Fetal heart rate in the cat averages about 228 beats per minute (range 193 to 263 beats per minute).[114] Unlike the dog, fetal heart rate remains stable during gestation in

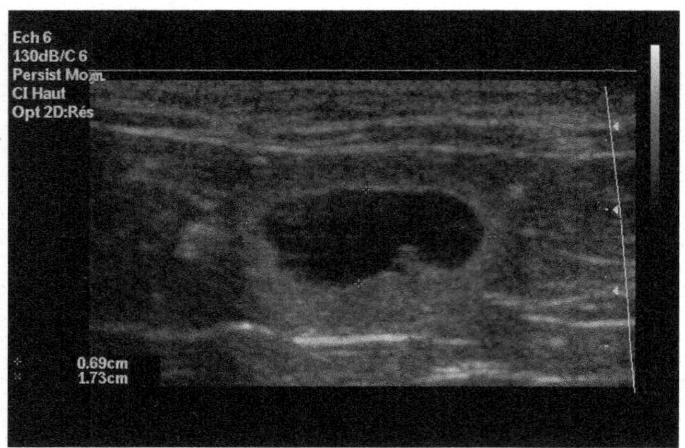

FIGURE 40-7 An empty and deformed gestational sac is visualized using ultrasonography in a queen experiencing early embryo loss. *(Courtesy Elise Malandain.)*

the cat. Sex determination is even possible, at about days 38 to 43 postbreeding.[119] Early fetal death is also identifiable, because examinations performed on consecutive days will show that the gestational sacs decrease in size (Figure 40-7). However, ultrasonography may not be as good as radiography for determining the number of fetuses present. Ultrasonography views each fetus individually, and movement of the queen or the uterus makes identification of individual fetuses confusing.

Many sonographers prefer that the hair coat is clipped, because it gives the best image quality. If the hair coat is not going to be clipped, alcohol or another wetting agent can be used in addition to the acoustic coupling gel to decrease the amount of air between the transducer and the skin and to improve the image quality. However, it is still possible to get a false negative pregnancy diagnosis early in pregnancy if the hair coat was not clipped. The queen ideally should have a full bladder to move the bowel out of the way and also move the uterine body out of the pelvic canal so that it is more readily imaged. It also helps to fast the queen for 12 hours before the ultrasound examination so that intestinal gas is less likely to obscure the views, especially in early pregnancy.

Traditionally, there has been no blood test available in the cat to detect pregnancy. Cats do not produce a placental hormone similar to human chorionic gonadotropin, which is the basis for some human pregnancy tests. However, the hormone relaxin is produced primarily by the placenta and is therefore a useful marker for pregnancy. Relaxin levels increase in pregnancy but not in pseudopregnancy. A commercially available test kit (Witness Relaxin, Synbiotics Corporation) has been developed as a rapid means of pregnancy detection for cats and dogs. The test requires a small volume of plasma, and results are available in about 10 minutes.

In a study designed to evaluate the commercially available relaxin test kit, 11 queens were mated and monitored for pregnancy.[93] All queens were confirmed pregnant and delivered kittens. In addition, 13 pregnant queens undergoing ovariohysterectomy were also tested. A group of 23 nonpregnant cats were tested as controls. The kit was able to detect pregnancy between days 20 and 25 of gestation. All pregnant queens tested negative within 5 days postpartum. In the control group, two cats tested false positive and both of these queens had large ovarian cysts. This suggests another possible source of relaxin production in some queens. The test was estimated to have 100% sensitivity and 91% specificity in cats after day 25 of gestation, with a positive predictive value of 93%.

Prediction of Due Date

The mean length of pregnancy in the queen is 65 to 67 days,[90,97] but it can be highly variable. It is influenced by breed (the longest gestations are in the Siamese and Oriental breeds) and litter size (larger litters are associated with shorter gestations).[97] Normal pregnancies lasting less than 54 days or more than 74 days are rare and are often associated with high neonatal mortality. During a breeding life, most queens will establish a fairly predictable pattern for length of gestation. If the breeding date is unknown, it is helpful to have an alternate method of estimating the queen's due date, especially if the queen may require assistance during labor and delivery. Due dates can be calculated using measurements obtained from radiography and ultrasonography.

There is a predictable sequence of bone mineralization in the feline, similar to that in the canine, but beginning about 1 week earlier in gestation. Prediction of the date of parturition within 3 days was possible for 75% of 32 cats (and within 7 days in all cats) using a schedule for bone mineralization developed in one study (Table 40-2).[44] Not all structures were reliable for prediction of parturition, however. Mineralization of the humerus and femur occur over the narrowest range, while the ulna, fibula, and pelvic bones have more variable mineralization times. The fibula, calcaneus, and phalanges may not become visibly mineralized before parturition.

Prediction of gestational age and date of parturition are also readily accomplished using fetal ultrasound measurements of head or body diameter (Box 40-3 and Figure 40-8). Using ultrasound measurements, the due date can be estimated ±2 days about 75% of the time. Ideally, the measurements should be taken between 23 and 28 days postbreeding.

Care of the Pregnant Queen

The nutritional requirements for reproducing queens are different from adult maintenance needs. In particular, lactation is the most demanding phase of reproduction; so, queens should be in good body condition in order to

TABLE 40-2 Number of Days Prior to Parturition for First Radiographic Detection of Fetal Skeletal Mineralization of Various Bones and Teeth in 17 Pregnant Cats

	First Day of Visible Mineralization	
Structure	**Mean ± SD**	**Range**
General mineralization	26 ± 1	25-29
Vertebral column	24 ± 1	22-27
Skull	22 ± 1	21-27
Ribs	22 ± 2	20-25
Scapula	20 ± 2	17-24
Humerus	20 ± 1	20-24
Femur	21 ± 1	19-23
Radius	19 ± 2	15-22
Tibia	19 ± 1	15-21
Ulna	17 ± 2	5-21
Pelvis	19 ± 1	8-20
Fibula	13 ± 3	0-17
Tail	15 ± 2	8-16
Metacarpals and metatarsals	8 ± 3	3-14
Phalanges	6 ± 3	0-11
Calcaneus	6 ± 3	0-10
Teeth	2 ± 1	1-6

SD, Standard deviation.
Reprinted with permission from the Journal of the American Veterinary Medical Association: Haney D, Levy J, Newell S et al: Use of fetal skeletal mineralization for prediction of parturition date in cats, *J Am Vet Med Assoc* 223:1614, 2003.

BOX 40-3

Prediction of Gestational Age in the Cat (Within 1 to 2 Days) from Ultrasonographic Measurements

Gestational age (GA) in days = 25 × HD + 3
or 11 × BD + 21
Days before parturition = 61 − GA

BD, Body diameter (transverse plane at level of liver) in centimeters; *HD*, head diameter (transverse plane) in centimeters.
Modified from Beck K, Baldwin C, Bosu W: Ultrasound prediction of parturition in queens, *Vet Radiol Ultrasound* 31:32, 1990.

meet the nutritional needs of nursing kittens. Unlike most other species, the queen gains weight linearly from conception to parturition.[68] Energy intake also increases linearly. Mean weight gain for queens during pregnancy is approximately 40% of pre-breeding weight.[68] At parturition, only 40% of the weight gained during

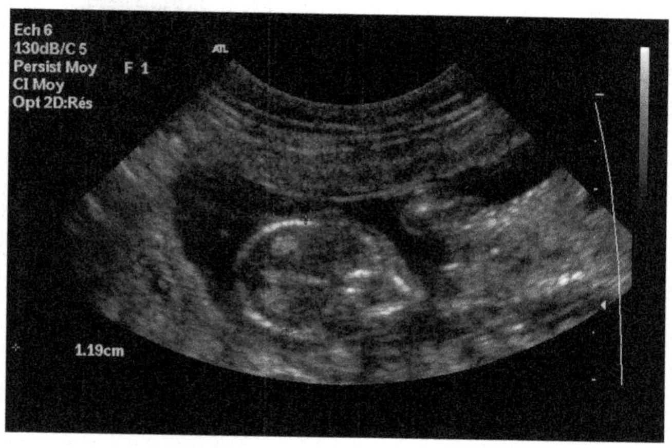

FIGURE 40-8 Prediction of gestational age and date of parturition are accomplished using fetal ultrasound measurements of head or body diameter. *(Courtesy Delphine Rault.)*

pregnancy is lost; the remaining weight is used for milk production.[68] In general, high-quality diets designed for growth or reproduction and lactation are appropriate for the pregnant queen.

During pregnancy, the queen should not be exposed to new cats or to sick cats. There is no need to restrict activity, although most queens become less active and eat smaller meals more frequently during the last trimester because of rapid abdominal enlargement. "Morning sickness" has not been documented in the queen, nor have diet cravings. During the last 2 weeks of gestation, the queen should be isolated from all other cats and provided with a safe, quiet maternity area for delivery. Stress should be avoided, because it has detrimental effects on normal labor and delivery and on normal maternal behavior. A nest box should be provided that is lined with absorbent material that can be laundered (e.g., towels or blankets) or that is disposable (e.g., disposable diapers or pads). Some queens will change nest sites as do feral queens, especially if they have access to the entire home or cattery.

The use of medications in a pregnant or lactating cat must be carefully considered in light of potential benefits versus potential risks. Most medications have not been specifically tested in pregnant or lactating queens; so, information may be scant about the safety of a given drug. More information is available in Chapter 4.

Normal Labor and Delivery

About 1 week before delivery, most queens will exhibit nesting behavior and will spend time in the nest box that has been provided or a site of their own choosing. Most queens wish to be secluded during delivery, but a few will want to be near the owner.

In dogs, the fetal heart rate shows a significant decrease in the 5 days before whelping, and this can be used to predict delivery. However, this cannot be used

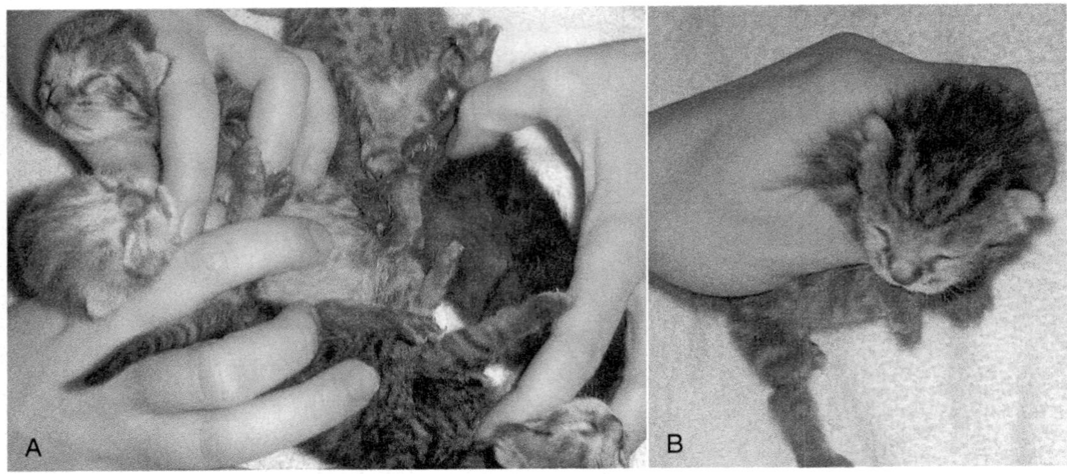

FIGURE 40-9 **A,** Kittens may become entwined by the umbilical cords as they crawl around the nest box. **B,** Entrapment of an umbilical cord around a distal limb may result in significant injury. This kitten eventually required amputation of the distal limb.

to predict delivery for queens, because the fetal heart rate of kittens is stable throughout gestation. Rectal temperature may be used to monitor for impending delivery, although it can be unreliable. The temperature can be monitored twice daily starting at about day 61. Labor typically begins when the temperature has dropped one full degree (usually to about 99° F [37.5° C] or less) and obvious signs should appear in 12 to 24 hours. Another sign that active labor will begin within 24 to 48 hours is the presence of milk in the mammary glands, although in some queens, milk comes in up to 8 days before delivery of the litter.

The first stage of labor may pass largely unnoticed. During this stage, the cervix dilates and the uterus starts contracting. Stage 1 labor may last for a few hours or for as long as 24 hours. Queens may be restless, exhibit overgrooming, pacing, panting, or even vomiting during this stage. Queens may not eat for up to 24 hours before active labor, although some queens eat normally through stage 1 labor. No visible contractions are seen, although there may be a clear mucous discharge from the vagina. As the end of stage 1 labor approaches, most queens will settle in the nest box, purr loudly, and scratch around to prepare the box. The location where the queen will give birth should be warm enough for the neonatal kittens (27° C to 32° C [80° F to 90° F]).

During stage 2 labor, the kittens are delivered, and during stage 3 labor, the placentas are delivered. The delivery of the litter is therefore a series of stage 2 and stage 3 labors. Strong, visible uterine contractions deliver each kitten from its uterine horn, into the uterine body and through the cervix and vagina. The queen can be seen bearing down, but crying out is uncommon. Both head first (two thirds of births) and hindquarters first (one third of births) presentations are normal in the cat. Presentation of the tail and rump before the hind legs is a more difficult delivery.

The time from the start of active labor to the birth of the first kitten is usually less than 60 minutes. A queen that is in active labor for more than 2 hours without delivering a kitten may need veterinary attention. Once delivery begins, kittens are generally born every 30 to 60 minutes, although they may be delivered more rapidly. In one survey of research colony cats, the average delivery time for the entire litter was 16 hours (range 4 to 42 hours).[90] In a large survey of pedigreed queens, the time from delivery of the first kitten to delivery of the last kitten was less than 6 hours in the majority of cases, but it was more than 24 hours in 1.6% of queens.[97] In extended deliveries, the queen may nurse the kittens already born, giving the appearance that delivery is finished. Queens are more likely to interrupt labor and delivery if something disturbing occurs in the environment. In general, the queen in labor should be monitored but interfered with as little as possible.

Kittens are typically born within the amniotic sac, and the queen will bite through the amniotic membrane and the umbilical cord and lick the kitten to stimulate breathing. Since stage 2 and 3 labor happen concurrently in the queen, delivery of kittens is interspersed with delivery of placentas. The queen may or may not eat the placentas; there is no evidence that it is necessary for the queen to do so.

If kittens are born in rapid succession, the queen may not be able to clear membranes from each kitten or sever the umbilical cords promptly. This may also be a problem for inexperienced queens delivering the first litter. Occasionally, kittens may be found dead still inside the amniotic sac, or several kittens may become entwined by the umbilical cords as they crawl around the nest box (Figures 40-9). Entrapment of an umbilical cord around a distal limb may result in significant injury. Gentle, calm intervention by the owner is necessary to ensure survival and prevention of injury in these situations. The

BOX 40-4

Indications for Veterinary Assistance in the Postpartum Period

Queen

1. Pyrexia or hypothermia
2. Foul-smelling, purulent vulvar discharge
3. Profuse hemorrhagic vulvar discharge
4. Lethargy, depression, poor appetite for more than 24 hours
5. Restlessness, panting, stiffness, or tremors
6. Inadequate milk production
7. Bloody or purulent discharge from mammary glands
8. Failure to produce milk
9. Hot, swollen, painful mammary glands
10. Profuse vomiting or diarrhea
11. Straining after all kittens and placentas are delivered

Kittens

1. Excessive crying, restlessness
2. Failure to gain weight
3. Death of any kittens

amniotic membranes should be removed and each kitten should be carefully cleaned and dried. The umbilical cord may be clamped, ligated, and transected about 1 inch from the body wall. Kittens should be kept warm and safe until the queen can attend to them.

Once delivery of the litter is complete, the queen will lie down on her side, curled around the kittens to protect and warm them and encourage them to nurse. Normal kittens have a strong suckle reflex and will knead the mammary gland while nursing to promote milk letdown. Kittens tend to develop a preference for a specific nipple.

Cannibalism of kittens is uncommon. Potential causes include pain (e.g., from mastitis, metritis, or postsurgical pain), stressful conditions, and overcrowding. Poor maternal behavior may account for queens that repeatedly cannibalize kittens without apparent reason. Queens may reject kittens that are unhealthy or unresponsive. Such kittens should be presented for veterinary examination. If the entire litter is rejected, the cause is more likely to be illness in the queen (e.g., mastitis, metritis, or eclampsia). Stressful environmental conditions may also lead some queens to reject an entire litter. A queen that is a poor mother for the first litter may well raise subsequent litters without problems.

Most queens begin eating within 24 hours of delivery and should be fed a diet intended for reproduction and lactation or growth. Fresh water should be provided *ad libitum*. Many queens are reluctant to leave the nest box for more than a few minutes at a time during the first week. The owner should ensure the queen has easy access to a litter box as well as food and water, and the queen should be monitored for adequate nutritional intake. By the time the kittens are about 4 weeks of age, the queen spends less time with them and often stands when they attempt to nurse.

Postpartum discharge (lochia) is typically scant in the queen. Because the queen cleans the vulva frequently, it may not even be noticed by the owner. Ultrasonographically, uterine involution is virtually complete by 28 days postpartum, much earlier than in the bitch.[26] The queen should be monitored for signs of abnormal vulvar or mammary discharge, fever, anorexia, or neglect of the kittens (Box 40-4). It is normal to be unable to express milk from the queen's mammary glands as long as the kittens are gaining weight.[56]

PROBLEMS WITH LABOR AND DELIVERY

Most queens deliver their kittens uneventfully, without the need of human intervention. On the occasions where the practitioner is presented with an apparent dystocia, it is important to understand the characteristics of dystocia in the queen, along with causes and effective treatments.

Dystocia

Dystocia (from the Greek "dys" meaning difficult or abnormal and "tokos" meaning birth) is defined as a painful, slow, or difficult delivery. It is not always easy to differentiate normal parturition from dystocia, especially in the queen, where prolonged time between the births of kittens is normal in a small percentage of cases (Box 40-5). Most commonly, birth of the kittens is difficult from the start in a dystocia, but it is possible for some kittens to be delivered without incident before difficulties are encountered.

Obstetrical monitoring is more commonly used for the bitch than the queen, but can be helpful in determining if labor is progressing normally in both species. External monitoring devices that detect and record uterine activity and fetal heart rates can be used in the home or veterinary clinic, starting about 1 week before the expected date of delivery.[15] Fetal heart rates of less than or equal to 150 to 160 beats per minute (bpm) indicate fetal stress.[114] Fetal heart rates less than or equal to 130 bpm are associated with poor survivability if not delivered within a few hours, and fetal heart rates less

BOX 40-5

Indications for Veterinary Assistance During Labor and Delivery

1. Queen is crying and biting at the vulvar area
2. Queen is more than 1 week overdue
3. Kitten and/or membranes are visible at the vulva for more than 15 minutes with no progress
4. Any systemic illness in the queen
5. More than 3 hours goes by between delivery of individual kittens
6. Abnormal vulvar discharge (e.g., profuse hemorrhage, green discharge with foul odor)
7. No kittens produced after 3 to 4 hours of stage 2 labor
8. Strong contractions present for more than 60 minutes with no kitten delivered
9. Failure to deliver all kittens within 36 hours

BOX 40-6

Causes of Dystocia in the Queen

Maternal

a. Primary or secondary uterine inertia
b. Familial predisposition
c. Stressors
d. Advanced age
e. Obesity
f. Systemic disease
g. Uterine overdistention (e.g., large litter size, large fetuses)
h. Uterine underdistention (e.g., small litter size, small fetuses)
i. Narrow pelvic canal
j. Uterine abnormalities (e.g., torsion, tear, rupture, prolapse)

Fetal

a. Malpresentation
b. Cephalopelvic disproportion (e.g., brachycephalic and dolicocephalic breeds)
c. Death of one or more kittens
d. Large fetuses
e. Congenital defects

than or equal to 100 bpm indicate immediate intervention is required.[114] Interpretation of the contractile patterns from uterine monitoring requires training and experience. At least one commercial service uses trained obstetrical personnel to interpret transmitted information and contact the veterinarian of record if labor is not progressing normally (Veterinary Perinatal Specialties, Wheat Ridge, Co., www.whelpwise.com). The time and expense of the service may be justified for a valuable litter or for a valuable queen with previous delivery problems.

The prevalence of dystocia in the queen has been evaluated in a few studies, although data is conflicting. The overall prevalence of dystocia in 2,928 litters in the United Kingdom was 5.8%.[42] Prevalence ranged from 0.4% in a research colony to 12.5% in Cornish Rex and 18.2% in Devon Rex cats. Prevalence of dystocia in Siamese-type cats was 10%. When breeds were grouped by head conformation, dolicocephalic (10%) and brachycephalic breeds (7.3%) were at higher risk than mesocephalic breeds (2.3%). Dystocia in mesocephalic breeds was more often resolved medically than surgically, whereas in dolicocephalic and brachycephalic breeds, surgical intervention was required in greater than 75% of cases. In brachycephalic cats, malpresentation and primary uterine inertia were the most common causes of dystocia. Primary uterine inertia was the most common cause of dystocia in dolicocephalic cats.

Another survey of pedigreed cat breeding in the United Kingdom was not designed to evaluate the prevalence or causes of dystocia, but it reported that 8% of 1,056 litters were born by cesarean section.[97] Breed was not identified as a risk factor in this study, although small litter size was significantly associated with risk of cesarean section.

A retrospective study of 155 cases of feline dystocia in Sweden found a higher incidence in Persians than other breeds.[22] In this study, litter size was not a significant risk factor. About two thirds of cases were of maternal origin, and medical treatment was successful in only 30% of cases.

There are several potential causes for dystocia in the queen, and accurate diagnosis is necessary to determine whether medical or surgical intervention is the most appropriate (Box 40-6). Causes are divided into maternal and fetal factors, and generally maternal factors are the most common. Dystocia may also be classed as obstructive or nonobstructive.

Maternal factors associated with nonobstructive dystocia include illness, malnutrition, parasitism, and obesity. Anatomic problems, such as a narrow pelvic canal or congenital or acquired abnormalities of the reproductive tract, are potential maternal causes of obstructive dystocia. Primary and secondary uterine inertia are the most common maternal factors and account for the majority of dystocia cases. Primary uterine inertia is complete failure of initiation of effective uterine contractions. Causes include obesity, inadequate uterine stimulation from small litters, overstretching of the myometrium from large litters, hypocalcemia, and uterine disease (e.g., infection, torsion, tear).[87] Familial tendencies are also suspected to play a role. It may be difficult to diagnose primary uterine inertia because of the variable gestation length in the cat and the fact that breeding dates are not always known. Veterinarians may intercede in some cases where queens would have delivered normally if left alone. Thorough evaluation of the status of the queen and ultrasound evaluation of the fetuses can help avoid unnecessary intervention.

Secondary uterine inertia occurs because of uterine fatigue and is typically seen after part of a large litter has been delivered. It may also occur during dystocia from another cause, such as obstruction resulting from fetal malpresentation. Although not strictly a type of inertia, delivery may be interrupted if a queen is disturbed or stressed, and will not resume until the queen feels calm and secure.

Fetal causes of dystocia include fetal defects, unusually large fetuses (often seen with one or two kitten litters), fetal death, and malpresentation. Cephalopelvic disproportion may occur in brachycephalic or dolicocephalic breeds and cause obstructive dystocia.

The diagnosis of dystocia involves certain criteria, such as interruption of a normal delivery (obstruction or secondary inertia) or failure of initiation of labor at term (primary inertia), maternal compromise (depression, shock) or fetal distress (decreased heart rate).[54] The diagnostic plan for dystocia includes collection of a reproductive and medical history, a physical examination (including abdominal palpation, rectal palpation of the pelvis, and vaginal examination), laboratory testing (minimum data required: complete blood count, serum calcium and glucose), and abdominal radiographs (to evaluate fetal size, number, and position). If available, fetal condition is evaluated with ultrasound examination (fetal movement and fetal heart rates) or Doppler examination (heart rates only).

If a kitten is visible at the vulva, it may be possible to deliver it with manipulation.[59] Copious amounts of sterile lubricant are necessary and can be applied around the kitten using a soft red rubber catheter. If the head is visible, clear the nose and mouth of membranes and fluid. The kitten may be grasped around the head and neck or around the pelvis and hind limbs with a clean, dry cloth. Traction should never be applied to an extremity, or avulsion may occur. Traction is applied in a posterior-ventral direction and can be coordinated with the queen's contractions. Gentle twisting or rocking may help free the kitten, and a lubricated finger can be used to free trapped extremities if necessary.

Pharmacologic treatment of dystocia is indicated if the queen is in good condition, there is no obstruction to delivery and the fetuses are not in distress. It is likely to be most effective in queens that have already delivered at least one kitten and where the litter size is not larger than average. Medical treatment is contraindicated if there is any obstruction of the birth canal, because uterine rupture may result. Abdominal radiographs should always be performed before medical treatment is instituted. Hypocalcemia and hypoglycemia, if present, should be corrected before treatment.

The drugs of choice for treatment of dystocia are oxytocin and calcium gluconate. The myometrium is particularly sensitive to oxytocin during pregnancy and at parturition. Oxytocin also promotes uterine involution and expulsion of retained placentas. Smaller, more frequent doses of oxytocin (0.5 to 2.0 U/cat, IM, every 30 minutes, maximum of 2 to 3 doses) are more effective than larger single doses (2 to 4 U/cat).[87] Larger doses of oxytocin may cause prolonged myometrial contraction, ineffective contractions, placental separation, and disruption of blood flow to the fetus. Postpartum treatment with oxytocin is not routinely needed for normal deliveries and should only be used if retained placentas are suspected.

Although oxytocin increases the frequency of uterine contractions, calcium is used to increase the strength of contractions. Criteria for use include weak and ineffective contractions, poor response to oxytocin alone, and the presence of hypocalcemia.[59] Calcium therapy has been shown to be effective in bitches that failed to respond to oxytocin alone, even in the face of normal serum calcium concentrations. Calcium therapy is used much less commonly in the queen, because it may stimulate very strong uterine contractions.[54] The recommended dose of 10% calcium gluconate is 0.5 to 1.0 mL/cat by slow intravenous infusion with concurrent auscultation of the heart.[87] Some queens may also benefit from administration of dextrose (0.25 mL 50% dextrose diluted to 2 mL in sterile water or saline by slow IV infusion).[117]

Uterine abnormalities, such as torsion or prolapse, are uncommon but present unique circumstances that may be life threatening. Uterine torsion typically involves only one horn and most often occurs during late gestation or parturition. Complete torsion may lead to uterine rupture and hemorrhage that is life threatening. Clinical signs of uterine torsion include abdominal pain, shock, hemorrhagic vaginal discharge, and obstructive dystocia.[59] Although radiography and ultrasonography may suggest the diagnosis, exploratory laparotomy is required for definitive diagnosis and treatment. The prognosis is favorable following ovariohysterectomy without correction of the torsion to avoid release of endotoxins and inflammatory mediators.[59,89]

Uterine prolapse is also uncommon in the queen, but more common in cats than dogs. The cervix must be open for prolapse to occur; so, the condition is seen during or immediately after parturition. Clinical signs include abdominal pain, straining, and a mass of tissue protruding from the vulva. The prolapsed tissue is often edematous and may be ulcerated and necrotic. If a uterine or ovarian blood vessel ruptures, life-threatening hemorrhagic shock may occur. The queen is stabilized with intravenous fluids before the prolapse is treated. If

BOX 40-7

Indications for Cesarian Section in the Queen

1. Failure of medical therapy
2. Complete primary uterine inertia
3. Secondary uterine inertia with a large litter
4. Systemic illness
5. Evidence of serious fetal distress (e.g., fetal heart rate <130 beats/minute)
6. Fetal death
7. Obstructive dystocia (e.g., malpresentation, narrow pelvic canal, large fetuses)
8. Uterine torsion, tear, rupture, or prolapse

significant hemorrhage has occurred, a blood transfusion is necessary. Systemic antibiotics are administered if the prolapsed tissue is necrotic. General anesthesia is induced, and if the uterus is in good condition, it is cleaned and manually replaced. Oxytocin is used to promote involution. An ovariohysterectomy can be performed if no further breeding is planned or the uterus is compromised. If the tissue cannot be replaced, surgical reduction may be necessary or tissue amputation may be required.[59]

Cesarean Section

Queens seem to respond to medical management of dystocia less often than bitches. Failure of medical therapy is a common indication for cesarean section. Other indications include systemic illness in the queen, evidence of fetal distress, and primary uterine inertia (Box 40-7). An anesthetic and surgical plan should be followed that maximizes the chances for survival of the queen and kittens. Prolonged induction and delayed delivery increase the chances of neonatal mortality resulting from hypoxia and depression. One recommended protocol is premedication with glycopyrrolate (to counteract vagal stimulation from handling the gravid uterus), induction with propofol, and maintenance with inhalant agents such as isoflurane.[17a] A local anesthetic line block can be applied to the skin and subcutaneous tissues at the incision site. Postoperative pain should be anticipated and opioids are the most commonly recommended drugs.

The queen should be prepared as much as possible before induction of anesthesia, including clipping of hair and surgical preparation. Intravenous fluid therapy should be administered before and during surgery, and any metabolic abnormalities should be addressed (e.g., hypocalcemia, hypoglycemia). The most common surgical technique is a ventral midline incision from umbilicus to pubis, with a single incision in an avascular area of the body of the uterus. Kittens are manipulated from the uterine horns and delivered through the incision one at a time. The placentas and fetal membranes are also removed as long as they are not firmly attached to the uterus, in which case they can be allowed to pass naturally. If future litters are desired, the incision in the uterine body is closed with absorbable suture in a continuous inverting pattern. After closure, oxytocin may be administered to facilitate involution, decrease bleeding, and assist in detachment of any placentas left in place.[105] It is also possible to perform ovariohysterectomy after hysterotomy and removal of the fetuses. Lactation is not adversely affected by ovariohysterectomy.

BOX 40-8

Suggested Equipment List for Resuscitation of Neonatal Kittens

1. Incubator set to 90° F (32° C) and 50% to 60% humidity (or warm water bottles covered by towels)
2. Hemostat and suture material for umbilical cords
3. Chlorhexidine solution or 2% tincture of iodine for disinfecting umbilical cords
4. Bulb syringe or mucus trap for cleaning fluids from airways
5. Soft towels for grasping kittens during delivery, rubbing, and drying
6. Appropriate drugs, diluted if necessary (e.g., naloxone, epinephrine, 50% dextrose)
7. Small anesthetic masks
8. Size 1 endotracheal tubes or 12- to 16-gauge IV catheters
9. Pediatric stethoscope
10. Doppler ultrasound blood pressure monitor
11. 25-gauge needles, 1-mL syringes

En bloc removal of the pregnant uterus and ovaries with subsequent hysterotomy and removal of fetuses has been recommended when speed is required because of the condition of the queen, but the technique is controversial because of concerns about high neonatal mortality.[54] Risks of ovariohysterectomy at the time of cesarean section for the queen include hypovolemia and hemorrhage.

Dystocia may produce significant distress in neonatal kittens, often indicated by meconium staining, apnea, and poor muscle tone at birth. Prompt attention after surgical delivery is critical for neonatal survival, and detailed protocols have been described.[104] The necessary equipment is simple and should be prepared beforehand (Box 40-8). Just as important as equipment is enough medical assistance to care for the newborn kittens. Ideally, one assistant should be available to assist each kitten. A modified Apgar scoring system has been described for routine evaluation of newborn puppies, but has not been evaluated in kittens.[108]

As soon as each kitten is born, it should be rubbed with a towel to dry it and stimulate respiration. Kittens

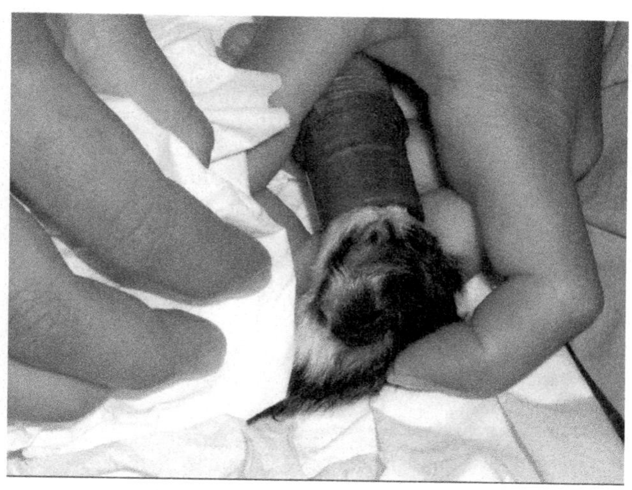

FIGURE 40-10 Oxygen may be administered using the end of a Bain circuit to assist in resuscitation of kittens born after dystocia or cesarean section. *(Courtesy Sandra Brau.)*

should not be allowed to become chilled, because neonates cannot regulate their body temperature, and hypothermia occurs rapidly. Normal body temperature for newborn kittens is 97° F to 98° F (36° C to 37° C). Weak kittens with poor body tone may benefit from a few drops of 50% dextrose solution under the tongue. "Swinging" kittens and puppies to clear airways of fluids is no longer recommended because of the risk of potentially lethal cerebral trauma.[40] Oxygen may be administered using the end of a Bain circuit (Figure 40-10). If vigorous rubbing and clearing the airways with a bulb syringe or mucus trap is not successful, the neonatal kitten may be intubated for oxygen administration and ventilation (slowly increasing up to 30 to 60 cm of water) with a large bore catheter (12 to 16 gauge) or a size 1 uncuffed endotracheal tube. The normal respiratory rate for newborn kittens is 10 to 18 breaths/minute.[39]

An acupuncture technique for resuscitation of newborn kittens has been described using the Renzhong acupressure point (GV26).[96] A 25-gauge hypodermic needle is inserted into the nasal philtrum at the base of the nose until bone is felt and gently rotated. Although no controlled studies have been performed to evaluate effectiveness, anecdotally the technique seems valuable.[104]

Drugs may be administered to neonates by several routes. Intravenous access is best achieved using the umbilical vein or the jugular vein in large kittens. Intraosseous needles or catheters can be placed in the proximal femur, especially if ongoing access is required for fluids or medications (see Chapter 41). The intramuscular and subcutaneous routes are the least desirable, especially for administration of emergency drugs.

Naloxone (0.1 mg/kg IV, SC or IM) may be administered to postcesarean section neonates to counteract opioids given to the queen.[104] Heart rate can be assessed with a pediatric stethoscope or a Doppler blood pressure monitor. Cardiac massage using lateral chest compressions (1 to 2 compressions/second, pausing for breaths) may be used if a heart beat is not detected, and epinephrine (0.1 mg/kg IV, intratracheal, or intraosseous) may be administered if cardiac massage is not successful.[104] Doxapram has been administered for many years as a respiratory stimulant for veterinary neonates, but there is no evidence to support its use. The effect of doxapram is reduced in hypoxic states, making it ineffective in most apneic neonates.[75]

POSTPARTUM PROBLEMS

Queens are rarely presented to practitioners for postpartum problems, but certain problems, such as mastitis, may be encountered in general practice. Features of many postpartum problems in the queen are different from similar problems in the bitch. Recognition of these differences is important for successful management of postpartum problems.

Eclampsia

Eclampsia or postparturient hypocalcemia is most commonly reported in queens that have had previous litters and are currently nursing a large litter. It has also been reported in pregnant queens 3 to 17 days before parturition.[24] Clinical signs include incoordination, stiff gait, vomiting, trembling and twitching, and panting.[56] If untreated, signs may progress to hyperthermia and seizures. Diagnosis is based on clinical signs in a lactating queen with total serum calcium less than 8 mg/dL (<2 mmol/L). Eclampsia is treated with a slow intravenous infusion of 0.5 to 1.5 mL/kg of 10% calcium gluconate, repeated as needed.[59] Electrocardiographic monitoring should be used during treatment to detect bradycardia or arrhythmias. After discharge, oral supplementation is started at 250 to 500 mg calcium gluconate daily[56] or 100 mg/kg calcium carbonate[59] daily in divided doses until kittens are weaned. Calcium supplementation before parturition is not recommended for queens at risk of eclampsia as it may down regulate parathyroid hormone secretion and actually increase the risk of eclampsia.[59]

Mastitis

Inflammation and infection of lactating mammary glands is typically caused by *Escherichia coli*, staphylococci, or streptococci.[59] Bacteria most commonly ascend into the gland through the nipple because of poor hygiene or trauma, although hematogenous spread is possible. Clinical signs include inflammation and pain

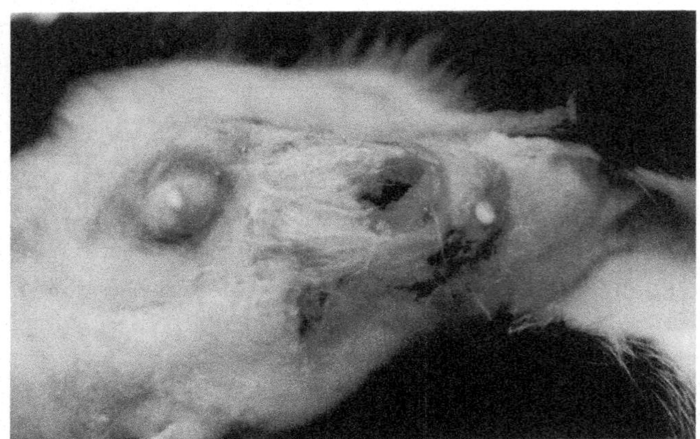

FIGURE 40-11 Severe mastitis in a young queen with abscessation and necrosis of skin and tissue.

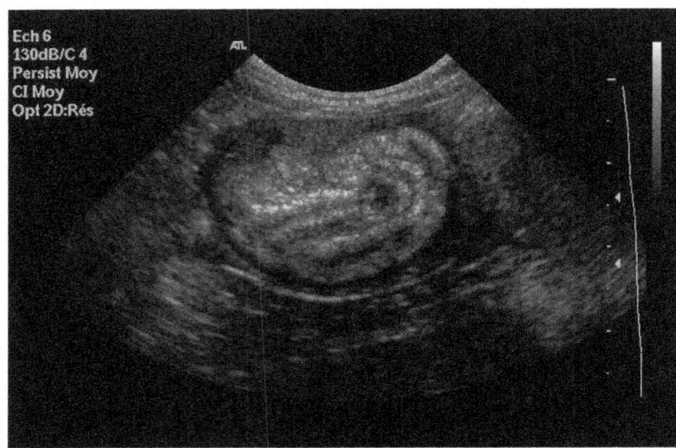

FIGURE 40-12 Ultrasonography is useful for detection of retained placentas. *(Courtesy Delphine Rault.)*

in one or more glands, fever, anorexia, depression, and neglect of kittens. Severe cases may progress to abscessation and necrosis of skin and tissue (Figure 40-11). Cytology of milk from an infected gland will show degenerate neutrophils and bacteria. Broad-spectrum antibiotics that are safe for neonates, such as amoxicillin-clavulanic acid or cephalexin, are good choices.[59] Warm compresses may also be helpful. If abscessation has occurred, surgical lancing and flushing to establish drainage is required. Large ruptured abscesses are managed as open wounds. If the mastitis is diagnosed early, kittens may continue to nurse.[56] The nursing kittens ingest some antibiotic in the milk and help drain the affected glands.

Metritis

Metritis, a bacterial infection of the postpartum uterus, is caused by bacteria ascending from the vagina into a compromised uterus and is most likely to occur in the first week postpartum. Risk factors for metritis include dystocia, especially with obstetric manipulation, dead fetuses, and retained placentas. Clinical signs include fever, anorexia, lethargy, purulent or sanguineous vaginal discharge, and neglect of kittens. A complete blood count typically shows leukocytosis with a left shift (although occasionally leukopenia is seen). The most common bacterial species involved are *E. coli*, staphylococci, or streptococci.[117] Cytologic examination of the vaginal discharge shows degenerate neutrophils with intracellular bacteria. Abdominal radiographs or ultrasound images should be obtained to look for fetal death, retained placentas or an enlarged uterus. Minimal or subtle changes to the uterus may be evident with imaging.

Prompt and aggressive treatment is indicated for queens with metritis. Broad-spectrum antibiotic therapy should be initiated and can be adjusted if necessary based on the results of culture and sensitivity testing of vaginal discharge. Appropriate choices include fluoroquinolones or a combination of amoxicillin-clavulanic acid and a fluoroquinolone. If the queen is nursing kittens, it is safest to avoid fluoroquinolones. However, the queen may be too ill to nurse kittens and hand-rearing may be required. If future litters from the queen are not desired, ovariohysterectomy can be performed once the queen is stable or the kittens are weaned. Antibiotic therapy should be continued for up to 4 weeks or for at least 10 days if ovariohysterectomy is performed.[117]

If the queen is intended for breeding, uterine evacuation is indicated if the uterus is not friable and thin walled and no retained fetuses or fetal membranes are present. Oxytocin (0.5 to 1.0 U/cat, IM, every 30 minutes for 1 to 2 doses) is only effective within 24 hours postpartum. After that time, uterine oxytocin receptors are no longer present. Other drug choices for uterine evacuation include prostaglandin F_{2alpha} (0.1 to 0.2 mg/kg, SC) or cloprostenol (1 to 2 μg/kg, SC) every 12 to 24 hours to effect.[117] Treatment to evacuate the uterus may take several days and is not recommended in severely ill queens.

Retained Placentas

The queen only occasionally suffers from retained placentas. It should be suspected if the number of placentas at delivery is less than the number of kittens (although occasionally, twin or triplet kittens will share one placenta). Abdominal palpation will usually reveal an enlarged uterus, although this is a subjective and unreliable test. Radiography or ultrasonography may confirm the diagnosis by detecting a placental mass (Figure 40-12). The treatment of choice is oxytocin (0.5 to 1.0 U/cat, IM, every 30 minutes, maximum of 3 doses) within the 24 hours following delivery. Prostaglandin F_{2alpha} (0.1 to 0.2 mg/kg, SC, every 12 to 24 hours to effect) can be used if oxytocin fails to evacuate the uterus or parturition occurred more than 24 hours previously. It is also possible for retained placentas to break down and pass with the normal lochia, but the owner should be instructed to monitor for signs of metritis.

Inadequate Milk Production

Prolactin, produced by the anterior pituitary, is the hormone responsible for the development of the mammary glands during pregnancy as well as initiating and maintaining lactation. Prolactin does not act alone, but through a complex interplay with other hormones, including oxytocin. Occasionally, young or nervous queens may have delayed milk letdown or poor milk production. Kittens should begin to nurse within 1 to 2 hours of birth. Hungry kittens will be restless and will tend to cry excessively. A maiden queen may be encouraged to settle down and allow the kittens to nurse with slow and patient introduction of the kittens. If this is not effective, treatment with oxytocin may be attempted. The effects of oxytocin are very short lived; so, the drug must be given frequently (0.5 to 1.0 U/cat, SC, every 30 minutes).[117] Metoclopramide (0.1 to 0.2 mg/kg, SC or IM) stimulates prolactin secretion from the anterior pituitary and will cause milk letdown within 15 minutes.[117]

Postpartum Intussusception

Intussusception is reported occasionally in young cats, and often occurs in association with gastroenteritis. Postpartum intussusception has been reported in five queens, occurring from birth to 8 weeks postpartum.[21] Queens ranged in age from 12 to 24 months, and all were primiparous. The most common clinical signs were lethargy, anorexia, and vomiting. An elongated abdominal mass was palpable in all queens. In four of the queens, the intussusception was located in the small intestine and in the ileocolic area in the remaining queen. All queens were treated surgically. No underlying reason could be found for the intussusception and histopathologic and cytopathologic examination of tissues failed to find significant abnormalities. Four of the five queens made an uneventful recovery, while the fifth queen died unexpectedly 36 hours postoperatively without postmortem examination. Although the etiology of postpartum intussusception in the queens remains unknown, it should be considered as a differential diagnosis for any postpartum queen with compatible clinical signs.

INFERTILITY IN THE QUEEN

An investigation into infertility in a queen may be prompted by an inability to be bred by a tom cat, an inability to conceive after successful breeding, or an inability to carry a pregnancy to term. There are many potential causes of infertility, ranging from inadequate daylight to breeding management problems (Box 40-9).

> **BOX 40-9**
>
> **Common Causes of Infertility in the Queen**
>
> **True Primary Anestrus**
>
> Abnormalities of sexual differentiation
>
> **Persistent Anestrus**
>
> Previous ovariohysterectomy or ovariectomy
> Inadequate daylight length or intensity
>
> **Infrequent Estrus**
>
> Silent heats
> Spontaneous ovulation and pseudopregnancy
> Concurrent diseases and stressors
> Medications
>
> **Prolonged Estrus**
>
> Normal phenomena
> Ovarian cysts and tumors
>
> **Infertility with Normal Estrus**
>
> Maternal abnormalities
> Male infertility
> Breeding management issues
> Failure to ovulate
> Inbreeding depression
> Cystic endometrial hyperplasia/pyometra
> Concurrent diseases and stressors
> Medications

Evaluation of infertility in the queen should begin with a complete physical examination, a thorough medical and breeding history, complete blood cell count, serum chemistries, and urinalysis. Feline leukemia virus and feline immunodeficiency virus testing should be performed if the queen's status is unknown. The stage of the queen's estrous cycle should be investigated by evaluating serum progesterone concentration and vaginal cytology. Patient-side test kits for canine serum progesterone have been validated for use in the cat.[6,43] Serum progesterone levels greater than 2 ng/mL confirm ovulation has occurred and may be associated with pregnancy or pseudopregnancy. A diagnostic plan for investigation of infertility in the queen is outlined in Box 40-10.

Culture of vaginal samples in queens without vulvar discharge is not informative as a wide variety of bacteria inhabit the normal feline vagina.[11,98] Relative numbers of vaginal bacteria are higher in young cats and increase

BOX 40-10

Diagnostic Plan for Investigating infertility in the Queen

1. Perform a complete physical examination, collect medical and reproductive history
2. Collect minimum laboratory database: complete blood count, serum chemistries, complete urinalysis, feline leukemia virus (FeLV) and feline immunodeficiency virus (FIV) infection status
3. Establish stage of estrous cycle with serum progesterone and vaginal cytology
4. Evaluate diet quality, especially taurine content; nutritional supplements
5. Investigate reproductive illnesses, especially cystic endometrial hyperplasia
6. Investigate nonreproductive illnesses, especially those causing debilitation and chronic ill health
7. Evaluate cattery conditions: population size and density, sanitation, lighting, temperature, ventilation
8. Identify stressors such as exhibition and travel, conflict in social interactions
9. Investigate the fertility of the tom cat
10. Determine if medications, nutritional supplements, or vaccines have been administered recently, especially anabolic steroids, glucocorticoids, progestins, and modified live vaccines containing feline panleukopenia virus

BOX 40-11

Stages of Estrus in the Queen and Their Corresponding Vaginal Cytology Changes

Anestrus

Numerous small round epithelial cells with large nuclei; occasional leukocytes; cellular debris

Proestrus

Increased number of intermediate epithelial cells; cornified cells begin to appear near estrus; cellular debris

Estrus

Large numbers of cornified epithelial cells; less debris; clearer background; no leukocytes or red blood cells

Diestrus

Degenerating cornified epithelial cells; sometimes bacteria and leukocytes seen; small epithelial cells begin to appear

during estrus and pregnancy.[11] Pure cultures of bacteria may be a normal finding so that antibiotic therapy should only be considered if clinical signs of infection are present.[98]

Vaginal Cytology

Although vaginal cytology is used less frequently in the queen than in the bitch, it can be useful as part of a diagnostic plan for infertility. The patterns seen on cytology are not always easy to relate to stage of estrous cycle, but the technique is generally useful for detecting estrus, especially silent estrus. Cells for cytology are collected by gently rotating a saline-moistened cotton-tipped swab on the dorsal wall of the vagina about ½ inch from the vulvar entrance. A human urethral swab is smaller and often easier to use in the queen than a standard cotton tip swab. The procedure is brief and painless. The swab is rolled on a microscope slide to deposit the cells; the smear is air dried and then stained with any product used to stain blood films. Use of a trichrome stain will color cells containing keratin red, and cells without keratin will appear blue.

The types of epithelial cells that are found on vaginal cytology in the queen include parabasal and intermediate cells, and nucleated and nonnucleated superficial (cornified) cells (Box 40-11). A smear consisting of more than 80% superficial cells is consistent with estrus (Figure 40-13). Estrogen has the effect of thinning the vaginal mucus, so that estrous smears have a clear background with little cellular debris and no red or white cells. Clearing of the background is a consistent indicator of estrus activity and may be noted just before estrus behavior is seen.[25]

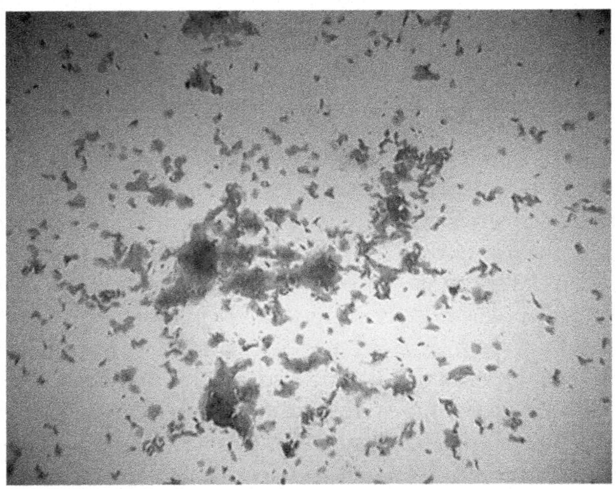

FIGURE 40-13 Superficial cells predominate in vaginal cytology smears made during estrus in the queen. The cells have been stained with Harris-Schorr stain, which stains keratin red. *(Courtesy Elise Malandain.)*

When investigating infertility in pedigreed catteries, breeders can be instructed in the method of collecting vaginal cytology specimens and making air-dried smears at home. The slides can be taken to the veterinarian for interpretation. If a queen is confirmed in estrus by vaginal cytology, the tom cat should be available for breeding immediately, because the collection technique may induce ovulation in some queens.

Causes of Infertility with Abnormal Estrus

A common presentation for infertility in the queen is failure to exhibit normal estrous cycles. Causes include immaturity or senility and primary anestrous or secondary anestrus. Signs of estrus vary widely among queens and among cat breeds. In general, the Oriental breeds, such as the Siamese and Burmese, will have more striking behavioral changes during estrus than the longhair breeds, such as the Persian. It may require close observation to ensure that estrous behavior is not going undetected.

The first estrus generally occurs between 5 and 9 months of age (range, 3.5 to 18 months). Because the age at first estrus is variable and influenced by many factors, such as breed and season, immaturity should be ruled out as a cause of failure to exhibit estrous cycles in young queens. After maturity, most queens will produce litters for 5 to 7 years before age-related changes diminish reproductive success. In queens older than 8 years of age, absent or infrequent estrous cycles may be a normal consequence of aging. The functional life span of the feline ovary is unknown. Senile or premature ovarian failure has not been well defined in cats.

Primary anestrus refers to failure to show the first estrus by 24 months of age.[50] Although hermaphroditism and abnormal gonadal development are rare in cats, primary anestrus has been associated with abnormal karyotype (e.g., 37,XO), true hermaphroditism and abnormal phenotypic sex. Male pseudohermaphrodites appear phenotypically female, but have a small vagina and vulva with an enlarged clitoris. Diagnosis of sex and gonadal abnormalities requires examination of any abnormal reproductive structures and karyotyping.

Persistent anestrus may occur in queens previously known or suspected to exhibit normal estrous cycles. If the queen's full medical history is unknown, previous ovariohysterectomy or ovariectomy should be ruled out with evaluation of serum luteinizing hormone concentration.

Secondary anestrus refers to prolonged interestrus intervals or infrequent estrous cycles and is more common in queens than primary anestrus. Inadequate daylight length or intensity may be a cause of infrequent estrous cycles in some queens. Breeding catteries should provide a minimum of 14 hours of bright artificial light per day. It may take several weeks for estrous cycles to resume once inadequate daylight has been corrected. Longhair queens, such as Persian cats, seem especially sensitive to low light levels and are more prone to infrequent estrous cycles. Evaluation and correction of daylight should always be performed before attempting hormonal induction of estrus. Housing anestrus queens with queens that are exhibiting regular estrous cycles may also be beneficial.

Queens that are timid or intimidated by other cats in the cattery may experience the hormonal events of estrus normally, but may not display overt estrous behavior. These "silent heats" may also occur in queens living in crowded or stressful conditions. This absence of overt estrous behavior may be erroneously interpreted as failure to cycle by the owner.

Silent heats may be diagnosed by evaluation of vaginal cytology once or twice weekly to detect cytologic signs of estrus. Queens confirmed with silent heats should be removed from their current situation and either housed separately or in a smaller group of cats. A queen that has been housed alone may benefit from exposure to other queens in estrus. Exposure to tom cats may also increase the chances that overt estrous behavior will be displayed. Successful management may include having the queen live with a tom cat until pregnancy is confirmed. Queens that fail to respond to these measures should be removed from the breeding program.

Spontaneous ovulation and subsequent pseudopregnancy is one important cause for infrequent estrous cycles in some queens. The interestrous interval for these queens is typically 40 to 50 days, rather than the normal average of 7 days. Queens that return to estrus 40 to 50 days after breeding may also have experienced a pseudopregnancy following ovulation and conception failure or early embryo loss. Pseudopregnancy is seldom associated with clinical signs in the queen and requires no treatment. Queens experiencing spontaneous ovulation and pseudopregnancy should be housed individually in a secluded area to avoid stimulation from other cats. Physical handling of these queens during estrus should be avoided. When estrus occurs, the queen is taken to the tom cat for breeding.

Nonreproductive illness may indirectly affect fertility in queens, especially conditions that cause debilitation or prolonged illness, such as chronic upper respiratory tract disease or diarrhea. However, unlike bitches, hypothyroidism has not been identified as a cause of infertility in queens. In some individuals, stressors may affect ovarian function and interrupt estrous cycles. Stressors that are common in catteries include frequent exhibition and travel, overcrowding, extremes of temperature variation and antagonistic social interactions. If more than one queen in a cattery is experiencing infertility, a site visit may uncover contributing management or environmental conditions.

The effect of many drugs on reproduction in cats is not known. Part of the medical history for a queen with infertility should include a list of any recently administered medications, including nonprescription drugs, nutritional supplements, and botanicals. Certain drugs are known as disruptors of estrous cycles by inhibiting secretion of gonadotropins (e.g., progestins, androgens, anabolic steroids, glucocorticoids). Herbal or botanical products may contain substances that act like or interfere with reproductive hormones.

Hormonal induction of estrus is not commonly required in queens. Every attempt should be made to document the cause of infrequent or absent estrous cycles before considering the use of exogenous hormone therapy. Only queens in good health between the ages of 1 and 5 years should be candidates for induction of estrus. Many reproductive hormones recommended for use in small animal theriogenology are not available in North America. Those products available are typically labeled for large animal or human use. Informed consent should be obtained from owners before using any treatments not licensed in cats. A variety of protocols using FSH or pregnant mare serum gonadotropin (PMSG) for estrus induction in the queen have been described and the reader is referred elsewhere for details.[64]

Both functional and nonfunctional cystic structures may affect feline ovaries, sometimes producing prolonged estrus. Ovarian cysts may be found incidentally during laparotomy (Figure 40-14). Most cystic structures are within the ovarian bursa, having originated from the mesonephric or paramesonephric duct systems, and are nonfunctional. Functional ovarian cysts may be either follicular or luteal. Luteal cysts are rare in cats, and the more common follicular cysts typically do not produce clinical signs. Follicular cysts derive from persistent follicles that have not ovulated. If the cysts produce estrogen, prolonged estrous behavior may result.

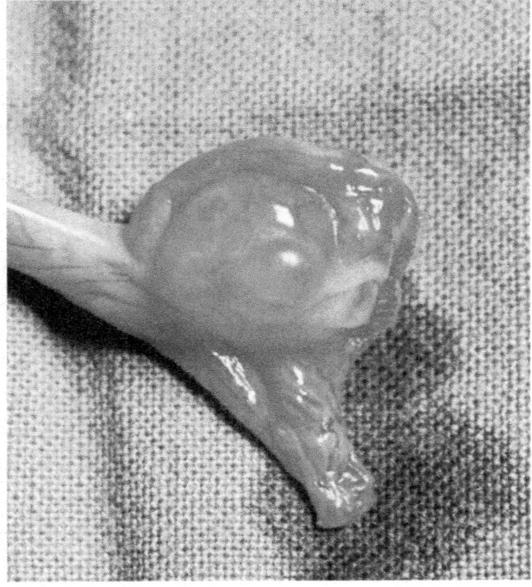

FIGURE 40-14 Ovarian cysts may be found incidentally during ovariohysterectomy.

Ovarian cysts may be identified using ultrasonography. The most effective treatment has not been determined. In some cases, ovulation or luteinization appears to occur spontaneously. If an ovarian cyst is associated with prolonged estrus, and natural breeding fails to induce ovulation, hormonal induction may be attempted. Recommended treatments include GnRH and hCG (see Table 40-1).[51] Surgical resection may also be attempted.

Primary ovarian tumors are uncommon in queens, and are typically found in older intact nulliparous individuals. Rarely, a primary ovarian tumor such as a teratoma may be identified in a spayed cat.[62] The most commonly reported ovarian tumor is the granulosa cell tumor.[51] The average age of affected queens is 9 years, and clinical signs include prolonged or irregular estrous cycles, aggression, and hair loss. These tumors are predominantly unilateral and less than 5 cm in diameter. A presumptive diagnosis is based on signalment, clinical signs, and ultrasonographic or radiographic findings. Granulosa cell tumors have been reported to metastasize to the lungs, liver, spleen, and kidneys. Surgical resection may be curative if metastasis has not occurred.

Causes of Infertility with Normal Estrus

Maternal abnormalities, such as inbreeding depression, congenital defects, and uterine disease, may cause infertility in a queen with normal estrous cycles. The fertility of the tom cat, although difficult to investigate, should also be considered (see Chapter 39). A queen should be bred to a proven sire (an experienced tom cat that has sired a litter within the previous 6 months) before being considered infertile.

Inbreeding (or linebreeding) is a common practice in pedigreed cat breeding and is necessary for breed development and fixation of desired traits. Intensive inbreeding, however, may perpetuate deleterious traits and contribute to loss of vigor and reproductive capacity. Inbreeding may be a cause of subfertility in queens with a normal estrous cycle. Queens that are difficult to breed may pass on undesirable reproductive traits to the next generation. Breeders should consider removing these individuals from the breeding program. One of the criteria for selecting new young queens as breeding stock should be normal reproductive performance in close female relatives.

Congenital defects, such as vulvar or vaginal abnormalities, are a rare cause of problems with intromission. Vaginal strictures secondary to trauma during parturition are possible but uncommon. These problems should be suspected if the tom cat makes repeated unsuccessful or prolonged attempts to achieve intromission. Vaginoscopy has been described in the queen for diagnostic purposes, but is not always feasible in practice because of the narrow feline vagina.

Failure to ovulate is suspected when a queen returns to estrus less than 18 days after breeding. It is associated with serum progesterone concentrations less than 1 to 2 ng/mL in the absence of a confirmed pregnancy. When failure to ovulate is suspected, breeding management should be reviewed with the owner (see above, Fertility and Breeding Management). Common causes include breeding too early or too late in estrus, unsuccessful intromission, and too few copulations. If problems with breeding management have been ruled out, hormonal induction of ovulation in queens in estrus may be attempted with GnRH or hCG (see Table 40-1), followed by natural breeding.[64] Treatment is most likely to be successful if given when mature ovarian follicles are present. These drugs should be used with caution; excessive use of hCG has been associated with ovarian hyperstimulation and formation of antigonadotropin antibodies.[100] Administration of hCG more frequently than every 6 months is not recommended.

Imaging methods, such as radiography and ultrasonography, may detect uterine abnormalities (e.g., abnormal wall thickness and morphology, accumulation of luminal fluid, retained fetal material, masses). A normal nonpregnant uterus is not usually visible on radiographs and may be difficult to detect with ultrasonography. Other methods, such as laparotomy and laparoscopy, allow for visualization of organs and structures as well as sample collection (e.g., tissue samples for histopathology, fluid samples for culture and sensitivity testing). During laparotomy, the uterus and oviducts can be assessed for impatency secondary to congenital defects, hyperplastic change, or scarring. Those more invasive methods may be appropriate for valuable breeding queens.

Uterine disease, especially cystic endometrial hyperplasia-pyometra (see below), is an important cause of infertility in queens.[4] Other less common uterine abnormalities include hydrometra (Figure 40-15) and mucometra. In these conditions, sterile, noninflammatory, clear or cloudy, watery or viscid fluid accumulates in the uterine lumen.[52] The fluid volume in the uterus may be up to 500 mL, leading to diffuse or segmental enlargement. Distention causes thinning of the uterine wall. Clinical signs are often absent or related to abdominal distention. Radiography, ultrasonography, or abdominal palpation may detect the enlarged uterus. Both conditions may progress to pyometra, and the only treatment is ovariohysterectomy.

Cystic Endometrial Hyperplasia-Pyometra Complex

Cystic endometrial hyperplasia (CEH) is characterized by proliferative and degenerative changes in the endometrium associated with aging and hormonal stimulation.[2] Endometritis and pyometra are forms of CEH

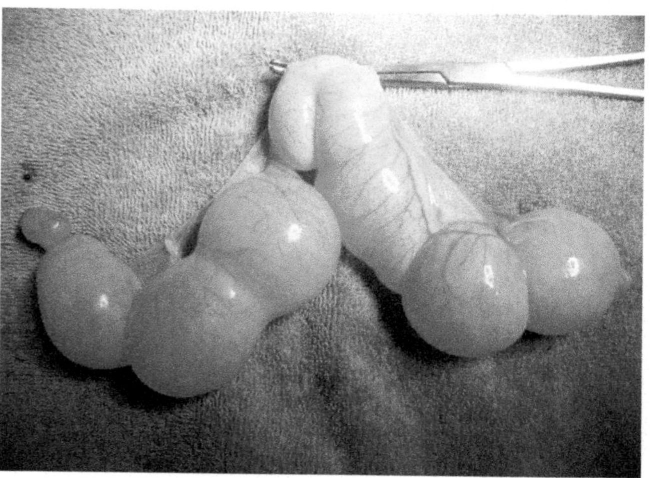

FIGURE 40-15 Hydrometra produces a distended, thin-walled uterus filled with noninflammatory, clear, sterile fluid.

associated with inflammation and secondary bacterial infection. Traditionally, CEH has been classified as a luteal phase disease in bitches and queens. Progesterone induces hyperplasia of the surface or glandular epithelium and cystic dilatation of the uterine glands.[85] Proliferation of the endometrial glands produces a wavy, coil-shaped appearance of the uterine lumen that may be seen with hysterography or ultrasonography.[9] Fluid present in cystic structures or in the uterine lumen readily supports bacterial growth. Progesterone also inhibits local leukocyte responses and decreases myometrial contractility, which increases the risk of ascending bacterial infection.[14,98] Bacteria are not normally found in the uterus, except in a small number of queens during estrus.[11] Endometrial hyperplasia may also be influenced by chronic estrogenic stimulation from recurrent estrous cycles that do not result in pregnancy.[85] In addition, estrogens increase progesterone receptors in the endometrium and dilate the cervix.[2,8]

In most published studies, older queens (average age 32 months to 7.6 years, range 1 to 20 years) and maiden queens greater than 3 years of age have the highest risk for CEH-pyometra.* Queens with uncomplicated CEH have no clinical signs of illness. Results of routine blood and urine testing are typically within normal ranges. CEH is associated with implantation failure and early embryonic death, resulting in small litter size or infertility.

Breeding catteries may have high rates of CEH, especially in queens greater than 3 years of age. This may be due to several factors, including spontaneous ovulation and the limitations imposed on the number and timing of pregnancies to accommodate exhibition schedules and planned breeding schedules.[65,85] Pregnancy appears

*References 16, 60, 65, 77, 84, 85.

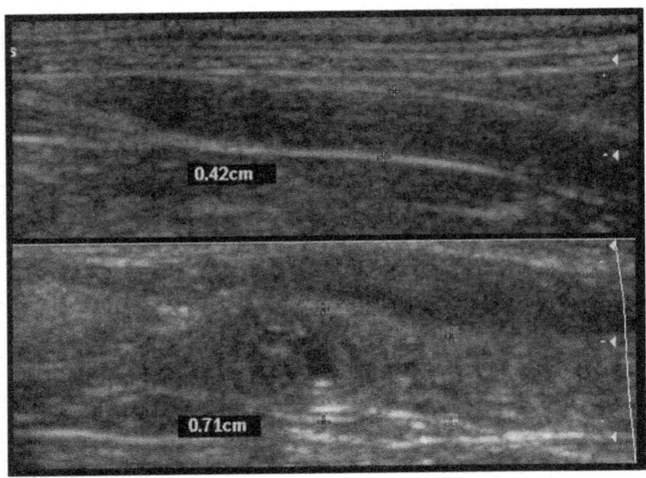

FIGURE 40-16 Ultrasonography shows endometrial thickening with focal anechoic structures representing dilated cystic glands in a uterus with cystic endometrial hyperplasia. *(Courtesy Delphine Rault.)*

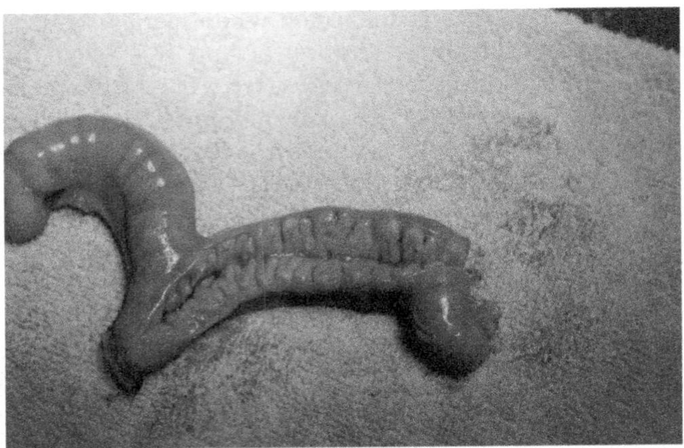

FIGURE 40-17 A uterus affected by cystic endometrial hyperplasia showing proliferative endometrium and thickening of the uterine wall.

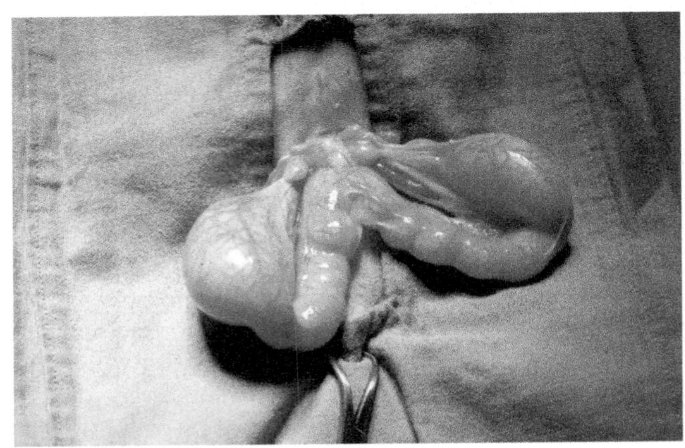

FIGURE 40-18 Pyometra may produce segmental uterine enlargement that may be mistaken for pregnancy on abdominal palpation.

to protect the uterus against pathologic changes. Many methods or medications used to control estrus in queens increase the risk of CEH and pyometra.

Endometritis is characterized by endometrial inflammation with the presence of neutrophils, lymphocytes, or plasma cells within the lamina propria. Bacterial infection is often present. The feline vagina hosts a wide range of normal bacterial flora, the most common of which are aerobes, such as *Escherichia coli* and *Streptococcus canis*, and is the source of ascending infections.[11,98] The only clinical sign of endometritis may be infertility as vulvar discharge may be scant or absent and the queen is typically otherwise well.

A definitive diagnosis of uncomplicated CEH or endometritis is difficult without uterine biopsy and histopathology. Ultrasonography may reveal endometrial thickening with focal anechoic structures representing dilated cystic glands and a small amount of luminal fluid (Figure 40-16).[17] However, there is no definitive set of ultrasound findings that distinguish between normal endometrial changes and CEH. A presumptive diagnosis is often made in queens that repeatedly ovulate after breeding but do not conceive, provided breeding management is appropriate and the fertility of the tom cat is proven. In many cases, the diagnosis is not confirmed until the uterus is examined after ovariohysterectomy (Figure 40-17). No definitive treatment is available for CEH, although some queens with endometritis may successfully carry a litter to term after treatment with a broad-spectrum antibiotic. In general, it is best to remove affected queens from the breeding program.

Pyometra is a severe endometrial infection with accumulation of purulent exudate in the uterine lumen. The most common bacterial species isolated in queens with pyometra is *Escherichia coli*.[16] Although one case report of pyometra associated with *Tritrichomonas foetus* has been published,[13] a study using microscopic, immunohistochemical and molecular methods found no evidence that the reproductive tract of cats is colonized by *T. foetus*.[35]

Diagnosis of pyometra is based on history, signalment, clinical signs, and physical examination findings. An intact queen with vulvar discharge should be assumed to have pyometra until proven otherwise. Pyometra has also been documented in queens with incomplete removal of the uterine body or horns.[18] The source of progesterone in these queens may be an ovarian remnant or exogenous progestins.

Clinical signs of pyometra in queens include sanguineous to mucopurulent vulvar discharge, lethargy, anorexia, abdominal distention, dehydration, polyuria, polydipsia, and pyrexia. The most important differential diagnosis for abdominal distention in an intact queen is pregnancy. Pyometra may produce either segmental or diffuse uterine enlargement, both of which may be mistaken for pregnancy on abdominal palpation (Figure 40-18). Queens with closed cervix pyometra have

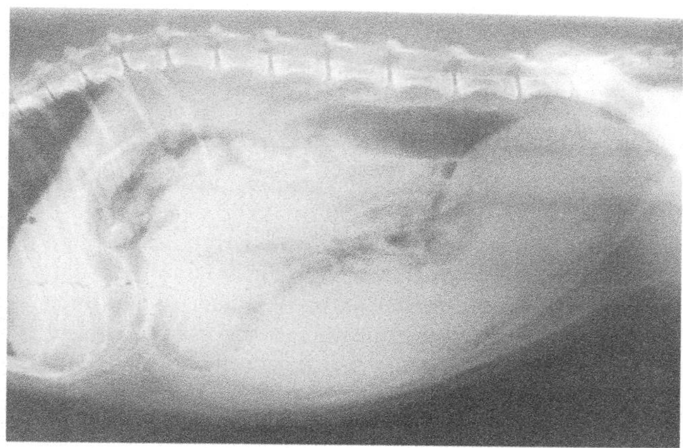

FIGURE 40-19 Radiography may demonstrate uterine enlargement in queens with pyometra but may not rule out pregnancy.

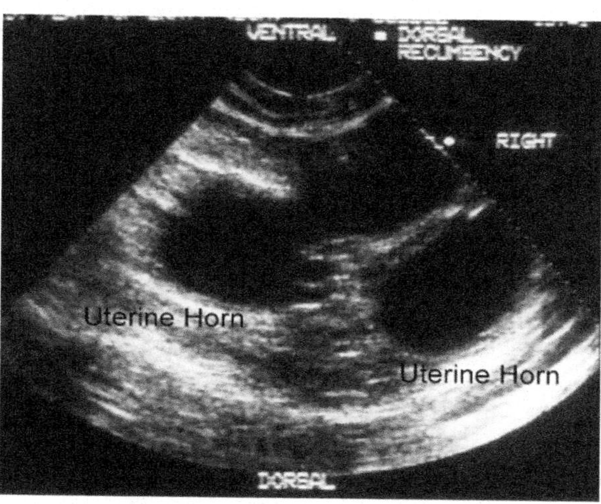

FIGURE 40-20 Typical ultrasonographic findings in queens with pyometra are an enlarged uterus with convoluted tubular horns filled with flocculent material of variable echogenicity.

abdominal enlargement with no vulvar discharge and may be severely ill due to septicemia. These queens have increased risk for uterine rupture and peritonitis.[16]

Laboratory abnormalities in queens with pyometra include mild anemia (normocytic, normochromic, nonregenerative), thrombocytopenia, leukocytosis with neutrophilia, as well as hyperproteinemia, hyperglobulinemia, hypokalemia, elevated alanine transaminase (ALT) and alkaline phosphatase (ALP), and azotemia.[16,60,77,85] Radiography may demonstrate uterine enlargement, but may not rule out pregnancy (Figure 40-19). Typical ultrasonographic findings are an enlarged uterus with convoluted tubular horns filled with flocculent material of variable echogenicity (Figure 40-20). Ultrasonography is preferred versus radiography for diagnosis and to rule out pregnancy. A queen may have pyometra in one uterine horn and viable fetuses in the other.[16]

Initial management of queens with pyometra depends on the status of the patient. Cats with closed cervix pyometra should be treated as emergency patients requiring urgent stabilization and surgical intervention. Cats with open cervix pyometra (diagnosed by the presence of vulvar discharge) are typically more stable and not in need of urgent intervention, although septicemia and endotoxemia are always a risk. Intravenous fluid therapy and correction of electrolyte imbalances may be necessary for some patients with open cervix pyometra. Broad-spectrum antibiotic therapy (e.g., a fluoroquinolone plus ampicillin) is initiated for all queens with pyometra and can be adjusted based on the results of culture and sensitivity testing of vulvar discharge.[117] Therapy should be continued for at least 3 weeks.

Antibiotic therapy alone will not resolve pyometra in the majority of queens. Therapeutic decisions should be based on the health status and age of the queen as well as reproductive value. Ovariohysterectomy is the treatment of choice for queens with closed cervix pyometra, critically ill queens, queens with uterine rupture or retained fetal material, and for queens without value to a breeding program. Surgical intervention is not without risk. In one study, 15 of 183 queens died or were euthanized after ovariohysterectomy for pyometra.[16] Postoperative complications, such as anorexia, lethargy, pyrexia, and vomiting occurred in 21% of the queens.

Young (<5 years of age), otherwise healthy nonpregnant queens with open cervix pyometra and reproductive value may be managed medically in an attempt to preserve fertility. In addition to broad-spectrum antibiotics, medical options for treatment include prostaglandins and antiprogestins.

Prostaglandin F_{2alpha} (Lutalyse, Pfizer Animal Health), also known as dinoprost tromethamine, is a naturally occurring prostaglandin administered to induce luteolysis and evacuation of uterine contents. However, luteolysis does not reliably occur with this drug in queens, especially early in diestrus. Prostaglandins are not recommended in closed cervix pyometra because of the risk of uterine rupture. Synthetic prostaglandins, such as cloprostenol and alfaprostol, have been used in the bitch, but experience with the use of these drugs in the queen for treatment of pyometra is lacking.

The most commonly recommended dose for PGF_{2alpha} is 0.1 mg/kg, SC, q12-24h although doses up to 0.25 mg/kg, SC, q12h have been published.[16,25] Smaller doses given more frequently have also been used to reduce side effects and increase the frequency of uterine contractions (e.g., 0.02 to 0.05 mg/kg, SC, 3 to 5 times daily).[110] The average length of treatment is 3 to 5 days, but treatment may be required for up to 10 days. Queens may be hospitalized during treatment for observation, especially during the first few days. The end point for treatment is reached when ultrasonographic examination shows a decrease in uterine size and no fluid in the uterine lumen, and the serum progesterone concentration is less than 2 ng/mL. Side effects from administration of PGF_{2alpha} are common, especially with the initial doses and when higher doses are used. Restlessness, panting, vomiting, defecation, tenesmus, salivation, and vocalizing have all been reported to occur within 60 minutes of administration.[16,25,52] The side effects are short lived and diminish with subsequent injections. Risks associated with PGF_{2alpha} in the queen are few when appropriate patients are chosen for treatment. The most serious risks are uterine rupture and leakage of uterine contents into the abdomen via the oviducts. These complications are very uncommon in queens with open cervix pyometra.

Queens should be reevaluated 1 to 2 weeks after therapy with a physical examination, ultrasonography, complete blood count, and serum chemistries. Abnormalities found on initial laboratory data should be resolved by 2 weeks posttreatment. A clear vulvar discharge may be present for several days after treatment. Affected queens should be bred at the next estrus. Most queens treated with PGF_{2alpha} have successfully delivered kittens following treatment.[16] Because most queens with pyometra have underlying CEH, recurrence has been noted in up to 14% of cases.[16] Queens with a recurrence of pyometra have been successfully re-treated, but the progressive and recurrent nature of the underlying disease warrants the removal of affected queens from the breeding program at the earliest opportunity.

More recently, the antiprogestin aglepristone (Alizin, Virbac) has been used in the queen for treatment of pyometra.[3,4,46,79] Antiprogestins are synthetic steroids that bind to progesterone receptors but lack the effects of progesterone. Intrauterine progesterone concentrations are reduced, allowing for increased myometrial contractility and opening of the cervix. Initially, serum progesterone concentrations are not affected. Aglepristone may be indicated for treatment of pyometra in queens with reproductive value and for queens that are a poor surgical risk. Compared with PGF_{2alpha}, aglepristone is an efficacious treatment without side effects that is administered less frequently. Disadvantages of the drug include cost, lack of licensing in cats, and limited availability.

In one study of 10 nulliparous queens with open cervix pyometra, aglepristone was administered at 10 mg/kg, SC on days 1, 2, and 7.[79] A fourth treatment was given on day 14 if necessary. A broad-spectrum antibiotic (trimethoprim/sulphadoxine) was also administered. The response to treatment was assessed by clinical signs, laboratory data and ultrasonographic findings 2 weeks after completion of treatment. No adverse effects were observed. Nine of 10 cats responded to treatment by day 14, with no recurrence in a 2-year follow-up period. Only two queens were subsequently bred, but both delivered live kittens.

BOX 40-12

Diagnostic Plan for Investigating Pregnancy Loss in the Queen

1. Collect a complete medical history, including vaccinations, control of internal and external parasites, past or current illnesses (reproductive and nonreproductive), and review prior laboratory data
2. Collect a complete reproductive history, including details of previous pregnancies and estrous cycles
3. Perform a complete physical examination
4. Collect preliminary laboratory data, including a complete blood count, serum chemistries, complete urinalysis, and feline leukemia virus (FeLV) and feline immunodeficiency virus (FIV) infection status
5. Evaluate diet quality, including nutritional supplements
6. Collect information on drugs (prescription and nonprescription) and supplements (e.g., botanicals, homeopathic products) administered
7. Evaluate breeding management, including breeding dates and method of pregnancy diagnosis
8. Evaluate cattery conditions, including population density, presence of disease, hygiene, and chemicals in use

Pregnancy Loss

Pregnancy loss in the queen includes all causes of pregnancy termination and may be characterized by fetal resorption, abortion of live or dead fetuses, stillbirths of full-term fetuses, or fetal death with retention of mummified or macerated fetuses in the uterus or abdominal cavity. Although pregnancy loss is a type of infertility, it must be investigated with specific etiologies in mind.

Ideally, the queen should be evaluated as soon after the event as possible to increase the chances of a definitive diagnosis. A definitive diagnosis allows for appropriate changes to management practices and use of specific therapies to reduce the risk of recurrence in future pregnancies or pregnancy loss in other queens in the cattery.

Preliminary investigation of pregnancy loss in the queen includes a complete medical and reproductive history, a full physical examination, and collection of laboratory data (Box 40-12). Breeding management and the queen's environment should also be evaluated. Information about herbal, homeopathic or traditional supplements that may have been administered to the queen or added to the diet should be sought. Breeders may use such products despite lack of scientific evidence of safety or efficacy.

Depending on the outcome of preliminary investigations, further diagnostic testing may be indicated. Radiography or ultrasonography is useful to detect retained fetal material and evaluate the uterus. Ultrasonography is preferred over radiography, because it provides more detailed information. Vulvar discharge, if present, can be sampled for culture and sensitivity testing as well as cytology.

Examination of any available fetal material can provide useful information, although this step is often omitted. Aborted fetuses and membranes may be refrigerated (not frozen) and submitted for histopathologic examination as soon as possible to a diagnostic laboratory with experience in reproductive and neonatal pathology. Additional testing, such as virus isolation or microbial culture, can be performed where indicated. Alternately, practitioners can perform a thorough neonatal necropsy and collect samples for laboratory analysis in a timely manner. The procedure for necropsy examination of neonates, including placentas and fetal membranes, has recently been described.[94]

The clinical signs associated with pregnancy loss are highly variable. Early fetal death and resorption usually do not result in clinical signs of illness. When fetal death occurs later in gestation, bloody or purulent vulvar discharge may occur, with or without clinical signs of illness (e.g., fever, anorexia, depression, vomiting, diarrhea). If spontaneous abortion of fetuses occurs, the queen may consume the fetal material before the owner notices.

Spontaneous abortion will result in the death of all or part of the litter, but the queen's life is rarely at risk. Systemically ill queens should be hospitalized for stabilization with intravenous fluids and other therapies as needed. Antibiotics are only administered if bacterial infection is likely based on clinical signs (e.g., purulent vulvar discharge), the complete blood count, and presence of fever. Hospitalization also allows for collection of diagnostic samples and evaluation of the uterus with radiography or ultrasonography.

Premature placental separation is associated with large amounts of bloody discharge late in gestation, and usually results in the loss of the litter. Excessive bleeding from the vulva is an indication for cesarean section in order to save the queen and possibly any live kittens.

If kittens are aborted, the uterus should be examined ultrasonographically to determine if any fetuses or fetal membranes are retained. The contents of the uterus can be evacuated with PGF_{2alpha} (0.25 mg/kg, IM) or ovariohysterectomy can be performed if the queen is not required for a breeding program. The queen should be treated with a broad-spectrum antibiotic for 2 to 4 weeks.

A variety of potential causes of pregnancy loss, both infectious (viral, bacterial, protozoal) and noninfectious, have been identified in queens (Box 40-13).[86,111] Although pregnancy loss is not as well studied in the queen as in the bitch, it appears the most important causes are noninfectious and viral.

BOX 40-13

Causes of Pregnancy Loss in the Queen

Infectious

1. Bacterial
   a. Coliforms
   b. *Streptococcus* spp.
   c. *Staphylococcus* spp.
   d. *Salmonella* spp.
2. Viral
   a. Feline panleukopenia virus (both natural and vaccine-induced)
   b. Feline leukemia virus
   c. Feline immunodeficiency virus
   d. Feline herpesvirus-1
3. Protozoal
   a. *Toxoplasma*

Noninfectious

1. Fetal factors
   a. Congenital and chromosomal anomalies
   b. Fetotoxic effects of drugs
2. Maternal factors
   a. Uterine disease
   b. Poor nutrition

Noninfectious causes of pregnancy loss include both maternal and fetal factors. Maternal factors include uterine disease and nutritional imbalances. Uterine disease, especially cystic endometrial hyperplasia, is an underestimated cause of pregnancy loss in queens because of the difficulty in obtaining a definitive diagnosis. As noted above, CEH is associated with implantation failure and early embryonic death without clinical signs of illness.

Because most owned cats are fed balanced commercial diets, nutritional causes of pregnancy loss are now uncommon. However, breeders may feed specialty commercial diets or home-prepared diets, either raw or cooked, that may not be appropriate for maintenance of pregnancy or that may contain pathogens. In addition, dietary supplements may contain substances harmful to the developing fetuses or that impair normal reproduction.

Taurine is an essential amino acid for cats and deficiency is classically associated with central retinal degeneration and dilated cardiomyopathy. The only sign of taurine deficiency in breeding queens may be fetal resorption, reduced litter size, and stillbirths. Fetal death occurs around day 25 of gestation, followed by resorption or abortion.[20] One study suggests that the effects of chronic taurine deficiency on reproduction may not be reversible.[20] Kittens born to taurine-deficient queens may have developmental abnormalities that include cerebellar dysfunction and abnormal hindlimb and thoracic anatomy.[99] Affected kittens are often born small and weak, with poor growth rates and low survival rates.[99]

Fetal factors associated with pregnancy loss include toxic effects of drugs, as well as congenital and chromosomal defects. Although many drugs are routinely administered to cats, the effect of most drugs on developing fetuses is not known. Most drugs cross the placenta, and some may achieve significant concentrations in fetuses. Some drugs are known to produce teratogenic or lethal effects during pregnancy and should be avoided.[83] These include certain antibiotics (e.g., chloramphenicol, metronidazole, tetracyclines, gentamicin), griseofulvin, nonsteroidal antiinflammatories, corticosteroids, misoprostol, testosterone and estrogen analogues, isotretinoin, antineoplastics, and organophosphate insecticides. In general, administration of any medication, prescription or nonprescription, should be avoided in pregnant queens unless benefits outweigh known or potential risks.

In domestic animals, genetic abnormalities are said to account for about 15% of pregnancy losses.[111] Known genetic defects associated with pregnancy loss include single-gene traits, such as Manx syndrome and polycystic kidney disease, where homozygotes die in utero. Fetal chromosomal errors, such as trisomy and 37,XO karyotypes, have been reported in the literature as causes of pregnancy loss.[55] Karyotyping of aborted fetuses is not commonly performed; so, the true prevalence of these defects is unknown.

The most important infectious causes of pregnancy loss in queens are viral diseases, such as feline herpesvirus-1, feline immunodeficiency virus, feline leukemia virus, and feline panleukopenia virus. Pregnancy loss may either be a direct effect of the virus or secondary to systemic illness and debilitation.

Feline herpesvirus-1 (FHV-1) is known to cause abortion in queens, probably resulting from debilitation rather than direct effects on the fetus or placenta.[111] Queens that become acutely ill during pregnancy, especially with fever, anorexia, and dehydration, are most at risk of pregnancy loss. FHV-1 may be enzootic in catteries, because control of disease is difficult. Breeders should have a well-designed vaccination program. However, vaccination can protect cats against severe disease but not necessarily against infection.

Feline immunodeficiency virus (FIV) can be transmitted to kittens by perinatally infected queens during both the prenatal and postnatal periods.[81] Transmission in utero may cause abortion, stillbirth, and low birth weights.[116] Feline leukemia virus (FeLV) can also be transmitted from an infected queen to kittens either in utero or in the postnatal period.[45] As for FIV, transmission in utero is associated with fetal or neonatal death. Breeding catteries should maintain rigorous testing programs for both FIV and FeLV, and infected cats should be removed from the cattery.

Infection of pregnant queens with feline panleukopenia virus (FPV) may have various outcomes.[36] The queen may not have classical signs of gastrointestinal disease, but the virus may infect rapidly dividing fetal cells. If infection occurs early in gestation, fetal death and resorption may occur. If infection occurs in midgestation, abortion may occur. Late gestation infections may cause neural damage, such as cerebellar hypoplasia, in liveborn kittens. All queens should be adequately vaccinated against FPV before breeding. The use of modified live virus vaccines against FPV should be avoided during pregnancy and in the first month of life, because the effects of vaccination on the developing fetuses or neonatal kittens may be similar to natural infection.

Feline coronavirus (FCoV) is a common pathogen in multicat environments. A virulent biotype of FCoV causes feline infectious peritonitis. In the older veterinary literature, reproductive failure, particularly resorption, was associated with FCoV in catteries. As the pathogenesis of this disease is better understood, it appears that FCoV infection is not a cause of pregnancy loss or neonatal mortality.[1]

Although pregnancy loss resulting from bacterial infection is uncommon in the queen, various bacterial species that ascend into the uterus from the vagina have occasionally been associated with pregnancy loss, including *Streptococcus*, *Staphylococcus*, and *E. coli*. *Brucella canis* is an important cause of pregnancy loss in the bitch but does not appear to be an important cause in queens.[86]

Chlamydial infections have been associated with reproductive disease in many species. *Chlamydophila felis* is an obligate intracellular pathogen that primarily infects the epithelial cells of the conjunctiva and upper respiratory tract. *C. felis* has long been suspected as a cause of infertility and abortion in queens, but definitive evidence is lacking.[102] Many catteries infected with *C. felis* do not have reproductive problems and attempts to isolate *C. felis* from the vagina of queens have met with variable success.

Cats are the definitive host for the protozoal parasite, *Toxoplasma gondii*. Experimental attempts to demonstrate transplacental infection of kittens following oral infection of queens have had variable outcomes.[86] Although toxoplasmosis does not appear to be an important cause of pregnancy loss in cats, infected queens may suffer abortion secondary to systemic illness and debilitation.

References

1. Addie D, Jarrett O: Feline coronavirus infections. In Greene C, editor: *Infectious diseases of the dog and cat*, ed 3, St Louis, 2006, Saunders Elsevier, p 88.
2. Agudelo CF: Cystic endometrial hyperplasia-pyometra complex in cats. A review, *Vet Q* 27:173, 2005.

3. Axner E: Catteries: reproductive performance and problems. In August J, editor: *Consultations in feline internal medicine*, ed 6, St Louis, 2010, Saunders Elsevier, p 834.
4. Axnér E, Ågren E, Båverud V et al: Infertility in the cycling queen: seven cases, *J Feline Med Surg* 10:566, 2008.
5. Axner E, Gustavsson T, Strom Holst B: Estradiol measurement after GnRH-stimulation as a method to diagnose the presence of ovaries in the female domestic cat, *Theriogenology* 70:186, 2008.
6. Baldwin C, Peter A, Evans L: Use of ELISA test kits for estimation of serum progesterone concentrations in cats, *Feline Pract* 24:27, 1996.
7. Chang J, Jung JH, Yoon J et al: Segmental aplasia of the uterine horn with ipsilateral renal agenesis in a cat, *J Vet Med Sci* 70:641, 2008.
8. Chatdarong K, Kampa N, Axner F et al: Investigation of cervical patency and uterine appearance in domestic cats by fluoroscopy and scintigraphy, *Reprod Domest Anim* 37:275, 2002.
9. Chatdarong K, Rungsipipat A, Axner E et al: Hysterographic appearance and uterine histology at different stages of the reproductive cycle and after progestagen treatment in the domestic cat, *Theriogenology* 64:12, 2005.
10. Church D, Watson A, Emslie D et al: Effects of proligestone and megestrol on plasma adrenocorticotrophic hormone, insulin and insulin-like growth factor-1 concentrations in cats, *Res Vet Sci* 56:175, 1994.
11. Clemetson L, Ward A: Bacterial flora of the vagina and uterus of healthy cats, *J Am Vet Med Assoc* 196:902, 1990.
12. da Silva TF, da Silva LD, Uchoa DC et al: Sexual characteristics of domestic queens kept in a natural equatorial photoperiod, *Theriogenology* 66:1476, 2006.
13. Dahlgren SS, Gjerde B, Pettersen HY: First record of natural *Tritrichomonas foetus* infection of the feline uterus, *J Small Anim Pract* 48:654, 2007.
14. Davidson A: Medical treatment of pyometra with prostaglandin F2alpha in the dog and cat. In Bonagura J, editor: *Current veterinary therapy XII: small animal practice*, Philadelphia, 1995, Saunders, p 1081.
15. Davidson A, Eilts B: Advanced small animal reproductive techniques, *J Am Anim Hosp Assoc* 42:10, 2006.
16. Davidson A, Feldman E, Nelson R: Treatment of pyometra in cats, using prostaglandin F2alpha: 21 cases (1982-1990), *J Am Vet Med Assoc* 200:825, 1992.
17. Davidson AP, Baker TW: Reproductive ultrasound of the bitch and queen, *Top Companion Anim Med* 24:55, 2009.
17a. Davidson A: Problems during and after parturition. In England G, von Heimendahl A, editors: *BSAVA manual of canine and feline reproduction and neonatology*, ed 2, Gloucester, 2010, British Small Animal Veterinary Association, p. 121.
18. de Faria VP, Norsworthy GD: Pyometra in a 13-year-old neutered queen, *J Feline Med Surg* 10:185, 2008.
19. DeNardo G, Becker K, Brown N et al: Ovarian remnant syndrome: revascularization of free-floating ovarian tissue in the feline abdominal cavity, *J Am Anim Hosp Assoc* 37:290, 2001.
20. Dieter JA, Stewart DR, Haggarty MA et al: Pregnancy failure in cats associated with long-term dietary taurine insufficiency, *J Reprod Fertil Suppl* 47:457, 1993.
21. Doherty D, Welsh E, Kirby B: Intestinal intussusception in five postparturient queens, *Vet Rec* 146:614, 2000.
22. Ekstrand C, Linde-Forsberg C: Dystocia in the cat: a retrospective study of 155 cases, *J Small Anim Pract* 35:459, 1994.
23. Erunal-Maral N, Aslan S, Findik M et al: Induction of abortion in queens by administration of cabergoline (Galastop) solely or in combination with the PGF2alpha analgoue alfaprostol (Gabbrostim), *Theriogenology* 61:1471, 2004.
24. Fascetti A, Hickman M: Preparturient hypocalcemia in four cats, *J Am Vet Med Assoc* 215:1127, 1999.
25. Feldman EC, Nelson RW: Feline reproduction. In Feldman EC, Nelson RW, editors: *Canine and feline endocrinology and reproduction*, ed 3, St Louis, 2004, Saunders, p 1016.
26. Ferretti L, Newell S, Graham J et al: Radiographic and ultrasonographic evaluation of the normal feline postpartum uterus, *Vet Radiol Ultrasound* 41:287, 2000.
27. Fieni F, Martal J, Marnet PG et al: Clinical, biological and hormonal study of mid-pregnancy termination in cats with aglepristone, *Theriogenology* 66:1721, 2006.
28. Georgiev P, Wehrend A: Mid-gestation pregnancy termination by the progesterone antagonist aglepristone in queens, *Theriogenology* 65:1401, 2006.
29. Georgiev P, Wehrend A, Penchev G et al: Histological changes of the feline cervix, endometrium and placenta after mid-gestational termination of pregnancy with aglepristone, *Reprod Domest Anim* 43:409, 2008.
30. Gimenez F, Stornelli MC, Tittarelli CM et al: Suppression of estrus in cats with melatonin implants, *Theriogenology* 72:493, 2009.
31. Goo M-J, Williams BH, Hong I-H et al: Multiple urogenital abnormalities in a Persian cat, *J Feline Med Surg* 11:153, 2009.
32. Goodrowe K, Howard J, Schmidt P et al: Reproductive biology of the domestic cat with special reference to endocrinology, sperm function and in-vitro fertilization, *J Reprod Fert Suppl* 39:73, 1989.
33. Gorlinger S, Kooistra HS, van den Broek A et al: Treatment of fibroadenomatous hyperplasia in cats with aglepristone, *J Vet Intern Med* 16:710, 2002.
34. Graham L, Swanson W, Wildt D et al: Influence of oral melatonin on natural and gonadotropin-induced ovarian function in the domestic cat, *Theriogenology* 61:1061, 2004.
35. Gray SG, Hunter SA, Stone MR et al: Assessment of reproductive tract disease in cats at risk for *Tritrichomonas foetus* infection, *Am J Vet Res* 71:76, 2010.
36. Greene C, Addie D: Feline parvovirus infections. In Greene C, editor: *Infectious diseases of the dog and cat*, ed 3, St Louis, 2006, Saunders Elsevier, p 78.
37. Griffin B: Prolific cats: the estrous cycle, *Comp Contin Edu Pract Vet* 23:1049, 2001.
38. Griffin B, Heath A, Young D et al: Effects of melatonin implants on ovarian function in the domestic cat [abstract], *J Vet Intern Med* 16:278, 2001.
39. Grundy SA: Clinically relevant physiology of the neonate, *Vet Clin North Am Small Anim Pract* 36:443, 2006.
40. Grundy SA, Liu SM, Davidson AP: Intracranial trauma in a dog due to being "swung" at birth, *Top Companion Anim Med* 24:100, 2009.
41. Gudermuth D, Newton L, Daels P et al: Incidence of spontaneous ovulation in young, group-housed cats based on serum and faecal concentrations of progesterone, *J Reprod Fertil Suppl* 51:177, 1997.
42. Gunn-Moore D, Thrusfield M: Feline dystocia: prevalence, and association with cranial conformation and breed, *Vet Rec* 136:350, 1995.
43. Hammer J: Use of a semi-quantitative canine progesterone test kit in the domestic cat, *J Am Anim Hosp Assoc* 30:50, 1994.
44. Haney D, Levy J, Newell S et al: Use of fetal skeletal mineralization for prediction of parturition date in cats, *J Am Vet Med Assoc* 223:1614, 2003.
45. Hartmann K: Feline leukemia virus infection. In Greene C, editor: *Infectious diseases of the dog and cat*, ed 3, St Louis, 2006, Saunders Elsevier, p 105.
46. Hecker B, Wehrend A, Bostedt H: Konservative Behandlung der Pyometra bei der Katze mit dem Antigestagen Aglepristone, *Kleintierpraxis* 45:845, 2000.
47. Howe LM: Surgical methods of contraception and sterilization, *Theriogenology* 66:500, 2006.

48. Ishida Y, Yahara T, Kasuya E et al: Female control of paternity during copulation: inbreeding avoidance in feral cats, *Behavior* 138:235, 2001.
49. Jochle W, Jochle M: Reproduction in a feral cat population and its control with a prolactin inhibitor, cabergoline, *J Reprod Fert Suppl* 47:419, 1993.
50. Johnston S: Premature gonadal failure in female dogs and cats, *J Reprod Fert Suppl* 39:65, 1989.
51. Johnston S, Root Kustritz M, Olson P: Disorders of the feline ovaries. In Johnston S, Root Kustritz M, Olson P, editors: *Canine and feline theriogenology*, Philadelphia, 2001, Saunders, p 453.
52. Johnston S, Root Kustritz M, Olson P: Disorders of the feline uterus and uterine tubes (oviducts). In Johnston S, Root Kustritz M, Olson P, editors: *Canine and feline theriogenology*, Philadelphia, 2001, Saunders, p 463.
53. Johnston S, Root Kustritz M, Olson P: The feline estrous cycle. In Johnston S, Root Kustritz M, Olson P, editors: *Canine and feline theriogenology*, Philadelphia, 2001, Saunders, p 396.
54. Johnston S, Root Kustritz M, Olson P: Feline parturition. In Johnston S, Root Kustritz M, Olson P, editors: *Canine and feline theriogenology*, Philadelphia, 2001, Saunders, p 431.
55. Johnston S, Root Kustritz M, Olson P: Feline pregnancy. In Johnston S, Root Kustritz M, Olson P, editors: *Canine and feline theriogenology*, Philadelphia, 2001, Saunders, p 414.
56. Johnston S, Root Kustritz M, Olson P: The postpartum period in the cat. In Johnston S, Root Kustritz M, Olson P, editors: *Canine and feline theriogenology*, Philadelphia, 2001, Saunders, p 438.
57. Johnston S, Root Kustritz M, Olson P: Prevention and termination of feline pregnancy. In Johnston S, Root Kustritz M, Olson P, editors: *Canine and feline theriogenology*, Philadelphia, 2001, Saunders, p 447.
58. Jurka P, Max A: Treatment of fibroadenomatosis in 14 cats with aglepristone—changes in blood parameters and follow-up, *Vet Rec* 165:657, 2009.
59. Jutkowitz L: Reproductive emergencies, *Vet Clin North Am Small Anim Pract* 35:397, 2005.
60. Kenney K, Matthiesen D, Brown N et al: Pyometra in cats: 183 cases (1979-1984), *J Am Vet Med Assoc* 191:1130, 1987.
61. Keskin A, Yilmazbas G, Yilmaz R et al: Pathological abnormalities after long-term administration of medroxyprogesterone acetate in a queen, *J Feline Med Surg* 11:518, 2009.
62. Kustritz M, Rudolph K: [Functional teratoma in a spayed cat], *J Am Vet Med Assoc* 219:1065, 2001.
63. Kutzler M, Wood A: Non-surgical methods of contraception and sterilization, *Theriogenology* 66:514, 2006.
64. Kutzler MA: Estrus induction and synchronization in canids and felids, *Theriogenology* 68:354, 2007.
65. Lawler D, Evans R, Reimers T et al: Histopathologic features, environmental factors, and serum estrogen, progesterone, and prolactin values associated with ovarian phase and inflammatory uterine disease in cats, *Am J Vet Res* 52:1747, 1991.
66. Lawler D, Johnston S, Hegstad R et al: Ovulation without cervical stimulation in domestic cats, *J Reprod Fert Suppl* 47:57, 1993.
67. Loretti A, Ilha M, Ordas J et al: Clinical, pathological and immunohistochemical study of feline mammary fibroepithelial hyperplasia following a single injection of depot medroxyprogesterone acetate, *J Feline Med Surg* 7:43, 2005.
68. Loveridge G, Rivers J: Bodyweight changes and energy intakes of cats during pregnancy and lactation. In Burger I, Rivers J, editors: *Nutrition of the dog and cat*, Cambridge, UK, 1989, Cambridge University Press, p 113.
69. MacDougall L: Mammary fibroadenomatous hyperplasia in a young cat attributed to treatment with megestrol acetate, *Can Vet J* 44:227, 2003.
70. Marcella KL, Ramirez M, Hammerslag KL: Segmental aplasia of the uterine horn in a cat, *J Am Vet Med Assoc* 186:179, 1985.
70a. Marti JA, Fernandez S: Clinical approach to mammary gland disease. In England G, von Heimendahl A, editors: *BSAVA manual of canine and feline reproduction and neonatology*, ed 2, Gloucester, 2010, British Small Animal Veterinary Association, p. 155.
71. Martin De Las Mulas J, Millan Y, Bautista MJ et al: Oestrogen and progesterone receptors in feline fibroadenomatous change: an immunohistochemical study, *Res Vet Sci* 68:15, 2000.
72. Mattoon J, Nyland T: Ovaries and uterus. In Nyland T, Mattoon J, editors: *Small animal diagnostic ultrasound*, ed 2, Philadelphia, 2002, Saunders, p 231.
73. Memon MA, Schelling SH: Non-patent left uterine horn and segmental aplasia of the right uterine horn in an infertile cat, *Vet Rec* 131:266, 1992.
74. Miller DM: Ovarian remnant syndrome in dogs and cats: 46 cases (1988-1992), *J Vet Diagn Invest* 7:572, 1995.
75. Moon P, Massat B, Pascoe P: Neonatal critical care, *Vet Clin North Am Small Anim Pract* 31:343, 2001.
76. Munson L, Bauman J, Asa C et al: Efficacy of the GnRH analogue deslorelin for suppression of oestrous cycles in cats, *J Reprod Fertil Suppl* 57:269, 2001.
77. Nak D, Misirlioglu D, Nak Y et al: Clinical laboratory findings, vaginal cytology and pathology in a controlled study of pyometra in cats, *Aust Vet Pract* 35:10, 2005.
78. Nak D, Nak Y, Seyrek-Intas K et al: Treatment of feline mammary fibroadenomatous hyperplasia with aglepristone, *Aust Vet Pract* 34:161, 2004.
79. Nak D, Nak Y, Tuna B: Follow-up examinations after medical treatment of pyometra in cats with the progesterone-antagonist aglepristone, *J Feline Med Surg* 11:499, 2009.
80. O'Brien CR, Wilkie JS: Calcinosis circumscripta following an injection of proligestone in a Burmese cat, *Aust Vet J* 79:187, 2001.
81. O'Neil L, Burkhard M, Hoover E: Frequent perinatal transmission of feline immunodeficiency virus by chronically infected cats, *J Virol* 70:2894, 1996.
82. Onclin K, Verstegen J: Termination of pregnancy in cats using a combination of cabergoline, a new dopamine agonist, and a synthetic PGF2 alpha, cloprostenol, *J Reprod Fertil Suppl* 51:259, 1997.
83. Papich M: Effects of drugs on pregnancy. In Kirk R, editor: *Current veterinary therapy X: small animal practice*, Philadelphia, 1989, Saunders, p 1291.
84. Perez J, Conley A, Dieter J et al: Studies on the origin of ovarian interstitial tissue and the incidence of endometrial hyperplasia in domestic and feral cats, *Gen Comp Endocrinol* 116:10, 1999.
85. Potter K, Hancock D, Gallina A: Clinical and pathologic features of endometrial hyperplasia, pyometra, and endometritis in cats: 79 cases (1980-1985), *J Am Vet Med Assoc* 198:1427, 1991.
86. Pretzer SD: Bacterial and protozoal causes of pregnancy loss in the bitch and queen, *Theriogenology* 70:320, 2008.
87. Pretzer SD: Medical management of canine and feline dystocia, *Theriogenology* 70:332, 2008.
88. Purswell BJ, Kolster KA: Immunocontraception in companion animals, *Theriogenology* 66:510, 2006.
89. Ridyard A, Welsh E, Gunn-Moore D: Successful treatment of uterine torsion in a cat with severe metabolic and haemostatic complications, *J Feline Med Surg* 2:115, 2000.
90. Root MV, Johnston SD, Olson PN: Estrous length, pregnancy rate, gestation and parturition lengths, litter size, and juvenile mortality in the domestic cat, *J Am Anim Hosp Assoc* 31:429, 1995.
91. Say L, Pontier D, Natoli E: High variation in multiple paternity of domestic cats *(Felis catus L.)* in relation to environmental conditions, *Proc Biol Sci* 266:2071, 1999.
92. Scebra L, Griffin B: Evaluation of a commercially available luteinizing hormone test to distinguish between ovariectomized and sexually intact queens [abstract], *J Vet Intern Med* 17:432, 2003.
93. Scebra L, Griffin B, Dodson A: Pregnancy detection in cats using a commercially available relaxin assay [abstract], *J Vet Intern Med* 17:432, 2003.

94. Schlafer DH: Canine and feline abortion diagnostics, *Theriogenology* 70:327, 2008.
95. Shille V, Munro C, Farmer S et al: Ovarian and endocrine responses in the cat after coitus, *J Reprod Fertil* 69:29, 1983.
96. Skarda R: Anesthesia case of the month, *J Am Vet Med Assoc* 214:37, 1999.
97. Sparkes AH, Rogers K, Henley WE et al: A questionnaire-based study of gestation, parturition and neonatal mortality in pedigree breeding cats in the UK, *J Feline Med Surg* 8:145, 2006.
98. Strom Holst B, Bergstrom A, Lagerstedt AS et al: Characterization of the bacterial population of the genital tract of adult cats, *Am J Vet Res* 64:963, 2003.
99. Sturman JA, Messing JM: Dietary taurine content and feline reproduction and outcome, *J Nutr* 121:1195, 1991.
100. Swanson W, Horohov D, Godke R: Production of exogenous gonadotropin-neutralizing immunoglobulins in cats after repeated eCG-hCG treatment and relevance for assisted reproduction in felids, *J Reprod Fertil* 105:35, 1995.
101. Swanson W, Roth T, Wildt D: In vivo embryogenesis, embryo migration, and embryonic mortality in the domestic cat, *Biol Reprod* 51:452, 1994.
102. Sykes JE: Feline chlamydiosis, *Clin Tech Small Anim Pract* 20:129, 2005.
103. Tamada H, Kawate N, Inaba T et al: Long-term prevention of estrus in the bitch and queen using chlormadinone acetate, *Can Vet J* 44:416, 2003.
104. Traas AM: Resuscitation of canine and feline neonates, *Theriogenology* 70:343, 2008.
105. Traas AM: Surgical management of canine and feline dystocia, *Theriogenology* 70:337, 2008.
106. Tsutsui T, Amano T, Shimizu T et al: Evidence for transuterine migration of embryos in the domestic cat, *Nippon Juigaku Zasshi* 51:613, 1989.
107. Tsutsui T, Stabenfeldt G: Biology of ovarian cycles, pregnancy and pseudopregnancy in the domestic cat, *J Reprod Fert Suppl* 47:29, 1993.
108. Veronesi MC, Panzani S, Faustini M et al: An Apgar scoring system for routine assessment of newborn puppy viability and short-term survival prognosis, *Theriogenology* 72:401, 2009.
109. Verstegen J: Physiology and endocrinology of reproduction in female cats. In Simpson G, England GCW, Harvey M, editors: *Manual of small animal reproduction and neonatology*, Cheltenham, UK, 1998, British Small Animal Veterinary Association, p 11.
110. Verstegen J: Contraception and pregnancy termination. In Ettinger S, Feldman E, editors: *Textbook of veterinary internal medicine*, ed 5, Philadelphia, 2000, Saunders, p 1542.
111. Verstegen J, Dhaliwal G, Verstegen-Onclin K: Canine and feline pregnancy loss due to viral and non-infectious causes: a review, *Theriogenology* 70:304, 2008.
112. Verstegen J, Onclin K, Silva L et al: Abortion induction in the cat using prostaglandin F2alpha and a new anti-prolactinic agent, cabergoline, *J Reprod Fert Suppl* 47:411, 1993.
113. Verstegen J, Onclin K, Silva L et al: Regulation of progesterone during pregnancy in the cat: studies on the roles of corpora lutea, placenta and prolactin secretion, *J Reprod Fert Suppl* 47:165, 1993.
114. Verstegen JP, Silva LD, Onclin K et al: Echocardiographic study of heart rate in dog and cat fetuses in utero, *J Reprod Fertil Suppl* 47:175, 1993.
115. Watson P, Glover T: Vaginal anatomy of the domestic cat *(Felis catus)* in relation to copulation and artificial insemination, *J Reprod Fertil Suppl* 47:355, 1993.
116. Weaver C, Burgess S, Nelson P et al: Placental immunopathology and pregnancy failure in the FIV-infected cat, *Placenta* 26:138, 2005.
117. Wiebe VJ, Howard JP: Pharmacologic advances in canine and feline reproduction, *Top Companion Anim Med* 24:71, 2009.
118. Zambelli D, Caneppele B, Bassi S et al: Ultrasound aspects of fetal and extrafetal structures in pregnant cats, *J Feline Med Surg* 4:95, 2002.
119. Zambelli D, Castagnetti C, Belluzzi S et al: Correlation between fetal age and ultrasonographic measurements during the second half of pregnancy in domestic cats *(Felis catus)*, *Theriogenology* 62:1430, 2004.
120. Zambelli D, Prati F: Ultrasonography for pregnancy diagnosis and evaluation in queens, *Theriogenology* 66:135, 2006.

CHAPTER

41

Pediatrics

Susan E. Little

OUTLINE

Most veterinarians have been presented with kittens that have failed to thrive, often called "fading kitten syndrome." These patients are challenging due to their small size, their unfamiliar physiology, and the tendency for their status to deteriorate quickly. Sick neonates should be examined as soon as possible with a systematic approach, including a complete history of the kitten, litter, and queen; examination of the kitten and queen; and diagnostic tests.[21,52]

KITTEN MORBIDITY AND MORTALITY

High-risk time points for kitten morbidity and mortality are at birth, in the first 2 weeks of life, and around the time of weaning. There is no specific disease entity attributable to "fading kittens," but rather a variety of causes have been identified. "Toxic milk syndrome" is often implicated when the cause of neonatal illness or death cannot be determined. There is no evidence that such a syndrome exists in kittens, and attention should be focused on finding the actual cause of illness or death. The most common causes of morbidity and mortality in kittens include[20,39]

- Perinatal events (e.g., dystocia, poor maternal care)
- Low birth weight
- Congenital defects
- Failure of passive transfer of immunity
- Neonatal isoerythrolysis
- Inadequate nutrition
- Environmental factors (e.g., poor ventilation, temperature fluctuations, overcrowding)
- Infectious diseases

In free-roaming populations, kitten mortality may be as high as 75%, with trauma and infectious disease accounting for most deaths.[60] The lowest mortality rates (less than 5%) are found in well-managed, specific–pathogen-free colonies. Pedigreed breeding catteries are a unique opportunity to collect feline reproduction data, including data on neonatal health and illness. In a study in the United Kingdom, data were collected using a convenience-sampling questionnaire on the births of 1056 litters (4814 kittens), representing 14 pedigreed breeds.[75] The breeds included in the study were Persian, Burmese, Siamese, British Shorthair, Oriental Shorthair, Birman, Devon and Cornish Rex (data analyzed together), Asian, Abyssinian, Korat, Somali, Maine Coon, Tonkinese, and Exotic Shorthair. Several parameters were affected by breed, such as mean stillbirth rate (highest in Persians and Exotic Shorthairs, lowest in Maine Coon) and mean kitten birth weight (highest in Maine Coon, lowest in Korat). Selected data from this study are summarized in Table 41-1.

In another study of 1191 litters (4804 kittens), data were collected prospectively using an Internet-based convenience-sampling submission system on 11 breeds

TABLE 41-1 Breed-Specific Reproduction Data Collected Using a Questionnaire-Based Survey in the United Kingdom

Breed	Number of Litters (Total = 1,056)	Mean Litter Size (No. Kittens)	Mean Birth Weight (Grams)*	Mean % Kittens Born Alive	Mean % Alive at 8 Weeks	% Litters with ≥1 Kitten Defects
Persian	212	3.8	92.8	89	75	9
Burmese	150	5.7	86.2	93	84	20
Siamese	138	4.9	92.4	92	82	19
British Shorthair	110	4.6	104.4	94	87	11
Oriental Shorthair	92	4.7	89.8	92	83	24
Birman	88	3.6	101.0	98	94	7
Devon + Cornish Rex	47	4.2	91.4	92	84	13
Asian†	41	6.5	84.7	95	93	19
Abyssinian	40	3.9	100.0	98	94	11
Korat	32	4.6	72.7	97	85	28
Somali	31	3.6	90.7	94	86	10
Maine Coon	27	4.6	116.1	99	90	15
Tonkinese	27	5.3	84.1	93	82	31
Exotic Shorthair	21	4.2	97.2	88	82	5
Overall means		4.6	93.5	93	84	14

*Kittens born alive.

†The Asian breed is similar to the Burmese but with a wider range of colors and patterns (tabbies, smokes, and solids or selfs). It also includes the Burmilla, Bombay, and Tiffanie.

Modified from Sparkes AH, Rogers K, Henley WE et al: A questionnaire-based study of gestation, parturition and neonatal mortality in pedigree breeding cats in the UK, *J Feline Med Surg* 8:145, 2006.

(S. Little, unpublished data, 2001 to 2005). Breeders submitting data were located primarily in the United States and Europe. The breeds included in the study were Bengal, Birman, Egyptian Mau, Havana Brown, Manx, Munchkin, Norwegian Forest Cat, Ocicat, Ragdoll, Devon Rex, and Sphynx. The mean stillbirth rate was highest in the Havana Brown and lowest in the Ocicat and Devon Rex. Mean kitten birth weight was highest in the Norwegian Forest Cat and lowest in the Havana Brown. Selected data from this study are summarized in Tables 41-2 and 41-3.

Data from such studies are very useful to help breeders evaluate their breeding programs and identify areas of poor performance. For example, mean kitten mortality by 4 to 8 weeks of age in these studies is approximately 15%. A study in Sweden involving 694 litters from various breeds calculated mean kitten mortality by 12 weeks of age as 18%.[76] Breeders experiencing greater losses should investigate possible causes. Caution must be exercised, however, because even though breeds may have the same name and similar phenotype in different countries, the genetic constitution may be quite different. A good example is the Burmese breed. The definition of this breed varies by country and registering organization, leading to genetically distinct populations with different disease risks.

EXAMINATION OF THE NEONATAL KITTEN

Neonatal kittens (up to 4 weeks of age) cannot be approached as small adults. Not only is their physiology different, but the basic approach to history and examination is different. Start with a complete medical history for the kitten in question as well as for littermates. It may also be helpful to have a medical history for the queen if available (e.g., illness, nutrition, vaccinations) and information about the labor and delivery, especially for kittens less than 2 weeks of age.

Investigate the kitten's home environment, noting temperature and humidity, sanitation, population size and density, and prevalence of infectious diseases and parasites. A home visit can gather important information, especially when working with breeders. However, if a home visit is not possible, the breeder can be asked to supply a floor plan and photos to help identify management issues. Unfortunately, little information exists on the optimum design of breeding catteries. Recommendations are often adapted from those designed for laboratory animals, or boarding facilities.[66] The Cat Fanciers' Association (http://www.cfa.org) has produced minimum requirements for catteries that address the environment (e.g., temperature, ventilation, lighting),

TABLE 41-2 **Breed-Specific Reproduction Data Collected Using an Internet-Based Survey from Breeders Primarily in the United States and Europe, 2001 to 2005**

Breed	Number of Litters (Total = 1,191)	Mean Litter Size (No. Kittens)	Mean Birth Weight (Grams)*	Mean % Kittens Born Alive	Mean % Alive at 4 Weeks
Ragdoll	232	4.4	98.8	95	90
Birman	204	3.6	95.3	93	87
Bengal	176	4.0	94.1	94	82
Ocicat	136	4.3	98.2	96	86
Norwegian Forest cat	124	4.5	105.3	95	89
Devon Rex	103	3.7	86.1	96	87
Munchkin	54	4.1	83.5	94	83
Egyptian Mau	52	3.7	104.9	94	89
Sphynx	50	4.0	95.5	95	80
Manx	39	3.1	93.4	92	82
Havana Brown	21	3.9	91.1	89	83
Overall means		4.0	95.1	94	85

*Kittens born alive.

TABLE 41-3 **Data on Congenital Defects in Selected Pedigreed Cat Breeds Collected Using an Internet-Based Survey from Breeders Primarily in the United States and Europe, 2001 to 2005**

Breed	No. Litters	% Litters with at Least One Congenital Defect	Examples of Congenital Defects
Bengal	181	18	FCK, PE, CP, UH, SYN
Birman	217	12	DER, UH, SYN, CP, GAS
Burmese: traditional	94	15	FCK
Burmese: contemporary	54	80	HD, DER, FCK
European Burmese	66	15	FCK
Devon Rex	204	13	FCK, CP, UH
Egyptian Mau	52	23	UH
Havana Brown	27	11	UH, FCK
Manx	31	13	GAS
Munchkin	54	11	CP, UH, GAS
Norwegian Forest cat	124	5	FCK, CP
Ocicat	128	25	FCK, PE, XIPH
Ragdoll	199	13	CP, COL
Sphynx	104	9	CP, PE, UH

COL, Eyelid coloboma; *CP,* cleft palate; *DER,* dermoids (nasal and ocular); *FCK,* flat chest defect; *GAS,* gastroschisis; *HD,* craniofacial (head) defect; *PE,* pectus excavatum; *SYN,* syndactyly; *UH,* umbilical hernia; *XIPH,* everted xiphoid process.

hygiene, and caging facilities. Although written about 20 years ago, valuable information on cattery design is found in *Feline Husbandry: Diseases and Management in the Multiple-Cat Environment* (http://www.vetmed.ucdavis.edu/ccah/felinehusbandry.cfm).[62]

Neonatal kittens should be examined with the queen and any available litter mates when possible, and in the home or cattery if problems are ongoing. Neonates should be handled gently, on a warm surface, such as a clean towel. Wash your hands and wear gloves. Simple

BOX 41-1

Developmental Milestones for Kittens

Umbilical cord falls off: 3 days of age
Eyelids open: 10 days of age (range 2 to 16 days)
Menace/pupillary light reflexes: 28 days of age or later
Normal vision: 30 days of age
Adult iris color: 4 to 6 weeks of age
Ear canals open: 9 days of age (range 6 to 17 days)
Functional hearing: 4 to 6 weeks of age
Crawling: 7 to 14 days of age
Walking: 14 to 21 days of age
Voluntary elimination: 3 weeks of age
Deciduous incisors/canines erupt: 3 to 4 weeks of age
Deciduous premolars erupt: 5 to 6 weeks of age

equipment will suffice: gram scale, pediatric digital rectal thermometer, otoscope with infant cones, penlight, and stethoscope with an infant bell and diaphragm.

One of the first challenges facing the clinician examining the neonatal kitten is to determine the age and sex. Unless the kitten comes from a breeding cattery, the exact birth date is often unknown. Several developmental milestones and parameters can be used to estimate the age of kittens (Box 41-1), such as dentition and body weight (see below). Sex may be surprisingly difficult to determine in very young kittens, especially without another kitten of opposite sex for comparison, because testicles are not readily visible until more than 6 weeks of age. In male kittens, the distance between the anus and genitals is greater (about 1.25 cm [0.5 inches]) than for female kittens. The genitals appear slitlike in female and appear rounded in the male. Coat color may also be a clue; almost all calico or tortoiseshell kittens are females, and orange kittens are most likely to be male (but not exclusively so).

Before handling the kitten, observe its body condition and response to the environment, including alertness, posture, locomotion, and respiratory rate. Healthy neonates will have strong righting, rooting, and suckling reflexes. Muscle tone should not be too flaccid or too rigid. Flexor muscle tone predominates for the first few days of life so that newborn kittens typically rest in a curled position. Once extensor tone develops, kittens rest on their side or chest with head extended. Normal kittens sleep about 80% of the time and are generally quiet when healthy, warm, and well fed. When stressed by hunger, the absence of the queen, or other reasons, normal kittens will cry and crawl around the nest box, moving the head from side to side in a searching motion. Pain perception is present from birth, but withdrawal reflexes are not well developed until about 1 week of age. Sick kittens have a limited number of clinical signs (e.g., crying, restlessness, failure to gain weight, weakness, respiratory difficulty, diarrhea), and therefore changes from normal should be investigated promptly.

Normal body temperature for newborns is 97° F to 98° F (36° C to 37° C). The rectal temperature rises slowly, reaching 100° F (38° C) by about 4 weeks of age. For the first few weeks of life, kittens are poikilothermic, relying on external sources of heat. Neonatal kittens are very susceptible to cooling because of their high surface area to body weight ratio, immature metabolism, immature shiver reflex, and poor vasoconstrictive abilities. The ability to shiver begins around 1 week of age. They gradually become homeothermic by 4 weeks of age.

The typical kitten birth weight is 90 to 110 g (range, 80 to 140 g), although there is considerable variation by breed (see Tables 41-1 and 41-2) and by sex (males typically weigh more than females).[75] Low birth weight is a common cause of mortality, with kittens weighing less than 75 g at birth at highest risk. Slight weight loss (less than 10%) can occur in the first 24 hours of life, but the kitten should then gain weight daily. Normal kittens gain 50 to 100 g per week (10 to 15 g/day) and should double their birth weight by 2 weeks of age. Breeders and other caretakers of newborn kittens should be instructed to weigh the kittens twice daily for the first 2 weeks of life, and then daily for at least the next 2 to 4 weeks. Often the earliest sign of illness is failure to gain weight in a 24-hour period.

Poor nutrition or inadequate nursing is a common cause of failure to gain weight. Smaller or weaker kittens may be excluded from nursing by stronger litter mates. Other causes of poor nutritional intake include congenital defects, such as cleft palate, or maternal factors, such as mastitis, systemic illness, or poor body condition.

The first deciduous teeth to appear are the incisors and canines at 3 to 4 weeks of age. The premolars erupt at about 5 to 6 weeks of age. The dental formula for deciduous teeth is 2(I3/3, C1/1, P3/2); there are no deciduous molars.

Inspect the kitten for gross anatomic abnormalities, such as cleft palate or lip, umbilical hernia or infection (omphalophlebitis), open fontanelles, limb deformities, chest wall deformities, and nonpatent urogenital or rectal openings. The normal umbilical cord is dry, with no redness, swelling, or discharge at the umbilicus (Figure 41-1). Umbilical cords will fall off at about 3 or 4 days of age.

Kittens younger than about 3 weeks of age cannot eliminate urine and feces voluntarily. The kitten's micturition and defecation reflexes can be evaluated by using a cotton ball with mineral oil to stimulate the anogenital area. Gastrointestinal function is well developed at birth, and normal flora is acquired within the first few days of life. Diarrhea is present in about 60% of sick neonatal kittens. Normal neonatal urine is dilute and pale in color. Hematuria or pigmenturia may

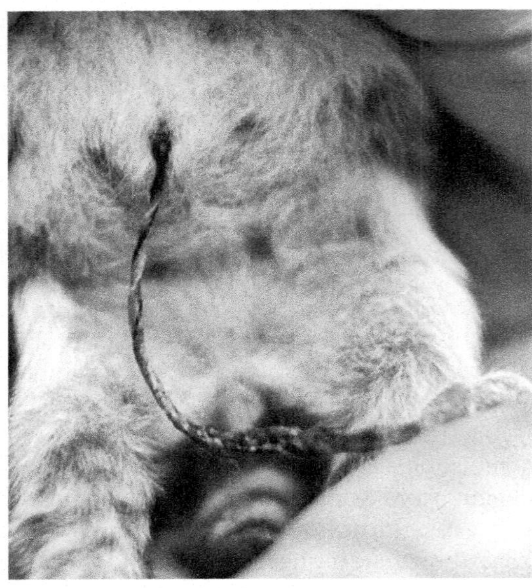

FIGURE 41-1 The normal umbilical cord is dry, with no redness, swelling, or discharge at the umbilicus and falls off at about 3 to 4 days of age.

> **BOX 41-2**
> **Normal Physiologic Values for Neonatal Kittens**
>
> *Birth weight:* 90 to 110 g
> *Rectal temperature (newborn):* 97° F to 98° F (36° C to 37° C)
> *Rectal temperature (1 month):* 100°F (38° C)
> *Heart rate:* 220 to 260 beats/minute for the first 2 weeks of life
> *Respiratory rate (newborn):* 10 to 18 breaths/minute
> *Respiratory rate (1 week):* 15 to 35 breaths/minute
> *Urine specific gravity:* <1.020
> *Urine output:* 25 mL/kg/day
> *Water requirement:* 130 to 220 mL/kg/day
> *Caloric requirement:* 20 kcal ME/100 g/day
> *Stomach capacity:* 4 to 5 mL/100 g
>
> *ME,* Metabolizable energy.

be signs of urinary tract infection, trauma, or neonatal isoerythrolysis. Dark yellow urine is typically a sign of dehydration in neonates.

The eyes should be inspected for abnormalities of the globe or eyelids and for neonatal conjunctivitis (ophthalmia neonatorum, see below). The eyelids typically open at about 10 days of age, but occasionally kittens are born with eyes already open, or the eyes open in the first day or two of life. Because tear production will not be normal for several weeks, a topical lubricating ophthalmic ointment should be applied for about the first week of life to prevent corneal damage. A menace reflex does not appear until 28 days of age or later. Pupillary light responses may appear as late as 28 days as well. A divergent strabismus may be present and may be normal until about 8 weeks of age. Evaluation of the fundus is difficult until after 6 weeks of age.

The pinnae should be inspected for evidence of trauma, parasites such as ear mites, and skin disease. The ear canals are not easy to inspect with an otoscope until after 4 weeks of age. The neonate's hair coat should be clean and shiny. Healthy neonatal kittens may have hyperemic mucous membranes until 7 days of age, whereas sick neonates often have pale, gray, or cyanotic mucous membranes.

Neonatal kittens may have lower blood pressure than adults, as well as greater cardiac output, and a faster heart rate in the first 2 weeks of life. Functional murmurs may be present in neonates because of anemia, hypoproteinemia, fever, or sepsis. Innocent murmurs not associated with disease are more common in puppies than kittens; murmurs still present after 4 months of age should be investigated. Congenital heart disease usually produces murmurs that are loud and accompanied by a precordial thrill. The normal neonatal heart rate can be more than 200 beats per minute in the first 2 weeks of life (range 220 to 260). By 4 weeks of age, once vagal tone has been established, the heart rate decreases to the normal adult range. The normal respiratory rate is 15 to 35 breaths per minute. See Box 41-2 for normal physiologic values for neonatal kittens.

A full abdomen is normal in a well-fed kitten, but an enlarged abdomen in an ill kitten may indicate aerophagia. The normal liver and spleen may not palpable; the kidneys are frequently palpable. The stomach may be palpable if it is full. The intestinal tract is palpable as fluid-filled bowel loops that should be freely moveable and nonpainful. The urinary bladder is also palpable, moveable, and should be nonpainful.

CONGENITAL DEFECTS

Congenital defects are abnormalities of structure, function, or metabolism that are present at birth. A defect may cause physical impairment, or it may cause the death of the kitten before or after birth. Congenital defects in stillborn kittens often go unrecognized, because few stillborns are submitted for complete necropsy. Many congenital defects are cosmetic or minor, while others may cause serious impairment of health (Box 41-3). Congenital defects may be of various types:

- Obvious at birth (e.g., cleft palate [Figure 41-2] or imperforate anus [Figure 41-3])
- Found only with diagnostic testing or at necropsy (e.g., diaphragmatic hernia)
- Subtle abnormalities found only with sophisticated testing (e.g., lysosomal storage diseases)

BOX 41-3
Selected Common Congenital Defects in Kittens

Eyes and Ears

- Glaucoma
- Colobomas
- Microphthalmia
- Corneal dermoids
- Congenital nystagmus

Neurologic

- Hydrocephalus
- Cerebellar hypoplasia
- Deafness

Skin and Musculature

- Hypotrichosis
- Umbilical hernia
- Gastroschisis/schistosoma (abdominal hernia)

Cardiac

- Patent ductus arteriosus
- Atrioventricular defects

Skeletal

- Radial hemimelia
- Polydactyly
- Syndactyly
- Flat chest defect
- Pectus excavatum ("funnel chest")

Urogenital

- Renal aplasia/hypoplasia
- Ambiguous genitalia/pseudohermaphroditism
- Cryptorchidism

Endocrine

- Congenital hypothyroidism/dwarfism

Gastrointestinal

- Cleft palate
- Atresia ani/anogenital fistula

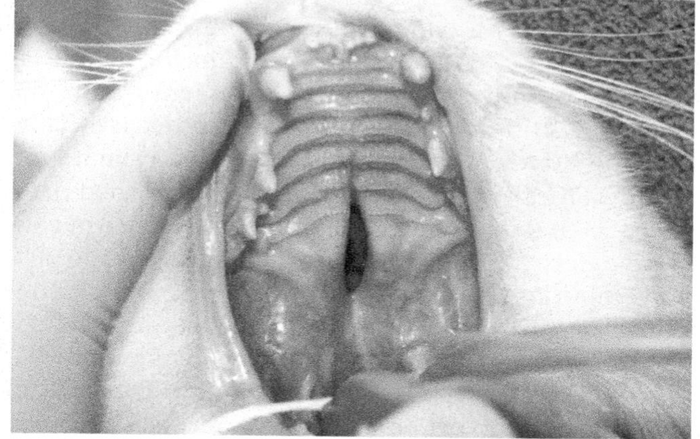

FIGURE 41-2 All kittens should be examined at birth for the presence of cleft palate, a common congenital defect. *(Courtesy Chris Carter.)*

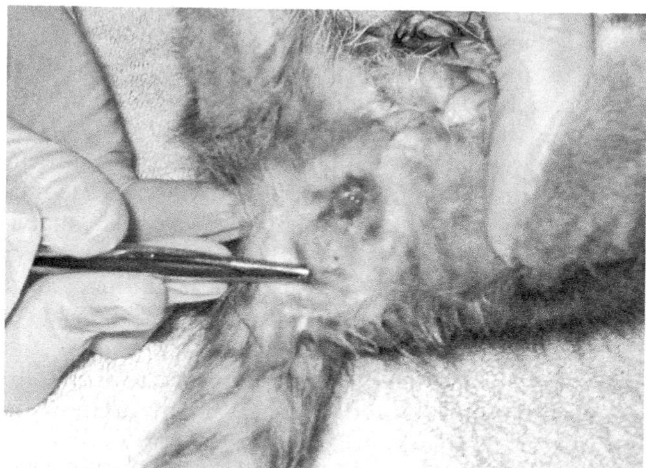

FIGURE 41-3 This female kitten has an imperforate anus and an anovaginal fistula. *(Courtesy Rosalyn MacDonald.)*

Feline fetal development can be divided into three stages: preimplantation (days 0 to 12), embryogenesis (days 12 to 24), and fetal growth (day 24 to term). The "critical period" is the stage during which each developing organ or structure is most sensitive to disruption. For most organs and structures, the critical period occurs during embryogenesis, in the third and fourth weeks of gestation. At the end of embryogenesis, the fetus is about ½ inch long. Developmental errors that occur during the first 2 weeks of gestation are usually lethal. It is also important to note that a defect in the development of one organ system or structure can result in the abnormal development of other organs or structures.

A teratogen is anything that disrupts normal fetal development (e.g., a drug or chemical). The timing of exposure of the fetus and the dose are important factors in determining outcome. Embryos are susceptible to teratogens, but this susceptibility tends to decrease as the critical developmental period for each organ system

BOX 41-4

Examples of Nongenetic Causes of Congenital Defects in Kittens

1. Infections in utero
   a. Usually viral, for instance, panleukopenia virus as a cause of cerebellar hypoplasia
2. Drugs
   a. For instance, griseofulvin as a cause of cleft palate
3. Chemicals, environmental toxins
4. Hyperthermia
   a. For instance, fever, high ambient temperatures, resting on heating pads, radiators or hot air vents, and so forth
5. Poor intrauterine environment
   a. For instance, inadequate development of the placenta, cystic endometrial hyperplasia/pyometra complex
6. Nutritional factors
   a. For instance, taurine deficiency as a cause of neurologic abnormalities[79]

passes. This makes the fetus increasingly resistant to the effects of teratogens with age, with the exception of structures that differentiate late in gestation, such as the cerebellum, palate, and urogenital system.

Congenital defects may be heritable, and the inheritance pattern or mutation(s) responsible may or may not be known (see Chapter 44). A few congenital defects are due to chromosomal abnormalities, such as pseudohermaphroditism. Many congenital defects are not heritable but caused by other factors (Box 41-4). In some cases, defects may be caused by interplay of both environmental and genetic factors. When pedigreed breeders encounter a congenital defect where no information is available on heritability, several factors can be evaluated. A defect is more likely to be heritable if there is evidence of a breed or familial predisposition and the problem has a consistent age of onset and clinical course. A defect is less likely to be heritable if more than one abnormality occurs in a kitten or a litter or there is potential exposure to teratogens. An informative fact sheet ("What to do if your cat produces a deformed kitten?") has been produced by the Feline Advisory Bureau to advise breeders on steps to take if a defect is observed (http://www.fabcats.org).

As in many other species, congenital defects are a significant contributor to neonatal mortality in the cat. Excellent reviews of congenital defects have been published,[31] including neurologic,[38] ocular,[25,56] renal,[26] cardiac,[45] and vertebral column defects.[57] There are also studies of congenital defects specifically in pedigreed cat breeds in the literature. One study noted that congenital disease was more common in pedigreed kittens than in the nonpedigreed kittens in a necropsy examination of 274 kittens aged up to 16 weeks.[9] However, the difference was not statistically significant and no individual breed of cat was significantly predisposed to congenital diseases in the data.

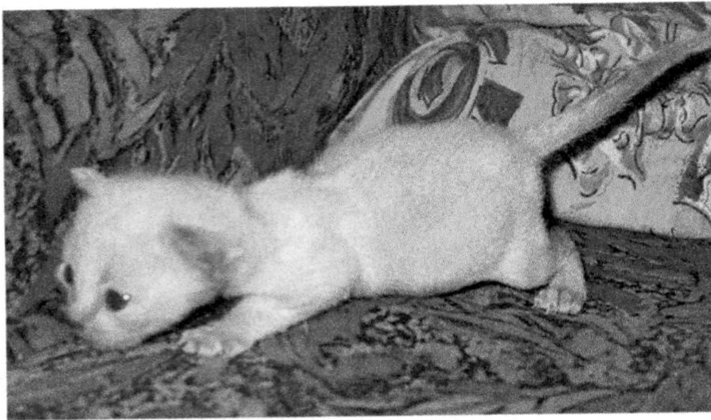

FIGURE 41-4 The flat chest defect is characterized by a dorsoventral flattening of the rib cage. *(Courtesy Barbara Hickmann.)*

In a survey of 3468 pedigreed kittens in the 1970s, 6.8% had malformations.[70] Individual breeds ranged from no defects reported to 17% (Colorpoint Shorthair) and 19% (Manx) of kittens affected. Another study from the same time period reported 4.2% of Burmese kittens from one cattery had congenital defects, as well as 12.7% of Persian kittens from four catteries.[71] The types of abnormalities reported included heart defects, open fontanelles, gastroschisis, eye and eyelid defects, and gastrointestinal tract defects.

In the United Kingdom analysis of reproduction data from 14 breeds,[75] 14.9% of the litters included one or more kittens with congenital defects, ranging from 6% of Devon Rex litters to 31% of Tonkinese litters (see Table 41-1). The survey of cat breeders conducted primarily in North America and Europe (S. Little, unpublished data, 2001 to 2005) found wide variation in prevalence of congenital defects, from 5% (Norwegian Forest Cat) to 80% ("contemporary" American Burmese) of litters demonstrating at least one defect (see Table 41-3). The high prevalence of congenital defects in "contemporary"-style American Burmese is due to a common craniofacial deformity caused by an autosomal recessive genetic mutation.[59] Congenital defects common to many breeds include thoracic wall deformities (e.g., pectus excavatum, flat chest defect), cleft palate, and umbilical hernia. Although certain common congenital defects of kittens are well described in the literature, others are less well documented.

Flat chest defect is one of the common thoracic wall deformities in kittens that are not well described in the literature. Although the defect may be seen in any kitten, it appears to be most common in Orientals, Burmese, and Bengals. The defect is characterized by a dorsoventral flattening of the rib cage and sharp angulation at the costochondral junction (Figure 41-4).[78] Curvature of the cranial thoracic spine may also be present (Figure 41-5).

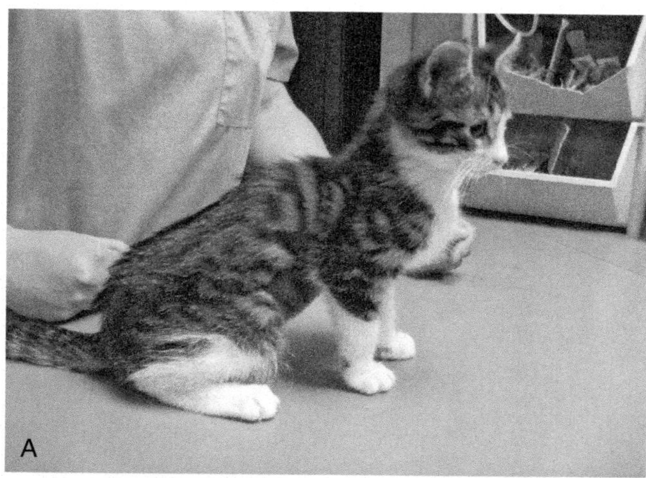

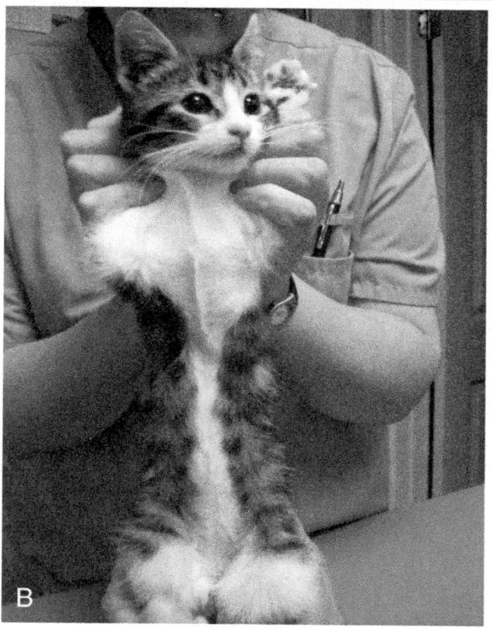

FIGURE 41-5 **A,** Kittens with flat chest defect may also have spinal curvature. **B,** Sharp angulation at the costochondral junction is evident.

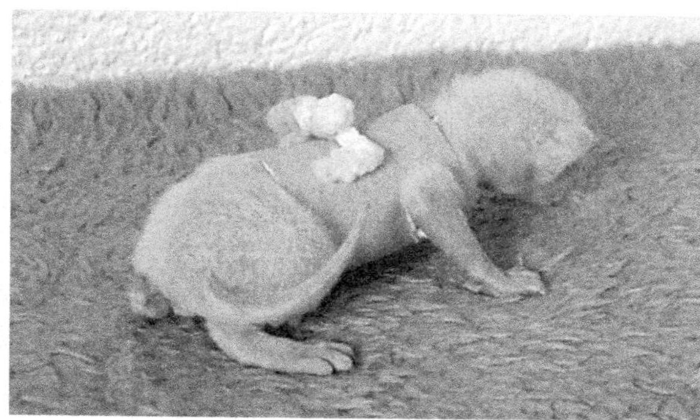

FIGURE 41-6 Owners of kittens with flat chest defect often apply temporary splints made of cardboard to help shape the compliant chest wall. *(Courtesy Barbara Hickmann.)*

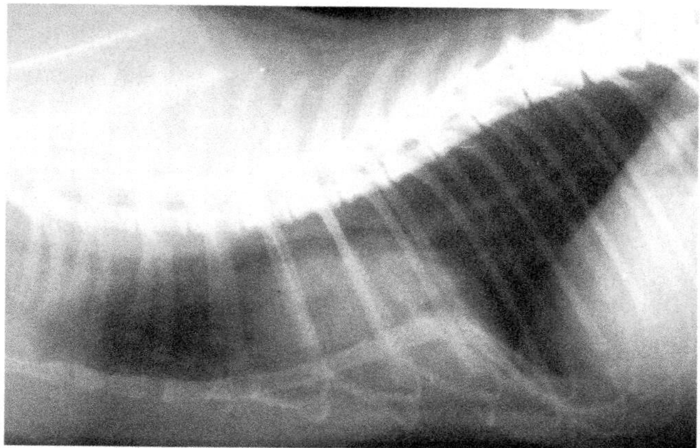

FIGURE 41-7 Pectus excavatum is characterized by dorsal deviation of the caudal part of the sternum. The defect reduces the size of the chest cavity and can lead to dyspnea and failure to grow.

The defect is not present at birth, but the mean age at which it is recorded is 9.5 days.[78] The defect has a variable presentation and is even transient in some cases. Mildly affected individuals may be difficult to detect. Moderate to severely affected kittens show poor weight gain, increased respiratory rate and effort, exercise intolerance, and they may die. In one study of Burmese kittens in the United Kingdom, 8.7% of the kittens with flat chest defect also had pectus excavatum, suggesting a possible association.[78] Although similar thoracic wall deformities have been reported in taurine-deficient kittens, affected Burmese kittens had higher whole blood taurine levels than unaffected kittens.[78] No investigation into the best treatment for kittens with life-threatening chest wall deformity has been published, but breeders and owners often apply temporary splints made of cardboard or plastic to force the compliant thoracic wall and sternum into a more normal confirmation until the ribs and sternum mature (Figure 41-6).

Pectus excavatum ("funnel chest") is characterized by dorsal deviation of the caudal part of the sternum (Figure 41-7). The sternal abnormality is noticed early in life, and the defect is usually progressive. The etiology in kittens and puppies is poorly understood, although reviews of the disease and its management have been published.[5,17] No breed or sex predisposition has been identified. The disease may be classified as mild, moderate, or severe based on radiographic measurements.[17,18] Mildly affected kittens typically have no clinical signs and do not require intervention. Severely affected kittens may be dyspneic, exercise intolerant, and fail to thrive. A heart murmur may be present, either resulting from congenital disease or secondary to abnormal positioning of the heart because of the sternal deformity.[18] The most commonly described surgical correction is percutaneous circumsternal sutures and external splinting (Figure 41-8).[18,19,50,72,85] This technique works well in kittens with a nonossified sternum (less than 4 months of age), because the goal is to pull the sternum outward and maintain the correct position while the sternum matures.

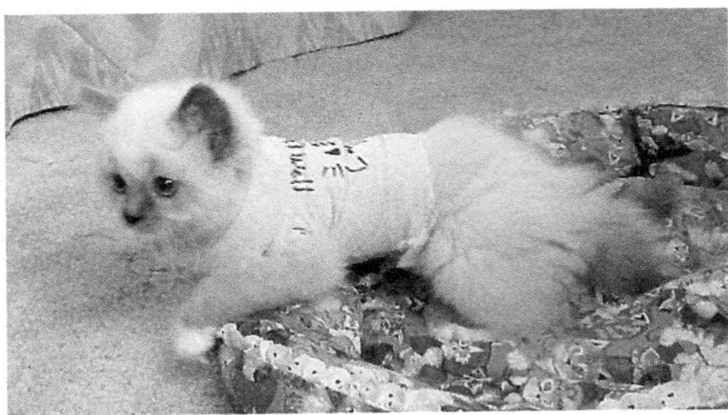

FIGURE 41-8 This Ragdoll kitten has had correction of pectus excavatum with circumsternal sutures and external splinting. *(Courtesy Sue Shorey.)*

Potential complications of the technique include inadvertent lung puncture or laceration and development of pneumothorax. One case of fatal reexpansion pulmonary edema has also been described.[72] Surgical approaches, such as wedge ostectomy,[72] trans-sternebral pinning,[13] and sternal wedge chondrectomy with internal splinting[64] have also been described.

Tarsal hyperextension (also known as "twisted legs," limb contracture, tendon contracture) is a recently described congenital defect in kittens.[7] The defect is obvious at birth and typically affects only one kitten in a litter. There is no breed or sex predisposition. The abnormality is characterized by severe tarsal hyperextension and metatarsal rotation (Figure 41-9). Typically both hind limbs are affected, but the condition can also be unilateral. No bone abnormalities or neurologic deficits are present. The etiology is unknown, but the defect appears similar to clubfoot in human infants. In the author's experience, the deformity completely resolves on its own in the majority of cases as the kitten begins to crawl and bear weight on the affected limbs. In some cases, delayed resolution has prompted the use of either soft molded splints or fiberglass casts for external coaptation.[7] If external coaptation is required, it should be instituted earlier rather than later to take advantage of the greater flexibility of the joints of young kittens. Splints and casts must be changed weekly as the kitten grows, and may be required for 6 weeks or longer. Physical therapy to gently manipulate the tarsal joint into normal configuration may also be helpful.

NEONATAL DIAGNOSTICS

Blood chemistry and hematology values for neonates differ from the adult; most values normalize to adult levels by 3 to 4 months of age (Tables 41-4 and 41-5). For several analytes, reference ranges change rapidly within the first few days and weeks of life so that using age-appropriate reference ranges is important. In one study

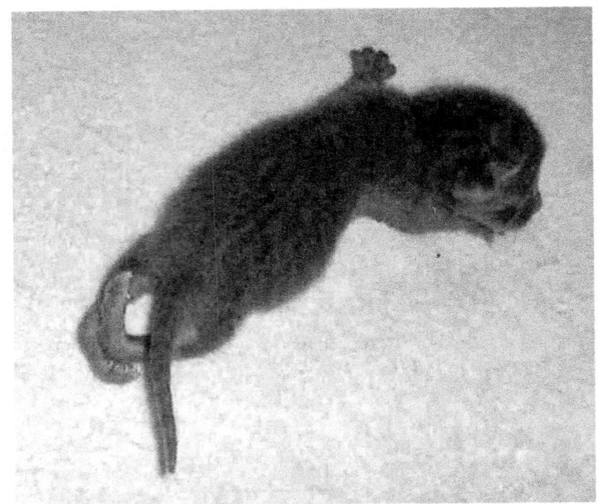

FIGURE 41-9 A newborn Korat kitten with tarsal hyperextension, showing the characteristic tarsal hyperextension and metatarsal rotation. *(Courtesy Carine Risberg.)*

TABLE 41-4 **Hematology Values for Kittens from Birth to 8 Weeks**

	2 Weeks	4 Weeks	6 Weeks	8 Weeks
PCV (%)	33.6-37.0	25.7-27.3	26.2-27.9	28.5-31.1
RBC (×10⁶/μL)	5.05-5.53	4.57-4.77	5.66-6.12	6.31-6.83
WBC (×10⁶/μL)	9.10-10.24	14.10-16.52	16.08-18.82	16.13-20.01
Neutrophils	5.28-6.64	6.15-7.69	7.92-11.22	5.72-7.78
Lymphocytes	3.21-4.25	5.97-7.15	5.64-7.18	8.02-11.16
Monocytes	0.0-0.02	0.0-0.04	0	0.0-0.02
Eosinophils	0.53-1.39	1.24-1.56	1.22-1.72	0.88-1.28

PCV, packed cell volume; *RBC,* red blood cell; *WBC,* white blood cell. Adapted from Moon P, Massat B, Pascoe P: Neonatal critical care, *Vet Clin North Am Small Anim Pract* 31:343, 2001.

of kittens up to 8 weeks of age, reference ranges for alkaline phosphatase (ALP), creatine kinase, triglycerides, calcium, and phosphorus were higher than for adults.[41] Reference ranges for aspartate aminotransferase (AST), bilirubin, urea nitrogen, and creatinine were higher in newborns, but similar to or lower than adults by 8 weeks of age. Reference ranges for albumin and total protein were lower than for adults for the entire 8 weeks, and values for calcium and phosphorus were higher.

For venipuncture, the holder positions the kitten in dorsal recumbency with the forelegs drawn back toward the abdomen and the head and neck extended. Blood is drawn from the jugular vein using a 1-mL syringe with a 25- or 26-gauge needle. Slow aspiration of blood is essential to avoid collapsing the vein. A small volume

TABLE 41-5 **Serum Chemistry Values for Kittens from Birth to 8 Weeks**

	2 Days	1 Week	2 Weeks	4 Weeks	8 Weeks
Albumin (g/dL)	1.6-2.6	2.0-2.5	2.1-2.6	2.4-2.9	2.4-3.0
ALP (U/L)	275-2021	126-363	116-306	97-274	60-161
ALT (U/L)	12-84	11-76	10-21	14-55	12-56
Bilirubin (mg/dL)	0-0.7	0-0.6	0-0.2	0-0.3	0-0.1
Calcium (mg/dL)	8.6-12.7	10.0-13.7	9.9-13.0	10.0-12.2	9.8-11.7
Cholesterol (mg/dL)	80-175	119-213	137-223	173-253	124-221
Creatinine (mg/dL)	0.5-1.1	0.3-0.7	0.4-0.6	0.4-0.7	0.6-1.2
GGT (U/L)	0-5	0-5	0-4	0-1	0-2
Glucose (mg/dL)	75-154	105-145	107-158	117-152	94-143
Phosphorus (mg/dL)	4.1-10.5	6.7-11.0	7.2-11.1	6.7-9.0	7.6-11.7
Total protein (g/dL)	3.9-5.8	3.5-4.8	3.7-5.0	4.5-5.6	4.8-6.5
Urea (mg/dL)	24-71	16-36	11-30	10-22	16-33

ALP, alkaline phosphatase; *ALT,* alanine aminotransferase; *GGT,* gamma-glutamyltransferase.
Adapted from Levy J, Crawford P, Werner L: Effect of age on reference intervals of serum biochemical values in kittens, *J Am Vet Med Assoc* 228:1033, 2006.

(0.5 mL) of blood can be used for the most critical tests (Box 41-5). Use of 0.5-mL microsample blood collection tubes is recommended and has been validated for evaluation of biochemistry and hematology samples.[82,83] Repeated sampling should be done cautiously, because the circulating blood volume of kittens is small (approximately 70 to 95 mL/kg). Daily blood sampling should not exceed 10% of the kitten's estimated total blood volume.

Urine is collected for chemistries, microscopic examination of sediment, and specific gravity by stimulating the perineum; cystocentesis should be performed with great care or avoided in the very young, because the bladder wall is easily lacerated. Urine specific gravity is 1.020 or less in the first few weeks of life; adult values are reached by about 8 weeks of age.[46] A fecal sample should be examined for common intestinal parasites, such as *Giardia* spp., *Isospora* spp., and roundworms, using both zinc sulfate centrifugation and a direct saline smear.

BOX 41-5

Minimum Database for Sick Neonatal Kittens

- PCV and total solids using microhematocrit tubes and refractometer
- Complete blood count: white blood cell count from one drop whole blood directly into Unopette, differential from blood smear
- Blood urea nitrogen with whole blood on reagent strip
- Blood glucose determined with drop of whole blood using glucometer (note these machines tend to underestimate blood glucose)

Radiography is a useful diagnostic tool, but is more difficult to perform than in adults because of the small size and often uncooperative nature of kittens. If required, the author prefers mask induction and maintenance with isoflurane as the safest method for immobilization. It is also difficult to interpret radiographic images of kittens, because contrast is poor from lack of body fat and mineralization of the skeleton is incomplete. The quality of images can be improved by setting the kilovoltage to about half of that used for an adult and using high-detail film or screens.

Quality thoracic images may be difficult to obtain because of the high respiratory rate of kittens and greater chest wall motion. Absence of motion and good positioning are critical. Common indications for thoracic radiographs are evaluation of heart murmurs and diagnosis of pneumonia. Thoracic radiographs of kittens show a generalized increase in pulmonary interstitial opacity because of the increased water content of the lung parenchyma. The thymus may appear as a sail sign in the cranial left hemithorax, and the cranial mediastinum will appear wider than in the adult. The heart appears proportionately larger in the thoracic cavity because of decreased alveolar volume.

Interpretation of skeletal radiographs presents difficulties because of decreased mineralization, open physes, and secondary centers of ossification. Trauma and infection are the most common lesions found, and are often associated with soft tissue swelling. It can be very helpful to radiograph the unaffected limb at the same time for comparison to aid in interpretation.

The usefulness of abdominal radiography in kittens is hampered by poor abdominal detail because of lack of intraabdominal fat, a small amount of normal peritoneal fluid, and a higher proportion of total body water. The liver appears comparatively larger than in the adult. The most common diagnoses are radiopaque foreign bodies and intestinal obstruction.

Ultrasonography is an effective modality for pediatric patients, especially for imaging the abdomen. Machines with a curvilinear variable frequency scan head (6.0 to 8.0 MHz) have been recommended.[3] Sedation is rarely required for the procedure, and the kitten is best positioned in dorsal recumbency in a padded trough. Techniques for examining the abdomen and the normal appearance of structures have been described.[3] Common indications for abdominal ultrasonography include gastrointestinal foreign bodies, intussusceptions, congenital hernias, congenital renal disease, and urolithiasis, among others.

Normal electrocardiographic values for kittens in the first 30 days of life have been described.[44] Changes in normal findings occur during the first month of life, such as shift of the electrical axis from right to left, a progressive increase in R wave amplitude, and a progressive decrease in S wave amplitude. Measurements for P wave, PR intervals, duration of QRS complexes, and the duration of the QT interval are similar to adult cats. Neonatal kittens have a sinus heart rhythm.

Necropsy is underutilized as a diagnostic tool for multicat environments, such as shelters or catteries. It is not uncommon for kittens to die or be euthanized before a definitive diagnosis can be established. Necropsy results may provide information necessary to save remaining littermates or a future litter, especially for infectious diseases. For the best results, the whole body should be submitted (refrigerated, not frozen) to a qualified pathologist. If necessary, freezing is preferable to autolysis, because some information can still be obtained.

BASIC THERAPEUTICS

Rapid identification of illness and prompt intervention are the keys to success when treating ill neonatal kittens. Intensive care of the sickest kittens can be very successful although intimidating. Often the exact cause of a kitten's illness is not apparent at the time of presentation, and therapy must be focused on supportive care. Initial therapy typically includes treatment of the "3 H" problems (hypothermia, hypoglycemia, and hydration) with supplemental warmth, hydration, glucose, and nutrition.[22,52] Awareness of physiologic differences between neonatal and adult cats is important, and recently published information should be reviewed.[29]

For newborn kittens, a fourth "H" can be added to the list—hypoxia. The main risk factor for hypoxia is dystocia, leading to prolonged time in the birth canal with placental separation and therefore decreased oxygen. Resuscitation of these neonates must be prompt and aggressive, involving rubbing to dry and stimulate breathing, and aspiration of airway secretions (see Chapter 40). Other factors that have a negative impact on the survival of kittens born during dystocia include the effect of drugs given to the queen for surgery, brain trauma from "swinging" to resuscitate (no longer recommended),[30] and hypothermia induced by the cool temperatures of most operating rooms. These kittens may survive the dystocia, but are often weak and unable to nurse effectively. The effects of hypoxia and hypothermia may cause death within a few days.

Rectal temperatures less than 34.4° C (94° F) are associated with depressed respiration, impaired function of the immune system, bradycardia, and ileus. Never attempt to feed a hypothermic kitten, because aspiration pneumonia is a significant risk. Hypothermic kittens should be re-warmed slowly, during 2 to 3 hours to a maximum rectal temperature of 38.3° C (101° F). Warming too rapidly may cause increased metabolic demand, resulting in dehydration, hypoxia, and loss of cardiovascular integrity. An incubator or oxygen cage is a good way to accomplish re-warming and has the benefit of providing humidified air. However, hot-water bottles, circulating warm-water blankets, and heating lamps can also be used with very careful monitoring. The kitten should be able to move away from the heat source. The environmental temperature for neonatal kittens should be about 27° C to 32° C (80° F to 90° F).

For severely hypothermic kittens, fluids warmed to 35° C to 37° C (95° F to 98.6° F) may be administered by the intravenous (IV) or intraosseous (IO) route. Bags of fluid can be warmed (but will cool quickly) or an in-line IV infusion warmer may be used. Another option is to place the portion of intravenous tubing nearest the kitten under a warming device, such as a heating pad or a circulating warm-water blanket. Monitor closely for recurrence of hypothermia after re-warming.

Clinical hypoglycemia occurs when the blood glucose is less than 3 mmol/L (50 mg/dL) and is a common problem for sick neonates because of immature liver function and rapid depletion of glycogen stores. Hypoglycemia may be caused by vomiting, diarrhea, sepsis, hypothermia, or inadequate nutritional intake. Kittens with hypoglycemia will be weak and lethargic, and may be anorexic. Prolonged hypoglycemia may cause permanent brain damage, because the neonatal brain depends on glucose and carbohydrates as energy sources. If the kitten is not hypothermic or dehydrated, administer 5% to 10% dextrose orally at 0.25 to 0.50 mL/100 g body weight periodically by gastric tube until the kitten is stronger and normoglycemic. Then begin feedings of kitten milk replacer. Critically ill neonates may require a bolus infusion of 12.5% dextrose IV or IO (0.1 to 0.2 mL/100 g body weight, or more) followed by a constant rate infusion of 1.25% to 5% dextrose in a balanced electrolyte solution to prevent rebound hypoglycemia.[51,54] Hypertonic dextrose solutions should not be administered subcutaneously, because tissue sloughing may occur.

Dehydration occurs easily in neonatal kittens with diarrhea, vomiting, or reduced fluid intake. Neonates have poor compensatory mechanisms and immature renal function so that both dehydration and overhydration during treatment are concerns. Daily urine output in 1-month-old kittens is 25 mL/kg compared with 10 to 20 mL/kg in the adult cat.[54] Neonates also have higher fluid requirements than adults because of a higher total body water content (about 80% of body weight, compared with 60% in adults), a greater surface area-to-body-weight ratio, a higher metabolic rate, and decreased body fat. Hydration status may be difficult to assess in the youngest patients. Skin turgor is not a reliable test of hydration for kittens less than 4 weeks of age, because their skin has decreased fat and increased water content compared with adults. The kitten's mucous membranes should be moist and either hyperemic or pink. Pale mucous membranes and a decreased capillary refill time indicate at least 10% dehydration. Neonatal urine is normally colorless and clear; in dehydrated kittens, the urine is dark with a specific gravity greater than 1.020.

If the kitten is minimally dehydrated and normothermic with no gastrointestinal dysfunction, warmed electrolyte solution may be given orally or warmed subcutaneous (SC) fluids can be administered. However, subcutaneous absorption of fluids is slower in hypovolemic kittens because of peripheral vasoconstriction. If the kitten is moderately to severely dehydrated, IV fluid administration is the most effective. A mini-set (60 drops/mL) is used with a fluid or syringe pump or a burette. The cephalic or jugular vein can be catheterized with a 24-gauge ¾-inch or 22-gauge 1-inch catheter (Figure 41-10). Small-gauge catheters develop burrs easily during placement. Making a small hole in the skin with a 20-gauge needle first may facilitate placement. Balanced crystalloid solutions are the preferred fluid therapy choices. Lactated Ringer's solution is ideal for rehydration, because lactate can be used as an energy source; 1.25% to 5% dextrose can be added if necessary.

Warmed fluids may be given as a slow IV bolus of 1 mL/30 g body weight (30 to 45 mL/kg body weight), followed by a maintenance infusion of 80 to 120 mL/kg/day (8 to 12 mL/100 g) plus any ongoing losses.[46,51] It is important to monitor fluid therapy closely, because it is easy to overhydrate young kittens. Hydration status can be monitored by several methods, but weighing the kitten every 6 to 8 hours on an accurate gram scale is

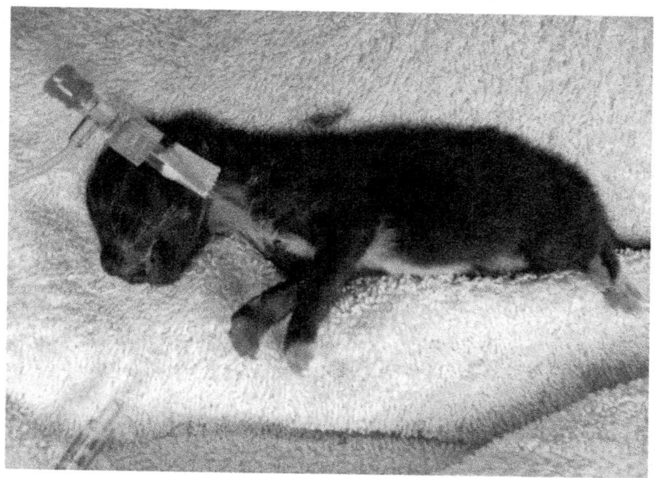

FIGURE 41-10 The jugular vein can be catheterized with a 24-gauge ¾-inch or 22-gauge 1-inch catheter. Lactated Ringer's solution is ideal for rehydration of neonatal kittens. *(Courtesy Jennifer Waldrop.)*

useful and easily accomplished. Other methods include serial packed cell volume (PCV)/total protein measurements, central venous pressure measurement, and urine output measurement with placement of a 3.5-Fr red rubber urinary catheter. Electrolyte and glucose status should also be monitored.

If it is difficult to achieve intravenous access, an alternate route for administration of fluids must be employed. The intraperitoneal route should not be used in neonatal kittens because of the risk of inducing peritonitis. Intraosseous access using the trochanteric fossa of the proximal femur is the best alternative to IV access; blood, fluids, and some medications can be administered in this way (Figure 41-11).[46] Contraindications to IO access are few, such as fracture or infection at the site. A 20- to 22-gauge 1-inch spinal needle or 18- to 25-gauge hypodermic needle may be used as a catheter.

The hair over the hip is clipped, and the skin is surgically prepared before the needle is inserted. The limb is positioned toward the ventral midline to rotate the trochanteric fossa laterally. The kitten's stifle can be supported in one hand while the needle is pushed and twisted into place. Resistance is felt initially as the needle penetrates bone. The spinal needle is firmly seated in the shaft of the femur, and the stylet is removed. If a hypodermic needle is used, the shaft may become clogged with bone debris. Placing a piece of surgical wire in the shaft of the hypodermic needle during placement will help avoid clogging.[49] If the needle still becomes clogged, it can be removed and another needle can be placed in the same location. A correctly placed catheter will move with the limb. Ideally, correct placement should be confirmed with a radiograph.

A T-port is inserted into the needle hub and the catheter is flushed with nonheparinized saline. If resistance

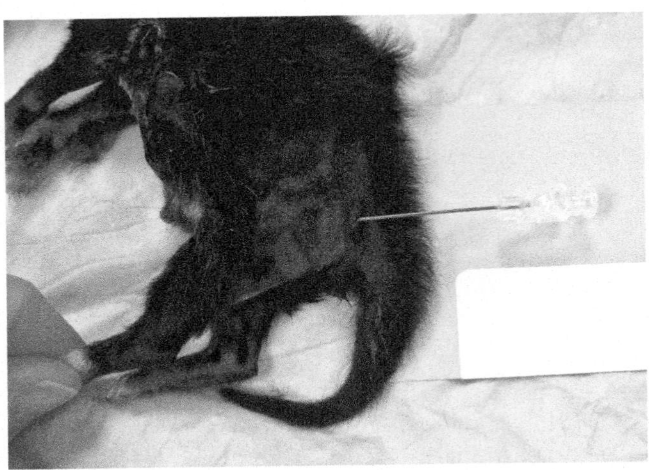

FIGURE 41-11 Placement of an intraosseous (IO) catheter in the femur is a quick way to administer fluids, whole blood, and some drugs. The IO catheter should be replaced with an intravenous catheter as soon as possible if ongoing fluid therapy is required. *(Courtesy Jennifer Waldrop.)*

to saline infusion is felt, rotate the needle 90 to 180 degrees to free the bevel from the wall of the femur. Fluid rates and amounts by the IO route are the same as for intravenous access. Administration can be with a syringe or a standard IV set. Use of cold fluids, rapid infusion, or hypertonic or alkaline solutions will cause pain. The IO catheter can be sutured in place with a stay suture through the skin for temporary use (typically less than 24 hours).[49] Bandaging IO catheters in small kittens is difficult and may not be necessary if excellent hygiene is maintained. IV access should be established as soon as possible. Once the kitten becomes more active, the catheter is easily dislodged. Complications of IO catheters include infection, extravasation of fluids, and bone and soft tissue trauma.

Blood transfusions may be necessary in some sick neonatal kittens, particularly those with anemia resulting from flea infestations or intestinal parasites. Indications for blood transfusion are weakness, tachycardia, pale mucous membranes, and a hematocrit less than 15%. Blood from a compatible typed donor is diluted 9:1 with a citrate anticoagulant and given using a Millipore blood filter by the IV or IO route at a rate of 20 mL/kg during a minimum of 2 hours.[46]

IMMUNITY

Queens have a colostral phase of lactation in which immunoglobulin concentrations are high, often exceeding their serum levels. The predominant immunoglobulin in both colostrum and milk is IgG. IgG concentrations are highest in the first 7 days of lactation and then steadily decrease, while IgA remains at a constant low level throughout lactation.[10] Kittens receive almost all their passive immunity during the first 12 to 18 hours of life (before gut closure) with the ingestion of colostrum; there is little or no transplacental transfer of immunoglobulins in the cat.[8] The amount of passively acquired immunity is determined by the amount of colostrum ingested, the time of ingestion, and the concentration of immunoglobulins in the colostrum. The kitten's serum IgG nadir is reached between 3 and 5 weeks of age because of catabolism of maternal IgG and correlates with a period of vulnerability to infection.[10,40] IgG levels then steadily increase as the kitten's own adaptive immunity develops.

Failure of passive transfer of immunity (FPT) is a well-documented concern in large animals and is diagnosed when neonates have serum IgG concentrations less than 400 mg/dL.[10] Several treatments, such as colostrum replacements, are commercially available for these species. Extrapolation from large animals would suggest that kittens with FPT may be at increased risk for infection. Although no studies on a correlation between FPT and susceptibility to infection in kittens have been published, neonatal sepsis is one of the most common causes of kitten mortality in the first few weeks of life. Kittens with uncorrected FPT start to produce IgG at about 4 weeks of age; they are therefore most vulnerable to infection from birth to at least 4 weeks of age. Adequate intake of colostrum during the first 18 hours of life may therefore be critical.

Many factors can influence whether a kitten ingests sufficient amounts of immunoglobulins, such as

- Birth order and litter size: In a large litter, kittens born later face increased competition to nurse.
- Suckling success: Weak kittens (e.g., due to low birth weight, effects of dystocia, congenital defects, disease) may not suckle effectively in the first day of life.
- Delayed ingestion: Queens recovering from cesarian section may not be well enough to nurse kittens effectively in the first day of life.
- Sick queens: An ill queen may not produce sufficient colostrum for the kittens, or it may be of poor quality with low IgG concentrations.
- Orphans: If the queen died during parturition or shortly afterward, orphan kittens may not have had an opportunity to ingest colostrum.
- Deliberate prevention of colostrum ingestion for prevention of neonatal isoerythrolysis: See below.

If a full history is not available for a kitten or litter, it may be difficult to know if FPT has occurred. No rapid assay for detection of FPT in cats is available. Definite diagnosis is by measurement of serum IgG concentration, a test only performed at some reference laboratories. One study evaluating surrogate markers for FPT in kittens found that adequacy of passive transfer correlated only with serum alkaline phosphatase activity, and then only for the first 2 days of life.[12]

A common recommendation for orphan kittens at risk of FPT is to foster the kitten on another lactating queen. However, colostrum-deprived kittens fostered on surrogate queens in the milk phase of lactation acquire insufficient levels of immunoglobulins.[10] Colostrum-deprived kittens fed milk replacer also fail to acquire sufficient levels of immunoglobulins.[10] Commercial milk replacers for kittens may be advertised as containing colostrum, but there is no evidence that the ingredient provides any immunity.

Correction of FPT can be accomplished by SC injection of adult cat serum from a cat with compatible blood type that has been screened for infectious diseases (15 mL/100 g body weight, divided into three doses during 24 hours).[40] This protocol requires collection of large volumes of blood and may be impractical, especially for more than one kitten at a time. Whether smaller amounts of adult cat serum may be effective in correcting FPT is not known. A commercially available equine IgG product licensed for treatment of FPT in foals was evaluated in kittens with FPT in an effort to find a more readily available solution.[11] Although treated kittens achieved adequate serum concentrations of the equine IgG, the equine antibodies failed to promote bacterial phagocytosis by feline neutrophils in vitro. Therefore equine IgG cannot be recommended for treatment of FPT in kittens.

INFECTIOUS DISEASES

The highest kitten mortality rates from infectious diseases are in the first 2 weeks of life and in the postweaning period. Common pathogens include those causing upper and lower respiratory tract disease, diarrhea, and systemic disease (Box 41-6).

Respiratory Tract Disease

Respiratory tract disease can cause significant morbidity and mortality in young kittens. Clinical signs in acute upper respiratory tract infections include fever, sneezing, depression, anorexia, and bilateral nasal and ocular discharge (mucoid, serous, or purulent) (Figure 41-12). Severe disease is characterized by dehydration, debilitation, and even death. Most infections involve feline herpesvirus (FHV-1), feline calicivirus, *Mycoplasma* spp., and/or *Chlamydophila felis*. Pathogens implicated in lower respiratory tract disease in kittens include *Bordetella bronchiseptica* and *Streptococcus canis* (see below). Treatment of respiratory tract disease in kittens is largely symptomatic and supportive, and aggressive nursing care is often required. The diagnosis and management of respiratory pathogens is found in Chapter 30.

BOX 41-6

Common Pathogens of Kittens

Upper and Lower Respiratory Tract Disease

Feline herpesvirus-1
Feline calicivirus
Bordetella bronchiseptica
Mycoplasma spp.
Chlamydophila felis

Gastrointestinal Tract

Parvovirus
Coliform bacteria
Tritrichomonas foetus
Giardia spp.
Isospora spp.
Ancylostoma spp.
Toxocara spp.

Systemic Disease

Feline leukemia virus
Feline immunodeficiency virus
Feline infectious peritonitis
Toxoplasma gondii
Gram-positive bacteria (e.g., *Streptococcus* spp., *Staphylococcus* spp.)
Gram-negative bacteria (e.g., *Escherichia coli, Salmonella* spp.)

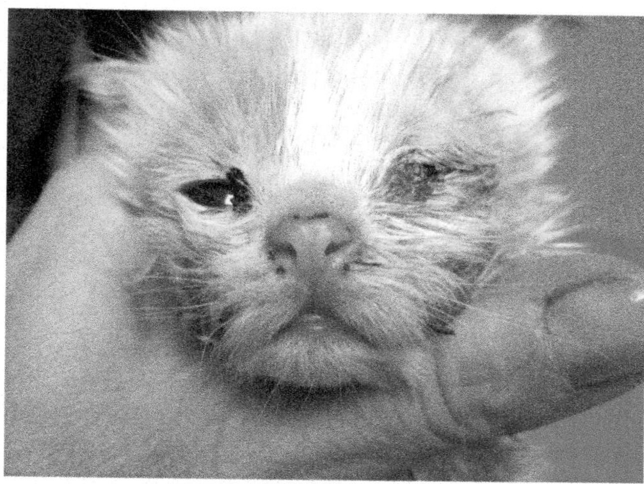

FIGURE 41-12 Conjunctivitis resulting from feline herpesvirus is common in young kittens. Clinical signs include fever, sneezing, and bilateral nasal and ocular discharges.

Ophthalmia neonatorum is conjunctivitis under the closed eyelids of neonatal kittens (Figure 41-13). Commonly implicated pathogens include FHV-1 and *Chlamydophila felis*.[47] Other possible pathogens include *Staphylococcus* spp., *Mycoplasma* spp., and *Bordetella*

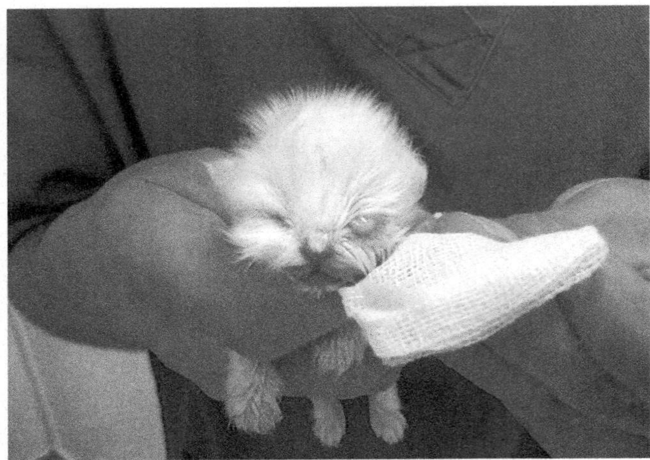

FIGURE 41-13 Ophthalmia neonatorum is conjunctivitis under the closed eyelids of neonatal kittens. Commonly implicated pathogens include feline herpesvirus and *Chlamydophila felis*. *(Courtesy Sandra Brau.)*

bronchiseptica. The eyelids are swollen from the accumulation of purulent material underneath, some of which may be discharging at the medial canthus. Drainage must be established by opening the eyelids using warm compresses and gentle traction. If this approach fails, the closed tip of a small mosquito forceps may be inserted at the medial canthus and gently opened to separate the eyelids. The forceps should never be returned to the closed position while inserted between the eyelids to avoid damage to ocular structures. Sharp instruments should never be used to separate the eyelids. The eyes should then be flushed with saline and the cornea should be stained with fluorescein for evidence of ulceration. A broad-spectrum topical antibiotic ointment should be applied 2 to 4 times daily for 1 week. When FHV-1 is suspected, topical antiviral therapy may be useful (see Chapter 29). Symblepharon (conjunctival adhesions) may be a sequel to severe or untreated cases.

Diarrhea

Although diarrhea in kittens is a common and frustrating condition facing clinicians, there is very little published research on the specific causes and treatments in this age group. Acute diarrhea is often self-limiting and may be managed with symptomatic and supportive therapy. For chronic diarrhea, a specific diagnosis should be made and treatment should be targeted (see Chapter 23). Inappropriate use of antibiotics to treat diarrhea should be discouraged. Indiscriminate use of antibiotics in young kittens may alter the commensal intestinal microflora, worsen the diarrhea, and induce antibiotic resistance. The most common causes of diarrhea in kittens are infectious agents, primarily parasites and viruses (see Box 41-6). Recently, enteroadherent *Enterococcus* spp. infection has been identified as a cause of diarrhea and failure to thrive in kittens.[58]

A comprehensive fecal examination is an important first step in diagnosis (see Chapter 23). Fecal examination should include a direct fecal smear (wet mount), a stained smear, and fecal flotation (zinc sulfate centrifugation with fresh feces). The next level of diagnostics would include immunoassays or polymerase chain reaction (PCR) testing for *Giardia* spp. and *Tritrichomonas* spp. The indications for performing fecal enteric panels on kittens with diarrhea are not well defined. Bacterial enteropathogens and toxins are commonly found in asymptomatic kittens as well as those with diarrhea, making interpretation difficult.[25a] Fecal cultures and toxin analysis are probably best reserved for specific situations, such as kittens with bloody diarrhea and evidence of sepsis. In general, for kittens with chronic diarrhea where no diagnosis has yet been made and response to therapy is poor, repeating previously negative diagnostic tests is more rewarding than intestinal biopsy (either by laparotomy or endoscopy).[48] Finding an inflammatory response on intestinal biopsy in kittens does not ensure a diagnosis of inflammatory bowel disease.

It is acceptable to administer a broad-spectrum anthelminthic to kittens with diarrhea even in the face of negative fecal examinations. Pyrantel pamoate (5 to 10 mg/kg, PO) can be started as young as 2 weeks of age. Most anthelminthics for kittens are labeled for use from 8 weeks of age, although a few are labeled from 6 weeks of age (e.g., Interceptor; Novartis Animal Health, Greensboro, NC). Another common empiric treatment is metronidazole (7 to 10 mg/kg, PO, every 12 hours for 5 days). This drug may resolve clinical signs by several mechanisms, such as altering intestinal microflora, moderation of cell mediated immunity, or treatment of a specific pathogen. The use of prebiotics and probiotics is receiving attention, although no studies on efficacy in kittens with diarrhea are yet available. In addition, there is little regulation or mandatory quality control for most commercial products, and label descriptions do not always match the contents.[81] Finally, some kittens with chronic diarrhea may develop vitamin B_{12} (cobalamin) deficiency. Empiric treatment can be safely instituted at 100 μg/kitten, SC, once weekly for 4 to 6 weeks.[48]

External Parasites

Fleas are the most common and most important external parasite affecting kittens (see Chapter 22). Severe flea infestations can lead to anemia and even death. Many effective flea control products are available, but most are labeled for use in kittens from 8 weeks of age. Exceptions include lufenuron (Program, Novartis Animal Health), which is labeled for use from 6 weeks of age, and nitenpyram (Capstar, Novartis Animal Health), which is labeled for use in kittens that are 4 weeks of age and weigh at least 0.9 kg (2 lb). Fipronil spray is labeled for use on kittens from 2 days of age in some countries, such as the United Kingdom. When treating very small kittens, it is safer to apply the spray to a cloth or cotton balls and wipe the kitten, avoiding the eyes and mucous membranes. Very young kittens should be flea-combed daily. Most pyrethrin flea shampoos are not labeled for use in kittens less than 12 weeks of age, and their efficacy is questionable. Anecdotally, hand dishwashing detergents are often used, although care must be taken to avoid hypothermia when bathing neonates. Many flea treatment products are safe for nursing queens (see Table 22-1); so, the queen and the environment should also be treated.

Neonatal Sepsis

Neonatal sepsis is a significant cause of death in kittens, and may be caused by a variety of pathogens. Risk factors may include failure of passive transfer of immunity, mastitis or metritis in the queen, prolonged delivery or dystocia, low birth weight, chilling because of low environmental temperature, and inappropriate use of antibiotics.

Pathogens that may be associated with neonatal sepsis include *E. coli*, *Staphylococcus* spp., *Pasteurella* spp., *Enterobacter* spp., *Clostridium* spp., *Salmonella* spp., and *Streptococcus* spp. These organisms typically enter through the umbilicus, but other points of entry include the gastrointestinal tract, the respiratory tract, and the urinary tract. Clinical signs will vary with the organ system involved, although death can occur quickly with few signs. Common syndromes include gastroenteritis (vomiting, diarrhea, dehydration), pyelonephritis (fever, dehydration, hematuria), and pneumonia (respiratory distress, cyanosis). Noncardiogenic pulmonary edema secondary to sepsis can lead to acute respiratory distress. Generic clinical signs associated with sepsis include failure to thrive, crying, restlessness, and hypothermia.

A diagnosis of neonatal sepsis is suspected based on clinical signs. Laboratory diagnostics may show anemia, neutrophilia, and hypoglycemia. A definitive diagnosis in the living animal requires blood or urine culture, but is rarely of use to the affected kitten because of the length of time required before culture results are received. However, culture results may help treat litter mates that also become ill. Therefore empiric treatment with a broad-spectrum antibiotic, such as a cephalosporin, is justified pending culture results. Unfortunately, a definitive diagnosis of neonatal sepsis is often made at necropsy. In addition to appropriate antibiotic therapy, treatment is mainly aggressive supportive care (Box 41-7). Antibiotics recommended for use in young kittens include the quinolones and beta-lactams (Table 41-6). More information on drug therapy for neonates in found in Chapter 4.

BOX 41-7

Summary of Therapeutics for Neonatal Septicemia in Kittens

Treat Dehydration

Fluid therapy through intravenous, intraosseous routes
Warmed balanced electrolyte solution (BES) with 1.25% to 5% dextrose
Slow bolus: 1 mL/30 g body weight
Maintenance rate: 80 to 120 mL/kg/day plus ongoing losses

Treat Hypoglycemia

PO: 0.25 to 0.50 mL/kg, 5% to 10% dextrose
IV bolus: 0.1 to 0.2 mL/100 g, 12.5% dextrose
IV CRI: 1.25% to 5% dextrose in BES

Treat Hypothermia

Rewarm during 30 minutes to 2 hours to maximum rectal temp of 101° F (36.3° C)
Environmental temperature for neonates should be 27° C to 32° C (80° F to 90° F)

Treat Infection

Start broad-spectrum empiric antibiotic therapy pending culture results

Monitor Treatment

Hydration: weigh every 6 to 8 hours, serial PCV/TP, central venous pressure, urine output, respiratory rate/effort, auscult chest
Serial electrolyte, glucose measurements
Rectal temperature every hour

CRI, Constant rate infusion; *PCV*, packed cell volume; *TP*, total protein.

Streptococci have been associated with severe infections in kittens, including sepsis.[27] They are typically beta-hemolytic infections, caused by the Lancefield group G organism, *Streptococcus canis*. Streptococci are commensal microflora of the feline skin, pharynx, upper respiratory tract, and genital tract. Neonatal kittens acquire infection from the vagina of the queen. The bacteria gain entrance through the umbilical vein, causing omphalophlebitis, peritonitis, and sepsis. A toxic shock–like syndrome has been reported in 8-week-old kittens,[80] and cervical lymphadenitis may be seen in kittens from 3 to 7 months of age. Untreated or undetected cases of lymphadenitis may progress to myocarditis or pneumonia (Figure 41-14). *S. canis* has also been associated with high-mortality disease outbreaks in shelters where

TABLE 41-6 **Antibiotic Choices for Neonatal Kittens**

Drug	Dose
Amoxicillin	6 to 20 mg/kg, q12h, PO
Amoxicillin + clavulanic acid	12.5 to 25 mg/kg, q12h, PO
Ampicillin	25 mg/kg, q8h, IV/IO/IM
Ceftiofur	2.5 mg/kg, q12h, SC; maximum 5 days
Cephalexin, cefazolin	10 to 30 mg/kg, q12h, PO
Enrofloxacin	2.5 to 5 mg/kg, once daily, SC or IV
Ticarcillin + clavulanic acid	15 mg/kg, q12h, IV or IM
Trimethoprim sulfa	30 mg/kg, once daily, PO

IM, Intramuscular; *IO,* intraosseous; *IV,* intravenous; *PO,* by mouth; *SC,* subcutaneous.

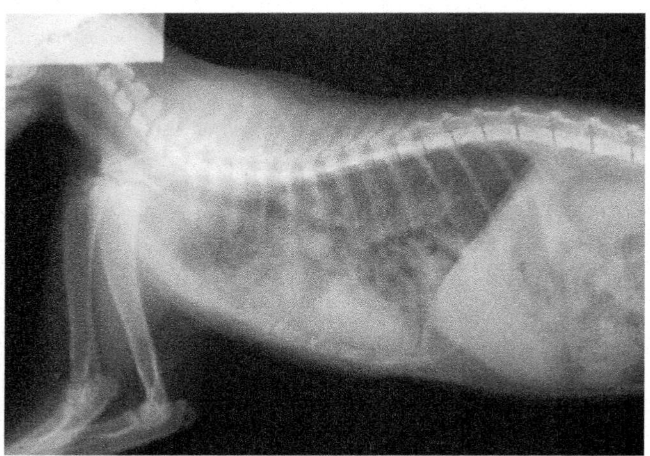

FIGURE 41-14 *Streptococcus canis* may be a cause of severe pneumonia in kittens.

affected cats may have skin ulceration, necrotizing sinusitis and meningitis, necrotizing fasciitis, toxic shock–like syndrome, and sepsis.[63]

Kittens born to queens less than 2 years of age are most at risk of streptococcal infections. Young queens maintain a carrier state with high numbers of bacteria in the vagina throughout pregnancy. Often, more than one kitten in a litter is affected, and mortality rates in the first 2 weeks of life may be high, especially when the organism is first introduced into a naïve population, such as a breeding cattery. Affected kittens fail to gain weight and may have an infected umbilicus. They may be found dead with minimal ante mortem clinical signs. Diagnosis may be made by culture of umbilical exudates or at necropsy, when the organism is most often isolated from liver, lung, umbilicus, and peritoneal cavity.

Kittens with lymphadenitis or omphalophlebitis should be treated with antibiotics and drainage of abscesses. Kittens with sepsis are treated with antibiotics and aggressive supportive care (see Box 41-7). *S. canis* is very sensitive to penicillins. Litter mates of affected kittens may be treated with oral amoxicillin. Prevention of infection in newborn kittens may be accomplished by disinfection of the umbilical cord in 2% tincture of iodine or 0.5% chlorhexidine solution at birth. In an endemic situation, routine antibiotic treatment of queen and kittens may reduce morbidity and mortality.[4] At the time of delivery, kittens are given a single injection of a combination benzathine penicillin and procaine penicillin product (both 150,000 IU/mL). The penicillin is diluted 1:6 with sterile 0.9% saline and administered at 0.25 mL/kitten, SC. The queen is given a single injection of the same undiluted product (1.0 mL/cat, SC).

NEONATAL ISOERYTHROLYSIS

Blood type is determined by antigenic, species-specific markers on the surface of red blood cells. In cats, blood type is characterized by an AB system.[2] It is believed that one gene with three alleles produces blood types A, B, and the rare AB. Blood type A is caused by the dominant allele and is found in 95% to 98% of nonpedigreed cats. Cats with blood type A have low titers of naturally occurring anti-B antibodies. Blood type B is recessive, and prevalence varies with geographic location and breed (see Tables 25-1 and 25-2).[23,24] Certain cat breeds have a high prevalence of blood type B individuals, such as the British Shorthair, Cornish and Devon Rex, and Birman. Cats with blood type B have high, *naturally* occurring titers of anti-A antibodies. No previous pregnancy or transfusion is necessary to induce antibody formation.

Neonatal isoerythrolysis (NI) may occur in kittens with blood type A or AB born to a queen with blood type B.[6] The queen's colostrum contains anti-A antibodies that are transferred when the kittens ingest colostrum. Kittens are typically born healthy, but stop nursing within a few days with suggestive clinical signs, such as failure to thrive, pigmenturia, icterus, and anemia. Affected kittens may be transfused with washed type B red cells, preferably from the queen, because she will not have antibodies against her own red blood cells.[46] The red cells are suspended in saline and administered at 5 to 10 mL/kitten, IV or IO, during a period of several hours. Despite aggressive intervention, the mortality rate is high.

Prevention of NI in breeding programs necessitates knowledge of the blood types of breeding cats in those breeds with a significant percentage of type B individuals. Breeders may choose to breed queens with blood type B only to males with blood type B to avoid producing kittens at risk of NI. In some cases, queens with blood type B must be bred with a male of blood type A or AB, and steps should be taken to prevent NI. Breeders can remove all the kittens from the queen immediately after birth for the first 18 hours of life to prevent ingestion of colostrum. The kittens are hand-fed milk replacer and cared for by the breeder until they are returned to the queen. Alternately, if the breeder can be present at the time of birth, patient-side blood typing cards (RapidVet-H, DMS Laboratories, Flemington, NJ) may be used to type umbilical cord blood from the kittens before they have a chance to nurse. Care must be taken to avoid cross-contamination with blood from the queen in birth fluids. Only kittens at risk of NI (blood type A or AB) are then removed from the queen for 18 hours, and kittens with blood type B are allowed to remain with the queen.

ORPHAN KITTENS

Veterinarians may be asked to evaluate and treat young kittens that have been orphaned or abandoned. Successful treatment can be accomplished with knowledge of the particular needs of these often fragile pediatric patients. If a foster queen is not available, the caregiver must replace physiologic needs normally provided by the queen, such as warmth, nutrition, elimination, sanitation, and social stimulation. The ideal housing for orphan kittens is an incubator, but any warm and safe enclosure will suffice, such as a pet carrier or cardboard box. Bedding should be absorbent, soft, warm, and either readily cleaned or disposable. The environmental temperature for kittens in the first week of life should be 30° C to 32° C (86° F to 90° F). The temperature can be gradually lowered to 24° C (75° F) during the next few weeks. If a heat source is used in a box or carrier, it should be placed so that a temperature gradient is created, allowing the kittens to move away from the warmest areas when needed. Humidity should be maintained at 55% to 60% to prevent dehydration and maintain the health of mucous membranes.

If a litter of kittens is orphaned, they will often try to nurse on each other. Skin trauma or genital trauma, especially of the penis and prepuce, may occur if the kittens are not separated. Social stimulation should be provided by regular but brief periods of handling. Protection against infectious diseases is important for orphaned kittens, especially if failure of passive transfer of immunity is possible (see above). Although it is tempting to expose young orphans to older kittens or adults for social interaction, this should be avoided until the kitten is immunized. All bedding and equipment should be kept clean and caregivers should wash hands before handling neonates.

Certain procedures should be followed for feeding orphans.[43] Orphan kittens should be fed a commercial milk replacer specifically designed for kittens to approximate the composition of the queen's milk. Homemade formulas are best reserved for short-term or emergency use. The manufacturer's directions should be followed for mixing, storage, and feeding quantities. Strict hygiene is necessary, and if milk replacer must be reconstituted, no more than a 48-hour supply should be prepared at a time. The reconstituted milk replacer can be divided into individual feedings and refrigerated until use. The energy requirement for kittens in the first few weeks of life is approximately 20 kcal metabolizable energy (ME)/100 g body weight/day.[14] The maintenance water requirement is about 180 mL/kg per day (range, 130 to 220 mL/kg/day).[35,46] Initially, only 50% of the recommended amount of milk replacer should be fed to avoid inducing diarrhea. Extra water or an oral electrolyte solution can be added to make up volume and provide fluid needs. Over several feedings, the concentration of the milk replacer can be increased to that recommended by the manufacturer.

Milk replacer should be warmed to 35° C to 38° C (95° F to 100° F) by immersing the container in a warm-water bath. Never microwave milk replacer, because overheating or uneven heating may result. Vigorous orphans with a good suck reflex may be bottle-fed or syringe-fed (Figures 41-15 and 41-16) while in sternal recumbency with the head elevated, simulating a normal nursing position. The hole or slit in the nipple should be made large enough to allow a drop of milk to form when the bottle is held upside down. A drop of milk is expressed from the bottle on the kitten's tongue to help initiate feeding. Milk should never be forced out of the bottle while it is in the kitten's mouth to avoid aspiration. Care should be taken to ensure no air is ingested while bottle-feeding.

Weaker kittens are best fed with a gastric tube (Figure 41-17).[46] Tube feeding is also efficient if more than one kitten must be hand-raised. Feeding tubes should be selected according to the size of the kitten: 5 Fr for kittens weighing less than 300 g, 8 Fr for kittens greater than 300 g. Measure from the tip of the kitten's nose to just before the last rib, and mark this position on the feeding

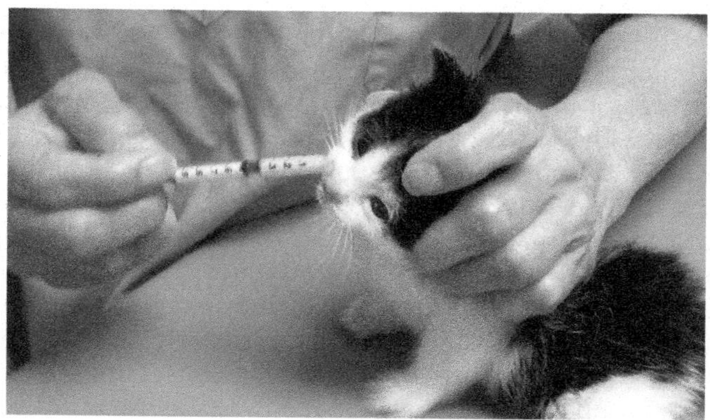

FIGURE 41-15 Orphan kittens can be fed milk replacer using a syringe.

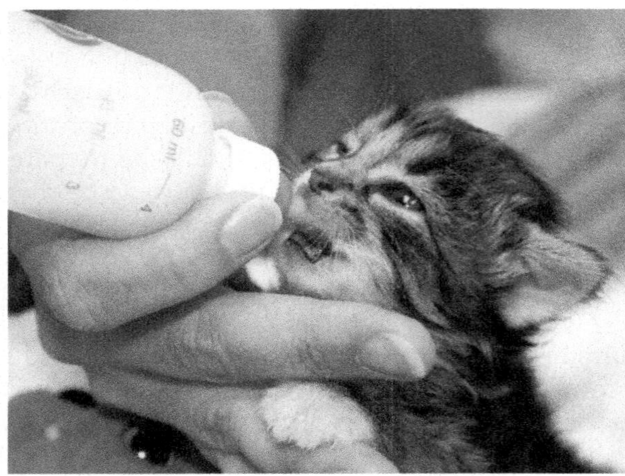

FIGURE 41-16 Orphan kittens that are otherwise healthy with a good suck reflex can be fed milk replacer from a pet nurser bottle. *(Courtesy Richard Young.)*

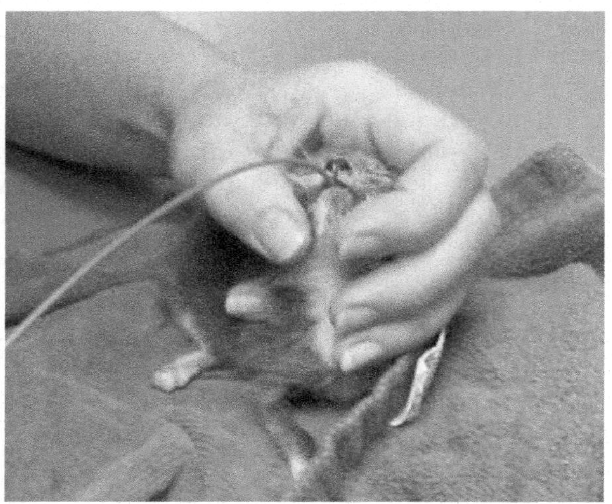

FIGURE 41-17 Weaker orphan kittens, or litters of orphan kittens, can be easily fed using a gastric tube. A size 5-Fr soft red rubber feeding tube is used for the smallest kittens.

tube. The tube will have to be remeasured and marked weekly as the kitten grows. With the kitten in a sternal position, the lubricated tube should pass easily down the left side of the mouth into the esophagus and is advanced to the mark. If resistance is felt or coughing occurs, the tube should be removed and repositioned. Kittens do not have a gag reflex until about 10 days of age. Proper placement of the tube can be confirmed by instilling a small volume of saline first and assessing the response. The milk replacer is drawn up in a 3- or 10-mL syringe that is then attached to the feeding tube. The tube is filled with milk replacer warmed to about 38° C (100° F). The milk replacer is slowly infused for several minutes. Before withdrawing, the tube should be kinked to prevent aspiration of formula. Avoid overfeeding; the maximum stomach capacity for kittens is about 4 to 5 mL/100 g body weight.[46] All tube feeding equipment should be cleaned thoroughly after use.

Kittens should be fed every 2 to 4 hours during the first week of life, and then every 4 to 6 hours until weaning. Diarrhea is the most common problem seen in kittens fed milk replacer. It can be treated by temporarily reducing the amount fed and by diluting the formula by 50% with water or oral electrolyte solution for a few feedings. Orphan kittens should be weighed every 12 hours in the first 2 weeks of life and at least daily thereafter to ensure nutrition is adequate to support growth. Daily records should be kept of weight, feedings, elimination, and general behavior. Identification of individuals in a litter is important for monitoring weight and health, and if kittens appear similar, different colors of nail polish can be applied to the claws for differentiation. Orphans less than 3 weeks of age must have the anogenital area stimulated after every feeding to induce defecation and micturition. At least twice a week, orphan kittens should be cleaned gently with a soft moistened wash cloth.

At 3 to 4 weeks of age, kittens can be taught to drink milk replacer from a shallow saucer. Then solid food can be introduced by mixing a small amount of canned kitten food with milk replacer and offering it for 30 minutes at a time, several times per day. Once the kitten has learned to eat from a saucer, the amount of formula fed can be slowly decreased until only solid food is being ingested. By 5 to 6 weeks of age, kittens are able to chew dry food. Weaning is usually completed by 6 to 8 weeks of age.

PEDIATRIC SPAY AND NEUTER

Although elective gonadectomy is one of the most common veterinary surgeries performed in North America, little data exist to suggest the optimal age.[37] Prepuberal gonadectomy refers to spay or neuter before the onset of puberty, which may occur in female cats between 4 and 21 months of age and in male cats between 8 and 10 months of age. Early spay and neuter (ESN) refers to gonadectomy between 6 and 16 weeks of age and is now more commonly practiced as veterinarians gain experience with pediatric anesthesia and surgery. ESN is one useful approach for control of pet overpopulation, because it enables shelters and pedigreed breeders to perform pre-adoption/pre-sale gonadectomy and avoids the risk of owner noncompliance with spay/neuter contracts. Increasingly, it is recognized there are also health benefits to ESN. Several veterinary organizations support ESN, such as the American Veterinary Medical Association, the Canadian Veterinary Medical Association, the International Society of Feline Medicine, and the Winn Feline Foundation.

Veterinarians have varying attitudes about when to spay and neuter cats. In one survey, small animal veterinarians in New York state were asked about their beliefs and practices regarding gonadectomy and their attitudes to surgery performed before 4 months of age.[73] The majority (70%) recommended gonadectomy for all owned animals, and 90% supported routine gonadectomy of shelter animals before adoption. Most respondents believed shelter animals should be gonadectomized at an earlier age than owned animals. The minimum age reported for gonadectomy ranged from 1 to 12 months. Just more than one third of respondents believed the earliest age for gonadectomy of owned animals should be at or more than 6 months of age. Opinions were affected by variables that included the veterinarian's age, sex, and date of graduation.

In a recent U.K. study, a questionnaire designed to obtain data on the age at which gonadectomy was recommended for cats was sent to over 4,000 veterinarians.[55] Information was also collected on the perceived advantages and disadvantages of gonadectomy in cats between 8 and 20 weeks of age. The mean age recommended for gonadectomy among respondents was 22.6 weeks, despite the fact that the British Small Animal Veterinary Association recommends the surgery be performed at approximately 16 weeks. Just more than one half of veterinarians believed gonadectomy should not be performed before 6 months of age. Only 28% of veterinarians believed it was appropriate to gonadectomize cats between 12 and 16 weeks of age. Beliefs were influenced by several factors, such as time since graduation, perceptions about cat overpopulation, and perceptions about surgical and anesthetic risks.

In addition to avoiding unwanted litters of kittens, the benefits of ESN include safe anesthetic and surgical techniques, shorter surgical and recovery times, and avoidance of the stresses and costs associated with spaying female cats while in estrus, pregnant, or with pyometra.[28] In addition, the risk of mammary adenocarcinoma is reduced by 91% when female kittens are spayed before 6 months of age.[61] Objections to ESN include concerns about effects on growth, increased fracture risk, obesity, behavioral changes, increased disease risk, and safety of anesthesia and surgery in pediatric patients. Several long-term studies have been performed to assess health risks of ESN. These studies confirm that ESN is not associated with any increased risk of disease, but rather is associated with a lower risk of some diseases, such as asthma, gingivitis, and mammary carcinoma.[34,61,74]

The most persistent health concerns associated with ESN are potential effects on urinary tract health. Lower urinary tract disease in cats is a diverse collection of conditions caused by a wide variety of factors, such as diet, water intake, and stressors. The diameter of the male urethra is no smaller in ESN cats than in intact cats.[67] Age at castration does not influence risk of urinary tract disease; in fact, one study showed a decreased risk of lower urinary tract disease in ESN male cats.[74]

Testosterone and estrogen assist maturation of the physes in long bones. Growth stops when physeal closure occurs. Intact cats have distal radial physeal closure at 1 year of age or older. Cats altered at 7 weeks and 7 months of age had distal radial physeal closure about 8 weeks later than intact cats.[69,77] The effect of this delay in physeal closure is unknown, but adult size in cats is not significantly affected by age at altering. It has been suggested that delayed physeal closure may predispose cats to Salter fractures of the femoral capital physes. The femoral capital physis normally closes between 7.5 and 10 months of age. Other risk factors for this type of fracture include obesity and sex/reproductive status (neutered males are at highest risk).[53] The risk of fracture would be the same for cats altered at any age that results in delayed physeal closure, not just cats spayed or neutered at an early age. These fractures appear to be rare in the general cat population. One large study failed to find any association between ESN and physeal fracture risk in cats.[74] Given the development of unwanted sexual behaviors in both male and female cats after puberty, it is not feasible for most owners to delay surgery until after physeal closure (e.g., after 10 months of age), and risk of other diseases such as mammary carcinoma would be increased.

Obesity is a multifactorial problem involving diet, exercise, age, and other factors. Gonadectomized cats have a lower metabolic rate than sexually intact cats regardless of the age at surgery. Castrated male cats require 28% less calories than intact male cats, and spayed female cats require 33% fewer calories than intact female cats.[68] However, one study found a significant increase in food intake in male and female cats after gonadectomy.[16] Therefore when cats are allowed to eat the same amount of food after surgery, or food intake increases because of surgical sterilization, weight gain will inevitably occur. Clients should be counseled on dietary and exercise needs for altered cats before surgical sterilization to avoid obesity.

Compared with gonadectomized cats, sexually intact cats show less affection to humans and more aggression to other cats. An early study showed that ESN male cats are less aggressive to veterinarians and exhibit fewer problems with urine spraying.[77] Other long-term studies have shown there is no difference in the prevalence of serious behavior problems based on age at surgery, although hiding and shyness (at a level not considered serious enough by owners to relinquish the pet) may be more common in cats gonadectomized at less than 5.5 months of age.[74,84] In fact, behavior problems are common in most kittens in the first month after adoption, emphasizing the importance of early owner counseling.[84]

Pediatric patients have unique perioperative, anesthetic, and surgical issues.[36] Kittens should have a complete physical examination as well as at least the first vaccination and treatment for parasites if in a shelter or rescue situation. Client-owned cats can be scheduled for surgery following the last vaccination at approximately 16 weeks. The minimum laboratory data that should be collected before surgery includes packed cell volume and total solids, blood glucose and blood urea nitrogen, and urine specific gravity. Postpone surgery if any illness or abnormality is found. Anesthesia and surgery do not affect response to vaccination so that kittens can be vaccinated at the time of surgery if required.[42]

With the use of safe and effective techniques, it has been shown that ESN does not increase morbidity or mortality associated with anesthesia and surgery.[1] In fact, in one study, kittens gonadectomized at less than 12 weeks had lower postoperative complication rates than those that had surgery at more than 23 weeks of age.[32] Surgical benefits of ESN include less bleeding, improved visualization of organs, shorter surgery times, and more rapid recoveries. Many veterinarians are comfortable with a 2-lb (1-kg) rule as a minimum weight for pediatric spay/neuter patients.

Pediatric patients distribute and metabolize drugs differently; so, the clinician must be careful with drug selection and doses. Weigh each kitten to the nearest 100 grams and calculate drug doses carefully. Renal and hepatic function does not reach mature levels until about 3 to 4 months of age. Certain anesthetic concerns must be addressed:

- Maintenance of breath rate is important because pediatric patients have limited ability to respond to elevated carbon dioxide in blood or tissues and have little oxygen reserves in the lungs; yet they have high oxygen needs (2 to 3 times that of adult cats). Use anesthetic equipment with minimal dead space and resistance.
- Cardiac output is believed to be dependent on heart rate, and there is poor tolerance for both volume overload and hypotension.
- Kittens are less able to compensate for blood loss than adults; therefore care should be taken when handling tissues and blood vessels. Even small volumes of blood loss may result in clinical anemia in kittens less than 8 weeks of age.

Hypothermia occurs easily because of the greater surface area to volume ratio of the neonate, less subcutaneous fat, and reduced ability to shiver. Hypothermia can cause bradycardia and prolonged recovery from anesthesia. The preparation, surgery, and recovery areas should be kept warm. Ensure kittens are never placed on cold metal surfaces. Use warmed towels, circulating water blankets, or other methods to maintain body temperature. Plastic "bubble pack" wrapping is also useful for maintaining warmth. Warm the surgical preparation solutions, and replace alcohol with sterile saline. Minimize the amount of hair coat that is clipped, and the surgical incision should be appropriate for the size of the patient to reduce the risk of hypothermia. Rectal temperature should be monitored during surgery and postoperatively.

Hypoglycemia occurs easily in neonates because of small hepatic glycogen reserves; so, the youngest patients should not be fasted for more than 1 to 2 hours before anesthesia. Water should never be withheld. Within 1 hour of recovery, patients should be offered a small meal. Kittens unwilling to eat after 1 hour or more can be given oral dextrose to prevent hypoglycemia.

Equipment suitable for pediatric gonadectomy is simple and includes

- Cuffed/noncuffed endotracheal tubes, 2 to 3.5 mm
- Clear, snug face mask
- Kit with small surgical instruments
- Stainless steel hemostatic clips for ligation if desired
- Absorbable suture material, such as 4-0 or 5-0 Vicryl (Johnson & Johnson; New Brunswick, NJ) or chromic gut; nylon may be used for closure of linea alba

Stress and anxiety may lead to unpredictable results of premedication and anesthesia. Decrease stress by keeping litter mates together before surgery in a warm quiet environment, minimize patient handling, avoid IV injections, and reunite litters of kittens as soon as possible after recovery. Certain anesthetic drugs should be avoided in pediatric patients. Xylazine may cause bradycardia and decreased cardiac output. Thiobarbiturates require IV administration, which is more stressful than other routes of administration. These drugs are also protein-bound, and neonates are easily saturated, because they have lower plasma protein levels than adult cats.

Several drugs and drug combinations using inhalant anesthesia are safe and effective for pediatric anesthesia.[15,32,36] Brief mask induction may be required with some protocols, then maintenance on isoflurane or sevoflurane (intubate females, use a snug-fitting mask for males). Examples of suitable protocols include

- Midazolam (0.22 mg/kg IM), ketamine (11 mg/kg IM), butorphanol (0.2 to 0.4 mg/kg IM), ±glycopyrrolate (0.011 mg/kg IM)
- Ketamine/diazepam (0.1 mg/kg IM of 1:1 mixture), butorphanol (0.2 to 0.4 mg/kg IM), ±glycopyrrolate (0.011 mg/kg IM)
- Tiletamine/zolazepam (11 mg/kg IM) for castration of male kittens
- Acepromazine (0.055 mg/kg IM), butorphanol (0.22 mg/kg IM), glycopyrrolate (0.011 mg/kg IM)
- Injectable only protocol for both spays and neuters: medetomidine (40 μg/kg), ketamine (20 mg/kg)

and buprenorphine (20 μg/kg), combined and given subcutaneously[65]; atipamezole (0.5 mg IM) is given at the end of surgery

Anesthetic monitoring is necessary and should include assessment of level of anesthesia, color of mucous membranes, Doppler monitoring of heart rate and blood pressure, pulse oximetry, and breath rate. Prolonged recovery is most often caused by hypothermia, but can also be caused by residual effects of drugs or hypoglycemia. Corrective measures for prolonged recoveries include warming, using reversal agents if available, and providing 50% dextrose for hypoglycemia.

Certain surgical concerns must be addressed.[33] Meticulous hemostasis is necessary because tissues are more friable than in adults; handle tissues gently and avoid the use of spay (Snook) hooks in young female kittens. For males, perform closed castration through a single or double scrotal incision, ligate the spermatic cord with absorbable suture or use hemostatic clips. Leave the scrotal incision open. For females, the ovariohysterectomy or ovariectomy technique is the same as for a mature cat. Close the skin with subcuticular sutures or tissue adhesive and avoid skin sutures. A small amount of serous fluid in the abdomen of kittens is normal.

Postoperative analgesia for spays can be addressed with splash blocks. One suggested protocol mixes two parts 0.5% bupivacaine, one part 2% lidocaine, and one part 0.9% NaCl.[28] Splash 0.22 mL/kg onto the incision after closure of the linea alba but before closure of the subcutaneous tissue and skin. A single postoperative dose of meloxicam (0.1 to 0.2 mg/kg, SQ) may be used for kittens more than 6 weeks of age; butorphanol or buprenorphine are also good analgesic choices.

ESN surgeries are safe and easily performed. Providing routine surgical sterilization for kittens less than 6 months of age also allows clinicians to become confident and proficient with anesthesia, surgery, and supportive care that can be applied to other surgical situations in this age group.

References

1. Aronsohn MG, Faggella AM: Surgical techniques for neutering 6- to 14-week-old kittens, *J Am Vet Med Assoc* 202:53, 1993.
2. Auer L, Bell K: The AB blood group system of cats, *Anim Blood Grps Biochem Genet* 12:287, 1981.
3. Baker TW, Davidson AP: Pediatric abdominal ultrasonography, *Vet Clin North Am Small Anim Pract* 36:641, 2006.
4. Blanchard P, Wilson D: Group G streptococcal infections in kittens. In Kirk R, editor: *Current veterinary therapy X: small animal practice*, Philadelphia, 1989, Saunders, p 1091.
5. Boudrieau R, Fossum T, Hartsfield S et al: Pectus excavatum in dogs and cats, *Comp Contin Edu Pract Vet* 12:341, 1990.
6. Bucheler J: Fading kitten syndrome and neonatal isoerythrolysis, *Vet Clin North Am Small Anim Pract* 29:853, 1999.
7. Buote N, Reese C: Congenital tarsal hyperextension in three cats, *J Amer Vet Med Assoc* 228:1200, 2006.
8. Casal M, Jezyk P, Giger U: Transfer of colostral antibodies from queens to their kittens, *Am J Vet Res* 57:1653, 1996.
9. Cave T, Thompson H, Reid S et al: Kitten mortality in the United Kingdom: a retrospective analysis of 274 histopathological examinations (1986 to 2000), *Vet Rec* 151:497, 2002.
10. Claus MA, Levy JK, MacDonald K et al: Immunoglobulin concentrations in feline colostrum and milk, and the requirement of colostrum for passive transfer of immunity to neonatal kittens, *J Feline Med Surg* 8:184, 2006.
11. Crawford P, Hanel R, Levy J: Evaluation of treatment of colostrum-deprived kittens with equine IgG, *Am J Vet Res* 64:969, 2003.
12. Crawford P, Levy J, Werner L: Evaluation of surrogate markers for passive transfer of immunity in kittens, *J Am Vet Med Assoc* 228:1038, 2006.
13. Crigel M-H, Moissonnier P: Pectus excavatum surgically repaired using sternum realignment and splint techniques in a young cat, *J Small Anim Pract* 46:352, 2005.
14. Debraekeleer J: Data for neonatal, pediatric and orphaned puppy and kitten care. In Hand MS, Thatcher CD, Remillard RL et al, editors: *Small animal clinical nutrition*, Topeka, Kans, 2000, Mark Morris Institute, p 1012.
15. Faggella AM, Aronsohn MG: Anesthetic techniques for neutering 6- to 14-week-old kittens, *J Am Vet Med Assoc* 202:56, 1993.
16. Fettman MJ, Stanton CA, Banks LL et al: Effects of neutering on bodyweight, metabolic rate and glucose tolerance of domestic cats, *Res Vet Sci* 62:131, 1997.
17. Fossum T, Boudrieau R, Hobson H: Pectus excavatum in eight dogs and six cats, *JAAHA* 25:595, 1989.
18. Fossum T, Hedlund C: Surgery of the lower respiratory system: lungs and thoracic wall. In Fossum TW, editor: *Small animal surgery*, ed 3, St Louis, 2007, Mosby Elsevier.
19. Fossum TW, Boudrieau RJ, Hobson HP et al: Surgical correction of pectus excavatum, using external splintage in two dogs and a cat, *J Am Vet Med Assoc* 195:91, 1989.
20. Freshman J: Causes of fading puppy and kitten syndrome, *Vet Med* 100:781, 2005.
21. Freshman J: Evaluating fading puppies and kittens, *Vet Med* 100:790, 2005.
22. Freshman J: Initially treating fading puppies and kittens, *Vet Med* 100:800, 2005.
23. Giger U: Blood-typing and crossmatching. In Bonagura JD,Twedt DC, editors: *Kirk's current veterinary therapy XIV: small animal practice*, Philadelphia, 2009, Saunders, p 260.
24. Giger U, Griot-Wenk M, Bucheler J et al: Geographical variation of the feline blood type frequencies in the United States, *Feline Pract* 19:21, 1991.
25. Glaze MB: Congenital and hereditary ocular abnormalities in cats, *Clin Tech Small Anim Pract* 20:74, 2005.

25a. Gow AG, Gow DJ, Hall EJ et al: Prevalence of potentially pathogenic enteric organisms in clinically healthy kittens in the UK, *J Feline Med Surg* 11:655, 2009.

26. Greco D: Congenital and inherited renal disease of small animals, *Vet Clin North Am Sm Anim Pract* 31:393, 2001.
27. Greene C, Prescott J: Streptococcal and other gram-positive bacterial infections. In Greene CE, editor: *Infectious diseases of the dog and cat*, ed 3, St Louis, 2006, Saunders, p 302.
28. Griffin B, DiGangi B, Bohling M: A review of neutering cats. In August J, editor: *Consultations in feline internal medicine*, ed 6, St Louis, 2010, Saunders Elsevier, p 775.
29. Grundy SA: Clinically relevant physiology of the neonate, *Vet Clin North Am Small Anim Pract* 36:443, 2006.
30. Grundy SA, Liu SM, Davidson AP: Intracranial trauma in a dog due to being "swung" at birth, *Top Companion Anim Med* 24:100, 2009.
31. Hoskins J: Congenital defects of cats, *Compend Contin Edu Pract Vet* 17:385, 1995.

32. Howe LM: Short-term results and complications of prepubertal gonadectomy in cats and dogs, *J Am Vet Med Assoc* 211:57, 1997.
33. Howe LM: Surgical methods of contraception and sterilization, *Theriogenology* 66:500, 2006.
34. Howe LM, Slater MR, Boothe HW et al: Long-term outcome of gonadectomy performed at an early age or traditional age in cats, *J Am Vet Med Assoc* 217:1661, 2000.
35. Kirk C: New concepts in pediatric nutrition, *Vet Clin North Am Small Anim Pract* 31:369, 2001.
36. Kustritz M: Early spay-neuter: clinical considerations, *Clin Tech Small Anim Pract* 17:124, 2002.
37. Kustritz MV: Determining the optimal age for gonadectomy of dogs and cats, *J Am Vet Med Assoc* 231:1665, 2007.
38. Lavely JA: Pediatric neurology of the dog and cat, *Vet Clin North Am Small Anim Pract* 36:475, 2006.
39. Lawler D, Monti K: Morbidity and mortality in neonatal kittens, *Am J Vet Res* 45:1455, 1984.
40. Levy J, Crawford P, Collante W et al: Use of adult cat serum to correct failure of passive transfer in kittens, *J Am Vet Med Assoc* 219:1401, 2001.
41. Levy J, Crawford P, Werner L: Effect of age on reference intervals of serum biochemical values in kittens, *J Am Vet Med Assoc* 228:1033, 2006.
42. Levy J, Reese MJ, Patterson EV et al: The effect of anesthesia and surgery on serological responses to vaccination in kittens, *J Vet Intern Med* 20:759, 2006.
43. Little S: How I treat orphaned kittens, *Waltham Focus* 16:2, 2006.
44. Lourenco M, Ferreira H: Electrocardiographic evolution in cats from birth to 30 days of age, *Can Vet J* 44:914, 2003.
45. MacDonald KA: Congenital heart diseases of puppies and kittens, *Vet Clin North Am Small Anim Pract* 36:503, 2006.
46. Macintire DK: Pediatric fluid therapy, *Vet Clin North Am Small Anim Pract* 38:621, 2008.
47. Maggs DJ: Eyelids. In Maggs DJ, Miller P, Ofri R, editors: *Slatter's fundamentals of veterinary ophthalmology*, ed 4, St Louis, 2008, Saunders Elsevier, p 106.
48. Marks S, Willard M: Diarrhea in kittens. In August J, editor: *Consultations in feline internal medicine*, St Louis, 2006, Elsevier Saunders, p 132.
49. Mazzaferro E: Intraosseous catheterization: an often underused, life-saving tool, *NAVC Clinician's Brief* 7:9, 2009.
50. McAnulty JF, Harvey CE: Repair of pectus excavatum by percutaneous suturing and temporary external coaptation in a kitten, *J Am Vet Med Assoc* 194:1065, 1989.
51. McMichael M: Pediatric emergencies, *Vet Clin North Am Small Anim Pract* 35:421, 2005.
52. McMichael M, Dhupa N: Pediatric critical care medicine: physiologic considerations, *Comp Contin Edu Pract Vet* 22:206, 2000.
53. McNicholas WT Jr, Wilkens BE, Blevins WE et al: Spontaneous femoral capital physeal fractures in adult cats: 26 cases (1996-2001), *J Am Vet Med Assoc* 221:1731, 2002.
54. Moon P, Massat B, Pascoe P: Neonatal critical care, *Vet Clin North Am Small Anim Pract* 31:343, 2001.
55. Murray JK, Skillings E, Gruffydd-Jones TJ: Opinions of veterinarians about the age at which kittens should be neutered, *Vet Rec* 163:381, 2008.
56. Narfstrom K: Hereditary and congenital ocular disease in the cat, *J Feline Med Surg* 1:135, 1999.
57. Newitt A, German AJ, Barr FJ: Congenital abnormalities of the feline vertebral column, *Vet Radiol Ultrasound* 49:35, 2008.
58. Nicklas JL, Moisan P, Stone MR et al: Molecular and histopathological characterization of enteroadherent bacteria in failure to thrive kittens [abstract], *J Vet Intern Med* 23:757, 2009.
59. Noden D, Evans H: Inherited homeotic midfacial malformations in Burmese cats, *J Craniofac Genet Devel Biol Suppl* 2:249, 1986.
60. Nutter F, Levine J, Stoskopf M: Reproductive capacity of free-roaming domestic cats and kitten survival rate, *J Am Vet Med Assoc* 225:1399, 2004.
61. Overley B, Shofer FS, Goldschmidt MH et al: Association between ovarihysterectomy and feline mammary carcinoma, *J Vet Intern Med* 19:560, 2005.
62. Pedersen N, Wastlhuber J: Cattery design and management. In Pedersen NC, editor: *Feline husbandry: diseases and management in the multiple cat environment*, Goleta, Calif, 1991, American Veterinary Publications, p 393.
63. Pesavento PA, Bannasch MJ, Bachmann R et al: Fatal *Streptococcus canis* infections in intensively housed shelter cats, *Vet Pathol* 44:218, 2007.
64. Risselada M, de Rooster H, Liuti T et al: Use of internal splinting to realign a noncompliant sternum in a cat with pectus excavatum, *J Amer Vet Med Assoc* 228:1047, 2006.
65. Robertson S, Levy J, Gunkel C et al: *Comparison of isoflurane and butorphanol with medetomidine, ketamine and buprenorphine for anesthesia of 7-12 week old kittens for surgical sterilization*, Doorwerth, The Netherlands, 2003, Association of Veterinary Anaesthetists.
66. Rochlitz I: Recommendations for the housing of cats in the home, in catteries and animal shelters, in laboratories and in veterinary surgeries, *J Fel Med Surg* 1:181, 1999.
67. Root M, Johnston S, Johnston G et al: The effect of prepuberal and postpuberal gonadectomy on penile extrusion and urethral diameter in the domestic cat, *Vet Radiol Ultrasound* 37:363, 1996.
68. Root M, Johnston S, Olson P: Effect of prepuberal and postpuberal gonadectomy on heat production measured by indirect calorimetry in male and female domestic cats, *Am J Vet Res* 57:371, 1996.
69. Root M, Johnston S, Olson P: The effect of prepuberal and postpuberal gonadectomy on radial physeal closure in male and female domestic cats, *Vet Radiol Ultrasound* 38:42, 1997.
70. Scott F, Geissinger C, Peltz R: Kitten mortality survey, *Feline Pract* 8:31, 1978.
71. Scott F, Weiss R, Post J et al: Kitten mortality complex (neonatal FIP?) *Feline Pract* 9:44, 1979.
72. Soderstrom MJ, Gilson SD, Gulbas N: Fatal reexpansion pulmonary edema in a kitten following surgical correction of pectus excavatum, *J Am Anim Hosp Assoc* 31:133, 1995.
73. Spain C, Scarlett J, Cully S: When to neuter dogs and cats: a survey of New York state veterinarians' practices and beliefs, *J Am Anim Hosp Assoc* 38:482, 2002.
74. Spain C, Scarlett J, Houpt K: Long-term risks and benefits of early-age gonadectomy in cats, *J Amer Vet Med Assoc* 224:372, 2004.
75. Sparkes AH, Rogers K, Henley WE et al: A questionnaire-based study of gestation, parturition and neonatal mortality in pedigree breeding cats in the UK, *J Feline Med Surg* 8:145, 2006.
76. Ström Holst B, Frössling J: The Swedish breeding cat: population description, infectious diseases and reproductive performance evaluated by a questionnaire, *J Feline Med Surg* 11:793, 2009.
77. Stubbs W, Bloomberg M, Scruggs S et al: Effects of prepubertal gonadectomy on physical and behavioral development in cats, *J Am Vet Med Assoc* 209:1864, 1996.
78. Sturgess C, Waters L, Gruffydd-Jones T et al: Investigation of the association between whole blood and tissue taurine levels and the development of thoracic deformities in neonatal Burmese kittens, *Vet Rec* 141:566, 1997.
79. Sturman J, Gargano A, Messing J et al: Feline maternal taurine deficiency: effect on mother and offspring, *J Nutr* 116:655, 1986.
80. Taillefer M, Dunn M: Group G streptococcal toxic shock-like syndrome in three cats, *J Am Anim Hosp Assoc* 40:418, 2004.
81. Weese JS: Evaluation of deficiencies in labeling of commercial probiotics, *Can Vet J* 44:982, 2003.
82. Whittemore JC, Flatland B: Comparison of biochemical variables in plasma samples obtained from healthy dogs and cats by use of standard and microsample blood collection tubes, *J Am Vet Med Assoc* 237:288, 2010.

83. Whittemore JC, Flatland B: Comparison of complete blood counts in samples obtained from healthy dogs and cats by use of standard and microsample blood collection tubes, *J Am Vet Med Assoc* 237:281, 2010.
84. Wright JC, Amoss RT: Prevalence of house soiling and aggression in kittens during the first year after adoption from a humane society, *J Am Vet Med Assoc* 224:1790, 2004.
85. Yoon H, Mann F, Jeong S: Surgical correction of pectus excavatum in two cats, *J Vet Sci* 9:335, 2008.

SECTION IX

THE FELINE GENOME AND CLINICAL GENETICS

Editor: Leslie A. Lyons

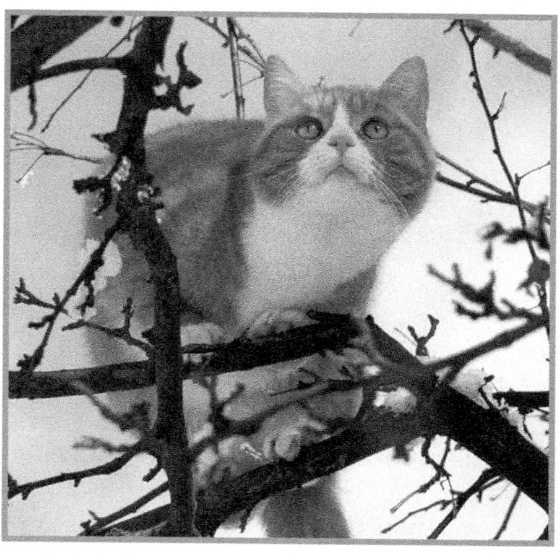

CHAPTER

42

A Short Natural History of the Cat and Its Relationship with Humans

Leslie A. Lyons and Jennifer Dawn Kurushima

OUTLINE

More than 71.1 million homes in the United States, approximately 59.5%, contain pets, and many owners have more than one pet.[3] According to the 2007-2008 National Pet Owners Survey, 38.4 million households in the United States, 54% of pet owners, own a cat. There are 88.3 million cats, compared with 74.8 million dogs, implying roughly 13.5 million more cats than dogs in U.S. households. A survey conducted by the American Veterinary Medical Association (AVMA) reported a 12.4% increase in pet ownership from 2001, when 61.1 million households contained a pet, to 2006, when 68.7 million households were estimated to include a pet.[4] Although the estimate of pet owners is slightly different in the two surveys, the trends are the same: Cats are increasing in popularity as companion animals in the United States. In the United Kingdom, households with dogs appear to be more common than those with cats; however, the number of owned cats and dogs is about the same.[48] Worldwide, domestic cats are clearly gaining in popularity, perhaps being more conducive pets to the modern lifestyle, and, as the cat's status upgrades from mere pet to family member, cat health care has become a common family value.

In tandem with human migrations, cats have traveled around the world, generally to work as vermin control on boats and farms; thus their population management has generally been unrestricted. The cat's co-migrations with humans have resulted in large feral cat populations in both highly populated cities and remote islands that have or previously had human occupation.[50] Because cats, as non-native species, severely threaten native wildlife species,[29] their management is a matter of significant debate, even though the resulting feral populations are due to human negligence. Many cats from the feral populations are captured and transferred to shelters. People are increasingly concerned about the welfare of cats in shelters, and shelter managers must balance kill versus no-kill strategies to ensure adequate population control.[29]

Currently, cats continue to travel the world but more commonly as our valued companions, thus contributing less to feral populations. Although migrant cats confuse the identity of a population's original genetic composition, the origins of the domestic cat can be traced to the dawn of human civilization by following human migrations back through time and sampling the random-bred, remote, and feral cat populations of the world.

DOMESTIC CAT ORIGINS

The domestic cat, *Felis catus*,[24,37] is one of 38 species in the cat family *Felidae*, being a member of the *Felis* lineage.[51] The *Felis* lineage is composed of three small African felids and four small felids that may be the progenitors of the domestic cat, including *Felis lybica* (African wildcat), *Felis silvestris* (European wildcat), *Felis ornata* (Asian wildcat), and *Felis bieti* (Chinese desert cat).[27,31] The domestic cat and the wildcat species can interbreed, producing fertile hybrids[25]; thus their demarcation as subspecies and even distinct species can be disputed. Because the common housecat is a domesticated derivative, the term *Felis catus* has been re-adopted and does not clearly denote the genetic relationship to the progenitor wildcats or their subspecies.[24] The relationship of the African, European, and two Asian wildcats is somewhat controversial; currently, 21 subspecies are defined within these groupings.[33] Other than the South African subspecies of African wildcat, *Felis lybica cafra*, most species of wildcat and their associated subspecies may be the progenitors of domestic cat populations,[21,39] *Felis lybica* having the most scientific support. The African wildcat definitely influenced the origins of the domestic cat[21]; however, detailed examinations of other wildcat species and subspecies have not been possible because of poor access to appropriate samples. For two wildcat subspecies, European and Scottish wildcats, introgressions with domestic cats may be an ongoing process,[7,55-57] threatening the existence of "pure" wildcat populations in Europe and the United Kingdom. Conservation efforts to protect the wildcat populations in Scotland, Italy, the Iberian Peninsula, and other regions fight the encroachment of domestic cats—household pets that may be returning to their feral states, obscuring and perhaps reversing the domestication process.[43,54]

Domestic cats likely participated actively in their own domestication; humans and felines developed a symbiotic, commensal, mutual tolerance. Several independent sites of early civilizations are known to have developed between 8000 and 3000 BCE, including the Huang He River region of China, the Indus Valley in Pakistan, and the Fertile Crescent region, which extends from Iraq, into Turkey, south along the Levant region of the Mediterranean coast, and, arguably, into the Nile Valley of Egypt.[8] As humans made the transition from hunter–gatherers to the more sedentary lifestyle of the farmer and permanent settlements subsequently developed, villages produced refuse piles and grain stores, attracting mice and rats,[11] a primary prey species for the small wildcat. To obtain these easy meals, bold wildcats perhaps began to tolerate humans, and humans accepted the cat because of its utility in vermin control.

Arguably, the domestication of the cat can be considered incomplete and in flux, because abandoned cats and feral populations can quickly adapt to a wildcat lifestyle.[19,20] The cat has behavioral and social attributes recalcitrant to domestication, such as being highly agile and a mainly solitary species; these very traits may be part of the reason that many humans find cats so fascinating and endearing. A combination of self-selection by the cat and selection by humans has led to a variety of aesthetically pleasing coat colors and traits specific to domesticated cats and behaviors that are conducive to companionship. A comprehensive review of coat color frequencies,[40,61] such as those performed in Great Britain,[26] have corroborated cat migrations and human selection preferences by indicating clines of higher and lower coat color frequencies across the world. These clines suggest some degree of controlled breeding or selection by humans, which probably began with the cat seeking human affection and companionship in the Fertile Crescent region and later became more systematic with the first controlled cat breeding programs, possibly in Egypt.[44]

DOMESTIC CAT BREEDS

The creation of cat breeds has been a significantly different process than breed development in other companion animal and agricultural species.[12,63] These nuances are important for an understanding of the appropriate genetic tools, resources, and techniques that will be the most beneficial and efficient for cat genetic research and health programs (see Chapter 43). Random-bred and feral cats represent the overwhelming majority of cats throughout the world, not fancy cat breed populations,[3] although most genetic studies have focused on cat breeds to date. Considering the worldwide distribution of cats, the United States likely has the highest proportion of pedigreed cats. However, the proportion of pedigreed versus random-bred cats is still fairly low; only 10% to 15% of feline patients at the University of California, Davis Veterinary Medicine Teaching Hospital is represented by pedigreed cats.[41] A general understanding of cat breed development and a more in-depth understanding of a limited number of foundation cat breeds will help the veterinarian predict health care problems on the basis of each patient's genetic background. A knowledge of cat breed relationships also helps the veterinarian prioritize differentials for health care management.

Some of the earliest descriptions of different "types" of cats were documented in Siam (now known as Thailand) by monks during the Ayutthaya period (1350-1767).[62] Korats, Burmese, and Siamese were clearly defined according to their coat colors. These same colorations define the same cat breeds today. The naturalist Georges-Louis Leclerc (Comte de Buffon) described races of domestic cats, identifying some of the current breeds, such as the Angora and the Chartreux, on the basis of coat colorations and fur length.[36] Early taxonomists used the coat variants to define domestic cats according to their different variants and subspecies.[37,52,53] The aesthetic value of the coat color and type variants led to competitive showing and breeding. The first documented cat show that judged cats on their aesthetic value occurred in London, England, at the Crystal Palace in 1871.[1] This competition presented only a handful of breeds, including the British, Persian, Abyssinian, Angora, and Siamese. Thus, these early documented cat breeds likely represented genetically distinct populations insofar as strict breeding programs were not established at the time.

Within a few years, cat shows began taking place in the United States, and the homegrown Maine Coon cat was added as a specific breed. The Maine Coon developed from western European random-bred cats that had traveled to the New World with the pilgrims and colonial settlers. By the early 1900s, several cat fancy registries were established and stricter breeding practices were developed. In contrast, a wealth of dog breeds were well established by the twentieth century, having been in development for several hundreds of years.[23,64] A variety of cattle[14] and horse[12] breeds also existed, domesticated from various regional wild populations of the world. Several modern encyclopedic volumes pertaining to the domestic cat list approximately 50 to 80 cat breeds worldwide.[46,47] However, a majority of breeds were developed in the past 50 years, and many listed breeds did not develop into viable populations; some no longer exist, in fact.

Another major difference between cats and other domesticated species lies in the selection process for cat breeds. Cats were originally, and continue to be, selected for aesthetic traits, such as coat colors and fur types, which are mainly single-gene traits. Cats performed their required function, vermin control, naturally. Dog breeds, however, have been selected for morphologies that support diverse functions and behaviors.[63] The breeds of agricultural species are selected for meat and milk quality and quantity.[13] These behavioral and production traits involve complex interactions among many genes, which suggests that more selection has been applied to the genome of dogs, cattle, pigs, and chickens than to the genome of the domestic cat. Less selection likely results in more genetic diversity for cats, which may mean comparatively fewer health problems for cats than for other species.

However, significant distinctions are now apparent among the structural morphologies of current cat breeds. On one end of the spectrum is the cobby and robust body of the Persian, which has extreme brachycephalia; on the other extreme is the slender and fine body of the Siamese, which has extreme dolichocephalia. The severity of these extremes, particularly in the facial structure, has led to certain feline health problems and resultant criticism[34,59] for the cat fancy. A greater emphasis on selection, drawing on more complex genetic interactions, may soon lead to more health concerns.

Today's most pertinent cat breeds and their genetic relationships are listed in Table 42-1. Most worldwide cat fancy associations, such as the Cat Fanciers' Association (CFA),[16,17] The International Cat Association (TICA),[60] the Governing Council of the Cat Fancy (GCCF),[2] and the Fédération Internationale Féline (FIFe),[22] recognize approximately 35 to 41 cat breeds, although only a few breeds overwhelmingly dominate the census of the registries. Persian cats and related breeds (e.g., Exotics, a shorthaired Persian variety) are among the most popular cat breeds worldwide and represent an overwhelming majority of pedigreed cats. Although not all cats produced by breeders are registered, perhaps only 20% to 30%, the CFA, one of the largest cat registries worldwide, generally registers approximately 40,000 pedigreed cats annually.[18] Approximately 16,000 to 20,000 are Persians, and approximately 3000 are Exotics; thus the Persian group of cats represents more than 50% of the cat fancy population. Common breeds that generally have at least 1000 annual registrants are Abyssinians, Maine Coons, and Siamese. Other popular breeds include the Birman and Burmese, which are more prevalent in other areas, such as the United Kingdom. Most of these popular breeds also represent the oldest and most established cat breeds worldwide. However, because of different breeding standards in different registries and population substructuring, not all cats identified as the same breed are genetically alike. Disease frequencies may be different

TABLE 42-1 **Domestic Cat Breeds of the World: Their Origins and Relationships**

Breed	Place Founded	Breed (Family) Grouping*
Abyssinian	Founder—India?	Somali
American Bobtail	Mutation	United States—random breds
American Curl	Mutation	United States—random breds
American Shorthair	Founder—United States	American Wirehair
American Wirehair	Mutation	American Shorthair
Australian Mist	Hybrid	Burmese derived
Balinese	Variant	Colorpoint, Havana Brown, Javanese, Oriental, Siamese
Bengal	Species hybrid	Leopard cat × Egyptian Mau and Abyssinian
Birman	Founder—Southeast Asia	
Bombay	Variant	Burmese, Singapura, Tonkinese
British Shorthair	Founder—Europe	Scottish Fold

TABLE 42-1 **Domestic Cat Breeds of the World: Their Origins and Relationships—cont'd**

Breed	Place Founded	Breed (Family) Grouping*
Burmese	Founder—Southeast Asia	Bombay, Singapura, Tonkinese
Burmilla	Hybrid	Burmese, Persian
Chartreux	Founder—Europe	
Colorpoint Shorthair	Variant	Balinese, Havana Brown, Javanese, Oriental, Siamese
Cornish Rex	Mutation	United Kingdom—random breds
Devon Rex	Mutation	United Kingdom—random breds, Sphynx
Egyptian Mau	Founder—Mediterranean	
European	Founder—Europe	
Exotic	Variant	Persian
Havana Brown	Variant	Balinese, Colorpoint, Javanese, Oriental, Siamese
Japanese Bobtail	Founder	
Javanese	Variant	Balinese, Colorpoint, Havana Brown, Oriental, Siamese
Korat	Founder—Southeast Asia	
Kurilean Bobtail	Mutation	Eastern Russia, Kuril Islands
LaPerm	Mutation	United States—random breds
Maine Coon	Founder—United States	
Manx	Mutation	United Kingdom—random breds
Munchkin	Mutation	United States—random breds
Norwegian Forest	Founder—Europe	
Ocicat	Crossbred	Siamese × Abyssinian
Oriental	Variant	Balinese, Colorpoint, Havana Brown, Javanese, Siamese
Persian	Founder—Europe	Exotic
Peterbald	Mutation	Russian—random breds, Don Sphynx
Pixie-bob	Founder—United States	United States—random breds
Ragdoll	Founder—United States	United States—random breds
Russian Blue	Founder—Europe	
Savannah	Species hybrid	Serval × domestic
Scottish Fold	Mutation	United Kingdom—random breds, British SH, Persian
Selkirk Rex	Mutation	United States—random breds, Persian
Siamese	Founder—Southeast Asia	Balinese, Havana Brown, Javanese, Colorpoint, Oriental
Siberian	Founder—Europe	Russian—random breds
Singapura	Variant	Bombay, Burmese, Tonkinese
Sokoke	Founder—Africa	African—random breds
Somali	Variant	Abyssinian
Sphynx	Mutation	Devon Rex
Tonkinese	Variant	Bombay, Burmese, Singapura
Turkish Angora	Founder—Mediterranean	
Turkish Van	Founder—Mediterranean	

*Modified from genetic studies based on 29 tetranucleotide short tandem repeat markers,[45] 39 dinucleotide short tandem repeat markers,[39] and unpublished data (Lyons).

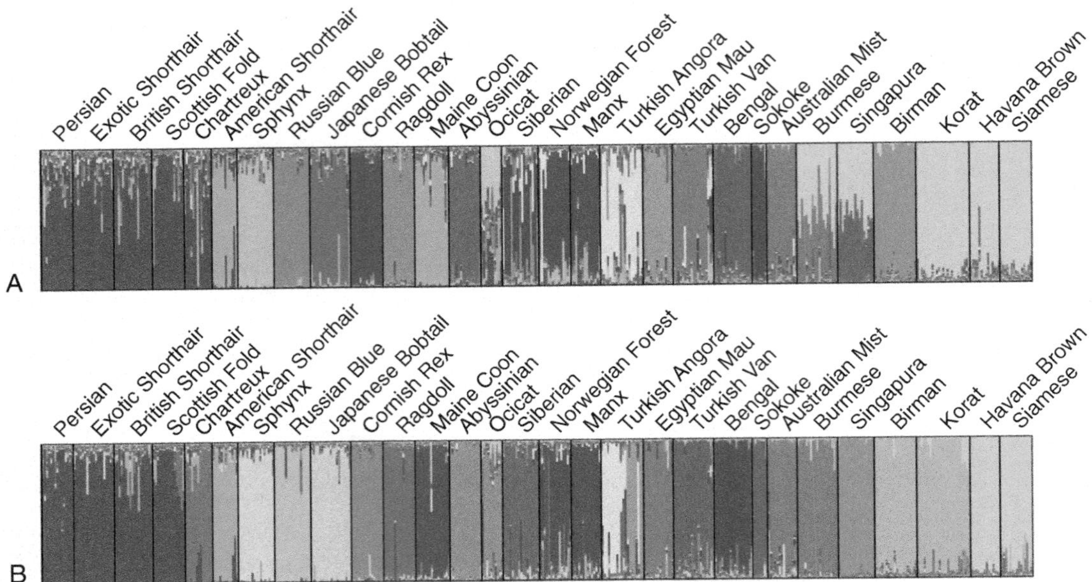

FIGURE 42-1 Population structuring of domestic cat breeds. The colors correspond to predicted genetic clusters. Each column represents an individual cat. **A,** Breed clustering defined by single nucleotide polymorphisms (SNPs). The slower mutation rate of SNPs resolves older breed relationships. There are 29 cat breeds that form only 17 distinct populations. Asian breeds, such as Burmese, Singapura, Birman, and Korat, are genetically distinct, but Korat, Havana Brown, and Siamese cluster. **B,** Breed clustering defined by short-tandem repeat, microsatellite markers (STRs). The faster mutation rate of STRs resolves more recent breed relationships. There are 29 cat breeds that form 21 distinct populations. Havana Browns and Siamese, and Burmese and Singapura are not genetically differentiated. Persian, Exotic Shorthair, British Shorthair, and Scottish Fold cannot be clearly defined. The Ocicat and Abyssinian relationship cannot be separated, nor can the Burmese and the Australian Mist.

for breeds in different parts of the world. For example, polycystic kidney disease has been shown to have about the same prevalence in Persian cats around the world,[5,6,10,15] but hypokalemia in the Burmese is more limited to cats in the United Kingdom and Australia[9,35] and not found in populations in the United States. Some lines of Burmese in the United States segregate for a craniofacial defect, which is not commonly found in Burmese cats outside the United States.[49] The breed substructuring may be partially due to rabies control measures that reduce migration of cats among countries, but it is also likely that the known health concerns in the breeds have led to strong restrictions of imports and exports of fancy-breed cats.

A more recently developed cat breed, the Bengal,[30] which is a hybrid between the Asian Leopard cat, *Prionailurus bengalensis*, and the domestic cat, has gained significant popularity throughout the world, even though some registries currently do not recognize the breed. The Bengal exhibits remarkable colorations and tabby patterns, but their temperament is generally a bit more fractious than that of other breeds. Several other hybrid breeds exist,[60] including crosses with Servals *(Felis serval)*, known as Savannahs, and Jungle cats *(Felis chaus)*, known as Chaussies. Because of limited wildcat founders, the hybrid cats may have decreased genetic variation. These hybrid cats may also have allelic incompatibilities for a given gene; the genes between the two species, leopard cat and domestic cat, have millions of years of evolutionary divergence, which allows differences at the DNA sequence level of a gene. Hence an accumulation of different genetic variants that are functional within the species, but nonfunctional across the felid species, are likely present in some Bengal cats. Thus hybrid cat breeds may have unexpected health problems and infertility, creating a challenge for both genetic studies and primary health care.

Many modern cat breeds derived from an older "foundation" breed, thereby forming breed families or groups (see Table 42-1). Approximately 22 breeds can be considered foundation or "natural" breeds. Genetic studies have also shown that the foundation breeds have either significantly different genetic pools or sufficient selection and inbreeding that created significant genetic distinction (Figure 42-1). Cat breeds derived from the foundation breeds are often based on single gene variants, such as longhaired and shorthaired varieties, or even a hairless variety, as found in the Devon Rex and Sphynx grouping. Color variants also tend to demarcate breeds, such as the "pointed" variety of the Persian, known as the Himalayan by many cat enthusiasts and as a separate breed by some associations, such as TICA.[60] These derived breeds are not genetically significantly different and therefore share health concerns. Selkirk Rex, American Shorthair, and British Shorthair all use Persians to help define their structure; thus these breeds also suffer from polycystic kidney disease,[42] and their genetic signatures are very similar to that of Persians, nearly obscuring their original population foundations of U.S. and U.K. cats.

Many cat breeds originated from single gene traits found in western European random-bred, feral cat populations, such as the folded ears of the Scottish Fold[28] and the dorsally curled ears of the American Curl.[58] Controlled breeding and selection of these cats slowly developed the populations into a unique breed, based on conformation as well as the original unique trait. Many newly identified spontaneous mutations that produce unusual traits, such as ear folding or curly fur, are generally recognized in random-bred, feral cat populations, followed by morphologic molding using various desired combinations found in other breeds. Thus many new and some established breeds have allowable outcrosses to influence their "type" and to support genetic diversity in the breed foundation. For example, genetic differentiation of the Scottish Fold and the British Shorthair is difficult because the two are allowed to interbreed to maintain diversity and to modify type. Because Persians have a highly desired brachycephalic head type, this breed tends to influence many other newer breeds. Breeds in which the dolichocephalic type is desired are often outcrossed with the Siamese family of cats. Hence the newly developing breeds can inherit health problems from the foundation breeds. For example, newer breeds such as Burmilla and Asian will likely have the same concerns for polycystic kidney disease as the Selkirk Rex and British Shorthair because of outcrossing with the Persian, which is desired for the production of the brachycephalic head type.

The outcrosses that are valid for any breed can vary among cat registries, and the same breed may even have a different name depending on the country or registry. For example, the Burmese registered by the GCCF[2] in the United Kingdom and FIFe[22] in Europe is known as the Foreign Burmese breed in the United States, and these cat "breeds" have significantly different craniofacial type among the countries. The Havana Brown has developed into a distinctive breed in the United States, also with a significantly different craniofacial structure than its foundation breeds, the Siamese and Oriental Shorthairs. However, in Europe the chestnut color variety of the Oriental Shorthair is similar to (basically identical to, in fact) the Havana Brown. Some breeds, such as Korats and Turkish Vans, have very similar standards across almost all countries and registries. However, breeds with similar standards may be different in different countries because their breeding histories are different, even though similar-looking cats have resulted from the selection process.

During the world wars cat breeding was not a priority, and many breeds became nearly nonexistent in Europe. To reconstitute the breeds in the early 1950s, many European breeds have been re-established with substantial crossbreeding and outcrossing using a concoction of breeds and feral populations as stock. Thus the genetics of breeds in the United States, which did not suffer such an extreme population crash, may be quite different from that of the same breeds in other parts of the world. For example, Burmese in the United Kingdom and Australia suffer from a heritable hypokalemia, whereas American Burmese do not[32,35] but instead have a recessive craniofacial defect in some prominent lines.[49] The worldwide regional differences of the cat breed histories should be considered with their health care management.

ORIGINS AND BREED HEALTH

Overall, from a phylogenetic point of view, cat breeders are "splitters" instead of "lumpers," and a few foundation breeds encompass most variation of cat breeds. More cat breeds are documented than can be genetically defined. In addition, the world's cat populations can be defined as only approximately eight populations (Figure 42-2). These world cat populations still mimic human migrations, some populations being distinct in areas of the world that have less European and Asian migration, such as Iran. The early descriptions of some cat breeds are genetically supported even today. Cats from Siam and Burma are represented by breeds such as the Korat, Siamese, Burmese, and Birman. Individuals from these breeds show strong genetic relationships with feral cats from Southeast Asian but not Western Europe, which strongly suggests that these breeds did originate in the Far East. For some breeds, such as the Japanese Bobtail, the origin of the tail trait does seem to be in Japan, although genetic influences from western cats have obscured its true origins. Like breeds within a breed family, genetically influenced health concerns could originate and be prevalent in the feral cat populations that are the origins of some modern breeds.

Some cat breeds are going "back to their roots"; the breeders have become concerned with genetic health and are proactively improving the size of their gene pools. Because genetic testing now allows the identification of cats that carry undesired aesthetic traits, such as certain coat colors and fur lengths, cat breeders are more open to outcrossing cats and then using genetic tests to prevent the undesired qualities. Breeders are now more willing to import cats from the countries of origin to add needed genetic diversity for health and also to help the selection process of type, behavior, and other important qualities of a cat breed. Two studies have presented the genetic diversity and inbreeding levels in domestic cats,[39,45] and both suggest that some breeds have more diversity than others and some breed management from the genetic point of view may be necessary (Figure 42-3).

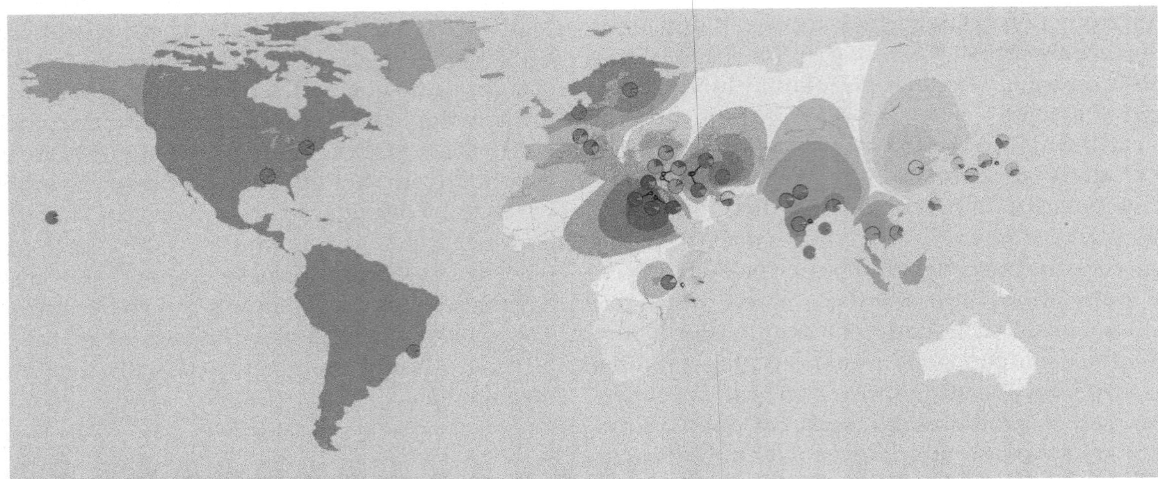

FIGURE 42-2 Population structuring of the world's random-bred cats. Bayesian clustering was used to define the world's cat populations. By using both single nucleotide polymorphisms and short tandem repeat markers (STRs; microsatellites), eight modern random-bred lineages can be defined from the world's random-bred cat populations. The pie charts represent the percentage of the eight worldwide lineages found at each location. The shading indicates the strength of the predominating lineage for each region of the world. The world's cat populations are parsed into the following categories: European/Americas *(green)*, Eastern Mediterranean *(light blue)*, Egypt *(blue)*, Iraq/Iran *(purple)*, West Indian Ocean *(pink)*, India *(red)*, Southeast Asian *(orange)*, and East Asian *(light orange)* cats.

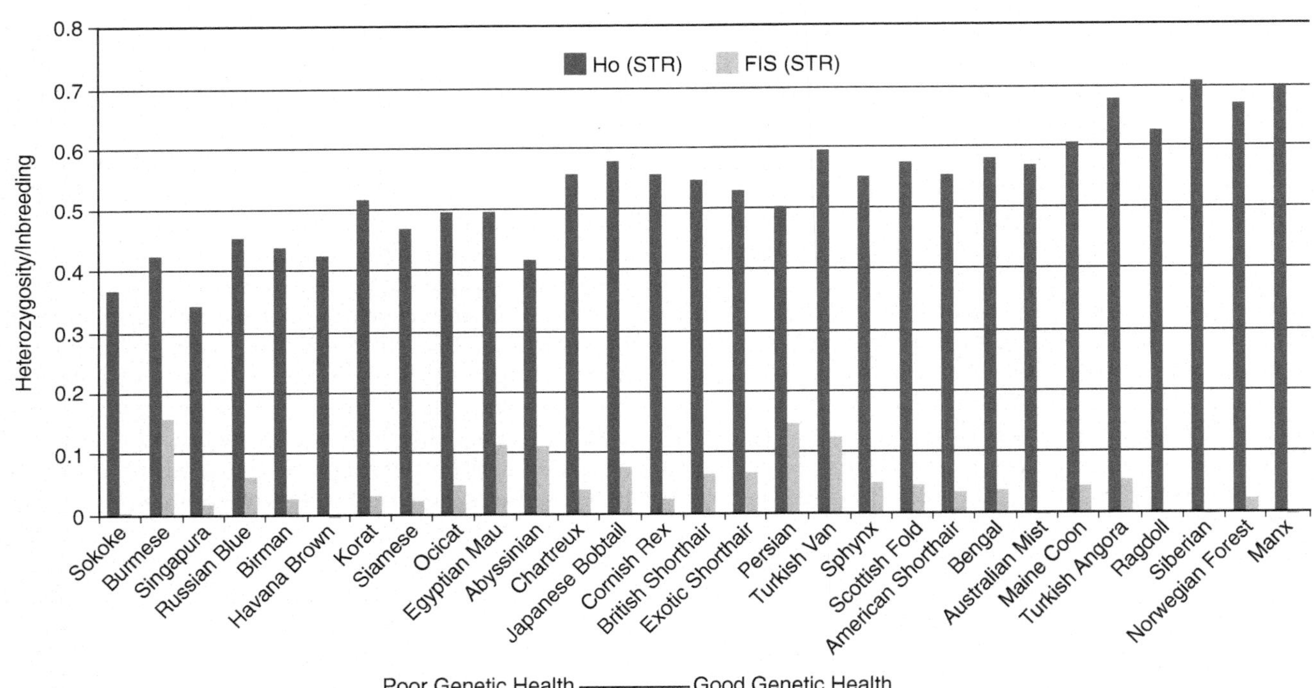

FIGURE 42-3 Relative genetic health of domestic cat breeds. A variety of genetic markers and population statistics are used to measure a population's genetic diversity. Short tandem repeat markers (STRs; microsatellites) and single nucleotide polymorphisms (SNPs) were used to calculate the genetic variation of cat breeds, measured as heterozygosity and inbreeding Wright's coefficients (F_{IS}). Presented are the heterozygosity values and inbreeding coefficients based on STRs for the breeds. Additional statistics were also calculated, including the SNP-based heterozygosity and inbreeding coefficients and the effective number of alleles for each type of genetic marker. The relative rank for each measure was determined for each breed and then averaged to determine "overall genetic health." The overall genetic health is represented from poor health on the *left* to good health on the *right*.

The availability of genetic tests and standardized markers for parentage testing[38] supports outcrossing and cat breed management. These same tools can be assets to veterinarians as they assist clients with the health management of their cats.

In conclusion, veterinarians should be knowledgeable about the relationship of cat breeds in their country and also be aware of regional differences in breeding practices. Many cat breeds are genetically distinct and genetically diverse, leading to fewer health problems. However, other breeds do harbor low genetic variation, which may be detrimental if the population is susceptible to a new viral or bacterial strain. Inbreeding depression can lead to a distinct health concern or just the overall poor health of the population. Knowledge of breed relationships and cross-breeding programs can help predict the potential spread of breed-related or breed-specific diseases across the cat fancy.

References

1. The Cat-Show, *Penny Illustrated Paper, The Naturalist*, July 22, 1871, p 511.
2. The Governing Council of the Cat Fancy (GCCF). http://www.gccfcats.org, 2010. Accessed June 22, 2011.
3. American Pet Product Manufacturing Association: *National pet owners survey*, Greenwich, Conn, 2008, The Association.
4. American Veterinary Medical Association: *US pet ownership and demographics sourcebook*, Schaumburg, Ill, 2007, The Association.
5. Barrs VR, Gunew M: Prevalence of autosomal dominant polycystic kidney disease in Persian cats and related-breeds in Sydney and Brisbane, *Aust Vet J* 79:257, 2001.
6. Barthez PY, Rivier P, Begon D: Prevalence of polycystic kidney disease in Persian and Persian related cats in France, *J Feline Med Surg* 5:345, 2003.
7. Beaumont M, Barratt EM, Gottelli D et al: Genetic diversity and introgression in the Scottish wildcat, *Mol Ecol* 10:319, 2001.
8. Bellwood P: *First farmers: the origins of agricultural societies*, Oxford, 2005, Blackwell Publishing.
9. Blaxter A, Lievesley P, Gruffydd-Jones T et al: Periodic muscle weakness in Burmese kittens, *Vet Rec* 118:619, 1986.
10. Bonazzi M, Volta A, Gnudi G et al: Prevalence of the polycystic kidney disease and renal and urinary bladder ultrasonographic abnormalities in Persian and Exotic Shorthair cats in Italy, *J Feline Med Surg* 9:387, 2007.
11. Bonhomme F, Martin S, Thaler L: Hybridation en laboratoire de *Mus musculus L.* et *Mus spretus lataste*, *Experientia* 34:1140, 1978.
12. Bowling AT, Ruvinsky AO: *Genetics aspects of domestication, breeds and their origins*, New York, 2000, CABI.
13. Bradley DG, Cunningham EP: *Genetic aspects of domestication*, New York, 1999, CABI.
14. Buchanan DS, Dolezal SL: *Breeds of cattle*, New York, 1999, CABI.
15. Cannon MJ, MacKay AD, Barr FJ et al: Prevalence of polycystic kidney disease in Persian cats in the United Kingdom, *Vet Rec* 149:409, 2001.
16. CFA: *The Cat Fanciers' Association cat encyclopedia*, New York, 1993, Simon & Schuster.
17. CFA: *The Cat Fanciers' Association complete cat book*, ed 1, New York, 2004, Harper Collins Publishers.
18. CFA: Cat Fanciers' Association registration totals by color and breed—2003, and 1/1/58 to 12/31/03, *Cat Fanciers' Almanac* 20:72, 2004.
19. Driscoll CA, Clutton-Brock J, Kitchener AC et al: The taming of the cat. Genetic and archaeological findings hint that wildcats became housecats earlier—and in a different place—than previously thought, *Sci Am* 300:68, 2009.
20. Driscoll CA, Macdonald DW, O'Brien SJ: From wild animals to domestic pets, an evolutionary view of domestication, *Proc Natl Acad Sci USA* 106(Suppl 1):9971, 2009.
21. Driscoll CA, Menotti-Raymond M, Roca AL et al: The Near Eastern origin of cat domestication, *Science* 317:519, 2007.
22. FIFe. Federation Internationale Feline. http://fifeweb.org/index.php, 2010. Accessed June 22, 2011.
23. Fogle B: *The encyclopedia of the dog*, London, 1995, Dorling Kindersley Limited.
24. Gentry AS, Clutton-Brock J, Groves CP: The naming of wild animal species and their domestic derivatives, *J Archaeol Sci* 31:645, 2004.
25. Gray AP: *Mammalian hybrids: a check-list with bibliography*, Farnham Royal, England, 1972, Commonwealth Agricultural Bureaux.
26. Gruffydd-Jones TJ, Jaffe P, Lloyd AT et al: *Carnivore Genetic Newsletter* 4:13, 1979.
27. Hemmer H: The evolutionary systematics of living Felidae: present status and current problems, *Carnivore* 1:71, 1978.
28. Jackson O: Congenital bone lesions in cats with folded ears, *Bulletin Feline Advisory Bureau* 14:2, 1975.
29. Jessup D: The welfare of feral cats and wildlife, *J Am Vet Med Assoc* 225:1377, 2004.
30. Johnson G: *The Bengal cat*, Greenwell Springs, La, 1991, Gogees Cattery.
31. Johnson WE, Eizirik E, Pecon-Slattery J et al: The late Miocene radiation of modern Felidae: a genetic assessment, *Science* 311:73, 2006.
32. Jones BR, Gruffydd-Jones TJ: Hypokalemia in the cat, *Cornell Vet* 80:13, 1990.
33. Kratochvil J, Kratochvil Z: The origin of the domesticated forms of the Genus Felis (Mammalia), *Zoologicke Listy* 25:193, 1976.
34. Kunzel W, Breit S, Oppel M: Morphometric investigations of breed-specific features in feline skulls and considerations on their functional implications, *Anat Histol Embryol* 32:218, 2003.
35. Lantinga E, Kooistra HS, van Nes JJ: [Periodic muscle weakness and cervical ventroflexion caused by hypokalemia in a Burmese cat], *Tijdschr Diergeneeskd* 123:435, 1998.
36. Leclerc G-L: *Histoire naturelle, generale et particulière, avec la description du cabinet du roi: description du chat*, Paris, 1756, L'Imprimerie Royale.
37. Linneaus C: *Systema naturae per regna tria naturae, secundum classes, ordines, genera, species, cum characteribus, differentiis, synonymis, locis*, ed 10, Holmiae, 1758, Laurentii Salvii.
38. Lipinski MJ, Amigues Y, Blasi M et al: An international parentage and identification panel for the domestic cat *(Felis catus)*, *Anim Genet* 38:371, 2007.
39. Lipinski MJ, Froenicke L, Baysac KC et al: The ascent of cat breeds: genetic evaluations of breeds and worldwide random-bred populations, *Genomics* 91:12, 2008.
40. Lloyd AT: Cats from history and history from cats, *Endeavour, New Series* 11:1987, 1987.
41. Louwerens M, London CA, Pedersen NC et al: Feline lymphoma in the post-feline leukemia virus era, *J Vet Intern Med* 19:329, 2005.
42. Lyons L, Biller D, Erdman C et al: Feline polycystic kidney disease mutation identified in PKD1, *J Am Soc Nephrol*, 2004.
43. Macdonald D, Daniels M, Driscoll C et al: *The Scottish wildcat: analyses for conservation and an action plan*, Oxford, 2004, Wildlife Conservation Research Unit.
44. Malek J: *The cat in ancient Egypt*, Philadelphia, 1993, University of Pennsylvania.
45. Menotti-Raymond M, David VA, Pflueger SM et al: Patterns of molecular genetic variation among cat breeds, *Genomics* 91:1, 2008.
46. Morris D: *Cat breeds of the world*, New York, 1999, Penguin Books.

47. Morris D: *Cat breeds of the world: a complete illustrated encyclopedia,* New York, 1999, Viking Penquin.
48. Murray JK, Browne WJ, Roberts MA et al: Number and ownership profiles of cats and dogs in the UK, *Vet Rec* 166:163, 2010.
49. Noden DM, Evans HE: Inherited homeotic midfacial malformations in Burmese cats, *J Craniofac Genet Dev Biol Suppl* 2:249, 1986.
50. Nogales M, Martin A, Tershy B et al: A review of feral cat eradication on islands, *Conserv Biol* 18:310, 2004.
51. Nowak RM: *Walker's carnivores of the world,* Baltimore, 2005, Johns Hopkins University Press.
52. Pocock RI: *On English domestic cats,* London, 1907, P.Z.S.
53. Pocock RI: *Catalogue of the genus Felis,* London, 1951, British Museum.
54. Randi E: Detecting hybridization between wild species and their domesticated relatives, *Mol Ecol* 1:285, 2008.
55. Randi E, Pierpaoli M, Beaumont M et al: Genetic identification of wild and domestic cats *(Felis silvestris)* and their hybrids using Bayesian clustering methods, *Mol Biol Evol* 18:1679, 2001.
56. Randi E, Ragni B: Multivariate analysis of craniometric characters in European wild cats, domestic cat, and African wild cat (genus *Felis), Z Saugetierkd* 51:243, 1986.
57. Randi E, Ragni B: Genetic variability and biochemical systematics of domestic and wild cat populations *(Felis silvestris: Felidae), J Mammal* 72:79, 1991.
58. Robinson R: The American curl cat, *J Hered* 80:474, 1989.
59. Schlueter C, Budras KD, Ludewig E et al: Brachycephalic feline noses: computed tomography and anatomical study of the relationship between head conformation and the nasolacrimal drainage system, *J Feline Med Surg* 11:891, 2009.
60. TICA. The International Cat Association, 2010. http://www.tica.org/ 22 June 2011
61. Todd NB: Cats and commerce, *Sci Am* 237:100, 1977.
62. Unknown: Cat book poems of Siam (Tamara Maew), circa 1350-1767.
63. Wayne R: *Consequences of domestication: morphological diversity of the dog,* New York, 2001, CABI.
64. Wayne R, Vila C: *Phylogeny and origin of the domestic dog,* New York, 2001, CABI.

CHAPTER

43

The Feline Genome and Clinical Implications

Leslie A. Lyons

OUTLINE

Genomics is a field of genetic study focusing on the organization and formulation of the DNA sequence of a species' chromosomes and the order, distance, and structure of the genes within the chromosomes. Several early and prominent geneticists recognized that many visual, phenotypic, mammalian traits such as pelage colors and fur types, including those of the cat, had simple modes of inheritance and followed the same segregation rules noted by Gregor Mendel regarding pea traits. One of the first loci ever mapped in a species, the first genomics, was the *Orange* coat color of cats, which was recognized to be sex-linked to the X chromosome. Since that time the inheritance patterns of many phenotypic traits in the cat have been defined, the loci localized to chromosomes, and now the causative genes and mutations are under investigation. The feline karyotype and early gene mapping studies indicated that the cat has a genome organization more similar to that of humans than to that of the mouse or the domestic dog. Now that the limitations of the use of murine models in human studies have been realized and the cost of genomic and genetic resource development is within a feasible range, genomic studies in the cat have significantly advanced. The advances of the genetic tools and resources support the investigation of feline health, improving the direct health of the cat and facilitating the use of the cat as a model for human disease. This chapter presents an overview of the evolution of genetic tools for the domestic cat and highlights their use and value for improving feline health.

CYTOGENETICS

Early studies of mitotic chromosomes of the domestic cat revealed an easily distinguishable karyotype consisting of 18 autosomal chromosomes and the XY sex chromosome pair, resulting in a 2N complement of 38 chromosomes for the cat genome (Figure 43-1).[57-60] Cat chromosomes are fortuitously easily distinguishable, clearly defined by size, centromere position, distinctive giemsa banding patterns of the short *(p)* and long *(q)* arms of each chromosome, and the presence of only a few small acrocentric chromosomes, which have no *p* arms and are traditionally hard to distinguish. Various cytogenetic techniques, such as R-, RBG-banding and fragile site studies, have also helped distinguish and characterize the cat chromosomes.[47-49,52] For example, cats do not have a significant fragile X site on the X chromosome that is found in humans and is associated with mental retardation. Although a sequential numbering of the chromosomes has been suggested,[3] the historical classification of chromosomes into morphologic groups has been retained in the cat. Hence cats have three large metacentric chromosomes (A1 to A3), four large subtelomeric chromosomes (B1 to B4), two medium-size metacentrics (C1 and C2), four small subtelomerics (D1 to D4), three small metacentrics (E1 to E3), and two small acrocentrics (F1 and F2). The X chromosome is midsize and subtelomeric, similar to chromosome B4.

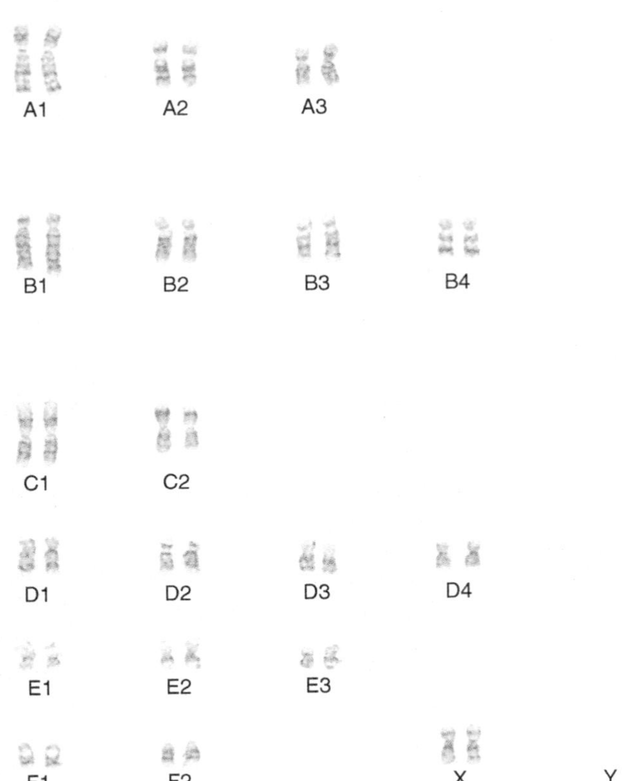

FIGURE 43-1 Karyotype of the domestic cat. Domestic cats have 38 chromosomes, including 18 autosomal pairs and the sex chromosomes, X and Y. This karyotype depicts a female cat and therefore has two X chromosomes. Cat chromosomes have retained the historical nomenclature of being grouped into alphabetical categories that reference the size and position of the centromere. *(Courtesy Roscoe Stanyon.)*

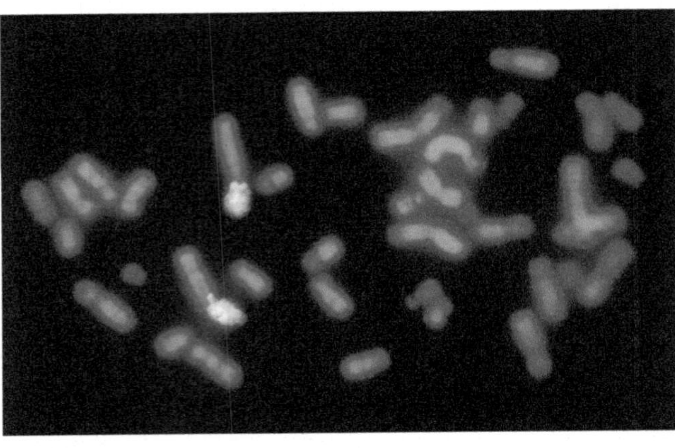

FIGURE 43-2 Chromosome painting of domestic cat chromosomes. DNA from flow-sorted human chromosome 13 was dye labeled and hybridized to a mitotic spread of cat chromosomes. The DNA for all of human chromosome 13 localizes to the short arm of cat chromosome A1, A1p. This comparative approach indicates that if a gene of interest is known to be on human chromosome 13, its location can be predicted to be on chromosome A1p of the cat. *(Courtesy Roscoe Stanyon.)*

Early chromosome staining recognized some major alterations in the felid genome, particularly the Robertsonian translocation of F1 and F2 to form chromosome C3 in the ocelot lineage of cats from South America (2N = 36).[59] Minor pericentric inversions, additions, or deletions of the small chromosomes cause variation in the felid karyotype. The pericentric inversion of chromosome F1 produces a small, more centromeric chromosome and represents as E4 in many cat species. Overall, domestic cats have a chromosomal architecture that is highly representative for all felids and ancestral for most carnivores.[34,44]

Historically, the first genetic consideration to explain reduced fertility or intersex cats is chromosomal differences, especially the loss of one of the sex chromosomes. Karyotypic and now gene-based assays are common methods to determine if a cat with ambiguous genitalia[50] or a poor reproductive history has a chromosomal abnormality. Karyotypic studies of male tortoiseshell cats have shown that they are often mosaics, or chimeras, being XX/XY in all or some tissues.* The minor chromosomal differences that are cytogenetically detectable between a domestic cat and an Asian leopard cat are likely the cause of fertility problems in the Bengal cat breed, which is a hybrid between these two species. Other significant chromosomal abnormalities causing common "syndromes" are not well documented in the cat.

The sufficient variation of cat chromosomal sizes also allowed for the easy flow sorting of cat chromosomes.[56] The DNA in the flow-sorted pools of each chromosome could be individually dye labeled. The dye-labeled DNA from each chromosome could then be hybridized to mitotic chromosomes of another species, such as humans, which provided a gross overall view of which chromosomes between the two species had the same DNA (Figure 43-2). For example, the *p* arm of human chromosome 1 (1p) is largely composed of the same genes that are on the cat chromosome defined as C1, whereas human chromosome 1q is composed of genes that are found on cat chromosome F1. The chromosome painting technique could also be performed reciprocally, implying painting cat chromosomes onto human mitotic chromosome spreads and human chromosomes onto cat mitotic chromosome spreads, revealing the high conservation of chromosomal arrangement of cat to humans,[56,61] specifically compared to mice.[53] Thus chromosome painting gave an excellent overview of cat genome organization,[38] which greatly facilitates candidate gene approaches because the location of particular genes could be anticipated in cats from comparison with the genetic map of humans.[55] This additional confirmation of conservation to human, with regard to genome organization, further supported additional genetic resource

*References 2, 4, 7, 10, 14, 19, 20, 42, 54.

development for the cat as a valuable animal model for human disease.

GENETIC MAPS

Somatic Cell Hybrid

The aesthetically pleasing karyotype supported the early somatic cell hybrid genetic maps of the cat.[35,37] A somatic cell hybrid is a fusion of the cell lines, generally fibroblasts, of two different species. The cell line of one species—usually a rodent, such as a mouse or Chinese hamster—is compromised in some way, such as by having an enzyme deficiency that causes growth incompatibility in non-supplemented media. The cell line from the species of interest, in this case the cat, is damaged by a different, chemical means. The fusion of the two compromised cell lines leads to the chromosomes of the cat integrating into the nucleus and sometimes the chromosomes of the rodent cell line, which then rescues the rodent cell line as a functional enzyme is now present to support the growth of fusion cells. Many different fusion lines are maintained and propagated; however, the entire complement of cat chromosomes is never completely retained in a given cell line. Thus a given cell line will have all the rodent chromosomes, which happen to be mainly acrocentric chromosomes, and only one or a few cat chromosomes. A proper somatic cell hybrid panel would have a representation of at least each of the cat chromosomes in the set of fusion cell lines. Analysis of the mitotic chromosomes of the cell lines can often show which specific cat chromosome may be present because the cat chromosomes are clearly distinguished from those of rodents by size and shape. These cell lines can then be assayed for the presence or absence of specific proteins, or DNA sequences, thereby indicating that the genes that create the proteins or are represented by the DNA segments must reside on the cat chromosome that is within the cell line. This mapping approach provided the first rudimentary genetic map of the cat with 105 different loci,[35] including the association for the genes for *hemoglobin beta (HBB)* and *tyrosinase (TYR)*.[36] The *HBB* polymorphism was shown to be associated with the Siamese coloration, also known as *points*. Recently, this coloration has been proved to be a mutation in *TYR*.[13,23,51]

The first cat map also provided the first indication that the cat genomic structure was very conserved to that of humans as many of the genes were clustering on the same chromosomes in a similar fashion to the human genetic map. This conservation to humans helped to promote the cat as a model for human diseases, insofar as finding genes in the cat would be drastically easier than in a species with a more rearranged genome.

Recombination Map

Interspecies Hybrids

During the late 1960s and early 1970s, the role of viruses in cancer etiologies was under intense investigation, and the cat figured largely in these studies. Feline leukemia had been shown to be caused by a virus (FeLV); hence the cat became an important model for viral carcinogenesis. Because leopard cats, a small and rather abundant type of wildcat from Asia, were shown to be resistant to FeLV infection,[43] genetic studies relating to viral carcinogenesis initiated with domestic and Asian leopard cats.[1] Although viral carcinogenesis did not play as significant a role in cancer etiology as was initially anticipated, the role of the leopard cat in cat genetics and genomics was crucial.

Genetic recombination–based maps of the cat are an improvement in resolution over somatic cell hybrid maps, with the added benefits of estimating gene order and distance between genes on a chromosome, not just presence or absence. The Bengal cat breed has been influential in the construction of the first genetic maps of the cat. Bengals are a hybrid between domestic cats, primarily Abyssinians and Egyptian or Indian Maus, and a different species of felid, the Asian leopard cat *(Felis [Prionailurus] bengalensis)*. The breed was developed in the late 1960s[15] and is now one of the most popular breeds in the world, although not all registries recognize it. The evolutionary distance between the parental type cats of the Bengal breed is significant.[16,17] The millions of years of evolution between a leopard cat and a domestic cat have made the DNA sequence of each gene more genetically diverse than the gene sequence found between any two domestic cats or any two leopard cats. Thus a pedigree consisting of the first-generation Bengals (F1) and a second-generation backcross to one of the parental-type cats was the basis of the first recombination map for the cat.[26] Genetic variation is required to build a genetic map based on recombination, and because these Bengal crosses would generate offspring with very high genetic polymorphism, the interspecies cross was efficient. The first version of feline interspecies hybrid-based linkage map contained approximately 250 microsatellite markers (also known as short tandem repeats [STRs]).[26] This map was effective for the initiation of pedigree studies for families segregating for particular phenotypic traits or diseases. Although rudimentary, the interspecies backcross map assisted targeted candidate gene approaches—in particular, the discovery of the mutation that causes feline polycystic kidney disease (PKD).[62] The genetic map also led to the discovery that a chromosomal rearrangement involving the gene *LIX1* causes spinal muscular atrophy in the Maine Coon cat.[8,12]

Intraspecies Families

Three different extended pedigrees have been developed from domestic cats to also produce recombination-based linkage maps of the cat. Although less efficient than interspecies hybrid maps, intraspecies families often segregate for more than one trait of interest, and they can more readily be produced or ascertained. An autosomal genetic linkage map based on a large (n=256) multigenerational intraspecies cat family, which was maintained by the Nestlé Purina PetCare company, contains 483 STRs.[28] Cat families from WALTHAM and the University of California, Davis have supported the pedigree studies for traits in the cat, such as *Tabby*,[22] *Spotting*,[5] and *Orange*.[9] Once these family studies help find a locus for a trait of interest, gene-scanning techniques are used to find the specific causative mutations. The causative mutations for the two different forms of progressive retinal atrophy in Abyssinian cats have been located in this manner.[27,29] These mutations are now assayed by commercial services to help identify cats that may develop blindness and help determine carriers so that affected cats will not be produced in breeding programs.

Radiation Hybrid

Another form of a gene map is termed a radiation hybrid (RH) map. RH panels are a variation of the somatic cell hybrid technique.[6] Radiation is used to fragment the DNA from the cat cell line, which is then rescued by the fusion process with the rodent cell line. Because the radiation fragments the DNA, smaller fragments get retained readily throughout the rodent chromosomes in the hybrid cells, not complete chromosomes. When the hybrid cells are tested for the presence or absence of a gene, genes must be in very close proximity to be found in the same cell line. Thus RH panels can map genes that are within 1 Mb or less on a chromosome. This level of resolution is a great improvement over a somatic cell hybrid panel and slightly better than a genetic map derived by recombination events in cat families. The current 5000_{Rad} radiation hybrid map of the cat has had several reiterations and currently has a 1.5 Mb resolution, consisting of 1793 markers.[24,25,30-33] The RH map has also proved useful for assisting with sequence assembly for the feline genome sequencing project.

FELINE GENOME PROJECT

The cat's importance in human health, comparative genomics, and evolutionary studies supported the decision of the National Institutes of Health—National Human Genomics Research Institute (NIH—NHGRI) to produce a low coverage (2×) sequence of the cat genome (http://www.genome.gov/Pages/Research/Sequencing/SeqProposals/CatSEQ.pdf). Led by the Broad Institute and AgenCourt, approximately 327,037 DNA variants termed single nucleotide polymorphisms (SNPs) were identified in the sequence from a solitary, highly inbred Abyssinian cat.[41] Because it was a small-scale sequencing effort, only approximately 65% of the euchromatin (gene-coding) sequence was identified. The sequence assembly suggested the identification of 20,285 feline genes that have counterparts (orthologs) in the human genome. This sequencing effort reiterated the conservation between human and cat chromosomal organization by identifying 133,499 regions of conservation and also identified additional introgression sites of endogenous retroviruses, such as FeLV.[45,46]

Recently, an additional approximate 10× genome coverage has been completed for the cat (http://www.genome.gov/19517271), and the work is in preparation for publication as of this writing. The more in-depth sequencing, which will provide a deeper coverage draft sequence of the cat, will improve the euchromatin coverage to approximately 90% to 95%. The better coverage implies that more cat-specific genetic sequence will be known for any gene of interest. Mutation screening methods will be more efficient, leading to the identification of causative mutations more rapidly and more efficiently. In addition to more genetic variation being identified in the Abyssinian cat used for the feline genome project, additional cats were partially sequenced as well. Four representatives from six breeds, including Birman, Maine Coon, Norwegian Forest Cat, Egyptian Mau, Japanese Bobtail, and Turkish Van, were sequenced. A pool of wildcats was also included, as well as four random-bred cats from Southeast Asia. In addition, Hill's Pet Nutrition, Inc. supported a private sequencing effort, which included Sanger-based sequencing of single cats from five different breeds (Persian, Siamese, Ragdoll, Cornish Rex, Burmese) and also a western random-bred cat and an African wildcat. These combined sequencing efforts helped identify the normal genetic variation that is found across cat breeds and populations, especially the SNPs.

CAT DNA ARRAY

An important by-product of the DNA sequencing effort is the identification of the normal genetic variation in the cat genome, SNPs. The SNPs can be verified to be specific to one breed or common across many breeds and populations. The genome assembly supports the proper positioning of the SNPs across the genome. A resource called a DNA array or DNA chip can then be produced that contains assays for the highly polymorphic and evenly dispersed SNPs; thus these arrays can assess the entire genome of the cat in one experiment. Hill's Pet

Nutrition, Inc. has also provided funding to support feline genome resource development[12a]; a cat SNP-based DNA array was commissioned and is due for release in early 2012. Each DNA chip, which is about the size of a microscope slide, has 12 regions; each region is used to test one cat. Each region has the assays for approximately 63,000 SNPs. The major benefit of the arrays is that they allow assessment of the entire genome; these are known as *genome-wide association studies (GWASs)*. Because the SNPs are at such a high density, the cats used for a GWAS can be from a population, not direct relatives. Thus individual cases of diseases or traits can be examined from a population or across breeds and populations; cases (cats with the trait) and controls (cats without the trait) are required. In addition, because there is less concern for the mode of inheritance of the trait, a GWAS can be performed even with traits that may have complex inheritance but a high heritability or relative risk in a population. Fewer cases are required to investigate a recessive trait, more for a dominant trait, and even more for complex traits that cause an increased relative risk—the lower the relative risk, the more cases required.

A second factor, linkage disequilibrium (LD), is considered when determining the number of cases and controls required for a GWAS. LD is often different among breeds, as seen in dogs and horses, and generally nearly absent in large random-bred populations, such as humans and random-bred cats. The lower the LD, the lower the power of the SNPs to identify an association with a trait of interest. Thus either more SNPs are needed, *or* more cases and controls are required if LD is low, to have effective association studies. Because the chip will have a defined set of SNPs, the LD estimates will predict the number of cases and controls for a study. For a recessive trait, perhaps 30 cases and 30 controls will be required (typical for the dog),[18] but if the population under consideration has high LD, fewer samples will be required. If the population has lower LD, more samples will be required. A more extensive LD study is under evaluation for the domestic cat and its breeds to assist with the proper development of the feline SNP chip.

FUTURE OF CAT GENETICS

The deeper sequencing of the cat genome and the investigation of variation by resequencing in different cat breeds have allowed a great deal of progress in feline genetics, from the analysis of single gene traits to the investigation of more complex traits. However, many of the common diseases that plague humans and are also found in cats will likely be examined in the outbred populations of nonpedigreed housecats because only 10% to 15% of cats in the United States are representatives of a fancy breed, a proportion that is higher than most other nations.[21] Our random-bred/alley/moggy housecats are sharing our sedentary and indoor lifestyle as well as the associated health problems, such as diabetes, obesity, and asthma. Cats are obligate carnivores and require very high protein levels for normal nutrition. Increased fats and carbohydrates in pet foods lower the cost but can jeopardize the cat's health. Increases in the prevalence of feline inflammatory bowel disease and feline lower urinary tract disease are affected by commercial food qualities. Even though pet food companies do make enormous efforts to provide balanced nutrition for our companion animals, cats seem to be having complications with the transition from a wild-prey diet. Food allergies are of particular concern in cats, leading to the development of a wealth of alternative protein diets. Thus genes involved in complex dietary interactions will be important in future studies.

Disease resistances and susceptibilities are also important to the future of feline genetics. Susceptibility to feline immunodeficiency virus (FIV) and particularly to disease caused by feline coronavirus are likely to be of particular interest. Although FIV has low morbidity and mortality rates in the cat, the genes influencing the cat's tolerance of FIV could shed light on interactions in humans and other species with similar immune-compromising pathogens.[40] Feline enteric coronavirus is nearly ubiquitous in domestic cats.[39] As an enteric pathogen, the virus may cause some malaise and diarrhea, but it is otherwise innocuous. However, mutated viral forms cause feline infectious peritonitis (FIP), which has a nearly 100% mortality rate in domestic cats, regardless of race, color, or breed. Deciphering the genes involved with infection and disease progression for FIP would be a major advancement for feline health. The cat genome sequence and the DNA arrays will greatly facilitate these studies.

Once causative mutations for heritable conditions are identified in the cat, cats become a more important asset to human health. Gene therapy approaches are already being explored for several inborn errors of metabolism in cats.[11] Cats will become a more useful alternative and supportive animal model than rodent models for many heritable conditions for reasons such as the following:

- Cats provide a balance between cost and efficiency.
- Drug dosages are more easily translated between cats and humans.
- The longer life span of the cat allows repeated therapy trials and longer term studies.
- Cats have strong conservation of biology, anatomy, and physiology with humans.
- Cats provide a second animal for validation and efficacy.
- The larger size of the cat and its organs are more amenable to therapies.

Finally, cats are intermediate with regard to genetic variation, mimicking human populations and ethnic groups more closely than inbred strains of mice. For example, many murine models exist for the study of cystogenesis, the hallmark of PKD; however, each rodent model has its shortcomings. PKD in cats is similar to human autosomal dominant PKD in several important aspects, including the following: (1) a causative mutation in *PKD1*; (2) a similar type of mutation that causes a similar protein disruption; (3) similar variability in disease progression; (4) cystogenesis in other organs, including the liver and pancreas; and (5) the fact that homozygosity for the mutation is lethal.

CONCLUSION

The available genetic resources for the cat are no longer a research bottleneck for feline studies; however, the acquisition of appropriate patients for sufficient cases and controls remains a rate limiting step. Hence the primary care veterinarian, veterinary specialists, and veterinary researchers need to join forces to properly characterize diseases and routinely collect research materials so that patients are not lost to important studies and health investigations. The development of the DNA tests for parentage and identification (http://www.isag.org.uk/), coat colors, and the prominent diseases (e.g., PKD and hypertrophic cardiomyopathy) has encouraged cat breeders to explore genetic research more openly and has encouraged their participation in research studies. For these reasons more cat breeders are banking DNA material from their animals and providing DNA to service and research laboratories. Many veterinary hospitals and large clinical conglomerates are developing electronic database systems that could facilitate the identification of proper patients, cases, and controls. Combined with DNA banking and specialty health care, the veterinary world stands to enhance the possibilities of complex disease research in the cat by leaps and bounds. Even though the origins of the cat remain a mystery and *domesticated* may not be the most appropriate term for the domestic cat, researchers are unlocking its genetic secrets to explain its form and function.

References

1. Benveniste RE, Todaro GJ: Segregation of RD-114 AND FeL-V-related sequences in crosses between domestic cat and leopard cat, *Nature* 257:506, 1975.
2. Centerwall WR, Benirschke K: Animal model for the XXY Klinefelter's syndrome in man: tortoiseshell and calico male cats, *Am J Vet Res* 36:1275, 1975.
3. Cho KW, Youn HY, Watari T et al: A proposed nomenclature of the domestic cat karyotype, *Cytogenet Cell Genet* 79:71, 1997.
4. Chu EHY, Thuline HC, Norby DE: Triploid-diploid chimerism in a male tortoiseshell cat, *Cytogenetics* 24:1, 1964.
5. Cooper MP, Fretwell N, Bailey SJ et al: White spotting in the domestic cat *(Felis catus)* maps near *KIT* on feline chromosome B1, *Anim Genet* 37:163, 2006.
6. Cox DR, Burmeister M, Price ER et al: Radiation hybrid mapping: a somatic cell genetic method for constructing high-resolution maps of mammalian chromosomes, *Science* 250:245, 1990.
7. Doncaster L: On the inheritance of tortoiseshell and related colours in cats, *Proc Camb Philol Soc* 13:35, 1904.
8. Fyfe JC, Menotti-Raymond M, David VA et al: An approximately 140-kb deletion associated with feline spinal muscular atrophy implies an essential *LIX1* function for motor neuron survival, *Genome Res* 16:1084, 2006.
9. Grahn RA, Lemesch BM, Millon LV et al: Localizing the X-linked orange colour phenotype using feline resource families, *Anim Genet* 36:67, 2005.
10. Gregson NM, Ishmael J: Diploid triploid chimerism in three tortoiseshell cats, *Res Vet Sci* 12:275, 1971.
11. Haskins M: Gene therapy for lysosomal storage diseases (LSDs) in large animal models, *Ilar J* 50:112, 2009.
12. He Q, Lowrie C, Shelton GD et al: Inherited motor neuron disease in domestic cats: a model of spinal muscular atrophy, *Pediatr Res* 57:324, 2005.

12a. Hill's Press Release, Topeka, Kansas, July 20, 2008.

13. Imes DL, Geary LA, Grahn RA et al: Albinism in the domestic cat *(Felis catus)* is associated with a *tyrosinase (TYR)* mutation, *Anim Genet* 37:175, 2006.
14. Ishihara T: Cytological studies on tortoiseshell male cats, *Cytologia* 21:391, 1956.
15. Johnson G: *The Bengal cat,* 1991. Gogees Cattery, Greenwell Springs, LA.
16. Johnson W, O'Brien SJ: Phylogenetic reconstruction of the Felidae using 16S rRNA and NADH-5 mitochondrial genes, *J Mol Evol* 44:s98, 1997.
17. Johnson WE, Eizirik E, Pecon-Slattery J et al: The late Miocene radiation of modern Felidae: a genetic assessment, *Science* 311:73, 2006.
18. Ke X, Kennedy LJ, Short AD et al: Assessment of the functionality of genome-wide canine SNP arrays and implications for canine disease association studies, *Anim Genet*, 2010, in press.
19. Kosowska B, Januszewski A, Tokarska M et al: Cytogenetic and histologic studies of tortoiseshell cats, *Med Weter* 57:475, 2001.
20. Kuiper H, Hewicker-Trautwein M, Distl O: [Cytogenetic and histologic examination of four tortoiseshell cats], *Dtsch Tierarztl Wochenschr* 110:457, 2003.
21. Louwerens M, London CA, Pedersen NC et al: Feline lymphoma in the post-feline leukemia virus era, *J Vet Intern Med* 19:329, 2005.
22. Lyons LA, Bailey SJ, Baysac KC et al: The *Tabby* cat locus maps to feline chromosome B1, *Anim Genet* 37:383, 2006.
23. Lyons LA, Imes DL, Rah HC et al: *Tyrosinase* mutations associated with Siamese and Burmese patterns in the domestic cat *(Felis catus)*, *Anim Genet* 36:119, 2005.
24. Menotti-Raymond M, David VA, Agarwala R et al: Radiation hybrid mapping of 304 novel microsatellites in the domestic cat genome, *Cytogenet Genome Res* 102:272, 2003.
25. Menotti-Raymond M, David VA, Chen ZQ et al: Second-generation integrated genetic linkage/radiation hybrid maps of the domestic cat *(Felis catus)*, *J Hered* 94:95, 2003.
26. Menotti-Raymond M, David VA, Lyons LA et al: A genetic linkage map of microsatellites in the domestic cat *(Felis catus)*, *Genomics* 57:9, 1999.
27. Menotti-Raymond M, David VA, Schaffer AA et al: Mutation in *CEP290* discovered for cat model of human retinal degeneration, *J Hered* 98:211, 2007.
28. Menotti-Raymond M, David VA, Schaffer AA et al: An autosomal genetic linkage map of the domestic cat, *Felis silvestris catus*, *Genomics*, 2008.
29. Menotti-Raymond M, Deckman K, David V et al: Mutation discovered in a feline model of human congenital retinal blinding disease, *Invest Ophthalmol Vis Sci* 51:2852, 2010.

30. Murphy WJ, Davis B, David VA et al: A 1.5-Mb-resolution radiation hybrid map of the cat genome and comparative analysis with the canine and human genomes, *Genomics*, 2006.
31. Murphy WJ, Menotti-Raymond M, Lyons LA et al: Development of a feline whole genome radiation hybrid panel and comparative mapping of human chromosome 12 and 22 loci, *Genomics* 57:1, 1999.
32. Murphy WJ, Sun S, Chen Z et al: A radiation hybrid map of the cat genome: implications for comparative mapping, *Genome Res* 10:691, 2000.
33. Murphy WJ, Sun S, Chen ZQ et al: Extensive conservation of sex chromosome organization between cat and human revealed by parallel radiation hybrid mapping, *Genome Res* 9:1223, 1999.
34. Nash WG, O'Brien SJ: Conserved regions of homologous G-banded chromosomes between orders in mammalian evolution: carnivores and primates, *Proc Natl Acad Sci U S A* 79:6631, 1982.
35. O'Brien SJ, Cevario SJ, Martenson JS et al: Comparative gene mapping in the domestic cat *(Felis catus)*, *J Hered* 88:408, 1997.
36. O'Brien SJ, Haskins ME, Winkler CA et al: Chromosomal mapping of beta-globin and albino loci in the domestic cat. A conserved mammalian chromosome group, *J Hered* 77:374, 1986.
37. O'Brien SJ, Nash WG: Genetic mapping in mammals: chromosome map of domestic cat, *Science* 216:257, 1982.
38. O'Brien SJ, Wienberg J, Lyon LA: Comparative genomics: lessons from cats, *Trends Genet* 13:393, 1997.
39. Pedersen NC, Allen CE, Lyons LA: Pathogenesis of feline enteric coronavirus infection, *J Feline Med Surg* 10:529, 2008.
40. Pedersen NC, Barlough JE: Clinical overview of feline immunodeficiency virus, *J Am Vet Med Assoc* 199:1298, 1991.
41. Pontius JU, Mullikin JC, Smith DR et al: Initial sequence and comparative analysis of the cat genome, *Genome Res* 17:1675, 2007.
42. Pyle RL, Patterson DF, Hare WC et al: XXY sex chromosome constitution in a Himalayan cat with tortoise-shell points, *J Hered* 62:220, 1971.
43. Rasheed S, Gardner MB: Isolation of feline leukemia virus from a leopard cat cell line and search for retrovirus in wild felidae, *J Natl Cancer Inst* 67:929, 1981.
44. Rettenberger G, Klett C, Zechner U et al: ZOO-FISH analysis: cat and human karyotypes closely resemble the putative ancestral mammalian karyotype, *Chromosome Res* 3:479, 1995.
45. Roca AL, Nash WG, Menninger JC et al: Insertional polymorphisms of endogenous feline leukemia viruses, *J Virol* 79:3979, 2005.
46. Roca AL, Pecon-Slattery J, O'Brien SJ: Genomically intact endogenous feline leukemia viruses of recent origin, *J Virol* 78:4370, 2004.
47. Ronne M: Localization of fragile sites in the karyotype of *Felis catus*, *Hereditas* 122:279, 1995.
48. Ronne M, Storm CO: The high resolution RBG-banded karyotype of *Felis catus*, *In Vivo* 6:517, 1992.
49. Ronne M, Storm CO: Localization of landmarks and bands in the karyotype of *Felis catus*, *Cytobios* 81:213, 1995.
50. Schlafer DH, Valentine B, Fahnestock G et al: A case of *SRY*-positive 38,XY true hermaphroditism (XY sex reversal) in a cat, *Vet Pathol* 2010 Sep 22. [Epub ahead of print].
51. Schmidt-Kuntzel A, Eizirik E, O'Brien SJ et al: *Tyrosinase* and *tyrosinase related protein 1* alleles specify domestic cat coat color phenotypes of the albino and brown loci, *J Hered* 96:289, 2005.
52. Shibasaki Y, Flou S, Ronne M: The R-banded karyotype of *Felis catus*, *Cytobios* 51:35, 1987.
53. Stanyon R, Yang F, Cavagna P et al: Reciprocal chromosome painting shows that genomic rearrangement between rat and mouse proceeds ten times faster than between humans and cats, *Cytogenet Cell Genet* 84:150, 1999.
54. Thuline HC: Male tortoiseshell, chimerism and true hermaphroditism, *J Cat Genet* 4:2, 1964.
55. Wienberg J, Stanyon R: Chromosome painting in mammals as an approach to comparative genomics, *Curr Opin Genet Dev* 5:792, 1995.
56. Wienberg J, Stanyon R, Nash WG et al: Conservation of human vs. feline genome organization revealed by reciprocal chromosome painting, *Cytogenet Cell Genet* 77:211, 1997.
57. Wurster-Hill DH, Centerwall WR: The interrelationships of chromosome banding patterns in canids, mustelids, hyena, and felids, *Cytogenet Cell Genet* 34:178, 1982.
58. Wurster-Hill DH, Doi T, Izawa M et al: Banded chromosome study of the Iriomote cat, *J Hered* 78:105, 1987.
59. Wurster-Hill DH, Gray CW: Giemsa banding patterns in the chromosomes of twelve species of cats (Felidae), *Cytogenet Cell Genet* 12:388, 1973.
60. Wurster-Hill DH, Gray CW: The interrelationships of chromosome banding patterns in procyonids, viverrids, and felids, *Cytogenet Cell Genet* 15:306, 1975.
61. Yang F, Graphodatsky AS, O'Brien PC et al: Reciprocal chromosome painting illuminates the history of genome evolution of the domestic cat, dog and human, *Chromosome Res* 8:393, 2000.
62. Young AE, Biller DS, Herrgesell EJ et al: Feline polycystic kidney disease is linked to the *PKD1* region, *Mamm Genome* 16:59, 2005.

CHAPTER

44

Genetics of Feline Diseases and Traits

Leslie A. Lyons

OUTLINE

The inherited diseases and traits currently described in the cat are more likely to be identified in a specific breed than in random-bred cats. More than 88 million owned cats are estimated in the United States.[2] Only a small percentage of this cat population is represented by cats of a specific breed, perhaps at most 15%.[63] Many traits that can also be considered diseases are actually the hallmarks or identifiers of some cat breeds. Inbreeding does not cause mutations to occur at a higher rate within a breed, although inbreeding, popular sire effects, and population bottlenecks will allow rare mutations to occur more frequently within the population. Usually, recessive mutations, which can go unrecognized for many generations because they require the causative mutation to be present on both chromosomes, are the traits and diseases that tend to suddenly appear in inbred populations. The higher likelihood of an undesired trait appearing in a breed population gives the impression that breeds are unhealthier than random-bred populations. Fortuitous and deleterious mutations occur at the same rate in cats, regardless of whether the cat is pedigreed or random bred. Fancy-breed cats are more likely to have a higher standard of health care and are more likely to be closely observed than the random-bred alley cat or housecat. Thus ascertainment bias contributes to the identification of deleterious traits that are presented to the veterinarian. However, many mutations have been found in random-bred domestic shorthairs. This chapter reviews the known inherited diseases of the cat from the genetic point of view. Additional details regarding the diagnosis and treatment of the specific diseases can be found in other chapters in this volume. A list of common genetic terms can be found in Box 44-1.

Diseases or conditions that are caused by genetic abnormalities cannot be cured, but the associated health problems may be manageable. An overall goal for identifying the genetic mutations for genetic conditions is the correction of the defect by way of gene or stem cell therapies or better management by way of designer drug therapies. Genetic testing is currently an effective preventive medicine because proper breeding can prevent the birth of diseased individuals; moreover, genetic testing may lead to the potential ultimate cure.

HALLMARKS OF GENETIC DISEASES

A cat's appearance, its phenotype, is a combination of visible traits and morphologic types. Attributes of the phenotype can be desirable or undesirable. As in breeds of other species, a disease or health concern can sometimes be considered part of the cat's desired phenotype. For example, a Manx cat is tailless, but incontinence and lameness are associated with the characteristic of having no tail. Because phenotypes can be a result of a single gene, the interaction of several genes, the accumulation of environmental exposures, or a combination of interactions, a veterinarian may choose different types of therapy or clinical management or make different prognoses if a phenotype is known to have mainly a genetic cause. If the same condition is found in a different species, a veterinarian may have opportunities to try novel approaches for health care by considering comparative medicine. Several characteristics are common to genetic diseases that will help distinguish sporadic, idiopathic occurrences from inherited conditions.

BOX 44-1

Glossary of Genetic Terms

Allele: Alternative form of a gene. One of the different forms of a gene that can exist at a single locus.

Base pair: The nucleotides that constitute a strand of DNA are also known as *bases*. A base pair implies the nucleotide from one strand of DNA and the pair with which it forms hydrogen bonds on the second strand of DNA, such as cytosine binding with guanine or adenine binding with thymine. The two strands of DNA are bound together by the hydrogen bonds of base pairs to form the double helix of DNA.

Common ancestry: The state of two individuals when they are blood relatives. When two parents have a common ancestor, their offspring will be inbred.

DNA (deoxyribonucleic acid): An antiparallel double helix of nucleotides (having deoxyribose as their sugars) linked by phosphodiester (sugar–phosphate) bonds to adjacent nucleotides in the same chain and by hydrogen bonds to complementary nucleotides in the opposite chain. The fundamental substance of which genes are composed.

Dominant allele: An allele that expresses its phenotypic effect even when heterozygous with a recessive allele; thus if **A** is dominant over **a**, then **AA** and **Aa** have the same phenotype.

Exon: A region of a gene that is present in the final functional transcript (mRNA) from that gene. Any non-intron section of the coding sequence of a gene; together the exons constitute the mRNA and are translated into protein.

Gene: Segregating and heritable determinant of the phenotype. The fundamental physical and functional unit of heredity, which carries information from one generation to the next. A segment of DNA, composed of a transcribed region and regulatory sequences that make possible transcription.

Gene interaction: The collaboration of several different genes in the production of one phenotypic character (or related group of characters).

Gene locus: The specific place on a chromosome where a gene is located.

Gene mutation: Mutation (point or larger change) that results from changes within the structure of a gene.

Genetic polymorphism: The occurrence together in the same population of more than one allele or genetic marker at the same locus with the least frequent allele or marker occurring more frequently than can be accounted for by mutation alone.

Genetic variance: Phenotypic variance resulting from the presence of different genotypes in the population.

Genetics: (1) The study of genes through their variation. (2) The study of inheritance.

Genome: The entire complement of genetic material in a chromosome set. The entire genetic complement of a prokaryote, virus, mitochondrion, or chloroplast or the haploid nuclear genetic complement of a eukaryotic species.

Genotype: The specific allelic composition of a cell, either of the entire cell or more commonly for a certain gene or a set of genes. The genes that an organism possesses.

Heritability: A measure of the degree to which the variance in the distribution of a phenotype is due to genetic causes. In the broad sense, it is measured by the total genetic variance divided by the total phenotypic variance. In the narrow sense, it is measured by the genetic variance due to additive genes divided by the total phenotypic variance.

Heterozygosity: A measure of the genetic variation in a population; with respect to one locus, stated as the frequency of heterozygotes for that locus.

Heterozygote: An individual having a heterozygous gene pair. A diploid or polyploid with different alleles at a particular locus.

Inbreeding: The mating of genetically related individuals. Mating between relatives.

Inbreeding depression: A depression of vigor or yield due to inbreeding.

Incomplete dominance: The situation in which both alleles of a heterozygote influence the phenotype. The phenotype is usually intermediate between the two homozygous phenotypes. The situation in which a heterozygote shows a phenotype somewhere (but not exactly halfway) intermediate between the corresponding homozygote phenotypes. (Exact intermediacy is not dominance.) *See also* dominance, co-dominance, and recessivity.

Intron (intervening sequence): A DNA segment of largely unknown function within a gene that specifically interrupts the coding (exon) sequences of that gene. Introns are transcribed as part of the normal gene primary transcript, but intron sequences are not found in the functional mRNA. Intron sequences are removed from the primary transcript by a splicing mechanism.

Locus (plural, loci): The position of a gene, DNA marker, or genetic marker on a chromosome.

Mosaic: A chimera; a tissue containing two or more genetically distinct cell types, or an individual composed of such tissues. Individual made up of two or more genetically distinct cell lines.

Mutant allele: An allele differing from the allele found in the standard or wild-type organism.

Mutation: (1) The process producing a gene or a chromosome differing from the wild-type. (2) The gene or chromosome that results from such a process.

Mutation rate: The number of mutation events per gene per unit of time (e.g., per cell generation). The proportion of mutations per cell division in bacteria or single-celled organisms or the proportion of mutations per gamete in higher organisms.

Nucleotide: One of four bases that constitute DNA, including adenine, guanine, cytosine, and thymine.

Pedigree: A family tree drawn with standard genetic symbols, showing inheritance patterns for specific

Continued

BOX 44-1

Glossary of Genetic Terms—cont'd

phenotypic characters. A representation of the ancestry of an individual or family; a family tree.

Penetrance: The proportion of individuals with a specific genotype who manifest that genotype at the phenotype level.

Phenocopy: A phenotype that is not genetically controlled but looks like a genetically controlled phenotype. An environmentally induced phenotype that resembles the phenotype produced by a mutation.

Phenotype: (1) The form taken by some character (or group of characters) in a specific individual. (2) The detectable outward manifestations of a specific genotype. (3) The observable attributes of an organism.

Pleiotropy: The phenomenon whereby a single mutation affects several apparently unrelated aspects of the phenotype.

Point mutation: A mutation that can be mapped to one specific site within a locus. A small mutation that consists of the replacement (transition or transversion), addition, or deletion (frameshift) of one base.

Popular sire: A specific male in a population whose genetics becomes overrepresented in the next generation as a result of excessive breeding. Popular sires are determined by some quality desired in the population and generally represent high-winning individuals for a breed in competition. A undesired recessive trait can quickly spread in a population as a result of the popular sire effect.

Recessive: (1) An allele that is not expressed in the heterozygous condition. (2) The phenotype of the homozygote of a recessive allele.

Selection: Genetic breeding methods start with selecting particular desirable phenotypes as parents for the next generation.

Sex chromosome: A chromosome whose presence or absence is correlated with the sex of the bearer; a chromosome that plays a role in sex determination. Heteromorphic (different-shaped [e.g., X and Y]) chromosomes whose distribution in a zygote determines the sex of the organism.

Sex linked: The inheritance pattern of loci located on the sex chromosomes (usually the X chromosome in XY species); also refers to the loci themselves.

Silent mutation: Mutation in which the function of the protein product of the gene is unaltered.

X chromosome inactivation: In female mammalian embryos, the early random inactivation of the genes on one of the X chromosomes, leading to mosaicism for functions coded by heterozygous X-linked genes.

The following are six common hallmarks for inherited diseases:

1. Early age of onset
2. Bilateral or multiple presentation (or both)
3. Presence in a closed or small population
4. Indications of inbreeding
5. Uniformity in presentation
6. Advanced parental age at birth

Only advanced age of parents at birth has not been shown to have an effect in feline inherited diseases to date. Examples of parental age effects in humans include older or very young mothers having a higher frequency of children with trisomy 21 (Down syndrome)[77] and certain types of dwarfism being associated with advanced paternal age.[78]

Two examples of diseases that present as sporadic and inherited forms are kidney cysts[13] and lymphosarcoma.[63] Each of the five characteristics that define genetic diseases can help differentiate cats with polycystic kidney disease (PKD) from cats with sporadic kidney cysts. Kidney cysts can occur in any cat, but not all cystic presentations are indicative of PKD. PKD can sometimes be detected by ultrasound as early as 6 to 8 weeks of age, consistently by 10 months of age.[26] Both kidneys are generally affected, and multiple cysts are generally present (see Figures 32-4 and 32-5). The cysts are not similar in size but are similar in etiology. PKD is rampant in Persian cats and therefore must be considered a health concern in related breeds, such as Exotic Shorthairs and Himalayans. Surprisingly, this genetic problem has a very high frequency in one of the oldest and largest cat breeds, which is not a small or closed population, but the early onset, the bilateral presentation, and the high prevalence in a breed clearly demarcate this condition as a heritable problem. An older, random-bred cat with one or a few cysts in one kidney would not be a candidate for heritable PKD and genetic testing.

Lymphosarcoma is also common in cats but generally found in older cats and cats that have been infected with feline leukemia virus (FeLV).[33] Mediastinal lymphosarcoma has been specifically identified in Oriental Shorthairs that are FeLV negative and generally younger than 2 years of age,[31,32] although a genetic cause has not yet been identified. Other related breeds, such as Siamese, Colorpoint Shorthair, and the longhaired varieties of Siamese, have an increased prevalence of this type of lymphoma. The tumors respond well to chemotherapy, but reoccurrence is high, and the disease generally carries a very poor prognosis. This disease is found in a closed, inbred population; it has an early onset and a generally uniform presentation; and the tumor is found in areas not common to older-onset forms of lymphosarcoma. These hallmarks strongly suggest that mediastinal lymphoma is a heritable condition in the Oriental cats.

Non-genetic components (e.g., toxins, infections, infestations, sporadic damage and changes to the DNA, and environmental influences such as diet, exercise, and social surroundings) can produce a phenotype that looks just like an inherited characteristic or disease; this is termed a *phenocopy.* Detailed examinations of cats with heart murmurs may reveal different presentations of heart disease, one that may be genetic and one that may be environmentally induced, such as by insufficient dietary taurine resulting in dilated cardiomyopathy.[82] Some diseases may present differently in different tissues, which is termed *pleiotropic effects* of the same gene. For example, some completely white cats show only the white coat color; others have blue eyes or one blue and one green eye, and some may be deaf.[4,10,99] The variations in eye color and hearing are pleiotropic effects of the *White* gene for cats. Genetic testing can help the clinician rule out the common and environmental causes of clinical presentations as opposed to a condition caused by a heritable defect in the cat's DNA.

SIMPLE GENETIC TRAITS

A cat's phenotype and its health can be influenced by both genetic (inherited) and nongenetic (environmental) influences. The diseases and traits that have known mutations—hence clearly heritable and genetic—are generally called *simple,* or *single, gene traits,* because the presentations are controlled mostly by a specific mutation in a specific gene. Environment may play some role in the overall presentation of a simple genetic trait, but the major contribution to the phenotype is from the single gene defect. Most of the early identified mutations for any species have been single gene traits, mainly because the presentation is similar to that found in another species. Comparative genetics and comparative medicine work in a similar fashion; the genetic knowledge for one species can be transferred to another species. Through comparative genetics genes that cause defects in one species, such as humans, dogs, or mice, can be scanned for causative mutations when a similar disease presentation or phenotype is discovered in the cat.

Genetic Traits with Known Mutations

The comparative genetics approach is also often termed a "candidate-gene" approach. Discovered in the early and mid-1990s, the first mutations identified in cats were for lipid and lysosomal storage diseases[100,102] because these diseases have well-defined phenotypes and known genes with mutations that were as found in humans (see reviews by Banks and Chamberlain,[6] and Valayannopoulos et al[97]). Most of the common diseases, coat colors, and coat types have been deciphered in the cat following the same candidate-gene approach, by finding a replicate trait in another species, usually mice, and checking the same gene for causative mutations.

Once a mutation is known, a genetic-based test can be established. DNA testing for domestic cat diseases and appearance traits is a rapidly growing asset for the veterinary community. Approximately 33 genes contain approximately 50 mutations that cause feline health problems or alterations in the cat's appearance (Tables 44-1 and 44-2). To date, other than the muscular dystrophy mutation,[100] all mutations in the cat are autosomal, not found on the X or Y chromosomes. A variety of commercial laboratories can now perform feline genetic diagnostics, allowing both the veterinary clinician and the private owner to obtain DNA test results. DNA is easily obtained from a cat by buccal swab using a standard cotton bud or cytologic brush, after which DNA samples can be sent to any laboratory in the world because the DNA is stable at room temperature. The DNA test results identify carriers of the traits, predict the incidence of traits in breeding programs, and influence medical prognoses and treatments. Once a genetic test proves that an animal has a genetic trait, preventive therapies and dietary restrictions could be implemented to slow or prevent the onset and progression of the associated disease. Thus genetic testing should not be viewed as an alternative to veterinary care but instead as a tool for veterinary care, part of a cat's overall health management plan.

Phenotypic Mutations of the Domestic Cat

Domestic cats have been selected to produce breeds mainly on the basis of aesthetic qualities, especially coloration, fur length and type, and some morphologic types such as folded or curled ears. Most of the genes controlling these traits are simple, and many of the causative mutations have been identified. Tables 44-1 and 44-3 present the common genes and loci that affect feline phenotypic traits. A trait is initially given a locus name, such as *Brown,* before the actual gene has been identified. The locus name usually is a descriptor of the trait, although the location in the genome for the locus will not be initially known; however, the mode of inheritance of the different alleles is usually determined. The alleles are given single- or two-letter designations, lower case implying a recessive allele. Once the gene is identified, such as *tyrosinase-related protein 1* (*TRYP1*) for *Brown,* the mutations are written to describe the genetic alteration within the gene, and the gene will be designated with the alleles, such as *TRYP1*^{b} for the brown allele.

Several of the cat coat color loci have only one mutant allele, such as *Agouti, Dilute,* and *Extension.* Because the phenotypic mutations are of value to cat breeders for

TABLE 44-1 **Common Commercialized DNA Tests for Domestic Cats**

Disease/Trait	MOI*	Phenotype	Breeds	Gene	Mutation
Agouti[27]	AR	Banded fur to solid	All breeds	*ASIP*	del122-123
Amber[81]	AR	Brown color variant	Norwegian Forest	*MC1R*	G250A
Brown[65,90]	AR	Brown, light brown color variants	All breeds	*TYRP1*	b = -5IVS6, b^l = C298T
Color[47,66,90]	AR	Burmese, Siamese color pattern, full albino	All breeds	*TYR*	c^b = G715T, c^s = G940A, c = C975del
Dilution[48]	AR	Black to gray/blue, orange to cream	All breeds	*MLPH*	T83del
Gloves[34]	AR	White feet	Birman	*KIT*	c.1035_1036delinsCA
Hairless (Naked)[35]	AR	Atrichia	Sphynx	*KRT71*	c.816_1G_A
Long fur[25,52]	AR	Long fur	All breeds†	*FGF5*	c.356insT, C406T, c.474delT, A475C
Rexing (curly fur)[35]	AR	Curly hair coat	Devon Rex	*KRT71*	c.1108-4_1184del, c.1184_1185insAGTTGGAG
AB blood type[11]	AR	Determines type B	All breeds	*CMAH*	18indel-53, G139A
Gangliosidosis 1[23]	AR	Lipid storage disorder	Korat, Siamese	*GLB1*	G1457C
Gangliosidosis 2[14]	AR	Lipid storage disorder	Burmese	*HEXB*	15bp del (intron)
Gangliosidosis 2[76]	AR	Lipid storage disorder	Korat	*HEXB*	C39del
Glycogen storage disease IV[28a,68]	AR	Glycogen storage disorder	Norwegian Forest	*GBE1*	230bp ins 5′-6kb del
Hypertrophic cardiomyopathy[75]	AD	Cardiac disease	Maine Coon	*MYBPC*	G93C
Hypertrophic cardiomyopathy[74]	AD	Cardiac disease	Ragdoll	*MYBPC*	C2460T
Progressive retinal atropy[72]	AR	Late onset blindness	Abyssinian	*CEP290*	IVS50 + 9T > G
Progressive retinal atropy[73]	AD	Early onset blindness	Abyssinian	*CRX*	n.546delC
Polycystic kidney disease[64]	AD	Kidney cysts	Persian	*PKD1*	C10063A
Pyruvate kinase deficiency‡	AR	Hemopathy	Abyssinian	*PKLR*	13bp del in exon 6
Spinal muscular atrophy[30]	AR	Muscular atrophy	Maine Coon	*LIX1-LNPEP*	140kb del, exons 4-6

AD, Autosomal dominant; *AR,* autosomal recessive; *ID,* incomplete dominance; *AS,* allelic series.
*Mode of inheritance of the non–wild-type variant.
†Long fur variants are more or less common depending on the breed.
‡Unpublished test, presented only as abstract.

managing their breeding programs, the phenotypic mutations generally have genetic tests readily available from commercial services. Because most of the mutations for the aesthetic traits are recessive, the mutant alleles must be present in both copies for the effect to be visible, and cats can carry the mutation without detection. Recessive mutations tend to be found in the genes that produce the enzymes of biological pathways. Thus most of the coat color mutations are recessive because they are usually part of disrupting the pigment production pathways. Many genes that affect pathways also tend to have more than one mutation that cause different effects; this is termed an *allelic series.* The locus for brown color variants, *Brown,* has two mutations in the causative gene, *TRYP1.* The wild-type allele, *B,* which causes normal black pigment, is dominant to the brown allele, *b,* which causes a reduced amount of black pigment, producing a more brownish hue to the fur. The brown allele, *b,* is considered dominant to light brown, whereas b^l imparts a cinnamon-color or reddish effect on the fur. The allelic series is written as: $B > b > b^l$ to indicate the dominance of one allele over the other. In the case of the *Color* locus, *C,* which is also an allelic series, the sepia coloration, c^bc^b, which is fixed in the Burmese (Figure 44-1) and Singapura (Figure 44-2) breeds, is co-dominantly expressed with the Siamese points, c^sc^s, producing an additive affect. Thus compound heterozygous cats, c^bc^s, have an intermediate coloration compared with that of the Burmese and the Siamese; this is usually referred to as a *mink Tonkinese* (Figure 44-3). Complete albinos, which have an additional allele at the *Color* locus, have been identified. The locus is controlled by the gene

TABLE 44-2 **Other Mutations for Inherited Domestic Cat Diseases***

Disease	Gene	Mutation	Disease	Gene	Mutation
Gangliosidosis 2[69]	*HEXB*	inv1467-1491	Mucopolysaccharidosis VI[22,101]	*ARSB*	G1558A
Gangliosidosis 2[51]	*HEXB*	C667T	Mucopolysaccharidosis VII[29]	*GUSB*	A1052G
Gangliosidosis 2[68]	*GM2A*	del390-393	Muscular dystrophy[100]	*DMD*	900bp del M promoter -exon 1
Hemophilia B[40]	*F9*	G247A	Niemann–Pick C[91]	*NPC*	G2864C
Hemophilia B[40]	*F9*	C1014T	Polydactyla[58]	*SHH*	A479G
Hyperoxaluria[39]	*GRHPR*	G>A I4 acceptor site	Polydactyla[58]	*SHH*	G257C, A481T
Lipoprotein lipase deficiency[38]	*LPL*	G1234A	Porphyria[19-21]	*HMBS*	c.842_844delGAG
Mannosidosis, alpha[9]	*LAMAN*	del1748-1751	Porphyria[19-21]	*HMBS*	c.189dupT
Mucolipidosis II[70]	*GNPTA*	C2655T	Vitamin D–resistant rickets[37]	*CYP27B1*	G223A, G731del
Mucopolysaccharidosis I[45]	*IDUA*	del1047-1049	Vitamin D–resistant rickets[42]	*CYP27B1*	G637T
Mucopolysaccharidosis VI[102]	*ARSB*	T1427C			

*The presented conditions are not prevalent in breeds or populations but may have been introduced into research colonies.

TABLE 44-3 **Simple Phenotypic Traits and Diseases of the Cat and Its Breeds: Mutations Are Unidentified**

Locus	Phenotype	MOI	Locus	Phenotype	MOI
Bobtail	Curly and kinked tail	AD, variable expression	*Orange*	Orange hue to pigment	X-linked
Craniofacial Defect	Skull structural closure abnormality common to Burmese	AR	Peterbald	Brush coat, hairless	ID
Ear curl	Pinnae curl rostrally	AD	Rexing	Curly coat	AD
Ear fold	Pinnae folds ventrally	AD	Rexing	Curly coat	AR
Hypokalemia	Potassium insufficiency	AR	*Spotting*	Bicolor white	AD
Inhibitor	No pheomelanin	AD	*Tabby*	Type of tabby pattern	AS
Lymphoma	Mediastinal in Oriental breeds	AR	*Ticked*	Production of a tabby pattern	AD
Manx	Tailless, short tail	AD, variable expression	*White*	Dominant white, no pigment	AD
Myopathy	Generalized muscle weakness	AR	Wirehair	Wired coat	ID

MOI, Mode of inheritance (of the mutations as compared to the wild-type allele); *AD,* autosomal dominant; *AR,* autosomal recessive; *ID,* incomplete dominance; *AS,* allelic series. Orange is the only X-linked phenotypic trait.

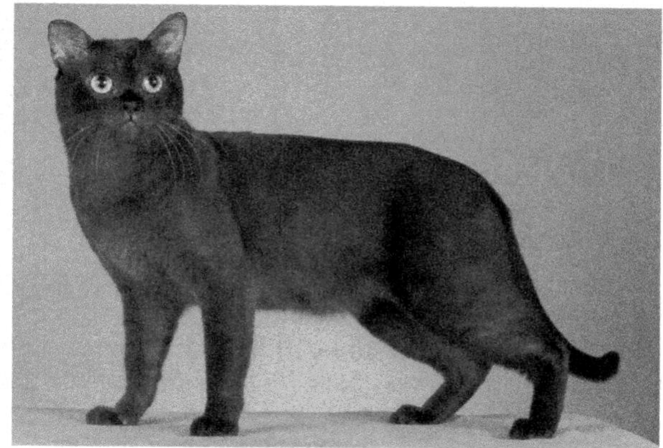

FIGURE 44-1 Burmese. *(Photo copyright 2011 Richard Katris.)*

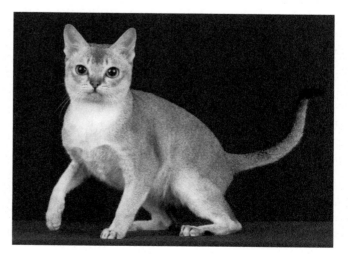

FIGURE 44-2 Singapura. *(Photo copyright 2011 Richard Katris.)*

FIGURE 44-3 Tonkinese. *(Photo copyright 2011 Richard Katris.)*

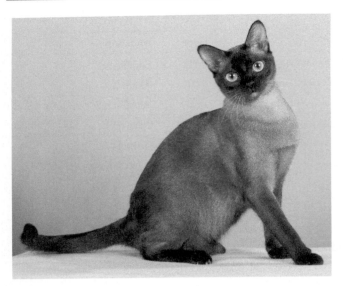

FIGURE 44-4 Cornish Rex. *(Photo copyright 2011 Richard Katris.)*

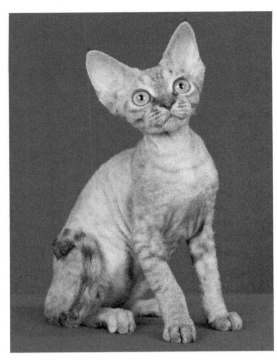

FIGURE 44-5 Devon Rex. *(Photo copyright 2011 Richard Katris.)*

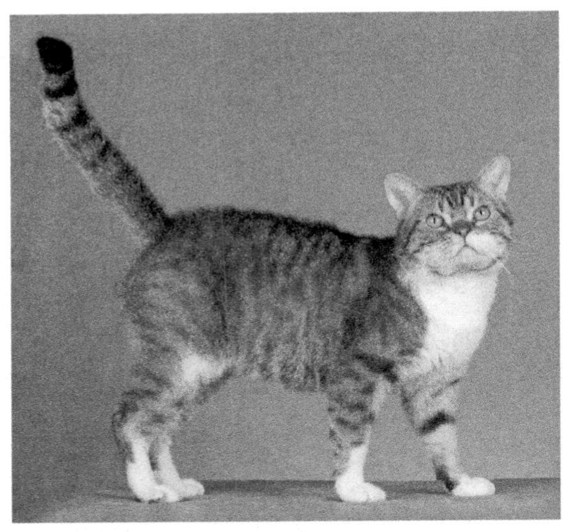

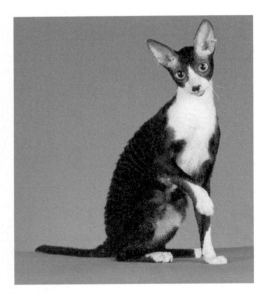

FIGURE 44-6 American Wirehair. *(Photo copyright 2011 Richard Katris.)*

tyrosinase; *TYR* and the allelic series is written as $C > c^b = c^s > c$.

The coat color mutations are common to all cats and are effective for genetic typing in all breeds and populations. However, even though long fur is common in pedigreed and random-bred cats, long fur is an exception because four different mutations in the gene *fibroblast growth factor 5 (FGF5)* can cause a cat to have long fur.[25,52] One mutation is common to almost all breeds and populations, which suggests that this mutation is the most ancient and present before breeds developed, but the other long fur mutations are more specific to particular breeds.[3] Some cats can have long fur because of two different mutations in the gene *FGF5*. These cats would be considered compound heterozygotes. Thus all four mutations must be genotyped to determine whether a cat carries a mutation for long fur.

Rexing is an interesting set of mutations for the domestic cat. At least six different types of rexoid mutations have been noted in the cat, including Cornish Rex (Figure 44-4) and Devon Rex (Figure 44-5), as well as several unpublished varieties, including American Wirehair (Figure 44-6), Selkirk Rex (Figure 44-7), LaPerm (Figure 44-8), and Tennessee Rex. The Devon Rex and

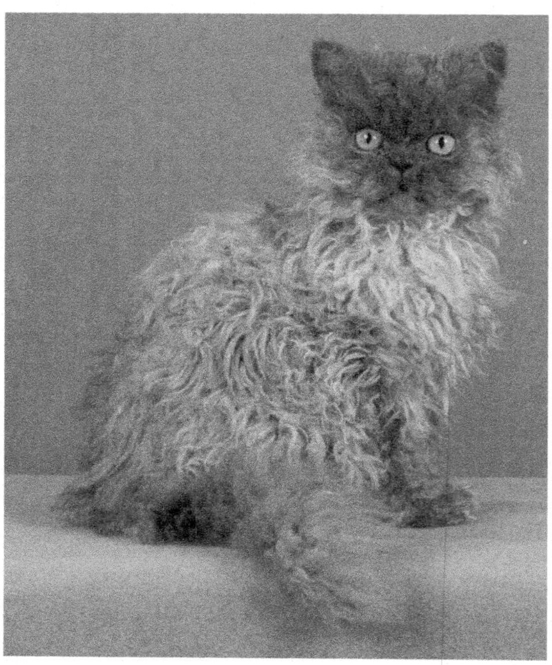

FIGURE 44-7 Selkirk Rex. *(Photo copyright 2011 Richard Katris.)*

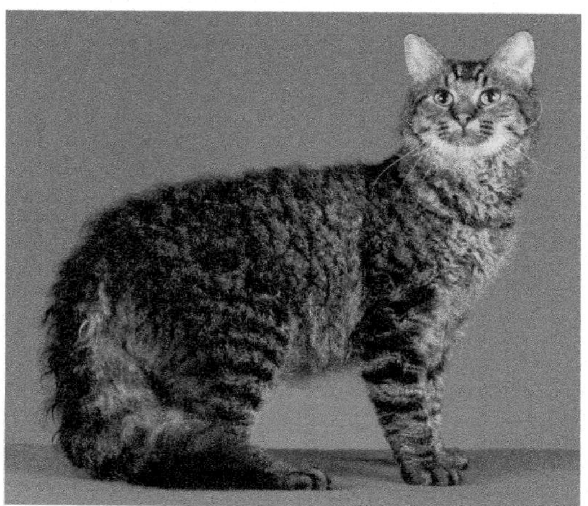

FIGURE 44-8 LaPerm. *(Photo copyright 2011 Richard Katris.)*

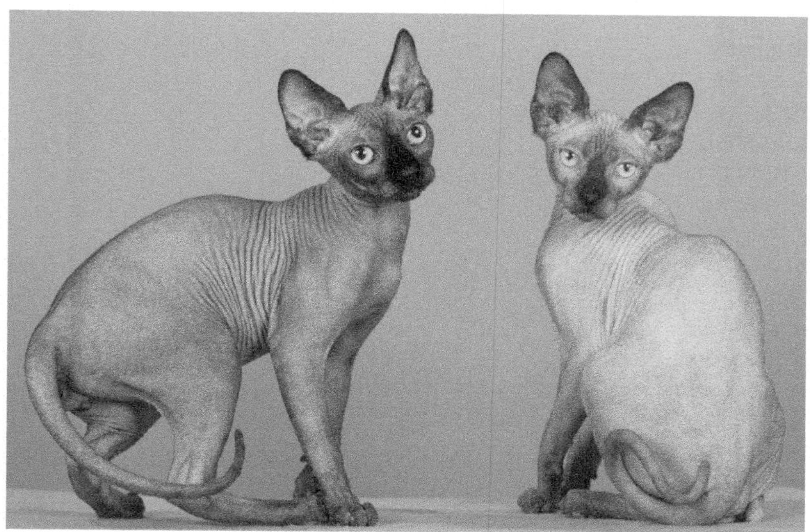

FIGURE 44-9 Sphynx. *(Photo copyright 2011 Richard Katris.)*

Cornish Rex had been known to be caused by different genes after cross-breeding experiments and genetic studies.[85] The genetic studies have ruled out the Devon Rex gene, *keratin 71 (KRT71),* as causative for the other rexoid cats.[35] The Selkirk and LaPerm have dominant mutations, Devon and Cornish are caused by recessive mutations, and the wirehair appears to be a dominant mutation with variable expression and even incomplete penetrance, wherein sometimes cats thought to have the mutation are not wirehaired. Sometimes two traits are not initially known to be caused by the same gene, such as hairlessness of the Sphynx and rexing in the Devon Rex.[35,86] Thus the hairlessness of the Sphynx (Figure 44-9) has had the locus name *Hairless* with alleles *Hr* and *hr,* whereas Devon Rex has had the locus name of *Rex* with alleles *Re* and *re* defining Devon Rex as a separate locus from *Rex,* with alleles *R* and *r* for the Cornish Rex. Both Sphynx and Devon Rex have been proved to be caused by mutations in *KRT71.*[35]

Orange is the only trait known to be on the X chromosome for the domestic cat.[5,24,46,62] Because the X chromosome is subject to X inactivation in females, female cats that are heterozygous for the *Orange* and wild-type black alleles will express the coloration associated with the allele that is on the active X chromosome. Because X inactivation is random and occurs early in

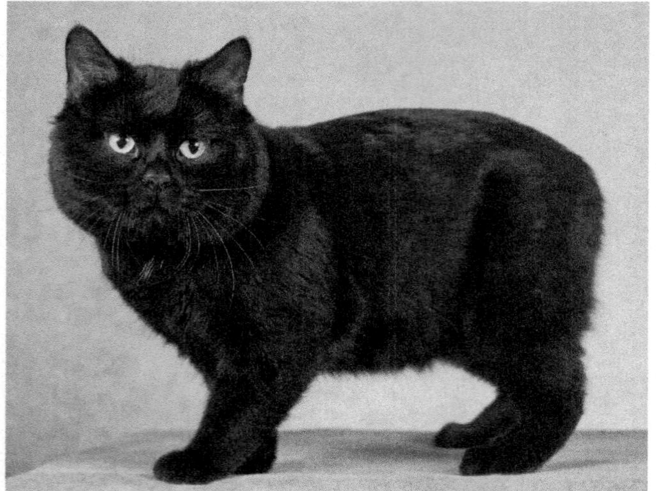

FIGURE 44-10 Manx. *(Photo copyright 2011 Richard Katris.)*

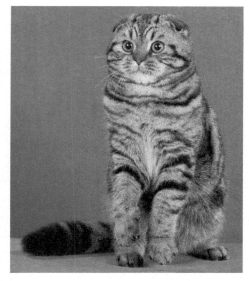

FIGURE 44-11 Scottish Fold. *(Photo copyright 2011 Richard Katris.)*

embryogenesis, the melanocytes in the skin will have different inactive X chromosomes, leading to the brindled black and orange of a tortoiseshell cat. Combined with the *Spotting* locus, which affects melanocyte migration and distribution, larger patches of skin will be covered by a clonal melanocyte population that has the same X inactivation, leading to large patches of orange or black or white coloration. Thus only female cats should be tortoiseshell or calico. Calico and tortoiseshell male cats are discovered fairly frequently, but they are usually sterile because they are genetic chimeras, having some cells as XX and some as XY. Chimeras are likely to be caused by the fusion of two embryos very early after fertilization.*

Mutations that affect structural traits, such as Manx (Figure 44-10) and ear fold (Figure 44-11) or curl (Figure 44-12), have a tendency to be dominant mutations. Two copies of a dominant mutation are often highly detrimental. Kittens that are homozygous for the Manx mutation die in utero,[87] and many cats homozygous for ear fold suffer from osteochondrodysplasia.[17,67,80,92] However, cats homozygous for ear curl have no known detrimental health effects, nor do homozygous Japanese Bobtails (Figure 44-13). Most of the dominant mutations have only one known allele, except for polydactylism, in which several causative alleles have been noted in the gene *sonic hedgehog (SHH)*.[58] Compound heterozygote cats for polydactylism mutations have not been identified, so the effects of having two different mutations that cause polydactylism are not known. Homozygote cats for a polydactyl mutation have been identified and do not necessarily have a more severe presentation, such as several extra toes or additional abnormalities to the digits (Lyons LA, unpublished data).

*References 16, 18, 43, 49, 55, 56, 83, 94.

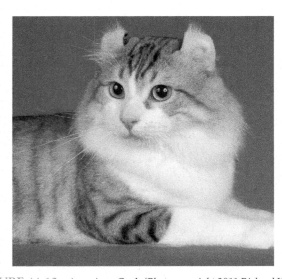

FIGURE 44-12 American Curl. *(Photo copyright 2011 Richard Katris.)*

Two genetic mutations of the domestic cat are not associated with a disease or a phenotypic trait. Cats have been shown to have mutations in a gene, *TAS1R2*, that disrupts the sweet receptors.[60,61] This mutation can be used to determine if an unknown DNA sample is of feline origin. Another example is the mutation that causes B blood type in cats.[11] Blood type incompatibilities obviously can lead to transfusion reactions and neonatal isoerythrolysis for the cat, but inherently this characteristic is not necessarily a disease. A point mutation and an 18 base pair deletion have both been implicated in the gene *CMAH* as indicating the presence of the B blood type, or a B blood type carrier. Because both mutations are on the same allele, a clear indication of the

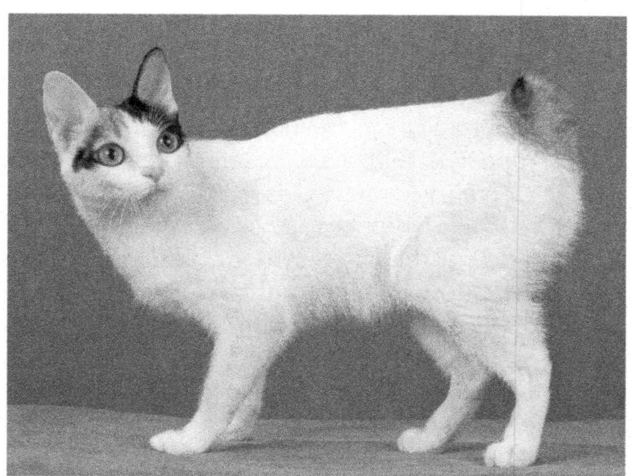

FIGURE 44-13 Japanese Bobtail. *(Photo copyright 2011 Richard Katris.)*

true causative mutation could not be determined. Thus both mutations should be examined in cats to genetically determine blood type.

Disease Mutations of the Domestic Cat

Many cat mutations that cause heritable diseases have been identified by way of the candidate-gene approach. Often, different biomarkers can identify possible inborn errors of metabolism, which lead to lysosomal storage diseases, such as gangliosidosis and mucopolysaccharidosis. Interesting, both gangliosidosis 1, caused by *GLB1* mutations, and gangliosidosis 2, caused by *HEXB* mutations, both found in the Korat breed, were some of the early discoveries of genetic mutations in the cat.[23,76] The clinical presentations strongly suggested conditions that were similar to those found in humans and other species. Because causative mutations had already been identified in these other species, the genes became obvious candidates for the cat. These mutations were identified at a time when significant genome sequence was not available for the cat; therefore, although a strong candidate was indicated, the studies were tedious. *Dystrophin,* the gene that causes Duchenne and many other types of muscular dystrophy, is a significantly large gene, and early studies discovered a feline mutation causing a similar dystrophy in the cat.[1,100] Cats having several of the diseases that were discovered early are actively retained in colonies because they are important models for gene therapies and many young children suffer from the same diseases as found in the cat.

Many of the disease mutations in the cat were identified in random-bred cats, such as hemophilia B[40] and vitamin D–resistant rickets,[37] or in a specific individual of a breed and are not a concern to the breed population in general, such as Niemann–Pick type C[91] and mannosidosis in Persians.[9] These breed-identified genetic mutations should not be part of routine screening by cat breeders and registries, but clinicians should know that genetic tests are available for diagnostic purposes, especially from research groups with specialized expertise, such as at the University of Pennsylvania (http://research.vet.upenn.edu/penngen). Unlike coat color mutations, which are common in the random-bred cat, the disease mutations are infrequent and should not be considered for genetic typing unless a clinical presentation is indicative of the disease. Even then, the clinical presentation may be more accurate for defining the disease as a new mutation in a known gene could be as likely in a random-bred population as the rediscovery of an already identified mutation. Several independent mutations have been identified in *HEXB* for gangliosidosis,[14,51,69,76] in *ARSB* for mucopolysaccharidosis VI,[22,101,102] and *HMBS* for porphyria.[19-21] A genetic test could rule out these mutations, although other mutations could also be present.

Like the Korat with gangliosidosis, the Abyssinian breed has had two different disease forms identified for a specific type of disease: progressive retinal atrophy (PRA). Mutations for both an early-onset, rapidly progressing autosomal dominant PRA, *CRX,*[73] and a late-onset, slowly progressing autosomal recessive PRA, *CEP290,* have been identified in Abyssinians.[72] Abyssinians also have a recessive trait causing deficiency of the enzyme pyruvate kinase in red blood cells, as well as cats in the breed population with different blood types. Therefore Abyssinian breeders commonly use genetic testing in breeding programs. The Abyssinian is one of the oldest cat breeds, present during the early foundations of cat registries. This breed's genetic heritage is obscure; it is not clearly a cat of eastern or western origins, although some evidence suggests that it may have originated in India. Historically, the breed has been fairly popular around the world, and genetic population statistics do not indicate that the Abyssinian breed is of any more or less concern for inbreeding depression than any other cat breed. Thus the detection of these various diseases in the Abyssinian may be an ascertainment bias or just sporadic bad luck for the breed.

Other diseases, such as PKD, are prevalent; PKD in Persians is estimated at 30% to 38% worldwide.[7,8,15] Because of cross-breeding with Persians, many other breeds, such as British Shorthair, American Shorthair, and Scottish Fold, also should be screened for PKD.[12,26,64] Thus veterinarians need to be aware of cross-breeding practices, which vary among different cat registry organizations, so that genetic tests can be placed as high or low priorities for differentials and diagnostics.

Unidentified Genetic Diseases and Traits of the Domestic Cat

Hundreds of traits and diseases that have been recognized to be genetic in other species have been documented in the domestic cat and its breeds (see Online Mendelian Inheritance in Animals: http://www.ncbi.nlm.nih.gov/omia). However, an increased incidence and prevalence must be documented before accepting that a single case report or case series of a condition constitutes a genetic problem for a breed or a population. Those traits with as yet unidentified mutations and a strongly suggestive mode of inheritance are presented in Table 44-3.

Breed dispositions to diseases, which may be due to genetics, environment, or both, have been reviewed for dogs and cats.[41] Common environmental factors are often difficult to identify and consider. Veterinarians should note that populations change genetically over time, and breeders have an impact on undesired traits through selection; thus conditions documented in the past may not be of present concern or risk. As previously mentioned, because breed populations vary greatly in different parts of the world, breed risks for diseases and health conditions vary accordingly. Many cat breeders and registries are proactive and openly list and discuss health concerns for their breeds. Overall, effective genetic studies to find mutations that cause health issues and traits require a sufficient sample size, which generally means active participation from the breed group.

Many of the morphologic and structural presentations of the domestic cat breeds may influence the presentation of conditions that are then noted to have a higher prevalence in a breed. Already mentioned are incontinence in the Manx and osteochrondrodysplasia of the Scottish Fold. These health conditions are actually secondary effects of the primary genetic mutation. The brachycephalia of Persian cats and related breeds has caused significant concern on account of the secondary structural abnormalities and chronic health problems caused by the extreme shortening of the skull.[57,89,90] Anecdotally, the fine, elegant structures of Abyssinians and Siamese exacerbate patellar luxation. The largest breed, the Maine Coon, may be affected by hip dysplasia, a very common problem in large dog breeds.

GENETIC RISK FACTORS AND COMPLEX TRAITS

All the mutations influencing a disease may not be identified at any given time; usually the mutations that influence a condition the most and have the highest heritability are identified first. Because multiple mutations may act additively to cause a disease, each mutation may be said to confer a "risk" for disease development. Thus some mutations may be considered risk factors, predisposing an individual to a health problem. These risk-conferring mutations are neither necessary nor sufficient for causing disease. An excellent example of a mutation that confers a risk are the DNA variants associated with cardiac disease in cats.

Hypertrophic cardiomyopathy (HCM) is a recognized genetic condition in cats.[53] In 2005, Meurs, Kittleson, and colleagues reported that a DNA alteration in the gene *cardiac myosin-binding protein C 3 (MYBPC3)* was strongly associated with HCM in a long-term research colony of Maine Coon cats at the University of California, Davis.[75] The DNA mutation is commonly referred to as *A31P* because this DNA mutation changes codon 31 from an alanine to a proline in the amino acid sequence (i.e., protein) of *MYBPC3*. The data clearly show that not all cats with the mutation had HCM and that some cats with HCM did not have the DNA mutation. Age of onset, variable expression, and disease heterogeneity were mentioned in this report. These aspects suggest that the identified DNA variant should be considered more of a risk factor than a directly causative mutation. Two recent papers have shown that not all Maine Coon cats with the A31P mutation develop HCM,[88,98] and one of those papers has mistakenly interpreted this lack of penetrance as being evidence that the A31P mutation is not causal.[98] This interpretation is misleading, causing debate about the validity of the Maine Coon HCM test.

To date, most cat genetic tests have been for traits that have nearly complete penetrance, have little variability in expression, and are early in onset. However, some imperfect examples do exist in cats that have not caused as much controversy as the HCM test. The *CEP290* PRA mutation in Abyssinians has a late age of onset, and some cats with subclinical disease have been identified.[71] Some cats with pyruvate kinase deficiency have very mild and subclinical presentations.[54] The interplay of various coat color genes often muddles the determination of the true coat color of cats. As is true in humans with cardiac disease, the finding that not all cats with the A31P mutation in *MYBPC3* develop HCM is actually more commonplace in the field of HCM genetic testing. Because disease- or trait-causing mutations may not be 100% penetrant, they do not always cause clinically detectable disease. Presence of clinical disease in an individual cat and the severity of disease (expression) are likely affected by the known genetic aspects presented in the subsequent sections.

Incomplete Penetrance

For some traits and diseases, even though a known causative mutation has been identified, an individual with that mutation does not present with the condition. Incomplete penetrance is an extreme of variable expression (discussed in more detail later in this chapter). In general, the reason that a condition associated with a mutation would not be present is unknown, but other genetic, biologic, and environmental interactions certainly play a role in the overall appearance and health of an individual and its organs. The sensitivity of clinical diagnostics may also influence the determination of penetrance. In the case of HCM, echocardiography can be considered an insensitive tool for detecting mild forms of the disease in cats; thus many cats with mild changes do not clinically appear to have cardiac disease. Experience and bias also play a role in diagnosis. For example, individuals who do not have expertise in the use of ultrasonic examinations for HCM or PKD are less likely to be able to provide an accurate diagnosis for these diseases.

Age of Onset (Age-Related Penetrance)

Some diseases have a slow progression and may not present until later in life. In humans HCM caused by *MYBPC* mutations is clearly a disease that has slow progression and commonly does not express until the individual is over 50 years of age. HCM in Maine Coon cats can also develop in older cats, especially in cats that are heterozygous for the mutation and, for some unknown reason, in females. Often, an autosomal dominant disease may be more severe if two copies of the risk mutation are present in an individual, leading to earlier and more severe disease, which appears to be the case with the A31P mutation. The definitive age as to when a cat is past the risk of developing HCM is not precisely determined.

Variable Expression

Most traits and diseases have some amount of variable expression depending on the individual. For example, not all cats with the mutation for blue dilution have the same color of blue–gray fur. Obviously, the background genetics and environment of the individual influence the overall presentations of traits and diseases. Thus the level of presentation can be variable in regard to left ventricular wall thickness in cats with HCM. Cats can have mild, moderate, or severe HCM. Only those cats with severe HCM show clinical signs, although a few cats with lesser severity of disease may die suddenly. Cats with HCM may fall in the "equivocal" range for wall thickness; therefore definitive disease status is difficult to declare. These equivocal cats may progress to more severe disease with time, or the equivocal status may be as severe as the disease gets. Some cats with PKD have only a few cysts and never progress to renal failure while others have severe and fast progression of disease and succumb to renal failure in a few years.

Disease Heterogeneity

More than one mutation in the same gene or mutations in different related genes can cause the same disease. Genetic heterogeneity for HCM in humans is well established, and there is no reason to think the same situation is not true for cats. Currently, more than 1000 mutations in more than 10 genes are known to cause HCM in humans. Only two mutations have been identified that cause HCM in cats, the A31P mutation in Maine Coon cats and the R820W mutation in Ragdolls,[74,75] which also causes disease in humans.[84] Both mutations are in *MYBPC3*, the most commonly mutated gene in humans with HCM (see review by Tsoutsman et al[96]). Other breeds of cats, including the Bengal, Siberian, Devon Rex, and Sphynx, and random-bred cats either do not have or have an extremely low prevalence of the A31P or the R820W mutation. However, because there are Maine Coon cats that have HCM and do not have the A31P mutation, there must be at least one more cause of HCM, most likely another mutation, in this breed. The long fur mutations in the cat are also examples of trait heterogeneity.

Accuracy of Genetic Testing

Even though a specific genetic mutation may be identified for a trait or disease, research laboratories use different methods to assay for the mutation. Errors in genetic assays may produce inaccurate DNA results, leading to confusion in genetic test interpretation. Direct DNA sequencing is considered the most robust method, "the gold standard," but it is also one of the more costly methods of analysis. Because DNA primers must bind to the DNA sequence flanking a specific mutation, other, unimportant mutations may be in the areas where the primers bind, causing poor or no amplification of one or both alleles for a given individual. This condition is known as allelic dropout, and all testing laboratories are aware of this potential source of error for a genetic test. Even direct DNA sequencing can suffer from allelic dropout, but because a larger portion of the gene that may have other DNA variants is generally amplified, a higher likelihood of detecting allelic dropout is present. Laboratories will place polymerase chain reaction (PCR) primers in different locations surrounding the mutation of interest, which is often proprietary information, in attempts to lower the risk of allelic dropout. Thus some laboratories have better assays than others, even if they are doing the same assay method and testing for the same mutation. The different DNA assay methods are usually developed to reduce cost and fit the laboratory's expertise and instrumentation. However, some assays may have, in general, an increased risk of test failure. Common methods for DNA testing include real-time PCR (TaqMan), restriction fragment length polymorphism (RFLP), allele-specific oligonucleotides (ASOs), or even mass spectroscopy–based methods. Just as a veterinarian may want to know if a feline immunodeficiency virus (FIV) test is performed by enzyme-linked immunosorbent assay (ELISA), PCR, or Western blot because each method has different sensitivities and specificities, this is also true for DNA-testing methods. Veterinarians will need to become familiar with the different genetic testing approaches and not hesitate to ask testing laboratory staff members about their methods and sensitivity and specificity for their approaches.

Inaccurate Clinical Diagnosis

Echocardiography is the most common and currently the only useful method for diagnosing cardiac disease in cats. Several studies have evaluated HCM in domestic shorthair and Maine Coon cats.[28,44,79] Not all cardiac disease is HCM, and even the definition of HCM can be debated. A consistent definition for HCM is not used by all cardiologists, which creates difficulty when correlating a genetic test result with an ultrasound report, especially if detailed diagnostic criteria are not presented in the report. Misinterpretations in ultrasound examinations may lead to different interpretations with disease status.

Overall, the only way to determine the true risk conferred by some mutations is to follow cats over the course of a lifetime with common diagnostic procedures and compare outcomes to the genetic test results. Only time and continued follow-up will help determine the true relative risk that mutations convey for complex diseases. In the case of HCM, various studies have indicated higher or lower risks in different populations of cats, but none has been able to follow cats throughout a lifetime. These studies are important and are of great value to the community. Other mutations must be found, and the cooperation of breeders must be positive and enthusiastic for these studies to succeed.

GENETIC TESTING

Breeding Recommendations

Cat breeders are very knowledgeable about weighing different factors to produce healthy cats that are of good physical type and temperament. Many genetic tests help a breeder make a clearer, more educated decision. Cats with a positive genetic test for a disease should be screened by another diagnostic method, such as ultrasound in the case of HCM and PKD, to determine disease status, and this overall information should be used in breeding decisions. Other health, physical type, and behavioral attributes should certainly be considered in the overall breeding program. However, breeders should work hard to reduce the risks with any health issue. Every cat that has the HCM A31P mutation is at risk for developing HCM, and every cat with the mutation will pass it on to some or all offspring. Cats that are homozygous for the A31P mutation will definitely pass the mutation to all offspring. The homozygous cats are at higher risk of developing severe HCM. Cats that are heterozygous for the mutation should not be bred unless they have other qualities that are either highly beneficial or necessary to the breed. Kittens that test negative for the mutation should be used to replace affected parents in the gene pool. A slow eradication of disease is recommended for highly prevalent diseases, such as HCM and PKD, because the quick elimination of a high number of cats could lead to other effects of inbreeding depression. Breeders of cat breeds with very low population sizes, such as the Korat, have learned to manage the gangliosidoses by never breeding carriers together. It is to be hoped that all the disease mutations can eventually be eradicated, but good breeding decisions and balancing population diversity must be considered.

Recently, estimated breeding values (EBVs) have been suggested as a means to apply selection to companion animal populations.[59,93] EBVs are not a new concept; they are used to assign a value to an animal based on selected qualities. Cat and dog breeders inherently assign EBVs to their breeding stock, but not in a preset and defined numeric fashion. The dairy and beef industries have used EBVs for decades to produce herds that have higher milk yields, milk fat content, or different carcass qualities. Generally, some industry standard has to be developed and routinely followed in the same direction of positive or negative selection for the trait(s) of interest. EBVs usually pertain to traits that are complex and have some quantitative measurement, such as weight, height, or tail length. Thus standard quantitative genetic techniques can be used to estimate the extent of inheritance of the disorder (heritability), followed by the development of a metric that can be used to assess the genetic merit of individual animals for the purpose of selection for reproduction and subsequent breed improvement. In the simplest form, cats that carry undesired traits, such as a disease, should be assigned a low EBV. However, other desired traits may outweigh the negative value of a disease or condition, giving a cat an overall high EBV. EBVs are a concept to consider as more genetic tests are developed because breeders now have more informative data to consider when selecting mating pairs for the propagation of a breed. Standards and a unified effort would need to be developed, as well as retrospective trials to model the effects of the EBVs before they are implemented.

Genetic Testing Concerns in Different Breeds or Populations

Once a mutation is identified for a gene that causes a particular coat color or disease, a service laboratory, either in association with the investigator who found the mutation or an independent commercial laboratory, will establish a genetic test for that mutation to offer to the public (Table 44-4). Over a dozen laboratories around the world now offer genetic testing for PKD in cats. All the laboratories may be technically accurate, but not all of them "know their cats" equally. Some of the concerns with specificity and sensitivity of genetic tests, particularly in regard to testing in hybrid cat breeds, are due to a lack of knowledge of how cat breeds are developed and cat evolutionary relationships.

Tables 44-1 and 44-2 contain all the currently known genetic mutations in the cat that have been published and may be of concern for genetic testing. Genetic diseases usually present in a specific breed and thus are associated only with that breed. However, some breeds are allowed to outcross with others, and some are legally

TABLE 44-4 **Domestic Cat DNA Testing Laboratories**

Lab/Website	Region	University Research Affiliate	ID	*Cat Test** *Disease*	*Color*	*Blood*	*Coat*
Animal DNA Testing www.animalsdna.com	Australia		Yes	4	Some	Yes	No
Animal Health Trust www.aht.org.uk	UK	Animal Health Trust	Yes	PKD	No	No	No
Antagene Immeuble Le Meltem www.antagene.com	France		Yes	4	Color	Yes	No
BioAxis DNA Research Centre Ltd. www.dnares.in	India		Yes	PKD	No	No	No
DNA Diagnostics Center www.dnacenter.com	U.S.		No	PKD	No	No	No
GENINDEXE www.genindexe.com	France		Yes	7	5	Yes	No
Genoscoper www.genoscoper.com	Finland		Yes	No	No	Yes	No
Gribbles www.gribblesvets.com	Australia		No	PKD	No	No	No
IDEXX www.idexx.ca	Canada		No	PK def.	No	No	No
Laboklin www.laboklin.de/	Germany		Yes	9	5	Yes	Long
Langford Veterinary Services, Molecular Diagnostics Unit, Langfordvets.co.uk	UK	Bristol	No	3	No	No	No
PennGen research.vet.upenn.edu/penngen†	U.S.	Pennsylvania	No	PK GSD	No	No	No
PROGENUS S.A. www.progenus.be	Belgium		Yes	HCM PKD	No	No	No
Van Haeringen Laboratory www.vhlgenetics.com	Netherlands		Yes	9	5	Yes	Long
Veterinary Cardiac Genetics Lab www.cvm.ncsu.edu/vhc/csds/vcgl	U.S.	North Carolina State	No	HCM	No	No	No
Veterinary Genetics Lab www.vgl.ucdavis.edu	U.S.	California, Davis	Yes	7	All	Yes	All
VetGen www.vetgen.com	U.S.	Michigan	Yes	No	Brown dilute	No	Long
Vetogene www.vetogene.com	Italy	Milan	Yes	HCM PKD	No	No	No

PKD, Polycystic kidney disease; *GSD,* glycogen storage disease; *HCM,* hypertrophic cardiomyopathy; *ID,* individual genetic identification; *PK def.,* pyruvate kinase deficiency.

*Tests reference to those listed in Table 44-1. If a laboratory offers only one or two tests, those tests are listed. PKD and HCM are the most popular tests to offer.

†PennGen also offers tests for diseases in Table 44-2 that are not of concern to the cat breeds or population in general.

or illegally used to help refine the appearance of another breed. The Siamese and Persian have influenced a host of other cat breeds. Hence any mutation found in one breed can be found in others if cross-breeding has occurred. In addition, cats are bred all over the world, and the rules of various registries and associations are not always the same. An outcross that may be acceptable for The International Cat Association[95] in the United States may be unacceptable for the Cat Fanciers' Association or perhaps the Governing Council of the Cat Fancy[36] in the United Kingdom. Thus the personnel of testing laboratories must understand cat breed dynamics to know whether a test is valid for a given breed in any part of the world and to offer the appropriate tests for the breeds at risk.

Why does one care if a genetic test developed in one breed is valid in a different breed? The concern is disease heterogeneity. Owners, breeders, and veterinarians may identify a clinical presentation that is abnormal in the cat, but they also may jump to conclusions too quickly. For example, there are many causes of renal failure besides PKD. There are different types of cardiac disease; not all cardiac disease is HCM. Even when a diagnosis of HCM is definitive, not all HCM is caused by the same mutation. Herein lies the concern. An unknowing veterinarian, owner, or breeder may want a cat to have a genetic test for HCM or PKD because the cat has clinical signs consistent with these diseases. If the test shows a negative result, this result does not necessarily mean the cat does not have HCM or PKD, if the test has not been proved effective in that selected breed. The result does imply that the cat does not have the mutation causing Maine Coon or Ragdoll HCM or Persian PKD. A laboratory may very well run the test, but laboratories have different capabilities and skills with genetic counseling. Veterinarians may be on their own when it comes to interpreting the meaning of a negative test. This is why a test is generally listed as pertaining to a specific breed. Until clinical data (e.g., ultrasound diagnoses and genetic test results) is available from a sufficient number of cats, a test cannot be valid for the breed unless clear outcrossing to the risk breeds is apparent.

Genetic Testing Concerns in Hybrid Cat Breeds

Some domestic cat breeds are hybrids of two species of cats. According to the biological species concept, organisms are classified in the same species if they are potentially capable of interbreeding and producing fertile offspring. The production of hybrid cat breeds generally has required a female domestic cat to be bred with a male cat from another wild felid species because of temperament concerns. For example, domestic cats have been bred to Asian Leopard cats to produce the Bengal and to the Serval to produce the Savannah. For the first-generation offspring, or first filial (F1) generation, of hybrid cat breeds, the male F1 is sterile; the subsequent generations cannot be produced by crossing a male F1 with a female F1. Thus the female F1 offspring are generally mated with a full-blooded domestic male or a lower-generation hybrid male that is fertile. Cat breeders will term the subsequent generations of offspring as F2, F3, and so on; however, these designations are actually genetically incorrect, and they should be considered backcross generations (e.g., BC1, BC2). The F1 females are also difficult to mate and may have reduced fecundity. Fertility may take several generations to re-establish in hybrid breeds. The infertility is due to problems with chromosomes aligning during cell reproduction for the production of the gametes, as well as allelic incompatibilities at different genes. Because the inheritance of the allelic incompatibilities is difficult to predict, many hybrid cats can have reproduction problems, even in the lower generations that can be shown in competition.

A normal level of genetic variation among cats is expected, typically far less than 1% of a sequence that codes for a protein. Herein lies a problem for hybrid cat breeds. The evolutionary time between the appearances of different cat species is millions of years,[50] not the hundreds to thousands of years between the appearance of cat breeds and populations. An Asian Leopard cat had a common ancestor with the domestic cat about 6 million years ago, the Bobcat about 8 million years ago, and the Serval about 9.5 million years ago. The Jungle cat is more closely related to the domestic cat than the Asian Leopard cat is. In addition, for some of these wild felid species, different subspecies have been incorporated into the breed. The DNA sequence of a domestic cat and one of these wild felid species will have many genetic differences, maybe a several percentage difference, less for the jungle cat, more for the Serval compared with that of a domestic cat. The genetic differences are most likely silent mutations, but the variation will interplay with genetic assays and may cause more allelic dropout than what would be normally anticipated. No genetic tests have been validated in the hybrid cat breeds, although they are used frequently. As mentioned, these allelic differences can cause allelic incompatibilities, which could produce reproduction problems and other health issues.

Most laboratories recognize that disease mutations are specific to breeds but not the coat colors. The coat color mutations occurred during the early domestication of the cat, before the breeds were developed, so all breeds tend to have the same mutation. This is true for all the coat color tests so far but for the hybrid breeds, such as the Bengal, Chausie (produced from the jungle cat), and Savannah, some oddities in coat color and disease testing may occur. The normal DNA sequence around each of the mutations for coat colors must be evaluated in many individuals from each wild felid species to find the normal, silent mutations that occur between the wild felids and the domestic cats. At any given gene, in a Bengal, it cannot be determined whether one Asian Leopard cat sequence or two are present. Thus the accuracy for any genetic test is not known for hybrid cat breeds. If the domestic cat alleles are present, the test will perform as expected. However, one never knows when one allele or both are from the Asian Leopard cat. Selection generally favors the wild felid colorations, so inherently the breed is selected for the DNA sequences that may cause the genetic tests to fail.

Inappropriate Genetic Testing Laboratory Procedures

Genetic testing laboratories attempt to provide the best service for the lowest cost. Many of the newer technologies allow for higher throughput of samples and also performance of more than one genetic test per assay, greatly lowering costs of reagents and human labor. Many testing laboratories aspire to be as complete as possible, providing all available genetic tests for any given species. However, in the zeal of competition, a few genetic tests that are offered in the cat do not have sufficient scientific support. Any genetic test should be based on a reference publication to determine the genetic sequence surrounding the mutation and provide the statistical support for the accuracy of the mutation for conferring disease or the trait of interest in specific breeds and populations. Published abstracts are not peer-reviewed articles and do not provide sufficient information to determine the accuracy of a test; thus abstracts are not appropriate references for genetic tests. Some universities or researchers own associated companies, the discoveries of which may be protected by licensure or patent, and the data may never be published for competitive advantage. Some genetic tests therefore can be found only with specific testing companies. Currently, the patented tests for cats include PKD, HCM, the mutations for *Tyrosinase* at the *Color* locus that confer Siamese and Burmese style "points," and blood type B.[11] However, licensure is available for each of these tests and the patents pertain only to the United States. Some companies will violate these patents because the overall income to the patent holder is generally very low and the likelihood that a university would enforce a patent would be low relative to the prohibitive cost. However, violation of genetic test patents is not encouraged and is generally considered inappropriate.

In addition to violating patents, some laboratories offer genetic tests that are not scientifically sound in an attempt to gain a competitive advantage. Another mutation in *MYBPC3* for HCM was reported in an abstract but was never presented in a peer-reviewed publication. Support for the risk this mutation confers for HCM in cats has not been well documented, but some laboratories nonetheless offer testing for this DNA variant. Laboratories often post disclaimers, leaving the veterinarian, owner, and breeder to speculate about a test's true diagnostic utility.

Some laboratories offer a single method, such as a type DNA array method, to genetically test all mutations for the cat. As noted in Tables 44-1 and 44-2, the mutations that cause traits and diseases of the cat come in a variety of types. Many mutations are point mutations: a single nucleotide difference in the DNA. Others are deletions of one or more bases, and some are very complex alterations that can disrupt several exons of a gene, such as the mutation that causes spinal muscular atrophy in the Maine Coon cat. The genetic sequence surrounding a mutation is also important because some regions may be rich in particular bases, such as a GC-rich region or a region with repeat elements of stretches of similar nucleotides, such as polyadenosine stretches. This information is less important to the veterinarian, but very important to the development of an assay that is sound and efficient. A single testing method, such as size variation, RFLP, real-time PCR (TaqMan), or any array method cannot effectively test all the different mutations. Thus a testing laboratory must be proficient in several methods to test all types of mutations for the cat or any other species. Veterinarians should be skeptical of any laboratory that offers one testing method for all mutations of the cat.

CONCLUSION

Genetic testing is an important diagnostic tool for the veterinarian, breeder, and owner. Genetic tests are not 100% foolproof, and the accuracy of the test procedure and the reputation and customer service of the genetic testing laboratory must be considered. Some traits are highly desired, and genetic testing can help breeders determine appropriate pairings more accurately. This may encourage more efficient breeding programs, thereby lowering costs and excessive cat production. Other traits or diseases are undesirable, and genetic testing can be used to prevent and potentially eradicate them from the population. Genetic tests for simple genetic traits are more consistent with predicting the trait or disease presentation, but as genomics progresses for the cat, tests that confer risk will become more common. Veterinarians will have to weigh the relative risks of having a mutation versus having disease as part of the differential diagnosis, and breeders will have to consider risk factors along with the other important attributes of a cat in making breeding decisions.

References

1. Allamand V, Campbell KP: Animal models for muscular dystrophy: valuable tools for the development of therapies, *Hum Mol Genet* 9:2459, 2000.
2. American Pet Product Manufacturing Association: *National pet owner's survey*, Greenwich, Conn, 2008, The Association.
3. Bach L, Gandolfi B, Grahn R et al: The distribution and possible origins of FGF5 mutations affecting fur length in cats, *submitted for publication*, 2011.
4. Bamber RC: Correlation between white coat colour, blue eyes, and deafness in cats, *Journal of Genetics* 27:407, 1933.
5. Bamber RC, Herdman EC: The inheritance of black, yellow and tortoiseshell coat colour in cats, *J Genet* 18:87, 1927.
6. Banks G, Chamberlain J: The value of mammalian models for duchenne muscular dystrophy in developing therapeutic strategies, *Curr Top Dev Biol* 84:431, 2008.
7. Barrs VR, Gunew M, Foster SF et al: Prevalence of autosomal dominant polycystic kidney disease in Persian cats and related-breeds in Sydney and Brisbane, *Aust Vet J* 79:257, 2001.
8. Barthez PY, Rivier P, Begon D: Prevalence of polycystic kidney disease in Persian and Persian related cats in France, *J Feline Med Surg* 5:345, 2003.
9. Berg T, Tollersrud OK, Walkley SU et al: Purification of feline lysosomal alpha-mannosidase, determination of its cDNA sequence and identification of a mutation causing alpha-mannosidosis in Persian cats, *Biochem J* 328 (Pt 3):863, 1997.
10. Bergsma DR, Brown KS: White fur, blue eyes, and deafness in the domestic cat, *J Hered* 62:171, 1971.
11. Bighignoli B, Niini T, Grahn RA et al: Cytidine monophospho-N-acetylneuraminic acid hydroxylase (CMAH) mutations associated with the domestic cat AB blood group, *BMC Genet* 8:27, 2007.
12. Biller DS, Chew DJ, DiBartola SP: Polycystic kidney disease in a family of Persian cats, *J Am Vet Med Assoc* 196:1288, 1990.
13. Biller DS, DiBartola SP, Eaton KA et al: Inheritance of polycystic kidney disease in Persian cats, *J Hered* 87:1, 1996.
14. Bradbury AM, Morrison NE, Hwang M et al: Neurodegenerative lysosomal storage disease in European Burmese cats with hexosaminidase beta-subunit deficiency, *Mol Genet Metab* 97:53, 2009.
15. Cannon MJ, MacKay AD, Barr FJ et al: Prevalence of polycystic kidney disease in Persian cats in the United Kingdom, *Vet Rec* 149:409, 2001.
16. Centerwall WR, Benirschke K: Animal model for the XXY Klinefelter's syndrome in man: tortoiseshell and calico male cats, *Am J Vet Res* 36:1275, 1975.
17. Chang J, Jung J, Oh S et al: Osteochondrodysplasia in three Scottish Fold cats, *J Vet Sci* 8:307, 2007.
18. Chu EHY, Thuline HC, Norby DE: Triploid-diploid chimerism in a male tortoiseshell cat, *Cytogenetics* 3:1, 1964.
19. Clavero S, Bishop DF, Giger U et al: Feline congenital erythropoietic porphyria: two homozygous UROS missense mutations cause the enzyme deficiency and porphyrin accumulation, *Mol Med* 16:381, 2010.
20. Clavero S, Bishop DF, Haskins ME et al: Feline acute intermittent porphyria: a phenocopy masquerading as an erythropoietic porphyria due to dominant and recessive hydroxymethylbilane synthase mutations, *Hum Mol Genet* 19:584, 2010.
21. Clavero S, Haskins M, Giger U et al: Molecular basis of acure intermittent porphyria in the cat, *Proc Adv Canine Feline Genomics Inherit Dis*, St Malo, France, 2008.
22. Crawley AC, Yogalingam G, Muller VJ et al: Two mutations within a feline mucopolysaccharidosis type VI colony cause three different clinical phenotypes, *J Clin Invest* 101: 109, 1998.
23. De Maria R, Divari S, Bo S et al: Beta-galactosidase deficiency in a Korat cat: a new form of feline GM1-gangliosidosis, *Acta Neuropathol* 96:307, 1998.
24. Doncaster L: On the inheritance of tortoiseshell and related colours in cats, *Proc Cambridge Philosophical Soc* 13:35, 1904.
25. Drogemuller C, Rufenacht S, Wichert B et al: Mutations within the FGF5 gene are associated with hair length in cats, *Anim Genet* 38:218, 2007.
26. Eaton KA, Biller DS, DiBartola SP et al: Autosomal dominant polycystic kidney disease in Persian and Persian-cross cats, *Vet Pathol* 34:117, 1997.
27. Eizirik E, Yuhki N, Johnson WE et al: Molecular genetics and evolution of melanism in the cat family, *Curr Biol* 13:448, 2003.
28. Fries R, Heaney AM, Meurs KM: Prevalence of the myosin-binding protein C mutation in Maine Coon cats, *J Vet Intern Med* 22:893, 2008.

28a. Fyfe JC, Kurzhals RL, Hawkins MG et al: A complex rearrangement in GBE1 causes both perinatal hypoglycemic collapse and late-juvenile-onset neuromuscular degeneration in glycogen storage disease type IV of Norwegian forest cats, *Mol Genet Metab* 90:383, 2007.

29. Fyfe JC, Kurzhals RL, Lassaline ME et al: Molecular basis of feline beta-glucuronidase deficiency: an animal model of mucopolysaccharidosis VII, *Genomics* 58:121, 1999.
30. Fyfe JC, Menotti-Raymond M, David VA et al: An approximately 140-kb deletion associated with feline spinal muscular atrophy implies an essential LIX1 function for motor neuron survival, *Genome Res* 16:1084, 2006.
31. Gabor LJ, Canfield PJ, Malik R: Immunophenotypic and histological characterisation of 109 cases of feline lymphosarcoma, *Aust Vet J* 77:436, 1999.
32. Gabor LJ, Canfield PJ, Malik R: Haematological and biochemical findings in cats in Australia with lymphosarcoma, *Aust Vet J* 78:456, 2000.
33. Gabor LJ, Malik R, Canfield PJ: Clinical and anatomical features of lymphosarcoma in 118 cats, *Aust Vet J* 76:725, 1998.
34. Gandolfi B, Bach L, Beresford L et al: Off with the gloves: mutation in KIT implicated for the unique white spotting phenotype of Birman cats, *submitted for publication*, 2011.
35. Gandolfi B, Outerbridge C, Beresford L et al: The naked truth: Sphynx and Devon Rex cat breed mutations in KRT71, *Mamm Genome* 21:509, 2010.
36. The Governing Council of the Cat Fancy (GCCF): http://www.gccfcats.org. Accessed June 22, 2011.
37. Geisen V, Weber K, Hartmann K: Vitamin D-dependent hereditary rickets type I in a cat, *J Vet Intern Med* 23:196, 2009.
38. Ginzinger DG, Lewis ME, Ma Y et al: A mutation in the lipoprotein lipase gene is the molecular basis of chylomicronemia in a colony of domestic cats, *J Clin Invest* 97:1257, 1996.
39. Goldstein R, Narala S, Sabet N et al: Primary hyperoxaluria in cats caused by a mutation in the feline GRHPR gene, *J Hered* 100:S2, 2009.
40. Goree M, Catalfamo JL, Aber S et al: Characterization of the mutations causing hemophilia B in 2 domestic cats, *J Vet Intern Med* 19:200, 2005.
41. Gough A, Thomas A: *Breed predispositions to disease in dogs and cats*, ed 2, Oxford, England, 2010, Wiley-Blackwell.
42. Grahn R, Ellis M, Grahn J et al: No bones about it! A novel CYP27B1 mutation results in feline vitamin D-dependent Rickets Type I (VDDR-1), *J Feline Med Surg, in press*, 2012.
43. Gregson NM, Ishmael J: Diploid triploid chimerism in three tortoiseshell cats, *Res Vet Sci* 12:275, 1971.
44. Gundler S, Tidholm A, Haggstrom J: Prevalence of myocardial hypertrophy in a population of asymptomatic Swedish Maine coon cats, *Acta Vet Scand* 50:22, 2008.

45. He X, Li CM, Simonaro CM et al: Identification and characterization of the molecular lesion causing mucopolysaccharidosis type I in cats, *Mol Genet Metab* 67:106, 1999.
46. Ibsen HL: Tricolor inheritance. III. Tortoiseshell cats, *Genetics* 1, 1916.
47. Imes DL, Geary LA, Grahn RA et al: Albinism in the domestic cat *(Felis catus)* is associated with a tyrosinase (TYR) mutation, *Anim Genet* 37:175, 2006.
48. Ishida Y, David VA, Eizirik E et al: A homozygous single-base deletion in MLPH causes the dilute coat color phenotype in the domestic cat, *Genomics* 88:698, 2006.
49. Ishihara T: Cytological studies on tortoiseshell male cats, *Cytologia* 21: 391, 1956.
50. Johnson WE, Eizirik E, Pecon-Slattery J et al: The late Miocene radiation of modern Felidae: a genetic assessment, *Science* 311:73, 2006.
51. Kanae Y, Endoh D, Yamato O et al: Nonsense mutation of feline beta-hexosaminidase beta-subunit (HEXB) gene causing Sandhoff disease in a family of Japanese domestic cats, *Res Vet Sci* 82:54, 2007.
52. Kehler JS, David VA, Schaffer AA et al: Four independent mutations in the feline fibroblast growth factor 5 gene determine the long-haired phenotype in domestic cats, *J Hered* 98:555, 2007.
53. Kittleson MD, Meurs KM, Munro MJ et al: Familial hypertrophic cardiomyopathy in maine coon cats: an animal model of human disease, *Circulation* 99:3172, 1999.
54. Kohn B, Fumi C: Clinical course of pyruvate kinase deficiency in Abyssinian and Somali cats, *J Feline Med Surg* 10:145, 2008.
55. Kosowska B, Januszewski A, Tokarska M et al: Cytogenetic and histologic studies of tortoiseshell cats, *Med Weter* 57:475, 2001.
56. Kuiper H, Hewicker-Trautwein M, Distl O: [Cytogenetic and histologic examination of four tortoiseshell cats], *Dtsch Tierarztl Wochenschr* 110:457, 2003.
57. Kunzel W, Breit S, Oppel M: Morphometric investigations of breed-specific features in feline skulls and considerations on their functional implications, *Anat Histol Embryol* 32:218, 2003.
58. Lettice LA, Hill AE, Devenney PS et al: Point mutations in a distant sonic hedgehog cis-regulator generate a variable regulatory output responsible for preaxial polydactyly, *Hum Mol Genet* 17:978, 2008.
59. Lewis T, Rusbridge C, Knowler P et al: Heritability of syringomyelia in Cavalier King Charles spaniels, *Vet J* 183:345, 2010.
60. Li X, Li W, Wang H et al: Cats lack a sweet taste receptor, *J Nutr* 136:1932S, 2006.
61. Li X, Li W, Wang H et al: Pseudogenization of a sweet-receptor gene accounts for cats' indifference toward sugar, *PLoS Genet* 1:27, 2005.
62. Little CC: Colour inheritance in cats, with special reference to colours, black, yellow and tortoiseshell, *J Genet* 8:279, 1919.
63. Louwerens M, London CA, Pedersen NC et al: Feline lymphoma in the post-feline leukemia virus era, *J Vet Intern Med* 19:329, 2005.
64. Lyons LA, Biller DS, Erdman CA et al: Feline polycystic kidney disease mutation identified in PKD1, *J Am Soc Nephrol* 15:2548, 2004.
65. Lyons LA, Foe IT, Rah HC et al: Chocolate coated cats: TYRP1 mutations for brown color in domestic cats, *Mamm Genome* 16:356, 2005.
66. Lyons LA, Imes DL, Rah HC et al: Tyrosinase mutations associated with Siamese and Burmese patterns in the domestic cat *(Felis catus)*, *Anim Genet* 36:119, 2005.
67. Malik R, Allan GS, Howlett CR et al: Osteochondrodysplasia in Scottish Fold cats, *Aust Vet J* 77:85, 1999.
68. Martin DR, Cox NR, Morrison NE et al: Mutation of the GM2 activator protein in a feline model of GM2 gangliosidosis, *Acta Neuropathol* 110:443, 2005.
69. Martin DR, Krum BK, Varadarajan GS et al: An inversion of 25 base pairs causes feline GM2 gangliosidosis variant, *Exp Neurol* 187:30, 2004.
70. Mazrier H, Van Hoeven M, Wang P et al: Inheritance, biochemical abnormalities, and clinical features of feline mucolipidosis II: the first animal model of human I-cell disease, *J Hered* 94:363, 2003.
71. Menotti-Raymond M, David VA, Pflueger S et al: Widespread retinal degenerative disease mutation (rdAc) discovered among a large number of popular cat breeds, *Vet J* 186:32, 2010.
72. Menotti-Raymond M, David VA, Schaffer AA et al: Mutation in CEP290 discovered for cat model of human retinal degeneration, *J Hered* 98:211, 2007.
73. Menotti-Raymond M, Deckman K, David V et al: Mutation discovered in a feline model of human congenital retinal blinding disease, *Invest Ophthalmol Vis Sci* 51:2852, 2010.
74. Meurs KM, Norgard MM, Ederer MM et al: A substitution mutation in the myosin binding protein C gene in ragdoll hypertrophic cardiomyopathy, *Genomics* 90:261, 2007.
75. Meurs KM, Sanchez X, David RM et al: A cardiac myosin binding protein C mutation in the Maine Coon cat with familial hypertrophic cardiomyopathy, *Hum Mol Genet* 14:3587, 2005.
76. Muldoon LL, Neuwelt EA, Pagel MA et al: Characterization of the molecular defect in a feline model for type II GM2-gangliosidosis (Sandhoff disease), *Am J Pathol* 144:1109, 1994.
77. Nakata N, Wang Y, Bhatt S: Trends in prenatal screening and diagnostic testing among women referred for advanced maternal age, *Prenat Diagn* 3:198, 2010.
78. Orioli I, Castilla E, Scarano G et al: Effect of paternal age in achondroplasia, thanatophoric dysplasia, and osteogenesis imperfecta, *Am J Med Genet* 59:209, 1995.
79. Paige CF, Abbott JA, Elvinger F et al: Prevalence of cardiomyopathy in apparently healthy cats, *J Am Vet Med Assoc* 234:1398, 2009.
80. Partington BP, Williams JF, Pechman RD et al: What is your diagnosis? Scottish Fold osteodystrophy, *J Am Vet Med Assoc* 209:1235, 1996.
81. Peterschmitt M, Grain F, Arnaud B et al: Mutation in the melanocortin 1 receptor is associated with amber colour in the Norwegian Forest Cat, *Anim Genet* 40:547, 2009.
82. Pion P, Kittleson M, Rogers Q et al: Taurine deficiency myocardial failure in the domestic cat, *Prog Clin Biol Res* 351:423, 1990.
83. Pyle RL, Patterson DF, Hare WCD et al: XXY sex chromosome constitution in a Himalayan cat with tortoiseshell points, *J Hered* 63:220, 1971.
84. Ripoll Vera T, Montserrat Iglesias L, Hermida Prieto M et al: The R820W mutation in the MYBPC3 gene, associated with hypertrophic cardiomyopathy in cats, causes hypertrophic cardiomyopathy and left ventricular non-compaction in humans, *Int J Cardiol* 145(2):405, 2010.
85. Robinson R: The rex mutants of the domestic cat, *Genetica* 42:466, 1971.
86. Robinson R: The Canadian hairless of Sphinx cat, *J Hered* 64:47, 1973.
87. Robinson R: Expressivity of the Manx gene in cats, *J Hered* 84:170, 1993.
88. Sampedrano C, Chetboul V, Mary J et al: Prospective echocardiographic and tissue Doppler imaging screening of a population of Maine Coon cats tested for the A31P mutation in the myosin-binding protein C gene: a specific analysis of the heterozygous status, *J Vet Intern Med* 23:91, 2009.
89. Schlueter C, Budras K, Ludewig E et al: Brachycephalic feline noses: CT and anatomical study of the relationship between head conformation and the nasolacrimal drainage system, *J Feline Med Surg* 11:891, 2009.
90. Schmidt-Kuntzel A, Eizirik E, O'Brien SJ et al: Tyrosinase and tyrosinase related protein 1 alleles specify domestic cat coat color phenotypes of the albino and brown loci, *J Hered* 96:289, 2005.
91. Somers K, Royals M, Carstea E et al: Mutation analysis of feline Niemann-Pick C1 disease, *Mol Genet Metab* 79:99, 2003.

92. Takanosu M, Takanosu T, Suzuki H et al: Incomplete dominant osteochondrodysplasia in heterozygous Scottish Fold cats, *J Small Anim Pract* 49:197, 2008.
93. Thomson PC, Wilson BJ, Wade CM et al: The utility of estimated breeding values for inherited disorders of dogs, *Vet J* 183:243, 2009.
94. Thuline HC: Male tortoiseshell, chimerism and true hermaphroditism, *J Cat Genet* 4:2, 1964.
95. TICA: The International Cat Association, 2010. http://www.tica.org/. Accessed June 22, 2011.
96. Tsoutsman T, Bagnall R, Semsarian C: Impact of multiple gene mutations in determining the severity of cardiomyopathy and heart failure, *Clin Exp Pharmacol Physiol* 35:1349, 2008.
97. Valayannopoulos V, Nicely H, Harmatz P et al: Mucopolysaccharidosis VI, *Orphanet J Rare Dis* 5:1, 2010.
98. Wess G, Schinner C, Weber K et al: Association of A31P and A74T polymorphisms in the myosin binding protein C3 gene and hypertrophic cardiomyopathy in Maine Coon and other breed cats, *J Vet Intern Med* 24:527, 2010.
99. Wilson TG, Kane F: Congenital deafness in white cats, *Acta Oto-laryngolica* 50:269, 1959.
100. Winand NJ, Edwards M, Pradhan D et al: Deletion of the dystrophin muscle promoter in feline muscular dystrophy, *Neuromuscul Disord* 4:433, 1994.
101. Yogalingam G, Hopwood JJ, Crawley A et al: Mild feline mucopolysaccharidosis type VI. Identification of an N-acetylgalactosamine-4-sulfatase mutation causing instability and increased specific activity, *J Biol Chem* 273:13421, 1998.
102. Yogalingam G, Litjens T, Bielicki J et al: Feline mucopolysaccharidosis type VI. Characterization of recombinant N-acetylgalactosamine 4-sulfatase and identification of a mutation causing the disease, *J Biol Chem* 271:27259, 1996.

SECTION X

POPULATION MEDICINE

Editor: Brenda Griffin

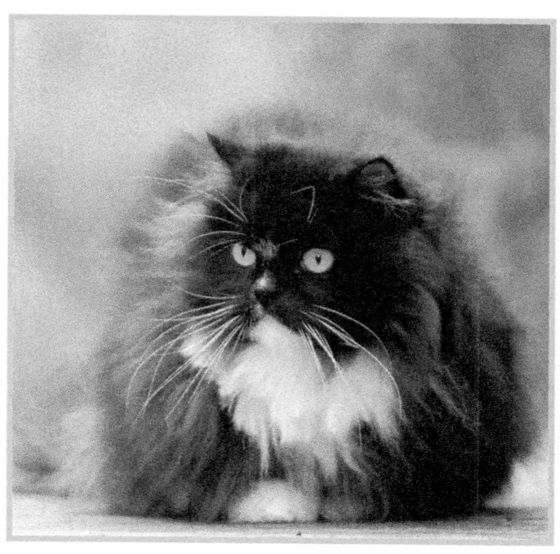

CHAPTER

45

Care and Control of Community Cats

Brenda Griffin

OUTLINE

In addition to the estimated 82 million owned pet cats in the United States,[6] there are an estimated 30 to 60 million free-roaming stray and feral cats.[27,40,48] In fact, these cats may represent as much as 50% of the total cat population in a given community. In addition, they are estimated to produce up to 80% of the kittens born annually in the United States.[27] Despite the lack of exact estimates of their numbers, there is no doubt that millions of these cats exist in communities across the United States, and millions of Americans feed them.[27]

A continuum of lifestyles exists between socialized house cats, free-roaming, previously socialized, or "loosely owned" strays and truly unowned, unsocialized feral cats.[36] Feral cats are "wild" offspring of domestic cats and result from pet owners abandoning and/or failing to control their pets' reproduction.[16] Like wildlife species, when raised without human contact, feral cats remain extremely wary of humans and flee if approached. They generally do not allow handling and must be trapped in order to be presented to a veterinarian for care. In contrast, stray cats are at least somewhat socialized to people and include those cats that may have been previously owned as well as those that are "loosely owned" neighborhood or barn cats.[36] Free-roaming stray and feral cats form colonies surrounding a "home base," which includes a source of food and shelter. Locations with garbage dumpsters, such as housing or shopping complexes, or those with livestock barns, are prime locations in which cat colonies form because they offer a supply of discarded foodstuffs and rodents.[16] Cats typically seek shelter in crawl spaces beneath buildings or other nearby structures (Figure 45-1). Because both stray and feral cats frequently co-exist within the same colonies, the term community cats is often used to refer to all of these outdoor-dwelling cats, regardless of socialization status.

Unlike wildlife species, cats cannot fully fend for themselves in most instances. Unattended, they survive and reproduce, yet frequently suffer from exposure, disease, and trauma. The mortality rate of kittens born outdoors is high, with fewer than 25% typically surviving beyond 4 to 6 months of age.[39,51] However, beyond 6 months of age, the odds of survival are much greater. The life span of free-roaming cats varies depending at least in part on the colony's location. Trauma is the most common cause of death.[39,51] In some cases, these cats become public nuisances, and many are euthanized at animal shelters each year. Because their reproduction frequently goes unchecked, community cats represent not only a result of feline overpopulation, but also a significant source of the problem.

Substantial debate surrounds the appropriate response to the presence of community cats. Scientific reviews of their control and its impact on both the cats themselves

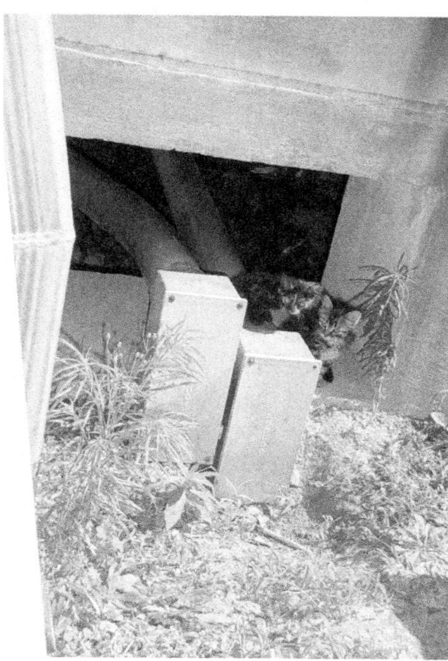

FIGURE 45-1 Three feral kittens observe the world from the safety of a crawl space. Such spaces under buildings are typical locations in which feral cats seek shelter and are popular sites for queens to nest and raise kittens.

as well as the environment have been published.[27,31,40,43] Numerous stakeholders have issued policy statements regarding this issue, representing many different and often polarized opinions.[1,3,5,52] The traditional approach to controlling free-roaming cats has been extermination by trapping and euthanasia. However, large-scale trap and kill programs, which would be necessary for even temporary population control, have not been widely implemented, and even small-scale attempts at trapping and euthanizing cats frequently result in public outcry.

There is little doubt that public sentiment is influential in policy making, and numerous examples exist whereby pressure exerted by the public and animal welfare organizations has been instrumental in stopping euthanasia of cat colonies.[2] In the author's opinion, trapping cats for euthanasia perpetuates the message that cats are disposable. In contrast, the provision of affordable services to neuter free-roaming cats raises awareness that cats require and deserve responsible care and enables people to "do the right thing" when cats take up residence on their property or in their neighborhood.

In addition to preventing reproduction, neutering cats also serves to promote their welfare. Studies have shown that feral cats roam less and have higher body condition scores following neutering.[46,51] In addition, urine marking, fighting, breeding, and roaming are rapidly and dramatically reduced, making these cats less likely to be targeted as public nuisances. Finally, cats in managed colonies are no more likely than pet cats to harbor common infectious and zoonotic diseases.[30,34,50]

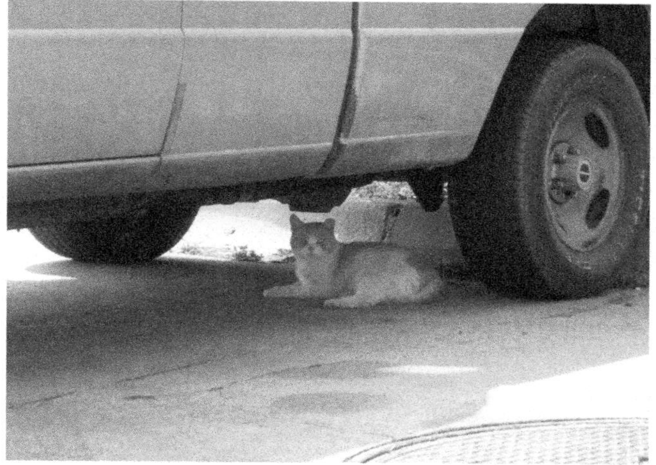

FIGURE 45-2 A feral cat rests under the shade of a parked car. His cropped left ear tip identifies him as a neutered member of a managed colony. This distinctive mark is the universally recognized symbol of a sterilized free-roaming cat.

"Trap-neuter-return" (TNR) is a humane, nonlethal method of managing existing colonies of free-roaming cats and represents a legitimate response to existing colonies of cats with caregivers.[29,38] Cats are trapped, vaccinated, neutered, and then returned to their "home" for release. The tip of the left ear is cropped to identify the cats as having been sterilized. This is the universal symbol for a sterilized free-roaming/feral cat (Figure 45-2). Caregivers take responsibility for feeding and monitoring the health of the cats in the future. TNR may not be appropriate in all circumstances; for example, colonies should not be located in wildlife refuges or where endangered wildlife species are known to reside.

TNR has become an increasingly popular method of managing existing colonies of community cats during the past 2 decades. Neutered cats display fewer "nuisance" behaviors, such as spraying and fighting, and they cannot reproduce. With time, colony size should decrease because of attrition. However, it is crucial to realize that emigration of new cats is always a possibility, and in many cases, a likelihood; thus ongoing vigilance and management are required. Therefore a dedicated caregiver is crucial for long-term cat control, as well as to ensure cat welfare.[16,17,51] TNR has also been purported to be more cost effective than trapping and euthanizing cats.[21] This is because most states require impoundment and holding of cats prior to euthanasia, and private volunteers are more likely to trap cats for surgery versus euthanasia.

Individuals caring for community cats frequently seek veterinary advice and services. The purpose of this chapter is to provide the veterinary clinician with current recommendations for providing care of free-roaming cats during the process of TNR. A general summary of these recommendations is found in Table 45-1.

TABLE 45-1 **General Veterinary Medical Care Protocol for Trap-Neuter-Return of Community Cats**

Procedure	Rationale
Short-term holding prior to surgery (e.g., 12 to 48 hours)	Provides time for acclimation; some cats that were initially reactive and feral-behaving may be determined to be tame
Balanced anesthesia administered by intramuscular injection	Essential to ensure smooth induction and proper analgesia with minimal handling to decrease stress and optimize staff safety
Physical examination, including scanning for a microchip	To identify any physical problems and to help determine if the cat might be owned
Subcutaneous fluid administration for cats that are pregnant, lactating, or dehydrated	Promotes normal hydration and prevention of complications related to dehydration
Ear tipping	Identifies cats as neutered, vaccinated members of a managed colony
Rabies vaccination (3-year product)	Affords protection against an important endemic disease of public health significance
Modified live FVRCP vaccination	Affords cats protection against common and life-threatening infections
Ivermectin 1% solution (0.3 mg/kg subcutaneously)	Treats ear mite infestations and temporarily limits round and hookworm infestations (cost effective at only pennies per dose)
Holding overnight after surgery prior to release	Ensures cat are fully alert and physically coordinated for safe release
Return to original colony site	Cats possess strong homing instincts, and release to a foreign location is not humane unless careful relocation procedures are followed

FVRCP, Feline viral rhinitis–calicivirus–panleukopenia.

SAFE AND HUMANE CAPTURE, HOLDING, AND HANDLING

Because of their lack of socialization, capture and handling is extremely stressful for feral cats. Proper education and equipment are keys to minimizing the feline stress response and keeping caregivers and cats safe. In most instances, cats should be humanely trapped using commercially available live traps (Figure 45-3). For those cats that are elusive, a drop trap is a humane alternative, but generally requires substantial time and patience (Figure 45-4).

Once captured, cats should be held securely in their covered traps. Transferring them to larger enclosures is neither necessary nor recommended for short-term holding (e.g., 2 to 3 days), because it increases the risk of human injury as well as cat escape. Indeed, if provided an opportunity, most cats will successfully escape, and serious injury can occur if individuals must recapture them. In addition, escaped cats can be destructive as they attempt to hide and resist recapture.

Another advantage of keeping cats confined in traps is that the administration of anesthetics is simple and can be done without extensive handling, minimizing stress, and enhancing safety for both cats and personnel. For all of these reasons, feral cats should not be removed from a trap until heavily sedated or anesthetized. Furthermore, at the completion of surgery and before awakening, they can be returned to their traps for recovery. With this system, cats are never handled while conscious, and there are no opportunities for escape or injury. And, importantly, they do not sustain any additional stress from unnecessary handling.

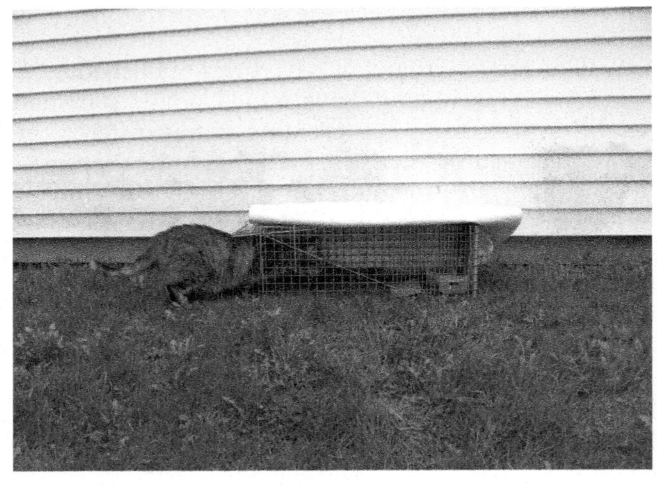

FIGURE 45-3 A cat enters a commercially available humane box trap (Tomahawk Live Trap, Tomahawk, Wis.).

Field Capture

Before trapping, attaching two small bowls to the back corners of each trap is helpful. Plastic bowls work well and can be secured using zip ties (Figure 45-5). Having these in place before trapping makes it possible to safely feed and water cats without opening the trap once they are captured. Water can be poured into the bowl from a watering can with a long spout, and food can be dropped

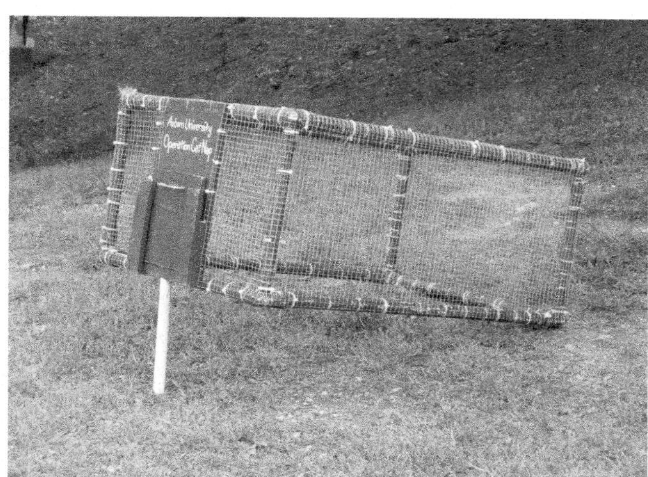

FIGURE 45-4 A drop trap can be used to humanely capture cats that will not enter a box trap. Strong-smelling food is placed on the ground beneath the trap, and the caregiver waits covertly nearby until the cat takes the bait. From the remote location, the caregiver pulls a string to remove the prop stick, causing the trap to drop, capturing the cat. A transfer door is used to safely transfer the cat from the drop trap into a regular box trap for transport.

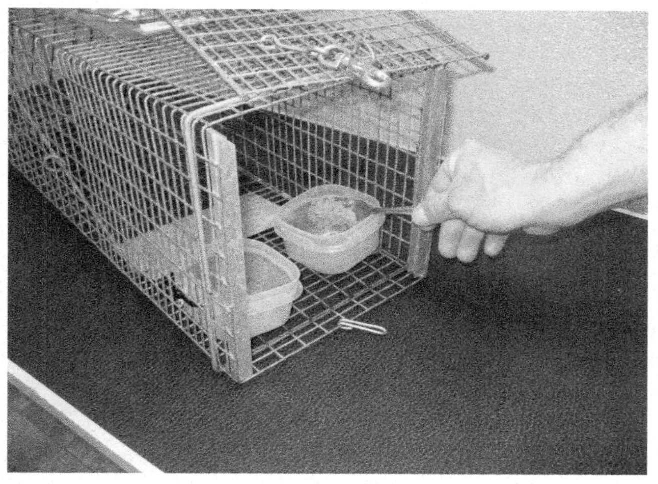

FIGURE 45-5 A trap is outfitted with small plastic bowls prior to use. The bowls are secured in place with zip ties. Canned cat food is placed in one of the bowls to bait the trap.

through the wire into the bowl from a safe distance (Figure 45-6).

Most live traps are activated by a foot plate: As the cat enters the open door of the trap to reach the food bowl at the opposite end, the footplate is depressed, which, in turn, unhooks the trap door, causing it to drop and lock in the closed position (Figure 45-7). Traps should always be covered with towels or other suitable materials: This serves to make them more inviting, increasing the likelihood of a cat entering and becoming trapped (Figure 45-8). More importantly, covering the trap serves to calm the cat, decreasing stress upon capture.

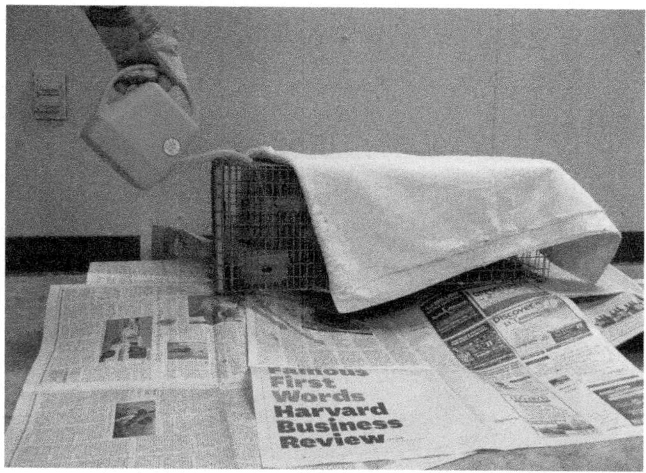

FIGURE 45-6 Proper holding procedures for feral cats. For safety and security, cats remain in their covered traps before and after surgery. Water is poured into the bowl in the trap from a safe distance using a watering can.

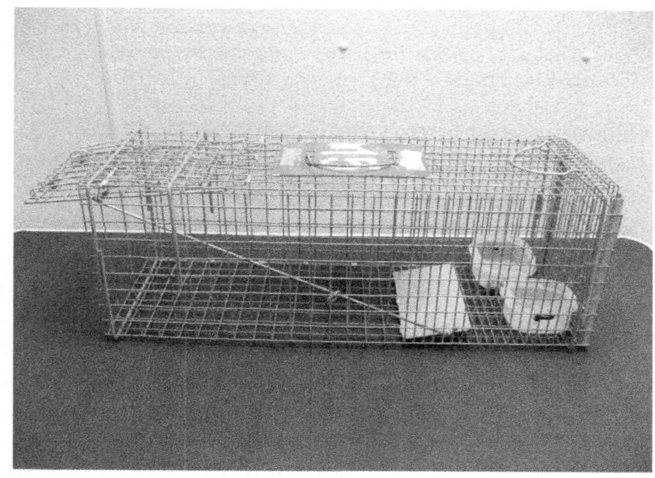

FIGURE 45-7 A commercially available box trap (Tomahawk Live Trap, Tomahawk, Wis.). When a cat steps on the spring-loaded footplate to reach the bait, the trap door will close and lock.

It is not uncommon for cats to initially panic once trapped. They may lunge and claw in their attempts to free themselves. Torn claws, scraped noses, and nosebleeds are common injuries that can occur in the trapping process. Although minor, these can be disturbing to caregivers, particularly if they are unaware of this possibility. Fortunately, most cats settle down physically within a few minutes of capture. However, emotionally they remain stressed, as evidenced by their tense body posture and dilated pupils. Many trapped cats tuck their feet under themselves and try to hide or back into the farthest corner of the trap. Some freeze, appearing nearly catatonic, while others strike out defensively if approached, particularly feral tomcats. Even the tamest house cats that are trapped or otherwise very stressed may exhibit the same behaviors as feral cats.[15]

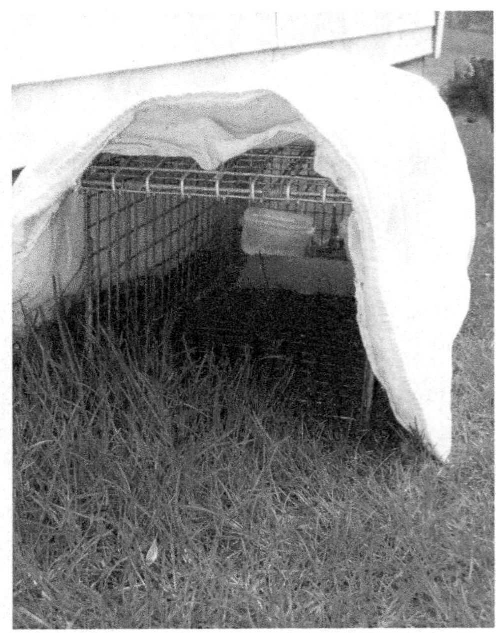

FIGURE 45-8 Covering the trap serves to make it more inviting. In addition, it helps to decrease the stress response by providing cover and security, helping to calm the cat once it is captured.

Clients planning to implement TNR should be instructed to contact people around the area where they intend to trap to explain their intentions. Caregivers should discontinue feeding of cats for 24 to 48 hours prior to trapping to ensure they are hungry enough to enter baited traps. Setting traps as much as 2 days before a surgery appointment is usually the best approach to ensure successful capture. Trapping further in advance is not recommended, because it leads to prolonged holding times, increasing stress. Every attempt should be made to capture all cats in a colony at the initiation of TNR. Whenever possible, trapping should continue until all members of a colony have been captured. When only a few members of the colony are captured at the outset, the remaining members may prove very difficult to capture in subsequent attempts, prolonging the process and complicating successful management.

Clients must be cautioned about the importance of safe handling. Ideally, they should receive rabies pre-exposure vaccination for their own protection. At a minimum, they should be advised that if they are scratched or bitten, they should not release the animal and should immediately contact their physician as well as the local health department or other appropriate agency for advice. Additional client instructions for trapping and holding cats are provided in Box 45-1.

In-Clinic Procedures

Most often, the veterinarians' role in TNR begins with the arrival of a trapped cat at their practice. Caregivers should be required to present cats for surgery in their covered traps. From the time they arrive at the clinic, care should be taken not to place cats within spatial, visual, or auditory range of other species, especially dogs. Traps containing cats should be placed in quiet holding areas until the time of surgery.

Prior to surgery, injectable anesthetic agents should be administered to the cat while it remains in the trap. This is accomplished by quietly but quickly standing the trap on end and using a commercially available "trap divider" to confine the cat. This allows an intramuscular injection to be administered to the cat between the wire bars of the trap (Figure 45-9). Recommendations for injectable anesthetic agents for feral cats are discussed in Chapter 7.

Feral cats should be returned to clean traps following surgery and monitored until they are sternal. A safe heat source, such as warm air or a carefully monitored heat lamp, should be used to ensure adequate body warming during recovery (Figure 45-10). Placing shredded paper in the trap will help to insulate and protect the cats during recovery.

Cats should be hospitalized in their traps overnight. At the veterinarian's discretion, they may be discharged the same day as surgery, but caregivers should be instructed to hold them overnight to allow for a full recovery (e.g., return of normal mental status and motor coordination) prior to being returned to their environments. Additional discharge instructions for caregivers are provided in Box 45-2.

Returning Cats to Their Colonies

It is imperative that caregivers understand the crucial importance of returning cats to their original home sites. Release of cats to other areas, even those that may seem protected, such as a private barn site, should only be done as a last resort and with careful consideration and planning (see Relocation of Cats). Releasing a cat in an unfamiliar area is analogous to a person being lost without a map or other method of communication to get home. Originally, the phrase "trap-neuter-*release*" was commonly used; however, the name quickly changed to "trap-neuter-*return*" to reflect the importance of returning a cat to its home colony. Emphasizing that the "R" stands for "return" remains important today, because well-meaning caregivers often consider release of cats in novel locations, not understanding the implications of their actions. In addition to creating serious welfare issues for cats, random release of cats constitutes abandonment and is illegal.

In Case of Escapes

When care is taken to adhere to the practices for handling and holding feral cats as described, escapes should not occur. However, accidents do happen and being

BOX 45-1

Trapping and Holding Instructions for Clients

Before Trapping

- Establish a routine of feeding the cats at the same time and location each day. Cats that are accustomed to a routine will be easier to capture. If possible, placing traps in the area before trapping begins will allow the cats to acclimate to their presence and facilitate trapping. The door of each trap can be secured in an open position and food placed in the trap so that the cats learn to go inside to eat.
- Try to determine the number of cats present and make plans to trap them all. The best trapping success always occurs during the first trapping session. If only a few members of the group are captured, subsequent attempts will be more difficult because cats quickly become savvy to the process.
- Prepare a warm, sheltered area (such as a garage) for holding the cats before surgery. Prepare an area to place the traps by spreading newspapers or disposable tarps on the floor to catch urine, stool, and food that will fall from the trap. Bricks or other items can be used to elevate the traps off the ground so that the cats are not sitting in their waste.
- Prepare to transport the cats by putting a plastic liner in the vehicle that will be used. This will prevent urine damage in the vehicle while traveling to and from the trap site and veterinary clinic.
- Contact neighbors around the area in which trapping will take place. Inform them of the plans and ask them not to feed the cats during this time. In addition, ask that they keep their pet cats indoors during the planned trapping period.
- Stop feeding the cats 1 to 2 days before beginning to trap: Hungry cats are much easier to capture.

Setting the Traps

- Begin trapping at the established feeding area up to two nights before the surgery appointment.
- Weather conditions should dictate when it is safe to trap. Trapping should not be done in temperature extremes. In hot weather, trapping is best accomplished in the evening and early morning hours. In very cold climates, trapping in the daylight hours when it is warmer is generally preferred.
- Traps should be set in secure, level areas scattered around the feeding area. Cats are unlikely to enter a trap if it is unsteady. If the traps are set in a public area, it is best to place them such that they are hidden from view to avoid attracting unnecessary attention.
- Whenever possible, set at least as many traps as there are cats to maximize the odds of trapping the entire colony at once.
- The traps should be baited with smelly food such as canned mackerel or the cat food that the cats are accustomed to eating. Most traps have a back door that must be securely latched to prevent escapes and ensure safety during transport of captured animals. Ensuring that this latch is secured is a crucial step.
- Each trap should be covered with a large towel or other suitable material when it is set. The cover helps to keep the cat calm in the trap. Cats should remain covered in the trap throughout transporting and holding procedures. For safety, wear protective gloves when carrying any animal in a trap.
- If trapping at multiple colony sites, traps should be carefully labeled in order to ensure that cats are not accidentally returned to the wrong colony site following surgery.
- Traps should be checked frequently. If a previously neutered cat or a wild animal (such as an opossum) is captured, carefully open the back door of the trap, stand back at a safe distance, and allow the animal to leave.

Holding Procedures

- Cats should be held in their traps before and after surgery. Opening the traps or transferring cats to other enclosures poses a safety risk and must be strictly avoided.
- Place the traps in the prepared area and keep them covered. If it is more than 12 hours before the surgery appointment, drop a small amount of cat food through the top of the trap into the food bowl and pour a small amount of water into the other bowl from a safe distance outside of the trap. If the surgery appointment is less than 12 hours away, only water should be given.
- Check the cats periodically and change dirty newspapers beneath the traps as needed. The cats will likely stay relatively calm and quiet as long as the traps are covered. Be sure the holding area remains at a comfortable temperature with adequate air ventilation.

prepared with appropriate equipment and knowledge is essential in order to reduce the chances of injury or damage should a cat escape and need to be contained. When working with cats, exit doors should always remain securely closed to prevent outdoor escapes. Nets are the safest and most humane tool for capture of a loose cat indoors. Alternatively, it may be possible or even necessary to use a live trap to recapture a loose cat. However, many cats will resist entering a trap once they have been previously captured this way.

When used properly, nets minimize stress, prevent injury of the animal, and ensure staff safety. In contrast,

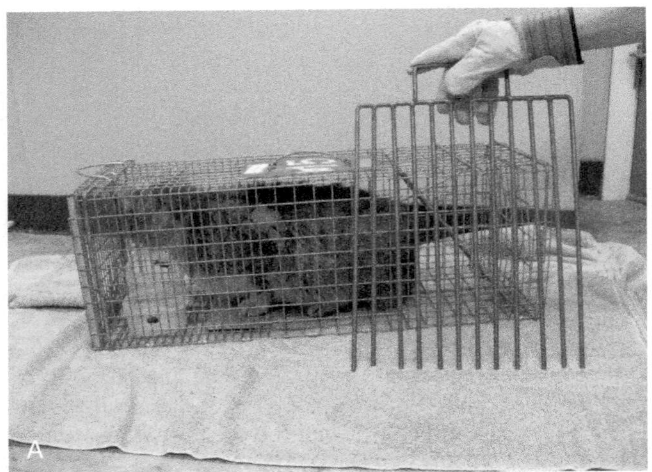

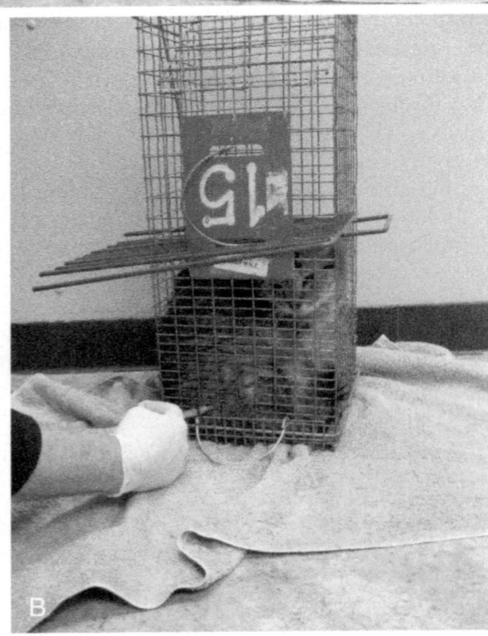

FIGURE 45-9 **A,** A commercially available "trap divider" (Animal Care and Equipment Services [ACES], Boulder, Colo.) is used to humanely restrain a cat in a box trap to facilitate intramuscular injection of an anesthetic agent. **B,** The trap is gently and swiftly turned on one end, and the device is inserted, confining the cat for the injection.

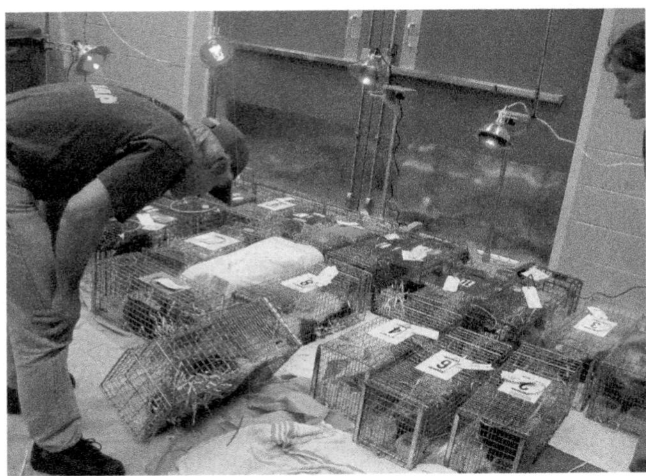

FIGURE 45-10 Carefully monitored heat lamps are used to provide warmth as staff members monitor feral cats during anesthetic recovery at a large-scale TNR clinic.

BOX 45-2

Discharge and Release Instructions for Clients*

- Following surgery, cats should be held in their traps overnight prior to return to their colony site. This is essential for their safety.
- Keep the cats covered in their traps in a quiet, warm area until the next morning. Check on them periodically during this time. Normal behaviors include sleeping, head bobbing, and wobbly movements.
- Some mild oozing of blood from the cropped ear tip may occur, but is not cause for concern unless it continues the day following surgery.
- There should be no bleeding from the spay or neuter surgery site.
- The morning following surgery, cats should be fed and watered. To feed or water the cats, do not open the traps. Water should be poured into the bowl and food dropped through the wire into the bowl from a safe distance.
- If the cats are fully alert the next day, they can be released at the same location from which they were trapped. To release the cat, point the back of the trap away from danger, such as a busy street. Take off the cover, unlock the back door, and lift the door away from the trap. Stand back and patiently and wait for the cat to leave—most run away immediately.

*Instructions for the provision of emergency care during the postoperative period should also be provided, as with any surgery patient.

the use of control poles to capture cats poses significant risk of injury to the animal and exacerbates stress. For these reasons, their use is considered inhumane and must be strictly avoided.[19,22]

Several commercially available cat nets are available. In some cases, the design allows the user to close the opening of the net using a special sliding mechanism on the handle (Figure 45-11). This type of net (often called a cage net) is designed for use when a cat is enclosed in a cage or other confined space. Other nets have a flexible rim that will allow the operator to press the opening of the net flat against the floor without placing the handle on the floor, as is required when using a net with a rigid rim. Such nets are more useful for capture in an open space. Although less sophisticated, fishing nets can also be used to humanely capture cats. In this case, the net should be placed over the cat and the rim held firmly against the floor. As the cat backs away, he will step over the rim of the net. The net can then be lifted and the weight of the cat will effectively close the opening, securing the cat and preventing escape (Figure 45-12). Conversely, leaving the net open at the top with the cat hanging in the bottom will likely result in a second escape and is not safe for the cat or handler (Figure 45-13).

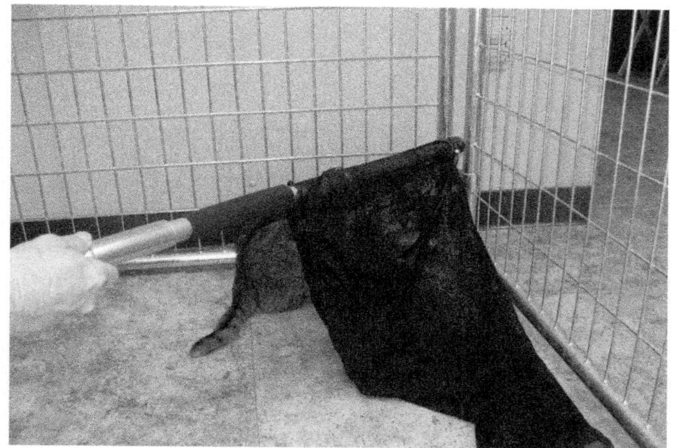

FIGURE 45-11 A Freeman cage net (Animal Care and Equipment Services [ACES], Boulder, Colo.) is used to humanely capture a cat in an enclosure. The design of the net allows the user to close it using a special sliding mechanism on the handle.

Once a cat is securely netted, chemical restraint may be administered through the netting. Covering the cat with a thick towel or blanket will aid in safe and humane restraint while an injectable anesthetic is administered. Once the cat is immobilized, it can be removed from the net. Alternatively, the cat can be transferred in the net to an enclosure without the use of sedatives. Returning a netted cat to a trap can be very tricky. Instead, the cat can be released into a larger cage containing a commercially available cat den. Cat dens are designed as secure hiding boxes for feral or reactive cats. They can be securely closed from a safe distance (Figure 45-14) and used to transport the cat. Alternatively, they have a guillotine door on one end that allows for safe transfer to a trap or other squeeze cage as needed (Figure 45-15).

Although it is best to use a net or live trap to capture an escaped cat, in some instances this may not be feasible. It may be physically impossible, for example, to retrieve a cat that has escaped into a narrow space using a net. In this case, commercially available cat tongs can be used to grasp and retrieve the cat (Figure 45-16). However, care must be taken to prevent the use of

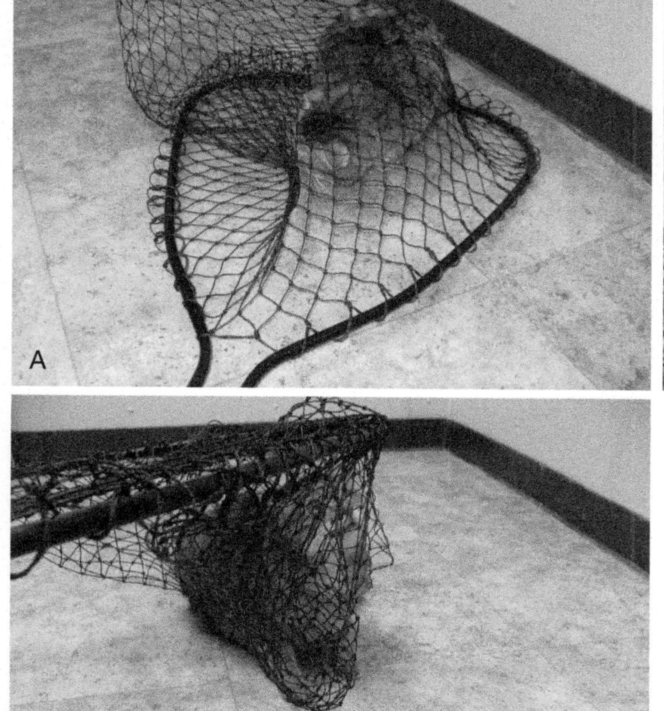

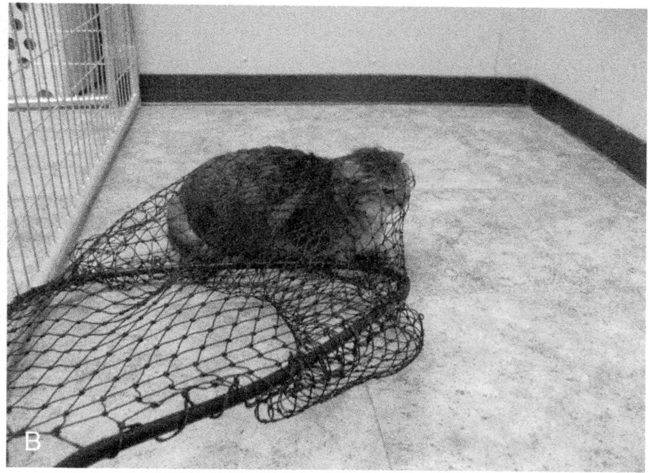

FIGURE 45-12 A rigid fishing net is used to capture a cat in an open space. **A,** The net is placed over the cat. **B,** As the handler moves closer, the cat backs away, stepping over the rim of the net. **C,** The handler lifts the net, safely entrapping the cat.

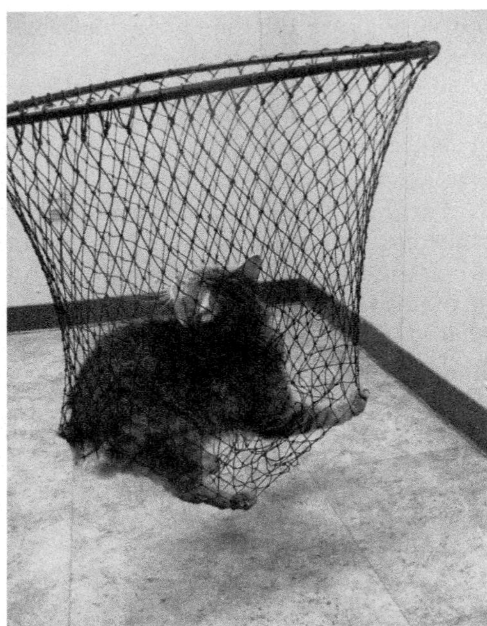

FIGURE 45-13 Improper use of a net. The top of the net is open as the cat hangs in the bottom. As he struggles to escape, there is risk of injury for both the cat and handler.

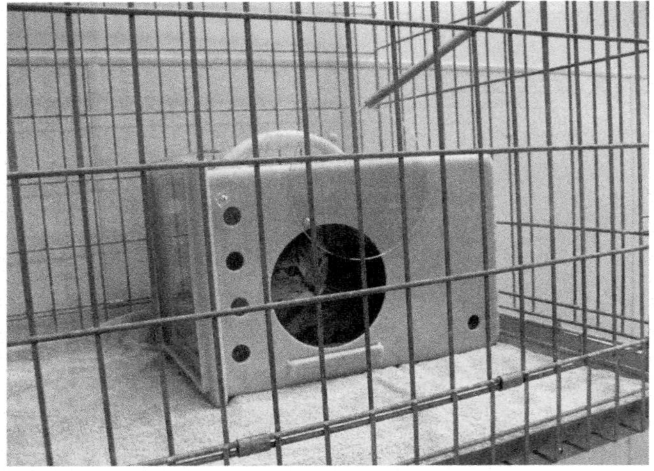

FIGURE 45-14 A commercially available feral cat den (Animal Care and Equipment Services [ACES], Boulder, Colo.) serves as a secure hiding place for a cat. The circular door can be closed from a safe and nonthreatening distance while the cage is spot cleaned as needed. The cat can also be securely transported in the den.

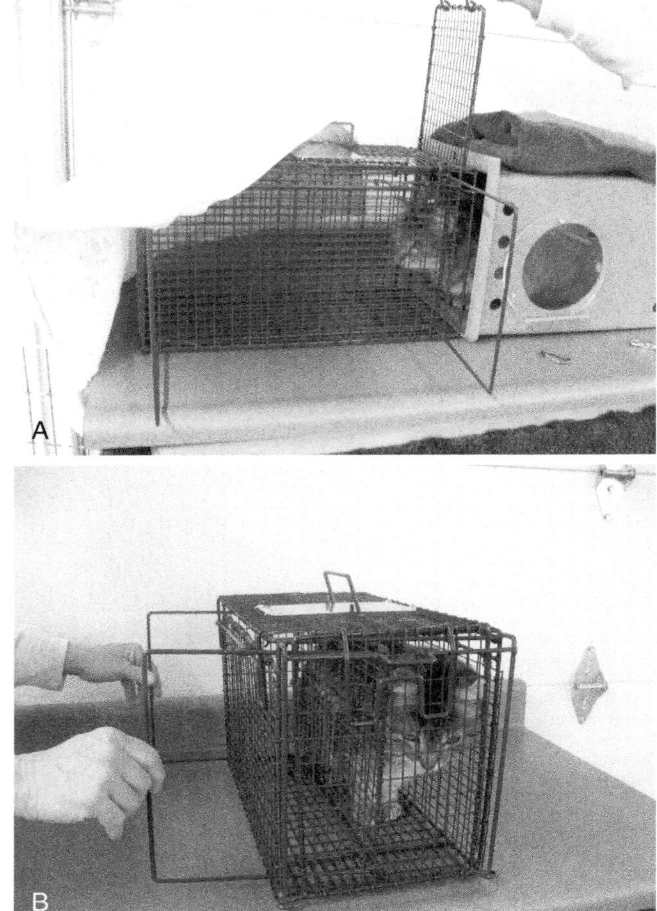

FIGURE 45-15 **A** and **B,** By raising and lowering the guillotine doors, a cat is safely and humanely transferred from a feral cat den to a squeeze cage for restraint.

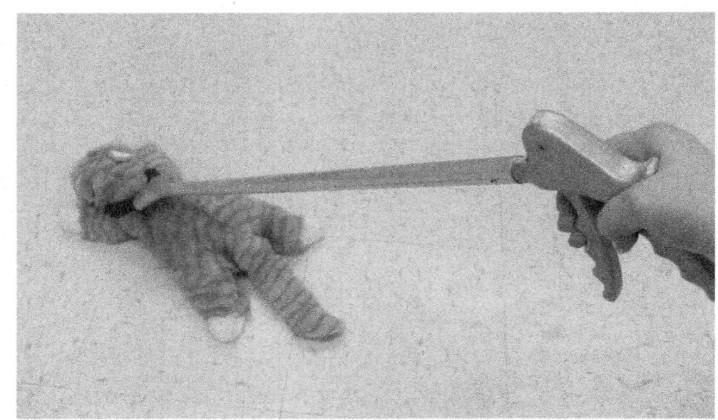

FIGURE 45-16 Commercially available cat tongs (Animal Care and Equipment Services [ACES], Boulder, Colo.) can be used to capture a cat when a net is not feasible. The cat should be grasped and transferred into a cage or other enclosure as quickly as possible, taking care to avoid injury and unnecessary stress.

unnecessary force when using cat tongs in order to prevent injury.

DIFFERENTIATING TRULY FERAL CATS FROM REACTIVE TAME CATS

It is important to remember that cats that are trapped and feral-behaving are not necessarily feral. In reality, it can be challenging to differentiate truly feral cats from those that are tame but very frightened and reactive.[15] Indeed, once highly stressed or provoked, cats frequently remain reactive for a prolonged time and may become more reactive if they are stimulated again before they have been allowed a period of time to cool down.[7] For this reason, special care should be taken to provide a calm and quiet environment during the time in which cats are being held awaiting surgery. Certainly, it is prudent to determine the cat's true level of sociability and tractability whenever possible. This information can help caregivers provide the best possible care for cats. Tame cats may be lost, and efforts to reunify them with owners may be warranted. Careful scanning for a microchip should be performed and other measures, such as posting signs in the area where the cat was trapped, should be taken to locate an owner. If an owner is not located, tame cats may be placed in homes rather than returned to their colony. If reunification and adoption efforts are not successful, the best option may be to return the cat to the colony as long as ongoing care will be provided by a caregiver. Relinquishment to an animal shelter may not be in the cat's best interests because approximately 70% of cats entering shelters in the United States are euthanized.[4] If the cat appears to be well adapted to its outdoor life and will receive ongoing care, return is appropriate regardless of socialization status.

In order to increase the odds of determining their true socialization status, trapped cats should be allowed "chill out time" to acclimate—preferably at least overnight. Fearful cats, whether feral or tame, may resort to overt aggressive behavior or may "teeter on the edge" of defensive aggression when stressed. Given time, some tame cats will relax. Caregivers can readily recognize these cats, because they will usually stand in the trap, rubbing, mewing, pawing, and chirping as they attempt to solicit attention. However, not all tame cats will relax in a short period of time; some remain reactive and fractious for prolonged periods. Caregivers should be cautioned that even when cats do not exhibit outward aggression in the trap and appear merely "shy" or "nervous," it is not safe to open the trap or to attempt to touch the cat. These are common behaviors for both fractious and feral cats, and opening the trap will likely result in escape or alternatively, defensive aggression.

In addition to behavior, certain physical characteristics may be helpful to distinguish feral cats from those that are tame but behaviorally reactive. When cats are not suspected to be feral, based on their physical characteristics, it may be desirable to allow a longer period for acclimation to see if they become less reactive and "show their true colors." Although it is not often possible to determine a cat's true status based on physical features alone, careful visual inspection of the cat in the trap may prove helpful. The following features should be noted:

- *Ear tip:* Removal of the tip of one of the ears is the universal symbol for a sterilized free-roaming cat. The presence of an ear tip alone should not be used as a singular designation for feral; the ear tip only truly means that the cat has been spayed or neutered. It likely signifies that the cat is a part of a managed colony. Caution must be taken not to mistake frostbite of the ear for a tipped ear.
- *Reproductive status:* Unless they are ear tipped, feral cats should be assumed to be reproductively intact. Females may be pregnant or lactating, especially between April and October (in the northern hemisphere). A large abdomen on a female may indicate pregnancy. If mature, males will have "tomcat urine odor," a wide neck, and well-developed jowls. In addition, they often have scars on their face and ears or torn ear flaps. In contrast, reactive tame cats may be spayed or neutered. Neutered adult toms will lack the typical secondary sex characteristics.
- *General body condition:* Prior to spaying or neutering, feral cats are usually in lean, wiry body condition. In contrast, reactive tame cats may be overweight, particularly if they have been spayed or neutered.
- *Age:* Feral cats are usually young (frequently less than 3 years of age), unless they are part of a managed colony. In contrast, reactive tame cats may be middle-aged or even geriatric. In fact, pampered adult house cats, including those that are geriatric can become very reactive in stressful situations.[12,41] An experienced practitioner may recognize the subtle aging changes that are suggestive of an older cat, especially in the eyes and face.

SPECIAL MEDICAL AND SURGICAL CONSIDERATIONS FOR FREE-ROAMING CATS

Patient Selection and Perioperative Care

Detailed veterinary medical guidelines for spay-neuter programs have been published.[32] Cats undergoing elective surgery should appear to be in reasonably good health and body condition. However, veterinarians must weigh the risks and benefits of spaying and neutering patients with apparent physical abnormalities (e.g., evidence of mild infectious disease or decreased body condition). In the context of feral cats, future opportunities for that animal to receive care may not be available, and the alternative outcome may be release without surgical sterilization or euthanasia. Although some conditions may increase the risk of complications, the benefits of neutering likely outweigh these risks in feral cats. Cats that are pregnant, in estrus, or have pyometra, as well as those that are thin or have mild upper respiratory infection, can be safely spayed or neutered.[32]

Injectable anesthetic protocols with a wide safety margin are preferred, because body weight must be estimated or determined based on an in-trap measurement and because physical examination must be performed following anesthetic induction for feral cats. It is imperative that balanced anesthesia, including proper analgesia, be used. Cats that are pregnant or lactating and those that are dehydrated should receive fluid supplementation. Warmed fluids can be administered subcutaneously postoperatively prior to recovery. Chapter 7 discusses anesthetic recommendations for feral cats.

Surgical Sterilization

Aseptic surgical technique is required, and separate sterile instruments must be used for each patient. Surgeries should be performed by experienced veterinarians, because free-roaming cats are returned to their environments the day following surgery and close follow-up is not generally possible. For this reason, most surgeons prefer to make small incisions and ensure that they are securely closed without the use of skin sutures.

For spaying female patients, some surgeons prefer a flank approach rather than the traditional ventral midline incision (Figure 45-17).[11,24,26,35,53] The flank approach allows caregivers to monitor a cat's incision from a distance and may help to prevent evisceration should dehiscence of the surgical wound occur. The flank approach has also been recommended for lactating queens, to prevent the possibility of incising mammary tissue and causing leakage of milk into the surgical wound. However, it is not recommended for pregnant cats because of the attendant morbidity associated with a large incision in the lateral abdominal wall. If pregnancy or pyometra is discovered upon entering the abdominal cavity, closing the flank incision and using a ventral midline approach is generally advisable.

Another limitation of this approach is that the small size and dorsal location of the incision render thorough abdominal exploration impossible; therefore, if it becomes necessary to locate a dropped pedicle, a ventral midline incision may also be necessary. Increased postoperative pain has also been reported in queens spayed

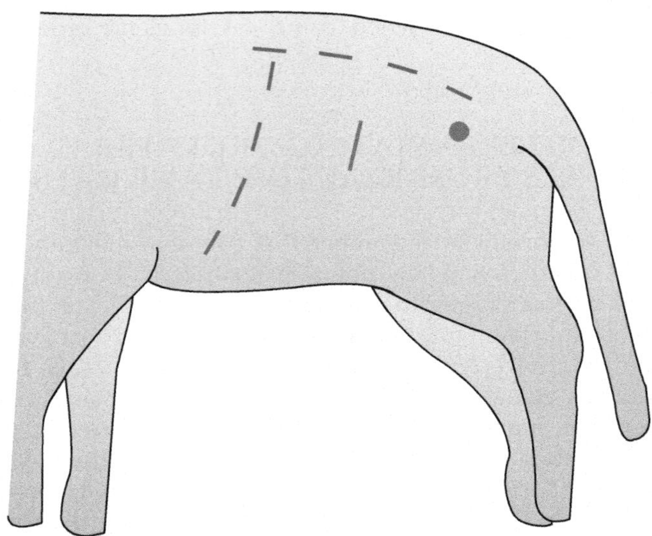

FIGURE 45-17 Location and landmarks of the flank spay incision. The incision should be located midway between the dorsal and ventral midline and approximately 3 cm cranial to the greater trochanter, or 3 to 4 cm caudal to the last rib.

by a flank approach compared with those spayed using a ventral midline approach.[8,20] Depending on the surgeon's preference, the flank approach can be performed with the patient in either right or left lateral recumbency. Box 45-3 describes the procedure.

Ear Tipping for Identification

As previously discussed, removal of the tip of one of the ears (or pinna) is the accepted global standard for marking or identifying a neutered free-roaming community cat. Alley Cat Allies (a national humane organization that serves as a resource on feral cats) recommends removal of the left ear tip, and this standard is widely used. However, some organizations identify cats by removing the right ear tip or by removing the tip on one side or the other, depending on the sex of the cat. Whichever ear is selected for tipping, it is best to be consistent with the standard in your community.[18]

Ear tipping is performed to clearly and permanently visually identify neutered, vaccinated cats that are being humanely managed by TNR. It is often impossible to get close enough to a feral cat to see a subtle mark or tattoo; thus such methods of identification are not useful because they are frequently ineffective. Similarly, other visual means of identifying cats have not been effective. Collars are impractical, because young cats will continue to grow, and collars are frequently lost with time. Ear tags and bands are also not useful, because they may become infected or be torn out. Microchips are not visible and even if a cat is trapped, proper scanning cannot be performed without removing the cat from the trap because of interference from the metal bars.

BOX 45-3

Lateral Flank Spay Technique

- Patient preparation: Shave and prepare the skin beginning at the last rib and extending caudally to the greater trochanter, dorsally to the vertebral transverse processes, and ventrally to the midline.
- Positioning: Place the cat in right or left lateral recumbency, according to the surgeon's preference. A small rolled-up towel may be placed under the lateral lumbar area to remove the concavity of the flank, improving visualization.
- Incision location: Midway between the dorsal and the ventral midline and approximately 3 cm cranial to the greater trochanter, or 3 to 4 cm caudal to the last rib (see Figure 45-17).
- Incision length and orientation: Approximately 1.5 to 2 cm in length—vertical, horizontal, or oblique.
- Entering the abdomen: After making the skin incision, grasp the body wall with thumb forceps and bluntly separate the fibers of the external abdominal oblique, internal abdominal oblique, and transversus abdominus muscles to enter the abdomen. If the left lateral approach is used, special care should be taken to elevate the body wall while separating the muscle layers to avoid trauma to the spleen beneath the incision. Tagging the body wall with a suture will ensure that it can be readily located for closure.
- Locating the uterine horn and ovary: The uterine horn should be readily visible and can be gently withdrawn from the abdomen and retracted to identify the ovary. The remainder of the procedure is performed as in the standard ventral midline approach.
- Closure: The body wall is closed with one or two cruciate mattress sutures passed through all three muscle layers; the subcutaneous and intradermal layers are closed according to the surgeon's preference.

When cats are ear tipped, animal control officers, shelter workers, and caregivers can easily and reliably identify cats that are graduates of a TNR program.[18] This is important to ensure that all cats in a colony are humanely managed and to prevent shelter euthanasia of feral cats that are part of managed colonies. Ear tipping should be performed even in colonies of cats with dedicated caregivers who believe they "know" all of the cats in their colony by sight, because it is very common for several cats in a colony to possess similar coat colors and patterns, making it difficult, if not impossible, to distinguish which cats have already been trapped and neutered. It is very important that ears be tipped rather than notched, because notching may occur as the result of fighting, especially in tomcats, and may be mistaken as a sign of previous TNR (Figure 45-18, *A* to *C*).

Ear tipping is an antiseptic procedure rather than an aseptic one. It should be performed under clean surgical conditions. Separate sterile scissors and hemostats should be used for each cat. Clean exam gloves or sterile surgical gloves should be worn. Hair removal or shaving of the pinna is unnecessary and is not recommended to avoid abrasion of the tender skin of the earflap. Antiseptic solution, such as chlorhexidine or Betadine, may be used to gently swab both sides of the pinna. Care should be taken to avoid introducing moisture into the ear canal, which could predispose the cat to otitis externa. The distal tip of the pinna may be removed using sharp dissection or, if available, electrocautery or laser, taking precautions not to induce thermal damage. Most veterinarians perform the procedure using a pair of hemostatic forceps and scissors (Figure 45-19). Scissors are preferred rather than a scalpel blade, because their crushing action aids in hemostasis. Straight scissors and straight hemostats should be used to crop the ear in a straight line. This is very important to ensure the desired visual effect: The ear should have a distinct straight edge that is easy to recognize from a distance. Box 45-4 describes the procedure for ear tipping using straight hemostat and straight scissors. Healing is rapid and complications are rare. This procedure is humane and represents a potentially life-saving permanent form of identification for community cats.[18]

Vaccination

Rabies is a core vaccination for all cats and is an absolute necessity for community cats. Rabies is endemic throughout the mainland United States, and vaccination is the most effective method of control. For this reason, all cats should be vaccinated against rabies virus using an approved 3-year vaccine at the time of surgery.[44] In addition, the administration of a modified live feline viral rhinitis–calicivirus–parvovirus (FVRCP) vaccine is also recommended. In particular, immunity against panleukopenia is especially important for cats, because of the widespread nature and severity of this disease.

Historically, scientists have debated both the effectiveness of vaccines given at the time of surgery and whether or not a single vaccination alone can confer clinically significant immunity. Recent studies have investigated these concerns. In one study of 61 cats undergoing TNR, cats were vaccinated against feline panleukopenia virus, feline herpes virus, feline calicivirus, and rabies virus at the time of surgery.[13] Antiviral antibody titers were measured at the time of surgery and again approximately 10 weeks later. The results of this study demonstrated that feral cats had a robust serologic response following vaccination at the time of neutering. The authors concluded that incorporation of vaccination into TNR programs is likely to protect the health of individual cats and possibly reduce the disease burden

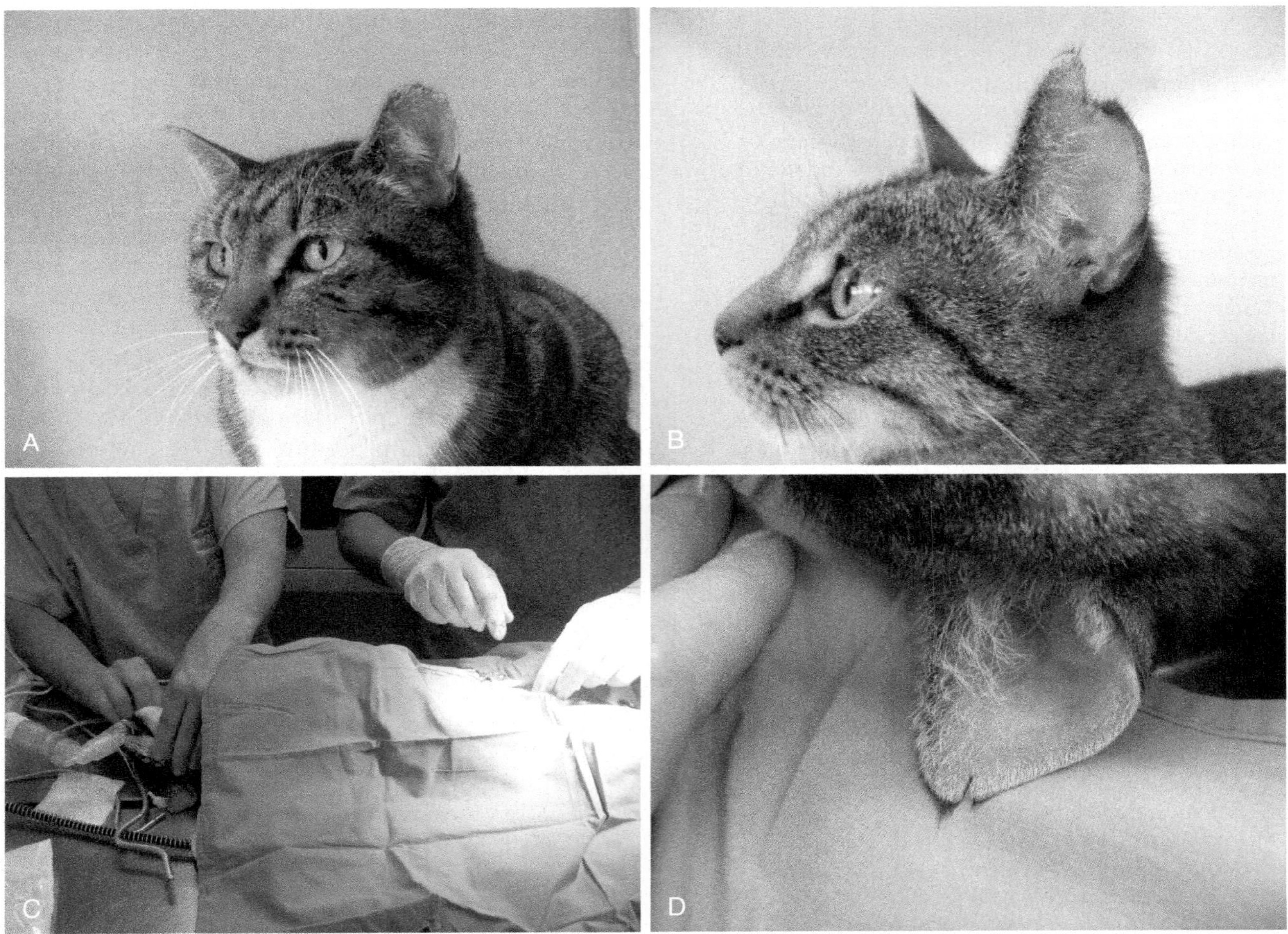

FIGURE 45-18 **A,** Correct appearance of a tipped ear. **B,** It is very important that ears be tipped rather than notched. This is because notching commonly occurs as the result of fighting or other injury, and may be mistaken as a sign of previous neutering. **C,** A female cat is anesthetized for ovariohysterectomy, but exploratory surgery revealed she is already spayed. **D,** Note the small ear notch, which unfortunately was not recognized as an identifying mark of a neutered cat, because it does not adhere to the universal standard.

in the community. Several other independent studies support these findings.[23,37,42]

Although the exact duration is unknown, immunity against rabies and panleukopenia following a single vaccination may persist for years.[14,44,49] Considering the relatively low medical risk and financial cost of vaccination compared with the potential benefits for feline health, community cats undergoing TNR should always be vaccinated against these important feline diseases. Periodically retrapping cats for revaccination is ideal, although it may prove challenging to recapture cats.

Feline Leukemia Virus and Feline Immunodeficiency Virus Testing

A common question regarding care of free-roaming cats is whether or not they should be routinely tested for feline leukemia virus (FeLV) and feline immunodeficiency virus (FIV). The American Association of Feline Practitioners recommends testing all cats for FeLV and FIV and confirming positive test results.[28] It is difficult, if not impossible, however, to apply these guidelines intended for pet cats to feral cats. When deciding whether or not to test feral cats, one must consider that based on surveys of thousands of free-roaming and feral cats, the incidence of these diseases is very low (e.g., less than 2% in healthy cats) based on screening tests.[30] In addition, community cats are no more likely to test positive than owned pet cats. When cats test positive on screening tests, confirmatory testing requires substantial time and monetary investment and is not generally feasible when cats need to be returned to their colony sites. Furthermore, one should keep in mind that neutering greatly reduces transmission of these viruses by decreasing fighting and preventing kitten births. Finally, one should consider that testing is generally expensive and that for successful cat control, the bulk of financial resources must be used to sterilize as many cats as possible. Although testing all cats for FeLV and FIV may be ideal, considering the cost of testing, the disease incidence, and

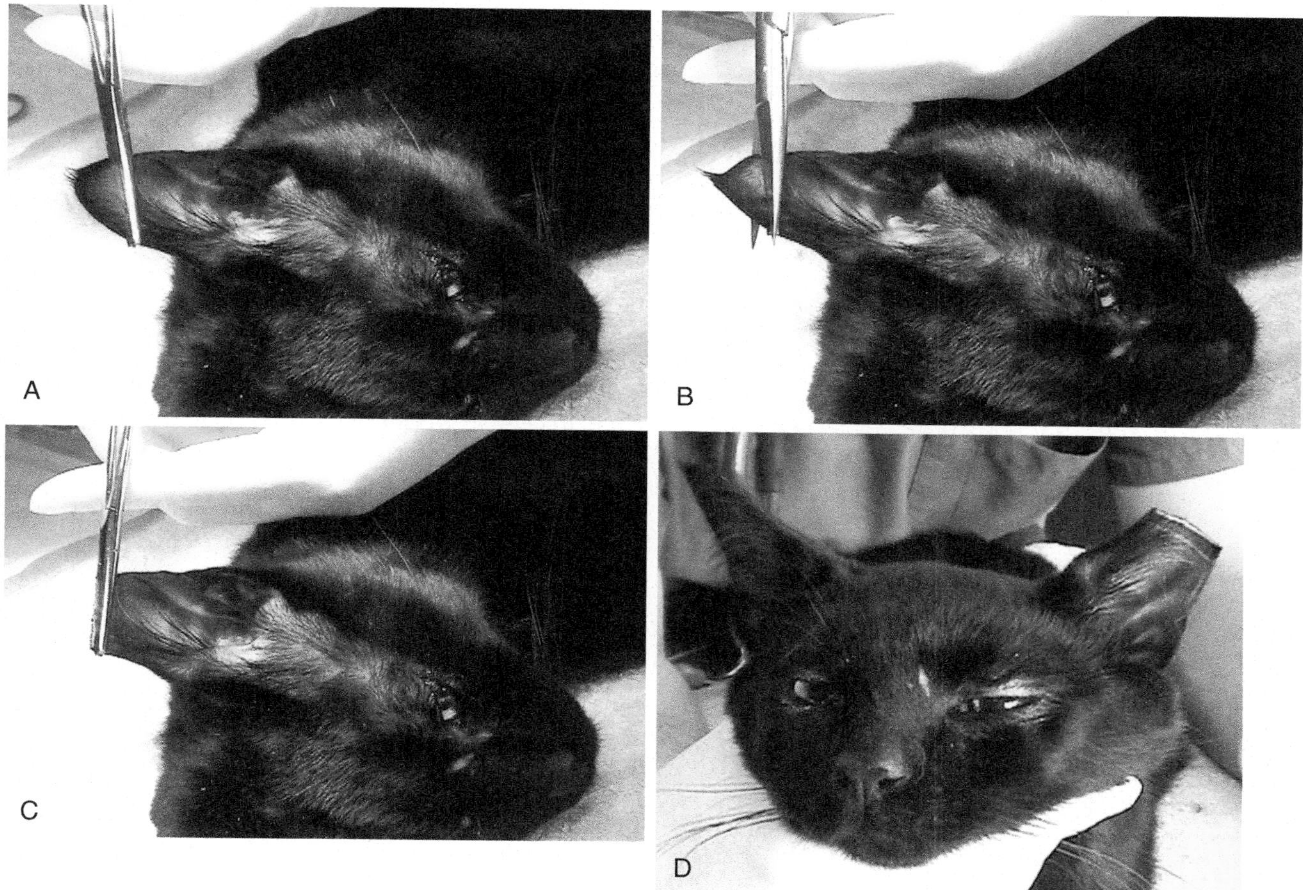

FIGURE 45-19 Ear tipping procedure. **A,** A straight hemostat is placed across the left pinna perpendicular to its long axis, exposing approximately 1.3 cm (0.5 inches) of the ear tip. **B,** Scissors are used to remove the ear tip by cutting over the top of the hemostat in a straight line. **C,** The hemostat is left in place until after surgical neutering to allow adequate time for hemostasis of the pinna to occur. **D,** Proper appearance of the ear following removal of the hemostat. Note the distinctive straight edge that is easily recognizable. *(Courtesy Brenda Griffin.)*

the effects of neutering on transmission, this approach is often not a feasible practice when working with community cats.[25,28]

Testing is recommended, however, when cats appear unthrifty at the time of presentation for TNR. Sick cats are more likely to test positive than apparently healthy cats. In addition, studies indicate that risk factors for infection include contact with other cats and living outdoors. In particular, intact adult tomcats are often at highest risk.[30] For these reasons, positive test results have a higher predictive value in community cats that appear to be in poor health and can be used to help guide decisions for return or euthanasia in the context of TNR programs. Tame cats that are identified as candidates for adoption should also be tested, preferably prior to making substantial investments in their care, because it is often very difficult to place cats in homes. If testing is not performed prior to adoption, adopters should be advised to have their new pet tested and kept separate from other cats prior to doing so.

Parasite Control

Both endoparasite and ectoparasite infestations occur frequently in community cats—fleas, ear mites, and roundworms are particularly common culprits.[17] To be successful for long-term control, repeated antiparasitical treatments are generally required, especially in the context of outdoor multicat environments where the risk of re-infestation is high. For these reasons, a single antiparasitical treatment at the time of TNR may be of limited or even questionable benefit in most cases. However, in the author's opinion, treatment may be of particular benefit to some cats, especially unthrifty juveniles, because even temporary reduction in parasite burdens may provide significant support in these maturing cats.

When considering products for use in unsocialized cats, selection should be limited to injectable and topical products to ensure safe and reliable administration. Imidacloprid/moxidectin (Advantage Multi, Bayer Animal Health, Shawnee Mission, Kans.) is an excellent

BOX 45-4

Procedure for Ear Tipping Using a Straight Hemostat and Straight Scissors (See Figure 45-19)

- Ear tipping is a quick and simple procedure. It should be performed after the cat has been anesthetized and reached a surgical plane of general anesthesia and prior to surgical sterilization. This will ensure adequate time for hemostasis to occur prior to recovery.
- The procedure is performed by placing a sterile straight hemostat across the designated pinna, exposing approximately 1.3 cm (0.5 inches) of the ear tip. The amount of the ear tip removed may be more or less depending on the size of the cat. Proportionately, approximately one third of the distal pinna is removed.
- Care must be taken to place the clamp perpendicular to the long axis of the pinna. This is necessary to ensure the desired visual effect—an easily recognizable, straight, cropped ear tip.
- Sterile scissors are used to cut the tip off, leaving the hemostat on the ear. The hemostat should remain in place until the cat is in recovery and is removed just prior to returning the cat to the trap.
- Some oozing of blood from the ear tip site may occur during recovery especially is the cat rubs or bumps the freshly clotted tissue against the trap.
- Gluing or suturing the ear is neither necessary nor recommended.
- Profuse, excessive, or prolonged bleeding is abnormal.
- Proper placement of the hemostat on the ear tip is critical for proper healing and appearance of the ear.
  - If the clamp is placed too high, the ear tip will be difficult to recognize from a distance.
  - If the clamp is placed too low, the skin may retract, exposing the ear cartilage, which may prolong healing and predispose to an incision site infection.
  - If the clamp is placed at an angle, the pinna will appear pointed from a distance and may be difficult to recognize as a tipped ear.
  - The use of curved hemostats and/or curved scissors should be avoided. If the ear tip remains curved, it may be difficult to recognize as a tipped ear from a distance.
- In very cold climates, mild frostbite of the ear tips is common and may be unilateral or bilateral. Frostbitten ear tips may appear to be cropped but often have a thickened, irregular border. However, it is often difficult to distinguish a frostbitten pinna from a tipped pinna, especially from a distance. In these climates, some programs apply green tattoo ink to the skin margins at the ear tip site to aid in identification.

choice for an effective single broad-spectrum treatment, because it can be administered topically, and a single dose is effective against fleas, roundworms, hookworms, and ear mites. Because of the cost associated with this and similar topical products, it may not be feasible to treat all cats. If flea treatment is desired, the author recommends topical treatment with fipronil (Frontline, Merial, Duluth, Ga.) as a spray or top spot. In particular, the spray is very cost effective. It is safe for use in cats of all ages, including pregnant and nursing mothers. In addition, fipronil also has activity against ear mites, *Cheyetiella* spp., chewing lice, and ticks.[9,45] Because it costs only pennies per dose, the author routinely administers injectable ivermectin to all cats at the time of TNR. A single subcutaneous injection of 1% ivermectin solution at a dosage of 0.3 mg/kg is highly effective against ear mites and also temporarily reduces roundworm and hookworm burdens.

PREGNANT AND LACTATING CATS

It is common to capture pregnant and lactating cats, particularly in the springtime. Veterinarians should discuss recommendations for these cats with caregivers before they begin trapping. In the author's experience, pregnant cats that are captured should be spayed, because it is the most humane course of action. This is for several reasons. First, delivering and raising kittens outdoors is stressful for both the mother and kittens. The mortality rate of kittens is high; often, more than 75% die within the first several weeks of life.[39,51] Secondly, pregnant queens frequently migrate prior to queening in order to find a secure nesting site. This is a familiar scenario to anyone who has discovered a mother and her litter on their property. Even if the queen chooses to deliver her litter nearby, it can be very difficult to locate her nest. Furthermore, if she perceives any threat from observation or other disturbance, she will likely attempt to move her kittens. This can make it extremely difficult to locate and capture the litter once they are born outdoors.

Some caregivers consider confining pregnant feral cats through delivery of their kittens; however, this is extremely stressful for them and cannot be recommended. Others choose to release pregnant cats that they capture, believing it will be in her best interest to allow her to deliver her kittens. Unfortunately, even if the cat remains in the area, she will likely prove to be difficult to retrap in the future and therefore will continue to reproduce for as long as she survives. Indeed, it is common for cats that have been previously trapped to quickly become "trap savvy" such that they will not enter traps on subsequent occasions.

For all of these reasons, caregivers should be advised that pregnant queens should be spayed. This will prevent unnecessary stress and suffering for the queen and her kittens and will prevent the possibility that she will relocate prior to giving birth. Even for those queens that are in an advanced state of gestation, spaying can be safely and humanely performed. In the author's experience, cats do not commonly experience signs of maternal loss following late-term spaying and quickly adjust to the less stressful lifestyle of a spayed cat.

When a lactating queen is trapped, caregivers should be advised to search for kittens. Even though they may look cute and innocent to caregivers, even small feral kittens can inflict serious injury if proper caution is not taken in their handling and capture. Kittens less than 3 to 4 weeks of age can sometimes be caught without a trap, although they may still be too wild to be easily handled. A thick towel can be used to pick them up, protecting the handler from scratching and biting, until they can be contained in a trap or carrier. Once kittens are coordinated enough to leave the nest (e.g., more than 3 to 4 weeks of age), it is safer and may be easier to trap them. Placing the trapped mother cat next to a baited trap will often facilitate capture of her kittens, because they will be attracted by her presence. Similarly, if small kittens are captured in an area, the mother cat will be attracted by their sound if they are placed near the trap. Obviously, frequent monitoring and common sense must be used to determine how long it is safe to leave trapped cats in an area, depending on such factors as the weather or other threats to their safety. Regardless of whether or not kittens are located, lactating queens should be spayed. Spaying will not interfere with the queen's ability to produce milk and nurse kittens. Efforts should be made to release mother cats as soon as it is deemed safe for her so that she can return to care for her kittens.

SMALL KITTENS

Because of their high mortality rate, if small kittens are captured, the author recommends that they be tamed and placed in homes as pets rather than being returned to their colony sites. If this is not possible, euthanasia may be a more humane option than return considering their poor odds of survival. A study of 70 feral kittens demonstrated that they can become good pets with friendly temperaments and that handling prior to 7 to 8 weeks of age improved socialization success.[33] In many cases, it is still possible to tame kittens up to 3 to 4 months of age; however, beyond this age range, taming is often not possible.

The process of taming involves confinement with daily handling sessions and requires patient and committed caregivers. Feral kittens can be absolute "spitfires," and clients should be counseled to wear gloves and use thick towels during handling sessions. In addition, they should be advised to contact their local health department and to seek medical care in the event of any bite. Despite the risks and time commitment required, many individuals are eager and willing to provide the care necessary to successfully tame these animals.

The taming process may take anywhere from a few days to several weeks to accomplish. In the author's experience, individual kittens, even within the same litter, may vary tremendously in their acceptance of human handling and their rate of progression in the process. Box 45-5 contains the recommended steps for taming feral kittens.

SICK AND INJURED CATS AND THE ROLE OF THE CAREGIVER

Minor physical problems are sometimes discovered once a cat has been anesthetized and a physical examination is performed. In the author's experience, common ailments include abscesses, wounds, tail tip injuries, dental disease, and *Cuterebra* infestation.[17] These can all be successfully treated at the time of surgical sterilization. In contrast, when cats present with signs of serious illness or injury, humane euthanasia should be considered. Although there are exceptions, ongoing treatment cannot typically be safely, reliably, and humanely administered to a feral cat. However, if treatment is attempted, it is imperative to have proper equipment for safe and humane handling and housing. Feral cat dens and squeeze cages are essential for this purpose (Figure 45-20).

In instances where the caregiver has had a long-term relationship with the cat (e.g., the cat has been part of a managed colony for years), the author has witnessed situations where cats accepted care when they were gravely ill despite the fact that they had never before allowed handling of any kind. In these instances, the caregivers found "their" cat in a state of shock (because of trauma or severe infection) and presented them for care. Therapy was initiated, and when the cats regained consciousness they readily accepted handling. Anecdotally, there are numerous stories of this kind because of the fluid nature of cat lifestyles. In the author's experience, cats that have been neutered and returned and are fed on a regular basis, may increasingly affiliate with their caregivers with time. Although they may not allow handling, they will interact from a closer and closer distance with time.

That being said, when cats do not accept handling, the provision of medical care can prove extremely stressful—and is not always in their best interest. In the context of population control efforts, financial resources are best spent by maximizing the number of cats that

BOX 45-5

Taming Feral Kittens

Step 1: Seclusion and Confinement

- Select a quiet room and set up a large pet carrier with a litter box, food, and water bowls and comfortable bedding in which to confine the kittens. Arrange the litter box and bowls so that they are within easy reach for cleaning and refilling.
- Allow the kittens strict "chill out" time to acclimate to their new surroundings without intrusion or disturbance. Check to be sure they are eating and using their litter box but otherwise do not disturb them for 1 to 2 days.

Step 2: Handling and Hand Feeding

- On the second or third day of confinement, begin handling sessions 3 to 4 times daily, or more often if possible. Wear protective gloves and use a towel to pick up each kitten. Start with the one that seems the least reactive and the most likely to accept handling. When one kitten exhibits a stressful response, its behavior may have a negative impact on the responses of the others. Likewise, some kittens may become less reactive as they observe calm and soothing handling of their littermates.
- Be sure to approach the kittens slowly; they will be less likely to react when movements are slow and deliberate. Securely wrap and fold the towel around the kitten's body and limbs, leaving only the head exposed. Holding the kitten so that the head is facing away from the handler will enable it to feel less threatened, making it less likely to struggle or fight to escape. Approaching from the back, carefully attempt to gently touch and rub the top of the kitten's head. Talk in a soothing tone. Put baby food* on a small spatula and hand feed it to the kitten.
- In general, the more often the kittens are handled, the more quickly they will be tamed. Eventually, progress to stroking the kitten's body during handling sessions.

Step 3: Ensuring and Continuing Progress

- Expect to see progress over the next several days. Kittens should begin to relax upon handling and may even begin to greet the caregiver at the front of the carrier. When the kittens are readily accepting handling and greeting caregivers, they can be released in a small room, such as a bathroom. Prior to their release, the room should be "kitten proofed." This should include putting away anything that could be broken or damaged or otherwise be harmful to the kittens, securely blocking off any places into which the kittens could crawl and, in the case of a bathroom, closing the toilet lid. Regular handling and feeding sessions should continue, and the kittens should be encouraged to interact with the handler by using toys such as feathers or wands. Play is a very important part of ensuring social bonding.
- It is not uncommon for one or more kittens in a litter to progress more slowly than the others. They may resist handling and remain frightened, reactive, or aggressive. In this case, solitary confinement can be extremely helpful. Without littermates for social companionship, the kitten will be more willing to interact with a human caregiver. This will greatly facilitate the taming process and can produce dramatic results.

Step 4: Continuing Socialization

- Ensure that the kitten's world does not "get too big, too fast." This is crucial to prevent the development of fear, which could hamper the taming process. If allowed too much room in which to explore too quickly, kittens may become stressed and overwhelmed, ultimately seeking a hiding place. They may be difficult to find and even more difficult to catch or retrieve, which, in turn, further induces stress and can compromise the progress they have made.
- As kittens progress, it is important to introduce different handlers: They need a healthy daily dose of positive attention from different human caregivers and reasonable amounts of exposure to the sights and sounds of household activities to become properly socialized pets.
- If adopted to a new home, new owners must take special care to introduce their new kitten very slowly into the new household. Confinement should be used to ensure the kitten continues to feel secure. Once the kitten is actively seeking to be let out of the carrier or small room, it is usually ready to venture forth.

*Baby food that contains onion powder should not be used because of the potential for toxicity from this ingredient.

can be sterilized rather than providing heroic care for individual cats. Nonetheless, in some cases, the human–animal bond will call for additional measures. Many caregivers are deeply bonded to the cats they care for despite their lack of direct physical contact with them.

HELPING CLIENTS SOLVE CONCERNS RELATED TO COMMUNITY CATS

When concerns arise regarding the presence of cats in managed colonies, clients sometimes reach out to their veterinarian for advice. In the author's experience, one

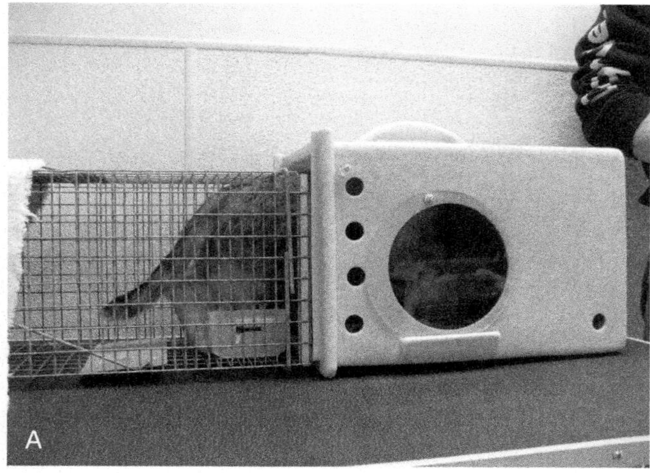

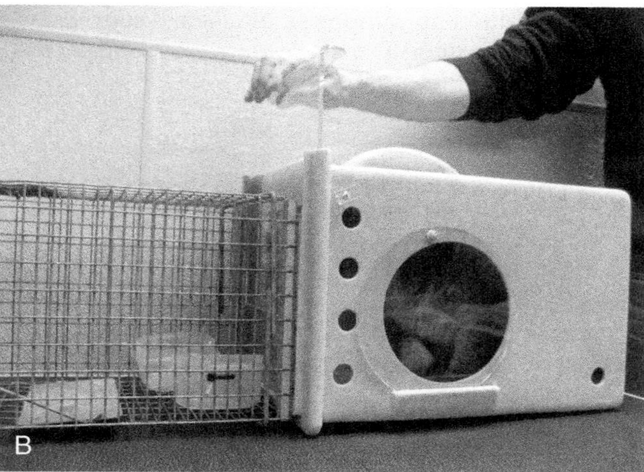

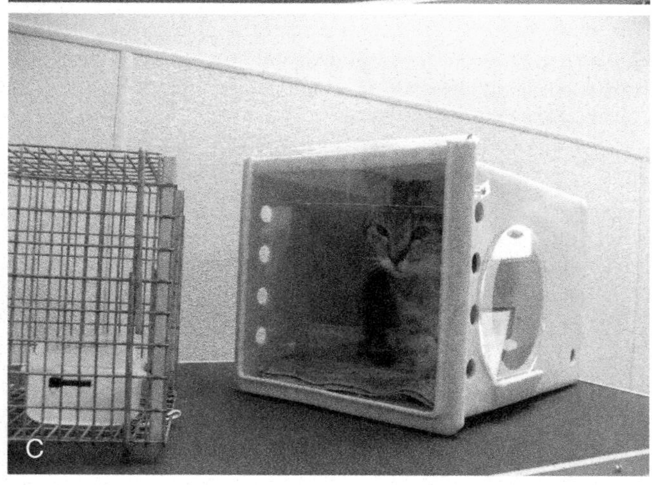

FIGURE 45-20 Proper equipment is essential when treating feral cats. **A, B,** and **C,** A cat is safely and humanely transferred from a box trap into a feral cat den. The den can be placed in a larger cage for longer-term holding during treatment. When necessary, transfer from the den into a squeeze cage can be accomplished to facilitate administration of medications.

of the most common concerns that arise occurs when cats take up residence in a crawl space beneath a home where they are not welcome. Whereas it is important for cats to have shelter available to them, it is sometimes necessary to prevent them from residing in certain locations. This is easy to do by simply eliminating access to this area. However, sealing off access without proper planning can result in accidental trapping of cats without a route for escape, creating serious welfare concerns for the animals. Such situations however can easily and humanely be avoided by using a one-way door: this will allow cats to leave the area, but makes it impossible for them to return to it (Box 45-6).

Another common concern arises when cats frequent gardens and/or sand boxes. Efforts to exclude cats from such areas are important for public health, especially because of the zoonotic risk posed from roundworms, hookworms, and toxoplasmosis as a result of contact with contaminated soil. In addition to community cats, pet cats also contribute to this potential risk.[10] Covers should be used for children's sand boxes, and gloves should be worn when gardening. Commercially available motion-activated sprinklers can be helpful in some instances. Spreading prickly textures around the garden, such as pinecones, holly leaves, chicken wire, or purpose-designed prickly mats, especially where there is newly turned dirt, can also be effective. To minimize risks, vegetables should always be washed thoroughly, and excellent hand hygiene should be

BOX 45-6

Using a One-Way Door

To safely exclude cats from a crawl space where their presence is problematic, use a one-way door. To make a one-way door, simply cut a piece of plywood to fit over the crawl space where cats are entering. Cut a cat-sized door in the board and attach it with a hinge that will only allow the door to open in one direction. Alternatively, attach a thin strip of wood along the bottom of the back of the board to prevent the door from opening inward. Secure the door over the entrance to the crawl space. This allows any cats to exit, yet prevents them from re-entering. After several days, any cats should have departed, and the one-way door can be replaced with a permanent covering. To safeguard the welfare of the cats, it is best to ensure than some alternate shelter is available in the area.

practiced. Additional resources for clients concerning all aspects of community cat care are included at the end of this chapter.

RELOCATION OF CATS

On occasion, individuals may wish to relocate feral cats to new sites, or major construction or some other event may necessitate relocation of a colony. However, the process of relocation is difficult and poses significant danger to cats, because they possess strong homing instincts and typically flee when released at a location other than their original colony site. In the author's experience, when caregivers have released cats at foreign sites, they have either readily disappeared or their remains have been discovered on a nearby roadside. In a few instances, cats have managed to return to their original home sites days or even weeks later. One investigator attempted to establish colonies of feral cats at a farm site in order to study them.[47] Following their release, all of the cats disappeared. For this reason, relocation of feral cat colonies must be viewed as a last resort.

If relocation cannot be avoided, cats must be confined for several weeks at their new "home" location prior to release. Cats should be confined in enclosures that are large enough to accommodate separate feeding and litter areas as well as a cat den or other suitable purpose-designed box. The enclosure should be situated in a secure location, such as inside a shed, barn, or other protected area. Caregivers should feed and care for the cats daily for a minimum of 3 weeks prior to release. This practice allows cats to acclimate to the new site and become entrained to a routine of feeding at this location. Following release, the cat should continue to be fed at the same location on a regular schedule. It is not unusual for a cat to "disappear" for days or more following release. However, most will come around in time and will ultimately be sighted, usually around the food bowl, as they anticipate feeding times. When more than one cat from a colony is relocated, the presence of familiar cats at the new location facilitates adaptation of others.

LARGE-SCALE TRAP-NEUTER-RETURN PROGRAMS

Large-scale programs to sterilize community cats in the United States have become increasingly commonplace during the past decade. Caregivers trap community cats for participation in large surgery clinics. In these clinics, cats are sterilized in an assembly line fashion that provides high-quality care to a high volume of patients.

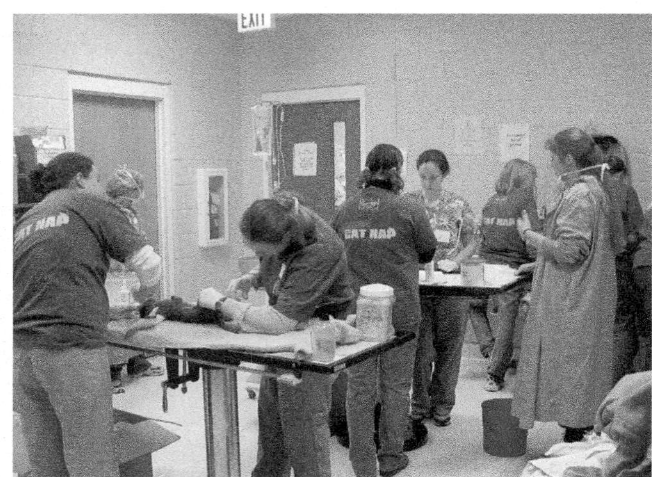

FIGURE 45-21 Veterinarians and volunteers care for cats at a large-scale TNR clinic. By using an assembly-line approach, high-quality care is efficiently delivered to a high volume of cats at various dedicated stations throughout the clinic.

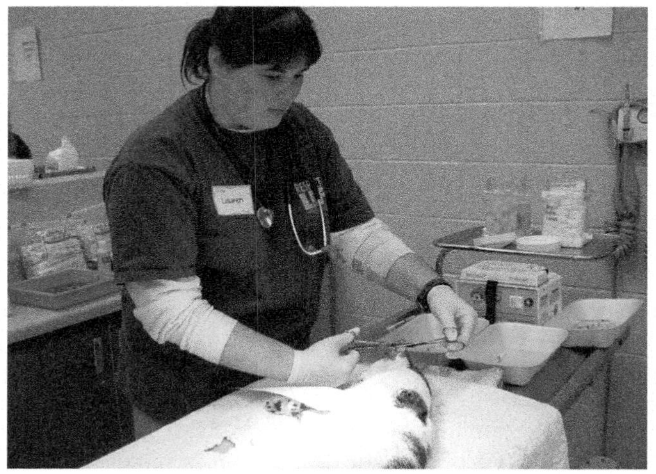

FIGURE 45-22 Ear tipping is antiseptically performed at a dedicated ear tipping station at a large-scale TNR clinic.

Most programs use trained volunteers to facilitate patient care and ensure constant monitoring of cats during the process. Following induction of anesthesia, cats are removed from their traps and identified by physically affixing a tag to their body, ensuring they are returned to the correct trap and caregiver at the end of the clinic. Cats are examined, ear-tipped, surgically sterilized, vaccinated, and then returned to their clean traps, where they are monitored until adequately recovered (see Figure 45-10). To maximize efficiency, these programs often establish "stations" that perform each task, using trained volunteers to transport and monitor cats between stations (Figures 45-21 and 45-22). Detailed protocols for establishing large-scale TNR clinics are available online (Box 45-7).

BOX 45-7

Resources for Care of Community Cats

Alley Cat Allies: http://www.alleycat.org
Neighborhood Cats:
http://www.neighborhoodcats.org
Operation Catnip: http://www.operationcatnip.org
Feral Cat Spay/Neuter Project:
http://www.feralcatproject.org
Feral Cat Coalition: http://www.feralcat.com

LIABILITY

As professionals, veterinarians should always be concerned about liability protection. It is always important to make clients aware of risks associated with any practices or procedures that are recommended and to obtain written consent prior to initiating them. Box 45-8 contains suggested statements for liability forms involving TNR programs, including the loan of traps. Some veterinary practitioners allow clients to "check out" traps as part of the service they provide, to facilitate spaying and neutering of community cats. It is important to discuss these services with your insurance provider to ensure coverage in the event of a claim. Despite the need to be aware of the potential liability concerns, such concerns should not prevent veterinarians from facilitating TNR. In fact, many veterinarians in communities throughout the United States work with individual clients performing TNR as well as with organized TNR programs on a regular basis.

CONCLUSION

As a sole measure, TNR programs cannot be expected to solve the problem of free-roaming cats in communities. However, they do hold great merit as a legitimate response to existing colonies of cats with caregivers and raise public awareness of the welfare issues surrounding cats. TNR programs emphasize to communities that cats require and deserve responsible care; including sterilization, vaccination, identification, and regular feeding, watering and shelter. The provision of accessible, affordable spay-neuter services for community cats helps individual cats and people, while promoting veterinary medical care for all cats and providing humane alternatives to sheltering and euthanasia.

Where emotions and controversies surround methods of community cat management, the goals of cat control and welfare should not be forgotten. Consideration should always be given to the messages we send with the methods we elect to use. Perhaps the greatest value of TNR is that it promotes both humane care and control of cats, setting an important example for responsible stewardship to all animals.

BOX 45-8

Suggested Statements for Liability Forms Involving Trap-Loan and TNR Services

- I understand that this spay/neuter service is for free-roaming community cats, and I certify that to the best of my knowledge these cats are unowned. I accept any liability that may occur secondary to the trapping and treatment of an owned cat.
- I understand that all cats will be "ear-tipped" by the surgical removal of the tip of the left ear under anesthesia so that they can be easily identified as having been sterilized and vaccinated.
- I recognize the risks feral cats face during handling, anesthesia, and surgery and hold __________ harmless should a cat experience complications, injury, escape, or death.
- I understand that trapped animals may be dangerous, and I agree not to open any trap or handle any trapped animal unless specifically instructed. I release __________ from any liability for any injuries or damages that I may incur or cause while trapping, confining, transporting, or releasing these cats.
- I promise to see that, following surgery, spayed/neutered cats will receive food, water, and necessary care on a regular basis when they are returned to the location from which they were taken. I commit to caring for these cats indefinitely and will secure a substitute caregiver if I am unable to provide adequate care. I acknowledge the possibility that once released, some cats may not return.
- I will not use the trap to capture any owned cat, or for any other unlawful act, and will only use it for the purpose of spay/neuter procedures or other necessary medical treatment. Under no circumstances shall this trap be used to capture a healthy animal for destruction or surrender to animal control agencies. I indemnify __________ from any liability based on my use of the trap.
- The value of each trap is $____. I will be responsible for said sum to secure its return or replacement. I agree that the traps I am receiving today are in good working order. I understand that if the traps are not returned in similar condition, I will forfeit my deposit for each trap not in good working order.

Acknowledgments

The author would like to acknowledge "Elmer," who fearlessly posed as a feral cat to demonstrate the various types of humane capture equipment for many of the illustrations in this chapter. Because of his unflappable good nature, he purred throughout most of his photo session, making it difficult to obtain shots where he actually "looked feral"!

References

1. American Association of Feline Practitioners (AAFP) position statement on feral cats. Available at http://www.catvets.com/professionals/guidelines/position/?Id=292, published 2007. Accessed April 17, 2010.
2. Alley Cat Allies: Feral cat activist archives. Available at http://www.alleycat.org/NetCommunity/Page.aspx?pid=439. Accessed April 8, 2010.
3. American Bird Conservancy: Resolution on free-roaming cats. Available at http://www.abcbirds.org/abcprograms/policy/cats/Resolution.PDF, published 1997. Accessed April 17, 2010.
4. American Society for the Prevention of Cruelty to Animals: Pet statistics. Available at http://www.aspca.org/about-us/faq/pet-statistics.html. Accessed January 12, 2010.
5. American Veterinary Medical Association (AVMA): Policy statement on free-roaming abandoned and feral cats. Available at http://www.avma.org/issues/policy/animal_welfare/feral_cats.asp, published 2009. Accessed April 17, 2010.
6. American Veterinary Medical Association (AVMA): *Center for information management: U.S. pet ownership and demographics sourcebook*, 2007 ed, Schaumburg, Ill, 2007, AVMA.
7. Beaver BV: Fractious cats and feline aggression, *J Feline Med Surg* 6:13, 2004.
8. Burrow R, Wawra E, Pinchbeck G et al: Prospective evaluation of postoperative pain in cats undergoing ovariohysterectomy by a midline or flank approach, *Vet Record* 158:657, 2006.
9. Coleman GT, Atwell RB: Use of fipronil to treat ear mites in cats, *Aust Vet Pract* 29:168, 1999.
10. Dabritz HA, Atwill ER, Gardner IA et al: Outdoor fecal deposition by free-roaming cats and attitudes of cat owners and nonowners towards stray pets, wildlife and water pollution, *J Am Vet Med Assoc* 229:74, 2006.
11. Dorn AS: Ovariohysterectomy by the flank approach, *Vet Med Small Anim Clin* 70:569, 1975.
12. Dybdall K, Strasser R, Katz T: Behavioral differences between owner surrender and stray domestic cats after entering an animal shelter, *Appl Anim Behav Sci* 104:85, 2007.
13. Fischer SM, Quest CM, Dubovi EJ et al: Response of feral cats to vaccination at the time of neutering, *J Am Vet Med Assoc* 230:52, 2007.
14. Greene CE, Addie DD: Feline parvovirus infection. In Greene CE, editors: *Infectious diseases of the dog and cat*, ed 3, Philadelphia, 2006, Saunders, p 78.
15. Griffin B: Scaredy cat or feral cat? *Animal Sheltering* Nov/Dec:57, 2009.
16. Griffin B: Prolific cats: the impact of their fertility on the welfare of the species, *Compend Contin Edu Pract Vet* 23:1058, 2001.
17. Griffin B: *unpublished data*. Scott-Ritchey Research Center, Auburn University, Auburn, Ala, 2004.
18. Griffin B, DiGangi B, Bohling M: A review of neutering cats. In August JR, editor: *Consultations in feline internal medicine*, ed 6, St Louis, 2009, Saunders Elsevier, p 776.
19. Griffin B, Hume KR: Recognition and management of stress in housed cats. In August JR, editor: *Consultations in feline internal medicine*, ed 6, St Louis, 2009, Saunders Elsevier, p 717.
20. Grint NJ, Murison PJ, Coe R et al: Assessment of the influence of surgical technique on postoperative pain and wound tenderness in cats following ovariohysterectomy, *J Feline Med Surg* 8:15, 2006.
21. Hughes KL, Slater MR, Haller L: The effects of implementing a feral cat spay/neuter program in a Florida county animal control service, *J Appl Anim Welf Sci* 5:285, 2002.
22. Humane Society of the United States: How-to series: how to use a control pole. Available at http://www.animalsheltering.org/resource_library/magazine_articles/sep_oct_1996/asmSO96_howto.pdf, published 2006. Accessed April 17, 2010.
23. Kelly GE: The effect of surgery in dogs on the response to concomitant distemper vaccination, *Aust Vet J* 56:556, 1980.
24. Krzaczynski J: The flank approach to feline ovariohysterectomy (an alternate technique), *Vet Med Small Anim Clin* 69:572, 1974.
25. Levy JK: Feline leukemia virus and feline immunodeficiency virus. In Miller L, Hurley KF, editors: *Infectious disease management in animal shelters*, Ames, Iowa, 2009, Blackwell, p 307.
26. Levy J: Feral cat management. In Miller L, Zawistowksi S, editors: *Shelter medicine for veterinarians and staff*, Ames, Iowa, 2004, Blackwell, p 377.
27. Levy JK, Crawford, PC: Humane strategies for controlling feral cat populations, *J Am Vet Med Assoc* 225:1354, 2004.
28. Levy JK, Crawford C, Hartmann K et al: 2008 American Association of Feline Practitioners' feline retrovirus management guidelines, *J Feline Med Surg* 10:300, 2008.
29. Levy JK, Gale DW, Gale LA: Evaluation of the effect of a long-term trap-neuter-return and adoption program on a free-roaming cat population, *J Am Vet Med Assoc* 222:42, 2003.
30. Levy JK, Scott HM, Lachtara JL, et al: Seroprevalence of feline leukemia virus and feline immunodeficiency virus infection in cats in North America and risk factors for seropositivity, *J Am Vet Med Assoc* 228:371, 2006.
31. Longcore T, Rich C, Sullivan LM: Critical assessment of claims regarding management of feral cats by trap-neuter-return, *Conserv Biol* 23:887, 2009.
32. Looney AL, Bohling MW, Bushby PA et al: The Association of Shelter Veterinarians veterinary medical care guidelines for spay-neuter programs, *J Am Vet Med Assoc* 233:74, 2008.
33. Lowe SE, Bradshaw JWS: *Effects of socialisation on the behaviour of feral kittens, Proc Third Int Congress Vet Behav Med*, Vancouver, British Columbia, 2001, p 68.
34. Luria BJ, Levy JK, Lappin MR et al: Prevalence of infectious diseases in feral cats in Northern Florida, *J Feline Med Surg* 6:287, 2004.
35. McGrath H, Hardie RJ, Davis E: Lateral flank approach for ovariohysterectomy in small animals, *Compend Contin Educ Pract Vet* 26:922, 2004.
36. Miller J: The domestic cat: perspectives on the nature and diversity of cats, *J Am Vet Med Assoc* 208:498, 1996.
37. Miyamoto T, Taura Y, Une S et al: Immunological responses after vaccination pre- and post-surgery in dogs, *J Vet Med Sci* 57:29, 1995.
38. Neville PF, Remfry J: Effect of neutering on two groups of feral cats, *Vet Record* 144:447, 1984.
39. Nutter FB, Levine JF, Stoskopf MK: Reproductive capacity of free-roaming domestic cats and kitten survival rate, *J Am Vet Med Assoc* 225:1399, 2004.
40. Patronek G: Free-roaming and feral cats: their impact on wildlife and human beings, *J Am Vet Med Assoc* 212:218, 1998.
41. Patronek GJ, Sperry E: Quality of life in long term confinement. In August JR, editor: *Consultations in feline internal medicine*, ed 4, Philadelphia, 2001, WB Saunders, p 621.
42. Reese MJ, Patterson EV, Tucker SJ et al: Effects of anesthesia and surgery on serological responses to vaccination in kittens, *J Am Vet Med Assoc* 233:116, 2008.
43. Robertson S: A review of feral cat control, *J Fel Med Surg* 10:366, 2008.
44. Richards JR, Elston TH, Ford RB et al: The 2006 American Association of Feline Practitioners Feline Vaccine Advisory Panel report, *J Am Vet Med Assoc* 229:1405, 2006.
45. Scarampella F, Pollmeier M, Visser M et al: Efficacy of fipronil in the treatment of feline cheyletiellosis, *Vet Parasit* 129:333, 2005.
46. Scott KC, Levy JK, Gorman SP et al: Body condition of feral cats and the effect of neutering, *J Appl Anim Welf Sci* 5:203, 2002.
47. Smith RE, Shane SM: The potential for the control of feral cat populations by neutering, *Feline Pract* 16:21, 1986.

48. Slater MR: *Community approaches to feral cats: problems, alternatives, and recommendations*, Washington, DC, 2002, Humane Society Press.
49. Soulebot JP, Brun A: Experimental rabies in cats: immune response and persistence of immunity, *Cornell Vet* 71:311, 1981.
50. Stoskopf MK, Nutter FB: Analyzing approaches to feral cat management—one size does not fit all, *J Am Vet Med Assoc* 225:1361, 2004.
51. Subacz KB: Impact assessment of a trap-neuter-return program on selected features of Auburn, Alabama feral cat colonies. Unpublished graduate thesis: Auburn Univeristy, Ala. Available at http://etd.auburn.edu/etd/handle/10415/1101, 2008. Accessed June 4, 2011.
52. Wildlife Society: Position statement on feral and free-ranging domestic cats. Available at http://joomla.wildlife.org/documents/positionstatements/28-Feral%20&%20Free%20Ranging%20Cats.pdf, published 2006. Accessed April 17, 2010.
53. Wilson FD, Balasubramanian NN: The lateral approach for the spaying of canines and felines, *Indian Vet J* 44:1052, 1967.

CHAPTER

46

Population Wellness: Keeping Cats Physically and Behaviorally Healthy

Brenda Griffin

OUTLINE

Whereas feline practitioners are usually well versed in the creation of wellness programs tailored to individual cats, optimizing the health of a population of cats requires additional knowledge and poses unique challenges. These challenges will vary depending on many factors, including the nature and purpose of the population itself. Indeed, veterinarians may be tasked with developing health care programs for cat populations in a wide spectrum of settings—from facilities housing laboratory animals, to animal shelters, home-based rescue and foster providers, care-for-life cat sanctuaries, breeding catteries, or large multicat households. Regardless of the setting, a systematic approach to the health of the clowder is crucial for success.

THE COMPONENTS OF WELLNESS

Merriam-Webster's Dictionary defines wellness as "the quality or state of being in good health especially as an actively sought goal."[80] Ensuring population health requires careful planning and active implementation of comprehensive wellness protocols that address both animal health and environmental conditions (Figure 46-1).[41] Addressing physical health alone is not sufficient to ensure wellness. For example, a cat may be in proper physical condition and free from infectious or other physical disease, yet suffering from severe stress and anxiety. In this case, the patient cannot be assessed as healthy, because its behavioral (emotional) state is compromising its health and well-being. Thus physical health and behavioral health are both essential components of wellness, and preventive health care must actively address each of these.

Addressing the environment of the population is also critically important when considering wellness. Even the best-designed facilities cannot favor good health in a multicat environment without thoughtful implementation of environmental wellness protocols. In small animal practice, environmental wellness is frequently not emphasized simply because many owners are accustomed to providing a reasonably healthy environment for their pets. In contrast, a structured program to address environmental wellness is essential in the

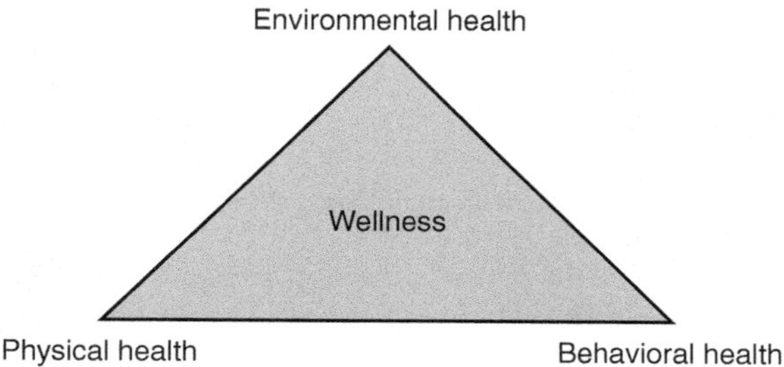

FIGURE 46-1 The inter-relationship among the components of population wellness. To optimize feline health, wellness programs must be carefully structured to address both the physical and behavioral health of the animals, which are intimately linked to their environment, making it crucial to systematically address environmental conditions as well.

context of a population, regardless of the actual physical facility. Proactive measures to maintain clean, sanitary environments that are not overcrowded—where cats are segregated by age and health status and provided with regular daily schedules of care by well-trained dedicated caregivers—are essential.[41]

GOALS OF A POPULATION WELLNESS PROGRAM

Simply stated, the overarching goals of a population wellness program are to optimize both the physical and behavioral health of the cats as well as preventing transmission of zoonotic diseases. In other words, a population wellness program should be designed to keep animals "healthy and happy" while keeping human caregivers safe.[41] It is not difficult to identify a healthy population of cats: When wellness protocols are successful, cats "look healthy" and "act like normal cats." In other words, they appear in good physical condition and display a wide variety of normal feline behaviors, including eating, stretching, grooming, scratching, playing, rubbing, resting, and if allowed, courtship and breeding. Just as changes in a cat's physical appearance should alert the clinician to potential problems, so should the absence of such normal feline activities and behaviors by members of the group.

Wellness goals must include maintaining the health of individual animals as well as that of the population as a whole. In the context of the population, the individuals that are physically or behaviorally ill serve as indicators or "barometers" of the health care and conditions of the population. When individuals are ill, their health and well-being is always a priority; however, it should also immediately trigger the clinician to ask, "Why is this individual sick? What is the cause of its illness, and how can I prevent this from affecting others?"

More specific goals will vary depending upon the given population and its purpose. For example, in an animal shelter, specific goals of the wellness program might include decreasing the incidence and prevalence of infectious diseases in the shelter and following adoption, decreasing the incidence of problem behaviors in the shelter, decreasing the rate of return of cats to the shelter for problem behaviors, increasing the adoption rate, and so forth. In the context of a breeding colony, the goals might include increasing kitten birth weights, decreasing neonatal mortality, or improving socialization of kittens. By identifying and tracking measurable factors (often called performance targets in large animal medicine), it is possible to measure progress toward these goals. Once baseline data (such as disease rates) are established, it is possible to measure the impact of protocol changes on population health by evaluating these performance targets. Both medical records and a system for regular surveillance and reporting are required to accurately track and access trends in animal health.[41]

HEALTH SURVEILLANCE (DAILY ROUNDS)

Early recognition is crucial for effective control of infectious disease and problem behavior in a group. Therefore a regular system of health surveillance must be in place to monitor every individual. In a population setting, daily "walk-through rounds" represent the foundation of an effective animal health care program. Rounds should be conducted at least once daily (preferably twice a day or more often, depending upon the needs of individual cats) for the purpose of monitoring and evaluating both physical and behavioral health. Medically trained caregivers should visually observe every animal and its environment, taking note of food and water consumption, urination, defecation, attitude, behavior, ambulation, and signs of illness, pain or other problems. Monitoring should take place before cleaning so that food intake and the condition of the enclosure, including the presence of feces, urine, or vomit can be noted. Alternatively, observation logs can be completed by caregivers at the time of cleaning and reviewed during walk-though rounds. Any cat that is observed to be experiencing a problem, whether it be signs of respiratory infection, diarrhea, anxiety, or obvious pain, suffering, or distress must be assessed and treated in a timely manner. Regardless of length of stay, regular daily assessment is imperative to identify new problems (medical or behavioral) that may develop so that they can be identified and addressed in a timely fashion to ensure the welfare of the individual animal as well as that of the population.

BOX 46-1

Suggested Topics for Health Care Policies and Protocols[41,51]

For each disease or problem in question, the following should be included:

- Definition or description (including cause, transmission [if applicable], and risk to other animals, including humans)
- Description of methods that will be used for diagnosis
- Criteria for notification and contact information for individual(s) to be notified
- General policy describing the handling and disposition of affected cats
- Description of housing/isolation procedures for affected cats
- Description of decontamination procedures, if necessary
- Criteria for treatment, if applicable
  - Who can initiate treatment?
  - Who is responsible for treatment?
  - How will recovery be monitored and defined?
  - How will treatment failure be defined?
- Description of medical record keeping and other documentation of cases

POLICY AND PROTOCOL DEVELOPMENT

In addition to early recognition of health problems, timely action is crucial to effectively limit their morbidity. Ideally, all facilities that house multiple cats should have written policies and protocols in place that detail how medical and behavioral problems will be handled.[41,51,54] A committee or team of individuals composed of medical staff, managers, and caregivers can establish and oversee these policies and protocols. Such protocols serve as guidelines for systematic triage and care of animals and help to prevent delays in care that may otherwise arise if such plans were not in place. Policies and protocols should be based on medical facts, taking into account the entity's purpose or mission and the availability of resources for care. They should include a definition or description of the disease or condition in question, a description of the methods that will be used for diagnosis, and a general policy regarding the handling and disposition of affected cats. In addition, protocols should include details on notification, housing, decontamination, treatment, and documentation (Box 46-1).

QUALITY OF LIFE AND THE FIVE FREEDOMS

Just as quality-of-life assessment is the responsibility of every veterinarian as they guide the medical care of individual animals, quality-of-life assessment is also a critical part of population health care and monitoring. The factors that affect physical and mental well-being are broad, complex, and often vary substantially among individuals.[76] Exacting criteria are lacking for the objective measurement of quality of life of cats. However, subjective assessments can and should be made by medical and behavioral personnel at regular intervals (weekly or even daily, as indicated) considering the most information possible.[76,109] The "Five Freedoms," which were originally described by the Farm Animal Welfare Council in the 1970s, represent a benchmark for ensuring quality of life or animal welfare[35] (Box 46-2). These principles provide a useful framework that is applicable across varying situations and species and have been widely accepted and endorsed by animal care experts.

BOX 46-2

The Five Freedoms[35]

1. Freedom from thirst, hunger, and malnutrition by providing ready access to fresh water and a diet that maintains full health and vigor
2. Freedom from discomfort by providing a suitable environment, including shelter and a comfortable resting area
3. Freedom from pain, injury, and disease by prevention or rapid diagnosis and treatment
4. Freedom to express normal behavior by providing sufficient space, proper facilities, and company of the animals' own kind
5. Freedom from fear and distress by ensuring conditions that avoid mental suffering

Many agencies have used the Five Freedoms as the basis of recommendations for minimum standards of care for many species, including cats housed in catteries, shelters, and research facilities.[7,13,54,87] The tenets of the Five Freedoms define essential outcomes and imply criteria for assessment but do not prescribe the methods by which to achieve those outcomes. Regardless of the setting, population wellness programs should ensure the Five Freedoms for all cats.

MEDICAL DECISION MAKING AND EUTHANASIA

Medical decisions must be weighed in the context of the health of the population as well that of the individual, while considering animal welfare and the availability of resources for care. When large numbers of animals are involved, situations may arise in which animal health and welfare cannot be managed in the case of every individual animal. This may be due to physical or behavioral illness, or environmental conditions that negatively impact animal health, such as crowding. Regardless of the cause, it may be necessary to euthanize affected individuals if no other remedies exist to relieve animal suffering or to protect population health. These decisions can be difficult and emotionally challenging, especially in instances where the individual could easily be treated or otherwise accommodated if adequate resources were available. However, such decisions may be crucial for disease control, animal welfare, and population health.

That being said, euthanasia should never be used as a substitute for providing proper husbandry and care. Indeed, a critical need for a comprehensive wellness program exists in every multicat setting. It is unacceptable to house animals under conditions likely to induce illness and poor welfare, and such conditions can be expected when wellness programs are not in place and carefully monitored.[41]

When facilities elect to house cats with medical or behavioral problems, appropriate veterinary care must be provided. It is imperative that a humane plan for diagnosis, treatment/management, monitoring, and housing be implemented in a timely fashion. When determining if cats with special needs can be humanely cared for in a population setting, the following goals and considerations should be addressed: What measures must be implemented to prevent transmission of disease to other cats or people? Can appropriate care realistically be delivered? Will the care provided result in a cure or adequate management of the disease or problem behavior? Can the facility afford the cost and time for care? How will it impact resources available for other cats? In the case of animal shelters, additional considerations should include Will the cat be adoptable? What steps can be taken to minimize the holding time required for treatment? If the cat is not adopted, do humane long-term care options exist in the shelter? What welfare assessment will be used to measure quality of life in the shelter?[41]

PROBLEM PREVENTION

Both infectious disease and problem behaviors are common in multicat settings. The old adage, "An ounce of prevention is worth a pound of cure" is certainly true. Wellness always starts with prevention: It is far more time and cost efficient than treatment, and it is kinder to the animals and their caregivers. With this in mind, population wellness programs should provide broad-based, holistic approaches to preventive care, rather than being based on the control of a single disease or problem, regardless of the setting.

Maintenance of good health or wellness is especially challenging in populations with high turnover and interchange of cats of varying ages and susceptibilities, such as animal shelters. Infectious diseases can become endemic in facilities where populations of animals are housed. Even in closed populations, certain pathogens can be difficult to exclude or to eliminate once introduced. Notably, upper respiratory viruses, dermatophytes, and coccidia are among the most difficult pathogenic agents to control because of their persistence in the environment through carrier states and/or resistance to environmental disinfection.

In particular, upper respiratory disease is the most common endemic disease in cat populations and is impossible to completely prevent in an open population. Feline herpes virus type 1 (FHV-1) and feline calicivirus (FCV) have been implicated as the causes of most infections: Both viruses induce persistent carrier states and are widespread in the cat population.[36] Cats that recover from FHV-1 remain latently infected and shed virus intermittently, especially following periods of stress. FCV carriers shed continuously for months to years following infection. A variety of other viral and bacterial pathogens may also contribute to feline upper respiratory disease, and *Bordetella*, *Chlamydophila*, and *Mycoplasma* are problematic in some populations. Feline infectious peritonitis (FIP) is another disease that is nearly impossible to eradicate from a multicat environment, and sporadic cases can be expected to occur, especially in young cats.[93] Fortunately, proper wellness programs can greatly limit the incidence and severity of diseases, even for pathogens that are difficult to control.

THE ROLE OF STRESS

The multicat environment also presents enormous opportunities for inducing stress. Because of their unique biology, cats are particularly prone to experiencing acute stress and fear in novel environments. Anything unfamiliar to a cat can trigger apprehension, activating the stress response. Confinement in a novel environment can result in a wide variety of behavioral indicators of stress including hypervigilance, feigned sleep, constant hiding, activity depression, and loss of appetite, among others. In the long term, if cats are unable to acclimate or cope in their environments, chronic stress, fear, frustration, or learned helplessness may result. In group settings, signs of social stress may also manifest with increases in problem behaviors, including urine marking, spraying, or other inappropriate elimination; constant hiding; and/or aggression.[46] Stress not only has the potential to negatively impact behavioral health but also physical health as well. The intimate link between stress and immunity has been well described. In fact, stress is a leading factor in the development of infectious disease and is particularly important in the pathogenesis of feline upper respiratory infections.[37,47] Wellness programs that reduce stress will also serve to minimize the morbidity of infectious disease.

CONSIDERATIONS REGARDING INFECTIOUS DISEASE TRANSMISSION

Despite the fact that infectious agents can never be completely eliminated from the environment, it is still possible to maintain good health. This is because the development of disease is determined by a complex interaction of many factors surrounding the host, the infectious agent, and the environment. Keeping these factors in mind provides a rational context for many of the recommendations in this chapter.

Some of the host factors that influence health and the development of disease include age, sex and reproductive status, immune status, body condition, stress, and genetics.[39] The amount and duration of exposure to an infectious agent (i.e., the "dose effect"), as well as its virulence and route of inoculation, also influence the likelihood and severity of disease. In addition, environmental conditions contribute to the development of infectious disease, including such factors as housing density, sanitation, and fluctuations in temperature or air quality. The fact that disease results from such a large combination of factors underscores the importance of a holistic and broad-based approach to population wellness.

GENERAL PRINCIPLES OF INFECTIOUS DISEASE CONTROL

When infectious disease does occur in a population, general principles of infectious disease control should guide the response. These include

- Removal of infected animals from the population
- Mass vaccination
- Mass treatment
- Quarantine of new arrivals or closure to admission
- Review of husbandry procedures (animals and environment)
- Staff education and communication

Coupled with vigilant surveillance to ensure early recognition of disease, these serve as the foundation of all disease control efforts when disease is present. However, the best method of disease control is always prevention.

ESSENTIAL ELEMENTS OF A POPULATION WELLNESS PROGRAM

When creating preventive medicine programs for a population, consideration must be given to all components of wellness: physical, behavioral, and environmental health.[41] With regard to promoting physical health, wellness programs should address the following essential elements:

- Patient history and physical examination
- Disease testing
- Vaccination
- Parasite control/prevention
- Spay/neuter
- Proper nutrition
- Grooming
- Periodontal disease prevention
- Breed-specific care

Likewise, to promote behavioral wellness, programs should include provisions for the following essential elements:

- History and behavioral care at intake
- Proper housing
- Social companionship
- Mental and physical activity
- Consistent daily routines

Finally, wellness protocols aimed at creating an environment that promotes health must take into account the following essential elements:

- Population density
- Cleaning and disinfection
- Segregation and traffic patterns
- Facility operations (e.g., heating–ventilation–air-conditioning [HVAC], noise and pest control, staff training)

MEDICAL RECORD KEEPING AND CAT IDENTIFICATION

Implementing population wellness protocols and ensuring quality and timely care require reliable systems for medical record keeping and animal identification. Regardless of the system used, medical record keeping procedures should comply with state and local practice acts, guidelines provided by state and national veterinary medical associations, and, in the case of laboratory animals, regulations as prescribed by federal law, the

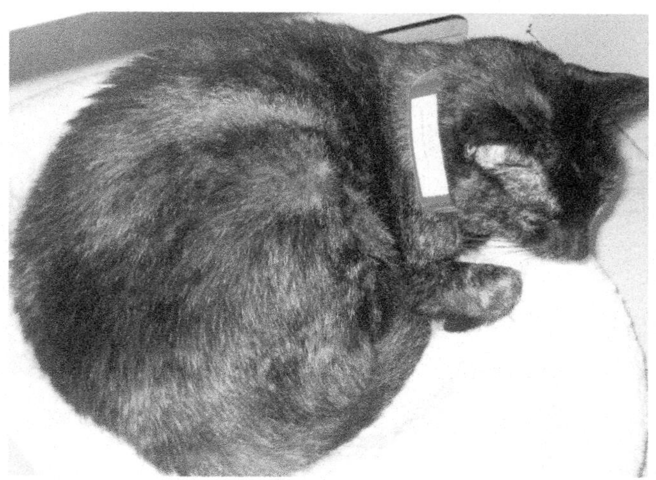

FIGURE 46-2 A plastic neckband designed for animals is used as an identification collar for this shelter cat (Safeguard 821, Precision Dynamics Corp., San Fernando, Calif.).

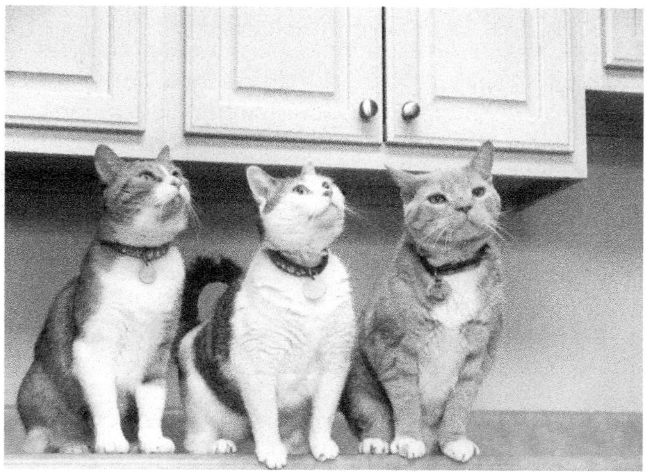

FIGURE 46-3 Cats in a private cattery wear collars with identification tags. Visual identification is essential for cats, regardless of the setting, and most cats can safely and reliably wear collars.

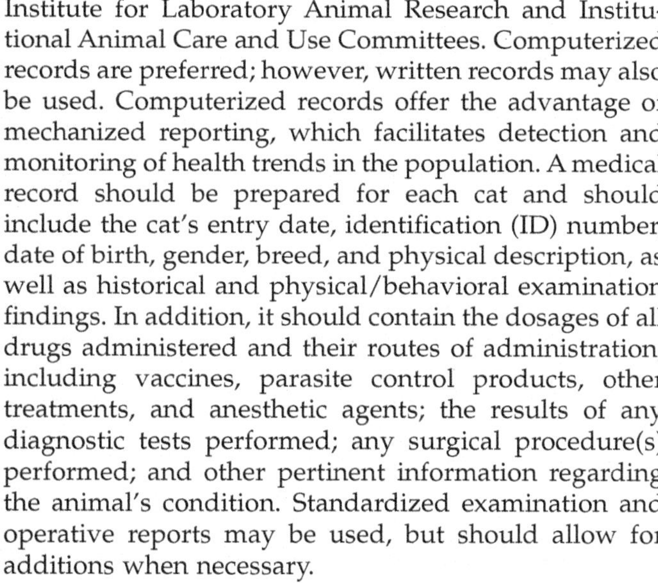

Institute for Laboratory Animal Research and Institutional Animal Care and Use Committees. Computerized records are preferred; however, written records may also be used. Computerized records offer the advantage of mechanized reporting, which facilitates detection and monitoring of health trends in the population. A medical record should be prepared for each cat and should include the cat's entry date, identification (ID) number, date of birth, gender, breed, and physical description, as well as historical and physical/behavioral examination findings. In addition, it should contain the dosages of all drugs administered and their routes of administration, including vaccines, parasite control products, other treatments, and anesthetic agents; the results of any diagnostic tests performed; any surgical procedure(s) performed; and other pertinent information regarding the animal's condition. Standardized examination and operative reports may be used, but should allow for additions when necessary.

Identification of cats in the form of a neckband, collar and tag, tattoo, earband, and/or a microchip is also essential for preventive health care and ongoing surveillance of individuals.[45] Whenever possible, some form of identification should be physically affixed to every individual cat. In addition, enclosures should be labeled with the cats' unique identification number and/or name.

Identification Collars

Contrary to popular belief, most cats can reliably wear collars safely and comfortably.[65] Many facilities use disposable collars, including commercially available plastic or paper neckbands made for animals or hospital-type wristbands made for human patients (Figure 46-2). Commercially available cat collars with an ID tag affixed are also a good option (Figure 46-3). Some facilities prefer to use safety collars that are designed to break away should the collar become caught on something. Even for kittens, collars can be used and may be especially beneficial, because they will learn to wear them from an early age.

Microchips

Microchips may also be used for identification and are safe and simple to implant (Figure 46-4). The procedure is well tolerated by the vast majority of cats without the need for sedation. Unlike visual means of identification, a scanner is necessary for positive identification of a microchipped animal. For this reason, microchips are often used in conjunction with a visual means of identification and serve as important permanent means of backup identification. Box 46-3 describes the proper technique for scanning for a microchip.

During the last 2 decades, microchips of varying radiofrequencies (125, 128, and 134 kHz) have been introduced in the United States.[4] The 125-kHz chips have historically been the most common, whereas the accepted standard in the rest of the world is the 134-kHz chip. Because some scanners read only certain radiofrequencies, it is possible to miss detecting a microchip that is present, depending on the scanner being used. Currently, there are efforts to standardize microchipping in the United States, including widespread distribution of universal (global) scanners to ensure that all implanted microchips can be reliably identified. Once global scanners are widely available, the American Veterinary Medical Association (AVMA) recommends adoption of the 134-kHz (ISO) microchip as the American standard, because this frequency is recognized as the international standard for microchips

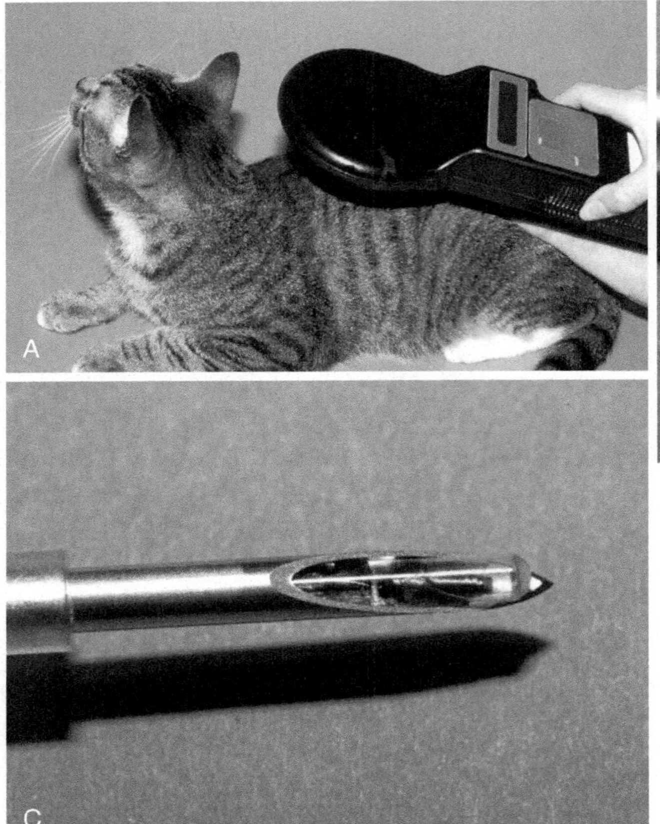

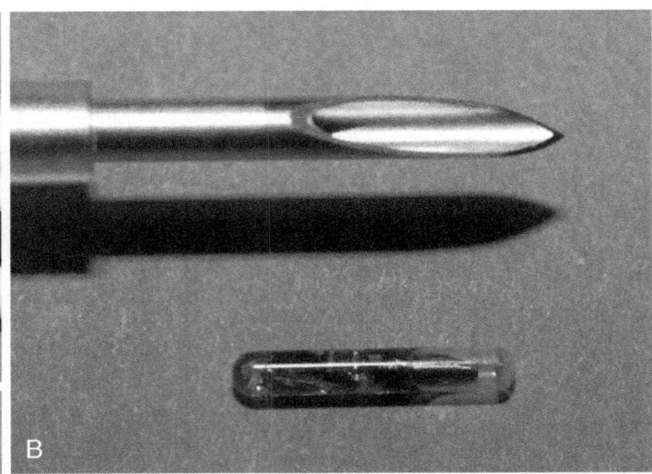

FIGURE 46-4 Microchip identification. Small (12- × 2-mm) microchips can be easily implanted in most cats, without sedation, using a needle. Cats may be scanned for reliable permanent identification. *(From Griffin B, Hume KR: Recognition and management of stress in housed cats. In August JR, editor:* Consultations in feline internal medicine, *vol 6, St Louis, 2006, Elsevier, p 717.)*

in the rest of the world. Efforts have also focused on improving, updating, and centralizing microchip registries. This is extremely important in the context of animal shelters. Box 46-4 contains information on the use of collars and microchips as tools for improving cat–owner reunification.

Tattoos

In laboratory settings, tattoos may be used as a means of permanent identification of cats (Figure 46-5).[45] Tattoos are most commonly applied to the inner pinna of the ear using a tattoo machine with multiple needles. Care must be taken to properly disinfect the needles between patients. A significant disadvantage of tattooing is that tattoos can sometimes be difficult to read because of the presence of hair, fading, or distortion that may occur as the cat grows. In addition, their application requires anesthesia or heavy sedation.

Earbands

Small stainless steel ear tags manufactured for wing banding of birds are especially useful for identifying newborn kittens in some settings and are highly economical (Figure 46-6).[45] They can be placed without the need for anesthesia or sedation when kittens are less than 10 to 14 days old. Placing earbands requires skill and experience. They must be positioned in such a way as to provide adequate space for growth of the ear, while seating them deeply enough in the ear margin to ensure a secure piercing far enough away from the edge. If placed too close to the ear margin, the ear flap may tear, resulting in loss of the band. Other complications include local inflammation or infection at the site of the piercing. Ear tags are a practical method for identifying individual kittens in institutional or commercial breeding colonies, because when applied skillfully, they are seldom lost and provide reliable, long-lasting visual identification.

In contrast, private breeding catteries and animal shelters generally prefer to use methods that will not alter the cat's cosmetic appearance long term. Colored ribbon, nail polish, or clipping of hair in various areas of the body can all be useful means of temporary kitten identification in the neonatal stage, especially when coat color or patterns do not easily allow individuals to be distinguished.

BOX 46-3

Microchip Scanning Technique

Every cat, including those surrendered by their owners, should be systematically scanned for the presence of a microchip at the time of intake, as well as prior to being made available for adoption or being euthanized. Proper technique and scanning more than once are crucial to avoid missing microchips.[67,68] A universal (global) scanner (e.g., one that will read all microchip frequencies that are currently in use) should be used to ensure that all microchip frequencies are detected. At this time, the only universal scanners available in the United States are the new Home Again Global World scanner (Schering Plough, Whitehouse Station, NY) and the iMax Black Label ResQ scanner (Bayer Animal Health, Shawnee Mission, Kans.). One of the most common causes of scanner failure is weak batteries; therefore it is imperative that batteries be checked and replaced regularly.

To ensure a thorough scan and avoid missing chips, cats must be removed from carriers or cages prior to scanning. Metal and fluorescent lighting may interfere with chip detection. Metal exam surfaces should be covered with a towel or other material prior to scanning to minimize interference. The entire animal should be scanned using a consistent speed, scanner orientation, scanning pattern, and distance.

- Scanner orientation: The scanner should be held parallel to the animal. Rocking the scanner slightly from side to side will maximize the potential for optimal chip orientation and successful detection. The button on the scanner should be depressed continuously during the entire scanning procedure.
- Scanning distance: The scanner should be held in contact with the animal during scanning such that it is lightly touching the hair coat.
- Scanner speed: The scanner should not be advanced any faster than 0.15 m/second (0.5 ft/second). Scanning slowly is crucial, because universal scanners must cycle through various modes to read all possible chip frequencies.
- Areas of animal to scan: The standard implant site is midway between the shoulder blades, and scanning should begin over this area. If a microchip is not detected here, scanning should proceed systematically down the back, on the sides, neck, and shoulders—all the way to the elbows in the front and the hindquarters in the rear.
- Scanning pattern: The scanner should be moved over the scanning areas in an "S"-shaped pattern in a transverse direction (from side to side). If no microchip is detected, the scanner should be rotated 90 degrees, and then the "S"-shaped pattern should be repeated in a longitudinal direction (e.g., the long way) on both sides of the animal. This pattern of scanning will maximize the ability of the scanner to detect the microchip, regardless of its orientation.

BOX 46-4

Use of Identification (ID) Collars and Microchips to Improve Cat–Owner Reunification

- Less than 2% of cats are reunited with their owners, compared to as many as 15% to 19% of lost dogs.[86]
- The use of collars and tags as visually obvious forms of identification is extremely valuable, although overlooked by many cat owners.[69]
- Cats wearing collars are more likely to be identified as owned and not mistaken for strays.
- Even indoor cats require identification in case they escape, and studies clearly demonstrate that visual identification improves the odds of pet–owner reunification.[69]
- The provision of permanent identification in the form of a microchip represents an important backup, further improving the odds of pet–owner reunification because collars and tags can be lost.[66]
- Because owners and shelter staff often describe cat coat color and patterns differently, photographs that can be posted online are a useful method of improving lost-pet matching and enabling owners to look for their pet, even if they are physically unable to come to the shelter.
- Adopted animals should be sent home with ID collars and microchips.
- Shelter staff should always register microchips before the cat leaves the shelter, because many owners will neglect to do so following adoption, making the microchip an ineffective means of identification.[66]
- Web-based search engines for pet microchip identification numbers (http://www.checkthechip.com and http://www.petmicrochiplookup.org) have been established in an effort to functionally centralize microchip registries by linking existing national databases.

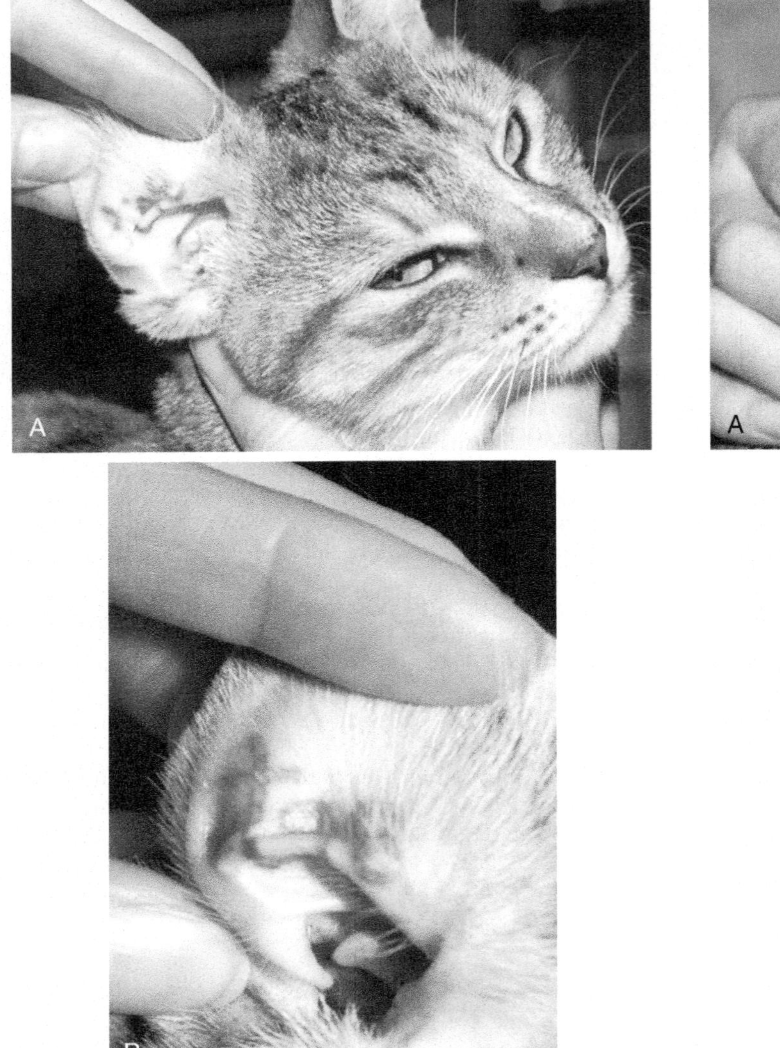

FIGURE 46-5 Permanent tattoo on the inner pinna of the ear of a laboratory cat. This form of identification requires heavy sedation with appropriate analgesia for placement. *(From Griffin B, Hume KR: Recognition and management of stress in housed cats. In August JR, editor:* Consultations in feline internal medicine, *vol 6, St Louis, 2006, Elsevier, p 717.)*

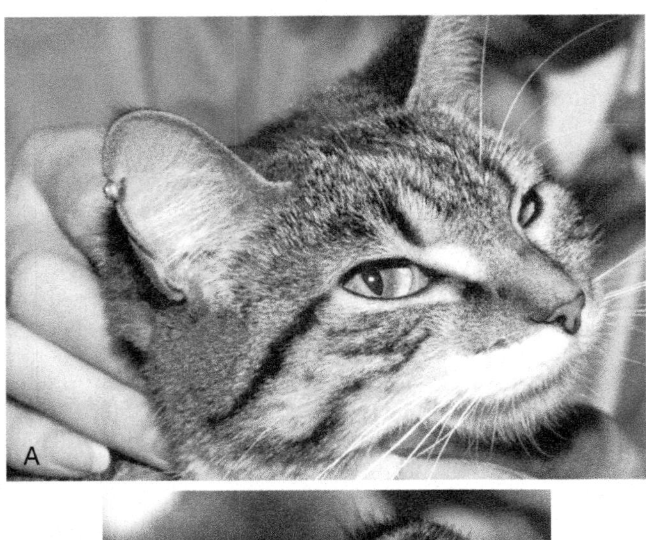

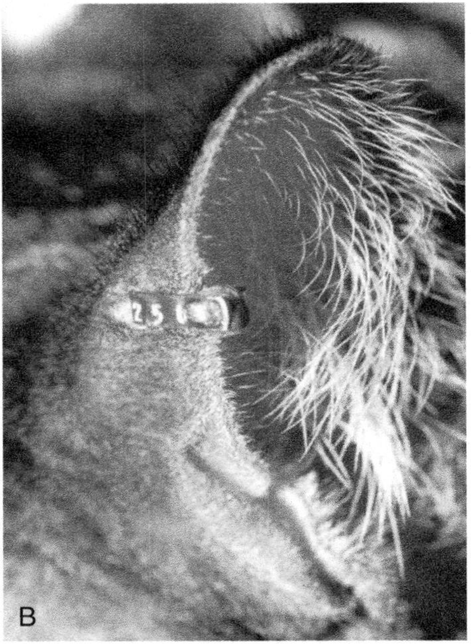

FIGURE 46-6 Earband identification. Small stainless steel bands manufactured for wing banding of birds are ideal for identification of young kittens in a laboratory setting. *(From Griffin B, Hume KR: Recognition and management of stress in housed cats. In August JR, editor:* Consultations in feline internal medicine, *vol 6, St Louis, 2006, Elsevier, p 717.)*

MANAGEMENT OVERSIGHT

The success or failure of a population wellness program hinges in large part on its implementation and oversight. A knowledgeable, cohesive, and dedicated team, where accountability, responsibility, and lines of authority are well defined, is crucial for management success.

As a part of the management structure and plan, veterinarians must be involved in the oversight of all aspects of animal care and must be given direct authority for the oversight of medical decisions. This requires that every facility that houses cats establish a formal relationship with one or more veterinarians who have direct knowledge of their animal population. This is essential to ensure that medical protocols are established with the proper professional oversight, and helps to ensure compliance with local veterinary practice acts that restrict the practice of veterinary medicine to licensed veterinarians. In facilities such as animal shelters, trained shelter staff can carry out preventive health care under the instructions of a veterinarian.[6]

DEVELOPING A POPULATION WELLNESS PROGRAM: CONSIDERATIONS FOR PHYSICAL HEALTH

The clinician should develop a program for physical health for the population that addresses all of the essential elements as noted. None of these should be considered as optional, but their implementation will depend on the setting, purposes, and resources of the group.

History

The value of obtaining an accurate medical history on any cat entering a population is immeasurable, because it will often alert the clinician to the presence of potential problems. In a laboratory setting, obtaining cats from commercial purpose-bred colonies or institutional breeding colonies ensures that an accurate history will be available, maximizing the odds that only healthy cats will be added to the population. Likewise, private breeding catteries should always strive to obtain an accurate medical history on any cat that may be accepted into the cattery. The introduction of cats from random sources to closed populations of cats risks the health of the population and should be avoided whenever possible.[45]

In contrast, by their very nature, animal shelters must frequently receive cats from multiple random sources, and it will not always be possible to obtain accurate histories. In some cases, cats are brought in by animal control officers or good Samaritans who have little if any information about them. Furthermore, some shelters provide a location (e.g., drop-off cages) where cats can be relinquished after business hours. This practice should be discouraged; however, if facilities elect to do this, every effort must be made to obtain a history through questionnaires that can be completed when the cat is left. The presence of staff to directly accept cats and obtain a history at the time of relinquishment is greatly preferred.[41] Even so, surrendering owners may or may not provide complete or accurate information, fearing that if they are honest about a pet's problems, the pet may be euthanized. Nonetheless, when available, a history can be extremely valuable, saving time and money as well as preventing unnecessary stress for cats and staff alike. Intake procedures should be in place to capture basic patient information, including both physical and behavioral data as well as the reason(s) for relinquishment. The importance of obtaining historical information cannot be overemphasized. In many cases, historical information may be used to expedite the disposition of the cat in the shelter.

Physical Examination

Physical examination is the clinician's single most important tool for evaluating health. Following a standardized physical examination form will ensure a complete and systematic review of all body systems. A veterinarian should carefully examine any new cat entering a closed population prior to admittance. In the context of animal shelters, every cat that is safe to handle should receive a physical examination at or as close to the time of admission to the shelter as possible. In many shelters, a veterinarian may not be available to examine incoming animals. However, staff can and should be trained to perform basic evaluations including sexing, aging, body condition scoring, and looking for evidence of fleas, ear mites, dental disease, overgrown claws, advanced pregnancy, or other obvious physical conditions. Of particular importance in the shelter physical examination are an accurate physical description of the animal and careful inspection for the presence of identification, both of which may aid in pet–owner reunification.[41]

Disease Testing

The gold standard for maintaining the health of a population is through exclusion of pathogens in combination with implementation of comprehensive wellness protocols. This requires that members of a population be free from specific pathogens when the group is established and that the colony be closed to any new individuals that do not meet the health standards of the group.[45] This is the foundation of disease control procedures in a laboratory animal setting, and these concepts should be applied to other population settings whenever possible. Consideration should be given to testing for the following: feline leukemia virus (FeLV), feline immunodeficiency virus (FIV), dermatophytosis, intestinal parasites and infections (e.g., *Campylobacter*, *Giardia*, coccidia), as well as other endoparasites and ectoparasites. The setting and resources available, as well as the individual's history and physical examination findings, should guide the clinician's decisions regarding selection of testing for cats entering a specific population. When new stock is added to a closed colony, disease testing is imperative.

Feline Leukemia Virus and Feline Immunodeficiency Virus

The American Association of Feline Practitioners (AAFP) maintains detailed professional guidelines for the management of FeLV and FIV infections. Identification and exclusion of infected cats is the most effective method of preventing new infections. Cats and kittens should always be tested prior to entry to a closed population. Those that test negative should be retested, because it may take as long as 60 days following exposure for a cat to test positive.[62,63]

In the context of animal shelters, testing decisions are often influenced by the availability of resources. The AAFP's guidelines include recommendations specifically for shelters. They state that all cats should ideally be tested at the time of entry and again in 60 days in case of recent exposure. When cats test positive on screening tests (e.g., point-of-care enzyme-linked immunosorbent assay [ELISA] tests), the AAFP recommends that the results be confirmed by additional testing, including testing over an interval of time, because false positives can occur. However, such confirmatory testing requires substantial time and monetary investment and may not be feasible in many shelters. In recognition of this, the Association of Shelter Veterinarians established a policy statement on "Management of Cats Who Test Positive for FeLV and FIV in an Animal Shelter," which states that the logistics and cost of holding and retesting unowned cats may be an ineffective use of resources.[5] In addition, it can be difficult to find homes for retrovirus-positive cats, which in many instances translates into stressful, prolonged shelter stays. Such long-term confinement may compromise quality of life and may compound the emotional stress of caregivers who may later be faced with euthanizing cats that have been held for long periods awaiting confirmatory testing or adoption opportunities. For all of these reasons, many shelters elect to euthanize cats that test positive on retrovirus screening tests.

Although it may be ideal for shelters to test cats on entry, it is not always feasible because of financial constraints. The next best practice might be to test cats prior to adoption as well as those that are housed in the shelter long term. In addition, cats should be tested prior to placement in group housing with unfamiliar cats and prior to investment, such as foster care, treatment, or spay/neuter surgery. However, given the limited resources of many shelters, the relatively low prevalence in healthy cats and the fact that transmission can be prevented by housing cats separately, it may not be cost effective for all shelters to screen every cat before selection for adoption. Each shelter should evaluate its own resources and determine their best use. When testing is performed, samples must never be pooled, and the negative results of one cat (such as a mother cat) should not be extrapolated to other cats (such as her kittens). These practices are invalid and can falsely lead to misidentification of a cat's true infection status.[62,63] If testing is not performed prior to adoption, adopters should be advised to have their new pet tested and to keep them separate from any other cats they may own prior to doing so.

Feline Heartworm Disease

Point-of-care heartworm tests for cats have recently become more widely available, but interpreting results can be problematic.[2] In relation to population health, testing is of little value, because infected cats pose no risk to other cats. Nonetheless, a clinician may elect testing as part of an initial database for individual cats, especially if they will be used for breeding. With heartworm tests readily available in combination with point-of-care FeLV/FIV tests, many animal shelters have been faced with determining whether or not to perform routine screening of cats in their care. To answer this question, it is helpful to consider the following:

- Infected cats pose no risk to other cats and usually remain asymptomatic.
- Even if infection is diagnosed in asymptomatic patients, definitive treatment is neither practical nor safe.
- Most infections resolve spontaneously with time and are not associated with a shortened life span.[38]
- Counseling owners about positive test results poses unique challenges.
- Positive test results may alter a cat's disposition in the shelter.

In consideration of these facts, the author does not recommend routine screening of cats for heartworm disease in shelters. Monthly chemoprophylaxis, however, is a safe and effective option for cats sheltered in areas where heartworm infection is considered endemic.

Dermatophytosis

Dermatophytosis or ringworm, the most common skin infection of cats, is a known zoonosis. It is caused by infection of the skin, hair, and nails with microscopic fungal organisms that cause varying degrees of hair loss and dermatitis. The dermatophyte that causes the majority of cases in felines is *Microsporum canis,* which is responsible for greater than 96% of all cases.[82] If left untreated, most infections will spontaneously resolve within 12 to 14 weeks postinfection. However, during this time, the infected cat will infect the surrounding environment and other animals or humans in the area. Not all cats infected with dermatophytosis develop lesions, and some may become chronic carriers. Control of dermatophytosis is difficult, because the spores formed by *M. canis* can survive in the environment for up to18 months or longer and are extremely resistant to disinfectants and detergents. In addition, the presence of asymptomatic carriers makes it difficult to readily recognize all infected cats. For this reason, consideration should be given to culturing all cats prior to entry to a closed colony. In particular, Persian cats may be predisposed to dermatophyte infection and can be particularly difficult to clear once infected. In closed colony settings, dermatophyte testing by culture is highly recommended unless the source of the cat excludes the possibility of infection (e.g., specific pathogen-free [SPF] cats, purpose-bred laboratory cats). To screen cats using cultures, samples should be collected using the McKenzie toothbrush method, where a new toothbrush is used to brush the cat's entire body, giving special attention to the face, ears, and limbs. In addition, if skin lesions are present, hair should be plucked around these areas for culture as well.

Enteric Pathogens

Campylobacter, Salmonella, Giardia, coccidia, *Tritrichomonas,* and other gastrointestinal parasites and pathogens are common in some cattery situations and can be very difficult to eliminate once they are introduced. In fact, in some settings, these pathogens may become endemic and nearly impossible to eliminate. Treatment of coccidia in shelter kittens is described in Box 46-5. Although clinical signs, such as diarrhea, may be associated with infection, some cats remain asymptomatic. These pathogens have the potential for high morbidity in a population (especially in young kittens), and some possess zoonotic potential. Therefore routine fecal examinations, cultures, and/or empirical treatments should be considered prior to the introduction of new cats.

Vaccination

It is well recognized that vaccination plays a vital role in the prevention and control of infectious diseases. Protocols should be established in the context of the population's exposure risk, which will vary depending upon the setting. In the context of population medicine, vaccination protocols are typically applied uniformly to all of the individuals comprising the population. This simplifies their application and helps to afford the best possible protection for the group. Detailed vaccination records should be maintained for each cat, including vaccine name, manufacturer and serial number, date, the initials of the person who administered it, and any adverse reactions.[96]

Proper vaccination can substantially reduce disease in cat populations, and serious adverse reactions are relatively rare. For this reason, vaccination against certain core diseases is recommended in all population settings. Although exclusion of infectious disease is always a goal of health management, certain pathogens are so widespread that even with careful biosecurity in a closed population, an infection may be introduced to susceptible cats. Only in the case of specific pathogen-free colonies, where there may be a compelling reason not to vaccinate as dictated by the purposes of the research, should vaccination be foregone. The AAFP maintains published guidelines for vaccination of cats in a variety of settings and includes detailed recommendations for cats in animal shelters.[96]

BOX 46-5

Ponazuril for Control of Coccidia in Multicat Environments

Ponazuril is a metabolite of toltrazuril that has proven activity against coccidia.* Because there is no approved product for use in cats, the equine product Marquis Oral Paste (15% w/w ponazuril; Bayer HealthCare) may be dosed at 50 mg/kg, PO, once daily for 1 to 5 days. Prophylactic treatment may be instituted in high-risk situations, such as young kittens in environments with documented infection. Proper hygiene, including the use of disposable litter boxes and frequent removal of feces, is also necessary. Oocysts survive in the environment and are not treated by routine disinfectants, such as bleach and quaternary ammonium compounds.

Preparation of the equine product for use in cats:
10 mL Marquis Oral Paste added to 20 mL water = 30 mL of 50 mg/mL oral suspension

*Data from Lloyd S, Smith J: Activity of toltrazuril and diclazuril against *Isospora* species in kittens and puppies, *Vet Rec* 148:509, 2001.

Core Vaccines for the Population: Feline Viral Rhinotracheitis, Calicivirus, Panleukopenia (FVRCP)

Although many vaccines are commercially available for cats, only a few are recommended for routine use in populations. Unnecessary use of vaccines should be avoided to minimize the incidence of adverse reactions and reduce cost. Core vaccines involve diseases that represent significant morbidity and mortality and for which vaccination has been demonstrated to provide relatively good protection against disease. Core vaccines for cats in a population setting include feline parvovirus (FPV or panleukopenia), FHV-1 (feline herpes virus type 1 or feline rhinotracheitis virus), and feline calicivirus (FCV).[96] These vaccines are usually given in a combination product commonly referred to as an FVRCP vaccine (feline viral rhinotracheitis, calicivirus, panleukopenia).

In most cases, timely vaccination against panleukopenia will prevent the development of clinical disease. In contrast, vaccination against the respiratory viruses (FHV-1 and FCV) does not always prevent disease. In many instances, it affords only partial protection, lessening the severity of clinical signs but not preventing infection. To optimize response, modified live vaccines (MLV) should be used in most cases, because they evoke a more rapid and robust immune response and are better at overcoming maternal antibody interference than killed products. This is especially important in multicat environments in which the risk of infection is high, such as animal shelters, foster homes, as well as any population setting where upper respiratory disease is endemic. A single modified live FVRCP vaccine will usually afford protection to cats that are at least 4 months of age. In contrast, killed products require a booster in 2 to 3 weeks to confer immunity, making their use largely ineffective in such environments.[96]

To ensure rapid protection against panleukopenia, injectable FVRCP vaccines are preferred, but intranasal vaccines may offer advantages for feline respiratory disease, because they have been shown to rapidly induce local immunity at the site of exposure. Furthermore, intranasal vaccines may be better at overriding maternal antibody in young kittens. For this reason, they are often used to reduce the morbidity and severity of upper respiratory infection (URI) in preweaning-age kittens. When intranasal vaccines are used in animal shelters, they should be used in combination with injectable FVRCP vaccines to ensure and optimize response against panleukopenia as well as the respiratory infections.[96]

Ideally, all cats should receive a MLV FVRCP vaccine at least 1 week prior to entering a population. In the context of an animal shelter setting, this is seldom feasible. Vaccination immediately upon entry is the next best practice and can provide clinically significant protection for the majority of cats. If neither maternal antibody nor another cause of vaccine failure interferes, modified live vaccinations against panleukopenia will often confer protection against disease in only 5 days.[12] Intranasal vaccines against respiratory infections, including FHV and FCV, typically provide partial protection within 2 to 4 days.[18,30]

In animal shelters, all incoming cats and kittens 4 weeks of age and older that can be safely handled should receive an injectable MLV FVRCP vaccine immediately upon entry. A delay of even a day or two significantly compromises the vaccine's ability to provide timely protection. Even injured cats, those with medical conditions, and those that are pregnant or lactating should be vaccinated on entry, because vaccination will likely be effective and the small risk of adverse effects is outweighed by the high risk of disease exposure and infection in the shelter.[96] When vaccination of all cats on entry is not financially feasible, the next best practice is to vaccinate all those that are deemed adoptable at the time of entry or that are likely to be in the shelter long term.[41] Whenever possible, vaccinated cats should be separated from those that will remain unvaccinated (e.g., those that will be euthanized following a brief holding period) as soon as that determination can be made.

In contrast, in lower-risk settings, ensuring that cats are in good health prior to vaccination should be a priority.[96] Vaccination of kittens with injectable FVRCP vaccinations may be delayed to 6 to 8 weeks of age. However, when respiratory disease is endemic, administration of intranasal vaccines beginning at 4 weeks of age may be beneficial. In breeding catteries, queens (especially those with a history of upper respiratory infection) may benefit from vaccination prior to breeding to maximize passage of maternal antibody to their kittens. For pregnant cats in such environments, administration of MLV should be avoided, because the potential risk of injury to the developing kittens may outweigh the risk of infection in this case. Vaccination of lactating queens should also be avoided in a low-risk environment.

A series of vaccinations should be administered to kittens less than 4 months of age to minimize the window of susceptibility to infection and ensure that a vaccine is received as soon as possible after maternal antibodies have decreased sufficiently to allow vaccine response.[96] For kittens, vaccines should be administered every 2 to 4 weeks until they are 16 weeks (e.g., 4 months) of age or their permanent incisors have erupted. The minimum interval of 2 weeks is recommended in high-risk settings to narrow the window of susceptibility as maternal antibody wanes. A vaccination interval of less than 2 weeks is not recommended, because it may actually blunt the immune response from previous vaccination.[40] In the case of an outbreak of panleukopenia, extending vaccination to 5 months of age may be warranted to ensure than no animal remains susceptible. Although the vast majority will respond by 4 months of age, a few may fail to respond, while others are provided with a boost to enhance the immune response.

Just as in owned pets, booster vaccines are generally not required until 1 year later for modified live vaccines but should ideally be administered once in 2 to 4 weeks whenever resources permit. This may be especially important for cats that were ill at the time of initial vaccination, as may be the case in an animal shelter. Revaccination in long-term shelter facilities should follow the guidelines set forth for pets: Boost at one year, then every 3 years for FVRCP.[96]

Rabies Vaccination

Vaccination against rabies virus is regarded as a core requirement for pet cats and is required by law in some jurisdictions.[96] Thus vaccination against rabies is recommended in the context of private catteries. In contrast, rabies vaccination may be considered optional in most closed laboratory settings, because the risk of exposure should be absent and legal requirements may not apply. In animal shelters, vaccination against rabies is not generally recommended at the time of admission, simply because there is no benefit in terms of disease prevention or public health.[96] Vaccination on admission will not provide protection against an infection acquired prior to entry, nor will it limit concern if a cat with an unknown health history bites someone soon after admission. Rabies vaccination is recommended for cats prior to adoption when a veterinarian is available to administer it (or as otherwise legally prescribed by state laws). Alternatively, rabies vaccination may be administered as soon as possible following adoption.[41] The latter may encourage new owners to establish a relationship with a private veterinarian. Rabies vaccination is warranted when cats are housed long term in shelter facilities. In addition, if individual cats must be held for bite quarantines, they should be vaccinated against rabies in accordance with the current Compendium of Animal Rabies Prevention and Control.[85]

Noncore Vaccines

Noncore vaccines include those that may offer protection against disease, but because the disease in question is not widespread or only poses a risk of exposure in certain circumstances, vaccination is only recommended based on the individual risk assessment of a population of animals. Noncore vaccines include FeLV, FIV, *Chlamydophila,* and *Bordetella.*[96]

FELINE LEUKEMIA VIRUS

Vaccination against FeLV is not warranted in a closed population of cats in which there is no risk of exposure (e.g., most laboratory animal settings). In private catteries, a risk assessment should be done to determine if vaccination is warranted (e.g., cats permitted in outdoor enclosures, frequent introduction of cats from external sources, other opportunities for exposure). Special consideration should be given to vaccinating kittens because of their high susceptibility to FeLV infection and the high likelihood that they will become persistently infected if exposed. In general, FeLV vaccination is not recommended in animal shelters when cats are housed short term. However, its use is warranted when cats are group housed when resources permit.[96]

FELINE IMMUNODEFICIENCY VIRUS

FIV vaccination is not generally recommended in population environments. A confounding feature of FIV vaccination is that vaccinated cats develop false-positive test results on most commercially available tests (see Chapter 33). If FIV vaccination is elected, vaccinated cats should be permanently identified (e.g., by use of a microchip) to help clarify their status.[96]

CHLAMYDOPHILA AND *BORDETELLA*

Chlamydophila felis (C. psittaci) and *Bordetella bronchiseptica* vaccines may be of benefit when clinical signs of these diseases are present in the population and diagnosis is confirmed by laboratory evaluation. Their efficacy is moderate, and reactions are more common than with most other feline vaccines; therefore ongoing use should be periodically reassessed.[96]

Vaccines Not Recommended

Some vaccines are not generally recommended for use because of undemonstrated efficacy, such as the feline infectious peritonitis (FIP) vaccine.[96]

Parasite Control and Prevention

Control and prevention of internal and external parasites represent another important component of a population wellness program. Common products used for their management are described elsewhere in this book. Of particular importance are roundworms and hookworms, common intestinal parasites with zoonotic potential (see Chapter 23). Although uncommon, the risk of human infection from contaminated environments is real and can result in organ damage, blindness, and skin infections. For this reason, the Centers for Disease Control and Prevention and the Companion Animal Parasite Council strongly advise routine administration of broad-spectrum anthelminthics for their control.[17,20] Pyrantel pamoate is one of the most cost-effective and efficacious drugs for treatment and control of roundworms and hookworms. In both shelter and cattery settings, the author recommends administration of pyrantel pamoate at a dosage of 10 mg/kg to all cats with re-treatment in 2 weeks and then at monthly intervals.[41] In shelters, if it is not possible to treat all cats at the time of entry, at a minimum, all cats that are deemed adoptable should be treated as soon as possible. In addition, kittens should be treated at 2-week intervals until 4 months of age. For cats with diarrhea, fecal examination (e.g., flotation or centrifugation, direct fecal smear and cytology) should be performed with treatment according to results. Even if results are negative, the administration of broad-spectrum anthelminthics should be strongly considered.

In animal shelters, ectoparasites, particularly ear mites and fleas, are also very common in cats and kittens. Shelter staff should be trained to recognize infestation and protocols should be established for treatment. In terms of shelter treatment protocols, the author recommends treating ear mites with ivermectin, because it is highly efficacious and costs only pennies per dose. The recommended dosage is 0.3 mg/kg subcutaneously. For fleas, the author recommends topical treatment with fipronil (Frontline, Merial, Duluth, Ga.) as a spray or top spot. In particular, the spray is very cost effective. It is safe for use in cats of all ages, including pregnant and nursing mothers and neonatal kittens. In addition, fipronil also has activity against ear mites, *Cheyetiella*, chewing lice, and ticks.[19,100]

Spaying and Neutering

Spaying and neutering is another important consideration in the context of population wellness.[41] Reproductive stress from estrous cycling in queens and sex drive in tomcats can decrease appetite, increase urine spraying/marking and intermale fighting, and profoundly increase social and emotional stress in the group. For these reasons, spaying and neutering cats that will not be used for breeding is recommended. In animal shelters, spaying and neutering cats prior to adoption will ensure that they do not reproduce and contribute to the surplus of community cats. This will also serve to enhance husbandry, because the procedures rapidly decrease spraying, marking, and fighting; eliminate heat behavior and pregnancy; and greatly mitigate stress. In addition to reducing stress and odor, spaying and neutering sexually mature cats will facilitate group housing, which is often beneficial for cats, especially when housed longer term (see below). The medical benefits of spay/neuter have also been well described, including dramatic reductions in the risk of mammary carcinoma, elimination of cystic endometrial hyperplasia, pyometra and ovarian cancer in queens, and decreased risk of prostate disease in toms.[55] Thus spaying and neutering favors both individual as well as population health.

Proper Nutrition

Proper nutrition has a profound impact on wellness. Not only is it essential for management of healthy body weight and condition, good nutrition is also known to support immune function. A regular diet of palatable commercial food consistent with life stage should be offered, and fresh water must always be available. Although some cats tolerate changes in food without apparent problems, it is important to recognize that for others, changing from one diet to another can cause loss of appetite and/or gastrointestinal upset. For this reason, it is generally best to provide the most consistent diet possible.[49] Whereas this may be relatively easy to do in a laboratory or cattery setting, it can be more challenging in a shelter environment. Some pet food companies offer feeding programs for animal shelters, providing a consistent food for purchase at a special rate for shelters. However, some shelters rely heavily on donations of food. In this case, by requesting donation of certain brands of food, shelters are able to provide a consistent diet whenever possible. It is also feasible to mix donated foods with the shelter's usual diet to minimize problems caused by abrupt diet changes while taking advantage of other donated products.

Free Choice versus Meal Feeding

The wild ancestors of domestic cats hunted to eat, feeding up to 30 times in a 24-hour period. This style of feeding behavior is preferred by many domestic cats that would nibble throughout the day and night, consuming many small meals if left to their own devices. Although this is true, most cats are capable of adapting to either free choice or meal feeding as their daily feeding pattern.[15,49] There are advantages and disadvantages to each in a population setting.

With free choice or *ad libitum* feeding, food is always available such that a cat can eat as much as he or she wants whenever he or she chooses. Dry food is used for this method of feeding, because canned products left at room temperature are prone to spoiling. The major advantage of free choice feeding is that it is quick and easy: Caregivers simply need to ensure that fresh dry food is always available. Major disadvantages include the fact that cats that are not eating may remain unrecognized for several days, especially when more than one animal is fed together, and some cats may choose to continually overeat and become obese. Free choice feeding is an excellent method for cats that require frequent food consumption. These include kittens up to 5 to 6 months of age, queens in late gestation, and those that are nursing. Unlike dogs, who are competitive eaters by nature, free choice feeding may benefit cats that are group housed, because it ensures that there will be ample time for all members to eat, provided that dominant members of the colony do not block the access of subordinate cats.[49]

Meal feeding using controlled portions of dry and/or canned food may be done as an alternative to or in conjunction with free choice feeding. When used alone, a minimum of two meals should be fed per day.[49] Meal feeding is ideal for any cat that requires controlled food intake and facilitates monitoring of appetite. Meal feeding also has the benefit of enhancing caregiver–cat bonding and provides a pleasant and predictable experience for cats when done on a regular daily schedule. Using a combination of free choice plus once daily meal feeding takes advantage of the positive aspects of both methods and works well for most cats in a population setting. Typically, dry food is available free choice, and a small meal of canned food is offered once daily. This combination approach accommodates the normal feeding behavior of cats by allowing them to eat several smaller meals throughout the day while allowing caregivers to monitor the cat's appetite at least for the canned food meal. As necessary for the individual cat, some may be fed additional meals of canned food to ensure adequate nutritional support.

Monitoring

Good body weight and condition and a healthy hair coat are evidence of an adequate nutritional plane and proper nutritional management. Both appetite and stool quality should be monitored daily. Normal stools should be well-formed and medium to dark brown. Adult cats typically defecate once daily, although healthy adults may defecate anywhere between twice a day and twice a week. Kittens tend to produce a larger volume of stool more frequently, which is often lighter in color and softer in form than that of adults. Simple scales can be used for monitoring appetite (e.g., good, some, none), and fecal scoring charts are available. The author recommends the Purina Fecal Scoring System chart available from Nestlé Purina PetCare Company (Figure 46-7).

Fecal Scoring System

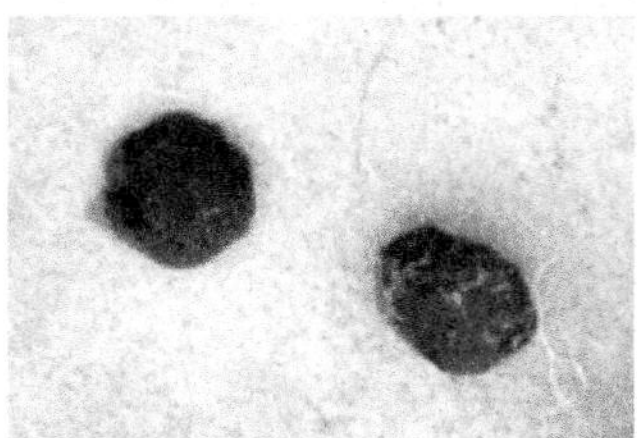

Score 1 - Very hard and dry; requires much effort to expel from body; no residue left on ground when picked up. Often expelled as individual pellets.

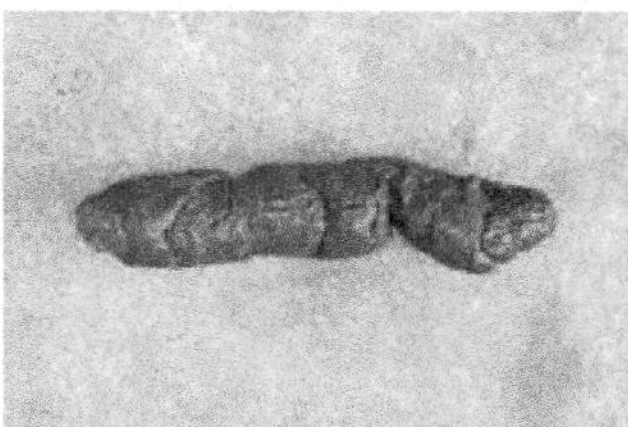

Score 2 - Firm, but not hard; should be pliable; segmented appearance; little or no residue left on ground when picked up.

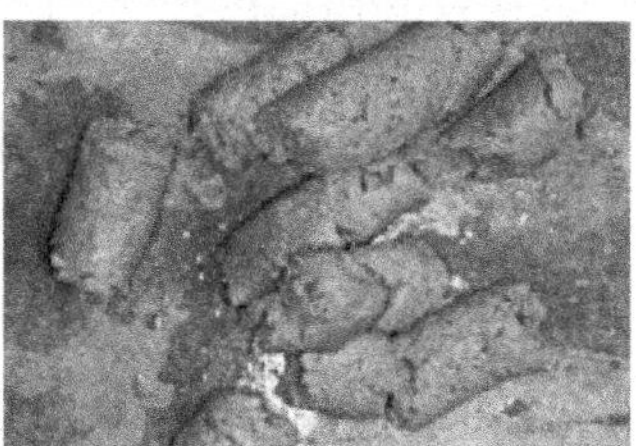

Score 3 - Log-like; little or no segmentation visible; moist surface; leaves residue, but holds form when picked up.

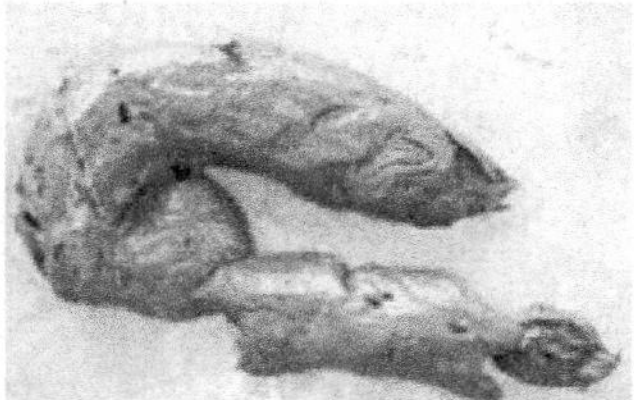

Score 4 - Very moist (soggy); distinct log shape visible; leaves residue and loses form when picked up.

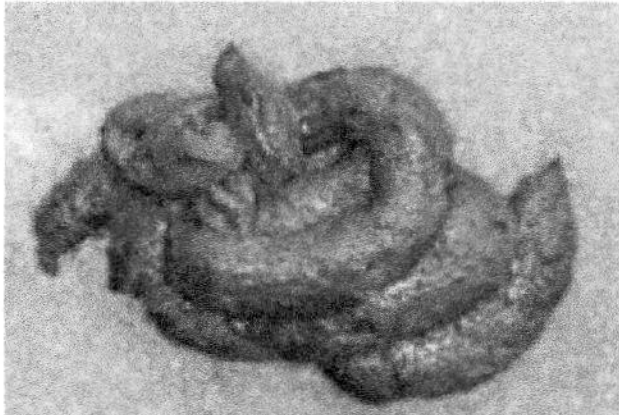

Score 5 - Very moist but has distinct shape; present in piles rather than as distinct logs; leaves residue and loses form when picked up.

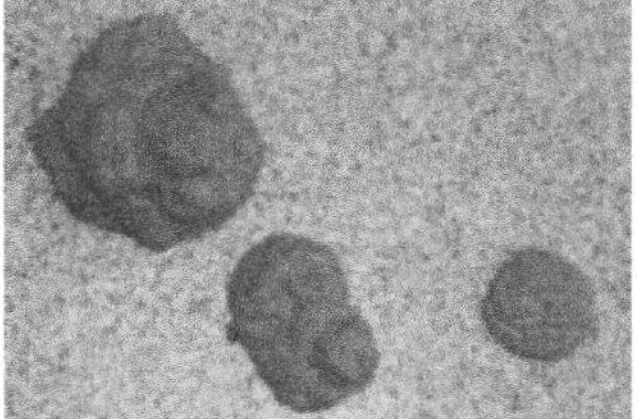

Score 6 - Has texture, but no defined shape; occurs as piles or as spots; leaves residue when picked up.

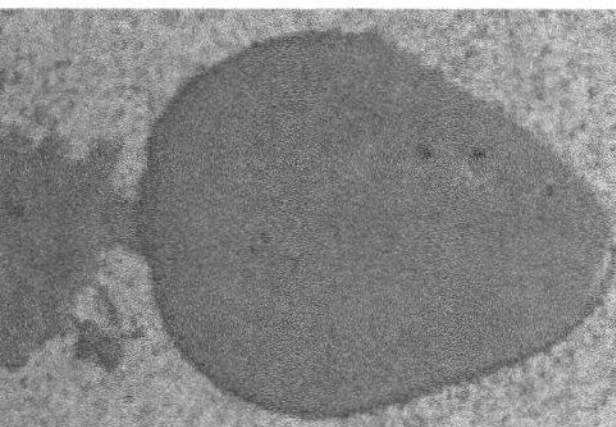

Score 7 - Watery, no texture, flat; occurs as puddles.

Nestlé PURINA
Trademarks owned by Société des Produits Nestlé S.A., Vevey, Switzerland

FIGURE 46-7 Fecal scoring system. *(Courtesy Nestlé Purina.)*

In addition to appetite and stool quality, it is essential to monitor body weight and condition. Body condition can be subjectively assessed by a process called body condition scoring, which involves assessing fat stores and, to a lesser extent, muscle mass. Fat cover is evaluated over the ribs, down the top line, tail base, and along the ventral abdomen and inguinal (groin) areas. Body condition score charts have been established on scales of 1 to 5 and 1 to 9. The author recommends use of the Purina body condition score chart which is based on a scale of 1 to 9 with 1 being emaciated and 9 being severely obese (see Figure 3-3).

Cats should be weighed and their body condition scored at routine intervals. Ideally, body weight should be recorded at entry to the population and then weekly during the initial month of care, after which it could be recorded once a month or more often as indicated based on the individual's condition. This is especially important for cats, because significant or even dramatic weight loss may be associated with stress or illness during the first few weeks of confinement in a new setting. On the other hand, in long-term–housed cats, excessive weight gain may occur in some individuals. Therefore protocols must be in place to identify and manage unhealthy trends in body weight, because both weight loss and gain can compromise health and well-being.

Grooming

Appropriate grooming is also essential to ensure wellness and must never be considered as optional or purely cosmetic. Most cats require minimal grooming because of their fastidious nature. However, long-haired cats are notable exceptions, often experiencing matting of the hair coat without regular grooming sessions. Matted hair coats are not only uncomfortable for the animal, but may lead to skin infection. Overgrown nails can also be a problem for some cats, particularly those that are geriatric or polydactyl. The provision of appropriate surfaces for scratching will encourage cats to condition their own claws; and a system for regular inspection of the hair coat and nails should be established. In addition to ensuring proper coat and nail maintenance, regular grooming sessions provide an excellent opportunity to monitor body condition; and some cats enjoy the physical contact and attention. In high-risk settings, the use of stainless steel combs or undercoat rakes that can be readily disinfected are generally preferable to the use of bristle brushes because the latter are impossible to disinfect and have the potential to spread common skin infections such as ringworm.

Periodontal Disease Prevention

Dental health is another component of wellness. In the context of population wellness, it may not be the highest priority; however, it should always be a consideration in terms of individual health care and well-being. This is important because periodontal disease will occur unless it is actively prevented, and plaque and tartar buildup may contribute to serious health concerns, ranging from oral pain to chronic intermittent bacteremia and organ failure. Feline tooth resorption and gingivostomatitis are also common conditions of the feline oral cavity that can lead to chronic pain, affecting the cat's appetite and ability to self-groom, and negatively impacting quality of life. When painful dental disease is present, a plan for timely treatment should be identified and implemented. Preventive dental care may include tooth brushing, dental-friendly diets, and treats and chew toys in combination with periodic professional dental care.[33] These should be tailored to meet the needs of individuals in the population to optimize dental health. Cats with stomatitis should be removed from breeding programs.[72]

Breed-Specific Care

Wellness protocols may also be dictated by the specific needs of certain breeds of cats. For example, Persian, Himalayan, and other brachycephalic cats are predisposed to respiratory disease and tend to be more severely affected than other cats because of their poor airway conformation. Because of the high likelihood of exposure in a shelter setting, these cats should be housed in highly biosecure areas that are well ventilated and should be prioritized for immediate adoption or transfer to foster care or rescue.[41] In the author's experience, even intranasal vaccination of these breeds can result in severe clinical signs of respiratory disease and is best avoided.

DEVELOPING A POPULATION WELLNESS PROGRAM: CONSIDERATIONS FOR BEHAVIORAL HEALTH

Just as a physical wellness program must be tailored to the population in question, a behavioral wellness program, composed of all of the essential elements, should be created to meet its specific needs as well. Even when animals will only be housed for short periods, considerations for behavioral care are essential to ensure humane care. Short-term confinement can induce severe stress and anxiety, and when confined long term, cats may suffer from social isolation, inadequate mental stimulation, and lack of exercise. A behavioral wellness program should strive to decrease stress from the moment cats arrive at a facility until the moment that their stay ends. As previously described, a thorough behavioral history will provide an important baseline for action and follow-up.

Behavioral Care at Intake

Understanding the importance of minimizing stress in cats and possessing the ability to recognize and respond to it are essential to facilitate a cat's transition into a population.[42,46] Staff should be trained to evaluate cats beginning at intake and to recognize and respond to indicators of stress. Active daily monitoring of cats for signs of stress or adjustment should be performed, and staff should record their findings daily, noting trends and making adjustments in the care of individual cats and the population as indicated.

In animal shelter environments, proper behavioral care of cats also requires an understanding of the wide spectrum of feline lifestyles and an approach tailored to the individual needs of each group. Domestic cat lifestyles and levels of tractability range from the most docile, sociable housecat, to free-roaming strays and truly unsocialized feral cats that will not allow handling. Stray cats include those that may have been previously owned or are "loosely owned" neighborhood or barn cats.[79]

Because of their lack of socialization, capture, handling, and confinement are especially stressful for feral cats. However, fearful cats may resort to overt aggressive or may "teeter on the edge" of defensive aggression regardless of their socialization status. In fact, even the tamest house cats may exhibit the same behaviors as feral cats when they are highly stressed (Figure 46-8).[29,42] These responses can compromise cat welfare and staff safety and hinder adaptation to a new environment.

Regardless of their demeanor, all cats and kittens should be provided with a hiding box in their enclosure at the time of entry, because the ability to hide has been shown to substantially reduce feline stress.[14] For those cats that are severely stressed or reactive, covering the cage front, in addition to providing a hiding box, and posting signage to allow the cat "chill out" time for several hours or even a few days can facilitate adaptation.[42] This is important because, once highly stressed or provoked, cats often remain reactive for a prolonged time and may become more reactive if they are stimulated again before they have been allowed a period of time to calm down.[9]

Soft bedding should be available for comfort and so that cats may establish a familiar scent, which aides in acclimation to a new environment. Care should be taken during cleaning procedures to minimize stress and noise,

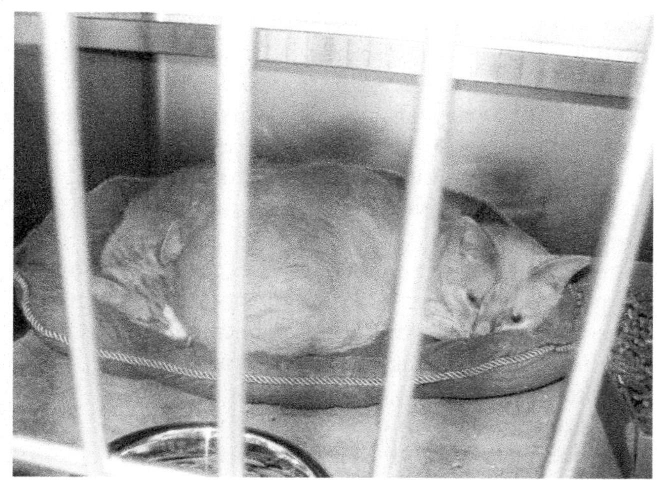

FIGURE 46-8 The behavioral responses of pampered house cats and feral cats may be indistinguishable at the time of intake to an animal shelter. Two cats exhibit signs of severe stress and fear—crouched and withdrawn in the back of a cage with dilated pupils, feigning sleep. Note the presence of the second cat hiding behind the first. The provision of an appropriate hiding box could greatly aid stress reduction for these cats.

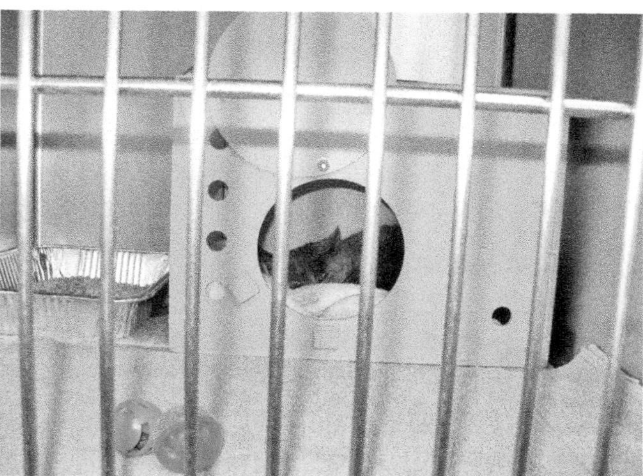

FIGURE 46-9 A commercially available feral cat den (ACES, Boulder, Colo.) serves as a secure hiding place for a cat. The circular door can be closed from a safe and nonthreatening distance while the cage is spot cleaned as needed. The cat can also be securely transported in the den.

and cats should be allowed to hide while their cage is quietly tidied and replenished around them as needed. Commercially available "cat dens" are ideal for this purpose, because they can be secured from a safe distance such that the cat is closed inside a secure, familiar hiding place during cleaning procedures (Figure 46-9). Cats should be returned to the same cage and only spot cleaning should be performed to preserve their scent, which is necessary for stress reduction. If it becomes necessary to house the cat in another location, the den and towel should accompany the cat to ease the transition. Finally, the use of commercially available synthetic analogues of naturally occurring feline facial pheromones (Feliway, Veterinary Product laboratories, Phoenix, Ariz.) have been shown to be useful for stress reduction in cats during acclimation to new environments and can be sprayed onto bedding and allowed to dry prior to use or dispersed in the room using plug-in diffusers.[48]

The way in which cats are handled at intake has a profound impact on their behavior, health, and well-being and will impact the cat's ability to adapt to its new environment. When stress is successfully mitigated, cats are more likely to adapt and to "show their true colors" rather than reacting defensively. During a period of a few days, many cats that did not appear to be "friendly" at intake will become tractable and responsive to their human caregivers, facilitating care.[42]

Behavioral Evaluation

Aside from informally "getting to know" cats during their initial acclimation period in a facility, a systematic behavioral evaluation may be useful, especially for cats that will be re-homed. Several evaluations have been recommended, but none are scientifically validated for predicting future behavior with certainty.[3,103,107] Nonetheless, this form of evaluation may be useful for determining behavioral needs while cats remain in a facility, as well as guiding appropriate placement. Box 46-6 describes common components of a feline behavioral evaluation (Figure 46-10).

Proper Housing

Housing design and operation can literally make or break the health of a population.[45] Regardless of the species in question, housing should always include a comfortable resting area and allow animals to engage in species-typical behaviors while ensuring freedom from fear and distress.[54] It is not sufficient for the design to address only an animal's physical needs (e.g., shelter, warmth). It must meet their behavioral needs as well, and both the structural and social environment are essential considerations for housing arrangements. Furthermore, the environment must provide opportunities for both physical and mental stimulation, which become increasingly important as length of stay increases.[54]

A sense of control over conditions is well recognized as one of the most critical needs for behavioral health.[77] Thus housing design must provide cats with a variety of satisfying behavioral options. Specifically, housing arrangements must take into account the following feline behavioral needs[46]:

- Opportunities for social interactions with humans and/or other compatible cats

BOX 46-6

Typical Components of a Formal Behavioral Evaluation for Cats[3,103,107]

Responses are observed and recorded for each of the following:

Cage Side Evaluation

- The tester approaches cage, stands quietly for 20 seconds, then offers verbal encouragement.
- If deemed safe to proceed, tester opens the cage door and calmly extends an open hand towards the cat, then attempts to gently touch the cat's head.
- If the caregiver is unsure if this is safe to do, a plastic hand may be used to gauge the cat's receptiveness to touch (see Figure 46-9).
- If the cat allows handling, the cat is gently lifted and carried to a secure, quiet room for further observation.

In-Room Evaluation

- The tester sits quietly on a chair and/or the floor; the tester calls and solicits the cat's attention.
- The tester pets the cat on the head.
- The tester strokes the cat down the back several times.
- The tester picks up the cat and hugs it for 2 seconds.
- With the cat standing on the floor, the tester strokes the cat down the back and firmly but gently grasps the base of the tail and lifts the cat off of its hind feet for 1 second. The tester repeats this a second time.
- The tester engages the cat in play with an interactive toy.

- The ability to create different functional areas in the living environments for elimination, resting, and eating
- The ability to hide in a secure place
- The ability to rest/sleep without being disturbed
- The ability to change locations within the environment, including using vertical space for perching
- The ability to regulate body temperature by moving to warmer or cooler surfaces in the environment
- The ability to scratch (which is necessary for claw health and stretching, as well as visual and scent marking)
- The ability to play and exercise at will
- The ability to acquire mental stimulation

Because these needs will vary depending upon such factors as life stage, personality, and prior socialization and experience, facilities should maintain a variety of housing styles in order to meet the individual needs of different cats in the population (Figure 46-11).[46]

Feline Social Behavior

Managing housing arrangements for a population of cats of varying ages, genders, personality types, social experiences, and stress levels requires knowledge of normal feline social behavior and communication.[46] During the past 2 decades, knowledge of feline social structure has evolved from the widespread belief that cats are generally an asocial and solitary species to the realization that they are social creatures.[24,25] With the exception of solitary hunting, free-roaming cats perform

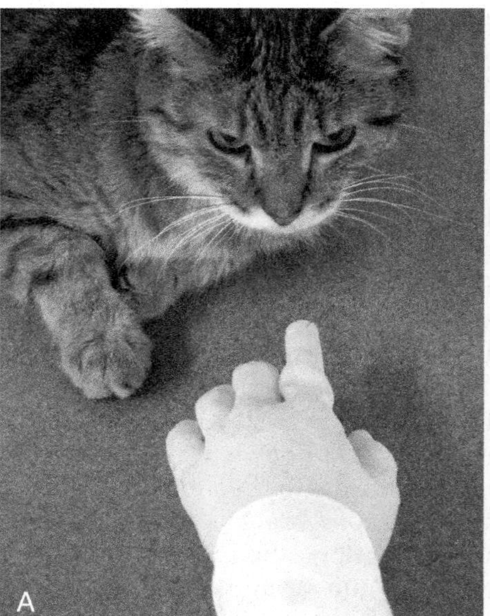

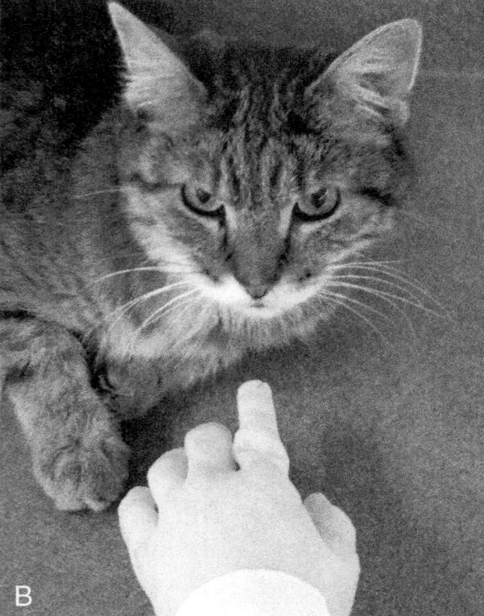

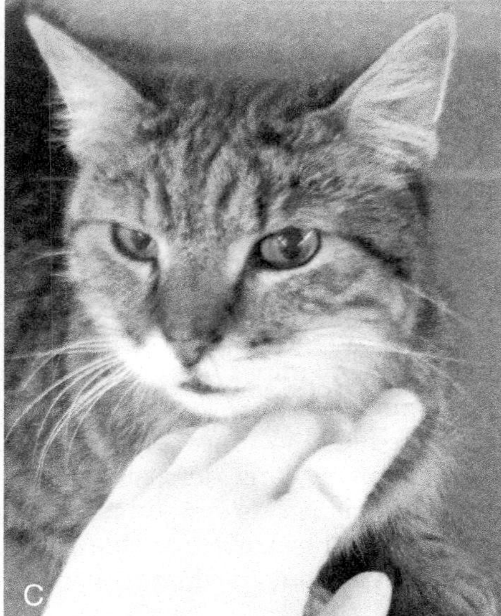

FIGURE 46-10 In some instances, it is difficult to determine if a cat will accept handling. To prevent injury to staff, a plastic hand (Assess-a-Hands; Great Dog Productions, Accord, NY) is used to approach this cat. As the hand approaches, the cat appears tense **(A)** but begins to relax and accepts petting (**B** and **C**).

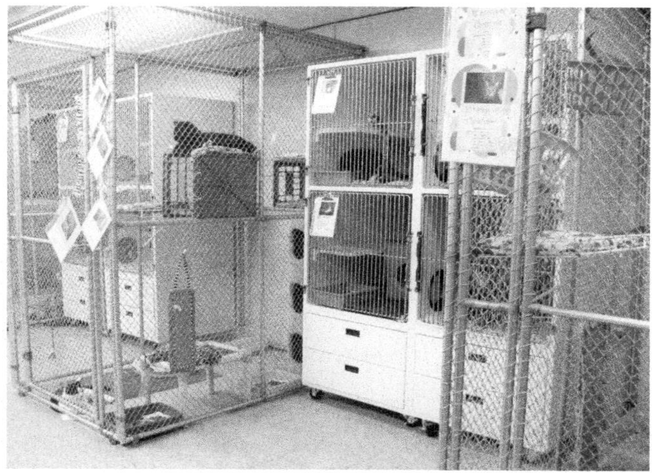

FIGURE 46-11 A combination of free-standing runs and condo units are used to house cats awaiting adoption in an animal shelter. The availability of a variety of housing styles facilitates meeting the individual needs of various cats in the population.

most of their activities within stable social groups where cooperative defense, cooperative care of young, and a variety of affiliative behaviors are practiced. Affiliative behaviors are those that facilitate close proximity or contact. Cats within groups commonly practice mutual grooming and allorubbing (e.g., rubbing heads and faces together). This may serve as a greeting or as an exchange of odor for recognition, familiarization, marking, or development of a communal scent. Cats of both genders and all ages may exhibit affiliative behaviors, and bonded housemates often spend a large proportion of their time in close proximity to one another.[8]

Maternal behavior is the primary social pattern of the female cat, and cooperative nursing and kitten care are common. If allowed, queens form social groups along with their kittens and juvenile offspring.[24,25] Tomcats typically reside within one group or roam between a few established groups. Within groups of cats, a social hierarchy or "pecking order" forms.[24,90] Once established, this hierarchy helps to support peaceful co-existence of cats within a stable group, minimizing agonistic behaviors between members. Social hierarchy formation occurs within groups of cats that are sexually intact, as well as in those that are neutered.

Feline Communication and Behavioral Signs of Stress

Knowledge of behavioral signaling is critical for successful management of housing arrangements. Manifestations of both normal and abnormal behavior indicate how successfully an animal is coping with its environment. Common behavioral expressions of feline anxiety may manifest with inhibited or withdrawal behavior, defensive behavior or disruptive behavior.[46,90] Inhibited or withdrawal behavior refers to activity depression or the absence of normal behaviors (e.g., grooming, eating, sleeping, eliminating, stretching, greeting people). Defensive behavior may involve characteristic postural and/or vocal responses, and is usually motivated by fear. Disruptive behavior involves destruction of cage contents and creation of a hiding place. Stereotypic behaviors (e.g., repetitive pacing, pawing, and circling) may also develop as a result of stress but generally occur less commonly. As an illustration of these feline behaviors, consider the responses of a typical social domestic cat when caged in a novel environment (Box 46-7 and Figures 46-12 to 46-15).

Behavioral signs of stress may be further classified as active communication signals or passive behaviors.[46,90] Signals of anxiety, fear, aggression, and submission may be subtle or obvious and include vocalization (growling, hissing), visual cues (facial expression, posturing of the body, ears, and tail), and scent marking (urine, feces, various glands of the skin).

Passive signs of stress include the inability to rest/sleep, feigned sleep, poor appetite, constant hiding, absence of grooming, activity depression (decreased play and exploratory behavior), and social withdrawal. High-density housing exacerbates these signs. Low-social-order cats in such an environment may exhibit decreased grooming, poor appetite, and silent estrus.[44] Cats that are consistently fearful or anxious may hide,

BOX 46-7

Typical Behavioral Responses of a Cat Caged in a Novel Environment[46]

- Fear is typically the initial response, and if threatened by the proximity of unfamiliar caregivers, defensive aggression may be displayed. Alternatively, the cat may freeze or appear catatonic.
- If provided with a box for concealment, the cat will hide or otherwise slink against the back of the enclosure, behind the litter box, or disrupt the cage and hide under the paper.
- Given time, most cats become more active and engage in greeting behaviors, coming to the front of the cage and pawing or mewing as caregivers approach.
- If the cat remains confined with time without adequate periods of exercise, mental stimulation, and social companionship, stress and frustration will manifest with activity depression and withdrawal (lying in the litter box, failure to groom, failure to greet caregivers, and, in some cases, displaying aggression towards caregivers).
- Displays of stereotypic behavior (such as pacing) may occur; however, inhibited or withdrawal behaviors are much more common (see Figures 46-12 to 46-15).

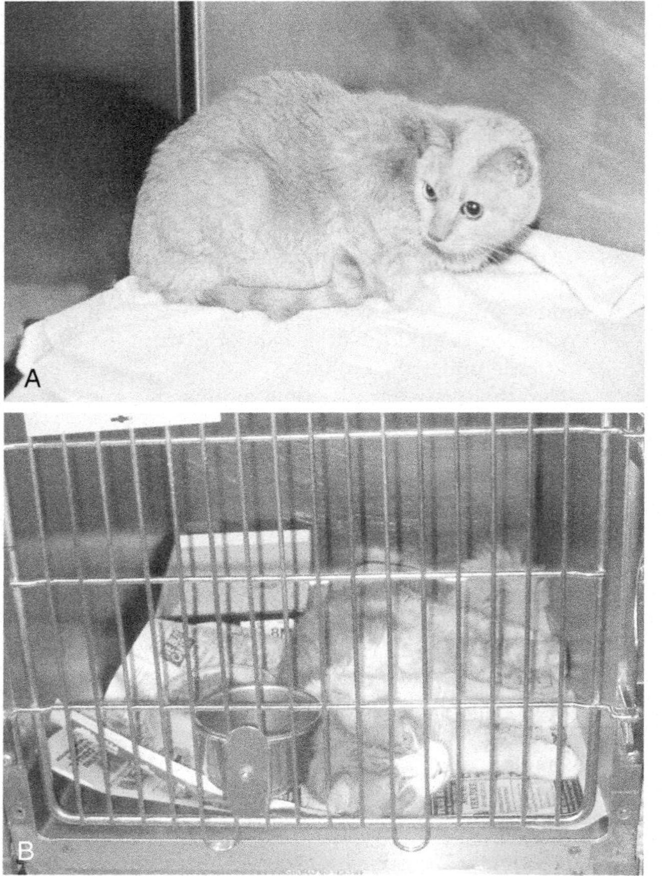

FIGURE 46-12 Feline stress commonly manifests with activity depression and social withdrawal. **A,** A caged cat exhibits signs of acute stress—crouched and withdrawn in the back of a cage with dilated pupils. **B,** Long-term cage confinement can result in frustration, activity withdrawal, and, in some cases, aggression. This cat lies helplessly in a cage with virtually no other behavioral options. Once friendly to caregivers, it may respond aggressively if handled. *(From Griffin B, Hume KR: Recognition and management of stress in housed cats. In August JR, editor:* Consultations in feline internal medicine, *vol 5, St Louis, 2006, Elsevier, p 717.)*

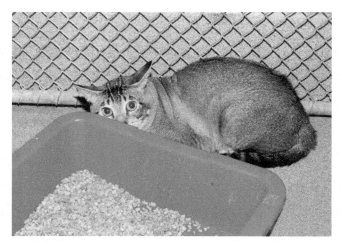

FIGURE 46-13 A stressed cat exhibits a marked fear response when caged and confronted. Note the frozen stance, dilated pupils, and sideways, flattened ears. If approached more closely, the cat would likely respond with defensive aggression if an escape route were not available. *(From Griffin B, Hume KR: Recognition and management of stress in housed cats. In August JR, editor:* Consultations in feline internal medicine, *vol 5, St Louis, 2006, Elsevier, p 717.)*

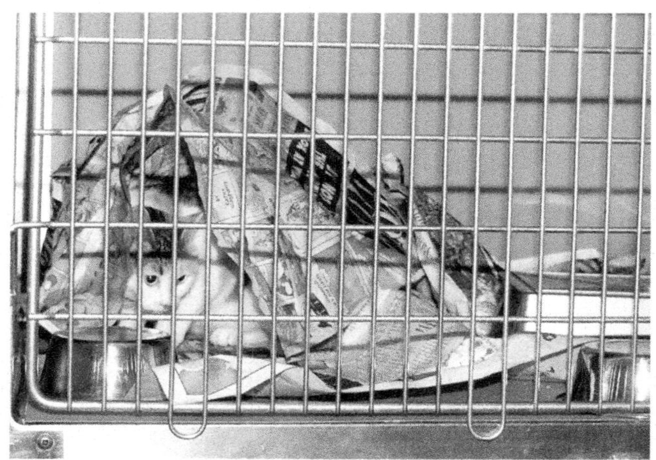

FIGURE 46-14 When caged in a novel environment, a typical response for a cat is to disrupt the cage contents and create a hiding place. *(From Griffin B, Hume KR: Recognition and management of stress in housed cats. In August JR, editor:* Consultations in feline internal medicine, *vol 5, St Louis, 2006, Elsevier, p 717.)*

turn their back, huddle, and avert their eyes from the gaze of other cats. Hiding is a normal and important coping behavior; however, when hiding is occurring with increased frequency or in response to stimuli that did not previously cause hiding, it should be recognized as a sign of stress.[46,90]

In group settings, the complexity of the social structure cannot be overestimated. The internal structure of social groups rarely represents a straightforward linear hierarchy, except in very small groups of less than four to five animals.[25] In larger groups of cats, there are usually one or two top-ranking individuals and one or two obvious subordinates, while the remaining cats share the middle space.[9,44] Most cats within the group form affiliative or friendly relationships; however, some may fail to form such relationships and remain solitary. Colony members commonly display aggression toward unfamiliar or new cats entering the group. Within an established group, however, most social conflicts are not characterized by overt aggression. Instead, the main mode of conflict resolution is avoidance or deference (Figure 46-16).[9,46,90] Deference behaviors include looking away, lowering the ears slightly, turning the head away, and leaning backward. Large numbers of cats peacefully co-exist together, using such strategies for avoidance provided ample space and resources are available for all members of the group.[10]

Signs of social stress within groups of cats may manifest with overt aggression, increased spraying and

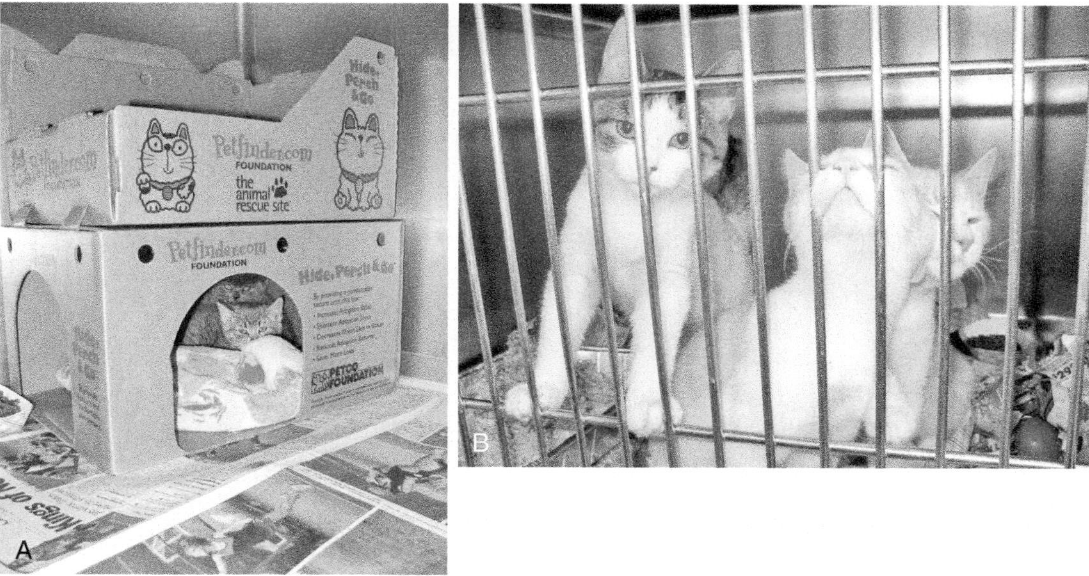

FIGURE 46-15 Hiding is frequently the initial response **(A),** but after a short period, many cats will solicit the attention of onlookers by pawing at the cage front **(B).**

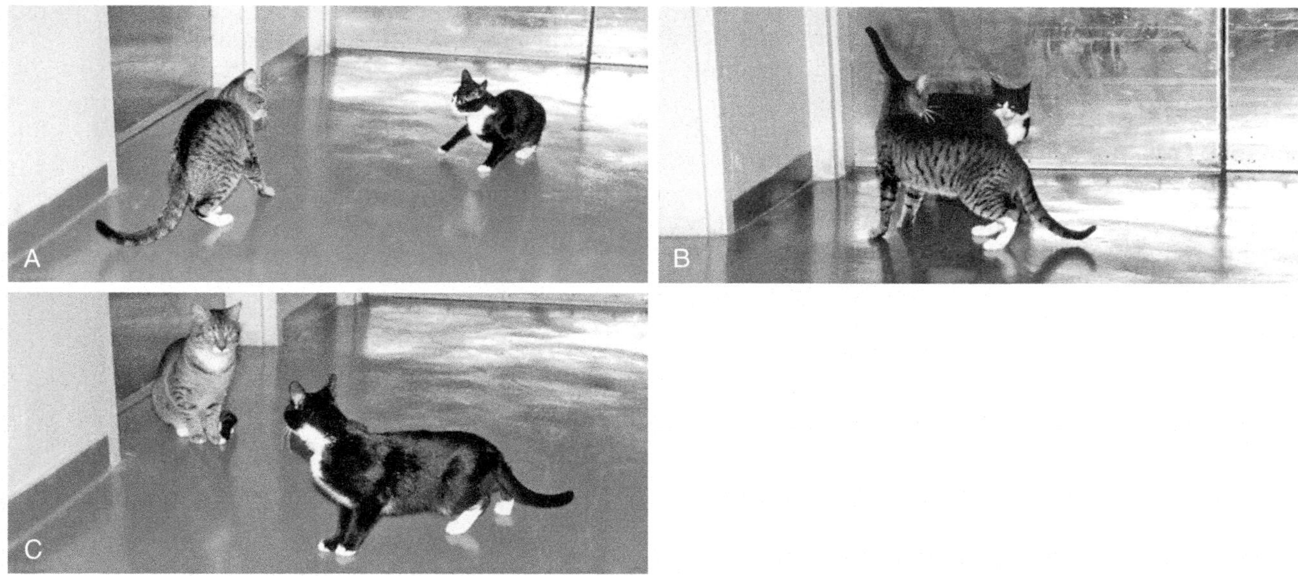

FIGURE 46-16 The major modes of conflict resolution for cats are deference and avoidance. **A,** An inquisitive cat *(left)* approaches a wary cat *(right).* **B,** The wary cat exhibits an offensive warning, signaling the approaching cat to stay away. **C,** Overt combat does not ensue, instead the cat on the left defers by simply sitting down a safe distance away. *(From Griffin B, Hume KR: Recognition and management of stress in housed cats. In August JR, editor:* Consultations in feline internal medicine, *vol 5, St Louis, 2006, Elsevier, p 717.)*

marking, or constant hiding.[46,90] Lower-ranking cats may spend little time on the floor, remaining isolated on single perches or other locations where they may even eliminate, while higher-ranking cats remain more mobile, controlling access to food, water, and litter resources.[44] High-density housing conditions frequently result in such abnormal behaviors and are associated with increases in transmission of infectious diseases and reproductive failure as well.[50]

Types of Housing Arrangements

Cats are commonly housed in three basic arrangements: cage or condo units, multiple runs within a room, or free ranging in a room.[45] Cage housing of cats should be avoided unless necessary for short periods for intake observation, legal holding periods in shelters as required by local ordinances, medical treatment or recovery, or to permit sample collection.[45] Although space recommendations vary substantially in the literature, common

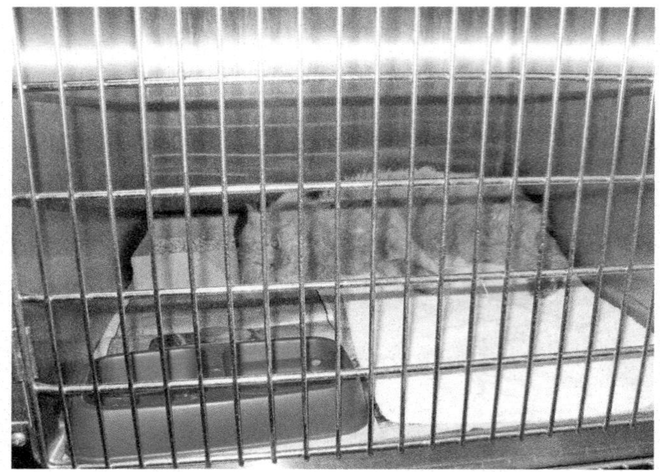

FIGURE 46-17 This housing arrangement is inadequate for the occupant. The small cage does not allow for an appropriately sized litter box, and there is not sufficient space for the cat to rest, move about, or hide.

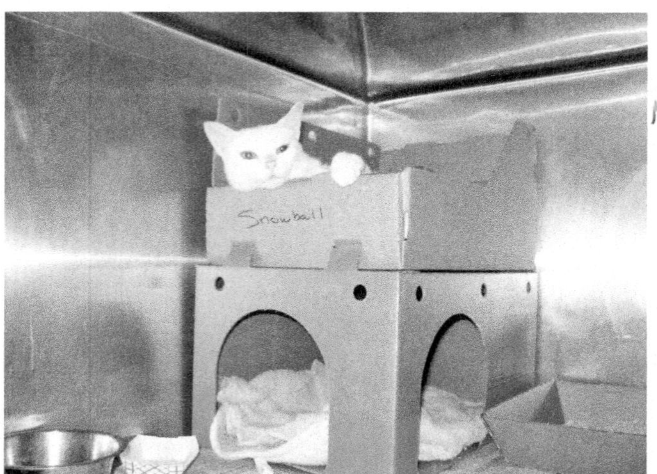

FIGURE 46-18 Traditional cage housing can be enhanced by the provision of proper resting perches and hiding places that divide the space into different functional living areas. Placement of a purpose-made cardboard box (Hide, Perch and Go Box, British Columbia Society for the Prevention of Cruelty to Animals) improves the quality of the space and the welfare of the cat. This box also folds into a transport carrier.

sense dictates that a determination of necessary housing space should take into account the cat's length of stay. In the author's opinion, it is neither appropriate nor humane to house cats in traditional cage housing long term (e.g., more than 1 to 2 weeks).

Short-Term Housing

The design of short-term housing should include provisions for housing individual animals, litters, families, or bonded housemates for intake evaluation and triage.[41] Housing must be easy to clean and sanitize, well ventilated, and safe for animals and caregivers. Short-term housing should provide sufficient space to comfortably stand, stretch, and walk several steps; sit or lay at full body length; and separate elimination, feeding, and resting areas. Litter boxes should be of appropriate size to comfortably accommodate the cats for which they are intended (Figure 46-17). Resting areas should include comfortable surfaces, soft bedding, and a secure hiding place to provide a safe refuge.[41] A hiding place is essential, because it reduces stress by allowing cats to "escape," facilitating adaptation to a new environment. The addition of a sturdy box to a cage will provide a hiding place as well as a perch (Figures 46-18 and 46-19). In addition, cages should be elevated off of the floor by at least 0.5 m (1.5 feet), because this serves to reduce stress as well.[73]

SIZE OF ENCLOSURES

In most instances, cage or condo style housing is used in most facilities for short-term holding at intake for observation, acclimation, and/or triage. Runs or small rooms are also appropriate for intake housing, and offer cats the obvious benefit of additional space to meet their behavioral needs (Figure 46-20). Regardless of their configuration, enclosures for short-term housing of cats should be large enough to allow them to stretch, groom, and move about while maintaining separate functional areas, at least 0.6 m (2 feet) apart, for sleeping, eating, and elimination.[41,58,98]

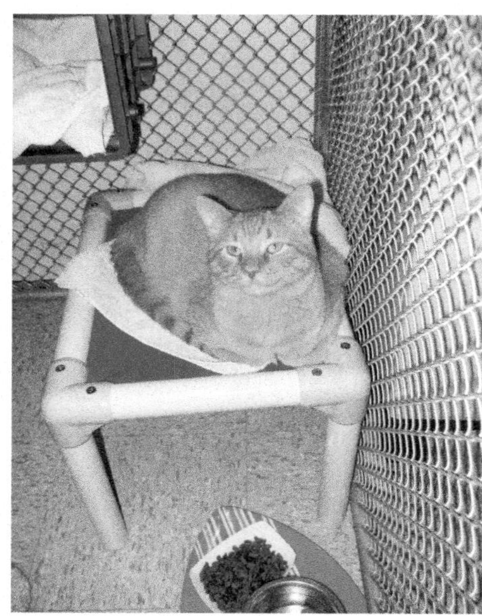

FIGURE 46-19 A perch and a bed are required for every cat, no matter what the housing arrangement. Portable perch-beds (Kuranda Cat Bed, Glen Burnie, Md.) can accompany the cat from intake cages to long-term housing to ease the transition to a new environment.

Laboratory guidelines in the United States call for a minimum floor area of 0.27 m^2 (3 ft^2) for cats weighing less than 4 kg and 0.36 m^2 (4 ft^2) for cats weighing 4 kg or more, with a minimum height 0.6 m (2 ft).[54] A resting

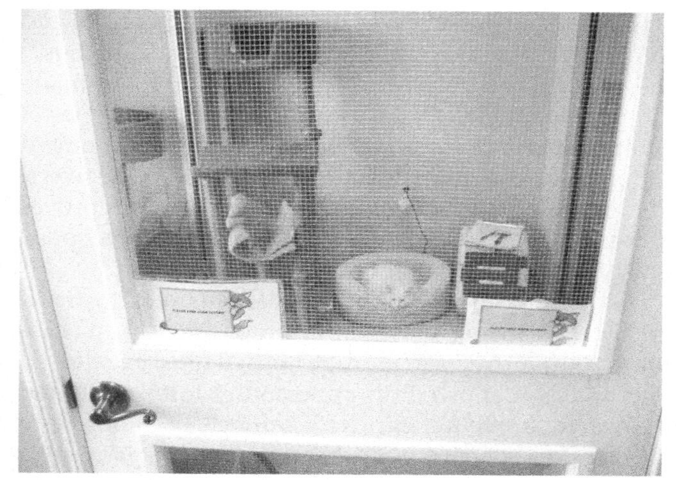

FIGURE 46-20 Single enriched housing in a 4 × 6 ft room for a shy cat during an acclimation period to a new facility. Note the multiple resting areas available and the use of a commercially available feline facial pheromone plug-in diffuser (Feliway, Veterinary Product Laboratories, Phoenix, Ariz.). The screen door facilitates ventilation as well olfactory exchange.

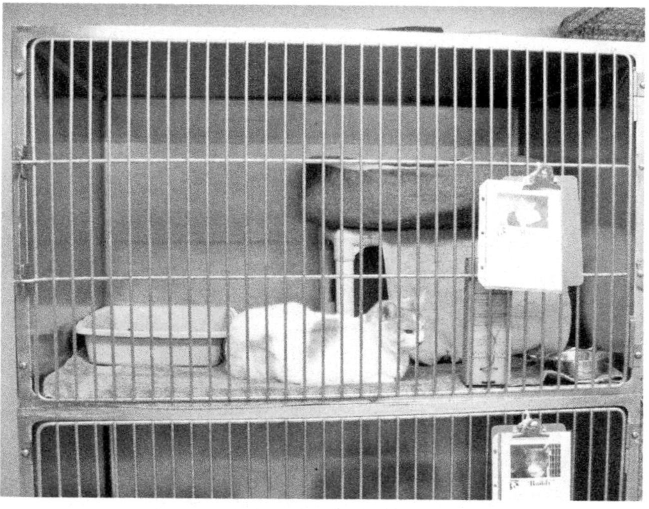

FIGURE 46-21 Appropriate short-term (e.g., less than 2 weeks) housing for a single cat. Note the large 4-ft long cage, provision of a secure hiding place and perch with bed, separation of litter from resting and feeding areas, and appropriately sized litter box for this large cat.

perch is also required. Current guidelines (European Convention for the Protection of Vertebrate Animals Used for Experimental and Other Scientific Purposes, ETS123) promulgated by the Council of Europe (http://www.coe.int) for laboratory cats are similar, but proposed revisions call for substantially more floor space for cats, at 1.5 m^2 (16.7 ft^2) per adult cat with a height of at least 2 m (6.5 ft).[21,22] The revisions, which have not been approved to date, also call for the provision of shelves, a box-style bed, and a vertical scratching surface. Animal shelter facilities in the United States have traditionally been equipped with small perchless cages (e.g., 0.5 to 0.75 m or 1.5 to 2.5 ft long) that are poorly designed for housing cats. The Association of Shelter Veterinarians (http://www.sheltervet.org) recommends a minimum enclosure size of 1 m^2 (11 ft^2) for adult cats.[7] Commercially available cages are typically approximately 0.75 m (2.5 ft) deep (e.g., an arm-length deep so that they can be readily accessed); therefore a cage with a length of 1.2 m (4 ft) is required to provide this approximate square footage, and it will also allow for adequate separation of food, water, and litter (Figure 46-21). Similarly, the Cat Fanciers' Association (http://www.cfa.org) recommends a minimum of 0.85 m^3 (30 ft^3) of space per cat for those weighing 2 kg or more.[16] Cubic measurements take into account the use of vertical space in addition to floor space, which is crucial for improving the quality of the environment. For example, a 0.85-m^3 (30-ft^3) enclosure would measure approximately 0.75 m deep × 1.2 m wide × 1 m high (2.5 ft deep × 4 ft wide × 3 ft high).

Larger enclosures also allow for better air circulation, which is an important consideration for control of feline upper respiratory infections. Double-sided enclosures (e.g., cat condos) are ideal for meeting these specifications and have the benefit of easily allowing cats to remain securely in one side of the enclosure while the opposite side is cleaned (Figure 46-22). This helps to minimize stress, prevent exposure to infectious disease,

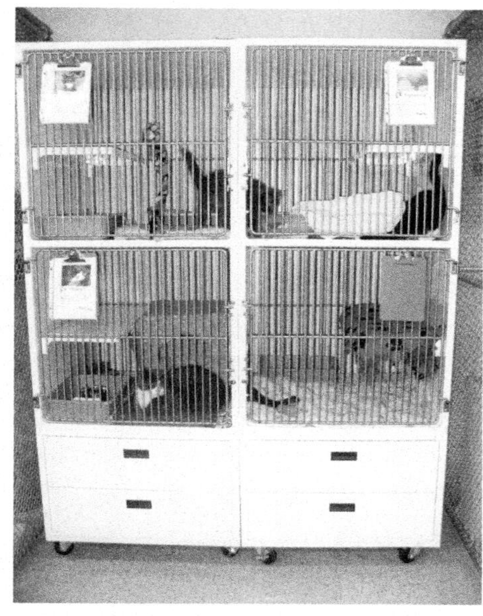

FIGURE 46-22 A variety of commercially available condo-style housing units are available for cats and serve to separate functional living areas and provide improved opportunities for exercise and exploration. This unit (Tristar Metals, Boyd, Tex.) is constructed of powder-coated stainless steel, which is highly durable and easy to disinfect but less noisy than uncoated stainless steel. Note the elevation from the floor and the grills on both the front and back, which allows flow-through ventilation.

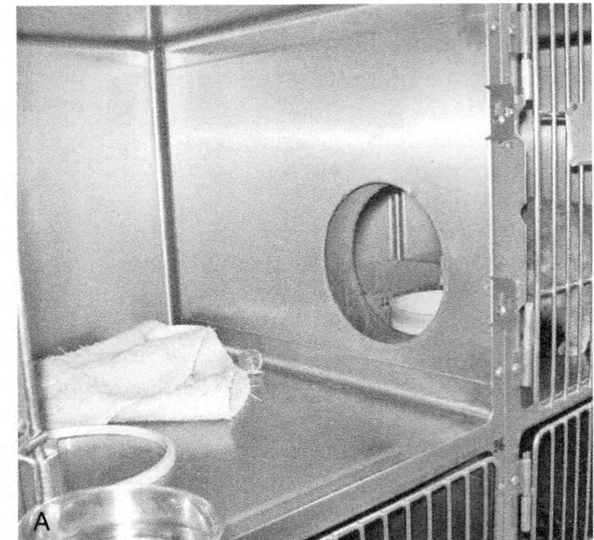

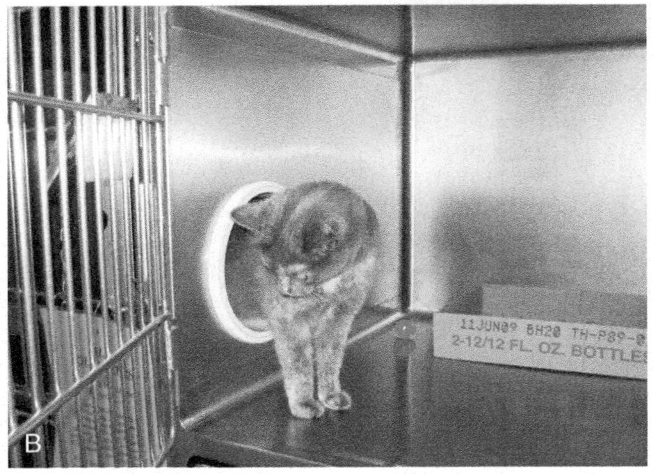

FIGURE 46-23 **A** and **B,** Conversion of existing cages into condo-style units. A hole is cut through the walls of adjacent cages and a section of polyvinylchloride (PVC) pipe with corresponding rims are used to create a safe portal for passage between the cages.

and preserve staff safety, which are especially crucial for newly arrived cats. Traditional cages can be modified into condo-style enclosures by creating portals to adjoin two or three smaller cages (Figure 46-23).

Regardless of the precise specifications of the enclosures, the importance of the overall quality of the living environment cannot be overemphasized. This includes a holistic approach to husbandry, with careful attention to the way in which cats are handled, noise levels, the provision of creature comforts, positive contact with caregivers, and strict avoidance of overcrowding, as well as good sanitation, medical protocols, and careful monitoring to ensure health and welfare.

Long-Term Housing

For long-term housing (e.g., greater than 2 weeks), consideration should also be given to providing space that is both mentally and physically stimulating for cats and preferably that which is esthetically pleasing to humans.[41] The latter is an important consideration to facilitate adoption in animal shelters. And, even in other types of facilities, it is important to create a pleasant environment not only for the animals, but also for their caregivers. Studies indicate that employee satisfaction improves animal care and staff retention, both of which may positively impact population health and well-being.[95]

For long-term housing of cats alternatives to traditional cage housing should be afforded.[41,45,46] At an absolute minimum, cats that are cage housed must be released each day and allowed an opportunity to exercise and explore in a secure enriched setting. For long-term housing, most cats will benefit from colony-style housing, provided there is sufficient space, easy access to feeding and elimination areas, an adequate number of comfortable hiding, and resting places and careful grouping and monitoring to ensure social compatibility among cats. Not every cat, however, will thrive in a group setting, and certain individuals will require enriched single housing, depending on their unique physical or behavioral needs. These may include cats that bully other cats or are otherwise incompatible and those with special medical needs. It is important to recognize that such singly housed cats will require more regular contact with their human caregivers and higher levels of mental and physical stimulation in order to maintain behavioral health during long-term confinement. Whenever possible, long-term housing of such individuals should be avoided. When cats are housed in amicable groups, it is easier to maintain proper behavioral welfare in the long term, because many of their social and emotional needs can be met by conspecifics.

Group Housing (Colony-Style Housing)

Group housing affords cats with opportunities for healthy social contact with others, which, in turn, provides additional mental and physical stimulation. When properly managed, this housing arrangement enhances welfare.* Insufficient space and crowding or poor compatibility matching of cats serves to increase stress and negates the benefits of the colony environment. Group housing should never be used as a means of simply expanding the holding capacity of a facility.

In animal shelters, the high turnover rate of cats contributes substantially to feline stress levels, especially in the context of groups of unfamiliar animals. Because it may take days to weeks to acclimate to a group environment, enriched individual housing may be preferable when a brief stay is anticipated. However, the benefits of enriched social group housing become evident when stays extend beyond a few weeks.[41]

---

*References 28, 45, 46, 57, 59, 70, 71, 74, 90, 98, 99.

SELECTION CRITERIA

Careful attention to groupings of cats is essential for success. Family groups and previously bonded housemates are natural choices for co-housing,[11,46] but unfamiliar cats may also be grouped using careful selection criteria. Many cats do have preferences for housemates, necessitating conscientious compatibility matching combined with the provision of a high-quality environment. Groupings of unfamiliar cats should always be given priority for the largest available enclosures. In addition, cats should always receive appropriate health clearances prior to admission to a group. These should be determined by the specific protocols of the facility; but in most cases, minimum requirements would include that cats be free of signs of contagious disease, tested for FeLV and FIV, vaccinated against FVRCP, and treated for parasites.

In addition to prior relationships, selection criteria for groupings should include age, reproductive status, and personality.

AGE Age is an important consideration regarding housing arrangements.[46] To ensure proper social and emotional development, kittens should be housed with their mother at least until they are weaned. Because it can be behaviorally beneficial, it is desirable for them to remain with her for a longer period of time when this is feasible. In fact, queens frequently do not fully wean their kittens until 12 to 14 weeks of age if left to their own devices. If older kittens are housed with their mother, it is important to provide a perch that allows her the option of periodically resting away from them if desired. Most queens will accept the kittens of another cat; therefore young orphan or singleton kittens should be housed with other lactating queens and/or kittens of similar age/size. In a shelter setting where there is a high turnover of cats, it may be beneficial to house young kittens up to 4 to 5 months of age in large cages or condos for biosecurity purposes. Juveniles and adults can be housed in colony rooms or runs but should be segregated by age (e.g., juveniles 5 to 12 months old, young adults, mature adults, geriatrics). Well-socialized juveniles tend to adapt quickly in a group setting with other cats of similar ages and exhibit healthy activity and play behavior. In contrast, mature adults and geriatric cats often have little tolerance for the high energy and playful antics of many younger cats, which can cause them substantial stress. For this reason, adult cats should be kept separate from juvenile cats, and aging or geriatric cats separate from other age groups. In animal shelters, compatible cats that enter the shelter together should be housed together regardless of age, whenever possible.

REPRODUCTIVE STATUS Unless cats will be used for breeding, group housing of sexually intact cats of breeding age should be avoided whenever possible. At a minimum, mature tomcats should be neutered to prevent intermale aggression, urine spraying, and breeding.[41] Reproductively intact females may be co-housed with other intact females or with neutered males. In contrast, in breeding colonies, harem-style housing may be used to facilitate breeding (e.g., a few queens with a tomcat). It is also advantageous to house compatible pregnant queens together before delivery, because they will usually share nursing and neonatal care (Figure 46-24).[45] After delivery, pairing of queens becomes more difficult. When tomcats are not breeding, they can usually be co-housed with a spayed female, a neutered male, or a compatible juvenile for companionship. Other recommended groupings in the context of a breeding colony include postweaning family groups, prepubertal juveniles, or compatible single-sex adults.

PERSONALITY TYPE There are two basic feline personality types: cats that are outgoing, confident, and sociable and those that are relatively timid and shy.[105] Cats with bold, friendly temperaments tend to cope and adapt more readily than shy, timid cats. A subset of the bold, friendly personality type is the "assertive" or "bully" cat.[90] Bully cats constantly threaten other cats in a group setting in order to control access to food, litter, perches, or the attention of human caregivers. To maintain harmony, removing cats of this personality type from a colony is usually necessary. Reassignment is possible, but may prove difficult, necessitating single housing. Shy, timid cats sometimes have difficulty interacting successfully with more dominant members of a group or may fall victim to a bully, resulting in chronic stress and increased hiding. Placement of shy cats in smaller groups or with calm juvenile cats, where they will not be intimidated or harassed, is generally rewarding and often helps them to "come out of their shells."[46,90] Similarly, dominant cats will often accept calm, younger cats, as opposed to other adults by whom they may feel threatened. And finally, in the case of some dominant males, the introduction of a female cat will be more likely to be successful.[46,64,90]

GROUP SIZE AND SPACE

The precise space requirements for long-term housing of cats will vary, because it is dependent on many factors (Box 46-8).[46,59] Of paramount importance is that group size must be small enough to prevent negative interactions among cats and to permit daily monitoring of individuals. Cats typically prevent social conflict through avoidance, and adequate space must be available so that cats can maintain social distance as needed. Crowding can make it impossible for animals to maintain healthy behavioral distance, creating situations where individuals may not be able to freely access feeding, resting, or elimination space because of social conflicts over colony

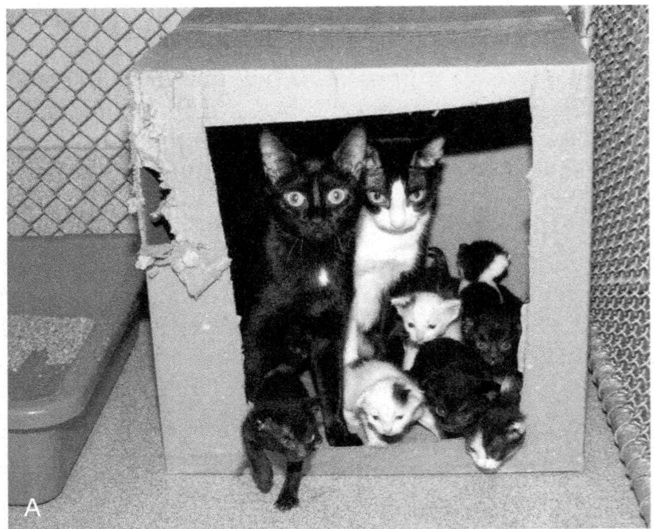

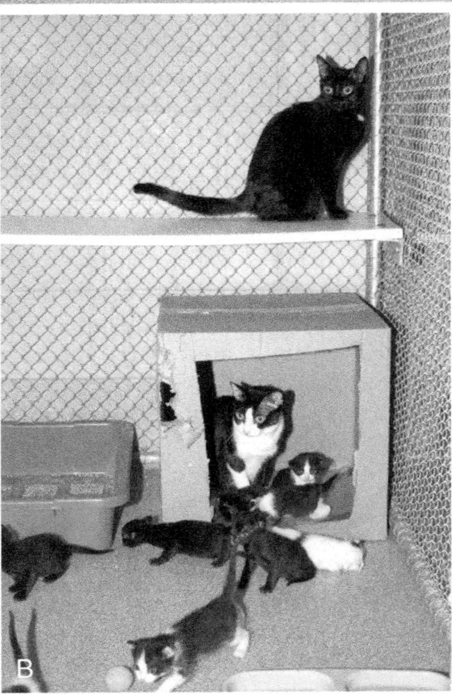

FIGURE 46-24 In breeding colonies, compatible pregnant queens may be housed together prior to delivery. **A,** Two queens share the care of their litters of kittens. **B,** Perches should be provided so that mother cats can periodically seek respite if they choose. *(From Griffin B, Hume KR: Recognition and management of stress in housed cats. In August JR, editor:* Consultations in feline internal medicine, *vol 5, St Louis, 2006, Elsevier, p 717.)*

BOX 46-8

Factors Influencing Spatial Needs of Housed Cats[46,59]

- Length of stay
- Overall quality of the environment, including use of vertical space
- Overall quality of behavioral care
- Physical and behavioral characteristics of the cat (e.g., age, personality type, prior experience, and socialization)
- Individual relationships between cats (e.g., family groupings, previously bonded housemates, versus unfamiliar groupings and degree of social compatibility among cats)
- Turnover of cats (e.g., frequency of introduction of new members)
- Total room size
- Absolute number of cats
- Individual needs and levels of enrichment being used to meet these needs

resources. Both crowding and constant introduction of new cats induce stress and must be avoided to ensure proper welfare. The addition of new cats always results in a period of stress for the group, and if there is constant turnover within the group, cats may remain stressed indefinitely. High turnover also increases the risk of infectious disease. If cat group numbers are small, disease exposure will be limited, facilitating control. For all of these reasons, housing cats in small groups is preferred.[41,45,46]

In most instances, the author recommends housing cats in compatible pairs or small groups of not more than three to four individuals. Housing cats in runs is ideal for this purpose (Figure 46-25). A well-equipped, 1.2- × 1.8-m (4- × 6-ft) run can comfortably house two to three adult cats depending on their familiarity and compatibility, or up to four juveniles (e.g., 6 to 12 months old). Juveniles tend to accept a slightly higher housing density than adults. Likewise, previously bonded housemates and families will generally peacefully co-exist at a higher density than will unfamiliar cats. When runs are used, they must have a top panel and should be at least 1.8 m (6 ft) high to allow caregivers easy access for cleaning and care. If chain-link is used, 2.5-cm (1-inch) mesh is ideal, but larger mesh can be used. Existing dog kennel runs can be converted into areas for cat housing. This is an important and practical consideration in animal shelters, because many shelters have experienced a decrease in dog intake, while the need for improved cat housing is great. Cats and dogs should never be co-housed in the same area; thus conversion should result in an exclusive cat housing area.

For colony rooms, the author recommends a minimum enclosure size of approximately 3 to 3.5 m × 5 to 5.5 m (10 to 12 ft × 16 to 18 ft) for colonies of up to a maximum of eight adult cats, or in the case of juveniles, a few more. Doubling the size of an enclosure does not necessarily allow a twofold increase in the number of cats that can be properly housed. Another author recommends 1.7 m^2 (18 ft^2) per cat as a general guideline for group housing,

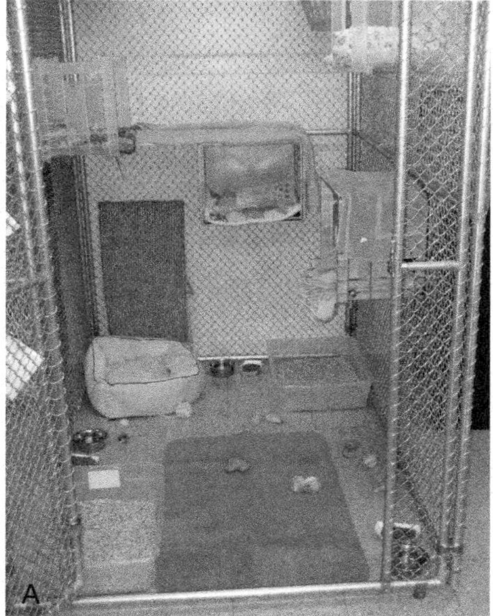

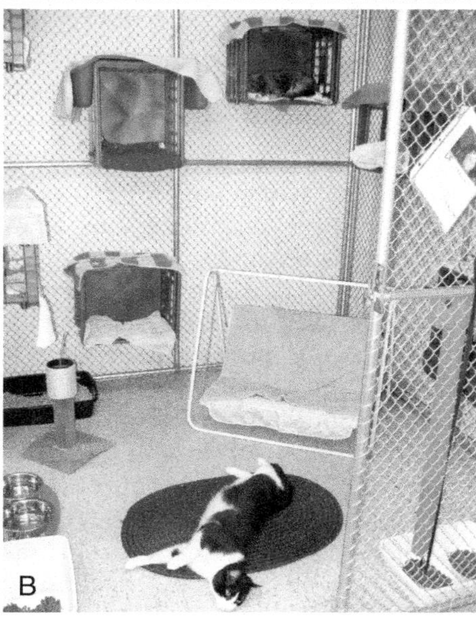

FIGURE 46-25 **A,** This 4- × 6-ft run has been appropriately outfitted for pair-housing of two adult cats. Note the multiple separate areas for resting, perching, hiding, feeding, eliminating, scratching, and playing. **B,** Cats enjoy the increased behavioral options provided by run-style housing.

acknowledging that many factors influence the spatial needs of cats, including the overall quality of the environment as well as the relationships of the individual animals.[59]

In sanctuary and laboratory situations where cats are housed for months to years in stable colonies, larger groupings of cats may be feasible, provided ample space is available.[46] Housing arrangements can also be created in which individual enclosures are maintained within a colony room. In this case, cats could be allowed to wander and interact freely in the colony room by day but be confined to their respective enclosures at night, enabling caregivers to better monitor individual appetites and litter box results while allowing cats a period of rest away from one another. Alternatively, individual enclosures may only be used for brief periods for meal feedings of canned food, with dry food available free choice in the colony. This sort of arrangement can also be used to facilitate introduction of new cats to the group and represents a desirable option. If design and biosecurity procedures permit, portable intake enclosures could even be transferred to group rooms to smooth the transition of new cats from intake to long-term housing areas.

INTRODUCTION OF NEW CATS

Tremendous individual variation exists among cats in the context of social relations with other cats. Although introduction of some previously unfamiliar cats will seem effortless and uneventful, introduction of others will result in considerable stress, not only for the new cat but for the entire group as well.[46] For this reason, introductions should always be done under supervision, and whenever possible, they should be gradual. To accomplish this, a new cat can be kept in a separate cage within or adjacent to the group enclosure equipped with food, water, litter, and a hiding box. Usually, within a few days, it will be evident by the behaviors of the cats whether or not the new cat can be transferred into the group enclosure without risk of fighting. Well-socialized kittens and juvenile cats frequently adapt readily to group accommodations, and prolonged introductions may not be necessary unless they are shy or undersocialized.

In established groups of cats, the introduction or removal of individuals will require a period of adjustment and may result in signs of social stress for members of the colony. These signs usually subside once a new social hierarchy and territorial limits (usually favored resting places) are established. In some cases, arrangement of incompatible cats, even within visible distance of one another, may create substantial anxiety, necessitating rearrangement (Figure 46-26). In the case of animal shelters, where population interchange is high, it is generally not feasible to maintain consistent groupings of cats. This underscores the absolute necessity of careful selection and compatibility matching, as well as maintaining a variety of housing styles. Even in modestly populated, carefully introduced, environmentally enriched colonies, behavior problems may occur. For this reason, some facilities elect to use an "all in–all out" approach to avoid repeated introductions of new cats into stable groups. In animal shelters, bonded pairs and family groupings of cats frequently enter the shelter together and are usually perfect choices for co-housing.[46]

Because cats do have strong preferences for new roommates, caregivers must expect to find many that are incompatible as roommates. If only one or two cats are responsible for social destabilization of a group, they can

FIGURE 46-26 In some instances, arrangement or location of enclosures where cats are within visual contact of others may induce stress and anxiety, even though they are not housed in the same enclosure. This caged cat has been isolated from the group, yet remains stressed and threatened by the stares of the on-looking cat.

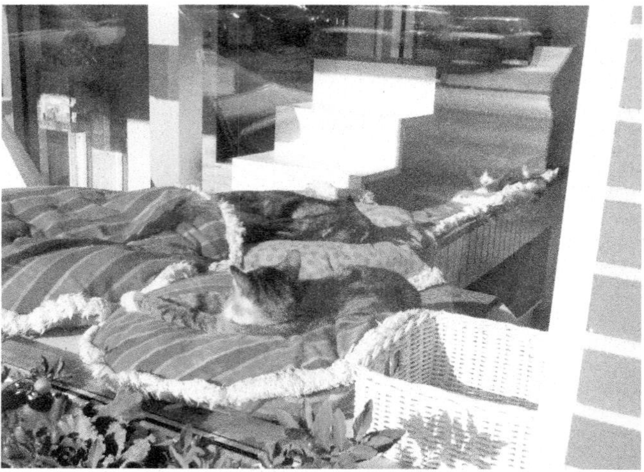

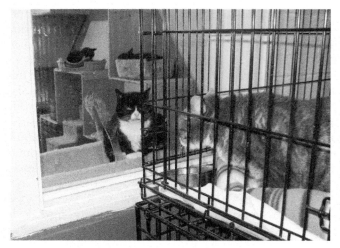

FIGURE 46-27 Cats enjoying a sunny window in a colony room at an animal shelter.

usually be reassigned to another colony, because it is often the social grouping, not the individual, that is the problem. If a cat shows persistent incompatibility with other cats, he or she should be housed singly. Studies indicate that cats that fight at the time of initial introduction are nearly 40 times more likely to continue fighting in the following weeks and months.[61] If overt fighting occurs, cats should be permanently separated. Co-housing of incompatible cats or cats that fight is unacceptable.

COLONY LIVING ENVIRONMENT

The success of group housing depends not only on selection of compatible cats and the size of the enclosure but also on the quality of the environment.* A variety of elevated resting perches and hiding boxes should be provided to increase the size and complexity of the enclosure and to separate it into different functional areas, allowing a variety of behavioral choices. The physical environment should include opportunities for hiding, playing, scratching, climbing, resting, feeding, and eliminating. Whenever possible, a minimum of 1 litter box and 1 food and water bowl should be provided per 2 to 3 cats and arranged in different locations of the colony space, taking care to separate food and water from litter by at least 0.6 m (2 ft). In addition, placement should allow cats to access each resource from more than one side, whenever possible, without blocking access to doorways. Litter boxes should not be covered, to allow easy access and to prevent entrapment or ambush by other cats. The number of resting boards and perches should exceed the number of cats and should be arranged in as many locations within the enclosure as possible. Open single perches should be separated by at least 0.6 m (2 ft) or staggered at different heights to ensure adequate separation, while larger perches should be available for cats who choose to rest together in close proximity. Many cats enjoy hammock-style perches or semienclosed box-style perches where they can hide. If there are not enough comfortable, desirable resting and hiding places, cats may choose to lie in litter boxes. Comfortable bedding (that is either disposable or can be easily laundered) should be provided. Not only do cats demonstrate preferences for resting on soft surfaces, they experience longer periods of normal deep sleep with soft bedding.[23] The environmental temperature should be kept comfortable and constant, and living quarters should be well ventilated, without drafts. By changing location within the colony (e.g., from the cooler surface of the floor to a sunny window), cats should be able to choose the environmental condition they prefer (Figure 46-27).[46]

In colony rooms, installation of stairs, shelves, and walkways are ideal for increasing the use of vertical space (Figure 46-28). In larger rooms, installation of free-standing towers provides additional living and activity space and contributes to functionally reducing overcrowding (Figure 46-29). Depending on the setting, it may not be desirable for cats to access areas above the level of an arm's reach so that cleaning is easy and cats can be easily retrieved from the highest perches if needed. Colony room design should also ensure that cats cannot easily escape. In some cases, constructing a foyer at the entrance to the room will be necessary to minimize the risk of escape when the room is entered (Figure 46-30). In addition, ceilings should be constructed of solid surfaces, because cats can easily dislodge the

*References 28, 45, 46, 57, 59, 60, 70, 71, 74, 89, 90, 97-99.

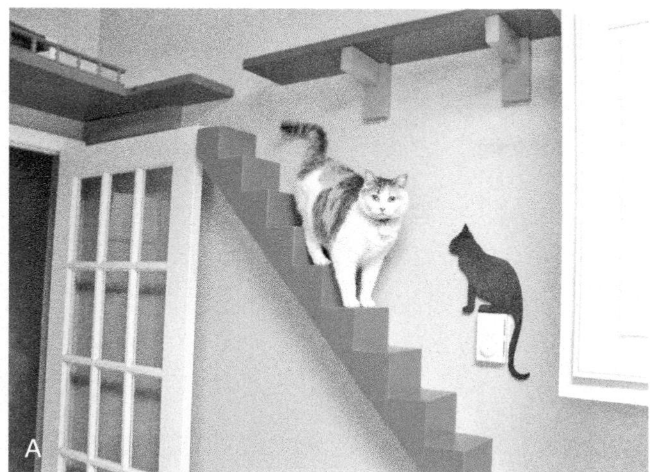

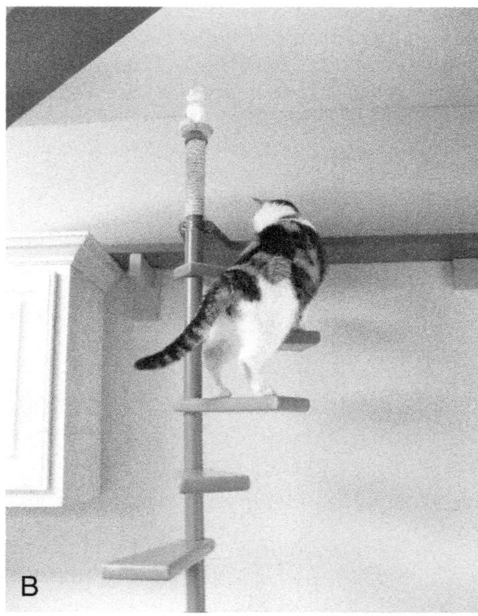

FIGURE 46-28 **A** and **B,** Installation of stairs, shelves, and walkways can be used to create additional function space and is visually appealing, creating an inviting environment for both cats and humans.

panels typically used for dropped ceilings, and escape into the rafters (Figure 46-31).[46]

Social Companionship

In addition to contact with conspecifics, cats must be afforded time for pleasant daily contact with human caregivers. As previously discussed, daily social contact and exercise sessions with humans are especially important for individually caged cats. Although social contact is usually highly desirable, it is not invariably pleasant for all cats. Personality, socialization, previous experience, and familiarity contribute to whether or not social interactions are perceived as pleasurable, stressful, or somewhere in between.[46,77]

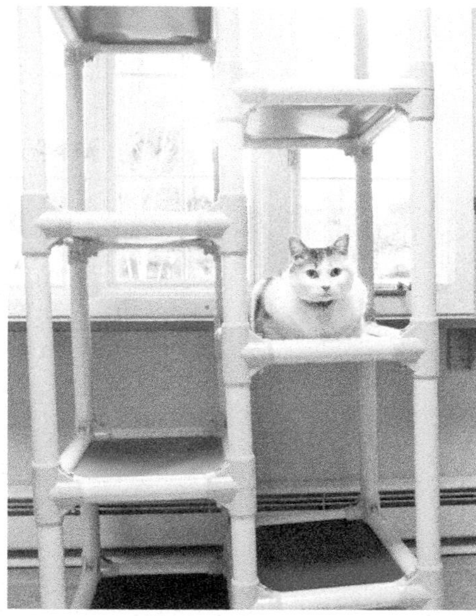

FIGURE 46-29 In larger colony rooms, free-standing towers (Kuranda Cat Tower, Glen Burnie, Md.) can be used to create additional functional space in the interior of the room.

Social Contact with Animal Care Staff

The importance of a cat-savvy staff that enjoys working with cats cannot be overemphasized. Animal care staff must be willing to spend quality time interacting with cats to assure socialization and tractability.[45,46] Whenever possible, caregivers should be assigned to care for the same cats on a regular basis so that they become aware of the personality of each individual cat, which is necessary for detection of health problems, incompatibilities between cats, and, in the case of breeding colonies, estrous cycling. This is also important, because not all cats uniformly enjoy human companionship and will be more likely to be stressed by the presence of different caregivers, rather than becoming familiar and more at ease with one. In general, regular daily contact and socialization is essential to ensure that cats are docile, easy to work with, and have no fear of humans. Caregivers should schedule time each day to interact with "their" cats aside from the activities of feeding and cleaning. Some cats may prefer to be petted and handled, while others prefer to interact with caregivers by playing with toys (Figure 46-32).

In particular, human contact is essential for proper socialization of young kittens. A sensitive period of socialization occurs during the development of all infant animals, during which social attachments to members of the same species and other species form easily and rapidly. In kittens, the sensitive period of socialization occurs between 2 and 7 weeks of age, and cats not properly socialized to humans during this time may never permit handling.[75,105] Beginning shortly after birth, kittens should be handled daily, talked to in a soothing

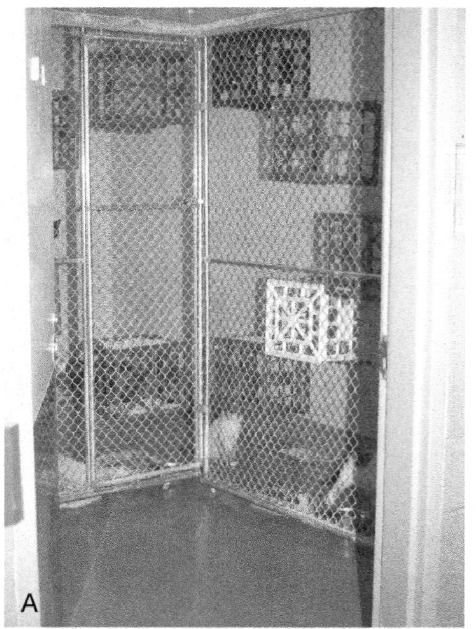
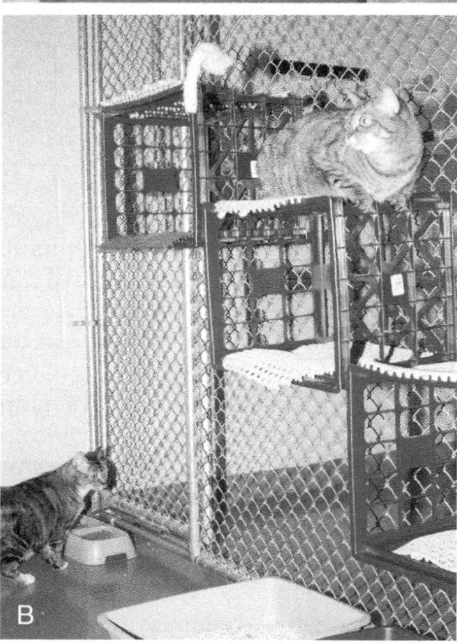

FIGURE 46-30 **A,** For colony room housing, the construction of a chain-link foyer at the entrance to the room prevents cats from escaping when the room door is opened. **B,** Inexpensive milk crates attached with zip ties create areas for climbing and perching on the chain-link wall. *(From Griffin B, Hume KR: Recognition and management of stress in housed cats. In August JR, editor:* Consultations in feline internal medicine, *vol 5, St Louis, 2006, Elsevier, p 717.)*

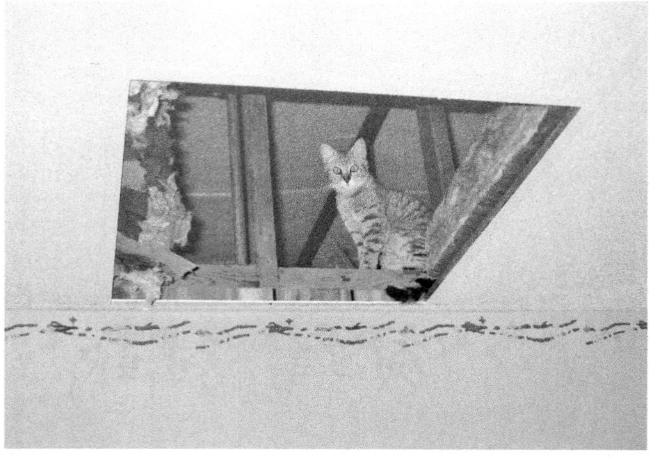

FIGURE 46-31 A solid-surface ceiling is essential in free-range housing rooms to prevent the escape of cats into the rafters. Once in the ceiling, cats may be difficult to recover, and injury and/or damage to the facilities may result. *(From Griffin B, Hume KR: Recognition and management of stress in housed cats. In August JR, editor:* Consultations in feline internal medicine, *vol 5, St Louis, 2006, Elsevier, p 717.)*

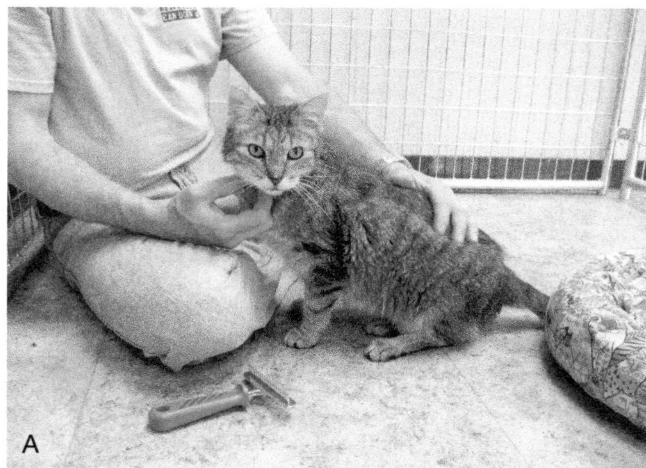
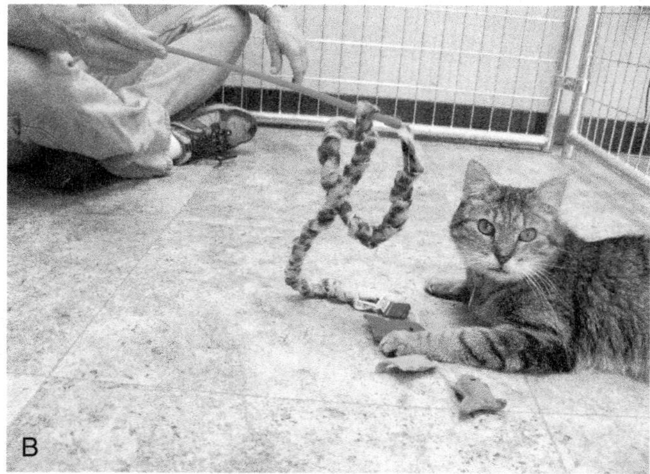

FIGURE 46-32 **A** and **B,** Daily social contact with humans aside from cleaning and feeding activities is essential for behavioral welfare. Cats may enjoy petting, grooming, or interaction with toys.

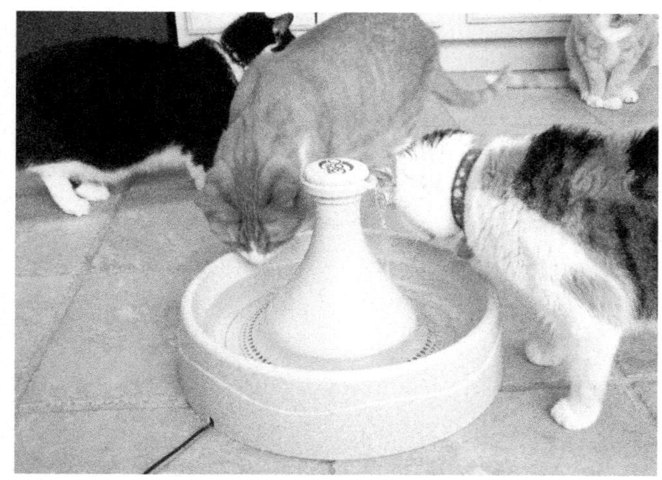

FIGURE 46-33 Cats surround a water fountain in this example of enrichment.

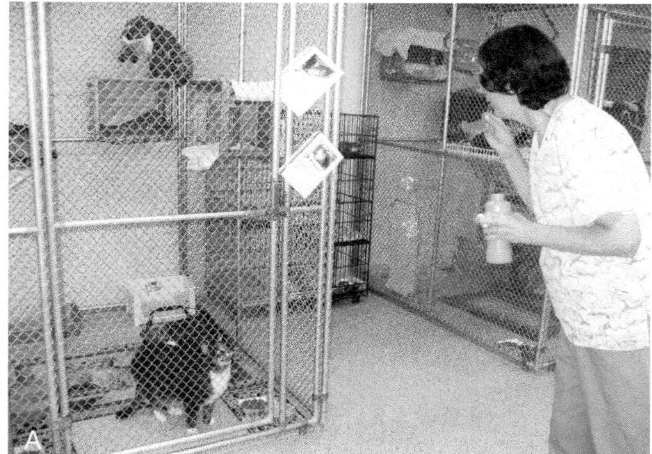

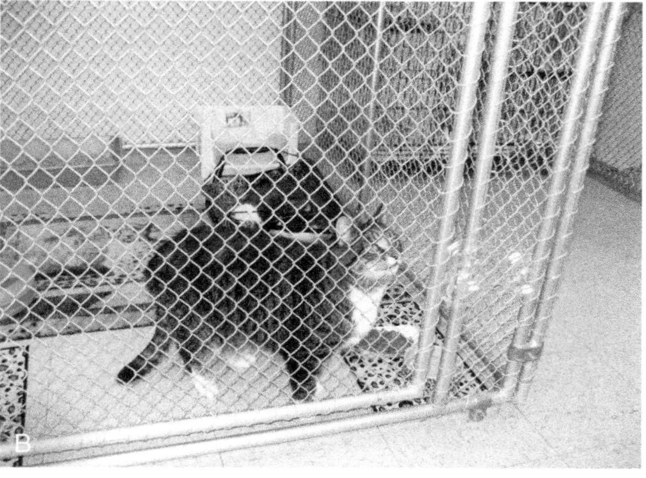

FIGURE 46-34 **A** and **B**, Enrichment does not have to be complicated or expensive. In this case, a cat enjoys watching soap bubbles blown by a caregiver.

voice, gently petted, and held. Interactions should include play (stimulated with toys) as the kittens become ambulatory. For kittens housed in a shelter, socialization must always be balanced with infectious disease control, and caregivers should take precautions accordingly.

Mental and Physical Stimulation

Other forms of stimulation, including those that engage the various senses, are important methods of enriching the living environment by promoting healthy mental and physical activity. For singly housed cats and long-term residents, appropriate levels of additional enrichment should be provided on a daily basis.

Visual Stimulation

The provision of birdfeeders, gardens, or other interesting stimuli in the external environment can enhance the internal environment of the colony. Resting perches in view of windows or other pleasant areas of the facility are especially desirable. Other novel and enriching visual stimuli include cat-proof aquariums with fish, water fountains, bubbles, perpetual motion devices, and videos especially designed for cats (Figures 46-33 to 46-35).[32]

Auditory Stimulation

A radio playing soft, low music in the room provides a welcome distraction and important source of

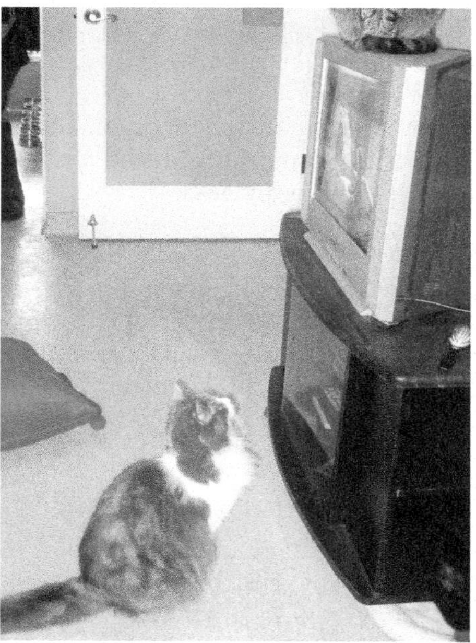

FIGURE 46-35 A shelter cat watches a specially produced feline video (Video Catnip, Pet Avision, Lyndon Center, Vt.). Provision of adequate mental stimulation is essential for behavioral wellness. *(From Griffin B, Hume KR: Recognition and management of stress in housed cats. In August JR, editor:* Consultations in feline internal medicine, *vol 5, St Louis, 2006, Elsevier, p 717.)*

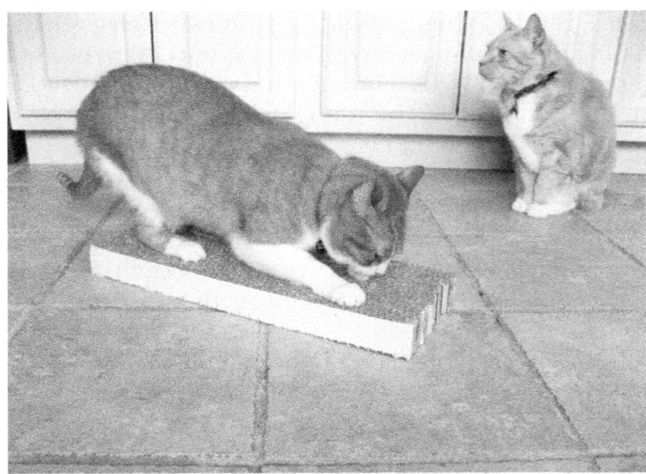

FIGURE 46-36 Disposable, corrugated cardboard cat scratcher. Scratching is an essential need of all cats. It conditions the claws and serves as an important means of feline communication through both visual and scent marking.

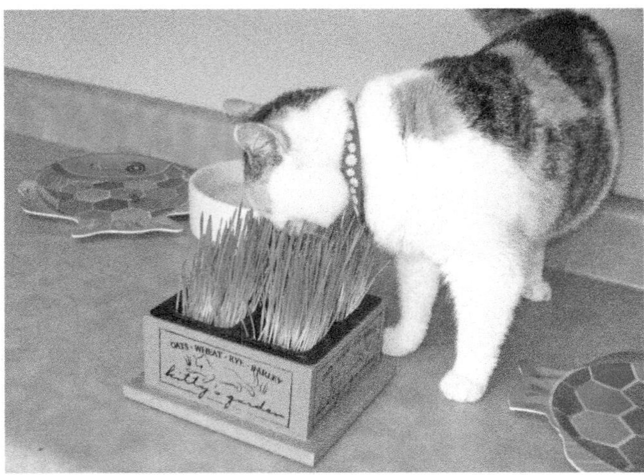

FIGURE 46-37 Olfactory stimulation is another important source of sensory enrichment. Many cats like to smell and chew grass, and containers of cat grass or catnip can be introduced for brief periods to stimulate activity.

stimulation. In addition, it may help to habituate cats to human voices and prevent them from being startled by loud noises. Most caregivers also enjoy listening to the radio, and happy caregivers create a relaxed environment.[45]

Tactile Stimulation

The provision of scratching boards is especially important, and a variety of sturdy surfaces, both horizontal and vertical, should be provided for scratching. Sisal rope, the backs of carpet squares, and corrugated cardboard are all useful (Figure 46-36).

Olfactory Stimulation

Many cats like to smell and chew grass, and containers of cat grass or catnip can be introduced for brief periods to stimulate activity (Figure 46-37).

Feeding Enrichment

Providing novel sources of food is another important source of stimulation and can be easily accomplished by hiding food in commercially available food-puzzle toys or in cardboard boxes or similar items with holes such that the cat has to work to extract pieces of food (Figure 46-38).[46,102]

Positive Reinforcement–Based Training

Obedience training using clickers with food rewards is an excellent form of enrichment, combining social contact with caregivers together with both mental and physical stimulation. Positive reinforcement training using a target stick is a powerful tool for teaching shy cats to approach the front of an enclosure. Teaching cats awaiting adoption to perform tricks is not only stimulating for them, but it often makes them more attractive to potential adopters (Figure 46-39).

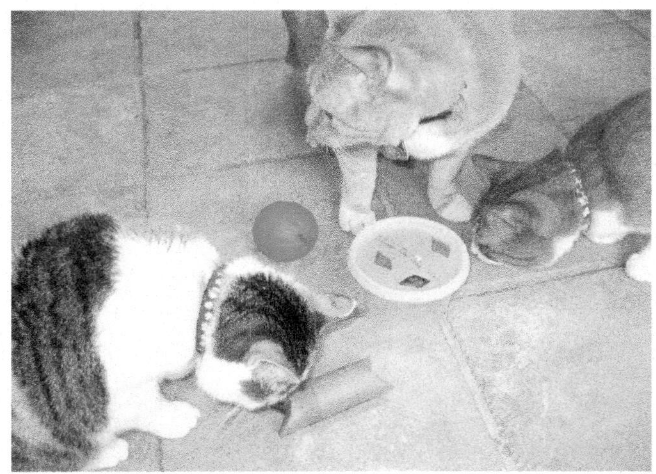

FIGURE 46-38 Cats surround a variety of food puzzle toys (a ball, a cardboard tube, and a plastic container with holes). Treats are hidden inside, and they will have to work to extract pieces of food. Novel feeding is an excellent source of enrichment for cats that are housed long term.

Physical Stimulation

Play items that stimulate prey drive and physical activity, such as plastic balls, rings, hanging ropes, spring-mounted toys, plastic wands, and catnip toys, should also be provided but must be either sanitizable or disposable. Empty cardboard boxes and paper bags are inexpensive, disposable, and stimulate exploration and play behavior as well as scratching. Cats tend to be most stimulated by active toys, including wiggling ropes, wands with feathers, kitty fishing poles, and toys that can be slid or rolled to chase.[81] Many cats enjoy chasing

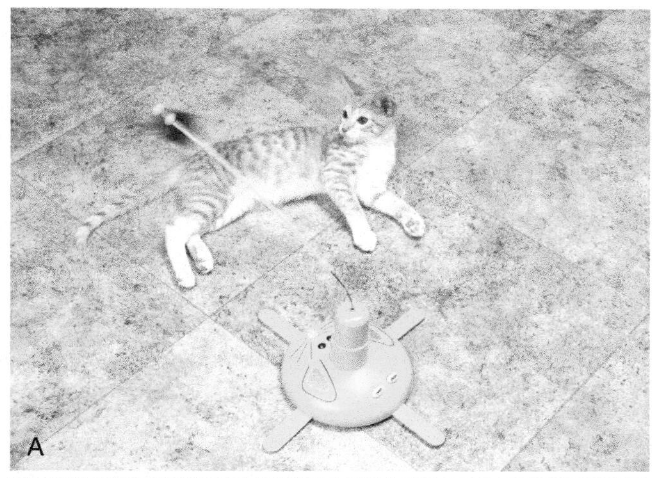

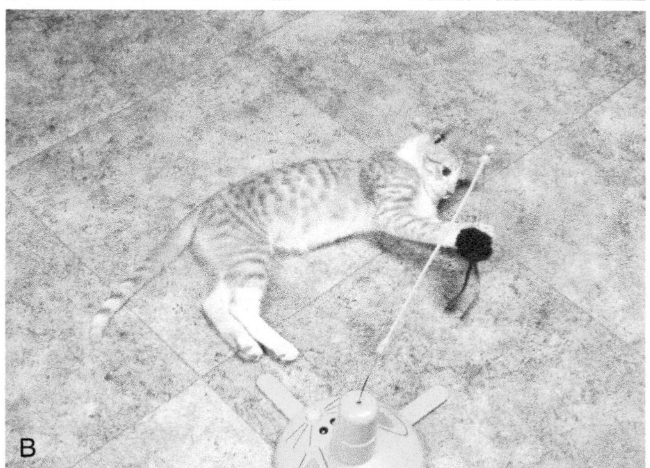

FIGURE 46-39 **A** and **B,** A juvenile cat watches and captures the toy at the end of the robotic arm. Commercially available electronic toys (Panic Mouse, Temecula, Calif.) may be used to stimulate mental and physical activity. By turning the toy on at the same time each day, cats can anticipate a predictable pleasant experience in their daily routine.

the beams of laser pointers, small flashlights, or suspended rotating disco balls. Commercially available electronic toys that stimulate play are especially useful in long-term settings (Figure 46-40). Varied toys should be substituted regularly to ensure continued interest.[46]

Outdoor Access

In some climates, cats may be housed comfortably in outdoor enclosures where fresh air, sunshine, and other stimuli can help to create a healthy environment (Figures 46-41 and 46-42).[46,60,71] When indoor group enclosures connect to outdoor enclosures, it is important to have ample space for passage between them (e.g., more than one doorway) so that cats can pass freely.

Daily Routine

Cats will also benefit greatly from consistent daily routines of care. They become entrained to schedules of care

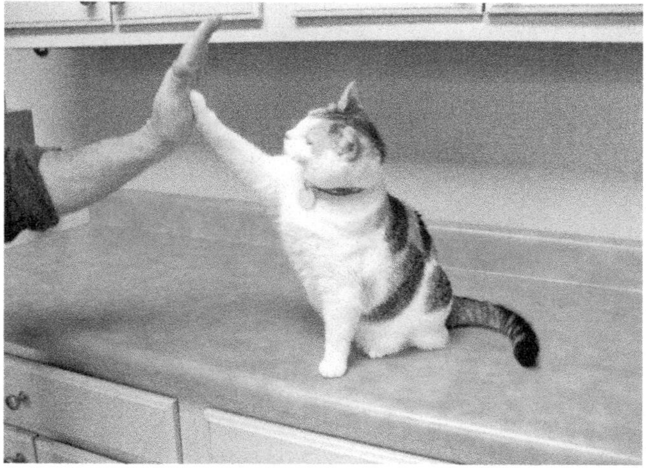

FIGURE 46-40 "High five!" A trained cat offers its paw to a caregiver. Positive reinforcement–based training combines pleasant social interaction, mental stimulation, and physical activity, making it a profoundly rewarding form of enrichment. It may also enhance the cat's appeal to adopters in a shelter setting.

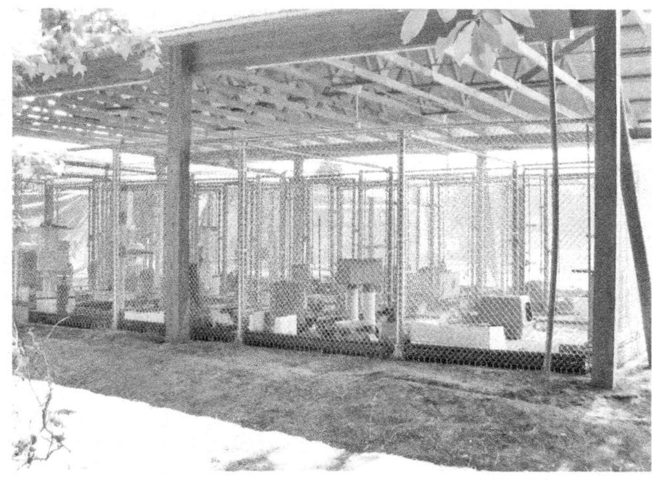

FIGURE 46-41 An open-air cattery with run-style housing may be feasible in some climates. Benefits include fresh air, sunshine, and a potentially enriching environment for residents.

(e.g., feeding, cleaning, enrichment activities), and unpredictable caregiving has been shown to dramatically increase stress.[14] If events that are perceived as stressful (such as cleaning time) occur on a predictable schedule, cats learn that a predictable period of calm and comfort will always occur in between. Cats also respond to positive experiences in their daily routines. For example, feeding and playtime may be greatly anticipated; thus scheduling positive daily events (e.g., a treat at 3:00 PM every day) should also be a priority.

Erratic periods of light and darkness are also known to be significant sources of stress for cats. Animals possess natural circadian rhythms and irregular or continuous patterns of light or darkness are inherently stressful. Lighting should be maintained on a regular

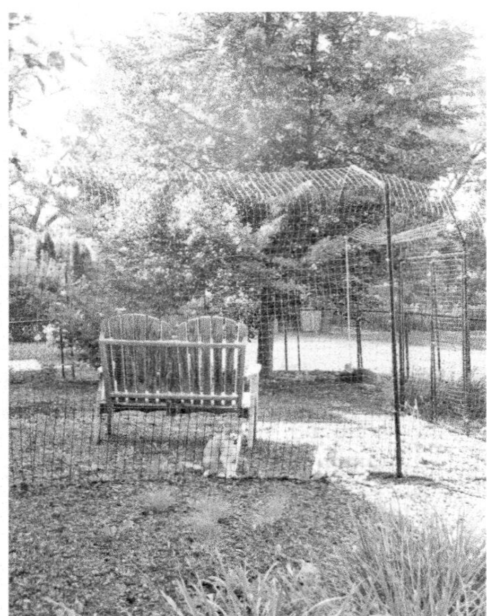

FIGURE 46-42 Purpose-designed cat fencing (Purrfect Fence, Conshohocken, Pa.) can be used to create outdoor enclosures. A mesh arc facing inward along the top of the fence prevents cats from climbing out.

schedule, with lights on by day and off by night. Whenever possible, full-spectrum and/or natural lighting is ideal.

Monitoring

Housed cats require active daily monitoring by staff trained to recognize signs of stress and social conflict. To the inexperienced observer, such signs may appear subtle (Figure 46-43). It is often the absence of normal behaviors (such as engaging in grooming or exercise) or subtle social signals (such as covert guarding of resources or dominant staring) that signify problems. Careful observers will note these behaviors and respond accordingly to ensure that stress or conflicts do not persist. When cats are well adjusted and housing arrangements meet their behavioral needs, they display a wide variety of normal behaviors, including a good appetite and activity level, sociability, grooming, appropriate play behavior, and restful sleeping (Figure 46-44).[44,46]

Ultimately, the success of adaptation of cats to a new environment will depend on both the quality of the environment and the adaptive capacity of the individual. Although most adapt to new environments with time, some never adjust and remain stressed indefinitely, ultimately resulting in decline of physical as well as emotional health. When cats fail to adjust to their environment and remain markedly stressed and fearful despite appropriate behavioral care, every effort must be made to prevent long-term stays. Depending on the circumstances, transfer to another colony room, foster care,

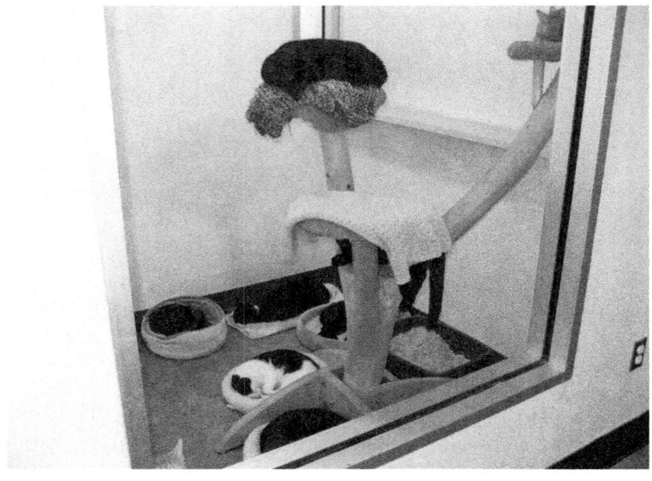

FIGURE 46-43 Signs of stress may be inapparent to the casual or inexperienced observer. In this 4 × 6 ft room, nine adult cats are seen with only a single litter box. Although they may appear to be resting comfortably at a glance, a skilled observer would quickly realize that the majority are sequestered in place, while more dominant members of the colony move about, accessing colony resources and controlling the most desirable resting areas.

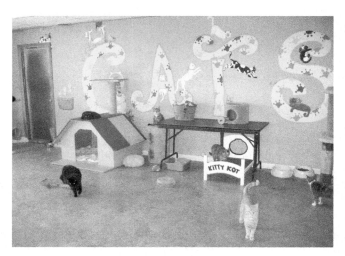

FIGURE 46-44 Group-housed cats in a free-ranging room. The fact that the residents are actively engaged in a variety of normal cat behaviors is evidence of a high-quality environment and a harmonious colony.

adoption, or euthanasia (when no other options exist) may be necessary to ensure cat welfare.

DEVELOPING A POPULATION WELLNESS PROGRAM: CONSIDERATIONS FOR ENVIRONMENTAL HEALTH

Achieving population wellness requires a healthy environment. Thus the clinician's final task in creating a population wellness program is to develop tailored protocols focused on optimizing environmental conditions that favor cat health. Once again, all essential elements as noted should be addressed.

Population Density

Perhaps the most critical aspect of environmental management is to ensure a modest population density. High population density increases opportunities for introduction of infectious disease while increasing the contact rate among members of a group. Both the number of asymptomatic carriers of disease, such as those with upper respiratory infection, as well as susceptible cats in a given group are likely to increase, enhancing the odds of disease transmission among group members through both direct contact as well as fomites. In addition, crowding also increases the magnitude of many environmental stressors (e.g., noise levels, air contaminants) and compromises animal husbandry, all of which induce unnecessary stress and further inflate the risk of disease in the population. Indeed, crowding is one of the most potent stressors recognized in housed animals.[77]

Although adequate space for animals is essential, it is crucial to recognize that crowding is not solely dependent on the amount of available space. It is also a function of the organization's ability to provide proper care that maintains animal health and well-being. Every organization has a limit to the number of animals for which it can provide proper care. When more animals are housed than can be properly cared for within the organization's capacity, caregivers become overwhelmed, and animal care is further compromised.[7,54,88]

In animal shelters, crowding may also negatively impact adoption rates, because potential adopters often find crowded environments to be overwhelming and uninviting. If disease spread results as a consequence of the environmental conditions, animal adoptions may be further disrupted. Although unexpected shelter intake may occasionally result in temporary crowding, a good wellness program dictates that protocols must be in place to alleviate crowding and maintain a modestly populated environment for the health and protection of the animals and staff.[41] Regardless of the setting, facilities must limit the number of animals housed to the number for which they can provide proper space and care.

There are three basic methods of reducing crowding: (1) limiting the admission (or births) of new animals into a population, (2) increasing release of animals from a population, and (3) euthanasia. In animal shelters, management practices that minimize each animal's length of stay and programs that speed or increase adoption, owner reunification, or transfer (e.g., to rescue or foster care) help to minimize crowding and maximize the number of animals that an organization can serve. It is a common misperception that housing more animals in a shelter will result in saving more lives. To the contrary, euthanasia rates are highly correlated to intake rates, regardless of the number of animals that a facility houses. In many instances, keeping more animals in the shelter may actually reduce the organization's ability to help animals, because time and resources are tied up caring for a crowded, stressed population, rather than focusing on adoption or other positive outcomes.

In shelter medicine, the term population management is used to refer to an active process of planning, ongoing daily evaluation, and responding to changing conditions as an organization cares for multiple animals.[7,88] The major goal of population management is to minimize the amount of time any individual animal spends confined in the shelter, while maximizing the organization's lifesaving capacity. Moving animals through the system efficiently is the foundation of effective population management. To move animals through the shelter more quickly, delays in decision making and the completion of procedures (e.g., intake processing, transfer from holding to adoption areas, spay/neuter surgery) must be eliminated or minimized whenever possible. In open-admission shelters, even delays of 1 to 2 days can have a dramatic effect on the shelter's daily census, particularly for shelters handling thousands of animals per year. This, in turn, affects the ability to provide adequate care. It is important to recognize that effective population management does not change the final disposition of an animal. It does mean that determinations are made as soon as possible, which serves both the individual animal as well as the population as a whole.

Cleaning and Disinfection

For wellness programs to be effective, a clean and sanitary environment must be maintained. Not only does this promote cat and human health, but it also promotes staff pride as well as public support. In addition to protocols for routine daily cleaning and disinfection procedures, protocols should be in place for periodic deep cleaning and disinfection as well as procedures to be used in the event of disease outbreaks.

When crafting protocols, it is important to recognize that cleaning and disinfection are two separate processes. The cleaning process involves the removal of gross wastes and organic debris (including nonvisible films) through the use of detergents, degreasers, and physical action. Although this process should result in a visibly clean surface, it does not necessarily remove all of the potentially harmful infectious agents that may be present. Disinfection is the process that will destroy most of these agents, but it cannot be accomplished until surfaces have been adequately cleaned.[27]

Disinfection is usually accomplished through the application of chemical compounds or disinfectants. The most commonly used of these are reviewed in Box 46-9.

BOX 46-9

Key Clinical Information Regarding Use of Common Disinfectants[27,53,92]

Alcohol Hand Sanitizers (70% Ethanol)

- Although commonly used, they must be applied to clean hands and allowed 20 seconds of contact time to be effective.
- They are highly effective against bacteria, but have only moderate activity against viral agents, including feline calicivirus (FCV).
- They should not be used as a substitute for hand washing or the use of gloves.

Biguanides

- Chlorhexidine is the most commonly used biguanide and is relatively expensive. Its major use is as a surgical preparation agent.
- Although biguanide compounds have broad antibacterial activity, they have limited efficacy against viruses and are ineffective against nonenveloped viruses, such as panleukopenia and FCV. Therefore they are not recommended as general-purpose environmental disinfectants.

Chlorine Compounds

- Household bleach (5.25% sodium hypochlorite) is the most commonly used chlorine compound and is an excellent, safe, and highly cost-effective disinfectant when used correctly.
- At a dilution of 1:32, bleach is highly effective against bacteria and viruses, including nonenveloped viruses, such as panleukopenia and FCV.
- Solutions must be made fresh daily and stored in opaque containers, because bleach is highly unstable once mixed with water and degrades in the presence of ultraviolet light.
- Surfaces must be thoroughly cleaned with a detergent, rinsed, and dried prior to the application of bleach, because it is ineffective in the presence of detergents and organic material.
- Proper disinfection requires 10 minutes of contact time with a bleach solution.
- Although bleach is not effective when mixed with detergents, it can be safely and effectively mixed with quaternary ammonium compounds, which do provide some cleaning activity.[101] Therefore this combination can be used for cleaning and disinfection, provided gross organic material is first removed and adequate contact time is allowed. The addition of bleach improves the disinfection properties of the solution, making it effective against nonenveloped viruses, including panleukopenia and FCV.[101]
- Concentrations stronger than a 1:32 dilution can result in respiratory irritation for both animals and people, as well as increased facility corrosion, and are therefore not recommended for routine use.
- At a dilution of 1:10, bleach will destroy dermatophyte spores. However, cats must be removed from the environment prior to application of this concentration.
- The use of calcium hypochlorite (Wysiwash, St. Cloud, Fla.) is becoming more common and offers the potential advantages of reduced contact time and a neutral pH, which prevents corrosion.[108]

Oxidizing Agents

- Potassium peroxymonosulfate (Trifectant; Vétoquinol, Buena, NJ) is a commonly used oxiding agent. A 1% solution is reliably bactericidal and virucidal (including nonenveloped viruses).
- Despite label claims, independent studies have demonstrated that potassium peroxymonosulfate does not effectively inactivate dermatophyte spores.[83]
- Trifectant contains a detergent; therefore it can be used as the primary agent for both cleaning and disinfection. However, periodic use of a degreaser will be necessary to remove ground-in dirt and buildup of organic debris.
- Trifectant retains activity in the presence of small amounts of organic material, making it ideal for use on porous surfaces, such as concrete and laminate. Once mixed, the solution is stable for 7 days. A 10-minute contact time is required to ensure complete disinfection.

Quaternary Ammonium Compounds

- Numerous products containing quaternary ammonium compounds are available, many of which contain detergents. At appropriate dilutions, as recommended by the manufacturer of a specific product, these compounds have activity against both bacteria and viruses; however, they do not reliably inactivate panleukopenia or FCV, despite label claims to the contrary.[31,34,56]
- A 10-minute contact time in the absence of organic material is required for proper disinfection.
- Although quaternary ammonium compounds may be safely used in cat housing areas, care should be taken to dry surfaces thoroughly before returning cats. Cats that lick quaternary ammonium compounds may develop ulcers of the tongue that can be severe.

Disinfectants Not Recommended Due to Toxicity

The use of products containing phenolic compounds (e.g., products such as Lysol [Reckitt Benckiser, Parsippany, NJ]) or pine oils (e.g., products such as Pine-Sol, The Chlorox Company, Oakland, Calif.) should not be used in areas housing cats. Exposure to these compounds can cause serious neurologic effects and liver damage.

Product selection should take into consideration the conditions present in a given environment (e.g., the type of surface and the presence of organic matter) and the compound's activity against the pathogens for which the animals are at greatest risk. The nonenveloped viruses, panleukopenia and feline calicivirus, are of particular concern. It is important to note that despite product label claims to the contrary, multiple independent studies have consistently shown that quaternary ammonium disinfectants do not reliably inactivate these important feline pathogens.[31,34,56] In addition to selecting effective agents, ensuring adequate contact time followed by thorough drying of surfaces is essential for achieving proper disinfection.

Protocols should include detailed methods for achieving both cleaning and disinfection. When performed properly and regularly, these practices decrease both the dose and duration of exposure to infectious agents. Box 46-10 outlines essential considerations for the development of cleaning and disinfection protocols.

Segregation of Cats

Segregation refers to the separation of animals from the main group or into subpopulations as necessary to promote health. Segregation of cats by physical and behavioral health status is essential for infectious disease control, stress reduction, and safety.[41] In animal shelters, segregation may also be required to ensure compliance with animal control procedures as prescribed by state or local ordinances. Depending on the setting, consideration should be given to separating cats by gender and reproductive status (e.g., intact, neutered, in heat, pregnant, nursing), physical and behavioral health status (e.g., apparently healthy, signs of contagious disease, reactive, feral), and life stage. A variety of separate areas will be necessary, depending on the needs of the given population and the context of the setting. The wellness program should define these areas in order to optimize cat health, while providing for the necessary functions of the facility.

Depending on the setting, consideration should be given to establishing areas for quarantine, isolation, general holding, adoption, and long-term housing, as well as to tailoring these by life stage.[106] For example, the very young and very old typically require more specialized care than healthy juveniles and adults. Kittens less than 4 to 5 months of age are particularly susceptible to infectious disease, and extra care must be taken to heighten biosecurity and limit their exposure. In particular, geriatric cats require comfortable, quiet quarters with careful attention to stress reduction[91] (e.g., the provision of a secure hiding place and a dedicated caregiver to enhance bonding and comfort). If cats are used for breeding, functional areas will be required to facilitate mating, queening, and kitten care.[45] And, as previously discussed, behaviorally fearful, highly reactive cats and feral cats should be separated from others—the stress responses of these cats can create fear in others.[42]

Quarantine

Quarantine involves the holding of healthy-appearing animals. It is most useful when animals enter a closed population to ensure that they are not incubating disease when they are introduced into the general population. Quarantine areas, with rigid biosecurity procedures in place, should be used to segregate healthy animals for observation. The use of such areas not only allows apparently healthy animals to be observed for developing signs of infectious disease, but it also allows time for response to vaccination in a highly biosecure environment where exposure risks are minimized.

The use of quarantine is a mainstay of effective infectious disease control programs and is intended to prevent the introduction of disease into a population. It should be used whenever it is feasible to implement effectively, such as in a laboratory setting, a private cattery, or a low-volume, limited-admission sanctuary setting. However, quarantine practices are not effective in most animal shelters, because the high volume and turnover of animals precludes proper implementation of a true quarantine where an "all in–all out" system is used.[41] Instead, incoming animals are usually added to the "quarantine group" on a daily basis, effectively defeating the purpose of true quarantine and simply prolonging the animal's stay. This is especially concerning given the fact that a cat's length of stay in a shelter is a major risk factor for development of upper respiratory infection.[26] For this reason, the use of quarantine is not recommended in most shelter settings. Instead, high biosecurity areas are recommended for housing the most susceptible animals (e.g., kittens less than 4 to 5 months of age). On the other hand, quarantine is warranted when a serious disease is discovered in a shelter population. If healthy-appearing animals are exposed during a serious outbreak, quarantine procedures should be used to stop the movement of animals and prevent further spread of disease. If possible, temporary closure to admittance is also recommended. Quarantine may also be required in bite cases to ensure compliance with state rabies laws.[41]

The particular population setting will guide the clinician's determination regarding implementation and length of quarantine, if any. A 14-day quarantine is sufficient to determine that cats are not incubating many common infectious diseases, including feline panleukopenia. However, other diseases, including feline leukemia virus and dermatophytosis, can have longer incubation periods and will therefore require a longer quarantine period.[63,82]

In breeding colonies, early weaning and quarantine have been advocated to prevent infection of kittens with feline coronavirus.[1] Pregnant queens are isolated, and

BOX 46-10

Key Considerations for Cleaning and Disinfection Protocols[27,53,92]

- Staff must wear personal protective equipment, as necessary, to prevent exposure to chemicals and/or pathogens.
- Thorough cleaning and disinfection of enclosures should occur between occupants and as part of periodic deep cleaning procedures.
  - Cats must be removed from enclosures during these procedures.
- "Spot cleaning" is generally sufficient for apparently healthy cats that will continue to occupy the same enclosure.
  - The cat remains in the enclosure while it is cleaned and soiled material is removed.
  - This method is often less stressful for cats (see Figure 46-8).
- Separate staff should clean and care for animals in areas with highly susceptible or sick animals, whenever possible.
  - At minimum, attention should be given to the order of cleaning.
    - The least contaminated areas should be cleaned before those that are the most contaminated.
    - The most vulnerable animals should be cleaned before the least vulnerable.
- Long-term residents that are housed in the same enclosure require less frequent disinfection of their enclosure, but daily cleaning remains essential.
- Protocols should always include practices to control fomite transmission.
  - Dedicated cleaning equipment should be available for each area.
  - Protective clothing should be worn to prevent cross-contamination.
  - Hand sanitation should be achieved through a combination of hand washing, hand sanitizers, and the use of gloves.
  - Protocols should include cleaning and disinfection of all equipment that comes into contact with cats and that cannot be discarded after use.
    - Scratched and porous surfaces are difficult to impossible to completely disinfect and should be used with caution or discarded (e.g., litter boxes, carriers, or bowls made of plastic).
- Equipment known to be contaminated by virulent or resistant pathogens (e.g., parvoviruses, ringworm) and that cannot be completely disinfected should be discarded.
- Protocols should include instructions for cleaning and disinfection of the following:
  - Transport cages and vehicles
  - Commonly touched surfaces (e.g., door knobs, cage handles, light switches)
  - Food and water bowls
  - Litter scoops
  - Buckets, squeegees, and other cleaning implements
- Vacuuming (with high-efficiency particulate air [HEPA] filtration) should be used whenever possible, to minimize airborne particles and dust.
- Mops should always be rinsed to remove organic debris before being returned to a bucket of disinfectant.
- Laundry/bedding should be discarded if heavily soiled; otherwise, it should be washed in hot water and thoroughly dried in a commercial washer and dryer.
- Periodic deep cleaning should be performed on a regularly scheduled basis (e.g., weekly, monthly, or quarterly, depending on the setting).
  - Cats must be removed for deep cleaning.
  - All disposable items in the room should be discarded.
  - Cages or enclosures should be removed or pulled out from the walls.
  - Thorough vacuuming should be done to remove all particles, dander, and hair present in the environment.
  - A degreaser should be used to remove organic buildup.
  - After a thorough mechanical scrubbing, everything should be rinsed prior to application of a disinfectant.
  - Adequate contact time with disinfectants must be allowed (e.g., usually 10 minutes).
  - All air-exchange filters should be changed at the time of deep cleaning.
  - The area must be thoroughly dried and ventilated before returning cats.

kittens are weaned as early as possible (e.g., 4 to 5 weeks of age) and placed in strict quarantine. In this manner, as maternal antibody wanes and kittens become susceptible to the virus, exposure and infection are prevented. However, it is important to note that the level of biosecurity required for success is difficult to achieve. Furthermore, eventual exposure and infection are highly likely because of the ubiquitous nature of coronaviruses.[93] In addition, because of the importance of the mother–kitten relationship to normal social and emotional development, this management practice may not always be desirable.

General Holding, Housing, Adoption, and Other Areas

In many settings, general holding areas are used for housing healthy juvenile and adult cats at intake. In animal shelters, it is important to consider that length of stay is associated with an increased risk of feline upper respiratory disease and that vaccination against core diseases often rapidly confers immunity. For these reasons, holding periods should be minimized whenever possible. In some cases, holding times will be influenced by legally required holding periods prescribed by state laws that allow owners a chance to reclaim lost pets. Legal holding periods are usually not required for owner-relinquished pets and preweaning-age animals, but a brief medical hold (e.g., 1 to 2 days) for evaluation and triage is usually warranted. Regardless, management practices that reduce length of stay are generally best for population health in a shelter setting.

Immunity is often strengthened with time through a combination of both active and passive immunity resulting from vaccination and exposure. Upper respiratory disease is often endemic in cat populations, and in open populations, constant introduction of large numbers of carriers and susceptible cats make exposure likely. As length of stay increases, many cats develop and recover from respiratory disease. As animals acclimate to their environment and gain immunity, less stringent biosecurity requirements may be required for long-term housing areas, depending on the particular setting. In animal shelters, the public is usually allowed to interact with cats in adoption areas, which is another management consideration.

Isolation

Isolation areas are used to segregate sick animals from the general population. Immediate isolation of animals with signs of infectious disease is critical to effective control. Isolation should be targeted by age and disease. For example, separate isolation areas should be available for cats and kittens with respiratory disease and those with gastrointestinal disease, whenever possible. In populations where upper respiratory infection is problematic, having two isolation areas for cats with respiratory infections is ideal: one area for those cats with moderate to severe signs that will require more intensive monitoring and treatment, and a separate area for those cats with only mild clinical signs and those that have been treated and are nearly recovered.[43] When mildly symptomatic cats can be housed separately from those that are very ill, staff compliance with isolation procedures are often improved. Cats with non-infectious conditions should also be housed in separate areas for treatment, and, in some cases, housing in the general population is appropriate.

Healthy environmental conditions in isolation areas promote recovery, and their importance cannot be overemphasized.[43] Crowding, noise, and stress must be avoided, and facilities must be easy to clean and disinfect. Room temperature should be warm and comfortable with good air quality. Windows are ideal, because natural sunlight is always beneficial to animal health and healing.

Biosecurity and Traffic Patterns

Strict biosecurity in quarantine and isolation areas, with attention to traffic patterns and the use of protective clothing, such as gowns and shoe covers, is essential. Footbaths are insufficient to prevent transfer of infectious agents on shoes. This is because disinfectants typically require 10 minutes of contact time and may be poorly effective in the presence of organic debris. In fact, footbaths may even contribute to the spread of disease. Dedicated boots or shoe covers should be used when entering contaminated areas.[84,104] In addition, separate, designated staff should care for animals in high biosecurity areas whenever possible.

By design, traffic patterns should move from the healthiest and most susceptible groupings to the least susceptible, and finally to isolation areas housing sick animals. Observation windows and signage are useful to reduce traffic flow into high-risk areas. Staff hygiene is extremely important, and the importance of diligent hand washing cannot be overemphasized.

Where space or facilities are not available, foster care may represent a viable and medically sound option for quarantine or isolation in some settings. For instance, in animal shelters, foster care is particularly useful for the care of preweaning-age kittens. Foster homes must be monitored to ensure that cats receive proper care and that resident animals are protected from disease exposure.[41]

Other Facility Operations

In addition to ensuring proper population density, segregation, and sanitation procedures, there are several other essential aspects of facility operations that must be incorporated into a population wellness program. These include heating, ventilation, and air conditioning (HVAC) considerations, noise and pest control, general facility maintenance, and staff training.[41]

Heating, Ventilation, and Air Conditioning

Extremes or fluctuations in temperature and humidity, as well as poor ventilation and air quality, can compromise animal health. Poor ventilation and high humidity favor the accumulation of infectious agents, while dust and fumes may be irritating to the respiratory tract. Many cats are particularly sensitive to drafts and chilling, both of which can predispose to upper respiratory infection. Heating, ventilation, and air conditioning (HVAC) specialists are uniquely qualified to help establish and maintain the environmental conditions required for animal health. When facilities are designed specifically for housing animals, these specialists should be consulted beforehand to ensure installation of the most effective and efficient systems possible. In reality, many facilities that house cats, including private catteries and shelters, among others, were not originally built for this purpose. Retrofitting existing facilities with the ideal HVAC system is often neither logistically nor financially feasible. Regardless, consultation with HVAC specialists is recommended in order to maximize the potential of the facility's existing system.

The recommended temperature range for cats is between 18° C and 29° C (64° F and 84° F) with a temperature setting in the low- to mid-20s Celsius (70s Fahrenheit) being typical.[54] The temperature setting should be determined according to the specific animals' needs. For example, neonatal kittens are more susceptible to hypothermia and generally require warmer temperatures than healthy adult cats. The location of the cats may also be a consideration. For example, enclosures located closer to floor level are often a few degrees cooler than those at higher levels. The exact temperature setting may also vary somewhat based on the season of the year. For instance, power companies typically recommend keeping the temperature between 25° C and 26° C (78° F and 79° F) during hot weather to conserve electricity and reduce power bills.[41]

Laboratory guidelines recommend 30% to 70% humidity for cats.[54] Higher humidity (e.g., 70%) may be advantageous in areas housing cats with respiratory disease because moist air may be beneficial to the respiratory passages, whereas lower humidity (e.g., 40% to 50%) may be beneficial in other areas in order to reduce survival of infectious agents in the environment. Although the range considered acceptable is large, a given room should have a relatively constant humidity (i.e., it should not have large fluctuations). Hosing or even mopping a room usually results in temporary spikes in humidity, but these will be short lived in a well-ventilated room.[41]

Adequate ventilation is crucial for good air quality. This is especially important for cats, because good air quality is essential for control of upper respiratory disease. Ten to fifteen air changes per hour is the standard recommendation for an animal room, but more or less airflow may be acceptable or necessary depending on the housing density.[54] Theoretically, the best case scenario, and what is typical in laboratory animal settings, is for the HVAC system to allow for 100% fresh (e.g., nonrecycled) air in each room so that the air entering a given room is exhausted out of the building and not recirculated to another room. Maintaining separate ventilation systems for various rooms or areas of a facility prevents exchange of air among them and is recommended, because air pressure gradients that recirculate or cause exchange of air between rooms have been associated with the spread of disease by aerosols.

When applying these standard recommendations to a particular setting, there are some practical considerations that should be taken into account.[41] First, even when ventilation systems provide 10 to 15 room air changes per hour, airflow may be restricted inside of cages or other enclosures within the room. In other words, the body of the room may be well ventilated, yet inside the cages, the air may remain relatively stagnant. In this case, ventilation may be improved by altering the housing design or arrangement; for example, the use of flow-through cages, runs, free-range rooms, or outdoor access may result in improved air quality. When considering the recommendations for 100% fresh, nonrecycled air with separate ventilation systems in various areas of the facility, consideration should be given to the fact that respiratory pathogens in cats are not aerosolized because of the cats' small tidal volume.[36] Although droplet transmission is possible, droplet spray does not extend more than 4 feet, and most transmission of respiratory disease in cats is through direct contact with infected cats, carriers, or fomites.[94] Although this recommendation seems prudent to consider, especially for isolation areas, it is very expensive to install and operate this type of ventilation system throughout a facility, especially in very cold or very hot climates. If air quality remains good and the facility maintains effective comprehensive wellness protocols, it may not be necessary for animal health.[41] More research is needed on the impact of such air exchange, but in the meantime, the author recommends consulting with an HVAC specialist to establish effective and efficient settings to suit the specific needs of the given population. In addition to ensuring good ventilation, it is imperative to use other strategies for maintaining good air quality, including regular maintenance of filters, control of dust and dander through routine vacuuming and periodic deep cleaning, and the use of dust-free litter.[52]

Noise and Pest Control

Noise control is another important consideration. It is crucial to keep cats out of auditory range of dogs, because many are profoundly stressed by the sounds of barking. Also, staff should be trained to reduce or avoid other sources of noise whenever possible. The installation of sound-proofing systems may be necessary for noise abatement and stress reduction.

Routine pest control may also be required, depending on the setting. It may be necessary to treat the environment for fleas, ticks, or other insects or ectoparasites. Products used to treat the environment must be selected carefully, because cats are extremely sensitive to the toxic effects of many insecticides.[78] In many instances, it will be necessary to remove cats during their application and only return them to the environment once it is thoroughly dried and ventilated. If rodent control is necessary, the use of rodenticide baits should be avoided, because cats can be exposed even if the bait is not within their reach. Rodents that have ingested the poisonous bait may enter an animal enclosure and, if the animal ingests the rodent, the poison will affect that animal. Humane live traps can be used to capture rodents for removal from a facility. Food containers should be kept tightly sealed, and clutter should be minimized to discourage pests in the environment.

General Facility Maintenance

General building maintenance procedures (e.g., regular inspection and servicing with repairs as needed) are also important considerations for the maintenance of a healthy environment. For example, periodic resealing of floors may be required as well as maintenance of plumbing fixtures to repair leaks or other problems. Developing and following written standard operating procedures and daily, weekly, monthly, and quarterly checklists will ensure that systematic schedules of maintenance are carried out in a timely fashion.[41]

Staff Training

Regular staff training is essential for implementing effective population wellness programs. Simply stated, staff caring for animals must be qualified to do so. To a large extent, their knowledge and skill will determine the success or failure of the wellness program. Embracing a culture of training promotes high-quality animal care as well as human safety. Both formal and on-the-job training should be provided to ensure that a staff has the knowledge and skills required to perform their assigned tasks. Protocols should be established for all levels of training, and a system should be in place to ensure proficiency. Staff training should be documented, and continuing education should be provided to maintain and improve skills. Finally, training must include the provision of information about zoonoses and other occupational health and safety considerations.[54]

CONCLUSION

Regardless of the setting, maintaining population health is essential for animal welfare as well as to meet the goals of the particular population. Population health depends on implementation of comprehensive wellness protocols, systematic surveillance, and excellent management. Facilities must establish goals for animal health, and wellness protocols must be regularly evaluated and revised to ensure that these goals are met. The bulk of efforts must focus on preventive strategies to ensure both the physical and behavioral health of cats, as well as a healthy environment. A proactive, holistic approach coupled with compassion is required. When these are combined with careful attention to the unique needs and stress responses of cats, the result will be "healthy, happy cats."

References

1. Addie DD, Jarrett O: Control of feline coronavirus in breeding catteries by serotesting, isolation, and early weaning, *Feline Pract* 23:92, 1995.
2. American Heartworm Society (AHS): Guidelines for the diagnosis, treatment and prevention of heartworm *(Dirofilaria immitis)* infection in cats (2007). Available at http://www.heartwormsociety.org/veterinary-resources/feline-guidelines.html. Accessed June 10, 2010.
3. American Society for the Prevention of Cruelty to Animals (ASPCA): *Mission possible, comfy cats. Shelter temperament evaluations for cats,* 2003, ASPCA, p 17.
4. American Veterinary Medical Association (AVMA). Microchipping of animals (2009). Available at http://www.avma.org/reference/backgrounders/microchipping_bgnd.pdf. Accessed June 10, 2010.
5. Association of Shelter Veterinarians (ASV): Board position statement on cats who test positive for FeLV and FIV (2008). Available at http://www.sheltervet.org/associations/4853/files/Management%20of%20Cats%20Who%20Tests%20Positive%20for%20FeLV%20and%20FIV.pdf. Accessed June 10, 2010.
6. Association of Shelter Veterinarians (ASV): Board position statement on veterinary supervision in animal shelters (2008). Available at http://www.sheltervet.org/associations/4853/files/Veterinary%20Supervision%20in%20Animal%20Shelters.pdf. Accessed June 11, 2010.
7. Association of Shelter Veterinarians (ASV): Standards of care for animal shelters (2010). Available at http://www.sheltermedicine.org. Accessed June 14, 2011.
8. Barry KJ, Crowell-Davis SL: Gender differences in the social behavior of the neutered indoor-only domestic cat, *Appl Anim Behav Sci* 64:193, 1999.
9. Beaver BV: Fractious cats and feline aggression, *J Feline Med Surg* 6:13, 2004.
10. Bernstein PL, Strack M: A game of cat and house: spatial patterns and behavior of 14 domestic cats *(Felis catus)* in the home, *Anthrozoos* 9:25, 1996.
11. Bradshaw JWS, Hal SL: Affiliative behaviours of related and unrelated pairs of cats in catteries: a preliminary report, *Appl Anim Behav Sci* 63:251, 1999.
12. Brun A, Chappuis G, Précausta P, Terré J: Immunisation against panleukopenia: early development of immunity, *Comp Immunol Microbiol Infect Dis* 1:335, 1979.
13. Canadian Veterinary Medical Association (CVMA): A code of practice for Canadian cattery operations (2009). Available at https://canadianveterinarians.net/Documents/Resources/Files/1316_CatteryCodeEnglishFINAL%20June8'09.pdf. Accessed June 10, 2010.
14. Carlstead K, Brown JL, Strawn W: Behavioral and physiological correlates of stress in laboratory cats, *Appl Anim Behav Sci* 38:143, 1993.
15. Case LP, editor: *The cat: its behavior, nutrition and health,* ed 1, Ames, Iowa, 2003, Blackwell.
16. Cat Fanciers' Association (2010): CFA cattery standard minimum requirements. Available at http://www.cfa.org/articles/cattery-standard.html. Accessed June 10, 2010.

17. Centers for Disease Control: Healthy pets, healthy people. Available at http://www.cdc.gov/HEALTHYPETS/browse_by_diseases.htm. Accessed June 10, 2010.
18. Cocker FM, Newby TJ, Gaskell RM, et al: Responses of cats to nasal vaccination with a live, modified feline herpesvirus type 1, *Res Vet Sci* 41:323, 1986.
19. Coleman, GT, Atwell RB: Use of fipronil to treat ear mites in cats, *Austr Vet Pract* 29:166, 1999.
20. Companion Animal Parasite Council (CAPC): General guidelines: controlling internal and external parasites in U.S. dogs and cats (2008). Available at http://www.capcvet.org/recommendations/guidelines.html#. Accessed June 10, 2010.
21. Counsel of Europe: Guidelines for accommodation and care of animals. Appendix A to the European Convention for the Protection of Vertebrate Animals used for experimental and other scientific purposes. Minimum cage floor area for cats. Available at http://conventions.coe.int/sécurité/EN/123-D7.htm. Accessed June 8, 2010.
22. Counsel of Europe: Guidelines for accommodation and care of animals. Proposed revision to Appendix A to the European Convention for the Protection of Vertebrate Animals used for experimental and other scientific purposes. Minimum cage floor area for cats. Available at http://www.ncbi.nlm.nih.gov/bookshelf/br.fcgi?book=nap11138&part=a2000b24cddd00081#a2000b24cddd00083. Accessed June 8, 2010.
23. Crouse MS, Atwill ER, Laguna M, et al: Soft surfaces: a factor in feline psychological well-being, *Contemp Topics in Lab Anim Med* 34:94, 1995.
24. Crowell-Davis SL: Social organization in the cat: a modern understanding, *J Feline Med Surg* 6:19, 2004.
25. Crowell-Davis SL, Barry K, Wolfe R: Social behavior and aggressive problems of cats, *Vet Clin North Am Small Anim Pract* 27:549, 1997.
26. Dinnage JD, Scarlett JM, Richards JR: Descriptive epidemiology of feline upper respiratory tract disease in an animal shelter, *J Fel Med Surg* 11:816, 2009.
27. Dvorak G, Petersen C: Sanitation and disinfection. In Miller L, Hurley KF, editors: *Infectious disease management in animal shelters*, Ames, Iowa, 2009, Blackwell, p 49.
28. Doweling JM: All together now: group-housing cats, *Animal Sheltering* Mar-April:13, 2003.
29. Dybdall K, Strasser R, Katz T: Behavioral differences between owner surrender and stray domestic cats after entering an animal shelter, *Appl Anim Behav Sci* 104:85, 2007.
30. Edinboro CH, Janowitz LK, Guptill-Yoran L, et al: A clinical trial of intranasal and subcutaneous vaccines to prevent upper respiratory infection in cats at an animal shelter, *Fel Pract* 27:7, 1999.
31. Eleraky NZ, Potgeiter LND, Kennedy M: Virucidal efficacy of four new disinfectants, *J Am Anim Hosp Assoc* 38:231, 2002.
32. Ellis SLH, Wells DL: Influence of visual stimulation on the behaviour of cats housed in a rescue shelter, *Appl Anim Behav Sci* 113:166, 2008.
33. Eisner ER: Feline dental prophylaxis and homecare, *Proc Western Vet Conf*, 2004.
34. Eterpi M, McDonnell G, Thomas V: Disinfection efficacy against parvoviruses compared with reference viruses, *J Hosp Infect* 73:64, 2009.
35. Farm Animal Welfare Council: Five Freedoms. Available at http://www.fawc.org.uk/freedoms.htm. Accessed June 11, 2010.
36. Gaskell RM, Dawson S, Radford A: Feline respiratory disease. In Greene CE, editor: *Infectious diseases of the dog and cat*, ed 3, Philadelphia, 2006, Saunders, p 145.
37. Gaskell RM, Povey RC: Experimental induction of feline viral rhinotracheitis in FVR-recovered cats, *Vet Record* 100:128, 1997.
38. Genchi C: Feline heartworm *(Dirofilaria immitis)* infection: a statistical elaboration of the duration of the infection and life expectancy in asymptomatic cats, *Vet Parasitol* 158:177, 2008.
39. Greene CE: Environmental factors in infectious disease. In Greene CE, editor: *Infectious diseases of the dog and cat*, ed 2, Philadelphia, 1998, Saunders, p 673.
40. Greene C: Immunoprophylaxis and immunotherapy. In Greene CE, editor: *Infectious diseases of the dog and cat*, ed 2, Philadelphia, 1998, Saunders, p 717.
41. Griffin B: Wellness. In Miller L, Hurley KF, editors: *Infectious disease management in animal shelters*, Ames, Iowa, 2009, Blackwell, p 17.
42. Griffin B: Scaredy cat or feral cat? *Animal Sheltering* Nov/Dec:57, 2009.
43. Griffin B: The lowdown on upper respiratory infections in cats, *Animal Sheltering* Jul/Aug:53, 2009.
44. Griffin B: Lessons on the importance of proper social housing in laboratory cats. In Griffin B: *A model of non-invasive monitoring of feline ovarian function in the domestic cat*, unpublished master's thesis, Auburn University, 2001.
45. Griffin B, Baker HJ: Domestic cats as laboratory animals. In Fox JG, editor: *Laboratory animal medicine*, San Diego, 2002, Harcourt Academic, p 459.
46. Griffin B, Hume KR: Recognition and management of stress in housed cats. In August JR, editor: *Consultations in feline internal medicine*, vol 5, Philadelphia, 2006, Saunders, p 717.
47. Griffin JFT: Stress and immunity: a unifying concept, *Vet Immunol Immunopathol* 20:263, 1989.
48. Griffith CA, Steigerwald ES, Buffington T: Effects of a synthetic facial pheromone on behavior of cats, *J Am Vet Med Assoc* 217:1154, 2000.
49. Hand MS, Novotny BJ, editors: *Small animal clinical nutrition*, ed 4, Topeka, Kans, 2002, Mark Morris Institute.
50. Hawthorne AJ, Loveridge GG, Horrocks LJ: Housing design and husbandry management to minimize transmission of disease in multi-cat facilities, *Proc Waltham Symposium Feline Infect Dis*, 1995, p 97.
51. Hurley KF: Implementing a population health plan in an animal shelter: goal setting, data collection and monitoring, and policy development. In Miller L, Zawistowski S, editors: *Shelter medicine for veterinarians and staff*, Ames, Iowa, 2004, Blackwell, p 211.
52. Hurley KF: Feline infectious disease control in shelters, *Vet Clin Small Anim* 35:21, 2005.
53. Hurley KF: Information sheet: cleaning and disinfection in shelters. Available at http://www.sheltermedicine.com/portal/is_cleaning.shtml. Accessed June 10, 2010.
54. Institute of Laboratory Animal Research, Commission on Life Sciences, National Research Council: *Guide for care and use of laboratory animals*, Washington, DC, 2006, National Academies Press.
55. Johnston SD: Questions and answers on the effects of surgically neutering dogs and cats, *J Am Vet Med Assoc* 198:1206, 1991.
56. Kennedy MA, Mellon VS, Caldwell G, et al: Virucidal efficacy of the newer quaternary ammonium compounds, *J Am Anim Hosp Assoc* 31:254, 1995.
57. Kessler MR, Turner DC: Stress and adaptation of cats *(Felis silvestris catus)* housed singly, in pairs, and in groups in boarding catteries, *Anim Welf* 6:243, 1997.
58. Kessler MR, Turner DC: Effects of density and cage size on stress in domestic cats *(Felis silvestris catus)* housed in animal shelters and boarding catteries, *Anim Welf* 8:259, 1999.
59. Kessler MR, Turner DC: Socialization and stress in cats *(Felis silvestris catus)* housed singly and in groups in animal shelters, *Anim Welf* 8:15, 1999.

60. Key D, editor: *Cattery design: the essential guide to creating your perfect cattery*, Cambridge, UK, 2006, Cambridge University Press.
61. Levine E, Perry P, Scarlett J, Houpt KA: Intercat aggression in households following the introduction of a new cat, *Appl Anim Behav Sci* 90:325, 2005.
62. Levy JK: Feline leukemia virus and feline immunodeficiency virus. In Miller L, Hurley KF, editors: *Infectious disease management in animal shelters*, Ames, Iowa, 2009, Blackwell, p 307.
63. Levy JK, Crawford C, Hartman K: American Association of Feline Practitioners feline retrovirus management guidelines, *J Fel Med Surg* 10:300, 2008.
64. Lindell EM, Erb HN, Houpt KA: Intercat aggression: a retrospective study examining types of aggression, sexes of fighting pairs and effectiveness of treatment, *Appl Anim Behav Sci* 55:153, 1997.
65. Lord LK, Griffin B, Levy JK, et al: Evaluation of collars and microchips for visual and permanent identification of pet cats, *J Am Vet Med Assoc* 237:387, 2010.
66. Lord LK, Ingwersen W, Gray JL, et al: Characterization of animal with microchips entering shelters, *J Am Vet Med Assoc* 235:160, 2009.
67. Lord LK, Pennell ML, Ingwersen W, et al: In vitro sensitivity of commercial scanners to microchips of various frequencies, *J Am Vet Med Assoc* 233:1723, 2008.
68. Lord LK, Pennell ML, Ingwersen W, et al: Sensitivity of commercial scanners to microchips of various frequencies implanted in dogs and cats, *J Am Vet Med Assoc* 233:1729, 2008.
69. Lord LK, Wittum TE, Ferketich AK, et al: Search and identification methods that owners use to find a lost cat, *J Am Vet Med Assoc* 230:217, 2007.
70. Loveridge GG: Provision of environmentally enriched housing for cats, *Animal Technol* 45:69, 1994.
71. Loveridge GG, Horrocks LJ, Hawthorne AJ: Environmentally enriched housing for cats when singly housed, *Anim Welf* 4:135, 1995.
72. Marretta SM: Managing oral health in breeding catteries. In August JR, editor: *Consultations in feline internal medicine*, ed 3, Philadelphia, 1997, Saunders, p 647.
73. McCobb EC, Patronek GJ, Marder A, et al: Assessment of stress levels among cats in four shelters, *J Am Vet Med Assoc* 226:548, 2005.
74. McCune S: Enriching the environment of the laboratory cat (1995). Available at http://www.nal.usda.gov/awic/pubs/enrich/labcat.htm. Accessed June 7, 2010.
75. McCune S: The impact of paternity and early socialisation on the development of cats' behaviour to people and novel objects, *Appl Anim Behav Sci* 45:109, 1995.
76. McMillan FD: Quality of life in animals, *J Am Vet Med Assoc* 216:1904, 2000.
77. McMillan FD: Development of a mental wellness program for animals, *J Am Vet Med Assoc* 220:965, 2002.
78. Merola V, Dunayer E: Toxicology brief: the 10 most common toxicoses in cats, *Vet Med* June:339, 2006.
79. Miller J: The domestic cat. Perspective on the nature and diversity of cats, *J Am Vet Med Assoc* 208:498, 1996.
80. Merriam-Webster's Online Dictionary 2010: Definition of wellness. Available at http://www.merriam-webster.com/dictionary/wellness. Accessed May 24, 2010.
81. Monte M De, Pape G Le: Behavioral effects of cage enrichment in single-caged adult cats, *Anim Welf* 6:53, 1997.
82. Moriello KA: Treatment of dermatophytosis in dogs and cats: review of published studies, *Vet Dermatol* 15:99, 2004.
83. Moriello KA, Deboer DJ, Volk LM, et al: Development of an in vitro, isolated, infected spore testing model for disinfectant testing of *Microsporum canis* isolates, *Vet Dermatol* 15:175, 2004.
84. Morley PS, Morris SN, Hyatt DR, et al: Evaluation of the efficacy of disinfectant footbaths as used in veterinary hospitals, *J Am Vet Med Assoc* 2005;226:2053.
85. National Association of State Public Health Veterinarians, CDC: Compendium of animal rabies prevention and control, 2008: National Association of State Public Health Veterinarians, Inc, (NASPHV), *MMWR Recomm Rep* 57(RR-2):1, 2008.
86. National Council on Pet Population Study and Policy: The shelter statistics survey (1994). Available at http://www.petpopulation.org/statsurvey.html. Accessed June 8, 2010.
87. New Zealand Ministry of Agriculture: Animal Welfare Advisory Committee: Companion cats code of welfare 2007. Available at http://www.biosecurity.govt.nz/animal-welfare/codes/companion-cats. Accessed June 14, 2010.
88. Newbury SP: Five key population management factors affecting shelter animal health, *Proc Western States Vet Conf*, 2009.
89. Ottway DS, Hawkins DM: Cat housing in rescue shelters: a welfare comparison between communal and discrete—unit housing, *Anim Welf* 173, 2003.
90. Overall KL: Recognizing and managing problem behavior in breeding catteries. In August JR, editor: *Consultations in feline internal medicine*, ed 3, Philadelphia, 1997, Saunders.
91. Patronek GJ, Sperry E: Quality of life in long-term confinement. In August JR, editor: *Consultations in feline internal medicine*, ed 3, Philadelphia, 1997, Saunders, p 621.
92. Petersen CA, Dvorak G, Spickler AR, editors: *Maddie's infection control manual for animal shelters*, Ames, Iowa, 2008, Iowa State University, Center for Food Security and Public Health.
93. Pedersen NC: A review of feline infectious peritonitis virus, 1963-2008, *J Fel Med Surg* 11:225, 2009.
94. Povey RC, Johnson RH: Observations on the epidemiology and control of viral respiratory disease in cats, *J Small Anim Pract* 11:485, 1970.
95. Reeve CL, Spitzmueller C, Rogelberg SG, et al: Employee reactions and adjustment to euthanasia related work: identifying turning points through retrospective narratives, *J Appl Anim Welf Sci* 7:1, 2004.
96. Richards JR, Elston TH, Ford RB, et al: The 2006 AAFP Feline Vaccine Advisory Panel report, *J Am Vet Med Assoc* 229:1405, 2006.
97. Rochlitz I, Podberscek AL, Broom DM: Welfare of cats in a quarantine cattery, *Vet Rec* 143:35, 1998.
98. Rochlitz I: Recommendations for the housing of cats in the home, in catteries and animal shelters, in laboratories and in veterinary surgeries, *J Feline Med Surg* 1:181, 1999.
99. Rochlitz I: Comfortable environmentally enriched housing for domestic cats (2000). Available at http://www.awionline.org/www.awionline.org/pubs/cq02/Cq-cats.html. Accessed June 10, 2010.
100. Scarampella F, Pollmeier M, Visser M, et al: Efficacy of fipronil in the treatment of feline cheyletiellosis, *Vet Parasitol* 129:333, 2005.
101. Scott FW: Virucidal disinfectants and feline viruses, *Am J Vet Res* 41:409, 1980.
102. Shepherdson DJ, Carlstead K, Mellen JD, et al: The influence of food presentation on the behavior of small cats in confined environments, *Zoo Biol* 12:203, 1993.
103. Siegford JM, Walshaw SO: Validation of a temperament test for domestic cats, *Anthrozoos* 16:332, 2003.
104. Stockton KA, Morley PS, Hyatt DR, et al: Evaluation of the effects of footwear hygiene protocols on nonspecific bacterial contamination of floor surfaces in an equine hospital, *J Am Vet Med Assoc* 228:1068, 2006.
105. Turner DC: The human-cat relationship. In Turner DC, Bateson P, editors: *The domestic cat: the biology of its behaviour*, Cambridge, UK, 2000, Cambridge University Press.

106. Vogt AH, Rodan I, Brown M, et al: AAFP–AAHA. Feline life stage guidelines, *J Am Anim Hosp Assoc* 46:70, 2010.
107. Weiss E: *Meet your match and feline-ality adoption program*, New York, 2006, American Society for the Prevention of Cruelty to Animals.
108. Wysiwash Product Information, St Cloud, Fla. Available at: http://www.wysiwash.com. Accessed June 8, 2010.
109. Wojciechowska JI, Hewson CJ: Quality-of-life assessment in pet dogs, *J Am Vet Med Assoc* 226:722, 2005.

Index

Pages followed by "f" indicate figures, "t" tables, "b" boxes.

E

I

J

M

O

S

T